Laryngitis 464.0
Lead poisoning 984
Legionnaires' disease 482.83
Leishmaniasis 085, 089
Leprosy 030
Lichen planus 697.0
Low back pain 724.2
Lyme disease 088.81
Lymphogranuloma venereum 099.1
Malabsorption 579
Malaria 084.6
Measles (rubeola) 055.9
Meconium aspiration 770.1
Melanoma 172
Meniere's disease 386.0
Meningitis..320–322
Menopause 627.2
Migraine headache.......................................346
Mitral valve prolapse...............................424.0
Monilial vulvovaginitis............................112.1
Multiple myeloma 203.0
Multiple sclerosis 340
Mumps 072.9
Myasthenia gravis 358.0
Mycoplasmal pneumonia 483.0
Mycosis fungoides 202.1
Nausea and vomiting 787.01
Necrotizing skin and soft tissue infections 785.4
Neoplasms of the vulva 239.5
Neutropenia 288.0
Nevi 216, 448.1
Newborn physiologic jaundice.................774.6
Nongonococcal urethritis..........................099.4
Non-Hodgkin's lymphomas 202
Nonimmune hemolytic anemia 283.1
Normal delivery 650
Obesity 278.0
Obsessive-compulsive disorders 300.3
Onychomycosis 110.1
Optic neuritis 377.3
Osteoarthritis 715
Osteomyelitis 730
Osteoporosis 733.0
Otitis externa 380.10
Paget's disease of bone 731.0
Panic disorder 300.01
Pap smear..V72.3
Parkinsonism...332.0
Paronychia 681.0
Partial epilepsy 345.4
Patent ductus arteriosus 747.0
Pediculosis 132
Pelvic inflammatory disease 614
Peptic ulcer disease 533
Pericarditis 423.9
Peripheral arterial disease.......................443.9
Peripheral neuropathies 356
Pernicious anemia and other megaloblastic anemias 281
Personality disorders 301
Pheochromocytoma 227.0
Phobia 300.2
Pigmentary disorders—vitiligo 709.01
Pinworms 127.4
Pityriasis rosea...696.3
Placenta previa 641.0
Plague 020
Platelet-mediated bleeding disorders 287.1
Pleural effusion 511.9
Polycythemia vera 238.4
Polymyalgia rheumatica 725
Porphyria 277.1
Postpartum hemorrhage...........................666.1
Post-traumatic stress disorder................309.81
Pregnancy V22.2
Pregnancy-induced hypertension...............642
Premature beats.......................................427.6
Premenstrual syndrome (PMS)................625.4
Prescribing oral contraceptive V25.01
Pressure ulcers 707.0
Preterm labor 644.2
Primary glomerular disease.................581–583
Primary lung abscess................................513.0
Primary lung cancer 162.9
Prostate cancer 185
Prostatitis 601

Pruritus 698.9
Pruritus ani 698.0
Pruritus vulvae 198.1
Psittacosis (ornithosis)..............................073
Psoriasis..696.1
Pulmonary embolism 415.1
Pyelonephritis 590
Q fever 083.0
Rabies 071
Rat-bite fever 026
Relapsing fever 087
Renal calculi 592
Reye's syndrome.....................................331.81
Rheumatic fever 390
Rheumatoid arthritis 714.0
Rib fracture 807.0
Rocky Mountain spotted fever................082.0
Rosacea 695.3
Roseola 057.8
Rubella 056
Salmonellosis 003.0
Sarcoidosis 135
Scabies 133
Schizophrenia 295
Seborrheic dermatitis 690.1
Septicemia 038
Sézary's syndrome...................................202.2
Shoulder dislocation 831.0
Sickle cell anemia 282.6
Silicosis 502
Sinusitis 473
Skull fracture 800, 801, 803
Sleep apnea 780.57
Sleep disorders 780.5
Snakebite..989.5
Stasis ulcers 454.0
Status epilepticus.....................................345.3
Stomach cancer 151
Streptococcal pharyngitis 034.0
Stroke 436
Strongyloides infection 127.2
Subdural or subarachnoid hemorrhage.........852
Sunburn 692.71
Syphilis 090–097
Tachycardias...785.0
Tapeworm infections 123
Telogen effluvium 704.02
Temporomandibular joint syndrome........524.6
Tendinitis 726–727
Tetanus 037
Thalassemia 282.4
Therapeutic use of blood components V59.0
Thrombotic thrombocytopenic purpura.........446.6
Thyroid cancer 193
Thyroiditis 245
Tinea capitis 110.0
Tinnitus 388.3
Toe fracture 826.0
Toxic shock syndrome 040.89
Toxoplasmosis 130
Transient cerebral ischemia 435
Trauma to the genitourinary tract 958, 959
Trichinellosis 124
Trichomonal vaginitis 131.01
Trigeminal neuralgia 350.1
Tuberculosis 011
Tularemia 021
Typhoid fever 002.0
Typhus fevers 080, 081
Ulcerative colitis 556
Urethral stricture 598
Urinary incontinence 788.3
Urticaria 708
Uterine inertia 661.0
Uterine leiomyoma...................................218
Varicella (chickenpox)..............................052
Venous thrombosis 453.8
Viral pneumonia.............................480.0–480.9
Viral respiratory infections 465.0
Vitamin deficiency.............................264–269
Vitamin K deficiency...............................269.0
Warts (verruca) 078.10
Wegener's granulomatosis.......................446.4
Whooping cough (pertussis) 033
Wrist fracture 814.0

Adapted from Jones MK, Castillo LA, Hopkins CA, Aaron WS (eds): St. Anthony's ICD-9-CM Code Book for Physician Payment, Vols 1 and 2, 5th ed. Reston, VA, St. Anthony Publishing, 1996.

LATEST APPROVED METHODS OF TREATMENT FOR THE PRACTICING PHYSICIAN

ROBERT E. RAKEL, M.D.

Professor, Department of Family and Community Medicine
Baylor College of Medicine, Houston, Texas

W.B. SAUNDERS COMPANY
A Harcourt Health Sciences Company
Philadelphia   London   Toronto   Montreal   Sydney   Tokyo

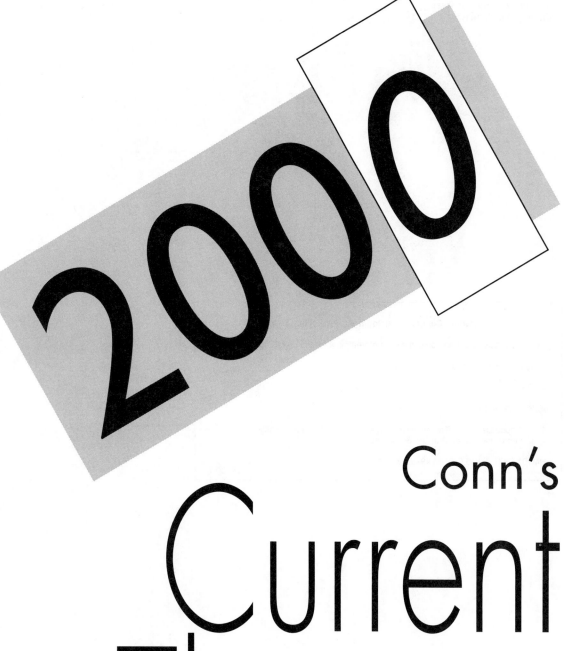

2000

Conn's
Current
Therapy

W.B. SAUNDERS COMPANY
A Harcourt Health Sciences Company

The Curtis Center
Independence Square West
Philadelphia, Pennsylvania 19106

Library of Congress Cataloging-in-Publication Data

Current therapy; latest approved methods of treatment for the practicing physician.

Editors: H. F. Conn and others

v. 28 cm. annual.

ISBN 0-7216-7225-6

1. Therapeutics.   2. Therapeutics, Surgical.   3. Medicine—Practice.
    I. Conn, Howard Franklin, 1908–1982 ed.

RM101.C87   616.058   49–8328 rev*

CONN'S CURRENT THERAPY 2000   ISBN 0-7216-7225-6

Printed in the United States of America.

Last digit is the print number: 9   8   7   6   5   4   3   2   1

Contributors

ANA ABAD-SINDEN, M.S.

Director/Instructor in UVA Health System, Dietetic Internship Program, University of Virginia, Charlottesville; Director, Dietetic Internship Program, and Neonatal Nutrition Specialist, University of Virginia, Charlottesville, Virginia
Normal Infant Feeding

BASSEL ABOU-KHALIL, M.D.

Associate Professor of Neurology, Vanderbilt University, Nashville; Director, Epilepsy Program, Vanderbilt University Medical Center, Nashville, Tennessee
Seizures and Epilepsy in Adolescents and Adults

DAVID ADAMSON, M.D.

Clinical Professor, Stanford University School of Medicine, Stanford, California; Associate Clinical Professor, University of California, San Francisco, School of Medicine, San Francisco, California; Active Staff, Good Samaritan Hospital, San Jose, California; Active Staff, Stanford University Hospital, Stanford, California
Endometriosis

PETER G. ADAMSON, M.D.

Pediatric Oncology Branch, National Cancer Institute, Bethesda, Maryland
Acute Leukemia in Children

MARK A. ADELMAN, M.D.

Assistant Professor, New York University School of Medicine, New York, New York; Director of Vascular Surgery, Bellevue Hospital, and Attending Surgeon, New York University Hospital, New York, New York
Acquired Diseases of the Aorta

MICHAEL J. ADLER, M.D.

Clinical Assistant Professor of Dermatology, Oregon Health Sciences University, Portland, Oregon; Attending Dermatologist, Legacy Health System, Portland, Oregon
Pruritus Ani and Vulvae

JOANN AHERN, M.S.N.

Diabetes Clinical Nurse Specialist and Co-ordinator of the Yale Pediatric Diabetes Program, Yale–New Haven Hospital, New Haven, Connecticut
Diabetes Mellitus in Children and Adolescents

DIANNE J. ALBRECHT, M.D.

Assistant Professor of Pediatrics, Division of Neonatology, Louisiana State University School of Medicine, New Orleans, Louisiana; Attending Physician, Medical Center of Louisiana, Children's Hospital, New Orleans, Louisiana
Care of the High-Risk Neonate

JEFFREY F. ALISON, M.B., B.S.

Honorary Lecturer, Department of Medicine, Monash University, Clayton, Victoria, Australia; Cardiologist and Director of Electrophysiology Program, Department of Cardiology, Monash Medical Centre, Clayton, Victoria, Australia
Premature Beats

JACK B. ALPERIN, M.D.

Professor, Departments of Internal Medicine, Pathology, and Human Biological Chemistry and Genetics, University of Texas Medical Branch, Galveston, Texas
Vitamin K Deficiency

BLANCHE P. ALTER, M.D.

Professor, Department of Pediatrics, Division of Hematology/Oncology, University of Texas Medical Branch at Galveston, Galveston, Texas; Attending Physician, University of Texas Medical Branch Hospital, Galveston, Texas
Aplastic Anemia

NAVIN M. AMIN, M.D.

Professor of Family Medicine, University of California, Irvine; Associate Professor of Internal Medicine, University of California, Los Angeles; Associate Professor of Family Medicine, Stanford, University, Stanford, California; Attending Physician, Kern Medical Center, Bakersfield, California
Infective Endocarditis

ROBERT J. ANDERSON, M.D.

Professor of Medicine and Biomedical Sciences, Creighton University School of Medicine, Omaha, Nebraska; Chief, Section of Endocrinology, Diabetes and Metabolism, Veterans Affairs Medical Center, Omaha, Nebraska
Hypopituitarism

KATHRYN M. ANDOLSEK, M.D., M.P.H.

Clinical Professor, Division of Community Health, Department of Community and Family Medicine, Duke University Medical Center, Durham, North Carolina; Attending Physician, Duke University Medical Center, Durham Regional Hospital, Durham, North Carolina
Contraception

KENNETH W. ANGERMEIER, M.D.

Attending Physician, Department of Urology, Cleveland Clinic Foundation, Cleveland, Ohio
Anterior Urethral Stricture

MAJOR M. ASH, Jr., D.D.S., M.D.

Professor of Dentistry, Marcus L. Ward Professor and Research Scientist Emeritus, University of Michigan School of Dentistry, Ann Arbor; Consultant, Veterans Affairs Medical Center, Ann Arbor, Michigan; St. Joseph Mercy Hospital, Ypsilanti, Michigan
Temporomandibular Disorders

BRENT R. ASPLIN, M.D.

Lecturer, Department of Emergency Medicine, University of Michigan Health System, Ann Arbor; Attending Physician, Department of Emergency Medicine, University of Michigan, Ann Arbor; Staff Physician, Department of Emergency Medicine, Foote Hospital, Jackson, Michigan
Cardiac Arrest: Sudden Cardiac Death

MICHAEL AUGENBRAUN, M.D.

Associate Professor of Medicine, State University of New York (SUNY), Brooklyn; Attending Physician, SUNY–Health Sciences Center at Brooklyn, Brooklyn, New York
Syphilis

ROBERT J. AWE, M.D.

Associate Professor, Pulmonary Section, Department of Medicine, Baylor College of Medicine, Houston, Texas; Attending Physician, Ben Taub General Hospital, Houston, Texas
Tuberculosis

JOHN BADALAMENTI, M.D.

Associate Professor of Medicine and Interim Director, Division of Nephrology, University of Texas Medical Branch, Galveston, Texas
Acute Renal Failure

DOUGLAS W. BALL, M.D.

Assistant Professor of Medicine and Oncology, Johns Hopkins University School of Medicine, Baltimore, Maryland; Attending Physician, The Johns Hopkins Hospital, Baltimore, Maryland
Thyroid Cancer

RICHARD R. BARAKAT, M.D.

Assistant Professor of Obstetrics and Gynecology, Cornell University Medical College, New York, New York; Associate Chief, Gynecology Service, Memorial Hospital, New York, New York; Associate Attending Surgeon, Gynecology Service, Memorial Hospital, New York, New York
Cancer of the Emdometrium

GRAHAM F. BARNARD, M.D., PH.D.

Associate Professor of Medicine and Biochemistry and Molecular Biology, University of Massachusetts Medical School, Worcester, Massachusetts; Associate Director, Center for Study of Disorders of Iron and Porphyrin Metabolism, Division of Digestive Disease and Nutrition, University of Massachusetts Memorial Health Care, Worcester, Massachusetts
The Porphyrias

FUAD M. BAROODY, M.D.

Assistant Professor, Section of Otolaryngology–Head and Neck Surgery and Department of Pediatrics, Pritzkin School of Medicine, University of Chicago, Chicago, Illinois; Staff Physician, University of Chicago Hospitals and Clinics, Chicago, Illinois
Allergic Rhinitis Caused by Inhalant Factors

THOMAS M. BASHORE, M.D.

Professor of Medicine and Director, Fellowship Training Program, Duke University Medical Center, Durham, North Carolina
Hypertrophic Cardiomyopathy

ROBERT G. BATEY, M.D.

Deputy Dean and Professor of Gastroenterology, University of Newcastle, Newcastle, Australia; Director, Gastroenterology, John Hunter Hospital, Newcastle, Australia
Alcohol-Related Problems

STEPHEN G. BAUM, M.D.

Professor of Medicine and Microbiology and Immunology, The Albert Einstein College of Medicine, Bronx, New York; Chairman, Department of Medicine, Beth Israel Medical Center, New York, New York
Viral and Mycoplasmal Pneumonias

ROY W. BECK, M.D., PH.D.

Director, Jaeb Center for Health Research, Tampa, Florida
Optic Neuritis

CHANDRA P. BELANI, M.D.

Professor of Medicine, University of Pittsburgh School of Medicine, and Co-Director, Lung Cancer Program, University of Pittsburgh Cancer Institute, Pittsburgh, Pennsylvania
Primary Lung Cancer

DAVID A. BENNETT, M.D.

Associate Professor of Neurological Sciences, Rush Medical College, Chicago, Illinois; Director, Rush Alzheimer's Disease Center, Rush–Presbyterian–St. Luke's Medical Center, Chicago, Illinois
Alzheimer's Disease

PAUL M. BENSON, M.D.

Associate Professor, Uniformed Services University of the Health Sciences, Bethesda, Maryland; Chief, Dermatology Service, Walter Reed Army Medical Center, Washington, D.C.; Residency Program Director, National Capital Consortium, Washington, D.C.
Donovanosis (Granuloma Inguinale)
Lymphogranuloma Venereum

DANIEL E. BERGSAGEL, C.M., M.D., D.PHIL.

Professor of Medicine, Emeritus, University of Toronto; Ontario Cancer Institute/Princess Margaret Hospital, Toronto, Ontario, Canada
Multiple Myeloma

VINOD K. BHUTANI, M.D.

Clinical Professor of Pediatrics, University of Pennsylvania School of Medicine, Philadelphia; Professor of Pediatrics, Jefferson Medical College, Philadelphia; Attending Physician, Pennsylvania Hospital and Children's Hospital of Philadelphia, Philadelphia, Pennsylvania
Hemolytic Disease of the Fetus and Newborn

AKHIL BIDANI, M.D., PH.D.

Professor, University of Texas Medical Branch, School of Medicine, Galveston, Texas; Division of Pulmonary and Critical Care Medicine, University of Texas Medical Branch Hospitals, Galveston, Texas
Acute Respiratory Failure

CAROLYN M. BLACK, PH.D.

Adjunct Assistant Professor, Department of Medicine, Emory University School of Medicine, Atlanta, Georgia; Chief, Chlamydia Section, Bacterial STD Branch, Division of AIDS, STDs, and TB Laboratory Research, National Center for Infectious Diseases, Centers for Disease Control and Prevention, Atlanta, Georgia
Chlamydia trachomatis Infection

JAMES R. BLACKMAN, M.D.

Assistant Dean, Regional Affairs and Rural Health, and Clinical Professor of Family Medicine, University of Washington School of Medicine, Seattle, Washington; WWAMI (Idaho/Wyoming) Office for Clinical Medical Education, Boise, Idaho; Staff Physician, Saint Alphonsus Regional Medical Center, Boise, Idaho
Spider Bites and Scorpion Stings

EUGENE S. BONAPACE, M.D.

Gastrointestinal Fellow, Temple University Hospital, Philadelphia, Pennsylvania
Dysphagia and Esophageal Obstruction

HERBERT L. BONKOVSKY, M.D.

Professor of Medicine, Biochemistry and Molecular Biology, University of Massachusetts Medical School, Worcester, Massachusetts; Director, Division of Digestive Disease and Nutrition, the Liver Center, and the Center for Study of Disorders of Iron and Porphyrin Metabolism, University of Massachusetts Memorial Health Care, Worcester, Massachusetts
The Porphyrias

WILLIAM Z. BORER, M.D.

Professor of Pathology, Jefferson Medical College of Thomas Jefferson University; Thomas Jefferson University Hospital, Philadelphia, Pennsylvania
Reference Intervals for the Interpretation of Laboratory Tests

PETER J. BOSTICK, M.D.

Clinical Assistant Professor, Louisiana State University Medical Center, New Orleans, Louisiana
Diseases of the Breast

EMILIO BOUZA, M.D., PH.D.

Professor of Medicine, Universidad Computense, Madrid, Spain; Servicio de Microbiologia Euferuedodes Infecciosas, Hospital General Universitario "Gregorio Marañón," Madrid, Spain
Brucellosis

SUZANNE L. BOWYER, M.D.

Associate Professor of Pediatrics, and Director, Section of Pediatric Rheumatology, James Whitcomb Riley Hospital for Children, Indiana University School of Medicine, Indianapolis, Indiana
Juvenile Rheumatoid Arthritis

ALAN S. BOYD, M.D.

Associate Professor, Departments of Dermatology and Pathology, Vanderbilt University, Nashville, Tennessee; Attending Physician, Vanderbilt University Medical Center, Nashville, Tennessee
Melanocytic Nevi

ROBERT W. BRADSHER, M.D.

Vice Chairman, Department of Medicine, and Professor of Medicine, University of Arkansas for Medical Sciences, Little Rock, Arkansas; Director, Division of Infectious Diseases, University Hospital of Arkansas and McClellan Veterans Affairs Hospital, Little Rock, Arkansas
Histoplasmosis

RICHARD D. BRASINGTON, M.D.

Associate Professor of Medicine and Director of Clinical Rheumatology, Division of Rheumatology, Washington University School of Medicine, St. Louis, Missouri
Hyperuricemia and Gout

DENISE F. BRATCHER, D.O.

Associate Professor, Department of Pediatrics, Division of Infectious Diseases, University of Louisville School of Medicine, Louisville, Kentucky; Staff Physician, Kosair Children's Hospital, Louisville, Kentucky
Rubella and Congenital Rubella Syndrome

KENNETH R. BRIDGES, M.D.

Associate Professor of Medicine, Harvard Medical School, Boston, Massachusetts; Director, Joint Center for Sickle Cell and Thalassemic Disorders, Brigham and Women's Hospital, Boston, Massachusetts
Iron Deficiency

GERALD K. BRISTOW, M.D.

Professor, Anesthesia, Faculty of Medicine, University of Manitoba, Winnipeg, Manitoba, Canada; Anesthetist, Health Sciences Centre, Winnipeg, Manitoba, Canada
Disturbances Due to Cold

KRISTINA K. BRYANT, M.D.

Kosair Charities Fellow in Pediatric Infectious Diseases, Department of Pediatrics, University of Louisville, Louisville, Kentucky
Rubella and Congenital Rubella Syndrome

FERNANDO CABANILLAS, M.D.

Professor of Medicine, Department of Hematology, University of Texas; M.D. Anderson Cancer Center, Houston, Texas
Non-Hodgkin's Lymphoma

MARLENE S. CALDERON, M.D.

Resident in Plastic Surgery, University of Michigan Medical Center, Ann Arbor, Michigan
Keloids

LOUIS B. CANTOR, M.D.

Professor, Indiana University School of Medicine, and Director, Glaucoma Service, Indianapolis, Indiana
Glaucoma

LOUIS R. CAPLAN, M.D.

Professor of Neurology, Harvard Medical School; Senior Neurologist, Beth Israel Deaconess Medical Center, Boston, Massachusetts
Intracerebral Hemorrhage

THOMAS R. CARACCIO, PHARM.D.

Assistant Professor of Emergency Medicine, State University of New York at Stony Brook Health Sciences Center School of Medicine, Stony Brook; Clinical Manager, Long Island Regional Poison Control Center, Winthrop University Hospital, Mineola, New York
Acute Poisonings

VICTOR J. CARDENAS, JR., M.D.

Associate Professor, University of Texas Medical Branch School of Medicine, Galveston, Texas; Staff Physician, Division of Pulmonary and Critical Care Medicine, University of Texas Medical Branch Hospitals, Galveston, Texas
Acute Respiratory Failure

DONALD O. CASTELL, M.D.

Kimbel Professor and Chairman, Graduate Hospital, Philadelphia, Pennsylvania
Gastroesophageal Reflux Disease

THOMAS R. CATE, M.D.

Professor of Medicine and Microbiology/Immunology, Baylor College of Medicine, Houston, Texas; Attending Physician, Ben Taub General Hospital, Houston, Texas
Viral Respiratory Infections

BARTOLOME R. CELLI, M.D.

Professor of Medicine, Tufts University, Boston, Massachusetts; Chief, Pulmonary and Critical Care, St. Elizabeth's Medical Center, Boston, Massachusetts
Chronic Obstructive Pulmonary Disease

EUGENIO CERSOSIMO, M.D., PH.D.

Assistant Professor of Medicine and Attending Physician, University Hospital, State University of New York at Stony Brook, Stony Brook, New York; Veterans Affairs Medical Center, Northport, New York
Diabetic Ketoacidosis

BONNIE P. CHAM, M.D.

Associate Professor, Department of Pediatrics, University of Manitoba, Winnipeg, Manitoba, Canada; Attending Staff, Manitoba Cancer Treatment and Research Foundation, Children's Hospital, Winnipeg, Manitoba, Canada
Neutropenia

STANLEY W. CHAPMAN, M.D.

Professor of Medicine, Vice-Chairman, Department of Medicine, and Director, Division of Infectious Diseases, University of Mississippi Medical Center, Jackson, Mississippi; Attending Physician, University Hospital, Department of Veterans Affairs Medical Center, Jackson, Mississippi
Blastomycosis

KANU CHATTERJEE, M.B.

Professor of Medicine and Lucie Stern Professor of Cardiology, University of California, San Francisco; Attending Physician, Division of Cardiology, Moffitt Long Hospital, University of California, San Francisco, California
Acute Myocardial Infarction

RUSSELL W. CHESNEY, M.D.

Professor, University of Tennessee, Memphis; Staff Physician, Le Bonheur Children's Medical Center, and Staff Physician, St. Jude Children's Research Hospital, Memphis, Tennessee
Parenteral Fluid Therapy in Infants and Children

LISA D. CHEW, M.D.

Acting Instructor, University of Washington School of Medicine, and Staff Physician, Harborview Medical Center, Seattle, Washington
Bacterial Infections of the Urinary Tract in Women

SUMANT S. CHUGH, M.D.

Instructor, Department of Medicine, Boston University School of Medicine, and Instructor, Department of Medicine, Boston Medical Center, Boston, Massachusetts
Diabetes Insipidus

DAVID A. CLARK, M.D.

Professor and Chairman of Pediatrics, Albany Medical College, and Director, Children's Hospital of Albany Medical Center, Albany, New York
Care of the High-Risk Neonate

HARRIS R. CLEARFIELD, M.D.

Professor of Medicine, MCP-Hahnemann University, and Section Chief of Gastroenterology, Hahnemann University Hospital, Philadelphia, Pennsylvania
Dyspepsia (Indigestion) and Gaseousness

ANTHONY J. COMEROTA, M.D.

Professor of Surgery, Temple University School of Medicine, Philadelphia, Pennsylvania; Chief, Vascular Surgery, and Director, Center for Vascular Diseases, Temple University Hospital, Philadelphia, Pennsylvania
Venous Thrombosis

JAMES D. COOK, M.D.

Phillips Professor of Medicine, Kansas University Medical Center, Kansas City, Kansas
Hemochromatosis

JONATHAN CORREN, M.D.

Assistant Clinical Professor of Medicine and Pediatrics, University of California, Los Angeles (UCLA); Attending Physician, UCLA Center for Health Sciences, Los Angeles, California
Asthma in Adolescents and Adults

JOSE A. CORTES, M.D.

Resident, Department of Pediatrics, University of South Alabama, Mobile, Alabama
Pediatric Head Injury

BRYAN D. COWAN, M.D.

Professor, Obstetrics and Gynecology, and Director, Division of Reproductive Endocrinology, University of Mississippi Medical Center, Jackson, Mississippi
Ectopic Pregnancy

J. THOMAS CROSS, JR., M.D., M.P.H.

Associate Professor, Department of Medicine and Pediatrics, Division of Infectious Diseases, Louisiana State University (LSU) Medical Center, Shreveport, Louisiana
Bacterial Pneumonia

JOHN G. CSERNANSKY, M.D.

Gregory B. Couch Professor of Psychiatry, Washington University School of Medicine, and Medical Director, Metropolitan St. Louis Psychiatric Center, St. Louis, Missouri
Schizophrenia

BURKE A. CUNHA, M.D.

Chief, Infectious Disease Division, Winthrop University Hospital, Mineola, New York; Professor of Medicine, State University of New York School of Medicine, Stony Brook, New York
Rocky Mountain Spotted Fever and Ehrlichiosis

GILBERT H. DANIELS, M.D.

Associate Professor of Medicine, Harvard Medical School, Boston, Massachusetts; Physician and Co-Director, Thyroid Clinic, Massachusetts General Hospital, Boston, Massachusetts
Hypothyroidism

IRA DAVIS, M.D.

Assistant Professor of Dermatology, New York Medical College, Valhalla, New York; Assistant Attending Physician, Westchester Medical Center, Valhalla, New York; Active Attending Physician, Sisters of Charity Medical Center, Bayley-Seton Campus, Staten Island, New York
Melanoma

OWEN K. DAVIS, M.D.

Associate Professor of Obstetrics and Gynecology, Weill College of Medicine of Cornell University, New York, New York; Associate Attending Obstetrician and Gynecologist, New York Presbyterian Hospital, and Associate Director of In Vitro Fertilization, Center for Reproductive Medicine and Infertility, New York, New York
Amenorrhea

LILLIAN G. DAWES, M.D.

Associate Professor of Surgery, Northwestern University Medical School, Chicago, Illinois
Cholelithiasis and Cholecystitis

ROSS M. DECTER, M.D.

Associate Professor of Surgery, Section of Urology, The Milton S. Hershey Medical Center, Hershey, Pennsylvania
Bacterial Infections of the Urinary Tract in Girls

C. M. De GEUS-WENCESLAU, M.D.

Staff Physician, Hospital São Lucas, Curitiba, Parana, Brazil
Ankylosing Spondylitis

VINCENT A. DeLEO, M.D.

Chairman, Department of Dermatology, St. Luke's/Roosevelt Hospital Center, New York, New York
Sunburn

PETER K. DEMPSEY, M.D.

Assistant Clinical Professor, Department of Neurosurgery, Tufts University School of Medicine, Boston, Massachusetts; Staff Physician, Lahey Clinic, Burlington, Massachusetts
Brain Tumors

RICHARD B. DEVEREUX, M.D.

Professor of Medicine, Weill College of Medicine of Cornell University, New York, New York; Director, Echocardiography Laboratory, New York Presbyterian Hospital, New York, New York
Mitral Valve Prolapse

PAUL T. DICK, M.D.C.M., M.Sc.

Assistant Professor of Paediatrics, Faculty of Medicine, University of Toronto, Toronto, Ontario, Canada; Attending Physician, The Hospital for Sick Children, Toronto, Ontario, Canada
Fever

ROGER R. DMOCHOWSKI, M.D.

Clinical Assistant Professor, Uniformed Services University of the Health Sciences, Bethesda, Maryland; Medical Director, North Texas Center for Urinary Control, Fort Worth, Texas
Urinary Incontinence

W. EDWIN DODSON, M.D.

Professor of Pediatrics and Neurology, Associate Vice Chancellor, and Associate Dean, Washington University School of Medicine, St. Louis, Missouri; Staff Physician, St. Louis Children's Hospital, St. Louis, Missouri; Staff Physician, Barnes-Jewish Hospital, St. Louis, Missouri
Epilepsy in Infants and Children

ANNE HAMILTON DOUGHERTY, M.D.

Associate Professor of Medicine and Director of Cardiac Arrhythmia and Pacing Services, Division of Cardiology, The University of Texas–Houston Health Science Center, Houston, Texas; Attending Physician, Memorial Hermann Hospital, Houston, Texas
Heart Block

J. DRESSNANDT, M.D.

Staff Physician, Bad Aibling Hospital for Neurology, Bad Aibling, Germany
Tetanus

R. M. Du BOIS, M.D.

Honorary Senior Lecturer, National Heart and Lung Institute at Imperial College, London, United Kingdom; Consultant Physician, Royal Brompton Hospital, London, United Kingdom
Sarcoidosis

MARTIN J. EDELMAN, M.D.

Associate Professor of Medicine, University of Maryland, and Attending Physician, University of Maryland Medical Center, Baltimore, Maryland
Nausea and Vomiting

RICHARD F. EDLICH, M.D., PH.D.

Distinguished Professor of Plastic Surgery and Professor of Biomedical Engineering, University of Virginia, School of Medicine, Charlottesville, Virginia
Necrotizing Skin and Soft Tissue Infections

MARYLENE J. EGHO, M.D.

Chair of Infection Control/Private Practice and Medical Director of HIV Clinic, Edward John Noble Hospital, Gouverneur, New York
Rat Bite Fever

HOWARD EIGEN, M.D.

Billie Lou Wood Professor of Pediatrics, Indiana University School of Medicine, Indianapolis; Director, Section of Pulmonology and Critical Care, and Associate Chairman for Clinical Affairs, Riley Hospital for Children, Indianapolis, Indiana
Cough

M. L. ELKS, M.D., PH.D.

Professor, Medicine and Medical Education, Morehouse School of Medicine, Atlanta, Georgia; Attending Physician, Grady Memorial Hospital, Atlanta, Georgia
Premenstrual Syndrome

WILLIAM J. ELLIS, M.D.

Associate Professor of Urology, University of Washington, Seattle, Washington
Malignant Tumors of the Urogenital Tract

JEFFREY P. ENGEL, M.D.

Associate Professor of Medicine, East Carolina University School of Medicine, Greenville, North Carolina; Chief, Infectious Diseases Division, Pitt County Memorial Hospital, Greenville, North Carolina
Gonorrhea

MILTON K. ERMAN, M.D.

Clinical Professor of Psychiatry, University of California, San Diego, School of Medicine; Adjunct Professor, Scripps Research Institute, San Diego, California
Insomnia

JEFF FAUNT, M.B.B.S.

Clinical Lecturer, Departments of Medicine and Clinical Pharmacology, University of Adelaide, Adelaide, South Australia; Staff Physician, Royal Adelaide Hospital, Adelaide, South Australia, Australia
Effects of Heat Stress

ARTHUR M. FELDMAN, M.D., PH.D.

Director of the Cardiovascular Institute of the UPMC Health System, Pittsburgh, Pennsylvania; Staff Physician, UPMC Presbyterian, Pittsburgh, Pennsylvania
Congestive Heart Failure

ANDREW FENVES, M.D.

Ralph Tompsett Professor of Medicine, Baylor University Medical Center, and Clinical Professor of Medicine, University of Texas Southwestern Medical Center, Dallas
Hypertension

CARACIOLO J. FERNANDES, M.D.

Assistant Professor of Pediatrics, Baylor College of Medicine, Houston, Texas; Attending Physician, Texas Children's Hospital and Methodist Hospital, Houston, Texas
Resuscitation of the Newborn

STEPHAN D. FIHN, M.D., M.P.H.

Professor, Departments of Medicine and Health Services, University of Washington, Seattle; Veterans Affairs Puget Sound Health Care System, Seattle, Washington
Bacterial Infections of the Urinary Tract in Women

THOMAS M. FILE, JR., M.D.

Professor of Internal Medicine, Northeastern Ohio Universities College of Medicine, Rootstown; Chief, Infectious Disease Service, Summa Health System, Akron, Ohio
Legionellosis (Legionnaires' Disease and Pontiac Fever)

DAVID R. FISCHER, M.D.

Resident, Department of Surgery, University of Cincinnati Medical Center, Cincinnati, Ohio
Parenteral Nutrition in Adults

JOSEF E. FISCHER, M.D.

Professor and Chairman, University of Cincinnati Medical Center, Department of Surgery, Cincinnati, Ohio
Parenteral Nutrition in Adults

LORRAINE A. FITZPATRICK, M.D.

Professor, Internal Medicine and Endocrinology, Mayo School of Medicine and Mayo Graduate School, Rochester, Minnesota; Director, Women's Health Fellowship, Rochester, Minnesota
Paget's Disease of Bone

CHARLES N. FORD, M.D.

Professor and Chair, Division of Otolaryngology–Head and Neck Surgery, University of Wisconsin, Madison; Attending Physician, University of Wisconsin Hospitals and Clinics, Madison, Wisconsin
Hoarseness and Laryngitis

MURRAY A. FREEDMAN, M.D.

Associate Clinical Professor, Department of Obstetrics and Gynecology, Medical College of Georgia, Augusta; Attending Physician, Medical College of Georgia University Hospital, Augusta, Georgia
Menopause

FAITH JOY FRIEDEN, M.D.

Assistant Professor, Mount Sinai School of Medicine, New York, New York; Director, Maternal-Fetal Medicine, Englewood Hospital and Medical Center, Englewood, New Jersey
Antepartum Care

JOSEPH H. FRIEDMAN, M.D.

Professor, Department of Clinical Neurosciences, Brown University School of Medicine, Providence; Adjunct Professor, School of Pharmacy, University of Rhode Island, Providence; Chief, Division of Neurology, Memorial Hospital of Rhode Island, Pawtucket, Rhode Island
Parkinson's Disease

RICK A. FRIEDMAN, M.D., PH.D.

Clinical Faculty, University of Southern California, Los Angeles; Attending Physician, St. Vincent's Medical Center and Cedar Sinai Medical Center, Los Angeles, California
Tinnitus

PETER C. FROMMELT, M.D.

Assistant Professor of Pediatrics, Division of Pediatric Cardiology, Medical College of Wisconsin, Milwaukee; Attending Physician, Children's Hospital of Wisconsin, Milwaukee, Wisconsin
Congenital Heart Disease

CLAIRE Y. FUNG, M.D.

Instructor, Harvard Medical School, Boston, Massachusetts; Radiation Oncologist, Massachusetts General Hospital, Boston, Massachusetts; Associate Medical Director, South Suburban Oncology Center, Quincy, Massachusetts
Hodgkin's Disease: Radiation Therapy

JOHN N. GALGIANI, M.D.

Professor of Medicine, University of Arizona, Tucson; Director, Valley Fever Center for Excellence, and Program Director for Infectious Diseases, Veterans Affairs Medical Center, Tucson, Arizona
Coccidioidomycosis

DAVID R. GANDARA, M.D.

Professor of Medicine, University of California, Davis; Staff Physician, Veterans Affairs Northern California Health Care System, Martinez, California
Nausea and Vomiting

BRUCE J. GANTZ, M.D.

Professor, Department of Otolaryngology–Head and Neck Surgery, University of Iowa School of Medicine, Iowa City; Department Head, University of Iowa Hospitals and Clinics, Iowa City, Iowa
Acute Facial Paralysis (Bell's Palsy)

NELSON M. GANTZ, M.D.

Clinical Professor of Medicine, MCP–Hahnemann School of Medicine, Philadelphia, Pennsylvania; Chairman of Medicine and Chief of Infectious Diseases, Pinnacle Health Hospitals, Harrisburg, Pennsylvania
Streptococcal Pharyngitis

MICHAEL A. GARDAM, M.Sc., M.D.C.M.

Lecturer, University of Toronto, and Associate Hospital Epidemiologist and Infectious Disease Consultant, University Health Network, Toronto, Ontario, Canada
Toxic Shock Syndrome

GREGORY C. GARDNER, M.D.

Associate Professor, Division of Rheumatology, and Attending Physician, Bone and Joint Center, University of Washington, Seattle, Washington
Polymyalgia Rheumatica and Giant Cell Arteritis

WARREN L. GARNER, M.D.

Associate Professor of Surgery, University of Southern California; Director, Los Angeles County and University of Southern California Burn Center; Attending Physician, University of Southern California, Los Angeles, California
Keloids

W. TIMOTHY GARVEY, M.D.

Professor of Medicine and Director, Division of Endocrinology, Diabetes, and Medical Genetics, Medical University of South Carolina, Charleston; Staff Physician, Medical University Hospital, Charleston; Staff Physician, Charleston Veterans Affairs Medical Center, Charleston, South Carolina
Diabetes Mellitus in Adults

MICHAEL J. GEHMAN, D.O.

MCP-Hahnemann School of Medicine, Philadelphia, Pennsylvania
Primary Lung Abscess

MARY L. GEMIGNANI, M.D.

Fellow, Department of Medicine, Division of Infectious Diseases, Gynecologic Oncology Fellow, Memorial Sloan-Kettering Cancer Center, New York, New York
Cancer of the Endometrium

TERRY GERNSHEIMER, M.D.

Assistant Professor of Medicine, Division of Hematology, Department of Medicine, University of Washington School of Medicine, Seattle; Director, Platelet Immunology Laboratory, Puget Sound Blood Center, Seattle; Puget Sound Blood Center Director of Medical Transfusion Services, University of Washington Medical Center, Seattle, Washington
Platelet-Mediated Bleeding Disorders

BERNARD J. GERSH, M.B.CH.B., D.PHIL.

Professor of Medicine, Mayo Medical School, Rochester, Minnesota; Consultant in Cardiovascular Diseases and Internal Medicine, Mayo Clinic, Rochester, Minnesota
Atrial Fibrillation

HARRIET S. GILBERT, M.D.

Clinical Professor of Medicine, Albert Einstein College of Medicine of Yeshiva University, Bronx, New York; Attending Physician, Department of Medicine and Division of Hematology, Montefiore Medical Center, Bronx, New York; and Mount Sinai Medical Center, New York, New York
Polycythemia Vera

ALLEN L. GINSBERG, M.D.

Professor of Medicine, George Washington University School of Medicine, Washington, D.C.; Attending Physician, George Washington University Hospital, Washington, D.C.
Inflammatory Bowel Disease

ARMANDO E. GIULIANO, M.D.

Clinical Professor of Surgery, University of California, Los Angeles; Chief of Surgical Oncology, Saint John's Health Center, and Director, Joyce Eisenberg Keefer Breast Center, Santa Monica, California
Diseases of the Breast

JOHN S. GOFF, M.D.

Clinical Professor of Medicine, University of Colorado Health Sciences Center, Denver; Staff Physician, Rocky Mountain Gastroenterology Associates, Denver, Colorado
Bleeding Esophageal Varices

BARRY S. GOLD, M.D.

Assistant Professor of Medicine, Johns Hopkins University School of Medicine and University of Maryland, School of Medicine, Baltimore; Attending Physician, Johns Hopkins Hospital and Sinai Hospital, Baltimore, Maryland
Snake Venom Poisoning

JAY L. GOLDSTEIN, M.D.

Associate Professor of Medicine, University of Illinois at Chicago; Staff Physician, University of Illinois at Chicago Medical Center; Staff Physician, Veterans Affairs Westside, Westside, Illinois
Peptic Ulcer Disease

ADRIAN J. GOLDSZMIDT, M.D.

Instructor, Johns Hopkins University School of Medicine, Baltimore, Maryland; Director, Stroke Center, Sinai Hospital, Baltimore, Maryland
Intracerebral Hemorrhage

DONALD E. GOODKIN, M.D.

Associate Professor, Department of Neurology, University of California, San Francisco (UCSF), School of Medicine, San Francisco; Director, UCSF/Mount Zion Multiple Sclerosis Center, San Francisco, California
Multiple Sclerosis

LUIGI GRADONI, PH.D.

Senior Researcher and Director, Section of Protozoology, Parasitology Department, Istituto Superiore di Sanità, Rome, Italy
Leishmaniasis

DAVID F. GRAFT, M.D.

Clinical Professor of Pediatrics, University of Minnesota School of Medicine, Minneapolis; Chairman, Asthma and Allergic Diseases, Park Nicollet Clinic, Minneapolis; Admitting Staff, Methodist Hospital, St. Louis Park, Minnesota
Allergic Reactions to Insect Stings

CLIVE E. H. GRATTAN, M.D.

Consultant Dermatologist and Honorary Senior Lecturer, Guy's, Kings and St. Thomas's Hospital Medical School, Norwich, United Kingdom; Consultant Dermatologist, West Norwich Hospital, Norwich, United Kingdom
Urticaria and Angioedema

JOSEPH GREENSHER, M.D.

Professor of Pediatrics, State University of New York at Stony Brook, Health Sciences Center School of Medicine, Stony Brook; Medical Director, Associate Director, and Chairman, Department of Pediatrics, Winthrop University Hospital; Associate Director, Long Island Regional Poison Control Center, Winthrop University Hospital, Mineola, New York
Acute Poisonings

MILTON D. GROSS, M.D.

Professor of Internal Medicine, University of Michigan, Ann Arbor; Attending Physician, University of Michigan Health System, Ann Arbor; Veterans Affairs Medical Center, Ann Arbor, Michigan
Pheochromocytoma

KLAUS E. GYR, M.D., M.P.H.T.M.

Professor of Medicine, University of Basel, and Attending Physician, Department of Medicine, University Hospital, Basel, Switzerland
Acute Infectious Diarrhea

DAVID W. HAAS, M.D.

Associate Professor of Medicine, Division of Infectious Diseases, Vanderbilt University School of Medicine, Nashville; Director, Clinical Infectious Diseases Services, Vanderbilt University Hospital, Nashville, Tennessee
Osteomyelitis

BRUCE W. HALSTEAD, M.D.

Private practice, Colton, California
Marine Animal Injuries

DOUGLAS H. HAMILTON, M.D., PH.D.

Director, Epidemic Intelligence Service, Centers for Disease Control and Prevention, Atlanta, Georgia
Cat-Scratch Disease and Bacillary Angiomatosis

A. F. HANEY, M.D.

Roy T. Parker Professor of Obstetrics and Gynecology, Duke University, Durham, North Carolina; Attending Physician, Duke University Medical Center, Durham, North Carolina
Leiomyomata

PHILIP HANNO, M.D.

Professor of Urology, University of Pennsylvania School of Medicine, Philadelphia; Attending Physician, Division of Urology, University of Pennsylvania School of Medicine, Philadelphia, Pennsylvania
Nongonococcal Urethritis

CATHERINE P. M. HAYWARD, M.D., PH.D.

Associate Professor, Pathology and Medicine, McMaster University, Hamilton, Ontario; Head, Regional Coagulation and Hemostasis Laboratory, Hamilton Health Sciences Corporation and the Hamilton Regional Laboratory Medicine Program, Hamilton, Ontario, Canada
Thrombotic Thrombocytopenic Purpura

CHARLES L. HEATON, M.D.

Professor of Dermatology, University of Cincinnati College of Medicine, Cincinnati, Ohio, Active Attending Physician, University of Cincinnati Hospital, and Active Attending Physician, Children's Hospital Medical Center of Cincinnati, Cincinnati, Ohio
Condyloma Acuminatum

ADELAIDE A. HEBERT, M.D.

Professor and Vice Chairman, Department of Dermatology, University of Texas Medical School, Houston, Texas
Atopic Dermatitis

ALFRED D. HEGGIE, M.D.

Professor of Pediatric and Associate Professor of Pathology, Case Western Reserve University School of Medicine, Cleveland, Ohio; Medical Director, Pediatric Family Clinic, Rainbow Rabies and Childrens Hospital, Cleveland, Ohio; Associate Director, Virology Laboratory, University Hospitals of Cleveland, Cleveland, Ohio
Measles

WAYNE J. G. HELLSTROM, M.D.

Professor of Urology, Tulane University School of Medicine, and Chief, Section of Andrology and Male Infertility, Tulane University Medical Center, New Orleans, Louisiana
Erectile Dysfunction

THOMAS N. HELM, M.D.

Assistant Clinical Professor of Dermatology and Pathology, State University of New York at Buffalo, and Attending Physician, Department of Dermatology, Buffalo Medical Group, Buffalo, New York
Hair Disorders

JEROME M. HERSHMAN, M.D.

Professor of Medicine, University of California, Los Angeles, School of Medicine, Los Angeles; Chief, Endocrinology and Metabolism Division, Veterans Affairs Greater Los Angeles Healthcare System, Los Angeles, California
Hyperthyroidism

DAVID R. HILL, M.D.

Associate Professor of Medicine, Division of Infectious Diseases, and Director, International Traveler's Medical Service, University of Connecticut, School of Medicine and Health Center, Farmington, Connecticut
Intestinal Parasites

KEITH HOOTS, M.D.

Pediatrician and Professor of Pediatrics, University of Texas Medical School at Houston; Professor of Pediatrics, University of Texas M. D. Anderson Cancer Center; Attending Physician, Hermann Children's Hospital, Houston, Texas
Hemophilia and Related Conditions

EMÍNA H. HUANG, M.D.

Assistant Professor of Surgery, Columbia-Presbyterian Medical Center, New York, New York
Tumors of the Colon and Rectum

WILLIAM J. HUESTON, M.D.

Professor and Chair, Department of Family Medicine, Medical University of South Carolina, Charleston, South Carolina
Acute Bronchitis and Acute Exacerbation of Chronic Bronchitis

WARNER K. HUH, M.D.

Clinical Instructor, Tufts University School of Medicine; Attending Physician, Department of Obstetrics and Gynecology, New England Medical Center, Boston, Massachusetts
Pelvic Inflammatory Disease

CHRISTOPHER D. HUSTON, M.D.

Fellow, Division of Infectious Diseases, University of Virginia School of Medicine, Charlottesville, Virginia
Amebiasis

GLENN R. JACOBOWITZ, M.D.

Assistant Professor of Surgery, New York University School of Medicine, New York University Medical Center, New York, New York; Attending Surgeon, Division of Vascular Surgery, New York University Medical Center, and Chief, Vascular Surgery, Manhattan Veterans Affairs Hospital, New York, New York
Acquired Diseases of the Aorta

LESLIE K. JACOBSEN, M.D.

Assistant Professor, Yale University School of Medicine, New Haven, Connecticut
Drug Abuse

ROBERT R. JACOBSON, M.D., Ph.D.

Director, Gillis W. Long Hansen's Disease Center, Carville, Louisiana
Leprosy (Hansen's Disease)

THOMAS W. JAMIESON, M.D.

Associate Professor of Medicine, Uniformed Services University of the Health Sciences, Bethesda, Maryland; Attending Physician, National Naval Medical Center, Bethesda, Maryland
Bursitis, Tendinitis, Myofascial Pain, and Fibromyalgia

STEPHANIE A. JOE, M.D.

Attending Physician, The Methodist Hospital and Texas Children's Hospital, Houston, Texas
Rhinosinusitis

DONNA D. JOHNSON, M.D.

Assistant Professor, Medical University of South Carolina, Charleston, South Carolina
Vaginal Bleeding in the Third Trimester

DEBORAH P. JONES, M.D.

Associate Professor, Department of Pediatrics, University of Tennessee, Memphis; Attending Physician, LeBonheur Children's Medical Center, Memphis, Tennessee
Parenteral Fluid Therapy in Infants and Children

PETER H. JONES, M.D.

Associate Professor of Medicine, Section of Atherosclerosis and Lipid Research, Baylor College of Medicine, Houston, Texas; Attending Physician, The Methodist Hospital, Houston, Texas
Hyperlipoproteinemias

CHRISTINE W. JORDAN, M.D.

Private practice, Metairie, Louisiana; Medical Staff, Lakeside Hospital and East Jefferson General Hospital, Metairie, Louisiana
Dysmenorrhea

WALTER H. A. KAHR, M.D., Ph.D.

Resident in Hematology, Department of Medicine, McMaster University, Hamilton, Ontario, Canada
Thrombotic Thrombocytopenic Purpura

MARTIN S. KARPEH, Jr., M.D.

Assistant Professor of Surgery, Cornell University Medical Center, New York, New York; Assistant Attending Surgeon, Department of Surgery, Memorial Sloan-Kettering Cancer Center, New York, New York
Tumors of the Stomach

PHILIP O. KATZ, M.D.

Associate Professor of Medicine, MCP-Hahnemann University School of Medicine; Vice Chairman, Department of Medicine, Graduate Hospital, Philadelphia, Pennsylvania
Gastroesophageal Reflux Disease

SCOTT H. KAUFMANN, M.D., Ph.D.

Associate Professor, Mayo Medical School, and Consultant, Department of Oncology and Division of Hematology, Department of Medicine, Mayo Clinic, Rochester, Minnesota
Acute Leukemia in Adults

ANDREW M. KAUNITZ, M.D.

Professor and Assistant Chair, Department of Obstetrics and Gynecology, University of Florida Health Science Center, Jacksonville; Attending Physician, University Medical Center and Methodist Medical Center, Jacksonville, Florida
Dysmenorrhea

WENDY ANNE KEITEL, M.D.

Associate Professor, Department of Microbiology and Immunology, and Department of Medicine, Baylor College of Medicine, Houston, Texas
Influenza

V. ANTOINE KELLER, M.D.

Fellow, Department of Cardiovascular and Thoracic Surgery, Carolinas Medical Center, Charlotte, North Carolina
Bacterial Diseases of the Skin

DAVID C. KEM, M.D.

Professor of Medicine and Geriatrics (Adjunct), University of Oklahoma School of Medicine, Oklahoma City; Attending Physician, University of Oklahoma Health Sciences Center and Veterans Administration Medical Center, Oklahoma City, Oklahoma
Primary Aldosteronism

STEPHEN F. KEMP, M.D.

Assistant Professor of Medicine and Pediatrics and Co-Director, Division of Allergy and Immunology, Department of Medicine, The University of Mississippi Medical Center, Jackson, Mississippi
Anaphylaxis and Serum Sickness

BRADLEY KESSER, M.D.

Clinical Fellow, House Ear Clinic, Los Angeles; Staff Physician, St. Vincent's Medical Center, Los Angeles, California
Tinnitus

KAMI KIM, M.D.

Assistant Professor of Medicine (Infectious Diseases) and of Microbiology and Immunology, Albert Einstein College of Medicine, Bronx, New York; Attending Physician, Montefiore Medical Center and Jacobi Medical Center, New York, New York
Toxoplasmosis

LOUIS V. KIRCHHOFF, M.D., M.P.H.

Professor, Department of Internal Medicine, University of Iowa College of Medicine; University of Iowa Hospitals and Clinics and Veterans Affairs Medical Center, Iowa City, Iowa
American Trypanosomiasis

MARIKO KITA, M.D.

Clinical Instructor, Department of Neurology, University of California, San Francisco, School of Medicine, San Francisco; Attending Physician, UCSF/Mt. Zion Multiple Sclerosis Center, San Francisco, California
Multiple Sclerosis

IRA W. KLIMBERG, M.D.

Director of Medical Affairs and Clinical Research, The Urology Center of Florida, Ocala; Medical Director, The Florida Foundation for Health Care Research, Ocala; Attending Physician, Ocala Regional Medical Center and Munroe Regional Medical Center, Ocala, Florida
Prostatitis

DAVID C. KLONOFF, M.D.

Clinical Professor of Medicine, University of California, San Francisco, California; Mills-Peninsula Medical Center, Burlingame, California
Chronic Fatigue Syndrome

SANDRA KNOWLES, B.Sc.Phm.

Lecturer, University of Toronto Faculty of Pharmacy, Toronto, Ontario, Canada; Drug Safety Pharmacist, Sunnybrook and Women's College Health Sciences Centre, Toronto, Ontario, Canada
Allergic Reactions to Drugs

STEVEN M. KOENIG, M.D.

Associate Professor of Medicine, University of Virginia, Charlottesville; Attending Physician, University of Virginia Health System, Charlottesville, Virginia
Obstructive Sleep-Disordered Breathing (Sleep Apnea)

JONATHAN E. KOLITZ, M.D.

Assistant Professor of Medicine, New York University School of Medicine, New York, New York; Associate Attending Physician, North Shore University Hospital, Manhasset, New York
Chronic Leukemias

NEIL J. KORMAN, Ph.D., M.D.

Associate Professor of Dermatology, Case Western Reserve University, Cleveland, Ohio; Attending Physician, University Hospitals of Cleveland, Cleveland, Ohio
Bullous Diseases

THOMAS R. KOSTEN, M.D.

Professor of Psychiatry, Yale University School of Medicine, New Haven, Connecticut; Chief of Psychiatry, Veterans Affairs Connecticut Healthcare System, West Haven, Connecticut
Drug Abuse

RICHARD A. KRASUSKI, M.D.

Fellow, Division of Cardiology, Department of Medicine, Duke University Medical Center, Durham, North Carolina
Hypertrophic Cardiomyopathy

BENJAMIN KREVSKY, M.D., M.P.H.

Professor of Medicine, Temple University School of Medicine, Philadelphia; Director of GI Endoscopy, Temple University Hospital, Philadelphia; Attending Physician, Temple University Hospital, Philadelphia, Pennsylvania
Constipation

LEONARD R. KRILOV, M.D.

Associate Professor of Pediatrics, New York University School of Medicine, New York, New York; Chief, Pediatric Infectious Disease, North Shore University, Manhasset, New York
Infectious Mononucleosis

MARSHALL K. KUBOTA, M.D.

Associate Clinical Professor, Department of Family and Community Medicine, University of California, San Francisco; Program Director, Family Practice Residency, Sutter Medical Center of Santa Rosa, Santa Rosa, California
Human Immunodeficiency Virus Infection and Its Complications

MANJUSHA KUMAR, M.D.

Assistant Professor, Department of Pediatrics, Division of Hematology/Oncology, University of Texas Medical Branch at Galveston, Galveston, Texas; Attending Physician, University of Texas Medical Branch Hospital, Galveston, Texas
Aplastic Anemia

DANIEL H. LACHANCE, M.D.

Senior Associate Consultant, Mayo Clinic/Mayo Foundation, Rochester, Minnesota
Brain Tumors

PAUL W. LADENSON, M.D.

Professor of Medicine, Oncology, and Pathology, Johns Hopkins University School of Medicine, Baltimore; Director, Division of Endocrinology and Metabolism, The Johns Hopkins Hospital, Baltimore, Maryland
Thyroid Cancer

STEVEN W. J. LAMBERTS, M.D.

Professor of Medicine, Erasmus University, Rotterdam, The Netherlands
Cushing's Syndrome

CAROL A. LANGFORD, M.D., M.H.S.

Senior Investigator, Immunologic Diseases Section, Laboratory of Immunoregulation, National Institute of Allergy and Infectious Diseases, National Institutes of Health, Bethesda, Maryland
Cutaneous Vasculitis

JENNIFER L. LARSEN, M.D.

Section Chief, Section of Diabetes, Endocrinology, and Metabolism, Department of Internal Medicine, University of Nebraska Medical Center, Omaha; Director, University Diabetes Center, and Director, Clinical Research Center, Nebraska Health System, Omaha, Nebraska
Adrenocortical Insufficiency

DONALD A. LEOPOLD, M.D.

Professor and Chairman, Department of Otolaryngology–Head and Neck Surgery, University of Nebraska Medical Center, Omaha, Nebraska
Rhinosinusitis

LOUIS LETENDRE, M.D.

Associate Professor, Mayo Medical School, Rochester, Minnesota; Consultant, Division of Hematology, Department of Medicine and Department of Oncology, Mayo Clinic, Rochester, Minnesota
Acute Leukemia in Adults

CHARLES LEVENBACK, M.D.

Associate Professor, Department of Gynecologic Oncology, University of Texas–M.D. Anderson Cancer Center, Houston, Texas
Cancer of the Uterine Cervix

MICHAEL A. LEVINE, M.D.

Professor of Pediatrics, Medicine, and Pathology and Director, Division of Pediatric Endocrinology, The Johns Hopkins University School of Medicine, Baltimore, Maryland
Hyperparathyroidism and Hypoparathyroidism

MATTHEW E. LEVISON, M.D.

Professor of Medicine and Public Health and Chief, Division of Infectious Diseases, Medical College of Pennsylvania, Philadelphia, Pennsylvania
Primary Lung Abscess

SUE LEVKOFF, Sc.D., S.M., M.S.W.

Associate Professor, Department of Social Medicine, and Associate Professor, Department of Psychiatry, Harvard Medical School, Boston, Massachusetts; Associate Professor, Department of Health and Social Behavior, Harvard School of Public Health, Boston, Massachusetts; Staff, Brigham and Women's Hospital, Boston, Massachusetts
Delirium

CHARLES S. LEVY, M.D.

Associate Professor of Medicine, George Washington University Medical Center, Washington, D.C.; Attending Physician, Infectious Diseases, Washington Hospital Center, Washington, D.C.
Food-Borne Illness

ROBERT M. LEVY, M.D., PH.D.

Associate Professor of Surgery and Physiology, Northwestern University Medical School, Chicago, Illinois; Northwestern Memorial Hospital, Chicago, Illinois
Trigeminal Neuralgia

KAREN B. LEWING, M.D.

Assistant Professor of Pediatrics, University of Missouri at Kansas City School of Medicine, Kansas City; Staff Hematologist/Oncologist, The Children's Mercy Hospital, Kansas City, Missouri
Sickle Cell Disease

BRUCE LEWIS, M.D.

Staff Physician, Loyola University Medical Center, Maywood, Illinois
Angina Pectoris

ERIC CHUN-YET LIAN, M.D.

Professor of Medicine, University of Miami School of Medicine; Attending Physician, University of Miami Hospital/Sylvester Cancer Center and Veterans Affairs Medical Center, Miami, Florida
Disseminated Intravascular Coagulation

MATTHEW H. LIANG, M.D., M.P.H.

Professor of Medicine, Harvard Medical School, Boston, Massachusetts; Attending Physician, Brigham and Women's Hospital, Boston, Massachusetts
Osteoarthritis

STUART M. LICHTMAN, M.D.

Associate Professor of Clinical Medicine, New York University School of Medicine, New York, New York; Associate Attending Physician, North Shore University Hospital, Manhasset, New York
Chronic Leukemias

MARK R. LITZOW, M.D.

Assistant Professor, Mayo Medical School, Rochester, Minnesota; Consultant, Division of Hematology, and Director, Blood and Marrow Transplant Program, Mayo Clinic, Rochester, Minnesota
Acute Leukemia in Adults

ELIZABETH LODER, M.D.

Instructor in Medicine, Harvard Medical School, Boston, Massachusetts; Attending Physician, Spaulding Rehabilitation Hospital and Massachusetts General Hospital, Boston, Massachusetts
Headache

DONALD P. LOOKINGBILL, M.D.

Professor of Dermatology, Mayo Medical School, Jacksonville, Florida; Chairman of Dermatology, Mayo Clinic, Jacksonville, Florida
Acne Vulgaris and Rosacea

CHRISTY A. LORTON, M.D.

Clinical Preceptor, Medical College of Ohio, Toledo; Clinical Preceptor, W. W. Knight Residency Program; Consultant, Toledo Hospital and St. Luke's Hospital, Toledo, Ohio
Pigmentary Disorders

DONALD F. LUM, M.D.

Assistant Professor of Medicine, University of California, Davis; Attending Physician, Veterans Affairs Northern California Health Care System, Martinez, California
Nausea and Vomiting

PATRICK D. LYDEN, M.D.

Professor of Neurosciences, University of California, San Diego (UCSD); Chief, Neurology, UCSD Medical Center; Staff Physician, Veterans Affairs Medical Center, San Diego, California
Ischemic Cerebrovascular Disease

DEBORAH S. LYON, M.D.

Associate Professor, University of Florida Health Science Center, Jacksonville; Active Staff, University Medical Center and Methodist Medical Center, Jacksonville, Florida
Dysmenorrhea

MAURIZIO MACCATO, M.D.

Assistant Professor, Department of Family Medicine, Baylor College of Medicine, Houston, Texas
Vulvovaginitis

NANCY E. MADINGER, M.D.

Assistant Professor of Medicine and Pathology, Division of Infectious Diseases, University of Colorado Health Sciences Center, Denver; Attending Physician, University Hospital and Denver Veterans Affairs Medical Center, Denver, Colorado
Relapsing Fever

JAMES A. MADURA II, M.D.

Assistant Professor of Surgery, Rush Medical College, Chicago; Attending Physician in Surgery, Rush–Presbyterian–St. Luke's Medical Center and Cook County Hospital, Chicago, Illinois
Chronic Pancreatitis

HIRALAL MAHESHWARI, M.D., PH.D.

Fellow, Department of Internal Medicine, University of Nebraska Medical Center, Omaha, Nebraska
Adrenocortical Insufficiency

BHAGIRATH MAJMUDAR, M.D.

Professor of Pathology and Associate Professor of Gynecology-Obstetrics, Emory University, Atlanta, Georgia; Attending Physician, Grady Memorial Hospital and Emory University Hospital, Atlanta, Georgia
Tumors of the Vulva

CHARLES M. MANSBACH II, M.D.

Professor of Medicine and Physiology, University of Tennessee, Memphis; Attending Physician, University of Tennessee Medical Center/William F. Bowld Hospital, Memphis; Veterans Affairs Medical Center, Memphis, Tennessee
Malabsorption Syndromes

JOHN F. MARCINAK, M.D.

Associate Professor of Pediatrics, University of Illinois College of Medicine, Chicago; Staff Physician, University of Illinois Hospital, Chicago, Illinois
Varicella (Chickenpox)

DAVID J. MARGOLIS, M.D., M.S.C.E.

Associate Professor of Dermatology, University of Pennsylvania School of Medicine, Philadelphia; Attending Physician, Hospital of the University of Pennsylvania, Philadelphia, Pennsylvania
Venous Leg Ulcers

PAULA MARLTON, M.B., B.S.

Senior Lecturer, Department of Pathology, University of Queensland; Assistant Director of Haematology, Princess Alexandra Hospital, Brisbane, Queensland, Australia
Non-Hodgkin's Lymphoma

THOMAS J. MARRIE, M.D.

Professor, Department of Medicine, and Associate Professor, Department of Microbiology, Dalhousie University, Halifax; Attending Staff, Division of Infectious Diseases, Queen Elizabeth II Health Sciences Center, Halifax, Nova Scotia, Canada
Q Fever

LAWRENCE F. MARSHALL, M.D.

Professor and Chair, Division of Neurological Surgery, University of California, San Diego, California
Acute Head Injuries in Adults

SHARON B. MARSHALL, M.D.

Assistant Clinical Professor of Surgery, Division of Neurological Surgery, University of California, San Diego, California
Acute Head Injuries in Adults

PATRICIA MARSHIK, PHARM.D.

Assistant Professor, Department of Pharmacy, University of New Mexico Health Sciences Center, Albuquerque, New Mexico
Cystic Fibrosis

ANN G. MARTIN, M.D.

Assistant Professor of Medicine, Washington University School of Medicine, Division of Dermatology, St. Louis, Missouri; Attending Physician, Barnes-Jewish Hospital, St. Louis, Missouri
Papulosquamous Diseases

JANICE M. MASSEY, M.D.

Professor of Medicine, Division of Neurology, Duke University Medical Center, Durham; Attending Physician, Duke University Medical Center, Durham, North Carolina
Acquired Myasthenia Gravis

GAYLE L. McCLOSKEY, M.D.

Resident in Dermatology, Mayo Graduate School of Medicine, Rochester, Minnesota
Diseases of the Mouth

MONICA L. McCRARY, M.D.

Chief Resident, Medical College of Georgia, Augusta, Georgia
Viral Skin Infections

PHILIP G. McMANIS, M.D.

Senior Lecturer, University of Sydney, Sydney, New South Wales, Australia; Senior Consultant in Neurology, Nepean Hospital and Royal North Shore Hospital, Sydney, New South Wales, Australia
Peripheral Neuropathies

J. SCOTT McMURRAY, M.D.

Assistant Professor, University of Wisconsin Medical School, Madison; Staff Physician, University of Wisconsin Hospital and Clinics, Madison; Staff Physician, University of Wisconsin Children's Hospital, Madison, Wisconsin
Hoarseness and Laryngitis

JESSICA N. MEHTA, M.D.

Resident Physician, Division of Dermatology, Washington University School of Medicine, St. Louis, Missouri; Resident, Barnes-Jewish Hospital, St. Louis, Missouri
Papulosquamous Diseases

JACK METZ, M.D.

Professorial Fellow, Department of Pathology, University of Melbourne; Head, Haematology, Royal Melbourne Hospital, Melbourne, Australia
Pernicious Anemia and Other Megaloblastic Anemias

DONALD J. MIECH, M.D.

Clinical Professor of Medicine (Dermatology), University of Wisconsin–Madison; Assistant Clinical Professor of Dermatology, University of Wisconsin, Marshfield, Wisconsin; Active Staff, St. Joseph's Hospital, Marshfield, Wisconsin
Parasitic Diseases of the Skin

MARIE E. MINNICH, M.D.

Clinical Assistant Professor, Thomas Jefferson University, Philadelphia; Staff Physician, Penn State Geisinger Health System and Geisinger Medical Center, Danville, Pennsylvania
Obstetric Anesthesia

JAMES E. MITCHELL, M.D.

President and Scientific Director, Neuropsychiatric Research Institute, Fargo, North Dakota; Professor and Chair, Department of Neuroscience, University of North Dakota School of Medicine and Health Sciences, Fargo, North Dakota
Bulimia Nervosa

HOWARD C. MOFENSON, M.D.

Professor of Pediatrics and Emergency Medicine, State University of New York at Stony Brook School of Medicine, Stony Brook; Professor of Pharmacology and Toxicology, New York School of Osteopathy, Westbury; St. John's University College of Pharmacy, Jamaica; Medical Director, Long Island Regional Poison Control Center, Winthrop University Hospital, Mineola, New York
Acute Poisonings

MARK E. MOLITCH, M.D.

Professor of Medicine, Northwestern University Medical School, Chicago; Attending Physician, Northwestern Memorial Hospital, Chicago, Illinois
Acromegaly

DAVID J. MOLITERNO, M.D.

Associate Professor of Medicine, Department of Cardiology, and Director, Angiographic Core Laboratory, Department of Cardiology, Cleveland Clinic Foundation, Cleveland, Ohio
Care After Myocardial Infarction

CRAIG H. MOSKOWITZ, M.D.

Assistant Professor of Medicine, Cornell University Medical College, New York, New York; Assistant Attending Physician, Memorial Sloan-Kettering Cancer Center, New York, New York
Hodgkin's Disease: Chemotherapy

LARRY C. MUNCH, M.D.

Assistant Professor of Surgery, University of Kentucky, Lexington; Staff Physician, University of Kentucky Medical Center and St. Joseph Hospital, Lexington, Kentucky
Renal Calculi

PATRICIA MUÑOZ, M.D., PH.D.

Assistant Professor of Medicine, Universidad Computense, Madrid, Spain; Servicio de Microbiologia, Euferuedodes infecciosas, and Staff Physician, Hospital General Universitario "Gregorio Marañón," Madrid, Spain
Brucellosis

HARLAN R. MUNTZ, M.D.

Associate Professor of Otolaryngology, Washington University School of Medicine, St. Louis; Attending Physician, St. Louis Children's Hospital and Barnes-Jewish Hospital, St. Louis, Missouri
Otitis Externa

JOHN J. MURRAY, M.D.

Assistant Clinical Professor of Surgery, Tufts University School of Medicine, Boston; Attending Surgeon, Department of Colon and Rectal Surgery, Lahey Clinic, Burlington, Massachusetts
Hemorrhoids, Anal Fissure, and Anorectal Abscess and Fistula

SARAH A. MYERS, M.D.

Assistant Professor, Duke University Medical Center, Durham, North Carolina
Pruritus

ROBERT B. NADELMAN, M.D.

Associate Professor of Medicine, Division of Infectious Diseases, New York Medical College, Valhalla, New York; Attending Physician, Westchester Medical Center, Valhalla, New York
Lyme Disease

VINODH NARAYANAN, M.D.

Associate Professor of Pediatrics, Neurology and Neurobiology, University of Pittsburgh; Attending Physician, Children's Hospital of Pittsburgh, Pittsburgh, Pennsylvania
Viral Meningitis and Encephalitis

THEODORE E. NASH, M.D.

Head, Gastrointestinal Parasite Section, Laboratory of Parasitic Diseases, National Institute of Allergy and Infectious Diseases, National Institutes of Health, Bethesda, Maryland; Clinical Center, National Institutes of Health, Bethesda, Maryland; National Naval Medical Center, Bethesda, Maryland
Giardiasis

NAIEL N. NASSAR, M.D.

Assistant Professor of Clinical Medicine, Division of Infectious Diseases, University of California, Davis, California
Bacterial Infections of the Urinary Tract in Men

DILIP NATHWANI, M.B.

Consultant Physician and Honorary Senior Lecturer in Infectious Diseases and Internal Medicine, Tayside University Hospitals NHS Trust, Dundee, Scotland
Salmonellosis

JERYL NATOFSKY, M.D.

Assistant Professor, University of South Florida College of Medicine, Tampa; Attending Physician, Tampa General Hospital, Tampa; Attending Physician, Bayfront Medical Center, St. Petersburg, Florida
Dysfunctional Uterine Bleeding

CATHERINE C. NEWMAN, M.D.

Clinical Assistant Professor and Director of Mycology Laboratory, University of Texas Medical Branch, Galveston, Texas
Fungal Diseases of the Skin

KHANH NGUYEN, M.D.

Attending Physician, Department of Internal Medicine, University of Texas–Houston Medical School, Houston, Texas
Atopic Dermatitis

RONALD LEE NICHOLS, M.D.

William Henderson Professor of Surgery and Professor of Microbiology and Immunology, Tulane University School of Medicine, New Orleans; Attending Physician, Tulane University Hospital and Clinic, New Orleans; Attending Physician, Medical Center of Louisiana at New Orleans, New Orleans, Louisiana
Bacterial Diseases of the Skin

JOHN M. NINOS, M.D.

Fellow, Transfusion Medicine, Department of Pathology and Laboratory Medicine, Hospital of the University of Pennsylvania, Philadelphia, Pennsylvania
Therapeutic Use of Blood Components

JOHN W. OGLE, M.D.

Professor and Vice Chairman, Department of Pediatrics, University of Colorado School of Medicine, Denver; Director of Pediatrics, Denver Health Medical Center, Denver, Colorado
Pertussis (Whooping Cough)

PETER M. OSHIN, M.D.

Associate in Medicine, University of Illinois at Chicago; Attending Physician, University of Illinois at Chicago Medical Center, Chicago, Illinois
Peptic Ulcer Disease

JEFFREY A. PAFFRATH, M.D.

Attending Physician, Middle Tennessee Medical Center and Centennial Medical Center, Murfreesborough, Tennessee
Otitis Media

THEODORE N. PAPPAS, M.D.

Professor of Surgery, Department of Surgery, Duke University School of Medicine, Durham, North Carolina; Vice Chairman, Department of Surgery, Duke Medical Center, Durham, North Carolina; Chief of the Surgical Service, Durham Veterans Administration Medical Center, Durham, North Carolina
Acute Pancreatitis

HENRY P. PARKMAN, M.D.

Associate Professor of Medicine, Temple University School of Medicine, Philadelphia; Staff Physician, Gastroenterology Section, Temple University Hospital, Philadelphia, Pennsylvania
Dysphagia and Esophageal Obstruction

GEOFFREY PASVOL, M.D., D.Phil.

Professor of Infection and Tropical Medicine, Imperial College School of Medicine, London; Consultant Physician, Northwick Park and St. Mark's Hospital, Harrow, Middlesex, United Kingdom
Malaria

AARON PERLMUTTER, M.D., Ph.D.

Assistant Professor of Urology, Weill Medical School of Cornell University, New York, New York; Attending Urologist, New York Presbyterian Hospital, New York, New York
Benign Prostatic Hyperplasia

SUSAN P. PERRINE, M.D.

Associate Professor, Boston University School of Medicine, and Attending Physician, Boston Medical Center, Boston, Massachusetts
Thalassemia

WILLIAM A. PETRI, Jr., M.D., Ph.D.

Professor of Medicine, Microbiology and Pathology, University of Virginia School of Medicine, Charlottesville; Attending Physician and Associate Director of Clinical Microbiology, University of Virginia Hospitals, Charlottesville, Virginia
Amebiasis

JOHN C. PETROZZA, M.D.

Assistant Professor of Obstetrics and Gynecology, Tufts University School of Medicine, Boston, Massachusetts; Department of Obstetrics and Gynecology, New England Medical Center, Boston, Massachusetts
Pelvic Inflammatory Disease

AGRON PLEVNESHI, M.D.

Research Volunteer, The Hospital for Sick Children, Toronto, Ontario, Canada
Fever

PAUL J. POCKROS, M.D.

Associate Clinical Professor of Medicine, University of California, San Diego, Medical School, San Diego; Head, Division of Gastroenterology/Hepatology, and Co-Director, Liver Disease Center, Scripps Clinic and Research Foundation, La Jolla, California
Cirrhosis

MARK H. POLLACK, M.D.

Associate Professor of Psychiatry, Harvard Medical School, Boston; Director, Anxiety Disorders Program, Massachusetts General Hospital, Boston, Massachusetts
Anxiety Disorders

CAROL S. PORTLOCK, M.D.

Professor of Clinical Medicine, Cornell University Medical Center, New York, New York; Attending Physician, Memorial Sloan-Kettering Cancer Center, New York, New York
Hodgkin's Disease: Chemotherapy

RICHARD A. PRINZ, M.D.

Professor of Surgery, Rush University, Chicago; Attending Surgeon, Rush–Presbyterian–St. Luke's Medical Center and Cook County Hospital, Chicago, Illinois
Chronic Pancreatitis

TIMOTHY A. PRITTS, M.D.

Resident, Department of Surgery, University of Cincinnati Medical Center, Cincinnati, Ohio
Parenteral Nutrition in Adults

NARAIN H. PUNJABI, M.D.

Research Scientist, U.S. Naval Medical Research Unit No. 2, Jakarta, Indonesia; Staff Physician, AEA International Clinic, Jakarta, Indonesia
Typhoid Fever

SUNIL K. PUROHIT, M.D.

Resident, Department of Urology, Tulane University School of Medicine, New Orleans, Louisiana
Erectile Dysfunction

EAMONN M. M. QUIGLEY, M.D.

Professor, National University of Ireland, Cork; Adjunct Professor, University of Nebraska Medical Center, Omaha, Nebraska; Consultant Gastroenterologist, Cork University Hospital, Cork, Ireland
The Irritable Bowel Syndrome

THOMAS C. QUINN, M.D.

Professor of Medicine, Johns Hopkins University School of Medicine, Baltimore, Maryland; Senior Investigator, National Institute of Allergy and Infectious Diseases, Washington, D.C.; Attending Physician, Johns Hopkins Hospital, Baltimore; National Institutes of Health Clinical Center, Bethesda, Maryland
Psittacosis (Ornithosis)

G. H. RABBANI, M.D., PH.D.

Scientist and Head of Physiology Laboratory, Clinical Sciences Division, and Head, Clinical Unit II, International Centre for Diarrhoeal Disease Research, Bangladesh
Cholera

C. VENKATA S. RAM, M.D.

Clinical Professor of Internal Medicine, University of Texas Southwestern Medical Center, Dallas, Texas; Senior Attending Physician, St. Paul Medical Center and Parkland Memorial Hospital, Dallas, Texas
Hypertension

RAMESH K. RAMANATHAN, M.D.

Assistant Professor of Medicine, University of Pittsburgh School of Medicine, and Attending Physician, University of Pittsburgh Cancer Institute, Pittsburgh, Pennsylvania
Primary Lung Cancer

FRANCISCO C. RAMIREZ, M.D.

Assistant Professor of Clinical Medicine, University of Arizona College of Medicine, Tucson; Associate Chair of Medicine for Gastroenterology and Chief of Therapeutic Endoscopy, Carl T. Hayden Veterans Affairs Medical Center, Phoenix, Arizona
Hiccup

HENRY W. RANDLE, M.D., PH.D.

Consultant, Department of Dermatology, Mayo Clinic–Jacksonville, Jacksonville, Florida; Professor of Dermatology, Mayo Medical School; Rochester, Minnesota
Diseases of the Mouth

P. SUDHAKAR REDDY, M.D.

Professor of Medicine, School of Medicine, University of Pittsburgh, Pittsburgh, Pennsylvania
Pericarditis

JOHN T. REPKE, M.D.

Chris J. and Marie A. Olson Professor of Obstetrics and Gynecology, University of Nebraska Medical Center, Omaha; Chairman, Department of Obstetrics and Gynecology, University of Nebraska Medical Center, Omaha, Nebraska
Hypertensive Disorders of Pregnancy

PHOEBE RICH, M.D.

Clinical Associate Professor, Oregon Health Sciences University, Portland, Oregon
Nail Disorders

ELLIOTT RICHELSON, M.D.

Professor of Psychiatry and Pharmacology, Mayo Medical School, Rochester, Minnesota; Consultant in Psychiatry and in Pharmacology, Mayo Clinic–Jacksonville; St. Luke's Hospital, Jacksonville, Florida
Mood Disorders

HAL B. RICHERSON, M.D.

Professor Emeritus, Department of Internal Medicine, University of Iowa College of Medicine, Iowa City; Attending Physician, University of Iowa Hospitals and Clinics, Iowa City, Iowa
Hypersensitivity Pneumonitis (Extrinsic Allergic Alveolitis)

THOMAS S. RILES, M.D.

Professor of Surgery, New York University School of Medicine; Director, Division of Vascular Surgery, New York University Medical Center; Attending Surgeon, Bellevue Hospital Center, New York, New York
Acquired Diseases of the Aorta

ROSS RISTAGNO, M.D.

Director of Pulmonary Medicine, Respiratory Care and Medical Intensive Care Unit, The Christ Hospital, Cincinnati, Ohio
Atelectasis

THOMAS E. ROHRER, M.D.

Director of Dermatologic Surgery, Department of Dermatology, Boston University Medical Center, Boston, Massachusetts
Cancer of the Skin

ALLAN RONALD, M.D.

Professor Emeritus, Department of Medicine, Section of Infectious Diseases, University of Manitoba, Winnipeg; Consultant, Infectious Diseases, St. Boniface General Hospital, Winnipeg, Manitoba, Canada
Epididymitis

LISA D. ROTZ, M.D.

Medical Officer, Bioterrorism Preparedness and Response Program, National Center for Infectious Diseases, Centers for Disease Control and Prevention, Atlanta, Georgia
Rabies

JEAN-CLAUDE ROUJEAU, M.D.

Professor of Dermatology, Université Paris XII, Paris; Department of Dermatology, Hôpital Henri Mondor Créteie, France
Erythema Multiforme, Stevens-Johnson Syndrome, and Toxic Epidermal Necrolysis

LARISSA ROUX, M.D., M.P.H.

Clinical Fellow, Department of Surgery, Sport Medicine Center, University of Calgary, Calgary, Alberta, Canada
Osteoarthritis

BRAD H. ROVIN, M.D.

Associate Professor of Medicine and Pathology, Ohio State University College of Medicine and Public Health, Columbus; Attending Nephrologist, Division of Nephrology, Ohio State University Hospitals, Columbus, Ohio
Primary Glomerular Diseases

CHARLES E. RUPPRECHT, V.M.D., Ph.D.

Chief, Rabies Section, Viral and Rickettsial Zoonoses Branch, Division of Viral and Rickettsial Diseases, National Center for Infectious Diseases, Centers for Disease Control and Prevention, Atlanta, Georgia
Rabies

R. SCOTT RUSHING, M.D.

Resident, Obstetrics and Gynecology, University of Missouri at Kansas City, Kansas City, Missouri
Postpartum Care

H. GIL RUSHTON, M.D.

Professor of Urology and Pediatrics, George Washington University School of Medicine, Washington, D.C.; Chairman, Department of Urology, Children's National Medical Center, Washington, D.C.
Childhood Enuresis

A. S. RUSSELL, M.B., B.Chir.

Professor of Medicine, University of Alberta, Edmonton, Alberta, Canada
Ankylosing Spondylitis

MICHAEL SACCENTE, M.D.

Assistant Professor of Medicine, University of Arkansas for Medical Sciences, Little Rock; Attending Physician, University of Arkansas Hospital and John L. McClellan Memorial Veterans Hospital, Little Rock, Arkansas
Histoplasmosis

RONALD A. SACHER, M.D.

Professor of Medicine and Pathology, Georgetown University Medical Center, Washington, D.C.; Chairman, Department of Laboratory Medicine, and Hematologist, Division of Hematology-Oncology, Georgetown University Medical Center, Washington, D.C.
Autoimmune Hemolytic Anemia

ROBERT L. SAFIRSTEIN, M.D.

Professor of Medicine and Vice Chair, Department of Medicine, University of Arkansas Medical School, Little Rock; Chief of Medicine, Veterans Affairs; Little Rock, Arkansas
Acute Renal Failure

WILLIAM E. SANDERS, Jr., M.D.

Director, Clinical Cardiac Electrophysiology and Pacing, Assistant Professor of Medicine, and Assistant Professor of Pathology, University of North Carolina, Chapel Hill, North Carolina
Tachycardias

CLAUDIO SARTORI, M.D.

Chief Resident, Department of Internal Medicine, Centre Hospitalier Universitaire Vaudois, Lausanne, Switzerland
High-Altitude Sickness

RALPH M. SCHAPIRA, M.D.

Associate Professor of Medicine, Division of Pulmonary and Critical Care Medicine, Medical College of Wisconsin, Milwaukee; Staff Physician, Milwaukee Veterans Affairs Medical Center, Milwaukee, Wisconsin
Silicosis

PAUL J. SCHEEL, Jr., M.D.

Associate Professor of Medicine, The Johns Hopkins University School of Medicine, Baltimore; Clinical Director, Division of Nephrology, The Johns Hopkins Hospital, Baltimore, Maryland
Chronic Renal Failure

URS SCHERRER, M.D.

Associate Professor of Medicine, Department of Internal Medicine, Centre Hospitalier Universitaire Vaudois, Lausanne, Switzerland
High-Altitude Sickness

JANET A. SCHLECHTE, M.D.

Professor, Department of Internal Medicine, University of Iowa, Iowa City, Iowa
Hyperprolactinemia

VIRGINIA M. SCHNEIDER, R.N.

The Cardiovascular Institute of the UPMC Health System; UPMC Presbyterian, Pittsburgh, Pennsylvania
Congestive Heart Failure

MITCHELL K. SCHWABER, M.D.

Staff Physician, Nashville Ear, Nose, and Throat Clinic; Staff Physician, Centennial Medical Center and St. Thomas Hospital, Nashville, Tennessee
Otitis Media

KATHY SCHWARZENBERGER, M.D.

Associate Professor of Dermatology and Medicine, Medical University of South Carolina, Charleston; Attending Physician, Medical University Hospital, Charleston, South Carolina
Skin Diseases of Pregnancy

MICHAEL D. SEIDMAN, M.D.

Assistant Clinical Professor, Department of Otolaryngology–Head and Neck Surgery, Wayne State University, Detroit; Regional Coordinator for Otolaryngology–Head and Neck Surgery, West Bloomfield Satellite; Co-Chair of Complementary-Alternative Initiative Henry Ford Health System, West Bloomfield, Michigan
Meniere's Disease

HEATHER SELMAN, M.D.

Resident, Department of Urology, Temple University Hospital, Philadelphia, Pennsylvania
Nongonococcal Urethritis

JESSICA L. SEVERSON, M.D.

Resident, Department of Dermatology, University of Rochester, Rochester, New York
Viral Skin Infections

AMY D. SHAPIRO, M.D.

Staff Physician, St. Vincent Hospital and Healthcare Center, Indianapolis, Indiana
Hemophilia and Related Conditions

BRAHM SHAPIRO, M.B., Ch.B., Ph.D.

Professor of Internal Medicine, University of Michigan, Ann Arbor; Attending Physician, University of Michigan Health Systems, Ann Arbor, and Veterans Affairs Medical Center, Ann Arbor, Michigan
Pheochromocytoma

KAUSHIK A. SHASTRI, M.D.

Assistant Professor of Medicine, State University of New York at Buffalo; Staff Hematologist/Oncologist, Veterans Affairs Western New York Healthcare System, Buffalo, New York
Adverse Reactions to Blood Transfusion

NEIL H. SHEAR, M.D.

Professor of Medicine, Pharmacology and Pediatrics, and Director, Drug Safety Research Group, University of Toronto Medical School, Toronto; Chief, Clinical Pharmacology, Sunnybrook and Women's College Health Sciences Centre, Toronto; Staff, Hospital for Sick Children, Toronto, Ontario, Canada
Allergic Reactions to Drugs

ROBERT L. SHERIDAN, M.D.

Associate Professor of Surgery, Harvard Medical School, Boston; Attending Physician, Massachusetts General Hospital and Shriners Burns Hospital, Boston, Massachusetts
Burns

MITCHELL L. SHIFFMAN, M.D.

Associate Professor and Chief, Hepatology Section, Medical College of Virginia Commonwealth University, Richmond, Virginia
Acute and Chronic Viral Hepatitis

LESLIE E. SILBERSTEIN, M.D.

Professor, Department of Pathology and Laboratory Medicine and Department of Medicine, University of Pennsylvania School of Medicine, Philadelphia; Director, Blood Bank and Transfusion Medicine, Hospital of the University of Pennsylvania, Philadelphia, Pennsylvania
Therapeutic Use of Blood Components

FREDRIC J. SILVERBLATT, M.D.

Professor of Medicine, Brown University, Providence; Chief, Managed Care, Providence Veterans Affairs Medical Center, Providence, Rhode Island
Bacteremia and Sepsis

NAOMI M. SIMON, M.D.

Instructor in Psychiatry, Harvard Medical School, Boston; Clinical Assistant in Psychiatry and Psychiatrist, Anxiety Disorders Program, Massachusetts General Hospital, Boston, Massachusetts
Anxiety Disorders

GARY L. SIMPSON, M.D., Ph.D., M.P.H.

Research Professor, Department of Biology, University of New Mexico, Albuquerque; Medical Director, Infectious Diseases Bureau, New Mexico Department of Health, Santa Fe, New Mexico
Plague

FREDERICK R. SINGER, M.D.

Clinical Professor of Medicine, University of Los Angeles, California, School of Medicine; Attending Physician, John Wayne Cancer Institute at Saint John's Health Center, Santa Monica, California
Osteoporosis

JAMES C. SISSON, M.D.

Professor of Internal Medicine, University of Michigan, Ann Arbor; Attending Physician, University of Michigan Health System, Ann Arbor, Michigan
Pheochromocytoma

JAMES W. SMITH, M.D.

Staff Physician, Section of Gastroenterology, Ochsner Foundation Hospital, New Orleans, Louisiana
Diverticula of the Alimentary Tract

JAMES W. SMITH, M.D.

Professor, Internal Medicine, University of Texas Southwestern Medical School at Dallas; Attending Physician, Dallas Veterans Affairs Medical Center, Dallas, Texas
Bacterial Infections of the Urinary Tract in Men

MICHAEL C. SNELLER, M.D.

Chief, Immunologic Diseases Section, Laboratory of Immunoregulation, National Institute of Allergy and Infectious Diseases, National Institutes of Health, Bethesda, Maryland
Cutaneous Vasculitis

STANLEY M. SPINOLA, M.D.

David H. Jacobs Professor of Infectious Diseases, Medicine, Microbiology and Immunology, Pathology and Laboratory Medicine, and Chief, Division of Infectious Diseases, Wishard Memorial Hospital, Indianapolis Clarion Health, Indianapolis, Indiana
Chancroid

J. PATRICK SPIRNAK, M.D.

Associate Professor of Urology, Case Western Reserve University, Cleveland; Director of Urology, Metrohealth Medical Center, Cleveland, Ohio
Trauma to the Genitourinary Tract

PETER C. SPITTELL, M.D.

Consultant, Department of Internal Medicine and Division of Cardiovascular Diseases, and Assistant Professor of Medicine, Mayo Medical School, Rochester, Minnesota; Active Staff/Consultant, Mayo Medical Center, Rochester, Minnesota
Peripheral Arterial Disease

RICHARD S. STACK, M.D.

Chief, Urology Service, Dwight David Eisenhower Army Medical Center, Augusta, Georgia
Acute Pyelonephritis

ROBERT STEFFEN, M.D.

Professor of Travel Medicine, Division of Epidemiology and Prevention of Communicable Diseases, Institute for Social and Preventive Medicine, University of Zurich, Zurich, Switzerland
Acute Infectious Diarrhea

FERNANDO STEIN, M.D.

Associate Professor of Pediatrics, Baylor College of Medicine, Houston; Deputy Director of Critical Care and Director, Progressive Care Unit, Texas Children's Hospital, Houston, Texas
Pediatric Head Injury

RICHARD K. STERLING, M.D.

Assistant Professor of Medicine, Medical College of Virginia of Virginia Commonwealth University, Richmond; Attending Physician, Medical College of Virginia and McQuire Veterans Affairs Medical Center, Richmond, Virginia
Acute and Chronic Viral Hepatitis

JOHN C. STEVENS, M.D.

Professor of Clinical Pediatrics, Section of Pulmonology, Indiana University School of Medicine, Indianapolis; James Whitcomb Riley Hospital for Children, Indianapolis, Indiana
Cough

SETH R. STEVENS, M.D.

Assistant Professor of Dermatology and Oncology, Case Western Reserve University, Cleveland; Attending Physician, University Hospitals of Cleveland and Louis Stokes Department of Veterans Affairs Medical Center, Cleveland, Ohio
Cutaneous T Cell Lymphomas

BRADFORD H. STILES, M.D.

Clinical Instructor, Department of Family and Preventive Medicine, University of California, San Diego; Staff Physician, Kaiser Permanente San Diego Medical Center, San Diego, California
Common Sports Injuries

BRENDON M. STILES, M.D.

General Surgery Resident, Department of General Surgery, University of Virginia School of Medicine, Charlottesville, Virginia
Necrotizing Skin and Soft Tissue Infections

MARK J. STILLMAN, M.D.

Staff Physician, Department of Neurology, Cleveland Clinic Foundation, Cleveland, Ohio
Pain

ELIZABETH A. STREETEN, M.D.

Assistant Professor of Medicine, The Johns Hopkins University School of Medicine, Baltimore, Maryland
Hyperparathyroidism and Hypoparathyroidism

PAUL M. SURATT, M.D.

John L. Guerrant Professor of Internal Medicine and Pulmonary and Critical Care Medicine, and Director, Sleep Disorders Center, University of Virginia School of Medicine, Charlottesville; Staff Physician, University of Virginia Hospital, Charlottesville, Virginia
Obstructive Sleep-Disordered Breathing (Sleep Apnea)

JAMES L. SUTPHEN, M.D., Ph.D.

Professor of Pediatrics, University of Virginia Health System, Charlottesville; Section Chief, Division of Gastroenterology and Nutrition, University of Virginia Children's Medical Center, Charlottesville, Virginia
Normal Infant Feeding

JEFFREY SVERD, M.D.

Associate Professor of Clinical Psychiatry, Department of Psychiatry and Behavioral Science, State University of New York at Stony Brook; Staff Psychiatrist, Sagamore Children's Psychiatric Center and New York State Office of Mental Health, Dix Hills, New York
Gilles de la Tourette Syndrome

ZBIGNIEW M. SZCZEPIORKOWSKI, M.D., Ph.D.

Instructor in Pathology, Harvard Medical School, Boston; Assistant Director, Blood Transfusion Service, Massachusetts General Hospital, Boston, Massachusetts
Autoimmune Hemolytic Anemia

WILLIAM V. TAMBORLANE, M.D.

Professor of Pediatrics and Chief, Pediatric Endocrinology, Yale University School of Medicine, New Haven; Attending Physician, Yale–New Haven Children's Hospital, New Haven, Connecticut
Diabetes Mellitus in Children and Adolescents

JAMES S. TAN, M.D.

Professor and Vice Chairman, Department of Internal Medicine, and Head, Infectious Disease Section, Northeastern Ohio Universities College of Medicine, Akron; Chairman, Department of Medicine, Summa Health System, Akron, Ohio
Legionellosis (Legionnaires' Disease and Pontiac Fever)

MANUEL E. TANCER, M.D.

Associate Professor of Psychiatry and Behavioral Neurosciences and Pharmacology, Wayne State University School of Medicine, Detroit, Michigan
Panic Disorder

DAVID R. THOMAS, M.D.

Professor of Medicine and Attending Physician, St. Louis University School of Medicine, St. Louis; Attending Physician, St. Louis University Hospital, St. Louis, Missouri
Pressure Ulcers

MARSHA M. THOMPSON, M.D., Ph.D.

Assistant Professor of Pediatrics, University of New Mexico School of Medicine, Albuquerque, New Mexico; Director, Cystic Fibrosis Center, University of New Mexico Health Sciences Center, Albuquerque, New Mexico
Cystic Fibrosis

JAMES A. THORP, M.D.

Associate Professor of Obstetrics and Gynecology, University of Missouri at Kansas City; Attending Physician, St. Luke's Hospital, Kansas City, Missouri
Postpartum Care

GREGORY C. TOMPKINS, Pharm.D.

Assistant Clinical Professor, University of Houston, College of Pharmacy, Houston; Memorial Hospital Southwest, Houston, Texas
New Drugs for 1998

WALTER TORDA, M.D.

Director, Central Pediatric Asthma Program, Harvard Vanguard Medical Associates, Boston; Clinical Instructor of Pediatrics, Harvard Medical School, Boston; Assistant in Medicine, Children's Hospital, Boston; Associate Pediatrician, Brigham and Women's Hospital, Boston, Massachusetts
Asthma in Children

CYNTHIA M. TRACY, M.D.

Associate Professor of Medicine, Georgetown University Medical Center, Washington, D.C.; Director, Cardiac Arrhythmia Service, Georgetown University Hospital, Washington, D.C.
Atrial Fibrillation

ALLAN R. TUNKEL, M.D., Ph.D.

Professor of Medicine, Associate Chair for Education, and Director, Internal Medicine Residency Program, MCP-Hahnemann University, Philadelphia, Pennsylvania
Bacterial Meningitis

RONALD J. TUSA, M.D., Ph.D.

Professor of Neurology, University of Miami; Anne Bates Leach Eye Hospital, Jackson Memorial Hospital, Miami, Florida
Episodic Vertigo

J. PETER VanDORSTEN, M.D.

Professor and Vice Chairman, Medical University of South Carolina, Charleston, South Carolina
Vaginal Bleeding in the Third Trimester

PETER D. VASH, M.D., M.P.H.

Assistant Clinical Professor of Medicine, Division of Endocrinology, University of California, Los Angeles; Executive Medical Director, Lindora Medical Clinics, Costa Mesa, California
Obesity

E. DARRACOTT VAUGHAN, Jr., M.D.

James J. Colt Professor of Urology, Cornell Medical School, New York, New York; Chairman, Department of Urology, New York Presbyterian Hospital, New York, New York; Attending Surgeon, Memorial Sloan-Kettering Cancer Center, New York, New York
Benign Prostatic Hyperplasia

CARLOS A. VAZ FRAGOSO, M.D.

Staff Physician, Gaylord Hospital, Wallingford, Connecticut
Pulmonary Thromboembolism

JOHN S. VENGLARCIK III, M.D.

Associate Professor of Pediatrics, Northeastern Ohio Universities College of Medicine, Youngstown; Director, Division of Pediatric Infectious Diseases, Tod Children's Hospital, Youngstown, Ohio
Mumps

RALPH S. VIOLA, M.D.

Clinical Assistant Professor of Ophthalmology, University of Rochester School of Medicine and Dentistry, Rochester, New York; Associate Attending Ophthalmologist, Strong Memorial Hospital, Rochester, New York
Conjunctivitis

HEIDI A. WALDORF, M.D.

Assistant Clinical Professor and Director of Dermatologic Laser Surgery, Department of Dermatology, Mount Sinai School of Medicine, New York, New York; Director of Dermatologic Laser Surgery and Attending Physician, Mount Sinai Medical Center, New York, New York; Clinical Assistant, Nyack Hospital, Nyack, New York
Premalignant Lesions

DANIEL J. WALLACE, M.D.

Clinical Professor of Medicine University of California, Los Angeles, School of Medicine; Attending Physician, Cedars-Sinai Medical Center, Los Angeles, California
Autoimmune Connective Tissue Disorders

ERIN M. WARSHAW, M.D.

Chief, Dermatology, Minneapolis Veterans Affairs Medical Center; Assistant Professor of Dermatology, University of Minnesota, Minneapolis, Minnesota
Contact Dermatitis

PETER C. WEBER, M.D.

Associate Professor and Interim Chairman, Department of Otolaryngology–Head and Neck Surgery, Medical University of South Carolina, Charleston, South Carolina
Acute Facial Paralysis (Bell's Palsy)

ANTHONY P. WEETMAN, M.D., D.Sc.

Professor of Medicine, University of Sheffield, and Honorary Consultant Physician, Northern General Hospital, Sheffield, United Kingdom
Thyroiditis

WILLIAM H. WEHRMACHER, M.D.

Clinical Professor of Medicine, Loyola University-Stritch School of Medicine, Attending Physician, St. Joseph Hospital, Chicago, Illinois
Angina Pectoris

BRYAN C. WEIDNER, M.D.

Chief Resident, Department of Surgery, Duke University School of Medicine, Durham, North Carolina
Acute Pancreatitis

RICHARD L. WHELAN, M.D.

Associate Professor of Surgery, College of Physicians and Surgeons, Columbia University, New York, New York; Director, Section of Colon and Rectal Surgery, Columbia-Presbyterian Medical Center, New York, New York
Tumors of the Colon and Rectum

THOMAS S. WHITECLOUD, III, M.D.

Ray J. Haddad Professor and Chairman, Department of Orthopaedic Surgery, Tulane University School of Medicine, New Orleans; Staff Physician, Tulane University Medical Center, New Orleans; Staff Physician, Medical Center of Louisiana at New Orleans, New Orleans, Louisiana
Low Back Pain

TIMOTHY E. WILENS, M.D.

Associate Professor of Psychiatry, Harvard Medical School, Boston; Attending Physician, Pediatric Psychopharmacology Unit, Massachusetts General Hospital, Boston, Massachusetts
Attention-Deficit / Hyperactivity Disorder

WILLIAM S. WILKE, M.D.

Department of Rheumatic and Immunologic Diseases, The Cleveland Clinic Foundation, Cleveland, Ohio
Rheumatoid Arthritis

MARTIN S. WOLFE, M.D.

Clinical Professor of Medicine, Georgetown University Medical School and George Washington University Medical School, Washington, D.C.; Attending Physician, Georgetown University Hospital and George Washington University Hospital, Washington, D.C.
Travel Medicine

GARY S. WOOD, M.D.

Professor of Dermatology, Pathology and Oncology and Vice Chairman of Dermatology for Veterans Affairs, Case Western Reserve University, Cleveland; Director of Multidisciplinary Cutaneous Lymphoma Program, University Hospitals of Cleveland; Chief of Dermatology, Louis Stokes Department of Veterans Affairs Medical Center, Cleveland, Ohio
Cutaneous T Cell Lymphomas

GERALD M. WOODS, M.D.

Professor of Pediatrics, University of Missouri at Kansas City School of Medicine; Chief, Section of Hematology-Oncology, The Children's Mercy Hospital, Kansas City, Missouri
Sickle Cell Disease

KIMBERLY A. WORKOWSKI, M.D.

Chief, Guidelines Unit, Epidemiology and Surveillance Branch, Division of Sexually Transmitted Diseases Prevention, Centers for Disease Control and Prevention, Atlanta; Assistant Professor of Medicine, Division of Infectious Diseases, Emory University, Atlanta, Georgia
Chlamydia trachomatis *Infection*

GARY P. WORMSER, M.D.

Professor of Medicine and Pharmacology, Chief of Infectious Diseases, and Vice Chairman, Department of Medicine, New York Medical College, Valhalla, New York; Chief of Infectious Diseases and Vice Chairman, Department of Medicine, Westchester Medical Center, Valhalla, New York
Lyme Disease

CAMERON D. WRIGHT, M.D.

Associate Professor of Surgery, Harvard Medical School, Boston; Associate Visiting Surgeon, Massachusetts General Hospital, Boston, Massachusetts
Pleural Effusion and Empyema Thoracis

HENRY M. YAGER, M.D.

Associate Professor of Medicine, Tufts University School of Medicine, Boston; Associate Chair of Medicine and Chief, Nephrology Service, Newton-Wellesley Hospital, Newton, Massachusetts
Diabetes Insipidus

YOSHIHITO YAWATA, M.D., Ph.D.

Professor of Medicine and Chief, Division of Hematology, Department of Medicine, Kawasaki Medical School, Kurashiki City, Japan; Chief, Division of Hematology, Department of Medicine, Kawasaki Medical School Hospital, Kurashiki City, Japan
Nonimmune Hemolytic Anemia

TIMOTHY R. YEKO, M.D.

Associate Professor, Department of Obstetrics and Gynecology, University of South Florida College of Medicine, Tampa; Attending Physician, Tampa General Hospital, Tampa, and Bayfront Medical Center, St. Petersburg, Florida
Dysfunctional Uterine Bleeding

KAREN E. ZANOL, M.D.

Assistant Professor, Division of Dermatology, University of Missouri Health Sciences Center, Columbia; Chief, Dermatology Section, Harry S. Truman Memorial Veterans Hospital, Columbia, Missouri
Warts

RICHARD KENT ZIMMERMAN, M.D., M.P.H.
Associate Professor, Department of Family Medicine and Clinical Epidemiology, School of Medicine, and Department of Health Services Administration, Graduate School of Public Health, University of Pittsburgh; Staff Physician, Shadyside Hospital, Pittsburgh, Pennsylvania
Immunization Practices

RICHARD D. ZOROWITZ, M.D.
Assistant Professor of Rehabilitation Medicine, University of Pennsylvania, Philadelphia; Medical Director, Piersol Rehabilitation Unit, and Director, Stroke Rehabilitation Hospital of the University of Pennsylvania, Philadelphia, Pennsylvania
Rehabilitation of the Stroke Survivor

Preface

This is the 52nd edition of *Conn's Current Therapy*. Our goal remains the same as for the first edition in 1949: to provide the busy physician with a concise reference to the most recent advances in therapy. Up-to-date information on the treatment of conditions frequently encountered in practice is presented by international authorities who see these problems frequently. The authors are on the leading edge of new developments because they have usually participated in the research leading to improved methods of care. The drugs recommended are the most effective according to their experience, even though some have not yet been FDA approved for the indication.

As in the past, this is a completely fresh and new edition in comparison to last year. Ninety-one percent of the authors are new, and the remaining 9% have updated their material. Often, varying methods of managing a problem can be appreciated by comparing the treatment methods of different authors in previous editions.

Thirty chapters have been written by authors outside the United States in places where the problems that they have written about are encountered more often. Examples are Disturbances Due to Cold (Canada); Disturbances Due to Heat (Australia); High-Altitude Sickness (Switzerland); Cholera (Bangladesh); Brucellosis (Spain); Leishmaniasis (Italy); Salmonellosis (Scotland); Erythema Multiforme (France); Cushing's Syndrome (Netherlands); Sarcoidosis (England); and Nonimmune Hemolytic Anemia (Japan).

Travel Medicine was added this year to assist in advising patients who are traveling internationally.

The full institutional affiliation of each contributor is given in the front of the book should more information be desired from the author.

Every topic undergoes thorough editorial review by a pharmacist, physician, and editors to ensure accuracy of the material. The person who manages the flow of manuscripts and makes sure that this annual book is published on schedule is Caroline Kosnik, my editorial assistant. I am grateful for her help and that of Ray Kersey and the excellent editorial staff at W.B. Saunders, whose commitment to accuracy ensures the continued quality of this publication.

ROBERT E. RAKEL, M.D.

Contents

SECTION 1. SYMPTOMATIC CARE PENDING DIAGNOSIS

Pain 1
Mark J. Stillman

Nausea and Vomiting 5
Martin J. Edelman
Donald F. Lum
David R. Gandara

**Dyspepsia (Indigestion)
and Gaseousness** 11
Harris R. Clearfield

Hiccup 13
Francisco C. Ramirez

Acute Infectious Diarrhea 15
Klaus E. Gyr
Robert Steffen

Constipation 18
Benjamin Krevsky

Fever 20
Paul T. Dick
Agron Plevneshi

Cough 22
John C. Stevens
Howard Eigen

Hoarseness and Laryngitis 25
J. Scott McMurray
Charles N. Ford

Insomnia 32
Milton K. Erman

Pruritus 35
Sarah A. Myers

Tinnitus 37
Bradley Kesser
Rick A. Friedman

Low Back Pain 39
Thomas S. Whitecloud III

SECTION 2. THE INFECTIOUS DISEASES

**Human Immunodeficiency Virus
Infection and Its Complications** 41
Marshall K. Kubota

Amebiasis 56
Christopher D. Huston
William A. Petri, Jr.

Giardiasis 59
Theodore E. Nash

Bacteremia and Sepsis 61
Fredric J. Silverblatt

Brucellosis 64
Emilio Bouza
Patricia Muñoz

Conjunctivitis 67
Ralph S. Viola

Varicella (Chickenpox) 69
John F. Marcinak

Cholera 72
G. H. Rabbani

Food-Borne Illness 74
Charles S. Levy

**Necrotizing Skin and Soft Tissue
Infections** 81
Richard F. Edlich
Brendon M. Stiles

Toxic Shock Syndrome 82
Michael A. Gardam

Influenza 85
Wendy Anne Keitel

Leishmaniasis 88
Luigi Gradoni

Leprosy (Hansen's Disease) 91
Robert R. Jacobson

Malaria 94
Geoffrey Pasvol

American Trypanosomiasis (Chagas' Disease) 101
Louis V. Kirchhoff

Bacterial Meningitis 103
Allan R. Tunkel

Infectious Mononucleosis 108
Leonard R. Krilov

Chronic Fatigue Syndrome 110
David C. Klonoff

Mumps 113
John S. Venglarcik III

Otitis Externa 114
Harlan R. Muntz

Plague 115
Gary Simpson

Psittacosis (Ornithosis) 116
Thomas C. Quinn

Q Fever 118
Thomas J. Marrie

Rabies 119
Lisa D. Rotz
Charles E. Rupprecht

Rat Bite Fever 122
Marylene J. Egho

Relapsing Fever 123
Nancy E. Madinger

Lyme Disease 125
Robert B. Nadelman
Gary P. Wormser

Rubella and Congenital Rubella Syndrome 130
Kristina K. Bryant
Denise F. Bratcher

Measles 132
Alfred D. Heggie

Tetanus 134
J. Dressnandt

Pertussis (Whooping Cough) 137
John W. Ogle

Immunization Practices 139
Richard Kent Zimmerman

Travel Medicine 145
Martin S. Wolfe

Toxoplasmosis 151
Kami Kim

Cat-Scratch Disease and Bacillary Angiomatosis 157
Douglas H. Hamilton

Salmonellosis 159
Dilip Nathwani

Typhoid Fever 161
Narain H. Punjabi

Rocky Mountain Spotted Fever and Ehrlichiosis 165
Burke A. Cunha

SECTION 3. THE RESPIRATORY SYSTEM

Acute Respiratory Failure 167
Victor J. Cardenas, Jr.
Akhil Bidani

Atelectasis 170
Ross Ristagno

Chronic Obstructive Pulmonary Disease 171
Bartolome R. Celli

Cystic Fibrosis 176
Marsha M. Thompson
Patricia Marshik

Obstructive Sleep-Disordered Breathing (Sleep Apnea) 180
Steven M. Koenig
Paul M. Suratt

Primary Lung Cancer 186
Ramesh K. Ramanathan
Chandra P. Belani

Coccidioidomycosis 193
John N. Galgiani

Histoplasmosis 195
Michael Saccente
Robert W. Bradsher

Blastomycosis 199
Stanley W. Chapman

Pleural Effusion and Empyema Thoracis 201
Cameron D. Wright

Primary Lung Abscess 203
Michael J. Gehman
Matthew E. Levison

Otitis Media 204
Jeffrey A. Paffrath
Mitchell K. Schwaber

Acute Bronchitis and Acute Exacerbation of Chronic Bronchitis 207
William J. Hueston

Bacterial Pneumonia 209
J. Thomas Cross, Jr.

Viral Respiratory Infections 213
Thomas R. Cate

Viral and Mycoplasmal Pneumonias 215
Stephen G. Baum

Legionellosis (Legionnaires' Disease and Pontiac Fever) 216
Thomas M. File, Jr.
James S. Tan

Pulmonary Thromboembolism 218
Carlos A. Vaz Fragoso

Sarcoidosis 224
R. M. Du Bois

Silicosis 228
Ralph M. Schapira

Hypersensitivity Pneumonitis (Extrinsic Allergic Alveolitis) 230
Hal B. Richerson

Rhinosinusitis 231
Stephanie A. Joe
Donald A. Leopold

Streptococcal Pharyngitis 236
Nelson M. Gantz

Tuberculosis 238
Robert J. Awe

SECTION 4. THE CARDIOVASCULAR SYSTEM

Acquired Diseases of the Aorta 243
Glenn R. Jacobowitz
Mark A. Adelman
Thomas S. Riles

Angina Pectoris 247
William H. Wehrmacher
Bruce Lewis

Cardiac Arrest: Sudden Cardiac Death 250
Brent R. Asplin

Atrial Fibrillation 256
Cynthia M. Tracy
Bernard J. Gersh

Premature Beats 260
Jeffrey F. Alison

Heart Block 264
Anne Hamilton Dougherty

Tachycardias 269
William E. Sanders, Jr.

Congenital Heart Disease 280
Peter C. Frommelt

Mitral Valve Prolapse 287
Richard B. Devereux

Congestive Heart Failure 291
Arthur M. Feldman
Virginia M. Schneider

Infective Endocarditis 297
    Navin M. Amin

Hypertension 303
    C. Venkata S. Ram
    Andrew Fenves

Acute Myocardial Infarction 315
    Kanu Chatterjee

Care After Myocardial Infarction 328
    David J. Moliterno

Pericarditis 333
    P. Sudhakar Reddy

Peripheral Arterial Disease 336
    Peter C. Spittell

Venous Thrombosis 339
    Anthony J. Comerota

Hypertrophic Cardiomyopathy 346
    Richard A. Krasuski
    Thomas M. Bashore

SECTION 5. THE BLOOD AND SPLEEN

Aplastic Anemia 351
    Manjusha Kumar
    Blanche P. Alter

Iron Deficiency 356
    Kenneth R. Bridges

Autoimmune Hemolytic Anemia 358
    Zbigniew M. Szczepiorkowski
    Ronald A. Sacher

Nonimmune Hemolytic Anemia 363
    Yoshihito Yawata

**Pernicious Anemia and Other
Megaloblastic Anemias** 366
    Jack Metz

Thalassemia 369
    Susan P. Perrine

Sickle Cell Disease 374
    Karen B. Lewing
    Gerald M. Woods

Neutropenia 381
    Bonnie P. Cham

**Hemolytic Disease of the Fetus
and Newborn** 383
    Vinod K. Bhutani

Hemophilia and Related Conditions 390
    Amy D. Shapiro
    Keith Hoots

**Platelet-Mediated Bleeding
Disorders** 397
    Terry Gernsheimer

**Disseminated Intravascular
Coagulation** 400
    Eric Chun-Yet Lian

**Thrombotic Thrombocytopenic
Purpura** 402
    Walter H. A. Kahr
    Catherine P. M. Hayward

Hemochromatosis 404
    James D. Cook

Hodgkin's Disease: Chemotherapy 406
    Carol S. Portlock
    Craig Moskowitz

**Hodgkin's Disease: Radiation
Therapy** 409
    Claire Y. Fung

Acute Leukemia in Adults 413
    Mark R. Litzow
    Louis Letendre
    Scott H. Kaufmann

Acute Leukemia in Children 421
    Peter G. Adamson

Chronic Leukemias 425
    Jonathan E. Kolitz
    Stuart M. Lichtman

Non-Hodgkin's Lymphoma 432
    Paula Marlton
    Fernando Cabanillas

Multiple Myeloma 440
Daniel E. Bergsagel

Polycythemia Vera 445
Harriet S. Gilbert

The Porphyrias 447
Herbert L. Bonkovsky
Graham F. Barnard

**Therapeutic Use of Blood
Components** 453
John M. Ninos
Leslie E. Silberstein

**Adverse Reactions to Blood
Transfusion** 458
Kaushik A. Shastri

SECTION 6. THE DIGESTIVE SYNDROME

Cholelithiasis and Cholecystitis 463
Lillian G. Dawes

Cirrhosis 465
Paul J. Pockros

Bleeding Esophageal Varices 471
John S. Goff

**Dysphagia and Esophageal
Obstruction** 473
Eugene S. Bonapace
Henry P. Parkman

Diverticula of the Alimentary Tract 479
James W. Smith

Inflammatory Bowel Disease 482
Allen L. Ginsberg

The Irritable Bowel Syndrome 488
Eamonn M. M. Quigley

**Hemorrhoids, Anal Fissure, and
Anorectal Abscess and Fistula** 492
John J. Murray

Peptic Ulcer Disease 496
Jay L. Goldstein
Peter M. Oshin

**Acute and Chronic Viral
Hepatitis** 501
Richard K. Sterling
Mitchell L. Shiffman

Malabsorption Syndromes 507
Charles M. Mansbach II

Acute Pancreatitis 514
Theodore N. Pappas
Bryan C. Weidner

Chronic Pancreatitis 518
James A. Madura II
Richard A. Prinz

Gastroesophageal Reflux Disease 524
Philip O. Katz
Donald O. Castell

Tumors of the Stomach 527
Martin S. Karpeh, Jr.

Tumors of the Colon and Rectum 532
Emina H. Huang
Richard L. Whelan

Intestinal Parasites 537
David R. Hill

SECTION 7. METABOLIC DISORDERS

Diabetes Mellitus in Adults 549
W. Timothy Garvey

**Diabetes Mellitus in Children
and Adolescents** 566
William V. Tamborlane
Joann Ahern

Diabetic Ketoacidosis 572
Eugenio Cersosimo

Hyperuricemia and Gout 576
Richard D. Brasington

Hyperlipoproteinemias 578
Peter H. Jones

Obesity 585
Peter D. Vash

Vitamin K Deficiency 592
Jack B. Alperin

Osteoporosis 593
Frederick R. Singer

Paget's Disease of Bone 597
Lorraine A. Fitzpatrick

Parenteral Nutrition in Adults 600
Timothy A. Pritts
David R. Fischer
Josef E. Fischer

**Parenteral Fluid Therapy
in Infants and Children** 607
Deborah P. Jones
Russell W. Chesney

SECTION 8. THE ENDOCRINE SYSTEM

Acromegaly 615
Mark E. Molitch

Adrenocortical Insufficiency 618
Hiralal Maheshwari
Jennifer Larsen

Cushing's Syndrome 621
Steven W. J. Lamberts

Diabetes Insipidus 624
Sumant S. Chugh
Henry M. Yager

**Hyperparathyroidism and
Hypoparathyroidism** 627
Elizabeth A. Streeten
Michael A. Levine

Primary Aldosteronism 634
David C. Kem

Hypopituitarism 635
Robert J. Anderson

Hyperprolactinemia 640
Janet A. Schlechte

Hypothyroidism 642
Gilbert H. Daniels

Hyperthyroidism 645
Jerome M. Hershman

Thyroid Cancer 648
Douglas W. Ball
Paul W. Ladenson

Pheochromocytoma 653
Brahm Shapiro
James C. Sisson
Milton D. Gross

Thyroiditis 657
Anthony P. Weetman

SECTION 9. THE UROGENITAL TRACT

**Bacterial Infections of the Urinary
Tract in Men** 661
Naiel N. Nassar
James W. Smith

**Bacterial Infections of the Urinary
Tract in Women** 662
Lisa D. Chew
Stephan D. Fihn

**Bacterial Infections of the Urinary
Tract in Girls** 666
Ross M. Decter

Childhood Enuresis 668
H. Gil Rushton

Urinary Incontinence 671
Roger R. Dmochowski

Epididymitis 674
Allan R. Ronald

Primary Glomerular Diseases 675
Brad H. Rovin

Acute Pyelonephritis 680
Richard S. Stack

Trauma to the Genitourinary Tract 682
J. Patrick Spirnak

Prostatitis 685
Ira W. Klimberg

Benign Prostatic Hyperplasia 687
E. Darracott Vaughan, Jr.
Aaron Perlmutter

Erectile Dysfunction (Impotence) 691
Sunil K. Purohit
Wayne J. G. Hellstrom

Acute Renal Failure 694
John Badalamenti
Robert L. Safirstein

Chronic Renal Failure 701
Paul J. Scheel, Jr.

**Malignant Tumors of the
Urogenital Tract** 705
William J. Ellis

Anterior Urethral Stricture 710
Kenneth W. Angermeier

Renal Calculi 712
Larry C. Munch

SECTION 10. THE SEXUALLY TRANSMITTED DISEASES

Chancroid 717
Stanley M. Spinola

Gonorrhea 718
Jeffrey P. Engel

Nongonococcal Urethritis 720
Heather Selman
Philip Hanno

Donovanosis (Granuloma Inguinale) 721
Paul M. Benson

Lymphogranuloma Venereum 722
Paul M. Benson

Syphilis 722
Michael Augenbraun

SECTION 11. DISEASES OF ALLERGY

Anaphylaxis and Serum Sickness 725
Stephen F. Kemp

Asthma in Adolescents and Adults 729
Jonathan Corren

Asthma in Children 735
Walter Torda

**Allergic Rhinitis Caused by
Inhalant Factors** 743
Fuad M. Baroody

Allergic Reactions to Drugs 748
Sandra Knowles
Neil H. Shear

Allergic Reactions to Insect Stings 753
David F. Graft

SECTION 12. DISEASES OF THE SKIN

Acne Vulgaris and Rosacea 757
Donald P. Lookingbill

Hair Disorders 759
Thomas N. Helm

Cancer of the Skin 763
Thomas E. Rohrer

Cutaneous T Cell Lymphomas 765
Gary S. Wood
Seth R. Stevens

Papulosquamous Diseases 770
Ann G. Martin
Jessica N. Mehta

**Autoimmune Connective Tissue
Disorders** 774
Daniel J. Wallace

Cutaneous Vasculitis 778
Carol A. Langford
Michael C. Sneller

Nail Disorders 780
Phoebe Rich

Keloids 783
Marlene S. Calderon
Warren L. Garner

Warts 785
Karen E. Zanol

Condyloma Acuminatum 787
Charles L. Heaton

Melanocytic Nevi (Moles) 788
Alan S. Boyd

Melanoma 790
Ira Davis

Premalignant Lesions 792
Heidi A. Waldorf

Bacterial Diseases of the Skin 794
V. Antoine Keller
Ronald Lee Nichols

Viral Skin Infections 799
Jessica L. Severson
Monica L. McCrary

Parasitic Diseases of the Skin 804
Donald J. Miech

Fungal Diseases of the Skin 806
Catherine C. Newman

Diseases of the Mouth 808
Henry W. Randle
Gayle L. McCloskey

Venous Leg Ulcers 817
David J. Margolis

Pressure Ulcers 819
David R. Thomas

Atopic Dermatitis 821
Adelaide A. Hebert
Khanh Nguyen

**Erythema Multiforme,
Stevens-Johnson Syndrome, and
Toxic Epidermal Necrolysis** 824
Jean-Claude Roujeau

Bullous Diseases 826
Neil J. Korman

Contact Dermatitis 830
Erin M. Warshaw

Skin Diseases of Pregnancy 831
Kathy Schwarzenberger

Pruritus Ani and Vulvae 833
Michael J. Adler

Urticaria and Angioedema 834
Clive E. H. Grattan

Pigmentary Disorders 837
Christy A. Lorton

Sunburn 841
Vincent A. DeLeo

SECTION 13. THE NERVOUS SYSTEM

Alzheimer's Disease 844
David A. Bennett

Intracerebral Hemorrhage 847
Adrian J. Goldszmidt
Louis R. Caplan

Ischemic Cerebrovascular Disease 850
Patrick D. Lyden

**Rehabilitation of the Stroke
Survivor** 853
Richard D. Zorowitz

**Seizures and Epilepsy in Adolescents
and Adults** 856
Bassel Abou-Khalil

Epilepsy in Infants and Children 867
W. Edwin Dodson

**Attention-Deficit/Hyperactivity
Disorder** 871
Timothy E. Wilens

Gilles de la Tourette Syndrome 874
Jeffrey Sverd

Headache 877
Elizabeth Loder

Episodic Vertigo 884
Ronald J. Tusa

Meniere's Disease 892
Michael D. Seidman

Viral Meningitis and Encephalitis 894
Vinodh Narayanan

Multiple Sclerosis 896
Mariko Kita
Donald E. Goodkin

Acquired Myasthenia Gravis 903
Janice M. Massey

Trigeminal Neuralgia 908
Robert M. Levy

Optic Neuritis 910
Roy W. Beck

Glaucoma 912
Louis B. Cantor

Acute Facial Paralysis (Bell's Palsy) 915
Bruce J. Gantz
Peter C. Weber

Parkinson's Disease 918
Joseph H. Friedman

Peripheral Neuropathies 924
Philip G. McManis

Acute Head Injuries in Adults 933
Sharon B. Marshall
Lawrence F. Marshall

Pediatric Head Injury 936
Fernando Stein
Jose A. Cortes

Brain Tumors 940
Daniel H. Lachance
Peter K. Dempsey

SECTION 14. THE LOCOMOTOR SYSTEM

Rheumatoid Arthritis 945
William S. Wilke

Juvenile Rheumatoid Arthritis 953
Suzanne L. Bowyer

Ankylosing Spondylitis 958
C. M. De Geus-Wenceslau
A. S. Russell

Temporomandibular Disorders 960
Major M. Ash, Jr.

**Bursitis, Tendinitis, Myofascial Pain,
and Fibromyalgia** 964
Thomas W. Jamieson

Osteoarthritis 967
Larissa Roux
Matthew H. Liang

**Polymyalgia Rheumatica and Giant
Cell Arteritis** 970
Gregory C. Gardner

Osteomyelitis 971
David W. Haas

Common Sports Injuries 974
Bradford H. Stiles

SECTION 15. OBSTETRICS AND GYNECOLOGY

Antepartum Care 979
Faith Joy Frieden

Ectopic Pregnancy 985
Bryan D. Cowan

**Vaginal Bleeding in the Third
Trimester** 986
Donna D. Johnson
J. Peter Vandorsten

**Hypertensive Disorders of
Pregnancy** 988
John T. Repke

Obstetric Anesthesia 995
Marie E. Minnich

Postpartum Care 999
R. Scott Rushing
James A. Thorp

Resuscitation of the Newborn 1001
  Caraciolo J. Fernandes

Care of the High-Risk Neonate 1007
  Dianne J. Albrecht
  David A. Clark

Normal Infant Feeding 1018
  James L. Sutphen
  Ana Abad-Sinden

Diseases of the Breast 1022
  Armando E. Giuliano
  Peter J. Bostick

Endometriosis 1029
  David Adamson

Dysfunctional Uterine Bleeding 1037
  Timothy R. Yeko
  Jeryl Natofsky

Amenorrhea 1040
  Owen K. Davis

Dysmenorrhea 1043
  Christine W. Jordan
  Andrew M. Kaunitz
  Deborah S. Lyon

Premenstrual Syndrome 1044
  M. L. Elks

Menopause 1047
  Murray A. Freedman

Vulvovaginitis 1053
  Maurizio Maccato

Chlamydia trachomatis Infection 1055
  Kimberly A. Workowski
  Carolyn M. Black

Pelvic Inflammatory Disease 1057
  John C. Petrozza
  Warner K. Huh

Leiomyomata 1060
  A. F. Haney

Cancer of the Endometrium 1063
  Mary L. Gemignani
  Richard R. Barakat

Cancer of the Uterine Cervix 1066
  Charles Levenback

Tumors of the Vulva 1069
  Bhagirath Majmudar

Contraception 1074
  Kathryn M. Andolsek

SECTION 16. PSYCHIATRIC DISORDERS

Alcohol-Related Problems 1090
  Robert G. Batey

Drug Abuse 1093
  Leslie K. Jacobsen
  Thomas R. Kosten

Anxiety Disorders 1098
  Naomi M. Simon
  Mark H. Pollack

Bulimia Nervosa 1102
  James E. Mitchell

Delirium 1105
  Sue Levkoff

Mood Disorders 1107
  Elliott Richelson

Schizophrenia 1117
  John G. Csernansky

Panic Disorder 1120
  Manuel E. Tancer

SECTION 17. PHYSICAL AND CHEMICAL INJURIES

Burns 1123
  Robert L. Sheridan

High-Altitude Sickness 1127
  Urs Scherrer
  Claudio Sartori

Disturbances Due to Cold 1130
  Gerald K. Bristow

Effects of Heat Stress 1135
  Jeff Faunt

Spider Bites and Scorpion Stings 1137
James R. Blackman

Snake Venom Poisoning 1139
Barry S. Gold

Marine Animal Injuries 1141
Bruce W. Halstead

Acute Poisonings 1144
Howard C. Mofenson
Thomas R. Caraccio
Joseph Greensher

SECTION 18. APPENDICES AND INDEX

**Reference Intervals for the
Interpretation of Laboratory Tests** 1205
William Z. Borer

New Drugs for 1998 1214
Gregory C. Tompkins

**Nomogram for the Determination
of Body Surface Area of Children
and Adults** 1217

Index 1219

Section 1
Symptomatic Care Pending Diagnosis

PAIN

method of
MARK J. STILLMAN, M.D.
Cleveland Clinic Foundation
Cleveland, Ohio

Pain is the most common reason why patients make appointments to visit a physician. In the United States, in addition to formal interaction with medical consultants, Americans spend a countless amount of money and effort to eradicate pain, through the use of over-the-counter medications, self-treatment, and alternative therapy. In spite of this, the U.S. medical system and medical education system lag far behind European counterparts in recognizing the fields of pain management and palliative medicine. National institutes of medicine in countries such as Italy and Sweden published guidelines and national policies on cancer pain management years before the U.S. Department of Health and Human Services' Agency for Health Care Policy and Research released the *Management of Cancer Pain** in March 1994. Only in the 1990s have state legislatures recognized the problem of intractable chronic (noncancer) pain as justification for the prolonged use of opioid medications. In spite of all this, patients continue to suffer from pain, because of much ignorance and bias.

DEFINITION OF PAIN

The International Association for the Study of Pain, whose American branch celebrated its 20th anniversary in 1998, defines pain as "an unpleasant sensory and emotional experience associated with actual or potential tissue damage, or described in terms of such damage. Pain is always subjective. Each person learns the application of the word through experiences related to injury in early life. It is unquestionably a sensation in a part or parts of the body, but it is always unpleasant and therefore an emotional experience." This definition is successful largely because it recognizes all dimensions of pain—physical, neurophysiologic, and emotional.

HISTORY TAKING AND PAIN ASSESSMENT

In an era in which the demands of practice administrators, insurers, and health maintenance organizations (HMOs) mandate that more patients be seen in shorter amounts of time, history taking and, in particular, pain assessment are easy casualties. Clinicians are prone to

---

*This book is available free to anyone from the National Cancer Institute at 1–800–4–CANCER.

forget that the patient with pain, if given enough time, will tell him the diagnosis. It is well worth rereading Cope's *The Diagnosis of the Acute Abdomen* (William Silen, ed.; Oxford University Press) as a refresher on pain history-taking skills and for its clear explanation of classification of pain. During the history taking, attention should be paid to the site and severity, the duration, and the quality of the pain. In research and in practice, many pain specialists assign a number, between 0 and 10, to the pain severity, but verbal qualifiers are also adequate (e.g., "mild," "moderate," or "severe"). A more useful task during the clinical interaction is to attempt to categorize the described pain to facilitate treatment.

One particularly useful classification divides pain into somatic (nociceptive), visceral, and neuropathic pain. *Somatic pain* has an aching or sharp quality, arising from stimulation of pain receptors (nociceptors) in the periphery and is easily localized. It may radiate to dermatomes, myotomes, or sclerotomes, and it is generally easy for the patient to describe in terms recognizable to the interviewer. *Visceral pain* is much more vaguely localized; it may have a diffuse, aching quality punctuated by cramps or waves of pain. What distinguishes visceral from other types of pain is its referral to distant, seemingly unrelated sites because of the site's shared embryologic origin with the distant dermatomal site. An example is shoulder (C4 dermatomal) pain associated with a subphrenic abscess and diaphragmatic irritation. *Neuropathic pain* follows damage to the central or peripheral nervous system; a classic example is postherpetic neuralgia. Patients experiencing this pain use descriptors such as "burning," "tearing," "numb," "dead," "cold," "woody," "shooting," and "jabbing," among others. There is much conjecture and research concerning the origin of this refractory type of pain; disinhibition of the nervous system can somehow lead to spontaneous pain symptoms of neuropathic character.

The importance of distinguishing one type of pain from another has to do with the ability to predict a clinical response to a specific drug class. For example, somatic pain tends to respond to nonsteroidal anti-inflammatory drugs (NSAIDs), whose mode of action is to block production of prostaglandin E_2, a mediator of pain transduction at the pain receptor. Opioid analgesics, such as morphine and related agents, work both peripherally at the level of the nociceptor and centrally in the spinal cord and brain stem, successfully relieving somatic pain. Somatic pain therefore is traditionally considered opioid-responsive pain. Visceral pain, the result of stimulation of pain receptors in the viscera, is also opioid responsive and may respond to other agents, such as NSAIDs. According to classical teaching, however, neuropathic pain is opioid resistant and may respond better to classes of drugs prescribed by neurologists, psychiatrists, and anesthesiologists —anticonvulsants, tri-

1

cyclic antidepressants (TCADs), and lidocaine derivatives—better known as adjuvant analgesics.

PRINCIPLES OF PAIN MANAGEMENT

The goals of all pain management are to eliminate the cause and, at the same time, palliate the pain and associated morbidity. The cause of pain may not be realized in chronic cancer and noncancer pain, and symptomatic pain control is the only reasonable goal. Much has been written on cancer pain management, and the tenets of cancer pain management are applicable to the office management of pain in general. As discussed in the literature, they are (1) by mouth (use the oral route, if possible); (2) by the clock (treat constant pain with time-contingent, and not as-needed, dosing of medications; (3) by the analgesic stepladder (mild pain is treated with mild analgesics; stronger or increasing pain is treated with larger doses of opioids or more potent opioids); (4) to make use of adjuvant analgesics, in addition to opioids, to enhance the pain relief; and (5) to reassess the patient often for analgesia and drug-induced side effects.

TREATMENT

The three classes of analgesics essential for the palliation of pain are the nonopioid analgesics, the adjuvant analgesics, and the opioid analgesics. As the field of pain and palliative medicine grows, new medications, routes of delivery, and techniques will continue to emerge. A strong basic foundation will, however, always remain integral to pain management in daily practice.

Nonopioid Analgesics

Acetaminophen (Tylenol), available worldwide, is a general-purpose analgesic with antipyretic properties. Its mechanism of action remains obscure, but when used alone or when added to other analgesics, it can be very useful. For the treatment of severe pain of cancer, it can be used as a co-analgesic with opioids. It has a ceiling dose effect, a dose above which no further analgesia, but increased toxicity, is achieved. This dose is approximately 650 mg every 4 hours, and particular attention should be paid to patients with impaired liver function. Clinicians need to keep in mind that acetaminophen is frequently combined with other analgesics in a number of over-the-counter pain relievers, and the amount of acetaminophen consumed may limit the number of pills the patient can safely take. Examples of such combinations are acetaminophen, aspirin, and caffeine (Excedrin Migraine); acetaminophen, butalbital, and caffeine (e.g., Fioricet); acetaminophen and oxycodone (e.g., Percocet); and acetaminophen and hydrocodone (e.g., Vicodin).

Nonsteroidal Anti-Inflammatory Drugs

The NSAIDs are classic examples of useful but potentially toxic nonopioid analgesics, and their widespread use has been fostered by the availability of over-the-counter, lower dose formulations of ibuprofen (Motrin, Advil), naproxen (Aleve), and ketoprofen (Orudis KT). Previous editions of this book have discussed the use of NSAIDs in detail, stressing their particular role in the management of metastatic and inflammatory bone and joint pain. Physicians have generally chosen NSAIDs on the basis of their efficacy, safety profile, cost, and ease of use, and have learned how to manage patients with several NSAIDs well. The development of highly specific NSAIDs heralds a new chapter of improved care with these agents.

NSAIDs exert their antipyretic and anti-inflammatory action by blocking the production of prostaglandins, particularly PGE_2 through the inhibition of the cyclooxygenase (COX) enzyme. COX exists in two isoforms: the constitutive form (COX-1) and inducible form (COX-2). COX-1 is essential for maintaining normal physiologic functions, such as renal blood flow, gastric mucosal integrity, endothelial antithrombogenic homeostasis, and platelet aggregability, whereas COX-2 is induced in a number of cells by proinflammatory stimuli, leading to the development of pain and inflammation. The pharmacologic goal has always been to find potent inhibitors of COX-2, not of COX-1, but traditional NSAIDs have been more potent inhibitors of COX-1 than of COX-2. A new subclass of NSAIDs is being introduced that preferentially inhibits COX-2, leading not only to the reduction of inflammation but also to the reduction of the risk of side effects. Meloxicam* in daily doses of 7.5 or 15 mg is as effective against pain and disability from osteoarthritis and rheumatoid arthritis as piroxicam (Feldene), 20 mg a day; naproxen (Naprosyn and others), 750 mg a day; or diclofenac (Voltaren and others), 100 mg a day. Celecoxib (Celebrex), a COX-2 inhibitor, has been approved by the FDA. The dose is 100 to 200 mg per day in one or two divided doses. This new class of anti-inflammatory drugs with analgesic properties and low gastrointestinal and renal side effects shows great promise.

Adjuvant Analgesics

This class of analgesics is distinguished from the opioids and the nonopioid analgesics by having been developed for purposes other than for pain. These drugs exhibit three important properties: (1) they have independent analgesic properties; (2) they augment the analgesia of opioids and may be opioid sparing; and (3) they have useful side effects, which relate to their original purposes for use. Among the members of this class are the tricyclic antidepressants, anticonvulsants, lidocaine derivatives, certain antihistamines, and central nervous system (CNS) stimulants. The adjuvant analgesics are especially well suited for treating neuropathic pain, and this is not surprising inasmuch as many were developed as

---

*Not available in the United States.

CNS drugs. Careful assessment of the patient's pain may aid the clinician in correctly choosing one of these agents.

Antihistamines

Hydroxyzine (Vistaril) has traditionally been the non-narcotic half of a parenteral mixture (with an opioid) used to treat acute pain in the emergency department. Studies have demonstrated its analgesic properties in doses of 25 to 50 mg every 4 to 6 hours intramuscularly, and hydroxyzine has been used orally with oral opioids, whereby it also functions as a mild antiemetic. Another antihistamine with analgesic properties is cyproheptadine (Periactin), useful as a migraine prophylactic in doses of 2 to 16 mg, or higher, orally at bedtime.

CNS Stimulants

When combined with opioids for the treatment of cancer pain, CNS stimulants counteract the sedating effects of opioids and augment their analgesic properties and clinical versatility. Studies have demonstrated that this group of agents has independent analgesic properties. Methylphenidate* (Ritalin) is used in doses of 2.5 to 20 mg orally twice a day (bid) (early in the morning and in the afternoon). Other effective agents include dextroamphetamine* (Dexedrine), 5 to 10 mg bid, which is also available as a parenteral preparation and as the less cardiostimulatory pemoline* (Cylert). Pemoline is prescribed in doses of 18.75 to 37.5 mg orally bid. The CNS stimulants have also found a niche as rapid-acting antidepressants in palliative medicine.

Anticonvulsants

Anticonvulsants remain a class of effective analgesics, particularly for neuropathic pain. In the United States, carbamazepine (Tegretol) was initially approved by the Food and Drug Administration (FDA) for managing trigeminal neuralgia and later was accepted as an anticonvulsant. Anticonvulsant therapy has generally been applied to lancinating and jabbing neuropathic pain (ticlike) but is also effective for other manifestations of neuropathic pain, such as cramping pain, aching pain, and even burning pain in such disorders as diabetic neuropathy. Dosages (100 to 200 mg bid and higher) tend to be lower than those used in seizure management. Phenytoin* (Dilantin) and valproic acid* (Depakote and Depakene) have a less established track record for the management of neuropathic pain disorders, but pain specialists employ them as a second resort. Valproic acid has a well-established role as a migraine prophylactic, and doses are similar to those used for antiepileptic activity. There has been intense interest in newer anticonvulsants, particularly gabapentin* (Neurontin), since the publication of anecdotal re-

ports of successful treatment of reflex sympathetic dystrophy and thalamic pain. There is substantial evidence that gabapentin is better than placebo for the management of diabetic neuropathic pain and postherpetic neuralgia (constant burning and intermittent shooting pain) in doses as high as 1200 mg three times a day. Specialists may push the dose higher than 3600 mg a day in more refractory cases, especially because sedation and dizziness are not as problematic with this drug as with other anticonvulsants.

Lidocaine Derivatives

Mexiletine* (Mexitil) and flecainide* (Tambocor) have been used as second-line agents for neuropathic pain. Mexiletine has the best studied track record for diabetic pain and is effective orally in divided doses as high as 900 mg a day. Dizziness and nausea can be problematic, and the risk from and side effects of overdosing are identical to those of intravenous lidocaine.

Antidepressants

Through modulation of descending and ascending antinociceptive pathways in the spinal cord and brain, antidepressants have been established as some of the most effective analgesics. In particular, the tricyclic class, developed in the 1950s, remains the standard against which all others are judged. Well-designed studies show that amitriptyline* (Elavil), nortriptyline* (Pamelor), and desipramine* (Norpramin) are more effective than either placebo or fluoxetine* (Prozac) for diabetic pain and postherpetic neuralgia. In smaller doses than those used to treat depression, these medications can rapidly alleviate burning and jabbing neuropathic pain, reduce the need for opioids, and promote appetite and sleep. Ten to 25 mg is the starting dose, usually given at night (desipramine is given in the morning), and the dose is titrated up to 75 to 150 mg, by 10 to 25 mg every 3 to 4 days, until analgesia or side effects intervene. Once the dose is above 50 mg, it is advisable to check levels if long-term therapy is anticipated, because individual metabolism rates are not predictable from one patient to another. Side effects such as sedation, confusion and hallucinations, dry mouth, urinary retention, orthostatic hypotension, and weight gain are the most worrisome and may preclude the use of TCADs.

The selective serotonin reuptake inhibitors (SSRIs) are a new class of antidepressants, which, with the exception of headache management and diabetic neuropathy, have no proven track record. Fluoxetine* (Prozac) in doses of 20 to 60 mg every morning, has been effective in the management of chronic daily headache, and the other SSRIs have been used for similar purposes by headache clinics. Paroxetine*

---

*Not FDA approved for this indication.

*Not FDA approved for this indication.

(Paxil) was effective for diabetic neuropathic pain in one study.

Opioid Analgesics

Opioids remain the cornerstone in the treatment of moderate to severe pain, especially acute postoperative and cancer pain. Morphine and related compounds have been valued for centuries, and yet ignorance, bias, and fear have curtailed the use of these essential drugs. Pain specialists readily admit that opioids are perhaps the safest, most effective, and most predictable of all the strong analgesics currently available. Several misconceptions, shared by many medical personnel, patients, and regulators, concerning the definitions of physical dependence, tolerance, and addiction impede the proper use of opioids. *Tolerance* is the need for larger doses or more frequent dosing of any medication in order to achieve the same effect. It is a manifestation of receptor-ligand physiology and is to be expected. It differs from *physical dependence*, manifested by the development of a withdrawal phenomenon either when too rapid a taper of an opioid ensues or when an opioid antagonist is administered. In contrast to common belief, the development of tolerance or physical dependence is not synonymous with addiction, also referred to as psychological dependence. *Addiction* is a form of sociopathic behavior in which a person uses opioids for purposes other than pain control and over which he or she has no control. This overwhelming desire for the opioid leads to self-destructive behavior, such as lying and theft, and continues in spite of legal and personal difficulties. In contrast to patients in pain who require opioid analgesia, the opioid addict uses the drug to escape life, not to reenter it.

Since the 1950s, morphine sulfate has been the standard against which all opioid analgesics have been compared and continues to remain the most versatile agent because it can be administered by mouth, under the tongue, parenterally (intramuscularly [IM], subcutaneously [SC], and intravenously [IV]), rectally, epidurally, or intrathecally. Clinicians should become familiar with the actions of morphine and several other commonly available opioid analgesics, such as hydromorphone (Dilaudid) and oxycodone (OxyContin, Oxy IR), if they plan to prescribe these medications. Table 1 compares the morphine-like opioids and provides a guide to dosing with morphine sulfate, 10 mg IM or IV, as the reference point. This chart allows the user to easily interchange doses of the drug when switching from one route of administration to another. For example, 5 mg of parenteral morphine every 4 hours (e.g., IV infusion or intermittent IV or SC bolus) is "equianalgesic" to 15 mg of oral morphine every 4 hours and to 30 mg of delayed-release morphine every 8 hours. In addition, one opioid can be switched to another according to this table, although it must be kept in mind that there is a phenomenon of incomplete cross-tolerance, referring to the fact that different opioids bind CNS opioid receptors differently and a smaller than equianalge-

TABLE 1. **Opioid Equivalency Chart for the Treatment of Chronic Cancer Pain***

Drug	Equianalgesic Dose	Relative Potency in Comparison with Parenteral MS	Approximate Duration of Action (Hours)
Morphine			
Parenteral	10 mg	1.00	3.5–4
Oral	30 mg	0.33	3.5–4
Hydromorphone			
Parenteral	1.5 mg	6.67	3.5–4
Oral	7.5 mg	1.33	3.5–4
Oxycodone			
Parenteral	—	—	—
Oral	30 mg	0.33	3.5–4
Levorphanol			
Parenteral	2 mg	5.00	>5
Oral	4 mg	2.50	>5
Meperidine†			
Parenteral	75 mg	0.13	3–3.5
Oral	300 mg	0.03	3–3.5
Methadone‡			
Parenteral	10 mg	1.00	>5
Oral	20 mg	0.50	>5
Fentanyl (patch)			
Transdermal	~50 µg	200.00	<1
Buprenorphine			
Parenteral	0.3 mg	25.00	6–8
Sublingual	0.4 mg	25.00	6–8

*Acute pain studies performed by Raymond Houde et al. in the 1950s did not demonstrate the analgesic potency of codeine or propoxyphene to be any greater than that of aspirin or actaminophen.

Switching a patient from one opioid to another opioid: With the exception of methadone and levorphanol, the clinician should use approximately ½ the equianalgesic dose, provided on a divided, time-contingent basis. With methadone, ¼ or ⅛ the equianalgesic dose should be provided on a q 6–8 h prn schedule for the first 48–72 h. The total daily requirements can then be given on a divided, time-contingent schedule.

†Meperidine is not recommended for chronic therapy of pain because its metabolite, normeperidine, is a central nervous system toxin and tends to accumulate in patients with renal insufficiency. Seizures and death have resulted from normeperidine toxicity.

‡The use of methadone should be undertaken by clinicians familiar with its use; the analgesic duration varies markedly in some patients with its serum half-life (18–36 h). Methadone may therefore accumulate and lead to side effects.

sic dose of the new opioid may be required. One half the equianalgesic dose, calculated from the table, is a reasonable starting point.

Several principles regarding opioid prescribing require emphasis. The opioids theoretically have no ceiling analgesic effect, and the smallest dose necessary to control pain is the dose that should be used. For a patient who has never been treated with opioids, 1 to 2 mg of parenteral morphine (or equivalent opioid) might suffice, whereas a patient treated chronically with opioids generally requires much higher doses. There is no formula to determine the correct dose for an individual, and experience and vigilance are necessary. Side effects from opioids are a major concern. Although pain is the best antidote to the sedating effects of opioid analgesics, first-time users should be observed for several hours for respiratory suppression. As a rule, if a patient can be easily aroused at the peak of the drug's effect, respiratory suppression should not be a concern. With time, the sedating and nauseating effects of opioids dissipate, but the constipating effects tend to persist. All patients should therefore be considered candidates for bowel regimens, such as bulking agents, stool softeners (docusate [Colace], 100 mg bid) and bowel stimulants (e.g., senna tablets, up to 6 to 12 per day). It cannot be overemphasized that constant pain warrants constant analgesia, and patients should receive opioid analgesics (and adjuvant analgesics) on a time-contingent—not as-needed—basis.

Methadone, although inexpensive and the center of a resurgence in clinical interest, should remain in the domain of physicians who understand its clinical pharmacodynamics. Its serum half-life is much longer than its clinical analgesic half-life and there may be a tendency to oversedate patients with it. Other opioid medications, such as meperidine (Demerol) and the partial antagonists/partial agonists pentazocine (Talwin), butorphanol (Stadol), and nalbuphine (Nubain), should be avoided in the management of chronic painful states. The latter group of medications can cause nightmares, hallucinations, and intense dysphoria and may induce withdrawal in patients who are physically dependent on a pure morphine-like agonist. Meperidine, when given in repeated doses over a period of time, is metabolized to a toxic metabolite that is excreted by the kidney. This metabolite, normeperidine, is a naloxone (Narcan)–unresponsive CNS toxin, and its accumulation may lead to seizures and death, especially in patients with impaired renal function. A similar phenomenon has been reported with propoxyphene (Darvon and others), the common weak oral opioid analgesic.

Nonmedicinal Approaches to Pain

Clinicians experienced in the management of pain readily admit that the treatment of chronic pain states, such as chronic noncancer pain, differs substantially from chronic cancer pain. As mentioned earlier, pain is an emotional experience that carries social, psychologic, and spiritual consequences and is likewise affected by a patient's past experiences. Multidisciplinary clinics that stress psychologic, physical, and occupational therapy, group therapy, and social work deemphasize medication as a "cure-all" and play a vital role in the reintegration of these patients into society. Expert consultation from pain management specialists should help initiate this therapy, if indicated.

NAUSEA AND VOMITING

method of
MARTIN J. EDELMAN, M.D.,
DONALD F. LUM, M.D., and
DAVID R. GANDARA, M.D.
University of California, Davis
Sacramento, California
VA Northern California Health Care System
Martinez, California

Nausea and vomiting are common symptoms that occur throughout life. These symptoms may reflect benign, self-limiting illnesses or more serious, debilitating diseases. Nausea is a vague sensation of sickness or "queasiness" that refers to the urge to vomit. Vomiting refers to the expulsion of gastric contents up through and out of the mouth. This occurs by a forceful, sustained contraction of abdominal muscles and the diaphragm through a relaxed lower esophageal sphincter and contracted pylorus. Retching is the rhythmic movement of vomiting without expulsion of gastric contents (dry heaves). It consists of spasmodic respiratory and abdominal movements and often culminates in vomiting. Vomiting should be distinguished from *regurgitation,* which refers to the act by which gastric contents are brought back into the mouth without the motor and autonomic activity that characterizes vomiting. Regurgitation is a symptom of free gastroesophageal reflux or an obstructed esophagus, whether obstructed mechanically from a benign or malignant stricture or physiologically from an esophageal motility disorder.

Control of vomiting occurs in the vomiting center, which is thought to arise within the lateral reticular formation, adjacent to the medulla oblongata areas, that coordinates respiratory, salivary, and vasomotor centers and the vagus nervous innervation of the gastrointestinal tract. The vomiting center can be stimulated by four different sources of afferent input, which include the following:

1. The chemoreceptor trigger zone: located in the area postrema on the floor of the fourth ventricle. This area has chemoreceptors that are responsive to various drugs and chemotherapeutic agents, toxins, hypoxia, uremia, acidosis, and radiation therapy. Evidence suggests that type 3 serotonin, dopamine D_2, and neurokinin-1 (NK-1) receptors as well as other neurotransmitters such as norepinephrine, glutamate, histamine, and endorphins play a role in mediating vomiting in the chemoreceptor trigger zone.
2. Higher central nervous system (CNS) centers: CNS disorders or certain smells, sights, or previously emotional experiences may result in nausea and vomiting.
3. The vestibular system: often stimulated by infections and motion. These fibers have high concentrations of muscarinic, cholinergic, and histamine H_1 receptors.
4. Afferent vagal fibers and splanchnic fibers from gastrointestinal viscera: often stimulated by gastrointestinal or biliary distention, peritoneal or mucosal irritation, or intra-abdominal infections.

Although nausea and vomiting may be evoked by disorders of the gastrointestinal tract, they may also reflect neurologic, psychogenic, endocrine, metabolic, toxic, or iatrogenic conditions and are common symptoms of pediatric illnesses (Table 1). Whereas nausea has few serious physical consequences, prolonged vomiting can lead to volume depletion, electrolyte depletion, acid-base disorders, malnutrition, pulmonary aspiration, esophageal rupture (Boer-

TABLE 1. **Causes of Nausea and Vomiting**

Acute Nausea and Vomiting

Pediatric

Atresia
Feeding disorder
Foreign body
Gastroesophageal reflux
Hirschsprung's disease
Intussusception
Meconium-ileus
Meningitis
Necrotizing enterocolitis
Peritonitis
Pyloric stenosis
Reye's syndrome
Subdural hematoma
Tracheoesophageal fistula
Volvulus or malrotation of gut

Infections

Viral gastroenteritis (Norwalk agent, rotavirus)
Toxin-mediated (food poisoning)
  Staphylococcus aureus
  Bacillus cereus
  Clostridium perfringens
Acute systemic infections
Infections in immunocompromised hosts

Central Nervous System

Motion sickness
Labyrinthitis (Meniere's disease)
Migraine headaches
Central nervous system (CNS) trauma
CNS tumors or pseudotumors
Meningitis, encephalitis, abscess
Epilepsy

Gastrointestinal Mechanical Obstruction

Acute gastric outlet obstruction
  Pyloric channel ulcer (peptic ulcer disease)
Constipation
  Fecal impaction
  Obstipation
Extrinsic small bowel obstruction
Incarcerated hernia
Volvulus
Adhesions
Internal hernias
Superior mesenteric artery syndrome
Ileus
  Postoperative
  Medical illness
  Gallstone

Visceral Pain

Appendicitis
Acute pancreatitis
Acute cholecystitis
Hepatitis
Peritonitis from any cause
Mesenteric ischemia

Systemic Conditions

Pregnancy
Myocardial infarction
Renal failure
Diabetic ketoacidosis
Hypercalcemia
Hyperparathyroidism
Graft-versus-host disease

Iatrogenic

Chemotherapeutic agents
Radiation therapy
Surgery
Heavy ethanol ingestion
Medications
  Nonsteroidal anti-inflammatory drugs
  Antibiotics
  Digoxin
  Theophylline
  Narcotics
  Niacin

Chronic Nausea and Vomiting

Gastrointestinal Mechanical Obstruction

Chronic gastric outlet obstruction
  Chronic peptic ulcer disease
  Gastric malignancy
  Crohn's disease with duodenal stricture
  Pancreatic malignancy
Small intestinal obstruction
Peritoneal carcinomatosis

Motility Disorders

Gastroparesis
  Diabetes mellitus
  Collagen vascular disorders (scleroderma)
  Postgastric surgery
  Idiopathic or iatrogenic
Small intestine motility disorders
  Chronic intestinal pseudo-obstruction
  Paraneoplastic syndromes
  Amyloidosis

Psychogenic

Anorexia nervosa
Bulimia
Psychogenic, anxiety

Miscellaneous

Increased intracranial pressure
Pseudotumor
Metabolic: hyperthyroidism, renal failure, Addison's disease
Medications (cardiac glycosides, narcotics, theophylline)
Pregnancy
Idiopathic cyclic vomiting

haave's syndrome), and gastrointestinal hemorrhage secondary to mucosal tear at the gastroesophageal junction (Mallory-Weiss tear).

CLINICAL FINDINGS

Symptoms and Signs

A thorough medical history and physical examination are essential to determine the etiology of nausea and vomiting. Acute onset of symptoms without abdominal pain is typically associated with infectious causes (gastroenteritis, food poisoning) or medications. In these instances, a careful history should be taken, focusing on recent medications; food ingestions; related viral symptoms of fever, diarrhea, and malaise; and similar illnesses in family members or coworkers. The acute onset of pain suggests visceral involvement associated with peritoneal inflammation, pancreatobiliary illnesses, or intestinal obstruction. Special attention to the physical examination may reveal tympany, focal tenderness, rebound, and guarding.

Chronic nausea or vomiting may suggest gastric outlet obstruction, gastroparesis, intestinal dysmotility, psychogenic disorders, CNS diseases, pregnancy, or other systemic disorders. In these instances, the timing of the emesis in relation to meals and the nature of the vomiting may provide clues to the specific etiology. Vomiting immediately after meals suggests bulimia or other psychogenic causes but may also occur in peptic ulcer disease with associated pyloric stenosis. Vomiting undigested food 1 hour or more after meals may be seen in esophageal dysmotility (achalasia), gastroparesis (diabetic, postvagotomy), or gastric outlet obstruction from malignancies (gastric or pancreatic) or peptic ulcer disease. Early morning vomiting may suggest pregnancy, alcoholism, or uremia. Vomiting associated with headache, neck stiffness, vertigo, paresthesias, or neuromuscular weakness may be related to CNS disorders and other causes of increased intracranial pressure. In these patients, careful neurologic and funduscopic examination are essential.

Orthostatic vital signs, along with skin turgor and appearance of mucous membranes, should be checked to rule out volume depletion. Malnutrition and weight loss suggest more chronic conditions such as malignancy, inflammatory bowel disease, or scleroderma. Tympany and abdominal distention raise the suspicion of small intestinal obstruction. A succussion splash is usually present with gastric outlet obstruction or severe gastroparesis. A check of hernia orifices should be performed with careful attention to previous surgical scars.

Laboratory Findings

Depending on the clinical presentation, laboratory studies should include serum electrolytes, glucose, calcium, amylase, lipase, creatinine, liver panel, and β-human chorionic gonadotropin for females of child-bearing age. Protracted vomiting may result in various metabolic imbalances, including metabolic alkalosis, hypokalemia, hyponatremia, and prerenal azotemia.

Special Examinations

In addition to routine laboratory data, flat and upright plain films of the abdomen may be indicated to look for intestinal obstruction or free peritoneal air. In patients with suspected obstruction, a nasogastric tube may be inserted to relieve symptoms. Aspiration of more than 200 mL of gastric fluid in a patient who has been fasting suggests gastroparesis or gastric outlet obstruction. One can confirm this with a saline load test (greater than 400 mL residual 30 minutes after 750 mL instillation via nasogastric tube) or, better yet, with upper gastrointestinal endoscopy. Nuclear scintigraphy should be performed when upper endoscopy or barium upper gastrointestinal testing is unrevealing to confirm gastroparesis. Abdominal ultrasound or computed tomography (CT) scanning can be performed if laboratory data suggest hepatobiliary or pancreatic pathology. Head CT or magnetic resonance imaging (MRI) should be considered for suspected CNS disorders.

TREATMENT

General Measures

The treatment of nausea and vomiting should be directed at the underlying cause as suggested by results of the history, physical examination, laboratory data, and other specific tests. The majority of acute causes are mild, self-limiting illnesses that often require no specific therapy. Patients should maintain hydration by ingesting clear liquids (broth, tea, carbonated beverages, sports beverages such as Gatorade) and small quantities of bland dry food. Hospitalization is required for more severe vomiting that leads to severe volume depletion and subsequent hypokalemia and metabolic alkalosis. Parenteral volume replacement using 0.45% saline with 20 mEq per liter potassium supplementation is often necessary. Placement of a nasogastric tube for suctioning promotes gastric decompression and enables a more accurate assessment of fluid losses.

Pharmacologic

If general measures fail to control the nausea and vomiting, pharmacologic therapy is given to prevent or control vomiting. Given the multitude of causes and various mechanisms involved in the control of nausea and vomiting, no single pharmacologic agent is effective for all patients. Table 2 lists many of the antiemetic agents available in the United States. Most of the agents listed are effective for nausea and vomiting due to a variety of causes. The type 3 serotonin antagonists are utilized primarily in the prevention and treatment of chemotherapy-, radiation-, and anesthesia-associated nausea and vomiting. They are relatively ineffective in the treatment of motion sickness. Conversely, transdermal scopolamine (Transderm Scōp) is primarily indicated for the treatment of motion sickness. Cisapride (Propulsid) and metoclopramide (Reglan), although effective in treating nausea and vomiting from a variety of causes, are particularly effective in treating gastroparesis-associated disease. Combination therapy with two or more agents from different drug classes is often required, and therapy should be individualized based on the cause of the vomiting. Most of the medications listed in Table 2 should be avoided in

TABLE 2. **Antiemetic Drugs**

Agents	Dose/Schedule	Route	Cost (U.S. $)*
Phenothiazines			
Prochlorperazine (Compazine)	5–10 mg q 6–8 h	PO, IV, IM	.66/5-mg tab
	25 mg q 6–8 h	PR	
Thiethylperazine (Torecan)	10 mg q 8 h	PO, IV, IM, PR	.54/10-mg tab
Butyrophenones			
Droperidol (Inapsine)	5–15 mg × 1, 2–7.5 mg q 2 h	IV	3.16/5 mg IV
Cannabinoids			
Dronabinol (Marinol)	5–10 mg/m² q 3–4 h	PO	3.16/5-mg tab
Corticosteroids			
Dexamethasone	10–20 mg q 2–6 h	PO, IV	30.55/20 mg IV
Antihistamines			
Diphenhydramine (Benadryl)	50 mg q 4–6 h	IV, PO	1.52/50 mg IV
Substituted benzamides			
Metoclopramide (Reglan)	1–3 mg/kg† q 2 h × 2–5 doses	IV	24.52/150 mg IV
	0.5–3 mg/kg† q 2–6 h	PO	
Benzodiazepines			
Diazepam (Valium)	5 mg q 4 h	PO, IV	2.08/5 ml IV
	1.5–2.5 mg/m² q 4 h	IV, SL	
Lorazepam (Ativan)	1–4 mg q 4 h	PO	12.01/2 mg IV
Type 3 serotonin antagonists			
Ondansetron (Zofran)	32 mg/24 h	IV	206.41/32 mg IV
	8 mg/24 h‡	IV	
	8 mg bid	PO	19.62/8-mg tab
Granisetron (Kytril)	10 µg/kg/24 h	IV	173.95/1 mg IV
	2 mg/24 h	PO	41.28/1-mg tab
Dolasetron (Anzemet)	1.8 mg/kg/24 h	IV	149.88/100 mg IV
	100 mg/24 h	PO	66/100-mg tab
Tropisetron (Navoban)§	5 mg/24 h	IV	
Prokinetic			
Cisapride (Propulsid)	10 mg 30 min ac and hs	PO	.75/10-mg tab
Anticholinergic			
Scopolamine	1 patch behind ear 30 min before travel	Transdermal	N/A

*Prices based on average wholesale price of brand name product in 1997 U.S. dollars.
†Exceeds dosage recommended by the manufacturer.
‡Recommended dose (see text).
§Not available in the United States.

pregnancy; however, the use of the dopamine antagonist droperidol and the antihistamine trimethobenzamide (Tigan) is common in pregnancy.

CHEMOTHERAPY-INDUCED EMESIS

Cancer chemotherapy is one of the most common causes of iatrogenic nausea and vomiting. Consequently, it is the best studied and serves as the model for other types of treatment-induced nausea and vomiting such as those that are induced by anesthesia or radiotherapy.

Significance of Chemotherapy-Induced Emesis

In addition to patient discomfort, chemotherapy-induced emesis may result in potentially life-threatening complications. Nausea and vomiting induced by chemotherapy may be so significant that patients may refuse to receive potentially curative chemotherapy. Before the introduction of the type 3 serotonin antagonist drugs, chemotherapy-induced nausea and vomiting was the most significant concern of cancer

patients. In addition, the adverse effects on nutritional status, already frequently compromised as a result of malignancy, may be severely aggravated and may lead to diminished muscle mass, fatigue, and increased susceptibility to infection, with potentially fatal consequences.

Types of Chemotherapy-Induced Emesis

Three patterns of emetic response are associated with chemotherapy. Anticipatory vomiting occurs before therapy and usually, although not always, occurs after an initial adverse outcome (in terms of nausea and vomiting) in a prior cycle of treatment. Immediate vomiting occurs minutes to 24 hours after administration of chemotherapy and is the best understood. It is a result of release of serotonin from enterochromaffin cells in the gut mucosa. The surge in serotonin acts peripherally through the vagus nerve and centrally at the chemoreceptor trigger zone. Delayed vomiting occurs 24 to 120 hours after treatment and is poorly understood. It appears to be mediated at least partially by type 3 serotonin receptors, as some, but not all, studies indicate amelioration of this problem with continued administration of type 3 serotonin antagonists. An accumulating body of evidence implicates substance P, a tachykinin distributed throughout the peripheral system and CNS that binds to NK-1 receptors in this problem. Trials of substance P antagonists in humans are under way.

Drugs Associated with Chemotherapy-Induced Emesis

There is enormous variation in the potential of various drugs to produce an emetic response. Many drugs have little or no emetic potential. In the case

TABLE 3. **Emetogenic Potential of Single Chemotherapy Agents**

Level	Frequency of Emesis (%)	Agent
5	>90	Carmustine >250 mg/m^2 Cisplatin >50 mg/m^2 Cyclophosphamide >1500 mg/m^2 Dacarbazine Mechlorethamine Streptozocin
4	60–90	Carboplatin Carmustine <250 mg/m^2 Cisplatin <50 mg/m^2 Cyclophosphamide >750 mg/m^2, <1500 mg/m^2 Cytarabine >1 g/m^2 Doxorubicin >60 mg/m^2 Methotrexate >1000 mg/m^2 Procarbazine (oral)
3	30–60	Cyclophosphamide <750 mg/m^2 Cyclophosphamide (oral) Doxorubicin 20–60 mg/m^2 Epirubicin <90 mg/m^2 Hexamethylmelamine (oral) Idarubicin Ifosfamide Methotrexate 250–1000 mg/m^2 Mitoxantrone <15 mg/m^2
2	10–30	Docetaxel Etoposide 5-Fluorouracil <1000 mg/m^2 Gemcitabine Methotrexate >50 mg/m^2, <250 mg/m^2 Mitomycin Paclitaxel
1	<10	Bleomycin Busulfan Chlorambucil (oral) 2-Chloro-2-deoxyadenosine Fludarabine Hydroxyurea Methotrexate <50 mg/m^2 L-phenylalanine mustard (oral) Thioguanine (oral) Vinblastine Vincristine Vinorelbine

Note: Proportion of patients who experience emesis in the absence of effective antiemetic prophylaxis.

From Hesketh PJ, Kris MG, Grunberg SM, et al: Proposal for classifying the acute emetogenicity of cancer chemotherapy. J Clin Oncol 15:103–109, 1997.

TABLE 4. **Algorithm for Defining the Emetogenicity of Combination Chemotherapy**

1. Identify the most emetogenic agent in the combination.
2. Assess the relative contribution of other agents to the emetogenicity of the combination. When considering other agents, the following rules apply:
   a. Level 1 agents do not contribute to the emetogenicity of a given regimen.
   b. Adding 1 or more level 2 agents increases the emetogenicity of the combination by one level greater than the most emetogenic agent in the combination.
   c. Adding level 3 or 4 agents increases the emetogenicity of the combination by one level per agent.

From Hesketh PJ, Kris MG, Grunberg SM, et al: Proposal for classifying the acute emetogenicity of cancer chemotherapy. J Clin Oncol 15:103–109, 1997.

of glucocorticoids (e.g., dexamethasone, prednisone), which are integral parts of regimens in lymphoma and myeloma, they are antiemetic. Table 3 lists chemotherapy drugs with their degree of emetic potential. Research in antiemetics has focused on the problem of the emetic potential of combination chemotherapy regimens. As it is relatively rare for a patient to be treated with a single agent, it is important to assess the potential of a combination of drugs to produce emesis and prescribe an appropriate antiemetic regimen. An approach for determining the emetic potential of combination chemotherapy regimens is presented in Table 4.

Factors Contributing to Chemotherapy-Induced Emesis

It has long been recognized that patient variables significantly affect the occurrence and severity of chemotherapy-induced emesis. Factors predicting for emesis include female sex, age younger than 40 years, history of emesis associated with pregnancy, emesis associated with prior exposure to chemotherapy, and poor performance status. Factors conferring relative protection are male sex, age older than 65 years, and alcohol ingestion of more than 10 drinks per week.

Treatment

Many medications have demonstrated some degree of effectiveness in the prevention and treatment of chemotherapy-induced emesis. Table 2 lists currently available medications. The availability of type 3 serotonin receptor antagonist drugs, of which ondansetron (Zofran) is the prototype, has revolutionized the management of chemotherapy-induced emesis. As single agents, these drugs are 50 to 70% effective in the total protection from nausea and vomiting due to highly emetogenic chemotherapy exemplified by regimens containing more than 50 mg per m^2 of cisplatin. The addition of steroids, most typically dexamethasone at an intravenous dose of 10 to 20 mg, enhances the effectiveness of the type 3 serotonin antagonists, with some investigators reporting greater than 90% protection. These drugs are even more effective in the prevention of emesis due to moderately emetogenic chemotherapy such as cyclophosphamide. For mildly to moderately emetogenic chemotherapy regimens, however, a phenothiazine, butyrophenone, or steroid—alone or in combination—may provide equal antiemetic efficacy to 5-hydroxytryptamine$_3$ (5-HT$_3$) antagonists. The addition of other antiemetic drugs such as prochlorperazine (Compazine) may result in additional protection.

Current Issues in Antiemetic Research

Despite the remarkable improvement in the prevention of chemotherapy-induced emesis in the past 5 years, several issues remain.

Appropriate Dose and Schedule of Type 3 Serotonin Antagonists

Remarkable variation in the approved dosage of type 3 serotonin antagonists exists between the United States and Europe. Ondansetron was initially approved at 0.5 mg per kg for 3 doses (or approximately 32 mg over 24 hours) in the United States. Further research determined that a single 32-mg dose was equivalent to the divided schedule and is currently recommended. The approved ondansetron dose in Europe, however, is 8 mg per 24 hours. Conversely, granisetron is approved at 10 μg per kg in the United States but at 3 mg (40 μg per kg) in Europe. These differences are a result of differences in pivotal studies employed by regulatory agencies. A consensus conference recommended that the lower doses of both drugs were appropriate for treating the effects of highly emetogenic chemotherapy. In addition, the divided dose schedule of the drugs appears to be unnecessary.

Route of Administration

All the serotonin antagonists were approved initially as intravenous formulations. Most now have an oral counterpart. Overwhelming evidence indicates that the oral versions of these drugs in bioequivalent doses are equally efficacious for the prevention of nausea and vomiting due to moderately emetogenic chemotherapy. Emerging evidence supports the use of oral serotonin antagonists for treating the effects of highly emetogenic chemotherapy.

The Problem of Delayed Emesis

Delayed emesis from chemotherapy remains a problem despite the advent of the type 3 serotonin receptor antagonists. The mechanism is unclear but likely involves a distinct pathophysiology in comparison with immediate nausea and vomiting. Current management of a patient with delayed emesis is uncertain. The serotonin antagonists, metoclopramide, and steroids all appear to have some activity in the prevention and treatment of this complication. Two randomized trials clearly demonstrated the value of

TABLE 5. **Prevention of Acute Nausea and Vomiting Due to Chemotherapy**

Emetogenic Potential	Regimen
Low (level 1 or 2)	No prophylaxis or single agent, e.g., dexamethasone (Decadron), 10–20 mg PO, or prochlorperazine (Compazine), 10 mg PO, or 15-mg spansule PO
Intermediate (level 3)	Dexamethasone (Decadron), 10–20 mg PO or IV, and/or prochlorperazine (Compazine), 10 mg PO, or 15-mg spansule PO
Intermediate to high (level 4)	Type 3 serotonin antagonist PO or IV plus dexamethasone (Decadron), 10–20 mg PO or IV
High (level 5)	Type 3 serotonin antagonist PO or IV plus dexamethasone (Decadron), 20 mg IV ± prochlorperazine (Compazine), 10 mg PO or IV, or 15-mg spansule PO

For all levels—consider the addition of lorazepam (Ativan), 1–4 mg PO or IV, for anxious patients to prevent anticipatory vomiting. Additionally, for levels 2–5, all patients should have medication available for use at home, e.g., prochlorperazine (Compazine), 10 mg PO, 15-mg spansule PO, or pr q 6 h prn.

NK-1 antagonists in this setting. At this time, however, no NK-1 antagonist is commercially available.

Practical Approach

Antiemetic regimens for low, moderate, and highly emetogenic chemotherapy are given in Table 5. Other drugs may be substituted depending on individual patient features. For example, many younger patients who are taking mild to moderately emetogenic regimens and who have experience inhaling marijuana may prefer the use of dronabinol (Marinol) to prochlorperazine (Compazine). Older patients frequently experience dysphoria with dronabinol, and its use is not recommended in that age group. Conversely, dystonic reactions are far more frequent in younger patients who use metoclopramide than in older patients.

The use of type 3 serotonin antagonists should be reserved for those on moderate to highly emetogenic regimens. Far less expensive alternatives usually suffice for regimens of lesser emetic potential. Should the patient experience nausea and vomiting despite appropriate prophylaxis, rescue medication in the form of phenothiazines and/or corticosteroids should be available. For patients with severe nausea and vomiting, intravenous hydration is indicated not only to replenish losses but also to relieve nausea by ameliorating orthostatic symptoms associated with dehydration. Furthermore, the patient with severe nausea and vomiting, particularly in the setting of advanced malignancy, should be evaluated for the possibility of non–chemotherapy-related causes. Specifically, electrolyte abnormalities (hyponatremia, hypercalcemia), gastrointestinal obstruction, and opiate intolerance should be considered.

DYSPEPSIA (INDIGESTION) AND GASEOUSNESS

method of
HARRIS R. CLEARFIELD, M.D.
Hahnemann University Hospital
Philadelphia, Pennsylvania

DYSPEPSIA

Definition and Etiology

Dyspepsia (indigestion) can be defined as chronic or recurrent upper gastrointestinal tract complaints. *Nonulcer* and *functional dyspepsia* are the labels often used to describe the symptoms if peptic ulcer disease, gastroesophageal reflux, malignancy, and pancreatic pathology can be excluded. Although the terms were applied principally to epigastric pain patterns, usage has broadened to include postprandial bloating, nausea, and vomiting. It is unlikely that a single etiology explains the discomfort. Approximately 40% of patients with the irritable bowel syndrome also have dyspeptic symptoms. Evidence derived from the inflation of gastric and rectal balloons indicates that many dyspeptic patients and patients with irritable bowel syndrome have a decreased threshold for visceral pain. Therefore, some patients with dyspeptic symptoms may be overly sensitive to stimuli, such as gaseous distention caused by delayed gastric emptying or exaggerated motility patterns originating from the upper gastrointestinal tract.

Another cause of dyspepsia is gastroesophageal reflux. Heartburn is usually defined as epigastric burning pain that radiates substernally. Some patients with reflux describe the epigastric component without the upward radiation, and thus their condition may be labeled dyspepsia. Endoscopic evaluation may fail to clarify the diagnosis, inasmuch as esophagitis is frequently not observed in patients with mild reflux.

Peptic ulcer accounts for approximately 15 to 25% of patients with dyspepsia, but the symptoms frequently cannot be distinguished from those of patients without organic pathology. There has also been interest in the role that *Helicobacter pylori* (found in 30 to 60% of dyspeptic patients) may play in the genesis of dyspepsia, either by its role in peptic ulcer disease or by inducing chronic gastritis.

Lowered visceral pain threshold, gastroesophageal reflux, peptic ulcer disease, delayed gastric emptying, abnormal motility patterns in the stomach and proximal small bowel, and *H. pylori* have each been considered to play a role in the symptom that patients call indigestion and that physicians refer to as dyspepsia. Although no significant pathology is identified in the majority of dyspeptic patients, those with functional dyspepsia are often significantly uncomfortable, frequently seek medical help (which results in many diagnostic studies), and may have considerable anxiety about the possibility of underlying malignancy or other organic diseases.

Diagnosis

The description of early satiety, postprandial bloating, or nausea may suggest the possibility of motility-related dyspepsia, such as delayed gastric emptying, but the correlation between these symptoms and the response to prokinetic agents is unimpressive. A therapeutic trial of cisapride (Propulsid), however, may prove useful. Isotope gastric emptying studies have not proved clinically helpful in this population. Burning epigastric and substernal pain may be secondary to reflux, but peptic ulcer should be ruled out. Physicians may elect to order an *H. pylori* antibody test with the intent to eradicate the bacteria if the test result is positive. Patients older than 45 years of age with new onset of dyspepsia should undergo upper endoscopy to rule out more serious disorders; they should also undergo biopsy for *H. pylori*. A negative radiograph or endoscopic finding may exclude active peptic ulcer disease but does not rule out reflux. The presence of "alarm" symptoms, such as pain radiating to the back, weight loss, anemia, dysphagia, and positive stool examination for occult blood mandate a thorough evaluation at any age. Failure to respond to empirical therapy should also prompt more extensive diagnostic efforts.

Therapy

Postprandial symptoms of bloating, nausea, and early satiety can be treated empirically in younger patients with a prokinetic agent such as cisapride (10 to 20 mg taken 30 to 60 minutes before meals) in an effort to enhance gastric emptying and proximal small bowel motility. Burning epigastric pain patterns, which suggest the possibility of reflux, can also be treated empirically with acid-reducing agents, such as twice-daily H_2-receptor antagonists, a daily dosage of a proton pump inhibitor, or a prokinetic drug taken before meals. The clinical usefulness of eradicating *H. pylori* in nonulcer dyspepsia is controversial, but if a serum antibody test or breath test yields a positive result, it is reasonable to provide empirical bacterial eradication therapy with three drugs. The current programs include a proton pump inhibitor taken twice daily plus two antibiotics—such as amoxicillin (500 mg twice daily), metronidazole (Flagyl; 500 mg twice daily), or clarithromycin (Biaxin; 500 mg twice daily)—also taken twice daily for 2 weeks.

If the patient is over 45 years of age, has alarm symptoms, or fails to respond to the aforementioned empirical therapeutic approaches, upper endoscopy should be performed. If the patient has no organic disease and fails to respond to these therapeutic strategies, antidepressive therapy may be beneficial with the older tricyclic agents, which also have a potentially helpful anticholinergic side effect.

GASEOUSNESS

Pathogenesis

The "gas" that is belched is generally similar in composition to atmospheric air: 79% nitrogen and

21% oxygen. Several milliliters of air are ingested in the process of swallowing food or saliva. Factors that decrease the efficiency of the swallowing mechanism or increase the frequency of swallowing are likely to result in increased air accumulation in the upper gastrointestinal tract. The volume of flatus passed daily usually ranges between 500 and 1500 mL, with marked variation, depending on dietary and other factors. Air swallowing has often been considered the predominant determinant of flatus volume, but the role of bacterial fermentation of undigested carbohydrate leading to excess colonic production of CO_2 and H_2 has also been shown to play a significant role in some patients. The transit time for intestinal gas is rapid, approximately 20 to 30 minutes from duodenum to anus. The midabdominal crampy pain frequently associated with gaseousness was thought to be directly related to the quantity of air propelled through the intestines, but studies have failed to show an increased total gas content in such patients. It appears that the discomfort may result from abnormal motility patterns induced by normal or slightly increased gas volumes in susceptible persons.

Symptoms and Syndromes Related to Gaseousness

Belching. Belching is a common symptom, resulting from the accumulation of swallowed air into a gastric air bubble. If a sensation of distention is perceived, spontaneous or induced belching may afford relief. The symptoms may become troublesome if excess air swallowing occurs. Some patients induce belching by purposely swallowing air in an attempt to gain relief from organic or functional disorders. This habit may become repetitive. An occasional patient has extremely loud belching (esophageal belching), which is almost always associated with a high degree of anxiety or other emotional disorders.

Magenblase Syndrome. A significantly enlarged air bubble may be experienced as epigastric or left upper quadrant pressure. The discomfort may radiate to the precordial area and may strongly suggest the possibility of angina. It generally occurs during or after eating, is relieved by belching, and is not related to exertion, which should help distinguish it from a cardiac process.

Splenic Flexure Syndrome. Left upper quadrant pressure and discomfort may occur if gas is trapped in the splenic flexure. Discomfort may radiate to the precordium and also simulate angina. Symptoms often occur after meals as the distended stomach presses on a gas-filled splenic flexure. Relief is often obtained by belching or passing flatus.

Hepatic Flexure Syndrome. Right upper quadrant discomfort may occur if gas is trapped in the hepatic flexure. This localization may be misinterpreted as biliary colic and may possibly lead to cholecystectomy. If the surgery is performed for the wrong reason, the pain may recur postoperatively and receive another erroneous diagnosis, the "postcholecystectomy syndrome," which is often the persistence of a functional disorder after biliary surgery, gallstones having played no role in the causation of the abdominal pain.

Abdominal Bloating and Distention. Bloating, in some instances, results largely from gastric gas accumulation from dietary or aerophagic causes; in other patients it represents decreased gastric emptying that results from a motility disorder at the pyloroduodenal area. Distention may result from relaxation of the rectus muscles, often occurring in women after one or more pregnancies. The lack of tone in these muscles leads to distention in the erect position, but the distention is absent when the patient is recumbent, which is a useful diagnostic observation. Explanation of the anatomic abnormality may spare the patient further diagnostic and therapeutic efforts.

Flatulence. The passage of flatus can be likened to belching, in that each is a normal response to gas accumulation and neither has been subjected to studies that would confidently distinguish between normal and abnormal. However, gas passage with a frequency exceeding 20 per day is probably abnormal. Patients concerned about their flatus frequency can benefit by keeping a diary of each gas passage and its relationship to meals over a 72-hour period. Some confidence may be gained if the gas passages fall into a "normal" range.

Gaseousness Associated with Organic Disease. Patients with organic disorders, such as hiatal hernia, peptic ulcer, or neoplasm may inadvertently swallow air in an effort to obtain relief from pain. Effective treatment of reflux, for example, may also reduce aerophagia. The new onset of gaseousness in a patient older than 45 years of age should raise the possibility of underlying organic disease.

Therapy

Diet. The mechanics of eating are important. Patients with ill-fitting dentures are likely to swallow excessive air. Meals should be taken in a reasonably relaxing atmosphere, preferably not at work, to reduce the potential for air swallowing. It is often helpful to spread the food intake into three meals rather than having a large meal in the evening. Liquid intake during meals should be reduced if postprandial bloating is a complaint. Carbonated beverages, chewing gum, and sucking on hard candies should be eliminated. If patients with crampy pain and flatulence are consuming milk or other dairy foods, withdrawal for several weeks may be a useful therapeutic trial. The "gas-forming foods" such as cabbage, cauliflower, broccoli, and baked beans should be eliminated. Bran and psyllium laxative preparations, which can also lead to excessive intestinal gas formation, should be reduced or avoided.

Pharmacologic Therapy. Promotility agents, such as cisapride or metoclopramide (Reglan), taken 30 to 60 minutes before meals may enhance gastric emptying and thus reduce postprandial bloating. Some patients with postprandial "gas cramps" may benefit from an antispasmodic medication taken before meals. Alpha-D-galactosidase (Beano) is a nonprescription agent that is probably most useful when taken with beans, but thorough studies for other applications are lacking. Charcoal preparations have been used to reduce flatulence, but the results of several studies are conflicting. Similarly, simethicone products have been offered to reduce gaseousness, but there is little objective evidence to support the claim. Patient who are significantly troubled by gas cramps have occasionally responded to antidepressive medications. The tricyclic agents have an anticholinergic side effect that may prove useful. Some patients require reassurance from diagnostic testing of the gastrointestinal tract in order to exclude organic disease.

HICCUP

method of
FRANCISCO C. RAMIREZ, M.D.
Carl T. Hayden Veterans Affairs Medical Center
Phoenix, Arizona
University of Arizona College of Medicine
Tucson, Arizona

Hiccup, or singultus, is defined as an abrupt, involuntary, repeated inspiratory muscle (diaphragmatic) contraction followed by closure of the glottis. It is usually unilateral, involving more often the left side, and affects men more frequently than women. Hiccup may be detected as early as the second trimester, increases in frequency during gestation, and continues throughout the neonatal period. The specific physiologic role of this event, however, is unknown. Hiccup is usually self-limited and temporary and may be considered a passing annoyance, but on occasions it may be chronic, persistent, and resistant to conventional forms of therapy, thus considered "intractable."

The side effects or complications of temporary hiccup are minimal or nonexistent. Physiologic changes, however, such as a decrease in the systemic arterial pressure due to transient decrease in the intrathoracic pressure during the hiccup episodes, have been described. Transient esophageal manometric changes, including aperistalsis, poor clearance in the distal esophagus, and a failure of the lower esophageal sphincter in response to swallowing—abnormalities similar to those observed in achalasia—have also been observed.

PATHOGENESIS

Although the exact pathogenesis of hiccup is unknown, there are experimental data from an animal model in which hiccups were evoked by electrical stimulation of the medullary region, suggesting that the hiccup reflex center is located within the lower brain stem. Further characterization of this hiccup-evoking site has shown it to contain GABA (B) receptors and indicates that the nucleus raphe magnus in the lower brain stem is likely to be the source of GABAergic inhibitory input to the hiccup reflex arc. Mechanical stimulation of the dorsal epipharynx has also been shown to evoke hiccup in the same animal model. The

reported effects of intravenous lidocaine* on the methohexitone-induced hiccup favor a decrease in the excitability of all nervous structures involved in the reflex by virtue of the membrane-stabilizing properties of lidocaine.

Hiccup is regarded by some authorities as an involuntary reflex mediated by sensory branches of the phrenic and vagus nerves as well as dorsal sympathetic afferents, with the main efferent limb mediated by motor fibers of the phrenic nerve. The center probably is located in the brain stem, with interactions among the respiratory center, phrenic nerve nucleus, medullary reticular formation, hypothalamus, and spinal connections. In one study, hiccup was consistently induced in 4 of 10 normal subjects upon rapid phasic distention of the proximal, but not distal, esophagus; resolution after deflation suggested that sudden rapid stretch of mechanoreceptors in this area may be an important trigger event of the afferent limb of the hiccup reflex.

On the basis of studies that demonstrate an organic cause at the level of the brain stem and cervical spine, hiccup is considered by other authorities, however, as a myoclonus rather than an abnormal reflex. The genesis of this myoclonus is proposed to be at the inspiratory solitary nucleus as a result of repetitive activity at that level due to release of higher nervous system inhibitory/regulatory control. Hiccup nevertheless is considered as a neurogenic dysfunction of the "valve function" between the inspiratory complex and the glottis closure complex. Hiccup must be differentiated from a rare condition named *diaphragmatic flutter* in which dyspnea, chest, and abdominal wall pain along with epigastric pulsations are present due to involuntary contractions of the diaphragm.

ASSOCIATED CONDITIONS

Hiccup has been associated with multiple clinical conditions, both metabolic/organic and medical/surgical. These conditions include, among others, sudden excitement, stress, cerebrovascular accidents, brain tumors, tuberculoma of the brain stem, sarcoidosis of the central nervous system, recent intra-abdominal or open heart surgery, subdiaphragmatic irritation, gastric distention, hiatal hernia, gastroesophageal reflux, esophagitis, achalasia, diabetes mellitus, uremia, alcohol intoxication, pleurisy, pharmacologic agents such as analeptics, short-acting barbiturates, antibiotics, and general anesthesia (Table 1). None of these associated conditions or drugs, however, have been consistently proved to be related in a causal manner to the development of hiccup and are mostly regarded as coincidental.

MANAGEMENT

The treatment of the occasional, self-limited hiccup includes mostly home remedies that range from breath holding, drinking water without stopping for breath, sudden fright, trying the Valsalva maneuver, swallowing granulated sugar, drinking water without turning the glass, coughing, and gasping or sneezing to hyperventilating, pulling hard on the tongue, and instilling irritants such as ammonia or vinegar. Because persistent hiccup not only causes embarrassment and disruption of the patient's private and social life, but may also be associated with impair-

---

*Not FDA approved for this indication.

TABLE 1. **Conditions Associated with Hiccup**

Metabolic
Uremia
Diabetes mellitus
Alcohol intoxication
Addison's disease
Gout
Hyperventilation
Electrolyte abnormalities

Pharmacologic
Corticosteroids (i.e., high-dose intravenous methylprednisolone)
Benzodiazepines
Short-acting barbiturates
Analeptics
Antibiotics (sulfonamides, ceftriaxone, cefotetan, doxycycline, imipenem/cilastatin)
Alpha-methyldopa
Anesthetics (i.e., methohexitone)

Central Nervous System
Cerebrovascular accidents
Tumors
Trauma (including surgical)
Infections (encephalitis, meningitis, tuberculoma)
Multiple sclerosis
Parkinson's disease
Sarcoidosis
Ventriculoperitoneal shunt
Syringomyelia

Other
Gastroesophageal reflux
Esophagitis
Achalasia
Hiatal hernia
Gastric distention
Gastritis
Peptic ulcer disease
Hepatitis
Cholecystitis
Pancreatitis
Recent intra-abdominal or thoracic surgery
Subdiaphragmatic irritation (subphrenic abscess)
Peritonitis
Pericarditis
Myocardial infarction
Open heart surgery
Pleurisy
Pneumonia
Tumors (ear, nose, and throat; cervical; pulmonary; mediastinal; abdominal)
Stress
Excitement
Anorexia nervosa
Idiopathic

ment of oral nutrition and its consequent weight loss and disruption of the sleep pattern, as well as potentially life-threatening complications such as severe hyponatremic episodes resulting from water intoxication due to psychogenic polydipsia or even severe respiratory alkalosis, multiple therapies have been proposed for its treatment without a clear understanding of its real mechanism. These therapies, however, in the vast majority of cases, are the result of anecdotal experience rather than have scientifically proved efficacy; therefore treatment of intractable hiccup remains vastly empirical, nonreproducible, and often unsatisfactory when employed by others than their reporting authors. It is not surprising then

that the number of medical therapies, so varied in the case of hiccup, is in direct relation to their inability to provide sustained and consistent control (Table 2).

Therapies used for the management of intractable hiccup have included pharmacologic and surgical manipulations such as implantation of phrenic pacemakers, phrenic nerve transection, phrenic crushing or blockage with alcohol or local anesthesia, and even rectal massages, acupuncture, and hypnosis but again without consistently proven results. Among the numerous pharmacologic agents reported to be effective in controlling hiccup, chlorpromazine (Thorazine) is the only approved drug for such purpose, but it may not work in all patients in a consistent and systematic manner.

The most promising pharmacologic therapeutic modality described in the literature has been the γ-aminobutyric acid beta (GABAB) agonist baclofen (Lioresal). This drug is used primarily for the treatment of muscle spasms and works at the cellular level by either inhibiting or releasing glutamate and aspartate (two excitatory amino acid neurotransmitters) or through an increase in the potassium flux in the neuronal cells resulting in a blockade of monosynaptic and polysynaptic reflexes. In addition to the multiple reports dealing with its efficacy for the treatment of intractable hiccup, baclofen is the only drug tested in a randomized, double-blind, placebo-controlled manner. Interestingly, in that study, contrary to the reported experience of decreasing the actual number of hiccup episodes and even the cessation of hiccup, baclofen was found not to affect the actual number of hiccups in comparison with placebo. The subjective improvement noted by the patients, however, was greater with the active drug than pla-

TABLE 2. **Pharmacologic Therapy of Hiccup***

Amantadine hydrochloride (Symmetrel): 100 mg PO qd
Amitriptyline hydrochloride (Elavil): 10 mg PO tid
Amphetamine sulfate (Adderall): 10–20 mg PO bid
Baclofen (Lioresal)†: 5–20 mg PO q 6–12 h
Carbamazepine (Tegretol): 200 mg PO qid
Chlorpromazine hydrochloride (Thorazine): 25–50 mg PO q 6 h; may be tried intravenously at same doses
Ephedrine sulfate (Marax): 25 mg PO tid
Lidocaine hydrochloride (Xylocaine): 2–4 mg/min continuous IV infusion
Magnesium sulfate: 2 mL of a 50% solution IM
Methylphenidate hydrochloride (Ritalin): 6–20 mg IV bolus
Metoclopramide hydrochloride (Reglan): 10 mg PO q 6 h or 5–10 mg IM or IV q 8 h
Midazolam (Versed): 5–10 mg IV bolus followed by 40–120 mg/24 h as continuous subcutaneous infusion
Nifedipine (Adalat): 10 mg PO bid up to 20 mg PO tid
Ondansetron hydrochloride (Zofran): 8 mg PO tid or 4–32 mg IV bolus
Phenytoin (Dilantin): 200 mg IV bolus, followed by 100 mg PO qid
Quinidine sulfate: 200 mg PO tid
Valproic acid (Depakene): 15 mg/kg/day PO or rectally

*No drug cited except chlorpromazine is FDA approved for hiccup treatment.

†Only drug tested in a randomized, placebo-controlled manner.

cebo. A central action of baclofen in somehow decreasing the perception of the severity of hiccup was postulated. There is some indirect evidence that baclofen induces central analgesia or antinociception, supporting the above hypothesis.

The reported inhibitory effect of baclofen on water intake along with its effect on the perception of hiccup severity may have a role in treating patients with intractable hiccup and severe hyponatremic episodes due to psychogenic polydipsia as it has also been reported in the literature. A more recent study in an animal model found that the injection of baclofen into the hiccup-evoking site in the medullary reticular formation of the cat rapidly suppressed its electrically induced activity.

A recent clinical report of the empirical use of a combination of a proton pump inhibitor (omeprazole [Prilosec] 20 mg daily), cisapride (Propulsid, 30 mg daily), and baclofen (45 mg daily) in patients with chronic idiopathic hiccup revealed that such combination arrested the hiccup in 38% of patients and significantly decreased its severity in an additional 24% of patients, suggesting that the combination should be used as first-line therapy for patients with chronic hiccup. Although the limitation of this study was the lack of randomization, its potential cost implications may be important as well for its use in clinical practice. Nevertheless, these studies again point toward a beneficial role of baclofen in the management of patients with chronic hiccup.

Given the lack of complete understanding of the pathophysiologic basis of hiccup and the consequent great variety of pharmacologic agents reported to be effective for hiccup, it is imperative now that these drugs be tested in a more scientific manner to probe their real efficacy.

ACUTE INFECTIOUS DIARRHEA

method of
KLAUS E. GYR, M.D., M.P.H.T.M.
University Hospital
Basel, Switzerland

and

ROBERT STEFFEN, M.D.
University of Zurich
Zurich, Switzerland

On a worldwide scale, spectacular progress has been achieved in reducing mortality in children younger than 5 years of age mainly by improved treatment of diarrhea. But diarrheal diseases in 1997 still cost the lives of 2.5 million persons. In some developing countries, diarrheal diseases remain the leading cause of death and account for the greatest proportion of years of potential life lost. The impact of acute diarrhea is less severe in our well-nourished population, but dehydration and electrolyte imbalance are potentially fatal anywhere, mainly in infants, the elderly, and malnourished patients. One third of the residents of industrialized countries who visit developing countries experience at least one episode of diarrhea.

Diarrhea is best defined as abnormal looseness of the stool, and this may include changes in stool frequency, consistency, urgency, and continence. Definitions of acute diarrhea vary depending on the age of the patient and occasionally depend on the diet. In adults, acute diarrhea is defined as a syndrome of no more than 2 weeks' duration with three or more stools with increased water content (watery or pasty stools) per 24 hours, when accompanied by at least one additional symptom such as abdominal cramps, tenesmus, nausea, vomiting, fever, and blood and/or mucus in stools. In some studies, an increased stool volume is used for definition, whereas in breast-fed infants, what mothers consider to be diarrhea is an acceptable definition according to World Health Organization (WHO) criteria. Diarrheal episodes lasting longer than 2 weeks are referred to as persistent; those lasting longer than 4 weeks are considered chronic diarrhea according to WHO. Bloody stools and fever indicate that inflammatory diarrhea has damaged the intestinal mucosa (dysentery), even if the stool volume is small.

No firm conclusions can be drawn from the symptoms or severity of the illness to the causative agent, because, for example, contrary to expectations *Shigella* may sometimes lead to mild watery diarrhea and some types of *Escherichia coli* may lead to severe bloody diarrhea. A careful history will indicate the severity and the chronology of the illness and will help distinguish infectious diarrhea from food poisoning (outbreak, often nausea, short incubation time, symptoms persist usually less than 24 hours); osmotic diarrhea secondary to saline laxatives, some antacids, carbohydrate and other malabsoption syndromes, or excessive ingestion of alcohol; and the secretory diarrhea caused by irritative laxatives (e.g., castor oil, cascara). Ulcerative colitis, Crohn's disease, and occasionally malignant tumors may also begin as acute diarrhea. A broader differential diagnosis has to be considered in persistent diarrhea.

GENERAL STRATEGY FOR THE EVALUATION AND LABORATORY WORK-UP

Most episodes of acute diarrhea are managed by the patient or by a family member. Only cases persisting after a few days of empirical treatment and, in industrialized nations, all patients with dehydration, dysentery, or with severe abdominal pain when older than 50 years of age require further assessment. Food handlers should always have their stools cultured. A positive test for fecal leukocytes (using a thin layer on a slide, with a drop of methylene blue added: 5 or more leukocytes per high-power field is positive) or for occult blood, rectal tenderness on examination, or very severe diarrhea also warrants a stool culture for invasive pathogens, such as *Campylobacter jejuni*, *Salmonella* species, *Shigella* species, *Yersinia enterocolitica*, *Vibrio parahaemolyticus*, *Aeromonas*, and *Plesiomonas*. In specific outbreaks, prompt assays for enterohemorrhagic *E. coli* O157:H7 may be indicated. If sheets of leukocytes are absent, the clinician should concentrate on the investigation of enterotoxigenic organisms. Diarrhea occurring after antibiotic therapy may necessitate stool cultures for *Clostridium difficile;* for a proper diagnosis, however, direct evidence of *C. difficile* toxin either in the stool or from isolated organisms is required. Diarrhea persisting after travel to developing countries should primarily be assessed for various types of *E. coli, Salmonella, Shigella, Campylobacter, Aeromonas, Plesiomonas,* and parasites. Parasitic infestation should also be considered in immunocompromised hosts and some occupations; this can be evaluated in watery stools immediately after voiding or in samples preserved in polyvinyl alcohol (PVA), merthiolate iodine formalin (MIF, obsolete in many countries because of its mercury content), or sodium acetate/acetic acid formalin (SAF) solutions. Serologic tests (e.g. for *Giardia)* cross react widely with other protozoa. So far, even with an elaborate and costly work-up, no more than two thirds of the microbial agents will be detected, but polymerase chain reaction for enterotoxigenic *E. coli* may result in higher detection rates. Adenoviruses, rotaviruses, and Norwalk viruses are not routinely investigated because they do not require special therapeutic measures.

CHARACTERISTICS OF THERAPEUTIC AGENTS

Oral Rehydration. Oral rehydration therapy (ORT) is the keystone of all national diarrheal disease control programs in developing countries, because it is simple, highly effective, and inexpensive. A solution prepared from Oral Rehydration Salts (ORS) is used both to treat clinically evident dehydration and to prevent dehydration. ORS contains (WHO/Pedialyte) sodium, 90/45 mEq per liter; carbohydrates, 20 grams per liter; potassium, 20 mEq per liter; and base bicarbonate, 30 mOsm per liter 310/270. ORT is effective because glucose-coupled sodium results in absorption of water by the small intestine during the course of infection. Although ORT is highly effective for combating dehydration and its consequences, it does not diminish the amount or duration of diarrhea, which leads to a lack of confidence, particularly in mothers and in rushed travelers. A more recently developed cereal-based generation of ORS has advantages over glucose-based brands in speeding recovery, at least in cholera. In contrast, administering solutions that contain too much sugar (cola drinks containing additionally some caffeine, which increases motility; fruit juices) creates an osmotic density in the intestine that draws fluid into the intestinal lumen.

The amount of ORT is about 5% of body weight in mild, 6 to 9% in moderate, and 10% in severe dehydration to be administered within 4 to 6 hours. Otherwise, ORT should be fed in small quantities at regular intervals. Plain water and food may also be given to minimize the monotony and the nausea or vomiting. After rehydration, the ongoing losses through stool or vomiting are corrected, using maintenance solutions with smaller amounts of sodium (40 to 50 mEq per liter; e.g., Infalyte, Lytren, Pedialyte, Resol). ORT should be replaced by intravenous therapy only in the initial hours when severe dehydration is present, in rare cases of incessant vomiting, or if the patient is unconscious.

Antimotility Agents. Opiates and their derivatives, such as codeine, paregoric, as well as loperamide (Imodium) and the less effective diphenoxylate (Lomotil) act primarily through their antimotility properties. None is recommended in infants and small children, because the benefits are modest and they may cause serious adverse reactions. If used for monotherapy in dysentery, such agents may prolong and worsen the symptoms; in severe diarrhea, they may cause fluid to pool within the bowel. On the other hand, loperamide given jointly with an antimicrobial agent may bring faster relief than an antimicrobial agent alone even in invasive travelers' diarrhea. For patients with nausea and bloating a combination with simethicone may be used.

Antisecretory Drugs. The following drugs have shown some benefit in experimental studies: chlorpromazine (Thorazine)* and nicotinic acid (Nicobid),* which inhibit adenyl cyclase; salicylic acid*; indomethacin (Indocin)*; somatostatin,* which inhibits prostaglandin synthesis or induced secretion; and berberine. However, because of important side effects and/or limited efficacy, none of these drugs can be recommended for routine treatment of acute diarrhea.

Aciduric Bacteria. Although normal aciduric bacteria in the human intestine inhibit the growth of certain bacterial pathogens, *Lactobacillus, Bifidobacterium, Saccharomyces boulardii,* and *Streptococcus faecium* have shown limited or no beneficial effect in the treatment of acute diarrhea.

Adsorbents. Charcoal, kaolin, and other adsorbents can bind and inactivate bacterial toxins, but results of clinical use have been disappointing. Moreover, some of these agents interfered with the beneficial effect of tetracycline.

Antimicrobial Agents. Infections in which antimicrobial therapy is clearly indicated include shigellosis, cholera, pseudomembranous colitis, and parasitic infections. The same probably applies to infections due to *Yersinia, Campylobacter, Aeromonas, Plesiomonas,* and enteropathogenic *E. coli* if they are severe. Fluoroquinolones are most effective against common enteric pathogens. When such agents are contraindicated, such as in children when they may affect cartilage formation or in pregnancy, trimethoprim-sulfamethoxazole (Bactrim, Septra) is the second choice. Bismuth subsalicylate (Pepto-Bismol), which may be considered a topical antimicrobial, results in only a modest improvement in acute diarrhea.

Antiparasitic Agents. Metronidazole (Flagyl) or possibly even more effective ornidazole† or tinidazole† may be used. These agents, besides causing some nausea, are well tolerated. In amebiasis, such therapy may be combined with the use of diloxanide furoate (Furamide). In giardiasis, quinacrine† or furazolidone [Furoxone] (particularly in children) may be used instead of nitroimidazoles.

TREATMENT

The therapeutic regimen of acute diarrhea depends on its severity, the age of the patient, and the patient's location. Dosages of common antidiarrheal agents are presented in Table 1. Except for fecal leukocytes and occult blood tests, all laboratory investigations require a few days for results to be available. Stool cultures are not routinely indicated, and it is reasonable to initiate empirical treatment in most patients because microbiologically confirmed diagnosis will not be available without a reasonable delay.

Diarrhea in Native Populations in Developing Countries. Oral or, if necessary, intravenous rehydration is the treatment of choice. Antibiotics and antidiarrheal agents are only necessary in patients with dysenteric symptoms and cholera. Otherwise, they may even be harmful and are a burden on the meager budget of poor families.

Diarrhea in Travelers Abroad. Travelers should have appropriate standby medication for self-therapy because they usually have a tight schedule and often

---

*Not FDA approved for this indication.
†Not available in the United States.

TABLE 1. **Dosage of Antidiarrheal Agents in Adults and Children**

Drug	Adult Dosage	Pediatric Dosage
ORS	See text	See text
Loperamide (Imodium) 2 mg capsules 1 mg/5 mL liquid	4 mg, then 2 mg after each loose stool to a maximum of 16 mg/day (OTC: ≤8 mg)	2–5 y: 1 mg three times on day 1
Bismuth subsalicylate (Pepto-Bismol)	30 mL q30 min for 8 doses (if needed, repeat on day 2) or equivalent tablet dosage	3–6 y: 5 mL q30 min for 8 doses 6–9 y: 10 mL q30 min for 8 doses 9–12 y: 15 mL q30 min for 8 doses; if needed, repeat on day 2
Ciprofloxacin (Cipro)	500 mg q12h for 3–5 days	
Norfloxacin (Noroxin)	400 mg q12h for 3–5 days	
Trimethoprim/sulfamethoxazole DS tablets 160/800 mg, suspension 40/200 mg per 5 mL (Bactrim, Septra)	One DS tablet q12h for 2–3 days	0.5 mL/kg q12h for 3 days, do not exceed adult dosage
Furazolidone (Furoxone) 100-mg tablets, 50 mg/15 mL liquid	100 mg q6h for 3–5 days	8 mg/kg/day in 3 doses for *Giardia* for 7 days
Metronidazole (Flagyl) For *Giardia* For *Entamoeba histolytica* (incl. drug to eliminate cysts)	250 mg qid for 7 days 750 mg tid for 5–10 days, plus diiodohydroxyquin (yodoxin), 650 mg tid for 20 d, or paromomycin (Humatin), 500 mg tid for 10 d, or diloxanide furoate (Furamide), 500 mg tid for 10 d	Use furazolidone 50 mg/kg/day in 3 doses for 10 d
Tinidazole* for *Giardia*	2 gm in single dose	Usually single dose

*Not available in the United States.

they prefer not to consult local doctors or buy over-the-counter drugs in developing countries. In all cases of travelers' (acute) diarrhea, the fastest cure is obtained by using loperamide (Imodium) and a quinolone, usually for 1 to 3 days only. For mild to moderate travelers' diarrhea without dysenteric symptoms, loperamide (Imodium) alone or bismuth subsalicylate (Pepto-Bismol) may be sufficient. Rehydration and electrolyte replacement can usually be achieved by fluid replacement (tea with little sugar) and by eating salted food. ORT is indicated for infants, children, and elderly patients. If travelers' diarrhea or other gastrointestinal symptoms persist after such empirical treatment over 1 to 2 weeks in a foreign country or for a few days after returning home, a laboratory work-up is indicated. This may reveal infection with *Entamoeba histolytica*, *Giardia lamblia*, or other pathogenic agents that necessitate specific treatment usually beyond the possibilities of self-medication.

Diarrhea in Patients in Industrialized Countries. In infants, small children, and elderly patients, ORT as described earlier is the keystone. In older children and adults it is usually sufficient to remind the patients to drink plenty of fluids. In mild to moderate acute diarrhea without dysenteric symptoms, loperamide will usually bring fast relief and often no further treatment is necessary. In severe or dysenteric diarrhea, a quinolone, trimethoprim/sulfamethoxazole (Bactrim DS, Septra DS), or furazolidone (Furoxone) may be given. Standard treatment for identified organisms is used if the respective organism is to be treated by antimicrobial agents. Although antibiotics are not always indicated, they should be used more generously in infants younger than 2 months of age and other patients with a high

risk of bacteremia and complications thereof (e.g., a patient with prosthetic valves).

NUTRITIONAL ASPECTS OF ACUTE DIARRHEA AND PROPHYLAXIS

Prophylaxis of Travelers' Diarrhea. The risk of travelers' diarrhea could be reduced by selecting food and drink carefully. Generally, safe foods include those served steaming hot, fruits that can be peeled by oneself, and bread; safe drinks include hot coffee or tea, carbonated beverages, bottled water, beer, and wine. However, most travelers succumb to the temptation of room temperature buffets including cooked food that may have been recontaminated, salads, sauces, or desserts and they use ice cubes in their drinks. Raw or undercooked shellfish, seafood, and meat are especially dangerous, because they may transmit hepatitis A, flukes, tapeworms, trichinosis, and so on.

Chemoprophylaxis of travelers' diarrhea is not routinely recommended because of the effective means for self-therapy. It is mainly prescribed for stays not exceeding 1 week abroad, particularly for travelers who are immunocompromised, who repeatedly suffered from severe diarrhea during previous travel, or in whom diarrhea might be dangerous. Bismuth subsalicylate (Pepto-Bismol) or a quinolone may be chosen, the latter being more effective but also having a higher risk of adverse events.

Food Consumption in Acute Diarrhea. A reduction of food consumption is frequently observed due to anorexia. However, except for milk and dairy products in the initial 24 to 48 hours, food should not be deliberately withheld during the diarrheal episode, because at least 60% of macronutrients are still absorbed and because children who were fed showed better and sustained weight gain than children who did not eat. After recovery, extra feeding should be encouraged.

CONSTIPATION

method of
BENJAMIN KREVSKY, M.D., M.P.H.
Temple University School of Medicine
Philadelphia, Pennsylvania

Constipation is common. It affects 2% of the U.S. population each year and costs millions of dollars for medications alone. A trip to the pharmacy quickly reveals the number and diversity of over-the-counter products that are available and readily used by patients. Although textbooks often describe objective criteria for constipation (e.g., fewer than three spontaneous bowel movements per week), patients have their own definitions. I listen carefully to them and give credence to their complaints of very hard stools, difficult or painful defecation, infrequent defecation, or incomplete defecation. On the other hand, many patients are concerned because they do not have a "regular" bowel movement every day. If their feces appear normal, they feel fine, they have no constitutional symptoms, and they have at least three bowel movements per week without the use of laxatives, the only treatment they need is reassurance.

ETIOLOGY

Constipation is caused by excessive dehydration of the stool, primarily because of inadequate propulsion through the colon. The absorption is normal, but contact time is increased, making stools harder and more difficult to pass. Interestingly, excessive absorption of fecal fluid across the colonic mucosa has not been described. There are many possible causes of this motor disorder, which will need to be investigated through a thorough history, physical examination, and selected laboratory tests. Constipation can be caused by systemic, gastrointestinal, or neurologic disorders. Systemic disorders include metabolic and endocrine disorders (e.g., diabetes, hypothyroidism, hyperparathyroidism, uremia), and drug effects (Table 1). Gastrointestinal disorders include colon cancer with obstruction, pseudo-obstruction, anal fissures, and hemorrhoids, to name a few. Both central and peripheral neurologic disor-

TABLE 1. Pharmaceutical Agents Associated with Constipation

Aluminum-containing antacids	Calcium-containing antacids
Analgesics	Diuretics
Anesthetics	Ganglionic blockers
Anticholinergics	Heavy metals
Anticonvulsants	Iron
Antidepressants	Major tranquilizers
Antihypertensives	Monoamine oxidase (MAO)
Antiparkinson drugs	inhibitors
Barium	Opioids
Bismuth subsalicylate	Sucralfate
Calcium channel blockers	Tricyclic antidepressants

ders can cause constipation. The classic disorder is Hirschsprung's disease; other disorders include brain tumors, pelvic floor dysfunction, and autonomic neuropathy. In a small subset of patients, no cause can be found, and the constipation is termed *idiopathic*.

PREVENTION

Whenever possible, physicians should be alert to the opportunity to prevent constipation. When a drug known to cause constipation is prescribed, alert the patient to the potential problem and make sure that fiber or other laxatives are available. Regular aerobic exercise, adequate fluids, and a fiber-rich diet should be recommended to most patients. Ignoring "the call of nature" (i.e., volitionally retaining feces for long periods of time) should be discouraged. In a similar vein, for patients with limited mobility, a bedside commode can provide both a degree of independence and relief.

INITIAL EVALUATION AND MANAGEMENT

When prevention fails, it is time for a first-level evaluation. This consists of a comprehensive history and physical examination in the search for the etiology of the constipation. Routine blood tests and a digital rectal examination complete the initial workup. If there is any suggestion of organic etiology of the constipation, colonoscopy or an air contrast barium enema study should be performed. Otherwise, the next step is to place the patient on a high-fiber diet (20 to 30 grams of dietary fiber per day), if there are no contraindications to fiber. Ensure that fluid intake is adequate and that constipating drugs are eliminated (if possible). A daily diary helps both the patient and physician evaluate progress (or lack thereof).

If this regimen is not successful, it is time for the second level of evaluation. If an imaging study of the colon has not been performed, it should be ordered now. An anorectal manometry will rule out Hirschsprung's disease, and a test of transit (radiopaque marker test or colonic transit scintigraphy) will give important clues to the severity and type of constipation. Transit tests are sometimes useful in determining that the patient has normal transit—and indeed normal bowel function. Fecal defecography may be useful to identify pelvic floor abnormalities such as rectocele or pelvic floor dyssynergia.

Many patients have severe constipation and fecal impaction. If present, an impaction must be cleared before any other therapy can be instituted. Enemas are often useful at this stage. The first to be used is the saline or phosphate enema (Fleet). This can be repeated, but if it is unsuccessful, a tap water enema should be administered. If there is still no response, then a mineral oil enema can be alternated with a tap water enema for two cycles. Soapsuds enemas should be avoided because they can occasionally precipitate an acute colitis. Oral purges are sometimes helpful, but a milk-and-molasses enema rarely fails. Digital disimpaction should be avoided if possible;

it is quite unpleasant for both the patient and the physician, and it can result in anal fissures, mucosal tears, and even Valsalva maneuver–induced arrhythmias. If all else fails, surgical disimpaction with spinal block, pudendal block, or general anesthesia can be performed.

Laxatives

Laxatives are the mainstay of therapy of chronic constipation. These work by many different mechanisms, including adding bulk, adding water, making stool more slippery, and increasing peristalsis to name a few. The use of one or more laxatives is often necessary to maintain adequate bowel function (Table 2).

Fiber, the bulk-forming laxative, comes in many forms. The most common are dietary supplements such as wheat bran, oat bran, psyllium, and calcium polycarbophil. It is available pharmaceutically as a powder (Metamucil), biscuit (Metamucil), tablet (FiberCon), and granule (Perdiem Fiber) and is even available for tube feedings (Ensure with fiber). Fiber absorbs water in the gut and swells to form an emollient gel. It is highly effective and generally well tolerated. Fiber is contraindicated in patients with bowel obstruction or strictures. Gassiness, bloating, and flatulence are common side effects but usually subside after a week or two of therapy. Warning patients about these side effects helps ensure compliance. The patient must read the labels to take appropriate doses; for example, 9 doses (teaspoons) of Metamucil are needed to ingest 30 grams of dietary fiber. Fiber supplements are generally considered safe for long-term use.

Emollients are commonly used over-the-counter agents. The most common is docusate (Colace). Although well tolerated, emollients are rarely effective, and I do not prescribe them.

Mineral oil is the classic lubricant (15 to 45 mL per day). It is not absorbed and, in essence, produces steatorrhea. It can interfere with the absorption of fat-soluble vitamins and fat-soluble drugs. Furthermore, accidental aspiration can lead to a potentially fatal lipid pneumonia. Mineral oil should be avoided in any patient at risk of aspiration.

Hyperosmolar agents such as lactulose (Chronulac) or 70% sorbitol are effective in many patients. These agents are not metabolized in the small intestine but are broken down by bacteria in the colon into highly osmotic constituents. These agents are associated with flatulence and bloating but are otherwise safe for long-term use. Patients typically require 15 to 45 mL of either agent daily. Sorbitol is substantially cheaper than lactulose.

Saline cathartics (e.g., milk of magnesia, citrate of magnesia) are effective for occasional use. Milk of magnesia is typically administered in doses of 30 to 45 mL at bedtime. These agents should be avoided in patients with renal insufficiency and congestive heart failure. They are generally not recommended for long-term use.

Lavage solutions have recently become more popular and are very useful in selected patients. These are balanced electrolyte solutions containing polyethylene glycol (GoLYTELY, CoLyte) that stay in the bowel and add significant fluid to the feces. Although they are not approved by the U.S. Food and Drug Administration (FDA) for this application, several studies have demonstrated their efficacy and safety. The patient mixes about ½ gallon at a time, stores it in the refrigerator, and drinks 250 to 500 mL daily.

Misoprostol* (Cytotec) is a prostaglandin analogue that induces small intestinal secretion through cyclic AMP. It is often a useful adjunct with other agents. Typical dosing is 200 μg before meals. In contrast to its use in nonsteroidal anti-inflammatory drug (NSAID) gastropathy, misoprostol works best for constipation when administered on an empty stomach. Patient selection is critical because misoprostol is a potent abortifacient.

Only one prokinetic that accelerates colonic transit and has proven efficacy is currently available: cisapride (Propulsid). However, it is FDA approved only for nocturnal reflux and has numerous drug interactions. In addition to drug interactions, it is contraindicated in the presence of QT prolongation, mechanical bowel obstruction, renal failure, hypokalemia, and other disorders. The usual dosage is 10 to 20 mg before meals and at bedtime.

Stimulant laxatives include the anthraquinones, diphenylmethanes, and castor oil. They are commonly found in over-the-counter preparations and are often touted because they are "natural." However, all these agents can become habituating and are associated with the development of melanosis coli. Although their association with "cathartic colon" is not certain, this class of agents should certainly be avoided for long-term use if at all possible. Tolerance is the major problem; increasingly higher doses are required. A typical agent is bisacodyl (Dulcolax), which is taken orally as 1 to 3 tablets at bedtime or as a rectal suppository. Ex-Lax used to contain phenolphthalein, the indicator that turns pink in an

TABLE 2. **Laxatives for Treatment of Constipation***

Laxative Class	Recommendation for Adults
Colchicine	Colchicine, 0.6 mg tid
Emollient	Docusate (Colace), 50–200 mg/d in divided doses
Fiber	Psyllium (Metamucil), 20–30 gm/d
Hyperosmolar agents	70% Sorbitol, 15–45 mL/d
Lavage solutions	Polyethylene glycol-electrolyte solution (GoLYTELY), 250–500 mL/d
Lubricants	Mineral oil, 15–45 mL/d
Prokinetic	Cisapride (Propulsid), 10–20 mg ac and qhs
Prostaglandin	Misoprostol (Cytotec), 200 μg ac and qhs
Saline cathartics	Milk of Magnesia, 15–45 mL qhs
Stimulant cathartics	Bisacodyl (Dulcolax), 2–4 tablets qhs

*See text for appropriate use of these agents and contraindications.

*Not FDA approved for this indication.

alkaline milieu. This property made it easy to detect in cases of laxative abuse, but the formulation was recently changed, and phenolphthalein is no longer used.

Colchicine* (0.6 mg tid) has been shown in small studies to ameliorate constipation. This finding is believed to be a microtubular inhibitory effect, resulting in improved smooth muscle function. Larger studies are needed to determine whether this observation holds up.

Combination therapy sometimes makes a lot of sense, inasmuch as different physiologic mechanisms are employed. When one agent (e.g., fiber) alone does not work, the addition of an osmotic (sorbitol) or a secretory agent may produce a satisfactory response.

Other Treatments

Enemas are often useful in the management of diarrhea. They are simple, inexpensive, easy to administer, quick in action, and effective. Although they are most useful for clearing an impaction, they can also be used to treat occasional relapses in patients on long-term therapy. A sodium phosphate (Fleet) enema administered about once a week can help to initiate a bowel movement. Patients who have congestive heart failure can absorb substantial amounts of sodium from these enemas.

Biofeedback training has gained increasing acceptance amongst gastroenterologists in the past few years. It is particularly useful in patients with poor rectal sensation or patients with pelvic floor dyssynergia. The latter disorder is thought to be a learned disorder in which patients paradoxically contract the pubococcygeus muscle during defecation rather than relaxing it. One to three biofeedback sessions are usually needed to effect a response.

Surgery is definitely a last-resort option in the management of constipation. Patients need a thorough work-up to rule out anorectal disorders, but in selected patients, long-term results are excellent. The typical procedure is an abdominal colectomy with ileorectal anastomosis. This procedure retains fecal continence, and the patient usually has four to six bowel movements daily. A less aggressive surgical option is the Malone antegrade continent enema (MACE). In this procedure, the appendix (or, if the appendix is not present, the cecum) is sutured to the anterior abdominal wall. Fluid is periodically introduced into the orifice via a catheter, and a controlled purge of the colon is accomplished.

---

*Not FDA approved for this indication.

FEVER

method of
PAUL T. DICK, M.D.C.M. M.Sc., and
AGRON PLEVNESHI, M.D.
The Hospital for Sick Children
Toronto, Ontario, Canada

Fever is a common manifestation of infectious and inflammatory illnesses. With the high prevalence of community-acquired respiratory and gastrointestinal infections, fever has been acknowledged as one of the leading triggers of medical advice–seeking behavior. In many instances, fever is perceived as a primary problem in itself, in addition to the significance it bears as a sign of underlying infection or disease. Accordingly, physicians are called on to respond to fever in a number of ways—as a sign, symptom, and source of anxiety and fear.

DEFINING FEVER

Although measuring and responding to fever is a common activity for health care practitioners, strictly defining fever and the body temperature corresponding to fever is far from straightforward. Fever is not merely an elevated body temperature but rather a complex physiologic response to disease. This response is characterized by an elevation of the hypothalamic temperature set point for the body, which is mediated by the release of cytokines and acute phase reactants. It involves recruitment of numerous physiologic strategies to increase the body temperature in response to this new set point. Fever should be clearly distinguished from hyperthermia, which is the abnormal elevation of body temperature in the absence of an elevated hypothalamic set point. Although the ranges in body temperature seen with both of these conditions might be similar, the physiology, causes, and significance of fever and hyperthermia are quite different.

The definition and measurement of fever is made complex by the variation in temperature by site of measurement and by time of day as well as between individuals. When measured simultaneously, an individual's axillary temperature is approximately 0.8 to 1.0°C lower, and oral temperature is approximately 0.4 to 0.5°C lower than the rectal temperature. When measured at different times of the day, an individual's rectal temperature will vary by approximately 0.5°C, with the lowest temperature in the early morning and the highest temperature in the late afternoon and early evening. Variations among individuals also appear to exist not only for the mean temperature but also for the degree of difference between axillary, oral, and rectal temperatures, and the extent of diurnal variation.

Temperature measurement and fever determination may also be affected by measurement error. Most physicians are aware of the pitfalls in using simple palpation for determination of fever and recommend the use of measured temperature with glass or electronic thermometers. With these devices a choice must be made between the three common sites for measurement, the axillary, the sublingual, and the rectal sites. The rectal site best reflects the core temperature and is preferable for accurate measurement, especially in young children. This method may be frightening, however, and psychologically harmful for older children and may in rare instances be associated with rectal perforation or other complications in newborns or premature neonates. Sublingual and axillary sites are more often used for older children and adults and for monitoring in younger children when accurate temperature measurement is not critical. For sublingual, rectal, and axillary site measurements, the careful maintenance of thermometer position for at least 3, 3, and 5 minutes, respectively, or until the temperature reading reaches a steady state is crucial for accuracy.

Newer methods for temperature measurement include infrared tympanic membrane thermometers and thermophototropic crystal-based plastic skin strip thermometers. Although some of the new tympanic membrane thermometers appear to produce reliable readings, their accuracy compared with rectal thermometry has not been demonstrated in all circumstances. Questions have also been raised about the reliability of plastic skin strips to measure temperatures near the critical value for fever. Even some of the standard glass and electronic thermometers may be poorly calibrated and produce biased temperature readings even when used properly. Accordingly, regardless of the method used, some degree of caution must always be used in interpreting measurement results.

When the presence or absence of fever in an individual is determined, the site and method of measurement, time of day, age and condition of the individual, and context may all be important, especially when the measured temperature lies close to the critical value. Temperature criteria based on the distribution of temperatures in healthy normal individuals are useful as a starting point, but the sensitivities and specificities of these criteria are likely enhanced by careful attention to the sources of variation in temperature as well as the potential for measurement error. With these issues in mind, fever should be considered present at and above these critical temperature values:

Rectal and tympanic temperature: 38.0°C (100.4°F)
Sublingual temperature: 37.6°C (99.7°F)
Axillary temperature: 37.2°C (99.0°F)

HARMS AND BENEFITS OF FEVER

Within the medical community, there exists much speculation and debate regarding the evolutionary benefit of the febrile response to infection. Although the febrile cellular and humoral response to infection as a whole plays an important role in defense against the infection, it is unclear how important the elevation of temperature is. There was some use of hyperthermia therapy in the preantibiotic era for treatment of some infections, such as gonorrhea and syphilis. There is currently little need for such an approach with the available antimicrobial armamentarium. Although laboratory studies suggest that the replication rate of a number of human pathogens may be adversely affected and that anti-infective mechanisms may be enhanced by increased temperature, these are not consistent findings, and their practical significance is unknown.

Febrile temperature elevation now appears to be almost an epiphenomenon associated with the cytokine and acute phase reaction. There is little evidence for a direct harmful or beneficial influence of moderate temperature elevation or antipyresis on the clinical outcome of disease within current practice. Research into the interactions and effects of the cytokines and acute phase reactants associated with the febrile response, however, may begin to explain whether and how these mediators and the resulting metabolic changes affect the outcome of infection and inflammation.

Although the temperature elevation in fever often generates fear and anxiety, it is rarely associated with significant harm. Anxiety that body temperature from a febrile response will continue to rise to the point of permanent brain or other organ damage is unfounded. There is a growing body of evidence regarding the mechanisms that brake the febrile response, and it is clear that the human core temperature is rarely allowed to rise beyond 41° to 42°C. Although the rise of temperature associated with the febrile response appears to trigger febrile convulsions in a significant proportion of children, it is only in exceptional circumstances that these convulsions are attended by significant morbidity or lasting harm. Furthermore, treatment with antipyretics has not been demonstrated to reduce the risk of febrile convulsions. Seizures often occur before the fever is detected. In addition, although high fever can trigger somnolence and delirium or confusion in a young child or a mentally fragile individual, this effect reverses with defervescence.

It appears that the only circumstances in which the temperature elevation with fever can really be predictably and significantly harmful is in critically ill or metabolically fragile individuals. This population would include individuals with critically impaired cardiorespiratory or metabolic function who cannot easily tolerate the increased tissue oxygen or energy substrate requirements or the increased metabolic waste associated with the accelerated metabolism of fever. This population would also include individuals with seizure disorders that are severe and difficult to control.

FEVER AS A SIGN

The temperature elevation of fever is of greatest significance as a sign of illness. In most instances of febrile illness, accompanying signs of inflammation and infection provide more helpful specific clues as to the etiology and focus of disease. In these cases the presence of fever may help the clinician to characterize the fever, gauge the systemic effect, and monitor the course of the illness. There are a number of circumstances, however, in which fever may play an important role as the only or the predominant clinical sign of disease. Prolonged fever without signs or symptoms to suggest a typical focal infection may suggest the presence of a significant underlying disease such as an indolent infection (e.g., tuberculosis), a connective tissue disease, or malignancy. Occasionally, the pattern of temperature rise and fall is suggestive of a specific infection or disease.

Special attention must be paid to fever in vulnerable and difficult to assess patients. In immunosuppressed individuals, a low-grade fever may be a crucial early warning sign of a serious infection and impending deterioration. In young infants fever is an important sign of illness that often triggers further investigation and empirical therapy. The presence or absence of specific signs of illness may be hard to detect, and these individuals are more susceptible to rapidly progressive bacterial infections, such as group B streptococcal sepsis.

All febrile infants younger than 1 month of age generally require investigation with cerebrospinal fluid, urine, and blood cultures and empirical treatment with antibiotics pending culture results. Infants 1 to 3 months of age with fever are usually also treated this way unless they have clear signs of a benign viral illness, lack risk factors for sepsis, are well looking on examination, can be closely followed up, and have no elevation of their white blood cell count. In all of these special cases, a careful understanding of the host and the host circumstances and exposures are as important as attention to the pattern of fever and associated signs and symptoms. A detailed discussion of the diagnostic aspects of fever is well beyond the scope of this discussion.

FEVER AS A SYMPTOM

The association between discomfort and febrile illness is well recognized. As a result of this association, antipyresis is often pursued for the sake of improving the comfort and quality of life for the affected individual. The cytokines involved in the febrile response can induce discomfort with rigors, sweats, aches, anorexia, and somnolence. In children the use of acetaminophen results in greater physical activity and less fussiness and somnolence. It should be noted, however, that the level of discomfort with febrile illnesses is not necessarily associated with the degree or timing of temperature elevation. Complete normalization of the body temperature is not an important or necessarily desirable objective of antipyretic therapy.

In some of the most common infections (e.g., viral respiratory tract infections such as influenza) much of the discomfort results from more direct focal involvement such as mucosal effects (e.g., sore throat and cough) and myalgias. Treatment with antipyretics, which happen to be potent analgesics, may therefore be beneficial because of their analgesic effect in addition to or instead of their antipyretic effect. Thus, regardless of the precise reason for efficacy, the use of antipyretic analgesics by individuals with febrile illnesses can be justified when symptom relief is desired, not just temperature reduction.

TREATMENT

Because the temperature elevation in the febrile response is not generally harmful and may possibly be beneficial, the rationale for antipyretic therapy hinges on the symptoms of discomfort with fever. Accordingly, the risks and discomfort in pursuit of temperature reduction must be minimized. The first choice of therapy for treating the discomfort associated with fever is acetaminophen (children, 10 to 15 mg per kg every 4 hours to a maximum of 65 mg per kg per 24 hours; adults 650 mg every 4 hours to a maximum of 4000 mg per 24 hours). It has been proved effective in reducing both temperature elevation and discomfort. It can be administered by the oral or rectal route and has an excellent safety record.

Ibuprofen is an equally effective alternative to acetaminophen. Although it also appears to be a safe antipyretic analgesic, it appears to have slightly more side effects. With the concerns regarding the association between Reye's syndrome and acetylsalicylic acid and the greater potential for toxicity, acetylsalicylic acid is not an appropriate antipyretic for children or a first-line antipyretic for adults. The only circumstance in which more aggressive antipyresis should be used is in the context of critical care when cardiorespiratory or metabolic fragility necessitate effective reduction of core body temperature. In these cases, tepid water sponge baths and application of cooling ice water packs may be necessary and justifiable as an adjunct to pharmacologic antipyresis. The use of alcohol sponging, ice water immersion, or enemas is not safe and should be avoided.

In addition to responding to fever, physicians are called on to respond to the distress it causes. Individuals with fever and their families need to be educated not to fear fever but to view it as a self-limited transient sign and symptom that rarely causes harm and appears to be part of an adaptive response to infection. Families and individuals can be encouraged to cope with fever by monitoring it using an accurate noninvasive method of measurement twice a day, encouraging increased fluid intake, avoiding overdressing or overbundling, and using acetaminophen for treatment of discomfort. They should also be instructed on when to contact their doctor for ongoing fever and other signs of illness.

COUGH

method of
JOHN C. STEVENS, M.D., and
HOWARD EIGEN, M.D.
Riley Children's Hospital
Indianapolis, Indiana

Patients seek medical treatment for cough more often than for any other complaint, and its treatment costs exceed $1 billion annually in the United States. Given today's medical economic climate, a physician's thorough understanding of the causes and treatment of cough are of the utmost importance.

Cough can be divided into acute (less than 3 weeks' duration) and chronic (more than 3 weeks' duration). Regardless of chronicity, therapy directed at the underlying cause results in controlling the cough 90% to 95% of the time. Therefore, our approach to cough therapy is first to identify its etiology and then to prescribe the appropriate treatment specific to the underlying cause. Nonspecific antitussive therapy directed at controlling (not eliminating) the symptom of cough is indicated only when specific therapy cannot be applied or is not immediately effective and when the patient would not be put at increased risk of complications from an underlying etiology.

Regardless of age, acute cough is most likely due to the common viral upper respiratory tract infection (URI). Cough associated with the common URI is most often secondary to stimulation of nasal, pharyngeal, and laryngeal mucosa receptors. This results from secretions of the nose and sinuses draining into the hypopharynx and is commonly referred to as *postnasal drip syndrome* (PNDS). Effective treatment of PNDS caused by acute URI is most often achieved by the use of an older generation of antihistamine/decongestant combination. The newer nonsedating antihistamines, even when combined with a decongestant, have been found to be ineffective in treating cough from the common cold. Intranasal steroids and ipratropium bromide (Atrovent) nasal spray are potential alternatives, but data regarding their effectiveness for cough in this situation are limited.

The approach to the diagnosis and subsequent prescription of appropriate therapy for chronic cough is best when carried out on an age-specific basis.

YEAR 1 OF LIFE

Any persistent cough in the first year of life is distinctly abnormal and warrants a thorough investigation to determine the appropriate treatment regimen. Congenital anomalies of the airway (e.g., laryngeal cleft, tracheoesophageal fistula, cleft palate, laryngomalacia, tracheomalacia, or vascular anomalies leading to airway compression, such as vascular rings or slings) often present in the first year of life with the symptom of cough. Appropriate therapy of these problems often includes surgical intervention; however, expectant management may suffice, as in the case of laryngotracheomalacia.

Infections are the most frequent cause of chronic cough of infancy. This is especially true of infants who have multiple older siblings or who attend a day care center. Children average five to seven URIs per year. Those in day care centers may get twice that amount. Subsequently, an infant's apparently chronic cough may come from a rapid series of viral URIs. A day care setting with only two or three other children may minimize this problem. Other infections that may in and of themselves lead to a chronic cough in infants include viruses such as respiratory syncytial virus, cytomegalovirus, and adenovirus. Cough may last for weeks after a serious lower respiratory infection from one of these agents. Studies show that 25 to 75% of infants hospitalized for respiratory syncytial virus bronchiolitis eventually have problems with asthma-like symptoms such as cough. Appropriate treatment in this case includes inhaled beta-agonist and anti-inflammatory agents such as cromolyn sodium (Intal) or inhaled steroids.

Bordetella pertussis continues to be seen despite widespread immunization. A number of children never receive the full complement of immunizations for this disorder, and some studies have found a rather high failure rate of both the cellular and the acellular vaccines for pertusis. Children usually contract the disease from an adult caretaker who has had a long-standing cough. The illness formerly referred to as the "100-day cough" is made up of three phases. Initially the illness consists of a 1- to 2-week catarrhal phase. Then a 2- to 4-week paroxysmal phase is noted during which the patient has a repetitive series of 5 to 10 forceful coughs followed by an inspiratory whoop. Finally, there is the convalescent phase, which lasts for 1 to 2 weeks, during which the paroxysms gradually decrease in severity and frequency. If the child contracts a simple viral URI during the convalescent phase, the paroxysmal phase can recur, prolonging the overall cough. Unfortunately, treatment with erythromycin, the antibiotic of choice, if not given early in the catarrhal phase only reduces the period of contagiousness and does not shorten the period of coughing. Infants with cough leading to apnea or cyanosis need to be observed in the hospital until this abates. Parents must be educated about the duration of cough and reassured that it will eventually resolve on its own.

Chlamydia trachomatis pneumonia, typically seen in the first 18 weeks of life, can occur in infants up to 6 months of age and can lead to coughing for 2 to 3 months. The infant is typically afebrile, has a congested staccato-type cough, and has physical findings of crackles on chest auscultation, peripheral eosinophilia, and hyperinflation on chest roentgenogram. Treatment consists of a 14-day course of erythromycin.

Mycobacterium tuberculosis needs to be considered if the infant has relevant household contacts.

Asthma often manifests in the first year of life even without the preceding severe lower respiratory tract viral infection as mentioned above. Approximately 25% of children diagnosed with asthma in our practice present with chronic cough alone and have never been noted to wheeze. Some investigators have found up to 57% of asthma cases

to be of the cough variant type. Treatment for the infant typically includes an inhaled beta agonist and an anti-inflammatory agent such as cromolyn sodium (first choice) or an inhaled steroid.

Other diagnoses that need to be considered in the infant with chronic cough that would allow for specific therapy include cystic fibrosis, foreign body aspiration (especially if there is a toddler in the household who might have fed the infant sibling), and aspiration either from an uncoordinated swallow, as in patients with underlying neurologic impairment, or from gastroesophageal reflux.

YEARS 1 TO 5

Infections are the most common cause of acute cough in toddlers and preschoolers. As with the infants who are repeatedly exposed in day care and to older siblings, children 1 to 5 years old with chronic cough, especially during the cold and flu months, may simply have consecutive viral URIs. Cough can persist after a URI with the development of PNDS or heightened airway reactivity. Treatment of the PNDS would be with an older generation antihistamine/decongestant preparation. If PNDS is complicated by chronic sinusitis, a 3-week course of an antibiotic in conjunction with a nasal steroid is needed. Asthma in this age range is most effectively treated with a nebulized inhaled beta agonist combined with an anti-inflammatory such as cromolyn sodium.

In children 1 to 5 years of age, foreign body aspiration needs to be at the forefront of diagnostic possibilities for chronic cough. Foreign body aspiration must also be considered because up to 20% of children will present for evaluation of symptoms such as cough 30 or more days after the aspiration. A simple chest radiograph, airway fluoroscopy, or a ventilation perfusion scan may aid in the diagnosis of this problem. Rigid bronchoscopy is needed for removal of the foreign body.

The effects of second-hand smoke in this age range have been well documented. Studies clearly show that children exposed to even one smoker in the household experience more problems with chronic cough. The physician should insist that there never be any smoking in the family's house or car.

Cystic fibrosis needs to be considered in this age range. The "gold standard" for diagnosis is a pilocarpine iontophoresis quantitative sweat chloride test preferably performed at a cystic fibrosis center. Congenital anomalies such as an H-type tracheoesophageal fistula or a pulmonary sequestration may cause chronic cough at this age and later.

YEARS 5 TO 18

The most common cause of chronic cough from ages 5 to 18 years is heightened airway reactivity. At least 25% of children with diagnosed asthma in our clinic have never been noted to wheeze and are described as having cough variant asthma. Diagnosis at this age is more easily established because the children can cooperate with pulmonary function testing. If reversible airway obstruction is not noted on baseline testing, then bronchial challenge testing with methacholine or exercise can be performed. Treatment for asthma at this age is again best accomplished with inhaled medications such as a beta agonist and an anti-inflammatory. The most common beta agonist employed is albuterol (Proventil); however, salmeterol (Serevent) is often helpful for the adolescent. Cromolyn sodium is the most often prescribed anti-inflammatory, but inhaled corticosteroids have been employed to a much greater degree in recent years. Metered-dose inhalers can be successfully used in this age range but a spacing device is usually needed to ensure maximum drug delivery to the distal airways.

PNDS is a frequent cause of chronic cough in elementary school–aged and adolescent children. This can be secondary to infectious or allergic rhinitis or sinusitis. Treatment is as discussed earlier with an older generation antihistamine/decongestant preparation and or a nasal steroid and at times an allergy evaluation with subsequent desensitization immunotherapy.

Mycoplasma infections are most prevalent in this age age and frequently lead to chronic cough. Diagnosis can be difficult, but is suggested by elevated cold agglutinins or *Mycoplasma* titres. Treatment consists of a 14-day course of erythromycin. Other macrolides such as azithromycin (Zithromax) or clarithromycin (Biaxin) may be used and are better tolerated.

Adolescents continue to take up cigarette smoking at an increasing rate, and this may lead to a daily cough. Although a teenager may not admit to smoking, indirect evidence may be noted, such as staining of the teeth and fingernails and a persistent conjunctivitis. Immediate cessation of smoking is advised for any patient with chronic cough who smokes cigarettes. This often is sufficient to resolve the problem.

Psychogenic or habit cough is most prevalent in the elementary school–age to adolescent age range. This often begins with a URI but then develops into an obnoxious barking, honking, or seal-like cough that is worse when attention is drawn to it and is typically not present with sleep. It is so disruptive that the children are often sent home from school. It is often accompanied by stereotypic hand movements. Treatment is through the power of suggestion. Once the diagnosis is explained to the parent in private, the physician tells the patient that the cause of the cough is known and that with a few simple measures it will improve, typically within the next 24 to 48 hours. We usually explain it to the child as a habit cough and use a cough suppressant with codeine and an inhaled corticosteroid to "soothe" the irritated vocal cords. If the child does not respond to this, as can be the case if they are receiving major secondary or tertiery gains, psychological counseling may be needed.

Cystic fibrosis still needs to be considered at this age as a possible cause of chronic cough.

ADULTS

In nonsmoking adults, PNDS, asthma, and gastroesophageal reflux disease (GERD) are the cause of chronic cough almost 100% of the time. PNDS can be caused by allergic or nonallergic rhinitis, vasomotor rhinitis, postinfectious rhinitis, chronic sinusitis, employment-related airborne irritants, or pregnancy. The patients often complain of the need to clear the throat or a tickle in the throat and nasal congestion. Examination of the patient often reveals cobblestoning of the oropharyngeal mucusa with mucus. Successful treatment of the cough with a first-generation antihistamine/decongestant preparation may be diagnostic. Treatment with an antibiotic for 2 to 3 weeks is needed if there is an accompanying sinusitis. For allergic rhinitis, allergy testing may be helpful, as may nasal steroids or cromolyn sodium or newer nonsedating long-acting oral antihistamines. Environmental controls to avoid the offending allergens or irritants should be instituted if feasible. Desensitization may be useful if avoidance is not possible for certain allergens. Nasal iprotropium bromide may be effective for vasomotor rhinitis.

The diagnosis and treatment of asthma in adults is the same as for that of the elementary school–aged and adolescent child as described earlier.

GERD can cause chronic cough by itself or in conjunction with an underlying process such as asthma, chronic bronchitis, or pulmonary fibrosis. The underlying mechanism may involve gross or microaspiration or simply the stimulation of a distal esophageal-tracheobronchial reflex mechanism. Not uncommonly, cough may lead to a vicious cycle of GERD, causing more cough, which in turn leads to more GERD. The most sensitive test for making the diagnosis of GERD is 24-hour esophageal pH monitoring. An empirical therapeutic trial of antireflux measures and medication may provide a diagnosis for a patient's chronic cough. Conservative management includes weight loss, when appropriate, elevation of the head of the bed, and elimination of caffeine-containing foods and beverages and smoking. H_2 antagonists such as cimetidine (Tagamet) and ranitidine (Zantac) have been shown to produce response rates as high as 80% in GERD-related chronic cough. Proton-pump inhibitors such as omeprazole (Prilosec) have also been successful. Adjunctive therapy with prokinetic agents such as cisapride (Propulsid) or metoclopramide (Reglan) may also be useful. On occasion, surgery with a fundoplication is needed when well-established GERD is unresponsive to conservative or medical management.

For the patient with a long-term smoking history, a cough productive of sputum on most days over a 3-month period for more than 2 years, chronic bronchitis is a likely diagnosis. Cough will respond to smoking cessation in nearly all of these patients; however, it may take 4 or more weeks to achieve results. During exacerbations of chronic bronchitis, treatment with antibiotics, corticosteroids, or ipratropium bromide may be useful.

Bronchogenic carcinoma, although not a common cause of chronic cough in adults, must be thought of especially for those patients with a significant smoking history.

NONSPECIFIC COUGH THERAPY

As stated earlier, the cough in 95% of patients given specific cough therapy will resolve, obviating the need for nonspecific antitussive treatment. If specific therapy, however, cannot be given either because the etiology is unknown or because specific therapy has not begun to work or is not expected to work and if antitussive therapy is not counterproductive, as with excessive sputum production, then antitussive treatment may be tried. Although all narcotics are effective at controlling cough, codeine is the most frequently prescribed for this indication.

Dextromethorphan is probably the most effective non-narcotic cough suppressant. Cough arising from local irritation of the pharynx may be relieved by local anesthetic and lozenges. Benzonatate (Tessalon Perles) capsules anesthetize the stretch receptors in the airway and may also provided symptomatic relief of cough.

Agents used to improve the effectiveness of cough include expectorants such as guaifenesin and water. Guaifenesin, despite being the most common constituent of cough medicines, has not been shown to be effective in the usual dose of 100 to 200 mg every 6 hours. Dornase alfa (Pulmozyme), studied in cystic fibrosis patients, has been shown to liquefy their sputum and to improve lung function with regular use.

HOARSENESS AND LARYNGITIS

method of
J. SCOTT McMURRAY, M.D., and
CHARLES N. FORD, M.D.
University of Wisconsin Medical School
Madison, Wisconsin

Hoarseness is a generic term often used to indicate any abnormality of the voice. *Laryngitis* refers to inflammation of the glottis. As medical science has shown, hoarseness can be completely unrelated to laryngitis. The more accurate term for an abnormal voice is *dysphonia*. Technical terms are also applied to the absence of voice *(aphonia)* and a voice generated at two pitch levels simultaneously *(diplophonia)*. Other related complaints include vocal fatigue, pitch breaks, reduced dynamic range, and inappropriate pitch. Hoarseness, which is dysphonia in all these forms, is an important symptom, the most frequent presenting complaint of patients with vocal fold disease or disorder. Laryngitis is just one of the conditions that hoarseness might indicate.

HOARSENESS

Hoarseness can be quantified for descriptive purposes. One method is to assign values to the parameters of grade of roughness, breathiness, asthenia, and strain (GRBAS). An overall value assessing the grade of hoarseness completes the five components of the GRBAS scale. Although this scale is helpful in following a patient's response to treatment, it is not helpful in establishing a diagnosis and deciding on treatment.

Treatment decisions for hoarseness must be based on specific diagnoses. The characteristics of the patient's hoarseness might provide clues to the diagnosis. A rough or raspy voice quality generally indicates a lesion of the vocal fold proper. Vocal fold lesions prevent smooth periodic vibration, disrupting the wavelike motion of the mucosa during phonation and creating turbulence as air moves across the glottis. A weak, breathy sound with fatigue and possible hyperventilation with extensive voice use indicates glottic insufficiency, the inability to approximate the vocal folds. Interrupted staccato-like speech that the patient may simply describe as hoarseness can indicate various movement disorders and focal dystonias.

Similarly, it is useful to learn about the onset of hoarseness and associated symptoms. A history of dysphonia from childhood suggests a congenital problem; progressive deterioration occurs with neoplasms; and abrupt onset of dysphonia is characteristic of traumatic, inflammatory, and functional disorders.

For all patients complaining of hoarseness, an attempt should be made to examine the larynx. Indirect laryngoscopy is usually sufficient to afford a working diagnosis and to monitor the patient after treatment is initiated. Fiberoptic nasopharyngoscopy may be easier for physicians unskilled in mirror examination technique, and it may be preferred by children and by adults with hyperactive gag reflexes. Rigid telescopes can be used for optimal optics, photodocumentation, and stroboscopic assessment of vocal fold vibration. Videostroboscopy is most helpful in establishing a diagnosis in the hoarse patient with a larynx that on indirect or nasolaryngeal examination appears normal.

Recognizing hoarseness as an important symptom and characterizing the nature of hoarseness aid the clinician in correctly diagnosing the cause and initiating the proper treatment.

VOCAL FOLD LESIONS

Papilloma

Hoarseness that worsens with time mandates careful examination and a search for neoplasms. The most common benign growths are polyps and papillomas. Squamous cell papilloma is a common laryngeal neoplasm that occurs typically in children but can occur at any age. The sites of origin are most often at squamous and mucociliary epithelial junctions such as the vocal folds. Severe hoarseness and stridor can result. The lesion is viral in origin and may be spread throughout the respiratory tract by inappropriate manipulation.

Treatment

Recurrent respiratory papillomas are usually self-limited and tend to disappear at puberty, but progressive symptoms mandate earlier intervention. Although many forms of therapy have been tried, the most successful has been careful microscopic ablation with the CO_2 laser. Maintenance of the airway to avoid tracheotomy while preserving laryngeal structures is the goal of therapy. Complete eradication of the disease is impossible because of its viral etiology. When the disease has become uncontrollable with surgery, interferon has proved helpful. Interferon* (Roferon-A), 3 million IU intramuscularly (for adults) given three times per week, is effective in suppressing the frequency and extent of recurrence. This drug must be administered with caution, and once it is started, it is important to maintain treatment for 6 to 12 months for maximal effect. Once discontinued, there is a tendency for the disease to recur in some patients. Other intralesional antiviral agents, such as cidofovir (Vistide), are beginning investigational trials. Tracheotomy should be avoided if possible because of the risk of spreading the disease lower into the trachea and bronchi.

Cysts and Sulci

Congenital epidermoid cysts, mucous retention cysts, and sulcus vocalis are conditions that are usually not noted during early childhood. These vocal fold lesions may be difficult to notice on routine examination but should be suspected in a patient who fails to respond to the usual treatment for disorders such as vocal nodules. A careful history might elicit the fact that the patient has never had a really nor-

---

*Not FDA approved for this indication.

mal-sounding voice. Laryngeal videostroboscopy is a helpful study to detect subtle areas of stiffness in a vocal fold that suggest the presence of such a lesion. A ruptured epidermal cyst may resemble an exophytic white vocal fold lesion and may be responsible for the formation of sulcus deformities and mucosal bridges.

Treatment

Cysts and sulci necessitate careful microsurgical dissection by a laryngologist skilled in this technique. It is important to maintain an index of suspicion and to refer such patients for appropriate diagnostic evaluation and treatment.

Polyps

Vocal fold polyps are often a response to chronic irritation. They might start out as focal edema in the lamina propria of the vocal fold and may progress to discrete, occasionally hemorrhagic, polyps. They are generally the result of phonotrauma with mechanical stresses that cause localized subepithelial edema. Increased permeability of vessel walls allows for the extravasation of edema fluid, fibrin, and erythrocytes. This may organize into a pedunculated lesion of the vocal fold. The polyp's mass may cause incomplete closure of the vocal fold and inhibition of mucosal wave formation, manifesting as hoarseness.

Treatment

Voice therapy is an essential adjunct but is less likely to be curative with this vocal fold lesion. Often, direct laryngoscopy with removal of the polyp by microlaryngeal techniques is required. Delineation and avoidance of future inciting events are important.

Granulomas

Granulomas generally occur in the posterior glottis, overlying cartilaginous structures such as the arytenoids. Histologically, they differ from polyps in that the epithelial covering is eroded and the connective tissue stroma is filled with abundant fibroblasts and collagen fibers. Mucosal injury from trauma, such as intubation or gastrolaryngeal reflux, causes exposure of cartilage and subsequent granuloma development.

Treatment

Identification and treatment of gastrolaryngeal reflux is important in the successful treatment of these lesions. In general, surgical removal of the granuloma is required, but the prevention of reformation is frequently dependent on successful treatment of gastrolaryngeal reflux.

Systemic Diseases

Many systemic diseases may manifest with hoarseness. Among the more common ones encountered are Wegener's granulomatosis, hypothyroidism, amyloidosis, systemic lupus, rheumatoid arthritis, and sarcoidosis.

Treatment

Treatment for hoarseness in these instances begins with a reasonable index of suspicion so that the disease itself is considered and the appropriate diagnosis is made. Direct laryngoscopy and biopsy are sometimes helpful in establishing the diagnosis.

Nodules and Reinke's Edema

Discrete lesions or diffuse edematous changes may result from chronic laryngeal irritation. Vocal nodules are one of the most common causes of dysphonia. A spectrum of histologic changes associated with the condition has been described, and there are some histologic similarities to vocal polyps. In both conditions, the changes are limited to the epithelium and superficial lamina propria (Reinke's space). Vocal nodules are the result of faulty or excessive vocal use. Excessive high pitch and loudness increase the mechanical trauma to the vibrating vocal fold tissues. Discrete nodule formation occurs at the midportion of the membranous vocal fold, where vibratory excursion is the greatest. *Reinke's edema* is the term used to describe diffuse edematous changes resulting from fluid accumulation in the superficial lamina propria.

Treatment

Each of these problems can be effectively treated by elimination of the irritant. Vocal nodules respond to voice therapy in most instances. The speech pathologist works with the patient on vocal hygiene measures and effective, efficient voice use. In the few patients who fail to respond to voice therapy, surgical excision might be indicated. Often, patients who fail voice therapy are found to have occult cysts, microwebs, or other pathologic processes. Reinke's edema occurs more commonly in older female smokers, and although microsurgical cordotomy and aspiration of contained fluid may improve the voice, continued smoking results in early recurrence.

Premalignant Lesions

The vocal folds are lined with nonkeratinized squamous epithelium. The ventricle and subglottis are generally covered with respiratory epithelium. The terminology of abnormal laryngeal histology has frequently been inconsistent and resulted in a confusing array of terms. Many clinician investigators use the terms *keratosis without atypia* and *keratosis with atypia* as two broad categories for the description of abnormal laryngeal histology. Physically these patches may manifest as whitish plaques (leukoplakia). If they are associated with the leading edge of the vocal fold, they can cause dysphonia or hoarseness.

Treatment

Malignancy cannot be ruled out by appearance, and the lesions should undergo biopsy. Cessation of smoking and of alcohol ingestion is important in preventing malignant transformation. Close follow-up with frequent laryngeal inspection to rule out recurrence or possible malignant transformation is often required.

Cancerous Lesion

Squamous cell cancer is the most common malignancy of the larynx. When it arises on the vocal fold, hoarseness is an early symptom, and the prognosis for patients with early vocal fold lesions is excellent. Lesions that arise in the supraglottis do not cause hoarseness until quite advanced; they are detected later, metastasize earlier, and have a much worse prognosis. Any patient with a smoking history who has chronic or progressive hoarseness should be suspected of having laryngeal cancer and should undergo careful endoscopic examination.

Treatment

The mainstay of treatment for laryngeal cancer remains surgery and radiation therapy. Advances in surgery and radiation oncology have resulted in removal of fewer larynges for cancer. Conservation laryngeal surgery allows removal of T2 and some T3 lesions with preservation of sufficient structures to preserve laryngeal functions. Small T1 lesions can be handled with laser cordectomy, microsurgery, or radiation therapy with excellent cure rates and voice results. Hyperfractionation radiotherapy techniques offer improved local control with less long-term regional tissue damage.

KINETIC LARYNGEAL PATHOLOGY ASSOCIATED WITH DYSPHONIA

Many neurologic diseases affect the larynx and produce characteristic dysphonias. Paralysis of the vocal folds can cause glottic insufficiency. Other neurologic disorders can be characterized as movement disorders: hypokinetic, hyperkinetic, or mixed. Nearly 90% of patients with Parkinson's disease develop laryngeal dysfunction, characterized by a weak, monotonous, breathy voice. Shy-Drager syndrome is a form of idiopathic hypotension characterized by loss of autonomic nervous system function and progressive vocal fold paresis as a result of lesions of the dorsal motor nucleus of the vagus and causes a mixed movement disorder. Essential tremor causes a rhythmic fluctuation in the voice that can be seen during respiration as well as during phonation.

Glottic Insufficiency

Congenital Vocal Fold Paralysis

Vocal fold paralysis may be present at birth or may become evident during the first few months of life.

As many as 15% of neonates with stridor may have laryngeal paralysis. Vocal fold paralysis suggests a central lesion such as Arnold-Chiari syndrome when bilateral and a peripheral lesion of the vagus or laryngeal nerves when unilateral. Interestingly, the patient with bilateral paralysis may well have a normal cry, whereas unilateral paralysis usually causes a weak cry. The diagnosis can be confirmed by flexible fiberoptic nasolaryngoscopy. The examiner must be alert to paradoxical movement of the vocal folds. They appear to adduct during inhalation as the vocal folds passively respond to decreased pressure in the glottic airway, and they appear to abduct during exhalation as they are blown apart.

TREATMENT

In the short term, airway management for bilateral vocal fold paralysis may necessitate intubation and tracheotomy while a search for the etiology is undertaken. In patients with bilateral paralysis in whom there is no return of function, various vocal fold lateralization procedures can be performed during preschool years.

Acquired Vocal Fold Paralysis

Vocal fold paralysis may arise spontaneously or from surgical injury. When the vocal fold is bowed and the palate droops on the paralyzed side, a central lesion should be suspected. In other cases, disease in the thyroid and mediastinum should be ruled out before the paralysis is considered idiopathic. A recent history of an upper respiratory tract infection before the breathiness may imply a viral cranial neuropathy. The symptoms of paralysis are breathy dysphonia and aspiration. Over time, many patients compensate without intervention, but if the symptoms do not improve within 6 to 12 months, surgical options are available.

TREATMENT

The standard treatment since the late 1950s has been injection of a suspension of polytef (Teflon) crystals in glycerin to passively medialize the vocal fold. Concern over the long-term fate of injected alloplasties and difficulty in restoring normal tissue characteristics to overinjected vocal folds have given rise to several options that appear to preserve the physiologic integrity of the tissues. These include injection of biologic materials such as bovine collagen and autogenous fat.

Modification of the laryngeal cartilaginous framework by thyroplasty allows medial displacement of the vocal fold without directly violating the soft tissues of the vibrating vocal fold. Arytenoid adduction techniques can be used to medialize the displaced arytenoid with wide posterior glottic gaps. Newer methods of nerve transfer, laryngeal pacing, and neuromuscular reinnervation are being developed.

It is now possible to design a treatment to address all aspects of the anatomic and function disorder (e.g., glottic insufficiency, atrophy, arytenoid fixation or dislocation, and scarring). There are also options for the patient with bilateral paralysis and airway impairment. Other than tracheotomy, most proven procedures for bilateral paralysis require some sacrifice of voice for improved airway. This loss might be minimized with some of the current laser arytenoidectomy and partial cordectomy procedures.

Movement Disorders

Presbylarynx

The most common cause of hoarseness in the elderly is presbylarynx. This is a normal aging phenomenon marked by soft tissue and skeletal changes of the larynx as well as neurodegenerative changes. The result is a weaker and more breathy voice that may be accompanied by some degree of tremor. The larynx reveals slight bowing of the vocal folds, and there is typically some edema in females. These changes contribute to creating the voice characteristics that are associated with the elderly.

TREATMENT

Treatment is generally not sought for presbylarynx. Patients often benefit from a short course of voice therapy. In patients sufficiently motivated, there have been some encouraging results from medialization thyroplasty and limited injection of collagen to correct bowing of the vocal fold.

Parkinson's Disease

Parkinson's disease is frequently associated with hypoadduction of the vocal folds. It is caused by nigrostriatal dopamine deficiency. Rigidity, tremor, and decreased range of motion are the primary physical findings. One in 100 persons older than 60 years and 1 in 1000 persons younger than 60 years are afflicted with some form of this disorder. The voice may be found to have decreased volume, monotony, hoarseness, and tremor. Decreased volume is generally the first presenting sign. There also may be a generalized dysarthria with imprecise articulation and short rushes of speech.

TREATMENT

A complete neurologic evaluation is important in treating patients with Parkinson's disease. It is important to maximize the medical treatment of the dopamine deficiency and to rule out Parkinson-plus syndromes such as Shy-Drager syndrome and progressive supranuclear palsy. Voice therapy may be beneficial. In some cases with severe hypoadduction, bilateral thyroplasty may also help closure of the glottis.

Parkinson-Plus Syndromes

A rare mixed movement disorder includes both hypokinetic and hyperkinetic features. Parkinson's disease represents 80% of the mixed movement disorders. Parkinson-plus syndromes constitute another 12%. The Parkinson-plus syndrome group routinely has features of hypokinesis and hyperkinesis. There

may be bowing of the vocal folds causing a breathy quality of the voice. Hyperadduction of the supraglottis may also be present. The voice may be described as breathy and monotone with uniformed loudness, with both strained- and strangled-sounding characteristics.

TREATMENT

Therapy is difficult in this group. Maximal medical treatment of the nigrostriatal disorder is most beneficial. Voice therapy may help maximize the current voice.

Spasmodic Dysphonia

Spasmodic dysphonia is a condition characterized by dysrhythmic involuntary contractions of laryngeal muscles during phonation. The result is a strangled- and strained-sounding voice that may at times be unintelligible. The etiology remains obscure, although it seems to occur after various emotional and physical traumas, and some patients exhibit multiple central nervous system (CNS) lesions. Although most patients have mainly laryngeal symptoms, spasmodic dysphonia may be associated with other regional or generalized dystonias, and a tremor component is often present.

TREATMENT

Treatment of spasmodic dysphonia is symptomatic. Some excellent results are obtained with voice therapy, and all patients should probably undergo at least a trial of therapy before considering other options. Initial success with recurrent nerve section has been tempered by long-term results showing a high incidence of recurrence. Thyroplasty procedures and various electrical stimulation techniques are being explored. Currently the most effective and widely used treatment is injection of botulinum toxin. In the typical patient with adductor spasmodic dysphonia, 2 to 5 units of botulinum toxin* (Botox) is injected into the thyroarytenoid muscle. After a period of a few days, during which the voice is a bit breathy, the voice often returns to near normal, and the patient can resume their normal activities. Symptoms tend to return in 3 to 4 months, at which time the injections are repeated.

Musculotension Disorder

One important condition must be mentioned because it is relatively common and often manifests without diagnosis. Muscle tension dysphonia is a condition most commonly seen in younger to middle-aged persons. Affected persons are often in stressful jobs and engage in extensive voice use. They may not exhibit any obvious laryngeal lesions, although careful examination often reveals an open posterior glottic chink during phonation. The cervical musculature around the larynx tends to be tight, and the chin juts forward. This condition predisposes the patient to the development of nodules.

---

*Not FDA approved for this indication.

TREATMENT

Treatment for tension dysphonia, as for nodules, is primarily voice therapy.

Essential Tremor

Essential tremor is the most common movement disorder. It afflicts 4 to 60 persons per 1000. It may manifest at any age but generally becomes more prevalent with increasing age. Inheritance of the condition is through autosomal dominance in 50% of cases. Tremors are most common in the hands and head. Voice disorders are present in 4 to 20% of patients with essential tremor. The voice is described as quavering or tremulous, more noticeable with vowel prolongation. Essential tremor may be confused with spasmodic dysphonia secondary to pitch breaks and voice arrest from large-amplitude tremor of laryngeal structures and from interrupted airflow.

TREATMENT

Voice therapy, although not curative, may help maximize the usable voice. Mixed results have been achieved with propranolol (Inderal), primidone* (Mysoline), acetazolamide* (Diamox), alprazolam* (Xanax), and phenobarbital.* Botulinum toxin* injected into the vocal folds has also been met with mixed results.

DEVELOPMENTAL DISORDERS

Laryngomalacia

Laryngomalacia accounts for 60% of laryngeal problems in the neonate. It is the most common cause of noisy breathing in infants. The symptoms are the result of a persistently infantile-shaped larynx with an omega-shaped epiglottis and shortened aryepiglottic folds. This configuration promotes inspiratory prolapse of the cuneiform and arytenoid cartilages, especially with feeding and agitation. Inspiratory stridor is the usual presenting symptom and begins typically during the first few weeks of life. Although the actual cry is not abnormal, the supraglottic structures are pulled during inspiration into the lumen of the larynx, generating turbulent airflow, noisy respiration, and a variable degree of airway obstruction.

Treatment

Laryngomalacia is a condition that improves as the patient grows. In most instances, no treatment is necessary. Positioning the child prone with the neck extended generally relieves the symptoms. When stridor is severe and especially when feeding is impaired, surgical options are available. Release of the shortened aryepiglottic folds by either CO_2 laser or microlaryngeal instruments is usually sufficient to relieve the airway obstruction. Tracheotomy is hardly ever required.

Subglottic Hemangioma

Subglottic hemangioma causes respiratory distress that tends to get worse with crying. Patients may function well for several months after birth until they have an upper respiratory tract infection. They then exhibit increased dyspnea and a harsh cry. Examination typically reveals an asymmetrical bluish subglottic fullness.

Treatment

Subglottic hemangioma has a natural history of regression after the first 18 months. If symptoms are not severe, no intervention is necessary. Laser surgery is a relatively safe and reliable way to buy time while incrementally ablating the lesion. Steroid therapy has not proved effective as a primary mode of treating these lesions, but perioperative dexamethasone sodium phosphate (Decadron Phosphate) probably reduces postoperative edema. In some select subglottic hemangiomas, surgical removal through a laryngofissure allows for successful excision and the avoidance of a tracheotomy.

Subglottic Stenosis

Subglottic stenosis is usually an acquired lesion, typically from intubation trauma. It manifests most commonly with respiratory difficulty and biphasic stridor. Other systemic diseases, such as Wegener's granulomatosis, can cause subglottic stenosis and should be a part of the differential diagnosis. Voice dysfunction may also manifest with subglottic stenosis by a change in the airflow over the vocal folds or by vocal fold motion disturbances associated with scarring from the subglottis. Aphonia may also be manifested if the stenosis is complete or nearly complete. The diagnosis is made by laryngeal examination, usually during laryngoscopy and rigid bronchoscopy.

Treatment

The treatment of subglottic stenosis depends on the character and the quality of the stenosis. Systemic disease processes should be treated or ruled out. Gastrolaryngeal reflux should be assessed and empirically treated. It has been shown in animal models that gastric secretions can cause subglottic stenosis, even with infrequent exposure. In general, the stenotic area is treated surgically with either expansion surgical techniques or by resection with primary anastomosis.

Congenital Webs

Congenital laryngeal webs are uncommon. They probably represent an incomplete form of laryngeal atresia, inasmuch as there is frequently a subglottic extension of the web. If the web does not cause severe airway obstruction, children may not come to medical attention until the age of 2 years with vocal dysfunction or less frequently aphonia. The cry or voice is

---

*Not FDA approved for this indication.

often described as high-pitched. Diagnosis is made by fiberoptic nasopharyngoscopy.

Treatment

Treatment entails release of the glottic web. If the web is thin, it is possible to perform the procedure transorally. More frequently, however, the web extends into the subglottis as a thickening of the cricoid cartilage for which open resection via a laryngofissure is required.

LARYNGITIS AND INFLAMMATORY CONDITIONS

Irritants

The vocal folds are susceptible to injury by vocal abuse and a variety of chemical and environmental factors. The most common form of irritative laryngitis is a product of brief periods of voice abuse such as shouting or speaking for prolonged intervals over background noise. Although gargling might be soothing initially, it is a leading cause of chronic laryngitis when continued over many days or weeks. This is in part mechanical, but gargled substances other than physiologic saline may act as chemical irritants as well. Inhalation of dry air and systemic dehydration predispose to vocal fold irritation. Smoke is a mechanical and chemical irritant with significant carcinogenic potential in the larynx. Gastroesophageal reflux is increasingly recognized as a source of chronic laryngitis and may also play a role in carcinogenesis, especially in nonsmokers.

Treatment

The best treatment for all forms of irritative laryngitis is to avoid the irritating agent. Susceptible persons should try to ameliorate dry environments by using humidifiers and vaporizers in the home whenever possible. Habitual travelers should be aware that the circulated air in airplanes is very dry, and they should maintain excessive hydration and avoid excessive talking over engine noise. Talking over background noise is also a cause of vocal abuse for the motorist. Consumption of liquids is important, but avoidance of caffeinated products is also helpful, to prevent diuresis and drying. Patients should be warned that frequent throat clearing is traumatic to the vocal folds. Repetitive nonproductive coughing should be voluntarily suppressed. Drinking liquids, sucking on lozenges, or creating a counterstimulus by rubbing the anterior neck should manage throat tickles.

Laryngitis

Laryngeal tissues might exhibit an inflammatory response to viral and bacterial infections and to allergic challenges. Unspecified, the term *laryngitis* usually refers to inflammation of the true vocal fold in response to a viral or, less commonly, bacterial infection. Onset is often associated with an upper respiratory tract infection. Hoarseness develops rapidly, and speaking may produce throat pain (odynophonia). The etiology is typically a rhinovirus, but persistence of symptoms beyond a few days is likely caused by a secondary bacterial infection. The most common secondary invaders are *Moraxella catarrhalis* and *Haemophilus influenzae; Pneumococcus, Streptococcus, Staphylococcus,* and *Mycoplasma* organisms are infrequent pathogens. Examination of the larynx reveals edema and erythema of the vocal folds.

Treatment

The best treatment is conservative and supportive, with an attempt to rest the vocal folds and increase ambient moisture. Relative voice rest, humidified air, systemic hydration, and rest may be sufficient. A decongestant such as phenylephrine and an expectorant such as guaifenesin are often helpful. An antitussive is indicated in the presence of an irritating cough.

Persistent symptoms warrant antibiotic treatment. Cefuroxime axetil (Ceftin) is an excellent choice because it is active against the principal pathogens, is well tolerated, and is effective in a dosage of 250 mg twice daily in adults. Alternatives include amoxicillin plus clavulanate potassium (Augmentin) and ampicillin plus sulbactam (Unasyn). Professional vocalists warrant special attention because performing with an inflamed larynx could threaten their careers; they should consult with a laryngologist. Persistence of hoarseness after 2 weeks suggests additional laryngeal pathologic processes and necessitates further evaluation.

Epiglottitis

Inflammation of the soft tissues above the glottis (supraglottitis or epiglottitis) can escalate to rapid airway compromise and death. It is important to make the diagnosis rapidly and to avoid aggravating the anxious patient. Previously, epiglottitis manifested most commonly in children. With the development of a vaccine against *H. influenzae* type B, the incidence of childhood acute epiglottitis has decreased. More frequently, adults and immunocompromised patients are coming to medical attention for acute epiglottitis, occasionally caused by other infectious pathogens. Epiglottitis characteristically results in a muffled dysphonia (not actual hoarseness, because there is no lesion creating turbulence at the vocal fold level), inspiratory stridor, and drooling. The patient prefers a sitting posture with the neck extended and head forward, and appears anxious and often moribund. A lateral neck radiograph reveals a thumb-shaped epiglottis and blunting of the aryepiglottic folds.

Treatment

A safe airway must be rapidly established. Ideally, the patient should have a nasotracheal tube placed in a controlled environment such as an operating room. Personnel should be available to perform rigid endoscopy and tracheotomy in the unlikely event that intubation fails. Once the patient is safely intubated, the larynx can be examined to confirm the diagnosis and obtain an epiglottic culture. During the processing of laryngeal and blood cultures, antibiotic therapy should be instituted against *H. influenzae*. Historically this has been one of the indications for chloramphenicol, and the combination of chloramphenicol and ampicillin remains a suitable backup regimen. Second- and third-generation cephalosporins are currently preferred; ceftriaxone (Rocephin) is effective in a dosage of 50 to 75 mg per kg per day given intravenously in divided doses every 12 hours. Resolution can be anticipated in 48 to 72 hours. Cessation of drooling and decreasing signs of toxicity suggest resolution, but fiberoptic examination should be performed before extubation. Sedation should be discontinued before extubation to ensure adequate cough. Extubation is performed after administration of 100% oxygen and careful suctioning of the endotracheal tube. After extubation, the voice may be a bit weak. A short course of aerosolized epinephrine might be helpful in the immediate postextubation period.

Candida-induced epiglottitis has become more prevalent in immunocompromised patients or in patients who have been treated with antibiotics for other respiratory complaints. Diffuse white fungal plaques cover the supraglottis. Diagnosis can be confirmed by potassium hydroxide (KOH) preparation and fungal culture at laryngoscopy. Treatment with antifungal therapy is useful.

Croup

A spectrum of problems falls under the umbrella of croup syndrome. The nature of croup hoarseness is typically raspy or brassy, and the accompanying cough has a barking quality suggestive of subglottic inflammation. The most benign form is spasmodic croup, which is probably allergic and usually occurs without prior upper respiratory tract infection. It is self-limited and usually resolves rapidly. Viral croup follows a respiratory infection and occurs in infants and children younger than 3 years of age. It is generally mild; symptoms are worse at night and respond to conservative home management.

Treatment

In children requiring hospitalization, racemic epinephrine (0.5 mL of 2.25% in 2.5 mL normal saline) may be administered by inhalation with mask and nebulizer. Failure to resolve, progressive toxicity, and airway obstruction are suggestive of bacterial tracheitis, a serious illness that necessitates aggressive management.

Bacterial Tracheitis

The pathogenesis of bacterial tracheitis is probably the evolution of a viral upper respiratory tract infection in a croup-susceptible person. The initial pathogens are typically parainfluenza virus, influenza A virus, and respiratory syncytial virus. Because patients are unable to clear secretions adequately from the lower airway, bacteria build up and coalesce with secretions to form a pseudomembrane. These infections are frequently of mixed bacterial origin, and the organisms cultured most frequently are *Staphylococcus aureus, H. influenzae, Streptococcus pyogenes,* and *M. catarrhalis.* Radiographically, the subglottic fullness creates a superiorly tapering airway that has been referred to as the steeple sign. The pseudomembranous thickening of the upper trachea and subglottis can often be appreciated on plain films of the neck.

Treatment

Treatment consists of early recognition, rigid bronchoscopy for diagnosis and clearance of obstructing pseudomembranes, and antibiotics. Affected patients have a great deal of retained tenacious secretions and require intubation for airway maintenance and suctioning of secretions. The antibiotic of choice is ceftriaxone (Rocephin), and a dosage of 50 to 75 mg per kg per day given intravenously in divided doses every 12 hours is adequate. An alternative is the combination of ampicillin and nafcillin (Unipen). Intubation should be discontinued as soon as toxicity resolves and the secretions diminish in quantity and viscosity.

Laryngopharyngeal Reflux

Reflux laryngitis is caused by gastroesophageal reflux. The posterior glottis typically appears hyperemic, and associated edema, ulceration, or granuloma formation may be present. Reflux laryngitis is recognized frequently by alert clinicians. A history of indigestion, regurgitation, heartburn, and globus sensation is not always elicited. Although the diagnosis can be confirmed only by pH monitoring, a suitable history or the presence of hiatal hernia should be sufficient to warrant a trial of antireflux measures.

Treatment

The three nonsurgical approaches in treatment of reflux are postural, dietary, and medical. The head of the patient's bed should be elevated 6 inches to reduce the spill of acid into the laryngopharynx. A weight-reduction diet is important for the obese patient with reflux. Acidic foods and those that promote reflux should be avoided; a partial list includes coffee, tea, beer, liquor, tomato products (pizza at bedtime is bad), milk, and citrus-based beverages. Medical management consists primarily of antacids taken 1 hour after meals and at bedtime. In refractory cases, proton pump inhibitors, such as omeprazole (Prilosec), in conjunction with prokinetic agents, such as cisapride (Propulsid), are indicated. These should be used in conjunction with dietary and behavioral modification. If reflux cannot be adequately controlled by these measures, surgical correction of the lower esophageal sphincter should be entertained.

INSOMNIA

method of
MILTON K. ERMAN, M.D.
*University of California, San Diego
and The Scripps Research Institute
and Pacific Sleep Medicine Services
La Jolla, California*

Insomnia is the most common sleep complaint in the general population, with prevalence rates of 30 to 50% reported in surveys of adult populations. That these rates appear high to practitioners is understandable, because only about 5% of patients who complain of chronic insomnia seek help from a physician for their problem. What drives the reluctance to report insomnia? Patients are not certain that their physician understands or is concerned about insomnia or that he or she has time to discuss their sleep problems with them. They feel responsible for the problem, believing that if they lived a healthier lifestyle that they would sleep better. They are frightened of "sleeping pills," associating them with dependency and addiction.

CAUSES OF INSOMNIA

To establish an accurate sleep diagnosis, specific data about sleep habits and pathologic processes must be obtained. Questions that should be included in a brief insomnia history are presented in Table 1.

Adjustment Sleep Disorder

Sleep is often disturbed by stress or emotional arousal. A transient "adjustment sleep disorder" may occur with conflict or major life change (marriage, divorce, birth of a child), with intense job or career demands, or even with "normal" events, such as the start of the school year or week, school examinations, and so on. When the stressor remits, the patient usually resumes normal sleep patterns. These patients usually have a history of prior normal sleep, but their insomnia may recur whenever stress levels are elevated. This disturbance may be viewed as "insomnia of everyday life," but individuals who are insecure and emotionally vulnerable are most often affected.

Circadian Rhythm Disorders

Jet lag, a circadian rhythm sleep disorder, occurs almost universally after rapid east-west travel across multiple time zones. It is characterized by complaints of disturbed sleep, altered sleep/wake schedules, and excessive sleepiness during desired waking hours. Similar problems may be seen associated with shift work.

Poor Sleep Hygiene

Habit patterns or the sleep environment may be arousing or may disrupt sleep rhythms. Examples include exercising too close to bedtime, engaging in intense mental activity late at night, using caffeine or cigarettes near bedtime, or a bedroom that is light, noisy, hot, cold, and so on. Sleep may also be disrupted by day-to-day variation in sleep and waking schedules, spending excessive time in bed, or daytime napping.

Chronic Hypnotic Use and Withdrawal

The sleep of patients who use barbiturate and barbiturate-like hypnotics nightly for months or years may deteriorate in association with their chronic medication use. If medications are stopped abruptly, the resulting withdrawal syndrome further disturbs sleep. Rebound insomnia—worsening of sleep immediately after medications are stopped—may be seen with the use of benzodiazepines with short and ultra-short half-lives, especially when used in high doses nightly for long periods of time. Rebound is less common with zolpidem and zaleplon* than with other short half-life compounds such as triazolam. Withdrawal from alcohol or sedative drugs produces insomnia and necessitates cautious, gradual reduction in dose, at times requiring a withdrawal schedule over several months.

Stimulants

Stimulants, including tea, coffee, or over-the-counter stimulants, can cause insomnia. Prescription of amphetamines and of methylphenidate is tightly controlled, but other stimulants are readily available and widely used. Use or abuse of these agents may lead to excessive stimulation and complaints of insomnia.

Medical Conditions

Medical problems of any type can cause insomnia. Any source of pain or physical discomfort such as arthritis, metastatic disease, pruritus, nocturia or polyuria, or the effects of trauma or surgery may lead to disturbed sleep. Other organic causes include endocrine disorders such as hyperthyroidism and hypoglycemia, gastroesophageal reflux, renal disease, chronic lung disease, and congestive heart failure.

Psychophysiologic Insomnia

Psychophysiologic insomnia is pervasive in general patient populations. Patients present with problems falling asleep, intermittent awakening, or early morning arousal. It develops due to negative conditioning to sleep and the sleep environment. Patients become anxious as bedtime approaches, and "try too hard" to fall asleep, increasing levels of arousal and anxiety, further interfering with sleep. They are frustrated as they lie in bed awake, and they establish negative associations between the bed, the bedroom, and their inability to sleep. As a result, these

---

TABLE 1. **Elements of a Brief Insomnia History**

1. What is the specific insomnia complaint—sleep initiation, sleep maintenance, or nonrestorative sleep?
2. What is the patient's perceived sleep quality? Is sleep sound and restorative?
3. How much sleep is needed on a daily basis to feel alert and energetic while awake? How often is that amount of sleep obtained? What are daytime symptoms related to poor sleep?
4. What is the sleeping and waking schedule? Does it vary between weekdays and weekends? Has it changed recently?
5. Are caffeine and alcohol used? If so, how much and when?
6. Does the patient snore? If so, how loudly? Are apneic pauses present in sleep?
7. Is the patient aware, or does a bed partner report, leg or body movements in sleep?
8. What is the sleep environment like, including temperature, bed comfort, noise, light and so on?

---

*Not available in the United States.

patients often sleep better elsewhere in the house or away from home.

As sleep worsens, the insomnia takes on "a life of its own," persisting for months or years. These patients focus their attention on their sleep condition, minimizing other mental and emotional concerns. They usually have relatively good family and work relationships, without the severity of interpersonal problems usually seen in psychiatric patients.

Primary Sleep Disorders

Periodic limb movement disorder (PLMD) and restless legs syndrome (RLS) occur most often in older patient populations. Many patients with PLMD are asymptomatic, but bed partners report being kicked at night or are aware of the patient's repetitive movements. RLS, which is usually accompanied by leg movements, is described as discomfort or pain in the legs at rest, leading to a need for leg movement for relief.

Patients with sleep apnea may complain of insomnia rather than excessive sleepiness. Apnea should be considered in patients with multiple awakenings of unclear origin without problems at sleep onset and in patients with primary complaints of nonrestorative sleep or daytime fatigue. PLMD and apnea require sleep studies for diagnosis.

Psychiatric Disturbances

Psychiatric patients are especially at risk for insomnia, and changes in sleep habits may alert the clinician to the development of depression or other psychiatric problems. These patients may complain of early morning awakening, disturbed midnocturnal sleep, or delayed sleep onset. Although most depressed patients report a decreased sleep time, a few patients, usually in the depressed phase of bipolar affective disorder, report increased sleep time and daytime sleepiness.

Relationships between insomnia and depression are complex. Insomnia is associated with depression; depression produces insomnia. Insomnia that persists for more than a year is associated with increased risk of depression. This causal relationship seems obvious to our patients: when sleep is poor, they feel more depressed; with good sleep, their mood is improved. Clearly, not all insomnia is caused by depression, nor does effective treatment with antidepressants prove that the insomnia complaint is caused by depression. Other causes should be considered and explored.

Manic patients have marked decreases in sleep time and time in bed, feeling well with 4 or 5 hours of sleep per night for long periods of time. Acute schizophrenia is also associated with a sleep disturbance, with delayed sleep onset, decreased sleep time, and increased time awake after sleep onset.

TREATMENT OF INSOMNIA

Effective treatment requires that disturbances in habits, circadian rhythm, mood, and underlying sleep physiology be identified. Although behavioral management is always a component of insomnia treatment, pharmacotherapy is often needed as well, at times combined with behavioral treatment.

Behavioral Treatments of Insomnia

Many approaches to insomnia are based on the observation that insomniac patients are tense, anxious, or excessively aroused. Various strategies can be used to combat this state of excessive arousal; among these are progressive relaxation techniques, self-hypnosis, meditation, abdominal breathing, biofeedback, and a host of other, similar approaches.

Stimulus Control Therapy

Stimulus control therapy assumes that the sleep environment has become associated with greater arousal, as demonstrated, for example, by the ability to fall asleep in the living room but not in the bedroom. To break this pattern, patients follow specific rules, promoting the capacity to sleep in the bedroom. A complete description and explanation of this approach is provided in Table 2.

Sleep Restriction Therapy

Sleep restriction therapy assumes that excessive time spent in bed may promote or perpetuate insomnia. By limiting time spent in bed, more consolidated sleep is generated. The sleep deprivation provoked by this approach also produces improved sleep efficiency. Sleep is consolidated, and sleep patterns become more regular and predictable. Total time in bed is allowed to increase as the patient experiences improved sleep over time.

Sleep Hygiene

"Sleep hygiene" refers to relatively neutral suggestions that should improve sleep in most patients with sleep problems. Most insomniacs should avoid naps, reduce or discontinue caffeine and alcohol intake, maintain a regular sleep and waking schedule, and not spend time in bed if awake.

Patients should try to implement one or two sleep hygiene rules at a time, with instructions to monitor progress until their next office visit. Improvement

TABLE 2. **Stimulus Control Instructions: "Rules" Patients Must Follow**

1. Lie down intending to go to sleep only when you feel sleepy.
2. Use your bed only for sleep.
3. If you are unable to fall asleep, get up and go into another room. Stay up as long as you wish and then return to the bedroom to sleep. Although we do not want you to watch the clock, we want you to get out of bed if you do not fall asleep immediately. Remember that the goal is to associate your bed with falling asleep quickly! If you are in bed more than about 10 minutes without falling asleep and have not gotten up, you are not following this instruction.
4. If you still cannot fall asleep, repeat rule 3. Do this as often as is necessary throughout the night.
5. Set your alarm and get up at the same time every morning irrespective of how much sleep you had during the night.
6. Do not nap during the day.

TABLE 3. Sleep Hygiene Instructions

1. Sleep only as much as you need to feel refreshed during the day.
2. A regular exercise program in the morning or afternoon may help to promote sleep.
3. Limit alcohol intake, especially in the evening.
4. Avoid caffeine use, especially in the late afternoon or evening.
5. Set aside time in the evening—at least an hour before bedtime—to deal with problems or thoughts that you have on your mind. Write down plans to cope with problems the next day. Don't let them bother you through the night.
6. A light bedtime snack may help sustain sleep.
7. Keep your bedroom as dark and quiet as possible. Maintain it at a comfortable temperature.
8. If you can't sleep and feel yourself getting more frustrated as you remain awake, get up, go to another room and do something relaxing—read or listen to the radio or a relaxation tape. When you feel sleepy go back to bed and go to sleep.
9. If you wake during the night, do not look at the clock. Try to just "roll over and go back to sleep."
10. Your wake-up time must be regular and the same on weekends as weekdays.
11. Do not nap during the day. Naps will only decrease your level of sleepiness at night and decrease the number of hours of sleep you may expect to obtain.
12. Don't worry about or focus on the amount of sleep you are obtaining. Focus instead on your level of daytime alertness and functioning. If this level is good (or at least improving), you are getting at least an adequate amount of sleep during the night.

from these changes is not immediate, and patients should be informed to expect gradual improvement in sleep rather than an immediate end to their insomnia. Sleep hygiene rules are listed in Table 3.

Medical Disorders and Primary Sleep Disorders

The treatment of medical causes of insomnia is, whenever possible, to treat the underlying medical problem. When insomnia is due to somatic pain, analgesics may help with sleep by their inherent sedating qualities, as well as by diminishing the noxious stimuli that tend to awaken a patient or keep him or her awake.

Treatment of sleep apnea usually includes nasal continuous positive airway pressure, surgery, or use of oral appliances to open the airway in sleep. Patients whose sleep apnea presents as insomnia require standard treatment, but they may need adjunctive treatment with hypnotics once apnea is adequately treated.

PLMS and RLS are treated with a variety of approaches. Dopaminergic agents such as carbidopa-levodopa (Sinemet)* and pergolide (Permax)* have been used effectively across a broad dosage range; early and limited experience with pramipexole (Mirapex)* suggests superior efficacy with fewer side effects and reduced likelihood of tolerance.

_____
*Not FDA approved for this indication.

Light and Circadian Rhythms

Light exposure plays an important role in regulating circadian rhythms. Light exposure at specific times of the day helps to maintain and establish circadian rhythms. Because exposure to morning sunlight plays an important role in maintaining a stable and desired rhythm of sleep and wakefulness, a regular morning hour of arousal (and light exposure) may help to establish or maintain sleep rhythms for insomniac patients. Both regular hours of arising and regular bedtimes are beneficial in maintaining stable and strong sleep-wake patterns.

Pharmacologic Therapy of Insomnia

The use of medications to treat insomnia dates to antiquity. Until the 1970s, agents most often used were the barbiturate and barbiturate-like agents and chloral hydrate. The release of the first benzodiazepine hypnotic, flurazepam (Dalmane), in 1970 established new standards for safety and efficacy in insomnia treatment. Flurazepam has a long half-life and is usually used at a dose of 15 mg for the elderly and 30 mg for other adults. Temazepam (Restoril), an intermediate half-life agent, is used at a dose of 7.5 to 15 mg for the elderly and 15 to 30 mg for other adults. Triazolam (Halcion), the first short half-life benzodiazepine, was the source of great (and largely unwarranted) controversy in the 1980s. It is usually used at a dose of 0.125 mg for the elderly and 0.25 mg for other adults.

The 1990s saw the introduction of new hypnotics such as zolpidem (Ambien). Zolpidem, a benzodiazepine agonist with a nonbenzodiazepine chemical structure, was the first compound of this type released in the United States. Zaleplon (Sonata), a similar benzodiazepine agonist with a half-life even shorter than that of zolpidem, has recently been approved by the U.S. Food and Drug Administration. Both these agents are generally used at a dose of 5 mg for the elderly and 10 mg for other adults.

The efficacy of hypnotic medications for short-term periods is well established. Although concerns are often expressed about use of these agents for longer than 4-week periods, data from long-term outpatient studies show low abuse liability and little risk of withdrawal symptoms. Benzodiazepine-agonist compounds are remarkably safe in overdosage, particularly when contrasted to the barbiturate and barbiturate-like agents and to chloral hydrate. Their toxicity is greatly increased, however, in combination with other agents that may suppress respiration (including alcohol).

The risk of carryover effects of long half-life agents has been a long-standing concern and has been demonstrated through performance measures and epidemiologic surveys. Increased risk of hip fracture is seen in elderly patients who use any of three classes of long half-life compounds—hypnotic-anxiolytics, tricyclic antidepressants, and antipsychchotics—compared with the risks in individuals who use short half-life hypnotic-anxiolytics.

Insomnia patients without mood disturbance often receive sedating antidepressants in treatment, although little published data support their safety and efficacy. Rationales for this practice include concerns that the benzodiazepines may lead to abuse, tolerance and habituation, rebound insomnia, daytime sedation, or disinhibition reactions. Although tricyclic and other antidepressants are alternatives to the benzodiazepines, their risks include anticholinergic toxicity, orthostatic hypotension and falls, cardiotoxicity, confusional states, and fatal overdosage.

Among the antidepressants often used to treat insomnia are amitriptyline (Elavil),* 10 to 50 mg; doxepin (Sinequan),* 10 to 50 mg; and trazodone (Desyrel),* 25 to 100 mg. Limiting factors to the use of these agents are typical side effects seen with tricyclic agents, including complaints of constipation, dry mouth, urinary retention, and orthostatic hypotension. Similar complaints may be seen with trazodone, as well as complaints of morning or daytime sedation.

Patients treated with selective serotonin reuptake inhibitors (SSRIs) often report disrupted sleep or insomnia, especially early in treatment. Benzodiazepine agonists or sedating antidepressants such as trazodone or doxepin are often given with the SSRIs to treat insomnia, with the hope that additive or synergistic effects may be seen.

Most over-the-counter sleeping aids contain sedating antihistamines. They are heavily promoted and are perceived as being safer than prescription agents, owing to their ready availability. Few data are available about their efficacy, but side effects, including hangover or anticholinergic effects, are common.

Herbal and other "natural" compounds are also quite popular and reflect increased interest in and reliance on "alternative" and "complementary" medical treatment approaches. Like agents purchased over the counter, little or no research data are available demonstrating the efficacy of such agents in the treatment of insomnia.

Melatonin is a hormone produced by most animals in the dark. It is not a sleep-promoting agent; in nocturnal animals, high melatonin levels at night are associated with wakefulness and physical activity. Melatonin's effects in mammals include controlling seasonal breeding in many species, with high melatonin levels in winter causing gonadal shrinkage and reduced sex drive. Human studies have shown limited effects of melatonin on sleep induction or sleep continuity, with the poor capacity to replicate positive results in repeat studies. Melatonin may be of benefit in re-entraining circadian rhythms disturbed in shift workers or patients with jet lag.

CONCLUSIONS

Insomnia is usually complex, multifactorial, difficult to understand, and difficult to treat. The better

*Not FDA approved for this indication.

we can identify the causative elements and define specific treatments for the individual patient, the higher the likelihood that we can provide successful treatment.

As a general rule, behavioral therapies are preferable to medications but take longer to teach, are not immediately effective, and are not universally accepted by patients. Although the combination of behavioral therapy and pharmacotherapy is somewhat controversial, it is always helpful to frame the treatment relationship with the patient in behavioral terms ("Our goal is to help you regain your ability to sleep well without medications") and to provide specific suggestions to the patient to improve sleep, even though medications are also being provided.

PRURITUS

method of
SARAH A. MYERS, M.D.
Duke University Medical Center
Durham, North Carolina

Pruritus, derived from the Latin word *prurire*, meaning "to itch," is the sensation in the skin that provokes one to scratch. Pruritus may be associated with a specific dermatologic condition and is the most common symptom in the dermatology setting (Table 1). In the absence of clinically evident primary skin disease, underlying systemic disease may be associated with generalized pruritus (Table 2). Skin lesions such as those created by rubbing, scratching, or infection are often present in this setting but are considered secondary to the underlying process and not a primary dermatologic condition. Treating pruritus can be frustrating to both the patient and the clinician, as scratching itchy skin is often inherently pleasurable and may lead to a vicious itch-scratch cycle that is very hard to break. Important aspects of management include accurate diagnosis, individualized treatment, and ongoing monitoring for new causes if the pruritus is persistent.

The precise neuroanatomy and neurophysiology of pruritus is not known. For years it was believed that itch was mediated through unspecialized C fibers. Recent studies, however, indicate a new class of fine cutaneous nerve fibers that appear to be itch specific. These fibers respond to histamine but not to heat or mechanical stimulation. Al-

TABLE 1. **Dermatologic Conditions Associated with Pruritus**

Inflammatory	Infestations
Atopic dermatitis	Insect bites
Bullous pemphigoid	Parasites
Contact dermatitis	Scabies
Dermatitis herpetiformis	**Neoplastic**
Dermatographism	
Drug hypersensitivity	Mycosis fungoides
Folliculitis	**Miscellaneous**
Lichen planus	
Miliaria	Xerosis
Psoriasis	Sunburn
Urticaria	Anogenital pruritus
	Notalgia paresthetica

TABLE 2. **Systemic Diseases Associated with Pruritus**

Hepatobiliary	Hematologic
Extrahepatic biliary obstruction	Iron deficiency anemia
Primary biliary cirrhosis	Polycythemia vera
Cholestasis of pregnancy	Paraproteinemia
Renal	**Malignancy**
Chronic renal failure	Hodgkin's and non-Hodgkin's
Endocrine	lymphoma
Hyperthyroidism	Multiple myeloma
Hypothyroidism	Visceral carcinoma
Diabetes mellitus	Mycosis fungoides
	Carcinoid syndrome
Infection	**Central Nervous System**
Human immunodeficiency virus	Multiple sclerosis
Autoimmune	Cerebrovascular accident
Sjögren's syndrome	Psychiatric disorders

though histamine is the classic mediator of pruritus, there is evidence for other nonhistamine mediators and/or modulators as well. They include various proteases, peptides such as kinins and substance P, prostaglandins, serotonin, and physical stimuli. Opioid peptides appear to be important central modulators, as opioid antagonists may benefit some patients with pruritus.

DIAGNOSIS

Careful history taking, skin examination (often requiring repeated inspections), and selected laboratory tests are the most important aspects of evaluating patients with pruritus. Duration and characteristics of the itch as well as initiating, exacerbating, and relieving factors are helpful clues in the patient's history. Drugs and environmental factors (such as exposures to fiberglass, chemicals, irritating dusts, infested pets, other itching people) are important causes of generalized itching and should be evaluated thoroughly before undertaking a major systemic work-up. Characteristic skin lesions are usually associated with pruritic dermatologic conditions, but skin biopsy may be necessary to make a definitive diagnosis. Two dermatologic conditions that are often overlooked as a cause for pruritus include generalized xerosis (dry skin) and dermatographism.

If no skin disease is evident to explain persistent pruritus (other than lesions produced by scratching), a work-up for underlying systemic disease should be performed. General history and review of systems and physical examination, with emphasis on adenopathy and organomegaly, are critical in this setting. Routine screening tests include complete blood count with differential, serum glucose, renal and liver panels, urinalysis, thyroid panel, sedimentation rate, serum protein electrophoresis, serum iron, stool for occult blood, and chest radiographs. A skin biopsy is rarely helpful if performed on normal skin. If laboratory test results are normal, conservative therapy can be initiated; however, the patient with persistent pruritus should be reassessed continually for the development of a primary dermatologic or systemic disease.

TOPICAL TREATMENT

Primary dermatologic conditions, when present, should be treated with therapy specific for the condi-

tion (e.g., permethrin [Elimite, Nix] for scabies infestation). Avoidance of causative or contributing factors involved in atopic, allergic, or other hypersensitivity dermatoses is important. Often, patients' behaviors such as taking long hot showers and self-treatments for pruritus (e.g., rubbing alcohol, witch hazel, or various over-the-counter products) may contribute to the problem even though they are temporarily soothing. Skin moisturization is critical, as dry skin frequently initiates pruritus or exacerbates other pruritic dermatoses such as atopic dermatitis and psoriasis. Mild, fragrance-free cleansing bars or liquids (Dove, Oil of Olay, Purpose, Basis, or Cetaphil) should replace harsh or deodorant soaps, and shorter, warm showers or baths should be stressed. Oatmeal baths (Aveeno) or baths with fragrance-free bath oils may also provide short-term symptomatic relief.

Patting dry with a towel and immediately applying emollients such as Eucerin, Aquaphor, petroleum jelly, Theraplex clear lotion, Dermasil cream or lotion, or Cetaphil lotion should be undertaken after bathing. Emollients with camphor and menthol (e.g., Sarna Anti-Itch lotion), phenol, or pramoxine (e.g., PrameGel, Pramosone, or Aveeno Anti-Itch lotion) may provide safe relief from pruritus. Cool compresses and shake lotions (calamine) may also be highly efficacious. The use of the topical anesthetic benzocaine and the topical antihistamine diphenhydramine (Benadryl, Caladryl) is generally discouraged because of significant development of allergic contact sensitization.

Topical corticosteroids (even in the absence of skin eruption) may be useful adjunctive agents for pruritus control. For widespread pruritus, hydrocortisone (1 or 2.5%) or triamcinolone (0.025 or 0.1%) preparations are generally effective. Capsaicin cream (Zostrix) may be of some benefit for selected patients with a wide range of severe pruritic disorders. It is most practical for localized or particularly problematic pruritic areas. Because capsaicin cream may produce burning or stinging sensations or superficial burns initially, careful patient instruction is required. In many cases, the burning sensation diminishes, and relief from pruritus follows. Topical doxepin (Zonalon) is indicated for short-term relief of pruritus. It may be applied four times per day to affected skin for up to 8 days. Sedation can result if Zonalon is applied to extensive areas; therefore, it too is more useful for localized pruritus. A eutectic mixture of the local anesthetics lidocaine and prilocaine (EMLA cream) may be helpful for recalcitrant pruritic conditions.

SYSTEMIC THERAPY

Treatment of any underlying disorder, such as decreasing serum bile concentration in cholestatic liver disease, correcting secondary hyperparathyroidism in uremia, or treating a malignancy with chemotherapy, often leads to improvement in or resolution of pruritus related to systemic disease. The use of systemic steroids, although often highly effective, is generally not recommended because of adverse sequelae associated with long-term use. As a result, symptomatic therapy with oral antihistamines is the mainstay of systemic therapy for pruritus.

The H_1 histamine antagonists constitute the treatment of first choice. Hydroxyzine (Atarax) is frequently beneficial when dosed 10 to 25 mg every 6 hours daily, with upward titration based on response and toleration of side effects. Alternative H_1 blockers include diphenhydramine hydrochloride (Benadryl), 25 to 50 mg every 6 hours, or cyproheptadine (Periactin), 4 mg every 8 hours. The use of H_1 antihistamines needs to be accompanied with warnings of sedation, mental status changes, and urinary retention, especially in the elderly. Cetirizine (Zyrtec), 10 mg once daily, is less sedating than hydroxyzine and may be a useful alternative. In conditions other than urticaria, the nonsedating antihistamines, including terfenadine (Seldane, 60 mg every 12 hours), fexofenadine (Allegra, 60 mg every 12 hours), astemizole (Hismanal, 10 mg once daily), and loratadine (Claritin, 10 mg once daily), may have only marginal therapeutic effects for pruritus. Because of potentially serious cardiac arrhythmias, the nonsedating antihistamines should not be used by patients also taking systemic agents, including azole antifungal agents and erythromycin. Another approach is to use tricyclic antidepressants, highly potent H_1 and H_2 antagonists. Doxepin (Sinequan),* 10 to 25 mg every 8 hours or in one nighttime dose (75 mg), can be highly effective in relieving pruritus.

A variety of other systemic agents have been used with some effect in specific disease states. Patients with cholestatic liver disease may experience relief from pruritus when serum bile concentration is lowered by oral cholestyramine (Questran), 4 g twice daily, or colestipol hydrochloride (Colestid),* which is less constipating. Activated charcoal can also be used as a potential binding agent to help reduce pruritus. Naloxone hydrochloride (Narcan),* an opiate antagonist, has demonstrated effectiveness in reducing pruritus and scratching activity in some patients with cholestasis. Erythropoietin therapy* (epoetin alfa [Epogen, Procrit]) (36 units per kg three times weekly) lowers histamine levels and relieves pruritus in patients with uremia.

Ultraviolet B phototherapy and, less commonly, ultraviolet A and psoralen photochemotherapy (PUVA) can be successfully employed in a wide range of pruritic disorders, including atopic dermatitis, renal disease, and human immunodeficiency virus infection. Doses of ultraviolet therapy are usually administered three times per week and increased until mild erythema is attained. Therapy is then adjusted to accommodate the patient's level of photosensitivity. It may take 20 to 30 treatments to attain symptomatic relief, and patients often need encouragement to continue therapy. Ultraviolet therapy is best utilized with the input or supervision of a dermatologist.

*Not FDA approved for this indication.

TINNITUS

method of
BRADLEY KESSER, M.D., and
RICK A. FRIEDMAN, M.D., Ph.D.
House Ear Clinic, Inc.
Los Angeles, California

"Any management which is based on a single panacea for the treatment of a symptom and not a disease will result in failure."

Victor Goodhill's statement on the management of tinnitus is just as accurate today as it was when he wrote it almost 50 years ago. It is estimated that 40 million Americans have experienced head noise, or tinnitus, at some point in their lives. Tinnitus seriously affects an estimated 10 million people; furthermore, it debilitates approximately 1 million. Nevertheless, almost every patient suffering from tinnitus can be helped. As Goodhill noted, tinnitus is in fact a symptom, not a disease, and an underlying etiology must be sought.

In evaluating the patient with tinnitus, a few important points in the patient's history will steer the physician toward a diagnosis or further testing. Is the tinnitus unilateral, bilateral, or "inside the head?" What is the character of the tinnitus (and, of importance, is it pulsatile)? Is it acute or chronic (i.e., what is the onset)? Are there any exacerbating or relieving factors? Has there been a history of noise exposure? Ear infections? Hearing loss? Stress? What is the degree to which the head noise has affected or debilitated the patient's life (does it keep the patient awake at night; does it awaken him or her from sleep; can the patient focus, concentrate, and perform daily activities)? The physician must address and gain insight into the psychologic status of the patient; many affected patients are depressed, anxious, and/or "stressed out." Stress plays a large role in these patients and is discussed later.

Physical examination should include tuning fork testing; otoscopic examination; neurologic examination with special attention to the cranial nerves; and auscultation of the ears, mastoids, and carotid arteries if the tinnitus is pulsatile. Objective tinnitus (noise heard by the patient and observer) necessitates a diagnostic work-up very different from that for subjective tinnitus (noise heard only by the patient).

The importance of audiometry cannot be overemphasized. Pure tone thresholds for air conduction, bone conduction, and speech testing are crucial in the evaluation of tinnitus; the answer often lies in the audiogram. If the audiogram is normal, reassurance of the patient is often all that is required.

Once this information has been collected, the diagnosis is usually apparent. If the diagnosis is unclear, a differential diagnosis is generated, and further testing may be needed. We have found that classifying tinnitus as pulsatile or nonpulsatile aids in evaluating the patient. Table 1 lists some of the more common etiologies of pulsatile tinnitus; Table 2 displays common causes of nonpulsatile tinnitus.

The treatment of tinnitus is based on the underlying pathology and on the diagnosis; further testing is occasionally necessary. In the category of pulsatile tinnitus, temporal bone computed tomographic (CT) scanning is the imaging study of first choice to evaluate a retrotympanic mass (glomus tympanicum or jugulare; CT scanning also picks up abnormalities of the jugular bulb and/or carotid artery). Carotid duplex scanning is indicated for patients

TABLE 1. Common Etiologies of Pulsatile Tinnitus

Benign intracranial hypertension ("venous hum" tinnitus)
Atherosclerotic carotid artery disease
Glomus tumor (tympanicum or jugulare)
Vascular malformation (dural arteriovenous malformation
  [AVM], carotid artery aneurysm)
Otosclerosis
Palatal myoclonus
Middle ear muscle (tensor tympani or stapedius) myoclonus
Hypertension

with a carotid bruit. Benign intracranial hypertension is an often overlooked but frequent cause of pulsatile tinnitus. Affected patients tend to be obese females; gentle compression of the jugular vein in the neck often relieves the symptoms. Referral to a neuro-ophthalmologist is appropriate for these patients. Magnetic resonance imaging/angiography (MRI/MRA) is an excellent first-line study if there is a suspicion of increased intracranial pressure (ICP) in the patient with pulsatile tinnitus and no mass behind the tympanic membrane. Myoclonus of either a middle ear muscle or the palate is generally described as an intermittent "clicking" sound, sometimes several times per second. Spasm of the soft palate can be observed when the patient is symptomatic. Muscle relaxants, botulinum toxin injection for the palate, or sectioning of the tensor tympani or stapedius muscles usually brings relief.

Eighty percent of patients with hearing loss have tinnitus at some point in their lives. More often than not, the tinnitus does not particularly bother them; they have gotten used to it over time. The audiogram is most helpful in diagnosing these cases, and most patients require only reassurance that nothing serious is going on and that their tinnitus is simply a manifestation of their hearing loss. Exposure to loud noises—either brief, high-intensity sounds (acoustic trauma) or prolonged exposure to medium- to high-intensity sounds (noise-induced)—will cause tinnitus. Hearing protection and counseling are important for these patients. Any patient with asymmetric sensorineural hearing loss should undergo retrocochlear evaluation (especially if the tinnitus is unilateral); MRI with gadolinium contrast is the study of choice for the diagnosis of acoustic neuroma. Infections of the outer, middle, or inner ear are often accompanied by tinnitus; diagnosis is made on the basis of the history and physical examination. Treatment of the infection relieves the tinnitus. Meniere's disease is characterized by the classic triad of fluctuating hearing loss, vertigo, and tinnitus. The diagnosis is a clinical one, usually based on the history and normal otologic examination. Meniere's disease can be difficult to manage

TABLE 2. Common Etiologies of Nonpulsatile Tinnitus

Hearing loss
Noise exposure/acoustic trauma
Acoustic neuroma
Otitis externa
Otitis media
Eustachian tube function or dysfunction
Labyrinthitis
Meniere's disease
Temporomandibular joint dysfunction
Tension headaches
Stress, depression, anxiety

TABLE 3. CAPPE Mnemonic for Tinnitus Evaluation

Chemical
Acoustic
Pathologic
Physical
Emotional

and generally warrants referral to an otologist or neurotologist.

In counseling patients on the possible causes of their tinnitus, we often use the mnemonic CAPPE (Table 3) to summarize and package this information. This mnemonic allows physician and patient to identify certain "stresses" in their lives that are causing or contributing to their tinnitus.

Chemical stresses that contribute to tinnitus include such medications as erythromycin and other macrolide antibiotics, vancomycin, aminoglycoside antibiotics, furosemide (Lasix) and other loop diuretics, high-dose aspirin or nonsteroidal anti-inflammatory drugs (NSAIDs), quinine/chloroquine, antineoplastic drugs (platinum-based regimens), caffeine, nicotine, and alcohol. We advise patients to reduce their caffeine intake (or switch to decaffeinated products) and alcohol consumption, to quit smoking, and to try alternative medications in consultation with their internists.

Acoustic stresses include chronic noise exposure, acoustic trauma, sensorineural hearing loss (presbycusis, noise-induced) or conductive loss. We strongly urge hearing protection for patients who are exposed to occupational noise, for people attending loud concerts, and for anyone exposed to loud noises.

Pathologic stresses include any infectious, inflammatory, vascular, or neoplastic process affecting the ear, including otitis externa, otitis media, labyrinthitis, acoustic neuroma, Meniere's disease, or glomus tumor. Diagnosis is usually made on the basis of the history and physical examination; further testing is occasionally indicated.

Physical stresses may be sequelae of natural events (you will hear your pulse in your ears after vigorous exercise) or nonotologic processes such as fever, upper respiratory tract infection, temporomandibular joint dysfunction (if you clench your teeth, you will hear noise in your ears), tension headaches, cervical muscle tension, or other major illness. Patients with normal or abnormal eustachian tube function describe a popping sound, the same sound you hear when you swallow.

Finally, emotional stress can be a significant contributor to tinnitus. Screening questions for problems at home, in the office, or with the family often reveal such stresses. Stress reduction is very helpful for these patients, and we have recommended biofeedback to help control symptoms. When patients hear the tinnitus, their stress level increases; in other words, tinnitus itself causes stress. The increased stress serves only to make the tinnitus louder, further increasing the stress. Such a vicious cycle leads to insomnia, depression, inability to focus, and malaise. Breaking the cycle is important in the management of these patients. For most patients, simple reassurance is all that is required. Patients may need a short course of a low-dose tricyclic antidepressant to help. We generally start with amitriptyline (Elavil), 25 mg orally at bedtime to help with symptoms of insomnia, stress, and depression. Consultation with the patient's internist is recommended. Stress management plays a large role in helping these patients.

In summary, tinnitus is a symptom, and an underlying disease process should be searched before simple reassurance of the patient. History, physical examination, and audiometry generally point to the correct diagnosis. Additional testing may be needed. Identification of various stresses in the patient's life helps physician and patient organize a differential diagnosis for head noise and helps sort out various possible causes. Most patients do well with education and reassurance; other patients go on to further testing and treatment.

LOW BACK PAIN

method of
THOMAS S. WHITECLOUD III, M.D.
Tulane University Medical Center
New Orleans, Louisiana

One of the most common musculoskeletal complaints for which patients seek the care of a primary physician is low back pain. Low back pain is a symptom not a diagnosis. In most instances, the actual pathologic cause of acute low back pain is not precisely diagnosed. This does not affect the care of the patient, because low back pain is generally a self-limiting condition that resolves within 4 to 6 weeks in 80% of patients. Their symptoms can be altered by treatment, but a precise diagnosis as to etiology is not always necessary.

The economic impact to society of low back pain is enormous. In the population of an industrialized country, approximately 80% of adults will experience back pain at some point in their life. In the United States, 50% of the adult population admits to back or leg discomfort in any given year. It is the most common cause of disability for patients younger than age 45. At any given time, 1% of the U.S. population is chronically disabled from back pain and 1% is temporarily disabled.

The direct cost to society is $18 to $20 billion per year. But when the indirect costs are included (e.g., lost time from work, compensation costs, the failed surgery patient) the costs are $50 to $80 billion per year. Obviously, it is extremely important to properly manage individuals with acute low back pain on initial presentation.

Back pain can be classified as acute, chronic, or recurrent. Acute back pain lasts up to 3 months, with the chronic condition beginning after 3 months. Recurrent back pain is pain that returns after a pain-free interval.

As in any patient with musculoskeletal problems, a routine should be developed for their evaluation. The evaluation should begin with a history, including the past history and psychosocial questions. Although it is not always possible, a questionnaire should be filled out by the patient before being seen by the health care provider. A standardized form should be available that provides information regarding referral source, work status, duration of symptoms, compensation and litigation status, past history of back pain, and response to treatment. Validated forms such as the SF36 and Oswestry scales, analogue pain scale, and pain drawing are useful for measuring response to treatment and clinical outcome.

Musculoskeletal or spondylogenic causes are not the only reason an individual has lower back discomfort. Other causes can be viscerogenic, vascular, neurogenic, and psychogenic. Careful questioning regarding the nature and duration of pain, what causes it to become worse, and what helps it to improve will help delineate the source of pain.

Musculoskeletal back pain in the younger patient often begins after a specific incident of trauma or strain. The pain varies in intensity and duration and should diminish with decreased activity. Bed rest should reduce the intensity of the symptom-complex.

There are certain "red flags" that should be looked for when obtaining a history from older patients. A history of trauma, cancer, constitutional symptoms, risk factors for infection, and pain that is constant and unremitting and persists at rest should warn the physician that a more serious cause of the patient's back pain is possible. Obviously, bowel and bladder dysfunction and or sudden onset of progressive neurologic deficit also are "red flags" that could indicate a possible fracture, metastatic disease, spinal infection, or cauda equina syndrome.

Once a detailed history has been obtained, a careful physical examination is performed. Musculoskeletal low back pain is not associated with neurologic deficits or root tension signs. However, there can be referred pain to the sacroiliac joints, posterior and lateral aspects of the hips, and down the posterior thigh. Referred pain should not extend below the knee. The examination should also include an evaluation of the hips, sacroiliac joints, and knees.

TREATMENT

Once the history and physical is completed and there is no indication of any other possible cause except a musculoskeletal one, treatment can be instituted. Treatment includes patient counseling with an emphasis on the natural history of low back pain—that it is a very common condition and almost all symptoms resolve in 80% of patients in 4 to 6 weeks. Although it has not been proven that any modalities can alter the natural history of this process, the purpose of treatment is to provide symptomatic relief and help ensure that the natural history of the condition is not altered.

Treatment should consist of alteration of activities, physical modalities (e.g., ice pack, then heating pad), and medication. There is no place for prolonged bed rest in the treatment of low back pain. Forty-eight hours is believed to be beneficial initially, but any longer period can be debilitating and lead to a slower recovery. Patients should be instructed regarding posture. Sitting places more strain on the lower back than standing or lying down. Even a slight degree of forward flexion increases low back load. Proper body mechanics should be used for lifting, utilizing hips and knees, and placing the load close to the body. Twisting of the trunk, especially when lifting, should be avoided.

A number of modalities have been recommended for treatment of low back pain. Very few have been scientifically validated. A short course of physical therapy is, however, beneficial. It should be of the active type, not passive, and the patient should be instructed to also perform the exercises at home. Low-impact exercises such as walking, elliptical trainers, and swimming should also be encouraged. Weight loss, when indicated, should be emphasized.

Three classes of medication are of value for acute

low back pain: analgesics, muscle relaxants, and non-steroidal anti-inflammatory drugs (NSAIDs). If possible, acetaminophen or aspirin should be used as an analgesic. In some patients, stronger analgesics are required, but they should be used short term and with caution. NSAIDs should also be used short term, and the side effects of both analgesics and NSAIDs drugs should be discussed with the patient, because the response to anti-inflammatory medications varies among patients. There are nine different subchemical groups, and failure to respond promptly to one category is an indication that another category of NSAIDs should be tried. The side effects of these medications can be deleterious, and NSAIDs must be used with caution. Muscle relaxants also should be used short term, and the patient should be warned of drowsiness.

Education is an important part of the treatment of the acute low back pain patient. The incidence and natural history of this condition should be emphasized. The patient should be kept active, encouraged to return to work, and told that he or she must be involved in the healing process. There is no indication for any imaging studies at the first encounter. Only in those few patients who are failing to improve at the 4- to 6-week interval should further diagnostic tests be done. In those patients who have chronic low back pain, an attempt should be made to identify an anatomic reason for the persistent symptoms. Because disks undergo biochemical and biomechanical changes with aging, most adults will have degenerative lumbar disk disease. Degeneration can lead to other causes of chronic back pain, such as spinal lateral and central stenosis, spondylolisthesis, disk herniation, degenerative scoliosis, and segmental instability.

These patients should be evaluated exactly as the acute low back pain patient is, but with the addition of imaging studies such as routine roentgenograms, magnetic resonance imaging (MRI), and possibly myelography/computed tomography. Caution must be observed in interpreting the results of these tests, because all adults have disk degeneration. Forty percent of people who are asymptomatic and older than age 40 will have abnormal findings on MRI. It is the duty of the clinician to correlate the results of the history, physical examination, and diagnostic studies to properly identify the source of chronic pain.

The management of chronic low back pain is quite similar to the method of dealing with acute low back pain. Modification of lifestyle, exercise, and medications are the mainstays of treatment. Surgery should be avoided if possible, and it must be remembered that an abnormal diagnostic test is not an indication for surgery.

The chronic back pain patient should be educated as to what has been shown to aggravate the condition, such as prolonged sitting, repetitive bending, repetitive lifting, and exposure to vibration (commercial driver). Job modification, if possible, might be of benefit.

Because disks are avascular and receive their nutrition by osmosis through small arterials at the vertebral endplates, it is not surprising that smoking worsens chronic back pain. The only proven modality of treatment is regular exercise, which results in cardiovascular fitness and good paraspinous and abdominal muscle tone. Exercise, obviously, will also improve obesity and its associated spinal loading.

The side effects of narcotics and NSAIDs are such that they must be used cautiously. The use of NSAIDs should be intermittent and liver enzymes monitored if used for 6 weeks or longer. Muscle relaxants are of little value in chronic back pain.

Other modalities of pain management such as biofeedback, transcutaneous electrical nerve stimulation (TENS) units, bracing, manipulation, acupuncture, and facet injections can be used in those patients who do not respond to the other methods of treatment.

When a patient has failed all modalities of treatment, surgery is an option if a specific diagnosis has been made that would respond favorably to spinal fusion.

There is a clear difference between a patient with low back pain and one who has both back and leg discomfort. If the leg pain follows a dermatomal pattern, it is most likely of nerve root origin. The most commonly involved nerve roots are the L4, L5, and S1. A careful neurologic evaluation can generally determine the level of root involvement. Tension signs such as a positive straight-leg raising test are diagnostic. A peripheral vascular examination is necessary to rule out a vascular origin for the leg pain.

Patients with back and dermatomal leg pain frequently have a herniated lumbar disk. This occurs most commonly in the fourth decade of life with equal male and female distribution. A detailed history and physical examination will provide a presumptive diagnosis, but confirmation and determination of the precise level of herniation necessitate an MRI.

Patients with herniated lumbar disks are not automatically surgical candidates. Only in those with a cauda equina syndrome secondary to a massive disk herniation is surgery urgent. Eighty percent of patients with herniated lumbar disks do not require lumbar surgery. Their leg pain can be managed with physical therapy, epidural corticosteroids, nerve root blocks, and short-term oral corticosteroids or NSAIDs. Only after these modalities are tried should surgery be considered. Good surgical results can be anticipated if the neurologic signs are constant, positive tension signs are present, and imaging studies correlate with the clinical findings.

The Infectious Diseases

HUMAN IMMUNODEFICIENCY VIRUS INFECTION AND ITS COMPLICATIONS

method of
MARSHALL K. KUBOTA, M.D.
University of California, San Francisco, and
Sutter Medical Center of Santa Rosa
Santa Rosa, California

In 1981, attention called to clusters of *Pneumocystis carinii* pneumonia (PCP) and Kaposi's sarcoma (KS) occurring among homosexual men living in large metropolitan areas defined the leading edge of the acquired immune deficiency syndrome (AIDS) epidemic in the United States. The syndrome includes opportunistic infections (OIs) associated with a decrease in CD4$^+$ (T helper) lymphocytes, a markedly increased risk for non-Hodgkin's B cell lymphomas (NHL) and Kaposi's sarcoma, dementia and disorders of the peripheral nervous system, and metabolic disorders resulting in wasting. Discovery of the putative agent of AIDS, the human immunodeficiency virus type 1 (HIV-1), led to a fuller understanding of the epidemiology, pathogenesis, and treatment of this syndrome.

EPIDEMIOLOGY

From 1981 through 1997, the Centers for Disease Control and Prevention had reported 632,999 adult and adolescent cases of HIV infection progressing to the stage of disease fulfilling the epidemiologic definition of AIDS. In 1996, for the first time, there was a decrease in the number of reported AIDS cases. In 1996, 56,730 cases fitting the definition of AIDS were reported, representing a 6% decrease compared with 1995. Women (1992—14%; 1996—20% by gender) and black non-Hispanics (1992—33%; 1996—41% by ethnicity) have shown the largest proportional increases in reported AIDS cases. Deaths due to AIDS also decreased 23% in 1996 (38,780) compared with 1995. These reductions have been greater for men than women (−25% vs. −10%), white non-Hispanics versus black non-Hispanics (−32% vs. −13%) and homosexual men versus heterosexuals (−30% vs. −8%). The overall improvements are due to the impact of prevention efforts of the mid-1980s, resulting in reduced transmission, and combination antiretroviral treatments, resulting in reduced progression to AIDS and death. An estimated 40,000 to 60,000 Americans are infected by HIV-1 annually. There are currently about 235,470 Americans living with AIDS, representing an 11% increase from 1995 to 1996.

TRANSMISSION

The modes of transmission of HIV are sexual transmission, transmission through significant exposure to infected blood or blood products, and vertical transmission in utero, intrapartum, and by breast-feeding. Blood, semen, and cervical/vaginal secretions contain enough HIV-1 to be infectious. Uncontaminated saliva has not been implicated in transmission. The susceptibility to transmission of portals of entry vary, with the rectum, vagina, penile urethra, and direct vascular and tissue exposure being of much higher risk than the mouth and other mucous membranes. Volume of infected fluid, exposure time, and concentration of HIV in the fluid are also factors in the risks of transmission. Direct intravascular injection of infected blood into the veins carries a high risk for infection, as occurs with injection drug users sharing needles, with infected individuals, or as might exist in occupational exposures (needlestick accidents). Infected men are more likely to transmit the virus to women during vaginal intercourse than infected women are to transmit the virus to men.

Vertical transmission from an infected mother to her child occurs in utero, intrapartum, and in the postpartum period through breast-feeding. The overall risk for transmission in utero and intrapartum ranges from 13 to 40%. The risk of transmission to an uninfected newborn by breast-feeding from an infected mother is about 14%. Reduction of transmission in pregnancy can be achieved through antenatal HIV testing, prenatal and intrapartum treatment of the mother to reduce HIV-1 titers, reduction (as possible) of blood exposure to the infant during birth, treatment of the newborn, and proscription of breast-feeding when safer alternatives exist.

HIV-1 KINETICS

Understanding the pathogenesis of HIV-1 infection and the kinetics of viral replication and mutation has aided in the development of logical treatment strategies. The ability to accurately measure HIV-1 in the plasma coupled with potent inhibitors of replication revealed that HIV-1 infection is a dynamic process of enormous levels of viral replication and immunologic destruction.

HIV-1 RNA in the plasma is measured by either branched DNA (bDNA) assay or quantitative polymerase chain reaction (PCR). A patient's viral titers (loads) could range from below limits of quantification (<25 to 50 copies of HIV-1 RNA/mL) to greater than 10^6 copies per mL. In an untreated state, higher titers are related to a more rapid deterioration in the immune system, as measured by CD4$^+$ counts and a poor prognosis. Daily virion production is in the range of 10^9 to 10^{10} particles.

Inherent in the replication of the virus is a high random mutation rate. Wild-type virus predominates, but within the diverse population of HIV-1 in any individual exist viruses with mutations predetermined to be resistant to simple regimens of antiretroviral treatment.

Rapid destruction of the immune system is prevented only by robust CD4$^+$ cell replacement. The initial HIV infection set point of viral production along with intrinsic immune repair mechanisms determines the long-term progression of HIV-1 (Figure 1).

Clinically, as long as immunologic replacement keeps

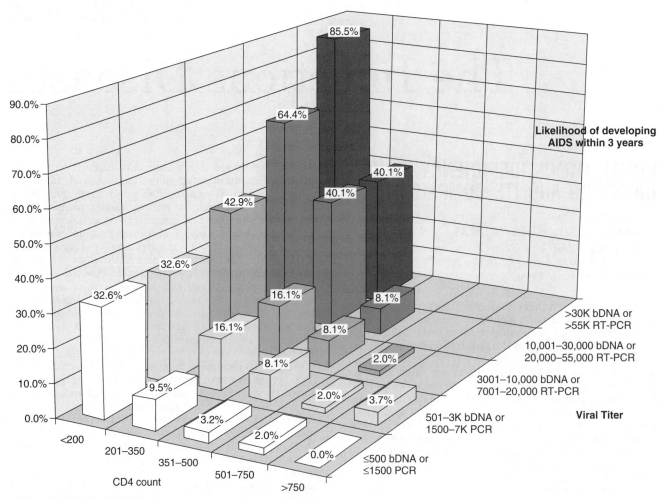

Figure 1. Progression of HIV-1. (Modified from Mellors JEW, Kinsley LA, Rinaldo CR, et al: Quantitation of HIV-1 RNA in plasma predicts outcome after seroconversion. Ann Intern Med *122*:573–579, 1995.)

pace with destruction, there is a prolonged asymptomatic period. Throughout this clinically uneventful time, viral burden grows and immunologic deterioration ensues, characterized by falling CD4$^+$ cell counts. Eventually, symptomatic HIV infection develops, leading to life-threatening opportunistic complications, neurologic dysfunction, and metabolic imbalances.

As the level of circulating CD4$^+$ cells declines, the immunologic protection afforded an individual passes down through succeeding layers of risk for specific OIs. Beginning at relatively normal levels of CD4$^+$ cells are conditions shared with the immunocompetent population but with greater frequency or severity (herpes simplex, herpes zoster, candidal vaginitis). If immunologic deterioration continues, OIs characteristic of AIDS become evident; and in an accumulation of risk, patients with very low CD4$^+$ cell counts are at risk for a large number of OIs.

The neurologic system is also the target of HIV-1 infection either directly or indirectly. Minor cognitive/motor disorder, HIV-associated dementia, and peripheral neuropathies are the common sequelae of HIV infection. A prominent metabolic disorder is wasting syndrome.

ACUTE RETROVIRAL INFECTION

The response to initial HIV-1 infection varies from asymptomatic to the acute retroviral syndrome experi-

enced by 50 to 90% of newly infected persons. The onset from exposure to symptoms is from 2 to 6 weeks. The duration of the acute illness is 1 to 2 weeks and can vary from mild to a severity requiring hospitalization. Heterophil testing commonly occurs in this setting and should trigger consideration of acute HIV infection. A large burst of viral replication occurs before the immunologic response, resulting initially in high plasma titers of virus. Widespread dissemination into lymphatic tissues occurs, and individual viral titer set points are established as antibody responses are developed. Within 6 to 10 weeks, most infected individuals have developed specific HIV antibodies, although for conservative counseling a 3- to 6-month seronegative window period is used (Table 1). Treatment dur-

TABLE 1. **Signs and Symptoms of Acute Retroviral Syndrome**

Fever	Headache
Lymphadenopathy	Nausea/vomiting
Pharyngitis	Hepatosplenomegaly
Maculopapular rash	Thrush
Mucocutaneous ulcerations	Weight loss
Myalgias, arthralgias	Central and peripheral
Diarrhea	neurologic signs

ing this acute period (positive HIV-1 RNA, negative antibody) may markedly improve long-term prognosis.

DIAGNOSIS OF HIV-1 INFECTION

Inquiries about risk behavior should be a routine part of history taking. There should be consideration of HIV-1 testing and counseling with patients whose behavior or medical history has put them at risk for exposure to HIV-1 (Table 2). Clinical conditions and laboratory abnormalities, although nonspecific, may be the consequence of HIV-1 infection or raise concerns about HIV-1 risk factors and should be followed by more specific tests for HIV-1 infection (Table 3).

The diagnosis of HIV-1 infection is made through the detection of specific IgG antibodies to HIV-1 viral proteins. These tests consist of screening with a sensitive enzyme-linked immunosorbent assay (ELISA), with positive results confirmed by the more specific Western blot technique. Testing is carried out on samples of blood, orally obtained oral mucosal transudate (OraSure), or urine (Sentinel) and is highly specific and sensitive for HIV-1 antibodies once they are formed. A window period of 6 months may exist after infection and before the formation of detectable HIV-1 antibody. Tests for direct detection of the virus such as HIV-1 RNA, although specific, lack sensitivity. The reliability of the test, the window period between infection and the development of detectable HIV-1 antibody, and the medical benefits of early detection of HIV-1 infection including treatment and transmission prevention should be discussed. Home testing kits are commercially available, and anonymous testing sites exist in many locales providing patients with discrete testing and results and counseling given confidentially.

MANAGEMENT OF PATIENTS WITH HIV-1 INFECTION

Management consists of baseline medical care, antiretroviral therapy, the prophylaxis and treatment of OIs, and treatment of neoplasms and metabolic disorders.

The treatment of HIV-1 infection is composed of the following decisions and activities:

- The decision to initiate antiretroviral therapy
- Design of a durable and individualized combination antiretroviral treatment regimen
- Monitoring for adequacy, maintenance, and failure of regimens
- Secondary treatment in the event of failure of the primary regimen

Baseline Medical Care

Initial data include a history or findings of current and past indicators of HIV-1 infection, how HIV-1

TABLE 2. **Risk Factors for HIV-1 Infection**

Illicit injection drug use
Male homosexual contact
Sexual contact with persons known to have HIV-1
  infection or at high risk for infection
Multiple or anonymous sexual contacts
Transfusion of blood or blood product from 1977 to 1985

TABLE 3. **Clinically Common Conditions Associated with or Aggravated by HIV-1 Infection**

Anemia
Lymphopenia
Thrombocytopenia
Elevated sedimentation rate
Elevated total protein (gamma globulin portion)
Bacterial pneumonia, tuberculosis
Shingles (herpes zoster)
Sexually transmitted diseases, including herpes simplex
  and hepatitis B and C
Persistent or frequent *Candida* vaginitis

infection was acquired and ongoing risk behaviors (unsafe sexual practices, injection drug use), psychosocial and family circumstances (knowledge of current condition and risk factors, support systems, presence of depression), concurrent medical conditions and medications, and baseline laboratory data (Table 4).

Antiretroviral Therapy

The decision to begin antiretroviral therapy is a cooperative agreement with commitment between the patient and the physician and is based on the following:

- The activity and trend of viral replication as measured by plasma HIV-1 RNA titers
- The degree and trend of immunologic damage as determined by CD4 cell count and patient symptoms
- Gauging the readiness and capability of a patient to adhere to demanding medication regimens

HIV-1 viral titer (viral load) is measured either by quantitative PCR or branched DNA. Because results vary depending on the methodology used, it is advisable to use the same test with any one patient. The same sample variance of HIV-1 titers can be as much as threefold. Both tests have active ranges from between 10^2 to 10^6 copies of viral RNA per milliliter. Ultrasensitive methodologies with active ranges from 25 to 80,000 copies ($\log_{10}$ 1.3 to 4.9) can be used in determining high-level viral suppression under treatment.

The statistical prognosis of patients with viral titers greater than 10,000 copies ($\log_{10}$ 4.0) per mL branched DNA or 20,000 copies ($\log_{10}$ 4.3) per mL PCR and/or CD4$^+$ counts below 500 per mL warrant consideration for treatment. The improved efficacy of antiretroviral medications allows for a more contemplative approach to the initiation of therapy. The patient's long-term trends in viral titer and CD4$^+$ count, the generally good short-term prognosis of persons with lower viral loads and higher CD4$^+$ counts (see Figure 1), the possibility of improved treatments, and the willingness of the patient to thoroughly commit to treatment should be factors in the decision to treat. Persistent constitutional symptoms attributed to HIV-1 infection (fever, weight loss, diarrhea, oral

TABLE 4. **Medical Database**

Current and Past Symptom History	Baseline Laboratory Data	Baseline Therapy
Persistent dermatoses, herpes zoster	HIV-1 titer (PCR or bDNA)	Cervical cytology screening
Oral thrush, hairy leukoplakia, gingivitis	CD4+ cell count	Polyvalent pneumococcal
Chronic sinusitis	Complete blood cell count	vaccine
Diffuse, persistent adenopathy	Basic chemistry panel	Influenza vaccine
Persistent fevers	Syphilis serology	Hepatitis vaccine as indicated
Chronic diarrhea	Tuberculosis skin testing	Contraception
Weight loss	Chest radiography	
Distal symmetrical sensory neuropathy	Hepatitis B, C serology	
Memory disturbances	*Toxoplasma gondii* antibody	
Recurrent and/or severe herpes simplex labialis or genitalis		
Bacterial pneumonia by history		

thrush, hairy leukoplakia) and more advanced disease are reasons to initiate antiretroviral treatment (Table 5).

Design of a Treatment Regimen

Initial regimens represent the greatest opportunity for maximum suppression of HIV-1 and must critically consider potency, tolerability, and adherence. The goal of antiretroviral treatment is to maximally reduce HIV-1 replication to levels that are below the quantifiable limits of HIV-1 plasma RNA tests (25–50 copies HIV-1 RNA/mL). In so doing there is partial reconstitution of the immune system, as evidenced by a rise in CD4+ cells and clinical improvement. This also reduces the rate by which the virus acquires the resistance. Successful regimens greatly reduce the rate of viral replication (mutation) and erect substantial genetic barriers to prevent the development of resistance. This combination of potency and genetic barrier endows a regimen with durability.

No single or two drug therapies are reliably durable. With the extensive inherent diversity of the virus, the mutations within target viral enzymes that result in high-level resistance to single drugs likely pre-exist before the administration of the drugs.

Antiretroviral Drugs

Antiretroviral drugs work by inhibiting the action of two HIV-1 specific enzymes. Reverse transcriptase is the enzyme responsible for the transcription of intracellular viral RNA into a DNA analogue that is then integrated into the host CD4+ cell chromosome. Drugs inhibiting this enzyme by a process of termination of DNA elongation are classified as nucleoside reverse transcriptase inhibitors (RTIs). Drugs targeting this enzyme through direct inhibition are referred to as non-nucleoside reverse transcriptase inhibitors (NNRTIs).

Protease inhibitors (PIs) target the viral protease enzyme that is responsible for the post-transcriptional modification of viral proteins during viral production.

Drug Combinations

In combining antiretroviral medications, the following factors should be considered:

1. Eliminate contraindicated medications (e.g., didanosine [ddI, Videx]; zidovudine, formerly azidothymidine [AZT Retrovir]; and marrow suppression for a patient on chemotherapy).
2. Eliminate medications for which prior resistance is expected (historically, possibly geno/phenotype).
3. Examine for toxicity, side effects, and drug interactions (see Table 10).
4. Develop potent combination candidates (Table 6).
5. Rank order according to adherence likelihood.

Durable Regimens

Initial regimens may reserve antiretroviral drug class(es) through the combination of compatible RTI

TABLE 5. **Indications for the Initiation of Antiretroviral Therapy in the Chronically HIV-1–Infected Patient**

Clinical Category	CD4+ T Cell Count and HIV-1 RNA	Recommendation
Symptomatic (AIDS, thrush, unexplained fever)	Any value	Treat
Asymptomatic	CD4+ T cells < 500/mL *or* HIV-1 RNA > 10,000 (bDNA) or > 20,000 (PCR)	Treatment should be offered. Strength of recommendation is based on prognosis for disease-free survival and the willingness of the patient to accept therapy.*
Asymptomatic	CD4+ T cells > 500/mL *and* HIV-1 RNA < 10,000 (bDNA) or > 20,000 (PCR)	Many experts would delay therapy and observe; however, some experts would treat.

*Some experts would observe patients with CD4+ T cell counts between 350 and 500/mL and HIV-1 RNA levels <10,000 (bDNA) or <20,000 (PCR).
From Department of Health and Human Services, 1997.

TABLE 6. **Common Antiretroviral Combinations**

Class	Advantages	Disadvantages	Secondary Regimens
2 Compatible RTIs + PI(s)	Longest history or success Utility in advanced disease demonstrated	PI side effects, in particular lipodystrophy	(2 novel RTIs) + (1 or 2 secondary PIs) *or* (1 or 2 novel RTIs) + (NNRTI and/or ABC [not if failure is AZT/3TC]) + (1 or 2 secondary PI[s])
EFV + AZT + 3TC	Reserves PIs and avoids PI side effects (lipodystrophy)	Shorter history of proven effectiveness Resistance to NNRTIs occurs as a class Utility in low CD4 patients not demonstrated as yet	(2 novel RTIs) + (1 or 2 PIs)
2 Compatible RTIs + NNRTI (EFV or NVP)	Reserves PIs and avoids PI side effects (lipodystrophy) EFV possible better than NVP	Utility in low CD4 patients not demonstrated as yet	(2 novel RTIs) + (1 or 2 PIs) *or* 2 novel RTIs + ABC (not if failure is AZT/3TC)
3 Compatible RTIs (currently applies to AZT + 3TC + ABC)	Reserves both PIs and NNRTIs	Shortest history of effectiveness (24 weeks) Must include ABC Utility in low CD4 patients not demonstrated as yet	Remaining RTIs, NNRTIs, and PIs in above regimens
1 RTI + 1 NNRTI + PI(s)	Untested but often used if no other alternatives		
ABC with non-AZT/3TC regimen	No substantial data Anticipated to work		
EFV with non-AZT/3TC regimen	No substantial data Anticipated to work		
NNRTI + PI(s)	No substantial data		
Combinations including 2 NNRTIs	No substantial data		

EFV = efavirenz (Sustiva); AZT = zidovudine (Retrovir); 3TC = lamivudine (Epivir); NVP = nevirapine (Viramune); ABC = abacavir (Ziagen).

pairs with (1) a PI(s), or (2) an NNRTI (efavirenz [EFV, Sustiva] or nevirapine [NVP, Viramune]), or (3) abacavir (ABC, Ziagen) and retain, respectfully, NNRTIs, PIs, or both classes for future use with other RTIs (see Table 6)

Pharmacologic and Pharmacodynamic Compatibility

Pharmacologic and pharmacodynamic compatibility takes into account interdrug antagonism, overlap in resistance profile, and drug interactions. Of particular importance is the high degree of cytochrome P-450 3A inhibition by ritonavir (RTV, Norvir) and, to a lesser extent, delavirdine (DLV, Rescriptor). Careful examination of current and any future drugs (e.g., terfenadine [Seldane], astemizole [Hismanal], cisapride [Propulsid]) for interaction with these drugs is imperative. Hydroxyurea (Hydrea), 500 mg twice daily potentiates ddI by increasing its intracellular concentration. It is marrow suppressive, so decreases in viral titers may be seen without CD4$^+$ cell increases. Incompatibility or antagonism exists between stavudine (d4T, Zerit) and AZT, d4T and zalcitabine (ddC, Hivid), ddC and lamivudine (3TC, Epivir), and possibly indinavir (IDV, Crixivan) and saquinavir (SQV, Fortovase), eliminating their concomitant use. The resistance profile of three sets of drugs (ddI/ddC, IDV/RTV, and NVP/DLV/EFV) overlap to the extent that when used together they add

little to the genetic barrier of a regimen. Similarly, virus resistant to one of the group will likely be resistant to the other(s). Although ABC works well with AZT or 3TC-resistant virus, it works less well against AZT and 3TC-resistant virus and works poorly for patients failing all NNRTIs. All PIs overlap to some extent with each other. If resistance develops to either RTV or IDV, subsequently used nelfinavir (NFV, Viracept) or SQV will perform suboptimally. Any not previously used PI may be used after SQV or NFV if changes are made as soon as treatment failure is suspected (Table 7).

Pharmacokinetics

Induction of hepatic cytochromes by some antiretroviral medications requires changes in dosing in

TABLE 7. **Antiretroviral Drugs with Substantial Resistance Profile Overlap**

ddC and ddI NVP, DLV, and EFV	RTV and IDV All PIs—partial overlap
ABC and AZT + 3TC dual resistance	

ddC = zalcitabine (Hivid); ddI = didanosine (Videx); NVP = nevirapine (Viramune); DLV = delavirdine (Rescriptor); EFV = efavirenz (Sustiva); ABC = abacavir (Ziagen); AZT = zidovudine (Retrovir); 3TC = lamivudine (Epivir); RTV = ritonavir (Norvir); IDV = indinavir (Crixivan).

TABLE 8. **Suggested Combination PI and NNRTI Doses**

	NVP	DLV	EFV	SQV	RTV	IDV	NFV
DLV	Not used						
EFV	Not used	Not used					
SQV	Same	Same	Caution				
RTV	Same	Same	No data	400 mg/400 mg bid			
IDV	IDV 1000 mg q 8 h	IDV 600 mg q 8 h	IDV 1000 mg q 8 h	Avoid	400 mg/400 mg bid* or RTV 200 mg/IDV 800 mg bid*		
NFV	Same	Caution	Same	NFV same or 1250 mg bid/SQV 1200 mg bid	NFV 750 mg bid/RTV 400 mg bid	IDV 1000 mg/ NFV 1250 mg bid	
AMP	No data	No data	Caution	Same	No data	IDV 1000 mg q 8 h	Same

NVP = nevirapine (Viramune); DLV = delavirdine (Rescriptor); EFV = efavirenz (Sustiva); SQV = saquinavir (Fortovase); RTV = ritonavir (Norvir); IDV = indinavir (Crixivan); NFV = nelfinavir (Viracept); AMP = amprenavir (Agenerase).

combination therapy. Some changes simplify dosing requirements and should improve adherence, whereas others require dose increases (Table 8).

Alternative dosing schedules have been suggested based on clinical and pharmacologic data, which may also simplify dosing (Table 9).

Adherence to Regimens

A high degree of adherence to antiretroviral regimens is required to prevent continued replication, mutation, and eventual development of drug resistance. Regimens under consideration should be examined for factors that will either promote or reduce adherence (Table 10). Factors that affect adherence can be inherent to the drug regimen, patient associated, or situation driven.

Failure of adherence will increase as the frequency of daily doses rises. Single daily dosing will be the most regularly taken, with thrice daily and every-8-hour dosing posing difficulties. Some medications must be taken with meals for adequate absorption (NFV, SQV), whereas others must be separated from meals by 1 hour before or 2 hours after (IDV, ddI). Further complicating this issue is the need to take IDV and ddI an hour apart.

The number of pills in a given regimen can become a psychologic barrier for some patients (e.g., SQV with 18 capsules daily and DLV with 12 capsules

TABLE 9. **Alternative Dosing Schedules**

Drug	Labeled Dosing	Altered Dosing	Comments
ddI	200 mg bid PO on empty stomach	400 mg/d PO on empty stomach	More convenient dosing
ddI + Mylanta DS Liquid		4 gm Videx powder + 200 mL Mylanta DS (powder + 100 mL—shake—add to 200 mL)	Makes 20 mg/mL shake mixture Refrigerate, stable 30 days—empty stomach
NVP	200 mg bid	400 mg/d	After 2-week introduction period
SQV	1200 mg tid PO with meals	1600 mg bid PO with meals	Only with Fortovase (Inverase obsolete)
NFV	750 mg tid with meals	1250 bid PO with meals	
NFV plus RTV		Nelfinavir, 750 mg bid Ritonavir, 400 mg bid	More convenient dosing and combined PIs—good early data
SQV plus RTV	1200 mg tid PO with meals 600 mg bid PO	400 mg bid ± meals 400 mg bid	More convenient dosing, and combined PIs
IDV plus RTV	800 mg q 8 h without food 600 mg bid	Indinavir, 400 mg/ritonavir, 400 mg bid PO ± meals	Combined PI regimen that relieves critical indinavir dosing Reduced incidence of kidney stones
IDV plus RTV	800 mg q 8 h without food 600 mg bid	Indinavir, 800 mg/ritonavir, 200 mg bid PO ± meals	Ritonavir being used only pharmacologically to relieve critical indinavir dosing Reduced incidence of kidney stones

ddI = didanosine (Videx); NVP = nevirapine (Viramune); SQV = saquinavir (Fortovase); RTV = ritonavir (Norvir); IDV = indinavir (Crixivan); NFV = nelfinavir (Viracept).

daily). Patients may poorly tolerate the taste and form of some of the drugs. The taste of chewable ddI or RTV is unacceptable for some patients. ddI and NFV are available in dissolvable powder (DLV tablets dissolve well). AZT, 3TC, d4T, ABC, and RTV are available in liquid forms.

The potential for drug toxicity requires that clinical or laboratory parameters are closely monitored. The toxicities for some combinations may be additive (e.g., peripheral neuropathy), and these combinations should be used with caution. ddI-related pancreatitis warrants special attention. Any persistent abdominal pain calls for an assessment of amylase and lipase levels to determine possible pancreatic injury. Patients should not be rechallenged. Neutropenia due to AZT is more frequent in advanced HIV infection. Levels down to 500 neutrophils per mL are protective. Filgrastim (Neupogen) can be used if AZT is continued. AZT causes macrocytosis with or without anemia. The anemia can be treated with recombinant erythropoietin (Procrit, Epogen). Prolonged AZT use (more than 9 months) can cause an aching myopathy with an elevated creatine kinase value. It resolves on withholding AZT, after which there can be a rechallenge. The rash caused by NVP, and to a lesser extent DLV and EFV, can become severe. With NVP, gradual introduction lessens the risk of rash. Hypersensitivity to ABC (3–5%), characterized by an accumulation and escalation of fever, nausea, vomiting, diarrhea, and malaise with or without rash, typically occurs in the first month of treatment, resolves quickly on discontinuation, and is a contraindication to further use. The use of adefovir (ADF, Preveon), commonly causes Fanconi's syndrome (hypophosphatemia, proteinuria, glucosuria, low serum bicarbonate, or elevations in serum creatinine concentration).

Patients should be advised to drink fluids to prevent IDV-associated kidney stones. Although painful, the stones of crystallized IDV usually pass unaided. All PIs, with the possible exception of amprenavir (AMP, Agenerase)* have been associated with the onset of glucose intolerance and non–insulin-dependent diabetes mellitus. These PIs have also been associated with elevations of cholesterol and triglycerides. Whether these abnormalities in lipids result in atherosclerotic disease or pancreatitis is not clear. An abnormal distribution of adipose tissue (lipodystrophy) with a loss of extremity and facial subcutaneous fat and deposition intra-abdominally, between the shoulders (buffalo hump), and in the breasts has been described in a significant number of patients on long-term PI-containing therapy. The risks of changing therapy (to other PIs or to non–PI-containing regimens) versus continued use recapitulates the principles of successful treatment of HIV-1 infection. Drugs used to treat non–insulin-dependent diabetes are effective. Although effective, drugs lowering triglycerides (gemfibrozil [Lopid]), and low-density lipoprotein-cholesterol (pravastatin [Pravachol] with the

least drug interactions) are of uncertain benefit and add to the complexity of regimens. Effective medical treatment of lipodystrophy is not yet clear.

Specific drug side effects and their frequency and the tolerance for them vary among patients. Patients should be warned about these possible side effects. Drugs may have additive side effects. Side effects may either ameliorate with time or become tolerated by the patients. Patients should be instructed to take all parts of the regimen and to call their physician if there are any medication difficulties. Intolerable side effects should prompt a stopping of the entire regimen and reassessment.

The critical patient-associated factor in the ability to adhere to a medication regimen is patient acceptance and commitment to therapy. Patients unconvinced of the need to be treated may adhere poorly to treatment schedules. This commitment to treatment should be firm regardless of the immunologic situation. Psychiatric disorders, drug abuse, or homelessness can make compliance unlikely or impossible. Adherence to regimens will be aided by

- A complete knowledge of medication names (generic, brand, alphanumeric) and dosing schedules
- Reminders for dosing or association with routine daily events (brushing teeth, meals)
- Medication sets, portable pill containers, emergency supplies
- Planning for irregularities in the routine schedule—weekends, vacations, holidays
- Special attention paid to mothers responsible for children (infected or not), midday doses for those working out of the home, shift workers, and changes brought on by intercurrent illness

Situational factors in adherence include the medical/financial status of the patient, which should ensure continuity of care and of medications, transportation and living situations, and reliable medication authorization and refill systems.

Therapeutic Monitoring

Reductions in HIV-1 titers of greater than 1 $\log_{10}$ and a concomitant rise in CD4 counts determine treatment effect. First measurements are usually made 2 to 4 weeks after the initiation of treatment. By 12 to 16 weeks, titers should be below 500 copies per mL and reach below 50 copies per mL by 24 weeks. The long-term durability of a regimen depends on reaching levels at least as low as 50 copies per mL (2.0 $\log_{10}$) as measured by ultrasensitive quantitation. This should be achievable in 60 to 80% of patients naïve to prior therapy and more so in those with titers less than 20,000 copies per mL (4.3 $\log_{10}$). If achieved, follow-up monitoring is done every 3 to 4 months. Any difficulties with adherence to a regimen should be sought and remedied.

Treatment Failure

Failure of a treatment regimen can be defined virologically as the existence of mutations or the stepwise acquisition of mutations resulting in HIV-1 drug re-

---

*Investigational drug in the United States.

TABLE 10. **Dosing and Prominent Side Effects of Antiretroviral Medications**

| Drug | Unit Size | Dosing Options (mg per dose) | | | Prominent Side Effects | | | | | | | | | | | | | | | | |
		qd	bid	tid or q 8 h	Nausea	Headache/Insomnia	Dizziness/Vivid Dreams	Diarrhea	Peripheral Neuropathy	Rash Hypersensitivity	Marrow Suppression	Pancreatitis	Aphthous Ulcers	Myositis	Oral Tingling	Kidney Stones	Increased Bilirubin	Renal/Fanconi's Syndrome	Glucose Intolerance/Lipid Abnormalities/Lipodystrophy	Decreased Carnitine
Reverse Transcriptase Inhibitors																				
AZT (zidovudine, Retrovir)	100 mg, 300 mg, 50 mg/mL, (300 mg + 150 mg 3TC)		300 mg	200 mg	x	x					x			x						
ddI (didanosine, Videx)	25 mg, 100 mg, 150 mg, buffered powder—100 mg, 167 mg, 200 mg	400 mg (>60 kg) 240 mg (<60 kg) empty stomach	200 mg (>60 kg) 120 mg (<60 kg) empty stomach		x			x	x			x								
ddC (zalcitabine, Hivid)	0.375 mg, 0.75 mg			0.75 mg					x				x							
d4T (stavudine, Zerit)	15 mg, 20 mg, 30 mg, 40 mg, 10 mg/mL		40 mg (<60 kg)	30 mg					x											
3TC (lamivudine, Epivir)	150 mg, 10 mg/mL, (150 mg + 300 mg AZT)		150 mg																	
AZT/3TC (Combivir)	AZT 300 mg + 3TC 150 mg		1 tablet		x	x					x			x						
ABC (abacavir, Ziagen)	300 mg, 20 mg/mL		300 mg		x					x										
ADV (adefovir, Preveon)*	30 mg, 60 mg	60 mg + carnitine			x													xx		x

	Formulation	Dose							
Non-nucleoside Reverse Transcriptase Inhibitors									
NVP (nevirapine, Viramune)	200 mg	200 mg/d × 2 weeks then 400 mg/d	200 mg/d × 2 weeks then 200 mg bid				xx		
DLV (delavirdine, Rescriptor)	100 mg	400 mg tid					x		
EFV (efavirenz, Sustiva)	200 mg	600 mg		x			x		
Protease Inhibitors									
SQV (saquinavir, Fortovase)	200 mg	1600 mg with food	1200 mg with food		x			x	
RTV (ritonavir, Norvir)	100 mg, 80 mg/mL	300 mg bid × 3 d, 400 mg bid × 4 d, 500 mg bid × 5 d, then 600 mg bid		xx	x			x	
IDV (indinavir, Crixivan)	200 mg, 333 mg, 400 mg	800 mg q 8 h on empty stomach, high fluid			x			x	x
NFV (nelfinavir, Viracept)	250 mg, 50 mg/gm powder	1250 mg	750 mg		xx			x	
AMP (amprenavir, Agenerase*)	150 mg	1200 mg		x				?	

*Investigational drug in the United States.

sistance. This occurs when there is continued replication and evolution of the virus toward drug resistance under selective drug pressure. Viral titers will be inadequately suppressed and subsequently rise. Treatment failure can also be defined as the inability of a patient to adhere to a treatment regimen or intolerance of side effects or toxicities. Clinically this is seen as

- Inadequate initial suppression of HIV-1
- Confirmed trend of rising HIV-1 titers after initial suppression
- Failure of CD4 cell response or loss of initial treatment gains
- Clinical deterioration
- Patient nonadherence or intolerable side effects or toxicities

Inability to reach target viral titers may signal an inadequate regimen. There can be early consideration of intensification by the adding of other antiretroviral agents to add potency. Patients beginning with very high HIV-1 titers ($>10^6$ copies per mL), with advanced disease, or with prior treatment and failure of antiretroviral therapy may be unable to achieve fully suppressed levels of HIV-1. The goal in this situation is to maximally suppress levels for as long as possible. A trend in HIV-1 titers rising from the nadir value under a treatment regimen signals the acquisition of drug resistance. This should take into account the variation in the precision of the HIV-1 viral titer testing, which can vary by threefold (0.5 $\log_{10}$). Repeated HIV-1 titer measurements may be required. Uncommonly, in spite of adequate suppression of HIV-1, a patient's CD4 gains may be lost or counts may decline. Although controversial, an alternative regimen might be considered. Remediable causes for clinical deterioration (e.g., OIs) should be considered before an otherwise effective regimen is abandoned as failing.

Secondary Treatment

During treatment, any residual viral titer represents either the ongoing replication of resistant populations or production of virus from long-lived latently infected cells. If allowed to continue, replication results in a stepwise acquisition of high-level resistance. Because of overlap in the mutations conferring viral drug resistance, prolonged administration of a failing antiretroviral regimen may result in viral resistance across a drug class. Remaining on a failing antiretroviral combination may threaten the durability of future regimens.

The addition or change of a single drug in a virologically failing combination regimen is tantamount to exposure of the residual HIV-1 to monotherapy, and resistance to the single new agent will arise quickly. When changes are necessary, residual HIV-1 should be treated with a regimen that contains at least two new antiretroviral agents. Preferably, the entire regimen is replaced. The order of preference is (1) a new class of antiretroviral agent, (2) a new drug with a novel resistance profile, and (3) historically drugs of

minimal prior use or possibly genotypically measured nonresistance. An exception to this is the ability to reuse AZT if not previously combined with 3TC. The mutations associated with 3TC resistance reestablish some sensitivity to AZT. A second exception is combining ddI with hydroxyurea (Hydrea),* 500 mg bid. Hydroxyurea increases the proportion of intracellular ddI and has the potential to overcome prior resistance. If a patient is able to adequately suppress viral replication but cannot tolerate or fully adhere to a regimen, replacement of only the offending antiretroviral drugs is acceptable.

As a result of shared resistance profiles, resistance to an NNRTI eliminates this class from further use. PI-containing regimens following other failing PI-utilizing combinations may perform poorly and might require combining PIs.

Genotyping and Phenotyping

The utility of viral genotyping and phenotyping for resistance to antiretroviral drugs is controversial. The ability to detect the resistance patterns of only dominant populations of virus leaves undetected minor populations of virus that may carry differing but potentially selectable (under drug pressure) geno(pheno)types. Typing of virus in the treatment-naïve patient may be important in determining whether the patient has been infected with resistant virus and in guiding initial treatment. Typing for treatment-experienced patients may direct away from some drugs but cannot ensure sensitivity to others. Typing early in failure may indicate single sentinel drug failure, allowing for consideration of the other drugs in the regimen for continued or future use. Consultation in interpretation of typing with treatment history is advisable.

Opportunistic Infections

With declining circulating CD4+ cells, the immunologic protection of patients pass down through succeeding layers of risk for specific OIs. At relatively normal levels of CD4+ cells are conditions seen in immunocompetent population but with greater frequency or severity (e.g., herpes simplex, herpes zoster, *Candida* vaginitis). If immunologic deterioration continues, OIs characteristic of AIDS become evident; and in an accumulation of risk, patients with very low CD4+ counts are at risk for a large number of OIs.

Although CD4+ cell counts rise with treatment of HIV-1 and antiretroviral treatment has been shown to reduce the incidence of OIs, the immunologic competence achieved is not equivalent to the CD4+ cell count attained. Unless the CD4 response is robust or prophylaxis is otherwise contraindicated (toxicity, adherance risk), the historic nadir CD4+ cell count establishes the indication for prophylaxis. Prophylactic regimens are available for many OIs, with those

---

*Not FDA approved for this indication.

for PCP and *Mycobacterium avium* complex (MAC) improving survival.

Although there is a large list of HIV-1–associated OIs, of greatest clinical importance are PCP, tuberculosis (TB), cryptococcal meningitis, toxoplasmosis encephalitis (TE), herpesvirus infections, mucosal candidiasis, and disseminated MAC. Other OIs are less common or will surrender to commonly utilized pathways of investigation and diagnosis.

Pneumocystis carinii Pneumonia

The risk for PCP begins at a CD4$^+$ cell count of 200 cells per mL. Prophylactic antibiotics are indicated at this level. Patients with unexplained fevers of 100.2°F or with thrush should also receive prophylaxis. Trimethoprim/sulfamethoxazole (Septra, Bactrim), one double-strength tablet daily, is highly protective and provides prophylaxis against TE and bacterial infections. Adverse reactions to this prophylaxis can occur 7 to 14 days after institution, evident as rash, nausea, and fevers. Severe reactions require discontinuing the drug; mild reactions may pass. A single-strength tablet daily may suffice, with fewer side effects. Every effort, including desensitization, should be made to institute this medication. Alternative prophylactic regimens are dapsone,* 100 mg daily; dapsone, 50 mg daily + pyrimethamine (Daraprim),* 50 mg daily + leucovorin, 25 mg daily; aerosolized pentamidine (Pentam), 300 mg monthly administered via Respirgard II nebulizer; or atovaquone (Mepron),* 750 mg twice daily orally.

As a nonpyogenic interstitial pneumonia, PCP presents as fever, night sweats, and dyspnea on exertion progressing to shortness of breath at rest. Spasms of nonproductive cough are triggered by deep inspiration. On examination, respiration is restricted but is usually clear to auscultation. The chest radiograph shows symmetrical interstitial infiltrates of varying amounts depending on degree of illness at presentation. Po$_2$ and oxygen saturation can be decreased or shown to decrease with exercise. Without antecedent prophylaxis, induced sputum may show cyst forms. Direct fluorescent antibody staining is more sensitive. Prior prophylaxis alters the presentation and reduces the sensitivity of laboratory tests. Specimens obtained by bronchoalveolar lavage are 85 to 95% sensitive. Rarely, transbronchial biopsy may be required for definitive diagnosis. Treatment can be given empirically when the diagnosis is evident; however, in questionable cases definitive diagnosis is preferred. Treatment is curative and is followed by indefinite prophylaxis.

Treatment Regimens for Acute PCP (21-Day Regimens)

- Trimethoprim/sulfamethoxazole, 15 mg per kg per day intravenously divided every 8 hours until improvement then orally
- Pentamidine, 3 to 4 mg per kg daily intravenously
- Clindamycin (Cleocin),* 600 mg intravenously or

orally three times a day plus primaquine,* 30 mg as base orally daily
- Dapsone,* 50 mg twice daily plus trimethoprim,* 15 mg per kg per day divided three to four times daily
- Trimetrexate (NeuTrexin), 45 mg per m², plus dapsone, 50 mg twice daily, plus leucovorin, 24 days at 20 mg per m²
- Atovaquone suspension, 750 mg orally twice daily, plus pyrimethamine,* 50 to 75 mg daily
- Adjunctive corticosteroids for Po$_2$ less than 70 mm Hg beginning at 40 mg prednisone or methylprednisolone (Solu-Medrol) and tapering over 2 weeks to reduce the risk of respiratory failure

Tuberculosis

Prompt identification and treatment of persons co-infected with HIV and TB (latent or active) decreases the chance of reactivation of TB and increases cure of active TB, reduction of mortality and infectivity, and ability to design dual regimens for the treatment of both. Because of TB susceptibility patterns, transmission concerns, treatment requirements, and drug interactions with antiretroviral agents, consultation with a specialist about the patient co-infected with HIV-1 and TB (active or latent) is advisable.

Most active TB in patients with HIV-1 infection is a result of reactivation, although the risk of development of acute TB after exposure is high. The risk for reactivation of TB in persons with HIV-1 infection is 2 to 7% per year. Purified protein derivative (PPD) testing (5 TU) should be done at baseline and yearly. Anergy testing is not necessary. A 5-mm or greater induration skin test, a history of untreated or inadequately treated prior past TB, and contact with an infectious TB patient are indications for preventive treatment regardless of age. Details of source case TB may influence the choice of preventive treatment, as will the patient's health status and current or planned medications. The concomitant use of rifampin (RIF, Rifadin) with protease inhibitors or NNRTIs is contraindicated owing to pharmacologic interactions. Rifabutin (RFB, Mycobutin) substitutions for rifampin or, when feasible, therapy for HIV-1 might be delayed. Two weeks are needed after discontinuation of rifampin before therapy with a PI or NNRTI is begun (Table 11).

Active TB

Knowledge of local and population-based TB epidemiology in conjunction with HIV-1 infection is important in the consideration of the possibility of any pulmonary infiltrate being TB. Pulmonary TB presents as cough and fever, but with greater immune suppression the presentation is atypical, with constitutional symptoms predominating and extrapulmonary disease common. Chest radiographs are variable with less cavitary and miliary disease. Mediastinal adenopathy, upper lobe disease, and pleural effusions as well as normal chest radiographs

---

*Not FDA approved for this indication.

*Not FDA approved for this indication.

TABLE 11. **Preventive Treatment for Adults with Latent Organisms Expected to Be Susceptible to Isoniazid and Rifampin**

HIV Therapy	Preventive Therapy	Duration of Therapy
PI or NNRTI (cannot be RTV, DLV, or hard-gel SQV [Invirase, obs.] if RIF is used	Daily INH	9 months (at least 270 doses) or 12 months if interrupted <2 months
	Twice weekly INH	9 months (at least 76 doses) or 12 months if interrupted <2 months by directly observed preventive therapy (DOPT)
	Daily RFB plus pyrazinamide (PZA)	2 months (at least 60 doses) or 3 months if interrupted <2 months (DOPT)
None	Daily INH	9 months (at least 270 doses) or 12 months if interrupted <2 months (DOPT)
	Twice weekly INH	2 months (at least 60 doses) or 3 months if interrupted <2 months
	Daily RIF plus (PZA)	2 months (at least 60 doses) or 3 months if interrupted <2 months

INH = isoniazid; RTV = ritonavir (Norvir); DLV = delavirdine (Rescriptor); SQV = saquinavir; RIF = rifampin (Rifadin); RFB = rifabutin (Mycobutin); PZA = pyrazinamide.

are seen. Extrapulmonary disease alone or with pulmonary infection occurs in 70% of cases, with a bias toward advanced HIV-1 disease. Blood, extrathoracic lymph nodes, and the genitourinary system are sites of infection and isolation of TB. Tuberculous meningitis presents as fever, headache and altered mental status, and other sites of infection. In contrast to cryptococcal disease, cerebrospinal fluid (CSF) pleocytosis is common. Radiometric isolation (Bactec) with DNA probes allows for faster isolation and identification of TB. Drug sensitivities should be determined for all isolates. Treatment consultation is advisable.

Because of drug interactions, RIF is replaced by RFB or streptomycin-based active TB treatments if the patient is also taking PIs or NNRTIs. RFB cannot be given concomitantly with RTV, DLV, or hard-gel SQV. The dose of RFB is decreased from 300 mg daily orally to 150 mg daily orally if given concomitantly with IDV, NFV, and AMP but unchanged if RFB is given in a twice-weekly regimen. If the patient is taking EFV, the dose of RFB is increased to 450 mg in all regimens with monitoring for RFB toxicity (uveitis, leukopenia) (Table 12).

Paradoxical TB reactions associated with antiretroviral therapy consisting of hectic fevers, lymphadenopathy, worsening of chest radiographs, and exacerbation of existing lesions may occur when antiretroviral therapy is begun in a patient with TB or under TB treatment. This is believed to be due to recovery of delayed hypersensitivity. The reactions are usually self-limited, and when they are severe short courses of corticosteroids are helpful.

Cryptococcal Meningitis

The risk for cryptococcal disease, which typically presents as meningitis, begins at a CD4+ cell count of about 100 cells per mL. Prophylaxis with azole antifungal agents is effective, but the overall incidence of cryptococcal meningitis in the AIDS population is low, making this optional. Baseline serum cryptococcal antigen testing is not useful. Persistent

headache with accompanying fever calls for a lumbar puncture. Meningeal signs are frequently absent. Combined cerebrospinal examination by India ink, cryptococcal antigen, and fungal cultures is highly sensitive. Cell counts and protein levels are commonly only slightly elevated. Elevated opening pressure, particularly if accompanied by altered mental status, is a poor prognostic sign and may require decompression by CSF removal. Serum cryptococcal antigen is also often positive, but this should not substitute for CSF sampling.

Preferred initial treatment is with intravenous amphotericin B (Fungizone), 0.3 to 1.25 mg per kg per day intravenously, or liposomal amphotericin B (Abelcet, AmBisome), which is further enhanced by the addition of flucytosine (Ancobon), 100 to 150 mg per kg per day, in divided doses. After 2 weeks of treatment or when clinical improvement is clear, long-term suppressive oral treatment with fluconazole (Diflucan), 200 to 400 mg daily, is necessary to prevent relapse.

Toxoplasmosis Encephalitis

The risk for reactivation of *Toxoplasma gondii*, presenting as encephalitis, begins below a CD4+ count of 100 cells per mL. Those at greatest risk are positive for *Toxoplasma* IgG antibodies. Trimethoprim/sulfamethoxazole provides prophylaxis for both PCP and TE. Alternatively, dapsone,* 50 mg daily, plus pyrimethamine, 50 mg weekly, plus leucovorin, 25 mg weekly, will provide prophylaxis. Reactivation occurs as multiple focal brain lesions. Presentation is dependent on location with focal neurologic deficits, altered mental status, and fever, leading to computed tomography or the more sensitive magnetic resonance imaging. Characteristic multiple ring-enhanced lesions are sufficient for a diagnostic/therapeutic trial of treatment. The primary differential diagnosis includes lymphoma and progressive multifocal leukoencephalopathy. Corticosteroids hasten recovery by reducing brain

---

*Not FDA approved for this indication.

TABLE 12. **Treatment of Active Tuberculosis in HIV-1–Infected Patients**

Therapy Base	Induction Phase	Maintenance Phase
RFB 6 months (may be extended to 9 months depending on response to therapy)	INH + RFB + PZA + EMB Daily for 8 weeks *or* Daily for 2 weeks then twice weekly for 6 weeks	INH + RFB Daily or 2 times weekly for 18 weeks
SM 9 months (may be extended to 12 months depending on response to therapy)	INH + SM + PZA + EMB Daily for 8 weeks *or* Daily for 2 weeks and then 2–3 times weekly for 6 weeks	INH + SM + PZA 2–3 times weekly for 30 weeks
RIF 6 months (may be extended to 9 months depending on response to therapy)	INH + RIF + PZA + EMB (or SM) Daily for 8 weeks *or* Daily for 2 weeks then 2–3 times weekly for 6 weeks *or* 3 times weekly for 8 weeks	INH + RIF Daily for 2–3 times weekly for 18 weeks *or* INH + RIF + PZA + EMB (or SM) 3 times weekly for 18 weeks

INH = isoniazid; RIF = rifampin (Rifadin); RFB = rifabutin (Mycobutin); PZA = pyrazinamide; SM = streptomycin; EMB = ethambutol (Myambutol).

edema but may lead to diagnostic confusion because central nervous system (CNS) lymphomas will also improve. Patients failing to show signs of improvement under treatment (7 to 9 days) may require brain biopsy for definitive diagnosis. Initial treatment consists of the combination of pyrimethamine, 200 mg loading dose followed by 100 mg* daily, and sulfadiazine, 4 grams daily in divided doses plus leucovorin, 10 to 20 mg daily. Alternatively, the same dose of pyrimethamine can be combined with clindamycin,† 600 mg four times daily intravenously or orally. The same combination with reduced pyrimethamine (25 to 50 mg daily) is used for long-term suppression.

Herpesvirus Infection

Herpes Zoster. Herpes zoster is a common early complication of HIV-1–related immunologic damage. Education for early recognition by patients leads to prompt antiherpetic treatment and reduction in morbidity.

Herpes Simplex. Herpes simplex labialis or genitalis recurs with greater frequency, length, and severity. If untreated, large erosive ulcerations can occur and extension of genital herpes into the rectum can result in debilitating proctitis. Genital herpes may increase the sexual transmission of HIV-1. Episodic or suppressive therapy with famciclovir (Famvir), 500 mg twice daily for 7 days acute or 250 mg twice daily* suppressive, or acyclovir (Zovirax), 200 mg five times daily acute or 400 mg twice daily suppressive, is effective. With repeated exposure to acyclovir, there is a small risk for the development of resistant herpes simplex virus requiring more intensive or alternative drug treatment.

Cytomegalovirus. Cytomegalovirus (CMV) infections reactivate at CD4+ cell counts below 100 cells per mL. Patients with CMV retinitis complain of fixed, progressive visual disturbances accompanied

at times by floaters. Ophthalmoscopic examination may visualize the retinal-based "cottage cheese and ketchup" hemorrhages and infarctions; however, with peripheral lesions ophthalmologic examination may be necessary. Prophylaxis is available, but the overall incidence of CMV retinitis, the toxicities, and the effectiveness of prophylaxis make this optional. CMV ulcers in the gastrointestinal tract from the oropharynx to the colon cause localizable pain, particularly in the esophagus, stomach, and fixed portions of the colon. CMV colitis of the cecum can be mistaken for appendicitis (or vice versa). CMV in body fluids turns any cultures positive, so a biopsy of involved gastrointestinal mucosa for histologic diagnosis is necessary. Initial treatment consists of either ganciclovir (Cytovene) or foscarnet (Foscavir) given intravenously. Ganciclovir can cause anemia and neutropenia. Absolute neutrophil counts (ANC) down to 500 cells per mL are protective. Filgrastim can be used to increase the ANC. Foscarnet can be nephrotoxic, and adjustment for serum creatinine or estimated glomerular filtration rate is necessary. For retinal disease, the insertion of a ganciclovir ocular implant (Vitrasert) supplies high-concentration, local treatment. This localized treatment does not provide for protection of other sites. Intraocular injections of fomivirsen (Vitravene) treat local disease in the same manner as implants. After initial suppression of CMV activity, long-term suppressive treatment with oral ganciclovir, 1 gram three times daily, provides a less effective alternative to maintenance intravenous doses of ganciclovir or foscarnet. Oral ganciclovir is commonly used to provide systemic coverage in combination with intraocular ganciclovir implants. In cases of CMV resistant to single drug therapy, the combination of ganciclovir with foscarnet can be used. Cidofovir (Vistide) can be used in cases of resistant CMV and other herpesviruses. Its high potential for nephrotoxicity requires the concomitant use of probenecid and hydration along with careful monitoring of renal function. Its infrequent dosing (every 2

---

*Exceeds dosage recommended by the manufacturer.
†Not FDA approved for this indication.

weeks) may alleviate the need for permanent vascular access.

Mucosal Candidiasis

Candida vaginitis is common at high CD4+ cell counts. Oropharyngeal candidiasis (thrush) can occur at about a CD4+ cell count of 400 cells per mL. Esophageal candidiasis can develop below a CD4+ count of 200 cells per mL. Because infection is generally uncomplicated and therapy is straightforward, prophylaxis is optional. Recognizable mucosal white patches of vaginal and oropharyngeal candidiasis may make confirmatory testing by potassium hydroxide prep or culture unnecessary for diagnosis. Thrush can be treated topically with nystatin, clotrimazole troches (Mycelex), or oral amphotericin B concentrate (Fungizone) or in persistent or severe cases systemically with ketoconazole (Nizoral), fluconazole (Diflucan), or itraconazole (Sporanox). In the presence of oropharyngeal *Candida* and odynophagia at low CD4+ cell counts, a diagnostic/therapeutic trial of systemic azole antifungal agents for the treatment of candidal esophagitis is warranted. Failure of clinical mucosal clearing or improvement may be due to a yeast other than *Candida albicans* and requires culturing or esophagoscopy for further treatment guidance. The need for suppressive therapy is made on a case-by-case basis.

Disseminated Mycobacterium avium Complex

MAC is the most common cause of fever without source in a patient with a CD4+ cell count of less than 50 cells per mL (others include subtle PCP, lymphoma, drug fever). Night sweats, weight loss, anemia with an elevated band count, an elevation of liver-associated alkaline phosphatase, and diarrhea may accompany the fever. In PI therapy, abdominal and other focal MAC adenitis occurs. Prophylaxis is recommended with a historic nadir CD4+ count of 50 cells per mL or lower. Clarithromycin (Biaxin), 500 mg twice daily, or azithromycin (Zithromax),* 1200 mg once weekly, have been shown to decrease the incidence of MAC. Rifabutin (Mycobutin), 300 mg daily orally, is effective but deleteriously interacts with PIs. IDV or NFV can be used with rifabutin at 150 mg daily. High blood levels of rifabutin are associated with uveitis. Active TB should be ruled out before the use of rifabutin. Diagnosis of MAC is most commonly made by isolation from the blood using specific media for acid-fast bacteria. Diagnosis of MAC can also be made by identification and culture from bone marrow, liver, lymph nodes, and intestinal mucosa. Life-prolonging treatment requires multiple antibiotics for an indefinite period. Azithromycin,* 250 mg once or twice daily, or clarithromycin, 500 mg twice daily, is combined with ethambutol, 15 mg per kg daily. Ciprofloxacin (Cipro),* 500 mg twice daily, may increase effectiveness. Amikacin

(Amikin),* 10 mg per kg daily intravenously, is given in 2-week courses to reduce the initial burden of MAC or in cases of relapse. Dose-related nephrotoxicity and ototoxicity could occur.

HIV-1–Related Neoplasms

Of the numerous candidates for association with HIV-1 infection, the three most clinically relevant are KS, NHL, and invasive cervical cancer. Before the HIV-1 epidemic, KS was rare. KS was one of the vanguard opportunistic processes bringing attention to the epidemic in 1981, resulting in 50% of the initial AIDS diagnoses. In subsequent years, the incidence has fallen dramatically. Because KS occurred primarily in homosexual men with HIV-1 infection, there is suspicion of a sexually transmitted cofactor. A likely candidate is human herpesvirus 8 (HHV-8), also referred to as the KS–associated herpesvirus (KSHV). KS presents as indurated, nonblanching pink-to-violaceous cutaneous nodules from 0.5 to 2 cm in diameter. Lesions are commonly distributed along Langer's lines, with a predilection for the inner aspects of the arms, thighs, and shins, where they may coalesce into large plaques. The tip of the nose and penis and palate are also commonly involved. Diagnosis is clinical to the experienced eye, but biopsy will yield definitive diagnosis and differentiate KS from the similar-appearing bacillary angiomatosis caused by the OI *Bartonella henselae*. If the infection is not treated, the course is variable—indolent in some but rapidly enlarging and becoming more numerous in others. Large plaques, particularly of the lower extremities, cause distal edema. Confluent involvement of the feet can be debilitating and painful. Extensive facial involvement can result in social isolation for the patient. Visceral involvement is common but rarely causes symptoms. The exception is pulmonary KS, in which there can be progression to the point of life-threatening respiratory failure. Pulmonary KS rarely occurs in isolation. Chest radiography shows variable patchy involvement and there may be pleural effusions, uncommon in PCP. Gallium scans are negative in KS, and computed tomography may show spread along bronchial pathways. Lesions can be seen at bronchoscopy, but transbronchial biopsy rarely obtains diagnostic tissue. For treatment, it has become apparent that highly suppressive antiretroviral regimens have resulted in regression of KS. Apart from this, the decision to treat is based on patient preference, rapidity of spread, pain, obstruction, peripheral edema, and cosmesis. Pulmonary KS should be treated to prevent respiratory complications. Therapy can be applied to local cutaneous lesions (cryotherapy, irradiation, topical alitretinoin [9-*cis*-retinoic acid, Panretin gel], intralesional vinblastine [Velban]*) or systemic treatment consisting of regimens containing various combinations of vincristine (Oncovin),* vinblastine, bleomycin (Blenoxane),* dox-

---

*Not FDA approved for this indication.

*Not FDA approved for this indication.

orubicin (Adriamycin,* Doxil), daunorubicin (DaunoXome), interferon alfa (Intron A, Roferon-A), etoposide (VePesid),* or paclitaxel (Taxol).

NHL occur 1 to 2% per year in patients with advanced HIV-1 disease. The incidence may rise as survival is prolonged with antiretroviral treatment. Factors in the development of NHL are not fully elucidated, but Epstein-Barr virus is implicated as a potential causative agent. Non-CNS, peripheral NHL occur at relatively high CD4$^+$ cell counts (~200 cells per mL), whereas those patients presenting with CNS lymphoma usually have CD4$^+$ cell counts below 50 cells per mL. Extranodal presentation of HIV-1–related NHL is common, with involvement of the marrow and CNS and gastrointestinal tract. Unusual sites outside the lymphatic system have also been noted. NHL isolated to the CNS varies in presentation with its location. Confusion, lethargy, and personality changes along with focal neurologic signs or seizures can be presenting symptoms. Solitary contrast medium–enhanced lesions on brain imaging are more likely NHL than toxoplasmosis, but solitary toxoplasmosis lesions are not rare. Conversely, CNS NHL is multiple in half the cases. In patients with positive toxoplasmosis serology, a diagnostic/therapeutic trial of toxoplasmosis treatment may be given, in a search for improvement within a week. The use of corticosteroids to reduce cerebral edema will result in improvement in either disease, a possible point of confusion. For definitive diagnosis, brain biopsy is necessary. With treatment, overall response rates range from 21 to 64% and vary by morphologic cell type. Median survival times range from 4 to 7 months, with predictors of poor survival being CD4 cell count less than 100 per mL, Karnofsky score less than 70, extranodal disease, and prior diagnosis of AIDS. Treatment regimens consist of variations to cyclophosphamide, doxorubicin, vincristine, and prednisone (CHOP); methotrexate, bleomycin, doxorubicin, cyclophosphamide, vincristine, and dexamethasone (m-BACOD); or the aggressive Adriamycin (doxorubicin), cyclophosphamide, vincristine, and bleomycin (ACVB). The effect of current antiretroviral therapy on survival with NHL is not determined.

The incidence of human papillomavirus infection and progressive cervical cytologic abnormalities is high in women with HIV-1 infection. Rates of invasive cervical cancer have not risen, but this may be an artifact of aggressive screening and treatment, premature death due to other HIV-1–related causes, or cervical cancer cases not recognized as HIV-1 related. False-negative rates of Papanicolaou smears become more important in populations of women with high cervical cytologic abnormality rates. At a minimum, there should be two initial normal Papanicolaou smears at 6-month intervals, followed by annual examinations thereafter. Treatment of cervical disease is less successful, and close follow-up is important.

---

*Not FDA approved for this indication.

Neurologic Disorders in HIV-1 Infection

Neurologic disorders due to HIV-1, opportunistic processes, or medications occur in most cases of progressive HIV-1 infection. Cerebral opportunistic processes of highest concern are TE, NHL, and progressive multifocal leukoencephalopathy (PML). Central neurologic conditions due to HIV-1 are HIV-1–associated minor cognitive/motor disorder (MCMD) and HIV-1–associated dementia. PML is an OI caused by the human papovavirus. Pathologically, there is demyelination of subcortical white matter without surrounding mass effect. Patients present with focal neurologic deficits. Computed tomography or magnetic resonance imaging is suggestive, but brain biopsy may be necessary for definite diagnosis. Prognosis is one of rapid deterioration. No successful treatments have been developed, although anecdotal regression has occurred with successful antiretroviral therapy.

HIV-1–associated MCMD occurs in up to 30% of patients and is more common in advanced HIV-1 infection. Neurologic deficits are minor and reflect minimal neuronal dysfunction. Forgetfulness, inattentiveness, and decreased concentration not disruptive to daily activity or work characterize this disorder. Only some will progress to frank dementia, but prognostic factors are lacking. Treatment is aimed at HIV-1, with consideration given to the CSF penetration of the antiretroviral agents used. However, saquinavir, which poorly penetrates into the CSF, has been effective at reduction of HIV-1 RNA in the CSF. HIV-1–associated dementia has an incidence of 15 to 20% and occurs in the setting of advanced HIV-1 infection. The most common complaint is that of memory impairment followed by gait impairment, mental slowing, and depressive symptoms. There can be a slowing of limb movement, hyperreflexia, hypertonia, and frontal release signs. The severity, as opposed to that seen in MCMD, is disabling. On CSF examination, beta$_2$-microglobulin levels may be elevated. Magnetic resonance imaging will show cerebral atrophy and abnormal white matter signals. Other causes of these symptoms should be ruled out, including depression, drug use, and CNS OIs. Zidovudine has reduced the incidence of this dementia in patients with advanced HIV-1 infection. The effect of using current potent antiretroviral medications has yet to be evaluated, but their use is advisable.

Of peripheral neuropathies seen in HIV-1 infection, a distal symmetrical neuropathy is the most common. Pathologically, a reduction in epidermal nerve fibers is seen. Although HIV-1 is directly implicated as causing the condition, medications (ddI, ddC, d4T, d4T plus ddC, isoniazid, vincristine, dapsone) can cause or worsen the condition. Patients complain of pain, tingling, or numbness in the ball of the foot, toes, and heel. Symptoms are worst in the mornings and again in the evenings. Symptoms move proximally and, in advanced cases, can interfere with gait and balance and involve the hands. Directed treatment is aimed at HIV-1 with consideration of medications that can cause the disorder. Gabapentin (Neurontin)* has not been fully evaluated for HIV-1–related peripheral neuropathy but is commonly used. Other treatments include tricyclic antidepressants in low dose, phenytoin,* analgesics, massage, and physical measures for comfort.

AIDS-Related Weight Loss

Weight loss is common at all stages of HIV-1 infection. Low levels of albumin, cholesterol, and transferrin are correlated with decreased survival. Death occurs as a total weight loss of 66% or a lean body mass loss of 54% is reached. Weight loss can be caused by inadequate nutrition, malabsorption, opportunistic processes, and HIV-1 infection itself. Nutrition can be affected by cognitive impairment, neurologic dysfunction, painful gastrointestinal tract conditions (aphthous or CMV ulcers, esophageal candidiasis), nausea, or anorexia caused by illness or medications. Malabsorption can be due to exocrine dysfunction, intestinal infection or parasitosis (cryptosporidia, microsporidia), and HIV-1 enteropathy. Opportunistic infections induce both a hypermetabolic state as well as a decreased caloric intake due to anorexia, resulting in rapid weight loss. HIV wasting, exclusive of the aforementioned causes of weight loss, occurs with altered metabolism and abnormal adaptive mechanisms due to cytokine dysfunction and results in a loss of lean body mass in excess of adipose tissue. Hypogonadism can be contributory. The treatment of weight loss is aimed at underlying causes. Diagnosis and treatment of OIs, neoplasms, and intestinal causes of malabsorption and manipulation of medications to reduce anorexia and nausea are therapeutic. Addition of medication to treat nausea or appetite stimulants such as megestrol (Megace) or dronabinol (Marinol) are helpful. Lean body mass loss due to testosterone deficiency responds to anabolic replacement through injection (testosterone, nandrolone [Deca-Durabolin]), orally with oxandrolone (Oxandrin), or with cutaneous patch application (Testoderm, Androderm). Effective treatment of HIV-1 infection reverses HIV wasting. PI use has been associated with lipid dysregulation and adipose deposits in the abdomen and across the shoulders. If treatment of HIV-1 infection is not adequate to reverse wasting, recombinant growth hormone (Serostim) is effective at increasing lean body mass; however, the cost may be prohibitive. Anabolic steroids have been used and may be effective in this circumstance.

---

*Not FDA approved for this indication.

AMEBIASIS

method of
CHRISTOPHER D. HUSTON, M.D., and
WILLIAM A. PETRI, Jr., M.D., Ph.D.
*University of Virginia Health Sciences Center
Charlottesville, Virginia*

Entamoeba histolytica, the cause of amebic dysentery and amebic liver abscess, is a protozoan parasite of global distribution. Two morphologically identical but genetically distinct amebae that infect the human colon are now recognized: *E. histolytica*, the cause of amebic liver abscess, and *Entamoeba dispar*, a noninvasive parasite.

EPIDEMIOLOGY

Approximately 500 million people worldwide are infected with *E. dispar* and/or *E. histolytica;* many of the asymptomatic infections are caused by *E. dispar. E. dispar* has not been shown to cause human disease. In Dhaka, Bangladesh, where diarrhea is the leading cause of death in children younger than 6 years old, approximately 50% of children have serologic evidence of exposure to *E. histolytica* by age 5. Amebiasis causes approximately 100,000 deaths annually, which makes it the third most common parasitic cause of death.

In the United States, travelers to and immigrants from endemic regions and institutionalized people are at increased risk of *E. histolytica* infection. The typical patient with an amebic liver abscess in the United States is a Hispanic male between the ages of 20 and 40 years who immigrated from an endemic country within the previous year. In rare cases, amebic liver abscess and ameboma have been documented as long as 12 years after emigration from an endemic country.

Several groups are at increased risk of fulminant amebiasis, including malnourished persons, the very young or old, pregnant women, and patients receiving corticosteroids. Expected increases in the severity or frequency of symptomatic infection in the setting of acquired immunodeficiency syndrome (AIDS) have, however, not been observed, and *E. dispar* appears incapable of causing invasive disease in this population as well.

PATHOGENESIS AND CLINICAL DISEASE SYNDROMES

E. histolytica is spread by fecal-oral transmission. After ingestion of the cyst form of the organism in contaminated food or water, excystation occurs in the small bowel lumen. Amebic trophozoites may then colonize the colon by adhering to intestinal mucous glycoproteins via an amebic adherence lectin. Alternatively, trophozoites may invade through the intestinal wall to cause amebic colitis and amebic liver abscess.

INTESTINAL AMEBIASIS

E. histolytica infection may be asymptomatic or may manifest with dysentery or extraintestinal disease. Asymptomatic *E. histolytica* infection is associated with a 10% risk of developing invasive amebiasis within 12 months and should therefore be treated.

Amebic colitis should be part of the differential diagnosis of diarrhea that contains gross or occult blood. Other diseases that need to be considered as part of the differential diagnosis include bacterial dysentery (e.g., caused by *Shigella, Salmonella,* or *Campylobacter* species and enteroinvasive and enterohemorrhagic *Escherichia coli*) and bloody diarrhea with noninfectious causes such as inflammatory bowel disease, ischemic colitis, diverticulosis, and arteriovenous malformation. In contrast to bacterial dysentery, which manifests abruptly, amebic colitis classically manifests with a gradual onset over 1 to several weeks of abdominal pain and tenderness, diarrhea, tenesmus, and bloody stools (Table 1). Because of the chronicity of illness, weight loss is common. Only a minority of patients (8 to 38%) have fever. Insidious onset and variable signs and symptoms, including gastrointestinal bleeding or abdominal pain without diarrhea, can make diagnosis difficult. Only occult blood is present in the majority of cases.

Of the unusual intestinal manifestations of amebiasis, the most feared is acute necrotizing colitis with toxic megacolon, which occurs in 0.5% of cases and is associated with a 40% mortality rate unless promptly recognized and treated surgically. Chronic intestinal amebiasis may occur and is clinically indistinguishable from inflammatory bowel disease. Other unusual manifestations of intestinal amebiasis include the formation of cutaneous, rectovaginal, and rectovesicular fistulas and ameboma. Ameboma, resulting from the formation of intraluminal granulation tissue, can mimic carcinoma of the colon.

EXTRAINTESTINAL AMEBIASIS

Amebic liver abscess is overwhelmingly the most common extraintestinal manifestation of *E. histolytica* infection. Amebic liver abscess is approximately 10 times more common in men than in women, and in children, although rare, it occurs in both sexes in equal proportions. Amebic liver abscess can manifest acutely with 1 to 2 weeks of onset of fever, cough, and abdominal and right upper quadrant pain. A subacute manifestation with less prominent fever, less prominent abdominal pain, and prominent weight loss is also common (Table 2). Most patients do not have coexistent dysentery, although frequently a history of dysentery can be obtained. On routine blood studies, the leukocyte count and serum alkaline phosphatase level are generally elevated, and chest radiographs usually reveal an elevated right hemidiaphragm. The differential diagnosis of a liver mass should include pyogenic liver abscess, which is less likely if the gallbladder and ducts appear normal; necrotic hepatoma; and echinococcal cyst, which would be an incidental finding and not a cause of fever and abdominal pain. Abscess location and number cannot be used to distinguish between pyogenic and amebic liver abscesses.

Infection at other sites typically results from direct ex-

TABLE 2. Amebic versus Pyogenic Liver Abscess

Characteristic	Amebic Abscess	Pyogenic Abscess
Age	20–40 years	>50 years
Male : female ratio	10 : 1	1 : 1
Epidemiologic risk factors	Immigrant/travel from developing world	Diabetes mellitus
Clinical characteristics	Amebic serology (+)	Biliary disease
	Circulating amebic antigen (+)	Jaundice
Aspirate	Sterile; amebic antigen (+)	(+) (also blood culture)

tension of liver abscesses (e.g., amebic empyema or pericardial abscesses) or hematogenous spread (e.g., brain abscesses).

DIAGNOSIS

The tests used to diagnose amebiasis are listed in Table 3. *E. histolytica* can be distinguished from *E. dispar* with a commercially available stool antigen test (Techlab *E. histolytica* test), polymerase chain reaction (PCR; investigational only), and stool culture with isoenzyme analysis. Of the commercial antigen detection kits available, only the Techlab *E. histolytica* test distinguishes *E. histolytica* from *E. dispar*. The simplest initial approach to diagnose amebic colitis is to use the *E. histolytica* stool antigen detection kit in conjunction with bacterial stool cultures and stool tests for bacterial toxins (e.g., *Clostridium difficile* toxin) to evaluate for bacterial dysentery. Both the sensitivity and specificity of the antigen test exceed 90%, and it can be performed rapidly and cheaply. PCR and stool culture with isoenzyme analysis are research tools only.

Stool microscopy is neither a sensitive nor a specific method for the identification of pathogenic amebae. The sensitivity of microscopy is only 33 to 60%, and microscopy cannot distinguish *E. histolytica* from *E. dispar*. The primary utility of stool microscopy is therefore to evaluate for other parasitic causes of diarrhea. Microscopy should be used to diagnose amebiasis only if the antigen test is not available. Although not common, erythrophagocytic trophozoites in stool are seen more frequently with *E. histolytica* than with *E. dispar* infection.

Seventy to 85% of patients with amebic colitis or amebic liver abscess have detectable antiamebic antibodies on presentation and more than 90% develop convalescent titers. In patients who have not spent time in endemic regions, a positive test result is strongly suggestive of amebiasis; a

TABLE 1. Clinical Characteristics of Amebic Colitis and Bacterial Dysentery

Characteristic	Amebic Colitis	Bacterial Dysentery
Immigration from or travel to endemic area	Yes	No
Duration of symptoms	most >1 week	2–7 days
Diarrhea	94–100%	100%
Heme-positive stools	100%	40%
Abdominal pain	12–80%	~50%
Weight loss	44%	Unusual
Fever >38°C	8–30%	56–72%

TABLE 3. Sensitivity of Tests for Diagnosis of Amebiasis

Test	Colitis	Liver Abscess
Microscopy (stool)	25–60%	8–44%
Microscopy (abscess fluid)	N/A	≤20%
Stool antigen detection	>90%	Usually negative
Serum antigen detection	65% early	~75% late, ~100% first 3 days
Abscess antigen detection	N/A	~100%
Serology (indirect hemagglutination)		
Acute	70%	70–80%
Convalescent	>90%	>90%

negative test result does reduce the likelihood of amebic infection. Antibody titers to *E. histolytica* can persist for years, however, and seropositivity rates of 25 to 50% in some regions limit the usefulness of serologic tests in patients with known risk factors for amebiasis.

Colonoscopy may confirm the diagnosis of amebiasis. Because amebic colitis is frequently localized to the cecum and ascending colon, sigmoidoscopy is inadequate. Amebic trophozoites can be identified on wet preparations of scrapings and aspirates from the base of colonic ulcers. Periodic acid–Schiff staining of biopsy specimens highlights the amebic trophozoites and aids in their identification. *E. histolytica* has been shown to invade colonic carcinomas, which can be a source of confusion.

The diagnosis of amebic liver abscess can be confirmed by a response to antiamebic therapy in a patient with antiamebic antibodies, a liver abscess, and a history of either recent travel to or emigration from the developing world. Aspiration, with its risk of bacterial superinfection, should be reserved to rule out a pyogenic liver abscess. Microscopy of fluid aspirated from an amebic abscess, even when done by the most skillful clinician, identifies amebic trophozoites only 20% of the time, but *E. histolytica* antigen can be detected in abscess pus from 100% of patients with hepatic amebiasis. Liver ultrasonography, computed tomography (CT), and magnetic resonance imaging (MRI) are equally sensitive for the identification of liver abscesses, but they cannot distinguish pyogenic abscesses and necrotic hepatomas from amebic abscesses. Dilatation of the biliary tree, especially in a diabetic patient, is suggestive of a bacterial process. Both the stool antigen test and stool microscopy findings are negative in most patients with amebic liver abscesses. In the serum, amebic antigen can be detected in nearly 100% of patients with hepatic amebiasis during the first 3 days of illness, which suggests a future role for serum and urine antigen detection to diagnose amebic liver abscess.

TREATMENT

The drugs currently available in the United States to treat amebiasis can be categorized according to the location of their amebicidal activity (Table 4). For invasive amebiasis, metronidazole (Flagyl) is the drug of choice. It is highly effective (>90% cure) for both amebic colitis and amebic liver abscess. Because of nearly complete absorption, however, metronidazole must always be followed by a regimen active against luminal infection. Three luminal amebicides are used to eradicate intestinal carriage of *E. histolytica*: diiodohydroxyquin or iodoquinol (Yodoxin), diloxanide furoate (Furamide), and paromomycin (Humatin). Paromomycin, a nonabsorbable aminoglycoside, is also active against amebic trophozoites that have invaded the intestinal mucosa. The recommended drug regimens for treatment of the different amebic syndromes are shown in Table 5.

Asymptomatic Infection

The stool antigen test discussed earlier allows rapid and accurate distinction between *E. histolytica* and *E. dispar*. Consequently, colonization by *E. histolytica* should be treated to eliminate the possibility of developing invasive amebiasis and to minimize

TABLE 4. **Current Amebicidal Agents Available in the United States**

Amebicidal Agent	Advantages and Disadvantages
Luminal Amebicides	
Paromomycin (Humatin)	7-day treatment course; may be useful during pregnancy; frequent GI disturbances; rare ototoxicity and nephrotoxicity
Iodoquinol (Yodoxin)	20-day treatment course; inexpensive and effective; contains iodine; rare optic neuritis and atrophy with prolonged use
Diloxanide furoate (Furamide)	Available in United States only from CDC; frequent GI disturbances; rare diplopia
For Invasive Intestinal Disease Only	
Tetracyclines, erythromycin	Not active for liver abscesses; frequent GI disturbance; tetracyclines should not be administered to children or pregnant women
For Invasive Intestinal and Extraintestinal Amebiasis	
Metronidazole (Flagyl)	Drug of choice for amebic colitis and liver abscess; anorexia, nausea, vomiting, and metallic taste in nearly one third of patients at dosages used; disulfiram-like reaction with alcohol; rare seizures
Chloroquine (Aralen)	Useful only for amebic liver abscess; occasional headache, pruritus, nausea, alopecia, and myalgias; rare heart block and irreversible retinal injury

Abbreviations: CDC = Centers for Disease Control and Prevention; GI = gastrointestinal.

spread of the infection; *E. dispar* infection does not necessitate treatment. All of the regimens listed in Table 5 are highly efficacious (>90% cure) and generally well tolerated. Paromomycin, although frequently associated with diarrhea, is safe, and only 7 days of treatment are required. Iodoquinol is difficult to obtain in the United States, and compliance with the 20-day course can be difficult. Diloxanide furoate is currently available in the United States only through the Drug Service at the Centers for Disease Control and Prevention.

Follow-up with the stool antigen test to confirm eradication should be performed 1 to 2 weeks after completion of treatment. Although data are lacking, patients with hematophagous trophozoites present on stool examination or with positive results of test for fecal occult blood should probably be treated for invasive disease, as described later.

Amebic Colitis

In patients with amebic colitis, metronidazole followed by a luminal agent is the treatment of choice (see Table 5). Nearly one third of patients develop side effects, including anorexia, nausea, and vomiting (in 11%) from metronidazole at the recommended dose of 750 mg orally three times a day. If this dose is intolerable, 500 mg orally three times a day may be effective, or doxycycline can be substi-

TABLE 5. **Drug Regimens for the Treatment of Amebiasis**

Type of Infection	Drug	Adult Dosage	Pediatric Dosage
Asymptomatic	Paromomycin (Humatin)	25–35 mg/kg/d in 3 doses × 7 d	25–35 mg/kg/d in 3 doses × 7 d
	or		
	Iodoquinol (Yodoxin)	650 mg tid × 20 d	30–40 mg/kg/d (max., 2 gm) in 3 doses × 20 d
	or		
	Diloxanide furoate (Furamide)	500 mg tid × 10 d	20 mg/kg/d in 3 doses × 10 d
Mild to moderate intestinal disease	Metronidazole (Flagyl)*	500–750 mg tid × 10 d	35–50 mg/kg/d in 3 doses × 10 d
	or		
	Doxycycline*	250 mg bid × 14 d	Doxycycline should not be given to children
Severe intestinal disease, liver abscess	Metronidazole (Flagyl)*	750 mg tid × 10 d or 2.4 gm once daily × 2 d	35–50 mg/kg/d in 3 doses × 10 d

*Treatment of invasive intestinal and extraintestinal amebiasis should be followed by treatment with a luminal agent.

tuted. Most patients respond promptly to metronidazole; bowel movements return to normal within 2 to 5 days of initiation of therapy. Patients with amebic infection and diarrhea are significantly more likely to be infected with *Shigella* organisms, however, so failure to respond rapidly to metronidazole should raise suspicion of a concurrent bacterial infection.

Fulminant amebic colitis may result in intestinal leakage and bacterial peritonitis, necessitating the addition of broad-spectrum antibiotics. In these cases, surgery is usually not necessary. Ameboma also usually responds to medical treatment alone. Acute necrotizing colitis with toxic megacolon mandates surgical intervention. Most affected patients have abdominal pain and distention with rebound tenderness (frank guarding is uncommon). The indications for surgery are free extraintestinal perforation, failure of intestinal perforation with a localized abscess to respond to medical treatment alone, and persistent abdominal pain and tenderness despite treatment. For localized colitis, partial colectomy may be adequate, but generalized colitis usually necessitates total colectomy. The most prudent surgical approach is to exteriorize the luminal ends and reconnect them after healing is complete; tissue friability makes intestinal leakage likely if the ends are reanastomosed immediately.

Because it is nonabsorbable and has activity in both the bowel lumen and mucosa, paromomycin may be useful for treatment of mild colitis during the first trimester of pregnancy. Despite conflicting reports about possible toxic effects of metronidazole on the developing fetus, however, treatment of severe disease during pregnancy with metronidazole should not be delayed.

To prevent recurrence, treatment of invasive disease must be followed by a luminal regimen. Although luminal and extraluminal amebicides can be used concurrently if necessary, this is generally inadvisable because of the high likelihood of gastrointestinal intolerance. The stool antigen test should be repeated 1 to 2 weeks after treatment is completed to confirm eradication, and for patients with continued symptoms despite treatment, colonoscopy with biopsies should be performed to reassess the diagnosis.

Amebic Liver Abscess

Metronidazole followed by a luminal agent is also the treatment of choice for amebic liver abscess (see Table 5). Right upper quadrant pain and fever usually resolve after 3 to 5 days of treatment, and complete resolution of symptoms occurs on average by day 8. Percutaneous or surgical drainage of liver abscesses does not speed recovery in most cases and should not routinely be performed because it increases the likelihood of bacterial superinfection. When pain and fever persist longer than expected, however, drainage may provide relief. Chloroquine may also be a useful adjunct to metronidazole when clinical improvement is slow. Some reports suggest a role for percutaneous drainage of very large amebic liver abscesses (>6 cm in diameter) or when an abscess is very close to the liver capsule (which carries a higher likelihood of rupture), but no controlled studies of this approach have been performed.

Because the lesions from amebic liver abscesses typically persist for many months, routine radiologic follow-up to document resolution only adds unnecessarily to the cost of treatment. Repeat imaging may be of use to reevaluate the initial diagnosis if symptoms persist after treatment. Eradication of intestinal infection should be confirmed with the stool antigen test after treatment is complete.

GIARDIASIS

method of
THEODORE E. NASH, M.D.
National Institute of Allergy and Infectious Diseases
Bethesda, Maryland

Giardiasis is caused by infection with the protozoan parasite *Giardia lamblia* (also known as *Giardia duodenalis* and *Giardia intestinalis*). It is one of the most common parasitic infections of humans and causes both epidemic and endemic gastroenteritis, manifested primarily as diarrhea. The parasite's development has two stages. An infectious cyst is excreted in the feces and is able to survive outside the host. When ingested by humans and other mammals, the cyst excysts in the upper small intestine, liberating motile trophozoites that multiply within the small intestine. This form is responsible for the manifestations of disease. As the trophozoites travel down the intestine, they develop into cysts. *Giardia* infections are common because very large numbers of cysts can be excreted in the feces, approaching 10 million per milliter of feces, and 100% of people become infected after ingestion of as few as 10 to 100 cysts. In addition, cysts may remain infectious in cold water for months, which is one reason why water-borne outbreaks are so common.

EPIDEMIOLOGY

The prevalence of *Giardia* infections varies, but giardiasis is the most commonly diagnosed parasitic infection in the United States and in most developed countries. *Giardia* is the most common parasite detected in stools submitted to state health laboratories; prevalences averaged from 5.6 to 7.2%. However, certain groups are more likely to become infected. Infections are frequent whenever fecal contamination occurs. Person-to-person, water-borne, and food-borne transmission have been well described. Giardiasis is most common in the young and more frequent in the summer in temperate regions. In the United States hospitalizations are about as common as for shigellosis. In many developing countries, infections are practically universal by the age of 2 years, and prevalences remain surprisingly high, although reduced, throughout adulthood. Because of the high level of endemic infections in these regions, travelers to these areas are at increased risk for infection.

Giardiasis is particularly common in day care settings, and prevalences can be 40% or higher. Infection in this setting is commonly cryptic or not appreciated until the infection is transmitted from children to their parents or other family members. Infected infants and toddlers contaminate recreational water supplies by indiscriminate defecation and are increasingly recognized as sources of epidemics in public swimming areas. Other groups more likely to be infected include homosexual persons and backpackers. The latter become infected because lakes and streams become contaminated with cysts from persons and/or animals such as beavers. Although contaminated foods have been vehicles in outbreaks, this has been recognized relatively infrequently. The parasite is one of the most common causes of defined water-borne outbreaks.

Although most people who become infected are immunocompetent, persons with hypogammaglobulinemia, nodular follicular hyperplasia without hypogammaglobulinemia, or lymphoma of the small intestine commonly develop debilitating and sometime life-threatening giardiasis. More recently, severe and difficult-to-treat giardiasis has been recognized in an increasing number of patients with acquired immune deficiency syndrome (AIDS).

INFECTION

The hallmark of *Giardia* infections is variability. The incubation period is commonly between 1 and 2 weeks but can be considerably longer. Infections may be aborted, transient, or prolonged, sometimes lasting years. Because

trophozoites inhabit the small intestine, signs and symptoms are related to alterations in the function of the small intestine and are to be distinguished from agents that cause colitis. Symptoms range from asymptomatic carriage, a relatively frequent occurrence, to fulminate diarrhea and vomiting, resulting in dehydration and hospitalization. Diarrhea without blood or mucus, cramping, foul-smelling flatus, belching, nausea and vomiting, anorexia, and weight loss are the most common symptoms. Fever is unusual. Malabsorption and failure to thrive are particularly serious problems in infants, in young children in developing regions of the world, and in others with marginal nutrition, such as in cystic fibrosis. In comparison with diarrheal illnesses caused by bacteria, giardiasis has a longer incubation period and is associated with fewer systemic symptoms, and therefore patients are less frequently acutely ill and have a more prolonged, intermittent course. Lactose deficiency may complicate giardiasis and contribute to continuing symptoms after therapy.

Extraintestinal manifestations such as uveitis, urticaria, and arthritis have been described. It is unclear whether the concurrence of these represents two independent processes occurring at the same time or a causal relationship.

DIAGNOSIS

The diagnosis is established by detection of cysts and occasionally trophozoites in the feces, trophozoites in the small intestines, or specific *Giardia* antigen in the stool. A good practice is to perform standard ova and parasite examinations, to rule out parasites other than *Giardia*, and a stool *Giardia* antigen test. A number of commercially available antigen detection tests have shown sensitivities and specificities higher than 95%. The advantage of the *Giardia* antigen test is that it detects infection even when cyst excretion is erratic or barely detectable, instances in which the diagnosis would likely be missed by microscopic stool examinations. A positive stool antigen test result is highly suggestive of the diagnosis. Previously, standard stool examinations for ova and parasites were unable to diagnose between 5 and 15% of *Giardia*-infected patients after three stool examinations. Diagnosis required invasive techniques to detect trophozoites in small intestinal mucus and fluid. These included a string test, duodenal intubation, and examination of touch preparations of small intestinal biopsy samples. However, in most cases, *Giardia* antigen detection tests should replace invasive techniques. Because both false-positive and false-negative results have been documented, more extensive evaluations are indicated in patients whose diagnosis is based solely on a positive *Giardia* antigen test result and who repeatedly fail to respond to therapy. Similarly, when the diagnosis is clinically suspected, repeated antigen tests and/or invasive tests may be indicated.

Giardiasis is both overdiagnosed and underdiagnosed. The symptoms of giardiasis are nonspecific, intermittent, and frequently of mild to moderate intensity, leading to both a reluctance of the patient or parent to seek medical attention and a failure of the physician to consider the diagnosis. Sometimes nausea and vomiting are the prominent manifestations of giardiasis and the diagnosis is not considered because diarrhea is not prominent. On the other hand, because the symptoms/signs caused by other conditions mimic those of giardiasis, *Giardia* infections are also overdiagnosed and, not uncommonly, treatment is offered without establishment of the diagnosis. Not unexpectedly, such patients frequently fail to respond to therapy. As mentioned earlier, *Giardia* infections are relatively frequent and commonly asymptomatic, which increases the possibility that two diseases coexist, leading to the attribution of symptoms and signs of other diseases to giardiasis.

TREATMENT

The drugs available for the treatment of giardiasis are listed in Table 1. All these drugs have significant side effects and drug interactions, and standard texts should be consulted before the drugs are used. Metronidazole, a nitroimidazole, is the most commonly used drug in the United States despite the fact that it has never been approved by the Food and Drug Administration (FDA) for the treatment of giardiasis. Another nitroimidazole not available in the United States, tinidazole, is usually superior to metronidazole and has fewer side effects. Metronidazole (Flagyl), although usually well tolerated, can cause troubling upper gastrointestinal upset, which occasionally limits its use. Alcohol ingestion should be avoided by patients taking metronidazole because it causes a disulfiram-like reaction. For many years, quinacrine (Atabrine) was the drug of choice for treating giardiasis, but it is no longer manufactured in the United States and not readily available, although it can be obtained through a few pharmacies (Panorama Pharmacy, Panorama City, California, 1-800-247-9767; Priority Pharmacy, San Diego, California, 1-800-487-7113). Major side effects include upper gastrointestinal symptoms, yellow discoloration of the skin and urine, and occasional psychosis or visual hallucinations.

Furazolidone (Furoxone), a broad-spectrum antibacterial nitrofuran, is less effective than either metronidazole or quinacrine. However, it is available as a liquid and therefore is more acceptable and effective than metronidazole or quinacrine in children.

TABLE 1. **Drugs for Treatment of Giardiasis**

Drug	Adult Dose	Pediatric Dose	Remarks
Metronidazole (Flagyl)	250 mg tid × 7 d	5 mg/kg tid × 7 d	GI upset, disulfiram-like effect, metallic taste
Quinacrine (Atabrine)	100 mg qid × 5 d	2 mg/kg qid × 5 d	Not generally available*; GI upset, yellow skin, urine, psychosis
Furazolidone (Furoxone)	100 mg qid × 7–10 d	6–8 mg/ kg/d in 4 doses × 7–10 d	Best tolerated in children; many potential side effects but usually well tolerated
Paromomycin (Humatin)	25–35 mg/ kg/d in 3 doses 5–10 d	—	Not absorbed; likely less effective; can use during pregnancy; GI upset

*See text for pharmacies.
Abbreviation: GI, gastrointestinal.

Although the drug is generally well tolerated, gastrointestinal upset is the most common side effect; there are a large number of less common but nevertheless reported other side effects, such as hemolysis, resulting from glucose 6-phosphate dehydrogenase deficiency; nitrofuran sensitivity reactions; and disulfiram-like reactions that follow ethanol ingestion. Furthermore, furazolidone is a monoamine oxidase (MAO) inhibitor, and so sympathomimetics and tyramine are contraindicated, and drugs metabolized by MAO require dose adjustments. Paromomycin (Humatin) is a nonabsorbable aminoglycoside less well studied than the other antibiotics with anecdotal reports of effectiveness. Because it is not absorbed, it has been suggested as treatment for symptomatic infections in pregnancy. Other less established drugs include albendazole, zinc bacitracin, and neomycin.

With the exception of paromomycin, none of these drugs should be used routinely during pregnancy. If the patient is able to clinically tolerate the infection and gains weight, the patient may not require treatment. Otherwise, in severe symptomatic giardiasis, metronidazole can probably be safely used in the second and third trimesters.

Treatment failures may result from immunologic impairment, reinfection, or drug resistance. In immunocompetent persons, treatment failures are more frequent than commonly reported and may result from biologic differences among isolates. However, organisms with proven drug resistance are unusual. In treatment failures, longer and/or increased dosing or a change to an alternative drug is usually effective. In immunologically impaired patients, therapy with combined quinacrine and metronidazole has been extremely effective. Patients who fail to achieve cure frequently respond transiently to treatment with lessening or abolition of symptoms but then experience relapse. Patients who continue to experience relapse should be questioned carefully about the possibility of reinfection, including source of water, presence of infected household members, and sexual practices.

BACTEREMIA AND SEPSIS

method of
FREDRIC J. SILVERBLATT, M.D.
Brown University
Providence, Rhode Island

Bacteremia is defined as the presence of viable bacteria in the blood. Bacteria can enter the bloodstream across a normally impervious mucosal or epithelial barrier during the course of daily activities such as vigorous tooth-brushing or as a consequence of medical instrumentalization. Bacteria can also enter the bloodstream from a severe adjacent infection, or can be introduced directly through an infected intravenous device. *Pseudomonas* species possess elastase, an enzyme that facilitates invasion of blood vessels. Severe granulocytopenia, whether as a result of leukemia or chemotherapy, weakens the mucosal barrier to the normal flora and permits transmigration of bacteria from the lumen into the bloodstream.

In most instances, bacteria are quickly cleared from the bloodstream by the reticuloendothelial system without further consequence. Occasionally however, transient bacteria adhere to the endothelium at sites of abnormal intravascular flow (e.g., heart valves damaged by rheumatic fever) and produce intravascular infections such as endocarditis or mycotic aneurysms. More commonly, the body responds to the presence of bacteria in the blood with fever and chills and progressive alterations in hemodynamic status. Surface substances found on many bacterial species interact with the host to initiate profound and progressive physiologic responses. The best-studied example is the lipopolysaccharide (LPS) of gram-negative bacteria. LPS interacts with receptors on macrophages to induce the release of tumor necrosis factor-α and interleukin-1. These two early-response cytokines stimulate a coordinated release of other cytokines to create a proinflammatory cascade that increases local perfusion, attracts polymorphonuclear leukocytes, activates complement, and promotes local thrombogenesis—all of which help limit the infection. This process affects cardiovascular function, temperature regulation, and oxygenation. Normal feedback loops engender the release of other cytokines that curtail the unregulated extension of these effects and bring the body back into homeostatic balance.

Under certain circumstances, however, the sequence escapes control and the proinflammatory limb functions autogenously with dire consequences for the individual. The microvasculature becomes increasingly permeable, leading to poor tissue perfusion, local ischemia, intractable hypotension, and multiple organ failure.

The clinical and physiologic events that accompany the presence of microorganisms in the blood are part of a generalized response of the body to a variety of stresses. This sequence of events, termed the *systemic inflammatory response syndrome*, can be triggered by infectious and noninfectious circumstances such as severe pancreatitis, multiple trauma, ischemia, immune-mediated organ injury, hemorrhagic shock, and the consequences of cardiovascular surgery. The American College of Chest Physicians/Society of Critical Care Medicine has developed a set of definitions to describe the various stages of the inflammatory response (Table 1). These definitions are intended to enable clinicians to recognize the signs of impending sepsis at an early stage so that patients can be admitted and treated before the condition progresses to more severe and less easily reversible, later stages of the process. In otherwise healthy people, the rate of recovery from the bacteremic/septic stage is over 90%, whereas with severe sepsis, septic shock, or multiple organ dysfunction syndrome, the survival rate is less than 50%.

The incidence of sepsis has not declined despite the introduction of powerful new antibiotics. In 1992, the Centers for Disease Control and Prevention reported that sepsis was the third leading cause of death due to infections. It is the leading cause of death among patients in intensive care units. During the 1960s and 1970s, sepsis was most commonly associated with bacteremia due to gram-negative bacilli. Beginning in the 1980s, the incidence of infections caused by gram-positive organisms started to become more prevalent, in part because of the greater use of intravenous catheters and the emergence of antibiotic-resistant isolates such as penicillin-resistant pneumococci, vancomycin-resistant enterococci, *Staphylococcus epidermidis*, and methicillin-resistant *Staphylococcus aureus*. Moreover, pa-

TABLE 1. **Definition of Terms Used in Bacteremia and Sepsis**

Bacteremia
  The presence of viable bacteria in the blood
Systemic inflammatory response syndrome (SIRS)
  Tachypnea (>20 breaths/min)
  Tachycardia (>90 beats/min)
  Temperature > 38.3°C (101°F) or < 35.6°C (96°F)
  Evidence of inadequate organ perfusion including one or more
      of the following:
    Elevated plasma lactate
    Hypoxemia (PaO_2 <75 mm Hg) without other pulmonary
        disease as a cause
    Oliguria (urine output <30 mL/h or 0.5 mL/kg of body
        weight)
    Poor or altered cerebral function
Sepsis
  SIRS caused by infection
Septic shock
  Sepsis with hypotension (systolic blood pressure <90 mm Hg
      or a reduction of 40 mm Hg from baseline) despite adequate
      fluid resuscitation, in conjunction with organ dysfunction
      and perfusion abnormalities in the absence of other known
      causes for the abnormalities
Multiple organ dysfunction syndrome (MODS)
  The presence of altered organ function in an acutely ill patient
      such that homeostasis cannot be maintained without
      intervention

tients were placed at greater risk for bacteremia because advances in medical technology exposed them to far more invasive therapeutic and diagnostic procedures than before.

The clinical presentation of the sepsis syndrome varies with the organism responsible and according to the patient's underlying physiologic state. Early signs include fever and chills. Body temperatures during infections with gram-negative organisms may reach 105°F. LPS stimulates centers in the brain that control breathing and can produce tachypnea. In the early stages of sepsis, patients may present with confusion or delirium. Hypotension may progress to shock with attendant impairment of tissue perfusion and oxygen delivery. There is a characteristic hemodynamic profile of progressive septic shock that includes tachycardia, hypotension, decreased systemic vascular resistance, elevated or normal cardiac index, and normal or decreased cardiac filling pressure. If the syndrome progresses to multiple organ dysfunction syndrome, the adult respiratory distress syndrome may develop, along with failure of the heart, kidneys, and liver.

Diagnostic testing should be guided by the likely source of the infection. Although bacteremia can arise from infections of any part of the body, the most common sites associated with sepsis are the genitourinary tract, lower intestinal tract, pelvic organs, and intravenous devices. Patients suspected of having sepsis should have cultures obtained from the appropriate site. Noninvasive imaging can be useful not only to identify the source of occult infection, but to guide aspirated cultures. Successful recovery of responsible organisms from the blood depends mainly on the volume of blood cultured. Each sample should contain at least 10 mL of blood. It is rarely necessary to take more than two samples. Timing of the cultures depends on the nature of the infectious process. Intravascular infections (e.g., endocarditis, infected intravascular devices, or arteriovenous fistulas) produce continuous bacteremia and it therefore does not matter when cultures are taken. In contrast, abscesses produce bacteremia episodically, and more widely spaced samples taken 15 to 20 minutes apart are more likely to be fruitful. It is also important to prepare the site adequately with an iodine-containing compound to reduce contamination with skin flora such as *S. epidermidis*. Isolation of a skin organism from more than one site is far more likely to be evidence of a true bacteremia than recovery from only a single culture. Organisms responsible for true bacteremia are also more likely to grow quickly in culture; growth after 48 or 72 hours of incubation is more commonly seen with a contaminant. Although most bacteria grow equally well under anaerobic conditions as in the presence of oxygen, some, such as *Pseudomonas* species, are obligate aerobes. It is therefore advisable to inoculate an aerobic bottle as well as an anaerobic one. Rarely, blood cultures are falsely negative because the responsible organism has fastidious growth requirements. This is particularly true for some causative agents of endocarditis. Collaboration with the staff of the microbiology laboratory before reculture may suggest alternative strategies to improve recovery of these "picky" eaters.

TREATMENT

The major determinant of successful outcome in sepsis that is under the control of the clinician is prompt institution of appropriate antibiotics. The choice of agents must be guided by the likely pathogens associated with infections from the suspected site (Table 2). Antibiotics must be given intravenously and in full therapeutic doses to achieve adequate levels in tissues that might be underperfused. Appropriate adjustments in dosage need to be made when sepsis impairs the function of organs involved in the elimination of antibiotics. Even under those circumstances, the amount of the initial or loading dose should be sufficient to achieve immediate therapeutic concentrations in the blood and in the tissue involved. Except in suspected *Pseudomonas aeruginosa* infection, there is little reason to provide double antibiotic coverage if the pathogen and its antibiotic sensitivities are known. Some sites, such as intra-abdominal abscesses, have a mixture of organisms that are challenging to cover with a single agent. Although there is controversy as to whether all isolated organisms need to be treated (e.g., enterococci from a biliary source), prudence dictates that all organisms isolated from the blood should be covered. Bacteremia in the febrile neutropenic patient can be treated with monotherapy, but my preference is to use two antibiotics because of the prevalence of *Pseudomonas* infection in these patients. Although the incidence of gram-positive infections is high in neutropenic patients, specific antistaphylococcal antibiotics such as vancomycin need not be a component of empiric therapy. Survival is no different whether vancomycin is included among the initial drugs given or if it is added after gram-positive organisms are identified in blood cultures.

TABLE 2. **Choice of Antibiotics in the Empirical Treatment of Sepsis**

Source	Likely Bacteria	Antibiotics	Alternative
Unknown	Gram-positive cocci, Enterobacteriaceae, *Pseudomonas* species, anaerobes	AP/B-LI *or* a carbapenem Vancomycin should be added if high probability of methicillin-resistant *Staphylococcus aureus*	Third- or fourth-generation cephalosporin *plus* either clindamycin or metronidazole *or* a fluoroquinolone plus clindamycin
Urinary tract	Enterobacteriaceae, enterococci	Aminoglycoside plus ampicillin	Vancomycin plus aminoglycoside or aztreonam
Biliary tract	Enterobacteriaceae, enterococci, anaerobes	Ampicillin/sulbactam plus an aminoglycoside (if enterococci isolated from blood)	Aztreonam plus clindamycin *or* third-generation cephalosporin plus clindamycin or metronidazole
Lower gastrointestinal tract or pelvis	Enterobacteriaceae, anaerobes	Metronidazole or clindamycin or ampicillin/sulbactam *plus* aminoglycoside	Metronidazole or clindamycin *plus* fluoroquinolone or aztreonam
Intravascular devices	*Staphylococcus aureus, Staphylococcus epidermidis*	Vancomycin	
Neutropenia	Enterobacteriaceae, *Pseudomonas* sp.	APP or ceftazidime *plus* aminoglycoside	Carbapenem or AP/B-LI

Dosages: All drugs are given intravenously.
AP/B-LI (antipseudomonal penicillin/beta-lactamase inhibitor combination): ticarcillin/clavulanic acid (Timentin) 3.1 g q 4 h; piperacillin/tazobactam (Zosyn) 3.375 g q 4 h
Carbapenem: imipenem/cilastatin (Primaxin) 0.5 g q 6 h; meropenem (Merrem) 1.0 g q 8 h
Third-generation cephalosporin: cefotaxime (Claforan), ceftizoxime (Cefizox) 2.0 g q 4 h; ceftriaxone (Rocephin) 2.0 g q 12 h; ceftazidime (Fortaz) 2.0 g q 8 h
Fourth-generation cephalosporin: cefepime (Maxipime) 2.0 g q 12 h
APP (antipseudomonal penicillin): ticarcillin (Ticar) 3.0 g q 4 h; piperacillin (Pipracil) 3.0 g q 4 h
Ampicillin/sulbactam (Unasyn) 3.0 g q 6 h
Aminoglycoside: gentamicin (Garamycin), tobramycin (Nebcin) loading dose 2 mg/kg followed by 1.7 mg/kg q 8 h; amikacin (Amikin) 7.5 mg/kg q 12 h
Ampicillin (Omnipen) 3.5 g q 6 h
Clindamycin (Cleocin) 900 mg q 8 h
Metronidazole (Flagyl) 1 g q 12 h
Aztreonam (Azactam) 2.0 g q 8 h
Vancomycin (Vancocin) 1.0 g q 12 h
Fluoroquinolone: ciprofloxacin (Cipro), ofloxacin (Floxin): 400 mg q 12 h

The response to antibiotic therapy of patients with bacteremia or sepsis should be re-evaluated daily and appropriate changes made when the results of culture and sensitivity tests are known. Antibiotics should be given for 10 to 14 days. The full course should be given intravenously; conversion to oral antibiotics once the patient stabilizes is not indicated with either bacteremia or sepsis. Closed abscesses often do not respond to antibiotics alone and must be surgically drained.

Patients with bacteremia or sepsis should be closely monitored for changes in blood pressure, urinary output, and oxygenation status. Hypotension should prompt a challenge with an intravenous fluid bolus. Although patients with hypotension controlled by intravenous fluids can be managed on a general medical-surgical ward, profound hypotension unresponsive to fluids is treated better in an intensive care unit, where hemodynamic status can be monitored by right heart catheterization and use of vasopressor agents and mechanical ventilation is available.

Despite our increased knowledge about the roles of cytokines in the pathogenesis of systemic inflammatory response syndrome, numerous studies have failed to find any utility for specific inhibitors in the treatment of sepsis. Indeed, some studies have shown a detrimental effect. Most likely, the inflammatory response to sepsis is so finely balanced between activators and inhibitors that therapeutic modulation of a single factor will have an unpredictable effect. Similarly, corticosteroids have not been shown to have any benefit in this clinical setting.

BRUCELLOSIS

method of
EMILIO BOUZA, M.D., Ph.D., and
PATRICIA MUÑOZ, M.D., Ph.D.
Hospital General Universitario
Madrid, Spain

Brucellosis is still an important endemic zoonosis in extensive areas of the world and one of the most frequent diseases acquired professionally by veterinarians, personnel in the meat industry, and microbiology laboratory workers.

Brucellosis may manifest initially as an unspecific febrile disease or as a disease with focal involvement, particularly of the bones and joints, the testes, the cardiovascular system, and the central nervous system. A definitive diagnosis is established when *Brucella* organisms are isolated from blood or other clinical samples. Brucellosis may be diagnosed with a high degree of probability in cases with a fourfold or greater rise in the titer of antibodies in the setting of a clinical manifestation compatible with this disease.

We discuss the antimicrobial susceptibility of *Brucella* in vitro, the medical treatment of brucellosis in humans, the current contribution of immunomodulators, the indications for surgery, and the therapy of choice in special circumstances.

ANTIMICROBIAL AGENTS WITH "IN VITRO" ACTIVITY

Tetracyclines, rifampin* (Rifadin), aminoglycosides,* co-trimoxazole* (Bactrim, Septra), fluoroquinolones,* azithromycin* (Zithromax) and other macrolides, and many beta-lactam drugs are highly active in vitro against *Brucella* species isolates. However, because of the intraphagocytic residence of this microorganism, the in vitro activity is a necessary but not sufficient condition to warrant clinical activity in the treatment of brucellosis in humans. Under those circumstances, only tetracyclines, rifampin, aminoglycosides, and co-trimoxazole have shown consistent results. Drug-resistant *Brucella* strains are rarely a cause of therapeutic failure.

Antimicrobial Therapy of Brucellosis in Humans

The 10 most important principles of treatment of brucellosis in humans are summarized as follows:

1. Doxycycline (Vibramycin) and other tetracyclines are the mainstays of treatment and should be included whenever possible.

2. Combination therapy is clearly better than monotherapy, and a second or third drug should be included when feasible.

3. Treatments of 6 weeks' duration are usually preferred to courses of 4 weeks.

4. The combination of doxycycline and an aminoglycoside, particularly streptomycin during the initial 2 to 3 weeks or gentamicin (Garamycin) during the initial 1 to 2 weeks, is better than oral rifampin during a 45-day period, in most circumstances.

5. In patients with focal involvement, longer therapeutic courses are usually required.

6. Co-trimoxazole alone during long periods of time (6 months) or the combination of co-trimoxazole and rifampin during shorter periods are a suitable alternative for treatment in children and pregnant women.

7. Data regarding the use of fluoroquinolones or macrolides in the treatment of brucellosis are discouraging, inconsistent, or insufficient to justify including them in regular therapeutic options.

8. Surgical treatment is usually required, among other circumstances, for most patients with brucellar endocarditis, for patients with undrained collections, and for patients with neurologic compression or column instability.

9. At present, immunomodulators and vaccines do not yet have a role in the regular management of brucellosis in humans.

10. Relapses are usually treated with the same regimens because they are not regularly a conse-

---

*Not FDA approved for this indication.

TABLE 1. **Therapeutic Regimens in Human Brucellosis**

Setting	Drug	Dose	Length	Comments
Regular cases in adults	Doxycycline + streptomycin*	100 mg bid 1 gm qd	6 weeks 2 weeks	Failures, 2%; relapses, 5%
	Doxycycline + rifampin* (Rifadin)	100 mg bid + 900 mg qd	6 weeks 6 weeks	Failures, 8%; relapses, 16%
	Doxycycline + gentamicin*	100 mg bid + 240 mg qd	6 weeks 1 week	Failures, 0%; relapses, 6%
	Doxycycline + gentamicin	100 mg bid + 240 mg qd	4 weeks 1 week	Failures, 0%; relapses, 23%
	Doxycycline + netilmicin* (Netromycin)	100 mg bid + 300 mg qd	6 weeks 1 week	Failures, 8%; relapses, 12.5%
	Co-trimoxazole* (Bactrim, Septra)	DS tid DS bid	1 week 3 weeks to 6 months	Failures, 6%; relapses, 3%
	Doxycycline	100 mg bid	6 weeks	Failures, 0%; relapses, 14%
Endocarditis	Doxycycline + rifampin + gentamicin and/or co-trimoxazole	100 mg bid 900 mg/d 240 mg qd	6–12 weeks	Hospital admission Consider surgery
Neurobrucellosis	Same as for endocarditis	Same as for endocarditis	At least 3 months or until CSF parameters improve	Hospital admission Imaging techniques commonly required
Focal disease, excluding endocarditis or neurobrucellosis	Doxycycline + streptomycin or gentamicin	100 mg bid 1 gm qd 240 mg qd	45 days to 3 months 2–3 weeks 1–2 weeks	Imaging techniques may be required for osteoarticular disease
Children <8 years old	Rifampin + co-trimoxazole or	15–20 mg/kg in 2 doses 10–12 mg/kg trimethoprim, 50–60 mg/kg sulfamethoxazole	6 weeks 6 weeks	Tetracyclines contraindicated
	Rifampin + gentamicin	5–6 mg/kg/d	6 weeks 5 days	
Pregnant women	Rifampin or	900 mg/d	6 weeks	Tetracyclines contraindicated
	Rifampin + co-trimoxazole	900 mg qd 10–12 mg/kg trimethoprim, 50–60 mg/kg sulfamethoxazole	4 weeks	

*Not FDA approved for this indication.
Abbreviations: CSF = cerebrospinal fluid; IM = intramuscularly.

quence of the development of antimicrobial resistance.

A summary of some therapeutic regimens is offered in Table 1.

For conventional (nonfocal) cases, the regimen of first choice is a combination of doxycycline (100 mg twice a day [bid]) for 45 days and streptomycin (1 gram intramuscularly [IM] per 24 hours) for 14 days. Gentamicin (240 mg in a single daily dose IM or intravenously [IV]) or netilmicin* (Netromycin; 300 mg in a single daily dose) for the first 7 days may be substituted for streptomycin.

Second-choice regimens consist of combinations of doxycycline and rifampin for 45 days or monotherapy with doxycycline for 45 days. In a study by Ariza and coworkers (Ann Intern Med 1992; 117:25–30), the combination of doxycycline and rifampin was less effective than doxycycline and streptomycin only in patients with spondylitis but not in cases with nonfocal brucellosis.

In children younger than 8 years, the preferred

regimen is rifampin with co-trimoxazole (trimethoprim-sulfamethoxazole) for 45 days. An alternative regimen consists of a combination of rifampin 15 mg per kg daily in two doses for 45 days with gentamicin, 5 to 6 mg per kg per day, for the first 5 days.

Data from experimental models suggest that the administration of aminoglycosides encapsulated in cationic liposomes have an enhanced effect in comparison with the conventional administration of aminoglycosides in the treatment of brucellosis, but clinical data to make any recommendation is lacking.

Co-trimoxazole has been reported for a long time to be inferior to the combination therapy, but it is effective when provided in very long courses and constitutes one of the drugs of choice for patients unable to receive tetracyclines and also a third drug in patients with meningitis or endocarditis.

Quinolones alone showed a very high rate of relapses and should not be considered adequate therapy for brucellosis in humans. Rifampin alone is also inadequate.

The results of treatment in animal models of acute brucellosis with azithromycin suggest that azithro-

*Not FDA approved for this indication.

mycin is less active than doxycycline and doxycycline plus streptomycin, and the new macrolides do not warrant a first-choice role in the treatment of brucellosis in humans.

IMMUNOTHERAPY

The role of immunomodulating agents such as levamisole* (Ergamisol) and interferon* is promising but is not a clinical reality at the present time. These agents can be considered only for patients with chronic anergic brucellosis.

Live attenuated vaccines, useful in animals, have not been applied in Western countries because of the fear of untoward complications and production of real brucellosis.

SURGICAL TREATMENT

As we mentioned, surgery in patients with brucellosis is usually required for infective endocarditis, in which a poor response to antimicrobial therapy is well known in most cases. It is also used for unstable vertebral columns and for drainage of paravertebral and other-site abscesses.

SPECIAL SITUATIONS

In a prospective study of 530 cases of brucellosis in humans, Colmenero and colleagues found that 169 patients (32%) older than 14 years had focal manifestations of the disease. The most frequent were osteoarticular complications (66%), genitourinary involvement (5% of males), neurologic disease (2%), and heart lesions (1.5%). Twenty-five patients with complications (14.5%) required surgical solutions. Rates of relapse were similar for patients with and without focal disease.

Infective Endocarditis

Less than 2% of all cases of bacterial endocarditis are caused by *Brucella,* and less than 2% of patients with brucellosis have endocardial involvement; however, *Brucella*-related endocarditis is a severe disease and probably the leading cause of death in patients with brucellosis.

Prosthetic valve endocarditis caused by *Brucella* species is a microbiologic indication for valvular replacement, because of the high rate of failures in patients treated only with antimicrobial therapy. Native valve brucellar endocarditis also frequently necessitates surgery, mainly in the presence of cardiac failure, abscesses, or persistent fever.

Table 1 includes therapeutic recommendations, such as the combination of doxycycline, rifampin, and co-trimoxazole for at least 6 to 12 weeks in patients with prior cardiac valve substitution and much longer otherwise. During the initial 2 to 6 weeks, co-

trimoxazole may be substituted for an IV aminoglycoside, particularly gentamicin.

Neurobrucellosis

Neurobrucellosis has occurred in only 2% of the cases of brucellosis in our experience, and it frequently mimics other neurologic diseases. The most common manifestation is chronic meningitis, followed by meningoencephalitis and polyradiculoneuritis. Demonstration requires the isolation of *Brucella* from cerebrospinal fluid (CSF) or neural tissues or the presence of anti-*Brucella* antibodies in the CSF in the setting of a compatible clinical syndrome.

There are no prospective and comparative studies from which to decide the optimal composition and length of medical treatment, but we recommend the same combination as for infective endocarditis, prolonged at least 3 months or until the altered CSF parameters have significantly improved.

Despite the absence of data regarding efficacy, the use of corticosteroids in tapering doses should be considered in patients with chronic meningitis, especially in children.

Osteoarticular Involvement

In cases of osteoarticular involvement, the treatment of choice includes doxycycline plus an aminoglycoside (streptomycin for 2 to 3 weeks or gentamicin for 1 to 2 weeks) because this has been shown to be superior to the combination of doxycycline and rifampin. The treatment should be prolonged at least 45 days, and some authors suggest continuing therapy for 3 months.

Children and Pregnant Women

In a prospective study, 113 children with brucellosis were treated with a combination of two oral agents: trimethoprim-sulfamethoxazole (10 to 12 mg of trimethoprim per kg, 50 to 60 mg of sulfamethoxazole per kg) and rifampin (15 to 20 mg per kg in two divided doses for 6 weeks). The treatment was well tolerated, and all patients responded with defervescence of fever and resolution of all symptoms within 1 to 3 weeks. Relapse after 6 months occurred in four children, all of whom responded to repeat therapy with the same agents.

In pregnant and nursing women, tetracyclines should be avoided. Streptomycin has been related to fetal eighth nerve damage, so it should not be used if possible. Therapy in these situations consists of rifampin for 6 weeks or rifampin plus co-trimoxazole for 4 weeks (see Table 1).

Relapses

At present, relapses after a well-selected antimicrobial regimen should occur in less than 10% of the cases. Relapses usually occur within the first year after therapy and may be clinically less significant

---

*Not FDA approved for this indication.

and less severe than the original episode. They should be treated with a second course of therapy selected within the same criteria and considerations previously mentioned for first episodes. There is no evidence that the incidence of recurrences is higher after the first episode than after subsequent episodes.

CONJUNCTIVITIS

method of
RALPH S. VIOLA, M.D.
University of Rochester School of Medicine and Dentistry and Genesee Valley Eye Institute Rochester, New York

Conjunctivitis, in its varying forms, is a frequent ocular occurrence involving all age and demographic groups. This inflammation of the conjunctiva is one of the most common causes of self-referral in eye care practices, with complaints of red eye and discharge. Permanent visual or structural damage is rare, but there is a great economic impact in terms of treatment costs and lost productivity.

Conjunctivitis can be classified as acute or chronic and infectious or noninfectious. The causes of infectious conjunctivitis include bacteria, viruses, fungi, parasites, and *Chlamydia.* Noninfectious conjunctivitis may be caused by allergies, mechanical irritants, toxins, and tumors. It is important to differentiate primary conjunctivitis from conjunctivitis that is secondary to systemic or ocular diseases because treatment of the latter usually involves correcting the underlying problem.

A detailed history is important in evaluating conjunctivitis. This should include signs and symptoms (discharge, pain, photophobia, itching, blurred vision), duration of the symptoms, and whether they are unilateral or bilateral. The clinician should also look at the possibility of trauma or recent exposure to an infected individual. Allergy, contact lens wear, medications, and cosmetic use are also important.

BACTERIAL CONJUNCTIVITIS

The principal causes of nonsevere bacterial conjunctivitis are *Streptococcus pneumoniae, Staphylococcus aureus, Moraxella,* and *Haemophilus* (in older children). More severe cases of bacterial conjunctivitis may be caused by *Neisseria gonorrhoeae* or *Neisseria meningitidis, Haemophilus influenzae* (in younger children), and *Streptococcus pyogenes.*

Bacterial conjunctivitis can be spread by a number of different means. Neonates most commonly are infected during vaginal delivery by an infected mother. As they grow, children may develop conjunctivitis secondary to a nasolacrimal duct obstruction, a bacterial otitis media, or contact with an infected individual. In adults, risk factors also include immunosuppression, trauma, oculogenital contact, and keratitis sicca.

The natural history of bacterial conjunctivitis is self-limiting in adults. Complications are rare but can include preseptal cellulitis or keratitis. Gonococ-

cal infections can rapidly progress to a hyperpurulent conjunctivitis, which can lead to corneal infection and perforation. Systemic complications include arthritis, septicemia, and urethritis.

Bacterial conjunctivitis can be unilateral or bilateral. There is usually marked injection of the bulbar conjunctiva. A purulent discharge is common. Gonococcal conjunctivitis can be accompanied by severe eyelid edema and preauricular lymphadenopathy. A corneal infiltrate may be seen that should be treated aggressively because corneal perforation is a real possibility in gonococcal disease.

Formerly, all conjunctivitis was cultured to determine the specific pathogen, and this is still considered the standard of care in many areas. With the development of topical broad-spectrum antibiotics, most cases are treated based solely on clinical appearance. Cultures are indicated in cases of neonatal conjunctivitis as well as recurrent or severe purulent cases and those that do not respond to medication.

Mild cases of bacterial conjunctivitis may resolve spontaneously, but topical antibiotic therapy does reduce the time course and morbidity. Gonococcal and neonatal conjunctivitis should receive systemic treatment as well as topical antibiotic therapy. In cases with severe purulent discharge, saline lavage may diminish the amount of discharge.

Nongonococcal infections can be treated with topical gentamicin or tobramycin to cover infection with gram-negative rods. Gram-positive infections are usually treated with polymyxin B/trimethoprim, erythromycin, or bacitracin. Drops are given every 2 to 4 hours (depending on severity) for 7 to 10 days. Patients with gonococcal conjunctivitis can be given one of the topical fluoroquinolones, but systemic treatment must be instituted. In children weighing less than 45 kg a single intramuscular dose of 125 mg of ceftriaxone (Rocephin)* is sufficient. Children weighing more than 45 kg and adults are treated with 1 gram of ceftriaxone given intramuscularly.

CHLAMYDIAL CONJUNCTIVITIS

Chlamydia trachomatis is the organism responsible for inclusion conjunctivitis. This is a sexually transmitted disease acquired through oculogenital spread. It is also a cause of ophthalmia neonatorum in infants secondary to vaginal delivery by infected mothers.

The disease in neonates can manifest in the first 20 days and, if untreated, can persist up to 1 year. Adults will have a similar duration. Complications include conjunctival and corneal scarring. Nasopharyngeal or genital infection can be associated.

Chlamydial cases are usually bilateral. Infants may have lid edema, bulbar conjunctival injection, and a purulent discharge. In adults, the clinician may also observe a follicular reaction of the tarsal conjunctiva as well as a superficial keratitis and preauricular lymphadenopathy.

---

*Not FDA approved for this indication.

Suspected chlamydial conjunctivitis should be confirmed by culture or immunodiagnostic tests. Systemic treatment is indicated, owing to the high rate of infections at nonocular sites. Neonates and children weighing less than 45 kg are given erythromycin, 50 mg per kg per day orally divided into four doses for 10 to 14 days. Children weighing more than 45 kg receive a single dose of 1 gram of oral azithromycin (Zithromax).* Adults and children older than 8 years old may take the same dose of azithromycin. Doxycycline (Vibramycin), 100 mg orally twice a day for 7 days, may be substituted.

VIRAL CONJUNCTIVITIS

The most common cause of epidemic viral conjunctivitis is adenovirus. Herpes simplex virus is responsible for most nonepidemic conjunctivitis. Other causes of viral conjunctivitis include Epstein-Barr, rubella, rubeola, and influenza viruses.

Viral conjunctivitis is most commonly spread by exposure (directly or indirectly) to an infected individual. Hand-to-hand contact under poor hygienic conditions can lead to rapid exposure. Ironically, many cases of conjunctivitis are contracted in the physician's office when examination rooms are not properly disinfected after examining a patient with conjunctivitis. Patients with a previous herpes simplex infection can undergo reactivation by stress, trauma, or an acute illness. Primary herpes simplex in young children often involves the cornea and lid and may be associated with systemic manifestations.

Adenoviral conjunctivitis is self-limiting. Signs and symptoms usually resolve within 5 to 7 days. Rare cases can last for weeks. Severe cases can lead to superficial keratitis, epithelial erosions, subepithelial infiltrates, and conjunctival scarring. Herpes simplex conjunctivitis can resolve without treatment in 4 to 7 days. Complications can include epithelial and stromal keratitis as well as conjunctival scarring.

Adenoviral infections can be unilateral or bilateral. Patients present with a watery discharge, injection of the bulbar conjunctiva, and a follicular reaction of the tarsal conjunctiva. Additional signs include preauricular lymphadenopathy, subconjunctival hemorrhage, and a multifocal epithelial punctate keratitis. Herpes simplex is usually unilateral. It also produces a watery discharge, bulbar conjunctival injection, and a follicular reaction of the tarsal conjunctiva. Herpes will usually produce an ulceration or vesicular rash of the eyelid as well as a dendritic lesion of the corneal epithelium or conjunctiva.

Viral cultures and diagnostic tests are not routinely used. Adenoviral conjunctivitis is self-limiting, and supportive therapy is usually given. Patients are warned that the uninvolved eye may become (or may already have become) infected. Good hygiene is stressed with frequent hand washing and laundry. Artificial tears and cool compresses can help reduce associated irritation. Topical corticosteroids may be

helpful in cases of severe adenoviral conjunctivitis but carry a risk of elevated intraocular pressure. Patients with severe conjunctivitis should be followed weekly whereas more routine cases can be monitored in 2 to 3 weeks.

Herpes simplex conjunctivitis is treated either with topical trifluridine (Viroptic) 1% solution eight times per day or with both vidarabine (Vira-A) 3% ointment five times per day and oral acyclovir (Zovirax),* 400 mg five times per day. Treatment is continued until resolution of the conjunctivitis. Patients should be seen within 1 week. Topical corticosteroids are contraindicated in herpes infections because cases may worsen. Consequently, in any case of suspected herpes simplex, corticosteroids should be withheld.

ALLERGIC CONJUNCTIVITIS

Allergic conjunctivitis is usually associated with exposure to environmental allergens. There may be a genetic predisposition. Some forms are more prevalent in hot, dry environments.

Seasonal allergic conjunctivitis is recurrent and produces minimal long-term complications. There is a vernal form that begins in childhood and gradually decreases in activity during the first three decades of life. It undergoes a chronic course with acute exacerbations. This can lead to eyelid thickening and ptosis. Patients can suffer from conjunctival or corneal scarring and, in rare cases, infection or ulceration.

Most allergic conjunctivitis is bilateral. Conjunctival injection and chemosis are present. There is usually a watery discharge and, in some cases, a mucoid discharge. In addition, vernal conjunctivitis may include giant papillary hypertrophy of the superior tarsus as well as conjunctival scarring. Corneal erosions, scarring, and neovascularization may be seen in cases of vernal conjunctivitis but rarely in seasonal allergic conjunctivitis.

Seasonal allergic conjunctivitis is best treated by avoiding the offending allergen. This is often impractical. Supportive therapy includes frequent use of artificial tears and cool compresses during exacerbations. Tears may be used as little as two to three times a day or as often as every hour. Patients using tears more than five to six times a day are advised to use preservative-free tears to avoid preservative-related complications. In cases in which tears alone are not sufficient, there are a number of over-the-counter allergy medications. These usually contain naphazoline (Naphcon-A, Opcon-A) and may be used up to four times a day. A number of topical nonsteroidal anti-inflammatory agents and mast-cell stabilizers can be used. These include ketorolac (Acular), cromolyn sodium (Crolom), and lodoxamide (Alomide) and can be given four times a day. More severe cases may require corticosteroids and should undergo careful ophthalmologic evaluation to look for corticosteroid-induced glaucoma. Patients with vernal con-

---

*Not FDA approved for this indication.

*Not FDA approved for this indication.

junctivitis can be treated in a similar fashion, but acute exacerbations are more likely to need topical corticosteroids.

MECHANICAL/MEDICATION CONJUNCTIVITIS

The most common type of mechanical conjunctivitis is contact lens–induced giant papillary conjunctivitis (GPC). Prolonged lens wearing time, poor lens hygiene, allergenic lens solutions or materials, and even poor fitting lenses can exacerbate GPC.

GPC involves a papillary hypertrophy of the superior tarsal conjunctiva, usually based on contact lens wear. There may be a mucoid discharge. Symptoms gradually increase with increased lens wear and may lead to corneal neovascularization and scarring.

Treatment involves reducing contact lens wear time in mild cases and discontinuation of lenses for several days to weeks in severe cases. Mast cell stabilizing agents and a short course of corticosteroids are sometimes beneficial. When patients return to contact lens wear, they are switched to preservative-free lens care systems and alternative lens materials. A change in lens wear habits to shorter wear schedules is recommended.

Medication-induced conjunctivitis can evolve after prolonged use of topical antiglaucoma drugs as well as neomycin and sulfonamides. The patient exhibits conjunctival injection and tarsal conjunctival follicles in the eye exposed to the medication. A contact dermatitis of the eyelids is also seen. Symptoms worsen with continuing drug use and can lead to corneal erosion and ulceration, deposition of the drug in the corneal stroma, and scarring of the conjunctiva.

Medication-induced conjunctivitis is treated by discontinuing the drug. In cases due to antiglaucoma medications, alternative drugs need to be prescribed to control intraocular pressure. In rare cases of severe conjunctivitis, a brief course of topical corticosteroids is used.

NEOPLASTIC CONJUNCTIVITIS

In cases of conjunctivitis that do not respond to conventional therapy, the clinician must include sebaceous cell carcinoma in the differential diagnosis. This is most common in the fifth to ninth decades of life.

Sebaceous cell carcinoma is unilateral with an intense injection of the bulbar conjunctiva. Conjunctival scarring may occur. There may be a hard, nonmobile yellow nodular mass in the eyelids. Progression to orbital invasion and metastases can be rapid.

A full-thickness lid biopsy is indicated in cases of suspected sebaceous cell carcinoma. If the diagnosis is confirmed, local excision is required.

VARICELLA
(Chickenpox)

method of
JOHN F. MARCINAK, M.D.
University of Illinois College of Medicine
Chicago, Illinois

Varicella-zoster virus (VZV), a common infectious exanthem of children, is the virus that causes varicella (chickenpox) and establishes latency in sensory ganglia after the primary infection. Reactivation of the virus causes herpes zoster (HZ), known as shingles. Chickenpox is usually a benign disease in immunocompetent children; the incidence of zoster increases with advancing age, as cellular immunity declines. Complications of chickenpox as well as of HZ can occur in normal children and adults; the risk of severe complications is highest in those with an immunodeficiency, particularly with impairments in cell-mediated immunity. Treatment includes antiviral chemotherapy, and prevention through passive and active immunization is now possible.

EPIDEMIOLOGY OF CHICKENPOX AND HZ

Chickenpox is a highly contagious disease, with secondary attack rates of 80 to 90% in susceptible household contacts. There are approximately 4 million cases each year in the United States. It is estimated from age-specific incidence data derived from the 1980–1990 National Health Interview Survey that 33% and 44% of chickenpox cases occur in preschool and school-aged children, respectively. More recent parent-reported incidence data indicate that the incidence of chickenpox is increasing in preschool children in the United States. Most cases in the United States are reported during the winter and early spring. According to the Centers for Disease Control and Prevention (CDC), from 1990 to 1994 an average of 43 children aged 15 years or younger each year had chickenpox as the underlying cause of death, and from 1988 to 1995 up to 10,000 children per year were hospitalized for chickenpox or its complications. In the United States during the 1980s, an increase in hospital admissions of young adults for chickenpox at army and navy military facilities suggests an increase in susceptibility of chickenpox among young adults.

The incidence rates of HZ increase dramatically among persons older than 60 years. Age and cancer are significant risk factors for HZ, whereas a recent study in North Carolina elderly residents found a lower-than-average incidence among black persons. Finally, the overall number of cases of HZ in the United States is also expected to increase, inasmuch as the average life span is increasing.

PATHOGENESIS

VZV is a double-stranded DNA virus of the herpes family. Initial infection begins through the conjunctivae and/or mucosa of the upper respiratory tract. Over the next 2 to 3 days, the virus replicates in regional lymph nodes, and a primary viremia occurs on days 4 to 6. Replication then occurs in the liver and spleen with a secondary viremia 10 to 14 days later that coincides with the appearance of the vesicular rash. After primary infection with VZV, the virus migrates to the dorsal root and trigeminal ganglia, where the virus establishes latency. Reactivation of the virus through waning of cellular immunity later in life or from immunosuppression is thought to cause the unilateral dermatomal and usually painful vesicular rash of HZ. Immunity to chickenpox appears to be lifelong after natural infection, although there are a few documented reports of second cases of chickenpox. Both humoral and cellular immunity are necessary in eliminating infection and maintaining persistent immunity. These cellular and humoral responses to VZV can be boosted after close exposure to the virus.

CLINICAL MANIFESTATIONS

Primary infection with VZV is an illness that occurs approximately 14 to 16 days after exposure and has virtually no prodrome. The first manifestation of the illness is the exanthem, the appearance of which is associated with contagiousness. Because the rash may go unnoticed for 1 or 2 days, it is best to consider a person exposed if there is contact with the index patient during the 2 days before the rash is observed. The exanthem begins as macules that become maculopapular and then vesicular, followed by crusting and scab formation. Lesions in different stages are observed with the rash and are always more prominent on the trunk than on the extremities. Most patients with chickenpox have a low-grade fever. Lesions can also be seen on mucous membranes such as the oropharynx and conjunctivae. In children the median number of lesions is 300. The diagnosis of chickenpox is extremely important when immunocompromised patients and pregnant women are exposed. Diagnosis can be made routinely in the virology laboratory by viral culture or direct identification of VZV antigen by fluorescent antibody staining of vesicular fluid scrapings. Multinucleated giant cells containing intranuclear inclusions can be demonstrated in a Tzanck preparation of scrapings from chickenpox lesions but can be positive from herpes simplex virus–infected cells.

Prenatal infection is uncommon in the United States because most women of childbearing age are immune to chickenpox. Pregnant women who develop chickenpox during the third trimester are at risk for severe pneumonia and death. Spontaneous abortion can occur in women infected during the first half of pregnancy. Chickenpox infection in the first 20 weeks of pregnancy confers a 2% risk that the fetus will develop congenital varicella syndrome. This syndrome involves congenital limb hypoplasia, dermatomal skin scarring, and damage to the eyes (chorioretinitis or cataracts) and central nervous system. The risk of HZ in infancy after maternal varicella in the second half of gestation is also approximately 2%. If maternal chickenpox develops from 5 days before delivery to 2 days afterward, the newborn is at risk for severe disseminated and fatal chickenpox, with an attack rate of from 20 to 50%.

VZV infection in the immunocompromised host can be severe and fatal. Because children with primary agammaglobulinemia have uncomplicated disease and those with immunodeficiency affecting cell-mediated immunity, such as leukemia or lymphoma, are at high risk for severe disease, cell-mediated immunity plays an important role in limiting spread of disease and clearing of infection. Risk is increased with concomitant administration of immunosuppressive therapy. In the immunocompromised child, the lesions are more numerous and larger and persist for a longer time than in the immunocompetent child. The lung is the organ most frequently involved in children with leukemia who develop chickenpox, but the liver or central nervous system can be involved. Children with bone marrow transplants are also at high risk for disseminated

disease. There have been reports of disseminated chickenpox in children with human immunodeficiency virus (HIV) infection, but a prospective longitudinal study found only a 3% rate of severe chickenpox in 30 children with HIV infection who developed chickenpox. The rate of subsequent HZ was high (70%) in the HIV-infected children with low CD4 cell counts at the onset of chickenpox.

COMPLICATIONS

The most common complication of chickenpox is secondary bacterial infection of the skin. *Staphylococcus aureus* and group A beta-hemolytic streptococci (GAS) are the usual pathogens. Impetigo, cellulitis, or skin abscess can be seen. Since the early 1990s, an increasing number of severe invasive infections from GAS complicating chickenpox have been reported in the United States. A population-based surveillance system of invasive GAS infection in Ontario, Canada, from 1992 to 1996 found chickenpox to be a highly significant risk factor for invasive GAS infection. These infections have included deep-seated infections such as necrotizing fasciitis, myositis, osteomyelitis and/or arthritis, and pneumonia with empyema, as well as systemic infections. Systemic infections include sepsis with or without focal infection and the streptococcal toxic shock syndrome. The diagnosis of necrotizing fasciitis is often delayed, and when the patient first comes to medical attention, the need for surgical intervention is not always clear. Severe pain, erythema, and induration are the most common signs in children requiring surgical débridement.

Central nervous system complications can also be seen with chickenpox. The most common neurologic complication is acute cerebellar ataxia. The incidence in children younger than 15 years is 1 in 4000. Cerebellar ataxia develops 5 to 10 days after appearance of the rash; truncal ataxia is a prominent sign. In rare cases, the ataxia may precede the development of the rash. The prognosis is excellent; the symptoms of ataxia resolve over days to weeks. Varicella encephalitis is a more serious and yet less common complication than cerebellar ataxia. The risk of encephalitis in children 1 to 14 years of age is estimated at 1.7 per 100,000 chickenpox cases. It usually manifests 7 to 10 days after development of the chickenpox rash but has been reported to occur as early as 1 day before or up to 20 days after the rash develops. The clinical manifestation of encephalitis includes fever with an altered level of consciousness. Convulsions, coma, and paralysis may also be present. Cerebrospinal fluid changes usually include pleocytosis with a predominance of lymphocytes. Detection of VZV DNA by polymerase chain reaction (PCR) has been used to diagnose varicella encephalitis. Other rare neurologic complications include aseptic meningitis, transverse myelitis, optic neuritis, and Guillain-Barré syndrome. Reye's syndrome may be difficult to differentiate from varicella encephalitis. Reye's syndrome, which manifests with vomiting and altered mental status, has been associated with chickenpox more frequently than with other viral infections. This syndrome as a complication of chickenpox has become rare because aspirin and other salicylate-containing products are contraindicated for treatment during chickenpox.

Pneumonia is the third most common complication of chickenpox and occurs more frequently in previously healthy adults and immunocompromised children. The chest radiograph shows characteristic nodular densities throughout both lung fields. The course of pneumonia is variable, from mild or no cough to severe respiratory compromise necessitating oxygenation and ventilation.

A number of hematologic complications have been described with chickenpox. These include hemorrhage at sites of pox lesions that may progress to purpura fulminans with or without disseminated intravascular coagulation, thrombosis, transient thrombocytopenic purpura, or thrombocytopenia in association with sepsis. Purpura fulminans and thrombosis in children with chickenpox have been associated with acquired protein S deficiency. Other rare complications of chickenpox are arthritis, glomerulonephritis, myocarditis, and orchitis.

TREATMENT

Chickenpox in most children is an uncomplicated self-limited disease. Control of pruritus may be achieved with use of calamine lotion, cool compresses, or oatmeal baths. Oral antihistamines can be administered to decrease intense itching. Children's fingernails should be kept trimmed and clean. Symptomatic therapy for high fever can include acetaminophen if needed. Salicylates (aspirin) should not be given because this may lead to the development of Reye's syndrome.

Acyclovir (Zovirax) is the antiviral drug of choice for treatment of chickenpox in immunocompromised and some immunocompetent patients. Acyclovir is currently not recommended for routine use in immunocompetent children younger 12 years who have chickenpox, because the benefits are marginal. Oral acyclovir at a dose of 80 mg per kg per day in four divided doses for 5 to 7 days (maximal dose, 3200 mg per day) should be considered for selected healthy persons who are at increased risk for severe chickenpox. These include adolescents, adults, and possibly secondary household contacts, in all of whom the disease is usually more severe. Oral acyclovir at a dose of 4000 mg per day in five divided doses for 5 to 7 days has been effective for the treatment of HZ in adults by relieving acute pain, promoting healing of skin lesions, and decreasing duration of postherpetic neuralgia. Intravenous acyclovir, 30 mg per kg per day (children 12 months of age or younger) or 1500 mg per m² per day (children older than 12 months) in three divided doses for 7 to 10 days, is recommended for immunocompromised patients with chickenpox or HZ. Intravenous acyclovir is recommended for the pregnant woman with serious complications of chickenpox, such as pneumonia. Famciclovir (Famvir) and valacyclovir (Valtrex) are licensed for the treatment of HZ only in adults. These two new oral antiviral compounds have mechanisms of action similar to those of acyclovir but are more bioavailable, with longer half-lives, resulting in dosing intervals of two or three times daily.

PREVENTION

Varicella-zoster immune globulin (VZIG) can be given to prevent or modify chickenpox after significant exposure in susceptible persons at high risk of developing severe chickenpox. Administration of VZIG should be given within 96 hours but is most effective if given as soon as possible after exposure. One vial (~1.25 mL) containing 125 U is given for each 10 kg of body weight (minimal dose is 125 U and maximal dose is 625 U) by intramuscular injection. Significant factors for exposure include residing in same household, face-to-face indoor play, and, in the hospital setting, being in the same two- to four-bed room, adjacent beds in a large ward, or face-to-face contact with a person who has chickenpox. Candidates for VZIG with significant exposure include immunocompromised children, susceptible pregnant women, newborns of mothers who acquire chickenpox 5 days before to 2 days after delivery, preterm infants born at less than 28 weeks' gestation or with 1000-gram or less birth weight, and preterm infants born at 28 weeks' gestation or later whose mothers have no history of chickenpox or are seronegative.

A live attenuated varicella vaccine was developed in Japan in 1974 and has been used in Japan and Korea since 1987. The vaccine was licensed in the United States in March 1995 for routine vaccination of healthy 12- to 18-month-old children with no reliable history of chickenpox as well as susceptible older children, adolescents, and adults. Children 12 months to 12 years should receive 1 dose of varicella vaccine; adolescents aged 13 years or older and adults require 2 doses 4 to 8 weeks apart. Vaccine efficacy is high: probably 100% for prevention of severe cases and 85 to 90% for prevention of all cases of chickenpox in children. Vaccinated children with breakthrough infections have mild disease of short duration with fewer than 50 lesions. The vaccine has been well tolerated in children. Approximately 20% of children and 25 to 35% of adolescents experience transient redness, pain, or tenderness at the injection site. A mild vesicular rash at the injection site or elsewhere occurs in 5% of vaccinees with a median of five lesions. Vaccinated healthy children who develop more than 10 lesions after vaccination should be examined for natural chickenpox.

The incidence of HZ in healthy children who are vaccinated is no higher than that after natural chickenpox and may be lower. Children with acute lymphoblastic leukemia (ALL) who receive varicella vaccine have a lower incidence of HZ than do children with ALL who experience natural chickenpox. Studies are being conducted in adults aged 55 years and older to determine whether boosting of cell-mediated immunity with varicella vaccine protects against or lessens the severity of HZ. Persistence of high concentrations of VZV antibodies in Japanese children vaccinated 20 years ago and children in the United States up to 10 years ago is evidence of persistent immunity. Studies are ongoing to study the issue of persistence of immunity, because as more children are vaccinated, there will be less likelihood of natural boosting of immunity by exposure to wild-type virus.

CHOLERA

method of
G. H. RABBANI, M.D., PH.D.
International Centre for Diarrhoeal Disease
Research
Dhaka, Bangladesh

Cholera is caused by infection of the human small intestine by *Vibrio cholerae*, serotypes O1 and O139. It is the most severe form of all secretory diarrheas. The illness is clinically characterized by vomiting, massive rice-water–like stool, dehydration, and metabolic acidosis; death occurs in severe cases if patients are not rehydrated. Since 1817, there have been seven pandemics of cholera. The first six originated from the delta regions of eastern India, particularly Bengal, and swept all over the world, taking heavy toll on human lives. The seventh pandemic started in an Indonesian island in the early 1960s and has spread to all continents. Resurgence of epidemic cholera in Latin America and Africa and the report of cholera cases from the Gulf Coast of the United States signify the global public health importance of the disease.

THE ORGANISM

The genus *Vibrio* contains several bacterial species, of which *V. cholerae* and *V. parahaemolyticus* are the two most important pathogens of humans. *V. cholerae* is a gram-negative, monoflagellate, short, straight or curved rod (0.5 μm × 1.5 to 3.0 μm). *V. cholerae* is classified antigenically (O-antigens) into 60 to 70 serovars (serotypes). The serovar O1 includes all strains responsible for epidemic and endemic cholera and has two major subtypes, Ogawa and Inaba; a Hikojima subtype has been reported rarely. All these subtypes can be further distinguished into two biovars (biotypes): classical and El Tor.

PATHOGENICITY

Infection occurs after oral ingestion of a large numbers of *V. cholerae* organisms (10^{11} per mL), some of which escape the gastric acid barrier and colonize the small intestinal mucosa. Successful colonization depends on the adhesion of the bacteria to the epithelial surface, which secures the bacteria against the effects of intestinal motility and facilitates the delivery of the toxin that is produced. The mucosal adhesion is aided by the possession of bacterial toxin coregulated pili antigen (TcpA) and other colonizing factors of *V. cholerae*.

V. cholerae O1 produce a potent enterotoxin that stimulates intestinal secretion, leading to massive watery diarrhea. The toxin molecule consists of two subunits: a single, "heavy" A subunit (28,000 Da), and an aggregate of five "light" B subunits, each with a molecular weight of 11,600 Da. The A subunit can be split into fragments A_1 (22,500 Da) and A_2 (5500 Da). The light subunits are responsible for cell binding (B subunit), and the heavy subunits for direct toxicity (A subunit). The B subunits bind strongly to GM_1 ganglioside of the intact cells, and the A subunit penetrates through the cell membrane into the cytosol, activating an enzyme, adenylate cyclase, and generates cyclic AMP, which leads to increased permeability of the apical membrane to chloride ions and inhibition of coupled NaCl absorption. Besides cyclic AMP, other mechanisms involved in cholera toxin–stimulated secretion include prostaglandins, 5-hydroxytryptamine (5-HT), vasoactive intestinal peptide (VIP), and nitric oxide.

Minimal morphologic and inflammatory changes occur in the small bowel, the site of production of fluid loss in cholera in response to *V. cholerae* or its enterotoxin. The electrolyte content of the intestinal fluid of cholera patients varies greatly from the duodenum, where the bicarbonate concentration is less than that of plasma, to the ileum, where it is two to three times that of simultaneously obtained plasma (Table 1).

CLINICAL MANIFESTATIONS

The clinical manifestations of cholera vary from asymptomatic infection to severe diarrhea. In a typical adult case, diarrhea starts abruptly; the first few movements normally contain fecal materials, but the stool rapidly becomes clear and liquid, containing flecks of mucus but no trace of blood (rice-water–like stool). Vomiting of clear fluid may accompany the initial stages of diarrhea and contribute to dehydration. However, vomiting rarely persists after adequate rehydration.

Most fluid loss in cholera occurs during the first 24 to 48 h of the illness. The loss of body fluids results in diminished skin turgor, sunken eyes, depressed fontanelle (in infants), dry mucous membranes, cold extremities, thready pulse, and orthostatic hypotension. The magnitude of fluid loss—that is, the severity of dehydration—can be clinically assessed and categorized as no dehydration (<5% deficit), some dehydration (5 to 10% deficit), and severe dehydration (>10% deficit). In severe cases, when adequate fluid replacement is given, the total weight of the diarrheal stool may exceed the body weight of the patient. Diarrhea tends to decline after 24 to 48 h and usually terminates within 1 to 5 days without leaving significant residual effects. Clinical complications are infrequently seen if fluid and electrolyte losses are efficiently replaced. However, without adequate rehydration, fatal complications may arise, including, (1) hypovolemic shock, (2) metabolic acidosis, and (3) hypokalemia. In rare instances, pulmonary edema occurs when severely acidotic patients are treated with

TABLE 1. **Electrolyte Composition of Stool of Cholera Patients and Different Rehydration Solutions**

Substance	Electrolyte Concentrations (mmol/L)				
	Sodium	*Potassium*	*Chloride*	*Bicarbonate*	*Glucose*
Cholera stool	80.0	21.0	68.0	45.7	2–5
Oral rehydration solution (WHO)	90.0	20.0	80.0	30.0	111
Normal saline	154.0	0.0	154.0	0.0	0.0
Half-strength Darrow's solution	61.0	17.5	52.0	26.0	150.0
Dacca solution	133.0	13.0	98.0	48.0	0.0

Abbreviation: WHO = World Health Organization.

normal saline containing no base. Paralytic ileus may occur as a consequence of hypokalemia. In the late stages of pregnancy, there is a risk of fetal death from acidosis and hypoxia.

LABORATORY DIAGNOSIS

In the laboratory *Vibrios* organisms can be grown on MacConkey's agar plates. A combination of thiosulfate, citrate, bile salt, and sucrose (TCBS) agar and tellurite, taurocholate, gelatin agar (TTGA) is considered very useful. The TCBS agar is a highly selective media for *Vibrio* species, with the exception of *V. hollisae*. TTGA is less selective than TCBS agar, and most *Vibrios* organisms are able to degrade gelatin in this medium, forming a turbid zone around the colony. Enrichment of media is not required for isolation of *V. cholerae* from fresh diarrheal stool, but it is useful for isolating the organisms from asymptomatic carriers. Alkaline peptone water (pH, 9.0) with 1% sodium chloride and alkaline tellurite–bile salt broth of Monsur are good selective enrichment media for isolation of *V. cholerae* O1. Stool specimens should be collected from patients as early as possible, preferably with cotton swabs treated with calcium alginate. If a delay in plating is anticipated, the swab should be placed in Cary-Blair transport medium, avoiding refrigeration.

TREATMENT

Oral Rehydration Solution (ORS)

The fundamental principle in treating watery diarrhea, including that of cholera, is to correct dehydration and to replace further losses by using ORS or intravenous infusions. Rapid intravenous infusions containing an appropriate amount of salts can be lifesaving in severely dehydrated patients. In less severe cases, rehydration can be achieved by drinking ORS that contains glucose and electrolytes. The electrolyte composition of ORS is based on the average electrolyte composition of the diarrheal stool (see Table 1), which may vary widely according to the severity of diarrhea and the age of the patient. The ORS recommended by the United Nations International Children's Emergency Fund (UNICEF) and the World Health Organization has the following composition: sodium, 90 mmol per liter; chloride, 80 mmol per liter; bicarbonate, 30 mmol per liter; potassium, 20 mmol per liter; and glucose, 111 mmol per liter. This solution is clinically useful and safe in the treatment of dehydration regardless of its etiology and age of the patients. ORS containing sucrose instead of glucose is also useful. An alternative source of glucose in ORS is the high carbohydrate-containing cereals, such as rice, which can provide more sodium-cotransporting substrate to the intestine without increasing luminal osmolality. In Bangladesh, rice-based ORS has been used with success and was superior to glucose-based ORS (WHO-ORS) in reducing stool losses in patients with cholera and *Escherichia coli*–induced diarrhea. A low-osmolality (249 mOsm) ORS containing reduced amounts of glucose (89 mmol) and sodium (67 mmol) has been shown to be clinically useful in children with cholera, although

there were some instances of asymptomatic hyponatremia.

Nevertheless, there are still certain limitations in using ORS. Initial concerns about the risk of hypernatremia in infants receiving ORS containing 90 mmol per liter of sodium has not been a significant clinical problem when mother's milk and free water are provided to infants. In addition to ORS, the importance of nutritional support during diarrhea has been increasingly emphasized. It has also been shown that, contrary to a belief common in many communities, food should not be withheld during diarrheal illness. Liberal feeding along with rehydration therapy has been shown to promote weight gain and positive nitrogen balance in children with diarrhea.

Antimicrobial Treatment

When used as an adjunct to fluid therapy in cholera patients, an appropriate antimicrobial agent can reduce the volume of stool and the duration of diarrhea and can shorten the period of fecal excretion of vibrios. *V. cholerae* organisms are sensitive (in vitro) to several antimicrobial agents, including tetracycline, chloramphenicol, trimethoprim, streptomycin, erythromycin, and quinolones. Table 2 lists effective antibiotics. Tetracycline is among the most commonly used antibiotics. *V. cholerae* are rapidly killed in the intestine by the antibiotic, and fecal cultures are usually bacteriologically negative after 24 hours. Erythromycin is useful for the treating of children and pregnant women if the infecting *V. cholerae* organisms are erythromycin-sensitive. The widespread use of antibiotics has led to the emergence of plasmid-mediated drug resistance in *V. cholerae*. Resistance to tetracycline and other antibiotics has been reported and is clinically important in specific regions. Quinolones, including ciprofloxacin, are useful in the treatment of resistant organisms. Single-dose antimicrobial regimens are advantageous in epidemic situations and disaster conditions.

EPIDEMIOLOGY AND CONTROL

Cholera is a disease of great epidemic potential. Humans are the only natural host of *V. cholerae* O1 and O139, and the disease is less common in adults than in children, probably because of lack of immunity in children. The seasonal incidence of cholera varies in different parts of the world and correlates more with poverty, poor sanitation, and overcrowding than with any particular climatic condition. Fecally contaminated water is the principal vehicle of transmission of cholera, although seafood, including shellfish, oysters, and shrimp, have been implicated in many outbreaks. The El Tor biotype has stronger epidemiologic potential than does the classical strain; however, both can survive in an aquatic environment in association with vegetation in the endemic areas. The association of cholera with *Helicobacter pylori* infection, particularly in malnourished children, has

TABLE 2. **Antimicrobial Agents in the Treatment of Cholera**

| Drug | Recommended Dosages | | Remarks |
	Adult	Children	
Tetracycline	500 mg qid for 3 days	12.5 mg/kg qid for 3 days	Tetracycline-resistant *Vibrio cholerae* has been reported. Tetracycline not recommended in children younger than 8 years of age.
Erythromycin	500 mg qid for 3 days	12.5 mg/kg qid for 3 days	Safe for use in pregnant women and children.
Doxycycline (Vibramycin)	100 mg bid for 3 days or 300-mg single dose		Recommended for patients with urinary suppression and shock.
Furazolidone (Furoxone)	100 mg qid for 3 days	5–7 mg/kg qid for 3 days	Safe for children and pregnant women
Ciprofloxacin (Cipro)	500 mg bid for 3 days or 1.0 gm single dose	Not recommended	Effective against *V. cholerae* O139. Resistance is rare.
TMP-SMX (trimethoprim-sulfamethoxazole) (Septra, Bactrim)	TMP, 160 mg, + SMX, 800 mg, bid for 3 days	TMP, 5 mg/kg, + SMX, 25 mg/kg, bid for 3 days	Also recommended for children.

also been suggested. In previously nonendemic areas such as the Latin America, cholera appeared, for the first time in the 20th century, in 1991, spreading fast from Peru to neighboring countries, affecting 640,000 persons and causing 5600 deaths. In the same wave of the epidemic, cholera entered the United States in association with the travelers who visited the Latin American countries. Sporadic cases of cholera, mostly caused by the O1 El Tor biotype and Inaba serotype, are commonly reported from the Gulf Coast reservoir and along the Louisiana Coast in the United States, which suggests that *V. cholerae* O1 strains persist as free-living organisms in these waters. The African continent had been free from cholera for many years; however, in 1994, severe cholera broke out among Rwandan refugees in Goma, Zaire, killing more than 20,000 people within a few weeks. This epidemic highlighted the global epidemic potential of cholera and the need for control and proper case management.

For controlling fecal-oral transmission of cholera, especially during an epidemic, several public health measures can be undertaken, including safe disposal of human excreta, adequate supply of safe drinking water, prevention of fecal contamination of food, and maintenance of good personal hygiene. For immunoprophylaxis, several types of vaccines, including whole cell, toxoid, and B-subunit (parenteral and oral), against cholera have been tested, but none have provided long-term protection. Newer vaccines are under development.

V. CHOLERAE O139

Beginning in 1992, a new strain of *V. cholerae* non O1, designated *V. cholerae* O139 (syn. Bengal), has been a cause of several cholera outbreaks in India, Bangladesh, and neighboring countries. This new strain is almost identical to, and probably represents a minor genetic variant of, *V. cholerae* O1 El Tor, possessing a different capsular antigen. Both strains O1 and O139 have similar characteristics with regard to clinical disease, antibiotic susceptibility (although tetracycline resistance in O139 is rare), and epidemic potential.

FOOD-BORNE ILLNESS

method of
CHARLES S. LEVY, M.D.
Washington Hospital Center and
   George Washington University Medical Center
Washington, D.C.

There are millions of cases of food-borne illness each year, and most cases go unreported. A number of microorganisms, microbial toxins, and chemicals are responsible. Food-borne illness is a result of toxin-mediated syndromes caused by the ingestion of microbial and chemical toxins and of enteric infection caused by ingestion of pathogenic microorganisms.

Clinical manifestations (Table 1) include gastrointestinal symptoms such as nausea, vomiting, abdominal pain, and diarrhea; neurologic symptoms from paresthesias to paralysis; and systemic symptoms of fever, chills, and rigor. A food-borne disease should be considered when an acute illness with gastrointestinal or neurologic manifestations affects two or more persons who have shared a common food within 72 hours. Although there are many causes of food poisoning, four organisms—*Salmonella*, *Shigella*, *Staphylococcus aureus*, and *Clostridium perfringens*—represent 90% of documented cases of food poisoning.

Symptoms, travel history, the season of the year, dietary history, the type of food and its preparation, incubation period, and similar symptoms in family members or other companions can provide clues to the etiologic agent. The local health department may be helpful. A helpful resource link is the Centers for Disease Control and Prevention's Food-borne Diseases Active Surveillance Network (Foodnet). This

TABLE 1. **Characteristics of Food-borne Disease**

Organism	Incubation	Symptoms	Foods	Season	Duration	Stool White Blood Cells	Geographic Area	Secondary Cases
Nausea and Vomiting								
Staphylococcus aureus	1–6 h	Nausea, vomiting, diarrhea	Ham, poultry, egg salad, cream-filled pastry	Summer	<24 h	−		
Bacillus cereus (emetic)	1–6 h	Nausea, vomiting	Fried rice	Year-round	<12 h	−		
Noninflammatory Diarrhea								
Clostridium perfringens	8–24 h	Abdominal cramps, diarrhea	Beef, poultry, gravy, Mexican food	Fall, winter, spring	<24 h	−		
B. cereus (diarrhea)	8–24 h	Abdominal cramps, watery diarrhea	Vanilla sauce, beef, pork, chicken	Year-round	<24 h	−		
Vibrio cholerae	6–120 h	Watery diarrhea	Shellfish		3–5 d	−	Gulf Coast, South America	
Norwalk virus	12–48 h	Abdominal cramps, nausea, vomiting, diarrhea, fever, headache	Shellfish, salads, ice	Year-round	24–48 h	−	Northeast	Yes
Enterotoxigenic *Escherichia coli* (ETEC)	<48 h	Watery diarrhea	Travel	Summer	5–7 d	−	Underdeveloped world	
Inflammatory Diarrhea								
Vibrio parahemolyticus	16–96 h	Watery diarrhea, vomiting	Shellfish	Spring, summer, fall	24–48 h	−/+	Coastal states	
Shigella	12–72 h	Fever, abdominal cramps, bloody diarrhea	Eggs, lettuce, salads	Summer	3–5 d	+		Yes
Nontyphoidal *Salmonella*	12–72 h	Diarrhea, abdominal cramps, fever, nausea	Chitterlings, beef, eggs, poultry, dairy products	Summer	3–5 d	+		Yes
Campylobacter	24–170 h	Headache, malaise, fever, diarrhea	Raw milk, poultry, beef	Spring, summer, fall	5–7 d	+		Yes
Yersinia enterocolitica	10–144 h	Fever, abdominal pain, diarrhea, vomiting	Pork, tofu, chocolate milk	Winter	1–30 d	+	Europe	Yes
Enterohemorrhagic *E. coli* (EHEC) *E. coli* O157:H7	48–120 h	Bloody diarrhea, hemolytic-uremic syndrome	Beef, cider, deer meat, dairy products, alfalfa sprouts		5 d?	+		Yes
Neurologic Symptoms								
Clostridium botulinum	12–80 h	Nausea, diarrhea, vomiting, paralysis	Vegetables, fish, fruits, baked potato	Summer, fall	Weeks–months	−	West, Northwest	
Systemic Symptoms								
Listeria monocytogenes	11–70 d	Fever, diarrhea, sepsis, meningitis fetal death	Milk, cheese, shellfish, vegetables, hot dogs			−		

network monitors the regional and seasonal differences in the incidence of certain bacterial and parasitic diseases. This resource is available with a computer at http://www.cdc.gov/ncidod/dbmd/foodnet/foodnt97.htm.

Most food poisoning syndromes are self-limited. Thus, the most important treatment for individuals with food-borne illness is supportive therapy. Adequate hydration needs to be maintained. Mild dehydration is indicated by thirst, dry mouth, and decreased urine output. Moderate dehydration can be assessed by monitoring vital signs, heart rate, and blood pressure in several positions and to demonstrate orthostatic changes. Fluid and electrolytes should be given to restore intravascular volume. Rehydration can be either oral or parenteral. Oral hydration therapy is a simple approach to mild dehydration. The World Health Organization–recommended replacement is 3.5 grams NaCl, 1.5 grams of KCl, 2.5 grams of NaHCO$_3$, and 20 grams of glucose in 1 liter of boiled water. Rehydralyte and Pedialyte, which have slightly lower sodium concentration, are useful for infants and remain a convenient available option. Hypotension, tachycardia, and, ultimately, confusion and shock suggest severe dehydration. For patients with severe dehydration, altered mental status, or uncontrolled vomiting, hospitalization and parenteral rehydration are essential.

In patients with mushroom poisoning, gastric emptying, administration of active charcoal, and cathartics are useful. An effective emetic is ipecac, 30 mg orally. In patients with botulism and ciguatera in which vomiting has not occurred, the remaining food should be removed from the gut.

Phenothiazine antiemetics may be useful for persistent nausea and vomiting. Oral, intramuscular, or rectal promethazine (Phenergan), 12.5 to 25 mg every 4 to 6 hours, or prochlorperazine (Compazine), 5 to 10 mg orally or intramuscularly or a 25-mg rectal suppository, may be used in adults.

The role of antidiarrheal agents is controversial. In patients with food-borne illness, diarrhea is brief and may aid in removing toxin and pathogenic microorganisms. The agents reduce peristalsis and are contraindicated in patients with fever and fecal leukocytes, suggesting *Campylobacter, Salmonella,* or *Shigella.* Patients with moderate diarrhea may be treated with agents such as loperamide (Imodium), 4 mg followed by 2 mg after each stool to a maximal daily dose of 16 mg per day; diphenoxylate hydrochloride with atropine (Lomotil), 5 mg every 6 hours; or paregoric, 4 mL every 2 hours. Bismuth subsalicylate (Pepto-Bismol), 2 tablespoons or 2 tablets every 30 to 60 minutes, not to exceed eight doses, has been used in patients with travelers' diarrhea.

CLASSIFICATION BY PREDOMINANT SYMPTOM

One useful way to classify food-borne illness is according to presenting symptoms: nausea and vomiting, noninflammatory diarrhea, inflammatory diarrhea, neurologic symptoms, and systemic symptoms.

Nausea and Vomiting

S. aureus, Bacillus cereus, and heavy metal poisoning can produce syndromes characterized by nausea and vomiting within hours of eating contaminated food. Diarrhea and absence of fever are common. A high attack rate is frequently seen. These individuals require only supportive care because the syndrome is shortlived. Most individuals do not seek medical attention.

Nausea, vomiting, and diarrhea within 1 to 6 hours of ingestion of a preformed toxin suggest enterotoxigenic *S. aureus.* Whereas vomiting and diarrhea are common, fever and other systemic symptoms are not present. The etiology is contamination of food by an infected or colonized food handler followed by improper storage of food at room temperature. High protein, salt, and sugar concentrations favor the growth of *S. aureus.* Dairy products, meats, salads, and cream-filled pastries are often implicated as vehicles of infection. Foods contaminated with enterotoxigenic staphylococci taste and smell normal. It is necessary to demonstrate a similar phage type in *S. aureus* from a food handler to make a firm diagnosis because *S. aureus* can be normal flora of healthy individuals. Quantitative culture of *S. aureus* at 10^5 colonies per gram of food strongly suggests this syndrome.

B. cereus can produce an emetic illness with a short incubation period, the result of a preformed toxin usually associated with fried rice. The vomiting of *B. cereus* food poisoning can resemble that of *S. aureus. B. cereus* less commonly can produce watery diarrhea with abdominal pain and nausea with a longer incubation period of 8 to 16 hours. The diarrheal syndrome is associated with a variety of unrefrigerated foods. Isolation of the organism from food in high concentration would be diagnostic, but stool examination is not usually helpful.

Gastric irritation by heavy metals such as copper, zinc, tin, and cadmium causes rapid onset of cramps, nausea, and vomiting. This is a result of defective vending machines that allow acidic beverages to leach metal from corroded tubing. Metal containers with acidic drinks such as citric juices can be associated with this syndrome.

Noninflammatory Diarrhea

Noninflammatory diarrhea is a syndrome of watery diarrhea and abdominal pain with little invasion of intestinal mucosa. Vomiting may occur. The most likely agents are Norwalk agent, *C. perfringens, Vibrio cholerae,* enterotoxigenic *Escherichia coli* (ETEC), *Cryptosporidium,* and *Cyclospora.* Infected individuals require supportive care. Antibiotics may be useful for *Vibrio,* ETEC, and *Cyclospora.*

Food-borne transmission of Norwalk agent and related small, round structural viruses is common.

Whereas abdominal cramps and diarrhea may suggest a bacterial etiology, vomiting and headache are prominent features of Norwalk agent infection and occur in a majority of cases. The occurrence of secondary cases in close contacts not exposed to the suspected food is also suggestive of Norwalk agent infection.

C. perfringens food poisoning is characterized by watery diarrhea and severe, crampy abdominal pain without vomiting 10 to 20 hours after ingestion. Fever is not usually present. The vehicle is almost exclusively meat or poultry. A diagnosis can be made by demonstrating *C. perfringens* in the food. The organism can be found in the stools of ill individuals.

V. cholerae is the classic secretory or noninvasive gastroenteritis. The infection can be the result of eating contaminated shellfish from Louisiana or travel to or food from an endemic area. Whereas massive oral rehydration is the mainstay of therapy, antibiotics can also be of benefit. Tetracycline, trimethoprim-sulfamethoxazole (Bactrim, Septra), or a quinolone will decrease the symptoms, stool volume, and duration of excretion of organisms. The organism cannot be grown on routine stool culture and requires thiosulfate-citrate-bile salts-sucrose (TCBS) agar.

ETEC is the most common cause of diarrhea in travelers to the Third World. Analogous to *V. cholerae*, ETEC causes a watery diarrhea that may require hydration. Symptoms are shortened by antibiotic therapy with a quinolone such as ciprofloxacin (Cipro), 500 mg twice a day; trimethoprim-sulfamethoxazole (Bactrim, Septra); or doxycycline (Vibramycin), 100 mg twice a day.

Cryptosporidium enteritis is marked with watery diarrhea accompanied by crampy, abdominal pain, weight loss, and flatulence. The incubation period is 2 to 14 days. Whereas in immunocompromised individuals the onset is insidious, in healthy persons, symptoms may be explosive and last 2 weeks with continued shedding of oocysts for several weeks. There is no effective therapy.

A new parasite, *Cyclospora,* has been associated with watery diarrhea in the spring and summer. Lettuce, raspberries from Guatemala, and basil have been associated with the outbreaks in this country. The incubation period is 1 week. Symptoms can be protracted with nonbloody diarrhea, which may remit and relapse, abdominal pain, nausea, and weight loss. If untreated, symptoms can continue for several weeks. *Cyclospora* can be seen in stool. Modified acid-fast stain facilitates the detection of the organisms. Trimethoprim-sulfamethoxazole (Bactrim, Septra), one double-strength twice daily for 7 days in healthy individuals, is associated with resolution of symptoms and eradication of parasites from stool.

Inflammatory Diarrhea

Salmonella, Shigella, Campylobacter, Yersinia enterocolitica, and enterohemorrhagic *E. coli* O157:H7 (EHEC) can cause inflammatory diarrhea. Fever, abdominal pain, and stool with blood and fecal leukocytes are the hallmark of this syndrome. These patients may benefit from antibiotic therapy (Table 2). Antimotility drugs may be contraindicated. Stool culture should identify the etiology, but special media will be necessary to grow *Vibrio, Campylobacter,* and EHEC.

Nontyphoidal *Salmonella* is the most common cause of food-borne enteric infection in the United States. Poultry, eggs, and dairy products are foods most associated with *Salmonella* in a healthy individual. Antibiotics are not indicated for *Salmonella* gastroenteritis. These agents are associated with prolonged carriage of the organism and do not shorten symptoms. In bacteremic patients or patients at risk

TABLE 2. **Antibiotics for Food-borne Illness**

Pathogen	Drug	Adult Dose
*Shigella**	Ciprofloxacin (Cipro)	500 mg PO bid × 3–5 d
	Trimethoprim/sulfamethoxazole (TMP-SMX) (Bactrim, Septra)	1 double strength (DS) tablet PO bid
Nontyphoid *Salmonella†*	Ciprofloxacin	400 mg IV q 12 h/500 mg PO bid
	Ceftriaxone (Rocephin)	1 gm IV q 12 h
Campylobacter	Ciprofloxacin	500 mg PO bid × 5–7 d
	Erythromycin	250–500 mg PO qid × 5–7 d
Enterotoxigenic *Escherichia coli*	Ciprofloxacin	500 mg PO bid × 5 d
	TMP-SMX	1 DS tablet PO bid × 3–5 d
	Doxycycline (Vibramycin)	100 mg PO bid
Vibrio cholerae	Tetracycline	500 mg qid × 3 d
	TMP-SMX	1 DS tablet PO bid × 3 d
Yersinia	Ceftriaxone	1 gm/d IV
	Ciprofloxacin	500 mg PO bid × 5 d
Listeria monocytogenes	Ampicillin	2 gm IV q 4–6 h
	TMP-SMX	20 mg/kg/d (of trimethoprim) in four divided doses

*Check sensitivities.
†Antibiotic therapy may prolong shedding. See text for indications.

for the complications of *Salmonella* (patients with hemoglobinopathy, human immunodeficiency virus infection, lymphoproliferative disorders, prosthetic valves and joints, transplant recipients, and those receiving immunosuppression), effective therapies are parenteral ceftriaxone (Rocephin), 1 gram every 12 hours; trimethoprim-sulfamethoxazole (Bactrim, Septra); and ciprofloxacin (Cipro), 500 mg twice a day.

Vibrio parahaemolyticus is the most common cause of food poisoning in Japan. It manifests as explosive watery diarrhea. Although the diarrhea is not as profuse with *V. cholerae*, it can have invasive features mimicking nontyphoid *Salmonella*. Antibiotics do not affect the outcome. Infection is a result of raw or inadequately cooked contaminated seafood, frequently found in coastal waters. As with *V. cholerae*, the organism requires TCBS agar for isolation.

Shigella is a common cause of food-borne disease in the United States and is most common in the summer and fall. Closely associated with cool, moist foods, it is highly contagious because of the small number of organisms necessary to cause disease. Antibiotic therapy is indicated because it decreases the number of organisms in fecal specimens, therefore lowering the infectivity. Antibiotics also decrease the duration of disease. Trimethoprim-sulfamethoxazole (Bactrim, Septra) and quinolones are effective therapy. Certain enteroinvasive *E. coli* organisms produce a similar syndrome. *Shigella* is also associated with the development of reactive arthritis.

Campylobacter is associated with milk and poultry contamination and is more common in the summer and autumn. Erythromycin, 500 mg every 6 hours, and ciprofloxacin (Cipro), 500 mg twice daily, are active against the organism. The use of antibiotics is limited to patients with early or severe symptoms and immunocompromise. The organism cannot be grown on routine stool culture and requires selective culture media (Campy-Bap). *Campylobacter* is associated with the development of Guillain-Barré syndrome.

Yersinia enterocolitica, common in Europe, is rare in the United States. Associated with dairy products and meat, it is common in the winter and more common in children. The clinical picture of mesenteric adenitis can mimic appendicitis. *Yersinia* has been associated with reactive arthritis.

Enterohemorrhagic *E. coli* (EHEC), *E. coli* O157:H7, causes a bloody diarrhea 3 to 5 days after ingestion of food such as undercooked hamburger or unpasteurized cider. Hemolytic-uremic syndrome is a potential complication with acute renal failure, microangiopathic hemolytic anemia, and thrombocytopenia. Unfortunately, the efficacy of antibiotics in preventing hemolytic-uremic syndrome is not clear. To isolate the organisms, stool should be plated on sorbitol-MacConkey medium and sorbitol-negative *E. coli* should be serotyped.

Neurologic Syndromes

Neurologic syndromes are a result of neurotoxins that accumulate in food. This includes monosodium glutamate (MSG) poisoning, botulism, mushroom poisoning, and seafood poisoning syndromes.

MSG ingestion may cause nausea, flushing, and a burning skin sensation. It is commonly used in Chinese food, with won ton soup containing large quantities, hence the name "Chinese restaurant syndrome." Symptoms occur and resolve within 4 hours.

Botulism, a rare illness caused by *Clostridium botulinum,* produces symmetrical descending paralysis from improperly canned foods. Infants have developed botulism from honey contaminated with *C. botulinum* spores. Early symptoms include blurred vision, photophobia, dry mouth, dysphagia, nausea, and vomiting. Subsequent symptoms include constipation, postural hypotension, and possible paralysis requiring respiratory support. Removal of unabsorbed toxin by cathartics and emetics may be helpful. Trivalent equine antitoxin can be obtained from the Centers for Disease Control and Prevention (phone: 404-639-2206). Whereas antitoxin prevents further paralysis, it does not reverse established symptoms. Antitoxin is associated with hypersensitivity reactions in 10% of patients.

Mushroom poisoning can manifest in several different syndromes (Table 3). Most of these syndromes produce nausea, vomiting, and abdominal pain ac-

TABLE 3. **Mushroom Syndromes**

Syndrome (Toxin)	Incubation	Symptoms	Mushrooms
Anticholinergic syndrome (muscarine)	30 min–2 h	Sweating, salivation, lacrimation, bradycardia, hypotension	*Inocybe* species *Clitocybe* species
Delirium (ibotenic acid, muscimol isoxazole)	20–90 min	Dizziness, ataxia, incoordination, hyperactivity	*Amanita* species
Hallucination (psilocin, psilocybin)	30–60 min	Mood elevation, hallucination	*Psilocybe* species *Panaeolus* species
Disulfiram-like (coprine)	30 min after alcohol	Headache, nausea, vomiting	*Coprinus* species
Hepatic failure (gyromitrin)	2–12 h	Nausea, vomiting, hemolysis, hepatic failure, seizures	*Gyromitra* species
Hepatorenal (amatoxins and phallotoxins)	6–24 h	Abdominal pain, vomiting, diarrhea, renal and hepatic failure	*Amanita phalloides*
Nephritis (orellanine)	3–5 d	Thirst, nausea, headache, abdominal pain, renal failure	*Corinarius* species

companied by neurologic symptoms. In all mushroom poisoning, gastric emptying and activated charcoal may be administered to aid in removal of toxin. Cathartics such as magnesium citrate or sodium sulfate speed transit through the gut. Atropine is the treatment for muscarine-containing mushrooms that produce an anticholinergic syndrome of sweating, salivation, lacrimation, and bradycardia. *Amanita* species cause confusion, restlessness, and dizziness. Ataxia, stupor, and convulsions are seen in severe cases. Physostigmine (Antilirium), 0.5 to 1.0 mg intramuscularly or intravenously, can be used in serious cases. Mood elevation, hallucination, and hyperkinetic activity seen with *Psilocybe* and *Panaeolus* species can be treated with benzodiazepines. *Coprinus* species associated with a disulfiram (Antabuse)-like effect requires only avoiding alcohol. *Gyromitra* species causes nausea and vomiting followed by hemolysis with methemoglobinemia and hepatic failure. Methylene blue 1% solution, 0.1 to 0.2 mL per kg over 5 minutes, can be given for symptomatic methemoglobinemia with central cyanosis. Convulsions may be treated with intravenous pyridoxine, 25 mg per kg. Amatoxins and phallotoxins produce vomiting and diarrhea followed by renal and hepatic failure several days later. Thioctic acid is a partial antidote. Hemoperfusion may be useful.

All seafood syndromes are a result of toxins produced in microorganisms and acquired by eating contaminated fish and shellfish. In fish, the toxin is a result of the fish food chain or spoiled fish. In shellfish, the toxins accumulate because shellfish are filter feeders and accumulate local toxin, bacteria, or virus. The toxins, which are not destroyed by cooking, do not affect the shellfish. Whereas seafood outbreaks can be related to red tides, seafood can be safe in the presence of red tide and contaminated in its absence. Seafood-related syndromes are reviewed in Table 4.

Ciguatera is marked by gastrointestinal symptoms of nausea, vomiting, and diarrhea followed by neurologic symptoms, (paresthesias, blurred vision, photophobia, hot-cold temperature reversal), which may progress to coma and respiratory failure. Ciguatoxin, an odorless, tasteless, colorless toxin, is produced by the *Gambierdiscus toxicus*. This toxin is propagated through the aquatic food chain and found in grouper, red snapper, amberjack, and barracuda. The syndrome is limited to fish within 30 degrees of the equator and is the most common cause of fish poisoning in the tropics. The toxin is not altered by heat or cold and is stable over weeks. Although most patients improve over several weeks, occasional individuals have neurologic symptoms for months. It is important to remove toxin from the patient by emetics or gastric lavage within 4 hours of ingestion. Cathartics and enemas may also be helpful. Bradycardia may be treated with atropine. Intravenous infusion of mannitol (1 gram per kg of 20% solution given over 45 minutes) may affect neurologic symptoms.

Scombroid occurs throughout the world and is the most common cause of toxicity related to ingestion of fish. Scombroid takes its name from Scombroidea, which includes tuna, mackerel, and skipjack, fish initially implicated in this disorder. Scombroid is a histamine-like reaction resulting from eating spoiled fish. Decarboxylation by marine bacteria of histidine produces scombrotoxicosis. Symptoms include flushing, tingling, and burning headache, abdominal cramps, nausea, and diarrhea. Severe disease can produce tongue swelling, hypotension, and bronchospasm. Patients may report a peppery taste from the affected fish. The syndrome is self-limited. Antihistamines such as diphenhydramine (Benadryl) are useful. H_2 blockers, such as cimetidine (Tagamet), may shorten the course of symptoms.

Puffer fish poisoning, a result of tetrodotoxin intoxication, produces weakness, paresthesias, and abdominal pain. Primarily seen in Japan, it is caused by improperly prepared puffer fish. Tetrodotoxin is one of the most potent nonprotein poisons in nature; it has no antidote and a 60% mortality. The treatment is supportive.

There are three types of shellfish poisoning: paralytic shellfish poisoning (PSP), neurotoxic shellfish poisoning (NSP), and amnesic shellfish poisoning. PSP is caused by saxitoxin produced by toxigenic dinoflagellates. Ingestion of mussels, clams, oysters, and scallops contaminated by saxitoxin leads to symptoms of nausea, vomiting, and paresthesias and those that are subsequential, such as ataxia, dysphagia, mental status changes, and paralysis. The toxin is heat stable and not affected by cooking. NSP is a result of shellfish from the Gulf of Mexico and the Atlantic coast of Florida. It is sometimes called brevetoxic shellfish poisoning. Symptoms are similar but less severe than those of PCP. Amnesic shellfish poisoning has been reported from the Atlantic coast of Canada. The etiology is domoic acid, which produces nausea, vomiting, diarrhea, headache, and loss of short-term memory after the ingestion of mussels. The memory loss may be chronic.

Systemic Symptoms

Nongastrointestinal, non-neurologic systemic symptoms can be seen with food-borne illness. Hepatitis A, listeriosis, streptococcal pharyngitis, and eosinophilia-myalgia syndrome are examples.

Hepatitis A is discussed in another chapter.

Listeria monocytogenes is an interesting cause of food-borne illness epidemics related to milk, cheese, and hot dogs. Immunosuppressed adults including pregnant women are the primary victims. Bacteremia and meningitis are common complications of listeriosis. Pregnant woman are susceptible, with transmission to the child causing premature delivery and fetal death. Because of a long incubation period, it may be difficult to pinpoint the responsible food. Parenteral ampicillin, 2 grams every 4 to 6 hours for 2 to 4 weeks, is necessary. Trimethoprim-sulfamethoxazole (Bactrim, Septra),* 20 mg per kg per day of

---

*Not FDA approved for this indication.

TABLE 4. **Seafood Syndromes**

Syndrome	Incubation	Symptoms	Foods	Season	Duration	Geography	Toxin
Ciguatera fish poisoning	1–6 h	Nausea, vomiting, diarrhea, paresthesias, hot-cold temperature reversal, respiratory paralysis	Barracuda, red snapper, grouper	Spring, summer	Days–months	Tropical Hawaii, Florida, Caribbean	Ciguatoxin
Scombroid fish poisoning	5 min–1 h	Facial flushing, headache, dizziness, nausea, cramps, numbness, tingling of the lips, diarrhea, urticaria	Tuna, mackerel, mahimahi		Hours	Hawaii, California	Scombrotoxin
Puffer fish poisoning	10 min–3 h	Weakness, paralysis, abdominal pain, respiratory paralysis	Puffer fish		Several days	Japan	Tetrodotoxin
Paralytic shellfish poisoning (PSP)	5 min–4 h	Paresthesias of the mouth and extremities, headache, cranial nerve dysfunction, muscle paralysis, respiratory paralysis	Shellfish	Summer, fall	Hours–days	West Coast, Alaska, Northeast Atlantic coast	Saxitoxin
Neurotoxic shellfish poisoning (NSP)	5 min–4 h	Paresthesias, nausea, diarrhea, vomiting	Shellfish	Spring, fall	Hours–days	Florida, Gulf Coast	Saxitoxin
Amnesic shellfish poisoning	15 min–36 h	Vomiting, cramps, diarrhea, confusion, respiratory failure, amnesia	Mussels		Indefinite	Northeast Canada	Domoic acid

trimethoprim in four divided doses, can be used in the penicillin-allergic individual.

Group A streptococcal pharyngitis usually spreads person to person and has been spread by milk and dairy products. Eggs and meat products have also been implicated as vectors.

The eosinophilia-myalgia syndrome was an illness marked with myalgia and eosinophilia related to an unknown contaminant in an L-tryptophan dietary supplement. This scleroderma-like illness was seen from 1988 to 1990.

NECROTIZING SKIN AND SOFT TISSUE INFECTIONS

method of
RICHARD F. EDLICH, M.D., Ph.D., and
BRENDON M. STILES, M.D.
University of Virginia School of Medicine
Charlottesville, Virginia

Necrotizing skin and soft tissue infections, although rare, have been associated with high morbidity and mortality rates. These dangerous infections differ from simple superficial infections in their bacteriology, clinical manifestation, coexisting systemic complications, and treatment strategies. Group A beta-hemolytic streptococcus (GABS) is the organism most often involved in necrotizing infections. It may be found alone or, more frequently, in combination with other organisms, particularly anaerobes and facultative coliform bacteria. The latter organisms may also be isolated in necrotizing infections without the presence of GABS. Clostridial species are another significant cause of tissue-damaging infections.

Necrotizing infections may involve skin and subcutaneous tissue, as well as underlying fascia or muscle. Clinical features that suggest tissue-damaging infection include severe pain out of proportion to localized inflammatory changes, rapid progression of local infection, gas in the soft tissues, and signs of systemic toxicity. Physicians must maintain a high index of suspicion for any patient exhibiting skin erythema or tissue tenderness. Risk factors for the development of necrotizing soft tissue infections include recent trauma or surgery, inadequately treated or unrecognized minor infections, insulin-dependent diabetes mellitus, peripheral vascular disease, intestinal tract abnormalities (e.g., colon cancer, diverticulitis, bowel infarction, volvulus), alcoholism, and intravenous (IV) drug abuse. More aggressive infections have become prevalent in humans who had previously been spared from such severe infections. Minor, even trivial trauma may predispose healthy young individuals to necrotizing tissue infections, particularly those of GABS origin.

Early intervention is essential for the successful treatment of necrotizing skin and soft tissue infections. A delay in diagnosis of soft tissue infections is common and may predispose to the development of streptococcal toxic shock syndrome (strepTSS), a syndrome of bacteremia, shock, acute respiratory distress, and renal failure that follows GABS infection. Magnetic resonance imaging (MRI) complemented by bacterial examination by needle aspiration may aid in establishing an early diagnosis of necrotizing infection. Lifesaving treatments of these infections include immediate and aggressive surgical débridement, IV antibiotics, and hemodynamic support. Adjunctive therapies such as IV gamma globulin and hyperbaric oxygen may also be useful.

CLASSIFICATION AND CLINICAL PRESENTATION

Classification schemes are based on the anatomic structure involved, the infecting organism or organisms, and the clinical picture. Necrotizing soft tissue infections may be divided into three groups: necrotizing fasciitis, synergistic necrotizing cellulitis, and clostridial myonecrosis. It is important to recognize, however, that some infections may involve several layers of soft tissue and that many different bacteria may produce infections with a similar clinical appearance.

Necrotizing fasciitis includes two bacteriologic entities. In type I, at least one anaerobic species is isolated, in addition to a facultative aerobic species, such as streptococci (other than group A) or Enterobacteriaceae. In type II disease, also known as hemolytic streptococcal gangrene, GABS is present either alone or in combination with other species. Necrotizing fasciitis involves the subcutaneous soft tissues, particularly the superficial or deep fascia. Infected tissue is often firm and exquisitely tender. Subcutaneous gas may be present. The overlying skin is erythematous, edematous, hot, and shiny. The process progresses rapidly; skin color changes from purple to dusky blue or gray patches, with eventual skin breakdown and formation of bullae or development of cutaneous gangrene. The involved area may become numb secondary to destruction of superficial nerves in the necrotic subcutaneous tissue. Systemic toxicity is often prominent with necrotizing fasciitis. In soft tissue necrotizing infections associated with GABS, strepTSS may rapidly develop.

Synergistic necrotizing cellulitis—also known as gram-negative anaerobic cutaneous gangrene, necrotizing cutaneous myositis, or synergistic nonclostridial anaerobic myonecrosis—is a highly lethal variant of necrotizing fasciitis, characterized by involvement of underlying muscle and fascia. It is a mixed aerobic-anaerobic infection whose microbiologic features typically consist of organisms found in the gastrointestinal tract, including *Bacteroides* species, peptostreptococci, peptococci, *Escherichia coli*, and *Klebsiella* species. Muscle involvement is always present in addition to extensive necrosis of the skin, subcutaneous tissue, and fascia. Scattered areas of necrosis appear on the skin, and a foul-smelling, dishwater-like exudate may be prominent. Pain and edema are marked. Systemic toxicity may progress rapidly.

Clostridial myonecrosis is an acute process, typically developing within 1 to 2 days, and is associated with significant signs of systemic toxicity. Pain and edema are marked. The wound emits serosanguineous drainage and a foul odor. In contrast to the lack of extensive skin changes seen in simple clostridial cellulitis, myonecrosis manifests with dark blebs and bronzing of the skin, as well as areas of green-black cutaneous necrosis. Crepitus may be evident, although perhaps not as prominent as in clostridial cellulitis.

DIAGNOSIS

The patient's clinical appearance, as well as a history of predisposing conditions, should make the physician suspect necrotizing skin and soft tissue infection. The diagnosis is obvious when skin necrosis is prominent. When infection is confined to deeper tissues with sparing of the skin, clinical features, such as pain out of proportion to localized inflammatory changes, rapid progression of local infection, gas in the soft tissues, or signs of systemic toxicity are cardinal signs of necrotizing infection. Probing the edges of an open wound with a blunt instrument may permit easy dissection of the superficial fascial planes when deeper structures are involved.

In addition to a thorough history and physical examination, appropriate radiologic and bacteriologic studies allow for an early diagnosis and classification of necrotizing infections. Plain radiographs may be of some value in detecting soft tissue gas that is often present in polymicrobial or clostridial necrotizing fasciitis. However, the absence of soft tissue gas does not rule out the presence of a necrotizing soft tissue infection and may lead to a delay in operative intervention. Although there has been no published, well-controlled, clinical trial comparing the efficacies of various imaging modalities in the diagnosis of necrotizing infections, MRI is the preferred technique for detecting soft tissue infection because of its unsurpassed soft tissue contrast and sensitivity in detecting soft tissue fluid, complemented by its spatial resolution and its multiplanar capabilities. Although MRI is able to differentiate necrotizing soft-tissue infections from non-necrotizing cellulitis, its impact on morbidity and mortality has not yet been addressed.

In addition, percutaneous aspiration followed by prompt Gram's stain study and culture of the necrotic tissue may provide a rapid bacteriologic diagnosis in soft tissue infections. A needle aspiration should be performed on the advancing edge of the infection. A frozen-section biopsy may also help establish the diagnosis on the basis of histologic findings of subcutaneous necrosis, polymorphonuclear cell infiltration, and fibrinous vascular thrombosis. Other laboratory findings that may suggest necrotizing infection include leukocytosis with a left shift; anemia, possibly caused by bacterial hemolysins; and, later in the disease course, hypocalcemia as a result of extensive fat necrosis.

TREATMENT

Successful treatment of necrotizing skin and soft tissue infections is dependent on early diagnosis and immediate institution of therapy. Because these infections spread rapidly, a delay in diagnosis of 24 hours may be fatal. Initial therapy should be instituted immediately after clinical and radiologic inspection of the patient and microscopic examination of the infected tissue or drainage. Aggressive fluid resuscitation and stabilization are essential. Appropriate tetanus prophylaxis is mandatory.

Surgery remains the cornerstone of treatment. Early surgical débridement of necrotic tissue is a lifesaving intervention. An aggressive radical débridement of the involved area should be undertaken. Total removal of all necrotic tissue should be performed. It may be necessary to excise normal tissue surrounding the site of infection if the viability of the skin and its underlying tissue is in doubt. Pale muscle that does not contract after stimulation should be removed as a single muscle group whenever possible to salvage a functional extremity. If the infection has caused irreversible changes in several muscle groups, guillotine-type amputation may be necessary. After

débridement, the wound should be packed open. Dressing changes should initially be performed on a daily basis. Repeat exploration is frequently necessary to ensure the adequacy of initial débridement.

Initial antimicrobial therapy should be broad-based to cover aerobic gram-positive and gram-negative organisms and anaerobes. We recommend penicillin G, 24 million units per day IV, divided into every-4- to 6-hour doses; clindamycin (Cleocin), 900 mg IV every 8 hours; and gentamicin (Garamicin), 1 mg per kg IV every 8 hours. A more specifically targeted antibiotic regimen may be begun after initial Gram's stain smears, cultures, and sensitivities are available. Although some GABS infections may still be susceptible to penicillin, clindamycin is the treatment of choice for GABS infections because it is a potent suppressor of bacterial toxin synthesis and because the inoculum size or stage of bacterial growth does not affect its efficacy. If staphylococci are involved, nafcillin (Unipen) or vancomycin (Vancocin) should be used in place of penicillin.

Adjunctive therapies for necrotizing skin and soft tissue infections include hyperbaric oxygen (HBO) and gamma globulin. Well-controlled, randomized clinical trials demonstrating a statistically significant benefit of HBO are lacking; consequently, HBO therapy for necrotizing infections continues to be controversial. However, in hospitals where it is available, HBO therapy continues to be recognized for its potential benefit in patients with these severe life-threatening infections, particularly those of clostridial origin. If HBO is to be administered, it should be done so only after initial débridement so as not to delay this lifesaving intervention. Recommended therapy ranges from 100% oxygen at 3.0 atmospheres absolute (ATA) for 90 minutes to 2.0 ATA intermittently for 5 to 12 hours. HBO exposure at 3.0 ATA for 90 minutes three times a day during the active phase of the infection is well tolerated with few side effects.

In addition, neutralization of circulating toxin is a desirable therapeutic measure in these patients. Unfortunately, appropriate antitoxins are not available. However, successful use of IV immune globulin* (IVIG) in a dose of 0.4 g per kg per day over 4 to 5 days has been reported in the treatment of strepTSS. We believe that antibody present in commercial IV immunoglobulin preparations may serve to neutralize toxins produced by the infecting organisms.

---

*Not FDA approved for this indication.

TOXIC SHOCK SYNDROME

method of
MICHAEL A. GARDAM, M.Sc., M.D.C.M
University Health Network
Toronto, Ontario, Canada

Toxic shock syndrome (TSS) is a rapidly progressive infectious syndrome characterized by profound hypotension associated with multiple clinical and laboratory abnormalities indicative of multisystem organ failure. TSS has been traditionally associated with toxin-producing *Staphylococcus aureus* strains; however, TSS may be caused by other bacteria as well. Group A streptococci (GAS) have become a well-recognized cause of TSS, and TSS secondary to infection with group B streptococci (GBS) has been described. Regardless of the cause, the development of TSS is almost invariably associated with the production of one or more bacterial toxins that have the ability to indiscriminately stimulate the production of cytokines, resulting in a systemic inflammatory response.

EPIDEMIOLOGY

Staphylococcal TSS was first recognized in the late 1970s, although, in retrospect, cases had been reported in preceding decades. In 1980, an epidemic of TSS was recognized in young menstruating women that was epidemiologically linked to the use of highly absorbent tampons. Since the withdrawal of these products from the market, the incidence of staphylococcal TSS has dropped only moderately to 1 to 5 cases per 100,000 menstruating women per year, which suggests additional causative factors. Staphylococcal TSS has been associated with gynecologic infections, abortion, childbirth, burns, soft tissue infections, and postoperative wound infections. Staphylococcal TSS is less common in children, nonmenstruating females, and males, which indicates the importance of vaginal colonization with toxin-producing strains during menses as a major risk factor for disease.

GAS TSS usually occurs in conjunction with invasive streptococcal skin infections (most often necrotizing fasciitis or myositis), although in a sizable minority of cases, there is no evidence of skin infection and no portal of entry can be found. As with staphylococcal disease, GAS TSS often occurs in otherwise healthy young adults, but it has been reported in all age groups and in both sexes. Severe streptococcal disease, including TSS, has been recognized as a potential complication after varicella infection in children. There is epidemiologic evidence from several centers that the incidence of invasive streptococcal disease, including TSS, has been increasing over the past three decades. This increase is likely multifactorial in origin but may be partially due to the relative predominance of virulent clones in association with waning population immunity to streptococcal virulence factors. As with other streptococcal diseases, TSS-causing strains of GAS are transmissible by close contact; and hospital, nursing home, daycare, and family outbreaks of invasive disease have been reported. GBS TSS is a newly described entity that tends to occur in older persons with underlying illness, especially diabetes mellitus and malignancy.

PATHOGENESIS

Whatever the bacterial cause, the clinical manifestations of TSS appear to be directly related to the production of toxin(s) by the inciting organism in hosts who do not have protective antibodies. TSS-causing strains of *S. aureus* have been shown to produce a number of toxins, including enterotoxins B and C and toxic shock syndrome toxin 1 and/or 2 (TSST-1, 2), which act as superantigens. Superantigens are molecules that, at extremely low concentrations, have the ability to indiscriminately activate the inflammatory cascade by bypassing the usual requirement for the presence of a specific antigen-receptor complex on the T cell surface. The toxin(s) binds to monocyte and macrophage major histocompatibility complex class II receptors, and this complex is then recognized by receptors present on the cell surface of certain T helper cells, resulting in the production of cytokines such as tumor necrosis factor, interferon gamma, and interleukin-1. These cytokines, in turn, cause widespread activation of the inflammatory cascade, producing the multitude of clinical manifestations of TSS, including hypotension, multisystem organ failure, and rash.

The majority of TSS-causing strains of GAS have been shown to produce similar toxins called streptococcal pyrogenic exotoxins, which can also act as superantigens. The presence of previously formed antibodies to these toxins along with antibodies against streptococcal M proteins appear to protect against the development of TSS. Recently, TSS-causing strains of GBS have been shown to produce exotoxins that cause TSS-like symptoms when injected into rabbits.

CLINICAL MANIFESTATIONS

TSS is characterized by an initial nonspecific prodrome followed by the rapid onset of severe and progressive systemic symptoms. The prodrome phase, when present, is often characterized by the abrupt onset of fever, chills, malaise, headache, anorexia, sore throat, myalgias, and other "flulike" symptoms. It is not unusual at this stage for the patient to seek medical attention and be discharged without a specific diagnosis. It is therefore crucial that all patients presenting with such symptoms be examined for suggestive physical findings, such as the presence of a tampon or potential skin entry points and/or evidence of skin edema or erythema. Prominent initial symptoms of staphylococcal TSS may also include vomiting and diarrhea. In the case of GAS TSS, the patient may often complain of pain in an extremity or, rarely, over the torso or face, which is often far more severe than the physical examination might suggest. Examination of the painful area may be normal or may reveal mild erythema and/or swelling. In more advanced cases, a bluish discoloration associated with vesicles or bullae may be present, which suggests the development of necrotizing fasciitis.

The prodrome phase is typically followed by the rapid onset of hypotension and associated multisystem organ failure. The patient is often listless or confused, but focal neurologic signs are typically absent. A diffuse erythematous desquamative rash appearing several days after the onset of symptoms is typical of staphylococcal TSS whereas streptococcal TSS is occasionally associated with an erythematous "sunburn-like" rash that may desquamate. The physical examination must include a vaginal examination in women and a meticulous examination of the torso and extremities for abrasions, cuts, or signs of infection.

DIAGNOSIS

There are no specific confirmatory laboratory tests for the diagnosis of TSS. The clinical and laboratory diagnostic criteria for staphylococcal and streptococcal TSS are shown in Table 1. Although the criteria are similar for the two causes, there are some important differences. The isolation of the causative organism is not required for the diagnosis of staphylococcal TSS while it is central to the diagnosis of streptococcal TSS. In staphylococcal TSS, the causative bacteria are rarely invasive, unlike streptococcal disease in which the causative organism is commonly obtained from sterile sites. This explains why the elimination of other causes, which may cause similar shock syndromes,

TABLE 1. **Criteria for the Diagnosis of Staphylococcal and Streptococcal Toxic Shock Syndrome**

	Staphylococcal	Streptococcal
Major Criteria	*All of the Following:*	*All of the Following:*
Organism	Not required for diagnosis	Isolation of group A streptococci from either a sterile or a nonsterile site*
Core temperature	>38.9°C	Not required for diagnosis but elevated temperature often present
Blood pressure	<90 mm Hg	<90 mm Hg or <5th percentile for age in children
Other diagnoses	Negative results of serologic tests for Rocky Mountain spotted fever, leptospirosis, and measles	Not required for diagnosis but should be ruled out if the case history is suggestive
Skin	Rash with subsequent desquamation, especially on palms and soles	See Minor Criteria
Minor Criteria	*Plus Three or More of the Following:*	*Plus Two or More of the Following:*
Renal function	BUN† or creatinine > twice the upper limit for age with pyuria in the absence of urinary tract infection	Creatinine > twice the upper limit for age or ≥177 mmol/L (2 mg/dL) or > twofold increase in creatinine over baseline if chronic renal failure
Coagulation	Platelet count < 100 × 10⁹/L	Platelet count < 100 × 10⁹/L or evidence of disseminated intravascular coagulation‡
Hepatic function	Laboratory evidence of hepatitis§	Laboratory evidence of hepatitis§
Respiratory system	Adult respiratory distress syndrome often present but not required	Evidence of adult respiratory distress syndrome‖
Central nervous system	Disorientation without focal neurologic signs	Not required for diagnosis but often present
Mucous membranes	Frank hyperemia of one or more of the following: vagina, conjunctivae, or pharynx	Not required for diagnosis
Musculoskeletal system	Severe myalgias or > fivefold increase in creatine kinase	Not required for diagnosis but often present
Gastrointestinal system	Vomiting and/or profuse diarrhea	Not required for diagnosis but may be present
Skin	See Major Criteria	Generalized erythematous macular rash that may desquamate and/or evidence of necrotizing fasciitis, myositis, or gangrene

*Isolation of group A streptococci from a sterile site and ≥ two minor criteria is defined as a "definite" case. Isolation of group A streptococci from a nonsterile site and ≥ two minor criteria is defined as a "probable" case if no other cause is found.

†Blood urea nitrogen.

‡As defined by prolonged clotting times, low fibrinogen concentration, and presence of fibrin degradation products (split products).

§As defined by a twofold or greater elevation in alanine aminotransferase, aspartate aminotransferase, or total bilirubin. In patients with pre-existing liver disease, a twofold or greater elevation over baseline levels.

‖As defined by acute onset of diffuse pulmonary infiltrates and hypoxemia in the absence of cardiac failure, or evidence of diffuse capillary leak manifested by acute onset of generalized edema, or pleural or peritoneal effusions with hypoalbuminemia.

Adapted from Mandell GL, Bennett JE, Dolin R (eds): Mandell, Douglas and Bennett's Principles and Practice of Infectious Diseases, 4th ed. New York, Churchill Livingstone, 1995; and Defining the group A streptococcal toxic shock syndrome. Rationale and consensus definition. The Working Group on Severe Streptococcal Infections. JAMA *269*:390–391, 1993.

is particularly important to secure the diagnosis of staphylococcal TSS. In addition, a desquamative rash is required for the diagnosis of staphylococcal TSS. Although there are no proposed criteria for the diagnosis of TSS caused by streptococci other than GAS, it is reasonable to apply the group A criteria pending further definition of these syndromes. An elevated creatine kinase value may be particularly helpful in suggesting the diagnosis of streptococcal TSS associated with necrotizing fasciitis or myositis.

TREATMENT

The general treatment of the patient with TSS is similar to that of any patient suffering from distributive shock. The use of large volumes of crystalloid and or vasopressors is typically required. Intubation is often necessary for the management of severe hypoxemia secondary to adult respiratory distress syndrome.

The current recommended therapies for staphylococcal and streptococcal TSS are listed in Table 2. It is extremely important to perform a gynecologic examination on women presenting with TSS so that if a tampon is present, it can be removed immediately and the vaginal contents evacuated and cultured.

There is currently no recommendation for the use of antiseptic douches in the treatment of menses-related TSS. Other potential foci for TSS-producing staphylococci such as wounds should be cleansed and débrided as necessary. Antibiotic therapy should include an antistaphylococcal penicillin or a first-generation cephalosporin for 10 to 14 days. Although it is not clear that such therapy significantly alters the course of the disease, it does appear to decrease the risk of recurrence of menses-related TSS from 65% to less than 5%. Those patients with a history of significant penicillin or cephalosporin allergy should receive either vancomycin or erythromycin. There is little epidemiologic evidence to support the routine use of intravenous immune globulin (IVIG), although theoretically it may be of value by binding toxin(s) and thus inhibiting the superantigen-mediated development of the systemic inflammatory response.

The treatment of GAS TSS is typically more invasive because the majority of cases are associated with serious soft tissue infections. Those patients with evidence of either necrotizing fasciitis or myositis should be managed with urgent surgical débridement and possible amputation (see "Necrotizing Skin and

Soft Tissue Infections"). The recommended antibiotic combination for streptococcal TSS is high-dose penicillin G and clindamycin (Cleocin). Although GAS are typically exquisitely sensitive to penicillin in vitro, penicillin monotherapy is inferior to either clindamycin alone or in combination with penicillin in both animal models and in case-control studies. The reason for this discrepancy between in vitro sensitivity data and clinical outcome is likely multifactorial. Experimental evidence suggests that clindamycin inhibits toxin synthesis by interfering with protein production whereas beta-lactam antibiotics such as penicillin have no effect. Furthermore, beta-lactam antibiotics, unlike clindamycin, are less effective in circumstances in which large numbers of bacteria slow down bacterial growth, such as is the case in necrotizing fasciitis. In those patients allergic to penicillin, alternative therapies include erythromycin and ceftriaxone. Ceftriaxone (Rocephin) should be avoided in patients with a history of anaphylaxis to penicillins. It is reasonable to treat GBS TSS in a similar fashion, bearing in mind that maximum doses of antibiotics should be used because GBS are inherently more antibiotic resistant than GAS.

Close contacts of patients who have contracted invasive streptococcal infections, especially TSS or necrotizing fasciitis, should be considered for oral prophylactic therapy for 10 days with one of the following (adult doses): penicillin, 500,000 units orally four times a day; cephalexin (Keflex), 500 mg orally four times a day; or erythromycin, 250 mg orally four times a day.

There is more epidemiologic evidence that IVIG* may be a more useful adjunct in the treatment of streptococcal TSS than for staphylococcal TSS, although a randomized controlled trial has not been performed.

PROGNOSIS

The case-fatality rate for staphylococcal TSS is currently less than 5%. GAS TSS has a much higher mortality rate (30 to 70%), which appears to be positively correlated with older age and the presence of chronic illness. The mortality rate of TSS when caused by GBS is not known because this entity has only recently been described; however, it is likely to be high.

---

*Not FDA approved for this indication.

TABLE 2. **Specific Treatment of Staphylococcal and Streptococcal Toxic Shock Syndrome in Adults**

Therapy	Staphylococcal	Streptococcal
Local care	Removal of tampon if present. Incision and drainage of abscess if present	Urgent surgical débridement of affected area if necrotizing fasciitis or myositis suspected*
Antibiotic therapy	Antistaphylococcal penicillin or first-generation cephalosporin: Nafcillin (Nafcil, Unipen), 2 gm IV q4–6h or Oxacillin (Bactocill), 2 gm IV q4–6h or Cloxacillin (Cloxapen), 2 gm IV‡ q4–6h or Cefazolin (Ancef), 1 to 2 gm IV q8h† or If penicillin allergic: Vancomycin (Vancocin), 1 gm IV q12h† or Erythromycin, 1 gm IV q6h Treatment is given for 10–15 days	Penicillin G, 3 to 4 million units IV q4h† and Clindamycin (Cleocin), 600 to 900 mg IV q8h If penicillin allergic, substitute: Erythromycin, 1 gm IV q6h or Ceftriaxone (Rocephin), 2 gm IV q12h§ for penicillin G Intravenous treatment is given for at least 10 to 14 days followed by oral therapy‖
Immuno-therapy	Not usually recommended but may be given as per streptococcal disease	Intravenous immune globulin (IVIG)¶, one dose of 2 gm/kg IV; repeat dose at 48 hours if remains unstable

*See "Necrotizing Skin and Soft Tissue Infections."
†Dosage assumes normal creatinine clearance. If renal failure is present, adjust dose accordingly.
‡Not available in the United States.
§If patient is anaphylactic to penicillins, the use of ceftriaxone is not recommended.
‖The final duration of antibiotic therapy will depend on the patient's response to treatment as measured by clinical and laboratory parameters and bacterial culture results.
¶Not FDA approved for this indication.

INFLUENZA

method of
WENDY ANNE KEITEL, M.D.
*Baylor College of Medicine
Houston, Texas*

EPIDEMIOLOGY, IMPACT, AND SURVEILLANCE

Annual epidemics of influenza are responsible for excessive morbidity and mortality throughout the world. Epidemics in the United States usually occur during winter months, and may be caused by one or more types (A or B) or subtypes (A/H1N1 or A/H3N2) of influenza. The appearance of influenza in the community is associated with an upsurge in school absenteeism and visits to health care facilities for acute respiratory disease (ARD), followed by rises in industrial absenteeism, hospitalization for pneumonia and influenza, and death rates. Attack rates are highest among children, and children are primarily responsible for the spread of influenza in the community.

The impact of interpandemic influenza, caused by viruses that have relatively small changes (*drift*) in the genes for the surface proteins (hemagglutinin [HA] and neuraminidase [NA]), is considerable, taking its greatest toll among infants, the elderly, and others at high risk for complications of influenza: 20,000 to 50,000 in excess of expected deaths were reported during recent influenza epidemics in the United States. Pandemic influenza, caused by viruses that have major genetic changes (*shift*) in the HA and NA, can overwhelm a community and is responsible for excess mortality among young adults, in addition to the very young and the elderly.

Traditional measures of these effects of influenza can be used as indirect indicators that influenza is in the community. Regional, national, and international networks also conduct systematic surveillance of influenza in human populations. Surveillance data can be used to guide empirical therapy of ARD and to prepare for the appearance of new variants. The occurrence in 1997 of severe and fatal influenza A/H5N1 infections in Hong Kong was a grim reminder of the unpredictable and potentially disastrous impact of influenza, and it stimulated renewed efforts to address control of pandemic and interpandemic influenza.

CLINICAL MANIFESTATIONS AND DIAGNOSIS

The clinical manifestations of influenza are nonspecific, and definitive diagnosis cannot be made on clinical grounds alone. Nevertheless, the classical manifestations of influenza in the adult are sufficiently characteristic to permit empirical diagnosis in the appropriate epidemiologic setting. After a several-day incubation period, there is an abrupt onset of malaise, fever, chills, headache, anorexia, and myalgias. Respiratory symptoms develop simultaneously or shortly thereafter. Most frequent and characteristic among these is nonproductive cough, which may become productive at later stages of illness. Runny nose and sore throat occur in most patients; hoarseness, chest pain, and gastrointestinal (GI) symptoms each occur in a minority of cases in most series. Influenza in children may be accompanied by croup, bronchiolitis, febrile seizures, otitis media, and more frequent GI complaints than in adults. Fever, confusion, and other nonspecific symptoms may predominate in elderly patients.

Complications of influenza include secondary bacterial infections (sinusitis, otitis media, bronchitis, and pneumonia), myositis/myocarditis, and rare central nervous system (CNS) manifestations. Secondary bacterial infections develop several days to a week after the onset of illness and may appear while the symptoms of acute influenza are resolving. Although pneumococci are the most common causes of secondary infections, *Staphylococcus aureus* infections occur more frequently during influenza epidemics. Recrudescent fever and localized symptoms and signs strongly suggest the development of secondary complications. Influenza poses a high risk for certain populations (to be described), and exacerbations of underlying conditions such as asthma and chronic obstructive pulmonary disease often complicate the clinical manifestations and contribute to influenza-associated morbidity and mortality. Severe primary influenza pneumonia is a rare complication that appears to be more common during influenza pandemics and among pregnant women and other patients who have conditions that are associated with pulmonary vascular congestion during periods of interpandemic influenza.

In most patients who have typical symptoms and signs of influenza during a recognized outbreak, the clinical diagnosis of influenza can be made with a high degree of accuracy. Specific diagnosis can be attempted for the management of individual patients and for the identification of outbreaks of influenza in institutions and communities. Isolation of influenza in embryonated hens' eggs or in cell cultures remains the gold standard for the diagnosis. Appropriate specimens for virus isolation include nasal wash samples, nasopharyngeal swabs, and throat swabs; sputum, gargle specimens, and nasal swabs are alternatives. A combination of a throat swab with either nasal wash or nasopharyngeal swab in a single sample is optimal for the diagnosis of influenza. Bronchoalveolar lavage specimens may be indicated for the diagnosis of ARD in some critically ill or immunocompromised patients. Samples of respiratory secretions should be placed in appropriate viral transport media and taken to the laboratory on wet ice as soon as possible. If the sample cannot be inoculated into culture immediately, it can be stored in the refrigerator for up to several days. Detection of other respiratory viruses, however, may be adversely affected by this delay. Isolation of influenza viruses typically requires 3 to 4 days.

More recently, rapid diagnostic kits have been developed for the diagnosis of influenza. Commercially available kits make use of direct or indirect immunofluorescence or enzyme immunoassay methods to detect the presence of viral proteins in respiratory secretions. Rapid and specific diagnosis enables institution of appropriate antiviral therapy early in the illness, and use of inappropriate therapy (such as antibiotics) can be avoided. Although these tests are quite specific, they are only moderately sensitive. Sensitivity is greatest when samples are collected early during the illness and among pediatric patients.

Finally, serologic diagnosis of influenza can provide useful epidemiologic information, but it rarely provides information that is of immediate use for the management of an individual patient. A fourfold increase in antibody titer between serum samples collected at the onset of illness and 2 to 3 weeks after illness onset is considered diagnostic.

PREVENTION AND TREATMENT OF INFLUENZA

The most important tool for prevention of influenza and its complications is trivalent inactivated influenza virus vaccine (TIV). The efficacy of TIV depends on the age of the patient, the status of the patient's underlying health, and the degree of antigenic match between vaccine and epidemic viruses. Immunization of healthy younger adults with a well-matched strain results in 70 to 90% protection against influenza. Immunization of elderly persons confers a higher level of protection against complications and death than against influenza-associated illness.

Each year TIV is reformulated to contain antigens of viruses predicted to be the most likely causes of epidemic influenza during the upcoming winter. Current vaccines contain antigens of each of the three contemporary influenza viruses: influenza A/H1N1, A/H3N2, and B viruses. TIV contains either whole viruses that have been grown in eggs and inactivated with formalin (whole virus vaccines [WVV; Fluzone]) or viruses prepared in a similar manner that have undergone additional processing that results in disruption of the virus particles (split or subvirion virus vaccines [SVV; Fluogen, FluShield, and Fluzone]) or purification of the HA and NA from the virions (purified surface antigen [PSA; Fluvirin]). Although the efficacy of each of these vaccines is similar, WVV produces more febrile reactions when given to children under the age of 12 years, and SVV or PSA should be used instead.

Annual immunization with TIV is strongly recommended for persons who are at least 6 months old who are at increased risk for complications of influenza. This includes persons 65 years of age or older;

residents of nursing homes and other chronic care facilities; persons with chronic cardiac or pulmonary conditions; persons with chronic medical conditions (such as diabetes, kidney disease, hemoglobinopathy, and immunosuppression) who required regular medical care or hospitalization during the preceding year; children receiving long-term aspirin therapy who may be at risk for developing Reye's syndrome after influenza; and women who will be in the second or third trimester of pregnancy during the influenza season. Health care workers and others who are in close contact with persons in high-risk groups should be immunized to reduce the risk of spread of influenza to high-risk patients. Finally, anyone who wishes to reduce his or her risk of influenza should be offered TIV.

The dosage and administration of TIV according to age are summarized in Table 1. Influenza vaccines should be given intramuscularly. For persons younger than 9 years who are receiving influenza vaccine for the first time, 2 doses given at least 1 month apart are recommended. Protective antibody responses are maximal several weeks after immunization and decline steadily thereafter; therefore, optimal timing of immunization is mid-October through mid-November. However, earlier opportunities to immunize patients during regular medical encounters should not be missed. Pneumococcal vaccine may be given simultaneously in a different site, if indicated.

The most common side effect of immunization is tenderness at the injection site lasting a day or two. Less than 5% of patients complain of fever, malaise, or other systemic symptoms, which start on the day of immunization and resolve within 1 to 2 days. These local and systemic reactions usually necessitate no therapy, but acetaminophen can be administered, if indicated. Immediate allergic reactions are rare and are usually attributed to residual egg protein. Anaphylactic hypersensitivity to eggs or other components of the vaccine is a contraindication to immunization, although certain patients who are at very high risk of influenza complications should be considered for allergy evaluation and desensitization. Recent studies have detected a small elevation in the risk of Guillain-Barré syndrome (GBS) during the 6-week period after immunization, but the potential benefits of influenza vaccination outweigh the possible risk of vaccine-associated GBS. Nevertheless, persons with a history of vaccine-associated GBS should not be given TIV.

TABLE 1. **Dose and Administration of Trivalent Inactivated Influenza Virus Vaccine (TIV)**

Age Group	Type of Vaccine	Dose	No. of Doses
6–35 months	SVV or PSA	0.25 mL	1 or 2
3–8 years	SVV or PSA	0.50 mL	1 or 2
9–12 years	SVV or PSA	0.50 mL	1
>12 years	WVV, SVV, or PSA	0.50 mL	1

Abbreviations: PSA = purified surface antigen; SVV = split or subvirion virus vaccine; WVV = whole virus vaccine.

Two drugs are available in the United States for specific treatment of influenza A (not influenza B) virus infections: amantadine (e.g., Symmetrel) and rimantadine (Flumadine). Both drugs interfere with an early step in the replication cycle, and drug resistance is associated with mutations in the M2 protein. Treatment with these drugs significantly reduces the duration and severity of clinical influenza A among adult influenza patients. Amantadine, unlike rimantadine, is also approved for treatment of influenza A in children who are at least 1 year old. Treatment should be initiated within 48 hours of disease onset. The efficacy of amantadine is similar to that of rimantadine, although there are differences in their pharmacokinetic properties. Amantadine is excreted unchanged in the urine, whereas 75% of rimantadine is metabolized in the liver, followed by urinary excretion. The major adverse effects of treatment include CNS toxicity (insomnia, nervousness, dizziness, and difficulty concentrating) and GI side effects (nausea and anorexia). More severe but rare side effects include delirium, hallucinations, and seizures, usually in association with high plasma levels in patients who have renal insufficiency. CNS side effects are more common with amantadine therapy and are related to higher plasma concentrations.

Amantadine and rimantadine also are approved for prophylaxis against influenza A in adults and in children older than 1 year. When taken on a daily basis, each confers 70 to 90% protection against influenza. Prophylaxis should be considered in the following circumstances: for temporary use after immunization when influenza A activity has begun; for protection of persons for whom vaccine is contraindicated or who are expected not to respond to vaccine; and to control outbreaks of influenza in institutions that house high-risk persons.

Recommended dosage for treatment or prophylaxis of influenza A with amantadine and rimantadine in healthy persons who are 10 to 64 years old and who weigh at least 40 kg is 100 mg orally twice daily. Persons who are 65 years of age and older should receive up to 100 mg of amantadine per day and 100 or 200 mg of rimantadine per day. For children between 1 and 9 years of age, the dose is 5 mg per kg per day, up to a total of 150 mg, given in two divided doses. Dosage reduction may be necessary for persons with renal or hepatic insufficiency. Treatment should be discontinued as soon as clinically indicated (usually 3 to 5 days total, or 24 to 48 hours after symptoms resolve) in order to reduce the frequency of the emergence of resistant viruses. Prophylaxis should continue for the duration of exposure. Although not approved by the U.S. Food and Drug Administration for this indication, aerosolized ribavirin can be used to treat hospitalized patients with severe influenza A or B.

Additional measures for management of acute influenza include bed rest, adequate fluid intake, and antipyretics for control of fever, headache, and myalgias. Aspirin therapy should be avoided in persons under the age of 18 years, because of the risk of

Reye's syndrome. Antitussives, decongestants, and air humidification may provide additional relief from cough and nasal obstruction. Appropriate antibiotics are indicated only for treatment of suspected or proven secondary bacterial infections.

Promising new live attenuated vaccines and drugs that are effective for the treatment of both influenza A and B virus infections (neuraminidase inhibitors) may be available for use in the near future; they will enhance our ability to control influenza in individuals and in populations.

LEISHMANIASIS

method of
LUIGI GRADONI, Ph.D.
Istituto Superiore di Sanità
Rome, Italy

Leishmaniasis is not a single disease but a variety of syndromes caused by infection with protozoan parasites of the genus *Leishmania*. The flagellated forms (promastigotes) are transmitted by the bite of phlebotomine sandflies and multiply as aflagellated forms (amastigotes) within cells of the mononuclear phagocyte system. Three main clinical syndromes—visceral leishmaniasis (VL), cutaneous leishmaniasis (CL), and mucocutaneous leishmaniasis (MCL)—are widespread in tropical, subtropical, and temperate zones and often represent zoonotic infections. For some *Leishmania* species, humans are the principal or sole reservoir (anthroponotic leishmaniases). In the late 1990s, the worldwide incidence of leishmaniases was estimated to be 2 million cases, of which 1.5 million were CL/MCL and 0.5 million were VL. The current interest in leishmaniasis is probably attributable to the increasing importance of travel medicine, the inclusion of VL as a complication of human immunodeficiency virus (HIV) infection, and the opportunistic behavior of *Leishmania* organisms in organ transplant recipients.

Advances in biochemical taxonomy of *Leishmania* have made it possible to identify the parasite to the levels of species and strain and to define nosogeographic entities by which each of the 13 *Leishmania* species of medical interest is characterized by geographic distribution, clinical syndrome or syndromes provoked, vector, and host species. This information is of great medical importance because different species that infect the same tissue may display different susceptibility to a drug, or the efficacy of a drug regimen against a viscerotropic *Leishmania* organism in one region does not ensure that such a regimen will be effective against dermotropic species in the same region.

CLINICAL LEISHMANIASIS

Visceral Disease

VL (kala-azar) results from multiplication of *Leishmania* in the phagocytes of the reticuloendothelial system. Anthroponotic VL is caused by *Leishmania donovani* in India, East Africa, and the Arabic peninsula; zoonotic VL is caused by *Leishmania infantum* in Mediterranean regions and *Leishmania chagasi* in Latin America. These two species, however, are virtually identical by biochemical genotyping. In the endemic situation, there are about 30 to 100 subclinical, self-healing infections for every case of acute VL. Healing is associated with the transient appearance of specific antibodies and a positive result on the leishmanin skin test (LST). In epidemic situations, as those caused by *L. donovani* in Sudan and India, subclinical cases are less common.

Classical VL manifests as fever, hepatosplenomegaly, pancytopenia, and hypergammaglobulinemia. The clinical incubation period ranges from 3 weeks to more than 2 years, but 2 to 4 months is average. Patients report a history of fever resistant to antibiotics, which is present at the time of medical consultation. On physical examination, the spleen is typically appreciated 5 to 15 cm below the left costal margin. Symptomatic VL is commonly fatal if left untreated. Post–kala-azar dermal leishmaniasis, a dermatologic complication characterized by macules, papules, or nodules, may develop months or years after treatment of Indian or African VL.

Other clinical manifestations of VL have been described. Mild VL cases not advancing to symptomatic disease were reported among U.S. soldiers deployed to the Arabian peninsula during Operation Desert Storm. Fever and organomegaly were frequently absent, and all affected patients had normal hemoglobin concentrations. The patients complained instead of chronic fatigue, malaise, abdominal pain, and diarrhea. In southern Europe, the coexistence of HIV and *L. infantum* leishmaniasis has resulted in a large number of dually infected persons (by the end of 1998 the total number of cases was approximately 1500). Although the clinical manifestation of the disease in HIV-infected hosts is comparable with that in classic VL, the gastrointestinal tract is frequently involved, and hepatosplenomegaly may be absent.

Cutaneous Disease

CL results from multiplication of *Leishmania* organisms in the phagocytes of the skin. Anthroponotic CL is caused by *Leishmania tropica* in the Old World; zoonotic CL is caused by *Leishmania major*, *Leishmania aethiopica*, and dermotropic *L. infantum* in the Old World and by members of the *Leishmania mexicana* complex (*L. mexicana*, *Leishmania amazonensis*, and *Leishmania venezuelensis*) and the *Leishmania braziliensis* complex (*L. braziliensis*, *Leishmania peruviana*, *Leishmania panamensis*, and *Leishmania guyanensis*) in the New World. In the classical course of this disease, lesions appear first as papules, advance to ulcers or nodules, and then spontaneously heal with scarring over months to years. The incubation period ranges from 1 week to 8 months; lesions caused by some species (e.g., *L. major* and *L. mexicana*) tend to evolve and resolve quickly, whereas those caused by other species (e.g., *L. braziliensis*, *L. tropica,* and dermotropic *L. infantum*) may have longer periods of incubation and spontaneous healing.

Mucosal Disease

MCL results from parasitic metastasis in the nasal mucosa that eventually extends to the oropharynx and larynx. It may develop from CL lesions caused by members of the *L. braziliensis* complex. Characteristically, MCL does not heal spontaneously and evolves slowly (mean time, 3 years) before it is first brought to medical attention.

IMMUNOLOGIC FEATURES

Leishmaniases have typical immunologic polarity: cure is associated with the presence of cellular immune responses, whereas chronic disease is associated with the absence of such responses and the presence of high levels of specific, nonprotective antibodies. Self-healing CL is characterized by positive LST results and high values for *Leishmania* antigen–induced lymphocyte transformation in vitro. Classical VL does not heal spontaneously, and LST and in vitro lymphocyte transformation are negative in cases of acute disease but convert to positive after successful chemotherapy. In spite of this polarity, analysis of cytokine patterns reveals a less polar situation. Both the Th$_1$ and Th$_2$ cytokines are secreted in specimens of CL or MCL lesions and in bone marrow, lymph nodes, and skin of patients with acute VL. For only two cytokines, the Th$_1$ cytokine interleukin-12 (IL-12) and the Th$_2$ cytokine interleukin-10 (IL-10), can a reasonable association between clinical course of VL and cytokine levels be made.

DIAGNOSTIC METHODS

The standard diagnosis of leishmaniasis is still made by classical microbiologic methods. Samples of infected tissue are obtained, and the organisms are either seen in Giemsa-stained impression smears or cultured from tissue. In general, both staining and culture should be performed to increase sensitivity. Cultured organisms can be identified by isoenzyme electrophoresis.

For VL, aspirates or biopsy specimens of the spleen, bone marrow, the liver, or enlarged lymph nodes are examined. Sensitivity is organ dependent; higher diagnostic yields of *Leishmania* are obtained with spleen aspirates (>98%), although bone marrow aspirates (80 to 98% of yield) are usually preferred. In Indian VL, as well as in Mediterranean HIV-VL, microscopy and culture of buffy coat from peripheral blood has 64 to 75% sensitivity.

For CL, material is obtained by scraping tissue juice from a nodular lesion or from the edge of an ulcer. By this method, *Leishmania* organisms may be isolated from about 80% of sores during the first half of their natural course. After that, parasitologic diagnosis becomes more difficult. Biopsy specimens may also be used to make impression smears and cultures. Culture is more sensitive than microscopy for diagnosing MCL.

Immunologic tests are useful when the diagnosis of the disease proves difficult with standard methods, and these can be employed in decisions for or against treatment. In CL and MCL, LST results are positive in more than 90% of cases, whereas serologic results are often negative. In acute VL, LST results are negative, whereas antibodies are readily detectable by several techniques. Indirect immunofluorescence, conventional enzyme-linked immunosorbent assay (ELISA), and direct agglutination test results are positive in 97 to 100% of patients (among HIV-VL patients, however, sensitivity of these tests may be as low as 40 to 60%). Specificity is also high (90 to 95%), although cross-reactions may occur with *Trypanosoma cruzi* infections in Latin America. A new recombinant antigen used for the ELISA, rK39, is sensitive enough to identify 98 to 100% of cases of acute VL and 75 to 80% of cases of HIV-VL but not to identify subclinical VL cases or nonleishmanial infections.

The use of polymerase chain reaction (PCR) assay on peripheral blood may eliminate the need for tissue samples. In patients with VL from India, Kenya, and Brazil, PCR assay on blood samples demonstrated high sensitivity (90%) and high specificity (100%).

TREATMENT

Pentavalent Antimonials

Organic salts of pentavalent antimony (Sb) are still the mainstay of therapy for all the leishmaniases. Two preparations are available: sodium stibogluconate (Pentostam), containing 100 mg of Sb per mL, and meglumine antimoniate (Glucantime), containing 85 mg of Sb per mL.* The drugs are given intramuscularly or intravenously, and they are equal in efficacy and toxicity when used in equivalent Sb doses. As the leishmaniases became treated more extensively and studied more carefully, treatment failures with Sb became recognized. Alternatives to Sb have been found for some syndromes, and they are now used as first-line drugs in some countries.

The recommended dosage of Sb for all the leishmaniases is 20 mg per kg per day for 21 to 28 days and for 40 days in regions (e.g., in Bihar State, India) in which high rates of Sb-resistant VL have been documented. Uncomplicated CL may be treated at the same daily dose but for 10 days. With the aim of reducing the dose-related toxic effects of Sb, a lower daily dose (5 mg per kg) for 30 days was used in patients with CL caused by *L. braziliensis* and found to be effective in 84% of cases.

Clinical response to antimonials is rapid in CL cases, but complete reepithelialization of lesions is observed in only one third of patients by the end of a 3-week treatment course. In VL patients, fever recedes by day 4 to 5 of treatment, and well-being returns by the first week, whereas spleen size normalizes 1 to 2 months after the end of therapy. These observations indicate that Sb treatment should not be continued until all clinical parameters normalize. Relapses may occur after apparent clinical cure of both CL and VL from 2 to 8 months after the Sb treatment has been discontinued. In general, if the treatment schedule has been appropriate, relapses rarely occur, but in patients with both HIV and VL, the frequency of relapses approaches 100%.

Systemic toxicity caused by the antimonials normally relates to total dose administered and includes anorexia, musculoskeletal pain, minor T wave and ST segment changes on electrocardiography, and slow rise in hepatic enzyme levels. Moderate cytopenia may occur. Pancreatitis, revealed by elevation of serum levels of amylase or lipase, has been recognized as the commonest side effect of antimonial therapy, and pancreatic inflammation is probably the cause of the nausea and abdominal pain experienced by many patients. Doses in excess of 20 mg Sb per kg per day necessitate monitoring, especially for prolongation of the Q-T interval, which may precede a dangerous arrhythmia. Sudden death has been reported among Sb-treated adults, who tolerate antimonials more poorly than do children.

---

*These are available only from the Centers for Disease Control and Prevention.

Amphotericin B and Lipid-Associated Amphotericin B

The antifungal agent amphotericin B has long been recognized as a powerful leishmanicidal drug. This activity results from the specific target of amphotericin B, which is ergosterol-like sterols, the major membrane sterols of Leishmania species as well as of fungi. However, amphotericin B was traditionally administered infrequently because of its infusion-related side effects (fever, chills, and bone pain) and delayed side effects (toxic renal effects) when administered at the usual daily dose of 1 to 1.5 mg per kg. Because of the increasing resistance of VL to antimonial therapy in different areas of the world and to the availability of less toxic formulations of the drug, amphotericin B has been increasingly used for VL and constitutes the major advance in antileishmanial chemotherapy since the early 1990s.

Amphotericin B deoxycholate (Fungizone) administered at the low dosage of 0.5 mg per kg every other day for 14 days (total dose, 7 mg per kg) cured Indian VL in 98 to 100% of patients who were either Sb resistant or had not been treated with drugs previously. In the same study area, primary Sb resistance was approximately 40%.

Liposomal amphotericin B (AmBisome) was shown to be effective and nontoxic at high daily doses of 2 to 4 mg per kg for VL treatment in immunocompetent patients. A dose-finding study in Mediterranean VL showed that a total dose of approximately 20 mg per kg of AmBisome in patients hospitalized 5 to 6 days was optimal and cost effective, especially for cases in infants. A similar study in Brazilian VL indicated that the same total dose of AmBisome administered during 10 days was highly effective. This regimen was found ineffective for patients co-infected with HIV and L. infantum, who had VL relapses even when treated with a total dose of 40 mg per kg administered over 1 month. In dose-finding studies in Indian and Kenyan VL, total doses of AmBisome as low as 6 to 10 mg per kg were shown to be 100% effective. These studies suggest that treatment of VL caused by L. infantum or L. chagasi requires twice the dose of AmBisome as does treatment of VL caused by L. donovani, probably because of differences in drug susceptibility of the parasites.

A colloidal dispersion of amphotericin B (Amphocil) was found to be effective in Brazilian VL at the dose of 2 mg per kg for 7 days (total dose, 14 mg per kg), but the drug produced serious side effects in patients younger than 6 years.

A third lipid-associated amphotericin B lipid complex (Abelcet) administered at the dose of 3 mg per kg for 5 days (total dose, 15 mg per kg) to Indian patients who had been unresponsive to Sb therapy resulted in full cure but also in significant adverse effects. Although producing some amphotericin B–associated toxic effects, both Amphocil and Abelcet have more rapid efficacy than does the conventional drug.

Paromomycin* (Humatin)

Paromomycin is an aminoglycoside licensed in Europe for the parenteral treatment of bacterial diseases. Because the drug has revealed leishmanicidal activity in experimental leishmaniasis, injectable paromomycin was used as monotherapy in patients with Sb-resistant VL in Kenya; the drug, given at the dosage of 14 to 16 mg per kg per day for a mean of 19 days, cured disease in 79% of patients. The efficacy of paromomycin was augmented by administering it in combination with antimony for 20 days (82% of cure), in areas in which Sb treatment alone had to be given for twice as long (40 days) to obtain the same cure rate. A comparative study in Indian VL showed that the first-line treatment with 16 or 20 mg of paromomycin per kg for 21 days was significantly more effective than treatment with 20 mg of Sb per kg for 30 days, for a cure rate of 77% or 93% versus 63%, respectively. In general, paromomycin monotherapy is probably not as effective as antimonial therapy in Sb-susceptible VL.

Other Parenteral Drugs

In Sb-resistant VL, pentamidine isethionate* (Pentam 300) may be used at the dose of 4 mg per kg intramuscularly three times per week for 9 weeks. At this dosage, however, side effects—myalgias, nausea, headache, and hypoglycemia—are common. A lower dosage of pentamidine (2 mg per kg) for a shorter course (every other day for 7 days) was found effective and less toxic in the treatment of New World CL.

Cytokine therapy is limited to studies on human recombinant interferon-γ (Actimmune). This cytokine was found to be only partially effective when used alone in VL patients. When used at the intramuscular dose of approximately 100 μg per m² per day in combination with Sb, 10 to 20 mg per kg for 20 to 30 days, interferon-γ could speed the elimination of parasites in previously untreated Kenyan or Indian patients with VL and in patients with Sb-resistant New World CL or MCL. Side effects consisting of fever, chills, fatigue, myalgias, and headache occur in 30% of patients.

Pentamidine (2 mg per kg) and interferon-γ (175 μg) have been used with some success in combination three times per week, 1 week per month, as maintenance therapy in HIV-infected patients with VL.

Oral and Local Agents

The ultimate goal for leishmaniasis treatment should be the replacement of long-term therapy consisting of parenteral and moderately toxic drugs with shorter courses of nonparenteral, less toxic, and more effective agents.

Treatment with orally administered agents has been attempted in Indian patients with untreated

*Not FDA approved for this indication.

VL. Atovaquone* (Mepron) at the daily dose of 30 mg per kg for 15 to 30 days, alone or in combination with fluconazole* (Diflucan) at the daily dose of 12 mg per kg, cured disease in only 7% of patients. Oral treatment was also investigated for CL. The drugs used are inhibitors of ergosterol or purine biosynthesis, which have *Leishmania*-specific pathways. Ketoconazole* (Nizoral) was found effective at the dosage of 600 mg per day for 4 weeks against rapidly self-resolving disease caused by *L. mexicana* or *L. major,* but not against "slow-evolving" species such as *L. braziliensis, L. tropica,* or dermotropic *L. infantum.* Itraconazole* (Sporanox), although more easily tolerated than ketoconazole, is probably less effective. Allopurinol* (Zyloprim) monotherapy at the dose of 20 mg per kg per day for 28 days was found to be ineffective against New World CL. Although this drug has been extensively used in VL patients in combination with antimonials, its role in the treatment of VL has yet to be definitively proved. Allopurinol and ketoconazole or itraconazole have been used together or in sequence for the treatment of complicated leishmaniasis cases or in the maintenance therapy for HIV and VL.

Standard local treatment of CL consists of intralesional administration of antileishmanial agents, usually antimony, given intermittently over 20 to 30 days on outpatient basis. The cure rate is approximately 75% in Old World CL. Use of this technique may cause problems when multiple lesions are present, when lesions are in areas of the face (which are not suitable for injections), or when medical care centers are not readily accessible. Major emphasis has been placed on topical application of paromomycin (aminosidine)–containing formulations. *L. major* lesions treated with 15% paromomycin plus 12% methylbenzethonium chloride† in soft white paraffin twice a day for 10 days cleared more rapidly than did untreated lesions in the same patients. On the other hand, treatment with this ointment did not augment the response of CL lesions caused by *L. panamensis* to a short course of treatment (7 days) with Sb. Another paromomycin formulation in which the methylbenzethonium chloride was replaced by 10% urea* was found to be ineffective against CL caused by *L. major.* Topical miconazole* (Monistat) (2%) and topical clotrimazole* (Lotrimin) (1%) were administered twice a day for 30 days to patients with *L. major* CL, but the cure rate was unsatisfactory. Therapeutic failures with antileishmanial ointments may result from the fact that CL is not a superficial problem as are infections caused by the dermatophytes. *Leishmania*-infected macrophages reside deep in the dermis and also disseminate to the lymphatic system and mucosal membranes. Even when topical agents are effective in vitro, they also must penetrate deeply to be effective against cutaneous lesions.

---

*Not FDA approved for this indication.
†Not available in the United States.

LEPROSY (HANSEN'S DISEASE)

method of
ROBERT R. JACOBSON, M.D., Ph.D.
Gillis W. Long Hansen's Disease Center
Carville, Louisiana

Leprosy is a chronic infectious disease caused by *Mycobacterium leprae*. Because of the mobility of modern peoples, it is seen at least occasionally in nearly every country, but it is common only in a number of developing countries in tropical or semitropical areas. As a result of the intensive effort by the World Health Organization (WHO) to eliminate leprosy as a public health problem (prevalence, <1 per 10,000) by the year 2000, its prevalence has fallen in recent years, so that there are now about 800,000 registered cases worldwide. The incidence, however, has changed very little, and more than 500,000 new cases are still detected annually. The number of new cases detected annually in the United States is currently about 150. These are found mostly among immigrants, particularly those from Southeast Asia, Mexico, and the Philippines. Cases among native-born U.S. residents currently constitute about 15% of the total.

Leprosy is best viewed as a spectrum of diseases, and the problems encountered in treatment vary considerably from one end of the spectrum to the other. Although most people (>95%) are not susceptible, those who are initially develop indeterminate (I) leprosy. This may be self-healing, but it is always treated if it is diagnosed. When self-healing or treatment does not intervene, the disease eventually progresses to one of the advanced forms. Patients with the most intact immune response keep the infection localized, manifesting tuberculoid leprosy, which is referred to as *polar tuberculoid disease* (TT in the Ridley-Jopling classification). In contrast, the disease becomes generalized in patients with a poor immune response to the infection; these patients exhibit polar lepromatous (LL) disease. Between the two extremes is a broad borderline region in which the disease may be classified as borderline tuberculoid (BT), midborderline (BB), or borderline lepromatous (BL).

Classification is based on findings of the physical examination, skin biopsy, and skin scrapings. The numbers of bacteria in biopsy sections and skin scrapings are quantified according to the bacterial index (BI). The BI is a semilogarithmic scale ranging from 0 (none found in 100 oil immersion fields) to 6+ (>1000 per oil immersion field). Indeterminate, TT, and most BT cases have a BI of 0 on skin scrapings at diagnosis, and only rare bacilli are detected on biopsy specimens. The BI on biopsy specimens and skin scrapings in BB, BL, and LL cases usually ranges from 2 to 3+, 3 to 5+, and 4 to 6+, respectively.

Although the Ridley-Jopling classification is still used to varying degrees in the United States, the simpler WHO classification is rapidly replacing it. This has three categories: a single lesion with sensory loss, which is referred to as a single-lesion paucibacillary (SLPB) leprosy; paucibacillary (PB) leprosy, in which there are two to five lesions; and multibacillary (MB) leprosy, in which there are six or more lesions. PB cases generally yield negative results on skin smears and positive results on MB skin smears. Patients in the United States with positive skin smears are considered multibacillary and treated as such, regardless of how many lesions they have.

TREATMENT
Antileprosy Drugs

At present, three drugs are widely used to treat leprosy: dapsone, clofazimine (Lamprene), and rifampin* (Rifadin). However, ofloxacin* (Floxin) and some other fluoroquinolones (clarithromycin* [Biaxin] and minocycline* [Minocin]) are also very effective. Rifampin is highly bactericidal for *M. leprae*, as are ofloxacin, minocycline, and clarithromycin, although less so than rifampin. Dapsone and clofazimine are weakly bactericidal alone, but together they are much more active. Technically, only dapsone and clofazimine are approved by the U.S. Food and Drug Administration (FDA) for the treatment of leprosy. However, rifampin is routinely used, both in the United States and throughout the world, for this purpose because there is no question as to its effectiveness against *M. leprae*. Because *M. leprae* has never been grown in artificial media, drug sensitivity testing is usually done through the mouse footpad technique. Because this is costly and requires 6 to 12 months, other methods based on the BACTEC or BUDDEMEYER system may eventually replace it.

Standard Treatment Regimens at the Gillis W. Long Hansen's Disease Center

Patients with newly diagnosed disease in the United States are generally infected with fully sulfone-sensitive *M. leprae* (no growth in mice treated with 0.0001% dietary dapsone). Bacilli from occasional patients show varying degrees of primary resistance to dapsone in mouse footpad testing. Clinically, however, those treated with dapsone monotherapy in the past have shown a normal initial response to standard dosages, unless their bacilli were fully dapsone resistant (i.e., there was growth in mice treated with 0.01% dietary dapsone). Such resistance is rare in new cases. Thus dapsone probably remains useful in essentially all newly diagnosed disease but should be used only in multidrug regimens.

Standard therapy for paucibacillary (I, TT, and BT) disease in adult patients seen at the Gillis W. Long Hansen's Disease Center is 100 mg of dapsone plus 600 mg of rifampin daily for 12 months. Patients with multibacillary (BB, BL, and LL) disease receive 100 mg of dapsone plus 600 mg of rifampin, plus 50 mg of clofazimine daily for 2 years.

These regimens should also be effective even in the unlikely event that the patient is infected with partially or fully dapsone-resistant *M. leprae*, but experience in this setting is limited.

If a patient does not accept the pigmentation produced by clofazimine, 100 mg of minocycline or 400 mg of ofloxacin daily may be substituted. However, patient acceptance of the clofazimine should be encouraged both because of its potent antibacterial activity when given with dapsone and because its antireaction activity appears to diminish the chances

that erythema nodosum leprosum (ENL) will develop.

World Health Organization Treatment Regimens

Because of a steadily increasing problem with dapsone resistance in 1981, the WHO organized a study group to make recommendations for the "chemotherapy of leprosy for control programs" (WHO Technical Report Series No. 675–1982). They proposed two regimens, which with experience have since been modified. Current recommendations for PB disease are 600 mg of rifampin once monthly, supervised, and 100 mg of dapsone daily, unsupervised. Therapy is given for 6 months (completed within 9 months). MB patients are given the same regimen plus 300 mg of clofazimine monthly, supervised, and 50 mg daily, unsupervised. Treatment for 24 months (completed within 36 months) was recommended until 1998, when, on the basis of results from an ongoing trial and other data, the recommendation was changed to 12 months (completed within 18 months). In 1998, it was also recommended that patients with SLPB disease could be treated with a single dose of 600 mg of rifampin plus 400 mg of ofloxacin plus 100 mg of minocycline.

These regimens have thus far proved to be highly successful, and follow-up for up to 9 years on MB patients who received 2 years of therapy and on PB patients has generally revealed a relapse rate of only about 1% overall. A few centers have, however, reported significantly higher relapse rates among patients with a high BI on skin smears. Fortunately, this is a relatively small portion of MB patients worldwide, but it is more common in the United States. Because rifampin appears to be more effective when taken daily than monthly, and because 2 years may be better than 1 year, a 2-year daily regimen is recommended in the United States to minimize the possibility of relapse. Nonetheless, the WHO regimens are now the standard antileprosy therapy nearly everywhere. Furthermore, bacilli from patients who experienced relapse anywhere have, almost without exception, remained fully sensitive to the drugs used. Thus if relapse occurs, the patient should be re-treated with the same regimen.

FOLLOW-UP OF PATIENTS

Patients are monitored at varying intervals, depending on the severity of their disease, complications, the drugs they are receiving, and so forth. For example, patients receiving standard therapy and who have no complications may be seen monthly, whereas those with severe reactions may require weekly or more frequent follow-up. Complications are most likely to occur during the first 1 to 2 years; later, after therapy is completed, the danger of reaction has diminished, and the patient has gained an understanding of his or her disease, the follow-up visits can be less frequent. After completion of therapy,

---

*Not FDA approved for this indication.

patients should be advised to return at once if there is any evidence of reaction, neuritis, motor or sensory loss, iritis, or new skin lesions. They should, however, be evaluated at least yearly for a minimum of 10 years for any evidence of relapse, and if it occurs, they should be re-treated.

Clinically, there is a gradual clearance of skin lesions, mostly within the first year. The BI on skin scrapings or biopsy specimens falls slowly (about 0.5 to 1 per year), and it might thus take a decade for a patient with very active disease to completely clear bacilli. Routine follow-up laboratory studies would include a complete blood count, urinalysis, and creatinine and liver function tests. Drug toxicity, however, is uncommon after the first year of treatment, and serious toxicity may manifest itself clinically before it is detected in the laboratory. If possible, skin scrapings should be done from three or four of the most active sites yearly. Routine follow-up biopsies are not necessary unless new lesions appear.

REACTIONS AND OTHER COMPLICATIONS

More than 25% of patients with leprosy may have reactive episodes of varying degrees of severity during the course of their disease. Some episodes occur before treatment is started or after therapy is completed, but most occur during therapy, particularly during the first year. They appear to be less common in patients treated with clofazimine. Reactions should not be regarded as side effects of any drug; rather, they are apparently caused by destruction of bacilli and the immune response to bacterial antigens released. Chemotherapy should be continued in spite of reactive episodes, and the episodes themselves should be suppressed by other therapy as needed.

Reactions can be broadly divided into two main categories: ENL (type 2 reactions), occurring almost exclusively in BL and LL patients, and reversal (type 1) reactions, occurring in BT, BB, and BL patients. A third type of reaction known as the Lucio phenomenon is relatively rare and may be an extreme variation of ENL. It occurs in patients with diffuse lepromatous leprosy who are from Mexico and some other areas. It is occasionally seen in the United States and is managed with corticosteroids. A fourth type, known as downgrading reactions, is also uncommon. It represents inflammation associated with progression of the disease process in untreated patients and is usually managed just by initiation of antileprosy therapy.

Erythema Nodosum Leprosum

ENL usually manifests with fever and painful erythematous nodules, but peripheral neuritis, orchitis, lymphadenitis, iridocyclitis, nephritis, periostitis, and arthralgias may also occur. Mild episodes may necessitate no therapy, or symptomatic measures such as aspirin administration may suffice. Several drugs are useful for the management of severe episodes.

Corticosteroids are effective in all patients and should always be used if an acute neuritis is present, to prevent permanent nerve injury. Usually, 60 mg of prednisone daily is sufficient. When the initial episode has been completely controlled for several days, an attempt may be made to taper the drug dosage over a period of 2 to 4 weeks. The reaction often recurs, however, and the dosage has to be increased again. If the process becomes chronic, prolonged therapy may be needed. In these patients it may be useful to try tapering the prednisone to alternate-day therapy. When an alternate-day schedule is reached, the dosage is reduced still more slowly until either the drug is eliminated or the lowest possible maintenance level is reached. However, because steroid-associated side effects are often a problem, other forms of therapy should be considered in chronic cases. Also, when regulating the corticosteroid dose is a significant problem, giving the rifampin only once monthly, as in the WHO regimens, should be considered in order to avoid its adverse effects on corticosteroid levels.

Thalidomide (Thalomid) is effective in most patients. The initial regimen is 100 mg four times daily, and the reaction is usually controlled within 48 to 72 hours. The dosage is then tapered over 2 weeks to a maintenance level, usually 100 mg daily. Regular attempts are made to discontinue it, but patients may need to continue taking thalidomide for months to years before it can be discontinued without recurrence of the reaction. Side effects are few, drowsiness being the most common. It cannot, of course, be given to fertile female patients because of its well-known teratogenicity, except under conditions outlined by the manufacturer.

Clofazimine is also effective for the control of ENL. A dosage of 100 mg two or three times daily is usually necessary, and the reaction should come under control during a period ranging from a few weeks to a few months, depending on its severity. Normally, reaction control is maintained with prednisone in these patients, and the dosage of prednisone is gradually diminished as the clofazimine begins to act. Because GI symptoms may develop with high doses, the dosage should be reduced to 100 mg daily within a year if possible. Pigmentation from the clofazimine is usually quite marked in these patients, and they should be fully cognizant of this before therapy is started.

Reversal Reactions

Clinically, reversal reactions are usually evidenced by edema and erythema of pre-existing lesions that may progress to ulceration. Neuritis and occasionally new lesions or fever may also occur. If there is neuritis or ulceration, high doses of corticosteroids must always be used (e.g., 60 mg or more of prednisone daily). The reaction usually is controlled within 24 to 48 hours, and only a short course of therapy may be necessary if the patient has minimally active disease and no neuritis. Patients with neuritis may, however, require prolonged treatment (3 to 6 months) if neural damage is to be reversed. Patients with prolonged reactions may sometimes be managed with alternate-day steroids as noted for ENL, and some investigators have found clofazimine to be useful in these patients.

Other Complications

Neuritis or silent neuropathies (neuritis without nerve pain or tenderness) may occur independently of any reactive episode. Immediate treatment with high doses of corticosteroids is necessary to avoid permanent injury and recover lost function insofar as possible.

Iridocyclitis is a medical emergency and is probably best managed by an ophthalmologist. Atropine drops and corticosteroid drops must be started at once if permanent damage is to be avoided. Tear substitutes are used in patients with lagophthalmos and/or decreased lacrimation.

Orchitis may occur with or independently of a reactive episode. It usually responds quickly to corticosteroids, but sterility may result.

Injuries are common in all patients with leprosy who have significant degrees of sensory and/or motor loss. The patient must be taught how to avoid them by frequent inspections of involved skin and the use of protective measures such as wearing gloves or special footwear. When an injury does occur in an insensitive area, it must be protected from further damage during healing.

CONTROL MEASURES

Control measures include appropriate patient education and management, evaluation of contacts, and prophylaxis. Patient education is vital if treatment is to be successful. Prolonged compliance with any regimen is unlikely unless the patient fully understands the necessity for it. The family's cooperation is also important. Educating the patient's family, employer, fellow workers, and even the general public about the disease may be necessary if these people become aware of the patient's diagnosis. The stigma associated with this disease is still a significant problem, and informing everyone that this is merely an infectious disease that is difficult to transmit and easily curable may be necessary to reassure them.

Evaluation of contacts in countries of low endemicity, such as the United States, is limited to the household. Household members should be checked for evidence of the disease annually for at least 5 years and know to seek immediate attention if ominous changes occur at any time. Antileprosy prophylaxis is generally not recommended by the WHO even for household contacts. Compliance is often a serious problem, drug toxicity may occur, and it is uncertain whether such prophylaxis prevents or only delays the onset of the disease in contacts destined to develop multibacillary disease.

FUTURE PROSPECTS

Research emphasis has been placed on improved use of existing drugs to shorten therapy, cultivation of *M. leprae* in artificial media, antileprosy vaccine development, serodiagnostic and other tests such as the polymerase chain reaction (PCR) for the early detection and follow-up of this disease, and the clarification of the immunopathology involved. For example, trials are under way evaluating regimens of 600 mg of rifampin plus 400 mg of ofloxacin daily for 1 month for all types of leprosy and 600 mg of rifampin plus 400 mg of ofloxacin plus 100 mg of minocycline monthly for 1, 3, or 6 months in PB patients and 12 or 24 months in MB patients. Results from these should become available soon.

MALARIA

method of
GEOFFREY PASVOL, M.D., D.Phil.
*Imperial College School of Medicine and
    Northwick Park and St Mark's Hospital
Harrow, Middlesex, United Kingdom*

Malaria in humans is caused by four species of the coccidian protozoan parasite *Plasmodium: P. falciparum, P. vivax, P. ovale,* and *P. malariae.* The infection is initiated when sporozoites are injected during a blood meal by the female anopheles mosquito into the host. The sporozoites find their way to the liver, where they multiply within the hepatocytes, giving rise to thousands of merozoites that invade red blood cells (and are then called *rings*). These small ring forms grow through the trophozoite stage to the schizont form, which ruptures the red blood cell, releasing further merozoites. This asexual cycle in the blood is responsible for the clinical manifestations of the disease and is of 48 hours duration in *P. falciparum, P. vivax,* and *P. ovale* infections and 72 hours in *P. malariae.* Because all parasites may not develop synchronously, however, the fever associated with schizont rupture may be continuous rather than periodic as is often the case with *P. falciparum* malaria.

EPIDEMIOLOGY

The diagnosis of malaria must always be thought of for any febrile patient living in, or from, an endemic area. Wherever temperatures are favorable, and humans and mosquitoes coexist, there is the potential for malarial transmission. The four species affecting humans differ in their geographic distribution. *P. falciparum* occurs especially in sub-Saharan Africa and Melanesia (Papua New Guinea and the Solomon Islands), whereas *P. vivax* is found mainly within the Indian subcontinent, Central and South America, North Africa, and the Middle East. *P. ovale* is found almost exclusively in West Africa, and the relatively few cases caused by *P. malariae* occur mainly in Africa.

PATHOGENESIS

The pathogenesis of malaria is quite different from that of other infections because *Plasmodium* is one of the few infective agents of humans that invade red blood cells. The clinical symptoms and signs are due to the asexual forms of the parasite in the blood that invade and destroy red blood cells, localize in critical tissues and organs in the body by binding to endothelial cells (cytoadherence), and induce the release of many proinflammatory cytokines, of which tumor necrosis factor-α (TNF-α) is currently thought to be the most important.

The initiating step in pathogenesis is when merozoites invade red blood cells (and occasionally platelets). Invasion is a highly specific, ordered, and sequential process. Once inside the cell, the ring matures via the trophozoite to the schizont stage, and these infected cells specifically bind (cytoadhere) to endothelial cells in postcapillary venules in critical organs such as the brain. In addition, cytoadherence of mature parasites obviates their passage through the spleen, a major site of parasite destruction, localizes maturing parasites at sites of reduced oxygen tension, which favors parasite growth, and may facilitate the invasion of uninfected red blood cells. Cytoadherent parasites presumably lead to microvascular obstruction, although the role and extent of this obstruction remain unclear. Cytoadherence may also serve to localize the effect of putative parasite toxins, which lead to endothelial cell activation and damage as a result of cytokine release. The mature malaria parasite is also capable of rosetting, a process in which red blood cells containing the more mature stages of parasite bind uninfected red blood cells to their surface. The mechanisms by which rosetting leads to disease remain obscure but may cause microcirculatory obstruction. Rosetting *P. falciparum* parasites have been associated with severe disease.

Finally, an important feature of malaria is the explosive increase in cytokines, notably TNF-α, during a febrile episode and coincident with rupture of schizont-infected red blood cells, which suggests the release of an as yet unidentified toxin. The abilities of malarial parasites to invade red blood cells, adhere to endothelial cells, rosette, and induce the paroxysmal release of cytokines appear to be central to pathogenesis.

CLINICAL FEATURES

The most frequent presentation of malaria is that of a pronounced febrile illness after a visit to, or residence within, an endemic area. The incubation period for malaria is variable but under optimal conditions may be as short as 7 days, on average 10 to 14 days, and in exceptional cases up to 20 years (as in the case of *P. malariae* infections). More than 90% of *P. falciparum* infections in travellers, however, occur within 6 weeks of leaving an endemic area and within 1 year in the case of *P. vivax*. There may be a relatively short prodromal period of tiredness and aching.

The classic paroxysm begins abruptly with an initial "cold stage," with dramatic rigors in which the patient visibly trembles, followed by a "hot stage" with a temperature over 40°C in which he or she may be restless and excitable and may vomit or convulse; finally, there is a "sweating stage" in which the patient defervesces and may fall asleep. Such a paroxysm may last from 6 to 10 hours followed by a prolonged asymptomatic period leading to further rigors in untreated cases. There may be accompanying headache, cough, myalgia (flulike symptoms), diarrhea, and mild jaundice. Malaria is rarely, if ever, the cause of lymphadenopathy, pharyngitis, or a rash; when these occur, another explanation needs to be considered. In *P. falciparum* malaria in particular, severe manifestations may intervene and rapidly prove fatal (Table 1).

DIAGNOSIS

Malaria needs to be excluded as the cause of fever in any patient living in, or returning from, an endemic country whether or not they have been taking antimalarial drugs and may have little to distinguish it from other febrile illnesses. Malaria may occur in "airport malaria" in which infected mosquitoes are brought from endemic areas on planes, and occasionally cases have occurred during the hot summers in nonendemic areas where infected individuals have passed the infection on to the local mosquito population. Malaria must also be considered in those puzzling cases in which a patient has a fever after blood transfusion, organ transplantation, or needlestick injury. A critical step in the diagnosis of malaria, especially outside endemic areas, is consideration of the possibility of the diagnosis; a travel history should now be a routine part of any clinical consultation.

Malaria must enter the differential diagnosis of a number of clinical presentations; the fever of malaria needs to be differentiated from typhoid, viral illnesses such as dengue fever and influenza, brucellosis, as well as respiratory and urinary tract infections. Less common causes of tropical fevers include leishmaniasis, trypanosomiasis, rickettsial infections, relapsing fever, and acute schistosomiasis (Katayama's fever). Malaria should be part of any work-up

TABLE 1. **Manifestations of Severe (Complicated)** ***P. falciparum*** **Malaria**

Complication	Definition
Cerebral malaria	Unrousable coma, with peripheral parasitemia and other causes of encephalopathy excluded
Severe anemia	Normocytic anemia with hemoglobin <50 gm/L (<15% hematocrit) in presence of parasitemia >10,000 mL
Respiratory distress	Pulmonary edema or adult respiratory distress syndrome
	Would now also include rapid labored breathing sometimes abnormal in rhythm
Renal failure	Urine output <400 mL in 24 h (or <12 mL/kg in children) and a serum creatinine level >265 mmol/L (>3.0 mg/dL)
Hypoglycemia	Whole blood glucose level <2.2 mmol/L (40 mg/dL)
Circulatory collapse (shock)	Systolic blood pressure >70 mm Hg or core-skin temperature difference >10°C
Coagulation failure	Spontaneous bleeding with or without laboratory evidence of disseminated intravascular coagulation
Parasitemia ≥2%; impaired consciousness of any degree; prostration; jaundice; or irretractable vomiting	In nonimmune individuals, should be managed as severe malaria (i.e., with parenteral antimalarias). The level of 2% parasitemia is a conservative one for nonimmune patients who can rapidly deteriorate

for a pyrexia of unknown origin when appropriate. Coma due to cerebral malaria needs to be differentiated from that due to meningitis (including tuberculous meningitis), encephalitis, enteric fevers, trypanosomiasis, brain abscess, and other noninfectious causes of coma. The anemia of malaria can be confused with other common causes of hemolytic anemia occurring in the tropics such as that due to the hemoglobinopathies (e.g., sickle cell disease, thalassemia), glucose-6-phosphate dehydrogenase (G6PD) deficiency, and the Melanesian form of ovalocytosis. The anemia of malaria must be differentiated from that in iron, folate, or vitamin B_{12} deficiency. Acute renal failure occurring in malaria must be distinguished from the renal impairment due to massive intravascular hemolysis seen in G6PD deficiency, sickle cell disease, leptospirosis, snake venoms, use of traditional herbal medicines, and chronic renal disease resulting from glomerulonephritis and hypertension. The jaundice and hepatomegaly of malaria must be distinguished from those in viral hepatitis (A, B, and E but also including cytomegalovirus and Epstein-Barr virus infections), leptospirosis, yellow fever, biliary disease, and drug-induced disease, including alcohol.

A definitive diagnosis of malaria is made by prompt microscopic examination of thick and thin blood films. There is no need to wait for a peak of fever before carrying out a blood film. Apart from confirming the diagnosis, the blood film allows accurate speciation of the parasite as well as determination of the parasite density. Occasionally the blood film may be initially negative, especially if chemoprophylaxis has been taken, and may need to be repeated if the clinical suspicion is high.

Malaria can be diagnosed with other methods, but each has its own setbacks with regard to time and cost and to being nonquantitative or nonspecific. With the quantitative buffy coat (QBC) method, blood is put into a small capillary tube containing a float and an acridine orange stain that stains the nuclear material of the parasites. This method increases the sensitivity of detection, but its expense and inability to accurately speciate or quantitate parasites are limiting. The *Para*Sight F antigen-capture test uses a monoclonal antibody to the histidine-rich protein 2 (HRP 2) of *P. falciparum*. This is a very useful test for those who have not had malaria before; minimal expertise is needed, but it is expensive and nonquantitative and can only detect the presence of *P. falciparum*. The polymerase chain reaction (PCR) is useful to make an accurate species diagnosis and to detect low-level parasitemias. The expense, time needed, and requirement for specialized equipment, however, make it impractical.

MANAGEMENT

Once a definitive diagnosis of malaria has been made, treatment with specific antimalarial drugs and supportive measures can be initiated.

Non–*Plasmodium falciparum* Malaria

Malaria due to *P. vivax, P. ovale,* or *P. malariae* requires a standard course of treatment with chloroquine, which usually leads to defervescence (Table 2). In the case of *P. vivax* and *P. ovale* malaria, the 8-aminoquinoline primaquine is given to eradicate the exerythrocytic forms (hypnozoites) responsible for relapses. G6PD levels should be measured in all patients before they are given primaquine because of the danger of oxidant-induced hemolysis. Chloroquine-resistant *P. vivax* malaria has now been documented and may require quinine treatment. Chloroquine can aggravate psoriasis and produces a severe itch in black Africans.

Plasmodium falciparum Malaria

Mild Cases

Because resistance to chloroquine is now widespread, the mainstay of treatment is oral quinine sulfate listed in Table 3 followed by pyrimethamine-sulfadoxine (Fansidar)* or doxycycline (Vibramycin) to eradicate the remaining asexual forms of the parasite. Pyrimethamine-sulfadoxine may occasionally cause rashes such as erythema multiforme and lead to Stevens-Johnson syndrome, and resistance to it is increasing, especially in East and Southern Africa.

An alternative to quinine is mefloquine (Lariam), and more recently drugs such as a combination of atovaquone and proguanil (Malarone)* and coartemether* (artemether and benflumetol) have been successfully used. Halofantrine (Halfan) has been used as a quinine alternative and as a standby treatment, but reports of a number of fatal cardiac arrhythmias have curtailed its widespread application. Whatever drug is used, parasitemia may paradoxically rise in the first 24 to 36 hours; this is not generally indicative of treatment failure and does not always need a change in therapy. No nonimmune patient should be treated for *P. falciparum* malaria with quinine alone because of the risk of recrudescence.

Severe Cases

Severe *P. falciparum* malaria constitutes a medical emergency. The diagnosis needs to be confirmed microscopically and intravenous access sought as soon

---

*Not available in the United States.

TABLE 2. **Antimalarial Drugs for the Treatment of Non–*P. falciparum* Malaria**

Drug	Dose	Comments
Chloroquine phosphate (Aralen) or sulfate (each tablet contains 150-mg base)	10 mg/kg, then 5 mg/kg 6 h later, then 5 mg/kg daily for 2 d (usual adult dose in 150-mg tablets: 4, 2, 2, 2)	Chloroquine and primaquine resistance now documented in *P. vivax* malaria. May require quinine and/or prolonged treatment with primaquine
Primaquine (for use in *P. vivax* and *P. ovale* malaria)	15 mg daily for 14 d; in cases of resistance (West Pacific and Southeast Asia) extend to 21 days	Not given in G6PD deficiency. Alternatively, 45 mg may be given weekly for 6 wk with monitoring for hemolysis. Not given in pregnancy

Abbreviations: G6PD = glucose-6-phosphate dehydrogenase.

TABLE 3. **Summary of the Oral Drugs and Dosages Used in the Treatment of Mild *P. falciparum* Malaria**

Drug	Dose and Schedule	Comments
Quinine sulfate	10 mg (salt)/kg (usual adult dose in 300-mg tablets: 2 tablets tid; at a practical level until parasite clearance has been achieved for 24 h)	Almost all patients will develop cinchonism (e.g., ringing in the ears, deafness, nausea, vomiting) to some degree, especially if liver or renal impairment present; reduce dose to twice daily if parasite count falling
Followed by		
Doxycycline (Vibramycin)	200-mg loading dose, then 100 mg daily for 6 d	Not for children younger than age 8 yr or in pregnancy
or		
Pyrimethamine-sulfadoxine (Fansidar)*	Pyrimethamine 1.5 mg/kg, sulfadoxine 30 mg/kg, as a single dose (usual adult dose, 3 tablets; each tablet contains 500 mg sulfadoxine and 25 mg pyrimethamine)	Mainly for malaria from West Africa. Doxycycline is preferred for malaria from elsewhere
Clindamycin (Cleocin)†	10 mg/kg twice daily for 3–7 d	An alternative to doxycycline
Alternative drugs‡		
Mefloquine (Lariam)§	15 mg/kg as a single dose, repeated after 6 h (usual adult dose: 3 250-mg tablets followed by 3 more 6 h later)	Contraindicated in early pregnancy and for patients with neuropsychiatric history; can cause minor gastroenterologic upset, abnormal sleep patterns and dreams, and in some cases incoordination
Halofantrine (Halfan)§	8 mg/kg q6h for three doses (usual adult dose: 2 250-mg tablets × 3); repeat same course after a week for nonimmune patients	Care should be taken with those with underlying cardiac disease; an electrocardiogram should be obtained before commencing treatment because of QT interval lengthening and arrhythmias
Atovaquone-proguanil (Malarone)*	Adult dose: 4 tablets daily for 3 d (each tablet contains 250 mg atovaquone and 100 mg proguanil hydrochloride)	Especially for *P. falciparum* malaria resistant to the other drugs
Artesunate/mefloquine*	4 mg/kg (or artemisinin 10 mg/kg) daily for 3 d plus mefloquine 15–25 mg/kg as a single dose on day 3	Especially for highly resistant malaria (e.g., from Thailand)

*Not available in the United States.
†Not FDA approved for this indication.
‡These can be used when resistance is suspected or the patient is unable to tolerate other drugs, such as quinine.
§Not approved for use in children.

as possible. Depending on the clinical manifestations, investigations as detailed in Table 4 should be carried out, and the necessary measures outlined should be implemented.

Patients with severe malaria should be transferred to the highest possible level of clinical care (e.g., a high dependency or intensive therapy unit). The measurement of glucose and, when possible, lactate and arterial blood gases should not be omitted in the initial assessment. An effective antimalarial, at the present time quinine for most cases, should be given intravenously* by slow infusion (Table 5). If it is impossible to use the intravenous route, quinine may be given by deep intramuscular injection into the thighs. The same dose as given intravenously is diluted 50 mg per mL in sterile water and can be split between two sites for injection and given through sterile technique. In the United States, quinidine is used.

Meticulous care must be given to maintain fluid balance because both dehydration and overhydration can occur as a result of the disease or treatment. Convulsions should be treated with intravenous diazepam and attention paid to hypoglycemia and hyponatremia. The routine need for prophylactic anticon-

vulsants has not been clearly established, although one study undertaken in a tropical setting has advocated a single intramuscular dose of phenobarbital (3.5 mg per kg).

Blood should be taken for cross-matching and coagulation studies. In endemic areas, a loading dose of quinine (20 mg per kg) should be given to young children and to fit young adults. Care needs to be exercised in the administration of quinine in the elderly, especially those with underlying cardiovascular disease. In these patients, particularly those with underlying heart disease, a baseline electrocardiogram should be obtained, with careful observation of the rhythm and corrected QT interval; when possible, a cardiac monitor should be set in place. The rate of infusion should be slowed in the event of marked prolongation of the corrected QT interval. Recent studies of childhood malaria have shown that a blood transfusion may benefit patients with respiratory distress and metabolic acidosis.

Each patient needs to be assessed individually. During the course of treatment useful parameters for monitoring progress include twice-daily parasite counts, regular pH and blood gas measurements, and, when appropriate, measurement of glucose, lactate, and C-reactive protein levels and renal function parameters.

---

*Not available in the United States.

TABLE 4. **Investigations Relevant in the Management of Severe Malaria***

Investigation	Relevance	Management
Full blood count		
Hemoglobin	Often not anemic on presentation, an indicator of duration of infection	Generally threshold for transfusion is high (e.g., <7.5 gm/dL in adults, <5 gm/dL with respiratory distress in children in an endemic area); self-recovery generally rapid once parasites removed
White blood cells	Normal in uncomplicated cases; often lymphopenic; in severe malaria, often neutrophil leukocytosis	Generally no specific measures required; secondary bacterial infection common in severe cases
Platelets	Often low	Bleeding in absence of disseminated intravascular coagulation uncommon; platelet replacement not necessary unless clinical evidence of bleeding
Blood film and parasite count	Essential for diagnosis and continuing management if high; more mature ring forms or pigment in ≥5% neutrophils indicates poor prognosis (see text)	Depending on setting and severity, might require exchange transfusion (see text)
Electrolytes		
Sodium	Often low; some cases due to syndrome of inappropriate antidiuretic hormone secretion, others due to inability to secrete free water	Self-correcting with treatment
Potassium	Normal unless high in presence of acute renal failure	Dialysis may be necessary
Creatinine	Normal or high	Dialysis may be necessary
Calcium	Often low in severe cases	May need replacement, especially if QT interval prolonged on ECG
Magnesium	Can be low	May need replacement, especially if QT interval prolonged on ECG
Glucose and lactate		
Glucose	Often low in severe cases in children, also during quinine administration in adults; often absence of classic symptoms and signs of hypoglycemia	Regular monitoring of glucose in severe cases; immediate administration of 50 mL 50% glucose (1 ml/kg in children) followed by a constant infusion of 10% dextrose
Lactate	Raised in severe cases; good prognostic and progress marker from hour to hour; important to measure if lumbar puncture performed	Important to ensure good tissue perfusion, especially by corection of any hypovolemia
Coagulation		
Prothrombin time, thrombin time, D-dimers (or fibrogen degradation products) and platelets	Activated in almost all cases of malaria to some degree	Might require fresh-frozen plasma and/or platelets if clinical evidence of bleeding
Liver function tests		
Albumin	Often low in acute infection and almost always in severe infection	Does not need correction unless clinically relevant; danger of fluid overload and pulmonary edema
Transaminases	Can be moderately raised; if very high, consider other concomitant infections (e.g., hepatitis)	May need modification of quinine dosage (e.g., to twice daily dosing)
Alkaline phosphatase	Not raised in malaria	If raised, think of other causes
C-reactive protein	Raised in acute attack	Useful for daily monitoring in severe cases
Blood gases		
pH	Acidosis important in prognosis of severe cases	Requires adequate fluid replacement, possible blood transfusion in anemic cases and avoidance (if possible) of epinephrine if inotropes are required
Po_2	Hypoxia uncommon unless pulmonary edema/infection present	Oxygen
Pco_2	Can be low in presence of acidosis with respiratory distress	
Bicarbonate	Low in acidosis	Replacement unlikely to help in acidemia
Others		
Quinine levels	Free, rather than total quinine levels relevant to efficacy and toxicity (alpha$_1$-acid glycoprotein [alpha$_1$-AGP] is the main quinine-binding plasma protein)	Not generally helpful in management because of variable binding to alpha$_1$-AGP; maintain between 10 and 15 mg/L according to parasite sensitivity; for quinidine, 4–6 mg/L
ECG monitoring: corrected QT interval	Can be prolonged in nonimmune patients, especially if underlying cardiac disorder	Reduction of quinine dosage may be necessary
Blood/urine culture	Patients often acquire a secondary infection (most commonly respiratory, renal tract, or septicemia) due to immunosuppression	May require systemic antibiotics
Lumbar puncture	Relevant in very young and elderly patients and when other causes of encephalopathy, especially meningitis, need to be excluded	Appropriate antimicrobial chemotherapy

*The feasibility of these investigations and their management depend on the severity of disease and the availability of facilities.
Abbreviations: ECG = electrocardiogram.

TABLE 5. **Drugs Used in the Treatment of Severe Malaria**

Drug	Dose	Comments
Quinine dihydrochloride* with ECG monitoring	10 mg (salt)/kg (equivalent to 8.3 mg/kg base) infused slowly over 4 h q 8 h until parasites cleared; then doxycycline, pyrimethamine-sulfadoxine,* or clindamycin as above when the patient can take by mouth	Can induce hypoglycemia and cardiac arrhythmias, the initial warning of which may be prolongation of the corrected QT interval on ECG; a loading dose, 20 mg/kg, may be given to young otherwise healthy patients and when hyperparasitemia cannot be treated by exchange transfusion
Quinidine gluconate with ECG monitoring	10 mg (base)/kg infused over 1 h (loading) followed by 0.02 mg/kg/min as a constant infusion until parasite clearance achieved; then doxycycline or pyrimethamine-sulfadoxine as for mild *P. falciparum* malaria when the patient can take by mouth	In an emergency and in the United States and where quinine may not always be available
Artemether* (a qinghaosu [artemesinin] derivative, oil soluble)	160-mg loading dose; then 80 mg daily for 6 d	Alternative to quinine (at present in exceptional circumstances); usually requires doxycycline as recrudescences are common
Artesunate* (a qinghaosu [artemesinin] derivative, water soluble)	2.4 mg/kg IV followed by 1.2 mg/kg at 12 and 24 h; then 1.2 mg/kg daily (usual adult dose: 120 mg followed by doses of 60 mg)	Used when quinine unsuitable (e.g., with cardiac arrhythmias and in the event of quinine-induced hemolysis as in blackwater fever)

*Not available in the United States.
Abbreviations: ECG = electrocardiogram.

During infusion of quinine, careful monitoring of blood glucose level is essential. Elective ventilation needs to be considered when facilities are available, especially in circumstances of severe acidosis, clear evidence of raised intracranial pressure, and respiratory failure of whatever cause. Further details with regard to investigations and management are given in Table 4.

Management of Specific Complications

Cerebral Malaria

The mainstay of treatment of cerebral malaria is antimalarial medication. A number of adjuvant therapies such as steroids and heparin have been tried but have not been shown to be effective. Some children and a few adults might show evidence of raised intracranial pressure, in which case an osmotic agent such as mannitol (e.g., 100 to 200 mL of 10% mannitol as a bolus in adults) may be attempted.

Hypoglycemia

All patients with cerebral malaria should be monitored for hypoglycemia, especially on admission and during quinine infusion. Hypoglycemia should be treated with a 50-mL bolus of 50% glucose followed by a 10% dextrose infusion.

Acute Renal Failure

Acute renal failure is usually the result of acute tubular necrosis and may necessitate dialysis or hemofiltration. The indications are similar to those for any other form of renal failure. Nonoliguric renal failure may be managed conservatively.

Acidosis

Adequate fluid replacement but avoidance of fluid overload is essential for acidosis. Aspirin should be avoided because it may contribute to the acidosis. Sodium bicarbonate has not been shown to be of any benefit and in fact may make acidosis worse. Transfusions in anemic patients have been shown to improve severe acidosis and reduce lactate in young children. Early hemodifiltration and ventilation may be used in situations according to availability. The inotrope epinephrine should be avoided unless absolutely necessary, as it, unlike dopamine, dobutamine, and norepinephrine, may make the acidosis worse.

Anemia

Anemia is mainly due to the rupture of infected cells and hemolysis by an as yet undetermined mechanism of uninfected cells. The hemoglobin should be monitored, but transfusion should rarely be required and only when the hemoglobin level falls below approximately 7.5 grams per dL because there is often a brisk reticulocyte response a day or two after parasites have been removed.

Bacterial Superinfection

Bacterial superinfection with organisms such as *Streptococcus pneumoniae* or *Salmonella* species is common in malaria and must be suspected particularly when fever remains high despite antimalarial treatment, hypotension supervenes, or there is evidence of focal sepsis (e.g., pneumonia or urinary tract infection). Antimicrobial agents as appropriate should be given.

Jaundice

Mild jaundice may be common and is mainly due to hemolysis. Deeper jaundice may be due to major liver involvement with malaria but may equally be due to a viral hepatitis. Impairment of liver function necessitates modification of the quinine dosage (e.g.,

TABLE 6. **Brief Guidelines for the Chemoprophylaxis of Malaria***

Chemoprophylaxis	Area to Be Visited	Dose/Comments
None	North Africa (Morocco, Algeria, Tunisia, Libya, tourist areas of Egypt); tourist areas of Southeast Asia (Thailand, Philippines, Hong Kong, Singapore, Bali, China)	Malaria could still occur in restricted areas, but the side effects and inconvenience of taking drugs outweighs the potential benefits
Chloroquine (Aralen) **or**	Middle East (including summer months in rural Egypt and Turkey), Central America, rural Mauritius	300-mg base (2 tablets) once per week
Proguanil* (Paludrine†)		200 mg (2 tablets) once per day
Mefloquine (Lariam)	Africa (Cameroon, Kenya, Malawi, Tanzania, Zaire, Zambia, Uganda); all rural areas of Southeast Asia, Papua New Guinea, Solomon Islands, Vanuatu	250 mg (1 tablet) weekly; use up to 1 year. Contraindicated in epilepsy and psychiatric disorders
Chloroquine **and** Proguanil†	Sub-Saharan Africa, Indian subcontinent, Afghanistan and Iran, rural areas of Southeast Asia, South America	Doses as above; less effective than mefloquine, but fewer neurologic side effects
Doxycycline	Mefloquine-resistant parts of Southeast Asia	100 mg daily; beware sensitization to ultraviolet light

*A specialist's advice should be sought for details and local advice.
†Not available in the Unites States.

to twice rather than three times a day) because the drug is mainly excreted via this route.

Hyperparasitemia

In hospital units with appropriate facilities, complicated hyperparasitemia may be treated with exchange transfusion. The use of exchange transfusion is controversial but, when safe blood is available, should be considered for all patients when the parasitemia exceeds an arbitrary 30% and for those in whom parasitemia is lower (e.g., more than 15%)

- When there are manifestations of severe complicated malaria (see Table 1)
- In the presence of medical complications such as diabetes and ischemic heart disease
- For elderly patients
- During pregnancy

Adjunctive Therapies

Many adjunctive therapies have been attempted for malaria, but few, if any, have been shown to be of benefit. The use of anti-TNF antibodies has been disappointing, and steroids are clearly not indicated in the treatment of acute cerebral malaria. The roles of iron chelators and heparin remain unresolved, as is the use of the anti-TNF agent pentoxifylline (Trental). The roles of mannitol for patients with evidence of raised intracranial pressure, dichloroacetate for patients with hyperlactatemia, and the free radical scavenger desferrioxamine remain unclear.

PREVENTION

Malaria is a risk for all travelers to an endemic area. There are a number of periods in the malaria parasite's life cycle when infection can be interrupted. Prevention generally involves reduction of mosquito contact and the use of antimalarial chemoprophylaxis. Vaccination against malaria is currently not a reality. Travelers need to take antimosquito measures and appropriate chemoprophylaxis compliantly and be aware that no prophylaxis provides full protection.

Antimosquito Measures

In endemic areas, those at risk should

- Sleep in properly screened rooms
- Use mosquito nets without holes, impregnated with permethrin, and tucked in carefully under the mattress before nightfall
- Wear long-sleeved clothing and long trousers when outdoors after sunset
- Use other adjuncts: insect spray (usually permethrin containing) and mosquito coils or repellents such as diethyltoluamide

Malarial Chemoprophylaxis

Recommendations with regard to antimalarial drugs is a changing field with national guideline differences. The spread of drug-resistant *P. falciparum* malaria has complicated chemoprophylaxis, as has the awareness that some of the more effective combination drugs such as pyrimethamine and sulfadoxine (Fansidar),* pyrimethamine and dapsone (Maloprim),* and amodiaquine (Camoquin)* may rarely have severe, and sometimes fatal, side effects. The risk of contracting malaria in any given country or situation needs to be weighed constantly against the risk of a serious adverse reaction due to any drug used. In the absence of adequate data, this becomes difficult. Compliance with the drug regimen is of extreme importance because those who comply poorly have a significantly greater risk of infection.

Travelers should start chemoprophylaxis 1 week before entering an endemic area (to ensure adequate

*Not available in the United States.

blood levels and to evaluate any potential side effects), continue chemoprophylaxis while within such an area, and use it again for 4 weeks after return (Table 6). Chloroquine, 2 tablets (150-mg base each) once a week, together with proguanil (Paludrine),* 2 tablets (200 mg) daily, is one of the safest and most inexpensive regimens but is of diminishing efficacy. These drugs have only minor side effects, the most common being gastrointestinal effects and difficulty in visual accommodation in the case of chloroquine and mouth ulcers in the use of proguanil.

Mefloquine (Lariam), 1 tablet (250 mg) weekly, used by travelers to sub-Saharan Africa, Papua New Guinea, and the Solomon Islands, is far more effective and the side effects tend to be neuropsychiatric. More detailed and specialist advice should be sought in special circumstances, including long-term visits, young ages (under 12 years), presence of drug allergies, immunosuppression because of disease or therapy, pregnancy, and epilepsy. In areas of chloroquine and mefloquine resistance or when mefloquine is not well tolerated, a tetracycline such as doxycycline 100 mg daily may be used.

---

*Not available in the United States.

AMERICAN TRYPANOSOMIASIS
(Chagas' Disease)

method of
LOUIS V. KIRCHHOFF, M.D., M.P.H.
University of Iowa College of Medicine
Iowa City, Iowa

American trypanosomiasis, or Chagas' disease, is a zoonosis caused by the protozoan parasite *Trypanosoma cruzi*, which is transmitted by triatomine insects. This organism is enzootic in Latin America and the southern and southwestern United States. Approximately 16 to 18 million people in Latin America are infected with *T. cruzi*, and 45,000 deaths per year are estimated to result from Chagas' disease. Only a handful of cases of insect-borne transmission of *T. cruzi* to humans in the United States have been reported. The number of *T. cruzi*–infected persons living in the United States has increased markedly since the 1960s, however, as several million persons have emigrated from endemic countries. These infected people present diagnostic and therapeutic challenges to the physicians who provide their medical care. In addition, because most *T. cruzi*–infected persons harbor the parasite asymptomatically and are unaware of being infected, there is a risk of transmission of the parasite by blood transfusion; several such cases have been reported.

CLINICAL MANIFESTATIONS

Acute Chagas' disease is usually a mild illness, and manifestations may include malaise, fever, edema of the face and lower extremities, hepatosplenomegaly, and generalized lymphadenopathy. Severe myocarditis develops in a small proportion of patients with acute infections, and meningoencephalitis is a rare complication. The death rate is less than 5%. In most patients, acute Chagas' disease resolves spontaneously over 4 to 8 weeks, after which the *T. cruzi* infection enters the indeterminate phase. This asymptomatic phase is characterized by subpatent parasitemias and the presence of easily detectable anti–*T. cruzi* antibodies.

Years or decades after the resolution of acute *T. cruzi* infection, symptomatic chronic Chagas' disease develops in approximately 10 to 30% of infected persons. The heart is most commonly affected, with rhythm disturbances, congestive failure due to cardiomyopathy, and thromboembolic events. In some patients, megaesophagus and/or megacolon develops and causes regurgitation, dysphagia, recurrent aspiration, and constipation. Immunosuppression of patients who harbor *T. cruzi* chronically can cause a recrudescence of acute Chagas' disease. This is particularly true in infected patients who undergo cardiac transplantation and in persons co-infected with *T. cruzi* and the human immunodeficiency virus.

DIAGNOSIS

The diagnosis of acute Chagas' disease is made by detecting parasites and should be considered in persons who have resided recently in an endemic area or in infants born to mothers at risk of harboring *T. cruzi*. In immunocompetent patients, examination of anticoagulated or Giemsa-stained blood is the cornerstone of diagnosing acute *T. cruzi* infection. In immunosuppressed persons suspected of having acute Chagas' disease, other specimens such as bone marrow, cerebrospinal fluid, pericardial fluid, and lymph nodes should be examined microscopically. Hemoculture and polymerase chain reaction–based assay are alternatives for cases in which the parasite cannot be seen, and both are available in my laboratory (telephone 319-335-6786).

Chronic Chagas' disease is diagnosed by detecting IgG antibodies to *T. cruzi*, and parasitologic studies are unnecessary. In the United States, enzyme-linked immunosorbent assay (ELISA)–based tests, manufactured by Abbott Laboratories (Abbott Park, Illinois), Gull Laboratories (Salt Lake City, Utah), and Hemagen (Waltham, Massachusetts), have been cleared by the Food and Drug Administration for clinical use. A persistent problem with serologic tests for chronic *T. cruzi* infection, however, is the occurrence of false-positive results, which typically occur with sera from persons who have other infectious or autoimmune diseases. A more specific radioimmune precipitation test is available in my laboratory for confirmatory testing.

TREATMENT
Antiparasitic Drugs

Current therapy for *T. cruzi* infection is unsatisfactory. Only two drugs have been shown to be useful. The first of these is nifurtimox (Lampit*), a nitrofuran derivative. Extensive clinical experience regarding its use has accumulated since the late 1960s, when nifurtimox first became available. Its mechanism of action is not known. In patients with acute or congenital Chagas' disease, nifurtimox reduces the severity and duration of the illness and lessens mor-

---

*Investigational drug in the United States; available from CDC.

tality, but parasitologic cures are achieved in only 50 to 70% of these patients. Infections that are not cured enter the indeterminate phase, and patients are at risk for symptomatic chronic Chagas' disease. Cure rates are less than 50% in patients with chronic *T. cruzi* infections. Nifurtimox can cause severe side effects, including gastrointestinal complaints such as nausea, vomiting, abdominal pain, anorexia, and weight loss. Some patients taking the drug also develop neurologic symptoms, such as restlessness, insomnia, twitching, paresthesias, polyneuritis, and seizures.

Nifurtimox can be obtained from the Centers for Disease Control and Prevention (CDC) Drug Service (telephone 770-639-3670 [working hours]; 770-639-2888 [off hours]). It is available in 30- and 120-mg tablets. For adults the recommended oral dosage is 8 to 10 mg per kg of body weight per day. For adolescents the dose is 12.5 to 15 mg per kg per day, and for children 1 to 10 years of age, it is 15 to 20 mg per kg per day. The drug should be given each day in four divided doses, and treatment should be continued for 90 to 120 days.

The second drug useful for treating *T. cruzi* infections is benznidazole (Rochagan), which is also available from the CDC Drug Service. The effect of benznidazole on the clinical course of acute Chagas' disease is similar to that of nifurtimox, and cure rates are similar to those of nifurtimox in both acute and chronic infections. Side effects can include granulocytopenia, rash, and peripheral neuropathy. The recommended oral dosage of benznidazole is 5 mg per kg of body weight per day for 60 days. The daily dose is given in two or three divided doses. I favor benznidazole over nifurtimox because its side effects are less bothersome and its schedule of administration is simpler.

In terms of who should be treated, I believe that all patients infected with *T. cruzi* should be treated with either benznidazole or nifurtimox, regardless of the stage of infection. This view is based on the results of studies of *T. cruzi*–infected experimental animals and humans, which show that treatment with either of these drugs reduces the appearance and/or progression of cardiac lesions.

The usefulness of fluconazole (Diflucan), itraconazole (Sporanox), allopurinol (Zyloprim), and interferon-γ has been studied extensively in experimental animals and to a lesser extent in patients with acute Chagas' disease. None of these agents has shown a level of anti–*T. cruzi* activity that warrants use in patients.

Treatment of Clinical Chagas' Disease

Beyond the use of nifurtimox and benznidazole, the treatment of both acute and chronic Chagas' disease is symptomatic. Patients with severe acute chagasic myocarditis should be supported in the same way as any patient with acute congestive cardiomyopathy. In patients with symptomatic chronic Chagas' heart disease, therapy is directed at ameliorat-ing symptoms through the use of cardiotropic drugs and anticoagulants. Pacemakers have been shown to be useful in patients with ominous bradyarrhythmias or heart block.

Heart transplantation is an option for patients with end-stage chagasic cardiac disease. Several dozen *T. cruzi*–infected patients have undergone cardiac transplantation in Brazil, and about a dozen have undergone the procedure in the United States. The degree of cardiac parasitization after transplantation and its impact on implant viability have not been defined. The experience with a handful of the U.S. patients suggests that intermittent prophylactic nifurtimox (three successive days of therapy each week) is useful in preventing recrudescence of acute Chagas' disease after transplantation. It must be kept in mind, however, that the efficacy and adverse effects of long-term administration of nifurtimox or benznidazole are unknown. These uncertainties suggest that cardiac transplantation in patients with end-stage chagasic cardiac disease should be approached with caution, especially in view of the extremely limited availability of donor hearts. This view should not be applied to kidney transplantation, however, because postoperative immunosuppression is less intensive and the risk of reactivation is minimal.

Megaesophagus associated with Chagas' disease should be treated as idiopathic achalasia. Patients with megaesophagus who fail to respond to repeated balloon dilatation are treated surgically. The procedure most frequently used is wide esophagocardiomyectomy of the anterior gastroesophageal junction, combined with valvuloplasty to reduce reflux. Patients with severe distal esophageal dilatation are often treated with esophageal resection with reconstruction by means of an esophagogastroplasty. Laparoscopic myotomy is being used with increasing frequency in industrialized countries to treat patients with severe idiopathic achalasia, and this procedure may become the approach of choice for chagasic megaesophagus as well.

Chronic Chagas' disease in the early stages of colonic dysfunction can be managed with a high-fiber diet and occasional laxatives and enemas. Fecal impaction necessitating manual disimpaction can occur, as can toxic megacolon or volvulus, both of which necessitate surgery at some point. Endoscopic emptying can be done initially in patients with volvulus who have no clinical, endoscopic, or radiographic signs of ischemia in the affected area. Cases that are complicated should be treated with surgical decompression. In either case, however, surgical resection of the megacolon is ultimately necessary because of the frequent recurrence of volvulus. Several surgical procedures have been used to treat advanced chagasic megacolon, and all of them include resection of the sigmoid as well as removal of part of the rectum. The latter is performed to avoid subsequent recurrence of megacolon in the segment anastomosed to the rectum. The Haddad modification of the Duhamel procedure has been used with considerable success.

BACTERIAL MENINGITIS

method of
ALLAN R. TUNKEL, M.D., PH.D.

MCP Hahnemann University
Philadelphia, Pennsylvania

Bacterial meningitis remains a common and devastating illness. In a surveillance study of 27 states in the United States from 1978 to 1981, the overall incidence for bacterial meningitis was approximately 3.0 cases per 100,000 population. More than 80% of cases of bacterial meningitis reported in this survey were caused by infection with *Haemophilus influenzae* type b, *Neisseria meningitidis*, and *Streptococcus pneumoniae*, with mortality rates of 6.0%, 10.3%, and 26.3%, respectively. In a subsequent surveillance study of five states and Los Angeles county during 1986, case fatality rates were somewhat lower (e.g., 19% for *S. pneumoniae*), which suggests that improvements in early detection and antibiotic treatment may have occurred during the 1980s. In a more recent surveillance study conducted during 1995 in laboratories serving all of the acute care hospitals in 22 counties of four states, the incidence of bacterial meningitis decreased dramatically. This decrease was a result of the vaccine-related decline in meningitis caused by *H. influenzae* type b (from 2.9 cases per 100,000 population in 1986 to 0.2 case per 100,000 population in 1995); thus in the United States, bacterial meningitis is now a disease predominantly of adults rather than of infants and children.

Earlier recognition of the meningitis syndrome with rapid institution of antimicrobial therapy and perhaps adjunctive agents (e.g., corticosteroids) may further reduce the morbidity and mortality among patients with bacterial meningitis. Current recommendations for the use of antimicrobial agents and adjunctive therapy in bacterial meningitis are reviewed in the following sections.

INITIAL APPROACH TO MANAGEMENT

Patients who present with a presumptive diagnosis of bacterial meningitis should undergo an emergency lumbar puncture to determine whether the cerebrospinal fluid (CSF) evaluation is consistent with that diagnosis. In virtually all cases, the opening pressure is elevated; values over 600 mm H_2O suggest the presence of cerebral edema, intracranial suppurative foci, or communicating hydrocephalus. The white blood cell count is elevated in patients with untreated bacterial meningitis, usually 1000 to 5000 per mm³ (range, <100 to >10,000/mm³), with a neutrophil predominance in most cases. A CSF glucose concentration of less than 40 mg per dL is found in about 60% of patients, with a CSF:glucose ratio of less than 0.31 in about 70% of cases. The CSF protein concentration is elevated in virtually all patients. The CSF Gram's stain is positive in 60 to 90% of cases (and correlates with the concentration of bacteria in CSF) and CSF cultures are positive in 70 to 85% of patients. In patients with CSF indices consistent with the diagnosis of bacterial meningitis but with a negative CSF Gram's stain, a latex agglutination study, which may detect specific antigens of meningeal pathogens, should be performed on CSF. The sensitivity of latex agglutination ranges from 50 to 95%, although the tests are highly specific; a negative test result does not rule out the diagnosis of bacterial meningitis.

On the basis of the results of Gram's stain and/or positive bacterial antigen tests, targeted antimicrobial therapy

TABLE 1. Targeted Antimicrobial Therapy for Bacterial Meningitis, Based on Presumptive Pathogen Identification*

Microorganism	Antimicrobial Therapy
Streptococcus pneumoniae	Vancomycin (Vancocin), plus a third-generation cephalosporin†
Neisseria meningitidis	Penicillin G or ampicillin, or a third-generation cephalosporin†‡
Haemophilus influenzae type b	Third-generation cephalosporin†
Escherichia coli	Third-generation cephalosporin†
Listeria monocytogenes	Ampicillin or penicillin G§
Streptococcus agalactiae	Ampicillin or penicillin G§

*Positive Gram's stain or latex agglutination test result.
†Cefotaxime (Claforan) or ceftriaxone (Rocephin).
‡Some authorities would use a third-generation cephalosporin if a resistant organism is suspected.
§Addition of an aminoglycoside should be considered.

should be initiated rapidly in patients with bacterial meningitis (Table 1). If no specific etiologic agent of the meningitis can be identified by these methods, antimicrobial therapy should be initiated on the basis of the patient's age and underlying disease status (Table 2). If the patient presents with a focal neurologic finding or there is suspicion of an intracranial mass lesion, computed tomography (CT) should be performed. However, if there is any delay (i.e., longer than 90 to 120 minutes) in obtaining the CT scan or in performing the lumbar puncture, empirical antimicrobial therapy should be started immediately (see Table 2) and before the lumbar puncture, because of the increased potential for morbidity and mortality in patients with bacterial meningitis in whom antimicrobial therapy is delayed. Once the infecting pathogen is isolated, antimicrobial therapy can be modified for optimal treatment (Table 3). Recommended dosages of antimicrobial agents for neonates, infants, children, and adults are shown in Table 4.

ANTIMICROBIAL THERAPY

Streptococcus pneumoniae

Penicillin G or ampicillin is no longer the drug of choice for the treatment of meningitis caused by *S. pneumoniae*, because of changes in pneumococcal susceptibility patterns. In the past, pneumococci were uniformly susceptible in vitro to penicillin with minimal inhibitory concentrations (MICs) of 0.06 μg or less per mL. Reports from several centers have now documented pneumococcal strains that are relatively resistant to penicillin (MIC range of 0.1 to 1.0 μg per mL) as well as highly resistant strains (MIC ≥ 2.0 μg per mL); the mechanism of this resistance involves alterations in the structure and molecular size of penicillin-binding proteins. In some areas of the United States, 25 to 30% of invasive pneumococcal isolates were found to have either relative or high-level resistance to penicillin. Emergence of these susceptibility patterns is of particular concern in the therapy of pneumococcal meningitis because it is difficult to achieve sufficient CSF concentrations of penicillin with standard parenteral dosages (peak CSF concentration of approximately 1.0 μg per mL).

TABLE 2. **Empirical Therapy of Purulent Meningitis***

Predisposing Factor	Common Microorganisms	Therapy
Age		
0 to 4 weeks	*Escherichia coli, Streptococcus agalactiae, Listeria monocytogenes*	Ampicillin plus cefotaxime
4 to 12 weeks	*E. coli, S. agalactiae, L. monocytogenes, Haemophilus influenzae, Streptococcus pneumoniae, Neisseria meningitidis*	Ampicillin plus a third-generation cephalosporin†
3 months to 18 years	*H. influenzae, N. meningitidis, S. pneumoniae*	Third-generation cephalosporin†
18 to 50 years	*S. pneumoniae, N. meningitidis*	Third-generation cephalosporin†‡
Older than 50 years	*S. pneumoniae, N. meningitidis, L. monocytogenes,* aerobic gram-negative bacilli	Ampicillin plus a third-generation cephalosporin†
Immunocompromised state	*S. pneumoniae, N. meningitidis, L. monocytogenes,* aerobic gram-negative bacilli (including *Pseudomonas aeruginosa*)	Ampicillin plus ceftazidime plus vancomycin
Basilar skull fracture	*S. pneumoniae, H. influenzae,* group A beta-hemolytic streptococci	Third-generation cephalosporin†
Head trauma; post-neurosurgery	*Staphylococcus aureus, Staphylococcus epidermidis,* gram-negative bacilli (including *P. aeruginosa*)	Vancomycin plus ceftazidime
Cerebrospinal fluid shunt	*S. epidermidis, S. aureus,* gram-negative bacilli (including *P. aeruginosa*), diphtheroids, *Propionibacterium acnes*	Vancomycin plus ceftazidime

*Vancomycin should be added to empirical therapeutic regimens when highly penicillin- or cephalosporin-resistant strains of *S. pneumoniae* are suspected.
†Cefotaxime or ceftriaxone.
‡Ampicillin should be added if meningitis caused by *L. monocytogenes* is suspected.

TABLE 3. **Antimicrobial Therapy for Bacterial Meningitis**

Microorganism	Standard Therapy	Alternative Therapies
Streptococcus pneumoniae		
Penicillin MIC < 0.1 µg/mL	Penicillin G or ampicillin	Third-generation cephalosporin,* chloramphenicol, vancomycin
Penicillin MIC = 0.1–1.0 µg/mL	Third-generation cephalosporin*	Meropenem (Merrem), vancomycin
Penicillin MIC ≥ 2.0 µg/mL	Vancomycin plus a third-generation cephalosporin*†	Meropenem
Neisseria meningitidis		
Penicillin MIC < 0.1 µg/mL	Penicillin G or ampicillin	Third-generation cephalosporin*
Penicillin MIC = 0.1–1.0 µg/mL	Third-generation cephalosporin*‡	Chloramphenicol; fluoroquinolone
Haemophilus influenzae		
Beta-lactamase–negative	Ampicillin	Third-generation cephalosporin,* cefepime (Maxipime),§ chloramphenicol, aztreonam (Azactam)§
Beta-lactamase–positive	Third-generation cephalosporin*	Cefepime, chloramphenicol, aztreonam, fluoroquinolone
Enterobacteriaceae	Third-generation cephalosporin*	Aztreonam, fluoroquinolone, meropenem, trimethoprim-sulfamethoxazole§ (Bactrim, Septra)
Pseudomonas aeruginosa	Ceftazidime‖	Aztreonam,‖ fluoroquinolone,‖ meropenem‖
Streptococcus agalactiae	Ampicillin or penicillin G‖	Third-generation cephalosporin,* vancomycin
Listeria monocytogenes	Ampicillin or penicillin G‖	Trimethoprim-sulfamethoxazole
Staphylococcus aureus		
Methicillin-sensitive	Nafcillin	Vancomycin
Methicillin-resistant	Vancomycin	Trimethoprim-sulfamethoxazole
Staphylococcus epidermidis	Vancomycin†	

*Cefotaxime or ceftriaxone.
†Addition of rifampin should be considered; see text for details.
‡Superiority of a third-generation cephalosporin over penicillin has not been established.
§Not FDA approved for this indication.
‖Addition of an aminoglycoside should be considered.
Abbreviation: MIC = minimal inhibitory concentration.

TABLE 4. **Recommended Dosages of Antimicrobial Agents in Bacterial Meningitis***

| Antimicrobial Agent | Total Daily Dose (Dosing Interval in Hours) | | | |
| | Neonates† | | Infants and Children | Adults |
	0–7 Days Old	8–28 Days Old		
Amikacin (Amikin)‡	15–20 mg/kg (12)	20–30 mg/kg (8)	20–30 mg/kg (8)	15 mg/kg (8)
Ampicillin	100–150 mg/kg (8–12)	150–200 mg/kg (6–8)	200–300 mg/kg (6)	12 gm (4)
Aztreonam (Azactam)	60–90 mg/kg (8–12)	90–120 mg/kg (6–8)	90–120 mg/kg (6–8)	6–8 gm (6–8)
Cefepime (Maxipime)	—	—	50 mg/kg (8)	—
Cefotaxime (Claforan)	100 mg/kg (12)	150–200 mg/kg (6–8)	200 mg/kg (6–8)	8–12 gm (4–6)
Ceftazidime (Fortaz)	60 mg/kg (12)	90 mg/kg (8)	125–150 mg/kg (8)	6 gm (8)
Ceftriaxone (Rocephin)§	—	—	80–100 mg/kg (12–24)	4 gm (12–24)
Chloramphenicol (Chloromycetin)	25 mg/kg (24)	50 mg/kg (12–24)	75–100 mg/kg (6)	4–6 gm (6)‖
Ciprofloxacin (Cipro)	—	—	—	800 mg (12)
Gentamicin (Garamycin)‡	5 mg/kg (12)	7.5 mg/kg (8)	7.5 mg/kg (8)	3–5 mg/kg (8)
Meropenem (Merrem)	—	—	120 mg/kg (8)	6 gm (8)
Nafcillin (Unipen)	100–150 mg/kg (8–12)	150–200 mg/kg (6–8)	200 mg/kg (6)	9–12 gm (4)
Penicillin G	100–150,000 U/kg (8–12)	150–200,000 U/kg (6–8)	250,000 U/kg (4–6)	24 mU (4)
Rifampin (Rifadin)¶	—	—	10–20 mg/kg (12–24)	600 mg (24)
Tobramycin (Nebcin)‡	5 mg/kg (12)	7.5 mg/kg (8)	7.5 mg/kg (8)	3–5 mg/kg (8)
Trimethoprim-sulfamethoxazole (Bactrim)**	—	—	10–20 mg/kg (6–12)	10–20 mg/kg (6–12)
Vancomycin (Vancocin)‡	20 mg/kg (12)	30–40 mg/kg (8)	50–60 mg/kg (6)	2–3 gm (8–12)

*For patients with normal renal and hepatic function.
†Smaller doses and longer intervals of administration for infants with very low birth weight (<2000 gm).
‡Peak and trough serum concentrations need to be monitored.
§Use in neonates is not recommended because it may displace bilirubin from albumin-binding sites.
‖Higher doses are recommended for pneumococcal meningitis.
¶Oral administration; maximal daily dose is 600 mg.
**Dosage is based on trimethoprim component.

On the basis of these trends, susceptibility testing should be performed on all CSF pneumococcal isolates.

Several alternative antimicrobial agents have been evaluated for the treatment of meningitis caused by penicillin-resistant pneumococci. Chloramphenicol has been studied, although clinical failures have been reported; an unsatisfactory outcome was noted in 20 of 25 children in one study. The third-generation cephalosporins (cefotaxime and ceftriaxone) have been considered the agents of choice in the treatment of patients with relatively penicillin-resistant pneumococcal meningitis, although there are reports of treatment failure with the third-generation cephalosporins, and pneumococcal strains that are resistant to these agents (MIC ≥ 2 μg per mL) have emerged. Vancomycin was evaluated in 11 adult patients with pneumococcal meningitis caused by relatively penicillin-resistant pneumococcal strains; clinical failure of therapy occurred in four patients. The concomitant administration of dexamethasone and the subsequent decreased inflammation and poor entry of vancomycin into CSF may have contributed to this negative outcome, which supports the concept that vancomycin should not be used alone for the therapy of pneumococcal meningitis.

On the basis of these data, penicillin can never be recommended as empirical therapy in patients with suspected pneumococcal meningitis. As an empirical regimen, the combination of vancomycin plus a third-generation cephalosporin (either cefotaxime or ceftriaxone) is recommended (see Table 1); this combination was synergistic in a rabbit model of penicillin-resistant pneumococcal meningitis and was at least additive in the CSF of children with meningitis. Some authorities also recommend the addition of rifampin (Rimactane) to this regimen, although rifampin should only be added if the organism is susceptible and if there is a delay in the expected clinical or bacteriologic response. Once the organism is isolated, susceptibility testing can be performed for optimal management (see Table 3). Other antimicrobial agents have been evaluated for their efficacy in pneumococcal meningitis. Meropenem (Merrem) has recently been approved by the U.S. Food and Drug Administration (FDA) for the treatment of bacterial meningitis in children 3 months of age and older. In comparative studies with either cefotaxime or ceftriaxone, therapy with meropenem demonstrated similar microbiologic and clinical outcomes, although further studies are needed to determine the efficacy of meropenem against pneumococcal meningitis caused by penicillin- or cephalosporin-resistant strains. Studies are also currently under way to determine the usefulness of newer fluoroquinolones (e.g., trovafloxacin) in patients with bacterial meningitis; these agents cannot be recommended until results are available from clinical trials.

Neisseria meningitidis

Penicillin G or ampicillin can be used for meningitis caused by *N. meningitidis*. Meningococcal strains (most from serogroups B and C) have been described from several areas, particularly Spain, that are relatively resistant to penicillin and whose resistance is mediated by a reduced affinity of the antibiotic for penicillin-binding proteins 2 and 3; relatively penicillin-resistant meningococcal strains have also been reported in the United States. The clinical significance of this finding, however, is unclear because patients have recovered with standard penicillin therapy. Rare strains of *N. meningitidis* that produce beta-lactamase have also been isolated, and these strains are absolutely resistant to penicillin (MIC $\geq$ 250 μg per mL); a third-generation cephalosporin should be used for therapy in this situation. Furthermore, high-level resistance to chloramphenicol has recently been described.

Haemophilus influenzae Type b

The therapy of meningitis caused by *H. influenzae* type b has been markedly altered by the emergence of beta-lactamase–producing strains; these strains accounted for approximately 24% of isolates overall in the United States from 1978 to 1981 and 32% of isolates in 1986. Chloramphenicol resistance in *H. influenzae* type b has also been described, accounting for less than 1% of isolates in the United States but more than 50% of ampicillin-resistant isolates in Spain. In addition, one study found chloramphenicol to be bacteriologically and clinically inferior to ampicillin, cefotaxime, or ceftriaxone in childhood bacterial meningitis caused predominantly by *H. influenzae* type b. On the basis of these findings and studies that have documented similar efficacy of the third-generation cephalosporins (cefotaxime or ceftriaxone) in comparison with the combination of ampicillin plus chloramphenicol, the American Academy of Pediatrics has endorsed the use of the third-generation cephalosporins as empirical therapy in children with bacterial meningitis. Recently, cefepime* (Maxipime) has been studied in the therapy of bacterial meningitis. In a prospective, randomized comparison of cefepime and cefotaxime (Claforan) for treatment of bacterial meningitis in infants and children, cefepime was found to be safe and therapeutically equivalent to cefotaxime.

Although initial studies suggested that cefuroxime, a second-generation cephalosporin, was as efficacious as ampicillin plus chloramphenicol, a recent prospective randomized study comparing ceftriaxone with cefuroxime for the treatment of childhood bacterial meningitis documented the superiority of ceftriaxone; patients receiving ceftriaxone had milder hearing impairment and more rapid CSF sterilization than did the patients receiving cefuroxime. Additional reports have documented episodes of delayed CSF sterilization with cefuroxime treatment as well as the development of *H. influenzae*–related meningitis in patients receiving cefuroxime for nonmeningeal *H. influenzae*–related disease.

Enteric Gram-Negative Bacilli

The treatment of meningitis caused by enteric gram-negative bacilli has been revolutionized by the third-generation cephalosporins. Previous mortality rates in this illness ranged from 40 to 90% with standard regimens (usually an aminoglycoside with or without chloramphenicol), in comparison with current cure rates of 78 to 94% when a third-generation cephalosporin is used. One particular agent, ceftazidime (Fortaz), is also effective for bacterial meningitis caused by *Pseudomonas aeruginosa*, resulting in cure in 19 of 24 patients in one study when administered either alone or in combination with an aminoglycoside. In another study of *Pseudomonas* organism–related meningitis in 10 pediatric patients, 7 patients were cured clinically and 9 were cured bacteriologically when treated with ceftazidime-containing regimens. In patients with enteric gram-negative bacillary meningitis who have no response to systemic antimicrobial therapy, intrathecal or intraventricular aminoglycoside therapy should be considered; however, this mode of therapy is rarely needed at present.

Other antimicrobial agents have also been studied in patients with enteric gram-negative bacillary meningitis. Imipenem has a broad antibacterial spectrum against many meningeal pathogens, including *P. aeruginosa*. In a recent study of 21 children with bacterial meningitis, imipenem* (Primaxin) was efficacious in bacterial eradication from the CSF but was associated with a high rate of seizure activity (33%), which limited its usefulness for the treatment of bacterial meningitis in children. Meropenem, a new carbapenem with less seizure proclivity than imipenem, has been found to be successful in several patients with *P. aeruginosa*–related meningitis. The fluoroquinolones (e.g., ciprofloxacin* or pefloxacin†) have been used in some patients with gram-negative bacillary meningitis but currently should be used only in patients with bacterial meningitis in whom conventional therapy fails or when the causative organism is resistant to standard antimicrobial agents.

Listeria monocytogenes

Despite the broad antimicrobial spectrum of the third-generation cephalosporins, they are inactive against *Listeria monocytogenes*, a possible etiologic agent of bacterial meningitis in the elderly, neonates, patients with malignancies, transplant recipients, diabetic patients, and alcoholic patients. Therapy in this situation should consist of ampicillin or penicillin G, and the addition of an aminoglycoside should be considered in proven infection, because of documented in vitro synergy. Trimethoprim-sulfamethoxazole,* which is bactericidal against *L. monocytogenes* in vitro, is an alternative agent. Despite in vitro activity against *L. monocytogenes*, chloram-

---

*Not FDA approved for this indication.

*Not FDA approved for this indication.
†Not available in the United States.

phenicol and vancomycin have been associated with an unacceptably high failure rate in patients with *Listeria monocytogenes*–related meningitis. Meropenem is active in vitro and in experimental animal models of *L. monocytogenes*–related meningitis and may be a useful alternative if found to be clinically efficacious.

Staphylococci

Patients with meningitis caused by *Staphylococcus aureus*, which is usually encountered after neurosurgical procedures or trauma, should be treated with nafcillin; vancomycin should be reserved for patients allergic to penicillin or when methicillin-resistant *S. aureus* is suspected or proven. Coagulase-negative staphylococci, the most common bacterial isolates in patients with CSF shunts, should be treated with vancomycin; rifampin is added if the patient fails to improve. Shunt removal is often necessary to optimize therapy.

Group B Streptococci

The standard therapy of meningitis caused by group B streptococci *(Streptococcus agalactiae)* in neonates has been ampicillin or penicillin G in combination with an aminoglycoside; this combination is recommended because of documented in vitro synergy as well as recent reports documenting the isolation of relatively penicillin-resistant strains of group B streptococci. The third-generation cephalosporins are alternative agents, with vancomycin reserved for patients who have a significant penicillin allergy.

DURATION OF THERAPY

The traditional duration of therapy for bacterial meningitis is 10 to 14 days for most cases of nonmeningococcal meningitis, although a shorter course of therapy may be efficacious for certain subsets of patients. Penicillin treatment for 7 days is effective treatment for meningococcal meningitis, although some authors have suggested that shorter courses (e.g., 4 days) are also adequate; these studies require confirmation, however, before a shorter course of therapy can be recommended for meningococcal meningitis. For the therapy of *H. influenzae* type b–related meningitis in infants and children, several studies comparing 7 with 10 days of therapy have documented that 7 days of treatment are effective and safe in this age group. However, therapy must be individualized, and some patients, depending on their clinical response, may require longer courses of treatment. In adults with enteric gram-negative bacillary meningitis, treatment with appropriate antimicrobial agents for 3 weeks should be used because of the high rate of relapse reported with shorter courses of therapy. Ten to 14 days of therapy are recommended for therapy of meningitis caused by *S. pneumoniae* and 14 to 21 days for group B *Streptococcus*. *L. monocytogenes*–related meningitis should be treated for at least 21 days.

ADJUNCTIVE THERAPY

Despite the availability of effective antimicrobial therapy for bacterial meningitis, the rates of morbidity and mortality from this disorder remain unacceptably high. Studies in experimental animal models of meningitis have elucidated the pathogenic and pathophysiologic mechanisms operable in bacterial meningitis, which has led to the development of new treatment strategies for this disorder. Once bacteria enter the subarachnoid space, an intense inflammatory response ensues; this reponse can be augmented by antimicrobial therapy, which causes rapid lysis of organisms and release of bacterial virulence factors into the subarachnoid space. In experimental animal models of bacterial meningitis, anti-inflammatory agents (specifically corticosteroids) have been evaluated as adjunctive therapy to reduce this inflammatory response and the subsequent pathophysiologic consequences of meningitis (e.g., cerebral edema, increased intracranial pressure).

Adjunctive dexamethasone therapy has been evaluated in many published trials in patients with bacterial meningitis. A recently published meta-analysis of these clinical studies confirms the benefit of adjunctive dexamethasone (0.15 mg per kg every 6 hours for 2 to 4 days) against *H. influenzae* type b–related meningitis and, if commenced with or before parenteral antimicrobial therapy, suggests benefit against pneumococcal meningitis in childhood. Evidence of clinical benefit was strongest for hearing outcomes. Dexamethasone therapy does not appear to be compromised by significant adverse effects if the duration of treatment is limited to 2 days, which is likely to be as effective as 4 days of therapy.

Despite this meta-analysis, controversy remains regarding the use of routine dexamethasone therapy in all patients with bacterial meningitis. Dexamethasone therapy is not routinely recommended in adults, until results of ongoing studies are available. The use of adjunctive dexamethasone is of particular concern in patients with pneumococcal meningitis caused by highly penicillin- or cephalosporin-resistant strains, in which patients may require antimicrobial therapy with vancomycin. In this instance, a diminished CSF inflammatory response after dexamethasone administration might significantly reduce vancomycin penetration into CSF and delay CSF sterilization, as shown in an experimental rabbit model of penicillin- and cephalosporin-resistant pneumococcal meningitis. However, CSF vancomycin penetration was not reduced by dexamethasone in a study in children. Despite these conflicting reports, many experts have expressed concern regarding the use of adjunctive dexamethasone in treating pneumococcal meningitis caused by penicillin- and cephalosporin-resistant strains. If dexamethasone is to be used, the timing of administration is crucial; administration before or concomitant with antimicrobial therapy is optimal to attenuate the subarachnoid space inflammatory response. For any patient receiving adjunctive dexamethasone who is not improving as expected or who has a pneumococcal isolate for which the cefotaxime or ceftriaxone MIC is 2 µg per mL or higher, a repeat lumbar puncture 36 to 48 hours after initiation of antimicrobial therapy is recommended in order to document sterility of CSF.

Critically ill patients with bacterial meningitis often require other adjunctive therapies. Patients who are stuporous or comatose and show signs of increased intracranial pressure may benefit from insertion of an intracranial pressure monitoring device; pressures above 20 mm Hg are abnormal and should be treated. Several measures are available to reduce intracranial pressure: (1) elevation of the head of the patient's bed to 30 degrees to maximize venous drainage; (2) hyperventilation to maintain the arterial carbon dioxide tension between 27 and 30 mm Hg, which causes cerebral vasoconstriction with reduction in cerebral blood volume; (3) hyperosmolar agents (e.g., mannitol), which make the intravascular space hyperosmolar to brain tissue with movement of water from brain tissue to the intravascular compartment; and (4) high-dose barbiturate therapy (e.g., pentobarbital) to decrease cerebral metabolic oxygen demands and cerebral blood flow. However, some experts have questioned the routine use of hyperventilation to reduce intracranial pressure in patients with bacterial meningitis. In infants and children with bacterial meningitis who have initially normal CT scans of the head, hyperventilation can safely reduce elevated intracranial pressure because it is unlikely that cerebral blood flow would be reduced to ischemic thresholds. However, in children with cerebral edema of CT, cerebral blood flow is likely to be normal or reduced, and hyperventilation might decrease intracranial pressure at the expense of a significant reduction in cerebral blood flow, possibly approaching ischemic thresholds.

Glycerol, an osmotic dehydrating agent that can be given orally, has been evaluated in a trial of 122 infants and children with bacterial meningitis. Glycerol-treated patients had a lower incidence of audiologic or neurologic sequelae, although further placebo-controlled, blinded studies are required before glycerol can be routinely recommended in patients with bacterial meningitis.

CHEMOPROPHYLAXIS

Chemoprophylaxis is indicated for contacts of patients with *N. meningitidis* meningitis or septicemia for prevention of secondary disease by eradication of nasopharyngeal carriage of the bacterial pathogen. Therefore, transmission to contacts is prevented, as is the development of disease in those already colonized. For contacts of a patient with meningococcal meningitis, chemoprophylaxis is administered to intimate contacts (e.g., family, roommates) and is usually not indicated for other groups unless there has been intimate contact (e.g., through kissing). However, school-aged children in crowded classrooms and in frequent contact during lunch or recess may be at increased risk of secondary meningococcal infection. Prophylaxis is not indicated for medical personnel unless there has been intimate contact, as in mouth-to-mouth resuscitation, endotracheal intubation, or endotracheal tube management. In addition, the index case must receive prophylaxis because the usual antibiotics (e.g., penicillin G) given for invasive meningococcal disease do not necessarily eliminate nasopharyngeal carriage. Chemoprophylaxis should be administered as soon as possible (ideally within 24 hours) after the case is identified; administration 14 days or more after onset of illness in the index patient is probably of limited value. The drug of choice recommended by the Centers for Disease Control and Prevention (CDC) for meningococcal chemoprophylaxis is rifampin at a dose of 10 mg per kg (not exceeding 600 mg) twice a day for 2 days. One dose of oral ciprofloxacin* (500 or 750 mg) is also efficacious in eradication of the meningococcal carrier state and may supplant rifampin for chemoprophylaxis in adults in the future. Ceftriaxone,* given once intramuscularly at a dosage of 250 mg in adults or 125 mg in children younger than 15 years of age, is also effective for eradication of the meningococcal carrier state.

Contacts of a case of *H. influenzae* type b–related meningitis should also receive chemoprophylaxis if exposure has occurred in the household or in a day care center containing children 4 years of age or younger (other than the index case); prophylaxis should be given within a week after exposure to *H. influenzae* type b. Chemoprophylaxis is not currently recommended for day care contacts 2 years of age or older unless two or more cases occur in the day care center within a 60-day period. For children in day care who are younger than 2 years of age, the CDC recommends prophylaxis and the American Academy of Pediatrics does not. The question of whether to administer prophylaxis in this setting needs to be individualized and should be considered more strongly in day care centers that resemble households in which children have prolonged contact. The drug of choice is rifampin* at a daily dose of 20 mg per kg (not exceeding 600 mg) for 4 consecutive days. Prior or pending *H. influenzae* type b immunization should not influence decisions regarding administration of chemoprophylaxis.

---

*Not FDA approved for this indication.

INFECTIOUS MONONUCLEOSIS

method of
LEONARD R. KRILOV, M.D.
North Shore University Hospital
Manhasset, New York
New York University School of Medicine
New York, New York

THE CLINICAL SYNDROME

Infectious mononucleosis is a clinical syndrome characterized by fever, malaise, tonsillopharyngitis, cervical lymphadenitis (tender posterior cervical adenitis being most characteristic), and hepatosplenomegaly. Three manifestations of infectious mononucleosis have been described: *glandular*, in which lymph node enlargement predominates; *angiose*, in which exudative swollen tonsils are the dominant finding; and *typhoidal* or *febrile*, in which fever, malaise, and possibly faint rash are the major aspects of the clinical manifestation. The acute course of infectious mononucleosis is typically 2 to 4 weeks, followed by complete recovery.

Respiratory complications of acute infectious mononucleosis may include upper airway obstruction secondary to tonsillar hypertrophy and, much less commonly, pneumonia. Spontaneous splenic rupture, which rarely occurs, is potentially life-threatening. Neurologic findings that may antedate or occur without other classical symptoms of infectious mononucleosis include meningoencephalitis, Guillain-Barré syndrome, transverse myelitis, Bell's palsy, or metamorphopsia ("Alice in Wonderland syndrome"). Hematologic findings in acute infectious mononucleosis include a relative lymphocytosis in which 10% or more of the lymphocytes are atypical. Hemolytic anemia and/or thrombocytopenia may also be seen. Elevated liver function findings are seen in most cases, but only approximately 5 to 10% of patients are visibly icteric. Cutaneous manifestations have been reported in up to 10% of patients; a number of erythematous rashes have been described. Amoxicillin or ampicillin administration precipitates a rash in 70 to 100% of patients with acute infectious mononucleosis.

Although in the 1980s several reports suggested a syndrome described as "chronic mononucleosis" associated with high-titer antibody responses to Epstein-Barr virus (EBV), subsequent research has failed to demonstrate differences in EBV responses or viral shedding between patients and controls. Thus, although possibly beginning with acute infectious mononucleosis in many such patients, this illness, characterized by prolonged fatigue and an array of other symptoms, is now considered under the rubric of chronic fatigue syndrome.

DIAGNOSIS

EBV causes 80 to 95% of cases of infectious mononucleosis. Other reported etiologies of mononucleosis-like illness include cytomegalovirus (CMV), *Toxoplasma*, adenoviruses, togavirus (which causes rubella), *Francisella tularensis* (which causes tularemia), *Borrelia burgdorferi* (which causes Lyme disease), and human immunodeficiency virus (HIV). For EBV-associated cases of infectious mononucleosis, heterophile antibodies that agglutinate red blood cells of other species (e.g., sheep, horses) are detectable within 2 weeks of the onset of illness. These IgM antibodies are not specific anti-EBV antibodies and are not readily detected in children younger than 4 years of age with acute EBV infection. In children older than 4 years of age and in adults, however, detection of these heterophile antibodies establishes the diagnosis of acute infectious mononucleosis. Specific responses to EBV can be measured as well (Table 1). These assays are generally not indicated in the routine evaluation of a patient with acute infectious mononucleosis, but they may be helpful in the child younger than 4 years of age or early in the course of the disease when heterophile antibodies are not detectable. Non-EBV causes of infectious mononucleosis can be confirmed by serologic studies and/or isolation of the specific agent in culture.

EPIDEMIOLOGY, PREVENTION

EBV is a ubiquitous virus; most people are infected by adulthood. There is no seasonality to this infection. Spread

TABLE 1. **Serologic Findings in Epstein-Barr Virus (EBV)***

Status	VCA IgG	VCA IgM	EA	EBNA
No infection	−	−	−	
Acute infection	+	+	+/−	−
Recent infection	+	+/−	+/−	+/−
Past infection	+	−	−	+

*Other patterns (e.g., positive VCA IgM or VCA IgM and EBNA IgM only) may be reported. These patterns are uninterpretable. Ten to 20% of people with resolved EBV infection do not make detectable EBNA (i.e., positive VCA IgG only).

Abbreviations: VCA = viral capsid antigen; EA = early antigen; EBNA = Epstein-Barr nuclear antigen. *Symbols:* + = present or positive; − = absent or negative; +/− = present or absent.

of EBV occurs through respiratory droplets, but shedding of the virus occurs in asymptomatic persons with previous infection as well as in patients with current infection; thus avoidance of exposure to actively ill people is ineffective in prevention. There is no specific isolation requirement for hospitalized patients with infectious mononucleosis.

Close person-to-person contact is required for transmission (which is why it is called the "kissing disease"). Endemic infection in group settings such as college dormitories is common. Rare transmission by blood transfusion has been documented. The incubation period after exposure is prolonged: believed to be 30 to 50 days. In lower socioeconomic groups and developing countries, primary EBV infection tends to occur in younger children, whereas in more developed areas of the world, primary infection is more delayed, peak infection occurring between 10 and 30 years of age. Primary EBV infection in this adolescent and young adult range tends to cause clinical infectious mononucleosis, whereas infection at younger ages usually causes a more nonspecific febrile illness or is asymptomatic.

TREATMENT

The treatment of uncomplicated infectious mononucleosis is primarily supportive, with attention to maintaining adequate oral intake and hydration, use of anti-inflammatory and/or antipyretic medication as needed, and gargling with salt water for relief from the pharyngitis. Concomitant streptococcal pharyngitis is detected in a small percentage of patients with infectious mononucleosis. Those patients should be treated with oral penicillin (not amoxicillin) or another appropriate antibiotic. Reduction of activity and bed rest are dictated by the individual's condition. Contact sports, vigorous exercise, and heavy lifting should be avoided during the period of splenic enlargement (on the basis of examination; typically about 1 month's time). Short-term, high-dose corticosteroids (e.g., 40 mg per m^2 per day of prednisone for 5 days with a subsequent 5-day taper) have dramatic benefit in patients with obstructive tonsillar hypertrophy. Steroids have also been used in patients with neurologic complications, although their efficacy in these cases is unproven. Although it has in vitro activity against EBV, acyclovir has not demonstrated benefit in the treatment of acute infectious mononucleosis.

CHRONIC FATIGUE SYNDROME

method of
DAVID C. KLONOFF, M.D.
University of California, San Francisco
San Francisco, California

Chronic fatigue syndrome (CFS) is a real illness. Many patients with this illness can be helped. In CFS, symptoms occur out of proportion to currently identifiable pathology. To work effectively with CFS patients, health care professionals must be comfortable with making a diagnosis based solely on history without abnormal physical findings or abnormal test results. The absence of objective measures of illness severity, functional limitations, and response to therapy is a challenge for CFS caregivers.

DEFINITION

Chronic fatigue syndrome is a new name for an old disorder characterized by fatigue and multiple somatic symptoms. Over the past 100 years the symptoms, now labeled as CFS, have been known as neurasthenia, chronic brucellosis, hypoglycemia, candidiasis, and environmental illness, which is also known as the "twentieth century syndrome." In the 1980s, because of reports linking fatigue, somatic complaints, and a positive Epstein-Barr virus (EBV) serology, the illness became known as chronic EBV syndrome or chronic mononucleosis.

The U.S. Centers for Disease Control and Prevention (CDC) devised a case definition for CFS in 1988 and modified the definition slightly in 1994. The 1994 case definition of CFS is known as the International Chronic Fatigue Syndrome Study Group (ICFSG) case definition (Table 1). According to this definition, CFS is excluded when fatigue can be explained by known medical or psychologic diagnoses (Table 2). Within the report that redefined CFS, the ICFSG also coined the term "idiopathic chronic fatigue" to mean a case of severe prolonged fatigue without sufficient associated symptom criteria to qualify as CFS.

DEMOGRAPHICS

Fatigue is usually found to be caused by one of three types of disorders. These disorders, along with their approximate relative frequencies, are psychiatric diseases

---

TABLE 1. **International Chronic Fatigue Syndrome (CFS) Study Group Case Definition of CSF**

In a patient with severe fatigue that persists or relapses for 6 months, classify as CFS if fatigue is severe and accompanied by at least 4 symptom criteria

Fatigue severity: Fatigue of new or definite onset (not life-long) and not substantially alleviated by rest, resulting in substantial reduction in previous levels of occupational, educational, or personal activities

Symptom criteria: Beginning at or after onset of fatigue and concurrently present after 6 months:
1. Impaired memory or concentration
2. Sore throat
3. Tender cervical or axillary lymph nodes
4. Muscle pain
5. Multijoint pain
6. New headaches
7. Unrefreshing sleep
8. Postexertional malaise

TABLE 2. **International Chronic Fatigue Syndrome (CFS) Study Group Criteria for Exclusion from a Diagnosis of CFS**

1. A documented fatiguing medical disease
2. A previously diagnosed fatiguing medical disease that has not fully resolved
3. A prior or current major depressive disorder with psychiatric features such as bipolar disease, schizophrenia, dementia, anorexia nervosa, or bulimia nervosa
4. Substance abuse within 2 years of the onset of fatigue

(usually anxiety, depression, or somatoform disorders), 60%; chronic fatigue syndrome, 30%; and medical diseases, 10%. The gender breakdown for CFS patients is approximately 70% female and 30% male. The mean age of onset is 38 years. The prevalence has been measured from 2 to 200 per 100,000. Cases of CFS usually occur sporadically, but several apparent epidemics of CFS have also been reported. An unanswered question about each epidemic of CFS is whether mass exposure to a triggering factor for the illness occurred or whether mass hysteria was responsible for the outbreak of symptoms.

OTHER NAMES FOR CHRONIC FATIGUE SYNDROME

A variety of poorly understood illnesses characterized by fatigue and somatic complaints are probably closely related to CFS. These illnesses appear to represent extreme forms of the same underlying disorder known as the "affective spectrum disorder." This disorder is associated with a neurochemical imbalance and dysfunction of the central nervous system. Affective spectrum disorder is characterized by a spectrum of presenting symptoms. Whichever symptom predominates determines the name of the illness. Examples of illnesses that constitute the affective spectrum disorder include CFS, fibromyalgia, premenstrual syndrome, irritable bowel syndrome, chronic hypoglycemia, and chronic muscle tension headaches.

Other illnesses that are probably closely related to or identical with CFS include multiple chemical sensitivities, the yeast connection, environmental illnesses, seronegative Lyme disease, silicone breast implant syndrome, and Gulf War syndrome. In each of these illnesses, there is often a conflict between patients who ascribe their symptoms to an organic cause (which may not be evident even after extensive investigation) and the medical establishment, which tends to affix a psychiatric diagnosis to these symptoms. Many patients with CFS and these other illnesses have founded activist organizations to lobby for increased funding into research that will demonstrate an organic cause for their illness. These patients believe that they are being unfairly stigmatized as having a psychiatric illness. A psychiatric diagnosis, compared with a medical diagnosis, may also confer lesser disability payments by insurance payers.

ETIOLOGY

The exact cause of CFS is not known. The illness is often triggered by an acute physical stress such as an infection, trauma, surgery, or even a long vacation. EBV is one of the possible triggers; however, the final pathways of symptoms for all acute-onset cases are similar. There is no reason to obtain EBV serology tests in the work-up for CFS. These tests are not specific enough to distinguish patients with

CFS from approximately 90% of the adult population with serologic evidence of a prior EBV infection.

Minor perturbations of the immune system have been reported in CFS. They are for the most part not severe, not consistent, and not apparently mechanistically linked to the symptoms of CFS. The acronym CFIDS (chronic fatigue and immune dysfunction syndrome) does not seem to be as accurate a description of the illness as CFS. The acronym CFIDS is usually not used by mainstream CFS researchers or clinicians.

Patients with CFS often report a hyperactive, "high-powered" lifestyle before developing the illness. They are often managing many projects and were disinclined to refuse taking on additional tasks. In this overcommitted, overworked state, an acute physical stress that would usually produce days or weeks of debility resulted in a prolonged state of physical decompensation. Although studies are being conducted on the organic changes that occur in patients after they develop CFS, additional research is needed into the premorbid physical and psychologic health of these patients. This research may identify attitudes or behaviors that predispose to or perpetuate the illness.

WORK-UP FOR THE FATIGUED PATIENT

CFS is a diagnosis of exclusion. In the evaluation of a patient with fatigue, every medical and psychiatric diagnosis must be excluded before conferring a diagnosis of CFS. If CFS is incorrectly diagnosed, then the patient will miss out on treatment for the actual undiagnosed disease, and that condition might irreversibly worsen during the time that treatment for CFS is being inappropriately prescribed.

The diagnostic work-up of fatigue consists of four parts: (1) a history, (2) a complete physical examination, (3) laboratory tests, and (4) psychologic testing. A history for a fatigued patient should include an estimate of what percentage of the premorbid energy is now present. Most CFS patients estimate 50% or less. They also complain of the eight CDC or four ICSFG symptom criteria of CFS.

The physical examination should include measurement of temperature (which is usually normal and always ≤101.5°F) and a search for exudative pharyngitis or palpable lymph nodes (which are usually not found). Laboratory tests in a fatigue work-up need to consist of only five tests: (1) a chemistry panel, (2) a complete blood count, (3) a sedimentation rate, (4) a thyroid-stimulating hormone level, and (5) a urinalysis. No other studies are needed unless the fatigue is accompanied by significant symptoms that require testing in their own right. Serologies for EBV, human herpesvirus 6, cytomegalovirus, *Borrelia burgdorferi*, and *Candida*, and magnetic resonance images of the brain are examples of tests that should not be performed in the routine work-up for fatigue, but should be reserved for selected patients. Psychologic testing can consist of a simple mental status examination to exclude a thought disorder.

TREATMENT

CFS is a chronic illness. The goal is not a "cure," which would be a return to the prior level of functioning. Instead, the goal is to accommodate the illness, minimize symptoms, and maximize performance. The premorbid lifestyle was generally unhealthy for the patient and should not be the target for rehabilitation. CFS patients need to recognize which activi-

TABLE 3. **Nonpharmacologic Treatment of Chronic Fatigue Syndrome**

Exercise	Support group
Relaxation methods	Individual psychotherapy
Diet	

ties increase symptoms and then modify their lifestyles to minimize symptoms.

The three principles of treatment for physicians who treat CFS are to (1) be optimistic, (2) aim for gradual improvement, and (3) recognize the mind-body connection. CFS treatment is directed at both the medical and psychologic aspects of the illness.

No matter what psychologic problems may have preceded the onset of CFS, a patient with CFS expresses symptoms referable to multiple organ systems and requires the same symptom relief as any patient with a recognized medical disease. Symptom relief alone, however, will provide only temporary relief if underlying psychologic problems are perpetuating the illness. Most CFS patients achieve the best results when a medical approach to relieve current symptoms is combined with a psychologic approach to prevent future symptoms. CFS treatments can be divided into two categories: nonpharmacologic (Table 3) and pharmacologic (Table 4).

Nonpharmacologic Treatment

Exercise is the most important treatment for CFS. Exercise has three purposes in CFS: (1) to reverse muscle atrophy, (2) to relieve anxiety and depression, and (3) to provide a metaphor for success when fatigued patients cannot perform simple tasks.

Patients with CFS are usually too fatigued to exercise. They typically end up in a negative cycle consisting of rest, muscle atrophy, decreased performance, pessimism, disinterest in exercise, and more rest. Daily exercise can replace that cycle with a positive cycle consisting of exercise, muscle hypertrophy, increased performance, optimism, interest in exercise, and more exercise.

Daily aerobic exercise such as walking, bicycling, or swimming is best. The duration can be as little as 5 minutes per day. The duration should be increased each week by 3 to 5 minutes up to 60 to 120 minutes daily. The patient should not exceed the prescribed amount of exercise. CFS patients tend to incorrectly estimate exercise performance. They may overdo

TABLE 4. **Pharmacologic Treatment of Chronic Fatigue Syndrome**

One or more agents:
Nonsteroidal anti-inflammatory drugs (NSAIDs)
Symptomatic medications
Tricyclic antidepressants
Selective serotonin reuptake inhibitors (SSRIs)

their exercise and then develop muscle pain the next day that will limit future performance.

Relaxation methods such as biofeedback, yoga, and hypnosis can decrease CFS symptoms. If patients want to read about CFS, they should be advised to select the material carefully. Printed material from the National Institutes of Health or the CDC are factual; however, many books, magazines, and Internet Web sites contain material that is incorrect or dangerous for patients. The physician should approve these materials before patients read them. The amount of material read by CFS patients has actually been shown to be inversely correlated with improvement.

A hypoglycemia-avoidance diet is helpful because it prevents the autonomic hyperactivity response that is similar in CFS and reactive hypoglycemia. Patients should avoid 5 types of foods: simple sugars, fruit juice, large meals, caffeine, and alcohol. There is evidence that evening primrose oil, 500 mg twice daily, decreases muscle and joint pains in CFS. Salt has been claimed to cure CFS symptoms by correcting neurally mediated hypotension in some CFS patients. This controversial recommendation is unproved and requires further testing before it should be carried out routinely.

A professionally led support group is very helpful for stress reduction. External stresses such as family, job, finances, or transportation problems affect everyone and generally exacerbate symptoms in CFS patients. For CFS patients, stress reduction improves CFS symptoms, and stress reduction requires preparation. A CFS support group can help patients to avoid certain stressful situations and to manage other stressful situations. Behavior patterns can be modified to create a healthier lifestyle. The process of identifying and modifying self-destructive behavior is known as cognitive-behavioral therapy.

Ongoing internal stresses such as conflicting goals, unmet expectations, low self-esteem, and childhood sexual abuse can perpetuate symptoms of CFS. These problems are not appropriate topics for a support group but may respond to individual psychotherapy.

CFS is not the same as depression. Many CFS patients are wary of being dismissed or demeaned by a referral to a psychiatrist because they believe they have a medical disorder that will be overlooked after they begin psychotherapy. The physician should not say, "There's nothing wrong with you," "The problem is in your head," or "You are depressed" because the patient will hear, "You are crazy" and further communication will be blocked. Individual psychotherapy can help CFS patients cope with the frustration of developing a chronic illness, and often this treatment is essential to recovery.

Pharmacologic Treatment

Nonsteroidal anti-inflammatory drugs are useful for the muscle and joint pains of CFS. Long-acting medications are preferable because CFS patients might forget to take short-acting medications that require several daily doses.

Symptomatic medications that are not habit-forming can reduce pain, muscle spasm, and bowel spasm in CFS. For pain, acetaminophen is obtained over the counter, and tramadol (Ultram) is obtained by prescription. For muscle spasms, cyclobenzaprine (Flexeril) is effective. It should be taken after dinner or several hours before bedtime because of its sedating properties. Nonsedating muscle relaxers such as carisoprodol (Soma) and metaxalone (Skelaxin) can be used in the daytime. If occipital and posterior cervical muscle tension headaches are severe, then patients may also use stretching exercises, heat, massage, relaxation, or, in selected cases, home cervical traction after pretreatment cervical spine x-ray films. For bowel spasm, antispasmodics plus insoluble dietary fiber, such as two heaping teaspoons of oat bran daily, are effective.

Tricyclic antidepressants are effective for the insomnia of CFS. The dosage used in this setting is far lower than for depression. Amitriptyline (Elavil) is the first choice in this family of drugs because of its sedating, pain-relieving, and mood-elevating properties. Doxepin (Sinequan) is even more sedating. Imipramine (Tofranil) and nortriptyline (Pamelor) are each less sedating and desipramine (Norpramin) much less sedating than amitriptyline. Dosages of these medications should begin with 5 to 10 mg 1 hour after dinner (and not at bedtime) daily with weekly dosage increases in 5- to 10-mg increments until either sleep is restored or side effects occur. The most common side effects with these medications include excessive sleep if the dose is too high, a dry mouth, and postural light-headedness. To minimize or prevent nocturnal orthostatic hypotension, patients on amitriptyline should be instructed how to arise from a sitting or lying position. They should arise slowly, sit on the edge of the bed for 1 minute, walk slowly, and hold onto the wall for support. Trazodone (Desyrel) and nefazodone (Serzone) are also effective sedatives but are not tricyclic antidepressants.

Selective serotonin reuptake inhibitors (SSRIs) are effective for the hypersomnia that is common in CFS. Many patients with CFS report excessive sleep both at night (more than 8 hours) and during the day (a nap of more than 15 minutes), as well as fatigue. SSRIs are very effective for these complaints, and they also provide mood elevation. These medications are activating or stimulating and are also useful for obsessive-compulsive traits. Protriptyline (Vivactil), bupropion (Wellbutrin), and venlafaxine (Effexor) are also effective stimulants for selected patients, but are not SSRIs.

PROGNOSIS

Whether the goal of treatment is rehabilitation from work disability or a less constricted lifestyle, adherence to treatment is the best prognostic factor.

Patients who are unwilling or unable to comply with treatments do not generally improve. When CFS results in work disability, the most favorable prognostic factors include disability duration of up to 4 months, age at onset of treatment of up to 30 years, not receiving disability payments, and an illness duration of up to 40 months. As is the case with other chronic illnesses, after 1 year of work disability due to CFS, rehabilitation is rare. When the patient with CFS is motivated to improve and the physician utilizes a combined medical and psychologic treatment approach, then great improvement is possible.

MUMPS

method of
JOHN S. VENGLARCIK III, M.D.
Tod Children's Hospital and Northeastern Ohio
  Universities College of Medicine
Youngstown, Ohio

Mumps is a systemic illness that typically produces a painful swelling of the parotid gland. As a matter of fact, the term "mumps" is most likely derived from the British verb *mump,* which means to grimace. The virus that causes mumps is a paramyxovirus and is easily transmitted in respiratory secretions. Infection occurs primarily in childhood, with cases seen most commonly in late winter and spring. When the infection is acquired in adulthood the disease is more severe. Although fatalities are rare at any age, more than half the deaths occur in individuals older than the age of 19 years. The incidence of mumps has declined dramatically since an effective vaccine was licensed for distribution in 1967. Currently about 1500 cases per year are reported in the United States.

The incubation period of mumps is typically between 16 and 18 days. However, cases have developed from as soon as 12 days to as long as 25 days after exposure. The onset of the disease is heralded by the development of fever, but temperatures are usually only modestly elevated. The febrile period lasts for 3 to 4 days. Parotid swelling is noted after several days of fever. The parotid enlargement most commonly is bilateral and peaks in 2 or 3 days, with the total length of swelling lasting for a week to 10 days. Occasionally, the enlargement of one parotid gland may precede the enlargement of the other by a few days, giving an asynchronous appearance to the process. At the peak of the swelling, the angle of the jaw is obliterated and the pinna can be pushed away from the head.

Parotid swelling can cause a great amount of pain and discomfort. The enlarged gland may be exquisitely tender to touch. Furthermore, the ingestion of certain types of food and drink that stimulate the salivary glands, especially acidic foods, may cause a great deal of discomfort. As a consequence, anorexia can complicate the clinical picture.

Not all individuals who become infected with the mumps virus will develop parotitis; as many as one third will not. Other manifestations can include vomiting and abdominal pain, which may indicate pancreatic involvement as well as headache and photophobia, which may indicate meningeal involvement.

Mumps can be associated with a variety of complications: meningoencephalitis, eighth nerve involvement with hearing impairment, orchitis, mastitis, pancreatitis, thyroiditis, arthritis, and renal involvement. Of all the complications, orchitis causes the most concern. Orchitis develops in about one third of those with mumps and is typically seen in postpubertal males. Despite popular misconceptions, sterility is a rare event, even with bilateral involvement. Meningoencephalitis is another complication that engenders concern; it usually presents as an aseptic meningitis syndrome and carries a good prognosis.

Parotid swelling associated with mumps must be distinguished from other viral causes of parotid enlargement, which include influenza, parainfluenza, and cytomegalovirus. Suppurative parotitis can be distinguished from mumps by the presence of warmth, erythema, and severe tenderness associated with purulent drainage from Stensen's duct. Lymphadenopathy and lymphadenitis can usually be differentiated on clinical grounds and anatomic location.

TREATMENT

In general, the treatment of mumps is entirely supportive. Antipyretic therapy with acetaminophen or ibuprofen should be instituted to control the fever if the temperature is greater than 100.4°F. Fluid intake should be closely monitored and adequate hydration maintained, especially if vomiting ensues. The choice of liquids is important because some patients will not tolerate certain items, such as citrus juices. A diet that contains bland food and includes the liberal administration of the appropriate fluids may be the one that is best tolerated.

Acetaminophen and ibuprofen can be used for the pain associated with parotid inflammation. The management of orchitis includes the use of stronger analgesics, such as codeine or meperidine (Demerol). Other measures that might supply relief include ice packs and support of the testes. Corticosteroids have not been proven to be efficacious, and more extreme interventions such as nerve block or surgery should be reserved for the most severe cases of orchitis. Although lumbar puncture is used as a diagnostic tool in patients with meningoencephalitis, it is often associated with immediate relief of the associated headache.

Because mumps is, in general, a mild infection associated with spontaneous recovery no specific therapy is indicated. In addition, no antiviral agent effectively suppresses viral replication. The very nature of the disease makes the use of antibiotics inappropriate. Immunotherapy with live virus vaccine is ineffective in altering the course of acute disease, as is the use of pooled antibody products such as intravenous immunoglobulin. Mumps immune globulin is no longer available.

Prevention is the key to a continued decline in the annual incidence of mumps. Currently, mumps vaccine, which is live attenuated virus, is administered with measles and rubella vaccines at 12 to 15 months of age, with a second dose given between 4 and 6 years of age. Adults who have not had mumps or mumps vaccine should be immunized.

OTITIS EXTERNA

method of
HARLAN R. MUNTZ, M.D.
Washington University School of Medicine
St. Louis, Missouri

Otitis externa is an inflammatory process of the external auditory canal. The special anatomy of the ear canal predisposes to disease. The outer ear is a complex structure of convoluted cartilage covered with an exceptionally thin skin. This unique architecture allows for its delicate beauty. This form is carried into the ear canal.

The cartilage of the pinna forms the lateral aspect of the canal. The medial portion is formed by bone. As in the pinna, the covering skin is very thin and has little subcutaneous tissue. The skin appendages of the lateral canal include not only hair follicles and sweat glands but also specialized eccrine glands to form cerumen. The loose attachment of the pinna to the side of the head affords flexibility in the pinna and hence in the lateral ear canal. Typically at the junction of the cartilaginous and bony ear canal is an isthmus, or narrowed area. At this point there is a definite change in the character of the skin to a thinner epithelium with a loss of normal appendages.

The ear canal is self-cleaning. The squamous debris from the skin lining the tympanic membrane through the ear canal migrates laterally. This joins the cerumen and is carried to the meatus. If this process is impeded, debris accumulates, and the risk of inflammation increases.

The tympanic membrane is the most medial aspect of the ear canal. This trilaminar membrane separates the external auditory canal from the middle ear cleft. It is composed of skin laterally, mucosa medially, and a fibrous central layer. In its healthy form it is nearly translucent. The landmarks of the middle ear should be observed through the membrane. The tympanic membrane should be mobile with the application of positive or negative pressure (pneumotoscopy).

Classic otitis externa is commonly referred to as "swimmer's ear." There are, however, many important inflammatory disease processes in the external ear canal, which are discussed as well. These may be mistaken for a classic otitis externa or are characterized by similar symptoms and must be considered in the differential diagnosis. This chapter briefly elucidates these.

INFECTION

The classic otitis externa process is a skin infection caused by organisms growing in the dark, moist environment of the ear canal. Water exposure usually precedes the infection, with retention of moisture in the external auditory canal and a subsequent overgrowth of bacteria. The most common organisms include *Pseudomonas* species and *Staphylococcus aureus*. The initial phase of inflammation causes increased accumulation of debris in the ear canal. The edema and further inflammation leads to intense otalgia as the periosteum of the ear canal bone is affected. The erythema and edema can affect even the skin of the tympanic membrane, causing the tympanic membrane to appear opacified, which is suggestive of an acute otitis media even in the absence of that process. If the disease progresses, the canal becomes obstructed by edematous soft tissue, which further impedes clearance of debris and increases purulence. The pain is excruciating, especially on touching or pulling of the pinna.

The diagnosis is made by finding (1) the swollen, inflamed external auditory canal, (2) debris in the canal, and (3) the characteristic ear pain. Postauricular edema and erythema may also be present with otitis externa even though true mastoiditis is not present.

TREATMENT

Treatment of the otitis externa is focused on removal of the debris and topical application of the appropriate antibiotic ear drop. A combination of neomycin, polymyxin, and hydrocortisone (Cortisporin) is classically used: a steroid to reduce edema and two antibiotics to combat the infection. Other drops have been useful and are receiving greater acceptance. These include the aminoglycosides gentamicin (Garamycin) and tobramycin (Tobrex), usually in an ophthalmologic preparation, and the fluoroquinolones, such as ciprofloxacin (Ciloxan) and ofloxacin (Floxin). Occasionally, an acidic solution such as acetic acid (VōSol) can be used, although it may be less tolerated. The drop therapy should be continued until the patient has been free of symptoms for at least 5 days. Occasionally, a broad-spectrum oral antibiotic may be helpful if there is a large degree of cellulitis. Controversy exists in using potentially ototoxic drops in the presence of a perforated tympanic membrane.

Pain control is imperative. Repeated débridement may be necessary. If the edema precludes delivery of drops to the medial ear canal, a wick should be placed through the edematous ear canal. As the edema subsides, the wick either will fall out or may be removed at a subsequent setting. The patient should restrict swimming. Bathing is permitted if water exposure to the ear is eliminated with an occlusive plug.

In the patient with brittle diabetes or who is immunocompromised, otitis externa can be a deadly complication. The process called malignant otitis externa may seem rather benign apart from granulation in the ear canal near the bone-cartilage junction. Deep, severe ear pain accompanies this *Pseudomonas* infection. Osteomyelitis of the temporal bone is common. Aggressive treatment with intravenous and topical antipseudomonal agents for at least 6 weeks is necessary to ensure control. Removal of the granulation tissue and debris is necessary on at least a daily basis. Strict control of diabetes and intervention if possible to reverse the immunodeficiency assists in the control of this severe infection. Although the infection is life-threatening, aggressive treatment has significantly reduced the rate of mortality from this process.

Fungal otitis externa usually manifests with itching in the ear canal. Diagnosis may be made from culture, but the characteristic hyphae with or without spore formation are often seen at microscopic evaluation of the ear. The fungus seems to reside in the ear canal debris and cerumen. Treatment includes both débridement of the fungus and topical ear drops. The acetic acid solutions such as VōSol are very effective, as are antifungal drops such as clotrimazole (Lotrimin).

A herpes zoster infection may manifest with external ear lesions and is associated with facial paralysis. This complex is called the Ramsay Hunt syndrome. Early treatment with steroids may assist in resolution of the facial paralysis. Antimicrobial drops can be used to reduce problems with superinfection.

Dermatitis

Occasionally, inflammation in the ear canal is a result of a dermatitis instead of infection. An allergic or contact dermatitis often results from a reaction to the topical treatment with ear drops or other irritants. If this happens, the drops should be discontinued or the irritant eliminated. One can use a non-antibiotic drop such as acetic acid with a systemic antibiotic for infection. A steroid cream or drop may be used to reduce the inflammation. The differential diagnosis includes pemphigus, scleroderma, and cancer of the ear canal. Biopsy may be necessary if there is no prompt resolution.

Other Lesions

Chronic ear drainage must be evaluated carefully. Cholesteatoma of the ear canal or of the tympanic membrane and middle ear can manifest with chronic suppuration and formation of granulation or polyp. A first branchial cleft sinus with an ear canal opening may result in chronic discharge. Failure of the self-cleaning aspect of the ear canal may result in a process called keratosis obturans in which the squamous debris is retained in the ear canal, forming a cholesteatoma-like mass. Microscopic evaluation of the ear canal and tympanic membrane is necessary to establish the diagnosis.

PLAGUE

method of
GARY SIMPSON, M.D., Ph.D, M.P.H.
New Mexico Department of Health
Santa Fe, New Mexico

Plague is an acute, febrile, and often fatal disease caused by the gram-negative bacillus *Yersinia pestis*. Human infection results primarily from the bites of infected rodent fleas. The incubation period is 2 to 8 days after the flea bite, and the clinical course can be rapidly fatal without prompt, appropriate antimicrobial chemotherapy. Plague is also a historic disease: in the mid-14th century it was known as the "Black Death" and caused the deaths of one fourth of the population of Europe (an estimated 25 million persons). Although plague is endemic in many areas of the world (especially Asia and Africa), it is predominantly restricted in North America to the western, and most specifically southwestern, United States. From 1944 through 1994, approximately 90% of the nearly 400 cases of human plague in the United States were reported from four west-

ern states: Arizona, California, Colorado, and New Mexico. During each successive decade of this period, the number of states reporting cases has increased from 3 (during 1944 to 1953) to 13 (during 1984 to 1993), indicating the spread of human plague infection eastward to areas where cases previously had not been reported. The ecology and the epidemiology of plague transmission are complex, and they differ for the epidemic urban form and the sporadic sylvatic form of disease transmission.

In the United States, plague is a seasonal sporadic infection concentrated in endemic, sylvatic foci throughout the Southwest, with ground squirrels, prairie dogs, and wood rats being important natural reservoirs. Although human infection can result from direct contact with infected wild rodents or hares, approximately 85% of human infections are associated with bites of infected rodent fleas. Of note, 60% of plague cases occur in persons younger than 20 years of age, and attack rates are disproportionally high in Native Americans living in endemic areas. Other groups at higher risk of exposure include hikers, hunters, and campers, but domestic pets (especially dogs and cats) can provide exposure risks by returning infected rodents or infected fleas to their owners or by becoming infectious risks themselves (e.g., pneumonic plague in domestic cats).

CLINICAL FEATURES

Plague can present as any one or a combination of the following syndromes. Classic bubonic plague has a distinctive clinical presentation, described by sudden onset of fever, chills, and headache, followed shortly by the appearance of exquisitely painful, localized lymphadenitis (bubo). Buboes are ovoid swellings, ranging from 1 to 10 cm, with edema and erythema of overlying tissues frequently present. The majority of buboes are found in the groin (femoral and inguinal), but bubonic plague may present in the axillary and cervical or epitrochlear regions. Gastrointestinal symptoms including nausea, vomiting, abdominal pain, and diarrhea are common. The liver and spleen may be tender and enlarged. Bubonic plague can progress from first onset of symptoms to rapid clinical deterioration and death in 2 to 4 days. In septicemic plague, bacilli disseminate rapidly from the initial focus of infection, resulting in the syndrome of septicemic plague. By definition, septicemic plague presents as fever and hypertension but without bubo, in contrast to bubonic plague with septicemia. The importance of this distinction is highlighted by the observation that 25% of all cases of plague occurring over a 5-year period in New Mexico, a state with a high prevalence of plague, were, in fact, the septicemic form. The case-fatality rate was 33%, even in a region where physicians are unusually sensitized to the possibility of human plague infections.

A remarkable feature of plague sepsis is high-density bacteremia, which premorbidly can reach concentrations of thousands of bacilli per milliliter of blood. Hematogenous dissemination of organisms to the lung with resultant, secondary pneumonia (pneumonic plague) is associated with mortality in excess of 75%. Plague transmitted by aerosols is highly contagious. Individuals exposed to the pneumonic form reportedly have become ill and died of primary inhalation plague pneumonia all in a single day. Unusual manifestations of plague infections include vesicular eruptions, eschar or ecthyma gangrenosum associated with a bubo, and a meningeal form usually seen as a late complication of inadequately treated bubonic plague. Risk of transmission of plague to close contacts (e.g., family, medical personnel) is related to exposure to respiratory aerosols from patients with pneumonia and to blood through needlesticks or aerosols in patients with high-density bacteremia.

From this discussion, it follows that the diagnosis of plague must be considered in certain clinical settings. If a patient has been in a plague-endemic region (New Mexico, Arizona, Utah, Colorado, or California) in the previous 10 to 14 days during the seasonal period of March to November and was exposed to rodents or mammals, plague must be included in the differential diagnosis of the following clinical manifestations:

Sudden onset of fever and painful, localized unilateral lymphadenitis
Clinical sepsis in an individual without obvious focus of infection or without underlying conditions predisposing to sepsis
Any community-acquired, gram-negative pneumonia

The differential, clinical diagnosis of bubonic plague includes staphylococcal and streptococcal lymphadenitis, tularemia, incarcerated inguinal hernia, acute appendicitis, cat-scratch disease, and sepsis of unknown origin.

DIAGNOSIS

A high index of suspicion in the context of the clinical settings just outlined leads to the timely diagnosis of plague. Routine laboratory evaluation will typically reveal an elevated white blood cell count (in the range of 10,000 to 20,000 cells per mm^3) with neutrophil predominance, thrombocytopenia, and elevated serum aminotransferase levels.

The bacteriologic diagnosis is made by smear and routine culture of a bubo aspirate, blood, sputum, or cerebrospinal fluid. Because the bubo does not contain pus, it may be necessary to inject sterile saline into it. Much care, including a mask and gloves for the clinician, is required in obtaining the specimens because of the highly contagious nature of Y. pestis. Also, the clinical laboratory should be notified if plague is suspected. A sample of the aspirate should be placed on microscopic slides and air dried. Gram stain will reveal gram-negative coccobacilli, and Wayson stain will demonstrate light blue bacilli with dark blue, bipolar staining. Blood cultures are positive in as many as 80% of cases but may become positive only after 2 to 3 days of incubation. A specific, direct fluorescent antibody assay is available through public health reference laboratories. A passive hemagglutination serologic test is also available.

TREATMENT

The successful treatment of plague is directly related to the timely institution of appropriate, empirical antimicrobial therapy. The mortality of untreated bubonic plague is estimated to be 50 to 60%, whereas early and effective antimicrobial therapy may decrease case-fatality rates to less than 10%. Streptomycin, 30 mg/kg body weight per day, given in two divided daily doses intramuscularly is the therapy of choice. Other aminoglycosides (e.g., gentamicin) have demonstrated in vitro activity, but cumulative clinical experience is limited. For septic patients or those with meningitis, intravenous administration of chloramphenicol is recommended at a loading dose of 25 mg per kg, followed by 60 mg per kg per day in four divided doses. Completion of a 10-day course of therapy is important to prevent relapse. Tetracycline is an effective oral agent and can be used to complete a 10-day course of therapy, after initial response to parenteral treatment. The dosage is 30 to 40 mg per kg per day in four divided doses (to a maximum of 2 grams per day). Specifically, penicillins, cephalosporins and macrolide antimicrobial agents are inadequate to treat human plague. All North American Y. pestis isolates have been shown to be uniformly susceptible to these antimicrobial agents. Notably, however, one report has described plasmid-mediated, multidrug resistance in Y. pestis isolated from a patient in Madagascar.

Clinical response to appropriate antimicrobial therapy is usually evident in 2 to 3 days, although fevers may persist for several days. Buboes may continue to enlarge despite optimal antimicrobial therapy and may remain swollen and tender weeks after successful treatment.

PREVENTION

Hospitalized, suspect plague cases should be placed in strict respiratory isolation until the possibility of pneumonic involvement has been excluded. Active surveillance for febrile illness should be maintained for 8 days for family members and close contacts of an index case. Contacts of patients with pneumonic plague should receive prophylaxis with tetracycline, or doxycycline, for 7 days. Trimethoprim-sulfamethoxazole (Bactrim, Septra) is an acceptable alternative chemoprophylaxis in children and pregnant women. A formalin-fixed vaccine is available for persons with high-risk, occupational exposures, including laboratory personnel.

Persons, particularly children, living in endemic areas should avoid contact with wild rodents, carnivores, and animal carcasses during summer months. Control measures to minimize rodent harborage in dwellings and outbuildings should be followed. Importantly, flea control should be rigorously practiced for household dogs and cats.

All suspect plague cases should be reported immediately to local and state public health authorities to facilitate diagnostic efforts and to manage contact investigations and chemoprophylaxis, when appropriate. Assistance can also be obtained from the Plague Branch Center for Disease Control and Prevention in Ft. Collins, Colorado.

PSITTACOSIS
(Ornithosis)

method of
THOMAS C. QUINN, M.D.
Johns Hopkins University School of Medicine
Baltimore, Maryland

Psittacosis is primarily a disease of birds caused by *Chlamydia psittaci*, and humans become infected through direct exposure to infected birds. The disease is therefore solely a zoonosis and is seen primarily in people with direct contact with birds, such as pet shop owners and employees, poultry workers, pigeon fanciers, falconers, taxidermists, veterinarians, and abattoir workers. Anyone in contact with an infected bird or animal is at risk. Human cases occur both sporadically and as outbreaks. Psittacosis attracted considerable attention as a result of a pandemic in 1929 to 1930. In the preantibiotic era, the case fatality rate approached 20%. Psittacosis is now recognized as an occupational hazard to those exposed to infected turkeys in poultry processing plants. C. psittaci is also an important pathogen in domestic mammals, causing a number of conditions, such as abortion and arthritis, that have considerable economic impact.

Chlamydia organisms are obligate intracellular bacteria that consist of four species: C. trachomatis, C. pneumoniae, C. psittaci, and C. pecorum. They are differentiated from other bacteria by their unique developmental cycle, which involves two morphologic forms: the elementary body, a metabolically inert form that is adapted to extracellular survival, and the reticulate body, a metabolically active form that replicates intracellularly by binary fission. C. psittaci infects primarily the upper respiratory tract and eventually disseminates to the reticuloendothelial cells of the spleen and liver. Invasion of the lung probably takes place by way of the bloodstream rather than through a direct extension from the upper air passages. Histologically, the infected areas of the alveolar spaces are filled with fluid, erythrocytes, and lymphocytes. The respiratory epithelium of the bronchi usually remains intact, whereas more infiltration is present within the alveoli and in the reticuloendothelial system of the liver and spleen.

Infected birds may be asymptomatic or severely ill. Infected birds may exhibit anorexia, emaciation, dyspnea, and diarrhea, frequently with closed eyes and ruffled feathers. The infection in the birds may spontaneously relapse or remit, although it is during periods of illness that the birds excrete large numbers of organisms. Discharge from their beaks and eyes, as well as from feces and urine, are all infective, and the feathers and the dust around their cages become contaminated. Humans become infected by the respiratory route, by direct contact, or by aerosolization of infected discharges or dust. Although most human exposure comes from birds, mammals also become infected. Disease has occurred in ranchers after exposure to infected cows, goats, and sheep. Abortion in sheep has been followed by abortion in women who assist in lambing, and endocarditis has occurred with both avian and nonavian strains. Human-to-human transmission is rare, and isolation of infected patients is not required.

CLINICAL MANIFESTATIONS

The clinical manifestations of psittacosis are extremely variable. The incubation period is 5 to 15 days after exposure. The onset may be either insidious or abrupt, and the clinical manifestations may be nonspecific. Fever is present in nearly all cases and may be as high as 40°C (104°F). Headache is almost always present and associated with a nonproductive cough, but the cough frequently appears 3 to 5 days after onset of fever. The patient may complain of myalgia, arthralgias, lethargy, mental depression, agitation, insomnia, and disorientation. Gastrointestinal complaints include abdominal pain, nausea, vomiting, and diarrhea.

Clinical signs most frequently reported are fever, pharyngeal erythema, rales, and hepatosplenomegaly. The pulse rate is slow in relation to the fever. Hepatosplenomegaly in patients with acute pneumonitis should suggest the possibility of psittacosis. Jaundice is a rare but ominous finding reflecting severe hepatic involvement. A faint macular rash referred to as Horder's spots simulate the rose spots of typhoid fever. Other dermatologic lesions are erythema multiforme, erythema marginatum, erythema nodosum, and urticaria.

Cardiac complications may include pericarditis, occasionally with effusion and tamponade; myocarditis; and culture-negative endocarditis. In cases of endocarditis, Chlamydia organisms have been demonstrated histologically in both aortic and mitral valves and grown from the blood. Thrombophlebitis is not unusual, and pulmonary infarction has been reported in rare instances. Neurologic consequences include cranial nerve palsy, cerebellar involvement, transverse myelitis, confusion, meningitis, encephalitis, transient focal neurologic signs, and seizures. Cerebrospinal fluid is usually normal, but a small number of white cells, predominantly lymphocytes, may be seen, and the protein may be elevated.

The white blood cell count is usually normal or slightly elevated with an increase in lymphocytes. Hepatic enzymes may be elevated in 50% of cases. Chest radiographs often show an infiltrate, usually confined to a single lower lobe, that is usually patchy in appearance but can be hazy, diffuse, homogeneous, lobar, atelectatic, wedge-shaped, nodular, or miliary.

DIAGNOSIS

Diagnosis of psittacosis should be considered in anyone with pneumonia or a severe systemic illness who has had a history of contact with birds. The differential diagnosis is extensive and depends on the manifestation. The typhoidal picture is suggestive of one of the etiologies of the mononucleosis syndrome, typhoid fever, brucellosis, tularemia, influenza, and subacute bacterial endocarditis. Respiratory signs and symptoms plus headache and myalgias are suggestive of etiologies of atypical pneumonia such as viral pneumonia; Q fever; Legionella, Mycoplasma, or Chlamydia pneumoniae pneumonia; or miliary tuberculosis. Helpful clues to psittacosis when present are relative bradycardia, rash, and hepatosplenomegaly. The diagnosis is confirmed by isolation of the causative microorganism or by serologic studies. C. psittaci is difficult to isolate and requires tissue culture in an experienced laboratory. Serologic diagnosis is confirmed by a fourfold increase in titer to at least 1:32 on a complement fixation assay. An acute specimen and a convalescent specimen should always be tested. C. trachomatis, C. psittaci, and C. pneumoniae share a common genus-specific group antigen that can cross-react serologically, which is a problem because C. pneumoniae is a more common cause of pneumonia. A microimmunofluorescent test can help differentiate antibody to each of the three species, and polymerase chain reaction of sputum can help detect and rapidly differentiate all three species, but both assays are available only in research laboratories at this time.

TREATMENT

The preferred treatment for adults with psittacosis is doxycycline (Vibramycin), 100 mg twice daily, or tetracycline, 500 mg four times a day for 10 to 21 days. Azithromycin* (Zithromax), 500 mg the first

_____
*Not FDA approved for this indication.

day followed by 250 mg daily thereafter for 10 days, or clarithromycin* (Biaxin), 250 to 500 mg twice daily for 2 weeks, may be efficacious, although there is little experience with these agents. Erythromycin,* 500 mg, four times daily, is an alternative treatment, but it is less effective than the tetracyclines. Penicillins, cephalosporins, and sulfonamides are ineffective. With appropriate treatment, patients generally improve within 24 to 48 hours, and the rate of mortality among untreated patients has dropped to less than 1%.

Preventive measures should include quarantine and long-term antibiotic prophylaxis for all imported birds. Many birds, however, are imported without adequate antibiotics. All cases of psittacosis should be reported and fully investigated, and all ill birds should be treated with antibiotics.

---

*Not FDA approved for this indication.

Q FEVER

method of
THOMAS J. MARRIE, M.D.
Dalhousie University
Halifax, Nova Scotia, Canada

Q fever is the illness that results from infection by the rickettsial organism *Coxiella burnetii*. This zoonosis is widely distributed in nature, but the main reservoirs for transmission of the organism to humans are infected cattle, sheep, goats, cats, and occasionally dogs. *C. burnetii* undergoes reactivation during pregnancy, and the placenta of an infected animal is heavily colonized. The organism is shed in large amounts into the environment at the time of parturition. Humans become infected after inhaling the microorganisms. The incubation period ranges from 4 to 30 days and is usually 2 weeks.

The most common manifestations of this infection are a self-limited febrile illness; atypical pneumonia (which ranges from mild to severe and includes a rapidly progressive form); hepatitis; and chronic Q fever, manifested mainly as endocarditis. In rare cases, Q fever complicates human pregnancy.

SUPPORTIVE TREATMENT

The severe headache that is part of Q fever often necessitates use of analgesics. Fever may persist for up to 10 days, although usually it lasts for only 3 to 4 days. During this period, antipyretics are useful. In some patients, parenteral fluid therapy is necessary to correct dehydration. Valve replacement may be necessary in patients with Q fever endocarditis.

SPECIFIC THERAPY

In 1962, it was demonstrated that the administration of tetracycline to patients with Q fever during the first 3 days of the illness reduced the duration of fever by 50%. In spite of this observation, tetracycline

has no activity against *C. burnetii* in an infected fibroblast cell line. In this setting, rifampin, difloxacin, and ciprofloxacin are most active. Clarithromycin and doxycycline were active against *C. burnetii* when tested in infected tissue culture.

Our approach is to treat patients with severe pneumonia (when Q fever is considered likely) with both a respiratory fluoroquinolone (levofloxacin* [Levaquin], trovafloxacin [Trovan], or sparfloxacin [Zagam]) and rifampin (Rifadin). For adults, we use 300 mg of rifampin* (Rifadin, Rimactane) every 12 hours for the first 72 hours and then 300 mg once daily to complete a 10-day course of treatment. This approach also allows us to treat most etiologic agents of severe pneumonia, such as *Mycoplasma pneumoniae, Legionella pneumophila,* and *Streptococcus pneumoniae.* For patients who cannot tolerate rifampin, doxycycline, 100 mg every 12 hours, is used.

Patients with endocarditis (chronic Q fever) exhibit the features of culture-negative endocarditis and have phase I titers that are severalfold higher than phase II titers, a situation that we have never found in acute Q fever. Controversy exists as to the proper treatment for Q fever endocarditis. We start therapy with ciprofloxacin* (Cipro), 750 mg orally every 12 hours, and rifampin,* 600 mg orally every day. These medications are continued for at least 3 years. During this period, the phase I and phase II antibody titers should be monitored every 3 months. We discontinue therapy when the phase I IgG titer has declined to 1:512 or less according to the indirect fluorescent antibody technique. (Some authorities recommend continuing therapy indefinitely.) If ciprofloxacin cannot be tolerated, we prescribe doxycycline (Vibramycin), 100 mg orally two times a day. Other fluoroquinolones such as levofloxacin and trovafloxacin could probably be used instead of ciprofloxacin, although there is little experience with their use in this setting. Patients with Q fever endocarditis need careful follow-up, and valve replacement is frequently necessary for hemodynamic reasons.

PREVENTION

All cattle, sheep, and goats used in research laboratories should be serologically tested for *C. burnetii* before being admitted to the facility. Several outbreaks of Q fever have occurred when infected animals have been brought into research institutions.

VACCINATION

A phase I vaccine has proved to be effective in Australia. When available, this vaccine should be offered to persons at high risk for infection, such as veterinarians, abattoir workers, livestock dealers and transporters, auctioneers, bulk milk transporters, and meat inspectors.

---

*Not FDA approved for this indication.

RABIES*

method of
LISA D. ROTZ, M.D., and
CHARLES E. RUPPRECHT, V.M.D., PH.D.

National Center for Infectious Diseases
Centers for Disease Control and Prevention
Atlanta, Georgia

Rabies, one of the oldest recognized zoonoses, was documented in ancient Mesopotamia and Egypt thousands of years ago. Today, although many developed countries have successfully controlled domestic animal rabies, the disease remains a major health risk for people in many of the world's underdeveloped nations. Although no effective treatment for clinical rabies exists, prompt and appropriate prophylaxis after exposure to rabies almost always prevents the development of the disease.

The worldwide magnitude of human rabies fatalities is essentially unknown, partly because of inadequate resources for surveillance and laboratory diagnosis and partly because of the reluctance of persons with rabies to seek medical care because of the social stigma associated with the disease. Approximately 50,000 to 100,000 cases of rabies in humans may occur worldwide each year, which represent approximately 5 to 10 times the number of reported cases. Only a fraction of the reported cases of human rabies occur outside of the tropic and subtropic regions. In developed countries, evaluation of exposure for rabies prophylaxis, control of stray animals, animal quarantine, and domestic animal vaccination have a much greater economic and emotional impact than does the overt mortality caused by the disease itself.

EPIDEMIOLOGY

Some geographic regions, particularly islands, including Antarctica, New Zealand, and Pacific Oceania, are free of indigenous rabies. Other areas, including the United Kingdom, Scandinavia, Japan, and a few locations in the Americas, have achieved secondary elimination. Aggressive control measures, focused on both domestic animals and wildlife, have successfully eliminated rabies in these countries, and strict international importation, vaccination, or quarantine regulations have prevented its return thus far.

All mammals are likely susceptible to rabies, but with different sensitivities. Natural reservoirs belong to the Carnivora or Chiroptera, but rabies spillover into other mammalian species, such as livestock, usually results in a dead-end infection. Animals in a specific geographic area are typically infected by a distinct variant of rabies virus, as documented by monoclonal antibody and genetic sequencing studies.

Rabies is enzootic regionally in the United States among wildlife, such as skunks, foxes, and bats, and has been epizootic in raccoons in the eastern states and in coyotes in Texas. Domestic, free-ranging dogs are among the animals that pose the greatest risk of rabies transmission in the developing world, together with wolves, jackals, and mongooses. Although cats are clearly capable of transmitting rabies, they do not appear to maintain the disease as a primary reservoir. Feline rabies cases often outnumber dog rabies cases in areas where canine rabies has been largely controlled through induced herd immunity with vaccination. Rodents, rabbits, and opossums are rarely rabid, and infections in such animals have not been documented in association with a case of human rabies. Knowledge of which animal species are reservoirs for rabies in a geographic region is important in assessing the probability of disease transmission to humans after a bite by an animal.

With the exception of eight human-to-human transmission cases caused by corneal transplantation, infected animals are the primary sources of all recent documented human rabies cases. From 1980 through 1998, there were 37 cases of human rabies diagnosed in the United States; 14 of these cases were associated with a canine variant of the virus, including 12 in which the infection was acquired abroad, where canine rabies is enzootic.

In the United States, bats have become the most common source of rabies transmission to humans in recent years. The bat variant of rabies virus has accounted for 22 (59%) of the 37 cases of human rabies since 1980; 17 (77%) of these bat-associated cases have occurred since 1992. The majority (73%) of the bat-related cases have been associated with the silver-haired/eastern pipistrelle bat variant of the virus (16 of 22 cases since 1980). A single bat-related case was associated with a definite bite, and only 10 of the cases had a history of bat contact. This suggests either an unawareness of the risks associated with an untreated bat bite or the possibility that minimal bite exposure may go unrecognized but may be sufficient for virus transmission from bats infected with rabies. Indeed, laboratory studies with the silver-haired/eastern pipistrelle bat rabies virus variant suggest that it may be transmitted more easily than are other variants.

Although raccoon rabies has become an increasing problem in the mid-Atlantic and northeastern United States, no cases of human rabies to date have been associated with this particular virus variant. As most bites from raccoons are treated promptly with postexposure prophylaxis (PEP), the greatest danger to humans from the raccoon rabies epizootic appears to be from spillover into the unvaccinated or improperly vaccinated domestic animal population.

MOLECULAR VIROLOGY

All variants of rabies virus are bullet-shaped, membrane-bound, single-stranded, negative-sense RNA viruses that belong to the Rhabdoviridae family, genus *Lyssavirus*. Monoclonal antibody and genetic sequence studies have demonstrated significant variation between strains of lyssaviruses. Besides rabies virus, at least six other lyssavirus genotypes (Mokola, Lagos bat, Duvenhage, two subtypes of European bat virus, and a recently recognized Australian lyssavirus associated with bats), all Old World in distribution, are known to cause the disease. All of these lyssaviruses are associated with an acute encephalitis; however, it is unclear whether these different strains cause otherwise distinct clinical manifestations. Although there is considerable antigenic variation among the lyssaviruses of major public health significance, studies suggest adequate cross-reactivity against most lyssaviruses as a result of PEP with rabies immune globulin (RIG) and modern potent cell culture vaccines.

Analysis of the molecular structure of the virus has revealed an inner nucleocapsid core of ribonucleoprotein and an outer surface glycoprotein. The exterior glycoprotein spikes are involved in attachment and fusion to nerve cells and are the targets of virus-neutralizing antibodies and

*All material in this article is in the public domain.

cytotoxic T lymphocytes. However, the internal proteins of the virus also play a role in induced immunity. The virus receptor molecules on nerve and muscle cells appear to be gangliosides, and the acetycholine receptor has been implicated.

PATHOGENESIS

The virus usually enters the host via contaminated saliva through breaks in the skin caused by a bite. Other rare routes of infection include contamination of lesions or mucous membranes (e.g., eyes, mouth, nose) with infectious material (saliva or nerve tissue), aerosolization of the virus in unusual situations in which large amounts of the virus are present (e.g., rabies laboratory accidents or, very rarely, bat-infested caves), and corneal transplants from infected persons. After transdermal inoculation, the virus undergoes a so-called eclipse phase lasting several hours to days, during which time it may replicate in muscle cells at the site of entry or invade the nervous system directly. The virus is vulnerable to host defenses and neutralization by specific antibodies during this period. Viremia does not occur to any significant extent.

Invasion of the virus into peripheral nerve tissue at the portal of entry initiates a sequence of events that will most likely lead to the death of the patient. If clearance does not occur, the virus may bind to specific receptors in the vicinity of peripheral nerves and ascend centripetally by retrograde axoplasmic flow to ganglia and into the central nuclei in the brain. Infection of the parenchyma is progressive, with the virus spreading to most parts of the brain, although there appears to be a predilection for the limbic system, the reticular formation, the pontine tegmentum, and the nuclei of the cranial nerves at the floor of the fourth ventricle.

Nonspecific microscopic lesions include perivascular infiltrates, neuronophagia, and gliosis. More specific eosinophilic, intracytoplasmic inclusions (Negri bodies) are identifiable in nerve cells at this stage and are pathognomonic of rabies. Histologic examination may detect spongiform encephalopathy, but there may be minimal inflammatory response and the absence of necrosis. The relative lack of structural neuronal damage in contrast to the profound encephalitic manifestations raises the issue of functional interference with neurotransmission as one potential pathogenic mechanism.

At the height of cerebral infection, the virus moves back to the peripheral nerves and centrifugally invades highly innervated areas such as the cornea, the skin (especially of the head and neck), the salivary glands, and the buccal mucous membranes. There is heightened secretion of the virus into saliva at a time when agitation and aggressive biting behavior may be present, which can increase the risk of viral transmission.

CLINICAL HUMAN RABIES

Although human rabies is rare in the United States, the differential diagnosis of any rapidly progressive viral encephalitis should include rabies, especially with a history of animal bite. The incubation period between exposure and the onset of disease is usually 30 to 90 days, but periods of less than 10 days and of more than a year have been documented. Bites to the head and neck or other highly innervated areas may result in a shorter incubation period. The disease typically progresses through a prodromal period of nonspecific symptoms to encephalopathy and death within 10 to 30 days of symptom onset. Local cutaneous symptoms may include paresthesia at the site of the exposure, probably caused by viral excitation of the sensory ganglia. Early nonspecific prodromal signs and symptoms may include lassitude, pharyngitis, anorexia, dysphagia, insomnia, cough, headache, fever, nausea, vomiting, and diarrhea. Patients who have developed rabies after corneal transplantation have also reported retro-ocular pain.

The acute period of disease follows the prodromal period by 2 to 10 days. This period may be characterized by a generalized increase in neurologic activity with agitation and aggressive behavior (agitated or "furious" rabies) or by an ascending symmetrical or asymmetrical paralysis, leading to respiratory failure and necessitating mechanical ventilation (paralytic or "dumb" rabies). The paralytic phase may also follow the agitated phase during the course of illness.

The most profound and characteristic clinical manifestations of the agitated stage are hydrophobia and aerophobia, exaggerated respiratory reflexes that result in violent contractions of the diaphragm and inspiratory accessory muscles triggered by attempts to swallow, the sight or sound of water, or air currents. Other clinical manifestations include choking, hypersalivation, and diplopia. There may be central nervous system excitation with anxiety, confusion, hallucinations, disorientation, photophobia, ataxia, and seizures. Autonomic dysfunction may result in labile hypertension, hyperventilation, priapism, panic attacks, palpitations, and hypothermia or hyperthermia. Ultimately, rabies culminates in coma and generalized multiorgan failure that almost inevitably leads to death.

LABORATORY DIAGNOSIS

Routine clinical laboratory test results are nonspecific. Computerized tomography and magnetic resonance imaging scans are also nondiagnostic because of the lack of inflammation and edema. The electroencephalographic patterns may reveal diffuse encephalitic and encephalopathic changes, but these findings are nonspecific for rabies.

Direct histologic and immunohistologic examinations of infected tissue, reverse transcription (RT) of viral RNA by polymerase chain reaction (PCR), or virus isolation from saliva or fresh neural tissue produces a definitive diagnosis of rabies. Specific antirabies antibody detected in cerebrospinal fluid, at any titer, is also diagnostic of rabies. Biopsy specimens of brain or skin from the neck area can be submitted for rabies antigen detection by immunofluorescent techniques or viral detection of nucleic acid by RT-PCR. Saliva (not sputum) can also be collected for rabies virus isolation or RT-PCR. A single positive test result for rabies antigen, nucleic acid, or viral isolation in brain, skin, or saliva samples has a high predictive value for rabies, and this result may be positive before serum antibody is detected. Serum neutralizing antibodies may develop within 1 to 2 weeks of the onset of the prodromal phase. Positive serum antibodies are diagnostic in patients who have not received RIG or previous rabies vaccination.

CLINICAL MANAGEMENT

Pre-exposure rabies prophylaxis is appropriate for high-risk groups, such as veterinarians, animal control officers, animal handlers, and rabies research, production, and diagnostic laboratory workers. In addition, any person who is likely to come into contact with potentially infected animals, such as spelunkers who spend time in bat caves or persons spending extended periods (>30 days) in countries with enzootic canine rabies (Africa, Asia, or Latin America) who may have inadequate access to modern biologic agents for PEP, should consider pre-exposure vaccination.

Pre-exposure prophylaxis in the United States consists of 1.0 mL of human diploid cell vaccine (HDCV; Immovax), purified chick embryo cell vaccine (PCEC; RabAvert), or rabies vaccine adsorbed (RVA), given intramuscularly (deltoid area) on days 0 (first day of treatment), 7, and 21 or 28 or 0.1 mL intradermally (HDCV only).* Booster doses are recommended on the basis of the results of serologic titers and the relative risk of continued exposure. For example, if the risk category is deemed continuous (such as with rabies laboratory workers), serologic tests should be conducted every 6 months and a booster dose administered when the virus-neutralizing antibody titer falls below an acceptable level. The period between serologic testing and booster administration extends to every 2 years for people in a category of frequent or common exposure. No routine serologic testing or booster administration is needed for those with an infrequent risk, such as workers in an area of low rabies activity. Pre-exposure vaccination simplifies PEP management by obviating the need for costly RIG and may provide some degree of protection from inapparent exposures.

When a person is bitten by an animal, the possibility of rabies should be addressed. The first step in evaluating the need for PEP in a patient with an animal bite is to determine whether the bite constitutes a risk for rabies. If the bite was from an animal species that is essentially rabies free in the wild (birds, cold-blooded vertebrates, or invertebrates), the patient should receive appropriate wound care and tetanus vaccination with reassurance that no specific rabies prophylaxis is required. In addition, bites by most rodents and lagomorphs (rabbits and hares) almost never necessitate PEP. If the bite or injury was caused by a domestic, rabies-prone animal, PEP should be initiated if the animal (domestic dog, cat, or ferret) has been observed and demonstrates signs of rabies (either initially or within a 10-day observation period), if the animal has been euthanized and the brain specimen is positive for rabies infection, or if the animal is highly suspected of being rabid but is unavailable for observation or testing. No PEP is necessary if the dog, cat, or ferret remains healthy over a 10-day observation period or if the brain material is negative for rabies. Recommendations regarding PEP may be made on a case-by-case basis and depend in part on the circumstances of the bite, the rabies vaccination history and husbandry of the animal, and the local epidemiology of the disease. Suspected wildlife should be euthanized and tested for rabies, because there is no recommended observation period. Rabies PEP should also be started immediately if the wound-inflicting wild

carnivore or bat is unavailable for testing. Because minor bite exposure to a bat may be sufficient for virus transmission, PEP may be administered in instances in which a bat is physically present and exposure cannot be reasonably excluded (e.g., persons sleeping in a room where a bat was found, an intoxicated or mentally impaired person, or a very young child present in a room with a bat), unless the bat can be submitted for laboratory diagnosis and is found negative for evidence of rabies virus infection. Consultation with local public health officials familiar with regional rabies epidemiology is highly encouraged in all cases of potential exposure.

Rabies PEP, when performed promptly and properly according to the following protocol, has been extremely successful in preventing human rabies:

1. While wearing gloves, thoroughly washing the wound with soap and water to remove residual saliva and devitalized tissue.
2. Administering human RIG (Hyperab, Imogam), 20 IU per kg, locally around the wound or wounds. If administration of the total dose of human RIG around the wounds is anatomically impossible, the remaining dose should be administered intramuscularly at a location away from the vaccine administration site.
3. Administering 1.0 mL of HDCV, PCEC, or RVA in the deltoid muscle on days 0, 3, 7, 14, and 28, day 0 being the first day of treatment.
4. For previously vaccinated patients, administering 1.0 mL of HDCV, PCEC, or RVA in the deltoid muscle on days 0 and 3; human RIG is unnecessary.

Although rabies PEP should begin as soon as possible after an exposure, patients at risk who appear for medical evaluation weeks to months after exposure should still receive PEP regardless of the length of the delay, as long as clinical signs of rabies are not present. After the development of clinical rabies, administration of PEP is no longer effective and will not alter the course of the disease.

Outside of the United States, several different schedules and routes for the use of alternative rabies virus vaccines (e.g., purified duck embryo cell vaccine,* purified Vero cell rabies vaccine* and purified equine RIG* or heterologous rabies antisera may be available. Vaccines prepared from nerve tissue should not be used unless absolutely necessary because of the risk of neuroparalytic complications.

Without PEP, the probability of developing rabies after the bite of a rabid animal depends in part on the location and severity of the wound and the dose of inoculated virus. Only eight people have been documented to have survived clinical rabies. All of these patients had previously received some type of pre-exposure treatment or PEP before the onset of symptoms, and all required prolonged supportive therapy, including mechanical ventilation. At least six had significant, permanent neurologic sequelae.

There is no effective antiviral treatment for clinical

---

*Use of trade names is for identification only and is not implied as endorsement by the U.S. Public Health Service.

*Not currently available for use in the United States.

rabies. The intraneuronal site of the infection is a barrier to the penetration of therapeutic agents. Limited trials with interferon-α have been unsuccessful, and steroids may cause a more rapid progression of disease and higher viral titers in the saliva. Supportive and symptomatic therapy may include mechanical ventilation, vasopressors, antiseizure medications, sedatives, analgesics, and neuroleptics.

INFECTION CONTROL

Rabies virus may enter the body through breaks in the skin, through intact mucous membranes, through inhalation as an aerosol, or by means of an infected corneal graft. Blood products and nonconcentrated urine do not constitute rabies exposure. The only recent confirmed cases of human-to-human transmission of rabies have been associated with corneal transplantation from an infected donor. There has never been a reported case of rabies transmission from a patient to a health care worker. Strict adherence to barrier methods to prevent contact with body fluids contact minimizes the chance of transmission and markedly reduces the need for PEP in health care providers.

The control and prevention of animal and human rabies is a great public health challenge for many areas of the world. Cost-effective prophylaxis must be made available for people who have suffered rabies-prone animal bites, and strict animal control measures and pre-exposure domestic animal vaccination need to be implemented. Bats should be safely barred from human dwellings. Oral rabies vaccines for free-ranging wildlife may provide an additional tool for rabies elimination worldwide.

RAT BITE FEVER

method of
MARYLENE J. EGHO, M.D.
Edward John Noble Hospital
Gouverneur, New York

Rat bite fever is an uncommon systemic illness caused by two organisms: *Streptobacillus moniliformis* and *Spirillum minus*. In the United States, the majority of cases are caused by *S. moniliformis,* whereas *S. minus* causes most of the cases in Asia. The disease is typically transmitted by the bite or scratch of a rat, but it has occurred after the bites of mice, gerbils, squirrels, and carnivores (such as cats, dogs, and weasels) that prey on rodents. The risk of developing the disease after a rat bite is 10%. In the United States, more than half of the cases occur in children younger than 12 years of age. Animal laboratory workers are also at risk of acquiring the disease.

CLINICAL MANIFESTATIONS

Streptobacillary rat bite fever has an incubation period of 2 to 10 days. The area of the bite is healing when the patient manifests fever, headache, myalgia, and general-

ized lymphadenopathy. A maculopapular or petechial rash over the extensor surfaces develops 1 to 8 days later; it typically involves the palms and soles. The rash desquamates in 20% of patients and may persist for 3 weeks. In more than 50% of cases, an asymmetrical migratory polyarthritis involving knees, elbows, ankles and shoulders develops in the first 2 weeks of the illness. Septic arthritis has also been reported. The fever usually resolves after 3 to 5 days but can recur at irregular intervals for weeks to months. Haverhill's fever is a rare epidemic form of the disease that occurs after the ingestion of food or water contaminated by rat secretions. Two large outbreaks have been reported, both of which resulted from consumption of infected milk. The manifestation of this disease is similar to that of rat bite fever except for an increased incidence of pharyngitis and severe vomiting.

Spirillary rat bite fever, also known as *sodoku,* has an incubation period of 1 to 4 weeks. Patients have a painful indurated lesion at the site of the bite that may form an eschar or may ulcerate. This lesion is often associated with lymphangitis and regional lymphadenitis. They also have relapsing fever, chills, headache, and a diffuse maculopapular rash. If untreated, the patient will experience recurrent fever with exacerbation of the rash for 3 to 8 weeks. In contrast to streptobacillary fever, arthritis and myalgia are not common.

Complications of both diseases include pericarditis, nephritis, myocarditis, epididymitis, pneumonia, and amnionitis. Abscesses have been found in many organs, including the brain, liver, spleen, and kidneys, and subcutaneously. Endocarditis is the most serious complication; it generally occurs in patients with pre-existing valvular disease. In young children, diarrhea and weight loss are prominent symptoms.

With a known exposure to a rat bite, the differential diagnosis of a febrile patient with a rash is limited to leptospirosis and rat bite fever. When an exposure is not identified, the diagnosis becomes elusive, and the differential diagnosis includes Rocky Mountain spotted fever, rheumatic diseases, vasculitis, disseminated gonococcemia, meningococcemia, secondary syphilis, drug reaction, viral exanthems, and Lyme disease.

BACTERIOLOGY AND DIAGNOSIS

S. moniliformis is a nonmotile, pleomorphic gram-negative rod that grows best in microaerophilic conditions. It has characteristic bulbous swellings and is arranged in chains and loosely tangled clumps. This organism is found in the nasopharynx and urine of more than 50% of healthy rats. The diagnosis is made by isolating the organism from the bite site, blood, joint fluid, or abscess. The growth of the organism is inhibited by the anticoagulant sodium polyanetholsulfonate (SPS) found in blood culture bottles. Thus if Q fever is suspected, blood specimens should be cultured in SPS-free or resin bottles. Optimal growth is achieved by enriching the media with 10 to 20% horse or rabbit serum and incubating the plates in a CO_2-enriched atmosphere. Gas-liquid chromatography yields a characteristic fatty acid profile of the organism, permitting rapid identification of the bacillus. Serologic tests for *S. moniliformis* are not available, and the slide agglutination test is no longer used.

S. minus is a short, spiral, gram-negative rod that cannot be isolated in culture media. Diagnosis is made by direct visualization of the spirochete in blood smears with Giemsa stain, Wright's stain, or darkfield microscopy. The organism can also be recovered in 1 to 3 weeks after intraperitoneal inoculation of mice or guinea pigs. About 25% of healthy rats carry the organism in their secretions. A false-positive syphilis serologic finding is obtained in 25% of streptobacillary cases and in 50% of spirillary cases. In both forms, anemia may be present, and the white blood cell count may vary from 10,000 to 30,000.

A high index of suspicion is crucial for making a diagnosis of rat bite fever. Alerting the laboratory about this diagnostic possibility will improve the yield of diagnostic tests.

TREATMENT

Penicillin is the drug of choice for both forms of rat bite fever. The recommended treatment is parenteral penicillin, 1.2 to 2.4 million units per day, followed by oral penicillin, 500 mg every 6 hours, for a 10- to 14-day course. In cases of endocarditis, 20 million units of penicillin G per day for 4 to 6 weeks should be given. Penicillin-resistant strains have been reported. In penicillin-allergic patients, tetracycline (500 mg every 6 hours) or streptomycin (7.5 mg per kg intramuscularly every 12 hours) are appropriate alternatives. Cephalosporins, clindamycin (Cleocin), and erythromycin have been used with some success. Among untreated cases of rat bite fever, the mortality rate is 10%. Deaths are usually from complications of endocarditis.

After a rodent bite, the wound should be cleaned thoroughly and tetanus prophylaxis should be administered. Although the efficacy of prophylactic antibiotics against rat bite fever remains unknown, it would be reasonable to recommend a 3-day course of penicillin (500 mg every 6 hours), and the patient should be advised to report to the physician if any symptoms develop.

RELAPSING FEVER

method of
NANCY E. MADINGER, M.D.
University of Colorado Health Sciences Center
Denver, Colorado

Relapsing fever is an acute, febrile illness caused by several different species of *Borrelia*. Spirochetes are transmitted by specific arthropod vectors, and organisms circulate within the bloodstream and the reticuloendothelial system. The disease is distinguished by the recurring nature of illness, in which several days of fever alternate with periods of apyrexia. This cyclical pattern corresponds to spirochetemia, clearance by the host immune response, antigenic shift of surface proteins to evade the immune system, and a return of spirochetemia. Recovery occurs when the immune response is sufficiently specific to eliminate the organisms.

Relapsing fever has been reported throughout the world except in Australia, New Zealand, and Micronesia. Although limited to specific regions, cases can occur in travelers who frequently develop symptoms outside of endemic areas. The nonspecific nature of the illness, coupled with geographic restriction of the arthropod vectors, undoubt-

edly contributes to lack of recognition and frequent delay in diagnosis.

ETIOLOGY

There are two forms of relapsing fever: louse-borne (epidemic) and tick-borne (endemic). Louse-borne relapsing fever (LBRF), caused by *Borrelia recurrentis*, is transmitted between humans by the human body louse, *Pediculus humanus humanus*. LBRF occurs in epidemics, typically after wars, famine, or other catastrophic conditions associated with crowding and poor hygiene. Lice become infected after a blood meal, and the organisms replicate within the hemolymph. *B. recurrentis* is transmitted to humans only when the lice are crushed onto skin (e.g., during scratching). LBRF is most often reported from Ethiopia and surrounding regions.

Endemic or tick-borne relapsing fever (TBRF) is caused by at least 15 *Borrelia* species. These borreliae infect small rodents such as mice, squirrels, and chipmunks, with the exception of *Borrelia duttonii* (East African TBRF) which is exclusive to humans. Soft (argasid) ticks belonging to the genus *Ornithodoros* become infected when feeding on their rodent hosts. Borreliae survive for years within the tick and are also transmitted transovarially. Humans become infected when they accidentally enter the tick habitat. *Ornithodoros* ticks feed only at night, and their painless bites usually go unnoticed.

In the United States, TBRF is limited to mountainous and semiarid plains west of the Mississippi River. *Borrelia hermsii*, *Borrelia turicatae*, and *Borrelia parkeri* are the causative organisms. Risk factors for infection include camping, sleeping in cabins or mountain homes, cleaning rodent-infested areas, handling old wood, and exploring caves. There is no seasonal variation of infection in warm climates. In temperate zones, cases predominate during warm months, although infections also occur during winter when dwellings are heated. Borreliae may also be transmitted through blood contamination, blood transfusion, intravenous drug use, and to laboratory personnel from clinical specimens or cultures.

CLINICAL MANIFESTATIONS

The clinical manifestations of TBRF and LBRF are indistinguishable, although LBRF is typically more severe. The incubation period is approximately 7 days. Fever and rigors begin abruptly, and the body temperature often reaches 104 to 106°F. Associated symptoms include headache, nausea, vomiting, diarrhea, cough, myalgias, arthralgias, eye pain, meningismus, febrile seizures, facial palsy, lethargy, and delirium. Although tachypnea and tachycardia are present during febrile periods, other findings such as hepatomegaly, splenomegaly, petechiae, macular rash, conjunctival suffusion, jaundice, hematuria, and iritis are variable. The white blood cell count is usually normal, although a left shift is common, as is thrombocytopenia. Elevations in liver transaminase and bilirubin levels and hematuria also occur.

Fever is usually present for 3 to 5 days and then resolves by acute worsening of symptoms (crisis). This corresponds to clearance of organisms from the bloodstream. After the crisis, systemic vascular resistance is decreased, and prolonged hypotension may occur. An intervening period of 7 to 9 days ensues, and then the 2- to 3-day febrile period recurs. Malaise and weakness may persist into the afebrile intervals. Relapses are typically less severe with each new episode of fever. The mean number of relapses is three; the range is one to five for LBRF and 0 to 13 for TBRF.

COMPLICATIONS

The principal causes of death are myocarditis, acute hepatic failure, gastrointestinal or central nervous system hemorrhage, disseminated intravascular coagulation, and the Jarisch-Herxheimer reaction (JHR; to be described). Death usually occurs during the hypotensive phase after the first crisis or JHR. The rate of mortality increases with extremes of age, with malnutrition, and/or with concomitant infection.

Relapsing fever is more severe during pregnancy. Pregnant women have a larger burden of circulating organisms, which may contribute to the severity of crisis or JHR. In addition, hemodynamic changes associated with fever and blood pressure fluctuations may be poorly tolerated, particularly during the last trimester. Preterm labor is common during febrile periods (80% in one study) and preterm delivery occurs in approximately one third of cases. Transplacental spread can lead to congenital infection.

The rate of mortality from untreated LBRF is 10 to 70%; with treatment, the rate is only about 5%. TBRF is fatal in 0 to 8% of cases, and death is almost always associated with comorbid conditions, pregnancy, or extremes of age. The rate of perinatal mortality is about 15%.

DIAGNOSIS

Diagnosis is made by observing spirochetes on a thick or thin smear obtained during a febrile period. In the past, borreliae were often found incidentally on the manual differential count. The *Borrelia* species associated with relapsing fever stain well with Romanowsky stains, such as Wright's, Giemsa, and Diff-Quick, as well as with silver-impregnation stains. Acridine orange has been used to facilitate screening of smears. Borreliae are highly motile and are visible on wet preparations viewed in dark field microscopy. Morphology is dependent on environmental conditions and cannot be used to speciate the organisms. Organisms may also be seen in cerebrospinal fluid and urine. The sensitivity of smears collected during a febrile period is about 70%. Serial smears may need to be collected.

Serologic tests are not helpful for diagnosis. Relapsing fever may cause false-positive results of the enzyme immunoassays used to diagnose Lyme disease. The Western blot pattern may help to distinguish between Lyme disease and TBRF. Culture of borreliae is limited to research laboratories.

The symptoms of relapsing fever are sufficiently vague to mimic numerous other diseases, although after several relapses the diagnosis should be obvious. Physicians must be aware of diseases endemic in their geographic region and maintain a high index of suspicion. In areas of overlapping endemicity, relapsing fever may be mistaken for malaria, typhus, yellow fever, dengue, meningitis, leptospirosis, and infectious hepatitis. TBRF has been attributed to mononucleosis, influenza, Q fever, bacterial sepsis, Colorado tick fever, acute abdominal infections, pneumonia, and Lyme disease. The Division of Vector-Borne Infectious Diseases (Centers for Disease Control and Prevention) assists physicians with diagnosis of borrelial infections.

TREATMENT

Patients should be admitted to the hospital for treatment or held in an observation area for the first 24 hours. Vascular access should be established and intravenous fluids administered if evidence of volume depletion is present. In regions of high endemicity in which partial immunity may be present, outpatient treatment is appropriate for some patients. If resources are limited, children and pregnant women should receive preferential hospital admission.

Relapsing fever can be treated with a variety of antibiotics, including tetracyclines, penicillin,* erythromycin,* ceftriaxone* (Rocephin), and chloramphenicol.* Although penicillin is associated with a lower incidence of JHR, it is also associated with slow clearance of organisms, prolonged symptoms, and a higher failure rate. Doxycycline has the added advantage of also treating epidemic typhus.

LBRF can be treated with a single dose of tetracycline, 500 mg; doxycycline (Vibramycin), 100 mg; erythromycin, 500 mg; chloramphenicol, 500 mg; or procaine penicillin G IM, 600,000 to 1,000,000 U. TBRF responds less readily to treatment, and 5 to 10 days of therapy are required for eradication. Doxycycline, 100 mg twice a day; tetracycline, 500 mg four times a day; or erythromycin, 500 mg four times a day, is effective. Equivalent doses may be given intravenously in patients who cannot tolerate oral medication. Tetracycline administration should be avoided in pregnant women and children.

JARISCH-HERXHEIMER REACTION (JHR)

Treatment of relapsing fever is associated with a severe Jarisch-Herxheimer reaction that may be life-threatening. This reaction appears to be an exaggeration of the crisis seen in untreated patients. JHR typically begins 1 to 2 hours after treatment has begun. Patients often complain of intense anxiety and restlessness, which is followed by rigors. Temperature, pulse rate, and respiration rate rise rapidly. As the fever resolves, hypotension develops and may last for 8 to 12 hours. JHR is associated with high levels of circulating tumor necrosis factor, interleukin-6, and interleukin-8.

Attempts to decrease the severity of JHR have been largely unsuccessful. Antipyretics have a modest effect in preventing temperature elevation. Neither pentoxifylline nor corticosteroids are of benefit. In high-risk patients, some investigators have advocated a first dose of penicillin, followed by tetracycline. Fluid resuscitation and/or systemic pressors may be necessary to control hypotension. Digoxin has been used for patients with myocarditis and evidence of low cardiac output.

PREVENTION

TBRF is best prevented by use of protective clothing and avoidance of sleeping areas that are likely to

---

*Not FDA approved for this indication.

be infested with rodents (and their ticks). In Africa, the tick vector for *B. duttonii* can be eliminated by improvements in housing. Barring such an investment, some villagers collect household ticks to repopulate new dwellings and ensure a level of immunity. During epidemics of LBRF, mass treatment with antibiotics is combined with delousing (DDT or 1% lindane). Clothing and bedding may be boiled for 30 minutes to rid them of lice. Doxycycline, 100 mg twice weekly, is effective prophylaxis for epidemic LBRF.

LYME DISEASE*

method of
ROBERT B. NADELMAN, M.D., and
GARY P. WORMSER, M.D.

New York Medical College and Lyme Disease Diagnostic Center, Westchester Medical Center Valhalla, New York

EPIDEMIOLOGY

Lyme disease (also called Lyme borreliosis) is an infection caused by the spirochete *Borrelia burgdorferi* sensu lato (henceforth referred to as *B. burgdorferi*), which is transmitted to humans by the bite of certain ticks of the genus *Ixodes*. Ticks acquire this borrelial infection in a complex tick-vertebrate transmission cycle that, in North America, involves primarily the white-footed mouse and the white-tailed deer.

Lyme disease occurs in northeastern, mid-Atlantic, north-central, and far western regions of the United States, in limited foci in Canada (primarily one section of eastern Ontario), and much of Europe and northern Asia. Despite reports of rashes resembling erythema migrans in other locations (e.g., the southern United States), isolation of *B. burgdorferi* from humans in these locations has not been documented to date, and thus these regions should not be considered endemic for this infection.

CLINICAL MANIFESTATIONS

The clinical features of Lyme disease may include skin, joint, neurologic, or cardiac manifestations. Some of these (e.g., erythema migrans rash) occur within 1 to 2 weeks after infection, whereas others (e.g., arthritis) occur after several months. The surveillance definition of Lyme disease developed by the U.S. Centers for Disease Control and Prevention (CDC) for epidemiologic purposes is very useful clinically. A modified version is depicted in Table 1. Many disease manifestations attributed to Lyme disease have been based on case reports, uncontrolled series of patients, or indirect (serologic) evidence rather than on microbiologic documentation of infection (i.e., isolation in culture of *B. burgdorferi*). Further study on causation is indicated.

At least three genospecies of *B. burgdorferi* are known to cause clinical disease in Eurasia, as opposed to only one in North America. This may explain the somewhat differ-

*Dr. Nadelman was supported in part by a grant from the New York State Department of Health, Tick-Borne Diseases Institute (C-015088).

TABLE 1. **Lyme Borreliosis Manifestations***

Cutaneous

Erythema Migrans
- Expanding (over days or weeks) erythematous patch ($\geq$5 cm in diameter). Systemic complaints including fever and secondary erythema migrans lesions may occur.
- Does not include lesions occurring within hours of a tick bite (which represent hypersensitivity reactions) or lesions that resolve (without antibiotics) within ~48 h of onset.†

Borrelial Lymphocytoma
- Painless bluish-red nodule or plaque, usually on earlobe, nipple, or scrotum. B lymphocytic infiltrate present on biopsy specimen. (Borrelial lymphocytoma occurs in Eurasia but virtually never in North America.)

Acrodermatitis Chronica Atrophicans
- Long-standing red or bluish-red discoloration, usually on the extensor surface of extremities, sometimes with dough-like swelling, ultimately becoming atrophic (and sometimes associated with peripheral neuropathy, adjacent periarticular nodules, and/or joint subluxation beneath lesions). (Acrodermatitis chronica atrophicans occurs in Eurasia but virtually never in North America.)

Extracutaneous (When No Alternative Explanation Is Found)

Carditis
- Acute onset of heart block that resolves in days to weeks and may be associated with myopericarditis.
- Does not include palpitations, bradycardia, bundle branch block, or myocarditis alone without other objective manifestations of Lyme borreliosis.

Nervous System
- Lymphocytic meningitis, cranial neuritis (particularly peripheral facial nerve palsy), radiculoneuropathy, and, rarely, encephalomyelitis (the last must be confirmed by demonstration of specific intrathecal antibody production to *Borrelia burgdorferi*).‡
- Does not include headache, fatigue, paresthesia, or stiff neck without other objective manifestations of Lyme borreliosis.

Musculoskeletal System
- Recurrent brief attacks (length of attack: weeks or months) of objective joint swelling in one or a few joints, sometimes followed by chronic arthritis, typically in one or both knees.
- Does not include chronic progressive arthritis not preceded by brief attacks, chronic symmetrical polyarthritis, or arthralgia, myalgia, or fibromyalgia without other objective manifestations of Lyme borreliosis.

*Laboratory evidence required for all manifestations except for erythema migrans occurring in an area endemic for *B. burgdorferi* infection. Laboratory evidence should consist of isolation of *B. burgdorferi* from a clinical specimen, identification of organism-specific genetic sequences by polymerase chain reaction in synovial or cerebrospinal fluid, or demonstration of antibodies to *B. burgdorferi* in serum in a two-step test (enzyme-linked immunosorbent assay [ELISA] or indirect immunofluorescence assay [IFA] followed by immunoblot). (An endemic area is defined as wooded, brushy, or grassy locations in a county [or equivalent district] in which at least two confirmed cases of Lyme borreliosis in humans have been previously acquired or in which established populations of a known tick vector are infected with *B. burgdorferi*.)

†Untreated erythema migrans resolves spontaneously in a median time period of 4 weeks in U.S. patients and in a median time period of 10 weeks in Swedish patients.

‡Requires simultaneous serum and cerebrospinal fluid (CSF) samples in order to determine whether the level of specific antibody to *B. burgdorferi* in CSF is greater than that in serum.

Adapted from Nadelman RB, Wormser GP: Lyme borreliosis. Lancet 352:557–565, 1998. Modified from the Centers for Disease Control and Prevention (CDC) and European Union Concerted Action on Lyme Borreliosis (EUCALB) recommendations.

ent clinical manifestations of Lyme disease in Eurasia in comparison with North America. For example, U.S. patients with erythema migrans caused by *B. burgdorferi* sensu stricto are more likely to have constitutional symptoms than are Europeans with erythema migrans caused by *B. afzelii*. Skin lesions such as acrodermatitis chronica atrophicans and lymphocytoma occur almost exclusively in Eurasia because *B. afzelii*, which causes this clinical feature, is not present in the United States. *B. garinii*, another Eurasian genospecies, appears to be closely associated with neurologic disease. Because of these differences, clinical and laboratory experience learned in Europe may not be applicable to the United States, and vice versa.

ERYTHEMA MIGRANS

The erythema migrans rash, the clinical hallmark of Lyme disease, is recognized in 90% or more of patients with objective evidence of *B. burgdorferi* infection. Erythema migrans typically begins at the site of an *Ixodes* tick bite that occurred an average of 7 to 10 days earlier (range, 1 to 30 days). The tick is no longer attached at the time of the onset of the rash. Only one of four patients recall the tick bite, because nymphal *Ixodes* ticks are extremely small (size of poppy seeds) and their bite is usually asymptomatic and often occurs on areas of the skin that are difficult to visualize (e.g., the popliteal fossa). Erythema migrans begins as a red macule or papule that expands over days to weeks. Central clearing may or may not be present and is largely a function of length of duration of the rash before treatment. Secondary cutaneous lesions may develop after hematogenous spread of spirochetes. Local symptoms (pruritus, tenderness, and paresthesia) are generally minimal in primary lesions and are absent in secondary lesions. Erythema migrans must be distinguished from local tick bite reactions, tinea, insect and spider bite reactions, bacterial cellulitis, and plant dermatitis.

Most U.S. patients with erythema migrans experience systemic symptoms, which in one series of 79 culture-confirmed cases included fatigue (54%), myalgia (44%), arthralgia (44%), headache (42%), fever and/or chills (39%), and stiff neck (35%). The presence of prominent respiratory and/or gastrointestinal complaints is infrequent enough to suggest an alternative diagnosis or co-infection. Objective physical findings other than the erythema migrans rash itself are uncommon except for regional lymphadenopathy (23%) and fever (16%). Occasional cases of febrile virus-like illness without erythema migrans have been attributed to Lyme disease. Some of these patients may have sought medical attention before the appearance of a rash or after the spontaneous resolution of an asymptomatic, unrecognized erythema migrans. Others probably had a different illness associated with a false-positive Lyme disease serologic finding (e.g., human granulocytic ehrlichiosis). In cases without erythema migrans, the certainty of Lyme disease is lower.

CARDITIS

Cardiac disease caused by *B. burgdorferi* develops within weeks to months after infection, manifested by fluctuating degrees of atrioventricular block (typically at or above the atrioventricular node) that may cause dizziness, palpitations, dyspnea, chest pain, or syncope. Pericarditis with effusion is less frequently observed. Carditis (as measured by electrocardiographically confirmed heart block) is present in less than 1% of patients with erythema migrans.

European but not U.S. investigators have associated a dilated cardiomyopathy with Lyme disease.

NEUROLOGIC DISEASE

Peripheral facial nerve palsy (occasionally bilateral) is the most common neurologic manifestation of Lyme disease in North America. Erythema migrans may or may not be present concomitantly. The development of facial nerve palsy during the first few days of treatment for erythema migrans does not constitute treatment failure. A lymphocytic meningitis (with mild or absent meningismus) may occur separately or with erythema migrans, cranial neuritis, and/or radiculopathy.

Months to years after initial (untreated) infection, more subtle neurologic symptoms and signs may appear. A peripheral neuropathy, characterized by paresthesias and (less commonly) radicular pain, often with normal findings on physical examination, has been reported. Diagnosis is supported by electrophysiologic studies showing a mild axonal neuropathy. After a similar time course, certain patients develop subtle memory and cognitive dysfunction associated with a subacute or chronic encephalopathy. Intrathecal antibody production and elevated cerebrospinal (CSF) protein may be present. Uncontrolled studies suggest that parenteral antibiotic therapy will arrest or reverse these clinical manifestations. Their pathogenesis is unclear.

B. burgdorferi infection is not the cause of multiple sclerosis, amyotrophic lateral sclerosis, or Alzheimer's disease. Anecdotal reports of psychiatric illness occurring in patients who are seropositive for *B. burgdorferi* antibodies have in general not provided compelling evidence of causation.

RHEUMATOLOGIC DISEASE

Arthritis is the most common extracutaneous manifestation of Lyme disease. In a study of 55 untreated patients with erythema migrans diagnosed between 1977 and 1979 and monitored for a mean duration of 6 years, more than half of patients developed objective arthritis, 90% within 1 year. Intermittent bouts of migratory monoarthritis or asymmetrical oligoarthritis occurred and, in untreated patients, lasted a mean of 3 months (range, 3 days to 11.5 months). Large and (less often) small joints were affected, but the knee was involved at some point in almost all patients. In another series of patients with Lyme disease and arthritis, temporomandibular joint involvement occurred in 11 (39%) of 28 patients. Lyme arthritis is characterized by large effusions with relatively mild joint pain and erythema. Baker's cysts may develop and rupture. Synovial fluid analysis typically reveals a modestly elevated protein and white cell count (median, 24,250 white cells per mm^3; range, 2100 to 72,250 white cells per mm^3) with a polymorphonuclear predominance and a normal glucose level. A minority of patients develop synovitis lasting 1 year or more (preceded by brief attacks), sometimes associated with joint destruction. *B. burgdorferi* DNA can be detected by polymerase chain reaction (PCR) in the synovial fluid of up to 85% of untreated patients with Lyme arthritis.

CHILDREN

Children account for a disproportionate number of Lyme disease cases, presumably because of increased exposure and decreased attention to prevention. Manifestations are similar to those in adults.

The risk of transplacental transmission of *B. burgdorferi* is probably minimal when appropriate antibiotics (Table 2) are given to pregnant women with Lyme disease. There are no published data to support a congenital Lyme disease syndrome (i.e., analogous to TORCH).

LABORATORY TESTING

In locations endemic for Lyme disease, the diagnosis of erythema migrans is purely clinical; laboratory testing is not recommended. However, in patients with suspected extracutaneous Lyme disease, laboratory support of the diagnosis is essential and is usually provided by detection of antibodies to *B. burgdorferi.*

A two-step approach to serologic diagnosis, to increase the specificity of a positive test, has been proposed by a number of authoritative U.S. organizations. A positive or equivocal first-stage test (usually an enzyme-linked immunosorbent assay [ELISA]) is followed on the same serum sample by a second stage test (immunoblot), which can detect IgM and IgG antibodies to individual *B. burgdorferi* antigens that have been separated by electrophoresis. A reactive ELISA with a negative immunoblot is likely to be falsely positive. For persons with an illness of more than 1 month's duration, a positive IgG blot is necessary to support a diagnosis of Lyme disease. Even two-step testing is not indicated for persons with little or no clinical evidence of Lyme disease because of the low positive predictive value. Because IgM and IgG antibodies to *B. burgdorferi* may persist in serum for years after clinical recovery, serologic testing has no role in measuring response to treatment.

Patients with extracutaneous Lyme disease almost always have diagnostic serum antibodies to *B. burgdorferi;* the exceptions are some patients with early seventh cranial nerve palsy and occasional patients in whom antibodies to *B. burgdorferi* are present in CSF only. The specificity and sensitivity of T lymphocyte recognition of *B. burgdorferi* antigens are controversial. Tests for detection of *B. burgdorferi* antigens or *B. burgdorferi*–associated immune complexes require validation and should not be used in clinical practice.

PCR techniques to detect DNA sequences in clinical specimens may be diagnostically helpful in CSF or synovial fluid but cannot distinguish between live and dead organisms, and results may remain positive after clinical cure. Also, use of inappropriate primers or contamination may yield false-positive PCR results.

CO-INFECTION

Ixodes scapularis ticks are also vectors for other human pathogens such as *Babesia microti,* a protozoan that causes a malaria-like infection, and a rickettsial agent that causes human granulocytic ehrlichiosis (HGE). These infections may be transmitted separately or simultaneously with *B. burgdorferi* and may affect the clinical manifestations and the choice of antibiotic therapy. Certain clinical features (e.g., thrombocytopenia or leukopenia) that are not characteristic of Lyme disease are suggestive of co-infection. Visualization of *B. microti* in red blood cells (on peripheral blood smear) or the HGE agent in granulocytes (on buffy coat smear) can facilitate diagnosis, but these techniques may lack sensitivity. Available assays to detect these organisms by PCR or by measurement of serum antibodies are of variable quality and should be used with caution.

TREATMENT

Although most manifestations of Lyme disease resolve spontaneously without treatment, antibiotics hasten the resolution of some manifestations and almost certainly prevent the progression of disease. An approach to treatment is summarized in Table 2. For patients with erythema migrans, we recommend a 2-week course of oral antibiotics. Doxycycline (Vibramycin),* amoxicillin,* and cefuroxime axetil appear equally efficacious. We prefer doxycycline, in the absence of contraindications (see Table 2), because tetracyclines are the only antimicrobials proven to be effective against HGE, which may be present simultaneously, and because of the convenience of twice-daily dosing. The macrolides azithromycin* (Zithromax) and erythromycin* appear to be less effective against *B. burgdorferi* but may be considered if tetracyclines or beta-lactam agents are contraindicated. Clarithromycin (Biaxin), another macrolide, has been inadequately studied and cannot be recommended at present. Approximately 15% of patients with erythema migrans develop a Jarisch-Herxheimer–like reaction, characterized by transient intensified signs (e.g., rash and fever) and symptoms (e.g., arthralgias), limited to the first 24 hours after initiation of antibiotics. Treatment is symptomatic.

For patients with cranial neuritis, mild carditis (i.e., first-degree heart block) or arthritis, oral antibiotics are also usually effective. Arthritis is generally treated for 4 weeks, although there are no comparison studies of shorter treatment durations. In general, we reserve intravenous antibiotics (i.e., ceftriaxone* [Rocephin], cefotaxime* [Claforan], or penicillin G*) for patients with meningitis, disease of the central nervous system, peripheral neuropathy, advanced (second- or third-degree) heart block, or arthritis that persists or relapses after one or two courses of oral therapy. Ceftriaxone is our first choice for intravenous treatment because of its once-daily dosing, which makes it convenient for outpatient therapy. There is no evidence that more than 2 weeks of intravenous antibiotics is necessary.

Currently available quinolones, sulfonamides, first-generation cephalosporins, rifampin, and aminoglycosides have no appreciable activity against *B. burgdorferi* and should not be used. In addition, there is no evidence to support combination antimicrobial therapy, prolonged (>1 month) or repeated courses of antibiotics, "pulse" or intermittent antibiotic therapy, or the use of antibiotics to "stimulate the release of borrelial antigens" in order to enhance diagnosis.

Most persons treated for Lyme disease have an excellent prognosis. Although some patients treated for erythema migrans in some series continued to have a variety of mild nonspecific complaints after antibiotic therapy, the development of objective extracutaneous disease after treatment is extremely rare. The cause of these complaints is unclear. One

---

*Not FDA approved for this indication.

TABLE 2. **Treatment of Lyme Borreliosis*†**

Manifestation	Antibiotic†	Route/Dose Adults	Route/Dose Children†‡	Duration§	Comments
CUTANEOUS DISEASE					
Erythema migrans (EM)					Amoxicillin, cefuroxime axetil, and doxycycline probably equally effective; treatment failure rate <5% (objective findings); no evidence that intravenous ceftriaxone is advantageous in "disseminated" early disease.
	Doxycycline† (Vibramycin)	PO: 100 mg bid	2–4 mg/kg/d in two divided doses	14 days	Includes coverage of HGE; increased risk of photosensitivity.
	Amoxicillin	PO: 500 mg tid	40–50 mg/kg/d in three divided doses	14 days	Not active against HGE.
	Cefuroxime axetil (Ceftin)	PO: 500 mg bid	30 mg/kg/d in two divided doses	14 days	Useful when cellulitis cannot be distinguished from EM (as is amoxicillin/clavulanic acid [Augmentin]); alternative for some penicillin-allergic patients; most expensive; not active against HGE.
	Phenoxymethyl penicillin (penicillin V)	PO: 500 mg qid	50 mg/kg/d in four divided doses	14 days	Has been given at an oral dose of $1–1.5 \times 10^6$ units tid in European studies. Not active against HGE.
	Tetracycline†	PO: 500 mg qid	25–50 mg/kg/d in four divided doses	14 days	Includes coverage of HGE; increased risk of photosensitivity.
	Azithromycin (Zithromax)	PO: 500 mg once daily	5–12 mg/kg once daily	7–10 days	Second-line choice; more objective failures for *B. burgdorferi* infection than in amoxicillin-treated patients; not active against HGE.
Borrelial lymphocytoma	First-line oral EM regimen†			14 days	
Acrodermatitis chronica atrophicans	First-line oral EM regimen†			21–28 days	Evaluation for concurrent neuropathy prudent; intravenous antibiotics (see meningitis regimens) may be effective, but regimen and advantages over oral therapy not established.
EXTRACUTANEOUS DISEASE					
Carditis	First-line oral EM regimen†			14 days	For first-degree heart block.
	Ceftriaxone (Rocephin)	IV: 2 gm once daily	75–100 mg/kg once daily	14 days	For advanced (second- or third-degree) heart block; no proof that intravenous treatment is more effective than oral therapy; patient may need temporary pacemaker.
Facial nerve palsy	First line oral EM regimen†			14–28 days	No clinical trials; treatment does not shorten course; perform lumbar puncture if clinical signs of meningitis are present.
Meningitis	Ceftriaxone	IV: 2 gm once daily	75–100 mg/kg once daily	14 days	
	Cefotaxime (Claforan)	IV: 2 gm tid	90–180 mg/kg/d in three divided doses	14 days	
	Penicillin G	IV: 20×10^6 units/d in six divided doses	3×10^5 units/kg/d in six divided doses	14 days	
	Doxycycline†	PO: 100 mg bid	2–4 mg/kg/d in two divided doses	14–28 days	Equivalent to IV penicillin in one European study but requires confirmation.
Radiculoneuritis	Meningitis regimen†			see above	Since concomitant meningitis frequent, regimen for meningitis appears prudent.
Peripheral (chronic axonal) neuropathy	Meningitis regimen†			see above	

TABLE 2. **Treatment of Lyme Borreliosis*†** *Continued*

Manifestation	Antibiotic†	Route/Dose		Duration§	Comments
		Adults	*Children†‡*		
Encephalomyelitis					Up to 6 weeks of therapy recommended by one expert panel, but no data available.
	Ceftriaxone	IV: 2 gm once daily	75–100 mg/kg once daily	14–28 days	
	Cefotaxime	IV: 2 gm tid	90–180 mg/kg/d in three divided doses	14–28 days	
	Penicillin G	IV: 20×10^6 units/d in six divided doses	3×10^5 units/kg/d in six divided doses	14–28 days	
Chronic encephalopathy	Ceftriaxone	IV: 2 gm once daily	75–100 mg/kg once daily	14–28 days	
	Cefotaxime	IV: 2 gm tid	90–180 mg/kg/d in three divided doses	14–28 days	
	Penicillin G	IV: 20×10^6 units/d in six divided doses	3×10^5 units/kg/d in six divided doses	14–28 days	
Arthritis					Oral therapy usually effective; some patients treated with oral agents develop late neurologic disease (e.g., peripheral neuropathy, encephalopathy); role of PCR in synovial fluid to determine treatment duration unclear; no comparison studies with shorter courses of therapy.
	Doxycycline†	PO: 100 mg bid	2–4 mg/kg/d in two divided doses	28 days	
	Amoxicillin	PO: 500 mg tid	40–50 mg/kg/d in three divided doses	28 days	
	Ceftriaxone	IV: 2 gm once daily	50–75 mg/kg once daily	14 days	
MISCELLANEOUS					
Lyme borreliosis in pregnancy†					No comparison trials; treatment duration should be appropriate for individual manifestation of Lyme borreliosis (see above).
	Penicillin G	IV: 20×10^6 units/day		See comments	
	Ceftriaxone	IV: 2 gm once daily			
	Amoxicillin	PO: 500 mg tid			
Tick bite (asymptomatic)					Efficacy of prophylaxis has not been demonstrated; risk of adverse effects for the 10-day antibiotic regimens studied is comparable with risk of contracting Lyme borreliosis.
Not pregnant	No treatment				
Pregnant	Amoxicillin or no treatment	PO: 500 mg tid		10 days	Antimicrobials have never been studied in this setting; an alternative would be not to treat unless illness developed, in which case amoxicillin, penicillin, or ceftriaxone would be recommended (see Lyme borreliosis in pregnancy above).

*Few regimens studied in published trials with children; selection of amoxicillin in preference to penicillin V, or doxycycline to tetracycline, is based on convenience (decreased dosing) and not on comparison studies.

†Pregnant or lactating women and children younger than 9 years should not receive tetracyclines; tetracyclines are the only antimicrobial agents known to be effective against the agent of HGE.

‡Pediatric dose should not exceed maximal adult dose.

§Limited data concerning treatment duration are available; the only studies comparing treatment duration in EM showed no outcome differences; duration of treatment for EM ranging from 10–30 days has been recommended. In one study of patients with objective late Lyme disease (mostly arthritis), there was no difference in outcome for patients treated with either 14 or 28 days of ceftriaxone.

Abbreviations: HGE = human granulocytic ehrlichiosis; PCR = polymerase chain reaction.

Adapted from Nadelman RB, Wormser GP: Lyme borreliosis. Lancet *352:*557–565, 1998.

study reported that most patients with Lyme disease who were unwell 3 months after treatment had laboratory evidence of co-infection with babesiosis. A combination of oral clindamycin* (Cleocin) and quinine* may be prescribed for patients with babesiosis.

Patients with carditis and neurologic disease also tend to do well but may sometimes have residual deficits (e.g., mild seventh cranial nerve palsy) after treatment. Lyme arthritis typically resolves after antibiotic therapy (often in conjunction with a nonsteroidal anti-inflammatory medication). For patients with Lyme disease–related arthritis who also have signs of peripheral neuropathy or encephalopathy, intravenous antibiotics are preferred over oral therapy. Occasional patients with Lyme disease–related arthritis and the HLA-DR4 haplotype who continue to have synovial inflammation for months or years after the apparent eradication of *B. burgdorferi* from the joint following antibiotic therapy have improved after synovectomy.

Healthy control groups have been lacking from virtually all treatment trials for Lyme disease. A preliminary study indicated that in comparison with persons with a history of Lyme disease, healthy controls had a similar incidence of assorted somatic complaints. In addition, Lyme disease, like other infections, may trigger a fibromyalgia syndrome that does not appear to respond to repeated courses of antibiotics but may improve with symptomatic therapy.

A sizable number of U.S. patients with pain or fatigue syndromes in the absence of a clear etiology have been labeled as having "chronic Lyme disease." In our experience, most of the patients so classified have not had well-documented Lyme disease. Unconventional treatments have often been prescribed, including months or even years of higher than normally prescribed doses of oral and intravenous antibiotics (some of them never previously tested for Lyme disease) singly or in combinations; hyperbaric oxygen; ozone; and even the intentional inoculation of malaria in an attempt to eradicate "persistent" spirochetes. These experimental treatments have not been shown to be effective and are potentially dangerous. In addition, their use may delay the diagnostic evaluation necessary to establish the correct diagnosis.

PREVENTION

The risk of developing Lyme disease may be decreased by avoiding exposure to *Ixodes* ticks by limiting outdoor activities in tick-infested locations, using tick repellents, tucking in clothing to decrease exposed skin surfaces, and frequent skin inspections for early detection and removal of ticks. Use of insecticides (which also kill ticks) on property and construction of deer fences have also been recommended.

Antibiotic prophylaxis, when given to asymptomatic persons after recognized *I. scapularis* tick bites, has not been shown to decrease further the low

*Not FDA approved for this indication.

(<5%) transmission rate of Lyme disease after these bites. In fact, one severe life-threatening drug reaction would be expected for every 10 cases of Lyme disease theoretically prevented by a prophylactic course of amoxicillin. Although the incidence of Lyme disease appears to be increased for persons on whom a tick has fed for more than 48 hours, antimicrobial prophylaxis has not been shown to decrease this risk. A different approach, use of an experimental recombinant outer surface protein (OspA) vaccine, appears to be safe, immunogenic, and effective in adults. Its safety and immunogenicity in children is currently being studied.

CONCLUSION

The most common manifestation of Lyme disease is erythema migrans. In endemic areas, the diagnosis of erythema migrans is clinical. For patients with objective extracutaneous clinical findings, the diagnosis of Lyme disease should be supported by results of two-stage serologic testing. Laboratory techniques such as PCR are a welcome development but are usually not necessary in clinical practice, and the results may be misleading. The possibility of co-infection with other tick-borne diseases should be considered. The overwhelming majority of patients with Lyme disease respond completely to short courses of oral antibiotics. Short courses of parenteral therapy should be reserved for selected patients with Lyme disease who manifest certain neurologic conditions or advanced heart block and for patients whose arthritis persists or relapses after treatment with oral antibiotics and anti-inflammatory agents. For those who remain ill after treatment (e.g., those with fatigue and arthralgias), consideration should be given to alternative diagnoses (e.g., fibromyalgia) and co-infection.

RUBELLA AND CONGENITAL RUBELLA SYNDROME

method of
KRISTINA K. BRYANT, M.D., and
DENISE F. BRATCHER, D.O.
University of Louisville
Louisville, Kentucky

Rubella causes a mild, self-limited febrile illness with an erythematous maculopapular exanthem (German measles). Intrauterine infection, however, can cause significant congenital abnormalities. Despite aggressive immunization programs, up to 10% of young adults in the United States remain susceptible to rubella. Sporadic cases of acute infection and congenital rubella syndrome continue to occur.

EPIDEMIOLOGY

Humans are the only known source of rubella infection. In susceptible populations, the incidence of infection peaks in the winter and early spring; epidemics occur in 6- to 9-year cycles. Postnatal infection occurs after direct or droplet contact with infected nasopharyngeal secretions. The incubation period ranges from 14 to 21 days but is usually 16 to 18 days.

Before the licensure of rubella vaccine in 1969, most cases of rubella occurred in children; the attack rates were highest among 3- to 9-year-olds. With universal immunization of infants and targeted vaccination of susceptible women of childbearing age, the incidence of rubella in the United States has declined more than 99%; residual cases occur primarily in unvaccinated adults.

In 1997, only 181 cases of acute rubella infection and 5 cases of congenital rubella infection were reported to the Centers for Disease Control and Prevention's National Notifiable Disease Surveillance System and the National Congenital Rubella Syndrome Registry. The United States Public Health Service has targeted the year 2000 for the elimination of all indigenous cases of congenital rubella syndrome.

CLINICAL MANIFESTATIONS

A prodromal illness, characterized by malaise, low-grade fever, and conjunctivitis may appear in the second or third week after exposure to rubella and may be followed by an erythematous exanthem. Rose-pink macules and papules appear on the face and scalp and progress caudally to involve the entire body in 1 to 3 days (hence the term "3-day measles"). This rash fades as it spreads, and flaky desquamation may develop. Occasionally, the rash appears scarlatiniform or morbilliform. Suboccipital lymphadenopathy almost always occurs with symptomatic rubella infection and may precede the rash by 1 week. Fever, headache, and myalgia are associated systemic symptoms. Forchheimer's sign—pinpoint or larger petechiae on the soft palate—occurs in approximately 20% of cases. Many cases of rubella, especially those in children, may be asymptomatic.

COMPLICATIONS

Transient arthritis and arthralgias are the most common complications of postnatally acquired rubella, and frequency increases with age. Females are four to five times more likely to develop arthritis than males. Thrombocytopenia lasting days to months is an uncommon complication. A late, progressive rubella pan-encephalitis is rare. The most serious complication of acute rubella infection is transmission of infection to a developing fetus with resultant congenital rubella syndrome.

CONGENITAL RUBELLA SYNDROME

Cardiac malformations, ocular abnormalities, and deafness constitute the classic triad of congenital rubella syndrome, but nearly every organ system in the developing fetus may be affected. The timing of maternal infection determines the frequency and severity of fetal involvement; significant sequelae are less common with increasing gestational age. Maternal infection in the first trimester results in fetal infection in 90 to 100% of cases; fetal death and miscarriage may result. Infection between the 16th and 20th weeks of gestation may result in isolated hearing abnormalities.

More than half of infants born with congenital rubella syndrome appear normal at birth. Symptomatic infants may exhibit transient, nonspecific manifestations of a con-

genital viral infection, such as intrauterine growth retardation, hepatosplenomegaly, jaundice, thrombocytopenia, and radiolucent bone lesions. A purpuric "blueberry muffin" rash, caused by focal dermal erythropoiesis, may be present. Sensorineural hearing loss is the most common permanent sequela of congenital rubella infection, occurring in two thirds of affected infants. Cardiac defects include patent ductus arteriosus, pulmonary artery stenosis, and pulmonary valvular stenosis. Ocular abnormalities include retinopathy, cataracts, and microphthalmia. Late-onset manifestations, identified after patients are 2 years of age, include endocrinopathies such as diabetes mellitus, learning and behavioral problems, and immunologic defects.

DIAGNOSIS

Primary Rubella

The clinical diagnosis of rubella is unreliable. Virus may be cultured from nasopharyngeal secretions and urine, but serologic assessment is preferred. Acute infection is confirmed by demonstration of a fourfold rise in rubella IgG antibody titer between acute and convalescent sera or by presence of IgM antibody in the acute specimen. Enzyme immunoassay, latex agglutination, fluorescence immunoassay, passive hemagglutination, and hemolysis-in-gel tests are all preferable to hemagglutination inhibition methods for antibody determination.

Congenital Rubella Syndrome

Increasing levels of rubella IgG demonstrated in serial samples of infant sera and persistent IgG at 4 to 6 months of age are diagnostic of congenital infection. The presence of rubella IgM in cord or infant sera is strongly suggestive of congenital infection, but false-positive and false-negative findings occur.

Methods of prenatal diagnosis of fetal infection include detection of rubella IgM in fetal blood, although these antibodies may not be present until 22 weeks of gestation. Rubella virus may be grown from tissue obtained from chorionic villus sampling. DNA-RNA hybridization may confirm the presence of rubella virus in culture. Reverse transcription nested polymerase chain reaction has been used to detect rubella virus in amniotic fluid. This may be a useful diagnostic modality in the future.

REINFECTION

Reinfection may occur after rubella immunization or, less commonly, after natural infection. Reinfection is usually asymptomatic. In rare instances, reinfection during pregnancy results in congenital infection.

TREATMENT

Treatment of postnally acquired or congenital rubella is supportive. Routine administration of immune globulin for postexposure prophylaxis of susceptible women early in pregnancy is not recommended, but it may be considered when pregnancy termination is not possible. Although 0.55 mL per kg (maximum dose, 15 mL) of intramuscular immune globulin* may modify infection in an ex-

---

*Not FDA approved for this indication.

posed, susceptible person, it has not been proved to prevent fetal infection. Vaccination of susceptible persons after exposure does not prevent infection.

RUBELLA VACCINE

The rubella vaccine (RA 27/3) contains live, attenuated virus. The vaccine is administered as a subcutaneous injection, preferably in conjunction with measles and mumps vaccines (MMR). Serum antibody to rubella is produced in at least 95% of recipients after a single dose given after 12 months of age and probably confers lifelong immunity in 90%.

Rubella immunization is currently recommended for children at 12 to 15 months of age, with a booster dose at 4 to 6 years of age. Postpubertal patients should be assessed for evidence of rubella immunity and immunized if susceptible. Serologic screening before immunization is not necessary. Special emphasis should be placed on immunization of college students, military recruits, health care workers, and any person who works in an educational institution or day care center. Women should be advised to avoid pregnancy for 3 months after immunization. Pregnant women who lack rubella immunity should be immunized immediately after parturition, before hospital discharge. Breast-feeding is not a contraindication to rubella immunization.

Pregnancy is an absolute contraindication to rubella immunization, although actual risk to the fetus is low. Experience with 226 women inadvertently immunized during the first trimester of pregnancy revealed that 2% of the infants had asymptomatic infections but none had congenital defects. Rubella vaccination is not an indication for pregnancy termination. Children of susceptible pregnant women may be safely immunized. Although rubella virus can be isolated in nasopharyngeal secretions for up to 4 weeks after vaccination, transmission to susceptible contacts does not occur.

Rubella immunization should be deferred for at least 3 months after the receipt of immune globulin or other blood products, because administered antibody may neutralize vaccine virus and prevent the development of protective antibody. Rubella vaccine may be given after parturition to women who received blood products or anti–Rh$_o$ immune globulin D (RhoGAM), but these women should undergo antibody testing 8 weeks after immunization to confirm an antibody response.

In general, rubella vaccine should not be administered to persons with congenital or acquired immunodeficiencies, including those receiving chemotherapy or high-dose steroids. Patients infected with the human immunodeficiency virus (HIV) who are not severely immunocompromised should, however, be immunized.

Adverse reactions to rubella vaccine, including fever, rash, and adenopathy, occur in up to 15% of vaccine recipients. Acute arthropathy, including arthritis and arthralgias, are rare in children and in men but have been reported in up to 30% of women after vaccination. The role of rubella vaccination in chronic arthropathy is debated. In 1991, the Institute of Medicine of the National Academy of Sciences, Washington, D.C., concluded that a possible relationship between rubella vaccination and chronic arthritis exists; subsequent studies have not supported this conclusion.

MEASLES
method of
ALFRED D. HEGGIE, M.D.
Case Western Reserve University School of Medicine and Rainbow Babies and Children's Hospital
Cleveland, Ohio

Measles (rubeola) was formerly a ubiquitous disease that infected almost all children worldwide. Because of effective immunization programs, it is now seldom encountered in the United States or other industrialized nations. However, measles continues to be a common childhood infection in the developing world, where it is often fatal to children with severe malnutrition or other untreated underlying diseases. It is estimated that more than 1 million measles-attributable deaths occur yearly in developing countries.

PATHOGENESIS AND CLINICAL COURSE

Measles virus is an RNA virus that belongs to the genus *Morbillivirus* in the family Paramyxoviridae. Although there are different strains of the virus, there is only one antigenic type. Therefore, infection with one strain induces immunity to all strains, and second cases are extremely rare.

Measles is a multiorgan system infection that is initiated in nonimmune hosts by inhalation of virus-containing droplets of nasopharyngeal secretions from an infected person. The virus infects and replicates in foci of cells of the respiratory epithelium, from which it spreads to regional lymph nodes, in which further replication takes place. Spread of virus from infected lymph nodes to the blood produces a low-level primary viremia that disseminates virus throughout the body. This process, during which the infected host remains asymptomatic, takes about 9 days and results in a secondary prolonged and high-titer viremia on about the 10th day after infection. Coincident with this secondary viremia is the onset of prodromal symptoms and signs, primarily fever, cough, coryza, and nonpurulent conjunctivitis. Although these signs and symptoms are termed "prodromal" because they precede the measles rash by 4 to 6 days, they reflect the important features of uncomplicated measles, which is primarily a respiratory disease.

Viral damage to the respiratory epithelium results in denuding of affected areas. During this period, the patient is highly contagious, and measles virus can readily be isolated from respiratory secretions, blood, and urine. Koplik spots, the pathognomonic enanthem of measles, transiently appear as tiny bluish-white papules with an erythematous base on the buccal mucosa 24 to 48 hours before the exanthem. After 4 to 5 days of prodromal signs, the measles exanthem appears on the face and neck and, in the next 24 hours, spreads over the rest of the body. It first consists of erythematous macules that soon become papular and confluent. The cytopathologic features of Koplik spots and the exanthem are similar and show viral inclusion bodies, giant cells, and intracellular edema. Onset of the exanthem coincides with the appearance of circulating antiviral antibodies in the serum. The virus is then rapidly cleared from the blood, and clinical improvement ensues. Within 4 to 5 days after onset of the rash, viral shedding ceases, and the patient becomes noncontagious. Three to 4 days after its appearance, the rash begins to fade, in the sequence that it appeared, leaving fine desquamation.

COMPLICATIONS

Denuding of the protective mucosal epithelium of the respiratory tract and its extensions, such as the sinuses and eustachian tubes, predisposes to bacterial invasion, often leading to otitis media, sinusitis, and pneumonia. If fever continues after full development of the measles exanthem or recurs after defervescence, the patient should be examined for these complications and treatment with appropriate antibiotics initiated. Although viral pneumonitis probably occurs to some degree in most patients with measles, immunocompromised children are prone to development of an interstitial, giant cell pneumonia that is frequently fatal. Electroencephalographic abnormalities, found in more than half of patients with measles, suggests that neurologic involvement without clinical evidence of encephalitis is frequent. Clinically apparent postmeasles encephalitis occurs in approximately 1 in 1000 cases and is considered to be an autoimmune phenomenon. It is a serious complication with appreciable mortality and morbidity rates. Subacute sclerosing panencephalitis is a rare complication of measles with a risk of 1 to 2 cases per 100,000 infections. In this disease, measles virus acts as a slow virus, causing persistent infection of the brain. Mean interval before onset of symptoms is 7 years after the acute infection. It results in progressive profound disability and eventually death over a period of 6 to 9 months.

MANAGEMENT OF MEASLES

There is no specific antiviral treatment for measles. Although ribavirin (Virazole) inhibits replication of measles virus in cell culture, no efficacy against the disease has been demonstrated. For uncomplicated measles, acetaminophen can be used to control fever and general discomfort. Fluid intake should be maintained, and activity beyond the comfort level should be discouraged. Cough may be alleviated by room humidification and judicious use of antitussive medications. A darkened environment is unnecessary, except to the comfort level necessary to ease photophobia.

Studies in developing nations have shown that administration of vitamin A is associated with a decrease in rates of mortality and morbidity from measles. Many children in these areas have vitamin A deficiency, and measles further depresses serum levels of this vitamin. Because vitamin A is essential to the integrity of epithelial cells, it is biologically plausible that a deficiency might render epithelial cells more susceptible to damage by measles virus. In the United States, where vitamin A deficiency

is infrequent, the American Academy of Pediatrics Committee on Infectious Diseases recommends that vitamin A supplementation be considered for

1. Patients 6 months to 2 years of age hospitalized with measles and its complications. Limited data are available regarding the safety and need for supplementation for infants younger than 6 months of age.
2. Patients older than 6 months with measles who have any of the following risk factors and are not already receiving vitamin A:

- Immunodeficiency
- Ophthalmic evidence of vitamin A deficiency
- Impaired intestinal absorption
- Moderate to severe malnutrition
- Recent immigration from areas where measles-related mortality rates exceed 1%

The recommended dose of vitamin A is a single dose of 200,000 IU of an aqueous solution by mouth for children aged 1 year and older (100,00 IU for children 6 months to 1 year of age). The dose of 200,000 IU may be associated with vomiting and headache for a few hours. Children with ophthalmic evidence of vitamin A deficiency should receive a second dose the next day and a third dose 4 weeks later.

ACTIVE IMMUNIZATION

Because measles is a serious disease with no effective treatment, prevention by active immunization is important. The vaccine currently licensed in the United States is a live, further attenuated measles virus strain prepared in chick embryo cell culture. It is available as a monovalent vaccine (Attenuvax) and in combination with rubella (MR) (M-R-Vax II) and mumps (MMR) (M-M-R II) vaccines. MMR is the vaccine of choice for routine vaccination of children. Serum antibodies against measles are induced in approximately 95% of children vaccinated at 12 months of age and in 98% of those vaccinated at 15 months of age. One dose of vaccine usually induces permanent immunity, but immunity wanes in a small number of persons. The current recommendation by both the Centers for Disease Control and Prevention and the American Academy of Pediatrics is that children receive one dose of MMR vaccine at 12 to 15 months of age and a second dose at 4 to 6 years of age at school entry. Older children and young adults who have not been immunized should receive 2 doses of vaccine separated by an interval of at least 1 month. Between 5% and 15% of nonimmune vaccine recipients develop fever that begins 7 to 12 days after vaccination and usually lasts 1 to 2 days. Approximately 5% of recipients develop a transient rash. Vaccinated persons are not contagious even if they develop fever and rash. Thrombocytopenia is a rare additional reaction, as are minor allergic reactions at the injection site.

Pregnancy, compromised immunity, and a history of an anaphylactic reaction to neomycin are contraindications to immunization with measles vaccine. Female recipients should not become pregnant for at least 30 days after immunization because of the possibility that vaccine virus may be transmitted to the fetus. Measles vaccine should not be administered to immunodeficient or immunosuppressed persons because these conditions may potentiate replication of the vaccine virus that has resulted in fatal outcomes. However, the vaccine can be given to persons with asymptomatic human immunodeficiency virus (HIV) infection and to symptomatic HIV-infected patients who are not immunocompromised. An anaphylactic reaction to neomycin is a contraindication to immunization because the vaccine contains trace amounts of neomycin. Low-grade fever associated with minor illnesses, pregnancy in mothers of children requiring the vaccine, and breast-feeding are not contraindications to measles immunization. Although measles vaccine is prepared in chick embryo cell cultures, it does not contain significant amounts of egg protein; egg-allergic children are at low risk for anaphylactic reactions. However, as in any immunization procedure, treatment for allergic reactions should be readily available.

PASSIVE IMMUNIZATION

Human immune globulin (IG) (Massachusetts Public Health Biologic Laboratories), if given to a susceptible person within 6 days after exposure to measles, will prevent or modify the disease. This method of prophylaxis is indicated for exposed susceptible household contacts of patients with measles, for pregnant women, and for immunosuppressed persons. The usual dose is 0.25 mL per kg of body weight given intramuscularly. The dose for immunocompromised children is 0.5 mL per kg. The maximum dose in either case is 15 mL. Passive prophylaxis should be followed by active immunization with measles vaccine, beginning 6 months after the dose of immune globulin, provided that the patient is at least 12 months old at that time and there are no contraindications to immunization.

Patients who regularly receive human intravenous immune globulin (IVIG) (Gamimune N, Gammagard S/D, Polygam S/D, Sandoglobulin, Venoglobulin-S) have protection against measles for 3 weeks after doses of 100 to 400 mg per kg and do not require additional immune globulin for passive immunization. Vaccine administration, if indicated, should not be initiated until 8 months after the last dose of immune globulin. Larger doses of IGIV necessitate intervals of 9 to 11 months before immunization with vaccine is initiated.

For control of outbreaks in schools and communities, active immunization with vaccine instead of immune globulin prophylaxis should be employed. If given within 72 hours after exposure to measles, the vaccine induces protection in some persons and should protect against subsequent infection in most recipients.

TETANUS

method of
J. DRESSNANDT, M.D.
Bad Aibling Hospital for Neurology
Bad Aibling, Germany

ETIOLOGY

Patients with tetanus develop noncontrollable muscle contractions of increasing duration. The disease is caused by a toxin from the gram-positive, spore-building bacterium *Clostridium tetani*, which proliferates under anaerobic conditions. The spores of this microorganism are widely distributed (soil, dust, feces), and thus every injury contaminated with unsterile material (e.g., from farming, from car accidents, but also through the navel in newborns under unhygienic circumstances) bears the risk of an infection. The bacteria produce different toxins, from which only the toxin tetanospasmin causes the characteristic symptoms. The genetic information for tetanospasmin resides upon a plasmid. The toxin is dispersed by the blood but cannot cross the blood-brain barrier. It consists of two subunits, from which the larger subunit binds to gangliosides within the nerve membrane of peripheral nerves and the smaller subunit crosses the nerve membrane. Within the axons of motor, sensor, and vegetative nerves the toxin is retrogradely transported to the nerve cell body and disseminates transsynaptically to the surrounding nerve cells and interneurons in the spinal cord and brain stem. There it interrupts the excretion of inhibitory neurotransmitters such as glycine and gamma-aminobutyric acid (GABA). The loss of inhibitory regulatory neuronal circuits causes the characteristic symptoms of spasms and tetanic muscle contractions.

SYMPTOMS

After an incubation time of 4 to 20 days, the first symptoms appear, usually within facial muscles, manifesting as difficulties in opening the mouth (trismus), hypomimic and rigid face (risus sardonicus), and increased excitability of the facial nerve (Chvostek's sign); thereafter, increasing numbers of muscles from the neck and trunk (opisthotonus) and extremities are involved. The slightest tactile, acoustic, or endogenous stimuli lead to spasms and tetanic muscle contractions. Swallowing and respiration are finally blocked by laryngeal, pharyngeal, and diaphragmatic spasms. The brain is usually not involved, but sometimes an encephalitis is also observed. Increased heart rate or bradycardia, arrhythmia, arterial hypertension and hypotension, and increased perspiration can be observed. Vegetative dysregulations are the main cause of the increased mortality of patients with tetanus in spite of intensive care treatment. The severity of the tetanus symptoms depends on the amount of *C. tetani* being inoculated and on the amount of tetanospasmin being produced by the bacteria. Tetanus is usually generalized but can also be focal, occurring only in the region of inoculation. The faster the symptoms develop, the more severe the tetanus will be. Recovery starts after 3 to 4 weeks and requires several weeks.

DIAGNOSIS

Tetanus is diagnosed on the typical succession of symptoms: increasing muscle tone, starting with difficulties in chewing, then increasing neck and trunk stiffness up to opisthotonus. *C. tetani* bacteria are difficult to detect in tissue. A positive animal test can be used for proof of the suspected infection. A loss of the silent period, tested with electrophysiologic methods, is evidence for a loss of inhibitory circuits at the spinal level. The differential diagnosis should include early dyskinesia related to dopamine blocking agents (confirmation of diagnosis by administration of an anticholinergic drug, e.g., biperiden-HCl [Akineton], 2 to 5 mg IV); strychnine poisoning (detected in urine or blood); stiff-man syndrome (usually facial muscles less involved, no silent period in electromyography); and meningitis and encephalitis (cell elevation in cerebrospinal fluid).

TREATMENT

Prophylaxis

To prevent tetanus an active immunization is recommended for children 2 months or older. The primary vaccination in patients older than 1 year is begun with 0.5 mL of tetanus toxoid, a second intramuscular injection with 0.5 mL of tetanus toxoid 4 to 8 weeks later, and a third one 6 to 12 months after the second vaccination. Thereafter, the vaccination should be repeated with booster injections of 0.5 mL tetanus toxoid every 10 years. Patients younger than 7 years of age usually receive a vaccination with diphtheria-tetanus-pertussis (Tripedia), and patients older than 7 get an immunization with tetanus-diphtheria toxoid (Tetanus and Diphtheria Toxoids, Adsorbed Purogenated). A higher frequency of immunization against tetanus bears the risk of a postimmunization plexus neuritis and other complications. On the other hand, the elderly have a shortened immunologic memory. Whether booster injections with tetanus toxoid should be done earlier than 10 years after the last vaccination in the elderly has yet to be determined.

Prophylaxis After Injury

The wound should be carefully washed to eliminate contaminated material, and necrotic tissue should be excised. After an injury an active immunization (0.5 mL tetanus toxoid adsorbed) may be considered when the last immunization was longer than 5 years ago (especially in elderly patients) and should be done when it was 10 or more years ago. When the immune status is unknown or the primary vaccination is incomplete or the last booster vaccination was done more than 10 years ago, an active immunization with tetanus toxoid (usually tetanus-diphtheria toxoid, e.g., Tetanus and Diphtheria Toxoids, Adsorbed Purogenated) and a passive immunization with human antitetanus immune globulin (Hyper-Tet) at a dose of 250 U (500 U if immune status is unknown) should be administered intramuscularly, contralateral to the injection site of the active immunization. Some experts recommend a second administration of antitetanus immunoglobulins in patients with severe burn injuries after 3 to 4 weeks.

Treatment of Tetanus

A patient who develops signs of tetanus should be hospitalized in an intensive care unit. The treatment aims at (1) safeguarding of respiration, (2) elimination of tetanus producing bacteria, (3) neutralizing of tetanus toxin (tetanospasmin), (4) treatment of symptoms (spasmolysis, vegetative dysautonomia), and (5) prevention of secondary complications.

Safeguarding of Respiration

Close monitoring of the patient is necessary to decide when artificial ventilation should start. If intubation is necessary, a preceding relaxation with a benzodiazepine and a peripheral muscle relaxation with neuromuscular blocking agents is advisable because the intubation triggers severe spasms.

Elimination of Tetanus-Producing Bacteria

The wound should be cleaned of contaminated material, and necrotic tissue should be excised. To eradicate *C. tetani* bacteria and inhibit further proliferation, metronidazole (Flagyl) should be administered intravenously in a dose of 500 mg every 8 hours for 7 to 10 days. The antibiotic penicillin G (Pfizerpen), 1 to 5 million U every 4 hours for 10 days, is a central GABA antagonist and should therefore not be considered as first choice. An open study comparing metronidazole with penicillin demonstrated an advantage for metronidazole. Alternative antibiotics are erythromycin (Ilotycin Gluceptate) and clindamycin (Cleocin Phosphate). In case of concomitant microbial infection, the antimicrobial therapy should be adapted.

Neutralization of Tetanus Toxin

Tetanus toxin can be antagonized only before it has entered the nervous system. Human antitetanus immune globulin (Hyper-Tet) should be administered intramuscularly once. The dose is arbitrary. Doses of 250 to 10,000 U are reported to be given. There is no superiority of the high dose to the low dose. Human antitetanus immunoglobulin (250 U) can also be administered intrathecally,* but this way of administration is not unequivocal. There is no clear advantage of infiltrating the wound or the wound's vicinity with immune globulin in comparison to administration of the immune globulin intramuscularly at the conventional body sites. The endogenous production of antibodies should be initiated with an active immunization with tetanus toxoid, because the amount of tetanospasmin that leads to the tetanus symptoms is too small to lead to a sufficient antibody production. Patients younger than 7 years of age usually receive a vaccination with diphtheria-tetanus-pertussis toxoid (Tripedia), patients older than 7 years of age receive an immunization with tetanus-diphtheria toxoid (Tetanus and Diphtheria Toxoids, Adsorbed Purogenated). The serum level of antibodies against

---

*Not FDA approved for this route of administration.

tetanus toxin being protective in most cases is 0.01 unit per mL or higher. Immune globulins should not be given repeatedly after active immunization, because this hinders the endogenous production of antibodies against tetanospasmin.

Spasmolysis

To prevent spasms a dim room is needed with prevention of noise and careful nursing.

Established Therapy. Spasm frequency and muscle tone can be reduced by administration of GABAergic substances. Benzodiazepines, which are GABA-A receptor agonists, such as diazepam or midazolam, are usually used. Midazolam (Versed injection) is begun with a 5- to 15-mg bolus, continued with a continuous infusion of 5 mg per hour, and increased as necessary. Diazepam (Valium) is begun with a 10-mg intravenous bolus and then continued with an infusion of 5 mg per hour and increased in steps as necessary.

If the dose of diazepam is high, there is a risk of acidosis because of the compounded solution with propylene glycol. Therefore, it is favorable to use or to switch to midazolam because it has a different compounded solution that does not lead to acidosis. Furthermore, the half-life of midazolam is shorter than that of diazepam and thus accumulation is less severe.

When spasmolysis with GABAergic drugs is insufficient, peripheral neuromuscular blocking agents such as vecuronium (Norcuron) (6 to 8 mg/hour), succinylcholine (Anectine injection), pancuronium (Pavulon), or other neuromuscular blocking agents should be used. A report described that spasmolysis could not be reached with rocuronium (Zemuron) but was sufficient after the peripheral muscle blocking agent was changed to alcuronium (Alloferin).*

Alternative Therapy. Baclofen (Lioresal), a GABA-B receptor agonist, can be administered intrathecally by continuous infusion through an implanted catheter-port-system connected to an external pump. Intrathecal baclofen is begun with a 300-µg bolus, continued with a continuous infusion of 500 µg per day, increased in steps of 300 to 500 µg per day as needed. An alternative for the administration of intrathecal baclofen is the bolus injection in doses of 500 to 1000 µg every day. After some days the bolus dose should be reduced according to the effect of the last bolus administration.

Magnesium sulfate is started as an intravenous 5-gram loading dose (slow injection) and continued with 2 to 3 grams per hour until a serum level of 2 to 4 mmol per liter is reached. Kidney function should not be impaired when magnesium sulfate is used.

In milder forms of tetanus, dantrolene (Dantrium

intravenous),* 1.0 to 2.5 mg per kg four times a day, has been used successfully. Dantrolene can cause hepatic dysfunction in high doses (above 300 mg per day) and is usually not sufficient in the treatment of severe forms of tetanus.

Spasmolysis either with intrathecal baclofen, intravenous magnesium sulfate, or dantrolene has the advantage that control of spasms may be reached without the necessity for artificial ventilation. Furthermore, intrathecal baclofen and intravenous magnesium sulfate reduce also vegetative dysregulations (see later).

Autonomic dysregulations are usually treated with beta-adrenergic blockers in doses as necessary (e.g., propranolol [Inderal] or labetalol [Trandate]), which blocks beta- and alpha$_1$-adrenergic receptors. The co-administration of clonidine (Catapres), 2 µg per kg three times a day, an alpha$_2$-receptor agonist, was reported to lower the mortality rate due to vegetative dysregulations. Fentanyl (Innovar), 4 to 6 µg per kg per hour given intravenously, was described to reduce cardiovascular instabilities. Intrathecal baclofen (Lioresal intrathecal) can reduce vegetative dysregulations, but it can also lead to bradycardia and hypotension with high doses (2000 µg per day). Magnesium sulfate prevents sympathetic but not parasympathetic hyperactivity. Intravenous infusion of trimethaphan camsylate (Arfonad), 50 to 300 mg per hour, reduces vegetative dysregulations, but habituation necessitates dose increases within days, and side effects usually hinder the administration over a longer time period. Continuous intrathecal infusion of 0.5% bupivacaine (Marcaine)† is proposed by some experts to block vegetative dysregulations; the aim is a blockade not only of the sympathetic but also of the parasympathetic system (no reaction to atropine injection).

Prevention of Secondary Complications. Pulmonary infection is the most often occurring secondary complication due to the long time required for artificial ventilation. By using intrathecal baclofen (Lioresal intrathecal) or intravenous magnesium sulfate or dantrolene (Dantrium intravenous) for spasmolysis, the necessity for artificial ventilation can be shortened or may not be necessary, and thus the risk for pulmonary infections can possibly be reduced (the reported numbers of patients having been treated by these alternative methods is still small). Feeding should be done by nasogastric tube, so that spasms are not triggered by chewing and swallowing and the risk for aspiration is reduced. Gastrointestinal problems can be different, and therapy should be specific; the prophylactic administration of omeprazole (Prilosec), 20 to 40 mg per day or H$_2$ blockers for protection from stress ulcer, is advisable. Prophylaxis of thrombosis with heparin, of joint contractures with physiotherapy, and of decubitus ulcers with changing positioning of the patient is essential.

---

*Not available in the United States.

*Not FDA approved for this indication.
†Not available in the United States.

PERTUSSIS
(Whooping Cough)

method of
JOHN W. OGLE, M.D.

Denver Health Medical Center and
University of Colorado School of Medicine
Denver, Colorado

Historically, pertussis was a prominent cause of death during childhood. Before the development of effective vaccines, pertussis resulted in many deaths and considerable morbidity. The largest number of pertussis cases in the United States was the more than 250,000 reported in 1934. The largest reported mortality rate was 9200 deaths, in 1923. Standardization of pertussis vaccines in the late 1940s and subsequent widespread immunization dramatically reduced the numbers of pertussis cases and deaths. Nonetheless, 4000 to 8000 cases are reported yearly, and epidemic increases occur every 3 to 4 years. In 1996 and 1997, 7796 and 6315 cases, respectively, were reported. These numbers are, moreover, believed to represent substantial under-reporting of cases. Deaths from pertussis are currently uncommon. In 1996 and 1997, 11 of 17 pertussis-related deaths in the United States occurred in infants younger than 6 months. As pertussis has been controlled by immunization during infancy, cases have been recognized more frequently in older children and adults. Of pertussis cases since 1990, 46% occurred in persons older than 10 years.

PATHOPHYSIOLOGY

Bordetella pertussis organisms attach to the ciliated epithelium of the respiratory tract and may be identified in respiratory specimens taken early in the course of the disease. The attached organisms produce toxins, which are thought to cause the clinical manifestations of the disease. Infection in childhood was believed to confer lifelong immunity. Currently, most children receive immunization vaccines; the immunity conferred by those vaccines is known to wane after a number of years, and most adolescents and adults are susceptible to infection with *B. pertussis*.

The precise role of the known toxins in the disease process and the basis of pertussis immunity is uncertain. Adhesins (filamentous hemagglutinin [FHA], fimbriae, and a 69-kilodalton protein termed pertactin) mediate epithelial attachment. An adenyl cyclase inhibits polymorphonuclear leukocyte function. A low-molecular-weight tracheal cytotoxin causes ciliostasis and necrosis of respiratory epithelial cells. Pertussis toxin (PT) inhibits cellular adenyl cyclase through a G-protein linked receptor and may interfere with hormone signaling by these receptors. Lymphocytosis and leukocytosis are caused by PT and represent a redistribution of cells from the peripheral lymphatic organs to the central circulation.

CLINICAL DISEASE

Typical pertussis progresses through three stages. The incubation period is usually 7 to 10 days; in rare cases, it may be as long as 20 days. During the initial, or catarrhal, phase, children appear to have a nonspecific upper respiratory tract infection. Fever is absent or minimal, rarely exceeding 100°F. Clear nasal discharge and cough are the predominant symptoms. Initially, the cough is minimal, but it gradually becomes more frequent and forceful and develops a repetitive character.

After a period of days to 2 weeks, the child enters the paroxysmal phase. There is no fever. The child experiences bouts of forceful, repetitive coughing, but usually no other symptoms are present between coughing spells. The coughing paroxysm may last 15 to 30 seconds or, more typically, as long as several minutes. The child seems to be unable to clear the airway despite the cough. The face becomes pale and then ruddy, plethoric, or frankly cyanotic. The child is often diaphoretic from the effort of coughing and breathing. Attempts to inspire during the paroxysm result in a whooping sound, which is followed by more coughing. The paroxysm often ends with apparent vomiting; the vomitus often fills, and may obstruct, the mouth and nares. Although this post-tussive vomitus may be stomach contents, it is often thick mucus from the respiratory tract. At the end of the paroxysm, the child is often damp, limp, and cyanotic, exhausted by coughing and efforts required to breathe and clear the airway. Coughing paroxysms may occur 15 to 20 or more times in a 24-hour period. The paroxysmal phase lasts 2 weeks or longer.

The recovery phase follows, and coughing paroxysms gradually become less frequent and severe. After several additional weeks up to 2 months, the child stops coughing. During the recovery period and for several months afterwards, a viral upper respiratory tract infection may cause a return of paroxysmal coughing.

Although diagnosis of pertussis is suggested by typical clinical findings, misdiagnosis is common, and children are often examined several times before the correct diagnosis is considered. During the catarrhal phase, children appear to have an uncomplicated viral respiratory tract infection. Between paroxysms, the child may be completely asymptomatic, and physical examination findings are normal. Unless the examining physician observes a coughing spell or the parents describe typical whooping, paroxysms, cyanosis, or vomiting, the patient's true condition may not be suspected.

ATYPICAL PERTUSSIS

Pertussis is mild or atypical in many cases. Whooping is not present in the majority of affected infants younger than 3 months or in the majority of affected adolescents and adults. Infants younger than 3 months may have apnea, seizures, or cyanotic episodes, and cough may not be identified as a major concern. Adults and older children with partial immunity are a reservoir for pertussis in the community. Their cases are relatively mild and may lack typical features of pertussis. In adults and older children, the disease is frequently misdiagnosed as bronchitis, sinusitis, or atypical pneumonia. Infection with *Bordetella parapertussis* is generally milder but cannot be distinguished from infection with *B. pertussis*.

COMPLICATIONS

Pertussis results in hospitalization for more than 50% of affected children younger than 1 year, and complications are most common in children less than 6 months. The presence of fever is suggestive of a bacterial superinfection, most commonly otitis media or pneumonia. Radiographically confirmed pneumonia is present in about 10% of cases. Nosebleed and subconjunctival hemorrhages are common but rarely serious. Seizures and encephalopathy occur in 1.5 and 0.1% of cases, respectively. Although the etiology of pertussis encephalopathy is unproven, prolonged hypoxemia resulting from persistent coughing is the most likely cause. Small hemorrhages in the central nervous system and hypoglycemia may also contribute. The presence of a specific neurotoxin is debated. The majority of pertussis deaths are associated with infection or encephalopathy. Inadequate nutrition increases the risk of complications, particularly if pre-existing malnutrition is present. Pertussis alone does not cause significant permanent lung injury, but bronchiectasis may result when superinfection and poor nutrition coexist.

DIAGNOSIS

Pertussis should be suspected in any patient with a significant cough lasting longer than 2 weeks. Suspicion should increase if paroxysmal coughing, whooping, or post-tussive emesis is reported or if family members are known to have pertussis or a prolonged coughing illness. The majority of adults and older teenagers are susceptible to pertussis regardless of prior immunization, as are incompletely immunized children. Pertussis is easily spread within households, and 80 to 90% of susceptible contacts develop symptoms. Knowledge of the local community epidemiology may help the clinician assess the risk of pertussis in relation to other viral or bacterial illnesses.

An elevated absolute lymphocyte count (20,000 to more than 100,000 per mm^3) is present during the late catarrhal and early paroxysmal phases and is suggestive of the diagnosis. Lymphocytosis may be absent in immunized patients, adults, and children younger than 6 months.

B. pertussis and B. parapertussis are the etiologic causes of pertussis, and culture has been the gold standard for diagnosis. Gengou, who used potato-glycerol media with added horse blood (Bordet-Gengou media), demonstrated laboratory isolation in 1906. The plates must be freshly prepared and have been largely replaced by other media, such as Regan-Lowe, which contains charcoal and horse blood, either with or without cephalexin to reduce overgrowth by normal flora. Pertussis-causing organisms are strictly aerobic, but plates must be well sealed to prevent drying of the media. Despite improvements in culture technique, recovery of B. pertussis is time consuming, and obtaining positive cultures usually requires 5 to 7 days of incubation. Properly obtained and processed cultures may be negative in otherwise typical clinical cases. Cultures are positive in the catarrhal and early (7 to 10 days) paroxysmal phases of disease, but negative cultures are obtained later in the course, in adults, in immunized patients, and in patients who have received an effective antimicrobial agent. Cultures obtained 3 or more weeks into the paroxysmal phase are seldom positive.

A rapid technique for the diagnosis of pertussis is direct fluorescent antibody (DFA) staining of respiratory secretions. Although the laboratory can perform this test rapidly, considerable technical expertise is needed, interobserver variability is high, and false-positive and false-negative results are common. Some commensal bacteria present in the respiratory tract stain positively in the DFA test. Secretions from culture-negative patients may test positive by DFA staining because of antimicrobial therapy or testing late in the course of the illness. Under these circumstances, differentiating a false-positive result from true infection is difficult.

Serologic testing was developed shortly after bacterial culture but has not been widely available until the 1990s. Enzyme-linked immunosorbent assays (ELISAs) are now available from several commercial reference laboratories. These assays vary widely between laboratories in target antigens (whole or sonicated bacteria, PT, FHA, or fimbrial antigens), in antibody isotype detected (IgG, IgA, and IgM), in laboratory technique, and in the quality of results. There is no accepted standard for the interpretation of serologic results, and therefore the clinician is dependent on the experience and qualification of the reference laboratory. It is not clear whether a single serum sample is sufficient or whether paired sera are required for accurate diagnosis. Pertussis infection causes elevation of IgG titers to PT and FHA in more than 90% of patients, but IgA titers are elevated in only 20 to 50%. Antibody to FHA, but not to PT, is detected after B. parapertussis infection. Antimicrobial therapy during the paroxysmal phase does not seem to diminish the antibody response. Interpretation of IgM titers has been difficult. Pertussis immunization usually does not increase IgA titers but causes significant IgG and IgM increases in most children. Therefore, elevated IgG or IgA titers indicate likely recent infection in nonimmunized children and in older adolescents or adults. Elevated IgA titers also indicate likely recent infection in immunized children. Serologic diagnosis is most useful in adults and nonimmunized children who have had symptoms for longer than 3 to 4 weeks or who have received an effective antimicrobial agent.

Detection of nucleic acid by polymerase chain reaction (PCR) is an excellent means of establishing a diagnosis of diseases such as pertussis, in which bacterial cultures are difficult and time consuming. Several commercial and reference laboratories offer PCR detection of pertussis with reported excellent sensitivity and specificity. These laboratories report many cases of culture-negative, PCR-positive pertussis with typical clinical features and positive serologic profiles. These findings suggest that PCR is more sensitive than culture, without loss of specificity. As a result, some laboratories no longer perform DFA and/or culture for pertussis. PCR is much faster than culture, depending on how frequently the test is offered. PCR is also superior to culture for patients treated with antimicrobial agents (56% vs. 0% after 7 days of therapy in one study). PCR may also be superior for testing immunized children, older patients, and those who are late in the paroxysmal phase and unlikely to be culture positive. There is no standard PCR assay, and sequences from the PT region, FHA, the region upstream of the porin gene, and repeated insertion sequences are used as the targets for amplification. FHA is present in both B. pertussis and B. parapertussis, but the other targets are specific for B. pertussis. Laboratory quality standards are essential for reliable PCR results. Laboratories that separate specimen processing from the PCR facility and that include positive and negative control specimens in each PCR run generally have more reliable results. The specific PCR targets, primers, and amplification strategy may affect specificity and sensitivity, but all of these factors may be difficult for the clinician to evaluate. PCR is more expensive than culture, but the cost is similar to the combined cost of culture and DFA. PCR is most useful when rapid diagnosis is needed and a positive culture is unlikely.

THERAPY

Therapy consists of good supportive care. Most hospitalized patients are infants, and careful monitoring of respiration and oxygenation are important. Administration of oxygen, suctioning of secretions from the airway, and occasional intubation and ventilation may be required. Frequent paroxysms may necessitate intensive care. Chest percussion, continuous oxygen, and aggressive suctioning may precipitate paroxysmal coughing. Good nutrition is essential, and parenteral nutrition should be given if enteral nutrition is not possible or if the child has pre-existing nutritional deficits. Fever is not present in uncomplicated pertussis, and the febrile infant should be carefully evaluated. Atelectasis and mucus plugging may be difficult to differentiate from bacterial pneumonia. Empirical antimicrobial therapy of suspected pneumonia or bacteremia is indicated, pending culture results and clinical improvement of the febrile patient. Droplet precautions should be maintained for 5 days after an effective antimicrobial regimen is begun, to prevent nosocomial transmission of pertussis.

Erythromycin estolate, 40 to 50 mg per kg per day (maximum, 1 gram per day) divided into two to four doses for 14 days, should be administered to the patient to reduce infectivity. Treatment does not improve symptoms of paroxysmal pertussis, but it may shorten the illness if given during the catarrhal phase. Family, household contacts, and others directly exposed to the patient's respiratory secretions should receive erythromycin in the same dosage and duration and should be monitored for symptoms consistent with pertussis. Erythromycin resistance has been documented in rare instances, and clinical laboratories do not test antimicrobial susceptibility. Studies show equal efficacy with 7 and 14 days of treatment with erythromycin estolate. Many patients do not tolerate erythromycin because of gastrointestinal symptoms. Clarithromycin (Biaxin; 15 mg per kg per day divided into 2 doses; maximum, 250 mg every 12 hours) and azithromycin (Zithromax; 10 mg per kg the first day, then 5 mg per kg for 4 days; maximum, 500 mg the first day, then 250 mg every day for 4 days) are better tolerated, although they are far more expensive. Limited studies have shown that the efficacy of clarithromycin for 7 days and azithromycin for 5 days is equivalent to that of erythromycin for 14 days. Trimethoprim-sulfamethoxazole (Bactrim, Septra; 8 to 12 mg per kg per day of trimethoprim divided into 2 doses for 14 days) is an alternative, but evidence of efficacy is lacking. The fluoroquinolone antimicrobials have excellent in vitro activity, but clinical trials are not available. Fluoroquinolones are currently not indicated for children.

Albuterol (Ventolin, Proventil; 0.3 to 0.5 mg per kg per dose every 6 to 8 hours) has reduced the frequency and duration of paroxysmal coughing in some, but not all, studies. In some young children, administration of aerosolized albuterol may precipitate paroxysmal coughing. Orally administered albuterol often causes tachycardia. In several small studies and in anecdotal reports, corticosteroids (e.g., dexamethasone, 0.3 mg per kg per day for 4 days, or hydrocortisone sodium succinate [Solu-Cortef], 30 mg per kg per day in decreasing dosage for 7 days) have been reported to reduce duration of cough and frequency of paroxysms. Steroids may mask the development of fever and other signs of bacterial superinfection and may confuse the interpretation of white blood cell counts. Steroid therapy should be considered in young infants with severe disease, in whom the potential benefit justifies the risks. Cough suppressants, mucolytics, antihistamines, expectorants, and sedatives have no benefit and may be harmful. Immune globulin is not useful.

PREVENTION

Control of epidemic pertussis has been achieved by universal childhood immunization, which confers 80 to 90% protection against the disease. Evidence of protection 10 to 12 years after vaccination is lacking. Immunization is initiated at 6 to 8 weeks of age, and additional doses are given at 4, 6, and 12 to 18 months. A booster is given at 4 to 6 years. Immunization with whole cell pertussis combined with diphtheria and tetanus toxoids (DPT) was the norm until the development of acellular pertussis vaccines (DaPT). Four different acellular vaccines are licensed in the United States and are preferred over whole-cell vaccine because of the reduced incidence of local swelling, erythema, fever, and other minor systemic reactions. The four licensed acellular vaccines differ in the amount of PT, FHA, pertactin and fimbrial antigens. Immunization may be initiated with any of these vaccines, but the series should be completed with a single vaccine whenever possible. Additional booster doses of pertussis vaccine are not currently recommended for older children or adults. The current immunization strategy does not protect infants at the highest risk of pertussis: those younger than 4 months. New vaccination strategies are needed to limit the circulation of pertussis in older adolescents and adults in order to reduce the incidence of severe pertussis in such young infants.

IMMUNIZATION PRACTICES

method of
RICHARD KENT ZIMMERMAN, M.D., M.P.H.
University of Pittsburgh School of Medicine
Pittsburgh, Pennsylvania

Vaccination has been tremendously successful in decreasing the incidence of vaccine-preventable diseases in the United States. For example, the total number of measles cases among U.S. children dropped from 458,083 in 1964, the year before widespread use of measles vaccine began, to 138 in 1997 (provisional total). Cases of *Haemophilus influenzae* type b (Hib) disease among children in the U.S. have also dropped dramatically, from an estimated 20,000 annually before introduction of Hib vaccine to fewer than 300 in 1996.

HEPATITIS B VACCINE

Between 128,000 and 320,000 persons are estimated to be infected annually in the United States with hepatitis B virus (HBV) according to the Centers for Disease Control

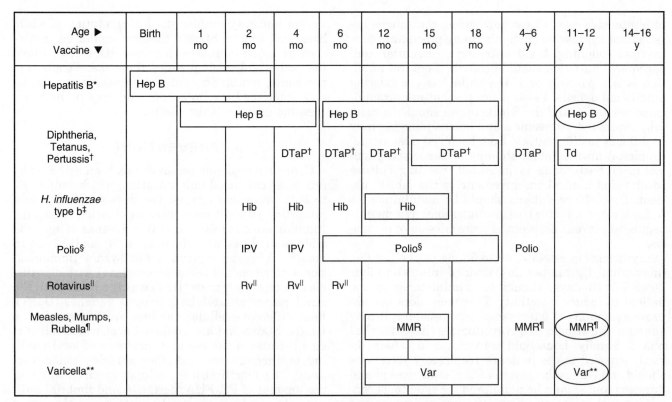

Figure 1. Recommended Childhood Immunization Schedule United States, January to December 1999. Vaccines are listed under routinely recommended ages. Bars indicate range of recommended ages for immunization. Any dose not given at the recommended age should be given as a "catch-up" immunization at any subsequent visit when indicated and feasible. Ovals indicate vaccines to be given if previously recommended doses were missed or given earlier than the recommended minimum age. This schedule indicates the recommended ages for routine administration of currently licensed childhood vaccines. Combination vaccines may be used whenever any components of the combination are indicated and its other components are not contraindicated. Providers should consult the manufacturers' package inserts for detailed recommendations.

*Infants born to HBsAg-negative mothers should receive the second dose of hepatitis B (Hep B) vaccine at least 1 month after the first dose. The third dose should be administered at least 4 months after the first dose and at least 2 months after the second dose, but not before 6 months of age for infants. *Infants born to HBsAg-positive mothers* should receive hepatitis B vaccine and 0.5 mL of hepatitis B immune globulin (HBIG) within 12 hours of birth at separate sites. The second dose is recommended at 1–2 months of age and the third dose at 6 months of age. *Infants born to mothers whose HBsAg status is unknown* should receive hepatitis B vaccine within 12 hours of birth. Maternal blood should be drawn at the time of delivery to determine the mother's HBsAg status; if the result is positive, the infant should receive HBIG as soon as possible (no later than 1 week of age). All children and adolescents (through 18 years of age) who have not been immunized against hepatitis B may begin the series during any visit. Special efforts should be made to immunize children who were born in or whose parents were born in areas of the world with moderate or high endemicity of hepatitis B virus infection.

†Diphtheria and tetanus toxoids and acellular pertussis vaccine (DTaP) is the preferred vaccine for all doses in the immunization series, including completion of the series in children who have received one or more doses of whole-cell DTP vaccine. Whole-cell DTP is an acceptable alternative to DTaP. The fourth dose (DTP or DTaP) may be administered as early as 12 months of age, provided 6 months have elapsed since the third dose and if the child is unlikely to return at age 15–18 months. Td (tetanus and diphtheria toxoids) is recommended at 11–12 years of age if at least 5 years have elapsed since the last dose of DTP, DTaP, or DT. Subsequent routine Td boosters are recommended every 10 years.

‡Three *Haemophilus influenzae* type b (Hib) conjugate vaccines are licensed for infant use. If PRP-OMP (PedvaxHIB or ComVax [Merck]) is administered at 2 and 4 months of age, a dose at 6 months is not required. Because clinical studies in infants have demonstrated that using some combination products may induce a lower immune response to the Hib vaccine component, DTaP/Hib combination products should not be used for primary immunization in infants at 2, 4, or 6 months of age, unless FDA-approved for these ages.

§Two poliovirus vaccines currently are licensed in the United States: inactivated poliovirus (IPV) vaccine and oral poliovirus (OPV) vaccine. The Advisory Committee on Immunization Practices (ACIP), the American Academy of Pediatrics (AAP), and the American Academy of Family Physicians (AAFP) now recommend that the first two doses of poliovirus vaccine should be IPV. The ACIP continues to recommend a sequential schedule of two doses of IPV administered at ages 2 and 4 months, followed by two doses of OPV at 12–18 months and 4–6 years. Use of IPV for all doses also is acceptable and is recommended for immunocompromised persons and their household contacts. OPV is no longer recommended for the first two doses of the schedule and is acceptable only for special circumstances, such as children of parents who do not accept the recommended number of injections, late initiation of immunization (which would require an unacceptable number of injections), and imminent travel to polio-endemic areas. OPV remains the vaccine of choice for mass immunization campaigns to control outbreaks due to wild poliovirus.

‖Rotavirus (Rv) vaccine is shaded and italicized to indicate that (1) health-care providers may require time and resources to incorporate this new vaccine into practice; and (2) the AAFP believes that the decision to use Rv vaccine should be made by the parent or guardian in consultation with the physician or other health care provider. The first dose of Rv vaccine should not be administered before 6 weeks of age, and the minimum interval between doses is 3 weeks. The Rv vaccine series should not be initiated at 7 months of age or older, and all doses should be completed by the first birthday.

Legend continued on opposite page

and Prevention (CDC), unpublished data. The number of persons chronically infected with HBV in the United States, each of whom is potentially infectious, is estimated at 1.25 million. HBV infection is much more likely to become chronic if acquired early in life than if acquired during adulthood: chronic HBV infection develops in 90% of those infected as infants, 30 to 60% of those infected before the age of 4 years, and only 5 to 10% of those infected as adults.

The hepatitis B vaccines currently produced in the United States are manufactured by recombinant DNA technology with baker's yeast and do not contain human plasma. The vaccination schedule is given in Figure 1.

For infants born to mothers with positive HBsAg status, postexposure prophylaxis, including both hepatitis B immune globulin (HBIG) and hepatitis B vaccine, should be initiated within 12 hours of birth, regardless of gestational age. These infants should receive their second and third doses of vaccine at ages 1 to 2 months and 6 months. If the mother is chronically infected with HBV, the infant should be tested for HBsAg and anti-HBs at 9 to 15 months of age.

For infants who weigh less than 2 kg at birth and whose mother is known to be HBsAg-negative, the first dose of hepatitis B vaccine should be delayed until the infant weighs 2 kg, because seroconversion rates are lower in infants born prematurely with birth weights less than 2 kg, and lower still in those with birth weights less than 1 kg.

PERTUSSIS VACCINE

Pertussis is transmitted primarily by respiratory droplets and is highly contagious: 70 to 100% of susceptible household contacts and 50 to 80% of susceptible school contacts will become infected following exposure. Pertussis complications include seizures, encephalopathy, and pneumonia, which occurs in about 15% of pertussis cases and is the leading cause of death from pertussis. Encephalopathy is fatal in approximately one third of cases and causes permanent brain damage in another one third.

In U.S. studies, diphtheria-tetanus-pertussis (DTP) vaccination was found to be between 70 and 90% effective in preventing pertussis disease. In studies conducted in Europe, diphtheria and tetanus toxoid and acellular pertussis (DTaP) vaccines demonstrated efficacies between 59 and 89% and DTP vaccines had efficacies from 36 to 98%.

DTaP vaccines have approximately one quarter to one half of the common adverse events associated with DTP vaccines; furthermore, the rates of adverse events are similar for DTaP and DT. Minor adverse events associated with DTP vaccination include localized edema at the injection site, fever, drowsiness,

and fretfulness. Uncommon adverse events are persistent crying for 3 or more hours after DTP vaccination, an unusual high-pitched cry, seizures, and hypotonic-hyporesponsive episodes. It is generally accepted that on rare occasions a child may have an anaphylactic reaction to DTP, and in these cases further doses of DTP or DTaP are contraindicated.

DTaP is recommended for all children because of the reduced reactions when compared with DTP. DTaP is strongly recommended over DTP for children with a family history of seizures. Premature infants should be vaccinated with full doses at the appropriate chronological age.

Completing the recommended series is important for optimal efficacy. For instance, one study found that the efficacy of whole-cell vaccine, based on a case definition of a cough of at least 14 days with paroxysms, whoop, or vomiting, is 36% after 1 dose, 49% after 2 doses, and 83% after 3 doses.

HAEMOPHILUS INFLUENZAE TYPE B VACCINES

Hib bacteria are spread by respiratory droplets and secretions. In unvaccinated populations, Hib is the most common cause of bacterial meningitis in preschool-aged children. Since the introduction of Hib vaccines, there has been a dramatic decrease (95%) in the rate of invasive Hib disease in children in the United States.

Three conjugate Hib vaccines—PRP-OMP (Pedvax-HIB), HbOC (HibTITER), and PRP-T (OmniHib/ActHIB)—approved for use in infants in the U.S. have estimated efficacies of 93 to 100% for a completed series. Adverse reactions to conjugate Hib vaccines are generally mild and include erythema, tenderness, or induration at the injection site.

All children younger than 60 months (after which time the risk of invasive Hib disease is significantly lower) should be vaccinated against Hib according to the recommended schedule shown in Table 1 for the particular Hib vaccine chosen. Hib vaccines should not be given before 6 weeks of age because they may induce immune tolerance, preventing adequate antibody response to further doses of Hib vaccine. Administration of Hib conjugate vaccines from different manufacturers results in as good or better antibody titers than does the same vaccine throughout the series; interchanging conjugate Hib vaccines is now considered fully acceptable.

Figure 1 *Continued*

¶The second dose of measles, mumps, and rubella (MMR) vaccine is recommended routinely at 4–6 years of age but may be administered during any visit, if at least 4 weeks have elapsed since receipt of the first dose and if both doses are administered beginning at or after 12 months of age. Patients who have not previously received the second dose should complete the schedule by the visit at 11–12 years of age.

**Varicella (Var) vaccine is recommended at any visit on or after the first birthday for susceptible children (i.e., those who lack a reliable history of chickenpox [as judged by a health care provider] and who have not been immunized. Susceptible persons 13 years of age or older should receive 2 doses, given at least 4 weeks apart.

Approved by the ACIP, AAP, and AAFP.

TABLE 1. **Detailed Vaccination Schedule for**
Haemophilus influenzae **Type b Conjugate Vaccines**

Vaccine	Age at First Dose (Months)	Primary Series	Booster
HbOC or PRP-T	2–6	3 doses, 2 mo apart	12–15 mo
	7–11	2 doses, 2 mo apart	12–18 mo
	12–14	1 dose	2 mo later
	15–59	1 dose	—
PRP-OMP (PedVaxHIB) (Comvax)	2–6	2 doses, 2 mo apart	12–15 mo 12–18 mo
	7–11	2 doses, 2 mo apart	2 mo later
PRP-D (Connaught) (ProHIBit)	12–14 15–59 15–59	1 dose 1 dose	— —

Hib = *Haemophilus influenzae* type b; HbOC = Hib vaccine conjugated with a pediatric dose of diphtheria toxoid; PRP-T = Hib vaccine conjugated with tetanus toxoid; PRP-OMP = Hib vaccine conjugated with *Neisseria meningitidis* group B; PRP-D = Hib vaccine conjugated with a pediatric dose of diphtheria toxoid.

Modified from Epidemiology and Prevention of Vaccine-Preventable Diseases. 4th ed. Atlanta, GA, Centers for Disease Control and Prevention, September 1997:110. Public domain.

POLIOVIRUS VACCINE

Poliovirus is quite infectious, and transmission to susceptible household contacts occurs in 73 to 96% of infections, depending on the contact's age. Poliovirus vaccination programs have resulted in dramatic decreases in disease incidence: circulation of indigenous wild polioviruses ceased in the United States in the 1960s and the last case of wild poliomyelitis contracted in the United States was reported in 1979. In 1994 the Americas were declared free of indigenous poliomyelitis.

Two vaccines are currently available in the United States for use to prevent poliomyelitis: inactivated poliovirus vaccine (IPV [IPOL]) and oral poliovirus vaccine (OPV [Orimune]). IPV cannot cause poliomyelitis but is administered by injection and offers less intestinal immunity. OPV has the advantage of easier administration, induces early intestinal immunity, and confers probably lifelong protection from poliomyelitis in almost all recipients. In one study of inner-city children unlikely to have been vaccinated, seropositivity rates ranged from 9 to 18% for poliovirus types 1 and 3 and from 29 to 42% for poliovirus type 2; thus secondary spread of OPV vaccine virus plays a modest role in increasing in inner-city populations. The main disadvantage of OPV is that the oral polioviruses can revert to a more virulent form and cause vaccine-associated paralytic poliomyelitis (VAPP). The overall risk of VAPP is quite small: 1 case per 2.4 million doses of OPV distributed. When VAPP occurs in healthy vaccine recipients, it is usually after the first dose of vaccine (1 case per 750,000 first doses). VAPP also occurs rarely in contacts of OPV recipients and among immunodeficient persons, especially those with B cell disorders, who are at highest risk of VAPP.

The Advisory Committee on Immunization Practices (ACIP), American Academy of Pediatrics (AAP), and American Academy of Family Physicians (AAFP) now recommend that the first 2 doses of poliovirus vaccine should be IPV, followed either by 2 more doses of IPV or by 2 doses of OPV; this later option is the sequential schedule. Most studies have shown that 2 doses of IPV induce protective levels of antibodies in greater than or equal to 90% of recipients. Thus, the sequential schedule avoids the risk of VAPP occurring when the first dose is OPV. For the sequential schedule, the ACIP recommends that the third dose be given at 12 to 18 months in order to delay administration of OPV until a later age, thereby increasing the likelihood that any immunodeficiencies, if present, would be diagnosed (in which case OPV would be withheld). OPV is recommended by the World Health Organization (WHO) for global eradication efforts and provides the earliest mucosal immunity.

Immunocompromised children and children with immunocompromised household contacts should receive IPV only. When an immunocompetent child starts the schedule after 6 months of age, the parents refuse the number of injections required for IPV use, or if the child is traveling to countries where poliovirus is endemic, then the all-OPV schedule is acceptable. IPV should be used for the primary vaccination of adults 18 years of age or older.

ROTAVIRUS VACCINE

Rotavirus is the most common cause of severe gastroenteritis in preschool-aged children in the United States. The annual number of hospitalizations in the U.S. range from 23,000 to 110,000 with recent data suggesting about 50,000: that is, 1 in 78. Rotavirus also results in about 160,000 emergency department visits and about 410,000 physician visits; 10.5% of children will be seen by a physician in the first 5 years of life for this illness. Rotaviruses are shed in very high concentrations in human feces (i.e., 10^{11} particles per gram) but a person can be infected by a low dose (i.e., about 10 viral particles); thus, rotavirus is highly contagious. It is spread by the fecal-oral route.

A live, tetravalent rhesus rotavirus vaccine (RRV [Rota Shield]), was licensed in 1998, based on a modified Jennerian (e.g., smallpox-like) approach to vaccination. In a U.S. trial over one season of observation was 49% (95% confidence interval of 31 to 63%) for gastroenteritis, 73% (95% confidence interval [CI] of 54 to 84%) for gastroenteritis resulting in physician intervention, and 100% against dehydration. Finnish data show that protection lasts several years. Based on cost-effectiveness analyses, RRV should be cost-saving to society.

Although most children do not have reactions to RRV, low-grade fever, diarrhea, and irritability sometimes occur. The incidence in the 5 days after administration of the first dose of a temperature greater than 38°C was 21% in vaccinees versus 6% in controls; for a temperature greater than 39°C, the rates were 2% versus 1%.

RRV is administered orally on a 2-, 4-, and 6-month schedule. The RRV series should not be started at 7 months of age or later and the third dose should be given before 12 months of age.

Contraindications include known or suspected immunodeficiency and anaphylaxis to a previous dose of RRV. It is reasonable to delay vaccination in a child who has been vomiting.

MEASLES, MUMPS, AND RUBELLA VACCINE (MMR)

Measles is transmitted person-to-person by respiratory droplets and also by smaller aerosolized droplets that can spread through ventilation systems within a building and are infective for at least 1 hour. Infected persons may transmit the disease 4 days before and 4 days after the appearance of the rash. After the introduction of measles vaccine in 1963, the incidence of measles dropped by more than 98%, although a major epidemic in 1989 to 1991 caused 55,467 reported cases and 136 deaths.

The measles vaccine contains live, highly attenuated virus. After measles vaccination, seroconversion rates are 95% for children vaccinated at 12 months of age and 98% for children vaccinated at 15 months of age.

When measles outbreaks occurred among school-aged children in the United States in the 1980s, despite high vaccination levels, measles vaccination guidelines were reassessed. Studies have found that failure of seroconversion after the initial dose of measles vaccine occurs at a rate of 2 to 5%. In 1989 the ACIP recommended a second dose of measles-containing vaccine at age 4 to 6 years (entry to kindergarten or first grade) in order to provide protection for most of those who did not respond to the initial measles vaccination.

VARICELLA VACCINE

Varicella in children is typically a self-limited, benign illness. However, complications can occur, and the disease is highly contagious, as indicated by secondary household attack rates as high as 90% in unvaccinated household contacts. Communicability (by the respiratory route) begins 1 to 2 days before the rash develops and lasts until all lesions have formed crusts. Most children who need hospitalization due to varicella were immunologically normal. Varicella is more severe in infants and adults than in children, as seen by age-specific hospitalization rates of 103, 23, and 65 per 10,000 cases in infants, 1- to 4-year-olds, and 20- to 29-year-olds, respectively. However, because the incidence of varicella is so high in young children, they suffer the highest hospitalization rate: the largest number of annual hospitalizations for varicella (2814) is in 1- to 4-year-olds. Routine vaccination of children 12 to 18 months of age was determined to be a cost-savings to society.

The varicella vaccine (Varivax), currently available contains live, attenuated virus and is highly immunogenic: almost all (97%) of children 1 to 12 years of age seroconvert after 1 dose. The ACIP concluded that varicella vaccination provides 70 to 90% protection against infection and 95% protection against severe disease for 7 to 10 years after vaccination. Furthermore, if children who have been vaccinated contract varicella, the clinical course is milder.

Adverse events after varicella vaccination consist principally of pain and erythema at the injection site. After vaccination, 4 to 6% of recipients report a generalized varicella-like rash consisting of a few (median 5) lesions. Children with leukemia who were immunized have transmitted the virus to others; however, the virus does not become more virulent. The risk of herpes zoster is lower after vaccination than after naturally acquired varicella.

Catch-up varicella vaccination is recommended for children between 18 months and 12 years old who do *not* have a history of varicella. Varicella vaccine is approved in adolescents (13 years of age or older) and adults without a history of chickenpox on a 2-dose schedule; the doses should be spaced 4 to 8 weeks apart. The vaccine is heat sensitive and must be stored at −15°C (+5°F) or colder. Vaccine not used within 30 minutes after being reconstituted should be discarded.

Vaccinees who develop a varicelliform rash after vaccination may be contagious; hence they should avoid contact with individuals at high risk for complications of varicella, such as immunocompromised persons. If contact does occur, however, it is not necessary to give the immunocompromised contact varicella-zoster immune globulin (VZIG) because the virus in the vaccine is attenuated.

INFLUENZA VACCINE

In each of the 10 most recent influenza epidemics in the United States, estimated deaths totaled more than 20,000. Furthermore, during some epidemics of influenza type A, approximately 172,000 hospitalizations were attributable to influenza and pneumonia. The cost of a severe influenza epidemic is estimated at $12 billion.

The elderly, partly because they have a higher incidence of chronic medical conditions, have the highest age-specific case-fatality rate from influenza: more than 90% of deaths due to influenza occur in persons 65 years of age or older. In one study of the elderly, influenza vaccination resulted in a 27 to 39% reduction in hospitalizations (depending on the year studied) due to acute or chronic respiratory conditions and, in 1 year, a 37% reduction in hospitalization due to congestive heart failure.

Beginning each September, when vaccine for the upcoming influenza season becomes available, all persons 50 years of age and older who are seen by health care providers should be offered influenza vaccine so that vaccination opportunities are not missed.

In addition, persons at high risk and those 6 months of age or older should receive influenza vaccine.

PNEUMOCOCCAL VACCINE

Pneumococcal disease causes an estimated 3,000 cases of meningitis, 50,000 cases of bacteremia, and 500,000 cases of pneumonia annually in the United States. Most (60 to 87%) cases of pneumococcal bacteremia in adults are associated with pneumonia and the rate of bacteremia is highest in persons 65 years of age and older. Despite appropriate therapy, the overall case-fatality rate for pneumococcal bacteremia is 15 to 20% among adults; this climbs to approximately 30 to 40% for elderly patients.

All persons 65 years of age and older should receive 1 dose of pneumococcal vaccine (Pneumovax 23), unless they are known to have received vaccination within the past 5 years. A prime opportunity for vaccination in this age group is at hospital discharge: in one study, 61 to 62% of persons aged 65 years or older who were hospitalized with pneumonia had been discharged from a hospital within the previous 4 years.

LATE VACCINATIONS

If the vaccination schedule is interrupted, it does not need to be restarted. Instead, the schedule should be resumed with minimal intervals between doses (Table 2).

VACCINATION PROCEDURES

Contraindications

There are two permanent contraindications to administering a dose of vaccine: (1) severe allergy to a vaccine component or anaphylactic reaction to a previous dose of the vaccine and (2) for pertussis vaccine, encephalopathy without a known cause within 7 days of a dose of pertussis vaccine. Contact dermatitis from neomycin, however, is a delayed-type (cell-mediated) immune response and is not a contraindication to vaccination. If the pertussis component is withheld because of a contraindication or precaution, then pediatric DT is administered instead, except in the case of true anaphylaxis, in which the diphtheria and pertussis components are permanently contraindicated.

Four conditions are temporary contraindications to vaccination: severe acute illness, immunosuppression, pregnancy, and recent receipt of blood products. *Severe acute illness* usually warrants postponement of vaccination until the patient has recovered from the acute phase.

Immunosuppression due to an immune deficiency disease or malignancy or therapy with high-dose corticosteroid drugs, alkylating agents, antimetabolites,

TABLE 2. **Minimum Age for Initial Vaccination and Minimum Interval Between Vaccine Doses, by Type of Vaccine***

Vaccine	Minimal Age for Dose 1	Minimal Interval from Dose 1 to 2	Minimal Interval from Dose 2 to 3	Minimal Interval from Dose 3 to 4
DTP/DTaP (DT)†	6 wk	4 wk	4 wk	6 mo
Combined DTP-Hib‡	6 wk	1 mo	1 mo	6 mo
Hib (primary series)				
HbOC	6 wk	1 mo	1 mo‡	
PRP-T	6 wk	1 mo	1 mo‡	
PRP-OMP	6 wk	1 mo‡		
Poliovirus§	6 wk	4 wk	4 wk‖	¶
MMR	12 mo‡	1 mo		
Hepatitis B	Birth	1 mo	2 mo‡	
Varicella	12 mo	4 wk		

*The minimal acceptable ages and intervals may not correspond with the *optimal* recommended ages and intervals for vaccination. For current recommended routine schedules see the annual Recommended Childhood Immunization Schedule, United States.

†DTP = pediatric dose of diphtheria toxoid and tetanus toxoid and whole-cell pertussis vaccine; DT = pediatric dose of diphtheria toxoid and tetanus toxoid. The total number of doses of diphtheria and tetanus toxoids should not exceed 6 each before the seventh birthday.

‡Hib = *Haemophilus influenzae* type b vaccine. The booster dose of Hib vaccine that is recommended following the primary vaccination series should be administered no earlier than 12 months of age *and* at least 2 months after the previous dose of Hib vaccine (See Table 1).

§Poliovirus vaccines include inactivated poliovirus vaccine (IPV) and oral poliovirus vaccine (OPV). Acceptable vaccination series include sequential IPV-OPV, all-OPV, all-IPV.

‖For unvaccinated adults at increased risk of exposure to poliovirus with less than 3 months but greater than 2 months available before protection is needed, 3 doses of IPV should be administered at least 1 month apart.

¶If the third dose is given after the third birthday, the fourth (booster) dose is not needed.

**Although the age for measles vaccination may be as young as 6 months in outbreak areas where cases are occurring in children less than 1 year of age, children initially vaccinated before the first birthday should be revaccinated at 12 to 15 months of age and an additional dose of vaccine should be administered at the time of school entry or according to local policy. Doses of MMR or other measles-containing vaccines should be separated by at least 1 month.

‡This final dose is recommended at least 4 months after the first dose and no earlier than 6 months of age.

MMR = measles, mumps, and rubella vaccine; HbOC = Hib vaccine conjugated with a pediatric dose of diphtheria toxoid; PRP-T = Hib vaccine conjugated with tetanus toxoid; PRP-OMP = Hib vaccine conjugated with *Neisseria meningitidis* group B.

Modified from Epidemiology and Prevention of Vaccine-Preventable Diseases, 4th ed. Atlanta, GA, Centers for Disease Control and Prevention, 1994. Public domain.

or irradiation is a contraindication to administration of a live vaccine, (although human immunodeficiency virus [HIV]-infected persons who are not severely immunosuppressed should receive MMR vaccine when indicated). Inactivated vaccines may be given to immunosuppressed persons because they do not contain live organisms that can replicate; however, immunosuppression may decrease the response to vaccination.

Pregnancy is a contraindication to administration of live-virus vaccines because of the theoretical risk of damage to the fetus. Women should avoid becoming pregnant within 3 months of receiving MMR or rubella vaccine and within 1 month of mumps or varicella vaccination. Inadvertent administration of a live-virus vaccine during pregnancy is not an indication for pregnancy termination because there are no data to link live-virus vaccination with increased risk of fetal malformations. Vaccines may be given to breast-feeding mothers.

Recent administration of blood products can interfere with development of an immune response to a live-virus (but not inactivated-virus) vaccine. CDC information that describes when various vaccines may be administered in such cases has been published.

Precautions

Precautions for vaccination are conditions that *may* increase the risk for a serious or life-threatening adverse event or may compromise the ability of the vaccine to produce immunity. Generally, the vaccine is withheld or postponed in such situations. However, the decision whether to vaccinate in such cases is made by weighing the individual patient's risk of acquiring the disease against the risk of the adverse event (or inability to produce immunity). Certain infrequent adverse events occurring after pertussis vaccination are precautions to further doses: (1) temperature of 40.5°C (105°F) or greater within 48 hours of a previous dose (not due to another identifiable cause); (2) collapse or shock-like state (hypotonic-hyporesponsive episode) with 48 hours of a previous dose; (3) persistent, inconsolable crying lasting 3 hours or more, occurring within 48 hours of a previous dose; or (4) convulsions within 3 days of a previous dose.

DTaP vaccination should be postponed for infants with an evolving neurologic disorder, unevaluated seizures, or a neurologic event between doses of pertussis vaccine. Vaccination should be resumed after evaluation and treatment of the condition.

Vaccine Information Statements for Patients

Under the Public Health Services Act, health care providers who administer any vaccine containing diphtheria, tetanus, pertussis, measles, mumps, rubella, poliovirus, varicella, hepatitis B, or Hib antigens are required to provide a copy of the relevant Vaccine Information Statements (VISs) to patients before vaccination. These VISs may be downloaded from www.cdc.gov/nip/vistable.htm.

Interchangeability of Vaccines from Different Manufacturers

Vaccines from different manufacturers can be given interchangeably if the disease has a serologic test that shows if a person is protected, as is the case for hepatitis B and Hib. No data are yet available on the safety or efficacy of acellular pertussis vaccination when different brands are administered for the first 3 doses. Thus, when possible, use of the same brand of acellular pertussis vaccine for sequential doses is preferred. However, when a child who started the series with one brand is due for another dose and the office stocks a different brand, it may be used.

Simultaneous Vaccination and Combination Vaccines

Most vaccines will be efficacious and safe when administered simultaneously with another vaccine, *except for* (1) yellow fever and cholera vaccine, which should be administered at least 3 weeks apart, and (2) cholera and plague vaccines, which should be given on separate occasions to avoid augmentation of adverse events.

TRAVEL MEDICINE

method of
MARTIN S. WOLFE, M.D.
Georgetown Medical School, George Washington University Medical School, and Traveler's Medical Service
Washington, D.C.

Of the approximately 15 million Americans who travel abroad each year, about half go to the developing world. Short-term consultants and tourists and, to a greater extent, longer term travelers and resident expatriates are exposed to diseases and environmental factors that are not present, or are at least rare, in the United States. In response to the hazards of travel to these millions of travelers, the medical specialty of travel medicine has evolved in recent years.

Travel medicine deals with both the prevention of travel-related disorders and the diagnosis and treatment of exotic, primarily tropical diseases. A focal point for travel and tropical medicine specialists is the American Society of Tropical Medicine and Hygiene (ASTMH) and this society's American Committee on Clinical Tropical Medicine and Travelers' Health. Although there are no specialty boards for travel or tropical medicine, the ASTMH prepares an annual examination to assess and recognize individual excellence in training and knowledge. Passing the examination leads to a Certificate of Knowledge in Clinical Tropical Medicine and Travelers' Health.* Another organization dealing with all aspects of travel medicine is the International Society of Travel Medicine (ISTM).†

Perhaps the most valuable general resource for information on preventive measures for travelers is *Health Hints for the Tropics*, published by the U.S. Public Health Service

---

*Information on ASTMH activities and the Certification Examination may be obtained from the American Society of Tropical Medicine and Hygiene, 60 Revere Drive, Suite 500, Northbrook, Illinois, 60062; phone: 847-480-9592; fax: 847-480-9282.

†Information on ISTM activities may be obtained from ISTM Secretariat, P.O. Box 871089, Stone Mountain, Georgia 30087-0028; phone: 770-736-7060; fax: 770-736-6732.

(for sale by the Superintendent of Documents, U.S. Government Printing Office, Washington, D.C. 20402; phone: 202-512-1800). Travel clinics have been established at many medical centers nationwide, as have numerous private travel clinics. Travel medicine information and, in some cases, expertise can be obtained from health departments at various government levels, which are in turn supported with information from the Centers for Disease Control and Prevention (CDC). Personal physicians should be the initial contact person for travelers in order to evaluate health and to regulate any existing health problems. In view of a certain amount of travel medicine knowledge on the part of the personal physician and a rather straightforward itinerary for the healthy traveler, the usual needs of the traveler may be satisfied at this level. More complicated needs should be provided by the nearest formal travel clinic.

PRE-TRAVEL ADVICE

A pre-travel physical examination is recommended for travelers with serious medical problems, for those planning a long or physically demanding trip, and for those planning to reside abroad. This examination is better accomplished by a personal physician who is familiar with the traveler and his or her health history. A medical summary and a copy of recent pertinent laboratory tests, electrocardiogram, or chest radiograph should be taken along by the traveler. Engraved bracelets or health cards with a brief summary of a serious medical condition can be obtained from a number of sources. The names of well-recognized English-speaking physicians overseas can be given to the traveler. The traveler's health insurance should be reviewed to determine whether coverage applies to conditions acquired while traveling, to hospitalization abroad, or to medical evacuation from foreign countries.

In some countries, over-the-counter drugs often lack label warnings. Travelers must be cautioned that potentially dangerous drugs may be included in such preparations, including chloramphenicol, sulfas, Butazolidin, and aminopyrine, among others. Travelers with chronic illnesses should carry a sufficient supply of required drugs.

PREPARATION OF AN INDIVIDUALIZED MEDICAL KIT

Components of a traveler's medical kit vary according to pre-existing and other potential needs. Useful general items include a thermometer, bandages, gauze, tape, a bactericidal soap solution, aspirin, antacids, anti–motion sickness drug, and a mild laxative or suppository for constipation. A nasal decongestant and saline nose drops may be useful during flight. An antihistamine may be taken for allergies. Cough medicine and other liquids should be carried in tightly stoppered plastic bottles. Antibiotic, antifungal, and anti-inflammatory ointments may be included. Salt tablets may be helpful in hot, humid climates. A sunscreen should be included. In general, antibiotics should not be given to the average traveler. If sufficiently ill, the traveler would be better served by consulting a local physician, except in remote areas where medical assistance is not readily available.

Suggested items for a traveler's medical kit and information on the use of specific products can be found in *Health Hints for the Tropics*.* Specific items are discussed in the following sections.

---

*Available from the American Society of Tropical Medicine and Hygiene at the address given earlier.

REQUIRED AND RECOMMENDED IMMUNIZATIONS

Vaccine requirements by country are published by the CDC in *Health Information for International Travel*. A number of commercial computer programs are also available.

Yellow fever vaccine is given only in travel clinics and other state-licensed official vaccination centers. Because this vaccine requires cold storage, it is viable for only 60 minutes after reconstitution. Certain other vaccines are difficult to obtain or come only in multiple-dose vials and are thus more cost-effective at busy travel clinics and government facilities; these include meningococcal meningitis, plague, Japanese encephalitis, and rabies vaccines.

Required Immunizations

Yellow Fever. Yellow fever occurs in parts of tropical Africa and South America, and the vaccine may be required for entry into countries in these regions or for travelers wishing to enter other countries if they have come from a country with regions where the disease is present. The vaccination must be validated in the specific section of the Yellow International Certificate of Vaccination. Yellow fever vaccine is contraindicated in anyone with altered immune status or a known hypersensitivity to eggs, in children below age 9 months, and in pregnant women. These persons should be given a letter of contraindication with an official letterhead and must be warned not to enter any area with active yellow fever infection. A single dose is valid for 10 years, and side effects are minimal.

Cholera. In 1988, the World Health Organization (WHO) dropped the requirement for cholera vaccine, and the International Certificate of Vaccination no longer has a special section for cholera. Cholera vaccine is not recommended for most travelers, even those going to cholera-epidemic areas, because the currently available, injectable, inactivated vaccine is not very effective in preventing cholera. Travelers should practice appropriate hygiene in handling food and water to prevent cholera, as well as numerous other diseases. Two new oral cholera vaccines have been developed, which are effective and better tolerated and provide high-level protection, at least for several months. Neither of these vaccines appears to offer protection against the O139 serogroup of *Vibrio cholerae*. These vaccines are not yet available in the United States, and recommendations for their use in travelers have not yet been formulated.

Smallpox. In 1983, the WHO deleted smallpox from the list of diseases subject to the International Health Regulations. The risk from smallpox vaccine exceeds the risk of contracting smallpox, and vaccination is not indicated for any international traveler.

Recommended Travel Immunizations (Table 1)

Certain vaccines are recommended for protection against diseases prevalent in many parts of the world. For children, routine childhood immunizations should be up to date before travel is undertaken (see the article on immunization practices).

Hepatitis A Vaccine. Hepatitis A is the most common type of hepatitis contracted by unprotected travelers to areas of endemicity. Two hepatitis A vaccines are now available in the United States. Havrix (SmithKline Beecham) and Vaqta (Merck) given in 2 two-dose series 6 to 12 months apart are expected to provide long-term

TABLE 1. **Dosing Schedules for Commonly Used Vaccines for Travel**

Vaccine	Primary Series	Booster Interval
Hepatitis A (Havrix, Vaqta)	1 dose for adults and children older than 2 y	1 dose 6 to 12 months after first dose One time only
Hepatitis B (Engerix-B) (accelerated schedule)	3 doses at 0, 30, and 60 d	A fourth dose is recommended at 12 months
Hepatitis B (Engerix-B) (standard schedule) or Hepatitis B (Recombivax) (standard schedule)	3 doses at 0, 1, and 6 mo	Need for further booster not determined
Immune globulin (IG) (hepatitis A protection)	1 dose IM in the gluteus muscle (2-mL dose for 3-mo protection; 5-mL dose for 5 mo); pediatric dose, 0.02 mL/kg for 3-month trip; 0.06 mL/kg for 5-month trip)	At 3- to 5-month intervals
Japanese encephalitis (JEV) (Japanese manufacturer, Biken)	3 doses on days 0, 7, and 30 (1 mL SC for children older than 3 y; 0.5 mL SC for children younger than 3 y)	After 3 years
Measles/mumps/rubella (MMR)*	1 dose† SC at 15 mo of age	Booster measles vaccine at 4–6 y old; boost measles vaccine *once* in adult life before international travel for people born in or after 1957
Meningococcus† (A/C/Y/W-135)	1 dose†	After 3 years
Plague†	First and second doses given 1–3 mo apart; third dose given 5–6 months after second dose	Booster if the risk of exposure persists
Poliomyelitis, enhanced-potency inactivated (eIPV) (killed vaccine; safe for all ages)	Single dose at ages 2, 4, and 6–18 months, and 4–6 years	*Once* before travel in areas of risk
Poliomyelitis, oral (OPV) (attenuated live virus)*	Single dose at ages 2, 4, and 6–18 months, and 4–6 years	*Once* before travel in areas of risk
Rabies, human diploid cell vaccine (HDCV) or Rabies, purified chick embryo cell vaccine (PCEC) or Rabies vaccine absorbed (RVA)	3 doses (1-mL doses IM in deltoid area) on days 0, 7, and 21 or 28	With frequent exposure risk, booster after 2 years or test serum for antibody level
Tetanus and diphtheria toxoids adsorbed (Td) (for children older than 7 y of age and for adults)	3 doses (0.5 mL SC or IM); first and second doses given 4–8 wk apart; third dose at 6–12 mo after second dose	Routinely every 10 years
Typhoid, oral (Vivotif)	1 capsule orally every other day for 4 doses (>6 y old)	5 years
Typhoid, Vi capsular polysaccharide vaccine (Typhim Vi)	Single dose (>2 y old)	2 years
Varicella (Varivax)	1 dose for children younger than 13 years of age; 2 doses for susceptible persons older than 13 y of age	None currently recommended
Yellow fever*	1 dose (0.5 mL SC); (for those 9 mo of age and older)	10 years

*Caution: may be contraindicated in patients with any of the following conditions: pregnancy; leukemia; lymphoma; generalized malignancy; immunosuppression due to HIV infection; or treatment with corticosteroids, alkylating drugs, antimetabolites, or radiation therapy.
†See manufacturer's package insert and text for detailed recommendations on dosage and schedule.
Adapted from Jong EC, McMullen R: The Travel and Tropical Medicine Manual, 2nd ed. Philadelphia: WB Saunders Co, 1995.

protection against infection. These vaccines are available in both adult and pediatric formulations. Children older than 2 years of age can receive the vaccine. After administration of an initial single dose of either vaccine, protective immunity can be assumed to be present by 4 weeks.

Hepatitis B Vaccine. Hepatitis B is more prevalent in the developing world and is a particular hazard for travelers having contact with blood or having sexual contact with local residents. If such contacts are possible, a recombinant hepatitis B vaccine series can be administered. Both available U.S.-licensed vaccines can be given in a standard three-dose series over a 6-month period. However, Engerix B (SmithKline Beecham) is approved for an accelerated course of three monthly doses, with a fourth booster given 12 months after the first dose. Hepatitis B vaccine is safe and effective, but its relatively high cost and extended course of doses are major inhibitors to its wide use in travelers.

Immune Globulin. This is an alternative to hepatitis A vaccine when only short-term protection is needed against hepatitis A. Persons traveling for less than 3 months are protected by a single intramuscular dose of 0.02 mL per kg. Those traveling for longer periods of up to 4 to 6 months should receive a 0.06 mL per kg dose. However, hepatitis A vaccine, although more expensive, is much more cost-effective and longer lasting for the longer term or frequent traveler.

Influenza Vaccine. Persons considered at high risk of contracting influenza who are traveling to areas of the world where epidemic influenza is present should receive the influenza vaccine.

Japanese Encephalitis Vaccine. Rare cases of Japanese encephalitis (JE) have occurred in resident expatriates and travelers in certain areas of the Far East and Southeast Asia where JE is endemic or epidemic. The risk of infection is much greater in rural agricultural than in urban areas and in some areas the risk is seasonal. A 3-dose JE vaccine series is recommended for persons spending more than 1 month in endemic areas during the transmission season, especially if travel includes rural areas, and for certain shorter term travelers to areas where epidemics occur and risk is high. JE vaccine is associated with moderately frequent local and mild systemic side effects and uncommonly with more serious allergic reactions. The rate of serious reactions in American citizens is approximately 2 to 6 per 1000 vaccine recipients. These reactions may be delayed in onset for 10 to 14 days.

Measles Vaccine. The risk of contracting measles is much greater in the developing world than in the United States, and for younger children traveling to measles-endemic areas, the age at immunization should be lowered from the usual 15 months to 6 months. A second dose of measles vaccine should be given at age 12 to 15 months. Adults born in the United States in or after 1957 are considered immune to measles, but persons born after 1957 who travel abroad should be protected against measles. Travelers who have not previously received 2 doses of measles vaccine and who do not have a history of measles infection should receive 1 dose of measles vaccine, unless there is a contraindication.

Meningococcal Meningitis Vaccine. Meningococcal meningitis is endemic worldwide, but in particular areas, seasonal epidemics caused by *Neisseria meningitidis* serogroup A and C occur. In the sub-Saharan Sahel region of Africa, epidemics occur almost yearly in the colder months. Meningitis is very uncommon in travelers, but immunization with the quadrivalent A,C,Y,W135 vaccine is recommended for all travelers to countries in this "meningitis belt" during the epidemic season. Pilgrims to Saudi Arabia for the Haj are required to have proof of this vaccine. Outbreaks of meningococcal meningitis serogroup B also occur, but there is currently no available vaccine against this serogroup.

Plague Vaccine. The usual traveler to plague-endemic countries is at very low risk of infection. Most outbreaks have occurred in remoter areas. Certain travelers at high risk for this disease should consider plague immunization. These include mammalogists, ecologists, and other field workers who have regular contact with wild rodents or fleas in plague-enzootic or plague-epizootic areas.

Polio Vaccine. Poliovirus transmission has been interrupted in the Americas, but wild poliovirus continues to circulate in other parts of the world. Polio remains a definite hazard to travelers to polio-affected areas of the world. Most adult travelers have had a basic polio vaccine series during childhood, and a single dose of either oral or injectable vaccine is recommended before travel. This is expected to give life-long protection, and the need for further supplementary doses has not been established.

Rabies Vaccine. Relatively few countries can be considered rabies free. For travelers to rabies-endemic countries who may be at high risk of infection, primarily from dog bites, a 3-dose intramuscular pre-exposure rabies vaccine series may be recommended. These might include young children, joggers, people working with animals, field workers, and persons in remote areas who are distant from facilities where adequate postexposure treatment can be obtained. Pre-exposure immunizations offers valuable added protection when rabies exposure occurs and the need for human rabies immune globulin, which is often difficult to obtain, is eliminated. However, administration of two post-exposure vaccine doses is still required. Three vaccines, all very expensive, are available in the United States: human diploid cell vaccine (HDCV); purified chick embryo culture vaccine (PCEC); and rabies vaccine adsorbed (RVA).

Tetanus-Diphtheria (Td) Vaccine. It is essential for all Americans, traveling or not, to maintain immunity against tetanus and diphtheria by getting a booster dose at 10-year intervals. Most travelers have had the basic diphtheria-pertussis-tetanus (DPT) vaccine during childhood. For boosters, persons older than age 7 years receive Td vaccine, which has a smaller amount of diphtheria toxoid. A particular risk of diphtheria infection is present in Russia and the new independent states, where epidemics occur.

Tick-Borne Encephalitis (TBE) Vaccine. TBE is a viral infection of the central nervous system that occurs in forested areas of central and eastern Europe and the former Soviet Union. This vaccine is unavailable in the United States, but an effective vaccine may be obtained in Europe and can be considered for travelers or residents who are at risk of exposure in forested areas of countries where the disease is endemic.

Tuberculosis–Bacille Calmette-Guèrin (BCG) Vaccine. BCG vaccine is rarely recommended for American travelers, but the worldwide increase in multidrug-resistant tuberculosis may reawaken interest in this vaccine.

Typhoid Vaccine. Typhoid fever is endemic in the developing world, and typhoid vaccine is recommended for travelers to those areas, where it is difficult to follow good hygienic practices with water and food. Two vaccines are recommended in the United States, and both provide only about 70% protection. An oral, live-attenuated vaccine is administered in capsules, with one capsule taken every other day for 4 doses; a booster series is required every 5 years for those still at risk. A parenteral capsular polysaccharide vaccine given in a single dose provides protection for 2 years.

Typhus Vaccine. Typhus vaccine is no longer recommended and is not available in the United States.

Varicella Vaccine. International travelers who do not have evidence of immunity to varicella virus should consider having this vaccine, especially if close personal contact with local populations is expected.

Immunization During Pregnancy and Breast-Feeding

Pregnancy is not a contraindication to the administration of toxoid vaccines, killed or inactivated vaccines, or immune globulin when risk of infection is present. Live measles-mumps-rubella, varicella, and live oral typhoid vaccines are contraindicated during pregnancy. Yellow fever vaccine is contraindicated unless exposure to yellow fever virus is unavoidable. Breast-feeding does not adversely affect immunizations and is not a contraindication for any vaccine. Neither killed nor live vaccines affect the safety of breast-feeding for mothers or infants.

Altered Immunocompetence

Killed or inactivated vaccines and immune globulin are not contraindicated for immunocompromised travelers. Measles vaccine is recommended for immunosuppressed travelers for whom it is indicated. Oral polio vaccine, however, should not be given to any immunocompromised person or to his or her household or other close contacts. Except in extremely unusual situations of high infection risk, yellow fever vaccine is contraindicated in immunosuppressed travelers.

PROPHYLACTIC MEASURES FOR MALARIA

With the emergence and continual spread of chloroquine and other drug-resistant *Plasmodium falciparum*–related malaria and the complexities involved with contraindications and toxic side effects of malarial prophylactic drugs, physicians may find it very difficult to offer appropriate advice to travelers. Travel clinics are better able to keep up to date on areas of resistance and to make decisions on the best drug and antimosquito measures for particular travelers. Malaria is probably the greatest hazard to travelers in many parts of the developing world, and expert opinion is required in order to give optimal protection. (See also the article on malaria.)

Drug Prophylaxis

P. falciparum is the species that causes the most serious malaria. This parasite is almost universally resistant to chloroquine and, to a lesser extent, to other available antimalarial drugs. *P. falciparum* remains sensitive to chloroquine only in Central America, Haiti, the Dominican Republic, and parts of the Middle East. In these areas, a weekly 500-mg dose of chloroquine phosphate (equal to a 300-mg base) can be used. In the United States, generic chloroquine phosphate is unavailable, and only oral Aralen Phosphate in a 500-mg salt tablet can be obtained. Other tablet and liquid preparations are available abroad. Chloroquine is considered safe in pregnancy.

For protection against chloroquine-resistant *P. falciparum* malaria, three available regimens are currently recommended by American experts.

Mefloquine (Lariam). This regimen is considered the most effective of the three. There is a high level of mefloquine resistance by *P. falciparum* parasites along the Thai-Cambodia and Thai-Myanmar borders, and rare confirmed cases of resistance in tropical Africa and other malarious areas have been reported. The adult dosage is a 250-mg tablet taken weekly; dosages for children and infants are reduced. Mefloquine is considered safe for use during the second and third trimesters of pregnancy and is most probably also safe in the first trimester when this drug is indicated because of significant infection risk. There has been considerable controversy over the safety of mefloquine, particularly in relation to the incidence of neuropsychiatric side effects, such as convulsions and hallucinations. However, comparative studies have shown that the adverse effects of mefloquine are similar in frequency and quality to those of chloroquine. Reported side effects of mefloquine include insomnia, bad dreams, dizziness, headache, anxiety, and gastrointestinal symptoms. The more serious toxic psychosis occurs in approximately 1 in 10,000 users. Long-term use of

mefloquine by Peace Corps Volunteers in Africa showed it to be well tolerated. Contraindications to mefloquine include a history of epilepsy, serious psychiatric disorder, or cardiac conduction system abnormalities.

Mefloquine is not recommended for emergency self-treatment of malaria because of the potential risk of the more frequent serious side effects (hallucinations and convulsions) that are associated with the high dosages used for treatment of malaria.

Doxycycline.* For persons unable to tolerate mefloquine or who have a contraindication to its use, and in areas where malaria has considerable resistance to mefloquine, doxycycline in a 100-mg daily dose can be used by adults and children older than 8 years of age. This drug cannot be used by pregnant women or by children younger than 8 years of age. Potential adverse effects include photosensitivity in about 2% of users, gastrointestinal effects, and vaginal moniliasis.

Proguanil† (Paludrine). When neither mefloquine nor doxycycline can be used, a weekly dose of chloroquine phosphate (as described earlier) plus a 200-mg daily dose of proguanil are recommended. Both these drugs are considered safe during pregnancy and in all age groups. Proguanil is not available in the United States, but it is available by prescription in Canada and Europe and usually over the counter in Africa. This combination is the least effective of the available regimens. It is recommended that travelers using this combination carry pyrimethamine-sulfadoxine (Fansidar) for indicated emergency self-treatment.

All these regimens must be followed regularly while the traveler is in a malarious area and for 4 weeks after departure from the area. With the exception of doxycycline, other regimens should be started 1 to 3 weeks before travel to a malarious area in order to ensure adequate blood levels of the drug on arrival. Because more than 75% of adverse reactions to mefloquine are apparent by the third dose, initial users of mefloquine should ideally begin taking the drug 3 weeks before departure.

Some new drug regimens for multidrug-resistant *P. falciparum*-related malaria are being evaluated but are not yet approved for use in the United States. These include a daily 30-mg base dose of primaquine and a daily dose of atovaquone plus proguanil (Malarone†).

Recently, chloroquine-resistant *Plasmodium vivax* malaria has been reported from Indonesia and Papua New Guinea and parts of Southeast Asia and Latin America.

Primaquine. Primaquine prophylaxis eliminates *P. vivax* and *Plasmodium ovale* parasites from the liver so that a future attack by these species will not occur after routine prophylaxis when administration of the earlier mentioned drugs is terminated. Primaquine in a dose of 15-mg base daily for 14 days is given after completion of routine drug prophylaxis. Primaquine for terminal prophylaxis is not indicated for all travelers, and the decision to administer it must be made on an individual basis. The intensity and duration of the traveler's exposure to *P. vivax* or *P. ovale* should be considered. Primaquine is not generally recommended for travelers with relatively short-term (less than 1 month's) exposure, because late relapses rarely occur in such persons. Before any use of primaquine, glucose-6-phosphate dehydrogenase deficiency must be ruled out. Primaquine is contraindicated during pregnancy. Terminal prophylaxis with primaquine is not universally effective: relative resistance to the drug by strains of *P. vivax* has

---

*Not FDA approved for this indication.
†Not available in the United States.

been documented in Oceania, Southeast Asia, and parts of Latin America.

Personal Protection Measures Against Mosquito Bites

Malaria transmission by mosquitoes occurs primarily between dusk and dawn. During these hours, measures to reduce contact with mosquitoes are an essential adjunct to drug prophylaxis in prevention of malaria. These measures include (1) remaining in well-screened areas; (2) using mosquito nets impregnated with permethrin; (3) wearing clothes that cover most of the body; (4) use of insect repellents containing diethyltoluamide (DEET; optimally a 20 to 35% concentration lotion) on all exposed body parts; (5) use of permethrin spray on clothing as a repellent; and (6) use of a flying-insect spray containing pyrethrum in living areas.

No present-day antimalarial drug regimen guarantees protection against malaria. Prevention of malaria infection requires greater attention to the personal protection measures against mosquito bites just listed. Even with the use of all these measures, particularly if they are not used religiously, it is still possible to contract malaria. Travelers in whom fever develops during travel and for up to 3 years after return from a malarious area should be promptly evaluated for possible malaria infection. Research is continuing on malaria vaccines, but one is not expected for some years.

TRAVELERS' DIARRHEA: PROPHYLAXIS AND TREATMENT

Travelers' diarrhea affects up to half of the travelers from industrialized countries who visit the developing world. Along with diarrhea, low-grade fever, abdominal cramping, or vomiting may also occur. Travelers' diarrhea is usually contracted by eating microbiologically contaminated food, drinking contaminated water, or coming into contact with the contaminated hands of an infected person. The syndrome can be caused by bacteria, viruses, and parasites. The most common cause is infection with enterotoxigenic *Escherichia coli*, and this is usually self-limited after several days. Other relatively common causes are *Campylobacter*, *Shigella*, and *Salmonella* species. Viruses and parasites are less common causes.

Recommended preventive measures include (1) eating well-cooked hot foods; (2) avoiding vegetable salads, unpeeled fruit, and ice cubes; (3) boiling drinking water for 3 minutes; (4) disinfecting water with iodine tablets or potable iodine resin filters; (5) avoiding dairy products whose safety is questionable; and (6) avoiding custards, cream pastries, mayonnaise products, and raw or poorly steamed shellfish.

Prophylaxis

Most authorities agree that prophylactic antibiotics should not be routinely recommended, because the potential risk may outweigh the benefit. Bismuth subsalicylate (Pepto-Bismol) in a dosage of two tablets four times a day for periods of less than 3 weeks is a safe and effective way of reducing the occurrence of travelers' diarrhea by approximately 65% of the persons at risk. Travelers already using salicylates should not use bismuth subsalicylate prophylaxis.

Treatment

The most important factor in treating travelers' diarrhea is the replacement of lost fluids and electrolytes. This can be accomplished by drinking tea, broth, or carbonated beverages. Better yet are oral rehydration electrolyte mixtures that are mixed with potable water to prepare a more ideal replacement fluid. For most patients, this is the only treatment necessary because of the usual short duration and self-limitation of diarrhea caused by enterotoxigenic *E. coli*. When bowel movements are frequent and abdominal cramps are troublesome, antisecretory or antimotility agents may be used. Bismuth subsalicylate liquid, taken in a dose of 1 ounce every half hour for a total of eight doses is effective because of its antisecretory effect. Loperamide (Imodium) is an over-the-counter synthetic opioid with a bowel antimotility effect, taken by adults in a 4-mg loading dose, followed by 2 mg orally after each loose bowel movement, to a maximal daily dose of 16 mg. Adding a single dose of a quinolone (i.e., 750 mg of ciprofloxacin) to loperamide may shorten the duration of symptoms to 24 hours. If significant diarrhea persists after these measures or is accompanied by blood or mucus in the stool or high fever, antibiotic treatment is indicated. If medical care is not available and the possibility of this situation has been discussed with a physician before travel, emergency self-treatment is appropriate. The most effective drugs against all of the usual causative bacterial agents are the fluoroquinolones in a 3-day course.

Diarrhea that develops after a traveler's return home from travel is likely to be caused by a pathogenic intestinal protozoan.

GENERAL ADVICE FOR TRAVELING

Flying. Jet lag is a major problem for international travelers. About 1 day for each time zone change is necessary to readjust the body clock. Sleeping pills such as benzodiazepine and melatonin help improve sleep during travel and after arrival.

Motion sickness can be prevented with dimenhydrinate, meclizine, or a scopolamine transdermal disk (Transderm Scōp). Abstinence from alcohol and from excessive heavy food will result in a more comfortable flight. Prolonged sitting should be avoided, to prevent venous stasis in the legs and potential pulmonary emboli.

Acclimatization. Gradual ascent is the cornerstone of prevention of altitude sickness. Current recommendations are to avoid abrupt ascents to altitudes higher than 3000 m (1000 ft) and to spend 2 or 3 nights at 2500 to 3000 m before further ascent. Initial moderate activity and avoidance of alcoholic beverages, tobacco, and excessive food are helpful in acclimatizing to high altitude. Increasing water intake is necessary at high altitudes. Acetazolamide (Diamox), at a dose of 125 mg twice a day taken 24 hours before ascent and continued for the first few days at the higher altitude, can prevent altitude illness.

Sun and Heat Disorders. Protection against strong sunlight can be obtained by applying a broad-spectrum sunscreen (one that protects against both ultraviolet A and B) to the skin 30 to 60 minutes before exposure to sunlight. Sunscreens with a sun protection factor (SPF) of 15 or higher offer a longer period of protection. Heatstroke and sunstroke can be avoided by limiting prolonged exposure to the sun, avoiding overly strenuous exercise, drinking extra fluids, and adding salt to food. Rapid cooling is the mainstay of treatment.

Water-Borne Diseases. In areas where schistosomiasis occurs, all bodies of fresh water must be considered infectious, and contact with this water must be avoided. Schistosomiasis cannot be contracted in salt water or chlorinated swimming pools. Attractive beaches near urban areas may be highly polluted. Jellyfish, corals, and other biting and stinging aquatic creatures are a hazard to bathers.

POST-TRAVEL CARE

A travel clinic should have the capability to recognize, diagnose, and treat unusual infections contracted during travel. Evaluation by a physician is usually unnecessary for persons who remain healthy during and after short-term travel. Travelers who have undertaken longer term travel, as well as expatriate residents from the developing world, should undergo a checkup if they are asymptomatic. Such a checkup should include a physical examination, complete blood count, blood chemistry profile, tuberculin skin test, and stool examinations for ova and parasites. If exposure has occurred, serologic testing can be performed for such infections as human immunodeficiency virus (HIV) and schistosomiasis. Both travelers and physicians must always consider previous travel in the evaluation of symptoms that appear months or, rarely, years after return home. Significant symptoms to be concerned about include fever, chills, sweats, fatigue, persistent diarrhea or other gastrointestinal symptoms, and weight loss. Differential diagnoses, diagnostic methods, and treatment for symptomatic returnees are fully described in textbooks on travel and tropical medicine.

TOXOPLASMOSIS

method of
KAMI KIM, M.D.
Albert Einstein College of Medicine
Bronx, New York

Toxoplasma gondii is a obligate intracellular protozoan parasite associated with opportunistic infections in immunocompromised persons and with congenital abnormalities (the *T* in TORCH syndrome). The parasite was first discovered in the gondi, a North African rodent, by Nicolle in 1908. *T. gondii* is member of the phylum Apicomplexa, which includes a number of important medical pathogens, including *Plasmodium* (which causes malaria) and *Cryptosporidium* (an important cause of diarrheal illness). This parasitic infection is not limited to humans; it is also present in most animal and bird species.

In the 1930s the association between congenital toxoplasmosis and retinitis was described; later, in the 1940s, severe disseminated toxoplasmosis was described. Shortly thereafter, a mononucleosis-like adenopathy syndrome and seropositive asymptomatic acute infection were recognized. Immunosuppressed persons with organ transplants were the first patients described with reactivation toxoplasmosis as a clinical syndrome. Currently patients with the acquired immunodeficiency syndrome (AIDS) are the persons most commonly affected by clinically apparent toxoplasmosis. In patients with AIDS, *T. gondii* is the most common opportunistic infection of the central nervous system, affecting at least 10 to 20% of patients.

T. gondii infection is one of the most prevalent parasitic infections in the world. Infection rates vary throughout the world; some countries, such as France, have a prevalence rate higher than 90%. In the United States, 20 to 70% of adults are seropositive. Humans and animals become infected by ingestion of food or water contaminated with oocysts, by ingestion of bradyzoites in inadequately cooked meat, or by transplacental transmission. Infection in vegetarians and in herbivorous animals is probably acquired by ingestion of food contaminated with oocysts (which contain sporozoites) or by exposure to cat feces that harbor oocysts. The highly infectious oocysts are products of a sexual cycle that occurs exclusively in feline species. Oocysts sporulate (become infectious) 1 to 21 days after passage, depending on temperature and availability of oxygen.

Transplacental transmission in humans results only when a seronegative women acquires toxoplasmosis during pregnancy. Seropositive women who become pregnant usually do not transmit toxoplasmosis to their children unless they are severely immunosuppressed (i.e., have AIDS or systemic lupus erythematosus [SLE]). A woman who has a documented seroconversion should wait at least 6 months before becoming pregnant. Transmission has also occurred through organ transplantation, blood transfusion, and laboratory accident.

After ingestion, sporozoites or bradyzoites invade the intestinal epithelium, differentiate into the rapidly growing tachyzoite form, and disseminate throughout the body. It is thought that the tachyzoite form (which is much less infectious than cysts or oocysts) is responsible for most of the clinical manifestations of toxoplasmosis.

The early stage of infection is characterized by replication of tachyzoites in the intestinal tract with subsequent hematogenous dissemination to every organ. Tachyzoites invade virtually any cell type. When the host has developed a immune response, infection with *T. gondii* reaches a latent or chronic stage during which tissue cysts (bradyzoites) are present in the tissues, especially in the brain and muscle, and parasitemia with tachyzoites disappears. Interferon-γ appears to be a critical factor in host defense against this organism. Tissue cysts persist for life. When a host with chronic toxoplasmosis (seropositive host) becomes immunosuppressed, reactivation of these latent foci (i.e., tissue cysts) occurs with the transformation of bradyzoites to tachyzoites and the development of reactivation disease, manifesting as either disseminated disease or focal abscesses.

In most persons, acute infection with *T. gondii* is asymptomatic or causes mild symptoms similar to those of a self-limited viral syndrome. Women who are infected during pregnancy generally do not develop clinically apparent disease, but they can pass the parasite to the fetus. Fetal death and severe congenital abnormalities are thought to result from damage caused by unchecked proliferation of the tachyzoite form.

Encephalitis, the most common clinical manifestation of *T. gondii* infection, is thought to result from reactivation of dormant bradyzoite forms. More than 90% of patients with AIDS who have *T. gondii* encephalitis have serologic evidence of prior *T. gondii* infection. In the early years of the AIDS epidemic, up to 40% of patients with AIDS with positive *Toxoplasma* serologic profiles developed encephalitis as a result of secondary reactivation of latent toxoplasmosis. The incidence of toxoplasmosis in patients with AIDS has decreased with the advent of effective antiretroviral treatment and routine prophylaxis for opportunistic infections. Chorioretinitis, a manifestation of congenital infection, is also ascribed to bradyzoite reactivation. Less common manifestations of toxoplasmosis include polymyositis and myocarditis, transverse myelitis, and pneumonia.

PREVENTION OF INFECTION

Patients at risk (e.g., persons infected with the human immunodeficiency virus [HIV] and pregnant women), particularly those who are seronegative, should be counseled as to sources of infection with *T. gondii*. Patient education appears to be effective in reducing cases of newly acquired *Toxoplasma* infection. Meat, particularly lamb, pork, and venison, should be thoroughly cooked (over 66°C [150°F]), smoked, or cured in brine. Freezing meat (−20°C [−4°F] for 24 hours) is also efficacious, but many home freezers cannot maintain temperatures cold enough. Hands, cutting boards, and knives should be washed thoroughly after meats are handled. Vegetables and fruits should be washed before being eaten raw. Cat litter box changes should be avoided or, if unavoidable, should be followed by thorough hand washing. Litter boxes can be disinfected with nearly boiling water for 5 minutes. Pet cats should be fed commercial food or thoroughly cooked table food. Patients should wash their hands thoroughly after gardening or other intensive contact with soil.

TREATMENT

The combination of pyrimethamine and sulfadiazine is the mainstay of clinical treatment. Unfortunately, this regimen is not always successful and is frequently associated with drug reactions, particularly to the sulfa component of the regimen. Patients with AIDS are particularly susceptible to drug allergies or reactions and are frequently forced to discontinue therapy because of adverse reactions. The combination of pyrimethamine and clindamycin is an alternative regimen but is also associated with side effects.

In contrast to a number of bacterial and protozoan infections, drug resistance is not a major reason for treatment failure. Typically, organisms that are recovered from patients in whom treatment fails are sensitive to the agents used. Failure may result from lack of adequate penetration or sustained levels of antimicrobial agents. The cyst wall surrounding bradyzoites probably provides a physical barrier to entry of antimicrobials, which may partially explain treatment failures. Because many chemotherapeutic agents are most effective against rapidly growing organisms, it is not surprising that bradyzoites are less sensitive to most chemotherapeutic agents. Patients treated for toxoplasmosis are thought to have a latent infection (tissue cysts) at the conclusion of treatment. Consequently, patients with prolonged immunosuppression, such as those with AIDS, usually require treatment indefinitely.

THE DRUGS USED IN TREATMENT

Pyrimethamine

Pyrimethamine (Daraprim), a substituted phenylpyrimidine, is effective in animal models and in in vitro studies against toxoplasmosis. It is a lipid-soluble folic acid antagonist that inhibits the dihydrofolate reductase (DHFR) of *T. gondii*. Pyrimethamine is metabolized by the liver. It is readily absorbed from the gastrointestinal tract and is found in the cerebrospinal fluid (CSF) as well as in other body compartments. The serum half-life of pyrimethamine is 35 to 175 hours, and the drug may persist in serum

for weeks. Unfortunately, serum levels for a patient are not predictable, because of the wide variation in absorption and serum half-life. Measurement of pyrimethamine levels by high-pressure liquid chromatography (HPLC) is reported, but HPLC is not commercially available. CSF levels of pyrimethamine are 10 to 25% of the corresponding serum levels.

Pyrimethamine has been shown to be teratogenic in animals and should not be given in the first trimester of infection. Teratogenicity has not been reported in women treated with pyrimethamine for malaria.

The usual adult dosage of pyrimethamine is 25 mg per day. In immunosuppressed hosts, a minimum of 50 to 75 mg per day is often used. Because of its long half-life, a loading dose of 100 to 200 mg (2 mg per kg) given in two divided doses can be administered for the first 2 days of therapy. When sulfonamides cannot be administered concurrently, the daily pyrimethamine dose should be 50 to 75 mg per day in adults. Monotherapy for *Toxoplasma* encephalitis with pyrimethamine, 100 mg per day, has been used in patients with AIDS who were sulfonamide intolerant.

Pyrimethamine may cause dose-related bone marrow suppression with thrombocytopenia, neutropenia, and anemia. Blood cell counts should therefore be checked regularly. Folinic acid (leucovorin) is routinely given at a dose of 5 to 10 mg per day orally to prevent these effects and should be given 1 week beyond the course of treatment. In cases in which there is significant neutropenia (absolute neutrophil count < 1000), folinic acid doses can be increased. In patients with AIDS and patients receiving more than 50 mg per day of pyrimethamine, 10 to 20 mg per day of folinic acid is routinely prescribed. Because folinic acid cannot be transported across the parasite plasma membrane, folinic acid does not inhibit the action of pyrimethamine on *T. gondii*. Folinic acid crosses mammalian cell membranes to limit the toxicity of pyrimethamine on mammalian cells. Folic acid should not be used because it can be utilized by *T. gondii* and therefore might interfere with the activity of pyrimethamine. Brewers yeast, 1 tablet three times a day (5 to 10 grams per day), is an effective alternative to folinic acid. Pyrimethamine can also cause nausea, headache, and an odd taste in the mouth. Although rash is a more typical effect of companion drugs, rash is reported to accompany pyrimethamine ingestion in patients with AIDS. Patients can frequently be rechallenged with pyrimethamine without recurrence of rash.

Sulfonamides (Sulfa)

Sulfonamides inhibit dihydropteroate synthetase (DHPS), which converts *p*-aminobenzoic acid (PABA) to dihydrofolic acid. Humans do not synthesize dihydrofolate from PABA but instead directly use dietary folic acid to generate dihydrofolate. Dihydrofolate is reduced to tetrahydrofolate by dihydrofolate reductase (DHFR). Because of their activities against sequential enzymes involved in folic acid metabolism, combinations of sulfa and DHFR inhibitors are commonly used. Combinations of sulfa with pyrimethamine are synergistic against *T. gondii* and are the treatment of choice for clinically significant toxoplasmosis. The most active sulfonamides are sulfadiazine or trisulfapyrimidines (sulfadimidine, sulfamerazine, and sulfadiazine). Sulfapyrazine, sulfapyrimidine, sulfamethoxazole, and sulfadoxine are less active in vitro against *T. gondii*. All other sulfa-based drugs are considered ineffective. The usual dose of sulfonamides for adults is 75 to 100 mg per kg per day (maximum, 8 grams per day) given in four doses. No loading dose is needed, because of the short half-life of most sulfa drugs. These drugs are well absorbed with good penetration into CSF.

Adverse reactions to sulfonamides are common, particularly in patients with AIDS. In some studies, adverse reactions to DHFR inhibitor/sulfa regimens have been as high as 60%; most of the adverse effects are ascribed to the sulfa component. Bone marrow suppression similar to that seen with pyrimethamine is seen, and this also responds to folinic acid. Hypersensitivity reactions with rash and Stevens-Johnson syndrome are seen; for this reason, many experts recommend avoiding long half-life sulfonamides such as combined pyrimethamine/sulfadoxine (Fansidar) in a 1:20 ratio, particularly in patients with AIDS. Some treatment trials for congenital toxoplasmosis have successfully used Fansidar (given every 15 days) for prolonged (1- to 2-year) treatment courses. Gastrointestinal effects with nausea, vomiting, and diarrhea are not uncommon. Nephrolithiasis and crystalluria occurs in 2 to 4% of patients treated with poorly soluble sulfonamides (such as sulfadiazine), and the incidence of nephrotoxicity is reported to be even higher in patients with AIDS. This can be prevented by an adequate fluid intake of 1 to 2 liters per day in adults (or intravenous hydration) and urine alkalinization (pH > 7.5).

Other Folate Metabolism Inhibitors

Trimethoprim, a DHFR inhibitor, in combination with the DHPS inhibitor sulfamethoxazole (TMP-SMZ; co-trimoxazole, Bactrim, or Septra) formulated in a 1:5 ratio, is not as effective as pyrimethamine/sulfa. A study of TMP-SMZ has demonstrated good response in patients with AIDS and *Toxoplasma* encephalitis. Patients given TMP-SMZ as *Pneumocystis* prophylaxis have a decreased incidence of cerebral toxoplasmosis as well. Because patients with AIDS have developed *Toxoplasma* encephalitis while receiving TMP-SMZ, it is not considered by most experts a treatment of choice. The folic acid antagonists piritrexim and trimetrexate (NeuTrexin) have demonstrated efficacy in vitro and in vivo in laboratory models of toxoplasmosis. In a limited trial of patients with AIDS who have sulfonamide intolerance, trimetrexate with leukovorin led to initial radiographic and clinical improvement that was transient. Dap-

sone, a sulfone that also inhibits DHPS, is reported to be effective against toxoplasmosis, particularly when given in combination with a dihydrofolate reductase inhibitor (pyrimethamine).

Macrolides

Spiramycin is a macrolide antibiotic that is available in many countries and has been used in France for the treatment of toxoplasmosis acquired during pregnancy. In the United States, spiramycin is available by request from the U.S. Food and Drug Administration (301-443-5680). In animal experiments, spiramycin has been shown to be active against toxoplasmosis and is reported to reach high levels in the placenta. Detection of parasites in the placenta is highly correlated with fetal infection, although there is a variable lag time before transmission to the fetus.

In French studies, spiramycin decreased both the severity of toxoplasmosis in children born to acutely infected mothers and the rate of transmission of toxoplasmosis to these children. Placental levels of 6.2 mg per liter and cord blood levels of 0.78 mg per liter are achievable with spiramycin, 3 grams per day orally. Studies suggest that it accumulates in tissues. Gastrointestinal symptoms such as nausea, vomiting, abdominal pain, and diarrhea are the most common side effects. Unlike many macrolides, spiramycin has little hepatic toxicity. No hematologic toxicity is found. Usually 50 to 100 mg per kg per day of spiramycin is given in three or four doses (2 to 4 grams per day).

Several of the newer macrolide antibiotics such as clarithromycin (Biaxin), azithromycin (Zithromax), and roxithromycin have in vitro activity and have been successfully used singly or in combination (usually with pyrimethamine) for treatment of patients who are intolerant of or failing conventional therapy (usually patients with AIDS).

Clindamycin

Clindamycin (Cleocin) is not as effective as pyrimethamine/sulfa in murine toxoplasmosis; however, it has been used successfully for treatment of toxoplasmosis. In ocular toxoplasmosis, clindamycin has been used in treatment, but definitive data about its use in chorioretinitis or congenital toxoplasmosis are not available. Clindamycin combined with pyrimethamine is an acceptable treatment in patients with AIDS who have *Toxoplasma* encephalitis. Side effects are diarrhea, pseudomembranous colitis, and rash. Because there is a slightly higher tendency for relapse with clindamycin/pyrimethamine, pyrimethamine/sulfa is still considered the treatment of choice.

Other Drugs

Atovaquone (Mepron) has shown an ability to eliminate tissue cysts in mice and has also been used as salvage therapy in patients with AIDS to achieve improvement or stabilization of clinical status. As single-drug therapy, it has been associated with high rates of relapse and therefore should probably be used in combination with another drug such as pyrimethamine. Other agents reported to work synergistically with atovaquone include clarithromycin, azithromycin, and rifabutin.

Tetracyclines are not effective at clinically achievable concentrations, but doxycycline (Vibramycin) or minocycline (Minocin) in combination with other agents may be efficacious. Quinolones such as trovafloxacin (Trovan) also have in vitro activity and are also reported to be more effective in combination with other drugs. Although bioavailability of orally administered macrolides and quinolones is generally very good, intravenous administration has been reported to be more efficacious in some cases.

Rifabutin (Mycobutin) has reported activity against T. gondii and has been used successfully in the mouse model of toxoplasmosis. It is reported to be synergistic with sulfadiazine, pyrimethamine, clindamycin, and atovaquone. Arprinocid, a purine analogue, is an anticoccidial agent that has shown efficacy in mice. 5-Fluorouracil (5-FU) has efficacy in vitro and was shown to have some effect on Toxoplasma encephalitis in a limited trial in France.

Immunomodulating agents may also eventually have a role in treatment of toxoplasmosis. Recombinant interferon-γ is effective in a murine model of toxoplasmosis. Therapy with interferon-γ has been effective in other human parasitic infections (Leishmaniasis and T. cruzi) and may prove useful in toxoplasmosis. Interleukin-12 and interleukin-4 have also shown promise in murine trials, particularly when given in combination with conventional antibiotics. Patients failing or intolerant of first-line therapy should probably be seen by either an infectious diseases consultant or a physician highly experienced in treating toxoplasmosis.

TREATMENT REGIMENS (Table 1)

Asymptomatic Infection or Latent Infection

Immunocompetent patients with latent toxoplasmosis as evidenced by positive serologic findings do not require treatment. In most immunocompromised patients, no treatment is indicated. In patients with AIDS who are seropositive for T. gondii, the risk of developing encephalitis has been estimated at up to 40%. Prophylactic treatment for Pneumocystis carinii pneumonia with TMP-SMZ (1 double strength orally every day = 160 mg TMP/800 mg SMZ) is effective against T. gondii and is the recommended prophylaxis regimen for patients at risk for P. carinii infection and toxoplasmosis (Toxoplasma seropositive with CD4 < 100 per μL). Dapsone/pyrimethamine (100 mg weekly dapsone with 25 mg biweekly pyrimethamine) is also effective for prevention of both P. carinii pneumonia and toxoplasmosis. Pyrimeth-

TABLE 1. Recommended Treatment for *Toxoplasma gondii* Infections

Syndrome	Treatment*
Asymptomatic infection: latent infection detected by positive serologic test	
AIDS	TMP-SMX prophylaxis if CD4 count < 100
Other immunocompromise	None
Immunocompetence	None
Adenopathy, fever, or malaise in the immunocompetent host	None†
Laboratory infection with tachyzoites; transfusion	PYR/sulfa
Disseminated disease (i.e., central nervous system disease, heart disease, or hepatitis) in the immunocompetent host	PYR/sulfa
Infection during pregnancy‡	
Fetal infection unknown	SPR§
Fetal infection documented	SPR-PYR/sulfa‡
Congenital toxoplasmosis	PYR/sulfa‖
Ocular toxoplasmosis	PYR/sulfa and steroids
Toxoplasmosis in immunocompromised hosts	PYR/sulfa
AIDS	PYR/sulfa for life
Transplantation	PYR/sulfa
Acute disease	PYR/sulfa

*Recommended primary treatments as described in the text.
†Painful adenopathy may respond to indomethacin; prolonged adenopathy may respond to PYR/sulfa.
‡Infection during pregnancy as determined by seroconversion of the mother is treated with SPR. If the fetus is confirmed to have toxoplasmosis by ultrasound, amniocentesis or cordocentesis then PYR/sulfa is given beginning week 18 (can alternate with SPR).
§Call the FDA: 301-443-5680.
‖Congenital toxoplasmosis is treated until the infant is 12 months old.
Abbreviations: AIDS = acquired immunodeficiency syndrome; PYR = pyrimethamine; sulfa = sulfonamides; SPR = spiramycin; steroids = corticosteroids; TMP-SMZ = trimethoprim-sulfamethoxazole.

amine/clindamycin probably does not prevent P. carinii pneumonia. In heart transplantation, seronegative recipients of a heart from a seropositive donor have been given 25 mg per day of pyrimethamine for 6 weeks after transplantation to prevent reactivation.

Acquired Toxoplasmosis

In immunocompetent patients, T. gondii infection is usually asymptomatic or manifests as a mild, self-limited illness characterized by adenopathy, fever, and malaise. Treatment is rarely needed. Lymphadenopathy can take months to resolve. In patients whose symptoms are persistent, treatment should be as described for disseminated disease. In an occasional patient, acute toxoplasmosis may manifest as severe disseminated disease with organ dysfunction. Myocarditis, encephalitis, a sepsis syndrome with shock, and hepatitis have been described. In these patients, treatment should be given with pyrimethamine (100-mg loading dose followed by 25 to 50 mg per day) and sulfadiazine or trisulfapyrimidines (4 to 8 grams per day) for 4 to 6 weeks or 2 weeks after signs and symptoms have resolved. Folinic acid (5 to 10 mg per day) should also be given.

Infections acquired through a laboratory accident or blood transfusion should be treated with pyrimethamine/sulfa or pyrimethamine/clindamycin for 4 to 6 weeks. Serologic studies should be done immediately to ascertain the immune status of the patient with regard to *Toxoplasma*. Laboratory workers with previous positive *Toxoplasma* serologic profiles can be treated for 2 weeks.

Acquired Toxoplasmosis During Pregnancy

Toxoplasmosis is transmitted to the fetus only when a women acquires the infection after the date of conception, except in cases in which a mother is severely immunocompromised. The risk of transmission of toxoplasmosis increases as pregnancy progresses. For women who are infected during pregnancy, the risk of fetal infection is 14% during the first trimester, 29% during the second trimester, and 59% during the third trimester. Although the risk of infection increases, the severity of the manifestations of infection falls with each trimester. In general, only fetal infections acquired in the first trimester result in severe congenital infections with mental retardation or blindness. Fetal infections in the third trimester are frequently asymptomatic at birth. The majority of congenitally infected children who are asymptomatic at birth develop clinical toxoplasmosis with retinitis and/or central nervous system effects later in life. Treatment of women who become infected with *T. gondii* during pregnancy decreases the incidence of fetal infection by approximately 60%.

Diagnosis of infection acquired during pregnancy requires documentation of (1) seroconversion, (2) a fourfold rise in *Toxoplasma*-specific IgG titer (i.e., two-tube rise in titer of samples drawn 3 weeks apart, run in parallel), or (3) the presence of significant amounts of *Toxoplasma*-specific IgM or IgA. IgM and IgA may be present only for a few weeks; on occasion, they persist for years. A single high IgG titer may not represent newly acquired disease, inasmuch as high titers can persist for years. A good review of the diagnostic tests can be found in *Infectious Diseases of the Fetus and Newborn Infant*, 4th edition (by Remington JS, Klein JO; Philadelphia: WB Saunders, 1995). A reference laboratory (e.g., Palo Alto Medical Foundation, Palo Alto, California, 650-326-8120) should be used if interpretation of screening tests is problematic. Many of the tests necessary for documentation of fetal infection are available only in reference laboratories. Screening for infection during pregnancy is standard practice in France and Austria.

Results of a French series suggest that acutely infected women should be given spiramycin, 3 grams in three divided doses per day, once maternal infection is suspected or diagnosed. Spiramycin should be continued during pregnancy. Amniocentesis, fetal blood monitoring, and fetal ultrasonography should be used to assess infection in the fetus. Ultrasonography should be performed every 2 to 4 weeks because ventricular dilation may develop in as little as 10 days.

If fetal toxoplasmosis is diagnosed (by demonstration of fetal *Toxoplasma* IgM, culture of *T. gondii* from amniotic fluid or fetal blood, PCR of amniotic fluid or fetal blood for *T. gondii*, or ultrasonographic evidence of ventricular dilatation), specific therapy with pyrimethamine (50 mg per day after loading with 100 mg per day for 2 days in 2 doses), sulfadiazine (100 mg per kg per day in 2 doses; 4 grams at most) and folinic acid (5 to 15 mg per day) should be administered to the mother for 3 weeks alternating with spiramycin (3 grams per day) for 3 weeks until delivery. This regimen significantly reduces the severity of disease seen at birth.

The majority of infants born to women treated with this regimen had subclinical disease at birth in a French study. Of note, the majority of women whose ultrasonograms demonstrated fetal hydrocephalus with ventricular dilatation in the second trimester elected to have abortions, and severe toxoplasmosis was found in these fetuses on autopsy examination. An alternative regimen of spiramycin (3 grams every day), sulfadoxine (1500 mg once every 10 days), pyrimethamine (75 mg once every 10 days) and folinic acid until delivery has been used in France with success. Pyrimethamine should not be used during the first 14 to 16 weeks of pregnancy, because of concerns about teratogenicity. Even if the mother receives pyrimethamine/sulfa, neonates with congenital toxoplasmosis should receive further drug therapy.

Spiramycin probably does not ameliorate disease in utero. For this reason, the investigators of the Chicago Collaborative Treatment Trial recommend pyrimethamine/sulfa with folinic acid continuously beginning week 18 of gestation if fetal infection is confirmed or if maternal infection is acquired late in pregnancy (with amniocentesis for diagnosis).

Congenital Toxoplasmosis

It is estimated that 1 per 1000 children born each year (approximately 3000 per year) in the United States have congenital toxoplasmosis. The cost of caring for all cases of congenital toxoplasmosis has been estimated to be $200 million to $400 million per year. Manifestations of congenital toxoplasmosis include cognitive and motor dysfunction, seizures, impaired vision, and hearing loss. Treatment of an infant with congenital toxoplasmosis during the first year of life probably mitigates tissue destruction and ameliorates sequelae. Children who are treated for the first year of life have better neurologic and developmental status than infants who are not treated or treated briefly (e.g., 1 month). Most neonates who appear normal at birth (who have subclinical disease) later demonstrate clinically apparent disease (primarily retinitis).

Documented congenital toxoplasmosis is treated

with pyrimethamine: a loading dose of 2 mg per kg per day for 2 days, followed by 1 mg per kg per day or 15 mg per m² for 2 months and then 15 mg per m² or 1 mg per kg 3 times a week for the next 10 months. In addition, sulfadiazine or trisulfapyrimidine at 100 mg per kg per day in 2 divided doses and folinic acid 5 mg every other day is administered. In France, spiramycin 100 mg per kg per day in 2 divided doses is used instead of pyrimethamine/sulfa/folinic acid for months 7, 9, and 11. Blood cell counts should be obtained twice weekly; they can be monitored weekly in cases in which counts and the patient are clinically stable. Neutropenia frequently occurs in the setting of viral syndromes. Neutropenia frequently responds to increased folinic acid dosage. For severely affected children, instead of 2 months of daily pyrimethamine, 6 months of daily pyrimethamine (1 mg per kg per day) followed by 6 months of every-other-day pyrimethamine (1 mg per kg per day) is often used. Corticosteroids (1 mg per kg per day) should be added for patients with active macular disease or active CSF profiles (CSF protein ≥ 1 gram per dL). Steroids should be tapered over 3 weeks once active disease or elevated CSF protein levels have resolved.

In all healthy-appearing infants born to mothers known to have had active toxoplasmosis in pregnancy, pyrimethamine/sulfa with folinic acid should be given for 6 weeks until results of laboratory tests for congenital infection are obtained.

Ocular Toxoplasmosis

It is believed that local reactivation of *Toxoplasma* cysts in the eye is responsible for ocular toxoplasmosis. Ocular disease can also occur with acute infection. Diagnosis is made if chorioretinitis is found on ophthalmologic examination and if there is serologic evidence of toxoplasmosis. Serologic titers may be low with this disease, and aqueous humor serologic testing is occasionally useful for diagnosis. There have been limited trials of the different regimens in this disorder. Because the chorioretinitis is self-limited, comparative trials are essential. Pyrimethamine/sulfa is effective in resolving active lesions. Corticosteroids (prednisone, 1 to 2 mg per kg per day) are indicated along with pyrimethamine/sulfa if the macula, optic nerve head, or papillomacular bundle is involved. Prednisone is tapered when pigmentation (healing) begins. Steroids should not be given without specific anti-*Toxoplasma* therapy. Clindamycin (1200 mg per day) has been used in place of pyrimethamine, but in a comparative trial it was inferior to pyrimethamine/sulfa. For ocular disease, treatment with pyrimethamine (25 mg per day) and sulfadiazine (4 grams per day in four divided doses) for 4 weeks is indicated. Folinic acid (5 to 10 mg per day) is also used. Improvement generally occurs within 10 days of starting treatment. Tetracycline and spiramycin are not effective.

Patients who are successfully treated have a lifetime risk of recurrence and should be monitored by an ophthalmologist. Early results of the Chicago Collaborative Treatment Trial suggest that early aggressive treatment of congenitally infected children may decrease the incidence of recurrences. Similarly, the incidence of retinal lesions was lower than expected in French infants treated in utero.

Toxoplasma Infection in Immunocompromised Hosts

In patients with AIDS, *Toxoplasma* encephalitis typically manifests with focal neurologic signs and radiographic evidence (computed tomography or magnetic resonance imaging) of ring-enhancing lesions (multiple or single) in the brain. Most patients with AIDS and encephalitis are seropositive for *T. gondii,* and negative serologic profiles are suggestive of another diagnosis. No specific serologic test can confirm this diagnosis. If a serologic test other than the Sabin-Feldman dye test is performed, low-titer positive evidence can be missed. Although in most patients disease develops as a result of reactivation of tissue cysts in the brain, acute infection has also been described. Therapy is often started empirically with pyrimethamine/sulfa, and the diagnosis is confirmed by an improvement with specific anti-*Toxoplasma* therapy. Radiographic improvement should be evident in 7 to 14 days. If improvement is not seen, brain biopsy should be performed for definitive diagnosis.

Treatment is with pyrimethamine (25 to 100 mg per day) and sulfa (4 to 8 grams per day). Folinic acid (10 to 20 mg per day) is also given. When 25 mg per day of pyrimethamine is used, a loading dose of 100 to 200 mg per day (divided into two daily doses) should be used because of the long half-life of pyrimethamine. Because of a wide variation in absorption and half-life, many authorities recommend using 75 to 100 mg per day of pyrimethamine combined with sulfa in the setting of *Toxoplasma* encephalitis with AIDS.

In patients with AIDS who are intolerant of sulfa, clindamycin (2400 to 4800 mg per day divided four times a day) with high-dose pyrimethamine (75 mg per day) is the best alternative. Clarithromycin (1.0 gram orally twice a day), azithromycin (1.2 to 1.5 grams orally every day), dapsone (100 mg orally every day), or atovaquone (750 mg orally every day with food) can be prescribed with pyrimethamine in a patient intolerant of both sulfa and clindamycin. Corticosteroids (e.g., dexamethasone [Decadron], 4 mg every 6 hours) are often used to control intracranial hypertension resulting from mass effect. Desensitization to sulfa has been reported to be successful in some sulfa-intolerant patients. In some patients, *Toxoplasma* encephalitis has progressed when sulfa was stopped, despite the use of high-dose pyrimethamine and clindamycin. These patients can have a decrease in neurologic symptoms after restarting sulfa after desensitization. Pyrimethamine alone at dosages of 75 to 100 mg per day can also be used with good results. Immunocompromised hosts are treated with pyrimethamine/sulfa as described above for 6 weeks. Patients with AIDS and *Toxoplasma* encephalitis are usually treated for life with pyrimethamine/sulfa or pyrimethamine/clindamycin at somewhat lower doses (sulfa, 500 mg to 1 gram four times a day; pyrimethamine, 25 to 50 mg every day; folinic acid, 10 mg every day; or clindamycin, 300 to 450 mg orally every 6 to 8 hours plus pyrimethamine/folinic acid). For patients taking pyrimethamine/sulfa, *P. carinii* prophylaxis is not necessary. It is not clear that patients other than those with AIDS are at high risk for relapse.

In heart transplantation, acute disease occurs only when a seronegative recipient receives a heart from a seropositive donor. Therapy for 6 weeks has been effective in these cases. In one transplantation center, pyrimethamine alone at 25 mg per day for 6 weeks after transplantation in seronegative recipients receiving seropositive hearts has prevented acute toxoplasmosis in the recipients.

CAT-SCRATCH DISEASE AND BACILLARY ANGIOMATOSIS

method of
DOUGLAS H. HAMILTON, M.D., Ph.D.
Centers for Disease Control and Prevention
Atlanta, Georgia

Cat-scratch disease (CSD) was first identified in 1930 by Robert Debré in Paris, who described a self-limited, regional lymphadenopathy occurring after a cat scratch or bite distal to the affected node. In 1983, researchers, using a Warthin-Starry silver impregnation stain, identified small, pleomorphic, gram-negative, non–acid-fast bacteria in the lymph nodes of patients with clinical CSD. Similar bacteria were later seen at the site of primary cat-scratch lesions, cultured from the tissues of CSD patients, and were subsequently identified as *Bartonella* (formerly *Rochalimaea*) *henselae*.

EPIDEMIOLOGY

Analyses of large national databases have documented that (1) 55% of persons with CSD are aged 18 years or younger, (2) 60% of cases occur in males, and (3) most cases occur in the fall and winter. An estimated 22,000 cases are diagnosed annually in the United States; more than 2000 of the patients require hospitalization; 90% have a history of contact with cats; and 57 to 83% have a history of a scratch from a cat. A case-control study of risk factors for CSD indicates that patients were more likely than controls to own a kitten aged 12 months or younger, to have been scratched by a kitten, or to have had at least one kitten with fleas. A study of *B. henselae* infection of cats revealed that 72% of the kittens tested were bacteremic, whereas the adult cats tested had serologic evidence of past infection but negative blood cultures. Fleas, implicated in the case-control studies, have been shown to harbor *B. henselae* and to be capable of transmitting the infection from cat to cat.

CLINICAL MANIFESTATIONS

Infection with *B. henselae* results in different clinical manifestations, depending on the immune status of the patient. Infection of an immunocompetent patient is likely to result in a classical CSD manifestation: 3 to 5 days after exposure to a bite or scratch from an infected cat, most patients develop a small, round, red-brown papule. This lesion progresses through a vesicular and crusty stage within 2 to 3 days and may persist for up to 2 or 3 weeks. Within 1 to 2 weeks after appearance of skin lesions, patients develop gradual enlargement of the regional lymph nodes that drain the site of the primary lesion. Eighty-five percent of patients come to medical attention with a solitary enlarged node. Multiple nodes are usually found in a regional distribution, and only 2% of patients have noncontiguous bilateral lymphadenopathy. The sites of lymph node involvement are most commonly an upper extremity (46%), the neck and jaw (26%), the groin (18%), a preauricular location (7%), and a clavicular location (2%). Additional constitutional symptoms noted in approximately 75% of patients include fever (39% of all patients with CSD), malaise or fatigue (34%), pharyngitis (13%), and headache (6%).

Unusual manifestations of CSD have been reported in 5 to 25% of patients. The most common complication is Parinaud's oculoglandular syndrome (POS), which occurs in 6% of patients. POS manifests as a unilateral granulomatous conjunctivitis with an ipsilateral preauricular lymphadenopathy. Ocular lesions are 2 to 10 mm in diameter and are usually located on the palpebral conjunctiva. These lesions resolve in weeks to months and do not result in permanent scarring. POS may also be caused by other infectious agents (e.g., those causing tuberculosis, tularemia, syphilis, and lymphogranuloma venereum), but CSD is believed to be the most common cause.

Neurologic manifestations are evident in 1 to 7% of patients with CSD. In one case series of 76 patients with neurologic symptoms, 80% had encephalopathy, and 20% had cranial or peripheral nerve involvement. Encephalopathy occurred 1 to 6 weeks after the onset of CSD and typically began with a headache and rapidly progressed to a change in mental status and to delirium and unresponsiveness. Convulsions occurred in 46% of these patients, and transient combative behavior occurred in 39%. In patients without a prior diagnosis of CSD, convulsions were often the initial symptom. Patients may become comatose for 1 to 4 days, but recovery is fairly rapid and complete without neurologic sequelae. Less common neurologic manifestations of CSD include persistent ataxia, transient hemiplegia, hearing loss, bilateral sixth cranial nerve palsy, and neuroretinitis with transient blindness.

Other rare complications of CSD in the immunocompetent host include hepatic and splenic abscesses (manifesting as abdominal pain of unknown etiology), osteolytic lesions, erythema nodosum, pneumonia or pleural effusions, and thrombocytopenic and nonthrombocytopenic purpura.

Infection of an immunocompromised person by *B. henselae* may result in a dramatically different clinical manifestation called bacillary angiomatosis (BA). BA is a vasoproliferative disorder with brown to violaceus or clear cutaneous and subcutaneous lesions. The BA lesions may be solitary but are usually multiple and tender and have been shown to involve essentially all organ systems of the body, including lymph nodes, bone, the brain, the liver, and the spleen. In patients infected with the human immunodeficiency virus (HIV), these lesions are often mistaken for Kaposi's sarcoma. Histologically, BA lesions consist of

TABLE 1. **Antibiotic Therapy for *Bartonella henselae* Infection**

Antibiotic	Dose/Route	Notes
Cat-Scratch Disease		
Azithromycin* (Zithromax)	Children (<45 kg): 10 mg/kg PO on day 1 and 5 mg/kg PO on days 2–5 Adults: 500 mg PO on day 1 and 250 mg PO on days 2–5	
Ciprofloxacin* (Cipro)	Adults: 500–750 mg PO bid for 7–14 d	
Rifampin* (Rifadin, Rimactane)	10–20 mg/kg PO divided into 2 or 3 doses/d for 7–14 d	600 mg is the maximal dose.
Trimethoprim-sulfamethoxazole* (Bactrim, Septra)	10 mg/kg of the trimethoprim component PO bid for 7 d	
Gentamicin* (Garamycin)	5 mg/kg/d IV or IM in divided doses every 8 h	For severely ill patients.
Bacillary Angiomatosis/Bacillary Peliosis		
Erythromycin*	500 mg PO qid for 2–4 wk	The duration of therapy depends on clinical response. Some HIV-positive patients may require long-term, even lifelong suppression.
Doxycycline (Vibramycin, Doryx, Monodox)	100 mg PO bid for 2–4 wk	
Clarithromycin* (Biaxin)	500 mg PO bid for 2–4 wk	
Azithromycin* (Zithromax)	250 mg PO qd for 2–4 wk	
Ciprofloxacin* (Cipro)	500–750 mg PO bid for 2–4 wk	

*Not FDA approved for this indication.
Abbreviations: HIV = human immunodeficiency virus; IM = intramuscularly; IV = intravenously; PO = orally.

proliferating small vessels with prominent endothelial cells and varying numbers of neutrophils and neutrophil debris. The epithelial cells of BA lesions are protuberant and are not spindle-shaped or form the slitlike spaces seen in Kaposi's sarcoma. Morphologically, three distinct types of BA lesions have been described. The most common type is a pyogenic granuloma, followed by subcutaneous nodules and indurated hyperpigmented plaques. Warthin-Starry staining of BA lesions reveals clumps of the characteristic small, pleomorphic, gram-negative bacteria seen in classical CSD lesions. Subsequent investigators have isolated *B. henselae* from the BA lesions of patients infected with HIV and have demonstrated high levels of antibodies to *B. henselae* in patients with BA. Laboratory studies have revealed that BA may also be caused by the related bacteria *Bartonella quintana*, the agent of trench fever.

B. henselae infection in the immunocompromised host may also manifest as bacillary peliosis, which is an extracutaneous form of BA found in solid organs with reticuloendothelial elements (e.g., liver [peliosis hepatitis], spleen, abdominal lymph nodes, and bone marrow). Symptoms include fever, nausea, vomiting, diarrhea, and abdominal distention. Patients often have hepatosplenomegaly.

B. henselae infection may also manifest as persistent or relapsing fever with bacteremia in the absence of lymphadenopathy or skin lesions. This condition has been observed in both immunocompetent and immunocompromised patients, although more commonly in the latter. These patients usually have fatigue, fever, and anorexia without an obvious source of infection.

DIAGNOSIS

Diagnosis of CSD has traditionally required the presence of three of four criteria: (1) history of animal contact (usually a cat) and an abrasion, scratch, or an ocular lesion; (2) a positive CSD skin antigen test result; (3) regional lymphadenopathy with a negative work-up for other causes of the lymphadenopathy; or (4) characteristic histopathologic changes consistent with CSD in a lymph node biopsy

specimen. For several decades, the CSD skin test antigen remained the sole diagnostic tool for CSD. The lack of an effective means of standardization and lingering doubts about the safety of the product led to the development and adoption of newer diagnostic tools. The first available serologic test was an indirect immunofluorescence assay (IFA) that was reported to be 88% sensitive and 94% specific. Published studies examining the performance of the IFA in a population of CSD patients who met the classical case definition have shown the test to be 98% sensitive and 98% specific. However, the ability to differentiate among *Bartonella* species using this test has not been well established.

Enzyme immunoassay (EIA) for either IgM or IgG antibodies to *B. henselae* have also been developed. Although the sensitivity and specificity of commercially available EIAs are not well established, it appears that the IgM EIA is more sensitive than the IgG EIA.

Polymerase chain reaction–based tests for detection of *B. henselae* DNA have been developed for investigational use and are not currently commercially available. These tests have been helpful in identifying the causative agent of CSD as *B. henselae* and not *Afipia felis,* as previously suspected.

Histologic findings on lymph node biopsy vary according to the stage of the disease. Early CSD lesions show lymphoid hyperplasia, arteriolar proliferation, and reticulum cell hyperplasia. This stage is followed by the development of granulomas with central necrosis and multinucleate giant cells. Late-stage lesions often show multiple stellate microabscesses. Bacteria, which are rarely seen on routine tissue stains, may be seen as clumps in samples stained with the Warthin-Starry technique. The characteristic findings of BA are as described above.

TREATMENT

In most immunocompetent patients with classical CSD, the disease is self-limited, and antibiotic therapy has not proved to be beneficial. The lymphadenopathy usually regresses spontaneously within 2 to 6 months but may last up to 2 years. Patients with severe symptoms or unusual manifestations may benefit from a trial of antibiotics. Several proposed treatment regimens, based on small sample sizes, have been published (Table 1). The only randomized, double-blind clinical trial of antibiotic therapy of CSD has involved azithromycin* (Zithromax). Incision and drainage of fluctuant lymph nodes is *not* recommended because of the tendency for these lesions to form chronic sinus tracts when managed surgically. If necessary, repeated aspiration of purulent material with a 16- or 18-gauge needle may provide symptomatic relief.

Managing patients with BA or bacillary peliosis, which if left untreated can be fatal, is different from managing immunocompetent patients with classical CSD. In contrast to CSD, for which treatment with antibiotics is of questionable efficacy, immunocompromised patients with BA have shown a dramatic response to antibiotic therapy. The current antibiotics of choice are erythromycin* and doxycycline, although other regimens have been published (see Table 1).

The reasons for the observed differences in clinical manifestations and response to therapy after *B. henselae* infection in immunocompromised and immunocompetent hosts are not known.

---

*Not FDA approved for this indication.

SALMONELLOSIS

method of
DILIP NATHWANI, M.B., FRCP
Tayside University Hospital
Dundee, Scotland

INTRODUCTION AND EPIDEMIOLOGY

In developed countries, many changes in human ecology and behavior have led to the emergence of food-borne diseases as a major source of public ill health. Factors contributing to this include commercialization of food production and service, increased importation of food from developing countries, linking of distant places by rapid intercontinental travel, and an increase in the population either attending child day care centers or institutions for care of the elderly.

Nontyphoid *Salmonella* infections occur worldwide and are the second most commonly reported infections in the United States, the United Kingdom, and Europe. For example, in the United States there has been a doubling of the incidence of salmonellosis in the last two decades, with an estimated 2 million cases annually and a mortality rate of 500 to 2000 annually. Under-reporting is believed to be common; up to 3.7 million cases annually are estimated. The attendant annual economic burden of all enteric infections has been estimated in the region of 5 billion U.S. dollars.

All salmonellae are now recognized as belonging to one of two species: *Salmonella enterica* or *Salmonella bongori*. The *S. enterica* species is subdivided into six subspecies, within which there are more than 2000 serotypes. Nearly all the salmonellae isolated from humans belong to the *S. enterica* subspecies *enterica*. The most prevalent of these (in the United States) in descending order are *Salmonella enteritidis*, *Salmonella typhimurium*, and *Salmonella heidelberg*. The emergence of infected eggs as the most important cause of *S. enteritidis* infections is related to the ability of this organism to infect the ovaries of egg-laying hens. This increase in *S. enteritidis* has been accompanied by the emergence of phage type 4 as the predominant phage type in human infections and is strongly linked to consumption of contaminated eggs. Apart from eggs, infection in humans occurs most frequently through consumption of poultry, red meats, and unpasteurized milk and other dairy products, although infection has more recently been associated with consumption of contaminated alfalfa sprouts, unpasteurized orange juice, tomatoes, and other fresh produce; with contact with animals on farms and at petting zoos; and with the care of household and exotic pets (especially turtles and lizards). These infections tend to peak in the summer months.

CLINICAL FEATURES

Salmonellosis can manifest as a broad range of clinical syndromes that range from asymptomatic carriage (*Salmonella* is usually harbored in the gallbladder) to gastroenteritis (~75%), bacteremia (~10%), vascular infections, enteric fever (~8%), and metastatic focal infections (central nervous system, cholecystitis, osteomyelitis, bone and joint sepsis: ~5%). Salmonellosis has an incubation period of 6 to 48 hours. Symptoms start with nausea and vomiting, are followed by abdominal cramps and diarrhea, and then resolve within 3 to 4 days. Fever is present in 50% of cases. However, more severe, invasive (bacteremia) or protracted diarrhea, often necessitating hospitalization, is not uncommon. For example, bacteremia occurs in about 10% of hospitalized patients. This is more common in patients at the extremes of age (particularly older than 60 years), in patients who are immunocompromised (receiving steroids, chemotherapy, or radiotherapy), in patients with AIDS, in those who have endovascular abnormalities (atheroma, aneurysm, or prosthesis), and probably in patients with underlying inflammatory diseases. Patients with hypochlorhydria, secondary to either surgery or acid-suppressing drugs, are susceptible to salmonellosis, which is also more severe in such patients. Finally, certain serotypes (e.g., *Salmonella virchow*, *Salmonella choleraesius*, *Salmonella dublin*, *S. typhimurium*) are more invasive, leading to bacteremia and metastatic infection (Table 1).

TREATMENT

General

The major goal is the replacement of fluid and electrolytes. Oral rehydration solutions remain the treatment of choice for mild to moderate diarrhea in both children and adults and can be used for severe diarrhea after some initial parenteral hydration. It is better to eat judiciously during an attack of diarrhea than to severely restrict oral intake. In an affected child, it is especially important to restart feeding as soon as the child is able to accept oral intake. Dairy products, tea, coffee, cocoa, and soft drinks

TABLE 1. **Risk Factors for Severe or Invasive Salmonellosis**

Age
>60 years
<3 months

Immunocompromised Status
Steroids
Chemotherapy
Radiotherapy
Underlying malignancy
AIDS
Transplant recipients

Endovascular Abnormalities
Atheroma
Aneurysm
Prosthesis

Hypochlorhydria
H_2 antagonists
Proton pump inhibitors
Gastric surgery

Inflammatory Bowel Disease (Possible Predisposing Condition)

Certain *Salmonella* Serotypes

Chronic Hemolytic Anemia
E.g., sickle cell disease

Schistosomiasis

should be avoided because they exacerbate cramps and diarrhea. Because most patients have a mild, self-limited course, neither stool culture nor specific treatment is usually required. If a reduction in bowel frequency is desirable, the addition (not to replace rehydration) of bismuth subsalicylate (Pepto Bismol) can give relief for mild to moderate diarrhea (three or fewer bowel movements daily). This drug possesses antimicrobial properties on the basis of the bismuth and antisecretory properties related to the salicylate moiety. In more severe disease (up to four loose movements a day), an antimotility drug such as loperamide (Imodium) should be considered. Loperamide induces rapid improvement, demonstrable even on the first day of treatment, and the results are significantly better than those for placebo or bismuth subsalicylate. Antimotility drugs should be avoided in elderly patients, for protracted periods, and in patients with diagnosed shigellosis or dysenteric symptoms (bloody, mucoid stools and fever).

Antimicrobial Therapy

Antibiotic treatment of uncomplicated noninvasive salmonellosis in a healthy host is not indicated. Therapy does not shorten the duration of the disease and can in fact prolong the shedding of *Salmonella* organisms. Indeed, an excellent systematic review published by the Cochrane Library (United Kingdom) on the role of antibiotics in culture-positive adults and children with symptomatic *Salmonella*-induced gastroenteritis confirmed this finding and also reported an increase in adverse drug-related effects. The studies in this review did not include immuno-

compromised hosts or neonates, and no information about quinolone therapy in infants and children was available. Despite this, quinolones remain an attractive and widely used option in adults with severe, metastatic, or invasive salmonellosis and in those who are at high risk for bacteremia or invasive disease. The quinolones have excellent in vivo activity and efficacy against *Salmonella* in humans and animals, penetrate macrophages well, and have been shown to be effective in shortening the duration of uncomplicated *Salmonella*-induced enterocolitis.

In the United Kingdom, these considerations have led a working party of the British Society for the Study of Infection to consider the role of quinolones for the empirical treatment of severe community-acquired diarrhea in adults (including salmonellosis) presenting primarily to the family practitioner or when hospitalized. The party recommends that in patients with dysenteric diarrhea (Table 2) and those at high risk for severe or invasive diseases, oral ciprofloxacin (Cipro) 500 mg twice daily (bid) for 5 days should be considered empirically after a stool sample is obtained, if possible. The recommended period of treatment is considered by some physicians to be too long and may be reduced to 3 days or less (single day). Most studies of antibiotics have required the presence of symptoms for at least 3 days before antibiotics are given, whereas others have shown benefit when the symptoms are treated within 48 hours of onset. In my opinion, antibiotics should be started as early as possible in severe disease. In children the evidence in support of antibiotics is limited although for cases when antibiotics are required (infants younger than 3 months of age, immunocompromised children, children with systemic or metastatic disease) trimethoprim (Trimpex) or co-trimoxazole (Bactrim) can be given orally for less severe cases, although the majority require ceftriaxone (Rocephin) or cefotaxime (Claforan). Many clinicians would safely prescribe a quinolone for severe or invasive disease on a compassionate basis with appropriate parental consent.

It is clear that patients with documented bacteremia without metastatic infection should be treated for 7 days with intravenous (IV) (400 mg bid) or oral (500 mg bid) ciprofloxacin or another quinolone,

TABLE 2. **Recommendations for Considering Empirical Therapy in Presumed Salmonellosis**

Definition of likely gastroenteritis:
diarrhea classified as 3 or more unformed stools/day plus one or more of the following clinical features:
  Abdominal pain
  Nausea, vomiting, or fever
  Blood in the stools or tenesmus
If the patient fulfills this definition and is either in the "high risk" group (see Table 1) and/or has dysenteric symptoms (fever, bloody diarrhea, and abdominal pain), consider empirical ciprofloxacin (or equivalent quinolone), 500 mg bid orally for 5 days. Obtain stool sample for culture if possible. Then review the patient's progress.

whereas those with metastatic infection should be treated with similar doses for 2 to 4 weeks, with focal drainage when appropriate. In the case of endovascular infection, therapy for 4 to 6 weeks is recommended, with excision of the infected sites when possible. Alternatives to the quinolones for severe or bacteremic (with or without localization) infection are IV ceftriaxone, 2 mg once daily, or trimethoprim-sulfamethoxazole, 960 mg bid. Interestingly, recent trends indicate that antibiotic susceptibility must be considered both for domestically and internationally acquired infection. For example, multidrug-resistant serotype *S. typhimurium* DT 104 is an emerging pathogen and is resistant to ampicillin, sulfonamides, streptomycin, chloramphenicol, and tetracyclines; thus the quinolones are the current agents of choice. However, the clinician must closely monitor for the emergence of quinolone resistance, which recently has been shown in *S. typhi* infection.

Persisting excretion of *Salmonella* may occur for weeks or months, especially in infants or adults with underlying gallbladder disease, gut disorders (such as diverticulosis), inflammatory bowel disease, ischemia, or AIDS. No action is generally necessary because *Salmonella* excretion does not compromise the health of an otherwise healthy patient and is only a minimal cross-infection hazard once the diarrhea has ceased and personal hygiene is easy to maintain. The physician must avoid the temptation of prescribing prolonged courses of antibiotics, because they are likely to prolong excretion. In these circumstances, it is important to reassure the patient or parent and to advise that the patient stop sending further stool samples. In rare circumstances, protracted (4- to 6-week) courses of quinolone antibiotics may be necessary to eliminate carriage, followed up by the requirement of three consecutive stool tests with negative findings.

PREVENTION AND CONTROL

A chapter on the therapy of salmonellosis would not be complete without emphasizing the need to promote prevention and control of infection. Adherence to good personal and food hygiene is crucial. Control measures require enhanced public health surveillance, which includes diagnosis, prompt reporting of cases, characterization of the isolates, and investigation of the sources of infection. There remains no effective vaccine for the prevention of non-typhoidal *Salmonella* transmission.

TYPHOID FEVER

method of
NARAIN H. PUNJABI, M.D.
U. S. Naval Medical Research Unit No. 2
Jakarta, Indonesia

DEFINITION

Typhoid fever is an acute systemic illness caused by the gram-negative bacillus *Salmonella typhi*. During an infection, this microorganism multiplies in mononuclear phagocytic cells and is continuously released into the bloodstream. Typhoid fever is characterized by prolonged fever, disturbance of bowel habits (constipation or diarrhea), and other systemic symptoms that include headache, malaise, and anorexia. Other serious complications, which are usually associated with a poor clinical outcome, include altered mental status, intestinal bleeding, and perforation of the bowel. Clinical illness that is indistinguishable from typhoid fever, although usually milder, is also caused by some strains of *Salmonella enteritidis*: *Salmonella paratyphi* A, *S. paratyphi* B (*S. schottmuelleri*), and *S. paratyphi* C (*S. hirschfeldii*); therefore, the name "enteric fever" is often used to describe the illness associated with this group of organisms.

EPIDEMIOLOGY

The Centers for Disease Control and Prevention (CDC) has reported 300 to 500 cases of typhoid fever annually in the United States, and almost all the cases are imported. There have been, however, several small epidemics of typhoid fever within the United States since the mid-1980s.

In developing countries, typhoid fever continues to be a significant cause of morbidity, with incidence rates up to 1000 cases per 100,000 persons per year in some areas. Children and young adults constitute the largest proportion of patients. Except for an increased frequency of disease in the postpartum period, there is no significant difference in incidence between males and females. In view of the fact that approximately 20 million Americans per year visit countries that are endemic for typhoid fever, the disease should be considered in the differential diagnosis of all febrile patients with a history of travel in endemic areas.

CLINICAL MANIFESTATIONS

Symptoms of typhoid fever vary from a mild illness with low-grade fever, malaise, and slight cough, to a severe condition with multiple complications. The clinical severity of typhoid fever has not been shown to be associated with specific host factors. Many general factors, however, may contribute to the severity and overall clinical outcome of the disease, including the duration of illness before therapy was initiated, choice of antimicrobial treatment, age, previous exposure or vaccination history, HLA type, bacterial strain, and the size of inoculum ingested.

Almost all typhoid fever patients report febrile episodes; fevers usually start insidiously, rise in stepwise fashion for a few days, and are then followed by a plateau. In the same pattern the fever gradually subsides over several days to a week. The febrile pattern can be significantly altered by antibiotic therapy.

Other constitutional symptoms are headache, weakness, malaise, myalgias, arthralgias, and anorexia. Many patients have abdominal pain or nausea; bowel function is almost always disturbed, constipation being reported more frequently than diarrhea. Patients often have a mild cough or sore throat.

Physical examination reveals a febrile, apathetic patient who is sometimes extremely ill. The patient may have mild bradycardia, coated or "furred" tongue, pulmonary rales or bronchi, or tender abdomen with mild hepatomegaly or splenomegaly or both. Some patients have rose spots: 2- to 4-mm maculopapular pinkish erythematous spots usually located on the lower thorax or upper abdomen and usually seen more easily on fair-skinned patients.

The clinical symptoms in pediatric patients are often milder and less specific than in adults and are often confused with other febrile illnesses. Nevertheless, pediatric patients can experience the same serious complications that occur in adults despite a seemingly mild clinical manifestation.

COMPLICATIONS

Depending upon the clinical setting and quality of available medical care, up to 5 to 10% of typhoid patients may develop serious complications. The presence of occult blood is a common finding in the stool of 10 to 20% of patients, but up to 3% may have melena. Intestinal perforation has also been reported in up to 3% of hospitalized cases. The patient develops increasing abdominal pain, often localized to the right lower quadrant, although it may be diffuse. The symptoms and signs of intestinal perforation and peritonitis sometimes follow, with a sudden rise in pulse, hypotension, marked abdominal tenderness, rebound tenderness and guarding, and subsequent abdominal rigidity. A rising white blood cell count with a left shift and free air on abdominal radiographs are usually seen.

Altered mental status in typhoid patients has been associated with a high mortality rate. Such patients generally have delirium or obtundation, although rarely with coma. Typhoid meningitis, encephalomyelitis, Guillain-Barré syndrome, cranial or peripheral neuritis, and psychotic symptoms, although rare, have been reported.

Other serious complications documented with typhoid fever include hepatitis, myocarditis, pneumonia, disseminated intravascular coagulation, thrombocytopenia, hemolytic uremic syndrome, genitourinary tract manifestations, relapse, and a chronic carrier state.

DIAGNOSIS

Isolation of the causative organism from blood or bone marrow aspirates provides a definitive diagnosis of acute illness. Cultures of rectal swabs or stool culture are less definitive, inasmuch as they can be positive in chronic carriers. Isolation rates from blood are increased when blood cultures taken during the week of acute illness, taken at multiple intervals, are of 10-mL volumes or greater and in a ratio of 1 part blood to 9 parts of culture. However, even with optimal technique, blood cultures are positive in only 55 to 75% of patients.

Cultures of bone marrow aspirates provide the highest rate of organism recovery (85 to 95%) and are the best clinical samples for definitive diagnosis. The culture recovery rate from bone marrow aspirates are less adversely affected by prior antibiotic use and by the time frame of sample collection than are blood cultures. S. typhi can be cultured from the stools of 40 to 55% of all cases, with higher rates of recovery after the second week of illness. The organism can also be isolated from duodenal fluid (the best culture site for detecting carriers), biopsy of rose spots, urine (low yield), and other body fluids and tissue such as lymph nodes, intestinal tissue, peritoneal fluid, bile, and cerebrospinal fluid (CSF).

Because 2 to 7 days are needed for bacterial culture and identification, a sensitive and specific rapid diagnostic test would be an important diagnostic adjunct. In 1896, Widal's test, which measures antibodies to the O and H antigens of S. typhi, was developed; however, this test has been shown to have little or no diagnostic validity in endemic areas. This is due to the presence of pre-existing antibodies from immunizations and previous exposure history or the presence of cross-reacting antibodies from infections with other gram-negative bacteria. Many other diagnostic tests have been developed to detect anti–S. typhi antibodies, antigens, or DNA. However, none of these diagnostic assays have been consistently shown to have the sensitivity, specificity, and predictive value to warrant widespread use.

MANAGEMENT

Supportive measures are important in the management of typhoid fever, such as oral or intravenous hydration, antipyretics, and appropriate nutrition and blood transfusions, if indicated. More than 90% of patients can be managed at home with oral antibiotics, a reliable caretaker, and close medical follow-up for complications or failure to respond to therapy.

First-line antibiotics used in developing countries where cost, availability, and efficacy are important criteria for their selection are chloramphenicol,* ampicillin, or amoxicillin and trimethoprim-sulfamethoxazole† (Table 1). These drugs are inexpensive and well-tolerated; ampicillin is safe in children and pregnant or nursing women.

The emergence of multidrug resistant (MDR) strains must be considered in the management of typhoid fever. Drug resistance is classified into two categories: resistance to first-line antibiotics such as chloramphenicol, ampicillin, and trimethoprim-sulfamethoxazole, and resistance to second-line antibiotics such as the fluoroquinolone drugs, also called nalidixic acid–resistant S. typhi (NARST) strain. A significant number of strains from Africa, the Indian subcontinent, and some Southeast Asia countries, except Indonesia, are MDR type. A small percentage of strains from Vietnam and the Indian subcontinent are NARST strains. Distinct patterns of drug resistance occur in each country affected.

Chloramphenicol, despite the risk of agranulocytosis (1 per 10,000 patients), is still widely prescribed in developing countries to treat typhoid fever. S typhi strains from Indonesia are still 98% sensitive to this drug. Chloramphenicol is reported to produce defervescence in a shorter time than any other first-line antibiotic. The disadvantages to using chloramphenicol include a slightly higher rate of relapse and the development of a carrier stage, due to its bacteriostatic mechanism of action. Dosage is 50 mg per kg per day (up to 100 mg per kg in children), divided into 4 doses, for 14 days, or for at least 5 to 7 days after defervescence. The usual adult dose is 500 mg four times a day. The oral route of administration gives greater bioavailability than intramuscular or intravenous (IV) administration.

Ampicillin, amoxicillin,* and amoxicillin/clavulanic acid†‡ (Augmentin) are used at 50 to 100 mg per kg per day, divided into 3 to 4 doses, orally, intramuscularly, or intravenously. No additional benefit has been

---

*Oral form not available in the United States.
†Not FDA approved for this indication.
‡Exceeds dosage recommended by the manufacturer.

TABLE 1. **Antimicrobial Therapy**

Antibiotic	Route	Adult Dosage/d	Pediatric Dosage: No./d
First-line antibiotics:			
Ampicillin/Amoxicillin	O‡, IM, IV	500 mg qid	50–100 mg/kg: 4
Trimethoprim-Sulfamethoxazole	O, IV	160–800 mg bid	4–20 mg/kg: 2
Chloramphenicol	O, IM, IV	500 mg qid	50–100 mg/kg: 4
Second-line antibiotics:			
Fluoroquinolones			
Ciprofloxacin (Cipro)	O, IV	500 mg bid	N/A
Norfloxacin (Noroxin)	O	400 mg bid	N/A
Pefloxacin*	O, IV	400 mg bid	N/A
Ofloxacin (Floxin)	O	400 mg bid	N/A
Fleroxacin*	O, IV	400 mg qd	N/A
Cephalosporins			
Ceftriaxone (Rocephin)	IM, IV	1–2 gm/bid	50–75 mg/kg: 1–2
Cefotaxime (Claforan)	IM, IV	1–2 gm/bid	40–80 mg/kg: 2–3
Cefoperazone (Cefobid)	IM, IV	1–2 gm/bid	50–100 mg/kg: 2§
Ceftizoxime (Cefizox)	IM, IV	1–2 gm/bid/tid	30–60 mg/kg: 2–3
Cefpirome*	IV	1–2 gm/bid	N/A
Cefixime (Suprax)	O	200–400 mg qd/bid	10 mg/kg: 1–2†
Other antibiotics:			
Aztreonam (Azactam)	IM	1 gm/bid–qid	50–70 mg/kg: 2–4§
Azithromycin (Zithromax)	O	1 gm/qd†	5–10 mg/kg: 1

*Not available in the United States.
†Exceeds dosage recommended by the manufacturer.
‡Oral.
§Not approved for use in children.

reported by the addition of clavulanic acid to amoxicillin.

Trimethoprim-sulfamethoxazole (TMP-SMZ) is used in adults at a dose of 160 mg TMP/800 mg SMZ twice daily, or 4 mg of TMP per kg and 20 mg of SMZ per kg for children, for 14 days, orally or intravenously.

Some second-line antibiotics such as the fluoroquinolones are able to achieve higher active drug levels in the gallbladder and bone marrow and are able to kill *S. typhi* in its intracellular stationary stage in monocytes. As a result of these qualities, the fluoroquinolones are considered to have excellent efficacy. The expense of fluoroquinolones limits their use by developing countries with limited health care resources. It should also be noted that fluoroquinolones are not recommended for children younger than 16 years of age or for pregnant or nursing females.

Ciprofloxacin (Cipro) is administered at a dosage of 500 mg twice daily; norfloxacin* (Noroxin), ofloxacin* (Floxin), and pefloxacin are administered at a dosage of 400 mg twice daily; and fleroxacin is administered at a dosage of 400 mg once daily. Ciprofloxacin, pefloxacin, and fleroxacin are also available for IV use. Most *S. typhi* isolates are highly sensitive to the fluoroquinolones but fluoroquinolone resistance has been reported. The recommended duration of treatment is 5 to 14 days; shorter courses may be associated with higher relapse rates.

Several cephalosporins are effective in the treatment of typhoid fever. The IV cephalosporins are given in the following doses: ceftriaxone* (Rocephin), 50 to 75 mg per kg per day (2 to 4 grams for adults)

in 1 to 2 doses; cefotaxime* (Claforan), 40 to 80 mg per kg per day (adults, 2 to 4 grams per day) in 2 to 3 doses; and cefoperazone* (Cefobid), 50 to 100 mg per kg per day (adults, 2 to 4 grams per day) in 2 doses. Other parenteral cephalosporins that are effective are ceftizoxime* (Cefizox), and cefpirome.† Oral cefixime* (Suprax), at 10 mg per kg per day (adults, 100 to 200 mg) twice daily has been shown to be 85% effective for treatment of typhoid fever in children.

Aztreonam* (Azactam) has also been shown to be effective in the treatment of typhoid fever. This antibiotic has been shown to be more effective than chloramphenicol in clearing the organism from the blood and was associated with fewer adverse reactions. Azithromycin*‡ (Zithromax) administered in a dose of 1 gram once daily for 5 days is also useful for the treatment of typhoid fever, although the disease takes longer to defervesce. The main advantage of aztreonam and azithromycin is that they can be used in children and in pregnant or nursing females.

Management of Complications

Typhoid fever patients, both outpatient and inpatient, need to be closely monitored for the development of complications. Timely intervention can prevent or reduce morbidity and mortality.

Typhoid fever patients with mental status changes should be immediately evaluated for meningitis by

---

*Not FDA approved for this indication.

---

*Not FDA approved for this indication.
†Not available in the United States.
‡Exceeds dosage recommended by the manufacturer.

TABLE 2. **Typhoid Fever Vaccines**

Vaccine	Age	Route	Dosage	Revaccination
Vivotif (Ty2la, live)	≥5 y	O*	1 capsule every other d, total of 4 capsules	5 y
Typhim Vi (ViCPS) P	≥2 y	SC	0.5 mL	3 y
Killed whole-cell vaccine	≥6 mo	SC	0.5 mL (0.25 mL for children <10 y of age) 2 times, 4 wk apart	3 y

*Oral.

CSF examination; if CSF examination findings are normal and typhoid menigitis is suspected, adults and children should immediately be treated, in addition to antimicrobials, with high-dose intravenous dexamethasone: a bolus of 3 mg per kg administered over 30 minutes, to be followed 6 hours later by 1 mg per kg every 6 hours a total of eight times. High-dose steroid treatment need not await results of typhoid blood cultures if other causes of central nervous system deterioration are unlikely. Dexamethasone therapy begun within 6 hours of clinical diagnosis can reduce mortality by approximately 80 to 90% in these high-risk patients.

Intestinal hemorrhage should be closely observed, and intervention is not needed unless there is significant blood loss. Monitoring of vital signs, hematocrit, and stool blood loss indicate the need for transfusion before hypovolemic shock occurs.

Surgical consultation for suspected intestinal perforation is indicated, and if perforation is confirmed, surgical repair should not be delayed longer than 6 hours. Parenteral antibiotics to treat leakage of *S. typhi* and other intestinal bacteria into the abdominal cavity should be administered before and after surgery.

Relapse of acute illness occurs in 5 to 20% of typhoid fever cases that have been successfully treated. It is heralded by the return of fever about 2 weeks after completion of antibiotics. Frequently the clinical manifestation is milder than the initial illness. Cultures should be obtained, and standard treatment administered. A shorter duration of antibiotic treatment of 3 to 5 days after defervescence could be considered.

Management of Carriers

An individual is considered a chronic carrier if he or she is asymptomatic and continues to have positive stool or rectal swab cultures for 1 year following recovery from acute illness. Overall, about 3% of typhoid fever patients become chronic carriers. The rate of carriage is slightly higher among female patients, patients older than 50 years of age, and patients with cholelithiasis or schistosomiasis. If cholelithiasis or schistosomiasis is present, the patient probably requires cholecystectomy or antiparasitic medication in addition to antibiotics to achieve bacteriologic cure. To eradicate *S. typhi* carriage, amoxicillin* or ampicillin (100 mg per kg per day) plus pro-

benecid (Benemid), 1 gram orally (23 mg per kg for children) or TMP-SMZ* (160 to 800 mg twice daily), is administered for 6 weeks; about 60% of persons treated with either regimen will have negative cultures on follow-up. Clearance of up to 80% of chronic carriers can be achieved with the administration of 750 mg of ciprofloxacin or 400 mg of norfloxacin twice daily for 28 days; other quinolone drugs may yield similar results.

PREVENTION

Sanitation

Typhoid is transmitted via the fecal-oral route through contaminated food and drinking water. Clean water, food inspection, proper food handling, and proper sewage disposal have allowed developed countries to virtually eliminate typhoid fever. Health care providers can educate susceptible populations, including travelers, about the importance of personal hygiene and avoiding foods and drinks that may harbor bacteria, such as improperly cooked foods, snacks prepared by street vendors, salads, ice, and tap water. A case-control study from Indonesia implicated eating at roadside stalls as an important risk factor in the development of typhoid fever.

Vaccines

Vaccines against typhoid fever provide 50 to 88% protection against disease and are recommended for people living in or planning travel to endemic areas, household contacts of cases, microbiology laboratory workers, and sanitation/sewage workers in endemic areas. Three vaccines are licensed in the United States and other countries: a live oral vaccine, a capsular polysaccharide vaccine, and a killed whole-cell vaccine. None of the vaccines provides complete protection, but they can be expected to provide at least 50% protection or more (Table 2).

The live oral vaccine Ty2la (Vivotif Berna) is available in enteric-coated capsule form. One capsule should be taken every other day for four times on an empty stomach. It is approved for use in children 5 years of age and older with revaccination every 5 years. Antibiotics should be avoided for 48 hours before or after the immunization series. Although the package insert allows simultaneous administration of mefloquine (Lariam) or chloroquine (Aralen) for

---

*Exceeds dosage recommended by the manufacturer.

*Not FDA approved for this indication.

malaria prophylaxis, it is recommended to keep 1 to 3 days' gap between completion of immunization series and the first dose of mefloquine.

It is recommended that the prospective traveler should complete the vaccination at least 1 week before departure. The vaccine produces a few side effects that include mild diarrhea and or abdominal pain. Because it is a live vaccine, it is not recommended for persons with compromised immunity.

The parenteral capsular polysaccharide vaccine (Typhim Vi) is given at a dose of 0.5 mL subcutaneously. This vaccine is well tolerated with only a few mild side effects reported. The vaccine is approved for persons above 2 years of age, with repeat doses recommended every 3 years. It is also recommended that the vaccine be given at least 2 weeks before exposure.

The parenteral killed whole-cell vaccine is given in two 0.5-mL doses, subcutaneously, separated by 4 weeks. For children younger than 10 years of age, the dosage is halved; it is not approved for children younger than 6 months. Side effects are frequent, can be disabling for 24 to 48 hours, and include fever, pain, and swelling at the injection site; headache; and malaise. The other two newer vaccines, if available, should be used instead of this vaccine.

ROCKY MOUNTAIN SPOTTED FEVER AND EHRLICHIOSIS

method of
BURKE A. CUNHA, M.D.
Winthrop-University Hospital
Mineola, New York

State University of New York School of Medicine
Stony Brook, New York

Rocky Mountain spotted fever (RMSF) is a tick-borne infectious disease caused by *Rickettsia*. RMSF is transmitted in the eastern United States by the dog tick *Dermacentor variabilis,* in the west by *Dermacentor andersoni,* and in the central states by *Amblyomma americanum.* RMSF also can be transmitted from wild rodents as well as from dogs. *Ehrlichia* are rickettsia-like organisms that belong to the family *Rickettsiae* and, although very similar to *Rickettsia,* have been accorded separate genus status. Ehrlichiosis is transmitted by the *Ixodes scapularis* tick and may be caused by different *Ehrlichia* species. The two predominant species in the United States are *E. chaffeensis* and *E. canis,* the causative agents of human monocytic ehrlichiosis (HME) and human granulocytic ehrlichiosis (HGE).

Both RMSF and ehrlichiosis manifest with very similar clinical pictures, which vary greatly in spectrum from a mild, self-limiting disease to a fulminant, life-threatening illness. Most patients requiring admission to the hospital have an acute febrile illness characterized by headache and myalgias, with or without a rash. Most patients with RMSF have an extremity maculopapular rash on the first day, which becomes petechial on days 3 to 5 and is most prominent on the ankles and wrists. Ehrlichiosis has been termed "spotless RMSF" and is clinically very similar to RMSF. A minority of patients with ehrlichiosis may have a rash similar to that seen in RMSF. RMSF causes a widespread vasculitis that is responsible for the characteristic multiple organ system involvement. A similar multisystem infection is seen with *ehrlichiosis* but without the vasculitic component. RMSF and ehrlichiosis often manifest with prominent neurologic manifestations, and both are characterized by early liver involvement. Cardiac involvement is common with RMSF but is not a feature of ehrlichiosis. Laboratory abnormalities in both RMSF and ehrlichiosis are similar. The most profound and consistent laboratory abnormalities in both infections are leukopenia and thrombocytopenia, which may be profound. Anemia is not a usual feature of RMSF but is commonly a feature with ehrlichiosis. Lactose dehydrogenase (LDH) levels may be elevated in ehrlichiosis but not in RMSF. The lungs are not involved early in the course of either RMSF or ehrlichiosis. Pulmonary edema or adult respiratory distress syndrome (ARDS) that occurs late in the infection and is associated with overzealous fluid replacement may complicate RMSF. Hypovolemia (i.e., relative intravascular volume depletion) may result in acute tubular necrosis (ATN).

Patients with RMSF are warm and dry and, because of fever, have become dehydrated. The fever pattern in early RMSF is that of a rapidly rising remittent fever with an appropriate pulse response that is also seen in ehrlichiosis. A pulse temperature deficit (i.e., relative bradycardia) may be seen in RMSF 1 week or more after the start of the fever. A "camel-back" fever curve has been described with ehrlichiosis.

For patients with an otherwise unexplained acute febrile illness from an area endemic for RMSF or ehrlichiosis, these infectious diseases should be considered in the differential diagnosis. The diagnosis of RMSF may be difficult if the association with a tick bite is not made. However, because the ticks transmitting RMSF are large, the patient is usually aware of the tick bite. In contrast, the tick that is responsible for the transmission of HGE/HME, *I. scapularis,* is very small. For this reason, co-infections with *Ehrlichia* and *Borrelia burgdorferi* are not uncommon, but RMSF and ehrlichiosis do not manifest as co-infections because the tick vectors are dissimilar.

The protean manifestations of RMSF and ehrlichiosis often present a difficult diagnostic problem. Nausea and vomiting are common to both and may suggest a primary intra-abdominal problem. RMSF with right lower quadrant pain may mimic appendicitis, leading the clinician away from the correct diagnosis. If, after 3 to 5 days, the characteristic rash is present on the wrists or ankles, a presumptive diagnosis of RMSF is possible. Ehrlichiosis unaccompanied by rash has no specific diagnostic features. The diagnosis of ehrlichiosis may be made if morulae are seen in monocytes or granulocytes in the peripheral smear. Morulae appear as cytoplastic inclusion bodies and, if present, are diagnostic of ehrlichiosis. RMSF, aside from the characteristic rash, may be confirmed later by serologic means (i.e., acute and convalescent titers).

If a patient is likely to have RMSF, doxycycline (Vibramycin) is the preferred antibiotic. Doxycycline may be administered orally to patients who are mildly ill, but it is best given parenterally to ill patients who require admission to the hospital. Doxycycline, because of its lipid solubility characteristics and long half-life, should be given initially in a loading dose of 200 mg intravenously (IV) every 12 hours for the first 72 hours. After steady-state blood levels have been achieved (72 hours), the dose may be decreased to the usual 100 mg IV or orally every 12 hours. Alternatively, doxycycline may be given as a 200-mg dose IV or orally every 24 hours, or chloramphenicol (Chloromycetin) may be given IV or orally as a 500-mg dose every 6 hours. Chloramphenicol, given IV, is associated with a lower incidence of aplastic anemia than when given orally. The fluoroquinolones* are probably effective against RMSF, but experience with these agents is limited.

*Not FDA approved for this indication.

TABLE 1. **Therapeutic Approach to Rocky Mountain Spotted Fever and Ehrlichiosis**

Empirical Treatment Group

Otherwise undiagnosed acute febrile illness in a patient from an endemic area, characterized by severe headache, myalgias with CNS, hepatic, or renal involvement with leukopenia and thrombocytopenia.

Antibiotic Options	RMSF Likely (Rash)	HGE/HME Likely (no Rash)
Preferred therapy	Doxycycline (Vibramycin)	Doxycycline (Vibramycin)
Alternative therapy	Chloramphenicol (Chloromycetin)	Rifampin* (Rifadin)
Probably effective	Fluoroquinolones*	Fluoroquinolones*
Clinically ineffective	Macrolides TMP-SMX (Bactrim-Septra)	Chloramphenicol (Chloromycetin)

RMSF or Ehrlichiosis
Doxycycline (Vibramycin)

Dosing Recommendations

Doxycycline (Vibramycin)	Parenteral	200 mg IV q 12 h × 72 h *then* 200 mg IV q 24 h *or* 100 mg IV q 12 h for 7–14 days
	Oral	200 mg PO q 12 h × 72 h *then* 200 mg PO for 24 h *or* 100 mg PO q 12 h for 7–14 days
Chloramphenicol (Chloromycetin)	Parenteral	500 mg IV q 6 h for 7–14 days
	Oral	500 mg PO q 6 h for 7–14 days
Rifampin (Rifadin)	Oral	600 mg PO q 24 h for 7–14 days
Fluoroquinolones	Parenteral	Ciprofloxacin (Cipro), 400 mg IV q 12 h *or* Levofloxacin (Levaquin), 500 mg IV q 24 h for 7–14 days
	Oral	Ciprofloxacin (Cipro), 500 mg PO q 12 h *or* Levofloxacin (Levaquin), 500 mg PO q 24 h for 7–14 days

*Not FDA approved for this indication.
Abbreviations: CNS = central nervous system; RMSF = Rocky Mountain spotted fever; HGE = human granulocytic ehrlichiosis; HME = human monocytic ehrlichiosis; TMP-SMX = trimethoprim-sulfamethoxazole.

Macrolides or sulfonamides should not be used to treat RMSF (Table 1). Erythromycin has activity in vitro, but in animal studies it kills *Rickettsia* at a very low rate or fails to eradicate the organism intracellularly; for these reasons, it should not be used to treat RMSF. RMSF rapidly defervesces after treatment with doxycycline or chloramphenicol, usually within 72 hours. Treatment is continued for 7 days in mild cases and for 14 days in severe cases. Children with RMSF may be treated with chloramphenicol or doxycycline. Children younger than 10 years of age are at risk of tooth staining from tetracycline drugs, which is a dose-related permanent side effect. Doxycycline is given at a lower dosage than conventional tetracycline and is less likely to stain the teeth of young children. It has been shown that a 5-day course of doxycycline does not stain the teeth of young children. Fluoroquinolones provide an alternative to doxycycline or chloramphenicol in the treatment of young children.

Relapse may occur with patients treated with shorter courses and is more likely with chloramphenicol than with doxycycline. Relapses should be treated with a 1- to 2-week course of doxycycline. Doxycycline is the preferred antibiotic for treating ehrlichiosis (HME/HGE). It is important to appreciate that chloramphenicol is ineffective in both HGE and HME. As with RMSF, fluoroquinolones may be used as alternative therapy in the rare patient who is unable to take doxycycline. Although experience is limited, rifampin* (Rifadin) is also effective against ehrlichiosis. If the clinical manifestations and laboratory features do not differentiate between RMSF and ehrlichiosis, doxycycline is the preferred antibiotic and is effective in treating both of these potentially life-threatening infectious diseases. The best alternative therapy in people unable to take doxycycline would be a fluoroquinolone.*

Non-antibiotic treatment of RMSF and ehrlichiosis depends on the degree and extent of end-organ dysfunction. Patients who develop ARDS need respiratory support until they are able again to breathe on their own. Patients with cardiac arrhythmias and myocarditis may require antiarrhythmic therapy. Patients with severe central nervous system complications may benefit from a short course of steroid therapy. Patients with ATN may be managed by judicious fluid management until the ATN resolves. Dialysis may be temporarily necessary to manage acute electrolyte problems (e.g., hyperkalemia).

The most common and important therapeutic mistake is overzealous rehydration. Patients are dry and hot from their fever and invariably have prerenal azotemia on presentation. Because RMSF causes a vasculitis and increased capillary permeability, overly aggressive intravenous fluid replacement, especially with hypotonic fluids, will result in generalized or pulmonary edema. Pulmonary edema may be an additional burden on a heart already compromised by myocarditis. The optimal therapeutic approach is to use isotonic fluids to judiciously replace volume, erring on the side of under-replacement so as to prevent ATN from developing as a result of oliguric renal failure.

Although most patients with RMSF or ehrlichiosis recover with prompt appropriate antimicrobial therapy, both of these infectious diseases are serious and potentially life-threatening. Early empirical treatment must be based on a high index of suspicion in acutely ill febrile patients from endemic areas. With the exception of finding morulae in the peripheral smear of patients with ehrlichiosis, definitive tests are not available during the early phases of RMSF or ehrlichiosis.

*Not FDA approved for this indication.

The Respiratory System

ACUTE RESPIRATORY FAILURE

method of
VICTOR J. CARDENAS, Jr., M.D., and
AKHIL BIDANI, M.D., Ph.D.
The University of Texas Medical Branch
Galveston, Texas

Acute respiratory failure (ARF) is a decompensating respiratory system that without rapid and effective treatment will result in cessation of function and ultimately death. Although it is often characterized by arterial blood gas criteria (arterial oxygen tension [PaO_2] < 60 mm Hg and/or alveolar carbon dioxide tension [$PacO_2$] > 50 mm Hg), it is a clinical syndrome in which signs and symptoms are often sufficient to establish the diagnosis and determine the severity of illness. ARF has multiple etiologies, and the course will depend on a variety of factors, including efficacy of available treatment, underlying medical conditions, and physiologic reserve. Inability to reverse the process ultimately results in the need for respiratory support, including mechanical ventilation. Up to 50% of patients admitted to intensive care units may require ventilatory support at some time during their stay, with significant impact both on local resources as well as the overall cost of health care nationally. Understanding the mechanisms underlying ARF and early recognition of the clinical manifestation may allow for effective intervention and prevent progression to mechanical ventilation. We examine primary hypoxic respiratory failure as represented by the acute respiratory distress syndrome and primary hypercapnic ventilatory failure as represented by obstructive airway disease.

ADULT RESPIRATORY DISTRESS SYNDROME

Epidemiology

The adult (or acute) respiratory distress syndrome (ARDS) is a clinical condition based on (1) history of a preceding associated event (pulmonary or extrapulmonary) with rapid onset of respiratory failure; (2) diffuse bilateral pulmonary infiltrates on the chest radiograph; (3) normal pulmonary capillary wedge pressure; and (4) refractory hypoxemia (PaO_2 < 60 for forced inspiratory oxygen [FIO_2] > 0.6; PaO_2/FIO_2 < 200). ARDS appears to be the common end point of a variety of disease processes, including physical trauma, sepsis, aspiration, drug or toxin exposure, diffuse pneumonia, oxygen toxicity, central nervous system disease, smoke and irritant gas inhalation, fat embolism, pancreatitis, burns, cardiopulmonary bypass, and multiple transfusions. Survival rates approximate 40 to 50% in most major series. Approximately 90% of all deaths in patients with ARDS occur within 2 to 3 weeks after the onset of the syndrome. The major determinant of outcome in ARDS is the failure of other vital organ systems (multiple organ failure syndrome).

Clinical Manifestations

Although ARDS may result from a variety of causes, the ultimate effect is the same; a loss of the functional integrity of the blood-gas exchange, leading to capillary leakage and noncardiogenic pulmonary edema. By definition, all ARDS patients have severe hypoxemia due to intrapulmonary shunting and, to a lesser extent, ventilation/perfusion ($\dot{V}/\dot{Q}$) mismatch. The onset of ARDS is characterized by severe dyspnea, tachypnea, and hypoxemia. The primary mechanism of hypoxemia is extensive right-to-left intrapulmonary shunting of blood flow. In ARDS the shunt fraction may approach 25 to 50% of cardiac output. Because blood flowing through a shunt is not exposed to alveolar gas, supplemental oxygen is ineffective in resolving the hypoxemia. In patients with severe intrapulmonary shunting, arterial hypoxemia may be exacerbated by conditions that lower the mixed venous oxygen saturation, because of either decreased peripheral oxygen delivery (e.g., severe anemia or low cardiac output) or increased oxygen consumption (fever, hard work of breathing).

Radiologic Findings

The chest radiographic findings, which may lag behind the pathology and symptoms of ARDS, can be divided into three stages according to the extent of lung injury. In stage I (radiographically latent), pathophysiologic changes are occurring, but the radiograph shows minimal abnormalities. Stage II (acute) usually develops about 24 hours after the initial injury and is characterized by bilateral, diffuse, "fluffy" interstitial and alveolar infiltrates that are the hallmark of ARDS. In contrast to "cardiogenic" pulmonary edema, the heart size is normal in ARDS. Fluid in the lung tissue highlights air in the airways and produces "air bronchograms." Stage III begins late in the first week after lung injury. Alveolar fluid diminishes, leaving interstitial edema. Pulmonary interstitial emphysema may also be seen.

Patient Management

The primary goals of ARDS management are to treat the underlying etiology (such as known infection), maintain adequate oxygenation, and maximize oxygen delivery to the tissues, while preventing treatment-associated complications such as oxygen toxicity, volume overload, gastrointestinal bleeding, local or systemic infection, and ventilator-associated problems (volutrauma/barotrauma, pneumonia, and so on). The initial approach to an ARDS patient is to rule out other causes of diffuse pulmonary infiltrates and severe hypoxemia, such as cardiogenic pulmonary edema, neurogenic pulmonary edema, diffuse alveolar hemorrhage, chronic interstitial disease, bronchiolitis obliterans with organizing pneumonia (BOOP), acute eosinophilic pneumonia, miliary tuberculosis, and bilateral pneumonia. In immunocompromised patients, *Pneumocystis carinii* pneumonia and other opportunistic infections must be considered.

Mechanical Ventilation

Mechanical ventilation is needed in most patients with ARDS to maintain adequate oxygenation. Mechanical ventilators neither prevent nor directly treat ARDS; rather, they keep the patient alive until the underlying problem resolves and the lungs heal enough to support the patient again. The use of positive-pressure ventilation in ARDS has undergone fundamental reevaluation on the basis of extensive human and animal studies. It is now recognized that regional overdistention of healthy alveoli can result in diffuse alveolar damage, indistinguishable from ARDS. As a consequence, ventilator management has veered away from the goal of maintaining normocapnia. Computed tomography of patients with ARDS has revealed that there are important regional differences in the distribution of noncardiogenic pulmonary edema. Dense, dependent consolidated regions are separated from apparently morphologically normal nondependent regions by regions of alveolar atelectasis. In such a heterogeneous lung, the optimal ventilation strategy avoids the cyclical opening and closing of atelectatic alveolar regions, while avoiding alveolar overdistention of the nondependent "normal" alveolar units. To accomplish this, a certain minimal level of positive end-expiratory pressure (PEEP) is required so as to avoid alveolar de-recruitment during expiration. The tidal volume is kept low (6 to 8 mL per kg) to avoid alveolar overdistention. It has been suggested that the end-inspiratory plateau-pressure (P_{plat}) be kept less than 35 cm H_2O as a lung-protective strategy to minimize ventilator-induced lung injury. Either pressure- or volume-controlled modes may be used.

Positive End-Expiratory Pressure

Recruitment of atelectatic alveoli by judicious use of PEEP increases functional residual capacity and pulmonary compliance. Although PEEP is an important part of maintaining adequate gas exchange in the lungs of the ARDS patient, side effects include decreased pulmonary compliance from overdistended alveoli, decreased venous return and cardiac output,

increased pulmonary vascular resistance, increased right ventricular afterload, and barotrauma.

Prone Position

There is growing interest in the use of prone positioning in ARDS patients. About half of ARDS patients demonstrate significant sustained improvement in arterial oxygenation when they are switched from supine to prone position. The primary mechanism appears to be a more uniform regional distribution of alveolar ventilation, resulting in improved $\dot{V}/\dot{Q}$ distribution and improved arterial oxygenation. Ventilating patients in the prone position, however, presents unique resuscitative and nursing challenges and may not be well tolerated by patients with marginal hemodynamics.

Tissue Oxygenation

Tissue oxygenation is dependent on adequate oxygen delivery, which is a function of arterial oxygen content and cardiac output. This means that both ventilation and cardiac function are vital to the patient's survival. Positive-pressure ventilation, however, may decrease cardiac output while improving arterial blood oxygenation. Efforts to improve tissue oxygen delivery by pressors is often necessary.

Nutritional Support

Malnutrition is common in patients who are severely ill, particularly in those receiving mechanical ventilation, and can result in iatrogenic immunosuppression. Enteral alimentation (i.e., food supplement via the nasogastric tube) is preferable whenever possible; however, if the bowel is not functional, parenteral (intravenous feeding) may be necessary for providing adequate protein, fat, and carbohydrate, along with minerals and vitamins.

Rescue Therapies

Current data do not support the routine use of new adjunctive measures such as partial liquid ventilation, intracorporeal and extracorporeal gas exchange, and inhaled nitric oxide. Instead, these experimental approaches should be considered as "rescue therapies" and used in circumstances in which the anticipated mortality risk is very high and routine therapies are failing. As our ability to stratify patients into well-defined risk groups improves in the future, there might well be a role for early initiation of rescue therapies in selected ARDS patients.

VENTILATORY FAILURE

Primary hypercapnic ventilatory failure is characterized by inability to maintain sufficient alveolar ventilation to excrete the metabolic carbon dioxide production at a normal P_{aCO_2}. Hypoxia occurs as elevated levels of alveolar CO_2 displace oxygen resulting in lower alveolar partial pressure of oxygen (P_{O_2}) and a normal alveolar-to-arterial oxygen gradient. Ventilatory failure can be acute and potentially life-threatening or chronic and compensated. The acidosis that accompanies the acute form helps distinguish it from the chronic form. In acute situations, for every 10–mm Hg increment in partial pressure of carbon dioxide (PCO_2), there is a fall in arterial pH of 0.08. In chronic situations, because of compensatory renal and intracellular mechanisms, the fall in pH is only 0.03 for each 10–mm Hg increment.

Failure of ventilation can be subclassified into primary disorders of the respiratory pump with normal lungs versus disorders with abnormal lung function. Primary disorders include central nervous system dysfunction (e.g., sedative overdoses, cerebrovascular accidents), impulse transmission (e.g., Guillain-Barré, organophosphate poisoning) or muscular causes (hypokalemia, hypophosphatemia, myositis). Management is directed at reversing the primary cause if possible and instituting assisted ventilation if needed. Because the lungs are normal, airway pressures are usually low and barotrauma/volutrauma is not a great concern. Mode of ventilation is primarily a matter of preference. Low PEEP (3 to 5 cm H_2O) is instituted to maintain resting lung volume and prevent atelectasis.

Ventilatory failure associated with intrinsic lung disease is more common. In this case, decompensation most often occurs as the result of excessive work of breathing, overloading the respiratory pump beyond its ability to adapt. Impedance to ventilation involves primarily two factors: resistive work and elastic work. Under normal physiologic conditions, work is minimized by breathing at a lung volume and frequency that balances the total amount of work required. Increases in resistive work are typical of obstructive diseases (decreased luminal radius), whereas increases in elastic work are typical of alveolar processes (stiff lungs). Even fit persons such as asthmatic athletes can deteriorate to failure if the work of breathing is sufficiently high. Frail, ill persons (e.g., emphysema patients) are more susceptible to failure at lesser loads.

Management of Obstructive Airway Disease

The general management of the patient with ventilatory failure may include bronchodilator therapy, corticosteroids, and theophylline. As in the ARDS patient, particular attention to nutrition and correction of electrolyte abnormalities are important. It is important to ascertain any underlying cause or precipitating factor that leads to decompensation. Infection with either pneumonia or acute bacterial bronchitis needs to be considered. Whether antibiotic therapy is helpful in acute exacerbations of chronic obstructive pulmonary disease without specific bacterial cause remains controversial. Recurrent pulmonary thromboembolism is often overlooked as a possible cause of failure, despite increased risk factors for many of these patients. Because the typical findings are often obscured by the underlying lung disease, a low threshold for initiating a work-up is often necessary to diagnose its presence. Similarly, non–Q wave myocardial infarction can often be missed unless looked for.

Treatment of nonventilated, chronically hypercapnic patients with severe hypoxia is somewhat problematic. The concern is that these patients are dependent on hypoxic drive to maintain respiration and that elimination of this drive will lead to higher CO_2 levels, narcosis, and respiratory suppression. More recent data indicate that for many such patients, elevation in PCO_2 does not result from a fall in minute ventilation but rather to a change in physiologic dead space caused by relief of hypoxic vasoconstriction as a result of supplemental oxygen therapy. These changes tend to be transient and return toward baseline as the patient's condition improves. Therefore, a rise in PCO_2 does not warrant a change in therapy if the patient's clinical condition improves. Nevertheless, there remains the possibility that overoxygenation may cause suppression of respiration in certain patients. The goal for PO_2 in these patients is the mid-50s mm Hg, approached from below by carefully titrating FIO_2 or increasing flow rates (i.e., via nasal cannula) by 0.5 to 1.0 liter per minute. If the patient continues to deteriorate, assisted ventilation is warranted. Often this deterioration is inevitable and is the result of muscle fatigue, not of overzealous administration of oxygen.

Ventilatory Management

Restoration of adequate gas exchange and relief of excessive work of breathing are the main end points for the institution of mechanical ventilation in hypercapnic failure. Relief of hypoxia is not problematic in most airway diseases unless there is another underlying process, such as pneumonia or pulmonary edema. Treatment of hypercapnia is somewhat more controversial. Acute hypercapnia and its accompanying acidosis is surprisingly well tolerated down to a pH of 7.2 and, according to some authorities, even lower. Patients with primary cardiac disorders or possible increased intracranial pressure are potentially more susceptible to side effects and intervention should occur earlier. Because pH seems to be a better marker for the deleterious effects of hypercapnia, maintaining a pH higher than 7.25 is a reasonable approach rather than focusing on the level of PCO_2. Overventilating the chronic hypercapnic patient is also to be avoided in order to avoid losing their compensatory bicarbonate stores.

Limitation of airway pressures has been demonstrated to reduce the incidence of barotrauma and improve mortality rates in asthmatics in small case series. Peak pressures less than 50 cm H_2O have been advocated as a benchmark. In addition, patients with expiratory flow resistance are very susceptible to the development of high levels of intrinsic PEEP. Ventilator settings that reduce expiratory flow time can prevent full exhalation of each delivered breath and lead to significant hyperinflation. If undetected, mean intrathoracic pressure may rise to a level that reduces venous return and results in significant hypotension. Disconnecting the endotracheal tube from the ventilator for a few seconds allows excess gas to escape, reducing intrathoracic pressure, and allows recovery of blood pressure.

Noninvasive Positive-Pressure Ventilation

The use of noninvasive positive-pressure ventilation is growing rapidly across the country. It is delivered via a nasal or full face mask connected to a bilevel pressure ventilator (e.g., BiPAP) that allows separate titration of inspiratory and expiratory pressures. In selected patients it has been found to reduce the need for intubation and has decreased length of stay in the intensive care unit. It is best used for the patient who has severe tachypnea but is still alert, is able to follow commands, and has stable vital signs. Patients with altered mentation, unstable hemodynamics, and falling respirations are not appropriate candidates for noninvasive ventilation.

Neuromuscular Blockade

Neuromuscular blockade may be needed in severe cases of patient agitation but is a method of last resort, given current concerns of significant postblockade myopathy in selected patients, particularly those taking high-dose corticosteroids.

Weaning

Weaning from mechanical ventilation remains an inexact science, and there is no factor that predicts with 100% certainty whether a patient will tolerate extubation and spontaneous breathing. Most important is resolution of the underlying process that led to respiratory failure. Significant electrolyte abnormalities can affect muscle strength and should be corrected. Patients must have a sufficient level of mentation to protect their airway and to produce an effective cough. Bronchial secretions, if too copious and tenacious, can result in extubation failure in marginal patients and should be controlled before weaning. If these factors are acceptable, pulmonary mechanics and spontaneous breathing trials can help predict whether a patient is ready. T piece trials, continuous positive airway pressure (CPAP) trials, or gradual reductions in pressure support are commonly used techniques, none of which is clearly superior to the others. Weaning by slow intermittent mandatory ventilation has been found to be inferior to these methods. Trials generally last from 30 minutes to several hours. Clinical signs such as tachypnea, tachycardia, hypotension, hypertension, or patient restlessness/anxiety indicate failure, as does desaturation or significant elevation in P_{CO_2}. The ratio of respiratory rate to tidal volume is used as a predictor of success during T piece trials; values less than 105 are suggestive of a good outcome after extubation. Maximal negative inspiratory pressure less than 20 cm H_2O is predictive of a poor outcome. In difficult cases, tracheostomy may be helpful. The timing of tracheostomy remains controversial.

ATELECTASIS

method of
ROSS RISTAGNO, M.D.
Tri-State Pulmonary Associates, Inc.
Cincinnati, Ohio

Atelectasis is collapse of lung parenchyma. Mild atelectasis may cause no symptoms and necessitates no specific therapy. In more severe cases, treatment for atelectasis that may include supplemental oxygen or even mechanical ventilation is required. The main causes of atelectasis are listed in Table 1. The underlying cause of atelectasis should always be treated vigorously.

Atelectasis often results from inadequate deep breathing. In most cases, atelectasis resolves when the patient increases physical activities, takes deeper breaths and coughs, or uses devices to assist spontaneous inspiratory efforts. Incentive spirometry (IS) is a device that helps teach the patient to take maximal sustained inspirations. The patient is instructed to take 5 to 10 deep, sustained breaths, using the IS device, each hour while awake. If atelectasis is not resolved, more aggressive treatment such as continuous positive airway pressure (CPAP) or intermittent positive pressure breathing (IPPB) may be attempted. CPAP is administered by face or nasal mask at 5 to 15 cm H_2O of pressure either intermittently or continuously. In IPPB, up to 20 cm H_2O of pressure is administered through a mouthpiece or a face mask. The use of CPAP and IPPB may be limited by discomfort or complications such as hypotension and pneumothorax. In recalcitrant cases of atelectasis (if expertise is available), catheter insufflation of air into a bronchus may be attempted.

Costochondritis, which may lead to severe chest pain and widespread atelectasis, responds to nonsteroidal antiinflammatory drugs (NSAIDs). When pleuritis results from a steroid-responsive process (e.g., postpericardiotomy syndrome, rheumatoid arthritis), the use of prednisone resolves the pain, pleural effusions, and atelectasis. For other etiologies, narcotic agents are necessary to reduce pain in the thoracoabdominal region that may limit inspiratory and cough efforts. Additional measures may include regional nerve blocks or intrathecal narcotics. Pulmonary

TABLE 1. **Causes of Atelectasis**

Failure to Generate a Deep Breath

Splinting from thoracoabdominal region pain with inadequate analgesia (surgery, trauma, rib fracture, costochondritis, acute abdomen)

External compression (pleural effusion, ascites, obesity, diaphragmatic hernia, pneumothorax, cardiomegaly, body brace or cast)

Neuromuscular weakness (diaphragm paralysis, cerebrovascular accident, coma, electrolyte abnormalities, malnutrition)

Splinting from pleuritis (viral, rheumatologic related, pulmonary infarction, postpericardiotomy syndrome, pneumonia)

Bronchial Tube Obstruction

Mucous plugs and/or blood clots (pneumonia, chronic obstructive pulmonary disease)

Malignant (primary lung or metastatic) or benign tumors

Foreign body aspiration

Compression of bronchus from hilar or mediastinal lymphadenopathy embolism (PE) should be treated with anticoagulants. PE, which causes chest pain and atelectasis, may be incorrectly attributed to viral pleurisy, pneumonia, or costochondritis.

Compression of lung parenchyma by pleural effusions or ascites limits the successful reversal of atelectasis. Thoracentesis should be considered when there is a moderate to large pleural effusion (except when it is a known transudate such as CHF). Paracentesis should be considered when there is massive ascites.

When the patient is on the mechanical ventilator, atelectasis is minimized by large tidal volumes, intermittent sigh breaths, and positive end-expiratory pressure (PEEP). The endotracheal tube should be positioned 2 to 5 cm above the carina to avoid atelectasis secondary to intubation of the right main bronchus. To clear secretions that may lead to endobronchial obstruction, the tube should be suctioned regularly, with the possible use of a directional catheter to reach the left bronchial tree.

Respiratory therapies, cough, and suctioning are the initial treatments for lobar atelectasis that results from mucous plugs. Bronchodilators such as albuterol (Proventil), 1.25 to 2.5 mg nebulized every 4 to 8 hours, or mucolytics such as acetylcysteine (Mucomyst), 10% 4 mL nebulized every 4 hours as needed, may be instituted. Adequate oral fluid intake helps avoid mucosal dryness, and mucosal drying agents such as antihistamines should be avoided. Moisture inhalational therapy (cool- or warm-mist aerosols) may be helpful, although bronchospasm may be a side effect. Gravity drainage and vibration are employed with percussion and postural drainage treatments, which may be used two to four times a day to dislodge mucous plugs. In a sitting patient who can generate a sustained exhalation, a Flutter device used for 2 minutes four times a day may generate tracheobronchial tree vibrations, move mucus to a more proximal location, and enhance expectoration. Intrapulmonary percussive ventilation (IPV) is an electric device that delivers through a mouthpiece a nebulized bronchodilator and vibration; these propagate through the tracheobronchial tree and mobilize retained secretions.

If these treatments are unsuccessful after 24 to 48 hours, fiberoptic bronchoscopy should be performed. Bronchoscopy should be performed sooner when the patient is immobilized in a supine position and has an ineffective cough, when atelectasis involves the entire left or right lung, or when endobronchial blood clots are anticipated. Nonresponse to treatment or a chest radiography or computed tomographic scan with a mass-like density suggests that the atelectasis is caused by tumor, a mucous plug, a blood clot, or a foreign body. The next diagnostic step should be bronchoscopy with biopsy of the tumor or removal of endobronchial obstructions.

Atelectasis is very common in the postoperative period and is caused by general anesthesia, splinting resulting from the surgical incision, prolonged bed rest, and mucous plugging. Treatment of atelectasis may incorporate many of the previously discussed modalities. Preoperative interventions should include smoking cessation (2 months or longer), treatment of obstructive airway disease, antibiotics for suspected respiratory tract infections, teaching the patient IS and cough techniques that will be used after surgery, and explaining early mobilization after surgery.

CHRONIC OBSTRUCTIVE PULMONARY DISEASE

method of
BARTOLOME R. CELLI, M.D.
Tufts University School of Medicine and
St. Elizabeth's Medical Center
Boston, Massachusetts

Chronic obstructive pulmonary disease (COPD) is characterized by the presence of airflow obstruction due to intrinsic airways disease (typified by chronic bronchitis) and parenchymal destruction (emphysema). The obstruction is generally progressive, may be accompanied by airway hyperreactivity, and may be partially reversible. Patients with nonremitting asthma who develop fixed airflow limitation suffer from COPD, but patients with chronic bronchitis and emphysema without airflow obstruction are not COPD sufferers. Airflow obstruction with a distinct specific pathology such as cystic fibrosis or bronchiolitis is not included as COPD. The interaction of the elements that partake in the genesis of COPD is shown in Figure 1.

The incidence, prevalence, health-related cost of COPD, and mortality rate are increasing. In the United States, COPD is the fourth leading cause of death, and the mortality rate has increased by 46% in men and 126% in women since 1979. In contrast, mortality from causes such as heart disease and stroke have declined.

Cigarette smoking is the single most important factor in the genesis of COPD and accounts for 80 to 90% of the risk of developing COPD. Other potential risk factors include bronchial hyperreactivity, passive smoking, air pollution and alpha-$_1$ antitrypsin (AAT) deficiency. Although only AAT deficiency is of importance comparable with that of tobacco smoking, this accounts for only less than 1% of COPD. Little is known about the factors that identify persons susceptible to develop COPD when exposed to those risk factors.

Although bronchial mucous gland enlargement is characteristic of COPD, the airflow obstruction is due largely to structural abnormalities in the smaller airways. Important causes are inflammation, fibrosis, goblet cell metaplasia,

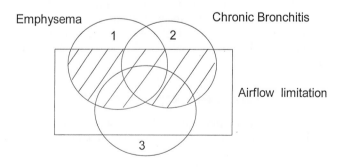

Figure 1. Nonproportional Venn diagram. Each circle represents a nosologic entity. The rectangle represents airflow limitation as documented in a forced spirometry. The striped area corresponds to patients diagnosed as having COPD. Notice that a patient (subset 1) may have emphysema without COPD (patient with bullae on chest roentgenogram without airflow limitation). Similarly, he or she may have sputum production and normal spirometry (subset 2), with simple bronchitis. Finally, an asthmatic patient may lack airflow limitation, and COPD will be diagnosed only after a bronchoprovocation test (subset 3).

and smooth muscle hypertrophy in terminal bronchioles. A major cause in emphysema is the loss of alveolar attachments to bronchioles. Part of the airflow obstruction may also be due to bronchoconstriction. Up to one third of patients demonstrate a significant increase in forced expiratory volume in the first second (FEV_1) after bronchodilator. This proportion increases to two thirds with repeated bronchodilator testing. There are no factors that predict response, and the response itself varies widely between tests.

DIAGNOSIS

In patients with the appropriate risk factors and history, lung function testing with a forced vital capacity is necessary for diagnosis, prognosis, and assessment of severity and response to therapy. Airflow obstruction is assessed by the FEV_1 of the forced vital capacity (FVC). The diagnosis is established when the FEV_1/FVC ratio is 70% or less. A chest roentgenogram is recommended since it helps rule out other pathologies leading to similar symptoms. There is no evidence to support computed tomography (CT) scans, other lung volume measurements, carbon monoxide diffusing capacity (DLco), and sputum examination in the routine investigation of these patients. Although it is desirable to include attributes such as dyspnea and health-related quality of life, the staging of COPD is based on FEV_1, as prognosis is intimately related to postbronchodilator FEV_1 (Table 1).

OUTPATIENT MANAGEMENT OF COPD

Once the diagnosis is established, the patient should be educated about the disease and encouraged to take an active part in its management (co-management).

Smoking cessation is the single most important goal. This can be achieved by physician intervention, strong support, behavioral modification, and pharmacologic intervention (Table 2). Well-implemented programs result in a 20 to 30% success rate in 1 year and in an improvement in FEV_1. As a result of our public and private campaigns, the smoking prevalence has decreased steadily over time, but it still stands around 29% of the population in the United States. More efforts in this area should result in a decrease in the prevalence of COPD in the near future.

STEPWISE PHARMACOTHERAPY

A stepwise approach to pharmacotherapy according to the severity of airway obstruction and the

TABLE 1. **Staging of COPD**

FEV₁ (% predicted value)	Stage	General Approach
≥49%	Stage I	Healthy lifestyle
≥35% but <49%	Stage II	Treatment and close supervision
≤34%	Stage III	Intense therapy

TABLE 2. **Protocol for Smoking Cessation**

1. Physician or health care worker should initiate discussion of smoking cessation. Explain risks of cigarette smoking. Offer strong admonition to quit; encourage a quitting date; offer referral for self-help or group program.
2. Physician or health care worker may arrange telephone follow-up. Call 3–5 d after quitting date. Review progress. Counsel regarding quitting date and recruitment of support individual. Call 1–2 wk after quitting date. Repeat above prn.
3. Physician or health care worker should arrange follow-up. Next regular visit should be <2 months after initial cessation. May assess the progress with CO and expired air and/or continue search in urine, blood, or saliva. If abstinent, should review and reward success. Continue follow-up at increasing intervals for 12 mo after quitting.
4. The use of nicotine replacement or buproprion (Zyban) in conjunction with a smoking cessation program has proved useful.

patient's symptoms is recommended for COPD. The initial approach relies on bronchodilator therapy, and symptomatic benefit may be obtained in the absence of significant spirometric changes. The improvement has been shown to include decrease in dyspnea, increase in timed walking distance, and health-related quality of life. The long-term response is not necessarily predicted by the short-term effect and the absence of an FEV_1 response during a single test does not justify withholding therapy. However, there is no evidence that regular use of bronchodilators will alter the natural progression of COPD (Figure 2).

Beta agonists work by increasing adenosine monophosphate in the bronchial smooth muscles, thereby decreasing muscle tone. They are usually administered with a metered dose inhaler (MDI) at a dose of 2 puffs as needed. They are indicated in mild-to-moderately obstructed patients (stage I) with intermittent symptoms. There are several beta agonists with similar therapeutic profiles. These include albuterol (Proventil, Ventolin, or generic), metaproterenol (Alupent, Metaprel), terbutaline (Brethaire, Bricanyl), bitolterol (Tornalate), and Pirbuterol (Maxair). The choice depends on the patient's and physician's preference, dosage, and cost. They are marketed usually as MDI, but powder inhaler and oral, subcutaneous, and nebulizer solutions are also available.

Treatment with bronchodilator on a continuous basis is required in patients with persistent symptoms, usually in stage II and certainly in stage III. Anticholinergic agents decrease 3′,5′-cyclic guanosine monophosphate in bronchial smooth muscle, which in turn decreases muscle tone. Ipratropium bromide (Atrovent) can be inhaled by means of MDI or by nebulizations. The onset of action is a little slower than the beta agonists, but its effect lasts longer. When given via MDI the recommended dose is 2 puffs four times daily (qid). If the response is not satisfactory it can be used at doses of up to 4 puffs qid. Some patients obtain more relief if administered with a nebulizer. Ipratropium bromide has little side effects, is well tolerated, and is not associated with tachyphylaxis. The other choice for these patients is long acting beta

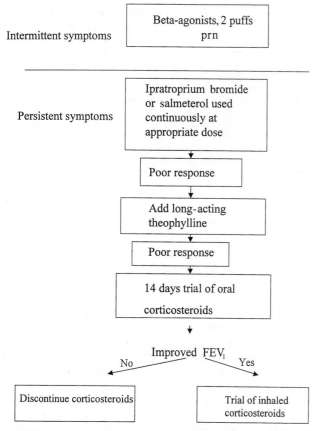

Figure 2. Stepwise pharmacologic management of a patient with COPD. See text for dose, frequency, and length of administration.

agonists such as salmeterol (Serevent) at 2 puffs twice daily (bid). This medication, recently approved for use in the U.S., has a more prolonged action, lasting up to 12 hours.

The combination of the beta-agonist Albuterol with Ipratropium bromide (Combivent) 2 puffs qid, can also be used. Besides being more efficacious than either agent alone, it has the advantage of providing both medications in one inhaler, thereby helping with compliance. This advantage may not be helpful if either component needs to be adjusted in terms of dose and frequency of administration.

With increasing symptoms the addition of theophylline may provide added benefit. Unfortunately the drug has a narrow therapeutic window, with important side effects occurring at serum levels not much higher than the upper limit of the normal range (20 mg per liter). The side effects include nausea, vomiting, insomnia, agitation, tremor, restlessness, seizures, and cardiac arrhythmia. Serum level of theophylline checked 4 to 6 hours after dosing must be frequently monitored as they will change in certain clinical conditions, such as elderly patients, congestive heart failure, and fever. In addition, the levels may fluctuate with the administration of certain medications, including macrolide and quinolone antibiotics, H_2 blockers, and propranolol. The current recommendation is to maintain serum levels between 8 and 12 mg per liter. The American Thoracic Society has recommended that any patient on theophylline evaluated for acute decompensation of COPD should have the serum level checked before additional theophylline is administered.

Inflammation may be an important contributor to the rapid functional deterioration in COPD. Neutrophils and lymphocytes (CD-8) are increased in patients with worsening airflow obstruction. Empirical evidence from several studies has shown that anywhere from 10 to 20% of patients with symptomatic COPD improve after the administration of corticosteroids. Patients more likely to respond are those that show reversibility after the administration of inhaled bronchodilator. The recommended approach is to measure an FEV_1 before and after treating the patients with a 2 to 3 week course of 40 mg daily of prednisone (0.6 mg per kg per day). If there is an improvement of 12% or more the patient may be a candidate for chronic steroid therapy. Data from two European studies show that inhaled budesonide (Pulmicort), at 400 μg a day or fluticasone (Flovent), at an equivalent dose may minimally slow down the decrease in FEV_1 over time. The best result appears to be in patients with stage II disease. In the study where side effects were carefully followed up, there was no increased evidence of bone loss when compared with placebo, but patients in the treatment group had a higher incidence of skin bruises. Care must be taken to taper the steroids as quickly as the clinical improvement allows it.

The use of mast cell stabilizing agents such as nedocromil (Tilade) and cromoglicates (e.g., Intal) have not been shown to be useful in COPD. The proven beneficial effect of leukotriene inhibitors in asthma has not been translated to COPD yet. Anecdotal evidence seems to support its use in selected patients.

Antibiotics may be used in patients with chronic infected sputum and during acute exacerbations, whereas yearly influenza vaccine and pneumococcal vaccine every 5 years should be administered routinely.

A healthy lifestyle is indicated for patients with COPD. Elements include regular exercise and weight control. Persistently symptomatic patients on optimal pharmacotherapy, those who are restricted in their daily activities, and those who otherwise have an impaired quality of life are candidates for a pulmonary rehabilitation program. Lower extremity and upper extremity exercise have proved to be beneficial. Ventilatory muscle training may help selected patients and breathing retraining and education help patients acquire self control.

Long-term oxygen prolongs life in hypoxemic patients with COPD. When long-term oxygen becomes necessary, ambulatory oxygen is the rule and patient must be encouraged to exercise. Oxygen must be started after arterial blood gases document a PaO_2 of 55 mmHg or less, or a PaO_2 between 56 and 59 mmHg, if there are signs of cor pulmonale. There are multiple forms of delivery and conserving devices for oxygen administration. The use of oxygen during special situations such as sleep and exercise has to be evaluated so that oxygen can be appropriately prescribed.

INPATIENT MANAGEMENT OF COPD

Increased dyspnea, cough, and sputum production, frequently associated with malaise and fever, are characteristic of acute exacerbation of COPD. The exacerbation is caused by intercurrent respiratory infections, although sometimes they may be due to congestive heart failure, pneumothorax, or rib fracture. The mortality rate varies and is frequently due to problems arising from hypoxemia (cardiac arrhythmia, renal failure, stroke) or from sepsis.

Although hospitalization of patients with acute exacerbations of COPD is very common, there is only limited information in this area. Patients who deteriorate in spite of therapy, who have co-morbid conditions, and who are without home support should be admitted to a hospital (Table 3). The objective is to manage the acute exacerbation and prevent further deterioration, while at the same time educating the patient on the nature of the disease, correct use of medications, and how to deal with the limitations presented by the disease and future exacerbations. Criteria for admission to the intensive care unit (Table 4) depend on the severity of the attack and the need to initiate mechanical ventilation. Noninvasive mechanical ventilation (NIV) is useful to prevent intubation and its complications. Current evidence indicates that it should be attempted in most patients in ventilatory failure especially if they present sig-

TABLE 3. Criteria for Admission in Chronic Obstructive Pulmonary Disease (COPD)

The patient has an acute exacerbation of COPD characterized by increased dyspnea, cough, and sputum production with one or more of the following features:

- Symptoms that do not adequately respond to outpatient management
- Inability of a previously mobile patient to walk between rooms
- Inability to eat or sleep because of dyspnea
- Family or physician assessment, or both, that the patient cannot not manage at home and supplementary home care resources are not immediately available
- Presence of high-risk co-morbid pulmonary (e.g., pneumonia) or nonpulmonary conditions
- Prolonged, progressive symptoms before emergency room visit
- Presence of worsening hypoxemia, new or worsening hypercarbia, or new or worsening cor pulmonale

Acute respiratory failure characterized by severe respiratory distress, uncompensated hypercarbia, or severe hypoxemia.
The patient has new or worsening cor pulmonale unresponsive to outpatient management.
Invasive surgical or diagnostic procedures are planned and necessitate analgesics or sedatives that may worsen pulmonary function.
Co-morbid conditions, such as severe steroid myopathy or acute vertebral compression fractures with severe pain, have worsened pulmonary function.

TABLE 4. Indications for Intensive Care Unit Admission of Patients with Acute Exacerbations of Chronic Obstructive Pulmonary Disease (COPD)

1. Patient with severe dyspnea who does not respond to initial emergency department therapy.
2. Patient with confusion, lethargy, or respiratory muscle fatigue characterized by paradoxical diaphragmatic motion.
3. Laboratory evidence of persistent/worsening hypoxemia despite supplemental oxygen or severe/worsening respiratory acidosis (e.g., pH < 7.30).
4. Patient requiring assisted mechanical ventilation by means of an endotracheal tube or noninvasive technique.

nificant hypercapnia, respiratory acidemia, adequate cognition, and are able to cooperate. NIV has a limited role in the treatment of chronic stable COPD. If NIV fails, the endotracheal intubation and conventional mechanical ventilation should not be withheld from first-time patients, since their prognosis is better than for patients presenting with any other single cause of respiratory failure.

The pharmacotherapy available for the treatment of inpatients is similar to that of outpatients except with the more frequent use of nebulized medications in patients incapable of using MDI. Because of their additive effect, beta agonists and ipratropium are usually combined and administered via nebulizers. Intravenous corticosteroids have also proven useful, decreasing dyspnea and improving FEV_1 and oxygenation. Methylprednisolone at a dose of 20 to 120 mg every 8 hours is recommended. The dose should be decreased as soon as possible because of the frequent side effects (anxiety, fluid retention, and in certain cases acute psychosis). The length of therapy depends on the response but should last no longer than 2 weeks. The intravenous therapy should be converted to the oral form once the patient is able to tolerate it. Theophylline may be added if the response is inadequate or in the most severe patients. As stated before, a level should be obtained in any patient on chronic theophylline. The medication is administered to aim at serum levels ranging from 8 to 12 μg per mL.

Antibiotics are administered because respiratory infections are frequently present. A recent meta-analysis has confirmed a small but significant benefit when compared with placebo. Most infections are viral but certain bacteria may follow a viral infection or may be present in the lower respiratory tract from the inception of the decompensation. Common pathogenic bacteria include *Streptococcus pneumoniae*, *Haemophilus influenzae*, and *Moraxella catarrhalis*. For these patients the use of tetracyclines, macrolides (including the new generation), beta-lactamase resistant penicillins, cephalosporins, quinolones, and trimethoprim-sulfamethoxazole is indicated. Recent evidence suggests a role of certain gram-negative organisms such as *pseudomonas aeruginosa* and enterobacteriacea in patients with the most severe form of COPD. If this is suspected, or the patient fails to respond to the usual antibiotics, more aggressive therapy following sputum culture guidance may be especially helpful. The use of inhaled nebulized antibiotics (aminoglycosides*) may be considered in certain patients who continue to produce sputum in spite of what seems adequate therapy.

Oxygen therapy during acute exacerbations requires titration by careful monitoring of carbon dioxide levels. Before discharge, the patient needs to have regained clinical and functional stability and to have adequate arrangement for home care and medical follow-up.

NUTRITION, SLEEP, AND AIR TRAVEL

Nutrition, sleep-related issues, and air travel all constitute important aspects of the care of patients with COPD. Optimal nutrition is an important goal for these patients, many of whom are malnourished. Malnutrition is associated with respiratory muscle wasting and weakness. The incidence of sleep-related disorders in COPD may be similar to that in normal persons, but the consequences are more severe, and one night without sleep can lead to small but statistically significant decreases in FEV_1 and FVC. Sleep disruption can be caused by night-time pulmonary symptoms, and it may be necessary to maximize drug therapy to prevent coughing and shortness of breath. Obstructive sleep apnea should be considered as a possible cause of daytime sleepiness. Supplemental oxygen should be used in patients who have significant desaturation (<88%) during sleep, which can generally be predicted from daytime hypoxia (PaO_2 <55 mmHg) (≤88%). Patients with COPD who are receiving supplemental oxygen and are considering air travel require increased oxygen levels, although the risk for complications during air travel is minimal. There are formulas that help predict the level of oxygen needed to prevent oxygen desaturation. As a practical rule, the oxygen flow may be increased 1.5 times over that used at sea level.

SURGICAL OPTIONS FOR EMPHYSEMA

In 1959, Otto Brantigan postulated that the tethering force that tends to keep the intrathoracic airways open were lost in emphysema, and that by resecting the most affected parts of the lungs, the force could be partially restored. In spite of significant morbidity and mortality rates (6%), 75% of his patients manifested clinical improvement for up to 5 years. Because of the lack of some of the technical material currently and because of the need for bilateral thoracotomy, the procedure was abandoned. Joel Cooper and colleagues reported the results of surgical resection of emphysematous lungs of patients with severe COPD. Operating on both lungs in the same procedure through a median sternotomy, they reported a 1 year 45% increase in FEV_1, a 25% decrease in total lung capacity and a significant improvement

in exercise performance. Although the results are preliminary, several groups have shown improvement in lung function, dyspnea, and quality of life. Recent reports indicate a postoperative increase in lung elastic recoil as one likely explanation. The decrease in lung volume lengthens the diaphragm and other respiratory muscles, placing them in a better contractile position of the length-tension curve. This results in less effort to produce the same ventilatory pressure. This decreases respiratory drive and hence reverses some of the factors associated with dyspnea in these patients. More studies are needed to be able to recommend this procedure for most patients with emphysema. Little is known about the factors that help select the best candidates for surgery. More needs to be learned about the best surgical technique and the optimal timing of the surgery. Nevertheless, for a disease with little therapeutic choices when it is advanced, the revival of this operation seems to offer a reasonable alternative to lung transplantation.

Lung transplantation, on the other hand, has become a feasible option for some patients with very advanced COPD. Today, COPD is the most common diagnosis for which lung transplantation is considered. Close to 40% of all patients undergoing single-lung transplantation have the diagnosis of COPD. The selection of patients for lung transplantation includes limited life expectancy (less than 3 years), age less than 60 years, failure of maximal medical therapy, and no extrapulmonary organ failure. Particularly for emphysema, most patients have an FEV_1 lower than 25% predicted, are oxygen dependent, experience limitation of activities of daily living, and are not candidates for lung volume reduction surgery. Patients are not candidates for lung transplantation if they continue to smoke, have coronary artery disease, are receiving long-term corticosteroid therapy, and are either very cachectic or obese. Single or bilateral lung transplantation can be performed for end-stage emphysema even if pulmonary hypertension is present. Mortality rates are low, and improvement in quality of life and exercise capacity is excellent with both procedures. The survival rate at 1 year is close to 75%; subsequent mortality rates are 3 to 6% per year.

ETHICAL ISSUES

The basic issues relate to directives regarding the application of extraordinary measures to treat respiratory failure. Self-determination and co-management are the most important components of the decision. Patients with poor baseline function, malnutrition, limited lifestyle, and late deterioration have a poor prognosis. Finally, withholding and withdrawing life-support measures are ethically indistinguishable; therefore, discontinuation of mechanical ventilation once initiated may be chosen by those patients who have opted for mechanical ventilation, manifest no improvement, and do not want to continue futile treatment.

---

*Not FDA approved for this indication.

CYSTIC FIBROSIS

method of
MARSHA M. THOMPSON, M.D., Ph.D., and
PATRICIA MARSHIK, Pharm.D.

University of New Mexico School of Medicine
Albuquerque, New Mexico

Enormous progress has been made in the understanding of the pathophysiology of cystic fibrosis since the discovery of the gene in 1989. Each advance leads to possible new therapeutic interventions. Cystic fibrosis is an autosomal recessive disorder found most commonly in the white population, but it also occurs in African Americans, Hispanics, and Pueblo Indians. The mutation in the cystic fibrosis protein (CFTR) affects multiple organ systems in the body, including the lungs, sinuses, sweat glands, pancreas, intestines, liver, gallbladder, and vas deferens. This lifelong chronic illness classically manifests in childhood with multiple pulmonary infections and failure to thrive. Meconium ileus is virtually pathognomonic for the disease. Many patients are not diagnosed until adulthood, especially those who exhibit more atypical manifestations. A clinician must always be alert when a patient exhibits any of the following features: recurrent pulmonary infection particularly with *Pseudomonas aeruginosa*, malabsorption with failure to thrive, nasal polyps, recurrent pancreatitis, rectal prolapse, or bilateral absence of the vas deferens.

The diagnosis of cystic fibrosis remains very much a clinical diagnosis in conjunction with one of several laboratory tests. A patient must have a clinical feature of the disease (unless an infant is too young to yet develop symptoms) and one of the following three criteria:

1. Two positive pilocarpine quantitative sweat tests. The pilocarpine sweat test is a tedious and time-consuming test generally not performed at community hospitals. A conductivity test (Westcor "SweatCheck") has been approved for screening. A physician must be aware of what type of testing the laboratory performs to know its reliability.

2. Two mutations in the *CFTR* gene. Testing for mutations can be performed on either buccal mucosal cells or peripheral white blood cells. A number of reliable laboratories perform this test.

3. Abnormal nasal potential difference measurements. This technique, which is generally only available at a few research institutions, measures the ion channel defect in the nasal mucosa. The use of this test is obviously reserved for difficult diagnoses.

MAINTENANCE THERAPY

Pulmonary

Patients with cystic fibrosis have chronic pulmonary infections, but the degree of clinical involvement depends on the stage of the disease. Young children may have recurrent cough and wheezing and more severe or prolonged viral lower respiratory tract disease with minimal findings on chest radiography. As the disease progresses, cough and sputum production become persistent and one finds crackles on chest auscultation with bronchiectasis and cystic changes on chest radiography. Spirometry is usually normal early in the disease, but an obstructive pattern develops with a decline in the forced expiratory volume in 1 second (FEV_1). Respiratory failure remains the predominant cause of death in cystic fibrosis; therefore, the goal of maintenance therapy is to slow the progressive nature of the lung destruction from chronic infection and inflammation. Commonly used drugs, their doses, and details are listed in Table 1.

Airway clearance of the thickened mucus is central to treatment. A number of techniques are available, although extensive comparison studies of these methods have not yet been completed. Patients should include one of these therapies twice daily as part of their routine, increasing their frequency during respiratory illnesses or with progression of the disease. Typically, postural drainage and chest physiotherapy are used in infancy whereas older children and adults may prefer methods that give more independence by allowing the patients to perform them without assistance. These methods include autogenic drainage, active cycle breathing, the Flutter device, high-frequency chest oscillation (ThAIRapy Vest), and other positive end-expiratory pressure devices. These techniques must be taught by a therapist trained in these techniques.

TABLE 1. **Pulmonary Maintenance Therapy**

Drug	Dose	Comments
Albuterol (Ventolin, Proventil)	2–4 puffs before chest physiotherapy and as needed 2.5 mg nebulized before chest physiotherapy and as needed	
Dornase alfa (DNase)	2.5 mg nebulized qd	Must be nebulized through selected nebulizers used in conjunction with a PulmoAide or PariProneb compressor. Do not dilute or mix with other drugs in the nebulizer.
Ibuprofen (Motrin)	20–30 mg/kg/dose q 12 h	Do not substitute generic products. Monitor renal function. Stop when using IV tobramycin. Peak levels vary from 0–4 hours after dose. Adjust dose to peak level of 50–100 μg/mL. Reassess patient kinetics every 2 years or when weight changes by 25%.
Tobramycin (TOBI)	300 mg nebulized q 12 h; cycle every 28 days (i.e., on 28 days, off 28 days)	Must be nebulized through a Pari-LC Plus nebulizer using a Pulmo-Aide or PulmoMate compressor. Do not dilute or mix with other drugs in the nebulizer.

Dornase alfa (Pulmozyme) (recombinant DNAse I) has been developed for use as a mucolytic agent in cystic fibrosis. This enzyme degrades the viscous DNA released by dying neutrophils in the airways, making the secretions easier to remove. Efficacy has been demonstrated in patients with 40 to 75% of normal FEV_1; however, it may also be effective in patients with more or less severe disease.

Therapy directed toward countering the destruction from the host immune response to the chronic bacterial infection is important in cystic fibrosis. Inflammation in the lungs is responsible for much of the tissue destruction and has been shown to be manifest in infants before the first infection. To avoid the side effects of oral corticosteroids, daily high-dose ibuprofen has been shown to be effective in slowing the decline in FEV_1 in children older than 5 years of age with mild lung disease. Inhaled corticosteroids have not been adequately studied in this population but are indicated when asthma complicates this disease. Many centers also prescribe inhaled cromolyn as a mild anti-inflammatory agent.

Once chronically infected with *P. aeruginosa*, a patient is begun on regular inhaled tobramycin therapy. TOBI, the only antibiotic formulation approved for inhalation, has been shown to improve FEV_1 and reduce hospitalizations when used on an every-other-month basis. Patients with more severe disease may require continuous use of the medication.

All inhaled medications must be delivered in the correct nebulizer, and these nebulizers must not be used for any other medications. The nebulizer must be rinsed and dried after each use to prevent aerosol transfer of molds and other bacteria. Some patients accomplish this task by having a dedicated nebulizer for each treatment during the day. Other preventative care includes yearly influenza vaccination.

Nutritional

Pancreatic enzyme supplementation is a mainstay of therapy for cystic fibrosis (Table 2). After pancreatic enzyme supplementation begins, parents quickly note the difference in their child's behavior and appearance. Even with optimum enzyme supplementation, only 85% of the oral intake is absorbed. This factor, along with the increased energy demands from chronic infection, give patients their high caloric demands—up to 150% of the recommended daily allowances for age. A high-fat diet with liberal salt supplementation is recommended for patients with cystic fibrosis.

Increased care in pancreatic enzyme dosing resulted from cases of fibrosing colonopathy seen in 1994 related to high doses of pancreatic enzymes. Guidelines now start dosing at 500 to 1000 units per kg per meal and are increased according to response, although the effective dose for a particular patient is empirical. Dosing above 2000 to 2500 units per kg per meal is done only after carefully looking at other factors that may influence enzyme effectiveness or compliance. The addition of an H_2 blocker may increase the effectiveness of pancreatic enzymes. Patients should be warned about titrating the dose above these levels without consulting a physician.

Fat-soluble vitamin supplementation is necessary. All patients should be given a daily multivitamin. Vitamin A and E levels must be monitored and are frequently found to be low at diagnosis. Multivitamin products are available designed specifically for cystic fibrosis patients in which preparations provide fat-soluble vitamins in a water-miscible form. These products may help increase patient compliance, because only one pill is taken daily, versus several different ones.

The importance of excellent nutrition in cystic fibrosis has become increasingly evident. Although the exact relationship between nutrition and pulmonary function is not completely delineated, life span is extended with improved nutritional status. Evidence from the Epidemiology Study of Cystic Fibrosis showed that weight for age in the lowest quartile (<25%) is a risk factor for rapid decline in pulmonary function.

With this knowledge, nutritional support has become much more aggressive. In addition to dietary

TABLE 2. **Nutritional Maintenance Therapy**

Drug	Dose	Comments
Multivitamins (ADEK, Vitamax)	1 tablet/d	
Vitamin A	1,500–10,000 IU/d	Monitor vitamin levels yearly.
Vitamin E	25–400 IU/d	Monitor vitamin levels yearly.
Vitamin K	2.5 mg once weekly up to 5.0 mg twice weekly	
Pancreatic Enzymes (Pancrease, Ultrase, Creon)	<4 years of age: 1000 units of lipase/kg/meal ≥4 years of age: 500 units of lipase/kg/meal	Do not substitute generic products. Give one half of usual dose with snacks. Adjust dose according to response. Do not exceed 2500 units of lipase/kg/meal.
Cimetidine (Tagamet)*	10–40 mg/kg/d in divided doses q 6 h; maximum dose: 1200 mg/d	
Ranitidine (Zantac)*	3–5 mg/kg/d in divided doses q 12 h; maximum dose: 300 mg/d	

*Not FDA approved for this indication.

education to choose high-calorie foods, a variety of supplements are available, some designed specifically for cystic fibrosis. Often, caloric needs exceed the patient's intake and enteral supplementation is required, most commonly through night-time gastrostomy feedings. Many patients and their families are initially resistant to gastrostomy tube placement but find that pressures are relieved to get adequate caloric intake and patients are overall healthier. Parenteral nutrition is usually reserved for short-term needs, such as during hospitalizations surrounding surgery.

COMPLICATIONS
Pulmonary Exacerbation

The definition of a pulmonary exacerbation will vary depending on the stage of the disease, but in general it is considered to be an increase in pulmonary symptoms from a patient's usual baseline status. A patient with mild pulmonary disease may display few symptoms other than a cough, failure to gain weight, or a decrease in FEV_1. Patients with more advanced disease may have increased or change in sputum, chest congestion, hemoptysis, and changes in chest radiography.

Antibiotic therapy is the mainstay of the treatment of this condition and is directed toward the bacteria most frequently seen: *Staphylococcus aureus*, *Haemophilus influenzae*, and *P. aeruginosa*. Bacterial culture of sputum or deep pharyngeal cultures guide therapy, and specific testing guidelines must be followed to detect these and other organisms. A course of oral antibiotic therapy may be tried initially, depending on the severity of the exacerbation, but many patients will require intravenous antibiotics. Cystic fibrosis patients typically have altered kinetics for many antibiotics and require higher doses (Table 3). Treatment of *Pseudomonas* requires two antibiotics to prevent rapid development of resistance by the bacteria. Duration of therapy is generally 10 to 21 days and is guided by clinical response. Many patients are now completing much of their therapy at home.

Continuous use of antibiotics for decreasing the bacterial burden in the lung is advocated by some centers. This practice does raise concerns about selecting for antibiotic resistant organisms, but it may be useful in patients with more advanced disease.

The bacterium *Burkholderia cepacia* has emerged as an important pathogen, secondary to exaggerated morbidity and mortality in the 3 to 4% of patients with this organism. Those infected with *B. cepacia* have significantly worse pulmonary function and reduced survival rates. Most strains of the organism are highly resistant to antibiotics, especially to aminoglycosides and beta-lactams.

Upper Airway Disease

Sinuses are almost always radiographically abnormal in cystic fibrosis. The degree of symptomatic involvement, however, is variable. Three to 5% of cystic fibrosis patients undergo endoscopic sinus surgery in a given year, but some patients have multiple surgeries over a number of years. Nasal polyps occur less often than sinusitis, yet still are frequent and may be a presenting symptom. They sometimes regress spontaneously, and surgical removal is only indicated if there is significant obstruction of the nasal airway. The finding of nasal polyps in any individual is an indication for cystic fibrosis testing.

Distal Intestinal Obstruction Syndrome

One of the most common problems requiring medical intervention is partial bowel obstruction or distal intestinal obstruction syndrome (DIOS), formerly known as meconium ileus equivalent. DIOS results from the thickened mucus secreted by the colon and occurs more commonly when patients become dehydrated. Patients may also experience constipation, large, bulky stools, or diarrhea. It may manifest subacutely or acutely as recurrent stomachaches or cramping, vomiting, and constipation. A fecal mass may be palpable in the right lower quadrant or throughout the abdomen. Differentiation from appendicitis, intussusception, or other complication of cystic fibrosis can be difficult. Radiographic studies of the abdomen will often show the colon filled with stool.

Therapy for DIOS consists of rehydration and cleaning out the bowel. Enemas are effective, but they will only help with the distal colon. GoLYTELY (20 mL per kg per hour) given via nasogastric tube is often required, and the problem may take days to resolve. Surgical consultation for complete obstruction is required, but fortunately this complication is less common.

Diabetes

The development of cystic fibrosis–related diabetes (CFRD) is becoming increasingly recognized as a complication as survival increases. The extent of pancreatic fibrosis may not be the only determinant of CFRD: other factors, including genetic factors, may play a role. The characteristics of CFRD are unique, and defy its classification as either type I (insulin-dependent) or type II (non–insulin-dependent) diabetes, because it has some features of both. Certainly, insulin secretion is delayed in response to a glucose load, and the total amount of insulin secreted may also be decreased. In addition, there is some evidence of peripheral resistance to insulin.

CFRD is diagnosed by performing an oral glucose tolerance test and is suggested to be part of the yearly screening for adolescents and adults. It is important to recognize this condition because it impacts overall health and survival. Hyperglycemia may be intermittent and particularly associated with stress, such as seen with a pulmonary exacerbation, or glucocorticoid use. Ketoacidosis is rare, probably because most cystic fibrosis patients make enough

TABLE 3. **Treatment of Complications**

Drug	Dose	Comments
Sinopulmonary Disease AMINOGLYCOSIDES		

Amikacin (Amikin)	30 mg/kg/d IV; given in divided doses q 8–12 h	Monitor for renal and ototoxicity.
		Monitor drug levels, adjust dose based on individual kinetics:
		    Peak: 25–40 µg/mL
		    Trough ≤ 10 µg/mL

Gentamicin (Garamycin)	9 mg/kg/d IV; given in divided doses q 8–12 h	Monitor for renal and ototoxicity.
		Monitor drug levels; adjust dose based on individual kinetics:
		    Peak: 8–12 µg/mL
		    Trough ≤ 2 µg/mL

Tobramycin (Nebcin)	10 mg/kg/d; given in divided doses q 8–24 h	Monitor for renal and ototoxicity.
		Monitor drug levels; adjust dose based on individual kinetics:
		    If given q 8–12 h:
		    Peak: 8–12 µg/mL
		    Trough ≤ 2 µg/mL
		    If given q 24 h:
		    Trough ≤ 2 µg/mL

PENICILLINS Amoxicillin/potassium clavulanate (Augmentin)	25–45 mg/kg/d; given in divided doses q 12 h; maximum dose: 875 mg/dose	
Nafcillin (Nafcil)	50–100 mg/kg/dose IV; given q 4–6 h; maximum dose: 12 gm/d	
Piperacillin (Pipracil)	400–600 mg/kg/d IV; given in divided doses q 4–6 h; maximum dose: 24 gm/d	
Ticarcillin (Ticar)	400–600 mg/kg/d IV; given in divided doses q 4–6 h; maximum dose: 24 gm/d	
Ticarcillin/clavulanic acid (Timentin) OTHER	400–600 mg/kg/d IV; given in divided doses q 4–6 h; maximum dose: 24 gm/d	
Aztreonam (Azactam)	200 mg/kg/d IV; given in divided doses q 6 h; maximum dose: 8 gm/d	
Ceftazide (Fortaz), Cefepime (Maxipime)	50 mg/kg/dose IV; given q 8 h, maximum dose: 6 gm/d	
Ciprofloxacin (Cipro)	10–15 mg/kg/dose IV; given q 12 h; maximum dose: 400 mg Oral dosage: <12 y: 500 mg bid ≥12 y: 750 mg bid	
Imipenem (Primaxin)	60–75 mg/kg/d IV; given in divided doses q 6 h; maximum dose: 4 gm/d	
Trimethoprim/sufamethoxazole (Bactrim, Septra) DIOS	10–20 mg/kg/d of trimethprim; given in divided doses q 8–12 h; maximum dose: 320 mg trimethoprim	
Polyethylene glycol/electrolyte solution (Colyte, GOLYTELY) *Hepatobiliary Disease*	25–40 mL/kg/h until rectal effluent is clear (usually 4–10 h); maximum of 4 L	
Ursodiol (Actigall)*	10–15 mg/kg/d; given in divided doses q 12 h; maximum dose: 300 mg	
Gastroesophageal Reflux Disease Cisapride (Propulsid)	0.15–0.3 mg/kg/dose; given four times daily; maximum dose: 10 mg	Dose is 15 minutes before each meal and at bedtime. Discuss drug interactions with patients.

*Exceeds dosage recommended by the manufacturer.
Abbreviation: DIOS = distal intestinal obstruction syndrome.

insulin to suppress ketone formation. Treatment of CFRD consists of chronic use of insulin depending on self-monitoring glucose levels with the help of an endocrinologist. Because of the special nutritional needs of cystic fibrosis patients, diabetic patients are not usually restricted in their intake but carbohydrates are taken into account for insulin dosing.

Pancreatitis

Low-grade inflammation in the lobules may manifest as acute pancreatitis in teens and young adults with cystic fibrosis, and this diagnosis must be considered in any patient with abdominal pain. Occasionally, pancreatitis may be seen as the presenting symptom and should be eliminated as the diagnosis in children with recurrent pancreatitis. Treatment consists of pain management and bowel rest.

Hepatobiliary Disease

Although 25 to 30% of patients have fatty liver changes or focal biliary cirrhosis on examination at autopsy, clinically significant liver dysfunction is uncommon. The incidence of liver disease may increase, however, as longevity increases. Portal hypertension and hypersplenism occur in only 2 to 5% of patients. Those patients, however, may have severe manifestations, including malnutrition and coagulopathy, due to abnormal liver synthetic dysfunction, and may develop esophageal varices. Liver transplant may be considered in the worst cases. Ursodeoxycholic acid (Actigall) has been shown to reduce elevated liver enzymes, but its long-term effect on prevention of liver failure is unknown.

Abnormalities of the gallbladder are common, and malabsorption of bile acids may favor formation of cholesterol gallstones, which occur in 10 to 25% of adult patients. Elevation of alkaline phosphatase concentration is often noted without evidence of clinical liver disease; it indicates a mild obstructive form of liver dysfunction.

Gastroesophageal Reflux Disease

This condition is common in cystic fibrosis patients for several reasons. The frequent and severe cough in more advanced patients contributes to the reflux. In addition, postural drainage and chest percussion may also increase the likelihood of reflux. Treatment for this condition includes a kinetic agent, cisapride (Propulsid), and an H_2 blocker.

Osteoporosis

Because patients with cystic fibrosis are reaching adulthood in increased numbers, an increased number of atraumatic fractures have been noted. Such a high prevalence of osteoporosis may be a result of long-term malnutrition and inactive lifestyle related to chronic illness, although its origins are unclear. A number of investigations of biochemical markers of

bone disease and potential therapies for this population are underway.

OBSTRUCTIVE SLEEP-DISORDERED BREATHING
(Sleep Apnea)

method of
STEVEN M. KOENIG, M.D., and
PAUL M. SURATT, M.D.
University of Virginia Health System
Charlottesville, Virginia

The term *obstructive sleep-disordered breathing* (OSDB) describes the entire spectrum of obstructive breathing abnormalities during sleep. Narrowing of the human pharynx or upper airway is responsible for all the consequences associated with OSDB. On one end of the continuum of upper airway narrowing and the consequent increased upper airway resistance is primary, asymptomatic snoring. This is followed by the upper airway resistance syndrome (UARS), the obstructive sleep hypopnea syndrome, and then the obstructive sleep apnea syndrome. The term "obesity hypoventilation syndrome" (OHS) is typically used to describe individuals with OSDB who also have daytime hypoventilation and who are typically morbidly obese. OSDB is not, however, an essential feature of OHS.

Obstructive apnea is defined as the complete or near-complete cessation of airflow that lasts for at least 10 seconds despite continuing respiratory effort. Hypopnea is reasonably defined as a decrease in airflow of 30 to 50% from baseline, lasting at least 10 seconds. Obstructive apnea and hypopnea often occur together in the same patient. The respiratory disturbance index (RDI) is the number of episodes of apnea plus hypopnea per hour of sleep. The UARS is a newly described syndrome in which patients have repetitive arousals from sleep due to the increased respiratory effort generated to overcome upper airway narrowing without a decrease in airflow. That is, there are no associated episodes of apnea, hypopnea, or oxyhemoglobin desaturation. Obstructive sleep apnea syndrome was once thought to be an uncommon disorder, but a community-based study estimated that 2 to 4% of randomly chosen middle-aged adults have the disorder.

Sleep-disordered breathing (SDB) may lead to arousal from sleep, oxyhemoglobin desaturation, and hypercapnia. The consequences of these abnormalities are listed in Tables 1 and 2. OSDB syndrome has also been associated with an increased prevalence of coronary artery disease, cerebrovascular accidents, and increased mortality. Those

TABLE 1. **Consequences of Arousal from Sleep**

Sleep fragmentation
Excessive daytime sleepiness
Personality changes
Intellectual deterioration
Visuomotor incoordination
Impotence
Insomnia
Restlessness
Choking, gagging, gasping, resuscitative snorting

TABLE 2. Consequences of Nocturnal Hypoxia/Hypercapnia

Polycythemia
Pulmonary hypertension
Cor pulmonale
Chronic hypercapnia
Morning and nocturnal headache
Left-sided congestive heart failure
Cardiac dysrhythmias
Nocturnal angina
Diurnal systemic hypertension

features most useful in determining the probability of OSDB are listed in Table 3.

The goals of treatment are the elimination of apneas, hypopneas, UARS, arousals due to SDB, and increasing oxyhemoglobin saturation to 88 to 90% or higher. Therapeutic options for OSDB can be divided into conservative, medical, and surgical (Table 4). Because narrowing of the upper airway is the underlying cause of OSDB, therapies for this disorder are directed at improving one or more of the determinants of pharyngeal caliber. These determinants include the baseline pharyngeal area, which is determined by both craniofacial and soft tissue structures; the collapsibility of the airway; the pressures inside and in the tissues surrounding the pharyngeal wall; the outward pressure exerted by pharyngeal dilating muscles; the shape of the upper airway; and lung volume.

CONSERVATIVE TREATMENT

Although the importance of avoiding factors that can increase the severity of SDB should be discussed with all patients, if the patient has mild disease and a clear predisposing factor, conservative therapy may be all that is required. Patients should avoid factors that can increase the severity of upper airway resistance such as sleep deprivation, alcohol, and sedative hypnotic agents. Sleep deprivation increases upper airway hypotonia and delays contraction of pharyngeal dilator muscles, leading to more frequent and prolonged apneas and hypopneas. Both alcohol and sedative hypnotic agents increase the frequency of abnormal breathing events during sleep by reducing upper airway muscle tone and prolonging abnormal respiratory events by increasing the arousal threshold. If complete abstinence from alcohol is unrealistic, the patient should be advised to consume mini-

TABLE 3. Features Most Useful in Determining the Probability of Obstructive Sleep-Disordered Breathing

Nocturnal gasping, choking, or resuscitative snorting
Witnessed apnea
BMI >25 kg/m² or neck circumference
  ≥17 in in males, ≥16 in in females
Habitual snoring
Male sex
Age >40 years
Systemic hypertension

Abbreviation: BMI = body mass index.

TABLE 4. Treatment of Obstructive Sleep-Disordered Breathing

Conservative
  Weight loss
  Sleep deprivation avoidance
  Alcohol avoidance
  Sedative hypnotic drug avoidance
  Positional therapy
  Nasal congestion treatment
  Hypothyroidism treatment
  Acromegaly treatment
Medical
  First-line
    Nasal positive airway pressure
      CPAP
      Bilevel
    Nasal volume ventilation
  Second-line
    Oral appliance
    Medications
      Fluoxetine (Prozac)*, protryptyline (Vivactil)*, medroxyprogesterone (Provera)*, acetazolamide (Diamox)*
    Nocturnal oxygen
      Mask or nasal cannula
      Transtracheal
Surgical
  Nasal surgery
  Adenotonsillectomy (in children)
  Upper airway reconstruction
    Uvulopalatopharyngoplasty
    Laser-assisted uvulopalatopharyngoplasty
  Maxillofacial surgery
    Inferior sagittal mandibular osteotomy + genioglossal advancement ± hyoid myotomy and suspension
    Maxillomandibular osteotomy and advancement
  Tongue reduction surgery
    Laser midline glossectomy
  Upper airway bypass
    Tracheostomy
  Bariatric surgery
    Gastric bypass
    Jejunoileal bypass
    Gastroplasty

*Not FDA approved for this indication.
Abbreviation: CPAP = continuous positive airway pressure.

mal quantities at a time that will allow the blood alcohol level to return to zero at bedtime.

In some individuals, SDB occurs only in the supine position. Training such patients to sleep in the lateral recumbent position may completely alleviate their SDB, although the long-term effectiveness of this intervention is unclear. One technique is to place one or more tennis balls (or a similar object) in a pocket sewn in the back of a nightshirt or in a sock that is then pinned to the garment. The hope is that in time, the person will be "trained" to sleep in the lateral recumbent position and therefore no longer require the tennis balls. Some patients may benefit from elevating the head of the bed at a 30- to 60-degree angle. The head-up or lateral recumbent position may also benefit the patient who is suboptimally treated with maximally tolerable positive-pressure therapy such as continuous positive airway pressure (CPAP; see later).

If present, treatment of increased nasal resistance

with a combination of nasal steroids, decongestants, and/or antihistamines should be undertaken. Likewise, hypothyroidism and acromegaly should be treated appropriately. Because treatment of hypothyroidism without concomitant treatment of OSDB may result in more severe oxyhemoglobin desaturation due to increased oxygen consumption, both should be treated concurrently (i.e., with nasal CPAP). Nasal CPAP treatment may be discontinued after treatment of the endocrine abnormality if a follow-up polysomnogram no longer demonstrates significant SDB.

In obese individuals with OSDB, weight loss can significantly decrease the number of abnormal respiratory events, oxyhemoglobin desaturation, sleep fragmentation, daytime performance, and cardiovascular and pulmonary function. Although all weight loss produces improvement, the amount of weight loss needed to eliminate OSDB varies from person to person. Weight loss is very desirable and should always be encouraged, but most obese people are unable to loose enough weight and keep it off to eliminate their OSDB.

MEDICAL TREATMENT

Nasal Continuous Positive Airway Pressure

For patients with moderate to severe disease, conservative treatment alone is rarely adequate, and treatment with nasal CPAP becomes the next therapeutic option. Nasal CPAP is the first-choice medical therapy for the treatment of OSDB. With this device, CPAP is applied to the upper airway with a nasal mask, nasal prongs, or an oronasal mask. Although there are numerous proposed mechanisms, CPAP acts predominantly by providing a "positive pressure" or "pneumatic splint" to the upper airway, preventing the airway narrowing that occurs when airway dilator muscle activity decreases at sleep onset. CPAP has been shown to completely reverse or at least significantly improve all of the symptoms due to sleep fragmentation, oxyhemoglobin desaturation, and hypercapnia mentioned earlier, including diurnal hypertension, daytime hypercapnia, pulmonary hypertension, and cor pulmonale.

If tolerated, nasal CPAP is effective in the majority of cases of SDB. Thus, the major limiting factor is compliance, with subjective estimates by the patient being much higher than objective measurements. In one study, only 46% of patients complied with treatment, with compliance being defined rather loosely as wearing the CPAP machine for at least 4 hours on at least 70% of the nights. Compliance appears more closely linked to relief of daytime symptoms such as decreased alertness than to the number of apneas and hypopneas. Some studies have indicated that intensive education about OSDB and the consequences of being untreated plus continued support after initiation of treatment result in improved compliance.

At least part of the reason for the poor compliance with nasal CPAP is side effects, which can be divided into nasopharyngeal and pressure-related symptoms. The inconvenience of being attached to a machine is also a problem. Although the precise cause of the nasopharyngeal symptoms is unknown, they likely result from the machine's cool, dry air injuring the lining epithelium and/or stimulating nerves in the nasopharynx. These symptoms are exacerbated when patients using CPAP open their mouths. Opening the mouth produces a leak, and the CPAP machine increases the flow through the nose in an attempt to maintain the set pressure. Tables 5 and 6 list the potential adverse effects and recommended treatments. The function of the ramp option found on most CPAP machines is to allow the CPAP pressure to gradually increase to the prescribed level over a period of 5 to 45 minutes.

An oronasal mask is associated with an increased risk of aspiration of gastric contents. To minimize the likelihood of aspiration, patients should avoid oral intake several hours before using the mask and not use it if they contract an illness associated with repetitive vomiting.

"Autotitrating," "self-adjusting," or "automatic" CPAP devices have been developed. With various computer algorithms, these devices automatically adjust the delivered pressure according to what they detect as abnormal upper airway resistance. As a result, the pressure varies throughout the night, and the patient is not subjected to a single high pressure. The objective of these machines is to subject the patient to the minimal amount of pressure that maintains acceptable pharyngeal patency at any given time. Some studies comparing "autotitrating" CPAP to "fixed" CPAP have demonstrated similar effectiveness in eliminating respiratory disturbances,

TABLE 5. **Adverse Effects of Nasal Continuous Positive Airway Pressure**

Nasopharyngeal symptoms
Congestion (20%)
Dry nose/mouth (25%)
Sinus discomfort (10%)
Headache
Ear discomfort/infection
Epistaxis
Pressure-related symptoms
Chest wall discomfort (<5%)
Ear discomfort
Difficulty exhaling
Cannot fall asleep
Awaken smothering
Barotrauma
Pneumothorax
Pneumomediastinum
Pneumoencephalus
Other
Mouth opening
Claustrophobia
Conjunctivitis
Bridge of nose bruise/ulceration
Allergic reaction

TABLE 6. **Treatment of Adverse Effects of Nasal Continuous Positive Airway Pressure**

Nasopharyngeal symptoms
  Humidification
    Nasal salt solution/spray
    Add humidifier (heated or passover) to machine
  Nasal steroids
  Other
    For nasal congestion
      Infrequent: alpha-adrenergic spray
      Frequent: alpha-adrenergic pill
      Intractable: oronasal mask
    For rhinorrhea
      Anticholinergic spray
      Nasal nedocromil
      Nasal cromolyn sodium
Pressure-related symptoms
  Ramp
  BiPAP
  Relaxation techniques
  "Autotitrating" CPAP
Mouth opening
  Chin strap
  Form-fitting mouth guard
  Oronasal mask
Claustrophobia
  Different mask
  Relaxation technique
  Desensitization
Conjunctivitis
  Adjust mask fit
  Different mask
Bridge of nose bruise/ulceration
  Reinforce area
  Different mask
Allergic reaction
  Different mask

Abbreviations: BiPAP = bilevel positive airway pressure; CPAP = continuous positive airway pressure.

but lower average airway pressure and better sleep quality and compliance with the "variable" devices. Additional studies, particularly in the home setting, are needed to determine the optimal role of "autotitrating" CPAP devices in the treatment of OSDB. At the present time, it is reasonable for patients having difficulty tolerating "fixed" CPAP due to pressure-related symptoms to use one of these devices.

In patients with OHS, including those associated with OSDB, therapy with nasal CPAP may be ineffective or only partially effective. In such individuals, significant oxyhemoglobin desaturation and hypercapnia due to hypoventilation persist, particularly during rapid eye movement (REM) sleep, despite the absence or elimination of upper airway obstruction. In such situations, the patient should be ventilated with either a nasal bilevel system (see later) or a nasal volume ventilator with or without supplemental oxygen (see later). If neither bilevel nor nasal volume ventilation is tolerated, the patient may require a tracheotomy and volume ventilation at night through a tube. If this is not accepted by the patient or possible, supplemental oxygen alone should be administered through nasal cannulas or a face mask.

Nasal Bilevel Positive Airway Pressure

With bilevel positive airway pressure one can set different pressures for inspiration (inspiratory positive airway pressure; the IPAP pressure) and expiration (expiratory positive airway pressure; the EPAP pressure). With nasal CPAP, the IPAP and EPAP pressures are the same. Some bilevel systems also allow the operator to set a back-up respiratory rate, change the percent IPAP (inspiratory time), and adjust the flow sensitivity needed to alert the machine to initiate the inspiratory pressure. Thus a bilevel device can be set to act as a pressure ventilator, unlike CPAP, which only provides a constant pressure. In addition, because a higher pressure is needed to maintain adequate upper airway patency during inspiration than expiration, if a bilevel system is utilized, the EPAP pressure can usually be decreased. It has been suggested that the lower EPAP pressure may diminish problems with exhaling or a "smothering" sensation and with the risk of barotrauma (due to a lower mean alveolar pressure). Studies have not shown, however, that compliance is better with bilevel devices than with CPAP. BiPAP is the trade name for a bilevel system manufactured by Respironics, Inc. (Murrysville, Pennsylvania). If hypercapnia persists with nasal bilevel pressure, one possibility is that the patient is rebreathing exhaled CO_2. Increasing the EPAP pressure to at least 8 cm H_2O or replacing the standard exhalation device with a special non-rebreather valve will alleviate this situation.

Nasal Volume Ventilation

Some patients with OHS with or without coexistent OSDB have very high chest wall impedance and cannot be adequately ventilated with bilevel systems to correct oxyhemoglobin desaturation and hypercapnia. For these patients, a volume ventilator attached to their nasal mask will generate high enough inspiratory pressures to adequately ventilate them. For many patients with OHS secondary to OSDB, once the hypercapnia has improved, which typically takes 7 to 18 days, nasal CPAP may then be employed.

Oral Appliances

Currently, dental appliances are considered useful for primary snoring but second-line therapy for all but mild OSDB. These devices can be considered for patients with mild OSDB who do not respond to conservative measures or who have moderate to severe disease if they are intolerant of, refuse to use, or are not candidates for nasal CPAP, a bilevel system, and surgery. Those devices that work appear to do so by increasing the posterior airway space by providing a stable anterior position of the mandible, by advancing the tongue or soft palate, and possibly by changing genioglossus muscle activity.

Close cooperation between physician and a dentist

experienced with these devices is necessary to ensure optimal patient selection and follow-up and to avoid potential side effects. Problems include tongue, gum, or temporomandibular junction soreness; hypersalivation; and orthodontic complications. Compliance ranges from 50 to 100%, and in a recent study this method was preferred over nasal CPAP. It is difficult to predict who will respond to these devices. Consequently, a follow-up sleep study is required for moderate to severe disease but not for primary snoring or mild OSDB syndrome.

Medications

Fluoxetine (Prozac)* and tricyclic antidepressants such as protriptyline (Vivactil),* which decrease the amount of REM sleep and increase the tone of upper airway muscles, may be useful for patients with mild OSDB who cannot tolerate CPAP or lose weight. These medications also may allow a decrease in high nasal CPAP pressures. Anticholinergic side effects with the tricyclic antidepressants are a significant problem.

Progestational agents such as medroxyprogesterone (Provera)* augment hypercapnic ventilatory chemosensitivity and resting ventilation. These medications are not useful for the majority of patients with OSDB. The drugs may have a role for patients with OHS, with or without coexistent OSDB, but the data are too limited to make firm recommendations.

There are also scant data on the use of acetazolamide (Diamox)* for OSDB and OHS, which stimulates respiration by inducing a metabolic acidosis. Although effects are unpredictable, and usually small, this drug may have a role for normocapnic patients with primarily central apneas. In addition, acetazolamide can actually induce obstructive apneas.

Overall, the respiratory stimulants theophylline and almitrine† are not useful for OSDB and OHS.

Supplemental oxygen, administered via nasal cannula, may improve nocturnal oxyhemoglobin desaturation in patients with sleep apnea and hypoventilation. Because it does not improve the associated sleep fragmentation and daytime sleepiness, however, oxygen alone is not an adequate treatment option for OSDB.

Compared with no therapy and nasal cannula oxygen, transtracheal oxygen delivery resulted in a decrease in the number of apneas and hypopneas, improved nocturnal oxygen saturation, no increase in mean apnea duration, and diminished daytime sleepiness. Although these findings suggest that transtracheal oxygen may be a safe and effective alternative treatment of OSDB, data are too sparse to make strong recommendations.

The role of anorexiant drugs in the treatment of OSDB is also unclear. In one uncontrolled study with 13 patients over 6 months, fenfluramine resulted in

*Not FDA approved for this indication.
†Not available in the United States.

a decreased, although still markedly abnormal, RDI and a reduction of required nasal CPAP pressures. Clearly, additional trials with anorexiant drugs in the treatment of SDB appears warranted. The association of fenfluramine and phentermine with cardiac valvulopathies and primary pulmonary hypertension, however, has resulted in their being removed from the market.

In summary, medications are not very effective in the treatment of OSDB or OHS. With the exception, *perhaps,* of fluoxetine and tricyclic antidepressants in patients with mild OSDB and oxygen for central apnea and hypoventilation, medications for the treatment of OSDB and OHS should be limited to patients who refuse, cannot tolerate, or have contraindications to nasal positive airway pressure, dental appliances, and surgery. Moreover, when utilized, follow-up nocturnal sleep studies in patients who appear to have responded to treatment is mandatory.

SURGICAL TREATMENT

Nasal Surgery

Nasal surgery alone is rarely curative, but it is often used in conjunction with other surgical procedures (i.e., as part of "phase 1" surgery for OSDB; see later).

Adenotonsillectomy

Although an adenotonsillectomy can be curative in children and adolescents with OSDB, alone it is not usually helpful in adults.

Uvulopalatopharyngoplasty

The most commonly performed surgical procedure for OSDB is uvulopalatopharyngoplasty (UPPP). The procedure involves removal of the tonsils, uvula, redundant soft palate, and pharyngeal folds. Its purpose is to enlarge the retropalatal air space. The overall success rate is less than 50%. Moreover, preoperative imaging studies and testing cannot reliably predict surgical success. This procedure is most likely to be successful if upper airway collapse is limited to the oropharynx and the RDI below 20 to 30, that is, with less severe disease. Patients who undergo UPPP should have a follow-up nocturnal sleep study to objectively determine the efficacy of the surgery because more patients feel improved after surgery than actually do improve. Potential complications include nasal reflux and speech problems. Postoperative pain is significant.

Laser-Assisted Uvulopalatopharyngoplasty

Laser-assisted uvulopalatopharyngoplasty (LAUP) has recently been introduced as an outpatient treatment for snoring and potentially for OSDB. It involves removing part of the uvula and associated soft palate with a CO_2 laser in one to seven sessions, performed at 4- to 6-week intervals. Unlike the surgical UPPP, neither the tonsils nor the lateral pharyngeal tissues are removed or altered. Although less painful than UPPP, 60 to 75% of patients report severe postoperative pain from 1 to 8 (on a scale of 1 to 10), for up to 21 days. Snoring is *subjectively* cured or softer in 76 to 78% of cases, with the best results occurring when a long uvula or a draping soft palate are present. LAUP is currently not recommended for the treatment of OSDB. If performed for this reason, however, a postoperative nocturnal sleep study is essential. One potential problem with LAUP is that the elimination of snoring removes one of the signs of OSDB and may provide a false sense of security.

Radiofrequency Volumetric Tissue Reduction of the Palate

Radiofrequency volumetric tissue reduction of the palate is a new procedure that has been shown to be effective for snoring, but we have not found a study that demonstrates that it is effective for sleep apnea. The manufacturer states, however, that the FDA has approved it for treatment of sleep apnea. It is performed by inserting an electrode needle into the submucosa of the soft palate and cauterizing the tissue. It is reported to be less painful than LUAP and, like treatment for snoring, often requires repeated treatments.

Maxillofacial Surgery

Because of the poor and unpredictable results with UPPP, a variety of other procedures have been developed to further increase the size of the upper airway. Inferior sagittal mandibular osteotomy plus genioglossal advancement, with or without a hyoid myotomy and suspension, enlarges the retrolingual airway. These procedures may be performed in conjunction with a UPPP and nasal surgery. With success being defined as an RDI below 20 and at least a 50% decrease, there is a 66 to 67% response rate to this surgery, which has been termed *phase 1 surgery*. Complications include need for a root canal, numbness, dysesthesia of the chin for 3 to 6 months, and facial contour changes.

If the patient has significant craniofacial abnormalities and/or has not responded to phase 1 surgery, maxillomandibular osteotomy and advancement is an option. This procedure further advances the tongue and enlarges the retropalatal airway as well. In the right hands, results have been quite good, with a more than 90% success rate being reported. Average hospital stay is 2 days; the major complications are dysesthesia and paresthesia of the face that last 6 weeks to 6 months.

Tongue Reduction Surgery

Laser midline glossectomy is also an option for those who fail the other surgical procedures. Tongue reduction surgery however, is associated with a long, difficult recovery, speech problems, and some persistent sensory loss. The substantial associated edema requires placement of a temporary tracheostomy tube.

Tracheostomy

With the many surgical options, and in particular the advent of nasal CPAP and BiPAP, tracheostomy is infrequently used to treat OSDB. This procedure should be required in less than 5% of cases. Nonetheless, there is a small subgroup of patients with severe OSDB who cannot tolerate or do not respond to other therapeutic options. For these individuals, tracheostomy, which completely bypasses the upper airway obstruction, can provide dramatic improvement and be life-saving. The potential for additional medical and psychological morbidity, however, needs to be taken into account.

Bariatric Surgery

For significantly obese individuals with either OSDB or OHS, surgical weight loss procedures are another option. Weight loss surgical procedures that have been studied include gastric bypass, jejunoileal bypass, and gastroplasty. Results have been quite impressive and include weight changes of 31 to 72.5%, a decrease in RDI of 89 to 98%, improved nocturnal oxyhemoglobin saturation, decreased cardiac dysrhythmias, improved subjective daytime somnolence, and improved sleep continuity and architecture (increased total sleep time, percentage of slow-wave sleep, percentage of REM sleep). Unfortunately, all studies of the effect of weight loss on SDB thus far are poorly designed and little more than series of case reports. Moreover, good data on the risks and benefits of surgery, the effects of bariatric surgery on waking performance, and long-term follow-up on either the weight loss or improvements in sleep and SDB are lacking. Clearly, more and better controlled studies are needed.

SURGERY AND CONSCIOUS SEDATION IN PATIENTS WITH OSDB

Medications such a narcotics and benzodiazepines are frequently employed in the perioperative period and for conscious sedation. These agents can precipitate and/or exacerbate OSDB by depressing ventilatory drive, increasing upper airway collapsibility, and prolonging abnormal respiratory events by increasing the arousal threshold. Consequently, the amount of these agents given should be reduced to the minimal amount needed, and the patients should be carefully monitored. An airway management team should be immediately available. If the patient is treated with nasal CPAP, it should be used before, during, and after the procedure as is practical. If the patient is not receiving CPAP, a machine should be available and empirically titrated if needed.

LEGAL ISSUES

The physician's legal obligations with regard to patients with OSDB who operate motor vehicles and perform occupations or activities that require vigilance for safety vary from state to state. In addition to expeditiously diagnosing and treating such individuals, health care providers should counsel those individuals whose alertness is questionable not to engage in such activities until they have been adequately treated. The physician and the patient should also notify all current and future health care providers about the diagnosis of OSDB. Such notification will avoid the prescription of inappropriate medications and ensure proper monitoring when surgical procedures are performed and conscious sedation is used.

PRIMARY LUNG CANCER

method of
RAMESH K. RAMANATHAN, M.D., and
CHANDRA P. BELANI, M.D.
University of Pittsburgh School of Medicine and
  University of Pittsburgh Cancer Institute
Pittsburgh, Pennsylvania

Lung cancer is a major public health problem in the United States. It is one of the most common cancers worldwide, and the incidence is increasing by about 0.5% every year. In the United States, 171,600 new cases and 158,900 deaths were estimated for 1999. Lung cancer accounts for 28% of all cancer deaths and is the most common cause of cancer-related death in both sexes. In men, the incidence and death rate for lung cancer have declined; in women, recent data show that the incidence has started to decline, although death rates are still increasing. The 5-year survival rate for lung cancer has shown a small but significant improvement over the last 30 years, with current 5-year survival rates of about 14% for Caucasians and 11% for African-Americans.

ETIOLOGY

Cigarette smoking accounts for most lung cancer cases, which are related to the duration and number of cigarettes smoked in a lifetime. In heavy smokers (those who smoke more than 40 cigarettes per day), the risk of developing lung cancer is increased 18- to 24-fold compared with nonsmokers. Exposure to environmental tobacco smoke or second-hand smoke has been implicated as a risk factor in epidemiologic studies and may account for 2 to 3% of all lung cancer cases. Other risk factors for developing lung cancer include exposures to arsenic, some organic chemicals, asbestos, radon, chromium, nickel, and vinyl compounds.

CLINICAL MANIFESTATIONS

Early diagnosis of lung cancer is difficult, because most patients do not have symptoms until the cancer is advanced. Screening for lung cancer with sputum cytology or chest x-ray studies is imprecise and has not been shown to be cost-effective. The signs and symptoms of lung cancer vary, and patients can present with cough, hemoptysis, chest pain, weight loss, or recurrent lung infections. Generalized malaise and the anorexia-cachexia syndrome are common in advanced cancer. In metastatic cancer, different organ systems may be involved and give rise to various symptoms. A variety of paraneoplastic syndromes can be present and are more common in small cell lung cancer, except for hypercalcemia, which occurs more often with squamous cell carcinoma.

PATHOLOGY

The World Health Organization (WHO) lung cancer histologic classification is widely accepted. The histologic types are squamous cell carcinoma, adenocarcinoma, small cell cancer, and large cell carcinoma. Over the last several decades the incidence of adenocarcinoma has increased, and this entity has surpassed squamous cell carcinoma as the most common histologic type, at present accounting for about 31% of all cases. Well-differentiated squamous cell carcinoma usually presents as localized disease and is associated with the best outcome. Bronchoalveolar cell carcinoma, a variant of adenocarcinoma, appears to be increasing in incidence; the characteristic pathologic pattern is proliferating growth along the alveolar septa. Among tumors classified as non–small cell lung cancer (NSCLC), two distinct subtypes—well-differentiated squamous cell carcinoma and bronchoalveolar cell carcinoma—can be identified in this heterogeneous group. Small cell lung cancer (SCLC) accounts for about 20 to 25% of cases, and its differentiation from NSCLC is important for prognostication and treatment decisions. In some cases distinction between SCLC and NSCLC is difficult; disagreement among pathologists occurs in 5 to 7% of cases. Inadequate or crushed specimens may be the reason for diagnostic confusion, and rebiopsy may be needed.

DIAGNOSIS AND STAGING

In patients suspected of having lung cancer, a thorough history and physical examination are essential. Lung nodules are frequently first noted on the chest radiograph, and a computed tomography (CT) scan of the chest can confirm abnormalities and provide information for accurate staging. Pathologic confirmation of malignancy is mandatory. In centrally located tumors visualized through a flexible bronchoscope, the diagnosis can be established with an accuracy of more than 90%. In patients with peripheral lesions, percutaneous fine-needle aspiration under fluoroscopic or CT guidance is useful to obtain tissue for pathologic analysis. Video-assisted minimally invasive thoracoscopy is increasingly being used in the diagnosis of lung cancer because, in addition to excision and biopsy of peripheral nodules, the mediastinum and pleura can also be examined by this procedure.

Once the diagnosis of lung cancer is made, the disease should be accurately staged. In the United States, most patients undergo CT scanning of the chest and upper abdomen, including the liver and adrenal gland. CT scans of the head and bone scans should be done if the history and findings on physical examination and biochemical tests suggest metastatic involvement. The International System for staging lung cancer, a classification for staging NSCLC, was first proposed in 1986 and is widely accepted throughout the world. Revisions to this staging system were made in 1997 (Table 1). The current guidelines differ from the previous version in that both stage I and stage II have been subdivided into A and B groupings. The group of patients who have T3N0M0 disease, previously included in stage IIIA, are now in stage IIA, as they have a better prognosis than other subgroups in stage IIIA.

The new staging system also clarifies the role of the satellite nodules in the same lobe, now designated T4. The evaluation of mediastinal lymph nodes is of critical importance in determining prognosis and in formulating a treatment plan. In general, patients who have a small primary tumor and mediastinal lymph nodes less than 1 cm in diameter in greatest dimension on chest CT scans are unlikely to have mediastinal involvement. In this group of patients, mediastinal sampling may not be necessary. In all other patients with NSCLC, mediastinal lymph

TABLE 1. **Tumor-Node-Metastasis (TNM) Staging in Non–Small Cell Lung Cancer**

Primary tumor (T)

TX	Malignant cells in sputum or bronchial washings but not visualized by imaging or bronchoscopy
T0	No evidence of primary tumor
Tis	Carcinoma in situ
T1	Tumor ≤3 cm in greatest dimension, surrounded by lung or visceral pleura, without bronchoscopic evidence of invasion more proximal than the lobar bronchus
T2	Tumor with any of the following features of size or extent: • >3 cm in greatest dimension • Involves main bronchus, ≥2 cm distal to the carina • Invades the visceral pleura • Associated with atelectasis or obstructive pneumonitis that extends to the hilar region but does not involve the entire lung
T3	Tumor of any size that directly invades any of the following: chest wall, diaphragm, mediastinal pleura, parietal pericardium; or tumor in the main bronchus <2 cm distal to the carina, but without involvement of the carina; or associated atelectasis or obstructive pneumonitis of the entire lung
T4	Tumor of any size that invades any of the following: mediastinum, heart, great vessels, trachea, esophagus, vertebral body, carina; or tumor with a malignant pleural or pericardial effusion; or with satellite tumor nodule(s) within the ipsilateral primary tumor lobe of the lung

Regional lymph nodes (N)

NX	Regional lymph nodes cannot be assessed
N0	No regional lymph node metastasis
N1	Metastasis to ipsilateral peribronchial and/or ipsilateral hilar lymph nodes and intrapulmonary nodes involved by direct extension of the primary tumor
N2	Metastasis to ipsilateral mediastinal and/or subcarinal lymph node(s)
N3	Metastasis to contralateral mediastinal, contralateral hilar, ipsilateral or contralateral scalene, or supraclavicular lymph node(s)

Distant metastasis (M)

MX	Presence of distant metastasis cannot be assessed
M0	No distant metastasis
M1	Distant metastasis present

Modified from Mountain CF: Revisions in the International System for staging lung cancer. Chest 111:1710–1717, 1997.

TABLE 2. **Stage Grouping in Non–Small Cell Lung Cancer**

Stage	Tumor-Node-Metastasis (TNM) Subset	5-Year Survival Rate (%)
IA	T1 N0 M0	67
IB	T2 N0 M0	57
IIA	T1 N1 M0	55
IIB	T2 N1 M0 T3 N0 M0	39
IIIA	T1–3 N2 M0 T3 N1 M0	23
IIIB	T1–4 N3 M0	5
IV	Any T, any N, M1	1

Modified from Mountain CF: Revisions in the International System for staging lung cancer. Chest 111:1710–1717, 1997.

node sampling gives useful information and should be done either preoperatively or intraoperatively by the thoracic surgeon.

TREATMENT

Non–Small Cell Lung Cancer

Stage I/II Lung Cancer

Early-stage lung cancer is potentially curable by surgery, and every effort should be made to make affected patients eligible for the operation. Patients who have potentially resectable disease but are found to have isolated adrenal or liver metastasis on staging studies should have biopsy of these lesions to confirm metastatic disease. Patients with poor performance status or impaired pulmonary function who initially appear to be poor candidates for surgery may improve with intensive physical and pulmonary therapy. Smoking cessation is mandatory before surgery. In general, patients with a forced expiratory volume in 1 second (FEV_1) and diffusion capacity for carbon monoxide ($DLCO$) of more than 60% of predicted values have sufficient pulmonary reserve to tolerate surgery. For patients who have suboptimal FEV_1 and $DLCO$ values, quantitative lung scans to predict postoperative lung function are needed. The operation of choice is a lobectomy or pneumonectomy, as limited resection has been shown to result in an increased incidence of local recurrence. The use of limited procedures such as segmental or wedge resection should be confined to patients with poor pulmonary reserve; these patients are also candidates for surgery by minimally invasive techniques such as video-assisted thoracoscopic surgery. The 5-year survival rate for resected stage I patients is 57 to 67% and for stage II patients is 39 to 55% (Table 2). Numerous studies reported in the literature have shown that chemotherapy or radiation therapy after surgical resection confers no benefit in overall survival. A recent randomized study from Japan utilizing UFT (uracil* and ftorafur*), an oral form of 5-

*Not available in the United States.

fluorouracil, showed improvement in overall survival after surgical resection. Confirmatory studies need to be done, however, and at present postoperative thoracic radiotherapy or chemotherapy cannot be recommended as standard care. The role of preoperative chemotherapy in resected NSCLC shows promise and is being evaluated in a large intergroup randomized trial.

Stage III NSCLC

Stage III disease can be divided into stage IIIA, which is potentially resectable, and stage IIIB, which is categorically unresectable. Patients who have stage III disease historically have had a poor prognosis, but, with the advent of combined-modality therapy, the outlook appears to have improved for selected groups of patients.

Stage IIIA patients are a heterogeneous group with variable prognosis. Stage IIIA patients who have clinically evident N2 mediastinal nodal involvement treated with surgery alone have a 5-year survival rate of less than 10%, and many clinicians would consider these patients ineligible for surgery. Patients with T3N0 disease previously classified as stage IIIA have been reclassified as stage IIA in the revised staging system, owing to a relatively favorable 5-year survival rate of 33% reported with surgery alone (see Table 2).

Pancoast tumors are superior sulcus tumors in the apex of the lung that are associated with pain in the ipsilateral arm or shoulder, atrophy of the intrinsic muscles of the hand, and Horner's syndrome. This entity is most often due to NSCLC, although a few cases of SCLC have also been reported to present in this fashion. In the early stages of Pancoast tumors, symptoms such as cough, hemoptysis, and shortness of breath are not seen, and the tumor may not be evident on the chest film. For this reason the clinician should have a high index of suspicion for Pancoast tumor in a smoker who has pain in the arm or shoulder that is not otherwise explained. Pancoast tumors can be stage IIIA or stage IIIB, depending on the extent of local invasion. For patients with stage IIIA disease, the traditional treatment has been with preoperative radiation therapy followed by surgical resection, with 5-year survival rates of 40 to 50% in those who have complete resection of tumor. Current treatment strategies combine chemotherapy and radiation therapy in the preoperative setting for patients with superior sulcus tumors.

The traditional treatment for stage III patients who are not surgical candidates has been radiotherapy (RT). The impact of RT alone in unresectable locally advanced NSCLC, however, has been minimal, and the use of this modality does not appear to prolong survival. This finding has led investigators to explore new modalities and to combine chemotherapy, aimed at controlling systemic disease, with radiation therapy or surgery for control of local disease. These studies of combined-modality therapy in stage III disease have yielded encouraging results, and

these regimens are increasingly being used in community oncology practices.

In stage IIIA disease, systemic failure is common in patients who undergo surgery as the only modality of therapy. For stage IIIA patients with potentially resectable disease, induction or neoadjuvant therapy consisting of chemotherapy, RT, or both chemotherapy and RT has been used in an effort to "down stage" primary tumors and to increase the resectability rate. Early administration of chemotherapy may also eradicate systemic micrometastasis and hence improve overall survival. This concept was tested in phase II trials, with response to induction therapy seen in approximately 50 to 70% of patients, resectability rates of about 60 to 80%, and 2- to 3-year survival rates in the range of 30%. The therapy was well tolerated, and induction therapy did not appear to increase surgical complications.

Two recent randomized studies have evoked enthusiasm among the oncology community for use of a multidisciplinary approach to the management of lung cancer. The first study, published by the M. D. Anderson Cancer Center, randomized 60 patients with stage IIIA disease to surgery alone or to preoperative chemotherapy followed by surgery. The estimated median survival in the patients who underwent preoperative chemotherapy was 64 months compared with 11 months in the surgery-only group. In the second study, reported from Spain, 60 patients were randomized either to chemotherapy followed by surgery or to surgery alone. All patients received postoperative RT to the mediastinum. The median survival was 24 months in the group of patients who underwent preoperative chemotherapy compared with 8 months in the surgery-only group. The results in both studies were highly significant and led to early termination at interim analysis before completing planned accrual. Based on these two studies, it appears that chemotherapy given before surgical resection in patients with stage IIIA N2 disease improves overall survival and should be offered to patients with good performance status outside of a clinical trial. Further research is needed to improve these results. New agents with activity in lung cancer, such as the taxanes, gemcitabine, and vinorelbine, need to be incorporated into induction regimens and tested in randomized studies.

In stage IIIB disease, which is categorically unresectable, combined-modality therapy with chemotherapy and RT appears to be of benefit in selected patients. As in stage IIIA disease, the exact sequence of chemotherapy and RT needs to be determined. Chemotherapy has been given sequentially followed by RT or given concurrently with RT. Chemotherapeutic agents with radiosensitizing properties are typically used in concurrent protocols to enhance the efficacy of RT. Most of the large randomized studies with concurrent or sequential chemoradiation therapy in inoperable NSCLC have shown a small survival benefit, although at the cost of increased toxicity. A meta-analysis of 52 randomized trials of RT with or without cisplatin-based chemotherapy revealed that the risk of death was reduced by 13% with the addition of chemotherapy. The absolute survival advantage at 2 years was modest (4%). Paclitaxel, a newer agent derived from the bark of the Pacific yew tree *Taxus brevifolia,* has radiosensitizing properties. Preliminary studies with paclitaxel and RT in locally advanced NSCLC have shown encouraging activity with tolerable side effects, and these results need to be confirmed in large studies, which have been instituted.

Stage IV NSCLC

Stage IV NSCLC has a particularly poor prognosis and is incurable with currently available therapy. In the past, nihilistic attitudes prevailed among oncologists, with most electing not to offer chemotherapy to patients in view of the poor response rates and associated toxic effects. Early chemotherapy studies reported 1-year survival rates in the range of 12 to 15% for patients with metastatic NSCLC, and these results were similar to those in patients treated with supportive care alone. Progress appears to have been made, and a number of new agents have been developed with promising activity in NSCLC. Use of the new generation of chemotherapeutic agents in combination with other established agents has yielded 1-year survival rates of 40 to 50% in recent trials.

Does chemotherapy improve survival in advanced NSCLC? Meta-analysis of randomized trials has shown that median survival is prolonged by about 2 months with the administration of cisplatin-based chemotherapy. Quality of life also may be improved by chemotherapy, with diminution of symptoms and fewer days in the hospital necessitated by complications of cancer. A Canadian randomized study found that patients who received chemotherapy had improved quality of life indices and that use of chemotherapy resulted in cost savings in the long term compared with use of supportive therapy alone. At present the absolute survival advantage is modest with available chemotherapeutic regimens, and patients and physicians must weigh the potential benefits and risks of therapy on an individual basis.

Combination chemotherapy results in higher response rates and better median survival than those achievable with single-agent chemotherapy and should be used as first-line therapy. Cisplatin-based regimens have been the most commonly utilized regimens in NSCLC, and, until recently, cisplatin (Platinol), in combination with etoposide (VePesid) or vinblastine (Velban), has been the reference regimen for randomized studies. Carboplatin (Paraplatin), an analogue of cisplatin, has the advantage of easy outpatient administration and has less ototoxicity and nephrotoxicity than cisplatin. The combination of carboplatin and etoposide appears to be as active as the cisplatin-etoposide combination in NSCLC and has gained popularity.

In the last decade a number of new agents have been tested and have shown impressive activity in NSCLC. These agents include the taxanes (paclitaxel [Taxol]* and docetaxel [Taxotere]*), vinorelbine, gemcitabine (Gemzar),* and irinotecan (Camptosar).* These agents have shown consistent activity as single agents and are being tested in combination with cisplatin* and carboplatin.* The Eastern Cooperative Oncology Group (ECOG) tested the combination of cisplatin and paclitaxel at two dose levels against the standard regimen of cisplatin and etoposide in 560 patients with advanced NSCLC. The groups receiving the paclitaxel-containing regimens had the highest response rates (27 to 32%) and median survival times (9.6 to 10.0 months). In patients who received cisplatin and etoposide, the response rate was only 12%, and median survival was 7.7 months. Patients who received cisplatin with the higher dose of paclitaxel had an increased incidence of neurotoxicity, and for future ECOG studies the reference regimen is cisplatin in combination with moderate-dose paclitaxel.

The combination of carboplatin and paclitaxel, has shown impressive activity in early studies and is being increasingly used in community practice. In 1999, this has become the most commonly used regimen in advanced and metastatic NSCLC and also is a reference regimen for most ongoing randomized trials. Vinorelbine, or gemcitabine or paclitaxel, in combination with cisplatin are approved regimens for patients with advanced and metastatic disease.

The "definitive" optimum regimen for advanced NSCLC is not known at present. Results of an ongoing ECOG trial that randomizes patients to one of four regimens (cisplatin-paclitaxel, cisplatin-gemcitabine, cisplatin-vinorelbine, or carboplatin-paclitaxel) will help decipher some of the management issues for this difficult disease. Elderly patients with NSCLC have survival rates similar to those of younger patients when treated with combination chemotherapy provided they have good performance status (ECOG 0 or 1).

Evidence-based medicine is developed systematically by review of the literature to assist patients and clinicians in selecting appropriate therapy and is increasingly being used in practice. The guidelines published by the American Society of Clinical Oncologists for management of patients with unresectable disease should help immensely with selecting appropriate therapy for this group of patients (Table 3). In the United States, only 2 to 3% of all patients receive treatment based on clinical protocols. Progress can be made only if new agents and therapies are tested in lung cancer, and patients should be encouraged to participate in clinical trials.

NSCLC: The Future

Although we have made advances in the overall management of NSCLC, we have not yet "hit a home run." The discovery of new and active chemotherapeutic agents must continue, and we must be cautious when incorporating these agents in combined-

---

*Not FDA approved for this indication.

TABLE 3. **Treatment Guidelines for Unresectable and Metastatic Non–Small Cell Lung Cancer (NSCLC)**

Modality	Comments	Modality	Comments
Chemotherapy		*Radiotherapy*	
Outcome	Chemotherapy in association with definitive thoracic irradiation is appropriate for selected patients with unresectable, locally advanced NSCLC. Chemotherapy is appropriate for selected patients with stage IV NSCLC.	Radiation for locally advanced unresectable NSCLC	Radiation therapy should be included as part of treatment for selected patients with unresectable locally advanced NSCLC.
Selection of drugs	Chemotherapy given to patients with NSCLC should be a platinum-based combination regimen.	Patient selection	Candidates for definitive thoracic radiotherapy with curative intent should have good performance status, adequate pulmonary function, and disease confined to the thorax. Patients with malignant pleural effusion and those with distant metastatic disease are not candidates for definitive thoracic radiotherapy.
Duration of therapy	In patients with unresectable stage III NSCLC who are candidates for combined chemotherapy and radiation therapy, and in patients with stage IV NSCLC, the duration of chemotherapy should be two to eight cycles.		
Timing of treatment	In patients with unresectable stage III disease and stage IV disease, chemotherapy may best be started soon after the diagnosis of unresectable NSCLC has been made.	Dose and fractionation	The definitive radiation dose in thoracic radiotherapy should be no less than the biologic equivalent of 60 Gy, in 1.8- to 2-Gy fractions. Local symptoms from primary or metastatic NSCLC can be relieved by a variety of doses and fractionations of external-beam radiotherapy. In appropriately selected patients, hypofractionated palliative radiotherapy (using 1 to 5 fractions instead of 10) may provide symptomatic relief with acceptable toxicity in a more time-efficient and less costly manner.
Second-line therapy	No current evidence either confirms or refutes that second-line chemotherapy improves survival in nonresponding or progressing patients with advanced NSCLC. Second-line treatment may be appropriate for good performance status patients for whom an investigational protocol is not available or desired, or for patients who respond to initial chemotherapy and then experience a long progression-free interval off treatment.		
		Surgery	
		Role of resection for distant metastases	In patients with controlled disease outside of the brain who have an isolated cerebral metastasis in a resectable area, resection followed by whole-brain radiotherapy is superior to whole-brain radiotherapy alone.
Role of investigational agents/options	Initial treatment with an investigational agent or regimen is appropriate for selected patients with stage IV NSCLC, provided that patients are crossed over to an active treatment regimen if they have not responded after two cycles of therapy.		

Modified from American Society of Clinical Oncologists: Clinical practice guidelines for the treatment of unresectable non–small cell lung cancer. J Clin Oncol *15*:2996–3018, 1997.

modality programs with radiation and/or surgery. Careful selection of doses and agents should be aimed at limiting the toxicity of therapy. Selective approaches such as trastuzumab (Herceptin), insertion of adenovirus p53 (gene therapy) or introduction of antisense oligodeoxynucleotides are being explored and in the future will be combined with the known active chemotherapeutic agents. Most if not all patients with NSCLC will be offered chemotherapy in the years to come.

Small Cell Lung Cancer

SCLC accounts for about 25% of all lung cancer cases, and most patients have had exposure to cigarette smoke. The incidence of SCLC appears to be increasing. This type of cancer is characterized by rapid growth, early systemic dissemination, and chemotherapy responsiveness. One third of patients diagnosed with SCLC have limited-stage disease, which is defined as tumor confined to one hemithorax and encompassable within a single RT portal, without evidence of pericardial or pleural involvement. The other two thirds of patients with SCLC have extensive-stage disease, which is disease extending outside of a hemithorax.

The aggressiveness and rapid growth of SCLC are evident in patients who do not receive treatment. The median survival with untreated limited-stage SCLC is about 12 weeks and with extensive-stage SCLC, little more than a month. SCLC is a systemic disease; in patients who undergo surgery or thoracic RT alone for limited-stage disease, the 2-year survival rate is less than 10%, with death due to systemic metastasis in most patients. There may be a role for surgery, however, in patients who have a small lung nodule without any evidence of mediastinal involvement or metastatic disease. These patients should receive postoperative chemotherapy and thoracic RT as for other patients with limited-stage SCLC.

The role of chemotherapy in the treatment of SCLC has evolved over the last three decades. As it became evident that hematogenous metastases were present early in the course of the disease, investigators explored the role of single-agent and combination chemotherapy in the treatment of SCLC. Many phase II trials have been conducted in patients with SCLC, and a number of drugs with single-agent activity have been identified. Combination chemotherapy results in a superior response rate and survival compared with single-agent therapy. Although studies have been done using two to four agents in combination chemotherapy for SCLC, it is not clear if there is an advantage to using more than two or three drugs in the therapy of SCLC.

The most commonly used regimen for the treatment of SCLC in the United States is etoposide in combination with either cisplatin* or carboplatin.* The other regimens such as CAE (cyclophosphamide,* Adriamycin [doxorubicin], and etoposide), ICE (ifosfamide,* carboplatin, and etoposide) and CAV (cyclophosphamide, Adriamycin [doxorubicin], and vincristine*) are less commonly used as first-line therapy.

Limited-Stage SCLC

Although response rates as high as 70 to 80% and complete responses of up to 50% can be achieved with combination chemotherapy in limited-stage disease, most patients have recurrent disease, which ultimately causes death. The median survival time of patients who receive treatment ranges from 16 to 20 months. Several randomized studies have explored the use of concurrent thoracic RT to improve overall survival, but with conflicting results. Toxicity was increased in patients who received combined chemoradiation therapy. However, a meta-analysis of randomized trials of chemotherapy with or without thoracic RT in patients with limited-stage SCLC revealed a 14% reduction in the mortality rate in the combined-modality groups. The survival difference is modest, with an overall 3-year survival rate about 5.4% higher in patients who receive combined chemoradiation therapy.

Early thoracic RT appears to be superior to late thoracic RT. A randomized study showed that patients who received chemotherapy with thoracic RT during the second cycle of chemotherapy had a significantly improved median survival of 21.2 months compared with 16 months in the group that received chemotherapy and thoracic RT starting with the last cycle of chemotherapy. The results of an ECOG randomized study lend further support to this observation. Based on these studies, most patients with limited-stage SCLC are given cisplatin or carboplatin in combination with etoposide and with the addition of early thoracic RT.

Although almost 50% of patients with limited-stage SCLC will exhibit a complete response to therapy, almost 70% of the complete responders will have recurrent disease within 2 years. The 5-year survival rate is only 15 to 20% for all patients with limited-stage SCLC.

Extensive-Stage SCLC

Systemic chemotherapy is the mainstay of treatment for patients with extensive disease. RT is useful for palliation of painful or symptomatic local disease. As in limited disease, combination chemotherapy employing etoposide with either cisplatin or carboplatin is commonly used as first-line therapy. These patients are also candidates for investigational protocols, as survival and overall prognosis do not seem to be affected by initial therapy with investigational agents if patients are crossed over to standard therapy at the first evidence of progression of disease. The response rate with use of combination chemotherapy is in the range of 60 to 80%, with a complete response seen in about 15 to 20% of patients. The median survival time for treated patients with extensive-stage SCLC is in the range of 7 to 9 months, and most patients will die of progressive or recurrent disease; 5-year survivors are rare.

Trials have been conducted with the addition of maintenance chemotherapy in patients who had a complete response to initial chemotherapy; however, use of maintenance did not yield a survival advantage but resulted in increased toxicity. Other studies have also shown that there is no advantage in administering more than 4 to 6 cycles of chemotherapy in patients with SCLC despite the fact that the median duration of response is short. Patients who do not respond to chemotherapy have a poor prognosis. There is a small group of patients who may respond to the combination of PE (cisplatin [Platinol] and etoposide) if they initially are given the CAV regimen. If patients have received prior therapy with PE, however, there is no advantage to administering CAV. In patients who relapse 3 months or more after response to initial therapy, the cancer may still be chemoresponsive to a salvage regimen such as PE or oral etoposide. All patients with recurrent disease should be considered for participation in clinical protocol trials. The newer agents such as paclitaxel,* docetaxel,* topotecan,* CPT-11,* gemcitabine,* and vinorelbine have shown promising activity in SCLC. Two of these new agents, topotecan and paclitaxel, are worthy of mention in the treatment of SCLC, as they have shown substantial activity. These agents are currently being tested in combination regimens such as cisplatin-etoposide followed by topotecan, cisplatin-etoposide-paclitaxel, and topotecan-paclitaxel.

The role of alternating non–cross-resistant chemotherapy has been explored in SCLC, based on the Goldie-Coldman hypothesis that exposure to multiple non–cross-resistant drugs early in the course of the disease will reduce the development of drug-resistant clones. Some evidence suggests a survival benefit with alternating non–cross-resistant therapy, but controversy exists, and confirmatory studies are

---

*Not FDA approved for this indication.

*Not FDA approved for this indication.

needed before this can be recommended as standard care.

Dose intensification of chemotherapeutic agents can be achieved by either increasing the doses of drugs or decreasing the interval between successive chemotherapy cycles. To achieve these goals and avoid toxicity, hematopoietic growth factor support may be necessary. This approach results in higher response rates, but overall survival appears similar to that achieved by conventional chemotherapy. Similarly, the use of high-dose chemotherapy with peripheral stem cell infusion or bone marrow transplantation can result in high response rates but without a clear survival advantage. In the absence of randomized trials comparing these dose-intensive approaches with standard chemotherapy, the role of dose-intensive approaches must remain investigational.

Prophylactic Cranial Irradiation

The role of prophylactic cranial irradiation (PCI) remains controversial. Brain metastasis is common in patients with SCLC; at diagnosis, 10 to 14% of patients have evidence of brain involvement, and at time of death, about a third of patients have clinically diagnosed brain involvement. Patients who present with brain metastasis after initial therapy have a very poor prognosis, as this finding is usually associated with systemic involvement. Although brain metastasis is associated with considerable morbidity, death is usually due to associated systemic disease. Randomized studies in SCLC patients have shown that PCI can reduce the incidence of brain metastasis by about 50%. Meta-analysis of these studies has demonstrated a reduction in mortality of 16% in favor of PCI and a 5.4% increase in 3-year survival. In addition, neurologic sequelae as a result of PCI, though rare, are known to occur in long-term survivors. At present, most oncologists would offer PCI to patients with limited disease who achieve a complete response to therapy.

SCLC in the Elderly Patient

SCLC is a disease of the elderly, with median age at diagnosis ranging from 60 to 65 years. The relevance of age as a prognostic factor in patients with SCLC continues to be debated. Elderly patients vary in their ability to tolerate chemotherapy; those who are able to tolerate standard doses of therapy have survival rates similar to rates for younger patients. Elderly patients with a poor performance status and laboratory abnormalities in the white blood cell count or renal function appear to tolerate chemotherapy poorly and have inferior survival rates.

To minimize toxicity, the role of single-agent chemotherapy has been explored in the elderly patient with SCLC. Oral etoposide has been extensively tested because it can be administered on an outpatient basis and is well tolerated. In a randomized study comparing oral etoposide with combination chemotherapy in elderly patients with SCLC, however, the use of etoposide alone was associated with inferior survival rates and yielded no advantage in palliation of symptoms. The elderly patient with SCLC should be offered combination chemotherapy with a regimen such as cisplatin and etoposide or carboplatin and etoposide, which is relatively well tolerated as initial therapy. In the patient with poor performance status or laboratory abnormalities, a reduced-dose combination regimen or single-agent therapy may be offered.

Future Directions

Vaccine strategies are also being explored in an attempt to decrease recurrence rates and increase overall survival of patients with SCLC. Other selective approaches such as use of monoclonal antibodies, inhibitors of angiogenesis, and gene therapy are being tested in ongoing studies. There will be continued efforts to refine present chemotherapeutic regimens and to develop new and active agents for treatment of this disease.

Chemoprevention

The rate of development of second malignancies in the lung and aerodigestive tract is about 10 times higher in persons with a history of smoking who have been treated for lung cancer than in other smokers. The risk of developing second malignancies is higher in SCLC patients (2 to 14% per patient per year) than in those with a history of NSCLC (1 to 2% per patient per year).

Smoking cessation is the most important factor in preventing second malignancies. Chemoprevention trials with 13-*cis*-retinoic acid (Accutane)* have shown promising activity in head and neck cancer in decreasing second malignancies, especially lung cancer, in these patients. A large randomized study evaluating the role of 13-*cis*-retinoic acid in resected stage I NSCLC patients in preventing second primary malignancies or recurrent lung cancer has completed data accrual and is awaiting final analysis. At present, apart from smoking cessation, other chemopreventive approaches remain investigational.

Palliative Care

Most patients who have locally advanced or metastatic disease eventually die from progression of cancer. Pain is a frequent symptom, occurring in about 70% of patients with advanced cancer, and increases in severity with progression. Cancer pain has a substantial impact on the patient's physiologic, psychological, and sociologic well-being and should be aggressively treated. Cancer pain is often underdiagnosed and undertreated by health care professionals. A multidisciplinary approach is essential, and patients should be questioned about symptoms of pain at every visit. In almost 90% of patients, cancer pain can be relieved with relatively simple measures such as oral, transdermal, or parenteral narcotics.

---

*Not FDA approved for this indication.

COCCIDIOIDOMYCOSIS

method of
JOHN N. GALGIANI, M.D.

Valley Fever Center for Excellence,
University of Arizona, and
Veterans Affairs Medical Center
Tucson, Arizona

Coccidioidomycosis is a systemic infection caused by the dimorphic fungus, *Coccidioides immitis*. It grows in the soil of the lower Sonoran deserts of California, Arizona, New Mexico, western Texas, and scattered parts of Central and South America. When the climate is dry, single-cell mycelial elements (arthroconidia) are inhaled and within tissue convert to spherules. Of the approximately 100,000 infections per year, only one third come to medical attention, usually as a subacute respiratory syndrome, and most resolve without specific therapy. However, a small proportion of patients are left with residual pulmonary lesions (nodules, cavities). Others experience chronic pulmonary symptoms, and some develop lesions outside of the lungs (extrapulmonary dissemination), most typically in the skin, joints, bones, or meninges. These complications require a variety of management decisions involving diagnostic evaluation, selection of antifungal treatments, and adjunctive surgery.

Coccidioidomycosis is diagnosed by one of four ways: (1) identifying the organism in tissue or secretions; (2) recovering it in culture; (3) detecting antibodies against the fungus in serum or other patient fluid; and (4) evoking delayed-type dermal hypersensitivity to coccidioidal antigens. Tests for coccidioidomycosis are not routinely performed, and thus clinical suspicion is a critical first step for prompt diagnosis. Outside of the endemic regions, a detailed travel history may afford the only hint that coccidioidomycosis should be considered. Because the spherule is a morphologic structure unique to *C. immitis*, the identification of a spherical structure ranging in size between 15 and 75 μm in diameter with a doubly refractile wall and containing multiple internal spherical structures (endospores) establishes the diagnosis. Spherules can be seen microscopically in KOH preparations, cytology smears, tissue stained with hematoxylin and eosin or other special stains. Cultures of *C. immitis* will grow in nearly all laboratory media, often within the first week. Because mycelia of *C. immitis* pose a biohazard to laboratory personnel, it is helpful when submitting clinical specimens to indicate that this organism is being sought and any growth should be handled with appropriate (CDC Biohazard Level 3) containment procedures. Anticoccidioidal antibodies are detected in a variety of ways. Tube precipitin antibodies are characteristically IgM early responses, and complement-fixing antibodies are IgG that develop later, are directed against a different fungal antigen, and are often reported quantitatively. Both tube precipitin and complement-fixing antibodies can be detected by double-agar diffusion techniques sold commercially as kits. A commercial enzyme-linked immunosorbent assay (ELISA) kit that measures undefined coccidioidal antibodies is also available. This ELISA is more sensitive to early infections, but its specificity is not fully defined. Delayed-type dermal hypersensitivity to coccidioidal skin testing antigens develops in most patients after infection, although it may be absent when infection is widely disseminated. Because skin test reactivity is lifelong, its presence may not be related to a specific current illness and therefore is not usually helpful in diagnosis of active infection.

USEFUL ANTIFUNGAL DRUGS

Amphotericin B

Amphotericin B (Fungizone) has been in clinical use for the longest time, and may be the agent with the most rapid onset of action. It is therefore the first-line choice in patients with rapidly progressive infections. Amphotericin B is administered intravenously for all infections except in the treatment of coccidioidal meningitis in which it is delivered directly into the cerebrospinal fluid by intracisternal, intralumbar, or intraventricular routes. Alternative lipid formulations of amphotericin B have not been studied carefully in coccidioidomycosis. Treatment is initiated with once daily dosing with rapidly increasing doses to 0.5 to 0.7 mg per kg per dose. After several days, dosing can be continued on an alternate day schedule. Amphotericin B is a very toxic drug. Common reactions include phlebitis at the injection site, nausea, and high fever. If any of these side effects occur, premedication with analgesics, antiemetics, or antipyretics may ameliorate the symptoms (Table 1). Blood pressure should be monitored during infusion. If hypotension is noted, treatment should be discontinued that day, although this does not preclude reinstitution of amphotericin B at a later time. Transient azotemia is frequent during therapy. Serum creatinine concentrations should be measured weekly or more frequently if the dose of amphotericin B has been changed recently. Permanent renal impairment has been reported in some patients who have received a total of 3 or more grams. Hemograms should be obtained at least weekly during therapy to monitor leukocyte, erythrocyte, and platelet counts. Although anemia is common, it often stabilizes at a level that does not necessitate transfusion. Potassium, magnesium, and other electrolytes should also be monitored weekly, and deficiencies resulting from renal wasting should be corrected.

Azole Antifungal Agents

Ketoconazole (Nizoral) has Food and Drug Administration (FDA) approval for treatment of coccidioidomycosis. Although fluconazole (Diflucan) and itraconazole (Sporanox) have not been approved for this

TABLE 1. **Amphotericin B Premedication**

30 to 45 min before infusion:
  Aspirin (600 mg) or acetaminophen (650 mg) *plus*
  Diphenhydramine (Benadryl) 50 mg orally *or*
  Promethazine (Phenergan) 50 mg orally or
    intramuscularly
If ineffective, add:
  Meperidine (25 to 50 mg intravenously) for fever
  Hydrocortisone (25 mg added to infusion or given
    intravenously just prior to starting infusion)

indication, published reports have demonstrated their efficacy. All drugs are currently available for oral administration. A parenteral form is available only for fluconazole. Ketoconazole is used at a dose of 400 mg per day. Higher doses have only a marginally increased rate of response and incur a greater chance of side effects. Itraconazole is initiated at 200 mg three times daily for the first 3 days and continues at 200 mg twice daily. Dose-limiting toxic effects, including hyperkalemia and water retention, are often encountered at 600 mg per day. Fluconazole is initiated at 400 mg twice daily for 2 days and continues at 400 mg per day. Doses greater than 800 mg per day have been used in some patients for prolonged periods without serious consequences. However, it is not known whether higher doses of fluconazole improve response for most patients.

Gastric acidity is important to promote absorption of ketoconazole and itraconazole but not of fluconazole. Significant drug interactions at the level of the P-450 pathways occur between the azoles (especially ketoconazole and itraconazole) and several other drugs. For example, all three azoles decrease the metabolism of cyclosporine and warfarin, whereas rifampin increases the metabolism of itraconazole. Because such interactions are possible, a careful review of all concurrent medications should be made before treatment with these drugs is initiated. The most common side effect of all agents is nausea and is dose related. Nausea occurs in 5% of patients receiving 400 mg per day of ketoconazole and is less frequent with fluconazole or itraconazole therapy. Gynecomastia and azoospermia occur with increasing doses of ketoconazole and can be treated with testosterone replacement. Hair loss and dry skin are frequently reported by patients receiving fluconazole. Hepatitis has been reported with ketoconazole at a frequency of approximately 1 in 10,000 treated patients. It appears to be significantly less frequent with itraconazole or fluconazole. Stevens-Johnson syndrome has been reported with fluconazole.

MANAGEMENT OF SPECIFIC CLINICAL SYNDROMES

Primary Pneumonia

The vast majority of initial infections resolve without treatment, and it is not known whether treatment of early infections with any currently available therapy either speeds recovery or prevents future complications. Diagnosis is still useful in decreasing patient anxiety by providing an explanation and a prognosis for the patient's illness, in reducing other unnecessary diagnostic testing or empirical antibacterial treatment, and in recognizing complications as early as possible. Specific antifungal treatment need not be prescribed for most patients with uncomplicated pneumonia, and management relies primarily upon periodic reassessment of the patient's status over the ensuing weeks and months. Follow-up should include repeated radiographic examinations of the chest to monitor the course of pulmonary infiltrates, effusions, or hilar adenopathy. Serum anticoccidioidal antibodies should also be measured periodically to demonstrate their decrease. On the other hand, some patients with unusually severe primary infections or risk factors for complications make therapy advisable. The most critical risk factors are T cell deficiencies such as occur with acquired immune deficiency syndrome (AIDS), organ transplantation, Hodgkin's disease, and chronic corticosteroid therapy. Such patients should always be treated once a coccidioidal illness is manifest. Coccidioidal infection during the third trimester of pregnancy is also likely to progress and should be treated. Amphotericin B can be used during pregnancy because of its lack of teratogenicity. Other indications for early therapy are weight loss of greater than 10%, intense night sweats persisting longer than 3 weeks, infiltrates involving more than half of one lung or portions of both lungs, prominent or persistent hilar adenopathy, anticoccidioidal complement-fixing antibody concentrations in excess of 1:16, inability to work, and symptoms that persist more than 2 months. Persons of African or Filipino descent have a higher risk for dissemination, and this may also may be taken into consideration. Commonly prescribed therapies include currently available oral azole antifungal agents at their recommended doses. Courses of typically recommended treatments range from 3 to 6 months.

Pulmonary Nodules

Nodules are common residua of the initial pneumonia, usually single, 1 to 4 cm in size. They typically cause no symptoms but may be impossible to distinguish from malignancy without a bronchoscopic or percutaneous aspirate or surgical specimen for examination and culture. If the nodule is resected for purposes of diagnosis, antifungal therapy is not recommended either before or after the procedure.

Pulmonary Cavities and Chronic Pneumonia

Coccidioidal cavities usually measure 2 to 4 cm on chest radiographs, 75% are in the upper lung fields and are often thin-walled, and the majority close spontaneously within 2 years of their detection. In patients with small cavities and no symptoms, no intervention is required. Patients whose cavities are associated with symptoms such as cough, sputum production, or mild hemoptysis may be treated with 400 mg per day of an azole. Fibrocavitary infections associated with more extensive infiltrates are often a source of symptoms, and should be treated similarly. If symptoms abate, therapy should be continued for many months or even years. If symptoms recur on discontinuing therapy, restarting the same therapy is often effective and may need to be continued indefinitely. If response is not obtained, a trial of amphotericin B is warranted and after 0.5 grams, consideration should be given to surgical resection if a well-demarcated lesion is identified. However, recurrence may occur after this approach as well. If a cavity ruptures into the pleural space, the primary therapy is surgical resection.

Diffuse Reticulonodular Pneumonia

Bilateral multiple infiltrates are most frequently the result of hematogenous spread in immunosuppressed patients or occasionally multicentric primary foci that can result from exposure to high densities of arthroconidia. Amphotericin B should be used as initial therapy. Once pneumonia stabilizes (several weeks to a few months of treatment), continuation therapy can be switched to an oral azole.

Extrapulmonary Dissemination

Even when many lesions are present, patients often follow a subacute or chronic course. In such patients, the safety and convenience of oral azole therapy make them preferable for initial therapy; amphotericin B should be reserved for more fulminant presentations or for patients who do not respond to an azole. In responding patients, azole therapy should be continued until all pretreatment abnormalities such as symptoms, lesion size, and serum complement-fixing antibody concentrations stabilize and show no further progression. This may require many months or years of treatment but increases the chances that disease will not relapse after therapy is stopped. Coccidioidal meningitis is a special case of disseminated infection. In one study, fluconazole at 400 mg per day produced a clinical response in approximately 70% of new infections, and patients for whom this dose fails may respond if the dose is increased. Itraconazole may also be effective, but there is less published experience with this agent. The necessity of treatment appears to be life-long because 75% of patients who have discontinued azole therapy have experienced relapse. Intrathecal amphotericin B is also effective and in some patients has been curative. However, such therapy is technically difficult and is prone to serious complications, and drug toxicity is common. These limitations currently make intrathecal amphotericin B second-line therapy for most patients with coccidioidal meningitis.

HISTOPLASMOSIS

method of
MICHAEL SACCENTE, M.D., and
ROBERT W. BRADSHER, M.D.
University of Arkansas for Medical Sciences
Little Rock, Arkansas

Histoplasma capsulatum is a dimorphic fungus that exists in nature as a mould in soil or other material rich in organic matter and as a yeast in tissue. Although the distribution of *H. capsulatum* is nearly worldwide, histoplasmosis is endemic in certain regions of North America and Latin America, including the Ohio and Mississippi River valleys of the United States. Infection occurs via inhalation of airborne microconidia with conversion to yeast forms in the lung and subsequent hematogenous dissemination. Skin testing indicates that up to 90% of people residing in endemic areas are infected with *H. capsulatum*.

CLINICAL FEATURES

Symptomatic disease occurs in less than 5% of individuals infected with *H. capsulatum*. Inoculum size and the effectiveness of the host immune response determine whether an infected person develops disease. Most exposures are of low intensity; in this circumstance, a person with normal cellular immunity is either asymptomatic or has a self-limited illness that resolves in conjunction with an effective immune response. Relatively few infected individuals develop acute pulmonary histoplasmosis, a "flu-like" illness with fever, chills, headache, cough, dyspnea, chest pain, myalgia, hypoxemia, and diffuse pulmonary opacities on chest radiograph. Bird and bat excrement favor growth of the fungus, and patients with acute pulmonary histoplasmosis sometimes have a history that suggests heavy inoculation with *H. capsulatum,* such as cutting down trees that had been bird roosts, destroying old chicken coops, or spelunking in caves inhabited by bats.

Chronic pulmonary histoplasmosis is seen in patients with pre-existing lung disease (emphysema). These patients are unable to effectively clear the fungus because of the distorted lung structure associated with emphysema. Symptoms include cough with sputum production, fever, sweats, and dyspnea. Apical pulmonary opacities and progressive cavitary disease radiographically indistinguishable from tuberculosis are typical.

Progressive disseminated histoplasmosis most commonly occurs in patients with cellular immune deficiency, particularly now in patients with the acquired immune deficiency syndrome (AIDS) but also in patients with other conditions. Manifestations reflect widespread dissemination of *H. capsulatum* with involvement of reticuloendothelial tissues. Fever, sweats, weight loss, lymphadenopathy, hepatosplenomegaly, and bone marrow suppression are typical features of disseminated histoplasmosis. The severity and pace of illness vary with the degree of immunosuppression. Chronic and subacute disseminated disease may be seen in patients with apparently intact immune systems whereas patients with AIDS may present with fulminant illness similar to bacterial sepsis.

Rarely, an excessive host response to a prior episode of histoplasmosis causes mediastinal fibrosis, a progressive and often ultimately fatal condition. Cough, dyspnea, pleurisy, hemoptysis, sweats, and complications associated with obstruction of thoracic structures characterize this disorder. Erosion of calcified mediastinal nodes into large airways causes broncholithiases, which are associated with wheezing, cough, fever, hemoptysis, and expectoration of calcified pieces of tissue.

DIAGNOSIS

Tests available for the diagnosis of histoplasmosis include culture, special fungal stains of clinical specimens and tissue obtained by biopsy, serologic testing, and detection of *Histoplasma* polysaccharide antigen in urine or other body fluids. In endemic areas skin tests are not useful for diagnosis in adults. Serology may confirm the diagnosis of acute, self-limited forms of histoplasmosis. In addition, nearly all patients with chronic pulmonary histoplasmosis have positive serologic test results. Problems with serologic testing include a 6-week time lag between infection and the appearance of antibodies, false-positive results from cross-reacting antibodies, persistent antibodies from previous infection with *H. capsulatum*, and false-negative results in immunocompromised patients.

H. capsulatum grows in fungal culture in up to 85% of patients with chronic pulmonary histoplasmosis (multiple sputum specimens) and in 85% of those with disseminated disease. Bone marrow cultures give the highest yield in disseminated disease, but blood cultures are positive in up to 70% of patients when the lysis centrifugation technique is used. Culture is much less useful in acute, self-limited forms of disease. Wright's stain of peripheral blood and Gomori's methenamine-silver staining of tissue specimens allow a firm diagnosis, but are less sensitive than culture for the diagnosis of histoplasmosis.

Histoplasma polysaccharide antigen testing, available at the Histoplasmosis Reference Laboratory at Indiana University, is useful in the diagnosis of disseminated histoplasmosis and severe acute pulmonary histoplasmosis with positivity rates in urine specimens of 90% and 75%, respectively. Less severe forms of acute histoplasmosis are associated with significantly lower rates of antigen positivity. Antigen levels fall with successful therapy, and increasing levels may predict relapse.

TREATMENT

General Considerations and Medications

Self-limited forms of histoplasmosis, including those manifestations related to immunologic phenomena (pericarditis, arthritis, erythema nodosa), generally do not require antifungal therapy (Table 1). Treatment with an antifungal agent is indicated for patients with (1) severe acute pulmonary histoplasmosis associated with respiratory insufficiency, (2) acute pulmonary histoplasmosis with symptoms lasting longer than 1 month, (3) mediastinal histoplasmosis with obstructive symptoms, (4) chronic pulmonary histoplasmosis, or (5) disseminated histoplasmosis. The drugs available for the treatment of histoplasmosis include the azoles (ketoconazole [Nizoral, oral formulation], fluconazole* [Diflucan, intravenous and oral formulations], and itraconazole [Sporanox, oral formulation]) and the polyene amphotericin B (Fungizone, intravenous formulation). Less toxic but more expensive formulations of amphotericin B including amphotericin B lipid complex* (ABLC; Abelcet), amphotericin B colloidal dispersion* (ABCD; Amphotec), and liposomal amphotericin B* (AmBisome) are available. Although it may be reasonable to use one of these products in patients with histoplasmosis who have underlying renal insufficiency or who cannot tolerate conventional amphotericin B, none of these formulations has been used extensively or studied for the treatment of histoplasmosis. No studies have prospectively compared

---

*Not FDA approved for this indication.

amphotericin B to azole therapy or one azole to another for the treatment of histoplasmosis.

Amphotericin B at a dosage of 0.7 to 1 mg per kg per day or 50 mg per day is the drug of choice for the initial treatment of life-threatening histoplasmosis. Drawbacks associated with the use of amphotericin B include the requirement for intravenous administration, and toxicity, including infusion-related side effects (fever, chills, and rigors), renal insufficiency, hypokalemia, hypomagnesemia, and anemia.

Ketoconazole is the oldest and least expensive of the azole antifungals currently used in the treatment of histoplasmosis. It is usually given at a dosage of 200 mg orally twice a day with food. Gastric acidity is necessary for absorption of ketoconazole, and therefore efficacy may be diminished in patients with impaired gastric acid secretion due to prior gastric resection, old age, human immunodeficiency virus–associated gastropathy, and the use of histamine type 2 receptor blockers, or proton pump inhibitors such as omeprazole (Prilosec). Adverse effects include dose-related gastrointestinal symptoms, hepatic inflammation, and inhibition of adrenal steroidogenesis with decreased libido, impotence, gynecomastia, menstrual irregularities, and rarely, adrenal insufficiency. The metabolism of ketoconazole is increased (and serum levels are decreased) in patients who take rifampin (Rifadin, Rifamate, Rifater), isoniazid, carbamazepine (Tegretol), or phenytoin (Dilantin) concomitantly. Levels of cyclosporine (Neoral, Sandimmune), tacrolimus (Prograf), digoxin (Lanoxin), phenytoin, sulfonylurea drugs, warfarin (Coumadin), cisapride (Propulsid), and the non-sedating antihistamines, terfenadine (Seldane), and astemizole (Hismanal) are increased by the concomitant administration of ketoconazole. The interaction between the nonsedating antihistamines and ketoconazole has caused fatal ventricular arrhythmias. Elevated cisapride levels are also associated with ventricular arrhythmias.

Of the azoles, itraconazole is the most active against *H. capsulatum*. It is the drug of choice for primary therapy of moderate disease not involving the central nervous system, for continuation of therapy for patients with more severe disease who respond to an initial course of amphotericin B, and for lifelong maintenance therapy in patients with AIDS. The usual starting dosage is 200 mg twice daily, although 200 mg thrice daily for 3 days is sometimes given to reach steady-state serum levels more quickly. As with ketoconazole, gastric acidity is required for optimal absorption of itraconazole, and it should be taken with food. The itraconazole oral solution has better bioavailability and does not require concomitant food. Drug interactions associated with itraconazole are similar to those associated with ketoconazole, including the potentially fatal interaction with nonsedating antihistamines and cisapride. Although itraconazole has a lesser effect on steroidogenesis than ketoconazole, impotence has been reported in rare instances. A syndrome of hyperten-

TABLE 1. **Recommendations for Antifungal Therapy of Histoplasmosis**

Condition	Antifungal Agent*	Usual Daily Dosage	Duration	Comments
Acute pulmonary				
Mild, localized, symptoms ≥ 1 mo	Itraconazole (Sporanox)	200 mg	6–12 wk	Not studied
Moderate, diffuse	Itraconazole	200–400 mg	12 wk	Not studied
Severe, diffuse	Amphotericin B (Fungizone)	0.7 mg/kg	Until improvement, then itraconazole as described under "moderate, diffuse"	
Chronic pulmonary				Nodular lung disease is more responsive to therapy than cavitary disease
Mild to moderate	Itraconazole†	200–400 mg	12–24 mo	
	Ketoconazole (Nizoral)	200–400 mg	12–24 mo	
	Fluconazole‡ (Diflucan)	400–800 mg	12–24 mo	
Severe	Amphotericin B	0.7 mg/kg	Until improvement, then itraconazole as described under "chronic pulmonary, mild to moderate"	If amphotericin B is used for the entire course, give ≥ 35 mg/kg total dose over 2–4 mo
Disseminated, non-AIDS				Therapy should be continued until *Histoplasma* antigen concentration is < 4 U in urine and blood
Mild to moderate	Itraconazole†	200–400 mg	6–18 mo	
	Ketoconazole	200–400 mg	6–18 mo	
	Fluconazole‡	400–800 mg	6–18 mo	
Severe	Amphotericin B	0.7–1.0 mg/kg	Until improvement, then itraconazole as described under "disseminated, non-AIDS, mild to moderate"	If amphotericin B is used for the entire course, give ≥ 35 mg/kg total dose over 2–4 mo
Disseminated, AIDS§				
Induction				Total duration of induction therapy is 12 wk
Mild to moderate	Itraconazole†	600 mg, then 400 mg	3 d / To complete 12 wk	
	Fluconazole‡	800 mg	To complete 12 wk	
Severe	Amphotericin B	0.7–1.0 mg/kg	Until improvement, then itraconazole as described under "disseminated, AIDS, mild to moderate"	Duration is typically 3–14 d
Maintenance	Itraconazole†	200–400 mg	Life	If serum itraconazole level is > 4 μg/mL, on 400 mg dose, 200 mg/d dose can be used. Lifelong amphotericin B is poorly tolerated.
	Fluconazole‡	400–800 mg	Life	
	Amphotericin B	50–100 mg, once or twice a wk	Life	

*Itraconazole (Sporanox), ketoconazole (Nizoral), and fluconazole (Diflucan) are given orally. Amphotericin B (Fungizone) is given intravenously.

†For forms of histoplasmosis shown in this table, itraconazole is preferred over ketoconazole and fluconazole. Ketoconazole is used if itraconazole is unavailable because of cost or other extenuating circumstance. Fluconazole is used only in patients who cannot take itraconazole.

‡Not FDA approved for this indication.

§Do not use ketoconazole in patients with AIDS.

Adapted from Goldman M, Wheat LJ: Histoplasmosis. *In* Rakel RE [ed]: Conn's Current Therapy 1996. Philadelphia, WB Saunders Company, 1996, p. 192.

sion, edema, and hyperkalemia is seen rarely in patients taking 600 mg of itraconazole or more daily.

Fluconazole* has less activity against *H. capsulatum* than itraconazole and has lower rates of clinical success for initial or maintenance treatment of disease; it may be used as an alternative at dosages of 400 to 800 mg per day in patients who cannot absorb or tolerate itraconazole or to avoid drug-drug interactions. Gastric acidity is not required for the optimal absorption of fluconazole. Like itraconazole, fluconazole has little effect on mammalian steroid synthesis. Although drug interactions are less common with it than with itraconazole and ketoconazole, concomitant use of fluconazole and nonsedating antihistamines or cisapride is contraindicated.

Acute Syndromes

Mild, self-limited acute pulmonary histoplasmosis is usually diagnosed only in retrospect and does not require antifungal therapy. However, occasional patients will have an illness that lasts a month or more, and although it has not been studied, these individuals may benefit from a 6- to 12-week course of itraconazole at 200 mg per day. Patients with severe pulmonary histoplasmosis and hypoxemia who require hospitalization should be treated initially with amphotericin B at a dosage of 0.7 mg per kg per day until ready for discharge, followed by itraconazole, 200 to 400 mg per day. Some experts suggest adjunctive corticosteroids (prednisone, 40 to 60 mg per day or equivalent). Less ill patients should receive itraconazole initially. Duration of therapy is 12 weeks.

Chronic Pulmonary Histoplasmosis

Very ill patients should be treated initially with amphotericin B at a dosage of 0.7 mg per kg per day or 50 mg per day. If amphotericin B is the only therapy given, patients should receive a total dose of 35 mg per kg over 2 to 4 months, the majority of which can be given on a thrice weekly dosing schedule. The response rate is approximately 75% (range 59 to 100%), but a substantial relapse rate of around 25% is found. Most patients, however, do not receive a complete course of amphotericin B, but rather, are switched to an oral azole after clinical improvement occurs. Amphotericin B can be avoided in patients with less severe disease who may be treated with an azole initially. Rates of response to ketoconazole and itraconazole are similar at approximately 80%, but ketoconazole is less well tolerated. Fluconazole at 200 to 400 mg per day appears less efficacious than either ketoconazole or itraconazole. Relapse is about the same with azole therapy as with amphotericin B.

Therapeutic response is difficult to assess in patients with cavitary pulmonary histoplasmosis because of the functional disability and radiographic abnormalities associated with the underlying paren-chymal lung disease present in these patients. The duration of therapy for patients with nodular lung disease is 6 to 12 months; those with cavitary disease are treated for at least 12 months to as long as 24 months. For patients that relapse a second course of an azole may be tried.

Disseminated Histoplasmosis in Patients Without AIDS

Amphotericin B at a dosage of 0.7 to 1.0 mg per kg per day is the initial treatment of choice for disseminated histoplasmosis complicated by respiratory failure, sepsis, other evidence of overwhelming disease, or central nervous system manifestations. When amphotericin B is used alone for disseminated histoplasmosis, cure rates of 75% are attained. Relapse is less likely when the total dose of amphotericin B exceeds 35 mg per kg.

After an initial clinical response (resolution of fever, lack of need for pressors or ventilatory support, ability to take oral medications), therapy should be switched from amphotericin B to itraconazole at 200 to 400 mg per day. Mild to moderate disseminated disease can be treated with itraconazole initially; success rates in this setting approach 100%. Ketoconazole is also effective. As an alternative fluconazole can be given to nonimmunosuppressed patients at a dosage of 400 mg per day and to immunosuppressed patients at 800 mg per day. The usual duration of therapy is 6 to 18 months.

Disseminated Histoplasmosis in Patients with AIDS

The therapy of disseminated histoplasmosis in patients with AIDS is divided into a 12-week induction phase and a lifelong maintenance (or chronic suppressive) phase. Without maintenance therapy, 80% of AIDS patients with disseminated histoplasmosis experience relapse. As in patients without AIDS, amphotericin B at a dosage of 0.7 to 1.0 mg per kg per day should be the initial therapy for AIDS patients with life-threatening histoplasmosis. Satisfactory clinical response occurs in as little as 3 days in patients with moderately severe manifestations to 14 days in patients with severe disease. Thereafter, therapy is switched to itraconazole. Patients with mild to moderate disease are treated initially with itraconazole at a dosage of 200 mg three times a day for 3 days, followed by 200 mg twice a day for 12 weeks. This approach is associated with a response rate of 85%. Fluconazole at 800 mg per day is less effective (response rate 74%) and should only be used in patients who cannot take itraconazole. Ketoconazole appears ineffective in patients with AIDS and should not be used in this group.

After either induction therapy with amphotericin B or "up-front" itraconazole therapy, AIDS patients with disseminated histoplasmosis should be given lifelong itraconazole. At a dosage of 200 to 400 mg per day, itraconazole prevents relapse in approxi-

---

*Not FDA approved for this indication.

mately 90% of patients. Amphotericin B given weekly or biweekly at a dosage of 50 or 100 mg prevents relapse in 80 to 95% of patients who respond to induction therapy. However, chronic amphotericin B therapy is poorly tolerated, inconvenient, and not well accepted by patients. Fluconazole at 400 mg per day and ketoconazole at 200 to 400 mg per day are less effective than either itraconazole or amphotericin B for maintenance therapy of histoplasmosis in patients with AIDS.

Fibrosing Mediastinitis

In general, it is believed that antifungal therapy is not useful in the management of patients with fibrosing mediastinitis. However, a 3-month course of itraconazole is probably worth trying in symptomatic patients with elevated serum complement fixation titers and high erythrocyte sedimentation rates. If the patient improves, therapy can be extended to a year. Surgery is sometimes necessary, but this approach is associated with a poor outcome.

BLASTOMYCOSIS

method of
STANLEY W. CHAPMAN, M.D.
University of Mississippi Medical Center
Jackson, Mississippi

Blastomycosis is an uncommon but often serious systemic fungal infection caused by the dimorphic fungus *Blastomyces dermatitidis*. Blastomycosis is endemic in North America in the southeastern and south-central states adjacent to the Mississippi and Ohio Rivers; the midwestern states and Canadian provinces that border the Great Lakes; and a small area in New York and Canada along the St. Lawrence River. Most cases are reported from Mississippi, Arkansas, Kentucky, Tennessee, and Wisconsin. Several studies have also documented smaller hyperendemic areas with unusually high rates of blastomycosis. Point source outbreaks have been reported in association with occupational or recreational activities along streams and rivers.

Blastomycosis grows in the environment as the mycelial form in warm, moist soil that is organically enriched with decaying vegetation and wood. The terminal conidia are easily aerosolized when the soil is disturbed, and most infections are a result of inhalation of these spores into the lungs. Although pulmonary illness is most common, hematogenous spread to extrapulmonary sites may occur, most frequently to the skin, bones, and male genitourinary tract. Dissemination and multiple-organ disease occur most commonly in patients who are immunocompromised.

The varied clinical spectrum of blastomycosis includes asymptomatic infection, acute or chronic pneumonia, and disseminated (extrapulmonary) disease. When sensitive serologic studies have been applied to the investigation of point source outbreaks, about one half of infected individuals have asymptomatic infection. Acute pulmonary blastomycosis develops after an incubation period of 30 to 45 days and clinically mimics influenza or bacterial pneumo-

nia. Symptoms include the sudden onset of cough, fever, chills, and pleuritic chest pain. Cough is often productive of purulent sputum. Chest radiographs usually reveal alveolar infiltrates or lobar consolidation. Spontaneous resolution of acute pulmonary blastomycosis is well documented, but the exact frequency of such cures is not definitively established.

Most patients diagnosed with blastomycosis have a chronic, indolent pneumonia that is clinically indistinguishable from tuberculosis or bronchogenic cancer. Symptoms include low-grade fever, productive cough, hemoptysis, chest pain, and weight loss. Chest radiographs usually reveal lobar or nodular infiltrates, sometimes with cavitation. Perihilar mass lesions that mimic cancer also occur frequently. A rare patient may have miliary disease or a diffuse pneumonitis associated with adult respiratory distress syndrome. Mortality in these patients exceeds 50%; death usually occurs during the first few days of treatment.

Extrapulmonary disease occurs in 25 to 60% of patients with blastomycosis. In some patients, extrapulmonary lesions, especially those of the skin, may be present in the absence of clinically overt pulmonary disease. Skin disease is the most common extrapulmonary infection, and two types of skin lesions are reported. The more common is the verrucous lesion that mimics squamous cell carcinoma. Less common is the ulcerative skin lesion, which bleeds easily. Osteomyelitis most frequently involves the long bones, vertebrae, and ribs. Well-circumscribed osteolytic lesions are the typical radiographic feature. Vertebral disease mimics tuberculosis, with large paraspinous abscesses. The prostate and epididymis are the most common sites of male genitourinary tract involvement with blastomycosis. Central nervous system (CNS) disease manifests as either mass lesions (abscesses) or meningitis and occurs most frequently in patients in the late stages of the acquired immunodeficiency syndrome (AIDS).

Blastomycosis is being reported increasingly as an opportunistic infection, especially in patients with late-stage AIDS, transplant recipients, and patients on immunosuppressive medications. Pulmonary disease is more likely to manifest as respiratory failure, and multiorgan dissemination (including the CNS) is common. Mortality rates of up to 40% are reported, often during the first few weeks of therapy. Even with an aggressive initial course of amphotericin, relapse frequently occurs and chronic suppressive therapy, usually with itraconazole, is recommended.

A definitive diagnosis of blastomycosis requires growth of the organism from a clinical specimen such as sputum, bronchoalveolar lavage fluid, pus from a skin lesion, or a biopsy specimen. Specimens should be cultured on enriched agar and incubated at 30°C. Although early identification of mycelial cultures is possible with the use of exoantigen test kits or chemiluminescent DNA probes, most laboratories confirm identification by conversion to the yeast phase at 37°C. A presumptive diagnosis may be made by visualization of the characteristic yeast form in a clinical specimen and, in the appropriate clinical setting, usually prompts the start of antifungal therapy. Sputum or purulent secretions can be directly examined as a wet preparation or after digestion with a 10% solution of potassium hydroxide. Papanicolaou or Giemsa stains of cytologic specimens facilitate recognition of the organism in bronchial washings, lavage fluid, or postbronchcoscopy sputum specimens. Pathologic specimens should be stained with Gomori methenamine-silver stain and periodic acid–Schiff stain. Current serologic tests, because they lack both sensitivity and specificity, are of limited value in the diagnosis

TABLE 1. **Treatment Guidelines of Various Forms of Blastomycosis***

Type of Disease	Recommended Treatment	Dosage
Pulmonary Blastomycosis		
Life-threatening disease or immunosuppressed host	Amphotericin B (Fungizone)	Total dose: 1.5–2.5 gm
Mild to moderate disease	Itraconazole (Sporanox)	200–400 mg daily for 6 months
Disseminated Blastomycosis		
Central nervous system disease	Amphotericin B	Total dose: at least 2 gm
Non-CNS disease		
Life-threatening disease or immunosuppressed host	Amphotericin B	Total dose: 1.5–2.5 gm
Mild to moderate disease	Itraconazole	200–400 mg daily for 6 months

*See text for detailed discussion and alternative treatment regimens.
Abbreviation: CNS = central nervous system.

of blastomycosis. No skin test reagent is available for the diagnosis of blastomycosis.

TREATMENT

Most patients in whom blastomycosis is diagnosed require treatment (Table 1). Spontaneous cure has been documented in some immunocompetent patients with acute pulmonary blastomycosis. Thus, in a few selected cases of blastomycosis limited to the lungs, therapy may be withheld and patients carefully monitored for spontaneous cure or progression of disease. Patients must, however, be carefully evaluated for the presence of extrapulmonary disease before the decision is made to withhold treatment. In contrast, all patients who are immunocompromised, have progressive pulmonary disease, or have extrapulmonary blastomycosis must be treated. Treatment options include amphotericin B (Fungizone), ketoconazole (Nizoral), and itraconazole (Sporanox). Fluconazole (Diflucan)* has been used successfully to treat mild to moderate forms of blastomycosis.

Amphotericin B was previously considered the treatment of choice for all forms of blastomycosis. Studies, however, have proved ketoconazole, itraconazole, and fluconazole to be effective alternatives in the treatment of immunocompetent patients with mild to moderate pulmonary and extrapulmonary disease. Azoles should *not* be used for patients with life-threatening disease or those with CNS infection. The azoles are contraindicated in pregnancy, and amphotericin B is the only drug approved for the treatment of blastomycosis in pregnant women. Amphotericin B is also the drug of choice for patients who are immunocompromised; those who have life-threatening disease, CNS disease, or progression of disease during treatment with an azole; and those who cannot tolerate an azole because of toxicity.

The Azoles

Ketoconazole was the first azole proven to be effective for the treatment of patients with mild to moderate blastomycosis. Cure rates of 80% or greater have been documented for patients treated in both retro-

spective and prospective clinical trials with 400 to 800 mg per day of ketoconazole. Although efficacy is improved with the higher dose, the rate of toxic drug reactions necessitating discontinuation of therapy is more frequent. Thus, ketoconazole is usually started as a single daily dose of 400 mg per day. If the clinical response is not satisfactory, the dose may be escalated in 200-mg increments up to a maximum dose of 800 mg per day. Treatment should continue for a minimum of 6 months.

Itraconazole has also proven highly effective for the treatment of blastomycosis. Studies show documented cure rates of 90% or greater for patients treated with 200 to 400 mg per day of itraconazole. Although no therapeutic advantage has been clearly documented for doses exceeding 200 mg per day, I often have patients with more advanced disease begin treatment with 400 mg per day. Thus, the recommended initial dose of itraconazole is 200 mg per day, which should be successful in most patients with blastomycosis. The dose can be escalated in increments of 100 mg per day based on clinical response to maximum dose of 400 mg. Treatment should be continued for at least 6 months. Although there are no comparative trials, itraconazole appears more efficacious and better tolerated than ketoconazole. Thus, itraconazole, despite its increased cost, has replaced ketoconazole as the drug of choice for treatment of non–life-threatening, non-CNS blastomycosis.

Several important points must be emphasized regarding the use of ketoconazole or itraconazole for antifungal therapy. First, gastric acid is necessary for absorption of both agents, and subtherapeutic blood levels have been seen in patients receiving concomitant antacids or H_2-receptor antagonists. Second, the use of rifampin, phenytoin (Dilantin), and carbamazepine (Tegretol) has been shown to increase the hepatic metabolism of both itraconazole and ketoconazole. Therefore, concurrent use of any of these agents may result in treatment failure. Other significant drug interactions have also been reported with oral contraceptives, cyclosporine (Sandimmune), digoxin, phenobarbital, cisapride (Propulsid), and the nonsedating antihistamines (e.g., terfenadine [Seldane] and astemizole [Hismanal]). Administration of either ketoconazole or itraconazole concur-

*Not FDA approved for this indication.

rently with cisapride or any of the nonsedating antihistamines is contraindicated because of the risk of life-threatening ventricular arrhythmias. Third, adverse drug effects seen with both agents may be treatment limiting. Nausea and vomiting are dose-related and can usually be controlled by taking keto-conazole and itraconazole with meals or by using a twice-daily dose schedule. Hormonal abnormalities are more common with ketoconazole and include gynecomastia, impotence, oligospermia, and abnor-mal uterine bleeding. Pedal edema and hypokalemia are more frequently reported with itraconazole. Al-though severe hepatic toxicity is uncommon, I still monitor liver function monthly while patients are on therapy. Finally, relapse rates after azole therapy are higher than after amphotericin and are reported in the range of 10 to 14%. Thus, careful follow-up is warranted for 1 or 2 years after completion of azole therapy.

Fluconazole has been used to treat only a limited number of patients. I believe that fluconazole is of limited value for the treatment of blastomycosis in comparison to itraconazole and ketoconazole. In one study involving a dosage of 400 to 800 mg per day, a successful outcome was documented in 87% of 39 patients. Adverse events due to fluconazole are usu-ally mild, and cessation of therapy owing to toxicity is infrequent. Dry skin, chapped lips, and reversible alopecia occur at the higher dose of fluconazole. Drug interactions are less frequent than for ketoconazole or itraconazole. Fluconazole is well absorbed in the achlorhydric patient whether the condition is due to medications or prior surgery. On the basis of these results, I consider fluconazole at doses of 400 to 800 mg per day as equivalent to ketoconazole but less toxic. Fluconazole, however, is not as efficacious as itraconazole. Fluconazole penetrates well into the CNS and may have a role in the treatment of blasto-mycotic meningitis or brain abscess in patients who are intolerant to amphotericin B.

Amphotericin

Amphotericin is the treatment of choice for pa-tients who are immunocompromised, have life-threatening or CNS disease, or fail azole therapy. Although the optimal dose and duration of amphoter-icin B have not been adequately established, relapse rates are lowest ($\leq$4%) in patients who receive a total dose of at least 1.5 grams. Thus, I usually recom-mend a total dose of 1.5 to 2.5 grams of amphotericin. Patients who have CNS disease or life-threatening disease (pulmonary or extrapulmonary) begin am-photericin at a dose of 0.7 to 1.0 mg per kg per day. Less seriously ill patients or patients whose disease progresses on azole begin amphotericin therapy at a dose of 0.5 to 0.7 mg per kg per day. For patients who are not severely immunocompromised and do not have CNS disease, I have achieved therapeutic success by switching to itraconazole after the patient has been clinically stabilized following an induction course of amphotericin, usually 500 to 1000 mg. Even

after a full course of amphotericin B treatment, fre-quent relapses occur in AIDS patients and those pa-tients who continue on immunosuppressive regi-mens. Therefore, I recommend chronic suppressive therapy with itraconazole for those patients who re-spond to a primary course of amphotericin. I do not recommend ketoconazole because of the higher re-lapse rates reported for this agent.

Amphotericin is frequently associated with sig-nificant toxicity that complicates therapy. Renal fail-ure is the most serious complication and the most common reason for interruption or premature cessa-tion of therapy. The likelihood of renal failure can be reduced by preinfusion of saline and by avoidance of other nephrotoxic drugs and diuretics. Infusion-related toxicities (e.g., fever, rigors, headache) usu-ally resolve after the first few days of treatment but can be lessened by premedication with acetamino-phen or ibuprofen. Intravenous meperidine is effec-tive for the control of rigors. Premedication with in-travenous corticosteroids may be necessary for a short time period in a few patients with severe infu-sion-related reactions.

PLEURAL EFFUSION AND EMPYEMA THORACIS

method of
CAMERON D. WRIGHT, M.D.
*Harvard Medical School and
Massachusetts General Hospital
Boston, Massachusetts*

Pleural effusion, an abnormal collection of fluid in the pleural space, is a common clinical problem most fre-quently caused by pathology of the lung or pleura. Extra-pulmonary disorders of the heart, kidneys, liver, and pan-creas also may cause a pleural effusion. Systemic illness and drugs also cause pleural effusions. Pleural effusion usually results from an imbalance in pleural hydrostatic and oncotic pressures or increased capillary permeability.

A careful history and physical examination will usually narrow the diagnostic possibilities and allow a differential diagnosis to be formulated. Chest radiographs (posterior-anterior, lateral, and decubitus views) define the problem and can suggest loculation of fluid if fluid is not in a dependent location. Computed tomography (CT) scans are helpful in assessing loculated effusions and defining under-lying lung, pleural, or mediastinal pathology. Ultrasonog-raphy is helpful in guiding drainage of small or loculated effusions. Office or bedside thoracentesis of moderate to large effusions is readily accomplished. Radiologic-guided (CT scan or ultrasonography) thoracentesis is usually per-formed for small or loculated effusions. Except for tran-sient effusions clearly associated with systemic disorders (i.e., congestive heart failure, nephrotic syndrome) all pleu-ral effusions require diagnostic evaluation beginning with a thoracentesis.

The combination of pleural fluid cellularity, appearance, and chemistry can establish the diagnosis in about 75% of patients. The tests requested on aspirated pleural fluid should be based on the suspected diagnosis and the appearance of the fluid. Effusions may be classified as transudates or exudates on the basis of the pleural fluid protein and lactate dehydrogenase (LDH). Exudative effusions are present if any one of the following is present: (1) The pleural fluid–to-serum ratio of total protein is greater than 0.5; (2) the pleural fluid–to-serum ratio of LDH is greater than 0.6; or (3) the pleural fluid LDH concentration is greater than two thirds of the upper limits of normal of the serum LDH. Transudative effusions are noninflammatory in nature and most commonly caused by congestive heart failure. Less than 15% of all transudative effusions are caused by malignancy. The treatment of transudative effusions is that of the underlying disorder. In rare instances, therapeutic thoracentesis is required to relieve dyspnea until the underlying condition is improved. Exudative effusions have a broader differential diagnosis and require additional tests of the pleural fluid to refine the diagnosis. Helpful tests include pH, glucose, cell count and differential, triglyceride level, amylase, culture (aerobic, anaerobic, fungal, and mycobacterial) and microbiologic stain (Gram's, fungal, and acid-fast). Culture- and cytology-negative exudative effusions usually require further evaluation, which usually begins with video-assisted thoracoscopy (VAT) examination of the pleural space.

PARAPNEUMONIC EFFUSION

Small, uncomplicated effusions associated with pneumonia often resolve with antibiotic treatment alone. Complicated parapneumonic effusions (pH < 7.1, glucose level < 40 mg/dL, loculations present, culture positive, gross pus present) necessitate prompt intervention with drainage to prevent further complications such as trapped lung. Usually a chest tube is inserted at the bedside and the radiologic and clinical responses are evaluated within a day or so. If there is an incomplete response, there are usually residual loculations present that must be drained. In general, the earlier an effusion is drained, the more likely the lung will reexpand completely. Failure to reexpand the lung (indicating a significant undrained pleural collection) necessitates prompt further drainage intervention. If prolonged chest tube suction does not reexpand the lung within 1 to 2 days, it should be discontinued. Effective lung reexpansion and pleural drainage usually result in prompt defervescence.

EMPYEMA

Empyema is an infection in the pleural space, usually from a pneumonia or lung abscess. Other causes include trauma, postoperative, esophageal rupture, sepsis, and subdiaphragmatic abscess. Gram-positive organisms still predominate, but anaerobic and gram-negative infections are also common. Empyema is present when pus is aspirated from the pleural space or a pleural fluid culture is positive. The goals of empyema treatment are evacuation of the pleural collection, reexpansion of the lung with obliteration of the pleural space, control of the infection with antibiotics, and elimination of the underlying disease process. Figure 1 provides an algorithm for the management of empyema and complicated parapneu-

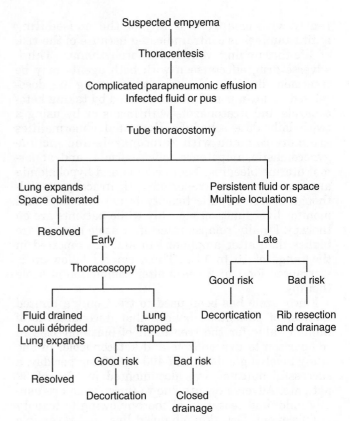

Figure 1. Treatment algorithm for empyema.

monic effusion. Many patients fail simple tube thoracostomy due to loculations. When diagnosed early (a few days) VAT can allow loculations to be broken up and drained as long as there is no significant rind on the lung. If the lung is trapped by a rind, the VAT procedure can be converted to an open thoracotomy to allow decortication. Patients at high risk for decortication include those with severe underlying lung pathology whose lungs do not reexpand and those rare patients with severe co-morbid diseases that would prohibit a thoracotomy. Rib resection and open drainage usually commit the patients to prolonged (months-long) daily wound care and so is reserved only for those patients that have a prohibitive operative risk. Recovery from decortication is usually quick as long as the lung completely reexpands.

MALIGNANT PLEURAL EFFUSIONS

The most frequent causes of malignant pleural effusions are lung cancer, breast cancer, lymphomas, and adenocarcinomas with unknown primary. The effusions are usually exudative and may be serous or bloody. About 50% of malignant effusions are cytology-positive on the first tap, and 70% are positive on the second. If cancer is suspected after two negative taps, VAT with pleural biopsy should be performed. Close to 100% of malignant effusions are correctly diagnosed with VAT. Large, symptomatic pleural effusions always require drainage (therapeutic thoracentesis or chest tube drainage). Small pleural effusions in chemotherapy responsive tumors (lymphoma, small cell lung cancer, nonseminomatous germ cell tumors) are treated with chemotherapy alone. Pleural effusions in more resistant tumors (nonsmall cell lung cancer, breast cancer) are treated by drainage and sclerosis. Many agents have been used to induce pleurodesis but talc is currently the agent of choice because of its high success rate (90%) and the cost (minimal). Other agents that can be used are doxycycline* (Vibramycin) and bleomycin (Blenoxane). Talc can be instilled as a slurry (5 grams in 100 mL of saline) through a chest tube at the bedside or insufflated (5 grams) at the time of VAT. Severe respiratory complications have been reported when 10 grams of talc have been used so it is important to limit the dose to 5 grams. A frequent problem in treating malignant pleural effusions is failure of the lung to reexpand after chest-tube drainage due to trapped lung. Decortication is usually not possible and unrewarding in these patients with limited survival. Treatment options include dyspnea palliation with narcotics and oxygen, repeated thoracentesis, or in occasional patients pleuroperitoneal shunts (which require constant pumping by the patients to maintain patency).

TUBERCULOUS EFFUSIONS

Tuberculosis may manifest with a pleural effusion alone or be associated with pulmonary parenchymal disease. If tuberculosis is suspected, the diagnostic yield is greatly enhanced with a closed pleural biopsy for both culture and histology. Besides appropriate antituberculous therapy, moderate or large effusions should be tapped dry to prevent chronic empyema and trapped lung. Tube thoracostomy of pure tuberculosis effusions should never be done, to avoid converting the effusion to a mixed bacterial and tuberculous empyema.

---

*Not FDA approved for this indication.

PRIMARY LUNG ABSCESS

method of
MICHAEL J. GEHMAN, D.O., and
MATTHEW E. LEVISON, M.D.
MCP/Hahnemann School of Medicine
Philadelphia, Pennsylvania

Lung abscess is a necrotizing infection that results in one or more discrete cavities, each 2 or more cm in diameter. If there are multiple, small cavities, each less than 2 cm in diameter, the process is usually referred to as *necrotizing pneumonia*, although the pathogenesis and microbiology of both lung abscess and necrotizing pneumonia are thought to be similar.

PATHOGENESIS

Respiratory pathogens can reach the lung by one of several routes: airways, the bloodstream, spread from contiguous infection, or traumatic entry (e.g., knife wound). The most common routes are the airways and bloodstream. Lung abscess developing as a consequence of bronchogenic spread to the lung is usually referred to as *primary*, and hematogenous lung abscess is referred to as *secondary*, because in the latter instance the primary infection (bacteremia, endocarditis, or suppurative thrombophlebitis) is usually clinically evident.

The most common risk factor for primary lung abscess is aspiration of oropharyngeal secretions. Aspiration occurs among normal people, especially during deep sleep, but in certain patients aspiration may be of sufficient magnitude or frequency, or the aspirated material may contain adjuvants (such as necrotic tissue, food or foreign bodies, or particularly virulent pathogens or synergistic combinations of microorganisms), to overcome lung defenses. Patients with lung abscess usually have underlying conditions that predispose to aspiration, such as loss of consciousness from any cause or neurologic or esophageal defects in swallowing.

Patients with primary lung abscess usually also have periodontal disease, which would be favorable for the presence of large numbers of potential pathogens and possibly necrotic periodontal tissue in aspirated oropharyngeal secretions. The development of primary lung abscess in patients who are edentulous should prompt a search for a neoplastic process in the oropharynx or the lower respiratory tract that would result in obstruction of the airways and provides a focus of anaerobic microbial proliferation in necrotic neoplastic tissue.

Initially the pathologic process that follows aspiration is infiltrative (aspiration pneumonia), but cavitation follows in about 1 to 2 weeks if there is no resolution at the infiltrative stage. The pathogenesis and microbiologic processes of aspiration pneumonia and lung abscess are similar.

MICROBIOLOGY

Multiple bacteriologic studies established that primary lung abscess is caused by polymicrobial anaerobic flora present in the oral cavity, particularly the gingival crevice. When oropharyngeal secretions are aspirated into the lower respiratory tract, there is a marked simplification of the flora, so that only the most virulent anaerobic species, such as *Prevotella melaninogenica, Fusobacterium nucleatum,* and *Peptostreptococcus* species, predominate. Microaerophilic and facultative streptococci are also frequently present.

In some patients, the anaerobes may be mixed with facultative respiratory pathogens, such as *Streptococcus pneumoniae, Staphylococcus aureus, Haemophilus influenzae,* or *Klebsiella pneumoniae.* The anaerobic bacterial etiology of primary lung abscess is often putative and based on the clinical presentation, especially the putrid odor of the breath or infected material, such as sputum or pleural fluid, that is characteristically produced by anaerobes.

Some aerobic pulmonary pathogens can cause primary lung abscess and should be suspected in certain clinical settings. For example, *S. aureus* can cause a necrotizing pulmonary infection, usually after influenza; gram-negative bacilli, such as *K. pneumoniae* or *Pseudomonas aeruginosa, Nocardia* species, or fungi, such as *Aspergillus,* can cause cavitary pneumonia in immunocompromised patients or in a nosocomial setting; *Histoplasma* or *Coccidioides* species can cause cavitary pneumonia in patients living in certain geographic areas of the United States; and

Mycobacterium tuberculosis can produce cavities that are usually located in the upper lobes.

CLINICAL PRESENTATION

About 75% of patients with primary lung abscess have an indolent febrile, wasting illness with respiratory symptoms (cough, sputum production, pleuritic chest pain, blood-streaked sputum) of several weeks' duration, similar to that of tuberculosis or lung cancer. One quarter of patients have a more acute illness similar to that of pneumococcal pneumonia.

DIAGNOSIS

Patients with typical features of lung abscess—which include a predisposition for aspiration, periodontal disease, sputum with a foul odor, and one or more thick-walled cavities in dependent bronchopulmonary segments with air-fluid levels—need little further initial diagnostic work-up and should be treated presumptively for a polymicrobial anaerobic infection. In these patients, expectorated sputum is of no value for detecting anaerobes because of contamination with oral flora, but it may be useful to exclude the presence of other organisms capable of causing necrotizing pulmonary infection.

Febrile patients should have blood cultures, and pleural fluid, if present, should be obtained for stains and cultures. Upper lobe cavities without air-fluid levels suggest tuberculosis and require exclusion of *M. tuberculosis* with three morning sputum collections for mycobacterial stains and cultures. For patients who fail to respond to empirical therapy for putative anaerobic lung abscess, are suspected of having a pulmonary neoplasm, or are immunocompromised, more rigorous diagnostic testing is usually indicated; this includes bronchoscopy, protected brushing, and collection of bronchoalveolar lavage fluid for stains and cultures for routine bacteria, *Rhodococcus equi* (in patients with AIDS), *Legionella* species, *Nocardia* species, and fungi, if expectorated sputum studies fail to disclose the presence of these organisms. Computed tomography (CT) of the chest may be important for defining pathologic anatomy in patients with a pyopneumothorax. CT and bronchoscopy are also necessary for exclusion of noninfectious conditions, such as cystic bronchiectasis, cavitating neoplasms, and Wegener's granulomatosis, all of which may be confused with lung abscess in some patients.

TREATMENT

Penicillin and tetracycline have been the standard antimicrobial agents used in empirical regimens to treat putative anaerobic lung abscess. However, most anaerobic gram-negative respiratory pathogens are now found to be penicillin resistant as a consequence of beta-lactamase production and are also tetracycline-resistant. Instead, clindamycin (Cleocin) can be used intravenously in doses of 600 to 900 mg every 8 hours initially in hospitalized patients unable to tolerate oral therapy, or orally in doses of 300 mg every 6 hours. Other agents that are active against both the oral anaerobes and microaerophilic streptococci include the carbapenems (imipenem [Primaxin] or meropenem [Merrem]), cefoxitin (Mefoxin), beta-lactamase/beta-lactam antibiotic combinations (e.g., amoxicillin/clavulanate [Augmentin], ampicillin/ sulbactam [Unasyn], ticarcillin/clavulanate [Timentin], or piperacillin/tazobactam [Zosyn]), or penicillin plus metronidazole (Flagyl) combination. Metronidazole alone has been found to be inadequate, apparently because it is inactive against microaerophilic streptococci, although it is reliably active against anaerobes.

Patients on effective therapy will defervesce within a week. Chest radiographic findings take weeks to resolve. The duration of therapy is controversial. The recommended duration of therapy for anaerobic lung abscess is usually at least 4 to 6 weeks to prevent relapse or until the abscess completely resolves or there is a small, stable residual scar. Failure to adequately respond should prompt more intensive investigation to exclude the presence of resistant pathogens or a noninfectious etiology.

Surgery is rarely indicated for putrid lung abscess, except for the rare complication of massive hemoptysis. Postural and bronchoscopic drainage and chest physiotherapy traditionally have been recommended to enhance antimicrobial therapy. However, caution should be exercised to avoid sudden massive emptying of pus-filled cavities into the airways and previously uninvolved bronchopulmonary segments.

OTITIS MEDIA

method of
JEFFREY A. PAFFRATH, M.D., and
MITCHELL K. SCHWABER, M.D.
Centennial Medical Center
Nashville, Tennessee

Otitis media is one of the most common conditions treated by practitioners caring for children, resulting in more than 30 million office visits per year in the United States. Although antibiotics have reduced the incidence of serious complications after an episode of acute otitis media, the emergence of antibiotic resistance has led to other problems, including recurrent otitis media, persistent middle ear effusion, and chronic otitis media. New treatment modalities, including once-a-day antibiotics, office-based tympanostomy, vaccines, and nasal inflation devices, are changing the treatment paradigms being used by practitioners.

In typical acute otitis media, an upper respiratory viral infection produces inflammatory swelling and collections in the nasopharynx with eustachian tube dysfunction. The resulting negative middle ear pressure and inhibited drainage produces an accumulation of fluid in the middle ear and predisposition to aspiration of virus or bacteria from the nasopharynx. This cycle thus produces an effusion and at times an acute suppurative event with otalgia, fever, and decreased hearing. Children remain predisposed due to frequent viral infections and developing immune systems and eustachian tubes.

Acute otitis media often results from infection caused by, in order of decreasing frequency, *Streptococcus pneumoniae*, *Haemophilus influenzae*, *Moraxella catarrhalis*, and *Streptococcous pyogenes*. Tympanocentesis with cultures have shown that there are no pathogenic bacteria in up to

30% of cases. Antigen identification techniques have yielded viruses in up to two thirds of affected ears, but there is not a clinically applicable test to date.

DIAGNOSIS

Complaints of otalgia, ear fullness, and decreased hearing are the most specific for the diagnosis of otitis media but are difficult to obtain from young children. Fever, irritability, and trouble sleeping are normally more obvious and yet nonspecific. "Pulling at the ears" and crying are highly inaccurate findings with respect to the diagnosis. Consideration should be given to risk factors such as recent viral illness, allergy, day care attendance, lack of breast feeding, maxillofacial abnormalities, or, rarely, immune deficiency.

Accurate diagnosis of otitis media relies on proper physical assessment. The tympanic membrane may be dull, thickened, erythematous, bulging with lack of landmarks, demonstrate bubbles of an effusion, or, most importantly, have decreased mobility. Pneumatic otoscopy or hand-held tympanometers are used to confirm the diagnosis.

MEDICAL TREATMENT

Current factors affecting treatment decisions include natural history, microbiology, antibiotic resistance, antibiotic spectrum, tolerability, expense, and prevention. Acute otitis media has a high spontaneous cure rate; 60 to 90% of episodes resolve spontaneously. This likely results from the local immune response and subsequent inflammatory reactions. In some countries such as the Netherlands and Iceland, children older than 2 years of age with "nonsevere" acute otitis media are treated without antibiotics. Antibiotics have been shown to have a statistically significant effect for one in seven children, producing faster symptom relief and clearance of the effusion. Thus, recommended antibiotic use has continued in the United States.

Although patients have come to believe that an antibiotic will provide rapid relief, the emergence of antibiotic-resistant pathogens is ever increasing. There are four general mechanisms of antibiotic resistance: decreased permeability, drug efflux, drug inactivation, and altered target. The phenomenon of decreased permeability is common in gram-negative bacteria such as *Pseudomonas aeruginosa* but has not been noted in either *M. catarrhalis* or *H. influenzae*. Drug efflux, in which the bacteria actively pump out penetrating antibiotics, has been demonstrated with macrolide resistance by *S. pneumoniae*. The most prevalent resistance mechanism currently is drug inactivation, seen as beta-lactamase production by *H. influenzae* and *M. catarrhalis*. This plasmid-transferred enzyme breaks down the beta-lactam ring present in penicillin and cephalosporins. Beta-lactamase production is present in 10 to 65% of *H. influenzae* and 80 to 95% of *M. catarrhalis*. The mechanism of resistance of most recent concern is the altered target in which *S. pneumoniae* have altered penicillin-binding proteins, present in the cell wall and serving a critical role in bacterial multiplication and division. The antibiotic usually binds to and in-

activates the penicillin-binding proteins. The alteration decreases binding ability, making the antibiotic less effective. Risk factors for a resistant organism include recent treatment with beta-lactam antibiotics, recurrent acute otitis media, day care attendance, age less than 3 years, and winter season.

ANTIBIOTIC SELECTION

In acute otitis media, antibiotics are given to produce faster symptom relief and to prevent suppurative complications (Table 1). First-line treatment continues to be amoxicillin (Amoxil). It is inexpensive, well tolerated, tastes good, and frequently results in resolution of infection. Trimethoprim-sulfamethoxazole (Bactrim, Septra) or erythromycin-sulfisoxasole (Pediazole) may be prescribed for the penicillin-allergic patient. Two clinical situations may require a beta-lactamase stable antibiotic as initial therapy for uncomplicated acute otitis media. These include children recently treated with a beta-lactamase stable antibiotic and those with otitis-conjunctivitis syndrome, which is the result of *H. influenzae* in more than 70% of cases.

Second-line agents should be limited to treatment failure in otherwise healthy children. Amoxicillin-clavulanate (Augmentin) remains a good choice but may result in diarrhea in more than 25% of patients. Of the macrolides, erythromycin is not recommended because it frequently produces gastrointestinal upset and has little activity against *H. influenzae*. The newer macrolides, azithromycin (Zithromax) and clarithromycin (Biaxin), provide better coverage, including *H. influenzae* and initially, intermediate-resistant *S. pneumoniae*. These are also well tolerated by most children.

Of the cephalosporins, cefprozil (Cefzil), cefuroxime axetil (Ceftin), cefpodoxime proxetil (Vantin), ceftibuten (Cedax), and cefixime (Suprax) may be considered for otitis media. Cefuroxime is well tolerated and

TABLE 1. **Preferred Antibiotics for the Treatment of Otitis Media in Children**

Antibiotic	Dosage
Amoxicillin (Amoxil)	40–80 mg/kg/d divided tid*
Amoxicillin-potassium clavulanate (Augmentin)	Amoxicillin 45 mg/kg + potassium clavulanate 7.5 mg/kg/d divided bid
Trimethoprim-sulfamethoxazole (Bactrim, Septra)	Trimethoprim 8 mg/kg + sulfamethoxazole 40 mg/kg/d divided bid
Azithromycin (Zithromax)	10 mg/kg on day 1 followed by 5 mg/kg/d on days 2–5 qd
Cefuroxime axetil (Ceftin)	30 mg/kg/d divided bid
Cefpodoxime proxetil (Vantin)	5–10 mg/kg/d divided bid
Ceftriaxone (Rocephin)	50–75 mg/kg IM†
Clindamycin (Cleocin)	16–20 mg/kg/d divided qid

*The double dose (80 mg/kg/d) of amoxicillin provides coverage of intermediate-resistant *Streptococcus pneumoniae*.

†Half-life in middle ear fluid is up to 25 hours. This one-time dose may need to be repeated.

has excellent beta-lactamase stability, but it is more expensive than most in this class. Cefixime, ceftibuten, and loracarbef (Lorabid) are highly active against *H. influenzae* and *M. catarrhalis* but are not particularly effective against *S. pneumoniae*.

The dilemma remains what to use against resistant *S. pneumoniae*. Amoxicillin (80 mg per kg per day), amoxicillin-clavulanate, cefuroxime, and cefpodoxime have intermediate activity against these organisms. Clindamycin, now available in suspension, is the most effective oral antibiotic against resistant *S. pneumoniae*. If used empirically, consideration must be made that it provides ineffective coverage of *H. influenzae*. Ceftriaxone (Rocephin) in multiple intramuscular doses may be required for highly resistant *S. pneumoniae* while having excellent activity against *H. influenza* and *M. cattarhalis*.

Children less than 3 years of age should be reassessed at 3 to 5 days to determine the status of symptoms and the findings on repeated examination. If significant clinical improvement is not observed, more aggressive therapy is required. Tympanocentesis, office tympanostomy, or intramuscular ceftriaxone may be indicated at this point.

OTITIS MEDIA WITH EFFUSION

An effusion is the expected outcome after initial successful treatment of an acute otitis media. This effusion usually lasts 3 weeks, and about 90% will resolve within 3 months unless re-infection occurs. An asymptomatic, newly diagnosed effusion may be treated with a first-line antibiotic, but if it is discovered 6 weeks after an acute infection, a second-line antibiotic is recommended. Day care alterations, avoidance of passive smoke exposure, and allergy management should also be instituted. If a middle ear effusion has been present for 3 months or more, hearing should be tested. If the child has a bilateral hearing deficit of 20 dB or greater, then tympanostomy with pressure equalization (PE) tube placement should be considered. Alternatively, close follow-up and treatment with another second-line agent might be considered. Most physicians, however, would recommend tympanostomy with PE tube placement if the effusions persist for more than 4 to 6 months with hearing loss. This procedure is recommended earlier in cases with speech delay, structural changes in the tympanic membrane (i.e., myringostapediopexy or significant retraction), or multiple antibiotic allergies or in high-risk patients such as those with cleft palate deformity (Table 2). Unilateral disease may be followed up longer, but tympanostomy with

TABLE 2. **Indications for Earlier Definitive Treatment of Otitis Media**

Speech delay
Deep retraction or myringostapediopexy
Multiple antibiotic allergies
Maxillofacial deformities (i.e., cleft palate)

PE tube placement may be required to prevent permanent structural change in the tympanic membrane or cholesteatoma formation.

Treatments for children 3 years of age or older include the combination of steroids, antibiotics, and autoinflation of the middle ear. Prednisone at 1 mg per kg per day for 5 days in combination with a 10-day course of a beta-lactamase stable antibiotic has been shown to result in clearing of the effusion in many cases, but it has a 40% relapse rate. Autoinflation of the middle ear with Otovent (Invotoc International, Jacksonville, Florida) has also produced improvement in up to 60% of ears. Otovent is an inexpensive method for encouraging children to autoinflate the middle ear and involves the use of a nasal tube to inflate a balloon. Decongestants and nasal steroids have not been shown to be effective and are not recommended in this age group.

RECURRENT ACUTE OTITIS MEDIA

Recurrent acute otitis media is defined as more than three episodes of acute otitis media in a 6-month interval or more than four episodes within 1 year. In these cases, preventive measures should be strongly encouraged, such as alternatives to group day care, avoidance of passive smoke exposure, influenzae vaccine, and pneumococcal vaccine (currently for children age 2 years and older). A protein conjugate *S. pneumoniae* vaccine, which has the potential to eliminate nasopharyngeal pneumococci, is currently under development. This vaccine may prevent up to 40% of episodes of acute otitis media in children, similar to the remarkable impact of the *H. influenzae* B vaccine.

Antibiotic prophylaxis for a period of 3 to 6 months may also be considered. The usual recommended drugs include amoxicillin 20 mg per kg per day or sulfisoxazole 35 to 75 mg per kg per day. Sulfisoxazole is favored due to a slightly higher efficacy and the lower possibility of induction of a penicillin-resistant *S.pneumoniae* infection. Two or more breakthrough infections on prophylaxis is an indication for tympanostomy with PE tube placement.

An alternative to the prolonged ventilation of tympanostomy tube placement is currently being studied, that is, office-based tympanostomy. This procedure is performed with a laser or radiofrequency probe with a local anesthetic and sedation. It provides an intermediate level of middle ear ventilation (2 to 4 weeks), which is between myringotomy (24 to 48 hours) and standard tympanostomy tubes (6 to 12 months). Preliminary results indicate a 75% rate of resolution of otitis media with effusion in short term follow-up studies. The procedure avoids the risks of general anesthesia and may decrease the rate of long-term complications associated with PE tubes, including otorrhea, granulation, and tympanic membrane perforation.

The main indications for tympanostomy and PE tube placement include persistent acute otitis media despite third-line antibiotic therapy, recurrent acute otitis media despite prophylactic antibiotics, and bilateral otitis media with effusion and conductive hearing loss.

COMPLICATIONS

The introduction of antibiotics has greatly reduced the incidence of serious complications of otitis media such as brain abscess, subdural empyema, meningitis, and mastoiditis. As the mastoid is a continuous space with the middle ear, subclinical inflammation does occur with each episode of otitis media. This phenomenon is frequently noted on computed tomographic and magnetic resonance imaging scans obtained for unrelated reasons, and it is of little significance. In contrast, true acute coalescent mastoiditis is a result of complicated acute otitis media producing bone destruction within the mastoid. Affected children present with the signs of acute otitis media and a bulging, tender mastoid with sagging or protrusion of the posterosuperior ear canal. This process (i.e., bone destruction) requires a complete mastoidectomy with parenteral antibiotics.

Facial paralysis is also a rare occurrence (0.2%) in association with acute otitis media. Most patients recover fully after immediate tympanostomy and PE tube placement in combination with parenteral antibiotics and steroids. Any evidence of cholesteatoma or granulation compressing the nerve in these patients necessitates mastoidectomy with parenteral antibiotics.

Much more commonly, otitis media can result in hearing loss, tympanic membrane perforation, or progression to chronic otitis media. By definition, acute otitis media is accompanied by an effusion, which typically produces a low-frequency conductive hearing loss of 20 to 30 dB. This loss is usually completely reversible with the spontaneous resolution of the effusion (90% by 3 months) or after tympanostomy tube placement. Tympanic membrane perforations may occur spontaneously or after PE tube placement. The size and location determine the amount of hearing loss, which can range from insignificant up to approximately 30 dB.

The chronic draining ear is usually due to a draining PE tube, a tympanic membrane perforation, granulation tissue, or a cholesteatoma. Initial treatment should include oral antibiotics combined with antibiotic-steroid ear drops (Table 3). The chronic draining ear is associated with multiple bacterial organisms, including *P. aeruginosa*, other gram-negative organisms, *S. aureus*, and anaerobes. These may be associated with a fetid odor, which is usually indicative of bone destruction. Culture guided therapy, frequent aural toilet and suctioning under microscopic guidance, and acetic acid irrigation are often beneficial in these cases. In most cases, surgical therapy is indicated to remove chronically infected bone, granulation tissue, and cholesteatoma.

ACUTE BRONCHITIS AND ACUTE EXACERBATION OF CHRONIC BRONCHITIS

method of
WILLIAM J. HUESTON, M.D.
Medical University of South Carolina
Charleston, South Carolina

ACUTE BRONCHITIS

Acute bronchitis is an inflammatory disease of the lower respiratory tract secondary to acute infection. Although *Mycoplasma pneumoniae* and *Chlamydia pneumoniae* (TWAR) are found in up to 10% of patients with acute bronchitis, viral agents are responsible for the overwhelming majority of cases. Acute bronchitis is a very common condition in primary care, ranking among the top five or six diagnoses seen in the primary care setting.

Pathophysiology

The symptoms of acute bronchitis are caused by excessive mucus production and airway narrowing associated with acute inflammation. Spirometry studies on patients with acute bronchitis demonstrate reversible airway obstruction similar to those seen in asthmatics. As the acute bronchitis episode resolves, these spirometry changes revert to normal. Complaints of shortness of breath, wheezing, and cough are similar to patients with an acute exacerbation of asthma. In fact, patients with new-onset early asthma may be misdiagnosed as having acute bronchitis.

Not all patients with viral respiratory infections develop acute bronchitis. There is probably an interaction between an infectious agent and a susceptible host. Patients with pre-existing bronchial irritation from sources such as cigarettes or occupational exposures and those with a predisposition to reactive airways are more likely to exhibit symptoms consistent with acute bronchitis during a viral respiratory infection.

TABLE 3. **Aural Antibiotics in the Treatment of the Draining Ear**

Antibiotic	Dosage
Neomycin and polymyxin B sulfates and hydrocortisone otic suspension (Cortisporin)	3–4 drops qid
Tobramycin and dexamethasone suspension (TobraDex)*	3–4 drops qid
Gentamicin sulfate solution (Garamycin)	3–4 drops qid
Ofloxacin otic solution (floxin Otic)	5–10 drops bid
Ciprofloxacin HCl solution (Cipro HC Otic)	5 drops bid

*More potent steroid is recommended when granulation tissue is present.

Diagnosis

The diagnosis of acute bronchitis relies on the clinical presentation. Symptoms of bronchitis often accompany those of upper respiratory tract infections and may include a low-grade fever. The hallmarks of acute bronchitis are a productive cough that worsens with exercise or reclining; night cough; and, occasionally, audible wheezing. The productive cough generally lasts between 1 and 2 weeks, although up to 25% of patients may cough for over a month.

Sputum produced in acute bronchitis is usually clear or white but may be yellow, green, or blood-tinged. The color of the sputum is not an accurate predictor of whether bacteria are involved in the infection. Hemoptysis with acute bronchitis is usually limited to minor blood-streaking of sputum and is caused by inflammatory changes in the bronchial tree. Large amounts of bleeding or a cough producing blood clots should prompt evaluation for other sources of bleeding.

The use of a chest radiograph in acute bronchitis should be limited to patients in whom pneumonia is strongly suspected. Routine chest radiographs are not indicated if the patient does not have a high fever or signs of pneumonia on physical examination. Chest radiographs also may be useful if the patient has hemoptysis and is at high risk for bronchogenic malignancies; however, in high-risk patients, cancer is not excluded by a normal chest film.

Routine evaluation of white blood cell count and Gram's stain of the sputum are not useful in making the diagnosis or guiding treatment.

Treatment

Because the vast majority of cases of acute bronchitis are caused by a virus, antibiotics are not an effective treatment. Double blinded placebo-controlled studies using a wide variety of antibiotics have failed to show consistent improvement in acute bronchitis patients.

Treatment of acute bronchitis should be directed toward symptoms. Because of the similarity between acute bronchitis and asthma in spirometry findings, bronchodilators have been investigated as treatment for acute bronchitis. Studies using albuterol and fentolol (not available in the United States) have demonstrated spirometric and clinical improvement in patients taking these beta agonists. In two studies using albuterol, patients treated with active drug were almost twice as likely to have stopped coughing in 1 week as those treated with antibiotics or placebo.

In addition to bronchodilators, cough suppressants may be useful in treating patients with cough that interferes with their ability to work or rest. Codeine-containing cough medications are effective agents at reducing cough in patients with bronchitis.

Complications

As indicated earlier, nearly all patients with acute bronchitis have resolution of their symptoms within 2 weeks. However, a small proportion continue to cough for 1 month or longer. In these patients, chronic use of a bronchodilator may alleviate their symptoms. Also, it has been suggested that these patients may have a *Mycoplasma* or *Chlamydia* infection, although there has been little evidence to substantiate that bacterial infections are more likely in patients with chronic cough. Nevertheless, empirical use of a macrolide when coughing for a month may be more cost effective than pursuing other laboratory or radiologic tests.

Another possible complication of *Chlamydia* bronchitis is adult-onset asthma. Investigations of patients with adult-onset asthma have noted that a large proportion have serologic evidence of previous *C. pneumoniae* infection. It has been hypothesized that asthma symptoms in these patients actually represent a chronic *Chlamydia* bronchitis infection. There are still many unanswered questions about *Chlamydia* and adult-onset asthma, however. Although a very small open-label trial did demonstrate some improvement in adult asthma patients treated with a macrolide antibiotic, there is little evidence that symptoms of adult-onset asthma can be permanently reduced with antibiotic use. Also, it is unclear whether early treatment of *Chlamydia* bronchitis confers any protective effect against subsequent development of asthma symptoms. For now, this is an intriguing possibility that requires additional research before clear recommendations for treatment can be offered.

ACUTE EXACERBATION OF CHRONIC BRONCHITIS

Patients with pre-existing chronic bronchitis frequently experience an exacerbation of their illness. Instead of their customary chronic cough and usual sputum, they experience increasing shortness of breath along with changes in the severity of cough or characteristic of the sputum. These types of episodes are categorized as an acute exacerbation of chronic bronchitis, which should not be confused with acute bronchitis in an otherwise healthy person.

Pathophysiology

Patients with chronic bronchitis have a daily productive cough for more than 3 months. In contrast to acute bronchitis, patients with chronic bronchitis experience irreversible bronchial wall thickening and hypertrophy of underlying mucous glands secondary to prolonged exposure to bronchial irritants such as cigarette smoke. Excessive mucus secretion results in the daily sputum production that typifies chronic bronchitis.

Because of the excessive mucus production and poor mucociliary clearance, patients with chronic bronchitis often experience superinfection with bacteria and are more susceptible to respiratory viruses. Because the mucus present in the bronchial tree is an ideal culture medium for bacteria, the bacteria found in sputum often do not represent an acute infection; rather, they are colonizers. There is no simple way to differentiate colonization from super-infection, however.

Diagnosis

Acute exacerbation of chronic bronchitis is defined as changes in respiratory status and sputum appearance without evidence of underlying pneumonia. Symptoms of respiratory distress or worsened dyspnea in the presence of a change in the color, consistency, or severity of cough usually are sufficient to make the diagnosis. Because of the compromised respiratory status of patients with chronic bronchitis, a chest radiograph may be useful to exclude pneumonia as the cause of these symptoms.

Because a large number of organisms may colonize the respiratory tract in patients with chronic bronchitis, Gram's stain of sputum is not useful in directing therapy. Organisms frequently found in sputum include *M. pneumonia, Haemophilus influenzae, Streptococcus pneumoniae,* and *Branhamella catarrhalis,* but, as noted earlier, it is difficult to assign causation in many acute exacerbations of chronic bronchitis. Many acute exacerbations actually may be viral in origin.

Treatment

Because of the underlying bacteria in the respiratory tract of patients with chronic bronchitis and the difficulty in deciding when a bacterial infection is present, most acute exacerbations of chronic bronchitis are treated with antibiotic therapy. Although small studies have yielded conflicting evidence regarding the effectiveness of antibiotic in acute exacerbations of chronic bronchitis, a meta-analysis did demonstrate improvement in symptoms when antibiotics were prescribed.

Antibiotic selection in acute exacerbations of chronic bronchitis is difficult because the offending organism is not usually identified. Although multiple suggestions have been offered to guide antibiotic selection, the original studies that demonstrated improvement all used either tetracycline analogues, amoxicillin, or sulfamethoxazole-trimethoprim (SMZ-TMP). Because there is no evidence that cephalosporins, quinolones, or macrolides are superior to these drugs and all are more expensive, treatment with tetracycline/doxycycline, amoxicillin, or SMZ-TMP is likely to offer the most benefit for the least cost.

In addition to antibiotics, short courses of corticosteroids (prednisone, 60 mg per day for 5 days) may shorten the course and reduce the severity of acute exacerbations of chronic bronchitis. Acute exacerbations may also afford another opportunity to counsel tobacco-using patients about the need to discontinue smoking.

Complications

Patients with severe chronic bronchitis may be significantly compromised by an acute exacerbation. Respiratory failure and the need for mechanical ventilation are rare but can occur in patients with very limited respiratory reserve.

Prevention

Physicians can encourage patients to do two things to reduce the likelihood or severity of an acute exacerbation of chronic bronchitis. Smoking cessation is the first key to reducing progression of chronic bronchitis and lessening the risk of an exacerbation. Second, annual influenza vaccination and a single vaccination against *Pneumococcus pneumoniae* are effective tools at preventing superinfection.

BACTERIAL PNEUMONIA

method of
J. THOMAS CROSS, JR., M.D., M.P.H.
LSU Medical Center–Shreveport
Shreveport, Louisiana

In the United States, community-acquired pneumonia is a common infection with an incidence of 1% in the general population per year. Pneumonia is the sixth most common cause of death. Estimated costs of treatment, including direct patient care costs and lost income from sick days, are more than $20 billion per year in the United States. Community-acquired pneumonia accounts for over 10 million physician visits per year. In patients older than 65 years of age, 1% a year in this age group will develop pneumonia severe enough to require hospitalization. Over 90% of deaths due to pneumonia occur in patients older than age 65.

Guidelines have been written by various expert panels to help with the selection of antibiotic therapy. Differing opinions exist within these panels as to what are the preferred ways to diagnose and treat this common infection.

ETIOLOGY

Studies conducted worldwide show that *Streptococcus pneumoniae* is the most common cause of community-acquired pneumonia. The incidence of *S. pneumoniae* as an etiology of pneumonia varies widely from 27 to over 55% in the United States. Today *S. pneumoniae* is still the primary concern of the physician when approaching a patient with community-acquired pneumonia. Concern has increased even though rates of infection with this organism are stable and newer antibiotics have become available. The rapid rise in resistance of *S. pneumoniae* to drugs in the 1990s has led to anxiety about covering this organism adequately.

The next most common pathogen varies depending on the study design. If viruses are isolated effectively, they generally are in second place. If serology is used as a diagnostic tool, then atypical pathogens such as *Chlamydia pneumoniae, Mycoplasma pneumoniae,* and *Legionella* become more prominent in incidence rates. If standard bacterial cultures are the means of detecting the etiology then *Haemophilus influenzae* follows *S. pneumoniae* as the next most common cause of community-acquired pneumonia. Other possible explanations besides laboratory techniques include geographical considerations and demographic differences in patient populations. In addition, co-infection with more than one organism varies between 10 and 40% of patients.

After these organisms, gram-negative rods generally are next most common. Other etiologies included *Mycobacterium tuberculosis*, fungal etiologies, and rare bacteria with these being discussed elsewhere.

In patients older than age 65, *S. pneumoniae* continues to be the most common etiology of community-acquired pneumonia. *H. influenzae*, gram-negative rods, respiratory viruses, and *Staphylococcus aureus* are more common in the elderly than in their younger cohorts. Many authors report that *M. pneumoniae* and other atypical pathogens occur less frequently in the elderly. However, data indicate that *M. pneumoniae* and *C. pneumoniae* may cause more infection in the elderly than previously thought.

Seasonal variation is thought to possibly be an important factor in the etiology of community-acquired pneumonia; however, no well-controlled trials have been able to confirm this. *S. pneumoniae* continues to be the most common cause of pneumonia throughout all seasons, although viral etiologies definitely increase during the winter and spring. In addition, in winter months, there are increased rates of *S. aureus* as an etiology of pneumonia in patients with recent influenza virus respiratory infection.

Even today, the etiology may not be determined in 25 to 50% of cases. As a result, many patients with community-acquired pneumonia must be treated empirically. Factors to consider in determining choice of antibiotic will be discussed next.

Nosocomial pneumonia is generally due to aerobic gram-negative rods. Frequently these infections are due to highly resistant organisms. Methicillin-resistant *S. aureus* has also become important in many centers as an etiology of hospital-acquired pneumonia.

HOST FACTORS

Predisposition to community-acquired pneumonia is increased in alcoholism, malnutrition, immunosuppression, and chronic disease states, and in persons with recent hospitalization. Smoking likely increases the risk of bacterial pneumonia by impairing pulmonary clearance of bacteria. Diabetics, chronic steroid users, cirrhotics, and renal dialysis patients have increased rates of pneumonia, possibly because of diminished neutrophil function and phagocytic activity. Patients with human immunodeficiency virus (HIV), malignancies (particularly lymphoma or myeloma patients), and other conditions with diminished immunoglobulin production are at increased risk. Splenectomized and sickle cell patients are at high risk for infection with encapsulated organisms such as *S. pneumoniae* and *H. influenzae*.

Of particular concern are patients with history of chronic obstructive pulmonary disease (COPD) who continue to smoke. These patients have a markedly increased rate of bacterial pneumonia. Organisms isolated frequently include *H. influenzae*, *Branhamella catarrhalis*, and *Legionella* infections. Gram-negative rods are more common in alcoholics and patients with chronic aspiration states. As stated previously, *S. aureus* is more common during influenza outbreaks and also in intravenous drug abusers.

Zoonotic, geographic, and occupational exposure can be important in the etiologies suspected. Pet shop owners and bird fanciers may be at risk for *Chlamydia psittaci*. Hunters in Arkansas/Missouri are at risk for *Francisella tularensis*. Cattle and cats have been implicated in *Coxiella burnetii* infections in the United States and Canada. Water storage areas used for heaters and air conditioners can harbor *Legionella*. Physicians should be familiar with local factors that may increase the likelihood of certain pathogens.

Nosocomial host factors generally follow those of the community. Patients who are hospitalized and debilitated are at high risk for development of hospital-acquired infections, including pneumonia.

CLINICAL PRESENTATION

Fever with cough, sputum production, dyspnea, and pleuritc chest pain are the presenting symptoms of bacterial pneumonia. Previously, medical students were taught that microbial etiology could be predicted reliably by the clinical presentation. However, well-controlled studies have revealed that presenting signs and symptoms cannot be used reliably to differentiate between "typical" and atypical pathogens.

Symptoms occurring outside of the respiratory tract can occur in 10 to 30% of patients with community-acquired pneumonia. These include headache, myalgias, arthralgia, and gastrointestinal symptoms. Interestingly, the elderly have fewer symptoms than do patients younger than age 65. It is not known whether this phenomenon is due to true physiologic effect of aging or diminished subjective response to symptoms.

Fever occurs in over 80% of patients. If careful clinical examination is undertaken crackles can also be heard in 80% of patients on auscultation. Consolidation can be documented on physical examination in 30% of patients.

DIAGNOSIS

Chest radiography should be used to confirm the clinical suspicion of pneumonia. Although findings on radiographs may suggest a particular bacterial pathogen, a microbiologic diagnosis should not be based solely on radiographic features. An important factor to consider is that patients who are substantially volume-depleted may initially present with a normal chest radiograph. Repeat radiography after hydration will show the evidence for pneumonia. Lobar infiltrates are common, but diffuse alveolar infiltrates can also occur. Cavitary lesions can be seen most commonly with *S. aureus*, *S. pneumoniae*, anaerobes, and obviously *M. tuberculosis*. Parapneumonic effusions occur with *S. pneumoniae* and *S. aureus*.

Resolution of disease on chest radiography can take weeks or months. It is controversial whether every patient with community-acquired pneumonia needs a follow-up chest radiograph. Most physicians would consider it for the elderly and those with underlying chronic conditions at a 6-week follow-up visit. Whether a healthy young adult needs a follow-up radiograph is debated among experts.

Hospitalized patients with community-acquired pneumonia should have a complete blood count, electrolytes, renal function tests (blood urea nitrogen [BUN], creatinine), liver function tests, and arterial oxygenation determination (arterial blood-gas analysis or pulse oximetry, depending on the severity of the patient's condition). The use of blood cultures in patients with pneumonia has been questioned; however, most authorities still recommend blood cultures be performed for those who require hospitalization. In addition, the Centers for Disease Control and Prevention recommend serologic testing for HIV-1 infection in young patients with pneumonia, among whom the rate of HIV-infected patients is at least 1 in 1000 for hospital discharges in the community.

Patients with pleural effusions who it is determined can undergo thoracentesis should have this performed. Some authors have suggested that 10 mm of fluid on a lateral decubitus film warrants diagnostic thoracentesis. Pleural fluid analysis should include Gram's stain and culture, cell count and differential, protein, lactate dehydrogenase, glucose, and pH measurements. Smears and cultures for mycobacterial and fungal pathogens should be considered. If an empyema is indicated by the fluid analysis, drainage and chest tube placement are indicated.

The controversy of Gram's stain and culture of expectorated sputum continues. This laboratory test is debated by pulmonologists and infectious disease experts. Guidelines for the management of community-acquired pneumonia from the American Thoracic Society in 1993 called for empirical antibiotic therapy without regard to Gram's stain findings. The British Thoracic Society believes that Gram's stain is useful but note that it is specific but not sensitive in determining the microbiologic etiology of community-acquired pneumonia. The Infectious Diseases Society of America supports the use of sputum Gram's stain, but the recommendation is based mainly on expert opinion without strong supporting evidence.

The latter two organizations believe that Gram's stain is useful in the initial selection of antimicrobial therapy and culture results can confirm or alter the initial choice of antibiotics. Most authorities believe that an adequate sputum sample should have fewer than 10 squamous epithelial cells and more than 25 polymorphonuclear leukocytes per low-power field. Culture can be helpful to determine presence of resistant pathogens, particularly the prevalence of penicillin- and cephalosporin-resistant pneumococcus. Culture, however, can frequently indicate colonization and not true infectious etiology; therefore correlation with Gram's stain results are recommended.

Some patients do not actively produce sputum or have poor quality production. Patient history of previous antimicrobial therapy must also be considered. Antibiotic therapy should not be delayed if Gram's stain interpretation is not an immediate option. In elderly patients, it has been shown that antibiotics started within 8 hours of presentation result in less mortality. Many authorities recommend starting empirical therapy if a sputum sample cannot be examined in this time period.

Use of fiberoptic bronchoscopy is generally reserved for severely ill or immunocompromised patients. This test with protected brush cultures can be of diagnostic value. The prior use of antibiotics in these patients, however, generally reduces the effectiveness of this invasive procedure.

For atypical pathogens, the best method in clinical practice is difficult to determine. Serologic evaluation can be made for *Legionella* species, *M. pneumoniae*, and *C. pneumoniae*, but the sensitivities of these serologic tests are quite variable and are retrospective in nature. *Legionella* can be cultured on special media with selective techniques frequently not found in community hospitals. Immunofluorescence techniques and a DNA probe for the detection of *Legionella* antigen in sputum have been developed. Urinary antigen detection by radioimmunoassay has a sensitivity of 80 to 99% and a specificity of 99%. This antigen can only detect *L. pneumophila* serogroup 1, which accounts for 70 to 90% of *Legionella* cases.

Mycoplasma cultures can take a week to return and require specialized techniques. *C. pneumoniae* is an obligate intracellular pathogen and therefore culture is not generally feasible. A polymerase chain reaction (PCR) test will likely allow more rapid diagnosis but is not yet clinically available. Currently, many authors do not pursue testing for atypical pathogens unless the patient is not responding to routine beta-lactam antibiotics, high rates of community-acquired *Legionella* exist, or epidemiologic information indicates that occupational or recreational exposure to water sources possibly contaminated with *Legionella* has occurred.

ANTIBIOTIC THERAPY

Because *S. pneumoniae* is the most common cause of pneumonia and the decline in its susceptibility has spread, particularly in the 1990s, treatment regimens focus on this organism. It should be noted however that virulence between the susceptible and nonsusceptible is no different. Isolates of *S. pneumoniae* are classified as penicillin susceptible if the minimum inhibitory concentration (MIC) is 0.1 μg per mL or less. They are considered intermediately susceptible if the MIC is between 0.1 and 1 μg per mL and resistant if the MIC is 2 μg per mL or more. Surveillance data from the United States show wide variation in the prevalence of resistant pneumococcus. In the mid- to late 1980s, only 5% of strains had intermediate susceptibility, and resistant pneumococcus was nonexistent. By the mid-1990s nearly 11% of strains nationwide showed intermediate susceptibility and 3 to 5% were penicillin resistant. Isolates of pneumococcus from pediatric day care attendees in the mid-1990s showed rates as high as 50 to 60% for intermediate susceptible and 20 to 30% for penicillin resistance.

Strains of *S. pneumoniae* with lowered susceptibility to penicillin generally have some cross-resistance to cephalosporins. However, third-generation cephalosporins such as ceftriaxone (Rocephin) and cefotaxime (Claforan) are still effective against most strains of *S. pneumoniae* that cause pneumonia. However, there are some strains of *S. pneumoniae* that are sensitive to penicillin but resistant to cephalosporins.

Cross-resistance to other antibiotics used in pneumococcal infections is also becoming more common. Erythromycin, the newer macrolides (azithromycin [Zithromax], clarithromycin [Biaxin]), clindamycin (Cleocin), doxycycline (Vibramycin), other tetracyclines, and trimethoprim/sulfamethoxazole (Bactrim) are seeing resistance rates rise. In some communities, erythromycin resistance is near 50% if penicillin resistance is already present.

Other antibiotics may be useful against beta-lactam-resistant pneumococci. All strains of *S. pneumoniae*, including those resistant to penicillin and cephalosporins, are susceptible to vancomycin. Activity of the quinolones has been looked at carefully in recent studies. Ciprofloxacin (Cipro) essentially has poor activity against many strains and is not recommended for empirical therapy for community-acquired pneumonia. The newer quinolones (trovafloxacin [Trovan], grepafloxacin [Raxar], sparfloxacin

[Zagam], levofloxacin [Levaquin]) have increased activity against *S. pneumoniae*. Quinolones tend to cause the selection of resistance to themselves and to other quinolones in most gram-positive bacteria that have been studied. It remains to be seen if the newer quinolones wil remain susceptible or follow in ciprofloxacin's path of resistance.

The other main bacterial pathogen in community-acquired pneumonia, *H. influenzae*, is generally susceptible to cefuroxime (Ceftin, Zinacef), third-generation cephalosporins (cefotaxime, ceftriaxone, ceftizoxime) and to all the fluoroquinolones. *H. influenzae* is less susceptible to the newer macrolides (azithromycin, clarithromycin). The newer fluoroquinolones and macrolides have in vitro activity against the atypical pathogens including *M. pneumoniae*, *C. pneumoniae*, and *Legionella*.

Currently penicillin resistance in strains of *S. pneumoniae* can be overcome with high-dose penicillins (at least 12 million units per day). Currently levels of resistance to penicillin and cephalosporins in *S. pneumoniae* do not preclude effective therapy for pneumococcal pneumonia and sepsis with high-dose penicillin. Highly penicillin-resistant *S. pneumoniae* can be treated with imipenem (Primaxin) or meropenem (Merrem) at present. Other options include vancomycin, and the newer quinolones. Each hospital should monitor its resistance rates of penicillin and determine whether MICs greater than 2 μg per mL are occurring in community-acquired pneumococcal infections in their setting. It is the responsibility of the physician to be aware of what resistance patterns are occurring in his or her community.

Initial Therapy of Community-Acquired Pneumonia

Many authorities would recommend using a penicillin or macrolide as empirical therapy. Doxycycline (100 mg twice daily [bid]) has been recommended by the Infectious Diseases Society of America as an appropriate agent. For the treatment of pneumococcal pneumonia in patients not admitted to the hospital, an antipneumococcal quinolone (levofloxacin, sparfloxacin, grepafloxacin, trovafloxacin) could be used if multidrug resistance is prevalent in the community. Other macrolides such as azithromycin (Azithromax) or clarithromycin may be alternatives especially for convenience (5 days of once daily therapy for the former). See Table 1 for a summary of antibiotic therapies.

For patients admitted to the hospital in the nonintensive care setting, a gram-stained smear of sputum or empyema fluid should be done. It this shows probable *S. pneumoniae* then high-dose penicillin (Penicillin G, 2 million units every 4 hours) could be adequate or a second- or third-generation cephalosporin. Patients with severe beta-lactam allergies could be treated with intravenous vancomycin (1 gram every 12 hours) or a quinolone. Levofloxacin and trovafloxacin are available for parenteral and oral use.

TABLE 1. **Initial Antibiotic Therapy for Community-Acquired Pneumonia**

Setting/Pathogen	Primary Treatment	Other
Outpatient		
S. pneumoniae	Amoxicillin Doxycycline (Vibramycin)	Quinolone*
H. influenzae	Cefuroxime (Ceftin) Amoxicillin/ clavulanate (Augmentin)	Quinolone* Azithromycin (Zithromax)
Unknown-young person	Doxycycline	Quinolone*
Unknown-high risk	Quinolone*	
Hospitalized (non-intensive care)		
S. pneumoniae	Penicillin G (12 million U/d)	Cephalosporin
H. influenzae	Cephalosporin	Quinolone
S. aureus	Nafcillin (Unipen)	Vancomycin (Vancocin)
Gram-negative rod	Cephalosporin + aminoglycoside	Imipenem (Primaxin) +/−, aminoglycoside
Unknown	Cephalosporin + macrolide	Quinolone*
Intensive care		
Cover all common organisms	Cephalosporin + macrolide Imipenem +/− aminoglycoside +/− macrolide	

*Quinolone: levofloxacin (Levaquin), sparfloxacin (Zagam), grepafloxacin (Raxar), trovafloxacin (Trovan).

If the sputum Gram's stain is nondiagnostic or if no sputum is available, then treatment should be aimed at *S. pneumoniae* and the other common pathogens. In these cases, many authorities recommend a second- or third-generation cephalosporin combined with a macrolide. An alternative is the use of a newer quinolone with antipneumococcal activity.

For intensive care patients who have a sputum consistent with *S. pneumoniae*, appropriate therapy could include a second- or third-generation cephalosporin combined with vancomycin or a quinolone (if concern of resistant pneumococcus is high). If the Gram stained smear is not helpful or available, then the use of a third-generation cephalosporin with erythromycin (500 mg to 1 gram intravenously [IV] every 6 hours) is generally recommended. Some authorities would add an aminoglycoside, although community-acquired pneumonia due to resistant gram-negative organisms is rare in most communities. Obviously if the patient has underlying conditions such as cystic fibrosis, then broader gram-negative coverage is definitely indicated. If diagnostic information becomes available that shows a specific pathogen (blood culture, empyema culture, *Legionella* urinary antigen positive) then the treatment can be narrowed accordingly.

Once the patient has improved in response to therapy and the patient can tolerate oral medications, therapy can be switched from intravenous to oral therapy. If the pathogen is known and susceptibility testing reveals its sensitivities, then oral therapy appropriate for the organism is recommended. If it is sensitive to amoxicillin (500 mg orally [PO] three times daily [tid]) or erythromycin (various formulations), these should be used. Otherwise, an oral cephalosporin, such as cefuroxime (250 mg PO bid) or cefpodoxime (Vantin), or a quinolone could be used. If the etiology of the pneumonia is unknown then the use of a quinolone might be appropriate for continued empirical therapy. The total course of therapy is generally 7 to 10 days, depending on the patient's severity of conditions. In cases of sepsis, longer therapy up to 14 days is indicated. For *Legionella*, some authorities recommend 21 days of therapy.

NOSOCOMIAL PNEUMONIA THERAPY

The mortality rate for nosocomial pneumonia remains high. The physician should base therapy for nosocomial pneumonia on the organisms that inhabit the hospital and ward setting where the patient becomes ill. Gram-negative bacteria, particularly *Pseudomonas*, *Enterobacter*, and *Acinetobacter*, are frequently seen as etiologies for nosocomial pneumonia. Empirical therapy usually includes a broad-spectrum cephalosporin such as ceftazidime (Fortaz), 1 gram IV every 8 hours, or broad-spectrum penicillins such as piperacillin/tazobactam (Zosyn, 3.375 grams IV every 6 hours) plus an aminoglycoside (gentamicin). If methicillin-resistant *S. aureus* is a problem in the hospital, vancomycin should also be added for empirical therapy; particularly if sputum or endotracheal secretions show evidence of this organism. After an organism is identified as the etiology, antibiotic coverage can be narrowed to cover the pathogen.

VIRAL RESPIRATORY INFECTIONS

method of
THOMAS R. CATE, M.D.
Baylor College of Medicine
Houston, Texas

Among the most common human infections are those associated with respiratory viruses. These agents spread from person to person by aerosol, droplets, fomites, or contact and cause infection and disease in various sites within the respiratory tract. The viruses involved belong to several groups, including orthomyxovirus (influenza), paramyxovirus (parainfluenza and respiratory syncytial viruses), picornavirus (rhinoviruses and enteroviruses), coronavirus, and adenovirus. Infections with these viruses occur more frequently in children than in adults and more often during colder months than warmer months in temperate climates. Manifestations of infection, although sometimes very minor, can include fever, malaise, myalgia, and symptoms caused by rhinitis, pharyngitis, laryngitis, laryngotracheobronchitis (croup), bronchitis, bronchiolitis, and pneumonia, alone or in various combinations. A likely

etiologic diagnosis can sometimes be made on the basis of clinical findings and epidemiologic data, but considerable overlap can occur in the illnesses caused by different viruses. Also, infection with any of them may increase airway reactivity to cold or pollutants or exacerbate preexisting asthma.

Respiratory virus illnesses are usually self-limited, but laryngotracheobronchitis, bronchiolitis, and pneumonia can be life-threatening. Specific antiviral medications are available for treatment of acute influenza A virus infections (see the article on influenza) and for severe bronchiolitis and pneumonia due to respiratory syncytial virus (see the article on viral and mycoplasmal pneumonias). Secondary bacterial infections involving paranasal sinuses, middle ear, bronchi, and/or lungs may develop a few days into the illness, often as the viral infection itself is fading, and necessitate antimicrobial therapy (see separate articles).

GENERAL PRINCIPLES OF TREATMENT

Most respiratory virus infections cause mild to moderate nasal obstruction, nasal discharge, hoarseness, cough, and/or malaise for only a few days. Maintaining good hydration to facilitate clearance of secretions, minimizing exposure to irritants such as smoke, and resting as much as possible are mainstays of treatment. Alcohol can transiently interfere with clearance of secretions and with cellular immune and phagocytic functions and should be avoided. With exception of the few specific antiviral agents, medications for treatment of respiratory virus infections are aimed primarily at alleviation of bothersome symptoms. Many products containing various combinations of decongestant, antihistamine, expectorant, antitussive, and/or analgesic medications are available for this purpose. I prefer to prescribe those containing one or a limited number of medications aimed at treating the most bothersome symptoms, so that possible complications are not obscured or perhaps are even promoted by interfering with clearance of secretions. Antibacterial agents should not be used unless signs, symptoms, and laboratory data suggest a secondary bacterial infection; earlier use risks unnecessary side effects and appearance of resistant organisms.

Isolation of infected, noninstitutionalized patients is not helpful for reducing transmission when respiratory virus illnesses are widespread in the community because unrecognized exposures will be frequent, but segregation or confinement may help reduce spread in an institutional environment. Also, staying home during the acute phase of a sporadic respiratory virus illness may spare a patient's work associates the infection. Covering coughs, avoiding close contact, and frequent hand washing are other measures that can reduce transmission.

TREATMENT OF SPECIFIC SYMPTOMS

Systemic symptoms of fever, malaise, and myalgias are often accompanied by headache; together with cough, they are typical components of the influenza syndrome. Although viruses other than influenza can cause this syndrome, it is probably attributable to an influenza virus when activity of these agents is high in the community, and it may be an indication for antiviral treatment (see the article on influenza). Whether caused by infection with influenza or another agent, the systemic symptoms themselves often necessitate treatment in order to facilitate rest. Reduction of high fever in infants and young children is also important for reducing the risk of febrile convulsions, and sponging with tepid water or alcohol may be required in addition to the medications listed subsequently.

Systemic symptoms can usually be alleviated by acetaminophen. Acetaminophen is preferred over aspirin, particularly in children, because of aspirin's association with Reye's syndrome in children when used during influenza or varicella virus infections. Acetaminophen is available in tablet, capsule, liquid, and suppository forms. Usual dosing for adults is 325 to 650 mg at 4- to 6-hour intervals as needed, with a maximal dose of 4.0 grams per day over a 10-day interval and 2.6 grams per day over longer intervals. Alcoholic beverages may increase this drug's potential for hepatotoxicity and should be avoided. Acetaminophen may be given to infants and children up to five times a day, at least 4 hours apart, in the following age-based doses as needed: 40 mg up to 3 months; 80 mg at 4 to 12 months; 120 mg at 1 to 2 years; 160 mg at 2 to 4 years; 240 mg at 4 to 6 years; 320 mg at 6 to 9 years; 320 to 400 mg at 9 to 11 years; and 320 to 480 mg at 11 to 12 years.

Ibuprofen can also be used for treating systemic symptoms in both adults and children. An advantage of ibuprofen is longer relief (1 or 2 hours more) of symptoms than with acetaminophen, but among potential disadvantages are gastric irritation and lack of a suppository form for patients in whom nausea and vomiting accompany the systemic symptoms. The dosages of ibuprofen are 200 to 400 mg at 4- to 6-hour intervals as needed for adults and, for children, 5 to 10 mg per kg at 6- to 8-hour intervals as needed, not to exceed 40 mg per kg. If it is desired, adults may substitute aspirin in a dosage of 325 to 650 mg every 4 to 6 hours as needed. If nausea and vomiting accompany the systemic symptoms, promethazine has antiemetic, antihistaminic, and sedative effects that can be useful in this setting and is available in tablet, syrup, and suppository forms. A common dosage of promethazine (Phenergan) is 25 mg for adults, given 1 to 4 times a day as needed, or 0.5 mg per pound for children weighing less than 50 pounds.

Nasal obstruction often accompanies respiratory virus infections and may force mouth breathing, prevent clearance of secretions, and interfere with feeding. When nasal obstruction is caused by thick secretions, saline nose drops, increased humidification in the room, and increased fluid intake may be effective at alleviating symptoms. When nasal obstruction is caused primarily by inflamed mucous membranes, temporary use of oral or topical sympathomimetic decongestants can be helpful. For oral administration, pseudoephedrine is available in capsule, tablet, and liquid formulations; the dosages are 30 to 60 mg at 4- to 6-hour intervals (maximum, 240 mg per day) for adults and 2 mg per pound per day in 4 divided doses as needed for children. Side effects of nervousness or insomnia, or both, may occur, particularly at higher doses of pseudoephedrine. A topical decongestant such as 0.25% phenylephrine, 2 or 3 drops into each nostril, relieves nasal obstruction for 3 to 4 hours and may be repeated at 4-hour intervals as needed. Longer acting (8- to 12-hour) preparations containing 0.1% xylometazoline (Otrivin) or 0.05% oxymetazoline (Afrin) are also available. A possible side effect of topical decongestants is rebound nasal congestion; also, they lose effectiveness and may cause burning, dryness, or stinging of the nasal mucosa with prolonged use.

Nasal discharge and sneezing during respiratory virus illness in adolescents and adults can be reduced, if believed necessary, through the anticholinergic activity of first-generation antihistamines such as chlorpheniramine, 4 mg every 4 hours, or clemastine (Tavist), 1.34 mg every 12 hours as needed, but may cause either drowsiness or more viscid secretions that are difficult to clear. More selective, nonsedating antihistamines are less likely to be effective unless allergies are contributing to the excess secretions. For infants and young children, a nasal suction bulb is helpful for removal of secretions.

Throat irritation can be soothed by gargling with warm salt water (½ teaspoonful of salt in 4 ounces or about one half glass of warm water). However, definite pain on swallowing together with fever might indicate streptococcal pharyngitis and necessitates diagnostic evaluation, particularly if it persists longer than a couple of days (see the article on streptococcal pharyngitis). Hoarseness is best managed by voice rest and breathing air with high humidity.

The urge to cough can also often be reduced and the clearance of secretions enhanced by breathing highly humidified air. The expectorant guaifenesin can loosen secretions, thus facilitating their clearance; it is available in tablets and capsules and in liquid preparations with and without alcohol. Alcohol-free Robitussin contains 100 mg of guaifenesin per teaspoonful, and the dosage that may be given every 4 hours as needed is ½ teaspoonful for children 2 to 6 years of age, 1 teaspoonful for those 6 to 12 years, and 2 teaspoonfuls for older persons. Cough suppression with the antitussive dextromethorphan is reserved for cough that interferes with rest or sleep but should generally be avoided in patients with chronic obstructive pulmonary disease. Dextromethorphan is available in strengths of 7.5 and 15 mg per teaspoonful (Robitussin Pediatric and Robitussin Maximum Strength Cough Suppressant), and doses administered every 6 to 8 hours as needed are 15 to 30 mg for persons older than 12 years, 7.5 mg for those aged 6 to 12 years, and 3.75 mg for those aged 2 to 6 years.

Croup in a child can be frightening because of the

inspiratory whoop as air is sucked past the subglottic narrowing caused by inflammation and spasm. Intense humidification of the air, perhaps in a shower stall or bathroom, often reduces the spasm and whooping, which then gradually clear over 3 to 4 days. However, air exchange can be so impaired during the acute illness as to cause hypoxemia, which necessitates hospitalization for therapy with oxygen, nebulized racemic epinephrine, and systemic corticosteroids (see the article on acute respiratory failure).

VIRAL AND MYCOPLASMAL PNEUMONIAS

method of
STEPHEN G. BAUM, M.D.
Beth Israel Medical Center
New York, New York
The Albert Einstein College of Medicine
Bronx, New York

Viral and mycoplasmal pneumonias constitute the majority of what used to be called "primary atypical pneumonias," a term used for pulmonary infections, the etiology of which could not be determined by culture or Gram's stain, and which did not respond to penicillin therapy. Other so-called atypical pneumonias are now known to be due to *Chlamydia* and *Legionella* (discussed elsewhere). It is important to establish the etiology of these pneumonias because there are effective therapeutic agents for many such infections.

VIRAL PNEUMONIAS

Etiologic Agents

Although many viruses can cause pneumonia, the most commonly identified agents in normal hosts are respiratory syncytial virus (RSV), influenza virus, parainfluenza virus, adenovirus, and some of the enteroviruses such as Coxsackie B and enterocytopathogenic human orphan (ECHO) viruses. In immu-nocompromised patients such as those with acquired immune deficiency syndrome (AIDS) or cancer, cytomegalovirus, herpesviruses, and adenoviruses are relatively common. A newly described agent, hantavirus, has caused life-threatening pneumonia outbreaks in the western United States and isolated cases on the East coast. Measles virus and varicella-zoster virus can cause pneumonia as part of their full-blown clinical syndromes. Unfortunately, the rest produce no clinical signs or symptoms that would point easily and certainly to an etiologic diagnosis. However, there are some epidemiologic and clinical factors that make one agent more likely than another, and these are listed in Table 1. Diagnosis can be aided by rapid culture and increasingly available molecular biologic methods (such as polymerase chain reactions) applied to sputum samples and, in severe and persistent cases, to bronchoalveolar lavage specimens to reveal nucleic acid of the etiologic agent.

Treatment

Agents such as influenza virus, respiratory syncytial virus, and adenoviruses most often cause upper respiratory disease that necessitates only supportive symptomatic therapy. When severe viral pneumonia supervenes, there are antiviral agents that may have efficacy; some of these are listed in Table 2. In these cases, an infectious disease consultation should be obtained to assist in the complex therapeutic decisions necessary.

MYCOPLASMAL PNEUMONIA

Etiologic Agent

Mycoplasma pneumoniae is one of the most common agents causing upper respiratory infection and may account for more than 100,000 cases of pneumonia a year in the United States. It is most common in young adults, particularly those in populations living in close quarters such as boarding schools and military recruit camps, but it can cause disease in

TABLE 1. **Clinical and Epidemiologic Aids in the Diagnosis of Viral and Mycoplasmal Pneumonia**

Virus	Patient	Season	Symptoms and Signs	Other
Respiratory syncytial virus	Infant, adult	Winter	Wheezing, persistent cough	
Influenza	Adult	Winter	Myalgias, headache	Epidemic
Adenovirus	Young adult military recruits, boarding students, transplant recipients	Winter		
Cytomegalovirus	AIDS patients, transplant recipients	Any	Cytomegalovirus retinitis	
Herpes simplex	Immunocompromised	Any		
Enterovirus	Adult	Summer-Fall	Rash, diarrhea, pleuritis, orchitis	
Hantavirus	Adult	Any	Renal failure, capillary leak	Mouse exposure
Mycoplasma pneumoniae	Young adult, adult, child	Any	Cough, insidious onset	10–21 d incubation period

TABLE 2. **Therapeutic Agents for Viral Pneumonia**

Virus	Specific Antiviral Therapy	Dosage
Respiratory syncytial virus	Ribavirin (Virazole)	Aerosol 12–18 h/d
Influenza type A	Amantadine (Symmetrel)*	Adult: 100 mg PO, bid for 5 d§ (>65 y, 100 mg PO daily)
		Child: 5 mg/kg/d PO divided Q 12 h (max 150 mg/d)§
	Rimantadine (Flumadine)*	Adult: 100–200 mg PO q d for 7 d§ (>65 y, 100 mg PO daily)
Influenza types A, B, & C	Zanamivir (Relenza)	FDA approval pending
Adenovirus	None	
Cytomegalovirus	Ganciclovir (Cytovene)†,‡ or	5 mg/kg IV q 12 h§
	Foscarnet (Foscavir)‡,‖	60 mg/kg IV q8h§
Herpes simplex	Acyclovir (Zovirax) or generic	10 mg/kg IV q 8 h§
Enterovirus	None	
Hantavirus	? Ribavirin	

*These agents can also be used prophylactically in unvaccinated patients at the onset of an epidemic.
†Can be used in conjunction with IV gammaglobulin given at a dose of 150 mg/kg/dose.
‡Not FDA approved for this indication.
§Doses should be reduced in the presence of decreased renal function; consult package insert.
‖To be used in cases of resistance to ganciclovir. Infectious diseases consultation is advised.

any age group. The hallmark of the syndrome is an insidious onset of cough and fever after a 10- to 21-day incubation period. Pleuritic pain, pleural effusion, myalgias, and bacterial superinfection are relatively rare. About half the patients have a positive result of a test for cold agglutinins (IgM antibodies directed against the I antigen on erythrocytes). Occasionally the titer of these antibodies is high enough to cause in vivo hemolysis. A small percentage of patients may exhibit Raynaud's phenomenon or Stevens-Johnson syndrome. In the absence of these findings, it may be impossible to differentiate this disease from that caused by any of the previously mentioned viruses or from Legionnaire's or chlamydial pneumonia. Definitive diagnosis is made by demonstrating a fourfold rise in complement-fixing antibodies or with the aid of some newer molecular biologic techniques to reveal mycoplasmal nucleic acid in sputum samples.

Treatment

Most often, therapy is empirical and based on suspicion of the disease. The organism lacks a cell wall and is therefore resistant to the beta-lactam antibiotics. The macrolides are very effective in the treatment of *M. pneumoniae* infection, and erythromycin (adults: 250 mg every 6 hours; children: 7.5 to 12.5 mg per kg four times daily [every 6 hours]) for 2 to 3 weeks is the therapy of choice. This, however, may be poorly tolerated because of gastrointestinal side effects. The newer macrolides, azithromycin (500 mg orally [PO] loading and 250 mg PO every day for 5 days) and clarithromycin (250 mg PO every 12 hours for 10 to 14 days), are also effective but are far more expensive. The fluoroquinolones are active as are the ketolides* (derivatives of macrolides) and the strepto-

*Not yet approved for use in the United States.

gramins,* a new class of combination antimicrobial therapy. The tetracyclines, including doxycycline, are effective, although somewhat less so than the macrolides and some of the fluoroquinolones, but are contraindicated in children because of their adverse effects on teeth.

LEGIONELLOSIS
(Legionnaires' Disease and Pontiac Fever)

method of
THOMAS M. FILE, Jr., M.D., and
JAMES S. TAN, M.D.
Northeastern Ohio Universities College of Medicine
Rootstown, Ohio
Summa Health System
Akron, Ohio

Legionella species are mainly intracellular organisms. In the environment, they live in flagellated amebas such as *Acanthamoeba* and *Hartmannella* species; in humans, they infect macrophages. Approximately 40 different *Legionella* species have been identified; less than half have been linked to human disease. *L. pneumophila* is the most common human pathogen. At least 15 different serogroups may be distinguished by antibody studies. The majority of the reported cases of *Legionella* pneumonia are caused by *L. pneumophila* serogroup 1.

EPIDEMIOLOGY

Water is the major reservoir for Legionellae. In natural water sources and municipal water systems, Legionellae may be found in low concentration; however, under certain circumstances within man-made water systems (i.e., water temperatures of 32°C to 45°C, stagnant water, and the presence of scale sediment biofilms or amebas) the concentration of organisms may increase markedly. Transmission to humans occurs when water containing the organism is aerosolized in respiratory droplets and inhaled or aspirated by a susceptible host. Aerosol-producing devices that have been associated with outbreaks include cooling towers, evaporative condensers, respiratory therapy equipment, showers and faucets, whirlpool spas, decorative fountains, and an ultrasonic mist machine in a supermarket. Epidemiologic risk factors for nonoutbreak, sporadic infection include recent travel with an overnight stay outside the home, recent domestic plumbing repairs, renal or liver failure, smoking, diabetes, systemic malignancy, and other immunosuppressive states.

CLINICAL MANIFESTATIONS

Legionellosis is primarily associated with two clinically distinct syndromes: Legionnaires' disease (LD), a potentially fatal form of pneumonia, and Pontiac fever, a self-limited, influenza-like illness. Most cases of Pontiac fever are diagnosed in outbreaks, wherein patients have a mild viral-like illness and share exposure from a common water source. Many of the clinical features of LD are indistinguishable from other pneumonias; however, certain features may be seen more commonly. Temperature often exceeds 40°C; gastrointestinal (especially diarrhea) and central nervous system (i.e., headache) symptoms are prominent. Some studies have found the following clinical features more likely associated with LD than other causes of pneumonia: high fever (>39°C), hyponatremia (<130 mEq/L), central nervous system manifestations (i.e., headache or confusion), and lactate dehydrogenase levels of more than 700 units per mL.

DIAGNOSIS

Microbiologic tests for Legionella must be specifically requested from the clinical microbiology laboratory because they are usually not routinely performed. The hallmark of diagnosis is culture; cultivation requires special media (buffered charcoal yeast extract agar) and technical expertise. Detection of growth often requires 3 to 5 days. Urinary antigen detection is a reliable and accessible rapid method of diagnosis. This test only detects antigens of *L. pneumophila* serogroup 1 and has a sensitivity of approximately 70% (specificity approaches 100%). Results become positive early in clinical disease and persist for weeks despite antibiotic therapy. Direct fluorescent antibody (DFA) stain of respiratory secretions is another rapid test but it requires substantial expertise for interpretation, and selection of reagents is critical. In addition this test has been shown to have low sensitivity and variable specificity especially outside of research laboratories. Polymerase chain reaction (PCR) is a potential rapid diagnostic test but presently is expensive and there are no Food and Drug Administration (FDA)–approved reagents. Serologic tests are useful for epidemiologic studies but are less valuable to physicians given the requirement for measurement during acute and convalescent specimens.

THERAPY

Pontiac fever is usually a self-limited illness for which specific therapy is rarely directed. On the contrary, prompt initiation of appropriate therapy is important for optimal management of patients with LD. Delay in instituting therapy significantly increases mortality. Therefore, empirical anti-*Legionella* therapy should be included in the treatment of severe community-acquired pneumonia and considered in selected cases of nosocomial pneumonia.

Erythromycin has generally been accepted in the past as the treatment of choice for LD although no controlled clinical trials have been conducted. However, intracellular models as well as animal models of *Legionella* infection indicate that the systemic fluoroquinolones (ciprofloxacin [Cipro], ofloxacin [Floxin], levofloxacin [Levaquin], sparfloxacin [Zagam], grepafloxacin [Raxar], trovafloxacin [Trovan]) and the newer macrolides (especially azithromycin) show superior activity compared with erythromycin. These newer agents have better pharmacokinetic properties: better bioavailability; longer half-life requiring fewer doses per day; and better intracellular penetration into macrophages. Also they are associated with fewer adverse effects; and the fluoroquinolones have fewer drug interactions with immunosuppressive therapy such as cyclosporine (Sandimmune) or tacrolimus (Prograf) than erythromycin. The addition of rifampin (Rifadin) to erythromycin has been suggested for patients who are more severely ill; however, there is no convincing laboratory data to show that adding rifampin to fluoroquinolones or the more active macrolide therapy improves bacterial killing. Although uncontrolled clinical reports show that ciprofloxacin and ofloxacin have effectively treated patients with LD, we prefer the newer fluoroquinolones (levofloxacin, sparfloxacin, grepafloxacin, trovafloxacin) because of greater activity in vitro against Legionella. In addition, they are more active against *Streptococcus pneumoniae* (including drug-resistant strains) and other common causes of community-acquired pneumonia that need to be considered for empirical therapy. Doxycycline (Vibramycin) has also been shown to be effective in limited, well-documented cases.

Although LD can undoubtedly cause mild disease amenable to outpatient therapy, in reality the large majority of documented cases are treated in the hospital with parenteral therapy initially. Our recommedations for initial parenteral therapy are listed in Table 1. Oral therapy for less serious cases or for step-down from intravenous (IV) therapy includes erythromycin, 500 mg every 6 hours; azithromycin

TABLE 1. **Parenteral Therapy for Serious** *Legionella* **Infections***

Preferred Antimicrobial	Alternative Antimicrobial
Fluoroquinolone	
Levofloxacin (Levaquin) 500 mg IV q 24 h	Erythromycin 1 g IV q 6 h +/− rifampin†,‡
Trovafloxacin (Trovan) 200 mg IV q 24 h	Doxycycline (Vibramycin) 100 mg IV q 12 h +/− rifampin
Azithromycin (Zithromax) 500 mg IV q 24 h	

*Requiring hospitalization or in immunocompromised patients; can change to PO when clinically stable and can take PO (see text).
†300–600 mg IV q 12 h.
‡Not FDA approved for this indication.

(Zithromax), 500 mg every 24 hours; clarithromycin (Biaxin), 500 mg every 12 hours; dirithromycin (Dynabac), 500 mg every 24 hours; ciprofloxacin (Cipro), 750 mg every 12 hours; ofloxacin (Floxin), 400 mg every 12 hours; levofloxacin (Levaquin), 500 mg every 24 hours; sparfloxacin (Zagam), 400 mg initially and then 200 mg every 24 hours; grepafloxacin (Raxar), 600 mg every 24 hours; trovafloxacin (Trovan), 200 mg every 24 hours; and doxycycline, 100 mg every 12 hours. Of the preceding agents, azithromycin, erythromycin, dirithromycin, levofloxacin, and trovafloxacin are currently licensed by the FDA for the treatment of LD. When the patient improves, the duration of treatment is usually 10 to 14 days for the fluoroquinolones and 10 days for azithromycin. If erythromycin (with or without rifampin) is used for more serious infection (or in immunocompromised patients), 21 days is recommended.

PULMONARY THROMBOEMBOLISM

method of
CARLOS A. VAZ FRAGOSO, M.D.
Gaylord Hospital
Wallingford, Connecticut

In the United States, pulmonary thromboembolism (PE) causes death in over 100,000 patients per year while contributing to the death of another 100,000 per year. Risk factors include age older than 40 years, immobility ($\geq$ 1 to 3 days), paralysis, previous venous thromboembolism (VTE), cancer, surgery, obesity (>175% of ideal body weight), congestive heart failure (New York Heart Association [NYHA] class 2 or greater), birth control pills, hormone-replacement therapy, varicose veins, and thrombophilia. These reflect underlying hypercoagulability, venous stasis, or endothelial injury, factors known to promote VTE.

WORKUP OF PULMONARY THROMBOEMBOLISM

Screening

The Prospective Investigation of Pulmonary Embolism Diagnosis (PIOPED) has established the prevalence of symptoms and signs in angiographically proven PE (Table 1). For example, of 117 patients with PE, 98% had dyspnea, tachypnea, pleurisy, or an abnormal chest radiograph. Oxygenation and the electrocardiogram (ECG) were also evaluated. Of those with PE, 74% had a PaO_2 less than 80 mm Hg, 86% had an abnormal alveolar, arterial O_2 difference greater than 20 mm Hg (room air), and 49% had nonspecific ST segment or T wave changes. In a more recent study of 80 patients with PE, anterior precordial T wave inversion was the most frequent (68%) ECG sign. Reversibility of this pattern before the sixth hospital day was consistent with a good outcome. This study also reported on other ECG signs including S1Q3T3 pattern (Q at least 1.5 mm; T wave inversion in lead III), low voltage, sinus tachycardia, right bundle branch block, P pulmonale, or a normal ECG; respective prevalences were 50, 29, 26, 22, 5, and 9%.

In summary, there is benefit in obtaining a history, physical examination, chest radiograph, ECG, and oxygen saturation in the evaluation of PE. Certain abnormalities have high prevalence and are associated with VTE. However, their lack of sensitivity and specificity precludes a definitive diagnosis. Instead, they serve to identify those patients who will need further diagnostic confirmation.

Ventilation/Perfusion ($\dot{V}/\dot{Q}$) Scan

The PIOPED investigators have assessed the value of a $\dot{V}/\dot{Q}$ scan in acute PE. The following are emphasized (see Table 2 for scan categories):

1. In patients without pre-existing cardiopulmonary disease, the sensitivity and specificity of a high-probability $\dot{V}/\dot{Q}$ scan is 41 and 97%, respectively. The sensitivity is reduced because of so few high-probability scans in the study population (e.g., 11% of 931 scans). Thus, most angiographically proven PEs are associated with a $\dot{V}/\dot{Q}$ scan other than high probability; for example, of 251 proven PEs, 105 scans were intermediate and 44 were low probability. The high specificity is beneficial as it yields a low false-positive rate and results in a lower risk of unnecessary treatment.

2. In patients with pre-existing cardiopulmonary disease, the sensitivity of a high probability $\dot{V}/\dot{Q}$ scan remains the same, but there is a higher prevalence of nondiagnostic indeterminate $\dot{V}/\dot{Q}$ scans.

3. The utility of $\dot{V}/\dot{Q}$ scans is improved by assessing concordance between clinical evaluation (history, physical examination, chest radiographs, ECG, and blood gases) and the $\dot{V}/\dot{Q}$ scan. Specifically, if a scan is concordant with the clinical suspicion, it is diagnostic. Surprisingly, in the PIOPED population, there was only a 28% concordance. This predicts that 72% of patients will require a definitive diagnostic procedure, namely a pulmonary angiogram.

4. The bleeding risk of anticoagulation is greatest when it is initiated despite the probability of acute PE being less than 80 to 90% on the basis of a $\dot{V}/\dot{Q}$ scan diagnosis. Thus, a pulmonary angiogram may also serve to justify the risk-benefit stratification before a decision to initiate anticoagulation for acute PE.

In summary, a high- or low-probability $\dot{V}/\dot{Q}$ scan is diagnostic when there is concordance with the clinical suspicion. Given that this occurs in only 28% of cases, noninvasive alternatives are required if one is to lower the pulmonary angiography rate.

Venous Duplex Scan

A venous duplex scan (VDS) of the lower extremities may facilitate the evaluation of PE by reducing the pulmonary angiography rate. This is achieved by documenting residual deep venous thrombosis (DVT) and thus precluding the need for an angiogram. It is reasonable to expect that if 30 to 50% of PEs have concurrent evidence of a DVT, a VDS may reduce the angiography rate to 33%. This strategy is summarized in Table 3.

The VDS, however, has limitations that may adversely affect diagnostic accuracy. Principally, in asymptomatic proximal DVT, a VDS has a reduced sensitivity of 40% in comparison with more than 95% in patients with leg symptoms. In distal DVT, the sensitivity of a VDS is also reduced at 50%. The diagnostic sequence is likewise problematic because of differences in false-positive rates. For example, if a VDS is ordered before a $\dot{V}/\dot{Q}$ scan, the percent of inappropriately treated patients may be doubled (4 versus 2%) relative to a $\dot{V}/\dot{Q}$ scan followed by a VDS. Clinical judgment is thus warranted.

TABLE 1. **Prevalence of Signs and Symptoms in Pulmonary Embolism (PIOPED)**

	PE Group (%) (n = 117)	No PE Group (%) (n = 248)	P Value
Risk factors			
Immobilization	56	33	P < .001
Surgery	54	31	P < .001
Malignancy	23	15	Not significant
Previous thrombophlebitis	14	8	Not significant
Lower extremity trauma	10	10	Not significant
Estrogen	9	10	Not significant
Stroke	7	4	Not significant
≤3 mo postpartum	4	3	Not significant
Symptoms			
Dyspnea	73	72	Not significant
Pleurisy	66	59	Not significant
Cough	37	36	Not significant
Leg swelling	28	22	Not significant
Leg pain	26	24	Not significant
Hemoptysis	13	8	Not significant
Palpitations	10	18	Not significant
Wheezing	9	11	Not significant
Nonpleuritic chest pain	4	6	Not significant
Signs			
Breathing at ≥20 min	70	68	Not significant
Crackles	51	40	P < .05
Pulse at >100 min	30	24	P < .05
S4	24	14	P < .05
Increased P2	23	13	P < .05
DVT	11	11	Not significant
Diaphoresis	11	8	Not significant
Fever (>38.5°C)	7	12	Not significant
Wheezes	5	8	Not significant
Homans' sign	4	2	Not significant
RV lift	4	2	Not significant
Pleural rub	3	2	Not significant
S3	3	4	Not significant
Cyanosis	1	2	Not significant
Plain chest radiograph			
Atelectasis or parenchymal abnormality	68	48	P < .001
Pleural effusion	48	31	P < .01
Pleural based opacity	35	21	P < .01
Elevated diaphragm	24	19	Not significant
Decreased pulmonary vascularity	21	12	P < .05
Prominent central pulmonary artery	15	11	Not significant
Cardiomegaly	12	11	Not significant
Westermark's sign	7	2	Not significant
Pulmonary edema	4	13	P < .05

Abbreviations: DVT = deep venous thrombosis; RV = right ventricular.

TABLE 2. V̇/Q̇ Scan Stratification

High Probability

≥2 large segmental perfusion defects (>75% of a segment) without matching ventilation or radiographic abnormalities or substantially larger than either matching ventilation or radiographic abnormalities.

≥2 moderate segmental perfusion defects (≥25 and ≤75% of a segment) without matching ventilation or radiographic abnormalities and 1 large mismatched segmental defect.

≥4 moderate segmental perfusion defects (≥25 and ≤75% of a segment) without ventilation or radiographic abnormalities.

Intermediate (indeterminate) Probability

Difficult to categorize either as low or high probability.

Low Probability

Nonsegmental perfusion defects (e.g., very small effusion causing blunting of the costophrenic angle, cardiomegaly, elevated diaphragm, and enlarged aorta, hila, and mediastinum).

Single moderate mismatched segmental perfusion defect with normal chest radiograph.

Any perfusion defect with a substantially larger radiographic abnormality.

Large or moderate segmental perfusion defects involving no more than four segments in one lung and no more than three segments in one lung region with matching ventilation defects either equal to or larger in size and chest radiograph either normal or with substantially smaller than perfusion defects.

Normal

No perfusion defects present.

Abbreviation: V̇/Q̇ = ventilation/perfusion.

Pulmonary Angiography

The gold standard for the work-up of PE is pulmonary angiography. The risks of the procedure are sufficiently low to permit its use as a diagnostic tool. In the PIOPED study, out of 1111 patients who underwent pulmonary angiography, there were 5 deaths (0.5%), 9 major nonfatal complications (1%), and 60 less significant complications (5%).

There are limitations to pulmonary angiography that merit emphasis. In the PIOPED study, angiography was nondiagnostic in 3.0% and incomplete in 1%. Surveillance after negative angiograms showed PE in 0.6%, suggesting that these were possible false-negative findings. Angiograms interpreted on the basis of consensus readings resulted in an unchallenged diagnosis in 96%. However, when lobar, segmental, and subsegmental PE were stratified, the concordance rate by two separate readers varied at 98, 90, and 66%, respectively.

In summary, although the angiogram remains the gold standard, it is imperative that the clinician review the angiogram with the radiologist to better ascertain its clinical contribution. A proposed diagnostic sequence for PE is outlined in Table 3.

Work-up of PE During Pregnancy

Of concern in the work-up of PE is possible radiation exposure during pregnancy. As a result, a VDS is ordered before a perfusion scan to avoid unnecessary radiation exposure to the fetus. However, if the VDS is negative, a perfusion scan only (no ventilation) employing 1 mCi has a favorable benefit/risk ratio during pregnancy. The estimated fetal radiation exposure would be 0.006 rads. In contrast, a pulmonary angiogram has an estimated fetal radiation exposure of up to 0.050 rads brachially or up to 0.221 rads femorally. Pulmonary consultation is recommended for a pregnant patient being evaluated for PE.

Future Directions in the Work-up of PE

Current research has investigated fast-scanning computed tomography (CT), magnetic resonance (MR) angiography, D-dimer evaluation, and transesophageal echocardiography (TEE) as alternatives to V̇/Q̇ scanning. A review of the literature suggests the following:

1. Spiral CT imaging is a volumetric, fast-scanning technique that employs contrast and permits evaluation of the pulmonary vasculature. In a study involving 75 patients who underwent spiral CT and angiography, spiral CT achieved a sensitivity of 98% and specificity of 90% for central emboli. However, with peripheral emboli, there were higher rates of inconclusive studies (10%), false-negatives (4%), and false-positives (18%). Some authorities pro-

TABLE 3. Diagnostic Confirmation of Pulmonary Embolism (PIOPED)

Diagnostic Sequence*	Probability of PE (%)	Further Work-up	Probability of PE if Negative VDS (%)	Pulmonary Angiogram
If after a detailed history, physical exam, SpO₂, ECG, and plain chest radiograph . . .				
Clinical suspicion is high and V̇/Q̇ scan is high probability	96	Not necessary	—	Not necessary
Clinical suspicion is indeterminate and V̇/Q̇ scan is high probability	88	VDS	88	Yes, if VDS negative
Clinical suspicion is low and V̇/Q̇ scan is high probability	56	VDS	56	Yes, if VDS negative
Clinical suspicion is high and V̇/Q̇ scan is indeterminate	66	VDS	49	Yes, if VDS negative
Clinical suspicion is indeterminate and V̇/Q̇ scan is indeterminate	28	VDS	16	Yes, if VDS negative
Clinical suspicion is low and V̇/Q̇ scan is indeterminate	16	VDS	9	Clinical judgment
Clinical suspicion is high and V̇/Q̇ scan is low probability	40	VDS	25	Yes, if VDS negative
Clinical suspicion is indeterminate and V̇/Q̇ scan is low probability	16	VDS	9	Yes, if VDS negative
Clinical suspicion is low and V̇/Q̇ scan is low probability	3	Not necessary	—	Not necessary

*If there is a need for a pulmonary angiography but there are significant contraindications, consider D-dimer _plus_ either a spiral CT scan, _or_ MR angiography, _or_ TEE. If these are unavailable, consider empirical anticoagulation and/or a follow-up V̇/Q̇ scan at day 7 and/or serial VDS at days 2 and 7. Please refer to text for abbreviations and discussion.

Please note an indeterminate V̇/Q̇ scan is analogous to an intermediate V̇/Q̇ scan.

Abbreviations: CT = computed tomography; ECG = electrocardiogram; MR = magnetic resonance; TEE = transesophageal echocardiography; V̇/Q̇ = ventilation/perfusion; VDS = venous duplex scan.

pose that spiral CT should replace $\dot{V}/\dot{Q}$ scans. This, however, has not been validated. For example, in the above study, only 25 of the 75 patients underwent $\dot{V}/\dot{Q}$ scanning precluding comparisons with spiral CT. Of further concern would be cost and, in cases where spiral CT is nondiagnostic, the prospect of additional contrast material from pulmonary angiography is disconcerting. As a result, spiral CT remains an investigational tool.

2. In a study of 30 patients, gadolinium-enhanced MR angiography of pulmonary arteries had an average sensitivity of 87% and specificity of 97% among three independent readers. This study is limited by the small number of patients but shows promise as a noninvasive method without ionizing radiation or iodinated contrast.

3. Plasma D-dimers are degradation products of cross-linked fibrin and are increased in acute PE. It has been proposed that D-dimer levels, measured by enzyme-linked immunosorbent assay (ELISA) technique, at less than 500 µg/L had a sensitivity of 99.5% but a specificity of 41%. Thus, if a D-dimer level is less than 500 µg/L, the likelihood of PE is extremely low. In a study of 671 patients with suspected PE, a D-dimer level of less than 500 µg/L allowed the exclusion of PE in 29%. Use of this assay could thus reduce pulmonary angiography rates even further. Caution, however, is advised. For example, in this study, only 164 of the 671 patients underwent a definitive pulmonary angiography. This lack of rigorous methodology places into question the validity of any D-dimer threshold level. Furthermore, the low specificity increases the risk for false-positives. As a result, D-dimer levels 500 µg/L or more are not specific for PE and are nondiagnostic.

4. Transesophageal echocardiography (TEE) as a tool in the evaluation of PE may have its greatest benefit in critically ill patients too unstable for transport. In a study of 24 patients with unexplained shock and distended jugular veins, 18 had right ventricle (RV) dilatation with global or segmental hypokinesis, 12 had direct visualization of central pulmonary thromboemboli, 1 had reduced flow in the right pulmonary artery, and 1 had RV free wall akinesis. The sensitivity and specificity for PE in patients with TEE documented RV dilatation was 92 and 100%, respectively.

Hypercoagulable Work-up

A history, physical examination, routine laboratory testing, and chest radiography is sufficient work-up for hypercoagulability (e.g., cancer) in "idiopathic" PE. However, a more detailed evaluation is indicated for recurrent PE or for a single episode when associated with a family history of VTE (first- or second-degree relatives), massive venous thrombosis, thrombosis at age 50 years or older, or thrombosis at an unusual site (mesenteric or cerebral vein). The work-up includes the following: antithrombin III, antiphospholipid antibodies (lupus anticoagulant, anticardiolipin antibodies), fibrinogen, homocysteine, and a protein C pathway test. The latter is valid only in the nonacute resting state, in the absence of anticoagulation, and is referred to as the phospholipid rich Russell Viper Venom Time [PRVVT]. It's reported as a ratio of PRVVT with protein C activator to PRVVT without activator. When the ratio is less than 2.0, levels of protein C, S, and factor V Leiden are ordered; when greater than 3.0, no abnormality is detected; when it is 2.0 to 3.0, the ratio is inconclusive and is repeated in 6 to 8 weeks in a nonacute state. Of the thrombophilias, the most prevalent is the factor V Leiden mutation occurring in 2 to 15% of patients of European descent. It may be found in up to 60% of cases of familial thrombophilia. The mutation results in glutamine replacing arginine at position 506 of coagulation factor V, making it more difficult for activated protein C to cleave and inactivate factor V. More recently, a new hereditary thrombophilia, a mutation in the prothrombin gene, has been identified by molecular genetic analysis. Its prevalence may be as high as 8% in unselected patients with VTE. It is associated with higher plasma prothrombin levels and may coexist with other forms of inherited thrombophilia, including the factor V Leiden mutation.

TREATMENT OF PULMONARY THROMBOEMBOLISM

The treatment of VTE begins with prevention (Table 4). Active treatment strategies are outlined in Table 5. The following are emphasized:

Supportive Therapy

The patient is admitted to a monitored setting. If the patient is in respiratory failure or with hemodynamic instability, the intensive care unit is preferred. At least two intravenous lines are established and arterial sticks are discouraged. Oxygen is titrated to a saturation 90% or greater and crystalloid resuscitation is judiciously administered for hemodynamic instability. Bed rest is ordered during the first 24 hours of therapeutic anticoagulation for DVT or during the first 24 to 72 hours for PE. While the patient is in bed, both the knees and feet are elevated. If upon ambulation there is dependent edema, graduated compression stockings are advised. Heating pads have no therapeutic effect but may provide comfort in symptomatic DVT.

Unfractionated Heparin

Unfractionated heparin by continuous infusion is the mainstay in the treatment of acute PE. A weight-based dose adjusted nomogram (Table 6) is helpful as it achieves prompt therapeutic anticoagulation (activated partial thromboplastin time [APTT] at 1.5 to 2.5X control); in general, a dose of 25,000 to 35,000 units per day is required. The APTT is drawn every 6 hours until within the therapeutic range and then daily while on heparin. Hemoglobin and platelet levels are followed every other day while on heparin.

Although confirmation is desirable, heparin may be started prior to diagnostic studies in the following settings: A test is not rapidly available; the likelihood of acute PE is extremely high; the presentation of the suspected PE is compromising; and the risk of bleeding with heparin is clinically acceptable.

It is reasonable to initiate warfarin and heparin together. The latter is discontinued on day 5 or 6 if the APTT has been stable and the international normalized ratio (INR) is therapeutic at 2.0 to 3.0 for two consecutive days. For massive PE or ileofemoral thrombosis, a longer period of heparin (5 to 10 days) may be considered.

TABLE 4. **Disease States Necessitating Deep Venous Thrombosis (DVT) Prophylaxis**

Low-Risk General Surgery:

Undergoing minor operations (anesthesia time <30–45 min), age <40 y, and have no clinical DVT risk:
Intervention . . . early ambulation.

Moderate-Risk General Surgery:

Undergoing major surgery (anesthesia time >30–45 min), age >40 y, and have no additional DVT risk:
Intervention . . . graded compression stockings, low-dose heparin SC (5000 units q12h), LMWH (dalteparin [fragmin] at 2500 IU SC qd, first dose at 2 h preop for 5–10 d), or intermittent pneumatic compression (IPC).

Higher-Risk General Surgery:

Undergoing major surgery (anesthesia time >30–45 min), age >40 y, and have additional DVT risks:
Intervention . . . low-dose heparin SC (5000 q8h), LMWH (enoxaparin [Lovenox] at 40 mg SC qd, first dose at 2 h preop for 5–10 d or dalteparin [fragmin] at 2500 IU SC qd, first dose at 2 h preop for 5–10 d), or IPC (if prone to wound infection or hematomas).

Very High-Risk General Surgery:

Major surgery (anesthesia time >30–45 min) with multiple DVT risks:
Intervention . . . low-dose heparin SC (5000 q8h) or LMWH (enoxaparin [Lovenox] at 40 mg SC qd, first dose at 2 h preop for 5–10 d; or dalteparin [fragmin] at 2500–5000 IU SC qd, first dose at 2 h preop for 5–10 d), *and* IPC.

Hip Replacement:

Perioperative warfarin therapy, adjusted dose heparin SC (target APTT 1.5–2.5X control), or LMWH (enoxaparin [Lovenox] at 30 mg SC bid, first dose at 12–24 h postop for a period of 7–14 d, or longer; prophylaxis may thus extend beyond hospital discharge).

Knee Replacement:

LMWH (enoxaparin [Lovenox] at 30 mg SC bid, first dose at 12–24 h postop for 7–14 d, or longer) *with* IPC. CPM's (continuous passive motion) with AV sequential boots may be more practical than IPC in knee surgery.

Intracranial Neurosurgery:

IPC with or without graded compression stockings.

Acute Spinal Cord Injury with Paralysis:

Adjusted dose heparin SC (target APTT 1.5–2.5X control) or warfarin.

Multiple Trauma:

IPC or warfarin.
Although not FDA approved, enoxaparin may have a favorable risk/benefit ratio as prophylaxis against DVT after major trauma.

General Medical Patient with VTE Risk:

If early ambulation is inadequate relative to the VTE risk, low-dose heparin SC (5000 SC q12h), or IPC, or graded compression stockings.

Myocardial Infarction:

Low-dose heparin SC (5000 q8–12h), IPC, or full-dose heparin.

Ischemic Stroke with Lower Extremity Paralysis:

Low-dose heparin SQ (q8–12h) or IPC.
Although not FDA approved, LMWH may become the agent of choice in the prevention of DVT in patients with acute ischemic stroke.

Long-Term Indwelling Central Vein Catheters:

Warfarin at 1 mg/d.

Abbreviations: LMWH = low molecular weight heparin; APTT = activated partial thromboplastin time; VTE = venous thromboembolism.

TABLE 5. **Treatment of Venous Thromboembolism**

Clinical Setting	Thrombolytics	Unfractionated Heparin	Warfarin*
Uncomplicated PE or DVT (including symptomatic distal DVT)	Not indicated	Yes and with a weight-based dose adjusted nomogram. Future: LMWH	Yes: see text for duration
PE complicated by hypoxemic respiratory failure or shock	Clinical judgment: TPA,† UK,‡ or SK§	Yes once TPA completed: see text	Yes: see text for duration
Ileofemoral DVT, or DVT complicated by severe leg edema, or Paget-Schroetter Syndrome¶	Clinical judgment: UK or SK	Yes once thrombolytic completed: see text	Yes: see text for duration

*Concurrent with heparin, start warfarin 5 mg PO qd on d 1 and 2, and thereafter estimated maintenance dose (1–9 mg) and frequency.

†TPA: if APTT or TT is ≤1.5X control, 100 mg loading dose is infused intravenously over 2 h. Thereafter, start a maintenance infusion of heparin when the APTT or TT is ≤1.5X control, usually within 30 min of terminating TPA (a loading dose of heparin is not recommended). TPA is not indicated for DVT.

‡UK: if APTT or TT is ≤1.5X control, 4400 IU/kg loading dose is infused over 10 min followed by a maintenance infusion of 4400 IU/kg/h for 12 h. Thereafter, start heparin when the APTT or TT is ≤1.5X control, usually 4 h after terminating UK infusion (a loading dose of heparin is not recommended).

§SK: if APTT or TT is ≤1.5X control, 250,000 IU loading dose over 30 min is followed by 100,000 IU/h maintenance for 24 h (PE only) or 72 h (PE + DVT). If thrombin time is not different from baseline control within 4 h of infusion, discontinue SK as excessive resistance is present. Otherwise, start heparin when the APTT or TT is ≤1.5X control, usually 4 h after terminating SK infusion (a loading dose of heparin is not recommended).

¶Paget-Schroetter Syndrome is spontaneous axillosubclavian vein thrombosis. As with other forms of complicated DVT, catheter-directed and systemic thrombolytic therapy may be required.

Please see text for discussion and abbreviations.

Abbreviations: DVT = deep venous thrombosis; APTT = activated partial thromboplastin time; LMWH = low molecular weight heparin; PE = pulmonary thromboembolism; TPA = tissue plasminogen activator; TT = thrombin time; SK = streptokinase; UK = urokinase.

Warfarin

The warfarin starting dose is 5 mg per day for the first 2 days. "Loading" doses are avoided as achieving an earlier "therapeutic" INR (at ≤ 3 days) does not reflect an antithrombotic effect. Early elevations in the INR primarily reflect reductions in factor VII (half-life of 6 hours) but do not account for a procoagulant effect due to continued elevations of prothrombin (half-life of 60 hours). On day 3, the estimated maintenance dose (range 1 to 9 mg per day) is started and subsequently titrated to a target INR of 2.0 to 3.0 (≥ 3.0 in the antiphospholipid syndrome). INR levels are followed daily during the first 5 to 7 days, and then 1 to 2 times per week depending on response. Adjustments for drug interactions and underlying hepatic function should be considered. If toxicity does develop, Figure 1 outlines several therapeutic options.

Warfarin is continued for 3 to 6 months in those

TABLE 6. **Unfractionated Heparin Dosing**

An initial heparin bolus of 80 U/kg, followed by a maintenance infusion of 18 U/kg/h. Check APTT every 6 h until within the therapeutic range, and, thereafter, qd. Adjustments are as follows:

APTT (sec)	Heparin Dosing
<35	80 U/kg bolus *and* increase infusion by 4 U/kg/h
35–45	40 U/kg bolus *and* increase infusion by 2 U/kg/h
46–70	No change (therapeutic)
71–90	Decrease infusion by 2 U/kg/h
>90	Stop infusion for 1 h and thereafter reduce infusion by 3 U/kg/h

Abbreviations: APTT = activated partial thromboplastin time.
Based on Raschke RA, Reilly BM, Guidry JR: The weight-based heparin dosing nomogram compared with a "standard care" nomogram. Ann Intern Med 119:874–881, 1993.

with a first presentation of VTE. In the setting of recurrent VTE or a continuing risk factor, such as inherited thrombophilia or active cancer, therapy is lengthened to 1 year or indefinitely, but is periodically reviewed. In the setting of a reversible risk factor, such as uncomplicated postoperative DVT without PE, 6 weeks of warfarin is adequate but clinical judgment is advised. A follow-up VDS or V̇/Q̇ scan at the end of therapy is warranted in those at risk for recurrence. This would serve as a baseline and assist in the determination of the duration of anticoagulation.

There are two specific settings that merit emphasis. First, warfarin is contraindicated in pregnancy but not in the nursing mother. Second, when there is heparin-induced thrombocytopenia, warfarin treatment of PE can lead to venous limb gangrene. In such situations, consultation is advised to assess alternatives to warfarin.

Fractionated Heparin

Depolymerization of standard heparin yields fragments with a low molecular weight of 4000 to 6000 (e.g., low molecular weight heparin [LMWH]). These have more anti-Factor Xa activity than standard heparin and result in an increased antithrombotic effect, less inhibition of platelets, and less vascular permeability. Of additional benefit is the lack of APTT monitoring requirements with LMWH.

Although only currently Food and Drug Administration (FDA) approved for VTE prophylaxis, it is expected that fractionated heparin will soon be approved for the treatment of VTE in the United States. Several studies have evaluated the treatment of VTE with unfractionated heparin administered in the hospital as compared with LMWH administered at home. The general consensus is that LMWH may have greater efficacy (reductions in thrombus size,

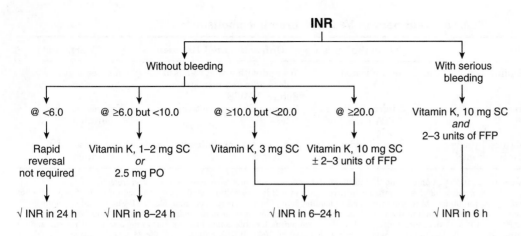

Figure 1. Treatment of warfarin-induced toxicity. (Based in part on Fourth ACCP Consensus Conference on Antithrombotic Therapy. Chest 108:238S, 1995; and Glover et al: Conservative treatment of overanticoagulated patients. Chest 108:987, 1995.

recurrence rates, and mortality), lower risk for bleeding, and may be safely incorporated into outpatient management of uncomplicated VTE.

Thrombolytics

The use of thrombolytics continues to be individualized. Consider the following: there is a lack of evidence that thrombolytics improve clinically relevant outcomes of patients with acute PE. Yet, in a survey of 100 pulmonologists, 100% used thrombolytics in PE associated with hypotension and 73% in PE associated with hypoxemia. Such a practice is not unreasonable as the stated lack of efficacy may be a function of the small sample size of clinical trials. In addition, recent work suggests that there may be a survival advantage to early thrombolysis (within 24 hours of diagnosis) in hemodynamically stable major PE. However, this study is limited by a selection bias in the comparison group.

Patient participation in the decision for thrombolysis is recommended. A prior study demonstrated that informed consent plays a role in the risk-benefit analysis of thrombolysis for DVT. Specifically, by the values attached to outcomes, these patients were unwilling to accept an increased risk of death with thrombolysis relative to heparin to avoid the postphlebitic syndrome.

Dosing recommendations for tissue plasminogen activator (TPA), streptokinase (SK), and urokinase (UK) and the appropriate clinical settings are detailed in Table 5. The FDA lists as indications for thrombolysis massive PE (lobar or multiple segmental involvement) and PE associated with hypotension.

Inferior Vena Cava Filter

An inferior vena cava (IVC) filter is considered appropriate in VTE in the following settings: when anticoagulation is contraindicated; when there is recurrence of VTE despite therapeutic anticoagulation; or when a severely compromised cardiopulmonary reserve would result in a patient being unable to survive any recurrent PE. An IVC filter may also be placed prophylactically in patients at high risk for VTE when anticoagulation is contraindicated.

Other

Alternatives such as catheter-tip embolectomy, catheter-tip fragmentation, or open pulmonary embolectomy are available at specialized centers. These are considered in patients with acute PE who are hemodynamically impaired and for whom thrombolytic therapy has failed or is contraindicated.

SARCOIDOSIS

method of
R. M. DU BOIS, M.D.
Royal Brompton Hospital
London, United Kingdom

Sarcoidosis is a systemic disorder that involves one or more organs (most commonly the lungs, liver, eyes, and skin) and most commonly affects young adults. The classical histopathologic features are chronic inflammatory cells that aggregate into epithelioid cell granulomas at disease sites. Although the cause is unknown, a granulomatous response is the result of persistent antigenic triggering of T cell immunity; numerous trigger agents have been suggested but never proven. Treatment has therefore been geared to suppressing the chronic immune response and cannot eradicate the as-yet-unknown initiating factor.

Treatment approaches have been hampered by the absence of high-quality prospective, controlled clinical studies. The studies that have been performed have largely suffered from poor design, heterogeneous groups of patients, unclear end points, or a lack of individualization of therapy and often a combination of these factors. Despite this, it is possible to distill from them certain conclusions about the drugs that are currently employed.

The most important issues regarding the treatment of sarcoidosis are as follows:

1. Which patients need to be treated?
2. When should treatment be started?
3. When should treatment be stopped?
4. Which drugs should be used as first-line therapy?
5. Which route of administration should be used?

The answers to these questions depend on the organ or organs involved, the severity of the involvement, and whether the patient is symptomatic. When there is evidence of disease in organs in which even a small granuloma load can have severe consequences, such as the eyes, central nervous system, or heart, treatment should be commenced immediately. In other organs, such as the lungs, skin, liver, or joints, the decision about treatment is driven more by the patient's symptoms and objective assessment of severity of disease rather than the presence of disease.

CORTICOSTEROIDS

Corticosteroid therapy remains the best anti-inflammatory approach currently available. Increasingly, the profile of the side effects that this drug can cause has become well known and this has resulted in a reluctance to use corticosteroid drugs. These concerns are appropriate, but they must be put in the context of possible benefit (i.e., for a particular individual, the potential for good must be weighed against the potential for side effects).

Corticosteroids suppress the up-regulation of a number of key cytokines that are involved in the process of granuloma formation, and thus the rationale for using these drugs in patients with sarcoidosis is sound.

There is widespread agreement that corticosteroids generally improve symptoms and improve indices of disease such as chest radiography and pulmonary function tests in the short term. There is, however, controversy about the effect of corticosteroids on long-term outcome. A number of studies have suggested that corticosteroids do not improve long-term prognosis in lung disease, but the majority of these studies have design flaws and were not set up to answer specifically whether corticosteroids prevent fibrosis. The British Thoracic Society's study of long-term corticosteroid efficacy in 149 patients, published in 1996, was better designed in this regard and concluded that long-term corticosteroids conferred a better long-term functional advantage in comparison to patients not receiving long-term corticosteroids, assessed by changes in a number of indices, particularly a combined clinical index derived from symptoms, radiography, and lung function.

Unless there are clear contraindications such as poorly controlled diabetes, hypertension, and peptic ulceration, corticosteroids should be first-line treatment for all forms of sarcoidosis. Treatment is typically by the oral route, although pulsed intravenous therapy may be used in selected situations. Oral treatment dosage varies from 40 to 100 mg per day, depending on the organ involved (see later discussion) for 1 month and then tapered over a 6-month period to a maintenance dose for a total of 1 year, at which point the drug is withdrawn slowly if stability has been maintained. Intravenous regimens can minimize side effects, particularly for patients with co-morbid conditions. Our regimen is up to 1 gram intravenously every week for 8 weeks, together with low-dose (10 to 15 mg per day) oral prednisolone.

Inhaled Corticosteroids

There have been three double-blind randomized controlled trials of high-dose inhaled corticosteroids in sarcoidosis. These trials showed few changes in objective indices, although there was a consistent trend toward improvement in some symptoms such as cough. It is reasonable to consider using inhaled corticosteroids as an adjunct to systemic therapy for predominantly airway disease, particularly when this is accompanied by cough; however, there is no evidence that inhaled treatment alone affects outcome.

Topical Steroids

In ocular and upper respiratory tract disease, topical corticosteroids are highly effective. This is first-line therapy for mild to moderate uveitis and nasal disease.

OTHER IMMUNOSUPPRESSIVE AGENTS

When corticosteroids are contraindicated, fail to achieve the desired result, or need to be maintained at unacceptably high doses, alternative forms of immunosuppression must be considered.

Methotrexate (Rheumatrex)

Methotrexate is a dihydrofolate reductase antimetabolite. At this time, methotrexate appears to be the most promising alternative to corticosteroids in the treatment of sarcoidosis. There is good evidence that lung, skin, and liver disease can be improved by the treatment, although the reports to date are largely anecdotal. Methotrexate is given weekly, starting at 7.5 mg per week, increasing, if necessary, to 15 mg per week or, rarely, 20 mg per week. It should be considered for patients with steroid-nonresponsive lung or liver disease and as a steroid sparer. It may also be considered first-choice treatment for skin disease.

The major side effects of methotrexate involve the bone marrow, liver, and lungs. Complete blood cell counts need to be checked on a regular basis. The evidence concerning the need for regular liver function testing is equivocal, but in my view, this testing should be performed at 6- to 8-week intervals. Some authorities suggest that liver biopsies need to be performed after a cumulative dosage of 1.5 to 2.5 grams. Toxic effects of methotrexate can be improved by folinic acid, and some centers use folic acid prophylaxis.

Azathioprine (Imuran)

The information on this drug is even more anecdotal than that for methotrexate. There have been no controlled studies, but there have been reports suggesting that it is also efficacious as a steroid-sparing agent and has been used for the treatment of neurosarcoidosis that is resistant to steroids. In my experience, azathioprine can improve lung function in patients with predominantly fibrotic lung disease. A small percentage of the population has a methyltransferase deficiency that impairs the metabolism of azathioprine. This can result in profound bone marrow suppression and hair loss. Therapy should therefore be initiated at 50 mg per day, with weekly complete blood cell counts for 4 weeks. If the white blood cell count remains stable, the dosage can be increased to 2.5 mg per kg per day, generally to a maximum of 150 mg. Thereafter, complete blood cell counts and liver functions tests should be monitored at approximately 6- to 8-week intervals.

Cyclophosphamide (Cytoxan)

Another cytotoxic alkylating agent, cyclophosphamide, has been used in uncontrolled studies as a steroid-sparing agent and also in steroid-resistant central nervous system disease. As with azathioprine, however, there have been no controlled studies and there are no clear indications of which patients should be treated with this agent. The side effect profile includes bone marrow toxicity, hemorrhagic cystitis, bladder neoplasia, and lymphocytic neoplasia. The side effect profile is worse than those of azathioprine and methotrexate; cyclophosphamide usage should therefore be restricted to patients for whom azathioprine and methotrexate were not successful. Complete blood cell counts and liver function tests should be monitored at 6- to 8-week intervals. Weekly testing of urine for blood is also mandatory.

Chlorambucil (Leukeran)

This drug is an alkylating cytotoxic agent widely used in patients with chronic lymphocytic proliferative diseases such as lymphocytic leukemia and lymphoma. It achieved popularity in the 1970s and 1980s for the treatment of sarcoidosis, but because of a high relapse rate on discontinuation and the risk of the development of secondary malignancies, this drug is no longer recommended.

Cyclosporine (Sandimmune)

This drug has a very specific anti–T cell activity that suggests that it would be an ideal drug for sarcoidosis when the initiation of the granuloma involves T cell activation. This promise was supported by in vitro studies, but use in humans has been extremely disappointing. Cyclosporine is therefore not recommended except in the most refractory disease.

Hydroxychloroquine (Plaquenil Sulfate)

The antimalarial drugs chloroquine and hydroxychloroquine have been used with success in some forms of sarcoidosis. Of the two, hydroxychloroquine has a better side effect profile and is therefore recommended by preference. Dosage is initially 200 mg per day, increasing if necessary to 400 mg per day. The most serious side effects are ocular, particularly corneal microdeposits and maculopathy. Symptoms from these side effects are haloes from the corneal changes and central field defects and impairment of visual acuity from the maculopathy. Retinal damage is unlikely if the dosage of hydroxychloroquine is less than 6.5 mg per kg of lean body weight per day.

Patients should have their eyes examined for baseline data before treatment is started.

Ketoconazole (Nizoral)

Ketoconazole and imidazole derivative antifungal agents inhibit the cytochrome P-450 complex and may inhibit synthesis of 1,25-dihydroxyvitamin D. It is a useful treatment of hypercalcemia in oral dosages of 600 to 800 mg per day. Its action is delayed for up to 2 days, which makes it inappropriate for the acute treatment of hypercalcemia, for which corticosteroids should always be first-line treatment.

Nonmedicinal Measures

In severe fibrotic disease of organs such as the lungs or liver, transplantation must be considered. Radiotherapy has been used with some success in localized central nervous system disease, especially in the spinal cord. Other supportive measures such as diuretics, oxygen, and treatment of infection also need to be instituted when necessary.

TREATMENT OF INDIVIDUAL ORGAN DISEASE (Table 1)

Lung Disease

Because sarcoidosis can remit spontaneously, the indications for treating lung disease are breathlessness and severe disease. Bilateral and/or mediastinal lymphadenopathy rarely necessitates treatment. Stage 2 (bilateral hilar lymphadenopathy together with pulmonary infiltrates) or stage 3 (pulmonary infiltrates without hilar lymphadenopathy) disease is not treated if the patient is asymptomatic with well-preserved lung function. In this situation, a 6- to 12-month period of observation is recommended for determining whether the disease will resolve spontaneously. If at the end of this period there is persistent parenchymal disease, treatment with corticosteroids is recommended. A suggested regimen is to commence treatment at 40 mg per day for 1 month and then to assess objective change at the end of that period. If there has been a response, the dosage should be tapered by roughly 5 mg every 7 to 10 days to a maintenance dose of 15 mg every other day (or a daily equivalent). This dosage should be continued up to a total treatment period of 1 year to make sure that remission has been maintained before tapering further with the goal of withdrawal.

TABLE 1. **Treatment Strategies for Sarcoidosis**

Clinical Features	First Line Strategy	Second Line Strategy
Fevers Night sweats Arthralgia Lofgren's syndrome	Observation and nonsteroidal anti-inflammatory drugs	Corticosteroids for severe or recalcitrant symptoms

Lung disease
  Stage 1
  Stages 2–4
	
	Observation
	Corticosteroids
		
		None

Ocular	Topical steroids Topical cycloplegics	Systemic steroids Immunosuppression
Upper respiratory tract	Nasal alkaline douche Topical steroids	Systemic steroids Hydroxychloroquine Methotrexate
Cardiac	Systemic steroids Antiarrythmics	Permanent pacemaker Automatic implantable cardiac defibrillator Heart transplantation
Skin	Systemic steroids Hydroxychloroquine Methotrexate	CO$_2$ laser (?) Isotretinoin* (?) Clofazimine* (?) Clobetasol (?)
Liver and spleen	Systemic steroids Methotrexate	Immunosuppression
Neurosarcoidosis	Systemic steroids	Immunosuppression Radiotherapy (?) Shunt (?)
Hypercalcemia/hypercalciuria	Low-calcium diet Low–vitamin D diet Rehydration Avoidance of sunlight Systemic steroids	Ketoconazole
Renal	Systemic steroids	Immunosuppression Transplantation

*Not FDA approved for this indication.
(?) indicates efficacy not established.

In extensive disease in which there is already evidence of fibrosis and contraction, it is still reasonable to consider a trial of corticosteroids because there is often ongoing inflammation even in the presence of evidence of chronicity. A positive gallium scan can be helpful in this context because it indicates persistent granulomas. The treatment approach is identical to that outlined in the previous paragraph. Inhaled corticosteroids may be used to improve cough.

Ocular Involvement

It is recommended that all patients with newly diagnosed sarcoidosis have an ophthalmologic evaluation. This is an absolute requirement if there are any ocular symptoms. Topical treatment with corticosteroid drops is first-line therapy, but posterior or recalcitrant anterior disease may necessitate oral corticosteroids in high dosage (often as much as 100 mg per day) or immunosuppression. Treatment is monitored by direct slit-lamp observation and is tapered to withdrawal once disease activity has been suppressed.

Skin

Nasal disease as part of lupus pernio, particularly at the earlier stages when induration is present only at the mucocutaneous junction, may respond to dexamethasone.

More widespread skin disease is treated with oral corticosteroids in doses similar to those used for the lung. Good alternatives include methotrexate, up to 15 mg (or, in rare cases, 20 mg) per week, and hydroxychloroquine, 200 to 400 mg per day. Local injection of corticosteroid may cause more severe skin disease and is not generally recommended.

Erythema nodosum usually necessitates no treatment, but if the lesions are persistently painful, nonsteroidal anti-inflammatory drugs often resolve the problem. If symptoms are more persistent and nonresponsive to nonsteroidal drugs, 20 mg of prednisolone daily is usually successful. This can be tapered rapidly.

Cardiac Disease

Arrhythmias and heart failure are the main complications of cardiac sarcoidosis. Disease is, however, often occult, manifesting for the first time with a terminal dysrhythmia.

High-dose corticosteroids (1 mg per kg per day) are indicated for suspected disease. The problem with treatment of heart disease that may manifest with intermittent dysrhythmia is how to monitor improvement. Magnetic resonance imaging (MRI) or gallium scans can be used to track progression of abnormalities at presentation, but in many instances, objective evidence of cardiac disease is more equivocal.

Central Nervous System

Neurosarcoidosis is often extremely difficult to treat. Prolonged courses of high-dose oral and/or intravenous corticosteroids may be necessary. In studies in the United States, cyclophosphamide has been shown to have a role in improving central nervous system disease. It should be considered in patients whose disease is refractory to corticosteroid treatment. Early treatment is critical because a low granuloma load can cause major neurologic deficits and should be reversed before fibrosis ensues.

Liver/Gastrointestinal Involvement

This is usually asymptomatic. It is rarely necessary to treat liver disease specifically, but progressive liver function impairment necessitates corticosteroid therapy.

Peripheral Lymphadenopathy

This is also asymptomatic. For large, often unsightly lymphadenopathy, corticosteroids may be given in the same dosages as for lung disease.

Hypercalcemia/Hypercalciuria

Uncontrolled hypercalcemia can be life-threatening and necessitates high dosages of intravenous corticosteroids together with rehydration. Patients must be warned not to ingest supplementary calcium or vitamin D because the granulomas themselves make large quantities of vitamin D. Prolonged exposure to direct sunlight should also be avoided because of the effect of ultraviolet radiation on vitamin D production by the skin.

For maintenance treatment of hypercalcemia or hypercalciuria, ketoconazole should be considered, particularly in more refractory situations.

SILICOSIS

method of
RALPH M. SCHAPIRA, M.D.
*Medical College of Wisconsin and Milwaukee
Veterans Affairs Medical Center
Milwaukee, Wisconsin*

Silicosis refers to the potentially fatal interstitial pulmonary fibrosis that results from the inhalation of crystalline silica (silicon dioxide [SiO_2]). Silica is a naturally occurring mineral oxide particle that is the cause of the most prevalent worldwide occupational lung disease, silicosis. The adverse health effects of silica exposure have been recognized for centuries, and legally enforceable limits on the exposure of industrial workers to airborne silica in the United States have been established. Nonetheless, nearly 15,000 silicosis-associated deaths were recorded in the United States during 1968 to 1994. Between the years 1987 and 1995, 577 people in the state of Michigan were reported to have met the clinical criteria of silicosis. Thus silicosis should always be considered in the differential diagnosis of an interstitial lung disease in a person who has had silica exposure, even if such exposure was in the distant past.

Several types of silica exist in both crystalline and noncrystalline structural forms. The noncrystalline forms of silica are not relevant to respiratory disease. Of the crystalline forms, quartz is the most common and is also the most important form of silica in terms of association with human pulmonary interstitial fibrosis. Numerous occupations are associated with the development of silicosis, including metal industries (foundries), surface and underground mining, construction (drilling and blasting), and sandblasting. Silica is related to asbestos in that asbestos is a naturally occurring fibrous mineral oxide particle that is associated with occupational interstitial pulmonary fibrosis (asbestosis). The parent structures of both silica and asbestos contain a silicon-oxide chemical group; both minerals also have associated transitional metals and similar chemical reactivity. However, silica and asbestos have important structural differences in size, shape, and chemical constituents.

After inhalation by humans, silica particles that are not trapped or cleared by the body's upper airway defense mechanisms accumulate in the lower respiratory tract, where the crystals mediate lung toxicity. Animal models of lung injury after exposure have been used to identify mechanisms by which silica causes lung injury and interstitial fibrosis. These studies demonstrate that silica exposure causes an accumulation of lung inflammatory cells composed of both neutrophils and macrophages. The inflammatory response can result in the generation of cytotoxic reactive oxygen products, including oxygen-based free radicals such as the hydroxyl radical, which may injure the lung epithelium, potentially resulting in interstitial pulmonary fibrosis. Other inflammatory mediators from lung inflammatory cells have also been implicated in lung injury after silica exposure, including arachidonic acid metabolites and various cytokines and growth factors. Most recent evidence from these animal models shows that lung inflammatory cells isolated from silica-exposed lungs increase the production of nitric oxide, the latest mediator identified that may play a proinflammatory role in the pathogenesis of silicosis.

CLINICAL DISEASE

Silicosis is clinically divided into three categories: simple (or nodular) silicosis, complicated silicosis, and acute silicoproteinosis. Simple silicosis manifests in persons who have a relevant occupational history of exposure to silica. Although most patients with silicosis have been exposed to silica for more than 20 years, silicosis can occur after far shorter exposures (termed *accelerated silicosis*). A study of silicosis in workers in Michigan (1985 to 1995) showed that 40 of the 567 reported cases of silicosis occurred in workers exposed to silica for less than 10 years. The intensity of exposure is believed to be related to the time course of disease expression (latency period) and progression. Patients with simple silicosis may be asymptomatic or have an occasional cough. Pulmonary function testing may be normal or demonstrate a mild restrictive abnormality (decrease in forced vital capacity [FVC] and total lung capacity [TLC]), usually in the absence of airway obstruction. The chest radiograph in patients with simple silicosis shows diffuse nodular opacities, usually most prominent in the upper lung zones. The opacities are small (<1 cm), in contrast to those in patients with complicated silicosis. Calcified hilar lymph nodes may be present. Computed tomographic scans confirm the presence of the nodular opacities, but these scans are not necessary to establish the clinical diagnosis. Histologic examination of the characteristic lesion in silicosis (the silicotic nodule) reveals concentric, acellular areas of collagen fibers, without necrosis, that may contain silica particles. The diagnosis of simple silicosis is usually based on clinical findings alone, and lung biopsy is needed only to evaluate for the presence of another interstitial lung disease when the diagnosis is in doubt.

Complicated silicosis (also termed *progressive massive fibrosis*) is characterized by symptoms that can include progressive dyspnea and cough and by physical examination findings such as clubbing, cyanosis, and evidence of right-sided heart failure (cor pulmonale). Chest radiographs demonstrate opacities larger than 1 cm in diameter. Pulmonary function testing shows a restrictive abnormality that may be severe and can be accompanied by airway obstruction (decrease in 1-second forced expiratory volume [FEV$_1$]/FVC ratio). The diffusion capacity for carbon monoxide is usually decreased. In addition, significant hypoxemia that is aggravated by exercise may be present. The large opacities may obscure the radiographic evidence of tuberculosis, and many authorities believe that the incidence of *Mycobacterium tuberculosis* and other nontuberculous mycobacteria is increased in patients with silicosis, particularly complicated silicosis. An increase in the incidence of bronchogenic carcinoma in patients with complicated silicosis has been suggested and is a matter of debate, because of the confounding issue of cigarette smoking. In any case, the opacities in complicated silicosis can obscure a coexisting lung cancer or pulmonary tuberculosis, and these diseases must always be considered carefully when a change in the chest radiograph is noted. Weight loss, malaise, a decrease in appetite, or hemoptysis may be additional clues to the development of tuberculosis or lung carcinoma in patients with silicosis. Fiberoptic bronchoscopy with biopsies may be needed as part of the evaluation of potential lung cancer or tuberculosis. Caplan's syndrome is the development of pulmonary nodules, which may cavitate, in patients with rheumatoid arthritis, pneumoconiosis, and silicosis.

Acute silicosis (also termed *silicoproteinosis*) clinically resembles pulmonary alveolar proteinosis and usually occurs within a few months after major, intense exposure to silica or years afterwards. As such, acute silicosis is not truly a classical interstitial lung disease. Many reported cases have occurred in sandblasters. Acute silicosis represents an unusual pathologic reaction to the massive deposition of silica particles in the lungs and is characterized histologically by the presence of abundant granular eosinophilic material that accumulates in the alveoli. It is hypothesized that the silica disrupts normal surfactant metabolism, resulting in the abnormal accumulation of the proteinaceous material that disrupts the normal surface

tension of the alveolar space and causes ventilation-perfusion mismatching and severe respiratory disease.

As is the case with most interstitial lung diseases, no specific treatment for the various forms of silicosis has proven efficacy. Thus silicosis is treated in much the same way as other interstitial lung diseases. The interstitial fibrosis characteristic of silicosis may progress even in the absence of continued exposure. Education and primary prevention is essential. Adherence to established occupational hygiene regulations, including legally enforceable limits of worker exposure, are mandatory in order to avoid concentrations of silica particles that can cause silicosis. The National Institute for Occupational Safety and Health (NIOSH) has set such exposure limits, and silicosis is reportable to the state health departments in many states. Patients at risk for silicosis as a result of type of employment should have a chest radiograph and pulmonary function testing at the start of employment and have these tests repeated every few years or sooner if clinically indicated. These tests are also important as tools for monitoring patients with an established diagnosis of silicosis in order to identify progression of the interstitial lung disease.

TREATMENT

Treatment of patients with silicosis is targeted at ameliorating symptoms; the physician must be vigilant for the development of tuberculosis, bronchogenic carcinoma (which may not be a direct effect of silica exposure), pulmonary arterial hypertension, and right-sided heart failure. Thus the treatment plan is not specific to patients with silicosis. In patients with silicosis and airway obstruction, inhaled bronchodilators, delivered by a metered-dose inhaler (MDI) should be used (beta agonists and anticholinergics). The use of a spacer device with the MDI, as well as patient education as to the proper MDI technique, are essential for maximizing the benefit from the use of the MDI. Acute bacterial infections (pneumonia or bronchitis) should be treated with antibiotic choices targeted according to local bacteriologic patterns and severity of illness. A pneumococcal vaccination and an annual influenza vaccination are highly recommended. Many authorities recommend that patients with silicosis receive an annual purified protein derivative (PPD) skin test and preventive therapy (chemoprophylaxis), if indicated. Because silicosis is a risk factor for the development of pulmonary tuberculosis, the Centers for Disease Control and Prevention (CDC) recommends that chemoprophylaxis be considered in patients with silicosis (regardless of age) and a positive skin reaction to 5 TU of PPD of 10 mm or more (or ≥5 mm if patient has had recent contact with a person with tuberculosis, is infected with the human immunodeficiency virus [HIV], or has radiographic evidence of healed tuberculosis). Because a positive skin reaction may be indicative of active pulmonary tuberculosis (in addition to latent [asymptomatic] infection), patients with silicosis and a positive skin reaction must be carefully evaluated for active disease. If active tuberculosis is established, treatment with appropriate agents, commonly including three or four drugs, is indicated. Prolonged therapy may be indicated, depending on the clinical response. Similarly, nontuberculous mycobacterial disease also warrants multidrug therapy. Patients with significant abnormalities in pulmonary function testing or evidence of cor pulmonale should be assessed for the need for supplemental oxygen therapy, both at rest and at exercise.

Pharmacologic therapy to interrupt the mechanisms of pulmonary inflammation and fibrogenesis in patients with silicosis is not well established. Glucocorticoids are widely used in interstitial lung diseases such as idiopathic pulmonary fibrosis, with mixed results. The role of glucocorticoids in silicosis is not well studied, and its use is reserved for patients with progressive pulmonary impairment. The use of other pharmacologic agents cannot be recommended. Another approach is bronchoscopic whole lung lavage, which can be performed safely and is successful in removing silica from the lungs. The long-term benefits of lavage in influencing the course of silicosis, however, are unclear.

HYPERSENSITIVITY PNEUMONITIS
(Extrinsic Allergic Alveolitis)

method of
HAL B. RICHERSON, M.D.
*University of Iowa Hospitals and Clinics and
College of Medicine
Iowa City, Iowa*

Hypersensitivity pneumonitis manifests with symptoms of dyspnea and cough that result from a susceptible host's repeated inhalation of a variety of antigenic organic dusts or other agents (Table 1 lists selected examples). Reports of putative new agents continue to appear. Pneumonitis resulting from exposure to medications or toxins is not included in this context; nor are eosinophilic pneumonias.

The clinical manifestation of hypersensitivity pneumonitis may be acute, subacute, or chronic, depending on the frequency, intensity, and duration of inhalational exposure and other factors. In the *acute* form, influenza-like symptoms of chills, fever, sweating, myalgias, lassitude, and headache often predominate. They begin 3 to 9 hours after exposure, peak between 6 and 24 hours after exposure, and last hours to days. (A similar manifestation occurs with organic dust toxic syndrome [ODTS], but pneumonitis is absent.) The *subacute* form appears gradually over several days to weeks and is characterized by increasing cough and dyspnea. Subacute hypersensitivity pneumonitis may advance to pulmonary consolidation and severe hypoxemia, necessitating urgent hospitalization. The *chronic* form often has an insidious onset; cough and dyspnea increase over a period of months. Fatigue and weight loss may be prominent.

Physical examination findings may be normal or disclose bibasilar or generalized crackles. A restrictive pattern is evident on pulmonary function testing,

and interstitial infiltrates are seen on chest radiographs. The presence of precipitating antibody (precipitins) to a suspected causative agent is helpful in confirming exposure. Pathologic studies typically show an interstitial granulomatous pneumonitis with bronchiolitis. Pathogenesis involves cell-mediated (type IV, Th1) hypersensitivity.

Diagnosis is established in most cases if the history and physical examination findings and pulmonary function test results indicate an interstitial lung disease, if the chest radiograph is consistent with hypersensitivity pneumonitis, if the patient has been exposed to a recognized etiologic agent or source, and if there is serum antibody (precipitins) to the suspected antigen.

TREATMENT

Management of hypersensitivity pneumonitis consists of environmental control to avoid further exposure to the causative agent and of the occasional use of glucocorticoids for severe symptoms.

Avoidance

Treatment depends primarily on identifying the source of the involved antigen and devising an appropriate plan for its avoidance in the workplace or other incriminated environments. The simplest way to avoid the causative agent is to remove the patient from the environment or to remove the source of the agent from the patient's environment. In some instances the source of exposure (birds, humidifiers) can be removed. If occupational exposure is suspected, however, specialty consultation (e.g., occupational medicine) must be considered in order to help address potential compensation and legal matters. It is rarely, if ever, justified to initially tell the patient that he or she must quit work and find a new job. Attempts at antigen avoidance should be least disruptive to the patient's livelihood. Avoidance of areas associated with heavy exposure, improved ventilation or filtration systems, or use of appropriate masks or ventilators may be sufficient. If symptoms recur or physiologic abnormalities worsen in spite of these measures, more therapy is required.

Drug Therapy

The only medication of demonstrable value against hypersensitivity pneumonitis is systemic prednisone or an equivalent glucocorticoid for symptomatic treatment of patients with severe disease. Inhaled steroids are not effective. The use of prophylactic glucocorticoids before antigen exposure in a patient with known hypersensitivity pneumonitis cannot be condoned because the disease may advance despite suppression of symptoms.

Patients with acute hypersensitivity pneumonitis usually recover without the need for corticosteroids. Subacute hypersensitivity pneumonitis may be associated with severe symptoms and marked physiologic impairment that may progress for several days de-

TABLE 1. **Hypersensitivity Pneumonitis (Extrinsic Allergic Alveolitis)**

Disease	Antigen	Source of Particles
Bagassosis	Thermophilic actinomycetes	Moldy bagasse (sugar cane)
Bird fancier's, breeder's, or handler's lung	Parakeet, budgerigar, pigeon, chicken, turkey proteins	Avian droppings or feathers
Chemical worker's lung	Isocyanates	Polyurethane foam, varnishes, lacquer, foundry casting
Coffee worker's lung	Coffee bean dust	Coffee beans
Compost lung	*Aspergillus* species	Compost
Detergent worker's disease	*Bacillus subtilis* enzyme	Detergent
Farmer's lung	Thermophilic actinomycetes	Mold hay, grain, silage
Hot tub lung	*Cladosporium* species	Mold on ceilings
Humidifier or air-conditioner lung (ventilation pneumonitis)	*Aureobasidium pullulans* or other microorganisms	Contaminated water in humidification and forced-air air-conditioning systems
Japanese summerhouse HSP	*Trichosporon cutaneum*	House dust?, bird droppings
Lycoperdonosis	Puffball spores	*Lycoperdon* puffballs
Malt worker's lung	*Aspergillus fumigatus* or *Aspergillus clavatus*	Moldy barley
Maple bark disease	*Cryptostroma corticale*	Maple bark
Miller's lung	*Sitophilus granarius* (wheat weevil)	Infested wheat flour
Mushroom worker's lung	Thermophilic actinomycetes, other	Mushroom compost
Sauna taker's lung	*Aureobasidium* species, other	Contaminated sauna water
Sequoiosis	*Aureobasidium, Graphium* species	Redwood sawdust
Suberosis	Cork dust mold	Cork dust
Tap water lung	Unknown	Contaminated tap water
Thatched roof disease	*Saccharomonospora viridis*	Dried grasses and leaves
Tobacco worker's disease	*Aspergillus* species	Mold on tobacco
Winegrower's lung	*Botrytis cinerea*	Mold on grapes
Woodman's disease	*Penicillium* species	Oak and maple trees
Woodworker's lung	Wood dust; *Alternaria* species	Oak, cedar, and mahogany dusts; pine and spruce pulp

HSP = hypersensitivity pneumonitis.

spite removal or avoidance of the causative agent. Urgent establishment of diagnosis and prompt institution of glucocorticoid treatment may be necessary in such patients. Prednisone, 1 mg per kg per day, is given for 7 to 14 days and then tapered over the next 2 to 6 weeks at a rate judged according to the patient's clinical status and response. Patients with chronic hypersensitivity pneumonitis may recover gradually without therapy after institution of environmental controls. For some patients, however, a prednisone regimen similar to that used for the subacute form may be useful for documenting maximal reversibility and a baseline for lung function. Transformation to a chronic fibrotic stage has been reported, but the frequency of this complication is uncertain, and the value of environmental control in preventing it is unproved. Glucocorticoids have not been shown to improve long-term prognosis.

RHINOSINUSITIS

method of
STEPHANIE A. JOE, M.D., and
DONALD A. LEOPOLD, M.D.
Johns Hopkins University
Baltimore, Maryland

Inflammation and infection of the nasal cavity and paranasal sinuses constitute a leading health care burden in the United States. They are major indications for the use of over-the-counter and herbal medicines, and it prompts numerous visits to physicians and providers of alternative medical care each year. Although it was previously thought that the common cold involved only the nasal cavity and that sinusitis was a rarer condition, studies have shown that both the nose and the sinuses are involved in colds, nasal allergies, and other nasal diseases. In addition, the mucous membranes of the nasal cavities and paranasal sinuses are continuous and similar. For these reasons, it is reasonable to define any inflammation or infection of these entities as rhinosinusitis. This was the conclusion in 1996 of the Task Force on Rhinosinusitis, sponsored by the American Academy of Otolaryngology–Head and Neck Surgery. Simply put, rhinosinusitis is defined as an inflammatory response involving the mucous membranes of the nasal cavity and paranasal sinuses. This usually results in membrane thickening and may or may not have an infectious component.

Healthy nasal and sinus function is illustrated in Figure 1. Normal ciliary function sweeps the mucous blanket toward the sinus ostia. As shown in Figure 2, if normal function is disrupted by inflammation, these ostia become blocked, ciliary clearance is prevented, and mucus stasis occurs. Along with reactionary mucus production, this provides an environment favorable for bacterial overgrowth and infection. Once obstruction is relieved and aeration is restored, healthy mucosa usually regenerates.

The etiology of irritation and/or inflammation of the nasal cavity and sinuses can be multifactorial. Sources include allergies; viral, bacterial, and fungal infection or irritation; anatomic factors; air pressure changes; systemic disease processes such as immune incompetence, immuno-

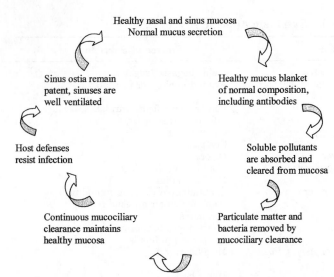

Figure 1. Normal nasal and sinus function. (Adapted from Kennedy DW, Gwaltney JM, Jones JG: Medical management of sinusitis: Educational goals and management guidelines. Ann Otol Rhinol Laryngol 104[Suppl 167]:22–30, 1995.)

globulin deficiencies, and disorders of mucociliary transport (such as cystic fibrosis and immotile cilia syndrome); air pollution; and chemical exposures. It is indeed often difficult to determine which of these possible factors is involved in the disease of a particular patient. The most common symptoms of rhinosinusitis are listed in Table 1.

For description, diagnosis, and treatment, it is easiest to think about rhinosinusitis in classes based on the duration of symptoms and their response to treatment. The classification of adult rhinosinusitis as approved by the Task Force on Rhinosinusitis in 1996 is outlined in Table 2.

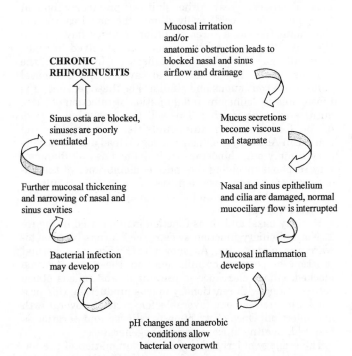

Figure 2. Development of chronic rhinosinusitis. (Adapted from Kennedy DW, Gwaltney JM, Jones JG: Medical management of sinusitis: Educational goals and management guidelines. Ann Otol Rhinol Laryngol 104[Suppl 167]:22–30, 1995.)

TABLE 1. **Signs and Symptoms Associated with Rhinosinusitis**

Major

Nasal obstruction and/or congestion
Rhinorrhea and/or purulent rhinorrhea and/or purulent postnasal drainage
Fever
Hyposmia or anosmia
Facial congestion and/or pain and/or pressure

Minor

Headache
Cough
Ear pain and/or pressure
Halitosis
Fatigue
Dental pain

Adapted from Report of the Rhinosinusitis Task Force Committee Meeting, Otolaryngology–Head and Neck Surgery, Vol. 117, No. 3, Part 2, September 1997.

Acute rhinosinusitis is almost always an infection (usually viral) and is characterized by the sudden onset of symptoms lasting up to 4 weeks. Manifestations strongly indicative of acute infections involve the presence of two or more major symptoms or one major and two minor symptoms (see Table 1). A history suggestive of such an infection includes one major or two or more minor symptoms. In the presence of possible viral infection, rhinosinusitis is suggested by a worsening of symptoms after 5 days, persistence of symptoms for more than 10 days, or the presence of symptoms of greater severity than those typically associated with viral upper respiratory infections. Purulence is usually present in bacterial infection. Symptoms of a bacterial infection usually resolve completely with or without treatment but resolve more quickly with antibiotic therapy.

The symptoms and history of recurrent acute rhinosinusitis are the same as those in the acute form but are typified by four or more episodes in one year. Between episodes, symptoms resolve completely and are absent without antibiotics. Subacute rhinosinusitis is the natural progression of acute rhinosinusitis with symptoms that are less severe and do not resolve within 4 weeks. It is distinguished from chronic rhinosinusitis in that with effective medical therapy, symptoms last less than 12 weeks.

Chronic rhinosinusitis is more of an inflammation than an infection and is defined as symptoms that last longer than 12 weeks. The conditions that the inflammation creates (e.g., edema, stagnant mucus, warmth), however, can be conducive to bacterial, viral, or fungal growth. Table 3 refers to the minor and major factors associated with its diagnosis. A strongly associated history involves two or more major factors or one major and two minor factors. A history suggestive of chronic rhinosinusitis includes two or more minor factors or one major factor. Acute exacerbations may occur and are characterized by a sudden worsening of the baseline condition, such as more membrane thickening. For comparison, Figure 3 graphically illustrates the various forms of rhinosinusitis. (Also refer to the diagnosis algorithm in Figure 4.)

The microbiology in rhinosinusitis varies, depending on the duration of the disease. In acute infection, *Streptococcus pneumoniae* and unencapsulated *Haemophilus influenzae* predominate. Other gram-negative bacteria, anaerobes, *Staphylococcus aureus*, *Streptococcus pyogenes*, and *Moraxella catarrhalis* are found much less frequently.

TABLE 2. **Classification of Adult Rhinosinusitis**

Classification	Duration	Strong Indication	Suggestive
Acute	Up to 4 weeks	Two or more major sx, or one major and two minor sx, or purulent rhinorrhea on examination	One major sx, or two or more minor sx
Recurrent acute	Four or more episodes per year; episodes last 7–10 days, and sx completely clear between episodes	Same as for acute form	Same as acute
Subacute	4–12 weeks	Same as for chronic form	Same as chronic
Chronic	12 weeks or more	Two or more major sx, or one major and two minor sx, or purulent rhinorrhea on examination	One major sx, or two or more minor sx
Acute exacerbations of chronic form	Sudden worsening over several days of chronic rhinosinusitis; returns to baseline with treatment in less than 4 weeks		

Abbreviation: sx = symptoms.

Adapted from Report of the Rhinosinusitis Task Force Committee Meeting, Otolaryngology–Head and Neck Surgery, Vol. 117, No. 3, Part 2, September 1997.

Viruses are often found in conjunction with bacteria in acute rhinosinusitis. The same bacteria are found in acute exacerbations of chronic disease.

Coagulase-negative *Staphylococcus* species are the prevalent organisms cultured in chronic rhinosinusitis. *S. aureus* is also found in a significant number of samples. Although anaerobic bacteria and *S. pneumoniae* are less common, they, along with microaerophilic streptococci and gram-negative bacteria, are more likely to be found with increasing duration of disease. On average, approximately 15% of cultures taken from patients with chronic rhinosinusitis grow multiple organisms, the incidence of which also increases with the duration of disease. The pathophysiologic significance of these bacteria and viruses as far as whether they are causing the chronic disease is uncertain.

Special consideration must be given to the growing emergence of antibiotic-resistant strains of bacteria. All the common bacteria found in acute sinusitis have developed strains resistant to beta-lactam agents. Resistance to other classes of antibiotics is also increasing. Since the early 1990s, drug-resistant pneumococci have become increasingly prevalent in many populations. Patients receiving frequent or prolonged courses of antibiotics, such as young children in day care centers, are particularly susceptible.

Studies have focused on the contribution of viral infection of the upper respiratory tract in the development of acute rhinosinusitis. The naturally occurring cold would be expected to cause inflammation of the nasal and sinus epithelium, leading to infection and blockage of the sinus ostia. Rhinovirus, coronavirus, respiratory syncytial virus, and influenza virus are among the most common viruses found in patients with the common cold. Viral rhinosinusitis is usually self-limited. Treatment with topical interferon and/or influenza vaccination in patients with chronic rhinosinusitis has been suggested.

TREATMENT

Therapy of rhinosinusitis is aimed at reestablishing the normal nasal and sinus environment by restoring airflow throughout the nasal and sinus cavities. Associated goals include improving mucociliary transport through reduction of swelling and inflammation, minimizing anatomic factors, eliminating infectious influences (in acute disease), moisturization,

TABLE 3. **Signs and Symptoms Associated with Chronic Rhinosinusitis**

Major

Nasal obstruction
Rhinorrhea (may or may not be purulent)
Hyposmia or anosmia
Cough not caused by lower respiratory disease (in children)
Facial pain or pressure

Minor

Cough (in adults)
Fatigue
Halitosis
Fever
Dental pain

Adapted from Report of the Rhinosinusitis Task Force Committee Meeting, Otolaryngology–Head and Neck Surgery, Vol. 117, No. 3, Part 2, September 1997.

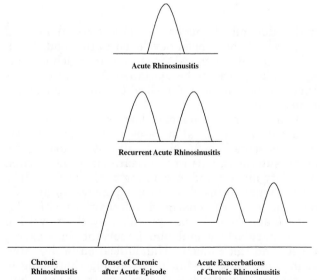

Figure 3. Comparison of forms of rhinosinusitis. (Adapted from the International Rhinosinusitis Advisory Board: Infectious rhinosinusitis in adults: Classification, etiology, and management. ENT J 76[Suppl]:1–22, 1997.)

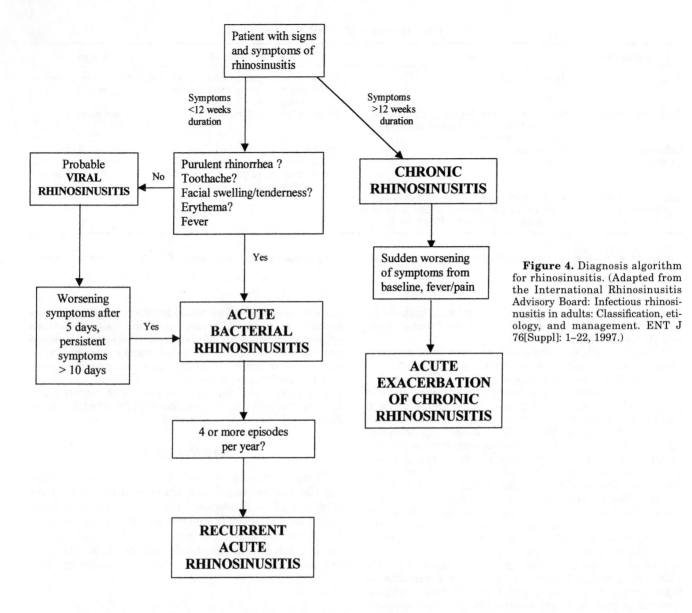

Figure 4. Diagnosis algorithm for rhinosinusitis. (Adapted from the International Rhinosinusitis Advisory Board: Infectious rhinosinusitis in adults: Classification, etiology, and management. ENT J 76[Suppl]: 1–22, 1997.)

and reduction of mucus viscocity. Several medical preparations have been developed to this end. Medical treatment is generally the first approach of therapy and may need to be continued chronically. Sometimes, a combination of medical therapy and surgery is necessary.

Because water transport has been shown to be deficient in some nasal diseases, moisturization therapy has some benefit. Nasal saline moisturizes, decreases dryness, aids in the clearance of inspissated or crusty mucus, and is soothing to the patient. It is most commonly used as an inexpensive spray, sold over the counter in pharmacies. Irrigations with solutions made from recipes provided by the physician are particularly useful and important for clearing crusts and thick mucus. Humidification in dry environments is also useful in preventing thickening of secretions, which slows mucociliary transport. Cautious use is warranted in patients with mold allergies; excessive humidification can trigger inflammation and precipitate rhinosinusitis. Any humidifier

used must also be cleaned regularly. Mucolytics also serve to thin mucus and thus, in theory, assist in mucociliary clearance and decrease mucus stasis.

The mode of action of decongestants is the stimulation of alpha-adrenergic receptors in the mucosa of the upper airways, leading to vasoconstriction of the capillaries with subsequent shrinkage of edematous mucosa. When mucosal swelling is decreased, obstruction of sinus ostia should be relieved and ventilation improved. Whether this has a beneficial effect on the treatment of rhinosinusitis has been debated. Decongestants could arguably interfere with normal defense mechanisms by decreasing mucosal blood flow. Nonetheless, topical decongestants provide rapid relief of symptomatic obstruction with minimal systemic effects. These should not be used longer than 3 to 5 days, however, in order to prevent the development of a rebound congestion and chemical irritation called rhinitis medicamentosa. Systemic decongestants similarly help alleviate symptomatic obstruction and drainage. Prescription forms are often combined with mucolytics. Their use is cautioned in the setting of certain medical conditions: hypertension, prostate hypertrophy, ischemic heart disease, hyperthyroidism, and with a regimen of monoamine oxidase inhibitors. Decongestants are most effective in acute forms of rhinosinusitis.

Antihistamines are prescribed by many physicians and used by many patients in the treatment of rhinosinusitis alone, despite the lack of studies clearly showing a positive effect. Antihistamines help prevent or alleviate the symptoms of allergy by reducing mucosal secretion and local edema upon exposure to an allergen. The development of these reactions could precipitate stasis within the nose or paranasal sinuses. Therefore, they are most useful in patients with both allergy and chronic rhinosinusitis in whom an acute allergic flare-up occurs. Their anticholinergic effects can cause side effects that include drowsiness and excessive drying of nasal and sinus secretions, leading to stagnation within the sinuses. Newer generations of antihistamines have fewer side effects. Immunotherapy should be considered in a patient in whom tests for inhalant allergies have yielded positive results. Remarkable success can sometimes be achieved when even one of the causes of the membrane inflammation is controlled.

Topical nasal sprays are considered mainstays in the treatment of acute allergic and chronic rhinosinusitis. Topical nasal steroids are applicable to allergic rhinosinusitis, nonallergic rhinosinusitis, and chronic rhinosinusitis. They reduce the sensitivity of cholinergic receptors, leading to decreased secretory response, reduction of the number of basophils and eosinophils in the epithelium and basophils on the mucosa, and inhibition of the late-phase reaction after exposure to allergens. In proper dosages, they do not have significant systemic effects. They ameliorate symptoms and decrease the volume of inflammatory cells.

Ipratropium bromide (Atrovent) is a topical anticholinergic and thus blocks glandular hypersecretion and sneezing in allergic rhinosinusitis, nonallergic rhinosinusitis, and the common cold. A possible effect is increased viscosity, but this is minimal in comparison with that caused by antihistamines. Similarly, cromolyn sodium (Nasalcrom) is more useful in allergic rhinosinusitis but has minimal efficacy in acute and chronic rhinosinusitis. Its action is the stabilization of mast cells and has no effect on the inflammatory process once it has occurred.

Systemic corticosteroids inhibit the production of the mediators of inflammation: prostaglandins, lymphokines, leukotrienes, bradykinins, serotonin, and interferon. Capillary permeability is decreased, thus minimizing tissue edema. Lysosomal membranes are stabilized, and circulatory eosinophils and T lymphocytes are redistributed to other compartments. Oral steroids are most useful in cases of allergic rhinosinusitis, nasal polyposis, chronic rhinosinusitis, and allergic fungal rhinosinusitis. Side effects include mucosal itching, superficial gastric ulceration, change in affect or temperament, sleep disturbance,

and premature ventricular contractions. Higher doses can alter insulin requirements in diabetic patients. Several disadvantages are also associated with long-term use of systemic steroids, including osteoporosis, myopathy, peptic ulcer disease, hypertension, ocular problems, weight gain, and increased susceptibility to infection. Steroids can suppress the hypothalamic-pituitary-adrenal axis, and thus abrupt cessation may result in adrenal insufficiency. A tapering dose is recommended for use longer than 1 to 2 weeks.

The treatment schemes for rhinosinusitis differ, depending on its duration. Acute rhinosinusitis is generally an infectious process, and antibiotics covering the most common bacteria are warranted. Nasal saline is recommended for moisturization, crust removal, and pathogen dilution. Decongestants provide symptomatic relief. Treatment is continued for up to 4 weeks. If the patient has concurrent allergy symptoms, these are treated as well with antihistamines, topical nasal steroids, avoidance of allergens, and immunotherapy.

Almost every patient who develops acute rhinosinusitis will improve whether they are treated with antibiotics or not. In general, patients treated with a regimen that includes antibiotics improve faster than do patients who do not receive them. Many studies indicate that empirical treatment with most antibiotic agents results in improvement in the majority of cases. Reasonable and cost-effective choices for first-line therapy to cover the most common organisms found in acute bacterial sinusitis include amoxicillin, trimethoprim-sulfamethoxazole (Bactrim, Septra), erythromycin-sulfisoxazole (Pediazole), and even doxycycline. Second-line choices are considered when there is no improvement with first-line therapy or when the risk for failure with such therapy is high. Amoxicillin-clavulanate (Augmentin), cefuroxime axetil (Ceftin), cefprozil (Cefzil), cefpodoxime proxetil (Vantin), and levofloxacin (Levaquin), are recommended for such cases. The addition of other choices such as clindamycin (Cleocin) and ciprofloxacin (Cipro), are considered in populations with high bacterial resistance rates and complicated cases. Culture-directed antibiotic selection is indicated in severe or complicated cases (e.g., orbit, intracranial, or soft tissue spread).

Chronic rhinosinusitis is treated with topical nasal steroids and nasal saline irrigations for more than 12 weeks and sometimes for life. Unlike acute disease, infection results from conditions created by chronic inflammation. Therefore, antibiotics are added only when there is evidence of bacterial infection. Antibiotic choice can be aided when cultures are obtained under endoscopic guidance from the middle meatus, although empirical therapy is usually recommended for the initial treatment. Leukotriene inhibitors can also be tried. One theory suggests that the pathophysiology of chronic rhinosinusitis is caused by the irritant, not allergic, effects of fungus on the mucosa. In the near future, oral antifungals and topical antifungal nasal sprays may be added to the regimen.

TABLE 4. **Absolute Indications for Surgery
in Rhinosinusitis**

Bilateral extensive and massive nasal polyposis
Complications of rhinosinusitis (orbital, intracranial, neurologic,
    soft tissue, bony)
Chronic rhinosinusitis with mucocele or mucopyocele formation
Invasive and noninvasive fungal rhinosinusitis
Tumor of the nasal cavity and/or paranasal sinuses

Adapted from Report of the Rhinosinusitis Task Force Committee Meeting, Otolaryngology–Head and Neck Surgery, Vol. 117, No. 3, Part 2, September 1997.

The most useful imaging study is a computed tomographic (CT) scan of the paranasal sinuses. It best illustrates nasal and sinus anatomy and associated disease. It is extremely useful to the surgeon and is essential in preoperative planning. It is best to obtain these imaging studies during a relatively quiescent period of the disease process. CT scans should be obtained only after one or two courses of empirical therapy have been ineffective in controlling the patient's symptoms. The full CT scan, not the abbreviated version, is recommended; the time to obtain it is only seconds longer and the radiation dose is only slightly higher. The advantage is that small areas of dysfunction such as the region around the frontal or maxillary ostia may be missed on an abbreviated study. Sometimes the cause of the patient's problems can be determined to be anatomic.

Indications for surgery are outlined in Table 4. Certain factors, including congenital variations in the anatomy of the nasal cavities and paranasal sinuses and the presence of systemic disorders, allergic fungal sinusitis, or invasive fungal sinusitis, may alter these indications. In general, surgery is recommended when maximal medical therapy has failed and the CT scan reveals blocked sinus spaces unable to ventilate properly and chronically thickened mucosa that needs more space.

STREPTOCOCCAL PHARYNGITIS

method of
NELSON M. GANTZ, M.D.
*PinnacleHealth Hospitals
Harrisburg, Pennsylvania
MCP Hahnemann School of Medicine
Philadelphia, Pennsylvania*

Sore throat is the third most common complaint for which people visit a health care provider in the United States. Despite the frequency of pharyngitis and the numerous articles on the subject, the approach to diagnosis and management remains highly controversial. Some of the controversial issues include the following: When is a throat culture indicated? How best can a patient with a sore throat and a positive culture for Group A beta-hemolytic *Streptococcus* be distinguished from a patient who is a streptococcal carrier with symptoms caused by some other organism, such as adenovirus? What is the role of rapid antigen detection tests in the diagnosis of group A beta-hemolytic streptococcal pharyngitis? How sensitive is a single throat culture in detecting group A *Streptococcus*? Should patients be treated without use of a rapid antigen detection test or a throat culture? What are the best treatment regimens? Should cultures be repeated at the end of a course of therapy? How should streptococcal contacts be managed? How should patients with recurrent streptococcal pharyngitis be managed?

A number of organisms have been implicated in pharyngitis, including viruses (adenovirus, coxsackievirus, herpes simplex, influenza, parainfluenza, rhinovirus, cytomegalovirus, and Epstein-Barr), bacteria (group A beta-hemolytic *Streptococcus*; non–group A *Streptococcus*, such as groups B, C, G, and F; *Neisseria gonorrhoeae; Corynebacterium diphtheriae; Arcanobacterium haemolyticum; Francisella tularensis*); and *Mycoplasma*. Pharyngitis can be an important feature of secondary syphilis, toxic shock syndrome, Vincent's angina (mixed infection with *Fusobacterium* and *Bacteroides* species), epiglottitis, chronic fatigue syndrome, and infections of the retropharyngeal space. *Haemophilus influenzae*, although frequently (60%) found on a pharyngeal culture, is an unusual cause of pharyngitis. Although *Staphylococcus aureus* and *Streptococcus pneumoniae* are frequently isolated from a patient with a sore throat, these organisms do not cause pharyngitis and should not be treated. *Chlamydia trachomatis* does not appear to cause pharyngitis. However, *Chlamydia pneumoniae* (TWAR) may be responsible for some cases of pharyngitis. For the clinician, however, the main problem is to determine whether the pharyngitis is caused by group A beta-hemolytic *Streptococcus* or whether the pharyngitis has a nonstreptococcal origin.

EPIDEMIOLOGY

The incidence of streptococcal pharyngitis peaks in the temperate zones during late winter and early spring; the lowest level is in the summer (during August). The organism is transmitted from person to person by large respiratory droplets, and crowding increases the attack rate. Streptococcal disease is most common in school-aged children, who are the main source of organisms introduced into a family. The incubation period is 3 to 5 days but can be as long as 3 months. Acquisition of the organisms is often associated with an asymptomatic infection. Foodborne outbreaks caused by group A *Streptococcus* and other nonstreptococcal organisms result from contamination of the food with the organism by a food handler. Milk and egg products are usually implicated. Streptococcal infection is unusual in children younger than 1 year of age. Specific antibiotic therapy after 24 to 48 hours reduces communicability of the organism, and the patient can return to school or work if symptoms are improved.

CLINICAL MANIFESTATIONS

Clinical findings are unreliable in predicting which organism will be identified by antigen detection or throat culture. The classical description of streptococcal pharyngitis in a school-aged child consists of an illness with an acute onset, fever, headache, sore throat, pain with swallowing, and painful or enlarged cervical lymph nodes. On examination, the throat is red, tonsils may have exudates (20%), and the cervical lymph nodes are tender and enlarged. Although the presence of pharyngeal exudates, enlarged cervical lymph nodes, temperature higher than 101°F (38.4°C), and a peripheral leukocytosis is consistent with a streptococcal etiology, these symptoms may be seen with all causes of pharyngitis. Moderate throat exudates are indicative of a *Streptococcus* infection but can occur with adenovirus or *Mycoplasma* infections. The rash of scarlet fever suggests a streptococcal etiology, but a rash can also occur with *A. haemolyticum* infections or with infectious mononucleosis. The presence of cough, hoarseness, diarrhea, conjunctivitis, and a runny nose suggests a nonstreptococcal etiology. Detection of pharyngeal vesicles or ulcers points to a diagnosis of herpes simplex virus or coxsackievirus infection.

DIAGNOSIS

The gold standard for diagnosis of group A beta-hemolytic *Streptococcus* is the throat culture, which has a 10% false-negative rate. The isolation of *Streptococcus* on a throat culture does not distinguish an acute infection with streptococcal pharyngitis from another cause for the pharyngitis in a patient who is a chronic streptococcal carrier. About half the patients with cultures that are positive for group A *Streptococcus* show a rise in antistreptococcal antibodies, and such patients are at risk for the development of nonsuppurative complications. The other half have elevated streptococcal antibody titers when first seen that do not subsequently increase, and they are streptococcal carriers. Because serologic studies are not usually done when patients have a sore throat, and because other simple tests to detect carriers are not available, all patients with a positive culture are treated similarly. Except for some nasal carriers of group A streptococci, chronic carriers are not a major source of spreading the streptococcal organism.

A number of tests to detect streptococcal antigens through the use of an enzyme immunoassay technique on the throat specimen have become available and are alternatives to a throat culture. The tests have 80 to 90% sensitivity and 95% specificity. The test is positive only with group A *Streptococcus* and does not detect other streptococcal groups. If the rapid antigen test result is positive, the organism is likely to be group A *Streptococcus,* and a culture can be omitted. If the rapid antigen test result is negative and a streptococcal infection is suspected, a throat culture should be done, and treatment should be based on the results. The rapid immunologic tests may fail to identify small numbers of streptococci, which may be associated with a rise in antistreptolysin O titer.

TREATMENT

There are four reasons to treat group A streptococcal pharyngitis. First, therapy begun within 48 hours of the onset of illness can result in a more rapid resolution of fever and symptoms. Second, antibiotic therapy can prevent the development of local suppurative complications such as cervical adenitis, peritonsillar abscess, or retropharyngeal abscess. Third, therapy, even if delayed for 9 days, can prevent acute rheumatic fever but probably not acute glomerulonephritis. Fourth, therapy can decrease the infectivity of the index case. Although non–group A beta-hemolytic *Streptococcus* organisms probably cause pharyngitis, the effects of treatment on the clinical course and on the incidence of sequelae need further study.

Because the clinical findings, even when several criteria are met, fail to distinguish a viral from a streptococcal sore throat, the question of whether to take a culture or treat without a culture is controversial. In the setting of a streptococcal epidemic, treatment without a culture is appropriate and is not controversial. In the usual nonepidemic setting, arguments can be made for (1) treating only patients with positive direct antigen tests or cultures (the currently recommended approach), (2) using antibiotic treatment for all patients who have sore throats but no culture, or (3) neither culturing nor treating any patient with a sore throat. The approach adopted depends on the clinician's weighing the rationale for treatment, the various costs to the patient (such as those for cultures and drugs), and the consequences of widespread antibiotic therapy (e.g., drug reactions, bacterial resistance). I suggest that the clinician swab the patient's throat with two swabs. If the rapid streptococcal test is positive, the second swab is discarded and therapy is begun. If the rapid test is negative, the second swab is cultured. Therapy may be instituted pending culture results or may be withheld until the diagnosis is confirmed.

TREATMENT REGIMENS (Table 1)

Penicillin is the drug of choice for streptococcal pharyngitis; most patients may be treated with oral penicillin V. The duration of therapy must be 10 days; 7 days is inadequate. Benzathine penicillin G is an alternative therapy that ensures compliance but is associated with considerable pain at the injection site for both children and adults. Penicillin V in adults is given in a dose of 500 mg twice or three times daily or in a dose of 250 mg three or four times daily for 10 days. In children weighing less than 60 pounds, penicillin V, 250 mg twice or three times daily, is effective. Amoxicillin at a dose of 40 mg per kg in three divided doses or 750 mg once daily is well tolerated in children and is also effective. Benzathine penicillin G, 1.2 million units, is given to adults intramuscularly into the buttocks. Erythromycin is the alternative drug in the United States for penicillin-allergic patients. Children may be given erythromycin estolate, 20 to 50 mg per kg per day orally in two to four divided doses. Adults can be given other erythromycin preparations such as the ethylsuccinate, 400 mg orally three or four times daily, or erythromycin base or stearate, 250 mg four times daily, for 10 days. Erythromycin preparations are better tolerated when they are taken with food.

Other drugs include cephalexin, 250 mg orally four times a day for 10 days, and, rarely, clindamycin (Cleocin). More expensive alternative drugs include cefuroxime axetil, 250 mg twice daily for 10 days in adults and 20 mg per kg per day given in two divided doses daily for 5 days in children. Cefdinir, 300 mg twice a day for 5 days, is also effective. The macrolides azithromycin and clarithromycin are alternatives for patients who cannot tolerate erythromycin. Cephalosporins are contraindicated in patients with an immediate hypersensitivity reaction to penicillin.

TABLE 1. **Selected Treatments for Streptococcal Pharyngitis**

Drug	Dosage	Frequency	Duration	Comments
Penicillin V	500 mg	bid or tid	10 d	Drug of choice in adults
Penicillin V (<60 lbs)	250 mg	bid or tid	10 d	Drug of choice
Penicillin G benzathine (Bicillin L-A)	1.2×10^6 U	once		Painful but ensures compliance
Penicillin G benzathine and procaine combined (Bicillin C-R)	900,000 U benzathine penicillin G 300,000 U procaine penicillin	once		Painful but ensures compliance
Amoxicillin (Amoxil)	40 mg/kg/day	tid	10 d	Pleasant taste
Erythromycin				Alternative for patients with penicillin allergy
Ethylsuccinate (E.E.S.)	400 mg	tid or qid	10 d	
Base or stearate (Erythrocin)	250 mg	qid	10 d	
Estolate (Ilosone)	20–50 mg/kg/day	qid	10 d max, 1 gm/d	Alternative for children with penicillin allergy
Cephalexin (Keflex)	250 mg	qid	10 d	Adults
Cefuroxime axetil (Ceftin)	250 mg	bid	10 d	Expensive
Cefdinir (Omnicef)	300 mg	bid	5 d	Expensive
Azithromycin (Zithromax)	500 mg day 1 250 mg days 2–4	daily	5 d	Causes less GI distress than erythromycin
Clarithromycin (Biaxin)	250 mg	bid	10 d	Causes less GI upset than erythromycin Expensive

Abbreviation: GI = gastrointestinal.

Drugs such as trimethoprim-sulfamethoxazole (Bactrim, Septra), tetracycline, and the quinolones (e.g., ciprofloxacin [Cipro]) have no role in treating streptococcal pharyngitis. Amoxicillin-clavulanate (Augmentin) is far more expensive and is no more effective than penicillin V, even in patients with penicillin-resistant staphylococci on throat culture. Adjunctive therapy consists of rest, saline gargles, warm liquids, aspirin for adults or acetaminophen, and lozenges.

The failure rate associated with penicillin is 15 to 20%. The role of pharyngeal penicillinase-producing organisms in contributing to this failure rate is controversial. For selected patients in whom conventional therapy fails, clindamycin, 600 mg per day in two to four divided doses, may be effective. The addition of rifampin (Rifadin),* 20 mg per kg per day (600 mg maximum) orally, to the last 4 days of a 10-day course of penicillin has been associated with improved bacteriologic cure rates.

There is no indication to treat or culture asymptomatic family contacts unless they have a history of rheumatic fever. Symptomatic contacts should obtain cultures and be treated.

RECURRENT PHARYNGITIS

Streptococcal carriers do not need treatment unless there is a history of recurrent streptococcal disease in a family with "ping-pong" spread of infection. There is no evidence that family pets contribute to recurrent streptococcal disease. Because patient compliance with an oral drug can be an issue, use of intramuscular benzathine penicillin G should be used for recurrences. Most recurrences are seen in

*Not FDA approved for this indication.

patients who are streptococcal carriers and have viral pharyngitis. Continuous antimicrobial prophylaxis for group A streptococci is not indicated. In rare cases, tonsillectomy may decrease the frequency of recurrent streptococcal infection.

FOLLOW-UP EVALUATION

Culture testing for cure is not indicated unless a patient is still symptomatic. Only symptomatic patients should be re-treated.

TUBERCULOSIS

method of
ROBERT J. AWE, M.D.
Baylor College of Medicine and Ben Taub General Hospital Houston, Texas

Despite the fact that most cases of tuberculosis are curable, this disease still kills more people worldwide than any other infectious disease, including malaria and AIDS. More than 10 million people develop active disease each year, and 3 million die annually. Hopes that tuberculosis could be eradicated from the world have been dashed by the rapidly spreading AIDS epidemic into areas already endemic for tuberculosis, especially Africa, India, and Southeast Asia. In addition, recent recognition of the increasing occurrence of mycobacteria resistant to isoniazid and rifampin and the widespread lack of national government interest and funding have made the potential conquest and eradication of tuberculosis unattainable in the near future. Thus although it is both preventable and curable in the overwhelming number of cases, tuberculosis will remain a major health threat to the world's population for decades to come.

However, the picture this year is not as bleak as it was in the mid-1980s, when the number of tuberculosis cases increased for the first time in 50 years. In fact, in 1998 there were some incredible advances in the battle against the disease. For the first time in 25 years, a new promising drug, rifapentine (Priftin), has been approved by the U.S. Food and Drug Administration (FDA). This medication can be given only once weekly instead of two or three times a week. This year, the entire genome of tuberculosis has been mapped, opening the way for better vaccines and more effective designer drugs to be developed. A new polymerase chain reaction (PCR) can identify *Mycobacterium tuberculosis* as soon as the smear is seen to be positive, allowing identification of organisms within hours rather than weeks. Last, a new fluoroquinolone antibiotic, levofloxacin (Levaquin), has demonstrated significant effectiveness against *M. tuberculosis* in the murine model and is one of the better second-line medications.

SYMPTOMS

The typical symptoms of tuberculosis are weight loss, night sweats, fatiguability, and fever, often up to 103 to 104°F. These symptoms usually have been present for several days to weeks by the time the patient seeks medical attention. The organ most commonly involved is the lung. Pulmonary tuberculosis manifests with a productive cough and often with streaking hemoptysis. Massive hemoptysis caused by rupture of a Rasmussen aneurysm may occur.

In most cases, a chest radiograph shows an apical fibronodular infiltrate, often with cavitation. In more advanced cases, tuberculosis can spread to involve any lobe of the lung. In AIDS, the radiologic picture is different; hilar lymphadenitis or middle or lower lobe infiltrates are often seen. Cavitation is uncommon. For this reason, all patients with AIDS and new pulmonary infiltrates should be placed in respiratory isolation until tuberculosis can be ruled out.

Up to 20% of smears for acid-fast bacilli (AFB) in patients with active pulmonary tuberculosis are negative. If the clinical suspicion for active disease is high (i.e., in the presence of fever, sweats, weight loss, and a chest radiograph showing apical disease), treatment should be commenced rather than waiting for cultures results to return. If the local mycobacteriology laboratory has a PCR test such as Amplicor, this should be ordered for smear-negative cases because the PCR may be positive even though the smear is negative.

EXTRAPULMONARY TUBERCULOSIS

Tuberculous Pleural Effusion

Symptoms. Cough, fever, pleuritis, chest pain.
Diagnosis. Exudate with lymphocyte predominance, low glucose. AFB smear is usually negative. Pleural biopsy is often needed to confirm diagnosis and obtain tissue for culture.

Tuberculous Lymphadenitis (Scrofula)

Most frequent form of extrapulmonary tuberculosis. Usually unilateral cervical node, firm, painless.
Diagnosis. Fine-needle aspiration or excisional node biopsy should be performed for AFB smear and culture.

Spinal Tuberculosis (Pott's Disease)

Pain over lower thoracic or lumbar spine. Paraspinal cold abscesses in 50%. Computed tomographic (CT) scan or magnetic resonance imaging (MRI) usually reveals diskitis. Biopsy should be performed for histologic study and culture.

Renal Tuberculosis

Low back or flank pain. Sterile pyuria and hematuria. Intravenous pyelogram is usually suggestive; 3 AM urine specimens should be cultured.

Tuberculous Meningitis

Headache, vomiting, lethargy. Lumbar puncture reveals lymphocytosis, elevated protein levels, low glucose. Smears for AFB are often negative; these findings should be confirmed by culture.

Miliary Tuberculosis

Hematogenous dissemination to multiple sites. Miliary infiltrates are visible on chest radiographs. Transbronchial lung biopsy should be performed for histologic study and culture.

TRANSMISSION

Tuberculosis is transmitted to a susceptible host with variable efficiency, depending on three things: (1) the infectivity of the source, (2) the immune defenses of the person exposed, and (3) the environment in which the contact occurs. Persons with large cavitary lesions who shed thousands of organisms into the air with each cough are obviously more contagious than a person with a minimal apical fibronodular infiltrate and negative sputum smears.

The host's immune defenses are also important. Alcoholic persons, intravenous drug abusers, and homeless persons are more susceptible than well-nourished healthy people. The population with the least defense is that of people infected with the human immunodeficiency virus (HIV). In the general population, only 5 to 10% of people infected with tuberculosis manifest the disease in their lifetime. Of persons with HIV infection, 8 to 10% per year develop disease. Black males with histocompatibility leukocyte antigen (HLA) type Bw 15 and genetic variation in natural resistance–associated macrophage protein (NRAMP) appear to be more susceptible to developing active disease. NRAMP defects lead to decreased production of nitric oxide, which increases susceptibility to tuberculosis.

Probably the most important factor in determining the transmission of tuberculosis is the air quality of the environment at the time of contact. In a calm, stale room with no significant air circulation, the source case may discharge large amounts of infectious droplet nuclei into the room. These particles remain suspended in the air and infectious for hours. The host may contract infection without even seeing the person who infected him or her. On a windy, sunny day outside, tuberculosis transmission rarely occurs, no matter how susceptible the host. Minimal air quality standards to reduce transmission are six air exchanges per hour. Virtually all of the droplet nuclei are removed from the air after 1 hour. With 12 air exchanges per hour, the air is considered safe after 30 minutes. Other environmental controls, such as ultraviolet lighting and negative-pressure rooms, which lessen the amount of contaminated air spilling into hallways, should be made available in today's hospitals. Health care workers should wear masks when in the presence of a patient with suspected newly active disease. Paper tie-on masks are not appropriate; a dust-mist cup–shaped mask with a tight face seal is necessary. The more elaborate high-efficiency particulate air (HEPA) filter masks are marginally more efficient at particle filtration but are bulky and uncomfortable and, in my opinion, not generally useful.

Public health clinics generally classify tuberculosis in these stages, which are internationally recognized:

TB 0: no exposure, no infection

TB I: exposure, no infection, insignificant reaction to purified protein derivative (PPD) test

TB II: infection, no disease (postive PPD reaction), greater than 10 mm of induration

TB III: active disease

TB IV: inactive disease, history of previous tuberculosis; residuum of granulomatosis disease visible on radiograph

TB V: abnormal chest radiograph but unclear about whether disease is active, pending sputum cultures; can keep this classification only for 3 months.

TREATMENT

The key to the successful treatment of tuberculosis is isoniazid and rifampin (Rifadin). These drugs are bactericidal to both rapidly growing and slowly replicating *M. tuberculosis* organisms. Cure rates are 95% when these two drugs are taken daily for 9 months.

Pyrazinamide (PZA) is effective mainly against rapidly replicating organisms and is beneficial mainly in the first 2 months of therapy. Studies have demonstrated that adding PZA to isoniazid and rifampin for the first 2 months can decrease the total treatment period to 6 months and still achieve a cure rate better than 90%.

Because of the increasing incidence of drug resistance in the United States, primarily among Hispanic and Asian immigrants, it is now recommended that initially four drugs be started—isoniazid, rifampin, PZA, and ethambutol—until it is documented that the organism is susceptible to all medications given. If the organism is a sensitive strain, the ethambutol can be stopped at once. The isoniazid, rifampin, and PZA are continued for a total of 2 months. Then the PZA can be discontinued and the isoniazid and rifampin continued for another 4 months, for a total of 6 months of therapy.

COMPLIANCE

The critical issue in successfully treating tuberculosis is to ensure that the patient takes all of the medication prescribed for the total period needed. It is very difficult to predict when patients will be compliant and when they will not. Thus it is recommended that in most cases, therapy be administered by a health care worker who ensures that the patient is ingesting the medication. It has been shown that intermittent twice weekly therapy is as effective as daily therapy, so in most cases, directly observed

therapy twice weekly has become the standard of care once the induction phase is completed. For pansensitive tuberculosis, therapy for a total of 6 months is recommended.

Induction Phase

Daily for 2 weeks:

Isoniazid, 5 mg per kg (300 mg maximum)
Rifampin, 10 mg per kg (600 mg maximum)
PZA, 15 to 30 mg per kg (2500 mg maximum)
Ethambutol, 15 mg per kg (1200 mg maximum)

Continuation Phase

Twice weekly for 2 months:

Isoniazid, 15 mg per kg (900 mg maximum)
Rifampin, 10 mg per kg (600 mg maximum)
PZA, 40 mg per kg (3500 mg maximum)

The PZA can be stopped after 2 months.

Final Continuation

Twice weekly for 4 months:

Isoniazid, 15 mg per kg (900 mg maximum)
Rifampin, 10 mg per kg (600 mg maximum)

Pyridoxine (vitamin B_6), 50 mg per day or 100 mg biweekly, should be added to lessen the chances of isoniazid-induced neuropathy in malnourished patients.

If the organism is reported to be resistant to one of the primary drugs, consultation with an expert is recommended. Rifapentine (Priftin) is a long-acting rifamycin that allows therapy to be given once weekly, after a 2-month twice-a-week induction phase is completed. The relapse rate with isoniazid and rifapentine once weekly is slightly higher than that with isoniazid and rifampin given twice weekly but the advantage of only once weekly therapy outweighs the disadvantage of a few more relapses.

The newer fluoroquinolones, levofloxacin (Levaquin) and sparfloxacin (Zagam), are becoming important second-line drugs for the treatment of multiple-drug–resistant tuberculosis. However, if the cultures show resistance to isoniazid and rifampin, a local public health expert should be consulted to help plan the therapy. Rifabutin is used primarily to treat tuberculosis in patients with AIDS who are taking protease inhibitors, because it does not lower the levels of protease inhibitors to the same degree as rifampin does. Rifabutin decreases levels of indinavir (Crixivan) and nelfinavir (Viracept) by 25 to 30%, whereas rifampin causes these levels to drop by 85 to 90%. Thus rifampin cannot be used to treat most HIV-infected patients who have tuberculosis because protease inhibitors are the key drugs in the management of people with HIV infection and AIDS. The reason for the interaction of rifampin with the protease inhibitors is the cytochrome P-450 enzyme system in the liver. Rifampin induces or stimulates this system, increasing the metabolism of the protease inhibitors, whereas the protease inhibitors inhibit the system, causing the serum concentration of rifampin to increase to toxic levels. Rifabutin decreases levels of the protease inhibitors by only 30%, but it is recommended that only half the usual dose (150 mg daily) be taken, to avoid the toxic levels of rifabutin that result when its metabolism is slowed by the protease inhibitors.

MONITORING

The most dangerous side effect of isoniazid is hepatitis. In patients younger than age 35, this complication is rare, but hepatitis occurs in 4.6% of patients older than age 65. Once hepatitis develops, the death rate is as high as 12%. In patients taking isoniazid, it is not uncommon for their baseline serum transaminase levels to increase slightly (i.e., 1.5 to 2.0 times normal levels), but these levels return to normal despite continuation of the isoniazid. If the liver enzyme levels rise three times or more above baseline, the isoniazid should be stopped. Routine monthly monitoring of liver enzymes is recommended for patients older than 35 years of age. In patients younger than 35, verbal monitoring of hepatitis symptoms is sufficient. The patient should be told to avoid alcohol and acetaminophen (Tylenol) and to stop taking isoniazid if nausea, vomiting, lethargy, or jaundice occurs.

Hepatitis is also the most serious side effect of rifampin. The incidence of hepatotoxicity is slightly increased if isoniazid and rifampin are used together. PZA also may cause hepatitis and, rarely, hyperuricemia. Monthly monitoring of visual acuity and red-green color discrimination are indicated in order to detect optic neuritis in patients taking ethambutol.

If signs or symptoms of hepatitis appear, all medication should be stopped. After the transaminase levels have returned to baseline, one drug should be started each week and liver enzymes checked until the offending agent is identified. As a rule, rechallenge with isoniazid is not attempted.

Sputums samples for AFB should be checked monthly. For 90% of patients, smears and cultures are negative by the end of the second month of adequate therapy. Smears and cultures that are still positive at the end of the third month indicate probable treatment failure. The primary reason for treatment failure is noncompliance. This is why directly observed therapy is so important, as it ensures ingestion of all medications. Unrecognized drug resistance and malabsorption of drugs are other explanations. Consultation with the local health department would be in order to help solve the problem.

OTHER MYCOBACTERIAL DISEASES

Mycobacterium avium complex (MAC) includes *Mycobacterium avium*, which causes tuberculosis in birds, and *Mycobacterium intracellulare*. Ninety per-

cent of disseminated disease in patients with AIDS is caused by *M. avium*. Of the cases of disease in patients without AIDS, half are caused by *M. avium* and the other half are caused by *M. intracellulare*. The manifestation of the disease is entirely different in patients with AIDS.

In patients without AIDS, the clinical and radiologic picture is similar to that of *M. tuberculosis* except that the patient is usually less ill. MAC tends to cause disease in older males with underlying chronic lung disease, but increasing numbers of older females with normal lungs have recently been seen with MAC disease, often in the form of middle lobe or lower lobe infiltrates rather than the usual apical fibronodular infiltrates.

MAC is ubiquitous in the environment, and colonization is common. To document infection, at least two strongly positive cultures of sputum or bronchial lavage are necessary. Other causes of apical infiltrates (*M. tuberculosis*, fungi) must also be excluded.

Treatment is usually successful with clarithromycin* (Biaxin), 1000 mg per day, or azithromycin* (Zithromax), 500 mg per day, plus ethambutol* (Myambutol) at 15 mg per day and rifabutin* at 300 mg per day. Therapy is generally needed for 18 to 24 months.

Disseminated MAC in patients with AIDS manifests with prostration, high fever, drenching sweats, diarrhea, and weight loss. Diagnosis is made with blood cultures, which are positive in 95% of the cases. Therapy is the same as that for patients without AIDS and should probably be continued for the rest of the patients' lives.

Another atypical organism that causes pulmonary disease virtually identical to that of *M. tuberculosis* is *Mycobacterium kansasii*. It is distributed worldwide and seems to be more prevalent in urban areas. It is a Runyon group I photo chromogen and, like all the atypical pathogens, is not transmitted from human to human. The environmental source is probably soil. Treatment is isoniazid, ethambutol (Myambutol), and rifampin daily for 18 months. *M. kansasii* is almost always resistant to PZA. Because *M. kansasii* is not contagious and thus not a threat to public health, directly observed therapy is not offered.

CHEMOPROPHYLAXIS

Isoniazid, 5 mg per kg up to 300 mg given daily for 1 year, will prevent up to 90% of infected patients from developing active disease. But the risk of developing disease must be balanced by the risk of developing isoniazid-related hepatitis.

Chemoprophylaxis is clearly indicated mainly for young patients; a cut-off of 35 years of age is standard. Before the age of 35 years, the risk of hepatitis toxicity is low and isoniazid is indicated in persons with a PPD reaction greater than 10 mm of induration. For patients older than 35 years, isoniazid prophylaxis is recommended only for certain high-risk

---

*Not FDA approved for this indication.

groups; patients with recent PPD conversion are given the highest priority. Recent conversion is defined as changing from a negative PPD reaction to one greater than 10 mm of induration within a 2-year period. Other high-risk groups include jail inmates, residents of nursing homes or other long-term care facilities, homeless persons, and health care workers. These persons should be offered chemoprophylaxis regardless of age if their PPD reactions are greater than 10 mm of induration. In the majority of cases, a positive PPD skin test result in a person older than 35 years does not warrant chemoprophylaxis. The group at most risk of developing active tuberculosis after being infected are those co-infected with HIV. These persons should be given high priority to receive isoniazid when their PPD reaction is 5 mm of induration. In many areas, to ensure compliance, directly observed preventive therapy is offered at 900 mg twice weekly for 1 year.

TUBERCULIN SKIN TEST

The multiprong PPD tests such as the tine are not satisfactory for tuberculosis screening. The gold standard is the Mantoux, an intradermal injection of 0.1 mL of PPD, usually into the ulnar surface of the forearm. The test is read at 48 to 72 hours by measuring the amount of induration, not erythema. Unfortunately, the test is not extremely sensitive or specific. False-negative findings can result from advanced tuberculosis, malnutrition, and, most important, HIV co-infection. False-positive results can be obtained from people infected with MAC organisms or from immigrants from countries where bacille Calmette-Guérin (BCG) vaccine is used to prevent serious tuberculosis in children. Thus a positive PPD reaction, defined in most cases as greater than 10 mm of induration, does not prove infection with *M. tuberculosis*, and a negative result does not rule out infection.

BACILLE CALMETTE-GUÉRIN

BCG is widely used in most developing countries. It is efficacious primarily in lessening the impact of *M. tuberculosis*–induced disease in children so that cases of miliary disease or meningitis are decreased. It does not prevent tuberculosis in children or adults; nor does it usually cause a strongly positive vesicular reaction to the Mantoux skin test. However, it can cause a PPD test result to be falsely positive, but it virtually never causes a PPD induration of more than 12 mm.

Two nucleic acid amplification (NAA) tests have been approved by the FDA since 1985. Gene-Probe developed the *Mycobacterium* direct test (MDT), which amplifies the RNA in *Mycobacteria*. Amplicor

TABLE 1. **Utility of Amplicor**

AFB Smear	Amplicor	Diagnosis
+	+	*Mycobacterium tuberculosis*
−	−	Not *M. tuberculosis*
+	−	*Mycobacterium* species other than *M. tuberculosis*

AFB = acid-fast bacilli.

(Roche) amplifies mycobacterial DNA by PCR. Nucleic acid amplification tests are close to 100% specific in establishing the presence of *M. tuberculosis* in the sputum, and culture results are available in hours rather than weeks. As noted in Table 1, if the AFB smear is positive but the Amplicor result is negative, isolation can be discontinued, because the smear is positive for a mycobacterium other than *M. tuberculosis* and the patient is not contagious.

PUBLIC HEALTH DEPARTMENTS

It is extremely important that suspected cases of tuberculosis be reported to the local health department. Without their essential contribution to identify contacts and the need for chemoprophylaxis in those infected, control of tuberculosis can never be achieved in this country. In addition, health departments screen high-risk persons, such as jail inmates, persons in homeless shelters or long-term institutions, and those with HIV, for infection. In most states, the treatment of tuberculosis is without cost to the patient. Medications and periodic screening are also free of charge. Private physicians who wish to manage tuberculosis cases almost always find a helpful partner in their local health department.

DRUG RESISTANCE

Primary drug resistance is very uncommon in the United States. Drug resistance almost always results from inadequate doses of drugs, inappropriate regimens, or patient noncompliance; that is, the physician is usually to blame if a patient becomes drug-resistant. The World Health Organization demonstrated that worldwide, 10% of organisms had primary resistance, usually to isoniazid. Treatment of drug-resistant tuberculosis is very expensive, has a success rate much lower than that in pansensitive cases, and often requires the use of second-line drugs and injectables such as streptomycin or amikacin* (Amikin), which have significant side effects. Treating physicians confronted with a drug-resistant case should ask for consultation from local health departments early and often.

*Not FDA approved for this indication.

The Cardiovascular System

ACQUIRED DISEASES OF THE AORTA

method of
GLENN R. JACOBOWITZ, M.D.,
MARK A. ADELMAN, M.D., and
THOMAS S. RILES, M.D.
New York University Medical Center
New York, New York

Acquired diseases of the aorta include aneurysm, aortic dissection, and atherosclerotic occlusive disease. These entities are usually associated with an underlying degenerative process that becomes more common with age. Other causes of aortic disease include connective tissue disorders, inflammatory processes, infections, and trauma. Multiple associated medical problems are often present with acquired aortic disease. Although the nature of aortic disease and associated problems has not changed over the years, the advent of endovascular techniques has enhanced the ability of the vascular surgeon to intervene for high-risk patients.

Risk factors associated with atherosclerotic occlusive or aneurysmal disease of the aorta include cardiac disease, hypertension, smoking, and other peripheral vascular occlusive or aneurysmal disease. Myocardial infarction remains the most common cause of mortality associated with aortic surgery. Therefore, before elective aortic surgery, thorough cardiac evaluation should be performed to minimize risk. The evaluation may include echocardiography, stress testing (dipyridamole thallium study, exercise, dobutamine echocardiography), and coronary angiography. Medical optimization, coronary angioplasty or stenting, and coronary artery bypass surgery may reduce the cardiac risk associated with aortic surgery.

Intraoperative invasive monitoring—including that for arterial blood pressure, central and pulmonary capillary wedge pressure with Swan-Ganz catheters, core temperature, and urine output—is essential during aortic surgery. Blood transfusion can be significantly reduced with autotransfusion devices that salvage blood lost at operation and process it for reinfusion. Postoperative care in the intensive care unit by an experienced team is essential.

ANEURYSMAL DISEASE

The incidence of aortic aneurysm disease is clearly increasing. Most aortic aneurysms are fusiform and are located in the infrarenal aorta. The incidence of abdominal aortic aneurysms is about seven times that of thoracic aortic aneurysms. The incidence increases with age in both men and women, peaking at 5.9% for men and 4.5% for women at age 90 for abdominal aneurysms. The pathogenesis of aortic aneurysmal disease is multifactorial. The predilection of the disease process for the distal aorta is suggestive of a hemodynamic component. Fewer medial elastic lamellae are present in the infrarenal aorta than in the suprarenal aorta, resulting in reduced elasticity, and the nutrient vessels of the aorta, the vasa vasorum, are diminished. Both of these factors may contribute to aneurysm formation. In addition, genetic factors have been implicated because of a tendency for aneurysmal disease to occur in several members of the same family, particularly males. Once an aneurysm begins to form, wall tension continues to increase, causing further dilation. At a given transmural pressure (p), the wall tension (T) is directly proportional to the radius (r) of the aorta according to the law of LaPlace (T = pr). Thus as radius or pressure increases, tension (and the risk of rupture) also increases. When mural tension exceeds the tensile strength of the vessel wall, rupture occurs.

Abdominal Aortic Aneurysms

Diagnosis of abdominal aortic aneurysms (AAAs) may be based on physical examination (pulsatile abdominal mass), plain radiography, ultrasonography, computed tomographic (CT) scan, or magnetic resonance imaging (MRI). Most are asymptomatic and are detected on routine physical examination or by diagnostic imaging performed for other reasons. The majority of AAAs are fusiform and are caused by atherosclerotic degeneration. A more rare manifestation is that of a mycotic (infected) aneurysm, which may be saccular in shape. The most common complication of AAA is rupture, which may manifest with a pulsatile abdominal mass, abdominal or back pain, and hypotension. Mycotic aneurysms may manifest with signs and symptoms of systemic infection. In addition, symptoms may be present with the more rare inflammatory aneurysm. Only 5% of AAAs have an inflammatory component, which is seen on CT scan as a thickening, usually over the anterolateral surface of the aneurysm. Although frequently symptomatic, these particular aneurysms rarely rupture.

Treatment

Elective repair of abdominal aortic aneurysms is based on a cost/benefit (perioperative mortality/prevention of rupture) analysis. The rate of perioperative mortality from elective AAA surgery is approximately 2 to 5%. The natural history of AAAs at various diameters has been well documented. Aneurysms less than 5 cm diameter have a less than 2% annual rupture rate. Aneurysms 5 to 5.9 cm have a

243

5-year rupture rate of about 25%. This rises to 35% for 6-cm aneurysms and 75% for aneurysms 7 cm or larger. The rate of mortality from a ruptured aneurysm is 50% for patients who arrive at a hospital alive and probably closer to 90% when prehospital deaths are included. Thus the current recommendation is for elective operative repair of AAAs larger than 5 cm in diameter. The annual growth rate of AAAs is 2 to 4-mm increase in diameter. For aneurysms less than 5 cm in diameter, yearly follow-up with abdominal ultrasonography or CT scan should be performed. Aneurysms that increase more than 5 mm over the course of 1 year should be considered for repair.

One treatment method is a standard open repair that includes laparotomy, aortic cross-clamping, and replacement of the aneurysmal segment with a prosthetic graft of either Dacron or polytetrafluoroethylene (PTFE). A retroperitoneal approach may also be used. This may be particularly useful with inflammatory aneurysms. An endoaneurysmorrhaphy approach is usually used, in which the aneurysm is opened and the synthetic graft is laid within the aneurysm sac, anastomosing proximally and distally to normal arterial wall. The aneurysmal disease often extends into the iliac arteries, necessitating a bifurcated aortic graft.

The other method of abdominal aortic aneurysm repair is placement of an endovascular stent. This was first described by Parodi in 1991 and has since been popularized on a global scale. The technique involves transfemoral access to the aorta. An aortic graft (Dacron or PTFE) is collapsed into an introducer system, passed into the aorta, and expanded across the aneurysm sac under fluoroscopic guidance. The graft is held in place by metal alloy hooks or friction-fitted stents. The attachment points are proximal and distal to the aneurysm, thereby diverting the flow of blood through the endoprosthesis and preventing the transmission of systemic blood pressure to the aneurysm wall. Several devices are currently approved by the U.S. Food and Drug Administration, and continued experience has enabled improvement in success rates and lowering of complication rates. Safety and efficacy have been proved in multicenter studies. Nevertheless, complication rates remain slightly higher than those with standard open repair. The benefit has been significant, markedly decreasing the number of hospital days and the recuperative time. Current limitations of endovascular repair include proximal extent of the aneurysm (an infrarenal neck of nonaneurysmal aorta is usually necessary to safely deploy the graft) and distal disease (iliac aneurysms preclude distal attachment, and iliofemoral occlusive disease may preclude introduction of the graft into the aorta). Treatment of mycotic aneurysms includes aortic resection, ligation, and extra-anatomic bypass (axillo-bifemoral graft) to revascularize the lower extremities.

Thoracic Aortic Aneurysms

These aneurysms may be divided into ascending, arch, and descending thoracic aneurysms. Risk factors are similar to those of AAAs, although there is sometimes an association with aortic dissection. Historically, syphilis was associated with ascending aortic aneurysms, but this association is now rare. Most thoracic aneurysms are caused by atherosclerotic disease. Aortic valvular disease may also be present, particularly with ascending aortic aneurysms. The natural history of thoracic aortic aneurysms is not as well defined as that of AAAs. Aneurysms larger than 5 to 6 cm should be considered for repair. Most are asymptomatic and are found on routine plain chest radiography. CT scan, MRI, or transesophageal echocardiography (TEE) may be used to further delineate the extent of these aneurysms.

Treatment

Ascending and aortic arch aneurysms necessitate surgical treatment. This includes resection of the aneurysm and replacement with a Dacron graft. Ascending aortic aneurysms may necessitate concomitant aortic valve replacement, and arch aneurysms often necessitate reimplantation of the brachiocephalic vessels on a patch of aorta. Cardiopulmonary bypass and hypothermic circulatory arrest are required in these procedures. Descending aortic aneurysms may be repaired with standard aortic replacement techniques in which the aorta is cross-clamped and the aneursymal segment is replaced with a synthetic graft. The main risk of descending aortic aneurysm repair is paraplegia or paralysis caused by spinal cord ischemia, which may occur in up to 5% of patients. This risk may be minimized by reimplantation of intercostal branches.

Thoracoabdominal Aneurysms

Aneurysms that extend from the thoracic aorta into the abdomen involve the visceral vessels. Etiology, risk factors, and indications for repair are similar to those of abdominal aortic aneurysms. Most are asymptomatic and are discovered either on routine chest radiographs or as proximal extensions of AAAs. Ultrasonography is less useful in the detection of thoracoabdominal aneurysms than with infrarenal aneurysms. The Crawford classification system divides these aneurysms into type I, which involve most of the descending thoracic and upper abdominal aorta; type II, which involve most of the descending thoracic aorta and most or all of the abdominal aorta; type III, which involve the distal descending thoracic aorta and most of the abdominal aorta; and type IV, which involve most or all of the abdominal aorta, including the visceral vessel origins. CT scans provide excellent imaging of the proximal and distal extent of these aneurysms. In most cases, preoperative angiography is needed to determine the anatomy of visceral arteries in relation to the aortic aneurysms. Appropriate cardiac evaluation is also necessary preoperatively.

Treatment

Operative treatment must include both replacement of the aneurysmal aortic segment and the reimplantation of renal, mesenteric, and intercostal vessels. A double-lumen endotracheal tube is inserted, which allows collapse of the left lung during exposure of the descending thoracic aorta. Some authors use an intrathecal catheter for drainage of cerebrospinal fluid and continuous monitoring of spinal fluid pressure intraoperatively and postoperatively. Patients are positioned in a right lateral decubitus position, and a thoracoabdominal incision is made in the fourth or fifth intercostal space for type I or type II aneurysms or in the seventh to ninth intercostal space for a type III or type IV aneurysm. The incision is carried down to the abdominal paramedian area. The diaphragm is divided, and the crus of the diaphragm to the left of the aorta is divided to allow exposure of the thoracoabdominal aorta. Visceral vessels are identified. In some cases, particularly types I and II aneurysms, atrial-femoral bypass may be employed to maintain distal perfusion during the proximal anastomosis. Large aortic patches that include critical visceral vessel orifices are sewn onto the main aortic graft. These may include intercostal vessels at the T7 to L2 level (from which up to 90% of spinal cord blood supply arises), the celiac artery, the superior mesenteric artery, and the renal arteries. Distal anastomosis is usually performed at the aortic bifurcation, although it may be extended to the iliac arteries if the aneurysmal disease extends to that level. The rate of overall mortality from this procedure has been steadily improving and is now about 5%. The incidence of paraplegia or paraparesis is about 7%. Other significant perioperative morbid outcomes include renal failure, pulmonary insufficiency, and cardiac complications. Although repair of thoracic aortic aneurysms is clearly a high-risk procedure, it may be performed by experienced surgical teams with low morbidity and mortality rates.

AORTIC DISSECTION

Acute aortic dissection is often a lethal entity. Because the signs and symptoms are so widely varied, delay in diagnosis is common. The hallmark of aortic dissection is the acute onset of severe tearing pain in the back, chest, or abdomen. However, because nutrient arteries to virtually all end organs may be sheared off by the dissection, arterial ischemia of almost any body part may be a presenting sign that obscures the diagnosis of dissection. Aortic dissection is more common in patients with Marfan's syndrome or Ehlers-Danlos syndrome because of the associated collagen defects. The most common classification systems are those of DeBakey and Stanford University. The Stanford classification is divided into type A, which involves the ascending aorta and arch, and type B, which involves the descending thoracic aorta (distal to the left subclavian artery). In the DeBakey classification, type I involves the entire aorta, usually originating in the ascending aorta, although the intimal tear may occur anywhere and extend proximally and distally; type II is limited to the ascending aorta; and in type III the dissection is distal to the left subclavian artery, extending distally to the thoracic or abdominal aorta.

As soon as the diagnosis of aortic dissection is entertained, medical management is indicated to control hypertension. Definitive diagnostic imaging is undertaken. Options include angiography, TEE, CT scan, and MRI. Once the diagnosis is made, the site and extent of the intimal tear determine the course of treatment. TEE has arguably become the test of choice in the diagnosis of acute aortic dissection. Sensitivity and specificity approach 100% in imaging the lead point and determining the extent of involvement of the ascending aorta, arch, and descending aorta. Unfortunately, TEE offers little in imaging below the diaphragm or in determining perfusion of aortic branches. Conventional biplane aortography has a sensitivity of approximately 80%, with a high false-negative rate. MRI offers up to 99% accuracy and may replace CT scanning for determining the extent of dissection below the diaphragm. If MRI is unavailable, CT scanning should be used as an adjunct to TEE.

Treatment

Type A dissections should be considered for emergency or urgent surgical repair. The mortality rate may be as high as 50% in the first 48 hours without surgical intervention. Mortality is often from free intrapericardial rupture with cardiac tamponade, from acute aortic regurgitation, and from intrapleural rupture. Even with distal organ ischemia, repair of the lead point of dissection often relieves the ischemic symptoms. Repair is performed via a sternotomy, and hypothermic circulatory arrest is commonly used, with either the distal or proximal anastomosis performed first; a synthetic graft is sutured to the two layers of aorta (intima and media-adventitia). The anastomoses may require reinforcement with additional prosthetic material because of the weakness of the dissected aortic wall. If the distal anastomosis is completed first, the graft may be clamped and cardiopulmonary bypass resumed while the proximal anastomosis is performed. Concomitant aortic valve replacement or valve resuspension may be necessary.

The treatment for type B dissections is not as well defined. The rate of operative mortality from repair of acute type B dissections is high, and medical management has been comparably effective. Surgical treatment for acute type B dissections is reserved for patients with complications such as distal or visceral ischemia, uncontrolled hypertension, contained rupture, or intractible pain. The cornerstone of medical treatment is blood pressure control. In patients undergoing nonoperative therapy, false aneurysms developed in 45% with ongoing hypertension and in only 17% with controlled blood pressure. These data illustrate the need for frequent follow-up (by CT scan or MRI) and continued blood pressure control.

ABDOMINAL AORTIC OCCLUSIVE DISEASE

Occlusive disease of the abdominal aorta is a common manifestation of advanced atherosclerotic disease. The iliac arteries are often involved, and the superficial femoral arteries may also have extensive disease. Risk factors include tobacco use, hyperlipidemia, hypertension, and diabetes mellitus. Co-morbid conditions are common, including coronary artery disease, cerebrovascular disease, and other associated vascular occlusive disease. The most recognized manifestation is Leriche's syndrome, which includes impotence, buttock pain and atrophy, and absence of femoral pulses. Other symptoms may include more moderate erectile dysfunction, more distal pain at rest (particularly when combined with more distal occlusive disease), and chronic colonic ischemia (from involvement of the mesenteric arteries and iliac arteries). Physical findings may include diminished or absent femoral pulses, distal extremity hair loss and skin desquamation, dependent rubor, and nonhealing ulcers. Occasionally, there is evidence of distal emboli, usually bilateral and confined to the toes (blue toe syndrome). These emboli are usually atheroemboli from ulcerated plaques.

Treatment is based on the severity of the ischemia. Patients with chronic lower extremity occlusive disease usually complain of claudication before the onset of either pain at rest or gangrene. Claudication represents the inability to mount an appropriate augmentation of blood supply in response to exercise. It consists of three essential features: pain in a functional muscle unit, pain reproducible by a consistent amount of exercise, and pain promptly relieved by the cessation of exercise. This pain is usually in the buttocks or upper thighs in patients with aortic occlusive disease. Most of these patients are treated with nonoperative measures, including regular exercise and cessation of smoking. Up to 80% of patients with claudication remain stable or improve over 2.5 to 6 years with nonoperative management. Limb-threatening ischemia occurs when the resting blood flow is unable to meet the baseline metabolic demands. Clinically this manifests as pain at rest (typically in the most distal portion of the extremity, such as the forefoot or toes), ulceration, or gangrene. Operative intervention is indicated for limb-threatening ischemia or for disabling claudication that leaves a patient with an unacceptable quality of life.

Most aortic occlusive disease manifests as a chronic process; symptoms progress from claudication to limb-threatening ischemia. In rare instances, acute aortic occlusion may result from thrombosis of an atherosclerotic aorta or from the lodging of a large embolus (usually cardiac in origin) in the distal aorta. In this setting, collateral flow is inadequate for sustaining adequate perfusion, and emergency surgical revascularization is necessary to prevent limb loss or death. Acute aortic occlusion may manifest as an acute neurologic deficit to both legs and is often misdiagnosed as spinal cord compression. In fact, these symptoms result from spinal cord ischemia. Absence of femoral pulses should alert the clinician to the diagnosis of acute aortic occlusion. In the acute setting, immediate surgery is indicated. In all chronic or subacute cases, preoperative imaging should be performed. This is usually conventional angiography, although advances in magnetic resonance angiography (MRA) with gadolinium enhancement have made that modality beneficial, particularly in patients with renal insufficiency. In addition, MRA eliminates the need for arterial cannulation, which may be more hazardous in patients with aortic occlusion that necessitates access via the axillary artery.

Treatment

Surgical treatment consists of aortic bypass with synthetic Dacron or PTFE grafts. These are bifurcated grafts, and they are anastomosed proximally to the infrarenal aorta (where the occlusive process typically begins) and distally to the iliac or femoral arteries. The rate of 5-year patency of aorto-bifemoral bypass grafts is about 90%. As noted earlier, these patients often have significant medical co-morbid conditions. Occasionally, axillofemoral or axillo-bifemoral bypass grafts may be used in high-risk patients who are unlikely to tolerate aortic bypass. Rates of 5-year patency are only 50 to 75% for axillofemoral bypass, but this is usually performed only in patients with limited life expectancies. Another treatment option is aortoiliac balloon angioplasty and stenting. Although data on aortic angioplasty and stenting are limited, the iliac arteries are particularly amenable to this treatment. Iliac artery stenoses or occlusions can be dilated by balloon angioplasty, and the placement of intra-arterial stents has improved long-term patency. This method of treatment of therapy has become so widespread that the number of aorto-bifemoral bypass procedures performed has been significantly reduced.

AORTIC INFECTION

Although rare, primary infection of the native aorta has been well documented. It is usually associated with an AAA, and the most common bacterium involved is *Salmonella*. The infection usually begins as a microbial aortitis and leads to formation of an aneurysm. For unclear reasons, the atherosclerotic aorta appears to have a unique susceptibility to *Salmonella* species. The manifestation may be similar to that of ruptured aneurysm with abdominal or back pain. Fever and elevated white blood cell count may also be associated. Diagnosis should be considered if there is air or air-fluid levels surrounding the abdominal aorta on CT scan. Treatment consists of aortic resection and débridement. The infrarenal aortic stump is oversewn and often reinforced with omentum. Axillo-bifemoral bypass is performed to revascularize the lower extremities.

Secondary aortic infection associated with a surgically placed graft (for aneurysmal or occlusive disease) is also rare but more common than primary aortitis. The manifestation may be as an aortoenteric erosion (usually into the duodenum) or an aortoenteric fistula. Aortoenteric erosion may manifest as recurrent sepsis; an aortoenteric fistula may manifest with a so-called herald bleed which is a low-volume upper gastrointestinal hemorrhage. Any such bleeding in a patient with a prior abdominal aortic graft should be evaluated for possible fistula. This is usually caused by inadequate separation of the aortic graft from the overlying aorta by retroperitoneal tissue. Diagnosis can be made by upper endoscopy (although visualization of the distal third portion of the duodenum is often necessary to establish the diagnosis). CT findings are similar to those of primary aortitis. An ill-defined area of inflammatory tissue may be seen between the aorta and overlying duodenum. Treatment is similar to that of primary aortic infection, with the addition of repair or resection of the segment of bowel involved with the fistula. An aortoenteric fistula should be considered a surgical emergency. The initial bleeding episode is usually followed by an exsanguinating, fatal hemorrhage if surgical intervention is not performed.

ANGINA PECTORIS

method of
WILLIAM H. WEHRMACHER, M.D., and
BRUCE LEWIS, M.D.
Loyola University Stritch School of Medicine
Maywood, Illinois

As the classic symptom complex resulting from myocardial ischemia, the chest distress of angina pectoris requires consideration of at least seven characteristics:

1. Location, substernal (50–75%)
2. Radiation, ulnar left arm or both arms, neck, jaw, and upper abdomen
3. Quality, 70% use pressure or some equivalent
4. Intensity, mild or minimal in 50%, moderate in 25%
5. Duration, 1 to 30 minutes in 90%
6. Fluctuation and periodicity, guide patient to describe pattern, including seasonal variation, circadian variation, and so forth, without reference to what seems to provoke or to relieve the distress. This relationship to be evaluated by the physician's correlation as the seventh characteristic, as follows;
7. Circumstances of occurrence and subsidence, provoked by effort or exertion in 90% and relieved promptly by rest and/or nitroglycerin.

First effort or "warm up" angina occurs in some patients who may be able to tolerate the same level of exertion after a little rest. Although individual cases vary substantially, eliciting all seven characteristics provides a giant step toward accurate diagnosis and prevents the use of noninformative terms, such as "atypical chest pain" or "atypical angina." There are more than 100 causes that can produce pain in the chest. One should not consider differential diagnosis as a dichotomy, distinguishing only between anginal and nonanginal pain. The key to diagnosis unlocks the pain.

Truly spontaneous attacks of angina, that is, attacks without any provocation, are unusual, although the patient's ability to recognize the provocative incident may be poor, but worth improving. Angina equivalent without pain, *angina sine dolore*, may account for some cases of sudden death and is worth considering when a patient has the primary sensation of expectation of sudden death. Sometimes this is a clue that surgeons should consider when a patient says "I will not survive this operation" when the outlook ordinarily would be good.

Unstable angina occurs with greater frequency than the patient had expected from previous experience or occurs in a patient who has not experienced it previously. It has a grave prognosis, although it cannot be characterized, as it once was, as *preinfarction angina*. Nonetheless, many instances do result in death or infarction if not intensively monitored and treated.

Unstable angina requires intensive therapy. Some consider episodes or dyspnea, palpitation, or dizziness as *anginal equivalents*. Diagnosis requires additional substantial evidence of intermittent myocardial ischemia correlated chronologically with the episode and usually with other episodes or ordinary angina. Associated with normal coronary angiograms, variant or Prinzmetal's angina is associated with focal or multifocal coronary spasm, and syndrome X produces angina-like chest pain probably associated with microvascular dysfunction. Both have an excellent prognosis.

Careful clinical inquiry and cardiologic examinations are routinely employed, and a wide variety of noninvasive tests are appropriate if the diagnosis remains obscure. Exercise or drug-induced stress testing with electrocardiographic monitoring, often combined with echocardiographic or radioisotope studies, are the most frequently employed noninvasive tests. They may also help identify particularly high-risk patients for special management. In the silent or asymptomatic patient with recurrent ischemia demonstrable on ambulatory electrocardiographic (AECG) monitoring of chronic stable angina, treatment may also be beneficial as shown by the Atenolol Silent Ischemia Study (ASIST) demonstrating substantial reduction in the number and duration of ischemic episodes detected after 4 weeks of treatment.

The general examination may demonstrate atherosclerosis in noncoronary vascular beds, corneal arcus, xanthelasma and other lipid deposits, elevated blood pressure, diabetes, and an abnormal earlobe crease. During the attack there may be an extra heart sound, parodoxical splitting of the second sound, dyskinetic cardiac activity, or rapid relief of the angina by carotid massage (vagal response). Signs of anemia, thyrotoxicosis, fever, infections, cardiac dysrhythmias, excessive weight, use of stimulant drugs (amphetamines, cocaine), and cardiac failure need special attention.

PATHOPHYSIOLOGY

Stable angina is ordinarily the result of chronic atherosclerotic coronary artery disease with *stable* atherosclerotic plaques, whereas the unstable variety and myocardial infarction are thrombotic-driven processes produced by *unstable* atherosclerotic plaques, with thin fibrous cap, apoptosis, lipid-rich atheromatous "gruel," content, collagen, and macrophages. In stable angina, the deposit of lipid lies within the coronary arterial wall of the larger epicardial vessels, and its interaction with various mediators of the endothelial wall results in chronic atherosclerosis, compromising the lumens of the vessels and thereby compromising the flow of blood through them.

The intramural vessels are less subject to atherosclerosis but are responsible for substantial resistance to flow. The sympathetic nervous system, histamine, serotonin, thromboxane, leukotrienes, and activators of smooth muscle influence this intramural resistance. The endothelium of the vessels is a responsive organelle productive of both endothelium-derived relaxation factor (EDRF) and endothelium-derived constrictive factors, the endothelins that substantially alter coronary vascular resistance to blood flow.

Autoregulation helps to maintain constant perfusion in the face of changing driving pressures but requires a well-functioning endothelium. Reductions in myocardial blood flow may be triggered by coronary vasoconstriction, platelet aggregation, and thrombosis—individually or in combination. Normally functioning endothelium regulates vascular tone and provides a nonthrombotic surface for the flow of blood; endothelial dysfunction becomes responsible for vasoconstriction and for the thrombotic and inflammatory reactions of atherosclerosis.

Pain is the result of inadequate coronary blood flow to supply myocardial demands. Myocardial hypertrophy and circumstances such as exercise, fever, sepsis, hyperthyroidism, catecholamine storms, and so forth increase myocardial demands that can provoke symptoms in stable angina and greatly increase the risks in both unstable angina and myocardial infarction. Inadequate oxygen-carrying capacity of the blood, as in anemia or carbon monoxide poisoning, as well as unfavorable cardiac rhythms and hypotension also jeopardize provision of adequate myocardial supply for its requirements. Cardiac catheterization and angiography can readily identify the coronary artery lesions and are usually necessary in the unstable variety or after myocardial infarction to access the damage and to guide correction of it by angioplasty, stents, or bypass surgery. In stable angina, there is no evidence to show improved life-expectancy after angioplasty, stents, or bypass surgery, although they are beneficial symptomatically if medical therapy fails to relieve the pain. The key to therapy must fit appropriately to correct pathophysiology.

ANTIANGINA THERAPY

Coexisting conditions that aggravate coronary artery disease should be identified and managed. The patient should lead as tranquil a life as possible and control both physical and emotional stresses that produce symptoms. Coitus may produce both stresses but need not be completely abandoned if counseling and adjustment is made to minimize these stresses during intercourse and the patient remains symptom free as a result. Inclement weather should be avoided. Meals and the post-absorptive state should not coincide with other stresses. Supervised exercise sessions are beneficial.

Circadian rhythm deserves special attention because stresses are less well tolerated in the morning hours and again in the late afternoon. The circadian rhythm should be considered in the exercise and activity prescriptions for patients. Tranquilizers often benefit anxious people. Unfortunately, patients seem to prefer prescriptions for pills to proscription of an unhealthy lifestyle, but this can be a poor choice for the patient with angina pectoris.

Management of underlying risk factors and low-dose aspirin ingestion are fundamental. Antioxidants may have some benefits. The patient should avoid unecessary drug use, particularly cocaine, sympathomimetic amines, and stimulants.

Nitrates

Nitrates have been the primary therapeutic agents for treating angina for over a century. They can be administered sublingually as a tablet or spray, transdermally, or intravenously. Their well-known use and actions, reducing oxygen consumption and relaxation of smooth muscles of vascular walls with resulting vasodilatation, continue to keep them in the forefront of antianginal therapy. Both the rapid-acting sublingual nitroglycerin for acute attacks and longer acting preparations for prophylaxis continue to be safe, effective therapies, but it is now necessary to monitor for tolerance that can occur from continued use in order to ensure action when needed.

For the longer action, isosorbide dinitrate (Isordil), isosorbide-5-mononitrate (ISMO), and topical nitroglycerin are appropriate. There appears to be less need for the 8- to 12-hour nitrate-free interval when isosorbide-5-mononitrate is used. The short-acting preparations automatically provide the nitrate-free interval. Nitrate tolerance is always worth consideration because nitrates tend to lose their effectiveness if administered continuously.

Beta-Adrenergic Blockade

Beta-adrenergic blockade of receptors on vascular and cardiac muscle cells has also become an important part of routine therapy, resulting in sympatholytic action and control of heart rate, blood pressure, and cardiac contractility along with symptomatic improvement. Beta-adrenergic blockade improves survival, particularly among patients with angina occurring after myocardial infarction. To decide which of the many beta-adreneric blocking agents to prescribe, one must consider the durations of action and availability in sustained-release formulations, hydrophilic and lipophilic properties, selectivity, intrinsic sympathomimetic activity, and available routes of elimination. Some agents provide alpha blocking, and some have effects on cardiac rhythm and vasodilation.

Sexual and central nervous system (sleep disturbances, depression, malaise) side effects vary among the drugs. For the diabetic, the loss of awareness of insulin reactions and lipid effects need consideration. For the patient with asthma or chronic obstructive pulmonary disease, beta blockade is inappropriate and can be dangerous. Dosage needs careful attention; starting doses should be low and increase slowly, reducing resting heart rate to 50 to 60 beats per minute and preventing a more than 20 beat increase with modest exercise but providing adequate pain control.

Angiotensin-Converting Enzyme Inhibitors

Angiotensin-converting enzyme inhibitors are clearly indicated if there is left ventricular dysfunction, but available studies are equivocal or still incomplete to demonstrate improvement in the severity of stable angina pectoris. These inhibitors are certainly of value for the angina pectoris that occurs after myocardial infarction. The cough that sometimes results from their use often discourages continuation of the therapy.

Calcium Blockade

Calcium blockade has become controversial despite initial enthusiasm because of clear symptomatic benefits and few side effects. Constipation, however, was disturbing for many patients. The short-acting agents, like nifedipine (Procardia), particularly have been suspected to increase risk after myocardial infarction, especially among patients with angina, and the longer acting agents seem to lack this risk, particularly those agents that reduce cardiac rate. Diltiazem (Cardizem) is an intermediate-acting drug between the cardiostimulant, nifedipine, and the cardiodepressant verapamil. Nifedipine is also available in a delayed-action form, which modulates its stimulant properties.

Newer agents include amlodipine (Norvasc), nicardipine, felodipine, and bepridil. The PRAISE study showed no increase in mortality with amlodipine use for pain relief, whereas rapid-acting nifedipine had increased mortality although it was effective for pain relief.

Phosphodiesterase Inhibitors

Theophylline and other phosphodiesterase inhibitors, popular in the remote past, have been virtually discarded from the ordinary recommendations for management of angina today. They can, however, frequently provide just enough additional smooth muscle relaxation to help with some residual symptoms in patients managed with the other agents. They are particularly useful among patients who also suffer from bronchospasm.

The use of the phosphodiesterase V inhibitor sildenafil citrate (Viagra) is contraindicated. Its availability has encouraged many patients to engage in sexual activity again although they had earlier abandoned it with resulting benefits because it eliminated strong emotional and physical stress. Restoration of strong sexual activity should be avoided like other provocative stresses; and sildenafil citrate should also be avoided because of its lethal incompatibility with nitrates and other aspects of angina management.

Combination Therapy

Combination therapy is almost always appropriate and certainly so when monotherapy fails. Careful consideration of potential drug interactions becomes essential. Both beta-adrenergic blockade and angiotensin-converting enzyme inhibitors provide double benefits for the control of angina and for the control of the hypertensive stress.

Myocardial Revascularization

Myocardial revascularization often provides symptomatic relief for patients who fail to respond adequately to medical therapy, but there is little evidence to suggest that it improves life expectancy for those with ordinary angina. Among patients with unstable angina or myocardial infarction, however, there are both symptomatic and life-prolonging benefits. The scope of revascularization has increased substantially since the original aortocoronary bypass procedures were first introduced and include percutaneous coronary angioplasty, stents, atherectomy, rotational ablation, and lasers. Unstable angina and myocardial infarction are likely to occur in the natural history of ordinary angina and may even present as the first manifestations of common coronary artery disease. The clinician must keep these possibilities clearly in mind during management.

CONTROL OF RISK FACTORS

Lipids

Current guidelines appropriately recommend that low-density lipoprotein level be lowered toward normal among all patients with coronary artery disease. Dietary therapy is fundamental to management and can be approached through the National Cholesterol Education Program, but it almost invariably needs pharmacologic supplementation.

Although apparently ludicrous, it is nonetheless true that patients accept prescription of pills more readily than proscription of an unhealthy life style. Bile acid sequestrants, nicotinic acid, and fibric acid derivatives are effective but have been virtually replaced by the statins, which are HMO-CoA reductase inhibitors, that limit the rate of cholesterol synthesis. Side effects, particularly myopathy, are increased if the HMO-CoA reductase inhibitors are combined with nicotinic acid or fibric acid derivatives, with cyclosporine, or with erythromycin. The AVERT trial clearly demonstrated not only an effective reduction of low-density lipoprotein cholesterol level after statin therapy (atorvastatin, Lipitor; 80 mg per day in that trial) but also an effective reduction in ischemic events. Antioxidants (vitamin E, beta-carotine, and flavanoids) have also been recommended, although their use remains controversial.

Hypertension

Hypertension (and pheochromocytoma, although rare) clearly needs to be controlled to reduce stress.

That control is also consequential to prevent the hypertrophy of the myocardium that increases the need for myocardial perfusion.

Hyperthyroidism and Hypothyroidism

Control of hyperthyroidism and resulting correction of metabolic demands is obvious and needs doing, and hypothyroidism, which once was considered as therapy for angina, now clearly needs correction because of its unfavorable influence on the lipids of the body and accelerating effect on the atherosclerotic process. For the hypothyroid patient, thyroid hormone must be initiated in very small doses and then increased gradually to avoid rapidly increasing metabolic demands, which the coronary circulation is ill-prepared to supply.

Other Risk Factors

Because adequate oxygen carrying capacity of the blood becomes particularly important when myocardial perfusion is marginal, anemia should be controlled. Hypoglycemia often triggers anginal episodes and must be avoided. This becomes particularly important in the diabetic person receiving beta-adrenergic blockade, which may conceal the ordinary symptoms of hypoglycemia but still allow its adverse, but perhaps unrecognized, effect on myocardial performace. Estrogen replacement therapy is generally recommended for anovulatory women, although this recommendation is still being debated. The National Cholesterol Education Program has endorsed it. Cigarette smoking must be abandoned, and obesity must be corrected.

Stimulant drugs must be avoided. Not only the obvious stimulants like adrenalin and cocaine but also a wide variety of drugs prescribed for other purposes but with stimulant side effects need interdiction. Sumatriptan (Imitrex), prescribed for migraine and cluster headaches, as well as some antiallergy medications, many psychotropic drugs, and others, should be recognized as stimulants so that they can be avoided because of their potential to aggravate coronary insufficiency.

Exercise programs are available with the presumption that the conditioning effect of exercise is as beneficial for the heart as it is for skeletal muscle. By retarding tachycardia induced by any level of exercise after conditioning, the myocardial efficiency is improved, as is the capacity for physical performance. Nonetheless, the lack of truly prospective studies of matched populations with and without an exercise program makes it difficult to know actual benefits. Exercise programs tend to promote useful health consciousness. People who like to exercise certainly do better; but whether this advantage is a result of greater fundamental fitness or of the exercise program remains for further evaluation. Exercise programs must be tailored for a specific patient and must avoid excesses that can produce angina.

Medical management is the key to treatment of stable angina. Medical management should ordinarily be sufficient; however, patients who continue to suffer with pain with a multidrug treatment regimen or who are at high risk, as determined by noninvasive and other methods of observation, should be considered for coronary angiography and revascularization by angioplasty or bypass surgery.

CARDIAC ARREST: SUDDEN CARDIAC DEATH

method of
BRENT R. ASPLIN, M.D.
University of Michigan Health System
Ann Arbor, Michigan

Each day in the United States, between 500 and 1000 people experience sudden and unexpected cardiovascular collapse that leads to cardiopulmonary arrest. Clinically, this condition is known as sudden cardiac death (SCD). Because SCD is a leading cause of death in the United States, its impact is devastating. Although the exact number of cases is unknown, SCD accounts for approximately 250,000 to 350,000 deaths annually. The vast majority of these deaths occur outside the hospital and are therefore classified as out-of-hospital cardiac arrests (OHCAs). The fundamental interventions for the successful treatment of SCD have been established since the late 1960s. Despite this knowledge and the tremendous growth in emergency medical services (EMS) in the United States, many experts estimate that the overall rate of survival of OHCA is only 3 to 5%. Furthermore, there is striking variation in survival between communities. Survival rates as low as 1 to 2% have been reported in Chicago and New York, but Seattle has reported rates as high as 18% for all patients with OHCA and more than 30% for patients who are found in ventricular fibrillation (VF). Smaller cities such as Rochester, Minnesota, have reported survival rates as high as 40% for patients found in VF. These disparities in survival, coupled with the fact that the major determinants of survival from SCD are established, illustrate the importance of viewing SCD as a public health challenge that can only be met with a systematic and community-based approach.

The electrophysiologic substrate for SCD in approximately 80% of patients is the sudden onset of a tachyarrhythmia, most commonly ventricular tachycardia (VT) that degenerates to VF. Bradyarrhythmias initiate SCD in less than 20% of patients. Although coronary artery disease (CAD) is usually present, SCD may or may not be accompanied by symptoms of coronary ischemia. In fact, the majority of cases of SCD are not accompanied by myocardial infarction. The treatment of SCD is based on the four links in the American Heart Association's (AHA's) chain of survival. These links include early access, early cardiopulmonary resuscitation (CPR), early defibrillation, and early advanced care. Although each link in the chain of survival is important, the most important determinant of survival is early defibrillation. To improve survival from SCD, a community-based approach is needed that recognizes the importance of the chain of survival and establishes a system that reliably provides these interventions within minutes of patient collapse. Because the majority of survivors of SCD are patients who receive prompt defibrillation, this report focuses on the systematic approach to treating victims of SCD initially found in VF or VT. Although patients found in pulseless electrical activity (PEA) or asystole can be resuscitated successfully, the number of survivors with these initial rhythms is low. Therefore, community and EMS system interventions focused on consistently delivering defibrillation within 6 to 8 minutes of patient collapse have the greatest likelihood of improving the chance of survival from SCD.

A description of the patient most likely to survive SCD without neurologic impairment is helpful: The person's collapse is witnessed; bystanders immediately call 911 to activate the EMS system and then begin bystander CPR. Within 6 to 8 minutes, a defibrillator arrives, and VF is terminated by initial shocks, leading to return of spontaneous circulation (ROSC). Paramedics are available at or shortly after the time of defibrillation to provide advanced cardiac life support (ACLS). This care may include endotracheal intubation, cardiac monitoring, capnography, and the administration of antiarrhythmic or vasoactive medications, or both, if needed. Failure in the delivery of any of these steps decreases the chance of survival. To illustrate the concept of the chain of survival, each of these steps is discussed in detail. Clinicians are encouraged to critically analyze the ability of their communities to deliver these interventions consistently and quickly. Improvement in SCD survival rates can occur only when communities identify breaks in the chain of survival and develop innovative strategies to overcome them.

EARLY ACCESS

The EMS system must be contacted as soon as possible after patient collapse. Because of the critical role of early defibrillation, bystanders should be instructed to call as soon as the patient is determined to be unresponsive (before performing CPR). In most U.S. communities, 911 serves as a universal access number for the public safety system. The establishment of a 911 communications system is an important goal for communities that currently lack this service, because delays in access obviously impair the effectiveness of the subsequent links in the chain of survival. Many communities have enhanced 911 service, allowing EMS dispatchers to immediately identify the location of the caller and improve the speed of EMS response.

EARLY CARDIOPULMONARY RESUSCITATION

The birth of CPR took place in William Kouwenhoven's laboratory at Johns Hopkins Hospital in Baltimore between 1958 and 1961. In 1960 Kouwenhoven, along with co-investigators James Jude and Guy Knickerbocker, reported the successful use of chest compressions as a temporizing measure until an external defibrillator arrived to treat victims of cardiac arrest in the operating room. By late 1960 Peter Safar had demonstrated the effectiveness of mouth-to-mouth resuscitation, which was coupled with chest compressions, forming the basis for CPR. Since that time, CPR has been widely promoted and documented as a life-saving intervention for the treatment of cardiac arrest.

Under ideal circumstances it is estimated that CPR generates approximately 30% of normal cardiac output. Undoubtedly there is wide variation in the effectiveness of bystander CPR technique; however, it is generally believed that some CPR is better than no CPR at all. Despite clearly documented survival improvements for patients who receive it, CPR primarily serves a life-sustaining role during the wait for more definitive interventions. VF is sustained longer when CPR is performed, prolonging the window of opportunity for defibrillation (Figure 1). Cerebral perfusion during CPR also improves the likelihood of survival without neurologic deficit. It is fundamentally important that all physicians be able to perform the basic steps of CPR. Furthermore, clinicians who are responsible for the treatment of SCD in their communities should take a leading role in the promotion of community-wide CPR training programs. Studies have shown that video-based instruction techniques may be as effective as standard CPR courses. Video instruction on television may enhance community efforts to promote the performance of CPR.

EARLY DEFIBRILLATION

Although it has been known for decades that early defibrillation is the most important determinant of survival in the treatment of cardiac arrest, most communities do not consistently provide defibrillation within a time window most likely to be effective (i.e., within 8 minutes of patient collapse). Therefore, it is important to identify alternative methods for delivering this life-saving treatment to the scenes of cardiac arrests. In response to this challenge, many EMS systems have placed defibrillators in the hands of personnel with less medical training, such as first responders. The technologic advance that has made this possible is the automated external defibrillator (AED). An AED is a device that interprets the electrocardiographic rhythm, determines the need for electrical therapy, and instructs the operator to deliver shocks when indicated. The sophisticated nature of AED technology has revolutionized the treatment of cardiac arrest. Once cardiac arrest is confirmed, an AED is attached by means of two monitor/defibrillator adhesive electrodes. A microprocessor interprets the patient's rhythm, and the device instructs the operator through a series of voice prompts. When VF or rapid VT (above a predetermined cutoff rate) is detected, the device charges automatically and the operator is instructed to deliver a shock (Figure 2). After shock delivery, the rhythm is automatically reanalyzed. If VF has not been terminated, the device charges again and delivers up to three consecutive shocks in rapid succession (all within 1 minute). Upon termination of VF or delivery of three shocks, the operator is instructed to perform CPR. After 1 minute, the AED instructs the

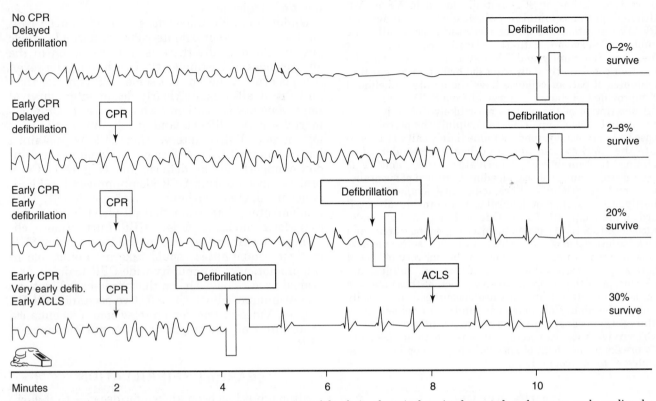

Figure 1. Improvements in survival occur as the components of the chain of survival are implemented: early access, early cardiopulmonary resuscitation (CPR), early defibrillation, and early advanced care. A primary function of bystander CPR is to prolong ventricular fibrillation and increase the likelihood of successful defibrillation. (Reproduced with permission from Textbook of Advanced Cardiac Life Support, 1997. Copyright by the American Heart Association.)

operator to stop CPR, and the analysis algorithm is repeated. The algorithms in today's AEDs exhibit very high specificity (≥98%) and sensitivity (>90%) for VF. Audio and electrocardiographic data are stored on data cards or in internal memory, enabling complete review of operator decisions and device performance. Along with these improvements in sophistication, today's AEDs are more compact, lightweight, and maintenance-free than earlier generations. The cost of an AED also has decreased to approximately $2500 to $4000.

Initially AEDs were used only by emergency medical technicians (EMTs) and other basic life support personnel working within EMS systems. The advances in technology discussed here have simplified AED operation so that laypeople have successfully been trained to operate the devices. The concept of layperson defibrillation, also known as public access defibrillation (PAD), is an exciting new possibility for improving survival from SCD. Security guards, fitness trainers, flight attendants, and other laypeople who work in public areas have been identified as potential "designated responders" for PAD. These persons have the potential to expand their role from delivering bystander CPR to performing "bystander defibrillation." There are reports of successful defibrillation by laypeople using AEDs, but the effec-

tiveness of widespread PAD is unknown. The cost effectiveness of such a program and the initial and ongoing training requirements of participants also require further study. Finally, it is not clear that widespread deployment of AEDs in public places would have a major impact on survival from SCD, because approximately 70% of cardiac arrests occur in the home. Nevertheless, despite these limitations, there is no question that targeted laypeople can be trained to provide defibrillation by using AEDs and that these programs can lead to improvements in survival in some settings.

AEDs should be readily available for any medical personnel expected to respond to medical emergencies. These devices have been deployed at outpatient clinics, occupational medicine sites, dental offices, and even noncardiac hospital wards. The simplicity of AED operation, ease of maintenance, and minimal training requirements make AEDs highly suitable for these environments, especially when the incidence of cardiac arrest is very low. Physicians, nurses, and other medical personnel should be trained to operate AEDs at these sites. In view of the effectiveness and affordability of AED deployment for medical personnel, outpatient medical facilities should no longer rely solely on EMS systems for defibrillation, because this constitutes an unneces-

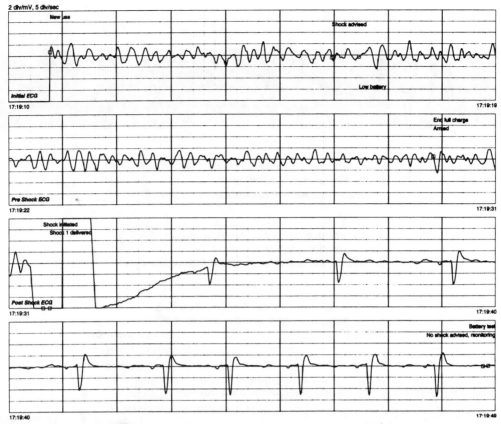

Figure 2. Restoration of sinus rhythm with a 150-J biphasic shock in a patient with ventricular fibrillation in out-of-hospital cardiac arrest.

sary delay and decreases the likelihood of patient survival.

EARLY ADVANCED CARE

The AHA's ACLS guidelines are the basis for advanced treatment of SCD patients (Figure 3). When patients receive early CPR and defibrillation that result in on-scene ROSC, advanced interventions can often be limited to the establishment of intravenous access, cardiac monitoring, and the administration of lidocaine to prevent recurrent VF. This, unfortunately, applies to only a small minority of SCD patients. The majority of patients require airway management and additional medications. The most effective method of airway protection is endotracheal intubation; however, this should be performed only by personnel who have been properly trained. Alternatives to endotracheal intubation include bag-valve mask ventilation, flow-restricted oxygen-powered ventilation devices, and ventilation devices that can be inserted without direct laryngoscopy, such as the Combitube. This device is inserted blindly and is equipped with two ventilation ports that allow the patient to be ventilated with either an endotracheal or esophageal placement. The Combitube can be used either as a primary airway management device or

as a backup device in cases of failed endotracheal intubation.

The pharmacologic management of VF primarily involves the use of antiarrhythmics and vasopressors. Antiarrhythmic therapy begins with intravenous doses of lidocaine (1.0 to 1.5 mg per kg, repeated to a maximum of 3.0 mg per kg) and continues with bretylium (Bretylol), 5 mg per kg for the initial dose, repeated if necessary with 10 mg per kg. If VF is refractory to these treatments, procainamide may be used (30 mg per minute to a maximum of 17 mg per kg). Amiodarone (Cordarone) is an antiarrhythmic medication that has recently been studied in the setting of OHCA. Although the data are inconclusive, patients receiving amiodarone may be more likely to survive to hospital admission than are patients receiving placebo. This benefit appears to be greatest for patients who have recurrent VF after transient ROSC. The dose of amiodarone for OHCA is an intravenous bolus of 150 mg. Epinephrine is the standard vasopressor for the treatment of cardiac arrest. The usual intravenous dose of epinephrine is 1.0 mg repeated every 5 minutes. Since the 1980s, much attention has been devoted to the use of high-dose epinephrine (e.g., repeated doses of 3.0 to 5.0 mg). Patients may have higher rates of ROSC and hospital admission with high-dose epinephrine; however, several large prospective trials have now conclusively

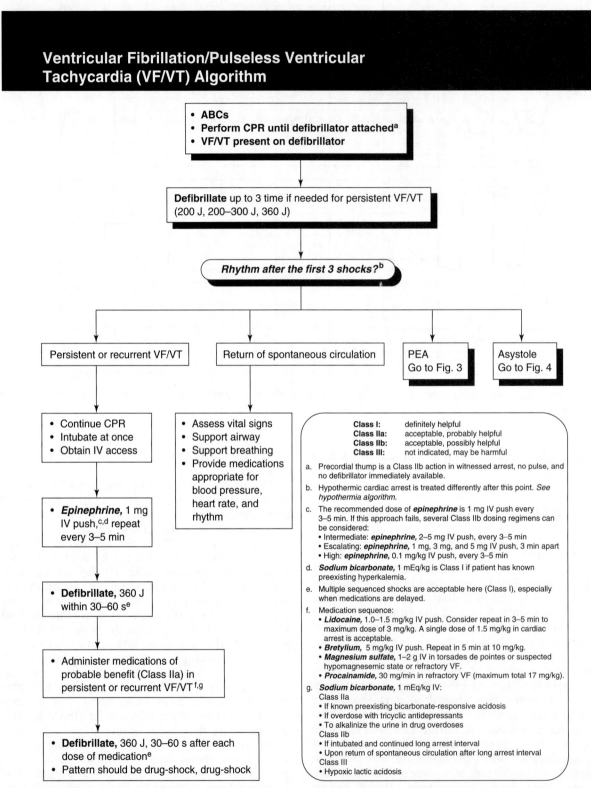

Figure 3. Advanced care for cardiac arrest is based on advanced cardiac life support algorithms from the American Heart Association. The standard treatment for ventricular fibrillation or pulseless ventricular tachycardia is demonstrated. (Reproduced with permission from Textbook of Advanced Cardiac Life Support, 1997. Copyright by the American Heart Association.)

shown that there is no long-term survival benefit from high-dose epinephrine, and its routine use should therefore be abandoned. All of the medications discussed thus far are ideally given intravenously. For patients without intravenous access, the endotracheal route can be used for the administration of lidocaine, epinephrine, and atropine. Typically the dose is doubled and then diluted with approximately 10 mL of saline.

TREATMENT OF ASYSTOLE AND PULSELESS ELECTRICAL ACTIVITY

The majority of survivors from OHCA are found in VF or VT; however, a small percentage of survivors may present in asystole or PEA. Almost all of the survivors in the latter two categories are people who experience a witnessed cardiac arrest. The key to management of asystole and PEA is to consider the potential etiologies of these rhythms. Most commonly, asystole develops after prolonged hypoxia and is therefore irreversible. Profound hyperkalemia occasionally leads to asystole, and patients have responded in this setting to aggressive treatment with intravenous calcium and sodium bicarbonate. PEA is defined as the persistence of any organized electrical activity in the absence of palpable pulses. Again, a search for correctable causes is justified. Hyperkalemia may cause PEA and should be suspected in patients with known renal disease. Hypoxia and profound acidosis are other metabolic etiologies of PEA. Mechanical causes of PEA include hypovolemia (from hemorrhage or profound dehydration), tension pneumothorax, cardiac tamponade, massive pulmonary embolism, and cardiac rupture after myocardial infarction. Although these conditions are rare, successful management relies on clinical suspicion and on

immediate interventions, such as needle decompression for tension pneumothorax and pericardiocentesis for cardiac tamponade.

CAPNOGRAPHY

Capnography is a monitoring technique routinely used in operating suites and other critical care settings. The most common application of capnography in emergency care settings is the use of qualitative end-tidal carbon dioxide (ETCO$_2$) detectors for confirmation of endotracheal tube placement. Quantitative capnography is defined as the measurement and display of ETCO$_2$ pressure. There is growing interest in the use of capnography during the management of cardiac arrest. The major determinants of ETCO$_2$ are tissue production of carbon dioxide, pulmonary blood flow, and alveolar ventilation. During cardiac arrest, ETCO$_2$ pressure is limited by flow; therefore, although changes in tissue production of carbon dioxide likely occur, ETCO$_2$ is determined almost entirely by pulmonary blood flow and alveolar ventilation. The significance of this physiology is that changes in ETCO$_2$ pressure correlate directly with pulmonary blood flow (and therefore cardiac output) when ventilation is constant. Clinically this means that capnography is a useful noninvasive indicator of changes in pulmonary blood flow during CPR. Studies have confirmed that capnography is the most sensitive and reliable noninvasive technique for detecting significant changes in hemodynamic status such as ROSC (Figure 4). Furthermore, it is known that patients with higher ETCO$_2$ pressure during CPR are more likely to have ROSC. Conversely, it is also apparent that patients with persistently low ETCO$_2$ pressure (i.e., < 10 mm Hg) are unlikely to be resuscitated. Capnography can therefore be a useful prognostic

Figure 4. Capnographic recording during out-of-hospital cardiac arrest. 1: Standard cardiopulmonary resuscitation (CPR). 2: Increased rate and depth of chest compression in CPR is followed by a small but immediate increase in end-tidal carbon dioxide pressure. 3: Return of spontaneous circulation is accompanied by a large increase and overshoot, which gradually levels off (4).

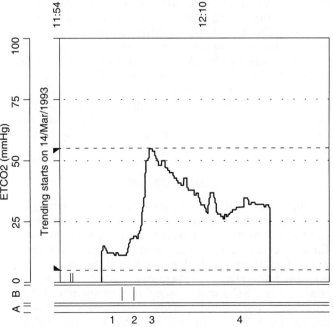

indicator of the likelihood of successful resuscitation. It can also be used as a diagnostic tool for patients in PEA. Extremely low $ETCO_2$ in the setting of PEA strongly suggests the presence of a mechanical (and likely irreversible) complication such as massive pulmonary embolism or cardiac tamponade secondary to contained cardiac rupture. Persistently low $ETCO_2$ pressure in the presence of PEA is in fact an indication for terminating resuscitation efforts. Of importance is that clinicians who use quantitative capnography in a patient in cardiac arrest must remember to maintain constant minute ventilation to ensure the reliability of this technique for assessing cardiac output during CPR.

INNOVATIONS IN CARDIAC ARREST MANAGEMENT

Much of the research in cardiac arrest management is currently focused on two areas: (1) mechanisms and prevention of neurologic injury and (2) improvements in defibrillation technology and delivery. The molecular basis of ischemic brain injury is rapidly being elucidated, and new therapies directed at preventing the cascade of events leading to neuronal cell death are being identified. Many of these therapies are still being tested in the laboratory and as yet remain a generation away from clinical practice. One neuroprotective therapy that may be promising is hypothermia. Animal studies have shown that hypothermia improves neurologic outcome, even when implemented after ROSC. It is not yet clear whether practical methods for implementing hypothermia in the prehospital setting (e.g., cooling packs around the head) can improve neurologic recovery after cardiac arrest.

Defibrillation technology is another area of intense research. Most defibrillators use monophasic waveforms to deliver defibrillatory shocks. Biphasic waveforms have been established as more efficient methods for shock delivery in implanted cardioverter-defibrillators. Some AED manufacturers are now evaluating biphasic waveform performance in the treatment of OHCA. The initial experience with these waveforms is promising. Defibrillation success with low-energy biphasic waveforms is comparable to traditional high-energy monophasic waveforms. The advantages of lower energy shocks include less potential for myocardial injury and the ability to use smaller capacitors and batteries.

CONCLUSION

Although technological innovations are exciting to consider, an immediate opportunity and challenge exists for improving survival from cardiac arrest. Early defibrillation is the most important determinant of SCD survival. Because VF is the most common initial rhythm, a substantial portion of patients experiencing SCD will respond to treatment if defibrillation is performed quickly. Strategies for providing earlier defibrillation include PAD and the deployment of AEDs in medical settings or other public venues where cardiac arrests are likely to occur. Advanced care for cardiac arrest includes airway management and pharmacologic interventions based on ACLS guidelines. Capnography is a useful noninvasive method for evaluating pulmonary blood flow during CPR and is especially helpful for identifying patients in PEA or asystole who may have potentially reversible causes of cardiac arrest. The public health challenge of SCD is formidable, but not insurmountable. The chain of survival outlines the necessary interventions for successful management of SCD. Physicians must take a leading role in promoting communitywide systems that consistently provide these interventions within a realistic therapeutic window.

ATRIAL FIBRILLATION

method of
CYNTHIA M. TRACY, M.D.
Georgetown University Hospital
Washington, D.C.

and

BERNARD J. GERSH, M.B., C.H.B., D.PHIL.
Mayo Clinic
Rochester, Minnesota

Atrial fibrillation is the most common sustained arrhythmic disorder seen in the population at large. Its prevalence is around 0.89%, and approximately 2.2 million people in the United States alone suffer from this rhythm disturbance. The incidence of atrial fibrillation increases with age and in the presence of structural heart disease, and congestive heart failure is possibly the most common associated condition. Atrial fibrillation is uncommon in patients younger than age 60 years, and the aging in the United States and other populations has resulted in a marked increase in the incidence and prevalence of atrial fibrillation since the 1950s. Moreover, for reasons as yet unexplained, in the Framingham study the age-adjusted incidence of atrial fibrillation has increased quite strikingly since the 1960s, particularly among men. The clinical manifestations are varied and include palpitations, fatigue, heart failure, and angina. However, many patients are asymptomatic or at least unaware of any abnormality in pulse rate or rhythm. Although atrial fibrillation is typically associated with another disease entity, lone atrial fibrillation is frequent in younger patients, particularly those with paroxysmal atrial fibrillation (Table 1).

In addition to the physical constraints imposed by symptoms, primarily rapid heart rate, atrial fibrillation imposes a potential risk of thromboembolism and, in a minority of patients, the development of a tachycardia-induced cardiomyopathy. In addition, among patients with pre-existing left ventricular dysfunction, atrial fibrillation is an independent predictor of mortality and further deterioration of left ventricular function. Regardless of the impact of atrial fibrillation on mortality, it is the most common underlying cause of embolic stroke, accounting for approximately 75,000 strokes annually in the United States. The eco-

TABLE 1. Conditions Associated with or Causing Atrial Fibrillation

Cardiac	Valvular heart disease
	Cardiomyopathy (dilated or hypertrophic)
	Coronary artery disease
	Hypertension
	Surgically repaired congenital heart disease
	Primary electrical
	Lone atrial fibrillation
	Wolff-Parkinson-White syndrome
	Reentrant arrhythmia degenerating to atrial fibrillation
Noncardiac	Thyrotoxicosis
	Diabetes
	Toxic-Alcohol
	Stimulant drugs
	Pulmonary disease
	Postoperative
Lone	Atrial fibrillation occurring without overt evidence of structural heart disease by physical exam, electrocardiogram, chest x-ray, and echocardiogram. Does not include toxic reactions. Can occur as an isolated event or may be paroxysmal, persistent, or chronic.

nomic impact of atrial fibrillation is damaging, particularly in the presence of the current demographic tide toward an increasingly elderly population.

Therapy is largely directed at the elimination of symptoms and prevention of the serious sequelae of this cardiac arrhythmia, in particular heart failure and thromboembolism. Treatments focus on (1) rate control, (2) anticoagulation, and (3) consideration of conversion/maintenance of sinus rhythm.

MANIFESTATION

When the patient initially comes to medical attention with atrial fibrillation, the cause of symptoms may not be clear and could be the consequence of the loss of atrial synchrony, rapid rates, or the irregularity of the heartbeat itself. Terminologies vary, but atrial fibrillation can occur as acute, paroxysmal, persistent, chronic, or postoperative (Table 2). The initial clinical assessment is directed not only to the underlying cause of atrial fibrillation but also

TABLE 2. Forms of Atrial Fibrillation

Acute	Initial presentation, frequently highly symptomatic.
	Can result in hemodynamic compromise that requires urgent intervention.
Paroxysmal	Short, repetitive, often self-limited episodes of atrial fibrillation lasting from minutes up to 7 d.
Persistent	Still intermittent episodes of atrial fibrillation but lasting over 2–7 d.
	Typically requires intervention for termination.
Chronic	Patient always remains in atrial fibrillation. Restoration of sinus rhythm not feasible.
Postoperative	Extremely common after coronary bypass surgery (25–30%) and valvular surgery (up to 50%). Prognostic impact is unknown and no one treatment strategy has proven much better than any other at prevention or treatment.

toward estimating the risks and benefits of anticoagulation for stroke prevention. A careful clinical history with attention to history of heart failure, prior transient ischemic attacks, prior stroke, or hypertension is crucial to the assessment of stroke risk, as is evaluation of comorbidity in regard to the risk of bleeding on anticoagulation. Laboratory investigations include thyroid function studies and other tests as clinically indicated. Valvular and structural heart disease can often be ruled out by history, physical examination, and electrocardiogram (ECG). Echocardiography and stress testing may be appropriate for determining the presence or absence of structural or ischemic substrates. Echocardiography may be also useful when stroke risk is considered.

RATE CONTROL

Initial Therapy

For the patient with angina or hemodynamic compromise, urgent cardioversion is usually indicated. However, for the patient who is stable but has a rapid heart rate, an initial goal is rate control. Although many patients are tachycardic when they come to medical attention, patients can display a wide range of heart rates. Those with rates slower than 90 beats per minute may have intrinsic atrioventricular (AV) node conduction disease, but the entity "vagally-induced atrial fibrillation" may be accompanied by a relatively slow ventricular rate in the absence of concomitant drug therapy. Pharmacologic rate control almost invariably requires the use of a beta blocker or a calcium channel–blocking agent, but a variety of medications can be used (Table 3). For the stable patient without heart failure, intravenous diltiazem (Cardizem) or verapamil (Isoptin) or a beta-blocking drug such as metoprolol (Lopressor), propranolol (Inderal), or atenolol (Tenormin) can be used. In patients who are potentially unstable and in whom a drug with rapid onset and offset of action is needed, esmolol (Brevibloc) is appropriate. Patients with thyrotoxicosis respond better to beta blockers than to calcium channel blockers. Patients with heart failure may benefit from digoxin (Lanoxin), but this is usually inadequate as the sole drug. Intravenous amiodarone* (Cordarone) has also been used for acute rate control in these patients. Often, patients require a combination of medications in order to slow the heart rate. Whenever rate control cannot be achieved or if a patient becomes hemodynamically unstable, cardioversion is appropriate.

Chronic Therapy

In patients with chronic atrial fibrillation, a resting heart rate of 60 to 90 beats per minute should be maintained. Rate control is defined by an average rate of 80 beats per minute or less over 24 hours on Holter monitoring or rates around 110 beats per minute with light to moderate exercise, such as a 6-minute treadmill walk. The same AV nodal blocking

---

*Not FDA approved for this indication.

TABLE 3. **Agents Used for Rate Control in Atrial Fibrillation**

Calcium channel blockers:

Diltiazem (Cardizem) — 0.25 mg/kg IV over 2 min. Repeat 0.35 mg/kg in 15 min if desired heart rate response not achieved. Continuous infusion can be started immediately after bolus dose at a starting rate of 10 mg/h and increased as necessary. Some patients may respond to lower bolus and infusion rates.

Verapamil (Isoptin) — 5–10 mg IV over 2 min. Repeat with 10 mg IV after 30 min if desired heart rate response not achieved.

Beta blockers:

Esmolol (Brevibloc) — 0.5 mg/kg/min IV over 1 min followed by a 4-min maintenance infusion of 0.05 mg/kg/min. A maintenance drip at 0.05 mg/kg/min can be infused if desired heart rate response is achieved. If the heart rate remains elevated, a loading dose can be repeated and the maintenance dose increased.

Inderal (Propranolol) — 1–3 mg IV at a rate of 1 mg/min. Repeat after 2 min if desired heart rate response not achieved. Drug administration should not be repeated for 4 h.

Metoprolol (Lopressor) — 5 mg IV over 2 min. Repeat every 5 min to a total dose of 15 mg if desired heart rate response not achieved.

Other:

Digoxin — 0.25–0.50 mg IV followed by 0.25 mg IV every 4–8 h not to exceed 1 mg in 24 h.

Amiodarone* (Cordarone) — 5 mg/kg IV over 30 min followed by 1200 mg over 24 h.

*Not FDA approved for this indication.

agents mentioned previously are suitable forms of therapy. Data do not support the use of sotalol (Betapace) or amiodarone chronically for rate control. Digoxin provides reasonable rate control at rest and is useful in patients with heart failure. However, the increases in sympathetic tone accompanying exercise typically necessitate addition of either a calcium channel blocker or a beta-blocking drug. Care should be taken to avoid excessive heart rate blunting in very active patients.

Because of underlying heart disease and ventricular dysfunction, patients may not tolerate pharmacologic efforts at rate control or rate control may be difficult to achieve. Clinical situations in which rate control can be difficult include decompensated heart failure; severe chronic obstructive lung disease; thyrotoxicosis; and conditions with diastolic dysfunction, such as hypertrophic cardiomyopathy. Similarly, patients with bradycardia-tachycardia syndrome may require permanent pacing early in their course to gain control over both ends of their heart rate spectrum.

ANTICOAGULATION

In every patient with atrial fibrillation, the issue of anticoagulation needs to be addressed. Although traditional concepts of stroke in atrial fibrillation logically implicated a dilated left atrium or left ventricle as the putative source of thrombus and subsequent embolism, more recent data require that this paradigm be expanded. In some patients, perhaps many, atrial fibrillation may be a marker of other vascular conditions that can independently result in stroke, such as aortic atherosclerosis, lacunar infarcts in hypertensive patients, or associated carotid artery disease in patients with mitral annular calcification. This may be particularly true in the elderly, among whom the prevalence of both atrial fibrillation and stroke is increased. However, in the elderly, in comparison with a younger population, atrial fibrillation imparts an even greater additional risk of stroke. In these patients the atrial fibrillation may be an indicator of other coexistent pathology.

Nearly all randomized trials have shown the benefits of anticoagulation in patients with nonrheumatic atrial fibrillation at reducing risk for stroke. The current indications for anticoagulation with warfarin (Coumadin) are based on five randomized trials that provided overwhelming evidence that warfarin is superior to placebo in reducing the risk of stroke. Less evidence is available regarding the benefits of aspirin, but the consensus is that warfarin is better than aspirin and aspirin is better than placebo. All patients with one or more risk factors or echocardiographic risks should undergo anticoagulation if possible, and the only groups who do not fulfill these criteria are patients younger than 65 years without clinical or echocardiographic risk factors (Table 4). The specific risk factors that must be sought are age older than 65 years, history of hypertension, prior myocardial infarction, prior stroke, and mitral valve stenosis. Other risk factors that need to be considered are a history of prior congestive heart failure, thyrotoxicosis, dilated or hypertrophic cardiomyopathy, prior surgical repair of atrial septal defects, and diabetes. In addition, there are two echocardio-

TABLE 4. **Recommended Anticoagulation Regimens for Prevention of Thromboembolism in Atrial Fibrillation**

Age	Risk Factors	Level of Risk	Therapy
<65 y	Present	Intermediate	Warfarin to maintain INR 2–3. If warfarin cannot be used, consider aspirin 325 mg/d.
<65 y	Absent	Low	None, or aspirin 325 mg/d.
≥65 y	Present	High	Warfarin to maintain INR 2–3. If warfarin contraindicated, aspirin 325 mg/d.
≥65 y	Absent (other than age)	Intermediate	Warfarin to maintain INR 2–3. If warfarin cannot be used, consider aspirin 325 mg/d.

INR = international normalized ratio.

graphic risk factors: left ventricular dysfunction and left atrial enlargement. In patients with atrial fibrillation who have clinical risk factors for stroke, the risk is around 7.2% per year, in comparison with 2.5% per year in those without clinical risk factors. If no clinical or echocardiographic risk factors are present, the risk of stroke is approximately 1% per year.

If warfarin is used, the recommended international normalized ratio (INR) range is from 2 to 3. At an INR of less than 2, the risk of stroke increases. Conversely, at an INR of more than 3, the risk of bleeding goes up particularly in the elderly. Decisions about anticoagulation must consider patient compliance both with taking the drug and with obtaining the necessary frequent follow-up laboratory evaluations.

ANTICOAGULATION FOR CARDIOVERSION

The recommendations for anticoagulation for cardioversion are dependent on the duration of the atrial fibrillation. The risk of thromboembolism with acute cardioversion from atrial fibrillation that has been present for 24 to 48 hours is quite low (approximately 0.8%). The risk of stroke is increased by a longer duration of atrial fibrillation—presumably, a function of mechanical atrial stunning after the restoration of sinus rhythm. The current recommendation from the American College of Chest Physicians is to anticoagulate patients with atrial fibrillation of over 48 hours' duration for 3 to 4 weeks before either electrical or chemical cardioversion.

The use of transesophageal echocardiography (TEE) to identify atrial thrombi has been advocated to allow earlier cardioversion in patients with atrial fibrillation of unknown duration. In patients among whom early conversion is desired, heparin administration is initiated and TEE is performed. If TEE demonstrates no evidence for atrial thrombi or spontaneous contrast, the patient can undergo cardioversion, and anticoagulation with warfarin is continued for several weeks or months. Around 15% of patients undergoing TEE in this setting are found to have thrombi. Anticoagulation is then accomplished with warfarin, and TEE is repeated in 3 to 6 weeks, or cardioversion is deferred indefinitely. It is critical to remember that anticoagulation must be continued for an extended period as the risk of recurrent atrial fibrillation is highest in the early postcardioversion weeks.

CARDIOVERSION/MAINTENANCE OF SINUS RHYTHM

Restoration and maintenance of sinus rhythm is an alternative approach but limited by the toxic effects, poor tolerance, and relative lack of efficacy of antiarrhythmic drugs. Moreover, anticoagulants must be continued until there is strong evidence that sinus rhythm has been maintained over a period of at least weeks but usually months. It is important to

TABLE 5. **Intravenous Agents Used for Conversion to Sinus Rhythm**

Amiodarone* (Cordarone)	5 mg/kg IV over 30 min followed by 1200 mg over 24 h.
Procainamide* (Pronestyl)	10–12 mg/kg (typically 1 gm) IV over 30 min.
Propafenone*,** (Rythmol tablets)	2 mg/kg IV over 10 min.
Ibutilide (Corvert)	1 mg IV over 10 min. Repeat in 10 min if sinus rhythm is not achieved and excessive QT prolongation has not occurred.
Digoxin	0.25–0.50 mg IV initial followed by 0.25 mg IV every 4–8 h not to exceed 1 mg in 24 h.

*Not FDA approved for this indication.
**Intravenous form not available in the United States.

recognize that cardioversion alone may not improve the clinical status, symptoms, or prognosis of the patient with atrial fibrillation. Also, many patients who have been in atrial fibrillation for more than 6 months to 1 year either fail to convert with antiarrhythmics or do not maintain sinus rhythm after electrical cardioversion, despite the use of antiarrhythmics. There are, however, many potential means by which to achieve sinus rhythm.

Acute Cardioversion

For the patient with a first episode of atrial fibrillation, we typically attempt cardioversion without the initiation of chronic antiarrhythmic therapy. For acute conversion of atrial fibrillation, synchronous direct-current shock is certainly a first line of therapy. Intravenous amiodarone* (Cordarone), procainamide hydrochloride,* propafenone hydrochloride,* ibutilide fumarate (Corvert), digoxin, and other agents have been used to accomplish acute cardioversion (Table 5). There are no studies directly comparing these drugs; however, it appears likely that the earlier they are used in the course of atrial fibrillation, the greater the likelihood of successful conversion. Approximate success rates for each are as follows: for amiodarone, 30% at 1 hour, 80% at 24 hours; for procainamide, 65% at 1 hour; for propafenone, 90% at 1 hour; for ibutilide, 50 to 60%; and for digoxin, 50%. It should be noted, however, that spontaneous conversion to sinus rhythm occurs in up to 50% of patients within 24 hours. With ibutilide, it is critical to remember not to use this drug in the presence of other agents that can prolong the QT interval, because the risk of torsades de pointes is excessive.

Studies have shown electrophysiologic changes caused by atrial fibrillation, including shortening of the atrial refractory periods and spatial dispersion of refractoriness that predisposes to the recurrence of atrial fibrillation or the resistance to cardioversion. Therefore, early recurrences after cardioversion are possible, and often a short course of antiarrhythmics

*Not FDA approved for this indication.

is given in this event in hopes that these changes will normalize as sinus rhythm is maintained. Agents that can be used include procainamide (Procan SR, 500 to 750 mg orally [PO] every 6 hours, or Procanbid ER); disopyramide (Norpace CR, 150 to 200 mg PO twice daily); propafenone (Rhythmol, 150 to 225 mg PO every 8 hours); or flecainide (Tambocor, 50 to 100 mg PO every 12 hours). The use of procainamide and disopyramide is guided by serum drug levels. The use of the class IC agents flecainide and propafenone is restricted to patients with structurally normal hearts. Our practice is to start these agents on an inpatient basis, particularly if the patient has structural heart disease. In general, we then stop antiarrhythmics after 6 to 8 weeks.

Chronic Antiarrhythmic Therapy

If the patient has had multiple recurrent episodes of atrial fibrillation and proves to be intolerant to rate control and anticoagulation, consideration is given to chronic antiarrhythmic therapy. The drug efficacy for the class IA agents is maintenance of sinus rhythm at 1 year in 50% of patients. The class IC agents have approximately a 50% maintenance of sinus rhythm at 1 year. Amiodarone, a class III drug, has approximately a 60% maintenance of sinus rhythm at 3 years.

Chronic use of aniarrhythmics can yield disappointing results because of limited efficacy and frequent drug intolerance. Potential proarrhythmic effects of the antiarrhythmics must be considered, particularly in patients with left ventricular dysfunction or QT prolongation. Deaths related to torsades de pointes and conduction abnormalities have been reported with virtually every antiarrhythmic agent currently used. There is an increased risk of cardiac death in patients with heart failure (relative risk, 4.7) and an increased risk of arrhythmic death (relative risk, 3.7) treated with antiarrhythmic drugs. Patients without heart failure fail to show this increased risk of cardiac death when treated with antiarrhythmics but remain susceptible to drug side effects.

It has been our practice to start class IA and IC agents while patients are in the hospital. The class III agents sotalol and amiodarone are potentially more effective than either IA or IC drugs. Sotalol is started as an inpatient. The beta-blocking effects are seen before the class III effects are noted, and frequently patients are intolerant of the higher doses of sotalol. Amiodarone may be the most effective antiarrhythmic agent for maintenance of sinus rhythm. Symptomatically, patients generally tolerate amiodarone well, but the side effects can be quite severe. Oral amiodarone can usually be initiated safely in an outpatient, but the patient must be evaluated frequently during the loading phase for bradycardia or QT interval prolongation.

NEW APPROACHES TO MANAGEMENT OF ATRIAL FIBRILLATION

In view of the limitations with available therapies, the current wave of interest in nonpharmacologic approaches to the management of atrial fibrillation is understandable. The most successful method of achieving rate control is through catheter ablation of the AV node and implantation of a permanent pacemaker. Because the atria continue to fibrillate, the need for anticoagulation persists. Surgical procedures such as the maze frequently achieve sinus rhythm, but open heart surgery is required, and some patients subsequently need a permanent pacemaker. In addition, the effects of extensive surgery on atrial contractility and thrombogenicity require further evaluation. Catheter-based techniques aimed at reproducing the surgically induced lesions are strictly experimental at present and by early appearances have yielded a high morbidity rate. Ablation of focal atrial tachycardia, which has been linked to atrial fibrillation in some patients, is an interesting technique and is highly promising. Typically, patients with focal atrial tachycardia are seen to have frequent premature atrial contractions preceding atrial fibrillation. The proportion of patients in whom this ablative technique is beneficial remains to be established.

Pacing techniques under evaluation include dual-site right atrial pacing, bicameral pacing, and coronary sinus pacing alone. The implantable atrial defibrillator is currently another focus of investigation. The device is highly successful in the restoration of sinus rhythm, but its widespread use is limited by the strength of current required to defibrillate, which is often quite painful to the patient.

PREMATURE BEATS

method of
JEFFREY F. ALISON, M.B.
Monash Medical Centre
Clayton, Victoria, Australia

A premature beat is a nonsinus cardiac electrical event, causing myocardial depolarization, that occurs earlier than expected in relation to the prevailing cardiac rhythm. Premature beats can originate from any site within the heart. They are generally classified as either supraventricular (from foci within the atria, atrioventricular [AV] node and His bundle) or ventricular (originating below the His bundle in the bundle branches and more distal Purkinje fibers or ventricular myocardium).

Premature beats of all varieties occur commonly and in most cases are asymptomatic and benign without evidence of underlying pathologic cardiac processes. However, they can be markers for cardiac or systemic disease or may act as triggers for sustained tachyarrhythmias. Hence a considered approach to the evaluation of premature beats is warranted.

ATRIAL PREMATURE BEATS

Clinical Features

Atrial premature beats (APBs) are usually asymptomatic and detected during examination or investigation for unrelated conditions. However, if they are particularly frequent or occur in repetitive forms such as couplets, triplets, bigeminy, or nonsustained runs, they may produce symptoms. Patients may report palpitations with features such as "fluttering" sensations in the chest or intermittent "pounding" in the chest or throat. In rare instances, there may be associated symptoms of dyspnea or lightheadedness.

APBs are common and not usually a marker of underlying pathologic processes. They often appear in response to various ingested stimulants such as caffeine, alcohol, nicotine, and sympathomimetic drugs. They may also be provoked by intrinsic stimuli such as increased sympathetic drive in the setting of physical or mental stress. APBs are sometimes a feature of hyperthyroidism, and this condition should be considered if other clinical markers are compatible with the diagnosis.

Acute ischemic syndromes (e.g., unstable angina, myocardial infarction) may be complicated by frequent APBs, which themselves may be triggers for atrial tachyarrhythmias such as atrial fibrillation or atrial flutter. Atrial ectopy is common in other cardiac conditions that result in atrial dilatation, such as valvular heart disease and all forms of cardiomyopathy (dilated, hypertrophic, and restrictive). APBs are often associated with chronic obstructive lung disease.

Electrocardiographic Diagnosis

The typical electrocardiographic (ECG) characteristics of APBs include an early P wave, QRS and T wave morphologic characteristics unchanged from sinus beats, and a subsequent R-R interval the same as or only slightly longer than the sinus cycle length. The P wave morphologic pattern is usually quite different from that of sinus P waves, and the waveform is often inverted. Occasionally the QRS morphologic pattern may differ from that of sinus beats as a result of "aberrant conduction." A bundle branch block or hemiblock conduction disturbance may result if the His-Purkinje system is activated while partially refractory (i.e., incompletely repolarized) after transmission of the preceding sinus beat. If an APB occurs very early, the AV node or His-Purkinje system may be sufficiently refractory to completely prevent conduction to the ventricles, resulting in absence of the QRS complex (nonconducted APB).

Management

Most patients with APBs are asymptomatic and have no pathologic cardiac processes. In this setting, no treatment, apart from reassurance, is required. When APBs are a marker of other disease states but still asymptomatic, these other diseases should be managed on their own merits.

In patients with asymptomatic APBs, an initial search for reversible causes should be made. Stimulants such as caffeine, nicotine, and alcohol should be avoided. Electrolyte disorders, anemia, and hyperthyroidism should be ruled out. Cardiac failure and chronic lung disease should be optimally treated. If symptoms of palpitations persist but are mild, reassurance and acceptance remain the best approach, in as much as all forms of antiarrhythmic therapy have drawbacks.

In highly symptomatic patients, antiarrhythmic drug therapy may be considered (Table 1). First-line antiarrhythmic therapy should be a beta blocker such as atenolol (Tenormin), 25 to 50 mg daily, or metoprolol (Lopressor), 25 to 50 mg twice daily. If beta blockers are contraindicated or not tolerated, the next choice should be a calcium channel antagonist, such as sustained-release verapamil (Isoptin SR), 180 to 240 mg daily; diltiazem (Cardizem), 60 mg three times a day; or sustained-release diltiazem (Cardizem CD), 180 to 240 mg daily.

Very occasionally, when other approaches have failed and the patient remains symptomatic, class IC antiarrhythmic drugs such as flecainide (Tambocor), 50 to 100 mg twice a day, or propafenone (Rythmol), 150 to 300 mg three times a day, and the class III antiarrhythmic drug sotalol (Betapace), 80 to 160 mg twice a day, can be used. However, these more potent antiarrhythmics have the capacity to produce major adverse effects, including proarrhythmia (see Table 1). Hence careful monitoring is vital.

When APBs act as triggers for sustained supraventricular tachyarrhythmias, management should be as described elsewhere in this section (see articles on atrial fibrillation and tachycardias).

JUNCTIONAL PREMATURE BEATS

The clinical features and management of junctional premature beats are identical to those of atrial premature beats.

Electrocardiographic Diagnosis

ECG characteristics vary according to the site of origin of the premature beat within the AV junction (AV node and proximal His bundle) and relative rates of conduction into the atria and ventricles. Typically, an early inverted P wave, with a very short P-R interval, precedes a normal QRS complex. The following R-R interval is less than fully compensatory. Atrial activation is often more delayed, coinciding with ventricular activation, and the resultant P wave is buried within or occurs shortly after the QRS complex. Junctional premature beats are more commonly associated with aberrant QRS conduction than with APBs.

TABLE 1. **Summary of Important Antiarrhythmic Drug Properties**

Drug Class	Cell Membrane Effects	Potential Electrocardiographic Effects	Examples	Relative Antiarrhythmic Efficacy*		Major Adverse Effects
				Supraventricular	*Ventricular*	
IA	Sodium channel blockers (moderate)	Prolonged QRS and QT interval	Quinidine	+ +	+ +	GIT, thrombocytopenia, TDP
			Procainamide	+ +	+ +	GIT, SLE, TDP
			Disopyramide	+ +	+ +	Anticholinergic, CCF, TDP
IB	Sodium channel blockers (weak)	Shortened QT, normal QRS	Lidocaine	0	+	Neuro.
			Mexiletine	0	+	GIT, neuro., hepatotoxicity
IC	Sodium channel blockers (strong)	Prolonged QRS and PR interval	Flecainide	+ +	+ +(+)	Blurred vision, headache, CCF, TDP
			Propafenone	+ +	+ +(+)	Blurred vision, headache, CCF, TDP
II	Beta receptor blockade	Bradycardia, AV block	Atenolol	+(+)	+(+)	Bradycardia, AV block, CCF, bronchospasm, exercise intolerance
			Metoprolol	+(+)	+(+)	
			Propranolol	+(+)	+(+)	
III	Prolonged repolarization	Prolonged PR and QT intervals	Sotalol	+ +	+ +(+)	Beta blocker effects, TDP
			Amiodarone	+ +(+)	+ +(+)	Skin, thyroid, hepatotoxicity, pulm., corneal microdeposits
IV	Calcium channel blockers	Prolonged PR interval/ AV block	Verapamil	+	0(+)	Bradycardia, AV block, CCF, constipation, edema
			Diltiazem	+	0	

*0 = no effect; + = effective; + + = very effective; (+) = intermediate.

Abbreviations: AV = atrioventricular; CCF = congestive cardiac failure; eyes = blurred vision; GIT = gastrointestinal effects, including nausea, diarrhea, abdominal pain; neuro. = tremor, ataxia, convulsions; pulm. = interstitial pneumonitis/pulmonary fibrosis; SLE = systemic lupus erythematosus–like syndrome; TDP = torsades de pointes (polymorphic ventricular tachycardia).

VENTRICULAR PREMATURE BEATS

In keeping with the nature of premature beats in general, ventricular premature beats (VPBs) are common, most patients are asymptomatic, and the majority have no associated heart disease. In studies with 24-hour ambulatory ECG (Holter) recordings, the prevalence of VPBs in normal persons tends to increase with age. VPBs were found in approximately 25% of persons in their early teens; this rate increased to approximately 80% among persons 70 years of age and older. The ventricular ectopy seen is generally monomorphic, isolated VPBs. Multimorphic VPBs are seen in approximately 10% of teenagers and young adults. Of persons older than 70 years, approximately 30% have multimorphic VPBs on Holter recordings. More complex forms of ventricular ectopy such as repetitive beats (couplets and nonsustained ventricular tachycardia [VT]) are very uncommon in normal persons, regardless of age. The presence and frequency of VPBs may be influenced by stimulants such as caffeine, nicotine, alcohol, and sympathomimetic drugs. Mental stress may also provoke VPBs. They may be aggravated by electrolyte disturbances such as hypokalemia, hypocalcemia, and hypomagnesemia.

Many studies have shown that VPBs may be major prognostic markers when underlying cardiac structure or function is abnormal. By far the most important association is that between VPBs and ischemic heart disease, particularly myocardial infarction. During acute myocardial infarction, VPB frequency may increase markedly. Short-coupled ("R-on-T") VPBs may occur and have been linked to the development of sustained VT and ventricular fibrillation (VF). Early post-infarct VPB frequency may remain high. The finding of frequent VPBs (>10 per hour) or repetitive forms in the subacute phase after in-

farction (2 weeks to 3 months) indicates increased risk for sudden cardiac death from malignant ventricular tachyarrhythmias (VT) and VF over the ensuing 2 to 4 years.

The extent of myocardial damage is an important predictor of prognosis; that is, the worse the left ventricular systolic function (as measured by left ventricular ejection fraction) after infarction, the higher the risk of mortality. Among patients in whom significantly impaired left ventricular function is associated with frequent or complex ventricular ectopy, the mortality rate over 2 years may be greater than 30%, of which at least half is due to arrhythmias.

VPBs are commonly associated with both dilated and hypertrophic cardiomyopathies. Although this premise is not as well established, it is generally accepted that frequent or repetitive forms of VPBs, in patients with these conditions, are markers for premature death.

Clinical Features

In most patients, VPBs are an incidental finding. Even when associated with severe forms of cardiac disease, isolated VPBs are usually asymptomatic. Patients with symptomatic ventricular ectopy usually report "missing" or "extra" beats and "thumps" or "flutters" in the chest or neck. Because there is loss of AV synchrony with VPBs, jugular venous cannon waves are produced by right atrial contraction against a closed tricuspid valve. These cannon waves can give rise to sensations of choking or a lump in the throat. Jugular venous cannon waves can sometimes be the cause of "dizziness." In a similar manner, pulmonary venous cannon waves can produce symptoms of dyspnea. Symptoms of presyncope and syncope are rare with ventricular ectopy but may be reported if the VPBs act as triggers for VT that spontaneously reverts to sinus rhythm.

Electrocardiographic Diagnosis

VPBs typically have bizarre, broad QRS complexes that occur earlier than the expected sinus beat, without a preceding premature P wave. ST segments and T wave vectors are usually opposite to the QRS complex. The following sinus beat is usually fully compensatory. Retrograde conduction from the ventricle to the AV node collides with anterograde conduction from the coincident, normal sinus beat, preventing perturbation of the following sinus beat, which occurs on time. Sometimes very early VPBs result in retrograde conduction through the AV node to activate the atrium and (prematurely) the sinus node. The early sinus node activation resets the sinus cycle so that the next sinus beat is earlier than expected, and therefore the post-VPB pause is not fully compensatory. VPBs that occur very late in the sinus cycle may activate a portion of the ventricle, whereas the remainder of the ventricle is activated by normal anterograde conduction of the sinus impulse through the AV node and His-Purkinje system. This results in the so-called fusion beat, in which the QRS complex is less broad than a typical VPB and retains some of the features of a normally conducted sinus beat.

VPBs originating from the same focus in the ventricle are identical in morphology and are described as monomorphic or unifocal. When QRS morphology is variable, the term *multimorphic* (or polymorphic or multifocal) *VPBs* is applied. VPBs may have a typical bundle branch block appearance. VPBs with right bundle branch block morphology originate in the left ventricle; those with a left bundle branch morphology originate from the right ventricle.

A discrete form of VPB with characteristic features of left bundle branch block and inferior frontal plane axis (QRS upright in ECG leads II, III, and AVF) originates from a focus in the right ventricular outflow tract. In most instances, the underlying cardiac structure and function are normal and the VPBs are benign. In rare instances, VPBs with a similar QRS morphology are associated with right ventricular dysplasia.

Initial Evaluation

Patients with VPBs should be evaluated with regard to possible underlying cardiac disease, as well as for electrolyte or metabolic disorders and drug toxicity. In most cases, a thorough history, examination, and ECG suffice. Useful investigations include blood biochemistry studies (electrolytes, thyroid function, and drug levels if indicated) and echocardiography. If correlation between VPBs and patient symptoms is required, 24-hour Holter monitoring is helpful.

Baseline evaluation of patients with known cardiac disease should include full biochemistry studies and appropriate tests of drug levels, chest radiography, echocardiography, and some form of functional assessment such as an exercise ECG, thallium scan, or stress echocardiography and Holter monitoring.

Treatment

No Cardiac Disease Present

In patients with normal hearts and asymptomatic VPBs, no intervention is required apart from reassurance.

When patients are symptomatic, aggravating factors such as stimulants and stress should be searched for and removed if possible. Beyond this, reassurance should remain the first choice of therapy. Often a clear explanation, in simple terms, of *why* the patient is experiencing symptoms and of the benign nature of the VPBs allays anxiety and diverts attention from the symptoms.

When patients are highly symptomatic, suppression of VPBs is indicated (see Table 1). The first choice antiarrhythmic drug should be a beta blocker. Either atenolol, 25 to 50 mg daily, or metoprolol, 25 to 50 mg twice a day, is a good choice, but other beta blockers are also appropriate.

Intervention beyond simple beta blockade is problematic, and a cardiologic/electrophysiologic opinion should be sought. Patients with VPBs of right ventricular outflow tract morphology that produce intolerable symptoms despite antiarrhythmic drugs should be referred to an electrophysiologist, because the VPB focus is amenable to catheter ablation.

Coexistent Cardiac Disease

Frequent or complex VPBs in the presence of cardiac disease are markers of an increased risk of sudden cardiac death. However, a direct causal link between VPBs and the onset of malignant ventricular tachyarrhythmias has never been established.

This perhaps in part explains why past studies designed around supression of VPBs have failed to show any mortality-related benefit of antiarrhythmic drug therapy. The Cardiac Arrhythmia Suppression Trial (CAST) clearly showed that suppression of asymptomatic VPBs in postinfarction patients with class I antiarrhythmic drugs does not confer any mortality-related benefit. In fact, this study showed that use of class IC drugs (flecainide and encainide) was associated with excessive mortality in comparison with placebo. The results of other studies have also supported the conclusion that class I antiarrhythmic drugs should not be used for treatment of VPBs, either asymptomatic or symptomatic, in patients with underlying structural heart disease, particularly ischemic heart disease.

The class III antiarrhythmic drug amiodarone (Cordarone) has been used to treat VPBs in the postinfarction setting and in patients with various forms of cardiomyopathy. Trials designed to evaluate this drug's efficacy in these various conditions have failed to show a statistically significant mortality-related benefit. Both the Canadian Amiodarone Myocardial Infarction Arrhythmia Trial (CAMIAT) and the European Myocardial Infarction Amiodarone Trial (EMIAT) showed a reduction in arrhythmia-related deaths but no overall benefit with regard to total mortality. The VPB suppression hypothesis has not been directly tested with sotalol, another drug with class III antiarrhythmic action. However, sotalol also has important class II (beta-blocking) effects, which are a major determinant of the drug's overall antiarrhythmic efficacy.

There is a wealth of data concerning use of beta blockers in cardiac disease. They have been clearly shown to reduce mortality rates over extended follow-up. The reduction in mortality rates relates to both arrhythmic deaths and total mortality rates. The greatest reduction in mortality rates appears to occur in patients at highest risk: that is, those with significantly reduced left ventricular function and those with high-grade ventricular ectopy.

In view of the foregoing findings, beta blockers should be the first and only choice of antiarrhythmic drug therapy for asymptomatic VPBs in patients with structural heart disease.

Symptomatic VPBs pose a difficult problem. Beta blockers should be the first choice. If pure beta blockers are ineffective, the next choice should be between sotalol (Sotacor, Betapace), 80 to 160 mg twice a day, and amiodarone (Cordarone), 200 mg daily (after initial loading consisting of 600 to 800 mg daily for 1 week followed by 400 mg daily for another 2 weeks), because neither of these drugs has been shown to produce excess mortality in comparison with placebo in large trials. It should be noted that optimal treatment of the underlying cardiac condition may reduce ventricular ectopy.

Because of the difficulties in satisfactorily treating VPBs in patients with cardiac disease, particularly when the VPBs are sufficiently frequent or complex to indicate an adverse prognosis, referral for electrophysiologic evaluation is often appropriate. The Multicenter Automatic Defibrillator Implantation Trial (MADIT) studied patients with previous myocardial infarction at high risk of sudden death. Entry criteria included left ventricular ejection fraction of less than 0.35; more than 10 VPBs per hour or nonsustained VT on Holter monitoring but no previous episodes of sustained VT; resuscitation from cardiac arrest; and syncope. Of this group, patients with VT inducible on electrophysiology study but not suppressible with procainamide were randomly assigned to treatment with either conventional antiarrhythmic drugs or an implantable cardioverter-defibrillator (ICD).

Among patients who received ICDs, the total mortality rate was reduced more than 50%, in comparison to conventional antiarrhythmic therapy, prompting the data monitoring committee to halt the trial prematurely. If further studies support the conclusions of MADIT, patients with adverse prognostic markers, such as frequent VPBs in association with moderate to severe structural heart disease, may be in the future routinely treated with ICD insertion.

HEART BLOCK

method of
ANNE HAMILTON DOUGHERTY, M.D.
University of Texas—Houston
Houston, Texas

The term "heart block" describes a group of bradyarrhythmias resulting from delay or block in propagation of excitatory impulses between the atria and ventricles. Conduction abnormalities may occur either at the level of the atrio-ventricular (AV) node or more distally in the His-Purkinje system. The consequences of the resultant arrhythmias may be benign or severe, even life-threatening, depending upon the level and severity of block.

ANATOMIC AND ELECTROPHYSIOLOGIC CONSIDERATIONS

Structure and Function of the AV Junction

A complex sequence of structures beginning with the AV node and extending through the penetrating bundle of His, the bundle branches, and the Purkinje fiber system, the AV junction forms an electrical bridge between atria and ventricles. In normal sinus rhythm, the sinus impulse excites adjacent atrial myocardium and is propagated to the AV node. Functional conduction slowing in the AV node provides an interval for active ventricular filling during atrial systole that augments cardiac output in a dynamic fashion. The impulse is then dispersed throughout the ventricular myocardium in a rapid uniform wavefront through the His-Purkinje system, resulting in synchronized ventricular systole.

The compact AV node lies in the interatrial septum at the apex of the triangle of Koch, an anatomic area bounded by the tendon of Todaro, the tricuspid valve annulus, and the Eustachian valve. Two primary approaches, anterosuperior and posteroinferior, funnel atrial impulses into the AV node. The AV node has been divided into three regions: AN, N, and NH, based upon differences in histologic and electrophysiologic properties; however, actual transitions from zone to zone and into the bundle of His are gradual.

The AV node action potential is characteristic of slow-response calcium channel–dependent tissue. The resting membrane potential is less negative than that of atrial or ventricular myocardium and the slow–inward calcium channel current produces the upstroke. Spontaneous diastolic depolarization during phase 4 provides latent pacemaker capability, which may become manifest during sinus node inactivity. AV node conduction is decremental; increasing heart rates or premature impulses produce progressive delay. With incremental atrial pacing, second degree AV block of the Mobitz I type can be demonstrated in normal individuals; however, the rates at which block occur vary widely. Rich sympathetic and parasympathetic innervation modulates nodal function significantly.

The AV nodal artery arises out of the posterior descending branch of the right coronary artery in 90% of the population; in others, it arises from the left circumflex. Thus, the node is vulnerable to ischemia in the event of inferior or posterior myocardial infarction; transient AV nodal block may occur. Collateral supply from other penetrating branches of the posterior descending artery and septal perforators usually restore function within a few days.

The common bundle of His lies within the connective

tissue of the central fibrous body at the apex of the membranous interventricular septum and measures approximately 1 cm in length. It emerges into the left ventricular outflow tract, at which point it bifurcates into the right and left bundle branches. The right bundle branch is a discrete structural extension of the penetrating bundle coursing toward the ventricular apex and crossing over to the right ventricular free wall in the moderator band. In contrast, the left bundle forms a broad fan over the subendocardial surface of the left ventricle, usually with two or three major divisions, or fascicles. The bundle branches arborize into fine Purkinje fibers that excite myocardial cells. Perhaps because of significant anatomic variability, surface electrocardiogram (ECG) patterns of left anterior and left posterior fascicular blocks correlate poorly with actual anatomic lesions. His-Purkinje cells are sodium-channel dependent with rapid conduction velocity. A dual blood supply is provided by the left and right coronary arteries. Innervation, less dense than that of the AV node, is predominantly sympathetic.

Electrophysiologic Considerations

The PR interval on the surface ECG normally measures 120 to 200 milliseconds in adults. More specific components of A-V conduction can be analyzed with an intracardiac His bundle recording (Figure 1). Intraatrial conduction time is represented by the P-A interval, from the onset of the surface P wave to the low right atrial (A) electrogram, recorded in the His region. The A-H interval on the His electrogram represents AV nodal conduction time, usually 50 to 130 milliseconds; the H-V interval, measured from onset of the His deflection to earliest surface QRS complex, reflects conduction time from the proximal bundle of His to ventricular myocardium, normally 35 to 55 milliseconds. Intracardiac His bundle recordings during sinus and paced rhythms can be helpful in identifying subclinical conduction system disease and in determining the level of AV block.

Pathologic Considerations

In adults, the most common causes of AV block are pharmacologic, autonomic, ischemic, and degenerative processes of the conduction system. Drugs that produce delay or block in the AV node include digitalis, beta blockers, and certain calcium channel antagonists. Class I and III antiarrhythmic agents and other membrane-active drugs may produce infranodal block. Neurally mediated block in the AV node may occur in vagotonic states, neurocardiogenic reflex syncope, or carotid sinus hypersensitivity. In these instances, AV block is almost always accompanied by sinus bradycardia. The most common degenerative diseases of the conduction system are Lev's (calcific or fibrotic) and Lenegre's (sclerodegenerative) diseases. Unusual causes of AV block include infiltrative and inflammatory myocardidites and muscular dystrophies.

AV block in children is usually congenital and is associated with structural heart defects in approximately one-half of cases. Maternal lupus, especially when antiribonucleoprotein antibodies are present, is a common etiologic factor. There is a higher incidence of concomitant ostium primum atrial septal defect and transposition of the great vessels in individuals with congenital heart block.

ELECTROCARDIOGRAPHIC DIAGNOSIS OF HEART BLOCK

First Degree AV Block

First degree AV block is defined as a PR interval exceeding 200 milliseconds in an adult (180 milliseconds in adolescents). A 1:1 A-V relationship is maintained throughout. Most often, the conduction delay occurs at the level of the AV node (prolonged A-H); however, intraatrial delay and His-Purkinje delay may in rare cases result in first-degree AV block. In patients with a widened QRS complex or bundle branch block, the likelihood of lower intra-His (H-H') and infra-His block (increased H-V interval) is substantially higher and implies a poorer prognosis. Invasive His bundle recordings are useful in identifying the level of block for risk stratification in patients with first degree AV block and wide QRS complexes.

Second Degree AV Block

Intermittent failure of normal sinus impulses to be propagated to the ventricles defines second degree AV block. Electrocardiographic patterns show regular P waves, only some of which are followed by a QRS complex. Second degree AV block is classified further into Mobitz I (Wenckebach) or Mobitz II types, terms useful in predicting the anatomic level of block and, thus, potential risk.

Wenckebach AV block is usually, but not always, due to decremental conduction in the AV node, resulting in cycles of progressive AV conduction delay punctuated by intermittent AV block. On surface leads, P-P intervals remain constant as the PR interval progressively prolongs until one P wave is not followed by a QRS; then the cycle may repeat, resulting in group beating (clusters of beats with decreasing R-R intervals, separated by pauses). The QRS complex is usually narrow. Intracardiac recordings during typical Mobitz I block show progressive prolongation in the A-H interval, then the nonconducted A wave is not followed by either an H or a V. As with first degree AV block, Wenckebach may be a benign finding in healthy individuals, especially under conditions of enhanced vagal tone.

Mobitz II AV block is characterized on surface ECG by sudden failure of a P to be followed by a QRS with constant P-P and PR intervals. Type II block usually occurs in patients with other evidence of His-Purkinje disease, especially bundle branch block, and confers a worse prognosis. The infra-His or intra-His level of conduction block can be documented on intracardiac recordings by demonstrating an A-H not followed by a V in the nonconducted beat. Sudden 2:1 AV block may not be classifiable into Mobitz I or II categories on the surface ECG, however, the presence of a widened QRS increases the likelihood of the latter. Intracardiac recordings to determine the level of block may be required.

Some authors refer to a more severe form of second degree AV block as high degree AV block. In this condition, two or more consecutive P waves are not conducted to the ventricle, but the A-V relationship is otherwise maintained.

Third Degree AV Block

Third degree, or complete, AV block results from total failure of propagation of atrial impulses to the ventricles. Atrial and ventricular rhythms are fully dissociated with the atrial rate exceeding a regular ventricular escape rate. The electrocardiographic appearance depends upon the anatomic site of block (Figure 2). Most congenital heart block

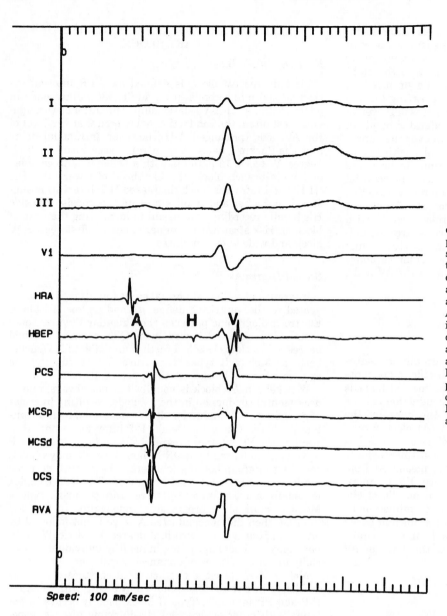

Figure 1. Normal intracardiac electrocardiograms recorded during invasive electrophysiologic study in a patient with normal sinus rhythm. A bipolar recording from the tricuspid valve area at the level of the bundle of His (HBEP) demonstrates a low right atrial potential (A), a low His potential (H), and a low right ventricular potential (V). The A-H interval is 78 msec and the H-V interval is 48 msec. Simultaneous surface electrocardiographic leads I, II, III, and V₁ are shown at the top of the page, along with a high right atrial recording (HRA); proximal and distal His recordings (HBEP and HBED); proximal, proximal-mid–, distal-mid–, and distal–coronary sinus recordings (PCS, MCSP, MCSD, and DCS); and a right ventricular apex (RVA) recording.

is due to block within the AV node (intranodal block). Like acquired blocks that arise from drugs or ischemia affecting the AV node, it is characterized by a narrow QRS complex rhythm with an escape rate of 40 to 60 bpm. The escape rate, originating from the AV junction, may increase with exercise, isoproterenol, or atropine. The intracardiac His bundle recording will show A complexes at a regular rate, but not associated with H or V complexes. Coupled H-V complexes are superimposed at an independent, slower rate. In contrast, acquired complete heart block usually occurs within the His-Purkinje system (infra-His or, rarely, intra-His block). The escape rhythm is ventricular in origin, resulting in a wide QRS rhythm between 20 and 40 bpm. Thus, the His bundle recording will show A-H complexes not succeeded by V complexes and dissociated V complexes at a slower rate. Long pauses may be seen if the ventricular escape rhythm is unreliable.

Bundle Branch Blocks

Conduction delay in one of the bundle branches or its fascicles, either absolute or relative to the other fascicles, may produce electrocardiographic criteria for bundle branch or fascicular block. The widened or distorted QRS complex results from inhomogeneous ventricular activation. Right bundle branch block is the most common and most benign. It is usually associated with little or no prolongation of the H-V interval. Left bundle branch block is more frequently associated with other heart disease and more frequently produces H-V prolongation. Because of the variability in the distribution of the left bundle and its fascicles, left anterior and posterior fascicular blocks correlate poorly with actual anatomic lesions of these structures. Nonetheless, the ECG criteria remain useful prognostically. The combination of right bundle branch block with either left anterior or left posterior fascicular block is termed a bifascicular block. Trifascicular block refers to the additional finding of first-degree AV block.

CLINICAL MANIFESTATIONS

Signs and Symptoms of AV Block

Symptoms due to first-degree AV block are extremely rare and only observed in cases where PR prolongation is

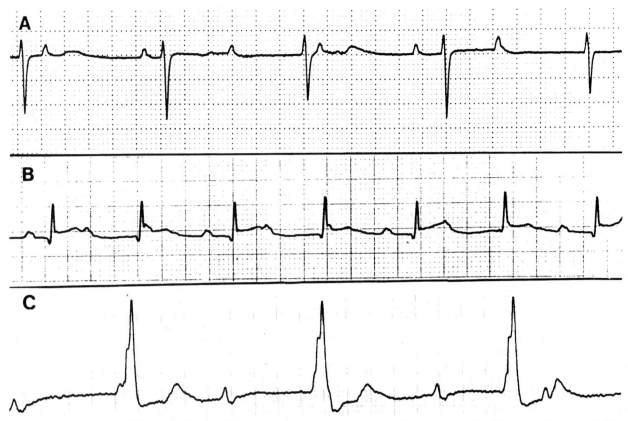

Figure 2. Electrocardiograms from three different patients with complete AV block. *A,* A V$_1$ recording from an asymptomatic 10-year-old girl with congenital complete heart block, showing a narrow QRS complex (junctional) escape rhythm at 51 bpm. A ventriculophasic sinus arrhythmia accounts for the slight irregularity in the P-P intervals. *B,* Transient complete AV block in a 33-year-old man with an acute inferior myocardial infarction involving the AV nodal artery. The lead II recording demonstrates small inferior Q waves and ST elevation. The junctional escape rhythm provides a rate of 75 bpm. *C,* Complete AV block in a 91-year-old man with syncope. Lead V$_3$ shows a wide QRS escape rhythm at 36 bpm that is ventricular in origin.

extreme (e.g., >.30 seconds). Fatigue or dyspnea may result from the equivalent of a pacemaker syndrome in which the hemodynamic benefit of AV synchrony is lost due to the excessive delay. Patients with significant systolic or diastolic ventricular dysfunction are most prone to this condition. Because of the rarity of causality between first-degree AV block and these symptoms relative to their incidence in the population, convincing proof of the relationship should be sought. Relief of symptoms with temporary dual chamber pacing and establishment of physiologic AV intervals suggests causality.

Dizziness, fatigue, presyncope, and syncope may result from second- or third-degree AV block. The severity of symptoms depends largely upon the degree of bradycardia produced, as well as underlying cardiac or cerebrovascular disease. Sudden and significant bradycardia due to complete heart block frequently results in a Stokes-Adams attack, a sudden and catastrophic loss of consciousness.

Hemodynamic consequences of significant bradycardia include pallor, hypotension, and shock. AV dissociation due to complete heart block produces variation in the intensity of the first heart sound due to the variable position of the mitral valve leaflets at the onset of ventricular systole. Careful examination of the jugular veins will also reveal intermittent cannon A waves due to the occasional atrial contraction against a closed tricuspid valve.

Natural History of AV Block

First-degree AV block and Wenckebach AV block are typically benign. Mobitz II AV block is more commonly associated with underlying cardiac disease; the incidence of symptoms and the probability of progression to complete AV block are high. Mobitz II block, left bundle branch block, and left posterior fascicular block occurring in the setting of acute anterior myocardial infarction each increase the likelihood of progression to complete heart block and increase mortality. On the other hand, even complete heart block associated with inferior myocardial infarction is usually self-limited due to collateral blood flow. Acquired complete heart block may be fatal if not treated swiftly and effectively.

In contrast, congenital complete heart block is better tolerated and carries a more favorable prognosis. Some affected children may develop symptoms in infancy or even in utero, but most remain asymptomatic until adolescence. Permanent pacemaker implantation at the first notice of effort intolerance or slowing of the escape rhythm, or both, helps to prevent syncope and myocardial dysfunction and improves mortality.

MANAGEMENT

Diagnosis

Electrocardiographic documentation of the arrhythmia and correlation with symptoms and the underlying cardiac status are necessary to guide management. Second- and third-degree AV blocks may be intermittent, eluding routine diagnosis. In symptomatic patients with suspected conduction system disease, documentation can frequently be achieved with ambulatory ECG monitoring or transient symptomatic event recording, especially in a loop format. This process may be too tedious, however, for patients with severe, asymptomatic, or infrequent events. In those patients, invasive electrophysiologic study is useful in identifying abnormalities in AV node and His-Purkinje function. It is also helpful in determining the site of AV block when prognosis cannot be determined with certainty from the surface ECG. The diagnostic use of intravenous procainamide as a provocative test for infra-His conduction disease has been advocated by some. Patients with syncope of undetermined etiology associated with structural heart disease can also benefit from electrophysiologic testing, not only to assess the conduction system, but also to determine whether ventricular tachyarrhythmias might account for symptoms.

Indications for Pacemaker Therapy

Although symptomatic AV block can frequently be palliated with emergency use of isoproterenol infusion, pacemaker therapy is the standard of care for symptomatic and high-risk patients. Guidelines for implantation of permanent pacemakers have recently been revised and published by a joint task force of the American College of Cardiology and the American Heart Association. They are summarized in Table 1. Indications are divided into the following classes:

Class I: Conditions for which there is general agreement that pacing is beneficial and effective.

Class II: Conditions for which there is conflicting evidence or divergence of opinion about pacing benefit.(Class IIa: Evidence or opinion favors benefit. Class IIb: Benefit is less well established.)

Class III: Conditions for which there is evidence or general agreement that pacing is ineffective.

Pacemaker Prescription

Whereas the most basic single chamber pacemaker can prevent bradycardia, modern pacemakers provide more physiologic pacing to optimize functional capacity. The most important options to be considered in pacemaker prescription are dual chamber pacing and rate-responsiveness. AV universal (DDD) pacing requires leads in both the atrium and ventricle and provides AV synchrony that contributes approximately 10% to cardiac output. The atrial contribution to ventricular filling is even more significant in patients with ventricular hypertrophy or congestive heart failure, thus, dual chamber pacing provides even more hemodynamic benefit in afflicted individuals. Dual chamber pacing has been shown to reduce the frequency of paroxysmal atrial fibrillation but is inappropriate in patients with chronic atrial fibrillation. Automatic mode switching to ventricular pacing may be a very useful feature in individuals

TABLE 1. **Indications for Permanent Pacemaker Implantation in Atrioventricular (AV) Block**

Class I

Symptomatic third-degree AV block
Persistent third-degree AV block resulting from AV junction ablation, cardiac surgery, or neuromuscular disease
Asymptomatic third-degree AV block with periods of asystole >3.0 sec, or with escape rates <40 bpm while awake, or with chronic bifascicular or trifascicular block
Any second-degree AV block with symptomatic bradycardia
Mobitz II second-degree AV block with bifascicular or trifascicular block
Transient second- or third-degree AV block with bundle branch block following acute myocardial infarction
Congenital third-degree AV block with a wide QRS escape rhythm or ventricular dysfunction
Congenital third-degree AV block in infants with ventricular rates <50–55 bpm, or with ventricular rates <70 bpm in the presence of congenital heart disease

Class IIa

Asymptomatic third-degree AV block with mean awake ventricular rates >40 bpm
Asymptomatic Mobitz II second-degree AV block, or demonstrated infranodal second-degree AV block with invasive electrophysiologic study
Symptomatic first-degree AV block and documented symptom relief with temporary AV pacing
Congenital third-degree AV block in children >1 y of age with ventricular rates <50 bpm or abrupt pauses 2–3 times basic cycle length
Bifascicular or trifascicular AV block with syncope not proven to be AV block after exclusion of other likely causes, especially ventricular tachycardia
Incidental finding of H-V >100 msec or pacing-induced infra-His block

Class IIb

Marked first-degree AV block (>0.3 sec) with congestive heart failure, when a shorter AV interval is demonstrated to result in hemodynamic improvement
Persistent second- or third-degree AV block at the AV nodal level following acute myocardial infarction
Transient postoperative third-degree AV block with residual bifascicular AV block after reversion to sinus rhythm in children and adolescents
Asymptomatic congenital third-degree AV block with an acceptable rate, narrow QRS complex, and normal ventricular function

with uncontrolled paroxysmal atrial fibrillation to prevent rapid atrial tracking and inappropriately rapid pacing rates.

Sensor-driven rate responsive pacing is particularly effective in patients with chronotropic incompetence. Physical activity, acceleration, minute ventilation, core blood temperature, and evoked responses have each been used in commercial biosensors as indices of metabolic activity to determine the appropriate pacing rate on a minute-to-minute basis. Devices can be programmed to tailor function to address the needs of the individual. Quality of life is improved with the appropriate use of these features, even in elderly patients. The arrhythmia history and hemodynamic profile of the individual patient should be considered in choosing a device to suit his or her needs.

TACHYCARDIAS

method of
WILLIAM E. SANDERS, JR., M.D.
University of North Carolina
Chapel Hill, North Carolina

Significant changes in the therapeutic options available for the treatment of most arrhythmias have resulted in a dramatic modification of the approach to the tachycardic patient. During the 1990s, the development and widespread use of radiofrequency catheter ablation provided actual cure to thousands of patients with debilitating symptoms from paroxysmal supraventricular tachycardias. In addition, the risk of mortality from ventricular tachyarrhythmias has been virtually eliminated by implantable cardioverter defibrillators (ICDs). Determination of the specific type of tachycardia is extremely important in discussions with the patient when considering long-term drug administration versus radiofrequency ablation or device therapy. As with any therapeutic approach, the likelihood of success and the risks encountered are best assessed when the origin of the tachycardia has been elucidated.

The cause of a particular tachycardia can usually be determined by careful history, physical examination, and 12-lead electrocardiography both in sinus rhythm (not always available) and in tachycardia. Any history of syncope, lightheadedness, palpitations, chest pain, previous coronary artery disease, or congestive heart failure should be carefully elicited. The manner in which the symptoms initiate and terminate (e.g., whether it is abrupt), as well as the rate and regularity of palpitations, is important to the appropriate diagnosis. Many patients who have experienced emergency department visits during an episode of arrhythmia can recall the drug used to eliminate their symptoms (e.g., intravenous adenosine, lidocaine). With these historical clues and basic electrocardiographic information, the type of arrhythmia can be established.

Regardless of their medical sophistication, patients frequently inquire, "Why does this happen?" In a simplistic model, most tachycardias can be considered extra wires that short-circuit the normal conduction (Figure 1). The mechanism responsible is reentry involving two distinct pathways ("wires") with different speeds of conduction (a "slow" and a "fast" wire) and varying recovery times (refractoriness). Early beats (premature atrial or ventricular beats), which fail to conduct in the refractory/fast-conducting (normal) wire, may travel down the recovered, slowly conducting (extra) wire. At the distal junction of the two wires, the arriving slow impulse can return in a retrograde manner up the recovered fast-conducting (normal) wire. This completes the short circuit and may result in a sustained arrhythmia. Radiofrequency ablation therapy successfully eliminates the extra wire by application of thermal energy, leaving only normal conduction. Drug regimens, when effective, modify conduction or refractoriness in the circuit, or reduce the number of premature beats, resulting in fewer occurrences of tachycardia. ICDs do not modify the substrate, but they are extremely effective in terminating ventricular arrhythmias and reducing mortality.

SUPRAVENTRICULAR TACHYCARDIAS

Supraventricular tachycardias (SVTs) are best classified on the basis of arrhythmia origin: nodal tissue (sinoatrial node and atrioventricular [AV] node), atrial tissue, or AV connection (accessory pathway bridging the mitral valve, tricuspid valve, or septum) (Table 1). This system allows general delineation of all possible arrhythmias (including atrial fibrillation and tachycardias with AV block) but is of little assistance in the determination of the specific type of tachycardia. A second method of classifying narrow complex, regular SVTs is based on the relationship between the preceding QRS and the observed P wave (Table 2). Tachycardias can readily be

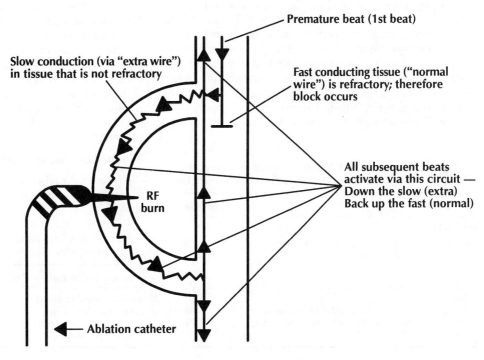

Figure 1. Model of initiation and circuit for reentrant tachycardia (see text for discussion). *Abbreviation*: RF = radiofrequency.

269

TABLE 1. **Classification of Supraventricular Tachycardias by Site**

Nodal	Atrial	Atrioventricular Connection (Accessory Pathway)
Sinus tachycardia	Atrial fibrillation	Atrioventricular reentry
Sinus node reentry	Atrial flutter	
Atrioventricular nodal reentry	(types I and II)	
	Atrial tachycardia	
Nonparoxysmal junction tachycardia	Multifocal atrial tachycardia	

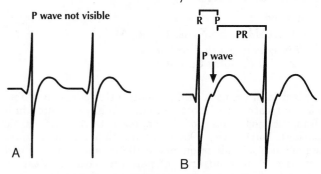

Short R-P tachycardias

P wave not visible

P wave

A

B

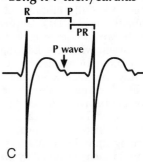

Long R-P tachycardias

P wave

C

Figure 2. Electrocardiographic patterns associated with most common forms of supraventricular tachycardias (SVTs). *A*, No observed P wave: "short R-P" rhythm. *B*, P wave observed in T wave and is less than half of R-R interval from preceding QRS: "Short R-P" rhythm. *C*, P wave occurs at more than half of the R-R interval from preceding QRS: "Long R-P" rhythm.

divided into short RP arrhythmias (the RP interval is less than the PR interval) and long RP tachycardias (RP interval is longer than PR interval), as illustrated in Figure 2. If no discernible P wave is observed, the tachycardia is considered a short RP rhythm. This implies that atrial activation and ventricular activation occur at the same time and the P wave cannot be observed because of the QRS complex. The electrocardiograms (ECGs) may be identical despite very different arrhythmic mechanisms, but attention to specific electrocardiographic findings, such as the QRS/P wave relationship (RP interval) and tachycardia rate, helps narrow the possibilities (Table 3; see also Table 2). In this chapter, SVTs are discussed by site of origin, with emphasis on electrocardiographic analysis.

Nodal Tachycardias

Sinus Tachycardia

A normal function of the sinoatrial node is to increase discharges in response to stress. The stress can be physiologic or pathologic and can result from exercise, anxiety, fever, anemia, hypokalemia, heart failure, myocardial infarction, pulmonary embolism, and hyperthyroidism. The observed heart rates in adults are usually less than 150 beats per minute (bpm) but in rare instances may exceed 200 bpm. There is no rapid onset or termination of the tachycardia, and the rhythm is therefore nonparoxysmal. The ECG shows a P wave with normal morphology

preceding each QRS complex, unless the rhythm is so fast that the P wave is buried in the preceding T wave. In these instances, the use of adenosine (Adenocard) can help demonstrate normal P wave morphology by slowing the rate of AV conduction and allowing the visualization of atrial depolarization. The lack of termination with adenosine suggests a non-reentrant mechanism. When hemodynamic compromise is secondary to elevated heart rate, beta-blocker therapy may be useful in alleviation of symptoms. The primary therapy for this arrhythmia is treatment of the underlying cause. A search for pulmonary embolism and metabolic causes (e.g., hyperthyroidism) may be warranted in the hospitalized patient.

Sinoatrial Nodal Reentrant Tachycardia

Sinoatrial nodal reentrant tachycardia (SANRT) is a relatively uncommon cause of sustained tachycar-

TABLE 2. **Diagnostic Characteristics of Narrow Complex, Regular Supraventricular Tachycardias**

Type	Incidence
Short RP	
Atrioventricular nodal tachycardia	56%
Atrioventricular reentry	27%
Long RP	
Atrial tachycardia	4%
Sinus node reentry	5%
Atypical atrioventricular nodal tachycardia	4%
Atrioventricular reentry with long conduction time	3%

TABLE 3. **Diagnostic Characteristics of Narrow Complex, Regular Supraventricular Tachycardias**

Tachycardia Rate > 160	Tachycardia Rate < 160
Atrioventricular nodal tachycardia	Atrial flutter (variable rate; 2:1 = 150)
Atrioventricular reentry	Sinus node reentry (usually < 140)
Atrial tachycardia	

dia, with a reported incidence of 1 to 16% of all paroxysmal supraventricular arrhythmias. SANRT is the clinical arrhythmia in 3% of patients referred for radiofrequency catheter ablation therapy. The tachycardia arises from the region of the sinus node, but it is extremely difficult to distinguish sinus nodal tissue from working atrial myocardium. Consequently, the specific role of sinus nodal and perinodal tissue remains unclear. P wave morphology similar or identical to that seen during sinus rhythm is a requirement for the diagnosis of this arrhythmia. The paroxysmal onset and termination help distinguish SANRT from sinus tachycardia. Specifically, heart rates during tachycardia of less than 130 bpm are typically observed. SANRT can consistently be terminated by vagal maneuvers and adenosine administration and is a "long RP" tachycardia. Beta-blocker and calcium antagonist therapy have proved effective in some patients with this arrhythmia. Radiofrequency catheter ablation is highly effective in eliminating the circuit for this tachycardia.

Atrioventricular Nodal Reentry Tachycardia

AV nodal reentry tachycardia (AVNRT) is by far the most common of the paroxysmal SVTs, occurring in up to 60% of patients with SVTs. AVNRT is not associated with underlying structural heart disease and can occur at any age. However, the usual patient is young to middle-aged, and there is a slightly higher prevalence among women. The arrhythmia is narrow complex and regular, and the rate is 160 to 250 bpm. In rare instances, AVNRT has been observed at heart rates between 100 and 160 bpm. The typical form of AVNRT is shown in Figure 1. A premature atrial impulse initially blocks in normal (fast-conducting) tissue, travels down a slow pathway, and then travels in a retrograde manner up the normal conducting pathway (reenters the normal system). The presence of two conducting routes is referred to as dual AV nodal physiology and can be demonstrated during electrophysiology study. This typical form represents 93% of all AVNRTs (Figure 3*A*). The P wave may occur just before, during, or just after the QRS complex during tachycardia. Most frequently, a P wave cannot be observed because atrial and ventricular activation occur simultaneously ("short RP"; see Figure 2). Chronic drug treatment relies on the use of beta blockers and calcium channel blockers. Radiofrequency catheter ablation has virtually eliminated the need for drug therapy by providing a safe, effective cure for this disorder (Figure 4).

The circuit can also function in a reverse manner, whereby the initial impulse goes down the fast (normal) wire and returns to the proximal end of the circuit via the slow (extra) wire. This represents "atypical" AVNRT and is observed in approximately 7% of all cases. The resulting atrial activation (P wave) occurs well after the preceding QRS complex, yielding a long RP arrhythmia (see Figure 2).

The patient reports that the arrhythmia occurs randomly, with no consistent relationship to exercise

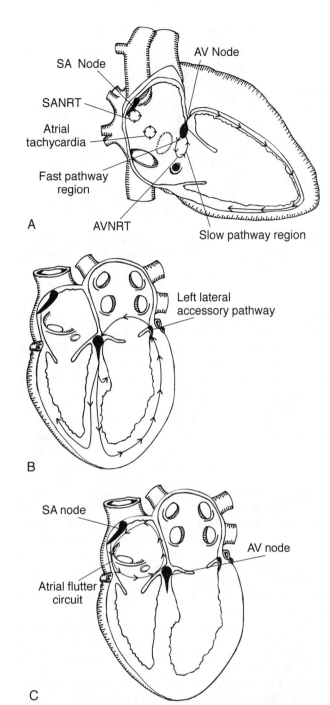

Figure 3. Possible origins of tachycardia. *A*, Reentry in the sinoatrial node (SANRT), atrioventricular node (AVNRT), and atrial myocardium (atrial tachycardia): right anterior oblique view. *B*, Orthodromic reciprocating tachycardia (ORT) in which accessory pathway is used for retrograde conduction: sagittal view. *C*, Typical atrial flutter conducting through the isthmus between the coronary sinus os and the tricuspid value annulus: right anterior oblique view. *Abbreviations*: AV = atrioventricular; SA = sinoatrial.

or posture. The most helpful historical point is the sudden onset and termination of the tachycardia. Other symptoms are nonspecific and vary widely among individuals. Palpitations—the sensation of forceful, rapid heartbeats—are extremely common.

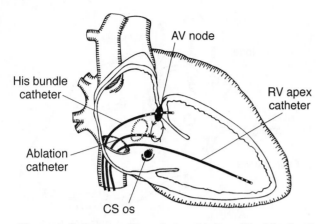

Figure 4. Catheter positions during ablation of the "slow" pathway for the treatment of atrioventricular (AV) nodal reentrant tachycardia (AVNRT): right anterior oblique view. *Abbreviations:* CS = coronary sinus; RV = right ventricular.

In AVNRT, the palpitations are frequently felt in the neck. On occasion, lightheadedness, near-syncope, chest pain, or dyspnea may be experienced. Syncope is rare but may occur with extremely rapid heart rates. Mild hypotension is common, but because most patients have structurally normal hearts, significant hemodynamic compromise is unusual. Once the diagnosis of AVNRT has been established, recurrence, despite medical therapy, is the rule. The duration of each episode and the frequency of recurrence vary markedly. Both types of AVNRT (typical and atypical) may be terminated by vagal maneuvers, including carotid sinus massage. Vagal stimulation results in further prolongation of conduction in the slow pathway with ensuing block, which interrupts the reentrant circuit. In the acute setting, adenosine (Adenocard) is extremely effective (>95%) in terminating AVNRT. Verapamil and diltiazem also terminate this tachycardia but should be employed only in narrow complex rhythms or if the diagnosis of AVNRT is firmly established.

Electrocardiographic analysis of the tachycardia reveals a regular, narrow complex rhythm with minimal oscillation in cycle length. The amplitude of the QRS on a beat-to-beat basis may change at more rapid rates (QRS alternans), but this finding is nonspecific. Bundle branch block can also occur at rapid rates, resulting in a wide complex tachyarrhythmia. P waves, when observed, are typically inverted in the inferior leads (II, III, and aVF), but usually P waves cannot be identified. In circumstances in which P waves are not visible, it is impossible to distinguish AV nodal reentry from AV reentry (from a retrograde accessory pathway) on the basis of the ECG. ST depression may be seen and is not associated with coronary artery disease. A rhythm strip or ECG of the initiation of an AVNRT shows that a premature atrial beat typically results in an abrupt PR prolongation (conduction down the slow pathway) and subsequent tachycardia. In addition, when termination of the arrhythmia occurs, it is usually in the antegrade (slow) pathway, and the final QRS is followed by a P wave (the final conduction in a retrograde manner of the fast [normal] pathway) with subsequent resumption of a normal sinus P wave morphology. This type of termination can occur with AV reentrant tachycardias as well.

Nonparoxysmal Junctional Tachycardia

This arrhythmia is observed in the settings of acute digitalis toxicity, myocardial infarction, myocarditis, and after a surgical procedure. Junctional tachycardia is not a reentrant arrhythmia; it manifests at relatively slow heart rates (70 to 130 bpm). Electrocardiographically, the QRS morphology is narrow complex, and AV dissociation is frequently seen. If bundle branch block is present, this may create the impression of idioventricular rhythm. The tachycardia rate may increase with exercise or isoproterenol and may decrease when beta blockers are administered. Rarely is therapy required for nonparoxysmal junctional tachycardia. This arrhythmia resolves with resolution of the primary inciting event.

Atrioventricular Connections (Accessory Pathways)

Atrioventricular Reentry

In normal cardiac physiology, the only electrical connection between the atrium and the ventricle occurs in the AV node. Congenital abnormalities may create "accessory pathways" that bridge from the atrium to the ventricular myocardium. These tissue connections can cross along the mitral annulus, tricuspid annulus, or septum. Accessory pathways (AV "extra wires") also allow the possibility of a reentrant loop ("short circuit"; see Figure 3*B*). Paroxysmal reentrant tachycardias involving accessory pathways are referred to as AV reentrant tachycardias (AVRTs) and account for 30% of all SVTs.

Preexcitation Syndrome

The Wolff-Parkinson-White syndrome (WPW) is defined electrocardiographically by the presence of a short PR interval, QRS prolongation (secondary to a delta wave), and symptoms related to tachycardia (Figure 5). The abnormal morphology of the QRS is caused by the fusion of the normal ventricular activation via the AV node and preexcitation of the ventricle by the accessory pathway. Therefore, the delta wave represents the small area of ventricular myocardium activated in an antegrade manner through the accessory pathway. Many of these pathways function in both an antegrade and a retrograde manner. In order to diagnose WPW from a sinus ECG, antegrade function of the accessory pathway is required. However, most tachycardias in this syndrome are the result of a macro-reentrant circuit conducting normally through the AV node and subsequently returning to the atrium by retrograde conduction through the accessory pathway. The resultant arrhythmia is known as orthodromic reciprocating tachycardia (ORT) (see Figure 3*B*). An un-

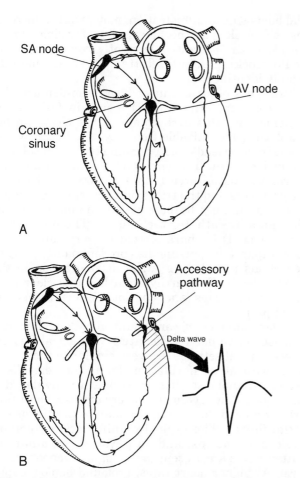

Figure 5. *A*, Activation originating from the sinoatrial node and normally conducted to the ventricles via the atrioventricular (AV) node and the His-Purkinje system: sagittal view. *B*, Activation originating from the sinoatrial node and conducted to the ventricles by both the AV node and the accessory pathway, resulting in a fusion beat with a delta wave: sagittal view. *Abbreviation*: SA = sinoatrial.

usual wide complex tachycardia with the appearance of the ventricular tachycardia can be observed when the circuit functions in reverse. This arrhythmia, antidromic reciprocating tachycardia (ART), occurs when ventricular activation is through the accessory pathway with atrial activation occurring in a retrograde manner through the AV node. Accessory pathways may be present in patients without manifest WPW syndrome. These pathways function only in a retrograde manner but may lead to the same ORT observed in WPW. In these persons, the baseline ECG shows a normal, narrow QRS complex with no evidence of preexcitation.

The ECG during AVRT may be identical to that observed in AVNRT. However, a P wave can typically be discerned in the T wave after the QRS complex in AVRT. Although this is a short RP tachycardia, the ability to detect a P wave remains a clue that AV reentry is the mechanism and that the arrhythmia is not of AV nodal origin. The tachycardia rate, which may range from 150 to 250 bpm, is usually slightly faster than that of AVNRT. Again, QRS alternans

may be observed but is a nonspecific rate-related finding. The electrocardiographic anomaly of WPW is found in 1 to 3 per 1000 individuals in the general population. The majority of these patients have structurally normal hearts and do not experience any symptoms. No specific therapy is required for WPW when the patient has no symptoms and the physical examination yields normal findings. Structural heart abnormalities may be present in association with WPW, such as Ebstein's anomaly (primarily associated with right-sided accessory pathways) and mitral valve prolapse. In contrast to asymptomatic patients, patients with palpitation, chest pain, dyspnea, light-headedness, or syncope represent a group that may be at risk for sudden cardiac death. Rapid atrial fibrillation in a patient with preexcitation can result in ventricular fibrillation. Consequently, patients with WPW who have experienced true syncope or markedly symptomatic palpitations require careful evaluation and electrophysiologic study.

Tachycardias Associated with Wolff-Parkinson-White Syndrome

A spectrum of arrhythmias may be observed in patients with WPW. These include both narrow complex (ORT) and wide complex tachycardias (ART, preexcited atrial fibrillation, or flutter). Preexcited atrial fibrillation may result in rapid ventricular rates and bizarre-appearing ECGs that mimic polymorphic ventricular tachycardia (Figure 6). It is essential to remember that with the exception of polymorphic ventricular tachycardia, all rhythms that are irregularly irregular without P waves must be atrial fibrillation, regardless of QRS morphology (wide or narrow complexes). Preexcited atrial fibrillation should be suspected in any young patient in an emergency department with an irregular, wide complex tachycardia. Atrial flutter in such patients can also conduct at very rapid rates (1:1 ventricular response) and lead to marked hemodynamic compromise. By

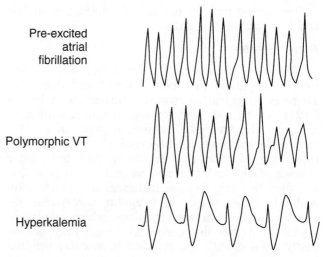

Figure 6. Common causes of irregular wide complex tachycardias. *Abbreviation*: VT = ventricular tachycardia.

far, the most common arrhythmia is ORT (described earlier). However, ART is frequently mistaken for ventricular tachycardia in this population. Other arrhythmias, including AVNRT, SANRT, and atrial tachycardias, can occur in association with WPW. Multiple accessory pathways can also occur in the individual patient.

Management of Atrioventricular Reentrant Tachycardia

Therapeutic modalities for ORT and ART are designed to block circuit function at either the AV node or the accessory pathway. If block can be achieved at either location, the tachycardia is terminated. Acute therapy is most easily directed toward the AV node. If vagal maneuvers do not result in termination of the arrhythmia, adenosine is highly effective. In the setting of a wide complex preexcited atrial fibrillation, procainamide is the drug of choice. This agent blocks conduction in the accessory pathway and may contribute to resolution of atrial fibrillation. Calcium channel blockers such as verapamil (Isoptin, Calan) are contraindicated in atrial fibrillation associated with preexcitation. The use of verapamil may result in ventricular fibrillation in this situation.

Use of chronic medications for patients with AVRT has declined dramatically with the introduction of curative therapy. Radiofrequency ablation is highly effective in eliminating accessory pathways, with extremely low morbidity and mortality rates. When patients desire continued drug therapy for AVRT and no preexcitation is present on a baseline ECG, therapy is similar to that for AVNRT. AV nodal blocking agents may be used. If a delta wave is present, these agents should be avoided, and drugs designed to modify conduction in the accessory pathway are indicated if the heart is structurally normal (types IA and IC agents).

Atrial Arrhythmias

Atrial Fibrillation

This arrhythmia is extensively discussed in the article on atrial fibrillation.

Atrial Flutter

Electrocardiographically, atrial flutter is characterized by an atrial rate between 250 and 350 bpm. There is a typical sawtoothed pattern seen in the flutter waves and best appreciated in the inferior leads II, III, and aVF. Several degrees of regular ventricular response are observed, the most common rate being 150 bpm (2:1 AV conduction), but higher degrees of AV block may also be seen at ratios of 4:1, 6:1, and so forth. In rare instances, nodal Wenckebach block can result in irregular ventricular response rates. P wave morphology, which is readily visible at higher degrees of AV block, may not be easily defined with 2:1 atrial-to-ventricular conduction.

Vagal maneuvers, such as carotid sinus massage and adenosine administration, may result in increasing AV block and the emergence of visible flutter waves. If the patient is currently treated with AV nodal blocking agents, flutter waves are usually readily identified.

Two types of atrial flutter have been defined. The most common form (type I) occurs in 90% of the patients with this arrhythmia and is electrocardiographically recognizable from negative flutter waves in the inferior leads corresponding to the typical sawtoothed pattern. The circuit of the arrhythmia involves the tissue area (isthmus) between the coronary sinus os and the tricuspid valve ring (see Figure 3C); thus it may be possible to eliminate this arrhythmia by catheter techniques. The uncommon form (type II) is characterized by very rapid atrial rates (up to 450 bpm) and has predominantly positive deflections recorded for atrial depolarization in the inferior leads. This arrhythmia has less clear anatomic boundaries and cannot be terminated by atrial pacing.

A vast number of cardiopulmonary and systemic diseases have been associated with atrial flutter. These clinical settings are very similar to those that occur with atrial fibrillation. Pulmonary embolism, excess ethanol use, hyperthyroidism, valvular disease, pericarditis, coronary artery disease, heart failure, and cardiac surgery appear to predispose to atrial flutter. The typical manifestations include rapid palpitations, and on physical examination, flutter waves are present in the jugular venous waveform. At higher heart rates, profound hemodynamic compromise, as well as syncope, can occur. In patients capable of 1:1 AV conduction during flutter, cardiac arrest may ensue if the rhythm degenerates to ventricular fibrillation. Most commonly, patients have decreased exercise tolerance, dyspnea, or congestive heart failure.

Acute management of this arrhythmia is similar to that of atrial fibrillation and involves initial rate control either by drug therapy or cardioversion. The subsequent maintenance of sinus rhythm may require antiarrhythmic therapy, and most patients with atrial flutter should receive anticoagulative agents. Rate control in this population is achieved by combination of AV nodal blocking agents, primarily calcium channel blockers and beta blockers. Once rate response is adequately controlled, the best method to achieve maintenance of sinus rhythm can be addressed. Direct current cardioversion may be employed acutely and without anticoagulation, if the duration of the arrhythmia is clearly less than 48 hours. However, if the arrhythmia duration is unknown, anticoagulation before cardioversion is recommended. Adequate anticoagulation for 2 to 3 weeks before cardioversion and 4 weeks after the procedure with an International Normalized Ratio (INR) of 2.0 or more ensures the lowest risk of thromboembolic events. The embolic complication risk with atrial flutter is not as well defined as that of atrial fibrillation. However, because these arrhythmias are frequently paroxysmal and both commonly occur in the same patient, chronic anticoagulation is recommended if the arrhythmia is persistent. Chemical cardioversion with the use of antiarrhythmic agents, which result in membrane stabilization, carries the same embolic risk. The maintenance of sinus rhythm after electrical cardioversion is significantly affected by the use of antiarrhythmic agents (primarily propafenone, sotalol, and amiodarone). Patients must be screened carefully in order to avoid side effects that are prevalent with certain agents (e.g., class IC drugs in patients with coronary artery disease). The efficacy of antiarrhythmic agents for the maintenance of sinus rhythm in atrial fibrillation and atrial flutter ranges from 30 to 80%; amiodarone achieves the highest rate of success.

It is imperative that routine monitoring for adverse effects be maintained. (The most common side effects for antiarrhythmics are listed in Table 4.) Proarrhythmia is the most important concern with these agents. QT interval prolongation and bradycardia-dependent polymorphic ventricular tachycardia can occur with type IA agents. Flecainide and propafenone may result in intracardiac conduction slowing and subsequent prolongation of the PR and QRS intervals. Although type IC agents tend to be better tolerated than type IA agents, they carry an increased risk of sudden cardiac death in patients with previous myocardial infarction or complex ventricular ectopy. Therefore, in patients with structural heart disease, type IC agents should be avoided.

Sotalol (Betapace) has been used for the maintenance of sinus rhythm in the population with atrial fibrillation and atrial flutter. QT interval prolongation with risk of polymorphic ventricular tachycardia increases in a dose-related manner with this drug. The QT interval should be closely followed and maintained at a QT_C of less than 550 milliseconds. This agent also may precipitate acute bradycardia as a result of beta blockade. Patients may not tolerate this therapy because of prior lung disease or the coexistence of heart failure. In some studies, sotalol has been shown to be more effective than type I agents.

Amiodarone (Cordarone) is an efficacious agent in preventing recurrence of atrial arrhythmias. The side effect profile has prompted great debate over its utility in non–life-threatening arrhythmias. At low doses, most side effects are easily controlled or reversible. The most commonly encountered problems include thyroid and liver abnormalities, skin discoloration, corneal microdeposits, and bradycardia. Pulmonary fibrosis occurs in a small number of patients on low-dose therapy and may be irreversible. In general, low-dose amiodarone is extremely well tolerated and quite effective in maintaining sinus rhythm in this population.

An approach to chronic atrial flutter may involve anticoagulation for several weeks, followed by attempted chemical cardioversion with the initiation of an antiarrhythmic agent and then, if sinus rhythm is not restored, direct current cardioversion. In contrast to atrial fibrillation, low-energy application (50

to 100 J) usually results in the restoration of sinus rhythm. The common form of atrial flutter can also be eliminated by overdrive pacing of the atrium. This is achieved by either direct intracardiac stimulation or the use of a transesophageal electrode. In an occasional patient with atrial fibrillation or flutter, sinus rhythm cannot be maintained, and medical regimens fail to provide adequate rate control. In this setting, AV junction ablation with permanent pacemaker implantation is indicated. This therapy has reversed tachycardia-induced cardiomyopathy in some patients.

TABLE 4. **Antiarrhythmic Agents**

Agent	Dose	Major Side Effects
Type IA		
Quinidine (Quinidex)	600–1600 mg qd PO (divided doses q 6 h)	GI disturbance, rash, cinchonism, proarrhythmia (↑ QT)
Procainamide (Procan)	2000–4000 mg qd PO (divided doses)	GI disturbance, lupus, proarrhythmia (↑ QT), agranulocytosis
Disopyramide (Norpace)	150–450 mg q 12 h	Anticholinergic disturbance (urinary retention), proarrhythmia (↑ QT)
Type IB		
Lidocaine	1.5 mg/kg bolus, IV only, then IV 1–4 mg/min	CNS disturbance (paresthesia, tremor, confusion, seizure)
Mexiletine (Mexitil)	150–300 mg q 8 h	GI, CNS disturbances
Type IC		
Flecainide (Tambocor)	50–200 mg q 12 h PO	CNS disturbance, CHF, proarrhythmia
Propafenone (Rhythmol)	150–300 mg q 8 h PO	GI disturbance, metallic taste, CNS disturbance, proarrhythmia
Type II		
Beta Blockers	Refer to specific agent	Bradycardia, CNS depression, sexual dysfunction
Type III		
Amiodarone (Cordarone)	200–600 mg qd PO	Bradycardia; pulmonary fibrosis; thyroid, skin, CNS, and liver abnormalities
Sotalol (Betapace)	80–240 mg q 12 h PO	Bradycardia, fatigue, and Torsades de pointes
Type IV		
Diltiazem (Cardizem)	240–360 mg qd PO	Hypotension, bradycardia
Verapamil (Calan)	240–480 mg qd PO	Bradycardia, constipation, peripheral edema
Others		
Digoxin (Lanoxin)	0.125–0.35 mg qd PO	GI and visual disturbances, proarrhythmia
Adenosine (Adenocard)	6–18 mg, IV only	Facial flushing, chest pain, dyspnea, anxiety (lasting <10 s)

Abbreviations: CHF = congestive heart failure; CNS = central nervous system; GI = gastrointestinal.

In isolated type I flutter, direct catheter ablation of the circuit is successful in up to 80% of selected patients. It is imperative that paroxysmal atrial fibrillation not be present along with atrial flutter. If both rhythms are known to occur in the same patient, catheter ablation of the flutter may not result in elimination of the symptoms.

Atrial Tachycardias

Atrial tachycardias are the result of depolarization of a focus within the atrial myocardium. The arrhythmia may be secondary to micro-reentry within the atrium or automatic firing of an isolated focus. These two etiologies account for approximately 4% of supraventricular arrhythmias. Sudden onset and sudden termination of atrial tachycardia suggest a reentrant mechanism, whereas a gradual progression (warm-up) is more typically observed in automatic arrhythmias. ECGs of atrial tachycardias show "long RP" rhythms with P wave morphologies different from that of the sinus rhythm (see Table 2). The heart rate ranges from 100 to 240 bpm. Vagal maneuvers again assist in the diagnosis by resulting in AV block and clear observation of the abnormal P wave. Therapy for this tachycardia consists of AV nodal blocking agents and, occasionally, the use of antiarrhythmic agents (atrial stabilizing drugs). Radiofrequency catheter ablation can be employed to eliminate the atrial arrhythmic focus. This procedure is rapidly becoming the treatment of choice.

Multifocal Atrial Tachycardia

Severe chronic lung disease underlies most cases of multifocal atrial tachycardia. However, this tachycardia may be observed in patients with diabetes, hypoxia, respiratory failure, acidosis, or electrolyte imbalance. Heart rates range from 100 to 160 bpm and frequently diminish as the patient's general condition improves. Electrocardiographically, the arrhythmia is defined by the presence of three or more different P wave morphologies and an irregular ventricular response. Beta blockers may reduce ventricular response but are frequently contraindicated in this population because of pulmonary disease. Verapamil and digoxin therapy may provide temporary symptomatic relief, but resolution requires improvement in the underlying lung disease or illness state.

VENTRICULAR ARRHYTHMIAS

Ventricular Tachycardia: Definitions

Three or more consecutive beats originating from ventricular myocardium are considered ventricular tachycardia. Two forms of ventricular tachycardia are recognized: (1) monomorphic ventricular tachycardia, in which each complex has uniform morphology and a constant cycle length, and (2) polymorphic ventricular tachycardia, in which the different morphologies are present, and the cycle length is not constant. A rhythm is considered sustained when it lasts more than 30 seconds. Hemodynamic compromise (hypotension) may occur with nonsustained, as well as sustained, arrhythmias. Of importance is that many patients with ventricular tachycardia are "stable," with normal blood pressures and full cognitive function. Hemodynamic state at initial evaluation provides very little information as to the origin of the arrhythmia. The most valuable clue in discriminating SVT from ventricular tachycardia lies in the patient's history. If the patient has had previous ischemic heart disease (previous myocardial infarction, coronary artery bypass grafting, percutaneous transluminal coronary angioplasty), the likelihood that a wide complex tachycardia represents ventricular tachycardia is more than 90%.

Wide Complex Tachycardia: Electrocardiographic Differentiation of Origin

The literature on the subject of differentiating wide complex tachycardias is extensive. The major criteria for diagnosis of ventricular tachycardia are reviewed in Table 5, but a relatively simple screen involves only the data from two common ECGs. If a wide complex arrhythmia is secondary to SVT with aberrancy, the QRS complex during the tachycardia must be compatible with some form of bundle branch block or fascicular block. If no combination of bundle branch block or fascicular block can result in the observed QRS morphology, then by default, ventricular tachycardia is the rhythm (Figure 7). As a consequence, left bundle branch/right axis, wide complex tachycardias are almost always ventricular tachycardias, whereas right bundle branch block with a normal axis is very rarely ventricular tachycardia.

There are several specific ECG features that may assist in establishing the diagnosis of ventricular tachycardia. The most powerful criterion is the manifestation of AV dissociation. If P waves continue on a regular, uninterrupted, slower rate through a regular wide complex tachycardia, AV dissociation is present. An equally useful finding is an AV ratio of less than 1. There exist only rare cases of SVT with aberrancy that could have fewer P waves than QRS complexes. Fusion or capture beats are also indicative of ventricular tachycardia (Figure 8). A fusion beat is a hybrid or combination of two QRS complexes from different areas of simultaneous ventricular activation. The colliding wave fronts from ventricular activation via the AV node and that of an abnormal circuit (ventricular tachycardia) result in fusion. A capture beat occurs

TABLE 5. **Recognition of Ventricular Tachycardia on Electrocardiogram**

Atrioventricular dissociation	Concordant pattern in leads V_1–V_6
Fusion complexes	Absence of RS in precordial leads
Capture beats	Atypical bundle branch block pattern
QRS complex > 140 msec	Left axis or extreme right axis

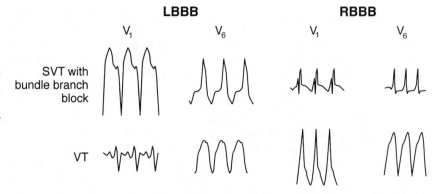

Figure 7. Commonly observed morphologies of regular wide complex tachycardia. *Abbreviations*: LBBB = left bundle branch block; RBBB = right bundle branch block; SVT = supraventricular tachycardia; VT = ventricular tachycardia.

when a narrow complex beat caused by atrial activation, normally through AV node, is conducted without interruption of the underlying wide complex tachycardia. Concordant precordial R wave progression (leads V_1 to V_6), in which all leads have either predominantly negative or predominantly positive deflection, is rare in SVT and is suggestive of a ventricular origin. QRS duration may also prove informative in that in most cases of ventricular tachycardia, the QRS complex exceeds 140 milliseconds. In general, a more leftward axis is also suggestive of ventricular tachycardia rather than of SVT. Other criteria that may aid in the discrimination of ventricular tachycardia from SVT are listed in Table 5.

For a patient experiencing wide complex tachycardia, an ECG during sinus rhythm may provide valuable information concerning the current tachyarrhythmia. The presence of a fixed bundle branch block with the exact same morphology of the arrhythmia points to a supraventricular origin. A delta wave present at baseline raises the possibility of ART. If Q waves are present in a previous ECG, a wide complex tachycardia is considered ventricular tachycardia until proven otherwise.

Acute Patient Evaluation

As previously stated, the overall appearance of the patient and hemodynamic stability of the rhythm are of little diagnostic value. Termination of a wide complex tachycardia by physical maneuvers (including Valsalva maneuver and carotid sinus massage)

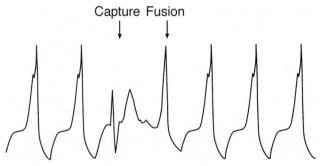

Figure 8. Ventricular tachycardia with capture and fusion beats.

or medications (adenosine) is highly suggestive of SVT but may also occur in nonischemic ventricular tachycardia. A history of previous ischemic heart disease is of marked utility, but beyond this, the most reliable distinctions can be drawn from electrocardiographic analysis.

Acute Management of Wide Complex Tachycardia

Any patient who is unstable in tachyarrhythmia should undergo immediate direct-current cardioversion. If at the time of initial evaluation the patient is hemodynamically stable without complaints of angina, pharmacologic management is the initial treatment of choice. Although lidocaine is recommended as a first-line therapy for suspected ventricular tachycardia, procainamide is safer in the settings of wide complex tachycardia not believed to be associated with acute ischemia. From an electrophysiologic standpoint, the use of procainamide to treat a wide complex tachycardia can never be criticized, regardless of whether the origin is ventricular or supraventricular. The use of calcium channel blockers in the setting of wide complex tachycardia of unknown etiology is specifically contraindicated; ventricular tachycardia, when treated with calcium antagonists, frequently deteriorates to ventricular fibrillation. In addition, the administration of verapamil during preexcited atrial fibrillation results in increased ventricular response and the possibility of ventricular fibrillation. If drug therapy with procainamide proves ineffective, or if the patient becomes hemodynamically compromised, direct-current cardioversion should be performed immediately.

Monomorphic Ventricular Tachycardia

After the establishment of ventricular tachycardia as the diagnosis, myocardial infarction should be ruled out. Monomorphic ventricular tachycardia should not be considered an ischemic rhythm. In order to maintain this reentrant circuit, the myocardial substrate must already be present. However, ischemia can indeed trigger this arrhythmia, and specific therapy may not be required for monomorphic ventricular tachycardia that occurs within the first 48 hours of myocardial infarction. However, after that time, in the setting of no obvious ischemia, ventricular tachycardia greatly increases the risk of subsequent sudden cardiac death and usually necessitates ICD placement. Further evaluation of the patient with monomorphic ventricular tachycardia should include echocardiography or radionuclide ventriculography, in order to assess structural heart disease, including wall motion abnormalities, hypertrophy, congenital abnormalities, valvular disease, and ventricular function. Most patients require cardiac catheterization to assess coronary anatomy. Monomorphic ventricular tachycardia that occurs in structurally normal hearts manifests with a left bundle branch pattern, and its origin is usually in the right ventricular outflow tract or is fascicular in location. Magnetic resonance imaging (MRI) is useful for ruling out right ventricular dysplasia or infiltrative disease that may not grossly affect left ventricular function. Holter monitoring may be used to assess arrhythmia burden with regard to frequency and duration of the tachycardia. Clinical electrophysiologic study is extremely effective in confirming the diagnosis in patients with coronary artery disease. Ventricular tachycardia can be induced at electrophysiologic study in more than 95% of these cases. In patients without known coronary artery disease, the ability of programmed electrical stimulation to reproduce a clinical arrhythmia is approximately 50%. Electrophysiologic study also provides a setting in which the ventricular tachycardia can be analyzed and the ability to terminate by overdrive pacing assessed.

Studies have clearly shown that ICDs reduce mortality rates in a population with sustained monomorphic ventricular tachycardia. This is true not only for hemodynamically unstable arrhythmias in a clinical setting but also for monomorphic ventricular tachycardia induced in the electrophysiology laboratory. The marked advantage of these devices over conventional drug therapy has significantly changed the traditional management of ventricular tachycardia. Currently, serial electrophysiologic studies and drug therapy are performed only in patients with stable ventricular tachycardia or in those whose arrhythmias may be slowed to the point that catheter ablation therapy is possible. Holter monitor–guided therapy may be used as an alternative to invasive electrophysiologic study. This method involves the use of type IA agents (quinidine, procainamide, and disopyramide), type IC agents (flecainide, propafenone), and type III agents (sotalol or amiodarone). Current data suggest that the risk of tachycardia-induced sudden death is less than 2% with an ICD in place. It is difficult to justify drug therapy alone in patients with hemodynamically unstable monomorphic ventricular tachycardia, in view of the efficacy of the device. However, in order to reduce activation/discharge of ICDs, many patients remain on low-dose antiarrhythmic therapy. Amiodarone and sotalol have proved to be useful agents in this regard.

The implantation of an ICD has now become as facile as the placement of a pacemaker. Most systems involve a lead with a distal right ventricular coil as one electrode, and the device itself serves as the other electrode. A shock is delivered between the right ventricular coil and the pulse generator ("hot can"). The lead system is placed via the subclavian vein in most cases. Current ICD technology allows tiered therapy, which involves the ability of the device to (1) pace-terminate the tachycardia; (2) cardiovert the tachycardia with the use of low energy; and (3) defibrillate faster rhythms. Most cases of monomorphic ventricular tachycardia can be eliminated by antitachycardic pacing from the ICD. In addition, all the defibrillators that are currently implanted have backup bradycardia pacing capabilities.

Nonischemic Cardiomyopathy

Monomorphic ventricular tachycardia is not an uncommon finding with severe left ventricular dysfunction but normal coronary arteries. Affected patients with nonischemic cardiomyopathy who have sustained ventricular tachycardia are at high risk of sudden cardiac death from arrhythmia. Treatment of the tachycardia is similar to the approach used in patients with coronary artery disease, in regard both to acute management and to the need for placement of ICD. However, these nonischemic patients differ dramatically in their response to programmed electrical stimulation at electrophysiologic study. Although they come to medical attention with monomorphic ventricular tachycardia, this clinical arrhythmia can be induced in the electrophysiology laboratory by programmed electrical stimulation in only 50% of the patients. ICD placement is warranted in patients with sustained ventricular tachycardia, regardless of results at electrophysiologic study.

In the nonischemic population, an unusual form of ventricular tachycardia referred to as bundle branch reentrant ventricular tachycardia may occur in up to 10% of patients. This tachycardia can be cured by radiofrequency ablation of the right bundle, which eliminates the tachycardia circuit.

Ventricular Tachycardia Without Structural Heart Disease

The occurrence of ventricular tachycardia in patients without obvious structural heart disease is an uncommon clinical scenario. The majority of these patients manifest a left bundle branch block (negative QRS complex in leads I and V_1) and an inferior axis (predominantly positive QRS complex in leads II, III, and aVF). Most tachycardias in this group are exercise related and catecholamine induced. This monomorphic ventricular tachycardia originates from the right ventricular outflow tract and may be suppressed by beta blockers or calcium channel antagonists. Radiofrequency catheter ablation offers cure for these patients; the success rate exceeds 90%.

A second form of ventricular tachycardia that occurs in normal hearts originates from the base of the posterior papillary muscle and has been referred to as idiopathic left ventricular tachycardia, or fascicular ventricular, tachycardia. Electrocardiographic findings include a right bundle branch block with left axis deviation (positive QRS complex in leads V_1, I, and AVL, and a negative QRS complex in lead aVF). This arrhythmia is responsive to verapamil therapy and is also approachable by radiofrequency catheter ablation.

Infiltrative heart disease is a rare cause of ventricular tachycardia, but mortality risks appear to be high. Sarcoidosis can result in clinical ventricular arrhythmias, as well as conduction system abnormalities. Rest/redistribution thallium scans show regions of myocardium with abnormal uptake, which is consistent with infiltration. These patients typically do not have coronary artery disease, and the observed lesions are in locations unusual for ischemic abnormalities. Electrophysiologic study frequently reveals inducible tachycardia. However, in a substantial number of patients, the tachycardia cannot be induced, and they remain at high risk. Device therapy has been recommended in those with clinical ventricular tachycardia. Another form of infiltrative heart disease involves primarily the right ventricle and has been termed "arrhythmogenic right ventricular dysplasia." Initially, the heart appears normal despite massive fatty infiltration of the right ventricle. This diagnosis is best confirmed by MRI scan, but wall motion abnormalities may be observed in an echocardiogram and a right ventriculogram. Right ventricular biopsy may provide information confirming the diagnosis but is a relatively insensitive method. There is a high risk of sudden cardiac death in this patient population, and ICD therapy is recommended.

Polymorphic Ventricular Tachycardia

Sustained polymorphic ventricular tachycardia is typically observed in acute myocardial infarction or ischemia but may also occur with QT prolongation in the form of torsades de pointes and digitalis toxicity. In addition, polymorphic ventricular tachycardia may be observed in up to 1.5% of patients with advanced heart failure. Anatomic substrate (old scar), which is the most common mechanism for sustained monomorphic ventricular tachycardia, may be present but is not necessary for the induction of polymorphic arrhythmia. Polymorphic ventricular tachycardia usually degenerates rapidly into ventricular fibrillation. Electrocardiographic evaluation shows a wide complex, chaotic rhythm with a varying axis (Figure 9; see also Figure 6). Preexcited atrial fibrillation in the setting of multiple AV pathways can resemble polymorphic ventricular tachycardia, but the clinical setting usually allows rapid differentiation between patients who experience these types of arrhythmias.

Rhythm strips and ECGs obtained before an episode of polymorphic ventricular tachycardia may reveal important clues to etiology. If QT interval is

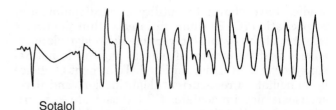
Sotalol

Figure 9. Acquired (drug-induced) development of torsades de pointes with prolonged QT interval.

markedly prolonged in sinus rhythm and bradycardia is present, polymorphic ventricular tachycardia is likely of the form referred to as torsades de pointes. The arrhythmia is triggered by early depolarizations occurring in a prolonged plateau phase of the cardiac action potential. Prolongation of the QT interval occurs in two distinct clinical settings. The first (acquired) form is most often induced by antiarrhythmic drugs that prolong repolarization. Common offenders include class IA and class III antiarrhythmic drugs, as well as tricyclic antidepressants, phenothiazines, haloperidol, antibiotics (erythromycin and trimethoprim-sulfamethoxazole), and antihistamines (astemizole and terfenadine) (see Figure 9). Hypokalemia and hypomagnesemia predispose patients to this arrhythmia. Therapy for this type of polymorphic ventricular tachycardia involves elimination of the precipitating factors (discontinuing all medication that might prolong QT) and increasing the heart rate with isoproterenol or cardiac pacing. The second form of torsades de pointes is idiopathic/congenital prolonged QT. This includes the autosomal recessive Jervell and Lange-Nielsen syndrome, which is accompanied by deafness, and the autosomal dominant Romano-Ward syndrome, without deafness. Sudden cardiac death and syncope are most commonly observed in association with physical, emotional, or auditory stress. The patient usually comes to medical attention after an episode of syncope, sudden cardiac death, or the cardiac-related death of a young relative. Beta blockers, pacemakers, and stellate ganglion blockade/resection have been used as therapy in this population. Because of the high risk of sudden cardiac death, implantation of ICDs is now frequent.

Ventricular Fibrillation

Ventricular fibrillation and most polymorphic ventricular tachycardia should be considered of ischemic origin. Evaluation of cardiac enzymes and cardiac catheterization are almost always necessary. These studies aid in assessing patients' risk for recurrence. Ventricular tachycardia may also degenerate into ventricular fibrillation; however, if the initial observed rhythm is ventricular fibrillation, ischemia is more likely. Ventricular fibrillation is easily recognized by course-undulating electrical activity without obvious organization on the ECG.

In the acute setting, ventricular fibrillation results in loss of consciousness within seconds. Multiple studies have shown the utility of cardiopulmonary resuscitation (CPR) when initiated within the first 4 minutes of the event. Irreversible neurologic damage ensues within minutes if normal rhythm is not restored or if CPR is not initiated. Treatment of choice is immediate direct-current defibrillation, and if response is not immediate, CPR (basic life support/advanced cardiac life support) protocol should be initiated until defibrillation is available. Survival rates remain poor (approximately <5%) for patients experiencing out-of-hospital cardiac arrest. If ischemia can be documented as the cause of ventricular fibrillation by temporally related ECGs consistent with acute myocardial infarction or positive cardiac enzyme findings (creatine kinase levels with isoenzyme MB), the patient requires only correction of the underlying coronary artery disease. No further electrophysiologic evaluation is necessary. However, in the setting of no obvious ischemia and negative cardiac enzyme findings, an ICD should be placed. Electrophysiologic study is useful in evaluating concomitant ventricular tachycardia, but drug therapy has proved less effective than ICD placement.

CONGENITAL HEART DISEASE

method of
PETER C. FROMMELT, M.D.
The Medical College of Wisconsin and Children's Hospital of Wisconsin
Milwaukee, Wisconsin

Congenital heart disease (CHD) is defined as structural or functional heart disease that is present at birth. The incidence of CHD is thought to be 8 to 10 per 1000 live births. This incidence, however, does not include three important cardiac lesions. Mitral valve prolapse and the patent ductus arteriosus of prematurity usually are not included in any estimate of CHD. In addition, a bicuspid aortic valve is thought to occur in at least 2% of the population. Finally, the incidence of CHD is likely underestimated because of the increased frequency found in fetuses that are aborted early and in those that are delivered stillborn.

This chapter discusses the common forms of CHD. The lesions are grouped by their primary physiologic consequence: (1) acyanotic lesions with a left-to-right shunt; (2) acyanotic lesions with outflow obstruction; and (3) cyanotic lesions.

ACYANOTIC LESIONS WITH A LEFT-TO-RIGHT SHUNT

Ventricular Septal Defect

With the exception of a bicuspid aortic valve, ventricular septal defect (VSD) is the most common congenital cardiac malformation, accounting for approximately 20 to 30% of all CHD. The ventricular septum can be divided anatomically into four major portions where defects occur. The most common location is in the membranous septum, where approximately 80% of VSDs are found. Defects in the trabecular muscu-

lar septum are the next most common, representing 5 to 20% of all defects. Outlet defects, which have also been called supracristal defects, are located in the infundibular septum beneath the aortic and pulmonary valves. These account for 5 to 7% of all isolated defects and are much more common in complex congenital lesions. Isolated defects in the inlet portion of the muscular septum below the atrioventricular (AV) valves are very rare and usually found in association with AV septal defects (AVSDs). Defects in the inlet and outlet septum usually do not decrease in size, whereas perimembranous and trabecular muscular defects frequently do.

The size of the VSD is of critical importance in determining its physiologic consequences. A small defect has little or no hemodynamic impact because the left-to-right shunt is negligible and pulmonary artery pressures are unaffected. Moderate-sized VSDs are also restrictive and rarely cause significant pulmonary hypertension. The predominant hemodynamic consequence of a moderate-sized defect is the significant volume of left-to-right shunt, and the chief risk associated with these defects is late development of left ventricular failure secondary to the chronic volume overload during adulthood. Large VSDs result in a large-volume left-to-right shunt and systemic right ventricular and pulmonary artery pressures. The infant with a large VSD is at greatest risk both for congestive heart failure and elevated pulmonary vascular resistance. There is a significant risk of irreversible pulmonary vascular changes if a large VSD is not closed by 1 year of age.

The clinical examination varies according to the size and physiologic consequences of the VSD. A small defect should present with no signs of heart disease except for a holosystolic murmur along the left sternal border. There sometimes can be a palpable thrill along the precordium as well because the high-velocity jet across the defect is directed into the right ventricle and anterior chest wall. A moderate-sized defect is also associated with a holosystolic murmur and thrill, but there is also a mildly increased and laterally displaced left ventricular impulse with a soft mid-diastolic apical murmur secondary to increased flow across the mitral valve. A dramatic increase in precordial activity, both of the left and right ventricles, is a constant hallmark of a large VSD. The pulmonic component of the second heart sound is frequently increased because of significant pulmonary hypertension; a loud mid-diastolic rumble and evidence of congestive heart failure with tachypnea, tachycardia, and hepatosplenomegaly are frequently appreciated.

The electrocardiogram (ECG) and chest radiograph also vary according to the size of the defect. Small defects should result in no changes on either study. A moderate-sized defect may result in left ventricular heart hypertrophy on ECG and mild to moderate cardiomegaly with increased pulmonary vascular markings on the chest radiograph. A large defect is usually associated with marked biventricular hypertrophy on ECG and significant cardiomegaly with increased pulmonary vascular markings on the chest radiograph.

Two-dimensional and Doppler echocardiography are the diagnostic studies of choice to identify both the location and the size of the VSD. The size of the left-to-right shunt can be estimated by the amount of left atrial and left ventricular volume overload, and right ventricular and pulmonary pressures can be well estimated by Doppler interrogation of the VSD jet. Late development of subaortic and subpulmonary obstruction can occur with some perimembranous VSDs, and this can be assessed by echocardiography. In addition, perimembranous and outlet defects sometimes can affect the support structure of the aortic valve, resulting in aortic valve prolapse and insufficiency. This also can be documented echocardiographically.

Small VSDs do not require surgical intervention, and many close spontaneously. Large defects with intractable congestive heart failure during infancy should be closed; occasionally, these defects can be palliated by surgically placing a constrictive band around the main pulmonary artery to control the left-to-right shunt and protect the pulmonary vascular bed. This is especially useful in the patient with multiple muscular VSDs because the hypertrophy generated by the band may facilitate spontaneous closure of many of these defects. Moderate-sized defects without evidence of congestive heart failure or significant pulmonary artery hypertension usually can be safely followed during early childhood, and they are usually electively closed before the child enters school if there is continued evidence of a significant-volume left-to-right shunt. All patients with a VSD require bacterial endocarditis prophylaxis before surgery and for 6 months after surgery if the defect is successfully closed. Finally, in patients in whom pulmonary vascular obstructive disease has developed, a right-to-left shunt with cyanosis develops. In such patients, the VSD cannot be closed. The survival rate after development of pulmonary vascular obstructive disease (Eisenmenger's complex) is poor, and palliative options are limited to lung transplantation.

Atrial Septal Defect

Atrial septal defects (ASD) are common (8% of all CHD) and are found twice as frequently in girls. There are four types of ASD. The most common is the ostium secundum defect, which is located in the region of the foramen ovale in the mid-portion of the atrial septum. The next most common is an ostium primum defect, which is part of the spectrum of AVSD. This defect is located at the inferior aspect of the atrial septum immediately above the AV valves, and there is always an associated abnormality of the anterior leaflet of the mitral valve. The third type of ASD is a sinus venosus defect. These defects usually are of the superior vena cava type, immediately inferior to the orifice of the superior vena cava as it enters the right atrium, and are frequently associated with partial anomalous pulmonary venous drainage. The last type, the coronary sinus ASD, which is very rare, is located at the mouth of the coronary sinus.

Atrial septal defects rarely cause significant symptoms in infants and children. In fact, many defects are missed for several years because of the subtle clinical findings. The classic finding on examination is a widely split second heart sound that remains fixed and split throughout the respiratory cycle. Because of the left-to-right atrial shunt, flow murmurs across the tricuspid valve in diastole and across the pulmonary valve in systole can frequently be appreciated. The parasternal precordial impulse can be increased secondary to the right ventricular volume overload. The murmur of mitral insufficiency may be appreciated in some patients with an ostium primum ASD.

The ECG can have a classic appearance characterized by an rSR' pattern in the right precordial leads. Ostium primum defects, as with all forms of AVSD, can also result in left axis deviation. The chest radiograph usually shows mild to moderate cardiomegaly with increased pulmonary vascular markings and a prominent main pulmonary artery segment. Two-dimensional and Doppler echocardiography can usually diagnose the size and type of ASD. Although pulmonary vascular disease is rare with an isolated ASD in childhood, it can develop in adults. Indirect estimates of right ventricular and pulmonary artery pressures can be made by Doppler techniques if tricuspid insufficiency is present.

All ASDs that result in a significant-volume left-to-right shunt (in general, those 5 mm in diameter or greater) should be closed. This can usually be done electively at 3 to 5 years of age if the child is asymptomatic. Surgical closure of ostium secundum defects is uniformly successful with very low morbidity. Closure devices that can be delivered through catheters and placed under fluoroscopy in the cardiac catheterization laboratory have been developed; the long-term efficacy and safety of these devices is unclear. Late complications after closure of an ostium primum defect are usually related to abnormalities in mitral valve function. Patients with sinus venosus ASDs frequently require repair of anomalous pulmonary venous drainage, but this usually is accomplished without complications. Patients with an isolated ASD do not require bacterial endocarditis prophylaxis except for the 6-month period after surgical closure.

Patent Ductus Arteriosus

The ductus arteriosus is a normal fetal structure, and it usually closes spontaneously during the first 72 hours of life. Isolated persistent patency of the ductus arteriosus accounts for approximately 2% of all CHD. Spontaneous closure is less likely in infants born prematurely or at high altitude, and it is unusual for spontaneous closure to occur after 3 months of age.

The classic clinical finding in the patient with patent ductus arteriosus (PDA) is a continuous murmur that peaks in late systole and can be heard throughout the cardiac cycle. The murmur usually is not appreciated in the newborn but develops only after neonatal pulmonary vascular resistance falls. If the left-to-right shunt is significant, associated findings include bounding peripheral pulses, a wide pulse pressure, and an increased apical impulse secondary to left ventricular volume overload. If the defect is large enough, congestive heart failure and failure to thrive can develop during infancy. If a large PDA persists into childhood, pulmonary vascular obstructive disease can develop.

The ECG usually is not helpful, but can show left ventricular hypertrophy. A chest radiograph can reveal cardiomegaly with increased pulmonary vascular markings if the shunt volume is significant. Two-dimensional and Doppler echocardiography can usually identify a PDA, and the volume of the shunt can be estimated by the size of the left atrium and left ventricle. Pulmonary artery pressures can be estimated by Doppler interrogation of the velocity of the shunt across the PDA.

All PDAs that can be auscultated should be closed, even if the infant or child is completely asymptomatic, because there is a risk of bacterial endocarditis that is greater than the risk of the closure procedure. Small defects can be followed during the first year of life because there is the possibility of late spontaneous closure. Any symptomatic infant should undergo closure at the time when symptoms develop because the procedure carries little risk and is well tolerated. Coil occlusion of restrictive PDAs has been performed successfully in the cardiac catheterization laboratory, and this appears to be a reasonable alternative to surgical closure. Bacterial endocarditis prophylaxis is necessary before surgery and for 6 months after the closure procedure.

Atrioventricular Septal Defect

AVSDs are found in 7% of all CHD and are very common in children with Down syndrome. These defects (also called endocardial cushion defects or AV canal defects) are characterized by a deficiency or absence of septal tissue at the crux of the heart, where the atrial septum, ventricular septum, and AV valves meet. AVSD has a spectrum of morphologic abnormalities, and it is simplest to divide this defect into the three components where deficiencies or abnormalities can be identified: (1) the atrial septum, (2) the ventricular septum, and (3) the AV valves. Almost all types of AVSD have an ostium primum ASD. In addition, when the deficiency of the inlet portion of the ventricular septum is significant, a VSD below the AV valves can develop. This is considered a complete AVSD. In all forms of AVSD, the AV valves are abnormal. Instead of separate mitral and tricuspid fibrous rings, the AV valves form as one common ring of tissue that sits above both ventricles.

AV valve insufficiency is frequently an associated finding.

Most infants with a complete AVSD have heart murmurs and significant congestive heart failure. The physical examination is usually striking because the congestive heart failure results in poor weight gain, tachypnea, retractions, and tachycardia. An increased impulse is felt over both the right and left ventricles, and a systolic heart murmur is usually appreciated at the left lower sternal border. A prominent apical diastolic murmur is frequently heard at the apex, related to the large-volume left-to-right shunt. If significant pulmonary hypertension has developed, the pulmonary component of the second heart sound is increased. Hepatosplenomegaly is common in those infants with congestive heart failure.

The ECG can be helpful because AVSD is usually associated with a counterclockwise frontal plane loop, left axis deviation, and biventricular hypertrophy. The chest radiograph usually shows cardiomegaly with increased pulmonary vascular markings. Two-dimensional and Doppler echocardiography are diagnostic because they can document not only the extent of the atrial and ventricular septal deficiency but the competence of the AV valves.

Surgical repair of complete AVSD is usually done between 6 and 12 months of age because of the risk of pulmonary vascular obstructive disease. This risk is higher in infants with Down syndrome, where the surgery is usually performed between 3 and 6 months of age. All patients with AVSD require bacterial endocarditis prophylaxis before surgery and afterward for life.

ACYANOTIC LESIONS WITH OUTFLOW TRACT OBSTRUCTION

Aortic Stenosis

Congenital obstruction to left ventricular outflow can be valvar, subvalvar, or supravalvar in origin. Most patients with left ventricular outflow tract obstruction have valvar aortic stenosis, usually associated with a bicuspid aortic valve. Valvar stenosis is much more common in boys. This lesion usually presents with a murmur from birth, and symptoms are uncommon except in the young infant with severe aortic stenosis and congestive heart failure. The systolic ejection murmur is usually heard best along the left sternal border with radiation to the right sternal border and suprasternal notch. A constant, early systolic ejection click is frequently heard both at the apex and right upper sternal border, and a thrill is always felt in the suprasternal notch related to transmission of turbulence into the carotid arteries. A thrill is sometimes also palpable on the precordium, and this usually means the peak systolic gradient exceeds 40 mm Hg. Peripheral pulse intensity is usually normal, although patients with severe aortic stenosis may have decreased pulses and a narrow pulse pressure. In patients with subaortic stenosis, the clinical findings are similar except for the absence of an early systolic ejection click; in addition, the subaortic turbulence frequently damages the aortic valve and causes aortic insufficiency, characterized by a high-frequency diastolic decrescendo murmur at the right upper sternal border and apex. Supravalvar aortic stenosis is frequently associated with Williams' syndrome, characterized by peculiar facies, mental retardation, infantile hypercalcemia, and branch pulmonary artery stenosis.

The ECG can show left ventricular hypertrophy, although correlation between ECG changes and severity of stenosis is poor. Resting ST-T–wave changes are unusual in a child with aortic stenosis, but evidence of left ventricular strain can sometimes be identified with exercise stress testing. The chest radiograph usually is not helpful, although a dilated ascending aorta may be evident. The diagnosis and severity of aortic stenosis can be made by two-dimensional and Doppler echocardiographic techniques, localizing the site of obstruction as well as the peak systolic gradient.

The need for intervention depends on the severity of the obstruction and the presence of symptoms. All patients with evidence of myocardial ischemia or exercise-induced syncope or arrhythmias should have relief of the obstruction. In the asymptomatic patient, a peak left ventricular outflow tract gradient greater than 80 mm Hg is usually considered an absolute indication for surgical intervention. In patients with moderate obstruction (gradient of 40 to 80 mm Hg), the indications are less clear and frequently depend on the type of obstruction, the presence of associated aortic insufficiency, and the finding of progressive left ventricular hypertrophy on cardiac imaging. Patients with discrete subvalvar obstruction and progressive aortic insufficiency are considered candidates for surgical resection, even if the gradient is mild, because this may prevent progressive aortic insufficiency. In the patient with valvar obstruction, both surgical valvotomy and balloon dilatation in the cardiac catheterization laboratory have been used with good results. These procedures to relieve valvar aortic stenosis are not curative, may result in significant aortic insufficiency, and have been traditionally associated with a mortality rate of approximately 10% in infants. Many patients with valvar aortic stenosis eventually require aortic valve replacement, and the indications and type of valve used vary according to the age and sex of the patient. All patients with aortic stenosis, even those with a bicuspid aortic valve and trivial aortic stenosis, should receive endocarditis prophylaxis.

Coarctation of the Aorta

Coarctation of the aorta (CoA) is an obstruction in the aorta usually related to a posterior shelf adjacent to the origin of the ductus arteriosus immediately distal to the left subclavian artery. It occurs in 5% of CHD, is much more common in boys, and is frequently seen in Turner's syndrome. Up to 80% of patients with CoA have an associated bicuspid aortic valve. CoA is likely to produce significant symptoms during early infancy. Infantile presentation is usually related to spontaneous closure of the ductus arteriosus because this vessel provides an additional pathway to maintain blood flow to the lower extremities. It is common for a newborn with CoA to do well for the first several days of life and then acutely manifest shock-like symptoms with acidosis and absent lower extremity pulses precipitated by ductal closure. If not identified during infancy, most children with untreated CoA are asymptomatic but have a significantly shortened life expectancy, with an average age at death of 33 years.

The hallmark of CoA by physical examination is decreased or absent lower extremity pulses in association with upper extremity hypertension and a differential blood pressure between the upper and lower extremities. A long systolic ejection murmur is frequently appreciated in the mid-scapular area of the back, and an apical systolic ejection click can also be appreciated if there is an associated bicuspid aortic valve. Claudication in the lower extremities with activity is occasionally a complaint in a child with unrepaired CoA.

The ECG is associated with striking right ventricular hypertrophy in infancy and left ventricular hypertrophy in the child or adolescent. Poststenotic dilatation of the descending aorta and rib notching from dilatation of thoracic collateral vessels can sometimes be appreciated on chest radiography in the child with long-standing CoA. Two-dimensional and Doppler echocardiography are useful in delineating both the site and the degree of obstruction, and magnetic resonance imaging is an excellent technique for outlining the aortic and brachiocephalic vessel anatomy.

Surgical repair of CoA is frequently an emergent procedure in the symptomatic neonate. Reopening the ductus arteriosus by continuous infusion of prostaglandin E_1 can stabilize these sick infants before surgery. In asymptomatic children, intervention is usually performed when the difference between upper and lower extremity blood pressure is greater than 20 mm Hg in association with upper extremity hypertension. Older patients with unrepaired CoA are at risk for persistent hypertension after repair, so there is little benefit in delaying surgery once CoA is identified. The arch obstruction recurs in approximately 10% of patients after surgery, and this frequently can be addressed by balloon dilatation in the cardiac catheterization laboratory. All patients with CoA require bacterial endocarditis prophylaxis for life.

Pulmonary Stenosis

Valvar pulmonary stenosis (PS) is a relatively common defect, representing approximately 10% of all cases of CHD. It has been associated with both Noonan's syndrome and the rubella syndrome. Valvar PS rarely causes symptoms except in the newborn with critical obstruction across the valve, persistent shunting of desaturated blood from the right atrium to the left atrium through a patent foramen ovale, and cyanosis.

The clinical examination tends to parallel the severity of the obstruction. There is a systolic ejection murmur heard along the left upper sternal border with radiation to both axillae and the back; the intensity and length of the murmur correspond in general to the severity of the obstruction. There may be a variable early systolic ejection click at the left upper sternal border with opening of the abnormal valve; this click is not appreciated in the patient with severe PS. The second heart sound usually is normal with mild PS, more widely split with moderate stenosis, and single with severe stenosis. A thrill at the left upper sternal border is usually present when the gradient across the valve exceeds 40 mm Hg, defining the obstruction as moderate.

The ECG may reveal right ventricular hypertrophy, and again the degree of hypertrophy usually is proportional to the severity of the obstruction. The chest radiograph may show prominent poststenotic dilatation of the main pulmonary artery. Two-dimensional echocardiography can define the defect well and can look for associated branch pulmonary artery stenosis or pulmonary annular hypoplasia. The peak gradient across the valve can be accurately estimated with Doppler techniques.

Patients with valvar PS and a peak gradient of 30 to 40 mm Hg should have intervention. This is now almost exclusively performed using balloon dilatation of the valve in the cardiac catheterization laboratory, and results have been uniformly excellent with this procedure. It is only the rare patient with severe annular hypoplasia or leaflet dysplasia who does not respond well to balloon dilatation. The long-term prognosis for patients after this procedure is excellent, and recurrence of the obstruction is rare. All patients with PS require bacterial endocarditis prophylaxis, although the risk is low.

CYANOTIC CONGENITAL HEART LESIONS

Many forms of CHD are associated with intracardiac shunting of desaturated blood back into the systemic circulation, resulting in cyanosis and hypoxxemia. Newborns presenting with cyanosis usually have either lung disease or CHD as the cause. It is critical to differentiate the etiology of the cyanosis rapidly to ensure proper management. Intrapulmonary shunting can frequently be differentiated from intracardiac shunting by hyperoxia testing. The infant is placed in 100% oxygen for 10 minutes and then an arterial Po_2 is measured. Infants with lung disease usually have an increase in Po_2 to 200 mm Hg or greater, whereas infants with CHD and cyanosis usually maintain a Po_2 less than 100 mm Hg. ECG and chest radiography are rarely definitive in identifying the etiology of the cyanosis, and therefore two-dimensional and Doppler echocardiography are

critical in any infant with cyanosis of unclear etiology. Because many newborns with CHD and cyanosis depend on a PDA to maintain pulmonary blood flow, accurate diagnosis should be considered a medical emergency. Some of the major forms of cyanotic CHD are reviewed.

Tetralogy of Fallot

Tetralogy of Fallot (TOF) is the most common congenital cardiac defect that results in cyanosis. It consists of four anatomic features: (1) an outlet VSD, (2) pulmonary valve or subvalvar stenosis, (3) an overriding aorta that straddles the VSD, and (4) right ventricular hypertrophy. All these features are related to one morphologic abnormality: anterior deviation or malalignment of the infundibular septum. The degree of cyanosis in TOF is variable and usually proportional to the severity of the right ventricular outflow tract obstruction. Infants with severe outflow tract obstruction present with marked cyanosis in the newborn period, whereas those with mild outflow obstruction can be acyanotic and act physiologically like the infant with a large VSD.

All patients with TOF have some degree of right ventricular outflow tract obstruction, and so the constant physical finding is a systolic ejection murmur along the left upper sternal border with radiation into the axilla and back. Because the VSD is almost always large and nonrestrictive, no murmur from the VSD is appreciated. With significant obstruction, an increased right ventricular precordial impulse can be appreciated along with a palpable thrill along the left upper sternal border. Some patients with severe stenosis may have continuous murmurs heard throughout the precordium and back related to development of abnormal aortopulmonary collateral vessels that become the major source of pulmonary blood flow.

The ECG is rarely helpful in the newborn, although it may show right ventricular hypertrophy and right axis deviation in the patient with severe obstruction. The chest radiograph usually shows a normal-sized heart with decreased pulmonary vascular markings in the cyanotic newborn. Right ventricular hypertrophy can elevate the apex of the heart, resulting in a "boot-shaped" appearance to the cardiac shadow. In addition, 25% of the patients with TOF have a right aortic arch. Two-dimensional and Doppler echocardiography are diagnostic and usually focus on the site and degree of right ventricular outflow tract obstruction. Branch pulmonary artery hypoplasia can be an associated finding, and cardiac catheterization may be necessary to visualize better the branch pulmonary arteries in some cases. Coronary artery anomalies are present in 5% of patients with TOF and are also sometimes best delineated at catheterization.

Severe cyanosis in the newborn with TOF can frequently be improved with maintenance of a PDA using prostaglandin E_1. In severely cyanotic infants, early surgical repair or palliation is necessary. Although complete repair, which involves closure of the VSD and relief of the right ventricular outflow tract obstruction, can be accomplished in young infants, many centers elect to create a palliative aortic-to-pulmonary artery anastomosis using a GoreTex graft between the subclavian and pulmonary arteries (Blalock-Taussig shunt) to augment pulmonary blood flow as an intermediate procedure. The shunt alleviates cyanosis and can encourage pulmonary artery growth, making the child a better candidate for complete repair at an older age.

Hypercyanotic spells can occur in patients with unrepaired TOF, characterized by a marked increase in cyanosis with agitation and hyperpnea. This is usually related to acute spasm of the right ventricular infundibular outlet, so that pulmonary blood flow is reduced and right-to-left shunting through the VSD is increased. These spells should be considered a medical emergency, although most respond to three interventions: (1) placement of the patient in a knee-to-chest position to increase systemic vascular resistance and decrease right-to-left ventricular level shunting, (2) supplemental oxygen to decrease the pulmonary vascular resistance, and (3) calming and sedation, with the use of morphine sulfate, 0.1 mg per kg by intramuscular/intravenous injection. Transport to an intensive care setting with intubation, hyperventilation, and initiation of alpha-adrenergic agonist agents is necessary if the cyanosis persists. Onset of hypercyanotic spells is a clear indication for surgical intervention.

Long-term prognosis in patients with TOF is good, although late arrhythmias and right ventricular failure can occur if residual right ventricular outflow tract obstruction or significant pulmonary insufficiency is a sequela of the surgical procedure. All patients require bacterial endocarditis prophylaxis for life.

Transposition of the Great Arteries

Complete or *d*-transposition of the great arteries (TGA) is a congenital defect in which the pulmonary artery arises from the left ventricle and the aorta from the right ventricle. This puts the pulmonary and systemic circulations in parallel rather than in series, so that the desaturated blood returns to the aorta without passing through the pulmonary circulation. Survival is possible only if there is a site of mixing between the pulmonary and systemic circulations; this can occur at the atrial level with an ASD, the ventricular level with a VSD, or the great artery level with a PDA. It is the second most common cyanotic defect, representing 5 to 8% of all CHD, and is much more common in boys.

This defect usually manifests during the newborn period with severe cyanosis. Clinical features are otherwise relatively subtle, with an increased right ventricular impulse at the left lower sternal border and a single accentuated second heart sound. Approximately one third of patients have some form of obstruction in the left ventricular outflow tract and can

have a systolic ejection murmur. An ECG is rarely helpful in the newborn. A chest radiograph usually shows cardiomegaly with increased pulmonary vascular markings and a narrow vascular pedicle ("heart on a string"). Two-dimensional and Doppler echocardiography can rapidly identify this defect, and the study usually focuses on adequacy of the atrial communication, the presence or absence of ventricular communications, and patency of the left ventricular outflow tract. In addition, coronary artery anomalies are common with this defect and can frequently be identified by echocardiographic imaging.

Infusion of prostaglandin E_1 can maintain patency of the ductus arteriosus and improve mixing in infants with TGA. This is usually effective, however, only if an adequate ASD also exists. Creation of an ASD can be performed by balloon atrial septostomy. A catheter is passed from the femoral vein into the left atrium under echocardiographic or fluoroscopic guidance; a rigid balloon at the tip of the catheter is then inflated with saline and pulled vigorously across the atrial septum into the right atrium, tearing the flap valve of the atrial septum and creating an ASD. This procedure is effective in stabilizing most newborns with TGA, allowing more elective surgical repair.

The procedure of choice to repair TGA is the arterial switch operation, where the great arteries are repositioned over the appropriate ventricle so that the aorta now comes off the left ventricle and the pulmonary artery off the right ventricle. The coronary arteries must be transferred to follow the aorta. This procedure usually is performed during the first week of life because delay until later infancy can result in a poorly prepared left ventricle that has grown accustomed to functioning against subsystemic pulmonary artery pressures. The PDA is ligated and atrial and ventricular communications are closed at the same time. Many older patients have been palliated with an atrial switch procedure (Mustard's or Senning's procedure) in which right atrial blood is redirected to the left ventricle and left atrial blood is redirected to the right ventricle. Although the success rate with this procedure has been excellent, late complications related to systemic right ventricular failure and atrial arrhythmias have been common in the second and third decades of life.

Tricuspid Atresia

Tricuspid atresia is a rare cardiac anomaly characterized by an atretic tricuspid valve, varying degrees of right ventricular hypoplasia, an interatrial communication, and a normally formed left ventricle. Because there is no egress of blood from the right atrium into the right ventricle, there is an obligate right-to-left shunt across the atrial septum. The great arteries can be normally related or transposed; patients with normally related great arteries usually have obstruction to pulmonary blood flow and cyanosis, whereas those with TGA usually have unrestrictive pulmonary flow and congestive heart failure.

Most patients with tricuspid atresia present during the newborn period with cyanosis, but some are not detected until later infancy if pulmonary blood flow is unrestricted. The ECG can be helpful in the diagnosis because there is commonly left axis deviation. The chest radiographic findings are variable; the heart is of normal size with decreased pulmonary vascular markings in the patient with PS and cyanosis, whereas cardiomegaly and increased pulmonary vascular markings are found in the patient without stenosis. Two-dimensional and Doppler echocardiography are diagnostic with this lesion.

Because of the tricuspid atresia and right ventricular hypoplasia, two-ventricle repair is not possible with this defect. Long-term palliation has been focused on creation of right heart bypass procedures, most commonly performed using the modified Fontan operation. This results in passive flow of all desaturated blood through the pulmonary circulation, so that only oxygenated blood returns to the single left ventricle and systemic circulation. Good short- and intermediate-term results have been achieved with this procedure, with the understanding that absence of a right ventricular pump results in decreased exercise endurance and activity. Transition of the circulation to this physiology is usually done in several steps. Patients with significant PS may have insufficient pulmonary blood flow, so creation of a Blalock-Taussig shunt or anastomosis of the superior vena cava to the pulmonary arteries (bidirectional Glenn procedure) can be performed as an intermediate step. Patients without PS frequently need pulmonary artery banding to control pulmonary blood flow, decrease congestive heart failure symptoms, and prevent the development of pulmonary vascular obstructive disease. The Fontan procedure is usually performed at 2 to 4 years of age. Late complications after this procedure include chronic systemic venous hypertension with resultant protein-losing enteropathy, systemic venous thrombosis, and atrial arrhythmias.

Truncus Arteriosus

Truncus arteriosus (TA) is characterized by a single great artery exiting the heart that gives rise to the coronary, pulmonary, and systemic arteries. This truncal artery straddles the ventricular septum and communicates with both ventricles by a nonrestrictive VSD. The pulmonary arteries usually arise unobstructed from the truncal artery distal to the origin of the coronary arteries. This frequently results in excessive pulmonary blood flow, minimal cyanosis, and severe congestive heart failure during infancy. TA has been associated with DiGeorge's syndrome, characterized by hypocalcemia and T cell immune deficiency.

The cardiac examination is remarkable for significantly increased apical and precordial impulses with a loud single second heart sound. Truncal valve stenosis and insufficiency are common, with a to-and-fro systolic/diastolic murmur at the cardiac base. Pulses are frequently full and bounding, and a wide pulse pressure can be appreciated. The ECG usually shows biventricular hypertrophy. Cardiomegaly and increased pulmonary vascular markings are appreciated on the chest radiograph, and a right aortic arch may be identifiable (present in 33% of patients with TA). Two-dimensional and Doppler echocardiography are diagnostic and usually focus on truncal valve anatomy and function as well as site of origin and size of the branch pulmonary arteries. In rare cases, the aortic arch is interrupted.

Complete repair of TA is usually performed in early infancy because of intractable failure symptoms and the risk of early pulmonary vascular obstructive disease. This repair includes closure of the VSD so that all left ventricular output is directed into the truncal artery. The pulmonary arteries are removed from the back of the trunk and connected to the right ventricle by placement of a right-ventricular–to–pulmonary-artery conduit. Outgrowth of the conduit necessitates multiple replacement procedures as the child ages. Surgical outcome and long-term prognosis are most influenced by truncal valve function, and truncal valve replacement may be necessary as part of the initial surgical procedure. All patients with TA require bacterial endocarditis prophylaxis before and after surgical correction.

Hypoplastic Left Heart Syndrome

The hypoplastic left heart syndrome is a spectrum of anomalies characterized by mitral, left ventricular, and aortic atresia or hypoplasia so that systemic circulation depends on right-to-left shunting through the ductus arteriosus. Because there is limited egress from the left atrium to the left ventricle, an interatrial communication is also necessary for survival. This CHD is not compatible with long-term survival, and the average life span is approximately 2 weeks. It is one of the commonest causes of neonatal death from CHD.

Neonates with hypoplastic left heart syndrome are usually critically ill after spontaneous ductus arteriosus closure, although fetal echocardiographic techniques have enabled prenatal diagnosis and early intervention. With ductal closure, systemic profusion becomes severely limited, and so the infant presents with tachypnea, acidosis, cyanosis, and absence of pulses. If a nonrestrictive ductal communication is present, these infants can appear quite healthy with mild to moderate cyanosis. A markedly increased right ventricular impulse is always present, and a single loud second heart sound is appreciated. The ECG can show striking right ventricular hypertrophy, right axis deviation, and absence of left ventricular forces. The chest radiograph usually shows cardiac enlargement with increased pulmonary blood flow. Two-dimensional and Doppler echocardiography are diagnostic and focus on the adequacy of the atrial communication, degree of left heart hypoplasia, and anatomy of the aortic arch and ductus arteriosus.

Effective surgical palliations for hypoplastic left heart syndrome have been challenging and only successful during the past 10 years. Provision of comfort measures without intervention is still considered a reasonable option with this lethal defect. Reconstruction of the aortic arch with the main pulmonary artery to re-create a systemic outflow with placement of a Blalock-Taussig shunt and resection of the atrial septum (the Norwood procedure) has been a successful initial palliation at some centers. Later Fontan palliation allows complete separation of the pulmonary and systemic circulations (see section on Tricuspid Atresia). Neonatal heart transplantation is another potential therapy, although the limited donor availability has made this an unpredictable option.

MITRAL VALVE PROLAPSE

method of
RICHARD B. DEVEREUX, M.D.
*The New York Presbyterian Hospital–Weill
Medical College of Cornell University
New York, New York*

The term "mitral valve prolapse" (MVP) describes displacement of the mitral leaflets in superior and posterior directions from their normal location during systole, in keeping with the dictionary definition of prolapse as "the slipping of a body part from its normal position in relation to other body parts." Mitral valvular function in MVP may range from mild leaflet displacement without regurgitation to marked leaflet "billowing" and severe regurgitation.

PATHOGENESIS AND ETIOLOGY OF MVP

The mitral valve motion abnormalities that characterize MVP result from enlargement of the valve's connective tissue elements (leaflets, annulus, and chordae tendineae) relative to the supporting papillary muscles and left ventricular myocardium. Generalized enlargement, localized distortion, and abnormal distensibility of the valve have all been documented in patients with MVP. Although MVP may be a secondary component of many conditions, these are uncommon; and the best documented of these—the Marfan syndrome—accounts for only about 1 in 500 cases of MVP. In most instances, therefore, MVP is a primary condition. Its frequency (2 to 3% of the general population) makes it the most common heart valve abnormality in the United States.

Although the precise cause of primary MVP remains undefined, most instances of MVP are inherited in an autosomal dominant mode. The MVP gene(s) appears to be fully expressed in adult women younger than the age of 50 years, with less consistent gene expression in adult men, older women, and children of both sexes. The genetic defects causing MVP are likely to involve an as-yet-undefined component of connective tissue.

The pattern of abnormal mitral leaflet motion in patients with MVP causing significant valvular regurgitation is characterized by systolic billowing of mitral leaflets into the left atrium while dynamic systolic expansion of the mitral annulus may cause posterior displacement of the leaflets in systole as well as systolic clicks and murmurs. Strong familiality of these patterns of MVP suggests that they reflect separate genetic entities. Mitral valve enlargement and leaflet thickening, markers of increased risk of complications, occur in a subset of MVP patients with leaflet billowing. The disproportionate occurrence of complications or severe pathologic abnormalities in older subjects with MVP suggests an additional role of "wear and tear" superimposed on the underlying gene defect(s).

DIAGNOSIS OF MVP

Because of the potential to induce anxiety about nonexistent heart disease or about the presence of a more serious condition if MVP is overdiagnosed or underdiagnosed, respectively, the most important step in patient management is determining whether MVP is present or not (Table 1).

The most useful auscultatory features of MVP are (1) midsystolic clicks that move earlier in systole with sitting, standing, or other interventions that reduce ventricular size or later with those that increase chamber size, such as squatting, and (2) late systolic murmurs in individuals too young to be at risk for mitral annular calcification or papillary muscle dysfunction. The clicks and murmurs caused by prolapsing mitral valves may be made louder by isometric handgrip exercise (clenching both fists), which raises arterial blood pressure and thus increases the intensity of left-sided heart auscultatory events. One must be attentive to the timing of auscultatory abnormalities, because we have found widely split first heart sounds and midsystolic, rather than late systolic, murmurs to be present in a high proportion of patients with false-positive diagnoses of MVP. It is also noteworthy that auscultatory manifestations are highly variable in subjects with echocardiographic MVP, with both fluctuation among audible clicks, murmurs, and combinations thereof, as well as shifts back and forth between typical auscultatory findings and "silent" mitral prolapse. As a result, several examinations are needed to determine whether an individual intermittently has a murmur of mitral regurgitation, an important consideration in determining whether to recommend antibiotic prophylaxis.

Role of Echocardiography

Because of its ability to visualize the anatomy and function of the mitral valve, echocardiography is a nearly ideal method to detect and characterize MVP. The initial mainstay of echocardiographic diagnosis of MVP was demon-

TABLE 1. **Diagnosis of Mitral Valve Prolapse**

Auscultation

DEFINITIVE

Midsystolic click(s) alone or with late systolic murmur that move(s) earlier with sitting/standing and become(s) louder with handgrip.

SUGGESTIVE

Midsystolic click that does not vary with maneuvers.
Late systolic murmur alone.

Echocardiography

DEFINITIVE

Leaflet billowing in long-axis (parasternal or apical views).
>2 mm late systolic prolapse by two-dimensionally guided M-mode echocardiography.

SUGGESTIVE

Marked late systolic billowing in other apical two-dimensional views.

stration on M-mode recordings of late systolic posterior motion, by at least 2 mm, of continuous mitral leaflet interfaces behind the line connecting the valve's closure and opening points. Diagnosis of mitral prolapse by this criterion has been shown to be reproducible, provided that tracings are of high technical quality, and to be more sensitive for detection of MVP in patients with typical systolic clicks and murmurs than currently accepted two-dimensional (2D) echocardiographic criteria.

Two-dimensional echocardiography now plays a central role in recognition of MVP. MVP should be diagnosed by 2D echocardiography only when systolic billowing of mitral leaflets is demonstrated in parasternal or apical long-axis views. This is because the mitral annulus is not flat, but rather has a saddle shape. The mitral annulus is farthest from the left ventricular apex in its anterior and posterior portions, where the hinging points of the anterior and posterior mitral leaflets are seen in long-axis views, and is closest to the apex in its medial and lateral portions, where it is seen in the apical four-chamber view. Because of this, mitral leaflets that lie clearly on the left ventricular side of the mitral annulus during systole in long-axis views may appear to protrude artifactually into the left atrium in the apical four-chamber view. This artifact has been found in up to one third of normal adolescents.

Diagnosis of MVP in 2D long-axis views is highly specific but is somewhat insensitive, because it detects billowing into the left atrium of enlarged central scallops of the posterior mitral leaflet but yields negative results in individuals with auscultatory evidence of MVP in whom there is isolated anatomic deformity of the medial or lateral portion of the posterior mitral leaflet. Correct recognition of such localized MVP requires expert echocardiographic interpretation.

CLINICAL FEATURES OF MVP

Although MVP was first recognized by its auscultatory features and by abnormal mitral valve motion revealed by angiography and echocardiography, reports soon appeared of a high prevalence of nonanginal chest pain, dyspnea, and anxiety-related symptoms in patients with MVP. The concept of an inclusive "MVP syndrome" has proved clinically useful because it provides an explanation for common, troublesome, and otherwise confusing, cardiovascular and psychologic symptoms that is acceptable to patients and physicians alike. However, controlled studies have documented similar prevalences of chest pain, dyspnea, and psychologic symptoms, as well as prolongation of the electrocardiographic QT interval among prolapse patients and cardiovascularly normal individuals evaluated in the same clinical or epidemiologic setting. MVP also appears to be no more common among patients with panic and anxiety disorders than control subjects when similar precautions are taken. Our own studies compared affected relatives (relatively unselected individuals with MVP) to unaffected relatives and spouses in over 100 families of patients with MVP (who constitute genetically related and unrelated control groups). Affected relatives were more likely than control subjects to have thoracic bony abnormalities (pectus excavatum, scoliosis, and "straight back"), low body weight and systolic blood pressure, and palpitations. In contrast, we found no difference between MVP and control subjects in the prevalence of nonanginal chest pain, dyspnea, panic attacks, high levels of anxiety, or electrocardiographic repolarization abnormalities. We showed that MVP and panic attacks were associated with contrasting patterns of autonomic dysfunction. More MVP than control

subjects exhibited orthostatic hypotension and syncope, possibly related to reduced blood volume, whereas the group with panic attacks exhibited hyperreactive heart rate and blood pressure increases in response to orthostatic stress. Thus, MVP and panic disorders are biologically distinct as well as statistically unassociated.

Thus, controlled studies show a relatively narrow spectrum of clinical features associated with MVP. Even features truly associated with MVP, such as thoracic bony abnormalities, low body weight, or palpitations, are not sufficiently specific to be useful diagnostic features. Furthermore, we found that patients in whom nonspecific symptoms led to consideration of MVP are particularly likely to have false-positive diagnoses due to misattribution to MVP of panic attacks and midsystolic murmurs.

COMPLICATIONS OF MVP

Patients with MVP are at risk for infective endocarditis, mitral regurgitation, serious arrhythmias, and sudden death; a possible association with stroke has been suggested. MVP has been found more commonly among patients with these complications than expected from its prevalence of about 3% in unselected populations. Among patients with severe mitral regurgitation in industrialized countries, from 38 to 64% have MVP as the underlying cause, whereas the proportion ranged from 11 to 29% among patients with infective endocarditis. The data for neurologic ischemic episodes have been quite variable, with MVP found in 2 to 35% of patients, leaving it uncertain whether this is a true association. Sudden death occurs with discernible frequency only among MVP patients with severe mitral regurgitation, although MVP has also been found in a disproportionate number of the small minority of sudden death patients who are free of obstructive coronary artery disease.

Identifying MVP Patients at Risk of Complications

By comparing the characteristics of MVP patients with infective endocarditis and a control group of adults found to have MVP in our family studies, we were able to show that male gender, age 45 years or older, and a history of a pre-existing heart murmur were independently associated with infective endocarditis. Compared with an average incidence of 1 per 20,000 per year in the general population, we estimated that infective endocarditis would occur each year in 1 in 1,920 MVP patients with a late or holosystolic murmur of mitral regurgitation versus 1 in 21,950 without a mitral systolic murmur. Similar calculations would suggest annual incidences of infective endocarditis of 1 in 3,640 among affected men and 1 in 2,930 among individuals 45 years of age or older with MVP. The facts that major morbidity occurred in one third of our MVP patients with endocarditis during short-term follow-up (three deaths, four valve replacements) and that endocarditis appeared to be of dental origin in one third suggests that infective endocarditis as a complication of MVP is both dangerous and partially preventable.

In long-term follow-up studies, we found the risk of complications of MVP, principally mitral valve repair or replacement but also including infective endocarditis, heart failure, and sudden death, to be increased by male gender, by age 45 years or older, and most markedly by a holosystolic murmur and left ventricular or left atrial dilatation. These findings result in overall rates of complications that ranged from well under 0.5% annually in MVP subjects with a midsystolic click and normal heart size to nearly

7% per year among MVP patients (principally men) with clinical and echocardiographic evidence of moderate or severe mitral regurgitation. Among all patients with MVP it has been calculated that the lifetime risk of needing mitral valve replacement is approximately 4 to 5% among men and 1.5% among women. For sudden, presumably arrhythmic, death, the estimated annual risk may be as high as 1 in 100 among MVP patients with important mitral regurgitation, but only 1 in 5000 or less in subjects with little or no mitral regurgitation.

TREATMENT

Appropriate care of an individual with MVP depends on accurate diagnosis of the valvular abnormality and on matching the intensiveness of evaluation and treatment to the level of risk (Table 2).

Initial Diagnosis and Screening

Auscultation remains the most common method by which MVP is recognized. When both a midsystolic click and late systolic murmur are present and vary appropriately in timing and intensity with maneuvers, or a loud midsystolic click exhibits appropriate mobility, the diagnosis is definitive. If there are less specific auscultatory features, such as a soft or immobile midsystolic click or a late systolic murmur in a middle-aged or older individual, echocardiographic confirmation of MVP is desirable. Diagnosis of MVP by echocardiography should be based on either unequivocal systolic billowing of one or both mitral leaflets across the mitral annulus in 2D long-axis views or on 2 mm or more late systolic posterior displacement of continuous mitral leaflet interfaces in high-quality 2D targeted M-mode recordings (which can have the advantage of visualizing the medial and lateral portions of the posterior mitral leaflet). Echocardiographic screening for MVP in un-

---

TABLE 2. **Matching Risk and Management in Mitral Valve Prolapse**

Lowest Risk

Subjects without mitral regurgitant murmurs or Doppler regurgitation, especially women <45 years.
Management: reassurance; no clear need for antibiotics; re-evaluation and echocardiogram at moderate intervals (5 years).

Moderate Risk

Subjects with intermittent or persistent mitral murmurs, mild Doppler regurgitation, and/or thickened valves.
Management: antibiotic prophylaxis (see doses in Table 3) with amoxicillin or clindamycin; treat even mild established hypertension; re-evaluation and echocardiography more frequently (2–3 years).

High Risk

Patients with moderate or severe mitral regurgitation.
Management: antibiotic prophylaxis with amoxicillin (unless allergic); optimize afterload (arterial pressure); re-evaluate with Doppler echocardiogram and other tests if needed annually. Consider valve repair or replacement for exertional dyspnea or decline of left ventricular function into low-normal range.

---

selected populations or symptomatic patients without typical auscultatory features is not cost effective because of its low yield and disproportionate identification of subjects at low risk. Echocardiography may, however, be useful as an objective means to expunge a dubious diagnosis of MVP and free a patient from unfounded concerns about heart disease and unwarranted treatment. Echocardiographic screening of adolescent and adult first-degree relatives of patients with unequivocal MVP is likely to be cost effective, because about 30% of such individuals also have MVP. MVP is too rare among children younger than 10 years of age to warrant screening.

Management of Uncomplicated MVP

Management of the patient with MVP should be matched to the risks of infective endocarditis and progressive mitral regurgitation. Because these risks are related to the presence of at least mild mitral regurgitation, no specific treatment may be needed for subjects with MVP, particularly women younger than age 45, who do not have a mitral systolic murmur on any of several examinations that include auscultation in multiple positions and with isometric handgrip exercise or evidence of more than trivial mitral regurgitation by Doppler echocardiography. We reassure such individuals that the outlook is benign and may even be enhanced if they have low body weight and blood pressure; antibiotic prophylaxis is not routinely recommended unless the individual wishes maximum protection against even the remotest risk; re-evaluation by auscultation and echocardiogram is recommended at moderate intervals (perhaps every 5 years) to be certain the patient has not passed into a higher risk group.

On the basis of current evidence, patients with echocardiographic MVP who even intermittently or with simple maneuvers such as sitting or handgrip exercise have soft late systolic murmurs of mitral regurgitation appear to be at modestly increased risk of endocarditis or progressive mitral regurgitation. We recommend antibiotic prophylaxis to such patients, following the 1997 American Heart Association's recommendations of amoxicillin (Amoxil and other brands), 2 grams orally 1 hour before dental procedures (Table 3). Clindamycin, 600 mg 1 hour before dental procedures, is recommended for patients allergic to penicillin. In view of suggestive evidence that elevated blood pressure may predispose to chordal rupture and progressive mitral regurgitation in patients with MVP, we recommend antihypertensive treatment for all MVP patients with mild mitral regurgitation with even very mild established systemic hypertension. Doppler echocardiography is an important adjunct to imaging techniques in defining precisely the extent of mitral regurgitation, and this evaluation as well as auscultatory examination is warranted at more frequent intervals (every 2 to 3 years) to assess possible progression of mitral regurgitation.

TABLE 3. **Endocarditis Prophylaxis: 1997 American Heart Association Recommendations for Dental Procedures**

Drug	Dose
Oral: amoxicillin (Amoxil and other brands)	2.0 gm PO 1 h before procedure
Parenteral: ampicillin (Polypen and other brands)	2.0 gm IV or IM within 30 min of procedure
Penicillin-allergic patients:	
Oral: clindamycin	600 mg PO 1 h before procedure
Parenteral: clindamycin (Cleocin)	600 mg IV within 30 min of procedure

MVP with Hemodynamically Important Mitral Regurgitation

MVP patients who have hemodynamically important mitral regurgitation are at greatest risk of endocarditis, sudden death, and need for mitral valve surgery. This group constitutes 2 to 4% of adults with MVP. Severe regurgitation is suggested on physical examination by a holosystolic or nearly holosystolic mitral regurgitant murmur, commonly accompanied by a left ventricular third heart sound and leftward displacement of a dynamic left ventricular impulse, and is confirmed by the demonstration of significant mitral regurgitation by Doppler color flow mapping and calculation of regurgitant volume in conjunction with imaging echocardiographic evidence of MVP and left heart chamber enlargement. Infective endocarditis prophylaxis is mandatory, with amoxicillin in the absence of a specific allergy, and it is theoretically attractive although not of proven value to treat even borderline systemic hypertension with antihypertensive drugs in such patients. Angiotensin-converting enzyme inhibitors (e.g., ramipril [Altace] starting at 2.5 to 5.0 mg daily) or other agents that reduce peripheral resistance and enhance arterial compliance may be especially valuable in reducing stress in prolapsed mitral valves. Regular follow-up is required, with annual imaging and Doppler echocardiograms and selected use of other methods such as nuclear angiograms and treadmill exercise tests being recommended. Corrective valvular surgery, by valve repair rather than by valve replacement in an increasing proportion of cases, is recommended when patients either develop dyspnea of class II or greater New York Heart Association severity or when left ventricular systolic performance falls into the lower part of the normal range in the absence of symptoms. A simple partition value for recognition of the latter is an M-mode echocardiographic left ventricular fractional shortening of less than 31%, reported to predict a suboptimal outcome after mitral valve surgery for severe mitral regurgitation. Frankly, subnormal ventricular performance should not preclude corrective valvular surgery, which may improve the poor survival associated with medical management of patients with severe mitral regurgitation and ventricular dysfunction.

Treatment of Arrhythmias

Arrhythmias in MVP may require treatment to relieve symptoms or to reduce risk of sudden death. Palpitations and salvos of atrial premature complexes and brief bursts of atrial tachycardia are found slightly more commonly in subjects with MVP than in normal individuals. Suggested mechanisms of arrhythmogenesis include (1) stimulation of atrial pacemakers by the impact of prolapsing leaflets or mitral regurgitant jets and (2) origin of impulses from electrically active cells, shown to have beta-adrenoceptors, in the mitral leaflets. However, many episodes of palpitation reflect forceful heart beating during sinus rhythm, and many episodes of atrial arrhythmia are asymptomatic. Awareness of palpitation in other prolapse subjects may coincide with simple ventricular premature complexes, but the prevalence of ventricular arrhythmias in controlled studies of MVP is not strikingly higher than in normal subjects.

In our experience, many cases of atrial arrhythmia and some instances of ventricular premature contractions will respond to treatment with beta-blocking drugs (e.g., nadolol [Corgard] beginning at a dose of 40 mg per day). However, periods of remission and of exacerbation of symptoms may continue to occur in these subjects, as often occurs in untreated subjects. Some patients with atrial arrhythmias may respond favorably to digitalization (digoxin [Lanoxin], 0.25 mg per day, or reduced doses in the presence of renal dysfunction) or to administration of verapamil (240 to 480 mg per day of long-acting Calan, Isoptin, or Verelan). Episodes of supraventricular tachycardia in MVP patients are usually due to reentry in the atrioventricular node. If episodes are recurrent and disruptive to the patient, we offer electrophysiologic study and potentially corrective ablation of the extra electrical pathway as a treatment option. Because of their frequent side effects and occasional proarrhythmic activity, we use type I agents (e.g., quinidine, procainamide [Pronestyl], flecainide [Tambocor], and amiodarone [Cordarone]) only when simpler regimens have failed in highly symptomatic subjects.

Whether and when to use antiarrhythmic drugs to prevent sudden death in patients with MVP remains controversial. Sudden death appears strongly concentrated in the 2 to 4% of patients with hemodynamically severe mitral regurgitation, but even in this high-risk group there is no evidence that antiarrhythmic drug treatment is beneficial. Individuals with MVP who experience sustained ventricular tachycardia or are resuscitated from near sudden death are best evaluated with electrophysiologic testing followed by use of medications shown to be protective or, more frequently, an implantable antitachycardia device. The occurrence of arrhythmic death among the larger population of subjects with otherwise uncomplicated MVP is too rare for either potentially toxic antiarrhythmic agents or expensive antitachycardia devices to represent cost-effective management strategies.

Treatment of Nonspecific Cardiovascular Symptoms

Management of the patient with MVP and symptoms other than palpitations or dyspnea related to mitral regurgitation may require varied approaches. Chest pain, palpitations, and dyspnea may occur concurrently with severe anxiety and other symptoms, including tremor, dizziness, and diaphoresis in repeated episodes termed panic attacks. If panic attacks occur spontaneously ("out of the blue") or in response to emotionally stressful situations such as elevators or crowded places, treatment directed toward either pharmacologic or behavioral therapy for panic disorder under the guidance of an experienced psychiatrist is often effective. Patients with these complaints generally do not respond well to standard cardiac medications. Meticulous attention to details of the clinical history is important, for in some anxiety-prone individuals the sudden onset of rapid palpitations due to paroxysmal atrial tachycardia or fibrillation may lead to other cardiovascular symptoms and secondary panic; this situation often responds well to appropriate medications (e.g., digoxin, beta-blockers) and reassurance. Both panic disorders and repeated paroxysms of atrial arrhythmia may remit spontaneously or recur after a period of quiescence. Other chest pain syndromes with features suggestive of angina, esophageal disorders, or a musculoskeletal origin should not be attributed to MVP but rather should lead to appropriate further evaluation and specific treatment if clinically indicated.

Management of Autonomic Dysfunction

A variety of autonomic dysfunction syndromes may occur in patients diagnosed or considered to have MVP. The most common of these in our experience consists of recurring episodes ranging from dizziness through presyncope, requiring the individual to sit or lie down, to even frank syncope that occurs most commonly with variably prolonged standing or with exercise on a hot day. These episodic symptoms may be associated with physical fatigue and a sense of being emotionally drained but occur in the absence of evidence of generalized autonomic failure or specific metabolic defects. In such patients, orthostatic hypotension (>10 mm Hg fall in diastolic blood pressure) or tachycardia (>10 beats per minute increase in heart rate) are usually provoked by 5 minutes of quiet standing. Nausea, mild chest constriction, and bradycardia may precede actual syncope. Detailed investigation commonly reveals a deficit in blood volume, and most such patients respond favorably to dietary supplementation or addition of NaCl tablets (1 gram, 1 to 4 tablets per day). Fludrocortisone acetate (Florinef), 0.05 to 0.1 mg per day, or clonidine hydrochloride (Catapres), 0.1 to 0.2 per day, may be added if necessary, with careful monitoring of blood pressure responses; individuals with features of neurocardiogenic syncope may benefit from treatment with atenolol (Tenormin), beginning at a dose of 25 mg daily. Orthostatic hypotension in women with MVP may also remit during the natural volume expansion that occurs during pregnancy.

A variety of other syndromes of autonomic dysfunction, characterized by evidence of sympathetic or parasympathetic overactivity, appear to occur with nearly equal frequency in individuals with and without MVP. Their evaluation commonly requires specialized testing, the results of which should guide therapy.

CONGESTIVE HEART FAILURE

method of
ARTHUR M. FELDMAN, M.D., PH.D., and
VIRGINIA M. SCHNEIDER, R.N.
University of Pittsburgh Medical Center
Health System
Pittsburgh, Pennsylvania

Congestive heart failure (CHF) is a disease that affects over 4 million people in the United States; over 400,000 new cases were expected to be diagnosed in 1999. The disease affects people of all races and genders equally; however, it is predominant in the elderly. Indeed, CHF is the number one discharge diagnosis in patients older than 65 years. Data from the Framingham study demonstrates that only 57% of men and 64% of women survive 1 year after their initial diagnosis. Furthermore, patients with CHF undergo frequent hospitalizations for worsening heart failure; older women have a worse prognosis than do older men. CHF is also associated with an enormous economic burden: Yearly costs for the care of patients with CHF exceed $18 billion. Interestingly, this cost is substantially higher than that for the care of all malignancies and myocardial infarctions. However, in contrast to that of many other human diseases, the incidence of CHF is increasing each year in the United States. Although this increase was originally attributed to better recognition of the disease, it is now recognized that the increased incidence is attributable to the aging of the U.S. population and to new and aggressive measures that allow patients to survive longer with significant coronary artery disease.

Although we refer to CHF as a "disease," in reality it is a triad of signs and symptoms (i.e., shortness of breath, edema, and fatigue) that can be caused by a variety of specific cardiovascular diseases. These include dilated cardiomyopathy, hypertrophic cardiomyopathy, constrictive heart disease, and restrictive heart disease. The most common cause of congestive heart failure in the United States is dilated cardiomyopathy. As the name implies, the pathognomonic feature of this disease is dilatation of the left ventricle, although in many cases there is an accompanying dilatation of the right ventricle. Furthermore, dilated cardiomyopathy is characterized by marked systolic dysfunction (although the dilated heart also demonstrates some degree of diastolic dysfunction). Cardiac dilatation can be caused by either ischemic heart disease or idiopathic dilated cardiomyopathy. In the case of ischemic myopathies, cardiac dilatation and systolic dysfunction can occur as a result of ventricular remodeling after a single large myocardial infarction or multiple small myocardial infarctions. Alternatively, dilatation and remodeling can follow chronic ischemia and myocardial hibernation. Less commonly, cardiac dilatation is seen in women shortly before, during, or within 6 months of parturition. However, these women have a much better prognosis than do other patients. In a small number of cases, a dilated cardiomyopathy can follow other diseases, including rheumatologic disease, thyroid dysfunction, hemachromatosis, and human immunodeficiency virus (HIV) infection. In addition, a dilated cardiomyopathy may result from excessive alcohol consumption or exposure to environmental toxins. Although heritable forms of dilated cardiomyopathy were originally considered rare, more recent studies suggest that as many as 20% of patients with idiopathic dilated cardiomyopathy have a positive family history. Of importance is evidence that patients may have a dilated cardiomyopathy and yet remain asymptomatic for relatively long periods of time.

In contrast, the hypertrophic heart is characterized by marked hypertrophy of the ventricular myocardium. Furthermore, the heart demonstrates a hypercontractile state that occasionally results in near obliteration of the ventricular cavity. Although the heart is hypercontractile, it is dysfunctional because of a marked decrease in diastolic compliance, which results in increased filling pressures. In most cases, hypertrophic cardiomyopathy results from prolonged hypertension; however, hypertrophic myopathies can also be secondary to inheritance of a gene mutation. Although hypertrophy is often concentric, some patients demonstrate focal asymmetrical hypertrophy with obstruction of the aortic outflow tract. Hypertrophic cardiomyopathy is most effectively treated with agents that reduce contractility and, in so doing, improve diastolic compliance. The two agents most commonly used for this disease are the calcium channel blocker nifedipine and the beta blockers. In patients with the heritable form of hypertrophic cardiomyopathy, sudden death is not uncommon and may be the initial manifestation in young athletes. Patients with familial hypertrophy should be evaluated by physicians who have expertise in cardiac genetics, because the risk of sudden death varies in different families and at different ages and appears to be mutation-specific. Antiarrhythmic drugs have varying degrees of effectiveness, and the potential efficacy of implantable defibrillators remains undefined. Less frequently, the compliance of the ventricular myocardium may be altered by either pericardial constriction or myocyte infiltration. Pericardial constriction can often be ameliorated with surgical intervention. However, infiltrative diseases are far less treatable. For example, amyloid heart disease, the most common form of infiltrative disease, is associated with a poor prognosis, and care is largely supportive.

When a patient comes to medical attention for the first time with signs and symptoms of CHF, it is imperative that a complete evaluation be performed to ascertain the specific disease that has caused those signs and symptoms (see Table 1). Dilated cardiomyopathies can be easily distinguished from hypertrophic cardiomyopathies by echocardiography. Evaluation of restrictive or constrictive myopathies may require magnetic resonance imaging to assess the pericardium, an endomyocardial biopsy with appropriate staining to confirm the presence of amyloid or other infiltrative diseases, or cardiac catheterization to distinguish restrictive from constrictive disease. In addition, laboratory investigations should be performed with special attention to analysis of thyroid function, indices of rheumatologic disease, serum ferritin, serum calcium, and HIV status. A thorough family history should be obtained from each patient, and when there is a suspicion of a familial inheritance, patients should be referred to heart

TABLE 1. Evaluation of the Patient Presenting with a First Episode of Congestive Heart Failure

Complete history/physical examination	Family history
	Toxic exposure
	Alcohol ingestion
	Drug abuse
Cardiopulmonary examination	Heart sounds
	JVD
	Carotid pulsations
	Hepatomegaly
	Peripheral edema
Echocardiogram	EF
	Valve morphology
	LVEDD
Chest radiograph	Heart size
	Vascular congestion
	Pulmonary infiltrates
Laboratory studies	ANA, Rheumatoid Factor, SED rate, Serum ferritin, TSH, Urinalysis, VMA, Metanephrines
Diagnostic catheterization	Right heart pressure
	Coronary anatomy
Endomyocardial biopsy	Infiltrative disease

Abbreviations: ANA = antinuclear antibodies; EF = ejection fraction; JVD = jugular venous distention; LVEDP = left ventricular end-diastolic pressure; SED = sedimentation; TSH = thyroid-stimulating hormone; VMA = vanillylmandelic acid.

failure centers that have expertise in molecular genetics. We believe that every patient with a first-time diagnosis of dilated cardiomyopathy should undergo left- and right-sided heart catheterization with coronary angiography. Furthermore, if coronary disease is identified, aggressive steps should be taken to assess the viability of the downstream myocardium, including dobutamine echocardiography or positron-emission tomography (PET) imaging, and revascularization should be pursued when appropriate. Although ischemic heart disease is less common in younger patients, we have seen patients in their early thirties who have high-grade coronary stenosis and hibernating myocardium that are amenable to revascularization. Furthermore, hemodynamic information can be useful in the development of initial therapeutic strategies. Endomyocardial biopsies have provided an important research tool in understanding the pathophysiology of dilated cardiomyopathies and can be performed with low risk by experienced operators. However, their role in the routine evaluation of patients with new-onset CHF remains undefined.

MANAGEMENT

After a thorough evaluation, the vast majority of patients with CHF are found to have a dilated cardiomyopathy. Once a dilated cardiomyopathy has been diagnosed and steps have been taken to address potentially reversible causes, it is imperative that patients receive thorough counseling regarding diet, medical compliance, and exercise. Patients with CHF should be maintained on a strict low-salt diet, and all members of the household should be instructed as to the salt content of commonly consumed beverages and foods. Care givers should ensure that patients have a scale in the home, that they weigh themselves at the same time each day, and that they call their physician if their weight increases by more than 3 to 5 pounds over a period of 1 week. Because compliance is of great importance, patients should understand what each of their medications does and the reasons for its use. Patients should be urged to exercise aerobically because maintenance of peripheral muscle tone is important in preserving exercise performance and quality of life. However, patients should markedly limit their anaerobic exercise, and we instruct our patients not to lift any item heavier than 10 pounds. Care givers should also assess the socioeconomic status of each patient to ensure that there is someone to help with their care and financial support to allow them to purchase their medications. Finally, it is imperative that patients with CHF be seen frequently by their physician or by physician-extenders.

Furthermore, we believe that the initial evaluation of every patient with new-onset CHF should be performed by a cardiologist and that subsequent care be performed in conjunction with physicians or physician-extenders who have an interest in the care of patients with CHF. This is supported by studies that have shown long-term improvements in outcomes and decreased costs and hospitalizations when patients receive careful and frequent outpatient follow-up. Of importance is that nurses with training and expertise in the management of patients with CHF provide an invaluable resource in caring for the many patients with CHF. Indeed, nurse-managed outpatient centers have demonstrated objective benefits in many clinical studies.

The first line of pharmacologic therapy for patients with symptomatic CHF is a diuretic (see Table 2). Although the long-term effects of diuretics on survival have not been assessed in large multicenter clinical trials, it is clear that diuretics are the best means of improving symptoms. Diuresis effects a rapid decrease in fluid volume, thereby causing a fall in left ventricular filling pressures. A variety of diuretics are available as initial agents; however, the loop diuretics appear to be the most beneficial. They can be given either once or twice a day and can be administered either orally or intravenously. Resistance may result from worsening renal function, and absorption may be affected by bowel edema secondary to right heart failure or diminished splanchnic perfusion. Diuretics are not without adverse effects; their use can be associated with hypotension, hypovolemia, hypokalemia, activation of the renin-angiotensin system, activation of sympathetic drive, hypomagnesemia, and azotemia. Therefore, their use should be accompanied by routine electrolyte surveillance, assessment of renal function, and potassium supplementation (if warranted and in the absence of potassium-sparing diuretics). However, many of the side effects of diuretic use can be abrogated by the concomitant use of an angiotensin-converting enzyme (ACE) inhibitor and a beta blocker.

In patients who develop resistance to diuretic therapy because of worsening renal dysfunction and hypoperfusion, the addition of a second diuretic can provide synergistic effects when its site of action differs from that of the loop diuretics. For example, whereas the loop diuretics exert their effects on the ascending limb of the loop of Henle, metolazone and the potassium-sparing diuretics affect diuresis at other sites in the nephron. Metolazone (Zaroxolyn) is a potent diuretic that may initiate a robust diuresis. For this reason, we often hospitalize patients when metolazone therapy is initiated or do follow-up on a daily outpatient basis to ensure that their doses are effectively titrated and that hypovolemia has not ensued. We have found the antialdosterone potassium-sparing diuretics particularly useful in patients with right-sided heart failure and passive liver congestion, because aldosterone is metabolized by the liver. Interestingly, one study has suggested that the use of spironolactone (Aldactone) is associated with improved survival in patients with CHF. However, it is important to assess potassium levels relatively frequently in these patients and to limit potassium supplementation, because hyperkalemia is a common side effect. The use of low doses of dopamine are also beneficial in patients with diuretic resistance, because dopamine improves diuresis by increasing renal blood flow. Finally, it should be noted that nonsteroidal anti-inflammatory agents can interfere with the actions of the loop diuretics and should be avoided whenever possible.

Activation of the renin-angiotensin system is a hallmark of CHF, and numerous studies have demonstrated a direct relationship between renin-angiotensin activation (as assessed by plasma levels of angiotensin II) and mortality. Thus, it is not surprising that a series of seminal clinical trials have demonstrated marked benefits of ACE inhibitors in patients with mild, moderate, and severe symptoms of CHF. However, the ACE inhibitors also have potent antiadrenergic effects and enhance tissue bradykinin. Thus the salutorious effects of the ACE inhibitors is likely multifactorial. In some but not all clinical trials, ACE inhibition has been associated with improvement in functional performance and quality of life. However, there are incontrovertible data demonstrating that ACE inhibitors lower both mortality and morbidity rates among patients with CHF, morbidity being defined as hospitalization (or therapy) for worsening heart failure. These beneficial effects can be seen in patients with idiopathic dilated cardiomyopathy as well as in those with diminished left ventricular function after a myocardial infarction. Furthermore, in patients with asymptomatic cardiac dilatation and in those with myocardial dysfunction after a myocardial infarction, the use of an ACE inhibitor is associated with delayed disease progression. Indeed, there is a general consensus that patients with both asymptomatic and symptomatic CHF should receive therapy with an ACE inhibitor.

The beneficial effect of ACE inhibitors appears to be a class effect because as many as five ACE inhibitors have shown survival benefits. These various agents differ in their dosing and cost. Although the vast majority of patients with CHF can tolerate an ACE inhibitor, they are not without side effects in-

TABLE 2. **Medications Commonly Used for Heart Failure**

Drug	Initial Dose	Target Dose	Major Adverse Reactions
Loop diuretics			Postural hypotension, hypokalemia, hyperglycemia, hyperuricemia, rash, rare severe reaction with pancreatitis, bone marrow suppression, anaphylaxis
Furosemide (Lasix)	10–40 mg qd	As needed	
Bumetanide (Bumex)	0.5–1.0 mg qd	As needed	
Torsemide (Demadex)	20 mg qd	As needed	
Thiazide-related diuretic			Same as Loop diuretics
Metolazone (Zaroxolyn)	2.5 mg	As needed (Not to exceed)	
Potassium-sparing diuretics			Hyperkalemia, especially if administered with ACE inhibitor; rash; gynecomastia (spironolactone only), anaphylaxis
Spironolactone (Aldactone)	25 mg qd	200 mg qd	
Triamterene (Dyrenium)	50 mg qd	200 mg qd	
Amiloride (Midamor)	5 mg qd	20 mg qd	
ACE inhibitors			Hypotension, hyperkalemia, renal insufficiency, cough, rash, angiodema, neutropenia
Enalapril (Vasotec)	2.5 mg bid	20 mg bid	
Captopril (Capoten)	6.25–12.5 mg tid	50 mg bid	
Lisinopril (Zestril, Prinivil)	5 mg qd	20 mg qd	
Quinapril (Accupril)	5 mg bid	20 mg bid	
Ramipril (Altace)	2.5 mg qd	10 mg qd	
Fosinopril (Monopril)	10 mg qd	10–20 mg qd	
Benazepril (Lotensin)	10 mg qd	10–20 mg qd	
Digoxin	0.125 mg qd	Not to exceed 0.250 mg qd	Cardiotoxicity, confusion, nausea, anorexia, visual disturbances
Beta blockers			Hypotension, dizziness
Carvedilol (Coreg)	3.125 mg bid	25 mg bid	
Hydralazine + isosorbide	10–25 mg tid	75 mg tid or qid	Headache, nausea, dizziness, tachycardia, lupus-like syndrome, hypotension, flushing
dinitrate (Isordil)	10 mg tid	40 mg tid (Not to exceed)	
Inotropes			Tachycardia, ventricular ectopy, phlebitis, hypotension
Dobutamine (Dobutrex)	1 µg/kg/min	10 µg/kg/min	
Milrinone (Primacor)	0.25 mg/kg/min	0.75 mg/kg/min	
Dopamine	1 µg/kg/min	5 µg/kg/min	

Abbreviations: ACE = angiotensin converting enzyme.

cluding: hypotension, renal dysfunction, hyperkalemia, and rarely, angioedema. The most common side effect of ACE inhibitors is a dry cough. Because patients with CHF have numerous reasons for the development of a cough, it is important to clarify that its etiology is the ACE inhibitor. Even if the ACE inhibitor is found to be causative, the patient should be urged to continue the medication if at all possible. In addition, although the side effects of the ACE inhibitors are thought to be class dependent, anecdotal information suggests that the incidence and/or severity of cough may differ among the different agents. Therefore, a trial of an alternative ACE inhibitor might be warranted. Of importance is that ACE inhibitors should not be used in patients with bilateral renal artery stenosis. Because of their potential side effects, ACE inhibitor therapy should be initiated with very low dosages with upward titration over a period of days to weeks, depending on an individual patient's ability to tolerate the initial doses. Upward titration should be based on signs and symptoms, the most useful end point being a decrease in blood pressure. Upward titration appears to be important because the Assessment of Treatment with Lisinopril in Heart Failure (ATLAS) study, assessing the combined risk of death or hospitalization, demonstrated that high doses of ACE inhibitors were superior to low doses. Therefore, the ideal doses of the various ACE inhibitors are those that proved efficacious in the large multicenter clinical trials. Finally, it is important to note that ACE inhibitors

should be used in conjunction with a diuretic in order to avoid fluid retention.

For those patients who are intolerant of ACE inhibitors, the combination of hydralazine and isosorbide dinitrate (Isordil) provides an alternative therapy. However, it must be recognized that this drug combination is not as beneficial as an ACE inhibitor in terms of decreasing morbidity and mortality. Furthermore, neither hydralazine nor isosorbide dinitrate are as well tolerated as are the ACE inhibitors and the use of both of these agents has been associated with the development of tolerance. Although some physicians have advocated the use of either hydralazine or nitrates as single agents for the management of CHF, controlled clinical studies have not substantiated these claims. Therefore, we add nitrates to the pharmacologic therapy of patients with CHF only when there is active concomitant ischemic heart disease and institute nitrate-free periods in order to avoid the development of tolerance. Angiotensin receptor antagonists have been developed for the therapy of CHF, and many physicians have used them as alternative therapy for the management of the ACE-intolerant patient. However, their potential benefits have not been assessed in large multicenter randomized studies, and thus their use cannot be recommended at the present time.

Like activation of the renin-angiotensin system, increased adrenergic drive is also associated with a worsened prognosis in patients with CHF. Seminal studies in the early 1980s led investigators to propose that high levels of norepinephrine in patients with CHF were both arrhythmogenic and cardiotoxic and that the use of beta blockade would be beneficial in the therapy of patients with CHF. However, in contrast to trials with ACE inhibitors, initial clinical trials with beta blockers were not impressive because the results were only suggestive of improvement in mortality and morbidity rates, and therefore their use remained controversial.

In contrast, a group of large and multicenter clinical trials have clearly demonstrated marked benefits of beta blockade. In a group of studies assessing the efficacy of beta blockade in patients with mild to moderate disease (U.S. carvedilol study; Australian and New Zealand study) as well as in patients with moderate to severe heart failure (Prospective Randomized Evaluation of Carvedilol on Symptoms and Exercise [PRECISE], Multicenter Oral Carvedilol Heart Failure Assessment [MOCHA] studies), treatment with carvedilol reduced all-cause mortality and reduced the risk of hospitalization in patients with CHF. These studies with carvedilol (Coreg) resulted in the drug receiving approval from the Food and Drug Administration (FDA) of therapy for patients with CHF. Furthermore, the carvedilol results were supported by recent studies with the beta blockers bisoprolol* (Zebeta) and metoprolol* (Lopressor). In a study of patients with moderate to severe heart failure, bisoprolol was associated with a marked reduction in mortality and a decreased risk of hospitalization for heart failure, results that led the Data and Safety Monitoring Board to recommend early termination of the study (Cardiac Insufficiency Bisoprolol Study [CIBIS] II). Similarly, a study assessing the efficacy of metoprolol in patients with New York Heart Association (NYHA) class II and class III symptoms of CHF was also discontinued prematurely at the suggestion of the Data and Safety Monitoring Board because of a significant reduction in mortality in the active treatment group. Beta blockers have also been shown to improve heart failure symptoms; benefits are most obvious in patients with moderate to severe symptoms. Thus, clinical trials strongly support the use of beta blockers in the therapy of CHF; however, it should be noted that in each of these studies, patients were receiving concomitant therapy with a diuretic and an ACE inhibitor.

Although clinical trials have shown great promise for beta-blocker therapy, several important caveats should be noted. First, beta-blocker therapy has not been assessed in patients with bradycardia, hypotension, or class IV symptoms. Therefore, beta-blocker therapy should not be used as rescue therapy in patients hospitalized for or coming to medical attention with worsening heart failure. Similarly, the effects of beta blockers have not been assessed in patients with left ventricular dilatation but compensated function and the absence of symptoms. In addition, as many as 6% of the patients in these clinical trials could not tolerate the administration of even

small amounts of a beta blocker, and as many as 30% of patients experienced dizziness or fatigue. Thus, the initial doses of beta blocker must be very low with gradual and careful upwards titration over a period of 3 to 6 months. During the titration period, patients must be closely monitored for changes in blood pressure and/or heart rate and for signs of worsening heart failure and should be seen at least weekly. These side effects can often be adequately treated by discontinuing the upward titration and/or by adjusting the doses of both diuretics and ACE inhibitors. Because of the complexities associated with the initial administration of beta blockers to patients with CHF, we believe that the early titration should be regulated by cardiologists and physician-extenders who have expertise in CHF; care can be taken over by the primary care physician once the patient's condition has been stabilized. Furthermore, consultative assistance by a cardiologist should be provided if patients receiving a beta blocker are hospitalized with worsening heart failure.

The oldest pharmacologic agent for the management of CHF is digoxin. It was first described in 1792; since then, it has been recognized that its inotropic properties come from an effect on sodium/potassium adenosine triphosphatase (ATPase) resulting in an increase in intracellular calcium. In addition, digoxin has also been shown to inhibit adrenergic drive. In patients with atrial fibrillation, digoxin also slows heart rate. Although the role of digoxin in the management of patients with CHF and normal sinus rhythm remained controversial for nearly 200 years, studies have demonstrated its efficacy in the management of patients with CHF. In the Randomized Assessment of the (effect of digoxin) on Inhibitors of the Angiotensin Converting Enzyme (RADIANCE) trial, patients chronically treated with digoxin were randomly assigned to having their digoxin maintained or replaced by placebo. Those patients in whom digoxin was withdrawn demonstrated increased hospitalizations for worsening heart failure and enhanced heart failure symptoms. In the digoxin trial, 6800 patients with mild to moderate CHF were randomly assigned to receive either digoxin or placebo while receiving baseline therapy with a diuretic and an ACE inhibitor. Although treatment with digoxin did not affect survival, it significantly reduced the risk of hospitalization for worsening heart failure. Therefore, we use digoxin in most patients with symptomatic heart failure. However, important caveats regarding the therapy of digoxin should be kept in mind: (1) digoxin should not be loaded except in patients with atrial fibrillation; (2) the digoxin level should be maintained less than 1.0 mg per dL; (3) levels should be measured periodically if changes are seen in renal function, the electrocardiogram, or symptoms; (4) patients taking medications affecting digoxin levels—including antibiotics, antiarrhythmic drugs, and spironolactone—should have their levels closely monitored; and (5) digoxin dosages should be decreased in elderly patients, in

---

*Not FDA approved for this indication.

patients with cachexia, or in patients with increasing renal dysfunction.

With the exception of digoxin, oral inotropic agents have not proved safe or effective in patients with chronic CHF. However, intravenous inotropic agents play a key role in the therapy of patients hospitalized for worsening heart failure. Three intravenous inotropic agents are FDA approved for the therapy of acute exacerbations of CHF: the adrenergic agonist dobutamine (Dobutrex), the phosphodiesterase inhibitor milrinone (Primacor), and the dopaminergic/adrenergic agonist dopamine (Intropin). Dobutamine effects a marked increase in contractility, has a short half-life, and has a relatively low cost. Milrinone increases myocardial contractility and also effects marked peripheral vasodilatation; however, it has a longer half-life and is substantially more costly than dobutamine. At low doses (<5 µg per kg per minute), dopamine activates dopaminergic receptors in the renal and splanchnic vasculature and, in so doing, improves renal diuresis and splanchnic blood flow. However, at higher doses it increases cardiac contractility via activation of beta$_1$-adrenergic receptors but also activates alpha$_1$-adrenergic receptors in the peripheral vasculature. Thus, the pharmacologic effect of high dosages of dopamine is a marked increase in afterload accompanied by a decrease in cardiac output. In patients with disease refractory to either dobutamine or milrinone, the two can be used together to take advantage of synergistic actions. Furthermore, we often administer dobutamine in combination with low dosages of dopamine, particularly in patients with right-sided heart failure and substantial ascites or peripheral edema. Alternatively, some physicians administer potent vasodilators, including intravenous nitrates and nitroprusside (Nipride), in the therapy of patients hospitalized with acute exacerbations of worsening heart failure. This approach appears particularly useful in patients with elevated peripheral vascular resistance. However, the relative usefulness of these two approaches (i.e., inotropes vs. vasodilators) remains undefined. Similarly, clinical trials have not established the relative efficacies of dobutamine and milrinone, and thus physicians usually choose between these two agents on the basis of their anecdotal experience.

Several other pharmacologic agents have been used with varying success in patients with CHF. Calcium channel blockers have generally been found to be of little benefit in patients with CHF. Indeed, diltiazem (Cardizem) was associated with increased mortality when used in patients with CHF. The only calcium channel blocker that has been shown to be safe in patients with CHF is amlodipine (Norvasc). Therefore, it is the agent of choice in patients with CHF and ongoing ischemic heart disease. A single trial has suggested a beneficial effect of amlodipine in patients with idiopathic CHF; however, this finding is currently undergoing further clinical evaluation. Antiarrhythmic therapy has also been shown to have little benefit in the management of patients with CHF, inasmuch as most of these agents have

significant proarrhythmic effects and they often have negative inotropic properties. However, amiodarone (at low dosage) has proved useful in some patients with recalcitrant atrial fibrillation. In patients with documented sustained ventricular tachycardia or fibrillation, internal cardiac defibrillators (ICDs) have been beneficial. However, the role of ICDs in the therapy for patients with nonsustained ventricular tachycardia is under active investigation. The use of anticoagulative agents, particularly warfarin (Coumadin), has engendered considerable controversy. Although there are no objective data supporting the use of warfarin in patients with heart failure and normal sinus rhythm, we administer warfarin in patients with a dilated cardiomyopathy and an ejection fraction less than 30% unless contraindicated by a history of a bleeding diathesis, gastrointestinal or cerebral hemorrhages, advanced age, or work or hobbies that involve potential risk of bleeding. However, heart failure specialists agree that patients with a dilated cardiomyopathy and atrial fibrillation should be treated with warfarin unless specific contraindications exist. Finally, all patients with CHF should receive an influenza vaccination and the pneumococcal vaccine.

In summary, neurohormonal modulators have been accepted as important new therapies for the treatment of CHF. In combination with diuretics and digoxin, they form the cornerstones of therapy for this important disease. However, despite the fact that far more medications for treating CHF are available now than were in the 1980s, the rates of morbidity and mortality associated with this disease remain at an unacceptable level. For this reason, we feel strongly that patients should be given the opportunity to receive new and novel therapies through participation in clinical investigations. A review of all heart failure clinical trials in the 1980s and 1990s reveals that the lowest mortality rate was seen in patients enrolled in the placebo groups of clinical trials. However, the mortality rate seen in the active treatment groups in these trials was still substantially lower than that reported in the Framingham population. Currently, several novel agents are undergoing clinical investigation in the United States. Perhaps the most interesting is etanercept, a recombinant-produced soluble receptor for tumor necrosis factor (TNF). Because TNF can induce the development of CHF in experimental animals and its levels are directly related to disease severity in humans, inhibition of TNF activity by etanercept would intuitively be beneficial for the failing heart. Indeed, several phase I and II studies have demonstrated the safety of etanercept in patients with CHF and suggest salutorious effects on both cardiac hemodynamics and heart failure symptoms. In addition, ongoing clinical trials are assessing the efficacy of a diverse array of therapeutic options, including angiotensin receptor antagonists, novel inotropic agents, and biventricular pacing in the treatment of patients with CHF. It is hoped that in the next millennium, new technologies that can actually reverse the disease process rather than simply providing palliation will be developed.

INFECTIVE ENDOCARDITIS

method of
NAVIN M. AMIN, M.D.
Kern Medical Center
Bakersfield, California

EPIDEMIOLOGIC CHANGES

Infective endocarditis denotes microbial infection of the cardiac valves and, less frequently, infection of the mural endocardium or of septal defects.

At present, infective endocarditis accounts for 1 case per 1000 hospital admissions. The age of patients with endocarditis has increased. In the preantibiotic era, the average age of patients with endocarditis was 32 to 39 years old; currently more than half the cases occur in patients older than 60 years of age. Men are affected twice as often as women; the ratio increases to 5:1 in men older than 60 years of age.

Three major changes have been seen in endocarditis:

1. Pattern of infective organisms: early in the antibiotic era group A *Streptococci* (β hemolyticus), *Pneumococci*, *Gonococci*, and *Meningococci* used to be the predominant pathogens. *Streptococcus viridans*, *Staphylococcus*, and gram-negative organisms are more common at present.

2. Signs and symptoms: peripheral lesions involving skin, nails, and eyes—petechiae, subungual hemorrhage, Janeway's lesions, Osler's nodes, or Roth's spots, once characteristic of endocarditis, are seen in less than 5% cases today.

3. Surgical procedures: can both be a "cause" and "cure" of endocarditis. Prosthetic valves inserted to improve mechanically malfunctioning valves can predispose recipients to endocarditis. Surgery, on the other hand, can be lifesaving in patients with refractory congestive heart failure (CHF), or resistant infection.

FORMS OF ENDOCARDITIS

Endocarditis has been classified as acute or subacute on the basis of its clinical course. The acute form evolves over days to weeks and is diagnosed within 2 weeks. It is usually caused by such invasive organisms as *Staphylococcus aureus*, *Streptococcus pneumoniae*, group A streptococci, *Neisseria gonorrhoeae*, *Haemophilus influenzae*, *Salmonella*, other Enterobacteriaceae, and *Pseudomonas aeruginosa*. Clinically acute endocarditis is associated with high fever, systemic toxicity, and leukocytosis with rapid destruction of the valves. It carries high morbidity and mortality.

Subacute endocarditis has a duration of more than 6 weeks and an indolent course. The most common agents are streptococcal species, *Streptococcus viridans* being the most predominant: *Enterococcus*, HACEK *(Haemophilus, Actinobacillus, Cardiobacterium, Eikenella, Kingella)* organisms, fungi, and *Coxiella burnetii*. Clinically subacute endocarditis is associated with prolonged, low-grade fever (FUO), night sweats, weight loss, and vague symptoms like generalized weakness, lethargy, and myalgia.

Infective endocarditis can also be grouped into three categories:

1. *Native valve endocarditis* usually develops when there is structural damage to the heart valve. Rheumatic/syphilitic valvular disease is responsible in 20 to 40% of the cases. The mitral valve is involved in 85% and the aortic valve is affected in 50% of the cases. In elderly patients, 30% of cases occurs with degenerative cardiac lesions such as calcified mitral valve annulus and calcified nodular lesions secondary to atherosclerosis or post-myocardial infarction thrombus. Twenty percent of cases with mitral valve prolapse (with thickened leaflets or significant mitral regurgitation) and obstructive cardiomyopathy can predispose to endocarditis. In 6 to 25% of cases, congenital heart disease is a risk factor as is evident in ventricular septal defect (VSD), patent ductus arteriosus (PDA), tetralogy of Fallot, or coarction of aorta. It can also occur with stenotic or regurgitant valve such as bicuspid aortic valve and pulmonary stenosis. Endocarditis is rare in patients with atrial septal defect (secundum type) because of low pressure gradient between the atria.

Finally there is a group of patients without any structural defect who are susceptible to endocarditis. Tricuspid valve endocarditis can develop in intravenous drug abusers and immunocompromised patients (with chronic renal failure, severe burns, chronic active hepatitis, collagen vascular disease, or neoplasm involving the pancreas, lung, or stomach).

2. *Prosthetic valve endocarditis* (PVE) at present constitutes 20% of all cases of endocarditis. It occurs in 2 to 4% of patients with prosthetic valve. It can be early or late. Early PVE occurs within 60 days of the valve replacement and predominant organisms are *Staphylococcus epidermidis* and *S. aureus*. In the case of late onset endocarditis, which occurs after 2 months, *Streptococcus viridans* are the main offending pathogens.

3. *Nosocomial endocarditis* commonly affects elderly and serious ill, hospitalized patients. These individuals are subjected to invasive procedures such as insertion of central venous pressure, monitoring lines, hyperalimentation catheters, or intracardiac pacemaker wires that represent nidus of infection. See Table 1 for a summary of factors predisposing to endocarditis.

MICROBIOLOGY

Any microorganism can cause endocarditis (Table 2). Certain pathogens have increased ability to adhere to valvular leaflets, thereby establishing infection. About 70% of the cases are caused by streptococci and staphylococci.

Staphylococci are encountered predominately in intravenous drug abuse (IVDA), in early PVE, in immunocompromised host, and in nosocomial endocarditis. *S. viridans* is more commonly seen in native valve endocarditis and in late PVE. Gram-negative bacilli commonly cause right-sided endocarditis as in IVDA and in patients with intravascular catheters.

About 10% of patients with endocarditis will have negative blood culture after 48 to 72 hours of incubation. Factors that produce culture-negative endocarditis are (1) antibiotic therapy before cultures are obtained; (2) a low level of bacteremia (common with right-sided and mural endocarditis); (3) infection with fastidious or nutritionally deficient bacteria that require prolonged cultures (2 to 3 weeks) or additional supplements (e.g., pyridoxine) for growth; this group includes HACEK organisms, *Brucella*, and nutritionally deficient streptococci; (4) nonbacterial infectious agents such as fungi, viruses, spirochetes, *Rickettsia*, *Chlamydia*, or parasites; and (5) noninfectious causes:

TABLE 1. **Factors Predisposing to Endocarditis**

Native Valve Endocarditis

Structural Damage	No Structural Damage
Rheumatic valvular disease	IVDA
Syphilitic valvular disease	Immunocompromised
Degenerative	
Calcified mitral/aortic valve	
Calcified post-MI thrombus	
Mitral valve prolapse	
IHSS	
Congenital heart disease	
Regurgitant or stenotic valve, bicuspid aortic valve, PS, Ebstein's anomaly, Marfan's syndrome	
High-pressure shunt, VSD, PDA, coarctation of aorta, tetralogy of Fallot	

Prosthetic Valve Endocarditis

Early (<2 mo)	Late (> 2 mo)
S. epidermidis	S. viridans
S. aureus	

Noscomial Endocarditis
Invasive procedures

Abbreviations: IHSS = Idiopathic hypertrophic subaortic stenosis; IVDA = intravenous drug abuse; MI = myocardial infarction; PDA = patent ductus arteriosus; PS = pulmonary stenosis; VSD = ventricular septal defect.

Adapted with permission from Amin NM: Infective endocarditis. Consultant *34*(3):319–343, 1994.

left atrial myxoma, Libman-Sacks endocarditis, systemic lupus erythematosus, Löffler's hypereosinophilic endocarditis, carcinoid syndromes, and marantic endocarditis associated with malignancies of the pancreas, stomach, or lung.

CLINICAL MANIFESTATIONS

The clinical manifestations of infective endocarditis are extremely diverse and can mimic pulmonary, neurologic, renal, or bones and joint disease. The classic manifestations of fever, heart murmur, splenomegaly, and petechiae of the skin and the mucous membranes help establish the diagnosis.

The onset may be abrupt or insidious. The early manifestations may be vague flulike symptoms that occur within 3 weeks after an invasive procedure. The patient may complain of malaise, fatigue, weakness, myalgia, arthralgia, low-grade fever, night sweats, or weight loss. Anorexia is almost universal. When the onset is acute, as in intravenous (IV) drug abuse, prosthetic valve endocarditis, or nosocomial endocarditis, there may be evidence of severe infection heralded by high fever (90 to 95%), shaking chills and rigors, or, more ominous, symptoms of frank heart failure or embolic phenomena.

In elderly patients, diagnosis is often delayed because 5% of the cases may not have fever or are admitted with diagnosis of cerebral vascular accident (CVA), pneumonia, occult neoplasm, degenerative joint disease, or osteomyelitis. Always consider infective endocarditis in elderly patients who have fever and associated unexplained CHF, CVA, renal failure, weight loss, anemia, new-onset murmur, or confusional state.

In 85% of the cases, cardiac manifestations include a heart murmur. In right-sided endocarditis and mural infection, murmur is absent. A new or changing murmur (usually of aortic regurgitation) occurs in 5 to 10% of the patients and is a very helpful diagnostic sign. Persistent or progressive CHF is indicative of serious complication that carries a high mortality rate.

Peripheral cutaneous manifestations take a variety of forms: skin pallor due to secondary anemia; petechiae found in 20 to 40% of cases concentrated on the conjunctiva, palate, buccal mucosa, and distal extremities; clubbing of nails in 10 to 20% if infection is long-standing; splinter hemorrhages as linear, red-to-brown streaks in the middle of the nail bed of fingers and toes; Osler's nodes (5 to 20% cases), which are small, painful, tender, purplish, subcutaneous nodules in pads of fingers and toes; and Janeway's lesions, which are small macular, painless, erythematous or hemorrhagic plaques on the palms of hands or soles of feet.

Ocular manifestations include Roth's spots, which occur in 5% of the patients and appear as oval or boat-shaped, white or pale retinal lesions surrounded by hemorrhage and located near the optic disk. In a few cases there may

TABLE 2. **Microbiology of Infective Endocarditis**

Type of Infection	Specific Associated Risk Factors
Bacterial	
Gram Positive	
Streptococci (40–60%)	
S. viridans, S. pneumoniae, S. bovis, S. pyogenes, S. sanguis	NVE, late onset PVE
Enterococci (Group D) (5–20%)	
S. faecalis, S. faecium, S. durans	Gastrointestinal malignancies
Staphylococci (17–40%)	IVDA, early PVE
S. aureus, S. epidermidis	IVDA, early PVE
Diphtheroids	
Listeria	
Gram Negative	
Cultured Easily	
Pseudomonas aeruginosa, Serratia marcescens, Salmonella, Proteus mirabilis, Shigella, Providencia, Enterobacter, N. gonorrhoeae, Escherichia coli	IVDA, immunocompromised, nosocomial endocarditis
Difficult to Culture (HACEK) (1–10%)	
Heamophilus, Actinobacillus, Cardiobacterium, Eikenella, Kingella, Brucella, Legionella	
Nonbacterial	
Fungi (2–4%)	
Candida, Aspergillus, Histoplasma, Coccidioides, Blastomyces	IVDA, PVE, cardiac surgery, IV catheters, immunosuppressed
Viruses	
Coxsackie B, adenovirus	
Spirochetes	
Borrelia burgdorferi	Tick bite
Spirillum minus	Rat bite
Rickettsiae	
Coxiella burnetii	Infected livestock or unpasteurized milk
Chlamydia	
C. psittaci	Infected birds
Parasites	
Trypanosoma cruzi (Chagas' disease)	Kissing bug bite

Abbreviations: IVDA = intravenous drug abuse; NVE = native valve endocarditis; PVE = prosthetic valve endocarditis.

Adapted with permission from Amin NM: Infective endocarditis. Consultant *34*(3):319–343, 1994.

be presence of cotton-wool exudates, petechiae, or flame-shaped hemorrhages.

Embolization can occur in 15 to 35% of cases. A cerebral emboli may produce hemiplegia, monoplegia, aphasia, or unilateral blindness. Mesenteric emboli can result in acute abdominal pain, ileus, or melena. Splenic emboli may cause left upper quadrant pain that radiates to the left shoulder or chest with a small pleural effusion or splenic frictional rub. Flank pain with hematuria indicates a renal infarction. Peripheral arterial emboli may produce pain or gangrene. Large arterial occlusions are frequently seen with fungal endocarditis. Very rarely, emboli to coronary arteries cause acute myocardial infarction, myocardial abscess, or mycotic aneurysm.

Neurologic complications (30 to 40%) include CVA from embolization, mycotic aneurysm causing cerebral or subdural hemorrhage and seizure, and brain abscess or toxic encephalopathy with confusion and nonspecific obtundation.

Renal manifestations are accompanied by microscopic or frank hematuria secondary to renal infarct, diffuse membranoproliferative glomerulonephritis, focal embolic glomerulonephritis, or renal abscess.

Splenomegaly occurs in 25 to 45% of the patients. This is more common in subacute than in acute endocarditis.

DIAGNOSIS

Infective endocarditis may mimic any systemic disorder. For this reason and because of its high morbidity and mortality, keep this disorder in mind whenever you encounter a high-risk patient with an unexplained fever, constitutional symptoms, or multiple systemic involvement with a changing or new heart murmur. A high index of suspicion to consider endocarditis in certain clinical situations will be very helpful: (1) IV drug abusers with high fever; (2) elderly patients with nonspecific, vague symptoms with a calcified mitral valve annulus; (3) unknown source of embolization; and (4) certain virulent infections with organism-like *Staphylococcus* or *Enterococcus*.

A thorough history, complete examination, and laboratory tests should establish the correct diagnosis. Various laboratory abnormalities in infective endocarditis are outlined in Table 3.

A baseline electrocardiogram (EKG) is helpful to detect chamber enlargement or possible conduction defect that may indicate underlying valvular or congenital anomalies. However, later development of first-degree atrioventricular (AV) block, new bundle branch block, or new ectopic beats may indicate a myocardial abscess, especially in aortic valve endocarditis.

Echocardiography (transesophageal [TEE], M-mode, two-dimensional, or Doppler) can confirm the diagnosis, detect complications, and help assess the prognosis. The echocardiogram can detect vegetations larger than 2 to 3 mm on mitral or aortic valves. Sensitivity in detecting vegetations is about 87 to 90% with TEE, 30 to 75% with M-mode, 40 to 50% with two-dimensional, and 50% with Doppler echocardiography. False-positive results are seen with old healed vegetations, myxomatous valvular degeneration, arterial myxoma, or a thrombus.

Complications such as torn or perforated valves, ruptured chordae tendineae, myocardial abscess, or pericardiac effusion that may require surgical intervention can be detected by echocardiogram. Large-sized vegetations in the left side of the heart or in the aortic valve, or myocardial abscess, suggest a relatively poor prognosis and surgery may be indicated.

TABLE 3. **Laboratory Abnormalities in Endocarditis**

Hematologic
  Leucocytosis
  Anemia of chronic disorder
  Thrombocytopenia (10% SBE)
  Elevated ESR
Urine analysis
  Hematuria, microscopic
  Proteinuria
Cardiac abnormality
  ECG: chamber enlargement, conduction defect
Chest x-ray
  Cardiomegaly
  Evidence of congestive heart failure
  Nodular infiltrate (staphylococcal endocarditis)
Diagnostic gold standards
  Echocardiography (transesophageal preferred)
  Three sets of blood (embolus) cultures
Immunologic abnormalities
  Rheumatoid factor (disappears after treatment)
  Hypergammaglobulinemia
  Cryoglobulinemia
  Circulating immune complexes
  Low complement levels

Abbreviations: ECG = electrocardiogram; ESR = erythrocyte sedimentation rate; SBE = subacute bacterial endocarditis.

Serial blood cultures are required to establish the diagnosis by isolating the offending bacterium or fungus. Minimum of three blood samples should be drawn 30 to 60 minutes apart before initiating empirical antibiotic therapy. If the patient has taken an antibiotic in the preceding 2 weeks, two or three additional sets of blood cultures should be taken. Cultures of arterial blood offer no additional advantage over venous blood. Ninety percent of the blood cultures become positive within 7 days of incubation. Negative blood cultures are likely to be seen in patients who have received prior antibiotics or who have endocarditis caused by fastidious gram-negative (HACEK) bacilli, fungi, or nutritionally deficient streptococci. Be sure to alert the microbiology laboratory that you suspect endocarditis, and include a report for prolonged incubation for 2 weeks.

In fungal endocarditis in which there is embolization of large arteries, a culture of the removed embolus can establish the diagnosis. Serologic studies can be helpful in fungal infection (histoplasmosis or coccidioidomycosis) or when rickettsial (Q fever) *Legionella* or *Chlamydia* infections are suspected.

TREATMENT OF INFECTIVE ENDOCARDITIS

The main goal is to eradicate the infecting pathogens as quickly as possible to reduce the risks of morbidity and mortality. This can be achieved with antibiotic therapy or surgical intervention, or both.

Antibiotic Therapy

Whenever you are using antibiotics to treat infective endocarditis keep in mind the following guidelines: (1) use parental antibiotics to sustain bactericidal activity; (2) employ bactericidal antimicrobials for complete eradication of the pathogens. Syner-

TABLE 4. **Antibiotic Regimens for Bacterial Endocarditis**

Infecting Organism	Antibiotic	Dosage, Route, and Frequency	Duration in Wk
Penicillin-susceptible *Streptococcus viridans,* and *S. bovis* (MIC <0.2 µg/dL)	*Preferred Regimen* Penicillin G	12–16 million U/d IV in 6 divided doses	4
	or Penicillin G *PLUS*	12–16 million U/d IV in 6 divided doses	4
	Gentamicin	1 mg/kg IM or IV q 8 h	2
	or Penicillin G *PLUS* Gentamicin	Dosages same as above regimen	2
	or Ceftriaxone	2 gm IV or IM q 24 h	4
	Alternative Regimen Vancomycin	0.5 gm IV q 6 h	4
Relative penicillin-resistant streptococci (MIC > 0.2 µg/dL)	*Preferred Regimen* Penicillin G *PLUS*	20–30 million U/d IV in 6 divided doses	4
	Gentamicin	1 mg/kg IV or IM q 8 h	4
	Alternative Regimen Vancomycin	0.5 gm IV q 6 h	4
Staphylococcus epidermidis	*Native Valve* Vancomycin	0.5 gm IV q 6 h	4
	Prosthetic Valve Vancomycin *PLUS*	0.5 gm IV q 6 h	4–6
	Gentamicin	1 mg/kg IV or IM q 8 h	2
	or Rifampin	300 mg PO/IV q 12 h	2
Enterococcus (S. faecalis, S. faecium, S. durans)	*Preferred Regimen* Penicillin G *PLUS*	20–30 million U/d IV in 6 divided doses	4–6
	Gentamicin	1 mg/kg IM or IV q 8 h	4–6
	or Ampicillin *PLUS*	2 gm IV q 4 h	4–6
	Gentamicin	1 mg/kg IM or IV q 8 h	4–6
	Alternative Regimen Vancomycin *PLUS*	0.5 gm q 6 h	4–6
	Gentamicin	1 mg/kg IM or IV q 8 h	4–6
Staphylococcus aureus (methicillin sensitive)	*Preferred Regimen* Naficillin or Oxacillin *OR*	2 gm IV q 4 h	4–6
	Naficillin or Oxacillin plus	2 gm IV q 4 h	4–6
	Gentamicin or plus	1 mg/kg IM or IV q 8 h	2
	Rifampin	300 mg PO/IV q 12 h	2
	Alternative Regimen Cefazolin *OR*	2 gm q 6 h	4–6
	Vancomycin	0.5 gm q 6 h	4–6
S. aureus (methicillin resistant [MRSA])	Vancomycin *PLUS*	0.5 gm q 6 h	4–6
	Gentamicin *OR / PLUS*	1 mg/kg IM or IV q 8 h	2
	Rifampin	300 mg PO/IV q 12 h	2
"HACEK Group" *(Haemophilus, Actinobacillus, Cardiobacterium, Eikenella, Kingella)*	Ampicillin *OR*	2 gm IV q 6 h	4
	Ampicillin *PLUS*	2 gm IV q 6 h	4
	Gentamicin *OR*	1 mg/kg IM or IV q 8 h	4
	Ceftriaxone	2 gm IV q 24 h	4
Culture negative	Vancomycin *PLUS*	0.5 gm q 6 h	6
	Gentamicin	1 mg/kg IM or IV q 8 h	6

Abbreviations: MIC = minimum inhibitory concentration.
Adapted with permission from Amin NM: Infective endocarditis. Consultant *34*(3):319–343, 1994.

gistic bactericidal activity is achieved with combination therapy such as ampicillin and aminoglycosides in treatment of entercoccal endocarditis; (3) tailor the drug regimen and prescribe appropriate duration of course, 2 to 6 weeks, to prevent relapse; (4) monitor the bactericidal activity of the antibiotic by determining the minimum inhibitory concentration (MIC) and the minimum bactericidal concentration (MBC) against the infecting organisms; and (5) initiate antibiotic therapy as quickly as possible. When endocarditis is severe and/or complicated, institute empirical treatment immediately with antibiotic effective against S. aureus and enterococci. Once a specific organism is identified, appropriate bactericidal antibiotic should be used.

Most streptococci other than entercocci are exquisitively sensitive to penicillin. If MIC is less than 0.2 μg per mL, high-dose penicillin alone or in combination with either gentamicin (Garamycin) or streptomycin or ceftriaxone (Rocephin) can be used for 4 weeks. If the MIC is below 0.1 μg per mL treat for 2 weeks. If MIC is greater than 0.2 μg per mL or MBC:MIC ratio exceeds 10:1, as it occurs in 15 to 20% of cases with S. viridans infection, use higher

dose of penicillin with aminoglycoside. In penicillin-allergic patients, vancomycin (Vancocin) is the best alternative with or without aminoglycoside (Table 4).

In enterococcal endocarditis, ampicillin is recommended in combination with an aminoglycoside. Gentamicin is preferred as 40% of the isolates are resistant to streptomycin. In penicillin-allergic patients, vancomycin with an aminoglycoside is the best choice.

In S. aureus infection semisynthetic penicillin or first-generation cephalosporins are the agents of first choice. Addition of gentamicin or rifampin* during the first few days rapidly reduces bacteremia. Vancomycin is recommended for patients allergic to penicillin or if the organism is methicillin resistant (MRSA.) Addition of rifampin, although controversial, is recommended in patients demonstrating poor bactericidal activity during therapy with beta-lactams or vancomycin and for patients with suppurative complication, such as a valve ring abscess.

Endocarditis with S. epidermidis, which commonly develops on prosthetic valves, is ideally treated with

*Not FDA approved for this indication.

TABLE 5. **Preprocedural Antibiotic Prophylaxis for At Risk Patients**

Type of Procedure and Situation	Antibiotic	Dosage, Route, and Frequency
Dental, oral respiratory tract, and esophageal procedures		
■ Standard prophylaxis	Amoxicillin	2 gm PO 1 h before procedure
■ Patient unable to take oral medication	Ampicillin	2 gm IM/IV within 30 min before procedure
■ Patient allergic to penicillin	Clindamycin (Cleocin) or	600 mg PO 1 h before procedure
	Cefadroxil (Duricef) or	2 gm PO 1 h before procedure
	Cephalexin (Keflex) or	2 gm PO 1 h before procedure
	Azithromycin (Zithromax) or	500 mg PO 1 h before procedure
	Clarithromycin (Biaxin)	500 mg PO 1 h before procedure
■ Patient allergic to penicillin and unable to take oral medication	Clindamycin (Cleocin) or	600 mg IV within 30 min of starting procedure
	Cefazolin (Ancef) or	1 gm IV within 30 min of starting procedure
	Vancomycin (Vancocin)	1 gm IV over 1–2 h within 60 min of starting procedure
Genitourinary/gastrointestinal procedures		
■ Moderate-risk patient	Amoxicillin or	2 gm PO 1 h before procedure
	Ampicillin	2 gm IM/IV within 30 min of starting procedure
■ Moderate-risk penicillin-allergic patient	Vancomycin	1 gm IV over 1–2 h infusion completed within 30–60 min of starting procedure
■ High-risk patient	Ampicillin PLUS	2 gm IM/IV given within 30 min of starting procedure
	Gentamicin	1.5 mg/kg given within 30 min of starting procedure
	6 h later	
	Ampicillin or	1 gm IM or IV
	Amoxicillin	1 gm PO
■ High-risk penicillin-allergic patients	Vancomycin PLUS	1 gm IV over 1–2 h
	Gentamicin	1.5 mg/kg given within 30 min of starting the procedure

Adapted from Dajani AS et al: Prevention of bacterial endocarditis: Recommendations by the American Heart Association. JAMA 277(22):1794–1801, 1997.

TABLE 6. **Indications for Endocardial Prophylaxis**

Cardiac Conditions	Procedures
High-risk category	Dental
Prosthetic valve	Dental extraction
Previous endocarditis	Peridontal procedures;
Complex cyanotic disease	surgery, scaling, root
Tetralogy of Fallot, single	planing
ventricle	Dental implant placement
Surgically conducted	Subgingival placement of
systemic-pulmonary	antibiotic fibers
shunt	Intraligamentary local
Moderate-risk category	anesthetic injection
Congenital heart disease	Cleaning of teeth or implants
VSD, PDA, AS, PS	Respiratory
Acquired valvular	Tonsillectomy/adenoidectomy
dysfunction	Rigid bronchoscopy
Rheumatic/syphilitic	Gastrointestinal
Hypertrophic	Sclerotherapy
cardiomyopathy	Esophageal stricture dilation
MVP with MR or thickened	ERCP with biliary obstruction
leaflets	Biliary tract surgery
	Surgery involving intestinal
	mucosa
	Genitourinary
	Prostatic surgery
	Cystoscopy
	Urethral dilation
	Septic abortion

Abbreviations: AS = aortic stenosis; ERCP = endoscopic retrograde cholangiopancreatography; MVP = mitral valve prolapse; MR = mitral regurgitation; PDA = patent ductus arteriosus; PS = pulmonary stenosis; VSD = ventricular septal defect.

Adapted from Dajani AS, et al.: Prevention of bacterial endocarditis: Recommendations by the American Heart Association. JAMA *277*(22):1794–1801, 1997.

vancomycin and rifampin.* An aminoglycoside may be added for 2 weeks.

Gram-negative infections causing high mortality are best treated with broad-spectrum penicillin or, preferably, a third-generation cephalosporin with an aminoglycoside. In most of these patients, valve replacement is necessary.

Surgical Interventions

About 25% of patients with severe or complicated endocarditis undergo surgery. The chief indications for surgery are (1) refractory moderate or severe CHF; (2) perivalvular invasion or myocardial abscess as evident by persistent fever despite antibiotics or electrocardiographic changes of conduction defects; (3) systemic or arterial embolization; (4) fungal endocarditis; (5) PVE of early onset; (6) large bulky vegetations that increase risk of CHF; (7) persistent infection (particularly with gram-negative bacilli) that does not respond to 7 to 10 days of antibiotic therapy; and (8) staphylococcal endocarditis in IV drug abusers that does not respond to antimicrobials.

Prevention of Bacterial Endocarditis

Transient bacteremia that develops after a variety of manipulations or surgical procedures in patients

*Not FDA approved for this indication.

with structural heart defects causes endocarditis. Prophylactic antibiotics in this situation can be highly effective when given before the procedure. Administration of these agents only once is required 30 minutes to 2 hours before the procedure (Table 5).

In choosing prophylactic therapy, consider the following questions (Table 6):

- Is your patient at increased risk for endocarditis with underlying structural defect?
- Is there a high risk that the procedure will produce bacteremia with organisms that cause endocarditis, such as *S. viridans* infection with oral cavity procedures, or enterococcal with gastrointestinal, or genitourinary procedures?

Antibiotic prophylaxis is recommended for patients with VSD, PDA, pulmonary or aortic stenosis, tetralogy of Fallot, or coarctation of aorta. Such therapy is needed for patients with rheumatic or syphilitic valvular defects, prosthetic valves, calcified valves, obstructive cardiomyopathy, or mitral valve prolapse with either regurgitant murmur or with thickened mitral valve leaflets.

Endocarditis prophylaxis is not advised for patients with isolated secundum atrial septal defect or those who have undergone surgical repair for VSD or PDA and who have no residual defect beyond 6 months. The same is true for those who have coronary artery bypass graft, previous rheumatic fever, or Kawasaki disease without any valve dysfunction.

TABLE 7. **Endocardial Prophylaxis Not Recommended**

Cardiac Conditions	Procedures
Isolated secundum ASD	Dental
Surgical repair of ASD,	Restorative dentistry
VSD, PDA (without	Local anesthetic injections
residue > 6 mo)	Intracanal treatment
Previous CABG surgery	Postoperative suture removal
MVP without valvular	Oral impression/radiograph
dysfunction	Fluoride treatment
Functional murmur	Shedding of primary teeth
Kawasaki disease without	Respiratory
valvular dysfunction	Endotracheal intubation
Previous rheumatic fever	Fibro-optic bronchoscopy
without valve dysfunction	Tympanostomy tube insertion
Cardiac pacemaker and	Gastrointestinal
implanted defibrillators	TEE*
Cardiac catheterization,	Endoscopy with/without biopsy*
balloon angioplasty	Genitourinary
Coronary stent placement	Vaginal delivery/hysterectomy*
	Cesarian section
	Urethral catheterization
	Uterine dilatation and
	curettage
	Insertion/removal of IUD
	Circumcision

*Prophylaxis optional for high-risk category.

Abbreviations: ASD = atrial septal defect; CABG = coronary artery bypass graft; IUD = intrauterine device; MVP = mitral valve prolapse; PDA = patent ductus arteriosus; TEE = transesophageal echocardiogram; VSD = ventricular septal defect.

Adapted from Dajani AS, et al.: Prevention of bacterial endocarditis: Recommendations by the American Heart Association. JAMA *277*(22):1794–1801, 1997.

Prophylaxis is not recommended for those who have MVP without MR and for persons with cardiac pacemaker or implanted defibrillator (Table 7).

Procedures for which antibiotic prophylaxis is needed are those where transient bacteremia will develop when mucosal surfaces colonized with microorganisms are traumatized. For example, bacteremia may occur following dental manipulation in 80% of cases or 20% of patients after urethral instrumentation. Prophylactic antimicrobials are recommended for high-risk patients who are scheduled to have certain dental, oropharyngeal, gastrointestinal, or genitourinary manipulations.

Standard antibiotic prophylaxis for patients undergoing oral, dental, or upper respiratory tract manipulations include oral amoxicillin. Give clindamycin* (Cleocin), cefadroxil* (Duricef), cephalexin* (Keflex) or azithromycin* (Zithromax) or clarithromycin* (Biaxin) for those who cannot tolerate or are allergic to penicillin.

Parenteral ampicillin is recommended for patients who cannot take oral antibiotics and for those at high risk for infective endorcarditis, such as patients with prosthetic valve, previous endocarditis, or surgical systemic pulmonary shunts. Clindamycin or cefazolin (Ancef) can be used as an alternative. Give vancomycin in patients undergoing gastrointestinal or gastrourinary instrumentation.

It is important to emphasize that as per American Heart Association's recommendations, all prophylatic antibiotics need to be used only once before the procedure. There is no need for additional anitibiotic administration except in high-risk patients undergoing gastrointestinal or gastrourinary manipulation and who are given the ampicillin and gentamicin combination.

---

*Not FDA approved for this indication.

HYPERTENSION

method of
C. VENKATA S. RAM, M.D.
*Texas Blood Pressure Institute and
    University of Texas Southwestern
    Medical Center*
Dallas, Texas

and

ANDREW FENVES, M.D.
*Baylor University Medical Center and
    University of Texas Southwestern
    Medical Center*
Dallas, Texas

Systemic hypertension is one of the most common disorders in clinical practice. Over a lifetime, hypertension develops in most people. Because of widespread awareness of hypertension as a major cardiovascular risk factor, it has become the leading indication for the use of prescription drugs in the United States. Although this is an impressive statistic, hypertension is poorly controlled in many patients. Consequently, hypertension is a frequent cause of morbidity and mortality. Despite its arbitrary nature, hypertension is defined as systolic blood pressure (SBP) of 140 mm Hg or greater and diastolic blood pressure (DBP) of 90 mm Hg or greater. The principal reason for diagnosing and treating hypertension is to reduce the risk of cardiovascular and other related complications. The linear relationship between cardiovascular risk and systemic blood pressure is well recognized. This risk is predictive, independent, and continuous. Therefore, it is useful to follow the classification of blood pressure and hypertension as defined in the Sixth Report of the Joint National Committee on Prevention, Detection, Evaluation, and Treatment of High Blood Pressure, often referred to as the *JNC report*. The classification is shown in Table 1. These criteria are for people older than 18 years of age, based on the average of two or more readings. When SBP and DBP fall into different categories, the higher category should be chosen to make therapeutic decisions. To record the blood pressure accurately, the following methodology should be adopted:

Patients should be comfortably seated, having refrained from tobacco or caffeine consumption for at least 30 minutes before the measurement.

An appropriate cuff (bladder within the cuff should encircle at least 80% of the arm) should be used on all occasions.

If a mercury sphygmomanometer is not available, calibrated aneroid or electronic devices are acceptable.

The first appearance of sound (phase 1) is SBP, and the disappearance of the sounds (phase 5) is the DBP.

Two or more readings taken 2 minutes apart should be averaged.

Under special circumstances, such as in elderly, ill, or symptomatic patients, blood pressure should be measured in the supine and standing positions as well.

On the basis of the initial set of measurements, follow-up recommendations should be made per the JNC report (Table 2).

INITIAL EVALUATION OF THE PATIENT WITH NEWLY DISCOVERED HYPERTENSION

Evaluation of patients with hypertension includes assessment of target organ function/damage, identification of concomitant risk factors (Table 3) and co-morbid conditions (Table 4), and detection of possible secondary forms of hypertension.

TABLE 1. **Classification of Blood Pressure for Adults**

Category	SBP (mm Hg)		DBP (mm Hg)
Optimal	<120	and	<80
Normal	<130	and	<85
High-normal	130–139	or	85–89
Hypertension			
Stage 1	140–159	or	90–99
Stage 2	160–179	or	100–109
Stage 3	≥180	or	≥110

When SBP and DBP fall into different categories, use the higher category.
Abbreviations: DBP = diastolic blood pressure; SBP = systolic blood pressure.

TABLE 2. **Recommendations for Follow-up Based on Initial Blood Pressure Measurements**

Initial Blood Pressure (mm Hg)		
Systolic	Diastolic	Follow-up Recommended
<130	<85	Recheck in 2 years
130–139	85–89	Recheck in 1 year, give lifestyle advice
140–159	90–99	Confirm within 2 months, give lifestyle advice
160–179	100–109	Evaluate/refer to care within 1 month
≥180	≥110	Evaluate/refer to care within 7 days

A complete medical history is an important step in the evaluation and treatment of patients with hypertension. Proper details of medical history should include the following points: family history of hypertension, renal disease, heart disease, stroke, hyperlipidemia, and endocrine/metabolic disorders; duration and degree of hypertension, symptoms of coronary artery disease, heart failure, cerebrovascular disease, peripheral vascular disease, and diabetes; history of tobacco or alcohol consumption; dietary history of sodium, potassium, and fat intake; intake of prescribed, over-the-counter, or illicit drugs that could increase the blood pressure; psychosocial history; results or effects of current/previous antihypertensive therapy; sexual dysfunction; and symptoms suggestive of secondary hypertension.

The physical examination of a patient with newly discovered hypertension should include the following: correct measurement of blood pressure according to the recommendations described earlier; waist and weight measurements; funduscopic examination for hypertensive retinopathy; detection of carotid or peripheral vascular disease; complete cardiopulmonary examination; assessment of neurologic and endocrine function; abdominal examination for bruits and kidney enlargement; and evaluation of extremities for vascular disease, arthritis, and edema. The standing blood pressure should also be measured.

In patients who may exhibit labile or unsteady hypertension or in whom there is considerable discrepancy between blood pressure readings, it is appropriate to obtain ambulatory 24-hour blood pressure recordings with an automatic device to document the degree of hypertension or its variability. For some patients, home blood pressure measurements may be useful in assessing blood pressure control and for tailoring the treatment. When the accuracy of the home blood pressure monitor is in doubt, it should be tested against a standard mercury sphygmomanometer.

Blood pressure measurements obtained outside the physician's office may provide information about the accuracy of the blood pressure readings and can be used to assess the response to treatment and improve patient participation in the treatment program. Although the mercury sphygmomanometer is the most reliable means of measur-

TABLE 3. **Major Cardiovascular Risk Factors in Patients with Hypertension**

Smoking
Dyslipidemia
Diabetes mellitus
Age older than 60 years
Gender (men or postmenopausal women)
Family history of cardiovascular disease

TABLE 4. **Clinical Risk Factors for Stratification of Patients with Hypertension**

Heart diseases
Stroke or transient ischemic attack
Nephropathy
Peripheral arterial disease
Retinopathy

ing the blood pressure, it is not possible to apply this method for home use. Therefore, either an electronic device or an aneroid sphygmomanometer is acceptable.

INITIAL LABORATORY TESTS

Certain "routine" laboratory tests are recommended in the initial evaluation and treatment of hypertension. These include a complete blood cell count; blood chemistry profiles; electrolyte, glucose, and lipid measurements; and an electrocardiogram. On the basis of clinical need, additional tests such as creatinine clearance, microalbuminuria, and thyroid studies and an echocardiogram can be obtained.

Further special testing is indicated when a secondary (identifiable) cause of hypertension is suspected. The important subject of secondary hypertension is discussed later in this article.

MANAGEMENT OF HYPERTENSION

The overall initial management of hypertension should be based on the risk stratification (Tables 5 and 6) proposed by the JNC. The aim of treating hypertension is to prevent its complications and reduce the associated morbidity and mortality. This goal is achieved by maintaining SBP below 140 mm Hg and DBP below 90 mm Hg. The published results of the Hypertension Optimal Treatment (HOT) trial suggest that a further reduction of DBP to 80 mm Hg or lower could be highly cardioprotective, especially in diabetic patients. Other concomitant cardiovascular risk factors must also be controlled at the same time. For most patients with uncomplicated hypertension, lifestyle modifications are strongly recommended as the initial step in managing hypertension. Although we realize that lifestyle changes may not be satisfactory, they often complement the effects of antihypertensive drug therapy. The following nonpharmacologic modalities, either singly or in combination, have been shown to be helpful in the treatment of hypertension.

TABLE 5. **Risk Stratification in Hypertension**

Risk group A
　No risk factors
　No target organ disease/clinical cardiovascular disease
Risk group B
　At least one risk factor, not including diabetes
　No target organ disease/clinical cardiovascular disease
Risk group C
　Target organ disease/clinical cardiovascular disease or diabetes
　With or without other risk factors

TABLE 6. **Treatment Strategies and Risk Stratification in Hypertension**

Blood Pressure Stages (mm Hg)	Risk Group A	Risk Group B	Risk Group C
High-normal (130–139/85–89)	Lifestyle modification	Lifestyle modification	Drug therapy* Lifestyle modification
Stage 1 (140–159/90–99)	Lifestyle modification (up to 12 months)	Lifestyle modification (up to 6 months)†	Drug therapy Lifestyle modification
Stages 2 and 3 (≥160/≥100)	Drug therapy Lifestyle modification	Drug therapy Lifestyle modification	Drug therapy Lifestyle modification

*For those with heart failure, renal insufficiency, or diabetes.
†For those with multiple risk factors, clinicians should consider drugs as initial therapy plus lifestyle modifications.

Restriction of Sodium Intake

Sodium intake has been linked to blood pressure levels and several prospective studies have demonstrated the value of sodium restriction in the treatment of hypertension. Several clinical trials have shown that a reduction of 100 mmol in sodium intake lowers blood pressure over a variable period of time. Even a moderate restriction of sodium intake may offer therapeutic benefits and reduce the need for high dosages of antihypertensive drugs. Our studies have shown that salt restriction offsets diuretic-induced hypokalemia by limiting the amount of sodium available for exchange with potassium in the distal renal tubule. A substantial amount of the sodium intake is derived from processed food, and therefore the patients should be counseled accordingly. Although alarm has been raised about the dangers of sodium restriction, there is no evidence that a sensible, moderate salt restriction is harmful. A vigorous salt restriction can trigger the renin-angiotensin system (thereby potentially causing coronary ischemia), but this is not a realistic consideration with the modest reduction of sodium intake advocated by the JNC.

Weight Reduction

Obesity (body mass index > 27) correlates with increasing blood pressure levels and is associated with diabetes, dyslipidemia, and coronary mortality. Weight reduction reduces the blood pressure in obese, hypertensive patients and may enhance the efficacy of antihypertensive drug therapy. Therefore, overweight, hypertensive patients should be counseled about caloric restriction and increased physical activity.

Physical Fitness

Blood pressure levels can be reduced by regular physical conditioning such as 20 to 40 minutes of brisk walking daily. Intense physical activity (approximately 50% of maximum oxygen consumption) can produce significant blood pressure reductions. Regular physical activity (aerobic) can lower the blood pressure, enhance weight loss, and modify cardiovascular risk factors.

Moderation of Alcohol Consumption

Alcohol abuse is an important common contributing risk factor for hypertension and also can minimize the effectiveness of antihypertensive drug therapy. Hypertensive patients should be clearly instructed to limit their daily alcohol consumption to no more than 1 ounce of ethanol (720 mL of beer or 300 mL of wine). Women absorb more alcohol than do men; therefore, they should be counseled to limit their alcohol intake to no more than 15 mL (½ ounce) of ethanol per day. Such amounts do not affect hypertension and may even be associated with cardiovascular protection.

Potassium Intake

Inadequate intake of potassium may raise blood pressure levels, and a high potassium intake can improve blood pressure control. Therefore, sufficient intake of potassium (50 to 80 mmol daily), preferably from natural food sources, should be encouraged. Diuretic-induced hypokalemia should always be prevented or treated.

Magnesium and Calcium Intake

Although there is no firm proof that magnesium is directly linked to blood pressure regulation, magnesium deficiency in patients with cardiovascular disorders can be hazardous and should be prevented. Similarly, the calcium–blood pressure connection is not sufficiently established to warrant broad therapeutic recommendations. However, calcium supplementation is suggested in pregnancy and calcium-deficient conditions.

Miscellaneous Considerations

Because of the inconclusive nature of the evidence, no recommendations can be made about the value of omega-3 fatty acids or protein supplementation to treat hypertension. Biofeedback and stress relaxation techniques have received mixed reviews in the published literature, but may provide an adjunct in certain patients. Those who consume tobacco are at a high risk for cardiovascular disease and may not get the full degree of protection from antihypertensive drug therapy. Tobacco avoidance should be emphasized to all patients with hypertension.

All patients with hypertension should be counseled about the previously discussed lifestyle measures, although most will need pharmacologic therapy sooner or later. For those with advanced or complicated, severe hypertension, lifestyle modifications should not delay the implementation of antihypertensive drug therapy.

PHARMACOLOGIC TREATMENT OF HYPERTENSION

There is general agreement and overwhelming evidence to suggest that antihypertensive drug therapy decreases cardiovascular morbidity and mortality. Clear-cut evidence demonstrates that antihypertensive drug therapy protects against congestive heart failure, coronary events, stroke, and progression of renal disease. Furthermore, early treatment prevents progression to more severe hypertension. Sustained blood pressure reduction is beneficial to all patients with hypertension regardless of age, race, or sex.

General Considerations

Most antihypertensive drugs are equally effective in the treatment of hypertension. The only drugs that are not indicated for initial monotherapy are the direct vasodilators, such as hydralazine and minoxidil. A low dose of the drug should be chosen and titrated upward depending the clinical response and the patient's needs. Ideally, a long-acting formulation should be chosen to allow for improved compliance and smooth control of hypertension. An abrupt rise in blood pressure in the morning hours may contribute to cardiovascular and cerebrovascular ischemic events. Therefore, every effort should be made to secure adequate control of hypertension around the clock. A combination of low dosages of two different pharmacologic compounds has been shown to provide excellent blood pressure control while minimizing the dose-dependent side effects. For example, low doses of a diuretic can augment the therapeutic effects of nondiuretic antihypertensive drugs.

Nearly 60% of hypertensive patients respond to any given drug. However, individual patients do not respond in a predictable manner. Thus, the treatment choices should be individualized. If a therapeutic response is not observed with adequate dosing of the first drug, it can be substituted for a different drug. This "substitution approach" is preferable to the old-fashioned, "stepped-care" method. But if the response to the initial choice is only partial, a second (or third) drug from another class should be added in a sequential manner (Figure 1).

As mentioned previously, the goal of therapy is to achieve and maintain an SBP of 140 mm Hg or less and a DBP of 90 mm Hg or less. With gradual reduction in systemic blood pressure, tissue hypoperfusion is unlikely to occur in clinical practice. We believe

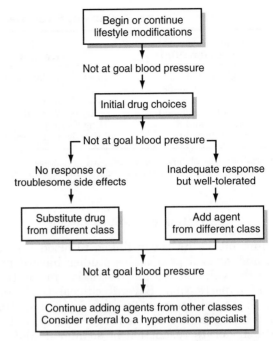

Figure 1. Algorithm for treatment of hypertension.

that myocardial ischemia as a result of blood pressure reduction—the J curve phenomenon—does not occur with gradual treatment of hypertension that follows the current guidelines. Nevertheless, rapid treatment of chronic hypertension should be avoided unless the situation is truly urgent.

Patients with target organ damage should be treated vigorously to prevent progression of the underlying complication. In particular, adequate blood pressure control should be achieved in patients with diabetic renal disease and in African-American patients with nephrosclerosis. In elderly patients with isolated or disproportionate systolic hypertension, the goal of treatment should be an SBP of 140 mm Hg or less.

Although responsiveness to a prescribed drug is not predictable, African-Americans and the elderly are more responsive to therapy with diuretics and calcium antagonists than to drugs that block the renin-angiotensin system. However, if a beta blocker, angiotensin-converting enzyme (ACE) inhibitor, or an angiotensin receptor antagonist is needed for a specific therapeutic advantage, differences in efficacy can be overcome by adding a diuretic or with reduction in salt intake. With any antihypertensive regimen, attention should be given to the effects on quality of life, cost, concomitant diseases and risk factors, and consequences for target organ function. Before choosing a drug, the physician should be familiar with positive as well as negative interactions with concurrent therapies. This clinical point cannot be overemphasized. When, and if, the blood pressure is well controlled for at least a year, careful consideration should be given to decreasing the dosage and the number of antihypertensive drugs. But this step-down approach has to be undertaken with caution and with a supervised follow-up program.

Initial Drugs for Hypertension

As mentioned previously in this chapter, most antihypertensive drugs are equally efficacious and offer important therapeutic benefits to the population at large. Although the JNC guidelines state that "a diuretic or beta-blocker should be chosen" for initial drug therapy, we subscribe to the recognized notion that other classes of drugs can be selected to achieve the goal of therapy. It is true that the large therapeutic trials showing the benefits of cardiovascular and stroke protection used a diuretic- or a beta blocker–based regimen. Other classes of antihypertensive drugs may offer certain potential advantages because of their mechanism of action, metabolic effects, and target organ protection. The choice therefore has to be individualized on the basis of the patient's demographic and risk profile, concomitant and co-morbid conditions, lifestyle, and vocational factors. Table 7 provides a brief summary of various antihypertensive drugs.

Diuretics

The thiazide and other diuretics have been widely used in the treatment of hypertensive disorders. Although the role of diuretics has been supplanted by nondiuretic drugs to some extent, they are commonly used in clinical practice either as monotherapy or in combination with other drugs. Patients with edematous conditions such as heart failure and renal insufficiency frequently require the use of a diuretic for optimal blood pressure control. The antihypertensive response to diuretics is seen at lower doses, which produce a small but optimal natriuretic effect; higher doses should be avoided because of the risk of unnecessary volume depletion, electrolyte disturbances, and other biochemical adverse effects. We use a higher dose only when indicated by the clinical circumstances, such as resistant or severe hypertension, congestive heart failure, renal failure, and edema. Diuretics initially reduce the cardiac output, but in the long run, the peripheral vascular resistance falls. For patients with normal renal function, a thiazide diuretic is preferred. For those with renal insufficiency, a loop diuretic should be used. Diuretics are used as monotherapy or as adjuncts to other classes of antihypertensive drugs. Potassium-sparing drugs like triamterene and spironolactone combined with a thiazide diuretic minimize the potassium losses caused by the latter. Potassium-sparing agents should be used with considerable caution, if at all, in patients with significant renal failure or other potassium-retaining conditions.

Any diuretic can cause side effects such as dehydration, hypokalemia, hyponatremia, hypomagnesemia, hypercalcemia, hyperlipidemia, and hyperuricemia. These adverse effects can occur with high doses, and appropriate corrective steps should be implemented.

Beta Blockers

Beta blockers continue to be used in the management of hypertension and coronary artery disease. Their major advantage is secondary protection in patients with coronary artery disease, a characteristic not established for other antihypertensive drugs. A large number of beta blockers are available with more or less equal antihypertensive efficacy. Although the short-term hemodynamic effects of beta blockers are achieved mainly through a reduction in cardiac output, in the long run they decrease peripheral vascular resistance through several mechanisms, including anti-adrenergic effects, renin inhibition, central nervous system action, and a peripheral action in the circulatory system.

The important pharmacologic properties that distinguish the beta blockers are lipid solubility, cardioselectivity, and intrinsic sympathomimetic activity. Beta blockers that are less lipid soluble and are cardioselective are advantageous in many respects. Beta blockers that possess intrinsic sympathomimetic activity tend to cause less bradycardia and less bronchospasm.

Beta blockers are suitable as initial monotherapy for younger and middle-aged patients. Contrary to earlier belief, beta blockers have been shown to be effective even in the elderly population. African-American patients, however, are less responsive to beta-blocker therapy. These drugs work much better in combination with a diuretic, and many combination products are available. Beta blockers are necessary to counteract the reflex cardiac stimulation that occurs with direct vasodilators such as hydralazine or minoxidil. Beta blockers can cause bronchospasm and should be avoided in susceptible patients. Traditionally, congestive heart failure was an important contraindication to the use of beta blockers, but studies have shown their usefulness in this condition; additional safety data are awaited. Central nervous system effects and sexual dysfunction can occur with beta blockers, particularly at high doses. The nonselective beta blockers can have an unfavorable effect on lipid metabolism. Decreased physical capacity, including fatigue, is an expected side effect of beta blockade. Rebound angina is a potential problem when beta blockers are suddenly discontinued in patients with coronary artery disease.

Alpha Blockers

Selective alpha$_1$ blockers have been recommended by the JNC for the initial treatment of hypertension. Although not very popular, alpha blockers provide certain special advantages, including their ability to improve the lipid profile and insulin resistance. In addition to the short-acting drug, prazosin (Minipress), two long-acting preparations (doxazosin [Cardura] and terazosin [Hytrin]) are available for

TABLE 7. **Oral Antihypertensive Drugs**

Drug	Trade Name	Dose Range (mg/d [frequency])	Side Effects (other considerations)
Diuretics (partial list)			
Hydrochlorothiazide	Hydrodiuril, Esidrix	12.5–50 (1)	Biochemical abnormalities:
Chlorthalidone	Hygroton	12.5–50 (1)	↓ potassium, ↑ cholesterol,
Metolozone	Mykrox	0.5–1.0 (1)	↑ glucose, ↑ uric acid
	Zaroxolyn	2.5–10 (1)	Rare: blood dyscrasias, photosensitivity,
Indapamide	Lozol	1.25–2.5 (1)	pancreatitis, hyponatremia
			(Less or no hypercholesterolemia)
Loop diuretics			
Furosemide	Lasix	40–240 (2–3)	(Short duration of action)
Bumetanide	Bumex	0.5–4 (2–3)	Same as above
Torsemide	Demadex	5–40 (1–2)	(Longer duration of action)
Ethacrynic acid	Edecrin	25–100 (2–3)	
Potassium-sparing agents (plus thiazide)			
Spironolactone	(Aldactazide)	25–100 (1)	Hyperkalemia, gynecomastia
Dyrenium	(Dyazide, Maxzide)	25–100 (1)	Hyperkalemia
Amiloride	(Moduretic)	5–10 (1)	Hyperkalemia
Adrenergic inhibitors			
Peripheral			
Reserpine	Serpasil	0.05–0.25 (1)	Sedation, depression
Guanethidine	Ismelin	10–150 (1)	Orthostatic hypotension, diarrhea
Guanadrel	Hylorel	10–75 (2)	Same as above
Central alpha agonists			
Clonidine	Catapres	0.2–1.2 (2–3)	Sedation, dry mouth, "withdrawal"
Guanabenz	Wytensin	8–32 (2)	Sedation, dry mouth
Guanfacine	Tenex	1–3 (1)	Same as above
Methyldopa	Aldomet	500–3000 (2)	Hepatic and "autoimmune" disorders
Alpha blockers			
Doxazosin	Cardura	1–20 (1)	Postural hypotension, lassitude
Prazosin	Minipress	2–20 (2–3)	Same as above
Terazosin	Hytrin	1–20 (1)	Same as above
Beta blockers			
Acebutolol	Sectral	200–800 (1)	Serious: bronchospasm, congestive heart
Atenolol	Tenormin	25–100 (2)	failure, masking of insulin-induced
Betaxolol	Kerlone	5–20 (1)	hypoglycemia, depression
Bisoprolol	Zebeta	2.5–10 (1)	
Carteolol	Cartrol	2.5–10 (1)	
Metoprolol	Lopressor, Toprol XL	50–300 (2:1)	
Nadolol	Corgard	40–320 (1)	Less serious: poor peripheral
Penbutolol	Levatol	10–20 (1)	circulation, insomnia, fatigue,
Pindolol	Visken	10–60 (2)	decreased exercise tolerance,
Propranolol	Inderal, Inderal LA	40–480 (2:1)	hypertriglyceridemia, decreased high-
Timolol	Blocadren	20–60 (2)	density lipoprotein (except with intrinsic sympathomimetic activity agents)
Combined alpha and beta blockers			
Labetalol	Normodyne, Trandate	200–1200 (2)	Postural hypotension, beta-blocking side
Carvedilol	Coreg	12.5–50 (2)	effects
Direct vasodilators			
Hydralazine	Apresoline	50–300 (2)	Headaches, tachycardia, lupus-like syndrome
Minoxidil	Loniten	5–100 (1)	Headaches, fluid retention, hirsutism
Calcium channel blockers			
Verapamil	Isoptin, Calan; Verelan, Covera	90–480 (2:1)	Constipation, conduction defects
Diltiazem	Cardizem; Dilacor, Tiazac	120–360 (2:1)	Nausea, headache, conduction defects
Dihydropyridines			
Amlodipine	Norvasc	2.5–10 (1)	Flush, headache, local ankle edema
Felodipine	Plendil	2.5–20 (1)	Same as above
Isradipine	DynaCirc	5–20 (2)	Same as above
Nicardipine	Cardene	60–90 (2)	Same as above
Nifedipine	Procardia XL, Adalat CC	30–120 (1)	Same as above
Nisoldipine	Sular	20–60 (1)	Same as above

TABLE 7. **Oral Antihypertensive Drugs** Continued

Drug	Trade Name	Dose Range (mg/d [frequency])	Side Effects (other considerations)
Angiotensin-converting enzyme inhibitors			
Benazepril	Lotensin	5–40 (1)	Common: cough
Captopril	Capoten	25–150 (3)	Rare: Angioedema, hyperkalemia, rash, loss of taste, leukopenia
Enalapril	Vasotec	5–40 (2)	
Fosinopril	Monopril	10–40 (1)	Same as above
Lisinopril	Prinivil, Zestril	5–40 (1)	Same as above
Moexipril	Univasc	2.5–10 (2)	Same as above
Quinapril	Accupril	5–80 (1–2)	Same as above
Ramipril	Altace	1.25–20 (1)	Same as above
Trandolapril	Mavik	1–4 (1)	Same as above
Angiotensin II receptor blockers			
Losartan	Cozaar	25–100 (1–2)	No cough, but angioedema may occur: hyperkalemia
Valsartan	Diovan	80–320 (1)	
Irbesartan	Avapro	150–300 (1)	
Candesartan	Atacand	8–32 (1)	

Courtesy of Dr. Norman Kaplan.

clinical use in hypertension. These drugs block the postsynaptic alpha$_1$-adrenergic receptor, thereby blunting catecholamine-induced vasoconstriction. The decrease in blood pressure usually is not accompanied by a significant change in cardiac output or heart rate. The decrease in preload with simultaneous blockade of alpha$_1$ receptors prevents the sympathetic stimulation seen with direct vasodilators such as hydralazine and minoxidil. The efficacy of the alpha blockers rivals that of diuretics and beta blockers. Alpha blockers can be combined with diuretics, beta blockers, or calcium antagonists. The initial dose should be 1 mg, preferably given at bedtime (to avoid first-dose hypotension), and can be titrated up gradually over several weeks.

Although alpha blockers are in general well tolerated, first-dose hypotension can occur with a short-acting drug like prazosin, particularly in volume-depleted patients, and can be prevented with proper precautions. Alpha blockers exert a favorable effect on lipid metabolism and insulin resistance. In addition, these drugs relieve the urinary obstructive symptoms in patients with benign prostatic hypertrophy.

Alpha and Beta Receptor Blockers

Labetalol (Normodyne), a combined alpha- and beta-receptor–blocking drug, is recommended for use either as monotherapy or in combination with other agents like diuretics and direct vasodilators. In the dosage range of 200 to 1000 mg daily (given in two divided doses), labetalol provides sufficient 24-hour blood pressure control. Unlike classic beta blockers, labetalol has been shown to be effective in African-Americans and the elderly. The side effects of labetalol are similar to those of beta blockers; at high doses, alpha-blocker–induced adverse effects like postural hypotension and nasal stuffiness can occur.

Central Alpha Agonists

The centrally acting alpha agonists lower the systemic blood pressure by inhibiting sympathetic activity in the cardiovascular system. Examples of this class include methyldopa, clonidine, guanfacine, and guanabenz. They all share the same hemodynamic profile and therapeutic and adverse effects. The antihypertensive response to central alpha agonists is accompanied by a modest reduction in heart rate and cardiac output. They are usually used for uncomplicated hypertension singly or in combination with other drugs like diuretics. Reflecting their central mechanism of action, the side effects of these drugs include sedation, dry mouth, decreased alertness, and sexual dysfunction. Abrupt discontinuation of central alpha agonists (clonidine in particular) can cause rebound hypertension. Methyldopa has been associated with autoimmune derangement. Rarely, heart block has been reported with these drugs.

Other Sympathetic Blocking Drugs

There are other sympathetic inhibiting drugs that are effective in the treatment of hypertension, such as reserpine, guanethidine, and guanadrel. None of these drugs is used for the routine treatment of hypertension because of a number of bothersome side effects like depression, nasal stuffiness, postural hypotension, diarrhea, and impotence. The alpha-adrenergic agent, phenoxybenzamine, is reserved for the treatment of pheochromocytoma.

Calcium Antagonists

Calcium antagonists are widely used in the treatment of hypertension and other cardiovascular conditions such as coronary artery disease. All calcium antagonists reduce systemic vascular resistance and thereby lower the SBP and DBP in patients with hypertension. These drugs are heterogeneous in their chemical structure as well as in their cardiac actions. In general, the dihydropyridine calcium antagonists are more powerful than verapamil (Isoptin) or diltiazem (Cardizem) in the treatment of hypertension. Short-acting dihydropyridines (nifedipine capsules) produce a rapid hypotensive response accompanied by reflex tachycardia, and should be avoided for chronic hypertension. Longer-acting, slow-release preparations of nifedipine (Procardia XL) and other dihydropyridines like amlodipine (Norvasc) and felodipine (Plendil) are less likely to cause tachycardia and reflex stimulation of the sympathetic nervous system. Verapamil and diltiazem may reduce the heart rate modestly.

Calcium antagonists are used to treat all grades of hypertension. Besides their efficacy in hypertension, calcium antagonists offer certain beneficial effects in cardiovascular diseases. They can be used singly or in combination with other drugs such as beta blockers or ACE inhibitors. In contradistinction to other classes of antihypertensive drugs, sodium restriction or diuretic use does not appear to potentiate the antihypertensive actions of calcium antagonists, for reasons not entirely clear. One study suggested that antihypertensive therapy using a dihydropyridine calcium antagonist reduced the cardiovascular morbidity and mortality rates in the elderly population. Although the effectiveness of calcium antagonists in hypertension is well documented, they are particularly potent in African-American patients and others with volume-dependent or low-renin hypertension.

An important adverse effect of short-acting dihydropyridines is rapid onset of effect associated with reflex increases in heart rate and cardiac output; they may also cause headache and flushing. Co-administration of beta blockers attenuates these so-called "vasodilator" side effects. Gingival hyperplasia is a reported adverse effect of calcium antagonists. Leg edema can occur with all calcium antagonists. This is a local hydrostatic effect and does not respond to diuretics. The vasodilator side effects are not seen with verapamil or diltiazem. Verapamil use can cause constipation. Atrioventricular conduction disturbances have been reported with verapamil and diltiazem in patients with pre-existing cardiac conduction defects. Both verapamil and diltiazem can produce a negative inotropic effect in patients with heart failure.

Angiotensin-Converting Enzyme Inhibitors

Angiotensin-converting enzyme inhibitors block the activity of ACE, which converts the inactive angiotensin I to the potent vasoconstrictor hormone angiotensin II. There are several ACE inhibitors available and all are equally effective in the treatment of hypertension. The pharmacologic differences among the ACE inhibitors are related to duration of action, tissue binding, site of metabolism, and drug elimination. Besides decreasing the formation of angiotensin,

ACE inhibitors also potentiate the activity of bradykinin. The real clinical significance of this ancillary action is not known.

Angiotensin-converting enzyme inhibitors are useful in the management of all degrees of hypertension. Although the therapeutic response to ACE inhibitors is markedly superior in patients with high renin levels, renin profiling is not needed in the selection of antihypertensive drug therapy that has to be individualized. If the decrease in blood pressure in response to an ACE inhibitor is not adequate, a diuretic should be considered for additional therapy. This combination is particularly necessary in patients with low renin levels such as African-Americans and the elderly. In patients with evidence of volume depletion, ACE inhibitors should be used with considerable caution, if at all, and then in small doses, to avoid an unwanted degree of hypotension.

Angiotensin-converting enzyme inhibitors provide important advantages in patients with congestive heart failure (or reduced ejection fraction), diabetic nephropathy, and other renal disorders. Studies have clearly shown that ACE inhibitors decrease the morbidity and mortality rates in patients with congestive heart failure. Similarly, ACE inhibitors retard the progression of diabetic nephropathy. Thus, ACE inhibitors are the drugs of choice for hypertensive patients with congestive heart failure or diabetic nephropathy (unless the disease is advanced). In uncomplicated hypertension, ACE inhibitors are used as monotherapy or in combination with other agents, diuretics in particular.

The published incidences of side effects may differ among various ACE inhibitors, but in general they are similar. Significant hypotension may occur in volume-depleted patients, more so with the short-acting ACE inhibitors. By inhibiting the release of aldosterone, ACE inhibitors may cause hyperkalemia, particularly in patients with underlying renal insufficiency or in those receiving potassium-sparing agents or potassium supplements. Acute deterioration of renal function can occur after administration of ACE inhibitors in patients with significant renovascular disease. Dry, nonproductive cough is probably the most common side effect of ACE inhibitors. The onset of cough is quite variable. Angioneurotic edema is a rare but dangerous adverse effect of ACE inhibitors. Both the cough and angioneurotic edema are related to the bradykinin effects of ACE inhibition. Taste disturbances, skin rash, and leukopenia have been reported rarely with ACE inhibitors. Because of the potential fetal toxicity, ACE inhibitors are contraindicated in pregnancy.

Angiotensin II Receptor Blockers

Angiotensin II receptor blockers (ARBs) are a new class of drugs approved for use in hypertension. As their name implies, ARBs block angiotensin II, resulting in decreased peripheral vascular resistance and blood pressure. By reducing the aldosterone output, ARBs also promote sodium excretion. These dual mechanisms explain the antihypertensive efficacy and advantages of ARBs. All the ARBs appear to share similar hemodynamic and other actions. The differences lie in their duration of action, receptor binding, and pharmacokinetics (e.g., half-life and volume of distribution). Like ACE inhibitors, ARBs are effective as monotherapy or in combination with diuretics. The new, longer acting ARBs (e.g., irbesartan [Avapro] and candesartan [Atacand]) permit once-a-day administration of the drug. Preliminary clinical investigations suggest that ARBs (like ACE inhibitors) provide beneficial effects in patients with congestive heart failure and diabetic renal disease, but long-term results are awaited.

The principal advantages of ARBs accrue from their mechanism of action. Because of their mechanism of action, ARBs are not likely to cause cough or angioneurotic edema. They are well tolerated and offer freedom from side effects. Although ACE inhibitors and ARBs produce synergistic and additive effects, the safety of their combination is not known. As of this chapter's writing, ARBs are being used increasingly in hypertension. Their precise role, however, is not fully known. Additional clinical experience and research will reveal the therapeutic spectrum of ARBs.

Direct Vasodilators

The direct vasodilators, such as hydralazine and minoxidil, are to be used only when hypertension is not controlled on an adequate trial with sufficient doses of other agents described previously. The direct vasodilating drugs act predominantly on the resistance vessels, causing a substantial drop in blood pressure. These drugs cause reflex tachycardia and marked fluid retention and activate the renin-angiotensin and sympathetic nervous systems.

Hydralazine and minoxidil are indicated and may be necessary to control severe and refractory hypertension. They should not be used as initial or even secondary therapy. Only when blood pressure is not controllable with a combination of at least two or three different antihypertensive drugs do we consider direct vasodilator drug therapy. First, we try an optimal dose of hydralazine. When hydralazine treatment fails, we use minoxidil. Both hydralazine and minoxidil cause pronounced tachycardia and fluid retention. Hence, a beta-blocking drug and a diuretic should always be co-administered when using minoxidil or hydralazine. Minoxidil is more potent than hydralazine. The choice of diuretic depends on the extent of fluid retention and the status of renal function. In patients with considerable edema and in those with renal insufficiency, a loop diuretic is used rather than a thiazide. In fact, with minoxidil, we consistently use loop diuretics as needed.

The side effects of direct vasodilators are reflex tachycardia (and palpitations), fluid retention, headache, and flushing; these have to be countered with a beta-blocking drug and a diuretic. A lupus-like syndrome has been reported with long-term use of high doses of hydralazine. The risk of this reaction depends on the acetylator and HLA phenotype status of susceptible patients. Minoxidil use causes hypertrichosis, which limits its use in women. Hair growth reverses after stopping the medication. Very rarely, one of us (Ram) has observed and reported pericardial effusion with minoxidil use.

SUMMARY OF THERAPEUTIC APPROACH TO UNCOMPLICATED HYPERTENSION

The decision to initiate treatment of hypertension requires several considerations, including multiple measurements of blood pressure to confirm the diagnosis. The other factors include the degree of hypertension, target organ damage, and the presence of other cardiovascular risk factors. The overall treatment plan should be made on the assessment of risk stratification, as discussed in the introductory paragraphs of this chapter. For patients with complicated or advanced hypertension, drug therapy should not be delayed. For others, a trial of nonpharmacologic therapy should be attempted before instituting drug therapy. Although the JNC guidelines favor the choice of a beta blocker or a diuretic for initial therapy, we believe that other classes of antihypertensive agents, like ACE inhibitors, calcium antagonists, or ARBs, can be selected for initial therapy and may even be advantageous under certain clinical circumstances. If there is no response whatsoever to the initial drug, it should be substituted for another from a different class. If only a partial response is observed, a second and, if needed, a third drug should be added to achieve the goal blood pressure. Before proceeding to each additional treatment, the physician should evaluate the reasons for inadequate response (Table 8). When the blood pressure is well controlled for at least 1 year or longer, consideration should be given to step-down therapy under careful supervision and follow-up.

SPECIAL SITUATIONS

Resistant Hypertension

In general, hypertension is considered resistant or refractory if the blood pressure is not normalized in patients who are compliant with a regimen of at least three drugs in combination used in appropriate doses. Based on clinical judgment, patients with resistant hypertension should be considered for a work-

TABLE 8. **Causes for Inadequate Response to Antihypertensive Drug Therapy**

Pseudoresistance
Nonadherence to therapy
Volume overload
Drug-related causes
Associated conditions
Identifiable causes of hypertension

up of possible underlying secondary causes such as renovascular hypertension (RVH), pheochromocytoma, primary hyperaldosteronism, and renal disease. If no correctable or reversible cause for refractory hypertension is found, treatment should be modified to include a direct vasodilator such as hydralazine or minoxidil. As discussed previously, a beta blocker and a diuretic should always be used in conjunction with a direct vasodilator. Patients with refractory hypertension should be followed closely. Sodium restriction and volume contraction are important factors in managing refractory hypertension.

Hypertensive Crises

Hypertensive emergencies and urgencies are unusual situations that require immediate blood pressure reduction. Examples include malignant hypertension, hypertensive encephalopathy, coronary artery disease syndromes, eclampsia, acute aortic dissection, and acute left ventricular failure. It is the extent and degree of target organ damage that determine the development of a hypertensive crisis. Elevated blood pressure alone in the absence of acute or progressive target organ damage should not be subjected to urgent therapy. The scope of this chapter does not permit us to discuss hypertensive crises in detail. Drugs useful in the acute management of severe hypertension are listed in Table 9.

SECONDARY FORMS OF HYPERTENSION

Thus far, we have discussed the approach used to evaluate and treat patients with essential or primary hypertension. The balance of this chapter deals with secondary causes of hypertension. Although Table 10 lists the various secondary causes of hypertension, our description is restricted to the renovascular and adrenal forms of secondary hypertension.

Secondary forms of hypertension are much less common than essential (or primary) hypertension, but recognizing an underlying cause is important in terms of prognosis and management for the individual patient. Only approximately 5% of patients with hypertension have a secondary cause, but the overall number of these patients is by no means small. Assuming that 60 million Americans have hypertension, approximately 3 million people have secondary hypertension. In some, there is specific medical therapy for their hypertension, and for some a cure may be possible.

There has been an ongoing debate over the aggressiveness with which clinicians should pursue secondary causes of hypertension because of their low incidence and the high cost of the work-up. Clues suggestive of secondary hypertension are given in Table 11. There are a number of new screening procedures to detect secondary forms of hypertension that make evaluation less expensive than in the past. A careful medical history, physical examination, and brief laboratory evaluation can often guide the clinician on whether to pursue further studies to exclude or confirm secondary hypertension.

Two common causes of secondary hypertension are renal parenchymal disease and RVH; two other important, unusual causes include primary hyperaldosteronism and pheochromocytoma. In the ensuing discussion, we elaborate on the clinical diagnosis and management of selected secondary forms of hypertension.

Renal Parenchymal Disease

Hypertension is quite common in patients with renal disease. In acute renal failure, hypertension is

TABLE 10. Secondary Causes of Hypertension

Renal parenchymal disease
Renin-producing tumors
Renovascular hypertension
Pheochromocytoma
Primary hyperaldosteronism
Cushing's syndrome
Congenital adrenal hyperplasia
Hyperthyroidism or hypothyroidism
Hyperparathyroidism
Exogenous hormones (e.g., glucocorticoids, mineralocorticoids, and sympathomimetic drugs)
Pregnancy-induced hypertension
Alcohol abuse
Miscellaneous drugs (e.g., cyclosporin A, cocaine, erythropoietin, and oral contraceptives)

TABLE 11. Clues Suggesting Secondary Hypertension

Age <30 years
Sudden onset of hypertension at >50 years of age
Epigastric, abdominal, or flank bruits in a patient with severe hypertension
Proteinuria or microscopic hematuria
Palpable kidney
Symptomatic hypertensive patient
Unexplained weight loss
Metabolic abnormalities such as hypokalemia, hypercalcemia, or hyperglycemia
Absent or delayed peripheral pulses
Clinical features of endocrine disorders such as hypothyroidism or hyperthyroidism or Cushing's syndrome
Features of acromegaly
Angiotensin-converting enzyme inhibitor–induced renal dysfunction
Unilaterally small kidney
Extensive occlusive disease in the coronary, cerebral, or peripheral vessels

TABLE 9. Drugs Available for Hypertensive Emergencies

Vasodilators	Adrenergic Inhibitors
Nitroprusside (Nipride)	Labetalol (Normodyne)
Nicardipine (Cardene)	Esmolol (Brevibloc)
Fenoldopam (Corlopam)	Phentolamine (Regitine)
Nitroglycerin (Tridil)	
Enalaprilat (Vasotec I.V.)	
Hydralazine (Apresoline)	

chiefly mediated by expansion of the extracellular fluid volume. Therefore, volume control usually normalizes blood pressure, and hypertension usually resolves with improvement in renal function. Because hypertension is often transient in acute renal failure, therapy should be guided to decrease the consequences of hypertension.

Hypertension is a common accompaniment of chronic renal disease. Renal hypertension is more likely to progress to an accelerated or malignant phase than is essential hypertension at any given level of blood pressure. Underlying kidney disease is a risk factor for cardiovascular events, ventricular hypertrophy, and further progression of the kidney disease, and therefore aggressive blood pressure control is essential in this setting. The overall strategy in terms of pharmacologic therapy is not very different from that with essential hypertension. However, because increased intravascular volume is often a feature of renal insufficiency, diuretics play an important therapeutic role. By the time patients with chronic renal failure reach end-stage renal disease, nearly all have some degree of hypertension. It has been demonstrated that proper blood pressure control significantly delays the progression of renal disease.

Renovascular Hypertension (RVH)

Renovascular hypertension (RVH) is among the most common secondary causes of hypertension. It is a potentially correctable form of high blood pressure. Angioplasty, renal artery stenting, or surgical bypass procedures provide the clinician with the opportunity to prevent cardiovascular morbidity and mortality related to sustained hypertension and to preserve renal function. RVH is defined as high blood pressure secondary to renal ischemia as a result of renal artery stenosis. The presence of renal artery stenosis (e.g., as found by renal arteriography), however, does not always equate with the presence of RVH. In clinical practice, the diagnosis of RVH is made retrospectively as hypertension resolves or improves after repair of a renal artery lesion. The mere presence of renal artery stenosis in a hypertensive patient does not establish the diagnosis of RVH. Some patients simply have concurrent essential hypertension.

The true incidence of this condition remains unknown. However, a fair estimate might be that 1 to 2% of the hypertensive population has RVH. In some selected populations, especially among older patients and those with grade 3 or 4 hypertensive retinopathy, the prevalence is much higher.

In patients with RVH, blood pressure initially rises because of activation of the renin-angiotensin-aldosterone system. Ischemia to the kidney leads to the release of renin from the juxtaglomerular apparatus. This in turn promotes the conversion of angiotensinogen to angiotensin I. ACE converts angiotensin I to angiotensin II. Angiotensin II is a potent vasoconstrictor that also stimulates aldosterone release, which leads to salt and water retention. Vasoconstriction and increased intravascular volume through salt and water retention result in sustained hypertension.

Atherosclerotic renal artery disease is the most common cause of RVH, followed by fibromuscular dysplasia. Fibromuscular dysplasia usually occurs in younger patients, especially women in their twenties and thirties. Atherosclerotic lesions, on the other hand, usually occur in older people, with a male-to-female ratio of approximately 2 to 1. Atherosclerotic lesions often occur at the ostium of the renal artery and represent an extension of the disease process from the aorta. The lesions are bilateral in one third of cases. Tobacco use is associated with an increased prevalence of both atherosclerotic and fibromuscular renal artery lesions.

Although renal artery stenosis alone does not equal RVH, it is a precondition for the diagnosis. Consequently, it is important to screen for renal artery stenosis. A hypertensive intravenous pyelogram or selective renal vein or peripheral renin estimation are rarely used anymore for this purpose. The gold standard for this diagnosis remains the conventional renal arteriogram. Unfortunately, it is an invasive procedure with significant risks and cost. More recently introduced screening procedures include captopril scintigraphy, intravenous or intra-arterial digital subtraction angiography, duplex ultrasound, and magnetic resonance angiography.

Intravenous digital subtraction angiography uses a considerable amount of intravenous contrast material but it avoids an arterial puncture. Unfortunately, obesity and excessive bowel gas can make this test uninterpretable. We prefer an intra-arterial digital subtraction angiogram because of the markedly decreased dye load and its high index of sensitivity. Duplex ultrasound is probably the least expensive noninvasive test to screen for this condition. Among its drawbacks, it is a highly operator-dependent procedure and requires considerable skill to perform. An emerging new technique is magnetic resonance angiography, but so far only a small number of studies have been reported; preliminary experience with this technique, however, is very encouraging.

Renal nuclear scans have been used in the past as a screening tool, but this test may miss bilateral renal artery lesions. A more sensitive technique is captopril renal flow scanning. This test is based on the premise that in RVH, glomerular filtration rate and renal plasma flow depend on angiotensin II–mediated glomerular afferent arterial vasoconstriction. With acute administration of the ACE inhibitor, captopril, the renal flow scan demonstrates renal ischemia. This test is one of the most useful noninvasive screening tests for RVH. One drawback is that patients must stop their chronic ACE inhibitor therapy several days before this scan is performed. The accuracy of this screening study is reduced in the setting of renal parenchymal disease.

The management of RVH continues to be debated. Some continue to advocate medical therapy even though it is often very difficult to maintain adequate blood pressure control. Even when blood pressure is well controlled, renal function declines with time. Definitive therapies include surgery, percutaneous transluminal angioplasty, or renal artery stenting. Surgical correction of renal artery stenosis is superior to other corrective techniques. We usually recommend surgical correction in patients with bilateral, severe ostial atherosclerotic lesions. Percutaneous transluminal angioplasty is an excellent therapy in experienced hands, especially for fibromuscular dysplasia. It is a more technically difficult procedure in atherosclerotic ostial lesions. Restenosis occurs in approximately 20% of patients, and the incidence may be higher in patients with atherosclerotic lesions. The advent of more sophisticated stenting procedures has improved on the results from angioplasty, and stenting may eventually be the equivalent of surgical therapy for the definitive management of RVH.

Pheochromocytoma

Pheochromocytoma is a rare disease accounting for less than 0.5% of cases of hypertension. The symptoms that patients with pheochromocytoma experience represent the effects of tumoral hypersecretion of catecholamines. Classically, patients have hypertension, headache, hypermetabolism, hyperhydrosis or excessive sweating, and hyperglycemia. Other features may include palpitations, anxiety, tremulousness, weakness, weight loss, paroxysmal hypertension, tachycardia or, rarely, bradycardia, and orthostatic hypotension. Many patients, however, simply present as if they have essential hypertension, with pheochromocytoma discovered only accidentally or with a catastrophic rise in blood pressure during surgery or anesthesia induction.

Approximately 95% of pheochromocytomas are intra-abdominal, and approximately 90% are found in the adrenal glands. Ten percent of these tumors occur in both adrenal glands, and less than 10% are malignant tumors. Malignant lesions are histologically and biochemically the same as benign tumors. The only clue to the presence of a malignant tumor is either local invasion or metastatic spread. It is essential that the diagnosis of pheochromocytoma be made first using biochemical tests rather than by obtaining a computed tomography (CT) scan of the abdomen, because many adrenal masses are incidental and do not represent a pheochromocytoma. Only after an appropriate biochemical work-up has been completed should the tumor be localized by radiologic techniques.

Most pheochromocytomas are sporadic, but in a few patients the disease is part of a familial disorder. The diagnosis of pheochromocytoma is usually established by biochemical assays of blood and urine. A spot urine test for metanephrines is an excellent screening procedure that correlates well with total metanephrine measurement from a 24-hour urine collection. An overnight urine collection for metanephrines can also be obtained, and this is an accu-

rate and more convenient test for the patient. Plasma catecholamines can be used to confirm the diagnosis of pheochromocytoma. A total plasma catecholamine (norepinephrine + epinephrine) concentration above 2000 pg per mL in a hypertensive patient who has been at rest for at least 30 minutes is essentially diagnostic of a pheochromocytoma, whereas values above 950 pg per mL are highly suggestive. When diagnostic plasma catecholamine levels are not seen, a clonidine suppression test should be performed. This test consists of an oral administration of 0.3 mg of clonidine given at least 12 hours after antihypertensive medications have been discontinued. The total plasma catecholamine concentration is measured both before therapy and 3 hours after the clonidine is administered. Patients without pheochromocytoma should suppress their plasma catecholamine concentration to less than 500 pg per mL. This test is approximately 92% accurate in making the biochemical diagnosis of pheochromocytoma.

After biochemical confirmation of a pheochromocytoma, a radiologic evaluation to locate the tumor is warranted. Although any site containing periganglionic tissue may be involved, the most common extra-adrenal locations include the superior and inferior periaortic areas, the bladder, the thorax, the neck, and the pelvis. CT or magnetic resonance imaging is preferred to locate these tumors. The clinician must be aware that arteriograms can precipitate hypertensive crisis in these patients. If an imaging method fails to localize the site of tumor, a metaiodobenzylguanidine (MIBG) nuclear scan is indicated.

Pheochromocytomas are potentially curable forms of hypertension, and therefore surgical resection should be the aim. It is important to prepare the patient appropriately before surgery. It is standard to use an alpha-adrenergic blocker such as phenoxybenzamine 10 mg orally once per day, and raise the dose every few days until symptoms and blood pressure are well controlled. A beta blocker may then be added, but should never be started before alpha blockade is achieved. If a beta blocker is used initially, the patient could have unopposed alpha-mediated vasoconstriction and might experience severe hypertension. An alternative is to use α-methyl-paratyrosine, an inhibitor of catecholamine synthesis. If a hypertensive crisis develops during surgery in a patient with an unsuspected pheochromocytoma, intravenous phentolamine is the preferred immediate therapy. After surgical removal of the tumor, some patients may experience significant postoperative hypotension or hypoglycemia. This can be avoided by adequate fluid replacement and glucose infusion. Successful surgery often normalizes catecholamine secretion in approximately 1 week and usually cures hypertension.

Primary Hyperaldosteronism

Primary hyperaldosteronism is characterized by hypertension, hypokalemia, elevated plasma aldosterone (PA) levels, and suppressed plasma renin activity (PRA). This syndrome stems from hyperfunction of the adrenal cortex, leading to excessive hormonal secretion. Such hyperfunction may be caused by either a solitary adrenocortical adenoma (in approximately 70% of the patients) or by bilateral adrenal hyperplasia. Although its true incidence is unknown, this condition probably accounts for fewer than 0.5% of all cases of hypertension.

Patients with primary hyperaldosteronism are nearly always hypertensive. Some may also have headaches or symptoms associated with their hypokalemia, such as muscle weakness, tetany, paralysis, or polyuria. Despite the notion that this disorder is associated with only mild elevations in blood pressure, in our experience hypertension may be quite severe and is often refractory to therapy. This syndrome should be suspected when there is spontaneous hypokalemia in a hypertensive patient, or when there is profound hypokalemia on relatively small doses of diuretics. Patients with an adenoma frequently have sustained hypokalemia, whereas those with bilateral hyperplasia tend to have intermittent hypokalemia or even normal potassium levels. A high salt intake tends to aggravate the hypokalemia because this allows increased sodium delivery to the more distal parts of the tubule, where the excess aldosterone can result in increased potassium and hydrogen ion secretion.

When this syndrome is suspected, it is reasonable to measure a 24-hour urine for potassium excretion on a normal diet while the patient is hypokalemic. In primary hyperaldosteronism, the 24-hour urinary potassium excretion exceeds 30 mEq per day. A useful first diagnostic test is the measurement of PRA and PA levels. In patients with primary aldosteronism, the PRA is very low and PA levels are usually greater than 10 ng per dL. In some institutions, a PA:PRA ratio of greater than 30 to 40 is used to suggest the diagnosis of primary hyperaldosteronism. If the PA:PRA ratio is not diagnostic, an aldosterone suppression test is performed. A simple way to perform this test is to obtain a baseline aldosterone level in the morning. The patient then receives 2 liters of intravenous normal saline over a period of 4 hours, and a repeat aldosterone level is drawn. If the aldosterone level does not suppress below 6 to 10 ng per dL, then the diagnosis of primary hyperaldosteronism is likely. Once the biochemical diagnosis of this condition is made, it is very important to establish whether the patient has an adrenal adenoma or bilateral hyperplasia. The procedure of choice is CT of the adrenal glands using 3- to 5-mm cuts so that small tumors are not missed. Solitary adenomas are usually unilateral, whereas the adrenal glands appear normal or enlarged bilaterally in patients with adrenal hyperplasia. Measurements of aldosterone concentration in the adrenal venous effluent have been the gold standard for differentiating adenomas from bilateral hyperplasia. Unfortunately, considerable skill and experience are required for this procedure, and it is not available in every institution.

The therapy of choice for adenomas is surgical excision. This can sometimes cure the hypertension and lead to the resolution of the hypokalemia. Even if blood pressure does not completely normalize, blood pressure control often markedly improves after surgery. The treatment of bilateral adrenal hyperplasia, however, is not surgical, but medical. Surgery in bilateral adrenal hyperplasia does not cure hypertension. Medical therapy in primary hyperaldosteronism includes control of blood pressure and potassium balance. Spironolactone is a rational choice because it antagonizes the action of aldosterone at the distal renal tubule. Patients may not tolerate long-term treatment with spironolactone, however, because of side effects such as gastrointestinal disturbances or gynecomastia. Other potassium-sparing agents could be used to treat hypokalemia in this condition.

ACKNOWLEDGMENTS

The authors thank Jan Leaf, Marcie Gonzales, and Estella Gomez-Lopez for assistance in preparing the manuscript and Dr. Norman Kaplan, University of Texas Southwestern Medical Center, Dallas, Texas, for providing the table on antihypertensive drugs.

ACUTE MYOCARDIAL INFARCTION

method of
KANU CHATTERJEE, M.B.
University of California, San Francisco
San Francisco, California

INCIDENCE AND PATHOGENESIS

In the United States, over 900,000 persons each year have an acute myocardial infarction. Approximately 25% of these patients die as a result. Between 40 and 60% of these deaths occur within 1 hour of the onset of symptoms, and the acute ischemic syndrome is the most frequent cause of all sudden cardiac deaths.

Although atherosclerotic coronary artery disease is the most common cause of acute myocardial infarction, myocardial necrosis can also result in absence of atherosclerotic coronary artery disease. Nonatherosclerotic coronary artery disease such as coronary anomalies, nonatherosclerotic coronary artery aneurysms, collagen vascular disease involving the coronary arteries, spontaneous or traumatic coronary artery dissection, coronary artery embolism, coronary vasospasm in absence of coronary atherosclerosis, drug abuse such as cocaine-induced coronary artery thrombosis and spasm, and type I aortic dissection involving the coronary arteries are the rare causes of acute myocardial infarction. Myocardial infarction can also occur in patients with valvular heart disease, such as severe aortic stenosis and aortic regurgitation, hypertensive heart disease, and hypertrophic cardiomyopathy, as a result of prolonged myocardial ischemia resulting in both excessive increased myocardial oxygen demand and impaired myocardial perfusion. Myocardial contusion and acute myocarditis may also be associated with myocardial necrosis and infarction. Some of the nonatherosclerotic causes of myocardial infarction

TABLE 1. **Some of the Causes of Myocardial Infarction Not Resulting From Atherosclerotic Coronary Artery Disease**

Coronary vasospasm	Variant angina, drug-induced coronary vasospasm (cocaine, amphetamine)
Coronary embolism	Atrial fibrillation with mitral valve disease and prosthetic mitral valve disease, infective endocarditis, paradoxical embolism
Coronary artery dissection	Traumatic, spontaneous (more frequently during pregnancy), associated with type A thoracic aortic dissection, various arteritis, Marphan's and marphanoid disease
Prolonged myocardial ischemia	Due to imbalance between myocardial oxygen demand and supply; aortic stenosis, aortic insufficiency, hypertension with severe left ventricular hypertrophy, hypertrophic cardiomyopathy
Thrombotic coronary artery disease	Homocystinemia, polycythemia, thrombocytosis, thrombotic thrombocytopenic purpura, disseminated intravascular coagulation, hypercoagulable states, sickle cell anemia and other hemoglobinopathies, macroglobulinemia and hyperviscosity states, blood dyscrasia including leukemia, infectious diseases including *Falciparum* malaria, drug overuse such as cocaine overdose, rarely oral contraceptives, systemic vasculitis involving the coronary arteries (systemic lupus erythematosus, scleroderma, rheumatoid arthritis, Takayasu's disease, Kawasaki's disease, and polyarteritis nodosa)
Metabolic and degenerative coronary vascular disease	Amyloidosis, pseudoxanthoma elasticum, lipid storage disease, and mucopolysaccharidosis, homocystinemia
Cardiomyopathy with muscular dystrophies	Pseudohypertrophic muscular dystrophy and other muscular dystrophies, Friedreich's ataxia, and specific cardiac muscle diseases
Congenital coronary anomalies	Anomalous origin of the left coronary artery from the pulmonary artery (Bland-White-Garland syndrome)
Coronary artery venous fistulas	Congenital coronary artery aneurysms
Trauma	Myocardial contusion secondary to coronary artery dissection

that can be encountered in clinical practice are summarized in Table 1.

In adults, the atherosclerotic coronary artery disease is the most common cause of myocardial infarction, and hence this etiology should be suspected in all patients with evidence of myocardial necrosis. Acute myocardial infarction is one of the consequences of acute ischemic syndrome, which also includes unstable angina and sudden cardiac death. The essential pathologic substrate of acute ischemic syndrome is a vulnerable atherosclerotic plaque that usually consists of large, soft lipid core and a thin fibrous cap. Fissuring, ulceration, and plaque rupture after injury to the endothelium lining the fibrous cap is the initial event in the pathogenesis of acute myocardial infarction in approximately 70% of patients. Endothelial injury and ulceration of the surface of the cap without rupture and fissuring accounts for acute ischemic syndrome in about 30% of patients. The precise mechanism for the endothelial injury of the vulnerable plaque in individual patients remains unclear. It may be precipitated by various stimuli such as flow or sheer stress, increased blood pressure, hyperlipidemia, vigorous exercise, a surge in catecholamines, or a combination of these factors.

Changes in intraplaque stress, such as alteration in the shape of the plaque and longitudinal and circumferential stresses may also be contributory to endothelial injury and plaque rupture. After the rupture of the vulnerable plaque and formation of intraplaque fissures, blood enters into the fissures, and concurrently the thrombogenic intraplaque material is exposed to the flowing blood. Platelet aggregation, adhesion, and formation of nonocclusive intraluminal thrombi are the principal mechanisms for primary unstable angina syndrome. The nonocclusive thrombi in unstable angina are also platelet rich (white thrombi). When fibrin-rich occlusive thrombus forms, causing complete interruption of blood flow to the ischemic myocardium, myocardial infarction is precipitated. When there is spontaneous and rapid dissolution of the occlusive thrombus and recanalization of the infarct-related artery, usually non-Q wave or nontransmural myocardial infarction occurs. If the total occlusion persists without prompt recanalization of the infarct-related artery, Q wave or transmural myocardial infarction is the usual outcome.

The thin fibrous cap, an important anatomic component of the vulnerable plaque, is deficient in smooth muscle cells as well as collagen fiber content. Simultaneous increased degradation and decreased synthesis of collagen appears to be the predominant mechanism for the formation of the thin fibrous cap. It has been also suggested that activation of the various proteolytic enzymes (matrix metalloproteinase) contribute to disruption and ulceration of the fibrous cap. The fissuring or breakdown of the fibrous cap usually occurs at the shoulder region of the plaque, and in these regions activated T lymphocyte macrophages and mast cells are aggregated that appear to be the source of the various proteolytic enzymes. In the acute ischemic syndromes, the existence of a pro-inflammatory state is also suggested by the presence of increased C-reactive protein and fibrinogen. A prothrombotic state is suggested by the presence of increased fibrinopeptide A and plasminogen activator inhibitor and decreased tissue plasminogen activators. Infection has also been suggested in the pathogenesis of acute ischemic syndrome in patients with atherosclerotic coronary artery disease. Increased antibodies to *Chlamydia, Helicobacter pylori,* and cytomegalovirus have been detected in higher concentration in patients with acute ischemic syndrome and who had adverse cardiac events. The precise role of infection in the pathogenesis of acute ischemic syndrome, however, has not been clarified. The importance of the tissue factor in the pathogenesis of acute ischemic syndrome has also been recognized. The important pathophysiologic mechanisms for myocardial infarction are summarized in Table 2.

CLINICAL MANIFESTATIONS

Symptoms

Approximately 50% of patients who suffer from acute myocardial infarction have a history of a precipitating factor. Severe emotional stress, moderate or heavy physical activity, lack of sleep, overeating, tiredness, and fatigue

TABLE 2. **The Pathogenetic Mechanisms for Acute Myocardial Infarction**

Presence of a vulnerable plaque with a thin fibrous cap and a large, soft lipid core; the plaque may be small or large and hemodynamically nonobstructive lesion

Presence of prothrombotic and hypercoagulable states

The external and intrinsic triggers, including changes in blood pressure, catecholamines, and vasoconstriction

Fissuring, ulceration, and disruption of the vulnerable plaque after endothelial injury and disruption of the thin fibrous cap

Platelet activation and adhesion and formation of nonocclusive thrombi resulting in unstable angina

Formation of occlusive thrombus with interruption of blood flow to the ischemic myocardium

Prompt recanalization and establishment of blood flow to the ischemic myocardium results in non-Q wave myocardial infarction

Persistent occlusion of the infarct-related artery with occlusive thrombus results in Q wave and transmural myocardial infarction

---

may precede the onset of myocardial infarction. It needs to be emphasized that in approximately 50% of patients no precipitating mechanism is identified. In some patients, progressively worsening angina or recurrent episodes of rest angina can be present. Acute myocardial infarction occurs more often in the morning, shortly after waking, than at other times of the day or night. Surgery, septic shock, increased metabolic demand, and hypoxia may be precipitating factors for acute myocardial infarction.

Chest pain is the most frequent symptom. The character, location, and radiation of chest pain of acute myocardial infarction are similar to those of angina. The intensity in myocardial infarction, however, is usually more severe, and the duration is longer than 30 minutes. The character of the chest pain may be crushing, constricting, pressing, or heaviness. The chest pain, however, may be mild, and it may feel like indigestion. It is usually located retrosternally but may be located parasternally, particularly over the left precordium. The pain may or may not have radiation. Radiation to the arms, back, throat, and epigastrium are common. If pain radiates to the lower jaw, however, it is more likely due to myocardial ischemia. In approximately one third of patients with acute myocardial infarction, particularly in elderly patients and in patients with diabetes, acute myocardial infarction can occur without chest pain. Chest pain may also be absent in patients with stroke, syncope, or severe pulmonary edema at the onset of infarction. In elderly patients, unexplained confusion, light headedness, dyspnea, and gastrointestinal upset may be the manifestations of acute myocardial infarction instead of chest pain. The other associated symptoms are dyspnea, nausea, vomiting, and light headedness. Vomiting is more common in patients with acute myocardial infarction than in those with unstable angina. Anxiety, nervousness and apprehension, and a sensation of impending doom are voiced by some patients with evolving myocardial infarction.

Physical Examination

The physical examination can be entirely normal in patients with uncomplicated myocardial infarction. With persistent chest pain, however, the patient may appear restless and anxious and unable to find a comfortable position in bed. In contrast, patients with angina usually lie still because physical movement may enhance the ischemic

pain. Patients may appear pale, sweaty, and clammy due to increased adrenergic activity. Mental obtundation or confusion may be a manifestation of cardiogenic shock. Patients appear dyspneic and gasping for breath when pulmonary edema complicates acute myocardial infarction.

A paucity of abnormal physical findings is the rule rather than the exception in patients with uncomplicated myocardial infarction. In most patients, heart rate remains in the normal range. At the onset of myocardial infarction, however, sinus bradycardia may be present. In patients with heart failure and cardiogenic shock, sinus tachycardia is present. When pulsus alternans is present, left ventricular systolic dysfunction (reduced ejection fraction) should be suspected. Irregular pulse due to premature ventricular beats or nonsustained ventricular tachycardia may be present. Irregular pulse due to atrial fibrillation or flutter is an uncommon complication at the onset of acute myocardial infarction. Systemic blood pressure is usually normal in patients with uncomplicated myocardial infarction. Transient hypertension, however, may be observed in patients with persistent chest pain, and in these patients sinus tachycardia is also frequently encountered. Hypotension with a systolic blood pressure of 90 mm Hg or less is one of the diagnostic criteria of cardiogenic shock. Relative hypotension, however, is also a feature of hypovolemic shock, inappropriate autonomic response, and decreased stroke volume due to bradyarrhythmias and tachyarrhythmias complicating acute myocardial infarction.

The jugular venous pressure and pulse are normal in patients with uncomplicated myocardial infarction. Transient elevation of jugular venous pressure is common in patients with pulmonary edema who also frequently develop transient systemic hypertension. The mechanism of elevated jugular venous pressure, which reflects elevation of right ventricular diastolic pressure in these patients, is not entirely clear. Transient right ventricular failure due to pulmonary hypertension and increased right ventricular afterload, as well as decreased right ventricular diastolic compliance, are the most likely mechanisms. Patients with severe left ventricular systolic dysfunction with or without manifestations of cardiogenic shock may also have elevated jugular venous pressure due to secondary right ventricular failure. In patients with right ventricular myocardial infarction with right ventricular failure, jugular venous pressure is elevated. In these patients usually there is no evidence of left ventricular failure like signs of pulmonary venous congestion. In patients with right ventricular myocardial infarction, Kussmaul's sign may also be detected.

Pulsus paradoxus is encountered rather rarely in patients with right ventricular myocardial infarction. Analysis of the carotid pulse characteristics does not usually reveal any specific abnormality except that the pulse volume may be decreased in patients with low cardiac output due to reduced stroke volume, and in these patients the pulse pressure is also decreased. The palpation of the precordium may not reveal any abnormal finding. In patients with right ventricular myocardial infarction and overt right ventricular failure, a lower left parasternal systolic impulse may be appreciated. The left ventricular apical impulse may be sustained in some patients with overt left ventricular systolic dysfunction, and a presystolic wave indicating increased left ventricular end diastolic pressure may be present. Palpable S_3 gallop is a rare finding in patients with acute myocardial infarction.

Auscultation may not reveal any abnormal findings. An S_4 gallop over the cardiac apex, however, may be present. In patients with pulmonary edema and cardiogenic shock due to left ventricular systolic dysfunction, left ventricular

S_3 gallop is present but may not be appreciated because of the difficulty of auscultation in the presence of pulmonary edema. In patients with right ventricular myocardial infarction and right ventricular failure, S_3 gallop is appreciated along the lower left sternal border. The first heart sound is usually normal. The decreased intensity of the first heart sound most frequently indicates increased left ventricular diastolic pressure. First-degree atrioventricular block, however, is also associated with decreased intensity of the first heart sound. The second heart sound is normal in the majority of patients. The intensity of P_2 may be increased due to postcapillary pulmonary hypertension secondary to left ventricular failure. The second heart sound is paradoxically split in patients who present with left bundle branch block.

An early systolic murmur or a late systolic murmur due to papillary muscle dysfunction may be detected in up to 50% of patients with acute myocardial infarction. These murmurs, however, may not represent severe mitral regurgitation. A new loud pansystolic murmur over the cardiac apex or along the left sternal border indicates either severe mitral regurgitation or ventricular septal rupture. One- or two-component pericardial friction rub is frequently appreciated in patients with episternal pericarditis. Three-component friction rub, however, is more frequently observed in patients with Dressler's syndrome (postmyocardial infarction syndrome). The pericardial friction rub is also a finding of subacute free wall rupture.

DIFFERENTIAL DIAGNOSIS OF CHEST PAIN

The differential diagnosis for patients who present with severe chest pain should include acute thoracic aortic dissection, primary pericarditis, acute myocarditis, mediastinitis, mediasternal emphysema, ruptured esophagus, acute massive or submassive pulmonary embolism, left-sided tension pneumothorax, and, rarely, acute cholecystitis, pancreatitis, and other upper abdominal catastrophes.

Electrocardiography

A 12-lead electrocardiogram (ECG) should be obtained in all patients with suspected acute myocardial infarction, not only for diagnosis but also for making decisions regarding reperfusion therapy. Localized ST segment elevation and hyperacute T waves overlying the ischemic myocardium are early ECG findings of transmural myocardial ischemia. With persistent ischemia, there is loss of R waves and development of Q waves overlying the affected myocardial segments. Without reperfusion of the ischemic myocardium, the magnitude of ST segment elevation decreases by approximately 50% within 24 hours of onset of symptoms. ST segment elevation, however, may persist for several days. When ST segment elevation declines and becomes isoelectric, T wave inversions occur in the same leads. When Q waves develop, it is termed Q wave myocardial infarction. Although in the vast majority of patients Q wave myocardial infarction indicates transmyocardial necrosis, Q wave infarction may be seen in patients with nontransmural myocardial infarction.

The infarct location can be identified by detecting ST-T wave changes in the precordial and the limb leads; when the ECG changes of infarction and ischemia are localized in leads V_1 to V_3, left ventricular anteroseptal myocardial infarction is diagnosed. If these changes are observed only in leads V_4 to V_6, apical myocardial infarction is diagnosed. In apical myocardial infarction frequently there is ST segment depression in the right arm lead (aV_R). When the electrocardiographic changes of ischemia and infarction are localized in leads V_5 and V_6 and in the left arm lead (aV_L), lateral wall myocardial infarction is suspected. It should be emphasized, however, that true lateral wall myocardial infarction may be electrocardiographically silent when a conventional 12-lead ECG is employed. When electrocardiographic changes of ischemia and infarction are localized in leads II, III and aV_F, left ventricular inferior wall myocardial infarction is diagnosed. Acute true posterior wall myocardial infarction is suspected when there is a prominent R wave in V_1 and V_2 along with ST segment depression and T wave inversion in the same leads. The duration of an R wave of more than 0.04 seconds in V_1 and an R/S ratio of greater than 1 also suggest true posterior wall myocardial infarction. The ECG findings of right ventricular myocardial infarction are (1) evidence of left ventricular inferior wall myocardial infarction, (2) ST segment elevation in leads V_1 and V_4R, (3) when the magnitude of the Q wave in lead III is greater than the magnitude of the Q wave in lead aV_F.

The ECG findings in non-Q wave myocardial infarction are ST segment depression with or without T wave inversion. T wave inversions may persist even when ST segment depression resolves. In patients with shell myocardial infarction, widespread persistent ST segment depression with T wave inversions are seen in the precordial leads. The shell infarction indicates extensive subendocardial myocardial infarction, which may also involve the papillary muscle and produce mitral regurgitation. The prognosis for patients with shell infarction is poorer than for patients with other types of non-Q wave myocardial infarction. In the presence of right or left bundle branch blocks, discordant ST-T changes may indicate myocardial ischemia or acute myocardial infarction.

Serum Enzyme Levels

Elevated serum enzyme levels that may suggest myocardial necrosis are creatine kinase (CK) and the MB isoenzyme of creatine kinase (CK-MB), the CK isoform MB2 (a subtype of the MB isoenzyme), myoglobin, and cardiac-specific troponin T (CTNT) and troponin I (CTNI). These enzymes should be measured at the time of presentation and again 6 to 8 hours later. The enzymes CK and CK-MB begin to rise above normal levels approximately 4 to 6 hours after the onset of symptoms and peak in approximately 24 hours, returning to baseline within 72 to 96 hours. Although CK-MB is widely used for the diagnosis of acute myocardial infarction, it can be present in extensive skeletal muscle damage, hypothyroidism, and renal failure. The CK isoform MB2 may be released into the circulation by 2 to 3 hours after the onset of infarction; however, estimation of this CK isoform enzyme has not gained popularity.

Myoglobin, being a smaller molecule, is rapidly excreted into the urine, and therefore estimation of myoglobin may not allow diagnosis of myocardial infarction late after the onset of symptoms. Furthermore, myoglobin is very nonspecific, and it can be released from skeletal muscle necrosis.

Elevation of CTNT and CTNI above the normal values of the individual laboratories is diagnostic of myocardial damage, although elevations do not establish the cause of cardiac damage. CTNT and CTNI can be elevated in patients with Q wave and non-Q wave myocardial infarction and myocarditis. The release of CTNT and CTNI is increased by reperfusion of the ischemic myocardium whether the reperfusion occurs spontaneously or by therapeutic intervention. Of all the serum enzymes that are currently used for the diagnosis of myocardial necrosis, CTNT and CTNI are regarded as the most specific. For patients with low suspicion of acute myocardial infarction, normal serum enzyme levels, including CTNT and CTNI levels, and no ECG evidence of myocardial ischemia, the diagnosis of acute myocardial infarction can be excluded with about a 99% certainty. For patients with a high suspicion of myocardial ischemia, however, 24-hour observation with repeated ECG monitoring and measurement of serum enzyme levels are indicated to exclude the diagnosis of acute myocardial infarction.

Echocardiography

Two-dimensional echocardiography is indicated to assess changes in left ventricular systolic function. For all patients with pulmonary edema or when assessment of left ventricular systolic function is required for establishing the diagnosis of acute ischemic syndrome, two-dimensional echocardiography is the noninvasive investigation of choice. For patients with suspected acute myocardial infarction and uninterpretable ECG, assessment of left ventricular systolic function may help to establish the diagnosis of ischemic syndrome as well as to determine appropriate therapeutic intervention. Echocardiography can be useful in the differential diagnosis of right ventricular myocardial infarction, cardiac tamponade, and subacute free wall rupture. Two-dimensional echocardiography is also useful for the diagnosis of mural thrombi. It should be emphasized, however, that abnormal left ventricular regional and global function detected by two-dimensional echocardiography does not establish the cause of such dysfunction. Acute ischemia, old myocardial infarction, and acute and chronic ischemic heart disease can produce similar changes in ventricular function. Two-dimensional echocardiography may also be used for the diagnosis of left ventricular pseudoaneurysm.

Doppler echocardiography is extremely useful for the diagnosis of complications of acute myocardial infarction such as mitral regurgitation and ventricular septal rupture. Doppler echocardiography can also be used to assess right ventricular systolic pressure by estimating the tricuspid regurgitation velocity jet. Doppler echocardiography combined with two-dimensional echocardiography and hemodynamic monitoring may be useful for the differential diagnosis of the complications of acute myocardial infarction and the etiology of cardiogenic shock.

Nuclear Imaging

Nuclear imaging techniques such as radionuclide ventriculography, myocardial perfusion imaging, infarct avid scintigraphy, and positron emission tomography can be used to assess changes in left ventricular function, myocardial perfusion, and myocardial metabolic changes in patients with acute ischemic syndrome. Radionuclide imaging modalities, however, are seldom used for the diagnosis of acute myocardial infarction and its complications.

Transesophageal Echocardiography, Magnetic Resonance Imaging, and Computed Tomography

Transesophageal echocardiography is the investigation of choice for the rapid diagnosis of type A thoracic aortic dissection. Magnetic resonance imaging and cine-computed tomographic techniques, however, can also be used for the diagnosis of diseases of the aorta, including dissection. To exclude the diagnosis of pulmonary embolism, ventilation perfusion scintigraphy and spiral computed tomography may be useful in specific clinical circumstances.

Chest Radiography and Other Laboratory Tests

Chest x-ray studies should be performed routinely in all patients with suspected myocardial infarction. Chest x-ray films can reveal the degree of pulmonary venous congestion and also help to exclude the diagnosis of spontaneous pneumothorax and acute pulmonary embolism in patients with severe dyspnea. Other laboratory tests such as liver function tests and complete blood count are routinely performed, although they are not very useful for routine management of patients with acute myocardial infarction. The lipid profile within 24 hours of onset of acute myocardial infarction symptoms is a valid measurement.

MANAGEMENT

Management of Patients with Acute Myocardial Infarction with ST Segment Elevation (Q Wave Myocardial Infarction)

Because a total occlusion of the infarct-related artery with a fibrin reach thrombus is the mechanism for complete interruption of blood flow to the ischemic myocardium, a major goal of therapy is to establish adequate blood flow to the myocardium at risk as early as possible by recanalization of the infarct-related artery. As soon as the diagnosis of evolving myocardial infarction is suspected from the ECG changes (i.e., ST segment elevation with or without Q waves), aspirin, 160 to 325 mg, should be given immediately. The first dose of aspirin should be chewed rather than swallowed because, when aspirin is chewed, it increases the blood level rather rapidly.

Sublingual nitroglycerin (0.3 to 0.4 mg) should be given to exclude vasospastic angina, which is usually promptly relieved with sublingual nitroglycerin, and there is rapid resolution of ST segment elevation. It should be emphasized that in patients with acute ischemic syndrome, a paradoxical response to nitroglycerin may occur, which is characterized by hypotension and sinus bradycardia or junctional escape rhythm. This paradoxical response is more frequently observed in patients with inferior wall myocardial infarction but can occur in patients with anterior or lateral wall myocardial infarction. This response is mediated by activation of the Bajold-Jarish reflex (baroreceptor-mediated and central nervous system–mediated cardioinhibitory and vasodepressor response). In patients with documented right ventricular myocardial infarction, nitroglycerin should be given with caution because it can produce hypotension due to the reduction of right and left ventricular preload. For patients who do not get relief of chest pain with nitroglycerin, an analgesic such as morphine sulfate should be administered. Morphine 5 to 15 mg is administered intravenously every 5 to 15 minutes until the chest pain is relieved. It is unusual for the infarct-related pain to be relieved by nitroglycerin, and almost all patients require analgesic therapy.

Oxygen is usually administered with nasal prongs to patients with suspected acute myocardial infarction, although its benefit has not been established. When the clinical evaluation is being made and initial therapies are being administered, a decision should be made about reperfusion therapy. Reperfusion therapy consists of either intravenous thrombolytic agents or catheter-based recanalization of the infarct-related artery. As the facilities for the primary angioplasty and stenting of the infarct-related artery are limited, most patients with evolving myocardial infarction with ST segment elevations should be considered for intravenous thrombolytic therapy as soon as the diagnosis is made. A hospital mortality rate as low as 1.2% has been reported with institution of the thrombolytic agent tissue plasminogen activator (t-PA) within 70 minutes of symptom onset.

An early and adequate reperfusion within 6 hours of symptom onset is usually associated with preserved left ventricular ejection fraction. Left ventricular remodeling, an important determinant for development of progressive heart failure, is less likely to occur in the presence of preserved left ventricular ejection fraction. A delay in institution of the reperfusion therapy significantly reduces the magnitude of benefit of decreasing the risk of mortality and preservation of left ventricular function and development of congestive heart failure. The maximum benefit is achieved if perfusion therapy can be instituted within 1 hour of symptom onset; a significant benefit is retained if reperfusion therapy is instituted within 6 hours of symptom onset, and some benefit is still obtained if reperfusion therapy is instituted between 6 and 12 hours after symptom onset. The benefit of reperfusion therapy after 12 hours of symptom onset has not been established. For those patients who continue to have symptoms such as infarct-related pain and whose ECG demonstrates persistent ST segment elevation, however, reperfusion therapy is still indicated. Patients with new left or right bundle branch block with typical symptoms of acute myocardial infarction are also candidates for reperfusion therapy.

The relative benefits of reperfusion therapy with various thrombolytic agents have been observed in both men and women, in patients with and without previous myocardial infarction, and in younger and older patients. The magnitude of benefit, however, is greater in patients with evolving anterior wall than with inferior wall myocardial infarction. The benefit is also greater in patients with diabetes mellitus, hypertension, tachycardia, and complicated myocardial infarction. The major complication of thrombolytic therapy is hemorrhage, and intracranial hemorrhage is the most serious complication. Patient age older than 74 years, body weight less than 75 kg, hypertension (over 180/100 mm Hg), and the use of t-PA as opposed to streptokinase are the risk factors for intracranial hemorrhage. Primary angioplasty in-

stead of thrombolytic therapy may be preferable for these high-risk patients.

The choice of thrombolytic agent for reperfusion therapy for patients with acute myocardial infarction depends on the availability of the specific thrombolytic agent, the cost of therapy, and the indications for the use of a specific thrombolytic agent in a given clinical circumstance. The thrombolytic agents in clinical use are streptokinase, t-PA (Activase), recombinant tissue plasminogen activator (rt-PA) (reteplase), and anisoylated plasminogen streptokinase activator complex (APSAC) (Eminase). The front-loaded t-PA regimen is most frequently used in the United States. It consists of a 15-mg bolus followed by 0.75 mg per kg per 30 minutes (maximum 50 mg) and then 0.50 mg per kg per 60 minutes (maximum 35 mg). rt-PA (reteplase) has similar efficacy as t-PA. The advantage of rt-PA is that two bolus injections of 10 IU are administered at 30-minute intervals, and therefore the ease of administration is greater than with t-PA. When either t-PA or rt-PA is used, intravenous heparin should be used concurrently. A bolus of heparin, 60 to 70 units per kg, followed by an infusion of 12 to 15 units per kg per hour is used for approximately 48 hours. The activated partial thromboplastin time (aPTT) is maintained between 50 and 75 seconds.

Intravenous streptokinase therapy for recanalization of the infarct-related artery is used in many parts of the world. The dose of streptokinase is 1.5 million units per 100 mL given as a continuous infusion over 60 minutes. The disadvantage of streptokinase therapy is that the rate of recanalization of the infarct-related artery is significantly lower than that when t-PA is used. With front-loaded t-PA and heparin therapy, approximately 50% of the infarct-related artery is recanalized with normal flow (TIMI 3) to the ischemic myocardium. The use of t-PA is also associated with a slightly better ventricular function and with a 1% lower absolute 30-day mortality rate than streptokinase.

The major disadvantage of t-PA is a slightly greater risk of intracranial hemorrhage compared with streptokinase. The other disadvantage is that t-PA therapy is more expensive than streptokinase. Streptokinase may be ineffective in patients with streptococcal antibodies and who have received previous streptokinase therapy. The hypersensitivity reaction occurs more frequently with streptokinase than with t-PA. The incidence of hypotension appears to be relatively equal between t-PA and streptokinase therapy. In elderly patients with hypotension, streptokinase may be more effective than t-PA in reducing the risk of mortality.

Primary, Nonpharmacologic, Catheter-Based Reperfusion (Primary Angioplasty)

Instead of thrombolysis, recanalization of the infarct-related artery can be achieved by mechanical means such as balloon angioplasty with or without a stent. Primary angioplasty compared with thrombolysis has a greater potential to reduce the risk of 30-day mortality for patients with acute myocardial infarction. Better survival is observed particularly in high-risk patients with anterior myocardial infarction, patients with previous myocardial infarction, and patients with evidence of left ventricular dysfunction. With primary angioplasty, the recanalization rate of the infarct-related artery is over 90%, and the incidence of establishment of normal blood flow to the ischemic myocardium is also significantly higher than with thrombolysis. Furthermore, the incidence of life-threatening bleeding complications, including intracranial hemorrhage, is negligible with primary angioplasty. With the introduction of stents, as well as glycoprotein IIb/IIIa platelet antagonists, the incidence of acute reocclusion has markedly declined after angioplasty. After successful reperfusion by angioplasty compared with thrombolysis there is decreased incidence of recurrent ischemia and need for repeated revascularization therapy.

Although primary angioplasty provides several advantages over thrombolysis, a number of problems need to be considered when catheter-based reperfusion therapy is contemplated. The facilities for cardiac catheterization and angioplasty are available only in a few institutions. Furthermore, even when cardiac catheterization laboratories and experienced interventional cardiologists are available, a considerable delay may be encountered in transferring patients from the emergency department to the cardiac catheterization laboratory. This delay is considerably longer when a patient is transferred from an emergency department from the institution without cardiac catheterization facilities for angioplasty. This delay will substantially reduce the benefit of reperfusion therapy in terms of both reducing the risk of mortality and preserving ischemic myocardium and maintaining ventricular function. Thus, if a considerable delay is anticipated before primary angioplasty can be performed, thrombolysis is preferable. If prompt angioplasty is feasible, however, it should be considered, particularly for patients with anterior wall myocardial infarction, patients with complicated inferior and right ventricular myocardial infarction, patients with evidence of pump failure, and in high-risk patients such as those with previous myocardial infarction.

Primary angioplasty should also be considered when use of thrombolytic agents is contraindicated, such as in patients with bleeding diathesis, known intracranial aneurysm, recent major thoracoabdominal surgery or recent stroke. Primary angioplasty is preferable to thrombolysis for elderly patients (75 years or older) and for persistent hypertension.

Cardiac catheterization and rescue angioplasty with or without stents are also considered for patients who have received thrombolytic therapy but develop either persistent or recurrent ischemia, evident from unrelieved or recurrent ischemic pain and persistent or recurrent ST segment elevation. Cardiac catheterization should also be considered for patients whose history is very suggestive of acute myocardial infarction but whose ECG changes are nondiagnostic. Such intervention is particularly useful when noninvasive investigations such as echocardiography or thallium perfusion scintigraphy reveal a large area of myocardium at ischemic risk.

Adjunctive Therapy

Supplemental oxygen therapy is routinely used although its beneficial effects in absence of hypoxia have not been well documented. Supplemental oxygen therapy is clearly indicated for patients with pulmonary venous congestion. Although adequate reperfusion of the ischemic myocardium after recanalization of the infarct-related artery is the most effective treatment of infarct-related pain, patients who have not received reperfusion therapy or who had inadequate reperfusion of the ischemic myocardium require analgesics such as morphine sulfate for relief of infarct-related pain. Some patients may also benefit from anxiolytics.

Although all patients with acute ischemic syndrome with ST segment elevation should initially receive sublingual nitroglycerin to distinguish between vasospastic angina and evolving myocardial infarction, routine use of intravenous or nonparenteral nitroglycerin or nitrates by all patients with acute myocardial infarction do not appear to provide any survival benefit. Furthermore, nitroglycerin may produce hypotension and a low-output state in patients with right ventricular myocardial infarction. Nitroglycerin may also be associated with a paradoxical response characterized by bradycardia and hypotension mediated by activation of Bazold-Jarish reflex. The paradoxical response to nitroglycerin may be encountered in about 15 to 20% of patients with acute myocardial infarction. Nitroglycerin or nitrate therapy, however, is useful for treatment of ischemic pain and pulmonary venous hypertension.

Beta-blocker therapy should be considered for all patients with evolving myocardial infarction if no contraindication exists. The contraindications for beta-blocker therapy are overt severe heart failure, persistent hypotension with a systolic blood pressure of 100 mm Hg or less, bradycardia and heart block, cardiogenic shock, and bronchospastic disease. For patients who do not receive reperfusion therapy, beta-blocker therapy provides a survival benefit particularly for the high-risk subset of patients, which include elderly patients and patients with previous myocardial infarction and mild pulmonary venous congestion. For patients receiving reperfusion therapy, immediate administration of beta-adrenergic blocking agents does not decrease the risk of immediate mortality. However, immediate beta-blocker therapy has the potential to reduce the incidence of reinfarction and recurrence of angina. Usually beta blockers are given intravenously initially, such as metoprolol (Lopressor) 15 mg or atenolol (Tenormin) 5 mg. This intravenous therapy is followed by oral beta-blocker therapy, usually metoprolol 50 to 100 mg twice daily or atenolol 50 to 100 mg once daily. During beta-blocker therapy it is desirable to monitor changes in hemodynamics such as heart rate and blood pressure and to assess any evidence of heart failure such as pulmonary congestion and development of S_3 gallop. Most patients, however, tolerate beta-blocker therapy without experiencing adverse effects.

Angiotensin-converting enzyme (ACE) inhibitors such as captopril (Capoten), lisinopril (Prinivil), and ramapril (Altace), given orally during the acute phase of myocardial infarction, can potentially decrease the risk of immediate mortality. The beneficial effect of ACE inhibitors is observed with or without concomitant reperfusion therapy. The immediate survival benefit, however, is greatest in those patients who have some evidence of left ventricular systolic dysfunction or mild congestive heart failure.

ACE inhibitors can be administered soon after the onset of symptoms provided that the patient is hemodynamically stable. The initial oral dose should be low and should be gradually increased to the maximum tolerated dose. Treatment should be continued for approximately 4 weeks. For patients with depressed left ventricular systolic function, however, ACE inhibitor therapy should be continued indefinitely to attenuate ventricular remodeling. ACE inhibitor therapy is contraindicated for patients with significant hypotension with or without clinical features of cardiogenic shock. The mechanism for the decrease in early mortality with ACE inhibitor therapy may be due to a decreased incidence of ventricular rupture rather than to prevention of remodeling.

The benefit of the routine use of intravenous magnesium in patients with acute myocardial infarction has not been established. In some prospective randomized clinical trials, the beneficial effect of magnesium given soon after the onset of myocardial infarction has been associated with decreased mortality. Other studies, however, have demonstrated potential deleterious effects on survival after routine use of intravenous magnesium. Thus, intravenous magnesium therapy should be reserved for selected patients with polymorphous ventricular tachycardia or patients who develop arrhythmias due to digitalis toxicity.

Prophylactic use of lidocaine is not recommended for patients with acute myocardial infarction. Prophylactic use of amiodarone to decrease the risk of arrhythmic death is also not recommended. Intravenous amiodarone (Cordarone) therapy, however, is indicated for patients with ischemic polymorphous ventricular tachycardia. Long-term oral amiodarone may also be of benefit for some patients with impaired left ventricular systolic dysfunction and nonsustained ventricular tachycardia.

Determination of the lipid profile and assessment for other risk factors of coronary artery disease such as diabetes, obesity, and hypertension should be performed concurrently. Treatments to modify these risk factors should be considered for all patients with acute myocardial infarction resulting from atherosclerotic coronary artery disease. The treatment of hyperlipidemia with low-density lipoprotein–lowering agents, particularly statins, is useful to reduce the risk of reinfarction and fatal myocardial infarction and the need for angioplasty or coronary artery bypass surgery. All patients should be advised to refrain from smoking.

Before discharge from the hospital, assessment of left ventricular systolic dysfunction is indicated and usually done noninvasively by two-dimensional echocardiography or radionuclide ventriculography. Patients with depressed left ventricular systolic function with an ejection fraction of 40% or less should be considered for long-term treatment with ACE inhibitors and a beta-adrenergic antagonist. Aspirin and low-density lipoprotein–lowering agents, particularly statins, are indicated for all survivors of acute myocardial infarction.

Assessment of risk of sudden death for patients recovering from myocardial infarction is indicated and can be accomplished by many investigations, including ECG testing, Holter monitoring, signal average ECG, heart rate variability studies, and determination of baroreceptor sensitivity. Currently, signal average ECG is used the most. A negative signal average ECG is associated with a very low risk of sudden death. Patients with an abnormal signal average ECG but without symptomatic ventricular tachyarrhythmia should be treated with beta-adrenergic antagonists.

For the survivors of acute myocardial infarction, myocardium at ischemic risk can be assessed by various noninvasive investigations, including stress ECG, exercise or persantine thallium perfusion scintigraphy, exercise echocardiography, and dobutamine stress echocardiography. If significant residual myocardial ischemia is identified, catheter-based or surgical revascularization therapy is considered. The therapeutic approach for uncomplicated myocardial infarction is summarized in Table 3.

Complications of Acute Myocardial Infarction

Bradyarrhythmias

Transient sinus bradycardia is common at the onset of acute ischemic syndrome. Persistent sinus bradycardia with a resting heart rate of less than 60 beats per minute, however, is uncommon. It can be observed in patients who had been taking large doses of beta blockers. Sinus bradycardia does not require any specific treatment unless it is associated with hypotension and a low cardiac output state. Initially, intravenous atropine should be administered, and the dose of atropine should not exceed 0.8 mg because a higher dose may cause a sudden increase in heart rate and precipitate myocardial ischemia and ventricular tachyarrhythmia.

Persistent sinus bradycardia unresponsive to atropine may require transvenous temporary pacemaker therapy. Atrial pacing is preferable to ventricular

TABLE 3. **Therapy for Uncomplicated Myocardial Infarction (ST Segment Elevation and Q Wave Present)**

Chewable aspirin followed by oral aspirin

Sublingual nitroglycerin except in patient with suspected right ventricular infarction and hypotension

Reperfusion therapy with intravenous thrombolytic agents or by catheter-based techniques (angioplasty)

Intravenous heparin (in patients receiving t-PA) and glycoprotein IIb/IIIa antagonists in patients undergoing primary angioplasty with or without stents

Supplemental oxygen and analgesics

Beta-adrenergic blocking agents, initially intravenously and then orally—if not contraindicated

Oral angiotensin-converting enzyme inhibitor therapy for approximately 4 weeks in patients with normal left ventricular systolic function and indefinitely in patients with depressed left ventricular systolic function

Low-density lipoprotein (LDL) lowering agents, particularly statins, in patients with elevated total cholesterol and LDL cholesterol

Cessation of smoking, control of diabetes, and treatment of obesity and hypertension

Assessment for risk of sudden death, left ventricular systolic function, and residual myocardial ischemia

pacing, particularly in patients with suspected or documented right ventricular myocardial infarction. Ventricular pacing may be adequate, however, when an increase in heart rate is required to suppress ventricular tachyarrhythmia precipitated by bradycardia. First-degree atrioventricular (AV) block and Mobitz type I second-degree AV block usually does not require any specific treatment. Some patients with anterior myocardial infarction complicated by persistent Mobitz type I AV block and significant bradycardia, however, may need temporary pacemaker therapy. Temporary transvenous pacemaker therapy is also indicated for Mobitz type II, advanced, and complete AV block.

Complete AV block, however, needs to be differentiated from AV dissociation in which ventricular response is faster than the atrial rate which usually indicates functional AV block. AV dissociation is frequently observed in patients with inferior wall myocardial infarction and does not require transvenous pacemaker therapy. Temporary transvenous pacing is recommended for patients who had brief episodes of asystole, bilateral bundle branch block, new or age indeterminate bifascicular block-like right bundle branch block with left anterior fascicular block or left posterior fascicular block, or left bundle branch block with first-degree AV block. For patients with only right bundle branch or left bundle branch block, or stable bradycardia without any hemodynamic compromise, a standby transcutaneous pacing system can be used.

Tachyarrhythmias

Atrial fibrillation occurs in approximately 15% of patients with acute myocardial infarction. It may occur at the onset of infarction when it is usually transient and more frequently occurs in inferior wall myocardial infarction due to right coronary artery occlusion. Sustained atrial fibrillation or flutter occurs less frequently (approximately 7% incidence) and often reflects left ventricular failure, which occurs more frequently in patients with anterior myocardial infarction. In the absence of hypotension or left ventricular failure, beta-adrenergic antagonists may be appropriate treatment to control ventricular response. In many patients beta-blocker therapy alone may convert atrial fibrillation to sinus rhythm and also maintain sinus rhythm.

For patients with hypotension, heart failure, or evidence of myocardial ischemia, immediate cardioversion electrically or with pharmacologic agents such as ibutilide (Corvert) should be attempted. After cardioversion to maintain sinus rhythm, intravenous procainamide (Pronestyl) therapy is frequently useful. When procainamide is used, usually a loading dose of 500 to 1000 mg (100 mg every 5 minutes) followed by a maintenance infusion rate to 2 to 4 mg per minute is administered. It should be emphasized that procainamide can cause depression of cardiac function. Most patients also require digitalization. Intravenous digoxin is administered, usually 0.5 mg in 10 minutes to avoid digitalis-induced vasoconstriction. The intravenous digoxin at a dose of 0.125 to 0.25 mg a day may be required for a few days. In refractory patients and for long term maintenance of sinus rhythm, amiodarone therapy is more effective. Amiodarone can be given intravenously initially 1 gram every 24 hours for 4 or 5 days and then continued orally 200 mg two times daily for 3 to 6 weeks, then usually 200 mg daily.

Cardioversion for atrial flutter or fibrillation is usually achieved with direct electrical countershock. The initial energy used is usually 50 to 100 volts and then gradually increased if the first shock is not successful. Pharmacologic cardioversion can be achieved with ibutilide, which is a short-acting class III antiarrhythmic agent and is given intravenously in a 1-mg dose in 10 minutes. If the 1-mg dose is ineffective, another 1 mg is repeated in 30 minutes. For patients with recent onset of atrial fibrillation or flutter, ibutilide is effective in cardioversion in 60% of instances. When ibutilide is used for cardioversion, it is essential to assess changes in the QT interval. If there is prolongation of the QT interval, ibutilide should not be used as it can induce polymorphous ventricular tachycardia.

Ventricular Arrhythmias

Unifocal or multifocal premature ventricular contractions or short runs of monomorphic nonsustained ventricular tachycardia do not require immediate antiarrhythmic drug therapy. Sustained monomorphic ventricular tachycardia is frequently associated with hypotension and should be promptly treated with direct current cardioversion. To prevent recurrence, lidocaine is given intravenously. Initially, a bolus dose of 75 to 100 mg is given, which can be repeated every 5 to 10 minutes to a maximum dose of 3 mg per kg. The maintenance dose of lidocaine is usually

TABLE 4. Therapy for Bradyarrhythmias

Dysrhythmia	Therapy
Transient sinus bradycardia or junctional rhythm	No therapy
Persistent sinus bradycardia or junctional rhythm	
No hemodynamic compromise	No therapy
Hemodynamic compromise	Atropine; if unsuccessful, transvenous pacing
First degree, Mobitz I AV block, vagotonic block	No therapy
AV dissociation	No therapy
Mobitz type II, advanced and complete AV block	Transvenous pacing
Bifascicular or trifascicular block	Prophylactic transvenous pacing
Right bundle or left bundle branch block	Transcutaneous standby pacing

Abbreviation: AV = atrioventricular.

between 1 and 3 mg per min. If monomorphic ventricular tachycardia recurs despite lidocaine therapy, intravenous procainamide should be considered. The dose and method of administration of procainamide is similar to that for treatment of atrial fibrillation.

For resistant monomorphic ventricular tachycardia, intravenous amiodarone should be considered. A 100-mg bolus infusion is followed by 1 gram every 24 hours. Ischemic polymorphous ventricular tachycardia whether nonsustained or sustained should be treated aggressively. For patients with acute ischemic syndrome polymorphous ventricular tachycardia is usually not pause dependent, and there may not be prolongation of the QT interval. The typical torsades de pointes is also rarely encountered in acute myocardial infarction. Initially, intravenous magnesium, 2 to 4 grams, should be given, and hypokalemia should be corrected. The antiarrhythmic drug of choice for treatment of polymorphous ventricular

tachycardia complicating acute myocardial infarction is intravenous amiodarone. A loading infusion of 100 to 150 mg in 30 minutes is administered, followed by 1 mg per minute for 6 hours and then 1 gram every 24 hours. The amiodarone therapy should be continued for 3 to 4 days.

Ventricular Fibrillation

Three forms of ventricular fibrillation are encountered during the acute phase of myocardial infarction. The primary ventricular fibrillation occurs early within a few hours of onset of symptoms and is not associated with left ventricular failure. Secondary ventricular fibrillation occurs in association with severe left ventricular dysfunction. Ventricular fibrillation may also be the agonal rhythm. Ventricular fibrillation, primary or secondary, should be treated promptly with unsynchronized electric shock and the energy used initially should be 200 to 360 volts. If ventricular fibrillation persists, 1 mg of epinephrine is given intravenously, or intracardiac epinephrine is administered, 5 to 10 mL as a 1/10,000 concentration. Intravenous lidocaine, procainamide, or amiodarone may also be necessary to prevent recurrence of ventricular tachycardia and fibrillation. Management approaches for dysrhythmias are summarized in Tables 4 and 5.

Acute Heart Failure Complicating Myocardial Infarction

The management approach for acute heart failure can be outlined based on clinical presentation and, in some instances, hemodynamic profile. Mild pulmonary congestion is common, and, clinically, bilateral pulmonary rales are present with mild or no dyspnea. Occasionally an S_3 gallop is appreciated, and chest x-ray films may reveal evidence of mild to moderate pulmonary venous congestion. The hemody-

TABLE 5. Therapy for Tachyarrhythmias

Dysrhythmia	Therapy
Sinus tachycardia	Beta blockers if not contraindicated
Transient paroxysmal atrial tachycardia, atrial flutter or fibrillation	No therapy
Nonparoxysmal, sustained supraventricular tachycardia, atrial flutter, or atrial fibrillation	
No hemodynamic compromise and stable	Beta blocker and/or digoxin
Hemodynamic compromise and/or ischemia	Cardioversion
	IV Procainamide; if refractory, IV amiodarone (digoxin to decrease ventricular response)
Premature ventricular beats and nonsustained monomorphic ventricular tachycardia	No therapy
Accelerated idioventricular rhythm	No treatment
Sustained monomorphic ventricular tachycardia	
No hemodynamic compromise	IV lidocaine; if ineffective, IV procainamide; if ineffective, IV amiodarone
Hemodynamic compromise	Cardioversion
Sustained or nonsustained ischemic polymorphous ventricular tachycardia	IV magnesium, IV procainamide; if ineffective, IV amiodarone (cardioversion and adequate reperfusion therapy may be required)
	Pacemaker therapy is not effective and contraindicated
Ventricular fibrillation (primary and secondary)	Unsynchronized electric shock
	IV lidocaine, procainamide, or amiodarone to prevent recurrence

namic abnormality in such patients is usually a modest increase in pulmonary capillary wedge pressure, 18 to 25 mm Hg, without hypotension or decrease in cardiac output. Hemodynamic monitoring is not required for the diagnosis or for initial therapy of these patients. The treatment consists of maintenance of adequate arterial oxygenation with supplemental oxygen and reduction of pulmonary venous congestion with diuretics and nitroglycerin.

The diuretic of choice is furosemide (Lasix) 20 to 40 mg administered intravenously. Furosemide can decrease pulmonary venous pressure due to its extrarenal effect of increasing systemic venous capacitance. Diuresis of course reduces intracardiac volume and causes further reduction in pulmonary capillary wedge pressure. Intravenous or nonparenteral nitroglycerin and nitrates also decrease pulmonary venous pressure by causing venodilatation and venous pooling. When intravenous nitroglycerin is used, the initial dose should be low, 10 to 20 μg per minute, and the dose should be increased by 5 to 10 μg per minute every 10 to 15 minutes until an adequate clinical and hemodynamic response is achieved. Usually not more than 200 μg per minute of intravenous nitroglycerin is required for treatment of pulmonary venous congestion or pulmonary edema.

Sodium nitroprusside is another vasodilator that can be used to decrease pulmonary capillary wedge pressure. Sodium nitroprusside (Nipride) has a balanced effect on venous capacitance and arterial resistance vessels. The hemodynamic responses of sodium nitroprusside are a substantial decrease in pulmonary venous pressure, right atrial pressure, and systemic vascular resistance and an increase in cardiac output. Arterial pressure also tends to decrease. Sodium nitroprusside should not be used in the absence of heart failure in patients with acute myocardial infarction because of its enhanced risk of myocardial ischemia. The initial dose of sodium nitroprusside is also very low, 10 μg per minute, and the dose should be increased by 5 μg every 15 to 20 minutes until the desired clinical or hemodynamic response is achieved. Arterial pressure should be constantly monitored. If there is significant hypotension, nitroprusside therapy should be discontinued. Most patients with mild pulmonary venous congestion do not require continued nitroglycerin or nitroprusside therapy, as they usually respond to intermittent diuretic and nitroglycerin therapy.

Acute Pulmonary Edema Without Shock

Patients with acute pulmonary edema without shock have acute respiratory distress with tachypnea, tachycardia, and extensive bilateral pulmonary rales with or without bronchospasm. Chest x-ray films reveal frank bilateral pulmonary edema. Moderate to severe hypoxemia (decreased arterial Po_2) and retention of carbon dioxide (increased CO_2) are also common. The hemodynamic profile in these patients is characterized by marked increase in pulmonary capillary wedge pressure exceeding 25 mm Hg

with normal or slightly decreased cardiac output. Sinus tachycardia, marked elevation of systemic vascular resistance, and elevated blood pressure are also frequently observed. In all patients with acute pulmonary edema complicating myocardial infarction, transthoracic and Doppler echocardiography should be performed to exclude significant mitral regurgitation due to papillary muscle dysfunction or infarction.

Therapy consists of administration of supplemental oxygen, 60 to 100% by face mask, intravenous morphine, and sublingual nitroglycerin or nitroglycerin spray. Intravenous diuretics should be administered concurrently. If arterial Po_2 is 60 mm Hg or less, endotracheal intubation should be considered. Intravenous nitroglycerin should be administered, along with intravenous diuretic therapy. For some patients, hemodynamic monitoring to guide aggressive supportive therapy is required.

Hypoperfusion Without Pulmonary Congestion

In patients with hypoperfusion without pulmonary congestion, there is clinical evidence of hypoperfusion such as decreased urine output, mental obtundation, and cool periphery and hypotension without signs and symptoms of pulmonary venous congestion. In patients with this clinical profile, hypovolemic shock or predominant right ventricular infarction should be considered. Hypovolemic shock can be confirmed by hemodynamic monitoring, which reveals decreased right atrial and pulmonary capillary wedge pressures with low cardiac output. In patients with right ventricular myocardial infarction, in addition to characteristic changes in the ECG, the hemodynamic profile reveals decreased or normal pulmonary capillary wedge pressure with disproportionate elevation of right atrial pressure.

The treatment of hypovolemic shock consists of rapid administration of intravenous fluids 50 to 100 mL every 15 to 20 minutes under close clinical and hemodynamic observation until the pulmonary capillary wedge pressure is elevated to 14 to 18 mm Hg. In some patients, low cardiac output persists despite maintaining adequate filling pressure. For these patients, inotropic therapy such as dobutamine should be considered to maintain adequate cardiac output.

Cardiogenic Shock

Cardiogenic shock is the most serious complication of acute myocardial infarction and carries a very poor prognosis. Left ventricular systolic dysfunction without mechanical defects accounts for 75% of patients with cardiogenic shock and can occur very quickly, within a few hours (6 to 24 hours) of the onset of symptoms. Patients with cardiogenic shock require hemodynamic monitoring, which reveals hypotension (systolic blood pressure) 90 mm Hg or less, low cardiac index (usually 2.2 liter per minute per m²), and elevated pulmonary capillary wedge pressure exceeding 18 mm Hg.

Vasopressor and inotropic therapy and intra-aortic balloon counterpulsation therapy alone without adequate reperfusion of the ischemic myocardium does not appear to improve prognosis. The mortality with such supportive therapy alone is close to 100%. The intravenous thrombolytic therapy with streptokinase also has not been shown to improve prognosis. Uncontrolled studies have suggested that primary angioplasty, if successful to establish adequate blood flow to the ischemic myocardium, can improve prognosis of patients with cardiogenic shock, and the survival rate may be as high as 70%.

It should be emphasized, however, that if the facilities for cardiac catheterization and primary angioplasty are not available, intravenous thrombolytic therapy, preferably t-PA, should be administered, and, if possible, patients should be transferred to an institution with facilities for cardiac catheterization and angioplasty.

Supportive therapy is still required after reperfusion therapy. The most effective supportive therapy is intra-aortic balloon counterpulsation, which maintains diastolic perfusion pressure (diastolic augmentation) and unloads the left ventricle (systolic unloading), which is associated with improved cardiac performance. Furthermore, effective intra-aortic balloon counterpulsation has the potential to keep the infarct-related artery open after the reperfusion therapy. Supportive therapy also consists of vasopressors such as norepinephrine (Levophed) or phenylephrine (Neo-Synephrine) or dopamine to maintain arterial pressure and inotropic agents such as dobutamine or phosphodiesterase inhibitors such as milrinone to maintain forward cardiac output. Diuretics, nitroglycerin, and nitroprusside may also be added to maintain adequate cardiac performance. Such combination therapy, however, can only be performed with hemodynamic monitoring.

The usual dose of dobutamine is between 2 and 10 μg per kg per minute. The dose of intravenous milrinone (Primacor), is between 0.3 and 0.7 mg per kg per minute. For patients with hypotension, dopamine is also used, and the dose varies between 5 and 20 μg per kg per minute. The dose of norepinephrine is also variable and is between 2 and 10 μg per minute.

Mitral Regurgitation Due to Papillary Muscle Infarction With or Without Rupture

Severe mitral regurgitation resulting from papillary muscle infarction with or without rupture and infarction of the left ventricular wall anchoring the papillary muscle is a catastrophic complication that occurs in approximately 1 to 2% of patients. The diagnosis is confirmed by transthoracic or transesophageal echocardiography. Hemodynamic monitoring, if performed, reveals severe elevation of pulmonary venous pressure with a giant V wave and a reflected V wave in the pulmonary artery pressure

tracing. Cardiac output is frequently reduced. Rupture of the posteromedial papillary muscle occurs 6 to 12 times more frequently than rupture of the anterolateral papillary muscle. It is more frequent in patients with inferior or interoposterior myocardial infarction. In approximately 50% of patients with papillary muscle infarct, there is single-vessel coronary artery disease, and the size of the infarction is relatively small. Papillary muscle infarct producing severe mitral regurgitation can occur soon after the onset of symptoms.

With conservative treatment without surgery, mortality is 50% in 24 hours and 94% within 8 weeks. With early surgery, a salvage rate of 60 to 70% of patients may be expected. Supportive therapy consists of intra-aortic balloon counterpulsation to maintain arterial pressure and to reduce the severity of mitral regurgitation. Vasodilators such as sodium nitroprusside with or without inotropic agents such as dobutamine may be required as supportive therapy before corrective surgery is undertaken. Surgical treatment should not be delayed, however, and should be performed as soon as the patients are stabilized.

Ventricular Septal Rupture

Ventricular septal rupture occurs in 0.5% to 2% of patients with acute myocardial infarction. A considerable number of patients develop ventricular septal rupture within a few hours of onset of symptoms. Ventricular septal rupture produces a left to right shunt that increases the volume load on the right and left ventricle and increases the left ventricular diastolic pressure, left atrial pressure, and pulmonary artery pressure. There is also a substantial increase in right atrial and right ventricular diastolic pressure. The systemic cardiac output is reduced as the magnitude of left to right shunt increases. Clinical presentation is characterized by the appearance of a new pansystolic murmur as in patients with mitral regurgitation and worsening congestive heart failure. Two-dimensional echocardiography is the investigation of choice for diagnosis of ventricular septal rupture. It also reveals regional wall motion abnormalities and changes in right and left ventricular systolic function. Doppler studies demonstrate transseptal flow across the defect. Hemodynamic monitoring is not required for the diagnosis of ventricular septal rupture, but it is usually useful for assessing the response to therapy. Right heart catheterization reveals step up in the oxygen saturation in the pulmonary arterial blood compared with right atrial blood.

With conservative therapy, the mortality rate of postinfarction ventricular septal rupture is approximately 25% during the first 24 hours, and up to 80% of patients die within 2 months. Early surgical repair is preferable, although the operative mortality rate may be as high as 30%. Overall survival in patients with ventricular septal rupture after corrective surgery is 50 to 70%. The supportive therapy of choice

TABLE 6. **Therapy for Pulmonary Congestion Without Hypoperfusion**

Mild pulmonary congestion
  Supplemental oxygen by nasal cannula or face mask
  Chewable aspirin (160 mg)
  Sublingual nitroglycerin
  Intravenous furosemide (20–40 mg)
  Intravenous nitroglycerin (5–10 μg/min) increasing by 5–10
    μg/min every 5–10 min until 200 μg/min dose is reached
    or there is 10% decrease in mean blood pressure in
    normotensives or 30% decrease in blood pressure in
    hypertensives
  Avoid hemodynamic monitoring in the absence of clinical
    deterioration
Pulmonary edema without hypotension
  Supplemental oxygen (60–100%) by face mask, early
    mechanical ventilation if arterial $Po_2 < 60$ mm Hg
  Sublingual nitroglycerin followed by IV nitroglycerin
  Chewable aspirin (160 mg)
  Intravenous furosemide (40 mg), may be repeated depending
    on response
  Reperfusion therapy
  Hemodynamic monitoring in refractory patients

is intra-aortic balloon counterpulsation, which reduces the magnitude of left to right shunt and increases the forward stroke volume and systemic cardiac output. The management strategies for treatment of pulmonary edema and cardiogenic shock are summarized in Tables 6 and 7.

Right Ventricular Myocardial Infarction

Right ventricular myocardial infarction is usually seen in association with inferior or inferoposterior myocardial infarction. The ECG characteristically demonstrates evidence of inferior wall myocardial infarction and ST segment elevation in lead V_1 and right precordial leads such as V_4R. Occasionally ST segment elevation can be seen in precordial leads V_1

TABLE 7. **Management Strategies for Cardiogenic Shock**

Left ventricular systolic dysfunction without mechanical defects
  Reperfusion therapy, preferably by primary angioplasty
  Vasopressors to maintain arterial pressure
  Intra-aortic balloon counterpulsation
  Supportive pharmacotherapy according to hemodynamics
  Left ventricular assist device as a bridge to cardiac transplant
    in refractory patients
Severe mitral regurgitation due to papillary muscle infarction
  with or without rupture
  Supportive therapy with intravenous vasodilators (sodium
    nitroprusside or hydralazine) in absence of hypotension
  Intra-aortic balloon counterpulsation (particularly in
    hypotensive patients)
  Addition of inotropic agents for further hemodynamic
    improvement
  Corrective surgery as early as possible
Ventricular septal rupture
  Intra-aortic balloon counterpulsation
  Add vasodilators, preferably hydralazine
  Add inotropic agent for further hemodynamic improvement
  Corrective surgery whenever feasible

to V_5. Clinically these patients may not have any symptoms of low-output state. The incidence of sinus bradycardia and second-degree and complete AV block are higher in patients with right ventricular infarction. Complete AV block should be treated by AV sequential pacing rather than by ventricular pacing. Approximately 10% of patients with right ventricular infarction develop low-output state in the absence of bradyarrhythmia. The mechanism of decreased systemic output is decreased left ventricular preload, which results from right ventricular pump failure, the constraining effect of the pericardium, diastolic shift of the intraventricular septum toward the left ventricle, and right atrial and ventricular septal dysfunction.

All patients with right ventricular infarction should be considered for adequate reperfusion therapy. For patients with low-output state, intravenous fluid therapy is indicated if the right atrial pressure or pulmonary capillary wedge pressure is less than normal. If the right atrial pressure or pulmonary capillary wedge pressure is already elevated above 15 mm Hg, intravenous fluid therapy is not effective in improving systemic output. For these patients, inotropic therapy with dobutamine or dopamine may be effective. Vasodilator therapy such as sodium nitroprusside is rarely effective in improving systemic output in patients with a low-output state complicating right ventricular myocardial infarction. For patients with refractory heart failure and a low-output state, a right ventricular assist device may be required. The therapeutic approach for the management of low-output state, complicating right ventricular infarction is summarized in Table 8.

Acute and Subacute Rupture of Left Ventricular Free Wall

Rupture of ventricular free wall is a sudden, usually fatal complication of acute myocardial infarction. It is the most common form of ventricular myocardial rupture and is 8 to 10 times more frequent than papillary muscle rupture. The overall incidence of free wall rupture is approximately 3%, and it occurs in 10 to 20% of patients who die from complications of acute myocardial infarction. Rupture occurs most

TABLE 8. **Right Ventricular Myocardial Infarction Management Approach**

Asymptomatic
  Aspirin, reperfusion therapy
  Avoid diuretics and nitroglycerin
Symptomatic and normal systemic venous pressure
  Volume loading; if ineffective, hemodynamic monitoring,
    dobutamine, or dopamine
Symptomatic and elevated systemic venous pressure
  Hemodynamic monitoring, dobutamine or dopamine depending
    on the level of blood pressure
  Right ventricular assist device in refractory patients
Atrioventricular block
  Atrioventricular sequential pacing

frequently in the free wall of the left ventricle (80 to 90%) and less commonly of the right ventricle. Female gender, past infarction, advanced age, infarct expansion, uncontrolled hypertension, absence of collaterals, and thrombolytic therapy have been thought to predispose to free wall rupture. Approximately 90% of free wall ruptures occur during the first week of the onset of myocardial infarction, but approximately 30% of all ruptures occur within the first 24 hours of onset of symptoms. Most frequently, rupture occurs abruptly and unexpectedly and produces cardiogenic shock due to tamponade. Abrupt free wall rupture is almost always fatal. Subacute rupture, however, if diagnosed can be repaired surgically and a considerable number of patients can be salvaged. Subacute rupture also occurs more frequently in women older than 55 years old, with persistent hypertension and past myocardial infarction. Persistent chest pain, not characteristic of myocardial ischemia or pericarditis, repetitive vomiting and nausea, and restlessness and agitation are frequently encountered. The ECG changes of regional pericarditis are frequently associated with subacute rupture.

The treatment of choice is surgical repair. A new treatment has been suggested, however, that involves the application of a Teflon patch to the epicardium with adhesive glue similar to commercially available household glues. The procedure has been done with and without cardiopulmonary bypass. The potential also exists for use of a pericardioscope to apply the adhesive glue. At the present time, however, surgical repair is preferable if the diagnosis can be made before the cardiac tamponade develops.

Postinfarction Pericarditis

Three forms of postinfarction pericarditis are recognized. The pericarditis associated with transmural myocardial infarction, episternal pericarditis, is common and is observed in approximately 30% of patients. Pericarditis also may accompany acute or subacute free wall rupture. Postinfarction autoimmune pericarditis (Dressler's syndrome) occurs in approximately 3 to 5% of patients with myocardial infarction. Recurrent pericarditis with pericardial pain can occur in the absence of any other manifestations of pericarditis. Dressler's syndrome, however, is characterized by pericardial pain, arthralgia, occasionally fever, pulmonary infiltrates, pleural effusion, and occasionally pericardial effusion.

Most patients will respond to nonsteroidal, antiinflammatory agents. Corticosteroid therapy should be avoided as it is associated with increased incidence of recurrence of chronic pericardial pain. Recurring chronic pericarditis with pericardial pain may respond to colchicine therapy.

Recurrent Ischemia or Reinfarction

Myocardial ischemia or reinfarction recurs in approximately 20 to 25% of patients after acute myocardial infarction. Patients with recurrent myocardial ischemia require aggressive anti-ischemic therapy along with antiplatelet and antithrombotic therapy. Most patients will require coronary arteriography with a view to reperfusion therapy by angioplasty or by surgical revascularization.

Non–Q Wave Myocardial Infarction

Management of non–Q wave myocardial infarction is similar to that of primary unstable angina. As the pathophysiologic mechanisms are similar, aggressive antiplatelet and anti-ischemic therapy are recommended. The antiplatelet therapy consists of aspirin if not contraindicated. Those patients who are intolerant to aspirin are treated with clopidogrel (Plavix). The glycoprotein IIb/IIIa platelet receptor antagonists have been found to be effective to reduce the risk of fatal and nonfatal myocardial infarction in patients with primary unstable angina and non–Q wave myocardial infarction. Thus, patients with non–Q wave infarction, like high-risk patients with primary unstable angina, should be considered for glycoprotein IIb/IIIa antagonists.

Aggressive anti-ischemic therapy consists of intravenous nitroglycerin and beta-adrenergic blocking agents. Patients with non-Q wave myocardial infarction also may benefit from heart rate regulating calcium channel blocking agents such as diltiazem (Cardizem). It should be emphasized, however, that calcium channel blocking agents are not useful for treatment of Q wave or ST segment elevation myocardial infarction. Controversy exists for the indication of immediate aggressive therapy (cardiac catheterization or revascularization). A conservative approach (i.e., cardiac catheterization and revascularization only when indicated) is preferred as it is associated with a better prognosis.

CARE AFTER MYOCARDIAL INFARCTION

method of
DAVID J. MOLITERNO, M.D.
The Cleveland Clinic Foundation
Cleveland, Ohio

In the United States, as in nearly all industrialized nations, the leading cause of adult hospitalizations is acute coronary syndromes and the leading cause of death is ischemic heart disease. An estimated 1.5 million Americans will have a myocardial infarction (MI) this year, and for two thirds of these patients it will be their first attack. One third will die within minutes to hours of symptom onset, and for the majority of those dying suddenly, there were no symptoms before this first and final event. Fortunately, with the widespread establishment of emergency medical services, coronary intensive care units, and novel medical therapies, the death rate from coronary heart disease has decreased approximately 25% since the late 1980s. Currently, 12 million living Americans have a history of MI or angina pectoris. With this, it is easily understood why the primary and secondary prevention of atherosclerotic heart disease remains so important to contemporary health care. As will be explained, the medical care of MI survivors is filled with opportunities to improve the likelihood of survival and the quality of life of these patients.

POSTINFARCTION PATHOPHYSIOLOGY AND TREATMENT GOALS

Therapies, both pharmacologic and nonpharmacologic, for survivors of infarction are directed at three main intervals in the postinfarction setting: acute (in-hospital), subacute (early weeks to months of outpatient recovery), and chronic (months to years later). Another way to view the backdrop of this care is to consider the three underlying treatment goals: (1) prevent recurrent ischemia and infarction, (2) minimize ventricular dysfunction, and (3) protect against new atherosclerotic events and premature death. Each of the main time intervals in the post-MI setting contains the three treatment goals, but to differing extents. For example, heparin may be needed in the acute setting but has no benefit in chronic therapy. In contrast, lipid-lowering agents serve little benefit in the acute setting but are paramount for chronic therapy.

Acute Phase

The pathophysiology of MI is the result of excessive demand or inadequate supply of nutrients, primarily oxygen. The overwhelming majority of infarctions are caused by abrupt cessation of coronary blood flow at the site of a ruptured plaque. Less commonly, episodes of excessive demand can outstrip the usually adequate blood supply, although these conditions are not subtle: severe aortic stenosis, thyrotoxicosis, cocaine use, acute anemia or hypoxemia, and perioperative hemodynamic events. More commonly, plaque rupture exposes the inner vessel wall, resulting in activation of platelets, initiation of the coagulation cascade, thrombin generation, and thrombus formation. Thus, the most initial therapy for myocardial infarction (use of anticoagulants) is aimed at restoring and maintaining coronary vessel patency (i.e., maximizing supply). At the same time, it is of benefit to minimize myocardial oxygen demand by decreasing wall stress and the heart rate/blood pressure product (nitrates and beta blockers). This phase can be considered one of plaque stabilization.

Subacute Phase

In the days to months after an MI, the ruptured arterial plaque usually becomes quiescent and heals. Important changes also occur at the myocardial level. Early after an infarction the area of myocardial necrosis is replaced by scar. Often after large, anterior wall infarctions the ventricle dilates and undergoes structural changes referred to as remodeling. These changes can help to preserve ventricular stroke volume but can become pathologic. If the left ventricular (LV) wall stress (internal pressure × volume) is unfavorably high, infarct expansion or excessive ventricular dilatation may occur. Both result in worsened myocardial efficiency and an increased risk of heart failure, ventricular arrhythmias, and death. Indeed, among the leading predictors of survival are LV ejection fraction and end-systolic volume. The mainstays of therapies during this stage are aimed at reducing ventricular afterload, cavitary pressure, and volume, thereby optimizing remodeling and mechanical efficiency. Hence, this stage can be considered as modulation of ventricular remodeling.

Chronic Phase

For the long term, efforts are shifted more heavily toward the prevention of new atherosclerotic events. During this stage the original plaque should be fully quiescent and ventricular remodeling should be complete. A greater emphasis can now be placed on risk factor modification even though it has been a part of the earlier stages. For example, while angiotensin-converting enzyme (ACE) inhibitors, nitrates, and beta blockers all have essential roles in the early phases of therapy, agents affecting remodeling (ACE inhibitors) likely lose relative importance in the longer-term treatment plan except among patients with persistent LV dysfunction. Similarly, further improvements in myocardial efficiency are primarily derived from physical conditioning, whereas additional plaque stabilization is gained by lipid-lowering therapies and perhaps antioxidants.

DRUG THERAPY AFTER MYOCARDIAL INFARCTION

Antiplatelets

Because the pathophysiologic cornerstone of acute coronary syndromes is the formation of thrombus, all postinfarction patients should be treated with an antiplatelet, an anticoagulant, or, in some situations, both. Aspirin is a relatively weak but effective, pathway-specific, platelet inhibitor. Aspirin in an acute phase dose of 160 to 325 mg and a lifelong daily dose of 81 to 325 mg is inexpensive and relatively safe, and pooled data from prospective trials have shown long-term aspirin use to reduce cardiovascular mortality by 15%, nonfatal MI by 30%, and nonfatal stroke by 40%. For patients intolerant of aspirin, ticlopidine (Ticlid), 250 mg twice daily, or clopidogrel (Plavix), 75 mg per day, should be used. Ticlopidine and clopidogrel inhibit adenosine diphosphate–mediated platelet aggregation and antagonize the interaction of fibrinogen with the platelet's IIb/IIIa receptor. These mechanisms are distinctly different from the actions of aspirin and require 48 to 72 hours to become fully manifest. Clopidogrel is favored over ticlopidine because it has fewer major and minor side effects. Clopidogrel was tested against aspirin in more than 11,000 post-MI patients and was found to be similarly effective. Because of its greater expense relative to aspirin, it has not become a front-line therapy unless concomitant cerebrovascular or peripheral vascular disease is present. On the other hand, clopidogrel would be favored over oral anticoagulants, such as warfarin (Coumadin), for patients unable to take aspirin. The most potent antiplatelet agents are IIb/IIIa receptor antagonists. During the final stage of platelet aggregation, so-called IIb/IIIa receptors on adjacent platelets link to one another by binding an interposing fibrinogen molecule. By blocking this final common pathway, IIb/IIIa antagonists inhibit platelet aggregation irrespective of initiating stimulus or pathway. Several large-scale studies are ongoing testing these agents for secondary prevention in the first 3 to 12 months after MI.

Anticoagulants

Use of low-molecular-weight heparins or warfarin beyond hospital discharge has not shown to be beneficial except in specific subgroups (e.g., those with atrial fibrillation, pulmonary or systemic embolization, or prosthetic valves, and those unable to take aspirin). For secondary protection against ischemic events, several trials have compared warfarin alone or in combination with aspirin to aspirin therapy alone, and no clear benefit over aspirin alone has been observed. Patients suffering an anterior wall MI should undergo predischarge echocardiography to assess ventricular function and to discern the presence of intracavitary thrombus. Among patients with large anterior wall infarctions, LV aneurysm, or echocardiographically evident thrombus, a 1- to 3-month course of warfarin is likely prudent.

Nitrates

Nitrates, the oldest category of antianginal agents, are used at some point in nearly every patient with an acute coronary syndrome. Through endothelium-independent smooth muscle relaxation in the vasculature, nitrates lower systemic arterial pressure and decrease venous return to the heart, both of which reduce myocardial wall stress. Similarly, nitrates are excellent coronary vasodilators. On the other hand, there is little to no evidence that nitrates alone lower the incidence of recurrent infarction or death in secondary prevention. Therefore, whereas every patient discharged after a myocardial infarction should be given and instructed on the use of sublingual nitroglycerin, chronic oral nitrate therapy is mainly for patients with residual myocardial ischemia or important LV systolic dysfunction. For patients with depressed LV function who are unable to take ACE inhibitors, an alternative of lesser benefit is the combination of direct vasodilators, such as hydralazine, with nitrates. For such patients and those with residual ischemia, isosorbide mononitrate (Imdur, 30 to 90 mg per day; Ismo, 20 mg twice daily) or isosorbide dinitrate (Isordil, 10 to 40 mg three times a day) can be used, maintaining a nitrate-free interval at night.

Beta-Adrenergic Blockers

Beta blockers serve a number of important roles in the treatment of myocardial ischemia. Their main function, blocking adrenergic receptors, serves to blunt heart rate increases, which occur in response to physical exertion, chest pain, or as a reflex to vasodilators. By decreasing blood pressure, heart rate, and myocardial contractility, beta blockers lower myocardial oxygen demands and ischemic events. In addition, beta blockers have antiarrhythmic properties. Clinical trials of beta blockers among post-MI patients have shown a decrease in subsequent hospitalizations, nonfatal MI, and sudden and nonsudden cardiac death. After pooling multiple studies including over 37,000 total patients, beta blocker therapy was found to reduce mortality 24%. Despite these benefits, many clinical trials and registries have found that beta blockers are prescribed to only 50 to 60% of patients discharged after MI. Although patients with clinically important bronchospasm, hypoglycemic events (from poorly controlled diabetes), uncompensated heart failure, bradycardia, or hypotension should not receive beta blockers, all other post-MI patients should. Indeed, patients at highest risk for adverse outcome (e.g., large or anterior wall infarctions, electrical complications, moderate or worse ventricular function, residual ischemia) receive the greatest benefit. Even patients with congestive heart failure, once stabilized and compensated (i.e., without S_3 or rales) benefit from low-dose beta blockade. Cardioselective beta blockers, such as metoprolol (Lopressor, 25 to 100 mg twice daily; Toprol XL, 50 to 200 mg per day) and atenolol (Tenormin, 50 to 100 mg per day), are preferred to the nonselective beta blockers because they produce fewer unwanted (noncardiac) effects. In patients with severe ventricular dysfunction, metoprolol, 6.125 to 12.5 mg twice daily, or metoprolol XL, 12.5 to 25 mg per day, or carvedilol (Coreg), 3.125 mg twice daily, can be cautiously initiated with gradual titration to higher maintenance doses over a period of weeks to months.

ACE Inhibitors

ACE inhibitors favorably affect left ventricular wall stress and remodeling and should be used early in the course of nearly all post-MI patients. Many large-scale studies have shown ACE inhibitors to reduce episodes of congestive heart failure, rehospitalizations, and perhaps reinfarctions. Beyond this, mortality is reduced 20 to 25%, and patients at highest risk (e.g., anterior infarctions, prior history of congestive heart failure, ejection fraction less than 40%) appear to receive the greatest benefit. ACE inhibitors can be discontinued after the subacute phase in patients with normal or minimally depressed ventricular function but should be continued indefinitely in all others. Contraindications to ACE inhibitors include bilateral renal artery stenosis, significantly worsening renal function, and hypovolemic hypotension. A nuisance cough is the most common side effect, and consideration can be given for switching to an angiotensin receptor blocker, such as losartan (Cozaar), although these agents have not been well studied in the post-MI setting. ACE inhibitors should be started orally at a low dose in the first post-MI days, and the dose should be quickly increased. Numerous ACE inhibitors are available, and common regimens include captopril (Capoten), 12.5 to 50 mg three times a day; enalapril (Vasotec), 5 to 20 mg twice daily, and lisinopril (Prinivil, Zestril), 5 to 20 mg per day.

Calcium Channel Blockers

Calcium channel antagonists are effective in lowering blood pressure and decreasing chest pain frequency in patients with stable angina. On the other hand, current guidelines do not recommend the use of calcium channel antagonists in the postinfarction setting because some (nifedipine) have been associated with an increased mortality risk. Rate-limiting calcium channel blockers (verapamil [Calan, Verelan] and diltiazem [Cardizem, Tiazac]) can be of benefit in patients with preserved or mildly impaired ventricular function who are unable to take beta blockers but need rate control of atrial fibrillation. Agents free of chronotropic or inotropic effects, such as amlodipine (Norvasc) and felodipine (Plendil), have been shown to be safest among patients with depressed ventricular function.

RISK FACTOR MODIFICATION

Identifying High-Risk Patients

Although seemingly intuitive, among the first tasks while planning care for the MI survivor is a careful consideration of risk for adverse outcome based on demographic and manifesting characteristics as well as early post-MI signs and symptoms. Several large prospective studies and registries have identified such key variables (Figure 1). Importantly, age, vital signs, ventricular function, extent of coronary artery disease, and presence and severity of recurrent angina provide the overwhelming majority of predictive value. Despite this, the elderly (in particular), women, minorities, and those at highest risk (prior MI, congestive heart failure, or known decreased ventricular function) all too often receive the least aggressive care. Based on simple consideration of demographic variables and residual LV function, patients can be broadly categorized as relatively low or high risk and level of subsequent care and assessment can be initiated (Figure 2). For example, a patient younger than age 65 years with mild ventricular dysfunction has a less than 5% risk of death through the subacute phase, whereas a patient older than 75 years with more than mild ventricular dysfunction has a greater than 30% risk of death during this time.

Exercise and Cardiac Rehabilitation

Regular exercise training is an important part of the care after MI. Most patients suffering an MI should have received phase I cardiac rehabilitation and instruction before hospital discharge. Although

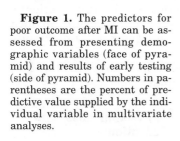

Figure 1. The predictors for poor outcome after MI can be assessed from presenting demographic variables (face of pyramid) and results of early testing (side of pyramid). Numbers in parentheses are the percent of predictive value supplied by the individual variable in multivariate analyses.

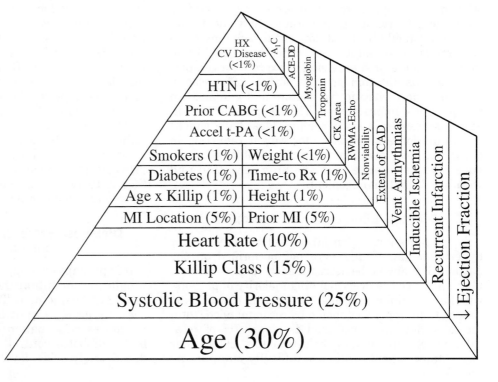

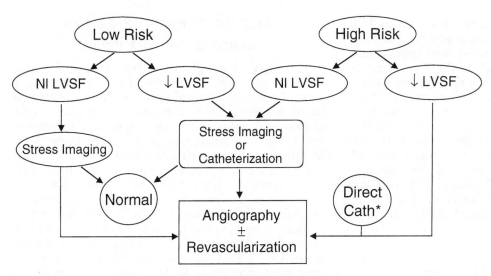

Figure 2. An algorithm of an assessment strategy for post-MI patients based on their level of risk for adverse outcome and their residual left ventricular systolic function. (↓ = decreased; Nl = normal; LVSF = left ventricular systolic function.)

* (Re) MI or CP, VT, CHF, Prior MI, Prior Revascularization

the majority of MI patients need lifestyle modification and can benefit from phase II (outpatient) cardiac rehabilitation, only a minority currently enter a formal program after discharge. Patients at increased risk for subsequent cardiovascular events should especially be encouraged to complete a prescriptive program. Beyond physical conditioning, exercise improves muscle efficiency, which reduces the cardiac output required for these activities and those of daily living. Moreover, a regular exercise program will improve blood lipid levels, assist with weight loss and blood pressure control, and give an improved sense of well-being.

Physical exercise should be performed a minimum of three times weekly for 20 minutes or more per session. Low-impact, aerobic exercise (e.g., walking, swimming, bicycling) is preferable, and the target heart rate should be about 85% of the safe maximum determined at baseline exercise testing. In addition to instruction and supervision of exercise, a comprehensive rehabilitation program should offer assessment of atherosclerotic risk factors and guidance on the patient's improvement. This would include dietary assessment and counseling, ideal body weight determination and guidance for weight reduction in obese patients, serial measurements of blood pressure, and assistance with smoking cessation and with blood lipid management.

Diet and Lipid-Lowering Therapies

All patients having an MI should be screened for hyperlipidemia. If this were not performed on the day of MI, it should be assessed early in the subacute phase because the overwhelming majority of patients will have a lipid abnormality. An American Heart Association Step 2 diet should be recommended (total fat to < 30% and saturated fat to < 7% of total caloric needs and dietary cholesterol to < 200 mg per day). Many patients will have difficulty maintaining

such a strict diet or lowering the low-density lipoprotein value to below the target of 100 mg per dL. Even a very prudent diet can only lower the cholesterol levels by 10 to 15%, and thus medical therapy will be needed for many patients. Dietary supplements of antioxidants, such as vitamin E, have been associated with improved cardiovascular prognosis in primary prevention registries and surveys but have not been consistently shown to be beneficial in prospective trials. Because of their believed safety, some have chosen to recommend 400 IU of vitamin E daily. Likewise, hormone replacement therapy among postmenopausal women has been shown to favorably affect the lipid profile and risk for osteoporosis, but prospective evidence for lowering adverse cardiovascular events is lacking.

In contrast, because most of the concern for lipid lowering focuses on low-density lipoprotein-cholesterol, HMG-CoA reductase inhibitors are a clear mainstay of therapy. By lowering low-density lipoprotein levels, HMG-CoA reductase inhibitors over a several-year period have been shown to reduce the occurrence of death, MI, and stroke by 20 to 40%. A single evening dose is effective for most patients, although the highest doses are commonly divided given twice daily: lovastatin (Mevacor, 20 to 80 mg), pravastatin (Pravachol, 10 to 80 mg), simvastatin (Zocor, 10 to 40 mg), and atorvastatin (Lipitor, 5 to 80 mg) are common examples.

Diabetes, Hypertension, Weight Loss, and Smoking Cessation

It is perhaps even more difficult for patients to lose weight and maintain the weight loss by following a prudent, low-fat diet. The rewards are great, however. By losing weight by means of proper diet and regular exercise, patients will almost invariably have better diabetes control, lowered blood pressure, reduced triglyceride levels with a corresponding increase in high-density lipoproteins, and improved self-esteem. The only more important goal would be smoking cessation for tobacco users. Post-MI smokers who quit smoking halve their likelihood of death in the subsequent 5 years (from about 30% to 15%). Nicotine substitutes are not recommended in the early post-MI period, although they deliver a fraction of the nicotine usual smokers intake and are likely a safe alternative if patients do not smoke cigarettes concomitantly. Several studies have shown that health care professionals who send a personal, strong, and clear message about smoking cessation make an important impact. The highest rate of smoking cessation without relapse is with a stepwise, combination approach using behavioral techniques, nicotine substitutes, and formal counseling.

TESTS AND PROCEDURES

Stress Testing, Cardiac Imaging, and Revascularization

A substantial amount of prognostic information is obtained from assessment of cardiac function, both at rest (e.g., echocardiography or radionuclide imaging) and with stress (treadmill or pharmacologic provocation). Because LV function is a strong predictor of survival post MI, all post-MI patients should have an assessment of LV function and inducibility of recurrent ischemia before or very early after hospital discharge. Coronary angiography is a reasonable early step for patients deemed likely to benefit from revascularization (i.e., those with prior history of MI, depressed ventricular function, or prior revascularization) based on noninvasive clinical evaluation. Patients with post-MI angina, mild ventricular dysfunction, and believed multivessel coronary artery disease, spontaneous or inducible ischemia despite medical therapy, or hibernating myocardium should be strongly considered for early coronary angiography and revascularization. For patients with an otherwise uncomplicated post-MI course, there are no data to support "routine" coronary angiography.

PERICARDITIS

method of
P. SUDHAKAR REDDY, M.D.
University of Pittsburgh School of Medicine
Pittsburgh, Pennsylvania

Pericarditis may produce disease in the following three respects:

1. Pain
2. Cardiac tamponade
3. Constrictive pericarditis

Cardiac tamponade and constrictive pericarditis stiffen the ventricles necessitating higher filling pressures. In spite of the compensatory rise in filling pressures to maintain stroke volume, the cardiac output may decrease.

Therefore, the signs and symptoms of cardiac tamponade and constrictive pericarditis are related to elevated ventricular filling pressures (systemic and pulmonary venous pressures) and decreased cardiac output. A chronic decrease in cardiac output causes fatigue; an acute decrease in cardiac output can result in cardiogenic shock and death. Systemic venous hypertension manifests as elevation of jugular venous pressure, enlargement of the liver, and edema of the feet. In severe cases, it may cause ascites and generalized anasarca. Because cardiac tamponade is usually not a chronic state, the elevated venous pressure is manifested as elevated jugular venous pressure not associated with other features. Although pulmonary venous hypertension usually causes pulmonary congestion, shortness of breath, and pulmonary edema, cardiac tamponade and constrictive pericarditis almost never cause pulmonary edema. It is not exactly known why pulmonary venous hypertension does not cause pulmonary edema when it is associated with equivalent systemic venous hypertension.

TREATMENT

The treatment of pericarditis is directed toward the underlying causes (Table 1): relief of pain and a reduction in the stiffness of the ventricles, so as to facilitate filling of the ventricles without a significant increase in the filling pressures. Pericardiocentesis and pericardiectomy decrease the stiffness of the ventricles.

Pain

The treatment of pain is based purely on symptoms. Stepwise therapy for pain starts with simple analgesics such as aspirin. If pain is not relieved, more powerful analgesics (nonsteroidal anti-inflammatory drugs, meperidine, or opiates such as morphine) are prescribed. In rare instances, corticosteroids may be required to suppress inflammation and pain. Corticosteroids should be used as a last resort because withdrawal is difficult.

Stepwise therapy for relief of pain is as follows:

1. Aspirin, 325 to 1000 mg every 4 to 6 hours.
2. Ibuprofen, 400 to 800 mg 6 to 8 hours. (Ibuprofen is preferred to indomethacin [Indocin] because the latter is known to reduce coronary flow.)

TABLE 1. **Etiology of Pericarditis**

Idiopathic
Infectious
Viral
Bacterial
Tuberculous
Parasitic
Fungal
Connective tissue diseases
Metabolic: uremia, hypothyroidism
Neoplasm, radiation
Hypersensitivity: drugs
Postmyocardial injury syndrome
Trauma
Dissecting aneurysm
Chylopericardium

3. Morphine sulfate, 5 to 15 mg intramuscularly every 4 to 6 hours. Other analgesics, such as pentazocine (Talwin), codeine, and meperidine (Demerol), may be used in doses recommended by manufacturers and guided by the treating physician's experience.

4. Prednisone, 60 mg daily in four divided doses, to be reduced every few days to 40, 20, 10, and 5 mg daily. Steroids should be used as a last resort because relapses are common on withdrawal. If a relapse occurs, the dose should be increased to at least one step higher than the dose at which the relapse occurred and then reduced more gradually.

Cardiac Tamponade

The filling pressures necessary to distend the ventricles to any given volume are determined by the stiffness of the ventricles. In the intact heart, the stiffness of the ventricles is determined by the endocardium, myocardium, and pericardium. Normally, the pericardium does not significantly contribute to ventricular stiffness. In normal people pericardiectomy results in minimal decreases in the ventricular filling pressures. However, the fluid-filled pericardium can considerably stiffen the ventricles, depending on the rate and amount of accumulation. Rapid accumulation of a small amount of fluid (e.g., after trauma or secondary to cardiac catheterization or steering wheel injury) can cause a severe elevation of filling pressures and a severe decrease in cardiac output. However, a large amount of pericardial fluid that accumulates slowly causes only minimal hemodynamic compromise.

The treatment of cardiac tamponade is straightforward: pericardiocentesis. Because cardiac tamponade is not an all-or-none phenomenon but a spectrum of hemodynamic changes, it is crucial to know when to intervene. Accumulation of pericardial fluid contributes to the stiffness of the ventricles, thereby necessitating higher filling pressures. The hemodynamic changes induced by pericardial effusion can be categorized into three phases (Figure 1). During the first phase, intrapericardial pressure, right ventricular filling pressure, and left ventricular filling pressure become elevated. However, left ventricular filling pressure is higher than the right ventricular filling pressure, which is higher than the intrapericardial pressure. Cardiac output is not compromised. Pericardiocentesis can be avoided unless required for diagnosis. During the second phase, the elevated right ventricular filling pressure is equal to elevated intrapericardial pressure but less than the left ventricular filling pressure. Cardiac output is decreased significantly in some patients but not in others. The inspiratory fall in arterial systolic pressure is exaggerated, but the quantitative definition of pulsus paradoxus (decrease of 10 to 12 mm Hg with inspiration) is fulfilled in some patients but not others. This phase can be called right ventricular tamponade. Echocardiographically, inferior vena caval plethora (i.e., failure of inferior vena caval collapse with inspi-

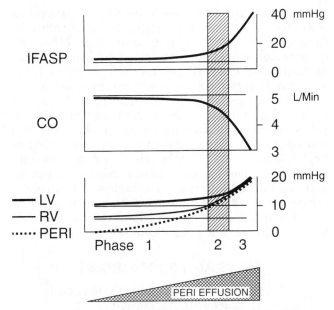

Figure 1. Hemodynamic changes induced by pericardial effusion. See text for explanation. CO = cardiac output; IFASP = inspiratory fall in arterial systolic pressure; LV = left ventricular end-diastolic pressure; PERI = pericardial; RV = right ventricular end-diastolic pressure.

ration) is present, but right atrial collapse and right ventricular collapse may or may not be present. Pericardiocentesis is not urgent but can be postponed to a convenient hour. Phase three represents severe tamponade. Hemodynamically, such patients have *elevated* intrapericardial, systemic venous and pulmonary venous pressures which are *equal* to each other. Cardiac output is significantly compromised. The inspiratory fall in arterial systolic pressure fulfills the quantitative definition of pulsus paradoxus in all cases. Pulsus paradoxus of 20 mm Hg or more requires urgent pericardiocentesis.

In evaluation of pericardial effusion, the clinician should not ask whether cardiac tamponade is present; rather, the clinician should determine the degree of hemodynamic embarrassment, particularly with regard to the decrease in cardiac output. The severity of decrease in cardiac output is best estimated from the severity of systemic venous pressure rise and inspiratory fall in arterial systolic pressure. Again, the clinician should not ask whether pulsus paradoxus is present; rather, the clinician should measure the amplitude of the inspiratory fall in arterial systolic pressure. One note of caution: If the compensatory rise in venous pressure in pericardial effusion is prevented by venous dilatation, as in septicemia, or artificially decreased with diuretics, severe cardiac tamponade may coexist with a low venous pressure (low pressure tamponade). This happens very rarely.

Until pericardiocentesis is performed, stroke volume and cardiac output can be temporarily increased with the following measures: First, ventricular filling may be increased by administration of intravenous fluids. Second, ventricular emptying may be improved by increasing contractility and decreasing afterload (arterial pressure). Both results can be achieved by isoproterenol (Isuprel) infusion. Third, increasing the heart rate increases the number of times the heart fills and empties. Isoproterenol also increases the heart rate. Because isoproterenol decreases the filling pressures by venodilatation, it should be administered in conjunction with measures to increase filling pressure, such as volume load. Dobutamine (Dobutrex) exhibits actions similar to those of isoproterenol.

Constrictive Pericarditis

The pericardium may be thickened and become adherent to the myocardium. The thickened and adherent pericardium may be very stiff and result in a requirement for high pressures to fill the ventricles. In spite of high venous pressures, the filling may be inadequate, and cardiac output may be decreased to a varying degree. The severity of constriction is proportional to the elevation of venous pressure and the decrease in cardiac output. If the pericardium is thickened but does not contribute to the stiffness of the ventricles, it is clinically inconsequential, and no treatment is required. In rare instances, the epicardium may be thickened and adherent to the myocardium but, at the same time, there may be an excessive accumulation of fluid between the epicardium and parietal pericardium. Such patients exhibit elements of both constriction and tamponade. This condition is known as effusive-constrictive pericarditis. After pericardiocentesis, if venous pressures continue to remain elevated, constrictive pericarditis should be suspected and treated accordingly. The commonest cause of effusive-constrictive pericarditis is malignancy. If prognosis of the underlying condition is poor, minimal elevation of venous pressure may be accepted without treatment.

Pericardiocentesis

The procedure is safe when performed by experienced clinicians, particularly if done in a cardiac catheterization laboratory under hemodynamic monitoring or echocardiographic guidance. The subxiphoid approach is preferred. Local anesthetic is infiltrated about 2 cm below the xiphoid process just to the left of the midline. A 17-gauge long needle with beveled tip is advanced toward the left shoulder with or without electrocardiographic monitoring while applying gentle suction. If unsuccessful, the needle direction may be changed toward the midline or right shoulder. If the returning fluid is blood, the needle may have entered one of the cardiac chambers. A sample should be taken and subjected to oximetry analysis. A hemoglobin content or oxygen saturation that is significantly lower than that of systemic venous blood indicates pericardial fluid. If uncertainty still exists, injection of dye under fluoroscopic or echocardiographic monitoring helps confirm the position of the needle. If the needle enters one of the chambers, the clinician should slowly withdraw the needle under pressure monitoring until it enters the pericardial cavity. Pericardiocentesis via needle is very useful only when the amount of pericardial fluid is small. Once needle position in the pericardial cavity is confirmed, an appropriate-size guide wire should be advanced into the pericardial cavity. A No. 5 or 6 French catheter with multiple side holes arranged spirally close to the tip of the catheter (although a pigtail catheter is preferable, a straight catheter is easier to advance) is advanced over the guide wire, which is then withdrawn. The fluid can be withdrawn under controlled conditions. Pressures can be measured and the adequacy of pericardiocentesis can be confirmed by noting a subatmospheric pressure during inspiration. The catheter can be left in situ for further drainage. The longer the catheter is left in place, however, the greater the risk of infection. If the fluid is loculated, pericardiocentesis under echocardiographic guidance is preferable.

Pericardial Window

If pericardial fluid continues to reaccumulate or recurs, surgical creation of a pericardial window should be considered. This procedure drains the pericardial fluid into the pleural cavity. Unfortunately, the windows eventually close. A window can also be created with a balloon: percutaneous balloon pericardiotomy. After the fluid is partially drained, 20 mL of dilute contrast medium (50%) is injected into the pericardial cavity. A 0.038-inch stiff J-tip guide wire is advanced through the pericardiocentesis catheter. The pericardiocentesis catheter is withdrawn and replaced with a 20-mm-diameter, 3-cm-long balloon catheter. Once the balloon is positioned to straddle across the pericardial border, the balloon is inflated. The balloon catheter is then replaced with the original pericardiocentesis catheter. About 100 mL of dilute contrast medium is rapidly injected to confirm the escape of dye through the window. The remaining fluid is then withdrawn.

The procedure is not without complications. Twenty percent of the patients may develop pneumothorax; the majority require thoracentesis. The balloon procedure is no more effective than a surgically created pericardial window. Experience with the pericardioscope in creation of a pericardial window is limited.

In view of the tendency of pericardial windows to close, partial or total pericardiectomy may be needed for recurrent accumulation of pericardial fluid.

Uremic Pericarditis

The treatment of pericarditis in patients with chronic renal failure is no different from the general principles just outlined. Treatment includes relief of pain, intense hemodialysis, and treatment of tamponade. Affected patients may have elevation of jugular venous pressure just on the basis of volume overload secondary to renal failure. They may also have right-sided cardiac tamponade with equilibration of elevated pericardial pressure with systemic venous pressure but not with (pre-existing) markedly elevated left ventricular filling pressure due to hypertension, anemia, and volume overload. In right-sided tamponade, cardiac output may be significantly compromised without satisfying the quantitative definition of pulsus paradoxus. In this group of patients, whenever there is moderate to large accumulation of fluid with elevation of jugular venous pressure, pericardiocentesis should be performed regardless of the degree of pulsus paradoxus. If pericardiocentesis is followed by recurrent pericardial effusion, pericardiectomy is the treatment of choice.

PERIPHERAL ARTERIAL DISEASE

method of
PETER C. SPITTELL, M.D.
Mayo Clinic and Mayo Foundation
Rochester, Minnesota

Peripheral arterial disease, because it most commonly results from atherosclerosis, is a relatively common disorder in current medical practice. Occlusive and aneurysmal disease are the most frequently encountered disorders, but less common types of arterial disease can present an interesting diagnostic challenge. Although the clinical findings of peripheral arterial disease are often characteristic, readily available noninvasive tests provide objective quantification of both the location and severity of disease. Effective medical therapy and surgical therapy for most types of peripheral arterial disease are widely available, which further emphasizes the importance of familiarity with these diseases.

CHRONIC OCCLUSIVE PERIPHERAL ARTERIAL DISEASE

Occlusive peripheral arterial disease is usually caused by atherosclerosis; therefore, men are more commonly affected, particularly those with recognized cardiovascular risk factors (tobacco use, hyperlipidemia, and/or diabetes mellitus). The lower extremities are affected more frequently than the upper extremities, but in view of the diffuse nature of atherosclerosis, coronary artery disease and carotid occlusive disease are commonly also present. In younger patients without identifiable risk factors, hyperhomocysteinemia should be suspected and appropriate tests performed.

Patients with lower extremity arterial occlusive disease ordinarily come to medical attention with intermittent claudication. Intermittent claudication is described as a discomfort (aching, cramping, or tightness), is always exercise-induced, and may involve one or both legs, and symptoms occur at a fairly constant walking distance. Relief is obtained by standing still. When more severe ischemia develops, pain at rest (ischemic rest pain) and, even with minor trauma, ischemic ulceration can occur.

Pseudoclaudication, which is caused by lumbar spinal stenosis, is the condition most often confused

TABLE 1. Intermittent Claudication: Differential Diagnosis

	Intermittent Claudication	Pseudoclaudication
Onset	Walking	Standing, walking, other
Character	Discomfort (muscular)	"Paresthetic"
Bilateral	+/−	+
Walking distance	Fairly constant	Variable
Relief	Standing still	Sit down, lean forward
Cause	Atherosclerosis	Lumbar spinal stenosis
Diagnosis	ABI pre- and postexercise*	CT, MRI lumbar spine Electromyography

*Treadmill exercise (1–2 mph, 10% grade, symptom-limited or 5 min).
Abbreviations: ABI = ankle:brachial systolic pressure index; CT = computed tomography; MRI = magnetic resonance imaging.

with intermittent claudication. Pseudoclaudication causes "paresthetic" discomfort or pain, or both, that occurs with standing and walking (variable distances). Symptoms are almost always bilateral and are relieved by sitting, leaning forward, or both. A history of prior chronic back pain or prior lumbar spinal surgery is common. The diagnosis of lumbar spinal stenosis can be confirmed with computed tomography or magnetic resonance imaging of the lumbar spine, often in conjunction with electromyography. Ankle:brachial systolic pressure indices before and after treadmill exercise are usually normal in the patient with lumbar spinal stenosis unless the patient has concurrent lower extremity arterial occlusive disease (Table 1).

Reduced or absence of one or more peripheral pulses is the classic physical finding in occlusive arterial disease. Proximal arterial narrowing may cause audible systolic bruits over large arteries (carotid, subclavian, and femoral arteries and the aorta), and when the lumen becomes severely narrowed, creating a gradient in diastole (>80% stenosis), the bruit may extend into diastole. A useful clinical estimate of the degree of lower extremity ischemia can be obtained by observing the development of pallor on elevation of the extremity and the time required for the return of color to the skin and the superficial veins to fill on dependency of the extremities after elevation (Tables 2 and 3). In the upper extremities, brachial blood pressures should be determined bilaterally to detect subclavian artery stenosis or occlusion. In the presence of a significant subclavian artery stenosis, si-

TABLE 2. Elevation Pallor Testing in Peripheral Arterial Disease

Grade of Pallor	Duration of Elevation*
0	No pallor in 60 s
1	Pallor in 60 s
2	Pallor in 30–60 s
3	Pallor in less than 30 s
4	Pallor on the level

*Elevation of the lower extremities to 60° for 1 min.

TABLE 3. **Color Return and Venous Filling Time in Peripheral Arterial Disease**

	Time for Color Return (s)	Venous Filling Time (s)
Normal	10	15
Moderate ischemia	15–20	20–30
Severe ischemia	>40	>40

multaneous radial artery palpation reveals a delay in the radial pulse ipsilateral to the subclavian stenosis. Allen's test to evaluate the circulation in the hand and the thoracic outlet maneuvers to uncover dynamic subclavian artery compression are additional useful tests in patients with symptoms of upper extremity or digital arterial disease.

Noninvasive diagnosis of peripheral arterial occlusive disease, using supine ankle:brachial systolic pressure indices (ABI), taken with a standard blood pressure cuff and a hand-held Doppler probe, can provide an objective measure of the severity of lower extremity arterial occlusive disease. Normally, the systolic blood pressure at the ankle level (posterior tibial and dorsalis pedis artery) is equal to or exceeds the brachial systolic blood pressure. The ratio of the ankle systolic pressure to the brachial systolic pressure provides a measurement of disease severity in patients with occlusive peripheral arterial disease (resting ABI > 1.0 normally, = 0.8 to 0.9 in mild disease, = 0.5 to 0.8 in moderate disease, and < 0.5 in severe disease). ABI testing before and after exercise testing (treadmill or active-pedal plantar flexion) is the screening test of choice for patients with intermittent claudication, providing both a functional and a semiquantitative assessment of the severity of occlusive arterial disease. Duplex ultrasonography is able to accurately provide both anatomic and functional information regarding the location and severity of peripheral arterial disease. More recently, magnetic resonance angiography has been demonstrated to be an accurate alternative to standard angiography, especially in preoperative planning for patients with contraindications to invasive angiography (e.g., renal insufficiency or allergy to contrast media, or both). Duplex ultrasonography and magnetic resonance angiography are useful in patients with established peripheral arterial disease before revascularization and in postoperative follow-up. Angiography is indicated when surgical or endovascular intervention is being considered or an unusual type of occlusive arterial disease is suspected. Angiography is not necessary for establishing a diagnosis of peripheral arterial disease.

The overall rate of 5-year mortality in patients with intermittent claudication is 29%, the increase largely resulting from complications of associated coronary artery disease and carotid artery disease. The rate for major lower extremity amputation in patients with intermittent claudication over 5 years is 4%; 55% of patients have stable or improved symp-

toms. Concurrent use of tobacco results in a 10-fold increase in the risk for major amputation and a more than twofold increase in mortality. The effect of diabetes on patients with intermittent claudication is also significant, resulting in a 12-fold increased risk of below-knee amputation and a cumulative risk of major amputation exceeding 11%. Additional clinical features that predict an increased risk of limb loss in patients with peripheral arterial occlusive disease include ischemic rest pain, ischemic ulceration, and/ or gangrene (Table 4).

Initial medical management of intermittent claudication includes discontinuation of tobacco, control of other modifiable cardiovascular risk factors (e.g., hypertension, diabetes, hyperlipidemia), weight reduction (if patient is obese), foot care and protection, avoidance of vasoconstrictive drugs, a walking program, antiplatelet agents, and hemorrheologic agents.

A regular walking program (level ground, walking the distance to claudication, stopping to rest for relief, repeatedly for 30 minutes per session, 4 or more days a week) for patients with intermittent claudication can result in a 100 to 400% increase in initial claudication distance over 3 months in many patients. Aspirin (325 mg once daily) is effective primary and secondary prevention in patients with peripheral arterial disease, resulting in a decreased risk of limb loss and reduced need for vascular surgery, as well as a decreased incidence of major coronary and cerebrovascular events. More recently, clopidogrel (Plavix, 75 mg once daily) has been shown to be more effective than aspirin in preventing major atherosclerotic vascular events. Pentoxifylline (Trental), a methyl-xanthine, has vasoactive properties that result in the relaxation of vascular smooth muscle, inhibition of platelet aggregation, and decreased blood viscosity. Patients with intermittent claudication who are most likely to benefit from pentoxifylline are those with stable symptoms present more than 1 year and a resting ABI less than 0.8. Only one dosing regimen of pentoxifylline (400 mg three times daily) is used clinically.

Patients with peripheral arterial occlusive disease who have disabling symptoms, diabetes mellitus, rest pain, ischemic rest pain, ischemic ulceration, and/or gangrene should be considered for surgical or endovascular intervention if their general medical condition permits.

Percutaneous transluminal angioplasty (PTA) is often effective in patients with proximal arterial occlusive disease; short, partial occlusions; and good distal runoff. The "ideal" lesion for PTA is an iliac stenosis

TABLE 4. **Indications for Revascularization in Peripheral Arterial Occlusive Disease**

Lifestyle limiting (disabling) claudication
Diabetes mellitus
Ischemic rest pain
Ischemic ulceration, gangrene

less than 5 cm in length or a femoropopliteal occlusion or stenosis less than 10 cm in total length (excluding lesions involving the origin of the superficial femoral artery and those affecting the distalmost 2 cm of the popliteal artery). An initial good result is obtained with PTA in over 80% of patients and lasts 2 to 3 years in 70% of patients. Advantages of PTA over surgery include lower morbidity and mortality rates, shorter convalescence, lower cost, and preservation of the saphenous vein for the future. PTA for aortic or iliac disease may also allow for an infrainguinal surgical procedure to be performed at reduced perioperative risk (as compared with procedures requiring aortic cross-clamp application). Selective stent placement in iliac artery stenosis is used when the results of angioplasty are insufficient (residual mean pressure gradient > 10 mm Hg). Surgical therapy remains the treatment of choice for most patients with diffuse symptomatic atherosclerotic disease of the lower extremities.

ACUTE ARTERIAL OCCLUSION

The symptoms of acute arterial occlusion are sudden in onset (<5 hours) and include pain, numbness, and coldness of the involved extremity (or extremities). On examination, additional findings include pallor, absence of pulses, and neurologic deficits (decreased fine touch or motor deficits, or both).

An embolic cause of acute arterial occlusion is suggested by the presence of cardiac disease, atrial fibrillation, proximal aneurysm, and proximal atherosclerosis.

Features suggesting a thrombotic cause of acute arterial occlusion include prior occlusive disease in the involved limb, occlusive disease involving other extremities, acute aortic dissection, hematologic disease, arteritis, inflammatory bowel disease, neoplasm, and ergotism.

After confirmation by angiography, initial therapeutic options for acute arterial occlusion include intra-arterial thrombolysis and surgical therapy (thromboembolectomy). If thrombolytic therapy is used, PTA or surgical therapy is often indicated to treat the underlying stenosis, if present, to improve clinical outcome and long-term patency rates.

PERIPHERAL ARTERY ANEURYSMS

Like occlusive peripheral arterial disease, arterial aneurysms most commonly result from atherosclerosis. Therefore, peripheral arterial aneurysms are more frequent in men and more commonly occur in the lower extremities than in upper extremities. Other predisposing factors for aneurysmal disease are systemic hypertension, inherited disorders, connective tissue disease, trauma, infection, chronic obstructive pulmonary disease, and inflammatory diseases.

Most aneurysms are asymptomatic, frequently incidentally discovered during a test being performed for another reason (e.g., abdominal ultrasonography, computed tomography). The sensitivity of the physical examination in detecting an aneurysm depends on the location of the aneurysm. Abdominal aortic aneurysms are often occult on examination unless they have achieved a diameter greater than 4 cm and the patient is not obese. Aneurysms of the subclavian, femoral, and popliteal arteries are frequently palpable as a pulsating mass.

Complications of aneurysms include peripheral embolization, pressure on surrounding structures, infection, and rupture. Aneurysms of certain arteries develop certain complications more often than others; for example, the most common complication of aortic aneurysms is rupture, whereas embolism is a more common complication of femoral and popliteal artery aneurysms.

Abdominal aortic aneurysms can be accurately diagnosed through ultrasonography, computed tomography, or magnetic resonance imaging. Angiography is not required unless visualization of the renal or peripheral arterial circulation is needed to plan surgical treatment. In a patient with few risk factors, selective surgical treatment of abdominal aortic aneurysm is advisable for aneurysms more than 4.0 cm in diameter, to avoid the excessive risk of surgical treatment when an aneurysm is ruptured. Elective surgical repair is definitely indicated when aneurysm diameter is between 4.5 cm and 5.0 cm in such patients. Surgery is also indicated for abdominal aortic aneurysms that are symptomatic, traumatic, or infectious in origin or are rapidly expanding (>0.5 cm per year)(see Table 5). In patients with other significant diseases (e.g., pulmonary, cardiac, renal, and/or hepatic disease), surgical therapy should be individualized. In patients who have a large and/or symptomatic abdominal aortic aneurysm and whose general medical condition makes them a poor surgical candidate, exclusion of the aneurysm by placement of an intraluminal stent–anchored Dacron prosthetic graft via retrograde transfemoral cannulation has produced encouraging results.

Inflammatory abdominal aortic aneurysm is suggested by the triad of back (or abdominal) pain, weight loss, and an elevated sedimentation rate. Obstructive uropathy may occur with ureteral involvement. The findings on computed tomography are diagnostic. Treatment is surgical resection.

Iliac artery aneurysm usually occurs in association with abdominal aortic aneurysm but may occur as an isolated finding. Iliac artery aneurysm may cause obstructive urologic symptoms, unexplained groin or

TABLE 5. **Abdominal Aortic Aneurysm: Indications for Surgery**

Aneurysm diameter 4.5–5.0 cm*
Symptomatic
Traumatic or infectious etiology
Rapid expansion (>0.5 cm/y)
Inflammatory etiology

*Selective repair when 4.0–4.5 cm in "good risk" patients.

perineal pain, iliac vein obstruction, or embolization. Computed tomography with intravenous contrast is the preferred diagnostic procedure. Surgical resection is indicated when an iliac aneurysm is causing symptoms or exceeds 3.0 cm in diameter.

Popliteal artery aneurysms are bilateral in 50% of patients; 40% of patients have one or more aneurysms at other sites, most often the abdominal aorta. Untreated popliteal artery aneurysms frequently produce complications, most often thromboembolic, that may threaten the limb. Additional complications include venous obstruction, venous thrombosis, popliteal neuropathy, infection, and, in rare instances, rupture. The diagnosis is readily made with ultrasonography, but angiography is necessary before surgical treatment to evaluate the proximal and distal arterial circulation. When a popliteal aneurysm is diagnosed, surgical therapy is the treatment of choice to prevent serious thromboembolic complications.

Atheroembolism secondary to a peripheral arterial aneurysm is characterized by livedo reticularis, blue toes, palpable pulses, hypertension, renal insufficiency, elevated sedimentation rate, leukocytosis, and peripheral eosinophilia (transient). Atheroembolism can occur spontaneously or can follow medication (warfarin or thrombolytic therapy), angiographic procedures, or surgical procedures. Atheroembolism in a lower extremity is most commonly caused by an abdominal aortic aneurysm or diffuse atherosclerotic disease. In such patients, livedo reticularis and blue toes are bilateral. Unilateral blue toes suggest that the embolic source is distal to the aortic bifurcation. Treatment of choice for atheroembolism is identification of the source of embolism and surgical resection, if feasible.

UNCOMMON TYPES OF PERIPHERAL ARTERIAL DISEASE

The less common types of occlusive peripheral arterial disease include thromboangiitis obliterans (Buerger's disease), arteritides (giant cell arteritis and connective tissue disorders), extrinsic arterial compression (popliteal artery entrapment and thoracic outlet compression of the subclavian artery), and traumatic (repetitive blunt type) arterial occlusive disease in the hand. An uncommon type of occlusive arterial disease is suggested by occurrence in young persons and by acute, often digital, ischemia or associated systemic symptoms or both. In connective tissue disorders, the occlusive disease is usually digital; giant cell (temporal, cranial) arteritis affects persons older than 60 years of age whose dominant symptoms are headache and those of a systemic illness, whereas Takayasu's arteritis typically affects the branches of the aortic arch of young women. In occlusive arterial disease caused by arteritis, the frequency of limb loss depends on the severity of ischemia at the time of diagnosis and the control of the arteritis achieved.

Management should include therapy of the systemic process and general measures to protect the ischemic limb. In thromboangiitis obliterans, the risk of limb loss is greater than that of atherosclerosis and depends mainly on the severity of the ischemia at the time of diagnosis and on tobacco use. In chronic occlusive arterial disease caused by repetitive blunt trauma to the hand, loss of digits can occur if the cause is not recognized and corrected. Measures to protect the hand (regular use of gloves and avoiding blunt trauma) are important in preventing progression. If ischemic ulceration has already occurred, an alpha-adrenergic blocking agent (e.g., doxazosin [Cardura], 1 mg once daily at bedtime) or sympathectomy can be used to hasten healing and provide better long-term protection of the ischemic digit. Limb or digital loss can occur with arterial compression syndromes as a result of embolization from mural thrombus that develops in the poststenotic aneurysm that chronic arterial compression can cause. The appropriate management of arterial compression syndromes is surgical relief.

VENOUS THROMBOSIS

method of
ANTHONY J. COMEROTA, M.D.
Temple University School of Medicine
Philadelphia, Pennsylvania

Venous thrombosis refers to blood clot formation in veins anywhere in the body. For the purpose of this discussion, treatment will focus on deep vein thrombosis (DVT) of the lower extremities.

Although the spectrum of acute DVT ranges from asymptomatic calf vein thrombosis to venous gangrene, many physicians choose to treat the entire range of DVT similarly, with intravenous unfractionated heparin followed by oral anticoagulation with warfarin. Since the mid-1980s, studies have expanded our understanding of the natural history of DVT, of the pharmacology of anticoagulation and its effect on DVT, and of the impact of fibrinolysis on the management of DVT. Refinement in the mechanical removal of venous thrombi and the results of prospective clinical trials have put operative intervention into proper prospective.

The signs and symptoms of DVT occur because of obstruction of the deep venous system, an associated inflammatory response of the vessel wall and surrounding tissue, or fragmentation of the thrombus with embolization to the pulmonary arteries. The diagnosis of acute DVT remains elusive in many patients. The physical examination can be helpful in selected patients having a constellation of high-risk factors but always must be confirmed with objective testing before committing a patient to long-term therapy.

Once diagnosed, treatment can have a major impact on outcome, both short and long term. After a brief look at the natural history of acute DVT, the details of anticoagulation, thrombolytic therapy, and venous thrombectomy are reviewed. This is followed by suggested treatment strategies based on the location and severity of the venous thrombosis.

NATURAL HISTORY

The early complication of DVT is pulmonary embolism, which is universally recognized as an important consequence of acute DVT. The late complication of acute DVT is the post-thrombotic syndrome. The post-thrombotic syndrome is frequently not associated with acute DVT by many physicians, who often believe that this long-term complication cannot be avoided. Interestingly, when post-thrombotic sequelae occur, they are frequently attributed to the patient's "disease" rather than inadequate treatment of the acute DVT.

Insight into appropriate treatment of acute DVT can be obtained by an understanding of the pathophysiology of the post-thrombotic syndrome, which is ambulatory venous hypertension. The two components leading to ambulatory venous hypertension are residual venous obstruction and valvular incompetence. Recanalization of thrombosed venous segments can occur, restoring at least partial patency. Physiologic studies of maximal venous outflow may fall within normal ranges; however, the fact that recanalization allows a normal maximal venous outflow does not mean that the veins are free of luminal obstruction, because maximal venous outflow tests are insensitive in detecting less than complete venous obstruction. The additive effects of venous obstruction and valvular incompetence on ambulatory venous pressure in post-thrombotic patients have been well documented. Patients with the highest ambulatory venous pressures have the most severe post-thrombotic syndrome. Therefore, if either obstruction or valve incompetence can be minimized or avoided, the severity of the post-thrombotic syndrome can be reduced. Natural history studies of acute DVT demonstrate progressive valvular dysfunction over time. Valve reflux occurs more commonly in patients with occlusive venous thrombosis. However, patients who spontaneously lyse the clot in their venous system are likely to preserve normal valvular function. These patients tend to have early and complete recanalization, frequently lysing their clot within 3 months of diagnosis. These observations erase previously erroneous concepts that valves are irreparably destroyed within 3 to 5 days of venous thrombosis.

The accelerated morbidity of combined venous obstruction and valve reflux becomes apparent after observations that after acute DVT limbs with the post-thrombotic syndrome had more than three times the odds of having combined reflux and obstruction than did limbs without the post-thrombotic syndrome. Observations from natural history studies are consistent with results of studies evaluating both thrombolysis versus anticoagulation and venous thrombectomy versus anticoagulation for acute DVT, which show that by successfully clearing the deep venous system of thrombus, valvular function can be maintained and post-thrombotic symptoms reduced.

ANTICOAGULATION

Heparin

Anticoagulation by unfractionated heparin followed by oral warfarin compounds has been the mainstay of therapy for acute DVT. Anticoagulation is essentially prophylactic, because these agents interrupt thrombus formation but do not actively dissolve the thrombus. However, effective anticoagulation will prevent clot propagation and allow the body's endogenous fibrinolytic system the opportunity to reduce the thrombus burden and recanalize the occluded vein.

With the exception of aspirin, heparin is likely to be the most commonly used drug by vascular surgeons and other physicians commonly involved in the care of patients with thrombotic disorders. The biologic half-life of unfractionated heparin does not follow simple first-order kinetics. With increasing doses of unfractionated heparin, the biologic half-life increases; therefore, the dose-response relationship is not linear. Heparin is bound by platelets, vascular endothelium, and antithrombin III and is neutralized by platelet factor 4 and other plasma proteins such as histidine-rich glycoprotein and vitronectin. Complicating matters further, heparin will be bound by intravascular thrombus, which thereby further reduces its biologic activity in those patients.

The adequacy of initial anticoagulation is critical for reduction of future venous thromboembolic events. Inadequate anticoagulation is associated with significantly higher recurrent thromboembolic events. Early aggressive anticoagulation, maintaining the activated partial thromboplastin time greater than 100, is associated with significantly fewer recurrent thromboembolic complications without an increased risk of bleeding (in the absence of associated co-morbidities for bleeding). Prospective randomized trials have shown a 15-fold increase in recurrent DVT when early anticoagulation fell below therapeutic levels. Such findings emphasize the necessity for early, consistently therapeutic anticoagulation and also point to the safety of "supratherapeutic" early anticoagulation in the absence of a co-morbidity for bleeding.

Randomized trials have shown that oral anticoagulation alone, without initial and concomitant heparin anticoagulation, is associated with a significantly higher risk of recurrent venous thrombosis.

Some believe that the hemorrhagic risk of anticoagulation increases as the dose increases and that patients with an increased risk can be identified by in vitro anticoagulation tests used to monitor heparin therapy (activated partial thromboplastin time [PTT]). There is some merit to this observation in patients who have co-morbid risk factors, which can identify this high-risk group. However, in patients without co-morbid risk factors, a supratherapeutic activated PTT does not appear to be associated with an increased risk of clinically important bleeding complications. Audits of heparin anticoagulation indicate that large numbers of patients continue to be inadequately treated. Investigators have repeatedly confirmed that a prescriptive approach to heparin administration is more effective than the subjective, individual approach attempted by most clinicians (Table 1).

When ordering heparin anticoagulation for acute DVT in the absence of co-morbidities for bleeding, I prescribe a 10,000-IU bolus intravenously followed by 2000 IU per hour and check PTT 8 hours after the bolus, with the goal of maintaining the PTT at more than 90 seconds. If the PTT is supratherapeutic (>100 seconds), this dose will be continued if the patient does not have a co-morbidity for bleeding. This level of anticoagulation is required for only 4 to 5 days, at which time the heparin can be discon-

TABLE 1. **Prescriptive Approach to Intravenous Heparin Therapy: A Titration Nomogram for Activated Partial Thromboplastin Time (APTT)**

APTT	Intravenous Infusion		Additional Action
	Rate Change (mL/h)	Dose Change (units/24 h)*	
≤45	+6	+5760	Repeat APTT† in 4–6 h
46–54	+3	+2880	Repeat APTT in 4–6 h
55–85	0	0	None‡
86–110	−3	−2880	Stop heparin sodium treatment for 1 h; repeat APTT 4–6 h after restarting heparin treatment
>110	−6	−5760	Stop heparin sodium treatment for 1 h; repeat APTT 4–6 h after restarting heparin treatment

*Heparin sodium concentration, 20,000 units/500 mL = 40 units/mL.
†With the use of Actin-FS thromboplastin reagent (Dade, Mississauga, Ontario).
‡During the first 24 hours, repeat APTT in 4–6 h. Thereafter, the APTT will be determined once daily, unless subtherapeutic.

tinued because the warfarin is therapeutic. Using the prescriptive approach summarized in Table 1 is another good option. However, one must be cautious in using the prescriptive approach in patients with co-morbidities for bleeding.

Heparin-induced thrombocytopenia is a well-recognized and feared complication of heparin therapy caused by heparin-specific antibodies binding to the platelet membrane, stimulating platelet aggregation. It is usually recognized 2 to 10 days after heparin therapy is initiated, is reported in 2 to 20% of patients receiving heparin, and is more frequent with bovine heparin than with porcine heparin. Heparin-induced thrombocytopenia is an antigen-antibody immunologic response that is not dose related. Platelet counts should be monitored in all patients receiving heparin, regardless of the route of administration or the dose prescribed. A drop in platelet count by more than 30% indicates a high likelihood of heparin-induced thrombocytopenia; and if the platelet count decreases, heparin should be discontinued with alternative antithrombotic therapy initiated.

Warfarin Compounds

Oral anticoagulants inhibit the vitamin K–dependent clotting factors II, VII, IX, and X. They also inhibit vitamin K–dependent carboxylation of proteins C and S. Because proteins C and S are naturally occurring anticoagulants that function by inhibiting activated factors V and VIII, any vitamin K antagonist can potentially produce a hypercoagulable state before achieving its anticoagulant effect, because the half-lives of proteins C and S are shorter than the half-life of the clotting factors. Warfarin compounds do not have an immediate effect on the

coagulation system because the normal clotting factors present must be cleared. They generally require 3 to 5 days of administration to achieve a therapeutic effect; therefore, patients should be treated with heparin until this occurs. Primary anticoagulation with warfarin compounds alone is associated with an unacceptably high rate of recurrent thromboembolic complications.

The appropriate intensity of oral anticoagulation has been revised. Evidence from prospective studies indicate that less intense warfarin that achieves a prothrombin time 1.3 to 1.5 times control or an international normalized ratio (INR) of 2.0 to 3.0 is equally effective in preventing recurrent thromboembolic events compared with higher levels of anticoagulation and is associated with significantly fewer bleeding complications. Monitoring of oral anticoagulation has been critically evaluated, and the INR is now the standard by which all patients should be followed. Because prothrombin time ratios have shown remarkable variability depending on the thromboplastin used, the INR standardizes therapy and improves safety.

The major complication of oral anticoagulation is bleeding, which usually correlates with the degree of anticoagulation as predicted by the prothrombin time. Nonhemorrhagic complications include skin necrosis, which has been associated with a heterozygous protein C deficiency and malignancy. Coumadin (warfarin) compounds cross the placenta and have been associated with teratogenic effects when given during the first trimester of pregnancy. Because there are similar concerns in the second trimester as well as the risk of fetal bleeding during and after delivery, warfarin compounds should be avoided when treating a pregnant woman. All women of childbearing potential taking warfarin compounds should avoid pregnancy during treatment. If anticoagulation is indicated during pregnancy, subcutaneous heparin or low-molecular-weight heparin (LMWH) is recommended.

Low-Molecular-Weight Heparin

LMWHs function by inhibiting factor Xa activity and factor IIa activity, with relatively more anti-Xa activity (2:1 to 4:1). Compared with unfractionated heparin, LMWH preparations have a longer plasma half-life and substantially higher plasma levels after subcutaneous injection. As a result of their improved bioavailability, they have less variability in anticoagulant response to a fixed dose. Because of their pharmacokinetic properties, they can obtain a stable and sustained anticoagulant effect when administered subcutaneously once or twice daily and laboratory monitoring is not necessary.

LMWHs are approved in the United States for DVT prophylaxis in general surgical and orthopedic patients, for the treatment of acute DVT, and for prevention of ischemic complications of unstable angina and non–Q wave myocardial infarction. The evidence that these newer anticoagulants are safe and

TABLE 2. **Initial Treatment of Acute DVT with Low Molecular Weight Heparins (LMWH) compared with Unfractionated Heparin (UFH): A Meta-analysis of 10 Prospective Trials**

	UFH	LMWH	Risk Reduction	A-Value
Symptomatic	6.5%	3.1%	53%	<0.01
Venographic change				<0.01
Improved	52%	63%		
Worse	12%	6%		
Major hemorrhage	2.8%	0.8%	68%	<0.005
Mortality	7.1%	3.9%	47%	<0.04

Results from Lensing AWA, Prins MH, Davidson BL, Hirsh J: Treatment of deep venous thrombosis with low molecular weight heparins: A meta-analysis. Arch Intern Med 155:601–607, 1995.

effective for the treatment of acute deep venous thrombosis is impressive. A meta-analysis of randomized trials evaluating the treatment of acute DVT with LMWHs versus standard unfractionated heparin compared adjusted-dose unfractionated heparin with fixed-dose (weight adjusted) subcutaneous LMWH in patients with objectively diagnosed acute DVT. The incidence of recurrent symptomatic venous thromboembolism, venographic change of DVT, major bleeding complications, and mortality is summarized in Table 2. The subcutaneous injection of LMWH compounds once or twice daily without laboratory monitoring likely represents an important advance in the treatment of venous thrombosis. Their longer plasma half-life and high bioavailability when given subcutaneously offer obvious treatment advantages. Because laboratory monitoring is not necessary, the results included here indicate that anticoagulation for acute DVT will evolve to outpatient therapy for many patients.

The formulation approved for treatment is enoxaparin (Lovenox). It is anticipated that other LMWH compounds will be approved for this indication in the near future. Those receiving outpatient treatment of acute DVT without pulmonary embolism should receive 1 mg per kg subcutaneously every 12 hours. In inpatient treatment for patients with pulmonary embolism and for patients with acute DVT without pulmonary embolism who are not candidates for outpatient treatment, the recommended dose of enoxaparin is 1 mg per kg every 12 hours given subcutaneously or 1.5 mg per kg once daily subcutaneously the same time every day. In both outpatient and inpatient treatments, warfarin sodium therapy should be started when appropriate, usually within 72 hours. I prefer to start warfarin shortly after the first subcutaneous injection. LMWH should be continued for a minimum of 5 days and until a therapeutic oral anticoagulant effect has been achieved, with the INR in the 2.0 to 3.0 range.

Thrombolytic Therapy

Pharmacologic dissolution of thrombus from the deep venous system appears to be an ideal goal of treatment that has the potential of eliminating deep venous obstruction and maintaining valvular function. Practical questions regarding thrombolysis for deep venous thrombosis are

- Can venous thrombi be lysed?
- Is lysing venous clot important in preserving long-term valvular function?

Thirteen studies are reported in the literature that compared anticoagulation therapy to thrombolytic therapy for acute DVT. Each patient had the diagnosis confirmed with ascending phlebography, and the phlebogram was repeated to assess the results of therapy (Table 3). Of the patients treated with thrombolytic therapy, 45% had significant or complete clearing on post-therapy phlebography compared with only 4% of those treated with heparin. Although the precise level of venous occlusion was not known in each case, a reasonable number of patients were expected to have iliofemoral DVT. Considering that all patients treated with lytic therapy were given systemic intravenous infusion and that systemic thrombolysis is inadequate for iliofemoral DVT, a 45% lysis rate appears reasonable for the entire group. Prospective studies have shown that patients successfully treated with lytic therapy for DVT have fewer post-thrombotic symptoms and are more likely to retain normal valve function.

Patients with iliofemoral DVT represent a subset of patients who are not likely to respond to systemic lytic therapy. Because occlusive thrombus in the iliofemoral system has limited exposure to any circulating plasminogen activator, and because the thrombus burden is large, it is understandable why these patients are unlikely to respond to the systemic administration of plasminogen activators.

A number of reports have indicated improved success with the delivery of a thrombolytic agent directly into the iliofemoral clot through the catheter-directed approach. A number of reported series in addition to a prospective "venous registry" observed an 85 to 90% success rate, with patency being maintained in 60 to 80% at 1 year. Identifying and correcting an underlying iliac venous stenosis significantly improves long-term patency. It is apparent that clinical sequelae of iliofemoral deep venous thrombosis are related to patency of the iliofemoral venous segment.

TABLE 3. **Thrombolytic Therapy Versus Standard Anticoagulation for Acute DVT: Venographic Results of 13 Studies**

	Lysis		
Prescriptions (No.)	None/ Worse (%)	Partial (%)	Significant/ Complete (%)
Heparin (254)	82	14	4
Lytic prescriptions (337)	37	18	45

From Comerota AJ, Aldridge SA: Thrombolytic therapy for acute deep vein thrombosis. Semin Vasc Surg 5:76–81, 1992.

Venous Thrombectomy

Vascular surgical techniques have been remarkably refined since the 1970s, and results of surgical revascularization have improved in all areas of vascular surgery. This also is true regarding venous thrombectomy, although, unfortunately, many vascular surgeons are reluctant to apply these improved techniques to venous thrombectomy in clinical practice. Technical improvements include (1) accurate preoperative definition of the extent of thrombosis, which includes routine contralateral iliocavography; (2) completion phlebography after thrombectomy to ensure the adequacy of thrombectomy and examine the residual venous lumen; (3) correction of an underlying venous stenosis, which could be a precipitating factor for DVT; (4) construction of a small arteriovenous fistula to increase venous velocity and assist in maintaining patency of a thrombogenic iliofemoral venous segment; and (5) immediate and prolonged anticoagulation.

The steps of successful venous thrombectomy are listed in Table 4. If unobstructed ipsilateral venous drainage cannot be established, a cross-pubic venous bypass with a 10-mm externally supported polytetrafluoroethylene graft combined with an arteriovenous fistula is recommended. Endoluminal repair with angioplasty and stenting is the preferred method of correcting a short, segmental residual lesion in the ipsilateral iliac vein after thrombectomy.

Venous thrombectomy has been evaluated in a prospective randomized fashion and compared with standard anticoagulation in patients with iliofemoral venous thrombosis. Results indicated significantly better patency and fewer post-thrombotic symptoms in patients undergoing thrombectomy. As might be anticipated, long-term success is dependent on maintaining long-term patency.

A large review of patients undergoing thrombectomy for iliofemoral thrombosis confirmed the safety of the procedure, with less than a 0.5% operative mortality and no fatal pulmonary emboli. Pooled data from contemporary reports of iliofemoral venous thrombectomy indicate that the early and long-term patency of the iliofemoral venous segment is approximately 80%, contrasted to only 30% of patients treated with anticoagulation alone. Iliofemoral venous thrombectomy should now be considered in patients with symptomatic iliofemoral DVT who cannot be offered catheter-directed lysis or who fail lytic therapy.

Elastic Compression to Control Lower-Extremity Edema

Most patients with symptomatic DVT and many with asymptomatic DVT will develop swelling of the involved lower extremity once full activity is restored. The edema causes physical morbidity and psychological concern and should be controlled. Clinicians should assume that post-thrombotic edema will occur in all patients with proximal DVT and selected

---

TABLE 4. **Technical Considerations for Venous Thrombectomy**

1. Completely visualize the thrombus; include contralateral iliofemoral phlebography and a cavogram.
2. Draw blood for full hypercoagulable evaluation (before anticoagulation).
3. Patient is fully anticoagulated on heparin, which is continued throughout procedure and postoperatively.
4. Prepare operating room for fluoroscopy and radiography.
5. Preferentially use general anesthesia with positive end-expiratory pressure.
6. Type and crossmatch 2 to 3 units of blood.
7. Use an autotransfusion device during the procedure.
8. Perform inguinal incision to expose and control common femoral, saphenous, superficial femoral, and profunda femoris veins.
9. Use right retroperitoneal caval control and caval venotomy for removal of caval thrombus.
10. If a caval filter is in place, use fluoroscopy during thrombectomy, with contrast material used to inflate the venous thrombectomy catheter balloon.
11. Pass venous thrombectomy catheter part of the way into iliac vein for several passes before advancing into vena cava (use No. 8 or No. 10 venous thrombectomy catheter).
12. Consider intraoperative infusion of plasminogen activators after thrombectomy, with balloon occlusion of the iliac vein.
13. Exsanguinate leg with rubber bandage and expel clot from below to remove infrainguinal thrombus.
14. If lower leg extrusion maneuver does not clear infrainguinal clot, consider infrainguinal balloon catheter thrombectomy. Cut down to posterior tibial vein and advance No. 3 Fogarty catheter to femoral venotomy. Attach and guide No. 4 Fogarty catheter retrograde in leg, to allow balloon catheter thrombectomy in selected patients (especially patients with thrombus in or inadequate drainage from profunda femoris) and repeat as needed. Flush leg with high volume/pressure heparin-saline solution and infuse urokinase, 500,000 U, before ligating posterior tibial vein (consider leaving catheter in posterior tibial vein for heparin infusion).
15. After completing thrombectomy, evaluate iliofemoral system with completion phlebogram/fluoroscopy.
16. If iliac system has residual stenosis or small segment occlusion, balloon dilation with stenting (if necessary) is performed under fluoroscopic guidance. If the iliac system has persistent long segment occlusion, a cross-pubic venous bypass with a 10-mm externally supported polytetrafluoroethylene (PTFE) graft and associated arteriovenous fistula (AVF) is performed.
17. Construct a small-diameter AVF (4 mm) with the saphenous vein or one of its large proximal branches to the proximal superficial femoral artery (AVF is considered permanent). Slip piece of 5- to 6-mm diameter PTFE graft around saphenous vein segment and leave small loop of 0-prolene with clip in subcutaneous wound (in case closure of AVF becomes necessary).
18. Measure femoral vein pressure before and after AVF is open. If pressure increases, the problem is either the AVF is too large or there is persistent proximal iliac vein stenosis. Re-evaluate iliac venous system and correct lesion or band AVF to decrease flow and normalize pressure.
19. Apply external pneumatic compression devices in the recovery room.
20. Continue heparin throughout the postoperative period, switching the patient to oral anticoagulation.

patients with calf vein thrombosis. Elastic compression is important for controlling post-thrombotic edema and the long-term morbidity of the post-thrombotic syndrome. Simply put, the post-thrombotic syndrome is controlled by controlling lower extremity edema. The majority of patients require compression only to the knee, because thigh swelling is infrequent and when it occurs is associated with minimal morbidity. Long-leg compression is offered if it is the patient's preference. Occasionally, when thigh swelling is a problem, total-leg compression is best achieved by a panty style stocking.

Most patients will require a 30- to 40-mm ankle gradient below-knee compression stocking. They are instructed to wear the stocking from the time they awake in the morning until the time they go to bed at night. More severe post-thrombotic edema necessitates higher compression. Occasionally, patients will be unable to apply the 30- to 40-mm stocking and a 20- to 30-mm stocking will be used. If patients cannot apply any stocking, because of arthritis or other physical limitation, an elastic bandage firmly applied daily from the base of the toes to the knee is an effective alternative.

TREATMENT STRATEGIES FOR ACUTE DVT

The following treatment strategies are recommended according to the level and extent of venous thrombosis. They are proposed based on the known natural history of acute DVT and the known benefits of therapy.

Calf Vein Thrombosis

Venous thrombosis limited to the calf veins is an important clinical issue; however, treatment remains controversial. Taken alone, calf vein thrombi usually do not cause major sequelae and do not place the patient at high risk for pulmonary emboli. However, calf vein thrombi can embolize, and propagation to large veins substantially increases the risk for pulmonary embolism and the post-thrombotic syndrome.

Whether patients are symptomatic or asymptomatic, and whether the calf vein thrombi are found incidentally on screening examinations of high-risk inpatients or symptomatic outpatients, complicates the clinical question. A number of studies reviewing isolated calf vein thrombosis conclude that propagation rates of up to 30% occur in postoperative and hospitalized patients. Early propagation occurs in at least 10% of symptomatic patients. If not treated, recurrent venous thromboembolic complications are observed in up to 30% of patients.

In light of this information, it appears that treatment of patients with calf vein thrombosis is indicated, especially if their thrombotic risk continues or if the cause of their DVT has not been defined and eliminated (Figure 1). Outpatients with symptomatic calf DVT and inpatients with ongoing thrombotic risk should benefit from 3 months of anticoagulation. If

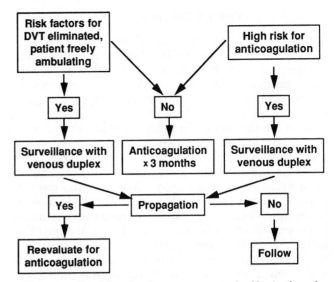

Figure 1. Algorithm for the management of calf vein thrombosis.

not treated because of concern for complications of anticoagulation, patients should be monitored with venous duplex imaging at 3- to 4-day intervals until the high-risk period has passed and the patient returns to full ambulation. If extension into the proximal venous system is demonstrated, the patient must be re-evaluated for definitive therapy.

Femoral-Popliteal Venous Thrombosis

Ventilation/perfusion lung scans should be considered as part of the routine initial evaluation of patients with proximal DVT. Up to 40% of these patients have asymptomatic pulmonary emboli. Approximately 25% of those with asymptomatic pulmonary emboli subsequently experience new signs or symptoms of pulmonary embolism during anticoagulation. These new symptoms might suggest failure of anticoagulation, unless the patient had prior documentation of the ventilation/perfusion mismatch. A repeat lung scan that fails to identify new perfusion defects indicates that the symptoms are a consequence of the prior pulmonary embolism; therefore, caval filtration is not indicated because primary anticoagulation has not failed.

DVT involving the superficial femoral and popliteal veins is the most common form necessitating therapy. Anticoagulation is the standard therapy, but it does not resolve thrombus in the deep venous system. However, effective anticoagulation will allow physiologic fibrinolysis to recanalize the occluded veins. Furthermore, even in the absence of recanalization, morbidity may be minimal if thrombosis is limited to the femoral vein in the thigh. It has been shown that ligation of the femoral vein below the origin of the profunda femoris causes minimal morbidity, because most patients have adequate venous collateral drainage around a mid thigh obstruction. In light of these observations, early effective anticoagulation is the preferred therapy.

Immediate treatment with intravenous heparin is recommended. Supratherapeutic anticoagulation early in the course of therapy is my preference compared with monitored anticoagulation. This is not accompanied by additional bleeding complications in the absence of a co-morbidity for bleeding. Oral anticoagulation is started immediately and continued over the long term, maintaining an INR of 2.0 to 3.0. Patients are allowed to ambulate normally. The appropriate duration of anticoagulation is under study; however, 1 year of oral anticoagulation is more effective than shorter courses of therapy. Longer therapy should be considered for patients with extensive DVT at the outset and those who have persistent venous obstruction on repeat duplex imaging 1 year after initiation of therapy. Maintaining the INR between 2.0 and 3.0 is associated with minimal bleeding complications, yet patients are effectively protected from recurrent thrombosis. Patients suffering recurrent DVT are evaluated for an underlying malignancy and hypercoagulable state and are treated indefinitely with oral anticoagulation.

With the approval of LMWHs by the U.S. Food and Drug Administration, they will become the preferred initial treatment of most patients with acute DVT. As stated earlier, a weight-adjusted subcutaneous injection of 1 mg per kg of enoxaparin every 12 hours or 1.5 mg per kg subcutaneously daily is recommended. This is continued until the patient has received oral anticoagulants for 4 or more days and the INR is therapeutic. Because the LMWH is given subcutaneously and does not necessitate monitoring, hospitalization is not mandatory for safe and effective treatment. An initial hospitalization period of 24 hours may be required for patient instruction and education and for planning the logistics of ongoing care.

Although superficial femoral vein ligation has been abandoned as primary treatment for DVT in patients with thrombus located distal to the profunda femoris vein, there still may be a place for this option in patients who cannot be anticoagulated. Superficial femoral vein ligation is effective in preventing pulmonary embolism and propagation to the more proximal venous system in patients with thrombus limited to the infraprofunda venous system. Interestingly, the long-term post-thrombotic sequelae are infrequent in these patients. This reinforces the importance of preserving drainage through the profunda femoris vein.

Patients with proximal vein thrombosis who have an absolute contraindication to anticoagulation, and those who have had pulmonary emboli while therapeutically anticoagulated, are treated with vena caval filtration. Percutaneous placement of vena caval filters is safe and effective. If the indication for caval filtration is failure rather than a contraindication to anticoagulation, anticoagulation should be continued after filter placement to treat the primary process, DVT.

Iliofemoral Venous Thrombosis

Iliofemoral venous thrombosis represents the most extensive form of acute disease, and these patients experience the most severe post-thrombotic sequelae. Eliminating thrombus from the iliofemoral venous system significantly improves short- and long-term venous function and reduces morbidity. The primary goals of therapy should be to prevent pulmonary embolism and eliminate the acute and chronic post-thrombotic morbidity.

These goals can be achieved if the clot is eliminated from the iliofemoral venous system, if unobstructed venous drainage is restored (at least from the profunda femoris vein to the vena cava), and if re-thrombosis is avoided.

Two treatment options offer the potential to achieve these goals (Figure 2): (1) catheter-directed thrombolysis and (2) venous thrombectomy.

In patients without contraindications to thrombolysis, catheter-directed thrombolysis is preferred, with multi-sidehole catheters positioned into the thrombus from the contralateral femoral vein or the right jugular vein or ultrasound guided percutaneous access to the ipsilateral popliteal or posterior tibial vein. A bolus of urokinase (Abbokinase)* of 250,000 to 500,000 units is given, followed by 250,000 to 400,000 units per hour by continuous infusion. This concentration is delivered in 25 to 50 mL of saline.

---

*Not FDA approved for this indication.

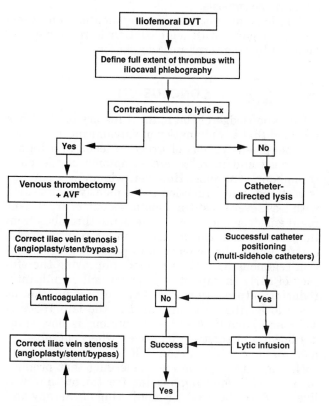

Figure 2. Algorithm for the management of iliofemoral deep vein thrombosis.

In particularly severe cases, 5- to 10-mg bolus doses of recombinant tissue plasminogen activator (rt-PA [Activase])* have been used, followed by urokinase infusion, to take advantage of potential lytic synergism with these two plasminogen activators. Lytic response is followed by repeat phlebography at 6- to 12-hour intervals. If catheters can be appropriately positioned, lysis is achieved in the majority. An underlying lesion in the iliac vein is commonly observed and must be corrected, usually with balloon angioplasty and occasionally with the addition of a stent. Patients who have free floating thrombus in their vena cava should have caval filters placed before catheter-directed thrombolysis.

Recently the FDA has restricted the use of urokinase. I have found that rt-PA infused as a 4- to 5-mg bolus into the thrombus, followed by a continuous infusion of 0.05 mg/kg/hour, is a good alternative.* This offers the opportunity for effective lysis with a low risk of bleeding complications.

If catheters cannot be positioned into the occluded iliofemoral venous system or if contraindications to thrombolysis exist, a venous thrombectomy with an adjunctive arteriovenous fistula is recommended. If ipsilateral patency cannot be restored, a cross-pubic venous bypass with a 10-mm externally supported polytetrafluoroethylene graft and a small adjunctive arteriovenous fistula should be performed. After restoring patency to the iliofemoral venous system, aggressive anticoagulation is required to prevent rethrombosis. External pneumatic compression devices are applied to further accelerate venous return and avoid re-thrombosis.

If patients are not operative candidates, supratherapeutic heparin with leg elevation is recommended followed by long-term anticoagulation.

CONCLUSION

Our knowledge of the natural history of DVT has revealed that a combination of valvular incompetence and persistent venous obstruction leads to a higher frequency and more severe symptoms of the post-thrombotic syndrome. However, when early patency is restored, valve function is frequently maintained with less severe post-thrombotic sequelae. Treatment regimens designed to eliminate acute thrombus from the deep system can achieve similar results if successful and if the veins remain patent. Anticoagulation regimens have been refined, improving the efficacy of early therapy with heparin and significantly reducing future recurrence. Oral anticoagulation at doses lower than recommended in the late 1980s is safer and equally effective. Treatment is now standardized, and safety is improved when patients are monitored according to the INR.

Newer anticoagulants are emerging that promise to offer additional options for treatment that will likely reduce the need for monitoring of therapy and hospitalization.

_____
*Not FDA approved for this indication.

ACKNOWLEDGMENT

The author gratefully acknowledges the capable assistance of Connie Presser in the preparation of this text.

HYPERTROPHIC CARDIOMYOPATHY

method of
RICHARD A. KRASUSKI, M.D., and
THOMAS M. BASHORE, M.D.
Duke University Medical Center
Durham, North Carolina

BACKGROUND

In the late 1860s at the Hôpital La Salpêtrière in Paris, Vulpian described a pathologic specimen of a heart with "retrecissment de l'orifice ventriculo-aortique," or "subaortic stricture." Several names have since been given to this condition; the most commonly used ones include "idiopathic subaortic stenosis," "asymmetric septal hypertrophy," and "hypertrophic cardiomyopathy" (HCM). Although occasional isolated descriptions followed, it was not until nearly a century later, with the reports of Brock and Teare in the late 1950s, that HCM began to attract widespread attention. HCM's ability to dramatically distort cardiac anatomy and lead to death and disability in an otherwise young, healthy person, has fascinated scientists and clinicians and led to rapid advances in its understanding.

DEFINITION

The growth of molecular genetics and cardiovascular imaging has complicated previous classification schemes. In its purest form, HCM is characterized by increased left and occasionally right ventricular wall thickness in the absence of an underlying etiology such as hypertension, aortic stenosis, intense athletic training, or coarctation of the aorta. HCM can be obstructive or nonobstructive at rest; the latter condition is about three times more common. It usually results in asymmetrical hypertrophy of the left ventricular (LV) septum in comparison with the LV posterior wall and is associated with microscopic evidence of cardiac myocyte disarray, particularly in the septum. The asymmetrical variants have different forms, including subaortic, midventricular, and apical; the subaortic form is the most common.

EPIDEMIOLOGY

The definition of HCM becomes critical when clinicians attempt to quantify its prevalence; guidelines for its diagnosis were developed before advances in imaging and genetics in the 1980s and 1990s. Most commonly quoted are echocardiographic studies, which estimate the prevalence to be between 0.1 and 0.3%. These studies also show an age dependency; the Framingham study has shown that nearly 2% of the elderly population (average age, 74) has HCM, in contrast to only 0.3% in the young (average age 47), and that the elderly are also more symptomatic. A retrospective review of the population of Olmstead County in Minnesota found a prevalence of only 0.02%. Unfortunately, epidemiologic data usually include only patients who go to their clinicians with symptoms and are therefore not a true screening of the generalized population. With the advancements in genetics, family members of large kindreds with HCM who have the genetic abnormality but no physical, electrocardiographic, or echocardiographic evidence of disease have been identified.

GENETICS

Davies first described the autosomal dominant mode of inheritance of HCM in 1952, and the first large pedigree of familial HCM was reported in 1960. Advancements in human genetics have allowed isolation of the genes responsible for several human disorders, and at present, mutations in at least seven genes have been reported to cause HCM. These include cardiac troponin I and T, α-tropomysin, cardiac myosin–binding protein C, β-myosin heavy chain, ventricular myosin essential light chain, and ventricular myosin regulatory light chain, all of which are determinants of sarcomeric structure. How these defects result in the pathophysiologic manifestations of HCM has not been fully explained. One popular hypothesis is that a gene mutation results in a "poison polypeptide" that incorporates itself into the sarcomere and results in an alteration of myocyte structure. This resultant interaction causes either hypofunctioning myocytes with dilatation, followed by compensatory hypertrophy, or a hypercontractile state with hypertrophy as a direct result.

PATHOLOGY

Gross pathologic examination demonstrates a primary myocardial process with hypertrophy and no obvious cause. Light microscopy and electron microscopy reveal cellular hypertrophy, disorganized myofibers with the appearance of whorls, and myocardial scarring. Although other diseases can produce focal areas with this pattern, it usually accounts for less than 2% of the total myocardium. In almost all patients with HCM, 5% of the myocardium is involved with the abnormal whorls; in half, at least 25% of the septum is involved. In 80% of HCM cases, medium-sized intramural coronary arteries are partially or completely obstructed by intimal and medial hypertrophy, even when epicardial coronary arteries are normal.

PATHOPHYSIOLOGY

The hemodynamic manifestations of HCM are based on three underlying features: diastolic dysfunction, ventricular outflow tract obstruction, and mitral regurgitation. Absolute wall thickness varies broadly from mildly increased (13 to 15 mm; normal, <12 mm) to the most substantial hypertrophy observed in any cardiac disease (>30 mm and up to 60 mm). Progressive degrees of hypertrophy result in a stiffer, less compliant left ventricle that requires higher pressures for chamber filling. Ischemia secondary to supply-demand mismatch (the increased muscle mass and enhanced inotropy demanding greater oxygen supply, and the elevated intracavitary pressures and narrowing in intramural arteries limiting oxygen supply) also contributes to stiffening the ventricle. The elevated ventricular diastolic pressures result in higher left atrial, pulmonary arterial, right ventricular, and right atrial pressures and manifestations of congestive heart failure.

Outflow tract obstruction, although not necessary for the diagnosis of HCM, is a characteristic feature of the disease. Two separate theories have evolved to explain the outflow gradient. According to the first, the mitral valve is simply a bystander and its motion has nothing to do with the gradient. During LV contraction it is drawn into the outflow tract by the Venturi effect. This is an attractive hypothesis because the LV is almost empty when systolic anterior motion (SAM) occurs. According to the second theory, the mitral valve must contact the septal wall in order for obstruction to occur. In its support is echocardiographic evidence that onset of the gradient is nearly simultaneous with the onset of mitral contact between the leaflet and the septum and that the time to onset and duration of contact determines the magnitude of pressure gradient. It is possible that elements of both theories are correct, inasmuch as replacement of the mitral valve in patients with HCM usually removes the gradient.

The outflow gradient is dynamic in nature, inasmuch as resistance to flow is highly dependent on inotropic state (contractile force), preload (filling pressures), and afterload (systemic pressure). All these factors greatly contribute to the outflow gradient, and certain physiologic conditions such as exercise can result in pressure drops of more than 100 mm Hg, resulting in hypotension and syncope.

Mitral regurgitation is believed to result from malpositioning of the mitral valve during midsystole, caused by SAM and leading to interference with normal valve function. This explanation is not complete, however; about 20% of patients with subaortic obstruction in HCM have mitral regurgitation that is independent of SAM. Of interest is that mitral annular calcification, a common cause of mitral regurgitation in the elderly population, has been shown to be more common in an age-matched population without HCM. The mitral regurgitation in HCM is usually mild but can be severe, particularly in association with large outflow tract gradients.

CLINICAL MANIFESTATIONS

Symptoms can develop at any age but usually do so in early adulthood. The predominant symptoms include dyspnea, chest pain, palpitations, and syncope. The most common of these is dyspnea, which results from elevated left ventricular diastolic pressure, leading to elevated left atrial pressure and pulmonary congestion. Other symptoms of congestion, including orthopnea and paroxysmal nocturnal dyspnea, may occur as well. Chest pain is common and may be secondary to coronary atherosclerosis or inadequate microvascular flow to the thickened myocardium. Palpitations usually result from atrial or ventricular arrhythmias and are fairly common in this population. Because of the dependence on atrial contraction for adequate ventricular filling in HCM, atrial fibrillation can result in reduced preload, reduced stroke volume, and increased outflow gradient. It is poorly tolerated in these patients. Syncope can result from a variety of processes, including severe outflow gradient and reduced cardiac output, atrial arrhythmias, or ventricular arrhythmias. Embolic stroke is rare, but patients with atrial fibrillation are at increased risk.

PHYSICAL EXAMINATION

The presence of right ventricular involvement can be detected by a prominent A-wave in the jugular venous pulse, a systolic murmur along the left sternal border reflecting obstruction to outflow, and possibly a right-sided fourth heart sound that indicates right ventricular diastolic dysfunction. This is occasionally best heard in the right subclavicular region. LV obstruction is detectable as a systolic ejection murmur along the outflow tract, from the apex to the carotid arteries. Maneuvers that increase ventricular contraction, diminish ventricular filling, or reduce afterload will accentuate the murmur. This helps distinguish HCM from conditions of fixed outflow obstruction such as aortic stenosis. A holosystolic murmur consistent with mitral regurgitation is often present. In obstructive HCM the initial carotid upstroke is brisk, followed by a plateau and often a secondary impulse (bifid pulse). Other findings of obstructive HCM can include a double systolic or triple apex beat, reversed splitting of the second heart sound, a mitral diastolic inflow murmur due to significant mitral regurgitation, and, rarely, the sound of contact between a mitral leaflet and the septum.

DIAGNOSTIC MODALITIES

The chest radiograph may be normal or show evidence of LV, left atrial, or right atrial enlargement with or without pulmonary venous redistribution. The aorta is typically small. A bulge on the left border of the heart, between the left atrial appendage and the left ventricular apex, can reflect anterolateral wall extension of anteroseptal hypertrophy.

Electrocardiographic abnormalities are found in about 90% of patients with HCM and are highly variable and often nonspecific. The most common findings are ST-segment alterations and T wave inversion, abnormal Q waves, signs of LV hypertrophy, signs of right or left atrial enlargement, and diminished R waves in the lateral leads. Although HCM usually involves the ventricular septum, complete bundle branch blocks are rare. Interestingly, the apical form of HCM has been associated with "giant" negative T waves in the precordial leads.

The wide availability and ease of performance have made echocardiography the gold standard in the diagnosis of HCM. The commonly used echocardiographic definition of HCM has been a left ventricular wall thickness of 15 mm or more or a ratio of septal to posterior wall thickness of 1.3 or more, in the absence of other causes (cardiac and systemic) of increased wall mass and without ventricular dilatation. However, studies have found wide variations in morphologic patterns and a significant overlap between wall thicknesses of genetically affected and unaffected patients. Problems also arise in distinguishing between HCM and the so-called athlete's heart. Echocardiographic findings in HCM that may be helpful in distinguishing HCM from athlete's heart include unusual patterns of hypertrophy, LV end-diastolic dimension of less than 45 mm, left atrial enlargement, and abnormal Doppler diastolic indexes of left ventricular filling.

Radionuclide angiography can demonstrate systolic and diastolic ventricular function in patients with HCM. Stress perfusion imaging can assist in demonstrating myocardial ischemia or infarction and can provide important prognostic information.

Magnetic resonance imaging (MRI) is a novel manner in which to study diseases affecting the myocardium. Myocardial tagging and ultrafast scanning techniques have greatly improved its application to HCM. Advantages include improved resolution over that of echocardiography, absence of ionizing radiation, ability to use inherent contrast, and ability to obtain three-dimensional spatial resolution. Unlike echocardiography, MRI is not limited by poor windows from distorted skeletal anatomy, by pulmonary disease, or by obesity (except by weight limits of the scanning table). MRI also shows significant advantages over echocardiography in imaging the apical septum. Disadvantages remain the absence of widespread availability, claustrophobia on the part of patients, the presence of implanted metal devices, and cost.

Cardiac catheterization, although no longer used routinely for the diagnosis of HCM, can provide additional details not obtainable by noninvasive means. The femoral pulse wave is notable for a spike-and-dome configuration characterized by an initial rapid rise in aortic pressure (spike) followed by a slight decrease (plateau) and a secondary peak (dome). Elevated LV diastolic pressure and elevated right heart pressures are often found. Signs of diastolic dysfunction such as a prolonged rapid filling phase and a larger percentage of ventricular filling provided by atrial contraction (leading to accentuated A waves) can be seen. An intraventricular gradient can often be demonstrated at rest or by provocation (e.g., a Valsalva maneuver or amyl nitrate) and can be carefully localized by a slow catheter pullback. Brockenbrough's sign can be demonstrated by inducing premature ventricular contractions and observing the failure of the pulse pressure to widen during the post-extrasystolic beat. This occurs as a result of augmented inotropy overcoming the preload and afterload changes. The post-extrasystolic beat also often demonstrates the classic spike-and-dome pattern. In addition, cardiac catheterization can help exclude coronary disease as the etiology of exertional chest pain or dyspnea in patients with HCM. Studies have also shown an increased incidence of myocardial bridging (tunneling into the myocardium) of the left anterior descending coronary artery. Some authors believe that left anterior descending artery bridging is associated with myocardial ischemia and a poorer clinical outcome.

NATURAL HISTORY

The most feared complication of HCM is sudden cardiac death, and HCM remains the most common cause of sudden death on the athletic field in young competitive athletes. Controversies exist in estimating the yearly incidence of sudden death in HCM. The greatest extent of data has been from tertiary referral centers, where mortality rates have been estimated as high as 3 to 6% per year. It is possible that these patients were referred because of their elevated risk for sudden death, and these studies could overestimate risk. In contrast, reports from large unselected populations estimate the yearly mortality rate to be 0.5 to 1.5%.

Sudden death can occur at any point in the disease process but is rare before the age of 10; it occurs most commonly between the ages of 12 and 35. It appears that a majority of these deaths occur during or just after vigorous physical exertion. The ability to predict which patients will die suddenly is poor, but several characteristics that portend a poor prognosis have been identified. They include previous history of resuscitated sudden death or family history of sudden death, exercise-induced hypotension, myocardial scarring and perfusion defects on nuclear imaging, inducible ventricular tachycardia by electrophysiologic study, and decreased LV ejection fraction and increased end-diastolic pressure. There also appear to be particular gene mutations that result in higher rates of sudden death in affected patients. Characteristics not found to be associated with an increased risk of sudden death include the severity of the outflow gradient, the presence of clinical symptoms, heart rate variability, and abnormal signal average electrocardiograms.

A small proportion of patients with HCM (~10%) progress to LV dilatation, which is believed to be secondary to scar formation from chronic myocardial ischemia as a result of microvascular disease.

UNUSUAL VARIANTS

Apical hypertrophic cardiomyopathy, although common in East Asia (accounting for up to 25% of all cases of HCM), is otherwise a very uncommon variant (accounting for less than 1% of all cases of HCM). The electrocardiogram reveals giant negative T waves (usually greater than 10 mm) in the precordial leads. On catheterization the right anterior oblique projection is notable for an "ace of spades" configuration due to the outline of the large papillary muscles on the LV angiogram. From epidemiologic data it appears that the clinical course of apical HCM is more benign, with a smaller incidence of sudden cardiac death.

Attention has been focused on the increasing frequency with which HCM is being diagnosed in the elderly population. Comparative studies have shown that presenting features and clinical outcome in the elderly do not appear to differ from those of HCM in a younger population. What appears to best predict outcome in these patients is New York Heart Association (NYHA) functional class. Asymptomatic patients had outcomes similar to age-matched controls, whereas patients with NYHA class III symptoms (dyspnea with low-level exertion) had a 1-year mortality rate in excess of 30%.

TREATMENT (Table 1)

The goals of therapy in HCM have been symptom palliation and the prevention of sudden cardiac death. Although many therapies that improve symptoms by reducing LV gradient and improving diastolic performance have been developed, no reduction in sudden death has been demonstrated with their use. For this reason, it remains controversial whether asymptomatic patients should receive any therapy.

Three classes of cardiovascular medications have been shown to relieve symptoms of HCM. Beta blockers such as propranolol (Inderal), metoprolol (Lopressor, Toprol XL), and atenolol (Tenormin) interrupt catecholamine effects on the myocardium and result in lowering of the inotropic state and slowing of the heart rate (resulting in increased diastolic filling time and a larger end-diastolic LV dimension). Calcium channel blockers such as verapamil (Calan, Isoptin, Covera-HS) and diltiazem (Cardizem, Tiazac) inhibit the influx of calcium ions into the cardiac

TABLE 1. **Treatment of Hypertrophic Cardiomyopathy**

Medical
Beta blockers (atenolol, propranolol, metoprolol)
Calcium channel blockers (verapamil, diltiazem)
Disopyramide
Diuretics (for congestive symptoms)
Anticoagulation (for atrial fibrillation)
Antiarrhythmics (amiodarone, disopyramide)

Percutaneous
ETOH ablation via first septal perforator
DDD pacemaker
AICD

Surgical
Myotomy
Myomectomy
Mitral valve replacement

Abbreviations: AICD = automatic implantable cardioverter-defibrillator; DDD = dual chamber pacing, sensing, and inhibition; ETOH = ethanol.

myocytes, smooth muscle cells of the coronary and systemic arteries, and into the cells of the cardiac conduction system. Verapamil and diltiazem are the preferred agents in this class, because they tend to have a more selective effect on the myocardium and less vasodilatory activity than do other calcium channel blockers. Anecdotal evidence has been used to designate calcium channel blockers as the drugs of choice for the treatment of diastolic dysfunction. Head-to-head comparisons with other drug classes, however, have failed to show any significant advantage. Despite its ability to slow conduction in the atrioventricular (AV) node, studies of verapamil have not shown it to be effective in preventing atrial or ventricular arrhythmias. Disopyramide (Norpace), a class IA antiarrhythmic agent with negative inotropic effects, has also been used with success in HCM. Unlike the other agents mentioned earlier, it does not have an antichronotropic effect. Because of clinical data from other facets of cardiology supporting a possible role of beta blockers in the prevention of sudden death, these agents have remained our first-line medications.

Diuretics in HCM are reserved for patients with congestive symptoms and should be used carefully, particularly in patients with documented obstructive physiology. Anticoagulation is not routinely recommended but should be used if atrial fibrillation occurs.

Although first described in the mid-1970s, dual chamber pacing for HCM has undergone significant reevaluation since the mid-1990s. The paradoxical septal motion created by pacing has been shown to reduce the resting outflow gradient and improve symptoms. It seems unlikely, however, that this action is solely responsible for the purported benefits. For pacing to be successful, complete ventricular capture must occur. This occurs readily in patients with a normal PR interval (120 to 180 milliseconds). However, when the PR interval is shorter, the time available for effective left atrial mechanical function is inadequate, and diastolic dysfunction can occur. These patients require either AV nodal-blocking agents (calcium channel blockers or beta blockers) or AV nodal ablation to lengthen the PR interval. Randomized crossover data have shown that not all patients achieve a favorable benefit from pacing and that further trials are necessary to determine which subgroups with HCM are most likely to benefit.

Percutaneous catheter-based septal reduction therapy has been proposed to reduce outflow gradient in HCM. The procedure involves injecting absolute alcohol into the first septal artery of patients in whom transient occlusion of the artery has been shown to reduce the intraventricular gradient. Preliminary results have shown successful reductions in outflow gradient and symptomatic improvement. Unfortunately, complete heart block can occur, necessitating permanent cardiac pacing. Patients also require hospitalization after the procedure, for postinfarction observation.

If a significant resting outflow tract gradient exists, three types of surgical procedures can be performed to reduce the gradient: myotomy, the creation of a slit in the septum; myectomy, the creation of two slits in the septum and removal of the myocardium between them; and mitral valve replacement. Overall the rate of mortality from these procedures has dropped to well below 3%. Although the gradient is abolished in these patients, up to 10% have recurrent or persistent symptoms, because these procedures do little to relieve diastolic dysfunction or ischemia.

Sudden death continues to be the greatest challenge in managing patients with HCM, and none of the interventions just mentioned have proved to reduce its occurrence. For patients with sudden death, documented sustained ventricular tachycardia (VT), or inducible VT on electrophysiologic study, the practice has been to implant a cardiac defibrillator. Randomized data are not available for this population of patients, and it seems unlikely that this approach is cost effective. Amiodarone has been shown to prevent atrial and ventricular arrhythmias in these patients, but its effect on mortality in HCM is as yet unknown.

APLASTIC ANEMIA

method of
MANJUSHA KUMAR, M.D., and
BLANCHE P. ALTER, M.D.
University of Texas Medical Branch at Galveston
Galveston, Texas

Aplastic anemia (AA) is characterized by peripheral blood pancytopenia and reduced or absent production of blood cells in the marrow. The disorder is rare and may be acquired (2 to 6 per million per year) or inherited, as in Fanconi's anemia (>1000 cases reported, incidence unknown) (Table 1). The clinical severity of acquired AA is important for prognosis and treatment decisions. In severe aplastic anemia (SAA), the patient has at least two of the following findings: a granulocyte count lower than 500 per mm³, a platelet count lower than 20,000 per mm³, and a corrected reticulocyte count of less than 1% (40,000 per

mm³), in addition to less than 25% cellularity on the bone marrow biopsy or moderate hypocellularity in which less than 30% cells are hematopoietic. Very severe aplastic anemia (VSAA) patients have absolute granulocyte counts of less than 200 per mm³.

Mild or moderate AA, also called *hypoplastic anemia,* has a variable and arbitrary definition in the literature and may be defined according to one of the following:

1. AA that does not meet criteria for severe disease.
2. Bone marrow hypocellularity with all of the following: an absolute neutrophil count (ANC) lower than 2500 per mm³, a platelet count lower than 120,000 per mm³, and a hematocrit of less than 38%.
3. At least 2 of the following: an ANC lower than 1500 per mm³, a platelet count lower than 40,000 per mm³, and an absolute reticulocyte count lower than 40,000 per mm³.

Many cases of acquired AA appear to result from immune-mediated destruction of marrow cells. A variety of factors, such as drugs, viruses, pregnancy, thymomas and graft versus host disease (GVHD), can activate the immune system, leading to marrow aplasia. Another pathogenetic mechanism of AA is direct marrow stem cell damage from agents such as chemotherapeutic drugs, radiation therapy, and benzene. In most cases, however, no associated factor can be identified, and the patient is said to have *idiopathic aplastic anemia.*

TABLE 1. A Classification of Aplastic Anemia

Acquired Aplastic Anemia	Inherited Aplastic Anemia
Secondary Aplastic Anemia	Fanconi's anemia
Radiation	Dyskeratosis congenita
Drugs and chemicals	Shwachman-Diamond
Regular effects: cytotoxic	syndrome
agents, benzene	Reticular dysgenesis
Idiosyncratic reactions	Amegakaryocytic
Chloramphenicol	thrombocytopenia
Nonsteroidal anti-	Familial aplastic anemias
inflammatory drugs	Preleukemia (e.g.,
Antiepileptics, gold	monosomy 7)
Other drugs and	Nonhematologic syndromes
chemicals	(Down's, Dubovitz's,
Viruses	Seckel's)
Epstein-Barr virus (infectious	
mononucleosis)	
Non-C (non-A, non-B) hepatitis	
Human immunodeficiency	
virus (acquired	
immunodeficiency syndrome)	
Immune diseases	
Eosinophilic fasciitis	
Hypoimmunoglobulinemia	
Thymoma and thymic	
carcinoma	
Graft-versus-host disease	
Paroxysmal nocturnal	
hemoglobinuria	
Pregnancy	
Idiopathic Aplastic Anemia	

From Young NS, Alter BP: Aplastic Anemia: Acquired and inherited. Philadelphia, W.B. Saunders Co., 1994, p 9.

CLINICAL AND LABORATORY FEATURES

The clinical manifestation is related to the severity of the underlying pancytopenia. Hemorrhagic symptoms from thrombocytopenia are usually the first manifestations of the disease. Fever, mouth sores, and fulminant sepsis can result from severe neutropenia. Severe anemia can lead to fatigue, palpitations, and shortness of breath, but often occurs late in the course of the disease because the life span of the erythrocyte (120 days) far exceeds those of platelets (10 days) and granulocytes (7 hours).

Laboratory findings are nonspecific; the peripheral smear reveals a paucity of platelets and leukocytes but normal red blood cell morphology. The anemia may be macrocytic or normocytic. The absolute reticulocyte count is decreased. Increases in fetal hemoglobin and red blood cell i antigen along with macrocytosis are manifestations of the fetal-like erythropoiesis seen in stress hematopoiesis and may be seen in long-standing aplasia. Results of the Ham or sucrose lysis test may be positive, as paroxysmal nocturnal hematuria may be associated with AA. Flow cytometric analysis of red and white blood cells for the presence of cell surface markers CD55 and CD59 (deficient glycophosphoinositol-linked protein expression) is a more sensitive and objective method for investigation of paroxysmal nocturnal hemoglobinuria in patients with AA. Peripheral blood chromosomes are normal, in contrast to increased breakage with clastogenic agents in patients with Fanconi's anemia. Vitamin B$_{12}$ and folate levels are normal.

Serum transaminase levels may be high in patients with hepatitis, and viral serologic studies for hepatitis A, B, and C viruses, Epstein-Barr virus, cytomegalovirus (CMV), parvovirus, and human immunodeficiency virus (HIV) may be helpful. Bone marrow aspiration and biopsy are useful for exclusion of other causes of pancytopenia (metastatic tumors, leukemia, granulomatous disease). The marrow cellularity is poor (<25%) with empty spicules, fat, reticulum cells, plasma cells, and mast cells. Sometimes a lymphocytic infiltration of the marrow is observed and correlates with poor prognosis if more than 70% of marrow cells are lymphocytes. Bone marrow cytogenetic findings are usually normal, thus excluding myelodysplastic syndrome.

THERAPY

Treatment of AA involves (1) specific therapy aimed at curing the disease and (2) ongoing supportive care to prevent complications of pancytopenia and its treatment. The choice of therapy depends on the severity of the disease and the age of the patient (Figure 1). Spontaneous recovery can also occur and has been reported anecdotally.

Bone Marrow Transplantation

In patients less than 40 years of age with newly diagnosed SAA, an urgent HLA typing of the patient's and first-degree relatives' lymphocytes should be instituted. There is a 25 to 30% probability of finding a fully compatible family member donor. Allo-

geneic bone marrow transplantation (BMT) from a fully HLA-matched related donor offers the best chance of cure of this disease (60 to 70% survival rates). Conditioning regimens for BMT currently involve non–radiation-based therapy: cyclophosphamide (Cytoxan), 50 mg per kg per day on days −5, −4, −3 and −2, in combination with antithymocyte globulin (Atgam), 30 mg per kg per day on days −5, −4, and −3 given 12 hours after the infusion of Cytoxan on each of these days. In patients younger than 20 years, survival rates higher than 90% are being achieved with current supportive care techniques and better GVHD prophylaxis in allogeneic BMT for SAA.

In the absence of a fully compatible related donor, other transplantation possibilities are blood from an unrelated matched donor, blood from a partially mismatched related donor, and matched or partially mismatched, related or unrelated umbilical cord blood. Each of these involves a higher risk of graft rejection, severe GVHD, and increased risks of morbidity and mortality. Results with unrelated donor transplants have been discouraging for these reasons, and survival rates are less than 30% in most series. Thus at this time it does not appear justified to offer a patient these alternative modalities of BMT as a treatment of first choice. Older patients (older than 40 years) appear to suffer significant toxic effects and GVHD from allogeneic BMT even with a sibling matched transplant; survival rates are 40 to 45%. Other treatments such as immunosuppression therefore offer

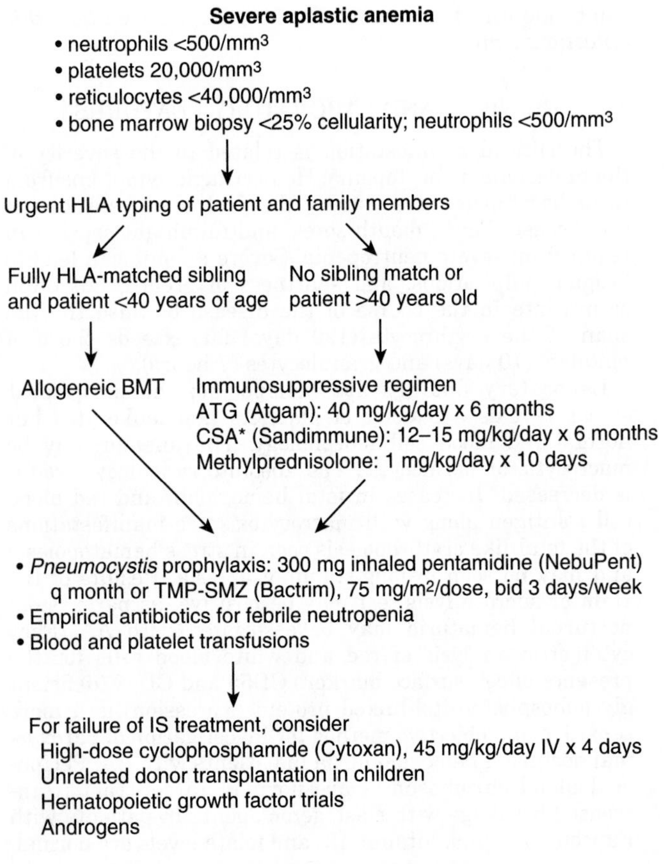

Severe aplastic anemia
- neutrophils <500/mm³
- platelets 20,000/mm³
- reticulocytes <40,000/mm³
- bone marrow biopsy <25% cellularity; neutrophils <500/mm³

↓

Urgent HLA typing of patient and family members

↙   ↘

Fully HLA-matched sibling and patient <40 years of age   No sibling match or patient >40 years old

↓   ↓

Allogeneic BMT   Immunosuppressive regimen
ATG (Atgam): 40 mg/kg/day x 6 months
CSA* (Sandimmune): 12–15 mg/kg/day x 6 months
Methylprednisolone: 1 mg/kg/day x 10 days

↘   ↙

- *Pneumocystis* prophylaxis: 300 mg inhaled pentamidine (NebuPent)
  q month or TMP-SMZ (Bactrim), 75 mg/m²/dose, bid 3 days/week
- Empirical antibiotics for febrile neutropenia
- Blood and platelet transfusions

↓

For failure of IS treatment, consider
High-dose cyclophosphamide (Cytoxan), 45 mg/kg/day IV x 4 days
Unrelated donor transplantation in children
Hematopoietic growth factor trials
Androgens

Figure 1. Approach to the management of aplastic anemia. *Abbreviations:* ATG = antithymocyte globulin; CSA = cyclosporine; IS = immunosuppressive. *Not FDA approved for this indication.

them a better chance of remission with significantly lower rates of morbidity and mortality.

Immunosuppressive Therapy

Several immunosuppressive regimens have achieved varying success in the treatment of AA, which suggests that this may be an immune-mediated disease. The most potent immunosuppressive regimen appears to be a combination of antithymocyte globulin (ATG) or antilymphocyte globulin (ALG) with cyclosporine* (Sandimmune) and methylprednisolone. This offers a 70% chance of response/remission and should be offered as first-line therapy to patients without a sibling matched donor for BMT and to those older than 40 years with SAA. We treat as per the National Institutes of Health (NIH) guidelines: ATG at 40 mg per kg per day† for 4 days and cyclosporine at 12 mg per kg per day in adults and 15 mg per kg per day in children, orally for 6 months. The dose of cyclosporine is adjusted to maintain serum levels of 200 to 400 ng per mL by radioimmunoassay. Subsequently cyclosporine is tapered slowly and discontinued over 5 months. Methylprednisolone, 1 mg per kg per day, is given for 10 days and tapered over 2 weeks. A test dose of 10 microliters of undiluted ATG (50 mg per mL) is given subcutaneously as a sensitivity test. Immunosuppressive treatment may ameliorate the disease and help the patient become transfusion independent and free of recurrent neutropenic infections. Rarely, however, is there a complete response with normalization of peripheral blood counts and bone marrow. There is a significant risk of development of clonal disease such as paroxysmal nocturnal hemoglobinuria, myelodysplastic syndrome, or acute myeloid leukemia (probability of clonal evolution is calculated to be 50% at 10 years).

Side effects of this regimen include anaphylaxis, urticaria, fever, chills, thrombocytopenia, and serum sickness from ATG. Cyclosporine may cause renal dysfunction, hypomagnesemia, hypertension, and neurotoxicity.

Another immunosuppressive regimen that has been shown to be promising in a small pilot study is high-dose cyclophosphamide. This is a potent immunosuppressive and cytotoxic drug and is used as conditioning preparation for BMT. Cyclophosphamide at 45 mg per kg per day for 4 days induced remission in 7 of 10 patients with SAA with a median follow up of more than 10 years. The beneficial effect of cyclophosphamide may be by potent immunosuppression and hence autologous recovery. Although these results appear promising, larger studies are needed to define the exact role and hierarchy of cyclophosphamide in the treatment of AA.

Transfusion Support

Patients with AA need frequent transfusions of blood and platelets during treatment whether ther-

apy is by BMT or immunosuppression. In addition, patients in whom all treatment modalities have failed need long-term transfusion support. Some key points in transfusing these patients are as follows:

- No family member should be used as a source of blood products if the patient with AA is a potential BMT candidate. This is to decrease the risk of alloimmunizations from minor histocompatibility antigens, which may impair the transplantation outcome (increased risk of rejection).
- To further decrease the risk of alloimmunization and possible graft rejection in transplantation candidates, these patients should undergo transfusion as little as possible. General guidelines are to transfuse for hemoglobin of less than 7 grams per dL or if the patient is symptomatic with tachycardia, lethargy, and subjective symptoms at higher hemoglobin values. Platelets should be given prophylactically for levels lower than 10,000 per mm³ in stable, nonfebrile patients.
- All blood products should be leukocyte-poor, irradiated, and CMV negative if the patient is CMV negative and is a potential transplantation candidate.
- Single donor platelets should be used as much as possible to decrease the exposure to multiple donors and decrease the risk of alloimmunization.

Infection Support

Patients receiving immunosuppressive regimens and undergoing BMT should receive *Pneumocystis carinii* prophylaxis, preferably with a nonmyelosuppressive agent such as pentamidine (NebuPent), 300 mg by inhalation once a month. In younger patients, trimethoprim-sulfamethoxazole (Bactrim, Septra) is used for prophylaxis (75 mg per m² per dose of trimethoprim, twice a day, 3 consecutive days a week). There is no role for other antibiotic prophylaxis in these neutropenic patients during the baseline state. With a febrile neutropenic episode (granulocyte count < 500 per mL), empirical broad-spectrum antibiotics should be started until infection is ruled out and the patient is afebrile. Several antibiotics have been used as either monotherapy or combination therapy for the initial fever. Important bacteria to be covered are the endogenous flora of the gastrointestinal tract such as *Escherichia coli, Pseudomonas* species, *Klebsiella* species, and anaerobic organisms. Both ceftazidime (Fortaz), a third-generation cephalosporin, and imipenem will cover any life-threatening gram-negative bacilli, especially *Pseudomonas,* and have been used as monotherapy. If a line infection is suspected, vancomycin (Vancocin) should be started empirically to cover any present coagulase-negative staphylococci. Anaerobic coverage with clindamycin (Cleocin) may need to be initiated if there are mouth sores or a perianal abscess. Depending on the type of organism in the blood culture, if any, the antibiotic therapy and duration may be changed accordingly. In patients who have a prolonged fever (>1 week) and are unresponsive to broad-spectrum antibiotics (covering

*Not FDA approved for this indication.
†Exceeds dosage recommmended by the manufacturer.

for gram-positive and gram-negative bacteria), especially if they have central lines, have mucocutaneous breaks, or have received prior antibiotics, empirical systemic antifungal therapy should be started with amphotericin B (Fungizone) while fungal cultures are examined.

Hematologic Growth Factors

Granulocyte colony-stimulating factor (G-CSF) (Neupogen) is commonly used in subcutaneous doses of 5 to 10 μg per kg per day in patients with AA during a febrile neutropenic episode, especially if they are very sick. It is also used to shorten the period of neutropenia in patients who have undergone transplantation. However, the sole use of growth factors as front-line therapy for treatment of newly diagnosed SAA offers no definite long-term benefit to the patient and may delay curative therapy. Because there is no established alternative treatment for patients who are not candidates for BMT and are primarily nonresponsive to ATG plus cyclosporine, growth factors have been used in phase I/II trials alone, in combination with immunosuppressive therapy, or as a combination of hematopoietic growth factors. There are reports of treatment of refractory AA with G-CSF, G-CSF plus immunosuppressive agents, granulocyte-macrophage colony-stimulating factor (GM-CSF), stem cell factor,* interleukin-3 (IL-3),* interleukin-1,† erythropoietin plus G-CSF, and erythropoietin alone. Responses are transient, monolineage, and generally limited to patients with nonsevere AA.

For patients with moderate AA who are transfusion independent, the "watch and wait" policy holds. Most patients with moderate AA require no therapy or minimal short-term transfusion support. In some patients in whom disease advances to SAA, the treatment is as detailed earlier for SAA.

Miscellaneous Treatments

Androgens no longer have a primary role in the management of AA unless all of the therapies discussed earlier are unavailable (as in several underdeveloped countries) or unsuccessful. Androgens may increase erythropoietin production, stimulate erythroid progenitor cells, and increase hemoglobin levels. The usual oral androgen is oxymetholone (Anadrol-50), 2 to 5 mg per kg per day, or nandrolone decanoate* (Deca-Durabolin), 5 mg per kg per week intramuscularly. Cholestatic jaundice and hepatomegaly can result, along with some masculinizing effects. Hepatic tumors are a serious risk, and liver function tests and abdominal ultrasonography should be performed for monitoring.

Splenectomy is currently done to facilitate supportive care when there is evidence of hypersplenism impacting on platelet and red blood cell transfusions.

In the past it had been used as a treatment modality for AA with occasional responses, but the risk of surgery, bleeding, and infection is difficult to justify.

In anecdotal reports, *plasmapheresis* and *lymphocytapheresis* ameliorated the disease, perhaps by removing immunoglobulins or soluble inhibitory factors and circulating lymphocytes.

Pooled human *immunoglobulin** at 0.4 mg per kg for 4 days every 3 weeks has rarely produced transient remission in this disease.

Antiviral treatment with acyclovir may result in temporary responses, perhaps because of the association of AA with viral infections (see Table 1). However, viral infection has not been documented in anecdotal reports of patients with AA who responded to acyclovir.

Lithium, a drug used in manic-depressive patients, can cause neutrophilia. There are rare reports of remissions in patients with AA.

Phytohemagglutinin, a plant lectin, was given intravenously in 6 patients with AA and ameliorated symptoms.

FANCONI'S ANEMIA

Fanconi's anemia (FA) is one of the important inherited causes of aplastic anemia and pancytopenia primarily but not exclusively in the pediatric age group. It is an autosomal recessive disease with at least eight complementation groups. Three of the FA genes have been cloned (FAC, FAA, and FAG), and a fourth (FAD) has been mapped but not yet cloned.

Clinical and Laboratory Features

FA was initially identified as an association between AA and a specific constellation of birth defects: hyperpigmentation and/or café au lait spots, short stature, and anomalies of the thumb and radius in more than half of affected patients. Other, less common physical stigmata are male hypogonadism, microcephaly, ocular and renal abnormalities, developmental delay, low birth weight, defects of the ear and lower limbs, and occasionally cardiopulmonary defects. However, up to one third of patients may not have birth defects, and hence it is important to rule out Fanconi's anemia in the work-up of all patients with AA.

Useful radiologic studies include skeletal radiographs, which may identify both obvious and occult abnormalities, and renal ultrasonography, to identify structural kidney defects.

The hematologic findings in FA are quite nonspecific; they begin to manifest at an average age of 8 to 9 years, but time of onset ranges from birth to the sixth decade. Patients commonly come to medical attention with thrombocytopenia or macrocytic anemia, which then advances to pancytopenia. Bone marrow appearances vary but generally are hypocellular with reduced or absent megakaryocytes. At

---

*Investigational drug in the United States.
†Not FDA approved for this indication.

---

*Not FDA approved for this indication.

least 10% of patients with FA develop leukemia (usually myeloid), and acute myeloid leukemia may be the first presentation in some FA patients. Myelodysplastic syndrome is also seen frequently.

The diagnostic laboratory test entails the use of metaphase preparations of phytohemagglutin-stimulated cultured peripheral blood lymphocytes. A high proportion of cells from FA patients have breaks, gaps, rearrangements, exchanges, and endo-reduplications. This breakage is dramatically increased in comparison to normal samples when clastogenic agents such as diepoxybutane or mitomycin C are added.

Therapy

Approximately 1000 patients with FA have been described in the literature. Because of improvements in supportive care in the 1990s, the median length of survival of patients with FA is projected to be more than 30 years. The major immediate causes of death are complications of pancytopenia: bleeding, fulminant sepsis, and, less frequently, malignancy (acute myeloid leukemia, liver tumors, squamous cell carcinomas). The same principles of transfusion support and infection control apply to these patients as for those with idiopathic AA. Hematopoietic growth factors (G-CSF, GM-CSF, IL-3) have shown some response in these patients in small pilot studies, but they are not yet standards of care in FA.

Androgens. About 50% of patients respond to androgen therapy, and we usually begin administering androgens when the platelet count is consistently below 30,000 per mm^3 and/or the hemoglobin is less than 7 grams per dL. Responses usually begin with reticulocytosis, with a rise in hemoglobin within 1 to 2 months. White blood cell counts increase next, although often inadequately; the platelet count rise is usually incomplete and, at androgren dosages of 2 to 5 mg per kg per day, may take 6 to 12 months to reach its maximum. Oxymetholone is most frequently used. Prednisone has been included at 5 to 10 mg every other day to possibly enhance the effect of androgens on the marrow, to counteract the growth acceleration of androgens, and to perhaps increase vascular stability.

Bone Marrow Transplantation. BMT currently offers the only possibility for cure of aplastic anemia in FA. Patients wth FA are very sensitive to alkylating agents and radiation therapy because of their DNA instability. Thus the standard cyclophosphamide and total body irradiation conditioning regimen has to be modified in FA patients, usually reduced to 20 mg per kg of cyclophosphamide over 4 days plus 5 Gy of thoracoabdominal irradiation. Survival rates are higher than 70% with a matched sibling donor transplant. It is mandatory to test the donor sibling for FA because this is an autosomal recessive disorder and not all patients may exhibit phenotypic features. Secondary cancers may develop in patients with FA because of their inherent risk and because of potentiation of the risk by immunosuppression for transplantation. For patients without a fully matched related donor, alternative donor transplants offer poor results. FA is now being diagnosed in adults with typical solid tumors, infertility, or late-onset aplastic anemia and should be considered in the evaluation of anyone with bone marrow failure at any age.

DYSKERATOSIS CONGENITA

Dyskeratosis congenita is a rare, inherited form of ectodermal dysplasia, characterized by reticulate skin pigmentation, mucosal leukoplakia, and nail dystrophy. Aplastic anemia occurs in at least 50% of patients with dyskeratosis congenita, usually during their teens, and cancer (predominantly squamous cell carcinoma) is seen in 10% of the patients during their twenties and thirties. The overall predicted median length of survival for patients with dyskeratosis congenita is 32 years, and death occurs from infection or malignancy. Treatment for patients with dyskeratosis congenita is at present unsatisfactory. For treatment of bone marrow failure, a combination of androgens and steroids may be tried. Transient responses to hematopoietic growth factors have been reported (erythropoietin, G-CSF, GM-CSF). Allogeneic sibling BMT has led to some engraftment, but rates of long-term survival have been poor. Compatible sibling donor BMT is still an experimental form of treatment for patients with dyskeratosis congenita, in contrast to patients with FA.

SHWACHMAN-DIAMOND SYNDROME

The Shwachman-Diamond syndrome consists of exocrine pancreatic insufficiency and neutropenia. Pancreatic insufficiency manifests in early infancy as steatorrhea and failure to thrive. Neutropenia occurs in early childhood, and recurrent skin infections and pneumonias may be present. Many patients develop anemia (15%), thrombocytopenia (7%), or both (20%). Physical examination reveals signs of malnutrition and short stature (50%), mental retardation (15%), and, in rare cases, dysmorphic facies, retinitis pigmentosa, syndactyly, and disordered skin pigmentation. Bone marrow cellularity is decreased in half the patients, the others showing an arrest of myeloid maturation. Chromosomes are normal, and there is no increased breakage after clastogenic stress. The malabsorption responds to treatment with oral pancreatic enzymes. Supportive care is given during infections (antibiotics, G-CSF, transfusions as needed). The projected median length of survival is 35 years for all patients with Shwachman-Diamond syndrome, and death is caused by hemorrhage or infection. There appears to be a malignant propensity in these patients, and acute leukemia has been reported. BMT has produced less than 50% survival in a small number of patients and is not strongly recommended.

SUMMARY

Severe aplastic anemia is more commonly acquired and idiopathic. The treatment of choice is matched related donor BMT, especially in children and young adults; survival rates exceed 90%. Immunosuppressive therapy offers a more than 70% overall remission rate in patients without a related matched donor and in older patients. High-dose cyclophosphamide may have potential as an immunosuppressive treatment, but larger trials are needed. Fanconi's anemia, dyskeratosis congenita, and Shwachman-Diamond syndrome are some of the inherited forms of aplastic anemia. Fanconi's anemia, by far the most common inherited AA, must be ruled out in all newly diagnosed cases of AA by chromosomal breakage studies of peripheral blood lymphocytes. There is a significant later risk of development of clonal disease such as acute myeloid leukemia, paroxysmal nocturnal hemoglobinuria, and myelodysplastic syndrome in idiopathic as well as inherited forms of AA. Solid tumors such as squamous cell carcinoma and liver tumors are also being seen in adults with FA. Patients with dyskeratosis congenita and Shwachman-Diamond syndrome moreover have a propensity for developing malignancies. Thus these inherited conditions (especially FA) must be kept in mind when young adults with refractory anemias or squamous cell carcinomas are evaluated.

IRON DEFICIENCY

method of
KENNETH R. BRIDGES, M.D.
Brigham and Women's Hospital
Boston, Massachusetts

Iron deficiency is a leading cause of anemia. In adults, the condition results almost exclusively from blood loss. Iron deficiency occasionally occurs in children because iron absorption fails to keep pace with the high demand created by neonatal and adolescent growth spurts. Body iron stores for women normally vary between 1 and 2 grams, whereas those of men average 3 to 4 grams. The liver is the source of most stored iron. Depletion of iron stores precedes a failure to produce iron-containing proteins—of most importance, hemoglobin. The two important stages of iron deficiency are thus (1) depletion of iron stores without anemia and (2) depletion of iron stores with anemia.

ETIOLOGY OF IRON DEFICIENCY

Treatment of iron deficiency cannot be efficiently undertaken until the cause of the iron deficit is discovered. Blood loss into the gastrointestinal tract is by far the most common cause of iron deficiency. A cautious physician should be aware of a couple of other possibilities, however.

Abnormal Iron Uptake from the Alimentary Tract

Impaired iron absorption from the gastrointestinal tract rarely causes iron deficiency. One etiology of increasing importance to internists is a high gastric pH. A high gastric pH reduces the solubility of inorganic iron, impeding its absorption. Surgical interventions, such as vagotomy or hemigastrectomy for peptic ulcer disease, were formerly the major causes of impaired gastric acidification. Iron deficiency developed as a secondary event. Today, the histamine H_2 blockers (such as cimetidine [Tagamet]) and the more recently introduced acid pump inhibitors (e.g., omeprazole [Prilosec]), used to treat peptic ulcer disease and acid reflux, are the most common causes of defective iron absorption. Although these medications infrequently produce iron deficiency, their widespread use means that most internists will encounter the problem at some time.

Peptic ulcer disease can itself produce iron deficiency as a result of bleeding into the gastrointestinal tract (described later). The use of agents that block gastric acidification and iron absorption by people whose iron stores are low or absent is an efficient means of producing iron deficiency anemia.

Some disorders disrupt the integrity of the enteric mucosa, thereby hampering iron absorption. Inflammatory bowel disease, such as Crohn's disease, can cause iron deficiency anemia by this mechanism. The diagnosis of Crohn's disease as the cause of iron deficiency is a straightforward exercise, however.

Celiac disease (nontropical sprue) can also impair iron absorption. Unlike Crohn's disease, celiac disease often disrupts iron absorption while manifesting only subtle clinical signs. Some patients with mild celiac disease experience minor symptoms such as bloating after eating a meal rich in gluten, such as bran cereal. Nonetheless, the condition sometimes substantially impairs iron absorption. Iron deficiency anemia occurs often when a concurrent predisposing condition exists, such as chronic use of aspirin or nonsteroidal anti-inflammatory agents. Some patients with deranged iron absorption lack gross or even histologic changes in the structure of the bowel mucosa. A gluten-free diet improves bowel function in many such patients, with secondary correction of the anemia.

Blood Loss

The gastrointestinal tract is both the site of iron uptake and the most common location of blood loss. This organ is unrivaled as a potential setting for occult bleeding. In adults, the chief cause is a gastrointestinal malignancy. A work-up of the gastrointestinal tract for malignancy is mandatory in men with iron deficiency anemia. Peptic ulcer disease, hiatal hernia, or other benign lesions are the most common findings. However, a malignancy must be searched for.

The problem is complicated in women, in whom menstruation is a physiologic source of blood loss. Iron deficiency anemia occurs in about 2% of premenopausal women solely as a result of menstruation. Iron stores are depleted in the absence of anemia in about 10% of premenopausal women. The key dilemma is whether to pursue the issue of gastrointestinal blood loss (with malignancy as the key target), despite menstruation as the probable cause.

No clear-cut answer to this quandary exists. Each situation must be considered carefully on it own merit. For example, in a 36-year-old mother of three children with a history of menorrhagia, gynecologic and obstetric blood loss alone are sufficient to explain iron deficiency anemia. Although gastrointestinal bleeding from a carcinoma could also contribute to the anemia, the chance of this is extremely small. Should stool guaiac cards over several days prove negative, iron replacement without further work-up is reasonable. In contrast, a 60-year-old postmenopausal woman with new-onset iron deficiency should be evaluated for gastrointestinal sources of iron loss because physiologic blood loss does not occur at this age.

DIAGNOSIS OF IRON DEFICIENCY

Laboratory evaluation is essential for the diagnosis of iron deficiency. Physical signs, such as koilonychia, glossitis, and angular stomatitis, are rare. These abnormalities manifest most commonly with severe, long-standing iron deficiency, which rarely occurs in industrialized nations. The most common symptom is easy fatigue caused by the anemia that accompanies advanced iron deficiency. Even fatigue is often absent in patients with moderately severe iron deficiency anemia. The anemia develops slowly, and many people subconsciously adapt their activity and expectations to fit their diminished stamina. Classical manifestations, such as geophagia, are rare.

The three key laboratory tests in the analysis of iron deficiency are the plasma ferritin, plasma iron, and the total iron binding capacity (TIBC). In uncomplicated cases, a low level of plasma ferritin is diagnostic of iron deficiency. The plasma iron level and TIBC are used together to determine the transferrin saturation (the ratio of the plasma iron to the TIBC.) With uncomplicated iron deficiency, the transferrin saturation is low.

Often, however, the diagnosis of iron deficiency must be made in the setting of potentially confounding conditions. The most common situation that presents a diagnostic dilemma is chronic inflammation. Chronic rheumatoid arthritis, for instance, frequently produces a moderately severe normochromic, normocytic anemia. In addition, this process raises the plasma ferritin level, which can mask coexistent iron deficiency. Chronic inflammation depresses both the plasma iron and the TIBC, complicating the interpretation of these parameters with regard to iron deficiency.

A common scenario features a patient with rheumatoid arthritis who takes nonsteroidal anti-inflammatory agents for pain control. These agents increase the likelihood of gastrointestinal bleeding as a result of irritation of the stomach lining and inhibition of platelet function. A review of the full panel of laboratory data, including a complete blood cell count (CBC), evaluation of the peripheral smear, and assay of plasma ferritin and transferrin saturation can sometimes provide a sense of whether iron deficiency, in addition to the chronic inflammation, plays a role in the anemia. If this approach fails, a definitive diagnosis of iron deficiency can be made only by bone marrow biopsy, with staining for iron.

Substantial iron deficiency produces a hypochromic, microcytic anemia. The most important alternate condition to rule out is thalassemia trait, also called thalassemia minor. A little-used datum that accompanies every electronic counter blood analysis called the red cell distribution width (RDW) can be extremely helpful in distinguishing between iron deficiency anemia and thalassemia trait. The RDW is normal in thalassemia trait (reflecting the uniformly small size of the red blood cells) but often is elevated in iron deficiency anemia, in which variation in red blood cell size is common.

Review of the blood smear is also helpful in distinguishing between these two conditions. Target cells are common in the smear of patients with thalassemia trait but are infrequent with iron deficiency. A further consideration in the use of the RDW and peripheral smear is that they add

nothing to the cost of the work-up. If the issue is still in doubt, hemoglobin electrophoresis usually settles the question. The hemoglobin A$_2$ (and often the hemoglobin F) level is elevated in patients with thalassemia trait.

TREATMENT OF IRON DEFICIENCY

Oral Supplementation

Although physicians commonly recommend ferrous sulfate to treat iron deficiency, frequent problems with the drug, including gastrointestinal discomfort, bloating, and other distress, make it unacceptable to many patients. Ferrous gluconate, which is approximately equivalent in cost, produces fewer problems and is preferable as the initial treatment of iron deficiency. Each 300-mg ferrous gluconate tablet contains 50 mg of elemental iron. Ascorbic acid substantially enhances iron absorption. Preparations that combine iron salts and ascorbic acid are significantly more expensive than separate tablets for each, however. A reasonable approach to oral iron supplementation is one ferrous gluconate tablet and one 250-mg ascorbic acid tablet twice a day.

Iron is best absorbed when taken between meals because some food components (for example, phytates in wheat products) complex with iron in the gastrointestinal tract and prevent its uptake. Abdominal distress is less common when iron supplements are taken with meals, however. Therefore, the pattern of replacement must be balanced between patient comfort and drug efficacy. Noncompliance with oral iron is one of the most common causes of therapeutic failure with oral iron supplementation (Table 1). Even with faithful use of oral iron, adequate replacement of body stores in patients with moderate iron deficiency anemia requires several months. With ongoing blood loss, replacing stores by means of oral iron supplements becomes an Olympian task.

Polysaccharide-iron complex (Niferex), a replacement form of iron that differs from the iron salts, is now available. The polar oxygen groups in the polysaccharide form coordination complexes with the iron atoms. The well-hydrated microspheres of polysaccharide-iron complex remain in solution over a

TABLE 1. **Causes of a Poor Response to Oral Iron**

Noncompliance
Ongoing blood loss
Insufficient duration of therapy
High gastric pH
   Antacids
   Histamine H$_2$ blockers (e.g., cimetidine [Tagamet])
   Gastric acid pump inhibitors (e.g., omeprazole [Prilosec])
Inhibitors of iron absorption/utilization
   Lead
   Iron-binding substances in food (such as phytates)
   Chronic inflammation
   Neoplasia
Incorrect diagnosis
   Thalassemia
   Sideroblastic anemia

wide pH range, which is a possible advantage for absorption. This has not been proven, however. Many patients tolerate this form of iron better than iron salts, even though the 150 mg of elemental iron per tablet is substantially greater than that provided by iron salts (50 to 70 mg per tablet).

Parenteral Iron Replacement

Parenteral iron is available in the United States only as iron dextran (InFeD). This medication is indicated when (1) oral iron is poorly tolerated, (2) rapid replacement of iron stores is needed, or (3) gastrointestinal iron absorption is compromised. Intramuscular injection or intravenous infusion are the two potential routes of parenteral iron administration. Intramuscular injection of iron-dextran can be painful, and leakage into the subcutaneous tissue produces long-standing skin discoloration. A Z-track injection into the muscle minimizes the chance of subcutaneous leakage. Suboptimal muscle mass in patients with concomitant nutritional deficiency frequently further complicates this mode of replacement. Intravenous infusion of iron-dextran circumvents these problems altogether. With either route of administration, the physician should observe the patient for 30 minutes after the 10-mg test dose to make sure there is no anaphylactic reaction to the medication (such reactions are infrequent).

I routinely administer intravenous iron as a "total dose" replacement, replenishing all or most of the iron deficit at a single stroke. After the initial test dose, up to 3 grams of iron dextran are diluted into 500 mL of normal saline for the infusion. A rate-controlled pump regulates the infusion of the medication over the 4 to 5 hours required for administration. The physician need not be at the scene of the infusion but should be readily available. Table 2 outlines the procedure for total dose infusion of parenteral iron replacement.

This bulk infusion of iron dextran obviates the need for repeated clinic visits by patients to receive parenteral iron. One hundred milligrams of iron dextran is the maximal quantity of the drug that can be given either by a single intramuscular injection or by intravenous push infusion. A person with a 2-gram deficit would need 20 clinic visits to correct the iron deficiency. This level of compliance is uncommon. Also, the cost of this approach is much higher because of the number of outpatient visits required. The total dose infusion approach is not approved by the U.S. Food and Drug Administration. Nonetheless, the technique is used extensively in the United States and abroad to replenish iron stores of patients with substantial iron deficiency.

About 10 to 15% of patients experience transient mild to moderate arthralgias or myalgias the day after intramuscular or intravenous administration of iron dextran. Acetaminophen usually relieves the discomfort effectively. Iron dextran can be a particular problem for patients with rheumatoid arthritis who frequently have painful flare-ups of the disease

TABLE 2. **Total Dose Infusion of Iron Dextran**

- Nursing staff should obtain orders from physician and ensure her or his ability to be in attendance, to administer test dose, and to be available during the infusion of full dose

Dose Calculation
Amount of iron in milligrams =

$$\frac{0.3 \times \text{wt (lbs)} \times 100\,(14.8 - \text{Hb})}{14.8}$$

- Prepare full dose of iron dextran as ordered in a 10-mL syringe; use single-dose ampules
- Transfer 10 mg or iron dextran into a 1-mL syringe and inject into a 50-mL bag of 0.9 NS (or as ordered by physician)†
- Start an IV access and hang a bag of 500 mL of 0.9 NS, using an IMED cassette tubing, and regulate IV access to KVO
- With the physician present, hook the 50-mL bag with the 10-mg test dose of iron dextran into a side port of the main IV tubing set, and infuse the test dose over 10 to 15 minutes, carefully observing the patient's vital signs‡
- Monitor patient for 15 to 20 minutes for signs of adverse reaction
- Only after it is clear that the patient will not have an adverse reaction after the completion of the IV test dose should the remainder of the iron dextran be added to the 500-mL bag of 0.9 NS. Administer full dose of iron dextran via IMED pump over 2 to 6 hours as ordered by physician§

*Potential for anaphylactic reaction necessitates the administration of a test dose.
†The use of 5% dextrose as diluent is associated with an increased incidence of local pain and phlebitis. Between 250 and 1000 mL of 0.9 NS diluent is recommended for the full dose of iron dextran.
‡The physician must stay in attendance.
§The physician should be available during the infusion, but not necessarily at the patient's bedside. Administration rate should not exceed 250 mg/h.
Abbreviations: Hb = hemoglobin; IV = intravenous; KVO = keep vein open; LBW = lean body weight; NS = normal saline.

after receiving the drug. Administration of 60 mg of intravenous methylprednisolone before the iron dextran abrogates this problem, however.

In uncomplicated cases of iron deficiency, intravenous iron replacement improves symptoms in a few days. Peak reticulocytosis occurs after about 10 days, and complete correction of the anemia takes 3 to 4 weeks. The hematocrit rises sufficiently in a week or two to provide symptomatic relief for most patients.

AUTOIMMUNE HEMOLYTIC ANEMIA

method of
ZBIGNIEW M. SZCZEPIORKOWSKI, M.D., PH.D.
Massachusetts General Hospital and Harvard Medical School
Boston, Massachusetts

and

RONALD A. SACHER, M.D.
Georgetown Medical Center and Georgetown University Medical School
Washington, D.C.

All autoimmune hemolytic anemias (AIHAs) have two features in common: shortened red blood cell (RBC) survival in the circulation and detectable host antibodies di-

TABLE 1. **Classification and Basic Characteristics of Warm Antibody and Cold Antibody Autoimmune Hemolytic Anemias (AIHAs)**

	Warm Antibody Type	Cold Antibody Type	
		Cold Hemagglutinin Disease (CHD)	Paroxysmal Cold Hemoglobinuria
Percentage of AIHA (including drug-induced immune hemolytic anemia)	70–80% (60–70%)	20–30% (15–25%)	<1% Primary 2–4% Secondary
Incidence	1:50,000–80,000	1:100,000–200,000	1:600,000–800,000
Characteristics of involved antibody	Polyclonal, sometimes monoclonal	Monoclonal, polyclonal (secondary to postinfectious CHD)	Polyclonal
Class	IgG >> IgA, IgM	IgM >> IgG	IgG (biphasic hemolysin)
Antibody specificity	Rh, Kell, Kidd, phospholipids	I, i, Pr	P
DAT result			
IgG alone	40–50%		
IgG and C3	45–60%	10%	10%
C3 alone	0–15%	90%	90%
Negative	2–4%		
Disease associations	Primary (idiopathic) (30%) Secondary (70%): Collagen vascular disorders (SLE, RA, scleroderma, Sjögren's syndrome) Neoplasms of the immune system (CLL, NHL, HD, WM, MM, thymomas) Immunodeficiency states (hypogammaglobulinemia and dysgammaglobulinemia, Wiskott-Aldrich syndrome, others) Infectious diseases (postviral syndrome, infectious mononucleosis, cytomegalovirus infection, HIV infection, parasitic infections [babesiosis, malaria?]) Others (pregnancy, ovarian tumors, ulcerative colitis)	Primary Secondary Lymphoproliferative disorders (NHL,* CLL,* MGUS,† WM*) Infectious diseases (Mycoplasma† pneumoniae infection, infectious mononucleosis*)	Primary Secondary Infectious diseases (syphilis; measles; chickenpox; influenza; infectious mononucleosis; Mycoplasma pneumoniae infection; smallpox vaccination; mumps; cytomegalovirus; Escherichia coli, Haemophilus influenzae, and Klebsiella pneumoniae infections)

*Disease associated with antibodies directed against i.
†Disease associated with antibodies directed against I.
Abbreviations: CLL = chronic leukocytic leukemia; HD = Hodgkin's disease; HIV = human immunodeficiency virus; MM = multiple myeloma; NHL = non-Hodgkin's lymphoma; RA = rheumatoid arthritis; SLE = systemic lupus erythematosus; WM = Waldenström's macroglobulinemia.

rected against autologous RBCs. The presence of the autoantibodies usually can be demonstrated by a positive direct antiglobulin test, also known as Coombs' test.

The AIHA can be further subdivided into the warm antibody type and the cold antibody type on the basis of serologic characteristics of pathogenic autoantibodies. The autoantibody in the warm antibody AIHA binds optimally to the RBC membrane at 37°C. If the pathogenic antibody has the highest avidity at temperatures below 37°C, usually between 0 and 5°C, a diagnosis of cold antibody AIHA that consists of cold hemoagglutinin disease (CHAD) and paroxysmal cold hemoglobinuria (PCH) can be established. All three entities—warm antibody AIHA, CHAD, and PCH—can be either idiopathic (primary) or associated with one of many diseases (secondary).

The separate category of AIHA, the drug-induced immune hemolytic anemia, includes all the scenarios in which hemolysis can be attributed to the administered medication. The drug-induced immune hemolytic anemia is also caused by the binding of autoantibodies to a drug adsorbed on the surface of an erythrocyte (i.e., hapten-drug adsorption); to a new epitope formed by the drug and erythrocyte membrane (i.e., drug dependent antibody

mechanism); and to the RBC membrane without the drug's involvement or incidentally.

Table 1 and Figure 1 summarize basic facts about AIHAs.

CLINICAL DIAGNOSIS

The annual incidence of AIHA is 1 to 2 cases per 100,000, whereas the incidence of a positive direct antiglobulin test (DAT) result without hemolysis is at least 10 times higher in the normal population. The positive DAT result without hemolysis can be found in as many as 8% of all hospitalized patients. Thus the positive DAT result has low specificity for the diagnosis of AIHA. The AIHA is observed in all races and all age groups; however, the prevalence of idiopathic AIHA increases with age. The prevalence of secondary AIHA in different age groups reflects the prevalence of an underlying disease. More females than males are affected.

PRESENTING SYMPTOMS

The most common presenting symptoms in the patients with warm antibody AIHA are weakness, dizziness, fever,

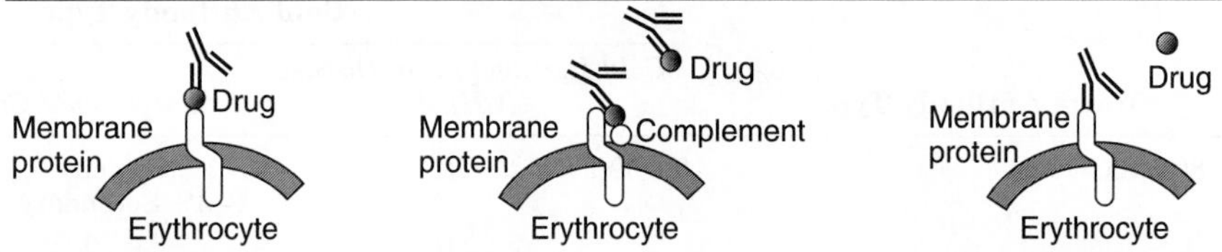

	Hapten-drug adsorption	Drug-dependent antibody mechanism (innocent bystander)	True autoantibody induction	Uncertain mechanism
Positive DAT	IgG>>IgG/C3d	C3d	IgG>>IgG/C3d	
Eluate	Reacts only with RBC coated with the drug	Nonreactive	Reactive with all RBC	
Antibody involved	IgG	IgG, IgM	IgG	
Hemolysis	Moderate Extravascular	Severe, abrupt Intravascular/extravascular	Mild to moderate Extravascular	Mild to moderate Extravascular
Examples of implicated drugs	Penicillins Cephalosporins Tolbutamide Streptomycin Tetracyclines	Quinine Quinidine Cephalosporins (cefotetan, cefotaxime, ceftriaxone, ceftazidime) Chlorpropamide Nitrofurantoin Diclofenac Phenacetin	Methyldopa Levodopa Cephalosporins Procainamide Mefenamic acid	Acetaminophen Thiazides Ibuprofen Erythromycin Omeprazole

Figure 1. The drug-induced immune hemolytic anemia. Only examples of medications causing the drug-induced immune hemolytic anemia are listed here. Any medication recently ingested should be considered an offending agent in a patient with a clinical picture consistent with hemolytic anemia. Some medications cause the drug-induced immune hemolytic anemia through two or more mechanisms (e.g., certain cephalosporins).

and jaundice. These symptoms usually develop over a few months, but sometimes they progress rapidly. In such instances, other symptoms of anemia such as dyspnea on exertion, progressive weakness and, in very rapidly progressive cases, angina can become reasons for seeking medical attention. Some patients may report dark urine. During the physical examination, splenomegaly, hepatomegaly, lymphadenopathy, and jaundice can be appreciated. Other, less frequent signs include thyromegaly, edema, cardiac failure, and pallor. The acuity of the disease process parallels its initial manifestation. Patients with low-grade hemolysis are usually well adjusted to a lower hematocrit, whereas patients with brisk hemolysis usually come to medical attention with signs and symptoms related to rapidly developing anemia.

Patients with CHAD, although typically anemic, commonly seek medical attention because of acute or chronic changes related to the intravascular hemolysis or agglutination. The acute process is significant for acrocyanosis, numbness, and pain, and exacerbations of hemolysis with or without jaundice, whereas chronic disease is limited to atrophic changes of the skin and, in rare circumstances, severe gangrene. More typical symptoms accompany the patients with PCH, who may experience malaise, muscle aches, cramps, headache, nausea and vomiting, diarrhea, chills, and fever, minutes to hours after exposure to cold. During or shortly after these symptoms appear, the patients pass dark urine, the sign of hemoglobinuria. Weakness, pallor, icterus, and organomegaly usually follow such episodes.

The spectrum of presenting symptoms with the drug-induced hemolytic anemia varies from very benign, almost asymptomatic, to rapidly progressive with very brisk destruction of RBCs. In some cases there is a history of recent change in medication or a newly prescribed medication. However, a number of medications may cause hemolytic anemia after a prolonged intake (e.g., methyldopa).

LABORATORY DIAGNOSIS

General Features

Patients' laboratory results usually reflect different features of hemolytic anemia. Hemoglobin levels can be as low as 4 to 5 grams per dL in both warm and cold antibody AIHA. Such severe anemia can also be seen in patients with drug-induced hemolytic anemia when the drug-dependent antibody mechanism is involved. A peripheral blood smear is usually significant for the presence of microspherocytes, reticulocytes, and, frequently, nucleated RBCs. Only few patients come to medical attention with leukopenia and neutropenia, and platelet counts remain stable except for patients with Evans' syndrome, in which AIHA is associated with immune thrombocytopenia. A bone marrow examination may be useful in cases in which a lymphoproliferative process is suspected.

As expected in all hemolytic anemias, the reticulocyte count is usually elevated. Some patients have a delayed response to a decreased RBC mass and have reticulocytopenia resulting from infection, from toxic insult to the bone marrow, or from nutritional deficiency. These patients should be evaluated carefully to assess their need for immediate transfusion of RBCs. The combination of ongoing hemolysis with an inappropriate bone marrow response as manifested by a relative reticulocytopenia may lead rapidly to severe, life-threatening anemia.

Other indicators of both intravascular and extravascular hemolysis may be abnormal. The total bilirubin level is usually below 5 mg per dL, most being in unconjugated form (i.e., direct bilirubin). Lactate dehydrogenase levels are almost always elevated, and serum haptoglobin commonly is significantly depressed.

Hemoglobinuria is detected in patients who suffered a very acute hemolytic episode. It is characteristic for patients with PCH and Donath-Landsteiner antibodies shortly after an exposure to cold. In other patients with

AIHA, only hyperacute hemolysis is accompanied by hemoglobinuria. Patients with drug-induced hemolytic anemia resulting from the drug-dependent antibody mechanism may have hemoglobinuria and acute renal failure related to hemoglobinemia, sometimes complicated by shock and disseminated intravascular coagulation.

Serologic Features

The presence of antibodies against autologous RBCs is a critical part of the diagnosis of AIHA. It is usually demonstrated either by positive direct antiglobulin test (Coombs' test) or from evidence of the presence of direct agglutinins or hemolysins in the patient's serum.

Warm Antibody AIHA

In warm antibody AIHA, the patient's RBCs are coated with nonagglutinating autoantibodies and/or components of the complement such as C3d. These autoantibodies are most commonly IgG, but IgA and IgM have also been reported. The presence of antibodies and complement bound to RBCs is confirmed by the use of the direct antiglobulin test. In this assay, the patient's RBCs are incubated with a polyspecific antiglobulin reagent. The presence of agglutination or hemolysis determines a positive test result. The antiglobulin reagent comprises immunoglobulins directed against IgG and against C3b and C3d. More specific reagents are used to distinguish which molecules are present on the RBC membrane. In the warm antibody AIHA, there are four possible patterns: a positive DAT result with only IgG present; a positive DAT result with only complement present; a positive DAT result with IgG and complement; and a negative DAT result. The negative result with a clinical picture consistent with warm antibody AIHA can be explained by a low sensitivity of the assay or a different antibody class (e.g., IgA or IgM) responsible for warm antibody AIHA. The negative DAT result for warm antibody AIHA is observed in less than 4% of cases.

Because the autoantibody in patients with warm antibody AIHA is in constant equilibrium between bound and unbound form, a certain fraction of it can be detected in such patients' serum in the indirect antiglobulin test (the indirect Coombs' test). However, if the antibody is detected only in the indirect antiglobulin test with a negative DAT, an autoimmune process should be questioned, and a search for more likely alloantibody should be initiated.

Cold Antibody Autoimmune Hemolytic Anemia

Two different antibody types, agglutinins and hemolysins, are implicated in the pathogenesis of cold antibody AIHA. Direct agglutinins present in CHAD are IgM antibodies that most efficiently agglutinate autologous RBCs at temperatures from 0 to 5°C. The serum agglutinin titers vary among patients with CHAD but may be as high as 1:1,000,000 in the most severe cases. The direct antiglobulin test is positive only for complement. Cold agglutinins dissociate from the RBCs during the washing steps in the antiglobulin test, whereas the complement molecules remain attached by the covalent linkage to the RBC membrane. Biphasic hemolysins, also called Donath-Landsteiner antibodies, are encountered in PCH. These are IgG antibodies that bind to RBC with cold-initiating complement activation that continues at higher temperatures, leading to RBC hemolysis. The direct antiglobulin test is positive for complement only briefly after the hemolytic

episode. The presence of these antibodies is confirmed by the biphasic Donath-Landsteiner test. In this test, the normal RBCs are incubated with the patient's fresh serum at 4°C and then warmed up to 37°C. The test result is positive if RBCs are hemolyzed.

Drug-Induced Immune Hemolytic Anemia

The method of detecting antibodies involved in the drug-induced immune hemolytic anemia is dependent on the suspected mechanism responsible for hemolysis (see Figure 1). In patients with the hapten-drug adsorption mechanism, the antibody binds only to RBCs coated with the implicated drug. Thus the DAT result is usually negative and the indirect antiglobulin test result is positive only when the RBCs coated with the drug are used.

When the autoantibody induction mechanism is implicated in the drug-induced hemolytic anemia, the direct antiglobulin test result is positive for IgG alone. In patients receiving methyldopa (Aldomet), the DAT result is positive in up to 30% of cases, but few (<1%) of these patients have hemolysis. Patients who develop hemolysis have also a positive result of the indirect antiglobulin test.

TREATMENT
Warm Antibody Autoimmune Hemolytic Anemia

Transfusion

The sole rationale for a transfusion in patients with warm antibody AIHA is a need to increase the oxygen-carrying capacity of the blood. Only patients with underlying heart disease, cerebrovascular ischemia, or life-threatening anemia should receive RBC transfusions. The difficulty of crossmatching blood is the major problem with transfusion of RBC components. The presence of an autoantibody may lead to a positive result of an antibody screening test and an apparently incompatible crossmatch. Unless the autoantibody has specificity for a defined blood group, almost all donor units are incompatible in the crossmatch. The detection of an alloantibody, which can be masked by the autoantibody, is the major task before the most compatible (least incompatible) units are issued to the patient. It is a good practice to phenotype the patient's RBCs at the time of diagnosis to help identify potential future alloantibodies or to select phenotypically matched RBCs if available. Transfusions should be administered slowly, and the patient should be monitoring continuously for signs of acute hemolysis. The transfused RBCs survive no longer in the patient's circulation than do the patient's own cells. In life-threatening situations, transfusions of RBC components help patients to survive an acute phase of disease.

Glucocorticosteroids

Glucocorticosteroids remain the mainstay of therapy for warm antibody AIHA. Their introduction in the late 1950s dramatically increased patients' survival rate. About 20% of patients achieve complete remission, and about 10% will show minimal or no response to glucocorticosteroids.

An initial daily dose of prednisone varies from 60 to 100 mg. Patients with very brisk hemolysis who are critically ill should be treated with intravenous methylprednisolone (Solu-Medrol), 100 to 200 mg in doses divided over the first 24 hours. Prednisone in high doses is usually required for 10 to 14 days. A rapid taper of steroids to 30 mg per day can be initiated once the hematocrit stabilizes or begins to increase. If improvement continues, the prednisone dose can be further decreased at a rate of 5 mg per day every week to a dose of 15 to 20 mg daily. This dose should be maintained for 2 to 3 months after the acute period of hemolysis subsides. If the patient remains in complete remission, prednisone can be tapered off completely over the course of 1 to 2 months, or an alternate-day schedule can be introduced (e.g., 20 to 40 mg every other day).

Relapses may occur after the glucocorticosteroids are discontinued. Patients who achieved full remission should be closely monitored for at least several years after treatment.

A relapse may necessitate repeated glucocorticoid therapy, splenectomy, or immunosuppression.

Splenectomy

Patients who either do not respond to the initial therapy or require chronic administration of prednisone in doses higher than 15 mg per day are candidates for splenectomy. About one third of patients with warm antibody AIHA belong to this category. The purpose of splenectomy is to remove the primary site of RBC destruction. But even after splenectomy, the RBCs can be continuously destroyed in the liver by hepatic Kupffer cells. The decision to proceed with splenectomy is based on clinical criteria. The results of splenectomy are variable. Up to two thirds of patients with warm antibody AIHA respond to splenectomy with a partial or complete remission. The relapse rate is nonetheless relatively high. In general, the rates of immediate mortality and morbidity from splenectomy are low, but they are closely related to the presence of an underlying disease and the preoperative clinical status. Splenectomy puts patients at an increased risk for pneumococcal sepsis; therefore, pneumococcal vaccine must be administered before surgery. It is also common practice to give prophylactic penicillin (250 to 500 mg daily) to all splenectomized children until they reach adulthood.

Immunosuppression

Cytotoxic drugs are sometimes also effective in warm antibody AIHA. They are reserved for patients unresponsive to glucocorticosteroids and splenectomy and for patients with a high risk for complications from surgical procedures. The most commonly used cytotoxic agents are azathioprine (Imuran)* at 1 to 2 mg per kg per day and cyclophosphamide (Cytoxan)* at 1 to 2 mg per kg per day. Close monitoring of a white blood cell count is necessary because these drugs can cause bone marrow suppression. If there is little or no response within the first 4 to 6 months, the cytotoxic agent should be tapered and discontinued. The prolonged use of these agents is associated with an increased risk for subsequent neoplasia.

Other side effects of cyclophosphamide include hemorrhagic cystitis. Women of childbearing age who receive cytotoxic agents should be warned of the teratogenic effects of these drugs on fetuses.

Other Therapeutic Options

Danazol* (Danocrine), a synthetic androgen, has been used in warm antibody AIHA with some success. The initial dose of 600 to 800 mg per day is tapered down to 400 mg per day after the patient has a clinical response. Mild masculinization and cholestatic jaundice are some of the reported side effects.

Intravenous immunoglobulins have also been effective in a number of patients. A typical dose is 0.4 grams per kg per day for 5 consecutive days. Additional single doses can be administered as needed.

Plasmapheresis alone is not indicated in the treatment of warm antibody AIHA. In combination with other therapies, it may be of some benefit in a highly selected group of acutely ill patients. Other therapeutic approaches such as antithymocyte or antileukocyte globulins, vinblastine-loaded platelets, and thymectomy have been reported with variable success.

Cyclosporine* (Sandimmune) has been also used at a dose of 4 mg per kg per day. Renal function should be closely monitored.

Cold Antibody Autoimmune Hemolytic Anemia

In many patients, disease can be managed by avoiding exposure to cold, thereby preventing bouts of hemolysis and anemia. This management is especially beneficial for patients with mild chronic hemolysis. Patients typically have a benign course. Secondary CHAD associated with lymphoproliferative disorders usually responds to the treatment of the primary neoplasm. Successful therapy of underlying neoplasm with alkylating agents such as cyclophosphamide,* chlorambucil (Leukeran), nucleoside analogues, or, more recently, rituximab* (Rituxan) has been reported. Neither splenectomy nor corticosteroids are particularly useful in treating cold antibody AIHA.

The transfusion of RBCs should be reserved for patients with severe anemia and the potential for compromised cardiopulmonary function. Washed RBCs are not routinely recommended except for patients with very active hemolysis and concurrent complement depletion. Plasmapheresis should be used only as an adjuvant to chemotherapy during the acute phase of disease. The use of plasmapheresis in the chronic phase of CHAD is not beneficial. Sec-

---

*Not FDA approved for this indication.

*Not FDA approved for this indication.

ondary CHAD caused by an infectious process is typically self-limited and resolves within several weeks. Hemodialysis may be required in some patients who experienced massive hemoglobinuria, which has led to acute renal failure.

The prevention of acute attacks in PCH is usually achieved by avoiding exposure to cold. As in CHAD, splenectomy and corticosteroids are of limited use. Treatment of the underlying disease (e.g., syphilis) frequently leads to the resolution of PCH. Life spans of patients with PCH can be normal despite occasional bouts of hemolysis. PCH, which is secondary to a viral infection, is usually transient and self-limited.

Drug-Induced Hemolytic Anemia

Once the drug responsible for the hemolytic process is identified, its discontinuation should lead to the resolution of hemolysis. Acute and severe hemolysis can be associated with medications acting through the drug-dependent antibody mechanism. Hemoglobinuria in such patients may lead to acute renal failure and a need for hemodialysis. There is no definitive role for corticosteroids in drug-induced hemolysis. The RBC transfusions are restricted to rare patients with profound and life-threatening anemia. A selection of appropriate RBC components can be complicated by a strongly positive DAT result. When the drug-dependent antibody or hapten-drug adsorption mechanisms are responsible for hemolysis, the direct antiglobulin test result becomes negative, usually a few days after the offending drug is cleared from the circulation. Incidentally, the patients with hemolysis caused by the hapten-drug adsorption mechanism should have a compatible crossmatch, inasmuch as the implicated antibody binds only to drug-coated cells. When the autoantibodies are involved (e.g., methyldopa), the hemolysis usually ends promptly after the drug is discontinued. Nonetheless, the direct antiglobulin test results may be positive over a year.

NONIMMUNE HEMOLYTIC ANEMIA

method of
YOSHIHITO YAWATA, M.D., PH.D.
Kawasaki Medical School
Kurashiki City, Japan

The diagnosis of nonimmune hemolytic anemia (NIHA) is established by negative direct Coombs' test results. However, NIHA is not a definite clinical entity but rather heterogeneous, including many disorders of congenital or acquired origin (Table 1). In the former category are membrane disorders, hemoglobin abnormalities, and enzyme anomalies. The latter category includes paroxysmal nocturnal hemoglobinuria (PNH), red blood cell fragmentation syndrome, and other acquired hemolytic anemias resulting from infections.

TABLE 1. **Nonimmune Hemolytic Anemias**

Hereditary Disorders

Membrane disorders resulting from membrane protein anomalies
    Hereditary spherocytosis
    Hereditary elliptocytosis
    Hereditary stomatocytosis
Membrane disorders resulting from membrane lipid anomalies
    Hereditary high red blood cell membrane phosphatidylcholine hemolytic anemia
    Congenital lecithin: cholesterol acyltransferase deficiency
    Abetalipoproteinemia (acanthocytosis)
    α-Lipoprotein deficiency (Tangier disease)
Enzyme disorders
    Glucose-6-phosphate dehydrogenase deficiency
    Pyruvate kinase deficiency
    Other enzymopathies
Hemoglobin disorders
    Sickle cell disease (see separate article)
    Unstable hemoglobinopathy
    Hemoglobin M disease
    Other hemoglobin anomalies (HbCC, HbEE, etc.)

Acquired Disorders

Paroxysmal nocturnal hemoglobinuria
Red blood cell fragmentation syndrome
    Mechanical heart valve or other prostheses
    Aortic or mitral valvular disease
    Thrombotic thrombocytopenic purpura
    Hemolytic uremic syndrome
    Disseminated intravascular coagulation
Infections
    Malaria
    Clostridium perfringens
    Other infections
Miscellaneous

HEREDITARY RED BLOOD CELL MEMBRANE DISORDERS

Red blood cell membrane disorders, which compose only 5% of cases of NIHA, consist mostly of membrane protein anomalies and membrane lipid anomalies. Red blood cell morphology in peripheral blood smears is extremely useful for identifying each category of these disorders: microspherocytes for hereditary spherocytosis, elliptocytes or ovalocytes for hereditary elliptocytosis, stomatocytes for hereditary stomatocytosis, and acanthocytes for abetalipoproteinemia. To detect these characteristic red blood cell shapes, a wet preparation from the patient's blood is also useful with phase contrast microscopy or even conventional light microscopy. Such a preparation yields stereotactic features more precisely than those obtained with a fixed and dry preparation of a regular blood smear. This procedure is especially helpful in making a diagnosis of hereditary stomatocytosis.

Hereditary spherocytosis is the most common and most important disorder of red blood cell membranes. Most cases (approximately three fourths) of hereditary spherocytosis are of autosomal dominant transmission, and the others are of autosomal recessive transmission. Clinically, the severity of hereditary spherocytosis varies, because its pathogenesis is heterogeneous. Of the cases of hereditary spherocytosis in Western countries, approximately 55% are related to ankyrin gene mutations of approximately 30 kinds, 20% are related to band 3 (B3) gene mutations of about 40 kinds, and 20% are related to β-spectrin gene mutations of 13 kinds. These mutations are mostly so-called critical mutations: frameshift, nonsense, or splicing mutations. In these mutations, the mutated allele is usually not expressed, and the amount of the determined membrane protein is compensated by the presence of one normal allele. Therefore, the membrane protein content is usually diminished. In contrast, the mutations of membrane protein 4.2 (P4.2) are mostly point mutations with autosomal recessive transmission. Therefore, patients with a P4.2 deficiency are homozygotes or compound heterozygotes of these mutations.

Diagnosis is established by the presence of microspherocytosis of a hereditary origin in the patient's peripheral blood. However, hereditary stomatocytosis, in which microspherocytosis is absent despite the presence of a marked stomatocytosis, should be differentiated critically from hereditary spherocytosis. A helpful hint for diagnosis is a markedly increased mean corpuscular hemoglobin concentration level (>36 grams per dL), which indicates a decreased surface area in relation to the cell volume. The osmotic fragility test, for which fresh blood or blood aseptically incubated for 24 hours is used, is useful for establishing the diagnosis of hereditary spherocytosis.

Clinically, patients with hereditary spherocytosis demonstrate persistent jaundice of various degrees with or without anemia, depending on the extent of compensation by erythroid hyperplasia in the bone marrow. During its clinical course, a sudden episode of severe anemia may occur as a complication, mostly resulting from pure red cell aplasia by parvovirus B19 infection (aplastic crisis) or from acute hemolytic crisis associated with flulike infection, pregnancy, parturition, or the administration of some drugs. The most frequent complication is gallstones (cholelithiasis) with or without cholecystitis. Ultrasonic examination detects more than 50% of these cases with gallstones.

Splenectomy is the best treatment for hereditary spherocytosis. After this procedure, jaundice (indirect bilirubin level, 3.41 ± 1.87 mg per dL) disappears within 1 or 2 days, the reticulocyte count ($12.2 \pm 10.0\%$) is nearly normalized ($1.4 \pm 0.8\%$) within several days, and anemia (red blood cell counts, $3.07 \pm 0.62 \times 10^{12}$ per L) will also be normalized (4.44 ± 0.64) after 2 to 3 months. Concomitantly, red blood cell survival, which is elevated as the apparent half-life ($T\frac{1}{2}$) of chromium (^{51}Cr)–labeled red blood cells, markedly improves (from 9.9 ± 4.0 days to 22.2 ± 6.2 days). If splenectomy is not effective, the diagnosis of hereditary spherocytosis should be reexamined. If a relapse of the clinical symptoms occurs, the presence of an accessory spleen should critically be considered.

The ideal time for splenectomy is no earlier than 5 years of age. Before this age, the risk of postsplenectomic sepsis is quite high because of a still incomplete immune system. Early splenectomy is recom-

mended for patients with frequent gallstone attacks, a lower hemoglobin level (<8 grams per dL), and a high reticulocyte count (>4%). At the time of splenectomy, cholecystectomy is preferentially carried out, especially in patients with frequent gallstone episodes. Laparoscopic splenectomy has been advised by several surgical specialists, mainly from the cosmetic standpoint. The disadvantages, however, should be also seriously considered: exposure of the patient to longer hours under anesthesia for operation, especially in cases with marked splenomegaly; the possibility of overlooking an accessory spleen, which would induce a relapse; and difficulty in controlling a hemorrhaging tendency. As pretreatment, polyvalent pneumococcal polysaccharide vaccine (Pnu-Imune 23 or equivalent, 0.5 mL intramuscularly or subcutaneously) should be given 1 month before splenectomy. Meningococcal vaccine (Menomune-A/C/Y/W-135, 0.5 mL intramuscularly) is also recommended for infantile hereditary spherocytosis. After splenectomy, long-term prophylaxis against pneumococcal infection may also be advisable, such as penicillin VK* (Pen Vec K; 125 mg orally twice a day). Folic acid (1 mg per day orally) is also useful prophylactically.

Hereditary elliptocytosis is characterized by elliptocytosis with or without increased hemolysis. Hemolytic anemia may develop in 10% of patients with hereditary elliptocytosis. Incomplete assembly of the cytoskeletal network of red blood cell membranes, which results from an impaired tetramer formation of spectrins (especially the binding of the N-terminal region of the α-spectrin to the C-terminal region of the β-spectrin, which is the αβ contact region), underlies the pathogenesis of hereditary elliptocytosis. In Western countries, two thirds of hereditary elliptocytosis cases are frequently associated with about 20 kinds of mutations of the α-spectrin gene corresponding to its N-terminal region (mostly point mutations), and one third are associated with mutations of the protein 4.1 (P4.1) gene. The mutations of β-spectrin, which are mostly critical mutations (exon skippings, nonsense mutations, and frameshift mutations), are limited to its C-terminal region. The disorder is transmitted autosomal recessively. Hereditary pyropoikilocytosis is assumed to be a homozygous disorder in this category. Splenectomy is effective for patients with hereditary elliptocytosis and increased hemolysis.

Hereditary stomatocytosis is characterized by the presence of prominent stomatocytosis. Some membrane lipid abnormalities, such as hereditary high red blood cell membrane phosphatidylcholine hemolytic anemia (HPCHA) and congenital lecithin-cholesterol acyltransferase (LCAT) deficiency, also demonstrate marked stomatocytosis. Hereditary stomatocytosis in the strict sense (without membrane lipid anomalies) is categorized as (1) hydrocytosis with increased cell water content (increased red blood cell sodium influx: 8.90 ± 3.39 mmol per liter of red blood cells per hour; normal: 1.29 ± 0.14);

---

*Not FDA approved for this indication.

(2) dehydrocytosis or xerocytosis with decreased cell water content (increased sodium efflux: 5.36 ± 2.52 mmol per liter of red blood cells per hour; normal: 2.40 ± 0.50), and (3) hereditary stomatocytosis with normal cell water content. Splenectomy is not effective against dehydrocytosis and is even contraindicated for HPCHA because it worsens the clinical picture.

Acanthocytosis is observed in several anomalies, especially in abetalipoproteinemia. In this disorder, the pathogenesis has been found to involve 15 mutations of the gene of a microsomal triglyceride transfer protein that transfers triglyceride and esterified cholesterol to B-apolipoprotein. In familial hypo-β-lipoprotein deficiency, 23 mutations of the apo-B-100 gene have been detected.

HEREDITARY ENZYME DEFICIENCIES

Glucose-6-phosphate dehydrogenase (G6PD) is a key enzyme of the hexose monophosphate shunt pathway in human red blood cells. A deficiency of this enzyme provokes a decrease in production of reduced nicotinamide adenine dinucleotide phosphate, leading to increased susceptibility of the patient's red blood cells to oxidative stress. To date, approximately 120 variants of the G6PD gene have been identified, mostly with one or two missense mutations. Affected patients are mostly male hemizygotes, because the enzyme deficiency is X-linked. Clinically, there are three major phenotypes: (1) an asymptomatic type, (2) a type with acute hemolysis, and (3) a type with chronic hemolytic anemia. The highest incidence (400 million affected persons in the African-American population) is observed with G6PDA+ (376 A→G; 126 Asn→Asp), in which no clinical symptoms and normal G6PD activity are expected. In G6PDA− in the African-American population, the enzymatic activity is about 10% of normal with four point mutations of the gene. In the Mediterranean type with favism, a moderate deficiency of G6PD activity is detected with the mutation of 563 C→T (188 Ser→Phe). The most severe type of this deficiency is associated with about 70 kinds of gene mutations. Diagnosis can be made by a simple screening spot test, but the results may not be reliable after acute hemolysis. Direct determination of G6PD activity is obligatory. Splenectomy is partially effective. Oxidative drugs should not be given to these patients.

Pyruvate kinase is the most important enzyme in the Embden-Meyerhof pathway. There are 97 kinds of pyruvate kinase gene mutations associated with chronic hemolytic anemia of autosomal recessive inheritance. Therefore, the probands are usually homozygotes or compound heterozygotes for these mutations. The increased hemolysis is linked to decreased adenosine triphosphate content and increased 2,3-diphosphoglycerate in the patient's red blood cells. Diagnosis is totally dependent on the enzyme assay. Splenectomy may raise the hemoglobin level by 2

grams per dL, which may reduce the frequency of red blood cell transfusion, if any. Red blood cell transfusion should be minimized to reduce the risk of hepatitis C virus infection.

Other enzymopathies in the hexose monophosphate shunt and in the Embden-Meyerhof, glutathione, and nucleotide pathways in red blood cells are extremely rare.

HEREDITARY HEMOGLOBIN ABNORMALITIES

The most prevailing hemoglobin anomaly is sickle cell anemia with hemoglobin (Hb) SS, which is described in detail in another part of this text. At present, there exist approximately 200 alpha-globin gene mutations, approximately 350 beta-globin gene mutations, 25 delta-globin gene mutations, 60 gamma-globin gene mutations, and approximately 30 chimeric globin genes. Clinically, *unstable hemoglobin disease* is defined by the presence of Heinz bodies, which are easily detected by the Heinz body formation test. The instability of this abnormal hemoglobin, which is detected by the diethylaminoethyl (DEAE)–high-performance liquid chromatography method or isoelectric focusing, can be examined by the isopropanol test or the heat denaturation test. More than 100 unstable hemoglobins have been identified. Treatment is red blood cell transfusion or splenectomy, depending on the clinical severity, although these methods are less effective than they are in hereditary spherocytosis.

Hemoglobin M diseases are usually silent, producing no clinical symptoms except cyanosis. Seven phenotypes of this disorder are known.

ACQUIRED DISORDERS

Paroxysmal Nocturnal Hemoglobinuria

PNH is an acquired clonal disorder with episodic intravascular hemolysis and venous thrombosis. This disorder is the only disorder associated with hemolytic anemia, pancytopenia, and/or a hypercoagulable state. The pathogenesis lies in mutation of the PIG-A gene, which codes glycosyl-phosphatidylinositol (GPI)–anchor proteins. The PIG-A gene acts at the first step of the synthesis of the GPI-anchor proteins. Therefore, the mutation abolishes various membrane functions assigned to the GPI-anchor proteins, such as acetylcholinesterase, CD55, CD59, neutrophil alkaline phosphatase, and lymphocyte CD48. Because CD55 and CD59 are abolished by the mutation, the patient's red blood cells become much more susceptible to complement attack, leading to complement-mediated lysis and further to hemoglobinuria with intravascular hemolysis. Clinically, this disorder is usually observed in young to middle-aged adults with episodic dark-colored urine (hemoglobinuria). Even without overt hemoglobinuria, the presence of Prussian blue–positive hemosiderin in the urinary epithelia is strongly suggestive of a history of intravascular hemolysis. The sucrose hemolysis test and the acid hemolysis test (more specific) are useful for establishing the diagnosis of PNH. Flow cytometric analysis has been introduced to clinical laboratories for CD59, CD55, or CD48 and is extremely valuable.

The complications of PNH—thrombosis and hemorrhage—are life-threatening. In the overall clinical course, PNH may lead to aplastic anemia, and 10% of patients with aplastic anemia may develop PNH. The occurrence of acute myelogenous leukemia or myelofibrosis has also been reported, which suggests that PNH is a clonal disorder.

The clinical course of PNH, however, is generally benign, although several supportive treatments are required, such as red blood cell transfusion with online white blood cell filter and iron administration, which may provoke acute hemolytic attack as a result of the newly developed complement-sensitive red blood cells. For acute hemolytic episodes, prednisolone (20 to 30 mg per day) or cortisone (10 to 150 mg per day) may be effective. For thrombotic attacks, thrombolytic agents (tissue plasminogen activator [30 to 60 × 10⁶ units], streptokinase [0.1 to 0.2 × 10⁶ units], and urokinase [0.5 to 0.6 × 10⁶ units]), should be administered immediately. Heparin, 5,000 to 10,000 units (including a low molecular weight heparin) can be used for 7 days. Warfarin, 1 to 5 mg per day, is one of the choices for 6 months, but hypoplasia or even aplasia in the bone marrow is a serious complication. Antithymocyte globulin* (Atgam; 15 mg per kg per day for 5 to 8 days) and/or cyclosporin (Sandimmune; 6 mg per kg per day orally for at least 3 months) may be effective for this hypoplasia. Bone marrow transplantation is another choice but is still controversial because most PNH cases are clinically mild, and there is even spontaneous recovery in about 15% of all PNH cases.

Red Blood Cell Fragmentation

The pathogeneses are categorized into two types: (1) abnormalities of the large vessels (prosthetic valve, severe aortic stenosis, or mitral valvular disease), and (2) microangiopathy (thrombotic thrombocytopenic purpura, disseminated intravascular coagulation, or hemolytic uremic syndrome). In the latter category, red blood cells are spliced by fibrin strands in small vessels, which leads to red blood cell fragmentation. Diagnosis is based on the presence of fragmented red blood cells in the peripheral circulation. Therapy is directed mainly at the underlying disease or event. Hemolytic uremic syndrome is a life-threatening disorder associated with *Escherichia coli* O-157:H7 infection, which may produce verotoxin (Shiga-like toxin). This may induce acute renal failure and neurologic symptoms. Plasma exchange or hemodialysis is highly recommended, and these procedures should be carried out before the appearance of acute renal failure or psychoneurologic symptoms.

---

*Not FDA approved for this indication.

Infection-Related Hemolysis

Malarial infections with increased hemolysis are observed with the infestation of *Plasmodium falciparum, Plasmodium vivax,* or *Plasmodium malariae. Clostridium perfringens* infection is also life-threatening with intravascular hemolysis. The infection may occur with septicemia, biliary tract infection, or anaerobic tissue necrosis. Management in these disorders is based solely on establishing the precise diagnosis.

PERNICIOUS ANEMIA AND OTHER MEGALOBLASTIC ANEMIAS

method of
JACK METZ, M.D.
The Royal Melbourne Hospital
Victoria, Australia

Most of the megaloblastic anemias are the result of deficiency of either cobalamin (vitamin B_{12}) or folate. The nature of the anemia must be established before therapy is instituted. Steps to be taken include the drawing of blood samples for blood cell counts and assays of cobalamin and folate levels. In most patients with megaloblastic anemia, the blood picture is diagnostic and there is no need for bone marrow biopsy. Ideally, specific therapy should be delayed until the blood levels of cobalamin and folate are known, and with modern radioisotope dilution techniques, the results of such assays need not delay therapy for more than a day or two. However, in severely anemic patients, particularly if elderly, and in patients with cardiac decompensation, treatment should begin immediately after blood samples are obtained. Situations necessitating immediate therapy are discussed as follows.

COBALAMIN-DEFICIENT MEGALOBLASTIC ANEMIAS

Humans obtain their cobalamin from animal protein found in such foods as liver, meat, fish, eggs, and dairy products. The daily requirement is very small. The average Western diet contains 3 to 9 μg per day, from which 2 to 3 μg is absorbed and easily provides the recommended dietary allowance of 1 μg per day. Total body stores of cobalamin are 7 to 15 mg, so that deficiency caused by dietary deprivation develops slowly over many years. When there is malabsorption of cobalamin, deficiency occurs more rapidly, for there is malabsorption of both dietary cobalamin and that excreted from the liver into the bile. The diagnosis of cobalamin deficiency is usually made from the finding of low serum cobalamin and normal serum folate levels. When the results of these assays are equivocal, measurement of serum levels of methylmalonic acid and total homocysteine, products of the biochemical pathways of cobalamin and folate metabolism, is useful.

Pernicious Anemia

Pernicious anemia is the commonest and most important example of cobalamin-deficient megaloblastic anemia. The disease is caused by autoimmune (type A) atrophic gastritis with intrinsic factor deficiency, which lead to cobalamin malabsorption. It is seen in all ethnic groups and occurs predominantly in older people, affecting about 2% of persons over 60. All the clinical features of the disease can be ascribed to deficiency of cobalamin. Administration of cobalamin is complete therapy for uncomplicated disease. Because the underlying cause of the cobalamin deficiency cannot be corrected, therapy is lifelong, and the patient should be informed that therapy must never be stopped. Without treatment, the patient dies of anemia or of progressive neurologic disease (peripheral neuritis and subacute combined degeneration of the spinal cord). Inadequate therapy may prevent severe anemia, but neurologic deterioration may be rapid and severe.

Cobalamin Therapy

The aim of therapy is to restore the blood picture and tissue cobalamin stores to normal and to maintain this state throughout life. Replenishment of stores is achieved by administering relatively large doses of the vitamin, in excess of those required to restore the blood picture to normal.

Available Preparations, Route of Administration, and Dosage

Hydroxocobalamin is preferred to cyanocobalamin because it is retained better in the body and is thus more effective in restoring and maintaining cobalamin nutrition. Cobalamin may be administered either by mouth or by subcutaneous or intramuscular injection. Oral cobalamin is effective even in pernicious anemia; 1% of the dose is absorbed by mass action in the absence of intrinsic factor. Most physicians still prefer to administer injections because of the potentially devastating complications of noncompliance often in elderly, forgetful patients who are prescribed tablets. The oral route is justified for patients who can be relied upon to take tablets or who refuse injections, develop sensitivity reactions to the injected vitamin, or have an unrelated bleeding disorder.

With injected cobalamin, the larger the dose, the more is excreted in the urine; only about 20% of a 1000-μg dose is retained. Retention is better when there is an interval between doses. The aims of therapy are fulfilled by cobalamin, 1000 μg by intramuscular or subcutaneous injection three times per week for 2 weeks, followed by maintenance therapy of 500 μg every 2 months for life. The total of 6000 μg of cobalamin administered during the initial 2 weeks of therapy contributes significantly toward the replenishment of body stores and is more than adequate to induce hematologic remission. In patients who cannot visit the physician regularly for injections, maintenance can be given as six injections of 1000 μg of cobalamin spread over a 2-week period once per year. In the patient in whom cobalamin is given orally, the dosage should be 1000 μg per day.

Monitoring the Response to Therapy

In the patient with untreated pernicious anemia, treatment with cobalamin produces an increase in well-being before hematologic changes are recognizable. The serum iron value falls within the first 48 hours, and the bone marrow becomes normoblastic by day 3. Reticulocytes reach a peak by days 5 to 7, and the hemoglobin concentration and red blood cell count return to normal within 6 to 12 weeks of commencing therapy. It is essential that in the initial response to treatment, serum potassium is monitored daily for the first 4 days. In some patients, hypokalemia occurs in the first few days after cobalamin therapy is instituted. Potassium in a dose of 40 mEq per day should be administered promptly to patients manifesting hypokalemia. Patients receiving diuretics for cardiac decompensation should be given potassium supplementation prophylactically during the first few days of treatment. The hemoglobin concentration and red blood cell count should be determined weekly until these values return to normal.

Absence of reticulocytosis and failure of the hemoglobin value and red blood cell count to rise after adequate cobalamin therapy are usually the results of incorrect diagnosis. A suboptimal response, such as poor reticulocytosis and failure of the hemoglobin value and red blood cell count to reach normal levels, are usually indicative of the presence of accompanying disease such as infection, renal disease, thyroid disease, malignant disease (particularly carcinoma of the stomach), rheumatoid arthritis, cardiac failure, or iron deficiency. Associated iron deficiency occurs in about one third of patients with pernicious anemia and becomes manifest especially after cobalamin therapy. Iron deficiency should be corrected by appropriate therapy.

Once hematologic remission has been achieved, all patients should undergo tests to confirm the diagnosis of pernicious anemia or reveal some other cause of cobalamin deficiency. Confirmation of the diagnosis of pernicious anemia is important because it reinforces the need for lifelong cobalamin therapy, alerts the physician of an increased risk of carcinoid and carcinoma of the stomach, and could assist in the elucidation of any unexplained anemia in other family members. In the past, tests of cobalamin absorption (the Schilling test) with or without intrinsic factor were commonly performed to confirm the diagnosis of pernicious anemia. The Schilling test involves the 24-hour collection of urine; in a significant number of patients, especially the elderly, urinary collection is incomplete, leading to spurious results. In about two thirds of patients with pernicious anemia, antibodies to intrinsic factor can be detected in the serum; for practical purposes, this confirms the diagnosis of pernicious anemia, and further tests are unnecessary. Parietal cell antibodies are present in 90% of patients, and in 80% there is significant hypergastrinemia; although these abnormalities are not specific for pernicious anemia, the diagnosis is most unlikely in patients in whom no antibodies are detected and the serum gastrin level is normal. It is only in this subgroup of patients that cobalamin absorption tests are needed mainly to establish an intestinal cause for the deficiency.

Careful supervision of maintenance therapy must be exercised throughout the patient's life. The hematocrit and neurologic status should be checked at 4-month intervals, as are any symptoms that may herald the development of carcinoma of the stomach. In the patient receiving cobalamin by mouth, closer supervision is required. In patients with pernicious anemia, there is a twofold increase in the relative risk for carcinoma of the stomach and a much greater risk of gastric carcinoid tumors, which are relatively benign. Regular gastroscopic surveillance is controversial but is generally regarded as unwarranted.

Patients with Cardiac Decompensation

Although the megaloblastic anemias are eminently treatable diseases, there remains an appreciable mortality rate. Among hospitalized patients, the mortality rate is on the order of 4%, and among severely anemic patients (hematocrit less than 25%), the figure may be as high as 14%. The mortality rate is directly related to age. More than half of the fatalities occur within 1 week of hospitalization, and one third are sudden and unexpected. More than three quarters of fatal cases show evidence of congestive cardiac failure. In patients with evidence of cardiac decompensation, conventional therapy for cardiac failure is instituted. When anemia is severe, the cardiac decompensation may be aggravated by the low level of hemoglobin, and blood transfusion may be life-saving. Blood transfusion is a hazardous procedure in the severely anemic patient, for it may readily induce circulatory overload with a fatal outcome. Fortunately, in most patients with pernicious anemia, blood transfusion is unnecessary and should be avoided.

Severe anemia per se is not an indication for transfusion, but the presence of circulatory collapse, cardiac failure with pulmonary congestion and dyspnea at rest, or severe intractable angina are situations necessitating immediate transfusion. The patient should be propped up in bed, and a diuretic (e.g., furosemide [Lasix], 40 mg) administered. Packed cells (never whole blood) in a volume not exceeding 250 mL should be administered *slowly* over a period of 4 to 6 hours. If there is severe congestive cardiac failure, approximately 100 ml blood should be withdrawn from the other arm, so that the patient receives a partial exchange transfusion. During the transfusion, signs of circulatory overload should be carefully monitored.

In severely anemic patients with cardiac decompensation or with bleeding caused by severe thrombocytopenia or with infection associated with severe neutropenia, the institution of vitamin therapy cannot wait for the establishment of the nature of the underlying deficiency. After withdrawal of a sample of blood for vitamin assays, immediate therapy should consist of cobalamin, 1000 μg by injection, and folic acid, 5 mg by mouth. The latter is given in case the megaloblastic anemia of undiagnosed cause is the result of folate deficiency and not cobalamin deficiency. Folic acid *alone* should never be administered to a patient with megaloblastic anemia in whom the underlying deficiency has not been established. However, there is no evidence that folic acid is harmful to patients with cobalamin deficiency when it is administered together with adequate doses of cobalamin.

In pernicious anemia, leukopenia and thrombocytopenia are common. Occasionally, the thrombocytopenia is so profound that bleeding ensues, and in these patients, platelet transfusions should be given as a matter of urgency.

Patients with Subacute Combined Degeneration of the Spinal Cord

In patients with neurologic complications, physiotherapy should be given, and the patients should get out of bed as soon as the physical condition permits. Higher doses of cobalamin have been administered to patients with neurologic complications, but there is no evidence that such doses are more effective than those cited in the regimen for uncomplicated pernicious anemia. The response of the neurologic complications to cobalamin therapy is inconsistent and unpredictable and is related to the duration of the process. In all patients, the progress of the neurologic disease is arrested; almost all patients show some improvement, but response to therapy is usually very slow. Improvement may continue for months, but little further improvement can be anticipated after 5 months' therapy.

Patients with Infection

Pulmonary or urinary infection is not uncommon in patients with pernicious anemia. In one third of fatal cases of megaloblastic anemia, pneumonia is found at autopsy. These infective complications should be treated with suitable antibiotics, but trimethoprim-sulfamethoxazole preparations (Bactrim, Septra) are contraindicated in patients with untreated cobalamin deficiency, because of the antifolate activity of the latter drug. Higher doses of cobalamin are required by patients with active infection.

Other Cobalamin-Deficient Megaloblastic Anemias

Dietary Deficiency

In strict vegetarians who rigidly exclude all sources of animal protein from their diet (vegans), cobalamin deficiency megaloblastic anemia may develop, usually after many years of dietary deprivation. The clinical and hematologic manifestations are similar to those of pernicious anemia, but there is no abnormality of gastric function, and cobalamin absorption is normal. These patients are treated with oral cobalamin. A daily dose of 10 μg per day is adequate, but it is advisable to begin with 100 μg per day for 1 month to replete cobalamin stores. If the patient cannot be persuaded to include some source of animal protein in the diet, oral cobalamin must be continued for life.

Breast-fed infants of cobalamin-deficient mothers may develop severe cobalamin-deficient megaloblastic anemia in early infancy. Treatment is with oral cobalamin until mixed feeding is established.

Intestinal Malabsorption

After combining with gastric intrinsic factor, cobalamin is absorbed in the terminal ileum. Malabsorption may result from lesions such as regional ileitis (Crohn's disease), gluten enteropathy, ileal resection, or a lesion that enables overgrowth of bacteria within the small intestine (stagnant loop syndrome). Cobalamin-deficient megaloblastic anemia may occur with all these lesions, and the intestinal malabsorption can be demonstrated by the Schilling test, in which the cobalamin malabsorption is not corrected by intrinsic factor. Treatment of the megaloblastic anemia is with parenteral cobalamin, as for pernicious anemia; although oral cobalamin therapy should be effective, there are no published data from controlled clinical trials to support oral treatment. Patients with cobalamin-deficient megaloblastic anemia associated with intestinal malabsorption require further investigation to establish the nature of the intestinal lesion. When the underlying lesion cannot be remedied, cobalamin treatment is lifelong.

Folate-Deficient Megaloblastic Anemia

Folate is found in nearly all natural foods, and the richest source is uncooked green vegetables and fruit. The daily requirement for folate is 100 to 200 μg. An average mixed diet contains 200 to 300 μg per day, so that the margin of safety is much less for folate than for cobalamin. Normal tissue folate stores are about 5000 μg, so that with dietary deprivation, deficiency may develop within 4 months.

Folate deficiency is most commonly the result of inadequate dietary intake (resulting from poverty or poor dietary habits) coupled with increased demand and occurs particularly in association with pregnancy, lactation, and the rapid growth period of infancy. Other vulnerable groups are the elderly, alcoholic persons, and patients with chronic hemolytic anemia. Deficiency may also occur in intestinal malabsorption syndromes affecting the upper small bowel, such as gluten enteropathy.

The clinical and hematologic features of folate-deficient megaloblastic anemia are similar to those of cobalamin deficiency, but the neurologic complications of cobalamin deficiency do not occur. The diagnosis of folate deficiency is established by the finding of low concentrations of both serum and red blood cell folate levels, with normal serum cobalamin levels. Some patients with folate deficiency have subnormal serum cobalamin levels, and this scenario could reflect dual deficiency.

Serum folate falls rapidly when dietary folate intake is restricted, and it may fall below the reference range while stores are still replete. Tissue deficiency should thus be confirmed by a low red blood cell folate concentration.

Initial treatment of folate-deficient megaloblastic anemia is with oral folic acid (Folvite). A dosage of 1 mg daily is adequate, although the tablets available usually contain 5 mg. In patients with malabsorption syndrome, the 5-mg daily dose is preferred. The special provision pertaining to patients with cardiac decompensation, infection, or thrombocytopenia associated with cobalamin-deficient megaloblastic anemia applies equally to folate deficiency, as does the need to monitor the response to therapy. Tissue stores are usually replenished after a few weeks of folic acid, and the need for subsequent treatment is dependent on the continued presence of the cause. Many conditions in which folate-deficient megaloblastic anemia occur are either self-limiting or correctable and necessitate only short-term therapy. Associated iron deficiency is probably more common in folate deficiency than in cobalamin deficiency, because of similar dietary factors.

THALASSEMIA

method of
SUSAN P. PERRINE, M.D.
Boston University School of Medicine
Boston, Massachusetts

PATHOPHYSIOLOGY: BASIC MECHANISMS OF HEMOGLOBIN SYNTHESIS

The sequential expression of the different globin genes results in production of specific types of hemoglobins at different stages of development. At approximately 12 weeks of gestation, a transition from embryonic to fetal hemoglobin ($\alpha_2\gamma_2$) occurs, and at 28 weeks of gestation, increasing amounts of beta-globin and of adult hemoglobin (Hb A, $\alpha_2\beta_2$) are produced. Alpha-like globin protein must equal beta-like globin proteins in order for intact hemoglobin tetramers to form. Thalassemia syndromes result from deficiencies in either alpha-globin (α-thalassemia) or beta-like globin (β-thalassemia) chains. The disease becomes apparent when the affected globin is required during development. Thus α-thalassemia is symptomatic during gestation, because alpha-globin is required for fetal hemoglobin (Hb F, $\alpha_2\gamma_2$). Because beta-globin is not required before birth, β-thalassemia is asymptomatic until 6 months after birth. Mutations that cause prolonged production of fetal gamma-globin chains may manifest later, at 2 to 4 years of age.

The major pathologic process of thalassemia is caused by the imbalance of alpha and non–alpha chain accumulation. The unaffected chains, produced in normal amounts, precipitate during erythropoiesis. In β-thalassemia, the precipitated alpha-globin damages cell membranes and causes rapid cell death in the bone marrow (ineffective intramedullary erythropoiesis). Red blood cell life-span is further shortened by premature removal of abnormal cells in the reticuloendothelial system. In response to the hypoxia, erythropoietin levels increase, causing erythroid hyperplasia. Marrow expansion causes osteopenia, pathologic fractures, and bone deformities. Hypersplenism leads to even more severe anemia. An increase in plasma volume, from marrow and splenic expansion, also lowers the effective level of hemoglobin.

In α-thalassemic fetuses, the unbalanced gamma-globin chains form tetramers (γ_4, hemoglobin Bart's); excess beta-globin (β_4, hemoglobin H) accumulates after birth. Hemoglobin Bart's and hemoglobin H result in milder ineffective erythropoiesis but have abnormal oxygen binding and sensitivity to oxidant stress. If all four alpha-globin genes are deleted, only hemoglobin Bart's is formed, with a massively left-shifted oxygen dissociation curve that provides almost no oxygen delivery to tissues and results in a lethal intrauterine condition, hydrops fetalis. Deletion of three alpha-globin loci, or decreased production of alpha-globin from four abnormal alpha-globin genes, results in a moderate hemolytic anemia, hemoglobin H disease. Deletion of only one (α-thalassemia-2) or two (α-thalassemia-1) loci is asymptomatic.

Thalassemia syndromes are graded according to severity of the anemia. *Thalassemia major,* in which severe anemia manifests during infancy, is caused by inheritance of two seriously impaired beta-globin alleles. This homozygous or doubly heterozygous state may have a milder manifestation when there is a higher than usual increase in fetal (gamma) chain production or when the co-inheritance of α-thalassemia decreases the net imbalance of the synthesis of alpha-globin to beta-globin. *Thalassemia trait* (inheritance of a single defective allele) is characterized by mild hypochromic, microcytic anemia. *Thalassemia intermedia* manifests as moderate anemia with total hemoglobin levels of 7.0 grams per dL or more. Affected patients require occasional transfusions when they have infections, but they do not require chronic transfusions for survival. The same clinical manifestations, including splenomegaly, gallstones, osteopenia, and iron overload in the liver and endocrine organs, develop more slowly in thalassemia intermedia, but cardiomyopathy does not typically develop in patients who have not undergone transfusion. Extramedullary hematopoiesis can result in thoracic and paravertebral masses and in spinal cord compression.

DIAGNOSIS

The diagnosis of severe thalassemia is usually straightforward in ethnic groups at risk (Italian, Greek, African, Asian, Middle Eastern, East Indian, Caribbean). Thalassemia major and thalassemia intermedia are marked by severe microcytic anemia; hyperbilirubinemia, elevation of lactate dehydrogenase levels, and splenomegaly appear during gestation (α-thalassemia) or in the first few years of life. Hydrops fetalis manifests as polyhydramnios and fetal distress during the second trimester. β-Thalassemia trait (β-thalassemia minor) is characterized by mild anemia (hematocrit of >30), low mean corpuscular volume (<75 fL), and erythrocytosis (red blood cell [RBC] count of >5 × 10^6 per mm^3). Quantitative hemoglobin electrophoresis demonstrates elevated hemoglobin A_2 and F levels, and an absence of hemoglobin A, in β^0-thalassemia but not in β^+-thalassemia. α-Thalassemia is best diagnosed from the presence of hemoglobin Bart's in umbilical cord blood. Hemoglobin H is unstable, and electrophoresis of fresh specimens is required for its detection. In most, but not all, β-thalassemia heterozygotes, hemoglobin A_2 levels are ele-

vated. Iron deficiency can mask β-thalassemia trait by decreasing hemoglobin A_2 levels. α-Thalassemia trait can be silent or microcytic and hypochromic. Microcytosis with anisocytosis and hypochromia, basophilic stippling, target cells, fragmented cells (schistocytes), and nucleated RBCs are typical of severe thalassemias. The reticulocyte count may be relatively low because of ineffective erythropoiesis. The mean corpuscular volume may eventually become high, rather than low, as a result of the rapid emergence of erythroid precursors that have skipped cell divisions. Prenatal diagnosis of thalassemia is usually accomplished by direct polymerase chain reaction analysis of fetal DNA obtained by amniocentesis or chorionic villus sampling in a few specialized laboratories.

TREATMENT (Table 1)

Transfusion Therapy

In β-thalassemia major, RBC transfusion is the mainstay of supportive therapy. Transfusions that achieve a hemoglobin level of at least 9 grams per dL suppress the erythropoietic drive. Maintaining the mean hemoglobin level above 10.5 to 11 grams per dL (range, 10.5 to 13 grams per dL) reduces marrow expansion, plasma volume, and the amount of blood required to achieve the same level of hemoglobin, especially after splenectomy. Bone changes regress, splenomegaly recedes, growth improves, and improvement in physical activity can be expected. Regular transfusions are generally started for a persistent and otherwise unexplained fall in hemoglobin below 7 grams per dL in children with two β-thalassemic mutations. Transfusion of 15 mL per kg of RBCs at 2- to 4-week intervals is feasible for most patients. Acetaminophen and diphenhydramine before transfusions usually prevent febrile reactions. Transfusion records should be meticulously maintained in order to assess the annual mean hemoglobin level and annual blood consumption. A complete genotype of the patient's RBCs before transfusions facilitates later identification of involved antigens in the event of isoimmunization. Fresh ABO- and Rh$_0$D-compatible crossmatched blood, filtered to remove white blood cells, is given. Leukocyte filtering also removes viruses that inhabit white blood cells. Cytomegalovirus (CMV)–negative preparations are optimal for bone marrow transplantation candidates. Indirect antiglobulin testing for antibodies to RBC antigens should be routinely performed. An increase in transfusion requirements is suggestive of hypersplenism, isoimmunization, or an accessory spleen.

Transfusions can transmit blood-borne infections, including hepatitis viruses, human immunodeficiency virus (HIV), and CMV, reflecting the incidences of infection in the general population. In regions where hepatitis C is endemic, 90% of patients who undergo chronic transfusion develop hepatitis C within 5 years; chronic infection eventually advances to cirrhosis in 85%. Patients should be vaccinated against hepatitis A and B and monitored for elevated transaminase levels and for hepatitis C antibodies, with referral to consultants for liver biopsy and man-

TABLE 1. **Recommended Monitoring of Thalassemia Patients**

Monitoring of Patients Undergoing Regular Transfusions

Red blood cell phenotype (before transfusions)
History, monthly physical examination
Pre- and post-transfusion CBC and record of amounts of each transfusion
Indirect antibody screen twice annually or with a positive Coombs' test result on crossmatch
Studies of ALT, AST, bilirubin, GGT, LDH, alkaline phosphatase, albumin, total protein, and ferritin every 3 months
Hepatitis A and B panels (before vaccine)
Hepatitis C antibody (messenger RNA by PCR if antibody-positive) and HIV test annually
INR and PTT annually
Liver biopsy, after 5 years of transfusions or with hepatomegaly

Cardiac Monitoring After 5 Years of Transfusions

Echocardiogram, ECG annually
24-hour Holter monitor (for patients aged >12 years)
Cardiology consultation, MRI, stress test (for patients aged >18 years)

Endocrine and Osteoporosis Monitoring

TSH, free T_4 parathormone, calcium, inorganic phosphorus, growth hormone levels annually
Glucose tolerance test, Cotrosyn stimulation test annually
Gonadotropins and estradiol or testosterone after age 12 years
Bone mineral density test, bone age, 24-hour urine calcium, creatinine, hydroxyproline annually
Serum calcium, inorganic phosphorus, alkaline phosphatase, 1,25-hydroxyvitamin D level twice annually

Monitoring of Effects of Deferoxamine Therapy

Ophthalmologic and hearing evaluation annually
Sitting and standing height, weight every 4–6 months until the age of 18 years
Zinc, copper, selenium, vitamin C, and vitamin E levels every 4–6 months
Urinary iron excretion annually or biannually

Abbreviations: ALT = alanine aminotransferase; AST = aspartate aminotransferase; CBC = complete blood cell count; ECG = electrocardiogram; GGT = γ-glutamyltransferase; HIV = human immunodeficiency virus; INR = International Normalized Ratio; LDH = lactate dehydrogenase; MRI = magnetic resonance imaging; PCR = polymerase chain reaction; PT = prothrombin time; PTT = partial thromboplastin time; TSH = thyroid-stimulating hormone.

agement if these are found. Interferon alpha-2a and ribavirin can produce sustained responses in 36% of hepatitis C–infected patients. Unfortunately, relapses are common. HIV testing should be performed annually.

Splenectomy

Massive splenomegaly is avoidable by a proper hypertransfusion regimen. However, splenic sequestration of donor cells can cause excessive transfusion requirements. Splenectomy should be performed (1) if a 40% or greater increase in the transfusion requirement occurs during a 1-year period or (2) for a transfusion requirement of more than 200 mL per kg per year of packed RBCs, without evidence of isoimmunization. Significant leukopenia and thrombocytopenia from hypersplenism are other indications. Splenectomy increases the risk of overwhelming sepsis, especially in young children, and so ideally it should be deferred until the patient is 4 to 5 years of age. The most frequent pathogens are pneumococci, *Haemophilus influenzae,* and *Neisseria meningitidis* (meningococcus). *Yersinia enterocolitica* is also common, especially with deferoxamine treatment. Polyvalent pneumococcal vaccine should be given 1 month before splenectomy. Prophylactic oral Penicillin VK (250 mg twice a day) should be used in children younger than 10 years; trimethoprim-sulfamethoxazole may be given to patients allergic to penicillin. Immediate medical attention should be sought for significant fever (≥101°F) because patients are at risk for a fulminant course and death within hours. Broad-spectrum antibiotics should be given immediately, even before the results of any laboratory investigations. Patients who have undergone splenectomy should be given prophylactic penicillin for 24 hours before and after invasive procedures (e.g., all dental work).

Treatment of Iron Overload and Related Complications

There is approximately 1 mg of iron per mL of packed RBCs. Hypertransfusion regimens encumber patients each year with four times the normal total body iron burden, with no mechanism for elimination. By adolescence, iron stores are often at toxic levels (transfusional hemosiderosis). Frequent monitoring of transfusion requirements, ferritin levels, and target organ function is critical. Before the advent of iron chelation therapy, the multiorgan toxic effects of iron were the major cause of death in patients with thalassemia who had undergone transfusion.

Hemosiderosis causes clinical dysfunction in the heart, liver, and endocrine organs, and a grayish-bronzed coloration of the skin commonly develops. Complications have a more subtle manifestation in patients who have received iron chelation therapy. Glucose intolerance with insulin-dependent diabetes mellitus is common. Laboratory evidence of primary hypothyroidism, hypoparathyroidism, and other endocrinopathies can often be detected before symptoms develop; digoxin refractoriness and arrhythmias result from hypocalcemia secondary to hypoparathyroidism. Diminished adrenal reserves may occur with metabolic stress. Delayed puberty and amenorrhea commonly result from iron deposition in the hypothalamus. Retarded growth may become apparent at puberty, and patients may respond to growth hormone before 13 years of age. Hepatic hemosiderosis and hepatitis C commonly lead to fibrosis and cirrhosis. Liver biopsy to measure iron deposition in hepatic tissue and to assess chronic infection and fibrosis should be performed after several years of transfusions. Cardiac dysfunction, detectable by reduced ejection fractions, often begins in the early teens. Clinical symptoms begin with fatigue, arrhythmias, or pericarditis, advancing to congestive heart failure and death in the third or fourth decade. Osteopenia may be severe, resulting in fractures, especially in thalassemia intermedia. Patients should be maintained on elemental calcium (1500 mg per day) and vitamin D (400 IU per day). Severe cases may be treated with bisphosphonates such as pamidronate (Aredia), 1 to 3 mg per kg dose in children or 15 to 30 mg in adults intravenously over 4 hours, every 1 to 4 months, or alendronate (Fosamax), 5 to 10 mg per day orally, and should be monitored with alkaline phosphatase, calcium, phosphate, 1,25-hydroxyvitamin D levels, 24-hour urinary calcium, and hydroxyproline, and bone mineral density measurements at 6- to 12-month intervals.

The iron chelator deferoxamine mesylate (Desferal) is effective when administered five to seven times per week as a continuous subcutaneous or intravenous infusion or as twice-daily bolus subcutaneous (not intramuscular) injections of the same total dose. Such regimens can maintain negative iron balance despite continuation of transfusions. Urinary iron excretion is used to adjust the dosage to maintain negative iron balance. When begun within 2 years of transfusions, such regimens can prevent cardiac disease and prolong survival. If a significant iron burden is present before chelation therapy, progressive cardiac dysfunction and hepatic fibrosis may not be completely prevented or reversed. Early initiation of therapy and compliance is thus critical.

Iron overload should be documented by a deferoxamine test or begun after 12 to 18 months of regular transfusions, because children require iron for growth and chelation is detrimental for non–iron-overloaded patients. The amount of iron in a 24-hour urinary collection after injection of 500 mg of deferoxamine should exceed 1 mg in order to begin chelation therapy, or the serum ferritin level should exceed 1000 ng per mL. A small infusion pump is used to administer doses of 25 to 40 mg per kg per day (depending on degree of iron overload) over 10 to 12 hours into the abdominal subcutaneous fat, with rotation of the sites. Doses should be rounded off to deliver the nearest whole vial of deferoxamine, which because of its expense should not be discarded. Hypertonicity can be prevented by increasing the volume of water diluent. Local allergic reactions can be suppressed by adding hydrocortisone (up to 2 mg per mL) to the solution or with topical diphenhydramine. A topical anesthetic cream can be applied 1 hour before insertion of the needle, to decrease needlestick discomfort. Many patients find intravenous administration of deferoxamine, through an indwelling port device, more tolerable than subcutaneous injection because such devices can be used with an indwelling needle for 1 week without repeated needlesticks. Furthermore, intravenous chelation is more effective than subcutaneous chelation, and so fewer days of therapy are often sufficient. Severe arrhythmias and congestive heart failure have been temporarily reversed with high-dose deferoxamine (15 mg per kg per hour maximum for 12 hours per day, 7 days per week). Anaphylactic reactions can be treated with desensitization; idiosyncratic acute respiratory distress syndromes, although rare, are life-threatening, necessitating rapid recognition and intensive care. Excessive doses can cause optic and acoustic neuritis, and so annual ophthalmologic and hearing evaluations should be performed. If abnormalities resolve after the drug is discontinued, lower doses can be cautiously reinstated. Iron overload causes depletion of vitamin C, which inhibits iron release from reticuloendothelial cells. Sudden availability of vitamin C can cause a massive release of iron and serious cardiotoxicity. Vitamin C (100 mg per day) should be given only after the first cycle of deferoxamine.

The major problem with deferoxamine therapy is noncompliance because of needlesticks, local reactions, pain and induration at infusion sites, and inconvenience. Psychologic support is thus important. Results of trials with an oral chelator (deferipone) have indicated particular clinical efficacy at high ferritin levels (>5000 mg per mL); further testing for long-term efficacy and safety is in progress in the United States. This drug is in use in India and in Europe.

Thalassemia Intermedia

Patients with β-thalassemia who do not develop debilitating anemia should not be committed to a lifelong transfusion regimen. When the hemoglobin levels remain above 8 grams per dL, patients generally lead a relatively normal life. Most experts avoid regular transfusions at hemoglobin levels above 7 grams per dL, particularly in regions where the blood supply predictably results in hepatitis C transmission. However, patients should be monitored closely for signs of marrow expansion, splenomegaly, or growth retardation. Hypertransfusion can usually be delayed or entirely avoided by splenectomy.

The hyperplastic marrow in thalassemia intermedia stimulates intestinal iron absorption and iron overload, which eventually necessitates chelation therapy. Avoidance of iron-rich meats and regular consumption of tea can reduce iron absorption. Other complications are relative folate deficiency, gallstones, leg ulcers, osteopenia, and spinal cord compression syndromes. Folic acid and antioxidant supplements should be given. If symptoms of cholecystitis develop, patients should be evaluated promptly. Spinal cord compression from thoracic or vertebral bone marrow expansion and paraspinal masses should be suspected in patients with acute or increasing weakness, numbness, and diminished reflexes in the lower extremities. Diagnosis is made by magnetic resonance imaging or computed tomography; radiation therapy and steroids should be instituted on an emergency basis. Osteopenia and facial deformity are most severe in this group. Cardiac hemosiderosis does not usually develop in patients who have not undergone transfusion, although pericarditis does occur in rare cases.

α-Thalassemia

The homozygous form is usually lethal in utero. However, prenatal diagnosis and milder variants have enabled fetuses to be supported to term with intrauterine transfusions, followed by postnatal transfusions. For milder forms such as hemoglobin H disease, only folic acid, antioxidants, and monitoring for severe anemia during infections or with increasing splenomegaly are necessary. Because hemoglobin H is sensitive to oxidant stress, drugs such as sulfonamides should be avoided, particularly with coexistent glucose-6-phosphate dehydrogenase (G6PD) deficiency. Iron status should be monitored.

Bone Marrow Transplantation

Allogeneic bone marrow transplantation is curative by replacing the patient's hematopoietic stem cells, which contain two thalassemic globin genes, with normal stem cells, which contain two normal genes or one normal and one thalassemic globin gene. Transplantation from an HLA-identical related donor in young patients without hepatomegaly or hepatic fibrosis and with a good iron chelation history (risk class 1) carries an excellent prognosis. Nonetheless, the rate of mortality among patients undergoing transplantation in experienced centers is 15%. Morbidity may result from conditioning regimens and graft-versus-host disease (GVHD) in 5 to 13% of patients. Nonetheless, transplantation is the only curative option and has become standard for families who accept the low incidence of admittedly serious risks. Unrelated donors and cord blood as sources of donor cells currently carry increased risks of GVHD and graft rejection but offer broader availability of transplants in the future. Relapses (graft rejection) occur in 8% of patients receiving related donor transplants. Many patients clinically do well even with mixed chimeric states. In risk class 1 patients with an HLA-matched relative, transplantation is ideally performed before 8 years of age. The low incidence of serious risks of this curative modality must be weighed against the lifelong burden of hypertransfu-sion and chelation. This balance may be shifted by further development of oral chelators and by refinement of preparative regimens and unrelated donor cells.

Activation of Fetal Globin Gene Synthesis

In three reports on five thalassemia patients who could not receive transfusions because of the presence of alloantibodies, gamma-globin expression has been induced by intravenous administration of the cytotoxic chemotherapeutic agent 5-azacytidine, resulting in a mean increase in hemoglobin of 2.6 grams per dL (range, 2.3 to 3.4 grams per dL) above baseline levels and significant clinical improvement. Uncertainty about the long-term side effects of a cytotoxic and mutagenic agent has limited this therapy so far to patients with no other therapeutic options. Hydroxyurea (Hydrea), although beneficial in sickle thalassemia, has been less effective in nonsickle thalassemia. Butyric acid derivatives also induce gamma-globin synthesis and are not mutagenic or cytotoxic to myeloid or platelet precursors. However, these agents have short half-lives, and so large numbers of tablets of sodium phenylbutyrate are necessary and intravenous infusions are required for arginine butyrate. Sodium phenylbutyrate (Buphenyl) therapy over several months increased mean total hemoglobin by 2.1 grams per dL above baseline in four of eight patients who did not receive transfusions. Intravenous arginine butyrate induces gamma-globin messenger RNA and protein within days; increases in total hemoglobin and hematocrit occur after several weeks of therapy in patients in whom transfusions are withheld, to allow endogenous erythropoiesis. A mean increase in total hemoglobin of 2.8 grams per dL (range, 2.0 to 4.0 grams per dL) over baseline values was observed in six of seven patients treated with weekly infusions of arginine butyrate, usually followed by intermittent treatment (800 mg per kg per dose for 4 nights) twice a month as home therapy. Intermittent, or "pulse," regimens have been more tolerable for patients and more effective than continuous infusions long term. A few previously transfusion-dependent patients became transfusion independent. This briefer therapy (8 nights per month) is preferable to some patients over infusion of deferoxamine, which requires 20 nights of therapy per month. This experimental modality is in phase II academic trials.

Gene Transfer

Gene therapy for thalassemia requires high-level expression of genes that are transferred into repopulating hematopoietic stem cells. No other type of gene therapy faces this challenge. Major DNA regulatory elements (locus control region) must be introduced with the structural globin sequences for high-level abundant expression, which cannot be accommodated by currently available viral vectors. Significant problems must be overcome for gene transfer to be applied curatively to human thalassemic hematopoietic stem cells. These include transcriptional silencing and extinction of transduced genes, which occur in vitro and in animal models; low-level expression of transferred genes; difficulty in transducing the rare pluripotent repopulating stem cells; and inability to selectively expand transduced stem cells in vivo. No definite time frame for curative gene therapy in thalassemia is currently anticipated.

SICKLE CELL DISEASE

method of
KAREN B. LEWING, M.D., and
GERALD M. WOODS, M.D.
The Children's Mercy Hospital
Kansas City, Missouri

Sickle cell disease (SCD) is a hereditary hemoglobin disorder that occurs primarily in people of African descent. Sickle cell anemia (SCA) and sickle cell trait (SCT) are two distinctly different clinical entities. SCA occurs in about 1 in 500 African-American newborns and can cause progressive disability and can shorten life expectancy. Approximately 75,000 African-Americans are afflicted with SCA. SCT is, under normal physiologic conditions, an asymptomatic or carrier form of the hemoglobinopathy. SCT has been observed to be a contributing cause of complications or death under conditions such as hypoxemia or acidosis. Approximately 3 million African-Americans have SCT.

GENETICS

Normal human hemoglobin consists of two pairs of globin chains, combined with four heme groups. Adult hemoglobin (HbA) is composed of two alpha-globin chains and two beta-globin chains. Sickle hemoglobin (HbS) is the result of the substitution of valine for glutamic acid at the sixth position of the beta-globin chain. The inheritance of one HbS allele and one HbA allele produces the heterozygous state of sickle trait (AS). SCA is the result of inheriting two HbS alleles (SS). Other commonly seen genotypes arise from the combination of HbS with HbC (substitution of lysine for glutamic acid at position six of the beta-globin chain) or with β-thalassemia.

The incidence of SCT correlates with the worldwide distribution of malaria. SCT provides some protection against *Plasmodium falciparum* malaria; rates of morbidity and mortality from malaria are reduced in this group of patients. The mechanism of protection against malaria provided by HbS remains unclear but likely results from a lower parasite load. This lower parasite load is possibly secondary to more rapid clearance of infected cells or to inhibition of parasite invasion by the sickle cells.

PATHOPHYSIOLOGY

At the molecular level, the hydrophobic valine at the sixth position is exposed with deoxygenation of the hemoglobin. The hydrophobic valine fits into neighboring hydrophobic pockets of the beta-globin chains and results in polymer formation. Other interactions stabilize the polymer and form an HbS gel. The HbS gel distorts the red blood cell (RBC), increasing viscosity of the RBCs and causing sludging in the microvasculature. After deoxygenation, the time to gel formation in vitro may be hastened by elevation of the mean corpuscular hemoglobin concentration (MCHC) or temperature, decrease in pH, or increases in ionic strength. Elevations in HbA or fetal hemoglobin (HbF) may delay the time to gel formation, HbF having a greater effect than HbA. Both HbF and HbA increase the solubility of HbS with decreased HbS polymer formation. The knowledge of these interactions and influences on sickling has led to novel approaches for treatment. The combined effects of HbS polymerization, oxidant production by the denatured hemoglobin, and deposition of iron have detrimental effects on the RBC membrane. The abnormalities include increased membrane rigidity, abnormal membrane permeability with resulting erythrocyte dehydration, promotion of adhesion to endothelial cells, and accumulation of surface immunoglobulin. The end result of the molecular and cellular abnormalities of the sickle cell is a chronic hemolytic anemia and episodic vaso-occlusion. These vaso-occlusive events lead to tissue ischemia and organ damage.

DIAGNOSIS

Prenatal diagnosis can be made with polymerase chain reaction (PCR) amplification of DNA obtained through chorionic villous biopsy or amniocentesis. Counseling by a professional well versed in SCD should accompany prenatal diagnosis, because the severity of the disease varies from person to person. Although this technique is available, improvements in supportive care have greatly improved survival with SCD, making prenatal diagnosis less of an issue.

Neonatal screening is now done routinely with electrophoresis. With early identification of patients at risk, parental education, and institution of penicillin prophylaxis, infant mortality rates have been greatly reduced. Evaluation of the smear may not be helpful in the newborn period, because the typical peripheral blood smear for SCD is usually not evident at this early age. The characteristic sickled cells, target cells, spherocytes, and nucleated RBCs are usually apparent by the age of 3 years. The anemia of SCD usually manifests as the fetal hemoglobin level begins to fall at about 4 months of age.

The sickle preparation and solubility tests are both rapid means of detecting the presence of HbS, but they do not differentiate between SCT and SCD. These tests may be useful in an acute care setting. However, a definitive diagnosis should be made by means of hemoglobin electrophoresis or other methods that can identify additional abnormal hemoglobins. Typical electrophoresis patterns for newborns and adults are shown in Table 1, along with the representative hemoglobin and mean corpuscular volume (MCV) range for the most common syndromes. Identification of SCT is important in order to ensure appropriate genetic counseling.

No increases in morbidity or mortality rates have been found in large studies of patients with SCT. However, rare reports of sudden death and vaso-occlusion in patients with SCT are noted in the literature. SCT is associated with hyposthenuria and may also result in hematuria. Extreme changes in altitude have been correlated with splenic infarction in patients with SCT.

CLINICAL MANIFESTATIONS

Clinical manifestations of SCD vary greatly with the various disorders and among patients with the

TABLE 1. **Hemoglobin (Hb) Electrophoresis Patterns for the Most Common Sickle Cell Syndromes, with Typical Hb Concentrations and Mean Corpuscular Volume (MCV)**

Syndrome	Neonatal Electrophoresis Pattern	Adult Electrophoresis Pattern (%)	Hemoglobin (gm/dL)	MCV (fL)
Normal (HbA)	FA	HbA >96 HbF <2 HbA$_2$ <3.5	Normal (12–16)	Normal (80–95)
Sickle trait (HbAS)	FAS	HbA 60 HbS 40 HbF <2 HbA$_2$ <3.5	Normal	Normal
Sickle cell anemia (HbSS)	FS	HbS >80 HbF 2–20 HbA$_2$ 2–3	6–10	80–100
Sickle β^0-thalassemia	FS	HbS >80 HbF 2–15 HbA$_2$ 3.5–7	6–10	60–80
Sickle hemoglobin C (HbSC)	FSC	HbS 45–50 HbC 45–50	9–12	70–90
Sickle β$^+$-thalassemia	FSA	HbS 70–90 HbA 5–30 HbF 2–10 HbA$_2$ >3.5	8–12	65–75
Sickle–hereditary persistence of fetal hemoglobin (HbS-HPFH)	FS	HbS >70 HbF 13–30 HbA$_2$ <2.5	Normal	80–100

same disorder. Patients with SCA or S-β°-thalassemia are generally troubled with the most severe clinical courses, with more severe hemolysis and more episodes of vaso-occlusion. Patients with sickle hemoglobin C (HbSC), sickle cell β$^+$-thalassemia, or S-hereditary persistence of fetal hemoglobin (S-HPFH) usually have milder courses. Even within the group of patients with SCA, severity can range from rare episodes of vaso-occlusion treated primarily at home, to frequent severe painful episodes with complications necessitating hospitalization.

The clinical manifestations of SCD may be acute or chronic, and the underlying cause is increasing hemolysis, worsening anemia, or vaso-occlusion.

Acute Complications of Anemia

Aplastic Crisis

Aplastic crisis, or transient erythroblastopenia, is often secondary to infection with parvovirus but can occur with other infections. Aplastic crisis is a result of diminished RBC production in addition to the underlying chronic hemolytic anemia. RBC survival in SCA is shortened to 10 to 50 days, in comparison with the normal RBC survival of 120 days. Patients with SCA compensate with increased hematopoietic activity. In the wake of parvovirus or other infections, erythroid differentiation is halted, and the precarious balance between RBC production and destruction is lost. Reticulocytosis drops, with a resulting fall in hemoglobin. Symptoms of aplastic crisis are those of any acute anemia, including pallor and lethargy. Parvovirus infection can be documented with viral titers. Patients usually show signs of recovery within approximately 10 days but may require treatment with transfusion if the anemia is severe.

Splenic Sequestration

Splenic sequestration is the syndrome of rapid entrapment of RBCs within the spleen, with splenic enlargement and a fall in the hemoglobin by more than 2 to 3 grams per dL. This is the cause of death in approximately 5 to 10% of patients with SCD. This syndrome can occur as early as 2 months of age and is rarely seen after the age of 5 years in patients with SCA. Sequestration may occur later in children with HbSC or sickle cell β-thalassemia in whom autosplenectomy is delayed. Episodes of splenic sequestration may occur alone or in combination with acute chest syndrome, a painful episode, or infection. Symptoms include pallor, weakness, abdominal distention, and left-sided abdominal pain. Patients are noted to be tachycardic and dyspneic with splenomegaly and may deteriorate rapidly to hypovolemic shock. Laboratory evaluation reveals an acute drop in hemoglobin below the patient's baseline, with reticulocytosis. Thrombocytopenia is often present and is caused by splenic entrapment of platelets. Episodes of sequestration of the spleen may be mild, necessitating no definitive therapy, or can progress rapidly and lead to death. Adequate hydration with intravenous fluids at 1.5 times maintenance levels may reverse less severe episodes. Patients should be closely monitored for signs of progression. Hypovolemia and lack of oxygen-carrying capacity should be corrected rapidly with transfusion of packed RBCs or whole blood.

Approximately half the patients who survive the first episode have a recurrence of splenic sequestration. This recurrent episode often occurs within 4 months after the first event. Approaches to maintenance care include close monitoring by instructing parents to monitor spleen size, institution of a maintenance transfusion program, or surgical splenectomy. Some authorities advocate splenectomy after the first episode of splenic sequestration; others promote splenectomy after repeated episodes. The current plan of care in our institution is to defer splenectomy until age 5 if possible, because the risk for postsplenectomy infection is lower after this age.

Vaso-occlusive Events

PAINFUL EPISODES

Acute painful episodes are the most common symptom of SCD. Pain is caused by infarction of bones, bone marrow, or other organs. The most common sites for painful episodes after the third or fourth year of life are the long bones (more frequently in the humerus, tibia, and femur), the vertebrae, the abdomen, and the chest. In infancy, dactylitis, or "hand-foot" syndrome, is the most common manifestation of SCD. Infarction of the metacarpals and metatarsals causes this syndrome and results in swelling and pain in the hands and feet. Patients may refuse to bear weight on them. Fever and leukocytosis may accompany dactylitis. Treatment for dactylitis is the same as for other painful episodes.

Painful episodes in the abdomen may mimic peritonitis or appendicitis. An elevation of the WBC count, fever, or lack of response to the usual measures make a diagnosis that requires surgical exploration more likely. In this case, the patient should take nothing by mouth, and a surgical consultation should be obtained. Obstruction of the biliary tree may be the cause of right upper quadrant pain. Abdominal ultrasonography and evaluation of bilirubin and liver function tests are performed if this is suspected.

Signs and symptoms of painful episodes include tenderness to palpation and swelling over the affected site. Warmth, erythema, and diminished range of motion may be present. Painful episodes can mimic osteomyelitis, and it may be difficult to differentiate the two. A culture is needed for a definitive diagnosis of osteomyelitis. However, it is important to remember that painful episodes due to infarction are much more common than osteomyelitis in the patient with SCD. If the pain is typical for a patient and is responding to the usual measures for episodic pain, osteomyelitis is less likely.

Painful episodes have been attributed to infection, fever, dehydration, stress, and climate changes. However, no cause is identified in most patients. The severity of pain varies widely from mild events that can be managed at home to severe events necessitating hospitalization. Episodes usually last 3 to 5 days but may be prolonged in some patients.

The diagnosis of a painful episode is best made with a careful history and physical examination. Older children and adults can determine whether the pain is typical for their SCD. Pain level should be documented with numerical or visual analogue scales for older children and adults. Face scales for younger children help determine the severity of pain. In infants, parental ratings or behavioral indicators are used. There is no objective method for measuring pain, and so the report of the patient or parent should be accepted. Radiographs of the affected area are usually not helpful in acute episodes. Likewise, painful episodes are not associated with definitive changes in the complete blood count. Hemoglobin levels or amount of sickled cells on the smear cannot predict severity of an episode.

Treatment for painful episodes depends on the severity of the event. Attempts at home therapy can be made initially. Combinations of acetaminophen (10 to 15 mg per kg per dose every 4 to 6 hours; 24-hour maximum of 5 doses per day) and a nonsteroidal anti-inflammatory drug (ibuprofen, 10 mg per kg per dose every 6 hours) are used for milder episodes. Acetaminophen with codeine (0.5 to 1.0 mg codeine per kg per dose every 4 to 6 hours) may be used to strengthen the home regimen. Sufficient oral hydration should be stressed.

If treatment at home fails, the patient is evaluated in the clinic or emergency department. Adequate hydration is ensured with hypotonic intravenous fluids given at a rate of 1.5 times the maintenance level. Parenteral narcotics are the next line of therapy for patients with moderate to severe pain. The drug of choice in our institution is nalbuphine (Nubain) with a bolus dose of 0.3 mg per kg intravenously (maximal dose, 20 mg). This bolus may be repeated every 20 minutes for two additional doses. If adequate pain control is achieved, the patient is discharged to home with a sufficient supply of oral narcotics, NSAIDs, and acetaminophen. The patient should be instructed to take the oral pain medications on a scheduled basis for at least 48 hours. Oral fluid intake is again stressed.

If pain is not tolerably controlled in the emergency department or clinic, the patient is admitted for continuous parenteral narcotics. Nalbuphine is the first choice, at a starting dose of 0.075 mg per kg per hour. This infusion may be gradually increased to a maximum of 0.15 mg per kg per hour. The maximal daily dose for nalbuphine, 160 mg, must also be considered when this drug is used: Some patients cannot receive the hourly maximum without surpassing the daily limit. Although nalbuphine is preferred in our institution as a means of lowering the incidence of acute chest syndrome, therapy must be individualized. Some patients prefer certain medications. Hydromorphone hydrochloride (Dilaudid) and fentanyl (Sublimaze) are other options, followed by morphine. The dosage of narcotic is routinely divided between a continuous infusion and additional patient-controlled analgesia (PCA). PCA empowers patients, gives them more control in their treatment, and allows for an immediate bolus when required (within set parameters). This method is also a useful tool for monitoring a patient's course, because the PCA demands decrease as the pain improves. PCA is helpful in allowing a patient to self-wean as well.

Adjuvant therapies are used in addition to intravenous narcotics. Acetaminophen (Tylenol) and a nonsteroidal anti-inflammatory drug are scheduled every 6 hours. Hydroxyzine (Atarax) at a dose of 0.5 mg per kg orally every 6 hours may be used to potentiate the effects of the narcotics. Heat, transcutaneous electrical nerve stimulation (TENS) units, whirlpool, and relaxation techniques are other measures that may be beneficial. Transfusion of packed RBCs and provision of oxygen at the onset of painful episodes do not shorten the course of the event and are not indicated.

ACUTE CHEST SYNDROME

The syndrome of acute chest is the leading cause of death in patients over 10 years of age with SCD. The simplest definition of acute chest syndrome is a new infiltrate on chest radiograph. Some clinicians, including the authors, require that the patient show signs of hypoxia. Fever, tachypnea, and chest pain are other presenting symptoms. Abdominal pain may be the initial complaint in some patients. Acute chest syndrome is seen more commonly in patients with higher hemoglobin levels and lower fetal hemoglobin levels. The cause of acute chest syndrome may be infection, infarction, or a combination of factors. The source of the event is usually difficult to detect. In most cases, an infectious cause is not proven. When infection is documented, *Pneumococcus, Mycoplasma, Salmonella,* and *Klebsiella* species and *H. influenzae* are the organisms most commonly involved. Pulmonary fat embolization may be a significant cause of acute chest syndrome. In a study of 27 patients with acute chest syndrome, pulmonary fat embolus (thought to be secondary to bone marrow necrosis) was identified in 12 of those patients.

In evaluation of a patient for acute chest syndrome, the complete blood cell count (CBC) may reveal a drop in the hemoglobin level in comparison with baseline levels. The WBC count is often increased, and reticulocytosis may be present. The chest radiograph may not be abnormal initially. However, an infiltrate may appear or become more prominent as the patient is hydrated. An arterial blood gas measurement with room air is needed if acute chest syndrome is suspected. If the baseline oxygen saturation for the patient is known, trends in transcutaneous oxygen saturation may provide some assistance.

Treatment involves the use of supplemental oxygen if the patient is hypoxic. Incentive spirometry, percussion therapy, and albuterol nebulizations may be useful in preventing further atelectasis. Another means of preventing atelectasis is to ensure that the patient is out of bed several times a day when possible. Intravenous fluids are given at a rate of 1.5 times the maintenance level until the patient is rehydrated. At that time, the infusion is decreased to maintenance levels to prevent fluid overload. Empirical antibiotic therapy is given to cover the typical organisms. Cefuroxime sodium (Zinacef; 50 mg per kg intravenously every 8 hours) and erythromycin are chosen in our institution. Analgesics are administered carefully to avoid oversedation or undersedation, either of which may cause atelectasis. In milder episodes and when the hemoglobin level is below baseline, patients are treated with a simple transfusion. More severe or progressive episodes necessitate exchange transfusion. One article promoted the use of intravenous dexamethasone (0.3 mg per kg every 12 hours for 4 doses) in patients with mild to moderately severe acute chest syndrome. The patients who received dexamethasone had shorter hospital stays, a reduced need for blood transfusion, and shorter duration of analgesic and oxygen therapy than did patients who received placebo.

Acute Central Nervous System Events

Cerebrovascular accidents (CVAs) are responsible for devastating morbidity and are the second leading cause of death in one study of patients with SCD. The incidence of CVAs in children with SCA is approximately 7 to 8%. The Cooperative Study of Sickle Cell Disease reported a 4% overall incidence of CVAs. This complication is less common in patients with HbSC or sickle cell β^+-thalassemia but should be considered. CVA recurs in approximately 70% of untreated patients, usually within 3 years of the previous attack and with a more severe outcome. CVA usually occurs without warning but may manifest with painful episodes, aplastic crisis, or infectious illnesses. CVA occurs in patients after the age of 1 year; infarctive events are more common in children, and hemorrhagic events are most common in adults aged 20 to 29 years. A combination of the two types of stroke can also take place. Infarctive stroke usually occurs in larger vessels, secondary to stenosis or obstruction. The underlying pathophysiologic process consists of thrombus formation, embolization, or proliferation of smooth muscle and fibroblasts over damaged endothelium. The middle cerebral, anterior cerebral, and distal internal carotid arteries are often involved with infarctive CVA. Hemorrhagic stroke may be secondary to aneurysms of collateral or weakened vessels.

Risk factors for infarctive CVA include a prior episode of a transient ischemic attack (TIA), a recent episode of acute chest syndrome, and elevated systolic blood pressure. Patients most commonly come to medical attention with dysarthria, dysphagia, focal seizures, gait difficulties, hemiparesis, or hemiplegia. With hemorrhagic stroke, a severe headache, syncope, meningismus, or photophobia may be the initial complaint. A physical examination with a thorough neurologic evaluation is indicated in any patient with SCD and potential neurologic symptoms. Computed tomography or magnetic resonance imaging should be performed to rule out intracranial hemorrhage. Noninvasive magnetic resonance angiography allows definition of cerebral vessels without the use of hypertonic radiocontrast and its associated risk of sickling.

Treatment for CVA includes immediate hydration,

frequent neurologic assessment, and antiepileptic medications if seizures are present. Exchange transfusion is the standard initial therapy. Alternatively, simple transfusion may be used primarily in stable patients with no progressive symptoms and a hemoglobin level below steady state. A hemoglobin level of more than 12 grams per dL must be avoided in order to avert further difficulties from hyperviscosity. Simple or exchange transfusion is followed by a program of maintenance transfusion therapy every 3 to 6 weeks to maintain an HbS level of less than 30%. Up to 50% of patients may have complete or nearly complete recovery with rapid, aggressive transfusion therapy. The risk of CVA recurrence is approximately 70% in untreated patients and is highest in the first 3 years after the initial event. Maintenance transfusion therapy reduces this risk to 10%; most of these events consist of TIAs. Maintenance transfusion therapy clearly improves the mortality rate as well. Patients with a history of stroke should be maintained on a routine transfusion program indefinitely. Attempts have been made to liberalize the HbS level to 40 to 50% or to stop transfusion therapy after a period of time. However, CVA has recurred after completion of 5- to 12-year maintenance transfusion programs. The dangers of maintenance transfusion include infection risks, sensitization, and iron overload. Partial exchange transfusions decrease the overall iron burden. Iron chelation should be included in the maintenance transfusion protocol once iron overload is established.

One of the greatest difficulties has been identifying patients at risk for stroke and preventing the first CVA. Significant advances have been made in this area. Elevated velocities in the internal carotid or middle cerebral artery as evaluated by transcranial Doppler (TCD) ultrasonography have been strongly associated with an increased risk of stroke. This knowledge has been used in the Stroke Prevention Trial in Sickle Cell Anemia (STOP) to combine TCD evaluations with blood transfusions to identify patients at risk and evaluate the utility of maintenance transfusions to prevent CVA. Criteria for identifying patients at risk for stroke were defined as having two TCDs with an elevated mean blood flow velocity. Patients were randomly assigned to prophylactic transfusions that maintained the HbS below 30% or to standard care. Maintenance transfusion therapy was shown to significantly reduce the incidence of first stroke in patients with abnormal TCD. Patients with SCA disease or S-β°-thalassemia should therefore be screened beginning at age 2 years to determine the need for prophylactic transfusions.

Priapism

Priapism can occur at any age in males with SCD. In one study, the median age at onset was 21 years. The pathophysiologic process consists of obstruction of venous outflow from the corpora cavernosum. Two forms of priapism are seen: stuttering priapism, which consists of multiple short episodes, and severe prolonged priapism, in which painful erection lasts more than 24 hours. In one study, stuttering priapism was shown to advance to prolonged episodes in 28% of patients. Acute urinary retention may complicate priapism. In a study of Jamaican patients with a history of priapism, a 46% incidence of sexual dysfunction was reported.

Initial treatment for priapism consists of hydration with hypotonic fluids and analgesia. If no improvement is seen in 4 to 6 hours, simple or exchange transfusion is warranted. Surgical procedures are available and should be considered if the patient is unresponsive to less aggressive measures. The approaches include corporal aspiration and irrigation or construction of a fistula between the glans and corpora cavernosum. Patients with frequent episodes of priapism may benefit from a short course of maintenance transfusion therapy.

Infections

Bacterial infections are the leading cause of death in children with SCD. These patients are at highest risk for infection with *Pneumococcus,* a polysaccharide encapsulated organism. Other commonly seen pathogens include *H. influenzae* type B, *Staphylococcus aureus, Streptococcus viridans, Escherichia coli,* and *Salmonella* species. The increased rate and severity of infections in this population result from splenic dysfunction with abnormal clearance of bacteria from the intravascular space and impaired antibody synthesis. Sepsis, pneumonia, meningitis, urinary tract infections, and osteomyelitis are seen most frequently.

Immediate evaluation is recommended for patients with SCD and a fever of 101.5°F or higher or the presence of other symptoms indicative of sepsis (lethargy or poor feeding). A complete evaluation includes a thorough history and physical examination; CBC and reticulocyte count; urinalysis; blood, urine, and throat cultures; and a chest radiograph. Stool cultures and a lumbar puncture with cultures of spinal fluid should be obtained if indicated by the history and physical examination. In ill-appearing patients, pneumococcal sepsis should be presumed. These patients should receive appropriate antibiotics on arrival to the emergency department or clinic, before cultures or other laboratory studies are obtained. On the basis of the initial assessment of the patient, CBC, and chest radiograph, patients may be categorized into two treatment groups: toxic and nontoxic. Nontoxic patients have a temperature of less than 40°C (104°F), WBC count of less than 30,000 with no left shift, and no infiltrate on chest radiograph; they generally may be managed as outpatients. These patients are given ceftriaxone (Rocephin), 50 mg per kg, and then are monitored for several hours. If such a patient is stable and reliable transportation is established, the patient is discharged with follow-up the next day for a second dose of ceftriaxone and evaluation of culture results.

Patients are considered potentially toxic if the WBC is greater than 30,000 or less than 5000, a left shift is noted on the differential, or the temperature is greater than 40°C (104°F). Patients who have a pulmonary infiltrate or have no reliable transportation generally require admission to the hospital for intravenous antibiotics and monitoring. Cefuroxime sodium (Zinacef), 50 mg per kg per dose every 8 hours, provides broad-spectrum coverage for the common infecting organisms. However, the institutional sensitivities should be considered in the choice of a specific regimen, especially in areas with known penicillin- and cephalosporin-resistant *Pneumococcus* strains. Antibiotics are continued until the patient has been afebrile for 24 hours and cultures have been negative for 48 hours. Prevention of infection in the population with SCD has been previously discussed in the section on preventive care.

Chronic Manifestations of Sickle Cell Disease

Growth and Development

Growth curves generated by the Cooperative Study of Sickle Cell Disease (CSSCD) demonstrate delays in both weight and height, with greater improvement in height by the end of adolescence. Delays are greater in patients with SCA and S-β°-thalassemia. Growth delays have been attributed to increased caloric requirements as a result of amplified hematopoietic activity and cardiac output. Delayed sexual development has also been noted in patients with SCD. Decreased fertility has not been reported in females. However, abnormal sperm motility and lower sperm counts have been documented in some males.

Eyes

Proliferative retinopathy is a serious ocular complication of SCD. Manifestations range in severity from stage I retinopathy with peripheral arteriolar occlusion to stage 5 with retinal detachment. In a Jamaican investigation, 20% of the eyes examined showed evidence for proliferative retinopathy during the course of the study. Treatment with laser therapy may be helpful but remains controversial because blindness may be a complication of therapy. Painless vision loss is a rare complication of occlusion of a central retinal artery.

Heart

Systolic and diastolic ejection murmurs, a split S_1, and an S_3 may be auscultated in patients with SCD. Cardiomegaly is present in the majority of older patients, and left ventricular hypertrophy is seen on electrocardiograms in approximately 50% of patients. These findings usually result from compensation for the chronic hemolytic anemia. Myocardial infarctions are surprisingly rare in patients with SCD. Increased sickling is not noted in the coronary arteries, possibly as a result of the short transit time for the RBCs in the coronary vessels. SCD also appears to confer a protective effect toward development of atherosclerosis.

Lung

Chronic lung disease secondary to recurrent infarction ranges in severity from a chronic cough to severe pulmonary hypertension. Patients with SCD maintain a lower resting arterial partial oxygen pressure. These patients also have lower vital and total lung capacities.

Renal System

An inability to produce concentrated urine results in hyposthenuria in patients with SCD and SCT. This promotes dehydration and prohibits the use of the urine specific gravity for assessment of hydration status. Nocturia or enuresis ensues in approximately 50% of patients with SCD. Nephrotic syndrome may also be seen in association with SCD. Affected patients are often unresponsive to therapy, and the condition may advance to renal failure.

Hepatobiliary System

Gallstones are noted frequently in patients with SCD as a result of the chronic hemolytic anemia. In one investigation, 42% of 15- to 18-year-old patients with SCA were reported to have gallstones. Another study reported an overall incidence of gallstones in 13% of patients between the ages of 5 and 13 years. Prophylactic cholecystectomy is not recommended for asymptomatic patients. Cholecystectomy may be performed in a patient with recurrent right upper quadrant pain and gallstones, but it does not resolve the pain episodes in every patient. Moderate hepatomegaly is often noted in patients with SCD. Hepatitis related to transfusion is also seen in the population with SCD.

Skin

Leg ulcers usually occur in regions of the medial tibia and posterior to the medial malleolus. This is a complication in as many as 75% of patients in certain geographic areas. Skin breakdown may be secondary to elevations in the venous pressure of the legs with increased hematopoietic activity and expansion of the bone marrow volume. Impairments in wound healing may also contribute to the process. Treatment involves routine wound care with rest, elevation of the lower extremities, and débridement if necessary. Compression hose may be used to prevent the occurrence of ulcers. Oral zinc has been reported to improve healing.

Bones

The characteristic "hair on end" and flattened "codfish" vertebrae result from the marrow expansion in patients with the chronic hemolytic anemia. The more serious bony complication of SCD is avascular necrosis (AVN), usually of the femoral head but also occurring in the head of the humerus. SCD is the most common cause of AVN of the femoral head in the pediatric population. By one report, AVN occurs in 19% of patients with SCA and 9% of patients with HbSC. Approximately half the affected patients are symptomatic with pain and decreased mobility. AVN may develop as a result of elevations in pressure within the bone marrow after ischemic events. Vaso-occlusive infarctions within the femoral head may affect the vascular supply. Bone is remodeled, and resorption occurs with collapse of the femoral head.

The diagnosis of AVN is made with radiographs, showing a widened joint space, flattened epiphysis, and widening of the femoral neck. Treatment for mild cases involves avoidance of weight bearing. Patients who have completed growth with severe AVN may benefit from prosthetic hip replacement.

Spleen

Functional asplenia occurs by 5 to 36 months of age. Continued infarction leads to autosplenectomy, in which the spleen is reduced to a small, fibrotic piece of tissue. The consequences of asplenia are discussed in the section on infections.

PREVENTIVE CARE AND HEALTH MAINTENANCE

Comprehensive medical care has been shown to contribute to increased life expectancy in patients with SCD. Patients for whom a neonatal electrophoresis screen is suggestive of SCD should be referred to a center knowledgeable in sickle cell syndromes. Early teaching about the implications of SCD and confirmation testing are performed, preferably before the patient is 2 months old. These measures allow physicians to begin penicillin prophylaxis, greatly reducing the risk of morbidity and mortality in children. Penicillin prophylaxis in SCA patients has been shown to reduce the incidence of pneumococcal infection by 84%, in comparison with placebo. For SCA or sickle cell β°-thalassemia (S-β°-thalassemia), prophylactic penicillin is given in dosages of 125 mg orally twice a day for patients younger than 3 years, 250 mg orally twice a day for patients aged 3 to 12 years, and 500 mg orally twice a day for patients older than 12 years. Erythromycin ethylsuccinate is given to patients allergic to penicillin. Patients should remain on penicillin or erythromycin prophylaxis until 5 years of age. If pneumococcal infection is documented, penicillin or erythromycin prophylaxis is continued indefinitely. Parents are taught the signs and symptoms of sepsis, aplastic crisis, splenic sequestration, and vaso-occlusive episodes. A plan of care should be identified for the parents. Specifically, any child with SCD and a temperature above 101.5°F, an enlarging spleen, or new onset of pallor should be examined on an emergency basis.

Routine comprehensive clinic visits are scheduled on a yearly basis. These visits should include a thorough physical examination to document the spleen size, baseline murmurs, and jaundice. Laboratory evaluation at a well visit can define a patient's typical hemoglobin, platelet count, white blood cell (WBC) count, and reticulocyte level. This information can be extremely helpful when the patient seeks emergency care with possible acute chest or splenic sequestration syndrome. Renal and liver function are monitored yearly after the age of 5. Eye examinations are performed yearly after 7 years of age. Chest radiographs and pulmonary function should be considered every 3 to 5 years after the age of 5.

Patients are immunized against *Haemophilus influenzae* and hepatitis B as infants, on the standard schedule. Pneumococcal vaccine is given at age 2, with a booster at 5 years of age.

Anticipatory guidance is an important component of the regular clinic visit. The symptoms of infection, aplastic crisis, and splenic sequestration should be reviewed. Plans for coping with painful episodes at home will reduce hospital admissions and emergency room visits. Monitoring of growth and nutrition, yearly dental screening, genetic counseling, and birth control are other significant issues to include in the visit. Psychologic aspects, such as fear of death, chronic pain, and worry about growth delays should be addressed. As the patient reaches adulthood, a smooth transition from the pediatric facility to an adult center is essential.

TREATMENT

Transfusion Therapy

A simple transfusion usually suffices for patients with aplastic crisis and splenic sequestration. Simple transfusions are sometimes indicated in milder cases of acute chest syndrome or for central nervous system events if the hemoglobin level is below baseline. A hemoglobin level of more than 12 grams per dL should be avoided in patients with SCD in order to reduce the effects of hyperviscosity. Simple transfusion is also used in preparation for surgery, as discussed later. Partial exchange transfusion is conventionally employed with most central nervous system events and with more severe or progressive episodes of acute chest syndrome. Maintenance transfusion programs are indicated for patients at risk for CVA and for patients with recurrent acute chest syndrome, splenic sequestration, or debilitating painful episodes. The goal of maintenance transfusion therapy is to reduce and maintain a lowered HbS level, usually less than 30%. This lessens the frequency of vaso-occlusive events. Iron overload is a complication of maintenance transfusion therapy and should be monitored closely. Treatment consists of chelation with desferrioxamine. Alloimmunization, another complication of maintenance transfusion, occurs in less than 25% of patients. Antigen-matched packed RBCs would therefore be preferred but are expensive and more difficult to obtain. Some authors suggest antigen matching for the most common antibody-inciting antigens (K, C, E, S, Fy^a, Fy^b, and Jk^b).

Surgery

Complications of surgery are known to occur in patients with SCD. However, with careful management, these problems may potentially be avoided. A simple transfusion should be given to reach a preoperative hemoglobin level of 10 grams per dL. Strict attention to oxygenation, avoidance of temperature extremes, and provision of maintenance intravenous fluids are important prophylactic measures in the perioperative period. Even with preoperative transfusion, a 10% incidence of acute chest syndrome was noted after surgery in a multi-institutional study. A history of acute chest syndrome was noted to be a risk factor for postoperative episodes.

Bone Marrow Transplantation

Allogeneic transplantation is a potentially curative treatment for SCD. An ongoing multicenter trial reports promising data. Of the 34 children with SCD who have received transplants from HLA-identical siblings, 32 have survived; 28 of these patients had stable engraftment. A 93% survival rate and a 79% event-free survival rate are reported. Patients who underwent transplantation had a history of CVA, recurrent acute chest syndrome, or recurrent vaso-occlusive crises. Despite the encouraging results, difficulties with transplantation exist. Only a low percentage of patients have a matched-sibling, sickle cell–negative donor. Furthermore, older patients do not tolerate the complications of allogeneic bone marrow transplantation as well as do younger patients without significant organ toxicity. However, it is difficult to identify which patients with severe disease would benefit most from transplantation. Further studies are needed to identify early which patients are at risk for complications of SCD.

Hydroxyurea

As previously discussed, higher levels of HbF inhibit HbS polymerization in vitro. Patients with higher HbF levels have less severe disease. This knowledge is the basis for the use of hydroxyurea* (Hydrea), which increases HbF production. Use of hydroxyurea in adults has been shown to reduce the frequency of painful episodes, acute chest syndrome, and transfusions. Concerns regarding the potential teratogenicity and carcinogenicity of the drug warrant limited pediatric use until ongoing studies are completed. A phase II multicenter trial is currently under way to evaluate the effects of hydroxyurea in children with SCD.

Antisickling Agents

With increasing knowledge of the molecular pathophysiologic processes of SCD, numerous agents are being evaluated for potential antisickling effects. Medications are being studied for possible inhibition of the transport pumps that cause erythrocyte dehydration. Purified poloxamer 188 (Flocor), a surfactant with hemorrheologic and antithrombotic properties, is currently under investigation. Preliminary studies show evidence of shorter duration of painful episodes, shorter hospital stays, fewer analgesic requirements, and less pain intensity in patients receiving Flocor.

PROGNOSIS

The overall life expectancy for patients with SCA is 42 years for males and 48 years for females. With HbSC, the life expectancy is 60 for males and 68 years for females. Most childhood deaths are a result of sepsis, the highest mortality rate occurring between the ages of 1 and 3 years. Other causes of death in pediatric patients include acute chest syndrome, acute splenic sequestration, and stroke. Most adult deaths were not associated with a diagnosis of chronic illness. The majority of adult deaths in patients with SCD occurred in conjunction with acute chest syndrome, stroke, or painful episodes.

NEUTROPENIA

method of
BONNIE P. CHAM, M.D.
University of Manitoba and Manitoba Cancer Treatment and Research Foundation, Health Sciences Centre
Winnipeg, Manitoba, Canada

Neutropenia is defined as a decrease in the number of absolute circulating neutrophils. The age and, to a certain extent, race of the patient defines the normal absolute neutrophil count (ANC). The ANC is calculated as the total white blood cell count (WBC) multiplied by the percentage of neutrophils and bands. A normal ANC between 2 weeks and 1 year of age is more than 1000 per dL and after the first year, the normal count is more than 1500 per dL. Black persons have somewhat lower neutrophil counts, the lower limit of normal being 1200 per dL.

The number of circulating neutrophils depends on the rate of entry from the marrow and the rate of migration into the tissues. Therefore, neutropenia can result from failure of neutrophils to develop or egress from the marrow, from increased consumption or pooling in the tissues or circulation, or from a combination of both. Severe neutropenia (ANC < 500 per dL) can be associated with life-threatening infections, because neutrophils are important in protecting from invasive bacterial infections. Certain neutropenias may also be associated with abnormalities of neutrophil function or with abnormalities of other immune parameters. It is therefore important to attempt to characterize the etiology of the neutropenia in order to develop an appropriate plan for management.

CLINICAL MANIFESTATIONS

There are no particular symptoms associated with neutropenia other than the propensity for infections. Neutropenia may therefore be noticed on a routine laboratory test or as part of a work-up of either a significant infection or recurrent infections. Neutropenia may occur as an isolated finding or in combination with other cytopenias suggestive of more generalized marrow disease. In this setting, associ-

---

ated symptoms such as hemorrhage or fatigue may be among the manifestations.

DIFFERENTIAL DIAGNOSIS

Neutropenia may be either congenital or acquired. In general, the congenital neutropenias occur owing to decreased production of neutrophils. The congenital neutropenias usually manifest in childhood; the more severe forms manifest in infancy. Severe congenital neutropenia may occur as a result of an isolated failure of marrow production of neutrophils, such as that seen in Kostmann's congenital agranulocytosis, or occur in association with other abnormalities of the immune system, such as reticular dysgenesis. Other congenital disorders associated with severe neutropenia include Shwachman-Diamond syndrome, myelokathexis, and inborn errors of metabolism (e.g., glycogen-storage disease type Ib). In addition, neutropenia may be the manifesting sign of Fanconi's anemia. Severe neutropenia may also occur on a 19- to 21-day cycle as part of cyclic neutropenia. A more benign, often familial, neutropenia with associated monocytosis and neutrophil counts in the range of 250 to 1500 per dL has been termed *chronic benign neutropenia*.

Acquired neutropenias may be short-lived or chronic. Neutropenia associated with viral illness is often self-limiting and may be associated with viruses such as Epstein-Barr virus, the common childhood exanthems, and influenza A and B viruses, among others. Neutropenia may also be associated with human immunodeficiency virus (HIV) infection. It may follow exposure to drugs such as analgesics, antithyroid drugs, phenothiazines, sulfonamides, synthetic penicillins, and certain anticonvulsants on an idiosyncratic basis, or it may follow exposure to cytotoxic cancer chemotherapy and therapeutic irradiation. Neutropenia has also appeared after exposure to toxins, including heavy metals and organic compounds such as benzene. It may occur on a nutritional basis in relation to specific deficiencies of vitamin B_{12}, folate, and copper. Neutropenia may also be the manifesting symptom of infiltrative marrow disorders such as leukemia, metastatic malignancy, or metabolic storage diseases such as Gaucher's disease.

Acquired neutropenia related to decreased survival, rather than to marrow dysfunction, may be related to an autoimmune neutropenia that may be isolated or associated with other connective tissue diseases such as systemic lupus erythematosus or rheumatoid arthritis. Autoimmune neutropenia of infancy most often occurs within the first few years of life, after a viral infection, and tends to resolve by the age of 5 or 6 years. Immune destruction of neutrophils may also occur after multiple transfusions because of the development of antibodies directed against HLA or neutrophil-specific antibodies. Finally, splenomegaly may cause a mild neutropenia that usually is accompanied by anemia and thrombocytopenia.

EVALUATION

A thorough history with attention to recent exposure to drugs, radiation, or chemicals capable of inducing neutropenia is important. Any history of antecedent viral infection should be noted. A history of prior bacterial infections should be obtained, with particular attention to periodontal disease, mouth infection, perirectal or skin cellulitis, pneumonia, or sepsis. The family history may reveal recurrent infection or bone marrow failure syndromes in other family members. In the physical examination, particular attention should be paid to growth parameters in children, any physical anomalies that can be associated with disorders such as Fanconi's anemia or Shwachman-Diamond syndrome, and acute or chronic foci of infection.

In the absence of severe infectious complications or of clinical or historical findings suggestive of significant abnormalities, neutropenia may necessitate only observation. Medications that may be associated with neutropenia should be discontinued if possible. Serial blood cell counts will reveal whether the neutropenia is transient or persistent. Blood cell counts obtained two to three times weekly for 6 weeks will show whether a persistent neutropenia is cyclic or chronic.

If the neutropenia persists longer than 6 to 8 weeks, additional testing, such as serum studies for antineutrophil antibodies, serum copper, B_{12}, and folate levels and serologic investigations for connective tissues diseases, may be in order. A work-up of the humoral immune system may reveal associated abnormalities. HIV serologic study should be considered in the appropriate clinical setting. Bone marrow aspiration, which should be performed early if there are associated cytopenias or other worrisome clinical findings, may reveal the typical "maturation arrest" of a severe congenital neutropenia, the morphologic abnormalities associated with myelokathexis, or an abnormal infiltrate. If a bone marrow examination is undertaken, samples should undergo cytogenetic analysis as well as standard morphologic study, because certain neutropenias may be associated with preleukemic states and typical cytogenetic abnormalities, such as monosomy 7.

TREATMENT

Supportive Management

Management of the patient with neutropenia depends on the degree of the neutropenia, its etiology, and the patient's previous history of infections. General preventive measures should include good hand-washing, regular dental care with professional cleaning, and careful cleansing with antiseptic soaps of any skin punctures or lacerations. Rectal examinations and rectal temperature taking, as well as suppositories and enemas, should be avoided if possible.

Patients who are neutropenic but whose ANC is greater than 1000 per dL generally exhibit normal defense against infection and can be treated in the same manner as non-neutropenic patients with infections. Patients whose ANC is less than 500 per dL are at serious risk of bacterial infection, particularly from pathogens such as *Staphylococcus aureus* and gram-negative organisms. The onset of fever in these patients should be regarded as a medical emergency. By virtue of their low neutrophil counts, they may have few signs of inflammation and must be hospitalized and empirically treated with antibiotics while awaiting culture results. The antibiotics, which should be selected on the basis of local pathogens and susceptibility patterns, often include an aminoglycoside and a third-generation cephalosporin or penicillin with antipseudomonal activity (such as piperacillin). Patients with a neutrophil count between 500 and 1000 per dL may have difficulties with recurrent local infections (particularly oropharyngeal and periodontal disease) but generally do not require urgent hospitalization for fever.

For patients with recurrent infections, preventive medical therapy is desirable. Before the cytokine era, prophylactic antibiotics were the most effective means of attempting to prevent infections. The most popular antibiotics chosen in this setting are the penicillins and trimethoprim-sulfamethoxazole (Bactrim, Septra). Although antibiotics are thought to be effective in diminishing the frequency of infections, there can be significant problems associated with their continuous use. These include gastrointestinal complaints, a shift in organisms on the body's surfaces to be resistant to the antibiotic given, and allergic reactions.

Specific Therapy

In general, cytokines are reserved for patients who have frequent infections, a single life-threatening infection, or significant chronic gingivitis or periodontal disease. Granulocyte colony-stimulating factor (G-CSF) is the cytokine that has been used most frequently to treat severe chronic neutropenia, although there is a body of literature regarding the use of granulocyte-macrophage colony-stimulating factor (GM-CSF) after high-dose chemotherapy and in the setting of stem cell transplantation. A dose of 5 µg per kg per day given subcutaneously is generally recommended as a starting dose. Initially, frequent blood work (twice weekly) should be obtained in order to titrate the dose to the amount required to maintain the ANC between 1,500 per dL and 10,000 per dL. A range of doses from 1 µg per kg given two times a week to as high as 20 µg per kg* per day has been needed to achieve the desired effect. More than 90% of patients respond to G-CSF. Once a stable dosing regimen has been established, blood work can be obtained less frequently. Side effects include bone pain, splenomegaly, thrombocytopenia (which appears to be related to splenomegaly), and osteoporosis. In addition, patients with congenital severe chronic neutropenia have developed myelodysplastic syndromes and leukemia while receiving G-CSF, and thus this subgroup of patients should be monitored with yearly bone marrow aspirations with cytogenetic evaluations. This subgroup of patients had been observed to develop leukemia before the cytokine era, and it is thought that they represent a group of preleukemic patients. The G-CSF has not been shown to be causative in the development of leukemia. Patients in whom G-CSF fails may benefit from another cytokine, such as GM-CSF, either alone or in combination with G-CSF.

G-CSF is marketed as filgrastim (Neupogen) by AMGEN; GM-CSF is marketed as sargramostim (Leukine) by Immunex and distributed by Hoechst-Roussel Pharmaceuticals.

---

*Exceeds dosage recommended by the manufacturer.

HEMOLYTIC DISEASE OF THE FETUS AND NEWBORN

method of
VINOD K. BHUTANI, M.D.
*Pennsylvania Hospital
Philadelphia, Pennsylvania*

Hemolysis in the newborn results in increased bilirubin production and concomitant anemia and is associated with profound hypoalbuminemia in the fetus. The causes of hemolysis are (1) isoimmunization, (2) erythrocyte enzymopathies, (3) erythrocyte membrane disorders, and (4) hemoglobinopathies. Of these, isoimmunization is encountered in the fetus and the newborn most frequently. Fetal isoimmunization is likely related to Rh hemolytic disease, whereas, in the neonate, the more frequent and less severe cause of hemolysis is ABO or minor blood group incompatibility between the mother and her child. In this article, the focus is on immune-mediated hemolysis caused by Rh and ABO blood type incompatibilities.

Even with the approval of commercially prepared Rh D immune globulin (RhoGAM) in 1968 as a potent and effective weapon against hemolytic disease of the fetus and newborn, Rh isoimmunization remains a significant cause of neonatal morbidity and mortality. Hemolytic disease of the newborn (HDN) at one time was classified as individual diseases: erythroblastosis fetalis, congenital anemia, icterus gravis neonatorum, and hydrops fetalis. The clinical manifestations of HDN are mild disease in the form of anemia, affecting 50% of alloimmunized newborns; moderate disease with signs of hepatomegaly with moderate anemia, increasing jaundice and even kernicterus, affecting 30% of alloimmunized newborns; and severe disease in the form of hydrops, erythroblastosis fetalis, severe fetal anemia, and progressive neurotoxic hyperbilirubinemia, affecting 20% of alloimmunized newborns. In half these cases, hydrops develops before 30 weeks of gestation, and the fetus may die in utero without prenatal intervention.

Rh ISOIMMUNIZATION

In 1940 Landsteiner and Weiner developed rhesus monkey red blood cell antisera that, when added to blood from other monkeys and injected into rabbits, caused agglutination. The antisera were also found to cause agglutination in 85% of a tested white population in New York City, thus indicating that this proportion of subjects was Rh-positive and that the nonreactive 15% were Rh-negative. In comparison to an incidence of 15% in the white population, Rh antigen is absent in 8% of African-Americans and about 1% of Asians.

The five major Rh antigenic loci are C, D, E, c, and e; each class has many variations. The D antigen is more immunogenic than C, c, E, and e antigens and accounts for severe HDN. Most Rh D–negative (designated as dd) individuals have only Rh Cc and Rh Ee genes and no RhD gene. The d phenotype, classically Rh-negative, occurs because of a mutation deleting the D locus. Thus, no antiserum can be used to identify the heterozygous Rh-positive (Dd) individual. When the D antigen is present, the carrier is

Rh-positive. The Rh locus has been determined to be on the short arm of chromosome 12, and these antigens are inherited independently of ABO type. Of Rh-positive persons, 45% are homozygous (DD) and 55% are heterozygous (Dd). The risk of recurrent sensitization is 100% for homozygous persons and 50% for heterozygotes. It is possible to predict whether the father is homozygous or heterozygous, despite the lack of anti-d antibody, by using the serologic tests for the C, c, E, and e antigens and by considering phenotypes of the racial and ethnic populations to which the father belongs. The c antigen is found in 60% of white persons. Only a few cases of c-incompatibility have been described in the literature. The management of c-antigen sensitization is similar to that for anti-D sensitization.

Incidence, Risk, and Pathogenesis

Maternal sensitization and RhD alloimmunization occur when paternally inherited Rh D–positive blood cells cross the placenta and enter the circulatory system of an Rh D–negative (dd) mother. Initial exposure to D antigen leads to production of the IgM antibody. Because IgM is a larger immunoglobulin (molecular mass, 900,000 D), it cannot cross the placenta. Subsequent exposures (brief and very small) result in production of IgG (molecular mass, 155,000 D), which, unlike IgM, can cross the placenta. This is a frequent occurrence, particularly near or at the time of the delivery. The risk of isoimmunization in all Rh-negative ABO-compatible women after the first Rh-positive pregnancy is 8%. By the subsequent second pregnancy, the risk rises to 16%; if there are subsequent multiple deliveries with infusion of small exposures to Rh D–positive blood cells (<30 mL), the risk increases to about 50%. If there are multiple deliveries combined with large volumes of exposure (about 200 mL), the risk climbs to 80%. There appear to be no circumstances in which there is a 100% certainty of developing isoimmunization. Antibodies usually appear late in the pregnancy or after delivery, and the sensitizing fetus therefore rarely develops hemolysis. In subsequent pregnancies, however, the Rh antigen is expressed early in gestation and antibodies cross the placenta to cause persistent fetal hemolysis. Hydrops, the most severe symptom, manifests as subcutaneous edema and anasarca with hepatosplenomegaly (protuberant abdomen). Additional signs include a thickened, edematous placenta; anemia; hypervolemia; umbilical venous hypertension; and areas of ectopic erythropoiesis. Laboratory indices include very low hemoglobin, resulting from hemolysis; hypoproteinemia; hypoalbuminemia; hyperbilirubinemia; hepatic dysfunction; reticulocytosis; and normoblastemia.

Maternal exposure to fetal cells occurs during insidious or overt fetal-to-maternal hemorrhage. Fetal cell exposure occurs in 7% of pregnancies in the first trimester, in 16% of pregnancies in the second trimester, and in 29% of pregnancies in the third trimester. Of normal deliveries, 50% of the mothers during or after delivery have measurable evidence of fetal blood in their circulation. In half of these mothers, 0.1 mL of fetal blood enters the mother's circulatory system and may result in a 3% risk of isoimmunization. Thus, in the United States, the potential risk of Rh sensitization could be about 6 per 1000 births but has actually been reduced to about 6 per 10,000 births because of RhoGAM prophylaxis. Similarly, fetal-neonatal mortality has declined from 25% in the pre-RhoGAM era to about 2% or less currently.

Modulating Factors for Rh Sensitization

ABO incompatibility (in which the mother has blood type O and the fetus has blood type A, B, or AB) confers protection upon the fetus. For example, if the fetus has blood type B and is Rh-positive and the mother has blood type O and is Rh-negative, the anti-B antigen in the mother's plasma destroys the fetal cells by hemolysis before the Rh immune reaction occurs. Thus, if the mother has blood type O and is Rh-negative and the father has blood type A, B, or AB and is Rh-positive, there is a possibility of ABO incompatibility. In this case, the risk of Rh disease (otherwise 14 to 16%) is reduced to 1 to 3%.

With regard to amniocentesis and the risk of isoimmunization, the risk of Rh sensitization during amniocentesis with ultrasound guidance is 2.6% at 16 to 18 weeks and 2.3% at 32 to 34 weeks of gestation; without ultrasound guidance, the risk climbs to 11.2%.

With regard to the effect of fetal loss, fetal circulation begins 4 weeks after conception, and fetal D antigen is evident about 6 weeks after conception; it is therefore imperative that prophylactic treatment for fetal loss begin as early as 6 weeks after conception. The risk of sensitization is about 2 to 3% after a spontaneous fetal (Rh-positive) loss and about 5.5% after an operative intervention.

The so-called grandmother theory postulates sensitization without known exposure to fetal cells. It suggests that if an Rh-negative female fetus is exposed to maternal Rh-positive cells in utero, she may already be sensitized when she reaches adulthood and is in her first pregnancy. This theory is currently speculative and has not been confirmed through empirical research.

Prevention of Rh Sensitization

The administration of RhoGAM to an Rh-negative mother of an Rh-positive newborn at the time of delivery results in the lysis of fetal cells within the mother's circulation and prevents sensitization. This practice of postpartum prophylaxis is routine in many countries and has reduced the incidence of Rh immune disease. In addition, antepartum prophylaxis at 28 to 32 weeks of gestation further reduces the incidence of isoimmunization from 2 to 0.2%. It is probably cost effective in specific population groups. Thus, routine prenatal care includes a mandatory blood typing (including Rh) and an evaluation of the antibody screen (indirect Coombs' test). RhoGAM prophylaxis is also given in situations and during procedures with attendant risks of fetal-to-maternal hemorrhage: fetal loss, amniocentesis, chorionic villus sampling, percutaneous blood sampling, abdominal trauma, and abruption or manual removal of the placenta.

Dosage. The recommended dosage of RhoGAM is 50 μg before 13 weeks of gestation and 300 μg after 13 weeks of gestation and may be adjusted by the severity of the fetal-to-maternal hemorrhage, as determined by the Kleihauer-Betke test. At 300 μg dosage, RhoGAM prevents sensitization from 30 mL of fetal blood or 15 mL of fetal red blood cells. Also, RhoGAM should be administered at 300 μg for every additional exposure of 25 mL of fetal blood. Up to 4 doses (1200 μg) can be given every 12 hours until the required dose is obtained. It is recommended that RhoGAM, when administered after delivery, be given within 72 hours, but this should not be considered a hard-and-fast rule, because benefits have been reported after its administration up to 14 days after delivery. In many cases, treatment continues up to 28 days after delivery. RhoGAM has been effective in preventing Rh D isoimmunization and has shown no risk of hepatitis, and there have been no reported cases of human immunodeficiency virus (HIV) transmission. Certain allergic reactions are possible because of traces of IgA, IgM, and plasma proteins. Anaphylaxis is rare.

Although there has been a dramatic decrease in Rh sensitization since 1968, Rh disease has not been eradicated. Among the causes are inadequate prenatal care to screen for Rh sensitization, failure to give RhoGAM at prescribed intervals or at adequate dosages, failure to provide postpartum protection, and failure to recognize other forms of Rh antigen such as the Du antigen.

Maternal-Fetal Management of Rh Sensitization

Intensive maternal-fetal strategies are essential for the successful management of an Rh-sensitized pregnancy. Identification of an Rh-negative mother, the presence and quantification of maternal anti-D antibodies, and assessment of fetal involvement by ultrasonography, amniocentesis, and cordocentesis help determine the need for comprehensive evaluation and strategized intervention plans. The optical density of the amniotic fluid (to assess fetal hyperbilirubinemia) and the fetal hemoglobin concentration correlate with the degree of hemolysis and the level of fetal risk. Interventions include intrauterine fetal transfusions (intraperitoneal or intravascular) to correct fetal anemia, maternal plasmapheresis to reduce circulating antibodies, and planning for early fetal delivery. It is feasible to identify an affected fetus as early as 10 weeks of gestation by chorionic villous sampling for fetal blood type. The clinical relevance for each of the diagnostic techniques is described as follows.

Antibody titers are measured as an indirect Coombs test. The maternal serum is incubated with D-positive cells. Titers higher than 1:8 are indicative of Rh sensitization; titer values lower than 1:16 are not associated with fetal death. Titer values higher than 1:16 do not correlate with the degree of sensitization and hemolysis but do denote increased fetal risk. Thus if the antibody titer exceeds 1:8 during the first pregnancy or in a subsequent pregnancy with associated maternal history of sensitization or fetal abnormality suggestive of hydrops, an amniocentesis is indicated for further evaluation.

Amniotic fluid analysis should be performed at about 28 weeks of gestation but can be conducted as early as 18 weeks. Optical density at 450 nm is used to measure amniotic fluid bilirubin (indicated by the yellow portion of the spectrum). Optical density normally peaks at 23 to 25 weeks of gestation and then decreases with gestational age and maturation. In pregnancies affected by Rh factor, there is a rise at the 450-nm wavelength by spectrophotometer. Connecting points plotted at 550 and 365 nm on the spectrophotometric reading quantitate this rise. The vertical distance at 450 nm between the connected lines and the peak is measured in units of optical density. High values of this vertical distance are indicative of severe hemolysis. These have been characterized by zones, as described by Liley in 1961 and subsequently modified: zone I is associated with low risk; zone II, with moderate risk; and zone III, with severe fetal hyperbilirubinemia and hydrops (Figure 1). Rising values in zone I after 26 weeks of gestation and any value in zone II are the usual indication for more detailed fetal evaluation. In addition, amniocentesis also allows for fetal Rh typing from the amniocytes.

Ultrasonography allows for evaluation of fetal structural well-being and detection of polyhydramnios and evidence of various manifestations of hydrops. The assessment of fetal hemodynamics by Doppler flow velocity have not been as predictive of fetal hypervolemia. However, a sinusoidal pattern of fetal heart rate has been associated with fetal anemia and impending fetal decompensation.

Cordocentesis for fetal blood sampling allows for fetal Rh typing, especially when the father is heterozygous (Dd). In the event of any ultrasonographic evidence of hydrops, blood sampling is useful for hemoglobin measurement, karyotyping, and other appropriate investigations. Other indications include rising values of optical density 450 in the amniotic fluid.

Fetal transfusions include intraperitoneal and intravascular transfusions. Intraperitoneal transfusion was first described by Liley in 1963. Slow intraperitoneal absorption of erythrocytes from subdiaphragmatic lymphatic vessels increases the fetal hemoglobin concentration. It can be performed as early as 23 weeks of gestation and has clearly saved fetal lives. Other causes of fetal anemia—such as fetal-to-maternal hemorrhage, parvovirus infection, and syphilis—must be diagnostically evaluated. Intra-

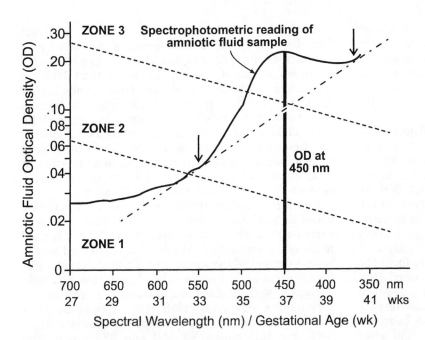

Figure 1. Schematic of the Liley curves with the designated zones for optical density of amniotic fluid as a function of gestational age (weeks) with a superimposed spectrophotometric reading of an amniotic fluid sample as a function of the wavelength (nm). This also shows the technique to measure the optical density at 450 nm (see text; *arrows* indicate the intersection points at 365 nm and 550 nm).

uterine intravascular transfusion was introduced in the early 1980s. It requires a sonographically guided needle to be inserted into the umbilical vein. The site of insertion is usually at the placenta, as opposed to the umbilicus, although some perinatologists have inserted the needle at the hepatic insertion of the umbilical vein. Combined with fetal blood sampling and induction of fetal paralysis, the procedure may be performed as early as 19 weeks of gestation and combined further with intraperitoneal transfusion. The risks include fetal bradycardia, fetal distress, cord hemorrhage, cord tamponade from extravasation, increasing maternal sensitization, and risk of fetal emboli.

Decision Making for Optimal Timing of Delivery

A joint consultation of the obstetrician, the perinatologist, the neonatologist, and the family is recommended in order to consider the optimal timing of delivery. On the basis of the ability to enhance fetal lung maturation with prenatal glucocorticoids and the feasibility of achieving neonatal survival with minimal neurologic sequelae, delivery may be considered as early as 28 weeks of gestation but is preferred after 34 weeks, after the maturation of germinal matrix and thereby invoking the least risk for neurologic injury. Each decision must be individualized after judicious assessment of risk versus benefits to the mother and the fetus. Mothers-to-be and families should be kept informed of mother's and baby's conditions; the appropriate family members are strongly encouraged to participate in perinatal decision making.

Postnatal and Neonatal Management

Delivery Room Management. Hydrops is considered a neonatal emergency, necessitating a delivery room cardiorespiratory care plan with teams of neonatologists, pediatricians, and nurse practitioners; the planning must be such that at least two to three skilled professionals are in attendance. Intensive cardiorespiratory support, removal of any tamponading fluid in the pleural spaces and/or the pericardial sac, restoration of normal hemoglobin concentration, and removal of bilirubin are the important interventional strategies. A prospective plan should be devised for the management of acute and chronic neonatal anemia, as well as for aggressive management of hyperbilirubinemia and hypoalbuminemia. A follow-up evaluation for delayed anemia should be conducted routinely, as should a follow-up evaluation for complications if fetal therapy was initiated. In newborns with milder hemolysis, the initial studies with the cord blood and during the first 6 hours after delivery should include those for bilirubin, hemoglobin, complete blood cell count, peripheral smear, reticulocyte, serum albumin, glucose, and calcium. Because of associated fetal hyperinsulinism, these infants need to be observed closely for hypoglycemia, hypocalcemia, and risk of respiratory distress syndrome.

Intensive Cardiorespiratory Support. Pulmonary complications include respiratory distress syndrome, pleural effusions, and pulmonary edema. Pulmonary hypoplasia may be present in some newborns with hydrops and associated long-standing pleural effusions. These infants need to be provided with appropriate ventilatory support and transferred for continued neonatal intensive care. Use of surfactant, both conventional or high-frequency ventilation, and neonatal analgesics to maintain optimal oxygenation and CO_2 elimination necessitate close bedside management. Air leakages from air trapping may be associated with severe respiratory distress syndrome or pulmonary hypoplasia. Ventilatory strategies should be adjusted to reduce the risk of air-trapping. The infants who survive acute respiratory problems are prone to development of bronchopulmonary dysplasia and chronic lung disease. Poor left ventricular function or cardiomyopathy may also be evident with chronic fetal anemia. Management of hypotension and hypervolemia is often challenging, and pressors may be used with judicious caution.

Removal of Any Tamponading Fluid. In the presence of any clinical signs of tamponade, thoracentesis for pleural effusion and pericardiocentesis may be considered during resuscitation, if these lesions were evident by prenatal ultrasonography. In general, paracentesis for ascites is not necessary. After resuscitation, needle aspiration of any the serous sacs is also not necessary, because a gradual drainage occurs as the neonatal hemodynamics and oncotic pressures improve. Placement of drainage tubes add to the risk of sepsis as well as continued serous drainage and loss of protein.

Restoration of Normal Hemoglobin. In the presence of severe anemia, tissue gas exchange is impaired, and the resulting metabolic acidosis must be corrected early. Restoration of hemoglobin necessitates red blood cell transfusion. Rh-negative blood needs to be used with either type O or a type matched to the baby's type. When anticipated, packed red blood cells should be available for immediate delivery room use, and when feasible, the family may consider the availability of donor-directed blood. A bedside decision to perform corrective transfusion or partial exchange transfusion is based on the extent of hypervolemia and an intention to minimize the circulatory overload. Maintenance of circulatory volume is often challenging because of the associated hypoalbuminemia. Clinically, the use of colloid agents such as fresh-frozen plasma in aliquots of 10 mL per kg have been helpful.

Removal of Bilirubin. Kernicterus is the cause of the significant neurologic morbidity in the infants who survive the complications of fetal anemia, pulmonary disease, and the risks of prematurity. The clinical risk factors for bilirubin-induced neurologic dysfunction include rising levels of unconjugated bilirubin, hypoalbuminemia and the concomitant high bilirubin-albumin ratio, increasing values of unbound bilirubin and presence of prematurity, asphyxia, or any disruption of the neonatal blood-brain barrier. The values that lead to a threshold of concern are listed in Table 1.

Phototherapy. Clinical use of phototherapy to control bilirubin has been effective, and its use in Rh-sensitized babies has been shown to reduce the need for exchange transfusions. The goals of phototherapy are to convert the bilirubin deposited in the subcutaneous tissue to a more excretable compound that is a photoisomer of bilirubin. The dosage of light is based on its irradiance, its spectral wavelength, and the surface of skin exposure. The irradiance of light may be increased from a standard dosage of 10 μW per cm per nm to intensive levels of 35 to 40 μW per cm per nm. Blue lights are more effective than white lights. Using a fiberoptic blanket in conjunction with overhead lights so that all exposed areas of skin

TABLE 1. Vectors Suggestive of Increased Risk of Bilirubin-Related Neurotoxicity

Vector that May Indicate Risk	Threshold for Increased Risk
Clinical examination	Progressive changes in muscle tone, cry, and mental (behavioral) status
Hour-specific total bilirubin value	A value above the 95th percentile
Bilirubin-albumin ratio	
Molar ratio	>0.8 molar ratio
mg:gm ratio	>7.0 mg:gm ratio
Unbound bilirubin	>0.8 μg/dL
Brain-stem auditory evoked response (BAER)	Abnormal latencies of waves I, III, and V; decreasing amplitude

are illuminated can increase the surface of area of exposure. Phototherapy needs to commence early as jaundice is evident within the first 24 hours after birth and more intensively as the hour-specific bilirubin is above the 95th percentile on the bilirubin nomogram or with an increasingly high rate of rise (>0.25 mg per hour or >6 mg per day). Thus far, no significant neonatal morbidity has been documented with over 3 decades of use with phototherapy. Techniques to consider means of reducing the enterohepatic circulation of unconjugated bilirubin and intestinal excretion of bilirubin need to be used. Of these, enteral feedings are the most effective. Pharmacologic approaches are discussed later.

Exchange Transfusion. This has been one of the most significant of interventions. The primary objectives of this procedure are to remove the neurotoxic bilirubin, to remove the antibody-sensitized erythrocytes, to concurrently restore hemoglobin, and to correct the oncotic pressure. The procedure involves an exchange of twice the blood volume of the newborn (blood volume = about 80 mL per kg) performed over a 1.5- to 2-hour period. This exchange may be conducted in an isovolumic, simultaneous process involving withdrawal from an arterial line (peripheral or umbilical) and an equivalent infusion rate through an umbilical vein (catheter tip preferably in the inferior vena cava) or a large-bore catheter in a major peripheral vein. The withdrawal and infusion are best conducted by infusion pumps and more infrequently by manual syringe infusions. Alternatively, the withdrawal from an arterial line may be done by regulating the spontaneous arterial blood flow into a graduated cylinder to match the intravenous pump infusion rate. Effectiveness of an exchange is based on the 85% removal of red blood cells or a reduction of the bilirubin to about 60% of its pre-exchange value. Complications include hypocalcemia, hypoglycemia, electrolyte abnormalities, thrombocytopenia, infection or emboli, and catheter-related events.

Pharmacologic Therapy. These approaches have been considered, and to date no randomized controlled trials have been deemed conclusive. The

TABLE 2. **Role of Pharmacologic Interventions in Rh-Sensitized Newborns**

Drug	Mechanism	Clinical Use
Phenobarbital	Induction of glucoronyl transferase enzyme	No conclusive evidence; potential use in severe hemolysis
Intravenous immune globulin	Fc receptor blockade to prevent erythrocyte lysis	No conclusive evidence; successful anecdotal reports
Heme-oxygenase inhibitors	To block bilirubin production	Experimental
Bilirubin oxidase	To oxidize bilirubin in the gut	Experimental

Abbreviation: Fc = crystallizable fragment.

agents currently used in a clinical setting or in trials are listed in Table 2.

Follow-up

In view of the continued hemolysis secondary to the persistence of IgG antibodies in the neonate, late anemia between 4 and 10 weeks of age is likely. This anemia does not respond to iron supplementation. Booster transfusions (15 mL per kg) may be indicated for hemoglobin values of less than 6 grams per dL or if the infants are symptomatic, as evidenced by poor feeding, retardation in weight gain, or early signs of congestive cardiac failure (tachycardia and/or tachypnea at rest). In addition, these infants need to be monitored by close neurologic evaluation of their extrapyramidal function and brainstem auditory evoked response (signs of bilirubin-induced neurologic dysfunction [BIND]) and also for any sequelae of fetal interventions.

ABO INCOMPATIBILITY

ABO incompatibility is the commonest cause of maternal-to-fetal blood group incompatibility. The clinical manifestations range from mild to severe but are difficult to predict; thus management is based on the rapidity of the rise of bilirubin level. Although 15% of all pregnancies are ABO incompatible, wherein the mother has blood type O and the fetus has type A, B, or AB, the actual hemolytic disease occurs in only about 3% of all pregnancies. The lower incidence is probably related to the variation in maternal levels of IgG antibodies to A or B antigen, binding of these antibodies to the antigens in the placenta and limited manifestations of antigens on the red blood cell surface, or the lowered immunogenicity of the fetal antigens in the neonatal period.

Although there are differences between ABO incompatibility and Rh disease, the interventional guidelines are likely to be similar on the basis of the severity of hyperbilirubinemia and anemia. The similarities and differences are compared in Table 3.

The steps that may be used in developing a strategic interventional approach to the postnatal management of HDN that is based on the percentile values of bilirubin in normal and healthy full-term neonates (hour-specific bilirubin nomogram) are outlined in Table 4. A case example of tracking a newborn with ABO incompatibility on this nomogram is shown in Figure 2.

MINOR BLOOD GROUP INCOMPATIBILITY

Whenever a direct Coombs' test result is positive during a screening evaluation of a neonate with hyperbilirubinemia, a potential diagnosis of minor blood group incompatibility should be considered. Isoimmunizations caused by Kell, Kidd, Duffy, M, N, and c antigens may cause severe fetal and neonatal hyperbilirubinemia and hemolytic disease. The management is similar to that discussed in the section on postnatal and neonatal management.

TABLE 3. **Comparison of Clinical Issues in Newborns with ABO Incompatibility and Rh Sensitization**

Study	ABO Incompatibility	Mild Rh Disease	Moderate Rh Disease	Severe Rh Disease
Mother's blood	O group	Rh-negative	Rh negative	Rh negative
Baby's blood	A, B, or AB group	Rh-positive	Rh positive	Rh positive
Antibody screen	Often negative	Positive	Positive	Positive
Prenatal intervention	None	Surveillance	May need intervention	Necessary
Direct Coombs' test	+	+ +	+ + +	+ + +
Anemia	Unusual	May be present	Present	Severe
Serum albumin level	Normal range	Low normal	Low values	Very low
Hydrops	None	None	None	Present
Jaundice	Variable	Significant	Severe	Fulminant
Phototherapy	As needed	Standard	Intensive	Intensive
Need for exchange transfusion	<10%	~20%	40–50%	100%
Mortality	None	None	Unusual	About 30%

TABLE 4. **Proposed Steps for the Bedside Management of a Full-Term Newborn at Risk for Hemolytic Disease According to Universal Neonatal Bilirubin Screen and Hour-Specific Bilirubin Nomogram**

Steps in Bedside Evaluation	Recommended Investigations	Intervention
Prenatal maternal screening History of previous hemolytic disease Routine blood type and antibody screen	Newborn at risk for HDN if Mother's blood type O or Rh-negative Mother's antibody screen is positive	Screen or save cord blood for neonatal blood type and direct Coombs' test if hyperbilirubinemia develops
Universal newborn bilirubin screen	Total serum bilirubin at same time as the routine metabolic screen before discharge	Determine whether hour-specific bilirubin is above the 40th percentile: in intermediate- or high-risk zone
Screen if jaundice is noted in first 24 h after birth	Bilirubin test on visual jaundice detection	Determine whether hour-specific bilirubin is above the 40th percentile: in intermediate- or high-risk zone
Bilirubin above the 75th percentile for age in hours at <72 h after birth	Diagnostic hemolysis work-up (see text) Serum albumin End-tidal CO measurement (if available) Follow serial bilirubin values q 6–8 h	Check cord blood type, Coombs' test, and bilirubin Consider early use of phototherapy (if rate of rise of bilirubin is >0.25 mg/h) Examine potential role of drugs to decrease bilirubin production
Second bilirubin screen > 95th percentile (<72 h after birth)	Stepwise investigation for hemolysis	Intensive phototherapy (document irradiance)
Persistent bilirubin levels >95th percentile (>72 hours after birth) with intensive phototherapy	Rate of rise of bilirubin, serum albumin Unbound bilirubin (if available) Assess for acute clinical signs of bilirubin-induced neurologic dysfunction (BIND)	Consider exchange transfusion on the basis of Level and rate of rise of bilirubin value (>0.5 mg/h) Bilirubin:albumin > 6.3 (gm:mg) or unbound bilirubin (if available) Early clinical signs of neurotoxicity
Persistent bilirubin levels > 95th percentile (>72 h after birth) with intensive phototherapy	Assess for acute clinical signs of BIND Assess for bilirubin elimination through changes in stooling pattern and color	Consider exchange transfusion and Minimize enterohepatic circulation (such as with feedings) Encourage enteral and hepatic clearance of bilirubin (?drugs)
Decreasing bilirubin values to <40th percentile for age (low-risk zone)	Assess for any residual signs of BIND Assess for late anemia	Wean to low-intensity phototherapy and discontinue Follow-up for any sequelae

Nomogram adapted from Bhutani V, Johnson L, Sivieri E: Predictive ability of a predischarge hour-specific serum bilirubin for subsequent significant hyperbilirubinemia in healthy term and near-term newborns. Pediatrics *103*:6–14, 1999.

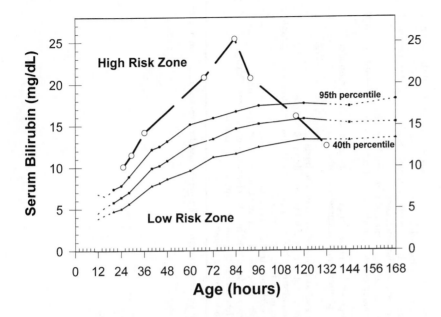

Figure 2. Case example of a newborn with ABO incompatibility, as monitored on an hour-specific bilirubin nomogram, who was treated with intensive phototherapy (40 μW/nm irradiance) about 28 hours after birth. Percentile tracks mark the risk zones. (Adapted from Bhutani V, Johnson L, Silvieri E: Predictive ability of a predischarge hour-specific serum bilirubin for subsequent significant hyperbilirubinemia in healthy term and near-term newborns. Pediatrics *103*:6–14, 1999.)

ERYTHROCYTE ENZYMOPATHIES

Deficiency of intracellular enzymes of the erythrocyte can also cause hemolysis and generally manifest as a postnatal problem. Specific enzyme deficiencies include those of glucose-6-phosphate dehydrogenase (G6PD), pyruvate kinase (PK), and glutathione peroxidase. Of these, G6PD deficiency is more frequent and is more prevalent in the Mediterranean, Africa, the North Indian subcontinent, and the East Asian population. A greater incidence of severe hyperbilirubinemia occurs with exposure to oxidant drugs and to bacterial or viral infections. The management of these neonates is similar to management of hyperbilirubinemia.

ERYTHROCYTE MEMBRANE DISORDER

Membrane disorders are uncommon causes of neonatal hyperbilirubinemia. Of these, the likely disorders are hereditary spherocytosis, elliptocytosis, and infantile pyknocytosis. Acquired disorders may occur with hepatic or lipid abnormalities.

HEMOGLOBINOPATHIES

These are a rare cause of HDN. Abnormalities in alpha- or gamma-globin chains of hemoglobin, rather than in the beta-globin chain, may lead to neonatal problems. Defects in the gamma-globin chains have been reported with a variant: hemoglobin F Poole (congenital Heinz body hemolytic anemia). Alpha-globin chain variants are usually silent. Bart's hemoglobin manifests as neonatal hyperbilirubinemia and lifelong anemia. Persistence of the embryonic hemoglobin (with no alpha-globin chain production) manifests with severe fetal hemolytic disease. Unexplained severe hemolysis in the neonatal period should include an evaluation for hemoglobinopathies.

Management guidelines are the same as described in the section on neonatal and postnatal management.

CONCLUSIONS

Proper management of hemolytic disease of the fetus and newborn requires a well-orchestrated effort of an interdisciplinary team in order to prevent a potentially tragic outcome. Meticulous first-trimester screening and antepartum care are essential in prevention. Effective prophylaxis against Rh sensitization may be achieved by RhoGAM; postnatal screening for neonatal blood type when a mother has blood type O or is Rh-negative is also helpful. Intensive fetal therapy combined with neonatal care has been effective for Rh sensitization but remains poor once hydrops is evident before 19 weeks of gestation. Patient education, screening, and prepregnancy planning are essential in reducing the incidence and complications of HDN.

HEMOPHILIA AND RELATED CONDITIONS

method of
AMY D. SHAPIRO, M.D.
Indiana Hemophilia and Thrombosis Center
Indianapolis, Indiana

and

KEITH HOOTS, M.D.
Gulf States Hemophilia Center
Houston, Texas

The hemophilias are a group of related bleeding disorders that are most commonly congenital. Many bleeding disorders are now recognized; however, "hemophilia" is a specific term representing three deficiency states listed below in the most common order of observation:

1. Factor VIII deficiency: hemophilia A
2. Factor IX deficiency: hemophilia B or Christmas disease
3. Factor XI deficiency: Rosenthal's disease

Von Willebrand's disease (vWD) is the most frequently observed bleeding disorder in the general population and is caused by a deficiency or abnormality in von Willebrand factor (vWF).

Deficiencies of other procoagulants (clotting factors that promote formation of the fibrin plug) and some of the fibrinolytic components (those factors that aid in dissolution of the clot once formed) may also lead to a bleeding diathesis. Therefore, although factor VIII, IX, and XI deficiencies are the classic hemophilias, there exist a group of uncommon, but clinically significant, bleeding states caused by genetically regulated decreases or absence of specific coagulation factors. These include deficiencies of factors VII, X, V, II, and XIII; afibrinogenemia; alpha$_2$-antiplasmin deficiency; and plasminogen activator inhibitor-1 (PAI-1) deficiency.

In this chapter the classic hemophilias and vWD are discussed in some detail. Although it is beyond the scope of this chapter to describe all bleeding diatheses, the signs and symptoms of bleeding disorders are reviewed as a guide to aid development of a differential diagnosis and decisions regarding referral of patients for further evaluation.

SIGNS AND SYMPTOMS OF BLEEDING DISORDERS

Severe bleeding disorders commonly present within the first 2 years of life. Abnormal bleeding in association with procedures (e.g., circumcision), with injury (frequently in the oral cavity), or as excessive bruising; and hematomas or hemarthroses with activities considered normal for age are the common manifestations of severe bleeding disorders. Despite the presence of severe factor VIII or factor IX deficiency, the vast majority of newborns traverse delivery and the first few months of life without detection of hemophilia. However, about 5% of cases of hemophilia may present as significant subgaleal or intracranial hemorrhage in the perinatal period. Approximately 50% of undiagnosed hemophiliacs bleed in association with circumcision.

Moderate and mild bleeding disorders may go undetected for significant periods of time, including well into adulthood, and present as abnormal bleeding associated with intercurrent injury or with medical interventions such as surgery or dental extractions.

Unlike hemophilia A and B, the clinical bleeding pattern for vWD is primarily localized to the mucous membrane surface, with epistaxis, menorrhagia, and postdental, surgical, and gastrointestinal bleeding representing the common manifestations. Postsurgical bleeding or hemorrhage secondary to significant trauma may occur, depending on the qualitative or quantitative defect in the circulating vWF.

Other symptoms of bleeding disorders include intracranial bleeding in a full-term newborn, excessive petechiae or ecchymosis, bleeding with circumcision, hematoma development with immunization, and so on.

GENETICS AND PREVALENCE

Hemophilia A and B are X-linked recessive inherited bleeding disorders. In contrast, vWD is an autosomal domi-nant trait with males and females equally affected. Factor XI deficiency, and the majority of other coagulation factor deficiencies leading to a bleeding tendency, are inherited as autosomal recessive disorders.

Both hemophilia A and B are coded for on the long arm (q) of the X chromosome. The factor VIII gene codes for a glycoprotein that is substantially larger than the factor IX protein (about 340,000 daltons vs. about 70,000 daltons) and has been demonstrated to be highly susceptible to deletions, insertions, and missense and nonsense mutational events. In addition, an inversion sequence of intron 22 of the *FVIII* gene is now known to account for more than 34% of mutations giving rise to hemophilia A. This inversion involves a crossover between the intragenic and extragenic copies of *FVIII* on the X chromosome, the "flip-tip" inversion. Although significantly smaller than the *FVIII* gene, the *FIX* gene also has been shown to be prone to new mutation events, particularly missense and nonsense types. In practical terms, this results in 25 to 30% of newly diagnosed cases of either hemophilia A or B representing new mutational events within a family and accounts for the consistency of incidence of these disorders across all racial and ethnic groups.

The incidence of hemophilia A and B together is 1 in 5000 live male births. Approximately 80% of affected neonates have hemophilia A, with approximately two thirds of affected individuals having severe disease. In contrast, almost half of individuals with hemophilia B have factor IX levels more than 1%. Patients with hemophilia A and B of comparable severity bleed with similar frequency.

vWD results when there is a defect in the gene for vWF located on chromosome 12. vWD is among the most prevalent of genetic diseases, with as high as 1% of certain genetically analyzed cohorts revealing abnormalities.

PATHOPHYSIOLOGY

Factors VIII and IX are essential cofactors for activating factor X to factor Xa and are primarily produced in the liver. Factor IX is a serine protease, and factor VIII is a large glycoprotein essential for configuring the clotting enzymes on the platelet surface so that enzyme-substrate reactions occur at optimal maximal kinetics.

The glycoprotein coded for by the vWF gene is a subunit of approximately 226,000 daltons that multimerizes into a large adhesive molecule essential for both platelet aggregation through cross linking of glycoprotein IB receptors between platelets and for platelet adhesion to the site of blood vessel endothelial cell injury. In addition, these vWF multimers, secreted from both endothelial cells and platelets, are essential for stabilization and protection against proteolysis of factor VIII in plasma. When vWF is either quantitatively or qualitatively abnormal, factor VIII activity levels may be decreased, despite the fact that both the *FVIII* gene and its coded protein are normal.

SEQUELAE OF HEMOPHILIA

Hemophilia A and B present as clinically identical conditions, with joint bleeding (hemarthrosis) and joint destruction constituting the primary morbid manifestation. Other sequelae of disease include transmission of blood-borne infections, such as hepatitis A, B, or C, human immunodeficiency virus (HIV), parvovirus, and so on. In about 28% of severe factor VIII–deficient and 3 to 5% of severe factor IX–deficient patients, an inhibitor develops. Inhibitors are antibodies, commonly IgG, that develop against the coagulation factor in which the patient is deficient, are measured in Bethesda units, and are classified as either high responding or low responding depending on the patient's historical anamnestic response. Development of an inhibitor is a severe complication of disease and may lead to uncontrolled hemorrhage. Optimal treatment for patients with inhibitors must start with referral to a comprehensive hemophilia treatment program. Inhibitors generally develop within the first 30 infusion exposure days, but they have been documented to occur anywhere in a particular patient's course. Inhibitors should be suspected when any bleeding episode is refractory to normal treatment. Inhibitors in moderately and mildly deficient patients have been reported. Inhibitor development in factor IX deficiency poses particular problems in that its presence may be heralded or associated with development of anaphylactic reactions to infusion of any factor IX–containing product. Individuals with hemophilia B caused by deletion mutations are at increased risk of inhibitor formation.

LABORATORY ABNORMALITIES

Decreased levels of prekallikrein, high-molecular-weight kininogen, and factors XI, XII, VIII, and IX will prolong the partial thromboplastin time (aPTT) but not the prothrombin time (PT). Bleeding symptoms are associated with deficiencies of factor VIII, IX, and XI. In contrast, factor XII deficiency, while prolonging the aPTT, produces no clinical bleeding. The degree of prolongation of the aPTT does not predict bleeding, rather the level and specific factor deficiency do.

vWD may be associated with a prolonged aPTT, bleeding time, and abnormal platelet function analysis. However, approximately 50% of affected type 1 individuals may have entirely normal screening tests and, therefore, one normal evaluation in the presence of clinically suspicious symptoms warrants re-evaluation or more specific testing. vWF is an acute phase reactant, and normal specific assays such as factor VIII activity, vWF:Ag, and vWF activity may be seen. Accurate diagnosis may be difficult, and underdiagnosis is common.

Factor VII deficiency is associated with a prolonged PT with normal aPTT and bleeding time. Severe factor X, V, and II deficiency and afibrinogenemia are associated with both a prolonged aPTT and PT.

A number of clinically severe, uncommon bleeding disorders are associated with a normal aPTT, PT, and bleeding time. These include factor XIII, alpha$_2$-antiplasmin, and PAI-1 deficiencies.

CLASSIFICATION OF DISEASE AND CLINICAL COURSE

Hemophilia A and B exhibit a range of clinical severity that correlates well with assayed factor levels. Severe disease is defined as less than 1% factor activity, whereas 1 to 5% and more than 5% of normal are defined as moderate and mild disease, respectively. Males within a family have the same level of deficiency because they share the same genetic defect.

The categorization of vWD is based on the amount, functional capacity, and structure of the vWF protein. Abnormalities have been divided into three major types.

Type 1 vWD is a heterozygous disorder in which the genetic defect is partially compensated for by vWF production directed by the normal gene. Laboratory, studies measuring quantitative vWF (vWF:Ag) are abnormal, and vWF functional studies (vWF activity) are proportionally reduced. Furthermore, the factor VIII level is frequently ab-

normal owing to diminished vWF binding capacity and subsequent decreased plasma half-life.

Type 2 vWD consists of multiple genetic defects, which result in defective functional vWF. A comprehensive discussion of all the type 2 variants of vWD is beyond the scope of this chapter; however, examples include abnormalities in the multimerization, defective factor VIII binding, and defective vWF secretion from platelets despite normal plasma vWF structure and function. Furthermore, as with vWD in general, there is often substantial clinical heterogeneity between individuals of the same type 2 variant.

Individuals with type 3 vWD have defects in both genes coding for vWF. In many cases, neither parent will have a clinically significant bleeding history because subclinical type 1 heterozygotes are common. In contrast, the individual with type 3 vWD will have severe clinical bleeding because there is little, if any, vWF, resulting in rapid proteolysis of factor VIII despite normal production. Hence, individuals with type 3 vWD may experience both the mucous membrane hemorrhages seen with vWD as well as bleeding into deep tissue or organs (e.g., hemarthroses) noted more commonly in hemophiliacs. Chronic morbidity is much more commonly observed in these individuals.

Autosomal inherited factor VII, V, X, and prothrombin deficiencies are rare but may produce a significant hemorrhagic state, the severity of which correlates inversely with the circulating plasma concentration of the deficient protease (factors II, VII and X) or glycoprotein (factor V).

The clinical course of factor VII deficiency is often very severe, and infants are at significant risk for intracranial hemorrhage. Afibrinogenemia, the incidence of which is approximately 1 in 1 million live births, may present in the neonatal period with life-threatening hemorrhage necessitating replacement therapy.

Both factor XIII and alpha$_2$-antiplasmin deficiencies are associated with spontaneous intracranial bleeding in 25 to 35% of affected patients. These bleeding events may be prevented with accurate diagnosis and life-long prophylactic replacement therapy. PAI-1 and alpha$_2$-antiplasmin deficiencies result in excessive fibrinolysis, with clinical bleeding after tissue injury. Inherited disorders of platelet and endothelial cell function cause clinical bleeding and are discussed elsewhere.

TREATMENT

Replacement Therapy

For the majority of inherited coagulation disorders, primary therapy consists of infusing a protein product to replace the deficient coagulation factor. Historically, the source for these replacement products was human plasma based. For the majority of these clotting factor concentrates, their hemostatic activity is defined in units of clotting activity, where 1 unit equals the amount of factor activity present in 1 mL of pooled normal plasma.

The strategy for improving replacement therapy for hemophilia has been to increase the concentration and purity of clotting factor concentrates and, ultimately, to develop recombinant products free of human and animal proteins in both the final formulation and in the manufacturing process.

In plasma fractionation, similar proteins co-purify. Commercial fractionation of cryoprecipitate yielded the first generation of lyophilized factor VIII concentrates, which resulted in an approximate 100-fold increase in concentration of factor VIII over fresh-frozen plasma. Convenient home infusion for hemophilia-associated hemorrhage became feasible. Unfortunately, because of the number of donors contributing to the commercial plasma pool, transfusion-transmitted viral disease (particularly hepatitis and HIV infection) became a common complication in the hemophilia A and B population.

For therapies used in the 1970s and 1980s, production of factor IX concentrate resulted in co-purification of all the molecularly similar vitamin K–dependent factors (II, VII, IX and X), yielding a final product called prothrombin complex concentrates (PCCs). Co-purification was also compounded by inadvertent activation of these proteases to their active enzyme (e.g., factor VII converted to factor VIIa), both of which contributed to a thrombogenic risk associated with the use of PCCs. PCCs administered in high and recurrent dosing schedules have produced significant and sometimes fatal events, notably in association with (1) orthopedic surgery, (2) sustained crush injuries, (3) large intramuscular hemorrhages (e.g., psoas or thigh), (4) the treatment of hemophilic neonates with immature natural anticoagulation, and (5) the treatment of individuals with severe chronic hepatitis (impaired production of antithrombin III and proteins C and S). In its most severe manifestations, PCCs have resulted in disseminated intravascular coagulation, acute myocardial infarction, and death. Fortunately, advanced purification technologies have resulted in the production of single component factor IX products, free of significant trace activated proteases, which now provide the mainstay for therapy of hemophilia B patients and are obligatory when high dose, recurrent infusion therapy is required.

Therapeutic Options for Treatment of Hemophilia A and B

Factor VIII Products

Initially, factor VIII concentrates were heat-treated to decrease the risk of transmission of HIV and, to a lesser degree, hepatitis and were first licensed in 1983. Subsequent viral inactivation methods included pasteurization, solvent-detergent washing, sepharose chromatography, affinity chromatography with monoclonal antibodies directed against the factor VIII/vWF complex, and, most recently, production of recombinant factor VIII products in transfected mammalian cell systems. Each non-recombinant clotting factor concentrate presently produced in the United States is made from a donor pool screened for HIV, hepatitis B, and hepatitis C, which in conjunction with viral inactivation procedures previously mentioned, effectively has eliminated HIV transmission and, to varying degrees, greatly reduced transmissible hepatogens.

Blood components such as cryoprecipitate and fresh-frozen plasma, do not typically undergo viral attenuation other than donor screening and therefore may present a risk of viral transmission. A new solvent detergent fresh-frozen plasma product is available and should be considered for use in individuals who require repeated exposure. Despite the low relative risk of transmission of HIV (between 1 in 40,000 and 1 in 100,000 per donor unit) and hepatitis C (≤0.03% per donor unit) in individuals treated with any plasma-derived product (including single donor or pooled attenuated product), it is recommended they receive the hepatitis B and A vaccines to completion.

Plasma-derived factor VIII concentrates currently available are considered relatively safe in regard to viral transmission; nonetheless, transmission of hepatitis viruses C and A and human parvovirus B19 has been documented. It is imperative for the physician prescribing these replacement products to be acutely aware of these issues and use the safest available therapy for any particular patient's circumstances.

Products may be stratified based on purity as follows: (1) intermediate purity, (2) high purity, and (3) ultra-high purity products. Intermediate purity factor concentrates, despite aggressive viral inactivation with heat or pasteurization, and/or solvent detergent washing, result in a final concentration of the coagulation factor representing a small percentage of the total protein present (6 to 10 units of factor activity per mg of total protein excluding albumin). High purity products are those with at least 50 units (range: 50 to 150) activity per milligram of protein (excluding albumin for stabilization). Ultra-high purity products are the monoclonal antibody affinity-purified plasma-derived factor concentrates and the recombinant products. Nonetheless, effective elimination of hepatitis C from the plasma-based monoclonal products has required subsequent treatment with either pasteurization or solvent detergent. The specific activity of the monoclonal preparations (before the addition of human serum albumin) is 3000 units of factor VIII per milligram of protein. This is essentially identical to the effective purity of the licensed recombinant products, which also require addition of albumin to maintain stability.

Presently licensed recombinant factor VIII products are purified from the cell culture of transfected hamster–derived cell lines; therefore, there is no requirement for further viral attenuation. The addition of human serum albumin constitutes the sole theoretical source for human viral contamination. There remains a theoretical risk for other nonhuman, mammalian viruses or other infective species.

Use of ultrapure products has been shown to stabilize the CD4 count in HIV-infected hemophiliacs, whereas infusion of intermediate clotting factor concentrates does not. These products are the preferred products for HIV-infected hemophiliacs and previously untreated and minimally treated patients.

Clinical trials have been conducted and are ongoing with the use of (1) a recombinant factor VIII preparation from which the B domain of the gene has been removed before transfection of the hamster cell lines and (2) an albumin-free recombinant factor VIII concentrate. The portion of factor VIII coded for by the B domain of the gene is not required for clotting activity; furthermore, its deletion confers greater stability on the resultant smaller factor VIII molecule. Hence there is no requirement for stabilization with human serum albumin. A change in formulation has allowed stabilization without added albumin to the second product. These products may provide a higher level of confidence against any future microbiologic contamination.

Factor IX Products

The clotting factor concentrates available for treating hemophilia B require scrutiny for potential complications, including (1) viral safety and purity and (2) thrombogenicity. Factor IX concentrates free of thrombogenic risk are those that have purified the factor IX away from the other vitamin K–dependent coagulation factors. Two technical strategies have been employed to purify factor IX: chromatographic partitioning and monoclonal antibody affinity purification. Both of these products are further subjected to viral inactivation processes, such as solvent detergent, thiocyanate treatment and ultrafiltration. The product produced by the former process contains minor residual plasma proteins, whereas the monoclonal product is free of other plasma proteins. Viral attenuation to remove HIV and hepatitis is effective for both processes. However, studies using surrogate viruses imply greater safety from hepatitis C or similar viruses with the monoclonal factor IX concentrate.

The other plasma-derived clotting factor concentrates available for treating hemophilia B patients are PCCs and, as previously mentioned, may be associated with thrombotic complications. Viral attenuation strategies for PCCs are either solvent detergent treatment or heating to 80°C for more than 10 hours. PCCs are no longer the replacement therapy of choice in hemophilia B.

Recombinant factor IX concentrate, Benefix, was licensed in 1997. Unlike the presently licensed recombinant factor VIII preparations, recombinant factor IX has no added albumin in the final product. The theoretical advantages of recombinant factor IX are similar to those of the B-domain–deleted recombinant factor VIII discussed earlier. The in-vivo half-life of recombinant factor IX concentrate is identical to plasma-derived concentrates; however, the volume of distribution is larger, owing to a difference in charge conferred by decreased/lack of phosphorylation and sulfation at two sites compared with the plasma species. Therefore, replacement therapy with recombinant factor IX requires calculation of doses based on an estimated volume of distribution of 1.2 and awareness that the volume of distribution in individuals is variable and may require adjustment of higher doses.

Treatment of Patients with Inhibitors

PCCs have been used since the 1970s in individuals with high-titer factor VIII or IX inhibitors for whom the normal replacement products no longer provide hemostasis. Subsequently, manufacturers of PCCs increased the concentration of active proteases resulting in production of activated prothrombin complex concentrates (APCCs). Unfortunately, there is no in vitro assay for the PCCs and APCCs that can be used to correlate with in vivo hemostatic efficacy. Hence, it is often difficult to predict the hemostatic efficacy of these products; individual response to and therapeutic efficacy for specific hemorrhagic episodes and of specific products in any one given clinical situation vary. An individualized therapeutic plan needs to be established and is best designed by a hematologist expert in the care of these complicated patients. However, certain general guidelines may be used for initial treatment and stabilization of these patients: (1) effective dosing of APCCs is within the range of 75 to 100 IU per kg; (2) dosing frequency should be every 12 hours up to three doses because more frequent infusion increases thrombotic risk; (3) because the activated proteases that account for the procoagulant activity of APCCs are short lived, initial hemostasis may be followed by breakthrough bleeding between doses that may create difficulty for maintenance of hemostasis. Therapy with APCCs is expensive, is less than reliable, and carries risk of significant complications. Experience and expertise in their use help to mitigate these risks and to differentiate the appropriate use of APCCs from other therapeutic alternatives for patients with inhibitors.

An alternative therapy for treating patients with high-responding, high-titer factor VIII inhibitors is porcine factor VIII. The human anti–factor VIII antibody may cross react with shared epitopes on the porcine molecule. Therefore, before use of this product is attempted, it is necessary to quantitate the neutralizing capacity of the antibody against both the porcine and human factor VIII product using the Bethesda assay. The use of porcine factor VIII may be associated with hypersensitivity reactions and development of anti–porcine factor VIII antibodies typically around the 7th to 10th day of use. The dose of porcine factor VIII is calculated based on the weight of the patient and the titer of the antiporcine antibodies. It is essential to monitor factor VIII levels in patients undergoing therapy with porcine factor VIII. As with most therapies for hemophilia A patients with inhibitors, therapy with porcine factor VIII is expensive.

Recombinant factor VIIa (rFVIIa, NovoSeven, Novo Nordisk) was licensed in 1999 in the United States for treatment of hemophilics with inhibitors to factor VIII (FVIII), IX (FIX), or VII (FVII). NovoSeven has been used effectively in both adults and children, and the response is independent of inhibitor titer. The risk of anaphylaxis or anamnestic response to FVIII or FIX with NovoSeven is minimal. As a recombinant protein, the risk of blood-borne disease transmission is near zero. NovoSeven's mode of action is through tissue factors exposed at the site of injury and results in induction of *local* hemostasis and minimizes the risk of systemic activation of the coagulation system. The usual dosage is 90 μg per kg per dose given in intervals of approximately 2 hours to achieve hemostasis. The average number of injections required is approximately three per bleeding episode. The infusion interval may be lengthened if maintenance of hemostasis is desired. The indications for use of other therapeutic interventions in patients with inhibitors, such as immune tolerance induction, antibody depletion by means of a *Staphylococcus* protein A sepharose column, or plasmapheresis, are beyond the scope of this discussion.

Specific problems exist for the factor IX–deficient patient with an inhibitor, including anaphylactic reactions and nephrosis associated with immune tolerance regimens. Comprehensive hemophilia treatment centers provide expertise for these specialized patients and should be consulted for the development of any treatment plan in a hemophilic patient with an inhibitor.

Therapies for von Willebrand's Disease

Patients with type 1 vWD often may be treated with desmopressin (DDAVP), a synthetic analogue of the antidiuretic hormone 9-arginine vasopressin. Desmopressin will increase circulating vWF/factor VIII on average two to four times the baseline level. Therefore, it becomes a treatment of choice for mild to moderate bleeding in most individuals with both mild hemophilia A (e.g., > 5% factor VIII activity) and type 1 vWD.

Desmopressin may be administered intravenously or subcutaneously at a dose of 0.3 μg per kg. Intravenous administration may be associated with an increased rate of reported side effects. A highly concentrated (1.5 mg per mL) intranasal form of desmopressin is available for use in vWD and mild hemophilia A. Two puffs in a single nostril in patients weighing more than 50 kg and 1 puff in those weighing less than 50 kg are used. As with the intravenous preparation, facial flushing, mild to moderate blood pressure elevation, and antidiuretic side effects may be experienced. Concomitant fluid restriction is considered especially in the surgical setting, where monitoring of urine output and electrolytes is also advised, to prevent water retention, hyponatremia, and seizures. Tachyphylaxis after repeated dosing with desmopressin can occur because of depletion of the vWF stores. Therefore, monitoring of levels in individuals requiring repeated dosing (e.g., daily or more often) is required.

Correct subtyping of vWD is mandatory in determining the appropriate therapeutic intervention. For example, in type 2b vWD, in which the largest vWF multimers are missing from plasma but are released in excess after desmopressin, there is risk of paradoxical thrombosis with the use of desmopressin, which is relatively contraindicated.

Other therapeutic options are indicated (1) in individuals with type 3 vWD; (2) in those with types 1 and 2 vWD who either fail to respond to desmopressin or do so to a degree inadequate to achieve complete and predictable hemostasis; (3) in those in whom desmopressin is contraindicated because of subtype or concomitant medical conditions (e.g., hypertension, heart disease, stroke); and (4) for those who experience tachyphylaxis precluding repeated therapy. Traditionally, cryoprecipitate has been the most effective means for achieving hemostasis in such patients. However, cryoprecipitate has an associated risk for transmission of blood-borne viral disease. Therefore, one of three intermediate or high purity factor VIII concentrates demonstrated to have most sizes of vWF multimers has been employed to treat vWD patients in these circumstances. Several studies have shown clinical efficacy to be good even when individuals with severe disease have experienced life-threatening hemorrhage or undergone surgical interventions.

Adjunctive Therapies/Antifibrinolytic Agents

Tranexamic acid (Cyklokapron) and epsilon-aminocaproic acid (EACA; Amicar) act by inhibiting fibrinolysis though plasminogen activation, thereby enhancing clot stability. These two agents are useful therapeutic adjuncts to stabilize clots in areas of increased fibrinolysis such as the oral cavity. These agents may also be useful for adjunctive therapy in patients with difficult episodes of epistaxis and menorrhagia. Dosing for tranexamic acid is 25 mg per kg every 8 hours; for EACA it is 75 to 100 mg per kg every 6 hours (maximum dose is 3 to 4 grams every 6 hours). For patients with hemostatic defects, treatment with antifibrinolytics may be required for 7 to 14 days after initial infusion therapy, depending on the amount of tissue injury. In hemophilia B, it is recommended to use a purified factor IX preparation when concomitant antifibrinolytic therapy is employed owing to additive thrombotic risks of PCCs and antifibrinolytics.

Other adjunctive therapies include use of microfibular collagen, especially for bleeding in the oral cavity, and fibrin glue. A highly effective fibrin glue, Tisseel, was licensed in 1998 and has been used for epistaxis, gastrointestinal bleeding, and neurosurgery and can be an important adjunctive therapy in appropriate patients.

PREVENTIVE CARE

Male infants born to known or suspected hemophilic carrier mothers should not be circumcised until hemophilia has been excluded. Blood for assay for aPTT and factor VIII or IX assay can be obtained from cord blood. When a cord blood sample is not available, venipuncture should be performed from a superficial limb vein to lessen the risk of hematoma development requiring replacement therapy. Femoral, arterial, and jugular sites must be avoided.

Routine immunizations, such as diphtheria-pertussis-tetanus or measles-mumps-rubella, may be given in the deep subcutaneous tissue or via the usual route when the smallest gauge needle is used and pressure and ice are applied to the site for 3 to 5 minutes after the injection. Hepatitis B vaccine should be given as soon after birth as possible to all infants with hemophilia. The live oral polio attenuated vaccine is contraindicated in any infant when there is an immunocompromised household member (e.g., HIV-infected hemophiliac). In these instances, the Salk vaccine is used. Hepatitis A vaccine should also be administered to unexposed hemophiliacs.

Early infant dental intervention is recommended to teach proper tooth brushing and ensure adequate household water fluoridation. The teeth should be cleaned routinely, and anticipated problem areas for causing bleeding discussed. In addition to education about hemophilia, both genetic and psychosocial counseling is important for the family with a newborn with hemophilia, especially for the approximately 30% for whom there is no previous family experience with the disease. Normal socialization and development is encouraged, and experienced personnel should discuss what minimum limitations are reasonable. An appropriate exercise regimen that excludes contact sports (e.g., tackle football) should be encouraged as a daily routine. Furthermore, the role of such an exercise program for the child and adult after episodes of bleeding is best discussed before the child has a joint hemorrhage.

IMPORTANT ISSUES IN HEMOPHILIC BLEEDING

Early treatment decreases the duration of therapy, predisposition to rebleeding, and morbidity experienced and improves the quality of life. Early signs and symptoms of bleeding may not be notable on physical examination, and patient report of pain should be used as a guide for institution of early therapy. Early bleeding episodes may be treated with a 30 to 40% factor correction.

More complicated bleeding episodes or bleeding in areas such as the face, neck, hip, and iliopsoas requires a higher correction level: 80 to 100%. Dosage may be calculated using the following formula:

Number of units required = weight (kg)
× level desired × volume of distribution

The level desired should be placed into the formula as a whole number (e.g., 40 representing 40%). The volume of distribution for factor VIII is about 0.5, and that for factor IX is about 1.0, except in the case of recombinant factor IX, when 1.2 is used.

Intervention strategies include on-demand (therapy instituted after a bleeding episode has been experienced/identified) and prophylactic therapy (therapy used to prevent bleeding). Prophylactic therapy has been demonstrated to prevent essentially all spontaneous hemarthroses. A decision to undertake a prophylactic regimen should be made in conjunction with the parent/patient and professionals in the comprehensive hemophilia treatment center.

Hip joint or acetabular hemorrhages may result in increased intra-articular pressure and lead to aseptic necrosis of the femoral head. Twice-daily infusion therapy designed to sustain a factor level above 10 units per dL for at least 3 days should be given, along with enforced bed rest. Hip hemarthrosis may be difficult to differentiate from an iliopsoas hemorrhage. The latter limits primary hip extension, whereas hemarthrosis makes any motion of the hip excruciatingly painful. Furthermore, an iliopsoas hemorrhage may lead to decreased sensation over the ipsilateral thigh because of compression of the sacral plexus root of the femoral nerve. Ultrasonography may demonstrate a hematoma in the iliopsoas region. Treatment of the two is similar, although rehabilitation from the hip hemarthrosis is more protracted. Both benefit from physical therapy.

Closed compartment muscle and soft tissue hemorrhages, often in the upper arm, forearm, wrist, volar hand, and anterior or posterior tibial compartment, may result in impingement on the neurovascular bundle. Swelling and pain precede tingling, numbness, and loss of distal arterial pulses. Infusion must maintain an adequate hemostatic factor level. Surgical decompression is undertaken only if medical therapy fails to forestall progression and in consultation with a comprehensive hemophilia treatment center.

For life-threatening bleeding in a hemophiliac, the exigency for immediate infusion is superseded only by resuscitative requirements. The factor level should be maintained more than 50% in these circumstances. An acutely hemorrhaging hemophiliac should be transported, if possible, to an emergency center that stocks appropriate replacement products. All head injuries must be considered nontrivial unless proved otherwise by observation and computed tomography/magnetic resonance imaging. Late bleeding after head trauma can occur up to 3 to 4 weeks after the event. Hence, patients with head and neck injuries should be infused immediately unless the injury is insignificant. Nonhospitalized patients and their families should be instructed in neurologic signs and symptoms of central nervous system bleeding so that repeat infusion, clinical and radiologic assessment, and hospitalization occur at the earliest manifestation of bleeding.

Bleeding in the floor of the mouth, pharynx, or epiglottic region may result in airway compromise or obstruction and is treated with an aggressive infusion program and extended clinical follow-up to ensure resolution. Such bleeding may be precipitated by coughing, tonsillitis, oral or otolaryngologic surgery (e.g., extraction of wisdom teeth, tonsillectomy, adenoidectomy), or regional block anesthesia. For surgery and anesthesia, prophylaxis with appropriate infusion therapy before the procedure is mandatory.

Continuous infusion regimens to maintain normal circulating factor activity are often used in patients postoperatively, in those with complicated or serious bleeding episodes, or in those with gastrointestinal lesions, such as ulcers, varices, or hemorrhoids.

COMPREHENSIVE CARE

Designated treatment centers have been established in the United States and many other countries to provide multidisciplinary care of hemophilia and related disorders. The multidisciplinary care team provides optimal chronic disease management and lowers associated morbidity and mortality.

The comprehensive hemophilia centers provide voluntary testing for blood-borne viral infections, counseling of patients found seropositive, and access to appropriate care and therapy. Risk reduction counseling and education are essential elements of comprehensive care. Comprehensive centers are the mainstay for ongoing education of patients and families for management of the bleeding disorder. The centers coordinate home therapy and preventive services and work closely with hemophilia consumer organizations. Further information about hemophilia care, hemophilia centers, and HIV risk reduction and counseling is available through the National Hemophilia Foundation, 116 W. 32nd St, 11th floor, New York, NY 10001 (800-424-2634), on the internet at www.hemophilia.org, or from your local hemophilia chapter.

PLATELET-MEDIATED BLEEDING DISORDERS

method of
TERRY GERNSHEIMER, M.D.
Puget Sound Blood Center and
  University of Washington Department of
  Medicine
Seattle, Washington

Platelets are necessary to maintain the integrity of the vascular system and to stop blood loss from a disrupted blood vessel. Platelets adhere to exposed subendothelium, both directly and by binding with von Willebrand factor (vWF). Platelets then go through the processes of activation, release, and aggregation into a platelet plug, setting the stage for fibrin formation and eventually repair and resolution of vascular injury. Platelet glycoprotein Ib/IX/V is the initial binding site. The platelet is stimulated by thrombin and collagen and is activated to release agents stored in its granules. These agents, including adenosine diphosphate, serotonin, and thromboxane A_2, activate additional platelets. Substances released by the platelet are also important in promoting coagulation (e.g., factor V) and fibrin formation. With platelet activation, the platelet glycoprotein receptor IIb/IIIa is expressed and binds fi-

brinogen, resulting in aggregation. Abnormalities in platelet numbers, platelet glycoproteins, or granule content may interfere significantly with this initial step of clot formation.

CLINICAL MANIFESTATION AND EVALUATION

The focus here is on the approach to platelet disorders in adult patients. The treatment of some of these disorders differs in children, and the reader is referred to another source for the care of pediatric platelet disorders.

Symptoms and signs of thrombocytopenia are dependent more on the platelet count than on the underlying cause unless platelet function or coagulation abnormalities are also present. In general, there will be no notable hemostatic abnormality above platelet counts of 100,000 per mm^3. Below that level the bleeding time begins to increase and patients may begin to note easy bruisability, which worsens as the count falls. Most patients are asymptomatic unless thrombocytopenia is severe ($<30,000/mm^3$) or they are hemostatically challenged. Below this level, patients may note some petechiae on the legs and bleeding when brushing their teeth. Serious mucosal bleeding is rare above platelet counts of 5000 to 10,000 per mm^3. Spontaneous intracranial bleeding does occur, but it is usually preceded by other mucosal bleeding manifestations or occurs in conjunction with other clotting abnormalities. Medications such as aspirin or cephalosporin antibiotics may exaggerate the manifestations of thrombocytopenia.

Intrinsic platelet defects may be either inherited or acquired and will manifest in a manner similar to thrombocytopenia, depending on the severity of the abnormality. The first manifestation of a platelet function abnormality may be excessive bleeding after a surgical procedure.

Frequently, mild to moderate thrombocytopenia is found on routine testing as part of a general health check. On questioning, patients may report mucosal bleeding from the gingiva, nares, or rectum. Menorrhagia and excessive bruising are common complaints and should be quantitated as objectively as possible. Patients should be closely questioned as to their response to day-to-day challenges as well as surgeries, dental procedures, and history of spontaneous bleeding episodes. A careful history of any exposure to licit or illicit drugs, including over-the-counter medications, is imperative.

Table 1 lists common causes of thrombocytopenia. Thrombocytopenia is usually divided into three etiologic categories. The platelet count may be low due to decreased platelet production, accelerated platelet destruction, or an increase in the number of platelets sequestered in an enlarged spleen. A combination of any of these mechanisms will result in further reduction of the platelet count. Decreased platelet production can be seen as an isolated abnormality or in association with failure of other cell lines. With splenomegaly, other cell lines are not as severely affected. Platelet destruction is usually an isolated phenomenon but occasionally may be associated with either immune or mechanical red blood cell destruction. A fourth cause of thrombocytopenia is dilutional due to massive blood and fluid resuscitation in a bleeding patient.

Physical examination may reveal increased numbers of bruises that are not readily accounted for. Petechiae, if present, will be found in dependent areas (e.g., on the flanks in a patient who has been bedridden). Mucosal surfaces also may be covered with petechiae or hemorrhagic bullae. Careful examination of the lymphatic system for any enlarged lymph nodes or organs is required. The spleen is frequently easily palpable when moderate or se-

TABLE 1. Platelet-Mediated Disorders

Decreased Platelet Production

Aplastic anemia or marrow hypoplasia
Myelodysplasia
Hematopoietic malignancy
Vitamin deficiency (B_{12}, folate)
Myelophthisis (solid tumor malignancy,
  lymphoproliferative disorders, granulomas,
  myelofibrosis)
Drugs (chemotherapy, thiazide diuretics, ethanol)
Radiation

Increased Splenic Pooling

Portal hypertension
Lymphoproliferative disease
Myeloproliferative disease
Metabolic storage disease

Accelerated Platelet Destruction

Nonimmune
  Disseminated intravascular coagulation
  Isolated platelet consumption
    Thrombotic thrombocytopenic purpura
    Hemolytic-uremic syndrome
    Vascular malformations
    Artificial or severely deformed heart valves
    Intraventricular assist devices
Immune
  Primary autoimmune thrombocytopenia (ITP)
  Secondary autoimmune thrombocytopenia
    Collagen vascular disease
    Lymphoproliferative
    Infection (human immunodeficiency virus, hepatitis B,
      hepatitis C, cytomegalovirus, Epstein-Barr virus)
  Drug-induced immune thrombocytopenia
  Post-transfusion purpura

Dilutional

Qualitative Platelet Defects

Hereditary
  Storage pool deficiency
  Bernard-Soulier syndrome
  Glanzmann's thrombasthenia
Acquired
  Drug-induced (aspirin, ticlopidine [Ticlid], some
    cephalosporin antibiotics, nonsteroidal anti-
    inflammatory drugs)
  Uremia
  Hepatic failure

vere thrombocytopenia is due to increased splenic pooling. The patient may have other signs of portal hypertension as well. Patients with platelet dysfunction will have similar manifestations of bleeding despite normal platelet counts.

Thrombocytopenia should be confirmed by examination of the peripheral blood smear to rule out an artifact due to clumping in the collection vessel. The blood smear is also helpful in diagnosing disorders of nonimmune destruction such as thrombotic thrombocytopenic purpura or hemolytic-uremic syndrome and will show the presence of red blood cell fragments (schistocytes) on the peripheral blood smear. Large and/or hypogranulated platelets can be seen in some inherited disorders of platelet function, but frequently the platelets and megakaryocytes appear normal by light microscopy. The bleeding time and platelet aggregation studies can demonstrate the severity and nature of the abnormality. Coagulation tests, including a prothrombin time and a fibrinogen level, are helpful in the diagnosis of disseminated intravascular coagulation. The bone marrow examination can differentiate between hypoplastic dis-

orders, marrow infiltration with malignancy or granulomas, and thrombocytopenia due to ineffective marrow production (e.g., myelodysplasia and vitamin B_{12} deficiency). Patients with increased platelet destruction will have increased numbers of normal-appearing megakaryocytes in their bone marrow.

THERAPY

The overall need and rapidity with which a response is necessary, either in platelet count or improved hemostasis, must be considered in choosing a therapeutic approach. Most patients can tolerate mild to moderate thrombocytopenia or platelet dysfunction unless they experience trauma or have a need for surgical intervention. If the thrombocytopenia or bleeding is such that the risks and expected time to response are unacceptable, then transfusion and/or other approaches to prevent/stop bleeding may be necessary.

Nonspecific Therapy

Platelet Transfusion

Platelet transfusions are indicated for the patient who is bleeding or requires an invasive procedure and has significant thrombocytopenia, usually considered to be less than 30,000 to 50,000 per mm³. The patient who is not bleeding and is otherwise stable should not be transfused unless the platelet count is below 5000 to 10,000 per mm³ and is continuing to fall or other risks for bleeding are present. Transfusions are also indicated for the patient with congenital or acquired platelet function disorders not caused by intrinsic factors that will render the transfused platelets abnormal as well (e.g., renal failure). The usual dose of platelets is either a single platelet apheresis component or 6 to 8 units of pooled whole blood platelets. Patients who are expected to require recurrent transfusions should receive only blood components that have been filtered to reduce their white blood cell content. This will reduce the risk of alloimmunization and refractoriness to platelet transfusion. Transfusions can be used to increase the platelet count, but disorders with increased platelet destruction will likely result in a shortened life span of the transfused platelets as well. Transfused platelets are rapidly destroyed in immune thrombocytopenias, severely limiting this approach to treatment. Patients with severe immune thrombocytopenic purpura may never have a significant rise in platelet count, and transfusion is avoided unless the patient has life-threatening bleeding. Treatment with intravenously administered IgG before the platelet transfusion may result in an improved increment in patients with immune thrombocytopenic purpura. Patients who have been alloimmunized because of prior transfusions may require apheresis platelets from an HLA-matched donor to increase their platelet count.

Epsilon-Aminocaproic Acid*

Epsilon-aminocaproic acid (Amicar) inhibits fibrinolysis. Although it does not specifically improve platelet function, it probably shifts the balance toward clot formation and can work quickly to slow or stop persistent bleeding in a patient in whom specific therapy or transfusion is not effective. It is occasionally used in patients with severe thrombocytopenia with recurrent bleeding refractory to platelet transfusions. In patients with uncontrolled bleeding, 500 mg to 1 gram orally every 4 to 6 hours is recommended as a starting dose. Up to 24 grams per day may be given. Epsilon-aminocaproic acid is contraindicated in the presence of bleeding in the urinary tract.

Desmopressin

Desmopressin (1-deamino-8-D-arginine vasopressin, DDAVP) is a synthetic analogue of vasopressin. It raises circulating levels of vWF and factor VIII from endothelial stores. It has been shown to be effective in patients with platelet dysfunction secondary to renal failure and in some patients with inherited intrinsic platelet dysfunction. The intravenous dose of 0.3 gram per kg can be repeated every 2 days to allow stores of vWF and factor VIII to reaccumulate.

Specific Therapy

When thrombocytopenia is due to consumption or destruction associated with another disorder, treatment of the underlying disease is mandatory. This includes, for example, antibiotics for sepsis or treatment of a hematologic malignancy. Pathophysiology of the thrombocytopenia should govern both the approach to diagnosis and the treatment plan.

Disorders of Platelet Production

Any possible offending agents such as drugs or alcohol must be discontinued. For most other causes of hypoproliferative thrombocytopenia, treatment of the underlying disease process is crucial and nonspecific therapy can be used until recovery.

Increased Splenic Pooling

It is rare that thrombocytopenia associated with splenomegaly requires therapy. Some of the platelets pooled in the spleen are probably available for hemostasis at times of vascular challenge. Splenectomy can be helpful if thrombocytopenia is severe, but in the case of myelofibrosis it may be followed by acceleration of hepatic involvement.

Disorders of Platelet Destruction

Nonimmune Disorders

Thrombocytopenia associated with disseminated intravascular coagulation should be approached by treating the underlying cause and supporting clot-

---

*Not FDA approved for this indication.

ting with nonspecific measures. Patients with thrombotic thrombocytopenic purpura require specific therapy, including plasmapheresis or plasma infusions. These disorders are considered in more detail in their respective sections. Mild thrombocytopenia may be due to indwelling vascular devices or abnormalities of a cardiac valve. The thrombocytopenia is rarely severe enough to warrant therapy.

Immune Disorders

DRUG-INDUCED THROMBOCYTOPENIA. Drug-dependent antiplatelet antibodies are responsible for most drug-related platelet destruction. The most commonly implicated drugs include quinidine, quinine, sulfa, valproic acid, procainamide, and gold. In most cases, recovery occurs 7 to 10 days after withdrawal of the offending agent. Occasionally, severe thrombocytopenia will require corticosteroid therapy and intravenous IgG. Persistent drug-related thrombocytopenia may respond to plasmapheresis. The immune thrombocytopenia induced by gold therapy for arthritis can persist for months to years; and although it sometimes responds to chelation therapy, it may require more definitive therapy like that for immune thrombocytopenic purpura.

Heparin-associated thrombocytopenia is defined by at least a 50% drop in platelet count. Its occurrence has been reported with all heparin preparations, administration routes, and doses as small as heparin flushes for intravenous lines. In previously unexposed individuals the onset is usually 7 to 10 days after beginning heparin exposure, but it can occur in 2 to 3 days if the patient has received heparin previously. The antibody associated with heparin-associated thrombocytopenia causes platelet aggregation and can be associated with thrombosis with significant morbidity and mortality. In patients with suspected heparin-associated thrombocytopenia, heparin must be stopped immediately. If anticoagulation is required, hirudin (lepirudin) [Refludan]) or danaproid (Orgaran) can be used successfully. A rapid switch to warfarin therapy before instituting other anticoagulant therapy may result in sudden, severe thrombosis. Low-molecular-weight heparin is contraindicated in patients with heparin-associated thrombocytopenia.

POST-TRANSFUSION PURPURA. Individuals differ in specific platelet surface antigens. Rare individuals may develop profound thrombocytopenia after reexposure to a foreign platelet antigen. Initial exposure is usually through pregnancy, and therefore the majority of patients are women, but the first encounter with the antigen may be through a transfusion. When transfused even years later with any cellular blood component, patients recall the antibody. This results in rapid destruction of the transfused platelets and, by a poorly understood mechanism, destruction of autologous platelets as well. The PL^{A1} antigen is most commonly implicated. Treatment with intravenous IgG (1 gram per kg per day for 2 days) with or without high-dose corticosteroids usually results in rapid recovery. Plasmapheresis may be effective in refractory cases. Individuals in whom the disease is suspected should have platelet antibody and antigens characterized. Confirmed cases should undergo genetic counseling as well as be identified as requiring antigen-typed blood components for future transfusions.

SECONDARY AUTOIMMUNE THROMBOCYTOPENIA. Autoantibodies may be associated with a broad variety of diseases, including other autoimmune disorders, malignancy, lymphoproliferative disorders, and infections. Treatment of the thrombocytopenia is usually directed at the underlying disease. If the underlying disorder cannot be cured, therapies for immune thrombocytopenic purpura are sometimes effective in controlling the thrombocytopenia.

AUTOIMMUNE THROMBOCYTOPENIC PURPURA. Immune thrombocytopenic purpura is the most common type of isolated thrombocytopenia in adults. It is a chronic disease in 90% of cases. Platelets are destroyed in the reticuloendothelial system at an accelerated rate owing to an autoantibody directed against one of the major platelet glycoprotein complexes (GPIIb/IIIa or GPIb/IX/V).

Initial Therapy

Treatment should be instituted when the platelet count falls below 30,000 per mm³ or if signs of bleeding are present. Patients should receive prednisone, 1 to 2 mg per kg per day orally. After an increase in the platelet count above 75,000 per mm³, the prednisone can be gradually tapered over 6 to 8 weeks. For severe thrombocytopenia (<5000 to 10,000 per mm³) with signs of significant bleeding, an IgG preparation (1 gm/kg) or anti-RhD (WinRho at 75 µg/kg) should be administered intravenously daily for 2 days. For life- or organ-threatening bleeding emergencies only, platelet transfusions should be administered every 6 hours. Response to transfusion may improve after the administration of IgG. Epsilon-aminocaproic acid may be helpful for intracranial bleeding.

Therapy for Chronic Immune Thrombocytopenic Purpura

The majority of patients will respond to the therapy just discussed but will either fail at attempts to taper the prednisone regimen or relapse weeks or months later. Upper respiratory tract infection or other biologic stress frequently precedes a relapse. For recurrent episodes or failure to maintain a safe platelet count (>30,000 per mm³) off chronic corticosteroid or IgG therapy, splenectomy is indicated. This can often be performed safely by laparoscopy, if necessary after a course of intravenous IgG to raise the platelet count above 50,000 mm³. All patients should be immunized with pneumococcal, *Haemophilus influenzae,* and meningococcal vaccines before surgery to reduce the risk of overwhelming sepsis that can occur in splenectomized individuals. There should be a low threshold for antibiotic therapy of upper respiratory infections for life, and patients should be counseled in this regard.

Patients who are poor surgical risks, or who have strong objections to splenectomy, may achieve remission after pulse dexamethasone therapy. Decadron is administered in an oral dose of 40 mg for 4 consecutive days at 4-week intervals. A total of six cycles is given. Most patients show some response after one or two cycles, but the occasional patient may take as many as four cycles before thrombocytopenia improves. Patients dependent on prednisone can be continued on daily therapy between cycles, tapering the dose as tolerated to maintain the platelet count above 30,000 per mm³.

Up to 25% of patients will have persistent thrombocytopenia after splenectomy. Treatment options for these refractory patients include pulse dexamethasone therapy, pulse cyclophosphamide (Cytoxan)* therapy, danazol (Danocrine),* low-dose immunosuppression with cyclophosphamide or azathioprine (Imuran),* and vincristine* among others. All of these treatment modalities are associated with significant side effects and should be considered only in the context of persistent severe thrombocytopenia.

---

*Not FDA approved for this indication.

DISSEMINATED INTRAVASCULAR COAGULATION

method of
ERIC CHUN-YET LIAN, M.D.
*University of Miami / Sylvester Cancer Center
Miami, Florida*

Disseminated intravascular coagulation (DIC) is an intermediary disease reaction that is initiated by the local or generalized activation of hemostatic systems, leading to the formation of systemic microthrombi and hemorrhage associated with the consumption of platelets, plasma clotting factors, and inhibitors. The process is usually accompanied by secondary fibrinolysis. DIC usually begins with subtle intravascular coagulation, manifesting as a hypercoagulable state. When intravascular coagulation continues to intensify, the equilibrium between hemostatic processes and homeostatic defense mechanisms (such as cellular clearance of activated clotting intermediates by the liver and reticuloendothelial system, inactivation of activated clotting factors by antithrombin and other naturally occurring inhibitors, and fibrinolysis) becomes unbalanced. Depending on the local and circulatory conditions and the degree of hemostatic activation and consumption, the intravascular coagulation may manifest as local or systemic thrombosis, chronic compensated DIC, or fulminant DIC with both thrombosis and hemorrhage.

DIC is caused by excessive entrance of activating substances into the bloodstream. The process is enhanced or facilitated by excessive reactivity of platelets and clotting factors and defective control mechanisms. Triggering mechanisms can be divided into three types: (1) contact activation of the intrinsic clotting pathway by agents that affect the contact phase of blood clotting, such as antigen-antibody complexes, particulate matter from amniotic fluid embolism, and collagen and basement membrane exposure after endothelial damage resulting from viremia, heat stroke, and septicemia; (2) activation of the extrinsic clotting pathway by release of tissue thromboplastin into the circulating blood from leukocytes, cancer cells, and endothelial cells (tissue thromboplastin is also released in trauma, burn, surgery, sepsis, and abruptio placentae to cause DIC); and (3) direct activation of factor X, prothrombin, and fibrinogen by proteolytic enzymes, such as trypsin, thrombin or thrombin-like substances, venoms, and extracts of mucin-producing adenocarcinoma.

The clinical pictures depend on the balance of opposing reactions of the coagulation processes and the limiting factors. In some patients, thrombotic features dominate, especially in the early stages. Clinical clues include oliguria, renal dysfunction, respiratory distress syndrome, liver dysfunction, mental confusion, and neurologic deficits. Bleeding may occur in the skin or mucous membrane (petechiae or ecchymosis). Hematuria and gastrointestinal bleeding may be observed. Bleeding on the venipuncture sites or sites of surgical drainage tubes is common. In severe cases, shock frequently exists, and microangiopathic hemolytic anemia may be observed.

In the early stages of DIC, clotting factors are still normal or even elevated; prothrombin time and partial thromboplastin time are either normal or shortened. More sensitive tests are required for the detection of DIC. These include elevation of D-dimer, prothrombin fragments 1 and 2, fibrinopeptide A or B, fibrin/fibrinogen degradation products, circulating soluble fibrin, thrombin-antithrombin complex, plasmin-antiplasmin complex, platelet factor 4, beta-thromboglobulin, and shortened half-life of platelets and fibrinogen. In the late stages of DIC, consumption of clotting factors, inhibitors, and platelets develops, along with the occurrence of secondary fibrinolysis. Laboratory studies may reveal a decreased platelet count; fragmented red blood cells; prolonged prothrombin time and partial thromboplastin time; abnormal clot formation and dissolution; decreased fibrinogen, factor II, factor V, factor VIII, and factor XIII levels; prolonged thrombin time; and depressed plasminogen, antithrombin, protein C, and protein S levels. Disseminated intravascular disorders should be differentiated from other acquired bleeding disorders such as vitamin K deficiency, liver disease, and acquired inhibitors. Many patients with DIC are debilitated, may not have eaten well for several days, and have been placed on antibiotics. Hence patients may have vitamin K deficiency as well.

THERAPY

The aims of therapy for DIC are to prevent the further formation of microthrombi, to remove the microthrombi already formed, and to correct the hemostatic defects.

General Measures

Treatment should be started as early as possible once DIC is suspected or in disease states that predispose the patient to DIC. The primary treatment should be directed toward the removal of underlying causes, such as evacuation of the uterus for abruptio placentae and antibiotics for septicemia. Supportive treatment for the correction of the hypoxia, shock, acidosis, and electrolyte imbalance is very important in order to slow down the intravascular coagulation process.

Anticoagulant Therapy

Heparin therapy used for DIC is based on the facts that it removes thrombin, interrupts the intravascular generation of thrombin, and prevents the further deposition of fibrin in the microvasculature. The choice of heparin dose should be individualized, depending on the underlying disease, vascular integrity, and hemostatic functions. A dose ranging from 5 to 25 units per kg per hour is usually sufficient. For acute DIC, continuous intravenous infusion is perhaps the safest way of attempting to treat DIC and prevent its complications. In my experience, low-dose heparin (5 to 10 units per kg per hour) minimizes the intensity of DIC to improve hemostatic function without causing bleeding. For subacute or chronic DIC, heparin can be given intravenously every 4 hours or subcutaneously every 8 to 12 hours. The prophylactic use of heparin in septic abortion and preeclampsia has been shown to be beneficial. For prophylactic use, low-dose heparin, 10,000 to 20,000 units per day, is recommended and given by either intravenous infusion or subcutaneous injection. In addition, prophylactic use of heparin has also been recommended for patients with sepsis, severe burn, or other disease states predisposing to the development of DIC. In heparin therapy for DIC, it is desirable to maintain a heparin level between 0.15 and 0.25 units per mL. The effectiveness of heparin therapy is best monitored by fibrinogen level, D-dimer, fibrin degradation products, and fibrinopeptide A assay if available. Other thrombin inhibitors, low-molecular-weight (LMW) heparin,* heparinoid,* hirudin,* and argatroban,† have also been used for DIC. There is evidence that LMW heparin is as effective and safe as unfractionated heparin. Instead of a thrombin inhibitor, warfarin (Coumadin) may be used for chronic DIC.

Replacement of Natural Anticoagulants

Antithrombin, protein C, or tissue factor pathway inhibitor concentrate has been used individually for DIC. High-dose antithrombin with or without low-dose heparin has been shown in limited studies to improve DIC and increase survival of patients with severe sepsis, but its benefit remains controversial. Combined use of inhibitor concentrates with or without low-dose heparin is theoretically more promising, and further clinical trials are warranted.

Replacement of Hemostatic Elements with Plasma and/or Platelets

When patients have active bleeding as a result of decreased levels of clotting factors or platelets,

---

*Not FDA approved for this indication.
*Investigational drug in the United States.

plasma infusion, platelet transfusion, or both are indicated. Replacement therapy for hemostatic components can be given simultaneously when heparin therapy is initiated. Plasma contains not only clotting factors to stop bleeding but also all the natural inhibitors to counteract the clotting processes. In obstetric complications, such as abruptio placentae, evacuation of conceptive product and massive transfusion with fresh blood and plasma without heparin have proved to be beneficial. In a few cases of DIC, plasma exchange has been shown to be helpful.

Activators and Inhibitors of the Fibrinolytic System

Secondary fibrinolytic activation is a protective mechanism against microthrombosis. During the intravascular coagulation process, plasminogen activator is decreased. The failure to activate fibrinolysis would favor persistence of microthrombi. Therefore, it is logical to use the thrombolytic enzymes streptokinase,* urokinase,* or tissue plasminogen activator* for DIC. Because of the high incidence of bleeding complications, their clinical application is limited. The use of streptokinase may be beneficial in hyaline membrane disease in premature infants and in the hemolytic-uremic syndrome.

Epsilon-aminocaproic acid (EACA; Amicar) and tranexamic acid (Cyklokapron) are potent antifibrinolytic agents. The administration of EACA alone in patients with DIC and secondary fibrinolysis is contraindicated. In patients with massive hemorrhage caused by secondary hyperfibrinolysis and defibrination, EACA, 20 to 50 mg per kg every 6 hours, may be considered if heparin is given simultaneously.

---

*Not FDA approved for this indication.

THROMBOTIC THROMBOCYTOPENIC PURPURA

method of
WALTER H. A. KAHR, M.D., Ph.D., and
CATHERINE P. M. HAYWARD, M.D., Ph.D.
*Hamilton Health Sciences Corporation and
McMaster University
Hamilton, Ontario, Canada*

Thrombotic thrombocytopenic purpura (TTP) is a rare disorder characterized by an acute onset of petechial bleeding, fever, anemia, and a microangiopathy involving terminal arterioles and capillaries. The introduction of plasma exchange as standard TTP therapy reduced its mortality from 90% to 10 to 30%. Although TTP is rare (approximate incidence of 1 per 1 million), it is important to diagnose this condition early, so that life-saving therapy can be administered.

CLINICAL FEATURES

TTP should be considered in the diagnosis of patients presenting with acute thrombocytopenia (platelet count

TABLE 1. Differential Diagnosis of Thrombotic Thrombocytopenic Purpura (TTP)/Hemolytic-Uremic Syndrome (HUS)

TTP/HUS
  Idiopathic TTP/HUS
  TTP associated with collagen vascular disorders
  Verotoxin-associated HUS
  Drug-induced TTP
  Transplantation-associated TTP
  HIV-associated TTP
  Malignancy or chemotherapy-associated TTP
Disseminated intravascular coagulation (infection, malignancy)
Preeclampsia or HELLP syndrome
Vasculitis, including systemic lupus erythematosus and
  polyarteritis nodosa
Disseminated carcinoma
Malignant hypertension
Dysfunctional prosthetic heart valve
Catheters or artificial vascular grafts
Kasabach-Merritt syndrome
Acute renal allograft rejection

< 100,000/μL), especially if they have concomitant anemia, red cell fragmentation, neurologic symptoms, or renal dysfunction. The differential diagnoses of TTP are shown in Table 1. The minimal criteria for diagnosing TTP are thrombocytopenia and microangiopathic hemolytic anemia in the absence of alternative diagnoses. The classic features of TTP include (1) microangiopathic hemolytic anemia, (2) thrombocytopenia, (3) neurologic dysfunction, (4) fever, and (5) renal dysfunction. However, only 20 to 30% of patients present with this pentad, and 60% present with microangiopathic hemolytic anemia, thrombocytopenia, and neurologic dysfunction (Table 2). Often, it is difficult to distinguish TTP from hemolytic-uremic syndrome (HUS), and they are considered by many to be overlapping conditions (TTP/HUS).

Patients with TTP commonly have malaise and weakness, and 25% have fever. Their bleeding commonly involves the skin and retina, but patients can also have gastrointestinal and genitourinary tract bleeding. Sixty percent of patients have neurologic manifestations that range from subtle behavioral changes, irritability, confusion, headaches, transient visual disturbances, focal neuro-

TABLE 2. Checklist for Suspected Thrombotic Thrombocytopenic Purpura (TTP)/Hemolytic-Uremic Syndrome (HUS)

- Fatigue, malaise, fever
- Bleeding symptoms
- Thrombocytopenia with evidence of a schistocytic hemolytic anemia
- Neurologic symptoms
- Oliguria or laboratory evidence of renal dysfunction
- Previous episode(s) of TTP/HUS
- Familial history of TTP/HUS
- Prodromal symptoms suggestive of HUS (abdominal cramps, bloody diarrhea, or known exposure to verotoxin-producing organisms)
- Concomitant conditions, (e.g., pregnancy, hypertension, transplant, malignancy, autoimmune disorders, prosthetic heart valves or vascular grafts, human immunodeficiency virus infection)
- Exposure to ticlopidine, quinine, quinidine, cyclosporine, tacrolimus, mitomycin C, other chemotherapeutic agents

logic deficits, seizures, coma, and death. Fifty to 60% of patients have renal dysfunction (elevated urea nitrogen and creatinine, hematuria, proteinuria, and, less commonly, acute renal failure), and 20% require dialysis support. Other complications of TTP include bowel infarction and perforation, heart failure, cardiac arrhythmia, myocardial infarction, and pulmonary edema. Patients with prodromal symptoms of severe abdominal cramps and bloody diarrhea should be investigated to determine if they have HUS caused by verotoxin-producing enteric organisms.

ETIOLOGY

The etiologies of TTP and HUS are poorly understood. Platelet-rich microthrombi form in capillaries and arterioles of many organs in TTP and can cause hemorrhage and tissue necrosis. Platelets and platelet-activating factors are believed to play a major role in the pathogenesis of TTP and HUS, but how these factors are generated is unknown. Abnormalities in plasma von Willebrand factor (vWF), a protein important for platelet adhesion and aggregation, are extremely common in TTP and include increases in the ultra-high-molecular-weight forms of vWF or a relative loss of high-molecular-weight forms. Although these changes may be due to endothelial cell injury, they may also be due to abnormal proteolysis of vWF by calcium-dependent proteases or an acquired deficiency of a plasma enzyme that cleaves the large, platelet reactive multimers of vWF into less-reactive forms. Some patients with TTP have IgG antibodies that inhibit the vWF-cleaving protease in normal plasma, suggesting an immune pathogenesis.

Familial forms of TTP and HUS are rare and can result in chronic or intermittent TTP/HUS. Many require long-term maintenance therapy with plasma to control their microangiopathy. The inheritance appears to be autosomal recessive. Some familial forms are associated with a deficiency of the plasma vWF-cleaving protease, but the identity of this protease and the genetic causes of familial TTP/HUS are not yet known.

Although TTP is commonly idiopathic, HUS can develop after exposure to verotoxin-producing strains of enteric pathogens such as *Escherichia coli* O157:H7, *Shigella dysenteriae*, and *Salmonella typhi*. These toxins are lethal to endothelial cells and are believed to initiate a cascade of events, culminating in platelet aggregation and microangiopathic hemolysis. Fortunately, not all patients exposed to these toxin-producing pathogens develop HUS. Another important infection associated with TTP/HUS is the human immunodeficiency virus (HIV). Because patients with HIV infection can also develop immune thrombocytopenia, it is important to exclude TTP/HUS in patients who present with thrombocytopenia in association with HIV infection.

TTP can manifest during or after pregnancy, and it is often difficult to differentiate from preeclampsia and HELLP syndrome (*h*emolysis, *e*levated *l*iver enzymes, *l*ow *p*latelets), owing to overlap in their clinical features. TTP is the most likely cause of thrombocytopenia and microangiopathy in the first half of the pregnancy. If the clinician cannot determine whether a pregnant patient has TTP or preeclampsia, it is best to treat both disease entities. The outcomes for mother and fetus are often good if the treatment is begun early.

It is important to identify patients who develop drug-induced TTP and HUS and discontinue the offending agent. The drugs commonly associated with TTP/HUS include ticlopidine (Ticlid), quinine, and quinidine. Re-exposure may trigger a relapse. TTP/HUS can occur after transplantation, and it is associated with the use of antirejection drugs such as cyclosporine (Sandimmune) or the related compound tacrolimus (Prograf). These patients may improve if treated and switched to different antirejection drugs.

TTP/HUS can manifest as a complication of malignancy and/or treatment with some chemotherapeutic agents (especially mitomycin C). In these patients, it may be difficult to distinguish from disseminated intravascular coagulation. The outcomes in chemotherapy and malignancy-associated TTP are much poorer.

LABORATORY INVESTIGATIONS

Patients with TTP are typically thrombocytopenic and have evidence of intravascular hemolysis. Their platelet counts are usually less than 100,000 per mm³, and 90% have hemoglobin levels of less than 100 grams per liter. Schistocytes (fragmented red cells) are a characteristic finding in TTP, but they may not appear until several days after the onset of symptoms, and they may be present before anemia develops. Manual platelet counts should be performed because schistocytes artifactually raise the platelet counts measured by automated cell counters.

Other laboratory abnormalities in TTP include elevated levels of lactate dehydrogenase (LDH) and indirect bilirubin. Blood urea nitrogen, creatinine, and urinalyses are abnormal if there is renal involvement. Most patients have normal prothrombin times and partial thromboplastin times, unless there is an accompanying disseminated intravascular coagulation. Platelet counts and LDH levels are useful in assessing ongoing disease activity.

THERAPY AND OUTCOMES

TTP/HUS should be considered a medical emergency. The mainstay of therapy is plasma exchange, which is more effective than plasma infusion. Plasma (100 to 150 mL per hour for an average-sized adult) should be infused while emergency plasma exchange is arranged, especially if the patient requires transfer to a plasmapheresis center. Care should be taken to avoid fluid overload. Patients should be exchanged with one plasma volume daily until they achieve a platelet count (150,000 per μL) and a decrease in their LDH value. Although cryosupernatant (which contains less vWF) is often preferred over fresh-frozen plasma, its superiority is not yet established. Patients may require plasma exchange for days to months before a remission is achieved, and improvements in LDH and platelet counts may be delayed. Most patients will achieve a remission with continued therapy, and larger volume exchanges or twice-daily plasma exchanges should be considered for patients with severe disease or deteriorating status. Once platelet counts normalize, plasmapheresis should be tapered to every second or third day for an additional 1 to 2 weeks. Exacerbations are frequent during the tapering and can be managed with renewed plasma exchange until platelet counts improve and are sustained. Red cell transfusions are frequently required to treat the hemolytic anemia. Platelet transfusions are of no benefit in TTP and, because of anecdotal reports of deterioration after platelet transfusions, they are contraindicated.

Corticosteroids are routinely administered as part of the initial treatment at many centers, but their benefit has not been evaluated in randomized clinical trials. Data implicating antibodies against a vWF-cleaving protease in the pathogenesis of TTP have led to a renewed interest in evaluating the roles of corticosteroids, intravenous gammaglobulin, and other immunomodulatory treatments. Antiplatelet agents (e.g., aspirin, 325 mg daily) can be given once the platelet count is more than 50,000 per mm^3, but their benefit, if any, is probably small. Splenectomy has been used as part of the treatment for acute TTP, but similar outcomes can be achieved with continued aggressive plasma exchange. The roles of other therapies, including intravenous immune globulin and vincristine, are uncertain.

With current therapy, around 90% of patients recover, but many patients are left with significant, permanent sequelae, which can include persistent renal dysfunction or failure (around 8% will be dialysis dependent), hypertension, and neurologic impairment, in addition to relapses, which occur in about 35% of patients within 10 years. Patients should be made aware of these risks so that they understand the urgency of seeking medical attention if they experience symptoms suggestive of a relapse. Isolated, transient thrombocytopenia can occur after remission, and it may resolve spontaneously or herald a relapse. Relapses should be treated in the same manner as an initial episode of TTP; and, if frequent, splenectomy (in remission) can be considered as a preventive measure. Relapses in women can occur during or after pregnancy and with the use of oral contraceptives. Because these relapses can be fatal, the potential risks of pregnancy and hormonal therapies should be discussed with patients as part of their long-term management.

HEMOCHROMATOSIS

method of
JAMES D. COOK, M.D.
Kansas University Medical Center
Kansas City, Kansas

Hemochromatosis refers to heavy iron accumulation in parenchymal cells that commonly results in progressive tissue damage, involving in particular the liver, heart, pancreas, and joints. The most common and important cause is an autosomal recessive disorder that is estimated to affect as many as 1 of every 200 white persons of Western European descent. This disorder has been referred to variously as primary, idiopathic, genetic, or hereditary hemochromatosis but is called simply hemochromatosis in this discussion. Similar clinical manifestations can result from a variety of diseases, the most important being chronic anemias associated with marked ineffective erythropoiesis. Thalassemia major and sideroblastic anemia are the prime examples. In these anemias iron chelation therapy is usually needed to reduce body iron. Secondary hemochromatosis can also be produced by repeated blood transfu-

sions, by excessive parenteral iron administration, and occasionally in association with hemolytic anemia, porphyria cutanea tarda, excessive oral iron ingestion, and chronic alcoholism.

The recent discovery of the HFE gene on chromosome 6 marked the beginning of a new era with regard to the diagnosis, epidemiology, and pathophysiology of hemochromatosis. Important clues about the nature of the underlying inherited defect in regulation of iron absorption by the intestinal mucosal cell are already emerging from studies of this gene. There are two relatively common mutations in the HFE gene, termed C282Y and H63D, that have been identified in patients with hemochromatosis. Approximately 80% of patients are homozygous for the C282Y mutation; an additional 5 to 10% of patients are doubly heterozygous for the C282Y and H63D mutations. Preliminary studies indicate that the frequency of these mutations in the population is far higher than the number of persons who develop clinical manifestations. In addition, because of the iron losses associated with childbearing and menstruation, the risk of clinical manifestations is considerably lower in women than in men.

The clinical manifestations of hemochromatosis are highly varied. Nonspecific complaints include weight loss, fatigue, abdominal discomfort, impotence, and arthritis. Symptoms resulting from diabetes or heart failure are not uncommon. The important physical findings include jaundice, increased skin pigmentation, hepatosplenomegaly, and testicular atrophy. A family history of hemochromatosis or its characteristic clinical manifestations in a pattern consistent with autosomal recessive inheritance is often obtained.

The initial approach to the laboratory diagnosis is now firmly established. The degree of iron saturation of plasma transferrin as measured by the ratio of the serum iron to total iron-binding capacity is the key measurement. In the absence of known causes of secondary iron loading, transferrin saturation values greater than 60% in men and 50% in women are diagnostic if confirmed on a second specimen obtained in the morning after an overnight fast. Because an elevated transferrin saturation reflects the inherent metabolic abnormality in hemochromatosis rather than the degree of iron loading, the latter should be assessed by measuring the serum ferritin concentration. If this concentration is elevated above 200 μg per liter in women and 300 μg per liter in men, genetic testing should be performed as a further aid in diagnosis and to assist in family screening. For patients whose liver test results are abnormal, many authorities still recommend a liver biopsy and a quantitative nonheme iron determination to detect fibrosis and thereby evaluate the risk of developing hepatocellular carcinoma. Magnetic resonance imaging can detect moderate to severe iron excess less invasively than liver biopsy but does not provide the same prognostic information. The most reliable method of determining the degree of iron excess is to maintain accurate records of the amount of iron removed during therapeutic phlebotomy.

TREATMENT

All patients with an elevated transferrin saturation and serum ferritin concentration should undergo therapeutic phlebotomy to fully deplete body iron reserves. The only possible exceptions are patients with debilitating medical illnesses such as an advanced malignancy, severe heart disease, or liver failure. Treatment of older patients should not be withheld because of age. Before treatment is initiated, detailed baseline investigations should be performed to evaluate the degree of organ dysfunction resulting from parenchymal iron deposition. Abnormalities detected in the history or on physical examination should be pursued with appropriate laboratory and radiologic studies to further assess the possibility of liver, cardiac, joint, endocrine, and sexual function abnormalities. All patients should be cautioned against the use of alcoholic beverages, iron-containing supplements, and foods heavily fortified with iron. The number of phlebotomies required for induction or maintenance therapy can be slightly reduced by eliminating the dietary intake of red meat, but in general, no alteration in the patient's customary diet is required.

The objective of the *induction* phase of phlebotomy therapy of hemochromatosis is to reduce body iron levels by repeated venesection. The goal is to induce mild iron deficiency to ensure complete exhaustion of iron stores. The program should be performed under medical supervision at a local blood bank, an outpatient clinic, the physician's office, or a hospital laboratory. From 400 to 500 mL of blood, equivalent to 200 to 250 mg of iron, is removed at each session, although lesser amounts can be withdrawn in the beginning in patients who experience postphlebotomy weakness, in elderly patients, and in patients who are initially anemic. The typical frequency of blood removal is weekly, but a frequency ranging from three times a week to twice a month has been used successfully. Patients should be encouraged to drink extra fluids before and after each phlebotomy and to avoid vigorous activity for a day or two.

A hemoglobin determination should precede each phlebotomy. It is wise to delay blood removal for a week if the baseline hemoglobin falls more than 30 grams per liter in men and 20 grams per liter in women or below 110 grams per liter at any time in patients who were not anemic initially. Typically, 1 to 2 months of regular phlebotomy is required to achieve maximal enhancement of red blood cell production. Consequently, problems with an excessive reduction in hemoglobin concentration during the initial weeks of therapy usually resolve with continued phlebotomy. It is important to record the hemoglobin concentration and the volume or weight of blood removed at each session. The amount of iron removed is calculated on the basis of an iron content of 3.38 mg of iron per gram of hemoglobin. I encourage patients to maintain a personal phlebotomy log with the date, hemoglobin concentration, and amount of blood and/or iron removed on each occasion. This record is useful if there is a change in physicians and, importantly, for determining the total amount of iron removed during the induction phase. A suitable definition of clinically significant iron loading is the removal of more than 4 grams of iron after subtracting 3 mg of iron daily over the duration of the phlebotomy program to account for the continued absorption of dietary iron.

The most reliable method for monitoring the progress of the induction phlebotomy program is to obtain serum ferritin measurements at monthly intervals. Although the initial ferritin level is not a reliable indicator of the total units of blood that will need to be removed, monitoring the rate of decline in serum ferritin is helpful. The serum ferritin determination is also the best method of determining the end point of induction therapy. A desirable end point is a reduction in serum ferritin below 10 μg per liter sustained for at least 3 weeks without further blood removal. In patients with liver damage or associated inflammatory disease, both of which elevate the serum ferritin independently of iron stores, it is seldom possible to achieve a subnormal ferritin level, which necessitates the use of a higher ferritin end point. An alternative method of determining the end point is to use the hemoglobin concentration, which begins to fall with each blood-letting once iron stores are exhausted. A significant reduction in hemoglobin should be sustained for 3 to 4 weeks without further blood-letting to establish mild iron deficiency anemia. With reliance on the hemoglobin, other laboratory indices of iron deficiency erythropoiesis such as a low mean corpuscular hemoglobin, elevated total iron-binding capacity, low transferrin saturation, elevated free erythrocyte protoporphyrin, or increased serum transferrin receptor are useful in establishing the end point of regular phlebotomies.

The *maintenance* phlebotomy program is started when the hemoglobin concentration returns to prephlebotomy levels. The objective of this phase is to maintain a serum ferritin concentration in the low normal range below 50 μg per liter. The number of phlebotomies necessary to achieve this varies considerably between patients, depending on the severity of the absorptive defect and, to a lesser extent, on the intake of heme and nonheme dietary iron. I initially recommend the removal of 4 units of blood annually. A serum ferritin determination should be performed yearly and the rate of phlebotomy adjusted to maintain the target ferritin concentration. The transferrin saturation usually returns to elevated levels soon after entering the maintenance phase of therapy and often before the serum ferritin level begins to increase. Attempts to maintain the transferrin saturation within the normal range by continuing phlebotomies can result in symptoms of mild iron deficiency such as weakness, fatigue, and malaise. Consequently, periodic measurements of transferrin saturation are of no apparent value in monitoring the adequacy of maintenance therapy.

Long-term management of patients with significant iron excess as determined by the total amount of iron removed should focus on the iron-related organ damage detected during the initial medical evaluation. The two most important complications are diabetes and cirrhosis, which reduce survival significantly. The clinical manifestations that are often ameliorated by phlebotomy therapy are heart failure, cardiac arrhythmias, diabetes, and liver impairment. On the other hand, cirrhosis, arthropathy, impotence, and sterility are usually unaffected by phlebotomy therapy. Treatment of these complications does not differ from their management in patients without hemochromatosis. The dreaded complication of iron excess in patients who have cirrhotic changes on liver biopsy at the outset is the development of hepatocellular carcinoma, the leading cause of death in patients with hemochromatosis. Medical examinations with particular attention to alteration in liver function, unexplained weight loss, and abdominal pain should be performed regularly. Abdominal sonograms at 6-month intervals should detect a limited proportion of early malignancies, but regular measurements of alpha-fetoprotein are not of proven benefit in surveillance.

One of the most important obligations of physicians caring for patients with hemochromatosis is to test family members who may be similarly affected, using strategies based on the known autosomal recessive transmission. Those at highest risk are siblings, but all first-degree relatives should be tested; because of the high frequency of the C282Y mutation, approximately 5% of the offspring of patients are affected. Measurements of transferrin saturation have been the mainstay of family screening, but there is mounting evidence that genetic screening may ultimately prove to be the most cost-effective strategy. The reason is that heterozygous siblings of patients may have an elevated transferrin saturation. Moreover, homozygous patients have a normal transferrin saturation during the first two decades of life, and the optimal age for definitive screening with the transferrin saturation is unknown at present. Many affected parents are reluctant to accept the continued uncertainty about whether their children have the disease. These limitations can be avoided by establishing the nature of the genetic mutation in the patient and using this information to search for affected family members. When screening for the disease in the children of large families, it is more efficient to test the other parent rather than all of the children. If the mate has a normal HFE gene, the children do not have to be tested.

HODGKIN'S DISEASE: CHEMOTHERAPY

method of
CAROL S. PORTLOCK, M.D., and
CRAIG MOSKOWITZ, M.D.
Memorial Sloan-Kettering Cancer Center
New York, New York

Hodgkin's disese (HD) is a highly curable malignancy of the immune system whose treatment has gradually evolved since the 1960s. Both radiotherapy and combination chemotherapy may be options for management, and the choice of strategy is tempered by the expected curability of the regimen employed, its acute toxicities, and its late effects. These recommendations have generally been developed with the successful completion of prospective, randomized phase III studies. Attention continues to be

TABLE 1. Staging of Hodgkin's Disease

Stage I: Involvement of a single lymph node region
Stage II: Involvement of two or more lymph node regions on the same side of the diaphragm
Stage III: Involvement of lymph node regions on both sides of the diaphragm
 E: Involvement of a single extranodal site that is contiguous to the known nodal region
Stage IV: Involvement of noncontiguous extranodal sites
 A: No symptoms
 B: Fever (temperature >38°C), drenching night sweats, unexplained loss of >10% body weight within the preceding 6 months

placed on decreasing toxicities, maintaining efficacy of established treatments, prognostic factors to identify poor-risk subsets for investigative therapy, and prevention of late effects whenever possible.

Although the cause of, and cell of origin in, HD is still uncertain, it appears to be a disease of lymphocyte origin with both genetic and environmental influences. The Reed-Sternberg cell must be identified in nodal tissue within the appropriate reactive cellular milieu to confer a definitive diagnosis. Immunostains for CD15 and CD30 are often positive, whereas B cell markers are negative. An exception is lymphocyte-predominant HD, which has now been separated clinically and pathologically from other cases and is often managed as a B cell indolent lymphoma. Lymphocyte depletion HD has disappeared as an entity. Nodular sclerosing and mixed cellularity HD are the two most common subtypes.

Non-Hodgkin's lymphomas that should be excluded when HD diagnosis is confirmed include anaplastic (CD30$^+$ or Ki-1$^+$) large cell lymphoma, mediastinal large cell lymphoma with sclerosis, and T cell–rich B cell lymphoma.

HD staging has been simplified, as chemotherapy is more commonly utilized in early stages (Table 1). All patients should have a careful history taken and undergo a physical examination, including complete blood count and sedimentation rate, routine liver and renal function, lactic dehydrogenase; posteroanterior and lateral chest radiographs; computed tomography (CT) scan of chest, abdomen, and pelvis; gallium scan; and bone marrow biopsy. Lymphangiography, bone scanning, and magnetic resonance imaging may be indicated under certain circumstances. Clinical stage must be confirmed pathologically only if it will change therapy.

CHEMOTHERAPY REGIMENS (Table 2)

Mechlorethamine, Oncovin, procarbazine, and prednisone (MOPP) chemotherapy was the first combination regimen with reported curability in HD. It has been abandoned since the 1980s because of its high incidence of infertility and the late development of myelodysplasia and acute myelogenous leukemia. Randomized studies have generally shown equivalent or slightly decreased efficacy of MOPP compared with doxorubicin-based regimens (see Table 2). With the introduction of ondansetron (Zofran), it became possible to easily administer Adriamycin, bleomycin, vinblastine, and dacarbazine (ABVD), and recent randomized studies have clearly demonstrated its superiority—not necessarily in efficacy, but in lack of

TABLE 2. **Selected Combination Chemotherapy Regimens for Hodgkin's Disease**

ABVD		
Doxorubicin (Adriamycin)	25 mg/m² IV	days 1, 15
Bleomycin	10 U/m² IV	days 1, 15
Vinblastine	6 mg/m² IV	days 1, 15
Dacarbazine	375 mg/m² IV	days 1, 15
(Repeat cycle q 28 d)		
MOPP		
Nitrogen mustard (Mustargen)	6 mg/m² IV	days 1, 8
Vincristine (Oncovin)	1.4 mg/m² IV	days 1, 8
Procarbazine	100 mg/m² PO	days 1–14
Prednisone	40 mg/m² PO	days 1–14
(Repeat cycle q 28 d)		
STANFORD V		
Doxorubicin	25 mg/m² IV	days 1, 15
Vinblastine	6 mg/m² IV	days 1, 15
Mechlorethamine	6 mg/m² IV	day 1
Vincristine	1.4 mg/m² IV	days 8, 22
Bleomycin	5 U/m² IV	days 8, 22
Etoposide	60 mg/m² IV	days 15, 16
Prednisone	40 mg/m² PO	qod
(Repeat cycle q 28 d)		
BEACOPP		
Bleomycin	10 mg/m² IV	day 8
Etoposide	100 mg/m² IV	days 1–3
Doxorubicin (Adriamycin)	35 mg/m² IV	day 1
Cyclophosphamide	650 mg/m² IV	day 1
Vincristine (Oncovin)	1.4 mg/m² IV	day 8
Procarbazine	100 mg/m² PO	days 1–7
Prednisone	40 mg/m² PO	days 1–14
(Repeat cycle q 21 d)		
VBM		
Vinblastine	6 mg/m² IV	days 1, 8
Bleomycin	10 mg/m² IV	days 1, 8
Methotrexate	30 mg/m² IV	days 1, 8
(Repeat cycle q 28 d)		
NOVP		
Mitoxantrone (Novantrone)	10 mg/m² IV	day 1
Vincristine (Oncovin)	1.4 mg/m² IV	day 8
Vinblastine	6 mg/m² IV	day 1
Prednisone	100 mg/m² PO	days 1–5
(Repeat cycle q 21 d)		

infertility and secondary myelodysplasia and leukemia.

Today ABVD is considered the "gold standard" of combination chemotherapy regimens against which all others will need to be judged. A complete response rate of approximately 80% and a disease-free survival rate of 50 to 60% can be anticipated in advanced disease.

Advanced Hodgkin's Disease

Advanced HD is classically defined as clinical stages IIIB and IV disease. In these stages, HD is only curable with a systemic approach, and ABVD is the standard combination chemotherapy. This regimen is generally administered for six cycles, often with restaging after four cycles. Interim images may assist in the assessment of chemoresponsiveness and in identification of patients for whom a second salvage regimen with autologous transplantation may

need to be considered. If the disease becomes gallium negative, even in the presence of uncertain complete response, no further therapy may be indicated after six cycles of chemotherapy.

It remains controversial whether postchemotherapy adjuvant irradiation improves outcome in advanced HD. If it is to be utilized, radiotherapy field sizes should be minimized, doses kept low, and sites to be irradiated limited to "bulky" areas.

New combination chemotherapy regimens under investigation for advanced HD include Stanford V and BEACOPP (see Table 2). Both are short-course, dose-intense, combined-modality regimens with promising early results. Randomized trials are underway to elucidate their real value compared with ABVD.

Early-Stage Hodgkin's Disease

As ABVD has gradually gained acceptance as standard therapy for advanced HD, this drug regimen has also had increasing use for early-stage disease (stages I, II, and IIIA). The advantages of combined-modality therapy in this setting include (1) disease below the diaphragm can be controlled without the need to proceed with laparotomy staging; (2) radiotherapy fields can be minimized because only the postchemotherapy disease volume is irradiated; and (3) late effects of both chemotherapy and irradiation can be minimized by the strategic use of both. More than 80% of all patients can be expected to achieve durable complete remission with this approach.

Randomized studies from the Milan group have demonstrated excellent disease-free survival rates and overall survival outcomes utilizing four cycles of ABVD followed by involved-field irradiation. This combined-modality regimen is becoming the gold standard by which other early-stage treatment approaches must be measured. It exposes the patient to only limited chemotherapy and limited irradiation, and it appears to maximize benefit while minimizing the potential for late effects.

Many other chemotherapy programs are being studied for early-stage HD in conjunction with radiotherapy. Vincristine, bleomycin, and methotrexate (VBM) and Novantrone, Oncovin, vinblastine, and prednisone (NOVP) are two such examples (see Table 2). It is unclear what advantage these regimens have over four cycles of ABVD except the lack of doxorubicin (Adriamycin; a cardiac toxic agent, although rarely so in clinical practice).

A pivotal question for the future is the role of chemotherapy alone for early-stage HD. This is the subject of several ongoing prospective studies.

Bulky Hodgkin's Disease

HD may present with a large mass, most often in the anterior mediastinum. According to the Cotswold staging criteria, this presentation is represented by the designation "x" and connotes the need to receive combined-modality therapy.

A "bulky" site is defined as a mass greater than 10 cm or greater than one-third the chest diameter.

Retrospective studies have shown that neither radiotherapy alone for bulky early-stage disease nor chemotherapy alone for advanced-stage disease with a bulky site is adequate treatment to control relapse at the bulky site. In these circumstances, both chemotherapy and radiotherapy are needed.

Combined-modality programs utilize chemotherapy to shrink the mass and then radiotherapy for consolidation. This strategy is particularly useful in the anterior mediastinum where large radiotherapy fields may expose the normal lungs and heart to unnecessary radiation. Some groups utilize a "sandwich" technique of interposing radiotherapy between courses of chemotherapy. This approach has not been proved superior and may entail a greater risk of drug-radiotherapy interactions.

How many cycles of chemotherapy to administer for the patient with early-stage HD with a bulky mediastinal component remains unsettled. Many groups will give six cycles followed by consolidative radiotherapy. A restaging gallium scan or CT scan is often performed at the end of chemotherapy or even as an interim study to measure disease response. The dose of consolidative radiation ranges from approximately 2000 to 3600 cGy in most series. The trend is to lower the dose and limit the field size, as in other settings of early-stage HD.

COMBINATION CHEMOTHERAPY: SIDE EFFECTS

ABVD chemotherapy may be generally well tolerated if the antinausea medication ondansetron is used. The primary side effects are fatigue (which is cumulative); moderate hair loss; some susceptibility to infection (myelosuppression is brief); autonomic and peripheral neuropathy complaints associated with vinblastine (Velban); and, potentially the most severe, pulmonary toxicity related to bleomycin (Blenoxane). It is wise to obtain pulmonary function test results before therapy, midway during therapy, and before consolidative radiotherapy.

Bleomycin should always be withheld if the patient has more than a 25% fall in diffusing capacity on serial pulmonary function tests or if the patient is clinically symptomatic. If stopped according to these guidelines, the drug is relatively safe; however, if bleomycin is continued, pulmonary toxicity may be life-threatening. Doxorubicin cardiotoxicity is rare; however, all patients should have their left ventricular ejection fraction measured before therapy.

Infertility is not a major concern with ABVD. All men, however, should be advised to bank sperm. In women younger than 30 years, little effect of ABVD is noted generally on the menstrual cycle. For women 30 to 35 years old, menstrual irregularities may be appreciated; and for those older than 35 years, menopausal symptoms may develop. ABVD has rarely been administered during the second and third trimesters of pregnancy. In the small numbers treated, no significant adverse effects on the fetuses or healthy children delivered have been reported.

All women of childbearing age should have a pregnancy test before therapy, and they should be advised to delay pregnancy for 2 years after treatment, to avoid the coincidence of pregnancy and relapse. Men should also avoid fathering children during therapy. Sperm counts may remain low for 1 to 2 years after treatment.

RELAPSED AND REFRACTORY HODGKIN'S DISEASE

Treatment options for patients with primary refractory (never achieving a remission) HD and relapsed HD depend on the history of prior therapy. In general, for patients who experience failure or relapse with radiotherapy alone, disease is highly curable with standard-dose chemotherapy such as ABVD. However, patients who have previously received chemotherapy will most likely require high-dose chemoradiotherapy with autologous stem cell transplantation (ASCT) to achieve a long-term remission.

Two randomized studies were designed to determine the role of high-dose therapy for patients with primary refractory and relapsed HD. The first was conducted by the British National Lymphoma Investigation and the second by the German Hodgkin's Disease Study Group. Both studies compared standard-dose second-line chemotherapy with high-dose chemotherapy with stem cell support and demonstrated the superiority of the high-dose approach.

Data from both the European and American bone marrow transplant registries demonstrate a continuous improvement in the overall survival rate of patients undergoing high-dose therapy since 1991. The increment in survival, however, resulted entirely from a 10% decrease in treatment-related mortality and not an improvement in disease-free survival after ASCT. These data emphasize that, although 35 to 50% of patients are cured with high-dose therapy and ASCT, the need to determine prognostic factors to predict survival is vital. In addition, physicians at many medical centers are attempting to design more effective transplantation conditioning regimens with the hope of improving curability.

LATE EFFECTS OF THERAPY AND FOLLOW-UP

Because HD is a highly curable malignancy, it is very important to select treatment with an eye to possible late complications. The many prospective studies that compare MOPP with hybrid or alternating regimens and with ABVD alone have led to the conclusion that ABVD should be considered the gold standard of combination chemotherapy—not so much because of dramatic differences in efficacy but rather because of decreased toxicities.

The most important decreased late effect is that of secondary myelodysplasia and acute myelogenous leukemia. ABVD, however, has both possible cardiac and pulmonary effects (as discussed above), and these may have late manifestations.

Second solid tumors are a risk of both chemotherapy and radiotherapy. As combined-modality regimens are refined in early-stage disease, attention is being paid to reductions in both chemotherapy duration and radiation field size and dose.

In the follow-up management of HD patients, prevention plays a key role. This includes

1. Breast cancer screening for all women who received radiation at sites within the upper torso. Mammography is generally initiated 5 to 7 years after treatment, regardless of patient's age at diagnosis. In fact, the younger the female, the higher the risk of secondary breast cancer.

2. Quitting smoking.

3. Avoiding sun exposure and sunburn, particularly in the areas of prior radiation.

4. For those irradiated below the diaphragm, undergoing regular colonoscopy and obtaining prompt evaluation of gastrointestinal tract complaints. Although less common, secondary cancers of the gastrointestinal tract may be devastating.

5. Regular testing of thyroid function and prophylactic suppression of chemical hypothyroidism secondary to neck irradiation. This will reduce later thyroid neoplasia risk.

6. Maintaining a heart-healthy diet, exercising, and managing lipid intake. An increased risk of coronary artery disease is associated with mediastinal irradiation, and doxorubicin is potentially cardiotoxic.

7. Recognizing and treating early menopause in young women exposed to chemotherapy or pelvic irradiation. Although menstrual function may recover fully after treatment, a risk of premature ovarian failure may be likely for many.

8. Pneumovax before splenectomy or splenic irradiation. Updating vaccinations regularly.

The outlook for patients treated for HD is excellent. As the biology of the Reed-Sternberg cell is elucidated, new treatment strategies will become available for those who do not experience a curative outcome with initial or salvage therapy. For the majority of HD survivors, the emphasis must be on successful secondary prevention and enjoyment of good health provided by careful initial treatment selection and administration.

HODGKIN'S DISEASE: RADIATION THERAPY

method of
CLAIRE Y. FUNG, M.D.
*Massachusetts General Hospital and
Harvard Medical School
Boston, Massachusetts*

In the United States, Hodgkin's disease is diagnosed in 7 of every 100,000 people annually. The age distribution is bimodal, with a median of 26. The management of Hodgkin's disease has evolved dramatically since the 1950s, with advances in diagnosis, staging, and treatment. The majority of patients with Hodgkin's disease can now experience cure with current treatment modalities, which may include radiotherapy, chemotherapy, or both. As the number of long-term Hodgkin's disease survivors increases, it has become apparent that treatment is associated with significant and sometimes fatal late sequelae. The choice of therapy is tailored according to specific clinical scenarios, designed not only to maximize the chance of cure but also to minimize the risks of short- and long-term side effects.

Hodgkin's disease involves primarily lymph node sites, the most common being the neck and the mediastinum. It can also involve non-nodal organs such as the spleen, liver, and bone marrow, but extranodal involvement without nodal disease is rare. The disease tends to spread in a contiguous fashion, from one nodal group to the next, and has a high propensity to involve axial nodal groups along the cervical, mediastinal, and para-aortic distribution.

A thorough staging work-up is important because the disease extent strongly influences the choice of therapy. The physical examination should include a thorough lymph node examination. The presence or absence of B symptoms (fever > 101° F, weight loss of >10% of baseline, and drenching night sweats) should be documented. Standard radiographic studies include a chest radiograph and computed tomography (CT) of the chest, abdomen, and pelvis. A gallium scan is often helpful in defining sites of disease and monitoring patients after treatment. A bipedal lymphangiogram is sometimes a helpful complement to abdominopelvic CT in the delineation of subdiaphragmatic disease. Bone marrow biopsy is generally recommended, although it is rarely positive in the patients with very favorable prognostic factors. Routine laboratory studies include a complete blood cell count, erythrocyte sedimentation rate, chemistries, and liver function tests. An exploratory laparotomy and splenectomy provides pathologic staging of the spleen, the para-aortic and pelvic lymph nodes, and the liver. This procedure has been for some time a part of routine staging in many centers in the United States. However, its popularity has waned because of refinements in radiographic studies, improved definitions of clinical prognostic factors, and better recognition of the potential morbidity and mortality associated with the procedure. A staging laparotomy and splenectomy should be performed only if the surgical findings would alter treatment and if the patient would be a suitable candidate for radiotherapy alone after a negative laparotomy.

TECHNIQUES

Radiotherapy is the single most effective agent in the treatment of Hodgkin's disease. A megavoltage linear accelerator is essential in the delivery of optimal radiotherapy. The preferred beam energy is in the range of 6 MV to allow for relatively homogeneous dose distribution of the more superficial nodal groups such as in the neck and the deeper ones such as in the mediastinum. Before starting treatment, patients undergo simulation for proper immobilization and design of the radiation field. Customized blocks are made to maximally protect normal structures such as the heart and lungs. Meticulous technique and good understanding of the disease distribution on the part of the radiation oncologist are prerequisites for a good treatment outcome.

The radiation fields can be divided into three parts: the mantle, the para-aortic region, and the pelvis. The mantle field covers in continuity the nodal chains in the submandibular, cervical, supraclavicular, infraclavicular, axillary, mediastinal, and hilar regions. The patient lies in a supine position with the neck hyperextended and arms akimbo. Parallel opposed anterior and posterior fields are employed. The superior border of the field is at the base of the tragus. The lateral border is determined clinically to cover the axillary nodes. The inferior border depends on the inferior extent of disease in the mediastinum and is generally at the T9–10 or T10–11 intervertebral space. Multiple measurements are taken for complex dosimetric calculations for all sites of interest. Customized irregularly shaped blocks are inserted into the machine to shield normal structures. Chin and humeral head blocks are used. Lung blocks are designed to shield as much lung as possible without underdosing adjacent nodal regions. The left ventricle of the heart is generally shielded throughout treatment. A subcarinal block is introduced later in the course to limit the dose to the right side of the heart to approximately 3000 cGy. If the entire cardiac silhouette is to be treated, such as for pericardial involvement by lymphoma, the dose to the whole heart is limited to 1500 cGy at 150 cGy per fraction. An anterior larynx block is added at 1800 to 2000 cGy if the distribution of disease allows. A posterior cervical cord block is added at 3000 cGy.

The para-aortic field covers the para-aortic nodes down to the level of the aortic bifurcation, at the disc space between the fourth and fifth lumbar vertebral bodies. The lateral borders cover the transverse vertebral processes. If the spleen is being treated, then the left border is extended; a CT scan is used to determine the location of the spleen and enable maximal blocking of the left kidney. In the patients who had a negative laparotomy, coverage of the splenic pedicle is optional. Placement of surgical clips at the time of laparotomy allows visualization of the splenic pedicle during radiation planning.

The pelvic field is used for coverage of the common, internal, and external iliac nodes. Sometimes the inguinal and proximal femoral nodes are included. Care is taken to shield as much of the iliac wing as possible to preserve bone marrow. A central block shields the bladder and central pelvic structures. In females, the ovaries may be shielded after surgical transposition. In males, if the testes lies within the field borders, they are shielded by the central block. A testicular shield is used to further reduce scatter radiation.

Total nodal irradiation (TNI) refers to treatment of all just-mentioned areas. Subtotal nodal irradiation (STNI) refers to treatment of the mantle and para-aortic (± splenic) regions. The "inverted Y" is a single field covering the para-aortic and pelvic regions. When two adjoining fields are treated sequentially, gap calculations are undertaken to avoid overlap between fields while ensuring an adequate dose distribution to the target structures.

When a patient is treated with radiotherapy alone, the radiation field covers the areas of gross disease as well as adjacent nodal sites considered to be at risk of harboring microscopic (subclinical) disease. In the patients who are treated with combined modality therapy, chemotherapy usually precedes radiotherapy. In this setting, the radiation field may be reduced to cover only the original sites of gross disease (involved field).

Because of its radiosensitivity, Hodgkin's disease requires only moderate doses of radiation for disease eradication. Radiation doses are tailored for involved sites versus subclinical sites. When radiation therapy is the sole modality of treatment, sites of gross disease can be controlled with doses of 3500 to 4000 cGy with greater than 95% probability. For subclinical disease, 3000 cGy is considered adequate. When radiation therapy is given after four to six cycles of chemotherapy, doses in the range of 3000 to 3500 cGy are given, depending on the response after chemotherapy.

Radiation therapy is generally given 5 days a week, at 180 cGy per fraction. A full course of mantle irradiation takes about 4.5 weeks to complete. If a para-aortic field is to follow, it starts after a 2-week interval.

TREATMENT STRATEGIES

In the selection of the optimal treatment for each patient, multiple prognostic factors come into consideration. Involvement of four or more sites and bulky mediastinal adenopathy are adverse prognostic signs. (Bulky mediastinal adenopathy is defined as the ratio of the mediastinal mass to the maximal intrathoracic diameter on an upright posteroanterior chest radiograph being greater than one third.) Other unfavorable variables include presence of B symptoms, erythrocyte sedimentation rate greater than 40 to 50 mm, older age (older than 40 to 50 years), male sex, and histologic subtypes of mixed cellularity and lymphocyte depletion. The following is a discussion of a risk-based approach to the treatment of Hodgkin's disease.

Early-Stage Disease

Stage I to II disease is considered early stage, whereas stage III to IV disease is considered advanced. Patients with early-stage disease can be divided into favorable versus unfavorable subgroups according to their prognostic factors. Those with clinical stage I to II disease, no B symptoms, no bulky mediastinal adenopathy or other bulky sites, less than four involved sites, and age younger than 40 are considered to be in a favorable group. These patients generally undergo an exploratory laparotomy and splenectomy. If the laparotomy is negative, they are treated with radiation therapy alone, consisting of mantle and para-aortic fields. Long-term results of large single-institution studies indicate that with such an approach, over 80% of patients would remain free of relapse and less than 10% would die of Hodgkin's disease.

Within this laparotomy-negative favorable subgroup, certain patients may be treated with mantle irradiation alone (without irradiation of the para-aortic region). These include patients who have nodular sclerosis or lymphocyte predominant histology and disease limited to above the carina. Furthermore, a select group of clinical stage IA patients have an extremely low risk of subdiaphragmatic disease: clinical stage IA lymphocyte predominant and clinical stage IA female with nodular sclerosis. Results from Europe and the United States support treating these patients with mantle irradiation alone, without a laparotomy.

The patients with clinical stage I and II disease who do not fall into the just discussed favorable treatment groups are treated with combined modality therapy. A staging laparotomy is not necessary in this circumstance. Radiation therapy follows four to six cycles of chemotherapy. Although the optimal radiation volume and dose are still under investigation, coverage of initially involved sites to 3000 to 3500 cGy is acceptable.

In the patients with involvement of the preauricular and/or very high neck areas, the radiation field is extended to cover the preauricular region. Patients who have disease extension to the pericardium or pericardial nodes, the pleura, or the pulmonary parenchyma are not appropriate candidates for radiotherapy alone.

Advanced-Stage Disease

Chemotherapy is the mainstay of treatment for stage III and IV patients. The most commonly used regimens are ABVD, consisting of doxorubicin (Adriamycin), bleomycin (Blenoxane), vinblastine (Velban), and dacarbazine; MOPP, consisting of nitrogen mustard, vincristine (Oncovin), procarbazine (Matulane), and prednisone; and a hybrid of the two. In a number of multicenter studies of advanced-stage patients treated with multidrug chemotherapy, the relapse-free survival is in the range of 65 to 75% and the overall survival is 75 to 84%. The role of additional radiotherapy after chemotherapy in advanced disease is controversial. Data from the International Database on Hodgkin's Disease Overview Study Group meta-analysis demonstrated that additional radiotherapy conferred an 11% improvement in tumor control rate but no survival benefit. Additional radiotherapy was associated with an increase in mortality from causes other than Hodgkin's disease, presumably related to treatment. However, certain subgroups of patients with advanced disease, such as those with bulky mediastinal adenopathy, may still benefit from consolidative radiotherapy.

Pediatric Hodgkin's Disease

Among children with Hodgkin's disease, cure rates and survival rates are high. The management of pe-diatric Hodgkin's disease is made particularly challenging by the musculoskeletal growth impairment caused by full-dose radiotherapy. Full mantle irradiation in a growing child can cause a short stature (particularly short sitting height), scoliosis, thin neck, and shortened interclavicular distance. Para-aortic irradiation may cause a short sitting height, and splenic irradiation may cause underdevelopment of the abdominal wall. The severity of the impairment is directly correlated with the radiation dose and is especially devastating in the very young patient. When the radiation dose is limited to less than 2500 cGy, the musculoskeletal effects are less apparent.

Treatment of pediatric Hodgkin's disease is tailored according to the age, sex, stage, and prognostic factors, as in the adult. However, full-dose radiotherapy alone is rarely used except for favorable patients with early-stage disease who have reached physical maturity. The majority of children are treated with combined modality therapy or chemotherapy alone. Disease-free and overall survival rates as high as 100% have been reported for children with early-stage disease treated with six cycles of combination chemotherapy and 1500- to 2500-cGy involved-field radiotherapy. For children with advanced disease, the disease-free survival rate is in the range of 70 to 90% after chemotherapy alone or combined modality treatment.

SIDE EFFECTS OF RADIATION THERAPY

Acute Side Effects

Radiation side effects are directly related to the areas being treated and the radiation dose. Acute side effects gradually appear during the course of treatment; they are usually transient, and most of them resolve within 3 to 4 weeks after completion of therapy. Mantle irradiation causes xerostomia, which may be relieved with oral pilocarpine. Occasionally, mild parotiditis produces pain at the angle of the jaws during the first week of radiation therapy. Patients have a change in taste and develop sore throat and dysphagia from pharyngitis and esophagitis. The esophagitis may be particularly severe in patients who received prior chemotherapy. Helpful remedies include a soft diet, viscous lidocaine, sucralfate (Carafate), and analgesics. Hair loss occurs within the irradiated areas such as the posterior lower scalp. Men may lose their beards and chest/body hair. Skin reaction manifests as erythema and possibly dry desquamation, sometimes accompanied by pruritus and tenderness. Patients are given a petrolatum-based ointment (Aquaphor) or an aloe-based lotion (Hydrogel), which are emollients that provide symptomatic relief and promote healing. Patients are advised not to shave and not to use deodorant. Men may use an electric shaver sparingly if they are compelled to shave. Other possible reactions include nausea, vomiting, dry cough, and fatigue. The blood cell count may fall if a significant amount of bone marrow is being irradiated.

Para-aortic and/or splenic irradiation may cause fatigue, anorexia, nausea, vomiting, and abdominal discomfort.

Subacute and Late Side Effects

Recovery of salivary function after mantle irradiation may take 6 to 12 months and sometimes longer in older patients. Patients are more prone to developing dental carries because of the change in salivary function and should be encouraged to see their dentists frequently to maintain good dental hygiene.

Thyroid disease is prevalent after mantle irradiation, affecting about 50% of patients by 20 years after treatment. The most common thyroid abnormality is hypothyroidism, which may be overt or subclinical (biochemical). Hypothyroidism is most often identified during the second or third year after treatment. There is evidence to suggest that thyroid hormone replacement reduces the incidence of thyroid nodules. Even patients who have only biochemical hypothyroidism without overt clinical manifestations are recommended to go on thyroid hormone replacement if the biochemical abnormalities persist. Other thyroid abnormalities include Graves' hyperthyroidism, silent thyroiditis, Hashimoto's thyroiditis, and thyroid nodular disease. Although the majority of thyroid nodules are benign, there is an increased risk of thyroid cancer in patients irradiated for Hodgkin's disease relative to the normal population.

Lhermitte's syndrome, considered a transient radiation myelopathy, consists of an "electric shock" sensation that radiates down the spine and extremities brought on by neck flexion. The mean time at onset is 3 months after irradiation, and it lasts for an average of 6 months. It is self-limited and is not associated with permanent transverse myelitis.

Symptomatic radiation pneumonitis occurs in less than 5% of patients after mediastinal irradiation. The time of onset is usually within the first 4 months after treatment. Symptoms include a nonproductive cough, dyspnea on exertion, and a low-grade fever. In the patients with these symptoms after radiation therapy, an infectious cause should be ruled out before attributing them to radiation pneumonitis. The characteristic radiographic finding is pulmonary infiltrates limited to the shape of the mediastinal radiation field. Radiation pneumonitis is often self-limited, but more severe cases require treatment with corticosteroids. Apart from pneumonitis, patients may develop chronic pulmonary fibrosis that tends to be subclinical but is evident only on radiographic studies.

The risk of radiation carditis is 1 to 2% with careful treatment technique. Radiation-related pericardial disease generally occurs during the first 6 months after treatment and may manifest as an acute pericarditis, a chronic pericardial effusion that may be asymptomatic, or both. Acute pericarditis manifests as chest pain and fever accompanied by a friction rub and electrocardiographic changes typical of pericarditis. Patients are managed with nonsteroidal anti-inflammatory agents and corticosteroids if necessary. Asymptomatic pericardial effusions detected on a follow-up chest radiograph should be further evaluated by an echocardiogram. The effusions generally resolve over several months, but large ones may require pericardiocentesis. Constrictive pericarditis is rare.

Mediastinal irradiation for Hodgkin's disease has been associated with an increased risk of death from acute myocardial infarction. The relative risk has dropped with the use of modern radiation techniques and careful blocking of the heart. Other late cardiac effects include myocardial dysfunction and valvular thickening, although these abnormalities tend not to be hemodynamically significant. Patients should be educated about modifiable cardiovascular risk factors such as diet/cholesterol, obesity, smoking, and exercise.

Survivors of Hodgkin's disease are at risk for treatment-related secondary neoplasms, a major contributor to the excess mortality rates in treated patients. The incidence of secondary neoplasms in Hodgkin's survivors exceeds the expected incidence of primary tumors in the general population, reaching an actuarial risk of 20% at 20 years after treatment. Excess second cancers include leukemia, non-Hodgkin's lymphoma, lung cancer, breast cancer, gastrointestinal cancer, urogenital cancer, melanoma, thyroid cancer, and sarcomas of bone and soft tissue. Solid tumors account for the largest component of second cancers in absolute numbers, whereas the highest relative risks are found in leukemia and non-Hodgkin's lymphoma. Both chemotherapy and radiation are associated with secondary malignancies. Chemotherapy is the main culprit in secondary leukemia, the alkylating agents (such as nitrogen mustard) being the most notorious. Secondary solid tumors are observed primarily in irradiated patients, and many of the secondary solid tumors arise within or at the margin of the radiation field. The most frequently seen solid tumor is lung cancer. One report indicated that patients who smoked more than 10 pack-years *after* the diagnosis of Hodgkin's disease had a sixfold increase in the risk of lung cancer, compared with those who smoked less than 1 pack-year. It is essential to advise patients not to smoke after treatment for Hodgkin's disease.

In women, there is an increased risk of breast cancer after radiotherapy for Hodgkin's disease. The increased risk only becomes apparent 15 years or more after treatment. The relative risk is 11 for women irradiated at age 30 or younger and as high as 42 for women irradiated at age 20 or younger. Female patients treated with mantle irradiation should be advised to do monthly self breast examinations, have periodic breast examinations by their physicians, and start screening mammography 10 years after treatment or by age 40. Women who have been irradiated in childhood should undergo mammography every 2 to 3 years, starting at age 25 to 30, and then yearly after age 40.

The effects of radiation on fertility are directly related to the radiation dose to the reproductive organs. In a course of standard mantle and para-aortic radiotherapy, the total scatter dose is approximately 13 cGy to the testes in a man and 82 cGy to the ovaries in a woman. These doses are unlikely to have any significant impact on fertility. If the pelvis is irradiated, special care should be taken to shield the gonads as much as possible. If the testes are below the inferior field border, testicular doses may be limited to approximately 135 cGy or less with specially designed testicular shielding. Oligospermia or azoospermia resulting from such doses is often transient, with recovery of the sperm count after 2 years. In women who require pelvic irradiation, the ovaries may be transposed to the midline to be shielded by a midline block. With appropriate protective measures, ovarian function is more likely to be preserved in younger women than in older women.

FUTURE DIRECTIONS

Great progress has been made in the treatment of Hodgkin's disease. However, the success has been tempered by the recognition of fatal late complications. Long-term outcome analyses show that Hodgkin's disease survivors have an excessive risk of death from second cancers, cardiac disease, and infection. Current treatment approaches are designed to minimize the extent of treatment while maintaining a high probability of cure. For example, the trend in the treatment of early stage disease is toward combined modality therapy, which eliminates the need for an exploratory laparotomy and splenectomy. Furthermore, it is hoped that reduction in the dose of chemotherapy and radiotherapy will lead to fewer long-term complications associated with each modality. Clinical studies are in progress to optimize the treatment outcomes for patients with Hodgkin's disease. Areas of active investigation include the optimal treatment combinations for various stages of disease, radiation therapy fields and doses, and chemotherapy regimens and doses.

ACUTE LEUKEMIA IN ADULTS

method of
MARK R. LITZOW, M.D.,
LOUIS LETENDRE, M.D., and
SCOTT H. KAUFMANN, M.D., Ph.D.
Mayo Clinic
Rochester, Minnesota

The acute leukemias are malignant disorders characterized by the clonal expansion of immature hematopoietic cells. These disorders are broadly divided into acute myelogenous leukemia (AML) and acute lymphoblastic leukemia (ALL), a distinction that has important therapeutic

and prognostic implications. Based on biologic features of the leukemic cells, AML and ALL can be further subdivided into various subsets, as described later. Accordingly, AML and ALL should be considered two groups of diseases rather than two homogeneous disease entities.

In considering the clinical behavior of these diseases, several concepts are helpful. First, mutations giving rise to the malignant clone can occur in cells at varying levels of maturation and, thus, can give rise to an acute leukemia with cells committed to a particular lineage (e.g., an erythroleukemia) or to very immature cells that have not yet committed to a particular lineage (e.g., a stem cell leukemia). Second, these leukemic cells share many properties (e.g., drug resistance mechanisms) with their normal counterparts. This can have a significant impact on the outcome of therapy. Third, although the leukemic cells in any particular patient might appear to be morphologically homogeneous, biologic studies indicate that the leukemic population contains cells at various developmental stages, much like the developmental hierarchy seen during normal hematopoiesis. This discovery is consistent with the postulated existence of a leukemic stem cell that, like a normal bone marrow stem cell, is capable of surviving during chemotherapy, only to proliferate months or years later and cause relapse.

ETIOLOGY

The initiating events in the development of leukemia involve alterations in the structure and expression of various genes in the putative leukemic stem cell. These genetic alterations, which vary with the leukemic subtype, result in clonal expansion of cells that have an enhanced ability to proliferate and a diminished ability to differentiate.

Many, but not all, of the epidemiologic associations elucidated in the past can be explained by the relationship between gene mutations and leukemogenesis. Increased incidences of AML have been noted in people of eastern European Jewish origin; in patients with a number of genetic disorders, including ataxia-telangiectasia, Bloom's syndrome, Down syndrome, and Fanconi's anemia; and among family members of patients with AML, although family clustering is still a rare event in this disease. The genetic disorders listed, several of which involve alterations in enzymes implicated in DNA repair (Down syndrome being the notable exception), also carry an increased risk of ALL, suggesting that failure to repair DNA damage can contribute to both groups of diseases. Industrial exposure to benzene-based solvents and petroleum products is associated with an increased risk of acute leukemia (especially AML), as is accidental exposure to high doses of ionizing radiation (e.g., the atomic bomb blasts during World War II and the Chernobyl nuclear reactor accident). Less striking from a relative risk perspective, but probably more clinically relevant, is the increased risk of AML observed in smokers and in patients who receive DNA-damaging cancer chemotherapeutic agents for neoplastic or non-neoplastic conditions. The latter effect has generally been observed with two classes of drugs. The alkylating agents (e.g., nitrogen mustard, melphalan, and cyclophosphamide) typically cause loss of part or all of chromosome 5 or 7 and precipitate a myelodysplastic syndrome (preleukemic state) or AML 2 to 10 years after exposure. In contrast, agents that target the nuclear enzyme topoisomerase II (e.g., etoposide and doxorubicin) are associated with AML that has a shorter latency and displays characteristic translocations involving the mixed lineage leukemia (*MLL*) gene at band q23 of chromosome 11. Finally,

RNA tumor viruses (retroviruses) can cause the development of acute leukemia in animals, and the human T cell lymphotropic virus type I is associated with acute T cell leukemia/lymphoma in humans.

DEMOGRAPHICS

The age-adjusted incidence of acute leukemia in the United States increases from less than 1/100,000 for people younger than 30 years of age to 14/100,000 at age 75 years. These figures translate into approximately 10,000 new AML cases (and 7000 deaths) per year; 90% of these cases occur in adults. It is important to keep in mind, particularly in regard to therapeutic alternatives, that the median age of patients with AML is 60 to 65 years. Approximately 3000 cases of ALL are also diagnosed per year. Although 60% of these ALL cases occur in children, the incidence of ALL in adults also increases with age.

CLASSIFICATION

Because of differences in the approach to managing various types of acute leukemia, it is essential to establish the type of leukemia as accurately as possible before starting treatment. The current classification scheme, referred to as the French-American-British (FAB) classification, divides leukemia into ALL and AML. The latter group is further subdivided using cytochemistry and immunologic analysis (by flow cytometry) into undifferentiated AML (M0), AML with granulocyte differentiation that lacks (M1) or contains (M2) evidence of granulocyte maturation, progranulocytic leukemia (M3), myelomonocytic leukemia (M4), monoblastic leukemia (M5), erythroleukemia (M6) and megakaryoblastic leukemia (M7). This classification not only describes the differentiation status of the predominant cells in the leukemic clone, but conveys some therapeutic and prognostic information. As described later, patients with M3 AML have a uniquely high incidence of disseminated intravascular coagulopathy (DIC), but also respond extremely well to induction therapy consisting of all-*trans*-retinoic acid (ATRA). In contrast, patients with M5 to M7 leukemia often have a history of prior hematologic disorders or exposure to DNA-damaging chemotherapy and tend to have a poorer response to conventional chemotherapy.

Although the original FAB classification also included three morphologic subtypes of ALL (L1 to L3), this scheme has fallen into disuse for ALL because of lack of reproducibility. Instead, an immunologic classification based on whether the leukemic cells have features of B cells or T cells is more widely used. Once again, the classification conveys prognostic information, with T cell leukemias carrying a somewhat better prognosis (up to 90% complete remission [CR] and 50% disease-free survival) in some series.

Although useful in classifying most acute leukemias, the FAB classification scheme does not take into account some of the rarer subtypes. These include acute basophilic, acute eosinophilic, and hybrid or biphenotypic leukemias that express both myeloid and lymphoid markers.

CLINICAL MANIFESTATIONS

The clinical manifestations of acute leukemia relate in general to decreased production of normal hematopoietic cells and invasion of various organs by leukemic cells. Patients come to medical attention with constitutional symptoms (malaise, weakness, fatigue, anorexia); symptoms related to anemia (dyspnea, palpitations, orthostatic hypotension), neutropenia (mucocutaneous or pulmonary infections), or thrombocytopenia (bruising and bleeding); and symptoms related to tissue infiltration by the leukemic clone (adenopathy, hepatosplenomegaly, gingival hypertrophy, bone pain related to invasion of the periosteum or expansion of the intramedullary space by leukemic cells, cranial nerve deficits related to leukemic meningitis). In patients with leukostasis (see later discussion), symptoms related to plugging of pulmonary or cerebral capillaries may predominate.

Patients in whom a diagnosis of acute leukemia is suspected should undergo a thorough physical examination to search for sites of infection or bleeding and to document sites of organ involvement with leukemic cells. If the patient is febrile, the differential diagnosis should include sinusitis, pneumonia, an impending rectal abscess, occult bacteremia or fungemia, and the underlying disease process. Although the evaluation for possible sinusitis or pneumonia is often straightforward, the usual clinical and radiographic signs of infection might be masked if the patient is neutropenic. The perianal area should be carefully inspected to exclude an impending rectal abscess or rectal fissure, but digital rectal examination should be omitted in neutropenic patients to avoid bacteremia.

Tissue infiltration by the leukemic clone is often encountered. Lymphadenopathy is common in patients with ALL or M5 AML. Leukemic soft tissue tumors, which are known as chloromas, granulocytic sarcomas, or myeloblastomas, can precede the presence of leukemia in the bone marrow or blood and lead to initial misdiagnosis, most frequently of lymphoma. Some of the more common sites of these extramedullary leukemic collections include the ovaries, testes, breasts, gastrointestinal tract, sinuses, and orbits. Cutaneous involvement (leukemia cutis), which occurs in up to 10% of patients with AML, typically consists of multiple, raised, violaceous, nontender subcutaneous plaques or nodules. These lesions should be distinguished from lymphoma cutis and Sweet's syndrome (acute neutrophilic dermatosis), a paraneoplastic syndrome that accompanies AML and consists of red, tender nodules or plaques infiltrated by mature granulocytes. Both leukemia cutis and Sweet's syndrome can precede the diagnosis of AML by several months or longer.

Leukemic involvement of the central nervous system (CNS), although uncommon at diagnosis, occurs in 30 to 50% of patients with ALL unless appropriate prophylaxis is administered. In contrast, neurologic involvement develops in only 5 to 7% of patients with AML, leading to the current practice of foregoing CNS prophylaxis in this disease. Nonetheless, CNS involvement should be suspected in any patient with focal neurologic signs at diagnosis or relapse. Patients with AML at highest risk for development of CNS leukemia are those with a monocytic subtype, a high peripheral blast count, or an elevated serum lactate dehydrogenase. There is controversy as to whether every patient with AML needs a spinal tap. All patients with ALL, however, should have an initial spinal tap performed early in the course of treatment, followed by prophylactic or definitive therapy. If patients are neurologically asymptomatic, a spinal tap can be deferred until the number of blasts in the peripheral blood is low to avoid the possibility that a traumatic tap will cause contamination of the cerebrospinal fluid with leukemic blasts or lead to misdiagnosis.

Medical Emergencies Encountered at the Time of Presentation

Several clinical manifestations encountered in patients with acute leukemia are medical emergencies. Patients with more than 50,000 blasts per mm³ in the peripheral blood can develop leukostasis. The organs most susceptible to capillary occlusion by large numbers of poorly deformable blasts are the lungs and CNS. Clinical features of leukostasis include dyspnea (often with a clear chest radiograph), neurologic signs and symptoms, and funduscopic findings of hemorrhage, papilledema, and distended vessels. Treatment requires immediate cytoreduction. This can be accomplished by emergent leukapheresis and simultaneous institution of hydroxyurea (Hydrea) at 1.5 grams per m² every 6 hours in addition to the supportive care measures (allopurinol, hydration) described in greater detail later. If this approach is used, systemic antileukemic therapy should be instituted as soon after the diagnosis is confirmed as practical. Alternatively, cytoreduction can be achieved by prompt institution of a chemotherapeutic regimen appropriate for the type of leukemia (see later).

Patients with high white blood cell counts and leukostasis have an elevated whole-blood viscosity. Because of this, red cell transfusions should be deferred even in anemic patients (if possible) to avoid aggravating the capillary sludging. These patients are also at increased risk of bleeding because of ischemia resulting from capillary occlusions. Accordingly, platelets should be transfused to maintain platelet counts in excess of 50,000 per mm³ in this setting.

Another common manifestation involves bleeding or clotting as a consequence of DIC. This syndrome is most commonly encountered in patients with acute progranulocytic leukemia (APL), but can also be seen with virtually any acute leukemia subtype, particularly if the initial therapy results in massive tumor lysis. Patients with leukemia-associated DIC are at high risk of life-threatening bleeding, including intracerebral hemorrhage. Because of the frequency with which this syndrome occurs, all patients with acute leukemia should be checked for clotting factor abnormalities or fibrinolysis. For patients with laboratory or clinical evidence of DIC, the current practice is to replace clotting factors if the fibrinogen is low and maintain platelets at more than 50,000 per mm³ until the fibrinolysis abates. The use of low doses of heparin to interrupt the aberrantly active intrinsic pathway is favored by some hematologists but remains controversial.

DIAGNOSTIC EVALUATION

Although most patients have a total white blood cell count of 5000 to 30,000 cells per mm³ at the time leukemia is diagnosed, the count can range from less than 1000 to more than 200,000 cells per mm³. Diagnosis is not difficult in patients with elevated counts, but acute leukemia should also be suspected in any patient with unexplained pancytopenia.

Ninety percent of patients with acute leukemias have blasts in their peripheral blood at diagnosis. Accordingly, the diagnosis can often be made by examining the peripheral smear. Nonetheless, a bone marrow aspirate and biopsy, along with marrow cytogenetics, should be obtained as part of the diagnostic evaluation whenever possible. Because a biopsy cannot be obtained with a sternal marrow, aspiration of the posterior iliac crest is preferred. The aspirate and biopsy are used not only to exclude a myelodysplastic, myeloproliferative, or myelophthisic process but also to provide a baseline with which subsequent post-treatment marrows can be compared. The results of the cytogenetic analysis convey additional prognostic information that is often used to guide postremission therapy.

To meet the FAB criteria for the diagnosis of acute leukemia, more than 30% of all nucleated cells in the marrow must be blasts. In most instances, this percentage is much higher because the marrow is usually hypercellular with a predominance of leukemic blasts and a marked decrease in normal precursors. A definitive diagnosis of the precise subtype of acute leukemia requires the use of cytochemical, histochemical, or immunologic analysis. This subtyping provides some important clues to complications that are likely to be encountered, as well as information regarding the patient's overall prognosis.

The result of the cytogenetic analysis performed at the time of diagnosis has emerged as the single most important prognostic indicator. The cytogenetic abnormalities that are encountered in the acute leukemias can, in most instances, be classified as translocations (exchange of genetic material between two chromosomes, e.g., t[9;22]), deletions of a portion or all of a chromosome (e.g., 5q− or del [5]), or inversions of genetic material on the same chromosome (e.g., inv[16]). At diagnosis, acute leukemias can express a single cytogenetic abnormality or multiple abnormalities, and additional abnormalities can emerge as treatment selects for resistant subclones. Some of the more common karyotypic abnormalities associated with particular subtypes of acute leukemia are listed in Table 1.

Chromosomal abnormalities, which reflect somatic mutations, can be detected by routine cytogenetic techniques in 60 to 70% of the cases of de novo acute leukemia. With more sophisticated molecular biology techniques, some of the cases that lack overt chromosomal abnormalities are found to have submicroscopic abnormalities. Ongoing studies in this area are identifying more and more of the genes involved in different subtypes of acute leukemia. With the improved understanding of the molecular basis of these diseases, new targets for therapeutic intervention are also likely to be identified.

TREATMENT

The complications of the acute leukemias, along with the side effects of their treatment, often result in profound and prolonged morbidity. Accordingly, the administration of antileukemic therapy should be undertaken only by physicians with advanced training in the care of patients with leukemia. That said, however, other physicians often diagnose leukemia (see earlier) or discuss its treatment with patients and their families. Accordingly, the following sections are intended to provide an overview of leukemia treatment rather than a step-by-step guide.

As noted earlier, acute leukemia can be thought of as a group of related disorders that vary in therapeutic response and overall prognosis. The major adverse prognostic factors in patients with AML and ALL are listed in Table 2. These prognostic factors are of essential importance in guiding therapy, especially in patients who achieve a CR.

Acute Myelogenous Leukemia

Induction Therapy

Before the initiation of systemic chemotherapy, all patients, regardless of white blood cell count, should be adequately hydrated and started on allopurinol

TABLE 1. **Acute Leukemia Syndromes**

Type	Clinical Findings	Morphology	Karyotype	Prognosis
Philadelphia chromosome positive ALL	Older age, high WBC	Pre–B cell	t(9;22)	Poor
Burkitt's type ALL		B cell	t(8;14)	Good
Biphenotypic leukemia	Infants or adults, splenomegaly, high WBC		t(4;11)	Poor
M2 AML	Splenomegaly—25%; Chloromas—20%	Myeloblasts with frequent Auer rods	t(8;21)	Good
M3 AML	Disseminated intravascular coagulopathy, bleeding, thrombosis		t(15;17)	Good
M4 AML with abnormal eosinophils		Myelomonocytic blasts, abnormal eosinophils	inv(16)	Good
M5 AML	Frequent skin or gum infiltration	Monocytic	t(9;11)	Poor
M7 AML	Antecedent or coincident thrombocytosis	Megakaryocytes often abnormal	t(3;3) or inv(3)	Poor
Therapy-related leukemia	Occurs after alkylating agent		5q−, 7q−	Poor
Therapy-related leukemia	Occurs after topoisomerase II poison		Translocations involving 11q23	Poor

Abbreviations: ALL = acute lymphoblastic leukemia; AML = acute myelogenous leukemia; WBC = white blood cell count.
Adapted from Koeffler H: Syndromes of acute nonlymphocytic leukemia. Ann Intern Med *107*:748–758, 1987, with permission.

(Zyloprim). These measures are used to reduce the risk of tumor lysis syndrome, a constellation of metabolic abnormalities that begins with hyperuricemia, hyperkalemia, or hyperphosphatemia and can lead to renal failure. Although more common in patients with ALL, this syndrome can also occur in AML.

Cytosine arabinoside (ara-C) and anthracyclines (e.g., daunorubicin, idarubicin) individually induce remissions in AML, but the remissions achieved with single-agent therapy are short-lived. Standard therapy for initial treatment of patients with newly diagnosed AML at Mayo Clinic and many other institutions combines 7 days of continuous infusion ara-C (100 mg per m² per day) with three daily boluses of an anthracycline. CR rates of approximately 65% are observed in patients younger than 55 years of age. Based on randomized trials showing a slight im-

provement in CR rate with idarubicin compared with daunorubicin, idarubicin (12 mg per m² per day) is currently preferred at our institution. This dose of idarubicin, which might be somewhat more dose intensive than the usual doses of daunorubicin, results in a somewhat higher CR rate after the first cycle of therapy. Although idarubicin and other newer anthracycline derivatives (e.g., mitoxantrone) were synthesized with the hope that they would produce less cardiotoxicity, this benefit has not been realized.

Three to 7 days after the completion of initial chemotherapy, a repeat bone marrow aspirate and biopsy are obtained. If this marrow is aplastic or severely hypoplastic without morphologic evidence of residual leukemia, further therapy is withheld pending recovery of the bone marrow. If significant residual leukemia remains, however, a second course of the same induction chemotherapy can be given in the expectation that some of these patients will achieve morphologic evidence of complete tumor clearance and marrow aplasia with the additional therapy.

If a patient does not achieve marrow aplasia after a second course of induction therapy, the disease is considered refractory to induction chemotherapy. Overall prognosis in this situation is understandably poor. Alternate salvage regimens (e.g., high-dose ara-C with mitoxantrone or etoposide) can sometimes induce CR in this setting, but such remissions usually are short-lived. Approximately 20% of the patients with refractory disease also have prolonged remissions after allogeneic bone marrow transplantation (BMT) from an HLA-identical sibling if this treatment can be coordinated quickly.

If patients achieve marrow aplasia after induction chemotherapy, another 2 weeks or more is required for recovery of normal hematopoiesis. After recovery of their blood counts, patients undergo another bone

TABLE 2. **Adverse Prognostic Factors in Acute Leukemia**

Factors related to the host
  Older age
  Infection at diagnosis
  Co-morbid conditions
Factors related to the leukemia
  Acute myelogenous leukemia
    WBC > 100,000 per mm³
    Chromosomal findings other than normal cytogenetics: t(8;21), inv(16), or t(15;17)
    Antecedent hematologic disorder (e.g., myelodysplastic or myeloproliferative syndrome)
  Acute lymphoblastic leukemia
    Common acute lymphocytic leukemia antigen–positive
    WBC ≥ 50,000 per mm³
    Structural chromosomal abnormalities, especially t(9;22) and t(4;11)
    Not achieving complete remission within 4 weeks

Abbreviation: WBC = white blood cell count.

marrow aspirate and biopsy. By definition, a CR requires the presence of 20% cellularity in the marrow with fewer than 5% blasts; circulating neutrophils and platelets of at least 1000 and 100,000 per mm³, respectively; and absence of circulating blasts. This definition depends on morphology, not on cytogenetic results. As might be expected, a patient with a morphologic CR but persistent cytogenetic abnormalities is at increased risk of relapse.

Postremission Therapy

If no further therapy is given after a CR is achieved, over 85% of patients relapse, with a median disease-free survival of 4 months. Low doses of maintenance therapy with oral 6-thioguanine and weekly subcutaneous ara-C can increase the median remission duration to 8 months. In patients younger than 60 years of age, a randomized trial has demonstrated that postremission therapy with high-dose ara-C (3 grams per m² twice a day every other day for six doses) results in a 40% disease-free survival rate at 4 years. The patients who did the best with this consolidation regimen were those with favorable cytogenetic abnormalities, including t(8;21) and inv(16). For these subsets of patients with AML, results with this consolidation therapy are so good that BMT should be deferred until the time of relapse (if it occurs).

After reports from the 1970s indicating that allogeneic BMT was able to cure a small percentage of patients with refractory or relapsed AML, the role of BMT in first remission was studied. Induction therapy followed by allogeneic BMT using marrow from an HLA-identical sibling results in disease-free survival rates of 40 to 60%. Collection and transplantation of autologous marrow in first remission produces similar survival rates. Simultaneously, improvements in outcomes after postremission chemotherapy were demonstrated. In the late 1980s, several large, randomized trials were initiated to compare the results of autologous or allogeneic BMT with postremission chemotherapy in younger patients (<55 years of age) with AML in first remission. Since 1995, many of these studies have been reported in preliminary or final form. Unfortunately, the results of these trials have been somewhat difficult to compare because of variations in the eligibility criteria, types of consolidation chemotherapy, and strategies used to remove residual leukemia cells from autologous marrow. These trials have uniformly demonstrated that as many as half of the enrolled patients cannot complete the entire treatment program because of excessive toxicity, early relapse, or preference by physician or patient for a particular form of therapy. Relapse rates and treatment-related mortality were found to vary depending on the type of postremission therapy administered. Relapse rates were highest with chemotherapy and lowest with allogeneic BMT. Conversely, treatment-related mortality rates were highest with allogeneic BMT (20 to 40% treatment-related mortality rate at 1 year) followed by autologous BMT (10 to 15%) and intensive consolidation

chemotherapy (3 to 5%). In general, these trials have also demonstrated equivalent or slightly improved relapse-free survival rates with either form of transplantation compared with chemotherapy, but overall survival has been similar because patients who relapse after chemotherapy can be salvaged with BMT. Therefore, many investigators now advise that an allogeneic or autologous transplant source should be identified as soon as possible after diagnosis, but that many patients should receive intensive consolidation chemotherapy in first CR and reserve BMT for use in the event of relapse.

The decision regarding the advisability and timing of transplantation depends on many factors, including the biology of the AML, the condition and age of the patient, and the availability of an HLA-matched sibling. For a patient with AML whose blasts have cytogenetic abnormalities that are associated with a good prognosis, the decision to administer intensive consolidation chemotherapy in first CR and reserve transplantation for possible use at a later date seems reasonable. For a patient with AML whose blasts have intermediate- or poor-risk cytogenetic abnormalities and other adverse risk factors, transplantation in first CR might be reasonable depending on patient and physician preference. A suggested approach is outlined in Figure 1. For patients who lack an HLA-matched sibling, deciding between an allogeneic transplant from an HLA-matched, unre-

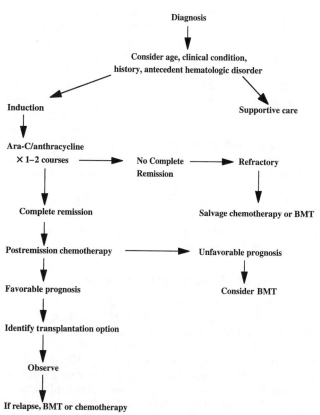

Figure 1. Acute myelogenous leukemia: treatment options. *Abbreviations:* Ara-C = cytosine arabinoside; BMT = bone marrow transplantation.

lated donor versus an autologous transplant is difficult. One retrospective study showed no difference in long-term disease-free survival rates for matched cohorts undergoing autologous or unrelated donor allogeneic BMT, but the toxicities and relapse rates differed.

Acute Myelogenous Leukemia in the Elderly

Optimal therapy in elderly patients with AML remains a difficult and unanswered question. The trials described earlier excluded patients older than 55 to 60 years of age, who comprise more than half of the AML population. Whereas CR rates in younger patients approach or exceed 70%, CR rates in elderly patients with standard induction chemotherapy are approximately 50%. This poorer response is related to a higher incidence of poor prognostic factors (e.g., poor-risk cytogenetics and prior myelodysplastic syndrome) as well as increased deaths during induction chemotherapy as a presumed consequence of poorer performance status and abnormal organ function.

Before considering therapy in an elderly patient with AML, it is important to carefully assess the patient's performance status and co-morbid conditions. Patients with significant co-morbidities should probably receive supportive care (e.g., broad-spectrum oral antibiotics, transfusions, and hydroxyurea to control leukocytosis) rather than intensive chemotherapy. Some elderly patients can survive for several months to a year or more with supportive care alone, although all of these patients eventually die of their disease. For elderly patients who have no significant co-morbidities, enrollment in a clinical trial or treatment with a combination of ara-C and an anthracycline as described for younger patients can be considered. At our institution, we have found that treatment with ara-C, 750 mg per m^2 every 12 hours for 12 doses, results in CR rates of 40% with 2-year disease-free survival rates of 15% in patients with AML older than age 65 years. The use of hematopoietic growth factors and broad-spectrum antibiotics after induction chemotherapy may reduce the morbidity of chemotherapy in elderly patients, but clinical trials with these agents have yielded mixed results (see later). For elderly patients who are candidates for more intensive therapy, autologous BMT has been successfully performed in carefully selected patients up to the age of 70 years.

Acute Progranulocytic Leukemia

The therapeutic options outlined previously apply to all AML subtypes except APL (M3 AML). During the 1980s, pharmacologic doses of ATRA were found to induce CRs in 70 to 90% of patients with APL. Although this subtype makes up only 10 to 15% of all cases of AML, this therapy has generated intense interest because of its unique mechanism of action. Nearly all cases of APL have a balanced reciprocal translocation between chromosomes 15 and 17 that results in the juxtaposition of a portion of the promyelocytic leukemia gene (*PML*), which encodes a tran-

scription factor, with a portion of the gene for retinoic acid receptor-alpha (*RARα*). The fusion protein that results from this translocation appears to prevent progranulocytes from differentiating, but pharmacologic doses of ATRA overcome this resistance and induce differentiation of leukemic progranulocytes into mature granulocytes. Because ATRA does not induce lysis of the progranulocytes, with leakage of their primary granules and activation of the intrinsic coagulation pathway, the risk of inducing or aggravating the coagulopathy commonly associated with M3 AML appears to be lower with ATRA than with conventional induction chemotherapy. Although the induction of remission with ATRA appears to be safer than with chemotherapy, it has also become clear that ATRA alone is rarely curative. After induction of remission with ATRA, postremission chemotherapy is required to maintain remission. A unique complication of ATRA therapy has been the development of the retinoic acid syndrome, which is characterized by pulmonary infiltrates and effusions, weight gain, and fever. Its development requires discontinuation of ATRA and rapid institution of dexamethasone therapy, followed by administration of standard induction chemotherapy.

Acute Lymphoblastic Leukemia

Chemotherapy can cure up to 70% of children, but fewer than 35% of adults with ALL. This difference reflects a higher incidence of adverse prognostic factors and a lower tolerance of intensive therapy in adults.

The approaches used to treat ALL in adults have been adapted from the successful pediatric experience. Induction therapy with prednisone, vincristine, and an anthracycline results in CRs in 70 to 90% of patients. The addition of L-asparaginase, cyclophosphamide, or etoposide increases the duration of these remissions. This induction therapy is usually followed by multiple cycles of intensive consolidation therapy with high-dose ara-C, methotrexate, and other agents. Low-dose 6-mercaptopurine and methotrexate are then administered for prolonged periods as maintenance therapy. In addition, therapy is delivered to the CNS in the form of cranial or craniospinal irradiation as well as intrathecal therapy with methotrexate or ara-C. Because ALL regimens, like AML regimens, are complicated to administer, specialists experienced in the treatment of ALL should care for these patients.

The role of BMT is less clearly defined in the treatment of ALL than in AML. For adult patients with ALL, randomized trials from France and retrospective comparisons of matched patients receiving chemotherapy and BMT have not shown a clear-cut advantage for BMT. As in AML, relapse rates are higher and treatment-related mortality rates lower with chemotherapy, whereas the converse holds for allogeneic BMT. Autologous BMT appears to carry a higher relapse rate in ALL than AML. In one French trial, allogeneic BMT was shown to be of benefit in a subgroup of patients with high-risk ALL. Most investigators would now recommend a related or unrelated allogeneic BMT in first CR for patients with high-risk ALL, especially those with Philadelphia chromosome–positive ALL (t[9;22]), t(4;11), or marked leukocytosis at presentation. To examine further the role of transplantation in the treatment of ALL, a large study conducted by the Medical Research Council of Britain and the Eastern Cooperative Oncology Group in the United States is prospectively comparing results obtained after postremission chemotherapy versus BMT using unpurged autologous marrow or marrow from an HLA-matched sibling. It is hoped that the results of this trial will further define the optimal therapy for adults with ALL.

In the past, patients with the L3 (Burkitt's) type of ALL were thought to have a particularly poor prognosis. However, the outlook for patients with this entity is gradually improving. New combination chemotherapy regimens that include very intensive short courses of chemotherapy with cyclophosphamide, high-dose methotrexate, vincristine, an anthracycline, and high-dose corticosteroids have been shown to produce CR rates exceeding 60 to 70%. Although the toxicities of this intensive chemotherapy can be severe, disease-free survival rates of 50% have been reported.

SUPPORTIVE CARE

Patients with the acute leukemias are at increased risk of infection and bleeding as a consequence of the cytopenias that accompany these diseases and their treatments. Intensive supportive care is required to prevent or treat these complications.

In the 1960s, it was clearly shown that a neutrophil count below 500 per mm^3 was associated with an increased risk of infection. Subsequent studies identified the pathogens that are commonly encountered in profoundly neutropenic patients. More recently, randomized trials have defined approaches that diminish the frequency of sepsis and death in patients with leukemia undergoing intensive chemotherapy.

Patients with neutropenia in whom fever develops (>38.5°C on one occasion or >38.0°C on three or more measurements within 24 hours) require prompt evaluation and treatment. Multiple factors, including disruption of normal epithelial barriers in the gastrointestinal tract, respiratory system, and skin, as well as the presence of long-term indwelling right atrial catheters, contribute to the development of bacterial and fungal infections in these patients. In the past, gram-negative aerobes that colonized the respiratory or gastrointestinal tracts were the predominant organisms isolated from patients with neutropenia and fever. With the increasing use of right atrial catheters for administration of chemotherapy, hydration, and blood products, gram-positive bacteremias and infections involving the subcutaneous tunnels of the catheters have become more common at the time of

first neutropenic fever. Infections with *Candida* and *Aspergillus* species also continue to be prominent problems, particularly at the time of second and subsequent fevers in neutropenic patients. Hepatosplenic candidiasis, for example, is increasingly recognized in patients who receive intensive regimens that cause prolonged neutropenia. The herpesviruses, including herpes simplex virus, cytomegalovirus, and varicella-zoster, can also cause morbidity and mortality in patients with acute leukemia. The realization that herpes simplex virus contributes to chemotherapy-associated mucositis in some patients has led to use of prophylactic acyclovir (Zovirax) with antileukemic therapy.

Because neutropenic patients frequently die of sepsis during the period required for pathogens to be isolated from blood cultures, antibiotic therapy should be promptly initiated in all patients with fever and neutropenia. Treatment with empirical broad-spectrum antibiotics that cover gram-negative aerobes, especially *Pseudomonas aeruginosa*, has been shown to be lifesaving in this setting. The choice of initial therapy depends on the pattern of bacterial isolates and their antibiotic sensitivities at a particular institution. At our institution, a late-generation cephalosporin, such as ceftazidime (Fortaz), 1 to 2 grams intravenously (IV) every 8 hours, or cefepime (Maxipime), 2 grams IV every 12 hours, is used as initial therapy. Although these agents are combined with vancomycin at some centers, the emergence of vancomycin resistance, coupled with the realization that gram-positive infections frequently involve coagulase-negative staphylococci of relatively low virulence, has led infectious disease experts to discourage the use of empirical vancomycin therapy.

If a patient has persistent fever with negative cultures after 3 to 4 days of initial antibacterial therapy, empirical therapy with amphotericin B (Fungizone) should be initiated and continued until resolution of the neutropenia and fever. If a patient experiences excessive toxicity from amphotericin B, one of the liposomal amphotericin preparations should be considered.

Typhlitis (necrotizing enterocolitis), a necrotic inflammatory process involving the wall of the colon, is increasingly recognized in patients receiving intensive chemotherapy. Clinically, patients have fever, abdominal pain and distention, and decreased bowel sounds. Computed tomography demonstrates characteristic bowel wall thickening. Although its etiology is unknown, typhlitis is most likely related to occult infection. Conservative management includes broad-spectrum antibiotics that cover anaerobes as well as aerobes, and total parenteral nutrition with bowel rest. If signs of peritonitis or perforation are present, surgical resection is required, although it is risky in the setting of neutropenia.

Because the infectious complications in patients with leukemia relate to the duration as well as depth of granulocytopenia, the use of the hematopoietic growth factors granulocyte/macrophage colony-stimulating factor (GM-CSF; Leukine) and granulocyte colony-stimulating factor (G-CSF; Neupogen) in patients receiving chemotherapy has been extensively investigated. G-CSF has been convincingly shown to reduce morbidity and length of hospitalization for patients with ALL. Results of similar trials in patients with AML have been more controversial. Multiple randomized trials have demonstrated that these agents can be safely administered after antileukemic treatment, do not appear to accelerate regrowth of AML cells, and are able to shorten the period of neutropenia. Nonetheless, the clinical benefits in terms of diminished infections, decreased antibiotic use, and reduced hospitalization have been less apparent in these trials. GM-CSF is approved for use in elderly patients with AML after induction chemotherapy as a result of one trial showing that the cytokine-associated reductions in the duration of neutropenia and incidence of severe infection were associated with improved survival.

Ongoing studies are examining another potential role for GM-CSF and G-CSF. In these studies, the growth factors are administered *before* the initiation of induction chemotherapy in an attempt to "prime" AML cells—that is, drive them into the cell cycle and thereby increase their susceptibility to S phase–specific agents such as ara-C. This approach remains investigational.

Transfusion therapy represents an essential component of the care of patients with acute leukemia. Several studies have shown that, under ordinary circumstances, platelet transfusions are essential only when the platelet count falls below 10,000 per mm^3. If there is evidence of increased platelet consumption (e.g., as a result of fever or hypersplenism), transfusion should be considered at a count of 20,000 to 30,000 platelets per mm^3. In the presence of bleeding, DIC, or a high blast count with an associated risk of bleeding, we routinely transfuse platelets to keep the count above 50,000 per mm^3.

Development of antibodies against allogeneic HLA antigens (alloimmunization) is a major problem in up to 50% of patients receiving repeated platelet transfusions. Patients who become alloimmunized must receive crossmatched or HLA-matched platelets, which are more difficult and expensive to provide. Alloimmunization is induced by residual leukocytes in blood products. Trials have demonstrated that the use of leukocyte filters with transfusions can decrease the risk of febrile transfusion reactions and the incidence of alloimmunization.

Patients with leukemia also require red cell transfusions. Although most patients can tolerate hemoglobin levels down to 8 grams per dL, patients with coronary or cerebrovascular disease, high fever, pneumonia, or hypoxemia should be transfused to higher levels. As indicated previously, red cell transfusions should be administered cautiously to patients with high circulating blast counts because of the risk of worsening rather than improving tissue perfusion.

Granulocyte transfusions play a more limited role in the management of patients with leukemia. Empirical antibiotic and antifungal therapies are usu-ally effective in controlling infections until the patient's neutrophils can eradicate them. A patient who has persistent bacteremia or fungemia despite treatment with appropriate antibiotics at effective doses can sometimes benefit from the institution of granulocyte transfusions, although this is only a temporizing measure until the patient's own marrow begins making neutrophils.

NEW DIRECTIONS IN THE TREATMENT OF ACUTE LEUKEMIA

Despite the progress made in the treatment of acute leukemia, the disease in most patients relapses and becomes refractory to all forms of therapy. This is exemplified by the poor results achieved with autologous BMT when the procedure is performed after the first remission. Various mechanisms of drug resistance have been identified. Overexpression of the multiple drug resistance gene *mdr1*, which encodes a polypeptide that is capable of transporting anthracyclines, epipodophyllotoxins, and *Vinca* alkaloids out of cells, has been demonstrated in leukemic cells, particularly at relapse and in the elderly. Other mechanisms of resistance include enhanced ability to repair DNA damage, qualitative or quantitative alterations in the enzymes targeted by various drugs, and changes in the complex signaling pathways that initiate the cell death process (apoptosis) after cells have sustained potentially lethal damage. Regarding this last mechanism of resistance, studies performed in a number of research laboratories have indicated that aberrantly high expression of the apoptosis regulatory protein Bcl-2 or certain of its homologues appears to render leukemia cells resistant to a wide variety of chemotherapeutic agents.

The discovery of these mechanisms of resistance has led to new treatment strategies. For example, drugs that inhibit the pumping capability of the mdr1 transporter are being tested clinically in conjunction with various antileukemic regimens. Likewise, antisense oligonucleotides, small molecules complementary to the RNA encoding a particular protein of interest, have been designed to selectively decrease expression of the Bcl-2 protein. These molecules are also being tested in conjunction with conventional chemotherapy.

The empirical development of new agents also continues. In APL, for example, research is focused on arsenic trioxide, a molecule that can induce progranuloblast differentiation at low concentrations and trigger apoptosis at high concentrations. Preliminary results have shown that this agent can induce remissions in patients with ATRA-resistant APL. Additional new agents and regimens continue to be tested for other variants of AML and ALL as well.

Immunotherapeutic approaches also show promise in the therapy of acute leukemia. Interleukin-2, a potent T cell cytokine, has demonstrated antileukemic activity in relapsed AML and may prolong remission when given after autologous BMT for AML. Conjugates containing monoclonal antibodies linked to protein toxins (e.g., diphtheria toxin), tyrosine kinase inhibitors (e.g., genistein), or radioisotopes (e.g., iodine 131) have the potential to target therapy to leukemia cells with less systemic toxicity. Animal data and preliminary trials in humans suggest a promising role for these therapies in the future.

ACUTE LEUKEMIA IN CHILDREN*

method of
PETER G. ADAMSON, M.D.
National Cancer Institute
Bethesda, Maryland

Acute leukemia is the most common malignancy during childhood, with an approximate incidence of 4 cases per 100,000 children younger than 15 years of age. Acute lymphoblastic leukemia (ALL) accounts for 80% of cases, with 2500 to 3000 new cases diagnosed annually in the United States. The peak incidence of ALL is at 4 years of age. Acute nonlymphocytic leukemia (ANLL) represents 15% of annual cases, with a stable incidence throughout the first 10 years of life, which then slowly rises during adolescence. The chronic myeloid leukemias account for the remaining 5% of childhood leukemias, and chronic lymphocytic leukemias occur only rarely in children.

Extraordinary advances made in the treatment of childhood ALL since the 1950s are such that today almost four in five children diagnosed with this disease can be expected to be cured. During the 1990s, the genetic alterations that appear critical to the development of the leukemic process began to emerge, along with the hope that this increased understanding may ultimately result in more specific, effective treatments with less toxicity. Progress in the treatment of ANLL has been slower, with the exception of acute promyelocytic leukemia (APL), for which new therapy (all-*trans*-retinoic acid [ATRA]; Vesanoid) directly targeting the underlying genetic alteration, when combined with chemotherapy, dramatically improves outcome.

Despite the relative success in the treatment of childhood leukemia, therapy is complex and can carry significant risks for acute and long-term toxicity. Treatment is therefore best carried out under the direction of a pediatric oncologist at a treatment center with specific expertise and subspecialty support for the care of children with cancer. Institutions that participate in either of the two nationwide cooperative groups, the Children's Cancer Group and the Pediatric Oncology Group, are best prepared to care for children with leukemia, and enrollment in cooperative group studies can maximize a child's chances at cure while contributing to advances in the care of the disease.

DIAGNOSIS

The most common presenting signs and symptoms of childhood ALL include fever, bleeding manifestations (petechiae or purpura), lymphadenopathy, hepatosplenomegaly, and bone pain, which in young children may manifest as a limp or refusal to walk. The differential diagnosis of childhood leukemia includes both nonmalignant conditions (infectious mononucleosis, pertussis, parapertussis, other

*All material in this chapter is in the public domain, with the exception of any borrowed figures or tables.

viral illnesses, juvenile rheumatoid arthritis, idiopathic thrombocytopenic purpura, aplastic anemia) and other malignant conditions that can invade the bone marrow (non-Hodgkin's lymphoma, neuroblastoma, rhabdomyosarcoma, retinoblastoma, Ewing's sarcoma). Hematologic abnormalities include anemia, thrombocytopenia, neutropenia, and an elevated leukocyte count, which in 20% of patients is markedly elevated (>50,000 cells per mm^3).

The initial diagnostic work-up of a child with suspected acute leukemia is presented in Table 1. Additional tests based on presenting symptoms and initial laboratory results are often necessary.

CLASSIFICATION

Acute leukemias are classified based on a panel of morphologic, immunologic, cytogenetic, biochemical, and molecular genetic features. Classification allows for tailoring the type and intensity of therapy and for evaluating outcome of treatment regimens from clinical trials.

Acute lymphoblastic leukemia is broadly categorized into B lineage or T lineage based on immunophenotypic features. B-lineage ALL is further subclassified into early pre–B (60% of cases), pre–B (25%), and B cell (Burkitt's type, 1%). T cell leukemia constitutes the remaining 15% of cases. The expression of immunologic markers is far more diverse in ANLL, where seven subcategories are defined by the French-American-British (FAB) classification scheme (Table 2).

Childhood ALL is further characterized by other laboratory features as described in Table 3. The initial presenting white blood cell count and patient age remain the two most important prognostic features of this disease, with gender, cytogenetic and molecular genetic findings, and response to initial therapy affecting the prognosis and treatment of

TABLE 1. **Initial Diagnostic Studies**

Test	Assess for
History and physical examination	Organomegaly, lymphadenopathy Signs of bleeding Sites of infection
Complete blood count and differential	Need for transfusion support Presence of blasts Prognostic factors
Chemistry panel, including electrolytes, blood urea nitrogen, creatinine, calcium, phosphorus, uric acid, hepatic transaminases, bilirubin	Evidence of tumor lysis Renal or hepatic dysfunction
Coagulation studies: prothrombin time, partial thromboplastin time, fibrinogen	Evidence of disseminated intravascular coagulopathy
Viral studies: varicella, cytomegalovirus titers	Risk of infection Transplantation risks
Chest radiograph	Mediastinal mass, hilar adenopathy
Bone marrow aspirate: morphology, immunophenotype, cytogenetics, DNA index, cryopreservation (future laboratory studies)	Classification Prognostic factors
Lumbar puncture: cell count, differential, cytospin preparation, glucose, protein	Diagnosis of central nervous system leukemia

TABLE 2. **Classification of Acute Nonlymphocytic Leukemia**

FAB Type	Common Name
M1	Acute myeloblastic leukemia without differentiation
M2	Acute myeloblastic leukemia with differentiation
M3	Acute promyelocytic leukemia
M4	Acute myelomonocytic leukemia
M5	Acute monocytic leukemia
M6	Erythroleukemia
M7	Acute megakaryocytic leukemia

Abbreviation: FAB = French-American-British classification.

the disease. Prognostic factors for ANLL have not been as well defined, but elevated leukocyte count, secondary ANLL, myelodysplastic syndrome, and monosomy 7 are recognized as significant adverse features. Favorable remission rates for ANLL have been associated with certain chromosomal abnormalities, including t(8;21) and inv(16).

INITIAL MANAGEMENT

The child with newly diagnosed leukemia may have a number of serious and potentially life-threatening complications from the disease. As the diagnostic work-up proceeds, therapy to correct disease-related complications should be instituted promptly.

Tumor Lysis

Children may present with metabolic complications resulting from a high rate of cell turnover, including hyperkalemia, hyperuricemia, and hyperphosphatemia. Aggressive intravenous hydration with non–potassium-containing fluids should be initiated at a minimum rate of 3 to 4 liters per m^2 per day. Allopurinol (Zyloprim) at a dose of 100 mg per m^2 thrice daily, and alkalinization to maintain urinary pH at 7 or more should be instituted to correct hyperuricemia. Once hyperuricemia is corrected, alkalinization should be stopped before initiating chemotherapy to minimize the risk of calcium phosphate precipitation in the kidney. Electrolytes, creatinine, calcium, phosphate, and uric acid must be monitored closely, often several times daily, during the initial period of stabilization and therapy.

Infection

Neutropenia is common at diagnosis, and the presence of fever may be the sole indication of serious bacterial infection. In children with fever and neutrophil counts less than 500 per mm^3, broad-spectrum antibiotic coverage should be initiated promptly. Antibiotic coverage varies based on clinical signs and the local antibiotic susceptibility patterns, but in general should provide for broad coverage of gram-negative organisms, including *Pseudomonas aeruginosa*. Ceftazidime (Fortaz) 30 mg per kg every 8 hours is the antibiotic we choose for initial empiric coverage of febrile neutropenic patients. Antibiotics are continued throughout the neutropenic period.

Hyperleukocytosis

Peripheral leukocyte counts greater than 100,000 cells per mm^3 can result in increased blood viscosity and produce central nervous system (CNS), pulmonary, and metabolic complications. The risk is greater for ANLL because of the relatively large size of myeloblasts and is common in chronic myelogenous leukemia. Children may present with signs of hypoxia, blurred vision, agitation, or confusion. Physical examination may reveal plethora or cyanosis, papilledema or retinal vessel engorgement, and ataxia. Initial fluid management as described for tumor lysis should be instituted promptly and chemotherapy started as soon as the patient's life-threatening metabolic complications have been corrected. Leukapheresis can decrease the peripheral counts and reduce viscosity, but its benefits have not been proven.

ACUTE LYMPHOBLASTIC LEUKEMIA TREATMENT

The treatment of ALL is based on the recognition that it is a heterogeneous disease, such that treatment today is based on a stratification of risk factors. As shown in Table 3, a white blood cell count greater than 50,000 cells per mm^3 or age 10 years or older places a child into the higher risk strata. Other factors can influence risk stratification, with a critically important factor being early response to therapy as measured by bone marrow aspiration at day 7 or 14 or, as done in the Berlin-Frankfurt-Münster studies, by evaluating the peripheral blast count at day 7. Therapy for higher risk patients is more intensive than that for lower risk patients. With current risk-directed therapy, higher risk patients can expect long-term event-free survival (EFS) rates of 65 to 80%, and lower risk patients, EFS rates of 80 to 90%. Mature B cell leukemia (1% of childhood ALL) is treated using Burkitt's (non-Hodgkin's) lymphoma

TABLE 3. **Risk Classification of Acute Lymphoblastic Leukemia**

Lower Risk	Factor	Higher Risk
1.00–9.99 y and	Age	≥10 y or
<50,000 cells/mm³	WBC	≥50,000 cells/mm³

Modifying Prognostic Factors	Effect on Prognosis
DNA index > 1.16	Better
Hyperdiploid	Better
Gene rearrangement	
TEL-AML1 translocation: t(12;21)	Better
Philadelphia chromosome: t(9;22)	Worse
MLL gene: 11q23	Worse
Slow response to treatment	Worse
Cerebrospinal fluid cell count > 5 cells/mm³ with blasts	Worse

regimens, which use dose-intensive, alkylator-based chemotherapy treatments of short duration.

Induction

The combination of vincristine (Oncovin), L-asparaginase (Elspar), and prednisone can induce remission in more than 95% of newly diagnosed children with ALL, and thus these agents are the cornerstone of induction chemotherapy. For higher risk patients, anthracyclines such as daunorubicin (Cerubidine) or, less frequently, alkylating agents such as cyclophosphamide (Cytoxan) may be included in protocol induction regimens. The goal of this initial therapy is to induce complete remission, defined by absence of evidence of leukemia when evaluated by physical examination and morphologic assessment of the bone marrow, peripheral blood, and cerebrospinal fluid. Peripheral blood values must be within the normal range and the bone marrow must contain fewer than 5% lymphoblasts to qualify as a complete remission.

Consolidation: Central Nervous System Preventive Therapy

The recognition that disease recurrence in the CNS would prove to be the major obstacle to overall treatment success in two thirds of children led to a series of clinical trials aimed at prevention of disease at this sanctuary site. The combination of cranial radiation and intrathecal (IT) methotrexate (MTX) was found to decrease the incidence of CNS leukemia from 60 to 70% to less than 10%, and during the 1970s and early 1980s, this was the standard treatment approach. However, recognition of the significant long-term neurocognitive deficits that result from cranial radiation in young children led to the development of alternative approaches to CNS preventive therapy. Today, the combination of IT chemotherapy with risk-adapted systemic chemotherapy can prevent CNS relapse in approximately 95% of patients, and although some centers continue to administer 1800 cGy cranial radiation to their highest-risk patients, this practice is becoming less frequent.

After remission induction, a short period of systemic chemotherapy and more intensive IT chemotherapy is initiated. This consolidation phase of therapy usually includes weekly IT MTX; an ongoing study is investigating whether the use of "triple" IT medications (cytosine arabinoside [ara-C], hydrocortisone, and MTX) can further minimize the risk of CNS relapse.

Intensification

After remission is achieved, additional chemotherapy is required because the leukemic cell burden of a child after successful induction can be as high as 10^{10} cells. The intensification phases of therapy administered after recovery of normal hematopoiesis are designed to decrease the leukemic burden as rapidly as possible to minimize the risks of a chemo-

therapy-resistant clone emerging. Intensification chemotherapy is adapted to the risk of relapse. For lower risk patients, retreatment with agents used for remission induction, with additional agents that may include combinations of cyclophosphamide, ara-C, or intermediate-dose MTX, is used. More intensive regimens are used for higher risk patients and may incorporate combinations of high-dose ara-C, high-dose MTX, cyclophosphamide, an anthracycline, and an epipodophyllotoxin.

Intensification chemotherapy has clearly improved the overall survival of children with ALL. Treatment protocols have therefore moved to incorporate additional periods of intensification into therapy (delayed intensification), usually after short periods of maintenance chemotherapy (interim maintenance) to allow for hematopoietic recovery.

Maintenance Chemotherapy

After the intensification portion of chemotherapy, which lasts several months, a prolonged course of less intensive chemotherapy is administered to eliminate the small number of residual leukemic cells. The combination of daily oral mercaptopurine (Purinethol) and weekly MTX remains the foundation of maintenance chemotherapy. Many protocols incorporate monthly pulses of chemotherapy, usually vincristine and prednisone, to supplement the antimetabolite regimen. The use of mercaptopurine and MTX dates back to the 1950s, but evidence suggests that thioguanine may offer an advantage over mercaptopurine; a randomized, clinical trial is investigating this question. Maintenance chemotherapy continues for a total duration of 2.5 to 3 years.

Treatment of Relapse

Although approximately 70% of children with ALL can be cured of their disease with current therapy, 30% experience a relapse of their disease, making relapsed ALL the fourth most common childhood malignancy. For most patients who relapse, especially children who experience a bone marrow relapse, current treatment usually proves inadequate. Of children who relapse, approximately 70% have involvement of the bone marrow, with the CNS and the testes being involved in approximately 26% and 14% of cases, respectively. The timing of relapse is related to the site of relapse, with isolated CNS relapse occurring at a median of 19 months from diagnosis, isolated bone marrow relapse at a median of 26 months, and isolated testicular relapse at a median of greater than 36 months.

Bone Marrow Relapse

A second complete remission can be induced in 70 to 90% of patients after initial isolated bone marrow relapse. Remarkably, retreatment with the standard four-drug induction regimen of vincristine, prednisone, L-asparaginase, and daunomycin, with IT preventive treatment, results in a complete remission in approximately 80% of patients. More intensive regimens based on the vincristine, prednisone, and L-asparaginase chemotherapy backbone have added high-dose ara-C/high-dose MTX or teniposide (Vumon)/ara-C.

The long-term prognosis for children who relapse in the bone marrow is inversely related to the duration of the initial remission. For children who experience an early isolated bone marrow relapse (within 6 months of completion of chemotherapy), prognosis is poor, and there is general agreement that these patients should proceed to bone marrow transplantation. The outlook for children with late bone marrow relapses (>6 months after completion of therapy) is more favorable, and many pediatric oncologists administer an intensive chemotherapy-based regimen to these children, recommending transplantation only after a third remission.

Central Nervous System Relapse

The outlook for patients with CNS recurrence has improved with the recognition that bone marrow relapse almost invariably follows CNS disease unless intensive systemic chemotherapy is administered concomitant with CNS-directed treatment. The general treatment approach to a child with CNS recurrence is to administer IT chemotherapy to induce a remission, and then, after a period of systemic intensification treatment, to administer craniospinal radiation. Usually, a dose of 2400 to 3000 cGy is administered to the cranial vault and 1200 to 1800 cGy to the spinal axis, although more recent data suggest that lower spinal doses of radiation combined with IT chemotherapy may be sufficient. Because administration of craniospinal radiation limits the subsequent use of intensive chemotherapy because of marrow intolerance, administration of radiation is often delayed for a short time (4 to 6 months) to allow for delivery of intensive systemic chemotherapy. For intensive systemic chemotherapy, CNS-directed agents such as high-dose MTX or high-dose ara-C are often incorporated. This approach can cure 35 to 50% of children with an isolated CNS relapse who have not received radiation as part of their initial treatment regimen.

Testicular Relapse

The outlook for children with isolated testicular relapse of their leukemia is considerably more favorable than for any other type of relapse. After diagnosis of an overt testicular relapse, radiation is administered to both testes and the inguinal canal, usually to a total dose of 2400 to 2600 cGy. Intensive systemic retreatment is also administered, including additional CNS preventive treatment. Such an approach can result in an EFS rate greater than 80% in boys experiencing a late isolated testicular relapse.

ACUTE NONLYMPHOCYTIC (NON-M3) LEUKEMIA TREATMENT

With the exception of APL (M3) and children with Down syndrome, the myeloid leukemias are all treated with intensive chemotherapeutic regimens for induction and consolidation, with allogeneic bone marrow transplantation from a matched sibling donor often used during first remission. With current regimens, the long-term EFS rate for non-M3 ANLL is 40 to 60%. The outlook for children with Down syndrome, who typically have M6 or M7 ANLL, is significantly better than for other children with ANLL for reasons that have not yet been elucidated.

Induction

Administration of two consecutive courses of intensive chemotherapy results in remission in approximately 80% of children with ANLL. Administration of the second course of chemotherapy should be delayed neither for evaluation of the initial course of chemotherapy nor for recovery of hematologic parameters. Although remission induction rates are not improved by such an approach, long-term EFS rates appear to be. In addition to intensifying therapy by the timing of drug administration, additional agents (etoposide, thioguanine, and dexamethasone) may be added to the standard 7 days of ara-C plus 3 days of daunomycin. The use of the anthracycline idarubicin (Idamycin) in place of daunomycin during induction is under investigation. Current induction strategies all result in prolonged periods of marrow aplasia, and thus patients require intensive hematologic and antimicrobial support.

Consolidation

Induction chemotherapy is followed by repetitive courses of intensive chemotherapy. Similar to induction, a combination of an anthracycline and ara-C is often the backbone of consolidation chemotherapy. In place of the standard 7-day dosing of ara-C at 100 mg per m² per day, high-dose ara-C plus L-asparaginase often is used. Other agents often used include cyclophosphamide, etoposide, and thioguanine. In contrast to ALL, there is no proven role for maintenance chemotherapy after intensive consolidation treatment.

Many centers recommend transplantation from an HLA-matched donor for patients in first remission, but definitive data supporting such an approach over intensive chemotherapy remain elusive. Thus, some centers advocate transplantation in second remission. Because the data are not clear on this issue, both treatment approaches should be discussed with families.

Central Nervous System Preventive Therapy

Without CNS preventive therapy, meningeal leukemia develops in at least 20% of children with ANLL. IT chemotherapy can decrease the incidence of CNS relapse, but conclusive evidence that it improves EFS rates is lacking. Given the relatively low risk of toxicity from a short course of preventive IT chemotherapy, its use in the treatment of childhood ANLL is nearly universally accepted.

Treatment of Relapse

Bone marrow transplantation is the treatment of choice for children with relapsed ANLL (non-M3). An attempt to reinduce remission is often made but is not a prerequisite for proceeding on to transplantation. Remissions that cannot be consolidated with a transplant are invariably brief.

ACUTE PROMYELOCYTIC LEUKEMIA TREATMENT

Since the late 1980s, our approach to treatment of APL (M3 ANLL) has changed dramatically and, as a result, long-term EFS rates have improved significantly. The addition of the vitamin A derivative, ATRA, to treatment regimens has been responsible for this improvement in survival, and the responsiveness of APL to ATRA has stimulated biologic studies that have elucidated the molecular pathogenesis of this disease. As a single agent, ATRA can induce remissions in more than 90% of patients, and remission induction rates are greater than 95% for patients with the reciprocal 15;17 translocation, which fuses the gene encoding the retinoic acid receptor-alpha on chromosome 17 with the *PML* gene on chromosome 15.

As a single agent administered on a chronic daily schedule, ATRA cannot maintain patients in remission, and thus patients also receive cytotoxic chemotherapy. Although ATRA originally was used as a single agent for remission induction, more recent data suggest that the concomitant administration of ATRA with cytotoxic chemotherapy may result in improved EFS rates. One life-threatening complication of ATRA in patients with APL, which can occur within the first 3 weeks of initiation of therapy, is the retinoic acid syndrome, which consists primarily of fever and respiratory distress. Additional signs and symptoms include weight gain, lower extremity edema, pleural or pericardial effusions, and episodic hypotension. Often the onset of the syndrome is preceded by a significant increase in the peripheral blood leukocyte count. Administration of high-dose corticosteroid therapy early in the course of the syndrome is the recommended treatment.

FUTURE DIRECTIONS

Advances in the treatment of childhood leukemia allow for cure of more than 70% of children with ALL and approximately 40% of children with ANLL. Treatment of disease, however, may be accompanied by long-term sequelae, including effects on growth, development, cardiac function, and CNS function, and a risk of development of a secondary cancer. The primary treatment obstacle for childhood leukemia remains disease recurrence, and both improved methods of identifying patients at risk for relapse

and new approaches for the treatment of higher risk patients are needed. Our ability to detect minimal residual disease will continue to improve and may allow for refinement of therapy for lower and higher risk patents. Novel treatments under evaluation for childhood ALL include the administration of the immunotoxin B43 (anti-CD19) pokeweed antiviral protein and, for children with relapsed T-lineage ALL, 506U, a prodrug of the guanine analogue guanine arabinoside. For ANLL, extending differentiation therapy beyond APL is being investigated, as are novel therapies aimed at overcoming drug resistance. The use of arsenic trioxide may further improve the outlook for children with APL, and could potentially affect the treatment of other myeloid leukemias.

For children with the highest risk leukemias, our ability to overcome the HLA barrier will continue to improve and, it is hoped, allow for better transplantation options for the majority of children who do not have an HLA-identical sibling donor. Improvements in our understanding and treatment of graft-versus-host disease and improved methods to exploit the graft-versus-leukemia effect are also needed.

CHRONIC LEUKEMIAS

method of
JONATHAN E. KOLITZ, M.D., and
STUART M. LICHTMAN, M.D.
*North Shore University Hospital
Manhasset, New York*

CHRONIC MYELOGENOUS LEUKEMIA

Introduction

Chronic myelogenous leukemia (CML) is perhaps the malignant disease that has been most extensively characterized at the molecular level. It is a clonal disease arising in a hematopoietic stem cell that gives rise to all hematopoietic elements with the exception of skin and marrow fibroblasts and some T cell subsets. The clonality of myeloid, erythroid, B lymphoid, and megakaryocytic lineages in patients with CML has been established with a range of cytogenetic, enzymatic, and molecular technologies. Over time, the unregulated growth of marrow elements leads to the clinical manifestations of disease, ultimately culminating in blastic transformation or blast crisis, a lethal form of acute leukemia.

Incidence

Approximately 4000 new cases of CML occur in the United States yearly, representing an incidence of 1.3 per 100,000. A variable male predominance has been reported, ranging between 1.2 and 1.7. Incidence rises continuously with age, with a sharp increase beginning in the fifth decade.

Etiology

Most cases of CML are idiopathic, with rare concordance noted in identical twins. Radiation exposure, most infamously following the atomic bombings of Japan, has been definitely implicated as a causative factor. There have been reported associations with exposure to therapeutic doses of iodine 131 and after radiotherapy for malignant disease, especially Hodgkin's disease. On the other hand, exposure to benzene and to cytotoxic drugs such as alkylating agents, which are known to induce acute leukemia, have not been reproducibly linked to the development of CML. Another known cause of acute leukemia, cigarette smoking, may accelerate the evolution of CML into its terminal phase.

Molecular Biology

Most cases of CML are associated with a balanced translocation involving the long arms of chromosomes 9 and 22, known as the Philadelphia (Ph) chromosome: t(9;22)(q34;q11). This chromosomal construct involves the fusion of *c-abl*, a proto-oncogene on chromosome 9 with weak tyrosine kinase activity to segments of *bcr*, a gene on chromosome 22 encoding a kinase whose physiologic function remains to be fully clarified. The resultant fusion gene, *bcr-abl*, encodes a stronger tyrosine kinase of higher molecular weight (210 versus 145 kD) than the native *c-abl* product.

When incorporated into retroviral vectors, *bcr-abl* has been shown to have transforming properties in tissue culture. The consensus is that while the Ph chromosome is essential to the development of CML, the disease's ultimate lethality depends on the presence of multiple additional molecular perturbations. Presence of *bcr-abl* leads to growth factor–independent survival on the part of CML cells, while autonomous proliferation depends on the development of additional molecular events. About 5% of patients with CML lack the Ph chromosome. Careful analysis of many of these cases yields either the presence of the *bcr-abl* construct with molecular techniques or an entirely distinct diagnostic entity such as chronic myelomonocytic leukemia or chronic neutrophilic leukemia.

The Ph chromosome product may exert transforming effects through its impact on the ras signaling pathway. By upregulating antiapoptotic pathways that counter programmed cell death, activation of ras-mediated pathways may ultimately render CML cells growth factor independent. Pro-apoptotic signals mediated by genes such as *myc* and *p53* may be downregulated in this setting. Mutations that inactivate *p53* have been associated with disease progression in CML.

An additional effect of *bcr-abl* involves its binding to cytoskeletal proteins such as F-actin, leading to decreased adhesion to stromal elements. This impairment may also be attributable to a decrease in expression of adhesion molecules such as integrins.

Both effects lead to the ancorage-independent growth characteristic of CML.

At the cellular level, the accumulation of progeny of the transformed stem cell is associated with a decreased production of lactoferrin by neutrophils, which normally inhibits production of growth stimulatory cytokines such as granulocyte-macrophage colony–stimulating factor (GM-CSF) by monocytes and macrophages. In addition, CML cells are resistant to the growth inhibitory effects of prostaglandin E and acidic isoferritins. The results of these effects on apoptotic pathways, cell adhesion molecules, and growth regulatory pathways is an increase in stem cells in cell cycle and an inexorable accumulation of myeloid cells with prolonged survival, ultimately leading to the clinical manifestations of disease.

Functionally, the neutrophils in CML may display subtle impairments, but these tend not to lead to an increase in infectious complications during the early phases of the disease. Abnormalities in platelet aggregation in response to agonists such as epinephrine may occasionally lead to a bleeding diathesis.

Clinical Manifestations

CML progresses through chronic, accelerated, and terminal blastic phases over an average of 3.5 to 4 years. The disease is often diagnosed when patients are asymptomatic upon the finding of an abnormal blood count. Chronic phase disease can also manifest with signs and symptoms referrable to the expanded myeloid pool, especially splenomegaly and, less commonly, hepatomegaly. Lymphadenopathy is distinctly uncommon at presentation. Less often, vaso-occlusive effects of hyperleukocytosis may include cerebrovascular accidents, digital ischemia, priapism, and splenic infarction. Thrombotic and bleeding manifestations may occur as a result of thrombocytosis, impaired platelet function, and, far less often, thrombocytopenia. The hemoglobin level is usually either normal or mildly depressed. Symptoms due to hypermetabolism, such as fevers, sweats, and weight loss, may also occur at the time of diagnosis.

Laboratory findings include an often markedly elevated white blood cell count, with the platelet count frequently elevated as well. A left shift is seen in the myeloid series, but the blast percentage is usually less than 5. An increase in peripheral blood eosinophils and basophils is characteristic. The erythrocytes are usually normochromic and normocytic, but teardrops and nucleated red blood cells are occasionally noted and are due to varying degrees of marrow fibrosis. About 25% of patients develop secondary myelofibrosis with associated cytopenias, whereas about 50% of patients will display increased collagen in bone marrow reticulin stains.

Additional laboratory findings include a decreased leukocyte alkaline phosphatase (LAP) score, which may be due to both a relative increase in immature myeloid progenitors that do not elaborate LAP or a decrease in humoral factors known to induce LAP activity, such as granulocyte colony-stimulating factor. The serum vitamin B_{12} level and B_{12} binding proteins are generally elevated, as are the serum lactate dehydrogenase and uric acid levels.

When treatment does not lead to partial or complete suppression of the Ph^+ clone, CML progresses to an accelerated phase marked by wider fluctuations in the peripheral blood count, which becomes increasingly difficult to medically manage, development of progressive end-organ involvement, including more pronounced hepatosplenomegaly, and encroachment of the bone marrow space leading to anemia and thrombocytopenia. Increased basophilia and eosinophilia are common. Systemic symptoms may become more pronounced during this phase, which generally lasts several months, culminating in the development of a highly virulent form of acute leukemia. The likelihood of entering blast crisis is initially about 10% per year, with the risk starting to rise steeply by the third year of diagnosis. Before the development of therapies that suppress or eradicate the Ph^+ clone at the cytogenetic level, the median time to blast crisis ranged between 3.5 and 4 years. Prognostic models based on parameters present at diagnosis have been used to predict the probability of entering blast crisis over time (Table 1).

In tandem with multiple molecular events that occur during this fatal transition, several well-recognized additional cytogenetic aberrations develop, especially trisomy 8, isochromosome 17, and duplications of the Ph chromosome. When acute leukemia develops, it most often takes the form of acute myelogenous leukemia (AML). The 50% or so of patients who develop a myeloid blast crisis succumb to their disease generally within 3 months of diagnosis. Therapy with standard AML induction regimens with an anthracycline in combination with cytosine arabinoside induce a transient complete remission in less than half of treated patients, an outcome substantially inferior to that achievable in de novo AML. Because CML is a stem cell malignancy, it is not surprising that about one-third of patients develop a lymphoblastic crisis, almost always a B lineage acute lymphoblastic leukemia (ALL), with very rare cases of T-ALL noted. Such patients often achieve remission with ALL induction regimens with vincristine

and prednisone, among other agents, but remission duration and survival rarely exceed 6 months. Less often, other stem cell progeny predominate in the terminal leukemia, most often erythroid elements in acute erythroblastic leukemia, with occasional cases of megakaryoblastic, mixed lineage, and even basophilic, eosinophilic, and mast cell crises.

Therapy

The goal of therapy is to restore patients to their premorbid state by suppressing the expansion of the myeloid progenitor pool, thereby causing regression of organomegaly, resolution of systemic symptoms, and normalization of the peripheral blood count. Oral cytotoxic agents can achieve this goal relatively easily in most patients with minimal toxicity. Unfortunately, exerting this level of clinical control on the disease, which can render a patient entirely asymptomatic and fully functional, has no impact at all on the ultimate evolution to acute leukemia. Clinical and biological characteristics present at diagnosis, coupled with the inevitable accumulation of secondary molecular events, lead to blast crisis at a time that may well be pre-ordained for every individual. Only suppressing or eradicating the Ph^+ population leads to long survival and, in the setting of allogeneic bone marrow transplantation, cure.

It is usually reasonable to initially control the disease's manifestations with an oral cytotoxic agent. The two agents most often used for this indication are hydroxyurea (Hydrea) (HU) and busulfan (Myleran). Although busulfan in conventional doses can rarely induce a cytogenetic response, it is a significantly more toxic drug than HU. Unlike HU, busulfan can induce unpredictable, often severe, and occasionally irreversible myelosuppression, serious pulmonary fibrosis, and more benign but often cosmetically distressing cutaneous hyperpigmentation. HU has the advantage of causing myelosuppression that is almost always rapidly reversible while not affecting pulmonary function. Skin ulcerations are rare, while its lack of cross-resistance with alkylating agents is helpful for patients who are ultimately slated to receive alkylator-based transplantation conditioning regimens. Doses of HU ranging between 20 and 30 mg per kg given as a single daily dose usually suffice to control peripheral blood counts.

Until the white blood cell count (WBC) falls below 20,000, it is reasonable to include allopurinol (Zyloprim) in the regimen. Historically, practitioners have interrupted HU therapy when the WBC fell below 10,000 to 15,000 and restarted therapy as the WBC rose above 20,000. The experience with alpha interferon (IFN-α; Intron-A), which exerts a cytogenetic response and prolongation in survival in association with suppression of the WBC count to below 5000, and not infrequently to 2000 to 3000, has increased the clinical practice of treating patients with HU in a more intensive fashion, reducing the WBC to levels comparable with those observed in interferon-treated patients. This can be done safely, but requires more

TABLE 1. **Sokal Scores**

Hazard Ratio*	Sokal Group	Distribution (%)	Likelihood of a Major Response to Interferon (%)
<0.8	Low risk	30–40	50
0.8–1.2	Intermediate risk	30	30
>1.2	High risk	20–30	15

*Calculation of Sokal scores: 1. For patients 5 to 84 years old: hazard ratio = exp |0.011 (age − 43) + 0.0345 (spleen − 7.5 cm) + 0.188 [(platelets/700)² − 0.563] + 0.0887 (% blasts in blood − 2.1)|. 2. For patients 5 to 45 years old: hazard ratio = exp |0.0255 (spleen − 8.14 cm) + 0.0324 (% blasts in blood − 2.22) + 0.1025 [(platelets/700)² − 0.627] − 0.0173 (hct − 34%) − 0.2682 (sex − 1.4)|: male, 1, female, 0.

From Lee SJ, Anasetti C, Horowitz MM, Antin JH: Initial therapy for chronic myelogenous leukemia: Playing the odds. J Clin Oncol 16: 2897–2903, 1998.

frequent monitoring. Data validating such an approach tend to be more impressionistic than scientific at this point. With respect to inducing the relevant end point of cytogenetic response, it is clear that HU in conventional doses is ineffective.

Attempts to eradicate the Ph⁺ clone with intensive multidrug combination therapies used to treat AML have generally induced major responses, including cytogenetic responses, in substantial numbers of treated patients, but response duration has been distressingly brief, and the impact on overall survival has been modest at best. Reproducible and sustained cytogenetic responses with therapies short of transplantation have been most often associated with treatment with IFN-α.

The largest single institutional experience with IFN-α in CML is at the M. D. Anderson Cancer Center in Texas, where many hundreds of newly diagnosed patients with CML have been treated with complete hematologic response rates (CHR) of 80% and partial to complete cytogenetic response rates approaching 40%. Other single institution, multicenter, and international trials have reported comparable incidences of CHR as well as significant, albeit lower, levels of cytogenetic response, variably defined as consisting of the presence of at least 33 to 35% or more Ph⁻ metaphases in a bone marrow sampling. The median survival among cytogenetic responders in the M. D. Anderson series is 89 months, with an overall 5-year survival rate for all treated patients of 63%. Several international randomized studies have demonstrated that therapy with IFN-α is superior to HU or busulfan with respect to major end points such as overall survival. A U.K. national trial even suggested that IFN-α confers a survival advantage to patients who do not achieve cytogenetic response. The advent of IFN-α as a standard initial therapy for CML has increased the median survival by 1 to 1.5 years over what had been achievable with oral cytotoxic agents alone.

There are preliminary data suggesting that a small number of patients treated with IFN-α for more than 5 years can have therapy discontinued with maintenance of remission off all therapy. The bulk of the molecular evidence suggests, however, that even patients enjoying complete cytogenetic response harbor residual clonal progenitors detectable with highly sensitive methodologies such as quantitative polymerase chain reaction (PCR) assays. This observation is leavened by yet other data documenting the presence of *bcr-abl* transcripts in the peripheral blood of normal subjects.

The recommended dose of IFN-α is 5×10^6 U per m² subcutaneously (SC) daily. To reduce the likelihood of early toxicity, principally fever, fatigue, flulike syndrome, myalgias, and nausea, it is advisable to initially lower the WBC with HU to below 20,000 and then introduce IFN-α at a lower dose, 1×10^6 U per m² representing a reasonable starting point. The target dose can then be gradually achieved over 3 to 4 weeks. Hematologic end points that signal a need to reduce dose are falls in the WBC to below 2000 and platelet count less than 50,000.

With chronic administration, fatigue predominates as the principal subjective toxicity. Selective serotonin reuptake inhibitors such as sertraline (Zoloft) and venlafaxine (Effexor) can sometimes be helpful with respect to countering fatigue. Acetaminophen and nonsteroidal anti-inflammatory drugs can effectively control fever and musculoskeletal complaints. Corticosteroids should be avoided. Local irritation at subcutaneous injection sites is an occasional concern. With longer term use, uncommon but potentially serious neurotoxicity can develop, especially in the form of a parkinsonian syndrome. Autoimmune effects can include the development of hypothyroidism, and thyroid function should be evaluated every 6 months.

Lower dose regimens have been reported to induce comparable hematologic and cytogenetic responses. Complete cytogenetic response has been less frequently observed with such regimens, and insufficient numbers of patients have been treated in randomized trials to generate enough confidence to adopt lower dose therapies at this time.

Attempts to exploit initial hematologic and cytogenetic responses obtained with AML-type chemotherapy regimens by instituting therapy with IFN-α either after induction therapy or interspersed between cycles of such therapy have led to disappointing results. It appears that continuous exposure to IFN-α is essential to its ability to induce cytogenetic response. Patients who are destined to achieve a major cytogenetic response generally do so by 12 months of therapy, with some data suggesting that a response at 3 months is helpful in predicting subsequent response.

Early observations suggesting that low doses of cytosine arabinoside (LD ara-C) exert meaningful anti-CML effects in vivo and in vitro have led to a series of phase II and III trials to evaluate the efficacy and toxicity of combining IFN-α with LD ara-C in a variety of doses and schedules. The most persuasive evidence supporting such combination therapy has been reported by the French, who halted a randomized trial when superior survival (86% vs. 79%) at 3 years was noted for the combination therapy compared with IFN-α alone. The major cytogenetic response rate was 41% for the combination therapy versus 24% for the immunotherapy alone. Also supporting the potency of the combination therapy is the fact that patients with later, more advanced disease are significantly more responsive to LD ara-C plus IFN-α than to IFN-α alone, even including some patients resistant to IFN-α.

Enthusiasm for the regimen has been somewhat dampened by experience in the United States and Austria of difficulties with patient compliance and high drop-out rates attributable to subjective toxicity. Typical dosing schemes use the standard IFN-α dose of 5×10^6 U per m² SC daily along with ara-C 20 mg per m² SC 10 days per month or 10 mg per m² SC daily. The lower dose daily regimen may be better tolerated. Even while results of a multicenter U.S. randomized trial are awaited, it can at least be concluded that the combination regimen is at the very least equal to IFN-α monotherapy and may well ultimately prove to be superior in patients who are tolerant of the regimen. Subset analyses suggest that the patients most likely to derive a survival benefit from therapy with IFN-α–based therapies are those with favorable clinical risk factors at the time of diagnosis.

Newer agents that are showing promise include the plant alkaloid homoharringtonine,* which induces significant cytogenetic response even in late chronic phase. The combination of homoharringtonine and LD ara-C is especially promising and will be evaluated in previously untreated patients in a U.S. cooperative group trial. Less striking but encouraging results have been reported in a small number of patients receiving combination therapy with homoharringtonine and IFN-α. GM-CSF (Sargramostim [Leukine]) has been given in low doses in combination with IFN-α to patients who have failed to display cytogenetic response to IFN-α alone at 1 year, with some responses observed.

An interesting variant of the LD ara-C plus IFN-α approach has involved the use of an oral lipophilic prodrug of ara-C, cytarabine ocfosfate,* which may provide comparable efficacy with increased convenience and, possibly, reduced toxicity. Longer acting IFN-α preparations such as a PEGylated product has the advantage of weekly subcutaneous dosing, a prolonged half-life, lower toxicity, and the potential for overcoming IFN-α resistance in at least some patients. An oral preparation of the anthracycline idarubicin* has been undergoing clinical trials. Designer drugs aimed at inhibiting the arrant tyrosine kinase of CML have also begun clinical trials. Finally, immunologic manipulations aimed at fostering cytotoxic T cell responses to peptides corresponding to the most prevalent bcr-abl breakpoints are undergoing evaluation in ongoing vaccine studies.

Ultimately, CML is reproducibly curable only when myeloablative therapies are applied in conjunction with allogeneic bone marrow transplantation. All patients under age 50 should be considered for early allogeneic matched related or unrelated bone marrow transplantation. Autologous transplantation using either unmanipulated CML marrow or marrow maintained in long-term culture so that normal progenitors predominate in the infused product have been actively investigated. A small number of patients receiving autologous marrow rendered Ph⁻ through long-term culture have engrafted in complete cytogenetic remission, but follow-up has been brief. Autologous transplantation of unmanipulated marrow can occasionally prolong the chronic phase by re-establishing sensitivity to IFN-α in resistant patients. Peripheral blood is relatively enriched for Ph⁻ precursors after recovery from myelosuppressive therapy, and autologous transplantation with such stem cell collections can also induce cytogenetic remissions

*Investigational drug in the United States.

that can be potentially maintained with IFN-α. Again, follow-up has been brief. Ongoing efforts are being directed toward purging CML marrow with antisense bcr-abl transcripts and direct inhibitors of tyrosine kinase.

CHRONIC LYMPHOCYTIC LEUKEMIA

Introduction

Chronic lymphocytic leukemia (CLL) is the most common leukemia in adults in the United States and most of western Europe. It accounts for approximately 30% of all leukemias. The median age at diagnosis is 65 to 70 years and is rarely seen before the age of 35 years. There is a male to female ratio of 2:1. There has been a trend toward a higher median age at diagnosis, particularly among patients with early-stage disease. Therefore, there will be an increased number of patients with this disorder due to the aging of the population.

There is no known cause of CLL; however, some factors have been associated. There is a high familial risk, with family members having a two to seven times increased risk of developing the disease. There is no known association with exposure to radiation, alkylating agents, or leukemogenic chemicals.

Biology

The majority of CLL cells are derived from mature, naive B cells that immunophenotypically resemble fetal B cells with low immunoglobulin M positivity, expression of CD5 and CD23, as well as a variety of pan B cell markers such as CD19, CD20, and CD40, but lacking CD10. In most patients the fraction of leukemia cells actively proliferating is low, and more than 95% are in a G_0 resting state. CLL appears to be a prime example of a malignancy that is caused principally by defects that prevent cell turnover due to programmed cell death rather than by alterations in the regulation of the cell cycle. These abnormalities in programmed cell death can make neoplastic cells resistant to the cytotoxic effects of chemotherapy and radiation.

There are a number of genetic alterations in CLL. The single most common alterations are deletions on the long arm of chromosome 13 at band q14. The specific gene affected by this abnormality is not known, but presumably is a recessive tumor suppressor gene. The second most common abnormality is trisomy 12. This abnormality is associated with a worse prognosis for patients. Patients have a significantly shorter therapy-free survival rate than that associated with other cytogenetic findings. It has also been found to be associated with an increased proportion of leukemic prolymphocytes and atypical morphology and also by an increased proliferation rate as indicated by Ki-67 staining. Chromosomal translocations involving the bcl-2 gene on chromosome 18, band q21 and one of the immunoglobulin gene loci on chromosomes 2 (kappa chain), 14 (heavy chain),

TABLE 2. **NCI-WG Diagnostic Criteria of Chronic Lymphocytic Leukemia**

Absolute lymphocytosis consisting of mature-appearing cells of at least 5000/mm³
Phenotypes of the lymphocytes should reveal
  Predominance of B cells that are CD19⁺, CD20⁺, CD23⁺, and CD5⁺
  Monoclonality with respect to either κ or λ
  Low-density surface immunoglobulin expression
Bone marrow evaluation
  Not an absolute necessity if the above criteria are met
  More necessary when the absolute lymphocyte count is relatively low
  Bone marrow aspirate must show ≥30% of all nucleated cells to be lymphoid with normal cellularity or hypercellularity
  Pattern of lymphoid infiltration in bone marrow biopsy has prognostic importance
    Diffuse involvement correlates with progressive or advanced disease
    Nondiffuse (nodular or interstitial) patterns predict better response

From Cheson BD, Bennett JM, Grever M, et al: National Cancer Institute–Sponsored Working Group guidelines for chronic lymphocytic leukemia: Revised guidelines for diagnosis and treatment. Blood 87:4990–4997, 1996.

or 22 (lambda chain) occur in a few percentage of patients. Chromosomal translocations involving the *bcl-1* gene on chromosome 11, band q14 and the IgH locus at 14q32 are reported in approximately 5% of patients. Many believe that these t(11;14)-containing cells are B cell CLL variants such as mantle cell lymphoma.

Patients also manifest a multitude of immune abnormalities. A significant percentage of patients are affected with hypogammaglobulinemia leading to severe complications such as infections with *Streptococcus pneumoniae, Staphylococcus aureas,* and *Escherichia coli.* Cellular defects lead to impaired immune responses to intracellular bacteria or viral infections, autoimmune disorders, and secondary neoplasms. A variety of autoimmune disorders are reported, including systemic lupus erythematosis, rheumatoid arthritis, vasculitis, aplastic anemia, pure red cell aplasia, immune thrombocytopenia, and autoimmune hemolytic anemia.

Laboratory Features

CLL is characterized by marked lymphocytosis with a mean value of 30 to 50 $\times$ 10⁹ per liter. The lymphocytes are small and mature with little cytoplasm and clumped chromatin. Some larger nucleolated cells, which may represent prolymphocytes, may be seen, but should comprise no more than 10% of the cells. The diagnostic criteria have been established by the National Cancer Institute–Sponsored Working Group (NCI-WG) (Tables 2 and 3).

Differential Diagnosis

There are other chronic lymphoproliferative disorders that can be similar in presentation and morphology to CLL. Patients with prolymphocytic leukemia have more than 55% prolymphocytes in the peripheral blood smear and/or more than 15,000 per mm³ absolute count of prolymphocytes. These lymphocytes are CD5⁻ in approximately 50% of cases and usually are bright-staining surface immunoglobulin. Mantle cell lymphoma in the leukemia phase has cells that are CD5⁺ but CD23⁻. The lymph node architecture is characteristic of this disorder. The other chronic disorders include hairy cell leukemia, splenic lymphoma with villous lymphocytes, large granular lymphocytosis, Sézary cell leukemia, leukemic phase of follicular center cell lymphoma, and adult T cell leukemia/lymphoma.

Staging

The two most common and valuable staging systems are that of Rai and Binet (Tables 4 and 5). The NCI-WG recommends modification of the five-stage Rai system by using the three-risk group (Table 4). In addition, the low and high beta₂-microglobulin levels are associated with good and poor survival times, respectively. The lymphocyte doubling time (longer than 1 year is better) and bone marrow biopsy lymphocytic infiltration patterns are also important predictors. There are very good prognostic patients who are in the low-risk or Binet A groups who may be classified as having smoldering CLL. This includes a blood lymphocyte count of less than 30,000 per mm³, a lymphocyte doubling time of longer than 12 months, a hemoglobin level more than 12 grams per dL, and bone marrow biopsy material showing a nondiffuse lymphocytic infiltration pattern. Normal cytogenetics conferred a better outcome than the presence of any cytogenetic abnormality.

TABLE 3. **Diagnostic Criteria for Chronic Lymphocytic Leukemia (CLL) According to the National Cancer Institute (NCI) and International Workshop on CLL (IWCLL)**

Cells	NCI	IWCLL
Lymphocytes	≥5 $\times$ 10⁹/L + ≥1 B cell marker (CD19, CD20, CD23)	≥10 $\times$ 10⁹/L + B phenotype or bone marrow involvement
Atypical cells	<55%	—
Bone marrow lymphocytes	≥30%	>30%

From Cortes JE, Kantarjian H: Chronic leukemias. *In* Pazdur R, Coia LR, Hoskins WJ, Wagman LD (eds): Cancer Management: A Multidisciplinary Approach, 2nd ed. Huntington, NY, PRR, 1998, pp 306–328. With permission of PRR, Inc., Melville, NY.

TABLE 4. **Staging System for Chronic Lymphocytic Leukemia**

Rai Stage	Modified Rai Stage	Clinical Characteristics	Median Survival (Y)
0	Low	Lymphocytosis in peripheral blood and bone marrow only	>10
I	Intermediate	Lymphocytosis and enlarged nodes	6
II		Lymphocytosis and enlarged spleen and/or liver	
III	High	Lymphocytosis and anemia (Hgb <10 gm/dL)	2
IV		Lymphocytosis and thrombocytopenia (platelets <100 × 10⁹/L)	

From Cortes JE, Kantarjian H: Chronic leukemias. *In* Pazdur R, Coia LR, Hoskins WJ, Wagman LD (eds): Cancer Management: A Multidisciplinary Approach, 2nd ed. Huntington, NY, PRR, 1998, pp 306–328. With permission of PRR, Inc., Melville, NY.

Treatment of Chronic Lymphocytic Leukemia

The NCI-WG recommends initiating therapy if criteria of active disease are met. These criteria include the presence of disease-related symptoms (weight loss, fatigue, poor performance score, fever without infection, or night sweats), progressive anemia or thrombocytopenia, autoimmune anemia or thrombocytopenia not responding to corticosteroids, massively enlarged nodes or spleen, progressive or rapid rate of increase in blood lymphocyte count, and repeated infections with or without hypogammaglobulinemia.

Radiation to an enlarged spleen and bulky lymphadenopathy may also help selected patients. Splenectomy may be reasonable when the spleen is enlarged and there is evidence of hypersplenism, particularly if chemotherapy and radiation therapy have not been effective.

The standard treatment of CLL has been chlorambucil (Leukeran). The drug is most commonly used on an intermittent schedule with a single dose of 0.4 mg per kg every 2 weeks. There are, however, many variations on schedule. The response rate to single-agent therapy is approximately 75% with two thirds of patients responding to second and subsequent courses. Cyclophosphamide (Cytoxan) has also been used as a single agent, but more commonly is incorporated in combination with vincristine (Oncovin)* and prednisone (CVP). The response rates to CVP have varied from 44 to 77%, with higher response rates in previously untreated patients. Many regimens combine chlorambucil with prednisone. There are dangers to prolonged corticosteroid therapy, however, particularly in the elderly. Corticosteroids are used for the treatment of autoimmune phenomena

*Not FDA approved for this indication.

such as autoimmune thrombocytopenia and hemolytic anemia. No survival advantage is seen with any one permutation of the scheduling of chlorambucil and/or the addition of corticosteroids.

There have been trials comparing chlorambucil with combination regimens, particularly CVP. In one study no significant difference in survival was observed, with median values of 4.8 years for chlorambucil and prednisone and 3.9 years for CVP. Median survival for the Rai stage III and IV patients was 4.1 years. There is some question whether an increased dose intensity of chlorambucil is associated with a prolonged survival.

In the French Cooperative Group study, Binet stage A patients were randomized to immediate versus delayed continuous oral chlorambucil. Survival was slightly higher in the delayed treatment group. Other studies have shown no survival advantage for immediate treatment. For Binet stage B patients there was no difference with oral chlorambucil compared with CVP. The median survival was 5 years. There are some data that anthracyclines may improve survival. Some of these studies have been criticized, however, and multiagent regimens containing anthracyclines have not been frequently utilized.

Nucleoside Analogues

Fludarabine (Fludara) is a fluorinated derivative of 9-β-arabinofuranosyladenine (ara-A), which is relatively resistant to rapid deamination by adenosine deaminase. This compound, 9-β-arabinofuranosyl-2-fluoroadenine monophosphate (F-ara-AMP, fludarabine) also has improved aqueous solubility. It has shown significant activity in low-grade lymphoproliferative malignancies, including chronic lymphocytic leukemia, Waldenstrom's macroglobulinemia, hairy cell leukemia, and non-Hodgkin's lymphoma. Its re-

TABLE 5. **Binet System for Staging Chronic Lymphocytic Leukemia**

Binet Stage	Clinical Characteristics	Median Survival (Y)
A	Hemoglobin ≥10 gm/dL, platelets ≥100 × 10⁹/L, and <3 areas involved	>10
B	Hemoglobin ≥10 gm/dL, platelets ≥100 × 10⁹/L, and ≥3 areas involved	6
C	Hemoglobin <10 gm/dL, platelets <100 × 10⁹/L, or both (independent of areas involved)	2

From Cortes JE, Kantarjian H: Chronic leukemias. *In* Pazdur R, Coia LR, Hoskins WJ, Wagman LD (eds): Cancer Management: A Multidisciplinary Approach, 2nd ed. Huntington, NY, PRR, 1998, pp 306–328. With permission of PRR, Inc., Melville, NY.

sponse rate of up to 80% in previously untreated patients make it the most active drug in this disease.

The addition of prednisone does not improve the response rate but is associated with an increased incidence of opportunistic infections, including *Pneumocystis carinii* pneumonia and *Listeria* sepsis or meningitis. This complication is partially due to the suppression of the CD4 lymphocytes. With therapy, CD4 levels were uniformly depressed from a median 1015 per μL pretreatment to a median 159 per μL after 3 months of fludarabine therapy. Fludarabine has also been associated with an increased incidence of autoimmune hemolytic anemia. The cause of autoimmune phenomena in CLL is not known, but some findings reinforce the view that they are caused by a disturbance in immunoregulatory T cells.

Other nucleoside analogues have activity in CLL. Cladribine (2-chlorodeoxyadenosine, 2-CDA [Leustatin]*) is active at doses of 0.1 mg per kg per day for 7 days. The clinical experience with 2-CDA in CLL is limited, but the preliminary results suggest a similar efficacy as fludarabine, whereas DCF (Pentostatin*; 2'-deoxycoformycin [Nipent]) seems to be less effective. Whether fludarabine-treated patients have any advantage for overall or progression-free survival has to be answered by ongoing randomized trials. Currently, the place of fludarabine and 2-CDA as two extremely active single agents in CLL is in second-line therapy. Their appropriate indication in the first-line strategy of CLL has, however, still to be defined.

Although fludarabine is being increasingly used as front-line treatment, its efficacy has only been proven as a second-line agent after oral alkylating drugs. A study by the Cancer and Leukemia Group B has shown a higher complete response rate and longer durations of remission and progression-free survival with fludarabine compared with chlorambucil. There is no evidence of significant improvement in survival.

The efficacy of fludarabine as initial therapy for CLL has been demonstrated in a large cooperative group study that randomly assigned patients to therapy with fludarabine versus pulse chlorambucil. A third arm, which combined fludarabine and chlorambucil, was closed because it was associated with unacceptable hematologic toxicity and was not more effective than fludarabine alone. A significantly higher response incidence (70% vs. 43%) and duration (33 vs. 17 months) was seen in patients receiving fludarabine. Progression-free survival was also significantly better in the fludarabine arm. Because the study had a cross-over design, no conclusions can be drawn regarding overall survival, which was similar in both arms. As a result, the strongest inference that can be drawn is that initial therapy with fludarabine is clearly associated with a superior initial outcome. Planned studies will address the question as to whether the addition of a monoclonal antibody variably reactive with CLL cells (rituximab [Rituxan]) can enhance the efficacy of fludarabine in previously untreated patients.

Determination of which therapy to use for elderly patients involves a number of issues. For early stage patients, a period of observation is warranted. Chlorambucil is a safe initial treatment option for most patients. The combination of other drugs must be assessed on an individual basis. Prednisone may have significant complications in the elderly. It can exacerbate diabetes mellitus, osteoporosis, and cataracts. Elderly patients may also manifest neuropsychiatric disturbances while on corticosteroids. The drug may also increase the risk of infection, particularly opportunistic infection. Vincristine neuropathy is particularly disabling in an elderly person. It may affect gait and motor function. Fludarabine can be used, but the risks of opportunistic infection must be considered and the use of prophylactic antiviral and anti-*Pneumocystis* treatments should be considered. Growth factors and erythropoietin may be helpful for selected patients to avoid treatment complications.

CLL is not a curable disease, but patients can be maintained with an adequate quality of life with the appropriate use of drug therapy. The role of bone marrow transplantation is being evaluated for younger patients. Experimental approaches include UCN-01, a hydroxylated derivative of staurosporine, a potent protein kinase C inhibitor; topoisomerase I inhibitors; bryostatin; flavoperidol, a synthetic flavone that antagonizes several cell cycle proteins including CDK1, CDK2, and CDK4 and thereby inhibits cell cycle progression at G_1 and G_2M; and Campath 1-H.

NON-HODGKIN'S LYMPHOMA

method of
PAULA MARLTON, M.B., B.S.
Princess Alexandra Hospital
Brisbane, Australia

and

FERNANDO CABANILLAS, M.D.
M. D. Anderson Cancer Center
Houston, Texas

The non-Hodgkin's lymphomas (NHLs) constitute a clinically and biologically diverse group of malignant disorders involving lymph nodes and extranodal lymphoid tissue. The incidence of lymphoma in Western societies has been steadily increasing for more than two decades, with a more rapid rise noted in recent years. Acquired immune deficiency syndrome (AIDS)–related lymphomas and an aging population are both contributing to this rise, but other etiologic factors remain poorly understood. The introduction of chemotherapy dramatically improved outcomes for many subsets of patients with these previously untreatable disorders; however, despite the progressive introduction of new treatment strategies, the majority of lymphoma patients are not cured. Herein lies the challenge to hematologists and oncologists for the new millennium.

---

*Not FDA approved for this indication.

TABLE 1. REAL Classification: Non-Hodgkin's Lymphoid Neoplasms Recognized by the International Lymphoma Study Group

B Cell Neoplasms

Precursor B cell neoplasm: Precursor B-lymphoblastic leukemia/lymphoma
Peripheral B cell neoplasms
  B cell chronic lymphocytic leukemia/prolymphocytic leukemia/small cell lymphocytic lymphoma
  Lymphoplasmacytoid lymphoma/immunocytoma
  Mantle cell lymphoma
  Follicle center lymphoma, follicular
    Provisional cytologic grades: I (small cell), II (mixed small and large cell), III (large cell)
    Provisional subtype: Diffuse, predominantly small cell type
  Marginal zone B cell lymphoma
    Extranodal (MALT-type $\pm$ monocytoid B cells)
    Provisional subtype: Nodal ($\pm$ monocytoid B cells)
  Provisional entity: Splenic marginal zone lymphoma ($\pm$ villous lymphocytes)
  Hairy cell leukemia
  Plasmacytoma/plasma cell myeloma
  Diffuse large B cell lymphoma
    Subtype: Primary mediastinal (thymic) B cell lymphoma
  Burkitt's lymphoma
  Provisional entity: High-grade B cell lymphoma, Burkitt's-like

T Cell and Putative Natural Killer (NK) Cell Neoplasms

Precursor T cell neoplasm: Precursor T-lymphoblastic lymphoma/leukemia
Peripheral T cell and NK cell neoplasms
  T cell chronic lymphocytic leukemia/prolymphocytic leukemia
  Large granular lymphocyte leukemia (LGL)
    T cell type
    NK cell type
  Mycosis fungoides/Sézary syndrome
  Peripheral T cell lymphomas, unspecified
    Provisional cytologic categories: Medium-sized cell, mixed medium and large cell, large cell, lymphoepithelioid cell
    Provisional subtype: Hepatosplenic $\tau\delta$ T cell lymphoma
    Provisional subtype: Subcutaneous panniculitic T cell lymphoma
  Angioimmunoblastic T cell lymphoma (AILD)
  Angiocentric lymphoma
  Intestinal T cell lymphoma ($\pm$ associated-enteropathy)
  Adult T cell lymphoma/leukemia (ATL/L)
  Anaplastic large cell lymphoma (ALCL), CD30$^+$, T cell and null cell types
  Provisional entity: Anaplastic large cell lymphoma, Hodgkin's-like

Abbreviation: MALT = mucosa-associated lymphoid tissue.
Modified from Harris NL, Jaffe ES, Stein H, et al: Perspective: A revised European-American classification of lymphoid neoplasm: A proposal from the International Lymphoma Study Group. Blood 84:1361–1392, 1994.

CLASSIFICATION

Although all NHLs are clonal disorders of cells derived from the lymphoid lineage, they encompass a great diversity of diseases. Initial histologic classification is an essential first step in clarifying the diagnosis of NHL. This almost always requires an excisional lymph node biopsy, although in some institutions with extensive experience, computed tomography (CT)–guided needle core biopsy or fine-needle aspiration is a useful alternative to major surgery, particularly in very ill patients. Classification of the lymphoma provides useful clinical information about the likely natural history and prognosis of the disease. The interpretation of nodal histology is a challenging field, with several classification systems in use. The most recent of these is the Revised European and American Lymphoma

(REAL) classification (Table 1), which is gradually replacing both the Working Formulation (WF), entrenched in U.S. practice since 1982, and the Kiel classification, popular in Europe. Entities defined in the REAL classification are described in terms of several features in addition to the fundamental histology, including immunohistochemistry, flow cytometric characteristics, clinical features, and, where applicable, cytogenetic and molecular findings. It includes several categories that have been recognized as distinct entities since the advent of the WF system, providing greater accuracy in subset definition. Since its publication in late 1994, the REAL classification has been validated clinically in several retrospective analyses. The next major landmark in classification will be the completion of the WHO classification, described by many as a refined version of the REAL.

STAGING AND PROGNOSTIC FACTOR ASSESSMENT

After histopathologic classification, the next important assessment in lymphoma management is to determine the extent or stage of disease. Staging procedures define the anatomic sites of disease; the findings are then systematized into a shorthand notation. The almost universally used staging classification is the Ann Arbor system (Table 2) originally devised for use in Hodgkin's disease, which is imperfect in its application to NHL. However, it remains central to determining prognosis and appropriate treatment.

Augmenting our ability to predict prognosis has been the identification of a range of other pretreatment variables besides stage that have been shown to correlate with outcome. An extensive analysis of more than 2000 patients with aggressive lymphomas performed by the International Non-Hodgkin's Prognostic Factor Project culminated in the "International Index," presented in Table 3. This index defines four distinct risk categories based on five pretreatment characteristics. At M. D. Anderson Cancer Center a similar analysis led to development of a "Tumor Score System" that defines low-risk and high-risk aggressive lymphomas based on five parameters (see Table 3). Other variables known to correlate with outcome include certain cytokine levels (interleukins IL-6 and IL-14), S-phase fraction, and specific cytogenetic and molecular variables. With these aggressive lymphomas, the risk of central nervous system (CNS) disease must also be evaluated to define appropriate therapy. With indolent lymphomas, risk factor identification analysis has shown that the serum beta$_2$-microglobulin (beta-2M) fraction is highly predictive

TABLE 2. Ann Arbor Staging System

Stage I	One lymph node (LN) region or one extranodal organ or site (IE)
Stage II	Two or more LN regions on the same side of the diaphragm, or one localized extranodal organ or site (IIE) and one or more LN regions on the same side of the diaphragm
Stage III	LN regions on both sides of the diaphragm
Stage IIIE	Stage III plus localized involvement of one extranodal organ or site or spleen (IIIS) or both (IIISE)
Stage IV	One or more extranodal organs with or without associated LN involvement (diffuse or disseminated)

TABLE 3. **Alternative Prognosticating Systems for Non-Hodgkin's Lymphoma**

International Index

Parameter	Criteria	Score
Age	<60 y	0
	>60 y	1
Ann Arbor stage	I–II	0
	III–IV	1
Serum LDH level	Normal	0
	Higher than normal	1
Performance status	0–1	0
	>1	1
Extranodal sites	0–1	0
	>1	1

Score	Risk
0, 1	Low
2	Low intermediate
3	High intermediate
4, 5	High

Tumor Score System

Parameter	Adverse Feature
Ann Arbor stage	III–IV
Symptoms	Presence of B symptoms
Tumor bulk	Mass >7 cm, or detectable mediastinal mass on chest x-ray film
β-2M fraction	>3.0 mg/L
Serum LDH level	≥685 IU/L

Each adverse feature scores one point. Totals of 3 or greater define poor-risk status.

Abbreviations: beta-2M = $beta_2$-microglobulin; LDH = lactate dehydrogenase; B symptoms = weight loss >10 lb, fever, night sweats.

of outcome. Several groups of investigators have shown that the International Index can also be applied successfully in patients with indolent lymphomas.

A guide to appropriate evaluation of stage and prognosis is outlined in Table 4. Restaging or response evaluation is always undertaken at defined intervals during and after therapy and consists of repeating tests that had positive results at the time of diagnosis. Other patient evaluations are included to predict tolerance to treatment and to assess toxicity when indicated.

TABLE 4. **Staging Work-up**

History of B symptoms: fever, sweats, weight loss
Detailed physical examination
Adequate node biopsy
Blood work: complete blood count, biochemical profile including serum LDH and β-2M, serum protein electrophoresis, ESR, HIV serology
Bone marrow aspirate and biopsy (bilateral in indolent lymphoma)
Chest x-ray film
CT scans of chest, abdomen, and pelvis
Lymphangiogram
Gallium scan
± Bone scan, GI work-up, CSF examination

Abbreviations: CBC = complete blood count; LDH = lactate dehydrogenase; β-2M = $beta_2$-microglobulin; ESR = erythrocyte sedimentation rate; HIV = human immunodeficiency virus; CT = computed tomography; GI = gastrointestinal; CSF = cerebrospinal fluid.

MANAGEMENT

In the following discussion, approaches to management of NHL are considered for the broad categories of indolent, aggressive, and highly aggressive lymphomas.

Indolent B Cell Lymphomas

Representing 40 to 50% of all NHLs, indolent B cell lymphoma is the most common subtype in Western countries. Most of these tumors are follicular lymphomas (follicle center lymphoma or follicular lymphoma grade I or II in the REAL classification or follicular small cleaved cell and mixed small cleaved and large cell in the WF). Other entities encompassed in this category include small lymphocytic lymphoma and its subtypes and marginal zone lymphomas, including mucosa-associated lymphoid tissue (MALT) lymphomas. Characterizing the common indolent lymphomas (follicular lymphomas) are the following features: advanced stage at presentation, long median survival of 7 to 9 years; high response rates to initial chemotherapy; gradual development of chemoresistance with subsequent courses of therapy; propensity to transform to more aggressive histology subtypes over time; and low curability with stage IV presentation. Despite these generalizations, the prognosis for patients with indolent lymphoma is variable, and prognostic factor assessment may identify subgroups with better or worse outcomes.

Management of Localized Disease

For the small group of patients (15 to 20%) with localized indolent lymphoma, cure is a realistic treatment goal. In stage I and nonbulky stage II disease, involved field (IF) radiation therapy with small doses of 30 to 40 Gy will achieve long-term disease-free survival in at least 50% of cases. This has been most convincingly demonstrated in laparotomy-staged patients. Relapse within the radiation field occurs in less than 10% of cases, with the majority of recurrences therefore occurring outside the original sites of known disease. Thus, the use of systemic chemotherapy in combination with IF radiation therapy has been evaluated; although this approach is not definitively superior in terms of overall survival, relapse-free survival is improved. Our preferred approach is therefore chemotherapy based on the combination of cyclophosphamide (Cytoxan), doxorubicin (Adriamycin), vincristine (Oncovin), and prednisone—CHOP (Table 5)—followed by IF radiotherapy.

Management of Disseminated Disease

Advanced-stage disease has been approached from widely disparate treatment philosophies. On the one hand, advocates of a conservative approach have quoted the long median survival and incurability as justification for minimally toxic therapy (using a single-agent regimen) or no therapy until a symptomatic indication occurs (watchful waiting). On the other hand, investigators seeking curative treatment have

TABLE 5. **Chemotherapy for Indolent Lymphomas**

Regimen	Dose
Single-Agent	
Chlorambucil (Leukeran)	14–16 mg/m² daily × 5 d PO q 21–28 d, or 0.1–0.2 mg/kg daily for 4–6 wk
Cyclophosphamide (Cytoxan)	500–1000 mg/m² IV q 21–28 d, or 60–100 mg/m² PO q d
Combination	
CVP (21-day cycle)	
Cyclophosphamide	400 mg/m² daily PO d 1–5
Vincristine (Oncovin)	1.4 mg/m² IV d 1
Prednisone	100 mg/m² daily PO d 1–5
CHOP (21-day cycle)	
Cyclophosphamide	750 mg/m² IV d 1
Doxorubicin* (Adriamycin)	50 mg/m² IV d 1 or infused over 72 h
Vincristine	1.4 mg/m² IV d 1
Prednisone	100 mg/m² daily PO d 1–5
Purine Analogues	
Fludarabine (Fludara) (4-week cycle)	25 mg/m² daily IV d 1–5
Cladribine† (Leustatin)	0.14 mg/kg daily IV d 1–5

*Formerly hydroxydaunomycin.
†Cladribine is 2-chlorodeoxyadenosine (2-CDA).

considered the chemosensitivity of the disease and the poor long-term outlook as justification for investigational strategies.

Watchful waiting has not been shown to compromise overall survival in the limited studies available; however, disease-free survival rates are clearly much higher in patients who receive treatment, so that consequent quality of life may be improved. Minimally toxic therapy, once considered the standard approach, consists of administration of a single alkylating agent (chlorambucil [Leukeran] or cyclophosphamide) in varying schedules (see Table 5). Such conservative strategies are still useful in specific clinical situations, particularly in elderly patients. More aggressive approaches to therapy began with simple combinations of chemotherapy. The cyclophosphamide-vincristine-prednisone (CVP) regimen (see Table 5) has not been convincingly demonstrated to be superior to single agents. However, the additional use of doxorubicin as in the CHOP or CHOP plus bleomycin (CHOP-Bleo) regimen (Table 6) is associated with more rapid responses, but whether it leads to superior survival remains controversial. Relapse rates remain very high, however, and treatment intensification has been tested in an attempt to improve the continuous remission rate. We have used alternating regimens of aggressive non–cross-resistant chemotherapy and observed a very high remission rate; in many cases, this was confirmed even at the molecular level. The durability of the remissions appears better, but results of longer follow-up studies are awaited.

High-dose chemotherapy (HDCT) with autologous bone marrow or peripheral blood stem cell (PBSC) rescue is increasingly utilized as a therapeutic option in the treatment of indolent lymphomas. Data supporting this approach are gradually accumulating. The optimal timing for a potentially toxic therapy is a difficult issue in disorders with a long natural history. The inevitability of relapse and emergence of chemoresistance have encouraged its use earlier in the course of the disease. HDCT in first relapse or even in first remission in young patients or those with poor prognostic features is being studied extensively. Several high-dose regimens are in common use such as BEAM, which employs carmustine (BCNU [bis-chloroethyl-nitroso-urea]), etoposide (VePesid), cytarabine (Cytosar-U), and melphalan (Alkeran). One of the factors complicating the use of autologous PBSC rescue in the indolent lymphomas is the high frequency of bone marrow involvement with disease. Attempts to purge contaminating lymphoma cells from the stem cell harvest using monoclonal antibodies to remove B cells or to positively select stem cells have been successful in some studies.

Interferon-α has also found a role in the treatment of indolent lymphomas. Several studies since the early work at M. D. Anderson Cancer Center have confirmed the efficacy of interferon in prolonging remission duration when used in the minimal residual disease setting after initial chemotherapy. Interferon has also been shown to improve remission duration when used concurrently with initial chemotherapy and may have a favorable effect on overall survival in this setting.

Alternative chemotherapy agents have been studied. The most successful among these are the purine analogues fludarabine (Fludara)* and 2-chlorodeoxyadenosine (cladribine [Leustatin*]) (See Table 5). At the M. D. Anderson Cancer Center, after demonstrating initial single-agent activity, we studied fludarabine in combination with mitoxantrone (Novantrone)* and dexamethasone (Decadron), with excellent response rates in patients with recurrent disease. Other new approaches being investigated follow exciting developments in the immunotherapy field. Humanized monoclonal antibodies to CD20, which target B cells, have been used alone and in combination with CHOP chemotherapy. Early results indicate that the antibodies have activity in approximately 50% of patients with recurrent indolent lymphoma, with responses lasting a median of 12 months. Additional studies with murine monoclonal antibodies conjugated to toxins or radionuclides are ongoing and show early promising results. Finally, the explosive developments in dendritic cell immunotherapy in many areas of cancer medicine are also being applied to the treatment of indolent lymphomas.

Salvage therapies for relapsed indolent lymphoma include several options already discussed, including HDCT with autologous PBSC rescue, allogeneic bone marrow transplant in young patients with a matched

*Not FDA approved for this indication.

TABLE 6. **Chemotherapy for Aggressive Lymphomas**

Regimen	Dose
First-Generation	
CHOP	
Cyclophosphamide (Cytoxan)	750 mg/m² IV d 1
Doxorubicin (Adriamycin)	50 mg/m² IV d 1 or infused over 72 h
Vincristine (Oncovin)	1.4 mg/m² IV d 1
Prednisone	100 mg/m² daily PO d 1–5
CHOP-Bleo (CHOP plus bleomycin)	
Bleomycin (Blenoxane)	10 U/m² IV d 1
Second-Generation	
M-BACOD (21-day cycle)	
Bleomycin	4 U/m² IV d 1
Doxorubicin	45 mg/m² IV d 1
Cyclophosphamide	600 mg/m² IV d 1
Vincristine	1 mg/m² d 1
Dexamethasone (Decadron)	6 mg/m² daily PO d 1–5
Methotrexate	3 gm/m² IV d 14
Leucovorin (rescue agent)	10 mg/m² IV 24 h after methotrexate infusion, then 10 mg/m² PO q 6 h for 72 h
Third-Generation	
MACOP-B	
Methotrexate	400 mg/m² IV wk 2, 6, and 10
Leucovorin	15 mg PO q 6 h × 6 doses commencing 24 h after start of methotrexate
Doxorubicin	50 mg/m² IV wk 1, 3, 5, 7, 9, 11
Cyclophosphamide	350 mg/m² IV wk 1, 3, 5, 7, 9, 11
Vincristine	1.4 mg/m² IV wk 2, 4, 6, 8, 10, 12
Prednisone	75 mg/m² daily PO, taper wk 11 and 12
Bleomycin	10 U/m² IV wk 4, 8, 12
Alternating Triple Therapy (ATT)	
ASHAP (IdSHAP)*	
Doxorubicin	50 mg/m² over 48 h
Methylprednisolone (Solu-Medrol)	500 mg daily IV d 1–5
Cytarabine [ara-C†] (Cytosar-U)	1.5 gm/m² over 2 h after cisplatin d 5
Cisplatin (Platinol)	100 mg/m² over 96 h (25 mg/m² daily)
M-BACOS (M-BIdCOS)*	
Methotrexate	1 gm/m² IV d 2
Leucovorin (rescue agent)	15 mg PO q 6 h × 8 doses starting 24 h after start of methotrexate
Bleomycin	10 U/m² d 1
Doxorubicin	50 mg/m² over 48 h
Cyclophosphamide	750 mg/m² IV d 1
Vincristine	1.4 mg/m² IV d 1
Methylprednisolone	500 mg daily IV d 1–3
MINE	
Mesna (Mesnex)	500 mg/m² daily PO d 1–3 plus 1.5 gm/m² daily IV d 1–3
Ifosfamide (Ifex)	1.5 gm/m² daily d 1–3
Mitoxantrone (Novantrone)	10 mg/m² IV d 1
Etoposide (VePesid)	80 mg/m² daily IV d 1–3
Salvage Regimen	
ESHAP	
Etoposide	40 mg/m² daily IV d 1–3
Solu-Medrol	500 mg daily IV d 1–5
Cytarabine	2.0 gm/m² IV d 5
Cisplatin	100 mg/m² IV over 96 h (25 mg/m² daily)

*Idarubicin (Idamycin) is substituted for doxorubicin in the alternatives IdSHAP and M-BIdCOS.
†Ara-C is cytosine arabinoside (cytarabine).

sibling donor, monoclonal anti-CD20 antibodies, purine analogue–based therapy, or other active chemotherapy regimens including cytarabine and cisplatin (Platinol)* combinations.

Aggressive Lymphomas

The aggressive lymphomas include the following entities identified in the REAL classification: diffuse large B cell lymphoma (diffuse large cell lymphoma and immunoblastic lymphoma in the WF), primary mediastinal large B cell lymphoma, anaplastic large B cell lymphoma, anaplastic large cell lymphoma of T cell and null cell types, and peripheral T cell lymphoma. The cornerstone of treatment for essentially all patients with aggressive NHL is initial combination chemotherapy. Several principles have been established. First, chemotherapy is administered with curative intent in all cases, and the regimen must therefore achieve a high rate of complete response (CR). Second, dose intensity is very important for the attainment of durable CRs; thus, drugs must be delivered in full therapeutic doses without treatment delays, particularly in patients up to 60 years of age. Third, toxicities must be predicted and precautions taken to reduce these wherever possible.

Management of Localized Disease

Early-stage disease is less uncommon than in indolent lymphoma, accounting for approximately 40% of patients. Previous recommendations for radiation therapy alone in this group have gradually been abandoned. The best long-term disease-free survival rates of 70% or more with radiation therapy alone were originally attained in patients who had laparotomy-proven stage I disease. The unacceptably low survival rate of 30% or less for stage II patients treated with radiation therapy alone indicated their need for systemic chemotherapy. The morbidity associated with laparotomy staging can no longer be justified for this group of patients, however, and thus systemic chemotherapy has been used for all stage I and stage II patients. An update on the British experience has rekindled some interest in the use of radiotherapy alone for highly selected patients: An 80% 10-year survival rate was reported in younger patients with favorable prognostic features such as low bulk, early stage disease.

Chemotherapy has been combined with radiotherapy in a variety of ways, with excellent survival rates of greater than 80% in most series. Short-course combination chemotherapy (e.g., three courses of CHOP) followed by IF radiotherapy is currently the most widely used approach. This strategy proved superior in terms of overall survival to a full course of chemotherapy alone (eight courses of CHOP) in a recent randomized study. It is important to recognize, however, that patients with limited-stage disease but unfavorable associated prognostic features, such as raised serum lactate dehydrogenase levels or beta-2M fraction or large tumor bulk, will not share the same favorable outlook and must be considered for more aggressive therapy.

Management of Disseminated Disease

Front-line therapy for all advanced-stage patients consists of multiagent chemotherapy. Regimens in common use are outlined in Table 6. Still considered standard among these is the original CHOP regimen introduced more than 20 years ago. The subsequent second- and third-generation regimens were the fruit of attempts to improve on CHOP by incorporating additional active agents and intensifying dosing schedules. Early single-institution data yielded greatly improved CR rates (70 to 80%) and survival rates (50 to 60%) over those (58% and 30%, respectively) that CHOP had been shown to achieve. Disappointment was great, therefore, when more definitive randomized studies directly comparing CHOP with other regimens failed to detect any advantages in terms of CR rates or overall survival. Small differences have been reported with longer follow-up periods in specific patient subsets in a small number of studies; however, the great hopes for the more toxic regimens have not been realized.

Current investigation is focused less on new regimen design and more on dose intensification principles and patient stratification according to prognosis prediction. Our current studies utilize the Tumor Score System to select patients with poor-risk disease for intensive alternating triple therapy (ATT) with non–cross-resistant regimens. As outlined in Table 6, ATT consists of a course of doxorubicin, methylprednisolone (Solu-Medrol), cytarabine, and cisplatin, or ASHAP; followed by a course of methotrexate with leucovorin rescue, bleomycin (Blenoxane), doxorubicin, cyclophosphamide, vincristine, and methylprednisolone, or M-BACOS; followed by consolidation with mesna (Mesnex), ifosfamide (Ifox), mitoxantrone (Novantrone), and etoposide, or MINE. In alternatives to the ASHAP and M-BACOS regimens, IdSHAP and M-BIdCOS, respectively, idarubicin (Idamycin)* is substituted for doxorubicin. An integral part of this approach is thorough restaging to identify patients with residual active disease after four courses, who are then directed to investigational approaches incorporating HDCT and autologous PBSC rescue. The ATT regimen based on doxorubicin appears better than other regimens tested in patients younger than 61 years who have poor prognostic features (i.e., a tumor score of 3 or higher). On the other hand, the idarubicin-based ATT regimen has less toxicity than its doxorubicin-based counterpart, and for that reason the survival was better with regimens incorporating idarubicin when used in patients older than 60 years of age with poor prognostic features.

The role of high-dose therapy with stem cell rescue has been clearly established in recurrent aggressive NHL, where it is the treatment of choice in chemotherapy-sensitive relapse. Its position earlier in therapy remains less well defined. Two studies investi-

---

*Not FDA approved for this indication.

*Not FDA approved for this indication.

gating its usefulness as a consolidative procedure in patients with high-risk disease have yielded conflicting results. In two further studies it has failed to show a convincing impact on outcome when compared with further conventional chemotherapy in patients who have not achieved complete remission after initial response evaluation during standard front-line treatment. Thus, HDCT and autologous PBSC rescue should still be considered investigational in the front-line setting.

Salvage chemotherapy regimens for relapsed patients utilize additional active agents that have not been used in the front-line combination. Cytarabine-based and cisplatin-based combinations (e.g., ESHAP; see Table 6) are effective in patients who have received initial CHOP therapy. In those with responsive disease who are eligible, HDCT with autologous PBSC rescue improves survival over that achieved with standard chemotherapy alone. Paclitaxel (Taxol)* is a newer agent with modest activity in relapsed aggressive NHL.

Mantle cell lymphoma is now recognized as a distinct entity with very poor prognosis. Categorized histologically in the WF most often with the low-grade lymphomas, it has a vastly different median survival of 36 months or less, with only 8% of patients alive at 10 years. Standard therapies have not demonstrated any significant cure fraction among this group of patients, and thus investigation of more aggressive therapy is under way. HDCT with PBSC rescue is being explored in some centers. At M. D. Anderson Cancer Center, an intensive protocol incorporating cyclophosphamide, mesna, vincristine, doxorubicin, dexamethasone (Decadron), methotrexate, cytarabine, and granulocyte colony–stimulating factor (G-CSF—filgrastim [Neupogen]), termed HyperCVAD (Table 7), is being tested, with very encouraging early results.

Highly Aggressive Lymphomas

Highly aggressive lymphomas include Burkitt's lymphoma, Burkitt's-like lymphoma, and lymphoblastic lymphoma. Burkitt's lymphoma occurs in endemic (African—Epstein-Barr virus–associated) and sporadic forms. It is more common in children and in AIDS patients and is characterized molecularly by a unique translocation between chromosomes 8 and 14. Burkitt's lymphoma is among the most rapidly growing of all neoplasms, with very high S-phase fractions, rendering it exquisitely sensitive to chemotherapy. Consequently, tumor lysis syndrome not infrequently complicates initial management. Hydration, urinary alkalinization, allopurinol (Zyloprim) therapy, and careful monitoring are all integral to managing highly aggressive lymphomas.

Diagnosis and staging may need to be curtailed if a medical emergency supervenes demanding urgent definitive therapy. The highly aggressive lymphomas are also associated with a high propensity for CNS involvement. Cerebrospinal fluid (CSF) must be ex-

TABLE 7. Chemotherapy for Highly Aggressive Lymphomas

Regimen	Dose
HyperCVAD	
Cyclophosphamide (Cytoxan)	300 mg/m² IV q 12 h d 1–3 (6 doses)
Mesna (Mesnex)	450 mg/m² IV at 1 h pre-cyclophosphamide d 1–3 and d 4
Vincristine (Oncovin)	2 mg IV d 4 and d 11
Doxorubicin (Adriamycin)	50 mg/m² IV d 4
Dexamethasone (Decadron)	40 mg IV or PO d 1–4 and d 11–14
Methotrexate	12 mg intrathecally d 2
Cytarabine (Cytosar-U)	100 mg intrathecally d 7
G-CSF (filgrastim [Neupogen])	5 µg/kg SC d 5 until white cell recovery
Alternatives with HiDAC/MTX	
Methotrexate	200 mg/m² IV over 2 h d 1, then 800 mg/m² IV over 22 h d 1
Leucovorin (rescue agent)	60 mg IV or PO 12 h after methotrexate infusion completed, then 15 mg q 6 h × 8 doses
Cytarabine	3 gm/m² IV q 12 h × 4 doses d 2–3
G-CSF	5 µg/kg SC d 4 until white cell recovery

Intrathecal therapy as for HyperCVAD in high-risk cases

Abbreviations: ara-C = cytosine arabinoside; G-CSF = granulocyte colony–stimulating factor; HiDAC = high-dose ara-C; MTX = methotrexate.

amined before therapy and CNS prophylaxis incorporated into the treatment protocol. Staging systems in use for Burkitt's lymphoma differ from the Ann Arbor system. The Ziegler and St. Jude's systems are commonly used. These emphasize the importance of abdominal disease and bone marrow involvement as poor prognostic features.

Intensive multiagent chemotherapy is the only curative approach to nonendemic Burkitt's lymphoma. Much progress has been made in recent years with regard to outcome for patients with this disease. The pediatric experience has led the way, with cures in more than 80% of patients now reported in this previously fatal disorder. Therapeutic principles for Burkitt's lymphoma have largely been borrowed from acute lymphoblastic leukemia (ALL) treatments, with current emphasis on brief but very intense chemotherapy supported by administration of growth factors. Therapy is tailored according to individual risk assessment, with the use of alternating non–cross-resistant regimens in the highest risk groups. The most encouraging results to date have come from the National Cancer Institute studies of the CODOX-M protocol, which utilizes cyclophosphamide, vincristine, doxorubicin, and methotrexate, alternating with non–cross-resistant drugs (ifosfamide,* etoposide,* and high-dose cytarabine*), in high-risk patients. The 2-year event-free survival rate has been reported at 92%. At M. D. Anderson Cancer Center we have

---

*Not FDA approved for this indication.

*Not FDA approved for this indication.

used the HyperCVAD protocol (See Table 7), originally developed for the treatment of ALL, which utilizes the principle of hyperfractionated delivery of cyclophosphamide to overcome the very rapid cycling of tumor cells. Results are very favorable to date.

Lymphoblastic lymphoma is another rare subtype, accounting for only 5% of adult cases of lymphoma. This is usually a T cell disorder, and patients frequently present with a large mediastinal mass. It is generally considered indistinguishable from T cell ALL, and treatment principles are the same. Thus, identical or similar regimens to those used in Burkitt's lymphoma are employed (HyperCVAD at M. D. Anderson Cancer Center). Cure rates are variable, with approximately 50% of adult patients cured overall. As with the other diseases in this category, the highest risk patients fare less well, and adults invariably have inferior outcomes compared with children.

There is no well-established role for HDCT with autologous bone marrow or PBSC rescue as part of initial therapy. The superior cure rates observed with the newer treatment regimens have not been improved upon by this approach, although it is still being investigated in the highest risk patient groups.

AIDS-Related Lymphoma

AIDS-related lymphoma (ARL) is worthy of separate discussion, because NHL occurring in the setting of human immunodeficiency virus (HIV) infection manifests differences in both natural history and therapeutic outcome. The probability of the development of NHL in AIDS patients is clearly higher than in the general population. The distribution of histologic subtypes differs from that in the non-AIDS population and appears to vary with stage of HIV-related disease. Almost 75% of tumors are aggressive or highly aggressive tumors of diffuse large B cell or Burkitt's types. Widely disseminated extranodal disease is present in most patients at presentation.

Chemotherapy for patients with ARL is often compromised by poor bone marrow reserve exacerbated by antiretroviral therapy and by the development of intercurrent opportunistic infections. Consequently, the high CR rates as expected in the nonimmunocompromised population are diminished significantly. The CD4+ count, pre-existing opportunistic infections, and performance status all are important prognostic indicators. Overall median survival has been reported at less than 6 months. Attempts to improve therapeutic outcomes have used lower doses of standard regimens and hematopoietic growth factors. Reduced-dose M-BACOD (see Table 6) was tried with no reduction in median survival but less toxicity. This approach has been validated in a randomized study comparing full-dose and reduced-dose therapies, with improved outcome in the reduced-dose cohort. Growth factors to reduce the incidence of febrile neutropenic episodes, prophylaxis against *Pneumocystis* pneumonia, and concurrent antiretroviral therapy all are important aspects of treatment.

At M. D. Anderson Cancer Center, our own approach has been to utilize a novel, minimally myelosuppressive regimen for patients with CD4+ counts of less than 200 mm³. This incorporates continuous-infusion 5-fluorouracil (5-FU), leucovorin, and cisplatin with provision for use of G-CSF. For patients whose CD4+ counts are higher than 200 mm³ and who have no prior history of opportunistic infections, standard-intensity regimens are used. Patients with localized nonbulky disease and histologic subtype other than Burkitt's lymphoma are given abbreviated chemotherapy (three courses of CHOP-Bleo) and local radiotherapy.

Primary CNS lymphoma accounts for 17 to 42% of cases of lymphoma in AIDS patients but only 1 to 2% in nonimmunocompromised patients. The majority of patients have low CD4+ counts and prior AIDS-defining opportunistic infections. The diagnosis should be confirmed by brain biopsy, particularly important in distinguishing lymphoma from toxoplasmosis, which may have an identical appearance on CT scan. The lesions are usually multifocal and often disseminate to the CSF, and the prognosis is poor. Standard therapy has been with whole-brain irradiation and steroids. This has improved median survival from 42 days in untreated cases to 136 days in one series. Chemotherapy has proved extremely difficult to deliver effectively to this group of patients, and no consistently good results have been achieved. Chemotherapy may benefit those patients in the better prognostic categories with greater tolerance to toxicity. Non–HIV-positive patients with primary CNS lymphoma have been given cytarabine-* and methotrexate-based chemotherapy in combination with brain irradiation, with a better although still poor median survival of approximately 18 months.

Gastrointestinal Lymphoma

As many as 25% of NHLs are extranodal in origin. The most common site for extranodal lymphoma is the gastrointestinal (GI) tract, accounting for 30 to 40%, and the majority of these are gastric (in the Western world). The histologic subtype varies, ranging from indolent MALT lymphomas to the more common aggressive lymphomas, most of which are diffuse large B cell in type. Diagnostic material is usually obtained at endoscopic biopsy, and the remaining staging work-up should proceed along standard lines.

Optimal management of aggressive GI lymphoma remains an equivocal issue with an absence of randomized trial evidence. In gastric lymphoma, the relative roles of surgery and chemotherapy have altered over time. Historically, surgery was the mainstay of treatment; however, its role more recently has been re-evaluated. For locally advanced or disseminated disease, when surgical resection is not possible or very difficult, combination chemotherapy is the treatment of choice. Response rates in patients with advanced gastric lymphoma are comparable with those

---

*Not FDA approved for this indication.

in patients with advanced nodal disease, with a survival rate of approximately 40%. The regimens used are the same as for nodal aggressive lymphoma. For localized gastric lymphoma, curability with surgery alone has been well established; however, even partial gastrectomy remains a procedure with considerable attendant morbidity, and alternative nonsurgical management has therefore been advocated.

This approach has been validated by the observation that the majority of recurrences after surgery are at distant sites, suggesting that local treatment may not be sufficient. Extensive experience with stomach conservation and front-line chemotherapy has now accrued at M. D. Anderson Cancer Center and elsewhere, with very favorable outcomes, and this is our recommended approach. Few patients require subsequent surgical intervention, and perforation has been an uncommon complication. Survival rates upwards of 70% can be expected in stage I patients. Radiotherapy was traditionally used as an adjuvant to surgery in patients with early-stage disease. It has not been shown definitively to improve outcome in patients who have received chemotherapy but is a useful modality in patients unable to tolerate chemotherapy or as an adjunct in bulky disease. It can also be used to complement a brief chemotherapy protocol (three courses of CHOP) in very limited and localized disease.

The indolent MALT lymphomas are characterized by a long natural history and prolonged confinement to the site of origin. Local surgical treatment has been used with excellent results; however, there is increasing evidence that surgery may not be necessary. A strong association between the presence of *Helicobacter pylori* and the development of gastric MALT lymphoma has been shown. Eradication of the organism with appropriate antibiotic therapy has been associated with regression of MALT lymphomas, both histologically and on molecular studies, in more than half the patients. In view of the long natural history and feasibility of close endoscopic monitoring, this is now considered appropriate initial treatment. In the majority of patients, this approach will avert the need for surgical intervention. Current studies are exploring the combination of *H. pylori* eradication and chlorambucil therapy in an attempt to improve regression rates.

MULTIPLE MYELOMA

method of
DANIEL E. BERGSAGEL, C.M., M.D., D.Phil.
Princess Margaret Hospital / Ontario Cancer Institute and University of Toronto
Toronto, Ontario, Canada

Multiple myeloma is initiated by the malignant transformation of a B lymphocyte that has differentiated to the stage that it is committed to the production of a unique immunoglobulin. The neoplastic clone resulting from the proliferation of this B lymphocyte grows in the marrow and must increase to approximately 5×10^9 cells before it produces enough of the monoclonal protein (M-protein) to be recognized as an M-spike in a serum protein electrophoresis pattern (SPEP). A screening study detected an M-protein by paper SPEP in 1% of normal Swedes older than 25 years of age; the incidence increases markedly with age to 19% in nonagenarians. Most patients with a serum or urinary M-protein are asymptomatic. If there are no bone lesions, and marrow plasmacytosis is less than 10%, patients with an M-protein have a monoclonal gammopathy of undetermined significance (MGUS); annually, 1 to 2% of these people progress to symptoms and signs of a plasma cell neoplasm. Without treatment, most remain stable and asymptomatic. An investigation of an unexplained elevation of the erythrocyte sedimentation rate or of rouleaux on a blood film should include SPEP, which reveals the M-protein. In patients with MGUS who progress to multiple myeloma, the expanding plasma cell mass produces osteoclast-activating cytokines, leading to bone destruction, either as discrete lytic lesions or diffuse osteoporosis, with bone pain or fractures. Anemia, hypercalcemia, and renal failure develop in many patients with myeloma. In North America, the annual incidence of myeloma is 4 to 5 per 100,000 in whites, at least twice this in African-Americans, and only 1 to 2 per 100,000 in populations of Chinese or Japanese origin. The median age at diagnosis is 72 years; only 3% are younger than 40 years. In the United States, myeloma accounts for 1% of all cancers, and slightly more than 10% of the hematologic malignancies.

Weakness, fatigue, bone pain, recurrent infections, or symptoms of hypercalcemia (anorexia, nausea, vomiting, thirst, polyuria, confusion, and constipation) suggest the possibility of myeloma. Conventional radiographs are best for detecting the typical "punched-out" lytic lesions, fractures, osteoporosis, and vertebral collapse that are present at diagnosis in 75% of patients. At diagnosis, two thirds of patients are anemic, 99% have an M-protein in the serum or urine, serum calcium is elevated in 20%, and the serum creatinine is greater than 2 mg per dL in 20%.

DIAGNOSIS

The tests shown in Table 1 are used in the evaluation of a patient with an M-protein. In addition to more than 10% marrow plasma cells, at least one of the following is required to confirm a diagnosis of multiple myeloma: (1) a serum M-protein, (2) a urine M-protein, or (3) lytic bone lesions. A soft tissue biopsy of a mass (or lymph node) demonstrating a monoclonal plasmacytosis confirms the diagnosis of an extramedullary plasmacytoma. It is very important to differentiate asymptomatic patients with MGUS or smoldering myeloma from active myeloma. If the indications for treatment are not clear at the completion of the initial evaluation, the clinician should pause and follow the patient with repeat SPEP and urine protein electrophoresis at 1- to 2-month intervals to ensure that the M-protein is stable. Treatment should not be started unless there is a progressive increase in the serum or urinary M-protein or other significant manifestations of disease progression, including weight loss, bone pain, anemia, or renal failure.

TREATMENT OF SYMPTOMATIC MYELOMA

The first responsibility of a physician is to the patient; we are duty-bound to answer their questions

TABLE 1. The Evaluation of a Patient with an M-Protein

1. Measure the M-protein:
   a. Serum M-proteins are best measured (gm/L) by serum protein electrophoresis.
   b. Urine M-protein—measure the total protein excreted in a 24-hour urine collection (gm/24 h), then determine the light chain fraction by electrophoresis of concentrated urine (UPEP) and calculate the gm/24 h of M-protein.
2. Identify the light and heavy chain of the M-protein by immunoelectrophoresis or immunofixation.
3. Do not bother with specific immunoglobulin assays for IgG, IgA, or IgM. Serum protein electrophoresis provides more useful information.
4. Measure the hemoglobin, leukocyte, platelet, differential, and reticulocyte counts.
5. Determine the percentage of marrow plasma cells.
6. Take needle aspirates of a solitary lytic bone lesion, extramedullary tumors, or enlarged lymph nodes to determine if these are plasmacytomas.
7. Evaluate renal function with serum creatinine. UPEP differentiates between proteinurea resulting from *glomerular* lesions (the urine contains an unselected mixture of all serum proteins) and *tubular* lesions (the urine protein consists of light chains, which cannot be reabsorbed by damaged tubular cells, and albumin).
8. Measure serum levels of calcium, alkaline phosphatase, lactate dehydrogenase, and, when indicated by clinical findings, cryoglobulins and serum viscosity.
9. Obtain radiographs of the skull, ribs, spine, pelvis, shoulder girdle, arms, and legs.
10. Perform magnetic resonance imaging if a paraspinal mass is detected or symptoms suggest spinal cord or nerve root compression.
11. If amyloidosis is suspected, examination of a needle aspiration of abdominal fat is the easiest and safest way to confirm the diagnosis.
12. Measure serum albumin and beta$_2$-microglobulin as useful, independent prognostic factors.
13. If available, the plasma cell labeling index and serum soluble interleukin-6 receptor are also useful prognostic factors.

Abbreviation: UPEP = urine protein electrophoresis.

and to determine which treatment choice they favor. Most patients are frightened and depressed. They do not know much about the disease and they do not know how it is going to affect their lives or what the treatment options are. Education helps to relieve their anxiety. Learning about the disease is an ongoing process as the patient gathers information from his or her physician, friends, other patients, reference books, libraries, the internet, and support groups like the International Myeloma Foundation.

Physicians can make every patient with myeloma feel better and can prolong the lives of most. Cures are rare, but because myeloma is a disease of the elderly, many patients die from other causes with the myeloma still under good control. The key decision with asymptomatic patients is to determine whether they require any treatment. Starting treatment early does not benefit asymptomatic patients, and patients with stable myeloma can remain asymptomatic for many years.

General Measures

Bone pain is a major problem for most patients by the time they come to medical attention. This pain must be controlled as quickly as possible so that the patient can be ambulated. Chemotherapy is more effective than radiation in relieving the acute spasms of back pain precipitated by a sneeze or attempting to get out of bed. This type of pain is often associated with diffuse osteoporosis. This treatment must be supplemented with effective analgesics to control the frightening spasms of back pain and allow the patient to relax and rest. Patients should be gradually ambulated as soon as a measure of pain relief has been achieved. All patients should be encouraged to take long walks, and to be as active as possible so that continued demineralization of the skeleton does not occur. Lumbar corsets can improve back pain by preventing rapid rotational movements that may precipitate microfractures that cause the back pain and muscle spasms. Radiation therapy in a dose of 20 to 30 Gy is better for treating *localized* lytic lesions.

Patients should be encouraged to increase their fluid intake to 3000 mL per day to maintain the increased urine output required for the excretion of light chains, calcium, uric acid, urea, and other metabolites. A fever should be treated as an emergency, with appropriate investigations and antibiotics.

Treatment Plan

Patients and their families must be consulted carefully in the development of a treatment plan for a chronic disease for which there is no known cure. Treatment options range from high-dose chemotherapy with hematopoietic rescue by allogeneic or autologous hematopoietic stem cell (HSC) transplantation, conventional chemotherapy (CC), and localized radiation therapy. Some patients (especially patients 65 years of age or younger) are anxious to have aggressive, experimental treatment, such as high-dose chemotherapy followed by autologous HSC transplantation. Patients like this are risk-takers; they want to "beat the disease." At the other extreme are those who do not want the disease or its treatment to interfere with what is left of their lives. The less time they have to spend with doctors, the better. These patients are adverse to risk; they want to receive appropriate, but not extreme, therapy. The treating physician must adjust the treatment plan to fit the patient.

High-Dose Chemotherapy with Autologous Hematopoietic Stem Cell Transplantation

This form of treatment is best reserved for patients 60 years of age or younger who have responded to remission-induction chemotherapy, or at least achieved disease stabilization. Alkylating agents such as melphalan (Alkeran) should not be used for remission-induction because these drugs may damage HSCs and reduce the chance of harvesting enough of these cells for a successful transplant. The usual remission-induction is with three courses of VAD: vincristine (Oncovin) 0.4 mg per m² per day and doxorubicin (Adriamycin), 9 mg per m² per day by continuous intravenous infusion for 4 days, plus dexamethasone (Decadron), 40 mg each morning for 4 days (days 1 to 4, 9 to 12, and 17 to 21) of each 28-day cycle. HSCs are harvested by leukapheresis from the blood of responding patients; these cells are frozen and stored in liquid nitrogen. The HSCs are reinfused to promote hematopoietic recovery after high-dose melphalan plus cyclophosphamide (Cytoxan) and busulphan (Myleran), or total-body radiation. The mortality rate secondary to the toxicity of this treatment is less than 5%. A randomized comparison of CC with high-dose chemotherapy (HDC) and autologous HSC rescue in patients aged 65 years or younger has shown that HDC induced more complete responses and improved progression-free survival. The overall survival rates of patients treated with CC and HDC are similar during the first 30 months. Thereafter, HDC patients survive better, with 52% alive at 5 years versus 12% for CC patients. Patients 60 years of age or younger benefited more from HDC than those aged 61 to 65 years. HDC patients continue to relapse at a constant rate, indicating that this treatment is not curative.

High-Dose Chemotherapy with Allogeneic Hematopoietic Stem Cell Transplantation

Hematopoietic stem cells obtained from another person with a closely matched tissue type are used to regenerate the marrow in an allogeneic HSC transplantation. The donor is usually a sibling who fully matches the HLA type of the patient. The transplantation-related mortality rate associated with allogeneic HSC transplantation is unacceptably high. However, trials of this form of treatment have shown that in some patients, grafted lymphocytes can mount a strong graft-versus-myeloma reaction, capable of controlling the disease. Many investigators are looking for safer methods of using the graft-versus-myeloma therapeutic potential of donor lymphocytes.

Conventional Chemotherapy

Conventional chemotherapy is indicated as primary therapy for most patients older than 60 years of age, and also for many younger patients with poor prognostic features such as a markedly elevated serum beta₂-microglobulin, other serious illnesses, or an aversion to aggressive therapy. Melphalan and prednisone are the drugs of choice as the initial form of treatment. I start with a melphalan (Alkeran) dose of 9 mg per m² (0.25 mg per kg) before breakfast daily for 4 days every 4 to 6 weeks, along with 100 mg of prednisone in 1 dose with breakfast for 4 days. The melphalan should be administered in 1 dose 1 hour before breakfast, on an empty stomach (giving melphalan with food greatly reduces the absorption of this drug). Blood counts should be repeated weekly. When an effective dose has been administered, the leukocyte and platelet counts fall to a nadir at ap-

proximately 3 weeks, with recovery by the fourth to sixth week. If a significant fall in leukocytes or platelets is not observed, the next course of melphalan should be increased by 2 mg per day. If necessary, melphalan should be increased by an additional 2 mg per day in subsequent courses until a transient fall in leukocytes or platelets or a definite clinical response occurs, to indicate that therapeutic amounts of melphalan have been absorbed. Most patients can tolerate repeat courses of melphalan and prednisone every 4 weeks, but marrow recovery is delayed in some. If the leukocyte or platelet count has not started to recover by the fourth week, the next course should be delayed by 1 or 2 weeks to prevent the development of cumulative hematologic toxicity. The dose of prednisone can be reduced or discontinued in patients who are bothered by the acute stimulatory effects (hyperactivity, insomnia, dyspepsia) of this hormone. I do not prescribe allopurinol (Zyloprim) with CC. An elevated serum uric acid is more likely the result of dehydration or renal failure rather than increased myeloma cell death, and is better treated with fluids. The administration of pamidronate (Aredia), 90 mg as a 4-hour intravenous (IV) infusion, once a month, reduces bone resorption and delays the progression of bone disease.

With this therapy, 46% of patients achieve a stable response, with the serum M-protein decreasing to reach a plateau (at <50% of the initial value) that is stable for at least 4 months, a greater than 90% fall in the urinary excretion of M-protein, and relief of bone pain, weight gain, and improved performance status. An additional 10% become asymptomatic but do not achieve a sufficient decrease in the M-protein to qualify as a responder, and 44% progress and require an alternate form of treatment.

Attempts to improve therapy by adding vincristine and other alkylating agents to melphalan and prednisone have failed to improve survival. There is some evidence that combining doxorubicin (Adriamycin) with alkylating agents may lead to a marginal improvement in survival.

Maintenance chemotherapy does not improve survival. My practice is to continue melphalan and prednisone as long as the M-protein level continues to fall. When the M-protein level reaches a plateau that is stable for 4 months, I discontinue melphalan and prednisone but continue to see the patient at 2-month intervals to follow the course of the response. Maintenance interferon alfa,* 3 million units subcutaneously three times a week, does prolong the duration of remission, but the effect on overall survival is minor because the interval between relapse and death is shortened. I do not recommend interferon maintenance therapy because the small effect on the course of the myeloma does not justify the considerable impact that interferon has on the patient's quality of life.

A chronologic treatment flow-chart to record the results of the tests outlined in Table 2 is essential in

---

*Not FDA approved for this indication.

TABLE 2. **Tests for Following the Response to Treatment**

1. On each visit record the date, weight, height, temperature, symptoms, signs, and the treatment prescribed.
2. Take blood counts once a week until an acceptable pattern of toxicity is established, then only before each treatment.
3. Measure the M-protein every 1 to 2 months:
    a. *Serum M-protein*—if an M-spike is visible, the M-protein is best measured by SPEP. Specific immunoglobulin assays always overestimate the M-protein because they measure a combination of normal immunoglobulin and the M-protein; furthermore, if only specific assays are followed, it is impossible to determine when the M-spike disappears. Because IF is 100 times more sensitive in detecting small amounts of M-protein, the modern definition of a CR requires that no M-protein be detected by IF. Thus, if the M-protein disappears from the SPEP, IF must be done to confirm a CR.
    b. *Urine M-protein*—measurement of the total protein excreted per 24 hours (gm/24 h) is usually sufficient, once UPEP has established that most of the urinary protein consists of monoclonal light chains. When urine protein falls below 1.0 gm/24 h, UPEP needs to be repeated to determine the amount of M-protein that is being excreted. Again, the definition of CR requires that no urinary M-protein be detected by IF.
4. Serum calcium and creatinine should be checked with a frequency determined by the clinical status; for example, check the serum calcium whenever the patient manifests nausea, vomiting, polydipsia, polyuria, constipation, somnolence, or confusion.
5. Radiographs are required to investigate new sites of bone pain. Lateral skull films are useful for deciding whether skeletal disease is healing, stable, or progressive.
6. Inspect spinal radiographs for evidence of a paraspinal mass whenever a patient complains of back pain radiating in a dermatome. Magnetic resonance imaging or a myelogram should be done to determine the location of the spinal cord or nerve root compression. Look for myeloma cells and the M-protein in the spinal fluid if myelography is done.
7. Marrow aspiration or biopsy should be done if pancytopenia develops. A hypocellular marrow suggests that the cytopenias may be the result of treatment, and further therapy should be withheld until recovery occurs. A cellular marrow, however, suggests that the cytopenias may be secondary to progressive myeloma and indicates a need for additional treatment.

Abbreviations: CR = complete response; IF = immunofixation; SPEP = serum protein electrophoresis; UPEP = urine protein electrophoresis.

monitoring the effectiveness of treatment. Patients who achieve a stable plateau in the M-protein response remain in remission for a median of 10 to 12 months after melphalan and prednisone are stopped, but some do not progress for 5 years or more. The aim of therapy is to *achieve disease stability.* The remissions are just as long in patients who achieve a stable plateau in the M-protein, without a significant decline in the serum level, as they are in those with a decrease greater than 50%. Patients must be monitored carefully so that treatment can be restarted at the first sign of relapse (usually a *progressive* increase in the serum or urinary M-protein), preferably before bone pain signals progressive disease.

The median survival of patients treated with melphalan and prednisone is approximately 30 months. Those who progress despite melphalan and prednisone induction therapy have the poorest prognosis, with a median survival of 15 months. Patients who achieve a stable response with a decrease in the M-protein level of greater than 50% have a median survival of 48 months, and those who reach a stable plateau in the M-protein level without a significant decrease in the M-protein also survive well, with a median of 49 months.

Second-Line Therapy

The prognosis is poor if the myeloma progresses during melphalan and prednisone induction therapy (primary resistance); only 10% respond to alternative therapy. If the myeloma responds initially to melphalan and prednisone and then progresses despite reinstituted melphalan and prednisone, the prognosis is better; from 25 to 30% respond to second-line therapy. If the disease progresses on melphalan and prednisone, I change to cyclophosphamide (C) 300 mg per m², orally or IV, once a week, combined with prednisone, 100 mg with breakfast, on alternate days. This treatment gives the patient the advantage of high-dose prednisone, which is well tolerated without signs of hypercorticism when administered on alternate days, as well as changing the alkylating agent to C, in a schedule that is well tolerated even by patients with pancytopenia.

Patients who progress during weekly cyclophosphamide and prednisone (CP), with severe bone disease and pain, are difficult management problems. The bone pain is best managed with irradiation; when the lesions are widespread, this may require wide-field or even half-body irradiation. VAD in the doses described previously or high-dose corticosteroids alone may be tried.

TREATMENT OF COMPLICATIONS

Hypercalcemia

Serum calcium should be measured weekly in hospitalized patients with myeloma, and on every follow-up visit, because hypercalcemia is present in 20% of patients at diagnosis and develops in an additional 30% during the course of the disease. This complication can usually be controlled in patients with myeloma by hydration (using normal saline to promote the excretion of calcium, whenever possible), prednisone (25 mg four times a day), and chemotherapy for the myeloma. Pamidronate is useful if these measures fail.

Renal Failure

Conscientious hydration by the patient (3000 mL of fluid per day) is the best way to reduce the risk of renal failure. Acute renal failure must be treated promptly with the maintenance of fluid and electrolyte balance. Plasmapheresis is more efficient than hemodialysis in clearing light chains from the plasma and reducing the risk of protein precipitating in the distal tubules. If severe renal failure is the major problem, and other manifestations of myeloma are under good control, renal transplantation has been followed by prolonged survival.

Hyperviscosity

High levels of M-protein can lead to an expanded plasma volume, which may precipitate congestive heart failure. M-proteins that form polymers can also cause hyperviscosity, manifested by headaches, epistaxis, blurred vision, neurologic symptoms, sludging of the blood (causing retinal veins to look like link sausages), and coma in extreme cases. Acute symptoms are quickly relieved by plasmapheresis, but this must be followed by chemotherapy to lower the M-protein concentration.

Anemia

Almost every myeloma patient becomes anemic eventually. Treatment with erythropoietin (Epogen) should be considered for every patient with myeloma with hemoglobin values that are chronically less than 12 grams per dL.

Spinal Cord or Nerve Root Compression

The sudden onset of severe radicular pain in the lower lumbar region is an early warning sign of spinal cord compression. The development of leg weakness, a Babinski plantar reflex, or difficulty in voiding or defecation all but confirms the diagnosis. This complication develops in approximately 10% of patients with myeloma and must be handled as an emergency if the devastating consequences of paraplegia are to be avoided. Dexamethasone, 20 mg four times a day, should be started immediately to reduce the edema and possibly shrink the plasma cell mass. Magnetic resonance imaging is the best way to determine the location of the cord compression. Radiation therapy with approximately 30 Gy should be delivered to the plasmacytoma causing the cord compression. Surgical decompression is rarely required.

Meningeal Myelomatosis

Late in the course of disease, some myeloma cells acquire the ability to grow outside of the marrow in many soft tissue sites. These myeloma stem cells circulate in the blood and can form plasma cell infiltrates anywhere they land. Growth of myeloma cells in the meninges releases the M-protein and myeloma cells into the cerebrospinal fluid, resulting in increased intracranial pressure, headaches, papilledema, and a stiff neck, as occurs with meningeal leukemia. If the site of the meningeal infiltrates can be identified, radiation therapy may be helpful. These patients are usually very ill and must be treated gently. Dexamethasone and weekly cyclophosphamide may be helpful. I never prescribe intrathecal methotrexate or arabinosyl cytosine (cytarabine), because these drugs have not been shown to be effective in the treatment of myeloma.

VARIANT FORMS OF MYELOMA

Solitary Osseous Plasmacytoma

Approximately 3% of patients with myeloma have an apparently solitary osteolytic lesion. These patients require a needle biopsy of the solitary lesion to establish the diagnosis of a plasmacytoma because marrow aspirations from other sites do not show a plasmacytosis. The solitary lytic lesion should be treated with radiation therapy, using approximately 35 Gy. Approximately one third of these patients have a serum M-protein, which should disappear completely after irradiation. Persistence of the M-protein means that myeloma cells persist, presumably outside of the irradiated area. These patients must be followed carefully; the disease eventually progresses to widespread myeloma in most.

Extramedullary Plasmacytoma

Approximately 3% of patients with plasma cell neoplasms have extramedullary plasmacytomas, usually in the nose, nasopharynx, or paranasal sinuses. Because the usual spread of these tumors is to lymph nodes, the radiation field should include the regional lymph nodes, using a dose of about 35 Gy. One third of these patients have a serum M-protein, which should disappear after irradiation. If the M-protein persists, along with residual tumor, the residual tumor should be resected. The M-protein often disappears if the tumor can be resected. Extramedullary plasmacytoma can usually be controlled with local irradiation and surgical resection. Melphalan and prednisone are useful in the management of those that are not controlled by local measures.

Osteosclerotic Myeloma (POEMS Syndrome)

Polyneuropathy, organomegaly, endocrinopathy, M-protein, and skin changes (POEMS) characterize this syndrome. The major clinical findings are a chronic demyelinating polyneuropathy with predominantly motor disability, and sclerotic bone lesions. Hepatosplenomegaly, lymphadenopathy, hyperpigmentation, hypertrichosis, gynecomastia, and testicular atrophy may occur. Radiation therapy (35 Gy) is recommended if the bone lesions are localized, but melphalan and prednisone are used for generalized disease. More than half of the patients treated with radiation or melphalan and prednisone are substantially improved, with relief of bone pain and healing of skeletal lesions. The polyneuropathy improves, with recovery of muscle strength, if the patient responds well to treatment. The overall survival of patients with myeloma with POEMS syndrome is substantially longer than for other forms of myeloma.

POLYCYTHEMIA VERA

method of
HARRIET S. GILBERT, M.D.
Albert Einstein College of Medicine
Bronx, New York

DIAGNOSIS

Polycythemia vera (PV) is a myeloproliferative disorder (MPD) in which clonal expansion of the pluripotential hematopoietic precursor cell (PHPC) with preservation of lineage commitment and differentiation results in the production of increased numbers of mature progeny of the hematic trilineage. The presence of increased erythroid proliferation with a demonstrable increase in the circulating red blood cell mass is the sine qua non of PV. However, to fulfill the criteria for PV and exclude conditions causing isolated erythrocytosis, this must be accompanied by some involvement of other hematic progeny (megakaryocytes/platelets, granulocytes, and monocytes) and/or splenomegaly due to extramedullary hematopoiesis (myeloid metaplasia [MyM]). Diagnostic criteria have changed little since they were first codified in 1967 by the Polycythemia Vera Study Group (PVSG) for purposes of conducting a randomized study. Major (A) criteria now consist of a red blood cell mass raised to greater than 25% of the mean normal predicted value, absence of a cause of secondary polycythemia, palpable splenomegaly, and a clonality marker (abnormal marrow karyotype). Minor (B) criteria are thrombocytosis to greater than 400×10^9 per liter, neutrophil leukocytosis to greater than 10×10^9 per liter, splenomegaly demonstrated by imaging techniques, and characteristic erythroid burst-forming unit (BFU-E) growth or reduced serum erythropoietin. A diagnosis of PV is established by A1 + A2 + A3, A4, or A1 + A2 + two B criteria. Before a measurement of red blood cell mass any occult bleeding or iron deficiency, or both, that might mask PV should be corrected.

COURSE AND COMPLICATIONS

Complications of PV are determined by the cell progenies involved in the proliferative process. Thrombosis is the major complication of untreated PV. This is attributable to increased proliferation of red blood cells and platelets. Erythrocythemia produces increased blood viscosity, which increases exponentially as the hematocrit exceeds 50%. Thrombocythemia is present in 30% of patients with PV at diagnosis. Platelets in MPD show increased in vivo adhesiveness and ability to aggregate. Stasis in small vessels of the digits, vestibular apparatus, and retina may be experienced as erythromelalgia, vertigo, and scotomata. Because the platelet aggregation that precipitates these episodes is reversible, these symptoms are usually transient. With more severe hyperviscosity and thrombocythemia, the arterial circulation may be involved with transient ischemic attacks, angina, or bowel ischemia. Atherosclerotic changes in the cardiovascular system of older patients increases the incidence of stroke and myocardial infarction in PV. Patients with uncontrolled PV are also prone to deep venous thrombosis of the extremities and venous thrombosis of the hepatic, portal, and splenic veins.

Abnormalities of coagulation and hemostasis have a mitigating effect on thrombotic and hemorrhagic complications of PV. Congenital hypercoagulable states, such as activated protein C resistance, or hypocoagulable states, such as acquired von Willebrand disease that occurs in thrombocythemia, can increase the likelihood of thrombosis or hemorrhage in the setting of PV and should be sought, because their presence will affect therapy.

Significant arterial or venous thrombosis occurs in one third to one half of patients with uncontrolled PV. Hemorrhage occurs in 20% of patients. Survival of patients with uncontrolled disease varies from 1.5 to 3 years after onset of the first symptoms. Phlebotomy has a significant impact on survival but does not eliminate the risk of thrombosis. The phlebotomy recipients in the PVSG had a significantly increased rate of life-threatening thrombosis in comparison with the myelosuppression recipients, especially in the first 3 years of study. The introduction of myelosuppressive therapy has had a major impact on the incidence of thrombosis and hemorrhage. However, myelosuppressive therapy with radioactive phosphorus or alkylating agents places the patient at risk for acute leukemic transformation. Patients who do not die of thrombosis or hemorrhage face complications of chronic myeloproliferative disease such as progressive myeloid metaplasia, fibrosis, bone marrow failure, and acute leukemic transformation. Proliferation of basophils and mast cells results in hyperhistaminemia with resulting pruritus, gastrointestinal symptoms of pyrrhosis, epigastic distress, diarrhea, and peptic ulcer. Clinical features of generalized bone marrow proliferation include hypermetabolism with fatigue, weight loss, and sweats. Hyperuricemia may cause gout and renal stones.

TREATMENT

PV is a hematopoietic malignancy that carries an excellent prognosis for longevity conferred by management and control of the proliferative process. Removal of the products of proliferation is feasible only for the red blood cells because of their long life span. For other types of proliferation, the therapy must be directed at the pluripotential stem cells. The history of therapy for PV has been a search for agents that have specificity for the clonally affected PHPC or for products of the proliferation. Because of the need for chronic therapy the optimal therapies should not be leukemogenic, carcinogenic, or mutagenic. The only curative therapy is bone marrow transplant, which is currently reserved for patients with aggressive disease that is not responsive to conventional therapies.

Phlebotomy

Control of the hematocrit (Hct) with phlebotomy is a mainstay of management in PV. It allows for rapid restoration and maintenance of a normal Hct once the diagnosis is made. Because it has been demonstrated that optimal cerebral circulation is attained at a Hct of 42%, the goal of phlebotomy should be a Hct of less than 45%. Phlebotomy may be performed twice weekly at the outset and reduced to 1 to 3 month intervals for maintenance. One of the objectives of phlebotomy therapy is to create iron deficiency in order to inhibit erythropoiesis. Thus, oral intake of vitamins and other supplements that contain iron must be avoided.

Phlebotomy is the management of choice in young patients, especially women in the childbearing age, who have not had a thrombotic complication and who do not have pronounced proliferative features of MPD, other than erythrocythemia, that would require treatment. The increased incidence of thrombotic complications in patients treated solely with phlebotomy may be mitigated by the addition of platelet antiaggregating agents such as low-dose aspirin. In such patients the concomitant use of nonsteroidal anti-inflammatory drugs or other platelet inhibitors is contraindicated, in order to avoid bleeding complications. Another helpful prophylactic measure in patients with increased hematopoietic cell turnover is the administration of allopurinol (Zyloprim) at a dose of 300 mg daily to avoid hyperuricemia-induced gout or renal stones. There are rare patients who have inadequate venous access or do not tolerate the hemodynamic changes or iron deficiency produced by phlebotomy. For these patients, those older than 60 years of age, and those with prior thrombotic or hemorrhagic complications, the use of myelosuppression is necessary.

MYELOSUPPRESSION AND CYTOREDUCTION

The demonstration by the PVSG of leukemogenicity and bone marrow failure as complications of long-term management of PV with radioactive phosphorus and alkylating agents was discouraging in view of the observed advantages of myelosuppressive therapy in decreasing the major complications of thrombosis and hemorrhage and prolonging survival. This led to a search for nonalkylating and nonradioactive agents that are myelosuppressive and cytoreductive. Since the 1970s, several new agents and approaches have become available; they provide flexibility in the choice of management that takes into consideration age, risk factors, and co-morbidities. In the absence of randomized, controlled studies of the newer agents, the management of PV remains controversial, but the armamentarium is expanding. The properties of current therapies are summarized in Table 1 and detailed subsequently.

Hydroxyurea

Since 1980 the myelosuppressive agent of choice has been hydroxyurea* (HU). This is a potent, nonalkylating myelosuppressive agent that inhibits cell growth by decreasing DNA synthesis through the inhibition of the enzyme ribonucleotide diphosphate reductase. It suppresses proliferation of the PHPC and causes generalized reduction in Hct, platelet count, and neutrophil count. Its effect on the PHPC is nonselective for the MPD clone, thus decreasing normal, as well as malignant stem cells. A PVSG protocol was initiated in 1977, and 51 patients who had never received prior myelosuppressive therapy were studied. A starting dose of 15 mg per kg daily was used to obtain myelosuppression. The dose was titrated to obtain optimal control of the blood count while avoiding cytopenias. Supplementary phlebotomy was employed to maintain the Hct below 45%. In this population with a median follow-up of 9.6 years and a maximum of 15.3 years, the judicious use of HU provided excellent control of the Hct and platelet count. The incidence of thrombosis was reduced significantly below that in the phlebotomy recipients in the original PVSG. Long-term safety studies showed that patients on HU fared less well than those treated with phlebotomy alone, in that the incidence of leukemic transformation was 5.9%. Other investigators have reported a leukemic transformation of 10% or higher with chronic HU therapy. In a suitable population of elderly patients with a high risk of thrombotic complications HU still offers the advantages of a well-tolerated oral agent. Side effects include rashes, oral ulcerations, nail changes, and gastrointestinal disturbances. A small number of patients have developed extremely painful and intractable leg ulcers that require withdrawal of HU to achieve healing. Patients who respond to HU require chronic administration and monitoring of the blood count every 6 weeks.

---

*Not FDA approved for this indication.

TABLE 1. **Current Therapeutic Modalities for PV**

	Hydroxyurea (Hydrea)	Interferon (Roferon-A, Intron A)	Anagrelide (Agrylin)
Route of administration	Oral	Subcutaneous	Oral
Ease of dose titration	Fair to poor	Good	Good
Duration of effect after stopping	Short with rebound	Long, no rebound	Short, no rebound
Effect on other MPD proliferation	WBC 4+	WBC 2+	None
	Hb 2+	Hb 3+	Hb ↓ by <10%
	Spleen 1+	Spleen 4+	None
Effect on MPD clone	Nonselective	Selective	None
Effect on megakaryocytes	Decreases polyclonally	Decreases monoclonally	Prevents budding
Effect on fibrosis	None	Potentially inhibits	Potentially inhibits
Side effects	1–2+	2–4+	2–3+
Cost	$1.00/cap	$8.00/MU	$6.00/cap
Use during pregnancy	No	Yes	No
Acute leukemia	5–10%	Unknown-unlikely	Unknown-unlikely

Abbreviations: Hb = hemoglobin; MPD = myeloproliferative disorder; MU = million units; PV = polycythemia vera; WBC = white blood cell.

Interferon-alfa

The success of interferon-alfa-2a and 2b* (Roferon-A, Intron A) in the management of chronic myelocytic leukemia (CML) and the demonstration of a selective effect of this agent on the malignant clone suggested that it might be efficacious in non-CML MPD. This has been demonstrated by numerous studies showing reduction of elevated Hct, platelet count, and neutrophil populations by using doses of IFN-α ranging from 3 to 5 million units (MU) daily, administered subcutaneously. Smaller starting doses may enhance tolerance as the patient develops tachyphylaxis to the flulike symptoms. Control of circulating counts occurs during the first 2 to 3 months of therapy. A unique property of IFN-α is its ability to reduce MyM and shrink the spleen and liver. This occurs after 3 months of therapy. Another unique finding is that a durable remission may be seen when IFN-α is discontinued after a 6-month to 1-year course of therapy. The duration of unmaintained response may be months to years. The best results have been seen in PV and in post-PV MyM. When relapse occurs a second or subsequent courses will reestablish remission in most cases.

The side effects of chronic IFN-α therapy, such as fatigue, anorexia, diarrhea, and neurologic symptoms, may be difficult to control and are responsible for a dropout rate of 7 to 10%. Older patients are less tolerant of IFN-α in which case lower doses must be used for longer courses.

Leukemic transformation has not appeared to be a problem, as would be expected from a naturally occurring biologic response modifier. IFN-α is not teratogenic and may be the agent of choice for young women who wish to conceive. Treatment before conception may induce a durable remission that could facilitate conception and maintain the platelet count at desired levels until the reduction in platelet count that is seen in PV during the second and third trimesters occurs, so that the pregnancy may progress without medication. If platelets increase during pregnancy, IFN-α may be introduced, inasmuch as it does not appear to harm the fetus.

Anagrelide

Anagrelide (Agrylin) is a unique agent that has been approved by the Food and Drug Administration (FDA) for the management of thrombocythemia in essential thrombocythemia (ET) and in other myeloproliferative disorders. It is a quinazoline that inhibits cyclic nucleotide phosphodiesterase. Among its actions is the ability to inhibit megakaryocyte maturation and platelet budding. This effect occurs at doses below those that inhibit platelet aggregation. At doses of 0.5 mg to 1 mg four times daily, the platelet count is reduced by 50% of baseline or to less than 600,000 per μL in 2 to 4 weeks. Response occurs in 80 to 90% of patients. Once an effective dose has

been determined, it continues to be effective without adjustment of dosage. There is no direct effect on other progeny of the PHPC except for a modest decrease in hemoglobin of less than 10% in one third of patients.

Side effects are cardiovascular, neurologic, and gastrointestinal. Anagrelide is a vasodilator, has a positive inotropic activity, and reduces renal blood flow. These actions are responsible for palpitations, forceful heartbeat, and tachycardia. One in four patients develops fluid retention or edema, or both. This may be controlled with diuretic therapy. The major neurologic side effect is headache, which responds to acetaminophen and usually subsides after 2 weeks of therapy. Dizziness is frequent but mild. Gastrointestinal effects are nausea, bloating, and diarrhea, generally mild and transient. Anagrelide is formulated with lactose and the use of a lactase supplement is effective in controlling gastrointestinal symptoms. The dropout rate due to side effects is 10 to 15% and can be minimized by judicious adjustments in dosing and symptomatic therapy of side effects.

The effect of anagrelide on the platelet count is reversible on cessation of therapy within 2 to 4 weeks. Thus, this agent must be administered on a chronic basis. It is believed to be teratogenic and should not be administered to women who are trying to conceive. During anagrelide therapy, attention must be directed at other features of MPD that will not be controlled by this drug. Supplementary phlebotomy may be required to control the Hct and IFN-α may be necessary to treat MyM. The concomitant use of anagrelide is acceptable to attain the desired platelet count and permit reduction of dosages of hydroxyurea or IFN-α to minimize their undesirable side effects.

THE PORPHYRIAS

method of
HERBERT L. BONKOVSKY, M.D., and
GRAHAM F. BARNARD, M.D., PH.D.
University of Massachusetts Memorial Health Care
Worcester, Massachusetts

The porphyrias are metabolic diseases caused by defects in normal heme synthesis (Table 1). They manifest clinically in two major ways: (1) with symptoms and signs of neurovisceral dysfunction, especially abdominal pain, constipation, and weakness; and (2) with cutaneous symptoms and signs. In two forms of porphyria, hereditary coproporphyria and variegate porphyria, patients may have both kinds of manifestations; in the other forms of porphyria, patients have only one or the other of the two cardinal manifestations of disease.

In considering therapy of the porphyrias, it is useful to classify the specific forms into two major categories: (1) the acute or inducible porphyrias, and (2) the chronic cutaneous porphyrias (see Table 1). Regardless of the specific

*Not FDA approved for this indication.

TABLE 1. **Classification and Major Features of Human Porphyrias**

Disease	Primary Enzymatic Defect	Autosomal Inheritance	Clinical Features	
			Neurovisceral Symptoms	*Photosensitivity Dermatosis*
Acute or inducible porphyrias				
ALA dehydratase deficiency porphyria	ALA dehydratase	Recessive	+	−
Acute intermittent porphyria	PBG deaminase	Dominant	+	−
Hereditary coproporphyria	Coproporphyrinogen oxidase	Dominant	+	+
Variegate porphyria	Protoporphyrinogen oxidase	Dominant	+	+
Chronic cutaneous porphyrias				
Congenital erythropoietic porphyria	Uroporphyrinogen III (co)-synthase	Recessive	−	+ +
Hepatoerythropoietic porphyria	Uroporphyrinogen decarboxylase	Recessive	−	+ +
Porphyria cutanea tarda	Uroporphyrinogen decarboxylase	Dominant or no inherited defect	−	+
Protoporphyria	Ferrochelatase	Dominant (perhaps sometimes recessive)	−*	+

*A neurovisceral syndrome reminiscent of those observed in the acute porphyrias was described in a few patients with protoporphyria and hepatic failure, around the time of orthotopic liver transplantation.

Abbreviations: ALA = 5-aminolevulinate—the first intermediate in the heme biosynthetic pathway; PBG = porphobilinogen—the second intermediate in the heme biosynthetic pathway.

form of acute porphyria or associated enzymatic defect, all of the acute porphyrias may produce similar neurovisceral manifestations and should be managed in similar ways. Although there are features peculiar to management of each type of cutaneous porphyria, there are also general principles of management for all of these disorders.

How to establish a firm diagnosis of porphyria is beyond the scope of this article. However, a correct and definitive diagnosis is of paramount importance before the initiation of therapy. Because of the complicated and unfamiliar tests often required for diagnosis, it is recommended that physicians without special training in the porphyrias discuss possible patients with, or refer patients to, physicians who have such expertise. Our experience with hundreds of referrals since the late 1960s has been that most patients thought to have acute porphyria do not; rather, they have one of the disorders that may produce secondary porphyrinuria (mainly coproporphyrin) or have totally normal porphyrin metabolism. We have also seen numerous patients who have been thought to have a cutaneous porphyria, but in whom porphyrin metabolism was normal. Of course, there are also many patients with porphyria in whom the diagnosis has been missed. References with up-do-date descriptions of how to diagnose or exclude porphyria are available.*

TREATMENT

Acute Hepatic Porphyrias

Management of Acute Attacks

Nearly always, the cardinal symptom is severe, colicky abdominal pain. Nausea, vomiting, constipa-

---

*See Bonkovsky HL, Barnard GF: Diagnosis of porphyric syndromes: A practical approach in the era of molecular biology. Semin Liver Dis *18*:57–65, 1998; Hahn M, Bonkovsky HL: Disorders of porphyrin metabolism. *In* Wu G, Israel J (eds): Diseases of the Liver and Bile Ducts: A Practical Guide to Diagnosis and Treatment. Totowa, NJ, Humana Press, 1998, pp 249–272; Bonkovsky HL, Barnard GF: The hepatic porphyrias. *In* Brandt L (ed): Clinical Practice of Gastroenterology. Philadelphia, Current Medicine, 1998, pp 947–960; and Kappas A, Sassa S, Galbraith RA, Nordmann Y: The porphyrias. *In* Scriver CR, Beaudet AL, Sly WS, Valle D (eds): The Metabolic and Molecular Bases of Inherited Disease, 7th ed. New York, McGraw-Hill, 1995, pp 2103–2160.

tion, and pain or paresthesias in the extremities are present in approximately half of patients. The most frequent signs are tachycardia and dark urine. The pathogenesis of acute porphyric attacks involves a deficiency of hepatic heme and induction of hepatic 5-aminolevulinate (ALA) synthase with resultant overproduction of ALA, which is neurotoxic. The approach to therapy is outlined in Table 2.

General measures should include parenteral administration of meperidine (Demerol), 50 to 150 mg, or morphine, 3 to 10 mg, for pain. Addition of a phenothiazine (e.g., chlorpromazine [Thorazine], 25 to 50 mg) enhances the analgesic and sedative effects of the narcotic. Propranolol (Inderal) may be given for control of severe tachycardia or arterial hypertension. The dose should be titrated carefully because serious bradycardia and hypotension may develop in some patients from propranolol. Frequent checks (every 6 hours) of neuromuscular function, looking specifically for developing weakness of crucial muscles such as the diaphragm, are important.

Specific treatment is directed at correcting the de-

TABLE 2. **Therapy of Acute Attacks of Porphyria**

Remove inciting factors: drugs, toxins, chemicals (see Table 3)
Nutritional supplementation: at least 300 gm glucose/d
Intravenous heme: 3–5 mg/kg/d for 3–5 days
Frequent checks of neurologic status: especially watch for development of paresis of muscles of respiration
Monitor for hyponatremia or hypomagnesemia and treat vigorously, if found
Parenteral meperidine (50–150 mg) or morphine (3–10 mg) for pain, every 4–6 hours
Chlorpromazine (25–50 mg every 4–6 hours) for nausea, agitation, and to enhance effects of opiates
Propranolol (10–40 mg every 6 hours) for tachycardia, hypertension
Magnesium sulfate, gabapentin, or vigabatrin* for seizures

*Not available in the United States.

ficiency of hepatic heme and decreasing activity of ALA synthase. One way to decrease ALA synthase is to administer glucose or other readily metabolized carbohydrates, taking advantage of the phenomenon of carbohydrate repression of the enzyme, the so-called glucose effect. In practice, this is accomplished by giving patients at least 300 grams per day of glucose. If patients do not have paralytic ileus or vomiting, this can be administered enterally; however, most patients who require hospitalization are too ill for adequate enteral nutrition and volume replacement, and intravenous feeding is required. Usually, 10% glucose can be administered into peripheral veins for a few days, after which adequate enteral nutrition can be instituted. Some patients have elevations of antidiuretic hormone and profound symptomatic hyponatremia and hypomagnesemia may develop rapidly, especially when dextrose in water is given intravenously. As a rule, it is best to give dextrose in normal saline. Serum electrolytes and magnesium should be checked every 12 hours for the first 2 days.

A large number of drugs and chemicals are known to exacerbate acute porphyrias, and many others are theoretically risky because they induce hepatic cytochrome(s) P-450, deplete hepatic regulatory heme, and induce ALA synthase, especially in animals with a partial block in heme synthesis (Table 3). Among dangerous drugs, the worst offenders are barbiturates, ethanol excess, hydantoins, and sulfonamides. These drugs should not be given at all to patients with acute porphyric attacks. The others listed in columns 1 and 2 of Table 3 should be avoided if possible. Column 3 of Table 3 lists numerous drugs thought to be safe; however, a wise practice is to use as few systemically absorbed drugs as possible.

If the patient is not clearly better within 36 hours of treatment as outlined earlier, or if the patient worsens appreciably, intravenous heme should be administered. The usual dose is 3 to 5 mg per kg of body weight per day, given once or in divided doses 12 hours apart. In the United States, only one Food and Drug Administration (FDA)-approved form of heme is available—hematin (Panhematin). Each vial of hematin contains 313 mg of heme, supplied as a lyophilized powder that also contains sodium carbonate. The manufacturer recommends dissolving the powder in sterile water. In this form, the resultant hematin (hydroxy heme) solution is unstable and must be administered within an hour of preparation. It is also irritating to veins, often producing thrombophlebitis, and causes a mild coagulopathy because of adverse effects on clotting factors and platelets. We have found that the heme is more stable (at least for 24 hours) and has fewer unwanted side effects when prepared as a 1:1 molar complex with human serum albumin. To prepare such a solution, add 132 mL of 25% human serum albumin (33 grams) to a vial containing lyophilized Panhematin and mix gently. Heme given in this form has biochemical and clinical effects on porphyria that appear equivalent to those of freshly prepared aqueous solutions of Panhematin and superior to those of aged aqueous solutions of Panhematin.*

In some other countries, another effective form of heme is available: heme arginate (Normosang). This preparation consists of heme complexed to arginine and is supplied as a solution that should be diluted in isotonic saline or dextrose just before administration. Usual doses are as for Panhematin.

Therapy of Seizures in Patients with Acute Porphyria

There is a broad spectrum of clinical manifestations of acute attacks of porphyria, ranging from abdominal or extremity pain to severe and global central nervous system dysfunction. Treatment of seizures in porphyric patients has been particularly problematic because most of the commonly used anticonvulsants produce induction of cytochrome P-450 and can precipitate or worsen acute attacks (see Table 3). Indeed, carbamazepine (Tegretol, Atretol, Epitol) may be porphyrogenic in anyone (even in subjects without defects in heme synthesis). Another difficulty is distinguishing whether the seizures are part of the acute porphyric attack (which can occur in approximately 20% of hospitalized patients with acute hepatic porphyria) or are due to a primary seizure disorder. Seizures in acute attacks may occur because of hyponatremia or hypomagnesemia, as already described, or as a manifestation of the porphyria per se. Seizures in patients with acute porphyria have been treated with bromides, which are effective and do not exacerbate porphyria but have a narrow therapeutic window. High doses of magnesium sulfate (3-gram loading dose; then 1 gram per hour in 0.15 M NaCl, with or without 5% dextrose) have been of benefit. A suggested therapeutic range for the serum magnesium level is 4 to 8 mEq per liter. Clonazepam has helped some patients, but in large doses has made others worse. Clonazepam must be considered a potential hazard because it induces cytochrome P-450 and ALA synthase in cultured hepatocytes (see Table 3).

In the 1990s, several newer anticonvulsants have appeared on the market, among them felbamate, gabapentin, lamotrigine, tiagabine, and vigabatrin, all of which are effective in seizure management. The safety of newer anticonvulsant medications has been studied in cultured liver cells. Phenobarbital, felbamate (Felbatol), lamotrigine (Lamictal), and tiagabine (Gabitril), but not gabapentin (Neurontin) or vigabatrin† (Sabril), increased levels of porphyrins and the mRNA of ALA synthase, the first and rate-controlling enzyme of porphyrin synthesis. The use of vigabatrin or gabapentin (but not felbamate, lamotrigine, or tiagabine) was therefore recommended in patients with acute porphyria and seizures. In the model system, tiagabine was mildly porphyrogenic

---

*See Bonkovsky HL, Healey JF, Lourie AN, Gerron GG: Intravenous heme-albumin in acute intermittent porphyria. Am J Gastroenterol 86:1050–1056, 1991.

†Not available in the United States.

TABLE 3. **Drugs and Chemicals in Acute Hepatic Porphyrias**

Reported to Exacerbate Disease	Theoretically Risky	Believed to be Safe
Aminoglutethimide	Alcuronium	Acetaminophen
Antipyrine	Alfadolone acetate†	Amitriptyline
Aminopyrine	Alfaxalone†	Aspirin
Barbamazepine	Allyl-containing compounds	Atropine
*Barbiturates**	Amphetamines	Bromides
Bemegride	Bupivacaine	Calcium salts
N-butylscopolammonium bromide	Bupropion	Chloral hydrate
Carbamazepine	Camphor	Chlorpromazine
Carbromal	Chloroform	Colchicine
Chloramphenicol	Clonazepam (large doses)	Corticosteroids
Chlordiazepoxide	Clonidine	Cyclopropane
Chloroquine	Colistin	Dezocine
Chlorpropamide	Diazepam	Dicumarol
Danazol	Dramamine	Digoxin
Dapsone	Enalapril	Diltiazem
Diazepam	Etidocaine	Diphenhydramine
Diclofenac	Etomidate	Droperidol
Enflurane	Erythromycin	Ethylenediaminetetraacetic acid (EDTA)
Ergot preparations	Felbamate	Epinephrine
Estrogens	Fluroxene†	Ether
Ethanol excess	Food additives (selected)	Fentanyl
Ethchlorvynol	Furosemide	Fluoxetine
Ethinamate	Heavy metals	Gabapentin
Eucalyptol (in mouthwash)	Hydralazine	Gallamine
Glutethimide	Lamotrigine	Guanethidine
Griseofulvin	Lidocaine	Heparin
Halothane	Mepivacaine	Hyoscine
Hydantoins	Methychlothiazide	Ibuprofen
Imipramine	Metoclopramide	Indomethacin
Isopropylmeprobamate	Metyrapone	Insulin
Mephenytoin	Mitotane	Labetalol
Meprobamate	Nefazodone	Lisinopril
Methyldopa	Nalidixic acid	Lithium
Methylprylon	Nifedipine	Losartan
Methsuximide	Nitrazepam	Mandelamine
Nikethamide	Nortriptyline	Mefenamic acid
Novobiocin	Pargyline	Meperidine
Oral contraceptives	Pentylenetetrazole	Methadone
Pentazocine	Phenoxybenzamine	Methylphenidate
Phensuximide	Prilocaine	Morphine
Phenylbutazone	Pyrocaine	Naproxen
Phenytoin	Rifampicin	Narcotic analgesics
Primidone	Sulfonylureas	Neostigmine
Progestagens	Spironolactone	Nitrofurantoin
Pyrazinamide	Terpenes	Nitrous oxide
Pyrazolone derivatives	Tiagabine	Oxazepam
Succinimides	Tramadol	Oxylate/sodium
Sulfonamides	Tranylcypromine	Pancuronium
Sulfonethylmethane†	Triazolam	Paraldehyde
Theophylline and derivatives		Paroxetine
Tolazamide	All agents known to induce cytochromes P-450 or to	Penicillamine
Tolbutamide	increase hepatic heme turnover	Penicillin
Trimethadione		Pentamethonium†
Troxidone		Pentazocine
Valproate		Phenothiazines
		Procaine
		Promazine
		Promethazine
		Propanidid†
		Propoxyphene
		Propranolol
		Prostigmin
		Rauwolfia alkaloids
		Reserpine
		Streptomycin
		Succinylcholine
		Tetracycline
		Thiouracil
		Thyroxine
		Vigabatrin
		Vitamins A, B, C, D, and E

*Chemicals shown in *italics* are the worst offenders.
†Not available in the United States.
A more complete list may be found in Hahn M, Bonkovsky HL: Disorders of porphyrin metabolism. *In* Wu G, Israel J (eds): Diseases of the Liver and Bile Ducts: A Practical Guide to Diagnosis and Treatment. Totowa, NJ: Humana Press, 1998, pp 249–272.

even without the addition of an iron chelator, which produces a defect in heme synthesis, and it was a more potent inducer of porphyrin production than phenobarbital. These results suggest that tiagabine may be porphyrogenic even in normal people and, like carbamazepine, may rarely cause porphyric symptoms in such people. Certainly, tiagabine is contraindicated for use in acute porphyria. The use of gabapentin in acute porphyria without precipitation of acute disease has been reported. Administration of gabapentin should be individualized; the usual dose range for adults is 900 to 1800 mg per day, given in three equal doses of 300 to 600 mg.

Management of Frequent Recurrent Attacks

Some women with acute porphyria have attacks nearly every month during the luteal phase of their menstrual cycles. Some have been helped by oral contraceptives, which are thought to act by interrupting the endogenous, cyclical production of sex hormones. However, such therapy is a two-edged sword, because exogenous estrogens and progestagens may induce ALA synthase (see Table 3). Minimally effective doses should be used and patients should be followed closely, particularly in the first 3 months of such treatment. Regular infusions of heme have also been of benefit but require frequent intravenous access. Also, chronic heme therapy may lead to iron overload because heme is approximately 9% iron by weight.

For most women with cyclical attacks of acute porphyria, the treatment of choice is a luteinizing hormone-releasing hormone (LHRH) analogue. Leuprolide (Lupron) has been used most often and is now generally available, although not FDA approved for therapy of acute porphyria. The usual daily dose is 1 mg (0.2 mL), subcutaneously, although higher doses may occasionally be required. LHRH analogues have initial partial agonist effects, followed by chronic antagonist effects. Thus, they may produce initial worsening of porphyric symptoms during the first month or two of therapy. Therapy with LHRH analogues usually must be continued for at least a year and sometimes longer. They produce symptoms of estrogen deficiency (menopause) and may produce osteopenia. Thus, after a year of therapy, efforts should be made to taper the dose. Throughout the period of LHRH analogue administration, patients should get regular exercise and maintain adequate intakes of calcium and vitamin D. There may also be a role for diphosphonates (e.g., alendronate [Fosamax]) to minimize development of osteopenia in such patients. Their use is advised whenever prolonged LHRH analogue therapy is used.

Prevention of Attacks

Patients should be counseled not to abuse ethanol and to avoid use of drugs not known to be safe (see Table 3). The use of herbal remedies and "alternative" therapies is also to be discouraged because many such preparations are likely to contain porphyrogenic compounds (see Table 3). They should also avoid very-low-calorie diets or prolonged periods of fasting and should receive prompt and vigorous management of intercurrent illnesses or other stressors. Pregnancy does not usually cause acute porphyria to worsen, and termination of pregnancy is not usually indicated on medical grounds, even if both mother and fetus have acute porphyria.

A small proportion of patients have frequent attacks and others complain of nearly constant symptoms. (In some of the latter, it may be difficult to tell whether symptoms are truly due to porphyria.) Some such patients require chronic infusions of heme. In some, the heme may need to be given only three to five times per month (usually menstruating women, treated around the time of ovulation and shortly thereafter). In others, heme must be given two to four times per week. In such cases, a chronically indwelling central catheter that can be accessed at home by the patient or caregivers is usually required. Development of iron overload may occur during chronic, frequent heme therapy because heme is 9% iron by weight. This may require iron reduction therapy by phlebotomy or by chelation with deferoxamine (Desferal).

Relatives at risk should be evaluated thoroughly, and all probands and relatives found to carry the genetic defect should be educated and encouraged to wear MedicAlert bracelets and to carry MedicAlert cards indicating their diagnosis and that barbiturates, hydantoins, progestagens, and sulfonamides should be avoided.

Chronic Cutaneous Porphyrias

Porphyrin accumulations in the skin, red cells, and liver cells are responsible for the pathophysiologic changes of the chronic porphyrias. Thus, the general principles of therapy of chronic cutaneous porphyrias are to decrease the overproduction and increase the excretion of porphyrins as much as possible. Protection of the skin from light (opaque sunscreens or clothing and avoidance of strong sunlight) and physical trauma should also be recommended, although many patients find it difficult or impossible to follow this recommendation with the assiduousness needed for achievement of convincing benefit. In several diseases, the chronic blistering and ulcerating skin lesions are prone to secondary infection, which requires prompt treatment to minimize further damage (Table 4).

Congenital Erythropoietic Porphyria

This disease is quite rare and usually manifests in infancy with red urine, erythrodontia, anemia, and a severe, blistering dermatosis. The marked overproduction of uroporphyrin I characteristic of congenital erythropoietic porphyria (CEP) arises from erythroid precursors. Elevated levels of porphyrins have been improved by large oral doses of activated charcoal (30 to 60 grams every 6 hours), by hypertransfusion, and by infusions of heme. Unfortunately, long-term therapy with any of these is difficult, and chronic

TABLE 4. **Therapy of Chronic Cutaneous Porphyrias**

General measures: Protect skin from light and trauma; treat secondary skin infections
Congenital erythropoietic porphyria: Oral activated charcoal; hypertransfusion; heme infusion; splenectomy for hemolysis; glucocorticoid trial for anemia; bone marrow transplantation; gene therapy in future
Hepatoerythropoietic porphyria: Uncertain; probably the same as for congenital erythropoietic porphyria
Porphyria cutanea tarda: Stop ethanol, estrogen, or other precipitating chemicals; iron depletion by venesection; treat chronic hepatitis C, if present; chloroquine or hydroxychloroquine; urinary alkalinization
Protoporphyria: Beta-carotene; adequate iron; oral charcoal; cholecystectomy for gallstones; plasmapheresis; intravenous heme; hypertransfusion; liver transplantation; gene therapy in future

transfusions of heme exacerbate iron overload, often a pre-existing problem related to ineffective erythropoiesis and increased iron absorption. Some patients with hemolysis have responded to splenectomy, and glucocorticoids have also been reported to improve anemia. Because of the rarity and phenotypic heterogeneity of CEP, a consensus regarding therapy has not emerged. A few patients have been cured by bone marrow transplantation. In future, gene replacement therapy will deserve serious consideration for treatment of severely affected patients.

Hepatoerythropoietic Porphyria

This disease is even more rare than CEP, which it resembles clinically. Hepatoerythropoietic porphyria (HEP) is due to a homozygous, severe deficiency of uroporphyrinogen decarboxylase. Infants with this defect manifest severe skin fragility and extensive vesicle and bulla formation, leading to scarring and mutilation of sun-exposed skin. They also have hypertrichosis, erythrodontia, anemia, and hepatosplenomegaly.

The general and specific measures outlined earlier for therapy of CEP are rational in HEP as well, although none has been shown to be clearly effective in HEP.

In HEP, unlike porphyria cutanea tarda (PCT), which shares a defect in uroporphyrinogen decarboxylase, no response to therapeutic venesection has been observed.

Porphyria Cutanea Tarda

Porphyria cutanea tarda is the most common form of porphyria. It is characterized by an inherited or acquired defect in activity of hepatic uroporphyrinogen decarboxylase. In the common inherited forms of PCT, there is a 50% decrease in activity of the decarboxylase, usually identifiable in nonhepatic tissues as well as in the liver. A defect in the decarboxylase is not sufficient to produce clinical manifestations; other factors, such as iron overload, chronic hepatitis C, ethanol abuse, estrogens, and porphyrogenic toxins, are important pathogenic elements. The typical patient is a middle-aged man with a vesiculo-bullous eruption on the dorsa of the hands. Patients usually abuse ethanol and have evidence of modest iron overload and liver injury. In some parts of the world, including the United States, most patients with PCT also have chronic hepatitis C. General measures of therapy of PCT are as listed in Table 4 and already discussed.

Patients with mild PCT often respond simply to the general measures and removal of the precipitating agent such as estrogen, ethanol, or halo-aromatic chemical exposure. For those with more severe disease, the treatment of choice is venesection for depletion of hepatic iron stores. The initial treatment regimen should be removal of a pint of blood each week, continued until the patient has a mild degree of anemia with decreased serum transferrin saturation and erythrocytic mean corpuscular volume. Although most patients with PCT have moderate iron overload (approximately 3 to 4 grams), venesection therapy is effective even when hepatic iron stores are not increased.

Unfortunately, the response to iron removal or other therapy of PCT is slow, and evidence of improvement in the skin may not appear for months. It is important to let patients know this and to encourage them to persist in therapy, for it eventually succeeds. Patients should, of course, not take medicinal iron and may also be encouraged to decrease their intake of red meats, which contain relatively large amounts of heme iron, a form of iron particularly well absorbed.

Results from our and other centers showed that most patients with active PCT also have chronic hepatitis C infection and one or both of the mutations of the *HFE* gene associated with HLA-linked hereditary hemochromatosis. Both may contribute to hepatic iron deposition, as may alcoholism or alcoholic liver disease. All patients with PCT should be screened for hepatitis C infection (test for anti-hepatitis C virus [HCV] antibodies, HCV RNA in serum) and for *HFE* gene mutations (search for C282Y and H63D mutations by reverse transcriptase and polymerase chain reaction and restriction fragment length polymorphisms).

Chloroquine* (Aralen) and hydroxychloroquine* (Plaquenil) form water-soluble complexes with uroporphyrin, increasing porphyrin removal from tissue stores and excretion in the urine. However, in previously untreated PCT, the doses of these drugs usually used for other disorders may cause acute hepatic injury with fever, jaundice, and right upper quadrant pain. This is due to excessively rapid mobilization of porphyrin from the liver. For this reason, such drugs should be started slowly at low doses (125 mg two or three times per week) with gradual increase to 500 mg per day. Monitoring for possible retinal damage, a major unwanted side effect of therapy, is advisable whenever chronic chloroquine or hydroxychloroquine therapy is used. Urinary excretion of uroporphyrin may also be enhanced by alkalinization of the urine,

---

*Not FDA approved for this indication.

conveniently achieved by administration of baking soda or Shohl's solution (sodium citrate and citric acid).

Porphyria cutanea tarda may occur in association with end-stage renal disease. Because the chloroquine-porphyrin complex is poorly dialyzable, chloroquine is ineffective. Because of anemia, venesection is relatively contraindicated in such patients. However, administration of recombinant human erythropoietin (Epogen) stimulates iron mobilization for red cell production sufficient to support therapeutic venesections.

Protoporphyria

This disease is usually clinically manifested in infants and children who experience intense, burning pain of sun-exposed skin after brief exposure in the spring and summer. A few hours later, erythema, edema, and itching become prominent. With more prolonged and repeated exposure, involved skin may become leathery and hyperkeratotic. This is especially prominent in a malar "butterfly" distribution on the face and over the knuckles of the hands. Vesicles, bullae, hypertrichosis, and severe mutilation, as seen in CEP, HEP, or PCT, rarely occur with protoporphyria (PP); when they do, they are milder than in the diseases due to uroporphyrin excess. Diagnosis of PP requires demonstration of increased amounts of protoporphyrin, without increased coproporphyrin, in the stool, red cells, or both. It is the only form of clinically manifested porphyria in which urinary heme precursors are normal. A common complication of PP is development of pigment gallstones, which contain a high content of protoporphyrin. A rare, but serious, complication is development of severe liver disease because of precipitation of protoporphyrin in hepatocytes and biliary radicles. Such disease may progress and produce liver failure with all its usual complications.

In addition to the usual general measures, PP is treated with beta-carotene. The usual adult dose is 120 to 180 mg per day. The recommended therapeutic serum beta-carotene level is 600 to 800 µg/dL. Drugs or chemicals that may increase protoporphyrin production or decrease its utilization should be avoided. Griseofulvin is the most obvious example because it can cause a protoporphyric condition in mice. Any drug or toxin that produces cholestasis is a risk because protoporphyrin must be excreted through the bile. Avoidance of iron deficiency is important because iron deficiency may exacerbate overproduction of protoporphyrin. Oral cholestyramine and activated charcoal have been suggested as treatment to prevent the enterohepatic circulation of protoporphyrin, which appears to be substantial. They have seemed to be effective in small numbers of patients. Patients with symptomatic gallstones are best treated by cholecystectomy, as long as they do not have severe liver disease or other contraindications to surgery.

Patients with evidence of liver disease require regular and frequent monitoring because decompensation can occur quickly. Those with abnormal liver chemistries or very high red cell (>1500 µg per dL) or plasma (> 150 µg per dL) protoporphyrin concentrations should undergo liver biopsy. Patients with liver injury must avoid ethanol or other hepatotoxins that may act synergistically to accelerate liver damage. Liver transplantation is an option for those with advanced liver disease, although it does not correct the biochemical abnormality because ferrochelatase deficiency in the bone marrow persists, and recurrent protoporphyric liver disease is a continuing possibility.

Unfortunately, in some patients with PP who have undergone liver transplantation, pigmentary fibrosis has redeveloped quite rapidly. Thus, transplantation of bone marrow before, during, or after liver transplantation is being considered. In future, gene therapy (the normal ferrochelatase gene targeted to the bone marrow stem cells) would be a major advance. Transient improvements in PP have been achieved by plasmapheresis followed by intravenous heme infusions. The dosage of heme used has been 3 to 5 mg per kg per day. Such therapy is recommended particularly as a way to stabilize hepatic function while awaiting transplantation or to decrease plasma protoporphyrin concentrations just before transplantation. Without such therapy, several patients have had severe neuromuscular complications requiring prolonged and expensive convalescence.

THERAPEUTIC USE OF BLOOD COMPONENTS

method of
JOHN M. NINOS, M.D., and
LESLIE E. SILBERSTEIN, M.D.
Hospital of the University of Pennsylvania
Philadelphia, Pennsylvania

The science of transfusion medicine today reflects the biology and physiology of the individual cellular and liquid components of whole blood (WB). With a sound understanding of the nature and characteristics of individual blood components, clinicians can better serve their patients by prescribing the proper component. Transfusion should be undertaken only if the anticipated benefit outweighs the potential risk. A thorough knowledge of the many blood components can help the physician make this important decision.

ADMINISTRATION OF BLOOD COMPONENTS

The transfusion process begins when a physician writes an order specifying the component and the amount to be given. The physician must explain the treatment's benefits and risks to the patient and obtain informed consent in accordance with the institution's guidelines. The transfusionist must confirm that the identity of the blood unit and the patient are correct and record the patient's pretransfusion vital signs. All blood components must be administered through a macroaggregate particulate filter (170 to 260 μm) within 4 hours of the time of release from the blood bank.

If desired, units can be divided by the blood bank into split units, allowing transfusion of a given volume over a greater time period. Solutions that can be co-administered with blood products are normal saline (0.9% USP) and 5% albumin. Hypotonic or hypertonic saline, lactated Ringer's, 5% dextrose, and medications must not be administered with blood products. There are devices available specifically designed for the safe warming of blood products to a temperature of 37°C, but not more than 42°C. These devices are indicated for adults receiving rapid and multiple transfusions of more than 50 mL per kg per hour, infants receiving rapid transfusions of more than 15 mL per kg per hour, adults or infants receiving exchange transfusions, and patients with cold agglutinin disease. Clinical personnel should periodically monitor the patient throughout the transfusion.

RED BLOOD CELL PRODUCTS

Whole Blood

Allogeneic WB units are rarely used in U.S. medical centers because they lack the advantages that component therapy offers. Blood units collected for autologous use, however, are often prepared as WB units. The standard single unit of WB contains 450 mL of WB collected into 63 mL of anticoagulant/preservative solution. The hematocrit is 36 to 44%, and it must be stored at 1 to 6°C. The shelf life depends on the anticoagulant/preservative solution and ranges from 21 to 35 days. After 24 hours of storage, there are few functional platelets or granulocytes and significantly decreased amounts of factors V and VIII.

WB units may be used in patients actively bleeding with massive volume loss (>25%) who need both oxygen-carrying capacity and blood volume expansion. Allogeneic WB should not be used for patients who are normovolemic; red blood cells (RBCs) are preferred in this setting. In an average-sized adult, 1 U WB should increase the hemoglobin concentration by 1 gm per dL and the hematocrit by 3 to 4%.

Red Blood Cells

RBCs are prepared by removal of 200 to 250 mL of plasma from 1 U WB. A variety of anticoagulant/preservative solutions are used that influence the shelf life and hematocrit. Units prepared in citrate/monobasic sodium phosphate/dextrose (CPD) are approximately 250 mL in volume with a hematocrit of 70 to 80% and a 21-day shelf life when stored at 1 to 6°C. Units prepared in citrate/monobasic sodium phosphate/dextrose/adenine (CPDA-1) have a longer, 35-day shelf life with a similar volume and hematocrit as CPD units. Additive solutions such as AS-1 (Adsol: dextrose, adenine, mannitol, sodium chloride) and AS-3 (Nutricel: dextrose, adenine, monobasic sodium phosphate, sodium chloride) can be added to the above units to further extend the shelf life to 42 days at 1 to 6°C. Units prepared with 100 mL of additive solution are approximately 350 mL in volume with a hematocrit of 50 to 60%.

RBCs are indicated for patients with anemia requiring an increase in oxygen-carrying capacity and red cell mass. As with 1 U WB, 1 U RBCs in an average-sized adult will usually raise the hemoglobin concentration by 1 gm per dL and the hematocrit by 3 to 4%. In pediatric patients, a volume of 3 mL per kg can be anticipated to raise the hemoglobin concentration by 1 gm per dL.

Leukocyte-Reduced Red Blood Cells

One unit of RBCs contains 1 to 3×10^9 white blood cells (WBCs). Current third-generation leukocyte reduction filters can provide 3 log or 99.9% reduction of WBC content to less than 5×10^6 WBC per product. The leukocyte reduction step can be performed at the bedside or, preferably, shortly after collection at the blood center. *Prestorage* leukocyte reduction offers the potential advantage of lower levels of cytokines, which would otherwise be generated by WBCs during storage of the product.

Leukocyte-reduced RBCs are indicated for patients with repeated febrile nonhemolytic transfusion reactions (NHTRs) to cellular blood components or to minimize alloimmunization to foreign HLA antigens. Febrile NHTRs are typically caused by reactions to donor WBCs or to cytokines present in the product. Patients having persistent febrile NHTRs to bedside leukocyte-reduced products may benefit from the lower levels of cytokines present in prestorage leukocyte-reduced products. Alloimmunization to foreign HLA class I antigens is of significant concern for patients who may require platelet transfusions. Because platelets also possess HLA class I antigens, patients sensitized to such antigens can become refractory to platelet transfusions. If the decision is made to use leukocyte-reduced RBCs to prevent alloimmunization, it should be made before the first transfusion, and leukocyte-reduced platelets should also be used.

Washed Red Blood Cells

RBC washing involves the use of sterile saline to rinse away the plasma remaining in an RBC unit. The procedure removes more than 98% of the plasma, including the plasma proteins, microaggregates, and cytokines, as well as 10 to 20% of the RBCs. The procedure takes approximately 1 to 2 hours with an automated cell washer, and the resultant product (about 180 mL) is suspended in sterile saline at a hematocrit of 70 to 80%. This product is indicated for severe, recurrent allergic reactions to blood components that are not prevented by premedication with an antihistamine. Typically, such reactions are caused by an allergy to plasma proteins. Patients known to be severely IgA-deficient may have anaphylactic reactions to IgA present in blood components and should receive either RBCs from IgA-deficient donors (must be scheduled in advance) or washed RBCs. Because the washing process creates an open system, this component has a shelf life of only 24 hours at 1 to 6°C.

Frozen-Deglycerolized Red Blood Cells

A freezing process is utilized for long-term storage (up to 10 years at −65 to −120°C) of RBC units with rare phenotypes. After the RBCs are thawed, the glycerol cryoprotectant is washed out with a series of saline-glucose solutions. Once thawed, the unit has a shelf life of 24 hours at 1 to 6°C.

PHYSIOLOGIC BASIS FOR RED BLOOD CELL TRANSFUSIONS

Because of the risk of adverse reactions to blood transfusions, the American College of Physicians has stated that transfusion of allogeneic blood should be avoided whenever possible. The primary indication for RBC transfusions is to restore or maintain oxygen-carrying capacity to meet tissue demands for oxygen. Oxygen delivery (DO_2) is the product of arterial oxygen content and the cardiac output. The critical DO_2 is the oxygen delivery below which organ function can no longer be maintained. Thus, the overall goal is to maintain a DO_2 reserve such that the critical DO_2 is never reached and oxygen demand never exceeds supply in any critical tissue.

The ability of each individual to compensate for acute anemia and an alteration in oxygen demand by increasing oxygen delivery to organs cannot be adequately determined in a practical manner aside from invasive monitoring. A National Institutes of Health panel in 1988 concluded that the traditional perioperative practice of transfusing red cells at hemoglobin levels less than 10 grams per dL should be replaced in the stable patient with no signs of end-organ hypoxia with a standard of 7 grams per dL. Hemoglobin levels between 7 and 10 grams per dL may require RBC transfusion if there are signs of tissue hypoxia, such as tachycardia, chest pain, shortness of breath, or electrocardiographic changes consistent with ischemia.

PLATELET PRODUCTS

Whole Blood–Derived Platelets

Platelets prepared by centrifugation of individual (often termed "random donor") units of WB must contain at least 5.5×10^{10} platelets in 50 to 70 mL of plasma. They must be stored at 20 to 24°C under constant agitation because storage at cold temperatures has been shown to be detrimental to platelet function. As a result of these warmer storage temperatures, the shelf life of these products is only 5 days because the risk of bacterial contamination rises sig-

nificantly with longer storage. WB-derived (WBD) platelet transfusions are indicated for (1) bleeding caused by insufficient numbers of normal platelets or platelets with abnormal function, and (2) prophylactic use in patients with severe thrombocytopenia who are at risk for spontaneous hemorrhage or scheduled for an invasive procedure.

Thresholds for prophylactic transfusions vary depending on the circumstance and have recently come under increased scrutiny. In general, maintaining a platelet count of more than 50,000 per μL is sufficient to obtain adequate primary hemostasis for most surgical or other invasive procedures. A threshold of 100,000 per μL may be indicated for procedures in which even minute bleeding can prove deleterious, such as neurosurgery and surgery of the retina or trachea. Prophylactic transfusion of platelets may be considered for patients with platelet counts of less than 20,000 per μL associated with marrow hypoplasia as a result of primary disease or myeloablative chemotherapy. Recent studies have shown that hospitalized patients with platelet counts of more than 10,000 per μL who are otherwise stable and have no symptoms of clinical bleeding may not need prophylactic transfusions. Many medical centers are now adopting this lower threshold of 10,000 per μL for prophylactic platelet transfusions in stable patients. Modification of this policy may be necessary if a patient has other risk factors that may deleteriously affect platelet function, such as fever, sepsis, or antibiotic therapy.

Platelet transfusions are often not effective in certain conditions associated with accelerated platelet destruction or consumption, such as immune thrombocytopenic purpura (ITP), disseminated intravascular coagulation (DIC), sepsis, uremia, and hypersplenism. Platelet transfusions in these conditions may be attempted, however, in the setting of active bleeding. Platelet transfusions are contraindicated except in life-threatening hemorrhage for patients with thrombotic thrombocytopenic purpura (TTP)/hemolytic uremic syndrome (HUS) and heparin-induced thrombocytopenia. Platelet transfusions in these patients may promote platelet thrombus formation and serious thrombotic complications.

The conventional wisdom is that 1 U WBD platelets raises the platelet count by 5000 per μL in an average-sized adult in the absence of factors leading to increased platelet consumption or destruction. A standard adult dose of 1 U per 10 kg and a pediatric dose of 5 to 10 mL per kg are common. Traditionally, hospitals pool individual units of WBD platelets into a single bag for ease of administration. The pooling process decreases the shelf life to 4 hours. The standard number of units pooled at a given institution is often determined more by custom than science. Standard pools of 6, 8, or 10 U are typical. Some hospitals, however, are decreasing the standard pool size to 5 or even 4 U.

Pheresis Platelets

Pheresis platelets are collected from an individual donor during a 2- to 3-hour cytapheresis procedure in which platelets are selectively removed in a volume of 200 to 400 mL plasma, while the rest of the blood components are returned. This allows an increased yield of platelets from that single donor. A single pheresis platelet unit contains approximately the same number of platelets as 6 to 8 U WBD platelets (minimum of $>3 \times 10^{11}$ platelets) but are generally more expensive than the latter. Clinicians often prefer these products for the patient who requires long-term hemotherapy (i.e., those receiving high-dose chemotherapy) because they expose the recipient to fewer donors, presumably decreasing the risk of acquiring transfusion-transmitted diseases and reducing the risk of alloimmunization to foreign HLA antigens. Recent scientific studies, however, do not support these theoretical advantages of pheresis platelets. The indications for the use of pheresis platelets are essentially the same as for WBD platelets.

Leukocyte-Reduced Platelets

Current third-generation leukocyte reduction filters provide 3 log or 99.9% reduction of leukocytes present in either a pool of WBD platelets or a pheresis platelet unit. After leukocyte reduction, these platelet products should contain less than 5×10^6 WBCs. Now available via current pheresis technology are *prestorage* leukocyte-reduced pheresis platelets in which the leukocyte reduction step is accomplished during the collection procedure. As with leukocyte-reduced RBCs, leukocyte-reduced platelets help prevent febrile NHTRs and alloimmunization to HLA antigens.

Platelet Refractoriness

Patients who fail to obtain an adequate increment in response to two sequential platelet transfusions are termed *refractory*. It is useful to calculate the corrected count increment (CCI) with the following formula:

$$\frac{[\text{Post-transfusion } (\leq 60 \text{ minutes after transfusion}) \text{ platelet count } (/\mu L) - \text{pre-transfusion platelet count } (/\mu L)] \times \text{BSA } (m^2)}{\text{Platelet dose (in multiples of } 10^{11})^*}$$

Two consecutive transfusions with a CCI less than 7500 per μL are presumptive evidence for the refractory state. This may be a result of either immune or nonimmune causes. Nonimmune causes (i.e., increased platelet sequestration, consumption, or destruction) include splenomegaly, fever, sepsis, DIC, bleeding, antibiotic therapy, and immunosuppressive agents. No special platelet product can improve platelet increments in cases of nonimmune refractoriness. The underlying cause must be resolved, if possible, while the patient is supported with the

---

*BSA = body surface area. For platelet dose, use 3.3 for a pheresis platelet unit; use 0.6 for each WBD platelet unit.

usual platelet products. Immune causes include autoantibodies (ITP) or alloantibodies to HLA class I antigens (more common) or platelet-specific antigens (less common). Patients with ITP generally have broadly reactive autoantibodies that rapidly destroy transfused platelets as well. No special platelet products offer any improved benefit, and these patients should be supported with usual platelet products if the patient is actively bleeding. Patients shown to have alloimmune refractoriness can be supported with special platelet products, as discussed later.

To distinguish immune from nonimmune causes, it is important to obtain post-transfusion platelet counts no later than 60 minutes after a platelet transfusion. Immune causes typically result in rapid destruction of transfused platelets, whereas nonimmune causes typically lead to lowered platelet counts over a period of hours. If an alloimmune refractory state is suspected, serum from the patient should be sent to the laboratory to screen for alloantibodies to HLA class I antigens. If the screen is negative, it is likely that the patient has a nonimmune cause of the refractory state, and the patient should be supported with the usual WBD or pheresis platelet products. Rarely, the patient may have an antibody to a platelet-specific antigen. If this is suspected, patient serum can be sent to reference laboratories to screen for antibodies to implicated platelet antigens.

If the screen for HLA alloantibodies is positive, the specificity of these can be determined. If the number of specificities detected is limited, pheresis platelets that lack the antigens corresponding to the patient's alloantibodies (*HLA antigen-negative pheresis platelets*) may be tried. If the number of specificities detected is great, then pheresis platelets that possess HLA antigens closely related or identical to the patient's (*HLA-matched pheresis platelets*) should be tried. It is important to realize that not all HLA-matched pheresis platelets are equivalent, and their degree of identity with the patient is graded on a scale of A (most identical) to D (least identical). This must be considered when judging responses to HLA-matched pheresis platelets. Excellent communication between the clinicians and the transfusion medicine specialists is critical for success in managing refractory patients.

PHERESIS GRANULOCYTES

Granulocytes are the least utilized blood component owing to the logistics of collection and limited benefit with current collection methods. This component has limited storage viability and is prepared only when requested by the clinician through the recruitment and cytapheresis of a volunteer donor. Depending on the collection facility, hydroxyethyl starch and corticosteroids may be administered to the donor to increase yield. The component contains at least 1×10^{10} granulocytes with variable numbers of lymphocytes, platelets, and RBCs in 200 to 300 mL plasma.

Granulocytes should be infused as soon as possible,

but no later than 24 hours after collection (stored at 20 to 24°C). They are indicated for patients with severe neutropenia, infection, a lack of response to antibiotic therapy, and marrow showing myeloid hypoplasia with a chance for recovery in the future. Although there is no general standard as to the dose and duration of granulocyte transfusion therapy, most believe that a minimum of 1 to 2 × 10^{10} granulocytes per day are necessary for clinical benefit. Some studies at these dosage levels have shown clinical benefit in selected settings such as neonatal sepsis. Studies of the use of recombinant granulocyte colony-stimulating factors in normal donors to increase yield are exciting and enable the collection of up to 6 to 8 × 10^{10} granulocytes per procedure. The efficacy and potential toxicity of growth factor–stimulated products still await randomized clinical trials.

PREVENTION OF TRANSFUSION-ASSOCIATED GRAFT-VERSUS-HOST DISEASE

Foreign T lymphocytes present in all of the cellular blood components discussed previously have the potential to cause transfusion-associated graft-versus-host disease (TA-GVHD) in immunocompromised or HLA-related recipients. This disease has up to 90% mortality and is characterized by fever, skin rash, diarrhea, hepatitis, and marrow aplasia. TA-GVHD can be prevented by gamma irradiation of cellular units with 2500 cGy. Donor units intended for blood relatives, intrauterine transfusions, neonatal exchange transfusions, immunocompromised patients, and solid organ or stem cell transplant recipients should be irradiated. All HLA-matched products should be irradiated as well. Leukocyte-reduced products do *not* prevent TA-GVHD because they still contain sufficient residual T lymphocytes.

PREVENTION OF CYTOMEGALOVIRUS DISEASE

Certain select immunocompromised populations at risk for severe disease caused by primary infection with cytomegalovirus (CMV) should receive products less likely to transmit the virus. Cellular components from CMV-seronegative donors are available. Furthermore, because the CMV virus resides within leukocytes, leukocyte-reduced (<5 × 10^6 WBC) blood components have been shown to be nearly equivalent to seronegative products in terms of preventing primary CMV transmission. Patients who should receive CMV-seronegative or, alternatively, leukocyte-reduced cellular blood components include CMV-seronegative stem cell or solid organ transplant recipients, CMV-seronegative pregnant women, low-birth-weight premature infants born to CMV-seronegative women, recipients of intrauterine transfusions, and those rare patients with acquired immunodeficiency syndrome who are CMV seronegative.

FRESH-FROZEN PLASMA

Plasma that is separated from a donated unit of WB and frozen within 8 hours of collection is termed fresh-frozen plasma (FFP). Plasma obtained via apheresis equipment can also be prepared into FFP. Each unit of FFP (200 to 250 mL volume) has a shelf life of 1 year when stored at −18°C or colder. These collection and storage conditions result in minimal loss of factors V and VIII.

FFP is indicated for patients with documented multiple coagulation factor deficiencies who are actively bleeding or at risk for bleeding before an invasive procedure. An unexplained prolonged prothrombin time (PT) or partial thromboplastin time (PTT) must be confirmed to be due to a factor deficiency before FFP infusion can be considered. Prolonged PT or PTT studies resulting from heparin therapy or a factor inhibitor are not indications for FFP therapy. FFP is, however, indicated for emergent reversal of bleeding associated with oral anticoagulant therapy after initiation of vitamin K replacement. FFP is also used during plasma exchange therapy for patients with TTP/HUS. FFP should not be used for patients with minimal prolongation of coagulation tests (<1.5 × midpoint of normal range) before invasive procedures. There is little evidence that FFP in this setting prevents bleeding. FFP should not be used for volume expansion, as a nutritional source, or to enhance wound healing.

Because normal plasma contains coagulation factors in excess, levels of coagulation factors needed to maintain hemostasis range from 10 to 50% of normal levels. Factor levels of 50% are generally considered adequate for surgical hemostasis. The FFP volume to infuse can be estimated from the following formulas:

$$\text{Estimated plasma volume (mL)} = \text{Weight (kg)} \times 70 \text{ mL/kg} \times (1.0 - \text{hematocrit})$$

$$\text{Volume FFP (mL)} = \% \text{ factor level desired} \times \text{estimated plasma volume (mL)}$$

FFP is thawed at 30 to 37°C. Thawed FFP has a shelf life of 24 hours when stored at 1 to 6°C. Posttransfusion assessment of coagulation status is critical for determining efficacy.

A solvent/detergent-treated pooled plasma product (PLAS + SD) is now available (200 mL per unit). Pools of FFP are obtained from a maximum of 2500 donors and treated to inactivate lipid-enveloped viruses including the human immunodeficiency virus and hepatitis B and C viruses. The risk of contracting nonenveloped viruses such as parvovirus B19 and hepatitis A is unknown. This product may not be suitable for selected populations at risk for serious complications of parvovirus B19 such as pregnant women and patients with chronic hemolytic anemia and chronic immune deficiency. Studies have shown an efficacy similar to that of FFP in treating coagulation factor deficiencies as well as acute and chronic TTP.

CRYOPRECIPITATE

When units of FFP are thawed at 1 to 6°C, a cryoprecipitate of select plasma proteins forms. After expressing off the cryo-poor supernatant plasma, the cryoprecipitate is refrozen at −18°C and has a shelf life of 1 year. This cryoprecipitate contains approximately 30 to 50% of the fibrinogen, von Willebrand factor (vWf), factor VIII, factor XIII, and fibronectin present in the original FFP unit.

Cryoprecipitate is indicated for patients with bleeding who have severe congenital or acquired hypofibrinogenemia (<100 mg per dL), dysfibrinogenemia, or factor XIII deficiency. It may also be used to form a topical fibrin sealant in certain surgical settings. It should only be used for hemophilia A or von Willebrand's disease if virus-inactivated concentrates containing factor VIII or vWf are not available. Cryoprecipitate is thawed at 30 to 37°C. Thawed cryoprecipitate has a shelf life of 6 hours when stored at 1 to 6°C. Typically, units of cryoprecipitate are pooled before transfusion, decreasing the shelf life to 4 hours. The dosage for treating hypofibrinogenemia (<100 mg per dL) can be estimated by the following formulas:

$$\text{Estimated plasma volume (in dL)} = \text{weight (kg)} \times 0.7 \text{ dL/kg} \times (1.0 - \text{hematocrit})$$

$$\text{Fibrinogen (mg)} = [\text{desired fibrinogen level (mg/dL)} - \text{initial fibrinogen level (mg/dL)}] \times \text{estimated plasma volume (in dL)}$$

$$\text{Units cryoprecipitate needed} = \text{fibrinogen (mg)} \div 250 \text{ mg fibrinogen/unit cryoprecipitate}$$

PLASMA DERIVATIVES

Plasma derivatives are concentrates of plasma proteins prepared from large pools of plasma from multiple donors. The specific protein of interest is purified, concentrated, and subjected to various procedures designed to inactivate or remove contaminating viruses. It is important for the clinician to realize that there are significant differences in plasma derivative preparation and viral inactivation/removal among the different manufacturers.

Methods of viral inactivation/removal include solvent/detergent (SD) treatment, 60 to 80°C dry heat, 60°C heat in solution (pasteurization), and immunoaffinity chromatography. There are rare reports of hepatitis B and hepatitis C transmission by 60°C heat-inactivated coagulation factor concentrates. There have been no reports of lipid-enveloped virus (human immunodeficiency virus, hepatitis B and C viruses) transmission with products inactivated by SD treatments. Transmission of nonenveloped viruses like hepatitis A, however, has been reported for SD-treated coagulation factor concentrates. Certain plasma proteins are now being produced by recombinant DNA technology with no known disease risk.

Human-derived and recombinant factor VIII preparations are available for treatment of bleeding episodes in hemophilia A patients. Certain human-derived factor VIII preparations, such as Humate-P, Alphanate, and Koāte-HP, contain significant amounts of vWf. They should be used for treatment of significant bleeding in von Willebrand's disease in place of cryoprecipitate.

Two different human-derived preparations of factor IX are available. *Factor IX complex* contains 1 to 5% of factor IX and some quantities of factors II, VII, and X. These additional factors, some of which become activated during preparation, increase the risk for thrombosis. *Coagulation factor IX* contains 20 to 30% of factor IX and only trace amounts of factors II, VII, and X, with less risk for thrombosis. Recombinant forms of factor IX are now available.

Recombinant factor VIIa is currently under study for the treatment of bleeding in cirrhotic patients and patients with inhibitors to factor VIII. *Antithrombin III* and *Protein C* concentrates are produced for patients with deficiencies of these proteins who are at risk for thrombosis. *Human albumin* (5% and 25%) preparations are commonly used to provide colloid replacement. They contain 96% albumin with 4% globulin and other proteins and are heated in solution at 60°C for 10 hours to inactivate viruses. The 5% solution is osmotically and oncotically equivalent to human plasma. Albumin given to correct nutritional hypoalbuminemia or to treat ascites in patients with portal hypertension is of questionable benefit. *Intravenous gamma globulin* preparations contain 90% IgG and trace quantities of IgA and IgM and are subjected to viral inactivation. They are administered to provide IgG replacement for patients with immune deficiencies and are also used as an immunomodulatory agent for autoimmune disorders such as ITP and Guillain-Barré syndrome.

ADVERSE REACTIONS TO BLOOD TRANSFUSION

method of
KAUSHIK A. SHASTRI, M.D.
State University of New York at Buffalo and Veterans Affairs Western New York Healthcare System
Buffalo, New York

Blood transfusions have become safer over the course of the past few decades. Identification of blood group antigens, techniques to separate and store blood components, better anticoagulants, and development of screening tests of donor blood for various infectious agents have all contributed to the safety of our blood supply. Clinicians should, however, be mindful that the risk of blood transfusion has not approached zero and that transfusion is in effect a form of tissue transplantation. Transfusion of blood components should be performed only when absolutely necessary. Many

TABLE 1. **Adverse Reactions to Blood Transfusion**

Immunologic Reactions

Immediate hemolytic transfusion reactions
Delayed hemolytic transfusion reactions
Acute febrile reactions
Acute urticarial/anaphylactic reactions
Graft-versus-host disease
Transfusion-related acute lung injury
Post-transfusion purpura
?Immune modulation (tumor recurrence, wound infections)

Transmission of Infections

Viruses
  Hepatitis viruses
  Retroviruses (human immunodeficiency virus, human T cell
    lymphotropic virus types I and II)
  Cytomegalovirus and others
Protozoa and other parasites; bacterial contamination

Miscellaneous Adverse Effects

Iron overload
Congestive heart failure
Complications of massive transfusions (citrate toxicity,
  hypothermia, dilutional coagulopathy, and thrombocytopenia)

states in this country now require the patient to sign an informed consent before transfusion of blood products.

Various adverse effects associated with blood transfusion are given in Table 1.

IMMUNOLOGIC REACTIONS

Immediate Hemolytic Transfusion Reactions

The most devastating hemolytic reaction occurs when ABO-incompatible red blood cells are transfused. Clerical errors account for most of the acute hemolytic transfusion reactions; hence, they are mostly preventable. Naturally occurring blood group antibodies of the recipient bind to the donor red blood cells, activate complement, and cause rapid intravascular hemolysis, producing hemodynamic shock, disseminated intravascular coagulation, and acute renal failure. The symptoms, which may begin after administration of only a few milliliters of blood, include pain at the transfusion site, back pain, chest pain, fever with or without chills, flushing, and generalized bleeding. In an anesthetized patient, hypotension, increased bleeding or oozing from the surgical site, and hemoglobinuria might be the only clues. Because only the donor cells are destroyed, the severity of the reaction depends on the amount of incompatible blood transfused. Hence, transfusion should be immediately stopped if a hemolytic reaction is suspected. A sample of blood should be drawn from the patient and sent immediately to the blood bank with the unused donor blood. After infusion of incompatible blood, there is usually hemoglobinemia and hemoglobinuria.

Treatment should begin at the mere suspicion of hemolytic transfusion reaction and not wait for laboratory confirmation of the diagnosis. A large-bore venous access should be established and vital signs

monitored. Therapy should be directed to maintain blood pressure, intravascular volume, and renal blood flow as reflected by adequate urine output. Hypotension should be treated with volume replacement with crystalloids such as normal saline. After adequate hydration, furosemide (Lasix), 40 to 80 mg, should be administered intravenously and repeated once, if necessary, to maintain a urine flow of greater than 100 mL per hour in adults at least for the first 24 hours. If, despite fluids and diuretic therapy, the urine output remains low, then it is likely that acute tubular necrosis has occurred. These patients may then require temporary hemodialysis. If the patient has laboratory and clinical features of disseminated intravascular coagulation with overt bleeding, therapy with cryoprecipitate to keep fibrinogen above 100 mg per dL, platelets to keep the platelet count above 50,000 per mm^3, and fresh-frozen plasma to correct elevated partial thromboplastin time is warranted.

Delayed Hemolytic Transfusion Reactions

Delayed hemolytic reactions occur in patients in whom alloantibodies to minor blood group antigens (most commonly Kidd system antigens) have previously developed, but whose antibody levels have fallen below the threshold of detection by routine screening procedures. After transfusion, an anamnestic response occurs within hours or days, resulting in IgG antibodies that bind to the transfused cells. Fever, a falling hemoglobin, and mild jaundice characterize these reactions. Sometimes, lack of the expected rise in hemoglobin after transfusion may be the only clinical clue. The direct antiglobulin test may become positive transiently, but plasma antibody against the antigen usually becomes detectable in 1 to 2 weeks. Specific treatment is seldom necessary, but it is wise to monitor urine output and coagulation parameters. It is important to identify delayed hemolytic transfusion reaction because the antibody may again disappear before the next transfusion and the blood bank records are the only method of identifying the antibody. An appropriate blood bank workup can ensure that the patient receives only the red blood cells lacking that particular antigen to prevent recurrent delayed hemolytic transfusion reactions.

Febrile Nonhemolytic Reactions

Febrile nonhemolytic reactions, which complicate approximately 1% of all transfusions, are defined by a rise in the patient's temperature by 1°C or more. Antileukocyte or antiplatelet antibodies of the recipient against the donor antigens cause most of these reactions, but the preformed cytokines in the donor component may be responsible in some. When fever occurs during a blood transfusion, the transfusion should be stopped temporarily and the patient studied for a hemolytic reaction. If a hemolytic reaction has not occurred, antipyretics such as acetaminophen (650 mg for an adult) may be given. Leukodepletion using filters can prevent febrile transfusion reactions in many instances.

Acute Urticarial/Anaphylactic Reactions

Systemic allergic reactions to blood components may range in clinical severity from minor urticarial reactions to severe anaphylaxis. Urticarial reactions (hives) occur during approximately 1% of blood transfusions and are usually caused by the recipient's allergy to some soluble antigen present in the donor plasma. The treatment consists of diphenhydramine, 25 to 50 mg orally or intravenously, and temporary interruption of transfusion.

Anaphylactic reactions are rare but occur mainly in patients with congenital IgA deficiency and high-titer, class-specific anti-IgA antibodies. The incidence of severe congenital IgA deficiency in the general population is approximately 0.1%, and 20 to 60% of these patients have class-specific anti-IgA antibodies. Symptoms related to the respiratory system (cough, dyspnea, bronchospasm), gastrointestinal tract (nausea, vomiting), circulatory system (syncope, hypotension), and skin (flushing, urticarial) may occur within seconds of starting transfusion, but may be delayed for up to an hour. Treatment consists of stopping transfusion, maintaining venous access with normal saline, and administration of epinephrine and oxygen with endotracheal intubation for significant airway obstruction. For patients with life-threatening anaphylactic reactions, autologous blood or blood from IgA-deficient donors should be used in the future.

Transfusion-Associated Graft-versus-Host Disease

Graft-versus-host disease, classically seen after allogeneic bone marrow transplantation, occasionally occurs after transfusion of cells that contain immunocompetent lymphocytes, which react with recipient tissues. This is most commonly seen in immunocompromised patients and in recipients of directed donation from first-degree relatives. Graft-versus-host disease is signaled by the appearance of fever, rash, mucositis, diarrhea, and abnormal liver function readings 3 to 30 days after transfusion and may not be recognized. There is no effective treatment, and over 90% of affected patients die. Graft-versus-host disease can be prevented by irradiation of blood products before transfusion. Immunodeficient patients and those receiving directed donations from first-degree relatives should receive irradiated blood.

Transfusion-Related Acute Lung Injury

Transfusion-related acute lung injury (TRALI) is an adverse effect of transfusion caused by interaction between the donor's leukocyte (HLA) or granulocyte antibodies with recipient antigens. Although the reported incidence of TRALI is 0.16%, less dramatic reactions probably occur more frequently. Activation of the complement system and neutrophils lead to neutrophil aggregation in small pulmonary vessels, resulting in increased capillary permeability, bilateral pulmonary edema, hypoxemia, and hypotension. The onset of TRALI usually occurs within a few minutes after transfusion, but it may be delayed for 4 to 8 hours. In severe cases, the mortality rate may be as high as 10%. Most patients recover completely in 2 days if appropriately managed. Treatment consists of adequate ventilatory and volume support until recovery ensues.

Post-Transfusion Purpura

Post-transfusion purpura is a rare cause of severe thrombocytopenia approximately 1 week to 10 days after blood transfusion. These patients, usually multiparous women, lack the common platelet antigen HPA-1a present in 98.3% of the population and have alloantibodies against this common platelet antigen. When they are transfused with blood products that contain the antigen, severe thrombocytopenia and bleeding develop. Treatment is empiric and includes the use of intravenous immune globulins (IGIV) and plasmapheresis. IGIV is given at 0.5 gram per kg body weight for each of 2 consecutive days, with infusions repeated according to platelet count response.

Immune Modulation

There is controversy regarding the role of transfusion of blood products in modulation of the recipient's immune system, leading to an increased incidence of postoperative infections and recurrence of certain types of tumors. This immune modulation is probably due to exposure of the recipient to donor leukocytes; hence, leukoreduction by filter devices might have a beneficial effect.

INFECTIOUS COMPLICATIONS OF BLOOD TRANSFUSION

Hepatitis Viruses

Among the hepatitis viruses, hepatitis B and C viruses, which are associated with chronic carrier states among the blood donor population, pose the greatest risk for transmission by blood products. Hepatitis D (formerly called the delta agent), although it can be transmitted by blood, requires prior infection with the hepatitis B virus. Because hepatitis A virus does not have a chronic carrier state, only collection of blood from the infected donor during the viremic period can lead to transmission. Donor blood screening programs for hepatitis B and C have greatly reduced the risks of transfusion-associated hepatitis. The risk of hepatitis B transmission by blood transfusion is estimated to be approximately 1 in 200,000 transfused units, and the risk for hepatitis C is estimated to be less than 1 in 3300 units transfused.

Retroviruses

Human immunodeficiency viruses (HIV-1 and HIV-2) and human T cell lymphotropic viruses (HTLV-I and HTLV-II) may be transmitted by blood products. Major advances have been made to prevent transmission of these viruses. Screening of donors with questionnaires and immunologic tests has made the blood supply fairly safe; application of newer screening techniques is expected to lower further the incidence of transmission of these viruses through blood products. The risk of transmission of HIV-1 is estimated to be 1 case per 450,000 to 660,000 units transfused. Better viral inactivation techniques and recombinant technology in preparation of coagulation factors have also contributed to blood product safety.

Other Viruses

Although over half of blood donors are seropositive for cytomegalovirus (CMV), it is estimated that less than 2% can transmit the virus. In immunocompetent recipients, CMV infection is in general of little clinical consequence. CMV-negative blood or high-efficiency leukocyte filters should be used in immunocompromised patients such as premature infants born to seronegative mothers and seronegative recipients of bone marrow transplants. Epstein-Barr virus can be transmitted by blood products and may very rarely cause hepatitis. Parvovirus B19, which produces erythroid hypoplasia in patients with chronic hemolytic states, may be transmitted by transfusion. There are no effective methods to screen transfusion products for these viruses.

Transmission of Other Infections

Rare diseases transmitted by transfusion therapy include malaria, babesiosis, trypanosomiasis, and syphilis. Transmission of malaria is controlled by deferring the donation of blood by potentially exposed individuals for 3 years. People with history of babesiosis are indefinitely deferred. Although not effective in preventing transmission of syphilis, standard serologic tests for syphilis are routinely performed in donor samples as an indicator of potentially high-risk behavior that makes transmission of other organisms more likely.

Bacterial contamination is an important cause of transfusion-associated morbidity and mortality, accounting for 16% of the transfusion-related deaths reported to the U.S. Food and Drug Administration between 1986 to 1991. Bacterial contamination can begin when the blood is drawn from the donor, either from the venipuncture site or from asymptomatic bacteremia, and the organisms can multiply in the rich culture medium of blood. Gram-negative organisms are seen in blood stored in the refrigerator, whereas gram-positive bacteria usually contaminate blood stored at room temperature. Septic transfusion reactions give rise to high fever, shock, renal failure, hemoglobinuria, and disseminated intravascular coagulation. Transfusion should be stopped and Gram's stain with culture obtained from the blood unit and the patient. Sometimes there is discoloration of the transfusion unit compared with the color of blood in the attached sealed segments. Immediate therapy with intravenous fluids and antibiotics should be begun along with other monitoring and supportive measures. Prevention of bacterial contamination includes thorough questioning of the donor, cleansing and sterilization of the venipuncture site, aseptic handling during separation of components, appropriate storage, and visual inspection for any color change before releasing the blood for transfusion.

MISCELLANEOUS ADVERSE EFFECTS OF TRANSFUSION

Iron Overload

Chronic transfusion therapy carries the risk of iron overload after red blood cell transfusions reach 50 to 100 units. The manifestations are similar to those seen with idiopathic hemochromatosis and include endocrine, hepatic, and cardiac failure. The iron chelation agent deferoxamine (Desferal) is available but difficult to use and not entirely effective.

Congestive Heart Failure

Circulatory overload leading to congestive heart failure may occur when blood is rapidly given to patients with compromised cardiovascular status. In such patients, packed red blood cells should be infused slowly with the patient in a semiupright position, and a diuretic such as furosemide should be given.

Complications of Massive Blood Product Transfusion

Among the complications of massive blood transfusions, coagulopathy and metabolic complications are prominent. Dilutional coagulopathy and thrombocytopenia are occasionally seen when massive amounts of packed red blood cells are transfused alone. To prevent this complication, it is useful to transfuse fresh frozen plasma and platelets along with red blood cells if the blood loss exceeds an entire blood volume. The potential for citrate toxicity and resultant hypocalcemia increases when large volumes of fresh frozen plasma, whole blood, or platelet concentrates are given at rates exceeding 100 mL per minute. Careful electrocardiographic monitoring should be performed and ionized calcium measured. If changes related to hypocalcemia occur, then small amounts of 10% calcium gluconate are given intravenously through a different venous access. Another complication of large-volume transfusion of cold blood is hypothermia, which can produce ventricular arrhythmias and can be prevented by warming the blood before infusion. Rarely, massive transfusion can produce hyperkalemia by potassium leakage from stored red blood cells; hence, careful monitoring is required.

The Digestive Syndrome

CHOLELITHIASIS AND CHOLECYSTITIS

method of
LILLIAN G. DAWES, M.D.
Northwestern University Medical School
Chicago, Illinois

Precipitation of components of bile into the formation of solid elements in the gallbladder results in gallstones. Millions of people develop gallstones. Approximately three quarters of patients who are found incidentally to have these aberrations continue to harbor them silently in their gallbladders. For the remaining patients, symptoms or complications lead them to seek medical attention.

The pathogenesis of gallstones is related to a combination of genetic and dietary factors. Certain populations have a very high incidence of gallstones. The incidence among the Pima Indians in the southwestern United States is extremely high; an estimated 70% develop gallstones. In addition to genetic predisposition, diet influences the risk of stone formation. High-fat and high-cholesterol diets are associated with a higher incidence of gallstones. Prolonged periods of fasting, intravenous feeding, and some diet plans promote the formation of stones in the gallbladder.

Gallstones occur at any age, but the risk of gallstone development increases with age. At any age, gallstones occur twice as often in women as in men. Hormonal therapy for birth control and hormonal replacement therapy increase the risk of gallstone formation; this suggests an association between female sex hormones and gallstones. Pregnancy also predisposes women to gallstones. Obesity, ileal resection, and intravenous nutrition are also known to increase the propensity to form gallstones.

There are several types of gallstones. Stones composed mainly of cholesterol, or cholesterol gallstones, are the most common gallstones in the United States. Twenty percent of all gallstones are pigment gallstones. Pigment gallstones are more frequent in hemolytic disorders, which increase the biliary secretion of bilirubin. Patients with sickle cell disease often develop pigment gallstones. Biliary infection, cirrhosis, and other liver disease are also conditions in which pigment gallstones are more common.

SYMPTOMS

Stones can reside in the gallbladder with no apparent symptoms. Once the stones start moving through the biliary system, there is usually associated discomfort. The resultant "attack" may be one of the first indications that a person has gallstones. This pain is referred to as "biliary colic." Biliary colic, although not typically a crescendo-decrescendo pain like colic from renal stones, is intermittent in nature. Biliary colic is usually described as right upper abdominal or epigastric pain that starts an hour or so after a fatty or spicy meal. This pain is constant while it lasts and usually resolves spontaneously in several hours. Pain that lasts more than 6 hours is more suggestive of acute cholecystitis. This pain may radiate to the back or to the right scapula. Nausea and vomiting often accompany the pain. Nonspecific chronic symptoms of gallstones may be fatty food intolerance, excessive belching, or flatulence. Diarrhea with certain foods may be a manifestation of impaired gallbladder function. Symptoms can be curtailed by controlling diet and avoiding spicy, fatty, and greasy foods. Once a person develops symptoms from the gallstones, however, it is likely that the stones will continue to manifest problems.

CHRONIC CHOLECYSTITIS

Once biliary colic is suspected, an ultrasonographic examination of the right upper quadrant is the most sensitive test. Ultrasonography, in addition to demonstrating the presence of gallstones, provides information about the liver and the biliary ductal system. Signs of acute inflammation may include thickening of the gallbladder wall, pericholecystic fluid, or a sonographic Murphy's sign (pain when the ultrasonographic probe approaches the gallbladder). Plain abdominal radiographs show calcifications in the right upper quadrant in 10 to 20% of patients with gallstones. Computed tomographic (CT) scans of the abdomen can show gallstones, but this imaging modality is not as sensitive as ultrasonography.

The treatment of choice for symptomatic gallstones or cholelithiasis is laparoscopic cholecystectomy. Placement of a laparoscope into the abdomen at the umbilicus with insufflation of the abdomen with CO_2 gas allows visualization of the intra-abdominal organs. Additional subxiphoid and subcostal ports allow for the dissection of the gallbladder. Laparoscopic removal of the gallbladder is possible in more than 95% of the elective cholecystectomies. The advantage of this technique over an open operation with a subcostal incision is the more rapid recovery. In uncomplicated cases, patients go home the same day of operation or the next day. Normal activity is resumed rapidly within a week or two of operation. The need for conversion to open operation is still occasionally necessary. This should be considered, not a complication, but rather good surgical judgment if the laparoscopic approach does not allow a safe operation. A small increase in common bile duct injuries has been seen since the introduction of laparoscopic surgery. Open operation is associated with a 0.2% incidence of bile duct injury; this incidence is approximately 0.4% with laparoscopic cholecystectomy.

Other nonsurgical methods have been used for the treatment of cholelithiasis. Gallstone dissolution agents such as bile salt therapy with ursodeoxycholate is safe but not as effective as cholecystectomy. The rate of recurrence of the gallstones after this therapy is high: approximately 50% within 5 years.

ACUTE CHOLECYSTITIS

If the episode of biliary colic persists longer than 6 hours, the disease process is probably acute cholecystitis. Patients with acute cholecystitis describe the pain as similar to previous symptoms, but this time the pain is more severe and persistent. In acute cholecystitis, the pain is usually in the right upper quadrant. The pain may radiate to the right scapula and remains constant. The physical examination reveals localized tenderness in the right upper quadrant. Murphy's sign is manifested when the patient is asked to take a deep breath while the examiner palpates the right upper abdomen: The patient will halt inspiration when the examiner's fingers approach the gallbladder. A tender palpable gallbladder can result from gallbladder distention, but most patients seek medical attention before the development of this physical finding. A nontender palpable gallbladder (Courvoisier's sign) is more indicative of a malignancy than of an inflammatory process in the gallbladder.

An elevated white blood cell count and a fever often accompany acute cholecystitis. Mild elevation in the serum liver function findings (i.e., aspartate aminotransferase [AST], alanine aminotransferase [ALT], and bilirubin) may also be seen. Any significant abnormality in these laboratory tests, however, should alert the physician to the possibility of bile duct obstruction. If a patient has jaundice with a fever and right upper quadrant pain, acute cholangitis or infection in an obstructed bile duct should be considered. If the obstruction is untreated, this can lead to sepsis, hypotension, and central nervous system depression. Imaging with endoscopic retrograde cholangiopancreatography (ERCP) is indicated, and this can be both diagnostic and therapeutic. If ERCP is unsuccessful or not available, transhepatic cholangiography and drainage can be performed. If the biliary obstruction is not relieved with either of these methods, operative decompression is needed.

Nuclear medicine scans can be used specifically to test for the presence of acute cholecystitis. The hallmark of acute cholecystitis is cystic duct obstruction. Biliary scintigraphy or nuclear scanning involves injecting an organic anion (iminodiacetic acid or a related compound) that is tagged with technetium Tc 99m. This organic anion can be visualized as it is rapidly taken up by the liver and excreted into the biliary tree. Abnormal scans do not show the gallbladder even with delayed imaging. This is a good test specifically for cystic duct obstruction if it is uncertain whether the clinical symptoms are attributable to the gallstones or if ultrasonography is not available and acute cholecystitis is suspected.

The first line of treatment of acute cholecystitis is intravenous fluids, bowel rest, and antibiotics. The antibiotic of choice should be a broad-spectrum antibiotic effective against the most common biliary tract organisms, such as *Escherichia coli*, *Klebsiella* species, and enterococci. If there is air in the gallbladder wall, or "emphysematous cholecystitis," an effective treatment for *Clostridium perfringens* should be part of the antibiotic regimen. Emphysematous cholecystitis is more common in diabetics and in males and necessitates early operation. Although uncommon, this infection is usually more virulent and is often associated with gallbladder gangrene.

Unless a patient is not a good surgical candidate, cholecystectomy is part of the recommended treatment for acute cholecystitis. Cholecystectomy is most often done during the hospitalization for acute cholecystitis. It has been suggested that earlier operation (within the first 72 hours after admission) leads to a reduction in the need for open operation. Although acute cholecystitis was previously considered a contraindication to the laparoscopic approach to remove the gallbladder, it is now known that laparoscopic cholecystectomy can be performed safely in this setting. The need for open operation occurs in 10 to 30% of the patients. Obesity, gallbladder wall thickening, and the presence of gangrene are associated with an increased risk for the need for laparotomy.

For patients who are at high risk for surgical complications and do not respond to medical treatment, a cholecystostomy can be considered. This can be done percutaneously with ultrasonographic guidance. In most cases, a percutaneous cholecystostomy leads to resolution of the symptoms, enabling an elective operation when the patient's medical condition improves.

A small percentage of patients with acute cholecystitis (less than 5%) do not have gallstones. The cause of "acalculous cholecystitis" is not known, but it may be related to a functional obstruction to the cystic duct or to gallbladder ischemia. This type of cholecystitis is most often seen in patients who are critically ill in the intensive care unit after trauma, burn injury, or acute medical illness such as myocardial infarction. Because many of these patients are intubated and sedated and therefore cannot describe symptoms, diagnosis can be difficult. This infection should be part of the differential diagnosis of sepsis of uncertain etiology in the intensive care unit. Gallbladder scintigraphy may be helpful for ruling out the diagnosis of acute cholecystitis, but nonfilling of the gallbladder in patients who are not enterally fed can be seen in the absence of cholecystitis. Ultrasonographic examination is often helpful; if the patient is a poor operative candidate, percutaneous gallbladder aspiration can be performed and a percutaneous cholecystostomy placed if the bile duct is infected. Cholecystectomy can then be performed if the infection does not clear with drainage and antibiotics or after the medical condition of the patient improves.

CHOLEDOCHOLITHIASIS

If the gallstones pass on through the biliary tree, they can become obstructed in the common bile duct. Common bile duct stones, or choledocholithiasis, occur in 5 to 15% of the cases of symptomatic gallstones. Obstruction of the bile duct can be the first sign of gallstones, and many affected patients have jaundice. This jaundice is usually accompanied by pain. If infection is also present with the obstructing stone, acute cholangitis or infection in the biliary ducts occurs, and urgent intervention is needed, as mentioned previously.

The differential diagnosis for a patient with common bile duct stones includes other causes of extrahepatic bile duct obstruction, such as pancreatic or bile duct malignancies. The diagnostic test of choice to confirm the extrahepatic bile duct obstruction is ultrasonography. If a malignancy is highly suspected (on the basis of associated weight loss, anemia, or blood in the stool), CT scan of the abdomen may be chosen instead to look for a mass. Both these modalities show dilated extrahepatic bile ducts and will most likely demonstrate stones in the gallbladder (CT scan is less sensitive than ultrasonograpy for gallstones). Only 30% of common bile duct stones are actually seen with ultrasonography. Although the clinical scenario, ultrasonography, or CT scan may suggest gallstone disease versus malignancy as the cause of the bile duct obstruction, other diagnostic imaging of the biliary tree is needed for confirmation.

ERCP is the test of choice because it can be both diagnostic and therapeutic. With an endoscope, the papilla of Vater is intubated, and dye is injected for a cholangiogram. Should a gallstone be found, it can usually be removed endoscopically and a sphincterotomy performed. If ERCP is unsuccessful or not available, a transhepatic cholangiogram can be performed to demonstrate the cause of the biliary obstruction. If common bile duct stones cannot be removed endoscopically, an operative exploration of the common bile duct is indicated.

Common bile duct stones can also cause pancreatitis. Biliary pancreatitis may rapidly abate, and these patients most likely have already passed the stone through the common bile duct into the gastrointestinal tract. Timing of cholecystectomy is dependent on the clinical situation, but a cholecystectomy can be performed during the same admission as for the pancreatitis, once the episode of pancreatitis has resolved. If an abnormality in serum liver function test results exists, a preoperative ERCP or intraoperative cholangiogram should be performed.

Not all stones in the common bile duct manifest with symptoms or laboratory abnormalities. Four percent of routine cholangiograms done at the time of cholecystectomy show unsuspected common bile duct stones. Small stones several millimeters in size usually pass spontaneously. If the stones are not removed intraoperatively, the patients should undergo postoperative ERCP. Postoperative ERCP is successful in removing more than 90% of stones.

GALLSTONE ILEUS

If a large gallstone is present in the gallbladder for prolonged periods, it can erode into surrounding structures and lead to formation of a cholecystenteric fistula. The most common place for this to occur is the duodenum, in which a cholecystoduodenal fistula is formed. The gallstone then either passes or becomes lodged in the intestine, causing a bowel obstruction. The point of obstruction is usually just proximal to the ileocecal valve. A typical patient with this problem is an elderly woman who comes to medical attention with a bowel obstruction but has had no previous surgery and does not have a hernia. Abdominal films show air in the biliary tree. Treatment is laparotomy with relief of the obstruction by removal of the stone.

SUMMARY

Cholelithiasis, or gallstone disease, is a common medical problem. Asymptomatic gallstones can be monitored, but once symptoms occur, a cholecystectomy is indicated. Acute cholecystitis, cholangitis, choledocholithiasis, biliary pancreatitis, and gallstone ileus are all potential complications of gallstone disease. Laparoscopic cholecystectomy can be performed in most cases, and endoscopic procedures are helpful in treating complications of gallstones such as cholangitis or common bile duct stones.

CIRRHOSIS

method of
PAUL J. POCKROS, M.D.
*Scripps Clinic and University of California, San
   Diego Medical School*
La Jolla, California

Cirrhosis is a pathologic process that results in nodular regeneration of hepatocytes separated by thick septi of scar tissue. The normal microscopic architecture of the liver, including the relationship between the portal tracts and the central veins, is distorted. The liver is firmer than usual, with a rounded leading edge, and is often smaller than normal with a diminished weight. Nodules may occur in sizes ranging from less than 3 mm in diameter (micronodular) to 20 mm in diameter (macronodular). The distinction between these two is of limited clinical value because most patients have a mixture of both large and small nodules.

The physiologic consequences of cirrhosis are basically the results of increased resistance of blood flow through the liver sinusoids and diminished function of the liver cells (hepatocytes). Increased blood flow leads to portal hypertension, which in turn leads to development of collateral vessels (including varices), resulting in reduction of

TABLE 1. **Causes of Cirrhosis in the United States**

Chronic hepatitis C	26%
Chronic hepatitis C plus alcohol	14%
Alcoholic liver disease	24%
Cholestatic and other liver disorders	22%
Chronic hepatitis B	11%
Chronic hepatitis B plus alcohol	3%

portal flow to the liver. This reduces the number of functioning hepatocytes as cirrhosis worsens and portal hypertension increases, ultimately leading to hepatic decompensation as a result of reduced synthetic and excretory function of the liver.

The classic physical findings of patients with cirrhosis include decreased muscle mass, especially in the face and upper torso; development of vascular spiders, usually on the face, chest, arms, and back; and development of organomegaly. The liver edge may or may not be palpable; if it is, it is quite firm. The spleen tip is often palpable with inspiration. Patients may or may not have shifting dullness on percussion or other features of ascites. Dilated superficial abdominal collateral veins are often present in patients with portal hypertension. Other stigmata of chronic liver disease include palmar erythema, opaque white fingernails, and gynecomastia, usually related to the use of spironolactone (Aldactone). Patients with well-compensated cirrhosis may have none of these findings on examination and often appear quite normal on physical examination.

The most common causes of cirrhosis in the United States have changed since the 1980s. Table 1 shows the frequency of these. Chronic viral hepatitis, especially hepatitis C, has emerged as a leading cause of chronic liver disease in the United States. This fact was unknown before the readily available testing for hepatitis C virus and the detection of the large prevalence (1.5%) of this virus in the blood donor population in the United States. More than 4 million people in the United States are infected, and nearly one third of patients whose condition was previously labeled as alcoholic liver disease have hepatitis C antibodies. The magnitude of this epidemic assumes larger proportions because of the frequency of this infection in the population aged 30 to 50. Most of these people acquired the infection in the late 1960s or early 1970s, when hepatitis C was epidemic in the United States. The incidence of new infections in the United States has decreased dramatically as a result of widespread screening for blood donors and the decreased frequency of high-risk behaviors (intranasal cocaine use, intravenous drug use, and sex with multiple partners).

TREATMENT AND GENERAL MEASURES

Liver Transplantation

It is virtually impossible today to discuss the management of patients with end-stage liver disease without at least a brief discussion of liver transplantation. Liver transplantation should be considered as a treatment option in any patient with cirrhosis who has evidence of decompensation, including (but not limited to) ascites, hepatic encephalopathy, muscle wasting with albumin loss, jaundice (especially in cases of cholestatic disorders), or disability caused by liver disease.

The management of patients who are considered candidates for transplantation is, by nature, somewhat different than that of patients who are not considered transplantation candidates. The attention to detail and meticulous care of patients awaiting transplantation has created a new specialty in hepatology because of the time, effort, and expertise necessary. In discussing the management of patients with cirrhosis, I attempt to specify the added care and attention required for patients awaiting liver transplantation.

At the time that this article is written, there are more than five times as many patients awaiting liver transplantation in the United States as will undergo transplantation this year, and the average waiting time is more than 12 months. As such, the care and attention to detail in maintaining these patients has taken on an increasingly important role. The United Network of Organ Sharing has attempted to prioritize the waiting status of patients according to severity of disease. The Child-Pugh staging score plays a fundamental role in determining the status and should be recalculated each time a patient is seen at follow-up visits (Table 2). For this reason alone, patients awaiting liver transplantation are seen at intervals no longer than 16 weeks.

Other Measures

In general, all patients with cirrhosis should be seen by the physician on a regular basis (every 4 to 12 weeks) for office visit, physical examination, and laboratory tests, including hepatic panel, electrolytes, creatinine, complete blood cell count, prothrombin time, and magnesium (Table 3).

All patients should receive vaccination for hepati-

TABLE 2. **Child-Pugh Staging Score**

Parameter	1	2	3
Ascites	None	Easily controlled	Difficult to control
Encephalopathy	None	Mild	Severe
Albumin (gm/dL)	>3.5	2.8–3.5	<2.8
Bilirubin (mg/dL)	<2.0	2.0–3.0	>3.0
Prothrombin time (seconds prolonged)	1.0–4.0	4.0–6.0	>6.0

Class A: 5–6 points; Class B: 7–9 points; Class C: 10–15 points.

TABLE 3. General Measures for All Cirrhotic Patients

Vaccinations
Hepatitis A (Havrix), 2 doses
Hepatitis B (Recombivax HB), 3 doses
Influenza, annually

Monitoring Serum Tests Regularly
Electrolytes and creatinine
Hepatic panel
Complete blood cell count
Prothrombin time
Magnesium

Monitoring for Hepatocellular Carcinoma
Serum AFP level and abdominal ultrasonography every 6 months
Dual-phase CT scan or MRI with ferumoxides (Feridex) more frequently if listed for liver transplantation or if AFP level rises

Monitor for Gastrointestinal Bleeding Risk
Endoscopy for varices annually if they have never bled; every 6 months after band ligation or sclerotherapy
Endoscopy and/or duplex ultrasonography every 6 months after TIPS
Flexible sigmoidoscopy or colonoscopy for colon cancer screening

Monitor for Cardiopulmonary Risk
Echocardiogram every 6 months for patients at risk for pulmonary hypertension
Contrast-enhanced echocardiography or radioactive macroaggregated albumin study for patients at risk for orthodeoxia
Angiography for patients at risk for progression of coronary artery disease or with coronary stents (every 6 months if listed for liver transplantation)

Monitor for Bone Disease (Males with Cholestatic Disorders; All Females)
Bone density measurement of spine annually
Bone disease prevention (see Table 4)

Avoid or Limit
Raw seafood (*Vibrio vulnificus*)
Excessive sodium intake
Elective surgery and dental extractions
Vitamin K or fresh-frozen plasma, unless invasive procedures are planned
Limit acetaminophen to 2000 mg/24 hours
Avoid aminoglycosides and nonsteroidal anti-inflammatory drugs

Abbreviations: AFP = alpha-fetoprotein; CT = computed tomographic; MRI = magnetic resonance imaging; TIPS = transjugular intrahepatic portosystemic shunt.

tis A (2 doses) and hepatitis B (3 doses). There is evidence that influenza virus can result in decompensation of liver function in patients with underlying cirrhosis, and all patients should therefore receive influenza vaccination annually. Patients should be monitored on a regular basis for hepatocellular carcinoma, with serum alpha-fetoprotein monitoring and abdominal ultrasonography every 6 months. This is especially important in patients with chronic hepatitis C or chronic hepatitis B, because they seem to be at strikingly increased risk of development of hepatocellular carcinoma. Data suggest that up to 30% of patients undergoing liver transplantation for chronic viral hepatitis C are found at the time of transplantation to have an incidental hepatocellular carcinoma in the explanted liver. The Scripps Clinic uses dual-phase computed tomographic (CT) scan or magnetic resonance imaging with ferumoxides (Feridex) con-

trast at frequent intervals if patients are believed to be at increased risk for development of liver cancer while awaiting liver transplantation. These methods are also used if a rise in alpha-fetoprotein level is identified.

Patients with cirrhosis should undergo upper gastrointestinal endoscopy initially to check for the presence of esophageal or gastric varices. If varices are identified and are of significant size, patients should begin prophylactic beta blocker therapy in the form of propranolol (Inderal), 10 to 80 mg twice daily. The dosage should be started slowly because postural hypotension will occur. Endoscopy should be repeated annually for patients at increased risk for variceal hemorrhage. If patients have undergone band ligation or sclerotherapy, follow-up endoscopy for surveillance should be done every 6 months. Patients who have received a transjugular intrahepatic portasystemic shunt (TIPS) should undergo upper gastrointestinal endoscopy and duplex ultrasonography of the TIPS at 6-month intervals. For further details regarding management of these patients, see the article "Bleeding Esophagogastric Varices." Flexible sigmoidoscopy or colonoscopy for colon cancer screening should be done at the time of initial evaluation and repeated at 3- to 5-year intervals.

Patients at risk for pulmonary hypertension should be monitored by echocardiography every 6 months. Contrast-enhanced echocardiography or radioactive macroaggregated albumin studies should be done for patients at risk for orthodeoxia, and this is done in the Scripps Clinic in all patients undergoing liver transplantation evaluation. Angiography is reserved for patients at risk for progression of coronary artery disease and those with coronary stents who are awaiting liver transplantation. Patients with coronary stents should undergo repeat angiography at 6-month intervals.

All female patients should be monitored for bone disease, as should males with cholestatic disorders or who have taken corticosteroids. Bone density measurement of the spine is done at the time of transplantation evaluation and annually thereafter. Bone disease prevention measures should be taken in patients at risk (Table 4).

Cirrhotic patients should avoid raw seafood because of the risk of *Vibrio vulnificus* infection. Patients without ascites and edema should avoid excess

TABLE 4. Managing Bone Disease of Cirrhotics Through Prevention

Condition	Prevention Technique
Osteomalacia	Oral calcium supplements
	Vitamin D supplements
	Exposure to ultraviolet light
	Calcitriol (Rocaltrol)
Osteoporosis	Low-impact exercise
	Oral calcium supplements
	Estrogen or testosterone replacement
	Alendronate sodium (Fosamax)

sodium intake, and patients with ascites and/or edema should be placed on a diet with sodium restricted to 22 to 44 mEq per day. Elective surgery and dental extractions should be avoided because of the risk of primary fibrinolysis in cirrhotic patients with prolonged euglobulin clot lysis times. If hematomas occur spontaneously, the euglobulin clot lysis time should be checked. Vitamin K and fresh-frozen plasma are generally avoided unless invasive procedures are planned. The Scripps Clinic recommends limitations of acetaminophen (Tylenol) to 2000 mg per 24 hours to avoid the possibility of exceeding a critical dosage in patients with underlying liver disease; it is known that patients with cirrhosis have glutathione depletion and are therefore at increased risk for acetaminophen hepatotoxicity. Aminoglycosides and nonsteroidal anti-inflammatory drugs must also be avoided because of the risk of inducing renal insufficiency in cirrhotic patients. Special care must be taken in management of drugs whose pharmacokinetics are altered in cirrhotic patients. These include phenytoin sodium (Dilantin), chlordiazepoxide HCl (Librium), and all diuretics (to be discussed later in this chapter).

DISEASE-SPECIFIC THERAPIES

Alcoholic Liver Disease

The mainstay of treatment for alcoholic liver disease is abstinence from alcohol. The Scripps Clinic requires that patients with a history of alcohol abuse be abstinent for 6 months before evaluation for liver transplantation. In addition, most are required to have documentation of 6 months of abstinence before acceptance for transplantation. This usually requires attendance at Alcoholics Anonymous and a log documenting this attendance to be brought to the office during follow-up appointments. In addition, periodic spot alcohol levels are checked during routine laboratory testing. Many patients with alcoholic liver disease who show evidence for decompensation recover during this period of abstinence and may ultimately not require transplantation. Unfortunately, some alcoholic patients die from fatal complications of liver disease before satisfying this period of abstinence. Despite this fact, because of the competition for organs at the current time, we strictly adhere to these principles.

Patients with alcoholic hepatitis may have underlying cirrhosis, or they may have a precirrhotic lesion that predisposes them to development of cirrhosis. These patients differ clinically in that they often have jaundice, fever, profound leukocytosis, and a markedly enlarged liver, often with tenderness and a bruit present on examination. Management of patients with alcoholic hepatitis differs from that of patients with cirrhosis primarily because of the usefulness of corticosteroid therapy in patients who have evidence of severe disease (i.e., patients with a history of hepatic encephalopathy or a Maddrey index of >32 [Maddrey index = serum bilirubin concentra-

tion in mg per dL + prothrombin time prolongation in seconds × 4.6]). Results of one trial have suggested that the use of pentoxifylline* (Trental), 400 mg three times a day, as an inhibitor of tumor necrosis factor is an effective treatment for alcoholic hepatitis.

Primary Biliary Cirrhosis

All patients with a confirmed diagnosis of primary biliary cirrhosis in the Scripps Clinic have undergone liver biopsy and usually have a positive result of an antimitochondrial antibody test. Patients are staged by liver biopsy at regular intervals, usually every 3 years. My patients are treated with ursodeoxycholic acid (Urso or Actigall) at a dose of 10 to 15 mg per kg for all stages of disease. In patients with more advanced disease, it is unlikely that the use of ursodeoxycholic acid will defer liver transplantation, but the drug may be useful for itching and the bilirubin elevations seen in more advanced stages of liver disease. These patients, usually female, are at increased risk for bone disease and therefore require careful monitoring, with bone density tests of the spine done on an annual basis. The Scripps Clinic places patients on bone disease prevention measures as soon as bone density examinations show any evidence for developing osteoporosis. Low-impact exercise and oral calcium supplements in the form of calcium carbonate (Tums), 2 to 3 tablets daily, are most effective. Postmenopausal women are placed on the estradiol transdermal patch system (Estraderm patch, 0.05 mg applied twice weekly). Patients with more severe disease may be placed on calcitriol, OH vitamin D (Rocaltrol), 0.25 μg per day, or alendronate sodium (Fosamax), 10 mg daily (see Table 4).

Primary Sclerosing Cholangitis

The managing physician should be amenable to the use of oral antibiotics or hospitalization with intravenous antibiotics for patients with this condition. If fever or other signs of acute cholangitis occur, the Scripps Clinic usually places patients on antibiotics immediately. Endoscopic retrograde cholangiography (ERCP) with stent placement is useful in many cases in which a dominant stricture causes cholestasis. Stents are usually changed prophylactically at 3- to 6-month intervals. The Scripps Clinic often places patients on ursodeoxycholic acid at a dose of 15 to 30 mg per kg if stents are in place, in order to benefit from the choleretic effect of this drug. Older patients, those with a history of colon carcinoma, and those with a dominant stricture are at increased risk for development of cholangiocarcinoma. Screening tests are sometimes, but not always, helpful in showing evidence of cholangiocarcinoma (serum tests of cancer antigen [CA] 19–9 and carcinoembryonic antigen [CEA]). Abdominal CT scan and ERCP tests are sel-

---

*Not FDA approved for this indication.

dom confirmatory of this diagnosis. Patients at risk of cholangiocarcinoma should undergo transplantation, if at all possible, before the development of this tumor. Once cholangiocarcinoma has been documented, the patient is not a candidate for transplantation, because of the universal recurrence of this disease after transplantation. Patients with a history of sclerosing cholangitis are at increased risk for colon carcinoma and should undergo screening colonoscopy annually.

Autoimmune Hepatitis

Liver biopsy is done routinely in the Scripps Clinic when a diagnosis of autoimmune hepatitis is established. A number of patients have cirrhosis at the time of diagnosis. In rare instances, the disease advances to cirrhosis if patients are maintained on adequate immunosuppression. Although liver biopsy reveals significant necro-inflammatory activity, we rarely use this to monitor the disease. Instead, elevation of aminotransferase levels is used as a surrogate of necro-inflammatory activity. Immunosuppression is usually started with prednisone, 20 to 40 mg daily, and the dosage is gradually reduced to 10 mg or less daily. Patients are placed on azathioprine (Imuran), 50 to 100 mg daily, in order to spare corticosteroid dosage. Approximately 75% of patients are eventually able to stop taking corticosteroids and be maintained on azathioprine, 100 to 200 mg daily. In my experience it is rare, although possible, that patients may stop all immunosuppression.

Patients who are resistant to conventional immunosuppression in the Scripps Clinic often have type 2a autoimmune hepatitis. This diagnosis is confirmed by a positive anti–liver/kidney microsomal antibody test (anti-LKM), and most of these patients come to medical attention with cirrhosis. They are generally young females in their late teens or early 20s. These patients may have decompensated liver disease and sometimes require liver transplantation. A number of these patients require immunosuppression with cyclosporine (Neoral), 100 to 200 mg per day, or tacrolimus (Prograf), 1 to 4 mg daily.

Chronic Viral Hepatitis

Patients with chronic hepatitis C and cirrhosis are candidates for antiviral therapy as long as they have not shown evidence of hepatic decompensation. Current data suggest that these patients do not have virologic responses to interferon therapy at the same rate as do patients with less severe histologic disease. However, studies with combination therapy of interferon and ribavirin has shown success in a number of patients with cirrhosis. Furthermore, long-acting interferons (pegylated interferon) may be more effective in patients with cirrhosis. Oral therapies with milder or no toxic effects are expected ultimately to be given to this sizable group of patients. Of great concern in the Scripps Clinic are patients with chronic hepatitis C and cirrhosis who are older than 55 years and in whom disease has had a significant duration. These patients have an increased risk for development of hepatocellular carcinoma and may be treated with interferon to diminish this risk. One study from Europe has suggested that interferon therapy may diminish the risk of hepatic decompensation in patients with cirrhosis, although a larger trial must be done to confirm these data.

Patients with chronic hepatitis B who have cirrhosis have a 5-year survival rate of approximately 50% if they remain viremic. These patients should be treated with antiviral therapy. If they have not shown evidence of hepatic decompensation, they may be suitable candidates for a 16-week treatment trial of interferon alfa-2b (Intron A) at 5 MU daily or 10 MU every other day. Alternatively, nucleoside analogue therapy is now available and has been approved by the U.S. Food and Drug Administration (FDA) for patients with chronic hepatitis B, in the form of lamivudine (Epivir) at a dose of 100 mg daily. Other nucleoside and nucleotide analogue treatments are currently in clinical trials (adefovir,* lobucovir,† and famciclovir†) and may be useful in the treatment of chronic hepatitis B in the future. Patients with chronic hepatitis B are also at risk for development of hepatocellular carcinoma and should be monitored with serum alpha-fetoprotein measurements and abdominal ultrasonography at 6-month intervals.

MAINTENANCE OF COMPLICATIONS OF CIRRHOSIS

Ascites

The mainstay of management of patients with ascites and edema is a diet in which sodium intake is restricted to 22 to 44 mEq daily and oral diuretics. I prefer to avoid spironolactone in favor of a potassium-sparing diuretic with a shorter half-life, such as amiloride (Midamor), 10 to 25 mg daily. If necessary, I add a loop diuretic such as furosemide (Lasix), 20 to 80 mg in divided doses, when edema appears or ascites is resistant to potassium-sparing diuretics alone. Plasma volume contraction should be avoided because renal insufficiency develops easily in patients with end-stage liver disease. Serum electrolytes, especially serum sodium and potassium, as well as serum creatinine, should be monitored frequently during periods in which the dosage of diuretics is changed or when new medications are added.

When ascites becomes diuretic-resistant, the Scripps Clinic prefers the use of large-volume paracentesis for management. The use of 25% human serum albumin (100 mL) after paracentesis is expensive but probably helpful in cases in which paracentesis is repeated frequently. Paracentesis fluid should be analyzed for cell count and culture after every procedure performed, because infections can develop during the intervals between paracentesis.

*Not available in the United States.
†Not FDA approved for this indication.

The experience of the Scripps Clinic with the use of TIPS, when done solely for management of diuretic-resistant ascites, has been poor, and we avoid this alternative in most cases. We prefer to reserve TIPS for patients with variceal hemorrhage for which conventional management has failed.

Although effective for ascites, we rarely use peritoneovenous shunts that are surgically placed for management of ascites. Many problems have occurred in the past with use of these shunts, including occlusions of the shunt valve and occasionally fatal disseminated intravascular coagulation (DIC).

Spontaneous Bacterial Peritonitis

Whenever suspected, paracentesis should be performed to rule out spontaneous bacterial peritonitis (SBP). Patients who are hospitalized for renal failure, hepatic encephalopathy, gastrointestinal bleeding, or other complications of liver disease should routinely undergo paracentesis to rule out this diagnosis. A cell count of more than 250 polymorphonuclear cells per mm^3 indicates infection, and treatment should be initiated. Ascites cultures in blood culture bottles inoculated at the bedside for aerobic and anaerobic cultures should be sent immediately. Blood cultures are often positive and should be drawn simultaneously.

Gram's stain of ascites is rarely helpful because of the low bacterial counts present. Most common organisms seen in bacterial peritonitis are either gram-negative from translocation across the bowel wall or *Streptococcus pneumoniae*. Patients with cirrhosis who are hospitalized for any reason and who have ascites should undergo paracentesis at the time of admission.

Patients with suspected bacterial peritonitis should be started on cefotaxime (Claforan), 1 to 2 gm every 8 hours intravenously. If needed, a repeat paracentesis should be done 48 hours after treatment is started. This should produce at least a 50% fall in the polymorphonuclear cell count and negative cultures. If it does not, resistant organisms such as *Enterococcus* species or secondary bacterial peritonitis (more than one organism cultured, low ascites glucose, and ascites protein level > 2 gm per dL) should be sought.

Initial episodes of SBP can be prevented in patients with ascites protein levels of 1 gm per dL or less, as can the recurrence of SBP in patients who have had previous episodes, with the use of norfloxacin (Noroxin), 400 mg daily, or trimethoprim-sulfamethoxazole (Septra), 1 DS tablet daily. The Scripps Clinic does not often maintain patients on these drugs longer than 30 to 60 days because of the risk of development of fungal superinfection.

Hepatic Hydrothorax

Hepatic hydrothorax should be suspected whenever shortness of breath develops suddenly in a patient who has a known diagnosis of cirrhosis. The diagnosis of hepatic hydrothorax is usually made easily in auscultatory examination in the physician's office and from chest radiograph. New cases may respond to diuretics initially but quickly become refractory with the development of hyponatremia and renal insufficiency.

Management of this condition is not ideal, and patients should undergo liver transplantation as soon as possible. The development of hydrothorax usually is predictive of a poor outcome. Repeat ultrasonography-guided thoracentesis is effective but poses a risk of puncture of intercostal blood vessels when done repeatedly. TIPS is effective but poses a risk of liver failure, which in our experience is unacceptable.

The risk of pneumothorax is added to possible complications of bleeding and infection in patients with repeat ultrasonography-guided thoracentesis. Spontaneous bacterial empyema may occur in patients with hepatic hydrothorax and is similar to the development of SBP, although it may occur without the development of SBP. For patients with ascites and hydrothorax, both fluids should be analyzed when infection is suspected.

Variceal Bleeding

In the Scripps Clinic, patients are managed by band ligation or endoscopic sclerotherapy unless previous endoscopic therapy has failed or the patients have bleeding gastric varices. In such cases, TIPS is effective and usually successful. Post-TIPS hepatic encephalopathy may occur and normally responds to lactulose therapy (Cephulac) at a dosage of 30 mL every 3 to 6 hours as needed. Surgical shunts are usually avoided in patients who are candidates for liver transplantation but may be placed on occasion when transplantation can be successfully delayed or deferred by the shunt. In such cases, the distal splenorenal shunt is preferred over portacaval surgery.

Prophylactic beta blockade may be indicated for patients who have not previously experienced bleeding but in whom moderate esophageal varices are detected on endoscopy. More details are available in the article "Bleeding Esophagogastric Varices."

Hepatic Encephalopathy

Cirrhotic patients with hepatic encephalopathy should be carefully examined for signs of infection, including bacterial peritonitis, gastrointestinal bleeding, severe hyponatremia, and other electrolyte disturbances. In the Scripps Clinic, the most common cause of hepatic encephalopathy is excessive diuretic therapy or the use of sleeping medications. All patients should be carefully questioned with regard to the use of these drugs. In patients in whom excessive diuretic therapy is suspected, the plasma volume contraction is usually treated by rapid hydration with normal saline or human serum plasma (Plasmanate) at 500 to 1000 mL over 2 to 3 hours.

All patients with hepatic encephalopathy are

treated with lactulose (Cephulac), 30 mL one to three times daily as needed to induce loose stools two to three times per day. Antibiotics such as neomycin, 500 mg daily, or metronidazole (Flagyl), 250 to 750 mg daily, may be useful additional treatments for the prevention of recurrent hepatic encephalopathy. Severe protein restrictions are rarely needed, in our experience, and lead to protein-calorie malnutrition if used indiscriminately in patients with cirrhosis.

Hepatopulmonary Syndrome

This condition occurs in approximately 5 to 10% of patients with cirrhosis who are awaiting liver transplantation, and it may be difficult to detect. Patients who complain of shortness of breath at elevation or high altitude or with exertion should be investigated for orthodeoxia. The diagnosis of hepatopulmonary syndrome may be confirmed by contrast-enhanced echocardiography or radioactive macroaggregated albumin particles in the brain or kidney, rather than the lung, after injection into an arm vein.

Treatment with oxygen supplementation and rest are the usual mainstays of therapy until liver transplantation can be performed. Symptoms of orthodeoxia often take months to fully resolve after completion of liver transplantation.

BLEEDING ESOPHAGEAL VARICES

method of
JOHN S. GOFF, M.D.
Rocky Mountain Gastroenterology Associates and
University of Colorado Health Sciences Center
Denver, Colorado

Esophageal and gastric varices are common complications of cirrhosis. The risk for bleeding from these varices is 25 to 35%. The rate of mortality from variceal bleeding has been reported to vary between 30 and 50%. Because the risk of bleeding is high and the rate of mortality from bleeding is significant, attempts at prophylactic measures to prevent bleeding have been employed with variable success. There is strong evidence that reduction of the patient's resting pulse by 25% with a beta blocker (propranolol, atenolol, or nadolol) prevents first-time bleeding because this correlates with a decrease in portal pressure. Isosorbide-5-mononitrate at 40 mg twice daily has been shown in small studies to be effective for preventing first-time bleeding. Better methods are still needed to determine who is at highest risk of bleeding and therefore most likely to benefit from prophylactic therapy. Better methods are also needed for assessing the effect of the drugs on portal pressure.

Endoscopic techniques have been used to prevent variceal bleeding. Endoscopic sclerotherapy (EST) has been used for many years to treat bleeding varices, but currently is not indicated for prophylaxis because of the lack of efficacy. Endoscopic variceal ligation (EVL) may be better than EST for managing acute variceal bleeding. Recent small studies have successfully used EVL for prophylaxis.

PATHOPHYSIOLOGY

Cirrhosis of the liver results in sinusoidal damage with resultant inability of blood to easily traverse the liver. This resistance results in increased portal pressure. When the pressure exceeds 12 mm Hg, the risk for variceal bleeding increases. Varices can be located in any part of the gastrointestinal tract, although the esophagus and proximal stomach are the most common sites. Isolated gastric varices are occasionally seen, particularly in patients with splenic vein thrombosis. Patients with large paraesophageal collateral veins are at increased risk of recurrent bleeding despite endoscopic therapy.

MANIFESTATION AND DIAGNOSIS

Patients with bleeding varices usually have obvious signs: hematemesis, hematochezia or melena, decreased blood pressure, and anemia. However, the simple presence of cirrhosis and thus of suspected portal hypertension does not exclude other possible sources of bleeding. Up to 50% of patients with portal hypertension have bleeding from nonvariceal sites. Some of these hemorrhages result from portal hypertensive gastropathy, which is related to increased portal pressure, but the majority are not related to the increased portal pressure. Therefore, these patients need to undergo urgent upper endoscopy to establish a diagnosis so that appropriate therapy can be initiated. Before endoscopy a nasogastric tube, preferably larger than No. 30 French, should be placed to aspirate and lavage the stomach. There is no significant increased risk in placing one of the tubes in a patient with varices. The procedure allows the physician to establish whether bleeding is still active and helps clear the stomach so that effective endoscopy can be performed.

INITIAL THERAPY

The first intervention for any patient with acute bleeding is to establish excellent intravenous access and then to begin volume replacement. This can start in most patients with crystalloid, followed by type-specific blood. If the patient is actively bleeding and the presence of portal hypertension is known or highly suspected, vasopressin or octreotide can be administered empirically to try to lower portal pressure acutely and thus reduce or stop the bleeding. Vasopressin* (Pitressin) is used at doses of 0.1 to 1.0 unit per minute; doses exceeding 0.6 unit per minute are of doubtful added benefit. This drug causes significant vascular constriction, which can lead to organ ischemia or necrosis. Patients with coronary artery disease or peripheral vascular disease should not receive this medication if possible. Nitroglycerin administerred intravenously at 0.3 mg per minute or through a patch can be added to vasopressin to reduce the cardiac and vascular risks. Octreotide* (Sandostatin), a synthetic analogue of somatostatin, lowers portal pressure without the side effects of vasopressin. Studies have shown considerable efficacy for octreotide in doses of 50 to 200 μg per hour† intravenously after a 50-μg bolus. Fresh-frozen

---

*Not FDA approved for this indication.
†Exceeds dosage recommended by the manufacturer.

plasma is indicated for patients with ongoing bleeding who have very prolonged prothrombin times. Similarly, platelets may be given if the platelet count is less than 50,000 and bleeding is persisting.

Patients who are encephalopathic, intoxicated, or otherwise mentally impaired need to be considered for endotracheal intubation before endoscopy or other invasive measures because of the high risk for aspiration. Any patient with variceal bleeding is at increased risk of an adverse outcome if complications such as aspiration pneumonia or infection develop. In fact, a study showed improved outcome in bleeding cirrhotic patients who were given prophylactic antibiotics (amoxicillin–clavulanic acid [Augmentin] and ciprofloxacin [Cipro]).

Definitive Initial Therapy

The Sengstaken-Blakemore (SB) tube with the Minnesota modification (an added suction port above the esophageal balloon) can be used to gain control of bleeding esophageal or proximal gastric varices, but it should be used only if the bleeding source is certain. The SB tube must be placed properly and monitored closely because there is moderate to high potential for doing harm. For most patients, it is recommended to inflate both the esophageal and gastric balloon initially and then to deflate them in 12 to 24 hours to avoid mucosal injury. Once the balloons are deflated, it is advisable to proceed with therapy that will prevent further bleeding, because the rebleeding rate after deflation of the SB tube is 80% or more. More definitive therapy includes endoscopic treatment (EST or EVL), transhepatic or transmesenteric (minilaparotomy) embolization, surgical interventions (shunts, ligation, devascularization), transjugular intrahepatic portosystemic shunts (TIPS), and orthotopic liver transplantation.

Preferential initial definitive therapy is either EST or EVL. Both injection of sclerosant (1.5% sodium tetradecyl sulfate [Sotradecol] or 5% ethanolamine oleate [Ethamolin]) and placement of rubber bands on esophageal varices have been shown to prevent rebleeding and prolong survival. To achieve this goal, patients must be treated initially and then at frequent intervals (1 to 2 weeks) until the varices are eradicated. The sooner eradication is achieved, the better are chances of preventing further bleeding. Unfortunately, EST is associated with many side effects (fever, chest pain, mediastinitis, pleural effusions, deep esophageal ulcers, esophageal perforation, and strictures). EVL is as efficacious as EST but has a much lower side effect profile and appears to actually result in less rebleeding and improved mortality in direct comparisons with EST. EVL requires the use of an overtube, which has been reported to cause esophageal perforations in a few patients. With the introduction of multiple ligators, the overtube needs to be used less frequently or not at all, which makes EVL even safer and quicker.

Radiologic embolization of the coronary vein and its collateral vessels, which feed the bleeding varices, can effectively stop bleeding. However, the transhepatic approach can be difficult with a very scarred, hard liver, and ascites makes the risk for complications too high to advise the transhepatic approach. An approach through the transmesenteric vein avoids these problems but adds the need for a small incision with its attendant complications. Surgical procedures have had variable success. Devascularization of the proximal stomach and esophagus with or without esophageal transection has had its proponents, but it has not been widely accepted as a very safe and effective method. Surgically created portosystemic shunts are very effective in controlling bleeding and preventing rebleeding, but they are associated with significant morbidity and mortality, especially in Child's class C patients. Mesocaval (H-graft) and distal splenorenal (Warren) shunts have been developed to try to reduce the postshunt encephalopathy rate. This has been successful to some degree, but these shunts are more prone to obstruction by clots, and thus encephalopathy may still develop, although with a more delayed time of onset.

The introduction of the TIPS procedure has greatly improved our ability to manage patients in whom endoscopic therapy has failed. The TIPS can be successfully placed by trained radiologists in up to 95% of cases. This shunt can effectively lower the portal pressure to less than 12 mm Hg and thus greatly reduce the rebleeding rate. The shunts are prone to obstruction by clots and to stenosis; monitoring for these by ultrasonography or, in many cases, by repeat venography is needed. Nonetheless, TIPS is often an excellent bridge to liver transplantation. It can be used in patients who are not transplantation candidates if they are willing to return for follow-up management. Unfortunately, encephalopathy is seen after TIPS, which can limit its utility in patients with poor liver function. Liver transplantation is still the ultimate solution for uncontrolled variceal bleeding.

The presence of gastric varices is a distinctly more difficult situation because these are not as easy to eradicate with EST or EVL alone. Large-volume sclerotherapy was shown to be a little better than standard dosing, but the results were still very poor in comparison with the results for treating esophageal varices. Combination therapy, EVL plus EST, has been effective in patients with isolated varices in the cardia of the stomach. These patients need very effective acid suppression after placement of bands, to avoid early dislodgment of the bands. Injecting glues (cyanoacrylate) into the gastric varices can be effective, but these materials are not yet available in the United States. These patients are to be considered for shunt placement earlier than those with only esophageal varices.

LONG-TERM TREATMENT

Although repeated endoscopic treatment eradicates varices, reduces rebleeding, and improves chances of survival in cirrhotic patients, these outcomes are limited primarily to Child's class A and B patients. No study has demonstrated improved survival for Child's class C patients, and some have not even been able to show less rebleeding. Cost issues come into play when physicians try to decide on repeated endoscopic therapy versus a shunt procedure in Child's class C patients. It is not clear at this time which of these various choices is most cost effective. The available expertise and the patient's overall condition must be considered in the decision on which therapy to choose.

Lowering portal pressure medically has been shown to reduce rebleeding. This can be done as single-modality therapy, or it can be combined with endoscopic therapy to improve survival and reduce rebleeding. Beta blockers are usually used to reduce portal pressure, but their effect can only be estimated, because there is no easy way to noninvasively measure portal pressure. The standard is to aim for a 25% reduction in resting pulse rate by using propranolol (Inderal), atenolol (Tenormin), or nadolol (Corgard). Favorable results have also been demonstrated with isosorbide-5-mononitrate (ISMO), 40 mg twice daily. It may be more efficacious to combine a beta blocker with isosorbide. Once the varices have been eradicated with EST or EVL, medical therapy can be discontinued unless there are continued problems with portal hypertensive gastropathy.

DYSPHAGIA AND ESOPHAGEAL OBSTRUCTION

method of
EUGENE S. BONAPACE, M.D., and
HENRY P. PARKMAN, M.D.
Temple University School of Medicine
Philadelphia, Pennsylvania

Dysphagia is defined as the subjective sensation of difficulty in swallowing and is derived from the Greek roots *dys* (with difficulty) and *phagia* (to eat). Dysphagia is characterized by a spectrum of sensations ranging from difficulty initiating a swallow to the perception of a blockage in the propagation of food down the esophagus. The presence of dysphagia implies a problem with the anatomy (mechanical obstruction) or the motor function (functional obstruction) of the oral cavity, pharynx, esophagus, or cardia of the stomach. According to a survey of U.S. households, 7% of people experienced dysphagia at some time during their lives, with increasing prevalence during advancing years. In nursing homes, 30 to 40% of patients have swallowing disorders.

Dysphagia is conventionally divided into oropharyngeal and esophageal dysphagia on the basis of the different anatomic or functional areas involved. This article reviews the manifestations, diagnoses, and treatment of the various pathologic conditions that result in oropharyngeal and esophageal dysphagia.

CONDITIONS CAUSING DYSPHAGIA

Oropharyngeal Dysphagia

Oropharyngeal, or transfer, dysphagia is characterized by difficulty in the initial stages of the swallowing process and is manifested by impaired transfer of food from the mouth through the upper esophageal sphincter (UES) into the upper esophagus. It often involves abnormalities affecting the striated muscle that encompasses the pharynx and upper third of the esophagus, and/or innervation of the striated muscle. Typical symptoms include difficulty initiating a swallow, the sensation of food sticking in the throat during swallowing, and the need to use repeated swallows to pass food into the esophagus successfully. Nasal or oral regurgitation of swallowed material and coughing or choking during swallowing caused by aspiration are also characteristic. In addition, dysarthria and a nasal quality to the voice (dysphonia) may be present.

More than 75% of cases of oropharyngeal dysphagia are caused by neuromuscular disorders involving the central nervous system, peripheral nervous system, or striated muscle (Table 1). As a group, elderly patients are particularly susceptible to these conditions. The differential diagnosis is broad and ranges from cerebrovascular accidents, midbrain tumors, and cranial nerve disorders to neuromuscular impairments such as myasthenia gravis.

Cerebrovascular accidents, the most common cause of oropharyngeal dysphagia, may affect the brain stem swallowing center or motor nuclei controlling the striated muscle of the hypopharynx and upper esophagus. Degenerative neurologic disorders such as Parkinson's disease, amyotrophic lateral sclerosis, and multiple sclerosis can also result in dysphagia. Dysphagia in some patients may develop years after an attack of acute paralytic poliomyelitis from dysfunction of the bulbar muscles. Certain connective tissue disorders such as polymyositis or dermatomyositis may affect the striated muscle portion of the esophagus, causing

TABLE 1. **Causes of Oropharyngeal Dysphagia**

Neuromuscular Disorders
Central Nervous System Diseases
Cerebrovascular accident
Parkinson's disease
Brain stem tumors
Cranial nerve disorders
Degenerative diseases (amyotrophic lateral sclerosis, multiple sclerosis, Huntington's disease)
Postinfections (poliomyelitis, syphilis)
Peripheral Nervous System
Peripheral neuropathy
Motor End Plate Dysfunction
Myasthenia gravis
Skeletal Muscle Diseases (Myopathies)
Polymyositis
Dermatomyositis
Muscular dystrophy (myotonic dystrophy, oculopharyngeal dystrophy)
Cricopharyngeal (Upper Esophageal Sphincter) Achalasia
Obstructive Lesions
Intrinsic Structural Lesions
Tumors
Inflammatory disorders
Trauma/surgical resection
Zenker's diverticulum
Esophageal web
Extrinsic Structural Lesions
Anterior mediastinal masses
Cervical spondylosis and osteophytes

a decrease in UES tone and poor propulsion of the bolus from the pharynx into the esophagus. Cricopharyngeal achalasia, with incomplete UES relaxation, may be a cause of difficulty in propelling a food bolus through the UES into the esophagus.

Esophageal diverticula are among the intrinsic structural lesions that may cause oropharyngeal dysphagia. These diverticula are acquired abnormalities often caused by underlying esophageal motility disorders. Dysphagia may result from a diverticulum itself or from an associated motor disorder of the esophagus. Zenker's diverticulum, an outpouching of one or more layers of the distal pharyngeal wall just above the cricopharyngeus muscle, probably occurs as a result of UES dysfunction.

Esophageal Dysphagia

Esophageal dysphagia involves difficulty in passage of the bolus down the esophagus into the stomach and can result from mechanical obstruction of the esophagus or neuromuscular disorders affecting the smooth muscle (Table 2). The majority of cases of esophageal dysphagia are associated with structural abnormalities, the most common of which are peptic strictures, Schatzki's ring, and carcinoma. The most frequent esophageal motility disorders that lead to dysphagia are achalasia, diffuse esophageal spasm, and scleroderma.

Esophageal Rings, Webs, and Strictures

Patients who have only intermittent dysphagia for solid foods are most frequently found to have esophageal rings or webs. Esophageal webs are usually located in the cervical region (Plummer-Vinson syndrome); esophageal rings are narrowings found in the distal esophagus and gastroesophageal junction. The internal diameter of a mucosal ring is the most important factor in determining the occurrence of dysphagia. Rings less then 13 mm in diameter almost always cause dysphagia, whereas rings more than

TABLE 2. Causes of Esophageal Dysphagia

Obstructive Lesions
Intrinsic Structural Lesions
Tumors
Strictures
  Peptic
  Radiation-induced
  Chemical-induced
  Medication-induced
Lower esophageal ring (Schatzki's ring)
Esophageal web
Foreign body
Extrinsic Structural Lesions
Vascular compression
  Enlarged aorta or left atrium
  Aberrant vessels
Mediastinal masses
  Lymphadenopathy
  Substernal thyroid
Neuromuscular Disorders
Achalasia
Spastic Motor Disorders
Diffuse esophageal spasm
Hypertensive lower esophageal sphincter
Nutcracker esophagus
Scleroderma
Inflammatory Conditions
Gastroesophageal reflux disease

20 mm in caliber are rarely symptomatic. Dysphagia is typically episodic and not progressive, but it may be severe when it occurs acutely because of temporary obstruction from a large food bolus.

Peptic esophagitis from gastroesophageal reflux disease (GERD) can produce a marked inflammatory reaction that leads to fibrosis and stricture formation, often extending several centimeters into the distal esophagus. Most peptic strictures are circumferential, with a smooth or tapered appearance. Patients complain of episodic dysphagia that is slowly progressive and usually report a long history of heartburn or antacid use. In contrast, patients with esophageal carcinoma have a history of rapidly progressive dysphagia with anorexia and significant weight loss. Because malignant strictures cannot be reliably distinguished radiographically from benign ones, patients with esophageal strictures should undergo endoscopy with biopsy and brush cytology to rule out carcinoma or Barrett's esophagus.

Neoplasia

Neoplasms, both benign and malignant, may cause dysphagia as a result of obstruction. Patients tend to have anorexia, rapidly progressive dysphagia for solids, and weight loss. The two major esophageal neoplasms are squamous cell carcinoma and adenocarcinoma. Squamous cell carcinoma, the more prevalent of the two, is associated with the long-term use of alcohol or tobacco, especially in African Americans. Adenocarcinoma tends to occur in white males with a long history of GERD and is superimposed on an underlying Barrett's esophagus. It has been reported that adenocarcinoma may develop within an area of "short-segment Barrett's esophagus." The diagnosis of esophageal carcinoma is often strongly suggested on barium swallow radiography by the classic findings of nodularity, rigidity, abrupt luminal angulation or "shelving," ulceration, and stenosis of the lumen, which typically has asymmetrical margins. The best method for confirming the diagnosis of carcinoma is endoscopy with biopsy and cytology. Endoscopic ultrasonography may be employed to detect depth of invasion and local nodal status. This information as well as that obtained from abdominal/thoracic computed tomographic scan is used to determine potential surgical resectability.

Achalasia

In achalasia, dysphagia for both solid and liquid food is typically present from the onset of symptoms and slowly worsens with time. Although the onset of primary achalasia is usually insidious, with an average symptom duration of 5 years at the time of initial treatment, 16% of patients with primary achalasia come to medical attention within the first year of symptom development. The site of obstruction usually is recognized correctly by the patient as occurring at the xiphoid area. Patients often develop maneuvers that enable them to finish meals, such as repeated swallowing, eating only small quantities of food, or drinking large volumes of water in an attempt to facilitate emptying of the esophagus. The characteristic appearance of a barium esophagogram in a patient with achalasia is of a dilated, fluid-filled esophagus with a smooth, tapered distal portion ("bird's beak"). Manometry often is used to confirm esophageal aperistalsis, elevated lower esophageal sphincter (LES) pressure, and incomplete relaxation of the LES on swallowing.

Secondary achalasia, or pseudoachalasia, is the development of achalasia as a result of an underlying disorder, usually local gastric or esophageal carcinoma. Malignancies distant from the esophagogastric junction, such as lung cancer, pancreatic cancer, lymphoma, hepatoma, and prostate carcinoma, also have been associated with secondary achalasia. Distinguishing malignancy-induced achalasia from primary achalasia on clinical grounds can be difficult. Three features that suggest the possibility of malignancy include (1) age older than 55 years, (2) short duration of dysphagia (<1 year), and (3) significant weight loss (>15 pounds). These criteria are only guidelines because exceptions to each have been reported. Indeed, 15% of patients with primary achalasia come to medical attention after the age of 60, and some cases of malignancy-induced achalasia have occurred in patients as young as 15 years of age. Therefore, all patients with achalasia should undergo upper endoscopy to exclude malignancy. In patients older than 55 years, brushings of the gastroesophageal junction for cytology are often obtained. In South America, the most common cause of secondary achalasia is Chagas' disease, caused by infection with *Trypanosoma cruzi*.

Spastic Motor Disorders of the Esophagus

Dysphagia may be a prominent symptom in patients with spastic motor disorders of the esophagus, such as diffuse esophageal spasm. Although the mechanism of dysphagia is unknown, the disorder may result from ineffective peristalsis (caused by simultaneous contractions) or impaired relaxation of the LES. Diagnosis of diffuse esophageal spasm by manometry rests on the presence of simultaneous, high-amplitude esophageal contractions in at least 10 to 30% of wet swallows, interspersed with normal peristaltic contractions and occurring in symptomatic patients with chest pain and/or dysphagia. Diffuse esophageal spasm and achalasia may be different manifestations of a similar underlying disorder. In some patients, diffuse esophageal spasm has been reported to progress to achalasia.

Scleroderma (Progressive Systemic Sclerosis)

Scleroderma affects the smooth muscle portion of the esophagus. The classic manometric findings are diminished or ineffective peristalsis in the distal two thirds to three fourths of the esophagus, accompanied by a hypotensive LES. Patients typically are middle-aged women who have chronic heartburn associated with progressive dysphagia with liquids and solids. Dysphagia results from the marked peristaltic dysfunction and/or severe GERD with stricture formation.

Gastroesophageal Reflux Disease

Dysphagia occurs in up to 40% of patients with GERD and may arise from a host of obstructive causes, including peptic strictures from long-standing reflux esophagitis, esophageal carcinoma arising within Barrett's esophagus, and esophageal peristaltic dysfunction from the esophageal inflammation.

EVALUATION OF PATIENTS WITH DYSPHAGIA

History and Physical Examination

The history forms the framework for the diagnostic evaluation of patients with dysphagia. An algorithm frequently employed by gastroenterologists for the diagnostic evaluation of dysphagia is shown in Figure 1.

Patients may describe other symptoms that should be differentiated from dysphagia. Odynophagia, or pain on swallowing, implies an inflammatory process of the esophageal mucosa and should be distinguished from the usually painless dysphagia. Globus is the constant sensation of a lump in the throat associated with dry swallows or the need to swallow, with no readily identifiable cause. In contrast to true dysphagia, there is no difficulty when swallowing is actually performed. The symptom often is regarded as psychogenic and, in the past, was termed "globus hystericus." With appropriate testing, however, the majority of patients with globus sensation are found to have a variety of responsible organic factors. The diagnosis of globus therefore should never be made without investigation for an anatomic lesion or motor abnormality of the oropharynx, larynx, or esophagus.

The patient should be asked whether the difficulty with swallowing lies in initiating the swallow or whether the food stops or sticks after being swallowed. A patient's localization of the site of dysphagia may help determine the site of obstruction. When the sensation of dysphagia is at the level of the xiphoid process, an underlying stricture, malignancy, or ring frequently is found in the lower esophagus. In contrast, when the bolus sticks in the region of the suprasternal notch, an obstructing lesion can be found anywhere along the course of the esophagus.

Determining the type of bolus that is arrested and the temporal progression of dysphagia may help differentiate between an obstructive lesion and a motor disorder (Figure 2). In neuromuscular disorders, the patient typically notes dysphagia for solids and liquids from the onset, whereas in patients with mechanical obstruction, dysphagia initially involves solids alone and only later progresses to involve liquids. In motor disorders of the esophagus, the onset of dysphagia is usually gradual, with progression over many

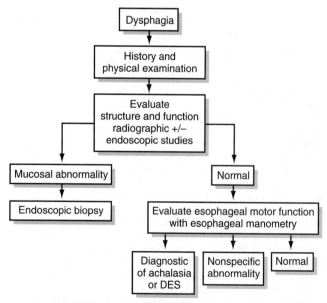

Figure 1. Flow diagram for the diagnostic evaluation of patients with esophageal dysphagia. The initial tests begin with an investigation for an anatomic abnormality of the esophagus with radiographic and endoscopic tests. The subsequent tests are conducted to define esophageal motility disorder. DES = diffuse esophageal spasm. (Modified from Trate DM, Parkman HP, Fisher RS. Dysphagia. Prim Care Clin Office Pract 1996; 23:417–432.)

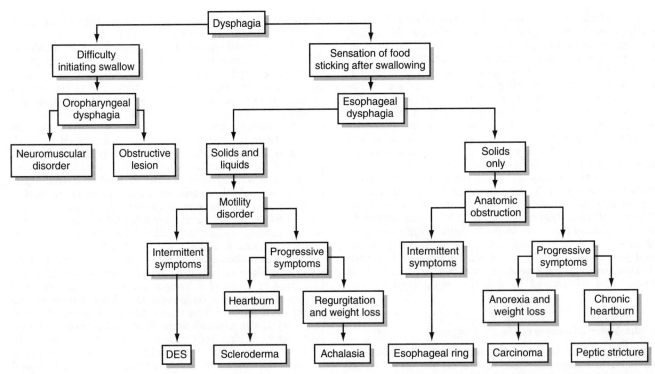

Figure 2. Flow diagram for history taking in patients with dysphagia to help arrive at a working diagnosis. The logic pattern depends on (1) the differentiation of oropharyngeal dysphagia from esophageal dysphagia, (2) whether the dysphagia occurs with solid food alone or with solids and liquids, (3) the presence of intermittent or progressive symptoms, and (4) associated symptoms of heartburn, regurgitation, or weight loss. (Modified from Trate DM, Parkman HP, Fisher RS. Dysphagia. Prim Care Clin Office Pract 1996; 23:417–432.)

months to years. An esophageal carcinoma should be suspected if the time course of the dysphagia is characterized by rapid progression of dysphagia for solids, especially in an older patient with anorexia and weight loss. Peptic strictures typically produce low-grade dysphagia for solids in a patient with long-standing heartburn or chronic antacid use. Episodic dysphagia for solids without other esophageal symptoms or weight loss may be produced by an esophageal ring. In the typical "beef house syndrome" caused by Schatzki's ring, a bolus of poorly chewed solid food sticks in the lower esophagus, producing the sensation of dysphagia. The food bolus eventually clears and the patient is able to finish the meal without difficulty.

Associated symptoms such as heartburn, regurgitation, and chest pain during eating may be suggestive of GERD. The presence of neuromuscular symptoms such as double vision, facial droop, change in voice, muscle weakness, and difficulty walking can imply a neurologic etiology. In particular, symptoms of a cerebrovascular accident and its temporal relationship to the development of dysphagia should be a subject of inquiry.

The patient should be asked directly about medications that may cause pill-induced esophagitis. These include tetracycline and its derivatives (doxycycline [Vibramycin] and minocycline [Minocin]), potassium chloride, iron preparations, vitamin C, quinidine and its derivatives, aspirin and other nonsteroidal anti-inflammatory drugs (NSAIDs), and alendronate (Fosamax). Characteristically, pill-induced esophagitis manifests initially with acute retrosternal pain exacerbated by swallowing (odynophagia) and, with continued use, may progress to dysphagia. Chronic esophageal injury may lead to the formation of esophageal strictures, usually located in the mid-esophagus. Pill-induced esophagitis is caused by local mucosal injury produced by a chemical burn. The pill often becomes lodged in the esophagus at the level of the aortic arch or left atrium. Treatment includes withdrawal of the offending medication, acid-suppressive therapy, viscous lidocaine for local anesthesia, and sucralfate (Carafate) slurry to coat the mucosa. As prophylaxis against a recurrence, patients should be instructed to ingest their medications after drinking 4 ounces of water, accompanied by an 8-ounce glass of water and followed by a 4-ounce chaser of water. Medications should be taken when the patient is sitting or standing and should not be ingested within 2 hours of going to bed. Other medications that may play a role in swallowing disorders include antihypertensive agents, tricyclic antidepressants, and anticholinergic agents, possibly by causing weakened esophageal peristalsis.

In general, physical examination findings in patients with esophageal dysphagia are normal. The presence of lymphadenopathy and malnutrition usually reflects serious underlying disease. Close attention should be paid to the mouth, pharynx, and neck because factors contributing to dysphagia can be found. A brief neurologic examination can be valuable in identifying abnormalities of the central or peripheral nervous system that may not have been recognized by the patient. Specifically, the physician should look for residual neurologic deficits from a previous cerebrovascular accident; the typical tremor, gait, or posture of Parkinson's disease; ptosis in patients with myasthenia gravis or oculopharyngeal dystrophy; the typical handshake, facies, or muscular wasting of myotonic dystrophy; and hyporeflexia, eyebrow changes, or skin and hair changes of hypothyroidism. In malignancies of the esophagus, cervical or supraclavicular lymphadenopathy, tylosis (hyperkeratosis of palms of hand and soles of feet), and/or cachexia may be noted. In patients with rheumatologic diseases, special attention is directed to manifestations of scleroderma or the CREST syndrome (calcinosis cutis, Raynaud's phenomenon, esophageal dysmotility, sclerodactyly, and telangiectasia).

DIAGNOSTIC STUDIES

Radiographic Evaluation

Barium radiographic studies should be the initial screening tests in patients with either oropharyngeal or esophageal dysphagia. Because the patient's subjective localization of dysphagia may be inaccurate, radiologic evaluation of the entire oropharynx, esophagus, and proximal stomach is often necessary. Several types of studies can be ordered, including the barium swallow, video esophagogram, modified barium swallow (MBS), and upper gastrointestinal series. The choice of examination should be directed by the patient's symptoms. Radiographic contrast studies are particularly valuable in detecting extrinsic structural lesions, such as thyromegaly, and some intrinsic obstructive lesions, such as esophageal rings and webs. The double-contrast technique provides good visualization of the mucosal surface. Liquid barium alone, however, may be insufficient to define rings and early strictures; a bolus challenge, such as a barium-coated tablet or marshmallow, may reveal a site of narrowing. Videofluoroscopic examination of the oral cavity, pharynx, and cervical esophagus can provide detailed information about swallowing function and allows slow-motion replay of the rapid and complex events that occur during the oropharyngeal phase of swallowing. Close observation of esophageal function during fluoroscopy may show esophageal aperistalsis, spasm, or gastroesophageal reflux. The modified barium swallow, performed with speech therapy, involves different consistencies and amounts of barium and is very helpful in evaluating oral and pharyngeal phases of swallowing. If no lesion is detected in the pharynx or esophagus, the study should be extended into an upper gastrointestinal series with careful attention to the gastric cardia, because tumors of the gastric fundus can manifest with dysphagia (pseudoachalasia).

Endoscopic Evaluation

If there is evidence of a lesion on radiologic evaluation such as an ulcer or mass, the patient should undergo esophagogastroscopy with biopsy and brush cytology. Radiographic and endoscopic studies are often complementary in the work-up of patients with dysphagia because each may identify abnormalities that the other may not detect. Thus, for persistent dysphagia, barium studies and endoscopy are often used together.

Endoscopy is preferable for the acute onset of severe dysphagia during eating. Affected patients may develop total esophageal obstruction from an impacted food bolus, which can usually be removed endoscopically. A previously undiagnosed esophageal abnormality may be found as the cause of the obstruction. Other advantages of endoscopy over radiographic studies are in the diagnosis of infectious esophagitis and ulcerations of the esophagus, stomach, and duodenum and in obtaining tissue samples from erosions, ulcers, and other esophageal lesions.

FLEXIBLE ENDOSCOPIC EVALUATION OF SWALLOWING AND SENSATION

Flexible endoscopic evaluation of swallowing and sensation (FEESS) is performed by otorhinolaryngologists and involves passing a small endoscope through the nares into the pharynx and feeding the patient various food consis-

tencies while directly visualizing the upper aerodigestive tract. It provides direct anatomic and physiologic information about the swallowing function, as well as an assessment of sensation, by observing the reflexes in response to controlled injections of air into the pharynx.

Esophageal Manometry and pH Monitoring

Esophageal manometry should be performed in patients with esophageal dysphagia if no anatomic abnormality is found on barium swallow or upper endoscopy. The primary goals of manometry are to assess the characteristics of esophageal contractions (peristaltic, simultaneous, or absent) and to define the LES and UES and their respective responses to swallowing. Occasionally, manometry can pick up early cases of achalasia that, because of a nondilated esophagus, may not have been recognized radiographically. Although esophageal manometry is the gold standard for diagnosing esophageal motor disorders, several studies using manometry in the evaluation of nonobstructive dysphagia have suggested that definitive abnormalities (e.g., findings considered diagnostic for achalasia or diffuse esophageal spasm) occur in only about 25% of patients with dysphagia. In another 25% of patients, the manometry reveals abnormalities of unclear significance (e.g., nonspecific esophageal motility disorder, hypertensive LES, and nutcracker esophagus), and findings are normal in the remaining 50% of patients. Provocative testing during esophageal manometry, including intravenous infusion of edrophonium, acid perfusion in the esophagus, and esophageal balloon distention, is usually reserved for patients with noncardiac chest pain but can also be useful in evaluating patients with dysphagia, especially if other esophageal symptoms such as heartburn are present. Some centers advocate having the patient swallow a solid bolus, such as bread, during manometry to help detect esophageal peristaltic dysfunction.

Ambulatory esophageal pH monitoring may aid in the study of patients with dysphagia, not only to look for increased acid exposure in the esophagus to suggest GERD, but also by determining the temporal association of acid reflux episodes and the patient's symptoms. Combined recording of esophageal pH and manometry may be useful for diagnosing reflux-induced esophageal spasm.

TREATMENT

Oropharyngeal Dysphagia

Treatment of oropharyngeal dysphagia is determined by the underlying cause. Medical treatment of systemic diseases such as myasthenia gravis, polymyositis, Parkinson's disease, and thyroid dysfunction may ameliorate the patient's dysphagia. In patients with dysphagia secondary to a stroke, the condition may improve with time but a residual swallowing defect often remains. The modified barium swallow provides an assessment of whether oral feedings can be given and whether swallowing rehabilitation by a speech therapist may help. These specialists can train patients to regain effective swallowing by adjusting food consistency, volume, and delivery rate; optimizing head posture during swallowing; coordinating breathing and coughing maneuvers to clear residual food from the pharynx; and exercising muscle groups involved in swallowing that are still functional. In the patients who do not recover adequate swallowing function and/or have evidence of aspiration on a barium swallow, enteral feedings with a Dobbhoff feeding tube or a percutaneous endoscopic gastrostomy (PEG) feeding tube may be necessary on a temporary or permanent basis.

Treatment of symptomatic Zenker's diverticulum requires resection or oversewing of the pouch along with a cricopharyngeal myotomy. There is a recurrence rate of 15% if the diverticulectomy is performed without myotomy. The main contraindication to cricopharyngeal myotomy is concomitant GERD, in which cutting the UES may increase the risk of pulmonary aspiration.

For some patients with oropharyngeal dysphagia without diverticula, empirical dilation with a large-bore (18- to 20-mm) dilating bougie may be helpful. Mechanical disruption of the cricopharyngeus by dilation or myotomy is thought to facilitate bolus transfer by reducing the UES resistance. Endoscopic injection of botulinum toxin into the cricopharyngeus muscle has been tried with some success in patients with cricopharyngeal achalasia. Botulinum toxin decreases the cholinergic neural input to the muscle, and this results in decreased UES pressure and/or improved UES relaxation. Usually, the effects of the treatment last only several months, and repeat injections are required. The close proximity of the injection area to the vocal cords, however, raises concern about possible acute respiratory complications. At present, this procedure is not performed routinely and generally should be performed by otorhinolaryngologists either endoscopically or transcutaneously with electromyographic guidance.

Esophageal Dysphagia

Treatment of esophageal carcinoma is, for the most part, palliative, consisting of chemotherapy and radiation therapy. Surgery, however, is occasionally curative in patients with early-stage esophageal cancer. In most patients with dysphagia who are not surgical candidates, palliative treatment options include esophageal dilation, esophageal prosthesis, and tumor ablation with electrocoagulation, laser therapy, or argon plasma coagulation. Often a PEG feeding tube is placed to maintain nutritional support during therapy and/or if the disease progresses.

Treatment of rings or webs consists of dilation with large-caliber bougie or through-the-endoscope balloon dilators. Peptic strictures often necessitate periodic bougienage along with aggressive acid suppression with a proton pump inhibitor. A Savary dilator over a guide wire and under fluoroscopic guidance offers controlled dilations.

Achalasia is best treated with pneumatic dilation or surgical myotomy (Heller myotomy). The overall success rate of pneumatic dilation is about 80%; however, esophageal perforation complicates pneumatic dilation in 2 to 5% of cases. The second, less troublesome complication of pneumatic dilation is GERD. Two new treatment options for achalasia include la-

paroscopic myotomy and botulinum toxin injection into the LES. The advantage of performing the myotomy laparoscopically is that the length of hospital stay and time until return to normal activity may be greatly reduced. With the short follow-up available, it appears that laparoscopic myotomy is as effective as an open procedure, which reportedly has success rates of 80 to 90%. A partial fundoplication is often used to prevent GERD. Botulinum toxin* (Botox) injection into the LES is an easy and relatively safe endoscopic procedure that has been shown to produce marked improvement of the patient's symptoms. Unfortunately, the effect tends to diminish during a 6-month period, necessitating repeat treatments. Early achalasia has been treated with calcium channel blockers, nitrates, anticholinergic agents, or intermittent bougie dilation. Medical therapy, unfortunately, is at best temporizing.

Treatment of spastic motor disorders is often performed with empirical treatment trials to assess for a response. Some patients may respond to smooth muscle relaxants, such as calcium channel blockers, nitrates, or anticholinergics, whereas others may respond to empirical bougie dilation, botulinum toxin injection into the LES, or even pneumatic dilation.

Treatment of severe peptic strictures secondary to scleroderma consists of periodic bougienage and long-term aggressive acid suppression with a proton pump inhibitor. There has been hesitancy to send patients with scleroderma for antireflux surgery because of the risk of worsening the dysphagia; however, this risk may be reduced by performing a loose fundoplication.

In patients with GERD with dysphagia but without an anatomic stricture, aggressive acid suppression with a proton pump inhibitor is the treatment of choice. We would hesitate to send a patient with GERD-induced dysphagia to surgery unless medical therapy improves the patient's symptoms. Patients with documented Barrett's esophagus secondary to GERD also should undergo periodic surveillance endoscopy with random biopsies to assess for dysplasia.

Occasionally, when no etiology of esophageal dysphagia is found, empirical bougienage is used with some degree of success.

SUMMARY

The description of difficulty swallowing by a patient should direct the physician to an orderly series of diagnostic tests of esophageal function to help determine the cause of the dysphagia (see Figures 1 and 2). Initial testing should begin with a videofluoroscopic barium examination of the oropharyngeal and esophageal swallowing process with liquid and then solid bolus challenges if no anatomic abnormalities are seen. Although esophagogastroscopy is performed most often in patients with esophageal dysphagia with abnormal findings on radiographic studies, endoscopy sometimes can provide additional

---

*Not FDA approved for this indication.

information in patients in whom barium examinations have been unrevealing. If no underlying cause of dysphagia is identified by these tests, esophageal manometry should be employed to determine whether an esophageal motility disorder is present. More sophisticated evaluation of esophageal function with ambulatory esophageal pH recording and occasionally pH/motility recording may provide additional information in patients with complex symptoms. An alternative way to implicate GERD as a cause of dysphagia in patients with negative evaluation is an empirical treatment trial of a proton pump inhibitor.

DIVERTICULA OF THE ALIMENTARY TRACT

method of
JAMES W. SMITH, M.D.
Ochsner Foundation Hospital and Clinic
New Orleans, Louisiana

Diverticula are epithelium-lined mucosal pouches of the intestinal tract and may be categorized as true or false. True diverticula contain all layers of the intestinal wall, including the mucosa, submucosa, and muscle, whereas false diverticula do not include the muscle layer. Diverticula may result from congenital abnormalities, motility disorders, or traction and pulsion forces. Although diverticula are often asymptomatic, a variety of complications can occur, some specific for the region of the gastrointestinal tract involved.

ZENKER'S DIVERTICULUM

The hypopharyngeal (Zenker's) diverticulum is the most common diverticulum of the esophagus. It is located posteriorly in the midline, protruding between the cricopharyngeous and inferior constrictor muscles. It is found in approximately 2% of patients with dysphagia; this percentage would be higher in a geriatric patient population. In fact, the typical patient with a Zenker's diverticulum is in the eighth decade of life. The cause is not precisely known and has been long debated. Most likely an underlying incoordination of the swallowing mechanism leads to the development of high pressure with subsequent pouch formation. Elongation occurs over time as a result of continued high pressure, peristalsis, and gravity. An association with gastroesophageal reflux has not been consistently found.

Dysphagia is the most common manifesting symptom. The patient may also complain of delayed regurgitation of undigested food. Other symptoms include halitosis, cough, hoarseness, and gurgling. Mild weight loss may ensue. Severe complications such as aspiration pneumonia, chronic pneumonitis, and lung abscess may occur. Squamous cell carcinoma has been reported in less than 1% of cases. Finally, the unanticipated diverticulum can be perforated by the passage of a nasogastric tube or endoscope. The physical examination would characteristically be unrevealing except for the rare patient with a large diverticulum that creates a neck mass.

The diagnosis is suspected from the history of dysphagia and regurgitation in an elderly patient and is confirmed by a barium swallow study. Upper endoscopy is not necessary for diagnosis, nor does esophageal manometry benefit the clinician.

Treatment

Most patients with symptomatic diverticula should undergo surgical treatment to relieve symptoms and prevent complications. A cricopharyngeal myotomy combined with diverticulectomy currently yields good results and a low risk of complications. An endoscopic approach of stapling the diverticulum has recently been reported. The truly asymptomatic patient may be observed.

DIVERTICULA OF THE ESOPHAGEAL BODY

Diverticula of the esophageal body occur typically in the mid- to distal esophagus. Mid-esophageal diverticula have been called traction diverticula because they were thought to be secondary to mediastinal granulomatous diseases (tuberculosis, histoplasmosis) with subsequent inflammatory response and adhesion formation. This entity is rare today in developed countries. Diverticula in the mid- or distal esophagus (epiphrenic) are associated with and likely caused by underlying motility disorders, such as achalasia or diffuse esophageal spasm. Symptoms usually are related to the motor disorder, but some patients regurgitate massive amounts of fluid while recumbent, which may lead to nocturnal cough, bronchitis, and recurrent pneumonia. Squamous cell carcinoma, although extremely rare, has been reported in patients with epiphrenic diverticula.

Diagnosis is based on barium swallow studies. Endoscopy is not needed for the diagnosis, although it can be used to pass a guide wire to facilitate the passage of motility catheters, which is often difficult by standard blind insertion technique. Esophageal manometry is needed before surgical treatment.

Treatment

The treatment of asymptomatic diverticula is controversial. Many authorities advocate observation, but surgical series have emphasized the potential for pulmonary complications, even in the absence of esophageal symptoms. Medical therapy for the underlying esophageal motility disorder is generally unrewarding and cannot prevent complications. Surgical treatment involves excision of the diverticulum and usually a myotomy of the distal esophageal body. Pneumatic dilatation of the lower esophageal sphincter in a patient with achalasia is considered to pose a greater risk of inducing perforation if an epiphrenic diverticulum is present.

ESOPHAGEAL INTRAMURAL PSEUDODIVERTICULA

The rare disorder of esophageal intramural pseudodiverticulosis is characterized by numerous 1- to 3-mm outpouchings protruding from the lumen into the esophageal wall. Pathologically, these are not true diverticula but represent dilated ducts arising from submucosal glands. These lesions are acquired, although the etiology is not clear. Many affected patients have gastroesophageal reflux, most have strictures, and a minority report prior ingestion of corrosive substances. Patients have dysphagia related to the underlying stricture, and the many tiny pseudodiverticula can be seen on either the barium swallow study or the endoscopic examination. Any stricture can be dilated in the standard manner, and there is no specific therapy for the pseudodiverticulosis.

GASTRIC DIVERTICULA

The gastric diverticulum is a rare entity; the most common location is the posterior wall of the cardia. In this position, it is termed *juxtacardiac*. Although usually asymptomatic, juxtacardiac diverticula may cause epigastric pain or a sense of fullness and in rare instances is complicated by bleeding, perforation, or torsion. Less common is the intramural gastric diverticulum, a rounded protrusion of gastric mucosa into the muscle layer of the antrum. In this location, symptoms or complications are not anticipated. Gastric diverticula do not necessitate treatment if asymptomatic.

DUODENAL DIVERTICULA

Duodenal diverticula occur in approximately 10 to 20% of the population; the incidence is higher in older patients. The most common location is in the region near the ampulla; diverticula in that area are known as periampullary. Most are asymptomatic, but a variety of potential complications can occur. Because of the periampullary position, the diverticula may cause partial obstruction and stasis in the common bile duct, leading to stone formation and subsequent pancreatitis or cholangitis. Diverticulitis (causing pain, fever, and leukocytosis) and hemorrhage are two potential, although rare, complications.

Treatment

Suspected biliary tract disease necessitates endoscopic retrograde cholangiography, which can be technically challenging when a periampullary diverticulum is present. Nonetheless, in most cases, the endoscopic therapy of sphincterotomy and stone extraction can be accomplished. In rare instances, surgery is needed to divert the biliary tract (e.g., Roux-en-Y choledochojejunostomy). Hemorrhage from a duodenal diverticulum is diagnosed endoscopically and managed with the usual supportive measures. Endoscopic treatment of active bleeding has been reported. Diverticulitis is diagnosed by computed tomographic (CT) scan demonstrating perforation, abscess, and inflammatory changes involving adjacent structures. Patients require antibiotics and drainage by percutaneous or surgical approaches.

JEJUNAL AND ILEAL DIVERTICULA

Jejunal and ileal diverticula are uncommon and considered to be acquired lesions. They are found along the mesenteric border of the intestines, usually the proximal as opposed to distal jejunum, and are more often multiple than solitary. The diverticula are frequently associated with disorders of small intestinal motility, such as pseudo-obstruction, scleroderma, and visceral neuropathy and myopathy.

Most jejunal diverticula are asymptomatic, but when symptoms occur, they reflect bacterial overgrowth and subsequent malabsorption, steatorrhea, weight loss, and deficiencies in fat-soluble vitamins. Symptoms such as abdominal pain and bloating are nonspecific and should be attributed to the diverticula only with caution. Rare serious complications include hemorrhage, diverticulitis, and mechanical obstruction. Diagnosis is established by barium studies.

Treatment

Bacterial overgrowth responds to antimicrobial therapy directed at aerobic and anaerobic organisms. Chronic therapy with cephalexin (Keflex), 250 mg four times a day (qid), metronidazole (Flagyl), 250 mg three times a day, or tetracycline, 250 mg qid for 1 to 2 weeks of each month is usually effective. Vitamin B_{12}, folic acid, and the fat-soluble vitamins should be supplemented. Surgery is required only for the severe complications listed earlier.

MECKEL'S DIVERTICULUM

Meckel's diverticulum is the most common true diverticulum of the gastrointestinal tract, with a reported incidence of 2% in autopsy series. It arises from the antimesenteric border of the ileum, usually within 100 cm from the ileocecal valve. Meckel's diverticula have a wide open mouth, are about 5 cm in length, and result from the incomplete closure of the omphalomesenteric duct. Most are asymptomatic.

Many of these diverticula contain ectopic gastric mucosa, and with the inherent capacity to secrete acid, this results in the most common complication, hemorrhage. The acid leads to ulceration of the diverticulum or adjacent small bowel mucosa, resulting in the characteristic passage of "currant jelly"–appearing bloody stools. This occurs in children and young adults and is not associated with abdominal pain. Diagnosis is established with a technetium Tc 99m scan, with pentagastrin (Peptavlon) used to stimulate the uptake of technetium by the gastric mucosa. Other potential complications include obstruction from intussusception and diverticulitis; the latter has a clinical manifestation indistinguishable from that of acute appendicitis.

Treatment

The diagnosis of Meckel's diverticulum should be pursued in any child or young adult with gastrointestinal hemorrhage, and a positive scan necessitates laparotomy and diverticulectomy. Surgical treatment is also necessary for any of the other complications.

DIVERTICULAR DISEASE OF THE COLON

The colon is the most common site of diverticular formation in the gastrointestinal tract; more than 50% of all people older than 50 years have colonic diverticula. These are not true diverticula but rather herniations of the mucosa and submucosa between muscle layers at the point where nutrient arteries penetrate the wall of the colon. Most colonic diverticula are found in the sigmoid colon, although all regions of the colon may be involved. The cause of diverticulosis is not known, although populations that consume low-fiber diets are more commonly afflicted. The "fiber hypothesis" suggests that a low-fiber diet reduces stool bulk and leads to increased colonic motility and intraluminal pressures.

Most patients with diverticulosis are asymptomatic; in fact, only 4 to 5% develop a complication. The diverticula are discovered incidentally by barium studies or flexible sigmoidoscopy. Asymptomatic diverticulosis does not necessitate specific treatment. Some patients have symptoms of irritable bowel syndrome, such as recurring abdominal pain and alterations of defecation. However, irritable bowel syndrome is a common entity, and it is difficult to determine how spastic diverticulosis differs. Therapy consists of dietary fiber supplementation and use of antispasm medications such as dicyclomine (Bentyl), 10 mg orally three times a day.

DIVERTICULAR BLEEDING

Hemorrhage from colonic diverticula manifests as a large-volume, maroon or red stool in a middle-aged or elderly patient. The patient may have mild cramps and an urge to defecate, but significant abdominal pain is not present. Bleeding is thought to be caused by erosion into an artery and it is not related to inflammation (e.g., diverticulitis). Although hemorrhage was initially believed to result primarily from diverticula in the right colon, recent reports have not supported this. Likewise, there have been recent reports that diverticular bleeding may be associated with the usage of nonsteroidal anti-inflammatory drugs (NSAIDs). Blood loss can be severe, although

spontaneous resolution occurs in most patients (80%).

Treatment

The management of the patient with suspected diverticular bleeding is similar to that of any cause of severe gastrointestinal bleeding. Supportive care and hemodynamic stability are of paramount importance. Appropriate volume replacement, judicious use of blood products, and surgical consultation are required. An upper source of bleeding (e.g., duodenal ulcer) must be excluded in any patient with hematochezia, either by the passage of a nasogastric tube and aspiration of gastric contents or by endoscopic evaluation. Once the patient is stable, consideration may be given to diagnostic tests to confirm the site of bleeding. Many physicians recommend colonoscopy as the initial diagnostic test, either acutely or after the bleeding ceases or slows. However, massive and ongoing bleeding makes this approach difficult; mesenteric angiography is then preferred. If a bleeding site is identified by extravasation of contrast into the colon lumen, selective intra-arterial vasopressin* (Pitressin), at 0.3 unit per minute, is administered. The selectively placed catheter is left in the patient, and the patient is slowly weaned from the vasopressin. Surgery is indicated for ongoing or recurrent bleeding and consists of resection of the involved portion of the colon. There have been reports of successful endoscopic treatment of actively bleeding colonic diverticula as well.

DIVERTICULITIS

Diverticulitis is the most common complication of diverticulosis and results from microperforation of a diverticulum by inspissated fecal material. Usually this occurs in the sigmoid colon and involves only one diverticulum. The perforation is contained and becomes a localized phlegmon or abscess. The patient has left lower quadrant pain and fever. Obstipation is common, and other associated symptoms are dysuria, nausea, vomiting, and back pain.

Physical examination reveals tenderness in the left lower quadrant. A mass may be palpable, in addition to guarding and rebound tenderness. Bowel sounds are variable but usually hypoactive. Distention may be present. An elevated white blood cell count and fever help confirm the diagnosis. The diagnosis is usually clinical and based on the symptoms as described. CT scanning of the abdomen and pelvis has emerged as the single best diagnostic test. Although not needed in mild cases, it should be ordered if the diverticulitis is of moderate severity, if it occurs in an immunocompromised patient, or if the diagnosis is unclear. It can be performed with oral, rectal, and intravenous contrast for excellent resolution. Diagnostic use of barium or diatrizoate (Hypaque) radiography can be performed safely but does not provide

---

*Not FDA approved for this indication.

as much information as does CT scanning. Endoscopic procedures should not be performed, because they add little information and may cause complications.

Treatment

Patients with pain and fever who require analgesics should be admitted to the hospital. Nasogastric suction is saved for those with obstruction; all patients receive intravenous fluids, and oral intake is restricted. Antibiotics should have a broad spectrum of action, and a number of regimens can be employed with success. An aminoglycoside such as gentamicin (Garamycin), 1.5 mg per kg every 8 hours with doses adjusted for renal insufficiency, can be combined with metronidazole (Flagyl), 500 mg every 6 hours, or with clindamycin (Cleocin), 600 mg every 6 hours. Single-drug therapy with cefoxitin (Mefoxin), 2 grams every 8 hours, is also effective, as are beta-lactamase antibiotics such as ticarcillin plus clavulanate (Timentin). Most patients improve after 3 to 4 days; others may require 1 to 2 weeks of medical therapy.

The most common complication of acute diverticulitis is abscess, which necessitates a specific approach. With CT guidance, the radiologist can often place a percutaneous drainage catheter. Most of these patients require surgery, and successful drainage enables the surgeon to provide a one-step resection of the involved colon. Other complications that generally necessitate surgery are fistula, obstruction, and peritonitis. Elective surgical treatment is appropriate in patients with recurrent bouts of diverticulitis. Patients 40 years old or younger with acute diverticulitis tend to develop more severe complications, and elective surgery should be considered after a single confirmed episode.

Patients with mild episodes of diverticulitis may not require admission. Oral therapy with ciprofloxacin (Cipro), 500 mg every 12 hours, and metronidazole, 250 mg every 8 hours, can be given for 10 days. Most patients should be restricted to a low-fiber diet as the acute episode is resolving, because any residual edema may limit the size of the colonic lumen. For long-term prevention after an episode, the use of high-fiber foods or the avoidance of seeds, nuts, corn, and other hard particles has not been proven effective.

INFLAMMATORY BOWEL DISEASE

method of
ALLEN L. GINSBERG, M.D
*George Washington University School of
    Medicine*
Washington, D.C.

The clinical course of inflammatory bowel disease (IBD) differs greatly from patient to patient. Because of such variables as disease location, extent, activity, and the presence or absence of complications such as strictures, fistulas, abscesses, bacterial overgrowth, anemia, and extraintestinal manifestations, therapy must be tailored to the individual patient. Patients also vary in response to specific therapeutic agents, and thus no single drug is successful in all patients.

The goals of therapy for IBD are to alleviate symptoms and induce complete remission when possible, while minimizing the toxic effects of therapy, especially those of corticosteroids. The benefits of therapy must always be weighed against the risks of adverse effects. For example, if a patient has only diarrhea, and the diarrhea can be controlled with loperamide or cholestyramine, this is preferable to the injudicious use of corticosteroids.

It is helpful in selecting therapy to consider the pathophysiology behind the symptoms. Diarrhea, for example, can be caused by several mechanisms, and treatment tailored to the pathophysiologic cause is the most effective.

Extensive colonic inflammation in ulcerative colitis or Crohn's colitis produces liquid stools because the diseased colon is incapable of efficiently absorbing fluids and electrolytes. Therapy should be focused at correcting the inflammation with sulfasalazine or mesalamine with or without corticosteroids, depending on disease severity.

Frequent, urgent, semiformed bowel movements, often with tenesmus, red blood, and mucus, should suggest rectal involvement. Disease is often limited to the rectum or rectosigmoid colon. After sigmoidoscopic confirmation, treatment with topical mesalamine (Rowasa enemas or suppositories) or topical corticosteroids (hydrocortisone [Cortenema]) is appropriate. Loperamide (Imodium) is a useful adjunct.

Watery diarrhea in a patient with a history of ileal resection or extensive ileal disease is likely to be caused by malabsorption of bile salts, which interferes with colonic absorption of fluid and electrolytes and which stimulates fluid and electrolyte secretion. This type of diarrhea is appropriately treated with the bile salt–binding resin cholestyramine (Questran), 4 grams in a glass of water, one to four times daily.

Diarrhea in Crohn's disease patients may be caused by bacterial overgrowth. Small intestinal strictures result in stasis in proximal loops of distended bowel. These patients respond best to antibiotics such as tetracycline, metronidazole, or ciprofloxacin. Fistulas between the small intestine and colon also result in bacterial overgrowth. In addition, fistulas may result in diarrhea by short-circuiting and bypassing large areas of small intestine. This problem is best treated surgically.

Pain in Crohn's disease patients may have several causes. Insidious development of crampy pain over weeks or months often associated with anemia and an elevated sedimentation rate is likely to be secondary to active disease and usually responds to mesalamine and corticosteroids. Additional therapy with antispasmodics such as dicyclomine (Bentyl) or hyoscyamine (Levsin) can help to provide symptomatic relief. In contrast, the abrupt onset of severe, often periumbilical pain associated with nausea and vomiting is likely to represent acute obstruction. This is confirmed with flat and upright abdominal radiographs and treated with bowel rest, intravenous administration of fluids, nasogastric decompression, and surgical consultation. If localized pain and fever are present, this should suggest an abscess. Antibiotics such as ciprofloxacin and metronidazole should be given and computed tomography done.

DRUG THERAPY

Aminosalicylates (sulfasalazine and mesalamine) form the foundation upon which therapy should be built in treatment of most patients with ulcerative colitis and Crohn's disease. Other therapies such as corticosteroids, antibiotics, and immunomodulatory agents are added to aminosalicylates, if needed, and are rarely used alone, unless aminosalicylates have totally failed or have been poorly tolerated.

Sulfasalazine

For many years the cornerstone of IBD therapy has been sulfasalazine (Azulfidine). Sulfasalazine is the combination of 5-ASA (mesalamine) and sulfapyridine connected to each other by a diazo bond. It is now known that 5-ASA is the active moiety of this compound and that sulfapyridine acts only as a carrier, transmitting the 5-ASA to the colon where it is released by colonic bacteria, which break the diazo bond liberating 5-ASA. In addition, the sulfapyridine moiety appears to be responsible for 90% of the adverse effects of sulfasalazine.

Indications for sulfasalazine are to treat active ulcerative colitis and to maintain disease remission. The usual therapeutic dose is 1 gram four times a day. Response rates are often dose related, and some patients who do not respond to 4 grams per day may respond to 6 grams daily of sulfasalazine in 4 divided doses. However, large doses of sulfasalazine are poorly tolerated. Large doses of mesalamine (1.2 grams 4 times a day), which delivers to the colon the amount of 5-ASA found in more than 10 grams of sulfasalazine, is a more effective and better tolerated approach. The usual maintenance dose of sulfasalazine is 1 gram twice a day; however, some patients experience breakthrough of disease activity at this dose and must be maintained indefinitely on 1 gram 3 to 4 times per day. Ulcerative colitis patients in remission who are maintained on sulfasalazine have only one fourth the number of flare-ups as patients who discontinue the drug.

Sulfasalazine should also be used to treat mild to moderate Crohn's disease. It is more effective in colitis then ileitis because most of the 5-ASA is released in the colon. Although the effectiveness of maintenance therapy in Crohn's disease has not been well documented, in patients whose disease has responded to sulfasalazine maintenance therapy is rea-

sonable. This is especially true if past sulfasalazine withdrawal has resulted in relapse.

Sulfasalazine is an excellent drug, is generic, and is relatively inexpensive. Although it crosses the placenta and appears in breast milk, it is safe in pregnancy, is not teratogenic, and does not cause kernicterus. Its use can be limited, however, by adverse effects. Ten to 15% of patients are allergic to the sulfa moiety and develop rash and/or fever 1 to 2 weeks after starting the drug. Many patients get dose-related nausea and gastric upset, which can be minimized by starting with a low dose of medication and gradually building up to a therapeutic dose. Giving sulfasalazine with food or using enteric-coated sulfasalazine can be helpful. Dose-related severe headaches from the sulfapyridine moiety can mimic migraine and limit the tolerated dose of sulfasalazine. Sulfapyridine is photosensitizing, and patients must be warned to use sunblock and to beware of sun exposure. Hematologic side effects include hemolysis, folate deficiency, and, rarely, agranulocytosis. Patients treated chronically with sulfasalazine should receive folic acid supplements, 1 mg per day. The sulfapyridine moiety depresses the sperm count in a dose-related fashion, which takes approximately 3 months to reverse. However, although sulfasalazine results in transient, reversible male infertility, it cannot be counted on as a reliable male contraceptive. Sulfasalazine can on rare occasion cause hepatitis, pneumonitis, and pancreatitis. The pancreatitis is caused by the 5-ASA (mesalamine) moiety.

Side effects of sulfasalazine often limit the ability to deliver 5-ASA to diseased bowel in sufficient quantity to achieve a complete clinical response. For this reason a number of mesalamine products devoid of the toxic sulfapyridine moiety have been developed.

Mesalamine (5-ASA) and Olsalazine

Mesalamine, the active therapeutic moiety of sulfasalazine comes in several distinct formulations. Asacol is 5-ASA encapsulated in a eudragit polymer that releases the 5-ASA at pH 7 in the colon and terminal ileum. Pentasa is 5-ASA encapsulated in slow release ethyl cellulose beads that release 5-ASA throughout the gastrointestinal tract, making it theoretically the drug of choice to treat Crohn's disease of the small intestine. Olsalazine (Dipentum) consists of two molecules of 5-ASA linked by a diazo bond. Colonic bacteria split the diazo bond, liberating 5-ASA in the colon. Olsalazine, in contrast to mesalamine, causes secretion of fluid in the small bowel. If there is active disease in the colon, this excess fluid may not be absorbed and secretory diarrhea results. For this reason, olsalazine is approved only for maintenance therapy of ulcerative colitis in a dose of 1 gram per day in two divided doses and is not approved to treat active ulcerative colitis.

Asacol is approved by the U.S. Food and Drug Administration (FDA) to treat active ulcerative colitis in a dose of 2.4 grams per day for up to 6 weeks. Published studies have indicated that at this dose approximately 50% of patients have clinical responses. On a higher dose of 4.8 grams per day,* however, 75% of patients respond. In my practice, sicker patients—namely, those also requiring corticosteroids—are treated with the larger dose until corticosteroids have been discontinued. Ulcerative colitis needs to be treated long term and not for only 6 weeks. Maintenance therapy with 5-ASA is safe and effective. Although low doses of mesalamine (1.6 grams per day) are often effective for this purpose, some patients require full therapeutic doses up to 4.8 grams per day to maintain remission.

Pentasa is approved in a dose of 4 grams per day (1 gram 4 times per day), for up to 8 weeks to treat active ulcerative colitis. Once again, ulcerative colitis cannot be treated for only 8 weeks, and maintenance therapy with this drug is also appropriate.

Although neither Asacol nor Pentasa nor even sulfasalazine is specifically approved by the FDA to treat Crohn's disease, several published placebo-controlled trials have demonstrated that all three drugs are more effective than placebo in treating active Crohn's colitis and ileitis. In Crohn's disease patients in remission, who were selected to have a high likelihood of relapse, both Asacol and Pentasa have also been shown to be more effective than placebo in preventing or delaying relapse.

Mesalamine is effective topically in the form of Rowasa suppositories (500 mg), taken twice daily after bowel movements and at bedtime, to treat proctitis. Rowasa retention enemas (4 grams) taken at bedtime are used in the treatment of proctosigmoiditis or left sided (distal) ulcerative colitis. These topical medications are sometimes needed in combination with oral mesalamine or sulfasalazine to treat pancolitis. Oral mesalamine effectively treats the ascending, transverse, and descending colon, but by the time it reaches the distal colon and rectum it may be encased in solid stool, which is rapidly and urgently expelled. Because the topical effect is important, adding mesalamine enemas or suppositories is often necessary to effect healing of the entire colon.

Mesalamine is usually well tolerated, with most studies showing a side effect profile not different from placebo. One to 2% of patients can paradoxically develop diarrhea and even colitis from mesalamine, and these patients usually experience the same reaction from sulfasalazine. Patients allergic to salicylates cannot use mesalamine. Occasional patients experience hair loss. Rare cases of hepatitis, pancreatitis, and pericarditis occur. In large doses in experimental animals nephrotoxicity can be seen, and rare cases of interstitial nephritis in humans have been reported. For this reason, it is my practice to obtain a urinalysis and serum creatinine determination at baseline and every 6 months. This is especially important because I often use these drugs in higher than the approved dosages, for longer periods than are approved, and often for unapproved indications (treatment of Crohn's disease).

*Exceeds dosage recommended by the manufacturer.

Corticosteroids

Corticosteroids can rapidly reduce inflammation and suppress disease activity and play an important role in the acute treatment of patients with moderate to severe disease activity. However, because of the myriad of serious corticosteroid-induced side effects, it is unacceptable for patients to be maintained indefinitely on toxic doses of corticosteroids without a plan for eliminating them. For this reason corticosteroids should rarely be used as monotherapy. When sulfasalazine or mesalamine has failed to induce remission in either ulcerative colitis or Crohn's disease, corticosteroids are added to the treatment regimen. Initially, doses of 40 to 60 mg of prednisone are added either to 4 grams of sulfasalazine or to 4.0 to 4.8 grams of mesalamine. It is better to suppress the disease initially with a large dose of prednisone followed by tapering of the corticosteroid dose than to give an inadequate dose followed by incremental dosage increases.

Side effects can be minimized by giving prednisone as a single morning dose. A small number of patients will have breakthrough of symptoms in the evening and will require splitting of the dose into morning and evening doses. If this can be avoided, however, it is preferable, because there is less adrenal suppression with a single dose and the morning dosing does not interfere with evening sleep. Once disease remission has been induced, I taper prednisone by 10 mg every 7 to 14 days until 20 mg per day is reached. I then reduce the dose in 5-mg increments to 10 mg per day. My last two tapering phases are 10 mg every other day, and then 5 mg every other day each for about 10 days. The idea is to find the minimal corticosteroid dose (hopefully zero) necessary to suppress disease. If the disease repeatedly flares on corticosteroid taper, despite maximal doses of mesalamine or sulfasalazine, then immunomodulatory agents or surgery should be entertained. Budesonide is an investigational corticosteroid metabolized in a single passage through the liver and thus has fewer side effects than other corticosteroids. Clinical studies have shown both budesonide enemas and enteric-coated budesonide, 9 mg once daily, to be clinically effective.

Hospitalized patients with severe ulcerative colitis or Crohn's disease should receive the equivalent of 300 to 400 mg per day of hydrocortisone intravenously by continuous infusion. Most studies show no advantage to therapy with adrenocorticotropic hormone. Solid foods initially should be withheld. Although controversial, I believe strongly that aminosalicylates should also be administered. I have seen patients who do not respond to corticosteroids until aminosalicylates are added to the treatment regimen. In fact, far too many patients have developed severe colitis simply because they have discontinued aminosalicylates on their own, thinking they were cured. Parenteral nutrition and transfusions should be provided when appropriate. Patients with ulcerative colitis who are sick enough to be hospitalized must be carefully monitored by daily physical examination by both gastroenterologist and surgeon. Abdominal radiographs should be obtained every 1 to 2 days, checking for development of megacolon. High-dose corticosteroid therapy can mask serious disease, produce a feeling of patient well-being, and lead the physician to a false sense of security. These patients are at risk of development of toxic megacolon or spontaneous life-threatening perforation. Patients who do not improve significantly after 1 week of intravenous corticosteroids should have surgery or therapy with intravenous cyclosporine (Sandimmune).*

Immunomodulatory Agents

Immunomodulatory agents can produce serious side effects and are not usually considered as initial therapy. Immunomodulatory therapy should be added to mesalamine and corticosteroids when these therapies have proven inadequate or when corticosteroids cannot be tapered and eliminated without a disease flare.

Extensive favorable experience has been obtained with 6-mercaptopurine (6-MP, Purinethol)* and its parent compound azathioprine (Imuran).* Approximately two thirds of patients with both ulcerative colitis and Crohn's disease have significant clinical improvement. Corticosteroids can be eliminated in more than 50% of patients while clinical well-being is maintained. Fistulas close in about one third of patients. It often takes 3 months or more before clinical response is seen. The usual therapeutic dose for 6-MP is 1.5 mg per kg per day, and for azathioprine, it is 2.5 mg per kg per day. I start with 50 mg of 6-MP and increase the dose to 1.5 mg per kg per day after the first month. Initially, the complete blood cell count should be monitored every 1 to 2 weeks. If the drug is well tolerated and the dose is not changed, after several months, monthly blood cell counts are sufficient. Patients on long-term maintenance therapy can be monitored every 3 months. If the white blood cell count drops below 3000 per mm³, the drug should be temporarily stopped or the dosage reduced. Open-ended prescriptions for more than 3 months are unwise, and refills should only be granted after laboratory studies have been obtained.

Adverse effects include marrow depression with leukopenia, which can lead to serious infectious complications. Pancreatitis, allergic reactions, and hepatitis may occur. Concerns about cancer and lymphoma have been raised but are overstated. Most physicians discontinue these drugs before pregnancy; however, when needed, they have been taken throughout pregnancy without teratogenicity or adversity. Although complications can be severe, it is important to keep in mind that only 5 to 7% of patients treated with these agents experience side effects. The drugs are usually well tolerated and with proper monitoring are relatively safe. In contrast, all patients treated with large doses of corticosteroids

for long periods will have adverse reactions. For these reasons, long-term maintenance therapy with 6-MP or azathioprine should be considered in patients with good therapeutic responses in whom corticosteroids have been successfully discontinued.

Methotrexate,* 25 mg intramuscularly for 12 weeks, has been demonstrated to produce clinical, endoscopic and histologic remission in patients with severe Crohn's disease. Improvement occurs within 2 to 8 weeks. When patients are switched to oral methotrexate and the dosage is lowered to 12.5 to 15 mg per day, disease activity ultimately recurs. Data for the treatment of ulcerative colitis with methotrexate have been less convincing, and sigmoidoscopic healing has not been documented. Potential side effects include nausea, diarrhea, hepatotoxicity, leukopenia, teratogenicity, atypical pneumonia, and pulmonary fibrosis. If any pulmonary symptoms develop, the drug should be withheld and pulmonary status should be thoroughly evaluated.

Cyclosporine* has been used effectively in hospitalized patients with severe ulcerative colitis who have failed 1 week of intravenous corticosteroids. Dosage is 2 to 4 mg per kg by continuous intravenous infusion, which is added to ongoing corticosteroid therapy. Hypocholesterolemia is a relative contraindication to cyclosporine therapy and increases the risk of seizures. Whole blood cyclosporine levels must be monitored, with attempts to maintain trough levels between 200 and 400 µg per mL. Blood pressure, renal function, and potassium and magnesium levels must also be monitored. Sixty to 80% of patients may leave the hospital without colon surgery; however, at least half have colectomies within 1 year. One of my patients developed spontaneous colon perforation and another developed toxic megacolon while on intravenously administered cyclosporine; hence the lack of great enthusiasm for this agent. Responders are switched to oral cyclosporine (Neoral) initially at twice the intravenous dose with efforts to maintain the same trough levels. Monitoring must be performed weekly. Trimethoprim-sulfamethoxazole prophylaxis for *Pneumocystis carinii* should be provided. When the condition is stable, 6-MP or azathioprine is added and corticosteroids are tapered as clinically permitted. After 3 to 6 months, if the patient remains in remission, cyclosporine therapy is tapered and discontinued. Complications of cyclosporine are common, and major complications have been reported in 15% of cases. Side effects include irreversible renal dysfunction, hypertension, hyperkalemia, seizures, hypertrichosis, opportunistic infections, and lymphomas.

Intravenous cyclosporine, 2 to 4 mg per kg by continuous infusion, has been used for patients with severe refractory Crohn's disease and for patients with refractory fistulas. Oral cyclosporine, 5 to 7.5 mg per kg per day, may also be effective in patients with severe Crohn's disease. Because of the potential toxicity associated with cyclosporine, its use should be restricted to the sickest patients who have failed all therapy or who are experiencing unacceptable

---

*Not FDA approved for this indication.

toxicity from conventional therapy. Low-dose cyclosporine is ineffective for either treatment of active Crohn's disease or for maintenance of remission. In fact, in one study, relapse occurred more frequently and in a shorter period of time in patients treated with low-dose cyclosporine than in those treated with placebo.

NEW IMMUNOMODULATORY AGENTS

The use of cytokines such as interleukin-10 and interleukin-11, which down-regulate the immune system, as well as antibodies to proinflammatory cytokines such as tumor necrosis factor-α are being investigated and show much promise.

Chimeric antibody to tumor necrosis factor-α, known as infliximab (Remicade), is the first of such agents to be approved to treat patients with severe refractory Crohn's disease. After a single intravenous infusion, 65% of such patients had clinical responses and 33% achieved remission within 4 weeks. Clinical response persisted 12 weeks after the initial infusion. Infusions at baseline and at 2 and 6 weeks have been reported to heal intractable fistulas. Dosage is 5 mg per kg administered in 250 mL of normal saline intravenously over 2 hours using an in-line low-protein binding filter and a polyethylene-lined infusion set, as recommended by the manufacturer. Side effects appear to be mild and uncommon. However, there is a disturbing report of adverse reactions including myalgias, rash, fever, and polyarthralgia in 25% of patients reinfused with infliximab 2 years or more after the initial infusion. The long-term safety of repeated infusions of infliximab remains to be established. Infliximab is not useful in the treatment of ulcerative colitis.

ANTIBIOTICS

Antibiotics have been believed by experienced clinicians to provide useful primary as well as adjunctive therapy in Crohn's disease. Antibiotic therapy may treat the underlying disease as well as infectious complications such as abscesses and bacterial overgrowth. Metronidazole in doses of 10 to 20 mg per kg in three divided doses has been demonstrated to be more effective than placebo and as effective as sulfasalazine in treating Crohn's colitis and ileocolitis. Improvement in perianal Crohn's disease with metronidazole therapy has been well documented. Side effects of nausea, anorexia, and paresthesias limit the long-term use of this drug. Although less well studied, similar benefits have been observed with twice-daily administration of 500 mg of ciprofloxacin (Cipro) or clarithromycin (Biaxin). In general, antibiotics have not proven to be beneficial in patients with ulcerative colitis.

DIETARY THERAPY

General nutritional support should be emphasized. Patients with lactose intolerance, which can add to symptomatology, should be counseled to avoid milk products or to use Lact-Aid products. Calcium supplements are appropriate in patients who must avoid milk products or who must take corticosteroids. Iron supplements should be given if iron deficiency is present, although these can often cause abdominal cramping in Crohn's disease patients. Folic acid, 1 mg per day, is appropriate for patients maintained on sulfasalazine or 6-MP or azathioprine. Vitamin B_{12} injections are necessary for patients who have had an ileal resection or who have extensive ileal disease. In malnourished patients with hypoalbuminemia, enteral supplements may be helpful.

Restrictive Crohn's or colitis diets are usually not helpful. Some patients find that fiber is symptomatically helpful whereas others find that it aggravates symptoms. Liquid diets can be helpful in patients with obstructive symptoms. Individual patients may find that specific foods aggravate symptoms and certainly they should avoid those foods. However, no consistent patterns that fit all or even most patients have emerged.

In patients with steroid-dependent Crohn's disease who are either unwilling or unable to take immunomodulatory drugs, elemental diets or total parenteral nutrition can at times be useful. It has been documented that replacement of the normal diet with an elemental diet such as Vivonex, or total parenteral nutrition, can induce remission. This suggests the possibility that removal of unknown dietary antigens may provide effective therapy. In children, this approach, using nocturnal feedings of Vivonex through a pediatric nasogastric feeding tube, has been effective in both inducing remission and reversing growth retardation. In contrast, there is no evidence that eliminating oral intake and providing either an elemental diet or total parenteral nutrition has any value as primary therapy for ulcerative colitis.

OTHER MEDICAL THERAPIES

Ulcerative colitis is more common in nonsmokers and ex-smokers, and some patients experience onset of disease or disease flares coincident with cessation of smoking. In this subset of patients, the disease can often be turned off by resumption of smoking and turned back on by smoking cessation. These observations have led to a number of studies investigating the use of nicotine patches (Nicoderm/Nicotrol) for the treatment of flares of ulcerative colitis. When patients were treated with the highest tolerated doses, up to 22 mg per day, as therapy supplemental to conventional therapy, improvement was statistically more common than seen in the group treated with placebo patches. There was, however, a high incidence of side effects, including nausea, lightheadedness, headache, and sleep disturbances, especially in the subgroup of patients who had never smoked. For this reason, I have usually limited my use of nicotine patches to patients who have experienced flares of the disorder with cessation of smoking. In this subgroup, nicotine patches are often effective;

however, when they are stopped, disease activity usually recurs. Crohn's disease, in contrast, is more common in smokers. Furthermore, the amount of smoking often correlates directly with disease activity. Nicotine therapy therefore has no role in treatment of Crohn's disease.

Fish oils (omega-3 fatty acids) decrease leukotriene production and have been postulated on the basis of epidemiologic data to be useful in preventing or treating inflammatory bowel disease. Data with respect to ulcerative colitis have been conflicting. Fish oils may, however, be useful in preventing relapse in patients with Crohn's disease. In one well-designed study, Crohn's disease patients in remission, selected because of a high likelihood of flare (elevated sedimentation rate or C reactive protein), were randomized to receive enteric-coated fish oil (Purepa), 2.7 grams per day or placebo. No other therapy was allowed. Over the following year, the incidence of clinical relapse was reduced by more than 50% in the group taking fish oil. Although fish oil capsules are available in health food stores, enteric-coated Purepa is not available in the United States. It is unclear whether the enteric coating is essential for clinical response. Because the patients in this study were not taking mesalamine, which also interferes with leukotriene synthesis, it is unclear whether fish oil offers any therapeutic advantage over mesalamine.

BIPHOSPHONATES

Factors that contribute to bone loss in inflammatory bowel disease include systemic inflammation, poor nutrition, malabsorption, and use of corticosteroids. Corticosteroids cause both increased bone resorption and decreased bone formation. Corticosteroid-induced osteoporosis occurs rapidly with a mean loss of 15% of trabecular bone in 12 months while on 10 to 25 mg per day of prednisone. Bone loss is directly dependent on both dose and duration of prednisone therapy. Furthermore, patients on corticosteroids experience fracture at a higher bone density mass than postmenopausal women. In addition, Crohn's disease patients have a significant decrease in bone density even if they are not taking corticosteroids. Thus, preventive bone treatment for patients with IBD receiving ongoing corticosteroid therapy should be routine. For low-dose prednisone therapy (<10 mg/day), 1000 mg of calcium plus 500 units of vitamin D per day should prevent bone loss. On higher doses of prednisone this approach is inadequate alone and biphosphonate therapy, either in the form of alendronate (Fosamax) or etidronate (Didronel), is appropriate. Alendronate is administered in a dose of 5 to 10 mg daily with copious amounts of water on arising. No food is allowed for 1 hour and the patient must not lie down after taking the drug. Severe esophagitis is a serious complication if instructions are not followed religiously. Daily calcium and vitamin D supplements are also required. Etidronate is taken at a dose of 400 mg per day on an empty stomach for 2-week blocks of time. Because it

does not cause esophagitis it can be taken at bedtime. Calcium, 1000 mg per day, is then taken for the next 11 weeks after the completion of etidronate. The cycle is then repeated with 2 weeks of etidronate followed by 11 weeks of calcium throughout the year. On this regimen, lumbar spine and trochanteric bone density increased and the relative risk of vertebral fractures was decreased compared with patients treated with calcium alone. Newer biphosphonates are being evaluated.

CANCER SURVEILLANCE

Ulcerative colitis is a premalignant disease. The entire colon is at risk. After extensive colitis has been present 8 to 10 years, colonoscopic surveillance is indicated every 1 to 2 years. Random biopsy samples are obtained at 10-cm intervals, and any raised areas are sampled looking for dysplasia. Colonoscopic surveillance is best performed when the disease is in remission. Colonoscopy is better tolerated when the disease is quiescent and the possibility that the pathologist may confuse reactive atypia with dysplasia is minimized. The presence of confirmed dysplasia (even low grade) indicates that neoplastic change has occurred and is an indication for colectomy. Surgical specimens from such patients not uncommonly reveal the presence of carcinoma. In patients with disease limited to the left colon, surveillance usually begins after 15 years of disease; and if the proximal colon is endoscopically and histologically normal, it can subsequently be performed with the flexible sigmoidoscope. Patients with Crohn's colitis are also at risk for colon cancer, especially in extensively diseased areas of colon. Colonoscopic surveillance is performed periodically but is controversial and more difficult to perform because of frequent cobblestone nodularity and stricturing that are part of the inflammatory process. Sampling error makes it easy to miss dysplastic or malignant changes.

SURGERY

Surgery is indicated in ulcerative colitis, when either the disease is refractory to medical management or the when the burden of chronic disease and the side effects of corticosteroids or other therapy become unacceptable. Massive bleeding, megacolon (with threat of perforation), dysplasia, stricture, or suspected colon cancer are also indications for surgery. Total proctocolectomy usually with ileoanal anastomosis is the procedure of choice. In most cases this is curative; however, some patients develop pouchitis in the surgically created ileal pouch. This usually responds to therapy with metronidazole. Mesalamine, cholestyramine, and bismuth (Pepto-Bismol) have also been reported to be useful in the treatment of pouchitis.

Most patients with Crohn's disease ultimately have surgery. Surgical indications include obstruction, nonhealing fistulas, perforation usually with abscess formation, uncontrollable hemorrhage, and toxic megacolon. When the disease appears grossly limited, the diseased intestinal segment is removed and healthy bowel is anastomosed to healthy bowel. When there are multiple skip areas of involvement it is best to remove only the major area of involvement producing symptoms in an effort to preserve as much bowel as possible. When multiple strictured segments are present, strictureplasties can be performed. Surgery often gives the patient a new beginning and eliminates the need for medication for a time; however, it is not curative. Recurrences, usually at the anastomotic site, are to be expected and should be managed medically when possible, because repeated resections can lead to short bowel syndrome.

EMOTIONAL SUPPORT

Patients with inflammatory bowel disease suffer from a chronic disorder, the cause and cure of which are unknown. They may experience chronic diarrhea, embarrassing urgency and incontinence, abdominal pain, fistulas, and painful and disfiguring perianal disease. They face the prospect of noncurative surgery, cancer risk, and the possibility of an ostomy. They worry about transmitting the disease to their offspring. Although there is no evidence that ulcerative colitis or Crohn's disease are psychosomatic disorders or are caused by stress, living with these disorders can be extremely stressful, producing depression or anxiety. As with any disorder, if emotional problems are present, they should be treated. A positive, nonrestrictive, supportive approach by both physician and family is essential to enable these patients to live as normal a life as possible. Local chapters of the Crohn's and Colitis Foundation of America provide patient educational material and patient support groups, which can be extremely helpful.

THE IRRITABLE BOWEL SYNDROME

method of
EAMONN M. M. QUIGLEY, M.D.
Cork University Hospital
Cork, Ireland

University of Nebraska Medical Center
Omaha, Nebraska

The irritable bowel syndrome (IBS) is a very common clinical disorder whose definition rests entirely on clinical grounds; a clear definition of the pathologic or biochemical basis for this syndrome does not, as yet, exist. Therein lies the major challenge of this disorder; our understanding of its prevalence, epidemiology, and prognosis may be considerably influenced by the nature of its very definition. Similarly, studies of pathophysiology and therapeutic response will likely yield vastly different results, depending on the population surveyed and the definition of IBS employed.

DEFINITION

Although some authorities question even the very attempt to define IBS, most investigators and clinicians value the concept of a clinical definition of IBS. Those who object to this approach contend that attempts to define IBS represent no more than a refuge for the nominalist, that is, the temptation, in an attempt to shroud our ignorance, to give a name to a clinical problem for which we have no explanation. These purists propose, instead, that unexplained abdominal pain should be described as such; no more, no less.

On the basis of a variety of evidence, others have come to view IBS as a true syndrome defined by the presence of a constellation of symptoms that tend to aggregate. It is clear, however, that at the margins of this constellation, one particular symptom may dominate. To facilitate clinical research in particular, various attempts have been made to provide a relatively inclusive, sensitive, and specific definition for IBS. Among the various diagnostic criteria that have been proposed, the Manning and Rome criteria have achieved the greatest popularity. The Rome criteria are currently being re-evaluated and may well be updated.

Other studies have included a variety of "simple" laboratory tests in an attempt to further refine separation between functional and organic disease. For the moment, the Rome criteria have come to be regarded as the standard instrument for community studies, pathophysiologic investigations, and therapeutic interventions. Although a variety of studies have suggested reasonable sensitivity and specificity for these criteria, it must be remembered that we have no gold standard for the definition of IBS, and data on sensitivity, specificity, and positive predictive value for these criteria are inevitably "soft." Patients who fulfill the criteria may or may not reflect the true epidemiology of IBS. On the basis of these criteria, it has been suggested that in the developed world, IBS affects between 14 and 24% of women and 5 and 19% of men. IBS tends to decrease in prevalence in later life.

A very important concept in functional disorders relates to the differences observed between patients with functional disorders who seek help from a physician and those whose symptoms are detected only on community surveys. Patients with functional disorders who seek medical attention are different psychologically from those who live with their symptoms without medical assistance. Health care–seeking behavior must be taken into account in the evaluation of the IBS patient seen in the clinic. Studies of any aspect of IBS performed in a clinic population, and especially in tertiary referral practice, must take into account the factors that led the patients both to see the physician in the first place and then to find their way to a highly specialized clinic.

Another problem that complicates the interpretation of IBS studies is the considerable overlap between IBS, functional dyspepsia, chronic constipation, and idiopathic diarrhea. Most studies suggest that perhaps half of all IBS patients fulfill diagnostic criteria for functional, nonulcer dyspepsia. This overlap may have a significant influence not only on patient symptomatology, but also on the outcome of studies of pathophysiology or therapy.

Not only is there overlap between IBS and other functional disorders but there also appears to be considerable overlap between IBS and a variety of other "functional" complaints such as fatigue, headache, urologic symptoms, gynecologic problems, and "fibromyalgia." Gastroesophageal reflux–type symptoms, noncardiac chest pain, dysphagia, chronic pelvic pain, dyspareunia, and dysmenorrhea are all more common among IBS subjects. A relationship between IBS and hysterectomy has also been proposed, although it is unclear what role hysterectomy per se may play in the development of such symptoms, and constipation and defecatory dysfunction in particular.

NATURAL HISTORY

The typical clinical course of IBS is one of waxing and waning. Although some patients may deteriorate, most tend to remain stable or improve. Somewhat reassuringly, it has been found that once the diagnosis of IBS is established—on the basis of clinical evaluation and application of one of the diagnostic criteria systems—with confidence, the likelihood of a new diagnosis is distinctly uncommon.

PATHOPHYSIOLOGY

Motor Dysfunction and Irritable Bowel Syndrome

When attempting to explain IBS symptoms, the physician frequently invokes such terms as "spasm," which suggests a fundamental role for motility in the pathophysiology of IBS. Although time honored and, indeed, supported by a considerable volume of literature, this concept may be ill founded. Abnormalities in esophageal, gastric, small intestinal, and colonic motor function have been reported in IBS, but the basis for a primary motor abnormality in IBS is far from firmly defined. Thus, colonic and small intestinal dysmotility have not been consistently described in IBS, and comparisons of studies are often marred by variations in technique, interpretation, and subject selection. Basal patterns of colonic and small intestinal motility are similar in IBS and appropriate control subjects, "abnormalities" among IBS patients being more consistent in response to either meal ingestion or various forms of stress. Although jejunal "clustered" contractions have been reported in a number of studies, this phenomenon has not been universal and it is not specific for IBS. Dysmotility may not be universal in IBS, but abnormal patterns do occur. What, then, is the role of motor activity in the clinical presentation and pathophysiology of IBS?

I believe that this question needs to be addressed in the broadest context. First and foremost, our efforts in this area continue to be frustrated by an inability to clearly define IBS. Different diagnostic criteria lead to the inclusion of varying patient populations. It has been shown, for example, that IBS patients with either predominant constipation or diarrhea may exhibit quite dissimilar motility patterns. Current diagnostic limitations may also lead to the inclusion, among those groups of patients currently considered to have IBS, of subgroups who truly have primary, although as yet undefined, abnormalities of intestinal nerve or muscle.

Other factors, such as stress or coexistent psychopathology, for example, could also explain abnormal motor patterns in IBS. The ability of various types of stress to influence motor activity throughout the gastrointestinal tract, while amply demonstrated, is rarely taken into account in study designs despite the fact that IBS patients may indeed be unusually susceptible to the effects of stress. The influence of psychopathology on IBS patients, in general, also remains uncertain. It is clear that various psychiatric disorders may influence motility per se, and their inclusion in IBS study groups will further confound study interpretation.

Motility may also interact with other factors. The role of sensation and perception in the pathophysiology of various functional disorders is being increasingly appreciated. Thus, several lines of evidence suggest that IBS subjects are more sensitive to a variety of intraluminal stimuli. It is also evident that sensory afferents are capable of influencing motor activity through effects mediated not only via the central nervous system but also through local reflexes within the gut wall, thereby providing a mechanism whereby an intraluminal stimulus may directly produce motor changes. IBS subjects may thus be more likely both to perceive an intraluminal event and to develop "dysmotility" in response to the same stimulus.

We are now, therefore, experiencing a shift in emphasis in IBS from a preoccupation with "abnormal" motor patterns to a viewpoint that interprets motility in the broader framework of neuroenteric interactions. Motility has a role in IBS, but it appears more likely that motor phenomena represent a component of a response to either the luminal milieu or the external environment rather than that they reflect an intrinsic abnormality of intestinal nerve or muscle. One study has, indeed, demonstrated a heightened perception of normal motor activity along some IBS subjects. IBS and related disorders may thus come to be regarded as disorders of gut hypersensitivity or hyperresponsiveness rather than intrinsic hyperactivity.

Enhanced Visceral Sensitivity

Given the abovementioned limitations of studies of motor function in IBS and the development of a variety of methods that permit a more reproducible assessment of visceral sensation, emphasis has lately shifted to the role of visceral sensation and the perception of gut activity in IBS. It has been known for some time that patients with IBS are more sensitive to balloon distention of the colon. Several studies have now extended this concept of visceral hypersensitivity to the entire gastrointestinal tract. Esophageal hypersensitivity has been demonstrated in patients with "noncardiac" chest pain, gastric hypersensitivity in nonulcer dyspepsia, and hypersensitivity of the small intestine and colon in IBS. Not all patients with IBS, however, demonstrate visceral hypersensitivity. Indeed, one investigator has suggested that as many as 36% of IBS subjects have normal baseline rectal sensitivity. It has also been suggested that rectal hyperalgesia (the development of greater pain and higher intensity rates of discomfort at a particular stimulus level) and not hypersensitivity (a lower threshold for sensation of a particular stimulus) is the hallmark of IBS.

Another characteristic of IBS noted in these studies is an increased viscerosomatic referral in response to rectal distention. In a very recent intriguing study, Munakata and colleagues demonstrated that repetitive stimulation of sigmoid afferents resulted in the development of central sensitization manifested as hyperalgesia and increased viscerosomatic referral on rectal distention. These subjects also developed spontaneous rectosigmoid hyperalgesia in the absence of applied stimuli. Munakata and colleagues speculated that repetitive sigmoid contractions, such as those that are known to occur in IBS patients in response to stress, emotions, postprandially, and before a bowel movement, may induce rectosigmoid hyperalgesia to normal luminal stimuli in IBS patients. This concept provides a further example of the interaction between motility and sensation in pathophysiology.

Other evidence suggests that abnormalities in central perception or sensory processing occur in IBS. Although this is a relatively new area of study, certain lines of evidence suggest that there may indeed be abnormalities in the central nervous system in functional disorders. Studies in nonulcer dyspepsia, for example, have revealed evidence of abnormalities in central serotonergic neurotransmission, and elegant studies of IBS have demonstrated aberrant brain activation patterns during both painful rectal distention and in anticipation of rectal pain in IBS subjects. Others have shown that motor patterns, such as the migrating motor complex, normally subconscious, are experienced at a conscious level among irritable bowel subjects.

These studies of visceral sensation and central perception are extremely intriguing. It is too early, however, to determine whether they contain the ultimate answer to IBS.

The Role of Psychopathology

Although it has been traditional to regard IBS subjects as being, to a greater or lesser extent, psychologically abnormal, there is, in fact, little or no evidence to support the concept of a universal psychological abnormality in IBS. Here perhaps more than in any other area of medicine has referral bias led to the extrapolation of results from a highly selective group of (IBS) subjects to (IBS) patients in general. Critical reviews of studies of psychopathology in IBS have concluded that such studies are, for the most part, highly questionable, on the basis of either the study population examined or the instruments employed. Those studies that have been performed with truly unselected groups of IBS subjects and that have also employed appropriate instruments do not suggest either that IBS patients as a whole are psychologically impaired or that there is a single psychological trait that explains their symptomatology. Rather, these studies suggest that psychopathology plays a more important role in patients' decisions to seek medical care and further referral. This is not to dispute either that psychological stress may exacerbate gastrointestinal symptoms or that IBS symptoms can in turn impact psychological and physical well-being.

Infection, Inflammation, and Irritable Bowel Syndrome

Clinicians have long been familiar with patients with IBS or other functional gastrointestinal disorders who give a history of the sudden onset of their now chronic symptoms in relation to a "flu-like illness" or a "gastric upset." Although experimental studies of immune-motility interactions in the gastrointestinal tract have provided a pathophysiologic basis for this phenomenon, there were, however, until the 1990s, few data to support this anecdotal observation. Other studies provide a firm basis for a relationship between IBS and prior infective gastroenteritis. In Nottingham, England, 544 individuals were studied for at least 6 months after an episode of bacteriologically confirmed bacterial gastroenteritis. One-fourth reported persistence of an altered bowel habit 6 months after the episode of infective gastroenteritis, and 1 in 14 had developed IBS. Risk factors for the development of chronic symptoms and IBS were female gender and the severity of the initial illnesses. This study does not, of course, define the pathophysiology of infectious IBS nor does it clarify whether the development of IBS, in this context, represents its clinical expression in an individual who was already predisposed or the induction, by the infectious agent or the related immune response, of dysmotility or other disordered physi-

ology in individuals who previously had a normal gastrointestinal tract.

EVALUATION AND MANAGEMENT

It is depressing to report that there has been little progress in our approach to the diagnosis and management of IBS since the 1950s.

Two approaches to diagnosis IBS are used in clinical practice. The first arrives at a diagnosis of IBS by exclusion; the second attempts to make a positive diagnosis of IBS. The acceptance of the Manning and Rome, as well as other, diagnostic criteria and the relative integrity of an IBS diagnosis arrived at by these means over time have given considerable support to those who attempt the less interventional approach.

In practice, the approach to clinical evaluation is based on several clinical (and some nonclinical) factors. In the younger patient (i.e., younger than 40 years), the diagnostic work-up is primarily based on a full history and careful clinical examination; formal tests are restricted to such routine ones as a complete blood count, sedimentation rate, chemistry profile, and simple stool studies. For the older patient, most physicians would add a study of colonic morphology, such as flexible sigmoidoscopy or barium enema, although the benefits of this approach have not been prospectively studied. Although the colonic morphology studies, together with hemoccult tests, can be justified on the basis of colon cancer screening, there is little evidence to suggest a significant diagnostic yield in the patient with "typical" IBS symptoms.

The driving force behind investigations in IBS is the concern that organic disorders will be missed. In the evaluation of the patient with chronic abdominal pain (perhaps the most difficult patient subgroup), endometriosis, pelvic inflammatory disease, ovarian cancer, metastatic cancer of the upper abdomen (especially from breast), chronic mesenteric ischemia, and Crohn's disease should be borne in mind, in particular, and sought for if there are suggestive clinical features. Perhaps for these reasons, many physicians would suggest the addition of abdominal ultrasonography for the female patient with chronic IBS-type symptoms. For the patient with predominant diarrhea, my own belief is that the diagnostic work-up needs to be more rigorous as there are a number of "organic" disorders that may masquerade as IBS among this subgroup; diagnoses to consider include latent celiac sprue, carbohydrate intolerance, and lymphocytic-collagenous colitis.

The cornerstones of management remain reassurance and treatment of symptoms. For patients with mild intermittent symptoms, reassurance that they do not have a serious organic disorder, together with a thoughtful discussion of the nature of IBS, may be sufficient. Although the role of these approaches has been little studied in this disorder, there is some evidence that the establishment of a good patient-physician relationship is of considerable importance in the management of IBS in general.

The primary IBS symptoms that necessitate treatment are constipation, diarrhea, and abdominal pain. Although almost universally recommended for IBS, evidence for the efficacy of fiber and fiber supplements for this disorder is, in fact, inconclusive. Indeed, there is evidence to suggest that, while these approaches may improve stool frequency and consistency, pain may be exacerbated. The physician needs to be aware, therefore, that while the constipation may be helped by an adherence to general guidelines for the treatment of constipation, some of the other symptoms of this disorder may be exacerbated.

For the treatment of diarrhea, loperamide (Imodium A-D) is generally recommended as the first-line option. This preference is, in part, based on the lack of penetration of this compound into the blood-brain barrier and the demonstration, in controlled clinical trials, of its efficacy for this symptom in IBS. In one study, whereas stool frequency and consistency improved, nocturnal pain was exacerbated by loperamide. There has been a tendency to recommend a variety of dietary adjustments for the patient with IBS. There is, in fact, no good evidence from prospective studies that these dietary adjustments are of benefit. My approach is to advise patients to avoid the foods that they have found, from experience, exacerbate their symptoms.

Pain is a prominent symptom in IBS, and its management remains a major challenge. For many years, presumably because this disorder was thought to arise from muscle spasm, antispasmodics have been the basis of therapy. Although studies of antispasmodics in IBS have been criticized on the basis of inadequacy of study design and interpretation, a meta-analysis suggested that these agents do relieve pain and improve global assessment scores in IBS. In this review, a variety of anticholinergics were found to be effective in symptom relief; there is little evidence, however, that any of these agents affect the natural history of IBS. Gut-specific antimuscarinic anticholinergics have been developed, and their role in IBS is under evaluation.

Given the importance now attributed to altered visceral sensitivity in IBS, considerable emphasis has been placed on the development of compounds capable of influencing visceral sensitivity. Experimental studies in animal models and in humans have demonstrated that a wide variety of agents, including serotonin (5-HT$_3$) antagonists,* the somatostatin analogue octreotide (Sandostatin),* and opiate agonists such as fedotozine,† can diminish or modulate the sensory response to intestinal distention. Formal clinical trials of fedotozine in functional bowel disorders have produced conflicting results, but initial results from studies of 5-HT$_3$ antagonists such as alosetron† have been encouraging. Interestingly, alosetron appears particularly effective for females with predominant diarrhea.

On the basis of the assumption that anxiety and depression are common among patients with IBS, antidepressants have been widely used in the management of this disorder. As discussed previously, however, the basis for this assumption is now questioned; there is ample evidence of the efficacy of these agents in IBS. It is also evident, again from more recent studies, that these agents can also modulate visceral pain, and this may be their primary mode of action in this and other functional gastrointestinal disorders. Most studies to date have been performed with traditional tricyclic antidepressants, and these drugs have been shown to reduce abdominal pain and diarrhea. Preliminary data suggest that the serotonin reuptake inhibitors may also be effective and may have the additional benefit of relieving constipation.

Several studies have examined the role of a variety of psychological therapies, including hypnotherapy, group therapy, and psychotherapy, for IBS. These approaches are time and therapist intensive, and most studies have therefore involved relatively small numbers of patients. These limitations notwithstanding, it is clear that these therapies are effective in relieving anxiety and other psychological problems as well as in improving the symptoms of irritable bowel syndrome per se. In a review, Drossman and colleagues suggested that the following patients are most likely to respond to psychological approaches: those who see a clear relationship between exacerbations of bowel symptoms and exposure to stress, have the more typical IBS rather than chronic pain, are younger than 50 years of age, and have lower levels of trait anxiety.

Perhaps the most difficult patient management problem is intractable abdominal pain. Some authorities would argue that affected patients, by definition, do not belong under the umbrella of IBS given their lack of bowel dysfunction. In my experience, however, some cases of classic IBS evolved into a chronic pain syndrome that seemed intractable to conventional therapeutic approaches. The temptation to resort to narcotic analgesics for this patient group must be resisted. Not only may the patient become dependent, but these agents are not particularly effective in the management of visceral pain. Of all the various agents that have been studied for this group, those that have demonstrated the most consistent results have again been antidepressants.

A few studies have examined the influence of motility-altering drugs on small intestinal motility and symptoms in IBS. Adopting the prokinetic approach, one group found that cisapride (Propulsid)* produced a symptomatic improvement among those with predominant constipation, but it led to deterioration in those with predominant diarrhea. In a more acute study, cisapride was shown to increase motor activity during fasting and after a meal and to promote clusters in those with diarrhea but not with constipation-predominant IBS. In the latter study, symptom correlates were not examined. In other studies, it has

---

*Not FDA approved for this indication.
†Not available in the United States.

*Not FDA approved for this indication.

been suggested that the therapeutic efficacy of such agents as the antidepressant imipramine (Tofranil),* the antispasmodics mebeverine* and octylonium bromide,* the serotonin antagonists ondansetron (Zofran)* and granisetron (Kytril),* or even psychological approaches may be mediated in some part through motility effects. None of these observations has, as yet, translated into broad therapeutic efficacy.

Because of the apparent predominance of IBS among young females and of the frequent association of symptom exacerbations with menses, the gonadotrophin-releasing hormone antagonist leuprolide (Lupron)* has also been employed in motility disorders and IBS. Although some preliminary studies have demonstrated apparent efficacy, this has not as yet been confirmed in large-scale multicenter studies.

SUMMARY AND CONCLUSIONS

IBS is a common clinical disorder of unknown pathophysiology that is responsible for considerable morbidity and health care usage. Its definition remains entirely clinical, although considerable progress has been made in developing clinical definitions that are widely accepted. Concepts in pathophysiology have moved from the search for a single "magic bullet" to one of complex interactions between luminal factors, environmental agents, motor function, visceral perception, central processing, and central nervous system modulation. Although one or more of these factors may be predominant in an individual patient, we have not yet reached a stage where we can define, with confidence, patient subgroups based on investigations of pathophysiology.

Our therapeutic success for IBS remains limited. The primary role of the physician is to reassure the patient and to relieve the symptoms. An approach to IBS that is based on pathophysiology and specific and effective therapies for patients with IBS will hopefully be developed in the future.

---

*Not FDA approved for this indication.

HEMORRHOIDS, ANAL FISSURE, AND ANORECTAL ABSCESS AND FISTULA

method of
JOHN J. MURRAY, M.D.
Lahey Clinic
Burlington, Massachusetts

HEMORRHOIDS

Despite popular misconception, hemorrhoids are a normal feature of anal anatomy and probably contribute to anal continence. They consist of a network of arterioles and dilated venules in a supporting matrix of smooth muscle and fibroelastic connective tissue that serves to anchor the hemorrhoid to the internal anal sphincter. Hemorrhoids appear typically as discrete submucosal cushions in the left lateral, right anterior, and right posterior quadrants of the proximal anal canal. The pathogenesis of symptomatic internal hemorrhoids is uncertain but may be a consequence of caudal displacement of these vascular cushions as a result of repeated straining at defecation. There is a decided lack of convincing evidence to support this hypothesis, however. Vascular engorgement develops as the supporting connective tissue framework is disrupted. Anal manometry has disclosed elevated anal sphincter resting pressures in some patients with symptomatic hemorrhoids, but it is unclear whether this is a primary or secondary phenomenon.

Bleeding, the most common feature of symptomatic internal hemorrhoids, may be quite brisk because of the presence of arteriovenous communications within the hemorrhoidal plexus. Progressive displacement of the internal hemorrhoids promotes prolapse of the engorged vascular cushions beyond the anal verge. This protrusion is responsible for mucus seepage and minor soiling that promote perianal dermatitis in individuals with symptomatic hemorrhoids. Progressive dilation of internal hemorrhoids causes engorgement of a subcutaneous venous plexus distal to the dentate line. These veins, constituting the external hemorrhoid network, have a tendency to thrombose. In the absence of acute thrombosis, pain is not a characteristic symptom of hemorrhoids. Patients complaining primarily of anal pain should be evaluated for the presence of anal fissure, abscess, or neoplasm.

Classification in internal hemorrhoids by degree of prolapse aids in selecting appropriate therapy. First-degree hemorrhoids bleed but do not prolapse. Second-degree hemorrhoids prolapse during defecation and reduce spontaneously, whereas third-degree internal hemorrhoids require digital reduction to relieve protrusion. Fourth-degree internal hemorrhoids are chronically prolapsed and cannot be reduced.

Evaluation of patients with symptomatic hemorrhoids should include sigmoidoscopy and anoscopy. Examination of the more proximal colon with flexible sigmoidoscopy or air-contrast barium enema should be undertaken in patients whose symptoms are atypical or whose age or medical history places them at risk of developing colorectal carcinoma.

Treatment

Options for treating internal hemorrhoids range from dietary and topical measures to a variety of office and operative procedures designed to shrink or eradicate the enlarged vascular cushions. Selection of the appropriate treatment is governed by the severity of symptoms, extent of hemorrhoid protrusion, and patient preference. Patients who are infrequently or minimally symptomatic may respond to a high-fiber diet augmented with a fiber supplement. This regimen alleviates symptoms by reducing the need for excessive or prolonged straining at defecation. Perianal dermatitis associated with symptomatic internal hemorrhoids will respond to treatment with topical ointments containing hydrocortisone.

Office procedures for treating symptomatic first-, second-, and small third-degree internal hemorrhoids include sclerotherapy, rubber band ligation, and infrared photocoagulation. Each of these procedures produces a focal area of inflammation and subsequent fibrosis at the apex of the hemorrhoid that decreases vascular engorgement and restores fixation of the hemorrhoid to the internal sphincter. When performed properly, these procedures do not necessitate anesthesia because the apex of the hemorrhoid is devoid of sensory innervation. Injection sclerotherapy is used infrequently in the United States because it is more cumbersome than the alternatives and has been shown to produce poorer long-term results in comparative trials with rubber band ligation. Rubber band ligation involves the use of a special applicator to encompass a tuft of mucosa and submucosa within a rubber band at the apex of the hemorrhoid. The tissue ensnared in the rubber band necroses and sloughs, producing focal ulceration. One or more hemorrhoids may be treated at a single time. Treatment of larger hemorrhoids may necessitate application of two or more sets of bands to achieve the desired symptomatic response. Patients may experience mild to moderate discomfort for 24 to 72 hours. Care must be taken to avoid encroaching on the dentate line during repetitive banding of a single hemorrhoid because there is intact sensory innervation at this level. Bands should be removed if a patient experiences acute pain with rubber band ligation. Discomfort associated with rubber band ligation usually responds to mild analgesics and sitz baths. Serious complications include delayed hemorrhage (1%) and thrombosis of external hemorrhoids (2 to 3%). Rare cases of potentially life-threatening soft tissue infection of the perineum were reported during the early experience with rubber band ligation. The cause for this complication has not been clearly defined. Patients who complain of severe anal pain, fever, or symptoms of urinary retention within 7 to 10 days of rubber band ligation warrant careful evaluation. Eighty to 90% of patients experience appreciable improvement in symptoms after rubber band ligation. Approximately 40% of patients develop recurrent symptoms within 5 years, but the majority will respond to additional rubber band ligation. Infrared photocoagulation uses infrared radiation to produce a focal area of protein coagulation and necrosis at the apex of the hemorrhoid. The procedure is associated with minimal discomfort and is particularly effective for treating patients with symptomatic hemorrhoids that are too small to be treated easily by rubber band ligation.

Bipolar diathermy and direct-current electrocoagulation have been promoted as alternative procedures for treating symptomatic third-degree internal hemorrhoids in the outpatient setting. Both approaches use electrical current to produce coagulation necrosis of the hemorrhoid. Three or four treatments may be needed to achieve the desired response. No anesthesia is necessary because treatment is confined to the apex of the hemorrhoid, but 12 to 15% of patients refuse further treatment because of discomfort. With direct-current electrocoagulation the probe must remain in contact with the hemorrhoid for 8 to 10 minutes. The duration of treatment is difficult for some patients to tolerate. Although some authors report successful results in 80% of patients with third-degree hemorrhoids, others have been unable to replicate these results.

Less than 10% of patients with symptomatic internal hemorrhoids require operative intervention. Although options include cryotherapy, anal dilatation, and internal sphincterotomy, hemorrhoidectomy is the preferred treatment for patients with third-degree hemorrhoids that fail to respond to rubber band ligation and for all patients with fourth-degree internal hemorrhoids. Elective hemorrhoidectomy is currently performed as an outpatient or same-day discharge procedure under local, regional, or general anesthesia. Inpatient hospitalization may be necessary for individuals who require emergency hemorrhoidectomy to treat acutely prolapsed, thrombosed, or gangrenous hemorrhoids. Delayed hemorrhage (1%), acute urinary retention (10%), and anal stenosis (1 to 2%) are the more common complications associated with the procedure. Depending on the extent of the procedure, postoperative convalescence is usually complete within 3 to 4 weeks. Long-term follow-up reveals a high degree of patient satisfaction, but 5 to 8% experience recurrent symptoms.

Laser Therapy

Enthusiasm for the use of lasers to treat internal hemorrhoids has been promoted for many years. Laser therapy has been advertised as being less painful and less traumatic. Both carbon dioxide and neodymium:yttrium-aluminum-garnet lasers have been used to excise internal hemorrhoids or to restore fixation to the internal sphincter. The few comparative trials with standard treatment measures have shown no benefit to laser therapy.

Treatment of External Hemorrhoids

External hemorrhoids necessitate treatment only when complicated by acute thrombosis. Most commonly this results from excessive straining at defecation or from atypically strenuous physical activity. Patients presenting with severe discomfort are best treated by excising the thrombosed hemorrhoid under local anesthesia. Simple incision and evacuation is prone to early recurrence and is not recommended. Patients seen several days after onset of symptoms, when the acute discomfort is beginning to subside, are best treated with sitz baths and dietary fiber supplements. Complete resolution will occur in 6 to 8 weeks. In this circumstance the patient may be left with a residual skin tag.

ANAL FISSURE

Anal fissure, a linear tear in the anal canal extending from the dentate line to the anal verge, is the most common cause of painful defecation. Traumatic injury during passage of a large, hard bolus of fecal material is the usual cause. Progression to a chronic fissure results in a fibrotic, scarred anal ulcer containing exposed fibers of the internal anal sphincter in its base. Fissures typically develop in young and middle-aged adults and are confined to the posterior midline of the anal canal in at least 90% of cases. Fissures in the anterior midline are more common in women than in men. Anal fissure may be a secondary manifestation of other diseases. Eccentric location of an anal fissure should suggest the possibility of Crohn's disease, tuberculosis, syphilis, leukemia, or anal carcinoma.

Pain with defecation is the most common symptom. The pain may become continuous and disabling in patients with chronic anal fissures. Surface bleeding is usually minimal in quantity but is frequently the symptom that leads patients to seek medical attention. Anal seepage, pruritus, dysuria, and dyspareunia may be additional symptoms of a chronic anal fissure. In most cases an anal fissure can be demonstrated by gently separating the buttocks to expose the anal margin. Examination under anesthesia is occasionally necessary to confirm the diagnosis and exclude other pathologic conditions in patients who are too uncomfortable to permit evaluation in the outpatient setting.

Acute anal fissures heal spontaneously in the majority of patients. Factors responsible for progression to a chronic anal fissure are uncertain. Anal manometry has demonstrated a tendency for spastic contraction of the internal anal sphincter with subsequent increase in anal resting pressure in patients with chronic anal fissures. Whether this abnormality is a primary or secondary phenomenon is unproved. Evidence suggests that impaired perfusion of the anoderm caused by hypertonic contraction of the internal anal sphincter may perpetuate ischemic injury and prevent spontaneous healing.

Treatment

Initial treatment should focus on interrupting the cycle of constipation, repetitive traumatic injury, internal anal sphincter spasm, and suppression of the urge to defecate. This is best accomplished with a high fiber diet combined with a dietary fiber supplement to optimize stool consistency. Sitz baths alleviate spasm of the internal anal sphincter and relieve pain. Narcotic analgesics should be avoided because of the risk of exacerbating constipation. Regimens employing topical corticosteroids, topical anesthetics, suppositories, or anal dilators are generally ineffective.

Previously, most individuals who failed to respond to nonoperative therapy were referred for lateral internal sphincterotomy or anal dilation under anesthesia. Although these procedures promote successful healing of chronic anal fissures, minor alteration of anal continence has been reported in as many as 30% of patients. This potential morbidity has prompted a search for alternative pharmacologic measures to produce temporary alteration of internal anal sphincter function. Physiologic relaxation of the internal anal sphincter is mediated by release of nitric oxide. Application of topical nitrate preparations to the anal canal produces the same response and may reduce anal canal resting pressure by 20 to 25%. Randomized prospective trials have documented successful healing of anal fissures within 6 to 8 weeks in 68 to 82% of cases. At present there is no standard dose delivery system. In most studies, patients have applied 0.2 to 0.4% nitroglycerin ointment (Nitrol)* to the anal canal two to four times daily. The medication causes a headache in 10 to 50% of patients, but few discontinue treatment because of this side effect. Local injection of botulinum toxin (Botox)* causes chemical denervation of the internal anal sphincter that lasts 3 to 4 months. Injection of the internal anal sphincter with doses ranging from 5 to 25 units has produced healing of anal fissures within 2 months in 70 to 80% of patients. Temporary incontinence for flatus and minor fecal soiling have been reported in 4 to 7% of cases. The efficacy of topical nitrates or botulinum toxin as primary therapy for chronic anal fissures requires confirmation in larger series of patients.

Lateral subcutaneous internal sphincterotomy remains the most predictably curative treatment for patients with a chronic anal fissure. The procedure involves division of the distal portion of the internal anal sphincter through a puncture wound at the anal margin. By relieving hypertonic contraction of the internal anal sphincter, the procedure improves mucosal perfusion. Patients experience rapid resolution of symptoms. Healing of the fissure is complete within 3 to 4 weeks in 90 to 95% of patients. Internal sphincterotomy can be performed successfully under local or general anesthesia. The procedure may be complicated by hematoma (1%) or wound abscess (2%). Although minor problems with impaired continence have been reported after internal sphincterotomy, this has generally been recorded in fewer than 15% of cases. The risk of impaired continence with internal sphincterotomy may be related to operative technique, female gender, and the extent of internal sphincterotomy. Careful consideration is required before internal sphincterotomy is undertaken in patients with chronic diarrhea, irritable bowel syndrome, prior sphincterotomy, or advanced age because an existing tendency for fecal urgency or anal seepage in these patients may be exacerbated by surgery.

Anal dilation under general anesthesia is an alternative surgical option for bluntly disrupting the internal anal sphincter to relieve sphincter hypertonia and promote healing of anal fissures. The procedure is less precise and may be associated with extensive perianal hematoma formation, an increased risk of impaired continence, and a higher recurrence rate.

---

*Not FDA approved for this indication.

For these reasons it remains a less attractive treatment option.

ANORECTAL ABSCESS AND FISTULA

Anorectal abscess and fistula represent acute and chronic phases of the same disease process. Abscess develops from obstruction of one of the anal glands as it discharges into an anal crypt at the dentate line. Obstruction produces a mixed pyogenic infection that may extend cephalad, caudad, or laterally from the intersphincteric plane to present as an intersphincteric, perianal, or ischiorectal abscess, respectively. Other potential causes for perianal or perineal abscess include pilonidal disease, infected sebaceous cyst, furunculosis, inflammatory bowel disease, foreign body, bartholinian abscess, and hidradenitis suppurativa. Drainage of the abscess by intentional incision or spontaneous eruption relieves the acute symptoms. In the majority of cases, however, the offending anal gland serves as a focus of chronic infection, giving rise to a fistula in ano manifested by persistent or intermittent seepage from the original drainage site.

Patients with an anorectal abscess typically complain of progressive, throbbing perianal pain. Fever, constipation, and difficulty voiding may be associated symptoms. Perianal abscess presents as a focal area of erythema and fluctuance adjacent to the anal verge. Patients with an ischiorectal abscess demonstrate more diffuse induration in the involved buttock with a variable amount of erythema. Patients with an intersphincteric or postanal space abscess typically complain of more deep-seated pain and may have no external signs to suggest an underlying infection. Examination under anesthesia may be needed to confirm the diagnosis. Patients with a symptomatic fistula complain of feculent or purulent perianal drainage. The physician should be alert for symptoms of underlying inflammatory bowel disease when evaluating patients with fistula in ano because the presence of Crohn's disease will influence management of the fistula. Physical examination reveals an external sinus with associated induration that may extend toward the anal canal as a palpable cord. Rectal examination may identify a punctate defect in the dentate line at the internal opening of the fistula. Sigmoidoscopy is performed before surgery to exclude a neoplasm or inflammatory bowel disease as contributing factors.

Treatment

Use of antibiotics as primary or temporizing treatment for anorectal abscess is inappropriate. Effective treatment necessitates incision and drainage under local, regional, or general anesthesia. Although selected patients with perianal or ischiorectal abscess can be treated successfully in the outpatient setting using local anesthesia, inadequate drainage is frequently a contributing factor to the morbidity and mortality that may complicate treatment of anorectal abscess. Adjunctive antibiotic therapy is useful if patients have cellulitis, or if the situation is complicated by coexisting diabetes or other systemic disorders that compromise immune function. A residual fistula will be identified in only 50 to 67% of patients after resolution of the abscess. Although some authorities have recommended performance of anal fistulotomy at the time of abscess drainage, most prefer a two-stage approach in which fistulotomy is performed after the acute suppurative process has resolved. This strategy avoids unnecessary injury to the anal sphincter and prevents creation of a false passage during injudicious attempts to identify an internal communication at the time of abscess drainage.

Traditional treatment of fistula in ano requires that the entire fistula, including the origin in the offending anal crypt, be unroofed and débrided. In most cases this procedure involves division of a portion of the internal anal sphincter as well as a segment of the external anal sphincter in patients with transsphincteric fistulas. Healing of the wound by secondary intention generally requires 4 to 8 weeks. Frank fecal incontinence is a rare complication, but 20 to 40% of patients with transsphincteric fistulas will experience minor difficulties with anal seepage or incomplete control of flatus after fistulotomy. To minimize the risk of incontinence when treating high transsphincteric or suprasphincteric fistulas, a cutting seton drain can be passed along the course of the fistula and tightened over 3 to 4 weeks. The fibrosis and scarring that accompany gradual division of the encompassed sphincter muscle prevent wide separation of the muscle. Despite successful results with this technique the majority of patients experience some alteration in continence. The potentially deleterious functional consequences associated with anal fistulotomy have precipitated interest in alternative sphincter-preserving procedures for treating complex transsphincteric anal fistulas. The most commonly employed technique uses an endorectal advancement flap of mucosa and circular smooth muscle to obliterate the origin of the fistula. The external anal sphincter is preserved and the distal portion of the fistula is débrided and drained. Although this procedure has a higher failure rate (15 to 30%) than that reported with anal fistulotomy, it preserves continence more successfully. The procedure can be repeated successfully in a proportion of those whose original advancement flap repair fails. An endorectal advancement flap repair should be considered optimal treatment for patients with preexisting problems with continence, for women with anterior anal fistulas, and for patients with high transsphincteric, extrasphincteric, or recurrent fistulas.

PEPTIC ULCER DISEASE

method of
JAY L. GOLDSTEIN, M.D., and
PETER M. OSHIN, M.D.
University of Illinois at Chicago
Chicago, Illinois

Gastric and duodenal ulcers are common clinical problems in patients with various symptoms such as indigestion, bloating, nausea, vomiting, and epigastric pain and/or discomfort. Collectively, these heterogeneous symptoms, among others, constitute the major components of what is medically termed "dyspepsia." However, dyspeptic symptoms may be associated with lesser lesions of the upper gastrointestinal tract and are at times difficult to distinguish from symptoms associated with the use of various medications, cholecystitis, pancreatic or gastric cancer, pancreatitis, irritable bowel syndrome, esophagitis, and other disease states. Moreover, dyspeptic symptoms can be found in patients who have normal results of upper endoscopy (functional dyspepsia, nonulcer dyspepsia).

"Gastritis" and "duodenitis" are pathologic terms to describe histologic inflammation of the stomach and duodenum, respectively. Whereas these terms are commonly, albeit erroneously, used to describe dyspeptic symptoms, it remains unclear if these histologic lesions are actually associated with symptoms of dyspepsia. Erosions and erosive gastritis refer to damage limited to the superficial layers of the mucosa, where damage does not extend beyond the mucularis mucosa. In contrast and unlike erosions, frank ulcers are defined by their depth with extension of the ulcer base through the muscularis mucosa and into the submucosa. The clinical implications of these definitions are important because ulcers are associated with more significant complications such as bleeding and perforation. Unfortunately, clinicians often interchange these terms, adding confusion to the diagnosis and treatment of upper gastrointestinal related symptoms/dyspepsia. Although dyspepsia may be associated with ulcers, ulcers may or may not be present endoscopically when patients complain of dyspeptic symptoms.

Our purpose here is to present a clinically relevant diagnostic and therapeutic approach to patients with dyspeptic symptoms and to discuss the current approaches to patients with endoscopically proven gastroduodenal ulcers.

OVERVIEW

As our understanding of the nature of ulcers evolves, it is clear that at least two common causes of gastroduodenal ulcers exist: (1) ulcers associated with the use of nonsteroidal anti-inflammatory drugs (NSAIDs), such as aspirin, ibuprofen, and naproxen and (2) ulcers associated with the bacterium *Helicobacter pylori*. Less common causes of ulcers in the upper gastrointestinal tract include, among others: Crohn's disease, gastric cancer, hypersecretory states, opportunistic infections (e.g., herpes simplex virus or cytomegalovirus), vascular insufficiency, or iatrogenically induced ulcers associated with either chemotherapy or radiation therapy. Given the vast array of potential upper gastrointestinal pathologies associated with dyspeptic symptoms, with or without endoscopically proven ulcers, clinicians are often challenged not only to establish the presence or absence of endoscopic ulcers but also to define the specific pathologic state so that effective treatment methods can be accurately chosen.

DYSPEPSIA

"Dyspepsia" is a term used to describe a range or complex of heterogeneous symptoms thought to be of upper gastrointestinal origin. Many attempts have been made to distinguish specific sets of symptoms and classify dyspepsia into different pathophysiologic/etiologic states. Often terms such as "reflux-type" dyspepsia, "ulcer-like" dyspepsia, or "motility-like" dyspepsia are used to designate the possibility of a specific cause. Unfortunately, these designations are often difficult to use, and their relevance for day-to-day patient care is limited because they lack specificity.

The evaluation of patients with dyspeptic symptoms should be individualized based on several factors that are available through a good history and physical examination. Key findings include the location of pain/discomfort, the severity and duration of the symptoms, their association with eating and/or specific foods, their response to various medications, the presence of night-time symptoms, and their impact on the patient's activities and quality of life (severity). Whereas these factors may help the clinician focus on the significance and possibly the cause of the symptoms, the history is often vague and may not suggest a specific diagnosis or aid in generating a limited differential diagnosis; use of data obtained from the history may only aid the clinician in ascribing the symptoms to the upper gastrointestinal tract. Likewise, findings on physical examinations are often limited, and significant disease states are often seen in the absence of physical findings on abdominal examination.

We heavily weigh the importance of symptoms that cause night-time wakening. Patients with functional dyspepsia generally can sleep through the night, whereas pain that awakens patients from sleep is often associated with organic lesions. In certain subgroups of the population, such as the elderly, the manifestation and progression of disease is more likely to be symptomatically incomplete or even silent. It is important to recognize that symptoms that respond to over-the-counter doses of histamine receptor antagonists (H_2RAs) (e.g., ranitidine [Zantac], 75 mg orally twice daily) or even higher doses of H_2RAs and/or proton pump inhibitors (PPIs) do not confirm the absence of true pathology. It has been our experience that dyspeptic symptoms may respond to acid suppression in patients with or without endoscopically proven ulcer disease or even other more serious organic causes of symptoms (e.g., cancer).

If endoscopy is performed and there is no mucosal injury, epigastric symptoms occurring over a 3-month period without any structural or biochemical basis for disease are referred to as functional dyspepsia or nonulcer dyspepsia. The prevalence of functional dyspepsia ranges anywhere from 24 to 41% in Western countries.

Notably, the presence of what are referred to as "alarm signs and symptoms" are important to help guide the initial diagnostic management of patients with dyspepsia. The "alarm signs and symptoms" listed in Table 1 are the key features that warrant early diagnostic procedures such as upper gastrointestinal endoscopy. Despite the fact that these symptoms intrinsically make sense, and foster a sense of urgency, the use of a specific age of older than 50 years is relatively arbitrary. Whereas this age is commonly used in algorithms of care, there is little evidence to suggest that this is absolute. In concept, the use of this age "cutoff" is based on epidemiologic evidence that the incidence of malignancies in the upper gastrointestinal tract sharply increases at or near this age. It is important to recognize that these "alarm signs and symptoms" are

TABLE 1. Alarm Signs and Symptoms Associated with Dyspepsia

Age >50 y
Anorexia
Weight loss
Early satiety
Dysphagia
Protracted vomiting/volume depletion
Anemia
Positive fecal occult blood test
Melena
Hematemesis
Family history of upper gastrointestinal malignancies

meant to be used for patients with symptoms that are new in onset. For example, for patients with long-standing and stable dyspeptic symptoms, reaching age 50 is not necessarily an indication for immediate evaluation. Laboratory tests used in the initial workup of patients with dyspepsia should include a complete blood cell count at a minimum. Additional tests may be considered to include/exclude pancreatitis or biliary/liver disorders.

Endoscopic examination of the upper gastrointestinal tract may be strongly considered for patients with "alarm signs and symptoms" because endoscopy remains the "gold standard" for establishing (or excluding) peptic ulcer disease and other organic and more serious causes of dyspeptic symptoms. As compared with upper gastrointestinal barium studies, endoscopy should be considered as the "procedure of choice" when a diagnostic evaluation of the upper gastrointestinal tract is indicated because of the diagnostic superiority of endoscopy and the ability to perform biopsies, not only to obtain tissue for histologic diagnosis but also for establishing the presence of *H. pylori*. In addition, endoscopy allows for therapeutic interventions that can easily be performed when clinically indicated.

For patients with upper gastrointestinal bleeding from peptic ulcer disease or other causes, upper gastrointestinal endoscopy is the most useful initial diagnostic, prognostic, and therapeutic intervention. The examination can be performed after the patient has been medically stabilized to determine the cause or location of the bleeding source. Control of bleeding may be accomplished through endoscopic coagulation devices or injection sclerotherapy.

CLINICAL APPROACH

When faced with an individual with dyspeptic symptoms and in the absence of an absolute need for endoscopic intervention such as alarm symptoms, a clinician has three basic treatment options: (1) an empirical trial of acid suppression, (2) endoscopy, or (3) a "test and treat" strategy for the presence of *H. pylori* (Figure 1).

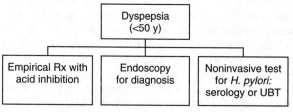

Figure 1. Possible approaches to dyspepsia.

Empirical Acid Suppression

Patients often visit their primary care physician or a specialist after trying (and failing) self-administered, over-the-counter trials of H₂RAs. If patients have not responded to self-medicated empirical therapy, further attempts with H₂RAs at even at higher doses (e.g., ranitidine, 150 mg orally twice daily) are often futile, delaying appropriate evaluation and therapy. If empirical therapy is still considered, a trial of PPIs (e.g., lansoprazole [Prevacid], 30 mg per day orally; omeprazole [Prilosec], 20 mg per day orally) would be a more reasonable approach.

However, whereas acid suppression (H₂RAs or PPIs) has been ingrained in the medical community as an initial therapy for patients with dyspepsia, it is not necessarily our first-line choice. The problem is that in the majority of patients a specific diagnosis is not made and dyspeptic symptoms often return after these short trials; response to acid suppression does not exclude the presence of significant organic lesions. Furthermore, if patients have *H. pylori*–associated ulcers, this treatment is not appropriate for the long-term management of these patients because *H. pylori* is not eradicated and there is a high probability of having recurrent ulcer disease.

Alternative empirical therapies such as prokinetic agents (e.g., cisapride [Propulsid], 20 mg orally twice daily) have been tried but again often lead to confusion in diagnosis, the need for further treatment interventions, or both. We generally reserve this empirical trial for patients who have symptoms suggestive of gastroparesis (early satiety, nausea, vomiting) and/or who have a higher probability of gastroparesis (e.g., long-standing diabetes mellitus). In the absence of "gastroparesis-like" symptoms, an empirical trial of a prokinetic agent is not commonly used.

In general, the duration of empirical acid suppression or prokinetic therapy should be no longer than 1 to 2 months before any further intervention is decided on. If patients do not respond or have incomplete resolution of their symptoms, then endoscopic intervention is warranted for diagnostic purposes. In addition, the use of endoscopy has been shown to alleviate fear and patient concerns regarding their specific state or condition.

Endoscopy

The second option for initial management of dyspepsia is endoscopy. Endoscopy is widely available and is becoming a cost-effective tool given the evolution of health care economics. The advantages of early endoscopy is that a specific diagnosis can be made and the presence of frank ulcer disease (and the presence of *H. pylori*) can be established or excluded in a timely manner. Even with the most detailed history, it has been estimated that only 20%, at most, of patients with dyspepsia have true ulcer disease. Moreover, an additional 20 to 40% will have other findings, such as esophagitis, which only further demonstrates the inaccuracy and low predictive value of the medical history in suggesting (or excluding) a diagnosis-specific mucosal lesion. Establishing a specific diagnosis of true ulcer disease and/or esophagitis allows targeted and specific therapies to be prescribed and allows the physician to better counsel their patients regarding long-term management. As mentioned earlier, early endoscopy is clearly warranted for patients with alarm symptoms (see Table 1).

Test and Treat Strategies for *H. pylori*

The third option consists of a "test and treat strategy" for *H. pylori* (Figure 2). It remains controversial whether *H. pylori* infection is found at increased rates above that in the general population of patients with dyspepsia or nonulcer dyspepsia. Furthermore, it is quite controversial in the literature whether *H. pylori* eradication will result in either short- or long-term relief of these symptoms in the absence of ulcer disease. Despite the lack of clear evidence supporting this approach, many physicians feel comfortable using this method. The rationale (or hope) for initial use of a "test and treat" strategy is that patients, if they test positive and if they respond to anti–*H. pylori* therapy, will not have to undergo endoscopy. Furthermore, the availability of inexpensive office-based serologic tests makes this an attractive option for primary care physicians because an intervention can be made at the time of the office visit. Currently available office-based serologic tests have sensitivities and specificities that range from 80 to 90%, and results are available within minutes. Economic modeling studies have suggested that a "test and treat" approach may be appropriate and as cost effective as

early endoscopy, in contrast to a trial of empirical acid suppression. However, it is essential to understand that this approach implies that an endoscopy will be performed if this initial "test and treat" approach fails.

The incidence of *H. pylori* in a dyspeptic population ranges from only 30 to 60%. As such, it is incumbent on any physician who uses this "test and treat" strategy to first confirm the presence of *H. pylori* by noninvasive (nonendoscopic) serologic testing (or possibly a urea breath test). Anti–*H. pylori* therapy should not be given "empirically" unless there is documentation of infection. Urea breath tests are becoming widely available but are more costly than serologic tests, and patients are required to return to the office (or laboratory) for additional visits. Urea breath testing is an excellent noninvasive test for follow up of eradication when clinically indicated. We reserve a "test and treat" strategy for patients who have not been treated for *H. pylori* in the past, because recurrent symptoms after anti–*H. pylori* treatment warrant further evaluation.

Based on the care map shown in Figure 2, if patients test positive, then treatment should ensue. If *H. pylori* testing is negative, endoscopy and/or empirical acid suppression should be considered. If patients have tested positive and have been treated and continue to exhibit or have recurrent symptoms, then endoscopy is warranted to evaluate for specific pathologic processes and for eradication of *H. pylori*. Because serologic tests usually remain positive even after successful eradication, serologic testing should not be repeated to confirm eradication. In patients who have tested positive and responded to a "test and treat strategy," follow up should be expectant management; patients should be reinvestigated only if symptoms recur or alarm symptoms develop.

The choice of these three approaches should be made in partnership with the patient and with full understanding of the action plan if they do or do not respond. Because there is little objective evidence to absolutely support one of these options over the others, we generally consider the costs, severity of symptoms, and the expected outcomes with our patients and include these factors in developing our plan.

TREATMENT OF NSAID-INDUCED ULCERS AND PROPHYLAXIS

Patients who use NSAIDs present a unique problem to physicians. With continued use, 10 to 20% of patients at any given time will have symptoms of dyspepsia. Unfortunately, these symptoms are often nondiagnostic or predictive of actual mucosal injury or ulcerations when evaluated endoscopically. In fact, among patients who are symptomatic while using NSAIDs, the incidence of ulcer disease is only approximately 20%. Conversely, patients who use NSAIDs are often asymptomatic even though frank ulcerations may be seen endoscopically in controlled clinical trials. Patients who use NSAIDs and do not have symptoms are placed in a sense of "false secu-

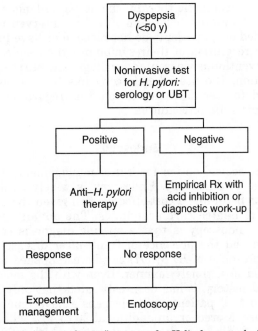

Figure 2. "Test and treat" strategy for *Helicobacter pylori* with initial noninvasive testing.

rity." The absence of symptoms does not preclude the fact that at any given time, 20% will have ulcerations in the stomach and/or duodenum.

Prophylaxis

NSAIDs are associated with an overall *annual* average incidence of symptomatic ulcers, bleeding, obstruction, and perforation in 2 to 4% of the patients who use them. Nearly all of these events (>80%) occur in the background of asymptomatic ulcers. For this reason, patients who are at high risk for NSAID-induced toxicity and specifically the complications mentioned previously are often proactively given co-prescribed medications to prevent ulcers and, more importantly, ulcer complications. The commonly reported risk factors listed in the Table 2 help predict those patients who are at greatest risk or above-average risk for these gastrointestinal events. Multiple risk factors have been identified and have been shown to act in concert to increase the rate of ulcer complications. Of these risk factors, a history of previous ulcer disease and a history of previous upper gastrointestinal tract bleeding are the most important factors that will predict NSAID-associated upper gastrointestinal toxicity. Increasing age also has been shown to be an independent factor for the development of NSAID-induced upper gastrointestinal complications. In regard to dose, patients who use supratherapeutic doses of prescribed NSAIDs do not have increased efficacy (reduction of pain and inflammation), but these doses are associated with increased toxicity in the gastrointestinal tract. In an interesting patient survey, we reported that approximately 38% of patients who use NSAIDs at prescribed doses given to them by physicians will add over-the-counter medications to their drug regimens. It is important to counsel patients to avoid the use of multiple NSAIDs because they are more likely to develop complications without increasing efficacy (pain relief/anti-inflammatory effect). Although intuitive, it is becoming increasingly clear that the cumulative incidence of NSAID-induced complications increases linearly with the duration of therapy and exposure. Several studies have shown that the occurrence of dyspepsia while NSAIDs are used is also an independent risk factor for NSAID-induced complications. Patients with rheumatologic disorders who are using co-prescribed corticosteroids also exhibit higher rates of upper gastrointestinal toxicities

TABLE 2. Risk Factors for Nonsteroidal-Induced Toxicity

Past history of gastroduodenal ulcers
Past history of upper gastrointestinal bleeding
Age (especially ≥ 65 y/o)
Dose (and duration)
Intolerance (dyspepsia) while using NSAIDs
Concomitant use of corticosteroids
Pre-existing debilitating illnesses

TABLE 3. NSAID-Induced Ulcer: Prophylaxis and Treatment

Prophylaxis
1. Misoprostol (Cytotec), 200 μg PO bid or tid*
2. Proton pump inhibitor: omeprazole (Prilosec), 20 mg, or lansoprazole (Prevacid), 30 mg PO qd
Acute Ulcer Treatment
1. Treat for *H. pylori* if there is documented infection
2. Reduce or discontinue the NSAID
3. Add proton pump inhibitor (4–12 weeks)†

* Misoprostol can be co-prescribed or used as a formulation of diclofenac plus misoprostol (Arthrotec).
† Alternatively, histamine receptor antagonists may be used (see text).

when using NSAIDs simultaneously. Whereas other factors have been reported to increase NSAID-associated gastroduodenal toxicity, their contribution is relatively minor as compared with those listed in Table 2.

Multiple formulas have been developed to quantify the absolute and relative risks of these factors especially when present together. Although these formulas that weight the importance of individual risk factors guide the physician in identifying patients at or above average risk, they are often cumbersome and difficult to use. As a rule of thumb, if patients have a history of previous ulcer disease or upper gastrointestinal bleeding or if they are elderly and/or if they have greater than one of these risk factors, we generally prescribe protective therapies.

For individuals at average or above-average risk, preventative therapies with agents such as misoprostol (Cytotec, 200 μg orally two, three, or four times daily) or PPIs (e.g., omeprazole, 20 mg per day orally; lansoprazole, 30 mg per day orally) are often co-prescribed with NSAIDs (Table 3). The "gold standard" of ulcer prophylaxis is misoprostol because it has been shown to actually reduce the incidence of ulcer complications by approximately 50%. Although this drug has been used at 200 μg orally four times a day in the past, an equally effective dose can be achieved with thrice-daily dosing and also possibly with twice-daily dosing. Four-times-a-day dosing is probably excessive and associated with an increased incidence of side effects (e.g., diarrhea). If patients develop side effects with misoprostol, we commonly (or at times proactively) titrate the dose up from 100 to 200 μg orally twice daily or thrice daily to 200 μg twice daily or thrice daily over 1 to 2 weeks.

In contrast to misoprostol and PPIs, H₂RAs (ranitidine, 150 mg orally twice daily) do little to reduce endoscopic ulcer rates or prevent ulcer complications. Whereas H₂RAs do reduce symptoms, they do not prevent overall ulcer formation or ulcer complications. Similarly, sucralfate (Carafate), 1 gram orally four times a day, is an ineffective preventative therapy. It is for this reason that when nonselective NSAIDs are prescribed, we recommend misoprostol or a PPI. Because compliance with co-prescribed protective medications may be an issue, physicians are advised to counsel patients about compliance to maximize the efficacy of these preventive therapies. Use of a formulation of diclofenac (50 or 75 mg thrice a day) and misoprostol (Arthrotec, 200 µg twice daily) ensures the concomitant use of protective therapy. Last, patients who are commonly prescribed NSAIDs are often told to take these medications with food. This may be an effective way of reducing drug-related dyspeptic symptoms, but this recommendation does not reduce the rate of endoscopic ulcers (or ulcer complications) in clinical trials.

Treatment of Acute Ulcers

For the treatment of ulcer disease that is endoscopically found in patients using NSAIDs, several issues come into play. First, at the time of endoscopy, an evaluation for *H. pylori* should be obtained. Despite the fact that patients may have a duodenal or gastric ulcer while using NSAIDs, there is still the possibility that *H. pylori* caused the particular lesion. For that reason, in the presence of documented ulcer disease, *H. pylori* eradication is always prescribed for these patients when it is found at the time of endoscopy. Second, studies have shown that discontinuing the NSAID in the presence of an ulcer is beneficial because it will improve the overall rate of ulcer healing. This is especially true if H$_2$RAs (e.g., ranitidine, 150 mg orally twice a day) are used in the treatment of an acute ulcer. For our patients who use NSAIDs and have documented ulcer disease, we try to discontinue or at the very least reduce the dose of the NSAID and try to substitute other analgesic agents for their pain. Equally and at the same time, we initiate acid suppressive therapy with a PPI for 4, but preferably 8 to 12, weeks (lansoprazole, 30 mg orally twice daily; omeprazole, 20 mg orally twice daily). Alterative therapies can include the use of H$_2$RAs. However, healing rates at doses such as ranitidine, 150 mg orally twice daily, tend to be less effective than those achieved with PPIs. For this reason we prefer to use a PPI. Studies suggest that higher doses of famotidine (Pepcid), 40 mg orally twice daily, may be equally efficacious as a PPI, but the cost-effectiveness of this treatment and the practical nature of using high doses of an H$_2$RA makes this less attractive.

Patients who have been using NSAIDs and have developed ulcers are at higher risk of developing recurrent ulcers with the continued use of NSAIDs. Therefore, after therapy for an acute ulcer and if NSAIDs are reinstated, patients are continued on a maintenance therapy of a PPI or misoprostol as described previously.

Many nonselective NSAIDs claim greater intrinsic gastrointestinal safety. These agents are often marketed as having lower rates of gastrointestinal ulcers in endoscopic trials. It has been our experience that this is difficult to evaluate because of the lack of "head to head" trials comparing one agent to another. In general, we discount these claims of relative safety.

Most recently a new class of agents has been identified for the treatment of pain, osteoarthritis, and rheumatoid arthritis that are now commonly referred to as COX 2 selective inhibitors (e.g., celecoxib [Celebrex], 200 mg per day orally [for osteoarthritis] or 200 mg orally twice daily [for rheumatoid arthritis]; rofecoxib [Vioxx], 12.5 to 25 mg per day orally [for osteoarthritis]). Whereas the literature is evolving about this new class of agents, "head to head" trials clearly show they are less ulcerogenic than traditional nonselective NSAIDs and are probably associated with lower rates of dyspepsia. Notably, initial studies suggest they are also associated with fewer ulcer complications (i.e., bleeding, perforation, obstruction) when compared with nonselective NSAIDs. Whenever possible use of these agents should be initiated (or substituted) to reduce the patient's risk for gastrointestinal toxicity. Unlike misoprostol or PPIs, these agents are not "protective" agents; they are intrinsically associated with lower ulcer rates approaching or not different from placebo.

HELICOBACTER PYLORI

Background

H. pylori is a bacterium that is transmitted by a fecal-oral or oral-oral route and colonizes the mucus layer of the gastric mucosa, causing a chronic active gastritis. Approximately 30% of the U.S. population is infected with this organism. Infection rates tend to be higher in the developing countries and in patients who were brought up in lower socioeconomic conditions. In the United States, the prevalence of infection increases with age.

H. pylori infection is found in 90 to 95% of patients with documented duodenal ulcer disease and 70 to 80% of patients with documented gastric ulcers. The lower rate in gastric ulcer patients is probably related to the use of NSAIDs, which cause gastric ulcers. However, not all patients with *H. pylori* will develop ulcers; the lifetime rate of ulcer disease in patients infected with *H. pylori* is only 30%. In other words, patients with ulcers are highly likely to be *H. pylori* positive but only 30% of *H. pylori*–positive patients will ever develop ulcer disease. Therefore, *H. pylori* should be tested for and be treated for only in the presence of a clinical indication such as active or history of previous ulcer disease, the unusual case of MALT lymphoma (mucosa-associated lymphoid tissue), and possibly in a "test and treat" strategy as described previously. *H. pylori* should not be tested for (or treated) in patients who are asymptomatic in the absence of ulcer disease. Even though *H. pylori* is recognized as a risk factor for gastric adenocarcinoma, it has not been demonstrated that proactive screening and treatment will reduce the rate of cancer. Conflicting data exist regarding the interaction of *H. pylori* and NSAIDs in causing ulcer disease. At best, it is commonly believed that there is no synergy of *H. pylori* and NSAIDs. Therefore, we do not recommend eradication of *H. pylori* before starting NSAIDs.

Diagnosis of *H. pylori*

Several tests are used to diagnose *H. pylori*. Noninvasive tests do not require endoscopy and include serologic tests and the urea breath tests. Serologic tests can be used in the "test and treat" strategy as discussed previously. They should not be used after eradication therapies have been given because immunologic evidence (positive test) may persist despite successful eradication (false-positive test for active infection). Urea breath tests are often used for follow up of eradication as medically indicated. Clinicians should be cautioned that because this test evaluates active infection, testing should not be performed for at least 2 to 4 weeks after bismuth, antibiotics, or PPIs have been used. Earlier testing may result in a false-negative result because the organism may be suppressed but not eradicated.

The invasive tests for *H. pylori* require endoscopy. Biopsy specimens may be obtained at the time of endoscopy for histologic staining and/or a rapid urease test. Rapid urease tests are assays for urease activity in gastric biopsy specimens, and a positive test correlates well (>90% sensitive and specific) with histologic staining for *H. pylori*.

Treatment

H. pylori therapy has evolved since the 1980s. At the current time, eradication regimens with less than 90% eradication rates in clinical trials should be avoided; there are several effective therapeutic regimens that can achieve greater than 90% eradication in most patients. *H. pylori* eradication should be initiated for patients who test positive for *H. pylori* and who have documented ulcer disease. The rationale for this strong statement is quite simple. Successful eradication of *H. pylori* in patients with ulcer disease dramatically reduces the rate of recurrent ulcer disease from 75% to less than 5 to 10% within 1 year. This has significant implications both economically and for quality of life. We prefer PPI-based triple therapies (Table 4), which include a PPI (omeprazole, 20 mg orally twice daily, or lansoprazole, 30 mg orally twice daily) *plus* two antibiotics: clarithromycin (Biaxin), 500 mg orally twice daily, *plus* either amoxicillin, 1 gram orally twice daily, or metronidazole (Flagyl), 500 mg orally twice daily. Although the duration of therapy is controversial, we generally use 14-day

therapies (see Table 4). Ten-day therapies may be equally efficacious. Alternatively, ranitidine bismuth citrate (RBC) (Tritec), 400 mg orally twice daily, may be substituted for the PPI with probably equal efficacy. LAC therapy (lansoprazole, amoxicillin, and clarithromycin) is available in a 14-day convenience pack (PrevPac).

Another effective therapy for the treatment of *H. pylori* includes a bismuth-based triple therapy as described in Table 4. These medications can be prescribed as individual components or in a compliance package (Helidac). Additional acid suppression is often used to control symptoms (e.g., omeprazole, 20 mg per day orally; lansoprazole, 30 mg per day orally) or an H_2RA (ranitidine, 150 mg orally twice daily). This regimen is quite effective when used over 2 weeks for the eradication of *H. pylori*. Patient compliance, however, needs to be stressed given the fact that patients are required to take multiple medications over a 14-day period of time. Whenever patients are prescribed these multiple medications for *H. pylori* therapy, we find it important to stress compliance. We have developed worksheets and patient instruction pamphlets for these regimens to ensure better patient education and understanding of their therapy.

There are multiple additional *H. pylori* regimens that are approved by the U.S. Food and Drug Administration for the treatment of *H. pylori*. These include dual therapies, such as omeprazole (20 mg orally twice daily) plus clarithromycin (500 mg three times a day for 14 days) *or* RBC (400 mg orally twice daily) plus clarithromycin (500 mg orally thrice daily). In both, we generally continue the PPI or RBC for an additional two weeks. Although these therapies have been used in the past, their eradication rates tend to be lower than PPI- or bismuth-based triple therapies, and they are not recommended.

A key element of the successful eradication of *H. pylori* lies in patient compliance. Patients should be counseled about the importance of compliance of these agents, because failure to eradicate the bacterium with the first round of therapy leads to higher rate of microbial resistance. We generally describe common potential side effects to proactively educate the patient and we hope ensure better utilization.

TABLE 4. *H. pylori* **Treatment (14-day regimens)**

1. Proton pump inhibitor (or RBC)-based triple therapy
   - Lansoprazole, 30 mg, or omeprazole, 20 mg, PO bid, or ranitidine bismuth citrate, 400 mg PO bid, *plus*
   - Clarithromycin, 500 mg PO bid, *and*
   - Metronidazole, 500 mg PO bid, *or* amoxicillin, 1 gm PO bid
2. Bismuth-based triple therapy
   - Pepto-Bismol: 2 tablets (chewed) PO qid *and*
   - Metronidazole, 250 mg PO qid *and*
   - Tetracycline, 500 mg PO qid

ACUTE AND CHRONIC VIRAL HEPATITIS

method of
RICHARD K. STERLING, M.D., and
MITCHELL L. SHIFFMAN, M.D.
Medical College of Virginia of Virginia Commonwealth University
Richmond, Virginia

Viral hepatitis is the most common of all liver disorders and can be caused by a number of human hepatotropic agents. More than 95% of all cases of viral hepatitis in the United States are caused by one of six viruses (referred to by the letters A through E plus G). In addition to these viruses, several others can cause acute hepatitis syndromes, including Epstein-Barr virus associated with mononucleosis, cytomegalovirus, and herpesvirus. These infections are usually self-limiting in immunocompetent individuals and are not discussed here.

ACUTE HEPATITIS

Acute hepatitis, by definition, is limited to 6 months from onset of symptoms. The spectrum of clinical presentations for acute viral hepatitis ranges from asymptomatic elevations in liver transaminase levels to fulminant hepatic failure and death. The incidence of acute infection, prevalence (reservoir), rate of chronicity, and other viral characteristics for the six common hepatitis viruses are listed in Table 1. Of note, nonenveloped viruses (A and E) are enterically transmitted and result in only acute hepatitis, whereas enveloped viruses (B, C, and D) are transmitted parentally and cause both acute and chronic disease. There are four phases of viral infection: an incubation period characteristic for each virus; a prodrome phase that may or may not be associated with symptoms; an icteric phase; and, finally, either resolution of acute infection or development of chronic infection.

During the viral prodrome, patients develop flulike symptoms, including anorexia, malaise, low-grade fever, nausea, loss of appetite, diarrhea, and tender hepatomegaly. Aminotransferases (aspartate aminotransferase [AST] and alanine aminotransferase [ALT] are elevated to a variable degree. The prodrome typically lasts 3 to 7 days and in approximately 25% of patients is followed by the appearance of jaundice. In general, these patients may remain icteric for 1 to 4 weeks. The symptoms of acute hepatitis, jaundice, and elevated serum ALT levels gradually improve, resolve, and return to normal, respectively. In contrast, most patients with acute hepatitis do not become icteric. These patients have resolution of flulike symptoms and are unaware that they had

acute disease and may present years later with serologic evidence of previous hepatitis infection or chronic disease.

Severe acute hepatitis is associated with progressive or prolonged jaundice, persistent elevations in serum transaminase levels, and development of coagulopathy. These patients must be closely monitored for the development of hepatic encephalopathy and fulminant hepatic failure (FHF). Survival of patients with FHF is only 10 to 50%. Therefore, these patients should be immediately considered for emergent liver transplantation. The risk of developing FHF for each virus is listed in Table 1.

Because most acute viral hepatitis infections resolve spontaneously in most patients, intervention is usually unnecessary. For patients who present acutely icteric, an ultrasound examination to exclude other liver and biliary tract pathology is often performed. For symptomatic patients, a carbohydrate-rich, low-fat diet may be better tolerated. Nausea and vomiting can usually be controlled with prochlorperazine (Compazine) or Promethazine (Phenergan). Acetaminophen (maximal dose, 2 gm per day) is preferred to aspirin for relief of flulike symptoms. Abstinence from alcohol and other hepatotoxic drugs is recommended until recovery. Patients with protracted nausea, vomiting, or evidence of dehydration should receive intravenous fluids. Because drug metabolism may be impaired, many medications should be monitored carefully.

Because the diagnosis of acute viral hepatitis is based on serologic studies (Table 2), liver biopsy is rarely necessary. After complete resolution of symptoms, patients with viral hepatitis B, C, and D should be followed up for either resolution of viral infection or development of chronic disease.

HEPATITIS A

Hepatitis A virus (HAV) is a small, nonenveloped RNA picornavirus distantly related to poliovirus that results in acute but not chronic hepatitis (see Table 1). HAV is transmitted enterically via contaminated

TABLE 1. **The Hepatitis Viruses**

Characteristic	HAV	HBV	HCV	HDV	HEV	HGV
Nucleic acid	RNA	DNA	RNA	RNA	RNA	RNA
Incubation (days)	15–45	30–180	15–160	21–140	14–63	15–160
Envelope	No	Yes	Yes	Yes	No	?
Fecal-oral transmission	+	−	−	−	+	−
Parenteral transmission	−	+	+	+	−	+
Incidence (thousand/year)*	125–200	140–320	35	?	?	0.9–2.0
Prevalence (million)*	n/a	1.25	4–5	?	n/a	10–15
Chronic hepatitis (frequency)	No	1–90%†	>85%	>50%	No	n/a
Fulminant liver failure rate	0.1%	<1%	No	≤17%	10–25%‡	?
Risk of HCC	No	Yes	Yes	Yes	No	?

*In the United States (recent Centers for Disease Control and Prevention data).
†Depends on age at exposure and immunocompetence of patient (see text).
‡In pregnant women.
Abbreviations: HAV = hepatitis A virus; HBV = hepatitis B virus; HCV = hepatitis C virus; HDV = hepatitis D virus; HEV = hepatitis E virus; HGV = hepatitis G virus; HCC = hepatocellular carcinoma; n/a = not applicable; + = present; − = absent.

TABLE 2. **Diagnostic Tests for Acute and Chronic Viral Hepatitis**

Virus	Status	Diagnostic Test
HAV	Acute	IgM Ab (+)
	Resolved	IgG Ab (+)
	Vaccinated	IgG Ab (+)
HBV	Acute	Surface Ag (+), core IgM Ab (+)
		Surface Ab (−), core IgG Ab (−)
	Chronic active	Surface Ag (+), core IgG Ab (+), E Ag (+)
		HBV DNA (+)
		Surface Ab (−), E Ab (−)
	Chronic persistent	Surface Ag (+), core IgG Ab (+), E Ab (+)
		Surface Ab (−), E Ag (−), HBV DNA (−)
	Resolved	Surface Ab (+), core IgM/IgG Ab (+), E Ab (+)
		Surface Ag (−), E Ag (−), HBV DNA (−)
	Vaccination	Surface Ab (+)
		Core IgM/IgG Ab (−), surface Ag (−), E Ag/Ab (−)
HCV	Active	Ab (EIA) (+), RIBA (+), HCV RNA* (+)
	Resolved	Ab (+), RIBA (+), HCV RNA (−)
HDV	Acute	IgM Antibody (+)
	Chronic	IgG Antibody (+)
HEV	Acute	Antibody (+)
	Resolved	Antibody (+)

*By polymerase chain reaction (PCR) or branched chain DNA (b-DNA) assay.

Abbreviations: HAV = hepatitis A virus; HBV = hepatitis B virus; HCV = hepatitis C virus; HDV = hepatitis D virus; HEV = hepatitis E virus; EIA = enzyme immunoassay; RIBA = recombinant immunoblot assay; DNA = deoxyribonucleic acid; RNA = ribonucleic acid; Ag = antigen; Ab = antibody; (+) = positive; (−) = negative.

food or water. The incubation period is 15 to 45 days, and the virus can be shed in stool for up to 2 weeks from the onset of illness. There are an estimated 125,000 to 200,000 HAV infections each year in the United States. Recent infection is indicated by the presence of anti-HAV IgM, which becomes detectable at the onset of symptoms, whereas anti-HAV IgG indicates past infection and confers immunity to reinfection (see Table 2).

Approximately 33% of Americans have evidence of past HAV infection. The pattern of infection varies around the world. In industrialized countries, mini-epidemics still occur in association with contaminated food or water supplies. Consuming raw shellfish harvested from contaminated waters is a common source of HAV infection. A major risk for HAV infection is to travel to underdeveloped areas of the world where HAV is endemic.

Most children with acute HAV are anicteric and have only mild, nonspecific, flulike symptoms. In contrast, the majority of adults become icteric after acute infection, accounting for 84,000 to 134,000 symptomatic HAV infections per year. After apparent resolution, approximately 15 to 20% of patients may develop biochemical or clinical relapse within 3 to 6 months. Chronic HAV, however, does not occur. Cholestasis with persistent jaundice and pruritus

may complicate 5 to 10% of patients and takes months to resolve. More than 99% of patients recover with no long-term sequelae. FHF develops from acute HAV in 0.2 to 0.5% of cases and contributes to approximately 100 deaths annually.

HAV infection can be prevented by vaccination. HAV vaccine (Havrix) is indicated for all persons at risk for being exposed to this virus. This includes people vacationing and working in endemic areas. Other individuals for whom vaccination should be considered include children who attend preschool centers and their parents, restaurant workers, institutionalized individuals, and intravenous drug users. Recent studies suggest that patients with chronic liver disease, especially cirrhosis, have an increased risk of mortality from FHF when they develop acute HAV. It is therefore recommended that all patients with chronic liver disease receive HAV vaccination.

Havrix is administered intramuscularly at a dose of 720 IU (0.5 mL) for children 2 to 18 years and 1440 IU (1.0 mL) for adults followed by a second injection 6 to 12 months later. A single injection of 1440 IU is effective at causing immunity to HAV in those patients traveling to endemic areas within 2 weeks of vaccination. This injection should be followed by a booster injection 6 months later. For persons without prior vaccination exposed to individuals with HAV, passive immunization is effective if administered early. Serum immune globulin (0.02 to 0.06 mL per kg) should be given within 2 weeks of exposure.

HEPATITIS B

Hepatitis B virus (HBV) is an incomplete double-stranded DNA virus composed of a lipoprotein envelope and a core of HBV DNA and several viral proteins (see Table 1). HBV DNA contains four genes: the surface gene, which encodes for surface antigen, which makes up the lipoprotein envelope; the polymerase gene, which encodes for a DNA polymerase; the core gene, which encodes two proteins, core antigen and e antigen; and the X gene, which encodes for a protein involved in viral transcription and replication.

HBV is transmitted parenterally. Major risk factors include intravenous drug use, sexual or intimate contact, tattoos or other needle stick injury from persons with chronic HBV infection, blood transfusion before 1975, hemodialysis, and vertical transmission (from mother to newborn). The incubation period for HBV is 45 to 180 days. The incidence of HBV in the United States is 140,000 to 320,000 cases per year. Approximately 5 to 6% of Americans have been exposed to HBV. The reservoir of chronic infection includes 1.25 million Americans and over 400 million people worldwide.

Serologic testing is directed at HBV antigens and antibodies that develop following exposure (Table 3). After acute infection, all patients develop S Ag and core IgM antibody. Patients with active viral replication are also positive for HBV e antigen (HBeAg) and

TABLE 3. **Serologic Testing for Hepatitis B Virus**

Phase	S Ag	E Ag	DNA	C IgM/IgG	S Ab	E Ab
Acute						
Acute active	+	+	+	+/−	−	+
Resolved	−	−	−	−/+	+	+
Window	−	−	−	+/+	−	+
Chronic						
Active	+	+	+	−/+	−	−
Nonactive	+	−	−	−/+	−	+
Pre-core mutant	+	−	+	−/+	−	−
Vaccination	−	−	−	−/−	+	−

Abbreviations: S Ag = surface antigen; E Ag = e antigen; DNA = deoxyribonucleic acid; C IgM/IgG = antibodies to core antigen; S Ab = antibody to surface antigen; E Ab = antibody to e antigen; + = positive; − = negative.

HBV DNA. Loss of active viral replication is marked by seroconversion of e antigen to e antibody coupled with loss of HBV DNA. Over time, core IgM antibodies decline and core IgG antibodies remain detectable. With resolution of infection, aminotransferase levels normalize and surface antigen is replaced by surface antibody. Surface antibodies are neutralizing. Therefore, development of surface antibodies and loss of surface antigen conveys lasting immunity. Patients who have been vaccinated against HBV will express isolated surface antibodies without other markers (i.e., core antibody) of past infection. Mutations in the pre-core region allow HBV to replicate without producing e antigen. These "pre-core mutants" are recognized serologically by the presence of surface antigen and HBV DNA and may be more virulent than wild-type HBV.

Approximately 45 to 60% of adults exposed to HBV will become symptomatic with jaundice and a 10- to 20-fold increase in ALT. Acute HBV accounts for 8400 to 19,000 hospitalizations per year. In 0.5% of cases, FHF can develop. The ability to resolve infection is dependent on the age of acquisition and inversely related to the intensity of the immune response against the virus. After acute exposure, neonatal infection from perinatal transmission is typically asymptomatic and results in low rates of viral clearance (<10%). In contrast, most adults with acute HBV are symptomatic with or without jaundice and infections resolve, with chronic hepatitis developing in less than 5%.

Prevention is the best strategy against HBV. It is currently recommended that all children be vaccinated against HBV before entering school. In addition, because the group at highest risk of HBV infection is between the ages of 15 and 30 years, all such individuals should also receive vaccination. Other populations at risk that should be vaccinated include health care professionals, hemodialysis patients, intravenous drug users, and those with high-risk sexual activity. The available vaccines are safe and confer long-lasting immunity. Recombivax HB (10 µg), or Engerix-B (20 µg) is administered as three intramuscular injections; the second and third injections are administered 4 weeks and 6 months after the first, respectively. The pediatric dose is 2.5 to 5 µg given at identical intervals.

Approximately 95% of patients develop protective levels of surface antibodies (>10 U per mL) in response to vaccine. Antibody response to vaccination need only be verified in individuals at high risk for HBV. In approximately 50% of patients, surface antibody levels may fall below detection of standard HBV surface antibody assays. The majority of these individuals, however, remain protected. Booster vaccination remains controversial but an option for high-risk populations such as health care personnel. Approximately 5% of the normal population are unable to mount an immune response to HBsAg and therefore do not respond to HBV vaccines. For these patients, a second series with 40 µg of vaccine has had some success of lasting immunity.

HBV vaccine has reduced efficacy in patients with compromised immune systems, such as those infected with human immunodeficiency virus (HIV), on hemodialysis, or with cirrhosis and transplant recipients taking immune suppression medication. When exposure to hepatitis B occurs in the absence of prior vaccination, passive administration of hepatitis B immune globulin (0.06 mL per kg intramuscularly) should be given within the first 48 hours after exposure followed by active vaccination.

HEPATITIS C

Hepatitis C virus (HCV) was first identified in 1989 as the primary agent responsible for post-transfusion non-A, non-B hepatitis. HCV is a positive, single-stranded RNA virus of the Flaviviridae family. Six major groups or genotypes have been identified. In the United States, genotype 1 is present in 70 to 75% of infected patients.

The major risk factors for HCV are transfusion of blood or blood products before 1992, intravenous or intranasal drug use, tattooing or body piercing, high-risk sexual contact, long-term hemodialysis, occupational exposure to blood (such as by health care workers), and recipients of organs or tissue transplants from an HCV-positive donor. The risk of sexual transmission in a monogamous relationship is low (<3%), as is the risk of perinatal transmission. This risk is increased, however, if the sexual partner or mother is co-infected with human immunodeficiency virus. There are no reports of transmission from nursing mothers to infants. The risk of developing HCV from a needle stick injury is 1 to 10% (median, 1.8%). The incubation period for HCV is 2 to 20 weeks. An estimated 36,000 new infections now occur annually, with an incidence of chronicity that exceeds 85%. As a result, the reservoir of chronic HCV infection is 4 to 5 million in the United States and over 175 million worldwide. At the present time, a vaccine for HCV is not available.

A number of diagnostic tests are available for HCV (see Table 2). The basic screening test is the anti-HCV enzyme immunoassay (EIA), which detects antibodies produced in response to HCV infection. In contrast to antibodies to HAV and surface antibody to HBV, HCV antibodies are not neutralizing and offer no long-lasting protection against current or subsequent infection. The current assay has a 95% sensitivity and a positive predictive value of 95% for identification of HCV in patients with elevated aminotransferase levels and risk factors for HCV. False-positive results, however, can occur. The positive predictive value is only 50% in healthy persons with normal liver chemistries and no risk factors for HCV. This test is therefore inappropriate for screening the general public.

Because false-positive results with anti-HCV testing can occur, supplemental tests for HCV were developed to confirm infection. One such test is the recombinant immunoblot assay (RIBA). This antigen-antibody assay conveys greater specificity than EIA HCV testing. Alternatively, HCV RNA can be measured directly. Two types of viral detection assays are available. Polymerase chain reaction (PCR) assays detect HCV RNA with the greatest sensitivity and can provide a quantitative measure of HCV RNA titer. Unfortunately, no universal standard exists for PCR-based assays. As a result, significant variations in viral titer may exist when this is measured by different laboratories. In contrast, branched chain DNA assays are highly reproducible when measuring HCV RNA. This assay, however, is limited by its inability to detect viral titers below 200,000 genome equivalents per mL. Thus, patients with undetectable virus by branched chain DNA may still be infected with HCV.

Acute HCV infection is accompanied by elevations in aminotransferase levels. Approximately 25 to 30% of infected people are symptomatic during acute infection. In contrast to HAV and HBV, FHF has not been reported during acute HCV infection. Antibodies to HCV develop 6 to 12 weeks after acute infection. Although 10 to 15% of cases of acute HCV infection resolve spontaneously, anti-HCV remains positive in the patients for decades. Patients with chronic HCV have fluctuations in serum ALT level, which can decline into the normal range for brief or prolonged periods of time. Several extrahepatic manifestations of HCV have been recognized. These include immune-related essential mixed cryoglobulinemia and membranoproliferative glomerulonephritis, porphyria cutanea tarda, corneal ulcers, B cell lymphoma, and non–insulin-dependent diabetes mellitus.

HEPATITIS D

The causative agent of hepatitis D (HDV) is an incomplete RNA virus that requires HBV (see Table 1). HDV can occur as a co-infection with acute HBV disease or as a super infection in patients with chronic HBV disease. Transmission is similar to that of HBV. The most important risk for HDV in the United States is intravenous drug use. HDV is also common in certain geographic areas, including Italy, South America, and certain parts of Africa. The clinical course of HDV is often more severe than with HBV alone and can result in acute liver failure. Diagnosis of HDV is based on the presence of antibodies to HDV (see Table 2), which should be measured in all patients with chronic HBV. HDV is prevented by preventing HBV infection.

HEPATITIS E

Hepatitis E virus (HEV) is a small nonenveloped RNA virus that, like HAV, is transmitted enterically. Although uncommon in the United States, HEV is responsible for both epidemic and sporadic outbreaks of hepatitis in Mexico, Central and South America, western China, India, Asia, and parts of Africa. Acute HEV is a self-limited hepatitis with no chronicity, similar to HAV (see Table 1). Unlike other hepatitis viruses, HEV carries a high incidence of fulminant liver failure in women who contract HEV during pregnancy. At present, anti-HEV testing is available only in reference laboratories (see Table 2).

HEPATITIS G

Hepatitis viruses A to E account for more than 95% of all cases of community-acquired hepatitis in the United States. Hepatitis G virus (HGV) was detected by PCR and found to be present in some patients with non-A, non-B, non-C post-transfusion hepatitis. HGV is an RNA virus with 25% homology to HCV. Studies have identified HGV RNA in 4% of blood donors. Studies suggest, however, that HGV may not contribute to chronic liver disease. Consequently, HGV testing is not recommended in blood donor screening or in the evaluation of patients with non–A to E hepatitis viruses.

CHRONIC HEPATITIS

When hepatitis continues beyond 6 months, it is termed *chronic hepatitis*. Of the six common hepatotropic agents, both HBV (with or without HDV) and HCV can progress to chronicity (see Table 1). Most patients with chronic viral hepatitis are asymptomatic. When symptoms do occur, they are nonspecific and include fatigue, malaise, loss of appetite, right upper quadrant discomfort, pruritus, and polyarthralgias. Physical examination of patients with chronic hepatitis is often unremarkable unless the patient has advanced to cirrhosis. As a result, most patients with chronic viral hepatitis are identified during routine blood testing, during application for health or life insurance, or during blood donation screening. It is suggested that patients with previous risk factors for HBV and HCV be screened for these viruses.

The diagnosis of chronic viral hepatitis is based on serologic testing. Patients with chronic HBV are persistently positive for HBsAg. These patients can have either chronic active HBV defined by the presence of e antigen and DNA or be chronic carriers with the presence of e antibody and absence of HBV DNA (see Table 2). Spontaneous seroconversion from the chronic active to the carrier state occurs in 5 to 10% of patients yearly. The rate of spontaneous loss of surface antigen and development of surface antibody with complete resolution of infection is much less frequent, being seen in 1% of patients yearly. All patients with chronic HBV should be tested for HDV.

Chronic HCV is manifested by persistence of HCV RNA. Testing for HCV RNA is useful for those individuals who test positive for anti-HCV, especially those with no identifiable risk factors, those with autoimmune antibodies, and those with normal aminotransferase levels. HCV RNA testing is also useful before treatment because loss of HCV RNA defines response to therapy. Liver biopsy is essential in chronic viral hepatitis because it determines the severity of underlying liver disease and is useful to assess the need for antiviral treatment. It is important to remember that liver histology does not correlate with the degree in elevation of serum ALT, HBV DNA, or HCV RNA levels.

The natural history of chronic viral hepatitis is insidious and variable. In HCV, approximately 10 to 15% of patients have persistence of mild hepatitis and an estimated 30 to 35% will progress to cirrhosis over 20 to 30 years. Cirrhosis develops in approximately two thirds of patients with active HBV or HBV/HDV co-infection. Factors that increase the rate of progression to cirrhosis include male sex, moderate to severe alcohol consumption, and other coexistent liver disorders.

One of the major complications of chronic viral hepatitis and cirrhosis is hepatocellular carcinoma (HCC). In the U.S. population, chronic HCV is the major risk factor for development of HCC. HCC appears to be limited to patients with cirrhosis and develops in 1 to 3% of patients per year. Unlike patients with HCV, patients with chronic HBV are at risk for development of HCC irrespective of the presence or absence of cirrhosis. Because of this increased risk, patients with cirrhosis secondary to HCV and all patients with chronic HBV should be routinely screened for HCC. Screening is performed by measurement of serum alpha-fetoprotein level every 3 to 6 months and by annual ultrasound examination of the liver.

The 5-year survival rate for patients with compensated cirrhosis exceeds 90%. Decompensation

marked by development of variceal bleeding, ascites, and hepatic encephalopathy occurs at the rate of 3 to 5% yearly. The survival of patients with decompensated cirrhosis is poor, only 10 to 50% after 3 years. The only long-term treatment option for these patients is hepatic transplantation. Viral hepatitis, primarily HCV, is the leading indication for liver transplantation.

Interferon-Based Therapy for Chronic Viral Hepatitis

The basis of therapy for chronic viral hepatitis is interferon. Interferons are a group of glycoprotein cytokines that possess both antiviral and immunomodulatory activity. These cytokines are produced by immune cells in response to viral and other antigens. Interferons inhibit viral replication, increase expression of HLA class I antigens on cell surfaces, enhance maturation of cytotoxic T cells, and promote natural killer cell activity. These actions promote viral clearance from infected cells. Three types of interferon have been recognized: α, β, and γ. Only interferon-α has been approved for treatment of chronic viral hepatitis.

Interferon treatment has two problems: route of administration and side effects. Interferon-α is administered subcutaneously and may cause local bruising. Unfortunately, side effects are common during treatment with interferon-α. The most common of these are flulike symptoms consisting of fever, myalgias, arthralgias, and headache. These symptoms occur primarily during the first few weeks of therapy but may last throughout the course of treatment. Patients can significantly reduce the flulike symptoms by administering the interferon injections before bedtime and by taking acetaminophen and/or nonsteroidal anti-inflammatory drugs at the time of injection and the following morning.

Mood changes, irritability, and mild depression can occur at any time throughout treatment. Serious depression with suicide ideation has been reported and should prompt immediate discontinuation of therapy. Other important side effects of interferon include hair loss, thyroid disease, and stimulation of autoimmune disorders. A decline in platelet and neutrophil counts is frequently observed. This can be pronounced in patients with cirrhosis and may require discontinuation of treatment. Contraindications for interferon-based therapy include significant thrombocytopenia (<80,000 per mL) or leukopenia (<3000 cell per mL), decompensated cirrhosis, autoimmune disorders, active drug or alcohol use, and ongoing psychiatric disease.

Recently, the oral nucleoside analogue ribavirin was combined with interferon-α for treatment of chronic HCV. Ribavirin is a guanosine nucleotide analogue that is thought to act by inhibiting viral replication. The most common side effect of ribavirin is hemolytic anemia, which reduces hemoglobin concentration by an average of 2 to 3 gm per dL in most treated patients. Severe hemolysis with a decline of

5 to 6 gm per dL of hemoglobin have been observed. In patients with profound hemolysis and a history of coronary artery disease or hypertension, coronary ischemia and myocardial infarction have been observed. Other common side effects of ribavirin include rashes and nausea. Ribavirin is also highly teratogenic. As a result, it is imperative that both men and women of childbearing age utilize adequate contraception during therapy and for at least 6 months after completion of treatment.

Treatment of Chronic HBV

Treatment of chronic HBV is restricted to those patients with active viral replication and active hepatitis determined by liver biopsy. In the past, treatment was limited to interferon-α administered at a dose of 5 MU daily for 16 weeks. The objective of therapy is seroconversion from HBeAg to HBeAb with loss of HBV DNA. This occurs in approximately 30% of patients. Asians and patients infected through perinatal transmission have a significantly lower rate of response. Before seroconversion, a flare associated with marked elevation in aminotransferase levels is frequently observed. Care must be taken during treatment of individuals with cirrhosis because the flare may be associated with hepatic decompensation and development of acute liver failure. Many patients who seroconvert in response to interferon treatment also lose surface antigens and develop surface antibodies over time.

Recently, the antiviral nucleoside analogues lamivudine (Epivir) and famciclovir (Famvir)* were shown to be effective in the treatment of chronic HBV. These agents suppress viral replication, which results in loss of HBV DNA, normalization of ALT, and decreased hepatic inflammation during treatment. Virus typically returns, however, once treatment is discontinued. A major limitation in the use of these antiviral agents is the development of specific mutations in HBV DNA that render these treatments ineffective.

Interferon-α has also been utilized to treat chronic HBV/HDV co-infection. Unfortunately, results of limited trials have been disappointing. Interferon is administered in similar doses as for chronic HBV and is associated with loss of HDV RNA and seroconversion in less than 10%.

Treatment of Chronic HCV

Treatment of chronic HCV is recommended for patients with active hepatitis on liver biopsy and presence of HCV RNA in serum. Treatment can be performed with either interferon-α monotherapy or interferon and ribavirin in combination. Interferon is administered at a dose of 3 MU (Intron A and Roferon A) or 9 μg (Infergen) thrice weekly for 12 months. Approximately 35% of patients become HCV RNA negative by the end of treatment. Unfortu-

---

*Not FDA approved for this indication.

nately, most of these patients relapse after therapy is discontinued. Long-term sustained response is observed in only 5 to 15% of patients treated with interferon alone. Patients who achieve a sustained response are uniformly HCV RNA negative within 3 months of initiation of therapy. Therefore, treatment can be discontinued if HCV RNA remains detectable after 3 months of treatment.

Interferon and ribavirin (Rebetron) therapy for chronic HCV has significantly increased sustained response compared with interferon monotherapy. Rebetron contains 3 MU Intron A administered three times weekly along with oral ribavirin (Rebetol) 1200 mg administered in two divided doses daily. In patients who weigh less than 75 kg, the dose of ribavirin should not exceed 1000 mg daily. Approximately 50% of patients achieve an end of treatment response with loss of HCV RNA. Sustained response is observed in 38% of patients treated with combination therapy. Rebetron can also be utilized by patients who have previously responded to interferon monotherapy and subsequently relapsed. Sustained response can be achieved in 50% of these patients. Unfortunately, patients who fail to respond to interferon monotherapy have only a 5 to 20% chance of sustained response when re-treated with combination therapy.

MALABSORPTION SYNDROMES

method of
CHARLES M. MANSBACH II, M.D.
University of Tennessee, Memphis
Memphis, Tennessee

"Malabsorption" is a generic term that covers both malabsorption and maldigestion. This term is most commonly used to refer to the impaired assimilation of dietary fat. This is because excessive fat excretion (>5% of the intake of a diet containing at least 100 grams of fat per day) is the most commonly used indicator of malabsorption. Protein and carbohydrate levels, which are malabsorbed concomitantly with fat, are usually not measured in the stool. Protein malabsorption is difficult to assess because large amounts of protein are normally excreted into the bowel each day. Assessment is further complicated by abnormal leakage of protein into the bowel in certain disease states. Carbohydrate malabsorption is also difficult to study because of the effective surface digestion of carbohydrate and because of the colonic bacterial transformation of malabsorbed carbohydrates to noncarbohydrate products. Specific defects in absorption of amino acids and carbohydrates, with the exception of lactase insufficiency, are rare. Therefore, excessive fat excretion remains the best indicator of malabsorption and maldigestion.

MALABSORPTION

Malabsorption should be considered in anyone with unexplained weight loss; production of stools suggestive of steatorrhea; the development of osteomalacia and/or a low serum calcium level; the development of a prolonged prothrombin time in the absence of liver disease; iron deficiency anemia not caused by blood loss, especially if it is difficult to control by oral iron replacement; or the development of lactase insufficiency in adulthood. The development of any of these symptoms is suggestive of (1) the establishment of the malabsorptive state and (2) the definition of the disease causing the malabsorption. Although there are screening tests for malabsorption in common use, such as the D-xylose test or the bentiromide (Chymex) test, the test involving 72-hour fecal excretion of fat coupled with a known fat intake remains the most secure way to establish the problem. A qualitative test of stool fat, in which the stool is examined for fat globules with the aid of Sudan III before and after being heated with acidic acid, may also be used.

Physical signs to be looked for include evidence of muscle wasting, edema, tetany, bruises and ecchymoses, and glossitis or cheilosis.

The establishment of the cause of malabsorption is crucial because therapy is directed in each instance to a specific diagnosis. If the diagnosis is correct and the treatment is appropriately tailored, stool output reduction and weight gain are to be expected.

Chronic Pancreatitis

The most common cause of malabsorption is lipase deficiency. This occurs when lipase excretion from the pancreas into the duodenum is less than 10% of normal output. The majority of cases are caused by chronic pancreatitis, usually because of excessive ethanol intake. Other causes of chronic pancreatitis include hypertriglyceridemia, the rare familial form of pancreatitis, cystic fibrosis, and the idiopathic form of pancreatitis. Gallstone-caused acute pancreatitis does not lead to the development of the chronic form. Not all cases of chronic pancreatitis are associated with abdominal pain; completely painless pancreatitis is well known. There are no tests to reveal subtle abnormalities of the pancreas. The most sensitive test to determine pancreatic insufficiency is the secretin-pancreozymin test, in which the hormones secretin and cholecystokinin are administered intravenously and duodenal fluid is collected for bicarbonate and enzyme measurement. Nearly 50% of the gland must be destroyed before results of this test become abnormal; a reduction in enzyme output is the most sensitive component. Particularly useful in establishing the diagnosis of chronic pancreatitis is the finding of pancreatic calcification on a flat plate of the abdomen. The sensitivity of identifying calcification can be enhanced by computed tomography or ultrasonography. Anatomic abnormalities in the pancreatic duct that are indicative of chronic pancreatitis can be identified by endoscopic retrograde pancreatography or magnetic resonance cholangiopancreatography. The development of diabetes without a family history and/or low serum trypsin-like immu-

noreactivity is also helpful in establishing the diagnosis.

Treatment

The treatment of the malabsorptive symptoms of chronic pancreatitis must often be individualized to optimize the results.

Pancreatic enzyme replacement therapy is either by tablet (such as Viokase) or microspheres (such as Pancrease or Creon). Microspheres are designed to release their encapsulated enzymes only when the bowel luminal pH approaches 6.0, thus avoiding the acid-based inactivation of the enzymes in the stomach. However, because of the size of the microspheres (1.2 to 2.0 mm), they are retained by the stomach longer than the meal itself. With either formulation, a disappointingly small amount of active enzyme reaches the duodenum in concert with the meal. Nevertheless, despite the theoretical problems, both tablets and microspheres provide symptomatic improvement, although rarely is the steatorrhea completely reversed.

Pancreatic enzyme replacement tablets or capsules should be given just before meals; tablets or capsules for adults should contain approximately 30,000 lipase units. If the patients' symptoms are not improved, a different formulation can be tried (tablet versus capsule), or an increase in the amount of lipase activity can be administered with each meal. Very high doses can result in colonic strictures or fibrosing colonopathy, which is seen mostly in children. Because of this, the capsules containing the highest dose have been removed from the market. Gout may also result from the large amount of purine administered with the enzymes. If no improvement results with dosage increase, gastric acid output should be reduced with either omeprazole* (Prilosec) or lansoprazole* (Prevacid). If this fails, smaller and more frequent meals can be tried, as can reducing the amount of fat in the diet to 50 to 75 grams per day.

Fat-soluble vitamins are usually not malabsorbed in chronic pancreatitis. This is because they do not require digestion before absorption. However, symptoms of vitamin deficiency occasionally result from poor intake, usually in the setting of chronic alcoholism. In these cases, vitamin supplementation can be given. Approximately 50% of patients with chronic pancreatitis have an abnormal result on Schilling's test for vitamin B_{12} absorption. Rarely, however, do these patients manifest clinical symptoms of vitamin B_{12} deficiency. Adequate pancreatic replacement therapy leads to restoration of vitamin B_{12} absorption.

Some patients demonstrating malabsorption from chronic pancreatitis continue to have the abdominal pain associated with this condition. These patients may also be helped by pancreatic replacement therapy. Pain relief is helpful in maintaining weight because some patients decrease food intake in an at-

---

*Not FDA approved for this indication.

tempt to avoid pain. Enzyme supplementation therapy for pain relief should be in the form of tablets instead of microspheres, and more tablets should be given than when treating chronic pancreatitis. In these cases, the development of hyperuricemia and hyperuricosuria should be considered, especially in patients with a history of gout. The presence of complicating factors in patients with chronic pancreatitis, such as the development of a pseudocyst or carcinoma of the pancreas, should also be considered.

A major problem in pain control is narcotic addiction. For this reason, only one physician should dispense these medications, and narcotics should be used as a last resort. A fentanyl patch (Duragesic) can also be tried. Other remedies are to stop alcohol ingestion, stent dominant pancreatic ductular strictures, and remove stones from the duct by endoscopic techniques.

Of importance is that the abdominal pain associated with chronic pancreatitis tends to wane over the years. In some patients, however, surgery is required for relief. Operations on the pancreas should be performed only by surgeons skilled in these procedures. In no case is pain relief always expected. Glandular destruction continues even after adequate surgical ductular drainage. Surgical therapeutic options include a modified Puestow procedure (longitudinal pancreaticojejunostomy) or a pylorus-sparing or duodenum-sparing Whipple operation. In highly selected cases with disease limited to the distal 50% of the pancreas, a distal pancreatectomy may be useful. Other patients may develop a stricture of the common bile duct, which, if persistent, must be bypassed. Endoscopic retrograde pancreatography is crucial in these settings. Celiac ganglionectomy and celiac block have been performed, but their use for pain control is, at best, uncertain. Some surgeons advocate 95% pancreatectomy as a last resort, but this operation is used infrequently. These patients are invariably left with diabetes as an outcome and require insulin replacement or the new approach of islet cell transplantation. Supplementation with digestive enzymes is always required.

MALDIGESTION CAUSED BY BILE SALT DEFICIENCY

Bile acids are secreted from the liver and conjugated to the amino acids glycine and taurine. Above a certain concentration, they aggregate to form micelles. These micelles have an exterior that is hydrophilic and an interior that is hydrophobic. The products of fat digestion are presumed to be found in the interior of the bile salt–mixed micelle. This property of bile salts optimizes fat absorption and is especially important for the absorption of vitamins D and E. Without any bile acids, approximately 50% of dietary fat can be absorbed. This percentage can be increased by maximizing the intake of polyunsaturated fatty acids, which, in the absence of bile acids, interact better with water than do saturated fatty acids.

Biliary Drainage

If bile is drained from the intestinal tract, the bile salt pool is quickly lost and the liver is stimulated maximally to synthesize bile acids. One way in which bile may be drained from the liver is the placement of a T tube in the bile duct, which enables bile to flow out of the long arm of the tube. In certain instances in which palliation for inoperable obstructive jaundice is desired, nasobiliary drainage or transhepatic drainage of the bile ductular system can be performed. When a transhepatic tube is placed, internal drainage may be possible, thus restoring bile drainage to the intestinal tract.

If malabsorption becomes a problem, a diet in which polyunsaturated fats are substituted for saturated ones should be consumed, or medium-chain triglyceride (MCT) oil should be substituted for normal dietary fat. The fatty acids of MCT are 8 to 10 carbons in length. They are essentially water soluble and thus do not require bile acids for absorption. On absorption, they go to the liver, where they are oxidized (which is not the normal fate of newly absorbed long-chain fatty acids). Patients who rely heavily on MCT oil should be observed for the development of essential fatty acid deficiency.

Bacterial Overgrowth

In this condition, bacteria, usually in the upper intestine, deconjugate bile acids that have reduced solubility at the slightly acidic pH present in the upper intestine. The precipitated bile acids are passively absorbed, and the lumen is therefore depleted of the bile acids necessary for optimal fat absorption. In addition, enzymes released by the bacteria hydrolyze portions of the luminal surfaces of absorptive cells, which, in turn, become dysfunctional. The bacteria primarily responsible for these abnormalities are anaerobes. The diagnosis is made most securely by intubating the duodenum, collecting duodenal fluid under anaerobic conditions, and finding more than 10^5 bacteria per mL. Alternatively, an increase in the amount of deconjugated bile acids in duodenal fluid is also diagnostic. Affected patients may have increased breath hydrogen in the fasting state and increased amounts of hydrogen appearing in the breath shortly after ingesting either glucose or the poorly absorbed sugar lactulose. An early increase in breath labeled carbon dioxide ($^{14}CO_2$) from ingested carbon ^{14}C–labeled xylose may also be found. This is a more specific and sensitive test than are the breath hydrogen tests. All of these absorptive tests depend on adequate gastric emptying.

Identification of the cause of the increase in intestinal bacteria is important because treatment varies, depending on the diagnosis made. An upper gastrointestinal series with small bowel follow-through aids in the diagnosis of multiple intestinal diverticula, Crohn's disease, radiation injury, and potentially impaired gastrointestinal motility. Scleroderma and diabetes, especially in the presence of peripheral neuropathy, are systemic diseases that may be associated with impaired intestinal motility. Achlorhydria produced either by gastric mucosal disease or injury or by the administration of a proton pump inhibitor may also be associated with this problem. A cologastric fistula is best diagnosed by means of barium enema study. Surgical correction of this condition is warranted.

Treatment

Treatment should first be directed to any condition that is surgically remedial. If there is no surgical option, antibiotic treatment should be started with tetracycline, 250 mg four times a day for 7 to 10 days. Often symptoms abate for months, but if not, the drug can be given 1 week per month or more often if necessary. More anaerobic bacteria are resistant to tetracycline, and so other regimens that are directed toward both anaerobes and aerobes need to be tried. Amoxicillin/clavulanate (Augmentin), 875 mg twice a day, or cephalexin (Keflex), 250 mg four times daily, or metronidazole (Flagyl), 250 mg three times daily, may also be used. For motility disturbances, a prokinetic drug such as metoclopramide (Reglan) or cisapride (Propulsid), 10 mg before meals and at bedtime for each, should be given. Serum folate levels are usually increased in this condition. If the vitamin B_{12} level is low, this vitamin should be replaced parenterally. Successful treatment should obviate the need for future B_{12} administration.

Impaired Bile Salt Reabsorption

The most common cause of this problem is intestinal resection. As little as 30 cm of the most distal ileum, including the ileocecal valve, can be associated with significant malabsorption of bile salts. Usually the resection is caused by Crohn's disease, which itself usually does not lead to bile acid malabsorption. Either stenotic Crohn's disease or resection of the ileocecal valve may result in bacterial contamination of the distal intestine. Excessive bile acid loss to the colon may result in diarrhea without the presence of steatorrhea. This is usually seen in ileal resections of 30 to 60 cm. Dihydroxylated bile salts cause the colon to secrete salt and water. A diagnosis of impaired bile salt reabsorption can be made by finding an increased proportion of bile salts conjugated with glycine compared to taurine or an increase in the amount of $^{14}CO_2$ excreted into the breath after ^{14}C-labeled bile salts are given by mouth. A more convenient method is to determine the retention of selenium 75–labeled HCAT ($^{75}SeHCAT$), a taurocholate analogue, by the body.

Treatment

Oral replacement of bile salts increases the diarrhea. Bile acid binders, such as cholestyramine* (Questran) or colestipol* (Colestid) should be given

---

*Not FDA approved for this indication.

as one packet (4 grams) before meals and at bedtime. The dose should be reduced if the patient becomes constipated.

For larger resections, especially those longer than 100 cm, vitamin B_{12} malabsorption can be expected, as well as more significant steatorrhea. In this setting, the diarrhea results from excessive fat in the stool rather than from the secretory stimulation of excessive bile acids in the colon. Although bile acid binders usually do not work in this condition, they should be tried first. If they are not successful, the patient should try a diet low in fat in which the proportion of fat eaten is high in polyunsaturates. MCT oil may also be used to provide calories. Four ounces of MCT oil equals 1000 calories.

MALABSORPTION SECONDARY TO PRIMARY INTESTINAL DISORDERS

The reasons for malabsorption are especially well documented in gluten-sensitive enteropathy (GSE). These include (1) a decreased intestinal surface area secondary to villous atrophy; (2) reduced amounts of the hormone cholecystokinin-pancreozymin (CCK-PZ) in the duodenum, resulting in poor CCK-PZ release on stimulation by food, which reduces the quantities of bile salts and lipase in the upper intestine after meals; (3) immature cells at the surface of the intestine that are unable to adequately perform the absorptive and transport functions of mature intestinal cells; and (4) the secretory state induced by the increased proportion of chloride-secreting cryptal cells to the sodium- and chloride-absorbing mature villous cells. This results in enlarged fluid volume in the upper intestine and reduces the effective concentration of bile acids, which in turn reduces the number of micelles available for lipid solubilization.

A small bowel biopsy is crucial for the specific diagnosis. Villous flattening can be present in GSE, collagenous sprue, immunoglobulin deficiencies, nodular lymphoid hyperplasia, and tropical sprue. Villus atrophy may be present in patients with intestinal irradiation, chronic intestinal ischemia, and Whipple's disease. A small bowel series may yield abnormal findings, demonstrating the disordered motility pattern or small bowel edema secondary to hypoalbuminemia. Nodules may be identified in nodular lymphoid hyperplasia. A specific diagnosis is necessary so that treatment may be appropriately directed.

Gluten-Sensitive Enteropathy

This disorder, also called celiac sprue, is probably an immunologic disorder in the appropriate genetic background caused by exposure of the intestine to gluten, which is found in wheat, rye, barley, and oats. Histologic examination of the intestine demonstrates cryptal hypertrophy and an increase in inflammatory cells, including plasma cells. Lymphocytes are seen infiltrating the abnormal-appearing surface cells.

Treatment

Dietary treatment of malabsorption secondary to GSE consists of avoiding all products containing gluten. Careful reading of the contents of all foods bought in cans or boxes is required. Information on gluten exclusion may be obtained from the Celiac Sprue Society, Internet sites, and gluten-free recipes from books such as *Luncheon with Laurie* (Carpenter Publishers, Rock Hill, South Carolina). Clinical improvement is expected within 1 to 2 weeks, but intestinal histologic improvement lags. If there is no improvement, the patient should be hospitalized to be certain that an adequate gluten-exclusion diet is being followed. If no improvement is apparent, the patient should be tested for pancreatic insufficiency and intestinal bacterial overgrowth as complicating factors. The establishment of the diagnosis is important because this is a lifelong problem that necessitates significant dietary changes. The diagnosis is based on the significant clinical improvement on dietary therapy. Usually patients, once improved, have a dietary indiscretion that leads to recurrence of symptoms.

Tropical Sprue

Patients who spend more than 1 month in a tropical area where the disease is endemic may be suspected of having this disease. Not all tropical areas are involved. The intestinal histologic characteristics of this condition are similar to those of GSE. Vitamin B_{12} and folate levels are often reduced.

Treatment

Any water and electrolyte abnormalities should be corrected first. Patients should be given oral folate replacement, 5 mg per day, and vitamin B_{12}, 1000 μg parenterally, followed in 1 week by tetracycline therapy, 250 mg four times a day. Improvement is quicker if folate deficiency is corrected. Folate should be given for 1 month and tetracycline for 6 months. This regimen prevents relapses.

Collagenous Sprue

In this condition, excessive collagen deposition is seen underneath the epithelial cells of the small intestine. There is no adequate treatment, although corticosteroids may be tried. The diarrhea may be decreased by reducing the amount of fat in the diet and increasing the percentage of polyunsaturated fatty acids in the fat eaten. Corticosteroids may be tried and are occasionally effective. MCT oil may be used. A low-calcium diet may also be helpful. Total parenteral nutrition (TPN) may be necessary to maintain the patient's weight.

Radiation Enteritis

After abdominal irradiation, diarrhea is common and may be treated by diphenoxylate hydrochloride with atropine sulfate (Lomotil) or loperamide (Imodium). This acute radiation-induced diarrhea is usually self-limiting. Many months or years later, chronic radiation enteritis may ensue. This is secondary to mucosal atrophy caused by the arteritis induced by the radiation.

Treatment

A low-fat diet with a high proportion of polyunsaturated fatty acids may be tried. MCT oil and a low-calcium diet may also be helpful. TPN may be necessary.

CHRONIC ISCHEMIC BOWEL DISEASE

This disease is caused by a decrease in blood supply to the intestine. At least two of the arteries supplying the intestine are stenosed. Patients complain of abdominal cramps after eating and learn to decrease food intake to avoid pain, causing weight loss. Diarrhea may be present.

SHORT-BOWEL SYNDROME

In this condition, usually caused by surgical resection, the surface area of the intestine is greatly reduced, with reduction in the contact time of nutriments with the intestinal mucosa. If the resection was recent, small oral feedings should be started because enteric nutrition helps to induce adaptation (hypertrophy of the remaining intestinal mucosa). Adaptation is not as great in the proximal intestine after distal resection as it is in the distal intestine after proximal resection.

Treatment

Chemically defined diets, especially those containing casein hydrolysates, should be used. Those containing crystalline amino acids should be avoided because small peptides are absorbed better than amino acids. These formulations may have to be diluted to avoid the effects of their high osmolar content. Multiple small feedings may be needed. Vitamin and mineral supplements are important and should be given orally if possible. Magnesium oxide is preferred to magnesium citrate or magnesium hydroxide because the latter two may enhance intestinal motility and thus further shorten the contact time. Calcium supplements should not be given with meals because the calcium may bind to fatty acids, reducing the likelihood of absorbing both the calcium and the fatty acids. In patients with distal resections, vitamin B_{12} malabsorption is expected and vitamin B_{12} supplementation should be given parenterally. Folate and other water-soluble vitamins should be given orally. TPN may also be required. A small amount of corn oil, given by mouth 30 minutes before eating, may delay gastric emptying enough to enable the patient to eat a modest meal.

DEFECTS IN DELIVERING ABSORBED LIPIDS TO THE SYSTEMIC CIRCULATION

Absorbed split triglycerides are resynthesized in the intestinal mucosa to triglycerides, which are transported out of the intestine into the lymph fluid in chylomicrons. Lymph fluid collects in the thoracic duct, which joins the general circulation. The chylomicrons have, on their surface, apolipoproteins that direct their delivery to specific bodily sites. Beta-lipoprotein synthesis is required for triglyceride transport out of the intestinal absorptive cell.

Impaired Lipoprotein Synthesis

Abetalipoproteinemia is a misnamed condition in which beta-lipoprotein is adequately synthesized but a genetic abnormality in the synthesis of a crucial protein (microsomal triglyceride transport protein) that delivers lipid to the developing chylomicron is defective or absent. The diagnosis is suggested by the finding of excessive fat in intestinal cells after an overnight fast. Serum cholesterol and triglyceride levels are low. The patients are usually young when they first come to medical attention and may manifest neurologic and red blood cell abnormalities, as well as growth deficiencies and steatorrhea. Reinfusion of beta-lipoproteins is not curative.

Treatment

Treatment consists of instituting a low fat diet with a high proportion of polyunsaturated fatty acids. MCT oil is usually required for caloric supplementation. Water-soluble vitamin E supplementation should be given.

ABNORMAL LYMPHATIC DRAINAGE

Abnormal lymphatic drainage may be seen in a variety of conditions that impede the normal flow of lymph fluid, such as retroperitoneal fibrosis, lymphoma, metastatic carcinoma, idiopathic lymphangiectasia, and severe right-sided heart failure. Intestinal biopsy reveals club-shaped villi caused by the dilated lymphatic vessels.

Treatment

Treatment should be directed to the specific condition. Chemotherapy for lymphomatous involvement is helpful, as is decortication of patients with constrictive pericarditis. Severe congestive heart failure may respond to appropriate therapy. In conditions such as retroperitoneal fibrosis or intestinal lymphangiectasia, for which no specific treatment is available, diarrhea may be greatly reduced by a low-fat diet, with MCT oil as caloric supplementation. Fat-soluble vitamins should be given. Over the long term, these patients should be observed for essential fatty acid deficiency.

WHIPPLE'S DISEASE

Whipple's disease is uncommon but is invariably fatal if not treated. It is found most often in middle-aged and older men. In addition to diarrhea and wasting, these patients usually have arthritis or arthralgias. They may also have fever and lymphadenopathy. The diagnosis is established by small intestinal biopsy, which demonstrates many periodic acid–Schiff (PAS)–positive macrophages infiltrating the lamina propria. In patients with the acquired immune deficiency syndrome (AIDS), infection with *Mycobacterium avium–intracellulare* may produce a similar picture. These organisms may be distinguished from the Whipple bacterium by electron microscopy or acid-fast stains.

Treatment

It is important to treat patients with antibiotics that cross the blood-brain barrier to prevent central nervous system manifestations of Whipple's disease, which are usually irreversible and occur later in the course of the disease. Trimethoprim-sulfamethoxazole (Bactrim, Septra), one double-strength tablet twice daily, may be given, or streptomycin with penicillin may be given for 10 days, followed by tetracycline, 250 mg four times a day. Patients receiving tetracycline alone or other antibiotics that do not cross the blood-brain barrier are at risk for central nervous system disease. Treatment should be continued for 1 year to prevent relapses. Clinical improvement is usually rapid (1 to 2 weeks). The rare patient whose condition does not improve with this regimen may require chloramphenicol. Severely malnourished patients may require TPN or other caloric supplements. Repeated intestinal biopsies should show a reduction in the number of PAS-positive macrophages. However, a few macrophages have been shown to exist as long as 25 years after successful treatment.

POSTGASTRECTOMY SYNDROMES

Weight loss and malnutrition are often seen after gastrectomy, especially if significant amounts of the stomach have been removed. The reduced gastric receptive relaxation leads to early satiety and a decrease in food intake. Reduction in food intake may also be caused by fear of inducing the dumping syndrome. In this condition, hyperosmolar food enters the small intestine more quickly than normal, which induces water secretion into the intestinal lumen to lessen the osmotic load. This reaction may be strong enough to induce hypotension with a feeling of faintness. Patients usually learn to lie down when these symptoms appear. Symptoms of hypoglycemia may also be found 2 to 4 hours after meals. This condition is caused by excessive insulinemia for the amount of glucose present in the blood. Symptoms of the early dumping syndrome are usually ameliorated by having the patient eat small, dry meals, followed later by liquids. Reduction in carbohydrate intake usually reduces the late manifestations of dumping.

Patients with Billroth II resections are likely (50%) to have steatorrhea. Steatorrhea is seen less often in patients with Billroth I resections or with a parietal cell vagotomy. The steatorrhea results from the poor synchronization of food and pancreaticobiliary secretions. This is because food is placed directly into the jejunum. The amount of CCK-PZ in the jejunal mucosa is much lower than in the duodenum, reducing its output, which further impairs digestion and absorption of the meal. Absorption sites for calcium and iron are also bypassed in patients with gastrojejunostomies.

Treatment

If the patient is symptomatic, pancreatin may be given with meals. If a blind loop syndrome develops as a result of obstruction of the afferent loop, surgical reconstruction should be performed. If this is not possible, treatment with tetracycline is usually efficacious. After gastrectomy, previously silent lactase insufficiency or GSE may become clinically manifest. It should be treated appropriately. Bacterial overgrowth may also result from low acid output in the stomach. In this condition, tetracycline should be given. In young or middle-aged patients, osteoporosis is expected as the patient ages. Careful attention to vitamin D and calcium supplementation in the intervening years is helpful.

PARASITIC INFECTION

The most common parasite associated with steatorrhea in the United States is *Giardia lamblia*. Contaminated water, even from mountain streams, is the usual cause. The reason for the malabsorption in this condition is not clear. The cysts of *G. lamblia* can be demonstrated in the stool, but only 50% of the time. Duodenal intubation to demonstrate trophozoites free in the lumen greatly increases the yield. The best way to identify *G. lamblia* is on the surface of the intestine. After biopsy of the small bowel, the luminal surface of the biopsy is applied to a glass slide and stained. Giardiasis is especially common in patients with AIDS and may be reacquired after treatment.

Treatment

Metronidazole (Flagyl), 250 mg three times a day for 10 days, or quinacrine (Atabrine), 100 mg three times a day for 7 days, is effective therapy for this condition. Patients with AIDS may have *Isospora belli* infection or cryptosporidiosis.

EOSINOPHILIC GASTROENTERITIS

In this condition the eosinophils, which are normally present in the lamina propria of the gastrointestinal tract, infiltrate the glands of the stomach or crypts of the small intestine. This may result in nodulation, which may be identified on gastrointestinal radiographic examination. Biopsy of the small bowel is helpful for diagnosis.

Treatment

Patients respond rapidly to prednisone, which should be begun at a dosage of 20 to 30 mg per day for 7 to 10 days, followed by a tapering dose. Patients who experience relapse may need additional treatment. If a partial response is seen, prednisone therapy may be continued at a dose of 10 to 15 mg per day.

CARBOHYDRATE AND PROTEIN MALABSORPTION

The complex carbohydrates seen in starch require breakdown by amylase secreted by the salivary glands, followed by breakdown by amylase secreted by the pancreas. This breakdown partially digests these complex sugars; final digestion is accomplished by specific hydrolases present at the luminal surface of the small intestine. The result is the production of monosaccharides that are absorbed by specific transport mechanisms present in the intestinal mucosa. In addition to these complex carbohydrates, disaccharides such as lactose and sucrose require hydrolysis before absorption.

Lactase Insufficiency

Lactase insufficiency is the most common malabsorptive condition in the United States. Lactase is localized to the tips of the villi and normally disappears after weaning. However, in people of Northern European descent and in certain tribes in Africa, the presence of lactase persists at a high level throughout life. Even in these people, after gastroenteritis, which reduces the height of the villi, transient lactase insufficiency may result. The symptoms occur rapidly after the ingestion of lactose-containing foods such as milk. They include abdominal bloating, cramps, and passage of gas. Acidic diarrhea may also occur, resulting from the increased osmolar load that passes into the colon. Usually the diagnosis is made most simply by having the patient avoid dairy products for 2 weeks and observing the effect on the symptoms. If symptoms persist and lactase insufficiency is suspected, a lactose tolerance test or a breath hydrogen test after ingestion of lactose may be performed.

Treatment

Patients who continue to drink milk may do so if the lactose in the milk has been reduced either by lactase enzyme (Lactaid) treatment or if they drink lactose-reduced milk, which is available at most stores. The amount of milk or other dairy products that can be ingested by these patients must be individualized because tolerance of lactose varies. Yogurt, especially natural vanilla-flavored yogurt, may be a good source of calcium for patients who cannot tolerate any milk products, because there is enough lactase activity associated with the bacteria present in the yogurt to digest the amount of lactose present. Calcium and vitamin D supplementation may be required for severely affected patients.

Selective Absorption Disorders

In rare cases, patients are congenitally unable to absorb glucose and galactose. Manifestations of diarrhea are first seen in infancy and result from the congenital absence of the specific transporter of these monosaccharides. Fructose should be substituted for glucose and galactose (the monosaccharides of sugar).

Several congenital defects in amino acid absorption also exist. Hartnup's disease and cystinuria are the ones most commonly seen. Protein deficiencies do not result from these rare entities because either dipeptides and tripeptides containing the neutral amino acids not absorbed in Hartnup's disease or basic amino acids, malabsorbed in cystinuria, are adequately absorbed.

ACUTE PANCREATITIS

method of
THEODORE N. PAPPAS, M.D., and
BRYAN C. WEIDNER, M.D.
Duke University Medical Center
Durham, North Carolina

Acute pancreatitis manifests in a variety of clinical settings with signs and symptoms ranging from mild epigastric pain and tenderness to severe pain with hemodynamic instability. Appropriate clinical suspicion can lead to early diagnosis and appropriate resuscitation and monitoring.

ETIOLOGY

Approximately 45% of cases of acute pancreatitis are caused by gallstones; alcohol accounts for 35%. Ten percent are idiopathic, and 10% are caused by other conditions (Table 1). Depending on the population studied, these ratios may be different. For example, inner city populations tend to have higher incidences of alcohol-induced pancreatitis.

PATHOGENESIS

The pathogenesis of pancreatitis is poorly understood. Diverse factors appear to be able to lead to a disturbance of cellular metabolism with inappropriate activation of zymogens within pancreatic cells, which leads to vascular damage, necrosis, and autodigestion of the pancreas. Numerous theories about the pathogenesis of acute pancreatitis have been advanced; however, no theory adequately explains the induction and severity of pancreatitis.

One classical theory holds that acute pancreatitis is caused by obstruction of the pancreatic duct, whereby con-

TABLE 1. **Causes of Acute Pancreatitis**

Biliary tract disease
Alcohol
Medications
Familial
Pancreatic duct obstruction
Tumor
Pancreatic divisum
Ampullary stenosis
Hyperlipidemia, hypercalcemia
Infection
Ischemia
Scorpion venom
Trauma
External
Iatrogenic: surgery, endoscopic retrograde cholangiopancreatography

tinued pancreatic secretions lead to ductal hypertension and ductal disruption. Subsequent extravasation of pancreatic enzymes into the parenchyma leads to autodigestion of the gland. Most experimental models of ductal ligation, however, lead only to pancreatic edema.

A long-standing hypothesis of acute biliary pancreatitis is the "common channel theory": A gallstone impacted in a common channel between the hepatic duct and the pancreatic duct allows reflux of bile into the pancreatic duct. However, bile by itself does not activate pancreatic enzymes. Another proposed theory is that intermittent obstruction of the pancreatic duct by the passage of multiple stones may lead eventually to acinar damage and pancreatitis. Decades of experimentation, however, have failed to prove the bile reflux theory of acute pancreatitis.

A third classical theory about pancreatitis is the reflux of duodenal contents into the pancreatic duct. This theory suggests that passage of a stone through the sphincter of Oddi renders the sphincter incompetent, which then allows the reflux of duodenal contents into the pancreatic ductal system. However, patients who receive sphincterotomies by endoscopic retrograde cholangiopancreatography (ERCP) or surgical sphincteroplasty do not suffer repeated bouts of acute pancreatitis.

Studies suggest that multiple initiating stimuli may lead to acinar cell dysfunction with co-localization of digestive enzymes within the cell. Enzyme activation leads to destruction of the acinar cell and intraparenchymal autodigestion. Ethanol has been shown to prevent fusion of secretory components to the cell membrane. The zymogens could then be activated and released intracellularly. Intense investigation into the pathogenesis of acute pancreatitis is ongoing, and many questions remain unanswered.

CLASSIFICATION

The terminology for the classification of acute pancreatitis is based on clinical findings and computed tomography (CT) and includes (1) acute pancreatitis, (2) severe acute pancreatitis, (3) mild acute pancreatitis, (4) acute fluid collections, (5) pancreatic necrosis, (6) pseudocysts, and (7) pancreatic abscess. The classification of severe pancreatitis is based on the presence of organ failure (shock, pulmonary insufficiency, and renal failure) and not upon the CT diagnosis of necrosis. This is important because CT may not be immediately obtained and because occasionally a patient with pancreatic necrosis may not be clinically ill. The classification also makes the distinction between an acute fluid collection (which occurs early in the disease, lacks a defined wall, and is likely to resolve without intervention) and a pseudocyst (which has defined walls and matures over 4 to 6 weeks). "Pancreatic phlegmon" has also been removed from the terminology because the term is too vague. It has been replaced by more specific terms such as "interstitial pancreatitis," "sterile necrosis," and "infected necrosis."

DIAGNOSIS

The clinical manifestations of acute pancreatitis are variable and range from mild complaints of midepigastric pain to circulatory shock. A history and physical examination are critical to the diagnosis, which is confirmed with radiographic and laboratory tests. The acute onset of constant, midepigastric pain, often radiating to the midback, is the most common manifestation; paroxysms of pain are rare. The patient typically cannot find a comfortable position and often sits rocking in a bent-over position. Nausea and vomiting are frequently associated findings. A history of gallstones, alcohol use, or prior pancreatitis may be obtained. Physical findings may range from mild upper abdominal tenderness to an acute-appearing abdomen with rigidity. An ill-defined upper or midabdominal mass may be palpable if the patient has an abscess or a pseudocyst. Bowel sounds are often diminished. Rare findings such as flank hematoma (Grey Turner's sign) or periumbilical discoloration (Cullen's sign) indicate severe pancreatitis with retroperitoneal hemorrhage. Vital signs range from mild tachypnea and tachycardia to postural hypotension, depending on the severity of the inflammatory process. Profound shock may be found in severe acute pancreatitis and is secondary to vomiting and hemorrhage, fluid loss in the intestine and retroperitoneum, and the vascular effects of kinins on the systemic circulation. Elevations in temperature may occur and do not necessarily signify infection, although sepsis is a potential complication of acute pancreatitis. The differential diagnosis would include perforated peptic ulcer, intestinal obstruction, and intestinal strangulation, as well as mesenteric infarction.

There is no laboratory value or marker that is 100% sensitive and specific for the diagnosis of acute pancreatitis, and all values must be interpreted in the context of the clinical presentation. Although serum levels of pancreatic alpha-amylase, phospholipase A, and C-reactive protein are touted as highly sensitive and specific, availability and application of these tests are not widespread. Measurement of serum amylase and lipase levels remains the most frequently used test in the diagnosis of acute pancreatitis. The serum half-life of amylase is shorter than that of lipase and returns to normal more rapidly. Typically, hyperamylasemia is observed within 24 hours of the onset of symptoms, with a gradual return to normal levels over the ensuing days. Persistent elevations in amylase levels may indicate the development of complications of pancreatitis, including necrosis or acute fluid collections. The degree of initial hyperamylasemia does not reliably predict the severity of the pancreatic injury. In addition, hyperamylasemia may also be found in other conditions (intestinal obstruction, mesenteric infarction, salpingitis, salivary gland disorders, renal failure, diabetic ketoacidosis). Although a normal amylase level (particularly in the case of a patient who seeks medical attention several days after the onset of symptoms) can be found in acute pancreatitis, it is elevated in 90 to 95% of cases of acute pancreatitis and is highest in gallstone pancreatitis. When compared to acute pancreatitis with elevated serum amylase levels,

normoamylasemic pancreatitis is often characterized by one of the following: (1) alcoholic etiology, (2) a greater number of previous attacks in alcoholic pancreatitis, and (3) a longer duration of symptoms before admission.

Serum lipase is a useful, easily obtained test for pancreatitis. The test is 90 to 97% specific for pancreatitis, and lipase levels stay elevated longer than do amylase levels. Some studies have found sensitivity as high as 100% and and specificity as high as 99% in cases of acute alcoholic pancreatitis. Serum lipase levels may be elevated in patients with nonpancreatic abdominal pain (e.g., ruptured aortic aneurysm, cholelithiasis, choledocholithiasis, small bowel obstruction, and nephrolithiasis). However, the levels with these nonpancreatic conditions are usually less than three times the normal values, whereas levels in acute pancreatitis usually are more than five times the normal values.

Leukocytosis, hyperglycemia, hypocalcemia, elevated lactate dehydrogenase level, and metabolic acidosis are not specific to pancreatitis and may not be present. They are predictive, however, of the severity and prognosis of pancreatitis, as discussed later.

Radiographic findings in acute pancreatitis are variable. The flat and upright abdominal films may reveal a segmental ileus (sentinel loop), colonic dilatation, obscured psoas margin, dilated duodenal loop, or pancreatic calcifications. A chest radiograph may reveal pleural effusions. The chief value of plain films is to exclude other causes of acute abdominal pain, such as free air from perforated viscus.

Although ultrasonography is inexpensive and can detect pancreatic enlargement and general reduction in parenchymal echogenicity, the study is often unsatisfactory because of poor beam penetration through air-filled loops of bowel. The main role of ultrasonography for patients with acute pancreatitis is to determine the cause of the pancreatitis by evaluating the biliary tree and gallbladder. In addition, ultrasonography may be the modality of choice for follow-up evaluation of known fluid collections.

CT scanning with rapid bolus intravenous oral contrast is currently the most sensitive noninvasive modality available for confirming the diagnosis of acute pancreatitis. CT can identify radiopaque gallstones, masses in the pancreas, and fluid collections, as well as diffuse enlargement of the gland. The advantage over ultrasonography is that overlying gas shadows do not obscure the pancreas. In addition, rapid bolus contrast–enhanced CT scan may reveal varying degrees of nonperfused, necrotic pancreas. Patients with necrosis and hemorrhage clearly have a higher risk of morbidity and a greater potential need for surgical intervention. The major disadvantages are cost and availability. Also, it is often undesirable for critically ill patients to be in a CT scanner away from appropriate monitoring equipment and personnel. It is not cost effective for all patients with pancreatitis to undergo CT scanning. However, CT scanning is appropriate for diagnosing acute pancreatitis when other tests are inconclusive, for detecting complications in patients with severe pancreatitis, or as an adjunct to therapeutic procedures such as CT-guided drainage of pseudocysts.

ASSESSMENT OF SEVERITY

Several classification systems have been developed to assess the severity of pancreatitis in order to predict outcome. The most well known are Ranson's criteria. Table 2 lists the 11 criteria, 5 of which are obtained on admission and 6 after 48 hours. Among patients with acute pancreatitis and one to two Ranson risk factors, the estimated mor-

TABLE 2. **Ranson's Criteria**

On Admission	At 48 Hours
WBC > 16,000 cells/mm³	Calcium < 8 mg/dL
Age > 55 y	Third space loss > 6 L
LDH > 350 IU/L	BUN rise > 5 mg/dL
Fasting glucose > 200 mg/dL	HCT fall > 10%
AST > 250 IU/dL	Base deficit > 4 mEq/L
	PaO₂ < 60 mm Hg

Abbreviations: AST = aspartate aminotransferase; BUN = blood urea nitrogen; HCT = hematocrit; LDH = lactate dehydrogenase; PaO₂ = arterial oxygen tension; WBC = white blood cell (count).

tality rate is 1%; among those with three to four risk factors, the mortality rate is 15%; and among those with six or more risk factors, the mortality rate approaches 100%. Other systems such as the modified Glasgow scale (based on the original Ranson factors) and the Apache II scoring system have been developed. Of note, the Glasgow scale and Ranson's criteria require 48 hours to complete and are not useful after 48 hours. Studies have shown that the highest predictor of mortality is the development of multiple organ system failure. In patients with severe acute pancreatitis, renal failure is the most common (10%), followed by cardiovascular and hepatic (8%), pulmonary (6%), and hematologic and neurologic failure (3%). Although all classification systems have varying sensitivity, specificity, and positive and negative predictive values, the most important aspect to monitor is the patient's clinical status. These patients have the potential to be extremely ill and may require aggressive support and monitoring.

MANAGEMENT

Acute pancreatitis can be viewed as analogous to a retroperitoneal burn injury that necessitates close attention to intravascular volume status. Management may be as simple as monitoring urinary output and capillary refill or more invasive, such as placement of central lines for monitoring of central venous pressures, Swan-Ganz catheters, and arterial lines. In addition, the patient should be closely observed for the development of complications such as multiple organ system failure, which occurs in patients with severe or necrotizing pancreatitis. An attempt should also be made to identify the etiology of the pancreatitis, especially treatable factors such as medication-induced pancreatitis and biliary pancreatitis.

Although mild cases of pancreatitis may be managed at home with careful follow-up, many patients demonstrate some degree of dehydration that necessitates admission and intravenous hydration. The rate and type of fluid given should be dictated by the electrolyte abnormalities and the volume status. Urinary output should be closely monitored and kept at 0.5 to 1 mL per kg per hour; this monitoring frequently requires a Foley catheter. Initially, all patients should take nothing by mouth. The use of a nasogastric tube depends on the clinical situation. Although gastric decompression has never been shown to alter the outcome of pancreatitis, it does decrease intestinal dilatation and relieves nausea and vomiting. In mild cases with minimal nausea and vomiting, the discomfort of nasogastric tubes may not warrant their placement. Ileus, however, frequently accompanies pancreatitis and would be an indication for nasogastric decompression. If a nasogastric tube is placed, its output should be strictly monitored and replaced with half-normal saline containing 20 mEq of potassium per liter of intravenous fluid.

Numerous electrolyte abnormalities may be encountered in acute pancreatitis. Hypernatremia from intravascular volume contraction can be treated with isotonic volume replacement and free water if necessary. Persistent emesis leads to hypochloremic, hypokalemic metabolic alkalosis and can be treated with normal saline infusions, as well as exogenous potassium administration. Abnormalities of magnesium and calcium are common and serum levels should be monitored and corrected accordingly. Hyperglycemia is a frequent occurrence secondary to the high catecholamine state and insulin insufficiency. Hyperglycemia should be treated with a combination of volume repletion and exogenous insulin administration.

Narcotic analgesics should be used cautiously to manage the abdominal pain that accompanies acute pancreatitis. Meperidine has been the narcotic of choice, mainly because of the possibility of spasm of the sphincter of Oddi, which may be caused by morphine. Patient-controlled pumps have been used for the purpose of pain control. However, any increase in pain or narcotic use should be viewed with suspicion and prompt a review of the patient's clinical status.

Moderate or severe disease (more than three Ranson criteria) should be managed in the intensive care unit because of the high risk of multiple organ system failure. Renal failure is the most common type of organ failure and is usually related to hypovolemia and shock. Although the azotemia is often prerenal, acute tubular necrosis or cortical damage may occur if the prerenal phase is not treated aggressively.

Respiratory failure is also common in patients with severe acute pancreatitis and is indistinguishable from adult respiratory failure secondary to other causes. Serial blood gas determinations are warranted in critically ill patients; hypoxemia is an ominous sign. Endotracheal intubation with mechanical ventilation and positive end-expiratory pressure (PEEP) may be necessary to maintain oxygenation.

The use of antibiotics to prevent septic complications in acute pancreatitis is debatable. Many studies have concluded that infections of injured pancreatic tissues are a secondary phenomenon and that secondary infections are at least theoretically preventable with antibiotics. However, prophylactic use of antibiotics also carries the theoretical risk of selecting out resistant organisms, and studies have shown that prophylactic antibiotics promote candidal infections. There is some evidence that the use of imipenem/cilastatin (Primaxin) in patients with necrotizing pancreatitis can reduce the rate of infectious complications. Mortality, however, is unaffected.

Review of multiple studies reveals some general guidelines for nutritional support of patients with acute pancreatitis. First, studies have shown that for a variety of disease processes, the average person can go for at least 2 weeks without any organized program of nutrition. The majority of patients with pancreatitis (80 to 90%) have a mild form of the disease (one or two Ranson criteria), have an uncomplicated course, and are expected to resume oral intake in 1 to 2 weeks. Such patients do not benefit from nutritional support. Typically, patients with severe pancreatitis (more than three Ranson criteria) may be expected to have a prolonged period of fasting and therefore benefit from nutritional support. Enteral nutrition through a nasojejunal tube or through a jejunostomy tube placed at surgery is warranted in patients who can tolerate this route of nutrition. For patients with prolonged ileus and abdominal distention, parenteral nutrition would be the preferred route.

Numerous medications have been given to patients with acute pancreatitis in an attempt to decrease the severity of the disease. Calcitonin (Calcimar), H_2 blockers, and atropine all have proved ineffective. Enzyme inhibitors such as aprotinin are under investigation. Somatostatin is an attractive agent because of its potential to inhibit pancreatic exocrine secretion. Some data suggest that it may be of more value if started early in the course of the disease, but large randomized trials are needed in order to clarify the issue.

Many studies have investigated the role of peritoneal lavage in acute pancreatitis. Although most have shown little effect from short-term (<2-day) lavage, one study has shown that longer term (8-day) lavage decreases the frequency of both pancreatic sepsis and death from sepsis. The efficacy of peritoneal lavage may be even more striking with increasing severity of acute pancreatitis (more than five Ranson criteria).

OPERATIVE TREATMENT

Nonoperative treatment is generally successful in non–biliary disease–associated acute pancreatitis. Operation is indicated for confirming diagnosis, for managing biliary disease, for managing complications of pancreatitis, or, in some cases, for continued clinical deterioration (Table 3).

It may be difficult to rule out other pathologic processes that mimic acute pancreatitis, such as per-

TABLE 3. **Indications for Surgery**

Uncertainty of clinical diagnosis
Treatment of biliary tract disease
Treatment of complications
  Infection
  Pseudocyst
  Fistula formation
  Hemorrhage
Continued clinical deterioration

forated viscus, gangrenous bowel, or small bowel obstruction, all of which may be associated with modest elevations in amylase. If the diagnosis is uncertain, laparotomy may be indicated to rule out potentially fatal but surgically correctable conditions. Fortunately, the sensitivity of modern CT has made this indication for laparotomy rare.

Approximately 30% of patients with gallstone pancreatitis suffer another attack in 6 to 8 weeks. Laparoscopic cholecystectomy during the first admission has proved to be safe and cost effective for the treatment of gallstone pancreatitis. The operation is typically performed once the patient has recovered from the acute event and enzymes have normalized or are clearly on the decline. Because in 95% of patients with gallstone pancreatitis the ducts clear without intervention, many surgeons do not routinely perform preoperative ERCP or intraoperative cholangiography if the enzyme levels have normalized. However, if the bilirubin or alkaline phosphatase level remains elevated, an intraoperative cholangiogram would be reasonable. Many surgeons attempt to laparoscopically clear a stone from the common bile duct discovered on cholangiography, with conversion to an open procedure should this attempt fail. Postoperative ERCP with clearance of a common bile duct stone is also an option, depending on the availability and experience of the gastroenterologist.

Infectious complications from acute pancreatitis are serious and potentially life-threatening, occurring in 2 to 5% of patients. These secondary infections include infected pancreatic pseudocysts, pancreatic abscess, and infected pancreatic necrosis. The development of infectious complications should be suspected in patients whose condition fails to improve clinically and in patients with documented bacteremia. An abdominal CT with aspiration of necrotic tissue for Gram's stain and culture is currently the procedure of choice for investigating possible infectious complications. In selected cases with a single, focal fluid collection, CT-guided catheter placement may be appropriate. However, any patient with documented infected pancreatic necrosis or whose condition fails to improve quickly after catheter drainage should undergo operative intervention. Surgical treatment includes débridement of all necrotic tissue as well as adequate drainage. Multiple débridements may be required.

Peripancreatic fluid collections are common and often resolve and reappear in different areas during the course of the acute event. Unless there is clinical deterioration with documented infection, these collections may be monitored, usually by ultrasonography. True pseudocysts require 4 to 6 weeks to form a mature capsule and should be treated if complications develop. Pain, mass effect on adjacent structures, and erosion into vascular structures are common indications for operation. Surgical management consists of internal drainage, usually into the stomach or a loop of intestine. Transgastric endoscopic drainage is becoming a potential option for the treatment of pseudocysts. Percutaneous drainage is most successful when communication with the main pancreatic duct has been ruled out by ERCP.

Life-threatening hemorrhage is an uncommon complication of acute pancreatitis. It is usually related to erosion of the necrotizing process into an adjacent vessel or bleeding into a pseudocyst. A rapidly falling hematocrit with shock may herald a severe hemorrhage, as may bleeding from surgically placed drains. Hemorrhage is best treated with arteriographic embolization. Emergency laparotomy is reserved for patients who cannot undergo embolization.

Fistula formation is a common complication of acute pancreatitis because of its necrotizing nature. Involved structures include the stomach, colon, small intestine, and skin in the case of surgery or percutaneous drainage. Supportive therapy is usually successful; however, persistent fistulas may be treated surgically in appropriate candidates.

Patients whose condition continues to deteriorate in spite of intensive support may be considered for laparotomy. These patients are extremely ill and may be coagulopathic, and thus the rate of operative mortality among them is high. Laparotomy is therefore extremely hazardous and should be undertaken only by surgeons expert in the care of pancreatic diseases. At the time of surgery, extensive necrosis of the pancreas and surrounding tissue is often found; resection of all necrotic tissue is indicated.

CHRONIC PANCREATITIS

method of
JAMES A. MADURA II, M.D.
Rush–Presbyterian–St. Luke's Medical Center and
  Cook County Hospital
Chicago, Illinois

and

RICHARD A. PRINZ, M.D.
Rush–Presbyterian–St. Luke's Medical Center and
  Rush University
Chicago, Illinois

Chronic pancreatitis (CP) is an irreversible, progressive inflammatory disease of the pancreas characterized by pain, progressive loss of exocrine parenchyma, fibrosis, and eventual loss of endocrine function. It is more common in men, and alcohol overconsumption is the main cause in developed countries. In 1988 a consensus conference revised the classification of pancreatitis (Table 1), taking into account abnormal imaging findings noted by computed tomography (CT), ultrasonography, and endoscopic retrograde cholangiopancreatography (ERCP). Admittedly, this Marseille-Rome classification does not always reflect the clinical manifestation or course of CP.

The incidence and prevalence of CP remain difficult to define. Worldwide estimates of its incidence range between 2 and 10 per 100,000 population per year, with a prevalence approaching 30 per 100,000 persons. These numbers appear to be increasing over time, concurrently with increases in alcohol consumption. However, some of the increase has been attributed to changes in disease coding as well as to increased diagnosis as a result of improved and more frequent use of imaging studies.

Among the digestive diseases, CP ranks as the 27th most common diagnosis encountered in the outpatient setting and is listed as the first diagnosis on more than 10 per 100,000 hospital discharges in the United States, according to estimates of the Commission on Professional and Hospital Activities. It is estimated that the prevalence of this disease is as much as threefold higher in black males in comparison to the overall population. Average hospital stay is estimated at 10 days for each admission related to CP. The majority of care is directed toward ameliorating the often disabling pain and acute exacerbations of pancreatitis; however, substantial resources are also spent on treating complications. Over half of all CP patients develop diabetes mellitus, one third of whom will be insulin dependent, and nearly 50% eventually require surgical intervention for pain or complications. Lost time from work and unemployment rates are extremely high. In addition, one quarter of all patients with CP die within 20 years of the diagnosis, a number much higher than in an age-matched healthy population.

Despite these figures, the underlying pathophysiologic process of CP remains elusive. Optimal management continues to rely on supportive treatment of endocrine and exocrine insufficiency and of pain. Surgical intervention is generally reserved for intractable pain and for specific complications such as pseudocysts, biliary or intestinal obstruction, and bleeding from splenic vein obstruction.

ETIOLOGY

The exact mechanism by which chronic pancreatitis develops is not known. It appears to be a multifactorial process involving both genetic predisposition and environmental factors (Table 2).

Alcohol use is by far the number one cause of CP in the

TABLE 1. **Marseille-Rome Classification of Pancreatitis**

Acute pancreatitis
Chronic pancreatitis
Chronic obstructive pancreatitis
Chronic calcifying pancreatitis
Chronic inflammatory pancreatitis
Complications
Diffuse fibrosis

TABLE 2. **Causes of Chronic Pancreatitis**

Alcohol	Toxic substances
Obstruction	Tropical pancreatitis
Pancreas divisum	Hypercalcemia
Congenital strictures	Hyperlipidemia
Acquired strictures	Autoimmune processes
Acute pancreatitis	Idiopathic processes
Trauma	
ERCP	
Neoplasm	
Pancreatic	
Periampullary	

Abbreviation: ERCP = endoscopic retrograde cholangiopancreatography.

western hemisphere, accounting for an estimated 70% of the cases in U.S. and European studies. Direct damage to the acinar cell with increased concentration of protein secretion, decreased production of bicarbonate, and decreased fluid volume has been demonstrated in experimental models and in patients with alcohol-induced CP. This combination appears to result in protein and calcium precipitation, ductal obstruction, activation of pancreatic enzymes, and autodigestion of the gland. The end result is patchy inflammatory lesions with intraductal protein plug formation, which progresses to calcification and stone formation. Over time, a fibrotic response to the inflammatory insult results in permanent ductal abnormalities, an irreversible component to the vicious cycle of autodestruction. The average age at diagnosis is 35 to 45 years, with an estimated 11- to 18-year history of alcohol consumption of approximately 150 to 175 grams per day.

Only about 10% of patients with chronic alcoholism develop CP, which is approximately the same percentage of those who develop hepatic cirrhosis. Nutritional factors may be involved. Diets high in fat and protein in the alcoholic population are associated with an increased incidence of CP. Several hypotheses have been proposed to explain the variable prevalence of CP in alcoholic patients. There are data to indicate the presence of a pancreatic stone protein (PSP), also known as lithostatin, which is thought to be an acinar cell product that acts to prevent precipitation of calcium salts. This theory is supported by evidence of decreased concentrations of PSP and decreased levels of PSP messenger RNA in the pancreatic juice and acini of patients with chronic calcific pancreatitis, regardless of origin (alcoholic, hereditary, tropical, and idiopathic). A second theory suggests that fatty degeneration of pancreatic cells with loss of zymogen content and periacinar fibrosis results from overstimulation of acinar cells and subsequent derangement of intracellular transport of secretory proteins. This may be the result of alcohol-induced toxic metabolites of lipid metabolism. A third hypothesis suggests that alcohol-induced disordered hepatic detoxification is the initiator of alcohol-induced CP. In this theory, oxygen free radicals and reactive intermediates produced in the liver during the process of ethanol detoxification are excreted into bile and cause damage to the pancreas when bile is regurgitated into the pancreatic ductal system. None of the theories accounts for all manifestations of CP. The range of experimentally identified abnormalities verifies the multifactorial nature of the disease.

A form of calcific pancreatitis that closely resembles chronic alcoholic pancreatitis is termed "tropical pancreatitis," because it occurs almost exclusively in equatorial countries. The clinical course of disease and histologic appearances are nearly identical to those of alcoholic CP except for the absence of a history of alcohol ingestion. Although it was once thought to be the result of protein malnutrition, more recent observations suggest that other dietary factors, such as cyanogens found in cassava root, may be responsible. It has been suggested that malnutrition, especially of trace elements, may impair the detoxification of dietary factors implicated in tropical pancreatitis.

Obstructive pancreatitis results from both congenital and acquired ductal obstruction, as in pancreas divisum, congenital and acquired strictures, and neoplasia. Unlike alcoholic pancreatitis, the obstructed pancreas shows uniform inflammatory changes with preserved ductal epithelium and rare protein plugs that do not tend to progress to calcification and stone formation. The hypothesis that high intraductal and intraparenchymal pressure results in CP

has been proposed partly on the basis of the finding of elevated pressures in this group of patients.

Additional causes of CP include hypercalcemia and hyperlipidemia, and there are autoimmune and hereditary forms of the disease. The mechanism by which CP develops in these situations is unclear. An additional 10 to 20% of patients have no clear predisposing condition to explain the development of CP.

DIAGNOSIS

The diagnosis of CP is often based on only a history of typical pain. Prior evidence of acute pancreatitis, a history of excessive alcohol use, and the presence of exocrine and endocrine insufficiency are frequently apparent when the patient seeks medical attention. Pancreatic calcification, diabetes mellitus, and steatorrhea constitute the classic triad of chronic pancreatitis, but all three occur in less than 25% of patients. Radiologic evidence of pancreatic calcification is pathognomonic in the 30 to 50% of patients in which it is present. Endocrine insufficiency in the form of diabetes mellitus is a sign of late disease, but even at initial diagnosis, two thirds of patients produce an abnormal result of a glucose tolerance test. Steatorrhea is commonly present and of multifactorial origin. Weight loss is common, occurring in three fourths of patients, and results from a voluntary decrease in food intake as a result of pain or steatorrhea, malabsorption, social issues, and dietary issues.

On the other hand, pain is present in more than 75% of patients. In the early stages of CP, the pain is characterized by recurrent acute attacks. The pain tends to become persistent later in the disease course. Variable periods of remission and even "burnout" (spontaneous remission of pain in advanced disease) complicate the reliability of pain as an objective measure of disease progression and success of treatment. The cause of pain in CP is uncertain. Table 3 lists some of the proposed factors. Ductal hypertension has been demonstrated in patients with painful CP and dilated ducts (average of 25 mm Hg, in contrast to 7 mm Hg in normal patients). However, not all patients with pain have dilated ducts, and not all patients with dilated ducts have pain. The most recent hypothesis to explain the pain of CP involves damage to local sensory nerves with subsequent exposure to irritants such as histamine, prostaglandins, and pancreatic enzymes. Pancreatic parenchymal hypoxia has been observed in experimental models of CP and is postulated to be another possible cause of pain.

Laboratory Evaluation

Laboratory evaluation for diagnosing CP is of limited value. Pancreatic enzyme (amylase, lipase) levels may be elevated in acute exacerbations but are not a measure of chronic disease, pancreatic function, or pancreatic reserve and do not correlate with symptoms. Functional studies are cumbersome and rarely necessary for diagnosing CP. However, stimulated pancreatic secretions collected from the duodenum (amylase, lipase, trypsin, chymotrypsin, and bicarbonate), urine (nitroblue tetrazolium–p-aminobenzoic

TABLE 3. **Proposed Factors Producing Pain in Chronic Pancreatitis**

Ductal hypertension	Parenchymal ischemia
Autodigestion	Perineural inflammation

acid [NBT-PABA] test and pancreolauryl test), or serum (P-isoamylase and trypsin) provide reliable estimates of pancreatic functional reserve and should be pursued in centers with such capabilities in which it is desirable to quantitate the results of treatment strategies in this patient population. Serum liver enzyme levels and leukocyte counts may delineate important information regarding the etiology, concomitant disease, or complications.

Imaging

Imaging of the pancreas is currently done most often by CT. Plain abdominal radiographs reveal pancreatic calcifications in less than 50% of patients and are otherwise nonspecific for pancreatic disease. Transabdominal ultrasonography of the pancreas has nearly 70% sensitivity in diagnosing CP. Skilled ultrasonographers can determine important information regarding the size and consistency of the gland, characteristics of the biliary tree, and the presence of peripancreatic complications. Ultrasonography can be considered an initial imaging study for patients suspected of having CP, because of the relatively low cost, ease of performance, and lack of radiation exposure with this modality. However, CT has proven 90% sensitivity and nearly 100% specificity in the evaluation of CP and should be considered in all suspected CP patients to help classify their disease and determine the possible presence of complications or surgically correctable lesions. CT may be the only imaging study required before surgical intervention. If CT is to be obtained, transabdominal ultrasonography is usually unnecessary.

ERCP is not mandatory but may provide important information regarding ductal anatomy in patients in whom surgical treatment is considered and in whom CT has not adequately demonstrated pancreatic ductal anatomy. Sensitivity and specificity for diagnosing CP approach 90% and 100%, respectively, but the ductal abnormalities can correlate poorly with pain and gland function. The small but persistent incidence of major complications related to ERCP should limit its use in CP patients to those who require anatomic definition for surgery and to those who are suspected of harboring ampullary or ductal obstruction amenable to ERCP treatment alone.

Magnetic resonance imaging (MRI) and magnetic resonance cholangiopancreatography (MRCP) are rapidly evolving and may eventually replace both CT and ERCP. These modalities provide definition of both soft tissue and ductal anatomy. Likewise, endoscopic and intraoperative ultrasonography are becoming more readily available and may have a role in the evaluation of patients with CP in whom surgical intervention is proposed.

TREATMENT

Medical

Treatment of CP consists primarily of supportive care. Relief of pain is often the primary concern of patients, but long-term management of endocrine and exocrine insufficiency is of equal importance.

Pain

The pain of pancreatitis may occur with only acute episodes early in the course of disease but often becomes more intense, persistent, and difficult to manage over time. A number of objective pain grading systems have been developed, and one system should be adopted and applied often when medication is prescribed for patients with CP. This will gauge the success of treatment and, to a limited extent, the progression of disease. Abstinence from alcohol consumption has correlated with improved pain relief, and continued alcohol consumption is an important predictor of recurrent pain even after surgical intervention. Of patients who were monitored after lateral pancreaticojejunostomy (LPJ), those who quit drinking alcohol had a 78% incidence of long-term pain relief; in contrast, only 43% of those who continued to drink alcohol sustained relief from pain. Abstinence is more likely to benefit patients with early disease but is poorly correlated with pain relief in advanced disease. Although there is no evidence that the progressive nature of CP is reversed by abstinence, patients should be strongly encouraged to avoid the use of alcohol early in the disease, in order to preserve as much glandular function for as long a time as possible.

There is some evidence that oral pancreatic enzyme supplementation provides pain relief. The mechanism of action is thought to be feedback inhibition of postprandial cholecystokinin release with a subsequent reduction in pancreatic stimulation. However, not all studies have shown the same promising results. One such study demonstrated no benefit in pain relief after 3 days of oral enzyme supplementation, whereas significant improvement in pain was noted after 7 days of supplementation in another study. Along the same lines, somatostatin* (Zecnil) is currently being evaluated for its role in relieving pain through the proposed mechanism of decreasing pancreatic activity.

Opiate addiction becomes more and more common in proportion to the duration of disease. Therefore, nonsteroidal anti-inflammatory drugs (NSAIDs) should be the mainstay of pain management; narcotics should be reserved for acute exacerbations and intractable disease. Once patients become addicted to narcotics, they are less likely to admit to being pain free for fear of discontinuation of their medication. Some authorities propose that surgical intervention should be considered before the chronic administration of narcotics for pain management.

Percutaneous nerve blocks with anesthetics and ethanol have been used with limited success and limited duration of pain relief. Less than half of the patients treated with percutaneous celiac plexus injection of 25% alcohol experienced pain relief with a mean duration of 2 months. Increased concentrations of alcohol have been used with marginally improved results. Side effects, including orthostatic hypotension, intercostal neuritis, and problems with ejaculation, can be severe. These complications are usually concentration dependent. Nerve blocks therefore have a limited role in the treatment of CP. Epidural and intrathecal continuous anesthetic techniques have shown some utility in patients who are incapacitated and for whom there are no alternatives.

---

*Not FDA approved for this indication.

A phenomenon of spontaneous remission of pain in advanced disease, "burned-out" pancreatitis, is well documented but an unreliable occurrence. It is thought to occur when secretory function is lost.

Exocrine Insufficiency

Steatorrhea is a common and troublesome problem in CP. It is, however, a complex problem, not purely the result of pancreatic exocrine insufficiency. Complete digestion of fat depends not only on adequate secretion of lipase from the pancreas but also on initial hydrolysis of lipids in the stomach by gastric and salivary lipases, adequate alkalinization of the duodenum from pancreatic bicarbonate secretion, and appropriate duodenal bile acid concentration. All of these factors may be diminished in alcoholic patients. The end result is incomplete lipolysis with decreased mucosal absorption of lipids. It has been estimated that pancreatic enzyme deficiency sufficient to produce protein malabsorption does not occur until 90% of the acinar mass is lost. However, enzyme supplementation may be necessary much earlier to treat the often disabling steatorrhea.

Early enzyme replacement agents consisted of crude porcine pancreatic extracts that lost nearly 90% of their activity as a result of gastric acidity. Currently, porcine extracts are encapsulated in enteric-coated tablets or microspheres, which markedly improve delivery of active enzymes to the duodenal lumen. Patients are instructed to start with two tablets or capsules with meals and increase the dose until diarrhea is controlled. Complete pancreatic insufficiency may necessitate 30 to 50 tablets per day. Large doses can be complicated by hyperuricemia, which results from the high purine content in the extracts. Pharmacologic intervention to decrease gastric acid secretion may also be necessary to raise duodenal pH, thereby achieving an adequate environment for enzyme activation.

Malnutrition

Weight loss, muscle wasting, and vitamin deficiencies are common in CP. Inadequate nutritional intake is the result of a number of factors, including fear of food-induced pain or diarrhea that follows meals, poor dietary habits, and metabolic problems in the alcoholic population. Every effort should be made to perform an adequate and regular nutritional assessment with professional dietary involvement. Special attention should be directed to providing a low-fat diet with adequate protein and calorie intake and vitamin supplementation. The presence of diabetes can make this task difficult but not impossible. Parenteral nutrition is rarely required in CP, but food-induced acute exacerbations and need for perioperative nutritional support may warrant its use.

Endocrine Insufficiency

Diabetes of chronic pancreatitis is not unlike other forms of type II diabetes in that it may be controlled by diet, oral hypoglycemic drugs, or insulin injections. In its extreme, it can be quite unpredictable

TABLE 4. **Indications for Surgery in Chronic Pancreatitis**

Pain refractory to medical management
Inability to exclude pancreatic malignancy
Complications
    Pseudocyst
    Biliary obstruction
    Duodenal obstruction
    Splenic vein thrombosis
    Pancreatic fistula
    Colonic obstruction
    Pancreatic ascites

and difficult to control. In general, lower insulin doses are required; hypoglycemia is more of a threat than ketoacidosis. This is the result of low levels of endogenous insulin, a low incidence of insulin resistance, and diminished glucagon secretion resulting in increased insulin sensitivity.

Surgical

Surgical intervention for CP is most commonly performed for intractable pain that is not responsive to medical management. Either inability to control pain without the use of narcotic medications or the occurrence of multiple relapses of pain should prompt surgical evaluation. At this stage of disease, the probability of benefit from surgery is greatest. Indications for surgical intervention are listed in Table 4. The ideal operation for CP would ameliorate the pain, correct and prevent complications, carry low operative mortality and morbidity risks, and stop the progression of disease. Unfortunately, no such operation exists. However, surgical procedures performed in properly selected patients result in marked alleviation of pain and improvement in quality of life (Table 5).

There is no evidence that surgery is able to improve pancreatic function, as was hoped by the pioneers of ductal drainage procedures. However, surgical decompression of the pancreatic duct can slow the progression of disease. In a series of 143 patients

TABLE 5. **Surgical Procedures for Chronic Pancreatitis**

Nerve interruption
Sphincterotomy/sphincteroplasty
Pancreatic drainage
    Lateral pancreaticojejunostomy (LPJ, or Puestow's)
    Local resection plus LPJ (LR-LPJ, or Frey's)
Pancreatic resection
    Distal pancreatectomy
    Pancreaticoduodenectomy (Whipple's, pylorus-preserving
      Whipple's)
    Local resection of pancreatic head (Beger's)
    Subtotal/total pancreatectomy
    Total pancreatectomy with islet cell autotransplantation
Complications
    Pseudocyst drainage
    Intestinal bypass

with mild to moderate pancreatitis reported by Nealon and coworkers in 1993, only 13% deteriorated to severe pancreatitis after LPJ, in comparison with 78% of those who did not undergo operative decompression. These patients were serially evaluated with ERCP, oral glucose tolerance testing, and measures of exocrine function to grade the severity of disease.

Improvement in perioperative care and surgical technique has enabled routine performance of surgical procedures on the pancreas with very low mortality and complication rates. Most contemporary series of operations for CP report perioperative mortality rates less than 3%. Late deaths average 16% at 5 years but are most frequently related to alcohol, accidents, suicide, and recurrent pancreatitis. Other series report the incidence of late deaths as more than 50% at longer follow-up, with cardiac disease, cirrhosis, cancer, and pulmonary disease the predominating causes. Complication statistics are more difficult to evaluate because of differences in reporting, follow-up, procedure performed, and progression of disease. In general, LPJ and pancreaticoduodenectomy (Whipple's) procedures carry less than a 20% rate of operative complications, including those specific to the pancreatic operation (fistula, pseudocyst, infection, sepsis), and morbidity related to any general anesthetic procedure (pulmonary, cardiac, genitourinary). This rate is comparable with that for other major intra-abdominal operations. Long-term endocrine function and exocrine function are universally reported as worse, regardless of the operation performed, but this outcome probably represents progression of the underlying disease. Early postoperative exocrine insufficiency is related to the extent of gland resected and has been reported to transiently improve after duct drainage procedures. Near total and complete resections carry significantly higher complication rates, from nearly 70 to 80%, and similar long-term rates of pancreatic insufficiency.

Patient Evaluation

Before undergoing an operation for CP, all patients should have a thorough evaluation to define the morphology of the gland and the pancreatic duct and to identify complications. A CT scan is usually sufficient for this evaluation. If ERCP is necessary, endoscopically placed stents should be discouraged before surgical intervention, because of the increased incidence of postoperative complications associated with their use.

Patients must be assessed for their ability to tolerate a major abdominal operation. Because of the association with alcohol, careful attention should be directed toward evaluation of hepatic function, in addition to the pulmonary and cardiovascular systems. Many patients with CP suffer from malnutrition and may benefit from preoperative efforts to improve nutritional status. In addition, psychologic factors must be taken into consideration. The hurdles of major surgery are demanding, but the potential long-term sequelae of CP and pancreatic insufficiency with or without surgery can be even more of

a challenge. Many patients have underlying psychosocial problems that contribute to their alcoholism and may render them unable to deal with the physical and emotional issues involved.

Operative Selection

Once patients are deemed operative candidates, decisions must be made regarding which operation to perform. A brief summary of procedures is presented in Table 6. The approach to pseudocysts, fistulas, and intestinal obstruction secondary to CP is relatively straightforward in the majority of patients. Similarly, when a neoplasm cannot be ruled out, adequate resection according to oncologic principles should be performed.

Unfortunately, no operation is uniformly successful in relieving pain. The best results in these patients are obtained when procedures are individualized according to pancreatic gland and duct morphology.

Pancreatic Duct Drainage

Lateral pancreaticojejunostomy (LPJ, or Puestow's) is the procedure of choice for patients with intractable abdominal or back pain related to CP who have dilated pancreatic ducts. The absolute degree of dilatation is a matter of debate. Historically, 8-mm dilatation was considered to be the required minimum. However, patients with dilatation of less than 8 mm have benefited from LPJ in several series, prompting many surgeons to perform the operation in patients with duct dilatation of 5 mm or more. Results have consistently demonstrated long-term pain relief in 80% of patients.

Concomitant procedures to address other complications, such as pseudocysts or biliary or intestinal obstruction, can be employed at the time of LPJ. Pseudocyst treatment can be incorporated into the ductotomy and jejunal anastomosis or by anastomo-

TABLE 6. **Selection of Operation for Chronic Pancreatitis**

Clinical Findings	Appropriate Procedure
Disease limited to tail of gland	Distal pancreatectomy
Masslike obstruction in head of gland	
Dilated duct	LPJ, LR-LPJ
Nondilated duct	Whipple's, PPW, DPPHR
No masslike obstruction in head of gland	
Dilated duct	LPJ
Nondilated duct	Whipple's or DPPHR (?)
Unable to tolerate major operation	Neurolysis (?)
Failure of primary drainage/resection	Neurolysis, subtotal resection, total resection (+ islet cell autotransplantation)
Inability to rule out malignancy in head of gland	Whipple's, PPW

Abbreviations: DPPHR = duodenum-preserving pancreatic head resection; LPJ = lateral pancreaticojejunostomy; LR-LPJ = local resection of the pancreatic head combined with LPJ; PPW = pylorus-preserving modification of Whipple's procedure.

sis to a separate area of the jejunal limb. Biliary obstruction can also be remedied during the same operation by performing a choledochoduodenostomy or bile duct anastomosis to the jejunal limb. Duodenal obstruction is easily treated with the addition of a gastrojejunostomy.

On the basis of the concept that the head of the pancreas may not be completely drained even with an adequate LPJ, the Frey procedure was developed. This procedure entails a "coring out," or local resection of the pancreatic head combined with LPJ (LR-LPJ). Results have been promising; only about 13% of patients report no relief of pain at 37 months of follow-up. Rates of complications, including pancreatic insufficiency, have been comparable with those of LPJ alone. Another proposed mechanism for the success of this operation in relieving pain may be related to the removal of damaged sensory nerves in the head of the gland.

Pancreatic Resection

Resections for CP are performed for pain, for complications of the disease, and as salvage procedures for patients who continue to experience pain after drainage procedures. Partial resections of either the head or tail of the gland address localized disease, whereas nearly complete and total resections, because of the attendant risk of morbidity, should be reserved for failure of a more conservative operation.

Disease limited to the tail of the pancreas most commonly occurs from obstruction of the main pancreatic duct in the midportion of the gland. Congenital strictures can account for this manifestation, but strictures are more often related to trauma from injury, instrumentation, and episodes of pancreatitis. When normal drainage of the proximal gland into the duodenum is preserved, resection of the diseased distal portion of the gland should be adequate. The Child procedure is an 80 to 95% distal pancreatectomy that can be performed for pain in CP with nondilated ducts. All but a small rim of pancreas adjacent to the duodenum that preserves the common blood supply is resected. Pain relief is expected in 80% of patients, but exocrine insufficiency and diabetes complicate the outcome, with more than a 70% incidence in some series. Equivalent results regarding pain relief and lesser morbidity after other operations has made more than 80% distal pancreatectomy obsolete as a first-choice operation for pain of CP.

Often most of the obstructive disease and a mass-like effect may be noted in the head of the gland. When this is not amenable to drainage, pancreatic head resection should be considered. Pancreaticoduodenectomy (Whipple's procedure) is the gold standard operation for comparison because it addresses both issues of ductal obstruction and local nerve irritation as the etiology of pain. The pylorus-preserving modification of Whipple's operation has ameliorated some of the long-term sequelae of the operation, notably dumping syndrome and marginal ulceration. However, the inflammatory nature of CP may make the operation difficult and even hazardous. Duodenum-preserving pancreatic head resection (Beger's procedure) and LR-LPJ have been shown to have equivalent long-term pain relief in series comparing patients who have undergone these procedures with those who have undergone traditional Whipple's operations; thus these alternatives are attractive. Devascularization of the duodenum with subsequent necrosis or stricture formation has been a limiting concern in the widespread use of Beger's procedure. Patients with substantial disease in the head of the gland and concomitant duodenal and biliary obstruction are ideal candidates for pancreaticoduodenectomy.

Because the apancreatic state after total pancreatectomy produces undue morbidity, this procedure should not be used as a first approach to pancreatic pain. Up to 20% of patients continue to have abdominal pain after total pancreatectomy. Even as a salvage procedure in patients who continue to have pain after less radical operations, it should be used rarely because of its effects on quality of life. Attempts at islet cell autotransplantation have resulted in preservation of some endocrine function in patients undergoing total pancreatectomy. The islet cells are harvested from the resected specimen and injected into the portal system, where they are deposited in the hepatic reticuloendothelial tissue in a functional state. Although initial reports of endocrine function have been promising, it appears that the effect is shortlived. Autotransplantation of a vascularized segment of the gland has also been attempted with limited success.

Sphincterotomy/Sphincteroplasty/ERCP Stenting

In the past, sphincterotomy and sphincteroplasty were performed for CP to relieve ductal obstruction at the level of the ampulla. Initial results revealed amelioration of pain, but this was shortlived and correlated with alcohol abstinence. Although these procedures are indicated for acute, recurrent bouts of pancreatitis in patients with pancreas divisum, no benefit has been obtained when performed in the presence of established CP caused by pancreas divisum. From this information, it is expected that endoscopic sphincterotomy and pancreatic duct stenting have little effect on the long-term management of CP. Trials comparing endoscopic pancreatic duct stenting to surgical pancreatic duct drainage have demonstrated superior long-term results in favor of surgery.

Nerve Ablation

On the basis of the theory that the pain of CP is related to inflammatory involvement of the splanchnic nerves, several approaches to surgical splanchnicectomy have been attempted, including extraperitoneal, intraperitoneal, thoracic, and thoracoscopic techniques. In addition, complete denervation procedures and combined splanchnicectomy and truncal vagotomy have been tried for treating the pain of CP. Results have been unpredictable, often unconfirmed, and limited in follow-up. The technical challenges of performing the procedures can be quite demanding in the presence of the chronically inflamed anatomy. Therefore, neurotomy is rarely considered at the present time but may be an option for patients who have not obtained relief of pain after surgical drainage or resective procedures.

GASTROESOPHAGEAL REFLUX DISEASE

method of
PHILIP O. KATZ, M.D., and
DONALD O. CASTELL, M.D.
Graduate Hospital
Philadelphia, Pennsylvania

Gastroesophageal reflux disease (GERD) is perhaps the most common problem seen in medical practice. Five to 10% of the U.S. population have heartburn daily and 40% at least monthly. Underscoring the frequency of GERD is the finding that almost 40 million people use over-the-counter antacids or H_2-receptor antagonists (H_2RAs) at least twice a week. Effective treatment mandates an awareness of the spectrum of GERD, its varied symptom manifestations and potential complications, an understanding of the pathophysiology of the disease, and an awareness of the multiple treatment options.

CLINICAL MANIFESTATION AND NATURAL HISTORY

Heartburn (substernal burning sensation after meals or upon bending over) is the most common symptom. Regurgitation, the spontaneous return of gastric contents into the esophagus or mouth, is the other frequent symptom. A patient with both heartburn and regurgitation is almost certain to have GERD and may be treated without any diagnostic testing. Heartburn is exacerbated by large meals, spicy foods, citrus products, and meals high in fat. Colas, coffee, teas, and beer have an acidic pH and may produce symptoms. Late-night meals, eaten before bedtime or taken with alcohol, make patients more prone to nighttime symptoms.

Neither the presence nor the frequency of heartburn is predictive of the degree of esophageal damage. Only about 50% of patients with heartburn who see a physician are found to have esophagitis when endoscopy is performed. Severe disease, including Barrett's esophagus and peptic strictures, may manifest with infrequent or no complaints of heartburn, whereas many patients with daily heartburn may have no endoscopic abnormalities.

Many atypical or extraesophageal symptoms are associated with GERD, including unexplained substernal chest pain without evidence of coronary artery disease (noncardiac chest pain), asthma, bronchitis, chronic cough, recurrent pneumonia, hoarseness, chronic posterior laryngitis, otalgia, aphthous ulcers, hiccups, and erosion of dental enamel. The frequency of these atypical or extraesophageal symptoms and their prevalence in the general population have not been studied as extensively as heartburn. One large survey of patients who had atypical heartburn or regurgitation found that at some point in a year, unex-plained chest pain was present in 23%, asthma in 9%, bronchitis in 20%, and chronic hoarseness in 15%.

On the other hand, the frequency of heartburn and regurgitation in patients who seek medical attention for these atypical symptoms is debated, but they may be absent in up to 50%. The clinician is cautioned that the absence of heartburn and regurgitation does not preclude a diagnosis of GERD in patients with atypical symptoms.

COMPLICATIONS AND NATURAL HISTORY

GERD may manifest with peptic stricture, ulceration, iron deficiency anemia, or Barrett's esophagus (which involves a change of the esophageal mucosa from normal squamous epithelial lining to a metaplastic intestinal type of epithelium with specific staining characteristics—a premalignant condition). Prevalence estimates range from 2 to 10% for stricture and 10 to 15% for Barrett's metaplasia. The presence of dysphagia, odynophagia (painful swallowing), early satiety, vomiting, or bleeding suggests complicated GERD and mandates early diagnostic intervention to search for a more serious condition.

Eighty percent of patients with reflux esophagitis have endoscopic and symptomatic relapse, in which symptoms are present 80% of the time, if therapy is discontinued or drug dosage is decreased. This observation has led to the clinical impression that GERD is a chronic condition. Most patients, especially those with erosive esophagitis or extraesophageal disease, require continuous medical therapy or surgery to achieve adequate symptom relief.

PATHOPHYSIOLOGY

Many factors can contribute to GERD; however, the primary underlying cause is abnormal motility. Reflux is usually prevented by a competent lower esophageal sphincter (LES), aided by the crural diaphragm. Some patients may have low resting LES pressures or reduced LES pressures during periods of increased intra-abdominal pressure; however, the most common abnormality is an increased frequency of transient relaxations of the LES.

Refluxed acid is normally rapidly cleared from the esophagus. Gravity and neutralization of acid by salivary bicarbonate help esophageal acid clearance. Delay in esophageal acid clearance may be caused by a reduction in the frequency or strength of peristaltic contractions. Patients with a hiatal hernia may develop GERD because of the loss of the contribution of the crural diaphragm to the antireflux barrier and because of ineffective clearing of acid trapped in the distal esophagus.

Delayed gastric emptying also may contribute to GERD. The composition of the refluxate (acid, pepsin, and bile) determines the severity of disease. The role of epithelial defense mechanisms in the esophagus is important; up to 50% of patients with nonerosive GERD and a smaller proportion of those with erosive disease have acid exposure times comparable with those of healthy persons and nonetheless have symptoms.

DIAGNOSTIC EVALUATION

When a patient with suspected GERD also has dysphagia, odynophagia, weight loss, bleeding, or anemia or has atypical GERD symptoms, early diagnostic evaluation is appropriate. Diagnostic evaluation is also warranted when GERD symptoms persist after a course of empirical treatment or when long-term daily proton pump inhibitors are needed. For patients who require long-term daily medical therapy, endoscopic examination should be considered in order to confirm or rule out Barrett's metaplasia.

On referral, patients are evaluated most often by endoscopy. At least half of patients with heartburn are found to have either normal endoscopic findings or mild to moderate esophagitis. In patients with symptoms who have negative endoscopic findings, some centers perform ambulatory pH monitoring to confirm the presence of abnormal gastroesophageal reflux. When endoscopy suggests a non-GERD diagnosis, such as cancer or peptic ulcer disease, further diagnostic testing and appropriate treatment are the next steps.

TREATMENT

Patient Education and Lifestyle Modification

Educating patients about the role of lifestyles in GERD is a key component of therapy. Simple changes in lifestyle and diet can help control heartburn and dyspepsia. We routinely instruct patients to lower daily fat intake, to eat small meals, not to eat within 3 hours before bedtime, to avoid lying down after meals, to stop smoking, and to elevate the head of the bed 6 inches, a maneuver that decreases esophageal acid exposure. An alternative measure is to place a foam rubber wedge (maximal elevation, 10 inches high) under the patient's head on top of the mattress. There is evidence that sleeping supine or on the left side results in less frequent reflux than does sleeping on the right side down or prone position. Esophageal irritants such as citrus juices, tomato products, coffee, colas, and alcohol should be reduced. Medications that decrease esophageal pressures and promote reflux—including anticholinergics, sedatives or tranquilizers (particularly benzodiazepines), tricyclic antidepressants, theophylline, prostaglandins, and calcium channel–blocking agents—should be avoided. In addition, gelatin capsules, potassium tablets, nonsteroidal anti-inflammatory drugs (NSAIDs), and alendronate (Fosamax) should be restricted because they may increase or cause injury. The intermittent use of antacids, alginic acid, or over-the-counter doses of H₂RAs are useful for symptom relief. Over-the-counter H₂RAs offer the advantage of prophylactic use before situations known to produce GERD symptoms.

Prescription H₂-Receptor Antagonists

The mainstays of therapy for patients with heartburn and dyspepsia have been the H₂RAs. Standard dosages of H₂RAs (equivalent of ranitidine [Zantac], 150 mg twice daily) can be expected to produce symptomatic relief in about 60% of patients and endoscopic resolution of documented esophagitis in about 50% after 8 to 12 weeks of therapy. In addition, lower doses are effective in symptom relief or prevention, thus supporting the over-the-counter availability of half-strength H₂RAs. Higher dose H₂RAs (ranitidine, 150 mg four times a day or equivalent) increase healing rates to 75% after a similar time period. The

current cost of this increased dosage, coupled with compliance issues, make this choice less efficacious than that of the proton pump inhibitors, which provide greater efficacy with once-a-day therapy.

Role of Promotility Agents

Therapy directed at correction of the motility abnormalities outlined earlier theoretically allows amelioration of GERD symptoms without suppression of gastric acid. Metoclopramide (Reglan) and cisapride (Propulsid) are two promotility agents currently available. Cisapride, the most commonly prescribed promotility agent, increases gastrointestinal motility, enhances buffering capacity and salivary flow, and has largely replaced metoclopramide because of the side effect profile. Daytime and nocturnal heartburn are alleviated with cisapride, 10 mg four times a day or 20 mg twice a day (bid). Symptoms suggestive of dysmotility, including postprandial bloating, feeling of fullness, early satiety, belching, and regurgitation, also are reduced with cisapride. Cisapride and H₂RAs produce comparable symptom relief and healing in patients with mild to moderate esophagitis. Cisapride in combination with cimetidine (Tagamet) or ranitidine enhances healing and symptom relief in comparison with H₂RA alone; however, cost and side effects in comparison with those of proton pump inhibitors discourage the use of this regimen. Cisapride, 10 mg bid or 20 mg at bedtime, is effective in preventing symptom relapse, particularly in patients with mild esophagitis. There is evidence that both H₂RAs and cisapride can provide long-term control of GERD in up to 50% of patients, especially in patients with less severe degrees of esophagitis.

The central nervous system side effects of metoclopramide (drowsiness, irritability, and extrapyramidal effects) make its use problematic, particularly in older people. Because cisapride does not cross the blood-brain barrier, these side effects are not seen, and so it has largely replaced metoclopramide as the motility agent of choice. The major side effects of cisapride are diarrhea (in about 10% of patients) and nausea. Prolongation of the QT interval and development of ventricular arrhythmias may be seen in rare instances in patients taking cisapride who are concomitantly treated with other drugs that are metabolized by a similar P-450 oxidase enzyme, including macrolide antibiotics (e.g., erythromycin) or antifungal agents. Use of these drugs in combination should be avoided.

Proton Pump Inhibitors

Proton pump inhibitors are the most effective medical therapy for controlling symptoms of GERD and healing esophagitis. Omeprazole (Prilosec), 20 mg daily, or lansoprazole (Prevacid), 30 mg daily, is more effective than either placebo or standard-dose H₂RA, producing symptomatic relief in more than 80% of patients and healing of esophagitis in more than 90% after 8 weeks of treatment. Omeprazole, 20 mg, and lansoprazole, 30 mg, have been shown to have equal healing rates. In patients with grades III and IV (severe) esophagitis, the healing rate is somewhat lower, often leading to the need for higher dosages. Some patients continue to secrete gastric acid and have gastroesophageal reflux even at doses as high as 20 mg bid of omeprazole or 30 mg bid of lansoprazole.

Continuous therapy with omeprazole, 20 to 60 mg per day, has been shown to maintain healing of esophagitis for up to 5 years. These observations emphasize the need for larger doses of proton pump inhibitors in some patients for effective long-term maintenance. Moreover, the potential to achieve effective long-term maintenance with appropriate doses of medical therapy in up to 100% of patients with GERD is supported by these observations. More recently, this observation has been extended to up to 11 years for continuous omeprazole, which has shown continued efficacy and safety. Proton pump inhibitors should be given 15 to 30 minutes before a meal (e.g., breakfast) for maximal efficacy.

The awareness of the need for higher doses of proton pump inhibitors in some patients has increased the use of combined intragastric and esopha-geal pH monitoring to evaluate the adequacy of acid suppression and control of reflux in patients with continued symptoms or those in whom profound acid suppression is desired (such as those with Barrett's esophagus). It is now recognized that this technique can be used to monitor the level of proton pump inhibitor therapy required for each patient and has redefined medical failure. This is important in the patient who fails to respond to treatment because of the high frequency of overnight recovery of acid secretion and accompanying reflux, which may not cause symptoms during sleep.

Proton pump inhibitors are remarkably safe. Few side effects, principally headache and gastrointestinal upset, are seen. Concern has been raised about the long-term safety profile of proton pump inhibitors, particularly for gastric malignancy. There is no evidence of development of gastric malignancy despite 11 years of continuous use. No long-term laboratory monitoring is currently recommended.

Antireflux Surgery

The use of laparoscopic approaches has changed the approach to antireflux surgery. Success rates ap-

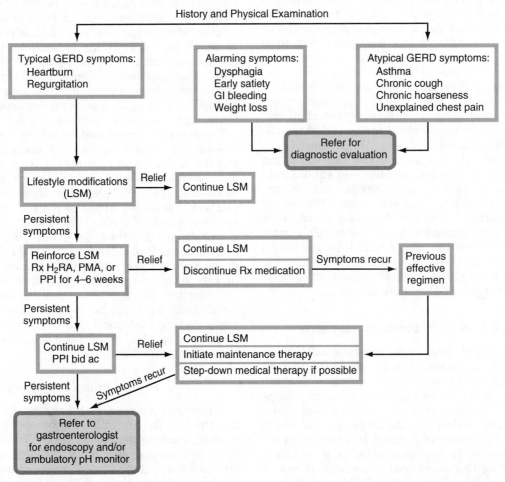

Figure 1. Algorithm for heartburn/gastroesophageal reflux disease (GERD) in adults: primary care approach. *Abbreviations*: ac = before meals; bid = twice a day; H₂RA = histamine H₂–receptor antagonist; LSM = lifestyle modifications, including over-the-counter antacid, alginic acid, or H₂RA; PMA = promotility agent; PPI = proton pump inhibitor.

proaching 90% after 3 years with minimal complications make fundoplication an attractive option for some patients. The use of a short, loose, "floppy" fundoplication has reduced the postoperative sequelae associated with antireflux surgery, including dysphagia and "gas bloat." Long-term dysphagia is less common (3 to 5%) after laparoscopic fundoplication. These benefits have been achieved without sacrificing the success in controlling reflux.

The indications for surgery in patients with GERD are controversial. The high success of medical therapy suggests that true medical failure is rare and in itself is not an indication for surgery. Antireflux surgery should be considered for the treatment of objectively documented, relatively severe GERD, including that accompanied by erosive esophagitis, stricture, and Barrett's esophagus and a consideration for patients without severe mucosal injury who require continuous high-dose proton pump inhibitors for long-term symptom relief. Patients with atypical or respiratory symptoms who have a good response to intensive medical treatment should be considered for surgery. The option of antireflux surgery should be discussed with patients who need long-term aggressive medical therapy, particularly if large doses of proton pump inhibitors are needed to control symptoms. Antireflux surgery may be the preferred option in young patients, those for whom medications are a financial burden, those who are noncompliant with their drug regimen, and those who prefer a single intervention to long-term drug treatment. Surgical approach should be based on an assessment of esophageal motility. Patients with normal contractions do well with a 360-degree Nissen fundoplication. If peristalsis is severely disordered (more than 50% simultaneous contractions) and ineffective motility is present (amplitude < 30 mm Hg or nontransmitted contractions in more than 30% of wet swallows), a partial fundoplication is the procedure of choice.

The experience and results obtained at a particular surgical center must be evaluated in the decision of whether to recommend surgical treatment. If expertise is not available, referral to a more experienced surgeon is suggested.

Approach to the Patient

An individualized approach to each patient is recommended. In patients with heartburn and regurgitation, empirical treatment is advised, with consideration given to the step care approach outlined in Figure 1. Each level of therapeutic trials should last from 4 to 8 weeks before the patient proceeds to the next step. Several options are available at each step, and the choices should be based on cost and side effects from drug interaction. Complete symptom relief should be the goal of acute therapy. Consideration should be given to a trial off medications (but continuing lifestyle modifications) to see whether symptoms recur. Maintenance should be attempted with the least costly agent available. Debate exists

regarding consideration of a "step-down" approach in which a proton pump inhibitor is used as initial therapy in an attempt to rapidly relieve symptoms and then switching to the least expensive therapy that produces satisfactory relief of symptoms. Cost-effectiveness studies are needed to assess the benefits of each approach.

Early diagnostic evaluation is suggested for patients with extraesophageal (atypical) symptoms or the warning symptoms of dysphagia, early satiety, weight loss, and bleeding. Patients with persistent symptoms after a course of empirical therapy and patients requiring continuous daily therapy should be referred to a specialist for consideration of endoscopy or pH monitoring (especially for patients with negative endoscopic findings or atypical symptoms). Patients who have erosive esophagitis or atypical symptoms are likely to require proton pump inhibitors for relief and may need increasing dosages if symptoms are refractory. There is no advantage to a step-up approach for these patients. Long-term continuous maintenance therapy is usually needed. Combination therapy with a motility agent can be considered, particularly in patients with abnormal gastric emptying. Data from studies using intragastric pH monitoring suggest that adding an H_2 blocker at bedtime may be useful in patients in whom proton pump inhibitors twice a day before meals are not effective. Antireflux surgery should be considered for these patients after documentation of adequate symptom relief with medical therapy.

Every patient should be treated with the goal of achieving complete long-term symptom relief. A careful, thoughtful approach to GERD should produce a successful outcome in essentially all patients.

TUMORS OF THE STOMACH
method of
MARTIN S. KARPEH, Jr., M.D.
Memorial Sloan-Kettering Cancer Center
New York, New York

The stomach epithelium is host to a variety of neoplasms, including adenocarcinomas, lymphomas, mesenchymal tumors, and endocrine tumors. Several non-neoplastic lesions, such as cysts, hyperplastic polyps, and hamartomatous polyps, have in the past been included in discussions of gastric tumors. This review will focus on true neoplasms of the stomach.

ADENOMAS

Adenomas are benign lesions defined as tubular and villous structures lined by a dysplastic epithelium. They are the most common type of neoplastic polyp found in the stomach. In contrast to those in the colon, adenomas of the stomach are uncommon. The exact incidence is, however, difficult to determine owing to changes in nomenclature over time and to the fact that adenomas are asymptomatic and usually found incidentally at endoscopy.

Adenomas are premalignant lesions that should be treated by complete polypectomy. Their endoscopic appearance is typically that of a raised, flat-topped lesion less than 1 cm in diameter usually located in the gastric antrum. They can also be pedunculated or viliform, but this is much less common. A depressed surface appearance has been associated with about a 15% incidence of carcinoma.

The dominant histologic pattern is tubular. In a large series from Germany, Manfred Stolte reported that of 600 tubular adenomas diagnosed with forceps biopsy, 10% had carcinoma when the entire polypectomy specimen was examined. Synchronous or metachronous carcinomas were identified in 11% of adenomas in this series. The association with carcinoma is thought to be even stronger for the tubulopapillary and papillary types. Less is known about the risk of malignant degeneration in the pyloric gland adenoma, but this type of adenoma should also be completely removed to rule out a small focus of carcinoma.

The risk of carcinoma is proportional to size and grade of dysplasia. Although high-grade dysplastic adenomas are associated with invasive carcinoma, the finding of low-grade dysplasia on forceps biopsy does not eliminate the risk of a focus of carcinoma in another part of the lesion. Complete polypectomy should be performed whenever clinically feasible.

ADENOCARCINOMA

Adenocarcinoma of the stomach continues to be a major cause of cancer deaths worldwide. In countries such as Japan, South Korea, Costa Rica, and the former Soviet Union, the death rates range between 38 and 55 per 100,000. In the United States, the incidence of gastric cancer declined steadily during the first half of the 20th century to its present level of 8.37 per 100,000 per year. The rate of new cases among U.S. white males and females has remained at approximately 22,000 and 13,500 per year, respectively, for the last two decades. Death rates have also been fairly stable at 7900 per year for men and 5600 per year for women. The decline has been predominately in the intestinal-type tumors involving the distal stomach. The incidence of proximal stomach cancers has increased at an alarming rate. Proximal tumors now make up close to 50% of the more than 2000 gastric cancers treated at Memorial Sloan-Kettering Cancer Center since 1985.

Histopathology

The World Health Organization has subcategorized adenocarcinoma into four main histotypes according to the growth patterns (Table 1). This classification is still the one most widely used. In 1965, Lauren classified gastric cancers into either intestinal or diffuse histopathologic types. There are epidemiologic and presumed etiologic differences between these

TABLE 1. **World Health Organization Classification of Histologic Types of Gastric Adenocarcinoma**

Tubular
Papillary
Mucinous
Signet-ring cell

types of adenocarcinoma. The intestinal type is commonly found in regions where gastric cancer is endemic in the population. The specific cause of these tumors is unknown. Environmental factors such as chronic *Helicobacter pylori* infection, dietary salt, and nitrosoamine intake and a diet lacking fruits and vegetables, however, are thought to have a cumulative carcinogenic influence over time.

A multistep process leading from atrophic gastritis to dysplasia and eventually frank carcinoma of the intestinal type requires years to develop. Diffuse-type cancers are associated with regions where the incidence of gastric cancer is seen in epidemic proportions. Tumors of familial gastric cancers are usually of the diffuse type, which supports the concept that genetics plays a more important role in the etiology of these tumors. Diffuse cancers are said to have a worse prognosis than the intestinal type, but none of the many classifications of adenocarcinoma has been found to have prognostic relevance independent of tumor stage.

Staging

Staging is based on the tumor, nodes, and metastasis (TNM) system (Table 2). The depth of tumor invasion (T) is an independent determinant of survival. Tumors confined to the mucosa and submucosa (T1) are referred to as *early cancers* regardless of lymph node status. Eighty percent or more of these lesions are cured at 5 years even in the face of lymph node metastases. Conversely, the presence of serosal invasion (T3) is a powerful negative factor associated with tumor recurrence and tumor-related death after complete resection.

The number of lymph node metastases is probably the single most significant prognostic factor found to

TABLE 2. **TNM Staging System for Adenocarcinoma of the Stomach**

Tis	Carcinoma in situ
T1	Invasion into the mucosa or submucosa
T2	Invasion into the muscularis propria or subserosa
T3	Invasion into or through the serosa
T4	Invasion into an adjacent organ
N0	No lymph node metastases*
N1	1–6 metastatic lymph nodes
N2	7–15 metastatic lymph nodes
N3	>15 metastatic lymph nodes
M0	No distant metastases
M1	Distant metastases

* A minimum of 15 lymph nodes should be evaluated for metastases.

date. The presence of more than 15 positive lymph nodes is equivalent to liver or lung metastases in terms of prognosis. In 1997, the Union Internationale Contre le Cancer and the American Joint Committee on Cancer (AJCC) changed the N stage to reflect the number of metastatic lymph nodes as opposed to their distance from the primary site. This change will, it is hoped, result in more accurate staging because few western surgeons or pathologists indicated the distance or location of resected metastatic lymph nodes. Validation of the new N stage is based on data collected prospectively from 477 uniformly treated patients in the German Gastric Cancer Group. When comparing the new and old N staging methods, they found that the new system provided better stratification of Kaplan-Meier survival curves than the old system. The new N stage essentially further subdivides the old N1 and N2 categories into three groups, thus creating an intermediate-risk group. The success of this new system depends on the removal and examination of at least 15 lymph nodes. Pathology reports should indicate the number positive nodes per the total number of lymph nodes removed. Without this information, consistent staging will be very difficult, if not impossible.

The presence or absence of systemic disease defines M stage. Distant visceral metastases, peritoneal disease, and/or the presence of more than 15 metastatic lymph nodes is considered M1 disease. A growing number of published reports have indicated that positive peritoneal washings are also an M1 equivalent. The final AJCC stage combines TNM to give an overall prognostic indicator of outcome (Table 3). It is only as good as the information that is entered into it. Currently, there are no universally accepted guidelines for surgical or pathologic staging of gastrectomy specimens. Standardization is needed to properly advise patients of their recurrence risk and to allow meaningful communication between collaborating centers.

Pretreatment Evaluation

The standard pretreatment evaluation involves a thorough physical examination, chest radiograph, and abdominal and pelvic computed tomography (CT) scan, in addition to a complete blood count and comprehensive chemistries, which include liver function studies. An elevated carcinoembryonic antigen (CEA) level is present in up to a third of adenocarcinoma patients. There is a modest positive correlation between CEA level and the extent of disease, but it rarely influences primary treatment.

The addition of laparoscopy to the standard workup has resulted in a change in the management of between 25 and 35% of patients. In most cases, small peritoneal implants that were not seen on CT scan are discovered. Although some of these patients benefit from a palliative gastrectomy, the majority will not suffer from the primary tumor before they succumb to the systemic effects of their disease and thus can be spared a gastrectomy. On occasion, patients respond or fail to progress with chemotherapy. The potential benefit of an incomplete resection in this setting is still unclear. There is good justification to perform laparoscopy on all patients with advanced gastric cancer before any therapy is begun.

Because of the generally poor results of postoperative adjuvant chemotherapy for gastric cancer, a number of medical centers are investigating neoadjuvant (preoperative) treatments. Not all patients are suitable candidates for this treatment approach. Patients with N3 disease, peritoneal implants, or any distant metastases have such a poor prognosis that chemotherapy in this setting is expected to be palliative. Laparoscopy has proved to be an invaluable pretreatment staging tool. In the absence of distant disease, the risk of tumor recurrence depends on factors that traditionally were available only after resection of the primary tumor (TNM). An accurate preoperative assessment of T and N stages allows for proper patient placement into protocols of neoadjuvant treatment. This would certainly include any T3 tumor. Endoscopic ultrasonography (EUS) is one reliable method used to visualize the depth of stomach wall invasion and determine N status. Most reports indicate that EUS for T staging is more reliable than for N staging. Although EUS has greatly improved our ability to preoperatively assess both T and M stages, it is not widely available. One can also use laparoscopy to determine T stage either by brushing the gastric serosa for cytologic analysis or by using laparoscopic ultrasonography. N stage is difficult to determine with any degree of accuracy by visual assessment alone; the combination of laparoscopic ultrasonography and selective biopsy improves the pretreatment identification of node-positive tumors.

Recommendations for treating early gastric cancer are straightforward because the vast majority of patients will be cured after a complete surgical resection. Similarly, most physicians would agree that the risk of recurrence after complete resection of a T3N tumor is sufficiently high to warrant entry of that patient into a protocol of adjuvant therapy. For the growing number of patients with intermediate risk

TABLE 3. **American Joint Committee on Cancer Staging System**

IA	IB	II	IIIA	IIIB	IV
T1N0M0	T2N0M0	T3N0M0	T4N0M0		T(any)N(any)M1
	T1N1M0	T2N1M0	T3N1M0	T4N1M0	T(any)N3M0
		T1N2M0	T2N2M0	T3N2M0	

tumors (pT2N0 or T2N1), recommendations for adjuvant therapy depend on a careful analysis of the individual tumor characteristics. For example, a pT2 tumor invading into the subserosa will do worse than a pT2 tumor confined to the muscularis propria, yet in the current staging system they are given equal prognostic weight. In addition to exact depth of invasion, the presence and number of positive nodes are also important factors to determine preoperatively.

Adjuvant Treatment

The standard treatment for gastric cancer is complete surgical resection. Because of the advanced stage at presentation, most patients experience recurrences and inevitably die of their disease. Postoperative therapy in the form of chemotherapy with or without irradiation therapy was for decades the principal form of adjuvant therapy. Few prospective randomized trials have shown a benefit of adjuvant chemotherapy with or without radiation over resection alone. In a meta-analysis of postoperative chemotherapy trials, the use of chemotherapy was associated with a risk ratio of 0.87. A large prospective randomized intergroup trial has just been completed in the United States that compared survival after surgery alone or surgery and postoperative chemoradiation. Follow-up should soon reach sufficient maturity to allow survival analyses. If this is a negative trial, the next major national trial will almost certainly focus on a preoperative treatment approach. For now, it is well accepted that postoperative adjuvant chemotherapy cannot be recommended as the standard of care after a complete surgical resection of gastric cancer.

Two promising doxorubicin (Adriamycin)–based chemotherapy regimens that were developed in the late 1980s were used in phase II trials for advanced and metastatic gastric cancer. The combination of etoposide (VePesid), Adriamycin, and cisplatin (Platinol) (EAP) was given to a group of gastric cancer patients who were deemed at operation to be unresectable. Seventy percent responded; the complete response rate was 21%. Similar findings were seen with the combination of 5-fluorouracil, Adriamycin, methotrexate, and leucovorin (FAMTX). The astonishing response rates reported in these two trials were, unfortunately, never duplicated. These regimens are, however, associated with a respectable 40% response rate, which has maintained great interest in the study of new neoadjuvant drug combinations. Numerous phase II neoadjuvant trials have now been completed that demonstrate the safety and efficacy of this approach both with and without radiation therapy. Reports of morbidity and mortality associated with radiation-containing regimens are acceptable but are higher than for those without radiation. At my institution, the approach has been to use chemotherapy alone.

Surgery

The goal of surgery is to remove all gross and microscopic disease by resection of the stomach omentum and surrounding lymph nodes. The extent of gastrectomy depends on the depth of invasion and location of the tumor. Small tumors of the mucosa and submucosa can be safely resected with a 2- to 3-cm margin. The exact depth is typically not known preoperatively, and it is generally suggested that 5 cm be the minimal margin for all tumors. The size and extent of infiltration determines whether a total or subtotal gastrectomy is necessary to obtain a negative microscopic margin. At least three randomized trials have shown that total gastrectomy for the treatment of gastric cancer provides no survival advantage over subtotal gastrectomy provided that a negative margin is achieved.

The extent of lymphadenectomy has been the source of controversy. A D1 lymphadenectomy is the removal of perigastric lymph nodes along the epiploic vessels of the stomach. The more extensive D2 lymph node dissection includes a D1 dissection plus removal of the entire omentum and lymph nodes along the celiac axis, and hepatic and splenic arteries. Early results of two large multicenter prospective randomized trials that compared survival after D1 or D2 lymphadenectomy suggest no difference in overall survival but increased morbidity and mortality after the D2 procedure. These increases in morbidity and mortality in the D2 group were higher than those reported from centers where the D2 is routinely performed. The increase was associated with a significantly higher rate of splenectomy and distal pancreatectomy, which is not needed to perform an adequate D2 dissection. Surgeons performing a D2 lymphadenectomy require experience, but the procedure is a logical approach to safely remove lymph nodes at risk for metastasis. Although there is no proven survival advantage of a D2 lymph node dissection, determination of the lymph node status provides valuable prognostic information for the patient.

LYMPHOMAS

There is no lymphoid tissue in the stomach, but lymphomas account for between 3 and 5% of all gastric malignancies. Twenty-five percent of all non-Hodgkin's lymphomas are extranodal, the stomach being the most common extranodal site of origin. The worldwide incidence of primary gastric lymphoma appears to be increasing. Whether this reflects a true rise in prevalence or a heightened awareness of gastric mucosa-associated lymphoid tissue (MALT) lymphomas is difficult to determine. Gastric lymphomas, however, are rare. A large international epidemiologic study of non-Hodgkin's lymphomas by Robert Newton and colleagues found a U.S. incidence of 0.4 per 100,000 for whites and 0.34 and 0.53 per 100,000, respectively, for blacks and Latinos.

Lymphomas originating in the stomach with no other solid organ or distant nodal site of involvement are considered primary gastric lymphomas. Nodal lymphomas (NL) involving the stomach as a secondary event are considered secondary gastric lymphomas. These distinctions have prognostic significance and are becoming increasingly important as our understanding of the differences between MALT lymphomas and NL improves. For example, CD5 and CD10 expression is absent in MALT lymphomas but present in NL. Rearrangements in the *bcl*-2 gene are found in MALT lymphomas but are absent in NL.

Primary gastric lymphomas are typically seen in patients in their sixth decade of life, with a slight male predominance. Epigastric abdominal pain with or without weight loss is the most common presenting symptom. Patients may present with chronic anemia, but significant bleeding is uncommon at presentation, and perforation is distinctly rare. The diagnosis is made by endoscopic biopsy. At endoscopy, lymphomas may appear as flat, polypoid, or ulcerated lesions of 10 located in the body or antrum. Lymphomas commonly involve the submucosa; therefore superficial biopsies may miss the tumor. The diagnostic yield is significantly improved by the taking of large forceps biopsies.

There is no universally agreed upon classification with which to classify gastrointestinal lymphomas. A modification of the Kiel classification is being used more frequently. This modification uses a high-grade versus low-grade distinction that appears to correlate better with treatment outcome than the low-intermediate and high-grade terminology used in the *Working Formulation*. Diffuse small centrocyte-like cells are considered low-grade MALT lymphomas; these lymphomas can be hard to distinguish from benign conditions. The large centrocyte-like cells seen in high-grade lymphomas should be diagnostic. Once the diagnosis has been confirmed, the extent of disease should be determined by physical examination, chest radiograms, blood chemistry, bilateral bone marrow biopsies, and CT scans of the abdomen and pelvis. Clinical staging is based on a modification of the Ann Arbor Staging System (see the AJCC Cancer Staging Manual).

Gastric lymphomas have traditionally been treated by surgical resection. Adjuvant irradiation and chemotherapy were usually added, depending on the presence or absence of lymph node involvement with or without positive resection margins. The trend now, based on reports of successful nonoperative therapy, is to attempt to preserve the stomach and reserve gastrectomy for treatment failures. Irradiation is increasingly replacing surgery as local therapy in combination with chemotherapy, depending on tumor grade and stage. Numerous reports have shown that for low-grade IE and IIE1 lymphomas, primary radiation without chemotherapy is adequate. In the case of MALT lymphomas, eradication of *H. pylori* with antibiotic therapy has resulted in regression of the lymphoma without additional therapy. The largest series to date included 50 patients treated with antibiotics alone with an 80% complete response rate. Follow-up is now 48 months. Careful continued follow-up is needed to assess the efficacy and long-term safety of all of these nonoperative approaches.

For the IIE2 patient, the risk of systemic lymphoma is sufficiently high to warrant chemotherapy in combination with a local therapy. Single-modality therapy is clearly inferior to combination therapy once intermediate- or high-grade stage IIE disease is present, but there are no controlled randomized trials comparing chemotherapy with either radiation or surgery to evaluate quality of life or long-term outcome in stage IIE patients. Stage III and IV patients clearly have systemic disease and benefit most from primary chemotherapy with or without irradiation.

MESENCHYMAL TUMORS

Tumors of mesenchymal origin represent approximately 1% of all gastric tumors. Traditionally, benign spindle cell tumors of the stomach were regarded as leiomyomas; they often contained elements that stained positive for smooth muscle markers and were thought to arise from muscle. Many of these tumors have now been reclassified on the basis of electron microscopic characteristics as *gastrointestinal stromal tumors* (GIST). Other less common mesenchymal tumors arising from the stomach include autonomic nerve plexus lesions known as gastrointestinal autonomic nerve tumors, lipomas, and glomus tumors.

The behavior of GIST is often unclear. Although many may have few mitotic figures and are considered low grade, a malignant potential still exists. The risk of developing metastasis and tumor-related mortality is increased for tumors larger than 5 cm and high-grade tumors of any size. The recommended treatment is complete resection with a 1-cm margin, which can often be accomplished by a wedge resection, depending on the size of the tumor. Unlike lymphomas and carcinomas, the malignant mesenchymal tumors (sarcomas) rarely ever metastasize to lymph nodes; therefore lymphadenectomy is not indicated in their treatment. Adjuvant therapy has not been proved to be of benefit and should be considered investigational. The pattern of recurrence is predominately intra-abdominal. Hepatic metastases are present in up to 65% of recurrences, with intraperitoneal

TABLE 4. **Characteristics of Well-Differentiated Neuroendocrine Neoplasia**

Type	ECL-like Cells	Gastrin	Multicentricity	Gastropathy
1	Hyperplastic	Hypergastrinemia	Present	Atrophic gastritis
2	Hyperplastic	Hypergastrinemia	Present	Hypertrophic
3	Hyperplastic	Normal	Absent	None

dissemination seen in about one third. As is true for extremity sarcomas, the lungs are also at risk for developing metastatic disease. Follow-up for a high-grade lesion should include an abdominal CT scan every 3 to 6 months for the first 2 years and then yearly at least through the fifth postoperative year or as symptoms dictate.

ENDOCRINE TUMORS

Endocrine cells exist throughout the stomach. Neoplasms found in the body and fundus are commonly called *carcinoid tumors* or *neuroendocrine carcinomas*. Their exact etiology is unknown. Classification is according to their degree of differentiation: well-differentiated tumors, predominately composed of argyrophilic enterochromaffin-like (ECL) cells or rarely antral G cells; and poorly differentiated tumors, which are considered neuroendocrine carcinomas. The type and presence of associated gastropathy further characterize well-differentiated tumors into three types (Table 4). The risk of malignant transformation in a well-differentiated neuroendocrine tumor is not fully understood, but it is generally accepted that well-differentiated tumors of type 1 and type 2 that are less than 1 cm follow a benign course and that malignant potential increases with increases in size to greater than 2 cm. Type 3 tumors have a higher malignant potential that also increases with size. Ideally, all tumors larger than 2 cm should be surgically removed with adjacent lymph nodes. Depth of invasion beyond the submucosa and the presence of angioinvasion can also be used as a guide to recommend removal. Metastases, however, have been documented in type 1 tumors as small as 1 cm, limited to the mucosa; thus more information is needed to establish clear guidelines for treatment and follow-up of these tumors. Neuroendocrine carcinomas are aggressive and should be treated as adenocarcinomas.

In 1996, Guido Rindi and associates published a collective series on 205 "gastric carcinoids and neuroendocrine carcinomas." They studied 144 type 1 patients and found no tumor-related deaths among 25 deaths that occurred after a mean follow-up of 23 months. Of the remaining 119 alive, 65% had persistent disease after a mean of 58 (0.5 to 252) months follow-up. No details regarding treatment were given. Of the 12 type 2 cases, lymph node metastases were present in 3 of 10 assessed; one patient died of disease after 49 months. Type 3 tumors tended to be larger than 1 cm (mean, 3.2 cm), more deeply invasive, and associated with metastatic disease. Seven of 26 died of disease, with a mean survival of 28 (2 to 120) months.

The vast majority of neuroendocrine tumors are type 1 and smaller than 1 cm and can probably be followed up with serial endoscopy. For larger multiple type 1 lesions, some surgeons have treated the associated hypergastrinemia by performing an antrectomy to remove the hypertrophic G cells. Documented regression in the proximal lesions has been reported, but others have reported persistent disease even with low gastrins after antrectomy. It is safe to assume that endoscopic surveillance to monitor size, depth of invasion, and level of differentiation is warranted for these patients until better markers of malignant potential are elucidated.

TUMORS OF THE COLON AND RECTUM

method of
EMINA H. HUANG, M.D., and
RICHARD L. WHELAN, M.D.
Columbia–Presbyterian Medical Center
New York, New York

After lung, breast, and prostate cancers, colorectal cancers are the most frequent cancers observed in patients in the Western Hemisphere. It was estimated that in the United States, in 1999, there would be about 129,400 new cases of colorectal cancer and approximately 56,600 deaths from colorectal cancer. The North American population has a 6% lifetime risk of developing colorectal cancer; 50% of those affected will ultimately die of this disease. Colorectal cancer accounts for 11% of all cancer deaths. Despite advances in the understanding of the molecular biology and pathophysiology of this cancer, only modest decreases in mortality rates have been noted.

EPIDEMIOLOGY

Racial differences exist in mortality rates. The mortality rate is higher among African-Americans than in the white population, which may be because of more limited health care accessibility or an increased incidence of this disease in this population. New cases of colon cancer are slightly more common in women than in men; the mean age at which patients seek medical attention is in the seventh decade. In contrast, rectal cancers are slightly more common in men than in women. Although these cancers can, in rare instances, manifest in patients younger than 30 years, the mean age at onset is 62 years of age and nearly 70% of patients are 50 or older. Although 60 to 70% of cancers occur in the descending colon, sigmoid colon, or rectum, an increasing incidence of proximal colorectal cancers has been noted since the 1960s.

ETIOLOGY

The adenoma-to-carcinoma sequence is a widely accepted concept that summarizes the transformation of a benign lesion to a malignant lesion. More than 95% of colorectal adenocarcinomas arise from adenomatous polyps, and the progression in this sequence from normal mucosa to adenoma and then to carcinoma is thought to occur over a 10-year period. According to the findings of autopsy series, adenomas have a prevalence of more than 30% among people older than 40 years. In the clinical setting, nearly two thirds of the polyps detected are adenomas. Adenomas are a monoclonal proliferation of neoplastic cells that are histologically classified into three groups: tubular, tubulovillous, and villous adenomas. There is considerable variability in regard to the frequency of malignant transformation and the length of time required for a benign adenoma to become a malignant lesion. The chance of cancer development is greater for villous lesions and is directly related to the size of the polyp. Other benign lesions include hyperplastic polyps, juvenile polyps, hamartomatous polyps, inflammatory polyps, and nonmucosal lesions. Although there are other malignant lesions of the colon and rectum, including carcinoids, lymphomas, and sarcomas, adenocarcinomas are by far the most common, constituting 98% of the malignant tumors of the colon and rectum.

Cancers of the colon and rectum are believed to have multiple etiologic factors, including genetic and lifestyle factors. Immigrant studies have documented an increased incidence of colorectal carcinoma in Puerto Ricans and Japanese who have moved from their native countries to the United States. Numerous dietary factors may play a role in the development of colorectal cancer. Numerous epidemiologic studies suggest that fat (especially animal fat), a diet low in calcium, and a low-fiber diet are associated with a higher incidence of colorectal tumors.

A diet high in fiber content may be protective against colon cancer. Fiber, which increases fecal bulk and thus decreases carcinogen concentration in the stool, changes the bacterial composition of the stool and decreases stool transit time. Not all types of fiber have the same protective effect. Cellulose and wheat bran may be more protective than corn and oat bran. Digestible fiber is broken down in the gut and therefore has no major effects on the stool bulk or transit time. Nondigestible fiber passes through the gut and obligates a certain amount of water to be contained in the stool, which has the effect of adding bulk to the stool and making it softer. The majority of fiber supplements on the market contain either psyllium or methylcellulose, both of which are nondigestible fibers.

A diet high in fat has been associated with an increased risk of colon cancer in animals. The belief is that dietary fat causes a change in the amount and composition of bile acids being secreted into the gut. The bile acids, in turn, are converted into potential carcinogens by the intestinal flora. Therefore, it is not surprising that a diet with a high meat content has been associated with an increased risk for colorectal carcinoma in the majority of case-control studies, to date. Unfortunately, data from epidemiologic studies concerning the effects of fat and fiber are not conclusive, because for populations from different countries with different types of diets, there are a great many other dietary factors that may affect the development of colonic neoplasms.

The majority of epidemiologic studies evaluating calcium intake have suggested that a significant inverse correlation exists; the higher the calcium intake is, the lower the incidence of colorectal cancer. Animal studies have demonstrated inhibition of colon carcinogenesis by calcium salts. However, a number of human case-control studies, far more meaningful than ecologic studies, have not documented a statistically significant effect. Similarly, with regard to vitamin D usage, contradictory results have been noted in the clinical studies carried out thus far.

Vitamin A, beta carotene, and vitamin E may be effective chemopreventive agents because of their antioxidant and free radical scavenging properties. Unfortunately, a randomized trial failed to document any efficacy with regard to vitamin A intake; however, the results of other trials are pending.

The impact of aspirin and other nonsteroidal anti-inflammatory drugs (NSAIDs) on the development of colonic neoplasia has been studied extensively. Animal experiments have shown that these drugs inhibit the growth of colon adenomas by altering arachidonic acid metabolism through inhibition of cyclooxygenase-mediated prostaglandin synthesis. Several agents, including aspirin, piroxicam, indomethacin, and sulindac, have been studied in clinical trials; the majority of these studies have demonstrated a positive, preventive effect. It is possible, however, that the lower-than-expected incidence of neoplasia in these patients results from associated changes in lifestyle that inhibit colorectal cancer. It is also possible that gastrointestinal blood loss facilitated by these agents may lead to earlier detection of neoplasms. Nonetheless, polyp regression has been noted in patients with familial adenomatous polyposis (FAP) who take NSAIDs. The association of NSAID use and lower-than-expected rates of neoplasia is less pronounced for patients with sporadic colon polyps, who are the great majority of those at risk for colorectal cancer.

A personal history of colon cancer, adenomas, or inflammatory bowel disease or a first-degree family history of colon or other cancers (particularly stomach, pancreas, ovarian, breast, or uterine cancer) predisposes affected persons to the development of colorectal cancer. Inflammatory bowel disease accounts for 1% of the new cases of colorectal cancer each year. The increased risk of colon cancer in patients with ulcerative colitis is dependent on the duration and extent of the disease. In patients with extensive or total colonic involvement, there is a significant increase in the incidence of colon cancer 8 to 10 years after the onset of symptoms. If the disease is limited to the left side of the colon, this increase begins 15 to 20 years after the onset of symptoms. Among patients with long-standing colonic Crohn's disease, the relative risk of cancer increases up to 20.9%.

Although the incidence of colorectal tumors is clearly increased among patients with FAP and hereditary nonpolyposis colon cancer (HNPCC), the effect of unnamed mutations that are genetically transmitted from generation to generation in non-FAP patients is unclear. Patients with a first-degree family member with a history of colon cancer, especially if the proband developed cancer before the age of 55 or if adenomatous polyps were diagnosed before the age of 60, are at a twofold increased risk. The FAP syndrome accounts for 1% of the new cancers diagnosed each year. Patients with this syndrome are commonly found as teenagers to have more than 100 colonic polyps. The best known phenotypic variant of this syndrome is Gardner's syndrome. Benign features of the syndrome include a pigmented fundal lesion, called congenital hypertrophy of the retinal pigment; epidermoid cysts; dental abnormalities; jaw cysts; fibromas; lipomas; and osteomas. Neoplastic features include gastric, duodenal, and endocrine adenomas, as well as periampullary duodenal carcinomas, papillary thyroid cancers, and hepatoblastomas. FAP is inherited in an autosomal dominant pattern with complete penetrance. The mutated gene in FAP is the APC gene. This is a tumor suppressor gene that has been localized to the long arm of chromosome 5 (5q21). The progression to colorectal cancer is inevitable; most affected patients have developed malignancies by the fourth decade of life.

HNPCC (Lynch's) syndrome accounts for 5% of new colorectal cancers. Also inherited in an autosomal dominant pattern, this syndrome is characterized by early age at onset (usually younger than 45 years), a propensity for the development of right-sided lesions, and an excess of synchronous and metachronous cancers. Lynch's syndrome type I is site specific for the colon, whereas patients with the type II syndrome are at risk for developing other cancers, such as gastric, small intestine, upper urologic tract, ovarian, and endometrial cancers. The Amsterdam criteria

TABLE 1. **Amsterdam Criteria for the Diagnosis of Hereditary Nonpolyposis Colon Cancer (HNPCC)**

Three or more relatives with colorectal cancer
One affected person is a first-degree relative of the other two
One or more cases of colorectal cancer diagnosed in the family
  before the age of 50

(Table 1) are currently the means by which type I and type II disease is defined. Interestingly, several genes involved in DNA repair have been found to be defective in patients with HNPCC: hMLH1, hMSH2, PMS1, and PMS2 (Table 2). Other genetic abnormalities in colon cancers that have been discovered, to date, include those in 17p (p53 gene), K-*ras*, and 18q (deleted in colon cancer).

DIAGNOSIS

Symptoms of a colorectal malignancy include fatigue related to anemia, bleeding per rectum, abdominal pain, weight loss, and a change in bowel habits. Any of these symptoms justifies and necessitates a comprehensive evaluation, including digital rectal examination, anoscopy, and total colonic evaluation. Total colonic evaluation can be accomplished through colonoscopy or flexible sigmoidoscopy combined with an air contrast barium enema study. The finding of hemorrhoids or another source of anorectal bleeding in a patient with persistent symptoms or with a suggestive history should not delay further assessment. Do all patients with rectal bleeding require a complete colonic evaluation? There is no consensus regarding when a sigmoidoscopy alone can be considered to be sufficient evaluation. Neoplasms, although rare, are occasionally found in seemingly average-risk patients in their thirties. For patients in their twenties who are without risk factors and in whom an anorectal source of bleeding is found, sigmoidoscopy should certainly be sufficient. However, if the bleeding persists despite treatment of the anal condition, patients should undergo a complete colonic evaluation.

Patients with advanced disease may have symptoms of obstruction, such as abdominal distention, obstipation, or vomiting. Such patients obviously require an urgent evaluation that would begin with supine and upright abdominal radiographs. A computed tomographic (CT) scan, a limited barium enema study, or limited lower endoscopy should enable identification of the source of the obstruction.

TABLE 2. **Genetic Alterations in Colon Cancer**

Oncogenes
  K-*ras* (12q)
Tumor Suppressor Genes
  APC (5q)
  DCC (18q)
  17p53
Abnormal DNA Methyltransferase and Hypomethylation
Abnormal DNA Mismatch Repair Genes
  hMLH1 (3p21)
  hMSH2 (2p22–21)
  PMS1
  PMS2

SCREENING

Clearly, the best way to improve survival in colon cancer patients and to decrease the overall incidence of the disease is through aggressive screening programs that allow for early diagnosis and treatment. Periodic endoscopic or radiologic evaluation of the asymptomatic adult population is the best means of achieving these goals. Despite much publicity regarding the need for colonic surveillance, both endoscopic and radiologic methods of colonic screening remain underused. Colonic screening allows for colonoscopic removal of benign adenomas before they have developed into invasive neoplasms. Cancers found in asymptomatic persons, in general, tend to be less advanced than those found in the symptomatic population.

Which screening method should be used? Each method of screening has its inherent virtues and problems. For example, fecal occult blood testing (FOBT) is inexpensive, has a sensitivity of 30 to 90%, and has a specificity of 96%. However, if FOBT is the only method used, approximately half of the colorectal cancers will be missed. Therefore, FOBT is far from the ideal screening test. Flexible sigmoidoscopy, which examines the terminal 60 cm of the large bowel, is a more invasive and expensive method and is often associated with some discomfort. A complete sigmoidoscopy should detect between 60 and 70% of all colonic neoplasms. Sigmoidoscopy also carries a small but definite risk of perforation or bleeding. Air contrast barium enema study has a complication rate lower than that of sigmoidoscopy and is nearly as sensitive as colonoscopy. However, it is purely a diagnostic tool, inasmuch as it is not possible to take biopsy specimens of or remove any polyps that may be found. Colonoscopy is currently the most sensitive screening modality and enables complete colonic evaluation in about 95% of patients. Biopsy specimens of polyps and lesions can be obtained and, if amenable, the polyps and lesions can be removed endoscopically. Therefore, colonoscopy is currently the gold standard of screening methods. However, it is the most expensive method and carries a small but significant risk of morbidity (perforation or bleeding).

It has been demonstrated, by large prospective studies, that routine endoscopic screening is associated with a lower-than-expected incidence of and rate of mortality from colorectal cancer. Although there is considerable controversy over when and how thoroughly patients should be evaluated, most authorities agree that for people at average risk annual FOBT with screening flexible sigmoidoscopy every 5 years, at the very least, should be carried out beginning at age 50. Any patient found to have adenomas would then undergo full colonoscopy. Persons with a first-degree family history of colon cancer or another risk factor should undergo colonoscopy every 5 years starting at age 40. Patients with a family history of either FAP or the HNPCC syndromes, as well as those with inflammatory bowel disease should begin colonic surveillance earlier and perhaps have more frequent examinations. These recommendations are summarized in Table 3.

Finally, patients with a personal history of colon cancer need regular full colonic screening for metachronous lesions. There is no clear consensus on the best schedule for follow-up examinations. The authors' practice is to perform the first full examination 12 months after the resection. The examination is repeated in 1 year's time. If no abnormalities are found on the second examination, the interval between examinations can be lengthened to between 3 and 5 years.

TABLE 3. **ACS Guidelines for Screening and Surveillance for Early Detection of Colorectal Polyps and Cancer***

Risk Category	Recommendation†	Age to Begin	Interval
Average Risk			
All people 50 years or older who are not in the categories below	Either FOBT plus flexible sigmoidoscopy‡ or TCE§	Age 50	FOBT every year and flexible sigmoidoscopy every 5 y Colonoscopy every 10 y or DCBE every 5–10 y
Moderate Risk			
People with a single, small (<1 cm) adenomatous polyp	Colonoscopy	At time of initial polyp diagnosis	TCE within 3 y after initial polyp removal; if normal, as per average-risk recommendations
People with large (≥1 cm) or multiple adenomatous polyps of any size	Colonoscopy	At time of initial polyp diagnosis	TCE within 3 y after initial polyp removal; if normal, TCE every 5 y
Personal history of curative-intent resection of colorectal cancer	TCE‖	Within 1 y after resection	If normal, TCE in 3 y; if still normal, TCE every 5 y
Colorectal cancer or adenomatous polyps in first-degree relative younger than 60 y or in two or more first-degree relatives of any ages	TCE	Age 40, or 10 y before the youngest case in the family, whichever is earlier	Every 5 y
Colorectal cancer in any other relatives (not included above)	As per risk recommendations (above); screening before age 50 may be considered		
High Risk			
Family history of familial adenomatous polyposis	Early surveillance with endoscopy, counseling to consider genetic testing, and referral to specialty center	Puberty	If genetic test result is positive or polyposis is confirmed, consider colectomy; otherwise, endoscopy every 1–2 y
Family history of hereditary nonpolyposis colon cancer	Colonoscopy and counseling to consider genetic testing	Age 21	If genetic test result is positive or if patient has not had genetic testing, colonoscopy every 2 y until age 40, then every year
Inflammatory bowel disease	Colonoscopies with biopsies for dysplasia	8 y after the onset of pancolitis; 12–15 y after the onset of left-sided colitis	Every 1–2 y

*Approximately 70–80% of cases are in average-risk patients, approximately 15–20% are in moderate-risk patients, and 5–10% are in high-risk patients.
†Digital rectal examination should be done at the time of each sigmoidoscopy, colonoscopy, or DCBE.
‡Annual FOBT has been shown to reduce the rate of mortality from colorectal cancer, so it is preferable to no screening; however, the ACS recommends that annual FOBT be accompanied by flexible sigmoidoscopy to further reduce the risk of colorectal cancer mortality.
§TCE includes either colonoscopy or DCBE. The choice of procedure should depend on the medical status of the patient and the relative quality of the medical examinations available in a specific community. Flexible sigmoidoscopy should be performed in instances in which the rectosigmoid colon is not well visualized by DCBE. DCBE would be performed when the entire colon has not been adequately evaluated by colonoscopy.
‖This assumes that a perioperative TCE was performed.
Abbreviations: ACS = American Cancer Society; DCBE = double-contrast barium enema [study]; FOBT = fecal occult blood testing; TCE = total colon examination.

MANAGEMENT

Colon Cancer

Once colon cancer is diagnosed, the routine screening evaluation for metastatic disease includes a chest radiograph and a CT scan of the abdomen. The latter is not absolutely essential for most patients at low risk, who would undergo resection of the primary tumor regardless of the presence of liver metastases. However, having a baseline scan is helpful, because most surgeons recommend yearly CT scans after resection. There may be a few patients at very poor risk with nonobstructing and nonbleeding cancers in whom the finding of distant metastases would prompt expectant monitoring without surgery. A complete colon evaluation through colonoscopy or barium enema study should be part of the preoperative evaluation in all patients with colorectal cancer, to rule out synchronous neoplasms.

Surgical resection is the only effective curative treatment for colon cancer. Patients who undergo an elective resection should complete a mechanical and antibiotic bowel preparation in order to decrease the chance of stool spillage (which is associated with postoperative intra-abdominal and wound infections) during surgery. An adequate segmental resection of the colon removes the tumor with decent proximal and distal margins of normal bowel as well as of the adjacent mesentery, which contains the supplying blood and lymphatic vessels. The mesenteric resection is an important component of the resection because invasive cancers spread via the lymphatic vessels to the regional lymph nodes or through vascular invasion to more distant sites. Direct extension of the tumor into adjacent structures or organs may also occur and, when feasible, necessitates en bloc resection of the tumor along with the involved structure. In elective cases, an immediate anastomosis is carried out to restore intestinal continuity and to avoid a colostomy.

Laparoscopically assisted colectomy techniques have been developed since 1990 and are currently well accepted for benign disease. The performance of curative laparoscopically assisted colon resection for adenocarcinoma, however, remains controversial. Fears of port wound tumors arose after a rash of early reports of such occurrences in 1992 and 1993. Although incisional tumors develop after open (large-incision) colectomy in about 0.75% of patients, there was concern that the incidence of wound tumors would be significantly higher after laparoscopic colectomy. Largely to settle this issue, a number of randomized and prospective trials were initiated and are still ongoing. Preliminary results of these and a number of nonrandomized prospective studies suggest that the incidence of port wound tumors is less than 1%, which is similar to the incidence after open surgery. Furthermore, 3-year survival and local recurrence data are, thus far, similar for patients who have undergone either laparoscopic or open procedures. Most authorities recommend that for the time being, cancers be treated in the setting of a randomized trial. It is crucial that surgeons gain considerable experience performing resections for benign disease before attempting curative resections for cancer.

Rectal Cancer

Rectal cancers are associated with a worse prognosis than are colon lesions. This is probably because two thirds of the rectum is extraperitoneal, which permits circumferential direct spread of tumors into the perirectal fat and into retroperitoneal structures such as the prostate, seminal vesicles, and vagina. This anatomy also makes complete rectal resection considerably more difficult than colectomy. Furthermore, for distal rectal cancers, the anal sphincter may need to be fully excised, which necessitates the formation of a permanent colostomy. Transabdominal "radical" surgical resection remains the gold standard of curative rectal cancer treatment; however, for select lesions, transanal local treatment may be a reasonable option. Thorough preoperative staging with abdominal CT scan (or magnetic resonance imaging or transabdominal ultrasonograpy) and, when available, transrectal ultrasonography (TRUS) is recommended by the authors. TRUS is performed for tumors in the middle and distal thirds of the rectum to determine the depth of invasion and to look for enlarged perirectal lymph nodes. TRUS also defines the relationship of the tumor to the sphincter and other extraperitoneal structures. This information determines whether definitive local treatment is an option and also demonstrates which patients may benefit from a course of preoperative radiotherapy. If the CT scan reveals distant metastases, radical

transabdominal proctectomy is usually not indicated. In these cases, palliative local treatment, which entails less morbidity and is better tolerated, is more appropriate.

For rectal cancers that are bulky or fixed or that on rectal ultrasonography are staged as T3 or T4 lesions, preoperative radiotherapy, possibly combined with chemotherapy, may be advantageous. Such treatment has been shown to increase the resectability of advanced lesions and is thought to allow for sphincter preservation in some patients with distal rectal lesions. It has also been shown to decrease the local recurrence rate and, in one study, to increase survival rates. Another advantage of preoperative radiotherapy is that there is a decreased incidence of small bowel complications in comparison to patients receiving postoperative radiotherapy, who are likely to have small bowel pelvic adhesions at the time of treatment.

Local, definitive, transanal therapies that avoid abdominal surgery are a reasonable alternative for selected patients with small tumors in the distal third of the rectum that are (1) mobile, (2) exophytic, (3) above the sphincter, (4) less than 4 cm in size, and (5) TRUS staged as T1 or superficial T2 lesions (deepest level of invasion being the submucosa or the muscularis propria). These lesions are not likely to have metastasized to perirectal lymph nodes, which makes local therapy a viable option. Patients electing to undergo local definitive treatment must be willing to accept a somewhat higher local recurrence rate and mortality risk. When faced with the prospect of a permanent colostomy, a fair percentage of patients opt for such treatment. Local treatment options include (1) transanal full-thickness local excision, (2) endocavitary radiotherapy, and (3) fulguration with either electrocautery or laser. Local excision can be combined with a course of pelvic radiotherapy in order to treat the pelvic lymph nodes.

The goal of radical transabdominal surgery is to remove the tumor-bearing segment of rectum along with the accompanying mesorectum, which contains the lymph nodes and blood supply. Reanastomosis of the proximal bowel to the rectum is performed if a 2- to 5-cm distal rectal margin can be obtained without resection of the anal sphincter. The anal sphincter can be preserved for most proximal-, middle-, and selected distal-third rectal cancers. Circular staplers facilitate low rectal anastomosis. Cancers that are at the level of or just above the sphincter still necessitate an abdominoperineal resection with permanent colostomy. For selected distal-third rectal cancers, the sphincter can be preserved and a coloanal anastomosis carried out.

Surgical Emergencies

Obstruction or perforation usually constitutes a surgical emergency. Malignant obstruction is more likely to occur with left-sided lesions but can occur with large cecal tumors. In the setting of a dilated and unprepared colon, surgical resection and pri-

TABLE 4. **TNM Staging System for Colon Cancer**

Stage	T	N	M
0	Tis	N0	M0
I	T1	N0	M0
	T2	N0	M0
II	T3	N0	M0
	T4	N0	M0
III	Any T	N1–N3	M0
IV	Any T	Any N	M1

Tis	Carcinoma in situ
T1	Tumor invades submucosa
T2	Tumor invades muscularis propria
T3	Tumor invades into serosa
T4	Tumor invades other organs or structures
N0	No regional lymph node metastasis
N1	Metastasis in 1 to 3 pericolic or perirectal lymph nodes
N2	Metastasis in 4 or more pericolic or perirectal lymph nodes
N3	Metastasis in any lymph node along course of a named vascular trunk, and/or metastasis to apical node(s) (when marked by surgeon)
M0	No distant metastasis
M1	Distant metastasis

mary anastomosis are associated with increased morbidity. In patients with complete obstruction, a staged approach may be necessary. Surgical options in this setting include (1) diverting proximal stoma, followed by resection and anastomosis weeks later; (2) resection, anastomosis, and proximal diverting stoma; and (3) subtotal colectomy with ileosigmoid anastomosis. In patients with partial obstruction, it may be possible to perform decompression in the patient with a nasogastric tube and to slowly carry out a mechanical bowel preparation. If this is possible, it should also be possible to perform a resection and primary anastomosis with increased risk.

Perforated cancerous colon constitutes a surgical emergency. Because this manifestation may mimic perforated diverticular disease, the primary process is not always clear. Surgically, the goal is to remove the perforated segment along with its mesentery and to drain any accompanying abscesses. Once this is accomplished, proximal diversion with or without distal anastomosis may be the safest option. In rare instances, primary anastomosis without diversion is possible. The prognosis for patients with this manifestation is poor; the overall 5-year survival rate is 30%.

Adjuvant Therapy

Adjuvant chemotherapy for colon cancer is, in the United States, routinely advised for patients found to have involved lymph nodes (Dukes C or stage 3 disease) (Table 4). Local and distant recurrences develop in 30 to 50% of these patients. Standard chemotherapy today includes 5-fluorouracil (5-FU) and levamisole (Ergamisole) (or leucovorin), although a number of other agents, including irinotecan (CPT-

11), are currently being evaluated in clinical trials. In this setting, adjuvant chemotherapy is usually given for 6 to 9 months.

For patients with T3 or node-positive rectal cancers who did not undergo preoperative radiotherapy, postoperative radiotherapy (usually 4500 to 5400 cGy) combined with chemotherapy (6 to 9 months) has been shown to significantly increase length of survival and decrease local recurrence rates. Postoperative radiotherapy alone is not as effective; although some trials have documented decreased local recurrence rates after its use, none have shown a survival benefit. Patients with node-positive high rectal cancers (tumor above the peritoneal reflection) are usually advised to undergo chemotherapy alone.

The frequency and type of follow-up of these patients after curative resection remain controversial. As mentioned, approximately 30 to 50% of patients experience a recurrence, and of these, 80% experience recurrence within 2 years of resection. Although these measures have not proved to improve survival in the trial setting, the authors recommend serial physical examinations, periodic determination of serum carcinoembryonic antigen levels, chest radiography, colonoscopy, and yearly CT scan of the abdomen for at least 5 years (pelvis as well for rectal cancer patients). In patients who are not monitored closely postoperatively, the development of new symptoms clearly warrants investigation.

SUMMARY

Of all the cancers, colorectal cancer, with the established adenoma-carcinoma sequence, is largely preventable. Although this measure is not fully proven, it makes sense to recommend low-fat and high-fiber diets as well as daily vitamin and calcium supplementation. Ideally, all adults should undergo routine colon screening examinations. Those found to have adenomas need periodic complete colonoscopy. Those found to have cancers require prompt surgery; adjuvant therapy should be reserved for appropriately staged disease. The authors predict a greater role for minimally invasive surgery in the future, pending the results of randomized prospective trials currently under way. Virtual colonoscopic methods are on the horizon and may possibly become the standard means of surveillance of the large bowel in the future.

INTESTINAL PARASITES

method of
DAVID R. HILL, M.D.
University of Connecticut School of Medicine
Farmington, Connecticut

Intestinal parasites account for millions to billions of infections throughout the world and cause frequent morbidity in the infected population. Although many of these parasites exist more commonly in developing, tropical regions of the world, others, such as *Giardia lamblia*, *Cryptosporidium*, and pinworm, are widely distributed in both temperate and tropical environments. International travel or immigration, poor fecal-oral hygiene, and the ingestion of raw or undercooked fish or meats may be risk factors for infection. In addition, immunosuppression caused by chemotherapy for neoplastic or inflammatory diseases and by human immunodeficiency virus (HIV) may allow the dissemination of some parasites such as *Strongyloides* and the persistence of others such as *Cryptosporidium* and *Cyclospora*.

Intestinal parasites can be divided into protozoa and helminths. Protozoa are single-celled organisms, whereas helminths are multicellular worms with complex digestive, neurologic, and reproductive organs. Intestinal protozoa are always transmitted by the fecal-oral route. Helminths, however, can be acquired not only by the fecal-oral route but also after ingestion of larval forms in raw or undercooked meats, fish, and other products or by penetrating the skin. Protozoan parasites multiply asexually within the host; thus ingestion of a single cyst may be sufficient to establish infection and cause severe disease. With intestinal helminths, adult worms usually reside in the lumen of the bowel and do not multiply, so clinical symptoms are directly related to the number of parasitic worms that are carried by the host. Occasionally, however, the errant migration of a single worm such as *Ascaris* entering the common bile duct can result in severe consequences.

Most protozoal or helminthic infections manifest with symptoms related to the gastrointestinal tract, such as nonspecific abdominal discomfort or diarrhea. Occasionally there is extraintestinal disease when the parasite spreads beyond the gut in the normal host (e.g., amebic liver abscess or central nervous system cysticercosis), disseminates in a compromised host (e.g., disseminated strongyloidiasis), or invades tissue as part of the normal life cycle (e.g., trichinosis).

The diagnosis of intestinal parasites is best accomplished by a careful examination of the stool for the ova or larvae produced by helminths or for the cysts produced by protozoa and occasionally for the protozoa itself. Increasingly, antigen detection tests are being employed for intestinal protozoa with either enzyme-linked immunosorbent assay (ELISA) techniques or direct fluorescence antibody (DFA); *G. lamblia* and *Cryptosporidium parvum* are usually detected by these methods. Serology may be helpful in diagnosis when parasites are in tissues; imaging techniques such as computed tomography (CT) scanning and ultrasonography may also be needed. Elevation of the eosinophil count usually occurs in helminth infection when there has been tissue invasion.

TREATMENT

Most of the drugs that are described are licensed and commercially available in the United States. Some are licensed for certain infections but not for others, however, and therefore are recommended for non–FDA-indicated conditions. Some agents manufactured outside of the United States can be obtained by contacting the parasitic disease drug service of the Centers for Disease Control and Prevention (CDC) in Atlanta, Georgia (telephone: 404-639-3670). In Canada, restricted drugs can be obtained by approval

of the Special Access Programme, Health Canada, Ottawa (telephone: 613-941-2108).

Recommended drugs and specific doses are listed in Table 1 for protozoa and in Table 2 for helminths. These are based on recommendations published in the *Medical Letter on Drugs and Therapeutics* (40:1–12, 1998). Further information on the agents used can be obtained from the *Drug Information for the Health Care Professional*, 18th ed (USP DI, Rockville, MD, the United States Pharmacopeial Convention, 1998).

Intestinal Protozoa

Giardia lamblia

Giardiasis is one of the most common intestinal parasitic infections and the most frequent cause of water-borne outbreaks of diarrhea in the United States. It is widely distributed throughout the world, and, although *G. lamblia* may be one of many pathogens to infect children in developing world settings, it can contribute to acute and chronic diarrhea in these children. Individuals at risk for *G. lamblia* infestation include those drinking untreated surface water, particularly in mountainous regions of the United States and Canada (e.g., hikers), international travelers, children in day care settings, sexually active gay men, and patients with hypogammaglobulinemia. Stool antigen detection is the most common mode of diagnosis.

Since the discontinuation of quinacrine production in the United States, agents of the nitroimidazole class have been preferred. Thus, although metronidazole (Flagyl) has never received FDA approval for therapy, it is the drug of choice and has an efficacy of 85 to 95% when given for a 5- to 7-day course. It is generally well tolerated in children, and, although there have been concerns about potential carcinogenicity, these have not been documented. Side effects include a metallic taste in the mouth, some nausea, dizziness, and headache, and, rarely, reversible neutropenia and neurologic problems of seizures and neuropathy. When metronidazole is taken with alcohol, a disulfiram-like reaction can occur. Metronidazole is an FDA pregnancy category B agent and can probably be taken safely during the final two trimesters of pregnancy. Although not available in the United States, another nitroimidazole, tinidazole (Fasigyn), has shown excellent efficacy in adults when given in a single 2-gram dose, and it may be better tolerated than metronidazole.

Quinacrine (Atabrine), although no longer manufactured in the United States, can be obtained through alternative sources (see Table 1). It has an efficacy of about 95% for a 5- to 7-day course but may be poorly tolerated in children. Common side effects are nausea, vomiting, and abdominal cramping. Yellow discoloration of the skin, urine, and sclerae occur, and exfoliative dermatitis and toxic psychosis are rare side effects.

Furazolidone (Furoxone), a nitrofuran, is an alter-

TABLE 1. **Drugs for the Treatment of Protozoal Infections**

Infection	Drug	Adult Dosage	Pediatric Dosage
Amebiasis (*Entamoeba histolytica*) Asymptomatic Drug of choice	Iodoquinol (Yodoxin)	650 mg tid × 20 d	30–40 mg/kg/d (max 2 gm) in 3 doses × 20 d
	or Paromomycin (Humatin)	25–35 mg/kg/d in 3 doses × 7 d	25–35 mg/kg/d in 3 doses × 7 d
Alternative	Diloxanide furoate (Furamide)*	500 mg tid × 10 d	20 mg/kg/d in 3 doses × 10 d
Mild to moderate intestinal disease Drug of choice†	Metronidazole (Flagyl)	500–750 mg tid × 10 d	35–50 mg/kg/d in 3 doses × 10 d
	or Tinidazole‡	2 gm/d × 3 d	50 mg/kg (max 2 gm) qd × 3 d
Severe intestinal disease and liver abscess Drug of choice†	Metronidazole	750 mg tid × 10 d	35–50 mg/kg/d in 3 doses × 10 d
	or Tinidazole‡	600 mg bid or 800 mg tid × 5 d	50 mg/kg or 60 mg/kg (max 2 gm) qd × 5 d
Balantidium coli Drug of choice	Tetracycline	500 mg qid × 10 d	40 mg/kg/d (max 2 gm) in 4 doses × 10 d (not recommended in children <8 y)
Alternative	Iodoquinol	650 mg tid × 20 d	40 mg/kg/d (max 2 gm) in 3 doses × 20 d
Blastocystis hominis infection§ Cryptosporidiosis (*Cryptosporidium parvum*) Drug of choice‖	Paromomycin¶	500–750 mg qid	
Cyclospora species Drug of choice	Trimethoprim (TMP)-sulfamethoxazole (SMZ; Bactrim, septra)¶,**	TMP 160 mg, SMZ 800 mg bid × 7 d	TMP 5 mg/kg, SMZ 25 mg/kg bid × 7 d
Dientamoeba fragilis infection Drug of choice	Iodoquinol	650 mg tid × 20 d	40 mg/kg/d (max 2 gm) in 3 doses × 20 d
	or Paromomycin¶	500 tid × 7 d	25–30 mg/kg/d in 3 doses × 7 d
	or Tetracycline¶	500 mg qid × 10 d	40 mg/kg/d (max 2 gm/d) in 4 doses × 10 d (not recommended in children <8 y)
Giardiasis (*Giardia lamblia*) Drug of choice Alternatives††	Metronidazole¶ Tinidazole‡	250 mg tid × 5 d 2 gm once	15 mg/kg/d in 3 doses × 5 d 50 mg/kg once (max 2 gm)
	or Quinacrine‡‡	100 mg tid × 5–7 d	2 mg/kg tid × 5–7 d
	or Furazolidone (Furoxone)	100 mg qid × 7–10 d	6 mg/kg/d in 4 doses × 7–10 d
	or Paromomycin	500–750 tid × 5–10 d	25–35 mg/kg/d in 3 doses × 5–10 d
Isosporiasis (*Isospora belli*) Drug of choice	Trimethoprim-sulfamethoxazole¶,§§	160 mg TMP, 800 mg SMZ qid × 10 d, then bid × 3 wk	
Microsporidiosis Intestinal (*Enterocytozoon bieneusi, Septata intestinalis*) Drug of choice‖‖	Albendazole (Albenza)¶	400 bid × 2–3 wk	

*Available from the CDC Drug Service, Centers for Disease Control and Prevention, Atlanta, Georgia; 404-639-3670.
†Treatment should be followed by a course of iodoquinol or paromomycin in the dosage used to treat asymptomatic amebiasis.
‡Not available in the United States. The higher dosage listed is for amebic liver abscess.
§Clinical significance of *Blastocystis* is controversial, but metronidazole 750 tid × 10 d or iodoquinol 650 tid × 20 d may be effective (as reported anecdotally) (Boreham PFL, Stenzel DJ: *Blastocystis* in humans and animals: morphology, biology, and epizootiology. Adv Parasitol *32*:1–70, 1993; Keystone JS: *Blastocystis hominis* and traveler's diarrhea [editorial]. Clin Infect Dis *21*:102–103, 1995; Markell EK: Is there any reason to continue treating *Blastocystis* infections? [Editorial]. Clin Infect Dis *21*:104–105, 1995).
‖Infection is self-limited in immunocompetent patients. Azithromycin in doses of 500 to 1000 mg initially and then 250 to 500 per day has been helpful in limited studies. Duration of treatment may need to be prolonged.
¶An approved drug, but considered investigational for this condition by the U.S. FDA.
**AIDS patients may need a higher dose (1 double strength tablet 4 times daily) and long-term maintenance therapy (Pape JW, Verdier RI, Boncy M, et al: *Cyclospora* infection in adults infected with HIV. Clinical manifestations, treatment, and prophylaxis. Ann Intern Med *121*:654–657, 1994).
††Albendazole 400 mg/d × 5 d may be effective (Hall A, Nahar Q: Albendazole as a treatment for infections with *Giardia duodenalis* in children in Bangladesh. Trans R Soc Trop Med Hyg *87*:84–86, 1993).
‡‡No longer produced in the United States. May be obtained from Panorama Pharmacy, Panorama City, CA; 800-247-9767.
§§In sulfonamide-sensitive patients, pyrimethamine 50 to 75 mg daily has been effective. AIDS patients may need long-term maintenance therapy.
‖‖Atovaquone, 750 mg tid × 1 mo, may control symptoms in some patients. Octreotide may also help to control the diarrhea.
Adapted from Medical Letter: Drugs for parasitic infections. Med Lett Drug Ther *40*:1–12, 1998.

TABLE 2. **Drugs for the Treatment of Helminth Infections**

Infection	Drug	Adult Dosage	Pediatric Dosage
Angiostrongyliasis (*Angiostrongylus costaricensis*) Drug of choice Alternative	Mebendazole (Vermox)* Thiabendazole (Mintezol)†	200–400 mg tid × 10 d 75 mg/kg/d in 3 doses × 3 d (max 3 gm/d); toxicity may require dosage reduction	200–400 mg tid × 10 d 75 mg/kg/d in 3 doses × 3 d (max 3 gm/d); toxicity may require dosage reduction
Anisakiasis (*Anisakis* and other genera) Treatment of choice	Surgical or endoscopic removal		
Ascariasis (*Ascaris lumbricoides*) Drug of choice	Albendazole† or Mebendazole or Pyrantel pamoate (Antiminth)†	400 mg once 100 mg bid × 3 d 11 mg/kg once (max 1 gm)	400 mg once 100 mg bid × 3 d 11 mg/kg once (max 1 gm)
Capillariasis (*Capillaria philippinensis*) Drug of choice Alternative	Mebendazole† Albendazole†	200 mg bid × 20 d 400 mg daily	200 mg bid × 20 d 400 mg daily
Cysticercosis; see Tapeworm infection			
Enterobius vermicularis (pinworm) infection Drug of choice	Pyrantel pamoate or Mebendazole or Albendazole†	11 mg/kg once (max 1 gm); repeat after 2 wk A single dose of 100 mg; repeat after 2 wk 400 mg once; repeat in 2 wk	11 mg/kg once (max 1 gm); repeat after 2 wk A single dose of 100 mg; repeat after 2 wk 400 mg once, repeat in 2 wk
Flukes (intestinal infection) *Fasciolopsis buski, Heterophyes heterophyes, Metagonimus yokogawai* Drug of choice	Praziquantel†	75 mg/kg/d in 3 doses × 1 d	75 mg/kg/d in 3 doses × 1 d
Nanophyetus salmincola Drug of choice	Praziquantel†	60 mg/kg/d in 3 doses × 1 d	60 mg/kg/d in 3 doses × 1 d
Flukes (liver infection) *Clonorchis sinensis* (Chinese liver fluke) Drug of choice	Praziquantel† or Albendazole†	75 mg/kg/d in 3 doses × 1 d 10 mg/kg × 7 d	75 mg/kg/d in 3 doses × 1 d
Fasciola hepatica (sheep liver fluke) Drug of choice‡	Bithionol (Lorothidol)§	30–50 mg/kg on alternate days × 10–15 doses	30–50 mg/kg on alternate days × 10–15 doses
Metorchis conjunctus (North American liver fluke) Drug of choice	Praziquantel†	75 mg/kg/d in 3 doses × 1 d	75 mg/kg/d in 3 doses × 1 d
Opisthorchis viverrini (SE Asian liver fluke) Drug of choice	Praziquantel†	75 mg/kg/d in 3 doses × 1 d	75 mg/kg/d in 3 doses × 1 d
Hookworm infection (*Ancylostoma duodenale, Necator americanus*) Drug of choice	Albendazole† or Mebendazole or Pyrantel pamoate†	400 mg once 100 mg bid × 3 d 11 mg/kg/d (max 1 gm) × 3 d	400 mg once 100 mg bid × 3 d 11 mg/kg (max 1 gm) × 3 d
Schistosomiasis (bilharziasis) *Schistosoma haematobium* Drug of choice	Praziquantel	40 mg/kg/d in 2 doses × 1 d	40 mg/kg/d in 2 doses × 1 d
Schistosoma japonicum Drug of choice	Praziquantel	60 mg/kg/d in 3 doses × 1 d	60 mg/kg/d in 3 doses × 1 d
Schistosoma mansoni Drug of choice Alternative	Praziquantel Oxamniquine (Vansil)‖	40 mg/kg/d in 2 doses × 1 d 15 mg/kg once (higher doses are used in some areas)	40 mg/kg/d in 2 doses × 1 d 20 mg/kg/d in 2 doses × 1 d
Schistosoma mekongi Drug of choice	Praziquantel	60 mg/kg/d in 3 doses × 1 d	60 mg/kg/d in 3 doses × 1 d

TABLE 2. **Drugs for the Treatment of Helminth Infections** *Continued*

Infection	Drug	Adult Dosage	Pediatric Dosage
Strongyloidiasis (*Strongyloides stercoralis*)			
Drug of choice¶	Ivermectin (Stromectol) or	200 µg/kg/d × 1 d	200 µg/kg/d × 1 d
	Thiabendazole	50 mg/kg/d in 2 doses (max 3 gm/d) × 2 d; ≥5 d for hyperinfection	50 mg/kg/d in 2 doses (max 3 gm/d) × 2 d; ≥5 d for hyperinfection
Tapeworm infection—adult (intestinal stage) *Diphyllobothrium latum* (fish), *Taenia saginata* (beef), *Taenia solium* (pork), *Dipylidium caninum* (dog)			
Drug of choice	Praziquantel†	5–10 mg/kg once	5–10 mg/kg once
Hymenolepis nana (dwarf tapeworm)			
Drug of choice	Praziquantel†	25 mg/kg once	25 mg/kg once
Cysticercus cellulosae (cysticercosis)			
Treatment of choice**	Albendazole†† or	400 mg bid × 8–30 d, repeated as necessary	<60 kg, 15 mg/kg/d (max 800 mg) in 2 or 3 doses × 8–30 d, repeated as necessary
	Praziquantel†	50 mg/kg/d in 3 doses × 15 d	50 mg/kg/d in 3 doses × 15 d
Echinococcus granulosus (hydatid cyst)			
Treatment of choice‡‡	Albendazole	400 mg bid × 28 d, repeated as 1 mo courses as necessary	<60 kg, 15 mg/kg/d (max 800 mg) × 28 d, repeated as necessary
Echinococcus multilocularis			
Treatment of choice§§	Surgery		
Alternative	Albendazole for inoperable disease		
Trichinosis (*Trichinella spiralis*)			
Drug of choice	Mebendazole† plus steroids for severe symptoms	200–400 mg tid × 3 d, then 400–500 mg tid × 10 d	
Alternative	Albendazole†,‖ ‖ plus steroids for severe symptoms	400 mg bid × 7–10 d	
Trichostrongylus infection			
Drug of choice	Pyrantel pamoate†	11 mg/kg once (max 1 gm)	11 mg/kg once (max 1 gm)
Alternative	Mebendazole† or	100 mg bid × 3 d	100 mg bid × 3 d
	Albendazole†	400 mg once	400 mg once
Trichuriasis (*Trichuris trichiura*, whipworm)			
Drug of choice	Mebendazole or	100 mg bid × 3 d	100 mg bid × 3 d
	Albendazole†	400 mg once; may require 3 d for heavy infection	400 mg once; may require 3 d for heavy infection

*Exceeds dosage recommended by the manufacturer.

†An approved drug, but considered investigational for this condition by the U.S. FDA.

‡Triclabendazole (Fasinex-Novartis), a veterinary fasciolide, has been safe and effective (79%) after a single dose of 10 mg/kg (Apt W, Aguilera X, Vega F, et al: Treatment of human chronic fascioliasis with triclabendazole: drug efficacy and serologic response. Am J Trop Med Hyg *52*:532–535, 1995).

§Available from the CDC Drug Service, Centers for Disease Control and Prevention, Atlanta, Georgia; 404-639-3670.

‖Oxamniquine may be effective in areas where there is a decreased response to praziquantel (Stelma FF, Sall S, Daff B, et al: Oxamniquine cures *Schistosoma mansoni* infection in a focus in which cure rates with praziquantel are unusually low. J Infect Dis *176*:304–307, 1997).

¶For disseminated infection, ivermectin is not FDA approved, and thiabendazole may be preferred.

**Corticosteroids should be given for 2 to 3 days before therapy and then during treatment for neurocysticercosis. Any cysticercocidal drug may cause irreparable damage when used to treat ocular or spinal cysts, even when corticosteroids are used (White AC: Neurocysticercosis: a major cause of neurological disease worldwide. Clin Infect Dis *24*:101–115, 1997). An ophthalmologic examination should be performed before treatment.

††Eight days of therapy with albendazole may be as effective as 30 days (Botero D, Uribe CS, Sanchez JL, et al: Short course albendazole treatment for neurocysticercosis in Colombia. Trans R Soc Trop Med Hyg *87*:576–577, 1993).

‡‡Some patients will benefit from or require surgical resection of cysts. Praziquantel or albendazole may be used preoperatively or in case of spillage during surgery. Percutaneous drainage under ultrasound or CT guidance, with instillation of a protoscolicide, plus albendazole has been effective for management of hepatic hydatid cysts (see text) (Khuroo MS, Wani NA, Javid G, et al: Percutaneous drainage compared with surgery for hepatic hydatid cysts. N Engl J Med *337*:881–887, 1997).

§§Surgical excision is the only reliable means of therapy; however, some cases may be inoperable. In these situations, high-dose albendazole or mebendazole may be tried (Hao W, Pei-Fan Z, Wen-Guang Y, et al: Albendazole chemotherapy for human cystic and alveolar echinococcosis in north-western China. Trans R Soc Trop Med Hyg *88*:340–343, 1994; World Health Organization (WHO) Informal Working Group on Echinococcosis: Guidelines for treatment of cystic and alveolar echinococcosis in humans. Bull WHO *74*:231–242, 1996).

‖ ‖There is limited information on albendazole efficacy (Cabié A, Bouchaud O, Houzé S, et al: Albendazole versus thiabendazole as therapy for trichinosis: a retrospective study. Clin Infect Dis *22*:1033–1035, 1996).

native drug for children because of its availability in a liquid suspension. However, it must be taken for 10 days and has an efficacy of only 80%. It may cause gastrointestinal side effects, turn urine brown, and cause mild hemolysis in glucose-6-phosphate dehydrogenase–deficient individuals. Although the drug has caused tumors in rodents, this was with long-term, high-dose administration.

Paromomycin (Humatin) is a nonabsorbable aminoglycoside that has been used during pregnancy, particularly in the first trimester by women who cannot be managed by symptomatic therapy alone. It has an efficacy of only 60% but may allow sufficient improvement either to complete the pregnancy or to enter the latter trimesters when metronidazole may be used. Paromomycin should not be appreciably absorbed, but it is prudent not to be used by persons with pre-existent renal insufficiency. Albendazole (Albenza), a benzimidazole, has limited experience in giardiasis, but, when given in a 5-day course, efficacy may approach 90%.

For the infrequent patients who experience failure of one drug course or relapse, a second course of the same drug or a switch to a drug of a different class is generally effective. Rare individuals may require a course of combined metronidazole and quinacrine.

Entamoeba histolytica

About 500,000,000 persons worldwide are infected with either *Entamoeba histolytica* or the morphologically indistinguishable but nonpathogenic *E. dispar*. Ninety percent of these infections are probably with *E. dispar*. Disease is caused by *E. histolytica* and ranges from asymptomatic passage of cysts to dysenteric colitis. Extraintestinal spread of ameba complicates infection in about 10% of patients with *E. histolytica*; amebic liver abscess is the most common site. Patients with amebiasis can be diagnosed by detection of hematophagous trophozoites in the stool or by sigmoidoscopy with scraping of a rectal ulcer. Serology is positive in about 80% of persons with intestinal disease and in more than 95% of those with liver abscess.

An important principle of therapy is to use drugs that are active in the lumen of the gut for the treatment of noninvasive infection and those that are active in the tissues for invasive disease (e.g., for dysenteric colitis and liver abscess). Use of only a tissue-active agent in cases of invasive disease can result in relapse of infection.

Luminal agents are iodoquinol (Yodoxin), paromomycin, and diloxanide furoate (Furamide). Iodoquinol is given for 20 days, paromomycin for 7 days, and diloxanide furoate for 10 days. Side effects with iodoquinol are rash, nausea, diarrhea, and, rarely, optic neuritis and peripheral neuropathy. A maximum dose of 2 grams per day should not be exceeded. It should also not be used by persons with iodine sensitivity. Diloxanide furoate can cause nausea, vomiting, diarrhea, and, rarely, diplopia, dizziness, and urticaria.

For treatment of either intestinal or extraintestinal invasive disease, metronidazole is the drug of choice. It is given in a higher dose (750 mg) than that used for giardiasis and for a longer period of time (10 days). If available, tinidazole is also effective. Immediately after metronidazole or tinidazole is administered, a luminal agent should be given. Medical therapy alone is usually sufficient for amebic liver abscess, with clinical improvement over 3 to 5 days. When the abscess may be in danger of rupture or the patient fails to improve clinically, percutaneous drainage may be needed.

Cryptosporidium

C. parvum is an intestinal coccidian parasite, which means that a portion of its replication cycle occurs within cells. It is transmitted by the fecal-oral route and resides on the surface of intestinal epithelial cells, under a host cell membrane, but external to the cytoplasm. It is widely distributed throughout the animal kingdom and is an important cause of water-borne outbreaks of diarrhea. In normal hosts it causes a watery, nonbloody diarrhea, often with nausea, cramping, and vomiting, but is self-limited, lasting days to a few weeks. In the immunocompromised host, usually patients with acquired immunodeficiency syndrome (AIDS), it is associated with voluminous (occasionally greater than 10 L), dehydrating diarrhea and leads to wasting and significant morbidity. Diagnosis is usually by DFA assays performed on the stool that detect the small, 2- to 6-μm cysts.

There is currently no reliable therapy to eradicate *Cryptosporidium* despite trials with many agents. For the normal host, treatment is supportive because diarrhea is self-limited. In the immunocompromised host, it is important to maintain hydration and electrolyte balance and to attempt to control the diarrhea. Antimotility agents may be helpful, but they should be used cautiously. Paromomycin has been successful in some patients in doses slightly higher than those used to treat giardiasis. If there is a response, paromomycin may need to be continued indefinitely in a maintenance dose of 1 to 2 grams per day. Azithromycin (Zithromax)* may also be effective, although there have been only limited clinical trials with this drug. Octreotide (Sandostatin)* has been given in an effort to limit intestinal fluid losses, but has had only variable efficacy. Efforts to improve the patient's immune system with highly active anti-retroviral therapy (HAART) may also help in clearing or controlling infection.

Cyclospora

Cyclospora cayetanensis is a recently recognized parasite. It was first thought to be a member of the blue-green algae or cyanobacteria but has now been identified as a coccidian protozoan. It causes prolonged diarrhea in normal hosts and was first described in travelers and expatriates in Nepal. In North America, there have been outbreaks of diar-

---

*Not FDA approved for this indication.

rhea associated with raspberries imported from Central America and also with lettuce and other fresh produce. A modified Kinyoun acid-fast stain of the stool can detect the 8- to 10-μm cysts. Treatment is effective with trimethoprim-sulfamethoxazole* twice daily for 1 week. HIV-infected patients may require longer treatment and then thrice-weekly suppressive therapy.

Isospora belli

Isospora belli is a coccidian parasite that undergoes asexual replication within human intestinal epithelial cells. It is a rare cause of diarrhea in the United States; however, the HIV epidemic has increased its recognition, primarily in patients from developing regions. Diagnosis is by demonstration of large, oval oocysts (~13 × 28 μm) containing two sporoblasts with the modified acid-fast stain. Treatment of the normal host is with trimethoprim-sulfamethoxazole.* If a patient has a sulfonamide allergy, pyrimethamine (Daraprim)* alone (50 to 75 mg per day for adults) may be tried. Long-term use of these medications may be accompanied by anemia and leukopenia, and folinic acid (5 to 10 mg per day) should be used to try to prevent marrow suppression. AIDS patients may require long-term prophylaxis with low-dose pyrimethamine (25 mg) or trimethoprim-sulfamethoxazole.

Microsporidia

Microsporidia are obligate intracellular protozoans with over 100 genera and 1000 species. Species of the genera Enterocytozoon and Encephalitozoon (Septata) are associated with diarrhea in humans. Nearly all cases are in immunosuppressed hosts, particularly those with HIV infection. Microsporidia cause chronic diarrhea and occasionally can extend into the biliary tree or disseminate to other organs such as the liver, muscle, central nervous system, and eye. A modified trichrome stain is required to identify microsporidia in the stool or duodenal contents by light microscopy; however, a duodenal biopsy with electron microscopy may still be needed. Albendazole* is the agent of choice to treat diarrhea caused by Enterocytozoon bieneusi and Encephalitozoon intestinalis. For compromised patients, it may need to be continued chronically. Atovaquone (Mepron),* 750 mg three times a day, has shown promise in preliminary trials for Enterocytozoon. Improvement in an AIDS patient's immune status with the use of HAART may also help to clear parasites.

Less Common Protozoa

Dientamoeba fragilis is a noninvasive amebo-flagellate existing solely in the trophozoite form and thus requires direct fecal-oral transmission for infection. Although it can be found in as many as 5% of stools, it frequently causes no symptoms. Symptomatic patients complain of mild diarrhea and abdominal discomfort. Treatment is with iodoquinol,* tetracycline,* or paromomycin.*

Balantidium coli is the largest intestinal protozoan of humans. It is ciliated and has a characteristic kidney bean–shaped nucleus. Although it is a rare cause of infection in the United States, it may be seen in tropical zones when humans are in association with pigs and, less commonly, with rats. It causes locally invasive disease in the colon, which may present asymptomatically as dysenteric colitis and, rarely, as colonic perforation. Treatment is with tetracycline.* Alternatives are iodoquinol* and metronidazole,* although the latter may not be consistently effective.

The role of Blastocystis hominis in symptomatic diarrhea is controversial. It is possible that this parasite can be a cause of diarrhea in patients for whom no other etiology can be found. In these cases, treatment is effective with amebicidal doses of metronidazole* for 10 days or iodoquinol* for 20 days.

Nonpathogenic Protozoa

Although it may be difficult to definitively classify a protozoan infection as nonpathogenic, there are several that have not been associated with symptoms. These infections generally occur in settings of poor fecal-oral hygiene and are often a marker of such. These protozoa include the amebae Entamoeba hartmanni, Entamoeba coli, Endolimax nana, and Iodamoeba bütschlii and the flagellates Chilomastix mesnili and Trichomonas hominis. Treatment of these infections is not required.

Intestinal Helminths

Intestinal helminths are classified as nematodes (roundworms) or platyhelminths (flatworms). Nematodes may reside in the lumen of the gut (e.g., hookworm and Ascaris) or the tissues of the human host (e.g., trichinella). Flatworms are subdivided into cestodes (tapeworms) and trematodes (flukes). When a human is the definitive host for cestode infections, the adult tapeworm (e.g., Taenia saginata) resides in the lumen of the gut. When a human acts as the intermediate host, larval forms of the cestodes (e.g., cysticercosis and echinococcosis) invade tissue, causing space-occupying lesions.

Therapy for intestinal helminths (Table 2) can be easily summarized: Each group of worms is treated by agents of only one or two classes of drugs. Albendazole plays a prominent role in therapy of nearly all helminths except trematode and intestinal cestode infections. Nematodes that live in the gut lumen are treated with benzimidazoles (albendazole and mebendazole [Vermox]) or pyrantel pamoate (Antiminth). Tissue nematodes are treated with the benzimidazoles; ivermectin (Stromectol) can be used for strongyloidiasis. Intestinal cestode infections are treated with praziquantel (Biltricide) and the larval

---

*Not FDA approved for this indication.

*Not FDA approved for this indication.

forms with albendazole or praziquantel. All trematode infections are treated with praziquantel.

Nematodes (Roundworms)

The most common intestinal roundworms are ascaris (*Ascaris lumbricoides*), hookworm (*Necator americanus* and *Ancylostoma duodenale*), whipworm (*Trichuris trichiura*), and pinworm (*Enterobius vermicularis*). Ascaris, hookworm, and whipworm are infections that occur in temperate to tropical climates when there is fecal contamination of the soil. In each of these infections, eggs that are passed in the feces need a period of time to mature in the soil before they either are ingested (ascaris and whipworm) or hatch and release larvae that penetrate the skin of the human host (hookworm). Although infections with these worms is most common in developing areas of the world, they are found in North America in immigrants, returned travelers, and residents of the southern United States. Children in all areas have the highest burden of disease and are often infected with more than one parasite. In contrast, pinworm is common in children from all socioeconomic groups in industrialized areas.

Ascaris is the largest (15 cm) of the nematodes. After the eggs are ingested, the larval form has a tissue phase, passing through the lungs before developing into an adult worm that lives in the small bowel. Treatment of ascaris is with a benzimidazole, mebendazole or albendazole,* or pyrantel pamoate. Mebendazole has been the traditional therapy and is given twice daily for three days. The advantage of albendazole and pyrantel pamoate is that they need to be given in only a single dose. Because albendazole also treats hookworm and whipworm, it has been used in mass treatment campaigns for children living in developing regions and resulted in improved weight and school performance. During therapy, *Ascaris* organisms may emerge from the nose or mouth. If an ascarid has migrated into the biliary tree, it can often be treated conservatively but may necessitate endoscopic retrograde cholangiopancreatography or surgery for removal.

Both albendazole and mebendazole are poorly absorbed, but this is not a major problem when they are being used to treat luminal worms. Albendazole absorption may be enhanced by ingestion of the drug with a fatty meal. The mechanism of action of these agents is likely to be inhibition of tubulin polymerization with loss of cytoplasmic microtubules. This also results in blockage of glucose uptake and subsequent glycogen depletion. Albendazole is metabolized to its active, primary metabolite, albendazole sulfoxide, which is widely distributed throughout body tissues, including the central nervous system and cyst cavities such as are present in echinococcosis. Mebendazole and albendazole are generally well tolerated, but can be associated with abdominal discomfort, particularly when in the treatment of individuals with large worm burdens. Other side effects are usually seen only when the drugs are used in high doses for prolonged therapy of larval cestode infections. These side effects include increased serum transaminases with albendazole and, rarely, bone marrow toxicity, rash, and renal toxicity with albendazole and hypospermia with mebendazole. Both drugs are category C agents and should not be used during pregnancy because of potential teratogenicity. Pyrantel pamoate is a neuromuscular blocking agent. It occasionally causes gastrointestinal symptoms, headache, dizziness, and rash.

Humans are infected by hookworms when larvae that are present in fecally contaminated soil penetrate the skin, migrate through the lungs, and develop to adulthood in the small bowel. Wearing shoes is, therefore, a helpful preventive measure. Most light infections are asymptomatic; however, heavy infections may be associated with nonspecific gastrointestinal upset, anemia, and hypoalbuminemia. Treatment of infection is with 3 days of mebendazole or pyrantel pamoate* or a single dose of albendazole.* In addition to anthelminthic therapy, iron should be given to correct any associated anemia.

Larvae of the dog or cat hookworm *Ancylostoma caninum* and *Ancylostoma braziliense*, respectively, can penetrate the skin of humans but are unable to complete their life cycle and, therefore, wander subcutaneously, causing an intensely pruritic, localized reaction. This illness, cutaneous larva migrans, can be treated with albendazole (400 mg daily for 1 to 3 days),* ivermectin (12 mg) in a single dose, or topical thiabendazole (15% for 3 to 5 days).* It should not be approached surgically or with topical freezing.

Most infections with whipworm are asymptomatic. Heavy infections are associated with colonic irritation with blood-streaked stool, abdominal pain, weight loss, anemia, and, rarely, rectal prolapse. Mebendazole and albendazole* are the drugs of choice.

Pinworm causes mild pruritus ani. Occasionally the adult female migrates to other sites such as the vagina, endometrium, or peritoneum and causes granulomatous disease. Pinworm is best diagnosed by touching the perianal region with a tongue blade covered with reversed scotch tape and examining the tape under the microscope for pinworm eggs. A single dose of pyrantel pamoate (available over the counter in the United States for treatment of pinworm), mebendazole, or albendazole is an appropriate therapy. A second dose of the agent is given after 2 weeks. Control of pinworm within the household may require family members to be screened and treated. Additional measures include better personal hygiene and laundering of bedclothes, sheets, and towels to kill ova.

Strongyloides stercoralis

Similar to hookworm, initial infection with *Strongyloides* is by larval penetration of exposed skin. Adult worms reside in the intestinal mucosa, where

---

*Not FDA approved for this indication.

*Not FDA approved for this indication.

they mate and produce eggs. Eggs hatch in the intestine, and larvae may mature sufficiently to reinfect the host rather than need a period of time in soil to fully mature. This autoinfection cycle accounts for persistent infection seen many years to even decades after the person departs from an endemic area. Symptoms in strongyloidiasis include nausea, diarrhea and occasionally vomiting, and an urticarial rash. In persons immunocompromised through organ transplantation, corticosteroids, or other immunosuppressive drugs, autoinfection can evolve into a hyperinfection syndrome with wide dissemination of larvae. AIDS patients have also presented with dissemination, particularly when they are co-infected with human T cell lymphotropic virus type I (HTLV-I). Diagnosis is by detection of larvae, not ova, in the stool or duodenal contents.

Ivermectin has now emerged as the treatment of choice for uncomplicated strongyloidiasis because it is well-tolerated compared with the traditionally used thiabendazole (Mintezol). It is given in a single dose (200 μm/kg or 12 mg in adults) for one day. For hyperinfection, thiabendazole may be preferred, and treatment needs to be continued for 5 to 7 days. If infection cannot be cleared or immunosuppression reversed, monthly 2-day courses of therapy may be necessary to prevent dissemination. Ivermectin has few side effects when used for this indication. In contrast, with thiabendazole, side effects are common and consist of headache, vertigo, weakness, nausea and vomiting, and pruritus. Erythema multiforme, leukopenia, neuropsychiatric effects, and, rarely, shock, cholestasis, and Stevens-Johnson syndrome have been documented with thiabendazole.

Trichinella spiralis

Trichinosis is acquired by ingestion of undercooked meat from domestically raised pigs, wild bear, boar, or other mammals. Larvae that have encysted in the muscle of infected animals are released, invade the intestinal mucosa, and mature to adult worms in the intestine, where they mate and produce larvae that invade human muscle and rarely the central nervous system. Initially there is nausea, vomiting, cramping, and diarrhea and then, during muscle invasion, myalgias, facial edema, fever, and mental status changes if there has been central nervous system invasion. Clinical symptoms are proportional to the number of larvae that invade the tissues. The need for treatment is controversial as antiparasitic therapy is not entirely satisfactory. Steroids (40 to 60 mg of prednisone daily) are usually given to reduce severe symptoms associated with larval invasion. In mild cases, antipyretics and analgesics may be sufficient. Traditional antiparasitic therapy is with mebendazole* in an escalating dose. Although data are limited, albendazole* may be an effective alternative.

Other Nematodes

When native or returned travelers from the Philippines and, less commonly, Southeast Asia, present with abdominal pain, diarrhea, and signs of malabsorption, capillariasis (*Capillaria philippinensis*) should be suspected. This filamentous nematode is acquired through ingestion of raw freshwater fish. Treatment is effective with mebendazole for 20 days or albendazole for 10 days.

Ingestion of raw marine fish such as mackerel, salmon, and herring or squid can lead to an infection of the stomach or upper small bowel with the larval forms of *Anisakis* nematodes. These infections are particularly common in Japan where ingestion of raw seafood in the form of sushi or sashimi is popular. There are no worms or eggs detected in the stool; therefore, one has to have a high index of clinical suspicion to detect such infections. In the gastric form, larvae can be detected endoscopically, often burrowing into the gastric mucosa. Treatment of this form is by endoscopic or surgical removal. In the intestinal form with abdominal pain and diarrhea, there is no effective drug therapy. Fish may be rendered noninfectious by being heated above 60°C or frozen at −20°C for 24 hours or −10°C for 7 days.

Trichostrongylus is a zoonotic nematode rarely causing infection in residents of the Middle and Far East. Most infections are light and asymptomatic. Heavy infections can produce gastrointestinal symptoms and should be treated. Treatment is with a single dose of pyrantel pamoate*; a single dose of albendazole* or 3 days of mebendazole* is an alternative.

Angiostrongylus costaricensis is a rodent nematode acquired in Latin America by ingestion of raw slugs (the parasite's intermediate host) or produce contaminated by the slug's secretions. The parasite can cause granulomatous, eosinophilic masses in the intestine after invasion of mesenteric arterioles. Patients may be thought to have appendicitis or a neoplasm until the diagnosis is made at surgery. Mebendazole* is the drug of choice. High-dose thiabendazole* is an alternative, but may be poorly tolerated.

Trematodes (Flatworms or Flukes)

SCHISTOSOMA SPECIES

The schistosomes are the most important of the trematodes that cause infections and account for over 200 million cases worldwide. *Schistosoma mansoni* is widely distributed throughout Africa and parts of Latin America and the Caribbean and is the most common of the intestinal schistosomes imported into North America. *S. japonica* from East Asia, *S. mekongi* from Southeast Asia, and *S. intercalatum* from Central Africa are rarely seen. The urinary form of schistosomiasis is caused by *S. haematobium* and originates from Africa and the Middle East. There have been cases of *S. haematobium* in persons exposed to river and lake water in East Africa.

Schistosomiasis (bilharziasis) is acquired when the larval forms, cercariae, penetrate the skin of humans

---

*Not FDA approved for this indication.

*Not FDA approved for this indication.

during exposure to fresh water. The larvae develop into adult worms that migrate and reside in either the venules of the mesenteric plexus (intestinal schistosomes) or the bladder (*S. haematobium*). Male and female worms mate and produce eggs. Eggs and egg products stimulate a host inflammatory reaction that results in extrusion of the eggs through the mucosa of the intestine or bladder and then passage into the environment via either the feces or urine. In intestinal infection, eggs are carried back to the liver, where a granulomatous reaction to them over a period of years can lead to periportal fibrosis, portal hypertension, splenomegaly, and esophageal varices.

All forms of schistosomiasis are treated with a 1-day course of praziquantel (Biltricide), although the dose varies depending on the species. Cure rates range from 60 to 100%. Although the exact mechanism of action for this agent is not known, detectable effects include flaccid paralysis of the worm and vacuolization and degeneration of the schistosome tegument. Both of these effects are associated with an influx of calcium ions into the worm. Praziquantel is tolerated well by most patients; however, some complain of headache, malaise, and abdominal discomfort. Rash and pruritus have also been described. An alternative agent for *S. mansoni* is oxamniquine (Vansil). This has been effective in areas where the population has a decreased response to praziquantel. Oxamniquine has caused neuropsychiatric disturbances, rash, elevation of liver enzymes, and electrocardiographic changes. Seizures have been rarely reported, and the drug should not be used during pregnancy.

OTHER INTESTINAL, LIVER, AND LUNG FLUKES

There are many other flukes that reside in the intestine and others that migrate to the liver and the lung. Praziquantel in a 1- or 2-day regimen is the treatment of choice for all of these except the sheep liver fluke, *Fasciola hepatica*. Acquisition of these infections occurs by ingesting uncooked freshwater plants (*Fasciolopsis buski*), raw crabs (*Paragonimus westermani*), and fish (*Heterophyes heterophyes, Metagonimus yokogawai, Nanophyetus salmincola, Clonorchis sinensis*, and *Opisthorchis viverrini*). Infections with the intestinal flukes *Fasiolopsis buski, H. heterophyes*, and *M. yokogawai* are rarely seen in North America. The liver flukes *C. sinensis* and *O. viverrini* are both acquired in Southeast Asia and usually occur in immigrant populations. The lung fluke *P. westermani* resides in the lung, producing eggs that are expelled in the sputum; illness may be confused with tuberculosis in immigrants from Southeast Asia. Bithionol (Bitin) is the drug of choice for *Fasciola hepatica*. It has been associated with urticaria, photosensitivity, vomiting, abdominal pain, diarrhea, and, rarely, leukopenia and hepatitis.

Cestodes (Tapeworms)

Most tapeworm infections are acquired when humans ingest undercooked meat or fish that contains encysted larvae. Larvae then develop into adult tapeworms within the intestine, and the person becomes the definitive host. Although the size of the *Taenia* worms is impressive (reaching 4 to 6 m) and patients may be disturbed by the passage of motile proglottids, there are usually few symptoms related to these helminths. The fish tapeworm *Diphyllobothrium latum* can compete for vitamin B_{12} in the host, causing a megaloblastic anemia. For *D. latum, Taenia solium* (pork), *T. saginata* (beef), and *Dipylidium canium* (an accidental infection when a dog or cat flea is ingested), a single dose of praziquantel is extremely effective and results in cures approaching 100%. For the dwarf tapeworm *Hymenolepis nana*, which is acquired when ova are ingested in fecally contaminated foods, higher doses of praziquantel* are needed. Purging is not necessary after treatment; there does not appear to be a danger of regurgitating and ingesting eggs or infective proglottids during treatment.

Tapeworm infections are a major problem when humans become the intermediate host and larval worms invade their tissues. This occurs with two tapeworms, *T. solium*, which causes cysticercosis, and *Echinococcus granulosus* and *E. multilocularis*, which cause echinococcosis. The most common site for dissemination in cysticercosis is to the brain where it causes space-occupying lesions with neurologic symptoms. The eye and muscle may also be invaded. Cysticercosis is seen where pigs and people coexist in areas of poor sanitation; it is a frequent infection in Mexico, Central and South America, and parts of Asia, Africa, and Eastern Europe. The variability in the clinical course and the lack of standardized clinical trials have led to controversy in management.

Treatment of cysticercosis may involve observation, specific antiparasitic therapy with albendazole or praziquantel,* corticosteroids to decrease the inflammatory response to parasites, and surgical removal of lesions that lie in critical sites of the central nervous system. Patients who are having seizures secondary to lesions require anticonvulsant therapy.

For active parenchymal lesions, albendazole and praziquantel are the drugs of choice. Albendazole should be taken with a fatty meal to aid in its absorption. Praziquantel levels may be decreased by steroid or anticonvulsant therapy. Many experts would use corticosteroids beginning 2 to 3 days before therapy and then during therapy to decrease an inflammatory response to dying larval worms. Because the reaction to dying larvae can cause irreparable ocular disease, a careful ophthalmologic examination should be done before initiating treatment. For single parenchymal lesions or lesions that are entirely calcified, antiparasitic treatment may not be necessary. For extraparenchymal infection with hydrocephalus, a shunting procedure or surgery may be required.

The definitive host for *Echinococcus* is the dog, although other mammals such as wolf, jackal, coyote, and fox (for multilocularis) may be infected. Infection in humans is seen when they are living in close

---

*Not FDA approved for this indication.

proximity to dogs that have access to the viscera of intermediate hosts. Sheep are frequently an intermediate host; thus in North America endemic infection is seen in sheep-raising areas of Utah, Arizona, and Nevada. In Alaska, human cases may be secondary to a parasite cycle in wolves, caribou, and moose. Nevertheless, most cases are in immigrants. In humans with cystic hydatid disease caused by *E. granulosus*, the liver is affected in two thirds of cases, the lung in nearly one fourth, and other sites less frequently. The more aggressive alveolar hydatid disease is caused by *E. multilocularis*.

Surgery has been the traditional mode of therapy for cystic hydatid disease. With the addition of benzimidazoles, however, medical therapy and combination treatments are becoming options. If open surgery is performed, a course of albendazole should begin at least 4 days before surgery and continue for a month to prevent the risk of peritoneal implantation if there has been spillage during the procedure.

Albendazole will decrease the viability of protoscolices, cysts, and larvae. Protoscolicides such as 15 to 20% hypertonic saline, 70 to 95% ethanol, or 0.5% cetrimide can be instilled at the time of surgery but are occasionally associated with systemic reactions. An alternative to open surgery is drainage percutaneously. The latter has acquired the acronym PAIR (puncture, aspiration, injection, reaspiration). The cyst is punctured, the contents aspirated with evacuation of the cyst, and then a scolicidal agent is instilled. This is then reaspirated.

Patients with cysts in multiple organs or with inoperable disease are usually treated medically with high-dose albendazole or mebendazole. Therapy needs to be cycled monthly for at least three cycles with regular follow-up of a patient's response by imaging techniques. For alveolar hydatid disease, radical surgery is usually the treatment of choice; if the disease is inoperable, prolonged medical therapy is needed with careful monitoring for hepatic, bone marrow, and renal drug toxicity.

Metabolic Disorders

DIABETES MELLITUS IN ADULTS

method of
W. TIMOTHY GARVEY, M.D.
*Medical University of South Carolina and
Charleston Veterans Affairs Medical Center
Charleston, South Carolina*

EPIDEMIOLOGY

Diabetes mellitus is a common disease and has been steadily increasing in prevalence in the western hemisphere since the 1950s. In the United States, the third National Health and Nutrition Examination Survey (1988 to 1994) found that the prevalence of diagnosed diabetes is 7.2% and that of undiagnosed diabetes is 4.0% among non-Hispanic white persons. Diabetes is even more common in other racial and ethnic populations; the prevalence of diagnosed and undiagnosed diabetes is 18% in African-Americans, 23% among Hispanic Americans, and 25 to 50% in various Native American tribal communities.* Approximately 5 to 8% of diabetic patients have type 1 diabetes resulting from autoimmune destruction of insulin-producing beta cells in pancreatic islets of Langerhans. This results in absolute insulin deficiency, and exogenous insulin therapy is needed to sustain life by preventing progressive hyperglycemia, catabolism, dehydration, and ketoacidosis. Most patients develop type 1 diabetes in adolescence or childhood; however, the disease can also develop in adults. This article does not discuss treatment for type 1 diabetes because therapeutic principles in adults with type 1 diabetes overlap with those discussed in the article "Diabetes Mellitus in Children." This article instead focuses on treatment of type 2 diabetes mellitus.

The majority of diabetic patients (90%) have type 2 diabetes, which also accounts for the high prevalence of diabetes in nonwhite populations. Type 2 diabetes can develop at any age; however, the incidence increases sharply as a function of aging between 40 and 70 years of life. Eighty percent of patients with type 2 diabetes are obese, which indicates that obesity is an important contributor to pathogenesis in many patients. The reason for the rising prevalence of diabetes is multifactorial, but this rise can be explained partly by the increasing frequency of obesity and sedentary lifestyle, the increasing mean age of populations, and higher birth rates in racial groups at increased risk of the disease.

The personal and public burden of diabetes results largely from the chronic complications of the disease. Diabetes is the most common cause of blindness in adults and is the leading cause of end-stage renal disease now responsible for 42% of all patients requiring hemodialysis for the first time. Diabetes increases the risk of lower extremity amputation by 10- to 15-fold and contributes heavily to stroke and coronary heart disease. Although the overall rate of mortality from cardiovascular disease is decreasing in the United States, the rate of cardiovascular mortality from diabetes is steadily increasing. The treatment of diabetes and its complications accounts for $1 in every $7 of health care expenses in the United States and one fourth of Medicaid expenditures. Thus diabetes accounts for a tremendous burden of patient suffering and public health expense. As discussed later, it is now clear that microvascular disease complications (retinopathy, nephropathy, and neuropathy) can be significantly prevented by good glycemic control and that macrovascular disease (coronary, peripheral, and cerebrovascular disease) can be prevented by aggressive management of risk factors. These goals can be accomplished effectively by intensive management programs employing a team of multidisciplinary health care professionals. Unfortunately, many health care systems have not invested resources for optimal management. Contributing to the problem are an endemic attitude among physicians in practice that diabetes is not a "serious" disease and the failure of medical school and residency program curricula to instruct trainees in principles of intensive diabetes and cardiovascular risk factor management. As a consequence, standards of care developed for optimal diabetes management are not achieved in many practice settings.

CLASSIFICATION AND DIAGNOSIS

A standard for the classification and diagnosis of diabetes mellitus was developed by the National Diabetes Data Group in 1979,* and modifications have been recommended based on newer data by an Expert Committee assembled by the American Diabetes Association (ADA).† The classification for diabetes recommended by the Expert Committee is shown in Table 1. "Type 1 diabetes" is the term used in place of "insulin-dependent" or "juvenile-onset diabetes," and "type 2 diabetes" is used in place of "non–insulin-dependent" or "adult-onset diabetes." The Expert Committee listed three criteria for the diagnosis of diabetes (Table 2): (1) presence of the classic symptoms of diabetes (polyuria, polydipsia, and unexplained weight loss) plus a random glucose level of 200 mg or more per dL; (2) fasting plasma glucose level of 126 mg or more per dL on more than one occasion; and (3) 2-hour plasma glucose value of 200 mg or more per dL during a 75-gram oral glucose tolerance test. Venous blood samples, rather than finger stick samples, are preferred for accurate plasma glucose determinations.

The most significant change from the previous criteria

---

*See Harris MI: Diabetes in America: Epidemiology and scope of the problem. Diabetes Care *21*(Suppl 3):C11–C14, 1998.

*See National Diabetes Data Group: Classification and diagnosis of diabetes mellitus and other categories of glucose intolerance. Diabetes *28*:1039–1057, 1979.

†See The Expert Committee on the Diagnosis and Classification of Diabetes Mellitus: Report of the Expert Committee on the Diagnosis and Classification of Diabetes Mellitus. Diabetes Care *21*(Suppl 1):S5–S22, 1998.

TABLE 1. **Etiologic Classification of Diabetes Mellitus**

Type 1 diabetes (beta cell destruction leading to absolute insulin deficiency)
    Immune-mediated
    Idiopathic
Type 2 diabetes (combined defects causing insulin resistance and relative insulin deficiency)
Other specific types
    Genetic defects of beta cell function (e.g., glucokinase mutation in maturity onset diabetes of the young)
    Genetic defects in insulin action (e.g., insulin receptor mutation in type A insulin resistance)
    Diseases of the exocrine pancrease (e.g., pancreatitis, cystic fibrosis, hemochromatosis)
    Endocrinopathies (e.g., Cushing's syndrome, acromegaly, pheochromocytoma)
    Drug or chemical-induced (e.g., pentamidine, diazoxide, glucocorticoids)
    Infections (e.g., cytomegalovirus)
    Uncommon forms of immune-mediated diabetes (e.g., anti-insulin receptor antibodies)
    Genetic syndromes associated with diabetes (e.g., Turner's syndrome, Friedreich's ataxia, Klinefelter's syndrome)
Gestational diabetes mellitus

was reducing the fasting glucose criterion from 140 to 126 mg per dL. The purpose of the less stringent criterion was to qualify patients with milder degrees of glucose intolerance for the diagnosis of diabetes because they are still at risk for diabetes-related complications. Two categories of abnormal glucose tolerance are recognized as intermediate between normal glucose tolerance and diabetes: "impaired fasting glucose" indicates a fasting glucose level of 110 to less than 126 mg per dL, and "impaired glucose tolerance" indicates a 2-hour glucose level of 140 to less than 200 mg per dL during an oral glucose tolerance test. Therefore, normal fasting plasma glucose concentrations are 109 mg or less per dL under fasting conditions and 139 mg or less per dL at 2 hours during an oral glucose tolerance test. In clinical practice, it is rarely necessary to perform an oral glucose tolerance test (except in the diagnosis of gestational diabetes), inasmuch as diabetes can reliably be identified on clinical grounds combined with measurement of the fasting plasma glucose concentration.

Screening for type 2 diabetes should involve measurement of the fasting plasma glucose level. The ADA recommends screening patients aged 45 years and older and younger patients in high-risk categories (i.e., obesity, diabetes in first-degree relatives, high-risk ethnic populations, previous gestational diabetes, hypertension, high-density lipoprotein [HDL] cholesterol level ≤ 35 mg [0.9 mmol] per dL, and triglyceride level ≥ 250 mg [2.8 mmol] per dL). However, there is evidence that it is cost-effective to screen younger persons regardless of risk, because if the disease is caught early, this will potentially result in more complication-free years in patients whose disease is managed intensively. Along these lines, epidemiologic data indicate that the disease is undiagnosed in approximately 40% of patients and that 25% of patients with newly diagnosed disease already have background retinopathy. Patients with undiagnosed disease are also predisposed to accelerated progression of atherosclerosis. Therefore, clinicians should set a low threshold for diabetes screening in an effort to facilitate early diagnosis and treatment.

A separate diagnostic and screening scheme is recommended for gestational diabetes. In the United States, most obstetricians employ a 50-gram oral glucose challenge

for screening between 24 and 28 weeks of pregnancy; a 1-hour value of 140 mg (7.8 mmol) per dL or higher is considered abnormal. This finding is followed by a 3-hour, 100-gram, diagnostic, oral glucose tolerance test in the fasting state. Gestational diabetes is diagnosed if two of four values are abnormal during the glucose tolerance test (abnormal values are as follows: fasting plasma glucose level, ≥105 mg per dL; 1-hour level, ≥190 mg per dL; 2-hour level, ≥165 mg per dL; and 3-hour level, ≥145 mg per dL). Efforts are being made to establish an international standard for the diagnosis of gestational diabetes through a 75-gram oral glucose tolerance test, as recommended by the World Health Organization.

PATHOPHYSIOLOGY

Both genetic and environmental factors are important in the pathogenesis of type 2 diabetes. The disease aggregates within families, and concordance rates are higher in monozygotic twin pairs (60 to 90%) than in dizygotic twins (30 to 40%). Transmission is consistent with a polygenic form of inheritance. Causal mutations have been identified in rare monogenic forms of type 2 diabetes: for example, mutations in the insulin receptor gene in patients with type A severe insulin resistance and acanthosis nigricans, and mutations in the glucokinase gene in some families with maturity onset diabetes of the young. Patients with single gene mutations exhibit a particular subphenotype of the disease and mild forms of diabetes. The polygenes that contribute to the common form of type 2 diabetes have not yet been elucidated. It is likely that type 2 diabetes is heterogeneous in that multiple polygenic forms of the disease share many characteristics of a common phenotype. Environmental determinants that predispose to the disease include physical inactivity, obesity, and high-calorie, high-fat diets. The presence of the insulin resistance syndrome (to be described) also signifies high risk for the development of diabetes, and this syndrome is epidemiologically related to low birth weight and nutritional stress in utero. The interaction between genes and environment is evident in the example of when groups of Africans, Australian aborigines, or Amerindians, who have a low prevalence of type 2 diabetes in their native cultures, adopt a western lifestyle and develop diabetes at higher rates than do other racial and ethnic groups in the same environment.

Although type 2 diabetes may be heterogeneous, several major metabolic defects consistently contribute to hyperglycemia. These major defects include (1) peripheral insulin resistance that results from decreased glucose transport activity in skeletal muscle; (2) impaired insulin secretion

TABLE 2. **Diagnostic Criteria for Diabetes Mellitus and Abnormal Glucose Tolerance**

Criteria for Diabetes Mellitus
Symptoms of hyperglycemia with random plasma glucose level ≥ 200 mg/dL (11.1 mmol)
Fasting plasma glucose level ≥ 126 mg/dL (7.0 mmol) on at least two occasions
2-hour plasma glucose level ≥ 200 mg/dL (11.1 mmol) after 75-gm oral glucose challenge
Abnormal Glucose Tolerance
Impaired fasting glucose: fasting plasma glucose level ≥ 110 mg/dL (6.1 mmol) but < 126 mg/dL (7.0 mmol)
Impaired glucose tolerance: 2-hour glucose ≥ 140 mg/dL (7.8 mmol) but < 200 mg/dL (11.1 mmol) after 75-gm oral glucose challenge

in response to glucose; and (3) elevated rates of hepatic glucose production. All three of these metabolic defects are present in overt diabetes and contribute importantly to the diabetic state. Thus amelioration of any single defect improves glucose tolerance. Multiple new classes of oral agents that differentially act to correct these various defects have been introduced. An understanding of the metabolic pathogenesis of diabetes can facilitate the rational use of these therapeutic agents.

An important question concerns which of these metabolic defects are primary and which are secondary (i.e., acquired) in the evolution of the diabetic state. In persons who are destined to develop diabetes (prediabetes), prospective studies have demonstrated that insulin resistance is the most prominent and earliest metabolic defect that can be detected and confers high risk for subsequent evolution to overt diabetes. Thus insulin resistance is not only critical to maintenance of hyperglycemia in type 2 diabetes but is also a primary and early defect in its development. In prediabetic patients, both fasting and postprandial serum insulin concentrations are elevated in an attempt to compensate for insulin resistance in peripheral tissues and to maintain normal glucose homeostasis. However, increased secretory responses in these patients primarily reflect second- or late-phase insulin secretion. Careful examination of glucose challenge test results shows that acute- or early-phase insulin secretion is impaired even during the prediabetic phase and that this reduction in early-phase insulin secretion is itself a risk factor for subsequent development of diabetes. Therefore, defects in both insulin resistance and early-phase insulin secretion can be detected early in prediabetic patients. Eventually, even late-phase insulin secretion begins to decrease and can no longer compensate for insulin resistance. At this point, blood glucose values begin to rise, and patients develop overt diabetes. Relative insulin deficiency (reflecting the sum of both early- and late-phase secretion) develops only once ambient glucose levels become elevated.

It has become clear that with the development of overt diabetes, chronic hyperglycemia itself may worsen insulin resistance and impair insulin secretion. This condition is referred to as "glucose toxicity" because these adverse effects appear to result from direct exposure of skeletal muscle and insulin-producing pancreatic beta cells to chronically elevated blood glucose concentrations. Glucose toxicity is a vicious cycle that leads to more severe diabetes. Conversely, a period of tight glucose control and near-euglycemia, produced by intensive medical therapy or weight loss, can partially reverse defects in insulin action and insulin secretion. This improves glucose homeostasis and can restore effectiveness of more conservative treatment such as diet or single-agent oral hypoglycemic therapy. The chronology described earlier has given rise to the "two-hit" hypothesis for genetic susceptibility to type 2 diabetes: The phenotypic expression of diabetes depends on the inheritance of at least two sets of genes; certain genes determine the early development of insulin resistance, and other genes predispose to beta cell defects under conditions of chronic metabolic stress.

INSULIN RESISTANCE SYNDROME

Insulin resistance is associated with a number of cardiovascular risk factors. This clustering of risk factors in insulin-resistant nondiabetic or prediabetic patients is referred to as the insulin resistance syndrome (IRS), or syndrome X. The IRS represents an important new concept in medicine that is critical for improved identification and management of cardiovascular risk. The central tenet of the syndrome is that insulin resistance occurs first, perhaps very early in life, and then produces the cluster of metabolic traits that increase risk for both diabetes and atherosclerosis later in life. Metabolic and cardiovascular risk factors that characterize the IRS include the following:

Hyperinsulinemia. Fasting and postprandial insulin concentrations are elevated in order to compensate for peripheral insulin resistance.

Glucose intolerance. Although some patients retain normal plasma glucose values as a result of compensatory hyperinsulinemia, others exhibit impaired fasting glucose (110 to 125 mg per dL) or impaired glucose tolerance (2-hour value, after oral glucose challenge, of 140 to 199 mg per dL).

Obesity. Many patients exhibit generalized obesity with body weights of 120% or more of normal, adjusted for height, frame, and gender. It should be noted that not all patients with the IRS are obese.

Upper body fat distribution or abdominal obesity. The relative distribution of fat to the upper body (apple shape, produced by abdominal obesity) in contrast to the lower body (pear shape, produced by increased fat deposition in hips and thighs) is a stronger indicator of insulin resistance than the degree of generalized obesity. Fat distribution is most readily quantified by circumferential measurements of waist and hips and calculation of a waist-to-hip ratio.

Elevated blood pressure. Both systolic and diastolic blood pressures tend to be higher in insulin-resistant persons and more often satisfy criteria for diagnosis of hypertension.

Lipid and lipoprotein abnormalities. The IRS is characterized by a consistent pattern of lipid abnormalities, including high triglyceride levels (fasting level ≥ 250 mg per dL), low HDL cholesterol (<40 mg per dL), and high levels of low-density lipoprotein (LDL). The IRS does not routinely result in alterations in total cholesterol; however, LDL particles are smaller and denser than normal as a result of relative enrichment in protein and triglyceride and a decrease in cholesterol ester content. These physicochemical alterations probably increase the atherogenicity of LDL even when LDL cholesterol levels are not increased.

Clotting abnormalities. The IRS is characterized by changes that promote thrombosis and inhibit breakdown of fibrin clots. This is important because there is always a balance between prothrombotic and antithrombotic processes in blood, and anything that tilts the balance toward thromboses could accelerate atherosclerosis and precipitate acute cardiovascular events. One example is that IRS patients have high circulating levels of plasminogen activator inhibitor-1, an inhibitor of fibrinolysis.

Many of these traits constitute independent risk factors for the development of both type 2 diabetes and atherosclerosis and thus predispose to the development of either or both of these diseases in individual patients. Support for the IRS hypothesis derives from the epidemiologic observation that hyperinsulinemia (or insulin resistance) is a risk marker for atherosclerosis and an independent predictor of fatal coronary heart disease. These prospective studies, which have largely involved men, have linked high fasting and/or post–glucose challenge serum insulin levels to myocardial infarction and cardiac death. These relationships were clearly demonstrated in the initial studies (the Helsinki Policemen Study, the Paris Prospective Study, the Brusselton Study); however, several subsequent investigations could not confirm that hyperinsulinemia was a risk factor for cardiovascular disease (the San Luis Valley Study, the Gothenburg Study, the Rancho Bernardo Study, and the Multiple Risk Factor Intervention Trial [MRFIT]). In resolving this controversy, it is important to keep in mind that elevated glucose values can suppress circulating insulin levels through glucose toxicity. Therefore, it is imperative to exclude patients with diabetes and even mild degrees of glucose intolerance from the analysis if hyperinsulinemia is used as the measure of insulin resistance. This concept was incorporated into the study design of the more recent Quebec study which demonstrated that hyperinsulinemia was a powerful and independent risk factor for cardiovascular disease.*

There is no single standardized laboratory test that indicates the severity of insulin resistance or the IRS. Even the fasting serum insulin level cannot be recommended because of the lack of a reference standard among laboratories and the overlap of values between insulin-sensitive and insulin-resistant patients. The overlap results partly from effects of glucose toxicity to suppress insulin secretion in patients with even mild degrees of glucose intolerance. Furthermore, rigorous clinical criteria for diagnosis of the IRS have not yet been established. Nevertheless, the IRS can be recognized clinically on the basis of the constellation of physical findings and laboratory characteristics described in the preceding section.

Detection and appreciation of the IRS are important for four reasons. First, recognition of the IRS leads the clinician to carefully screen the patient for other comorbid conditions. For example, the clinician would examine and test for the combination of glucose intolerance/diabetes, hypertension, lipid abnormalities, and cardiovascular disease in patients known to have any one of these conditions. Second, the clinician should more aggressively manage the cardiovascular risk profile in patients with the IRS. Medical and dietary treatment should be instituted at a lower threshold and used more aggressively to treat hypertension, obesity, glucose intolerance, and hypercholesterolemia in patients with the IRS than when these diseases occur in isolation. In addition, the imperative is greater in IRS patients to intervene with regard to other cardiovascular risk factors, including smoking cessation, regular exercise to counteract inactivity, treatment of homocystinemia with folic acid, treatment of hypertriglyceridemia, and use of aspirin and vitamin E. Third, patients can be identified at higher risk for subsequent diabetes and targeted for prevention through weight loss, exercise, and low-fat, high-fiber diets. Fourth, the presence of the IRS influences choice of drug therapy so as not to exacerbate other features of the IRS. For example, high-dosage thiazide diuretics or beta blockers may be avoided for treatment of hypertension because these agents can worsen the lipid profile, and niacin therapy for dyslipidemia should be used cautiously because it could worsen glucose tolerance.

TREATMENT OVERVIEW, SETTING OF TREATMENT GOALS, AND STANDARDS OF CARE

Treatment Objectives

Optimal therapy in diabetes is designed to prevent acute and chronic complications while achieving sat-

isfactory quality of life. Treatment has two specific aims. The first is to control glycemia in an effort to both eliminate the symptoms (polyuria, polydipsia, blurred vision, dehydration, and fatigue) and prevent acute complications (e.g., hyperosmolar nonketotic coma, infections, and ketoacidosis) of uncontrolled diabetes. Most patients with type 2 diabetes do not develop ketoacidosis except under severe physiologic stress. However, in high-risk racial and ethnic groups such as African-Americans and Hispanic Americans, it is not unusual for patients with an early onset variant of type 2 diabetes (atypical diabetes) to come to medical attention in diabetic ketoacidosis. The second specific aim is to prevent long-term microvascular and macrovascular complications. This requires maintenance of euglycemia to the fullest extent possible, routine monitoring for complications, and concerted management of cardiovascular disease risk factors.

Team Approach

Effective management of type 2 diabetes is best accomplished by a health care team that includes the patient as a full voting member, together with a physician, a diabetes clinical nurse specialist or practitioner, a nurse educator, a dietitian, a counselor/psychologist, and a readily accessible podiatrist and ophthalmologist. As many members of the team as possible should be certified diabetes educators. This multidisciplinary team is needed to assess each patient's clinical status, provide diabetes education to the patient and family, monitor the effects of treatment, make frequent short-term decisions regarding changes in medication dosage, develop exercise and dietary intervention, modify the treatment program to accommodate psychologic and socioeconomic factors, check for complications, and ensure appropriate referrals. These functions must be individualized for each patient and must occur on an ongoing basis with adjustments to changing circumstances over time.

It is helpful for the physician and health care team to jettison the traditional notion of patient noncompliance. To a large extent, "noncompliance" should be regarded, not as a failure on the part of the patient, but a failure of the health care team to develop a treatment regimen with which the patient will comply. It is counterproductive to unilaterally establish therapy and goals if the patient is not vested in the process and if barriers lead to frustration and disillusionment. Establishing an effective individualized treatment program is time-consuming and requires a complex of skills within the diabetes management team. It is difficult for an isolated physician to accomplish these tasks, especially when faced with a busy waiting room and constraints on time spent with each patient. In the absence of a multidisciplinary team approach, both the physician and patient are susceptible to frustration when goals are not achieved. The physician may then adopt a defeatist or accusatory attitude that affects the patient and leads to a vicious circle that ensures suboptimal man-

---

*See Depres JP, Lamarche B, Mauriege P, et al: Hyperinsulinemia as an independent risk factor for ischemic heart disease. N Engl J Med 334:952–957, 1996.

agement. Therefore, physicians should try to assemble the health care team as they develop a program for treating diabetic patients, and this team should include, at a minimum, a nurse or dietitian who is a certified diabetes educator.

Glucose Monitoring

Achieving goals for glycemic control requires two types of monitoring: (1) Home monitoring of capillary blood glucose is performed by the patient and measures instantaneous blood glucose level and daily fluctuations in glycemia. (2) Hemoglobin A_{1c} (HbA$_{1c}$), or glycohemoglobin, is measured by the physician and reflects the integrated glucose level over the previous 4- to 6-week period. Home glucose monitoring (HGM) has revolutionized diabetes management and made intensive glucose control possible. Essentially all diabetic patients should have the capacity for HGM. This technique enables patients to understand the impact of medical therapy, diet, and exercise on blood glucose levels and to be integrally involved in self-management. The physician and health care team should carefully review the HGM records with the patient, whether computerized or written in booklets, and use this information in selecting therapy and optimizing medication dosage.

For patients who have received diabetes education, HGM facilitates glycemic control by allowing them to make therapeutic decisions within prescribed guidelines. HGM is an important tool for enfranchising the patient in the therapeutic process and to reinforce adherence to therapy. The frequency of HGM is individualized to a large degree. More frequent measurements are needed during periods when changes are made in therapy to bring the patient's condition under better control. The author usually advises two to four times per day—before meals and at bedtime—until preprandial glucose levels are satisfactory. Once that is achieved, 2-hour postprandial measurements are helpful in addressing large glycemic excursions after meals. HGM frequency can be reduced when glycemic control is relatively stable, although this is highly individualized; a few fasting home glucose measurements per week may be all that is necessary in stable patients. At any stage, patients can use HGM to provide feedback on acute effects of specific meals or exercise, to verify hypoglycemic symptoms, and for guidance during periods of illness or stress.

Glycemia and Complications

HbA$_{1c}$ is the second form of monitoring and is used by the health care team as a chronic measure of glycemia. HbA$_{1c}$ can be related to an average glucose level, as shown in Table 3. HbA$_{1c}$ should be measured every 3 months in most patients and evaluated together with HGM in assessing glycemic control. It is helpful for the patient to know and understand this measure in the same manner that patients know their cholesterol level. A critical objective in diabetes management is to achieve a low target HbA$_{1c}$ value, because good glycemic control as measured by HbA$_{1c}$ prevents microvascular complications in both type 1 and type 2 diabetes. In the Diabetes Control and Complications Trial (DCCT), patients with type 1 diabetes randomly assigned to an intensively managed subgroup (mean HbA$_{1c}$ = 7%) experienced a 54 to 63% reduction in the development of retinopathy, nephropathy, and neuropathy in comparison with a conventionally managed subgroup (mean HbA$_{1c}$ = 9%). Furthermore, there was no glycemic threshold above which complications developed and below which patients were free of complication. Thus there is a continuous relationship between HbA$_{1c}$ and complications, so that risk is reduced for any lowering of HbA$_{1c}$.

In the United Kingdom Prospective Diabetes Study (UKPDS), patients with type 2 diabetes were randomly assigned to conventional therapy or to intensive therapy with sulfonylurea, metformin, or insulin. A moderate lowering of HbA$_{1c}$ markedly reduced risk for microvascular complications and had a tendency to diminish risk for myocardial infarction. The UKPDS showed that high HbA$_{1c}$, together with low HDL levels, high LDL levels, high blood pressure, cigarette smoking, age, and gender, was a risk factor for the development of macrovascular complications. Therefore, management of type 2 diabetes should achieve as low an HbA$_{1c}$ value as possible for each individual patient, taking safety into consideration. As was most clearly evident for patients with type 1 diabetes in the DCCT, but also true for patients with type 2 diabetes, the more intensive the glycemic control was, the greater the risk for hypoglycemia. These clinical trials support the general recommendation that HbA$_{1c}$ should be maintained at 7% or lower (normal is 4 to 6%) and that values higher than 8% merit concerted action, as shown in Table 4.

Cardiovascular Risk Factor Management

The treatment of type 2 diabetes is not confined to glycemic control and must include a comprehensive approach to overall risk factor reduction for macrovascular disease (i.e., coronary artery disease, stroke, peripheral vascular disease). Type 2 diabetes independently increases the risk for cardiovascular disease two- to threefold in men and three- to fivefold in women in comparison with their age-matched nondiabetic counterparts. Risk factors include those listed for the IRS. However, the superimposition of diabetes may interact with individual risk factors to alter their atherogenicity and exacerbate disease mechanisms in the vascular wall. For example, uncontrolled diabetes further raises triglyceride levels and lowers HDL cholesterol levels. Diabetes also promotes glycation of circulating lipoproteins, which can directly affect their interaction with vascular wall cells. Modified lipoproteins also induce autoantibody formation, which may indirectly promote atherogenesis as a consequence of altered metabolism of lipoprotein-antibody complexes. Diabetes increases oxida-

TABLE 3. **Relationship Between Hemoglobin A$_{1c}$ Value and Average Plasma Glucose Concentration**

Value	Normal	Desirable	Fair	Poor	
Average fasting glucose level	<110 mg/dL	≤140 mg/dL	~170 mg/dL	~200 mg/dL	~230 mg/dL
Hemoglobin A$_{1c}$ concentration	4–6%	≤7%	~8%	~9%	~10%

tive stress on proteins and lipids that may contribute to atherogenesis, although this remains an area under active investigation. Platelet plasminogen activator inhibitor-1 concentrations are also elevated in type 2 diabetes, which may contribute to dysfibrinolysis. Increased platelet aggregation and release of thromboxane are often present. The onset of microalbuminuria is itself a risk factor for future cardiovascular disease. Therefore, cardiovascular risk factors should aggressively be managed in patients with type 2 diabetes, and goals may differ from those established for patients without diabetes. These goals are delineated in Table 4.

One example of a condition for which more aggressive management is recommended is blood pressure, which should be controlled at 130/85 mm Hg or lower, as opposed to the more customary goal of less than 140/90 mm Hg. Another is elevated triglyceride levels, which may not contribute to cardiovascular disease in nondiabetic persons but may constitute an independent risk factor for coronary heart disease in patients with diabetes. A final example is LDL cholesterol. The National Cholesterol Education Project (NCEP) recommends an LDL cholesterol value of less than 160 mg (4.1 mmol) per dL in persons with one or no classic risk factors (diabetes represents one risk factor). The ADA recommends an LDL cholesterol goal of less than 130 mg (3.35 mmol) per dL in diabetic patients without active cardiovascular dis-

ease. Both the NCEP and ADA advise a target of less than 100 mg (2.6 mmol) per dL for patients with active cardiovascular disease. However, many diabetologists treat all patients with type 2 diabetes as if they have active cardiovascular disease and reduce the LDL cholesterol level to less than 100 mg per dL when this can safely be accomplished. The author endorses this latter approach. In this regard, several trials, including the Scandinavian Simvastatin Survival Study (4S) and the Cholesterol and Recurrent Events (CARE) Trial have demonstrated, using pravastatin, that lowering LDL cholesterol in diabetic patients dramatically reduces coronary heart disease end points, which greatly exceeds the benefit in nondiabetic patients, and that this benefit is continuous for LDL cholesterol levels below 130 mg per dL.

Standards of Care

Type 2 diabetes management is optimized by a systematic approach for routine examination, laboratory measurements, education, and referrals. In this context, the ADA has formulated "Standards of Care" that are based on complications and interventions data.* These standards facilitate prevention, timely identification, and treatment of diabetes complications and are listed in Table 5.

NONPHARMACOLOGIC THERAPY

Diet

Diet is an important component of management in all diabetic patients. A trained dietitian should be involved in assessing dietary history and lifestyle, reviewing dietary principles, and developing and executing the meal plan on an ongoing basis. Simply providing handouts with written dietary instructions is insufficient. The diet plan should be tailored to the individual and should account for personal preferences, age, gender, current nutritional and clinical status, degree of obesity, medications, and activity level. It is also necessary to accommodate cultural and ethnic food preferences, and to consider socioeconomic factors, for the meal plan to be successful.

Nutritional therapy for diabetes has two general goals: (1) to manipulate the composition of food to improve both glucose homeostasis and dyslipidemia and (2) to alter caloric intake so as to achieve ideal body weight. For caloric composition, recommendations have varied widely in the past with regard to

TABLE 4. **Goals and Thresholds for Medical Therapy in Type 2 Diabetes Mellitus**

Parameter	Goal	Action Required
Glycemia		
Glucose level		
Before meals	80–120 mg/dL	≥140 mg/dL
2-hour postprandial	100–160 mg/dL	>200 mg/dL
Bedtime	100–140 mg/dL	≥160 mg/dL
Hemoglobin A$_{1c}$ concentration	≤7%	≥8%
Blood pressure	≤130/85 mm Hg	≥130/85
Microalbuminuria	<30 mg/24 h	≥40 mg/24 h
Lipids		
Total cholesterol	<200 mg/dL	≥200 mg/dL
Triglyceride levels	≤200 mg/dL	>350 mg/dL
LDL cholesterol level	<100 mg/dL	>100 mg/dL*
HDL cholesterol level		
Men	>35 mg/dL	<35 mg/dL
Women	>40 mg/dL	<40 mg/dL

*This recommendation is more rigorous than that proposed by the National Cholesterol Education Project (NCEP) and the American Diabetes Association (ADA); see text.

Abbreviations: LDL = low-density lipoprotein; HDL = high-density lipoprotein.

*See American Diabetes Association Standards of Medical Care for Patients with Diabetes Mellitus. Diabetes Care 21(Suppl 1): S23–S31, 1998.

TABLE 5. **Standards of Care for Type 2 Diabetes**

Procedure	Initial Visit	Annual Visit	Quarterly Visit
History and Physical Examination	X	X	X
Blood pressure	X	X	X
Height and weight	X	X	X
Eye examination	X	X*	
Foot examination	X	X	X
Clinical Management			
Review home glucose record		X	X
Review therapeutic plan and goals (diet, exercise, medications, psychosocial)	X	X	X
Review self-management	X	X	X
Diabetes education	X	X	X
Ophthalmologist referral		X*	
Assess cardiovascular risk intervention	X	X	X
Laboratory Evaluation			
HbA$_{1c}$ concentration	X	X	X
Fasting lipid panel	X	X*	
24-h urine for albumin and creatinine clearance	X	X*	
Serum creatinine and blood urea nitrogen	X	X*	
ECG (adults)	X	X*	
Optional When Needed			
Podiatry referral			
Thyroid function tests			
Serum electrolytes			
ECG stress test			
Urine analysis and culture			

*To be performed more frequently if required or if results are abnormal. Also, annual and quarterly procedures are applicable once the patient's condition is stable; more frequent procedures are usually necessary after initial visit.

Abbreviation: ECG = electrocardiogram.

relative intake of carbohydrate and fat. With better characterization of dyslipidemia and the burden of vascular disease in diabetic patients, an appropriate emphasis is currently placed on reducing dietary fat. Thus, current recommendations of the ADA* and the NCEP should be followed. The basic prescription is 50 to 60% of daily calories as carbohydrates, 12 to 20% as protein, and 30% or less as fat, with restrictions on cholesterol and saturated fat intake. The traditional recommendation is that dietary carbohydrate should be composed primarily of complex carbohydrates, as opposed to simple sugars, in order to reduce postprandial glucose excursions. However, the glycemic response to sucrose can overlap with the response to ingestion of starches, and the glucose rise associated with fruit or milk can be less than the rise associated with many starches. Foods high in soluble fiber are recommended because they have

*See Franz MJ, Horton ES, Bantle JP, et al: Nutrition principles for the management of diabetes and related complications. Diabetes Care *17*:490–518, 1994. See also American Diabetes Association: Nutrition recommendations and principles for people with diabetes. Diabetes Care *21*(Suppl 1):S32–S35, 1998.

a beneficial effect on serum lipids and potentially slow glucose absorption in the gut. Saturated fat and polyunsaturated fat should each be limited to less than 10% of daily calories (i.e., <20% for both combined), and cholesterol intake should be less than 300 mg per day. This caloric distribution is consistent with both ADA recommendations and the NCEP step 1 diet. If the diet does not achieve targeted goals for LDL cholesterol level, an NCEP step 2 diet should be instituted. The step 2 diet reduces daily ingestion of cholesterol to less than 200 mg per day and saturated fat to less than 7% of calories.

These dietary prescriptions fix protein at 12 to 20%, saturated fat at less than 10%, and polyunsaturated fat at 10% or less, leaving 60 to 70% of daily calories as carbohydrate and monounsaturated fat. In individualizing diet to accommodate personal and ethnic preferences, monounsaturated fat can be increased at the expense of saturated and polyunsaturated fat or carbohydrate. The diet may contain acceptable daily intake of non-nutritive sweeteners (aspartame, saccharin). Nutritive and non-nutritive (olestra) fat replacers can be used to reduce saturated and total dietary fat when rationally incorporated into the overall meal plan. Patients may consume two alcoholic drinks per day (one drink equals 12 ounces of beer, 5 ounces of wine, or 1.5 ounces of spirits) with meals, because this can increase HDL; however, the effect on serum triglyceride levels and total calories should be monitored. Patients with triglyceride levels exceeding 400 mg per dL should generally refrain from drinking alcoholic beverages.

Weight loss can dramatically reduce (or sometimes eliminate) the need for diabetes medications, and can also ameliorate dyslipidemia and hypertension, in overweight patients. This is often best accomplished by moderate caloric reduction of 250 to 500 calories below the weight maintenance in the context of a nutritionally sound meal plan, proper caloric distribution, and an exercise regimen. Alternatively, a diet very low in calorie (500 to 800 kcal per day) can be used in selected patients. With either moderate reduction or diets very low in calories, weight loss is frequently achieved but is difficult to sustain. However, significant metabolic and cardiovascular benefits can be realized without achieving ideal body weight. Insulin sensitivity begins to improve within a few days after the patient is made hypocaloric, even before significant weight loss has occurred. A modest weight reduction of 5 to 10 kg significantly ameliorates glycemia, and improvement in insulin sensitivity is sustained if the patient maintains only a 10% reduction of the original body weight. Weight loss in the obese patient with the IRS can prevent progression to overt type 2 diabetes, lower blood pressure, and reverse the dyslipidemia (i.e., increase HDL cholesterol and decrease triglyceride levels). In patients with type 2 diabetes and more severe degrees of obesity (body mass index > 35 kg per m^2) that is refractory to diet and exercise, treatment with sibutramine (Meridia) should be considered. Sibutramine should be discontinued after 2 to 3 months if significant weight loss is not evident, and blood pressure should be monitored carefully because this neurotransmitter reuptake inhibitor can increase blood pressure. Gastric plication or reduction surgery should also be considered in morbidly obese patients and performed by experienced surgeons who monitor effectiveness and maintain a comprehensive health-maintenance program for these patients.

The timing of meals is also an important consideration in the dietary management of diabetes. In patients taking exogenous insulin and certain oral agents, the time course and peak absorption of nutrients should be coordinated to coincide with the dynamics of pharmacologic action. Between-meal or bedtime snacks, as components of total daily calories, may be needed to prevent hypoglycemia related to medication and exercise. However, in type 2 diabetes, postprandial glycemic excursions are prolonged, and meals should generally be spaced at least 4 to 5 hours apart (without snacks) to facilitate the return of blood glucose levels to baseline before another meal is ingested. Large meals should be avoided, in order to prevent exaggerated rises in blood glucose. Also, it is not imprudent for patients treated with diet alone or with metformin, troglitazone, or alpha-glucosidase inhibitors to skip meals entirely, particularly if this promotes weight loss in obese patients. In rare patients with a marked degree of insulin resistance or hypertriglyceridemia whose conditions have become increasingly refractory to medications, the author intermittently prescribes 1 to 3 days of fasting to restore metabolic homeostasis, taking special care to maintain hydration with water ingestion and to decrease or suspend administration of diabetes medications.

Exercise

Most diabetic patients should be prescribed some form of regular exercise. Exercise is an important adjunct in glycemic control, weight loss, and maintenance of weight reduction. Weight loss is more likely to be sustained if dietary recommendations are combined with a simple exercise plan. The timing of exercise can also be used to reduce glycemia at specified periods during the day: for example, walking after dinner or breakfast to blunt the increment in plasma glucose. Exercise training raises HDL cholesterol, lowers blood pressure, and leads to a 20 to 40% increase in insulin sensitivity by enhancing insulin action in skeletal muscle. In the past, the intensity of exercise needed for meaningful metabolic and cardiovascular benefits was unknown. There is now evidence that regular physical activity of even modest intensity, which for the most part comprised walking three to five times per week, significantly improved insulin sensitivity in a multiracial group of patients at high risk for diabetes.* The findings from this

study support recommendations by both the U.S. Centers for Disease Control and Prevention and the American College of Sports Medicine that all adults participate in at least 30 minutes of moderate-intensity physical activity on most days of the week. However, once exercise is stopped, the benefits gained from exercise disappear rapidly within days, which emphasizes the need for regular exercise. Therefore, in the absence of contraindications, all diabetic patients should be counseled to engage in 30 minutes of modest aerobic exercise (such as walking, light jogging, aerobics, swimming, or bicycling) 3 or 4 days a week. The intensity of the exercise should be gauged to produce an increase in pulse rate to approximately 60 to 70% of maximum, which can be calculated as 220 minus age. This level of exercise is referred to as "conversational exercise" because it is not intense enough to prevent the patient from conversing with a partner during the workout.

Exercise programs are ideally developed in collaboration with the patient, and instituted and followed by diabetes nurse educators, dietitians, or exercise counselors on the diabetes management team. All diabetic patients should be carefully examined and have resting electrocardiography performed before an exercise program is initiated. Selected patients older than 40 years, with multiple risk factors, or with disease of more than 20 years' duration should also first undergo stress testing. Patients with active coronary artery disease should undertake exercise in the context of a cardiac rehabilitation program, and patients with class III or IV symptoms may not be able to exercise. Lower extremity claudication or amputation and foot ulcers may limit types of exercise that can be performed; however, an appropriate exercise regimen can usually be devised (e.g., swimming, water aerobics, upper body exercise). Consultation with a physical or exercise therapist may be useful.

PHARMACOLOGIC THERAPY FOR GLYCEMIA

Oral Hypoglycemic Agents

The treatment of type 2 diabetes has been revolutionized by the availability of several new classes of oral hypoglycemic agents, listed in Table 6. These agents influence biochemical processes in different organs and differentially ameliorate multiple metabolic defects that cause hyperglycemia, as shown in Figure 1. Sulfonylureas and repaglinide (Prandin), a new non-sulfonylurea, interact with the sulfonylurea receptor/potassium channel complex on pancreatic beta cells and increase insulin secretion. The principal site of action of metformin (Glucophage) is the liver, and the drug acts to reduce hepatic glucose production. Thiazolidinediones, such as troglitazone (Rezulin), are insulin sensitizers and enhance the ability of insulin to stimulate glucose uptake in skeletal muscle. Therefore, these classes of oral agents ameliorate deficient insulin secretion, high hepatic glucose output, or insulin resistance, which are the

---

*Mayer-Davis EJ, D'Agostino R, Karter AJ, et al: Intensity and amount of physical activity in relation to insulin sensitivity. J Am Med Assoc 279:669–674, 1998.

TABLE 6. **Oral Hypoglycemic Agents Used in the Management of Diabetes Mellitus**

Class/Generic Name	Brand Name	Dose Range (mg/day)	Doses per Day	Tablet Sizes (mg)
First-Generation Sulfonylureas				
Tolbutamide	Orinase	500–3000	2–4	250, 500
Chlorpropamide	Diabinese	100–750	1	100, 250
Tolazamide	Tolinase	100–1000	1–2	100, 250, 500
Acetohexamide	Dymelor	250–1500	1–2	250, 500
Second-Generation Sulfonylureas				
Glyburide	Micronase, DiaBeta	1.25–20	1–2	1.25, 2.5, 5
	Glynase	1.5–12	1	1.5, 3, 6
Glipizide	Glucotrol	2.5–40	1–4	5, 10
	Glucotrol XL	2.5–20	1	5, 10
Glimepiride	Amaryl	1–8	1	1, 2, 4
Non-Sulfonylurea Insulin Stimulator				
Repaglinide	Prandin	0.5–4 mg before each meal to 16 mg max		0.5, 1, 2
Biguanides				
Metformin	Glucophage	500–2550	1–3	500, 850
Disaccharidase Inhibitors				
Acarbose	Precose	25–100 mg with each meal to 300 mg max		50, 100
Miglitol	Glyset	25–100 mg with each meal to 300 mg max		25, 50, 100
Thiazolidinediones				
Troglitazone	Rezulin	200–600	1	200, 400
Rosiglitazone	Avandia	2–8	1–2	2, 4, 8

three major defects that combine to produce hyperglycemia in nearly all patients with type 2 diabetes, as described in the section on pathophysiology. In addition, alpha-glucosidase inhibitors, which impede carbohydrate digestion and absorption in the gut, thus reducing the postprandial glycemic rise, have been introduced. The availability of multiple drug classes gives the physician more options for individualizing effective oral therapy, either as single agents or in combination with each other or with exogenous insulin.

Single-Agent Therapy

Each of the oral drugs can be used as single agents in patients with type 2 diabetes that is not ade-

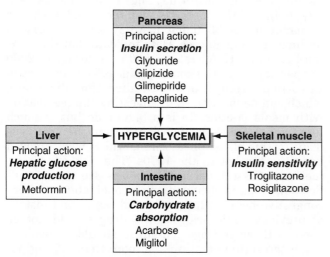

Figure 1. Different pharmacologic actions of oral hypoglycemic agents.

quately controlled by diet and exercise. The new criteria for the diagnosis of diabetes now include patients with milder degrees of glucose intolerance and lower fasting plasma glucose levels (126 to 140 mg per dL), as delineated in Table 2. These patients have a relatively large glycemic rise after meals in comparison with the more modest elevation of fasting glucose levels. In these patients with relatively mild and recent-onset diabetes and insulin resistance, alpha-glucosidase inhibitors and thiazolidinediones are rational choices for first-line oral agent therapy. Alpha-glucosidase inhibitors represent a drug class that does not induce weight gain and may be preferable in obese patients. Repaglinide, sulfonylureas, and insulin are also useful but induce a greater risk of hypoglycemia. Metformin may not be an optimal choice because basal hepatic glucose output is not markedly elevated in this phase of the disease.

In patients with more pronounced elevation of fasting glucose and/or longer disease duration, generic preparations of sulfonylureas (glyburide [Micronase] and glipizide [Glucotrol]) should be strongly considered because of their low cost. Long-acting sulfonylurea preparations reduce the number of doses, usually to once a day, and add to patient convenience. Metformin is an excellent choice for first-line therapy, especially in obese patients, because it is less likely to be associated with weight gain and may even promote a small weight loss. Metformin has also been shown to decrease the risk of cardiovascular events, diabetes-related deaths, and total mortality in the UKPDS. Thiazolidinediones like troglitazone may exert a lesser glucose-lowering effect in patients with chronic diabetes with markedly impaired insulin secretion caused by glucose toxicity, because this pure insulin sensitizer requires adequate circulating insulin for therapeutic efficacy. However, in patients with more severe or long-standing diabetes, thiazolidinediones or alpha-glucosidase inhibitors can be useful in combination with sulfonylureas or metformin.

Regardless of the choice of first-line oral agent, it is important to keep two principles in mind. First, physicians should not consider patients "treated" simply by placing patients on a drug. Patients require ongoing assessment of drug efficacy with HGM and HbA$_{1c}$ measurements to determine whether goals for the control of glycemia are achieved. Dosages of the oral agent may need to be altered, or combination therapy may need to be considered. With any oral agent, primary drug failure occurs in a significant proportion of patients. In addition, a patient's condition becomes refractory to oral agents over time (secondary failure), perhaps because of cumulative glucose toxicity, and combination therapy or insulin is then required. In general, if single-agent sulfonylurea or metformin therapy fails, replacement with an alternative single agent is not successful. Therefore, after primary or secondary failure of a single agent, combination therapy with another class of oral agent or insulin needs to be considered. The second point is that the oral agents do not obviate the need for continuing diet and exercise therapy. Diet and exercise synergize with effects of oral agents on metabolism and remain the most important determinants of oral agent efficacy. For this reason, even diabetic patients with a marked degree of hyperglycemia (i.e., fasting glucose level > 250 mg per dL) can be candidates for successful single-agent therapy in the context of appropriate diet, exercise, and weight loss.

Sulfonylureas

Sulfonylureas stimulate insulin secretion by binding to sulfonylurea receptors that regulate ion flux across the plasma membrane in beta cells. These drugs also act to increase insulin sensitivity through an unknown mechanism. The use of second-generation sulfonylureas, including glyburide, glipizide, and glimepiride (Amaryl), is recommended over that of first-generation sulfonylureas because of diminished untoward effects, such as hyponatremia, alcohol-induced flushing, and severe hypoglycemia. Glimepiride binds to a different site of the sulfonylurea receptor than other drugs in this class; however, it is not clear whether this translates into clinical advantages. These drugs should be initiated at a low or intermediate dosage, and the dosage increases on the basis of HGM information at 1- to 2-week intervals. Longer acting preparations given one to two times per day are more convenient but are currently more expensive and can entail higher risk of hypoglycemia than do short-acting preparations. Sulfonylureas are associated with approximately 30% of primary failures and with 3 to 5% of secondary failures per year, although this is dependent on intensity of diet and exercise and on duration of disease. Effective use of sulfonylureas is associated with some weight gain,

as demonstrated in the UKPDS. Other untoward effects of second-generation sulfonylureas are gastrointestinal symptoms, rashes, and rare hepatotoxicity. Results of the University Group Diabetes Program study in 1970 suggested that tolbutamide might be associated with increased risk of myocardial infarctions; however, this effect of sulfonylureas has not been supported by subsequent studies.

Repaglinide

Repaglinide is a new non-sulfonylurea oral agent that binds to the sulfonylurea receptor/potassium channel complex on beta cells and stimulates insulin secretion. Repaglinide-induced insulin secretion is dependent on ambient glucose and is increased by the rise in glucose levels after a meal. Thus postprandial serum insulin levels are increased to a much greater extent than preprandial or fasting insulin concentrations. The maximal blood level of the drug and its effects on insulin secretion peak 1 hour after ingestion, and the drug has a short half-life of approximately 1 hour. Because of these pharmacokinetics, repaglinide is taken only 0 to 15 minutes before meals. The action of the drug dictates its utility in managing postprandial hyperglycemia, and it can be an effective agent in patients with either recent-onset or long-standing diabetes. As a single agent, repaglinide's ability to decrease HbA$_{1c}$ is comparable with that of the sulfonylureas. Repaglinide has been shown to be effective in combination with metformin. It is cleared by the liver, which makes it a rational choice in patients with renal impairment, and the main side effect, as with sulfonylureas, is hypoglycemia.

Metformin

Metformin acts by reducing hepatic glucose overproduction that is directly responsible for elevated fasting glucose levels and is most appropriately used in patients with clear elevation in the fasting plasma glucose level. It also has a minor effect of increasing peripheral insulin sensitivity. The starting dosage is usually 500 mg once a day (qd) or 500 mg twice a day (bid), and the dosage is then increased weekly to a maximum of 2550 mg per day as necessary to optimize fasting glucose. Data indicate that the maximal effect on HbA$_{1c}$ is achieved at a dosage of 2000 mg per day. The most common side effects are gastrointestinal (cramps, nausea, indigestion, diarrhea), which can be minimized by ingesting the medication with meals. Metformin is a biguanide but is much less likely to cause lactic acidosis than the prototype drug in this class, phenformin, which was removed from the market in the 1970s. The risk factors for metformin-associated lactic acidosis are renal insufficiency, hepatic dysfunction, alcohol abuse, severe congestive heart failure or lung disease, and history of previous lactic acidosis; the drug should not be used in these settings. The drug should be avoided when the serum creatinine is more than 1.5 mg per dL in men and more than 1.4 mg per dL in women or when the creatinine clearance is less than 80 mL per minute. On average, metformin therapy is associated with a small degree of weight loss and is therefore a good choice for obese patients. In addition, metformin treatment leads to modest reductions in triglyceride and LDL cholesterol levels, and in the UKPDS it reduced the risk of cardiovascular events. It is useful as monotherapy as well as in combination with sulfonylureas, troglitazone, alpha-glucosidase inhibitors, repaglinide, or insulin.

Alpha-Glucosidase Inhibitors

These agents act in the brush border of the intestinal lumen to inhibit enzymes involved in the final stages of carbohydrate digestion to monosaccharides. This slows the adsorption of carbohydrate and blunts glycemic excursions after meals. Alpha-glucosidase inhibitors must be taken with the first bite of the meal to be effective, and the benefits are greatest after high-carbohydrate–containing meals (i.e., breakfast). These drugs are most appropriate as single agents in patients with pronounced postprandial hyperglycemia and modest elevation of the fasting glucose level; however, the HbA$_{1c}$-lowering effect has been comparable with that of any other class of oral agents in randomized studies, including all categories of type 2 diabetes. There is little or no systemic toxicity associated with alpha-glucosidase inhibitors. The side effect that most often limits therapy is flatulence. This can be minimized by starting the patient on low dosages (25 mg or even 12.5 mg of acarbose [Precose] or miglitol [Glyset]) with one or more meals and gradually increasing the dosage over a 12-week period to 50 to 100 mg three times a day (tid). Patients should be advised about this complication ahead of time, and instructed to decrease carbohydrates over periods of several days to manage a worsening of symptoms. In a properly informed and managed patient, the flatulence can be well tolerated and self-limited.

Alpha-glucosidase inhibitors are less likely to be associated with weight gain and can result in a small degree of weight loss in patients consuming high-carbohydrate diets. As single-agent therapy, alpha-glucosidase inhibitors do not cause hypoglycemia. These drugs are also highly useful in combination therapy with any other class of oral agent or with injections of intermediate- or long-acting insulin. Hypoglycemia in patients on combination therapy should be treated, not with oral sucrose or other disaccharides, but with glucose (dextrose) instead.

Thiazolidinediones

Troglitazone is the prototype for this new class of oral agents that act by increasing insulin sensitivity in skeletal muscle. The mechanism of action is not understood, although these drugs bind nuclear transcription factors (peroxisome proliferator-activated receptor γ) and enhance the activity of the insulin-responsive glucose transport system. Troglitazone is initiated at dosages of 200 to 400 mg per day and can be increased to 600 mg per day after 6 to 8 weeks to obtain full biologic effects in some patients. It is important to keep in mind that biologic action is not rapid and that 2 to 6 weeks, or more in some patients, are required to achieve full effects at any given dosage. As a single agent, troglitazone can be used in early-stage diabetes with mild fasting hyperglycemia when other agents are not effective or not tolerated. In patients with severe or long-standing disease, monotherapy is less effective because chronic glucose toxicity reduces beta cell insulin secretion, and insulin must be available if this pure insulin sensitizer is to be clinically efficacious. Troglitazone is, however, very useful in combination with sulfonylureas, metformin, and insulin injections. Due to hepatotoxicity, the FDA has restricted the indicated use of troglitazone. Troglitazone should be initiated in combination with insulin for those patients not achieving a targeted level of glycemic control on insulin alone.

The drug is well tolerated. As monotherapy in diabetes (or when ingested by normal control subjects in research studies), troglitazone does not cause hypoglycemia, inasmuch as endogenous insulin secretion decreases as peripheral insulin sensitivity increases. The drug is associated with some weight gain that is proportional to the HbA$_{1c}$-lowering effect. At least some of the weight gain results from fluid retention and expansion of plasma volume that can lower hematocrit a few percentage points. Troglitazone lowers levels of circulating free fatty acids and triglycerides and increases HDL cholesterol levels, but it is also associated with an approximately 5 to 10% increase in LDL cholesterol. The increase in LDL cholesterol may reflect the conversion of small dense LDL to normal-sized particles (i.e., there is no change in apolipoprotein B levels). Therefore, whether the effect on LDL cholesterol affects cardiovascular risk is not clear.

Troglitazone reduces estrogen levels by approximately 30% in patients taking oral contraceptives and should be used cautiously by patients on low-dosage estrogen preparations (<50 µg ethinyl estradiol). Co-administration of troglitazone with terfenadine reduces terfenadine levels by 50 to 70%. There are also rare cases of idiosyncratic severe hepatotoxicity (approximately 1 in every 60,000 treated patients). The drug should not be given to patients with baseline elevation of alanine aminotransferase (ALT) more than 1.5 times the upper limit of normal. In 2 to 3% of patients, troglitazone causes an elevation of liver transaminase levels; in most instances, this elevation is self-limited. After the drug is initiated, liver transaminase levels should be assessed every month during the first year and quarterly thereafter. If the ALT levels rise to three times above the upper normal limit, the drug should be discontinued.

Rosiglitazone (Avandia) is another insulin-sensitizer in the thiazolidinedione drug class that has become available for treating type 2 diabetes. It is effective as a single agent, and in combination with sulfonylureas, metformin, or insulin. As with other thiazolidinediones, rosiglitazone therapy can be associated with weight gain, edema, and a small decrease in hematocrit due to hemodilution. Rosiglitazone less frequently produces significant elevations in hepatic transaminases in comparison with troglitazone; however, the potential for severe hepatotoxicity and liver failure will not be known until there is a more broad and long-term experience with the drug. For this reason, as with troglitazone, hepatic transaminases should be carefully monitored in rosiglitazone-treated patients.

Insulin

The goals of insulin therapy differ between type 1 and type 2 diabetes. In type 1 diabetes, insulin therapy is designed to mimic physiologic daily fluctuation of serum insulin concentrations to provide for both basal regulation of hepatic glucose production and stimulation of glucose uptake after meals. In type 2 diabetes, the primary goal is to restrain hepatic glucose overproduction; the ability to effectively accelerate postprandial glucose disposal is variable, depending on the degree of insulin resistance, and is little affected by insulin injections in the most insulin-resistant patients. Although both the liver and skeletal muscle are insulin resistant in type 2 diabetes, dose-response differences dictate that at serum insulin levels produced by exogenous insulin therapy in many patients, hepatic glucose production can be partially or completely inhibited, whereas lesser degrees of glucose uptake stimulation are observed in skeletal muscle. Thus, in patients treated with insulin alone, multi-injection regimens to rigorously control preprandial and postprandial glucose values are often not the most effective way to achieve HbA$_{1c}$ goals in type 2 diabetes. Nevertheless, insulin is a valuable drug that can be used either as a single agent or in combination with oral agents to lower HbA$_{1c}$. With the availability of multiple classes of effective drugs, oral agents and not insulin have become the preferred choice for initiating medical therapy in many patients. However, insulin is indispensable once the disease becomes refractory to oral agents. Treatment often involves the addition of bedtime insulin in combination with an oral agent and, later, multiple daily insulin doses. Most studies showing that intensive therapy reduces vascular complications in diabetes have involved insulin treatment, and the physician should therefore not be reluctant to use large dosages of insulin if required for glycemic control.

Several other general features of insulin therapy in type 2 diabetes should be kept in mind. First, patients with type 2 diabetes need large dosages of insulin, when used as a single agent, as a consequence of insulin resistance. The average daily insulin dosage for achieving euglycemia in patients with moderate to severe hyperglycemia (fasting glucose level = ~250 mg per dL) is approximately 120 units per day, although the insulin dosage required to achieve this goal is extremely variable (50 to >300 units per day). Because of insulin resistance, physicians are sometimes too timid in making sizable dosage alterations in patients not actively losing weight. Second, insulin requirements can vary dramatically in a single patient, depending on dietary intake and physical activity level. This particularly applies to patients who are hypocaloric and losing weight. Insulin sensitivity improves soon after a hypocaloric diet is begun, and this may necessitate large decrements in insulin dosage, or even elimination of insulin, during weight loss. Third, it is futile to make pronouncements on insulin requirements on the basis of units of body weight in type 2 diabetes. These requirements are not predictable because of variability related to diet, activity level, degree of glycemic control, residual endogenous insulin secretion, and differences in insulin sensitivity that are independent of body weight. Finally, lean elderly patients sometimes respond to small daily doses of insulin (e.g., <20 units of NPH per day). For this reason, physicians should use insulin more cautiously in elderly patients. All these considerations point to the need to individualize insulin therapy on the basis of HGM and HbA$_{1c}$ measurements.

Several insulin treatment regimens can be useful in type 2 diabetes and are described as follows.

Single Daily Dose

As a first-line single agent or in combination with oral agents, insulin therapy is usually initiated in type 2 diabetes as a single daily injection of intermediate (NPH or Lente) or long-acting (Ultralente) insulin. Clinical studies have shown that this dosage is more effective, with regard to 24-hour glucose profiles and HbA$_{1c}$, when given at bedtime than in the morning before breakfast. This is because the bedtime insulin is better able to restrain hepatic glucose production through the night, which allows patients to begin their day with better fasting glucose concentrations. Therefore, 10 to 20 units of NPH insulin should be injected at bedtime, and the patients are instructed to increase the dosage by 5 units every 3 to 5 days until fasting HGM values before breakfast are consistently 80 to 140 mg per dL. There should be no surprise if this ultimately requires 60 to 100 units or more each night. When supper is by far the largest meal of the day, it might be useful to give the single daily injection before supper as NPH or as 70/30 insulin (a premixed preparation containing 70% intermediate and 30% short-acting regular insulin). The patient should be aware of symptoms of nocturnal hypoglycemia and should set the alarm for 3 AM glucose checks to test for this possibility if the concern is raised.

Multiple Daily Dose

If bedtime insulin controls the fasting morning glucose level but HbA$_{1c}$ goals are not achieved because of high postprandial glucose levels during the day, a decision must be made to add a morning dose of insulin, use more intensive diet and exercise, or add an oral agent. If the second daily injection of insulin is chosen, this can be accomplished by an injection of

70/30 or intermediate-acting insulin before breakfast and increasing the dosage by 5 units every 3 to 5 days until presupper glucose levels are consistently 80 to 140 mg per dL. Some reduction in the bedtime insulin dosage may be required because glucose levels during the evening hours will be reduced by the morning insulin injection. If this regimen (i.e., NPH insulin at bedtime titrated to the fasting morning glucose level and 70/30 insulin in the morning titrated to the presupper glucose level) is intensified to the point at which most prebreakfast and presupper glucose levels range between 80 to 120 mg per dL, an HbA_{1c} level of 7% or less can be achieved in many patients.

However, insulin therapy must be individualized, as with most aspects of diabetes therapy. Some patients do well on split/mixed and multidose regimens more characteristically used in type 1 diabetes. For example, in patients receiving prebreakfast and bedtime insulin injections, it may be advantageous to replace the bedtime NPH injection with a presupper injection of 70/30 insulin if the supper meal is relatively large. If presupper 70/30 insulin results in nocturnal hypoglycemia (caused by peaking of the NPH component at approximately 2 to 3 AM), it may be necessary to split the evening dose and take regular insulin before supper and NPH insulin at bedtime; this will shift the NPH peak to 5 to 7 AM, when more insulin may be required as a result of the "dawn phenomenon." The 70% intermediate and 30% regular composition for 70/30 insulin may not prove to be the optimal ratio in some patients, according to HGM measurements, and customized mixing of variable amounts of regular and intermediate insulin is necessary, as is the case for almost all patients with type 1 diabetes. Other patients with more erratic meal schedules may be treated successfully with Ultralente injections (qd or bid) to augment basal insulin levels, combined with regular or lispro insulin (Humalog) before each meal. Optimizing multidose insulin requires that the patient record the HGM measurement four times per day: before each meal and at bedtime. The fasting morning glucose measurement is used to adjust the evening dose of intermediate or long-acting insulin; the prelunch glucose measurement is used to adjust prebreakfast regular insulin; the presupper glucose measurement is used to adjust the morning dose of intermediate or long-acting insulin and/or the prelunch regular insulin; the bedtime glucose measurement is used to adjust presupper regular insulin. In patients treated with split/mixed bid insulin, it has been generally observed that patients do best if one half to two thirds of the daily insulin dosage is administered in the morning and one third to one half of the total daily dosage is given in the evening. Also, approximately 60 to 70% of daily insulin is given as intermediate- or long-acting preparations and 30 to 40% as short-acting preparations.

Combination Therapy

The principle guiding combination therapy is that when glycemic control becomes suboptimal on a single agent, it is helpful to add a second class of drug if better glycemic control would be achieved with the medications acting synergistically than with either drug alone. The availability of multiple classes of oral agents with different pharmacologic actions has greatly expanded the potential for combination therapy and has revolutionized the treatment of type 2 diabetes. This enhances the physician's ability to individualize therapy in achieving targets for low HbA_{1c} levels in a manner that is consistent with quality of life. Previously, when a patient's disease became refractory to a single oral agent, the only available option was either to intensify diet and exercise or to convert to insulin injection therapy (usually multiple daily doses). Now the physician and patient can achieve glycemic control by adding any one of a number of oral agents or bedtime insulin to the initial agent. The availability of these options forestalls or eliminates the need for multiple insulin injections and facilitates the maintenance of low HbA_{1c} values and prevention of vascular complications. Clinical data, now available for most possible drug combinations, show a lowering of HbA_{1c} values by 0.8 to 2.0 percentage points over that achieved with either agent alone.

In general, it is better to combine drugs that enhance insulin delivery (sulfonylureas, repaglinide, insulin) with drugs that lower hepatic glucose output (metformin) or with insulin sensitizers (troglitazone). However, this is not an absolute rule, inasmuch as the combination of metformin and troglitazone has been shown to be effective. In view of the pharmacologic synergism of these drug combinations, it can be cost-effective to use each drug at 50 to 75% of the maximal dosage without loss of therapeutic effectiveness. Alpha-glucosidase inhibitors are additive to the effects of sulfonylureas, metformin, troglitazone, and bedtime insulin and produce an additional lowering of HbA_{1c} values by ~1.0 percentage point. Clearly, the diabetes team can be flexible and creative in optimizing therapy with these multiple treatment modalities in combination with diet and exercise. However, these prescriptions need to be based on an understanding of the natural history and pathophysiology of type 2 diabetes, the pharmacologic action of drug therapy, and each patient's lifestyle.

Figure 2 shows a rational scheme for combination and step-up therapy. Appropriate first-line drugs are indicated for patients with either mild recent-onset diabetes or moderate or severe diabetes of longer duration. Once glycemic control is no longer achieved with the first single agent, a second oral agent or bedtime insulin is added. Ultimately, patients with severe insulin resistance or beta cell defects may progress to multidose insulin. The combination of insulin injections with troglitazone can dramatically reduce insulin requirements concomitantly with improved glycemic control. One example of an effective step-up program employing sulfonylureas and insulin maintained HbA_{1c} values of approximately 7% in the Veterans Affairs Cooperative Study of Diabetes. These patients progressed from sulfonylurea failure

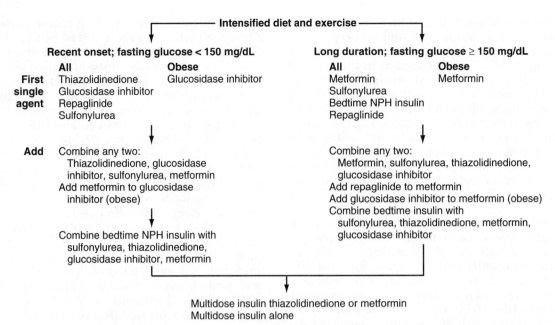

Figure 2. Scheme for combination and step therapy in type 2 diabetes.

to bedtime insulin alone, to a combination of bedtime insulin plus daytime sulfonylurea, to twice-a-day insulin, to multiple daily insulin injections.

A number of considerations may drive the choices of combination therapy for individual patients. The combination of bedtime insulin and daytime generic sulfonylureas is the most cost-effective. Metformin plus an alpha-glucosidase inhibitor is the combination least likely to promote weight gain and may even promote weight loss. Combinations with troglitazone, alpha-glucosidase inhibitors, and, to a lesser extent, metformin are the least likely to result in hypoglycemia. Repaglinide is metabolized entirely by the liver and can be used in patients with renal impairment. Troglitazone is a useful agent in refractory diabetes induced or exacerbated by adrenal-suppressive dosages of glucocorticoids. Triple combinations of oral agents can be used to avoid the need for insulin if patients are averse to injections. Although several studies are in progress, there are few data currently available for assessing the efficacy of three-drug combinations.

Pharmacologic Therapy of Cardiovascular Risk

Macrovascular Disease

Myocardial infarction is the leading cause of death in diabetic patients. Myocardial ischemia may not produce angina symptoms in patients with coexisting cardiac sensory neuropathy, and these patients may have "silent" myocardial infarctions. Diabetes patients with acute myocardial infarction are three times more likely to have a fatal outcome than are their nondiabetic counterparts and are more likely to have extensive involvement of coronary arteries with atherosclerosis. Diabetes also increases the risk of

thrombotic stroke by two- to sixfold and accelerates peripheral vascular disease, resulting in claudication, foot disease, and amputations. Good glycemic control per se may decrease risk of myocardial infarction, as was indicated by the UKPDS. However, for optimal prevention of macrovascular complications, drug therapy should be used aggressively to manage hypertension, hyperlipidemia, and dysfibrinolysis when lifestyle modifications are unsuccessful in controlling cardiovascular risk (Table 7). Total cardiovascular risk factor management is as integral to the care of diabetic patients as is glycemic control.

TABLE 7. **Treatment of Cardiovascular Risk Factors in Type 2 Diabetes**

Diet	Step 1 or 2 American Heart Association diet
Weight loss	Hypocaloric diet; lose at least 10–15% initial body weight and maintain loss
Regular exercise	30 min of modest exercise three to four times per week, aiming for 70% of maximal heart rate
Smoking cessation	
Dyslipidemia	Elevated LDL cholesterol → HMG-CoA reductase inhibitors, resins
	Elevated triglycerides → gemfibrozil, fenofibrate, niacin
	Combined hyperlipidemia → high-dose HMG-CoA reductase inhibitor (atorvastatin, 40–80 mg/d); HMG-CoA reductase inhibitor plus fibric acid derivative; niacin
Hypertension	ACE inhibitors, alpha$_1$-receptor blockers, calcium channel blockers, angiotensin II receptor antagonists
Aspirin	In high-risk patients (81–325 mg/d)
Consider vitamin E	400 IU/d

Abbreviations: ACE = angiotensin-converting enzyme; LDL = low-density lipoprotein.

Hypertension

Treatment of hypertension should be instituted at a blood pressure measurement of 130/85 mm Hg or higher. Preferred drugs used as single-agent therapy for hypertension include alpha$_1$-receptor blockers, angiotensin-converting enzyme (ACE) inhibitors, angiotensin II receptor antagonists, and calcium channel blockers. These drugs do not worsen the lipid profile or exacerbate glucose intolerance, and alpha$_1$-receptor blockers (e.g., prazosin [Minipress], doxazosin [Cardura], and terazosin [Hytrin]) may actually improve the lipid profile and increase insulin sensitivity. ACE inhibitor therapy is usually the first-choice antihypertensive agent for patients with microalbuminuria, because these drugs can prevent or retard progression of renal disease. Intraglomerular hypertension in the kidney, not always associated with systemic hypertension, is directly ameliorated by ACE inhibitor therapy. Serum creatinine and potassium levels should be closely monitored because ACE inhibitors can induce renal injury or precipitate hyperkalemia, particularly in patients with reduced glomerular filtration.

Another class of lipid-neutral agents for treating diabetic patients is the calcium channel blockers. The only caveat is that until more data are available, it is reasonable to avoid the use of short-acting dihydropyridine calcium channel blockers, such as nifedipine (Procardia), in patients who have already had a myocardial infarction. Low-dosage thiazides (e.g., hydrochlorothiazide at 25 mg per day or less) can also be used as single-agent or adjunctive therapy; hydrochlorothiazide in doses of 50 mg per day or more has adverse effects on the lipid profile. Cardioselective beta blockers can also be used effectively. However, beta blockers may worsen both lipid abnormalities and glucose tolerance and cause hypoglycemia unawareness. In both diabetic and nondiabetic patients who have already had a myocardial infarction, beta blockers are beneficial in reducing future cardiovascular events and should be considered in that setting.

Dyslipidemia

Lipid-lowering medication is recommended for hyperlipidemia that is unresponsive to a trial of weight loss, exercise, diet, and glycemic control. The first task is to identify the dyslipidemia as primarily an elevation of LDL cholesterol level, an elevation of triglyceride levels, or a mixed hyperlipidemia. Ideally, this is done after the patient is placed on a diet and is in good glycemic control, because hyperglycemia can have secondary effects on the lipid panel. The type of lipid disorder determines the class of drug that is used. Drug classes include the HMG-CoA reductase inhibitors ("statins") and the bile acid–binding resins, which are intended primarily for treatment of high cholesterol levels; fibric acid derivatives, which are intended primarily for the treatment of high triglyceride levels; and niacin, which can be used to treat both high cholesterol and triglyceride levels. The benefits of cholesterol

lowering with regard to coronary artery disease end points are twice as great in diabetic patients as in nondiabetic patients, according to several large trials. In diabetes, the total cholesterol level should be reduced to less than 160 mg per dL and the LDL cholesterol level to less than 100 mg per dL when these reductions can be accomplished safely. This is mandatory in patients with clinically evident macrovascular disease. High triglyceride levels independently increase cardiovascular risk in patients with diabetes. Treatment with fibric acid derivatives (gemfibrozil [Lopid], 600 mg bid; micronized fenofibrate [Tricor], 200 mg qd) is recommended when fasting triglyceride levels are more than 350 mg per dL despite good glycemic control.

In cases in which both LDL cholesterol and triglyceride levels are elevated, combination therapy with both statins and fibric acid derivatives may be employed, with the realization that risk for liver and/or muscle (creatine phosphokinase) enzyme elevation is increased. High dosages of statin drugs per se reduce serum triglyceride as well as cholesterol level; atorvastatin (Lipitor), for example, can be used to treat combined hyperlipidemia at dosages of 40 to 80 mg per day. Niacin in dosages of 2 to 4 grams per day also lowers both LDL-cholesterol and triglyceride levels and increases HDL cholesterol. Niacin therapy must be initiated in small dosages (100 to 250 mg per dL) and gradually increased to prevent flushing reactions, although new sustained-release preparations given at bedtime (Niaspan) are more easily tolerated. However, niacin increases insulin resistance, and its use may worsen glucose control. Therefore, diabetic patients treated with niacin must be monitored closely with HGM, and medication dosages must be increased if necessary.

Other Cardiovascular Risk Factors

The prothrombotic and antifibrinolytic alterations in type 2 diabetes warrant the use of aspirin (81 to 325 mg per day) in high-risk patients with no contraindications. In clinical trials, aspirin significantly reduces risk of myocardial infarction and thrombotic stroke as a primary or secondary prevention measure. In the U.S. Physician's Study, aspirin use was associated with a slight increase in hemorrhagic stroke in nondiabetic patients. Elevated blood homocysteine levels are known to augment cardiovascular risk. Therefore, blood homocysteine levels should be measured in high-risk patients and, if elevated, treated with folic acid alone or in combination with vitamin B$_6$ and vitamin B$_{12}$. Finally, aggressive measures should be taken to ensure cessation of cigarette smoking by diabetic patients.

Therapy for Microvascular Complications

Retinopathy

Diabetic retinopathy is the leading cause of new blindness in adults. After 25 years with the disease, approximately 80% of patients with type 2 diabetes have some form of retinopathy, classified as background, preproliferative, or proliferative. Most affected patients have background retinopathy characterized by microaneurysms, dot and blot hemorrhages, and hard exudates reflecting leakage of serous fluid from damaged vessels. Approximately 5% of patients with background retinopathy develop macular edema, which is a serious threat to vision. Macular edema cannot be visualized by direct ophthalmoscopy but can be inferred when hard exudates are close to the macula. This finding warrants immediate referral to an ophthalmologist. The preproliferative stage is an advanced form of background retinopathy distinguished by beading of retinal veins, soft exudates or cotton-wool spots from ischemic infarctions, and dilated tortuous capillaries. This signals possible progression to proliferative retinopathy and should also prompt referral to an ophthalmologist. In 4 to 6% of patients with type 2 diabetes (and 20 to 40% of those with type 1 diabetes), background retinopathy advances to proliferative retinopathy, which involves neovascularization on the retinal surface that may extend into the posterior vitreous. These fragile new vessels are at risk for bleeding, which becomes symptomatic as floaters, cobwebs, or painless loss of vision. Preretinal bleeding produces fibrous tissue that can contract, resulting in retinal detachment. Thus the two aspects of diabetic retinopathy detrimental to vision are macular edema and neovascular bleeding in the proliferative stage.

Loss of vision from proliferative retinopathy or macular edema can be prevented when laser retinal photocoagulation is used in a timely manner. Photocoagulation has been shown to reduce loss of vision by 50 to 60% when used to prevent neovascularization and retinal detachment. Therefore, all patients should, from the time of diagnosis of type 2 diabetes, have routine annual examinations by an ophthalmologist with experience in retinal diseases. These examinations should also include measurement of intraocular pressure to check for glaucoma, which more frequently occurs in diabetic patients, and to assess presence or progression of cataracts, another ocular diabetes complication. The patient should also be referred whenever key symptoms (decreased central visual acuity, floaters, blind spots) develop, if new hard exudates are detected near the macula, or if changes consistent with preproliferative or proliferative retinopathy are detected. The roles of the primary care physician are to ensure annual examinations by an ophthalmologist, to educate the patient about natural history and symptoms, to routinely question the patient about symptoms, to perform fundoscopic examinations, and to achieve therapeutic goals for control of glycemia and blood pressure. It is now certain that the development and progression of retinopathy are correlated with the degree of hyperglycemia. Recommended targets for glycemic control reflect the observation that maintaining lower HbA_{1c} values progressively decreases the risk of retinopathy and that proliferative retinopathy and macular edema can be dramatically prevented at HbA_{1c} levels of 7% or less.

Nephropathy

The prevalence of end-stage renal disease in patients who have had type 2 diabetes for 20 or more years ranges between 5 to 10% in white persons but is higher in other racial groups (~20%) such as Native Americans and African-Americans. The earliest indication of nephropathy is the development of microalbuminuria. Microalbuminuria is identified by measuring albumin in a 24-hour urine collection (30 to 300 mg per day) or by measuring the albumin/creatinine ratio in a spot urine sample, preferably with morning void urine (30 to 300 mg per gram of creatinine). Approximately one third of patients with microalbuminuria experience progressive nephropathy, characterized by persistent albuminuria (>300 mg of albumin per day) and proteinuria (>500 mg of total protein per day), followed by a steady decline in glomerular filtration and, ultimately, end-stage renal disease. As with retinopathy, good glycemic control can have a pronounced effect of preventing the development of microalbuminuria and progressive nephropathy in both type 1 and 2 diabetes. This again underscores the rationale and importance of the goals for glycemic control (see Table 4). To monitor patients for nephropathy, renal function should be assessed on an annual basis in every patient, including serum creatinine and urea measurements and 24-hour urine collection for quantification of creatinine clearance and albuminuria (see Table 5). Urine analysis with microscopic evaluation should also be performed frequently in patients prone to urinary tract infections.

There are three reasons why early recognition of microalbuminuria is a critical aspect of diabetes management. One reason is that the presence of microalbuminuria identifies patients at risk of progressive nephropathy, and therapeutic options that can prevent this progression exist. One intervention, of course, is intensified control of glycemia. In addition, ACE inhibitor therapy can reduce urinary albumin excretion and, in type 1 diabetes, slow the progression to end-stage renal disease. If patients are clearly found to have microalbuminuria on an initial and a repeated 24-hour urine collection, treatment with ACE inhibitors is recommended even in the absence of hypertension. Other factors can contribute to deteriorating renal function and necessitate vigilant attention, including urinary tract infections, nephrotoxic drugs (e.g., nonsteroidal anti-inflammatory agents), radiocontrast dyes, and neurogenic bladder.

The second reason is that microalbuminuria is associated with the onset of hypertension, and the presence of hypertension can accelerate the progression of nephropathy. Therefore, blood pressure should be measured frequently in microalbuminuric patients, both in the physician's office and with a home blood pressure cuff, and medical therapy should be instituted as soon as blood pressure rises above 130/85. This is done most appropriately with ACE inhibitor therapy, which is recommended in microalbuminuric patients without hypertension and in combination with other antihypertensive medications as needed. Blood pressure control per se is beneficial in slowing progression of nephropathy even when accomplished without ACE inhibitors. In treating hypertension, it is important to be cognizant of potential hyperkalemia. Many patients with type 2 diabetes and mild renal impairment have hyporeninemic hypoaldosteronism, which can cause hyperkalemia, and ACE inhibitors can unmask or exacerbate hyperkalemia in these patients.

The third reason is that the presence of microalbuminuria identifies patients at higher risk of developing macrovascular disease complications. Microalbuminuria is also more likely to be associated with an atherogenic lipid profile, including high total and LDL cholesterol, high triglyceride, and low HDL cholesterol levels. Therefore, with the identification of microalbuminuria, screening and therapy for cardiovascular risk factors, particularly those relating to hypertension and dyslipidemia, should be intensified.

When the serum creatinine level rises to 2 to 3 mg per dL, the patient should be referred to a nephrologist. At the appropriate time, the patient is readied for hemodialysis, chronic ambulatory peritoneal dialysis, or kidney transplantation. Among patients on hemodialysis, those with diabetes have higher mortality rates than do age-matched nondiabetic patients, and they continue to require aggressive treatment of hypertension, dyslipidemia, and hyperglycemia.

Neuropathy

Neuropathic complications are classified as either peripheral sensorimotor or autonomic, and both categories can be prevented with good glycemic control. Peripheral sensorimotor neuropathy includes distal symmetrical neuropathy, which affects the limbs in a "stocking glove" distribution; radiculopathies and mononeuropathies; and diabetic amyotrophy, characterized by symmetrical muscle weakness and wasting in the lower extremities and pelvic girdle. Therapy for these conditions involves intensified glycemic control and symptomatic treatment, and symptoms gradually diminish. Peripheral sensorimotor neuropathy can produce pain and hyperesthesia that gets worse at night. Several symptomatic treatment options for neuropathic pain are available, but none of these is effective in all patients. Patients may be given a trial of amitriptyline, 25 to 100 mg at bedtime, with the addition of fluphenazine (Prolixin), 1 to 2 mg at bedtime if needed; gabapentin (Neurontin), 300 to 1200 mg tid; or carbamazepine (Tegretol), 200 to 600 mg bid. Topical application of capsaicin (Zostrix) is particularly helpful for superficial burning pain and allodynia; this drug acts by depleting substance P from C-fiber nerve terminals. Capsaicin should be applied carefully with gloves, with care taken to avoid mucous membranes, and regular application is needed to maintain effectiveness. Opiates should be used for short periods of time

to treat severe pain, with close attention to the risk of addiction. Palsies caused by involvement of cranial nerves III and VI and of peroneal, median, and ulnar nerves usually remit spontaneously in 3 to 6 months. Muscle strength in diabetic amyotrophy returns gradually after 6 to 12 months and patients should receive physical therapy throughout its course.

Autonomic neuropathies tend to affect patients with poorly controlled long-standing diabetes and can be extremely troubling for patients. If the diagnosis of autonomic neuropathy is entertained, the clinician usually finds involvement of multiple organ systems, and cardiac examination reveals resting tachycardia and/or loss of beat-to-beat variations with deep breathing. *Gastroparesis* causes early satiety, bloating, and nausea, and diagnosis involves endoscopy or upper gastrointestinal barium series plus nuclear medicine scintigraphy after ingestion of a standard radiolabeled meal. The delay in gastric emptying can make postprandial glycemic control more problematic. Nonpharmacologic intervention includes small meals that avoid an excess of high-fat, spicy, and fibrous foods. Pharmacologic treatment includes elimination of drugs slowing gastric motility (opioids, anticholinergics) and institution of one of several possible drugs, all given before each meal, including cisapride (Propulsid), 10 to 20 mg; metoclopramide (Reglan), 10 mg; erythromycin, 125 to 250 mg; and domperidone,* 10 to 20 mg. Periods of metoclopramide administration should be intermittent because its effectiveness wanes when given chronically over long periods of time, and it can produce dystonic reactions and tardive dyskinesia.

Diabetic diarrhea can be persistent or alternate with periods of constipation. Bacterial overgrowth may be contributory and can be assessed with a 1- to 2-week trial of metronidazole (Flagyl), ampicillin, or tetracycline. High-fiber foods and/or psyllium supplements may help, and diarrhea can be controlled symptomatically with loperamide (Imodium), 4 to 16 mg per day, or diphenoxylate (Lomotil), 2.5 to 5 mg four times a day (qid). Some patients respond to clonidine (Catapres) or octreotide (Sandostatin), the latter requiring subcutaneous injection. *Neurogenic bladder* is manifested by symptoms of frequency and incontinence and can result in recurrent urinary tract infections. Demonstration of a large residual volume and abnormal cystometry is required for diagnosis, and evaluation may include prostate examination, cystoscopy, and intravenous pyelogram. Treatment can include either scheduling frequent voids (every 4 hours), with or without bethanechol (Urecholine), 10 to 50 mg tid or qid, or intermittent catheterization. Prophylactic treatment with trimethoprim-sulfamethoxazole (Bactrim) may prevent or suppress recurrent urinary tract infections. *Orthostatic hypotension* ranges in severity from asymptotic to disabling and life-threatening. Upright hypotension is not uncommonly associated with supine hypertension. Treatment should include support hose

---

*Not available in the United States.

or body stockings to increase venous return, rising to a supine position gradually, sleeping with the head of bed elevated to prevent supine hypertension, and avoidance of offending medications. Some patients require intravascular volume expansion with the mineralocorticoid fludrocortisone acetate (Florinef), 0.05 to 0.2 mg qd. Midodrine (ProAmatine), an alpha$_1$-receptor agonist, can help relieve hypotension in severe cases.

Erectile dysfunction is very common in diabetic men and can be caused by autonomic neuropathy or vascular disease related to diabetes, or it can be caused by the same psychologic, endocrinologic, or medicine-related factors operative in nondiabetic patients. When the cause is related to diabetes, libido is intact and there is an inability to generate or sustain firm erections while sleeping during the night or with any sexual partner. A history consistent with retrograde ejaculation is also common. In the past, external vacuum pumps or implantable penile prostheses were the only available therapies; however, quality of life has been enhanced by multiple new options for medical therapy. Many diabetic patients respond to sildenafil (Viagra), taken 1 hour before sexual intercourse. The penile erection is then dependent on sexual stimulation. Sildenafil should not be prescribed to patients who are prone to hypotension, who have active heart disease, or who are receiving nitrate therapy. Self-injection of drugs into the corpora cavernosa is an alternative approach; these drugs include papaverine, phentolamine (Regitine), or alprostadil (Caverject), or a mixture of all three, commonly known as trimix. Prolonged erection or priapism occurs 1 to 5% of the time, which may necessitate injection of phenylephrine or removal of blood with a needle and syringe. Chronic application can lead to corporeal fibrosis. Alprostadil can also be administered transurethrally (Muse) through a medicated urethral system; erections are obtained in approximately 65% of patients.

Diabetic Foot Disease

Diabetic foot disease accounts for most of the more than 50,000 nontraumatic limb amputations performed yearly in the United States. After one lower extremity amputation in a diabetic patient, there is a 50% likelihood that amputation in the contralateral limb will be necessary in 3 to 5 years and that death will occur within 5 to 10 years. The pathogenesis of diabetic foot disease is multifactorial and involves variable combinations of peripheral sensory neuropathy with loss of feeling; autonomic neuropathy, which causes dryness and cracking; peripheral vascular disease, which results in ischemia; microvascular disease, which reduces capillary blood flow; and structural deformities, such as Charcot's foot and bunions. These factors predispose to injury, pressure ischemia, and skin breakdown with subsequent development of ulcer, cellulitis, osteomyelitis, and necrosis. Of importance is that more than 75% of the amputations in diabetic patients can be prevented. Patients should be regularly educated about routine foot inspections

for recognition of early lesions. Daily cleaning, moisturizing creams, and proper footwear that provides protection, an even weight distribution, and absence of pressure points are necessary.

The diabetes health care team should include a podiatrist who provides regular care for nails and calluses and special shoe prescriptions in patients at higher risk. A trained member of the diabetes health care team, if not the physician, should inspect a patient's feet on every visit, and it is helpful to have patients remove shoes routinely after entering the examination room. The examination should include palpation of peripheral pulses, tactile and vibratory sensation testing, Achilles' tendon reflex, and careful inspection of the feet for ulcers, calluses, foreign bodies, skin cracking, and deformities. Once an ulcer develops, the site requires débridement, alleviation of pressure, and antibiotics if infected. Because these infections are often multibacterial, a broad-spectrum antibiotic is warranted (e.g., amoxicillin/clavulanate [Augmentin]) if a single offending pathogen cannot be cultured and analyzed for antibiotic sensitivities. For extensive or refractory infections, hospitalization should be considered in order to ensure immobilization, local wound care, and intravenous antibiotics. Radiographs and bone scans are necessary to assess for osteomyelitis. An orthopedic surgeon should be consulted when extensive débridement, foot-sparing surgery, surgical therapy for osteomyelitis, placement of walking casts to relieve pressure, or amputation is required. A vascular surgeon should be consulted to determine whether arterial revascularization may be beneficial.

ACKNOWLEDGMENTS

The author is grateful to Drs. John A. Colwell and Ronald Mayfield for critical review of the manuscript.

DIABETES MELLITUS IN CHILDREN AND ADOLESCENTS

method of
WILLIAM V. TAMBORLANE, M.D., and
JOANN AHERN, R.N., M.S.N.
Yale University School of Medicine
New Haven, Connecticut

Treatment of children and adolescents with diabetes mellitus provides a special challenge to clinicians. On the one hand, results of the Diabetes Control and Complications Trial (DCCT) indicate that the level of metabolic control has a profound impact on the risk of developing the microvascular complications of diabetes. On the other hand, the rapid physiologic and psychosocial changes that occur during childhood and adolescence make these patients the most difficult to manage.

DIABETIC KETOACIDOSIS IN CHILDREN

Because of the severe degree of insulin deficiency that commonly characterizes diabetes in childhood, the clinical onset of the disease in this age group is usually abrupt and the metabolic abnormalities at presentation are often profound. For children, a brief history and physical examination should readily suggest the diagnosis of diabetic ketoacidosis (DKA) even in patients with new-onset disease. The diagnosis of DKA should be quickly established at the bedside.

Capillary blood glucose values are elevated, and urine test results are positive for glucose and ketones. An intravenous line is placed to begin initial hydration, and additional studies are sent to the laboratory. The initial laboratory studies are for definition of the degree of metabolic derangement, not for diagnosis, and include plasma glucose, blood urea nitrogen, creatinine (creatinine values may be artificially elevated with certain methods), electrolytes, pH, PCO_2, serum calcium and phosphorus concentrations, and a lead II electrocardiographic rhythm strip. Other studies, such as complete blood cell count and blood and urine cultures, are obtained as needed for diagnosis of precipitating causes. Diagnosis, baseline laboratory assessments, and initiation of treatment should all be accomplished within minutes of arrival of the patient in the emergency department.

Goals of Therapy

The four general goals of treatment of DKA are (1) replacement of fluid and electrolyte deficits, (2) correction of the underlying metabolic disturbance, (3) identification and treatment of precipitating causes, and (4) avoidance of potential pitfalls. In most instances, treatment of DKA should be carried out in an intensive care setting and facilitated by a flow-sheet that charts physiologic data, clinical observations, intake and output, level of consciousness, and biochemical parameters. Each aspect of treatment of DKA is somewhat controversial. A consistent regimen, however, with careful follow-up monitoring and appropriate adjustments is probably most important.

Precipitating Causes and Potential Pitfalls

The most common precipitating cause of DKA in children is an intercurrent viral infection or failure by a patient with recurrent episodes of DKA to take prescribed insulin. The signs and symptoms of DKA may mask or mimic those of more serious precipitating causes, such as a systemic bacterial infection or an acute abdomen. Inadequate fluid replacement, hypoglycemia, hypokalemia-induced cardiac arrhythmias, and cerebral edema are the main pitfalls to be avoided.

Cerebral edema is an ominous complication to which children are especially prone; it accounts for 50% or more of the morbidity and mortality from DKA. Risk is increased by the degree and duration of the hyperosmolar state, in younger children, and in those with reduced consciousness on presentation. Overly vigorous rehydration and rapid fall in serum hyperosmolarity attributable to a rapid fall in plasma glucose levels also increase the risk of cerebral edema. Many of the aspects of treatment described later are aimed at reducing the risk of this catastrophic complication of treatment.

TREATMENT

Fluid Replacement

Fluid replacement should begin as soon as the diagnosis of DKA is made in the emergency room. A bolus of 10 to 20 mL per kg of body weight of an isotonic saline solution (0.9%) is given over the first hour to stabilize vital signs and improve peripheral perfusion. The infusion is then lowered to a rate calculated to replace maintenance plus deficit (usually on the order of 10%) over 48 hours. By this time, results of initial laboratory studies should by available to help with tailoring of electrolyte replacement. With mild to moderate DKA, 50% normal saline can be used, whereas normal saline or 50% normal saline with the addition of bicarbonate (see the section on bicarbonate) are used in more severe cases. Isotonic rather than hypotonic solutions are preferred in such cases for reducing the risk of cerebral edema caused by overly rapid reductions in serum osmolarity.

Adequate fluid replacement helps correct hyperglycemia and acidosis by improving the glomerular filtration rate and by increasing urinary excretion of glucose and ketones. Five percent dextrose solution is added to the regimen when the plasma glucose level falls below 400 mg per dL, with an aim of maintaining plasma concentrations between 200 and 300 mg per dL. In patients with marked hyperglycemia (i.e., >800 mg/dL), dextrose may need to be added earlier and in higher concentrations (i.e., 10 to 20%) to prevent too rapid a fall in plasma glucose levels.

Bicarbonate

For a variety of reasons, use of bicarbonate is not recommended routinely. Severe acidosis, however, may contribute to hypotension caused by peripheral vasodilation and impaired myocardial function. In addition, when the serum bicarbonate concentration falls below 10 mEq per liter, the buffering capacity of the blood is compromised, and ongoing hydrogen ion production can have profound effects on serum pH. Therefore, we use bicarbonate when the pH is less than 7.20 or the serum bicarbonate is less than 10 mEq per liter. Bicarbonate, 50 mEq, can be added to each liter of intravenous fluids after the initial fluid bolus is given. Bicarbonate is discontinued when the pH exceeds 7.20 in order to avoid overcorrection and late metabolic alkalosis owing to conversion of ketones to bicarbonate. We do not add bicarbonate if the initial serum potassium levels are low, because administration of bicarbonate with insulin in hyperglycemic patients may precipitate serious hypokalemia. For the same reason, bolus injections of bicarbonate are avoided in virtually all patients.

Potassium and Phosphate

All patients with DKA are depleted of total body potassium even though serum potassium level is usually modestly elevated owing to extracellular shifts of potassium with acidosis. In fact, a low serum potassium level when the patient is first seen is of great concern because almost all aspects of treatment of DKA work to lower serum potassium concentrations.

Assuming that serum potassium values are not excessively elevated (i.e., >7.0 mEq per liter), we begin potassium replacement after the initial fluid bolus at a dose of 20 to 40 mEq per liter, although more may be needed if serum levels are low. Subsequent doses are adjusted on the basis of frequent monitoring of serum levels.

Many experts suggest that about 50% of potassium replacement be given as phosphate. Controlled clinical trials, however, have failed to show that phosphate is beneficial, and its administration can induce hypocalcemic tetany owing to sluggish parathyroid hormone responses during DKA. Therefore, we do not routinely administer phosphate during correction of DKA.

Insulin Infusion

Continuous intravenous administration of regular insulin is the preferred method for correcting the underlying metabolic disturbance of DKA because of its simplicity and effectiveness. We use an initial bolus of 0.1 U per kg body weight, followed by a continuous rate of 0.1 U per kg per hour. It is the rare patient who requires more than 0.1 U per kg per hour, and a sluggish fall in plasma glucose during the early hours of treatment is more likely due to inadequate fluid than to inadequate insulin replacement. Intravenous insulin is continued until both hyperglycemia and acidosis are substantially corrected. Indeed, if stable plasma glucose values in the range of 200 to 300 mg per dL can be achieved with intravenous insulin and glucose, there is no compelling reason to switch to subcutaneous insulin until the patient is ready to resume oral intake.

Cerebral Edema

Failure of mental status to improve or any worsening of level of consciousness during the first 2 to 18 hours of treatment requires immediate evaluation. If possible, computed tomography of the brain to confirm brain swelling and an emergency neurosurgical consult for intracranial pressure monitoring should be obtained. Patients who develop cerebral edema require prompt intervention with intravenous mannitol (1 gram per kg of body weight), intubation, and hyperventilation. Additional doses of mannitol are given, as needed, according to intercranial pressure monitoring results. Early and aggressive evaluation is critically important because the response to treatment after the development of brain stem signs (e.g., dilated pupils, respiratory arrest) is usually poor.

LONG-TERM MANAGEMENT

We recommend hospital admission for the initiation of treatment for all children with newly diagnosed diabetes, even those who are reasonably well at diagnosis. An adjustment period is necessary for the child and family in a supportive environment because the diagnosis is a shock to the family. A comprehensive day treatment program staffed by a multidisciplinary diabetes team, however, can provide a suitable alternative to hospitalization for patients with newly diagnosed diabetes who are not in ketoacidosis.

Goals of Treatment

The traditional goals of treatment of children with diabetes were (1) to use insulin, diet, and exercise to minimize symptoms of hypoglycemia and hyperglycemia and promote normal growth and development and (2) to use intensive education to maximize independence and self-management in order to reduce the adverse psychosocial effects of this chronic disease. Since the DCCT occurred, another primary goal of therapy is to maintain plasma glucose and glycosylated hemoglobin as close to normal as safely possible. Practical considerations such as the age of the patient and acceptability of and compliance with the treatment regimens must be balanced appropriately in order to obtain all of these aims of therapy. Data suggest that an intensive approach to diabetes education and aggressive self-management by patients and families may reduce rather than increase the adverse psychosocial effects of this chronic illness.

Insulin Regimens

Subcutaneous insulin injections can begin when the child is well hydrated and able to tolerate regular meals. To avoid a rebound rise in plasma glucose levels, the intravenous insulin infusion should not be discontinued for at least 1 hour after subcutaneous insulin is given. A sampling of the variety of conventional and unconventional insulin regimens that can be employed is given in Table 1.

We start children who have newly diagnosed diabetes on two injections of insulin per day with a mixture of human Lente and lispro (Humalog) insulin at a total dose of 1 U per kg per day. Two thirds of the dose is given before breakfast and one third before supper. The dose is usually given as one-third lispro and two-thirds Lente. During the hospitalization, each component of the insulin regimen is adjusted on the basis of capillary blood glucose levels measured at the bedside six or more times per day (before each meal, at bedtime, at 12 AM and at 3 AM).

With aggressive management, most children enter a "honeymoon" or partial remission period after a few weeks as a result of increased insulin secretion by residual beta cells and improved insulin sensitivity with better glycemic control. Moreover, data from the DCCT indicate that therapy aimed at normalizing HbA_{1C} levels serves to prolong the period of residual beta cell function in patients with type 1 diabetes.

During the honeymoon phase, insulin requirements rapidly decrease. Commonly, the doses of rapid-acting insulin are sharply reduced or discontinued during this time; many children are well managed with two injections of intermediate-acting insu-

TABLE 1. **Insulin Injection Regimens**

Doses	Breakfast	Lunch/Afternoon Snack	Dinner	Bedtime
Two	Li/R* + Le/N		Li/R + Le/N	
	Li/R + Le/N		Li/R + U	
	Li/R + Le/N + U		Li/R + Le/N + U	
Three	Li/R + Le/N ± U		Li/R	
	Li/R + Le/N		Li/R + Le/N ± U	Le/N ± Li
Four	R	R (lunch)	R	Le/N ± R

*These insulins can also be mixed to give quicker onset and longer duration than either rapid-acting insulin alone.
Types of insulins: Rapid acting (Li = lispro, R = regular), intermediate-acting (Le = lente; N = neutral protamine Hagedorn), and long-acting (U = Ultralente). Slash (/) = either/or; ± = with or without.

lin, and some may not even require an evening injection. In the absence of symptomatic hypoglycemia, however, we are reluctant to lower the total daily dose of insulin below 0.20 to 0.25 U per kg of body weight per day because these are doses being employed currently in prediabetic children in the DPT-1 study.

A major reason why the two daily injections regimen is effective during the honeymoon phase is that endogenous insulin secretion provides much of the overnight basal insulin requirements, leading to normal fasting blood glucose values. Thus, increased and more labile prebreakfast glucose levels often herald the loss of residual endogenous insulin secretion. When residual beta-cell function wanes, problems with the two-injection regimen become apparent. One problem is that the peak of the predinner intermediate-acting insulin may coincide with the time of minimal insulin requirements (i.e., midnight to 4 AM). Subsequently, insulin levels fall off when basal requirements are increasing (i.e., 4 AM to 8 AM). Increasing the presupper dose of intermediate-acting insulin to lower fasting glucose values often leads to hypoglycemia in the middle of the night without correcting hyperglycemia before breakfast. Another problem with the conventional two-injection regimen is high presupper glucose levels despite normal or low prelunch and midafternoon values. This is due to eating an afternoon snack when the prebreakfast dose of intermediate-acting insulin is waning.

One way to deal with these problems without increasing the number of injections is to add Ultralente insulin to the prebreakfast and presupper mixtures of lispro and Lente. With this combination in the morning, lispro covers breakfast, Lente covers lunch, and Ultralente covers the late afternoon period. With the presupper dose, lispro covers supper, Lente covers the bedtime snack and part of the overnight period, and Ultralente helps limit the prebreakfast rise in plasma glucose. When strict control cannot be achieved with two daily injections, we do not hesitate to switch to a regimen involving three or more daily injections. A common approach to the problem in the overnight period is to use a three-injection regimen: lispro and Lente at breakfast, lispro only at dinner, and Lente at bedtime. In young children who go to bed early, we recommend that the parents give the third injection at their bedtime (i.e., 10:00 to 11:00 PM). Lispro can also be added to the bedtime dose, especially if glucose levels are elevated. For patients with elevated presupper glucose levels, a prelunch dose of regular or a preafternoon snack dose of lispro can be added. Such extra doses of insulin can be facilitated by the use of an insulin pen, which is small, light, and easy to carry.

Very few of our patients use a four-injection regimen (e.g., premeal regular and bedtime Lente). Over the past 2 years, however, many of our children have been started on insulin pump treatment. The pump delivers small amounts of rapid-acting insulin as a basal infusion with bolus doses given before each meal or snack. Although lispro is not yet labeled by the U.S. Food and Drug Administration (FDA) for use in pumps, most of our pump-treated patients use lispro rather than regular insulin. The pumps are battery powered and about the size of a beeper. The "basal" rate can be programmed to change each hour of the day, but it is unusual to need more than five or six basal rates. Variations in the basal rate can be particularly helpful in regulating overnight blood glucose levels, because it can be lowered for the early part of the night to prevent hypoglycemia and increased in the hours before dawn to keep glucose from rising. Some children seem to need a higher basal rate during the night, however, perhaps because of secretion of growth hormone at this time, and many need a lower basal rate in the late morning to avoid hypoglycemia before lunch. Bolus doses are given before meals on the basis of glucose level, exercise, and food intake.

The pump employs a reservoir (syringe) to hold the insulin and the infusion set, which consists of tubing with a small plastic catheter at the end. The insertion site can be the abdomen or hip area, except in the young child in whom there may not be sufficient subcutaneous tissue in the abdomen. Our patients are encouraged to change their catheters every other day. Because only a rapid-acting insulin is used in this pump, the child and parent must understand that the insulin infusion should not be discontinued for more than 4 hours at a time.

Monitoring Glucose Control

Insulin replacement for children and adolescents is a special challenge because insulin requirements increase as weight and calorie intake increase, as residual endogenous secretion declines, and as the patients progress through the hormonal changes of puberty. As a result, the average daily insulin dose for children with long-standing diabetes is about 0.6 to 1.0 U per kg of body weight, and doses of at least 1.5 U per kg or more may be required by well-controlled adolescents. Changes in total daily insulin requirements in a typical boy with onset of diabetes at 6 years of age are shown in Table 2.

Regular self-monitoring of blood glucose (SMBG) allows the family and clinicians to keep up with the child's steadily increasing insulin needs. We request that the patient check four times per day (before each meal and at bedtime), but many parents (especially those with very young children) check more often.

The most important component of SMBG is the interpretation of the results. The parent or child must be taught what the target value is and what the relationship is between diet, exercise, and insulin. If the parent and child grasp these concepts, they will make accurate adjustments aimed at achieving target goals. If they are unable to make accurate adjustments, they should be given guidelines of when to call the diabetes service for help. Day-to-day adjustments in the doses of rapid-acting insulin can be made on the basis of the premeal blood glucose value, amount of carbohydrate in the meal, and amount of anticipated exercise. In addition, patients and parents should be taught to look for repetitive patterns of hypoglycemia or hyperglycemia in order to make ongoing changes in their usual insulin doses. Patients and parents are instructed to check for ketones in the urine whenever a patient is nauseated or vomiting or if two successive glucose readings are more than 250.

SMBG is subject to a variety of problems, especially when a child makes up false numbers. These issues must be addressed with the child or adolescent. They must understand the reason for the tests and that the tests are used only to make proper adjustments to keep them healthy. Elevated glucose levels are not an indication of worsening of diabetes or that they have been cheating on their diet. Instead, we emphasize that the tests are being done primarily to determine when they have outgrown their current dose of insulin.

Glycosylated Hemoglobin

A variety of methods are available for assaying glycosylated hemoglobin The most widely accepted is the HbA$_{1C}$ method. A simple method that can be performed in the office in 6 minutes (Bayer DCA 2000) offers the opportunity to make immediate changes in the insulin regimen while the patient is being seen. The goal of treatment is to achieve HbA$_{1C}$ levels as close to normal as possible. On the basis of DCCT results, our general goal of therapy is to try to keep all patients under 8.0%.

Diet

Diet guidance for children with insulin-dependent diabetes mellitus is best provided by a nutritionist, who is an integral part of the treatment team and must be comfortable working with children. In addition to helping achieve optimal glucose levels and normal growth and development, nutritional management of diabetes is aimed at reducing the risk for other diseases such as obesity, high blood cholesterol level, or high blood pressure. Underlying all of these is the establishment of sound eating patterns that include balanced, nutritious foods and consistent timing of food intake.

The American Diabetes Association dietary guidelines are used for dietary counseling. In addition to incorporating sound nutritional principles concerning the fat, fiber, and carbohydrate content, the importance of consistency in meal size and regularity in the timing of meals is emphasized. The prohibition of simple sugar in the diet has been de-emphasized, but simple sugar should still be no more than 10% of total carbohydrate intake. The success of the nutritional program may ultimately depend on the degree to which the meal plans are individualized and tailored to well-established eating patterns in the family. Moreover, flexibility can be enhanced if blood glucose–monitoring results are used to evaluate the impact of change in dietary intake. As with other aspects of the treatment regimen, we preach consistency and teach how to adjust for deviations from the prescribed diet.

Carbohydrate counting is an increasingly popular way to increase flexibility in food intake, especially with patients using an insulin pump or multiple daily injections. The amount of insulin that is needed for each gram or serving of carbohydrate is used to calculate the amount of regular or lispro to be taken depending on the amount of carbohydrates in the meal. With instructions on how to use nutritional labels on food packages, even children can become expert at counting carbohydrates. An even simpler method is to vary the dose of regular or lispro by 1 or 2 U for a small, regular, or large meal. Some foods, such as pizza, that cause a prolonged increase in blood glucose levels may require an increase in the amount of intermediate-acting insulin.

Exercise

Regular exercise and active participation in organized sports have positive implications concerning the psychosocial and physical well-being of our pa-

TABLE 2. **Changes in Insulin Dose for an Average Boy (Onset Age 6 Years)**

Age (y)	Weight (kg)		U/kg/day		Total Daily Dose (U)
8	25	×	0.6	=	15
16	65	×	1.2	=	78

tients. Aerobic endurance exercise is preferred over weight lifting and other activities that involve straining and increased systemic blood pressure. Patients should be advised that different types of exercise may have different effects on blood glucose levels. For example, sports that involve short bursts of intensive exercise (e.g., hockey) may increase rather than decrease blood glucose levels. On the other hand, long-distance running and other prolonged activities are more likely to lower blood glucose levels. Patients also need to be warned that a long bout of exercise during the day may lead to hypoglycemia while they are sleeping that night.

Outpatient Care

Children and adolescents with type 1 diabetes should be routinely cared for at a diabetes center where a multidisciplinary team knowledgeable about and experienced in the management of young patients is used. This team should ideally consist of pediatric diabetologists, diabetes nurse specialists, nutritionists, social workers, psychologists, exercise physiologists, and referral resources for eye, neurologic, renal, and other problems.

In newly diagnosed patients with diabetes, the weeks following discharge from the hospital are critically important ones in the process of teaching self-management skills to the child and parents. The older child or parent is in daily contact with the diabetes clinical nurse specialist. Glucose levels, adjustment to diabetes, and diet and exercise are reviewed. The timing of the phone calls should be prearranged and ideally made to the same clinician. After making the insulin adjustment for the day, the clinician should explain the rationale to the child or parent. Usually within 2 to 3 weeks the parents and child are feeling more confident, and many are ready to attempt to make their own adjustments.

Once the child is stabilized, regular follow-up visits on a 2- to 3-month basis are recommended for each patient. The main purpose of these visits is to ensure that the patient is achieving primary treatment goals. In addition to serial measurements of height and weight, particular attention should be paid to monitoring of blood pressure and examinations of the optic fundus, thyroid, and subcutaneous injection sites. Signs and symptoms referable to diabetes complications are sought. Such surveillance is complemented by use of laboratory tests to measure lipids and circulating thyroid hormone levels, renal function studies (especially microalbuminuria), and retinal fundus photography after 5 years of duration. Routine outpatient visits provide an opportunity to review glucose monitoring and to adjust the treatment regimen. Follow-up advice and support should be given by the nutritionist, diabetes nurse specialist, and psychologist or social worker. Use of the telephone, fax, or electronic mail should be encouraged for discussions of adjustments in the treatment regimen between office visits.

Hypoglycemia

Severe hypoglycemia is a common problem in patients striving for strict glycemic control. In the DCCT, the risk of severe hypoglycemia was threefold higher in intensively treated than in conventionally treated patients, and being an adolescent was an independent risk factor for a severe hypoglycemic event. The majority of severe hypoglycemic events occur overnight, partly because of sleep-induced defects in counterregulatory hormone responses to hypoglycemia.

Monitoring glucose is critical to detect asymptomatic hypoglycemia, especially in the young child with diabetes. The older child is usually aware of symptoms such as weakness, shakiness, hunger, or headache and is encouraged to treat these symptoms as soon as they occur. The older child who can accurately recognize symptoms is taught to immediately treat with 15 grams of carbohydrate (e.g., three to four glucose tablets, 4 ounces of juice, or 15 grams of a glucose gel) without waiting to check a glucose level. By treating quickly, the child loses little time from the classroom by unnecessary trips to the nurse's office. Each episode should be assessed in order to make proper adjustments if a cause can be identified. Every family should have a glucagon emergency kit at home to treat severe hypoglycemia.

Particular care and attention must be given to adolescents who drive. They need to be instructed to check glucose levels before getting into the car and every 2 hours while on long trips. Careful instruction on the problems of alcohol use is also warranted because alcohol blunts the liver's response to hypoglycemia.

Sick Day Rules

Children with intercurrent illnesses, such as infections or vomiting, should be closely monitored for elevations in blood glucose levels and ketonuria. On sick days, blood glucose levels should be checked every 2 hours, and the urine should be checked for ketones every time a patient voids. Supplemental doses of short-acting insulin (0.1 to 0.3 U per kg of body weight) should be given every 2 to 4 hours for elevations in glucose and ketone levels. Because of its more rapid absorption, lispro lowers plasma glucose level faster than regular insulin. If the morning dose has not been given and the child has a modestly elevated glucose level (150 to 250 mg per dL), small doses of neutral protamine Hagedorn (NPH) can be given to avoid too rapid a fall in plasma glucose level. This works especially well in very young children whose glucose levels fall quickly with rapid-acting insulin. Adequate fluid intake is essential to prevent dehydration. Fluids such as flat soda, clear soups, popsicles, and gelatin water are recommended to provide some electrolyte and carbohydrate replacement. If vomiting is persistent and ketones remain moderate or large after several supplemental insulin doses, arrangements should be made for parenteral hydration and evaluation in the emergency department.

Children receiving Ultralente insulin seem to be prone to the development of hypoglycemia and ketonuria during episodes of gastroenteritis. If the child is unable to retain oral carbohydrate, then small doses of glucagon (i.e., 0.1 to 0.2 mg), given subcutaneously every 2 to 4 hours, can be used to maintain normal blood glucose levels.

DIABETIC KETOACIDOSIS

method of
EUGENIO CERSOSIMO, M.D., PH.D.
State University of New York at Stony Brook
Stony Brook, New York

Diabetes ketoacidosis (DKA) is a complex disturbance of carbohydrate, lipid, and protein metabolism secondary to a state of extreme insulin deficiency. Although the signs and symptoms are primarily related to carbohydrate and lipid abnormalities, DKA resembles the metabolic state of accelerated fasting with intense interorgan fuel mobilization and negative nitrogen balance. Hyperglycemia and hyperosmolality occur as a result of an increase in endogenous glucose production and a decrease in glucose utilization and storage, both induced by insulin deficiency. When plasma glucose concentration exceeds the capacity for renal tubular reabsorption, glycosuria and osmotic diuresis ensue. As water moves from the intracellular to the hyperosmolal extracellular compartment, there is a transient increase in glomerular filtration rate. Negative fluid balance, however, reduces total body water and results in hypovolemia, which is accompanied by a reduction in glomerular filtration rate. As a consequence, renal load, utilization, and excretion of glucose diminish and hyperglycemia becomes more severe. In response, circulating counterregulatory hormones—that is, glucagon, catecholamines, cortisol, and growth hormone—rise and further stimulate endogenous glucose production and adipose tissue lipolysis. Triacylglyceride hydrolysis leads to elevations in plasma fatty acid levels, which provide an alternative fuel for tissue oxidation and further impair glucose utilization. Overall, enhanced uptake and oxidation of fatty acids contribute to perpetuate the states of hyperglycemia and hyperosmolality.

With increased fatty acid extraction by the liver and inadequate insulinization of hepatocytes, fatty acids are directed toward beta oxidation with abundant formation of acetyl–coenzyme A (CoA) intermediates. The enzymatic conversion of excess acetyl-CoA into aceto-acetate, beta-hydroxy-butyrate, and acetone (keto acids or ketone bodies) is activated and ketone bodies are released into the circulation. Rising blood levels of ketone bodies due to overproduction and underutilization result in hydrogen ion accumulation, which increases consumption and depletes bicarbonate and other body pH buffers. Simultaneous limited formation of bicarbonate contributes to lowering of blood pH and an anion gap metabolic acidosis develops. In addition, ketonemia and ketonuria worsen hyperglycemia and hyperosmolality, exaggerate water and electrolyte disturbances, and, together with all other abnormalities, create a metabolic vicious cycle by further impairing insulin action and enhancing the secretion of counterregulatory hormone.

Although there is no uniformly accepted definition of DKA, most workers in the field agree that the syndrome consists of the triad of hyperglycemia, ketosis, and acidemia, usually documented in association with other clinical conditions. The major precipitating factors for DKA are infection, intercurrent illness, and omission of or inadequate insulin therapy. The fact that only about 25% of hospitalized patients with the diagnosis of DKA represent newly diagnosed diabetes mellitus underscores the need to pursue other potential precipitating factors for every episode of DKA. It should be recognized that with the introduction of insulin pumps to deliver fast-acting insulin formulations continuously in the subcutaneous tissue to treat diabetes, the use of intermediate- and long-acting insulin preparations is not necessary. Thus, patients can rapidly become insulin deficient and develop ketoacidosis during infection or unexpected stress. This is particularly important in the diagnosis of silent myocardial infarction, considering that patients with type 1 diabetes live longer than they used to and are vulnerable to coronary events at a younger age. Once the diagnosis of DKA is established, immediate aggressive therapy and evaluation of potential precipitating factor(s) are required.

INITIAL EVALUATION

Patients known to have type 1 diabetes mellitus who present with history of intercurrent illness, omission of insulin, abdominal pain, nausea, vomiting, and dehydration should be evaluated for DKA. If history cannot be obtained with certainty, as for example in dehydrated patients with altered mental status, findings that should raise suspicion of DKA include the presence of bracelets, necklaces, or identification cards indicating that patient has diabetes and evidence of subcutaneous insulin injection in areas of the skin. Gynecologic and obstetric history should be obtained in women in the reproductive age range, and pregnancy must be ruled out with appropriate blood/urine tests. A list of medications must be recorded for all patients, and blood and urine drug screening must be sought in those with a history or evidence of drug abuse. Initial assessment should include recording of body weight and vital signs and a complete physical examination to estimate severity of fluid deficit and document findings, which may help identify other associated clinical conditions. If the situation requires, airway, breathing, and cardiovascular stability must be established immediately. Nasogastric (or orogastric) tube placement may be necessary to evacuate the contents of the stomach and reduce likelihood of aspiration in a comatose patient. Urinary catheters are helpful in assessing urine output and fluid balance. Initial management is best if undertaken by properly trained personnel in the emergency room or intensive care unit setting. One or two peripheral intravenous lines for blood sampling, fluid replacement, and insulin infusion must be started immediately. Laboratory evaluation should include plasma glucose, urea, creatinine, electrolytes, and phosphate; complete blood cell count; blood gases and pH; serum amylase and ketones; dipstick urinalysis (to search for glucose and ketones); electrocardiogram; and plain chest film. In patients with suspected acute myocardial infarction, serum creatine phosphokinase (CPK) or troponin levels and continuous electrocardiographic monitoring are recommended (Figure 1). Bedside reflectance meter glucose monitoring should be available and used together

Diabetes Ketoacidosis Suspected

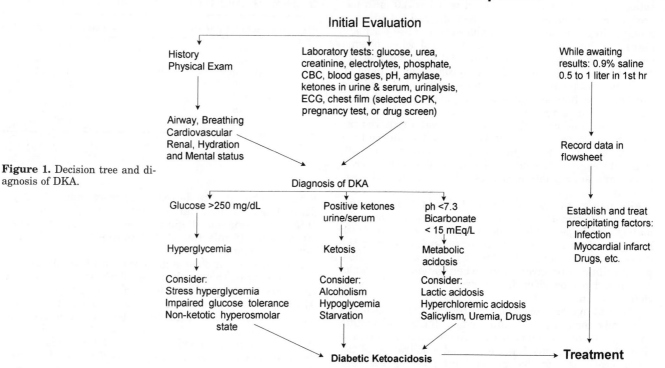

Figure 1. Decision tree and diagnosis of DKA.

with other laboratory values to guide fluid and insulin therapy, all recorded in a flowsheet (Table 1).

FLUID AND ELECTROLYTES

In severely ill patients, a central line with catheter introduced via jugular or subclavian vein must be placed. Nor-

TABLE 1. Recommended Monitoring Frequency of Clinical and Laboratory Parameters*

Fluid balance (intake/output)	Hourly, at least for initial 48 h
Vital signs and mental status	Every 4–6 h × 12 h; then twice daily
Body weight	Daily
Insulin therapy	Hourly rate and cumulative total
Electrolytes	Hourly rate and cumulative total
Laboratory parameters:	
Glucose (reflectance meter)	Every 1 h × 12 h; then every 2–4 h
Glucose (plasma)	Every 6 h × 24 h; then every 12 h
Sodium, potassium, chloride	Every 6 h × 24 h; then every 12 h
Bicarbonate, venous pH	Every 6 h × 24 h; then every 12 h
Urine, plasma ketones	Every 6 h × 24 h; then every 12 h
Phosphate, calcium	Every 12 h
Creatinine, urea	Every 12 h
Complete blood count	Daily
Chest film, electrocardiogram, creatine phosphokinase	As indicated
Blood, urine cultures	As indicated

*All clinical and laboratory parameters should be obtained at baseline.

mal saline (0.9% NaCl) and colloid solutions should be given at the rate needed to restore vital signs. During the initial 2 hours, most adults with DKA will tolerate normal saline infusion at the rate of 500 to 1000 mL per hour, and adolescents require approximately 500 mL per m² per hour. After the patient has received 1 to 2 liters of isotonic fluid, fluid replacement should be changed to a hypotonic fluid (0.45% NaCl). This enables repletion of the large intracellular volume deficit while minimizing chloride overload, which may induce nonanion gap metabolic acidosis. Although the total volume of fluid replaced during the first 24 hours may be as high as 5 to 10 liters in adults, or up to 4 liters per m² in adolescent patients, the rate of infusion varies according to patients' hydration status, which must be reassessed periodically. It is estimated that most patients with DKA have total body water loss that amounts to approximately 5 to 10% of their body weight. Complete restoration of the fluid deficit, in addition to daily water needs as dictated by urine output and insensible losses, can usually be accomplished safely over 2 to 3 days. When plasma glucose concentration decreases below 200 mg per dL, the addition of 5% dextrose in 0.45% NaCl or in water, depending upon plasma sodium concentration, is recommended. The use of dextrose infusion is intended to protect patients from developing hypoglycemia, because continued administration of large doses of insulin is required to overcome the state of insulin resistance associated with ketoacidosis.

Plasma potassium concentration in patients with DKA may be low, normal, or high, but total body potassium stores are usually depleted. Although the electrocardiogram can demonstrate low-voltage T waves and the presence of U waves (hypokalemia) or peaked T waves (hyperkalemia), intravenous potassium replacement should be guided by plasma levels. Except in rare emergencies, adequate urine output (at least 30 mL per hour) must be documented before potassium is given intravenously. A reasonable approach to initial replacement is to infuse 20 to 40 mEq of potassium per hour if plasma level is below 3.0 mEq per liter. When plasma levels are between 3.1 and 5.9 mEq per liter, the infusion rate may be reduced to 10 mEq per hour. Potassium infusion should be discontinued when plasma levels are equal to or greater than 6.0 mEq per liter. To further reduce chloride load, it is recommended that two thirds of total potassium be given as chloride salt and one third as phosphate salt, unless initial plasma phosphate is elevated. Periodic reevaluation of potassium concentration together with other electrolytes in plasma is required because rapid correction of acidosis and insulin infusion tend to increase potassium requirements. If acute renal insufficiency develops, potassium replacement should be discontinued and appropriate measures taken to prevent hyperkalemia.

Although an average total body deficit of approximately 90 mEq (50 mmol) of phosphate in adults and approximately 1 mEq per kg in adolescents has been reported in DKA, the need for replacement of phosphate during the initial 24 to 48 hours of treatment is controversial. Phosphate salts can be given orally when patients are awake but should not be given in the presence of renal insufficiency.

The acid overload associated with diabetic ketoacidosis is usually corrected with intravenous fluids and insulin therapy. In rare patients with extreme acidosis (pH less than 7.0), continuous intravenous administration of sodium bicarbonate at the rate of 1 mEq per kg per hour during 2 hours may be lifesaving. This is particularly important in critically ill patients with refractory cardiovascular dysfunction and hypotension.

INSULIN THERAPY

Intravenous insulin infusion should be started as soon as the diagnosis is confirmed (see Figure 1). Although subcutaneous and intramuscular injections are acceptable effective means of delivery, continuous intravenous infusion is the preferred route of insulin administration in the treatment of DKA. Because it takes approximately 30 minutes for peripherally administered insulin to begin lowering blood glucose, and its circulation half-life is only about 6 minutes, there is no need to administer bolus insulin before continuous infusion. Intravenous bolus of insulin may be appropriate, however, when insulin infusion solution is not readily available or when it is anticipated that preparation by pharmacy will take more than 30 minutes, or both. Recommended initial doses for intravenous insulin bolus range from 0.1 to 0.2 unit of fast-acting insulin (regular or Humalog) per kg body weight. A convenient solution can be prepared under sterile conditions by adding 50 units of fast-acting insulin to 500 mL of 0.9% or 0.45% saline. Theoretically, the use of Humalog, instead of regular insulin, may be more efficacious in patients with long-standing diabetes with large amounts of circulating insulin antibodies. There is no need to add albumin to the insulin solution, as suggested in earlier reports, although flushing all lines with a run of 10 to 20 mL may help reduce insulin absorption to tubing and provide more consistent delivery. The initial recommended rate of insulin infusion is 0.1 units per kg per hour, which should be adjusted hourly according to a sliding scale, as for example in Table 2. Occasionally, plasma glucose response is inadequate, and the insulin infusion rate must be increased above 0.1 unit per kg per hour. In these circumstances, I recommend doubling the dose every hour and monitoring plasma (blood) glucose every 30 minutes.

TABLE 2. **Suggested Rates of Intravenous Insulin Infusion During Treatment of Diabetic Ketoacidosis**

Plasma Glucose (mg/dL)	IV Infusion Rate (U/h)
>300	5–10
250–299	4.0
200–249	3.0*
150–199	2.0
120–149	1.5
100–119	1.0
<100	0.5†

*Add 10% dextrose infusion at 10–20 mL/h.
†Adjust 10% dextrose infusion upwards.

When plasma glucose decreases by more than 50 mg per dL in 1 hour, insulin infusion rate should be reduced by 50% and plasma (blood) glucose should be monitored every 30 minutes. If this rate of fall continues, 10% dextrose infusion should be added.

Rapid decline in plasma glucose concentration has been associated with the development of cerebral edema, especially in children, and with life-threatening hypoglycemia. Although the rate of insulin infusion must be reduced significantly at times, it should not be discontinued, except, perhaps, during severe hypoglycemia, when insulin infusion may be discontinued transiently (30 minutes) as 10% dextrose infusion is adjusted upwards. The use of intermediate- or long-acting insulin preparations (neutral protamine Hagedorn [NPH], Lente, Ultralente) should be avoided during treatment of DKA, and continuous subcutaneous insulin infusion with the assistance of a pump device should be restarted only after recovery is complete.

SPECIAL CONSIDERATIONS

Pregnancy and Ketoacidosis

Since the introduction of self-monitored blood glucose and frequent daily insulin injections, DKA has become rare during pregnancy. Nonetheless, when it occurs during midpregnancy, it is frequently lethal to the fetus; an episode of DKA carries a risk in excess of 50% for fetal death in utero. If DKA occurs in the third trimester of a pregnancy with a potentially viable fetus, aggressive medical therapy and continuous monitoring of fetal heart rate tracings are recommended. Fetal conditions tend to improve as the maternal DKA resolves. Emergency cesarean section should be avoided because it carries a very high maternal mortality risk. Once the mother's condition has stabilized after aggressive hydration, electrolyte replacement, and insulin therapy, cesarean section could be considered an alternative therapeutic option. Close monitoring of mother and fetus will eventually dictate the appropriate timing and mode of delivery in individual circumstances. To prevent these catastrophic events, patients with diabetes who become pregnant are routinely asked to monitor morning urine sample for ketones daily. Positive ketonuria indicates the presence of either starvation ketosis or diabetes ketoacidosis. Urine self-monitoring during pregnancy is an important practice that helps guide the nutritional assessment and review of dietary habits to ensure proper calorie and nutrient intake, and, at the same time, it enables early detection of developing ketoacidosis.

Type 2 Diabetes and Insulin Resistance

Although rare in patients with type 2 diabetes, DKA can be associated with critical illness reflecting extreme, albeit relative, insulin deficiency. Typical settings include hemo-dynamically unstable adult patients admitted to the intensive care unit for treatment of acute coronary events or sepsis who require large doses of pressor agents (dopamine, levofed, etc.) or steroids, or both. Intravenous insulin requirements may be as high as 100 units per hour, and resolution of ketosis and hyperglycemia can be accomplished only with improvement of the underlying condition. Reducing pressor agents and steroid doses to a minimum, eliminating unnecessary intravenous infusion of glucose and lactate solutions, and maintaining adequate renal function are helpful measures in the management of these critically ill diabetes patients. Some patients may actually have absolute insulin deficiency that manifests during adulthood, a disease category now recognized as adult-onset type1 diabetes. Unlike most adult patients with diabetes, who have predominantly insulin resistance, these patients tend to have insulin deficiency, which if untreated leads to DKA. On rare occasions, patients with DKA may be resistant to standard therapeutic doses of insulin. These patients may have an unrecognized, and thus untreated, precipitating cause of DKA, such as osteomyelitis, endocarditis, or silent myocardial infarction. Under these circumstances, it is always prudent to thoroughly ensure that the source of insulin and its delivery are adequate and that appropriate fluid balance has been achieved as originally anticipated. Although not yet approved in the United States, the use of insulin-like growth factor I has been associated with reduction in insulin requirements and correction of hyperglycemia in patients with "true" insulin resistance syndromes.

Transition and Hospital Discharge

Once the acute metabolic disturbance is corrected, and the patient is rehydrated and able to resume oral intake (3 to 5 days), the treatment program shifts to discharge and long-term planning. It is recommended that intravenous insulin infusion overlap with subcutaneous injection for approximately 1 to 2 hours. Introduction of subcutaneous insulin, short- and intermediate-acting and before meals, should be guided by patients' daily requirements recorded in conjunction with preadmission doses. It is often necessary to supplement short-acting insulin (regular or Humalog) with sliding scales in an effort to correct premeal blood glucose concentrations that are either higher or lower than a set goal range. For example, if desired premeal blood glucose is set for an individual patient between 70 and 120 mg per dL, then 1 additional unit of insulin must be given for every 60 mg per dL above 120 mg per dL. Keep in mind that blood glucose below goal range, that is, 70 mg per dL, would require subtraction of one or more units of insulin to avoid sustained hypoglycemia. Before hospital discharge, it is often necessary to monitor blood glucose between meals and administer supplemental insulin according to scale to achieve goal range. With the widespread utilization of Humalog, it has become necessary to self-monitor blood glucose 2 hours after a meal to ascertain that the desired blood lowering effect has been achieved. Because a given dose of Humalog injected subcutaneously has its full effect within 2 hours, measurement of blood glucose before the subsequent meal, usually 4 to 6 hours later, does not accurately reflect the action of Humalog alone. Intermediate-acting insulin (NPH, Lente) usually amounts to approximately two thirds of total daily requirements, and it should be given twice daily, preferably in the early morning and again before bedtime. Long-acting insulin (Ultralente) usually makes up half of daily needs and can be given in a single injection before evening meals. Daily Ultralente insulin doses in excess of 40 units are best tolerated if the total amount is divided in two equal doses every 12 hours, which reduces early morning hypoglycemic events.

Adjustments on intermediate- and long-acting insulin doses require time and thus cannot be completed during hospitalization. Health care providers should take advantage of the few days preceding hospital discharge to educate patients on self-monitoring, self-adjustment, and on supplementation of insulin. Maximal benefit is achieved with a team approach that should include dietitians, nurses, and social workers, although this is not always possible. Most patients admitted with DKA have limited resources and do not attend regular outpatient clinics and education programs. Follow-up arrangements should include a medical visit with a specialist after 2 to 4 weeks and a review of diabetes self-management practices and nutritional assessment with properly trained nurses and dietitians within 3 months after hospital discharge. Patients with underlying social or psychologic problems must be followed closely by a social worker and a clinical psychologist.

DIABETES OUTPATIENT MANAGEMENT

A considerable improvement in the management of patients with diabetes mellitus, resulting from widespread utilization of "diabetes education programs" in the outpatient setting delivered by a team of specialized health care professionals, has enabled a substantial fall in the incidence of and hospital admissions for DKA. Together with the advent of self-monitoring blood glucose, education to self-administer, adjust, and supplement insulin appropriately represents the greatest advance in the management of diabetes of modern times. Current recommendations for intensive insulin therapy with several daily insulin injections or continuous subcutaneous insulin infusion to achieve near-normoglycemia have been associated with a significant reduction in diabetes complications. Moreover, patients on intensive insulin therapy have more flexibility, a sense of well-being, and rare episodes of DKA, despite having more frequent episodes of hypoglycemia and mild weight gain in comparison with conventional insulin therapy.

The fact that "intensive insulin therapy" reduces the occurrence of DKA, however, has not been sufficiently emphasized. Self-administration of variable doses of short-acting insulin based on the carbohydrate content of a meal and the knowledge to be able to alter premeal insulin doses according to blood glucose concentration values have led to better glycemic control. As a consequence, most patients using these programs are comfortable with the concept of self-administering frequent additional insulin doses, as required during intercurrent illness ("sick-day rules"). During a period of several days, when these patients become ill, they are trained and capable of monitoring blood glucose and self-injecting supplemental subcutaneous insulin every 3 to 4 hours according to a scale. They are monitored closely over the telephone and through telefax in the outpatient clinic by members of the team, who provide orientation and support, thus preventing DKA, halting its progression, and avoiding hospitalization. Several patients with evidence of hyperglycemia and ketonuria have been successfully managed in the outpatient clinic. Persistent hyperglycemia above 300 mg per dL with moderate to severe ketonuria by dipstick urine self-test that is unresponsive to the described insulin supplementation regimen beyond 24 hours is one criterion that we frequently use to hospitalize patients. Immediate hospitalization is recommended for patients with severe dehydration, as evidenced by mental status changes, tachycardia, or orthostatic hypotension, or all three, and those with infectious processes. In-hospital treatment is also preferred in the management of uncontrolled diabetes for pregnant women and in patients with limited social contacts, especially elderly individuals and those unable to care for themselves.

The importance of education programs and the concept of team approach in the prevention and treatment of diabetes and its complications in the outpatient setting must be recognized. Unlike many other medical conditions, the ultimate goal in diabetes is self-management. This can be achieved only with honest dissemination of diabetes knowledge to patients and their families by using public and private education and awareness programs, all of which should be fully supported by health care providers.

HYPERURICEMIA AND GOUT

method of
RICHARD D. BRASINGTON, M.D.
Washington University School of Medicine
St. Louis, Missouri

Gout includes a number of clinical problems caused by the precipitation of excess amounts of monosodium urate (MSU) in body fluids and tissues. The four major manifestations are recurrent attacks of inflammatory arthritis, tophaceous deposits, kidney stones, and urate nephropathy. Gouty arthritis, with or without tophi, is the most common gout-related problem encountered by clinicians.

Adult males in the fifth decade of life are most commonly affected by gout. In fact, gout is the most common cause of inflammatory arthritis in men older than 30 years. Premenopausal females rarely experience gout, perhaps because estrogen promotes the renal excretion of urate.

PATHOPHYSIOLOGY

Gout is unusual among causes of arthritis in that its pathophysiology is well understood. Furthermore, understanding this pathophysiology is key to the rational diagnosis and treatment of gout. Uric acid is a normal product of the purine salvage pathway which recycles the nucleotides guanylic acid, inosinic acid, and adenylic acid. These are degraded through purine nucleoside intermediates to hypoxanthine and guanine, which are in turn converted to xanthine. Xanthine oxidase then catalyzes the conversion of xanthine to uric acid. Because the pKa of uric acid is 5.3, at physiologic pH the urate anion is the predominant circulating form.

Clinical problems develop as MSU crystallizes when present in the body in an oversaturated state. The theoretical limit of urate solubility in serum is 6.8 and is even lower at the reduced temperature of peripheral tissues such as the feet. The level of urate in the body is determined by the balance of production and excretion. In 90% of cases, hyperuricemia results from the inadequate renal excretion of urate, rather than from its overproduction. Whereas only one third of the body load of urate is degraded by intestinal bacteria, two thirds is excreted through a complex system of renal handling. Because only 5% of urate is protein-bound, it is readily filtered by the glomerulus, but then 90 to 95% is reabsorbed in the proximal tubule. About half of the urate is then resecreted into the tubular lumen (the source of most excretion), followed by postsecretory absorption. Thus medications that impair the tubular excretion of urate, such as diuretics, low-dose salicylates, and cyclosporine, can cause hyperuricemia, whereas agents such as probenecid reduce hyperuricemia by promoting urate excretion at the tubular level.

Only about 10% of cases of gout result from excessive production, defined as 24-hour urinary uric acid excretion of over 1000 mg. Myeloproliferative and lymphoproliferative diseases, psoriasis, and hemolytic anemia are among the more common causes of overproduction. Congenital enzyme deficiencies of hypoxanthine-guanine phosphoribosyltransferase (HGPRT; Lesch-Nyhan syndrome) or phosphoribosylpyrophosphate (PRPP) synthetase are rare.

Inflammatory arthritis occurs when the level of urate in the joint fluid exceeds its solubility and crystallizes. The phagocytosis of these crystals by neutrophils sets off a cascade of chemotactic recruitment of more neutrophils and secretion of inflammatory prostaglandins and cytokines. Intense inflammation of the joint ensues, sometimes accompanied by fever and leukocytosis. Periarticular tissue may be so inflamed as to suggest cellulitis or deep venous thrombosis, and exfoliation of the skin may follow. The first toe metatarsophalangeal (MTP) joint is the most commonly involved joint and is ultimately involved in 90% of affected patients. Indeed, the syndrome of podagra, in which this joint is intensely swollen and painful, is highly suggestive of gout, although the diagnosis is more certain when MSU crystals can be identified in the joint by compensated polarized microscopy. The ankle, foot, and knee may also be involved; less commonly involved are the wrist and fingers. Surgery, medical illness, trauma, alcohol excess, and medications sometimes precipitate cases of acute gouty arthritis.

An attack of acute gouty arthritis resolves spontaneously in a few days, although treatment hastens the resolution of symptoms. Initially, attacks of gout are punctuated by symptom-free intervals; this manifestation is referred to as "intercritical gout." After years of chronically elevated urate levels, subcutaneous masses of urate known as tophi develop. Tophi develop around joints, especially on extensor surfaces, and may be confused with rheumatoid nodules. They elicit a chronic granulomatous response and may erode into subchondral bone. Tophi can actually develop anywhere in the body except for the central nervous system, including such unlikely sites as the eye and the cardiac valves. The development of tophi is indicative of a heavy load of urate in the body.

DIAGNOSIS

The diagnosis of gout should be considered when a middle-aged patient has acute inflammatory arthritis of a single joint, especially the first toe MTP joint. Painful noninflammatory conditions of the first toe MTP joint, such as osteoarthritis (hallux rigidus) should not be mistaken for gout. Gouty arthritis occasionally manifests for the first time in multiple joints, especially in the elderly. Whenever possible, the diagnosis should be confirmed by the analysis of synovial fluid under the polarizing microscope. MSU crystals appear needle-shaped and bright under polarized light (strongly birefringent). "Negative birefringence" refers to the fact that the axis of the MSU crystal appears yellow when it is parallel to the axis of the microscope's first-order red compensator ("yellow-parallel gout"). Although aspiration of the first toe MTP may be difficult, the periarticular tissue sometimes contains diagnostic crystals; always leave some dead space in the syringe before attempting aspiration, which will allow you to expel a small amount of fluid from the syringe onto a microscope slide. It is also helpful to use a needle with a clear plastic hub, so that you can detect when fluid begins to flow upon aspiration. A 25-gauge needle is adequate for aspiration of this small joint, whereas a 21-gauge needle is more suitable for large joints such as the ankle or knee. A local anesthetic is recommended, especially for aspiration of the toe, which can be quite painful.

Once a patient has been shown to have crystal-proven gout, it may not be necessary to aspirate each swollen joint to document the diagnosis. However, sometimes it can be difficult clinically to distinguish gout from infection. Furthermore, decompression of an acutely swollen joint such as the knee often provides considerable relief of pain.

The serum uric acid level is of little value in diagnosis, inasmuch as the level may be normal during an acute attack.

Tophaceous gout can be strongly suspected from the presence of subcutaneous nodules, which may have a whitish hue. Aspiration of such tophi is usually quite easy, resulting in the expression of thick, white "milk of urate," which can be examined with the polarizing microscope. Radiographs of affected joints may show tophaceous erosion into subchondral bone, giving the classic appearance of a punched-out lesion with an overhanging osteophyte. The osteopenia that is so characteristic of rheumatoid arthritis is not seen in the radiograph of a gouty joint (Table 1).

TREATMENT

Treatment of acute gouty arthritis is straightforward in most cases. Response to maximal doses of

TABLE 1. Common Errors in Gout Management

Diagnosis
Failure to base diagnosis on presence of crystals in synovial fluid
Misdiagnosis of noninflammatory forefoot pain as gout
Diagnosis based on hyperuricemia
Misdiagnosis of chronic, tophaceous gout as rheumatoid arthritis (and vice versa)

Treatment
Initiating allopurinol during an acute attack
Failure to give a sufficient dose of allopurinol to lower the serum urate level to around 5 mg/dL
Treatment of asymptomatic hyperuricemia
Use of colchicine in renal insufficiency
Administration of allopurinol with azathioprine

TABLE 2. Alternatives to NSAIDs for Acute Treatment

Oral
Colchicine
COX-2 inhibitors?

Intra-articular
Triamcinolone hexacetonide (Aristospan)
Methylprednisolone (Depo-Medrol)
Betamethasone (Celestone)

Intramuscular
ACTH gel (Acthar)
Triamcinolone acetonide (Kenalog)

Intravenous
Colchicine

Abbreviations: NSAIDs = nonsteroidal anti-inflammatory drugs; COX-2 = cyclooxygenase-2; ACTH = adrenocorticotropic hormone.

nonsteroidal anti-inflammatory drugs (NSAIDs) is usually excellent in patients who can take these medications. Indomethacin may be considered the drug of choice but may not be well tolerated by elderly patients. After several days of high-dose NSAID therapy, the patient can gradually reduce the dose over a period of a week. Oral colchicine has a limited role because of its narrow therapeutic index: Diarrhea and abdominal cramping usually occur at doses necessary to adequately treat gout. The physician may prescribe 0.6 mg every 1 to 2 hours until a maximal dose of 6 to 8 mg is reached, although that cumulative dose is rarely tolerated.

Many patients are not good candidates for NSAID therapy for a variety of reasons: therapeutic anticoagulation, no oral intake status, volume depletion, congestive heart failure, or renal insufficiency. It should be remembered that ketorolac (Toradol) is pharmacologically an NSAID. Selective inhibitors of cyclooxygenase-2 (COX-2), such as celecoxib (Celebrex), do not inhibit platelet function and may prove useful in patients in whom anticoagulation contraindicates use of the traditional NSAIDs (Table 2). Whether the COX-2 inhibitors will prove to be safe in patients with renal insufficiency is unclear. Corticosteroid injection into a large joint such as the knee is often effective. Intramuscular therapies such as triamcinolone acetonide, 60 to 100 mg, or adrenocorticotropic hormone (ACTH) gel, 40 to 80 IU (which can also be given subcutaneously in the anticoagulated patient) are other options. Oral corticosteroids in a burst-and-taper manner may be effective, but several weeks of therapy may be needed.

Colchicine intravenously has a limited role and can produce excellent results. However, this is a potentially dangerous treatment if used inappropriately. Patients with renal or hepatic insufficiency or who have recently had oral colchicine therapy may suffer neutropenia, sepsis, and death without preceding gastrointestinal symptoms after receiving intravenous colchicine. A single dose of 2 mg of colchicine is reasonable in the absence of these contraindications. Great care must be taken to avoid extravasation, inasmuch as colchicine can produce substantial local toxicity.

Patients with fewer than three or four attacks of gout per year can be treated for acute events without chronic therapy. For recurrent attacks, prophylactic suppression with colchicine, 0.6 mg once or twice daily, or low-dose NSAIDs may be effective. Neither option would be ideal for patients with renal insufficiency. Treatment to lower the uric acid level is recommended for patients whose disease cannot be controlled with simple prophylaxis. Medication to increase the excretion of uric acid is an option for patients who excrete less than 600 mg daily into the urine, if they do not have renal insufficiency. Probenecid, 500 mg orally four times a day, inhibits tubular reabsorption of uric acid, but the need for multiple dosing, forcing fluids, and alkalinization of the urine are disadvantages of this treatment. Probenecid (Benemid) is generally not a good choice for patients with tophaceous gout and is ineffective when creatinine clearance is less than 50 mL per hour.

For most patients, allopurinol (Zyloprim) is simple to administer and effective. This inhibitor of xanthine oxidase reduces the production of uric acid and the concentration of urate in body fluids and tissues. For most patients, an initial dose of 100 or 150 mg is given, and the dose is subsequently increased to achieve a serum uric acid level of around 5, so that tissue and fluid levels of urate do not exceed the limits of solubility and formation of MSU crystals ceases. The dose of allopurinol must be reduced in the setting of renal insufficiency. Allopurinol has no role in the treatment of acute gout, and allopurinol therapy should not be initiated until an attack has subsided. Conversely, in a patient already taking allopurinol, it is not necessary to discontinue this medication during an attack of gout.

A severe hypersensitivity reaction to allopurinol with exfoliative dermatitis, vasculitis, hepatitis, fever, and eosinophilia is rare but more likely to occur in the setting of diuretic therapy or renal insufficiency. Ironically, most reported cases of this toxic effect have occurred in patients with asymptomatic hyperuricemia who were not appropriate candidates for allopurinol. A regimen for desensitization to allopurinol can be attempted with the assistance of an allergist or rheumatologist. Initiation of therapy to lower the serum uric acid level may be associated with an increased frequency of gout attacks, perhaps because polymorphonuclear leukocytes (PMNs) more effectively phagocytose crystals at lower serum urate concentrations. Use of colchicine or NSAID prophylaxis as described earlier is often effective in preventing this; treatment may be required for several months and occasionally for a year or more. Initiating prophylaxis should be routine when hypouricemic treatment begins, except for patients who should not take NSAIDs or colchicine chronically. Patients must be assured that continued administration of allopurinol will eventually result in the cure of their gout and should be reminded that allopurinol treatment

is usually lifelong. Recurrence of gout in a previously asymptomatic patient who has discontinued allopurinol is extremely frustrating.

A particularly challenging problem is the treatment of gouty arthritis in the organ transplant recipient. The cyclosporine therapy (Neoral, Sandimmune) used in most of these patients reduces tubular secretion of urate, and some patients develop hyperuricemia with recurrent gout attacks. Furthermore, allopurinol inhibits the metabolism of azathioprine (Imuran), which many transplant recipients take, and administering allopurinol necessitates reducing the dose of azathioprine substantially. Moreover, the tendency of cyclosporine to reduce renal function makes the use of NSAIDs problematic in transplant recipients. The COX-2 inhibitors may prove to be safe and effective in this setting.

Excess alcohol consumption may complicate gout management, because the resulting increase in lactic acid production reduces tubular clearance of urate.

HYPERLIPOPROTEINEMIAS

method of
PETER H. JONES, M.D.
Baylor College of Medicine
Houston, Texas

The strong relationship between lipid disorders and coronary heart disease (CHD), specifically high levels of low-density lipoprotein (LDL) cholesterol and low levels of high-density lipoprotein (HDL) cholesterol, has been well established for several decades. Five well-designed drug treatment trials published between 1994 and 1998 have firmly established that lowering LDL cholesterol reduces first and recurrent CHD events such as fatal and nonfatal myocardial infarctions, unstable angina, CHD death, and revascularizations. Some of these trials also demonstrated a reduction in the incidence of strokes, as well as a reduction in all-cause mortality. These trials have confirmed the guidelines of the National Cholesterol Education Program (NCEP) Adult Treatment Panel II (ATP II), which recommends interventional cut points for LDL cholesterol that are based on risk stratification.

GUIDELINES FOR TREATMENT

The ATP II guidelines provide LDL cholesterol cut points for implementation of lifestyle interventions and pharmacologic therapy (Table 1). These guidelines focus on the intensity of intervention on the basis of an individual's total risk for CHD. The presence of known CHD or other evidence of established atherosclerosis, such as peripheral and cerebrovascular disease, is the strongest risk factor. As demonstrated in the secondary prevention trials, affected patients derive great benefit from reducing LDL cholesterol. Primary prevention treatment is directed at persons without clinical CHD, principally in those with at least two CHD risk factors as defined by the NCEP (Table 2). In this group of people, termed the

TABLE 1. **NCEP Treatment Targets Based on Low-Density Lipoprotein Cholesterol**

Category of Patients	Initiation Level of LDL-C (mg/dL)		LDL-C Goal (mg/dL)
	Dietary Therapy	Drug Therapy	
PRIMARY PREVENTION			
Without CHD, <2 other risk factors	≥160	≥190	<160
Without CHD, ≥2 other risk factors	≥130	≥160	<130
SECONDARY PREVENTION			
With CHD or other vascular disease	>100	≥130	≤100

Abbreviations: CHD = coronary heart disease; LDL-C = low-density lipoprotein cholesterol.

Adapted from Expert Panel on Detection, Evaluation, and Treatment of High Blood Cholesterol in Adults: Summary of the second report of the National Cholesterol Education Program (NCEP) Expert Panel on Detection, Evaluation, and Treatment of High Blood Cholesterol in Adults (Adult Treatment Panel II). JAMA *269*:3015–3023, 1993. Copyright 1993, American Medical Association.

"high-risk primary prevention" group, benefit from LDL cholesterol reduction has been demonstrated in clinical trials.

For primary prevention, the NCEP ATP II guidelines recommend the screening of all adults aged 20 years or older for levels of total and HDL cholesterol. A person with a total cholesterol (TC) level of less than 200 mg per dL and an HDL cholesterol level of more than 35 mg per dL is considered at low risk for CHD. No intervention other than general health lifestyle education about such measures as exercise, low-fat diet, and weight control is recommended. Screening may be repeated at 5-year intervals. Persons with a TC level in the borderline range of 200 to 239 mg per dL, an HDL cholesterol level exceeding 35 mg per dL, and fewer than two CHD risk factors are also considered at low risk. Lifestyle education is highly recommended, and testing should be repeated within 2 years. For all patients with either a TC level of 240 mg per dL or more, a borderline TC level with up to two risk factors, or an HDL cholesterol level of less than 35 mg per dL, a complete fasting lipid profile is recommended. With these data, the LDL cholesterol can be calculated by use of the Friedewald

equation: LDL cholesterol = TC − HDL − (triglycerides/5). This estimation of LDL cholesterol can be done only if triglyceride levels are less than 400 mg per dL, in order to prevent miscalculation as a result of very-low-density lipoprotein (VLDL) remnants that are frequently present with very high triglyceride levels. The decision to intervene in primary prevention patients with diet and possibly medication depends on the LDL cholesterol level and cumulative risk factors, as outlined in Table 1.

For patients with established CHD or other vascular disease, a complete fasting lipid sample should be obtained, and LDL cholesterol calculated. Intervention is recommended at LDL cut points lower than those for primary prevention, and the goal of therapy (≤100 mg per dL) is also more stringent. Measurement of fasting lipids in patients with an acute coronary syndrome can be accurately made within 24 hours of onset. However, after this time, total and LDL cholesterol levels tend to drop substantially within the first week. This may lead the clinician to inappropriately decide that a patient surviving an acute event may not need lipid-lowering intervention. In this instance, fasting lipid sampling can be repeated 4 to 6 weeks after the CHD event or revascularization.

TABLE 2. **NCEP Risk Factors for Coronary Heart Disease**

Positive Risk Factors	
Age	Men: ≥45 y
	Women: ≥55 y
Family history of CHD	Premature CHD in first-degree family members (e.g., definite MI or sudden cardiac death in first-degree male relative <55 y or in first-degree female relative <65 y
Hypertension	Blood pressure ≥ 140/90 mm Hg or with treatment-controlled hypertension
Current tobacco use	
Low HDL-C	HDL-C < 35 mg/dL
Negative Risk Factor	
HDL-C ≥ 60 mg/dL	May subtract a risk factor

Abbreviations: CHD = coronary heart disease; HDL-C = high-density lipoprotein cholesterol; MI = myocardial infarction; NCEP = National Cholesterol Education Program.

Other Lipid Abnormalities

The NCEP ATP II has focused CHD preventive therapy based on the LDL cholesterol level and the associated CHD presence or risk. HDL cholesterol level is an important inverse prediction of CHD risk and, when low, can serve as one factor that may direct more aggressive primary prevention intervention on LDL cholesterol level. Conversely, a high HDL level (≥60 mg per dL) can be subtracted from a person's CHD risk factor total and therefore may serve to elevate the LDL cholesterol cut point level that necessitates intervention in that person. Elevations in fasting triglyceride levels can be associated with a risk for pancreatitis as well as a risk for CHD. The ATP II panel has provided cut points for defining importance of triglyceride levels: more than 1000 mg per dL is severely elevated, 400 to 1000 mg per dL is high, and 200 to 400 mg per dL is borderline high.

Pancreatitis risk is greatest for triglyceride levels exceeding 1000 mg per dL, lower but still important at 400 to 1000 mg per dL, and rare at 200 to 400 mg per dL. Treatment for high to severely high triglyceride levels should be considered for the prevention of pancreatitis. Whether triglyceride levels are directly related to CHD risk is controversial; as a result, recommendations for treatment to prevent CHD are lacking. It is generally accepted that triglyceride levels in the range of 200 to 400 mg per dL, in association with a TC level exceeding 200 mg per dL, should be considered for treatment if the patient meets NCEP LDL cholesterol criteria for either high risk primary prevention or secondary prevention, has diabetes mellitus, or has a strong family history of premature CHD.

Dietary Therapy

Dietary therapy should be the principal intervention in addressing hyperlipidemia and should be continued even if subsequent pharmacologic therapy is required. Dietary therapy focuses on caloric restriction to optimize weight and on reduction of saturated fat and cholesterol intake. Diet should be initiated in primary prevention for subjects with fewer than two other risk factors if the LDL cholesterol level exceeds 160 mg per dL, with a treatment goal to reduce LDL cholesterol levels below this threshold. Subjects without documented disease who have two or more risk factors and an LDL cholesterol value of greater than 130 mg per dL are advised to begin dietary therapy, with a treatment goal to reduce LDL cholesterol levels below this value. Secondary prevention has more stringent guidelines; the goal for dietary therapy is an LDL cholesterol level of less than 100 mg per dL.

The Step I diet of the NCEP recommends restriction of the percentage of dietary calories derived from total fat to less than 30% of the total caloric intake, with a goal of 8 to 10% of total calories from saturated fat. Polyunsaturated fats should not exceed 10% of total calories, and monounsaturated fats should not exceed 15%. Carbohydrates should constitute at least 55% of the total calories, with an emphasis on complex carbohydrates. The amount of protein in the diet should approximate 15%, and cholesterol should be restricted to 300 mg per day. Three months are allowed to assess the effects of the diet. However, a longer period may be necessary if substantial weight loss is needed. On the other hand, for secondary prevention after an acute CHD event or revascularization, diet and drug therapy may be instituted simultaneously. If dietary goals are not achieved, the Step II diet, which consists of further restriction of cholesterol to less than 200 mg per day in addition to a further reduction of saturated fats to 7% or less of total calories, may be initiated. Diet, exercise, and weight loss also have considerable benefit in diabetic subjects by reducing triglyceride levels, increasing HDL cholesterol levels, and improving glucose con-

trol, which further aids in the improvement of the dyslipidemia.

Pharmacologic Therapy

Drug treatment should be considered in high-risk primary prevention and secondary prevention subjects whose LDL cholesterol levels remain above the ATP II cut points (see Table 1) despite an adequate trial of lifestyle intervention. Men aged 20 to 35 years and premenopausal females with severe genetic disorders, such as familial hypercholesterolemia, may also be candidates for drug treatment if the LDL cholesterol level exceeds 220 mg per dL. If drug therapy is implemented, patients should be strongly encouraged to continue low-fat diets because the efficacy of drugs can be diminished by a return to high-fat intake.

A brief description of lipoprotein metabolism elucidates how lipid-altering drugs exert their effect. VLDLs are triglyceride-rich particles produced by the liver. After release into the plasma, they interact with lipoprotein lipase (LPL), an endothelium-based lipolytic enzyme that removes triglyceride from VLDL. The resulting lipid particle from this lipolysis is called a VLDL remnant, or intermediate-density lipoprotein (IDL), which can be removed from plasma by specific hepatic cell surface receptors. These receptors are called the LDL, or B/E, receptors. A certain number of VLDL remnant particles may not be removed by the liver; instead, they interact with hepatic triglyceride lipase to remove all remaining triglycerides, thereby converting the remnant into an LDL cholesterol–rich particle. LDL particles are removed from plasma principally by the hepatic LDL receptor. The amount of intracellular cholesterol within the hepatocyte inversely regulates the production of these LDL receptors. For example, a high level of cholesterol in hepatocytes down-regulates the number of LDL receptors, which decreases plasma LDL removal and results in a high LDL cholesterol level. Conversely, a reduced amount of hepatocyte cholesterol up-regulates receptor expression and decreases plasma LDL cholesterol.

The drugs that primarily reduce LDL cholesterol are the bile acid sequestrants (or resins), the hydroxymethylglutaryl-coenzyme A (HMG-CoA) reductase inhibitors (also called statins), and nicotinic acid (or niacin). The resins and statins lower LDL cholesterol by stimulating hepatic LDL receptor number, whereas niacin lowers LDL cholesterol by reducing the hepatic production of its precursor, VLDL. The drugs that lower triglyceride levels, and thereby increase HDL cholesterol level, are niacin and fibric acid derivatives (fibrate). As stated, niacin reduces hepatic VLDL synthesis, whereas fibrates primarily stimulate LPL lipolysis of triglyceride-rich lipoproteins with some decrease in VLDL production as well. The mechanism of action of these drugs can be complementary, so that combination drug treatment may be useful for selected dyslipidemias.

LDL Cholesterol–Lowering Drugs

HMG-CoA Reductase Inhibitors (Statins)

The statin class of drugs has revolutionized the prevention of CHD by providing well-tolerated, safe, convenient, and efficacious lowering of LDL cholesterol levels, as well as a wealth of clinical trial benefits. The members of this class of drugs competitively inhibit HMG-CoA reductase, the rate-limiting enzyme of cholesterol synthesis, within the liver. Very little of the active drugs are systemically available. The original three statins—lovastatin (Mevacor), simvastatin (Zocor), and pravastatin (Pravachol)—were isolated from fungal cultures, whereas the three newest statins—fluvastatin (Lescol), atorvastatin (Lipitor), and cerivastatin (Baycol)—are synthetically produced. Even though these drugs differ in chemical structure, they all share a common metabolic pathway directed at hepatic cholesterol synthesis.

MECHANISM OF ACTION

All of the statins produce partial, competitive inhibition of HMG-CoA reductase in the liver, which results in a decrease in hepatic intracellular cholesterol concentration. As a result, there is a compensatory increase in hepatic LDL receptor production and expression, which results in enhanced removal of apoprotein-B–containing lipoproteins—namely, LDL particles, but also, to a lesser degree, VLDL particles and their remnants, IDL—from plasma. Therefore, the statins primarily lower LDL cholesterol levels and may have a beneficial effect on triglyceride levels. There is also evidence that statins may have direct effects on hepatic lipoprotein synthesis; in particular, this effect may be seen with more potent statins, such as atorvastatin, or at higher doses of other statins.

EFFICACY

The six statins at their approved dose ranges have differing capacities for lowering LDL cholesterol levels. Some of these differences may result from one or more factors, such as chemical structure, half-life, and presence or absence of active metabolites. Because the synthesis of cholesterol in humans is diurnal, whereby most occurs in the evening hours, the most effective way to inhibit this synthesis is to administer single-dose statins at night. There is evidence that twice-a-day dosing of most statins produces slightly greater LDL cholesterol reductions than does administering the same dose once at night. Atorvastatin has active metabolites that extend the half-life of the parent compound, and as a result this drug has greater efficacy and can be administered any time of day. Both lovastatin (Mevacor), in dosages of 10 to 80 mg per day, and simvastatin (Zocor), in dosages of 5 to 80 mg per day, can reduce LDL cholesterol by 20 to 50%. Both pravastatin (Pravachol), approved at 10 to 40 mg per day, and fluvastatin (Lescol), at 20 to 80 mg per day, lower LDL cholesterol by 20 to 35%. Cerivastatin (Baycol), approved at 0.3 and 0.4 mg per day, achieves a 28% LDL cholesterol reduction. Atorvastatin (Lipitor), at 10 to 80 mg per day, produces LDL cholesterol reductions of 38 to 55%. All the statins produce a small but predictable increase in HDL cholesterol by 5 to 12%. The effects of statins on triglyceride levels are variable and depend on the baseline triglyceride values and the dosage of statin used. In general, high dosages of the statins can reduce triglyceride levels that are in the borderline high (200 to 400 mg per dL) and high (400 to 1000 mg per dL) ranges by 15 to 40%. Lipoprotein(a) levels do not appear to be altered by any of the statins.

SIDE EFFECTS AND DRUG INTERACTIONS

The three original statins—lovastatin, pravastatin, and simvastatin—have been used clinically all over the world since the late 1980s. In particular, these three statins have been extensively studied in more than 30,000 subjects randomly assigned to 5-year primary and secondary CHD prevention trials. The only clinically important side effects have been myositis and involved liver function.

The hepatotoxicity potential of all the statins appears to be quite low. Data from clinical trials suggest that the incidence of increased transaminase levels of more than three times the upper limit of normal is less than 2% and is related to the dosage of the statin used. At the approved starting dosages, all statins have less than a 0.7% incidence of significant transaminase elevation. The transaminase increases are completely reversible and usually resolve within a few weeks of discontinuation of the statin. Severe hepatic dysfunction or cirrhosis has not been reported. It is recommended that transaminases be measured before initiation of statin therapy, at 6 weeks and 12 weeks after initiation, and, if there are no adverse effects, periodically thereafter.

Clinically significant myositis, as defined by elevation of the creatine phosphokinase (CPK) level with or without symptoms of myalgia, is quite uncommon with statin monotherapy. The incidence of rhabdomyolysis, defined by a 10-fold or higher increase in CPK level, is less than 0.1% with all the statins. A syndrome of myalgia without CPK elevation can be seen with the statins, and although the long-term physical importance of this is not known, the patient may remain uncomfortable. Use of an alternative statin may reduce such myalgia complaints. The cause of myositis by statins is not known, but alteration of myocyte cell membrane stability by reducing cholesterol synthesis or decreases in mitochondrial levels of ubiquinone, a facilitator of electron transport, have been implicated. The incidence of myositis with statin use increases significantly (to nearly 30%) when these drugs are used in combination with immunosuppressives (cyclosporine [Sandimmune] and tacrolimus [Prograf]), azole antifungal agents (ketoconazole [Nizoral] and itraconazole [Sopranox]), fibric acid derivatives (gemfibrozil [Lopid] and fenofibrate [Tricor]), and erythromycin. The higher the dosage of statin used in combination with these agents, the greater the risk of myositis. Also, combinations of statins and the aforementioned medications are more likely to induce myositis in patients older than 70 years and in subjects with baseline renal insufficiency.

Bile Acid Sequestrants (Resins)

The resins have been clinically available for nearly 30 years and, as a result, have been tested in a variety of clinical trials to demonstrate their efficacy, safety, and benefit on CHD end points. These are nonabsorbable, quaternary amine compounds that irreversibly bind bile acids in the gastrointestinal tract. Two members of this class are clinically available: cholestyramine (Questran) and colestipol (Colestid).

MECHANISM OF ACTION

The resins bind bile acids and drastically reduce their reabsorption in the terminal ileum. This disrupts the normal bile acid enterohepatic recirculation; as a result, the intrahepatic bile acid pool is depleted. Hepatocytes respond to this deficiency by shunting cholesterol into bile acid synthesis, thereby reducing intracellular cholesterol levels. This, in turn, up-regulates hepatic LDL receptor activity, and the plasma level of LDL cholesterol declines. A byproduct of increased hepatic file acid synthesis is a concomitant increase in hepatic triglyceride and VLDL synthesis. In patients with baseline fasting hypertriglyceridemia, resins may increase triglyceride levels by this mechanism.

EFFICACY

Both cholestyramine and colestipol are available as powdered compounds; colestipol is also available in a tablet (one gram per tablet). The powdered resins must be mixed with cold liquids or combined with soft foods in order to enhance compliance with the treatment regimen. The LDL cholesterol–lowering capabilities of the resins are equivalent and dosage related. Cholestyramine (4 grams per dose) and colestipol (5 grams per dose) should be started as single-dose administrations of the powder per day, with an attempt to increase to two doses per day. At 8 grams of cholestyramine and 10 grams of colestipol per day, LDL cholesterol can be reduced by 15%. Progressive increases to a maximum of 24 grams of cholestyramine and 30 grams of colestipol per day may reduce LDL cholesterol by 30%. HDL cholesterol is variably increased, up to 5%, and triglyceride levels may increase by 20 to 30% if the patient has fasting hypertriglyceridemia. If more than two doses are titrated once per day, the doses should be divided to two or three times per day to enhance tolerability and compliance.

SIDE EFFECTS

Although the resins have proved safe, are desirable because of their nonabsorbable nature, and are reasonably efficacious for lowering LDL cholesterol, they are not first-line therapy because of their poor tolerability and the difficulty of compliance with their regimen. They commonly cause abdominal bloating, reflux, abdominal pain, constipation, and hemorrhoids. Using lower daily doses may allow patients to develop a tolerance to these gastrointestinal effects, and the use of fiber supplements and stool softeners may reduce the incidence of constipation. Because the resins are highly charged compounds, they have the capacity to bind to many co-administered medications, such as thyroxine, digoxin, diuretics, antibiotics, and warfarin. Therefore, it is recommended that any concomitant medications be given about 1 hour before or 4 hours after the dose of resin.

Nicotinic Acid (Niacin)

Niacin is a B vitamin that has beneficial effects on lipoprotein levels when used in much higher doses than its vitamin requirement. It is available in both immediate-release and sustained-release, over-the-counter preparations, as well as by prescription. Nicotinamide is sometimes marketed as niacin but does not have a significant effect on lipoproteins when used at doses similar to those of nicotinic acid. A sustained-release once-a-day preparation, called Niaspan, approved by the Food and Drug Administration (FDA), has shown better patient tolerance and compliance.

MECHANISM OF ACTION

Nicotinic acid has beneficial effects on all lipoprotein levels, including reductions in TC, LDL cholesterol, triglyceride, and lipoprotein(a) levels, as well as increases in HDL cholesterol level. The metabolic effect of nicotinic acid is directed at reduced hepatic production and release of VLDL particles. Because VLDL is the first step in endogenous lipid metabolism, a reduction in VLDL production results in decreased formation of its delipidated products, such as IDL and LDL particles. The increase in HDL cholesterol level results mostly from the concomitant reduction in high triglyceride levels; however, HDL levels can increase in patients without baseline hypertriglyceridemia by a mechanism that is not well understood. Although nicotinic acid can lower lipoprotein(a), the mechanism responsible for this has not been determined.

EFFICACY

Low dosages of nicotinic acid (<500 mg per day) have little predictable effect on lipoproteins. At dosages of 1000 to 1500 mg per day, niacin is most effective in reducing triglyceride levels up to 30% and increasing HDL cholesterol by 15 to 20%. At these dosages, LDL cholesterol is reduced about 15%. When dosages of 2000 to 4000 mg per day are used, the LDL cholesterol–lowering effect can be nearly 25%, and further reductions of triglyceride levels (up to 50%) and increases in HDL cholesterol level (up to 30%) occur. Lipoprotein(a) has been lowered by 25 to 40%, according to published reports, when at least 3000 mg per day is used. In most of the reports of niacin's effects at dosages exceeding 2000 mg per day, the immediate-release formulation, given in divided doses three times a day, was used. Data for Niaspan, a sustained-release preparation, at doses of 1000 to 2000 mg once a day at bedtime, suggest that LDL cholesterol can be lowered 15 to 18%, triglyceride levels lowered 25 to 30%, lipoprotein(a) level lowered 20 to 25%, and HDL cholesterol level increased by 20 to 25%. Compositional changes in LDL particles have also been shown with niacin therapy, converting small, dense particles to larger, less dense forms.

SIDE EFFECTS AND DRUG INTERACTIONS

The well-known, most common side effect of nicotinic acid is cutaneous flushing and pruritus. Although it is referred to as a side effect, the universal nature of the reaction makes flushing an "expected" effect of niacin. The reaction is most frequent and intense with immediate-release preparations, usually occurring within an hour of ingestion, lasting a variable time (usually 30 to 45 minutes), and completely resolving. The intensity and frequency diminish with time at a given dosage. Therefore, it is recommended to begin with a low dosage (e.g., 100 mg once to twice a day) and then to increase the dose slowly one week at a time. Because the flushing and pruritus may be prostaglandin mediated, one 325-mg aspirin per day can ameliorate the intensity of the reaction. Sustained-release preparations are less likely to produce the same intensity or frequency of flushing; however, it is still recommended that the dosage be slowly titrated upward and that the patient use aspirin. Niaspan is associated with a low incidence of flushing, and its bedtime dosing makes any flushing occurrence better tolerated as the patient sleeps. Proper patient education allows for a greater likelihood of long-term compliance with any formulation of nicotinic acid.

Other important side effects of nicotinic acid tend to be biochemical, such as increases in hepatic transaminases, elevations of blood glucose, and increases in uric acid. Transaminase elevations are frequently seen when more than 3000 mg per day of immediate-release and more than 2000 mg per day of sustained-release niacin preparations are used. These elevations are frequently near 10%. Reports of fulminant hepatic failure have also been noted with high doses of niacin. Most mild transaminase elevations (less than three times the upper limit of normal) are asymptomatic and completely reversible if the daily dose is reduced or if the drug is discontinued. If niacin is stopped because of elevated liver enzymes, a rechallenge can be done with up to 50 to 75% of the previous daily dose. Transaminase levels should be obtained every 6 to 8 weeks with initiation and titration of dose; if stable at a steady dose, they should be monitored 2 to 3 times per year. Elevations of fasting glucose levels can occur in diabetic patients and in persons who have impaired glucose tolerance, particularly in association with insulin resistance. Niacin is not contraindicated for use in diabetic patients if care is taken to tighten glucose control before initiation of the drug. Patients with poorly controlled diabetes usually do not do well with moderate to high dosages of niacin. Elevations of uric acid levels occur with niacin and may result in significant hyperuricemia. Occasionally, niacin may precipitate a gout attack. If niacin is considered for use or is currently being used in a patient with hyperuricemia or history of gout, concomitant administration of allopurinol may be considered as reasonable prophylactic therapy.

Finally, niacin has the potential to cause dyspepsia, epigastric pain, nausea, and, in rare instances, vomiting. Patients with active peptic ulcer disease or reflux esophagitis should not be given niacin until those diseases are treated or adequately controlled. Also, concomitant administration of niacin with food greatly reduces the incidence of these upper gastrointestinal complaints.

Fibric Acid Derivatives (Fibrates)

These drugs have been clinically available since 1970. The first to be marketed was clofibrate (Atromid-S), which is rarely used now. In the United States, gemfibrozil (Lopid) and fenofibrate (Tricor) are available, whereas bezafibrate is not but is used clinically in other countries. Gemfibrozil has been shown to reduce CHD events in trials of selected primary and secondary prevention subjects.

MECHANISM OF ACTION

The fibrates have a complex impact on lipid metabolism that affects all lipoproteins. The predominant effect of fibrates is to activate LPL, which catabolizes triglyceride-rich lipoproteins: mainly VLDL, but also chylomicrons. This results in a reduction in both fasting and postprandial triglyceride levels. This effect on LPL may be mediated through activation of peroxisome proliferator–activated receptors (PPARs). By enhancing the catabolism of VLDL through LPL, excess surface protein and cholesterol are transferred to HDL particles. Also, by reducing the plasma residence time of VLDL particles, there is less transfer of cholesterol out of LDL and HDL by cholesterol ester transfer protein (CETP). This results in the production of larger HDL particles, thus increasing the HDL cholesterol level as well as increasing the size and buoyancy of LDL particles. Fibrates may also decrease hepatic VLDL production and may enhance HDL formulation by PPAR-activated apoprotein AI production. The effect of fibrates on the LDL cholesterol level is variable and depends on the pretreatment triglyceride level. If fasting triglyceride levels are normal, LDL cholesterol usually declines from 10 to 25%, depending on the fibrate used. However, if fasting triglyceride levels are elevated, the LDL cholesterol level may stay the same or increase as a result of converting small, dense particles into larger, more buoyant ones. Some small studies have suggested that fenofibrate may lower lipoprotein(a) by a mechanism as yet undetermined.

EFFICACY

The fibrates are primarily used to lower triglyceride levels. Gemfibrozil, at 600 mg twice a day, and fenofibrate, at 200 mg once a day, may decrease triglycerides by 20 to 50% and increase HDL cholesterol by 10 to 25%. Fibrates can lower LDL cholesterol levels up to 25% in hypercholesterolemic subjects; however, LDL cholesterol levels may stay the same or increase in hypertriglyceridemic subjects. Fenofibrate has been shown to reduce fibrinogen levels as well as uric acid levels. Fibrates have no effect on blood glucose. The Helsinki Heart Study demonstrated primary CHD prevention benefits with gemfibrozil in patients with high LDL cholesterol, high triglyceride, and low HDL cholesterol levels. The HDL Intervention Trial showed that gemfibrozil had secondary CHD prevention benefit in males with low HDL cholesterol levels.

SIDE EFFECTS AND DRUG INTERACTIONS

The fibrates are generally well tolerated. The major side effects are gastrointestinal, which include dyspepsia, nausea, and cholelithiasis, the risk of which is increased. Mild hepatic transaminase increases have been noted but are very uncommon and reversible if the fibrate is discontinued. Myositis has been reported with fibrate monotherapy but is rare and usually seen in patients with renal failure. No adverse effects or malignancies have been noted in the trials with gemfibrozil. The fibrates may potentiate the action of warfarin, and the prothrombin time and international normalized ratio should be monitored when fibrates are initiated in a patient receiving warfarin treatment. The potential interaction of fibrates and statins used in combination is discussed later.

Other Treatments

Estrogen

The ATP II has suggested that oral estrogen replacement therapy in hypercholesterolemic postmenopausal women may be an adjunctive or alternative treatment option. Epidemiologic studies have shown that estrogen use is associated with a lower risk of CHD in postmenopausal women. Oral estrogens can lower LDL cholesterol levels by 15%, increase HDL cholesterol levels up to 15%, and lower lipoprotein(a) levels by 20 to 25%. However, oral estrogen may increase triglyceride levels in hypertriglyceridemic women. Secondary prevention data from the Heart Estrogen/Progestin Replacement Study have demonstrated that hormone replacement therapy (HRT) does not reduce recurrent CHD events. This has tempered the enthusiasm for HRT use in women with known CHD. Cutaneous estrogen administration has little effect on lipoprotein levels. The selective estrogen receptor modulators, such as raloxifene* (Evista), reduce LDL cholesterol levels 10 to 15% and have no effect on triglyceride or HDL cholesterol levels, and there are few epidemiologic data on CHD risk reduction.

---

*Not FDA approved for this indication.

Fish Oils (Omega-3 Fatty Acids)

High doses of omega-3 fatty acids reduce hepatic VLDL production and can reduce triglyceride levels by 20 to 30%. Over-the-counter preparations are available; in doses of 9 to 12 capsules per day, these products reduce triglycerides by the mentioned percentages. The effective amounts of docosahexaenoic acid (DHA) and eicosapentaenoic acid (EPA), which are the active fatty acids, are approximately 1 gram and 2 grams, respectively. Fish oils may be used as monotherapy or, more commonly, in combination with fibrates and niacin to treat hypertriglyceridemia.

Combination Drug Treatment

Combinations of lipid-altering drugs can be used in patients with severe elevations of LDL cholesterol level, severe hypertriglyceridemia, and combined hyperlipidemia. Bile acid resins, statins, and niacin can be used in two-drug (statin plus resin) or three-drug (resin plus statin plus niacin) regimens to treat severe elevations of LDL cholesterol level, such as that seen in familial hypercholesterolemia. Niacin plus fibrates may be necessary to lower triglyceride levels that exceed 1000 mg per dL. In combined hyperlipidemia, in which LDL cholesterol level is elevated, triglyceride levels are modestly elevated, and HDL cholesterol level is low, the use of resins plus fibrates or niacin is quite effective. Because of the compliance issues related to resins, combinations of statins with either fibrates or niacin have been implemented with great therapeutic success. However, there have been reports of significant myositis and even rhabdomyolysis when statins are combined with fibrates. It is generally recommended that these drug classes not be used together, particularly in patients with renal insufficiency. Statins combined with niacin have also been reported to increase CPK levels, but not as frequently as with statins plus fibrates. Use of statins with niacin should be confined to secondary prevention, and patients should be warned to report unusual muscle soreness immediately.

CONCLUSION

Clinical trials with statins have proved that lowering LDL cholesterol levels in high-risk patients with and without known CHD reduces the incidence of CHD events and improves rates of all-cause mortality. The NCEP ATP II guidelines provide LDL cholesterol cut points for initiation of lifestyle alterations and drug therapy, if necessary. Favorable alterations in triglyceride and HDL cholesterol levels may also provide benefit in selected patients. The challenge to primary care physicians and cardiologists is to implement cost-effective lifestyle and drug treatments for all high-risk patients and to encourage long-term compliance with these regimens.

OBESITY

method of
PETER D. VASH, M.D., M.P.H.
Lindora Medical Clinics
Costa Mesa, California

Obesity is a complex biopsychosocial disease that is characterized by an excess of body fat and a resistance to treatment. Obesity results from a sustained positive caloric balance caused by a complex interaction of underlying genetic factors, reduced physical exercise, and an environment that provides ready access to cheap, high-caloric, energy-dense, highly palatable foods and snacks. It is a chronically relapsing disorder that is closely associated with an increased morbidity and mortality from numerous chronic diseases such as hypertension, diabetes mellitus type 2, hyperlipidemia, cardiovascular disorders, sleep apnea, gallbladder disease, osteoarthritis, and certain cancers. It is now the leading nutritional problem in the United States, and more than 50% of all men and women in the United States are overweight or obese.

Obesity is also associated with increased health care costs, with the estimated direct and indirect costs totaling more than $65 billion in 1990. It has also been estimated that about 6% of all health care expenditures can be attributed to obesity and its related disorders in the western industrialized nations. Although the financial costs of treating obesity are high, the socioeconomic and psychosocial costs to obese individuals (usually women) are also especially burdensome and disabling.

MEDICAL CLASSIFICATION OF OBESITY WITH THE BODY MASS INDEX

A classification of obesity by degree of seriousness is helpful to identifying individuals at increased risk for obesity-related mortality and morbidity. Traditionally, the most commonly used index for body fat determinations was the Metropolitan Life Insurance Company's Height-Weight Tables, which were based on the weight at which adults have the greatest longevity. In 1985, the National Institutes of Health (NIH) Consensus Development Conference statement on the Health Implications of Obesity recommended that physicians use the body mass index (BMI) measurement as the preferred height-weight index for determining the degree of obesity.

The BMI is a relationship between height and weight that is expressed mathematically as follows: BMI = body weight in kilograms divided by height in square meters. It correlates more closely with precise measurements of body fat and is a reliable measure of body fat related to height. It permits the establishment of a standard measurement for the evaluation of normal, overweight, and obese adults. These measurements are helpful to distinguish between the degrees of overweight and obesity, to determine the need for specific therapy, and to evaluate the results of therapy. Care must be taken, however, to distinguish between a large BMI and a heavy body weight that is the result of an increased muscle mass rather than an increased fat mass. Because the BMI is independent of height—that is, its numerical significance is identical for all height measurements—it is a more meaningful measurement of the obese state than is weight alone.

To familiarize physicians with the calculation of the BMI, the NIH statement recommended the use of BMI nomograms. Figure 1 is an example of such a BMI nomogram currently in use by physicians. The virtue of the BMI nomogram is its simplicity. A line connecting height and weight crosses the BMI scale and the BMI is read as a whole number plus an estimate of the fraction, if any, between that number and the next higher number. The Frankel BMI graph (Figure 2) also facilitates the initial BMI calculation; in addition, it can be used to demonstrate graphically the decrease in the BMI that accompanies weight reduction. One line is drawn horizontally from the height column, and a vertical line is drawn from the weight scale. These lines intersect at the corresponding BMI line. When this determination is periodically performed in conjunction with weight changes, the clinician and the patient can easily observe the resultant changes in BMI levels.

In both the nomogram for BMI and the Frankel BMI graph, small errors can result because of the slight difficulty in estimating the location of height and weight when these two measurements are not exactly at scale intervals for pounds (or kilograms) and inches (or centimeters). A more precise determination of a patient's BMI, however, may be determined mathematically. The required calculations required are as follows:

1. Conversion of weight in pounds to kilograms either by division of weight in pounds by 2.2046 or with a pound to kilogram conversion table
2. Conversion of height in inches to meters
3. Squaring the meters
4. Division of the weight in kilograms by the meters squared

Each of these steps can be accomplished easily by a hand calculator. The one drawback is that the process is time-consuming, mainly because of step 3. The process can be considerably simplified by combining steps 2, 3, and 4. Table 1 is an inches–to–square meters conversion chart for all heights at ¼-inch intervals from 58 to 76 inches. With a calculator and this conversion table, the calculations for the BMI are shortened and simplified: (1) divide the weight in pounds by 2.2046 to give the weight in kilograms and (2) divide weight in kilograms by square meters to yield the BMI.

Once the figure for square meters is obtained from the conversion chart, the patient's weight in pounds for specific BMIs such as 35, 30, 27, and so forth can be quickly calculated by multiplying the desired BMI figure by 2.2046 and then by the square meters figure from Table 1. If the weight in kilograms, rather than in pounds, is desired for specific BMIs, simply multiply the BMI by the square meters figure.

The major limitation of the BMI in the past was that it was a difficult concept for physicians to interpret to patients and relate to a weight that needed to be reduced. Table 2 lists the weights in pounds for various grades of obesity for heights between 4 feet 10 inches and 6 feet 4 inches. The equivalence of a BMI of 27 and 120% of normal weight is derived from the 1985 NIH statement. At weight levels between normal and a BMI of 27, weight reduction therapy may not be medically required unless there is an associated disease such as diabetes, hypertension, hypercholesterolemia, hypertriglyceridemia, a family history of obesity-associated diseases, or upper body (abdominal) obesity.

The NIH statement strongly recommends treatment at weight levels associated with BMIs of 27 (grade 1 obesity) and above. The medical condition of obesity begins statistically at a BMI of 30, and medically significant obesity begins at a BMI of 35. At this level of obesity and above, almost all adults will have obesity-associated medical risk

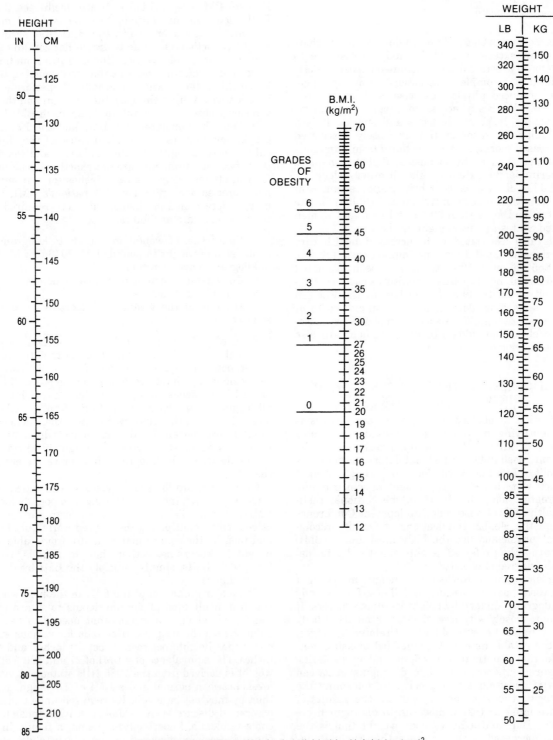

BODY MASS INDEX = Weight (kg) divided by Height (meters)^2

Figure 1. Nomogram for body mass index (BMI).

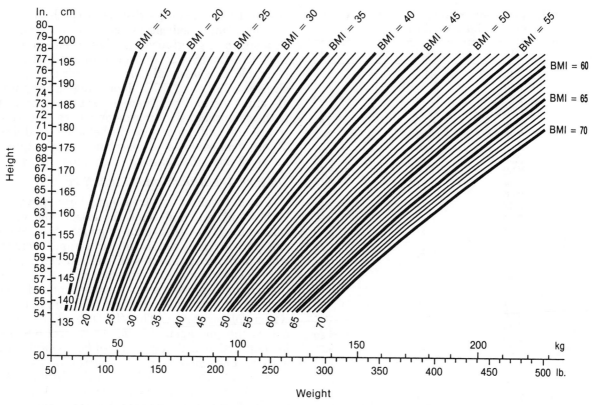

Figure 2. Body mass index (BMI) for specified height and weight, barefoot and unclothed. BMI is weight (kg)/[height (m)]². (Developed by the Portland Health Institute, Portland, Oregon.)

factors or diseases. There is a continuous relationship between an increasing BMI and morbidity; furthermore, the greater the degree of overweight, the higher the mortality in both smokers and nonsmokers.

HEALTH HAZARDS OF OBESITY

Obesity adversely affects the major organ systems, being directly responsible for accelerating the development of hypertension, coronary heart disease, diabetes mellitus (type 2), gallbladder disease, osteoarthritis, and certain cancers. Not only does the degree of excess fat contribute to the promotion of disease, but the regional distribution of the fat itself has been found to influence the adverse effects of obesity. Data suggest that obese persons whose fat is mainly in the upper body or abdomen (android) are at greater risk of morbidity and mortality than those whose fat is confined to the lower body or femoral gluteal region (gynoid). There is an increased prevalence of glucose intolerance, insulin resistance, hypertension, and hyperlipidemia in both men and women who have increased abdominal fat deposits.

TREATMENT

Goals of Obesity Therapy

The principal goals of obesity therapy should be to accomplish a reduction in obesity-related risk factors, to cause an improvement in physiologic health, and to foster an enhanced psychologic well-being. There is increasing evidence that a weight loss of 5 to 10% of total body weight can begin to reverse some of the

metabolic abnormalities associated with obesity and result in significant medical benefits for most obese patients. There is little medical evidence that weight reduction down to a "normal size" constitutes a reasonable or realistic goal. The misplaced emphasis on trying to achieve unrealistic goals in obesity treatment has led to the use of crash diets and diet fads, very few of which work for the long term. The combination of unrealistic goals and the use of medically unsound methods of dieting has led to the marked recidivism rates for most weight-reduction programs.

Meaningful short-term goals for most obese patients should be directed toward achieving an initial 10% weight reduction during a course of therapy, to be followed by a maintenance period at the new body weight. This gradual pattern of declining stepwise weight reduction may be repeated as many times as is needed to reduce the patient's total body weight into a healthy range. During the maintenance phase of treatment, the patient is checked periodically to help ensure against weight gain and a recurrence of risk factors. Patients who still have one or more obesity-related risk factors should continue therapy. The long-term goal of obesity treatment should be a reduction of sufficient excess body fat to achieve a BMI of 30 or below. For those with BMIs above 35, continued success will probably require long-term treatment programs with regular periods of follow-up to prevent a relapse into the lifestyle patterns that were initially responsible for the weight gain.

TABLE 1. **Height Conversion from Inches to Meters Squared (M²)**

Inches	M²	Inches	M²
58	2.17	68	2.98
¼	2.19	¼	3.01
½	2.21	½	3.03
¾	2.23	¾	3.05
59	2.25	69	3.07
¼	2.26	¼	3.09
½	2.28	½	3.12
¾	2.30	¾	3.14
60	2.32	70	3.16
¼	2.34	¼	3.18
½	2.36	½	3.21
¾	2.38	¾	3.23
61	2.40	71	3.25
¼	2.42	¼	3.28
½	2.44	½	3.30
¾	2.46	¾	3.32
62	2.48	72	3.35
¼	2.50	¼	3.37
½	2.52	½	3.39
¾	2.54	¾	3.42
63	2.56	73	3.44
¼	2.58	¼	3.46
½	2.60	½	3.49
¾	2.62	¾	3.51
64	2.64	74	3.53
¼	2.66	¼	3.56
½	2.68	½	3.58
¾	2.70	¾	3.60
65	2.73	75	3.63
¼	2.75	¼	3.66
½	2.77	½	3.68
¾	2.79	¾	3.70
66	2.81	76	3.37
¼	2.83		
½	2.85		
¾	2.87		

Developed by Robert E.T. Stark, M.D., Phoenix, Arizona, 1987.

Comprehensive Treatment of Obesity

Although the treatment of obesity has been disappointing to both the patient and the physician, with the currently advanced understanding of this disease and more sophisticated treatments, the therapeutic outlook now appears brighter. Although there is no one universal treatment for the obese patient, any effective weight loss program must at least incorporate these long-term behavioral changes: (1) a diet of reduced total caloric intake; (2) a diet of fat intake limited to below 30% of total calories; and (3) a lifestyle that includes physical activity on a regular and frequent basis. Weight loss depends on achieving a continued negative energy balance between total caloric and fat intake and energy expenditure. A compassionate and supportive therapeutic bond with the patient is a necessary part of a successful weight loss treatment. This is especially true within our highly stigmatized "anti-fat" culture, which maintains that obesity is a result of the patient's "lack of control."

Before the patient starts any form of therapy, a full history and physical examination should be conducted. A full laboratory evaluation should also be performed to rule out such common medical causes of obesity as Cushing's disease, hypothyroidism, insulinoma, and medication use that may promote fat deposition (e.g., glucocorticoids [prednisone]). The work-up should also include a urine analysis, complete blood count, full blood examination, and an electrocardiogram (ECG) depending on the individual's clinical situation. There are six basic components to the comprehensive treatment of obesity: (1) dietary treatment and education, (2) behavior modification, (3) physical exercise, (4) psychologic insight and cognitive change, (5) pharmacology, and (6) surgery.

Dietary Treatment and Education

A useful weight-loss treatment for achievement of both significant and rapid fat loss is the very-low-calorie diet (VLCD), which provides about 800 calories per day and can result in a rapid weight loss while minimizing the loss of lean muscle tissue.

A VLCD should consist primarily of high-quality protein, usually with a small amount of added carbohydrate, and adequate mineral, vitamin, and electrolyte supplementation. The VLCD should be employed not as the sole agent for weight control but instead in conjunction with a structured behavioral program with regular monitoring during the phase of rapid fat loss. VLCDs are available in the form of either a powdered formula based on egg or milk protein or regular "protein foods" such as lean meat, fish, and skinless fowl. These diets must be fortified with potassium replacement to offset obligatory renal losses of 30 to 50 mEq per day; a multiple vitamin and mineral complex; and small amounts of sodium chloride on an as-needed basis to prevent and treat dizziness, nausea, and orthostatic hypotension.

The VLCD is helpful in providing a dose of hopeful optimism to the obese patient. This generation of hope is needed if the patient is to survive the transition from a behavior of excessive eating into one of moderated fat and caloric intake and a routine of actively engaging in regular physical exercise. For example, a commercially available VLCD protein may be mixed with 10 ounces of nonfat milk and taken three to five times a day, depending on the patient's individual protein requirements. Potassium chloride is taken in tablet form of 10 mEq three to five times a day with the VLCD drink, and a multiple vitamin with minerals is taken twice a day. The patient is instructed to drink at least eight 10-ounce glasses of fluid (water or diet drinks preferably) each day. For the first 3 days, it is suggested that the patient take two aspirin tablets or acetaminophen (Tylenol) twice a day to prevent initial headaches.

The patient's initial clinical evaluation should include a complete history and physical examination, a 12-lead ECG, routine urinalysis, and complete blood examination, including electrolytes, fasting glucose, cholesterol (total, high-density lipoprotein [HDL], and low-density lipoprotein [LDL]), triglycerides, blood urea nitrogen, creatinine, liver function tests, calcium, and phosphorus. Blood chemistry profiles should be obtained every 4 weeks, depending on the individual patient's clinical situation, and an ECG

TABLE 2. **Medical Classification of Obesity Using Body Mass Index (BMI)**

Grade of Obesity	0	1	2	3	4	5	6
Description	Normal Weight*	Upper Limit of Normal Weight	Obesity†	Medically Significant Obesity	Morbid Obesity	Super Obesity	Super Morbid Obesity
PERCENT OF DESIRABLE WEIGHT	100	120	133	156	178	200	222
BMI	22.5	27	30	35	40	45	50
Height				*Weight in Pounds*			
4' 10"	108	129	144	167	191	215	239
4' 11"	112	133	149	174	198	223	248
5' 0"	115	138	153	179	205	230	256
5' 1"	119	142	159	185	212	238	265
5' 2"	123	147	164	191	219	246	273
5' 3"	127	152	169	198	226	254	282
5' 4"	131	157	175	204	233	262	291
5' 5"	135	162	181	211	241	271	301
5' 6"	139	167	186	217	248	279	310
5' 7"	144	172	192	224	256	288	320
5' 8"	148	177	197	230	263	296	329
5' 9"	152	182	203	237	271	305	338
5' 10"	157	187	209	244	279	313	348
5' 11"	161	193	215	251	287	322	358
6' 0"	166	199	222	259	295	332	369
6' 1"	171	205	228	265	303	341	379
6' 2"	175	210	233	272	311	350	389
6' 3"	180	216	240	280	320	360	400
6' 4"	185	222	247	288	329	370	411

*The figures for normal weight may not apply to men who have increased muscle mass due to physical conditioning. These men may be overweight without being obese, and, therefore, they may not have risk factors for obesity-related disease.

†Adults with lower body obesity consisting of excess abdominal and gluteal fat may have few, if any, risk factors associated with BMIs of 30 and above.

Developed by Robert E.T. Stark, M.D., Phoenix, Arizona, 1990.

should be obtained after each incremental 50 to 100 pounds of weight loss. Although VLCDs are safe and effective when used appropriately and with reasonable and responsible clinical judgment, there are several contraindications to their use, such as pregnancy; unstable renal, hepatic, or cardiovascular disease; substance abuse; and severe psychiatric disease. Because rapid weight loss has been associated with the aggravation of gallbladder disease and the possibility of gallstone formation, patients should be informed of this possibility and proper caution should be exercised. Patients on specific medications such as lithium or psychoactive medication and others whose serum levels must be closely regulated should be monitored with due caution because hepatic and renal metabolism of these medications may vary during the VLCD therapy. Above all, patients using a VLCD should be seen frequently (i.e., every 1 to 2 weeks) for follow-up.

Because blood pressure often decreases early in the course of the VLCD due to increased sodium loss balance and changes in sympathetic nervous system activity, diuretic medication should be reduced or stopped at the beginning of the program. Other antihypertensive medication may be gradually withdrawn and over time perhaps completely discontinued. Patients with adult-onset diabetes (type II), who may be on insulin to control the hyperglycemia, should have their insulin dosage lowered by 50% before starting the VLCD and should be closely monitored during the course of VLCD therapy. Very often, it is possible to further reduce or eliminate completely the use of insulin. There occurs an elevation in the serum uric acid during the early weeks of the VLCD that is due to an increased competition for its renal excretion during rising levels of ketone bodies as they are produced during fat metabolism. Therefore, patients who have a family history of gout, or established gouty disease, should use allopurinol (Zyloprim), 300 mg at bedtime, throughout the VLCD diet. When the patient achieves a weight loss at which physiologic functions are normalized (i.e., normotensive, euglycemic, and so forth) and at which the patient feels well and looks well, it is probably time to stop the VLCD.

Refeeding should commence with fish, chicken, lean meat, fruit, vegetables, and starches (rice, baked potato, and bread). Small portion sizes, with one or two such meals a day, provide an easy reintroduction to eating. Continued emphasis on behavior modification and regular physical exercise is necessary for successful weight maintenance. For example, the technique of self-reporting record keeping ("journaling") of calories taken in and calories expended is one of the behavior modification cornerstones for successful weight maintenance. Attention to limiting the percentage of calories from fat to below 30% of the total injested calories on a daily basis also helps to prevent fat regain. This experience with the VLCD serves to educate the patient to the fact that a low-calorie intake and a limited fat intake results in fat loss and is the basis for long-term weight management.

Behavior Modification

Many obese persons tend to use food as a form of coping mechanism, overeating in response to emotional cues such as stressful situations, social functions, or psychologic distress. This form of excessive or binge eating, however, has more to do with habit than with hunger. Because the eating environment has a direct effect on eating behavior, effective food cue control is a major part of the treatment of obesity. To help patients modify their eating behavior, they should be taught to (1) extinguish environmental cues that lead to overeating (e.g., television watching), (2) enforce a more conscious eating behavior (i.e., eating at scheduled times in a structured setting), (3) self-monitor (journaling of food intake and physical exercise), (4) set goals, (5) manage stress (i.e., use relaxation techniques), and (6) problem solve without food-related rewards. Only when inappropriate eating behaviors are stopped, and the stresses that led to overeating are managed, can patients really begin to control their weight.

Physical Exercise

Although regular physical activity is an essential part of any weight management program, its effects are probably more important for weight maintenance than for weight loss. The goal of a physical exercise program for weight management should be at least 30 minutes of moderate physical activity five to seven times per week. Aerobic activities such as walking, gentle aerobics, swimming, riding an exercise bicycle, or using a treadmill can be recommended. The intensity, duration, and frequency of activity should be gradually increased with time as the patient loses weight. This will help to offset the enhanced efficiency the body derives because of its weight loss. By increasing the level of exercise during the course of weight loss, weight plateaus can be prevented. Patients who start an exercise program early in their weight loss program and continue it on a regular basis are much less likely to regain their lost weight.

PSYCHOLOGIC INSIGHT AND COGNITIVE CHANGE

Eating is often used as a coping mechanism to deal with psychologic stress and discomfort. Any program of weight management should help patients to gain an insight into why they misuse food and help them to develop new non–food-related ways of coping so as to develop a new relationship with food and eating. Often a troubled marriage, an unfulfilling job, financial worries, low self-esteem, or a poor self-image may significantly contribute to a weight gain and the inability to lose weight. More people eat in excess to the point of obesity because of an "empty heart" than because of an empty stomach. Changing the patient's perspective on how to cope effectively with stresses without using food sets the stage for significant weight loss and long-term weight maintenance.

Pharmacology: Anorectic Medication

Anorectic medication can successfully be used to alter the patient's perception of hunger and fullness. Diet suppressant medication, however, is best utilized as part of an overall therapy, and it should not be used in place of the necessary changes in eating behavior and lifestyle. The major function of medication is to help patients adhere to their diet, use their behavior modification principles, and continue with a program of regular and frequent physical activity. In this way medication can help patients lose weight because to date current medications are unable to directly cause a fat loss. There is no currently available medication that acts directly on the fat cell to force the release of fat. Medication works only if it is taken properly, and its effect on weight loss and weight maintenance usually cease once it is stopped.

Anorectic medication should be reserved for obese patients with a BMI of 30 or more or for patients with a BMI of 27 or more with associated co-morbid diseases such as hypertension, hyperlipidemia, diabetes mellitus type 2, osteoarthritis, and so forth. Appetite suppressant medication can usually help patients lose about 10 to 15% of their initial body weight and often much greater amounts of weight, depending on individual patient motivation and compliance. About one third of patients treated with such medications, however, do not respond with any significant weight loss, and most patients will usually regain their lost weight after the anorectic medication is stopped. The major anorectic medications currently in use are listed in Table 3.

Phentermine can be used as a 15-mg dose every morning or twice a day or as a 30-mg or a 37.5-mg dose every morning, depending on the individual patient. Higher doses do not usually allow for greater weight loss, but do produce more side effects, such as tachycardia, dry mouth, premature ventricular contractions, mild elevations of blood pressure, insomnia, slight tremor, and a "hyper" feeling. Phentermine has been evaluated by the U.S. Food and Drug Administration (FDA) and found, to date, not to be implicated as a causative agent for cardiac valve disease. The role of phentermine as a causative agent for the generation of primary pulmonary hypertension is, to date, doubtful but not entirely certain. Although phentermine combined with serotonin selective reuptake inhibitor (SSRI) antidepressant (fluoxetine [Prozac] 20 mg; sertraline [Zoloft] 50 mg; paroxetine [Paxil] 20 mg) is off label and not recommended as such in the Physicians' Desk Reference, many clinicians have safely used this combination with good weight loss results. This combination appears to work well for those obese patients who have depression, stress-induced binge eating, obsessive-compulsive aspects to their eating, or problems with carbohydrate binge eating associated with their menstrual cycle. Although the combination of a phenter-

TABLE 3. **Anorectic Medication for Obesity Treatment**

Medication	Schedule	Trade Name(s)	Dosage (mg)	Common Use
Phentermine HCl	IV		8, 15, 30	Initial dose: 8–15 mg/d
		Adipex-P	37.5	Higher dose: 15 mg bid or 30 mg q AM Initial dose: ½ tablet/d
				Higher dose: ½ tablet bid or 37.5-mg tablet q AM
		Fastin	30	1 capsule q AM
		Obe-Nix 30	37.5	1 capsule q AM
Phentermine resin	IV	Ionamin	15, 30	Initial dose: 15 mg/d
Mazindol	IV	Sanorex	1, 2	Higher dose: 15 mg bid or 30 mg q AM Initial dose: 1 mg/d
Diethylpropion	IV	Tenuate	25	Higher dose: 2 mg q AM or 1 mg tid Initial dose: 25 mg/d
		Tenuate Dospan	75	Higher dose: 25 mg tid 75 mg q AM
Sibutramine	IV	Meridia	5, 10, 15	Initial dose: 5–10 mg/d
Orlistat	IV	Xenical	120	Higher dose: 15–25 mg/d Initial dose: 1 capsule with a fatty meal qd; bid; or tid

mine medication with an SSRI has not been found to date to cause cardiac valve disease, it should be used with caution and with a full disclosure to the patient of all potential side effects. Mazindol (Mazanor), an appetite suppressant related to the tricyclic antidepressants, can cause central nervous system stimulation similar to amphetamines. It does not, however, cause euphoria, and the abuse potential is low. The potential side effects are insomnia, dizziness, and mild agitation. Because there may be a mild tachycardia, mazindol should not be used by patients with marked hypertension or severe cardiovascular disease.

Diethylpropion (Tenuate) can be used as 25 mg two or three times a day or in a sustained release form of 75 mg per day with the potential side effects of dry mouth, restlessness, and constipation. There have been reported cases of psychologic and physical dependence, so it should be used with caution and not in combination with phentermine. Caffeine and over-the-counter cold medications that contain phenylpropanolamine and/or pseudoephedrine may interact with phentermine and diethylpropion to cause tachycardia, an elevation of blood pressure, and a sense of panic or agitation.

Sibutramine (Meridia) acts to block the reuptake of serotonin and norepinephrine and usually takes longer to effect a change in the patient's appetite and sense of fullness (at least 2 weeks). Some of the potential side effects are dry mouth, midsleep insomnia, headache, and a mild transient increase in pulse rate and an increase in diastolic and systolic blood pressure. To date, sibutramine has been found to be safe and effective, allowing about a 15% loss of total body weight without any association with primary pulmonary hypertension or cardiac valve disease.

Orlistat (Xenical) is a novel medication to treat obesity by blocking the intestinal action of gastric and pancreatic lipases to cause a decreased absorption of about 30% of any ingested fat. It does not have any effect on blocking the absorption of carbohydrates or protein. The nonabsorbed fat is expelled through the rectum as an oily discharge, but orlistat does not cause diarrhea or steatorrhea. Because it may reduce, by a small but not clinically significant amount, the serum level of fat-soluble vitamins, a daily multivitamin should be taken each day. Orlistat is not absorbed systemically and does not act on the central nervous system, and as such it does not affect appetite or satiety.

Surgery

Obesity surgery is recommended for those massively obese patients (BMI > 50) who have seriously tried but failed to lose weight with a comprehensive medical program. Surgery must be considered for those patients whose obesity is life-threatening or so massive that any quality of life is nonexistent. Although surgery has been shown to significantly reverse many of the chronic diseases associated with excessive obesity, there is still an increased risk for morbidity and mortality from such surgery. The surgical postoperative care of the massively obese patient is a demanding clinical challenge.

The two proven surgical procedures that are most often used for the treatment of morbid obesity are (1) vertical banded gastroplasty (gastric stapling) or laparoscopic gastric banding and (2) gastric bypass operations such as the Roux-en-Y gastric bypass or a more extreme gastric bypass such as the biliopancreatic diversion. Obesity surgery should be performed by those surgeons who are experienced with and regularly perform such procedures. Weight loss tends to plateau after about 12 months at a weight of about 60 to 70% above the patient's ideal body weight.

For additional resources, the treating physician can contact

1. North American Association for the Study of Obesity (301-563-6526)
2. American Society of Bariatric Physicians (303-770-2526)

VITAMIN K DEFICIENCY

method of
JACK B. ALPERIN, M.D.
University of Texas Medical Branch
Galveston, Texas

Vitamin K, a lipid-soluble vitamin, functions as a cofactor in the enzymatic gamma carboxylation of glutamyl residues in the vitamin K–dependent coagulation factors II (prothrombin), VII, IX, and X and in the regulatory proteins of coagulation, proteins C and S. Other vitamin K–dependent proteins, all with gamma carboxyglutamyl (Gla) residues, include protein Z, osteocalcin, the Gla-matrix protein in bone, and nephrocalcin. These Gla groups permit vitamin K–dependent clotting factors to bind calcium and phospholipid so that they may allow for normal coagulation. Failure of the vitamin K–dependent factors to bind calcium and phospholipid results in defective hemostasis and hemorrhage.

The estimated minimal daily requirement for vitamin K is 1 or 2 μg per kg body weight and comes primarily from the diet. Vitamin K_1 (phytonadione), the more important form of this vitamin for humans, occurs in highest concentrations in green, leafy vegetables (e.g., spinach, broccoli, mustard greens), but adequate amounts exist in nearly every diet. Before absorption, vitamin K_1 must be dissolved in fat that is solubilized by bile salts. Absorption occurs actively across the small intestinal mucosa and through the lymphatic system. Bacteria that normally inhabit the intestinal lumen also synthesize another form of the vitamin menaquinone, or vitamin K_2, that is absorbed passively from the colon.

CLINICAL FEATURES

Vitamin K deficiency causes a coagulopathy that leads to a bleeding disorder. Specific signs of deficiency include easy bruising, epistaxis, bleeding from the gastrointestinal or genitourinary tracts, menometrorrhagia, retroperitoneal bleeding, and intracranial hemorrhage. Bleeding may also follow trauma, needle punctures, and surgery.

ETIOLOGY

Factors leading to vitamin K deficiency include decreased intake of the vitamin, fat malabsorption, and inhibition of the vitamin K_2–synthesizing bacteria that live in the intestine. Failure to eat because of disease or surgery or parenteral nutrition that excludes vitamin K replacement contributes to vitamin deficiency. Fat malabsorption may occur because of cholestatic jaundice (e.g., obstruction of the common bile duct, cholestatic hepatitis), pancreatic insufficiency (e.g., chronic pancreatitis, cystic fibrosis), diffuse disease of the small intestinal mucosa (e.g., non-tropical spruce, regional enteritis), small intestinal or biliary fistulas, or short small bowel syndromes. Antibiotics contribute to vitamin K deficiency by inhibiting the intestinal microflora that synthesize vitamin K_2.

Therapy with warfarin and indanedione* anticoagulants, vitamin K antagonists, causes a coagulopathy identical to vitamin K deficiency. Warfarin is the active ingredient in some rodenticides. Other vitamin K antagonists, the superwarfarins (e.g., brodifacoum, difenacoum, chlorphacinone, bromodiolone), are preferred as rodenticides for their

---

*Not FDA approved for this indication.

592

effectiveness against warfarin-resistant rats. Rodenticide poisoning occurs accidentally or by attempted suicide. Poisoning has been observed after a mixture of marijuana and d-CON, a rodenticide containing brodifacoum, has been smoked.

Vitamin K deficiency can cause hemorrhagic disease of the newborn and infancy. Because the vitamin crosses the placenta poorly, body stores and serum levels of vitamin K are always low in the newborn. For unknown reasons, treating pregnant women with anticonvulsants (e.g., phenobarbital, phenytoin, primidone) contributes to vitamin K deficiency in the newborn and seldom causes vitamin K deficiency in the mother. Finally, human milk is so low in vitamin K that breast-feeding infants to the exclusion of other foods causes vitamin K deficiency in older infants.

Cephalosporin antibiotics with an *N*-methyl-5-thiotetrazole side chain (moxalactam,* cefamandole, cefoperazone) also contribute to the coagulopathy of vitamin K deficiency because they inhibit Gla synthesis in coagulation factors.

DIAGNOSIS

Prolonged values for the prothrombin time (PT) and the activated partial thromboplastin time (aPTT) typify a deficiency of vitamin K. Values for platelet counts, plasma fibrinogen level, thrombin time, fibrinogen degradation products or fibrinogen split products, and D-dimer are normal. Rarely are other laboratory tests necessary. Coagulation factors II, VII, IX, and X are be decreased, but all other coagulation factors are normal. The non–gamma-carboxylated precursor proteins of the vitamin K–dependent coagulation factors (e.g., des-gamma carboxyl prothrombin) or PIVKA (proteins induced by the absence of vitamin K) are present in plasma but are rarely necessary for diagnosis. The differential diagnosis should include disseminated intravascular coagulation and liver disease (Table 1). Diagnosis of vitamin K deficiency can be confirmed nearly always by demonstration that vitamin K replacement restores PT and aPPT values to normal.

FORMULATIONS OF VITAMIN K

Two formulations of phytonadione (vitamin K_1) are available for treatment and prevention of vitamin K deficiency. Phytonadione as Mephyton comes as a 5-mg scored tablet for oral use. AquaMEPHYTON, an aqueous colloidal solution of vitamin K_1, comes in concentrations of 10 mg/mL and 1.0 mg/0.5 mL for

---

*Not FDA approved for this indication.

TABLE 1. **Differential Diagnosis of Vitamin K Deficiency**

Test	VKD	Liver Disease	DIC
aPTT	Increased	Increased	Increased
PT	Increased	Increased	Increased
Platelets	Normal	Decreased	Decreased
Fibrinogen	Normal	Decreased	Decreased
D-dimer/FDP/FSP	Normal	Normal or Increased	Increased
PIVKA-II	Present	Absent	Absent

Abbreviations: aPTT = activated partial thromboplastin time; DIC = disseminated intravascular coagulation; FDP/FSP = fibrin degradation/split products; PIVKA-II = protein induced by vitamin K absence; PT = prothrombin time; VKD = vitamin K deficiency.

intramuscular and subcutaneous injection. Aqua-MEPHYTON may be given intravenously, but the dose should be diluted with a solution of 0.9% NaCl (1 mg/mL) and infused at a rate not to exceed 1.0 mg/min to minimize adverse reactions.

TREATMENT

Parenteral vitamin K_1 should be given to those patients with a deficiency who show evidence of bleeding or extremely abnormal PT and aPTT values. The initial dose is 0.5 to 1.0 mg for premature and term infants, 2 to 3 mg for children up to 12 months old, and 5 to 10 mg for ages 1 year to the mid-teens. The usual adult dose is 10 to 20 mg. Subcutaneous injection is preferred to the intramuscular route, which may result in hematoma formation. Slow intravenous infusion of vitamin K_1 ensures that the vitamin reaches hepatocytes where coagulation factors are synthesized but rarely causes hypotension or anaphylaxis. Within 24 hours after treatment, bleeding should cease, and values for PT and aPTT should be normal. A second dose of vitamin K_1 should be given 24 hours after the first. Failure to improve means that the diagnosis is incorrect or other coagulopathies are present. For those poisoned with a superwarfarin, the initial dose of vitamin K_1 should be 25 to 30 mg given intravenously, followed by a daily oral dose of 50 mg for weeks or months until the superwarfarin is no longer detected in blood and normal measurements of PT and aPTT persist.

For those with vitamin K deficiency with extremely severe bleeding manifestations (e.g., gastrointestinal or genitourinary tract bleeding, intracranial hemorrhage, retroperitoneal bleeding), treatment includes vitamin K replacement and fresh frozen plasma (10 to 20 mL per kg of body weight). Infusions of fresh frozen plasma provide immediate replacement of the vitamin K-dependent coagulation factors. Infusions of prothrombin-complex concentrates (e.g., Konyne 80, Proplex T) are rarely needed and should be avoided if possible because they carry a risk for thrombosis, especially in those patients who have associated liver disease. In addition, a risk of transmitting a viral illness always exists whenever blood products are given.

PREVENTION

All newborns should receive 0.5 to 1.0 mg of vitamin K_1 intramuscularly within the first hour after birth. Infants who are breast-fed exclusively need additional supplements of vitamin K_1. Pregnant women taking anticonvulsants or antibiotics should be given 10 to 20 mg mephenytoin (Mephyton) daily for 2 to 3 weeks before delivery.

Patients with a decreased intake of vitamin K or malabsorption of the vitamin should receive prophylactic supplements of vitamin K. Prophylaxis is needed especially for severely ill patients (often in intensive care units) who are not taking in vitamin K but are receiving antibiotics that may destroy the intestinal microflora that synthesize vitamin K_2 or may inhibit Gla synthesis in coagulation factors. Prophylactic treatments with vitamin K_1 may be given orally in doses of 2.5 to 5 mg daily or thrice weekly or subcutaneously as 10 mg once a week.

OSTEOPOROSIS

method of
FREDERICK R. SINGER, M.D.
John Wayne Cancer Institute
Santa Monica, California

Osteoporosis is a metabolic bone disease syndrome in which low bone mass and microscopic abnormalities of bone predispose the patient to traumatic and spontaneous fractures. It is estimated that more than 25 million white American women have low bone mass and that the cost of direct medical care for fractures in 1995 was approximately $13.8 million. About 50% of white women are expected to experience a fracture during their lifetime. Nonwhite women and men are also at risk, but not to the same degree. With aging, the risk of fractures increases; this phenomenon could certainly be reduced with appropriate use of existing diagnostic testing, modification of deleterious lifestyles, and medical therapy.

CLASSIFICATION

Numerous risk factors that can predispose a person to the development of osteoporosis have been identified; some are listed in Table 1. Those in the population who are most susceptible to osteoporosis are postmenopausal women not receiving estrogen replacement therapy. Prolonged therapeutic use of glucocorticoids is another major cause of osteoporosis. Hyperthyroidism, hyperparathyroidism, and androgen deficiency are other hormonal disorders associated with osteoporosis. Cigarette smoking and heavy alcohol usage are habits that can lower bone density. Chronically low calcium intake (particularly during childhood and adolescence) can also reduce bone density. A family history of osteoporosis is a major risk factor whose genetic basis is now the subject of considerable research. The vitamin D receptor, collagen type I, and estrogen receptor genes, among others, are receiving considerable scrutiny as contenders for the cause of osteoporosis in families.

TABLE 1. **Some Risk Factors Predisposing to Osteoporosis**

Family history of osteoporosis
Cigarette usage
Alcoholism
Endocrine disorders
Hypogonadism
Glucocorticoid excess
Hyperthyroidism
Hyperparathyroidism
Low calcium intake
Malabsorption
Malnutrition
Immobilization
Connective tissue disorder
Malignancy

Most patients with osteoporosis are asymptomatic but have a greater-than-normal risk for fractures because of reduced biomechanical integrity of the skeleton. A vertebral fracture is often the first sign of a problem. Fractures of the wrist or hip almost always occur with falls. Loss of height is associated with vertebral fractures and may progress to dorsal kyphosis if multiple wedge-type fractures occur. Occasionally, kyphosis occurs in the absence of episodes of acute back pain. Chronic and intermittent back pain after vertebral fractures may represent episodes of muscle spasm or recurrent fractures. Back pain may also reflect the presence of other common problems such as degenerative arthritis and degenerative disk disease.

DIAGNOSTIC TESTS

Skeletal Radiography

Although skeletal radiographs may bring to attention the possibility of osteoporosis in a given person, they are an insensitive means of detecting low bone density and should be used only to determine the existence of fractures.

Bone Densitometry

The standard means of establishing a diagnosis of osteoporosis is by measuring bone mineral density. The most common technique used is dual radiographic absorptiometry of the lumbar spine and/or hip. An alternative method is quantitative computed tomography of the lumbar spine, which measures the spongy bone within the vertebral bodies and thereby can avoid the artifacts of spine density measurement produced by degenerative arthritis and aortic calcification, seen with dual radiographic absorptiometry. Instruments that measure ultrasonographic parameters of the heel have become available and may be used as a less expensive screening test of the population at risk after adequate experience with the technique is obtained.

The World Health Organization has defined osteoporosis as a bone mineral density 2.5 standard deviations (SD) or more below the mean for young adults. Low bone mass, or osteopenia, is defined as 1 to 2.5 SD below the young adult mean. The term "T score" has been used to indicate these values and can be positive or negative. A "Z score," also provided by the instruments used to measure density, is the SD of the patient's bone density in comparison with those of sex- and age-matched normal subjects. A Z score in an elderly woman may be misleading in considering whether osteoporosis is present: A score that is average for the "normal" population at age 90 does not indicate adequate bone density, because the prevalence of osteoporosis among elderly estrogen-deficient women is high.

Because osteomalacia, a syndrome of impaired bone mineralization, is also associated with low bone mineral density, a diagnosis of osteoporosis requires that the existence of elevated total or bone alkaline phosphatase activity be ruled out. Depending on the underlying cause, osteomalacia is also usually associated with hypophosphatemia and, less frequently, hypocalcemia.

Bone Histology

Bone biopsies of the iliac crest have been used in the diagnosis of osteoporosis, but both the scarcity of physicians experienced in this technique and the discomfort associated with obtaining the specimen have restricted this diagnostic modality mainly to research studies of new drugs and to patients in whom osteomalacia or other unusual forms of bone disease are suspected.

Biochemical Testing

The biochemical profile includes calcium, phosphorus, alkaline phosphatase, renal function, and liver function. In addition, measurement of the complete blood cell count and serum immunoglobulins helps to exclude hematologic malignancies. Thyroid-stimulating hormone helps to exclude hyperthyroidism; parathyroid hormone to exclude primary hyperparathyroidism; free cortisol in a 24-hour urine collection to exclude Cushing's syndrome; and free testosterone in serum to identify androgen deficiency. Serum 25-hydroxyvitamin D to exclude vitamin D deficiency may be helpful in selected patients.

Measurement of the 24-hour urinary calcium/creatinine ratio may help detect malabsorption (low calcium excretion) or idiopathic hypercalciuria, both of which are sometimes associated with low bone density.

A number of biochemical tests reflect the rate of bone resorption and bone formation. Studies suggest that it may be possible to use these tests to predict future bone loss or gain, although the role of these tests in clinical practice is currently controversial. Biochemical markers of bone resorption such as deoxypyridinoline and N-telopeptide (reflecting collagen cross-link degradation) in urine are relatively specific markers of bone collagen destruction. Increased excretion of these markers may be predictive of bone loss over a several-year period. If drugs are given to inhibit bone resorption, a significant reduction of collagen cross-link excretion after 3 months may be predictive of an increase in bone density after one or more years of treatment. Bone formation markers include serum osteocalcin and bone-specific alkaline phosphatase and may also be predictive of future bone density after treatment. When anabolic agents become available these latter tests may have a larger role in patient follow-up.

PREVENTION AND TREATMENT OF OSTEOPOROSIS

Postmenopausal Osteoporosis

Estrogen deficiency at any age results in an increase in bone resorption through an increase in osteoclast activity. A secondary increase in bone formation by osteoblasts follows but is not sufficient to prevent bone loss. If the patient failed to achieve a peak bone mass during growth and development because of genetic influences or deleterious lifestyle habits, bone loss may lead to compression fractures of the spine after 10 to 15 years of estrogen deficiency or to hip fractures after 15 to 20 years. This reflects the greater metabolic activity in spongy bone than in dense cortical bone. Various types of therapy for osteoporosis now exist (Table 2). Because the efficacy of some agents does not extend across all stages of the disorder, it seems appropriate to consider their use with regard to early and later periods of the postmenopausal years.

Prevention of Early Postmenopausal Bone Loss

Several antiresorptive agents can prevent bone loss in the early postmenopausal years. Estrogen replacement therapy is highly effective in protecting against early postmenopausal bone loss and may of-

TABLE 2. Drugs Used in the Management of Postmenopausal Osteoporosis

Estrogens

Oral

Conjugated estrogens (Premarin)
Estradiol (Estrace)
Estropipate (Ogen)
Ethinyl estradiol

Transdermal

Estradiol (Estraderm)

Selective Estrogen Receptor Modulators

Tamoxifen (Nolvadex)
Raloxifene (Evista)

Bisphosphonates

Alendronate (Fosamax)
Etidronate* (Didronel)

Calcitonins

Salmon calcitonin (Miacalcin)
 Injectable and nasal

Vitamin D

Vitamin D_2
Calcitriol* (Rocaltrol)

Calcium Preparations

Calcium carbonate (Os-Cal)
Calcium citrate (Citracal)
Calcium phosphate (Posture)

*Not approved for this use by the U.S. Food and Drug Administration.

fer other potential benefits, including prevention of hot flushes (if present), cardiovascular disease, bladder dysfunction, and Alzheimer's disease. In women who fear cancer as a consequence of treatment or do not continue estrogen replacement therapy because of side effects, several alternative forms of therapy can prevent bone loss. The bisphosphonate alendronate (Fosamax), 5 mg daily, is highly effective in preventing bone loss. The drug must be taken with water only, in the upright position, and at least 30 minutes before breakfast. All this is necessary because bisphosphonates are poorly absorbed and alendronate may irritate the esophagus if it does not promptly pass into the stomach. More recently, the selective estrogen receptor modulator (SERM) raloxifene (Evista) also has been shown to prevent postmenopausal bone loss at a dose of 60 mg daily. It does not stimulate breast enlargement or uterine bleeding and can lower low-density lipoprotein cholesterol, although cardiovascular benefits have not been demonstrated as yet. Adverse effects of raloxifene include slight worsening of hot flushes and a threefold increased risk of blood clots, the same risk as that produced by estrogen. Although not approved by the U.S. Food and Drug Administration (FDA) for this purpose, intermittent etidronate (Didronel) can also prevent postmenopausal bone loss. This bisphosphonate is given as a 400-mg dose for 14 days every 3 months with water only and no food 2 hours before or after ingestion.

A calcium intake of 1000 mg daily from food and/or supplements and 400 units of vitamin D daily is recommended to potentiate the effect of the antiresorptive agents. A high daily calcium intake alone (1500 mg) is usually not sufficient to prevent bone loss in the early postmenopausal period. Nasal spray salmon calcitonin (Miacalcin) is also ineffective in preventing bone loss in the initial 5 years after the menopause.

Prevention of Late Postmenopausal Bone Loss

In women 65 years and older, estrogen, raloxifene, alendronate, and etidronate remain effective in control of bone loss. Numerous studies also document that a calcium intake of about 1500 mg daily with 400 units of vitamin D daily can prevent bone loss and may be a reasonable approach to preventing bone loss in women with mild to moderate osteopenia. Nasal spray salmon calcitonin at a dose of 200 units daily is also effective in preventing bone loss in postmenopausal women who have not had a menstrual period for at least 5 years. Bone density increases approximately 1.0% in the lumbar spine, but hip density does not change.

Reversal of Osteoporosis

In postmenopausal women who have a significant degree of bone loss with or without fractures, the reversal of osteoporosis is an ideal goal, but at this time, only a modest increase in bone density can be achieved with the drugs currently available.

Estrogen replacement therapy in a previously untreated woman can increase bone density of the lumbar spine by about 5% and that of the hip somewhat less. There have been no large prospective studies of fracture prevention by estrogen therapy, but retrospective studies indicate that hip fractures may be decreased by 50%.

Alendronate, 10 mg daily, can increase lumbar spine bone density by 6 to 7% over 3 years and hip density by about 4%. Lumbar spine and hip fractures are reduced by about 50%. Studies indicate that a combination of estrogen and alendronate can increase lumbar spine bone density by 2 to 3% more than can either agent alone. However, it is not known whether this further small increment in bone density translates into a greater reduction in fracture incidence.

Raloxifene, 60 mg daily, has been found to reduce the incidence of compression fractures by about 50% but does not significantly reduce the incidence of hip fractures. In the clinical trials of raloxifene therapy for osteoporosis prevention and treatment, breast cancer incidence decreased by 62% over 2½ years in treated patients, in comparison with placebo patients. Although these studies were not designed to demonstrate breast cancer prevention, trials to examine potential benefit have been implemented.

The results of a 5-year randomized trial of nasal spray salmon calcitonin, 200 units daily, revealed a 39% decrease in compression fractures but no significant decrease in the group who received 400 units daily. No reduction in hip fractures was found at either dose.

Although it has been believed that the therapeutic response to the antiresorptive agents (estrogen, SERMs, bisphosphonates, calcitonin) depends considerably on increasing bone density to reduce fracture incidence, the accumulating data from clinical trials suggest that this is not necessarily true. A reduction in the incidence of spinal fracture by 39 to 50% has been reported with an increase of bone density ranging from 1 to 7%. This modest increment in bone density almost certainly cannot completely explain the reduced incidence of fracture. The various treatments reduce biochemical markers of bone resorption, such as urinary N-telopeptide, by 20 to 60%, and the relative efficacy of the agents appears to correlate well with the suppression of bone resorption. Thus the concept has arisen that suppression of bone turnover is an important determinant of fracture prevention. This may be mediated through protection of the microarchitecture of the bone, a phenomenon that is not well delineated by bone densitometry.

In some countries, calcitriol, the most active form of vitamin D, has been advocated as a treatment of osteoporosis. It is not clear whether its main effect is to enhance intestinal calcium absorption or whether there is a direct beneficial effect on bone. If used, serum and urine calcium levels need to be carefully monitored to avoid hypercalcemia and hypercalciuria.

Patients with Breast Cancer

Postmenopausal women who have had breast cancer form a growing group of patients. Estrogen replacement therapy is not generally prescribed in these women. The first SERM, tamoxifen (Nolvadex), has been found to prevent lumbar spine and hip bone density loss in these patients with somewhat less potency than estrogen. In patients who are not receiving tamoxifen therapy, bisphosphonates offer a good alternative; nasal spray calcitonin instead of bisphosphanates may be effective in older patients. The safety of raloxifene in patients with breast cancer has not been studied.

Glucocorticoid-Induced Osteoporosis

Steroid therapy for disorders such as rheumatoid arthritis, polymyalgia rheumatica, systemic lupus erythematosus, asthma, and inflammatory bowel disease and for patients undergoing organ transplantation frequently produces a major loss of bone during the initial months of therapy, and fractures occur in a significant number of patients. This is particularly likely in patients with a severe chronic illness before steroid administration.

Prevention of bone loss has been attempted with calcium supplements, high-dose vitamin D, gonadal steroids, and calcitonin, but the efficacy of these therapeutic strategies has often been disappointing.

However, a growing literature has documented the general success of bisphosphonates in preventing or even partially reversing steroid-induced bone loss. Intermittent etidronate therapy, 400 mg daily for 14 days every 3 months, with calcium supplementation has proved effective in a high percentage of patients, and a 10-mg dose of alendronate has been perhaps even more effective. Many patients who had already been receiving steroid treatment for a period of time have been treated with etidronate and alendronate. It would seem more logical to institute bisphosphonate therapy simultaneously with the onset of high-dose steroid therapy in patients who are expected to be treated for more than several weeks. A baseline bone density study could identify patients in whom this preventive approach would be most likely to prevent fractures. Significant osteopenia (T score < −1.5) or pre-existing osteoporosis should prompt early use of bisphosphonates. Because patients with diseases associated with diarrhea may not tolerate bisphosphonate therapy, an alternative approach is intermittent intravenous administration of pamidronate disodium (Aredia).* A 30-mg infusion given over 1 hour every 3 months may protect against bone loss without irritating the gastrointestinal tract.

Experimental Agents

Sodium fluoride is an experimental agent that has been under investigation since the 1940s. It is well documented that this is an anabolic agent with regard to bone and can produce continuous increases in lumbar spine density in many patients for 4 years or more. Various forms of this agent are approved in other countries but not in the United States because of controversy over the quality of bone induced by fluoride and because of the uncertainty about fracture prevention during treatment. A slow-release form of sodium fluoride has produced promising results but is still under investigation.

Daily subcutaneous injections of recombinant human parathyroid hormone (PTH) or biologically active PTH fragments can also induce a substantial increase in lumbar spine density through an unexpected anabolic stimulation of osteoblasts. Uncertainties remain as to how long the anabolic response can be sustained and whether there is a deleterious influence on cortical bone. These questions should be answered by ongoing studies.

THE PATIENT WITH VERTEBRAL DEFORMITY AND BACK PAIN

Severe osteoporosis resulting in multiple fractures and deformity of the spine often produces a chronic pain syndrome that may be difficult to reverse. Dr. Harold Frost,† an orthopedist with extensive experience, recommends that after an acute fracture, bed rest is usually necessary for 4 to 8 days. After the

---

*Not FDA approved for this indication.

†Southern Colorado Clinic, Pueblo, CO.

patient can turn easily in bed, the patient can get up briefly, perhaps with a thoracolumbar back support, several times a day over about a 2-week period. For the next 10 weeks or so, the patient can be out of bed, but every 2 hours the patient should lie down or sit for 20 minutes. After this 3-month period, many patients can resume normal activities that do not place undue stress on the back. However, some patients experience low lumbar back pain in the afternoon or evening that disappears overnight and returns the next day. If this occurs, these patients generally do well if they return to the 20-minute rest period every 2 hours for about 10 days. If pain persists despite this regimen or if the pain radiates to the lower extremities, other causes should be sought and treated.

THE APPROACH TO AN INDIVIDUAL PATIENT

After a thorough history taking and careful physical examination in which osteoporosis is the focus, it is often apparent why a known low bone density is present. If the patient has not had a bone density test and significant risk factors exist, a lumbar spine and hip evaluation can be done by dual radiographic absorptiometry. If the patient has significant osteopenia or osteoporosis and the diagnosis is not apparent, the diagnostic tests discussed earlier can be applied.

The therapeutic regimen should include correction of underlying disorders, such as hyperparathyroidism, and then the addition of an agent such as estrogen or an alternative drug to prevent postmenopausal bone loss. Adequate calcium and vitamin D should be added. Follow-up evaluation could entail an annual bone density evaluation for several years or possibly the measurement of a biochemical marker of bone turnover. The latter test should be done both before treatment and at least 3 months after treatment is started. The advantage of these tests is the demonstration to the patient that the treatment is having a beneficial effect. If there is no apparent biochemical improvement, the problem may be noncompliance or malabsorption of the drug. In some patients, it may be necessary to change treatment. The effect of changing treatment is best evaluated in the short term by biochemical response.

The patient should be cautioned about how to avoid trauma and prevent fractures. This information is as important as the treatment program.

PAGET'S DISEASE OF BONE

method of
LORRAINE A. FITZPATRICK, M.D.
Mayo Clinic and Mayo Foundation
Rochester, Minnesota

Paget's disease is a localized disorder of bone remodeling with an incidence of 2 to 3% of persons in the United States older than 60. Abnormal bone architecture is initiated by an increase in osteoclast-mediated bone resorption. Because of the coupling between osteoclasts and the osteoblasts, this leads to an increase in new bone formation with deposition of disorganized woven bone mixed with lamellar bone. The result is highly vascular, mechanically incompetent bone.

The etiology of Paget's disease remains uncertain, although epidemiologic evidence has demonstrated a marked geographic distribution in the disease. Paget's disease is most common in Western Europe, Australia, New Zealand, and North America. It is rarely seen in Asia or most of Africa. Familial aggregation of patients with Paget's disease, with an autosomal dominant pattern of inheritance, has been described. Other studies have indicated a possible linkage of Paget's disease to HLA. A possible candidate susceptibility locus for Paget's disease has been identified on chromosome 18q. A second possibility involves a viral etiology, proposed on the basis of a description of nucleocapsid-like structures in the nuclei and cytoplasm of pagetic osteoclasts. Inclusions resemble the paramyxovirus family of viruses, and a variety of molecular techniques have been used to explore the possibility of the role of viral infection in the etiology of Paget's disease. The two theories together suggest a genetic predisposition to an infectious agent that leads to the development of Paget's disease.

Paget's disease can be monostotic or polyostotic and is most commonly found in the axial skeleton, skull, and long bones of the lower extremities. The bone may be enlarged and deformed in more advanced disease. Pagetic bone and overlying skin may be warm to the touch as a result of increased vascularity. In the earliest phase of the disease, the pathologic process is dominated by bone resorption and characterized radiographically by osteoporosis circumscripta in the skull or advanced osteolytic wedges in long bones. A second or intermediate stage is characterized by mixed remodeling, in which increased resorption is coupled with increased new bone formation. The abnormal remodeling causes enlargement of the marrow cavity, expansion of the bone, and mechanical weakening. In the later sclerotic phase, the bone becomes dense and sclerotic. Although pagetic bone may be denser than normal bone, it is more prone to fracture because of the woven nature of the deformed bone. This haphazard deposit of collagen fibers results in a structurally weak mosaic of woven and lamellar bone.

Approximately 90% of patients with Paget's disease are asymptomatic. Bone pain is the most common presenting symptom and is often described as a dull ache. Other potential causes of pain associated with Paget's disease include associated arthritis, fracture, and neurocompression. Deformity results from the abnormal remodeling and typically involves the long bones and the skull. Skeletal deformities can include frontal bossing, skull enlargement, kyphosis, and bowing deformities of the long bones. Involvement of the facial bones can result in cranial nerve entrapment. The bowing deformities of the femur or tibia produce limb shortening, gait disturbances, and abnormal distribution of mechanical forces with resulting arthritis of the joint. Fissures and stress fractures can often occur and may be a cause of local discomfort. Involvement of the skull is associated with a mixed sensory and conductive hearing loss. With long-standing skull involvement, patients may develop platybasia in which basilar invagination results in obstructive hydrocephalus and brain stem compression. High-output cardiac failure can occur with increased pulse pressure when there is extensive skeletal involvement. Malignant generation can occur, but the frequency is small (<1%). Most of the malignant complications are osteogenic sarcomas, although other tumor types have been described. Malignant degeneration typically manifests as a change in the patient's symptoms and a dramatic increase in serum alkaline phosphatase levels.

DIAGNOSIS

Diagnosis of Paget's disease is established in most cases from the appearance of the bone on a routine bone radiograph. Pagetic bone has a thick, coarse trabecular appearance with osteolytic and sclerotic lesions. Plain radiographs can also enable clinicians to assess involvement of weight-bearing areas, evaluate symptomatic areas, and confirm pagetic involvement suspected on bone scan. Radioisotope bone scanning is a sensitive means of identifying the sites of pagetic involvement and can be used to define the extent of involvement when the patient first comes to medical attention. Plain bone radiographs, however, are needed to confirm pagetic involvement in areas with increased radioisotope uptake. Repeat bone scans and radiographs are usually not necessary during follow-up unless new symptoms develop or current symptoms become worse or except to follow involvement of weight-bearing areas. Biochemical bone markers (bone-specific alkaline phosphatase, osteocalcin, pyridinoline, and deoxypyridinoline crosslinks or N-telopeptide) are useful for monitoring response to therapy.

TREATMENT OF PAGET'S DISEASE

With the development of new inhibitors of osteoclast-mediated bone resorption, the approach to Paget's disease has evolved, and many more therapeutic options are available. Several classes of medications are currently approved for use and include calcitonin, the bisphosphonates, plicamycin, and gallium nitrate (Table 1).

Bisphosphonates are analogues of pyrophosphates, and modification of the side chain alters potency and bioavailability. Bisphosphonates have high affinity for hydroxyapatite and localize to bone, where they inhibit osteoclast-mediated bone resorption. Intestinal absorption of the bisphosphonates is poor, and after resorption to bone, the rest is excreted in urine without metabolism to other products. All patients taking bisphosphonates should be provided supplementary calcium and vitamin D and instructed not to take these supplements with the bisphosphonates, which will bind to the calcium. The bisphosphonates are contraindicated in patients with hypocalcemia.

The first bisphosphonate to become available for the treatment of Paget's disease was etidronate (Didronel) (ethane-1-hydroxy-1,1-bisphosphonate). The usual dose for treatment is 5 mg per kg of body weight per day for 6 months. Some clinicians use high-dose therapy (10 to 20 mg per kg per day), but an increased incidence of fractures has been reported, and histologic evidence of osteomalacia has been noted in patients treated with this higher dosage. Because of the possibility that etidronate may impair mineralization, this drug is not recommended for patients who anticipate undergoing orthopedic procedures of fractures in the process of healing, in spite of the fact that no evidence exists to support this theoretical problem.

The availability of second-generation bisphosphonates, pamidronate and alendronate, for the treatment of Paget's diseases has reduced several concerns raised with etidronate. Pamidronate (Aredia) (3-amino-1-hydroxypropylidene-1,1-bisphosphonate) is an amino bisphosphonate available in intravenous form and is effective for the treatment of Paget's disease. Pamidronate is an antiresorptive agent, and although the mechanism of antiresorptive action is not completely understood, several factors contribute to this action. Pamidronate is adsorbed to hydroxyapatite crystals in bone and may directly block dissolution of the mineral component of bone. Inhibition of osteoclast activity contributes to inhibition of bone resorption. The amount and interval of administration is related to the severity of disease. Patients with mild disease may require a single 60-mg infusion; patients with polyostotic disease may benefit from higher doses (120 to 180 mg) administrated over a longer interval (weeks to months). Higher doses (>2.0 grams over 12 to 24 weeks) have been used in patients with extreme, resistant disease, but doses this high are unusual, and in patients with mild disease, high doses have been associated with

TABLE 1. **Pharmacologic Therapy for Paget's Disease**

Class	Name	Dose	Duration	Comment
Bisphosphonates	Etidronate (Didronel)	5 mg/kg/d PO	6 months	Associated with impaired mineralization at high doses.
	Alendronate (Fosamax)	40 mg/d PO	6 months	All bisphosphonates other than etidronate must be ingested 30–60 minutes before breakfast with water only.
	Pamidronate (Aredia)	60–90 mg IV	q 3–9 months	
	Tiludronate (Skelid)	400 mg/d PO	3 months	
	Risedronate (Actonel)	30 mg/d PO	2 months	
Calcitonin	Intranasal* (Miacalcin)	200–400 IU qd		
	Parenteral (Calcimar)	50–100 IU qod IM		
Gallium nitrate*	Gallium nitrate (Ganite)	0.25–0.5 mg/kg IV	14 days	
Plicamycin*	Plicamycin (Mithracin)	0.015–0.025 mg/kg/d, diluted in 1 liter of D5W or NS over 4–8 h	Repeat q 2–3 days as necessary.	High toxicity limits usefulness.

*Not FDA approved for this indication.
Abbreviations: D5W = 5% dextrose in water; IM = intramuscularly; NS = normal saline.

impaired mineralization. In one double-blind trial, patients receiving 90 mg over 3 days experienced an approximately 60% decrease in serum and urine biochemical markers. No change in bone pain or mobility was noted among groups, but improvement in the radiographic appearance of lesions occurred in patients in the 90-mg treatment group. Although no formal study exists, pamidronate has been used without any residual problems in patients undergoing orthopedic procedures. Adverse reactions include febrile reactions and influenza-like symptoms (musculoskeletal pain, dizziness, headache, and paresthesias). Transient mild elevation of temperature of more than 1°C above pretreatment baseline was noted within 48 hours after completion of treatment in 21% of the patients treated with 90 mg of pamidronate in clinical trials.

Alendronate (Fosamax) (4-amino-1-hydroxybutylidene bisphosphonate) is an orally administered bisphosphonate that is more potent than etidronate. Alendronate preferentially localizes to sites of bone resorption, specifically under osteoclasts. The osteoclasts adhere normally to the bone surface but lack the ruffled border that is indicative of active resorption. While incorporated in bone matrix, alendronate is not pharmacologically active and must be administered continuously to suppress osteoclasts on newly formed resorption surfaces. At 6 months, the suppression in alkaline phosphatase in patients treated with alendronate was significantly greater than that achieved with etidronate; in contrast, there was a complete lack of response in placebo-treated patients. Response (defined as either normalization of serum alkaline phosphatase level or ≥60% decrease from baseline levels of serum alkaline phosphatase) occurred in approximately 85% of patients treated with alendronate in the combined studies, in contrast to 30% in the etidronate group and 0% in the placebo group. Alendronate was similarly effective regardless of age, gender, race, prior use of other bisphosphonates, or baseline alkaline phosphatase within the range studied (at least twice the upper limit of normal).

Alendronate is not associated with abnormal mineralization and is usually provided in a dosage of 40 mg per day for 6 months. Because there is a remote possibility that alendronate causes esophageal problems, it is recommended that alendronate be administrated with at least 8 ounces of water and that the patient remains upright after taking the medication. The absorption of all of the bisphosphonates is relatively poor, so alendronate should be given after an overnight fast without any other food or drink (except water) for 60 minutes. Patients with esophageal stricture or other esophageal problems should not take this medication, because esophagitis and esophageal ulcerations have been reported.

Tiludronate disodium (Skelid) is a bisphosphonate characterized by a 4-chlorophenylthio group. In vitro studies indicate that tiludronate acts primarily on bone through a mechanism that involves inhibition of osteoclastic activity through at least two other mechanisms: (1) disruption of the cytoskeletal ring structure, and (2) inhibition of protein-tyrosine-phosphatase, thus leading to detachment of osteoclasts from the bone surface and the inhibition of the osteoclastic proton pump. In pagetic patients treated with tiludronate, 400 mg per day for 3 months, changes in urinary hydroxyproline, a biochemical marker of bone resorption, and in serum alkaline phosphatase, a marker of bone formation, indicate a reduction toward normal in the rate of bone turnover. The efficacy of 400 mg of tiludronate per day was demonstrated in two randomized, double-blind, placebo-controlled multicenter studies and one positive-controlled study. In all of these studies, the efficacy of tiludronate was assessed primarily by reduction of serum alkaline phosphatase activity after 3 and 6 months. Like alendronate, tiludronate must be ingested with no food, calcium, antacids, or indomethacin within 2 hours of administration. A single 400-mg daily oral dose of tiludronate, taken with 6 to 8 ounces of plain water only, should be administered for a period of 3 months. Side effects include nausea, vomiting, abdominal pain, and diarrhea. The more serious gastrointestinal side effects associated with alendronate have not been reported, but clinical use of tiludronate has been more limited than that of alendronate.

Risedronate (Actonel) is a potent pyridinyl bisphosphonate that is useful in the treatment of Paget's disease, especially in cases refractory to other treatments. Risedronate binds to hydroxyapatite and inhibits osteoclasts. The usual dosage is 30 mg per day for 2 months. Administration is similar to alendronate: It should be taken 30 minutes before breakfast with 6 to 8 ounces of water, and the patient is instructed to remain upright to prevent gastrointestinal reflux. In one comparison study, the remission rate was 77% with risedronate, in comparison with 11% with etidronate, in patients with moderate to severe Paget's disease. Risedronate decreased the radiographically evident osteolysis in pagetic patients. Side effects include arthralgias, nausea, abdominal pain, diarrhea, and headache.

Other bisphosphonates such as zoledronate and ibandronate are being studied in clinical trials and are effective at microgram doses. Improvements in drug delivery may circumvent some of the absorption problems associated with this class of compounds.

Calcitonin inhibits osteoclast-mediated bone resorption when administered in pharmacologic doses. Calcitonin interacts directly with receptors on osteoclasts to produce a rapid and profound decrease in ruffled border surface area, thereby diminishing resorptive activity. Currently, the only formulation of calcitonin available in the United States is synthetic salmon calcitonin (Miacalcin), in parenteral and intranasal forms. The usual dose is 50 to 100 IU subcutaneously daily with tapering to every-other-day administration. Nasal administration,* which is easier and less costly, requires 200 to 400 IU per day be-

---

*Not FDA approved for this indication.

cause of the reduced bioavailabity in this formulation. The usual response is a one-half to two-thirds' reduction in serum alkaline phosphatase or any of the other bone biochemical markers (urinary pyridinoline or deoxypyridinoline cross-links, N-telopeptide of type I collagen). Clear clinical improvement in terms of reduction of bone pain occurs. Over time, however, the disease may become refractory to treatment (manifested by the rise in bone markers), as a result of the development of neutralizing antibodies. Side effects, which are few, include flushing and nausea. Often the side effects can be attenuated by initial administration of lower doses, with a build-up to therapeutic doses over several days. Of the patients who use the nasal spray formulation, 10% experience rhinitis. The safety profile of this preparation, ease of administration of the nasal spray, and scarcity of side effects make calcitonin an excellent choice for elderly patients who cannot tolerate alternative therapies.

Plicamycin* (Mithracin) is effective in treating severe Paget's disease. Although the mechanism of action is not well understood, it has been suggested that plicamycin may lower calcium serum levels by inhibiting the effect of parathyroid hormone on osteoclasts. Inhibition of DNA-dependent RNA synthesis by plicamycin appears to render osteoclasts unable to fully respond to parathyroid hormone with the biosynthesis necessary for osteolysis. Plicamycin is available by intravenous administration, and its side effects are nausea and vomiting. The most common usage for this drug was in acute cases of nerve entrapment syndromes because of its rapid onset of action. Plicamycin is contraindicated in patients with thrombocytopenia, thrombocytopathy, coagulation disorders, or an increased susceptibility to bleeding from other causes. Plicamycin should not be administered to any patient with impairment of bone marrow function. For this reason, plicamycin is used rarely, and with the advent of the newer and more potent bisphosphonates, this medication may have limited use.

Gallium nitrate* (Ganite) is an inorganic metallic salt with hypocalcemic properties. It is used in the treatment of hypercalcemia associated with malignant neoplasms and has been investigated for use in other disorders associated with abnormally enhanced bone turnover, such as Paget's disease of bone. Gallium nitrate inhibits bone resorption by absorbing to hydroxyapatite and inhibits the ATP-dependent pump of osteoclasts. Cyclic, low-dose gallium nitrate has been demonstrated to effectively reduce bone turnover in patients with Paget's disease. Gallium nitrate may produce serious nephrotoxicity, especially when given as a brief intravenous infusion; administration by continuous infusion, with adequate hydration, may reduce the incidence of renal damage. Gastrointestinal disturbances, rashes, a metallic taste, anemia, hypophosphatemia, and hypocalcemia have also been reported. Beneficial results

---

*Not FDA approved for this indication.

were reported when gallium nitrate was given subcutaneously in doses of 0.25 or 0.5 mg per kg of body weight daily for 14 days to patients with advanced Paget's disease of bone. In a pilot multicenter study, 14 days of gallium nitrate injections were followed by 4 weeks off medication, and the cycle was repeated once. Gallium nitrate was effective in reducing bone turnover in patients with Paget's disease.

APPROACH TO THE PATIENT

There are several indications for treatment of Paget's disease. A patient who is symptomatic with bone pain can have significant relief from an antiresorptive agent. Asymptomatic persons who are likely to have an adverse outcome should also be targeted for therapeutic intervention. This includes patients with involvement at sites where complications are likely to develop (skull, weight-bearing areas such as spine and hip). It is generally not recommended that the serum alkaline phosphatase level be used as an indicator of disease activity, and the risk of complications should be carefully weighed.

The following indications have been proposed as guidelines for treatment of Paget's disease: (1) the presence of symptoms likely to respond to antiresorptive therapy, such as bone pain, increased warmth, or syndromes caused by neurocompression; (2) the prevention of local progression and of future complications; and (3) preoperative treatment for patients scheduled for elective orthopedic surgery that would involve pagetic bone. The overall goal of treatment is to reduce symptoms and biochemical indices of bone remodeling, and biochemical markers should be assessed at 3- to 6-month intervals.

Pharmacologic therapy may vary with severity of disease and side effects experienced by the patient. The second- and third-generation bisphosphonates are an excellent starting point because of their efficacy. In refractory cases, large doses of a bisphosphonate may be required. All patients should be treated with calcium and vitamin D supplementation. Some patients prefer the convenience of intravenous administration of pamidronate over oral preparations because of the necessity to wait before ingestion of food or drink. In patients who are unable to tolerate the bisphosphonates, calcitonin is an option because it has a long safety record and inhibits osteoclast-mediated bone resorption.

PARENTERAL NUTRITION IN ADULTS

method of
TIMOTHY A. PRITTS, M.D.,
DAVID R. FISCHER, M.D., and
JOSEF E. FISCHER, M.D.
University of Cincinnati College of Medicine
Cincinnati, Ohio

Since 1969, when Dudrick and Wilmore used total parenteral nutrition (TPN) to support an infant with intestinal atresia, parenteral nutrition has evolved from a rare and complicated therapy to a safe and commonly used intervention. Early enthusiasm for the widespread use of TPN has become justifiably tempered as an understanding of its risks, shortcomings, and expense has grown. TPN is now recognized to play an important and essential role in the management of several disease states. Advances in parenteral nutrition enable the clinician to provide adequate nutrients to patients in whom the enteral route is unavailable, nonfunctional, or incapable of furnishing full nutritional support. When used properly, TPN allows the metabolic support and survival of many patients who would otherwise die.

NUTRITIONAL REQUIREMENTS

Protein

Nutritional support, whether enteral or parenteral, depends on the clinician's ability to meet the metabolic needs of the patient at risk. Several classes of nutrients, of which protein may be the most important, need to be considered. The normal "safe" protein requirement is 0.8 grams per kg per day. In an affluent American society, the average daily intake may be twice this amount.

In states of metabolic stress, such as severe sepsis, burns, or multiple trauma, protein requirements may double. In these situations, both protein breakdown and synthesis are increased, but breakdown exceeds synthesis, so that a net catabolism of protein occurs. The catabolized protein, in the form of amino acids exported from skeletal muscle, connective tissue, intestine, and perhaps even from the liver itself, is used for gluconeogenesis, wound healing, and the inflammatory process. Although these processes are essential, there is no true storage form of protein. The failure to provide adequate substrate for these processes results in a rapid decrease in lean body mass, with resulting functional implications such as loss of skeletal muscle mass and strength.

The addition of excess protein to nutritional formulas does not blunt the increased catabolism seen in stressed states, but it does increase the rate of protein synthesis to more closely match protein breakdown. In addition, the provision of an adequate calorie-to-nitrogen ratio (see later section) helps minimize the use of protein for gluconeogenesis. A safe figure for protein intake under conditions of trauma and/or sepsis is 1.7 grams of protein equivalent per kg per day.

Calories

There are three sources of energy for bodily processes: protein, carbohydrates, and fat. Normally, 85% of daily energy expenditure is from fat and carbohydrates, and 15% is from protein.

Of the 15% of normal daily energy expenditure supplied by protein, half is from direct oxidation of the branched chain amino acids (valine, leucine, and isoleucine) to high-energy phosphate. The other half is derived from gluconeogenesis. Protein breakdown yields 4 kcal per gram. This is an inefficient source of energy, because four times as much energy is required for protein synthesis than is reclaimed through gluconeogenesis.

Ingested carbohydrates are converted into glucose, which yields about 4 kcal per gram through glycolysis. Glucose may be stored as glycogen in the liver and skeletal muscle. Glycogen breakdown yields 1 to 2 kcal per gram, but this source of energy is exhausted approximately 24 hours after the initiation of a fast. Most carbohydrates in parenteral nutrition are provided in the form of dextrose. Breakdown of dextrose yields 3.4 kcal per gram.

Fat may supply up to 45% of calories in the American diet. It is an energy-dense substance, and breakdown liberates about 9 kcal per gram. Nearly all tissues can use fat as an energy source, with the exception of the brain, red and white blood cells, and renal medulla, which are dependent exclusively on glucose in the early stages of a fast, although adaptation to ketone bodies may occur later in the renal medulla and brain.

Determination of Caloric Needs

A rough estimate of caloric needs is 25 to 30 kcal per kg per day. A more accurate estimate of basal energy expenditure (BEE) can be obtained from the Harris-Benedict equation:

$$\text{BEE (men)} = 66.47 + (13.75 \times W) + (5 \times H) - (6.76 \times A)$$

and

$$\text{BEE (women)} = 655.1 + (9.56 \times W) + (1.85 \times H) - (4.58 \times A),$$

where W is weight in kilograms, H is height in centimeters, and A is age in years.

To adjust for additional caloric needs during illness or metabolic stress, an injury factor is then used:

Minor operation	= 1.2 (20% increase)
Skeletal trauma	= 1.35 (35% increase)
Major sepsis	= 1.6 (60% increase)
Severe thermal injury	= 2.1 (110% increase)

Some of these injury factors may be excessive. For example, measurements by Kinney and coworkers after a minor operation (hernia repair) revealed no increased caloric need.

The patient's physical activity can be taken into account by multiplying by 1.2 for bedridden patients and 1.3 if the patient is not confined to bed. When these factors are integrated, caloric needs equal

$$\text{BEE} \times \text{injury factor} \times \text{activity factor}$$

A more accurate clinical determination of caloric requirements may be obtained through indirect calorimetry, in which a patient's carbon dioxide production (V_{CO_2}) and oxygen use (V_{O_2}) are measured and the respiratory quotient (RQ) is determined:

$$\text{RQ} = V_{CO_2} / V_{O_2}$$

An RQ of 0.8 to 1.0, indicating mixed substrate usage, is desirable. An RQ of 1.0 indicates pure carbohydrate usage. An RQ of less than 0.7 suggests ketogenesis. An RQ of more than 1.0, which is uncommon in clinical practice, suggests overfeeding.

Calorie-to-Nitrogen Ratio

An adequate number of calories in relation to nitrogen must be provided to permit protein synthesis and minimize protein catabolism for gluconeogenesis. A calorie-to-nitrogen ratio (nonprotein calories per gram of nitrogen) of between 100:1 and 150:1 is recommended for disease states. In uremic patients, less protein is indicated, and a calorie-to-nitrogen ratio of 300:1 to 400:1 is more appropriate. Septic patients require a relative increase in the amount of protein, and a ratio of 100:1 is appropriate.

Fat

As discussed previously, fat serves an important role in supplying and storing calories and supplying the caloric needs of most viscera. Fat is also required for growth, development, and normal immune responses. Two fatty acids, linoleic and α-linolenic acid, cannot be synthesized and must be supplied in the diet. Deficiency of these essential fatty acids may occur in patients receiving parenteral nutrition and may be prevented by administration of 4 to 6% of daily calories in the form of safflower or soybean oil emulsion.

INDICATIONS FOR NUTRITIONAL SUPPORT

There are no strict criteria to define the patient in need of nutritional support. Although the majority of patients undergoing elective procedures can tolerate brief periods of starvation without adverse sequelae, as many as 50% of patients in the hospital may be compromised nutritionally, depending on the definition. Adequate attention to nutritional status minimizes morbidity.

Several factors should be considered in determining the need for enteral or parenteral nutritional supplementation in patients. The need for nutritional intervention increases with the age of the patient and the duration of starvation. A previously healthy patient aged 60 years or younger may tolerate up to 10 days of starvation, but patients 70 years of age or older may tolerate only 5 days of starvation. The previous state of health of the patient should also be considered, because patients with chronic medical problems such as chronic obstructive pulmonary disease or hepatic insufficiency are probably at increased nutritional risk. The degree of metabolic insult should also be considered, as in burned or septic patients, and severely stressed patients should receive nutritional supplementation early in the hospital course.

Other factors suggestive of inadequate nutritional status include an involuntary weight loss of more than 10% of body weight over the previous 3 to 4 months or a current body weight of less than 85% of ideal body weight. Laboratory findings helpful in identifying the patient at risk include serum albumin level of less than 3 mg per dL, anergy to injected skin antigens (not commercial pinprick antigens), and serum transferrin level of less than 200 mg per dL. Impairment of normal functioning or of hand dynamometry is confirmatory. In identifying the patient at risk for complications related to nutritional status, it should be remembered that the overall impression of an experienced clinician may be as accurate as extensive laboratory testing.

ENTERAL VERSUS PARENTERAL NUTRITION

Once the need for nutritional supplementation has been determined, the route must be chosen. The enteral route should be used whenever possible. The benefits of enteral nutrition appear to surpass the simple nutritional value of the feedings given. Several studies in critically ill patients have demonstrated decreased rates of morbidity and mortality among enterally fed patients, in comparison with parenterally fed patients. Enteral nutrition maintains gut-associated lymphoid tissue, decreases atrophy of the gut mucosa, and theoretically protects against translocation of bacteria from the gastrointestinal tract. In addition, the enteral route is less expensive than parenteral nutrition. Even when delivery of a patient's complete nutritional requirements via the enteral route cannot be achieved, as much nutrition as possible should be given enterally. The advantages of enteral nutrition are probably obtained even when as little as 20% of nutritional needs are given enterally.

USES OF PARENTERAL NUTRITION

Parenteral nutrition can be used as either primary or supportive therapy in a variety of disease states. The efficacy of the use of parenteral nutrition has been established in some disease states, but not in others (Table 1). In still other areas, the use of parenteral nutrition remains under investigation. Indications for the use of parenteral nutrition are discussed in greater detail as follows.

Role in Primary Therapy

Efficacy Established

Gastrointestinal-Cutaneous Fistula. This is the classic indication for the use of parenteral nutrition. Parenteral nutrition allows bowel rest, which results in decreased fistula output. Parenteral nutrition also increases the spontaneous fistula closure rate, in comparison with enteral nutrition, and may obviate the need for operative closure. Malnutrition is a major cause of morbidity and mortality among patients with fistulas. With the use of parenteral nutrition, even if spontaneous fistula closure does not occur

TABLE 1. **Indications for Parenteral Nutrition**

Parenteral Nutrition as Primary Therapy

Efficacy Established

Gastrointestinal-cutaneous fistula
Short bowel syndrome
Acute renal failure
Hepatic insufficiency

Efficacy Not Completely Established

Inflammatory bowel disease
Anorexia nervosa

Parenteral Nutrition as Supportive Therapy

Efficacy Established

Radiation enteritis or chemotherapy toxicity
Hyperemesis gravidarum
Prolonged ileus

Efficacy Not Yet Established

Preoperative support
Cardiac cachexia
Pancreatitis
Respiratory insufficiency

Indications Under Investigation

Cancer
Sepsis

and operative intervention is needed, the patient will benefit from an improved overall nutritional status.

Short Bowel Syndrome. This condition may result from major bowel resection for such diseases as mesenteric vascular thrombosis or embolus, from resection for volvulus, and from multiple bowel resections for inflammatory bowel disease. The use of parenteral nutrition has enabled the survival of many patients who would otherwise die. Most patients with short bowel syndrome eventually adapt to the point that they can be managed entirely with enteral nutrition; for many patients, however, there is simply no alternative to long-term parenteral nutrition. In general, at least 60 cm of small bowel (45 cm if a competent ileocecal valve is present) is necessary for survival without parenteral nutrition. In the future, growth factors such as epidermal growth factor and glucagon-like peptide–2 may be used to stimulate adaptation or hypertrophy of small bowel in these patients.

Acute Renal Failure. In this setting, the goal is to provide maximal nutritional benefit in a minimal volume. In transient acute tubular necrosis, parenteral nutrition may result in earlier recovery from renal failure. Parenteral nutrition formulations consisting of essential amino acids and high concentrations of dextrose (up to 70%) can blunt increases in blood urea nitrogen and decrease the proteolysis that accompanies renal failure. This may delay the need for dialysis and may even help avoid dialysis altogether in patients with transient renal failure. This may be especially advantageous in acutely ill patients who, because of cardiovascular instability, may not tolerate hemodialysis. Many experts recommend that once the need for dialysis has been determined, the parenteral nutrition formulation be liberalized to include nonessential amino acids or at least the conditionally essential amino acids.

Hepatic Insufficiency. Decreased rates of mortality are seen in patients with hepatic failure who receive aggressive nutritional support. Patients with liver disease have decreased tolerance to stress and are frequently malnourished as a result of decreased food intake and excessive alcohol intake. These patients thus require protein to ameliorate their malnutrition and yet are relatively intolerant to protein because of the liver disease.

Patients with hepatic encephalopathy often have alterations in plasma amino acid levels, with increases in methionine and aromatic amino acids and decreases in branched chain amino acids. Patients with hepatic encephalopathy may benefit from the use of a parenteral nutritional solution with reduced aromatic amino acids and increased branched chain amino acids to correct plasma amino acid imbalances. In several studies, this solution has been shown to be as effective as lactulose or neomycin in the treatment of hepatic encephalopathy. In addition, morbidity is decreased in patients with cirrhosis who undergo liver resections for neoplasia and are supported aggressively with a modified amino acid solution.

Efficacy Not Completely Established

Inflammatory Bowel Disease. Patients with exacerbations of Crohn's disease or ulcerative colitis may tolerate oral nutrition poorly and may have diarrhea, bleeding, and protein-losing enteropathy. Although parenteral nutrition for inflammatory bowel disease has not been subjected to randomized prospective trials, this therapy may allow bowel rest and improved nutritional status. Patients with severe Crohn's disease may require long-term home hyperalimentation, chemically defined diets, or both for nutritional support. In patients with ulcerative colitis, parenteral nutrition may be necessary to optimize nutritional status before operative treatment of the disease.

Anorexia Nervosa. The use of parenteral nutrition for anorexia nervosa has not been evaluated in a prospective manner. Because these patients are prone to self-sabotage, they are difficult to treat, but they require nutritional support in conjunction with psychotherapy for a successful outcome. The use of parenteral nutrition in this condition is recommended only for patients with severe malnutrition in whom enteral nutrition is impossible.

Role in Supportive Therapy

Efficacy Established

Radiation Enteritis or Chemotherapy Toxicity. Severe enteritis resulting from chemotherapy and radiation therapy may prevent oral intake. In some patients, parenteral nutrition may be lifesaving, allowing nutrient delivery until the gut mucosa recovers. Patients with chronic radiation enteritis may require long-term parenteral nutrition because of multiple strictures.

Hyperemesis Gravidarum. In this circumstance, nutritional needs may not be met by oral intake. Parenteral nutrition may be necessary to supply nutrients for the mother and fetus. Fetal ultrasonographic studies may be useful for monitoring growth.

Prolonged Ileus. After abdominal operations, patients may develop a prolonged ileus (>5 days). If enteral nutrition is not possible, parenteral supplementation can be useful for minimizing catabolism until the gastrointestinal tract regains function.

Efficacy Not Yet Established

Preoperative Support. Many studies have examined the role of parenteral nutrition in malnourished patients who require major surgery. Studies indicate that metabolic end points may be improved in these patients, but only a few studies have shown statistically significant decreases in complications or mortality. The benefits of preoperative parenteral nutritional repletion must be weighed against increased rates of noncatheter infectious complications. It appears that the most severely malnourished patients receive the greatest net benefit from preoperative parenteral nutrition. Although it is possible to identify patients as a group, it is more difficult to identify individual patients at risk. Severe malnutrition may be evident from the history and physical examination. Supporting evidence includes a 10 to 15% loss of body weight and a serum albumin level of less than 3 grams per dL. The optimal duration for preoperative parenteral nutritional support is probably between 5 and 7 days.

Cardiac Cachexia. As with any other tissue in the body, the heart may suffer from the effects of malnutrition. Evidence for the use of parenteral nutrition under this circumstance is mainly anecdotal, but it suggests that at least a 2- to 3-week period of supplementation may help to restore cardiac function.

Pancreatitis. Many attacks of pancreatitis are self-limited and do not necessitate parenteral nutrition. Although parenteral nutrition does not alter the course of acute pancreatitis, it may be useful if exacerbation of symptoms renders enteral feeding impossible.

Respiratory Insufficiency. As with cardiac muscle, respiratory muscles are not immune to the effects of malnutrition. If enteral nutrition is not possible in severely ill patients, parenteral nutrition should be implemented until a transition to the enteral route is possible. Overfeeding with carbohydrates may lead to increased carbon dioxide production, making ventilator weaning more difficult. In practice, this rarely occurs and can be avoided by monitoring the patient's RQ, as previously discussed.

Indications Under Investigation

Cancer. Malnutrition is common in patients with malignancies. These patients may suffer directly from effects of the tumor and indirectly from the effects of chemotherapy, radiation therapy, and anorexia. Nutritional supplementation is not indicated in mildly malnourished patients who can support their nutritional needs orally. In fact, many experts are concerned that tumor growth may be stimulated by parenteral nutrition. Although formulations that actually inhibit tumor growth may be available in the future, current recommendations in cancer patients restrict parenteral nutrition to patients who would be unlikely to survive an upcoming operation or a course of therapy without it. Nutritional support before operation or other therapy should be limited to 5 to 7 days because of concern of nutrient stimulation of tumor growth.

Sepsis. In sepsis, altered plasma amino acid levels may be seen, as in hepatic encephalopathy. Solutions enriched with branched chain amino acids have been shown to decrease proteolysis in studies of septic animals. Clinical studies have thus far shown only marginal efficacy in blunting proteolysis and improving nitrogen balance in critically ill patients, and differences in clinical outcomes have not been demonstrated.

DELIVERY OF TPN

Peripheral Route. The peripheral route may be useful if the nutritional support is needed only for a very short time or if the need for parenteral nutrition has not been definitely established. It is used mainly in hospitals in which a nutrition support team does not exist. Veins are often quickly exhausted, but the incidence of thrombophlebitis may be decreased with meticulous attention to aseptic catheter insertion and use of large veins. The nutritional needs of severely ill patients are rarely met by this approach.

Central Route. In most institutions, the preferred route for delivering parenteral nutrition is via catheters placed in the central venous system. Percutaneous catheters, which may be placed at the bedside, are appropriate for most patients. Tunneled catheters (such as Hickman or Broviac) are placed operatively. These catheters are useful in patients with a prolonged need for parenteral supplementation, and the incidence of thrombosis and sepsis is lower with them.

COMPONENTS OF PARENTERAL NUTRITION

The traditional formulation of parenteral nutrition is based on a solution containing 25% dextrose, with 4.25 to 5% amino acids, vitamins, trace elements, and varying amounts of electrolytes. Lipids are given in emulsion as a separate infusion. A relatively recent advance has been the use of total nutrient admixture (TNA) solutions, in which all parenteral nutrition components, including lipids, are mixed in a single solution for continuous infusion. The components of various parenteral nutrition solutions available in our medical center are summarized in Table 2.

Carbohydrates. In the United States, dextrose is the exclusive carbohydrate source. The usual concentration is 15%, although higher and lower concentrations may be used.

Electrolytes. The amounts of individual electrolytes provided in parenteral nutrition vary and should be modified on the basis of each patient's needs. Standard amounts and ranges are shown in Table 2. Monitoring of patient serum electrolyte levels, especially when they are not stable, enables the clinician to determine the appropriate concentration for an individual patient.

Amino Acids. The usual concentration of amino acids is about 5% of the nutritional solution. The most common form of amino acids is a balanced solution, but special compositions are available in disease-specific formulations, such as enriched branch chain amino acid solutions.

Fat. Lipids may be administered either as TNA or in 10 or 20% solutions. Essential fatty acid deficiency is prevented by a single weekly infusion of 100 mL of a 10% solution. Between 20 and 60% of daily calories may be supplied as lipids; a 10% lipid emulsion provides 1 kcal per mL.

Vitamins and Trace Elements. Deficiencies of vitamins and trace elements can be prevented by the addition of these substances to parenteral nutrition. A multivitamin, 10 mL, is typically given daily. Vita-

TABLE 2. **Composition of Parenteral Nutrition Solutions Available at the University of Cincinnati Medical Center**

Component*	Range	Standard	High Dextrose	Hepatic	Renal	Cardiac	Peripheral
Dextrose (%)	10–47	15	20	25	46.7	35	5
Amino acids (%)	1.7–5	5	5	4†	1.7‡	5	3.5
Fat (grams; as TNA)	0–40	40	40	40	0	0	40
Sodium (mEq/L)	0–150	30	30	5	2	5	40
Potassium (mEq/L)	0–80	18	18	12	0	0	10
Calcium (mEq/L)	0–9.4	4.5	4.5	4.7	0	0	4.7
Magnesium (mEq/L)	0–12	5	5	8	0	8	8
Phosphorus (mmol/L)	0–15	10	10	5	0	5	5
Chloride (mEq/L)	0–150	37	37	13.5	1	2	40
Acetate (mEq/L)	14–80	55	55	31	14	45	52
Insulin (U/L)	0–60	0	0	0	0	0	0
kcal/mL		1.1	1.3	1.3	1.65	1.4	0.71

Formulations shown are TNA (total nutrient admixture), except renal and cardiac, which are not formulated as TNA.

*In addition to the listed components, a multivitamin solution (10 mL) and trace elements (Zn, 3.0 mg; Cu, 1.2 mg; Cr, 12 μg; Mn, 0.3 mg; and Se, 60 μg) are provided daily. Vitamin K, 5 mg, is given weekly.

†Amino acid solution in hepatic formula is enriched with branched chain amino acids–see text.

‡Amino acid solution in renal formula is essential amino acids.

min K, 5 mg, is given weekly to patients not receiving anticoagulant therapy. Zinc, copper, selenium, chromium, and manganese supplements are also typically given.

Insulin. Many patients receiving parenteral nutrition manifest abnormal carbohydrate metabolism. If the patient is hyperglycemic in a predictable manner, insulin can be added to the parenteral nutritional formula. Otherwise, intermittent injections of short-acting insulin are given as needed. If severe difficulties in glucose control exist, a concomitant continuous insulin infusion may be necessary.

Renal Formula. Renal formulations of parenteral nutrition are indicated in patients with renal failure who are not yet receiving dialysis. These solutions have an increased calorie-to-nitrogen ratio (between 300:1 and 400:1) and contain essential amino acids only. The volume of the formula is limited by use of a 47% dextrose base.

Hepatic Formula. The hepatic formulation of parenteral nutrition is for patients with hepatic encephalopathy, grade 2 (impending stupor) or higher, and for patients who manifest encephalopathy with conventional amino acid solutions. This solution is enriched with 35% branched chain amino acids and has relatively decreased amounts of aromatic and sulfur-containing amino acids.

Administration of TPN

Initiation. Before initiation of parenteral nutrition, placement of the infusion catheter must be confirmed by radiography. Baseline laboratory studies include electrolyte studies, blood urea nitrogen, creatinine, calcium, magnesium, phosphorus, liver enzymes, retinol-binding protein, transferrin, albumin, triglycerides, prothrombin time, and a complete blood cell count.

Infusion is begun at 40 mL per hour, with the exception of renal formulations, which should be initiated at 30 mL per hour because of the increased glucose content. As long as the patient does not be-

come hyperglycemic, the infusion rate can be increased by 20 to 25 mL every 8 to 24 hours until the target rate is reached. If parenteral nutrition infusion is temporarily interrupted, 5% dextrose in water should be infused at the parenteral nutrition infusion rate to prevent hypoglycemia.

Monitoring. Vital signs should be obtained before infusion is begun and then every 8 hours for at least the initial 24 to 48 hours. Intake and output should also be monitored. Serum glucose is measured twice daily for most patients; more frequent monitoring is necessary for diabetic patients. The patient's weight should be monitored three times weekly. A complete laboratory panel—including electrolyte studies, blood urea nitrogen, creatinine, calcium, magnesium, phosphorus, liver enzymes, retinol-binding protein, transferrin, albumin, and a complete blood cell count—is rechecked weekly. Serum electrolytes should be monitored more frequently: as often as every day if these parameters are unstable or if the patient is markedly catabolic.

Complications of TPN

Technical Complications. Most technical complications are related to the structures in the thoracic inlet and can be minimized with meticulous attention to proper technique during catheter placement.

Pneumothorax occurs typically in less than 5 to 6% of central catheter insertions. It is more common in elderly and cachectic patients, in whom an internal jugular, rather than subclavian, approach to catheterization may be indicated. The occurrence of this complication can be minimized with adequate hydration of the patient before placement, careful attention to technique, and ensuring that the procedure is performed in a comfortable, sedated patient with adequate help available.

Arterial lacerations are relatively rare and are minimized by initial use of a small finder needle to locate the vein and by not allowing the insertion needle past 10 to 15 degrees from the horizontal.

Air embolism may result from improper technique, inadequate hydration, failure to place the patient in the Trendelenburg position during insertion, and failure to cover the hub of the needle at all times.

Guide wire embolism may result from excessive manipulation of the guide wire through the insertion needle, causing a portion of the wire to shear off and embolize distally. Also, the guide wire must never be released, even momentarily, during insertion. Guide wire retrieval under fluoroscopy or by operation may be necessary. If the guide wire does not thread during insertion, both the guide wire and needle should be removed together.

Subclavian or vena caval thrombosis may occur in 5 to 10% of patients and may be clinically silent in one third of those affected. The patient may exhibit swelling in the upper arm and pain and swelling at the base of the neck in the supraclavicular fossa. If thrombosis is suspected, the catheter is removed, the diagnosis is confirmed with imaging studies, and the patient is heparinized until symptoms resolve. Long-term anticoagulation may be necessary if symptoms persist.

Septic thrombophlebitis is a potentially life-threatening event. If the condition is not ameliorated with antibiotics and anticoagulation, thrombectomy, catheter embolectomy, or even excision of the affected vein may be necessary.

Septic Complications. Most parenteral nutrition–related deaths are probably the result of infectious complications. Catheter care directly affects catheter sepsis rates. The incidence of catheter sepsis in our institution decreased from 27% to 4.5% with the establishment of a nutritional support team and adherence to strict protocols. The use of multilumen catheters, especially pulmonary artery catheters, may be associated with higher infection rates. If parenteral nutrition is not infused through a single-lumen catheter, one of the ports of the multilumen catheter should be dedicated solely to this purpose.

Quantitative skin cultures have indicated that the presence of 10^3 or more organisms on the skin surrounding the site is correlated positively with catheter infection. In order to minimize septic complications, meticulous attention must be paid to the skin surrounding the catheter site during placement of catheters and subsequent dressing changes. Protocols for catheter surveillance and site and dressing care should be established and administered by specially trained nursing personnel or the nutritional support team.

In addition to bacterial colonization of the skin, bacteria from distant sites may seed the fibrin sheath that often forms around catheters. This is more likely to occur with gram-positive organisms than with gram-negative organisms, because of the greater tendency of gram-positive organisms to become implanted on the catheter. If gram-positive bacteremia is present in a patient, the catheter should be changed over a guide wire and the tip sent for culture; however, this may not suffice, and catheter removal is often necessary. If the bacteremia organisms are gram-negative, antibiotic therapy directed at the primary infection may be sufficient.

Fungemia is a feared complication in patients receiving parenteral nutrition. Of fungal pathogens, *Candida* is the most common. It probably enters the bloodstream through the gastrointestinal tract. If cultures positive for *Candida* are obtained from two different sites, such as skin and urine, antifungal treatment should be initiated. If blood cultures are positive for fungi, administration of parenteral nutrition should cease, central lines should be removed, and therapy with amphotericin should be considered.

A suggested algorithm for work-up and management of suspected catheter sepsis is shown in Figure 1.

Metabolic Complications. Electrolyte abnormalities are relatively common in patients receiving parenteral nutrition. Markedly anabolic patients may require relatively large amounts of magnesium, potassium, and phosphorus. Electrolyte alterations may also be seen with altered excretion, as in renal failure, excessive administration, or inadequate replacement. The occurrence of electrolyte disturbances can be minimized with careful monitoring, especially in patients who are beginning parenteral nutrition or those who are seriously ill.

Hyperglycemia is another frequent metabolic alteration seen in patients receiving parenteral nutrition. Hyperglycemia most often results from too rapid an initiation and advancement of the parenteral nutrition infusion and can be minimized by careful monitoring of serum glucose levels during this time. Increasing the infusion rate is then based on the individual patient's glucose tolerance. Increased serum glucose levels can be treated by intermittent administration of short-acting insulin preparations or by addition of insulin to the parenteral nutrition formulation. The sudden onset of hyperglycemia in a patient previously tolerating a parenteral glucose load should prompt a work-up for an infectious source, because glucose intolerance may precede the onset of sepsis by 24 hours. Glucose in urine may be detected with initiation of parenteral nutrition and may result from a lowered renal threshold. Confirmation of elevated blood glucose levels must precede insulin therapy.

Hypoglycemia may result from a sudden slowing of the parenteral nutrition infusion or from excessive exogenous insulin administration. If the patient is symptomatic, glucose can be administered. If parenteral nutrition is suddenly discontinued or interrupted, administering 5% dextrose solution at the previous parenteral nutrition rate and then slowly decreasing the rate of infusion can prevent hypoglycemia.

The etiology of the hepatic dysfunction present in some patients receiving parenteral nutrition is not well understood and is probably multifactorial. An altered insulin-to-glucagon ratio is hypothesized by some authorities. Patients may have elevated liver function values, hepatomegaly, steatosis, and chole-

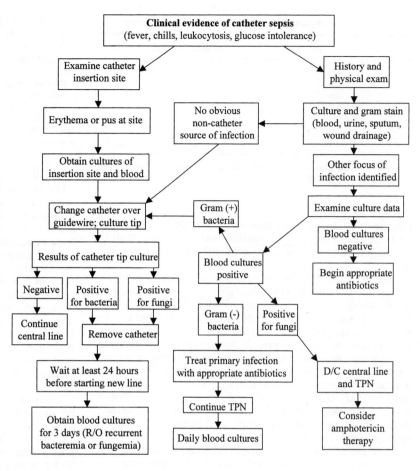

Figure 1. Suggested algorithm for the diagnosis and treatment of catheter-related sepsis. (Redrawn from Berry S: Nutrition. University of Cincinnati Residents [eds]: The Mont Reid Manual, 4th ed. St. Louis: CV Mosby, 1997.)

stasis. Elevated bilirubin levels are rare except when secondary to sepsis.

Deficiency States. Deficiencies of several nutrients may occur in patients receiving parenteral nutrition. A high degree of suspicion is necessary to diagnose them. Zinc deficiency may be seen in patients who have excessive diarrhea or who are markedly catabolic. It may manifest with darkened skin creases, impaired wound healing, taste disturbances, and perioral pustular rash. Between 3 and 6 mg of elemental zinc per day are required for patients with normal stool losses. If patients have excessive diarrhea, this amount may increase to 12 to 20 mg.

Chromium deficiency usually occurs only in patients receiving long-term parenteral nutrition who have little or no oral intake. Along with peripheral neuropathy and encephalopathy, patients with chromium deficiency may exhibit the sudden onset of refractory hyperglycemia, inasmuch as chromium is required for normal glucose usage. Suspected chromium deficiency is treated with 150 µg of chromium daily for several days.

Essential fatty acid deficiency may be prevented by parenteral administration of 4 to 6% of daily caloric needs in the form of safflower or soybean oil emulsion. An alternative, if the patient is able to tolerate any oral intake, is to administer 25 to 50 mL per day of corn, safflower, or sunflower oil or margarine on toast to increase palatability. Signs of essential fatty acid deficiency include dry, flaky skin, dermatitis, and alopecia.

PARENTERAL FLUID THERAPY IN INFANTS AND CHILDREN

method of
DEBORAH P. JONES, M.D., and
RUSSELL W. CHESNEY, M.D.
*LeBonheur Children's Medical Center and
    Crippled Children's Foundation Research Center
Memphis, Tennessee*

MAINTENANCE THERAPY

The goal of maintenance therapy is to maintain zero balance for water, and electrolytes, Na, K, Cl, and HCO$_3$. Maintenance therapy is most commonly prescribed based upon the expected metabolic demands and is indirectly related to body mass or surface area. The metabolic rate has a nonlinear relationship to body weight. For the average hospitalized child, the metabolic requirements allow 100 kcal per kg for the first 3 to 10 kg, 50 kcal per kg of body weight above 10 kg up to 20 kg. Beyond the weight of 20 kg, the metabolic requirement is 20 kcal per kg in addition to the 1500 kcal allowed for the first 20 kg. An alternative method allows 1500 kcal per square meter of body surface area. Preterm and low-birth-weight infants

TABLE 1. **Components of Normal Maintenance**

	mL/100 Cal
Insensible:	
Lungs	15
Skin	30
Stool	5
Kidney	40–70
Sweat	0–20
− Water of oxidation	−12

The sum of the above in a normal euvolemic individual is 100 mL/100 cal. (Insensible = 30–35% of maintenance.)

require special considerations, to be covered in a separate section, because their insensible water and electrolyte losses generally exceed those of healthy infants and children.

Daily ongoing fluid loss is largely due to insensible losses and urinary losses of water. Insensible loss from skin and lungs, which accounts for 45 mL of water for each 100 kcal expended, can be further subdivided into approximately one third from lungs and two thirds from skin losses (Table 1). Urinary volume is variable according to the obligate osmotic load to be excreted, the urinary concentrating ability of the individual, and the daily fluid intake. Therefore, a range of urinary volume per kcal is used to estimate daily urinary losses of fluid, and is designed to allow a comfortable range for the kidneys, which requires neither maximal concentration nor dilution. This value is approximately 55 mL per 100 kcal. In most cases, fluid losses from stool or sweat are small, and can be ignored as a component of maintenance, although stool is often estimated as 5 mL per 100 kcal. Diarrhea or excess water loss via the gastrointestinal tract should be treated as abnormal ongoing loss, which will be addressed later. Water of oxidation of fats, carbohydrates, and proteins is dependent upon the metabolic rate and averages 12 mL per 100 kcal expended. Thus, the maintenance water requirement is approximately 100 mL per 100 kcal expended. Insensible water loss, although 45 mL per 100 kcal, is usually estimated to be one third of total maintenance, or 30 to 35 mL per kg per day.

Electrolyte requirements are difficult to estimate. In the face of normal renal function, there is a wide range of comfort (Table 2). Usually expressed as mEq per body mass or surface area per day, they may also be expressed as mEq per calories expended. Sodium requirements are estimated to be 2.5 to 3.0 mEq per kg per day or 40 to 50 mEq per square meter per day, or 2.5 mEq per 100 kcal per day. Potassium requirements are estimated to be 2.0 to 2.5 mEq per kg per day, 30 to 40 mEq per square meter per day, or 2.5 mEq per 200 kcal per day. The maintenance sodium and potassium are typically administered as the chloride

TABLE 3. **Electrolyte Composition of Common Intravenous Solutions in mEq/L**

Solution	Na	K	Base	Cl	Ca
Lactated Ringer's solution	130	4	28	109	3
Normal saline	154	0	0	154	0
D5 ½ NS	77	0	0	77	0
D5 ¼ NS	38	0	0	38	0

salt. Glucose is generally provided as 5 grams per 100 kcal (D5W) expended; however, this does not meet daily caloric needs and is therefore of short-term use.

One should remember that the estimates of fluid and electrolyte losses and maintenance are based upon physiologic principles and are not to be viewed as exact calculations. Luckily, the kidneys are usually able to adapt to a comfortable range over which water and electrolyte maintenance are administered. Nothing substitutes for careful consideration of the patient's unique physiologic state as it compares with the average maintenance situation, which assumes normal renal function, minimal gastrointestinal losses, and average metabolic rate. Modifications in the estimated maintenance fluid requirements may be warranted in the setting of fever, which would increase the metabolic requirements by 10 to 12% for each degree over 38°C.

There are commercially available electrolyte solutions for parenteral administration in typical situations (Table 3). Derivatives of saline are commonly used for maintenance fluid therapy. In general, a solution of 5% dextrose plus ¼ normal saline is given for infants and children of 20 kg or less. Potassium is added at a concentration of 20 to 30 mEq per liter. Five percent dextrose with ½ normal saline will provide maintenance plus extra sodium for children over 20 kg. Potassium is added according to estimates based upon 2 mEq per kg per day, which gives a final potassium concentration of 20 to 30 mEq per liter. The daily fluid volume is estimated according to body mass or surface area, and is then divided by 24 hours to attain the hourly infusion rate.

Housestaff officers have derived a quick, yet reasonable, way to estimate intravenous (IV) fluid rate by the so-called 4-2-1 rule. This simply replaces the 100 mL per kg per day for the first 10 kg by dividing the daily need by 24 hours per day to arrive at 4 mL per kg per hour for the first 10 kg, with an additional 2 mL per kg per hour in place of 50 mL per kg per day for each kg body weight over 10 kg, and then an additional 1 mL per kg per hour instead of 20 mL per kg per day for each additional kilogram over 20 kg.

Abnormal Ongoing Losses

In certain situations there are fluid and electrolyte losses above those allowed in the normal maintenance calcula-

TABLE 2. **Maintenance Requirements for Water, Sodium, Potassium***

Method	kg	Water (mL/d)	Na (mEq/d)	K (mEq/d)
Per kg	3–10	100/kg		
	10–20	1000 + 50 (weight − 10)	3.0	2.0
	>20	1500 + 20 (weight − 20)		
Per m²		1500/m²/d	30–50	20–40

*Maintenance solution for patients ≤20 kg is D5W + ¼ NS + 20 mEq/L KCl. Maintenance solution for patients >20 kg is D5W + ½ NS + 20 mEq/L KCl.

tion. These losses are ideally replaced by estimating the volume and electrolyte content of the particular fluid lost. The most common setting for such a situation is nasogastric suction, which allows measurement of the volume of fluid in a volumetric container, thus administration of a similar volume as intravenous fluid. For gastric fluid, which is composed of HCl (150 mEq per liter) and a small amount of KCl, the appropriate replacement fluid would be NS plus 15 mEq per liter of KCl. Some have suggested that gastric fluid is more dilute and recommend an alternate solution containing 100 mEq per liter of sodium, 115 mEq per liter of Cl, and 15 mEq per liter of K. Small intestinal secretions differ in their composition from gastric or colonic fluids and contain approximately 15 mEq per liter of K, 40 mEq per liter of bicarbonate, 145 mEq per liter of Na, and 100 mEq per liter of Cl. Stool electrolyte content varies widely, is usually hypotonic with approximately 40 mEq each per liter of Na, K, Cl, and bicarbonate. Stool electrolyte content is higher in patients with cholera.

When excessive losses of water and electrolytes originate from excessive urinary losses, measurement of the electrolyte content of the urine can be helpful in guiding electrolyte content of the replacement fluid. One must be able to assess the volume and electrolyte content of intake. Collection of a timed urine with measurement of volume as well as Na, K, and Cl content is preferred, although a random urine for electrolytes with creatinine can also be helpful in designing fluid therapy to meet the individual's needs.

Occasionally normal maintenance allowances overestimate the needs of the individual. Such settings include oliguric renal failure, or edematous states such as nephrotic syndrome, glomerulonephritis, congestive heart failure, hepatic cirrhosis, or inappropriate secretion of antidiuretic hormone (ADH). In these situations, fluid and electrolyte administration should be based upon the desire for negative fluid balance. Estimates of insensible loss plus measured losses are helpful in guiding therapy in such situations.

Definition of the normal urine flow is dependent upon the total fluid balance of the individual over the recent past. Oliguria in and of itself does not always indicate renal disease or renal failure. If fluid losses are increased, the normal renal response is to conserve both sodium and water. Thus urine will become concentrated and decreased in volume. One useful measure of tubular integrity in the setting of oliguria is the fractional excretion of sodium. A random urine for sodium and creatinine with a recent plasma measure can be used to calculate the fractional excretion of sodium (FE_{Na}) (Table 4). If less than 1%, then the renal tubule is reabsorbing sodium and the oliguria is more likely to be related to decreased effective plasma volume. If greater than 2%, then the tubular epithelium may have been injured. Exceptions include recent administration of diuretics.

Normal urinary volume is equivalent to the total daily fluid intake minus the total fluid losses. One can measure urine and stool losses under controlled situations, and then estimate the insensible losses, subtracting the sum of losses from intake. The urine volume normally assigned as normal is 1 to 4 mL per kg per hour. However, this is merely a reference range and should never be viewed as an isolated parameter. In the normal child weighing less than 10 kg, assuming that insensible losses equal 35 mL per kg, the urinary loss would equal 60 to 65 mL per kg per day and the hourly urine volume would be expected to be 2.5 to 2.7 mL per kg per hour. In a 20-kg child, assuming

TABLE 4. Helpful Formulae

Fractional excretion of sodium (FE_{Na}):
$$\frac{(U\ sodium)(P\ creatinine)(100)}{(P\ sodium)(U\ creatinine)}$$

Premorbid weight:
$$\frac{X}{current\ body\ weight} = \frac{100}{100 - \%\ dehydration}$$

Na deficit:
Weight (kg) × 0.6 × (135 − P_{Na}) = mEq to raise P_{Na} to 135*

HCO_3 deficit:
Weight (kg) × 0.5 × (18 − P_{HCO_3}) = mEq to raise plasma bicarbonate to 18 mEq/L†

Hypertonic saline for the treatment of symptomatic hyponatremia:
3% NaCl 12 mL = 6 mEq/kg IV over a minimum of 60 min

---

*This is not the Na content of fluid lost, only current body extracellular fluid volume.
†Remember that administration of base can decrease Cai or K.
Abbreviations: P = plasma; P_{Na} = plasma sodium; P_{HCO_3} = plasma HCO_3; U = urine.

an insensible loss of 600 mL per day, and minimal stool losses, the expected urine output would be 800 to 900 mL per day and the hourly urine flow would be 1.5 to 1.9 mL per kg.

Maintenance for the Low-Birth-Weight Infant

Insensible water requirements are greater in the low-birth-weight infant and particularly in the infant of very low birth weight due to increased evaporative losses from skin particularly when radiant warmer or phototherapy is used. It is very difficult to estimate the needs of the low-birth-weight infant; however, estimates for insensible water loss range from 30 to 60 mL per kg per day and 15 to 35 mL per kg per day for infants less than 1500 grams and 1500 to 3000 grams, respectively. Total fluid needs range from 85 to 170 mL per kg per day and 70 to 145 mL per kg per day in infants of very low birth weight and low birth weight. An additional 20 mL per kg per day is added during phototherapy. A certain degree of weight loss occurs after birth, with relatively greater loss of ECV from the less mature infants of lower birth weight (15 to 20% of body weight) compared with full-term infants (5%).

Because of the immaturity of the renal tubule in sodium reabsorption, Na requirements are relatively greater in the low-birth-weight infant. The greater the fluid volume, however, the greater the sodium requirement, because of the inability of the immature infant to maximally excrete water or sodium. On the basis of daily weight, strict measurement of input and output, and monitoring of plasma sodium, the sodium intake can be adjusted to each infant's needs. There is a wide range of sodium requirements from 3 to 15 mEq per kg per day. Potassium requirements range from 1 to 2 mEq per kg per day.

DEFICIT THERAPY

When losses of fluid and electrolytes (sodium, chloride, bicarbonate, and potassium) exceed the intake, dehydration or volume contraction results. The etiologies of such dehydration include gastroenteritis, fever with decreased oral intake, increased urinary losses secondary to diabetes mellitus, diabetes insipidus, renal concentrating defect, or cystic fibrosis. In general, dehydration is the acute loss of mass as a result of negative balance between output and intake.

The management of the dehydrated infant or child is dependent upon clinical estimation of fluid and electrolyte deficits. Regardless of the etiology of the dehydration, restoration of the extracellular fluid compartment, which represents both plasma and interstitial spaces, is vital to care of the patient. Most schemes approach the treatment of dehydration with methodical estimation of fluid and electrolyte (primarily sodium) deficits and then aim to replace these deficits in addition to the provision of maintenance and ongoing excess losses. By using this approach with frequent clinical monitoring, morbidity and mortality are minimized. There is still much debate about the exact methods for rehydration because most use basic physiologic principles and a tincture of educated guesses to arrive at a treatment plan.

Determination of the fluid or volume deficit aims to estimate the volume "lost" so as to restore the child to his or her premorbid weight. One should question the caretakers about recent weights before the illness. Although there are differences among scales, subtraction of current weight from premorbid weight would allow some objective estimate of the volume of fluid lost. Unfortunately, recent weights are usually not available, and the child's volume deficit must be estimated on the basis of physical findings (Table 5). The so-called degree of dehydration is assessed and is conveniently divided into three categories of severity: mild, moderate, and severe. Classically, these accounted for 3 to 5%, 6 to 10%, and 10 to 15% acute volume loss as a percentage of total body weight, respectively. Older children and adults are allowed a relatively smaller percentage loss for equivalent physical findings, that is, 3, 6, and 9%, although no exact guidelines were given as to the age or size at which these were to apply. When the percentage of body weight lost is correlated to physical findings at presentation with dehydration, then mild is closer to 3 to 4%, moderate is 5 to 6%, and severe is 9 to 10%.

Of note, infants have a larger surface area to mass ratio and a higher heat exchange or metabolic rate relative to body mass when compared with adults. Infants exchange a greater percentage of their total body water during the average day with approximately 10% as compared with approximately 4% in adults. On the other hand, total body water as a percentage of body mass is greater in infants, and decreases to near adult levels by 1 year of life. This essentially means that although infants may lose a larger portion of their total body weight for equivalent signs of dehydration as older children and adults, they are at increased risk for negative fluid balance because of the mass of water exchanged each day.

The clinical manifestations of extracellular volume loss are the result of underfilling of the arterial vessels, in addition to renal and hemodynamic responses that attempt to compensate for extracellular volume contraction. Therefore, the first goal of therapy is to replenish the vascular volume and improve circulation. This rapid infusion phase allows for improved perfusion to organs and may be undertaken before a definitive plan of rehydration has been made. Isotonic fluids are recommended for restoration of the circulatory integrity. Choices include normal saline and lactated ringer's as the two most often used commercially available solutions. The volume infused will depend upon the clinical state of the child. The recommended initial volume is 10 to 20 mL per kg over 30 to 60 minutes; however, 40 mL per kg may be warranted in the severely dehydrated child. Saline or lactated Ringer's solution provide primarily extracellular fluid and serve as effective plasma volume expanders, whereas a glucose-containing solution (D5 ½ NS) would be expected to distribute between both intracellular and extracellular compartments, and, therefore, not to expand the plasma space to the same degree.

A commonly applied method for determination of the degree of dehydration is shown in Table 5. After examination of the child, the category that best fits the individual findings is chosen. From this, the volume deficit is calculated. Most methods prefer to use the current weight for such calculations as a way of simplification. An infant who presents at a weight of 10 kg and who is judged to have moderate dehydration has lost 600 to 900 mL according to this method, whereas calculation of the premorbid weight (see Table 4) would estimate the volume deficit to be 600 to 1000 mL if the premorbid weight is 10.6 to 11.0 kg, using moderate dehydration to be 6 to 9%. However, since the accuracy of clinical estimation probably does not allow one to discriminate between 1000 and 1110, it may provide no benefit to the child.

In addition, studies aimed at validating the clinical assessment of dehydration have indicated that the currently applied clinical schemes have limited accuracy. Mild dehydration is closer to 3 to 4%; moderate, 5 to 6%; and severe, 8 to 10%. Certain signs such as skin turgor and capillary

TABLE 5. **Clinical Evaluation of Volume Deficit**

	Mild (3–5%)*	Moderate (6–9%)*	Severe (≥10%)*
Estimated Volume Deficit Based Upon Physical Examination			
Pulses	Normal	Normal	Weak
Skin recoil	Instant	≤2 sec	>2 sec
Mucosae	Normal	sl dry	Very dry
Eyes	Normal	sl sunken	Very sunken
Mental status	Normal	nl/whimper	Lethargic/apathetic
Blood pressure	Normal	Normal	Normal to low
Estimated Volume Deficit According to Capillary Refill†			
Capillary refill	<1.5 sec	<5%	<50 mL/kg	Mild
	1.5–3 sec	5–9%	50–100 mL/kg	Moderate
	>3 sec	>10%	>100 mL/kg	Severe

*Some clinical studies indicate that mild dehydration is closer to 3%, moderate is closer to 5–6%, and severe is 8–10%.
†Using light pressure on the nailbed of the thumb.
Abbreviations: sl = slight; nl = normal.

refill are difficult to standardize, whereas the presence of a sunken fontanelle as an isolated finding was not found to be a particularly accurate indicator of the severity of dehydration in one study.

Estimation of the Sodium Deficit

Alterations in fluid tonicity may accompany the dehydrated state. One may distinguish between isotonic/isonatremic, hypotonic/hyponatremic, or hypertonic/hypernatremic dehydration by the level of plasma sodium upon presentation. Remember also that in some cases glucose or urea, or both, may be increased and result in increased plasma tonicity above that contributed by sodium. However, in most cases, the level of sodium is used to estimate the sodium deficit, guiding the sodium content of the rehydration solution. Unique alterations in the extracellular and intracellular fluid volumes accompany isonatremic, hyponatremic, and hypernatremic dehydration (Figure 1).

Isotonic dehydration is believed to result from loss of a relatively hypotonic fluid containing 70 to 80 mEq per liter of Na, with an equivalent loss of potassium. Sodium loss from the extracellular fluid (ECF) space is both out of the body and into the intracellular fluid (ICF) space when sodium enters the cell to compensate for potassium loss. Thus the primary loss in isotonic dehydration is from the ECF. Methods to estimate sodium deficit have assumed that the sodium content of the fluid lost is 70 to 80 mEq per liter. Therefore, one multiplies the volume deficit in liters by 70 to 80 to arrive at the sodium deficit expressed in milliequivalents.

Hyponatremic dehydration is associated with a relatively larger total body sodium deficit when compared with isotonic dehydration, and is accompanied by a marked decrease in ECF with an increase in ICF. Estimation of the sodium deficit combines the estimation of sodium required to bring the sodium up to normal plus an estimate of the sodium content of the fluid lost (similar to isotonic).

Isonatremic and Hyponatremic Dehydration

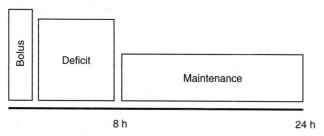

Hypernatremic Dehydration

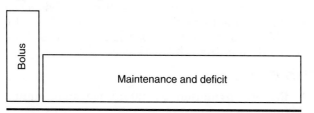

Figure 1. Treatment of isonatremic, hyponatremic, and hypernatremic dehydration.

$$Na\ deficit = weight\ (kg) \times 0.6 \times (135 - P_{Na})$$
$$= mEq\ Na\ required\ to\ raise\ sodium\ from$$
current level (P_{Na}) to 135 mEq per liter
$$+ volume\ deficit\ (liters) \times 80\ mEq\ per\ liter$$
or weight (kg) × % dehydration × 0.8

where P_{Na} = plasma sodium.

Hypernatremic dehydration results in both ECF and ICF volume contraction. The plasma volume is relatively spared compared with an equivalent volume loss in hyponatremic and isonatremic states. Similar clinical findings in isonatremic and hypernatremic dehydration indicate a greater total volume loss in the hypernatremic child, given the added loss from the cellular space. Treatment of hypernatremic dehydration requires care because of the risk for cerebral edema from rapid administration of hypotonic fluid. In some children with hypernatremic dehydration oral replacement fluids were hyperosmolar or rich in sodium. In the period between 1950 and 1970, when infants were commonly fed condensed milk, hypernatremic dehydration was more common and was attributed to relative salt poisoning.

One rule of thumb has been to aim to lower the sodium concentration slowly, no faster than 10 to 12 mEq per L per day. Estimation of the sodium deficit is more difficult in hypernatremic dehydration. The sodium deficit is estimated to be 2 to 5 mEq per kg in hypernatremic dehydration compared to 7 to 11 for isonatremic and 10 to 14 for hyponatremic dehydration. One may also use a formula to estimate the total body sodium derived from the premorbid weight and normal plasma sodium and the current weight and plasma sodium assuming ECV to maintain at 60% of body weight. Again, this provides merely a rough estimate upon which therapy can be designed.

Finberg has extensively studied therapies for hypernatremic dehydration and maintains that hypotonic fluid should be administered (0.225% NS = ¼ NS) after the restoration of the circulation. In practice the administration of ¼ NS may be accompanied by a rapid fall in the plasma sodium that demands either reduction of the IV rate or change in fluid composition closer to ½ NS. Continued sodium losses via the gastrointestinal tract or overestimation of the fluid deficit may explain, in part, the more rapid drop observed in some children. Oral fluid intake is often withheld due to the concern that hypotonic oral fluids may be difficult to regulate and result in a more rapid drop in the sodium than desired. Oral rehydration has been employed in underdeveloped countries in the treatment of hypernatremic dehydration with success, although also accompanied by seizures in some cases. The velocity of the decline in sodium concentration appeared to correlate with seizures.

Alternative methods have allowed relatively greater intracellular fluid deficit depending upon the length of illness leading to the state of dehydration. If the child has suffered losses for 48 hours or less, then the ECF deficit is 80% and the ICF deficit is 20%. If the illness has been ongoing for greater than 48 hours, then the ECF deficit is 60% and the ICF deficit is 40%. The author of this chapter prefers to calculate the individual fluid and sodium deficits using the current weight. The following examples illustrate one method for calculation of deficits.

PROBLEM SOLVING
Isotonic Dehydration

A 2-year-old child with vomiting and diarrhea has been unable to keep fluids down for 2 days. Mother does not know when she has last urinated. Her exam is remarkable for BP 80/38, HR 158, wt = 7.5 kg. She is lethargic and pale with markedly decreased perfusion. Mucous membranes are dry and capillary refill is greater than 3 seconds. She is judged to be severely dehydrated. Labs show Na 134 mEq per liter, K 3.2 mEq per liter, bicarbonate 15 mEq per liter, BUN 40 mg per dL and creatinine 1.2 mg per dL. One can consider severe dehydration in this child to represent an acute loss of 10% body weight.

Estimated fluid deficit using current body weight: (7.5 kg)(100 mL per kg) = 750 mL to be given over 8 hours, subtracting any bolus therapy given.

Estimated maintenance: (100 mL per kg)(7.5 kg) = 750 mL (to be given over the next 16 hours).

Total fluid for 24 hours: 1500 mL (1.5 liters).

Sodium deficit using rule of 80 mEq per liter as the sodium content of the volume lost: 0.75 liter × 80 mEq per liter = 60 mEq.

Maintenance sodium: 7.5 kg × 3 mEq per kg per day = 22.5 mEq.

Total sodium required: 22.5 mEq + 60 mEq = 82.5 mEq.

Sodium concentration of the fluid to be given for rehydration: 60 mEq per 0.75 liter = 80 mEq per liter.

Final Plan

1. Restore circulation and improve perfusion with NS 20 mL per kg = 20 mL per kg × 7.5 kg = 150 mL over 60 minutes. May repeat if indicated by clinical findings (Na = 20 mEq).

2. Rehydration to provide deficit and maintenance over the next 23 hours: D5 ½ NS at a rate designated by the original deficit of 750 mL − 150 mL = 600 mL in 7 hours = 86 mL/hour. If a metabolic acidosis is present, one may wish to use a fluid that contains one half of the sodium as the bicarbonate salt: ¼ NS plus 40 mEq per liter sodium bicarbonate (Na = 46 mEq).

3. Continue to rehydrate with D5 ¼ NS plus 20 mEq per liter of KCl to provide the remaining 750 mL over 16 hours = 47 mL per hour. In this phase, K acetate may be added if metabolic acidosis is present, or a portion of the sodium may be administered as the bicarbonate salt.

Hyponatremic Dehydration

A 3-month-old infant presents with vomiting and diarrhea for 3 days with T 38°C, BP 90/40, HR 146, dry mucous membranes, capillary refill 2 to 3 seconds, and poor skin turgor. Na = 123 mEq per liter, K 3.4 mEq per liter, bicarbonate 11 mEq per liter, BUN 30 mg per dL, creatinine 0.8 mg per dL. The baby's weight is 3.5 kg. He is judged to be moderately dehydrated, which is 6 to 9%, although some methods allow 10% for moderately dehydrated infants.

Deficit volume: (90 mL per kg)(3.5 kg) = 315 mL.

Maintenance volume: (100 mL per kg)(3.5 kg) = 350 mL.

Total volume to be given over 24 hours: 665 mL (0.67 liter).

Sodium deficit: (135 mEq per liter − 123 mEq per liter)(0.6)(3.5 kg) = 25 mEq (80 mEq per liter)(0.315 liter of volume) = 25 mEq = 50 mEq total sodium deficit.

Sodium maintenance = (3.5 kg)(3 mEq per kg per day) = 10.5 mEq.

Total sodium to be given = 60.5 mEq. Divide by the total volume of 665 mL (since we will replace this large sodium deficit over 24 hours rather than 8 hours as in the isonatremic patient) (0.67 liter) gives a fluid concentration of approximately 90 mEq/L, although NS given initially as a bolus may modify the Na concentration of the solution needed to replace the estimated Na deficit.

Final Plan

1. NS 20 mL per kg = (20 mL per kg)(3.5 kg) = 70 mL (11 mEq sodium).

2. Volume deficit 315 mL − 70 mL = 245 mL over 7 hours = 35 mL per hour. Use D5 ½ NS plus 20 mEq per liter of sodium bicarbonate at 35 mL per hour (24 mEq sodium).

3. Remainder of fluid: 350 mL over 16 hours = 22 mL/hour. Use D5 ½ NS + 20 mEq/L KCl at 22 mL/hour (sodium = 27 mEq). Total sodium = 62 mEq.

Hypernatremic Dehydration

A 4-year-old child with diarrhea for 2 days has been given chicken broth and Gatorade for replacement fluid. He is lethargic and presents with a weight of 14 kg, sodium 162 mEq per liter, K of 4 mEq per liter, bicarbonate 16 mEq per liter, BUN 28 mg per dL, and creatinine 1.0 mg per dL. He is judged to be moderately dehydrated, or to have lost 6% body weight. Due to his hypernatremia, we plan to correct his volume deficit over 2 days or 48 hours.

Fluid deficit: (14 kg)(60 mL per kg) = 840 mL (0.84 liter).

Fluid maintenance: 1000 mL for the first 10 kg, then (50 mL per kg)(4 kg) = 200 mL for a total of 1200 mL per day × 2 = 2400 mL total maintenance.

Total fluid to be given over 48 hours = 3.24 liters.

Deficit sodium using the estimate of 30 mEq per liter as the sodium concentration of the fluid lost: (0.84 L)(30 mEq per liter) = 25 mEq.

Maintenance sodium: (3 mEq per kg per day)(14 kg) = 42 mEq × 2 = 84 mEq.

Total sodium to be given = 109 mEq divided by the total volume to be given over 2 days = 109 mEq per 3.24 liters = 34 mEq per liter as the sodium concentration of the rehydration solution.

Final Plan

1. Restore circulation: NS 20 mL per kg minimum = 280 mL over 1 hour.

2. Rehydration begins after the NS: D5 ¼ NS at 77 mL per hour (3240 mL − 280 mL = 2960 mL divided by 47 hours gives an infusion rate of 63 mL

per hour over the next 47 hours. Potassium may be added at 20 mEq per liter as KCl or K acetate when urine flow is established. Some physicians prefer to start with a solution containing the equivalent of ½ NS in order to avoid lowering the plasma sodium level too rapidly. Most fluid and electrolyte models, however, estimate that ¼ NS provides adequate sodium.

It is important to monitor the plasma sodium during the initial rehydration phase. If the sodium drops too rapidly, then one may either reduce the infusion rate or increase the sodium concentration of the fluid to ½ NS. Infants with hypernatremic dehydration may also present with hyperglycemia. Insulin is rarely required as rehydration is usually accompanied by normalization of glucose levels. Hypocalcemia may also complicate the rehydration phase during hypernatremic dehydration. Therefore, the ionized calcium concentration should be measured if central nervous system symptoms occur.

Some authors have urged a more unified, simpler therapy for the treatment of dehydration and argue that the meticulous calculation of sodium and fluid deficits is unnecessary. Although this may be feasible for the treatment of hyponatremic and isonatremic dehydration, it is not recommended for hypernatremic dehydration. The simplified plan of treatment would allow 30 mL per kg of NS (or more if clinically indicated) to restore ECF over the first 2 to 3 hours, followed by D5 ½ NS, 60 mL per kg over the next 6 hours, and then the maintenance over the remainder of the day. Again, potassium may be added after urine flow is established.

In summary, administration of parenteral fluid and electrolytes is based upon fundamental physiologic principles. The aim of therapy is to provide adequate fluid and electrolytes to either maintain balance or to replace losses. This chapter uses calculation of fluid and sodium deficit to design therapy for dehydrated infants and children.

ACROMEGALY

method of
MARK E. MOLITCH, M.D.
Northwestern University Medical School
Chicago, Illinois

PRETREATMENT EVALUATION

Acromegaly is an insidious disorder, usually present for years before the diagnosis is made. It is important to establish the activity of the disease before instituting therapy, for two reasons. First, a small percentage of growth hormone (GH)–secreting tumors spontaneously infarct. This causes the condition known as "burned out" or "fugitive" acromegaly, in which GH levels are normal by the time the diagnosis is made and no therapy is indicated. Second, tumor activity after therapy can then be compared with that documented before therapy to determine whether additional treatment is needed.

The definition of an abnormal basal serum GH level has been difficult to ascertain in the past because of the poor sensitivity of GH assays and episodic secretion. Some patients with active acromegaly may have basal GH levels less than 5 ng per mL according to conventional radioimmunoassays (RIAs). However, normal GH levels have been shown to be even lower, according to immunoradiometric assay (IRMA) and enzyme-linked immunosorbent assay (ELISA). Except for the episodic secretory surges, a level of 2 ng per mL may well be the upper limit of normal for basal GH levels. For establishing the diagnosis and clinical activity of acromegaly it is necessary to document an elevated basal level of GH and the failure to suppress GH levels with an oral glucose load to less than 2.0 ng per mL by means of an RIA and less than 0.33 ng per mL by means of an IRMA or ELISA. Elevation of levels of insulin-like growth factor 1 (IGF-1), in comparison with age-adjusted normal values, has also become accepted as a criterion for the diagnosis of active acromegaly. IGF-1 levels correlate with indices of disease activity better than GH levels in most studies. IGF-1 binding protein 3 (IGFBP3) levels are also elevated in most patients with active disease, although there is some overlap with values in normal subjects.

Thirty-five to 40% of patients with acromegaly have elevated prolactin (PRL) levels. Uncommonly, patients will present with symptoms caused by the hyperprolactinemia, such as decreased libido, impotence, galactorrhea, or amenorrhea, rather than the normal presenting symptoms of acromegaly.

Almost all patients with acromegaly have GH-secreting pituitary adenomas. The size and degree of any extrasellar extension of the adenoma are assessed by magnetic resonance imaging (MRI) or, when that is unavailable, high-resolution computed tomography (CT). Compression of the optic chiasm by the adenoma can be determined with Goldmann visual field testing when MRI shows that the tumor abuts the optic chiasm. About 80% of patients have macroadenomas (more than 10 mm in diameter) and 15 to 20% have suprasellar extension of the adenoma. Large adenomas may cause hypopituitarism by directly compressing the normal pituitary or interfering with stalk function. A detailed evaluation of anterior and posterior pituitary function will determine whether hormone replacement is necessary.

Acromegaly may cause hypertension, diabetes mellitus, hypertrophic cardiomyopathy, and sleep apnea. Colonic adenomatous polyps and colon cancer occur more frequently than expected and colonoscopy is indicated. Should surgery be chosen as therapy, then these complications may need treatment preoperatively.

In rare cases, no evidence of pituitary adenoma is found, and if surgery is performed, hyperplasia of the somatotropes may be found. Such patients may have a syndrome in which GH-releasing hormone (GHRH) is being secreted by a pancreatic, carcinoid, hypothalamic, or other tumor. If one of these GHRH-secreting tumors is suspected, then GHRH blood levels can be measured.

Virtually all GH-secreting adenomas arise de novo in the pituitary and are not due to underlying hypothalamic dysfunction. In about 40% of cases, mutations have been found in the guanine nucleotide regulatory protein that couples the GHRH receptor to adenylyl cyclase, resulting in a constitutive, unregulated stimulation of the somatotropes to secrete GH. In other cases the specific mutations causing the tumors have not been identified. The clinical importance of these findings with respect to therapeutic goals lies in the fact that once a tumor is ablated in its entirety, it is not expected to recur because of some underlying hypothalamic dysfunction.

Goals of therapy include (1) elimination of effects due to the mass of the tumor (e.g., hypopituitarism, visual field defects); (2) reduction of elevated GH levels to normal; (3) amelioration of the end-organ effects of the elevated GH levels; (4) avoidance of damage to remaining normal hypothalamic or pituitary function; and (5) minimizing other potential adverse effects of therapy.

TREATMENT

Transsphenoidal Adenomectomy

Transsphenoidal surgery offers the patient a chance for cure. Even when "cure" is not achieved, surgery may effect a significant reduction in GH levels and considerable amelioration of clinical symptoms. As expected, the smaller the tumor and the lower the basal GH levels, the better the surgical result. The actual cure rates depend on the criteria used. According to the criterion of postoperative GH levels less than 5 ng per mL, "cure" rates of 60 to 80% can be expected for intrasellar lesions and 40 to 50% for larger tumors when the operation is performed by experienced neurosurgeons. Adding criteria such as suppressibility of GH to less than 2.0 ng per mL (RIA) by glucose, nonresponsiveness to thyrotropin-releasing hormone (protirelin [Thyrel TRH]), basal GH levels less than 2 ng per mL, and normal IGF-I levels substantially reduces these numbers. Relapses occur in 5 to 10% of patients who initially achieve GH levels of less than 5 ng per mL.

With microadenomas, the risks of surgery are very small. The mortality from surgery approaches that of anesthesia alone. Transient diabetes insipidus may occur in 10 to 20% of patients, but it is rare for the patient to need treatment after discharge from the hospital. Hypopituitarism occurs in less than 1%, and other complications such as meningitis and cerebrospinal fluid leak also occur in less than 1% of patients. The total complication rate for this surgery by an experienced pituitary neurosurgeon, except for transient diabetes insipidus, is less than 3%. The complication rate is higher for larger tumors, with risks for cerebrospinal fluid leak, meningitis, and permanent diabetes insipidus reaching 2% each. Loss of one or more anterior pituitary hormones occurs in 5 to 10% of patients.

Rarely, patients with very large tumors may need craniotomy and a subfrontal lobe approach. This may be necessary if the tumor has a large suprasellar extension with a dumbbell configuration. Risks are much higher with craniotomy, and mortality reaches 5% in some series.

Pituitary function tested 6 to 8 weeks postoperatively will determine whether the patient is cured or whether there is persistent GH hypersecretion. Testing involves obtaining basal GH and IGF-I levels and showing suppression of GH with glucose. Those patients who appear to be cured need to be followed to detect potential relapse. Testing of other pituitary function will detect other hormonal deficiencies that may need treatment. We routinely place patients with macroadenomas on maintenance glucocorticoids (prednisone, 5 to 7.5 mg daily) until this time of postoperative testing, in case loss of adrenocorticotropic hormone (ACTH) function has occurred. Because loss of ACTH is very unlikely after surgery for microadenomas, we usually do not prescribe maintenance glucocorticoids unless the patient is symptomatic or is found to be deficient on the formal testing carried out at 6 to 8 weeks.

Irradiation

Conventional irradiation, given at a dose of 4500 cGy through two or three fields over 5 weeks will lower GH levels substantially in over 80% of patients. The destructive effects of the irradiation are cumulative over time, with levels of GH continuing to decrease for up to 20 years of follow-up. GH levels decrease to less than 5 ng per mL in 15 to 20% of treated cases by 2 years, in about 40% by 5 years, and in about 70% by 10 years. Because the progressive reduction in GH levels appears to be a percentage function regardless of initial GH levels or tumor size, it is obvious that the lower the initial GH levels the faster GH levels will return to normal.

At the same time that irradiation affects tumor function, it also affects the normal pituitary. By 10 years after irradiation, about 20% of patients are hypothyroid, 35 to 40% are hypoadrenal, and about 50% are hypogonadal.

During irradiation therapy, some patients complain of fatigue. If a patient is deficient in ACTH and on glucocorticoid replacement therapy, a doubling of the glucocorticoid dose is sometimes needed during radiation therapy. In some patients, irradiation may cause subtle but permanent cognitive and short-term memory deficits. Patients may complain of difficulty concentrating, a poor memory, and lack of initiative.

Tumor infarction is more common after irradiation. It usually causes the sudden onset of severe headache and often coma and vascular collapse, a syndrome referred to as "pituitary apoplexy." CT or MRI usually show evidence of hemorrhage. Such patients must be supported with glucocorticoids in stress doses, and consideration should be given to emergency transsphenoidal decompression. Lesser degrees of tumor infarction may also occur, and the patient may have either no symptoms or a mild headache, with evidence of infarction being found only later on scan or at surgery.

A relatively new type of radiotherapy, called "stereotactic" radiosurgery involving the use of the "gamma knife" or linear accelerator (LINAC), may offer considerable advantages over conventional irradiation in that it requires only a single large dose of irradiation and may have a somewhat better therapeutic benefit-to-risk ratio. The irradiation is given through multiple ports and is "shaped" to correspond with the tumor visible on MRI. With this treatment, GH levels less than 5 ng per mL are achieved in about 20% of patients by 1 year and in about 50% by 3 years. Complications of this type of radiotherapy appear to be much less than with conventional radiotherapy, although the experience is much less and the follow-up periods are much shorter thus far. The cranial nerves that pass through the cavernous sinus (i.e., III, IV, V_1, V_2, and VI) appear to be resistant to this form of irradiation, and thus this technique is particularly useful for residual tumor in the cavernous sinus. The optic nerves, tracts, and chiasm appear to be more radiosensitive, and thus this form of radiotherapy is less useful for tumors with considerable suprasellar extension. The frequency of hypopituitarism appears to be less, but long-term follow-up studies are still lacking. Nonetheless, stereotactic "radiosurgery" appears to be the treatment of choice when radiotherapy is indicated for patients whose disorder is not cured by surgery.

Medical Therapy with Dopamine Agonists

Seventy to 75% of patients respond to bromocriptine (Parlodel) with some decrease of GH levels, albeit in only 10 to 20% do GH levels actually reach levels less than 5 ng per mL. Despite these modest reductions in GH levels, substantial clinical improvement may be seen, such as reduction in ring size and improvement in glucose tolerance. In contrast to its documented high efficacy in shrinking tumor size in PRL-secreting macroadenomas, bromocriptine has been found to be much less efficacious in shrinking GH-secreting tumors. The dose needed to lower GH levels is much higher than that used to lower PRL levels. The effective daily dose of bromocriptine is usually in the 10- to 40-mg range given in divided doses, although doses greater than 30 mg are rarely necessary. The starting dose is 1.25 to 2.5 mg daily, given with a snack at bedtime to avoid nausea and orthostatic hypotension. The dose is raised by 2.5-mg increments every 2 to 4 days, as tolerated. With each dose increase, nausea and lightheadedness may recur, but these symptoms usually resolve within 1 to 2 days. Constipation, digital vasospasm, nasal congestion, and alcohol intolerance may become problems at higher doses.

A much smaller number of patients with acromegaly have been treated with cabergoline (Dostinex), a long-acting dopamine agonist that has to be given only once or twice weekly.* The success rates appear to be higher than for bromocriptine, especially in those tumors that secrete both GH and PRL. The starting dose is 0.5 mg weekly, and this can be raised to as high as 8 to 10 mg weekly† if the patient continues to respond with progressively lower GH levels. Side effects are similar to those seen with bromocriptine, although cabergoline is generally better tolerated, even in high doses.

Medical Therapy with Somatostatin Agonists

A somatostatin analog, octreotide (Sandostatin), has a 40-fold greater activity in suppressing GH compared with insulin. In acromegalic persons, acute, subcutaneous octreotide administration results in a decrease in GH levels, the nadir occurring within 2 to 3 hours and the suppressive effects lasting for 6 to 12 hours. Long-term studies suggest that substantial reductions of GH and IGF-I occur in 90% of patients, and in over 60% IGF-I levels can be brought into the normal range. In most cases a dosing frequency of every 6 to 8 hours is usually necessary, beginning at 100 μg at each dose and increasing as necessary up to 1500 μg per day. Some patients respond better to the combination of octreotide plus bromocriptine than to either drug alone. MRI has demonstrated 10 to 20% tumor size reduction as a result of therapy in 20 to 30% of patients.

Side effects include mild abdominal bloating, nausea, moderate diarrhea, steatorrhea, and gastritis. Cholelithiasis and gallbladder sludge due to poor gallbladder contractility occur in up to 25% of patients. Cholecystitis occurs in less than 1% of patients and is treated by laparoscopic cholecystectomy

rather than stopping the drug if the patient is having a good GH/IGF-1 response.

Two long-acting preparations of somatostatin agonists have become available. Octreotide-LAR (Sandostatin-LAR) is given monthly intramuscularly in 20-, 30-, or 40-mg doses, depending on the GH and IGF-1 responses. Lanreotide-SR (Ipstyl)* is given every 7 to 14 days intramuscularly, the timing depending on the GH and IGF-1 responses. With both preparations, IGF-1 levels can be normalized in about 60% of patients and reduced considerably in most others. Complications are similar to those seen with octreotide. Thus, these long-acting preparations are greatly preferred to octreotide because of ease of use.

CONCLUSIONS

In patients with microadenomas and intrasellar macroadenomas, transsphenoidal surgery offers a 60 to 80% chance of cure, depending on the experience of the neurosurgeon. The recurrence rate after apparent cure is less than 10%. Thus, this would appear to be the best choice as primary therapy for such patients. In patients with larger tumors, surgery can cause a considerable debulking of the tumor with a concomitant reduction in GH levels, but the cure rate decreases as tumor size increases. Because radiotherapy appears to cause a fractional rate of decrease of GH levels, the lower the initial GH level, the more rapidly will this mode of treatment result in a decrease of GH levels to normal. This appears to hold true regardless of whether GH levels were low to begin with or as a result of prior surgery. Thus, an operation performed before radiotherapy also appears to be beneficial for larger tumors.

Because radiotherapy may take several years to bring GH levels to normal, I believe it should be regarded as second-line therapy to be used if an operation has not resulted in cure or is contraindicated. Stereotactic radiosurgery appears to cause a considerably faster reduction of GH levels with fewer adverse effects, especially when the residual tumor is in the cavernous sinus.

Medical therapy is best reserved for patients not cured by surgery and/or radiotherapy or in whom ablative therapy is contraindicated. In addition, these drugs may be useful while awaiting the eventual destructive effects of irradiation. Because of ease of use and lower cost, cabergoline should be tried first, although the success rates for dopamine agonists are relative low. In those patients in whom dopamine agonists are ineffective, a long-acting somatostatin agonist such as octreotide-LAR or lanreotide-SR can be given with good expectations of success at normalizing GH and IGF-1 levels.

---

*Not FDA approved for this indication.

---

*Not FDA approved for this indication.
†Exceeds dosage recommended by the manufacturer.

ADRENOCORTICAL INSUFFICIENCY

method of
HIRALAL MAHESHWARI, M.D., PH.D., and
JENNIFER LARSEN, M.D.

University of Nebraska Medical Center
Omaha, Nebraska

Adrenocortical insufficiency can result from either destruction of adrenal cortex (primary adrenocortical deficiency, or Addison's disease) or decreased hypothalamic or pituitary function due to declining adrenocorticotropic hormone (ACTH) or corticotropin-releasing hormone (CRH) secretion. The last two disorders are sometimes distinguished as secondary versus tertiary adrenal insufficiency, respectively. However, just as often they are grouped together under the heading of secondary deficiency, because it is often difficult to determine which of the hormones is deficient or deficiencies of both may be present. Adrenocortical insufficiency, although uncommon, can be associated with considerable morbidity and mortality if unrecognized, making it an important disorder to recognize and diagnose early. It should be considered in the differential diagnosis of many disorders because of the variety of vague complaints associated with it (e.g., weakness, fatigue, weight loss, and gastrointestinal symptoms).

PRIMARY ADRENOCORTICAL INSUFFICIENCY

Etiology

The clinical spectrum of primary adrenocortical insufficiency has changed over the past decade with the emergence of new causes, changes in distribution of causes, and the availability of molecular diagnostic testing in some cases. There are many causes of primary adrenal insufficiency (Table 1), but the most common cause remains autoimmune destruction, either isolated or as part of polyglandular autoimmune destruction. With autoimmune destruction, the onset is often gradual because signs and symptoms are not manifested until over 90% of the adrenal glands are destroyed. The one exception is when an overwhelming stress precipitates a more acute onset of symptoms or signs.

TABLE 1. Causes of Primary Adrenal Insufficiency

- Autoimmune adrenalitis (alone or as a component of polyglandular autoimmune failure syndrome)
- Tuberculosis and other mycobacterial diseases
- Systemic fungal infections (histoplasmosis, cryptococcosis, blastomycosis)
- Adrenal hemorrhage, necrosis or thrombosis in meningococcal or other sepsis, or with anticoagulation therapy or in antiphospholipid syndrome
- Congenital adrenal hyperplasia (most common: 21-hydroxylase deficiency)
- Acquired immunodeficiency syndrome (associated opportunistic infections such as cytomegalovirus, *Mycobacterium avium*, and, less commonly, Kaposi's sarcoma)
- Adrenoleukodystrophy
- Metastatic carcinoma, lymphoma
- Medications (decreased cortisol synthesis: mitotane, ketoconazole [dose dependent], aminoglutethimide, metyrapone; increased cortisol clearance: rifampin, phenytoin [Dilantin], phenobarbital, fluoxetine [Prozac])
- Surgical (bilateral adrenalectomy)
- Idiopathic

TABLE 2. Major Manifestations of Primary Adrenal Insufficiency

Symptoms
Weakness
Anorexia, weight loss
Gastrointestinal symptoms
   Nausea
   Vomiting
   Constipation
   Abdominal pain
   Diarrhea
Salt craving
Postural dizziness
Muscle or joint pain
Signs
Fever
Weight loss
Hyperpigmentation
Supine or postural hypotension
Vitiligo
Auricular calcification
Laboratory Findings
Hyponatremia
Hyperkalemia
Hypercalemia
Prerenal azotemia
Normochromic, normocytic anemia
Eosinophilia

Other causes of primary adrenal insufficiency include granulomatous diseases (e.g., tuberculosis and histoplasmosis), which have increased in frequency with the growing incidence of the acquired immune deficiency syndrome (AIDS). Metastatic malignancies (e.g., lung or breast carcinoma or Kaposi's sarcoma in AIDS), opportunistic infections associated with AIDS, hemorrhage (due to anticoagulant therapy or meningococcemia), hereditary disorders (e.g., congenital adrenal hyperplasia or adrenoleukodystrophy), and medications also can cause adrenal insufficiency.

Clinical Manifestation

In most cases, the synthetic functions of all three layers of the adrenal cortex (zona glomerulosa, zona fasciculata, and zona reticularis) are affected, resulting in inadequate secretion of mineralocorticoids, glucocorticoids, and androgens. However, many of the clinical manifestations (Table 2) are due to glucocorticoid deficiency, including decreased sense of well-being, anorexia, abdominal pain, weight loss, diarrhea, and relative hypoglycemia. Symptoms of mineralocorticoid insufficiency, such as orthostatic hypotension, are also often prominent. In a more fulminant presentation, vascular collapse and shock can be the sole presentation. Symptoms of adrenal androgen deficiency are often evident only in women (e.g., decreased pubic and axillary hair and decreased libido) because men usually retain their ability to secrete testicular androgens unless they experience considerable weight loss. Lack of negative feedback from adrenal corticosteroids increases secretion of pituitary ACTH, which, in turn, causes hyperpigmentation of skin and mucosa, especially in areas of recent trauma or injury or high turnover, such as buccal mucosa, gingiva, elbows, or palmar creases. Because many individuals with autoimmune destruction are at risk for other autoimmune diseases, vitiligo may also be present in addition to features of autoimmune thyroid disease (e.g., goiter, hypothyroidism). If the individual has type 1 (autoimmune) diabetes, hypoglycemia may be more frequent or insulin requirements may be decreased.

SECONDARY ADRENAL INSUFFICIENCY

Etiology

Secondary adrenal insufficiency is due to inadequate pituitary ACTH or, less commonly, decreased hypothalamic CRH secretion leading to inadequate cortisol production. Causes are listed in Table 3, but the most common is iatrogenic following the withdrawal (sudden or gradual) of supraphysiologic doses of glucocorticoids.

Clinical Presentation

Unlike primary adrenocortical insufficiency, symptoms of mineralocorticoid deficiency are rarely observed in secondary adrenocortical insufficiency, because aldosterone secretion can be regulated independent of the pituitary. In contrast to primary adrenal failure, pigmentation is not increased and can sometimes be reduced because ACTH concentration is often low, not high. Women may note a loss of pubic and axillary hair. In secondary adrenal insufficiency, symptoms of other hormone deficiencies may also be present.

ADRENAL CRISIS (ACUTE ADRENAL INSUFFICIENCY)

"Adrenal crisis" is the term used for acute presentation of adrenal insufficiency of any cause. It most commonly occurs in the setting of a major physiologic stress in a previously undiagnosed patient, or in a patient with established adrenal insufficiency who did not increase glucocorticoid replacement or could not take glucocorticoid medications due to persistent vomiting from any cause. Symptoms include nausea or vomiting; abdominal, flank, or back pain; joint pains; fever; weakness; fatigue; lethargy; confusion or coma; and late manifestations of vascular collapse and shock. Less commonly, adrenal crisis may result from sudden, bilateral infarction of the adrenals caused by hemorrhage, recent surgery, anticoagulant therapy, embolus, sepsis, or, very rarely, adrenal vein thrombosis in procoagulant states. Adrenal crisis is rare in patients with secondary adrenal insufficiency.

TABLE 3. **Causes of Secondary Adrenal Insufficiency**

- Pituitary or hypothalamic tumor including metastatic tumor to these areas
- Craniopharyngioma
- Central nervous system tumor
- Pituitary or central nervous system surgery or radiation
- Lymphocytic hypophysitis
- Empty sella syndrome
- Pituitary infarction (e.g., postpartum as with Sheehan's syndrome, post-traumatic, ischemic, or acute necrosis of a large pituitary tumor)
- Intermediate duration or long-term glucocorticoid treatment
- Miscellaneous infections: mucormycosis, meningitis, tuberculosis
- Infiltrative or basilar granulomatous diseases: sarcoidosis, histiocytosis X, hemochromatosis
- Isolated ACTH deficiency, familial
- Idiopathic

DIAGNOSIS

Diagnosis of adrenal insufficiency may be suspected based on the clinical presentation, known pathologic cause (e.g., recent pituitary surgery), or consistent laboratory findings (e.g., hyponatremia, hyperkalemia, eosinophilia, and prerenal insufficiency). Endocrine stimulation testing is required to establish the diagnosis. Stimulation testing is used to identify adequacy of cortisol secretion, and, depending on the test used, adequacy of the hypothalamic-pituitary response to distinguish primary from secondary causes. Radiologic procedures may help to establish the cause. All individuals with secondary adrenal insufficiency require a scan to identify or exclude a specific anatomic cause. Magnetic resonance imaging (MRI) is the most sensitive at identifying pituitary or other lesions, but lesions that cause pituitary or hypothalamic insufficiency are usually not small. Computed tomography (CT) of the brain has the advantage of identifying calcifications that are useful in identifying craniopharyngioma, one cause of secondary adrenocortical insufficiency. CT of the adrenal glands can be useful to confirm suspected causes of adrenal insufficiency such as metastatic tumor or bilateral adrenal hemorrhage, but anatomic scanning is not required to diagnose suspected autoimmune adrenal failure.

General Laboratory Testing

Hyponatremia, hyperkalemia, and prerenal azotemia can be observed in primary adrenal failure, particularly when volume depletion is noted on physical examination. Blood glucose levels can be low normal or low. The complete blood cell count often shows moderate eosinophilia, relative lymphocytosis, and a normocytic, normochromic anemia. Hypercalcemia can also occur. Electrocardiographic abnormalities can include peaked T waves, low P waves, and wide QRS complexes. In the extreme case, atrial asystole, intraventricular block, and, ultimately, ventricular asystole have been reported. In secondary adrenal insufficiency, hyperkalemia is less common and, when azotemia is present, is more likely secondary to diabetes insipidus or other causes. Hypercalcemia is also less common. Hypoglycemia is more common than in primary adrenal insufficiency perhaps because of accompanying hormone deficiencies (e.g., growth hormone and thyroid-stimulating hormone). ACTH will not be elevated but is often measurable.

A low 8 AM cortisol (<10 μg/dL) is suggestive for both types of adrenal insufficiency but is not diagnostic. However, an elevated random value (>20 μg/dL) virtually excludes the diagnosis. Plasma ACTH levels should be elevated in primary adrenal failure but are not observed in every random determination. Anyone with a suggestive history or with a condition known to predispose to adrenocortical insufficiency (primary or secondary) who does not have an elevated random serum cortisol value should undergo ACTH stimulation testing regardless of whether electrolyte abnormalities are found.

Short ACTH Stimulation Test

A short ACTH stimulation test is the first screening test for patients in whom a diagnosis of adrenocortical insufficiency is being considered. It can be performed in any setting at any time of the day. Baseline cortisol and ACTH values are evaluated, and the cortisol level is then checked at 30 minutes (and in some cases at 60 minutes) after administration of 0.25 mg of synthetic ACTH (Cortrosyn). A normal cortisol value 30 minutes after Cortrosyn administration is 20 μg per dL or more whether or not there was any increase from baseline. In the setting of an acute stress (e.g., hypotension in the emergency department), the stress itself is an adequate stimulus to determine whether the person has a normal hypothalamic-pituitary-adrenal axis. In this situation, a random cortisol (and ACTH) sample can be measured and a cortisol concentration of 20 μg per dL or more is considered an adequate adrenal response. A normal response to the short ACTH stimulation test virtually excludes either primary or significant secondary adrenal insufficiency because tonic ACTH secretion is required to maintain normal adrenal corticosteroid content required for a normal ACTH-stimulated cortisol response. Thus, although this test can identify adrenal insufficiency, it cannot distinguish primary from secondary causes. Further testing may not be required in some cases if the clinical presentation suggests the cause (e.g., hyperpigmentation in an individual with a bilateral, bulky adrenal mass and an elevated 8 AM ACTH level). However, in most cases further testing is required to determine the adequacy of the ACTH response and to distinguish primary from secondary failure. Those patients with suggested secondary adrenal insufficiency should also be screened for other hormone deficiency states.

Other Stimulation Tests

The insulin tolerance can be used as a stimulus for both cortisol and ACTH to distinguish between primary and secondary adrenal insufficiency and to screen for growth hormone deficiency if pituitary function is a concern. This test is performed after the patient having fasted by administration of a dose of insulin with a goal of inducing hypoglycemia (approximately 0.1 unit per kg unless the individual has obesity or known insulin resistance). Samples are drawn for determination of glucose, cortisol, and ACTH before and 30 and 60 minutes after administration of insulin. Capillary glucose should be sampled more frequently, particularly if the patient has symptoms or signs of hypoglycemia. A running intravenous line should be in place to quickly administer concentrated glucose solutions if needed for severe hypoglycemia. A glucose concentration less than 50 mg per dL is an adequate response for stimulation of the hypothalamic-pituitary-adrenal axis. Primary adrenal insufficiency versus secondary adrenal insufficiency is diagnosed if levels either of cortisol or of cortisol and ACTH, respectively, do not rise after hypoglycemia.

Other tests can also be useful in distinguishing primary from secondary insufficiency. Metyrapone, administered at bedtime, blocks 11-hydroxylase activity to cause a reduction in cortisol and a rise in ACTH and cortisol's precursor molecule 11-deoxycortisol (compound S) by 8 AM if the hypothalamus-pituitary unit is intact. The CRH test can also be used to differentiate specific causes of adrenal insufficiency. There is little or no ACTH response to CRH injection in patients with pituitary insufficiency, including individuals who have recently been on supraphysiologic corticosteroids. In patients with a hypothalamic or primary adrenal failure, there is a normal or exaggerated ACTH response. The prolonged ACTH stimulation test is usually used in the setting of previous adrenal corticosteroid therapy, where it is uncertain whether there is also underlying primary adrenal insufficiency. The prolonged ACTH test is performed by administering synthetic ACTH (Cortrosyn 0.25 mg) as a continuous infusion over 8 hours on 3 successive days. Increases in daily urinary free cortisol excretion and plasma cortisol concentrations before and after each

daily infusion are used to confirm normal adrenal gland function.

TREATMENT

Adrenal Crisis or Other Acute Stress

The initial goal of therapy is to reverse hypotension and electrolyte abnormalities. If onset is acute and diagnosis of adrenal crisis is suspected, treatment should not wait for the results from cortisol testing (Table 4). After a blood sample is drawn to determine cortisol, ACTH, and baseline electrolyte values, hydrocortisone sodium succinate (Solu-Cortef) (100 to 200 mg) should be administered intravenously along with 0.9% saline solution or 5% dextrose and 0.9% saline. If no intravenous access can be established immediately, the hydrocortisone can be administered intramuscularly, but this may take longer to have an effect. Thereafter, stress doses of hydrocortisone sodium succinate should be continued intravenously as 50- to 100-mg boluses every 6 hours or as a continuous infusion of 200 mg per day for the first 24 hours. The duration of continued high-dose corticosteroids will depend on the physiologic response of the individual (e.g., resolution of hypotension) and the nature of the precipitating cause. If a precipitating cause is identified and resolved, the patient is able to take food by mouth, and hypotension and electrolyte abnormalities resolve, the hydrocortisone dose can be tapered within 24 to 48 hours. Mineralocorticoids are not needed when large amounts of corticosteroids are given, but fludrocortisone acetate (Florinef Acetate), 0.05 to 0.2 mg orally per day, should be initiated when the dose is reduced and the patient is known or suspected to have primary adrenal failure.

Chronic Adrenal Insufficiency

Treatment of chronic adrenal insufficiency is the same whether the etiology is primary or secondary adrenal insufficiency, although any specific cause may require additional treatment. If the patient is established to have chronic adrenocortical insufficiency, treatment should include glucocorticoid (and mineralocorticoid in primary adrenal failure) replacement along with education about sick day corticoste-

---

TABLE 4. **Treatment of Suspected Adrenal Crisis**

1. Establish intravenous access.
2. Draw blood for stat serum electrolytes and glucose, routine plasma cortisol and ACTH measurements (if diagnosis of adrenal insufficiency not established). Do not wait for laboratory results.
3. Ensure 2 to 3 liters of 0.9% saline/5% dextrose as quickly as possible or as indicated based on blood pressure or central line monitoring.
4. Administer hydrocortisone sodium succinate (Solu-Cortef), 100 mg, intravenously immediately, and repeat 50 to 100 mg every 6 hours thereafter based on blood pressure response.
5. Identify cause of precipitating stress.

TABLE 5. **Treatment of Stress**

Minor Illness or Stress
- Increase glucocorticoid dose twofold to threefold (AM and PM) for duration of illness. Do not change mineralocorticoid dose.
- Inject contents of prefilled dexamethasone (Decadron), 4 mg, syringe intramuscularly if prolonged vomiting or symptoms of adrenal insufficiency.
- Contact physician if illness persists for more than 3 days, symptoms of adrenal insufficiency persist or worsen despite increased corticosteroid dose, or there is any change in level of consciousness.

Corticosteroid Coverage for Procedures or Hospitalization
- For most minor procedures under local anesthesia and most radiologic studies, no extra supplementation is needed.
- For moderately stressful procedures such as dental procedures, barium enema, endoscopy or arteriography, give a single 25- to 50-mg dose of hydrocortisone intravenously just before the procedure. In some cases the dose can be given orally the morning of the procedure.
- For major surgeries or other significant stress, hydrocortisone should be administered as a 100-mg intravenous injection on call to the operating room, before the induction of anesthesia. With a prolonged procedure, additional corticosteroids should be given during the operation. Increased corticosteroids will be required for the duration of a postoperative course or hospitalization.

roid coverage. All patients with adrenal insufficiency are advised to wear a medical alert bracelet. Hydrocortisone is the drug of choice because it has both glucocorticoid and mineralocorticoid effects. The general approach involves a maintenance dose of 15 to 40 mg orally per day; most patients require 15 to 25 mg per day, depending on weight and response to therapy. It is usually administered in two divided doses: two thirds in the morning and one third in the late afternoon or early evening. Fludrocortisone acetate in a dosage of 0.05 to 0.2 mg orally is required daily in most cases of primary failure. Prednisone has a longer half-life, with a 5- to 7.5-mg total dose required per day. Prednisone has less mineralocorticoid effect, so fludrocortisone is more likely to be required.

Stress doses of glucocorticoids should be given with trauma; surgery; stressful diagnostic or outpatient procedures, including dental work; fractures; fever; significant dehydration, as with heat stroke; or severe emotional stress (Table 5). Prefilled dexamethasone syringes can be prescribed for home use when there is protracted nausea or increased stress. The corticosteroid dose is increased proportional to the type of stress from two to three times usual replacement dose for small, planned procedures to larger doses of intravenous or intramuscular injections (50 to 100 mg) before and after larger planned procedures. Continued high-dose corticosteroids may be required for prolonged stress. The maximum hydrocortisone dose required for severe stress is 200 to 300 mg daily given as divided every-6-hour boluses or as a continuous infusion. The dose is reduced back to normal (as quickly as 50% reduction per day) as the stress subsides.

CUSHING'S SYNDROME

method of
STEVEN W. J. LAMBERTS, M.D.
Erasmus University
Rotterdam, The Netherlands

Cushing's syndrome is the clinical condition that develops after prolonged exposure of the body to excess levels of cortisol. This excess can result from the exogenous administration of adrenocorticotropic hormone (ACTH) or glucocorticoids, or from an endogenously increased secretion of cortisol, ACTH, or corticotropin-releasing hormone (CRH). A spectrum of physiologic and pathologic conditions is accompanied by prolonged activation of the hypothalamus-pituitary-adrenocortical (HPA) axis (Table 1). Although in some cases these states might represent the preclinical phase of Cushing's syndrome, clinically recognizable Cushing's syndrome is characterized by hypercortisolism accompanied by an escape of the normal regulatory mechanisms of the HPA axis; that is, an abnormal diurnal rhythm of ACTH and cortisol, an abnormal feedback control of the HPA axis; and an abnormal response to stress.

Endogenous Cushing's syndrome is ACTH dependent in 75 to 85% of all cases (Table 2). The two main causes are excessive pituitary ACTH secretion by a pituitary adenoma (Cushing's disease) and ectopic ACTH (or CRH) secretion. The ACTH-independent Cushing's syndrome is in most cases caused by unilateral benign or malignant adrenocortical tumors. A number of patients have been described with bilateral nodular adrenal hyperplasia and/or adenoma formation in which an increased expression of aberrant receptors for gastrin-inhibitory peptide, beta-adrenergic receptors, estradiol, or genetic factors (Carney complex) forms the pathogenetic basis.

DIAGNOSTIC STRATEGY

Cushing's syndrome is a deadly condition with limited survival. Causes of death include suicide, sepsis, peritonitis, and cardiovascular and cerebrovascular accidents. An accurate diagnosis is essential to initiate the appropriate treatment procedure promptly. In each patient the optimal diagnosis is made on the basis of a combination of clinical and biochemical assessments.

In the clinical recognition of patients with endogenous Cushing's syndrome, the presence of osteoporosis, muscle weakness and atrophy, easy bruisability of the skin, and

TABLE 1. **Classification of Hypercortisolism**

Chronic stress
Exercise
Severe disease
Psychiatric disorders
   Melancholic depression
   Anorexia nervosa
   Panic disorders
   Alcoholism
   Alcohol and narcotic withdrawal
Obesity
Diabetes mellitus
Pregnancy
Malnutrition
Glucocorticoid resistance
Cushing's syndrome

TABLE 2. **Causes of Endogenous Cushing's Syndrome and Their Relative Prevalence**

	% of Patients
ACTH Dependent	
Cushing's disease	65–70
Ectopic ACTH syndrome	10–15
ACTH Independent	
Adrenal adenoma	10
Adrenal carcinoma	10
Bilateral micronodular or macronodular hyperplasia	2–4

hypokalemia is most helpful in the differentiation from individuals with (truncal) obesity, hirsutism, hypertension, menstrual disorders, and/or glucose intolerance.

The laboratory assessment should be carried out in two steps, starting with establishing the presence of Cushing's syndrome and followed by the process of differentiating its origin.

Because many disease states as well as Cushing's syndrome are characterized by hypercortisolism (see Table 1), the demonstration of an increased excretion of free cortisol in a 24-hour urine sample has a low specificity. The most efficient screening tests include a low-dose dexamethasone suppression test, as well as the measurement of a sleeping midnight serum cortisol concentration that is invariably elevated (above 50 nmol per liter) in patients with Cushing's syndrome.

In terms of differential diagnosis, a persistently undetectable plasma ACTH concentration should lead to a search for an adrenal cause, and imaging (magnetic resonance imaging [MRI]) then differentiates between adrenal tumors (unilateral: adenomas or carcinomas) and the rare cases of bilateral micronodular or macronodular hyperplasia (see Table 2).

ACTH-dependent Cushing's syndrome is usually due to a pituitary adenoma (Cushing's disease), whereas occasionally very small ectopic sources ("occult" tumors) can be extremely difficult to diagnose. Results of high-dose oral or intravenous dexamethasone suppression tests and stimulation tests with CRH, desmopressin, or their combination, as well as the presence of very high ACTH levels, hypokalemia, and skin pigmentations, are helpful in the differentiation between a pituitary or ectopic source of ACTH production. Further support for either diagnosis can be given by imaging of the pituitary by MRI, computed tomography of the chest, or somatostatin-receptor imaging. Bilateral inferior petrosal sinus catheterization (with CRH stimulation) remains often vital to confirm the pituitary source of ACTH hypersecretion, however. This complicated diagnostic algorithm to establish the cause of Cushing's syndrome requires vast experience and skills. Because of the necessity of the prompt implementation of treatment, referral of patients with a clinical and biochemical diagnosis of Cushing's syndrome to specialized centers seems mandatory.

TREATMENT

Cushing's Disease

Most ACTH-producing tumors are microadenomas (90%). The treatment of choice of Cushing's disease is selective transsphenoidal adenomectomy by an experienced neurosurgeon after accurate preoperative localization of the corticotroph adenoma by MRI and/or a lateralization study at bilateral inferior petrosal sinus catheterization. The cure rate of this procedure is 75 to 85% for microadenomas but less than 50% for macroadenomas. The surgical procedure is complicated by meningitis, excessive bleeding (transient) diabetes insipidus, and/or cerebrospinal leaks in 3 to 4% of cases. Before surgery, patients should be prepared so that severe hypertension and hyperglycemia is controlled, whereas infected areas (especially in nose and sinuses) have been eradicated. Depending on the severity of the hypercortisolism some patients may benefit from a course of medical treatment to control hypercortisolism for a period of weeks to months preceding surgery.

All patients with Cushing's disease should receive glucocorticoid coverage intraoperatively and during the first 3 to 6 days postoperatively (e.g., 100 to 200 mg of hydrocortisone per day parenterally and orally thereafter) to prevent adrenal insufficiency after a successful and complete selective removal of the pituitary adenomas. It has become evident that ACTH secretion by the normal corticotrophs surrounding these adenomas is suppressed. This suppression often persists for many months after operation, after which the activity and regulation of the HPA axis gradually normalizes. This initial period after operation is accompanied by clinically and biochemically evident hypocortisolism (very low circulating serum cortisol levels, absence of a response to CRH or metyrapone stimulation). After a successful operative procedure the patient will be maintained on oral hydrocortisone replacement therapy (12 to 15 mg per m² per day) in two or three divided doses, which can only gradually be tapered off over a period of 6 to 12 months. During illness or severe stress the oral daily dose of hydrocortisone has to be tripled or be given parenterally. Recovery of the HPA axis can be monitored by measuring the morning serum cortisol concentrations before administering the morning steroid dose or by monitoring the response of the HPA axis to CRH.

The successful outcome of transsphenoidal surgery in patients with Cushing's disease (definition of "cure") characteristically includes a state of transient ACTH deficiency needing corticosteroid replacement therapy and initially (virtually) undetectable serum cortisol levels, which eventually return to normal.

In the case of a failure to achieve a "cure," reoperation of a microadenoma by means of the transsphenoidal route by an experienced neurosurgeon is successful in about 50% of patients.

Patients whose condition is not controlled by surgery are referred for external pituitary irradiation, which may cure 30 to 50% of patients after several years. Pendel rotation radiotherapy of 35 to 52 Gy with a daily fractional dose of 200 cGy by a linear accelerator seems optimal and especially in children with Cushing's disease has been reported to be successful as a primary treatment in about 50% of cases. Stereotactic radiosurgery with the gamma knife and with beams of cobalt-60 radiation is a promising

TABLE 3. **Drugs Used for Medical Therapy of Cushing's Syndrome**

Drug	Daily Dose	Complications and Restrictions
Ketoconazole (Nizoral)*	200–1200 mg	Liver toxicity, nausea, oligospermia
Aminoglutethimide (Cytadren)	1–2 gm	Drowsiness, rash, postural hypotension, dizziness, hypothyroidism
Metyrapone (Metopirone)*	1–4 gm	Hypokalemia, virilization, gastrointestinal disturbances
Mitotane (Lysodren)*	1–12 gm	Gastrointestinal disturbances, central nervous system depression, somnolence, dizziness, rash

*Not FDA approved for this indication.

treatment, especially in patients with adenoma remnants infiltrating or adjacent to the cavernous sinus.

Various drugs have been studied in the control of ACTH and/or cortisol hypersecretion. Drugs aimed at the pituitary level are largely unsuccessful; and an efficient control of ACTH release by pituitary adenomas by serotonin antagonists such as cyproheptadine (Periactin)* (12 to 24 mg per day), dopamine agonists such as bromocriptine (Parlodel)* (15 mg per day), or somatostatin analogues (octreotide [Sandostatin])* (300 μg per day), cannot be recommended in the routine treatment of patients with Cushing's disease. Also it remains unclear which factors determine the often transient and partial success of this pituitary-directed medical therapy in the limited (<10%) number of responders.

Drugs directly affecting cortisol production at the adrenal level are currently more successful (Table 3).

Ketoconazole

The best tolerated of these drugs is ketoconazole (Nizoral),* an imidazole-derivative antimycotic agent that inhibits various cytochrome P-450 enzymes, including the side-chain cleavage complex, 17,20-lyase, 11β-hydroxylase, and 17α-hydroxylase. Individual sensitivity to ketoconazole varies widely, necessitating close monitoring of steroid production and dose adjustment. Another approach is to administer 600 to 1200 mg per day and simultaneously replace the potential total suppression of cortisol secretion with low-dose dexamethasone (e.g., 0.25 mg twice daily). Interestingly, a ketoconazole-induced blockade of steroid synthesis in patients with Cushing's disease is not accompanied by an increase in ACTH levels, suggesting a glucocorticoid receptor–blocking effect of the drug as well. Substantial hepatic toxicity, which is in part dose dependent and mostly reversible is a common problem at higher doses of ketoconazole (see Table 3).

Aminoglutethimide

Aminoglutethimide (Cytadren), an anticonvulsant drug, inhibits several cytochrome P-450 steroidogenic enzymes. At three to four times daily administration of 250 to 500 mg orally an effective control of cortisol production in patients with Cushing's disease is reached in less than 50%, whereas a higher dose can often not be reached because of the dose-dependent sedation and rashes.

Metyrapone

Metyrapone (Metopirone)* (250 to 1000 mg four times daily) primarily inhibits 11β-hydroxylase activity and normalizes cortisol production in about 50% of patients with Cushing's disease. Side effects such as nausea, vomiting, acne, hirsutism, and hypokalemia limit its routine use in the medical control of hypercortisolism.

Mitotane

Mitotane (Lysodren)* is an adrenolytic agent that suppresses cortisol production by inhibiting 11β-hydroxylase and cholesterol side-chain cleavage enzymes, as well as by destroying adrenocortical cells. Mitotane (up to 12 grams per day), preferably given in milk or chocolate, induced a biochemical remission within a year after external pituitary irradiation in more than 80% of patients with Cushing's disease. However, in the follow-up, only about 50% of patients were cured after mitotane withdrawal. Severe gastrointestinal side effects often limit its use (see Table 3). The drug also induces mineralocorticoid deficiency in some patients, necessitating the simultaneous replacement with oral fludrocortisone (Florinef, 50 to 150 μg daily).

Ketoconazole, aminoglutethimide, metyrapone, and mitotane can be used separately or in combination with each other at lower individual doses. The advantage of such combinations at a lower dose is a lower incidence and severity of side effects. The main indications for their use in the treatment of Cushing's disease include temporary management of severe complex cases with muscle weakness, psychosis, or infections; the preoperative induction of eucortisolism to improve the patient's clinical condition; and after surgical failure to bridge the period before the optimal effect of radiotherapy is reached.

Mifepristone (RU 486),† at doses of 10 to 20 mg per kg per day, is a glucocorticoid receptor–blocking agent that has been used successfully to acutely block the deleterious effects of cortisol (e.g., in patients with Cushing's syndrome and severe psychosis). The efficacy of mifepristone therapy cannot be properly monitored, because cortisol production does not decrease.

In a minority of patients with Cushing's disease the effect of (repeated) transsphenoidal surgery followed by external pituitary irradiation and/or

*Not FDA approved for this indication.

*Not FDA approved for this indication.
†Not available in the United States.

gamma knife treatment, as well as medical treatment, is not effective to reach a normalization of cortisol secretion. In those few cases, bilateral adrenalectomy should be considered by laparoscopic intervention. In some patients with Cushing's disease, the changes in the negative feedback regulation after bilateral adrenalectomy are followed by the development of Nelson's syndrome, which comprises the development of rapidly and aggressively growing infiltrative ACTH-secreting tumors causing severe pigmentation.

Ectopic ACTH Secretion

In patients with ectopic ACTH secretion by tumors of causing Cushing's syndrome complete surgical extirpation of the neoplasm is mandatory. "Occult" tumors (mainly bronchial carcinoids or thymomas) often have to be removed by thoracotomy, whereas thyroidectomy of medullary thyroid cancers or (partial) pancreatectomy of islet cell cancers also involves major surgery. Most tumors secreting ACTH ectopically also express somatostatin receptors. Somatostatin receptor scintigraphy is often useful in the localization of the primary lesion, as well as often previously unknown (distant or local) metastases. A positive scan often predicts a good response of ACTH release to octreotide (300 μg per day SC), resulting in a temporary decrease in cortisol secretion and a (preoperative) improvement in the clinical condition. If the tumor is completely removed at operation, the patient generally undergoes prompt remission of Cushing's syndrome. Glucocorticoid replacement therapy in a tapering schedule (over weeks to several months) is necessary to wait for a return of normal ACTH secretion by the pituitary gland.

In many patients with ectopic ACTH secretion the tumor and its metastases cannot be completely removed. Radiotherapy (in the future possibly with radionuclide-coupled somatostatin analogues), chemotherapy, and embolization of the tumor and its (hepatic) metastases are treatment options in such individuals. Medical treatment with any, or combinations, of the drugs mentioned in Table 3 has to be initiated also in such patients, whereas in case of severe hypokalemia also spironolactone (Aldactone), 100 to 200 mg per day, is necessary. Despite this, bilateral adrenalectomy should be considered in some patients to acutely and definitively block cortisol production. A more rapid clinical improvement will thus be achieved, allowing aggressive surgical treatment of the primary tumor.

Adrenal Tumors

Unilateral removal of benign adenomas in patients with different forms of Cushing's syndrome (see Table 2) is currently done in most centers by laparojyscopic surgery. The advantages of this procedure include lower morbidity, less pain, shorter hospitalization, and more rapid return to work. In all patients, perioperative corticosteroid coverage and long-term glucocorticoid replacement therapy, which can be tapered when the HPA axis recovers, are mandatory.

Adrenal cancer is a rare tumor that generally carries a poor prognosis. The differentiation between adrenal cancer and adenoma is often difficult in the absence of metastases. In the case of incidentalomas, adrenal tumors larger than 5 cm in diameter should be resected surgically. Radical excision with en bloc resection of any local invasion offers the best chance for cure and prolongs life significantly. Mitotane (up to 12 grams per day) as an adjuvant treatment to surgery after the removal of the primary tumor and its known metastases offers advantages both regarding survival and remission.

DIABETES INSIPIDUS

method of
SUMANT S. CHUGH, M.D.
Boston Medical Center
Boston, Massachusetts

and

HENRY M. YAGER, M.D.
Newton-Wellesley Hospital
Newton, Massachusetts

The clinical features of diabetes insipidus (DI) result from a deficiency in the action of antidiuretic hormone (ADH) caused by reduced ADH production (central DI), excessive ADH degradation (excessive vasopressinase syndrome), or reduced renal tubular ADH response (nephrogenic DI). Accordingly, the major goals of treatment of DI are to replenish ongoing free water losses, reduce urine output by increasing ADH activity, and minimize nocturia to enable a normal sleep pattern. Whereas hormone therapy is the cornerstone of treatment in central DI, appropriate diuretics and modification of dietary solute load usually control nephrogenic DI.

GENERAL PRINCIPLES

The most important initial step in the treatment of DI is correction of the underlying water deficit. Hypotension must first be corrected by infusion of 0.9% saline, regardless of the presence of hypernatremia. Once this is done, the free water deficit can be calculated as follows:

$$\text{Free water deficit} = 0.5 \times \text{premorbid lean body weight} \times \left(\frac{\text{plasma Na}}{140} - 1\right)$$

Free water deficit is repleted either with intravenous (IV) 5% dextrose in water (D5W) or oral (PO) water. In addition to the free water deficit, the ongoing urinary free water loss and the estimated insensible losses (usually approximately 30 mL per hour) and gastrointestinal losses must be added before the hourly infusion rate is calculated. To calculate the electrolyte free water loss in urine, it is important to check urine Na + K concentration rather than osmolality, which includes electrolytes, urea, and ammonium excretion. For example, if the urine Na + K concentration is 50 mEq per liter in a patient with a serum Na concentration of 150 mEq per liter, every liter of urine can be viewed as one-third isotonic urine and two-thirds electrolyte free urine (i.e., one third of a liter has a Na + K concentration of 150 mEq per liter). The latter two thirds needs to be added to the calculation of replacement of free water. In order to reduce serum Na, the Na concentration of the IV fluids must be below the Na + K concentration of the ongoing fluid loss.

Most physicians supplement D5W infusions with infusions of 0.45% saline and PO or IV potassium chloride (appropriately diluted) to compensate for ongoing sodium and potassium losses. If one-quarter isotonic saline plus potassium chloride are used instead of the aforementioned regimen, the contribution of K to fluid osmolality needs to be recognized. For example, one-quarter isotonic saline plus 40 mEq per liter of potassium chloride has the same tonicity as half-normal saline and may be inappropriate for lowering serum Na if Na and K losses are not large. One major disadvantage of D5W at very high infusion rates is that the glucose load may exceed the body's metabolic capacity, resulting in hyperglycemia and an ADH-resistant DI-like condition caused by solute diuresis from glycosuria. This can be overcome by frequent blood glucose monitoring to avoid hyperglycemia and giving enteral rather than IV free water. For patients with hypernatremia and coma or seizures, the serum Na level may initially be lowered at a rate of 1 mEq per liter per hour to a level of 160 mEq per liter. If the patient is still symptomatic at this level of serum Na, the serum Na may be lowered at the same rate, but not below 150 mEq per liter. Most often, an initial decrease in serum Na of 3 to 4 mEq per liter stops the seizures. Once seizures are terminated, it is usually safe to correct the free water deficit over 48 hours, with serum Na declining at an hourly rate of 0.5 mEq per liter. In general, chronic hypernatremia should be corrected more slowly than acute hypernatremia.

TREATMENT OF CENTRAL DIABETES INSIPIDUS

Current literature favors the use of 1-desamino-8-D-arginine vasopressin (DDAVP or desmopressin), a synthetic long-acting analogue of arginine vasopressin (AVP) that lacks vasopressor activity, in the control of central DI. As indicated in Table 1, DDAVP can be administered via the intranasal, subcutaneous (SC), IV, or PO route. Conventional treatment in an alert and ambulatory patient is usually initiated with 10 μg of intranasal DDAVP at bedtime to control nocturia, with further increments of 10 μg as required. When the rhinal tube is used, increments of 5 μg can be made. Once nocturia is relieved, additional daytime doses are added to control polyuria. Most patients achieve adequate control with 10 to 20 μg once or twice daily of the nasal spray. A reasonable alternative is to initiate treatment with DDAVP tablets with 0.05 mg PO at bedtime (half of a 0.1-mg tablet), to be titrated upward to a maximal dose of 1.2 mg per day in two to three divided doses. Only about 5% of the oral form is absorbed from the gut. Accordingly, a 0.1-mg tablet is equivalent to about 5 μg of the nasal spray. Some patients taking intranasal DDAVP need to switch to oral DDAVP during episodes of nasal congestion because of erratic nasal absorption. Experience with the tablet form is more limited than that with the intranasal form. In a study comparing the antidiuretic effect of oral and intranasal forms of DDAVP, the bioequivalent intranasal/oral ratio was approximately 1:16. Whereas both duration and magnitude of the antidiuretic effect were greater for a PO dose of 0.2 mg than with 0.1 mg, increasing the dose from 0.2 to 0.4 mg increased only the duration of action. The tablets were well tolerated, and no major side effects warranting medication withdrawal were noted. Some patients find the tablets simpler to use.

The most important defense mechanism against metabolic complications in patients with central DI is intact thirst. Most patients are able to remain nearly euvolemic if they have full access to adequate amounts of water. Therefore, when therapy for DI is initiated, the patient should be instructed to make a conscious effort to drink less and only in response to thirst. The thirst mechanism gradually adapts to the new steady state. The perception of thirst, however, can be modified by drugs like anticholinergics and beta blockers, cigarette smoking, elevated angiotensin II levels, or mouth breathing; therefore, close initial follow-up and patient education are warranted.

Treatment of the unconscious or uncooperative patient is initiated with 1 μg of SC or IV DDAVP, because it is 5 to 10 times more potent than the intranasal form. Increasing the dose further increases the duration of antidiuresis more than the magnitude of its effect. The usual indication for the use of subcutaneous aqueous AVP is acute onset of DI, usually after head injury or neurosurgery. The short duration of action of AVP facilitates rapid withdrawal of the agent as pituitary function recovers, thereby avoiding hyponatremia in the patient receiving IV D5W. With both AVP and DDAVP, follow-up doses should be timed with the reappearance of polyuria. Because DI after head injury may be transient or triphasic, hormonal therapy should be periodically withheld and serial urine volume and urine osmolality measured to evaluate the patient for recovery of DI. The treatment of an alert, adipsic patient poses a major challenge to the patient, the patient's family, and health care providers. Constant monitoring of intake and output, daily weights, serial vital signs, and a regulated fluid regimen are often required. Appropriate fluid intake in such patients is calculated from the sum of the urine output and the sensible and insensible losses.

The perioperative patient, like the unconscious patient, is usually well managed with IV or SC DDAVP, with resumption of the baseline regimen as soon as possible after surgery. To avoid excessive intravenous hydration, weight, blood pressure, intake and output, and serum Na levels should be monitored serially. For patients with mild partial central DI not receiving DDAVP who need to have PO fluid restricted for a diagnostic procedure, intravenous hydration with

TABLE 1. **Pharmacologic Treatment of Diabetes Insipidus**

Trade Name	Chemical Composition	Concentration	Total Dose Range/24 h	Usual Duration of Action	Comments
DDAVP nasal spray	Desmopressin acetate	100 µg/mL	10–40 µg	8–12 h for single dose of 10 µg, 16–20 h for single dose of 20–40 µg	Delivers multiples of 10 µg per spray
DDAVP rhinal tube	Desmopressin acetate	100 µg/mL	10–40 µg	Same as for the nasal spray	Delivers multiples of 5 µg per dose
DDAVP tablets	Desmopressin acetate	0.1-, 0.2-mg scored tablets	0.05–1.2 mg	8–12 h for 0.2 mg, 16–20 h for 0.4 mg	
DDAVP injection	Desmopressin acetate	4 µg/mL	2–4 µg	10–14 h for 0.5–1 µg, 18 h for 2 µg	Subcutaneous or intravenous
Pitressin	Arginine vasopressin	20 USP U/mL	5–10 U	2–6 h	Prefer subcutaneous use; avoid intravenous use in view of pressor activity
HydroDIURIL	Hydrochlorothiazide*	25-, 50-, 100-mg tablets	50–100 mg	24–48 h	Other thiazide diuretics may be used in equivalent doses
Midamor	Amiloride hydrochloride*	5-mg tablets	5–20 mg	24 h	Drug of choice for lithium-induced nephrogenic diabetes insipidus
Indocin	Indomethacin*	25-, 50-mg capsules	100–150 mg	6–8 h	Anecdotally more effective in managing acute nephrogenic diabetes insipidus than thiazides or amiloride

*Not FDA approved for this indication.

hypotonic fluids to match the urine output should be started as soon as restriction of PO fluids is imposed. If high urine flow rates are desired, as in certain chemotherapy protocols, the hormone therapy may be discontinued for the period if vigorous PO or IV hydration can be maintained. Alternatively, antidiuretic therapy may be continued with concomitant administration of a loop diuretic and fluids. Close monitoring of physical and biochemical parameters as indicated earlier is imperative.

Hyponatremia may occur as a complication during the course of treatment of DI with DDAVP in the setting of vigorous PO hydration or treatment with hypotonic intravenous fluids, because the ADH activity is nonsuppressible. Mild to moderate hyponatremia is treated with volume restriction alone, whereas severe hyponatremia may necessitate hypertonic saline and furosemide (Lasix). In severe situations, interruption of DDAVP therapy may be justified to ensure a gradual rise in serum Na under closely monitored conditions; the level is not to exceed 12 mEq per liter per day. With the widespread use of DDAVP, the use of chlorpropamide (Diabinese), clofibrate (Atromid-S), and carbamazepine (Tegretol) in incomplete central DI has been on the decline. Both chlorpropamide* (usual dose, 125 to 250 mg once to twice a day; main side effect: hypoglycemia) and carbamazepine* (100 to 300 mg twice a day) enhance ADH effect, whereas clofibrate* (500 mg four times a day) enhances ADH secretion. Thiazide diuretics and solute restriction also help diminish urine output in central DI, as described in the next section.

DIABETES INSIPIDUS IN PREGNANCY

Pregnancy is associated with a reduced osmotic threshold for thirst and ADH release, and increased production of ADH and vasopressinase, an enzyme that degrades ADH. Unmasking of subclinical central and nephrogenic DI during pregnancy or the postpartum period are well documented. The excessive vasopressinase syndrome that occurs occasionally in pregnancy is treated appropriately with DDAVP, which, unlike AVP, is resistant to the effects of vasopressinase. Dosages of DDAVP required may be somewhat higher than those needed for central DI. Some pregnant patients may have a component of nephrogenic DI and may not respond to DDAVP, but they usually respond to treatment with thiazide diuretics.

TREATMENT OF NEPHROGENIC DIABETES INSIPIDUS

Treatment of nephrogenic DI is usually initiated with thiazide diuretics and a low-salt diet. Thiazide diuretics such as hydrochlorothiazide* (HCTZ; 25 mg once or twice a day) act by inducing mild volume depletion, thus increasing proximal tubular sodium absorption and reducing the delivery of tubular fluid to ADH-sensitive sites in the distal nephron. Thia-

*Not FDA approved for this indication.

*Not FDA approved for this indication.

zide diuretic–induced hypovolemia also leads to an increase in renal medullary interstitial osmolality by an unclear mechanism. Urine volume is often reduced by over 50%. Combination therapy of HCTZ and amiloride is beneficial, because it enhances the initial natriuresis and reduces the hypokalemia induced by HCTZ. For patients with lithium-induced nephrogenic DI, amiloride* (Midamor) is the drug of choice because its predominant effect is mediated by closure of Na channels through which lithium enters collecting tubular cells and interferes with the effect of ADH. Patients taking amiloride and lithium should be monitored for hyperkalemia and lithium intoxication. The latter develops in a minority of patients as a result of mild volume depletion caused by the diuretic, leading to increased proximal tubular reabsorption of lithium. Loop diuretics such as furosemide (Lasix) interfere with the generation of medullary hypertonicity, causing relative ADH resistance, and should not be used to treat nephrogenic DI.

Because reducing the net urinary solute excretion will decrease the urine output at a given urine osmolality, there is a role for salt and protein restriction in the treatment of nephrogenic DI. A low-salt diet should be prescribed at initiation of treatment with HCTZ. Mild protein restriction is also helpful in reducing the urinary solute load by reducing urea generation. Compliance with these measures can be evaluated by measuring 24-hour urinary excretion of Na and urea nitrogen. Because prostaglandins antagonize the action of ADH, inhibition of prostaglandin synthesis by nonsteroidal anti-inflammatory drugs (NSAIDs), such as indomethacin* (Indocin), may reduce the urine output by 25 to 50%. The effect of NSAIDs and HCTZ may be partially additive. However, not all NSAIDs are equally effective in a given patient, inasmuch as some patients respond to indomethacin (100 to 150 mg per day in two to three divided doses), but not to ibuprofen* (Advil). Sulindac (Clinoril) is also less effective, because in comparison with other NSAIDs, it tends to relatively spare renal prostaglandin synthesis. In general, the thiazide-amiloride combination has fewer side effects than the thiazide-NSAID combination and is therefore preferred. Some anecdotal evidence is suggestive of superiority of indomethacin over HCTZ or amiloride in the acute management of nephrogenic DI. Lastly, some patients with nephrogenic DI may have only partial resistance to ADH, and therefore DDAVP may be of some benefit in these patients if adequate response to the aforementioned measures is lacking.

---

*Not FDA approved for this indication.

HYPERPARATHYROIDISM AND HYPOPARATHYROIDISM

method of
ELIZABETH A. STREETEN, M.D., and
MICHAEL A. LEVINE, M.D.
The Johns Hopkins University School of Medicine
Baltimore, Maryland

HYPERPARATHYROIDISM

Primary Hyperparathyroidism

Incidence

Primary hyperparathyroidism (PHPT) is the most common cause of hypercalcemia in patients who are evaluated in the outpatient clinic. The incidence of PHPT has changed significantly since the mid-1970s. Before the routine measurement of serum calcium, the incidence of PHPT was 10 to 15 per 100,000 person years in the United States. However, soon after the inclusion of serum calcium measurement on the automated serum chemistry panel in July 1974, the incidence increased to more than 100 per 100,000 person years. Since that time, the incidence has been decreasing, for unknown reasons, such that the incidence of PHPT is currently estimated to be less than 10 per 100,000 person years. The prevalence of PHPT is slightly higher in women than men (3:2), with a peak incidence in the fifth to sixth decades. PHPT is far less common in adolescence and is unusual in childhood.

Etiology

Patients with PHPT may have single or multigland parathyroid disease (Table 1). In most patients (80 to 85%), PHPT is the result of a solitary parathyroid adenoma. Parathyroid adenomas are typically benign, monoclonal tumors. Occasional patients have double adenomas, which can be asynchronous, or parathyroid cysts. Most parathyroid adenomas are in the neck, but in some cases (1 to 5%) an adenoma is located ectopically in the thyroid, in the mediastinum, or at the angle of the jaw (an "undescended" gland). Approximately 10 to 15% of patients with PHPT have multigland disease, previously termed *parathyroid hyperplasia*, in which all four (or more) parathyroid glands are involved. Parathyroid enlargement in multigland disease can be asymmetric, and some glands may appear normal sized. Multigland disease occurs most commonly in patients with autosomal dominant forms of PHPT, such as familial hyperparathyroidism. PHPT also occurs as a component of the multiple endocrine neoplasia (MEN) type 1 syndrome, which also includes pituitary and pancreatic tumors, and results from defects in the *MENIN* gene. PHPT occurs less commonly in patients with MEN-2A, in whom medullary thyroid cancer and pheochromocytoma develop because of defects in the *ret* proto-oncogene. Familial benign hypo-

TABLE 1. **Causes of Hyperparathyroidism**

Primary hyperparathyroidism
  Single adenoma
  Multiple adenoma
  Multigland hyperplasia
    Sporadic or familial
    MEN-1 or MEN-2A
    Familial benign hypocalciuric hypercalcemia
  Parathyroid cancer
  Lithium
Secondary hyperparathyroidism
  Chronic renal failure
  Vitamin D deficiency
    Nutritional
    Gastrointestinal malabsorption
    Hepatobiliary disease
    Drug induced (phenytoin, phenobarbital, and glucocorticoids)
  Pseudohypoparathyroidism
  Renal hypercalciuria
  Untreated hypothyroidism
  Defective vitamin D action
    Defective calcitriol receptor
    Defective 1-alpha-hydroxylase activity
Tertiary hyperparathyroidism
  Renal osteodystrophy
  Prolonged administration of phosphorus

Abbreviation: MEN = multiple endocrine neoplasia.

calciuric hypercalcemia (FBHH) is also characterized by parathyroid hyperplasia, but differs from other forms of PHPT in that patients lack symptoms of hypercalcemia despite an onset during the first decade of life. Loss-of-function mutations in the gene encoding the parathyroid calcium-sensing receptor are present in most patients with FBHH. Heritable forms of multigland parathyroid disease are more likely to be diagnosed at a younger age (e.g., 20 to 30 years) than solitary adenomas. Parathyroid tumors are malignant in less than 1% of cases, and these patients tend to present with severe PHPT and a palpable neck mass (50%).

Although specific single-gene defects have been identified as the basis of most forms of inherited or sporadic multigland parathyroid disease, most solitary parathyroid adenomas lack an identifiable genetic cause. Acquired (i.e., somatic) mutations in the *MENIN* gene appear to be the most common genetic defects in solitary parathyroid adenomas, but are present in less than one third of these tumors, and other genes must be involved. Environmental factors also have been implicated in the development of PHPT, notably prior neck irradiation.

Clinical Manifestations

Because PHPT is frequently recognized only after the incidental discovery of hypercalcemia on a routine multichannel chemistry panel, at the time of diagnosis many patients lack the specific clinical signs and symptoms that have traditionally been ascribed to the disorder. However, some patients do experience consequences of either hypercalcemia or excessive parathyroid hormone (PTH), and may have one or more of the classic symptoms and signs of PHPT: "stones" (kidney stones), "bones" (low bone

mass or, rarely, radiographic evidence of osteitis fibrosa cystica), "abdominal groans" (pancreatitis, peptic ulcer disease, constipation), and "psychic overtones" (depression, lethargy, poor concentration). In addition, generalized "moans" may result from myalgias and arthralgias. Muscle weakness due to a neuropathic myopathy or arthritis due to pseudogout can also occur.

Laboratory/Radiographic Evaluation

Hypercalcemia is the biochemical hallmark of PHPT and is an essential diagnostic criterion. Several determinations of serum calcium may be required to confirm hypercalcemia because it may occur only intermittently. Routine determinations of serum calcium measure the concentration of total serum calcium, which can sometimes provide misleading information. For example, hypercalcemia may result from elevated or abnormal circulating proteins or from hemoconcentration induced by prolonged application of the tourniquet. By contrast, total serum calcium can be normal in patients with PHPT who have abnormally low concentrations of serum albumin. Determination of the ionized rather than total calcium concentration may be necessary in patients with serum protein abnormalities to avoid these diagnostic pitfalls.

The serum phosphate level is usually in the low or low normal range because of depressed renal tubular reabsorption. A mild hyperchloremic (Cl > 103 mEq per liter) metabolic acidosis is common. Additional biochemical features of PHPT include increased circulating concentrations of 1,25-dihydroxyvitamin D, increased urinary excretion of nephrogenous cyclic AMP, and decreased tubular reabsorption of phosphate (maximum tubular reabsorptive rate [TmP]/glomerular filtration rate). Several formulas that use the serum levels of calcium, phosphate, chloride, albumin, or alkaline phosphatase have been devised in an effort to distinguish between PHPT and other causes of hypercalcemia. None of these algorithms is entirely satisfactory, however.

A 24-hour collection (or at least a random sample) of urine should be obtained for determination of calcium and creatinine (Table 2). Patients with FBHH show relative hypocalciuria (a low 24-hour urinary calcium excretion or a ratio of calcium clearance to creatinine clearance that is less than 0.01) and serum levels of PTH are usually, but not always, nor-

TABLE 2. **Differential Diagnosis of an Elevated Parathyroid Hormone**

	Serum Ca	Immunoreactive Parathyroid Hormone	Urine Ca
Primary hyperparathyroidism	H	H	N or H
Familial hypocalciuric hypercalcemia	H	N/L or H	L
Secondary hyperparathyroidism	N/L	H	L, N, or H
Tertiary hyperparathyroidism	H	H	?

Abbreviations: L = low; N = normal; N/L = normal-low; H = high.

mal. FBHH is uncommon, but because patients seldom experience the consequences of hypercalcemia, it is important to distinguish this disorder from other causes of hypercalcemia. Tests that measure urinary excretion of breakdown products of type 1 collagen (e.g., deoxypyridine or N-telopeptide) can provide a sensitive index of bone resorption, and can be performed using the first or second urine void in the morning.

Primary HPT and malignancy account for over 90% of cases of hypercalcemia. The availability of highly sensitive and specific immunometric assays for the sequence of intact PTH, which has 84 amino acids, has greatly simplified the diagnosis of PHPT and makes extensive diagnostic evaluation unnecessary in most cases. The use of immunoassays for intact PTH and for PTH-related protein, the most common mediator of humoral hypercalcemia of malignancy, further refines the distinction between these two disorders. Circulating PTH is high in PHPT and low or undetectable in malignancy. Conversely, PTH-related protein is high in most patients with humoral hypercalcemia of malignancy and undetectable in PHPT.

With few exceptions, low serum levels of PTH accompany nonparathyroid causes of hypercalcemia. Chronic treatment with lithium may produce hypercalcemia associated with an elevated serum level of PTH, a picture indistinguishable from PHPT. Discontinuation of lithium therapy, if possible, may be necessary to determine the proper diagnosis.

Bone density measurements may reveal unsuspected osteoporosis in many patients with mild PHPT. Dual energy x-ray absorptiometry of the hip and spine is the recommended technique to detect reduced bone density, and can often help guide subsequent treatment. Excessive PTH tends to reduce cortical bone mass (e.g., hip) more than trabecular bone mass (e.g., spine). Consequently, analysis of the distal one third of the forearm, which is relatively enriched in cortical bone, may provide additional useful information.

In selected cases, a single abdominal radiograph or abdominal sonography can be useful to screen for calcium-containing kidney stones. Although computed tomography (CT) is more sensitive for detecting small stones or microcalcifications (nephrocalcinosis), the radiation involved makes its routine use imprudent. Parathyroid imaging studies (e.g., ultrasonography, technetium-labeled sestamibi scan, CT, magnetic resonance imaging [MRI]) are unnecessary in the patient who has not previously undergone a neck exploration.

Diagnosis

Patients with PHPT should have hypercalcemia and an elevated PTH; they often have hypercalciuria. An elevated serum level of intact PTH excludes virtually all nonparathyroid causes of hypercalcemia (e.g., malignancy, granulomatous disease). However, levels of intact PTH may be normal in up to 10% of patients with surgically proven PHPT. In these hypercalcemic patients, the "normal" concentration of intact PTH is inappropriate, and is consistent with the presence of nonsuppressible or autonomous parathyroid tissue (e.g., a parathyroid adenoma). Often, measurement of mid-molecule or carboxy-terminal PTH fragments provides the necessary biochemical confirmation of hyperparathyroidism in these cases. A 24-hour determination of urine calcium can identify patients with FBHH, in whom the urinary excretion of calcium (<100 mg per 24 hours) and clearance ratio of calcium/creatinine (<0.01) are lower than in other forms of PHPT.

Treatment

Despite significant advances in our understanding of the molecular pathophysiology of PHPT, surgical removal of hyperfunctioning parathyroid glands remains the only definitive treatment available. However, many patients do not require treatment, and not all patients benefit equally from surgery. Patients with PHPT who have neither signs nor symptoms of the disease are defined as having asymptomatic PHPT, a condition addressed by participants of a National Institutes of Health (NIH) Consensus Conference in 1990. The NIH Consensus Conference produced a set of guidelines that focused on the morbidity of PHPT, and concluded that patients older than 50 years of age be placed under medical surveillance if they failed to meet specific indications for surgery: (1) serum calcium 1 mg per dL or more above normal or a history of life-threatening hypercalcemia; (2) extreme hypercalciuria (>400 mg per 24 hours); (3) reduced bone density (>2 standard deviations below age-matched normal); 4) reduced creatinine clearance or history of kidney stones; and (5) the presence of typical symptoms of hypercalcemia (myalgias, arthralgias, epigastric pain, fatigue). Using these guidelines, approximately half of patients with PHPT have one or more indications for surgery. Young age (<50 years) and physician or patient choice are also accepted indications for parathyroid surgery once a definitive diagnosis of PHPT is made.

Preoperative localization studies (e.g., ultrasonography, sestamibi, CT, and MRI) are unnecessary before a first surgical exploration and are unlikely to reduce operative time or increase the likelihood of success when an experienced operator performs surgery. On the other hand, imaging studies of the neck and mediastinum play an important role in the preoperative evaluation of patients with persistent or recurrent PHPT. In these patients, the initial imaging studies should be noninvasive, and include sestamibi scanning and neck ultrasonography. If a suspected parathyroid lesion is co-localized with both techniques, additional imaging studies usually are not required. When a suspected parathyroid adenoma is identified only by ultrasonography, further confirmation can be obtained by sonographically guided needle aspiration. Aspirated material can be subjected to cytologic analysis and assayed for intact PTH. It is necessary to make special arrangements with the pathology laboratory before aspirating a lesion to ensure proper handling and processing of the specimen.

If ultrasonography and sestamibi scanning fail to localize parathyroid tissue, CT and MRI should be performed. If all noninvasive procedures fail to localize the abnormal tissue, selective arteriography and venous sampling can be considered for localization. These procedures should be performed only by radiologists who are experienced in the techniques.

Parathyroid surgery is typically performed under general anesthesia through a collar incision at the base of the neck. However, some surgeons now perform parathyroid surgery under local anesthesia using minimally invasive techniques, developments that are particularly appropriate for patients who are poor candidates for general anesthesia or protracted surgery. In cases of a single adenoma, at least one additional gland should be identified and sampled by biopsy to confirm that it is normal parathyroid tissue to exclude multigland disease. At the time of surgery, the size of the parathyroid gland often provides the best determination of whether it is normal ($7 \times 4 \times 2$ mm or less), because histologic study cannot always distinguish a normal gland from one that is mildly hyperplastic. If the second parathyroid gland found is enlarged, it is removed and the remaining two glands should then be located. If all four glands are enlarged at surgery, the preferred surgery is total parathyroidectomy with reimplantation of the most normal-appearing gland (minced and marked with surgical clips) into the forearm muscle. Additional parathyroid tissue should be cryopreserved, if possible. Approximately 2 to 3 months after implantation, fresh autografts perform as normal parathyroid tissue in over 95% of cases; cryopreserved autografts function in 50 to 70% of cases. In rare cases, hyperparathyroidism recurs years later in the forearm graft, at which time fragments can be removed under local anesthesia. If it is not possible to perform a simultaneous total parathyroidectomy and autograft, the surgeon should remove only three and one-half parathyroid glands, and leave in situ approximately 30 to 40 mg of the most normal-appearing parathyroid tissue. Although this subtotal parathyroidectomy is less difficult, the technique is associated with a 10 to 20% risk of recurrent PHPT with long-term follow-up.

Medical Management

Medical surveillance is appropriate for patients who are poor surgical candidates or who have mild PHPT and no surgical indications. No effective medical therapies are available to treat PHPT, and thus patients who require long-term treatment should be referred for surgery. Patients who are not referred for surgery should be followed conservatively and should have serum calcium measured every 6 months and bone density and renal function assessed annually. No firm guidelines have been established for the method of monitoring bone mass or for the duration of monitoring in patients who have apparently stable bone density. Although dual energy x-ray absorpti-

ometry of the spine and hip is the preferred technique to assess bone density, measurement of the distal one third of the forearm may be an acceptable alternative in patients with PHPT because preferential loss of cortical bone occurs in this disorder.

Patients should be advised that dehydration could worsen hypercalcemia and predispose to kidney stones. Thus, patients should be instructed to drink plenty of fluids (approximately 2 liters per day) and to avoid diuretics. Thiazide diuretics can reduce urinary calcium excretion through a direct action on the renal tubule. Although more potent loop diuretics such as furosemide (Lasix) produce a calciuretic effect at very high doses, at more typical doses these diuretics promote extracellular volume contraction and consequently lead to reduced renal calcium clearance. Calcium and vitamin D supplements should be avoided because they can worsen hypercalciuria or hypercalcemia. By contrast, a very-low-calcium diet can stimulate PTH secretion and may accelerate bone resorption. Therefore, patients should be advised to maintain a normal (approximately 1000 mg per day) calcium diet.

Efforts are ongoing to develop medical therapies. Specific PTH antagonists are undergoing evaluation, and calcimimetic compounds, which sensitize the calcium-sensing receptor on the parathyroid cell and can reduce PTH secretion, hold even greater promise. In postmenopausal women, estrogen replacement therapy can lower serum calcium by 1 mg per dL and prevent progressive bone loss, but PTH remains elevated. Newer-generation bisphosphonates such as alendronate (Fosamax), pamidronate (Aredia), and risedronate (Actonel) lower the serum calcium level during short-term therapy, but their beneficial effects on serum calcium or bone mass over longer periods of treatment remain to be demonstrated. Oral phosphate is a relatively reliable therapy, particularly in patients who have a serum phosphorus of less than 3.7 mg per dL. Administration of 1 to 2 grams per day of phosphate (e.g., K-Phos Neutral 250 mg tabs, two tabs three times per day) can reduce concentrations of serum and urinary calcium, but its usefulness is limited because it cannot be used safely in patients with renal insufficiency, and diarrhea develops in many patients. Oral phosphate can increase the serum phosphorus concentration, which can stimulate PTH release and cause soft tissue calcification if the calcium-phosphate product is exceeded.

Hypercalcemic crisis in severe or acute PHPT should be treated urgently. Intravenous infusion of 0.9% saline for rehydration and diuresis should be administered immediately at 200 to 800 mL per hour, depending on the severity of hypercalcemia and the cardiovascular status. Patients should be monitored closely because some may become hypernatremic. The combination of calcitonin (Calcimar) and pamidronate* (Aredia) is a rapid and effective way to treat hypercalcemia. Calcitonin acts within 12 hours, whereas the maximal effects of pamidronate may be

---

*Not FDA approved for this indication.

delayed for 48 to 72 hours. Pamidronate should be given as a single intravenous infusion of 15 to 90 mg, depending on the severity of the hypercalcemia, over 2 to 24 hours in 500 mL of 0.9% saline. Exploratory neck surgery should be undertaken, as described previously, as soon as an elevated PTH is confirmed and the patient is stable.

Secondary Hyperparathyroidism

Diagnosis

Secondary, or adaptive, HPT is characterized by an elevated concentration of PTH and a low or low-normal serum calcium level.

Etiology

The most common cause of clinically significant secondary HPT is chronic renal failure, and increased PTH secretion can be documented even in patients who have only mild renal insufficiency (i.e., glomerular filtration rate of 30 to 40 mL per minute). Multiple factors in renal failure contribute to the development of secondary HPT, including vitamin D deficiency (the kidney performs the final step in vitamin D production, 1-alpha hydroxylation, to produce 1,25-dihydroxyvitamin D_3), phosphorus retention (which further contributes to hypocalcemia), and skeletal resistance to PTH. In addition, parathyroid glands from patients with renal failure have decreased numbers of receptors for 1,25-dihydroxyvitamin D and calcium, which reduces the sensitivity of the parathyroid cells to the suppressive effects of these two ligands on PTH synthesis and secretion.

Other causes of secondary HPT include vitamin D deficiency and renal hypercalciuria. Nutritional deficiency of vitamin D, once considered to be uncommon in the United States because of supplementation of milk and other foods with vitamin D, is now diagnosed with alarming frequency in certain high-risk populations. Dark-skinned infants who are exclusively breast-fed for more than 6 months and who do not receive vitamin supplements are at greatest risk for development of vitamin D deficiency. In addition, vitamin D deficiency is common among the homebound elderly who avoid milk, sunlight, and vitamin supplements. Vitamin D deficiency also occurs in patients with hepatobiliary disease or gastrointestinal malabsorption and in patients who use medications that accelerate vitamin D metabolism (e.g., phenytoin, phenobarbital) or antagonize vitamin D action (e.g., glucocorticoids). Renal hypercalciuria is an uncommon cause of secondary HPT and calcium kidney stones, and likely represents a defect in proximal renal tubule reabsorption of calcium.

Treatment

The treatment of secondary HPT is guided by recognition of the underlying pathophysiologic process. In cases of nutritional vitamin D deficiency, treatment should consist of calcium and vitamin D. Doses of vitamin D_2 (ergocalciferol) that range from 10,000 to 60,000 IU (250 to 1500 µg) per month are similarly effective in children and adults. Higher doses, or parenteral treatment, may shorten the period of treatment needed to reverse vitamin D depletion, but may also increase the risk of vitamin D intoxication. Calcium conservation is very efficient during the early stages of treatment, but supplementation with additional calcium (1000 to 2000 mg elemental calcium per day in three divided doses for adults) restores mineralized bone and reverses secondary HPT more quickly. Several months of treatment may be necessary for complete resolution of secondary HPT and correction of all biochemical and skeletal abnormalities. In many patients, continued vitamin D supplementation is required to prevent a recurrence. A daily oral supplement of 10 µg (400 IU) of vitamin D_2 or vitamin D_3 is adequate for children and young adults, but studies support the recommendation that older people receive 15 to 20 µg (600 to 800 IU) of vitamin D per day.

In vitamin D deficiency due to fat malabsorption, higher doses of ergocalciferol (e.g., 1.25 mg or 50,000 IU one to three times per week) may be necessary to maintain normal plasma calcifediol levels, although higher levels are necessary in some patients to achieve normal calcium absorption. Alternatively, use of more polar compounds, such as calcifediol (Calderol; 25[OH]D_3, 20 to 30 µg per day) or calcitriol (Rocaltrol; 1,25-dihydroxyvitamin D_3, 0.25 to 1.0 µg per day) may be more efficacious. Parenteral preparations of vitamin D in oil are available, but absorption after intramuscular injection is unpredictable. The dose and frequency of administration of vitamin D or metabolite must be adjusted individually for each patient to achieve normal serum levels of calcium, phosphorus, alkaline phosphatase, PTH, and 25(OH)D_3. Frequent monitoring of serum and urinary calcium levels is necessary to avoid hypercalcemia or hypercalciuria and renal damage.

The treatment of secondary HPT related to renal failure requires administration of calcitriol and oral calcium salts plus restriction of dietary phosphorus intake. Although the resulting increased serum calcium level has a significant effect on reducing the serum PTH level, part of this response is independent of the change in serum calcium and likely reflects the direct action of calcitriol to inhibit PTH secretion. Calcitriol may be given orally or intravenously after each hemodialysis session. Doses of oral calcitriol typically range from 0.25 to 1.5 µg per day, but should be adjusted on an individual basis to achieve serum calcium levels between 10.5 to 11.0 mg per dL, concentrations that can suppress secondary HPT. Pulse therapy, given either orally or intravenously two or three times per week, can facilitate administration of greater cumulative weekly doses of calcitriol, with corresponding higher serum calcitriol levels, than daily therapy, with less risk of hypercalcemia. Thus, administration of calcitriol on an intermittent schedule may be superior to daily dosing in many patients with severe secondary HPT.

Calcitriol therapy is often limited by the development of intractable hyperphosphatemia or hypercalcemia, conditions that may signal the need for surgical intervention (see later). The development of hypercalcemia within the first few weeks of calcitriol therapy is common in patients with either nonsuppressible HPT (i.e., autonomous or tertiary HPT) or aluminum-related bone disease. By contrast, hypercalcemia may occur after many weeks or months of treatment when calcitriol therapy has reversed the skeletal changes of severe renal osteodystrophy. In renal failure, reducing the serum concentration of intact PTH to approximately two times the upper limit of normal is desirable.

Tertiary Hyperparathyroidism

The development of hypercalcemia in patients with long-standing secondary HPT indicates progression to tertiary HPT. Thus, tertiary HPT and PHPT share in common the presence of hypercalcemia due to nonsuppressible or autonomous parathyroid tissue. Serum concentrations of intact PTH can be extremely high in tertiary HPT, particularly in patients who have renal osteodystrophy. Administration of calcitriol to these patients often causes severe hypercalcemia despite partial suppression of serum PTH.

Treatment of tertiary HPT entails surgical removal of all abnormal parathyroid tissue, with simultaneous autograft, or subtotal parathyroidectomy, performed in cases of multigland disease. Before parathyroid surgery, patients with renal osteodystrophy must have aluminum-related bone disease excluded as a cause of hypercalcemia. In addition to severe hypercalcemia, other criteria for parathyroid surgery in patients with renal osteodystrophy and elevated serum levels of PTH include (1) persistent hyperphosphatemia despite appropriate use of phosphate-binding agents and a phosphorus-restricted diet; (2) extraskeletal calcifications; (3) development of calciphylaxsis; (4) progressive skeletal disease; and (5) intractable pruritus.

HYPOPARATHYROIDISM

Incidence

Hypoparathyroidism is an unusual (1 to 10%) complication of thyroid or parathyroid surgery, but is very common after more radical surgery for head and neck malignancies (e.g., laryngeal cancer). Nonsurgical hypoparathyroidism is rare.

Etiology

The most common cause of hypoparathyroidism is inadvertent removal or injury of the parathyroid glands during head and neck surgery (Table 3). Nonsurgical causes of hypoparathyroidism include autoimmune or infiltrative disorders; markedly elevated or reduced serum levels of magnesium; and genetic defects that impair development of the parathyroid glands (e.g., DiGeorge's syndrome) or that prevent syn-

TABLE 3. **Causes of Hypoparathyroidism**

Surgery (e.g., thyroidectomy, parathyroidectomy, head/neck tumors)
Genetic
  Dysembryogenesis (DiGeorge's syndrome)
  PTH gene defects
  Activating mutation of calcium-sensing receptor
  Developmental defects
Autoimmune
  Isolated
  Polyglandular failure syndromes
Infiltrative
  Malignancy
  Hemochromatosis
  Thalassemia (iron deposition from transfusions)
  Granulomatous diseases
  Wilson's disease (copper deposition)
Magnesium disorders (hypermagnesemia, hypomagnesemia)

thesis (e.g., PTH gene mutations) or secretion (activating mutations of the parathyroid calcium-sensing receptor) of PTH. Autoimmune hypoparathyroidism can be isolated or associated with other endocrine deficiencies (polyglandular failure), and is frequently associated with circulating parathyroid antibodies. Infiltrative disorders that cause hypoparathyroidism include malignancy, hemochromatosis, granulomatous diseases, thalassemia, and Wilson's disease.

Clinical Manifestations

Symptoms vary according to duration and severity of hypocalcemia. Mild to moderate hypocalcemia is associated with circumoral and distal paresthesias ("pins and needles") and occasional muscle cramps. More severe hypocalcemia can lead to spontaneous tetany, manifest as carpopedal spasm, laryngospasm, and generalized seizures, and requires urgent treatment. Muscle weakness, heart failure, prolongation of the ST segment and QT interval of the electrocardiogram, cardiac arrhythmias, hypotension, and papilledema are also indications for immediate treatment of hypocalcemia. Chronic hypoparathyroidism can be totally asymptomatic or can cause otherwise unexplained fatigue, depression, and irritability. Patients with mild hypocalcemia may have latent tetany, which may be revealed by gently tapping over the facial nerve and observing unilateral spasm of the mouth or face (i.e., Chvostek's sign). Chvostek's sign is positive in most patients with hypocalcemia, but is also slightly positive in approximately 10 to 30% of eucalcemic subjects. A more specific sign of latent tetany may be disclosed by the development of carpopedal spasm after compression of the upper arm by a cuff inflated to above systolic blood pressure for 3 to 5 minutes (i.e., Trousseau's sign).

Laboratory Evaluation

A low serum calcium and undetectable or inappropriately low intact PTH are diagnostic of hypoparathyroidism. Determination of the ionized calcium level may be necessary in patients with abnormal levels of serum proteins. In the absence of PTH, serum levels of phosphorus are elevated or high normal. Thus, measurement of serum phosphorus in patients who have protracted hypocalcemia after surgery for hyperparathyroidism (or hyperthyroidism) helps to distinguish hypoparathyroidism from "hungry bones" syndrome, in which serum levels of calcium and phosphorus are both low because of intense remineralization of the skeleton. The serum magnesium concentration should be determined in all patients with hypocalcemia because magnesium disorders are a common cause of hypocalcemia.

Treatment

Symptomatic hypoparathyroidism that is associated with tetany, seizures, or laryngospasm, or a markedly depressed ionized calcium (e.g., <0.75 mmol per liter) requires immediate administration of intravenous calcium and subsequent institution of vitamin D therapy (Table 4). One to two ampules of 10% calcium gluconate (93 to 186 mg of elemental calcium) should be given intravenously over 5 to 10 minutes. To prevent induction of cardiac arrhythmias, care should be taken to avoid overly rapid administration of intravenous calcium to patients who are receiving digitalis. Intravenous bolus administration of calcium corrects hypocalcemia rapidly, but the large volume of distribution of calcium results in the insidious recurrence of hypocalcemia within a few hours. Therefore, until vitamin D therapy takes effect, most patients require continuous intravenous infusion of calcium to maintain a normal serum calcium level. One common approach is to add 10 ampules of 10% calcium gluconate (93 mg of elemental calcium per ampule) to 1000 mL of 5% dextrose, and to infuse this solution at 50 to 100 mL per hour. This protocol provides 50 to 100 mg of elemental calcium per hour, and should be continued for at least 10 hours. The total or ionized serum calcium level should be monitored every 2 to 3 hours during the infusion. Oral calcium and vitamin D therapy should be started as soon as possible (see later).

Patients with mild to moderate hypocalcemia or with mild symptoms (e.g., circumoral paresthesias) can be treated initially with oral calcium and vitamin

TABLE 4. **Treatment of Hypoparathyroidism**

Hypocalcemic crisis (tetany, seizures, laryngospasm)
   10–20 mL 10% calcium gluconate intravenously over 10 min
Severe hypocalcemia
   10% calcium gluconate in 1000 mL 5% dextrose at 50–100 mL/h
Mild–moderate hypocalcemia
   Oral calcium carbonate (1–2 g elemental calcium in divided doses)
   Calcitriol (Rocaltrol) 0.25–1.0 μg p.o. bid or
   Ergocalciferol (Drisdol) (50,000–150,000 IU qd)

D. Oral calcium is usually administered in amounts from 1 to 3 grams of elemental calcium per day in 3 to 4 divided doses. To ensure optimal absorption, oral calcium supplements should be taken with water or other fluids, and with food in the stomach. Many considerations are involved in the selection of a calcium supplement, and none is unique to the treatment of hypoparathyroidism. Calcium carbonate is an inexpensive form of calcium that is very convenient owing to its high content of elemental calcium (40%). When taken with food, absorption of calcium from calcium carbonate is adequate even in achlorhydric patients. Because of the low content of elemental calcium in calcium lactate (13%) and calcium gluconate (9%), patients must take many tablets to obtain adequate amounts of calcium. Thus, these salts are inconvenient and are often not acceptable to the patients. Calcium citrate is 21% calcium and is well absorbed even in the absence of gastric acid. Although more expensive than many other forms of calcium, calcium citrate has the advantage of causing fewer gastrointestinal side effects. For those who prefer a liquid calcium supplement, calcium glubionate is very palatable and contains 230 mg calcium per 10 mL. Ten to 30 mL of a 10% calcium chloride solution (273 to 819 mg calcium) every 8 hours may be very effective in patients with achlorhydria. Hyperchloremic acidosis may occur and can be prevented by giving half of the calcium as chloride and half as carbonate simultaneously. Calcium phosphate salts should be avoided.

All patients with hypoparathyroidism who are hypocalcemic require vitamin D or analogues in addition to calcium. Calcitriol, the active form of vitamin D, is the most physiologic treatment choice and also the most rapidly acting, and therefore is often used as initial vitamin D therapy. Almost all patients with hypoparathyroidism can be effectively treated with calcitriol in the amount of 0.25 μg twice daily to 0.5 μg four times a day. Because of the expense of calcitriol and the need to administer the drug several times per day, other vitamin D preparations may be preferred. Ergocalciferol is the least expensive choice for vitamin D therapy, and provides a long duration of action (with corresponding prolonged potential toxicity). When initiating therapy with ergocalciferol (50,000 to 100,000 IU per day), it is reasonable to continue calcitriol for the first 3 to 4 weeks, with gradual tapering of the dose of calcitriol as ergocalciferol becomes effective. For the first week, the full dose of calcitriol should be continued, and the serum calcium levels should dictate the speed of the taper, monitored every 7 to 10 days. The goal of therapy is to maintain the serum calcium in the low-normal range without causing hypercalciuria. For chronic management of hypoparathyroidism, serum calcium should be measured every 3 to 6 months, and 24-hour urine calcium should be determined annually. Patients should see an ophthalmologist annually to screen for cataracts.

Treatment with calcium and vitamin D usually decreases the elevated serum phosphate to a normal level because of a favorable balance between increased urinary phosphate excretion and decreased intestinal phosphate absorption. In general, phosphate-binding gels such as aluminum hydroxide are not necessary.

Several issues require special attention. Because thiazide diuretics can increase renal calcium reabsorption in patients with hypoparathyroidism, the inadvertent institution or discontinuation of these drugs may respectively increase or decrease plasma calcium levels. By contrast, furosemide and other loop diuretics can increase renal clearance of calcium and depress serum calcium levels. The administration of glucocorticoids antagonizes the action of vitamin D (and analogues) and may also precipitate hypocalcemia. The development of hypomagnesemia may also interfere with the effectiveness of treatment with calcium and vitamin D.

Experimental treatments for hypoparathyroidism include transplantation of cultured human parathyroid cells and daily injection of synthetic human PTH(1–34). PTH(1–34) effectively normalizes serum concentrations of calcium and phosphorus while causing less hypercalciuria than treatment with comparable doses of calcitriol. Unfortunately, uncertainties regarding the future availability of human PTH(1–34), and the need to administer the drug by injection, lessen overall enthusiasm for this form of treatment.

PRIMARY ALDOSTERONISM

method of
DAVID C. KEM, M.D.
University of Oklahoma School of Medicine
Oklahoma City, Oklahoma

The incidence of primary aldosteronism (PA) ranges from 0.5 to 5%. Because PA shares certain signs and laboratory values with other forms of hypertension it is not surprising that PA may remain undiagnosed for years.

PATHOPHYSIOLOGY

PA is characterized by secretion of aldosterone due to adrenal neoplasia either from solitary or multiple cortical nodules or from biosynthetic variants of diffuse adrenal hyperplasia. The elevated blood pressure is generally attributed to expansion of the extracellular volume. There is a concomitant increase in potassium and magnesium secretion. Central nervous system mineralocorticoid receptors are also sensitive to aldosterone and translate this signal into an increased central adrenergic output, elevated cardiac output, and decreased renal blood flow. These changes lead to hypertension and suppression of renin and vasopressin.

PRESENTATION

Frequent headaches and vague malaise are common to both PA and hypertension. Additional symptoms of PA result from the hypokalemia and hypomagnesemia and include muscle cramps, weakness, nocturia, and/or isosthenuria and, more uncommonly, a metallic or bitter taste in the mouth. The hypertension ranges from mild to severe, encompassing classes 1 through 4. All sequelae of hypertension including congestive heart failure, stroke (cerebrovascular accident), malignant hypertension, and/or renal failure may obscure the underlying diagnosis. A notable increase in the frequency of cerebrovascular accident in patients younger than the age of 40 has been noted in the families of patients with glucocorticoid remediable hyperaldosteronism (GRA).

DIAGNOSTIC TESTING

The majority of patients demonstrate intermittent hypokalemia and relative hypernatremia, which remain the most frequently used screening test. The effectiveness of this approach requires a careful history and recognition that a low sodium diet, diuretic, or cathartic intake will alter the results. Hypokalemia in the absence of hypertension has confused a number of physicians. An elevated plasma renin activity (PRA) quickly identifies those patients having a volume deficiency. Urinary potassium values less than 10 mEq per 24 hours or more than 30 mEq per 24 hours may identify, respectively, patients with a primary gastrointestinal or urinary loss of potassium. Such testing, however, is not specific. It is desirable to take a patient off of a diuretic for 2 weeks and to replete him or her for 1 week with 20 to 40 mEq per day of oral potassium. Remeasurement of blood pressure and serum potassium level will identify those patients requiring further study for PA. This is generally desirable because diuretics and several other antihypertensive medications will also alter the plasma aldosterone concentration (PAC) and PRA in other diagnostic tests. Five to 15% of patients with PA, and a higher percentage of patients with familial GRA, may not demonstrate hypokalemia.

There is no clear distinction between suppressed PRA in patients having hypertension and PA. Finding a normal or elevated PRA, however, rules out PA. Measurement of a morning ambulatory or sitting PAC:PRA ratio either alone or 2 hours after ingesting a converting enzyme inhibitor (captopril-stimulated ratio) has provided sufficient discrimination between PA, secondary aldosteronism, and essential hypertension. Other methods involve suppression of PAC after rapid saline infusion (2 liters over 4 hours) or administration of an oral mineralocorticoid (Florinef, 0.3 mg three times a day for 3 days) or measurement of 24-hour urinary metabolites of aldosterone. Measurement of a 2-hour upright posture or furosemide (Lasix)–stimulated PRA is also important for interpretation of these data because evidence of renin suppression is required. We have noted several patients with suppressed PRA, borderline PAC:PRA ratio, and PAC whose ratio clearly became separated from normal after captopril administration and might have been missed through the use of an unstimulated ratio alone.

These studies may be inadequate for evaluating families of a patient with GRA because aldosterone secretion may be relatively low in some family members. It is likely that these and other variants may have relative hypersecretion of mineralocorticoids other than aldosterone.

DIFFERENTIAL DIAGNOSIS OF PRIMARY ALDOSTERONE AND MINERALOCORTICOID EXCESS SYNDROMES

Most patients with elevated PACs and suppressed plasma renin will have an aldosterone-producing adenoma

(APA) or a variant of idiopathic adrenal hyperplasia (IAH). In my experience, approximately 50% of our patients with PA have an APA and the rest have IAH. A higher proportion of black patients have IAH compared with the white population. Some confusion may exist if the patient has developed concurrent renal damage and a secondary increase in renin into the normal or slightly elevated range. The history, physical examination, and an abnormal PAC:PRA ratio greater 20 or another diagnostic test should exclude these entities. Once the diagnosis of PA is established, the subtypes should be identified. The cost of most of these tests mandates that the patient's medical care would be altered depending on their outcome. If surgery is not feasible, there is less need to proceed because medical therapy may be similar. I have generally obtained computed tomography without contrast medium enhancement by using 1.0- to 1.5-mm interval cuts through the adrenal itself to determine if a cortical adenoma greater than 1.5 mm is present. Magnetic resonance imaging is not satisfactory, owing to the difficulty of imaging cortical tissue with a high fat content. If an adenoma is present, there is still no definitive evidence that it is secretory or that it is not a variant of IAH with adenomatous changes. IAH may be present, and the adrenal size frequently is not enlarged. If there is no evidence for an adenoma, the presumptive diagnosis is IHA, but a small adenoma is still possible. Some experienced physicians would proceed to a trial of medical therapy to determine if control of both potassium and blood pressure can be achieved. Others would proceed with further testing if there were a particularly elevated PAC (greater than 50 ng/dL) or plasma 18-hydroxycorticosterone (over 100 ng/dL) characteristic of many patients with an APA. Another test used for this purpose is to measure an overnight recumbent PAC and plasma cortisol (PC) level at 8 AM and again after 4 hours of upright posture. Patients with IAH tend to have a rise is PAC and the expected drop in PC, whereas those with an APA tend to have a drop in both PAC and PC. In my hands, this test does not provide sufficient reliability on which to base a clinical decision. The other two tests that may provide specific data are listed below:

1. Iodocholesterol (NP59) radionuclide scanning after administration of 4 mg per day of dexamethasone (Decadron) for 2 days before and during the 3 to 5 days required for adrenal uptake. This is reasonably helpful when imaging provides adequate visualization because it provides a correlation between a functional and anatomic diagnosis. The two drawbacks are its cost and the evidence that physiologic localization is dependent on the size of the tumor.

2. Bilateral adrenal venous catheterization with concurrent ACTH infusion to measure the PAC:PC ratio in adrenal and peripheral venous blood. The PAC:PC ratio should be similar in the uninvolved adrenal and peripheral sample and be higher in the adenomatous adrenal effluent. This should be considered the most specific technique, but it suffers from its invasive nature, high cost, the need for an experienced selective radiographer, and the difficulty in identifying the right adrenal vein in up to one third of patients.

Most centers rely on the presence of two or more test results consistent with the same diagnosis.

The diagnosis of GRA should be entertained in patients with an IHA pattern and particularly in those with a family history of early strokes and intermittent hypokalemia or a history of already identified GRA. Identification of an elevated value for urinary 18-hydroxycortisol or 18-oxocortisol is helpful. This condition results from a chimeric gene derived from a crossover of the ACTH-sensitive promoter for 11-hydroxycorticosterone to the angiotensin II–controlled aldosterone synthase. Identification of the abnormal gene remains the most specific diagnostic method.

THERAPEUTIC CONSIDERATIONS

Surgical resection of an APA is curative for the hypermineralocorticoidism and its resultant hypokalemia. Successful reduction of blood pressure into the normal range is not as certain and in some studies may only reach 50 to 60%. The success rate appears to depend on the duration of the hypertension, the presence of renal sequelae of the hypertension, and the co-presence of essential hypertension. Lateralization of the adenoma permits a surgical flank approach and minimizes postoperative complications. Several centers have developed experience by using laparoscopic resection of the affected adrenal. This promises to reduce postoperative morbidity, but the experience from larger series has not been reported. Successful resection is frequently followed by a temporary mineralocorticoid deficiency due to long-term suppression of renal renin and aldosterone secretion of the uninvolved adrenal. Medical management of an APA or IAH is directed toward volume depletion with the use of hydrochlorothiazide in 25- to 50-mg dosages. I use the potent potassium antagonist amiloride (Midamor) in dosages of 5 to 20 mg per day or spironolactone (Aldactone) in dosages of 200 to 400 mg for such control. The majority of patients will achieve control of potassium, but additional medications are necessary for blood pressure control in over 25% of the patients. A calcium channel antagonist, which may further reduce aldosterone secretion and provide vasodilation, a beta blocker that diminishes cardiac output, or an angiotensin-converting enzyme inhibitor have all been used. Management of patients with GRA is remarkably similar. Although the aldosterone hypersecretion is suppressible by low-dose glucocorticoid therapy, the experience in several kindreds indicates this is insufficient for adequate blood pressure control, and it is now recommended their hypertension be controlled with antihypertensive agents with minimal use of glucocorticoid suppression.

HYPOPITUITARISM

method of
ROBERT J. ANDERSON, M.D.
*Veterans Affairs Medical Center and
Creighton University School of Medicine*
Omaha, Nebraska

Hypopituitarism implies the loss of one or more of the clinically important pituitary hormones. These include growth hormone (GH, somatotropin), adrenocorticotropic hormone (ACTH), thyroid-stimulating hormone (TSH), follicle-stimulating hormone (FSH), luteinizing hormone (LH), prolactin, and antidiuretic hormone (ADH). The picture of hypopituitarism is often one of a gradual cumulative loss of hormones with increasing debility, but the presentation can be widely variable. For example, a man may have the inexorable onset of fatigue, weakness, decreased libido, erectile dysfunction, and, finally, pressure symptoms of headache and visual disturbance associated with an expanding pituitary tumor. Soft, pale, waxy skin with fine facial wrinkles and female body habitus may suggest the diagnosis. Progression may be rapid and dramatic in pituitary apoplexy or after head trauma. Isolated loss of a hormone occurs less frequently. If it is found, care should be exercised to avoid missing progression to a multihormone deficiency. In the setting of large functioning tumors such as GH-secreting or glycoprotein-secreting adenomas, other pituitary hormone deficiencies should be sought. Common causes of hypopituitarism are pituitary adenoma, craniopharyngioma, traumatic injury, pituitary surgery, irradiation, ischemic necrosis, infiltrative disease, and autoimmune disease (Table 1). Loss of posterior pituitary ADH is not as frequent and suggests pituitary stalk or hypothalamic disease (see "Diabetes Insipidus").

There are several guidelines for treatment of hypopituitarism. Hormone deficiency should be documented by baseline testing and further stimulation testing if necessary. The picture is usually one of an endocrine target gland deficiency (e.g., low thyroxine)

TABLE 1. **Etiology of Hypopituitarism**

Tumors
    Pituitary adenomas—functioning + nonfunctioning
    Craniopharyngioma
Pituitary surgery
Traumatic injury
Infarction/vascular
    Ischemic necrosis
    (Sheehan's—postpartum, diabetes mellitus, sickle cell disease)
    Pituitary apoplexy—necrosis of tumor
Radiation of pituitary
    Usually gradual + progressive
Infiltrative + infectious diseases
    Sarcoidosis
    Hemochromatosis
    Meningitis
    Tuberculosis
Autoimmune
    Lymphocytic hypophysitis
Genetic diseases
    Gene mutations: *Prop-1* (deficiency of LH, FSH, GH, TSH,
        prolactin); *Pit-1* (deficiency of GH, prolactin, variable TSH)
Idiopathic
Iatrogenic
    Discontinuation of exogenous glucocorticoid treatment or
        inadequate glucocorticoid coverage during stress in patients
        on chronic or intermittent glucocorticoids by any route
Hypothalamic diseases
    Craniopharyngioma. Any hypothalamic tumor, injury,
        radiation, infarction, or infiltrative or infectious disease also
        can affect hypothalamic hormone secretion.

LH = luteinizing hormone; FSH = follicle-stimulating hormone; GH = growth hormone; TSH = thyroid-stimulating hormone.

without the corresponding increase in the pituitary tropic hormone (a "normal" or low TSH). Except for GH and ADH, hormone replacement is with the target hormones (such as L-thyroxine) because they are less expensive, they can be given orally or transdermally rather than parenterally, and they are not immunogenic. Finally, even though the replacement schedules are frequently the same as treatments of primary endocrine deficiencies, follow-up monitoring is not as ideal because the feedback response of the pituitary is lost. Specific treatments are detailed here. Stimulation test protocols are available in endocrinology textbooks.

GROWTH HORMONE DEFICIENCY

Diagnosis

GH deficiency in the adult patient is discussed. My practice is to document GH deficiency by demonstrating a failure to respond to a stimulation test such as insulin hypoglycemia (contraindicated in patients with coronary artery disease, seizure disorders, or cerebrovascular insufficiency) or L-dopa. Hypothalamic GH-releasing hormone (GHRH, Geref) given intravenously in conjunction with intravenous arginine may prove to be a less stressful method for detection of GH response. Insulin-like growth factor-1 (IGF-1) provides an averaged indication of GH presence but cannot be used as the sole diagnostic test because it may be in the normal range in some GH-deficient patients.

Treatment

Current practice is to replace GH in adults with documented GH deficiency. In aging adults with low IGF-1 levels due to decreased GH secretion, but without clear hypopituitarism, replacement of GH is investigational. Patients with hypopituitarism experience premature mortality from cardiovascular disease. Metabolic sequelae associated with the lack of GH may contribute to this. Subjects treated with GH have an improved sense of well-being and quality of life, increased muscle strength, decreased body fat, increased lean body mass, and increase in bone density. Because of the expense of the recombinant GH preparations, the deficiency must be documented. Baseline lipids, prostate-specific antigen (PSA), glucose, and bone mineral density are helpful for monitoring therapy. In my experience, lower doses are required to gain benefits and to avoid adverse effects. GH (Humatrope, Nutropin,* Genotropin*) is given as a single subcutaneous daily dose. The initial dose for men and for women taking transdermal estrogen preparations should be 2 μg per kg per day with increases of 1 μg per kg per day every 6 to 8 weeks to keep the IGF-1 level at the mid-normal range for age and sex. Women taking oral estrogens

*MedicAlert, P.O. Box 1009, Turlock, California, 95381-1009; telephone: 1-800-625-3788.

may start at 4 µg per kg per day with advances of 2 µg per kg per day every 6 to 8 weeks with the same IGF-1 goals. Older patients and obese patients require less. Doses above 4 µg per kg per day may not be needed in most men. Patients must be monitored for the more common side effects of peripheral edema, musculoskeletal pain, or aggravation of hypertension. The prostate gland should be monitored with digital rectal examination and PSA at least yearly in men older than age 50. Growth of persistent, but stable pituitary tumors is unlikely, but is under study. Use in the presence of any active cancer is contraindicated.

SECONDARY ADRENAL INSUFFICIENCY

Diagnosis

The diagnosis of secondary adrenal insufficiency is important because this condition is life-threatening. General malaise, fatigue, hypotension, and lack of skin pigmentation are suggestive findings. A careful history will detect exogenous glucocorticoid administration and subsequent unnoticed or inadvertent interruption of treatment. Exogenous glucocorticoid suppression of the hypothalamic-pituitary-adrenal axis is the most common cause of secondary adrenal insufficiency. The usual findings in secondary hypoadrenalism are a low or "normal" ACTH level (0–50 pg/mL) in association with a serum cortisol level of less than 10 µg per dL in the morning or during severe stress. The patient may present in an acute crisis with cardiovascular collapse. A serum cortisol level of less than 18 µg per dL in this situation is highly suggestive. To evaluate any patient suspected of secondary adrenal insufficiency a rapid adrenocortical screen with the synthetic ACTH cosyntropin (Cortrosyn) usually shows a less than adequate response (cortisol < 18 µg/dL at 30 minutes). A normal response does not exclude secondary (pituitary) adrenal insufficiency. The use of insulin-induced hypoglycemia or metyrapone testing to demonstrate lack of cortisol response associated with low ACTH is often not necessary and may be dangerous, owing to precipitation of a hypoadrenal crisis if not monitored carefully. Corticotropin-releasing hormone (CRH) stimulation of ACTH without the stress accompanying the previous two tests has not been as discriminatory for diagnostic purposes but may be helpful in some situations. If the patient has already been treated with glucocorticoids and the picture is not clear, the use of a 1- to 3-day intravenous ACTH infusion will document the presence of adrenal function.

Treatment

The major goal in treatment is to restore normalcy by attempting to reproduce the diurnal rhythm of cortisol production with a glucocorticoid preparation, not with ACTH. Our previous efforts at replacement have often used higher average doses that have increased risk for accelerated bone resorption. I prefer hydrocortisone at a dose of 10 mg in the morning, 5 to 10 mg at noon, and 5 mg in the late afternoon. The dose has to be individualized. Some patients prefer the entire dose in the morning. I avoid prednisone and other longer-acting preparations such as dexamethasone because of the inability to monitor dosing and the higher occurrence of exogenous Cushing's syndrome. A mineralocorticoid preparation is not required in most cases because the renin-angiotensin system should be intact. How do we know how much is enough? The 24-hour urine free cortisol test and a 9 AM cortisol sample should be in the normal range to avoid overtreatment. The blood pressure, serum electrolytes, and the clinical examination and history should be followed. Occasional patients will become cushingoid on the estimated doses and require a smaller twice-daily dose or a daily dose. In some situations, the afternoon doses can be given earlier or later in the day to allow the patient to function as normally as possible. The glucocorticoids may unmask underlying mild diabetes insipidus in some patients. I make certain that the patient understands the need to increase the dose during sick days. Each patient receives a detailed sheet that lists how to adjust the medicine. They double the dose during the 1 to 3 days of a moderate illness such as the "flu" with a low-grade fever (≤100°F) and triple the dose if fever (> 100°F) is present. They are given injectable dexamethasone (Decadron Phosphate, 4 mg/mL in 1-mL vials with syringes and needles) to use if they are vomiting and cannot get to medical care quickly. They give the contents of one vial intramuscularly (4 mg) and repeat the dose, if necessary, every 8 to 12 hours before arriving at the hospital. The patients must get a medical information bracelet or necklace* that details their need for cortisol.

Glucocorticoid coverage for surgery and stressful procedures is essentially the same for primary and secondary adrenal insufficiency. I give a depot of 100 mg of hydrocortisone sodium succinate (Solu-Cortef) intramuscularly on call to surgery and then 50 to 100 mg of hydrocortisone intravenously every 6 hours (starting in surgery) the first 24 hours. The dose is decreased by 50% each day as indicated by patient progress until the oral glucocorticoid can be resumed. Treatment of acute adrenal insufficiency requires intravenous glucocorticoid (Solu-Cortef), 50 to 100 mg every 6 hours, dextrose and saline intravenous fluids, and an aggressive review to define the precipitating event (see "Adrenocortical Insufficiency").

HYPOTHYROIDISM

Diagnosis

Patients are clinically hypothyroid but often not as severely myxedematous as patients with primary

---

*MedicAlert, P.O. Box 1009, Turlock, California, 95381-1009; telephone: 1-800-625-3788.

hypothyroidism. Clinical hypothyroidism with the finding of a low free and/or total thyroxine (T_4) level and a low or "normal" TSH gives the diagnosis of secondary (central) hypothyroidism (this includes hypothalamic hypothyroidism). An absent or blunted response of TSH to intravenous thyrotropin-releasing hormone (TRH, protirelin [Thyrel TRH]) is of limited usefulness because it occurs in only 21% of patients with central hypothyroidism.

Treatment

The great advances that have occurred in titrating thyroid hormone replacement doses with more sensitive TSH assays are lost in patients with hypopituitarism. In replacement therapy of primary hypothyroidism the goal is to keep the TSH within the normal range. With this measurement lost in patients with hypopituitarism, it is best to follow the free T_4 level, maintain it within the normal range, and adjust the dose carefully based on symptoms. I use synthetic levothyroxine (Synthroid, Levoxyl, Levothroid, Euthyrox) for replacement. Triiodothyronine (Cytomel) is not desirable for chronic replacement because of its short half-life. A general estimate for thyroxine replacement is 1.6 to 1.8 μg per kg per day. My target final doses are 100 to 125 μg per day in individuals younger than 60 and 75 to 100 μg per day in individuals older than 60. Variations in requirements occur, and individualization of the dose is necessary. In patients younger than 60 years of age in good health with a short duration of hypothyroidism, I usually start at 50 to 75 μg per day and increase by 25-μg increments every 6 to 8 weeks to normalize the free T_4. Younger patients may be given the full estimated daily dose without adverse effects. In patients older than 60, patients with prolonged hypothyroidism (longer than 6 months) and in patients with known ischemic heart disease, I start with 25 μg per day to avoid aggravation of cardiac disease. I increase by 25 μg in 4 weeks if there are no adverse symptoms and then increase by 25-μg increments every 6 to 8 weeks until the free T_4 level is normal. The patient is then followed every 6 to 12 months to maintain a normal level. Chronic overreplacement should be avoided to prevent potential accelerated bone loss in a patient with several problems that could contribute to loss of bone (GH and gonadal steroid deficiency and potential overreplacement with glucocorticoids). If the thyroid status is not clear from free T_4 measurements, the thyroid hormone sensitive proteins angiotensin-converting enzyme (ACE) and sex hormone–binding globulin (SHBG) may provide an indirect peripheral measure of T_4 effect. Both increase with elevated thyroid hormone levels. Care is taken to replace cortisol beforehand or concomitantly to avoid precipitating an adrenal crisis with increased metabolic demands of thyroid hormone replacement.

HYPOGONADOTROPIC HYPOGONADISM

Diagnosis

Because both LH and FSH are secreted from the gonadotrope, these glycoproteins are usually lost in tandem. The classic presentation in the adult is hypogonadotropic hypogonadism (secondary hypogonadism) with low or "normal" LH and FSH levels and low gonadal steroid levels (testosterone in men, estradiol in women). Both men and women experience loss of libido, decline in secondary sex characteristics, and decreased bone density. Women are amenorrheic. Men will be impotent. Testing with intravenous doses of gonadotropin-releasing hormone (GnRH, gonadorelin [Factrel]) has not provided the discrimination needed to diagnose a central lesion or to define pituitary LH/FSH reserve. Magnetic resonance imaging of the sella usually is necessary once biochemical evidence of secondary hypogonadism is documented. In men and in postmenopausal women the loss of LH and FSH may be sequential after the loss of GH and may be clinically silent until a pituitary adenoma expands to cause symptomatic defects and compression.

Treatment

Women

Replacement therapy with the gonadal steroid is required in premenopausal women. Premenopausal women with a uterus are given a full schedule to allow menstruation. I prescribe oral conjugated estrogens (Premarin, Menest) at 0.3 to 1.25 mg per day on days 1 to 25, with medroxyprogesterone (Provera, Amen, Cycrin), 5 to 10 mg per day, added from days 13 to 25. Five to 6 days are allowed for menses. An alternative treatment is an oral micronized estradiol (Estrace), 1 to 2 mg per day, or a transdermal system (Estraderm, Alora, Vivelle), 0.05- to 0.1-mg patches two times each week on days 1 to 25, in conjunction with medroxyprogesterone as noted on days 13 to 25. Pregnancy can be attained after induction of ovulation with human menopausal gonadotropins (menotropins [Pergonal, Humegon]) followed by human chorionic gonadotropin (hCG). A discussion of this procedure is beyond the scope of this article. The addition of small doses of intramuscular testosterone (enanthate or cypionate, 25 to 50 mg each month) can be considered if libido remains decreased owing to loss of adrenal androgen production stimulated by ACTH. Lower-dose testosterone patches and oral testosterone that does not affect liver function may be available options in the future. Side effects of acne, hirsutism, and virilization should be avoided. In hypopituitary postmenopausal women, the same considerations apply to the decision for gonadal steroid replacement as apply in a postmenopausal woman with normal pituitary function. Prescription of daily combined conjugated estrogen, 0.625 mg, and medroxyprogesterone acetate, 2.5-mg tablets (Prempro), is a useful option for women who wish to avoid menses. The treatment goal is to avoid osteoporosis and cardiovascular disease without causing side effects.

Men

Replacement therapy is given to men to attempt to normalize sexual function, increase the sense of well-being, maintain secondary sex characteristics, increase lean body mass, decrease fat mass, and prevent bone resorption. It is important to tell the patient that treatment will lead to progressive testicular atrophy if the hypopituitarism has not caused it already. In addition, it should be pointed out that fertility is usually lost. Treatment with pulsatile GnRH (if the defect is hypothalamic) or with hCG and human menopausal gonadotropin (hMG) can be attempted to recover fertility in appropriate cases. The usual therapy is chronic testosterone replacement in those who do not desire fertility. The three types of treatment available in the United States include oral, intramuscular, and transdermal. I avoid oral methyltestosterone preparations (Virilon, Android, Testred) because of the potential for hepatotoxicity presenting as cholestatic hepatitis, jaundice, peliosis hepatis, or hepatoma. The dose and frequency of testosterone are based primarily on the patient evaluation of improved strength, energy, libido, and sexual function and the goal of mid-normal range testosterone levels. Monitoring of testosterone replacement in secondary hypogonadism is less than ideal because adequate LH or FSH levels often are not available to allow an estimate of feedback response. Some patients prefer testosterone enanthate (Delatestryl) or testosterone cypionate (Depo-Testosterone, Virilon IM) intramuscularly every 2 weeks. This interval avoids the wide fluctuations in levels that can occur with 3- to 4-week intervals, but variations still occur. A family member or the patient can give the injections to avoid additional cost. I start with 50 to 100 mg for the severely hypogonadal individual and 100 to 200 mg every 2 weeks for most other patients. Men older than age 60 may require the lower doses. Testosterone levels are measured 7 days after injection for an estimate of the mid-normal range value and at 2 weeks to determine the nadir. I prefer the transdermal testosterone delivery systems because they mimic the diurnal pattern of testosterone secretion and they avoid the fluctuations inherent in intramuscular delivery. Both scrotal (Testoderm, 4 and 6 mg) and nonscrotal (Testoderm TTS, 5 mg, and Androderm, 2.5 and 5 mg) testosterone transdermal systems are available. Testoderm (usually the 6-mg patch) is applied to the shaved scrotum each morning. The Testoderm TTS patch is applied to nongenital skin each morning. The Androderm patch (one 5-mg or two 2.5-mg patches) is applied each evening. Testosterone levels can be monitored 6 to 8 hours after application of the patches to maintain a mid-normal range. Androderm has been reported to be associated with more frequent and more severe skin reactions. All transdermal systems are

more expensive than the intramuscular injections, but frequent visits to the physician's office for injections are inconvenient and costs can approach the daily patch treatment. Problems with acceleration of benign prostatic hyperplasia, occult prostate cancer, polycythemia, or sleep apnea are uncommon in my experience with carefully monitored replacement doses. Baseline digital rectal examination, PSA determination, and hemoglobin determination should be done and followed yearly in men older than 50 and as needed in younger men. Patients should be warned about the possible occurrence of acne, oily skin, and breast tenderness.

HYPOPROLACTINEMIA

Diagnosis

A well-known clinical setting of prolactin loss is postpartum pituitary necrosis and resultant failure of lactation (Sheehan's syndrome). Gradual progression to multihormone deficiency usually ensues. Any female with hypopituitarism can have failure of prolactin production if pregnancy is attained. Hypoprolactinemia occurs in men, but it is detected less often. The diagnosis is made by documenting a low baseline prolactin in the absence of any suppressing agent, and the lack of prolactin response to TRH. There is no clear clinical syndrome known in men without prolactin. The hormone may have an effect on sexual behavior and fluid balance, but the effect is not completely clear. Prolactin is not replaced.

ANTIDIURETIC HORMONE DEFICIENCY

Replacement of ADH in diabetes insipidus is usually required to maintain normal water balance. The vasopressin analogue desmopressin is used most frequently as nasal, oral and subcutaneous preparations (see "Diabetes Insipidus").

CONCLUSION

Documentation of pituitary hormone loss is essential before treatment. Selected stimulation tests (ACTH, CRH, insulin tolerance test, GHRH) can be done when appropriate. Glucocorticoids must be replaced first to avoid life-threatening deterioration. Cortisol is given before or with thyroid hormone to avoid precipitation of a hypoadrenal crisis. Gonadal steroids and GH can be replaced once contraindications are excluded. Periodic monitoring of replacement therapy is essential. Patients can live well with total replacement, but they will be inconvenienced. A patient with panhypopituitarism may need cortisol, L-thyroxine, gonadal steroids, GH, and desmopressin (Table 2), all of which can enhance the quality of life and potentially decrease long-term morbidity and mortality. The dose of cortisol must be adjusted during illness. The ability to fine tune the treatment to the best levels for each individual is

TABLE 2. **Treatment of Hypopituitarism**

| Hormone Lost | Treatment | | Monitor |
	Population / Drug	*Dosage*	
Growth hormone (somatotropin)	Men, and women (on transdermal estrogen)	2 μg/kg/day to start; increase by 1 μg/kg/d every 6–8 weeks as indicated by IGF-1	• IGF-1 • Lipids • Prostate-specific antigen • Bone mineral density • Body composition • Side effects
	Women (on oral estrogens)	4 μg/kg/day to start; increase by 2 μg/kg/d every 6–8 weeks as indicated by IGF-1	
Adrenocorticotropic hormone	Hydrocortisone	10 mg PO AM 5–10 mg PO noon 5 mg PO PM	• Sense of well-being, strength • Avoid cushingoid changes • 24-h urine-free cortisol, 9 AM cortisol levels • Blood pressure, electrolytes

Thyroid-stimulating hormone	L-Thyroxine (Synthroid)	1.6–1.8 μg/kg/d
		Target dose by age:
		  <60: 100–125 μg/d
		  >60: 75–100 μg/d
		  (may be lower as age increases)
			• Free thyroxine
			• Thyroxine-sensitive proteins (ACE, SHBG) if needed
			• Avoid hyperthyroid and hypothyroid signs and symptoms

Luteinizing hormone, follicle-stimulating hormone	Women:
	  Conjugated estrogens (Premarin)
	  Or estradiol (Estrace)
	  Or estrogen patch (Estraderm)
	  And medroxyprogesterone (days 3–25)
		0.3–1.25 mg/d
		
		1–2 mg/d
		0.05–0.1 mg twice/week
		
		5–10 mg/d
			• Menstrual cycle
			• Libido
			• Estrogen-sensitive tissue

	Men:
	  IM testosterone ester
	  Or scrotal patch (Testoderm)
	  Or nonscrotal patch (Androderm)
		100–200 mg every 2 weeks
		4–6 mg/d
		
		5 mg/d
			• Libido, sense of well-being
			• Strength, endurance
			• Sexual function
			• Testosterone levels, prostate-specific antigen

Prolactin	None		• Lactation
Antidiuretic hormone	Desmopressin: intranasal, oral, or subcutaneous (see "Diabetes Insipidus")		• Thirst • Intake and output • Weight • Serum sodium urine osmolality

Abbreviations: IGF-1 = insulin-like growth factor 1; ACE = angiotensin-converting enzyme; SHBG = sex hormone-binding globulin.

not optimal because the feedback centers are lost. Research into sensitive tissue indicators of adequate replacement will enhance our treatment of this important group of patients.

HYPERPROLACTINEMIA

method of
JANET A. SCHLECHTE, M.D.
University of Iowa
Iowa City, Iowa

Secretion of prolactin (PRL) from the anterior pituitary is under the inhibitory control of dopamine. PRL is secreted episodically, and serum levels are usually less than 20 ng per mL in females and less than 10 ng per mL in males. Although the primary action of PRL is to stimulate the development of mammary tissue it is the effect of PRL on the reproductive system that warrants clinical attention. Hyperprolactinemia suppresses pulsatile hypothalamic secretion of gonadotropin-releasing hormone, leading to amenorrhea in women and impotence and decreased libido in men.

CAUSES OF HYPERPROLACTINEMIA

PRL-secreting pituitary tumors are the most common cause of hyperprolactinemia. Other causes are listed in Table 1. A variety of medications elevate serum PRL by interfering with dopaminergic inhibition of PRL secretion. Neuroleptic agents and other dopamine receptor antagonists cause rapid elevation of PRL to levels that may reach 200 ng per mL. Metoclopramide (Reglan) may be associ-

TABLE 1. **Causes of Hyperprolactinemia**

Prolactinomas
Pregnancy
Hypothyroidism
Renal failure
Medications
  Phenothiazines
  Metoclopramide
  Estrogen
  Calcium channel blockers
  H_2 receptor antagonists
Nonfunctioning pituitary tumors
Hypothalamic disease
Nipple stimulation
Idiopathic

ated with a 15-fold increase in PRL concentration, and histamine type-2 receptor blockers produce hyperprolactinemia by a central mechanism. Administration of estrogen to normal women stimulates PRL secretion, and PRL levels increase substantially during pregnancy. In patients with primary hypothyroidism, hyperprolactinemia develops because of increased hypothalamic thyrotropin-releasing hormone (TRH) activity. PRL levels also rise after surgery, chest trauma, or chronic nipple stimulation. Psychic stress has a variable effect on PRL secretion but commonly causes a mild elevation.

DIAGNOSTIC EVALUATION

The diagnosis of hyperprolactinemia is confirmed by demonstration of sustained elevation of serum levels. Because PRL secretion is episodic and stress may raise PRL concentrations, a low or borderline level should be confirmed by obtaining several samples. Stimulation and suppression tests of PRL secretion with TRH, chlorpromazine (Thorazine), levodopa (Larodopa), or insulin-induced hypoglycemia are not valuable in the differential diagnosis of hyperprolactinemia.

If the cause of the hyperprolactinemia is not apparent after a careful history and physical examination, medication review, and measurement of thyroid hormone radiographic evaluation of the pituitary should be undertaken. Magnetic resonance imaging (MRI) is superior to computed tomography in delineating tumor size and determining whether there is lateral or suprasellar tumor extension. PRL-secreting macroadenomas (>10 cm) cause marked elevations of PRL (about 1000 ng/mL) and a macroadenoma that is accompanied by a PRL level of less than 200 ng per mL is unlikely to be a prolactinoma. Some patients with sustained hyperprolactinemia have no radiographic evidence of a tumor (idiopathic hyperprolactinemia).

TREATMENT OF PROLACTINOMAS

Women with hyperprolactinemia usually seek medical attention because of amenorrhea or infertility, whereas men with prolactinomas usually seek medical attention for headaches, visual loss, and neurologic defects. PRL-secreting tumors in women are usually microadenomas, and hypopituitarism is extremely rare. In contrast, prolactinomas in men are usually macroadenomas. Up to one third of men with a PRL tumor may have galactorrhea, and nearly one half will have visual impairment.

The two established indications for treatment of a prolactinoma are restoration of fertility and the presence of a macroadenoma. The goals of therapy are to normalize PRL, restore gonadal function, and decrease tumor size. The treatment of choice is a dopamine agonist.

Dopamine Agonists

All dopamine agonists inhibit PRL secretion by stimulating pituitary and neuronal dopamine receptors, and bromocriptine (Parlodel) is the prototype. Treatment with bromocriptine should begin with a dose of 1.25 mg administered at bedtime with a snack. After 1 week, 1.25 mg can be added in the morning. At weekly intervals the dose should be increased by 1.25 mg to a total of 5 to 7.5 mg daily. A PRL level should be checked about 1 month after starting the bromocriptine. If the level has not normalized, the dose should be increased slowly. Most patients will respond within 3 months. After treatment with bromocriptine 80% to 90% of women with a microprolactinoma will have normal serum PRL levels, regular menstrual periods, and restoration of fertility. Normalization of serum PRL may occur within 24 hours, and gonadal function may normalize as early as 3 months after treatment. Normalization of PRL is less likely to occur in a patient with a macroadenoma, but a dopamine agonist is still first-line therapy.

Bromocriptine in the range of 5 to 7.5 mg will decrease tumor size in 90% of women with microadenomas. Higher dosages (10 to 30 mg) may be necessary to obtain reduction in serum PRL and a decrease in tumor size in men and in women who have macroadenomas. Reduction in tumor size usually occurs within 4 to 6 weeks, and about 60% of women with macroadenomas will have more than a 50% reduction in tumor size. Bromocriptine must be given continuously to be effective, and discontinuation of the drug leads to a rapid return to pretreatment PRL levels and tumor re-expansion.

All of the dopamine agonists may cause nausea, vomiting, nasal stuffiness, and orthostatic hypotension. The side effects are lessened if the drug is started at a low dose. Transvaginal administration of bromocriptine has been reported to cause fewer gastrointestinal side effects. Patients who fail to respond to bromocriptine or who cannot tolerate that drug may respond to another dopamine agonist. Pergolide (Permax) has a longer duration of action, and dosages of 50 to 150 μg once daily are as effective as bromocriptine in normalizing PRL. Currently, pergolide is approved by the Food and Drug Administration (FDA) only for treatment of Parkinson's disease. Cabergoline (Dostinex) is a more potent dopamine agonist with a very high specificity for the dopamine D_2 receptor and a long half-life. Treatment with cabergoline normalizes PRL in patients with microadenomas and leads to normalization of PRL and tumor shrinkage in about one half of patients with macroadenomas. Dosages of 0.5 to 2 mg weekly are as efficacious as daily administration of bromocriptine and may be associated with fewer side effects. With the exception of one report of pulmonary fibrosis in patients with Parkinson's disease, long-term therapy with bromocriptine has not been associated with complications.

Other Therapeutic Options

If a dopamine agonist is ineffective or poorly tolerated, transsphenoidal surgery may be considered for treatment of a prolactinoma. Surgery performed by an experienced neurosurgeon will normalize PRL in 60 to 70% of patients with microadenomas and in about one third of patients with macroadenomas. Unfortunately, the recurrence rate of hyperprolactinemia is unacceptably high and the procedure should be used only in selected cases. Radiotherapy is not effective as primary therapy but may be useful as adjunctive therapy with large tumors or after surgery.

Treatment During Pregnancy

All of the dopamine agonists cross the placenta but are not associated with an increased risk of spontaneous abortion or congenital defects. A woman taking a dopamine agonist should stop the drug when pregnancy is documented. PRL normally rises during pregnancy, and it is not necessary to monitor serum PRL levels throughout pregnancy. Enlargement of the pituitary also occurs during pregnancy, but tumor expansion is rarely clinically significant. Fewer than 2% of women with microadenomas develop headaches or visual deficits, and less than 5% have radiographic evidence of tumor expansion during pregnancy. Because the risk of tumor growth with a microadenoma is very small, I do not recommend formal visual field testing or MRI examinations during pregnancy. In contrast, there is a risk of significant tumor enlargement during pregnancy with a macroadenoma. These patients should be followed closely with formal visual field testing and/or MRI. Although bromocriptine therapy has not been associated with congenital malformations, data related to its long-term fetal effects are limited, and continuous usage during pregnancy should be avoided unless symptomatic tumor enlargement occurs.

Fluctuations in serum PRL usually do not correlate well with tumor growth, so frequent MRI of a PRL microadenoma is not efficacious or cost effective. Patients with macroadenomas require close observation and radiographic evaluation at intervals to monitor for tumor growth and extrasellar tumor expansion.

When fertility is not an issue, it is controversial how to treat a PRL microadenoma. Microprolactinomas have a benign natural history, and treatment is not necessary to prevent tumor growth. If the hyperprolactinemia is associated with regular menses, no therapy is necessary. PRL-induced estrogen deficiency may lead to bone loss, and women with hyperprolactinemia have 25% lower spinal bone mineral than women with regular menses. Use of dual energy x-ray absorptiometry to measure spinal bone density may help with treatment decisions in individual patients.

Because estrogen increases PRL and has been associated with tumor formation in animals, the standard of practice has been to avoid estrogen in hyperprolactinemic women. New data suggest that estrogen may be administered without stimulating tumor growth. Nevertheless, estrogen should be administered with caution to women with macroadenomas, and radiographic follow-up should be undertaken to ensure that tumor growth is not enhanced.

HYPOTHYROIDISM

method of
GILBERT H. DANIELS, M.D.
Harvard Medical School
and Massachusetts General Hospital
Boston, Massachusetts

Hypothyroidism is a syndrome of decreased circulating thyroid hormone and its clinical consequences. Mild hypothyroidism, also called subclinical or biochemical hypothyroidism, is very common.

PATHOPHYSIOLOGY

The pituitary hormone thyroid-stimulating hormone (TSH) controls the synthesis, storage, and release of thyroid hormone, as well as thyroid gland size. The earliest sign of a failing thyroid is an elevated serum TSH concentration (primary hypothyroidism). Far less common is thyroid gland failure due to deficient TSH or its action (central hypothyroidism)

PRIMARY HYPOTHYROIDISM: ETIOLOGY

Primary hypothyroidism may be categorized by the presence or absence of a goiter (Table 1), although overlap occurs. Hashimoto's thyroiditis (HT) is the most common cause in the United States.

Hashimoto's thyroiditis is an autoimmune disorder with lymphocytic infiltration of the thyroid gland. The disease hallmark is antibodies against specific thyroid cell antigens, including the biosynthetic enzyme thyroid peroxidase (TPO), the thyroid hormone precursor thyroglobulin, and, less frequently, the TSH receptor or the iodide symporter (iodine transport protein). Anti-TPO antibodies (also known as antimicrosomal antibodies) are present in over 98% of patients with hypothyroidism, but their relationship to hypothyroidism is uncertain; cell-mediated immunity is a more likely culprit. The firm, nontender lobes may be confused with single or multiple nodules. A goiter with an elevated TSH in the United States usually means that HT is present. However, patients with HT need not be hypothyroid; a firm lobe or goiter with positive antithyroid antibodies is virtually diagnostic. Thyroid lymphoma, a rare disorder, often presents as relentless growth of a Hashimoto goiter.

Painless lymphocytic thyroiditis is a variant of HT. In the United States, this condition develops in 5 to 9% of all women after parturition (postpartum thyroiditis). The initial phase is transient hyperthyroidism (1 to 3 months) with zero radioiodine uptake because of leakage of thyroid hormone. Hypothyroidism follows but may occur without

TABLE 1. **Categories of Primary Hypothyroidism**

Goitrous Hypothyroidism	Atrophic Hypothyroidism
Hashimoto's thyroiditis	Post-radioiodine therapy for
Painful subacute thyroiditis	Graves' disease
Silent lymphocytic thyroiditis	Postthyroidectomy
Drugs	Postexternal radiation
Hereditary biosynthetic defects	Atrophic thyroiditis
Iodine deficiency	Thyroid-stimulating hormone
Postradioiodine therapy in	receptor–binding antibodies
Graves' disease (transient)	

antecedent hyperthyroidism. Most patients recover, but persistent hypothyroidism or goiter is found in 25 to 50% of patients after 2 years. Postpartum thyroiditis occurs in 35% of patients with HT and 25% of those with type I diabetes mellitus. Recurrent episodes are common and need not be related to pregnancy.

Iodide deficiency is not a problem in the United States but is the most common worldwide cause of goitrous hypothyroidism. Painful (postviral) subacute thyroiditis has a time course similar to that of silent thyroiditis but is not an autoimmune disorder. Severe pain or tenderness occurs in one or both lobes, often with radiation to the ear, an elevated sedimentation rate, fever, and systemic symptoms. Hereditary biosynthetic defects in thyroid hormone synthesis cause childhood goitrous or nodular hypothyroidism. Hypothyroidism may be caused by drugs that inhibit thyroid hormone biosynthesis (e.g., propylthiouracil [PTU] or methimazole [Tapazole]), release (lithium), or both (iodides, including saturated solution of potassium iodide [SSKI] and amiodarone [Cordarone]). Hypothyroidism is particularly likely when patients with HT are exposed to iodides or lithium.

Atrophic Hypothyroidism

Hypothyroidism without goiter is commonly an iatrogenic problem due to radioiodine therapy of Graves' hyperthyroidism, surgery, or neck external radiation for malignancy. Autoimmune thyroid atrophy may cause profound hypothyroidism, in some cases due to TSH receptor–inhibiting antibodies.

CLINICAL MANIFESTATIONS

The clinical manifestations of hypothyroidism include fatigue, lethargy, weight gain, decreased mental acuity, hair loss, dry skin, constipation, muscle cramps, arthralgias, depression, paresthesias, and menstrual irregularities, especially metrorrhagia. Signs include bradycardia, diastolic hypertension, cold skin, nonpitting edema (myxedema), carotenemia, hair loss, and delay in deep tendon reflex relaxation phase. Severe hypothyroidism may cause sleep apnea, reversible pituitary insufficiency, ileus, pericardial, pleural, or abdominal effusions, hyperprolactinemia, precocious puberty, arthritis, or carpal tunnel syndrome. Hypothyroid patients may also demonstrate iron deficiency or macrocytic anemia, concomitant vitamin B_{12} deficiency, hyponatremia, or hypercholesterolemia.

LABORATORY EVALUATION

Thyroid-stimulating hormone and thyroid hormone (thyroxine, T_4) concentration have an inverse logarithmic relationship. For example, a 50% decrease in free T_4 concentration causes a 90-fold increase in serum TSH concentration. Our clinic uses a TSH-based algorithm to screen for hypothyroidism. A normal serum TSH finding necessitates no additional studies. When serum TSH is elevated, a free T_4 concentration or index is performed. Measurement of serum triiodothyronine (T_3) concentration is rarely necessary. HT is diagnosed by the presence of a diffuse goiter and elevated serum TSH. When a similar goiter is present with normal serum TSH, antithyroid antibodies (e.g., anti-TPO antibodies) are measured to diagnose HT.

SUBCLINICAL HYPOTHYROIDISM

Although the range of thyroid hormone normal values is broad (e.g., for free T_4, 0.8 to 2.4 ng per dL), the hormone concentration is stable within a narrow range in a euthyroid person. The earliest sign of a failing thyroid is an elevated serum TSH. The combination of an elevated serum TSH concentration and a normal free T_4 (or free T_4 index) is called subclinical (or mild) hypothyroidism (SCH), provided other causes of elevated TSH are excluded. These include mouse antibodies, which give falsely elevated values, untreated adrenal insufficiency, and recovery from severe illness. SCH affects 10 to 20% of those older than 65 years of age.

What is the significance of SCH? The high prevalence of antithyroid antibodies in these patients confirms the presence of HT. Patients with both elevated TSH and positive antibodies become frankly hypothyroid at the rate of 4.3% per year. Either TSH elevation or antithyroid antibodies alone predicts a yearly hypothyroid incidence of just over 2%. Young patients with SCH are therefore at high risk to become seriously hypothyroid over time, but some patients spontaneously return to normal. When serum TSH rises above 10 μU per mL, significant low-density lipoprotein (LDL) cholesterol elevation occurs. When TSH is greater than 10 μU per mL, thyroid hormone therapy lowers LDL cholesterol by an average of 14 mg per dL, corresponding to a 28% decrease in cardiovascular risk. When levothyroxine therapy of SCH was compared with placebo in a double-blinded fashion, 50% of patients improved with therapy, compared with 25% with placebo, although patients with very high serum TSH concentrations were included. Therapy is recommended for SCH with TSH greater than 10 μU per mL, symptoms suggestive of hypothyroidism, strongly positive thyroid antibodies, absence of cardiac disease, or younger age. My colleagues and I are more inclined to follow patients with serum TSH between 5 and 10 μU per mL who are asymptomatic, older, antibody negative, and with concomitant heart disease.

THERAPY OF HYPOTHYROIDISM

The goal of thyroid hormone therapy is symptomatic improvement and TSH normalization. TSH concentrations slightly above or below the normal range (0.5 to 5 μU per mL) may be followed in asymptomatic patients. However, fully suppressed serum TSH (<0.1 or <0.01 μU per mL) may cause thinning bones or atrial fibrillation and is best avoided for most hypothyroid patients. Levothyroxine (Levothroid, Levoxyl, Synthroid), the therapy of choice, has a 7-day half-life and is administered once daily. Missed doses can be made up by doubling up the next day or, rarely, when compliance is poor, by taking a full week's therapy once weekly under supervision. Approximately 70% of an oral dose is absorbed. The full replacement dose of levothyroxine is 1.6 μg per kg per day. Initiate therapy in younger patients with near full replacement, whereas older patients and those with or at high risk for heart disease should receive lower doses (e.g., 12.5 to 25 μg per day). Because five to six drug half-lives are required for equilibrium, a meaningful TSH concentration is measured after 6 or more weeks at a given dosage. When thyroid function is absent, levothyroxine requirements remain stable over years, whereas the requirements are far less in mild hypothyroidism (e.g., 25 to

50 µg per day), but may require increased dosage with time.

Altered Thyroid Hormone Requirements

When compliance is variable, serum TSH may remain elevated despite escalating levothyroxine dosages. Increased requirements occur with

1. Drugs that increase levothyroxine metabolism, including rifampin, phenytoin (Dilantin), carbamazepine (Tegretol), and phenobarbital. The requirement may double.
2. Drugs that interfere with levothyroxine absorption, such as iron (including multivitamins containing iron), aluminum hydroxide (Maalox and others), sucralfate (Carafate), and cholestyramine.
3. Pregnancy, which may increase the levothyroxine requirement by 40% or more beginning in the first trimester, independent of iron administration. The mechanism is uncertain.
4. Drugs such as sertraline (Zoloft), estrogens, calcium, and lovastatin (Mevacor), whose effects on levothyroxine requirements are uncertain.

Less levothyroxine is required in women taking androgens (e.g., danazole [Danocrine]). Whether bran inhibits levothyroxine absorption is controversial. When possible, levothyroxine should be taken on an empty stomach without food or other medications. The price of different levothyroxine brands for 100 µg (100 pills) ranged from $10.99 to $31.59 at a local pharmacy. Although different brands are thought to be identical, brand interchange is often associated with significant TSH alterations. When a new brand is selected, thyroid function must be rechecked.

Other Thyroid Hormone Preparations

Liothyronine (Cytomel, T_3), with its rapid onset, high peak, and low trough concentrations, as well as the difficulty in thyroid function test interpretation associated with its use, is usually not recommended for chronic therapy. T_3 has a 1-day half-life. Direct comparisons between T_4 and T_3 potency are not possible, although T_3 is thought to be four times as potent as levothyroxine. Prescribed doses range from 12.5 µg daily to 25 µg twice or three times daily. Radioactive iodine therapy for thyroid cancer requires thyroid hormone withdrawal (to raise serum TSH); substituting liothyronine for levothyroxine for 4 weeks before withdrawal shortens the symptomatic period. After radioiodine therapy, 10 days of liothyronine added to levothyroxine decreases the symptomatic period and accelerates TSH normalization. The rapid onset of liothyronine action may be advantageous in hypothyroid emergencies (see section on Myxedema Crisis, later). Recent data suggest that some patients who do not feel well on levothyroxine alone improve when liothyronine, 12.5 µg per day, is added. In this situation, the levothyroxine dosage may be reduced by 50 µg per day.

Desiccated thyroid (USP Thyroid Tablets, Armour Thyroid) contains ground pork thyroid tissue with both levothyroxine and liothyronine in protein linkage. Although the relative amounts may vary, one grain of USP Thyroid contains approximately 40 µg of levothyroxine and 10 µg of T_3. Doses prescribed range from one-half to three grains. Some patients who have been on USP thyroid for many years note decreased energy or sense of well-being when switched to levothyroxine. Whether the T_3 content provides a physiologic advantage or a pharmacologic boost is uncertain. Liotrix (Thyrolar, Euthroid) contains levothyroxine and liothyronine in a fixed ratio of four to one (e.g., Thyrolar-1 contains 50 µg of levothyroxine and 12.5 µg of liothyronine). To some extent, the criticisms of T_3 extend to desiccated thyroid and liotrix.

Other Uses

Liothyronine and, less frequently, levothyroxine are successful adjuncts to antidepressant therapy in euthyroid people. Whether thyroid hormone itself has intrinsic antidepressant properties is uncertain. Levothyroxine suppressive therapy may benefit euthyroid, antithyroid antibody–positive patients with unexplained urticaria. Thyroid hormone should not be used for weight control. During critical illness, the conversion of T_4 to T_3 is inhibited; liothyronine has been prescribed for these patients to correct the T_3 deficiency. However, no improvement in mortality has been demonstrated in intensive care or cardiac surgical patients with low serum T_3. The use of liothyronine in cardiac transplant donors and recipients is experimental and of unproven benefit.

MYXEDEMA CRISIS (MYXEDEMA COMA)

Myxedema crisis occurs when a profoundly hypothyroid patient becomes severely ill (Table 2). Approximately half of these patients become comatose *after* hospital admission, possibly because of excessive fluid administration, sedating drugs, or unrecognized sepsis. With excellent medical management, patients usually improve, although the type, amount, and route of thyroid hormone administration is debated. Whether thyroid hormone per se is lifesaving is uncertain. Some advocate intravenous levothy-

TABLE 2. **Myxedema Crisis**

HYPOventilation
HYPOthermia
HYPOmetabolism of drugs
HYPOnatremia
HYPOmotility of bowel and bladder
HYPOtension
HYPOadrenalism
HYPOglycemia
HYPOresponsiveness to infection
HYPOthyroidism

roxine (e.g., 400 µg for 2 days followed by 100 µg daily) until patients are able to take medication by mouth. However, severely ill patients are unable to convert T_4 to T_3. I therefore prefer intravenous liothyronine (Triostat) in those rare cases in which profound hypothyroidism is life-threatening. I prescribe 10 to 25 µg twice to three times daily, reducing the dosage with tachyarrhythmia or ischemia and changing to the oral route and then levothyroxine with clinical improvement. Intravenous T_3 is expensive (hospital cost: $180 per 10-µg vial). Because glucocorticoid deficiency may accompany profound hypothyroidism, stress doses of glucocorticoids are also administered.

CENTRAL HYPOTHYROIDISM

Although hypothyroidism secondary to pituitary or hypothalamic disease is uncommon, it deserves special consideration. Adrenocorticotropic hormone (ACTH) and other pituitary hormone deficiencies may accompany TSH deficiency. Thyroid hormone therapy of hypothyroidism causes increased cortisol breakdown. The normal pituitary compensates by increasing ACTH secretion, whereas inadequate ACTH compensation may result in life-threatening acute adrenal insufficiency. Therefore, secondary hypothyroidism must be excluded before starting thyroid hormone.

The distinction between primary and secondary hypothyroidism seems easy: primary hypothyroidism is characterized by decreased T_4 and free T_4, and increased TSH; secondary hypothyroidism also has decreased T_4 and free T_4, but decreased TSH. The second pattern is commonly found with destructive pituitary lesions. However, with hypothalamic dysfunction, serum TSH may be normal or even slightly increased despite a very low free T_4 concentration, making TSH alone a misleading test in this situation. How does this occur? The hypothalamic hormone thyrotropin-releasing hormone (TRH) is required not only for coordinated TSH release but also for its glycosylation and hence biologic action. When TRH is absent (e.g., in patients with craniopharyngioma or after brain irradiation), the secreted TSH molecule is without biologic activity but is measured in TSH assays.

To distinguish the minimal TSH elevation of central hypothyroidism from SCH, recall the inverse logarithmic correlation between thyroid hormone and TSH. In contrast to mild primary hypothyroidism, where the free T_4 is normal or slightly decreased, with hypothalamic disease the free T_4 must be very low before TSH rises. The disparity between a very low free T_4 with minimal TSH elevation must alert the clinician to the dangers of central hypothyroidism. In this situation, cortisol should be administered with levothyroxine. Unfortunately, no early warning system exists to detect mild central hypothyroidism. With known pituitary or hypothalamic disease, a low normal free T_4 suggests hypothyroidism. Furthermore, TSH is not useful to monitor therapy of central hypothyroidism; clinical features and serum free T_4 must be followed.

HYPERTHYROIDISM

method of
JEROME M. HERSHMAN, M.D.
*West Los Angeles Veterans Affairs Medical
Center and University of California, Los
Angeles, School of Medicine*
Los Angeles, California

Hyperthyroidism is the condition resulting from the effects of excessive amounts of thyroid hormones on body tissues. The terms "hyperthyroidism" and "thyrotoxicosis" tend to be used interchangeably. At one time or another, approximately 1% of the population has hyperthyroidism.

Table 1 lists the various causes of hyperthyroidism. Graves' disease is the most common cause and probably accounts for over 80% of the cases. The serum IgG of patients with Graves' hyperthyroidism contains a thyroid-stimulating IgG (TSI). With sensitive assays, TSI is found in the serum of more than 90% of patients with active hyperthyroidism. Because thyroid hormone has many effects on different organ systems, there are numerous clinical features of the disorder. The principal clinical features are listed in Table 2.

DIAGNOSIS

Elevated serum levels of thyroid hormones are the hallmark of the diagnosis. Ordinarily, serum thyroxine (T_4), triiodothyronine (T_3), free T_4, and free T_3 levels are all elevated, and serum thyroid-stimulating hormone (TSH) is suppressed. The increased concentrations of T_4 and T_3 saturate the binding proteins so that the free T_4 and T_3 tend to be proportionally higher than the total hormone levels in relation to the normal ranges. In a small proportion of hyperthyroid patients (probably less than 5%), free T_4 level is normal and only serum T_3 and free T_3 levels are increased, leading to the term T_3-*thyrotoxicosis*. In some older patients with poor nutrition, free T_4 level is elevated while total and free T_3 levels are normal.

There is a high degree of correlation between the severity of the disorder based on clinical features and the thyroid hormone concentrations. This correlation does not hold for older patients who tend to have a paucity of typical clinical features.

With current sensitive TSH assays, the serum TSH level is less than 0.1 µU/mL (0.1 mU/L) in nearly all hyperthyroid patients. A normal or elevated serum TSH level in a clearly hyperthyroid patient should raise consideration of the rare forms of TSH-induced hyperthyroidism listed in Table 1.

Although thyroid radioiodine uptake is high in most forms of hyperthyroidism, it is low in patients who are thyrotoxic owing to lymphocytic thyroiditis, subacute thyroiditis, or ingestion of thyroid hormone. A large iodine load, such as contrast material for angiography, reduces thyroid uptake by increasing the pool of iodide. The thyroid scan in Graves' disease shows diffuse uptake of radioiodine. The scan is helpful if a solitary hyperfunctioning thyroid adenoma is being considered as the cause of hyperthyroidism in a patient with a palpable nodule.

TABLE 1. **Causes of Hyperthyroidism**

Cause	Etiology of Hyperthyroidism	Therapy
Graves' disease	TSI	See text
Hyperfunctioning solitary thyroid adenoma ("hot" nodule)	Activating mutation of TSH receptor	Radioiodine
"Toxic" multinodular goiter	Autonomy	Radioiodine
Lymphocytic thyroiditis with low thyroid radioiodine uptake	Inflammation	Beta blocker
Subacute (granulomatous) thyroiditis (early phase)	Inflammation	Prednisone or NSAID Beta blocker
Ingestion of excessive amount of thyroid hormones	Medication	Reduce dose
TSH-producing pituitary adenoma	TSH	Surgery
Pituitary resistance to suppression of TSH secretion by thyroid hormone due to mutation in the T_3 receptor	TSH	Experimental
Trophoblastic tumors (hydatidiform mole, choriocarcinoma)	Excessive production of HCG, a weak thyroid stimulator	Remove mole Chemotherapy
Hyperemesis gravidarum	HCG	Supportive measures
Follicular thyroid carcinoma with widespread metastases	Autonomy	Radioiodine and surgery
Struma ovarii (ovarian teratoma with thyroid elements)	Autonomy or TSI	Surgery

Abbreviations: TSI = thyroid-stimulating IgG; TSH = thyroid-stimulating hormone; NSAID, nonsteroidal anti-inflammatory drug; HCG, human chorionic gonadotropin.

Thyroid-stimulating IgG is measured in two ways, either as stimulation of cAMP generation in cultured thyroid cells (TSI) or as displacement of labeled TSH from the TSH receptor (TSH-R antibody), a simpler and less expensive method. Measurement of TSH-R antibody is useful in special situations. For patients with recent onset of hyperthyroidism who may have either Graves' disease or lymphocytic thyroiditis, a radioiodine scan will make the differentiation but is often inconvenient. Elevated TSH-R antibody indicates Graves' disease and makes the radioiodine uptake test unnecessary.

TREATMENT

Three definitive modes of treatment are available for the hyperthyroidism of Graves' disease: drugs, radioactive iodine ^{131}I therapy, and surgical thyroidectomy.

Antithyroid Drugs

E. B. Astwood introduced antithyroid drugs of the thionamide type for the treatment of hyperthyroidism in 1943. Propylthiouracil (PTU) and methimazole (Tapazole), the two drugs of this type presently used in the United States, block the synthesis of thyroid hormone by inhibition of thyroid peroxidase. The drugs are concentrated in the thyroid gland, where they have a much longer duration of action than the plasma half-life of 1 hour for PTU and 3 to 6 hours for methimazole. Inhibition of organic binding of iodine continues for 12 hours after a dose of methimazole, but much of this effect is lost after 24 hours. For this reason, a once-a-day dosage is not as effective as more frequent doses. Because the blocking action of PTU is slightly shorter than that of methimazole, it should also be given in divided doses, preferably every 8 hours. In humans, methimazole is 15 to 20 times as potent as PTU. PTU, but not methimazole, blocks the extrathyroidal conversion of T_4 to T_3 so that large doses of PTU cause a rapid fall in serum T_3 levels.

The initial dose of PTU is 300 to 600 mg per day given in divided doses at approximately 8-hour intervals. The initial dose of methimazole is 30 to 60 mg per day given in two divided doses. The initial dose should be based on assessment of the severity of the condition and the size of the goiter, with larger doses being used for those persons with severer disease and larger goiters. I follow patients initially at monthly intervals until the hyperthyroidism is controlled. At or before each visit, I obtain serum free T_4, free or total T_3, and TSH levels. After control of the hyperthyroidism based on clinical assessment and normalization of serum free T_4 and T_3 levels, the dose of the antithyroid drug can be reduced by one-third to one-half. Patients can then be followed-up at intervals of 2 to 3 months. To increase the possibility of achieving a permanent cure, I usually maintain the therapy with the antithyroid drug for 18 months before discontinuing it.

Side effects of antithyroid drugs include skin rash, hepatic reactions, arthralgia, serum sickness, vasculitis, and agranulocytosis. The incidence of agranulocytosis is about 0.4%; it usually appears within the first few months of therapy and is reversible. Most

TABLE 2. **Clinical Features of Hyperthyroidism**

System	Clinical Features
Nervous	Nervousness, emotional lability, tremor, brisk reflexes
Cardiac	Tachycardia, atrial fibrillation, congestive failure, flow murmurs
Gastrointestinal	Increased appetite and food intake, hyperdefecation, abnormal liver function tests
Musculoskeletal	Weakness, muscle atrophy, osteopenia
Eyes	Stare due to retraction of upper lid, proptosis, restricted ocular motility
Skin and hair	Warm, moist, velvety texture; hot sweaty palms, onycholysis
Reproductive	Oligomenorrhea, impaired fertility, gynecomastia, impotence
Metabolism	Weight loss, fatigue, increased sweating, heat intolerance

endocrinologists do not routinely follow the white blood cell counts, but instead warn the patients to have this test if an infection, such as pharyngitis, develops. It is important to obtain a baseline complete blood count and liver function tests for comparison with those measured subsequently, but I do not order these tests routinely when following up patients.

Treatment with antithyroid drugs results in long-term remission of hyperthyroidism in approximately 30 to 70% of patients. Long-term remission is defined here as remission persisting for 2 years after cessation of therapy. Most recurrences show up within 1 year after the drugs are stopped. Early reports showed remission rates that often exceeded 50%. In 1979, it appeared that remission rates had fallen to less than 20%, possibly in relation to high dietary iodine intake. More recent reports, however, showed long-term remission rates of more than 50%. The change may be related to more careful selection of patients and possibly to lower dietary iodine intake.

During the course of treatment with antithyroid drugs, there are no absolutely reliable indicators that a long-term remission will occur. The best evidence is that the disease remains under control on a low dose of drug, such as 50 mg of PTU or 5 mg of methimazole. Conversely, a requirement for a large dose of antithyroid drug to control the hyperthyroidism indicates that the disorder is active. Reduction of the size of the goiter suggests remission but is seldom apparent. Measurements of TSI have an 80% predictive value; that is, when the TSH-R antibody is no longer increased, there is about an 80% chance that the hyperthyroidism will not recur in the next year when therapy is stopped. However, I do not follow up the TSH-R antibody because of the expense, the uncertainty of the prediction, and the fact that cure of the disease is indicated by normal thyroid hormone measurements while the patient is on a low dose of drug.

Beta-Adrenergic Blocking Drugs

Beta-adrenergic blocking drugs have had considerable impact on the acute management of hyperthyroidism. Although propranolol (Inderal) may lower the elevated serum T_3 level of hyperthyroidism by inhibition of peripheral T_4 to T_3 conversion, other beta-adrenergic blocking drugs do not usually lower serum T_3 levels. Nevertheless, improvement of many of the clinical features of hyperthyroidism occurs. The efficacy of these agents is primarily through their inhibition of the action of catecholamines. Beta blockers cause rapid symptomatic relief and improve anxiety, nervousness, tachycardia, sweating, tremor, and muscle weakness. The use of a beta blocker is helpful for symptomatic patients until the serum T_4 and T_3 levels are normalized. I prefer either atenolol 50 mg twice daily initially or propranolol 20 to 40 mg two to three times daily. Metoprolol (Lopressor) or long-acting propranolol are also effective. I discontinue the beta blocker gradually over 1 to 2 weeks when the hyperthyroidism is controlled biochemically, usually after 6 to 12 weeks of the antithyroid drug.

Cholecystographic Agents

The cholecystographic agents sodium ipodate (Oragrafin)* and iopanoic acid (Telepaque)* are potent inhibitors of the conversion of T_4 to T_3 in peripheral tissues. This mechanism accounts for about one-half of the T_3 production in hyperthyroid patients. These drugs lower serum T_3 levels. In addition, the iodine released through the metabolism of these iodinated organic compounds blocks the release of hormone from the thyroid. Administration of sodium ipodate or iopanoic acid lowers serum T_3 and T_4 levels and causes rapid improvement of hyperthyroidism. Unfortunately, the results of chronic therapy with cholecystographic agents have been disappointing. These agents, combined with antithyroid drugs, are appropriate for acute management of severe hyperthyroidism that is not responding to conventional therapy.

Radioiodine ^{131}I

Radioiodine 131 (^{131}I) is the most common therapy in the United States for Graves' hyperthyroidism. Hypothyroidism is the main complication and occurs in the majority of patients, often years later, despite the attempt to tailor the dose to avoid hypothyroidism. Hypothyroidism within the first 6 months after ^{131}I may be temporary. Many endocrinologists prefer to use a larger dose with the expectation of certain hypothyroidism as the outcome. If the first dose of ^{131}I does not control the hyperthyroidism within 6 to 12 months, another dose is given. The dose of ^{131}I is calculated based on the 24-hour radioiodine uptake and the estimated size of the thyroid. Current doses are in the range of 5 to 20 mCi ^{131}I and deposit 7000 to 20,000 rad in the thyroid.

Therapy with antithyroid drugs reduces the therapeutic effect of the ^{131}I so that larger doses of ^{131}I are necessary to cure the hyperthyroidism in patients who have taken antithyroid drugs up to a few days before the ^{131}I dose. This radioprotective effect may last for 1 week after the antithyroid drug is stopped. PTU appears to be more potent than methimazole in this respect.

When patients are very ill from hyperthyroidism, it is preferable to control the disorder first with antithyroid drugs because ^{131}I therapy may result in a discharge of hormone from the gland resulting in a rise in both T_3 and T_4 levels by as much as twofold 10 days after the radiodine is administered. The antithyroid drug must be discontinued 2 to 3 days before the administration of the therapeutic dose, and a larger dose of ^{131}I (approximately 25 to 50% more than the usual dose) is given because of the radioprotective effect of the antithyroid drug. After administration of the ^{131}I, patients may begin taking the

---

*Not FDA approved for this indication.

antithyroid drug again 2 to 3 days later. Some of the manifestations of hyperthyroidism may be controlled with beta-adrenergic blocking drugs during the therapy with the radioiodine.

Because ^{131}I therapy may worsen pre-existing Graves' eye disease, patients with active Graves' eye disease should not be given ^{131}I until the eye disease stabilizes. If ^{131}I is given to a patient with active Graves' eye disease, a course of prednisone in a dose of 1 mg per kg tapered over 2 to 3 months prevents the deleterious effect of ^{131}I on the eye condition.

Surgical Thyroidectomy

Surgical thyroidectomy is dramatically effective for the eradication of hyperthyroidism. Unfortunately, there are a number of side effects and complications that limit its use so that only 1% of hyperthyroid patients are now treated by surgical thyroidectomy. Although some patients can be prepared for surgery with beta blockers alone to control tachycardia, common practice continues to be restoration of the euthyroid state with antithyroid drugs followed by stable iodine for 10 days before surgery. About 10% of patients develop a recurrence of hyperthyroidism, and 30% become permanently hypothyroid after this surgery. Permanent hypoparathyroidism occurs in 1%, and recurrent laryngeal nerve palsy occurs in about 1% of patients. These complications, as well as the trauma and expense of surgery, make it less appealing than radioiodine ablation. Surgical thyroidectomy is usually reserved for special situations, such as obstructing goiters, allergy to antithyroid drugs, noncompliance with medical therapy, or refusal to take [131]I.

Pregnancy

Hyperthyroidism occurs in about 1 per 1000 pregnant women. It can be treated effectively with antithyroid drugs, but, because these drugs cross the placenta, the lowest possible doses should be used to control the hyperthyroidism. Because pregnancy ameliorates autoimmune disease, the antithyroid drug can often be discontinued in the third trimester. Surgical thyroidectomy can be performed safely during the second trimester after control of the hyperthyroidism with antithyroid drugs but is a less desirable alternative for the reasons noted above. Care must be exercised to avoid postoperative hypothyroidism. Radioiodine should not be given to the pregnant woman because it crosses the placenta and could cause permanent hypothyroidism in the fetus, which has a functional thyroid by the 10th week of gestation.

Thyroid Storm

Patients with thyroid storm, or severe decompensated hyperthyroidism, have tachycardia, fever, agitation or psychosis, nausea, vomiting, and diarrhea. There is usually a precipitating factor, such as infection, gastroenteritis, severe trauma, or surgery. Supportive measures and treatment of the underlying causative factor are essential. Specific measures include propylthiouracil (600 mg) or methimazole (60 mg) stat and half this dose every 6 hours; propranolol, 40 to 80 mg every 4 to 6 hours; sodium ipodate, 1 gram stat and 1 gram daily for 14 days; or, alternatively, 0.5 mL of saturated solution of potassium iodide twice a day or 1 gram of sodium iodide intravenously over 8 hours. For patients who do not improve quickly, dexamethasone, 4 to 8 mg, is given daily.

THYROID CANCER

method of
DOUGLAS W. BALL, M.D., and
PAUL W. LADENSON, M.D.
Johns Hopkins University School of Medicine
Baltimore, Maryland

Thyroid cancer is a moderately common malignancy with higher survival rates than many other solid tumors. In 1997, there were 16,100 new cases of thyroid cancer in the United States, with a female/male ratio of 2.4:1. In women, the thyroid gland is the 11th most common cancer site, comparable to cervical and renal carcinoma in incidence. Thyroid cancer is most commonly detected in the fourth and fifth decades of life, although there is a significant incidence in both the young and the elderly. There has been a significant absolute increase in both thyroid cancer diagnoses and deaths since the 1970s. However, improvements in diagnosis and management have been associated with a better prognosis; 5-year survival rates among white Americans have increased from 83% in 1960 to 96% in 1992. In 1997, a total of 1230 Americans (780 females and 450 males) died of thyroid cancer.

Among known etiologic factors for thyroid cancer, the two most important are an inherited genetic predisposition and exposure to ionizing radiation. For the 20% of medullary thyroid cancer (MTC) cases inherited as part of the multiple endocrine neoplasia type 2 (MEN 2) syndromes, presymptomatic genetic diagnosis and prophylactic thyroidectomy have made this a surgically preventable form of thyroid cancer. The role of ionizing radiation has been underlined by the epidemic of pediatric thyroid cancer following the Chernobyl nuclear disaster in the Ukraine. From 1989 to 1991, the incidence of pediatric thyroid cancer, a previously rare tumor in this region, increased more than 50-fold. Much less dramatic cumulative increases in the United States have been attributed by some to the atomic weapons testing program, with peak exposures in the period of 1951 to 1957. Head and neck therapeutic radiation, especially in childhood, is also associated with an increased risk of thyroid neoplasms, both benign and malignant. In contrast, exposure to routine radiographic studies, including dental and chest radiographs and radioiodine scans, has not been shown to increase thyroid cancer risk. Patients with Graves' disease may have a modestly higher risk of developing thyroid cancer, particularly during the first 5 years after radioiodine therapy. Autoimmune thyroiditis does clearly confer a higher relative risk of thyroid lymphoma, but the absolute risk remains very low.

Benign follicular adenomas and multinodular goiters do not appear to progress to thyroid carcinoma at an appreciable rate.

The principal clinical challenges in thyroid cancer management include promptly identifying thyroid cancer patients from the much larger population harboring a thyroid nodule, correctly classifying the histopathologic type of thyroid cancer and choosing an appropriate surgical approach, deciding among multiple options for adjunctive treatment and long-term follow-up, and managing patients with recurrent or persistent disease. In deciding on the intensity of treatment and follow-up regimens for differentiated thyroid cancer (DTC), it is vital to appreciate prognostic factors that have been derived from the natural history of these tumors.

CLASSIFICATION OF THYROID CANCER

Thyroid cancer is conventionally classified according to the cell of origin. The great majority of thyroid cancers (~90%) are differentiated cancers of the follicular epithelium (Table 1). The remainder are medullary cancers (~5%), originating in the parafollicular C cells, undifferentiated or anaplastic cancers of uncertain origin, thyroid lymphomas, and miscellaneous tumors, including metastatic cancers to thyroid. DTC can be subdivided broadly into papillary and follicular groups. More than 70% of all thyroid cancers have papillary features (including tumors classified as follicular variant of papillary cancer or mixed papillary-follicular histology). The characteristic cytologic features of papillary cancer (nuclear inclusions and cellular grooves) can generally be identified both on fine-needle aspirate material and in surgical specimens, along with a distinctive frondlike architecture. Papillary thyroid cancer most commonly metastasizes to regional lymph nodes and frequently is iodine avid. Papillary microcarcinomas (<5 mm) are a common incidental finding in pathologic specimens, and when identified in this circumstance generally necessitate no treatment beyond postoperative thyroid hormone suppression therapy.

Less than 15% of thyroid cancers have a predominantly follicular histology, including minimally and frankly invasive tumors and Hürthle cell tumors. Follicular thyroid neoplasms generally cannot be effectively diagnosed as malignant or benign based on fine-needle cytology alone. The distinction between follicular cancer versus follicular adenoma rests on the presence or absence of capsular and vascular invasion. Many thyroid specialists distinguish microinvasive follicular carcinoma, which has a generally favorable prognosis, from follicular tumors with frank local and vascular invasion. The latter invasive follicular carcinomas are associated with relatively high rates of distant organ metastasis. Among follicular tumors, Hürthle cell tumors exhibit distinctive cells with abundant cytoplasm. The overall spectrum of Hürthle cell tumor behavior resembles follicular tumors in general, but they only rarely concentrate and respond to radioiodine.

MTC has distinctive clinical features and management challenges. MTC is the cardinal element of the multiple endocrine neoplasia (MEN) type 2 family of dominantly inherited disorders, which includes familial isolated MTC (FMTC), MEN 2A (MTC, pheochromocytoma, and hyperparathyroidism), and MEN 2B (MTC, pheochromocytomas, intestinal ganglioneuromas, and a marfanoid habitus). Among the most important clinical considerations in management of patients with MTC is recognizing the possibility of concurrent pheochromocytoma, selection of an appropriately aggressive primary surgical approach, and the limited nature of adjuvant treatments currently available.

CLINICAL MANIFESTATION OF THYROID CANCER

Patients with thyroid cancer typically come to medical attention with an asymptomatic or minimally symptomatic thyroid nodule. Their clinical histories and examinations are usually indistinguishable from patients with benign nodules. Potentially worrisome features include a history of head and neck radiation, local pain, dysphonia, hemoptysis, hard fixed masses, and the presence of regional lymphadenopathy. Overall, the risk of malignancy for an symptomatic thyroid nodule in an adult is approximately 5%. Nodules occurring in males and children have a relatively higher risk of malignancy than those identified in adult females. Undoubtedly, the most important tool in classifying thyroid nodules is fine-needle aspiration (FNA). For both solitary nodules as well as dominant nodules within a multinodular goiter, FNA is the diagnostic procedure of choice. Needle aspiration may be performed either with direct palpation guidance or, if necessary, under ultrasound guidance for nonpalpable nodules. Common benign diagnostic categories include adenomatoid and colloid nodules and autoimmune thyroiditis. Neoplastic categories include definite or suspected papillary carcinoma, follicular neoplasm (of which about 20% ultimately prove to be carcinoma), medullary carcinoma, lymphoma, other neoplasm, and tumors of indeterminate cause. Cytologic specimens that contain insufficient follicular epithelium for diagnosis should be distinguished from specimens that are adequate but diagnostically indeterminate. For the former category, the FNA is customarily repeated; for the latter, surgery or clinical follow-up may be elected, depending on associated clinical finding. For papillary carcinoma, FNA is highly sensitive (>95%) and specific (>95%). As previously noted, thyroid FNA cannot distinguish follicular adenoma from carcinoma. Although FNA is theoretically sensitive for MTC, success in practice has been disappointing, with 35 to 40% of U.S. patients going undiagnosed at primary presentation. Because the diagnosis of MTC can be readily confirmed by an elevated blood calcitonin level, it is important for the cytopathologist to convey any suspicion of this diagnosis to the clinician. Routine use of calcitonin levels in evaluation of thyroid nodule patients has not been widely accepted.

Serum TSH measurement is a useful adjunct, particularly when it is obtained before referral for FNA. Patients

TABLE 1. **Histologic Classification of Thyroid Cancer**

Differentiated thyroid cancer
  Papillary carcinoma
    Papillary microcarcinoma
    Conventional papillary carcinoma
    Mixed papillary-follicular carcinoma
    Follicular variant
    Tall cell variant
    Insular variant
  Follicular carcinoma
    Minimally invasive (encapsulated)
    Invasive
    Hürthle cell carcinoma
Medullary
Lymphoma
Anaplastic or undifferentiated carcinoma
Uncommon cancers: spindle cell, small cell, sarcoma, teratoma, metastatic

with a palpable thyroid nodule and a low serum TSH level (without obvious stigmata of Graves' disease) can be next evaluated by scintigraphy. Cold or "warm" nodules in this setting usually still necessitate FNA; but hot nodules have a very low risk of cancer despite sometimes exhibiting atypical cytology. Routine use of nuclear scintigraphy and thyroid ultrasound is not justified, however, because both studies have relatively modest independent predictive value. In selected instances, thyroid ultrasound can be helpful in determining whether multiple nodules or bilateral disease is present, accurately defining the size of poorly palpable nodules, detecting regional adenopathy, and guiding FNA for nonpalpable lesions. Measuring other serum thyroid hormone or thyroglobulin concentrations is not generally helpful in differential diagnosis.

For patients with MEN 2, at-risk first-degree relatives should be screened with DNA analysis for activating mutations in the *ret* proto-oncogene, typically obtained from blood mononuclear cells. Characteristic germline mutations can be detected in approximately 98% of such families. Detection of such a mutation, ideally between the ages of 4 and 6 years, enables prophylactic thyroidectomy, before development of a potentially metastatic cancer. All patients undergoing surgery for MTC should be screened for catecholamine excess to rule out a potentially unsuspected pheochromocytoma.

STAGING OF THYROID CANCER

Clinical staging of thyroid cancer is helpful for prognosis. The standard World Health Organization TNM Classification of DTC is shown in Table 2. In addition to standard classification by tumor size and the presence of nodal and distant metastases, several research groups have defined other criteria to stratify patient risk that have been based on thyroid cancer natural history data. Common features of these systems are patient age, tumor size, and the presence or absence of local invasion or distant metastases. An example of one commonly used scheme is the MACIS system (i.e., *m*etastasis, *a*ge, *c*ompleteness of resection, *i*nvasion, and *s*ize), which has prognostic value for DTC patients. Twenty-year survival rates for lowest to highest risk MACIS categories are 99%, 89%, 56%, and 24%, respectively.

SURGICAL TREATMENT OF THYROID CANCER

For patients with DTC as well as MTC, surgery is the initial treatment of choice. Complication rates for thyroid surgery are lower when the procedure is

performed by an experienced thyroid surgeon. Tumors with invasion, metastasis, or multifocality place even higher demands on operator skill and decision-making. Whether to perform unilateral or bilateral thyroid gland resection is guided largely by FNA results, tumor size, supplemental imaging studies if obtained, and the initial surgical findings. Blind resections without an FNA diagnosis should be discouraged. Knowledge of the patterns of local invasion and metastasis of each histologic subtype can be critical in formulating an appropriate surgical plan.

Controversies still exist among experienced surgeons regarding the optimal surgical procedure, especially for relatively small papillary cancers. For papillary cancers less than 1 cm in diameter, lobectomy appears to be sufficient. Survival is uniformly excellent and not influenced by subsequent treatments. For papillary cancers of more than 1.5 cm, survival appears to be significantly improved in patients who have a total or near-total thyroidectomy. Several factors favor total or near-total thyroidectomy. First, in papillary carcinoma, multifocal disease is common, leading to contralateral recurrences in a small but significant number of patients. Second, the use of adjuvant therapy with radioactive iodine is facilitated by a bilateral procedure. Third, patients who have undergone total or near-total thyroidectomy plus radioiodine ablation may be sensitively monitored with whole-body iodine-131 (^{131}I) scanning and serum thyroglobulin determinations. Recurrent or persistent disease may thus be detected at an earlier stage. Arguments against the routine use of total or near-total thyroidectomy are that there is increased risk of complications, particularly hypoparathyroidism, with a bilateral procedure. For experienced thyroid surgeons, the risk of permanent hypoparathyroidism is 3 to 5%, and recurrent laryngeal nerve injury rates are typically 1 to 3%. At our institution, we routinely perform total or near-total thyroidectomy in patients with papillary thyroid cancer greater than 1 cm in diameter.

In cases in which the preoperative diagnosis is follicular neoplasm, approximately 20% of such lesions will ultimately prove to be thyroid cancer. Unless there is gross local invasion or known lymphadenopathy or distant metastasis, such patients generally have an initial lobectomy and isthmusectomy. Frozen section has limited accuracy for intraoperative diagnosis of follicular cancer. If the permanent pathology sections reveal significant capsular or vascular invasion and a primary tumor size greater than 1.5 cm, patients typically undergo a completion thyroidectomy 1 to 3 weeks after their primary surgery. As a potential alternative, radioiodine ablation of an intact contralateral lobe can be done. However, the potential for painful radiation-induced thyroiditis and the frequent need for multiple radioiodine doses to ablate remnant tissue make this approach less attractive for most patients. If the permanent pathology sections indicate follicular adenoma, that is, no evidence for capsular or vascular invasion, the physician has an option to suppress thyroid-stimulating

TABLE 2. **TMN Classification of Papillary and Follicular Thyroid Cancer**

Stage	Age < 45 Years			Age > 45 Years		
I	Any	Any	M0	T1	N0	M0
II	Any	Any	M1	T2	N0	M0
				T3	N0	M0
III	—			T4	N0	M0
				Any	N1	M0
IV	—			Any	Any	M1

T1: <1 cm; T2: 1–4 cm; T3: >4 cm; T4: extending beyond thyroid gland.
N1: any regional lymph node metastasis.
M1: any distant metastasis.

hormone (TSH) with levothyroxine or follow the patient conservatively off of thyroid hormone therapy.

The extent of lymph node dissection required for cases of DTC remains controversial. Sampling and frozen section of adjacent lymph nodes in the thyroidectomy specimen is useful to detect unsuspected nodal metastasis. In the absence of clear-cut nodal involvement, formal neck dissections should not be performed routinely for DTC. The presence of obviously enlarged nodes generally mandates frozen section and at least a central neck dissection.

The surgical treatment of MTC requires several additional considerations. First, MTC patients should routinely undergo preoperative testing to rule out pheochromocytoma, as well as hyperparathyroidism, which can occur in patients with an otherwise unsuspected inherited syndrome. Second, the high rate of regional nodal metastases, even for small tumors, and the absence of effective adjuvant therapy for MTC makes the choice of operation critical. Third, the reduced sensitivity of FNA diagnosis of MTC in practice means that some patients are only identified after their primary surgery. In our institution, the typical approach for sporadic MTC without gross nodal involvement includes preoperative computed tomography or magnetic resonance imaging of the neck and chest, along with calcitonin and carcinoembryonic antigen levels to assess extent of disease. The minimal surgical procedure is a total or near-total thyroidectomy with central neck dissection down to the aortic arch and sampling of ipsilateral jugular lymph nodes. Presence of nodal metastasis generally directs the surgeon to perform an ipsilateral modified radical neck dissection. In patients with hereditary MTC, the potential for bilobar disease and bilateral nodal metastases must be considered.

The role of surgery in anaplastic thyroid carcinoma therapy is limited. The principal goals are to obtain adequate tissue for diagnosis and to secure the airway and enteral feeding access. More aggressive attempts to debulk tumor tissue are ineffective for this aggressive cancer.

ADJUVANT TREATMENT OF DIFFERENTIATED THYROID CANCER

Postoperative treatment of patients with DTC invariably includes TSH-suppressive thyroid hormone therapy and often radioiodine treatment. Although survival in DTC patients is generally excellent, it is important to recognize factors that confer a higher risk of recurrent or persistent cancer. These factors include older patient age, larger tumor size, the presence of local invasiveness, angiogenic invasion in the case of follicular lesions, the presence of multifocal papillary tumors, and local nodal involvement. There is general consensus supporting the use of levothyroxine (Synthroid) to suppress TSH and deprive remaining tumor cells of this growth stimulus. The optimal extent of TSH suppression for a given patient depends on a combination of factors: the perceived

risk of recurrence versus the potential for side effects of long-term excessive levothyroxine, particularly osteoporosis and atrial dysrhythmias. Patents with stage III or stage IV disease appear to have significantly better disease-free survival when their TSH is fully suppressed (e.g., <0.1 mU/L), as measured in a sensitive TSH assay. In contrast, patients with stage I disease probably obtain little benefit from aggressive TSH suppression. At our institution, patients with stage I and stage II disease typically are treated to obtain TSH levels in the reduced but detectable range (e.g., 0.1 to 0.5 mU per liter).

General consensus supports the use of adjuvant ^{131}I treatment of DTC tumors larger than 1.5 cm based on data from the studies of Mazzaferri and others, although radioiodine use in smaller tumors remains controversial. Some studies indicate improved disease-free survival in higher-risk patients when radioiodine treatment is performed. In the postoperative setting, the goal of radioiodine scanning is to enable sensitive detection of tumor tissue outside the immediate thyroid bed and distant metastasis.

To prepare patients for postoperative radioiodine scanning and ^{131}I therapy, thyroxine has traditionally been withheld for 4 to 5 weeks after surgery. Often, short-term triiodothyronine (T_3) therapy has been used for 2 to 3 weeks to shorten the period of thyroid hormone deprivation. During this period, patients should also be placed on an iodine-restricted diet and iodine-containing medications and contrast media should be avoided. After this period of hypothyroidism, the serum TSH concentration should be greater than 25 mU per liter. In women of child-bearing potential, a pregnancy test should usually be obtained before radioiodine is given for scanning and therapy. The majority of patients will have remnant tissue in the thyroid bed. In our institution, patients with a thyroid bed remnant alone are either admitted to hospital for treatment with 100 mCi of ^{131}I or given 29.9 mCi of ^{131}I as an outpatient dose. If distant metastases are detected on the initial postoperative scan, then a higher ^{131}I treatment dose, typically 150 to 200 mCi, is administered. In some institutions, a standard remnant ablation dose is administered without the preceding scan. Five to 10 days after the treatment dose, a post-treatment scan is obtained by using the treatment dose as tracer. The patient is then placed on levothyroxine therapy with a serum TSH measurement 5 to 6 weeks later to determine the adequacy of therapy.

After a remnant ablation dose, it has been customary to obtain one or more follow-up TSH-stimulated radioiodine scans coupled with serum thyroglobulin determinations. The time after ^{131}I ablation varies from 6 months to 1 year. Successful remnant ablation is indicated by the absence of thyroid bed uptake. A second ablative radioiodine dose is required in approximately 25% of patients who have received an initial 100 mCi ^{131}I dose and in approximately 40% of those who have received 29.9 mCi.

The optimal method for ^{131}I dose selection in treatment of locally invasive or metastatic disease is controversial. At some centers, formal dosimetry—entailing multiple uptake determinations or urinary radioiodine measurements over days—is performed to calculate the maximally tolerable radiation dose to bone marrow and tumor, theoretically permitting optimization of therapy. In a majority of centers, however, an empirical ^{131}I dose of 150 to 200 mCi is administered because the clinical superiority of formal dosimetry has not been unequivocally established. Radioiodine treatment is relatively effective for small lung metastases, especially in young patients with normal chest radiographs. More bulky lung disease in older individuals, bone metastases, and especially brain metastases, are less responsive to radioiodine. Lymph nodes larger than 1 cm in diameter are frequently resected when possible, reserving radioiodine therapy for microscopic and unresectable residual disease. Secondary surgical excision should also be considered for isolated brain and spinal cord metastases and for lesions in weight-bearing bones.

Radioiodine therapy obviously has no value in tumors that lack the ability to concentrate iodine. Progression to a non–iodine-avid phenotype is an adverse prognostic indicator in papillary and follicular cancer. Only a small minority of Hürthle cell carcinomas (~5%) have the ability to concentrate radioiodine from the outset. A relatively common circumstance is the patient who has a measurable serum thyroglobulin concentration but no detectable radioiodine uptake on diagnostic imaging. Several studies indicate that empirical radioiodine therapy (e.g., 200 mCi of ^{131}I) in such DTC patients permits detection of focal radioiodine uptake in at least 50% on the subsequent post-treatment scan. Furthermore, some of these patients have a later decline in their serum thyroglobulin concentration, suggesting an impact of the radiation on their residual thyroid tissue. However, the clinical importance of such empirical radioiodine treatment in thyroglobulin-positive scan-negative patients remains unclear. Radioiodine treatment is ineffective for medullary and anaplastic thyroid cancers.

Potential complications of radioiodine therapy include sialadenitis and xerostomia, gastritis, and transient, usually mild, leukopenia. A longer term reduction in salivary function is noted in approximately 30% of patients, although clinically significant xerostomia is less common. Amifostine (Ethyol), 500 mg per m^2 IV, administered before radioiodine, has been shown to offer effective prophylaxis against this complication. At high cumulative doses of radioiodine, there is probably increased risk of secondary hematologic malignancy. Small but apparently significant increases in leukemia as well as bladder and colon cancer have been observed in some follow-up studies. However, it is often just these patients for whom radioiodine has the most to offer in thyroid cancer treatment. Useful measures to minimize the risks of secondary malignancy include (1) limiting cumulative dose to less than 1000 mCi of ^{131}I whenever possible; (2) avoiding treating more frequently than every 6 months; and (3) encouraging fluid intake and frequent urination after the therapeutic dose. Pregnant patients must never be treated because of the risk of neonatal hypothyroidism and other anomalies.

External-beam radiation therapy has a limited role in thyroid cancer treatment. The principal applications for external radiotherapy are in patients with locally advanced DTC that is inoperable and causing local complications, such as pain, hemoptysis, bronchial obstruction, or impending fracture. The efficacy of external radiotherapy in preventing progression of incompletely resected tumor is controversial, but it is often employed because of a lack of alternatives. In a subset of MTC patients who have invasion beyond the thyroid capsule, adjuvant radiotherapy appears to confer a small but significant reduction in local recurrence rates. Because radiation treatment makes subsequent surgery extremely difficult, patients should undergo an expert neck dissection, when possible, before adjuvant radiotherapy. In thyroidal lymphoma, radiotherapy has a well-defined and often beneficial role to play.

Chemotherapy has proven relatively ineffective for DTC, MTC, and anaplastic thyroid carcinoma. In appropriately selected patients with advancing radio-resistant disease, investigational agents may be a rational choice.

EVALUATION FOR PERSISTENT OR RECURRENT DISEASE

Patients with a history of thyroid cancer require long-term surveillance to detect recurrent disease, which can arise even after long cancer-free intervals. Thyroid hormone suppressive therapy must also be monitored to ensure adequate TSH suppression while avoiding iatrogenic thyrotoxicosis. Generally accepted follow-up procedures include a periodic history and physical examination; serum thyroglobulin or calcitonin levels for DTC or MTC, respectively; and TSH and free thyroxine determinations. These evaluations typically occur every 6 months for the first 1 to 2 years after primary surgery and then annually thereafter for life. Periodic TSH-stimulated radioiodine scans and serum thyroglobulin measurements should also be performed in patients with treated DTC, either after withdrawal of thyroid hormone therapy or facilitated by recombinant TSH administration (see later). A number of other modalities have been employed for detection of persistent or recurrent DTC, particularly when it is non–iodine avid. Also shown to have value in some settings are anatomic imaging by ultrasonography, computed tomography, or magnetic resonance imaging; scintigraphy with thallium, sestamibi, and octreotide; and fluorodeoxyglucose positron emission tomography. Lesions identified by any of these techniques may then be sampled to confirm their thyroidal origin. Preliminary studies suggest a potential role in monitoring for circulating thyroglobulin messenger RNA.

This may avoid the interference in thyroglobulin immunoassays that is caused by the antithyroglobulin antibodies present in approximately 25% of thyroid cancer patients. Preoperative radioiodine administrative and intraoperative localization of disease with a radioiodine probe has been used to identify disease neck and mediastinal metastases.

The best studied of the new approaches to detect residual and recurrent DTC tissue is the use of recombinant human TSH (rTSH, thyrotropin alfa). rTSH circumvents the need for thyroxine withdrawal and avoids the morbidity of hypothyroidism that was previously associated with preparation for radioiodine scanning and stimulated thyroglobulin measurement. Combined radioiodine scanning and serum thyroglobulin measurement after 0.9 mg rTSH intramuscularly per day for 2 days has been shown to be sensitive in detecting residual disease that was not significantly less than that with thyroxine withdrawal testing. Guidelines for selection of the patients who will be best managed by conventional thyroid hormone withdrawal versus rTSH are still in evolution. At our institution, patients are deemed candidates for rTSH-mediated testing if there is no clinical evidence of normal remnant tissue and residual cancer, if a previous radioiodine withdrawal scan has been negative, and if the serum thyroglobulin concentration is undetectable on thyroid hormone therapy. Patients suspected of having significant thyroid remnants or known thyroid cancer that will probably require radioiodine treatment still undergo thyroxine withdrawal for diagnostic testing followed by ^{131}I therapy. rTSH is currently approved by the U.S. Food and Drug Administration only for diagnostic testing and not to facilitate radioiodine therapy. Nonetheless, rTSH has been used to permit ^{131}I therapy in certain special settings: patients with paraspinal or intracranial metastases that might grow during prolonged TSH exposure, patients with previous serious medical or psychiatric complications of hypothyroidism, and patients unable to surmount a TSH rise during primary hypothyroidism.

A major limitation of radioiodine treatment has been that the most aggressive tumors often lack or lose the ability to concentrate radioiodine. With cloning and characterization of the sodium-iodide symporter (NIS) responsible for cellular iodine uptake, it has become apparent that loss of NIS expression occurs in many radioiodine-resistant tumors. A number of cellular factors, including cyclic adenosine monophosphate and retinoic acid, are now known to upregulate NIS expression. Preliminary clinical trials to induce radioiodine uptake with retinoic acid have shown increases in uptake in 10 to 30% of patients, but these early findings must be verified. Progress in thyroid cancer diagnosis and management is needed in two other areas: (1) more accurate techniques for preoperative differential diagnosis of follicular neoplasms and (2) new approaches for treatment of radioresistant DTC, MTC, and anaplastic thyroid cancers, perhaps employing gene therapy or other novel approaches.

PHEOCHROMOCYTOMA

method of
BRAHM SHAPIRO, M.B., CH.B., PH.D.
University of Michigan and
    Department of Veterans Affairs Health System
Ann Arbor, Michigan

JAMES C. SISSON, M.D.
University of Michigan
Ann Arbor, Michigan

and

MILTON D. GROSS, M.D.
University of Michigan and
    Department of Veterans Affairs Health System
Ann Arbor, Michigan

The rational cost-effective management of pheochromocytomas and all hypersecretory endocrine neoplasms requires that the tumor be clinically suspected and diagnosed by hormonal measurements and all tumor deposits located before surgery. Catecholamine-secreting neoplasms have a confusing nomenclature. Some authors apply the term "pheochromocytoma" to all secretory tumors. Alternatively, "pheochromocytoma" is restricted to adrenal lesions, and "paraganglioma" is used for secretory or nonsecretory extra-adrenal tumors. These tumors arise from the neural crest; manifest chromaffin staining and amine precursor uptake and decarboxylation (APUD); and synthesize, store, secrete, and take up biogenic amines and peptide hormones.

Hypercatecholaminemia from pheochromocytoma leads to a dramatic, potentially lethal syndrome. Previous high perioperative morbidity and mortality has been strikingly reduced by modern integrated team management by endocrinologist, anesthesiologist, and endocrine surgeon in preoperative, operative, and postoperative phases.

CLINICAL FEATURES

Most symptoms and signs result from hypercatecholaminemia. The cardinal feature is hypertension, but only 0.1% of hypertensive patients harbor pheochromocytomas. Hypertension is usually sustained and often labile or even paroxysmal. Other features include early onset (age < 40 years), severity (malignant hypertension), poor response or exacerbation with hypotensive drugs (particularly beta blockers), episodic hypotension (particularly with epinephrine and dopamine hypersecretion), and episodic "spells" seldom lasting longer than 1 hour. Paroxysmal symptoms vary between patients but are stereotypical for individuals and may increase in severity and frequency. Most paroxysms are spontaneous but may be provoked by abdominal palpation, exercise, urination, defecation, anesthesia, and certain drugs (glucagon, histamine, tyramine, guanethidine, metoclopramide, phenothiazines, tricyclic antidepressants, intra-arterial radiographic contrast agents, opiates, corticotropin, saralasin, beta-adrenergic blockers, sympathomimetics such as phenylpropanolamine, pseudoephedrine, amphetamines, and cocaine). Symptoms include palpitations, pallor, throbbing headache, and sweating; less common features are chest and abdominal pain, nausea, vomiting, weight loss, cholelithiasis, and glucose intolerance.

Physical findings include hypertension (exacerbated by abdominal palpation), hypertensive retinopathy, vasoconstriction, and congestive heart failure.

Personal and family history and examination must specifically seek features of syndromes associated with pheochromocytomas (see later).

BIOCHEMICAL DIAGNOSIS

Biochemical diagnosis of pheochromocytoma requires documentation of autonomous hypersecretion of catecholamines and metabolites in urine and/or plasma.

Norepinephrine is synthesized from tyrosine through dopa and dopamine, and epinephrine is synthesized from norepinephrine, in the adrenal medulla. Only small amounts of free epinephrine and norepinephrine are excreted in urine. Greater quantities are conjugated, but the majority is metabolized to metanephrine and normetanephrine by catechol O-methyltransferase and then by monoamine oxidase and aldehyde dehydrogenase to vanillylmandelic acid. Biochemical diagnosis depends on demonstration of elevated excretion rates of these compounds in urine and/or plasma concentrations of norepinephrine and epinephrine. Optimal screening regimens favor 24-hour urine collections with creatinine measurement to confirm adequacy. Overnight (12-hour) collections may be substituted when prolonged collection is not practical and is less affected by posture and stress. Fractionated catechol amines and metanephrines are reported more efficacious than vanillylmandelic acid for diagnosis and are often twofold to fivefold elevated. Results must be interpreted in light of potential stimulation of endogenous catecholamine secretion by disease processes or drugs, administration of exogenous catecholamines, drugs altering catecholamine metabolism, and specific assay interference. Interference varies with the assay, and the pathologist performing the measurements should be consulted.

The classic pharmacologic provocative and stimulatory tests (histamine or glucagon) have low sensitivity and specificity, are potentially dangerous, and are obsolete. The clonidine suppression test is, however, an exception; the response of plasma norepinephrine to a single 300-μg oral dose of clonidine is measured over 3 hours. The hypercatecholaminemia of pheochromocytoma is autonomous, whereas in other causes it is suppressed. This test is most useful in patients with borderline plasma norepinephrine levels.

Noncatecholamine hormonal factors may lead to hypercalcemia (parathyroid hormone–related peptide), polycythemia (erythropoietin), flushing and hypertension (neuropeptide Y and endothelin), and hypotension (adrenomedullin). Chromogranin A and dopamine beta-hydroxylase are also measurable but offer little diagnostic advantage.

EPIDEMIOLOGY

Pheochromocytomas may occur at any age, including childhood (approximately 10%), with peak incidence between 30 and 50 years. It is unusual, with a population incidence of 1 to 2 per 100,000. Among hypertensive patients, the incidence is 0.1 to 0.4 per 1000.

FAMILIAL SYNDROMES

Approximately 10% of pheochromocytomas occur as part of autosomal dominant neurocristopathic disorders, including multiple endocrine neoplasia (MEN) type 2A (medul-

lary thyroid carcinoma; hyperparathyroidism; and pheochromocytomas, frequently bilateral and intra-adrenal); MEN type 2B (medullary thyroid carcinoma, multiple ganglioneuromatosis, and pheochromocytomas); von Hippel-Lindau disease (retinal hemangiomatosis, cerebellar hemangioblastoma, other tumors including renal carcinoma and pheochromocytoma); and neurofibromatosis (multiple neurofibromas, café-au-lait spots; and occasionally pheochromocytoma). Familial pheochromocytoma also occurs in isolation without associated tumors or syndromes. Other associations include islet cell and carotid body tumors and Carney's triad (pulmonary hamartoma, gastric leiomyosarcoma, multiple extra-adrenal pheochromocytomas). Modern molecular biology permits early diagnosis of many familial syndromes. Patients at risk can be identified and early surgery planned. This spares children at risk for MEN 2 syndromes from serial calcium and pentagastrin tests for diagnosis of medullary thyroid cancer. Sporadic pheochromocytomas seldom result from these syndromes if the family history is negative and there are no clinical features. In MEN 2, various mutations of the proto-oncogene ret cause activation of the ret receptor tyrosine kinase. In MEN 2A, mutations affect the extracellular domain; in MEN 2B, they affect the intracellular region. In von Hippel-Lindau disease there is loss of the VHL suppressor gene with resultant development of various characteristic tumors. The gene for neurofibromatosis has also been characterized.

TUMOR LOCATION

Accurate location of all pheochromocytoma deposits is essential in planning curative surgery or recognizing inoperable disease. Medical imaging is reserved for patients with a firm clinical and biochemical diagnosis and not for diagnostic screening purposes. Pheochromocytomas are derived from sympathoadrenal system chromaffin cells: 90% develop in the adrenal medulla, 5 to 10% of which are bilateral (the majority associated with familial syndromes). Extra-adrenal lesions are usually intra-abdominal, arising from para-aortic chromaffin tissue, including the organ of Zuckerkandl. Tumors arise from chromaffin tissue from the skull base to the scrotum, including neurovascular bundles of the neck, paravertebral paraganglia, cardiac atria and aorticopulmonary window, and bladder wall. Multicentric primary tumors are difficult to distinguish from metastatic disease, except when metastases occur in sites devoid of chromaffin tissue (bone and lymph nodes). Certain histologic criteria and/or aneuploid or polyploid DNA complement may predict malignancy, but histologically benign-appearing lesions may metastasize. Incidence of malignancy is 3 to 20%, with the most common sites for metastases being lymph nodes, bone, liver, and lung.

Computed tomography (CT) of the abdomen with attention to the adrenal regions correctly locates almost all intra-adrenal pheochromocytomas and many extra-adrenal lesions and is the most widely used initial imaging procedure.

Magnetic resonance imaging (MRI) can also effectively localize pheochromocytomas, and many of them manifest characteristic high-intensity T2-weighted signal.

Radionuclide imaging is also employed to locate pheochromocytomas. Iodine-131–meta-iodobenzylguanidine (^{131}I-MIBG) is actively accumulated by sympathetic tissues and images pheochromocytomas with a sensitivity of 85 to 90% and specificity approaching 100%. When available, ^{123}I-MIBG offers improved localization and single-photon emission tomography (SPECT) but is currently investigational. ^{131}I-MIBG is well suited to whole-body screening and is especially useful for locating occult extra-adrenal and metastatic disease, even when CT and MRI depict primary tumors. ^{131}I-MIBG uptake is inhibited by many drugs that interfere with catecholamine reuptake and/or secretory granule storage. Successful ^{131}I-MIBG imaging requires withdrawal of all interfering drugs, including non-prescription (phenylpropanolamine) and "recreational" drugs (cocaine). Fortunately, neither the alpha blocker phenoxybenzamine or beta blockers significantly affect ^{131}I-MIBG accumulation and can be used to protect against catecholamine hypersecretion.

The wide distribution of somatostatin receptors on neuroendocrine tissues, including pheochromocytomas, permits scintigraphy with the radiolabeled somatostatin analogue indium-111 (^{111}In)-pentetreotide. Localization efficacy for pheochromocytomas by means of ^{111}In-pentetreotide is similar to that of ^{131}I-MIBG. The biodistribution is more complex and studies are more challenging to interpret. Pentetreotide uptake by pheochromocytoma is not affected by drugs used to control hypertension.

More recently, epinephrine and carbon 11–labeled hydroxyephedrine and fluorine 18–labeled deoxyglucose have been used to locate pheochromocytomas by means of positron emission tomography (PET).

Arteriography and venography with venous sampling and assay of catecholamines can be used to delineate vascular anatomy and are especially useful in planning resection of large lesions. However, they have, in large measure, been replaced by noninvasive techniques. Administration of radiographic contrast media may provoke catecholamine release and life-threatening hypertensive crisis and should not be performed before adrenergic blockade.

There is now almost no role for exploratory surgery.

TREATMENT

Medical Management and Preparation for Surgery

Alpha-adrenergic blockade is the cornerstone of medical management and preoperative preparation of pheochromocytoma. Safe conduct of surgery requires adequate preparation started as soon as the diagnosis is made. Because almost all tumors may be removed electively, preparation may be gradual. The time-honored agent is phenoxybenzamine (Dibenzyline), an oral noncompetitive alpha-adrenergic blocker. Onset of action is slow, with a peak at 12 hours and a gradual cumulative effect. An initial dose of 10 mg every 12 hours may be increased by 10 mg every 2 days. Goals of therapy are elimination or blunting of paroxysms and normalization of blood pressure without symptomatic postural hypotension. The final dose may exceed 100 mg per day. It is well tolerated, and nasal congestion, diarrhea, and failure of ejaculation are indications of adequate alpha blockade. Treatment is continued for at least 1 week to permit restoration of plasma volume and re-regulation of adrenoreceptors. Longer therapy may be required with heart failure due to catecholamine-induced cardiomyopathy. Prazosin (Minipress), doxazosin (Cardura), and terazosin (Hytrin) are effective alternative selective alpha₁-receptor blockers with shorter duration of action and may be titrated more

rapidly but may cause more initial hypotension. Labetalol (Trandate/Normodyne), a combined alpha- and beta-adrenergic receptor blocker may be used to treat pheochromocytoma, but the relative degrees of blockade may not be optimal for all patients, and it interferes with ^{131}I-MIBG scintigraphy.

Beta-adrenergic blockade is occasionally necessary to control persistent tachycardia, supraventricular arrhythmias, and ventricular ectopy (rhythm disturbances may be more common with epinephrine hypersecretion). Although the risk may have been exaggerated, beta blockers should never be introduced until alpha blockade has been established because reduction in beta-receptor activity may lead to unopposed alpha agonism, vasoconstriction, and hypertensive crisis. Beta-receptor blockade may exacerbate catecholamine cardiomyopathy. Either nonspecific beta blockers such as propranolol or beta₁-selective blockers such as metoprolol (Lopressor) may be used. The therapeutic goal is to maintain the heart rate below 100 beats per minute and eliminate arrhythmias. Alpha blockade is also essential before angiography and percutaneous biopsy, and chronic therapy is central to managing malignant and inoperable disease.

If adrenergic blockade fails to control hypertension and other features or side effects are intolerable, synthesis of catecholamines can be reduced by alpha-methyl-paratyrosine (metyrosine [Demser]), which inhibits tyrosine hydroxylase, the rate-limiting enzyme for catecholamine synthesis. It seldom normalizes catecholamines but may eliminate the need for or reduce the dosage of alpha blockers. Initial doses are 250 mg twice daily, with progressive increases, guided by clinical response and side effects, to a maximum of 2 grams daily in divided doses. Side effects include sedation and parkinsonism, owing to inhibition of central nervous system dopamine synthesis. This may be controlled with Sinemet (a combination of carbidopa and levodopa) because the levodopa crosses the blood-brain barrier to correct metyrosine-induced deficiency while carbidopa inhibits the peripheral conversion of levodopa to dopamine in tissues outside the central nervous system.

There are reports of calcium channel blockers and angiotensin-converting enzyme inhibitors being useful. In addition to alpha and beta blockade and metyrosine, diuretics and digitalis may be required for treatment of the heart failure of catecholamine cardiomyopathy.

Operative Management

Complete surgical extirpation of all tumor foci remains the only cure for pheochromocytoma. Such operations are challenging and should be performed by experienced surgeons at centers of excellence. Stress-free, rapid induction of anesthesia is essential to minimize catecholamine release. We favor induction with pentobarbital followed by maintenance with enflurane (Ethrane) or methoxyflurane (Penthrane), oxygen, and nitrous oxide. These agents and avoidance of hypoxia minimizes cardiac sensitization to arrhythmogenic effects of catecholamines. Narcotics should be used with caution and only after alpha blockade. Adequate muscle relaxation, endotracheal intubation, and mechanical ventilation necessitate succinylcholine. Continuous monitoring of electrocardiogram, intra-arterial pressure, central venous pressure, and urine output is essential. With potentially impaired cardiac reserve a Swan-Ganz catheter to monitor pulmonary capillary wedge pressure is advisable.

Tumor manipulation causes sufficient catecholamine release to produce marked hypertension despite alpha blockade. This can be controlled by multiple small doses of phentolamine (Regitine) (1 to 5 mg), phentolamine drip, or nitroprusside (Nipride) infusion. The latter has the advantage of rapid clearance and easier regulation of blood pressure. After interruption of venous drainage from the tumor, hypertension ceases to be a major problem. Hypotension may occur, which may be controlled by generous fluid replacement guided by the central venous pressure. Response to pressor amines is blunted owing to receptor down-regulation and receptor blockade. Supraventricular tachyarrhythmias respond to beta blockers, and ventricular arrhythmias respond to lidocaine.

Long-accepted principles of surgical management include wide operative exposure, meticulous hemostasis, minimal tumor manipulation, early interruption of tumor venous drainage, and delivery of the tumor with capsule intact. Many tumors are cystic, and rupture may result in implantation of cells that, although benign, may result in new tumors. Malignant and unresectable tumors should be debulked when possible without major risk. Arteriographic tumor embolization may be a helpful prelude to surgery in some cases. Pheochromocytomas are highly vascular, and severe hemorrhage is a risk, especially during resection of extra-adrenal lesions. Blood loss must be closely monitored and corrected with blood and blood products if necessary.

The traditional approach for intra-adrenal lesions has been transabdominal through a transverse or bucket handle incision. Alternative approaches are thoracoabdominal or posterior incisions. For right adrenal lesions, early ligation of the short right adrenal vein is important and requires visualization of the entry point into the inferior vena cava. Left adrenal lesions are approached through the lesser omental space with mobilization of pancreatic body and tail, permitting ligation of the draining vein. Laparoscopic adrenalectomy has been performed for pheochromocytoma and other benign secretory and nonsecretory adrenal lesions but demands substantial expertise. Laparoscopic surgery substantially decreases operative time, reduces discomfort, and speeds discharge and recovery. Bilateral laparoscopic adrenalectomies have been performed for MEN 2. Currently, indications for laparoscopic adrenalectomy, particularly for pheochromocytoma are controversial, but it should be restricted to uncomplicated

small to moderate-sized intra-adrenal tumors. Randomized comparisons of laparoscopic adrenalectomy to other approaches are not yet available, and it should be considered investigational. Bilateral adrenalectomy requires intraoperative stress and postoperative replacement doses of glucocorticoids. Attempts to preserve adrenal function by partial adrenalectomy may be successful but often result in recurrence.

Special approaches and techniques are required for certain unusual lesions, such as lower abdominal incisions and partial cystectomy with or without ureteral reimplantation for bladder tumors. Posterior mediastinal lesions should be approached through posterior thoracotomies; and middle mediastinal tumors, including intrapericardial and left atrial tumors, necessitate median sternotomy and possibly cardiopulmonary bypass.

Postoperative Management and Follow-up

Catecholamine levels fall as soon as tumoral venous drainage is interrupted and normalize within hours. However, release of stored catecholamines from peripheral nerve terminals result in elevated urinary excretion of catecholamines and metabolites lasting days. Thus, biochemical normality should be documented 2 to 4 weeks postoperatively. Persistent elevation indicates residual tumor, second unappreciated primary tumor, or occult metastases. Normalization of catecholamines results in prompt reduction in blood pressure. Hypotension and hypovolemia are common, and close cardiovascular monitoring and generous fluid replacement are mandatory. Patients should be carefully assessed for hemorrhage, heart failure, adrenal insufficiency, and excessive adrenergic blockade. Successful tumor resection normalizes blood pressure in most patients and eliminates paroxysms and spells. A third of patients exhibit some mild, stable, residual hypertension (possibly due to hypertensive arterial damage or pheochromocytoma associated renal artery stenosis).

Early postoperative hypoglycemia may occur, and glucose-containing intravenous fluids should be administered. Patients rendered diabetic usually regain normal glucose tolerance after successful tumor resection. Adrenal cortical insufficiency after bilateral adrenalectomy necessitates glucocorticoid and mineralocorticoid replacement.

Pheochromocytoma recurs in 10% of patients operated on with curative intent but may not manifest for years or decades after apparently successful surgery and may result from regrowth after incomplete resection, distant metastases, or second primary tumors. This potential for late recurrence necessitates annual determinations of blood pressure, urine catecholamines, and metabolites for life.

Management of Unresectable and Malignant Pheochromocytomas

Local recurrences due to malignancy or residual tumor may be surgically extirpated. Malignant metastatic tumors or local vital organ invasion and even a minority of benign pheochromocytomas intimately related to critical structures (e.g., celiac axis) cannot be cured surgically. Angiographic embolization under alpha blockade may palliate selected unresectable or metastatic lesions. These patients have a highly variable clinical course. Five-year survival is approximately 50%, but some patients survive for decades without specific antitumor therapy. The cornerstone of management is control of hypercatecholaminemia effects by prolonged adrenergic blockade; addition of alpha-metyrosine may also be useful.

Pheochromocytomas tend to be radioresistant, and external-beam radiotherapy must deliver 4000 to 5000 cGy to shrink lesions. It is most useful for palliation of bone metastases. Experimental radiotherapy of malignant, metastatic pheochromocytoma with large doses of ^{131}I-MIBG has resulted in partial responses in a third of cases. Use of radiolabeled somatostatin analogues is also under investigation.

Combination chemotherapy with cyclophosphamide, vincristine, and dacarbazine is encouraging. Partial responses occur, and over half the patients treated have excellent biochemical improvements. Other combinations, similar to those used for neuroblastoma, may also be effective. Adequate pain management starting with nonsteroidal anti-inflammatory drugs escalating to long-acting high-dose narcotics is important for bone and visceral pain.

Other Special Circumstances

Pheochromocytoma in Pregnancy

Initial manifestation of pheochromocytoma may occur during pregnancy, labor, or delivery and must be differentiated from eclampsia. Even when recognized, prognosis for both mother and fetus is poor, and spontaneous abortion is common. Manifestation in early pregnancy may make termination preferable; alternatively, it may be possible to bring the fetus to viability under alpha blockade. Spontaneous delivery is to be avoided. Pretreatment with phentolamine should be followed by cesarean delivery and, when possible, tumor resection at the same operation. There have been no major fetal side effects of alpha blockade.

Pheochromocytoma Crisis

Severe crisis associated with malignant hypertension, cardiac arrhythmia, and intense vasoconstriction, in some cases sufficient to cause myocardial or mesenteric infarction or peripheral gangrene, occurs spontaneously or may be provoked by trauma, anesthesia, surgery, labor and delivery, and various drugs, all of which should be administered with great caution in patients with known or suspected pheochromocytoma.

Crisis should be managed in an intensive care setting with close hemodynamic monitoring similar to that for surgery. Intravenous infusion of nitroprusside or phentolamine (Regitine) in multiple 1- to 5-mg boluses is done to control hypertension and vasoconstriction. Beta-adrenergic blockers after alpha blockade and antiarrhythmics are used as appropriate.

PROGNOSIS

Prognosis is generally excellent. Modern anesthesia and surgery have reduced overall operative mortality to less than 1%. For certain subsets of extra-adrenal lesions, mortality may be significantly higher. After successful complete resection, survival is similar to that for the general population. Approximately a third of patients have some residual, nonparoxysmal hypertension. Recurrence due to residual, metastatic, or new primary lesions occurs in 10%. Mean survival for malignant metastatic disease is approximately 50%, but survival is possible for many years despite widespread disease. In MEN 2 syndromes, metastatic medullary thyroid cancer frequently determines survival.

THYROIDITIS

method of
ANTHONY P. WEETMAN, M.D., D.Sc.
University of Sheffield
Sheffield, United Kingdom

Thyroiditis simply means inflammation of the thyroid gland and arises from a number of different causes. Clinically these are best classified by the tempo of inflammation: acute, subacute, or chronic (Table 1). Mild to moderate focal thyroiditis, in which there is a patchy infiltration of the thyroid gland by lymphocytes, is so common (in around 15% of all autopsy specimens) that it has little clinical significance; in only a small fraction of such patients does disease progress to a chronic thyroiditis and destruction of thyroid tissue. Similarly, a focal thyroiditis is frequently found adjacent to (or even within) benign or malignant neoplasms of the thyroid. In the case of papillary carcinoma, the presence of focal thyroiditis, which is usually accompanied by serum antibodies against thyroglobulin and thyroid peroxidase, confers an improved prognosis.

ACUTE (SUPPURATIVE) THYROIDITIS

Background

This is a rare condition caused by a suppurative infection of the thyroid through the blood, lymphatics, trauma, a persistent thyroglossal duct, or, most commonly, extension from nearby infection. The latter usually arises through the piriform sinus, an anomalous remnant of the fourth branchial pouch, usually on the left side. This is the main cause of acute thyroiditis in children and young adults; a long-standing goiter, degeneration in a carcinoma, and immunosuppression are risk factors in the elderly.

Virtually any bacterium can cause acute thyroidi-

TABLE 1. **Clinical Features in Thyroiditis**

Condition	Incidence	Cause	Goiter	Course
Acute thyroiditis	Rare	Usually bacteria	Painful; usually localized and asymmetric	Recovery
Subacute thyroiditis	Uncommon	Usually viruses	Painful; usually small and diffuse	Recovery; relapses in 10%
Chronic thyroiditis	Common	Usually autoimmune	Painless; usually diffuse but variable size	Hypothyroidism
Drug-induced thyroiditis	Uncommon	Amiodarone, lithium, iodine	Small, sometimes painful	Hypothyroidism

tis. The most common are *Staphylococcus aureus*, *Streptococci* species, *Klebsiella pneumoniae*, and *Escherichia coli*. In immunosuppressed patients, including those with acquired immune deficiency syndrome (AIDS), unusual organisms can invade the thyroid, including *Aspergillus, Candida*, and *Coccidioides* species and *Pneumocystis carinii*. In rare instances, tuberculosis can affect the thyroid, but the picture then is usually one of a subacute thyroiditis.

The dominant clinical features are pain in the thyroid radiating to the ears, tenderness over the gland, fever, dysphagia, and malaise. Features of septicemia may be present, as may lymphadenopathy and a local thrombophlebitis. The differential diagnosis for thyroid pain includes subacute and, rarely, chronic thyroiditis, hemorrhage into a cyst, and lymphoma. Clinical features (see Table 1) help in the diagnosis, and simple investigations (Table 2) usually confirm the clinical suspicion.

Treatment

Treatment is with high-dose antibiotics selected on the basis of the microbiology results from fine-needle aspiration biopsy. Surgical drainage of any abscess is indicated when pus cannot be fully removed by aspiration. Complications of acute thyroiditis include tracheal obstruction, retropharyngeal abscess, mediastinitis, and internal jugular venous thrombosis. Any piriform sinus should be located (usually by barium swallow study) and excised to prevent a recurrence; a thyroid lobectomy is usually needed for this.

SUBACUTE (VIRAL OR GRANULOMATOUS) THYROIDITIS

Background

This condition has a variable frequency, depending on region. It appears to be more common in North America than in Europe, but it is possible that it is overlooked in areas of apparently low frequency. Three times more women are affected than men, with a peak incidence between the ages of 30 and 50 years, and HLA-B35 is a predisposing genetic factor. Many viruses have been implicated, especially Coxsackie, influenza, measles, mumps, and Epstein-Barr. There is no need to attempt identification serologically. The main clinical features are a painful and tender goitrous thyroid with fluctuating thyroid hormone levels. The pain can be in one or both thyroid lobes. Occasionally, a nodular form can be detected on palpation. Patients usually have a phase of thyrotoxicosis (caused by release of stored hormone from the damaged gland) lasting up to 4 weeks, followed by a phase of hypothyroidism of 1 to 3 months and then recovery, but recurrence occurs in approximately 10% of patients. Many patients describe a prodromal phase of systemic upset or upper respiratory tract infection. The diagnosis is confirmed by the high erythrocyte sedimentation rate and low isotope uptake (see Table 2).

Treatment

Mild cases necessitate no treatment except analgesics, usually aspirin. Severe disease warrants treatment with prednisolone at a dose of 40 to 60 mg a

TABLE 2. **Useful Diagnostic Tests in Thyroiditis**

Condition	Thyroid Function	Thyroid Antibodies*	Erythrocyte Sedimentation Rate	Leucocyte Count	Other
Acute thyroiditis	Normal	Negative	Elevated	Elevated	Fine-needle aspiration biopsy
Subacute thyroiditis	Thyrotoxicosis followed by transient hypothyroidism	Negative	Elevated	Elevated	Low isotope uptake
Silent thyroiditis	Thyrotoxicosis followed by transient hypothyroidism	Positive	Normal	Normal	Low isotope uptake
Chronic thyroiditis	Normal or sustained hypothyroidism	Positive	Normal	Normal	Fine-needle aspiration biopsy

*Thyroglobulin and/or thyroid peroxidase antibodies.

day initially. Depending on the clinical response and sedimentation rate, this is gradually tapered after 1 to 2 weeks so that steroids are stopped after 4 to 6 weeks. Patients' thyroid function should be monitored closely (every 1 to 2 weeks). During a phase of symptomatic thyrotoxicosis, propranolol,* 20 to 40 mg three to four times a day, is useful for controlling the signs. Antithyroid drugs (methimazole, propylthiouracil) are not effective in this situation. Subsequent symptomatic hypothyroidism is treated with levothyroxine (Synthroid, Levothroid, Levoxyl), 100 µg a day, but this should be withdrawn after 6 to 8 weeks because this phase is typically transient. However, patients with pre-existing thyroid abnormalities may develop permanent hypothyroidism after subacute thyroiditis, and therefore full recovery of thyroid function must be established by testing. Recurrences are dealt with in the same way as the initial attack, although prolonging prednisolone treatment by 2 to 4 weeks may be useful.

A similar pattern of thyroid dysfunction without thyroid pain is called "silent" thyroiditis. This has an autoimmune etiology and occurs most distinctly 3 to 6 months after pregnancy in women with thyroid peroxidase antibodies before delivery (see Table 2). Treatment for thyroid dysfunction is again with propranolol for thyrotoxicosis and thyroxine for the usually transient hypothyroidism; steroids are not needed. Postpartum thyroiditis is a risk factor for the development of future permanent hypothyroidism, and affected women should therefore be screened annually for this. The appropriateness of screening all pregnant women for thyroid peroxidase antibodies in the first trimester is not clear except in women with type 1 diabetes mellitus, who are at particular risk of developing postpartum thyroiditis. In such women, the presence of antibodies before delivery should lead to careful monitoring of postpartum thyroid function.

CHRONIC (AUTOIMMUNE) THYROIDITIS

Background

Hypothyroidism caused by autoimmunity affects approximately 1% of women and 0.1% of men. However, there is a much higher prevalence of subclinical autoimmune thyroiditis shown by the presence of sustained, elevated circulating thyroid-stimulating hormone (TSH) levels with normal free thyroxine levels, with or without accompanying thyroid peroxidase and/or thyroglobulin antibodies. This condition often comes to light during screening for nonspecific symptoms such as fatigue or weight gain. Some patients may have a goiter of variable size that is usually hard and often irregular (bosselated); this is Hashimoto's, or goitrous, thyroiditis. At the opposite end of the pathologic spectrum is atrophic thyroiditis or primary myxedema in which the thyroid is replaced by fibrous tissue and the only clinical sign of the destructive process is the development of hypothyroidism. These patients may have antibodies that block the TSH receptor, but these are neither frequent nor unique in atrophic thyroiditis.

Treatment

Overt hypothyroidism resulting from chronic thyroiditis is treated with levothyroxine. There is no role for thyroid extract or for liothyronine (triiodothyronine, T_3) supplementation (Thyrolar) or substitution (Cytomel), inasmuch as levothyroxine is always converted smoothly and physiologically to T_3, whereas the short half-life of liothyronine leads to peaks and troughs of circulating T_3. In otherwise healthy patients younger than age 60 with overt hypothyroidism, I start levothyroxine at 100 µg a day, but in those older than 60 or with ischemic heart disease, the usual starting dose is 12.5 to 25 µg a day, increasing every 2 weeks by 25-µg increments. In all cases the aim is to normalize the TSH level, although this in rare cases proves impossible in patients whose angina is worsened by thyroxine replacement. Propranolol or other beta blockers help minimize this adverse effect. If the TSH is maintained in the reference range, there is no adverse effect of thyroxine on bone metabolism. I check TSH levels only 2 to 3 months after changing dose because it can take this length of time for symptoms and TSH levels to normalize. The same applies if the commercial preparation of levothyroxine is changed. Once the desired dose is achieved, TSH levels need be checked only annually. It is unusual for patients to need more than 150 µg of levothyroxine a day. In my experience, an elevated (and usually fluctuating) TSH level in patients taking higher doses usually indicates poor compliance, although malabsorption syndromes and certain drugs (colestipol, cholestyramine, sucralfate, ferrous sulfate, aluminum hydroxide, phenytoin, activated charcoal) can interfere with absorption.

There is controversy about the optimal management of subclinical hypothyroidism. The risk of progression to overt hypothyroidism is highest in patients with both an elevated TSH and positive thyroid antibodies, and in my view it is worth treating these patients with levothyroxine (usually 50 µg initially) from the outset. In those with either an elevated TSH or thyroid antibodies, one option is a 3-month trial of levothyroxine and, if any symptomatic improvement occurs, to continue with this. If there is no improvement or the patient chooses not to have treatment, an annual check of thyroid function should be arranged to deal with the risk of progression to overt hypothyroidism.

The goiter of Hashimoto's thyroiditis usually shrinks with levothyroxine. Surgery is rarely needed to control the goiter. Any focal irregularity in the goiter raises the suspicion of malignancy, but such hard nodules are frequently found in Hashimoto's thyroiditis and should be investigated, initially by aspiration biopsy. Pain may be suggestive of lym-

*Not FDA approved for this indication.

phoma, which is a rare complication of autoimmune thyroiditis. Very rarely is the thyroid tender in uncomplicated Hashimoto's thyroiditis. Corticosteroids can be used but are sometimes unhelpful, and surgery may be needed in extreme cases.

DRUG-INDUCED THYROIDITIS

Autoimmune thyroiditis can be precipitated by lithium, excess iodide, or recombinant cytokines such as interferon-alfa, interleukin-2, and granulocyte-macrophage colony-stimulating factor (GM-CSF). Thyroxine replacement should be given and adjusted to maintain a normal TSH level. Amiodarone can cause both hypothyroidism, readily managed by levothyroxine, and thyrotoxicosis, the latter resulting either from a destructive process or from excess iodide supply that precipitates hyperthyroidism. Amiodarone-induced thyrotoxicosis can be very difficult to manage and necessitates specialist advice. Corticosteroids, potassium perchlorate, antithyroid drugs and even surgery may be needed to control the disease, whereas stopping amiodarone has little immediate impact because of the long half-life of the drug. A painful but transient thyroiditis may occur 1 to 2 weeks after radioiodine for hyperthyroidism. It responds to simple analgesics.

RIEDEL'S THYROIDITIS

This rare condition of unknown etiology is caused by fibrosis of the thyroid, leading to a wood-like, hard mass often extending outside the thyroid and involving any of the adjacent structures. There is an association with idiopathic fibrosis elsewhere (retroperitoneum, orbit, mediastinum, biliary tree, lung). The condition is often detected because of suspicion of thyroid malignancy. Aspiration biopsy typically yields no specimen, and diagnosis requires open biopsy. Thyroxine is useful only if there is hypothyroidism and corticosteroids are ineffective. The condition runs an unpredictable course, with a slow progression in many cases, and surgery should be reserved only for patients with esophageal or tracheal compression.

The Urogenital Tract

BACTERIAL INFECTIONS OF THE URINARY TRACT IN MEN

method of
NAIEL N. NASSAR, M.D., and
JAMES W. SMITH, M.D.
Veterans Affairs Medical Center
Dallas, Texas

Urinary tract infection (UTI) in otherwise healthy adult men between the ages of 15 and 50 years is uncommon, and the difference in prevalence compared with women in the same age group is striking. This difference is thought to be secondary to the antibacterial activity of the prostatic fluid and to the greater length of the male urethra. Invasive infections are most frequent in the very young (<3 months of age) and the elderly (>50 years of age). Identified risks for UTI in men include homosexuality, intercourse with an infected female partner, bladder outlet obstruction, and lack of circumcision. Local infection of the urethra is commonplace in young sexually active men.

The etiologic agents that cause uncomplicated UTI in men are similar to those in women, with *Escherichia coli* being the predominant causative organism. *Staphylococcus saprophyticus* is rarely found. Rarely, hematogenous spread to the urinary tract occurs during bacteremic episodes, particularly with *Staphylococcus aureus* or *Candida albicans*.

Dysuria is common to UTI and urethritis. As in females, frequency, urgency, suprapubic pain, flank pain, or hematuria suggests UTI. Urethritis must be ruled out in sexually active men. Older men may present with symptoms of dysuria, frequent urination, and, occasionally, isolated hematuria. Up to half of elderly men with UTI have prostate infection as well; and localization of symptoms to the lower urinary tract, prostate, or kidney by clinical symptoms alone can be difficult. The scrotum should be examined because epididymo-orchitis may be a complication of urinary tract or prostatic infection. Bacterial infection is suspected if the urine leukocyte esterase test and the nitrite test for gram-negative bacteria are positive. The prevalence of asymptomatic bacteriuria in institutionalized elderly men varies with the underlying degree of disability and is reported to be from 15 to 35%. Asymptomatic UTI in institutionalized men is frequently (10 to 25%) polymicrobial; however, this has not been reported to be associated with an increased likelihood of long-term adverse outcomes, such as renal failure, genitourinary carcinoma, or shortened survival.

TREATMENT

Because penicillinase-producing *Neisseria gonorrhoeae* is found throughout the United States, uncomplicated gonococcal infections are best treated with ceftriaxone (Rocephin), 125 mg intramuscularly in a single dose. Alternatively, single oral dose regimens with either cefixime (Suprax), 400 mg; ciprofloxacin (Cipro), 500 mg; or ofloxacin (Floxin), 400 mg, can be given. All patients given these regimens, as well as those with nongonococcal urethritis, should be treated with doxycycline, 100 mg orally two times a day for 7 days. Alternative treatments for chlamydial urethritis include azithromycin (Zithromax), 1 gram orally in a single dose (a 2-gram single oral dose is effective against gonococcal and nongonococcal urethritis); alternatively, ofloxacin, 300 mg orally two times a day for 7 days, or erythromycin base, 500 mg orally four times a day for 7 days, can be administered.

Chlamydia trachomatis may recur in patients who fail to comply with the treatment regimen or who are re-exposed to an untreated sex partner. Recurrent urethritis should be retreated with the initial regimen. In addition, a wet-mount preparation of a urethral swab specimen for *Trichomonas vaginalis* should be made, and, if possible, metronidazole treatment should be offered. Another possible cause of recurrent urethritis is tetracycline-resistant *Ureaplasma urealyticum,* which responds to a 14-day course of erythromycin base at a dose of 500 mg orally four times a day.

Men with UTIs and temperatures lower than 39.6°C (102°F) can usually be managed as outpatients with trimethoprim-sulfamethoxazole (Bactrim, Septra), one double-strength tablet twice a day for 10 to 14 days (short-course therapy has not been studied in men). If the patient is allergic to sulfonamides, the quinolones such as ciprofloxacin, 500 mg twice daily; ofloxacin, 400 mg twice daily; or levofloxacin (Levaquin), 250 mg once daily are other effective oral medications. Because oral cephalosporins or penicillin derivatives are excreted rapidly, they have reduced response rates in comparison with trimethoprim-sulfamethoxazole and the quinolones. Nitrofurantoin should not be used by men with UTI because it does not achieve reliable tissue concentrations and would be ineffective for occult prostatitis or pyelonephritis.

Patients with severe upper UTIs and temperatures higher than 102°F, volume depletion, and/or change of mental status should be hospitalized and treated with intravenous trimethoprim-sulfamethoxazole, 160/800 mg every 12 hours, combined with gentamicin (Garamycin), 5 mg per kg per day; ceftriaxone, 1 gram daily, or an intravenous quinolone also could be given. A patient who responds to these drugs can

661

be switched to an oral equivalent agent on the second or third hospital day to complete a 14-day course of therapy. One advantage of 2 to 3 days of a parenteral aminoglycoside is that the aminoglycoside persists in the kidney for up to 1 month after administration, providing continuous synergistic activity with the other administered agents.

If the patient continues to have fever after 72 hours of therapy, however, a urine culture should be repeated, and ultrasonography or computed tomography (CT) should be performed to rule out an intrarenal infection such as a phlegmon (nephronia) or a perinephric abscess. A perinephric abscess is more likely to occur in patients who have spinal cord injury, diabetes mellitus, or continuous urinary catheterization. Nephronia occurs in approximately 5 to 10% of those with the clinical diagnosis of pyelonephritis (fever, flank pain, and UTI). Patients with this intrarenal process generally respond to parenteral antimicrobial therapy continued for more than 2 weeks, with some patients requiring up to 6 weeks of parenteral therapy. Patients with multifocal masslike lesions on CT may require drainage, as this complication is associated with high mortality rates.

It is probably wise to obtain both pretreatment and post-treatment urine cultures routinely in all men with UTI. Early recurrence of cystitis or pyelonephritis with the same species suggests a prostatic or upper urinary tract source of infection and warrants a 4- to 6-week regimen of either trimethoprim-sulfamethoxazole or a quinolone. Urologic evaluation should consist of a careful history and physical examination to check for possible structural problems, including kidney stones and clinically significant benign prosthetic hypertrophy. If the patient has signs or symptoms of urinary retention, an in-and-out bladder catheterization should be done to check for residual. Other voiding studies, such as an intravenous pyelogram, are not indicated unless evidence of other abnormalities is found during initial evaluation. After patients respond clinically with a decrease in temperature and symptoms, they can be observed while taking antimicrobial medication. A urine culture 2 to 4 weeks after therapy is completed can be done to check for recurrence or persistence of infection. If the follow-up urine culture result is positive, a 4- to 6-week course of antimicrobial treatment is indicated. However, subsequent courses of therapy for asymptomatic bacteria are not indicated.

Epididymitis can occur after infection of either the urethra or the urinary tract in sexually active men younger than 35 years of age, usually by infection with *N. gonorrhoeae* or *C. trachomatis*. Both urethral discharge and urine with cultures are obtained to determine the causative agent. In men older than 35 years, epididymitis follows UTI with gram-negative organisms such as *E. coli*. Antimicrobial therapy is determined by the antimicrobial susceptibility of the bacteria recovered from the urinary tract. For patients younger than 35 years of age, treatment with ceftriaxone, 250 mg intramuscularly, plus doxycycline, 100 mg twice a day for 10 days, is indicated; for older men, treatment should include trimethoprim-sulfamethoxazole, 160/800 mg twice daily for 14 days, or a quinolone. If serious systemic infection is present, a combination of a cephalosporin and aminoglycoside is indicated until the patient responds. In addition, supportive measures, including elevation of the scrotum, are indicated.

Most episodes of bacteriuria associated with short-term catheters are asymptomatic; however, fever or other symptoms of UTI occur in up to 30% of patients. Less than 5% of catheter-associated bacteriurias are associated with bacteremia. Most bacteriurias in short-term catherizations are of single organisms, *E. coli* being most frequent, but as many as 15% may be polymicrobial, and most have accompanying pyuria. Long-term catheterization, on the other hand, is associated with polymicrobial bacteriuria in up to 95% of cases. Urine obtained from the catheter, however, may not always reflect bladder urine, suggesting that organisms colonizing the catheter, perhaps under a biofilm, may not in all cases colonize the bladder itself. Condom catheters have been used widely for men with urinary incontinence, and some studies suggest a lower frequency of bacteriuria with condom catheters. In the individual patient with positive urine culture and nonlocalizing symptoms (fever), it may be impossible to determine whether this is symptomatic UTI, and individual judgment with respect to whether antimicrobial therapy is warranted seems reasonable. In elderly men with asymptomatic bacteriuria, antimicrobial therapy is indicated within 12 hours before an invasive procedure, such as cystoscopy or transurethral prostatic resection. Antibiotic selection is based on the infecting organism and susceptibilities.

BACTERIAL INFECTIONS OF THE URINARY TRACT IN WOMEN

method of
LISA D. CHEW, M.D., and
STEPHAN D. FIHN, M.D., M.P.H.
*University of Washington School of Medicine
and Harborview Medical Center*
Seattle, Washington

Urinary tract infections (UTIs) are the most common bacterial infections in women. Approximately 20% of women will have a UTI during their lifetime, with 25% experiencing recurrent infections. The incidence rises quickly after sexual activity has begun and thereafter increases slowly. The cost of caring for women with UTIs probably exceeds $1 billion a year.

PATHOGENESIS

Uropathogenic bacteria from the fecal flora colonize the vaginal introitus and periurethral area, travel to the urethra and into the bladder, and, in some cases, ascend the ureters to cause pyelonephritis. Hematogenous and lymphatic spread, as well as direct extension of infection, is rare.

Factors such as host susceptibility and bacterial virulence, which predispose to bacterial colonization and enable organisms to ascend the urinary tract, are subjects of intense research. Sexual intercourse is a risk factor for UTI. In addition, contraceptive practices with spermicide and diaphragms or spermicide-coated condoms increase the risk of developing a UTI by altering the normal vaginal flora and possibly enhancing adherence of pathogens to the vaginal mucosa. Furthermore, women who have had a prior UTI are at increased risk for subsequent infections.

Bacterial strains with fimbriae or pili are more virulent because they have a higher degree of adherence. Other virulence factors include hemolysin, which degrades red blood cells, and aerobactin, which enhances iron uptake. These characteristics are more common when *Eschericia coli* is responsible for pyelonephritis and are usually absent in ordinary fecal isolates.

The most common causative organism is *E. coli* (80%), followed by *Staphylococcus saprophyticus* (10 to 15%). Other less common pathogens include gram-negative aerobic rods (e.g., *Proteus* and *Klebsiella* species) and *Enterococcus*.

CLINICAL SYNDROMES

In the female patient, UTIs can be broadly categorized as acute uncomplicated cystitis, acute uncomplicated pyelonephritis, recurrent uncomplicated UTI, complicated UTI, catheter-related UTI, pregnancy-associated UTI, and UTI in the elderly.

Acute Uncomplicated Cystitis

Acute cystitis, or lower UTI, results from a superficial bacterial infection of the bladder and/or urethra. Dysuria is the cardinal symptom of a lower UTI. Other symptoms include urinary frequency, urgency, hematuria, and suprapubic and pelvic pain. It is also important to consider other diagnoses with complaints of dysuria such as urethritis from *Chlamydia trachomatis*, *Neisseria gonorrhoeae*, herpes simplex virus, or vaginitis from *Candida* or *Trichomonas* species.

In the evaluation of a patient with a suspected lower UTI, a clinical distinction should be made between a lower and an upper UTI, which is suggested by fever (>38°C), flank pain, nausea, or vomiting.

Often, the history alone is sufficient to make a probable diagnosis of UTI, particularly in young women with a prior UTI. With an equivocal history, the diagnosis of a UTI is dependent on laboratory examination of a clean-catch midstream urine specimen, evaluating for bacteriuria and pyuria.

Quantitative urine for bacteriuria is the usual gold standard. Traditionally, patients with 10^5 or more bacteria per mL in the urine were considered to have significant bacteriuria and were given the diagnosis of a UTI. This is an insensitive standard, however, when applied to symptomatic women. A threshold of 10^2 or 10^3 bacteria per mL of urine provides a good combination of sensitivity (95%) and specificity (85%) for diagnosing acute cystitis. Microscopic evaluation

of the urine on wet-mount or Gram's stain for bacteriuria is a specific screen for infection but is insensitive for low levels of bacteriuria ($<10^4$ per mL).

Pyuria is present in most women with acute cystitis. The most accurate way to detect pyuria is to examine unspun urine with a hemocytometer and/or microscopic evaluation. The presence of greater than 10 white blood count (WBC) per mL or 10 WBC/high-power field with bacteria is 90% sensitive for a UTI.

Urine dipsticks for leukocyte esterase (LE) and bacterially generated nitrite are useful substitutes if urine microscopy is not feasible. The LE test is a practical screening test, with sensitivities and specificities ranging between 75 and 96% and 94 and 98%, respectively. The nitrite dipstick has reported sensitivities between 35 and 85% and a specificity of 98%. The accuracy of these rapid tests is lower in infections associated with colony counts less than 10^4 bacteria per mL. Therefore, if both the LE and nitrite testing are negative and suspicion of a UTI is present, a urinalysis and culture should be performed.

Because the causative organism and the antimicrobial susceptibilities are predictable in women with uncomplicated cystitis, a urine culture is generally not necessary. Unless the history is strongly compatible with a UTI, an abbreviated laboratory work-up, either by direct microscopy or rapid detection methods for pyuria or bacteriuria followed by empiric therapy, is recommended. If pyuria is absent or atypical symptoms are present, however, a culture should be performed before therapy is started.

Traditionally, therapy for acute cystitis included antimicrobial therapy for 7 to 14 days (Table 1). Single-dose therapy is a reasonable alternative, with the advantages of fewer side effects, lower cost, reduced emergence of resistant bacteria, and increased patient compliance. The major disadvantage of single-dose therapy is its failure to eradicate uropathogens from the vaginal reservoir, resulting in recurrent infections. To maintain the advantages of single-dose therapy but improve cure rates, 3-day courses of treatment have been advocated. With most antibiotics, a 3-day regimen appears optimal, with efficacy comparable to the 7-day regimen. Trimethoprim-sulfamethoxazole (TMP-SMZ) or trimethoprim can be used as a first-line agent with reported cure rates of approximately 80%. Amoxicillin/clavulanate (cure rates 78 to 87%) and fluoroquinolones (cure rates 88 to 98%) are effective, although they are more expensive alternatives and may promote bacterial resistance. No follow-up visit or urine culture after treatment is necessary unless symptoms persist or recur.

Acute Uncomplicated Pyelonephritis

Acute pyelonephritis is an infection involving the kidney parenchyma and renal pelvis, with the most common pathogen being *E. coli* (>80%). Patients frequently present with the triad of dysuria, flank pain, and fever. Pyuria is nearly always present. Urine cultures should be obtained in all women suspected

TABLE 1. **Common Medications Used in the Treatment of Urinary Tract Infections in Women**

Clinical Syndromes	Antibiotic Medication	Dose*	Notes
Acute cystitis	TMP-SMZ (Bactrim, Septra)	1 DS (160/800 mg) PO bid	Three-day therapy is adequate. Consideration should be given to 7- to 10-day therapy if the patient is pregnant, older than 65 years of age, or immunocompromised (e.g., diabetes). Single-dose therapy with TMP-SMZ (2 DS tablets) can be used but is associated with lower cure rates. Amoxicillin is not recommended owing to high rates of resistant *E. coli*.
	Trimethoprim	100 mg PO bid	
	Ciprofloxacin (Cipro)	250 mg PO bid	
	Norfloxacin (Noroxin)	400 mg PO bid	
	Ofloxacin (Floxin)	200 mg PO bid	
	Nitrofurantoin (Macrodantin)/ (Macrobid)	100 mg PO qid/100 mg PO bid	
	Amoxicillin/clavulanate (Augmentin)	875 mg PO bid	
Acute pyelonephritis Outpatient management	TMP-SMZ (Bactrim, Septra)	1 DS (160/800 mg) PO bid	Fourteen-day therapy should be given. Longer courses have not been shown to have additional benefit even if blood cultures are positive.
	Ciprofloxacin (Cipro)	250–500 mg PO bid	
	Norfloxacin (Noroxin)	400 mg PO bid	
	Ofloxacin (Floxin)	200–400 mg PO bid	
	Amoxicillin/clavulanate (Augmentin)	875 mg PO bid	
Inpatient management	Ampicillin/gentamicin	1 gm IV q 6 h/1 mg per kg q 8 h or 1 gm IV q 6 h/5 mg per kg IV q 24 h	Therapy should be given for 14 days. Intravenous therapy can be switched to oral therapy once patient is afebrile. Pregnant patients should be admitted. Fluoroquinolones and TMP-SMZ should be avoided in pregnancy owing to potential teratogenicity.
	Ciprofloxacin (Cipro)	400 mg IV q 12 h	
	Ceftriaxone (Rocephin)	1–2 gm IV q 24 h	
	Ampicillin/sulbactam (Unasyn)	1.5–3.1 gm IV q 6 h	
	Ceftazidime (Fortaz, Tazidime)	1–2 gm IV q 8–12 h	
	TMP-SMZ (Bactrim, Septra)	2 mg/kg IV q 6 h	
Recurrent urinary tract infections Continuous prophylaxis	TMP-SMZ (Bactrim, Septra)	1 SS (80/400 mg) PO qhs or thrice weekly	Regimen is initiated after eradication of an acute infection. Patients are placed on continuous prophylaxis for 6 mo and then observed for further infection. Factors that increase the risk of developing UTIs should be modified.
	Trimethoprim	100 mg PO qhs	
	Nitrofurantoin (Macrodantin)	50–100 mg PO qhs	
	Norfloxacin (Noroxin)	200 mg PO qhs	
	Cephalexin (Keflex)	250 mg PO qhs	
Postcoital prophylaxis	TMP-SMZ (Bactrim, Septra)	1 SS PO postcoitus	
	Nitrofurantoin (Macrodantin)	50–100 mg PO postcoitus	
	Cephalexin (Keflex)	250 mg PO postcoitus	
Pregnancy Asymptomatic bacteriuria	Amoxicillin	250 mg PO tid × 7 d or 3 gm single dose or 3 gm PO followed by 3 gm 12 h later	Single-dose therapy has lower eradication rates. Follow-up cultures should be obtained to ensure eradication of bacteriuria. Chronic suppressive antibiotic therapy is recommended if the patient has two or more episodes of recurrent bacteriuria.
	Nitrofurantoin (Macrodantin)	100 mg PO qid × 7 d 200 mg single dose 100 mg PO qid × 3 d	
	Amoxicillin/clavulanate (Augmentin)	250 mg PO tid × 7 d	

*Doses of drugs are based on normal hepatic and renal function.
Abbreviations: DS = double strength; SS = single strength.

of having pyelonephritis. Blood cultures should also be obtained in patients who are hospitalized because 15 to 20% are positive.

Patients with acute uncomplicated pyelonephritis can be stratified into those ill enough to require hospitalization and those able to be managed in the outpatient setting. Indications for admission include inability to maintain oral hydration or take oral medications, uncertain social situations, concerns about compliance, severe illness with high fevers, severe pain, and marked debility. Furthermore, for patients with co-morbidity such as diabetes, renal insufficiency, and immunosuppression, hospitalization should be strongly considered. Hospitalized patients should be started on intravenous antibiotics, usually ampicillin and gentamicin, a third-generation cephalo-

sporin (e.g., ceftriaxone, ceftazidime), a broad-spectrum β-lactam (e.g., ampicillin/sulbactam), or a fluoroquinolone (see Table 1). When signs and symptoms improve or resolve, usually within 48 to 72 hours, the remaining treatment can be given orally. Evaluation of the upper urinary tract with ultrasound or computed tomography to detect nephrolithiasis, renal or perirenal abscess, or other complications should be considered if fever persists 72 hours after treatment is begun. If the patient qualifies for outpatient treatment, acceptable regimens include TMP-SMZ, fluoroquinolones, and amoxicillin/clavulanate (see Table 1); however, in locations where resistance to TMP-SMZ is common, the other agents are preferred. Antibiotic therapy for 14 days is adequate, even if blood culture results are positive. Cultures should be obtained 2 weeks after treatment to ensure eradication of the infection.

Recurrent Urinary Tract Infections

Approximately 20% of women with an initial episode of cystitis have a recurrent infection. Recurrent UTIs are classified as either a reinfection or a relapse. Reinfections account for 90% of recurrences and represent a new UTI after successful eradication of a previous infection. A relapse is defined as the recrudescence of a prior, partially treated infection with a persistent focus of infection usually in the upper tract. A relapse should be considered if the infection recurs within 2 weeks after antimicrobial therapy. Most women with recurrent uncomplicated cystitis have no anatomic or functional abnormality of the urinary tract and therefore do not need urologic evaluation.

There are three effective approaches to managing recurrent UTIs: continuous prophylaxis, postcoital prophylaxis, or intermittent self-treatment (see Table 1). Prophylaxis is advocated for women who experience three or more symptomatic UTIs over 12 months and should be instituted only after an existing infection has been eradicated. Women who report a temporal association between infection and sexual intercourse are candidates for the postcoital approach, whereas others should receive continuous prophylaxis. The most common medications used are TMP-SMZ and nitrofurantoin. Women who do not want to take continuous antibiotics can treat themselves with a single-dose or 3-day regimen. It is important to alter those factors that may increase the risk of developing UTIs, such as contraceptive practices with diaphragms and spermicide. A 6-month trial of prophylaxis is usually prescribed after which the patient is observed for further infection. If necessary, however, treatment can be continued for years without the emergence of resistance.

One clinical trial of topical intravaginal estrogen among postmenopausal women with recurrent UTIs demonstrated a decrease of recurrent UTIs. Lack of estrogen induces changes in the vaginal microflora, including loss of lactobacilli and increased colonization with *E. coli*. The effect of oral estrogen replacement on recurrent UTIs, however, is unknown.

Complicated Urinary Tract Infections

Complicated UTIs encompass those patients with a structural or functional abnormality of the urinary tract or underlying co-morbidity such as diabetes and immunosupression. Complicated UTIs are often caused by pathogens that are resistant to first-line antibiotics. Risk factors include indwelling bladder catheterization, recent urinary tract instrumentation, functional or anatomic abnormality of the urinary tract, diabetes mellitus, symptoms that last longer than 7 days, immunosuppression, recent antibiotic use, and hospital-acquired infection. Clinical

presentations range from mild cystitis to life-threatening urosepsis.

Unlike the predictability of uropathogens in uncomplicated UTIs, a broader range of bacteria can cause complicated infections (e.g., *E. coli, Proteus* species, *Klebsiella* species, *Pseudomonas* species, *Staphylococcus* species). Urine cultures and susceptibility testing should be performed in all patients suspected of having a complicated infection. It is difficult to generalize the appropriate antibiotic regimen. Empirical therapy must take into account the setting, the medical history of the patient, the suspected organism, and any previous infecting organism and antimicrobial therapy. Usually a broad-spectrum antibiotic is administered for empirical therapy at least until resistance results are available. A 10- to 14-day course of therapy is usually necessary. Without correction of the underlying anatomic, functional, or metabolic defect, recurrent infections are common. Therefore, urine culture should be repeated 1 to 2 weeks after completion of therapy.

Catheter-Related Urinary Tract Infections

Catheterization is a risk factor for developing a UTI and is a common cause of nosocomial infections. The presence of a catheter in the bladder allows bacteria to adhere to the surface of the catheter and to initiate formation of biofilms that promote bacterial growth. Prevention is the best way to avoid morbidity and mortality from catheter-associated infection. Sterile insertion and care of the catheter, along with prompt removal, are effective preventive strategies.

Urine cultures from catheters that demonstrate bacterial growth higher than 10^2 colony-forming units (CFU) per mL are evidence of infection because these colony counts usually persist or increase within 48 hours. Systemic antibiotics prevent or delay the onset of bacteriuria but are not routinely recommended because of the cost and the emergence of antimicrobial resistance. Furthermore, there is little benefit in treating asymptomatic bacteriuria in chronically catheterized patients. Catheter-associated UTIs should be treated only if the patient shows signs or symptoms of a UTI (e.g., fever, hypotension, suprapubic pain, abdominal pain). Without removal of the catheter, prolonged or sequential courses of antibiotics for catheter-associated UTIs are usually unsuccessful.

Some authorities recommend giving a single dose of two double-strength TMP-SMZ tablets to women younger than 65 years of age who have persistent bacteriuria after catheterization for 1 week or less to prevent UTIs because many go on to have symptomatic UTIs.

Pregnancy-Associated Urinary Tract Infections

During pregnancy, hormonal and mechanical factors cause dilatation of the ureters and renal pelvis, referred to as hydroureter of pregnancy. The microbiology of pathogens is similar to that seen in nonpregnant women (*E. coli* > *Klebsiella* > *Enterobacter* > *Proteus* > group B *Streptococcus*). The approach to the pregnant patient with a UTI differs from that to the nonpregnant patient in the following manner: Asymptomatic bacteriuria is aggressively sought and treated, drugs that can be used safely are limited, and follow-up of bacteriuria during pregnancy is more intense.

Asymptomatic bacteriuria affects 4 to 7% of pregnant patients and is defined as recovery of 10^5 CFU per mL in two consecutive urinary midstream clean catches. The risk of bacteriuria is highest between the 9th and the 17th gestational weeks. Untreated bacteriuria during pregnancy is associated with adverse effects in the mother (symptomatic UTI) and the fetus (premature delivery, fetal infection, and perinatal death). Pyelonephritis occurs in 20 to 40% of pregnant women with untreated bacteriuria. Treatment of asymptomatic bacteriuria reduces the incidence of pyelonephritis by 80 to 90%. The serious implications of untreated bacteriuria justify screening all pregnant patients and treating asymptomatic bacteriuria. Screening is performed in the first trimester and no later than the 16th week. Acceptable drugs include beta-lactams (amoxicillin, amoxicillin/clavulanate, and oral cephalosporins) and nitrofurantoin (see Table 1). Single-dose therapies and 3- to 7-day treatments have been used. Regardless of the treatment regimen chosen, the important issue is not the length of therapy but the appropriate follow-up to ensure eradication of the bacteriuria. A follow-up culture should be performed 1 to 2 weeks after therapy. If short-course therapy fails to eradicate the infection, a 7- to 10-day regimen should be prescribed. Recurrence of asymptomatic bacteriuria after two courses of antibiotics is an indication for suppression therapy.

Symptomatic UTIs develop in 1 to 2% of pregnancies without treatment of asymptomatic bacteriuria. The usual duration of treatment for lower UTIs is 7 to 10 days. Shorter courses (i.e., single-dose or 3-day) have a 20 to 40% failure rate. Management of acute pyelonephritis in a pregnant patient should consist of hospital admission with intravenous antibiotics, usually ampicillin and an aminoglycoside or a third-generation cephalosporin. Acute pyelonephritis is associated with prematurity, low birth weight, and increased perinatal mortality. Furthermore, bacterial sepsis is associated with worse outcomes in pregnancy, compared with the nonpregnant state. Duration of treatment for acute pyelonephritis is 14 days. Follow-up cultures should be obtained every 4 to 6 weeks to rule out recurrence. Some authorities recommend placing patients on antibiotic suppression therapy until delivery after an episode of pyelonephritis.

Urinary Tract Infections in Elderly Women

The prevalence of asymptomatic bacteriuria in women older than 65 years of age has been reported to be between 8 and 25%. The prevalence is highest in women living in nursing homes and in women who require intermittent catheterization and have incomplete bladder emptying. The elderly may present with atypical symptoms (e.g., fever, altered mental status, incontinence, abdominal pain) and are generally more difficult to treat because of the increased incidence of abnormal bladder function, vaginal or urethral atrophy, and intermittent catheterization. Lower UTIs should be treated with a 3- to 7-day course. Generally, elderly patients are admitted for treatment of upper UTIs.

The management of asymptomatic bacteriuria in the elderly, defined as urine cultures greater than 10^5 CFU per mL, is controversial. Most authorities, however, believe that treatment of asymptomatic bacteriuria in elderly patients without indwelling catheters is not beneficial.

BACTERIAL INFECTIONS OF THE URINARY TRACT IN GIRLS

method of
ROSS M. DECTER, M.D.
The Milton S. Hershey Medical Center
Hershey, Pennsylvania

Urinary tract infections (UTIs) in girls manifest with a spectrum of severity. Severe infections of the upper urinary tract (pyelonephritis) may lead to irreversible renal damage, whereas lower urinary tract or bladder infections (cystitis) may cause only irritative voiding symptoms or be totally asymptomatic. Although the overriding objective in the management of urinary tract infections is to prevent renal injury, a secondary but significant goal is to allay the symptoms of cystitis. Renal injury due to pyelonephritis is more likely when the infection occurs in younger children, if it recurs, or if there is a delay in treatment.

DIAGNOSIS

The diagnosis of a UTI is predicated on the examination and culture of a properly collected, midstream urine specimen from the older child who is toilet trained. A catheterized specimen or suprapubic aspirate allows for the prompt diagnosis of an infection in the sick neonate or infant.

The concentration of bacteria in a voided urine specimen required to diagnose a UTI has classically been taught to be 10^5 colony-forming units per mL. If urine is obtained by urethral catheterization or suprapubic aspiration, most agree that a lower colony count of a single uropathogen indicates an infection.

The symptoms of a UTI vary greatly depending on the localization of the infection and the age of the patient. Symptoms of pyelonephritis in the neonate are nonspecific and may include lethargy, irritability, failure to thrive, jaundice, central nervous system symptomatology, and fever. The symptoms of an upper UTI in the infant in diapers may mimic those of a viral gastrointestinal illness. The mother of a toddler may comment that the urine in the diaper smells foul, the child seems irritable while voiding, or there is blood-stained urine in the diaper. Typical symptoms of cystitis in a girl who can verbalize them include urgency, frequency, dysuria, a sense of incomplete bladder emptying, incontinence, hematuria, and pelvic pressure or fullness. These complaints prompt a urinalysis, and a diagnosis is confirmed. Subtle changes in an older child's voiding pattern, especially new-onset enuresis, should prompt a urinalysis to confirm or rule out the possibility of a UTI.

INCIDENCE

The incidence of UTIs in neonatal girls is much lower than in neonatal boys. The prevalence of infection in girls increases until approximately the age of 2 years, when potty training begins, and peaks between the ages of 2 to 6 years. The incidence then gradually declines into the early teenage years. With the onset of sexual activity, the incidence of infections goes up to adult levels. Overall, bacteriuria will develop in at least 5% of girls during childhood; as many as 80% of these will have recurrent episodes.

PATHOGENESIS

The bacteria causing UTIs gain access to the urinary tract in most cases by ascending the urethra. The most important intrinsic bladder defense mechanism preventing infection is complete and regular bladder emptying. The few bacteria that enter the bladder are expelled during micturition and are unable to invade the bladder. The normal coordinated voiding pattern can be disturbed by a variety of processes, including inflammation of the bladder wall and compression from a rectal ampulla distended with stool. In addition, some bacteria possess factors that increase their pathogenicity. These factors, which have been best studied for *Escherichia coli*, include the presence of endotoxin, capsular antigens, and the adhesion factors known as pili. The pili of the *E. coli* confer on them the ability to invade the upper urinary tract in the absence of an anatomic abnormality.

EVALUATION

An integral part of the evaluation of the patient with a UTI is the examination. A particular element of the physical examination needs to be emphasized to avoid missing occult neuropathic states. The patient's back must be examined to detect a cutaneous manifestation such as a hemangioma or a hairy patch, which may aid in the discovery of the underlying neuropathic condition.

The radiologic evaluation should be tailored so that anatomic abnormalities that predispose to recurrent infections and renal damage will be promptly and precisely detected. On the other hand, when the clinical situation suggests that the likelihood of a significant anatomic abnormality is remote, the evaluation should not be invasive.

The imaging studies we recommend depend on the age of the patient at the time of infection and the nature of the infection. We routinely obtain a renal and bladder ultrasonogram and a voiding cystourethrogram in children younger than 10 years of age who have a febrile UTI. These studies allow us to diagnose vesicoureteral reflux (VUR) and any upper tract or bladder lesion that may predispose to recurring febrile infections. This evaluation is recommended at the time of the first febrile UTI to avoid unnecessary delay in the diagnosis of significant lesions. Because of the increased risk of renal injury in girls younger than 5 years of age, any UTI in this age group, regardless of whether the child is febrile, should be evalu-

ated with both the renal ultrasonogram and a voiding cystourethrogram. In the girl older than 5 years of age who has only urgency, frequency, and dysuria, it seems reasonable to obtain a renal ultrasonogram. A perfectly normal renal ultrasonographic study does not rule out the possibility of reflux, but it reassures the physician and parents if the kidneys are sonographically normal, because after this age the likelihood that a particular infection will significantly damage the kidneys is diminished. In the older, adolescent girl who has not had prior infections, the initial evaluation need consist only of a renal ultrasonogram.

Adjunctive radiologic evaluations, including renal imaging using nuclear medicine modalities or computed tomography scanning of the kidneys, can be valuable in complex cases when the diagnosis is confused by other issues or when treatment does not produce an appropriate response.

RESULTS OF EVALUATION

Significant anatomic problems are often detected in younger girls evaluated for UTIs. The most common abnormality revealed is VUR. VUR, the retrograde flow of urine from the bladder into the upper urinary tracts, places the patient at risk for pyelonephritis and renal scarring. Appropriate initial management for most patients with VUR consists of antibiotic chemoprophylaxis. The objective is to maintain sterile urine while waiting for spontaneous resolution of the VUR, which occurs in many patients.

Other anatomic abnormalities may be detected by the evaluation, including obstructive lesions at either the ureteropelvic or the ureterovesical junctions and duplication anomalies associated with either a ureterocele or an ectopic ureter. These require referral to a physician comfortable with their further evaluation and potential need for surgical management.

The radiologic evaluation does not reveal any obvious anatomic abnormalities in most toilet-trained girls with UTIs. In this subset of patients, the constellation of signs and symptoms of bladder and bowel dysfunction known as dysfunctional elimination are frequently encountered. Dysfunctional voiding symptoms include daytime urgency and frequency often associated with urinary incontinence of variable degrees. The bowel dysfunction associated with dysfunctional voiding may be manifest by constipation, large-volume stools, and encopresis. These patients require a plan of management directed toward both their bladder and bowel.

MANAGEMENT

If the patient with a UTI is toxic, cannot take fluids, and requires hospitalization, initial therapy after cultures are obtained and serum creatinine is assessed usually consists of a combination of ampicillin, 25 mg per kg every 6 hours, and gentamicin (Garamycin), 2 mg per kg every 8 hours, until the sensitivities of the infecting organism are reported. Culture-specific antibiotics are used at that time. Gentamicin peak and trough levels need to be monitored.

Most patients with UTIs are not ill enough to require hospital admission. Many physicians initiate therapy with a single injection of ceftriaxone (Rocephin), 25 mg per kg, in the younger child who comes to the emergency room with a presumed pyelonephritis, and send her home with a week to 10 days' supply of trimethoprim-sulfamethoxazole (TMP-SMX; Bactrim, Septra). If the sensitivities reveal the organism is not sensitive to TMP-SMX, therapy is changed when the sensitivities become available.

A logical choice for initial therapy of the outpatient with symptoms of cystitis is either nitrofurantoin or TMP-SMX. Although 7 to 10 days of therapy is usually prescribed, there is evidence that 3 days of therapy is very effective. Antibiotic chemoprophylaxis with either low-dose TMP-SMX, 2 mg of trimethoprim per kg daily, or nitrofurantoin (Furadantin), 1 to 2 mg per kg daily, is useful to try to prevent infections in girls with recurrent episodes of cystitis. Many of these children also benefit from medications such as oxybutynin chloride or propantheline bromide to treat their bladder instability. When bowel dysfunction is a component of the problem in girls with recurrent UTIs, a program to clean out the colon and provide adequate dietary fiber to prevent recurrent stool retention is useful. Several studies have shown that appropriate management of the bowel can improve symptoms of voiding dysfunction and even decrease the incidence of UTIs.

CHILDHOOD ENURESIS

method of
H. GIL RUSHTON, M.D.
Children's National Medical Center
and The George Washington University
Medical Center
Washington, D.C.

Enuresis is defined as the involuntary loss of urine beyond the age of anticipated control. The term is commonly used to refer to sleep wetting (nocturnal enuresis); however, it also applies to involuntary daytime (diurnal) wetting. Enuresis and voiding dysfunction represent the most common urinary disorders in children.

EPIDEMIOLOGY

Nocturnal enuresis occurs in 15 to 20% of 5-year-old children. An estimated 15% achieve control each year such that by age 15 years only 1 to 2% of adolescents remain enuretic. Secondary enuresis (onset of wetting after a 3- to 6-month dry period) accounts for 20 to 25% of the enuretic population. Furthermore, approximately 15 to 20% of young sleep wetters also have diurnal enuresis; this incidence rapidly decreases in children older than 5 years of age.

EVALUATION

Treatment of childhood enuresis must be preceded by a careful voiding history, physical examination, urinalysis, and urine culture. The voiding history should assess when (e.g., night only, day and night, before or after voiding, with giggling only) and how often wetting occurs, the typical amount of wetting (i.e., soaked or only damp), the frequency of daytime voiding and bowel movements, associated daytime voiding complaints (e.g., frequency, urgency, lack of sensation of bladder fullness), and history of urinary infection.

The physical examination includes an abdominal and genital evaluation to detect any physical abnormality that could be related to the child's voiding disorder, such as a palpably distended bladder. Epispadias, easily recognized in girls by the presence of a bifid clitoris, is a rare cause. If the child is constantly wet, pooling of urine in the vagina may be detected, the consequence of an ectopic ureter. If the history suggests an abnormal urinary stream, the clinician should observe the child voiding. The examiner should always visually inspect the lower back for evidence of sacral dimpling or cutaneous anomalies and asymmetry of the gluteal folds to rule out a neurologic cause. In most children with childhood enuresis and virtually all with nocturnal enuresis only, the physical examination is negative.

Urinary tract infection (UTI) is one of the most common and easily diagnosed and treated causes for daytime enuresis. Although microscopic analysis can be helpful, UTI can be reliably excluded only with urine culture. Urinalysis to exclude the rare nephrologic or metabolic cause, such as diabetes, should be done.

Based on an initial evaluation, enuresis can be categorized as either *uncomplicated* or *complicated*. Children with isolated nocturnal enuresis, a negative history for UTI, normal physical findings, and a negative urinalysis and urine culture have uncomplicated enuresis and comprise most of the enuretic population. Many also experience some daytime frequency or enuresis or a positive family history of nocturnal enuresis. In children with uncomplicated enuresis, the incidence of organic uropathology is not significantly higher than that of the normal population. Therefore, no further diagnostic studies are indicated. Even sonography cannot be routinely justified, and cystoscopy should not be performed unless an absolute indication exists.

In contrast, patients with a positive urine culture or a history of UTI, those with total urinary incontinence or a history of significant daytime voiding dysfunction associated with encopresis, and those with abnormal results of physical examination have complicated enuresis. These patients constitute an important, albeit small, minority of the enuretic population, most of whom have a history of UTI. Further evaluation of this group is indicated beginning with a renal and bladder sonogram with prevoid and postvoid views to assess bladder emptying. A history of UTI or abnormal sonographic findings such as a thickened bladder wall or hydroureteronephrosis warrants further evaluation with a voiding cystogram to exclude vesicoureteral reflux, a posterior urethral valve in boys, or evidence of neuropathic bladder dysfunction. Abnormal findings suggest the need for further urologic or neurologic evaluation because a very high incidence of urodynamic abnormalities is anticipated in this group of patients.

TREATMENT OF DIURNAL ENURESIS

A variety of voiding disorders can result in a child who wets while awake. Treatment is based on the underlying cause, age of the child, and severity of the wetting problem. One of the most common causes of day and night wetting, particularly in younger children, is persistence of a *small-capacity, uninhibited bladder*. Enuresis in this group is usually primary in onset and is associated with delayed toilet training. These children experience classic features of urgency incontinence. Urinary frequency, urgency, and posturing (squirming or squatting precipitated by the sudden urge to void) are caused by uninhibited bladder contractions associated with reduced functional bladder capacity. In some, this may be the consequence of prior and sometimes unrecognized UTI. Functional bladder capacity can be estimated by having the child void on several occasions when full and comparing the largest voided volume with the following formula, which predicts normal bladder capacity based on the age of the child:

$$\text{Age (years)} + 2 = \text{ounces} \times 30 = \text{mL}$$

For example, for a 3-year-old:

$$3 + 2 = 5 \text{ ounces} \times 30 = 150 \text{ mL}$$

The mainstay of treatment includes anticholinergics (oxybutynin or hyoscyamine) and timed voidings every 2 to 3 hours. The usual dosage for children older than 5 years of age is 2.5 to 5 mg of oxybutynin (Ditropan) three times a day or hyoscyamine (Levsinex) timecaps 0.375 mg twice daily. Anticipated side effects include facial flushing and dry mouth. Rarely, blurred vision or overheating may occur, necessitating stopping the medication or lowering the dose. If the child has a history of recurrent UTI, long-term antibiotic prophylaxis should be considered.

This type of voiding disorder must be distinguished from the *daytime frequency-urgency syndrome*. This is characterized by the abrupt onset of daytime frequency and urgency, sometimes voiding as often as every 10 to 15 minutes. This is most commonly seen in boys 4 to 8 years of age, but can occur in girls. Urine culture and physical examination are negative. Despite their excessive daytime voiding frequency, these children remain dry and sleep throughout the night without wetting the bed. These children do not actually have uninhibited bladder activity or reduced functional bladder capacity and do not respond to pharmacologic treatment. This is a self-limiting disorder that may persist for a few weeks or for several months. In many, it is thought to be stress or anxiety related. Imaging studies and evaluation beyond a urine culture are not indicated.

Another relatively common cause of daytime wetting is *infrequent voiding*. These children, mostly older girls, avoid urinating for extensive intervals. They typically awaken in the morning after having slept through the night, eat, and go off to school without urinating. Thus, the first time they void may be on coming home from school. They then often rush to get to the toilet and may dribble in the process or may already be wet. As expected, their bladder capacity is very large and emptying is often incomplete. Consequently, urinary infection or bacilluria is common. The diagnosis is made historically by asking whether the patient urinates on awakening in the morning, whether she uses the toilet at school, and

how many times a day she voids. Treatment involves the institution of a timed voiding schedule. It is advised that these children wear a wristwatch with a multiple alarm that can be set to go off every 3 to 4 hours, reminding them to urinate. Constipation is a frequent concomitant complaint and may even be associated with encopresis. Treatment may initially require a series of enemas or suppositories. Thereafter, these children are encouraged to have a bowel movement once a day. They typically require long-term increased dietary fiber on a daily basis (a fiber supplement is usually necessary) as well as continuous antibacterial prophylaxis to prevent UTI. This is a chronic problem that requires years of continuous attention to resolve.

A particularly difficult group of patients to treat are those with a *sensory-deficient bladder*. These children, almost always boys, soak themselves several times a day, are wet at night, and seem totally unaware of the need to urinate. In contrast to the infrequent voider, their bladder capacity is normal. Timed voidings every 90 to 120 minutes appear to be the only practical therapy because the patients do not respond to anticholinergics. Eventually, either maturation allows them to appreciate the status of their urinary bladders or timed voiding becomes a routine part of their lives.

Postvoid dribbling is a relatively common problem in prepubertal girls. These girls wet *only* immediately after voiding, usually resulting in mildly damp underwear. This results from vaginal pooling of urine caused by reflux of urine into the vagina during voiding. On standing from the toilet, the pooled urine in the vagina dribbles out. This type of wetting is treated by having the child spread her legs widely during voiding. In younger children, it may be necessary to place a stool in front of the toilet so that they can support their feet and sit securely on the family toilet. Alternatively, the child can sit backward on the toilet. On completion of voiding, the child should be encouraged to lean forward and use the Valsalva maneuver to push out any urine pooled in the vagina.

A more severe uropathologic process may exist in children in whom discoordinated voiding has developed. Failure fully to relax the voluntary sphincter during voiding interferes with emptying and results in a weak and stuttering or staccato urinary stream. These children have been labeled as *dysfunctional voiders*. Dysfunctional voiding, also known as detrusor-sphincter dyssynergia, results in a degree of bladder outlet obstruction that, if chronic, causes secondary bladder wall hypertrophy and high voiding pressures. This can result in secondary vesicoureteral reflux, bladder wall thickening, and hydroureteronephrosis. This extreme of dysfunctional voiding has been labeled the *non-neurogenic neurogenic bladder*, although a more appropriate term would be *non-neuropathic voiding dyssynergia*. Both daytime and nighttime enuresis, encopresis, recurrent UTI, and even renal damage are components of this problem. Emotional and behavioral problems are also common in this group of patients. Treatment is complex and usually involves both pharmacologic efforts and bio-feedback therapy after complete radiologic and uro-dynamic evaluation.

An *ectopic ureter* that drains into the distal urethra or vaginal introitus may cause *paradoxical incontinence*. These girls void normally but are still wet or damp all of the time. Because ectopic ureters do not bypass the urinary sphincter mechanism in boys, boys do not have this problem. Most ectopic ureters drain the upper segment of a duplicated collecting system. In rare instances, an ectopic ureter drains a hypoplastic kidney. The diagnosis of ectopic ureter is confirmed radiographically, and treatment consists of a partial nephrectomy or removal of a small ectopic kidney when present.

TREATMENT OF NOCTURNAL ENURESIS

Nocturnal enuresis is best thought of as a symptom, not a disease state. Although the etiology of nocturnal enuresis remains controversial, evidence supports the theory of maturational lag or developmental delay. This may be influenced by a number of factors, including stress, nocturnal polyuria, reduced functional bladder capacity, genetic predisposition, and, occasionally, infection. The role of inheritance is evidenced by the observation that when both parents have a history of nocturnal enuresis, their child has up to a 77% chance of being a bedwetter. Although psychopathology and enuresis may coexist, most enuretics do not have a psychological disorder. Evidence does not support the theory that enuresis represents a sleep disorder, although the possibility of an arousal disorder independent of sleep stage remains a possibility.

Treatment of nocturnal enuresis can be categorized into behavioral and pharmacologic modalities. The specific therapeutic approach should be based on the attitudes of the parents and child, as well as the family social structure and home environment. Timing of treatment is another important factor. It should rarely be necessary before age 5 or 6 years, and only then when it becomes a problem to the child as well as the family. Traditional home remedies such as limiting fluid intake before bedtime or waking the child at random during the night are usually ineffective.

Behavioral modification involves a combination of conditioning therapy and motivational therapy. Success rates approaching 80% can be achieved by using a moisture alarm and setting goals, monitoring progress, and rewarding success as a means of "response shaping." The moisture alarm is triggered when wetting occurs and, over time, the child can come to recognize bladder fullness before wetting and inhibit bladder contractions during sleep or awaken to void in the toilet. Unfortunately, some children do not awaken to the alarm, and it is often necessary for the parents to be involved initially to help wake the child. This may require applying a wet cloth to the child's face. Success depends on a cooperative and motivated family and child because it may take several weeks before positive results are seen. For this reason, conditioning therapy is usually reserved for patients older than 7 or 8 years of age. Several months of treatment may be required, and relapse occurs in up to one third of patients; however, retreatment is usually successful. Most moisture alarms cost between $60 and $75, and small, transistorized units are available (Wet-Stop alarm, Palco Labs, Santa Cruz, CA; Nytone alarm, Medical Products, Inc., Salt Lake City, UT; Potty Pager vibrator, Ideas for Living, Inc., Boulder, CO).

Pharmacotherapy has received heightened interest with the advent of antidiuretic therapy with desmopressin acetate (DDAVP). Other drugs that have been used to treat nocturnal enuresis include the tricyclic antidepressant imipramine (Tofranil) and anticholinergics such as oxybutynin (Ditropan). Pharmacologic treatment is best viewed as management therapy rather than as curative because relapse after short-term treatment is high. As a general rule, the author advises against implementation of medication for this problem until the child is 7 or 8 years of age.

Imipramine is the oldest of these drugs, but its exact mechanism of action is unknown. Theories include changes in sleep patterns (arousability), an anticholinergic effect in conjunction with its central nervous system activity, an antidepressant effect, and an antidiuretic effect. The usual dosage recommended by the author for bedwetting is 25 to 50 mg at bedtime for children 8 to 12 years of age, increasing to 75 mg in older children. Tofranil-PM, 75 mg, is released more slowly and may be more effective in the child older than 12 years of age. Noticeable improvement is reported in approximately one half of children; however, many children "escape" control while on treatment. Effectiveness is usually evident within the first few days of treatment, making use on an as-needed basis a possibility, such as for sleepovers or camp. Mild side effects are not uncommon, including anxiety, irritability, and insomnia. Imipramine has been reported to cause central nervous system and cardiac toxicity when overdosed, including potentially fatal arrhythmias, conduction blocks, and convulsions. Therefore, parents should be instructed to monitor the child closely, to administer the dosage carefully, and to *keep it out of reach of younger children*.

The newest form of treatment applies the antidiuretic effects of DDAVP. When given at bedtime, DDAVP reduces urine output, presumably below the level of the child's functional bladder capacity. Therefore, spontaneous bladder emptying does not occur. The drug is administered orally or by a nasal spray pump that delivers a dose of 10 µg of desmopressin per spray. The initial recommended nasal dosage for DDAVP for the treatment of nocturnal enuresis is 20 µg (one spray in each nostril) at bedtime. Dosage for nonresponders and partial responders can be increased over several days to a maximum of 40 µg. If no response is evident after 1 week of maximum dosage, treatment should be terminated and other alternatives pursued. The FDA has approved an oral tablet form of DDAVP (0.2 mg) with a recommended dose range of 0.2 to 0.6 mg.

Approximately 50% of children respond to DDAVP, with approximately half of these achieving complete dryness. Like imipramine, the effect of DDAVP is immediate, and it can be used occasionally or on a long-term basis without problems. Although rare instances of hyponatremia and water intoxication have occurred, reported side effects in all the clinical trials are minimal, and safety is not a real concern with DDAVP. Relapse can be anticipated in almost all patients on cessation of therapy. Similar to imipramine, long-term treatment with DDAVP should be interrupted at 4- to 6-month intervals to see if the problem has spontaneously resolved. If wetting recurs, patients can be successfully treated by resuming the most recent effective dose.

Reduced functional bladder capacity is associated with a lower response rate to DDAVP. Therefore, combination pharmacotherapy using DDAVP to reduce nocturnal urine output and an anticholinergic such as oxybutynin to increase nocturnal bladder capacity may be beneficial in select children with reduced functional bladder capacity. Otherwise, in patients with isolated nocturnal enuresis, anticholinergics alone are usually ineffective.

URINARY INCONTINENCE

method of
ROGER R. DMOCHOWSKI, M.D.
North Texas Center for Urinary Control
Fort Worth, Texas

Implicit to successful therapy for urinary incontinence is appropriate diagnosis of the underlying etiologic factors contributing to the patient's symptoms. Diagnostic accuracy is ensured by thorough history taking and physical examination, supplemented by adjunctive testing modalities that assist in defining lower urinary tract pathophysiology. A significant addition to the acquisition of the patient's history has been two tests to objectify the symptoms of incontinence for both the patient and the physician. A voiding diary is kept by the patient for 2 to 3 days and details the patient's normal voiding habit, including voiding times and amounts as well as incontinent episodes and associated symptoms. This instrument then becomes one method of monitoring the progress of therapeutic interventions and to counsel the patient regarding behavioral modifications. The second testing method is symptom score instruments that further objectify the physical and subjective emotional impact of incontinence. These tools also provide a longitudinal follow-up mechanism for evaluating incontinence interventions.

The most commonly used modality for evaluating lower urinary tract function is urodynamics. This modality provides graphic demonstration of pressure/volume relationships for urinary storage and voiding. Electromyography (EMG) is used in conjunction with intravesical pressure monitoring (performed with urethral catheters and pressure transducers) to allow observation of pelvic floor activity (sphincter behavior) during the cycle of bladder filling and emptying.

Other ancillary testing procedures that may be included in the evaluation of the lower urinary tract include ultrasonography (renal and pelvic), functional or anatomic radiographic studies (intravenous pyelography, nuclear renal scan), and cystoscopy. These modalities provide additional information in patients with unexplained hematuria or who may be at risk for renal functional compromise. Urine culture and voided urinary cytologic studies also provide key informational components to exclude complicating urinary tract infection or malignancy.

Normal lower urinary tract function depends on intact bladder and urethral function. Bladder or detrusor properties that promote continence include low-pressure urine storage during the capacitance stage of bladder function. Bladder storage capabilities are augmented by intact proximal urethral function, which provides coaptation or urethral closure and prevents urine loss. When bladder capacity is achieved, the second phase of urinary tract function is initiated. Bladder emptying is successfully completed with synergic or coordinated bladder and urethral function. This implies relaxation or opening of the urethra that occurs simultaneously with bladder contraction of adequate magnitude and longevity to empty the bladder, leaving little or no residual urine. This phase should be accompanied by voiding pressures that do not exceed values (40 cm H_2O) considered deleterious to renal function.

Incontinence and voiding dysfunction can be attributed to failure of either the filling (capacitance) phase or the emptying phase of the lower urinary tract. In some cases, a combination of storage and emptying abnormalities is present. These latter cases are often harder to manage successfully without intensive early evaluation and chronic therapy.

INCONTINENCE ASSOCIATED WITH BLADDER DYSFUNCTION

Bladder storage abnormalities may be related to detrusor muscular overactivity. The term *overactive bladder* has been used to describe urgency and frequency of urination that may or may not be associated with urinary loss. Affected patients are not a homogeneous group, however; they include patients with and without bladder muscular overactivity. In addition, some patients with pelvic pain disorders such as interstitial cystitis may also experience these symptoms as a component of their global symptoms.

Bladder storage disorders may result for diseases that produce detrusor motor overactivity (instability). Neurologic diseases, including spinal cord injury, dementia, cerebral infarction, multiple sclerosis, Parkinson's disease, diabetes (small sensory neuronal injury), and other systemic diseases with neurologic sequelae produce loss of integration between the central nervous system and lower urinary tract and result in detrusor muscular overactivity, which is referred to as *detrusor hyperreflexia* (implying a defined underlying neurologic pathology).

Disorders such as genuine stress urinary incontinence and pelvic prolapse in women also produce detrusor overactivity that occurs without neurologic abnormality. Detrusor overactivity in these patients is termed *instability*. Other patients who experience instability with urgency of urination and incontinence include those with bladder outlet obstruction (men with prostate enlargement and women with obstruction from previous incontinence surgery for pelvic organ prolapse) and menopausal women with inadequate estrogen replacement.

A third group of patients are those with urgency and frequency without detrusor overactivity that can be identified with urodynamics. These patients are described as having sensory urgency. They may complain of urge incontinence, but no bladder motor activity is apparently causative of these symptoms. These patients often have associated pelvic floor disorders such as fibromyalgia, urgency/frequency syndrome, interstitial cystitis, and other pelvic pain syndromes. The sensory nature of these disorders can complicate diagnosis and therapy.

Diagnosis

Symptomatic appraisal is crucial for elucidating other sensory complaints associated with urinary urgency. Postvoid residual measurement must be included as part of the initial evaluation to exclude poor bladder drainage as a complicating factor, especially in patients who may have a neurologic or obstructive etiology. Physical examination identifies coexistent stress urinary incontinence or pelvic organ prolapse.

Cystometrics are extremely useful for identifying definable motor dysfunction of the bladder. Also, a cystometrogram identifies functional or anatomic reduction of bladder capacity (sensory urgency or poor bladder storage secondary to anatomic abnormality). Finally, the pressure/volume relationship identified by cystometrics indicates which patients are at risk for renal functional compromise as a result of deleterious storage pressures (poor bladder compliance as seen in certain neurologic injuries; in patients with diseased detrusor musculature–radiation injury or chemical/toxic injury associated with use of intravesical chemotherapy such as doxorubicin [Adriamycin] and bacille Calmette-Guérin; and in patients with chronic bladder outlet obstruction with resultant detrusor muscular decompensation, as seen in men with long-standing prostatism and in patients with permanent indwelling urethral catheters).

In general, bladder pressures should not exceed a 15–cm H_2O change from baseline at bladder capacity. However, bladder compliance is best expressed by determining the ratio of total volume change to pressure change during filling. This ratio should not be less than 12 to 15 mL per cm H_2O; if it is, bladder compliance is poor and renal function is potentially at risk. Prolonged high-pressure storage can overcome the ureterovesical junction and allow pressure transmission directly to the nephrons. High pressure then alters renal blood flow and leads to renal functional deterioration. Bladder filling pressures exceeding 40 cm H_2O are extremely damaging and, in longitudinal studies of neurogenic populations, have been ascribed directly to higher incidences of renal deterioration.

Therapy

Before pharmacologic therapy is initiated for the patient with urgency incontinence, postvoid residual determination should exclude high residual volumes, because this circumstance can complicate effective control of urgency and convert a state of urgency and incontinence to one of urgency and retention. Once effective bladder emptying has been ascertained, first-line therapy begins with anticholinergics alone or in combination with the tricyclic agent imipramine hydrochloride (Tofranil). Oxybutynin (Ditropan), 2.5 to 5 mg three times a day, provides adequate initial effect. Side effects (xerostomia, heat intolerance, constipation) may limit patient adherence to the drug regimen. Alternative agents include tolterodine (Detrol), 2.0 mg twice daily, which is essentially equally effective with fewer side effects. The addition of the tricyclic agent is useful in patients with partial response and also in neurogenic patients. Imipramine is also particularly useful in postmenopausal women with mixed incontinence who demonstrate significant urgency as part of their symptoms.

In patients with elevated residual urine volumes, clean intermittent catheterization, either by patient or caregiver, in conjunction with drug therapy provides additive benefit. Catheterization frequency may vary from once to six times a day, depending on degree of urinary retention.

In patients who partially respond or who wish another therapeutic alternative, behavioral modification may be useful. Using a voiding diary, the patient can be instructed to modify fluid intake, adjust toileting frequency, and/or adjust interval to improve urinary habit. This technique is especially useful in patients with partial response to pharmacologic intervention and in patients with partial neurologic injury who have diminished bladder sensation (i.e., diabetic cystopathy).

More intensive behavioral and pelvic floor therapy involves biofeedback to enhance pelvic floor rehabilitation in patients with symptomatic urgency and bladder overactivity. Electrical stimulation with perineal, vaginal, and rectal probes has also been described as a modality for refractory urgency and detrusor instability. These modalities may also be useful for patients with associated pelvic pain disorders. The advent of selective needle electrode implantation into the sacral foramina has provided another option in electrical stimulation of the lower urinary tract. This option requires direct needle application to the sacral roots via a percutaneous technique. Direct sacral stimulation is used only after drug and other pelvic floor rehabilitative techniques have failed.

Direct neural ablation has also been described. Currently, deliberate bladder distention under anesthesia (hydrodistention) and vaginal denervation of the bladder base are used with varying rates of success. Surgical reconstruction is reserved for patients in whom the aforementioned modalities have failed. Reconstruction involves the use of a bowel segment, either small or large, to augment or increase the capacity of the bladder. Partial resection of the bladder muscle to create a pseudodiverticulum of the bladder has also been used for this purpose, although not with the reproducibility of results seen with bowel augmentation. Bladder augmentation is best used for patients with chronic, irreversible bladder wall changes secondary to muscular injury from obstruction, neural lesion, or toxic insult. In patients with dangerous bladder storage pressures, augmentation provides normalization of pressures and protection of renal function.

INCONTINENCE ASSOCIATED WITH URETHRAL DYSFUNCTION

Urethral dysfunction is diminished urethral resistance to urinary flow. The normal urethra does not leak with any activity. In women, incontinence resulting from an as yet not completely defined etiology (partially related to parturition, pelvic floor dysfunction, and hormonal deprivation) and associated with increasing abdominal pressure secondary to activities such as coughing, exercise, and, in severe cases, positional change is termed *stress incontinence*. Stress incontinence reflects a defect in urethral function manifested by diminished urethral resistance and an often associated hypermobility of the proximal urethra and bladder neck resulting from loss of musculofascial supports in that area. The primary defect, however, is intrinsic to the urethra, and the demonstrated incontinence may manifest as a spectrum of dysfunction from minimal (as defined by activity instigating the incontinence) to severe (urinary loss with trivial movements). Stress incontinence does occur in men in two circumstances: as a primarily iatrogenic entity resulting from prostatectomy (radical or simple) with associated damage to the smooth muscle sphincter, or as a result of neurologic disease with injury to the sympathetic innervation of the bladder neck and intrinsic smooth muscle sphincter.

Diagnosis

Physical examination must demonstrate urinary loss with typical stress maneuvers. The patient should be examined in the supine and standing positions. Coexistent pelvic prolapse should be identified in the female with stress urinary incontinence so as to plan effective therapies.

Many patients with stress incontinence have associated bladder storage abnormalities, which should be identified before therapy with cystometrics. Although these bladder abnormalities do not preclude successful intervention, these findings may be responsible for persistent symptoms after therapy has been administered for stress incontinence. In addition, findings from the cystometric study are useful for counseling the patient about the best modes of therapy to consider and reasonable expectations for therapy.

Cystoscopy is crucial in men with stress incontinence in order to exclude anatomic scarring or residual tissue from prior surgical intervention.

Therapy

In some patients, behavioral modification is useful, although many patients have already reduced fluid intake and increased frequency to compensate for their incontinence. Pelvic floor exercises and electrical stimulation can provide improvement for 30 to 50% of women; results are optimal in patients with lesser degrees of incontinence. Results of pelvic floor rehabilitation are less dramatic in men, but behavioral modification remains an option for men with less severe incontinence.

Drug therapy is founded on the rich adrenergic innervation of the proximal urethra and bladder neck in women and men. Alpha-stimulating agents containing phenylpropanolamine or pseudoephedrine (once-a-day, long-release formulation) produce stimulation of the bladder neck and may decrease incontinence in patients with lesser degrees of incontinence. Estrogen replacement (one third to one half applicator every other day for 6 weeks) is useful as an adjunct to these agents in postmenopausal women who demonstrate significant vaginal mucosal atrophy.

As with urgency incontinence, imipramine provides some benefit to elderly women with mixed incontinence who manifest stress incontinence. A combination of therapies, drug and behavioral, should also be presented as a therapeutic alternative to the patient.

Vaginal supportive devices, such as pessary variants, provide a nonsurgical option for patients who may also have pelvic organ prolapse.

Injectable therapy now occupies a significant place in the treatment of stress urinary incontinence. In men, the use of bovine collagen has provided some benefit, but only in patients with relatively minimal degrees of incontinence. Collagen provides substantial improvement or cure for 70 to 80% of women with little or no urethral hypermobility. However, the effect is not permanent, and reinjection is necessary; most patients require two or three injections within the first 12 months. Long-term results suggest that periodic reinjection will continue being required with this option.

Surgical options for men include the artificial urinary sphincter or male sling. The artificial sphincter provides substantial improvement in quality of life but with risk of device-related dysfunction on a long-term basis. Sling therapy for males is as yet not fully developed.

Surgery for women has evolved dramatically since 1993. Long-term results suggest that many standard procedures do not provide the success previously associated with needle suspensions. Retropubic suspensions and sling procedures appear to provide the most durable results, with slightly greater morbidity. New procedural modifications are currently being evaluated to decrease morbidity without affecting efficacy.

COMBINED INCONTINENCE

Overflow incontinence represents urinary dysfunction related either to detrusor failure (loss of contraction capability) or to outlet obstruction, from surgical intervention or physiologic process (prostate hyperplasia in males, uterine fibroids in females). Obstruction and detrusor decompensation can also coexist. The incontinence is often continuous.

Diagnosis can often be made from physical examination supplemented with postvoid residual documentation of high bladder volumes.

Initial therapy is bladder drainage and identification of underlying pathology. No effort should be made to obstruct bladder drainage, because postobstructive diuresis often complicates this manifestation.

EPIDIDYMITIS

method of
ALLAN R. RONALD, M.D.
St. Boniface General Hospital
Winnipeg, Manitoba, Canada

The epididymis is the accessory sex organ that stores and transports spermatozoa from the testes to the vas deferens. Infections of the epididymis are usually caused by organisms that ascend via the urethra. Ejaculation may protect against infection, but this is unproven. Infection elsewhere in the genitourinary tract, particularly in the urethra, bladder, or prostate, often precedes epididymal infection. The pathogenesis of epididymitis, however, is not known. The roles of humeral or cell-mediated immunity are undetermined, but the increased incidence of epididymitis among men with concomitant human immunodeficiency virus (HIV) infection suggests that cell-mediated immunity contributes to host defences.

CLINICAL FEATURES

Epididymitis usually manifests as a painful swelling within the scrotum that develops over 1 to 2 days. In more than 90% of patients it is unilateral. Patients may have concomitant symptoms in the urethra or prostate. Physical findings include a tender scrotal mass accompanied occasionally by erythema of the overlying skin. Although initially the epididymis can usually be clearly identified, testicular involvement leads to an epididymo-orchitis. A hydrocele may be present because of inflammatory fluid within the layers of the tunica vaginalis. Some patients have fever and other systemic symptoms due to localized or generalized sepsis. Imaging techniques are not essential in most instances. Color flow Doppler ultrasonography, however, can be useful for patients with complicated epididymo-orchitis to exclude testicular torsion or abscesses that require drainage.

EPIDEMIOLOGY

Epididymitis is common and accounts for more than 600,000 visits annually to physicians in the United States and for about 20% of urologic hospital admissions of men younger than age 35 years. Sexually transmitted urethritides and urinary infection are the major risk factors for epididymitis. Additional risk factors include urethral or prostatic manipulation and indwelling catheters or stents in the urethra. Anal insertive intercourse is a major risk factor for both urinary infection and epididymitis. Much less commonly, epididymitis is metastatic from a primary site during bacteremic illness. Patients with systemic or urogenital infections with mycobacteria, fungi, or parasites may have chronic epididymitis.

MANAGEMENT

Sexually Transmitted Epididymitis

Chlamydia trachomatis and *Neisseria gonorrhoeae* cause most episodes of epididymitis that occur in men younger than age 35 years. Before the antibiotic era, epididymitis occurred in about 20% of patients with gonococcal urethritis. The incubation period is variable and can be weeks, and epididymitis can occur in patients without active gonococcal urethritis. *C. trachomatis* now accounts for one half to two thirds of epididymitis cases in this age group. In about half of patients, no obvious urethral discharge is present. Urethral Gram's stain and investigation for both *N. gonorrhoeae* and *C. trachomatis* should be performed routinely.

All men with epididymitis who are at risk of sexually transmitted infections (STIs) should be treated empirically for both *N. gonorrhoeae* and *C. trachomatis*. My initial choice is a combination of cefixime (Suprax), 400 mg, together with azithromycin (Zithromax),* 1 gram each, taken in a setting where ingestion can be observed. This regimen will cure more than 98% of both *N. gonorrhoeae* and *C. trachomatis* epididymal infections. Other acceptable regimens include the combination of ceftriaxone (Rocephin), 250 mg parenterally, plus doxycycline (Vibramycin), 100 mg twice daily for 10 days; ofloxacin (Floxin), 400 mg daily for 10 days; and ciprofloxacin (Cipro), 500 mg as a stat dose, followed by doxycycline, 100 mg twice daily for 10 days. Other specific measures are essential. Be mindful of the six Cs of treating all patients with STIs: Exclude other *concomitant* STIs, particularly HIV; ensure *contact* tracing is carried out; review *compliance* with medication; provide for *counseling* about sexual risks; stress *condom* use; and do all this with the assurance of *confidentiality*.

Men with sexually transmitted epididymitis do not require routine urologic work-up, because underlying urologic disease is unusual. The course of acute epididymitis is one of rapid response, with acute symp-

---

*Not FDA approved for this indication.

toms resolving in 2 to 4 days. Chronic induration, however, may persist for weeks or months. Infertility is rare.

Epididymitis in Men with Urinary Infection

Urinary tract infection is a concomitant event with epididymitis in most men over the age of 35 years, particularly if they have no identified risk for STIs. All the pathogens responsible for urinary tract infections can cause epididymitis. It is common, however, in the presence of a urethral catheter or after urethral manipulation. Obtunded and cord injury patients are at high risk of complications. These include scrotal abscess, chronic draining scrotal sinuses, and testicular infarction.

Acute epididymitis must be differentiated from testicular torsion. Subacute and chronic epididymal orchitis must be differentiated from testicular cancer.

After a urine culture and, if necessary, a prostatic fluid culture, empiric antibacterial treatment should be prescribed. The regimen should treat both gram-negative and gram-positive pathogens. Epididymitis can be managed out of hospital after an initial clinical response to parenteral therapy. Ampicillin (2 grams every 6 hours) and gentamicin (5 mg per kg every 24 hours), ceftriaxone (2 grams every 24 hours) or a parenteral fluoroquinolone (ciprofloxacin, 400 mg every 12 hours) can be given for the first one or two doses. Ongoing oral therapy can be tailored to the specific etiologic agent cultured from the urine. The treatment course should be continued for at least 14 days. A fluoroquinolone (ciprofloxacin, 500 mg every 12 hours; or ofloxacin, 400 mg every 12 hours) or trimethoprim (160 mg)–sulfamethoxazole (800 mg) (Bactrim DS) every 12 hours are agents with proven efficacy. Surgery is seldom required unless an abscess develops. Response is often quite slow, and the epididymidis may be indurated for weeks or months.

Other measures, including scrotal support and analgesics, are often required. Urologic investigation may be necessary in the presence of concomitant bacterial urinary or prostatic infection or if epididymitis recurs. Urine and prostatic secretions should be cultured 2 to 3 weeks after completion of therapy to ensure that no focus of infection has persisted.

PRIMARY GLOMERULAR DISEASES

method of
BRAD H. ROVIN, M.D.
*The Ohio State University College of Medicine
and Public Health
Columbus, Ohio*

Glomerular diseases have a wide spectrum of clinical manifestations, from asymptomatic urinary abnormalities to severe renal failure requiring replacement therapy. Treatment of glomerulopathies may be divided into immunosuppressive therapies that interrupt the pathophysiologic mechanisms of glomerular injury, and adjunctive therapies designed to slow the tendency toward progressive renal failure that is often seen after renal injury. This chapter focuses on *primary glomerulopathies:* diseases that occur as a result of a process confined primarily to the kidney. In *secondary glomerulopathies,* the kidney is involved by an identifiable systemic disease that usually affects multiple organs. Treatment of secondary glomerulopathies is directed at the underlying process.

DIAGNOSIS OF GLOMERULAR DISEASE

A diagnosis of glomerular disease should be considered in the patient with hematuria, proteinuria, or an abnormal urinary sediment (dysmorphic red blood cells, erythrocyte casts, leukocytes in the absence of bacteria, or leukocyte casts). Urinary protein should be quantified with a 24-hour urine collection or a spot urine protein:creatinine ratio, and characterized by urine protein immunoelectrophoresis. Although nonglomerular processes such as interstitial nephritis may result in similar urinary abnormalities, proteinuria in excess of 2 grams per day, consisting of both low- and high-molecular-weight proteins (albumin or larger), is almost always indicative of a glomerulopathy. Serologic studies such as antinuclear antibody, antineutrophil cytoplasmic autoantibody (ANCA), or hepatitis profile may be helpful in reaching a specific diagnosis. A renal biopsy is commonly needed to establish a diagnosis, especially with primary glomerulopathies. A pathologic finding allows the selection of an appropriate therapeutic regimen. In addition, the renal biopsy usually indicates the likelihood of a response to therapy. For example, a biopsy showing severe glomerular sclerosis or interstitial fibrosis may suggest a poor outcome despite therapy. Such findings should decrease enthusiasm for using aggressive and potentially toxic immunosuppressive therapy.

THERAPEUTIC OPTIONS IN GLOMERULAR DISEASE

Because immune mechanisms have been implicated in the pathogenesis of most primary glomerular diseases, immunosuppressive agents are the main tools used to treat glomerulopathies. In conjunction with immunosuppression, a variety of maneuvers may be used to slow the progressive deterioration of renal function that is often seen even after resolution of an immune process. In this section, a general approach to immunosuppression and preservation of renal function is outlined. The application of these regimens to specific glomerular diseases is then discussed.

Immunosuppression

Corticosteroids

A number of steroid regimens have been used to treat glomerular disease. They vary primarily in the duration and intensity of treatment. I have divided these regimens into *standard* therapy and *intensive* therapy.

Standard therapy is initiated with oral prednisone, 1 mg per kg ideal body weight per day (maximum, 80 mg per day) for 6 to 8 weeks. A lower (75%) initial dose may be used in elderly patients. Prednisone may then be *rapidly* tapered over 16 weeks by changing to 1.6 mg per kg given on alternate days for 1 month and decreased by 0.4 mg per kg per month thereafter. Alternatively, prednisone may be *slowly* tapered over 32 weeks by changing to 1.6 mg per kg every other day for 1 month, and then reducing the dose by 0.2 mg per kg per month. A variation of standard therapy is to initiate prednisone at 2 mg per kg ideal body weight every other day (maximum, 160 mg) for 3 months, and subsequently taper by 20 mg per month.

Intensive therapy is often used in diseases that are associated with marked glomerular damage or rapid deterioration in renal function. Oral prednisone is started at 60 mg per day (<80 kg body weight) or 80 mg per day (>80 kg body weight) in two divided doses for weeks 1 to 4. In very severe disease (assessed clinically and by biopsy findings), oral prednisone may be preceded by 3 days of intravenous methylprednisolone (Solu-Medrol), 500 to 1000 mg per day, to maximize the anti-inflammatory effects of the glucocorticoid. Beyond 3 days, high-dose intravenous bolus corticosteroid therapy should be avoided because of increased risk of infection. At the beginning of weeks 5, 9, and 13, the daily prednisone dose is decreased by 10 mg. Patients who started with 80 mg per day should have their dose lowered by an additional 10 mg at the beginning of week 7. Prednisone may be given as a single morning dose when it has decreased to 50 mg per day. Starting at week 15, prednisone is reduced by 5 mg per week on alternate days until the patient is taking 20 to 25 mg of prednisone every other day. This dose is continued through week 52. Thereafter, prednisone is slowly withdrawn as tolerated. This regimen is associated with significant risk for infection and should be used only for patients with the most severe disease manifestations. In moderately severe disease a *modified intensive* approach can be used. Intravenous bolus therapy may be skipped, and the alternate-day taper should start on week 8, rather than week 15. To accomplish this, the daily prednisone dose should be reduced by 10 mg per week (rather than per month) during weeks 5, 6, and 7.

Drugs that induce the hepatic cytochrome P-450 system, such as phenytoin, phenobarbital, carbamazepine, and rifampin, increase the metabolism of glucocorticoids. To compensate, the prednisone dose has to be approximately doubled.

Alkylating Agents

For situations in which steroid resistance is encountered, or for treatment of severe glomerular disease, an alkylating agent such as cyclophosphamide* (Cytoxan), or chlorambucil* (Leukeran) may be required. Cyclophosphamide may be given intravenously or orally. We prefer oral cyclophosphamide because of its efficacy, convenience of administration,

and cost. The initial daily dosage is 1.5 mg per kg ideal body weight per day (maximum, 150 mg per day). Duration of therapy depends on the disease, but the frequency of malignancies (bladder, hematologic) is increased after the equivalent of 1 year of daily oral therapy. Therapy beyond 6 months should thus be carefully considered. To avoid bladder toxicity, patients are encouraged to take extra fluid (at meals and bedtime) to achieve at least 2 liters of daily urine output during therapy. Leukocyte count should be monitored weekly, and if the neutrophil count falls below 2000 cells per mm³, cyclophosphamide should be withheld until the neutrophil count rises above this level. Cyclophosphamide can then be restarted at one half to two thirds of the previous dose. To avoid irreversible gonadal failure, gonadal function may be suppressed during treatment using leuprolide beginning 2 weeks before cyclophosphamide, and continuing every 4 to 6 weeks, for not more than 6 months.

Chlorambucil* is an alternative to cyclophosphamide that has no bladder toxicity. Oral chlorambucil is given in doses of 0.15 to 0.2 mg per kg ideal body weight per day (maximum, 14 mg per day). Duration of therapy depends on the disease being treated. Leukocyte counts should be monitored, and the dose of chlorambucil adjusted as for cyclophosphamide.

Antimetabolites

When long-term administration of a cytotoxic agent is required, or for maintenance of remission after completing alkylating agent therapy, oral azathioprine* (Immuran) in a dose of 1 to 2 mg per kg ideal body weight per day is used. Experience with solid organ transplantation indicates that this drug may be safely administered for years. In addition, azathioprine has been used in pregnant patients. Leukopenia is the major side effect of azathioprine, so leukocyte counts should be monitored and the dose adjusted according to the white cell count. The dose of azathioprine must be decreased by 50% during concomitant allopurinol administration.

Mycophenolate mofetil* (CellCept) is receiving increasing attention as a cytotoxic agent that may be safer than cyclophosphamide. Mycophenolate mofetil is used orally in doses of 0.25 to 1.0 gram twice a day.

Calcineurin Inhibitors

Although mainly used in transplantation immunosuppression, cyclosporine (Neoral, Sandimmune) has also found utility in the treatment of primary glomerular disease, especially after other therapies have failed. Cyclosporine (3.5 to 5 mg per kg ideal body weight per day) is given in divided doses, usually for months. To minimize nephrotoxic effects, trough blood levels should be monitored by radioimmunoassay. Drugs that block the cytochrome P-450 system (e.g., erythromycin, clarithromycin, verapamil, diltiazem, amlodipine, fluconazole, ketoconazole) can increase the level of cyclosporine, so concomitant ad-

---

*Not U.S. Food and Drug Administration (FDA) approved for this indication.

*Not FDA approved for this indication.

ministration requires dose reduction. Conversely, drugs that induce the P-450 system enhance the metabolism of cyclosporine, and may require the dose to be increased.

Antiprogression Therapy

Renal function tends to decline once a critical number of nephrons are lost. Predictors of progressive renal failure include uncontrolled hypertension, proteinuria, and perhaps hyperlipidemia. The following therapies modify the risk of progression.

Blood Pressure Control

Strict blood pressure control is effective in slowing progressive renal disease in patients with renal insufficiency and proteinuria. The blood pressure goal for such patients is systolic blood pressure in the 120 to 130 mm Hg range, and diastolic blood pressure in the 70 to 80 mm Hg range. Certain antihypertensive medications may confer additional renal protection beyond that associated simply with blood pressure control. In this regard, angiotensin-converting enzyme (ACE) inhibitors* should be part of the antihypertensive regimen if possible, because of their antiproteinuric effects. The amount of ACE inhibitor needed to achieve renal protection is small (e.g., enalapril [Vasotec], 5 mg per day). It is not known whether larger doses of ACE inhibitor are more renal protective. It is suspected, although not proven, that angiotensin receptor type I antagonists, such as losartan* (Cozaar) may be renoprotective. Long-acting nondihydropyridine calcium channel blockers* (verapamil and diltiazem) also appear to have renal protective effects. These calcium channel blockers may be used in conjunction with an ACE inhibitor.

Diet

Dietary protein restriction may slow progressive renal disease and reduce proteinuria. Patients with moderate renal insufficiency (in general, a serum creatinine level of <3 mg per dL) who are not acutely ill or catabolic, should restrict daily dietary protein to 0.7 to 0.8 grams per kg of ideal body weight. In advanced renal insufficiency (in general, a serum creatinine level of >3 mg per dL), protein should be reduced to 0.6 grams per kg per day. These diets must have adequate calories, and more than 50% of the protein should be of high biologic value. Consultation with a dietitian is appropriate. Patients with heavy proteinuria should modify their protein restriction by adding 1 gram of dietary protein for every gram of protein lost in the urine exceeding 3 grams per day.

The antiproteinuric effects of an ACE inhibitor can be abolished if a high salt intake is maintained. Sodium must be restricted to 2 to 2.5 grams per day, unless renal salt wasting is present. This also helps control edema in nephrotic patients.

Hyperlipidemia, a common problem encountered in nephrotic patients, is difficult to control and usually requires both dietary and pharmacologic intervention. Hydroxymethyglutaryl–coenzyme A reductase inhibitors are recommended for hyperlipidemic patients with glomerular disease and heavy proteinuria.

SPECIFIC GLOMERULOPATHIES

Minimal Change Disease

Minimal change disease (MCD) accounts for 85% of idiopathic childhood nephrotic syndrome, but only approximately 15% of adult nephrotic syndrome. Long-term prognosis is good, with few patients progressing to chronic renal failure. Patients typically present with nephrotic syndrome. Urinary sediment tends to be bland, with evidence of lipiduria (oval fat bodies, fatty casts) and occasionally red blood cells or erythrocyte casts. Diagnosis is made by renal biopsy, which shows normal glomeruli by light microscopy but glomerular epithelial foot process fusion by electron microscopy. Systemic diseases (Hodgkin's lymphoma) and drugs (nonsteroidal anti-inflammatory drugs) may cause glomerular lesions similar to those of MCD. MCD is usually very responsive to therapy with corticosteroids. Although progression to renal failure is rare and spontaneous remission occurs, we favor treatment with prednisone to induce remission and avoid complications of the nephrotic syndrome, including infection, hyperlipidemia, and a hypercoagulable state. Treatment for adults should be initiated with *standard* prednisone therapy at 1 mg per kg per day until complete remission (urine protein <500 mg per day) occurs, or for 6 weeks (whichever comes first). If remission occurs, prednisone is tapered according to the rapid taper schedule. By 6 weeks, if there is no response, or only partial response (urine protein >500 mg per day but <3 grams per day), and the patient is tolerating prednisone, it should be decreased according to the slow taper protocol. If prednisone is poorly tolerated, patients may be switched to an alkylating agent. Most patients (80 to 90%) achieve remission. Patients who do not achieve remission after 3 to 4 months are termed "steroid resistant," and should be treated with an alkylating agent (plus prednisone, 10 mg per day) for 8 to 12 weeks. This should induce remission in 80% of steroid-resistant patients.

MCD has a high incidence (75%) of relapse (urine protein levels exceed 3 grams per day). The first relapse should be treated with prednisone, 1 mg per kg per day, until the urine dipstick for protein is less than 1+ for 3 consecutive days. Prednisone is then reduced to 0.6 mg per kg every other day until the patient has received a total of 6 to 10 weeks of therapy. Patients who relapse frequently need treatment with an alkylating agent for 8 weeks plus prednisone 10 mg per day. If steroids cannot be tapered without relapse of the nephrotic syndrome (corticosteroid dependence), 12 weeks of an alkylating agent is recommended to achieve a long-lasting remission. No more

---

*Not FDA approved for this indication.

than two courses of alkylating agent therapy are indicated in the treatment of MCD.

Patients who do not respond to steroids or alkylating agents should be treated with antiprogression therapy, and cyclosporine can be considered. Cyclosporine* is initiated at 4 to 5 mg per kg per day in two divided doses, and continued until complete remission has been maintained for 6 to 12 months. Relapse is high after stopping cyclosporine, so it is prudent to taper the dose by 25% every 2 months to determine the lowest dose needed to maintain remission. This dose can be continued for 1 year or longer. If the patient does not have a significant reduction in proteinuria within 4 months of initiating cyclosporine, it should be stopped.

Focal Segmental Glomerulosclerosis

Focal segmental glomerulosclerosis (FSGS) initially causes glomerular scarring that is segmental, and does not involve all glomeruli (focal). This histologic pattern is common, and may be seen in the advanced stages of other glomerulopathies, reflux nephropathy, human immunodeficiency virus (HIV) nephropathy, hypertensive nephrosclerosis, and heroin-abuse nephropathy. Idiopathic FSGS is a primary glomerulopathy that occurs in the absence of other renal disease. It is the most common form of idiopathic nephrotic syndrome in adults. Because juxtamedullary glomeruli are affected first, biopsy results early in the disease may be confused with those of MCD, with mainly glomerular epithelial cell foot process fusion seen on electron microscopy. As in MCD, most adults with FSGS have heavy proteinuria and the nephrotic syndrome. Unlike MCD, spontaneous remission is infrequent, FSGS is not as responsive to steroids, and in the setting of nephrotic-range proteinuria, progresses to renal failure. If complete or partial remission of the nephrotic syndrome can be achieved, renal survival is markedly improved. If chosen appropriately, approximately 30% of nephrotic patients may respond to corticosteroid therapy. Patients should ideally have a serum creatinine less than 2.5 mg per dL and a renal biopsy showing less than 25% interstitial fibrosis. *Standard* prednisone therapy should be started and continued until remission occurs, or for 8 weeks (whichever comes first). Prednisone may then be tapered according to the rapid taper schedule. If complete remission is not achieved by 8 weeks, continue prednisone at 0.5 mg per kg per day for an additional 8 weeks, and then taper according to the rapid schedule. If, after 16 weeks of therapy, the patient has not responded, treatment decisions are more difficult and long-term results tend to be less satisfactory. However, prednisone may be continued according to the slow taper schedule. Alternatively, cyclophosphamide* or chlorambucil* may be used for 8 to 12 weeks. Cyclosporine has shown efficacy in the treatment of patients with FSGS, and may be used as

outlined for MCD. All patients with unresponsive FSGS should be treated with antiprogression therapy. Relapse in patients who respond to prednisone should be treated as for MCD.

Membranous Glomerulopathy

Idiopathic membranous glomerulopathy (MGN) is an important cause of nephrotic syndrome in adults, especially in people older than 50 years of age. Clinical presentation is similar to that of MCD and FSGS, although the development of proteinuria can be more insidious. Microscopic hematuria is common. Renal biopsy, required for the diagnosis, demonstrates immune deposits in the glomerular basement membrane (GBM). Formation of new GBM around these immune deposits causes thickening of the GBM. A variety of systemic processes may result in MGN, including systemic lupus erythematosus (SLE), adenocarcinoma (lung, colon, breast, prostate), viral infections (hepatitis B, C, and G; HIV), and drugs (captopril, gold salts, penicillamine). These conditions should be excluded before instituting therapy for idiopathic MGN.

Treatment of MGN is complicated by its natural history. MGN is indolent, has a high rate of spontaneous remission (20 to 30%) and relapse, but can progress to chronic renal insufficiency (20 to 25%). All patients should be considered for antiprogression therapy. The use of specific immunosuppressive therapy is reserved for patients with risk factors for progressive renal deterioration. The factors most strongly associated with progressive MGN are persistent heavy proteinuria (>6 grams per day for >6 months), elevated serum creatinine, and greater than 20% interstitial fibrosis on renal biopsy. Moderate risk factors for progression are male gender, uncontrolled hypertension, and age older than 50 years.

Patients at moderate risk for progression can be offered treatment with the every-other-day prednisone protocol described under *standard* steroid therapy. For patients with strong risk factors for progression, I favor a combined prednisone and chlorambucil (or cyclophosphamide) regimen. Patients are treated with daily oral prednisone (0.5 mg per kg ideal body weight per day) for 1 month, followed by an alkylating agent for 1 month. Prednisone is continued (10 mg per day) during the alkylating agent month. This cycle is repeated twice more to complete 6 months of therapy. The effects of therapy may be delayed, and no decision regarding success should be made for 3 to 6 months after completion of initial therapy. If remission has been achieved, carefully follow the patient for relapse of proteinuria. Relapse may be treated once with a second round of cytotoxic therapy as outlined previously. Patients in partial remission should be continued on antiprogression therapy. Patients who have not responded to steroids alone can be treated with the prednisone/alkylating agent regimen. Patients who have failed this regimen may be tried on cyclosporine, 3.5 mg per kg per day for 1 year, or azathioprine for 1 year.

---

*Not FDA approved for this indication.

MGN with heavy proteinuria may be particularly associated with a thrombotic tendency, and thus use of low-dose aspirin (81 mg per day) seems reasonable.

Membranoproliferative Glomerulonephritis

Idiopathic membranoproliferative glomerulonephritis (MPGN) occurs as one of three histologic variants. In general, these nephritides show increased cellularity and matrix in the glomerular mesangium, and thickening of glomerular capillary walls. Patients with MPGN are usually young (<30 years) and present with hematuria and proteinuria, often in the nephrotic range. Urine sediment is more active (casts, cells) than in the previously discussed nephrotic glomerulopathies. Secondary MPGN, which is more common than primary MPGN in adults, may be seen in chronic bacterial infections (endocarditis, visceral abscess), chronic viral infections (hepatitis B, C), cryoglobulinemia, chronic lymphocytic leukemia, and B cell lymphoma. The prognosis of patients with primary MPGN and nephrotic syndrome is poor; 50% have renal failure within 10 years of diagnosis. Despite several trials, no clear therapy has emerged for adults with idiopathic MPGN. Because alternate-day prednisone is relatively safe, the alternate-day prednisone regimen described earlier under *standard* therapy may be tried. Patients with renal insufficiency or proteinuria (>1 gram per day) should receive antiprogression therapy.

IgA Nephritis

IgA nephritis is the most common form of glomerulonephritis (GN) in the world. It is characterized by hematuria, microscopic or gross, especially in association with a mucosal infection. The urine sediment may be nephritic with erythrocyte casts and moderate proteinuria, or patients may have nephrotic-range proteinuria. Prognosis is fair but the disease can slowly progress, and 20% of patients progress to end-stage renal disease over time (up to 2 decades). Biopsy demonstrates mesangial expansion and proliferation with mesangial deposition of IgA. IgA nephritis may show rapid progression to renal failure along with glomerular crescents on biopsy. Mesangial IgA deposition can also be seen in chronic liver disease, chronic infection with methicillin-resistant *Staphylococcus aureus*, HIV, inflammatory bowel disease, Henoch-Schönlein purpura (possibly a systemic form of IgA nephritis), and SLE. There is no consensus on the optimal therapy for slowly progressive idiopathic IgA nephritis. Risk factors for renal functional decline are uncontrolled hypertension, proteinuria (>1 gram per day), renal insufficiency at diagnosis, and glomerular or tubulointerstitial sclerosis on biopsy. Antiprogression therapy should be considered for high-risk patients. It is prudent to avoid or minimize situations that stimulate the mucosal immune system (i.e., limit contact with people who have upper respiratory infections or gastroenteritis). Because of the immunomodulating effects of omega-3 fatty acids, fish oil supplementation (Max EPA, 6 grams twice daily), has been used to treat IgA nephritis. Although fish oil is relatively safe, results of therapy have been mixed. Immunosuppressive therapy has not shown consistent benefit. We have successfully used *intensive* prednisone therapy for patients with IgA nephritis who have acute renal failure and severe crescentic GN.

Rapidly Progressive Glomerulonephritis

Rapidly progressive GN (RPGN) is a clinical syndrome in which renal insufficiency (>50% decrease in function) occurs quickly (<3 months) because of a GN. Biopsy, which is essential for the diagnosis, often reveals cellular glomerular crescents or necrosis. There may be other, more disease-specific findings on biopsy, such as linear GBM IgG deposition in anti-GBM GN. RPGN can complicate many of the nephropathies already discussed (i.e., MPGN, IgA nephritis, MGN). Idiopathic RPGN is usually divided into anti-GBM antibody disease, immune complex–mediated disease, and pauci-immune GN (showing few immune deposits on biopsy). Pauci-immune GN, which is more common than the other types of RPGN, is typically associated with the presence of ANCA, usually the perinuclear pattern type. RPGN may be considered a renal-limited form of a systemic process: anti-GBM disease (a limited form of Goodpastures's syndrome); immune complex disease (a limited form of autoimmune disease, such as SLE); or pauci-immune GN (a limited form of ANCA vasculitis, such as Wegener's granulomatosis). Treatment of these systemic diseases is similar to treatment of the renal-limited forms. Other systemic conditions must be excluded before starting the intense immunosuppression required to treat idiopathic RPGN. These include chronic infection, drug hypersensitivity, and malignancy. If RPGN is suspected, a renal biopsy must be performed urgently and treatment started as soon as possible to improve chances for recovery of renal function.

Anti-GBM GN should be treated with *intensive* prednisone therapy or *modified intensive* prednisone therapy (depending on the rapidity of renal functional deterioration) plus cyclophosphamide for 8 to 12 weeks. After the alkylating agent, azathioprine* (or perhaps mycophenolate mofetil*) should be given until the patient has been in remission for 1 year. In addition, plasmapheresis (daily for 10 to 14 treatments) is recommended to remove anti-GBM antibodies. Patients with oliguria, serum creatinine levels above 5 to 6 mg per dL, or extensive glomerular crescents (>50%) have a poor prognosis and rarely recover renal function. Intense immunosuppression may not be indicated in such patients. Immune complex GN is treated as for anti-GBM GN, except plasmapheresis is not usually necessary. Pauci-immune RPGN is also treated with prednisone plus cyclophos-

---

*Not FDA approved for this indication.

phamide, except cyclophosphamide is given for 4 to 6 months rather than 8 to 12 weeks, followed by azathioprine (or mycophenolate) to maintain remission for 1 year. If no renal response is seen by 8 to 10 weeks, remission of the RPGN is unlikely, and it is appropriate to taper and discontinue therapy. Relapse may occur in any type of RPGN, but is especially common in pauci-immune disease. Relapse should be treated aggressively using the same guidelines as for initial therapy.

ACUTE PYELONEPHRITIS*

method of
RICHARD S. STACK, M.D.
Dwight David Eisenhower Army Medical Center
Augusta, Georgia

Acute pyelonephritis is an infectious process involving the renal parenchyma and pelvis. Significant associated inflammation is usually present. The great majority of patients with this condition can be treated safely and efficiently as outpatients. There is no question that the diagnosis and treatment of pyelonephritis has greatly improved over the past two decades. This has resulted from a better understanding of the pathophysiology, coupled with improved oral antibiotics and imaging modalities.

When entertaining the diagnosis and treatment of acute pyelonephritis, the physician must remember that even one episode has the potential to contribute to significant complications, including permanent renal scarring and renal failure. Early and accurate diagnosis and therapy must be instituted promptly to avoid untoward sequelae. Management approaches differ based on the overall health of the patient, whether the patient has an uncomplicated or a complicated infection, and associated conditions such as diabetes or pregnancy.

EPIDEMIOLOGY

Pyelonephritis predominantly occurs in women. Except for cases of acute pyelonephritis in children (in whom there is a higher association of anatomic abnormalities), the average age at presentation is 30 years. Overall, women have a 50% lifetime risk of developing a urinary tract infection (UTI) in the lower urinary tract, which includes the bladder and urethra. However, ascending infection resulting in acute pyelonephritis occurs in less than 2%. Vesicoureteral reflux and the physiologic changes seen in pregnancy can significantly increase the risk of pyelonephritis. The association contributes to the recommendations that a prophylactic antibiotic regimen should be maintained in children with vesicoureteral reflux and that simple asymptomatic bacteriuria is treated with antibiotics during pregnancy.

ROUTES OF INFECTION

Ascending urinary tract infections contribute to over 90% of patients diagnosed with acute pyelonephritis. Hematogenous seeding is the cause in up to 5% of the pa-

tients, and lymphatic spread is rare. Lower urinary tract infections occur more often in women, therefore increasing the opportunity for an ascending infection to occur.

Gram-positive pyelonephritis, or the presence of diffuse, multiple, or bilateral lesions, should alert the clinician to the possibility of a blood-borne infection with hematogenous seeding. This route of infection is generally associated with decreased host immunity from other infections or chronic illness. The primary infection should be identified and eradicated when possible. Incompletely treated abscesses will likely result in a recurrent systemic infection once the antibiotic course is completed. Potential anatomic sources include virtually any organ, and evaluation must include possible sources such as oral, bone, and skin infections.

ETIOLOGY AND PATHOGENESIS

Aerobic gram-negative bacteria represent the most common pathogens of pyelonephritis. The bacterial organisms responsible for pyelonephritis generally mirror those causing lower tract infections, consistent with 95% of pyelonephritis episodes being due to ascending infections. *Escherichia coli* is the most common pathogen causing infections in the urinary tract. It represents 85% of community-acquired and 50% of the nosocomial infections. Other community-acquired organisms include *Proteus, Klebsiella, Enterococcus*, and *Staphylococcus saprophyticus*. The other prevalent nosocomial etiologic agents include *Enterococcus, Klebsiella, Enterobacter, Citrobacter, Serratia, Pseudomonas aeruginosa*, and *Staphylococcus epidermidis*.

Colonization of the perineum and external genitalia by uropathogens may be the initial source for progression to the bladder, which may then continue, in a retrograde fashion, to the level of the kidney to result in acute pyelonephritis. The retrograde progression of a lower UTI to the level of the kidney is related to the presence of bacterial cell surface fimbriae such as the P pili and type 1 pili seen on *Escherichia coli*. Over 80% of acute pyelonephritis episodes have fimbriated organisms as the etiologic agent. Host epithelial factors that either increase or decrease resistance are under study.

CLINICAL MANIFESTATION

The usual manifestation of acute pyelonephritis includes acute onset of fever and chills with flank pain and dysuria. It is also common to have associated gastrointestinal complaints, including nausea, vomiting, and diarrhea. Flank pain and/or fever are not reliable for the diagnosis and treatment of acute pyelonephritis. A study in 1984 showed that 50% of the patients in the series with flank pain and/or fever had infections limited solely to the lower urinary tract. In addition, patients with unquestionable pyelonephritis may lack associated flank pain entirely. Approximately 75% of the patients do have lower tract symptoms at the time of diagnosis.

On physical examination, the patient usually has fever and appears ill. Vital signs may range from slightly abnormal to that consistent with frank sepsis. As noted earlier, costovertebral tenderness can be elicited. In some cases, respiratory splinting may be noted on the affected side. The patient may also have abdominal tenderness.

LABORATORY FINDINGS

Specimens of blood and urine should be obtained before the institution of antibiotics. Although invasive techniques

---

*Note: The contents are the views of the author and are not necessarily the views of the Army Medical Department or of the United States Army.

such as ureteral catheterization with upper tract irrigation and urine sampling are not indicated, the clinician should ensure the urine specimen obtained is acceptable. If midstream urine is used, it should be spun down immediately and microscopic inspection carried out to ensure there is no epithelial cell contamination. Alternatively, a catheterized bladder urine specimen can be obtained for the urinalysis, Gram's stain, and culture. The typical urine evaluation is positive for pyuria, hematuria, and bacteriuria. It is not uncommon to note white blood cell casts in the urinary sediment. Gram's stain findings are usually positive. The usual threshold for the definition of infected urine is greater than 10^5 colony-forming units per mL. In patients with a properly collected urine specimen, a threshold of 10^2 colony-forming units per mL may be adequate.

Blood specimens will show leukocytosis with polymorphonuclear cells and a left shift. It is important to assess the serum creatinine level. Acute pyelonephritis may result in renal dysfunction. In an otherwise healthy patient, it is not common for the serum creatinine value to be significantly altered from baseline. However, it is important to define the serum creatinine, because it may impact on the potential tests and antibiotic course to consider. Positive blood cultures are found in 20 to 30% of patients diagnosed with pyelonephritis.

RADIOGRAPHIC FINDINGS

The majority of patients diagnosed with uncomplicated acute pyelonephritis do not require imaging studies. Imaging studies should be reserved for those patients who have not responded to the usual initial therapeutic steps or patients in whom there is increased suspicion for associated complications or co-morbidities. Factors or conditions that decrease the threshold to obtain imaging studies include pregnancy, a history of prior genitourinary surgery, a history of urolithiasis, recurrent episodes of pyelonephritis, prepubertal manifestations, increased age, and presence of fever for more than 5 to 7 days before the patient comes to medical attention.

If the clinical manifestation warrants an imaging study, the intravenous pyelogram (IVP) is considered the initial study to perform. It can identify global or segmental renal enlargement, delay in the nephrogram and/or excretion phase, anatomic abnormalities, and obstruction. It is essentially normal in 75% of patients diagnosed with acute pyelonephritis. Studies show that ultrasonographic evaluation may yield less information than the IVP, but there may be advantages due to availability and the fact that it is certainly less invasive. The ultrasound is quite helpful, however, to evaluate for an abscess, segmental changes, and hydronephrosis. It will also detect the great majority of significantly sized renal calculi. Computed tomography should be reserved for patients in whom the IVP or ultrasound evaluation does not yield adequate information or for patients who remain refractory to adequate treatment for more than 3 days.

MANAGEMENT

Once the diagnosis of pyelonephritis is entertained, one must determine if the patient has an uncomplicated or complicated pyelonephritis. In general, complicated infections occur in patients with anatomic or functional abnormalities of the urinary tract, or in individuals with underlying defects in natural host defenses. Pyelonephritis in prepubertal patients,

pregnant women, and adult men is treated by means of the complicated pyelonephritis pathway. In addition, patients with associated nausea and vomiting and patients with sepsis should be treated more aggressively. The treatment plan for diabetic patients having pyelonephritis should be determined on a case-by-case basis.

Patients with the signs and symptoms of clinical pyelonephritis, who appear ill but stable, and who lack the "complicated pyelonephritis" inclusion criteria (nausea, vomiting, or evidence of sepsis) can be treated through the "uncomplicated" pathway. The uncomplicated treatment pathway for pyelonephritis includes the following steps: (1) obtain urine for culture before initiation of antibiotics, (2) start the patient on an oral antibiotic regimen as listed in Table 1, and (3) if the patient shows improvement within the next 72 hours, continue the antibiotic course for 14 to 21 days. For most situations, an oral fluoroquinolone will be the best choice. If there is no significant improvement within the first 72 hours of treatment, the patient should be admitted for resuscitation, consideration for imaging and/or urologic consultation, close observation, and, in general, management along the "complicated" pathway. The results of the urine culture will direct adjustments in the therapeutic course. A urine culture should be obtained on the last day of therapy to ensure eradication of bacteriuria.

The "complicated" treatment pathway for pyelonephritis is used for those patients having the criteria previously outlined or who are ill enough to warrant admission to the hospital. I have a low threshold to aggressively treat patients with borderline findings. Blood and urine cultures should be obtained promptly; transfer or admission should not delay administration of parenteral antibiotics. The choice of coverage is listed in Table 2. Broad-spectrum coverage is continued until sensitivity directed changes are possible. Patients may require aggressive resuscitation and should be monitored appropriately for their respective conditions. The patient who responds favorably within 72 hours can be considered for the completion of therapy as an outpatient. The fever curve should show a declining trend. However, fever spikes usually continue for days. When patients appear stable and considered for transition to an outpa-

TABLE 1. **Outpatient Oral Antibiotic Regimens**

Drug	Dosage (mg)	Dosing Schedule
Fluoroquinolones		
Ciprofloxacin (Cipro)	500	q 12 h
Levofloxacin (Levaquin)	500	q 24 h
Ofloxacin (Floxin)	400	q 12 h
Trimethoprim/sulfamethoxazole (Bactrim, Septra)		
TMP/SMX	160/800	q 12 h
Cephalexin (Keflex)*	500	q 12 h

*Use is primarily limited to women who are pregnant

TABLE 2. **Parenteral Antibiotic Regimens**

Drug	Dosage	Dosing Schedule
Gentamicin and ampicillin*	5 mg/kg and 1 gm	q 24 h and q 6 h
Gentamicin and ampicillin†	1–1.5 mg/kg and 1 gm	q 8 h and q 6 h
Gentamicin and trimethoprim/sulfamethoxazole (Bactrim, Septra)‡	‡	‡
Ceftriaxone (Rocephin)	1–2 gm	q 24 h
Aztreonam (Azactam)§	1 gm	q 8 h
Fluoroquinolones		
Ciprofloxacin (Cipro)	200–400 mg	q 12 h
Levofloxacin (Levaquin)	250–500 mg	q 24 h
Ofloxacin (Floxin)	200–400 mg	q 12 h
Trimethoprim/sulfamethoxazole (Bactrim, Septra)	4–5 mg/kg/dose (based on trimethoprim component)	q 12 h
Ticarcillin-clavulanate (Timentin)‖	3.1 gm	q 4–6 h
Imipenem-cilastatin (Primaxin)‖	250–500 mg	q 6–8 h

*Daily dosing of gentamicin.
†Three times a day dosing of gentamicin.
‡For consideration in nosocomial infections. Dose each drug as listed on the table.
§May be substituted for gentamicin in patients with chronic renal insufficiency.
‖Not a first-line agent.

tient setting, they should be placed, while still an inpatient, on the planned outpatient antibiotic. They should remain afebrile (<100.5°F) for 24 hours on this regimen before discharge. The total antibiotic course can be extended to 4 or 6 weeks in certain cases. This decision is based on the patient's history, severity of disease, presence or absence of an abscess, and co-morbidities. For example, adult men with associated cystoprostatitis and severe diabetics are treated commonly for 6 weeks.

If the clinical course deteriorates in the first 24 hours, or does not improve within the first 72 hours, the patient should be fully reassessed. This includes reviewing the previous blood and urine culture and sensitivity results. The possibility of abscess or obstruction should be evaluated by imaging studies and urologic consultation. Repeat urine and blood cultures are obtained.

Special management issues apply to pediatric patients with pyelonephritis. These patients are likely to have anatomic abnormalities. Imaging studies, including voiding cystourethrography and renal ultrasound, are indicated. Urologic consultation should be obtained. Suppressive antibiotic therapy must continue beyond the initial therapeutic course until complete urologic and anatomic evaluation indicate this is not necessary.

Patients with indwelling urinary catheters should not be given antibiotics for the expected colonization of bacteria that usually exists. However, they should be treated when they are symptomatic. The foreign body (catheter) should, at a minimum, be changed to a new catheter. Conversion from Foley to clean, intermittent catheterizations or spontaneous voiding should be accomplished if possible. The post-void residuals should be ensured that they are acceptable in patients converted to a spontaneously voiding regimen.

COMPLICATIONS

Complications from acute pyelonephritis are uncommon with prompt diagnosis and treatment. How-

ever, the clinical course of patients can deteriorate quickly if the infection is not treated aggressively. Severe complications include sepsis and death, emphysematous pyelonephritis, and xanthogranulomatous pyelonephritis. Other complications include renal and/or perinephric abscess, chronic renal scarring, and possible hypertension.

Emphysematous pyelonephritis is a severe, acute, necrotizing infection. Although rare, it is life threatening. It is seen predominantly in diabetics, and the identified bacteria are usually *E. coli*. The hallmark finding is intraparenchymal gas noted on a simple abdominal radiograph. Intravenous pyelography does not usually add to the diagnosis because of the poor function of the involved kidney. The great majority of these patients require emergency nephrectomy, although a few selective cases have responded to percutaneous drainage.

Renal abscess formation should be evaluated by a urologist. With current antibiotics and imaging modalities to closely follow response to therapy, many can be treated with an antibiotic regimen alone. However, some patients require percutaneous drainage, surgical drainage, or nephrectomy.

TRAUMA TO THE GENITOURINARY TRACT

method of
J. PATRICK SPIRNAK, M.D.
Case Western Reserve University School of Medicine and MetroHealth Medical Center Cleveland, Ohio

RENAL TRAUMA

Renal trauma is classified according to the mechanism of injury into either penetrating or blunt. Penetrating renal injuries are further divided into those caused by gunshot and those caused by knife wounds. The incidence of penetrating renal injuries varies depending on the urban location and the number of violent crimes committed in that area. Blunt renal injuries are more common in a civilian population and account for most (80 to 90%) of all injuries. Although penetrating renal injuries are less common, they represent 80 to 90% of all renal injuries that require surgical exploration. Most blunt renal injuries occur as a result of either a direct blow or rapid deceleration sustained from motor vehicle accidents, falls, sports injuries, or physical assaults. Of these injuries, 85% can be classified as minor and are treated by observation. An additional 5% consist of shattered kidneys or pedicle injuries and, in many instances, require immediate surgical intervention. The remaining 10% of blunt renal trauma comprises major lacerations.

The indications for urologic evaluation in the trauma victim continue to evolve. In the past, it was not unusual for all blunt trauma victims to undergo emergency intravenous pyelography (IVP). The rationale for this shotgun approach was the fear of missing a significant renal injury that could occur in the absence of hematuria or other physical findings. It is known that the degree of hematuria does not correlate with the severity of the injury. Life-threatening renal pedicle injuries can occur in the absence of hematuria, whereas minor renal contusions can present with severe, gross hematuria. Urologic evaluation is recommended for all adult blunt trauma victims who present with either gross hematuria or microscopic hematuria with shock (systolic blood pressure < 90 mm Hg). In pediatric patients with microscopic hematuria alone, urologic evaluation is still performed.

Computed tomography (CT) has replaced arteriography and IVP as the gold standard for staging renal injuries in the clinically stable trauma victim. CT clearly defines the extent of parenchymal lacerations, hematomas, and the presence of urinary extravasation. It also allows assessment of the entire abdomen for the presence of other associated organ injuries. Helical (spiral) CT offers many advantages over conventional CT for the evaluation of the trauma victim. The ability of spiral CT to image the entire abdomen and pelvis through a series of 8-mm collimated helical scans minimizes potentially valuable time spent in the CT suite. However, the speed with which the scan is obtained after injection of contrast may allow for the detection of parenchymal injuries but may fail to identify injuries to the renal collecting system, which has not had adequate time to opacify. To avoid missing the presence of urinary extravasation, rescanning of the kidneys is routinely performed after completion of the initial scan. Patients who are hemodynamically too unstable to undergo a CT scan are evaluated by IVP performed in the trauma or operating room suite. Contrast is administered intravenously at a dose of 2 mL per kg (maximum, 150 mL). An abdominal film is obtained 5 to 10 minutes after the injection. Although the quality of these films may be poor, the presence of two functioning kidneys can usually be established. If the kidney cannot be visualized on IVP and the patient is stable, a renal arterial injury is suspected. Renal arteriography confirms the diagnosis.

Blunt Renal Trauma

The management and treatment of blunt renal trauma is based on the severity of the injury. Most injuries (80 to 90%) are minor parenchymal lacerations or contusions and are treated by observation. When gross hematuria is present, the patient is hospitalized with bed rest and serial monitoring of the vital signs and hematocrit until the urine clears. Single or multiple lacerations through the corticomedullary junction, with or without collecting system involvement, are findings typical of a major renal injury. Perirenal hematomas may or may not be present. If the patient is hemodynamically stable, treatment consists of observation. Bed rest is continued until the urine clears. A broad-spectrum antibiotic is administered in the presence of extravasation, and serial monitoring of hematocrit and vital signs is performed. The presence of urinary extravasation does not alter the management of major renal injuries. If sepsis, bleeding, or urinoma formation occurs, or the patient becomes clinically unstable, exploration is performed. Patients with lacerations to the renal pedicle or shattered kidneys usually present with hemodynamic instability and require prompt surgical exploration. Nephrectomy is usually required. The management of renal artery thrombosis is controversial. The presence of bilateral renal artery injuries requires prompt surgical exploration and attempted revascularization regardless of the time elapsed since the trauma. Patients with unilateral renal artery thrombosis are usually observed because it is rare to salvage renal function. These patients are followed closely because hypertension may develop.

Penetrating Renal Trauma

Penetrating renal injuries are divided according to the mechanism of injury into those caused by gunshot wounds and those caused by knife wounds. All patients with penetrating gunshot injuries to the chest or abdomen and a concomitant renal injury have at least one other significant organ injury; therefore, surgical exploration is required in all cases. At the time of surgery, the kidney is explored and repaired. Exceptions to this rule are those trauma victims who are clinically stable and have undergone complete staging of the renal injury by CT scan. Patients with only superficial injuries can be observed.

Renal stab wounds are more likely to occur without concomitant organ injury, and therefore a course of careful clinical observation may be warranted in selected patients. In general, renal stab wounds anterior to the anterior axillary line are associated with a high incidence of associated intra-abdominal organ injuries and require surgical exploration and repair. The treatment of renal stab wounds confined to the flank is controversial. When the entrance site is posterior to the anterior axillary line, there is a low incidence of intra-abdominal or retroperitoneal injuries. A nonoperative approach may be indicated in this select group of patients. Observation is considered appropriate when the peritoneal lavage is negative, there is no evidence of severe blood loss, the vital signs are stable, and CT findings suggest a superficial renal laceration. If hemodynamic instability should occur or signs of peritoneal irritation develop, surgery is immediately performed.

URETERAL INJURIES

Ureteral injuries can be divided into those caused by trauma and iatrogenic injuries. Ureteral injuries caused by external violence are rare and account for approximately 1% of all urologic trauma, with gunshot wounds accounting for approximately 95% of these injuries. Blunt ureteral injuries are rare and are most likely to occur in pediatric trauma victims who sustain severe deceleration-type injuries. The ureter can be injured by hyperextension with avulsion at the ureteral pelvic junction. Because up to 37% of all traumatic ureteral injuries may present with a normal urinalysis, a high index of suspicion should be maintained in the pediatric patient who has sustained a severe deceleration-type injury. Urologic evaluation consisting of either an IVP or CT scan is indicated in these patients, and failure to visualize the ureter suggests the diagnosis.

The exact incidence of iatrogenic ureteral injuries is unknown. However, an incidence ranging from 1 to 30% has been reported after gynecologic surgery. Iatrogenic ureteral injury can occur as a result of ligating or crushing the ureter with a clamp or ligature. Surgical transection, avulsion, devascularization, or angulation of the ureter may also occur. If recognized at the time of injury, simple deligation of the ureter with stenting may be appropriate. Transections or lacerations are surgically repaired. Injuries to the distal ureter are best managed by vesicoureteral reimplantation.

In the postoperative period, the presence of a prolonged adynamic ileus, persistent flank or abdominal pain, a palpable abdominal mass, an elevation in blood urea nitrogen, sepsis, prolonged and persistent drainage from operative drain sites, or the development of a spontaneous cutaneous fistula all suggest the presence of a missed ureteral injury. Evaluation by cystoscopy and retrograde pyelography confirms the diagnosis and allows for surgical correction.

BLADDER INJURIES

Traumatic bladder rupture may occur as a result of penetrating abdominal trauma or severe blunt injury. Penetrating bladder injuries are usually diagnosed at the time of abdominal exploration and require surgical repair. Bladder rupture associated with blunt injury occurs in approximately 5 to 10% of all patients with pelvic fractures. The perforation can be extraperitoneal (50 to 85%), intraperitoneal (15 to 45%), or, rarely, both (0 to 12%). Extraperitoneal bladder rupture associated with pelvic fracture usually occurs at the anterolateral aspect of the bladder near the bladder neck. It may occur as a result of direct perforation of a bony spicule associated with a pelvic fracture or by a burst mechanism that occurs when the bladder is empty. An intraperitoneal bladder rupture classically consists of a large horizontal tear in the dome of the bladder, and is usually associated with a direct blow to the lower abdomen in the presence of a full bladder. The intravesical pressure is acutely elevated and the bladder ruptures at its weakest point.

A cystogram is indicated in all patients with lower abdominal trauma and gross hematuria, an inability to urinate, or the absence of urine obtained on bladder catheterization. With a catheter in place, the bladder is filled by gravity to a capacity of 300 to 500 mL with a water-soluble contrast agent. Radiographs are obtained in the anteroposterior projection. Drainage films are also obtained. The characteristic finding on a cystogram of an extraperitoneal bladder rupture is extravasation of contrast confined to the pelvis. The extravasated material may appear as flame-like wisps or linear streaks that may assume a sunburst pattern. These findings are often more pronounced on the drainage film. Characteristic of intraperitoneal bladder perforation is diffuse extravasation of contrast throughout the peritoneal cavity with no discernible pattern or filling of the bladder.

All intraperitoneal perforations are surgically repaired at the time of diagnosis. The treatment of extraperitoneal bladder perforations is controversial; if the patient is undergoing abdominal exploration for other associated injuries, bladder repair is performed. If the patient is stable and does not require surgical exploration, a nonoperative approach is taken. Bladder drainage with a large Foley catheter (No. 24 French) is performed. A cystogram is performed after 7 to 10 days of bladder drainage, before catheter removal. Severe bleeding with clots, sepsis, or persistent extravasation are indications for surgical exploration.

URETHRAL INJURIES

Urethral disruption is an uncommon complication of blunt pelvic trauma and may be classified as partial or complete. Injury to the posterior urethra (posterior urethra) is often associated with a severe force delivered to the pelvis and occurs in 5 to 10% of men presenting with pelvic fracture. Urethral injuries to female trauma victims are rare because of the hypermobility of the urethra and lack of pubic bone attachments. Although not in itself life-threatening, urethral disruption is associated with significant long-term morbidity, including incontinence, erectile dysfunction, and urethral stricture.

The diagnosis of urethral injury should be suspected in all patients sustaining a pelvic fracture. Associated signs and symptoms suggestive of urethral trauma include gross hematuria or blood at the urethral meatus, an inability to urinate with a distended or palpable bladder, perineal or genital swelling, and an absent prostate on rectal examination. A retrograde urethrogram is performed in all male patients presenting with any of the aforementioned findings.

Extravasation of contrast with partial filling of the bladder on retrograde urethrography is diagnostic of a partial urethral disruption. Extravasation without bladder filling is diagnostic of a complete urethral disruption. Treatment of traumatic urethral injury is controversial. Patients with partial urethral injury are treated by catheter drainage. Catheter placement should never be performed in the emergency room by a physician other than a urologist. If a catheter does not go easily, suprapubic drainage is indicated.

Patients with complete urethral disruption who are clinically stable undergo immediate primary urethral realignment. By realigning the urethra, the resultant stricture is minimized, thereby making future reconstructive procedures more successful. Several principles must be adhered to: (1) the torn urethra is never surgically exposed and suture repaired; (2) the associated pelvic hematoma is never drained or violated; and (3) the realignment is performed by opening the bladder and by placing either a catheter or a metal sound through the urethra. Manipulation of the prostate is minimized to avoid trauma to the neurovascular bundles. If the patient is too unstable or alignment is not possible, a suprapubic catheter is placed. Endoscopic realignment is then attempted through cystoscopic techniques when the patient is stable, usually 3 to 10 days from the time of the injury. The urethral catheter is usually left in place for 6 weeks. Before catheter removal, a urethrogram is performed to ensure that complete healing has occurred. All patients are encouraged to perform urethral self-dilation with a No. 20 French catheter, which helps dilate and stabilize the site of the injury. The self-dilation is usually stopped after 3 months. It is believed that primary urethral realignment limits the incidence of stricture, impotence, and incontinence that has been associated with delayed urethral reconstruction. An alternative approach in patients with urethral disruption is to place a suprapubic tube and reconstruct the urethra in 6 months.

GENITAL INJURIES

The penis consists of the paired erectile bodies (corpora cavernosa) and the corpus spongiosum, through which the urethra runs. Penile trauma may involve any or all of these structures.

Avulsion of the penile skin calls for prompt surgical débridement and repair. Skin proximal to the injury is saved, whereas distal skin is excised. This technique is essential to avoid chronic penile edema due to scarring and obstruction of the superficial penile veins and lymphatics. A split-thickness skin graft may be necessary to cover the defect. Penetrating injuries involving the penis are best managed by surgical exploration with débridement of devitalized tissue and repair of the defect. Retrograde urethrography is indicated to rule out an associated urethral injury.

Blunt injuries involving the nonerect penis are usually limited in severity to contusions of the soft tissues and may be managed by immobilization, elevation, and ice. Corporeal rupture usually occurs when the fully erect penis is forcibly bent or severely angulated. Typically a loud cracking sound is heard, followed by detumescence, swelling, ecchymosis, and pain. Immediate surgical exploration with repair of the corporeal tear limits future morbidity.

SCROTAL TRAUMA

Penetrating scrotal trauma is best managed by surgical exploration with débridement and wound closure. If the testicle has been injured, the herniated testicular tissue is débrided and the tunica albuginea repaired.

Physical findings in patients sustaining blunt scrotal trauma may vary from a small area of ecchymosis to massive scrotal swelling and discoloration due to extensive hematoma formation. Scrotal ultrasonography is performed when adequate testicular examination cannot be performed because of either pain or swelling. Scrotal exploration with repair of the testicle is undertaken when the sonogram suggests a testicular injury or when scrotal bleeding persists.

PROSTATITIS

method of
IRA W. KLIMBERG, M.D.
Urology Center of Florida
Ocala, Florida

Prostatitis is one of the most common urologic problems. Nearly 50% of men experience the symptoms of prostatitis at some time. Prostatitis has been traditionally classified as acute or chronic bacterial prostatitis, nonbacterial prostatitis, granulomatous prostatitis, or prostatodynia (pelviperineal pain). In 1995, the National Institutes of Health (NIH) reclassified nonbacterial prostatitis and prostatodynia as "chronic pelvic pain syndrome."

Bacterial prostatitis, either acute or chronic, accounts for no more than 10% of cases in clinical practice and is readily diagnosed from the presence of pyuria and a positive urine culture. Nonbacterial prostatitis, an inflammatory process that mimics the symptoms of chronic bacterial prostatitis, accounts for 90% of cases. Granulomatous prostatitis is a histologic diagnosis, usually made after pathologic examination of a prostate biopsy specimen.

Prostatodynia is a term that causes urologists to shudder and has produced much of the confusion about prostatitis.

Prostatodynia defines symptoms that mimic prostatitis but are accompanied by negative urine cultures and no evidence of inflammation in expressed prostatic secretions (EPS). The term is used to describe any unexplained pelviperineal complaints in men. The NIH designation "chronic pelvic pain syndrome" is appropriate. Stamey referred to this spectrum of real or imagined prostatic diseases as a "wastebasket of clinical ignorance."

All patients with bacterial, nonbacterial, or granulomatous prostatitis have evidence of significant inflammation in their prostatic fluid. This is clinically defined as the presence of 10 or more white blood cells per high-power field of the EPS. The diagnosis of prostatitis cannot be rationally entertained in the absence of inflammatory cells in the EPS; it is the sine qua non for prostatitis. Meares and Stamey described segmented urine cultures to aid in the diagnosis of prostatitis. The patient collects the first 10 mL of voided urine (VB1), which represents the urethra, and a midstream specimen (VB2), which represents the bladder. Prostatic massage is then performed, and the patient collects the EPS. The first 10 mL of voided urine after prostate massage (VB3) is also collected. Each sample is subjected to microscopic examination and quantitative cultures.

In actual practice, urine specimens are obtained before the patient's examination. It is frequently painful to perform prostatic massage vigorously enough to recover EPS in all suspected cases of prostatitis. A valuable surrogate for the EPS is the VB3 specimen, which can be obtained easily and painlessly after digital prostate examination. Virtually all cases of bacterial prostatitis manifest with a concomitant urinary tract infection and are readily identifiable by the presence of pyuria in the midstream urine and a positive urine culture. If the VB1 and VB2 are negative, 10 white blood cells per high-power field in the EPS is diagnostic of prostatitis; if EPS are unobtainable, pyuria in VB3 is highly suggestive of prostatic inflammation. If inflammatory cells are absent from all of the specimens, then the diagnosis of prostatitis cannot be made.

ACUTE BACTERIAL PROSTATITIS

Acute bacterial prostatitis is usually manifested by the sudden onset of fever, urinary frequency, urgency, and dysuria. Low back, suprapubic, or perineal pain and varying degrees of bladder outlet obstruction often accompany these symptoms of bacteriuria. An extremely tender, enlarged, and indurated prostate are characteristic physical findings. Vigorous prostatic massage should be avoided because of the risk of bacteremia and patient discomfort. It is not necessary to obtain EPS, because the bacterial pathogen can be easily isolated from the voided urine. Escherichia coli and other members of the Enterobacteriaceae family predominate; Pseudomonas and Enterococcus organisms are less common.

Many men with acute bacterial prostatitis require hospitalization. Signs of bacteremia and urosepsis are frequent. Hydration, analgesics, antipyretics, and stool softeners are helpful supportive measures. Acute urinary retention is common, and suprapubic catheter placement is preferable to urethral catheter drainage in order to minimize prostatic inflammation. For toxic patients, I obtain blood and urine cultures and initiate therapy with ceftriaxone* (Rocephin), 1 gram intravenously every 24 hours, and a fluoroquinolone such as ciprofloxacin* (Cipro), 500 mg intravenously or orally every 12 hours, or ofloxacin (Floxin), 400

mg intravenously or orally every 12 hours. These patients usually respond dramatically to antibiotic therapy. By the time the urine culture and sensitivity results are available, patients can usually be treated with oral fluoroquinolone therapy alone. If the patient is not as acutely ill and does not require hospitalization, oral fluoroquinolone therapy such as ciprofloxacin, 500 mg orally twice a day (bid), or ofloxacin, 400 mg orally bid, is administered. Oral antimicrobial therapy is continued for a minimum of 14 days.

CHRONIC BACTERIAL PROSTATITIS

The hallmark of chronic bacterial prostatitis (CBP) is recurrent urinary tract infections caused by the same pathogen. The pathogenic bacteria persist unaltered in prostatic fluid during therapy with some antimicrobial agents because they accumulate poorly in prostatic secretions. Most patients complain of irritative voiding symptoms such as urgency, frequency, and dysuria during episodes of bacteriuria. Ill-defined pelvic or perineal discomfort, symptoms of bladder outlet obstruction, postejaculatory pain, and hematospermia may accompany these symptoms. In rare instances, men are found to have chronic bacterial prostatitis because of asymptomatic bacteriuria.

Prostate examination is vital in making the diagnosis. Although there are no findings on palpation of the prostate that are specific for CBP, the prostatic examination is required in order to perform bacterial localization studies. Meticulous microscopic examination and culture of the segmented urine specimens (VB2 and VB3) and the EPS establish the diagnosis. The likelihood of CBP is remote if urine cultures are sterile. As in acute prostatitis, E. coli, other Enterobacteriaceae, Pseudomonas species, and Enterococcus species are the prevailing pathogens.

CBP has become an exceedingly uncommon entity in recent years as a result of the proliferation of fluoroquinolone antibiotics that show excellent penetration into prostatic tissue and secretions. Long-term therapy (4 to 8 weeks) appears to be more effective than short-term therapy in achieving bacteriologic cures. Ciprofloxacin, 500 mg orally bid, or ofloxacin, 400 mg orally bid, for 4 weeks resolves most cases. Trimethoprim-sulfamethoxazole* (TMP-SMZ, Septra, Bactrim), one double-strength tablet (160 mg TMP and 800 mg SMZ) orally bid for 12 weeks, may be used alternatively or in cases of bacterial resistance to the quinolones. Antibiotic therapy should be tailored to microbiologic sensitivity results.

NONBACTERIAL PROSTATITIS (CHRONIC PELVIC PAIN SYNDROME)

Nonbacterial prostatitis, by far the most common prostatitis syndrome, is an inflammatory condition of unknown etiology. The symptoms vary but are indistinguishable from those of CBP. Physical findings are nonspecific; tender and boggy prostates are not reliable indicators of prostatitis. Examination of the urine usually yields normal findings. Pyuria is rare, and bacteriuria is never seen. The diagnosis of chronic nonbacterial prostatitis can be entertained only if there are excessive leukocytes in the EPS or VB3 specimens in the presence of negative cultures. The cause of the inflammatory changes in the prostatic secretions is unknown. Chlamydia trachomatis and Ureaplasma urealyticum, although frequent causes of urethritis, are no longer thought to be prostatic pathogens. If concomitant

---

*Not FDA approved for this indication.

*Not FDA approved for this indication.

urethritis is suspected, I recommend a course of doxycycline* (Vibramycin) or minocycline* (Minocin), 100 mg orally bid for 10 days.

An honest and frank discussion of the treatment that is afforded men diagnosed with nonbacterial prostatitis is difficult. Most affected men are initially treated with antimicrobial therapy and in fact respond to treatment. Treatment flies in the face of scientific reason, although clinical experience and the desires of our patients reinforce it. What is not clear is why this is so; it appears that we are treating the expectations of our patients and deluding ourselves about the efficacy of our treatment. The agents and duration of therapy follow those specified earlier for chronic bacterial prostatitis.

A major pharmaceutical manufacturer recently completed a fascinating and enlightening research project. The study was a randomized, double-blind, well-controlled, multicenter study conducted at experienced urologic research sites. A total of 502 patients with scrupulously documented nonbacterial prostatitis were enrolled and randomly assigned to treatment with one of two quinolone antibiotics for a month or to placebo. Clinical success was achieved by 66% of patients 1 week after the end of therapy and by 92% at 1 month after therapy. At 6 months, clinical success was sustained in approximately 75% of patients. There was no statistically significant difference in the response of patients treated with 1 month of antibiotic therapy or with placebo.

In the majority of men, prostatitis is a self-limited process, the symptoms of which resolve spontaneously within several weeks. The repetitive administration of antimicrobial drugs is unwarranted and uniformly ineffective in the treatment of recalcitrant prostatitis symptoms. Patient education and symptomatic treatment with nonsteroidal anti-inflammatory agents and hot sitz baths are advised. Avoidance of caffeine, alcoholic beverages, and spicy foods is occasionally beneficial. Patients with obstructive voiding symptoms often get relief with alpha-adrenergic blockers such as terazosin (Hytrin), 5 mg orally at bedtime, or doxazosin (Cardura), 4 mg orally at bedtime, both of which must be slowly titrated, or tamsulosin (Flomax), 0.4 mg orally every day, which does not require titration, because of its relative uroselectivity. Men with unrelenting symptoms should be referred for urologic evaluation.

GRANULOMATOUS PROSTATITIS

Granulomatous prostatitis caused by *Mycobacterium tuberculosis* may develop as a sequela of miliary tuberculosis, but it is more commonly encountered in patients undergoing intravesical immunotherapy with bacille Calmette-Guérin for bladder cancer. Fungi associated with systemic mycosis may also cause granulomatous prostatitis. Irritative voiding symptoms predominate in these patients. Urologic and infectious disease consultations are appropriate for defining and monitoring therapy.

Nonspecific granulomatous prostatitis occurs in two forms: an eosinophilic variety thought to result from a localized vasculitis, and a noneosinophilic form. Although uncommon, they may mimic acute prostatitis in their clinical manifestations. Prostate biopsy is required for diagnosis and to rule out carcinoma.

*Not FDA approved for this indication.

BENIGN PROSTATIC HYPERPLASIA
method of
E. DARRACOTT VAUGHAN, JR., M.D., and
AARON PERLMUTTER, M.D.
Cornell University Medical Center
New York, New York

EPIDEMIOLOGY

Benign prostatic hyperplasia (BPH) is an extremely common problem in aging men. Epidemiologic studies reveal that about 50% of men are bothered by lower urinary tract symptoms believed to be due to prostatic enlargement and 35% will eventually undergo some form of intervention to relieve these symptoms. Moreover, it is estimated that about 20% of men will experience acute urinary retention over a lifetime. The requirements for continued prostate growth, in men older than 60, estimated to be 0.6 to 2 grams per year, are simply aging and normal testicular function. Despite numerous studies, the role of other factors such as race, diet, frequency of sexual activity, or smoking remains unclear. There is growing evidence for a genetic inheritable component. Accordingly, there are no lifestyle changes that are recommended to ameliorate prostatic growth.

PATHOPHYSIOLOGY

The prostate strategically surrounds the posterior urethra from the bladder neck to just above the urogenital diaphragm. BPH is believed to arise from the transitional zone of the prostate. The initiation of BPH occurs at midlife; on autopsy studies, 50% of men aged 51 to 60 show hyperplasia. Thus, a change in hormonal status is an unlikely cause for initiation of BPH. The prostate is composed of glandular and stromal elements, and strong experimental data implicate secretion of a stromal protein factor that regulates epithelial cell proliferation and differentiation; this paracrine state has been termed "stromal-epithelial interaction." It is also clear that intraprostatic formation of dihydrotestosterone (DHT) is necessary for normal prostate development. Testosterone is converted to DHT by the enzyme 5α-reductase. There are two 5α-reductase isoenzymes; type 2 is critical for prostate growth, and, interestingly, it shows primarily stromal cell localization. This information again supports the importance of stromal cells for androgen-dependent prostatic growth. The observation that males born with a 5α-reductase deficiency had a paucity of prostatic glandular tissue led to the synthesis of finasteride (Proscar), one of two pharmacologic strategies to treat men with BPH.

The smooth muscle component of the prostate also plays a critical role in a patient's development of lower urinary tract symptoms. The smooth muscle and connective tissue component greatly outpopulate the glandular and luminal components by a 70:30 ratio. The active smooth muscle tone at the prostate is regulated by the adrenergic nervous system. Pharmacologic studies have identified the dominant alpha receptor in the prostate to be of the $alpha_1$-A subtype. Thus, the use of alpha-adrenergic blocking agents is the second strategy for combating the symptoms of BPH. There appear to be both active and passive factors that play a role in the lower urinary tract symptoms that affect men as they age. It is most likely that varying glandular/muscular pathologic components may be one reason that there is a poor correlation of prostatic size and lower urinary tract symptoms. However, there is evidence that patients with large prostates (>40 grams) are twice as likely to have symptoms and also more likely to experience acute urinary retention and/or the need for surgical intervention.

SYMPTOMS

BPH can lead to obstructive nephropathy and renal failure, chronic bacterial urinary tract infections, bladder calculi, and urinary retention. However, of all the procedures performed on patients for BPH, 90% are for the patient's symptoms. Thus, those symptoms become critically important in determining treatment. Unfortunately, lower urinary tract symptoms are not specifically due to BPH, and the astute clinician should look for coexisting symptoms referable to other diseases of the bladder and prostate.

Lower urinary tract symptoms are commonly divided into obstructive or irritative. The critical question is whether the symptoms interfere with the patient's daily activities or his quality of life. Fortunately, an American Urological Association Symptom Score (AUA-SS), also called International Prostate Symptom Score (IPSS), has been developed, validated, and accepted by the Agency for Health Care Policy and Research (AHCPR) and the World Health Organization (Figure 1). Thus, it is recommended that patients with mild symptoms (0 to 7) be assigned to watchful waiting whereas those with moderate (8 to 19) or severe (20 to 35) symptoms undergo evaluation and treatment. The AUA-SS is paired with a quality of life determination, and a moderate impairment (e.g., 3) indicates a need for treatment.

DIAGNOSIS

A detailed history is critical for diagnosing BPH. A symptom score is obtained and an inquiry is made looking for symptoms suggestive of neurogenic bladder disease, bladder carcinoma, urinary tract infection, diabetes, pelvic trauma, urethral stricture, past urologic surgery or prostatic carcinoma, or cardiac disease.

On physical examination, the rectal examination gives an approximate determination of size, although the anterior lobe and the intravesical median lobe tissue cannot be palpated. The size, consistency, and symmetry of the gland should be noted as well as the presence of any tenderness and the adequacy of rectal sphincter tone. If there is marked bladder decompensation, then a suprapubic mass or fullness is present.

Minimum laboratory data include a urinalysis, a serum creatinine determination, and urinary cytology if the patient has severe irritative symptoms. It is also recommended that all men older than 50 have a prostatic-specific antigen (PSA) test to rule out carcinoma of the prostate.

The AHCPR does not recommend examination of the upper urinary tract (intravenous, urogram, or renal ultrasonography) unless there are other indications, such as hematuria. Often before beginning pharmacologic intervention, a urinary flow rate coupled with abdominal ultrasonography to determine bladder residual urine is obtained as a baseline. More complex urodynamic tests such as a bladder pressure monitored flow-rate (pressure-flow) study are reserved for patients for whom pharmacologic management fails and who may require surgical intervention.

TREATMENT
Watchful Waiting

The AHCPR Guidelines recommend watchful waiting for patients with a symptom score of 0 to 7.

However, advice should be given to limit fluids at night and avoid coffee, tea, or alcohol if those beverages aggravate the patient's symptoms. In addition, some patients may realize that certain foods increase their lower urinary tract symptoms and thus they gain relief by dietary changes. Finally, the patient should be warned to avoid drugs that impair voiding, such as nasal decongestants and anticholinergic agents.

Phytotherapy

Numerous herbal preparations are available, and older male patients are bombarded by literature recommending prostatic drugs to improve urinary symptoms, restore sexual prowess, and improve general well-being. These agents are almost always compounded with multiple components, and the mechanism of their actions are poorly studied. The most common compound is saw palmetto (Serenoa repens), and randomized studies are available showing a modest effect decreasing symptoms and increasing flow rate. Side effects are minimal, and selected patients have a positive quality of life response while remaining on phytotherapeutic agents alone.

Alpha-Adrenergic Blocking Agents

Once a patient requires prescription drug therapy for lower urinary tract symptoms, the initial selection often depends on prostatic size, as shown in Figure 2. Alpha-adrenergic blocking agents (Table 1) have been shown in multiple placebo-controlled studies to significantly reduce symptoms and increase urinary flow rate. The response is quite rapid (within hours), and long-term (5 years) studies have been completed showing prolonged efficacy. The introduction of the selective alpha$_1$-A antagonist tamsulosin (Flomax) has eliminated the need for titration of the dose, as is required for the previously most commonly used drugs terazosin (Hytrin) and doxazosin (Cardura). Titration was necessary with these agents to avoid the most common side effect—postural hypotension. All patients should be warned of that possibility, as well as dizziness, fatigue, headache, and nasal stuffiness. Alpha-adrenergic blockers have not been associated with sexual dysfunction, although retrograde ejaculation is common, especially at higher doses.

The symptoms of BPH characteristically wax and wane. Therefore, patients sometimes prefer to take alpha blockers intermittently when their symptoms are aggravated by stress, traveling, or other factors. Alpha blockers are the treatment of choice for patients with a smaller (<35 gram) prostate. A carefully performed Veterans Cooperative study showed the efficacy of alpha blockers but not finasteride in these patients, and the addition of finasteride to alpha blockade gave no additional benefit. The effectiveness of combined therapy in patients with larger prostates is not known.

International Prostate Symptom Score (I-PSS)

Patient's Name

Date of Birth   Date Completed

	Not at all	Less than 1 time in 5	Less than half the time	About half the time	More than half the time	Almost always	Your score
1. Incomplete emptying Over the past month, how often have you had a sensation of not emptying your bladder completely after you finished urinating?	0	1	2	3	4	5	
2. Frequency Over the past month, how often have you had to urinate again less than two hours after you finished urinating?	0	1	2	3	4	5	
3. Intermittency Over the past month, how often have you found you stopped and started again several times when you urinated?	0	1	2	3	4	5	
4. Urgency Over the past month, how often have you found it difficult to postpone urination?	0	1	2	3	4	5	
5. Weak stream Over the past month, how often have you had a weak urinary stream?	0	1	2	3	4	5	
6. Straining Over the past month, how often have you had to push or strain to begin urination?	0	1	2	3	4	5	

	Not at all	1 time	2 times	3 times	4 times	5 times or more	
7. Nocturia Over the past month, how many times did you most typically get up to urinate from the time you went to bed at night until the time you got up in the morning?	0	1	2	3	4	5	
Total I-PSS Score							

Quality of Life Due to Urinary Symptoms

	Delighted	Pleased	Mostly satisfied	Mixed-About equally satisfied and dissatisfied	Mostly dissatisfied	Unhappy	Terrible
If you were to spend the rest of your life with your urinary condition just the way it is now, how would you feel about that?	0	1	2	3	4	5	6

Figure 1. The IPSS or AUA symptom score asks the patient to score, on a scale of 0 to 5, seven different urinary tract symptoms as well as provide a quality of life assessment of the impact of the symptoms on the patient's life, which can be an important aid for deciding about therapy.

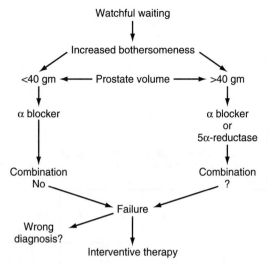

Figure 2. Treatment algorithm for patients with benign prostatic hyperplasia.

5α-Reductase Inhibition

Finasteride effectively prevents the conversion of testosterone to DHT in the prostate and lowers serum DHT. In randomized trials at 5 mg per day, there was a sustained 20% reduction in prostatic size accompanied by a significant decrease in symptoms and an increase in urinary flow rate. Although at least 6 months of treatment is required, chronic studies over 5 years reveal that the expected prostatic growth does not occur. Therefore, the drug changes the natural progression of prostatic growth. On review of the accumulated studies there is a direct correlation between efficacy of the dug and prostatic size. Moreover, in a 4-year randomized trial, finasteride reduced the probability of acute urinary retention by 57% and the risk of BPH-related surgery by 51%. Studies also have shown that the risk of urinary retention is three times greater if the patient's prostate is larger than 30 grams.

Other indications for finasteride include prostatic bleeding, neoadjuvant preparation for some minimally invasive technique, and adjuvant treatment if a patient's symptom score begins to rise after other treatments.

The most common side effect of finasteride is decreased ejaculatory volume, which is common, and sexual dysfunction, which occurs in 6 to 8% of cases. Breast tenderness may also occur.

TABLE 1. **Alpha$_1$-Adrenoreceptors**

Drugs
  Terazosin (Hytrin)
  Doxazosin (Cardura)
  Prazosin* (Minipress)
  Tamsulosin (Flomax)
  Alfuzosin†
  None are completely "uroselective"

*Not FDA approved for this indication.
†Not available in the United States.

Finasteride causes a 50% reduction of PSA. All patients on finasteride should have their PSA level monitored regularly; and if there is a documented rise, then further evaluation to determine prostate cancer should be performed.

Minimally Invasive Therapies

Since the late 1980s, a number of new minimally invasive therapies have been introduced to treat the lower urinary tract symptoms. Most patients choose pharmacologic therapy first because of the ease of oral drug administration. However, patients who have inadequate symptomatic improvement or side effects from alpha blockade or 5α-reductase inhibition, often require further therapy. Traditionally, this has been transurethral prostatectomy (TURP) for most patients and open surgery for the largest prostate glands. To offer therapies with less morbidity and hospitalization than surgical prostatectomy, the new minimally invasive therapies were introduced.

The new therapies are characterized by little or no hospitalization, minimal blood loss, and either local anesthesia or only sedation for anesthesia. These therapies do not substantially debulk the prostate, but most use heat to create coagulation necrosis in the obstructing transition zone tissue. Transurethral microwave thermotherapy (TUMT) is an outpatient therapy that involves the placement of a modified urethral catheter with a microwave antenna mounted in the intraprostatic portion of the catheter. The microwave antenna generates heat in the transition zone, and this results in coagulation necrosis. Although the mechanism of action is not completely understood, there may be some tissue loss as well as a change in alpha-receptor–mediated prostatic tone, resulting in an improvement in symptoms.

Sham controlled studies had shown that two thirds of patients have at least a 30% improvement in symptom score and one half of the patients have a 50% improvement. Peak urinary flow rate is improved slightly more than pharmacologic therapy, to 14 to 15 mL per second. Thus, there is not the magnitude of improvement with TURP, but the symptomatic improvement is often completely satisfactory for the patient.

Another method for creating regulation necrosis involves the placement of small needles that emit radiofrequency energy into the prostate via a cystoscope. This causes heating surrounding the needle tips, and this so-called transurethral needle ablation (TUNA) is another minimally invasive therapy option. The clinical outcome is again intermediate with oral medications and surgery.

If a patient has urinary retention secondary to a condition that is likely to improve, temporary urethral stents provide another minimally invasive option. For example, the immobility associated with hip surgery in the elderly often results in transient urinary retention. There are temporary prostatic stents that can be placed without surgery to restore voiding. Once the patient regains his strength and is

Table 2. **Treatment Plan**

IPSS 0–7			
QOL 1–2		Watchful waiting	
IPSS >7		Phytotherapy	
QOL 3–5		Alpha-Adrenergic blocker	
		5-Alpha Reductase Inhibitor	
	Response:	IPSS	decrease 25%
		Qmax	increase 20%
IPSS >7			
QOL 3–5		TUMT	
		TUNA	
	Response:	IPSS	decrease 50%
		Qmax	increase 50%
IPSS >7		TURP Thick Loop	
QOL 3–5		Interstitial Laser	
		IPSS	decrease 75%
		Q max	increase 100%

Abbreviations: IPSS = International Prostate Symptom Score; Qmax = maximum urinary flow rate; QOL = quality of life; TUMT = transurethral microwave thermotherapy; TUNA = transurethral needle ablation; TURP = transurethral prostatectomy.

no longer bedbound, spontaneous voiding is often again possible. These endoprostheses, although associated with irritative voiding symptoms or infection in some patients, avoid chronic urethral catheterization or suprapubic tube placement for such patients and improve their quality of life.

Prostate Surgery

TURP has been the gold standard for relieving prostatic obstruction for several decades. In general, patients in refractory urinary retention, with recurrent prostatic bleeding or bladder calculi or hydroureteronephrosis or who have inadequate symptomatic improvement with other therapies undergo TURP. This operation, done in the hospital under anesthesia, removes obstructing tissue. This surgery offers the best chance for symptomatic improvement of all therapies for BPH, with the average patient enjoying a 75 to 85% reduction in symptoms and a doubling of peak urinary flow rate. However, the complications of incontinence (1%), blood transfusion (3 to 5%), retrograde ejaculation (20 to 75% depending on the procedure), and stricture formation (5%) remain a problem.

Several new techniques, including prostatic vaporization (TUVEP) and introduction of loops that resect, vaporize, and coagulate simultaneously, have improved the safety of TURP while retaining its efficacy. Furthermore, laser surgery is now possible to remove prostatic obstruction. Although somewhat less effective than TURP, laser prostatectomy is appealing because there is a lower risk of bleeding complications. Complete resection is possible with the holmium:yttrium-aluminum-garnet (YAG) laser, and in situ coagulation necrosis is possible by means of the interstitial laser. Both of these procedures offer excellent alternatives for patients requiring anticoagulation or for those who are at high medical risk for TURP.

Open prostatectomy remains the surgery of choice for prostate glands that are too large to be removed safely by TURP. In general, these would include glands of greater than 80 to 100 grams. This represents a minority (<5%) of patients.

CONCLUSIONS

The currently available options for patients with lower urinary tract symptoms secondary to benign prostatic hyperplasia and their effects are summarized in Table 2. This table illustrates four categories of intervention, each of increasing efficacy as well as morbidity. Watchful waiting has the lowest associated morbidity and is appropriate for the minimally symptomatic patient. Pharmacologic therapy is the next tier of treatment, and patient selection now provides improved efficacy. The minimally invasive therapies (TUMT and TUNA) now allow patients to another option to improve their voiding pattern before opting for surgery. Finally, surgical removal of the prostate has become much safer with the advent of new electrosurgical devices and techniques as well as the application of lasers for prostatic tissue removal.

ERECTILE DYSFUNCTION
(Impotence)

method of
SUNIL K. PUROHIT, M.D., and
WAYNE J. G. HELLSTROM, M.D.
Tulane University School of Medicine
New Orleans, Louisiana

Male erectile dysfunction (impotence) is a condition defined by the inability to attain and/or maintain a penile erection sufficient for vaginal penetration and satisfactory sexual intercourse. The incidence of impotence is known to increase with age, affecting less than 5% of men younger than age 40 and up to 75% of men older than age 75 years. Although in the past it was believed that erectile dysfunction was primarily due to nonspecific psychologic causes or was secondary to the physiologic aging process, an organic etiology can be found in most cases. The treatment of this condition has evolved since the early 1980s with the emergence of highly effective surgical and nonsurgical modalities. The introduction of effective oral medications, such as sildenafil (Viagra), has certainly had a major impact on how society and the medical establishment now perceive the common complaint of sexual dysfunction.

PHYSIOLOGY OF ERECTION

Penile erection is a complex hemodynamic process that occurs under the regulatory control of the nervous system and is influenced by both hormones and components of signal transduction pathways operating at the intracellular and transcellular levels within the penis. Briefly, the penis is composed of erectile tissue (the cavernous smooth musculature and the smooth muscle of the arterial walls) that is covered by a tough connective tissue sheath called the tunica albuginea. In the flaccid state, this erectile tissue is tonically contracted, allowing for a small amount of arterial flow. Sexual stimulation causes the release of neurotransmitters (e.g., nitric oxide, vasoactive intestinal polypeptide) from the cavernous nerve terminals, which in turn causes relaxation of the corpora cavernosal smooth musculature and dilatation of the arterial vessels. This increased arterial inflow results in engorgement of the sinusoidal spaces, compressing the subtunical venular plexus beneath the tunica albuginea. As a result, venous outflow is restricted. Prerequisites for a normal erection are these three sequential events: neurotransmitter release, increased arterial inflow, and venous outflow restriction.

CLASSIFICATION

Erectile dysfunction has been traditionally classified into two major categories: psychogenic and organic. Although the pathogenesis of psychogenic impotence is poorly understood, sympathetic overactivity and inhibition of neurotransmitter release are likely causes. Only approximately 10% of impotent men are found to have a psychogenic problem as the primary cause of their dysfunction, and this usually occurs in younger people. Organic impotence can be further subcategorized into vasculogenic (arteriogenic or venogenic), neurogenic, hormonal, or other etiologies (e.g., drugs and systemic diseases).

Arteriogenic impotence results from poor blood flow into the penis. This can be caused by traumatic occlusion of the hypogastric-cavernous-helicine tree or by generalized systemic diseases (e.g., diabetes, atherosclerosis). Venogenic erectile dysfunction (venous leak) represents the inability to retain blood within the corpora cavernosa because of veno-occlusive dysfunction. This may be due to the presence of abnormally large venous channels draining the corpora cavernosa, degenerative changes (e.g., Peyronie's disease, aging, diabetes), trauma to the tunica albuginea (penile fracture), or priapism. Neurogenic impotence can be caused by disease or traumatic injury to the brain, spinal cord, or bony pelvis. Most frequently, direct injury to the pudendal or cavernous nerves from trauma or pelvic surgery causes this form of erectile dysfunction. Hormonal disorders inherent to primary or secondary hypogonadism may be due to various disease processes, including hypothalamic disorders, prolactin-secreting pituitary tumors, and Klinefelter's syndrome. In addition, many drugs (e.g., antihypertensives, antidepressants, H_2 blockers, antiandrogens, marijuana, alcohol) and various diseases (e.g., diabetes mellitus, renal disease) have been implicated in erectile dysfunction.

INITIAL WORK-UP

A detailed medical and sexual history and a thorough physical examination are the most important factors in diagnosing and determining the etiology of erectile dysfunction. This information often leads to a more efficient and cost-effective approach to diagnosis and treatment. A psychosexual history should include the level of desire (libido), the onset and duration of erectile dysfunction, the presence of morning erections, the quality of erection, and the presence of any psychologic conflict. Also, interviewing the sexual partner can be very helpful in eliciting a reliable history and planning treatment. All medical illnesses, past surgical treatments, injuries, and drug history (including alcohol and tobacco) should be documented. Examples of medical illnesses commonly associated with erectile dysfunction include vascular diseases (coronary artery or pe-

ripheral vascular), renal failure, diabetes, hypertension, multiple sclerosis, and hyperthyroidism. Radical pelvic surgery (abdominoperineal resection, radical prostatectomy), pelvic trauma, and pelvic irradiation can result in erectile dysfunction as well.

On physical examination, particular attention should be focused on sexual and genital development. The presence of microphallus, Peyronie's plaque, or penile curvature can often result in erectile dysfunction. A patient with gynecomastia or soft, atrophic testes needs to be worked up for possible endocrine disorders, such as hypogonadism or hyperprolactinemia. Specific genetic or developmental disorders (e.g., Klinefelter's or Kallmann's syndrome) can be suspected based on distinctive body habitus or obvious physical characteristics of hypogonadism. Finally, a careful neurologic examination may show evidence of peripheral neuropathy, which is common in the presence of certain degenerative neurologic diseases or diabetes.

The laboratory evaluation helps confirm a possible etiology of the erectile dysfunction suspected after the initial history and physical examination. It may include serum chemistries, complete blood count, renal function evaluation, or urinalysis. An initial early morning serum total testosterone level helps rule out a hormonal etiology. If the serum testosterone level is low, serum prolactin and luteinizing hormone levels are obtained to help differentiate a primary (testicular) from a secondary (pituitary) etiology of hypogonadism. If a high serum testosterone level is found, thyroid function tests are performed to help differentiate between possible hyperthyroidism or an androgen insensitivity disorder.

DIAGNOSTIC EVALUATION

The vascular status of the penis can be evaluated with a simple diagnostic office test by injecting a vasoactive agent into the corpora cavernosum. Alprostadil (prostaglandin E_1 [Caverject, Muse]), phentolamine* (Regitine), and papaverine* are the three most common pharmacologic agents used for this purpose. The injection of these agents mimics the release of natural neurotransmitters required for a normal erection. After intracavernosal injection and manual stimulation of the penis, if a full erection is evident by 15 minutes and lasts longer than 30 minutes, a vascular cause for erectile dysfunction is unlikely and further evaluation for vasculogenic impotence is not usually required.

A patient who fails to respond to the combined injection and stimulation test ideally should be further evaluated with high-resolution ultrasonography in combination with pulsed Doppler analysis of the penile arteries before and after injection with a vasoactive agent. This technique gives valuable information about penile architecture and can accurately measure the velocity of blood flow through individual penile vessels. As a result, arteriogenic (inflow) impotence can be diagnosed. Venogenic impotence, usually suspected after an arteriogenic etiology is ruled out, requires dynamic infusion cavernosometry and cavernosography. Cavernosometry is performed by measuring the intracorporeal pressure during infusion of saline into the corpora cavernosa, and cavernosography consists of infusing contrast material into the corpora and radiographically identifying the sites of venous leakage. The inability to attain or maintain an erection at even high rates of saline infusion suggests a venogenic (outflow) cause for erectile dysfunction.

*Not FDA approved for this indication.

Nocturnal penile tumescence testing has been advocated by some authorities, particularly in identifying psychogenic impotence. Unfortunately, this test lacks adequate specificity or sensitivity and is not a part of the routine evaluation of erectile dysfunction. Selective penile arteriography is reserved for younger patients who have traumatic injuries to their inflow vessels and who may benefit from an arterial bypass procedure.

TREATMENT

Treatment of erectile dysfunction involves the use of various nonsurgical and surgical therapies. The patient should be given adequate information about the risks and benefits of these various treatment approaches. Nonsurgical treatment should be offered initially to all patients, and only when conservative, noninvasive treatments are unsuccessful should surgical options be discussed. Treatment begins with the elimination of ongoing risk factors (e.g., smoking) and alteration of any medications or drugs (e.g., alcohol, marijuana, antihypertensives) that may be responsible for erectile dysfunction. Also, a healthy lifestyle, including daily exercise, healthy eating habits, and cessation of tobacco use, needs to be encouraged by physicians.

The vacuum constriction device (VCD) is a popular noninvasive method of treatment for impotence. This consists of a plastic cylinder that is placed over the penis. The cylinder is connected to a vacuum-generating source that induces a negative pressure, allowing for engorgement of the penis. A constricting ring is positioned around the base of the penis to maintain tumescence. The ring can be left in place for up to 30 minutes, after which ischemic injury can occur. Adequate arterial inflow to the cavernosal tissue is required for the successful use of the VCD. A patient's motor skills, strength, and vision must also be taken into consideration before prescribing a VCD because its operation requires basic hand-eye coordination.

Oral medications traditionally used for the treatment of erectile dysfunction include centrally and peripherally acting drugs such as trazodone* (serotonergic agonist) and yohimbine* (alpha-adrenergic antagonist). These medications, however, have only marginal beneficial effects on the erectile function. The most effective oral medication for treating erectile dysfunction is sildenafil citrate (Viagra). Sildenafil is a type 5 phosphodiesterase inhibitor that enhances cavernosal smooth muscle relaxation by nitric oxide during sexual stimulation. The initial dose for most patients is 50 mg taken approximately 1 hour before sexual intercourse. The dosage may be increased to a maximum dose of 100 mg or decreased to 25 mg, depending on effectiveness, side effects, and patient tolerance. Sildenafil is absolutely contraindicated in patients taking nitrates because it potentiates their hypotensive effects, and may not be recommended in patients with significant cardiovas-

---

*Not FDA approved for this indication.

cular disease. It can also cause transient symptoms such as headaches, flushing, and dyspepsia in some patients. Future oral medications nearing FDA approval include sublingual phentolamine (Vasomax) and apomorphine (Uprima).

Young, hypogonadal men with erectile difficulties benefit from testosterone replacement therapy by intramuscular injection or transdermal patches. Because testosterone therapy may be associated with lipid abnormalities, polycythemia, azoospermia, or possible prostate changes, it is important to obtain a baseline digital rectal examination, hemoglobin, lipid profile, and prostate-specific antigen. Parenteral preparations (testosterone cypionate [Duratest, Depotest] and enanthate [Delatestryl]) are safe, practical, and the least expensive. The injections are usually administered every 2 to 4 weeks, and the dose is adjusted according to clinical response. Customarily, 200 to 300 mg every 2 to 3 weeks is a satisfactory starting point. The two types of transdermal systems are the scrotal patch (Testoderm) and the nonscrotal body patch (Androderm and Testoderm TTS). The transdermal patches are much more expensive than the parenteral preparations and may cause local skin irritation.

The pharmacologic intracavernous injection program using prostaglandin E_1 (Alprostadil), papaverine with phentolamine, or a combination of all three drugs (tri-mix) has been a popular mode of treatment for erectile dysfunction since the mid- to late 1980s. This drug or drug combination is injected directly into the corpora cavernosum with a 28-gauge needle, resulting in vasodilation, penile smooth muscle relaxation, and subsequent tumescence. Intraurethral prostaglandin E_1 (Muse) has also been shown to be effective in selected patients. The drug is inserted into the urethral meatus through a special applicator and is quickly absorbed as the penis is gently massaged. It is an ideal local therapy for those patients who are contraindicated from taking oral (systemic) agents. Patients who are using vasoactive drug injections for erectile dysfunction need to be warned about potential hazards, such as dizziness, hypotension, pain, priapism, hematoma formation, and scarring at the injection site. Also, papaverine may cause hepatotoxicity.

Psychosexual therapy is reserved for patients who experience impotence because of anxiety, fear, or interpersonal conflicts without any organic etiology. Often, psychosexual therapy is used effectively in conjunction with nonsurgical treatments, such as oral medications, intracavernous injection pharmacotherapy, and VCDs.

Surgical treatment of impotence is usually reserved for the patient who has failed or exhausted the various nonsurgical modalities. Placement of a penile prosthesis provides the penis with excellent rigidity for vaginal penetration, thereby ensuring satisfactory coitus for both the patient and the partner. Studies have demonstrated high satisfaction rates for this form of therapy when it is indicated. Because there are many types of penile prostheses, the selection of the prosthesis to be used involves a detailed discussion of the advantages and disadvantages of each for both the patient and partner. Potential complications, such as pain, infection, erosion, mechanical failure, and the possible need for reoperation, need to be carefully explained.

Arterial microsurgical revascularization procedures are usually reserved for young, nonsmoking men with a specific traumatic disruption of the penile vasculature confirmed by selective pudendal arteriography. Venous ligation surgery directed at treatment of impotence secondary to veno-occlusive dysfunction has had limited long-term success because of the redevelopment of venous collaterals that continue to carry the leak.

Specialized tertiary referrals include penile reconstruction procedures using microvascular free flaps from the nondominant forearm. These efforts are indicated in cases of traumatic penile amputation, phallic malignancy, severe infections, or in stable gender dysmorphia, where restoration of body image is of paramount importance.

On the horizon, the progress made in the diagnosis and therapy of male sexual dysfunction will undoubtedly be applied to the fledgling field of female sexual dysfunction. Initial reports with gene therapies for the treatment of erectile dysfunction show promise.

ACUTE RENAL FAILURE

method of
JOHN BADALAMENTI, M.D.,
University of Texas Medical Branch
Galveston, Texas

and

ROBERT L. SAFIRSTEIN, M.D.
University of Arkansas and the
Central Arkansas Veterans Healthcare System
Little Rock, Arkansas

Acute renal failure (ARF) is defined as a rapid loss in renal function that is often reversible. As a result of the reduced glomerular filtration, there is an accumulation of nitrogenous wastes in the body and a rapid rise in serum urea nitrogen and creatinine levels. ARF is commonly seen in the practice of clinical medicine. Approximately 5% of patients admitted to the hospital develop a rapid rise in the serum creatinine concentration. The incidence of ARF is even higher in an intensive care setting, where as many as 25% of patients will develop some form of ARF. In the ambulatory setting, ARF is also frequently encountered and is the cause of as much as 1% of all hospital admissions in some studies. ARF is associated with significant in-hospital morbidity and mortality rates, increasing the relative risk of death by 6.2-fold and increasing the length of hospital stay by 10 days. Oliguric ARF is associated with a higher mortality rate, as high as 80%, as compared with nonoliguric ARF with a mortality rate of 10 to 30%. Many of these outcomes are related to the metabolic complications of ARF, such as volume dysregulation and elec-

trolyte disturbances. It is thus obvious that early recognition of ARF and its underlying cause, coupled with aggressive treatment of its pathophysiologic consequences, may have beneficial effects on patient outcomes. In the text that follows, these points will be amplified for the clinician in practice to aid in the identification and treatment of ARF.

ETIOLOGY

The etiology of ARF has been categorized according to the site of the pathophysiologic process leading to ARF (Table 1). Prerenal ARF implies a reduction in renal function due to a reduction of the effective arterial volume. Intrinsic renal ARF implies damage to one or more of the components of the nephron. Postrenal ARF is usually related to obstruction to urine flow, such as a bladder outlet obstruction, or nephrolithiasis. It is important to characterize the renal failure along these lines so that early correction can prevent subsequent irreversible loss of renal function.

Prerenal Acute Renal Failure

Prerenal causes of ARF are those associated with a reduction in renal perfusion either from decreased blood volume, cardiac output, or renal blood flow and/or increased renal vascular resistance with or without systemic vasodilatation. Therefore, reduced intravascular volume, heart failure, liver functional abnormalities, drug-induced vasoconstriction (cyclosporine, angiotensin-converting enzyme inhibitors, nonsteroidal anti-inflammatory drugs) and the

TABLE 1. **Etiology of Acute Renal Failure**

Prerenal

Hypotension
Volume depletion:
    Renal losses: diuretics, adrenal insufficiency
    Gastrointestinal losses: vomiting, diarrhea
    Cutaneous losses: excessive sweating, burns
Congestive heart failure
Hypoalbuminemic states: liver failure, nephrotic syndrome
Increased renovascular resistance: hypercalcemia,
    nonsteroidal anti-inflammatory drugs, cyclosporine,
    hepatorenal syndrome

Intrinsic

Inflammatory damage:
    Glomerulus: glomerulonephritis, small-vessel vasculitis
    Tubules: allergic tubulointerstitial nephritis
Noninflammatory damage
    Ischemia: systemic hypotension, sepsis,
        thromboembolism, atheroembolism, medium/large
        vessel vasculitis
    Toxins:
        Endogenous: myoglobin, hemoglobin, calcium-
          phosphorus complexes, uric acid
        Exogenous: aminoglycoside, vancomycin, pentamidine,
          amphotericin B, cephalosporins, cisplatin,
          radiocontrast dye

Postrenal

Bladder outlet obstruction: benign prostatic hypertrophy,
    prostate cancer, cervical cancer, bladder cancer,
    phimosis, urethral strictures
Ureteral obstruction: transitional cell cancer,
    nephrolithiasis, tumor encasement, retroperitoneal
    lymphadenopathy and/or fibrosis

presence of infection need to be considered in every patient with ARF.

Intrinsic Acute Renal Failure

Intrinsic causes of ARF are those associated with inflammatory or noninflammatory damage of specific components of the nephron (i.e., the glomerulus and/or tubules) and represents as many as 40% of patients with ARF. This form of ARF may have symptoms and signs of systemic disease with fever, arthralgias, rash, and multiorgan dysfunction. A history of recent ingestion of medications coupled with the presence of a systemic inflammatory process would make tubulointerstitial nephritis more likely. Acute tubular necrosis (ATN), on the other hand, is a process that stems from either severe hemodynamic insults or damage from endogenous or exogenous nephrotoxins without obvious systemic inflammatory processes. Often the medical history will provide evidence of episodes of hypotension, cell lysis, and/or administration of a known nephrotoxin.

Obstructive Acute Renal Failure

Obstructive ARF causes decreased renal function by increasing the hydrostatic pressure in the urinary tract and reducing the transglomerular hydrostatic pressure gradient responsible for glomerular filtration. Urinary obstruction itself causes vasoconstriction of the afferent arteriole, reducing perfusion and glomerular hydrostatic pressure further. Most patients have a medical history compatible with urinary obstruction (i.e., prostatism in males, cervical cancer in females) and/or a history of nephrolithiasis. Prostate and pelvic examinations are, therefore, essential in patients with ARF.

PREVENTION

Because a significant number of hospital-acquired ARF is due to diagnostic and therapeutic interventions, it is important to identify and correct as many risk factors as possible in patients undergoing procedures of known nephrotoxic potential. The two most important risk factors associated with the development of ARF are the presence of a sodium-avid state and pre-existing renal insufficiency. Sodium avidity is seen in volume depletion, congestive heart failure, liver disease, and the nephrotic syndrome. Pre-existing renal disease may be overlooked in patients with reduced muscle mass (i.e., the elderly population), because the serum creatinine value may be in the normal range despite significant renal compromise. It is, therefore, imperative to establish maximum hydration and cardiac output, before exposure to any nephrotoxin. It is also important to treat proteinuric states and liver failure when possible before such exposures, as well. Several strategies may be used to prevent ARF from developing in patients at high risk. Administration of 0.45% saline, 1 mL per kg per hour, 12 hours before radiocontrast exposure and/or surgical procedures has been shown to ameliorate the development of ARF. Every effort should be made to avoid potentially nephrotoxic medications in high-risk patients. The administration of allopurinol (Zyloprim) before chemotherapy may prevent or limit the development of cell-lysis–induced ARF.

APPROACH TO THE PATIENT WITH ACUTE RENAL FAILURE

The most important evidence of ARF is a rise in serum creatinine level above baseline. However, in many cases, this information may not be known or available. The medical history, physical examination, and selected laboratory and radiologic data may be helpful in identifying the presence and etiology of ARF.

History

Prerenal ARF is suggested by a recent history of hemorrhage, hypotension, congestive heart failure, renal sodium wasting from diuretics or adrenal insufficiency, gastrointestinal fluid losses from vomiting and/or diarrhea, and excessive skin fluid losses from sweating or burns. Intrinsic renal ARF of glomerular origin is suggested by recent fevers, rashes, joint pains, hemoptysis, new heart murmurs, and/or multiorgan failure and would be consistent with a systemic glomerulonephritis or vasculitis. Prolonged hypotension, muscle trauma, transfusion reaction, nephrotoxin administration, and/or recent radiocontrast procedure, on the other hand, would be consistent with ARF due to tubule damage. Renal failure after nonsteroidal anti-inflammatory drugs, allopurinol, or oxacillin administration is consistent with tubulointerstitial nephritis as a cause of intrinsic ARF. Elevation of serum creatinine after an invasive vascular procedure in a patient with known peripheral vascular disease is suggestive of atheroembolic renal disease. Lastly, a recent history of voiding problems, flank pain, nephrolithiasis, gross hematuria, and cervical cancer would suggest postrenal ARF.

Physical Examination

Physical examination may aid in providing clues to the cause of ARF. Orthostatic blood pressure and/or pulse changes, poor skin turgor, signs of congestive heart failure and pulmonary edema, and a gallop rhythm would be consistent with prerenal ARF. Skin changes, such as discoid lesions, malar erythema, splinter hemorrhages, palpable purpura, and/or petechiae may provide clues to the presence of a systemic inflammatory, infectious, and/or vascular disease. Skin necrosis and distal lower extremity ecchymoses would be consistent with atheroembolic renal disease. Lastly, the presence of a palpable bladder and/or flank pain on abdominal examination, an enlarged prostate on rectal examination, or a cervical mass on pelvic examination would suggest the presence of postrenal ARF.

Laboratory Studies

URINALYSIS

Examination of a freshly double-voided urine specimen may give insight as to the cause of ARF. The urine dipstick can measure specific gravity, blood, protein, bilirubin, nitrites, pH, and glucose. The urine specific gravity is an indirect measure of urinary osmolality. An elevated specific gravity suggests a high urinary osmolality from high urinary urea concentrations and is seen in prerenal causes of azotemia. Caution must be exercised, however, if there is reason to suspect the presence of radiocontrast dye and/or glucose, because these may increase urine osmolality. The urinary dipstick identifies heme pigments, either as a product of red blood cell breakdown or from the presence of free myoglobin or hemoglobin. Thus, it is imperative that the presence of red blood cells be verified by examination of the urinary sediment. The presence of high albumin concentration in the urine suggests glomerular disease. Urinary pH is usually less than 7.0, but if it is higher, then bicarbonaturia (renal tubular acidosis) or infection with urea-splitting organisms must be considered. A positive urinary dipstick for nitrite suggests pyuria, which may be vaginal as well as from the urinary collecting system or kidney. Pyuria without the presence of microorganisms in the urinary sediment suggests tubulointerstitial disease. Bilirubinuria suggests the presence of liver disease, whereas glucosuria suggests uncontrolled diabetes mellitus, all of which may be associated with ARF.

The urinary sediment examination is a very helpful tool in identifying the likely site of damage in ARF (Table 2). In the case of prerenal azotemia, because there is little structural damage to the kidney, the urine sediment is unremarkable. The presence of dysmorphic red blood cells, red blood cell casts, proteinuria, and oval fat bodies (fat-laden renal tubular cells) is characteristic of glomerular disease. In tubulointerstitial nephritis, the urine contains white blood cells and white blood cell casts along with renal tubular epithelial cells and renal tubular epithelial casts. Eosinophils can be found on a Wright or Hansel stain of the urine in patients with allergic interstitial nephritis. In ATN, renal tubular epithelial cells and renal tubular epithelial casts are present without significant pyuria. Coarse pigmented granular casts (muddy brown casts) are the hallmark urinary finding of ATN. Lastly, in obstructive uropathy, the urinary findings can range from minimal urinary abnormalities to varying degrees of tubulointerstitial damage and inflammation. Hematuria, if present in postrenal ARF, is usually eumorphic.

URINARY SODIUM, URINARY OSMOLALITY, AND FRACTIONAL EXCRETION OF SODIUM

In the setting of ARF and oliguria, certain urinary diagnostic indices can aid in differentiating the cause of a patient's renal dysfunction. Urine sodium, urine osmolality, and the fractional excretion of sodium (FE_{Na}) may each help to distinguish intrinsic from prerenal causes of ARF. In the prerenal state, the kidney attempts to restore the fullness of the arterial volume by conserving salt and water. Increased production and release of renin, aldosterone, and antidiuretic hormone and changes in filtration fraction each augment sodium reabsorption in both the proximal and distal tubules and reduce urinary sodium to less than 20 mEq per liter. Because of the increased production of antidiuretic hormone, the reabsorption of water in the collecting duct increases and urinary osmolality rises above that of serum. To increase the specificity of these urinary indices, it is helpful to calculate the fractional excretion of filtered sodium normalized to glomerular filtration, with

the use of creatinine clearance as an estimate of the latter. The FE_{Na} is calculated by the formula

$$\frac{U/PNa}{U/PCr} \times 100,$$

where U is urine, P is plasma or serum, Na is sodium concentration, and Cr is creatinine concentration. If the fractional excretion of sodium is less than 1%, prerenal ARF may be present. If the fractional excretion of sodium is 1% or more, then ATN is more likely. It must be emphasized, however, that there is much variability in sodium excretion in both prerenal azotemia and ATN, depending on the volume status of the patient and whether diuretics were administered before the urine was collected. Therefore, the index should be interpreted in the background of the history and physical examination. The fractional excretion of sodium, urinary sodium, and urinary osmolality should only confirm the clinical suspicion of prerenal or intrinsic causes of ARF. High fractional excretion of sodium may be most helpful in the oliguric patient as an indicator of intrinsic renal failure.

BLOOD STUDIES

A complete blood cell count that shows severe anemia would be more consistent with chronic, rather than acute, renal failure. However, gastrointestinal bleeding, hemolysis, and/or bone marrow failure may accompany ARF and severely reduce hemoglobin levels. The complete blood cell count is helpful when schistocytes and thrombocytopenia are present in a patient with ARF, because the diagnosis of hemolytic uremic syndrome can be made. Standard electrolyte panels may be similarly abnormal in both acute and chronic renal failure and are not helpful in distinguishing between them. For example, the presence of a serum blood urea nitrogen to creatinine ratio of more than 20:1, which is indicative of prerenal azotemia, is also affected by protein intake, the presence of hypercatabolism (glucocorticoids, tetracycline, malnutrition, and sepsis), or reduced production of urea by the liver during liver failure.

The serum creatinine concentration is a more specific measure of renal function. However, serum creatinine levels are affected by muscle mass and general nutrition. Furthermore, spurious elevations of serum creatinine levels are seen with ketoacidosis, which are chromogenic, and with drugs such as cimetidine (Tagamet) and trimethoprim (Proloprim), that interfere with the tubular secretion of creatinine. More specific laboratory blood analyses, on the other hand, are helpful in establishing the underlying cause of ARF. When glomerulonephritis is suspected, antinuclear antibodies, antineutrophil cytoplasmic antibodies (ANCA), antiglomerular basement membrane antibody titers, and serum complement may aid in establishing the diagnosis. C3 levels are extremely helpful in narrowing the differential diagnosis of ARF. A low C3 is associated with systemic lupus erythematosus, bacterial endocarditis, postinfectious glomerulonephritis, essential mixed cryoglobulinemia, membranoproliferative glomerulonephritis, and nonglomerular atheroembolic renal disease. In intrinsic ARF, elevated plasma hemoglobin and low serum haptoglobin, or elevated creatine kinase can establish the diagnosis of hemolysis or rhabdomyolysis, respectively, as the cause of ARF. Exogenous toxins causing intrinsic ARF are best diagnosed by measuring the serum levels of the toxins in question (e.g., aminoglycosides, vancomycin, lithium carbonate, and others).

TABLE 2. **Urinary Sediment Findings in Acute Renal Failure**

Prerenal

Normal or hyaline casts

Intrinsic

Glomerulonephritis: dysmorphic RBCs, RBC casts, marked proteinuria, oval-fat bodies, free lipids
Interstitial nephritis: pyuria, RTEs, RTE casts, WBC casts, granular casts, eosinophils
Acute tubular necrosis: pigmented granular casts, RTEs, RTE casts
Vascular disorders: Normal or hematuria, mild proteinuria

Postrenal

Normal or pyuria, eumorphic RBCs, RTEs, RTE casts, WBC casts, granular casts

RBC = red blood cell; RTE = renal tubular epithelial cell; WBC = white blood cell.

The most useful diagnostic tool in the investigation of ARF is renal ultrasonography. It is very helpful in distinguishing acute from chronic renal failure because chronic renal damage, for the most part, causes loss of renal mass, which can be quantified by renal ultrasonographic evaluation. There are only a few chronic renal diseases that do not reduce renal mass in the presence of progressive renal damage (i.e., diabetic glomerulosclerosis, malignant hypertension, polycystic kidney disease, and infiltrating diseases of the kidney, such as amyloidosis). The renal ultrasonogram is also helpful in determining whether urinary obstruction is present because it allows good visualization of the urinary bladder, renal pelvis, calyces, and kidneys in the nonobese patient. By identifying the presence of a dilated urinary collecting system (hydronephrosis), urinary obstruction can be identified in most cases. Exceptions to this rule are the very early stages of obstruction and/or encasement of the collecting system in tumor or fibrosis tissue, where dilatation of the ureter is restricted.

Other studies, such as Doppler ultrasonography and radionuclide scans with ^{99m}Tc-DTPA or ^{131}I-hippuran are only helpful when vascular obstruction or stenosis of the main renal arteries or its intrarenal branches is suspected.

RENAL BIOPSY

The renal biopsy can consistently provide both diagnostic and prognostic information, but since it is an invasive procedure, it should be used only when the benefits outweigh the potential risks (i.e., bleeding, infection, and/or bowel perforation). Because ATN may resolve spontaneously, it is hard to justify a renal biopsy in such cases. However, in cases in which the cause of ARF is not obvious, when there is a high suspicion of glomerular disease, or when the expected recovery is delayed, the renal biopsy is helpful in determining a proper therapeutic plan.

APPROACH TO THE PATIENT WITH ESTABLISHED ACUTE RENAL FAILURE

In established ARF, the patient becomes vulnerable to the complications of reduced excretory function. Close monitoring and early intervention when such complications become evident is imperative in reducing the morbidity and mortality rates associated with ARF.

Intervention in Maintaining Volume and Electrolyte Homeostasis

Volume Homeostasis

Careful daily assessment of volume status is required in ARF, especially if oliguria (<400 mL per day of urine output) is present. Monitoring daily weights, fluid intake and output, orthostatic blood pressure and pulse, jugular venous pressure, pulmonary congestion, edema, skin turgor, and/or direct measurements of central venous pressure or pulmonary capillary wedge pressure will aid in maintaining euvolemia. Hypovolemia can be corrected with intravenous isotonic saline or packed red blood cells if frank hypotension or orthostasis is present. Maintenance fluids of 0.45% normal saline in D5W is the fluid of choice in hemodynamically stable pa-

tients with continued fluid losses from the skin, gastrointestinal tract, urinary tract, or wounds. Volume overload should be treated with sodium restriction to at least 2 to 4 grams per day and with loop diuretics, such as furosemide (Lasix) or bumetanide (Bumex), titrated to achieve a diuretic response. If no response is achieved with loop diuretics alone, addition of oral metolazone may improve the diuretic response to these agents. The failure to achieve a diuresis in a patient with ARF and volume overload necessitates the initiation of renal replacement therapy.

Potassium Homeostasis

In established ARF, especially with oliguria, potassium excretion falls significantly. The development of hyperkalemia and its effect on the heart is one of the most serious complications of ARF. The cardiotoxic effects of hyperkalemia cause changes in cardiac conduction that can be monitored by electrocardiography. The first electrocardiographic evidence of serious hyperkalemic cardiotoxicity is peaked T waves. As serum potassium levels rise further, shortening of the QT interval ensues, followed by loss of P waves, widening of the QRS wave, bradycardia, ventricular tachycardia, ventricular fibrillation, and cardiac arrest. Treatment of hyperkalemia is outlined in Table 3. At the early stages of hyperkalemia, intervention with sodium polystyrene sulfonate (SPS, Kayexalate) given orally in sorbitol or rectally in saline retention enemas may help bring the serum potassium into the normal range through sodium-potassium exchange in the gastrointestinal tract. As electrocardiographic signs progress, intravenous calcium gluconate or calcium chloride, intravenous glucose and insulin, and/or intravenous or inhaled beta$_2$-adrenergic agonists will temporarily reduce serum potassium by intracellular movement. These temporizing measures should be followed by administration of sodium polystyrene sulfonate. Refractory hyperkalemia, as seen in massive cellular breakdown (i.e., rhabdomyolysis or tumor lysis syndrome), will necessitate initiation of hemodialysis because this modality of renal replacement therapy is most efficient in potassium removal.

Acid-Base Homeostasis

As renal function worsens, both the ability to generate bicarbonate and excrete an acid load diminish,

TABLE 3. **Treatment of Hyperkalemia**

Agent	Dosage
Calcium gluconate 10% IV	10 mL given over 1 min; repeat q 3–5 min
Sodium bicarbonate IV	1 or 2 ampules over 5 min
Glucose 50% IV and regular insulin IV	glucose 50 mL; regular insulin 10 units
Albuterol IV or nebulized	0.5 mg IV or 10–20 mg nebulized
Sodium polystyrene sulfonate PO or PR	15–30 gm PO q 2–4 h in 50–100 mL of 20% sorbitol 50 gm PR in 200 mL of 20% dextrose

resulting in a reduction in serum bicarbonate and the development of a metabolic acidosis. Acid generation continues in an individual with ARF because of the metabolism of dietary protein and/or catabolism of endogenous protein. Other acid-producing states, such as lactic acidosis or ketoacidosis, ingestion of methanol or ethylene glycol, or salicylate toxicity may contribute to the acidosis of ARF. Therapy for acidosis should be aimed at reducing acid generation by limiting protein intake to 0.6 to 0.8 gram per kg per day and treating any underlying acid-producing state. Bicarbonate replacement is only indicated when metabolic acidosis is severe (serum bicarbonate less than 15 mmol per liter). Bicarbonate replacement can be given as sodium bicarbonate either orally or intravenously. If intravenous bicarbonate is used, it should be given as an isotonic solution (i.e., three ampules [50 mEq per liter per 50 mL] added to 1 liter of D5W). Other oral or intravenous agents, such as sodium citrate or sodium acetate, may be used instead of bicarbonate. However, these agents are converted to bicarbonate by the liver and must be avoided in patients with liver failure. Administration of sodium bicarbonate may precipitate metabolic alkalosis, hypokalemia, hypocalcemia, and volume overload. Refractory acidemia in oliguric patients must be treated with renal replacement therapy.

Calcium and Phosphorus Homeostasis

Hyperphosphatemia is due to reduced phosphate excretion. In instances when ARF is associated with muscle or cell breakdown, the serum phosphorus level may rise to toxic levels. The development of ectopic calcification, especially when the $Ca \times PO_4$ product is more than 70, is most often seen in the cornea and conjunctiva. Calcifications at the limbic-corneal junction can be visualized by slit-lamp examination. Ectopic calcification may take place in the joints as chondrocalcinosis or pseudogout. Blood vessels and other soft tissues may also be the site of ectopic calcifications. Increased serum phosphorus reduces serum calcium levels by binding ionized calcium and by inhibiting the generation of 1,25-dihydroxyvitamin D. Reduced 1,25-dihydroxyvitamin D levels diminish intestinal calcium absorption and increase the set point for stimulation of parathyroid hormone production, further reducing serum calcium concentration. Hyperphosphatemia is treated by the administration of calcium-based phosphate binders such as calcium carbonate and calcium acetate. In cases of an elevated calcium-phosphate product, the use of aluminum hydroxide or aluminum carbonate avoids further calcium administration. Treatment of hypocalcemia is only necessary when symptomatic. Serum calcium levels should be restored to normal by intravenous calcium gluconate administration followed by supplementation with oral calcium and vitamin D. Care should be taken in attempting to improve the serum bicarbonate level in patients with hypocalcemia and acidemia, because symptomatic hypocalcemia can be precipitated by the administration of alkali to such patients. Frequent assessment

for the presence of Trousseau's and Chvostek's signs, the prelude to tetany, are warranted in any patient with severe hypocalcemia. Intravenous calcium followed by oral calcium and vitamin D supplementation is the mainstay of therapy.

Water Homeostasis

Disturbances in water homeostasis in ARF are manifested as hyponatremia or hypernatremia. Hyponatremia is usually related to excess water intake by administration of hypotonic fluids. Hypernatremia is unusual in ARF and can be precipitated either by aggressive diuresis without adequate water supplementation or by the administration of hypertonic fluids usually in the form of intravenous sodium bicarbonate for the treatment of acidemia. Close monitoring of serum electrolytes and appropriate adjustments of intravenous fluid administration will prevent the development of hyponatremia or hypernatremia.

Magnesium and Uric Acid Homeostasis

Hypermagnesemia and hyperuricemia are common manifestations of ARF because of impaired excretion. Severe hypermagnesemia occurs with excessive magnesium administration, usually in the form of magnesium-containing antacids, which should be avoided in ARF. Severe hyperuricemia is seen with massive cell breakdown in the tumor lysis syndrome. In this case, uric acid levels should be reduced with hemodialysis. Symptomatic gouty arthritis can be treated with colchicine and/or oral corticosteroids. However, nonsteroidal anti-inflammatory drugs should be avoided because these agents can prolong ARF by altering intrarenal hemodynamics or by causing the development of interstitial nephritis.

Nutrition Homeostasis

The main goals of nutritional therapy in ARF are to provide enough calories and protein to prevent the development of hypercatabolism and maintain optimal nutrition status. Total caloric intake should be at least 30 kcal per kg per day while protein intake should be restricted to 0.6 to 0.8 grams per kg per day in patients who are not wasted or on dialysis. Once dialysis is initiated, protein intake can be increased to at least 1 to 1.2 grams per kg per day. Nutrition should be administered orally or by nasogastric or gastrostomy tubes if possible. Total parenteral nutrition should be reserved for those patients who cannot tolerate enteral feedings because of bowel dysfunction.

Intervention in Other Complications Associated with Acute Renal Failure (Uremic Syndrome)

Hematologic Complications

As ARF progresses, uremic toxins accumulate and affect platelet function and red cell production and survival. The result is anemia and a bleeding tendency characterized by a prolonged bleeding time. Improvement in platelet function and red cell production and survival are variable with dialysis. Active bleeding unresponsive to renal replacement therapy should be treated with cryoprecipitate (10 U) or 1-deamino-8-D-arginine vasopressin (desmopressin [DDAVP], 0.3 μg per kg intravenously. Conjugated estrogens (Premarin), 0.6 mg per kg per day for 5 days, may also inhibit the bleeding tendency associated with ARF. The presence of anemia may necessitate transfusion of packed red blood cells and/or administration of erythropoietin (Epogen), 50 to 75 U per kg, if iron stores are adequate (i.e., transferrin saturation level > 20% and serum ferritin level > 100 ng per mL).

Neurologic Complications

As nitrogenous waste products accumulate in ARF, neuromuscular symptoms may develop. Asterixis, seizures, somnolence, stupor, and coma are central nervous system manifestations of advanced ARF. A sensory-motor neuropathy may also develop as ARF progresses. The presence of neurologic abnormalities in ARF are indications for the initiation of renal replacement therapy.

Gastrointestinal Complications

Anorexia, nausea, vomiting, and gastritis, often hemorrhagic, may be seen during the course of ARF. Gastrointestinal bleeding due to gastritis and stress ulcers may be prevented by the administration of aluminum-containing antacids, such as aluminum hydroxide, and/or the administration of H_2-receptor blocking agents, such as ranitidine (Zantac) or cimetidine. The dosage of these H_2-receptor blockers should be reduced in ARF. Initiation of dialysis may improve these gastrointestinal abnormalities and prevent the high morbidity and mortality rates associated with gastrointestinal bleeding in ARF.

Cardiopulmonary Complications

Heart failure, arrhythmias, pulmonary edema, pericarditis, and pneumonia may develop in patients with ARF. Sodium restriction and antihypertensive medications are indicated for those individuals with volume-dependent hypertension and volume overload. The development of pericarditis with or without tamponade is an indication for the initiation of dialysis in patients with advanced ARF. The use of heparin for anticoagulation on hemodialysis is contraindicated when pericarditis is present because the pericardial fluid in advanced ARF may be hemorrhagic. The use of anticoagulation may precipitate further bleeding into the pericardium and cardiac tamponade. Appropriate antibiotic administration is warranted in patients with pneumonia and ARF.

Infectious Complications

Infection complicates a majority of cases of ARF. Common sites of infection are the lungs, urinary tract, skin, and abdominal cavity. Most infections are related to trauma and surgery, but complications from indwelling vascular and urinary catheters are important sources. Early recognition and treatment of infections along with early removal of indwelling catheters are necessary to reduce the morbidity and mortality rates associated with infections in patients with ARF. Antibiotic dosages need to be adjusted in ARF when necessary to avoid complications such as ototoxicity and neurotoxicity that may accompany the use of some antibiotic agents. Nephrotoxic antibiotics should be avoided when possible to prevent any prolongation of the ARF episode.

Renal Replacement Therapy

Indications

If resolution of the acute renal insult does not take place, conservative measures to regulate sodium, water, and acid-base balance may no longer control the physiologic complications of ARF. Renal replacement therapy must then be initiated to maintain life. Because the optimal time to initiate dialysis is relatively unclear and the dialysis procedure itself has significant complications, renal replacement therapy must only be initiated when the potential benefits of dialysis are not outweighed by the risks. The accepted indications for the initiation of acute renal replacement therapy are shown in Table 4.

Different Modalities of Renal Replacement Therapy

Hemodialysis. Intermittent hemodialysis is the mainstay of renal replacement therapy. Percutaneous cannulation of a large vein (femoral, internal jugular, subclavian) is necessary to access the vascular space so that enough blood can be pumped through a dialyzer (300 mL per minute). Dialysis of blood occurs across a semipermeable synthetic membrane that separates the blood compartment from the bathing dialysate solution. Solutes are removed from the blood by diffusion driven by differences in concentration across the membrane. Removal of fluid by ultrafiltration is accomplished by hydrostatic pressure differences between the blood compartment and the dialysate compartment. Flow of dissolved solutes across the semipermeable membrane during ultrafiltration also removes solutes. A typical hemodialysis treatment is performed for 4 hours thrice weekly. The main advantages and disadvantages of hemodialysis are shown in Table 5. It must be emphasized that the hypotension and arrhythmias seen

TABLE 4. **Indications for Renal Replacement Therapy**

Refractory fluid overload
Refractory hyperkalemia
Refractory acidemia
Refractory severe hypermagnesemia, hyperuricemia, hyperphosphatemia
High serum levels of toxins or harmful drugs
Uremic syndrome
Severe azotemia (serum blood urea nitrogen > 100 mg/dL)

TABLE 5. **Different Modalities of Renal Replacement Therapy**

Hemodialysis

Advantages: less extracorporeal circulation by intermittent utilization, greater efficiency, direct access to circulation
Disadvantages: bleeding, anticoagulation necessary, hypotension, dialysis dysequilibrium, cardiac arrhythmias, hypoxia, infection

Peritoneal Dialysis

Advantages: no extracorporeal circulation, hemodynamic stability, no anticoagulation necessary, low costs
Disadvantages: peritonitis, low efficiency, protein losses, hypoxia

Continuous Renal Replacement Therapy

Advantages: hemodynamic stability, more physiologic solute and water exchange
Disadvantages: prolonged extracorporeal circulation, anticoagulation necessary, infection

in hemodialysis pose significant risks to the patient and, although infrequent, may cause death. The risk-benefit ratio of hemodialysis in each individual patient should always be favorable before initiating this procedure.

Peritoneal Dialysis. Peritoneal dialysis involves the same principles involved in the exchange of solute and plasma water as in hemodialysis. However, the semipermeable membrane separating blood from dialysate, in this case, is the peritoneal membrane and basement membranes of the peritoneal blood vessels. Although diffusion governs solute exchange as in hemodialysis, ultrafiltration is driven by osmotic pressure differences between blood and dialysate established by the concentration of glucose in the dialysate. As compared with hemodialysis, the peritoneal cavity is accessed by means of a catheter that is placed either surgically or percutaneously at the bedside. Furthermore, peritoneal dialysis is much less efficient than hemodialysis because of the inability to regulate peritoneal blood flow and adjust the surface area of the peritoneal space so that solute and plasma water exchange can be maximized. This inefficiency precludes its use in life-threatening electrolyte disturbances, such as severe hyperkalemia. The advantages and disadvantages of peritoneal dialysis are outlined in Table 5.

Continuous Renal Replacement Therapy. Continuous renal replacement therapies that are currently available are (1) continuous arteriovenous hemofiltration (CAVH) and continuous venovenous hemofiltration (CVVH) and (2) continuous arteriovenous hemodialysis (CAVHD) and continuous venovenous hemodialysis (CVVHD). These modalities are based on the same physical principles as in conventional hemodialysis, with the use of extracorporeal blood circulation and a hemofilter for solute and plasma water exchange. However, instead of being intermittent therapies, these are performed continuously, permitting slow, gradual exchange of solute and plasma water. As a result, continuous renal replacement therapies have less hemodynamic insta-

bility and cause less osmotic and electrolyte shifts than conventional hemodialysis. Besides differences in how the blood is accessed and replaced (artery to vein in CAVH and CAVHD; vein to vein in CVVH and CVVHD), the fundamental difference between hemofiltration and hemodialysis is how solute is removed. In hemofiltration, solute is removed by convection, that is, as plasma water moves across a semipermeable membrane so do dissolved solutes. In hemodialysis, solute is removed by diffusion down a concentration gradient. To make CAVH/CVVH more efficient, large volumes of ultrafiltration are necessary. This requires large volumes of replacement fluid to be administered. Although CAVHD/CVVHD are less efficient than conventional hemodialysis, the continuous performance of these procedures improves solute and plasma water clearances. The advantages of continuous renal replacement therapy are that slow, continuous exchange of solute and plasma water prevents dialysis disequilibrium and hypotension and that it can be used in the hemodynamically unstable patient. The disadvantages are bleeding from extracorporeal circulation and anticoagulation and infection due to prolonged indwelling intravenous catheters (see Table 5).

RECOVERY FROM ACUTE RENAL FAILURE

In general, patients who experience ARF from ATN usually improve their renal function quickly. In those patients who require dialysis support, renal function usually recovers within 2 weeks of the first dialysis procedure. Maximal recovery should be expected within 4 to 6 weeks. Only about 5% of patients require long-term dialysis. Poor prognosis for recovery and survival is related to the presence of multiorgan failure and solid organ transplantation. Although renal function usually recovers even in those patients requiring dialysis, there is some evidence that conventional hemodialysis may prolong renal recovery and affect overall prognosis. Small changes in blood pressure on conventional hemodialysis may affect renal perfusion in a damaged kidney that has lost its ability to autoregulate blood flow. New ischemic ATN lesions may develop, thus prolonging the episode of ARF. The use of continuous renal replacement therapies and peritoneal dialysis, which have only minor hemodynamic effects, may prove to accelerate recovery from ARF. There is also evidence that more biocompatible material used in hemodialyzer construction may affect recovery of renal function and survival from an episode of ARF. The use of more "biocompatible" synthetic-polymer hemodialyzers may improve outcomes in patients with dialysis-dependent ARF. Despite these advances, the rate of mortality from ARF remains high. New approaches to augment renal perfusion, to improve cytoprotection, and to hasten cellular recovery are undergoing clinical trials in an attempt to alter the morbidity and mortality rates among patients with ARF.

CHRONIC RENAL FAILURE

method of
PAUL J. SCHEEL, JR., M.D.
*The Johns Hopkins University School of
Medicine
Baltimore, Maryland*

Chronic renal failure (CRF) describes the slow progressive loss of kidney function over time. Diseases leading to renal damage may be localized to the kidney (i.e., glomerulonephritis, chronic pyelonephritis) or may be systemic, such as hypertension or diabetes, and affect multiple organs. Clinicians treating patients with this entity must have a clear understanding of the many functions of the kidney and how loss of these functions leads to a disruption of the normal physiology of their patients.

EPIDEMIOLOGY

There are little published data on the number of patients with CRF in the United States. There is, however, very detailed information on patients who progress to develop end-stage renal disease (ESRD) and require either dialysis or transplantation. It is from this second body of literature that we infer information about the epidemiology of CRF. Over the past decade, there has been a dramatic rise in the number of patients with ESRD. Data from the United States Renal Data Systems (USRDS) show that the number of patients with ESRD has risen from 74,000 in 1986 to 250,000 in 1996. This growth has been fueled by older Americans with diseases such as diabetes and hypertension. As can be seen from Table 1, hypertension and diabetes account for more than 65% of ESRD in the United States. It is estimated that for every patient with ESRD, there are eight patients with CRF. Therefore, conservative estimates on the number of Americans with CRF range from 1.5 to 3 million patients.

MEASUREMENT OF KIDNEY FUNCTIONS

The kidney is composed of millions of functioning units called nephrons. As kidney tissue is destroyed, the remaining nephrons have the ability to increase their functional capacity. It is for this reason that healthy individuals can donate a kidney to a friend or relative without adversely influencing their own kidney function and why a significant loss of kidney tissue can occur without the onset of symptoms.

Table 2 lists the primary functions of the kidney. Although each of these functions can be measured separately, it is more practical to use the combined glomerular filtration rate (GFR) of all nephrons as an indicator of overall kidney function. A normal GFR for an adult male is 130 ± 18 mL per minute, and for an adult female it is 120 ±

TABLE 1. Etiology of Chronic Renal Failure

• Diabetes	39%
• Hypertension	29%
• Glomerulonephritis	11%
• Cystic/hereditary/congenital	3%
• Vasculitis	2%
• Interstitial nephritis	4%
• Neoplasms	1%
• Other	12%

TABLE 2. Functions of the Kidney

- Elimination of nitrogenous wastes
- Hormone production
- Maintenance of acid-base homeostasis
- Regulation of volume status
- Regulation of electrolytes concentration

14 mL per minute. As one ages, this number may fall into the range of 75 to 80 mL per minute in those individuals in their seventh and eighth decades.

Patients are rarely symptomatic with a GFR greater than 50 mL per minute. As the GFR falls below this value, subtle physiologic changes occur that are measurable but rarely cause symptoms.

As the GFR falls below 30 mL per minute, there are significant changes that occur that lead to anemia, hyperparathyroidism, and eventually anorexia, malnutrition, and, without dialysis or transplantation, death. Thus, to efficiently assess and follow patients, it is imperative that tools be available that can rapidly estimate the GFR.

The clearance of inulin is the gold standard for measuring the GFR. Unfortunately, this test is not clinically available and the clinician is left using one or a combination of three tests that are surrogate markers of GFR.

Creatinine is a by-product of muscle metabolism that is excreted primarily by the kidney. Assuming breakdown of muscle is at a constant rate, any increase in serum creatinine would therefore be reflective of decreased elimination and, hence, kidney function. Although convenient and inexpensive, the serum creatinine level is a very crude estimate of GFR. Unfortunately, the relationship between serum creatinine and GFR is logarithmic and not linear; and, therefore, small changes in serum creatinine concentration in the low end of this scale represent large changes in GFR, whereas similar changes at higher creatinine values represent smaller changes in GFR. As a general rule, each time the serum creatinine doubles, the GFR is decreased by 50%. For example, an increase in serum creatinine from 1.0 to 2.0 mg per dL represents a 50% reduction in GFR, whereas a quantitatively similar rise in creatinine from 8 to 9 represents only a drop in GFR 1 to 2%. Therefore, small changes in serum creatinine in the low range need to be viewed as a serious event.

The second test available to estimate GFR is the clearance of creatinine. Although more accurate than measuring serum creatinine concentration alone, this test requires patients to collect their urine for a 24-hour period—a task that many patients find inconvenient. To calculate the clearance of creatinine, a 24-hour urine collection is obtained with a simultaneous measurement of serum creatinine. The creatinine clearance is calculated according to the following formula:

$$UV/P \div 1440$$

where U is the concentration of creatinine in mg per dL; V is the volume of urine in milliliters; and P is the plasma concentration of creatinine. This value is then divided by 1440, which equals the number of minutes in 24 hours, and the final product is expressed as the creatinine clearance in milliliters per minute.

It is important that when measuring creatinine clearance that the clinician also calculate the quantity of creatinine excreted per 24 hours. Adult males normally excrete 1.5 to 2.0 grams of creatinine, whereas females excrete 1.0

to 1.5 grams. Values less than that suggest an undercollection of and, hence, an underestimation of, GFR.

In addition to being difficult for the patient to perform, this test has other drawbacks. As the GFR falls, the concentration of creatinine in the blood rises and the percent of creatinine eliminated through tubular secretion increases. This increase in tubular secretion will artificially raise the value for creatinine clearance. Therefore, as the GFR falls below 20 mL per minute, creatinine clearance can overestimate the GFR by as much as 50%.

The final methodology used to measure GFR is the clearance of various radioisotopes. Agents such as pentetic acid (DTPA) or iothalamate are injected into a peripheral vein, and the disappearance of these isotopes is measured in serial blood samples or a traditional clearance formula is used by collecting the patient's urine.

These methods are believed to be the most accurate means of measuring GFR, but given the expense and complexity of the procedure, it is reserved for those situations in which it is crucial to have a precise measurement of GFR.

TREATMENT

The treatment of patients with CRF can be divided into five separate categories: (1) establishment of a diagnosis with treatment of those conditions that are reversible; (2) delaying the progression of renal failure; (3) treatment and prevention of complications of CRF; (4) avoidance of additional renal insults; and (5) ensuring a smooth transition between pre-ESRD and ESRD.

Establishment of a Diagnosis

In evaluating the patient with an elevated serum creatinine, it is essential to establish a cause for the patient's renal insufficiency. Although many renal diseases will progress independent of treatment, others, if identified early, can be treated, thus avoiding the inevitable path to ESRD.

The evaluation of the patient with CRF is beyond the scope of this chapter. Causes of renal insufficiency can be divided into three major categories: prerenal, intrarenal, and postrenal. Within each of these categories, there are pathophysiologic conditions that, if identified, can lead to full recovery of renal function. For example, patients with atherosclerotic renal vascular disease can undergo bypass surgery or percutaneous transluminal angioplasty with resolution of azotemia. Patients with vasculitis of the kidney can be effectively managed with immunosuppressive agents, and patients with outflow obstruction can be effectively managed with surgical or percutaneous decompression. Unfortunately, unless these types of conditions are identified early, the patient is destined to progress and suffer from the pathophysiologic consequences of CRF.

Delaying Progression

Once a diagnosis of renal insufficiency is established and no reversible component is identified, it is crucial to slow the progression of CRF and maintain the GFR as high as possible and for as long as possible. Strategies to delay progression include aggressive control of systemic hypertension, dietary protein restriction, and pharmacologic reduction of intraglomerular pressure through the use of angiotensin-converting enzyme (ACE) inhibitors.

Systemic hypertension is a common finding in patients with CRF. Hypertension in this setting may be secondary to the activation of the renin-angiotensin system or secondary to volume overload (a common finding in patients with CRF).

The reduction of systemic blood pressure into the "normal" range has been shown in multiple studies to slow the progression of CRF. Normal blood pressure has been defined as systolic blood pressure less than 160 mm Hg and diastolic blood pressure less than 90 mm Hg. Multiple different classes of antihypertensive agents have been shown to slow progression of CRF associated with reduction in systemic blood pressure. These agents include beta blockers, calcium channel blockers, ACE inhibitors, vasodilators, and, in the setting of volume overload, diuretics.

What has not been determined is how low blood pressure should be reduced to optimally retard the progression of CRF. In patients with proteinuric syndromes with 24-hour urine excretion of more than 1 gram of protein per 24 hours, a reduction of systemic blood pressure below that which has been defined as normal has shown an added benefit. This fact is countered by large studies in patients with cardiovascular disease that have shown that lowering blood pressure beyond the "normal" limit actually increased mortality. It is hypothesized that this increase in mortality is secondary to myocardial and cerebral ischemia associated with lowering mean arterial pressure. Until additional data are available, the aggressive lowering of blood pressure below normal should be undertaken with caution, especially in those individuals with proteinuric syndromes.

The selective decrease in intraglomerular pressure can be accomplished with the administration of ACE inhibitors and, to a lesser degree, with calcium channel blockers. This concept was first introduced in patients with diabetic nephropathy who had serum creatinine values less than 2.5 mg per dL. In these studies, the administration of the ACE inhibitor captopril (Capoten) significantly delayed the progression of the underlying diabetic nephropathy. This reduction in the rate of decline in GFR was independent of the systemic blood pressure effect of these agents. Subsequent studies have shown similar results with CRF from many different causes.

These agents must, however, be used with caution. As GFR falls, these agents may actually accelerate the decline in GFR and lead to the development of life-threatening hyperkalemia. Serum creatinine and potassium concentrations should be assayed within 48 to 72 hours after starting these agents. Depending on the level of renal in sufficiency, these values may need to be rechecked on a monthly or quarterly basis.

Since the 1940s, dietary protein restriction has been shown to delay the progression of renal insufficiency in animal models. It is postulated that by lowering dietary protein, there is a decrease in intraglomerular pressure, thus providing a favorable change in renal hemodynamics.

Human studies have strongly suggested that in highly motivated individuals, the restriction of dietary protein not only limits uremic symptoms but likely slows the progression of CRF. There are two nutritional prescriptions used to slow progression of CRF. The most widely used protocol is to restrict dietary protein to 0.6 gram of protein per kilogram of body weight. Others believe that an additional benefit can be achieved by further reduction in dietary protein to 0.3 gram of protein per kilogram of body weight with supplemental essential amino acids.

For patients opting for nutritional therapy, the input and close monitoring of a registered dietitian is essential. This close monitoring will be necessary to monitor compliance while ensuring that patients do not become malnourished.

Treatment and Prevention of Complications

Anemia

As CRF progresses and GFR falls below 40 mL per minute, there is a parallel decrease in the production of erythropoietin by the kidney. This decrease in erythropoietin production results in a normochromic, normocytic anemia. When evaluating patients with chronic renal insufficiency and anemia, it is important not to assume that all anemia is related to decreased erythropoietin production and ignore other potential causes of anemia. Initial evaluation of anemia includes a complete blood cell count, peripheral blood smear, and reticulocyte count.

Once other potential causes of anemia have been excluded, patients with hematocrits less than 30% should be considered for treatment with recombinant erythropoietin. Normalization of the hematocrit improves patients' functional status while improving many parameters of cardiac performance, including an increase in exercise tolerance, normalization of cardiac output, a decrease in the potential for myocardial ischemia, and a decrease in left ventricular hypertrophy.

Erythropoietin is administered through either the intravenous or the subcutaneous route. For patients not yet on dialysis the subcutaneous route is more practical. Erythropoietin is administered at an initial dose of 50 to 75 units per kg subcutaneously once to twice weekly. Hemoglobin and hematocrit values need to be checked within 2 to 4 weeks of initiating therapy. The initial target hematocrit is 33 to 37%. Hematocrit values should be checked weekly until a stable hematocrit has been achieved. Once stabilized, monthly hematocrits are then acceptable. In patients where the hematocrit fails to rise to the target range after 4 weeks, the dose of erythropoietin should be increased by 20%. Similarly, in patients whose hema-

tocrit exceeds the target range, the dose can be reduced by 20%.

Patients receiving erythropoietin therapy universally will require concurrent iron therapy. There are many iron preparations available, but no one preparation appears to be more efficacious than others. Ferrous sulfate (300-mg tablets) supplies 65 mg of elemental iron, and it is this preparation that is typically given three time daily. Side effects of oral iron are common, and 20% of patients will have gastrointestinal disturbance. These side effects can be diminished by taking iron therapy with food, but this strategy reduces the absorption of oral iron. Patients who cannot tolerate oral iron will require intravenous iron administration several times per year. For patients who require intravenous iron, iron dextran (InFeD), 500 mg, is typically given intravenously after a 1-mg test dose.

Iron stores should be assayed at the start of erythropoietin therapy and quarterly thereafter. The goal is to maintain the percentage saturation of transferrin greater than 20% and the ferritin level greater than 100 ng per mL.

Metabolic Bone Disease

As GFR falls below 30 mL per minute, two simultaneous physiologic processes begin that will ultimately lead to renal osteodystrophy if they are not managed appropriately. Because ingested phosphorus exceeds the ability of the failing kidney to excrete this mineral, hyperphosphatemia develops. Initially, this hyperphosphatemia may not be evident on routine biochemical testing, because circulating phosphorous complexes with serum calcium to form calcium phosphate. This chemical reaction decreases serum phosphorus toward normal levels. The resulting hypocalcemia is masked by the release of parathyroid hormone, which stimulates bone reabsorption and thus normalizes the serum calcium concentration.

Simultaneous with this process is a decreased production of 1,25-dihydroxyvitamin D from the kidney. As circulating levels of vitamin D fall, there is a reduced absorption of dietary calcium from the gastrointestinal tract. This process also leads to hypocalcemia and subsequent release of parathyroid hormone with resultant bone reabsorption.

This appropriate response of the parathyroid gland to hypocalcemia leads to hypertrophy of the parathyroid gland. The increase in circulating levels of intact parathyroid hormone, and subsequent remodeling of cortical bone if left untreated, leads to renal osteodystrophy. The management of renal osteodystrophy in patients with CRF is twofold. First, it is important to limit the quantity of dietary phosphorus that is available for absorption; and, second, it is crucial to supply an adequate quantity of 1,25-dihydroxyvitamin D.

As renal failure progresses, dietary phosphorus should be limited to 700 mg per 24 hours. This usually requires the patient to meet regularly with the registered dietitian. If hyperparathyroidism persists, dietary phosphorus should be bound in the gastrointestinal tract to prevent absorption. This process is performed preferably with calcium-containing compounds. Table 3 lists the various products available as phosphate-binding agents. These products should be taken with food and should not be taken with iron, because iron will also bind to this product, eliminating its absorption. Historically, aluminum-containing products were used to bind dietary phosphorus. Unfortunately, aluminum can also be absorbed and deposited in bones of patients with CRF, leading to a second form of metabolic bone disease, namely, osteomalacia or low-turnover bone disease.

1,25-Dihydroxyvitamin D, along with parathyroid hormone, should be measured two to three times yearly in patients with a GFR less than 30 mL per minute. If 1,25-dihydroxyvitamin D levels are low or if intact PTH levels are elevated, patients should be treated with 1,25-dihydroxyvitamin D. Initial therapy is typically 25 μg orally each day. Once treatment is initiated, serum calcium levels need to be followed to avoid hypercalcemia. PTH levels should be followed quarterly with a goal of maintaining an intact level less than 200 pg per mL. If subsequent measurements indicate a rise in immunoreactive PTH despite treatment, the dose should be increased by 25 μg at quarterly intervals.

Acidosis

The kidney is responsible for elimination of "titratable" acids. These acids are a by-product of metabolism of dietary proteins, typically in the form of phosphoric and sulfuric acid. As the kidney fails and is unable to excrete these acids, blood pH and serum bicarbonate values fall. This decrease in pH can be buffered by bony hydroxyapatite, once again leading to a disturbance in the normal bony architecture. To prevent this occurrence, patients with carbon dioxide levels of less than 20 mEq per liter should be treated with either sodium bicarbonate or sodium citrate. Sodium bicarbonate is typically administered in the form of 650-mg tablets, one to two three times daily. Primary side effects are early satiety and belching. Sodium citrate is usually better tolerated and is given in a dose of 1 tablespoonful one to three times daily. Care must be taken to avoid the prescription of potassium citrate, because patients cannot tolerate this potassium load.

Hypervolemia

Patients with CRF experience retention of both sodium and water, leading to edema and hypertension. This problem can be aggravated by underlying hypoalbuminemia from either malnutrition or the nephrotic syndrome. Therapy should be aimed at decreasing dietary intake of sodium and water. Patients with a GFR of 15 to 30 should be placed on a 2- to 4-gram sodium-restricted diet with 1500 to 2000 mL of fluid restriction. Diuretics should be titrated to affect. When GFR is less than 30 mL per minute, mono-therapy with thiazide diuretics is not efficacious. However, when these agents are combined with agents such as bumetanide (Bumex), furosemide (Lasix), or torsemide (Demadex), these agents are synergistic and provide a significant diuresis. Care must be taken to avoid hypovolemia, because this may accelerate the progression of renal insufficiency.

Malnutrition

CRF is associated with the retention of uremic toxins. These toxins may lead to a significant reduction in nutritional intake and to a resistance to anabolic hormones, a decrease in insulin and growth hormone, and an increase in the level of catabolic hormones.

In addition to protein caloric malnutrition, patients with CRF also are at risk for deficiencies of vitamin B_6, folic acid, vitamin C, iron, and carnitine.

Therefore, dietary intervention is crucial in the management of patients with CRF. The issue of protein restriction was covered elsewhere in this volume. The decision to opt for a very low protein diet is one that needs to be agreed on by the patient and his or her physician. Crucial to success to this program is compliance and close monitoring. For patients who do not wish to pursue such a program, protein restriction (moderate) is used to limit symptoms. For patients with GFR of less than 30 mL per minute, a protein restriction of 0.6 gram per kg is reasonable and tolerated by most patients. This amount of protein restriction usually limits dietary phosphorus to less than 700 mg per 24 hours. Thirty-five kilocalories per kg per day is appropriate for patients with CRF. Patients with CRF are at high risk for atherosclerosis; therefore, it is recommended that patients' diet be limited to less than 30% of calories from fat and less than 10% from saturated fat with less than 300 mg per day of cholesterol. As part of the initial evaluation, total cholesterol, high-density lipoproteins, low-density lipoproteins, and triglycerides should be assayed and managed accordingly.

Hyperkalemia

The kidney is the main route for potassium elimination. As the kidney fails, life-threatening hyperkalemia may develop. This hyperkalemia may develop as a result of (1) decreased excretion; (2) cellular shifts; (3) metabolic acidosis accompanying CRF; (4) administration of drugs, such as ACE inhibitors, beta blockers, or aldactazide (Aldactone); or (5) excessive dietary intake.

Patients with CRF should receive no more than 70 mEq of dietary potassium per day. If hyperkalemia develops, dietary intake should be reviewed. Drugs that lead to hyperkalemia, such as ACE inhibitors or

TABLE 3. **Products Used to Bind Dietary Phosphate**

• Calcium citrate	• Aluminum hydroxide
• Calcium carbonate	• Aluminum carbonate
• Calcium acetate	

beta blockers, may need to be changed. As mentioned earlier, the acidosis of CRF should be aggressively treated. For patients with evidence of volume overload, diuretics can be added to increase tubular secretion of potassium. Potassium-binding resins can be used in the gastrointestinal tract to bind potassium. Sodium polystyrene sulfonate (SPS) is typically mixed with 70% sorbitol to avoid constipation. Depending on the degree of hyperkalemia, sodium polystyrene, 15 to 30 grams one to three times daily, may be given.

Prevention of Additional Insults

The patient with CRF has little renal reserve. Care must be taken to avoid additional insults to the kidney. It is imperative to avoid hypovolemia either from the aggressive use of diuretics or secondary to a gastrointestinal illness, manifested as diarrhea or vomiting. The physician caring for these patients should have a lower threshold for the intravenous administration of fluids than for those patients who possess normal kidney function.

Nephrotoxic drugs need to be avoided if at all possible. Patients with CRF depend on the presence of vasodilatory prostaglandins to maintain renal blood flow. The use of nonsteroidal anti-inflammatory agents will block the production of these prostaglandins leading to acute renal failure. If not discovered, this may lead to a rapid need for dialysis. Alternative agents must be used in this patient population. Other nephrotoxic agents such as radiocontrast agents and aminoglycosides should be avoided if at all possible. Urinary tract infections should be treated aggressively so as not to compromise any remaining GFR.

Ensuring a Smooth Transition

Patients with CRF will progress to ESRD unless age or intercurrent illness intervenes. As GFR progresses, it is important for the patient and the patient's family that a smooth transition occur between the pre-ESRD years and those that necessitate either dialysis or transplantation.

As the patient's native kidney fails, attention should focus on which type of renal replacement therapy the patient will require in the future. For those patients who are otherwise healthy, especially for those individuals younger than 65 years of age, renal transplantation is the treatment of choice. Historically, patients were started on either hemodialysis or peritoneal dialysis before initiating the transplant evaluation process. This does not make practical, physiologic, or economic sense. Patients with a GFR less than 20 mL per minute who may be potential candidates for renal transplantation should be referred to a transplant center for evaluation. In some areas of the country, the waiting time for a cadaveric renal transplant is 4 to 5 years; thus it is advantageous to accumulate waiting time before the need for dialysis. For those patients who have a family member or friend who wishes to donate a kidney, they,

too, should be evaluated at this time. It is preferable to perform the evaluation on the recipient and the donor far in advance of the time of anticipated transplantation.

Once evaluation is complete, the surgery should be performed on an elective basis before the patient becomes symptomatic from uremia. This typically occurs with GFRs between 8 and 15 mL per minute. For patients who are not candidates for renal transplantation or for those patients who do not have a donor available before dialysis, the education process on dialytic modality selection should be initiated well in advance of the need for dialysis. Ideally this should occur 12 to 18 months before the need for dialysis therapy. For patients who chose hemodialysis, every effort should be made to place an arterial venous native fistula in the nondominant arm. This process should be started approximately 12 months before the need for hemodialysis. This time allows for adequate maturation of the fistula and for repetitive attempts if the initial access fails. For patients who elect hemodialysis, the patient should be instructed not to allow phlebotomy or blood pressure measurements on the nondominant arm so as to avoid irreversible damage to these veins—thus precluding placement of an arteriovenous native fistula.

For patients who cannot have an arteriovenous native fistula placed because of poor arterial inflow or poor venous outflow, a synthetic bridge graft should be placed 6 to 8 weeks before the start of hemodialysis.

Patients who chose peritoneal dialysis should have all inguinal and ventral hernias repaired preferably 12 to 18 months before needing peritoneal dialysis. A peritoneal dialysis catheter is usually inserted 4 to 6 weeks before starting treatment.

If managed appropriately, patients will undergo transition from the pre-ESRD years to the ESRD years without requiring hospitalization. The patient's venous access should be in place and functioning, a dialysis center should be selected, and therapy should be initiated on an elective basis.

This approach has been shown to decrease the patient's anxiety, to decrease the morbidity associated with the initiation of dialysis, and, in this era of cost containment, to have a substantial cost savings during the first year of the dialysis therapy.

MALIGNANT TUMORS OF THE UROGENITAL TRACT

method of
WILLIAM J. ELLIS, M.D.
University of Washington School of Medicine
Seattle, Washington

PROSTATE CANCER
Epidemiology

Prostate cancer is the most common cancer in men and the second leading cause of cancer death in men.

Histologic evidence of prostate carcinoma is found in approximately 30% of men at age 60 years and in more than 50% of men at age 80 years. The natural history of prostate cancer is long. Most men with prostate carcinoma do not die of their disease. Due to the high prevalence of this disease, however, the death rate is significant. By far the most common histologic pattern of prostate carcinoma is that of adenocarcinoma. Other histologic variants, such as small cell carcinoma or endometroid carcinoma, can originate in the prostate. As those tumors are quite rare, they are not discussed in this article.

Diagnosis

Most men with clinically localized prostate carcinoma are asymptomatic. Locally advanced disease presents with bladder outlet obstruction. Symptomatic bone metastases are a late presentation of prostate cancer. For most of the past century the mainstay of prostate cancer detection has been digital rectal examination. Unfortunately, many tumors are not detected by digital rectal examination until they are locally advanced or have developed metastasis and are not amenable to cure by local therapy. There are no digital rectal examination–based screening studies that show a survival benefit for those patients screened.

In the 1980s, the prostate-specific antigen (PSA) test was developed. PSA is a 33 kDa serine protease specific to prostate epithelial cells. The function of this enzyme is to lyse the seminal coagulum. Levels of PSA in the ejaculate are approximately 1 million times those in the serum. Serum PSA can be used as a marker of prostate disease. An elevated PSA level increases a patient's risk for prostate carcinoma. As the marker is not specific for prostate cancer, however, there are many false-positive results with this test. PSA velocity, free/total PSA ratios, age-specific PSA levels, and PSA density can all give additional insight concerning the risk of prostate cancer. Controversy surrounds the use of PSA for prostate cancer screening. The introduction of PSA into clinical practice has resulted in a stage migration, with most prostate cancers now detected at an earlier stage than those in previous decades. After the initial use of PSA in clinical practice, there were concerns that overdetection would result. Indeed, in the early 1990s prostate cancer detection skyrocketed. The incidence of prostate cancer has now stabilized, however, at a level consistent with the historical incidence of prostate carcinoma. Sufficient time has not yet passed to determine if earlier detection will lead to lower death rates for prostate cancer. An entire discussion of the pros and cons of PSA screening for prostate carcinoma is beyond the scope of this article.

Digital rectal examination and PSA are complementary tests for the diagnosis of prostate cancer. Either an abnormal digital rectal examination or an abnormal PSA level should be followed by biopsy in those patients who are candidates for treatment. Biopsy of the prostate is performed under transrectal ultrasound guidance. For those patients with a life expectancy of less than 10 years, prostate cancer screening is not warranted.

Staging

Prostate cancer typically spreads locally to the periprostatic soft tissue and seminal vesicles or through lymphatic and hematogenous routes to regional and distant lymph nodes or the bone marrow. Visceral metastases are less common. Estimates of the extent of the disease can be made from nomograms or tables based on the digital rectal examination, serum PSA level, and Gleason grade of the tumor. When the probability of metastatic disease is high, computed tomography (CT), magnetic resonance imaging (MRI), or bone scans may be obtained to rule out distant disease. In general, bone scans are not warranted unless the Gleason score is greater than 8 or the PSA level is greater than 10 mg per mL. CT and MRI scans are not indicated unless the PSA level is greater than 20 mg per mL. Radiolabeled antibody scans (Prostascint) are available to look for distant metastases. The relatively poor sensitivity and specificity of these scans, however, do not warrant their use in routine clinical staging of prostate carcinoma.

Treatment Options

Local Disease

A wide variety of options are available for the treatment of clinically localized prostate carcinoma. For men with a life expectancy of less than 10 years, observation or watchful waiting is a very reasonable option as relatively few men with clinically localized prostate carcinoma will die of the disease within a 10-year period. On the other hand, most men with life expectancies of greater than 10 years will opt for definitive local therapy. There is a subset of men with low-volume, low-grade cancer for whom close observation is a reasonable course of action. As these men are candidates for treatment should their disease become more significant, they should be monitored every 6 months with a serum PSA level test and every 1 to 2 years with repeat prostate needle biopsies.

Radical Prostatectomy

Radical prostatectomy is complete removal of the prostate and seminal vesicles. Radical prostatectomy may be accomplished through either a retropubic or a perineal approach. The retropubic approach is often combined with a pelvic lymphadenectomy for staging purposes. If metastatic disease is identified in the pelvic lymph nodes, cure with radical prostatectomy is rare, so the prostate is rarely removed in this situation.

The major complications of radical prostatectomy are incontinence and impotence. The technique of prostatectomy has evolved significantly over the past 20 years and has resulted in decreased blood loss, shorter operating times, shorter hospital stays, and fewer long-term complications. Incontinence rates after radical prostatectomy range from 5 to 40%. In most series from experienced surgeons, the rates are in the 5 to 10% range. The type of incontinence observed is stress incontinence. This means that men are continent during most normal activities but exhibit incontinence during coughing, sneezing, lifting, and vigorous physical activity. In patients with severe incontinence, artificial urinary sphincters can be implanted around the bulbous urethra to provide continence.

Before 1980, essentially all men undergoing radical prostatectomy were impotent after the procedure due to damage to the cavernosal nerves. A nerve-sparing technique was subsequently developed that allowed reservation of potency. Because the nerves are closely applied to the prostatic capsule, the point of dissection is very close to the prostatic capsule. This technique should not be performed on a side of the prostate where the prostate nodule deforms the shape of the capsule or where biopsy specimens indicate that extensive disease is present. In these situations, the nerve-sparing approach increases the likelihood of incompletely resecting a tumor. The rates of potency following nerve-sparing prostatectomy range from 30 to 70%. Rates are higher with the bilateral nerve-sparing than with the unilateral nerve-sparing procedure. The age of the patient and preoperative erectile function also are associated with postoperative potency. The perioperative mortality rate of this operation is less than 0.5%.

After radical prostatectomy, patients are monitored with digital rectal examination and PSA testing semiannually for 5 years and annually thereafter. Because PSA is produced only by cells of prostatic epithelial origin, the serum PSA level should decrease to undetectable levels after successful prostatectomy. With rare exceptions, detectable PSA levels after radical prostatectomy indicate residual or recurrent disease. Digital rectal examinations are included to detect those rare cases of non-PSA–producing recurrences that are primarily small cell (neuroendocrine) tumors.

External Beam Radiation

Prostate cancer may also be treated with external beam radiation therapy. External beam radiation is delivered in small fractions over a 5- to 7-week period. Photons are used for standard radiation therapy. Traditional application of external beam radiation has been with a four-field technique, with beams being directed in the anteroposterior and lateral directions. Damage to adjacent organs, namely, the bladder and rectum, is the dose-limiting factor for external beam radiation. Most patients experience some transient cystitis and proctitis near the end of their treatment course. In 10 to 15% of patients these symptoms may be permanent. Impotence develops in approximately 50% of men after external beam radiation therapy. Newer conformal techniques include additional portals and decreased dose of radia-

tion to the rectum. Conformal radiation allows a higher dose of radiation to be applied to the prostate while minimizing the side effects. It appears that this higher dose of radiation is associated with higher long-term cure rates for clinically localized carcinoma.

Heavy particle irradiation with protons and neutrons has also been evaluated in recent years. Proton radiation is associated with a Bragg's peak of energy release that allows the photon energy to be focused very precisely. Although this tight focusing does have advantages in terms of limiting the dose of radiation to nearby structures, the tight margins may not provide adequate dosimetry to the entire prostate. Standard photon irradiation is usually combined with proton irradiation to provide wider radiation fields. There are no published reports of long-term cancer control after the proton irradiation of the prostate. At this time, this treatment should still be considered investigational. Neutron irradiation of prostate cancer improves cell kill in vivo. Clinically, this treatment results in greater damage to normal tissues. This modality should be limited to patients with bulky disease for whom there may be a therapeutic advantage over standard photon therapy.

After external beam radiation, patients should be followed up with digital rectal examination and PSA determination as after radical prostatectomy. Because the prostate remains in place, there is usually some residual prostate epithelium that secretes PSA. The precise level of the PSA nadir that corresponds to a favorable outcome is not known, but a PSA nadir below 1.0 ng per mL is desirable. A stable PSA level should be maintained once the nadir is reached. The current definition of biochemical failure after radiation treatment is three consecutive rises in serum PSA.

Prostate Brachytherapy

Prostate brachytherapy as now practiced in most medical centers involves the transperineal placement of permanent iodine or palladium seeds into the prostate under ultrasonic guidance. The radiation sources can be delivered in a single outpatient session. With the radiation source directly in the prostate, the irradiation dose to the prostate can be maximized while the radiation to the adjacent structures can be minimized. In men with high-grade disease, higher PSA levels (>10 to 15 ng per mL), or bulky disease, who are thought to be at higher risk for extracapsular extension or seminal vesicle invasion, treatment with external beam radiation for 4 to 5 weeks followed by seed implant "boost" to the prostate is the preferred brachytherapy technique. Although studies have not documented an improved cancer control rate with the combined therapy, the technique does provide therapeutic radiation dosimetry to a larger area than monotherapy seed implants.

The major morbid features of prostate brachytherapy are obstructive and irritative voiding symptoms. The prostatic urethra receives a much higher dose of radiation with this technique than with external beam therapy. All men experience these symptoms to some degree, usually for several months. From 10 to 20% of men will develop transient urinary retention. Proctitis is generally less than that seen with external beam radiation. Impotence ranges from 20 to 50%, depending on a patient's age and pretreatment erectile status. These data appear to be improved over standard external radiation, possibly due to the younger age of men seeking brachytherapy treatment.

Advanced Disease

Hormonal therapy has been the main treatment for advanced prostate cancer for the past 60 years. Androgen withdrawal produces a clinical response in 80 to 90% of men with advanced prostate cancer. Bilateral orchiectomy effectively reduces the serum testosterone levels because approximately 90% of systemic androgens are produced by the testicles and another 10% by the adrenal glands. Medical castration can also be attained through the administration of estrogen or luteinizing hormone–releasing hormone (LHRH) agonists. Both of these treatments suppress LH release, resulting in suppression of serum testosterone levels into the castrate range. Higher dose estrogen treatment has been associated with cardiovascular side effects. Oral antiandrogens are available to block the 10% of androgens produced by the adrenal glands. These agents may be useful in the first month of LHRH therapy to block the testosterone flare associated with LHRH therapy. These agents, however, do not improve patient survival when used in conjunction with orchiectomy. The major complications of hormone therapy are hot flashes, impotence, loss of libido, weight gain, decreased energy levels, and osteoporosis. Hot flashes are best controlled by oral megestrol (Megace).*

Ultimately, all advanced prostate cancers progress to androgen independence. There is great debate about whether the physician should begin hormonal therapy as soon as a patient fails local therapy or is detected with advanced disease or whether one should wait until the patient develops symptomatic metastasis. There are no available studies that adequately address this question. The current trend is to treat men earlier. Whether early treatment prolongs survival or hastens the onset of androgen independence is unknown. A relatively recent concept is that of intermittent androgen suppression. Prostate cancer is driven into remission with approximately 9 months of hormonal suppression. Therapy is then withdrawn until the disease reappears. This therapy is currently undergoing clinical trials.

When patients develop hormone refractory disease, they are treated with second-line therapies, primarily chemotherapy and further hormonal manipulation. Most of these agents show only modest efficacy with prostate carcinoma and rarely produce complete remissions. Life expectancy after the patient develops hormone refractory disease is less than 2 years.

---

*Not FDA approved for this indication.

TRANSITIONAL CELL CARCINOMA

Epidemiology

Transitional epithelium lines the urinary tract from the renal calyces to the penile urethra. The most common site of transitional cell carcinoma is the urinary bladder. This is thought to be due to prolonged contact with carcinogens in the urine. The major risk factor for transitional cell carcinoma is smoking. Synchronous and metachronous tumors are common in transitional cell carcinoma.

Diagnosis

Transitional cell carcinoma may be broadly categorized as upper tract, including the renal pelves and ureters, and lower tract, comprising the bladder and urethra. Transitional cell carcinoma typically presents with hematuria, although some patients present with persistent irritative voiding symptoms. Evaluation of hematuria involves an intravenous pyelogram and cystourethroscopy. Suspicious lesions in the bladder can be biopsied during cystoscopy. If an upper tract filling defect is noted on intravenous pyelogram, then the diagnosis can be confirmed with urethroscopy. If the filling defect is clearly a tumor, however, and not a benign condition, then ureteroscopy is not necessary.

Treatment

Lower Tract Tumors

For papillary transitional cell carcinoma, transurethral resection of the bladder tumor is the mainstay of treatment. Although complete excision of the primary lesion is generally possible in low-grade superficial tumors, the rate of recurrence is on the order of 50 to 70%. For this reason, patients must be monitored for recurrence with periodic urinalysis, cystoscopy, and intravenous pyelograms. The newer tests of urinary antigens associated with bladder tumors may also play a role in monitoring for recurrent disease. For those patients with multiple recurrences of superficial bladder cancer, intravesical therapy may be warranted. Approximately 10% of patients progress to invasive disease.

Carcinoma in situ of the bladder is a flat, high-grade tumor that exhibits an aggressive behavior. Diagnosis can be difficult and is often made only after biopsy prompted by a positive cytology in an otherwise normal-appearing bladder. These flat lesions cannot be resected. Some form of intravesical therapy is required to eradicate this disease.

Intravesical therapy may be either immunotherapy or chemotherapy. The immunotherapeutic agent currently used is bacille Calmette-Guèrin (BCG). This treatment is believed to stimulate an immune response in the bladder that eradicates existing tumor and prevents the development of recurrent disease. Most initial courses of intravesical therapy involve one treatment every week for 6 weeks. There is evidence that maintenance therapy with periodic

3-week courses of BCG for up to 2 years may decrease recurrence of carcinoma in situ. BCG therapy can be associated with severe frequency and dysuria. If the bacillus is disseminated into the bloodstream, systemic infection results, and patients require treatment with antituberculous drugs. The chemotherapeutic and intravesical agents include thiotepa, mitomycin,* doxorubicin, and valrubicin (Valstar). Valrubicin is indicated only in cases of BCG failure. The other agents appear to be less efficacious than BCG, but are better tolerated.

Muscle-invasive tumors, select high-grade tumors invading the lamina propria (T1 tumors), and refractory carcinoma in situ are indications for a radical cystectomy. If the tumor involves the prostatic urethra, then a urethrectomy should also be performed. The simplest technique of urinary diversion is ileal conduit. These patients require an ostomy bag to collect the urine. For those patients in good health, a variety of alternative urinary diversions are available in which a larger segment of small or large bowel is used to create new urinary reservoirs. The reservoirs are then connected to the abdominal wall by means of a continent catheterizable urinary stoma or to the urethra in which case the patient voids by a Valsalva maneuver. Approximately 20% of patients with an orthotopic bladder connected to the urethra experience nighttime incontinence. In addition, some of these patients will require intermittent catheterization as they are unable to generate sufficient pressure to completely empty the neobladder. The longer bowel segments required for creation of all types of urinary reservoirs can produce permanent loose stools.

Combined chemoradiation approaches have been explored for muscle-invasive bladder cancer. Some efficacy has been demonstrated with this approach, which preserves the bladder. The approach should be considered investigational, however, until randomized clinical trials can be completed comparing the treatment with radical cystectomy.

Upper Tract Disease

Upper tract transitional cell carcinoma tends to seed downstream into the lower ureter and bladder. A distal ureteral tumor may be treated with distal ureterectomy and ureteral reimplantation. Proximal ureteral tumors and renal pelvic tumors, however, usually require a nephroureterectomy with complete removal of the ureter and a small cuff of bladder for adequate treatment. When the patient has a solitary kidney, additional effort is made to preserve the remaining kidney. In select cases, papillary tumors may be treated with endoscopic or open excision and fulguration. BCG therapy may be delivered to the upper tracts by means of a percutaneous nephrostomy tube to treat high-grade lesions or carcinoma in situ, although the risk of systemic BCG dissemination is considerably higher than that associated with intravesical treatments.

Metastatic Disease

Systemic chemotherapy is administered to patients with evidence of metastatic disease. The most common regimen used currently is one of methotrexate,* vinblastine (Velban)*, cisplatin (Platinol), and doxorubicin. Unfortunately, many elderly patients with metastatic transitional cell carcinoma are unable to tolerate the full dose of the treatment with these agents. Paclitaxel (Taxol)* based therapies are less toxic, but the efficacy of these treatments is still being defined.

RENAL CELL CARCINOMA

Renal cell carcinoma is a clear cell tumor originating from the proximal tubule cells. The disease occurs more frequently in males. Smoking is the major environmental risk factor associated with renal cell carcinoma. The genetics of renal cell carcinoma are in the process of being characterized. Those patients with von Hippel-Lindau disease, an autosomal dominant trait, are at increased risk for the development of renal cell carcinomas. Mutations in chromosome 3p have been identified in patients with von Hippel-Lindau disease, as well as in patients with sporadic renal cell carcinoma.

Diagnosis

Traditionally patients with renal cell carcinoma presented with the triad of flank pain, hematuria, and an abdominal mass. With widespread availability of modern imaging techniques, many renal cell carcinomas are discovered incidentally or during evaluation of vague abdominal complaints. Distinction between complex cysts and cystic renal neoplasms can be difficult. Fine-cut CT scans with and without contrast are invaluable in making this distinction. If the suspicion of malignancy is low, serial evaluation with CTs or ultrasound imaging is warranted. If the suspicion for malignancy is high, then renal exploration is indicated.

Treatment

The treatment of localized renal cell carcinoma is radical nephrectomy. Nodal tissue along the renal hilum should be excised with the nephrectomy specimen. The tumor may extend as a tumor thrombus into the renal vein or vena cava. In most cases this tumor does not invade into the wall of the vessels and can be surgically removed. Removal of tumors with vena caval thrombi can be curative. The risk of metastatic disease, however, increases with the extent of the tumor thrombus. Metastatic renal cell carcinoma is a difficult treatment problem. The tumor is very refractory to traditional chemotherapeutic drugs. Radiation is only modestly effective for palliation of local symptoms. Interferon-α* and in-

---

*Not FDA approved for this indication.

*Not FDA approved for this indication.

terleukin-2 show modest efficacy against this tumor. In most cases these treatments are administered in the setting of a protocol.

PENILE CARCINOMA

Penile carcinoma is a relatively rare malignancy in the United States and Europe, but comprises approximately 10% of male malignancies in South America and Africa. The peak incidence of this tumor is in the seventh decade and beyond. Circumcision appears to have a protective effect, as the disease is extremely rare in those who have been circumcised in infancy. There is also an association with herpes simplex virus and human papillomavirus 18 infection. Penile carcinoma presents as an exophytic mass on the penis. Often there is a delay of presentation to the physician because of embarrassment on the part of the patient. Extensive lesions colonize with anaerobic bacteria and may be foul-smelling. The tumor can sometimes be confused with condyloma acuminatum, bowenoid papulosis, and Buschke-Lowenstein giant condylomata. Erythroplasia of Queyrat and Bowen's disease are premalignant lesions.

Treatment of the primary disease is local excision. For those lesions confined to the prepuce, circumcision alone is adequate. Small, noninvasive lesions are treated with local excision. Buck's fascia provides a productive barrier against invasion into the corporal bodies. Tumors that invade Buck's fascia must be treated with a partial penectomy. A 2-cm margin beyond all gross disease should be obtained, and the presence of a clear histologic margin should be confirmed by examination of frozen sections. If the resection will leave only a minimal amount of penis, then total penectomy is indicated.

Penile tumors drain through the inguinal lymph nodes. Invasive tumors or high-grade superficial tumors require superficial inguinal lymph node dissections. Patients with palpable nodes or positive superficial inguinal nodes require deep inguinal lymph node dissections as well as pelvic lymph node dissections. Attention to detail in this lymph node dissection is crucial, as this is one of the few tumors in which metastatic disease can be cured by surgical excision alone.

More advanced disease is treated with chemotherapeutic agents. Bleomycin (Blenoxane), 5-fluorouracil,* and methotrexate* have all been used with some success. Radiation therapy can also be used for palliation and locally recurrent disease.

---

*Not FDA approved for this indication.

ANTERIOR URETHRAL STRICTURE

method of
KENNETH W. ANGERMEIER, M.D.
Cleveland Clinic Foundation
Cleveland, Ohio

In the male, the anterior urethra is the segment encompassed by the corpus spongiosum and consists of three divisions: glanular, pendulous (penile), and bulbous. The membranous and prostatic divisions make up the posterior urethra (Figure 1). Within the pendulous urethra, the urethra lies near the central portion of the corpus spongiosum. More proximally, the bulbous urethra is located progressively closer to the dorsal aspect of the corpus spongiosum up to the bulbomembranous junction. A stricture is a urethral scar that occurs as a result of tissue injury. Scars tend to contract over time. Because the urethra is a tubular structure, circumferential contraction may occur and lead to luminal narrowing. The degree of scarring of the corpus spongiosum (spongiofibrosis) associated with a urethral stricture is an important factor in determining the probability of success of various treatment modalities.

The cause of anterior urethral strictures has changed over the years. In the past, gonococcal urethritis was most commonly implicated. With the advent of more effective antibiotic therapy, external trauma to the penis or perineum and urethral instrumentation have emerged as the most frequent causes today. Many times the trauma may be unrecognized or forgotten, and the patient presents years later with the insidious onset of voiding symptoms. Alternatively, acute trauma can result in significant urethral injury or disruption, leading to a dense or obliterative stricture.

A patient generally begins to notice urinary symptoms when the urethral caliber decreases to approximately No. 14 to 15 French, which represents a luminal diameter of 4.5 to 5 mm. The most common symptom described by a patient with a urethral stricture is a decreased urinary stream. When this happens gradually, a patient may not pay much attention for many years, with the belief that this is "normal" for him. Urinary retention can occur but is relatively uncommon. Unexplained or recurrent epididymitis, particularly in a young patient, may also be a presenting complaint. This often indicates an anatomic abnormality of the urinary tract, and a urethral stricture should be considered in the differential diagnosis. Recurrent urinary tract infections may also occur in patients

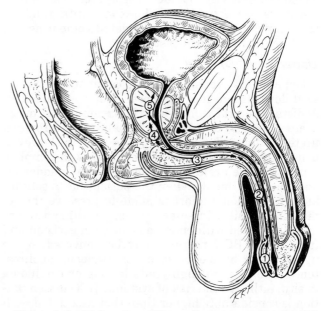

Figure 1. Sagittal section of the urethra enumerating the divisions of the urethra: (1) glanular, (2) pendulous or penile, (3) bulbous, (4) membranous, and (5) prostatic. (From Devine CJ Jr, Angermeier KW: Anatomy of the penis and male perineum. AUA Update Series, *13*:11, 1994, with permission.)

with a urethral stricture, but this is not a consistent finding as some patients will have no documented infections by history. Evaluation for a possible stricture seems reasonable if other causes have not been identified.

Postvoid dribbling or a bloody urethral discharge after voiding may also be reported by some patients. Postvoid dribbling may occur due to pooling of urine in a potentially dilated segment of urethra proximal to the stricture. Urethral bleeding may be seen when high pressures are generated during voiding in the urethra proximal to a narrow stricture, resulting in acute dilation and small lacerations of the mucosa. Spraying of the urinary stream or a "split" stream has often been considered to be a hallmark of a urethral stricture. This occurs most commonly, however, as a consequence of a decreased urinary stream, which can obviously occur for a variety of reasons. It does not seem to be specific for a urethral stricture.

A patient suspected of having a urethral stricture should be referred to a urologist. Evaluation includes a detailed history and physical examination, as well as a urinalysis. A voiding flow rate and postvoid bladder ultrasonography may be considered to document the severity of voiding dysfunction. The definitive diagnosis is made with a retrograde urethrogram or cystoscopy. Flexible cystoscopes have greatly facilitated evaluation of the lower urinary tract in the male, making cystoscopy readily available in the office with minimal patient discomfort. If enough contrast is instilled into the bladder during the retrograde urethrogram, a voiding urethrogram should be obtained to confirm the upper extent of the stricture and to better assess the status of the urethra proximal to it. Transperineal ultrasonography has also been used at some medical centers to image urethral strictures. Its primary role seems to be in establishing the precise length of the stricture and the depth of spongiofibrosis, which may be useful to formulate a treatment plan.

TREATMENT

In the past, patients with a urethral stricture were often managed with the "reconstructive ladder" approach, which implies that treatment begins with the simplest procedure (dilation) and proceeds sequentially as needed to more involved techniques. Internal urethrotomy would usually be employed next, followed by formal urethral reconstruction as a last resort. Further experience and study has shed light on the outcomes of various treatment modalities and correlated them with the initial characteristics of the stricture. This has allowed an "anatomic" approach to the treatment of urethral strictures in which the stricture is initially matched to the procedure with the best chance of providing a good outcome. This approach has improved the outlook for patients with this difficult problem, allowing them to be treated more promptly with a higher rate of success.

For many years, urethral dilation was the mainstay of urethral stricture treatment. It usually required repetition on a regular basis, often with incomplete resolution of symptoms between dilations. We now know that urethral dilation is primarily a method of management for patients who are not candidates for more aggressive surgical intervention. Although the interval of dilation varies, in most cases it must be continued indefinitely to avoid recurrence of the stricture. Infrequently, a patient with minimal

stricture in the form of a urethral mucosal scar and minimal to no spongiofibrosis may be cured by dilation alone. The development of balloon dilating catheters has simplified the dilation of mild to moderately dense strictures. The radial forces exerted by the balloon catheter may lead to less urethral trauma than the shearing forces generated by traditional dilators.

A significant advance in the treatment of urethral strictures occurred in 1972 when Sachse described the technique of direct vision internal urethrotomy (DVIU). This procedure gained popularity rapidly and remains one of the most common procedures used to treat a urethral stricture. An endoscopic urethrotome is passed transurethrally and the stricture visualized. A small knife is then used to incise the stricture, usually at the 12 o'clock position. Ventrolateral incisions are sometimes preferred in the proximal bulbous urethra due to the paucity of corpus spongiosum dorsally. The incision needs to be carried completely through the stricture into healthy corpus spongiosum to be effective. A catheter is left indwelling for 1 to 5 days.

Early on, it was recognized that there were some patients who did not respond to DVIU or who needed to have it done repeatedly. More recent studies have tried to clarify which patients are optimal candidates for this procedure. In 1996, Pansadoro and colleagues and Albers and coworkers reported long-term success rates of 42% and 65.7%, respectively, for bulbous urethral strictures treated with DVIU. In both studies, the success rate increased to approximately 70% if the stricture was less than 1 cm in length. Success rates diminish significantly with repeat procedures and longer strictures. Therefore, DVIU seems to be best suited for relatively short strictures with mild spongiofibrosis.

If the initial attempt at DVIU fails, the patient should be reassessed radiographically and endoscopically. If these studies show some improvement from baseline, the procedure may be repeated. If there is significant scarring of the mucosa and deep spongiofibrosis, however, open urethral reconstruction should be considered. For patients who are not good medical candidates for open surgery, DVIU followed by intermittent self-dilation may help maintain patency of the urethra for a longer period of time.

The intraurethral stent (Urolume Endoprosthesis, American Medical Systems, Minnetonka, Minnesota) is an option for patients with a recurrent anterior urethral stricture. The stent is a braided mesh cylinder made of biocompatible superalloy wire, which exerts gentle radial pressure to keep the urethral lumen expanded after either urethral dilation or DVIU. It may be used for strictures in the bulbous urethra that are no longer than 3 cm in length (up to 5 cm with two stents) and at least 1 cm away from the external urethral sphincter. Suboptimal results seem to occur when the stent is used in areas of dense spongiofibrosis and possibly in the setting of post-traumatic and posturethroplasty strictures. For properly selected patients, the overall success rate is approximately 80%. Although there are certainly those who may benefit from the intraurethral stent, its role in the long-term management of patients with a recurrent urethral stricture remains to be determined completely.

Open urethral reconstruction remains the procedure of choice for urethral strictures associated with dense spongiofibrosis and those that have recurred after more conservative forms of treatment. There are a variety of surgical techniques available to the reconstructive surgeon, depending on the length, location, and density of the stricture. The optimal procedure, when feasible, is excision of the urethral scar with a primary urethral anastomosis. Because of restrictions on mobilization of the two ends of the urethra, this procedure is limited to bulbous urethral strictures of 2.5 cm or less in length. As with most operations on the bulbous urethra, the patient is carefully placed in the exaggerated lithotomy position to expose the perineum. Through a perineal incision, the corpus spongiosum is mobilized and the stricture identified with a bougie or sound. The corpus spongiosum and urethra are then transected at the site of the stricture, and all scar tissue is excised. The proximal and distal ends of the urethra are mobilized and spatulated. A tension-free urethral anastomosis is then performed. A urethral catheter is left indwelling for 3 weeks, and the patient may also have a suprapubic catheter for urinary diversion during the same time. With this approach, long-term success rates approaching 95% can be reliably achieved.

For patients with longer strictures of the bulbous urethra or disease involving the pendulous urethra, some form of substitution urethroplasty is performed. This technique consists of initial exposure of the urethra, followed by longitudinal incision through the entire length of the stricture to open it. The incision is carried into healthy urethra proximally and distally. The urethral wall is then reconstructed with a graft or a flap, depending on the situation. The most commonly used grafts are a buccal mucosa graft or a full-thickness penile or preputial skin graft. Grafts are most useful when a well-vascularized host bed is available. Flaps are developed as penile skin islands, which are mobilized and transferred along with their underlying blood supply in the form of a dartos fascia pedicle. Penile island flaps may be configured in a variety of ways, depending on the length and location of the stricture, and can be used throughout the entire anterior urethra. If a graft is not feasible due to a scarred host bed and local penile skin is not available, a hairless scrotal island flap may be effective as well. It is generated in similar fashion with an intact underlying dartos fascia pedicle. The long-term results with scrotal skin, however, do not seem to be quite as good as those with penile skin.

On the basis of the aforementioned principles, the majority of patients with an anterior urethral stricture can now be treated with a high degree of success, sparing them the discomfort and inconvenience of repeated procedures. With ongoing clinical and research efforts, new treatment techniques will undoubtedly continue to emerge in the future.

RENAL CALCULI

method of
LARRY C. MUNCH, M.D.
University of Kentucky Medical Center
Lexington, Kentucky

Renal and ureteral stones develop in nearly 10% of Americans and are the third most common affliction of the urinary tract (behind urinary tract infections and prostate disease). Signs and symptoms of stone disease usually develop in the fourth and fifth decades. Approximately two times as many males as females are afflicted with urolithiasis. White people develop stones nearly three times as often as African-Americans. In patients in whom no adjustments are made after a first stone passes or is otherwise removed, the recurrence rate is approximately 50%. Although long-term morbidity is uncommon, short-term disability is significant. With the development of shock wave lithotripsy, fiberoptic ureteroscopes, lasers, and other minimally invasive techniques and devices, morbidity of stone removal has been significantly reduced. Unfortunately, the cost of treating stones with this technology has increased and now approaches $1 billion annually. Understanding the factors that can lead to stone formation and finding ways to modify them should be a part of the evaluative process in patients with stones.

DIAGNOSTIC EVALUATION

Signs and Symptoms

The most common symptom in patients with ureteral calculi is severe, colicky flank pain, often acute and intermittent in nature caused by the spasm of the obstructed ureter. Stones in the lower ureter cause pain radiating around to the groin or testes. Stones near the entrance to the bladder often cause urinary urgency and frequency. Nausea and vomiting are commonly encountered. Hematuria (either gross or microscopic) is found in over 90% of patients with urinary stones. Low-grade fever usually implies a coincidental urinary tract infection, whereas high fevers imply a more serious condition such as pyelonephritis or an intra-abdominal process such as cholecystitis or appendicitis. Unlike patients with an acute abdomen, patients with stone colic move around constantly, unable to get comfortable. The pain can wax and wane as the stone moves down the ureter. Because stone passage can take hours to days, it is not unusual to see patients seemingly get instant pain relief but return with additional bouts of colic.

Unlike stones in the ureter or ureteropelvic junction (UPJ), most stones in the renal pelvis or calyces do not cause pain. These stones rarely cause obstruction and are often incidentally discovered during evaluation of asymptomatic hematuria. Although dull or burning localized discomfort can be caused by stones in calyces, severe colic is not common, and other causes for pain should be considered.

Physical examination usually reveals an increased pulse rate and blood pressure as a result of the pain. Patients may splint to the affected side. Bowel sounds are often decreased; peritoneal signs are usually absent. Costovertebral angle (CVA) tenderness is usually present but is often not as impressive as the degree of pain experienced by the patient. Rebound tenderness usually indicates an intraabdominal process or pyelonephritis and should be evaluated accordingly.

Laboratory Evaluation

Urinalysis uniformly reveals red blood cells. The presence of significant numbers of white blood cells or bacteria is often indicative of an associated urinary tract infection. Urinary pH above 7 might indicate the presence of ureaseproducing bacteria that cause an infection stone. Crystals can be found on microscopic examination and are often representative of the stone composition. A urine culture should be obtained if infection is suspected, both to identify the organism and to direct therapy if standard treatment is ineffective.

A complete blood cell count and a basic metabolic profile should be obtained. The white blood cell count ordinarily is mildly elevated as a result of the pain. A significantly elevated white blood cell count could represent an intraabdominal process or pyelonephritis; a low white blood cell count might be indicative of urosepsis. Serum chemistry studies might identify the hypokalemic, hyperchloremic metabolic acidosis of Type I renal tubular acidosis. Half of affected patients initially present with urolithiasis; this condition usually warrants more urgent medical intervention. A significantly elevated serum calcium level might be indicative of hyperparathyroidism and may also necessitate more urgent medical attention. Results of renal function studies (blood urea nitrogen [BUN], creatinine) are generally normal or slightly elevated because of vomiting and dehydration. Significant elevation is indicative of severe underlying renal disease, an obstructed solitary kidney, or bilateral ureteral obstruction. Even a completely obstructed kidney should not cause a significant rise in creatinine if the contralateral kidney is functioning normally.

Radiographic Evaluation

Spiral computed tomographic (CT) scans have markedly improved the diagnostic accuracy in evaluating flank pain. These noncontrast studies can be performed in minutes with few false-negative results. All urinary stones (except those associated with the AIDS drug indinavir) are radiopaque on CT scan. Stones as small as 2 mm can be identified. Hydronephrosis and perinephric standing are characteristic secondary findings consistent with acute ureteral obstruction. CT scanning immediately identifies congenital absence of a kidney as well as provides a relative assessment of renal size and parenchymal thickness. In addition to detecting urolithiasis, this study can also identify nonurologic causes of pain, including cholelithiasis, appendicitis, and diverticulitis. With a positive CT study, a patient with a urinary calculus can be treated for pain in a much more timely manner. The main limitations of this study are that it does not provide functional information of the kidneys (intravenous pyelography [IVP] can be performed electively after proper preparation at a later time) and it is usually more costly than IVP. Smaller hospitals or physician offices may not have ready access to the high-speed scanners and should continue to rely on IVP.

Until the mid-1990s, the intravenous pyelogram (IVP) was considered to be the gold-standard diagnostic study for the evaluation of possible urinary stones. It remains the study of choice for evaluating function of kidneys and provides an anatomic road map that assists in monitoring patients with known stone disease. In the emergency setting, however, it is of more limited value than CT scanning. False-negative findings occur in 10 to 15% of patients with only minimal obstruction and may delay appropriate therapy. Patients with chronic renal disease and diabetes should probably not be given intravenous contrast.

Ultrasonography is usually not a desirable test in the acute setting, but it can be useful for monitoring the progress of a stone that had previously been associated with obstruction.

MANAGEMENT

Initial management of urolithiasis depends primarily on the severity of symptoms and presence of comorbid factors such as associated fever or infection. The degree of obstruction and the location and size of stones should be documented but are less important in the immediate management. The finding of urinary extravasation caused by a forniceal rupture brought on by high pressures in the upper collecting system also does not necessitate acute intervention unless associated with a urinary tract infection. This condition almost uniformly resolves spontaneously.

In the acute setting after the diagnosis has been made, standard therapy comprises intravenous hydration and pain control. Small distal stones can sometimes be flushed out with the initiation of a brisk diuresis. Acute pain control can be achieved with opioid analgesics such as morphine or meperidine (Demerol) given intravenously. Nonsteroidal anti-inflammatory drugs (NSAIDs) such as ketorolac (Toradol) work synergistically with narcotics. Antiemetics should be used for nausea. If pain can be adequately controlled, the patient is able to tolerate fluids, and no other significant comorbid factors are present, the patient can be managed on an outpatient basis. Oral narcotics such as oxycodone, hydrocodone, and NSAIDs such as naproxen usually decrease the intensity and duration of subsequent colicky attacks. Antibiotics are not routinely given unless a coexisting lower urinary tract infection is being treated. Patients with significant obstruction should be monitored on an outpatient basis weekly or until the hydronephrosis resolves. Patients with persistent hydronephrosis for 3 to 4 weeks should be referred for definitive treatment to prevent significant permanent renal loss from obstruction.

Patients whose pain can be controlled only with parenteral medications, who have a solitary kidney, or who have fever should be admitted for observation. Patients with fever and obstruction should have a urologic consultation for consideration of percutaneous nephrostomy drainage or ureteral stent placement to facilitate drainage of the system. Patients who are unable to achieve adequate pain control while in the hospital after 1 or 2 days should be referred for urologic evaluation.

Factors that determine the outcome of a stone event depend on the stone size and location, anatomic considerations, and stone composition. In general, 85% of stones less than 5 mm in diameter are passed spontaneously with conservative measures. Larger stones or stones that are initially located in the upper ureter (above the pelvic brim) have a much smaller chance of spontaneous passage. Few stones greater than 6 mm are able to pass. However, patients with a history of previous passage of larger stones may well be able to pass stones as large as 8 to 10 mm. Stones associated with obstructive processes such as ureteropelvic junction obstruction or ureteral stricture (usually secondary to previous surgery) have a much lower incidence of spontaneous passage. Most radiopaque stones (>90%) contain calcium and cannot be dissolved. However, patients with stones that are radiolucent (on plain radiographs) or who have passed uric acid stones in the past might be candidates for medical dissolution with alkaline therapy.

Surgical Management

The most common indications for urologic intervention are for treatment of pain that cannot be adequately controlled by either oral or parenteral analgesics and for persistent obstruction. Nearly all stones can be treated with noninvasive modalities, such as shock wave lithotripsy, or with minimally invasive treatments, such as ureteroscopy or percutaneous nephrostolithotomy. The technique chosen depends on many factors such as stone size and location, suspected composition, availability of equipment, and surgical expertise.

Shock wave lithotripsy is a technique employing external acoustic energy that can be focused onto the stone. These forces act on the crystalline substance of the stone to break it apart. These small particles can then pass down the ureter. This technique causes little injury to surrounding tissues and has not been associated with any significant renal damage after long-term follow-up. Occasionally the particles are too large to pass, and a secondary modality is needed either to break them up further or to remove them directly.

Ureteroscopy employs passage of fiberoptic endoscopes directly into the ureter via the bladder. Smaller stones can be grasped in wire baskets and removed intact or can be fragmented into very small particles with laser or electrohydraulic probes.

Percutaneous nephrolithotomy requires insertion of a nephroscope through the flank directly into the renal collecting system. Stones can be removed directly or fragmented into smaller pieces. These smaller pieces can then be directly removed or flushed out of the collecting system. In addition, conditions such as UPJ obstruction can be treated at the same time. This modality usually requires 1- to 2-day hospitalization.

Stones located in the lower ureter (below the pelvic brim) that require intervention can be treated effectively with either shock wave lithotripsy or ureteroscopy. Ureteroscopy is successful 98% of the time but is slightly more invasive than shock wave lithotripsy.

Stones that are in the upper ureter are usually treated with shock wave lithotripsy, although the newer ureteroscopes enable the experienced urologist to treat stones throughout the urinary tract. Stones in the renal pelvis or calyces that are less than 2 cm in diameter are best treated with shock wave lithotripsy. Larger stones or those in the lower pole of the kidney often require multiple shock wave lithotripsy treatments and are not as efficiently passed, and so they are often treated with percutaneous nephrolithotomy, which, although more invasive, is a very efficient method of removing stones. Open surgery is now reserved for large staghorn calculi or for repair of a congenital abnormality such as UPJ obstruction. These procedures are much more invasive and necessitate a significantly longer convalescent period.

Passage of a ureteral stent is often performed in conjunction with any minimally invasive procedure, or it can be employed in a more urgent setting, such as when the stone is associated with infection, pregnancy, or a solitary kidney or when pain cannot be controlled in an acute setting. The stent relieves obstruction, eases colic, and passively dilates the ureter to facilitate stone passage.

Medical Evaluation and Treatment

All patients who pass a stone or require surgical intervention should be counseled in basic preventive measures against recurrences. The most important factor in preventing recurrent stones is to maintain a dilute urine. This can be accomplished by drinking enough fluids to produce 2 to 2.5 liters of urine a day. Maintaining dilute urine alone can reduce recurrences by 50 to 75% in patients with no other risk factors. Unfortunately, most patients lose interest in drinking fluids, and many of these subsequently develop recurrent stones.

Patients who have formed recurrent stones or have bilateral stones, children with stones, African-Americans with stones, patients with a family history of stones, patients with concurrent medical conditions predisposing to stone formation (sarcoidosis, gout, Crohn's disease, or other inflammatory intestinal conditions), and patients with skeletal diseases such as osteoporosis should undergo a metabolic evaluation. All patients with noncalcium stones (e.g., uric acid, cystine, struvite) should also undergo a more thorough evaluation. Studies have shown that the best time to perform this evaluation is approximately 1 month after stone passage or intervention.

A metabolic evaluation consists of at least one 24-hour urine collection with measurements of volume, calcium, oxalate, uric acid, sodium, citric acid, and creatinine with the patient on a regular diet. Blood studies should include serum electrolytes, BUN, creatinine, calcium, phosphorus, and intact parathyroid hormone (PTH) levels. An adequate collection of urine should exhibit 15 to 20 mg per kg per day creatinine excretion for females and 20 to 25 mg per kg per day creatinine excretion for males. If the patient has a personal or family history of cystine stones, a quantitative cystine level should also be obtained.

Hypercalciuria (>250 mg of calcium per 24 hours or 4 mg per kg per day in children) can be subclassified as absorptive, renal leakage, or primary hyperparathyroidism. Patients with hyperparathyroidism need a surgical referral for possible subtotal parathyroidectomy. Treatment of other causes of hypercalciuria initially involves the administration of a thiazide diuretic, which increases calcium reabsorption in the distal tubules. Excessive urinary sodium overcomes this effect; patients must be counseled in the importance of a low-sodium diet. Thiazide treatment results in sustained lower urinary calcium levels in patients with renal leakage hypercalciuria, whereas patients with absorptive hypercalicuria (90% of patients with hypercalciuria) lose this effect over time. A more selective therapy employing a slow-release potassium phosphate preparation (UroPhos-K) appears to maintain normal urinary calcium levels in patients with absorptive hypercalciuria for extended periods of time and may be a useful adjunct in these patients.

Citrate is now recognized as one of the most potent urinary inhibitors of urolithiasis. It combines with urinary calcium to form a very soluble compound, limits calcium oxalate crystal aggregation, and raises urinary pH to increase solubility of both uric acid and cystine crystals. Hypocitraturia (<350 mg of citrate per 24 hours) is commonly identified in patients with recurrent stones and may be associated with other metabolic abnormalities. Currently, preferred treatment of hypocitraturia is with potassium citrate (Urocit-K) supplementation. The sodium-containing forms of citrate (Bicitra, Polycitra) do not have the same beneficial effects because the excess sodium in these preparations actually aggravates both hypercalciuria and hyperuricosuria. Natural sources of citrate are citrus fruits. Lemons contain the most concentrated form of citrate and, when provided as lemonade, can increase both fluid volume and citrate excretion.

Hyperuricosuria (>750 mg per day) can result both in primary uric acid stones (when the urine pH is <6) and in calcium oxalate crystallization by the process of heterogeneous nucleation. Patients with excessive urinary uric acid can reduce levels by taking allopurinol. Patients with normal uric acid levels but who form uric acid stones should be treated with potassium citrate at doses that maintain urinary pH between 6 and 7. In this range, 90% of urinary uric acid is in the soluble urate form. Higher pH levels may precipitate calcium phosphate deposition and so should be avoided. Many uric acid stones can be dissolved by urinary alkalinization after 4 to 6 weeks.

Struvite or infection stones are caused by the precipitation of magnesium ammonium phosphate and carbonate apatite crystals associated with urease-producing bacteria such as *Proteus* and *Klebsiella* organisms. Treatment of struvite stones involves complete removal of all stones (usually by percutane-

ous nephrolithotomy), correction of conditions leading to urinary tract infections, and appropriate antibiotic administration. Patients with neurogenic bladders or chronic indwelling catheters may be unable to maintain sterile urine. These patients may be able to decrease recurrent stone formation with the addition of acetohydroxamic acid (Lithostat), which is a competitive inhibitor of urease. Dosing is dependent on renal function; numerous side effects limit its use.

Cystinuria is an autosomal recessive disorder in which dibasic amino acids (cystine, ornithine, lysine, arginine) are poorly absorbed in the gut and excreted in the urine. Only cystine is clinically significant, because it is extremely insoluble at physiologic urinary pH. Treatment involves fluid intake sufficient to produce 4 liters of urine per day, urinary alkalinization with potassium citrate, and the addition of chelating compounds that render cystine more soluble. Alpha-mercaptoproprionylglycine (tiopronin [Thiola]) and penicillamine (Cuprimine) are currently employed but are associated with significant side effects. Captopril (Capoten) can be effective in patients who have cystinuria and hypertension. The disulfide-chelating agent bucillamine is currently being tested in clinical trials and may be a very useful adjunct for treating this very difficult condition.

Normocalciuric calcium stone disease (idiopathic stone disease) can occur in persons with hyperoxaluria. Treatment is usually directed at maintaining adequate fluid intake and empirical addition of potassium citrate. A new preparation containing potassium magnesium citrate has been shown in clinical trials to decrease recurrent calcium stones in patients with idiopathic calcium urolithiasis.

Although most patients with hyperoxaluria (>40 mg per day) have no underlying medical conditions, patients with inflammatory or surgical bowel conditions may benefit from dietary restriction of oxalate-containing foods, urinary alkalinization with potassium citrate, and additional fluids to replace the excessive intestinal losses associated with these conditions. Patients with primary oxaluria, a genetic condition resulting in massive hepatic overproduction of the metabolic end product oxalate, usually have stones in childhood. If untreated, these patients can develop oxalosis, which results in renal failure and pathologic bone fractures. Treatment of mild cases involves dietary oxalate reduction and pyridoxine replacement. More serious cases necessitate liver transplantation to correct the enzyme deficiency, vigorous hemodialysis to eliminate the excess oxalate, and subsequent renal transplantation.

All patients undergoing treatment of metabolic conditions should have follow-up 24-hour urine collections in 3 to 4 months to assess the effectiveness of therapy and to rule out secondary conditions. Treatment success can be assessed by absence of new stone formation or lack of growth of existing stones on plain radiographs over time. Patients who pass pre-existing stones should be encouraged to continue therapy, inasmuch as this does not represent active disease.

The Sexually Transmitted Diseases

CHANCROID

method of
STANLEY M. SPINOLA, M.D.
Indiana University School of Medicine
Indianapolis, Indiana

Chancroid is caused by the gram-negative bacillus, *Haemophilus ducreyi*. Chancroid is a common genital ulcer disease (GUD) in Africa, Asia, the Caribbean, and South America. Only 386 cases of chancroid were reported in the United States in 1996. However, during the late 1980s, up to 5000 cases of chancroid were reported annually because of sporadic urban outbreaks. In the 1990s, outbreaks occurred in New Orleans and Jackson, Mississippi. Patients with chancroid were significantly more likely to report sex with a crack cocaine user, exchange of drugs or money for sex, and multiple sexual partners than those without chancroid.

H. ducreyi and the human immunodeficiency virus (HIV) facilitate the transmission of each other. *H. ducreyi* infection enhances HIV transmission by providing a more accessible portal of entry, by promoting viral shedding, and by recruiting CD4 cells and macrophages into the skin. HIV infection enhances *H. ducreyi* transmission because co-infected patients are frequently less responsive to single-dose antibiotic therapy for chancroid. This cycle may be partially responsible for the heterosexual transmission of both diseases in endemic areas.

H. ducreyi enters the skin through breaks in the epithelium that occur during sex, and erythematous papules form at each entry site within hours to days. Papules evolve into pustules in 2 to 3 days. After several days to weeks, the pustules ulcerate, and one to four soft, painful ulcers usually develop. The most frequent sites of the ulcers are the foreskin and the entrance of the vagina. Internal vaginal and cervical ulcers may be painless and go unnoticed by infected women. Suppurative inguinal lymphadenopathy may occur in up to 50% of patients with ulcers.

The clinical diagnosis of chancroid is neither sensitive nor specific, and chancroid cannot be reliably distinguished from syphilis or herpes on clinical grounds. Co-infection with these agents can occur. Laboratory confirmation of chancroid is difficult because culture is not very sensitive and most laboratories do not have the capacity to grow the organism. A multiplex polymerase chain reaction assay, which simultaneously detects *H. ducreyi*, herpes simplex, and *Treponema pallidum* from a single swab, is more sensitive than culture for the diagnosis of *H. ducreyi*, but it is not yet available commercially. In practice, the diagnosis of chancroid is frequently made by exclusion. If treatment failures for primary syphilis or patients with GUD and inguinal buboes appear in a community, the clinician should consider treating patients who do not have obvious herpes empirically for both syphilis and chancroid. Public health authorities, such as state health departments, should be notified so that proper diagnostic testing can be initiated.

H. ducreyi has acquired antimicrobial resistance factors, and several formerly effective agents such as penicillin, tetracycline, sulfonamides, and trimethoprim-sulfamethoxazole are no longer useful. The Centers for Disease Control and Prevention recommends azithromycin (Zithromax), 1 g orally in a single dose; ceftriaxone (Rocephin), 250 mg intramuscularly in a single dose; ciprofloxacin (Cipro), 500 mg orally twice a day for 3 days; or erythromycin* base, 500 mg orally four times a day for 7 days. Patients who are uncircumcised or who are HIV seropositive may not respond as well to single-dose regimens; some experts suggest using multidose regimens for these patients. Patients should be re-examined 1 week after initiation of therapy. If treatment is successful, the ulcers should have improved both symptomatically and objectively. If treatment fails, the diagnosis may be incorrect, the patient may be co-infected with another sexually transmitted disease or may be HIV seropositive, or the strain may be resistant. Large ulcers may require several weeks to heal completely. Fluctuant buboes may be treated with repeated needle aspirations or with incision and drainage; the latter lessens the need for repeated procedures. All patients with chancroid should undergo HIV testing at the time of diagnosis. If results are negative, patients should be retested within 3 months. All sexual partners of patients with chancroid should be examined and treated regardless of whether GUD is present.

---

*Not FDA approved for this indication.

GONORRHEA

method of
JEFFREY P. ENGEL, M.D.
East Carolina University School of Medicine
Greenville, North Carolina

HISTORY AND MICROBIOLOGY

Gonorrhea is one of the oldest known human infections; ancient literature contains numerous references to it. Galen (AD 130) introduced the term *gonorrhea*, which means "flow of seed," presumably due to the confusion of the purulent penile urethral discharge with semen. The causative organism was first described by A. L. S. Neisser in 1879 and was first cultivated in 1882. In the preantibiotic era, untreated infections were known to heal spontaneously over weeks to months. It was not until the advent of sulfonamides in the 1930s and penicillin in 1943 that effective therapy was available.

The bacterium *Neisseria gonorrhoeae* is a nonmotile, non–spore-forming, gram-negative coccus that grows in pairs (diplococci) with adjacent sides flattened. It closely resembles *N. meningitidis* and many other nonpathogenic *Neisseria* species. Gonococci are strict aerobes and grow ideally on chocolate agar media at 35 to 37°C with a requirement of added carbon dioxide (5%) to the atmosphere. The organism does not tolerate drying, so patient samples should be inoculated immediately onto appropriate media. Although Gram's stain and culture remain the "gold standard" for diagnosis, several nonculture methods are available with high sensitivity and specificity in the proper clinical setting. Nonculture methods, including immunoassays, genetic probes, and nucleic acid amplification, can be used when culturing patient specimens is impractical.

EPIDEMIOLOGY

According to Centers for Disease Control and Prevention (CDC), gonorrhea is the second most commonly reported sexually transmitted disease (STD) in the United States (chlamydial infections being the first). Genital herpes, which is not reportable, is probably the most prevalent STD; one in five people over the age of 12 years is seropositive for herpes simplex virus type 2. In the post-antibiotic era, gonorrhea incidence rates saw a resurgence in the mid-1970s, peaking at 470 cases per 100,000 population in 1975. After the introduction of a national control program, the reported incidence of gonorrhea in the United States has been steadily declining. The 1997 rate, however, for the first time in 22 years showed a leveling off at 123 cases per 100,000 population, equal to the 1996 rate. Factors associated with increased rates include urban residence, black race, unmarried status, lesser education, lower socioeconomic status, and illicit drug use. Higher rates in these groups may be due in part to bias introduced by the reporting primarily from public health departments to the CDC.

Antimicrobial resistance in *N. gonorrhoeae* remains an important epidemiologic and management problem. In 1997, the CDC reported that 33.4% of isolates were resistant to penicillin, tetracycline, or both. Penicillinase-producing *N. gonorrhoeae* (PPNG) declined from a peak of 11% in 1991 to 3.9% in 1997. In the same period, however, chromosamally mediated resistance to penicillin increased from 1.8% to 3.9%. With the introduction of fluoroquinolones as alternative therapy for gonorrhea, resistance to this class of antibiotics soon emerged. Resistance to ciprofloxacin was first observed in 1991 but remains rare (0.1% in the United States) in 1997. More common is the incidence of isolates with reduced susceptibility (but not full-blown resistance) to ciprofloxacin, which decreased from a high of 1.3% in 1994 to 0.5% in 1997.

CLINICAL MANIFESTATIONS

In men, gonorrhea manifests as a urethritis with dysuria and a purulent discharge after a short incubation period of 2 to 5 days. In women, gonorrhea is more likely to be asymptomatic, as often as 90% in some clinical settings, and has a more variable incubation period. In the asymptomatic patient, the diagnosis is made only when screening cultures are performed. In symptomatic cases, women usually present with a vaginal discharge or dysuria with evidence of a mucopurulent cervicitis and/or urethritis on examination. It is impossible to separate gonorrhea from *Chlamydia trachomatis* infection on clinical grounds, so testing to determine the specific disease is recommended because both of these infections are reportable to state health departments, and a specific diagnosis may improve compliance and partner notification. Other sites of local gonococcal infection in men and women include the rectum, the pharynx, and, rarely, the conjunctivae.

Complications of gonorrhea include pelvic inflammatory disease (PID) in women and disseminated gonococcal infection (DGI). PID refers to the ascending spread of infection from the endocervix, resulting in endometritis, salpingitis, and sometimes peritonitis, and presents with vaginal discharge, dyspareunia, pelvic and abdominal pain, and fever. The differential diagnosis includes ectopic pregnancy and appendicitis, and women often require hospital admission for both evaluation and management. The most common long-term sequela of PID is infertility due to tubal scarring. DGI, which can occur in both men and women, is the result of hematogenous dissemination of *N. gonorrhoeae* from the local mucosal site. Manifestations of DGI include the characteristic purpuric skin lesions with or without pustules, tenosynovitis, and arthritis. In rare instances, hepatitis, endocarditis, or meningitis occurs.

MANAGEMENT OF ADULTS

Uncomplicated Local Infection

The management of adults with urogenital, rectal, or pharyngeal gonorrhea often depends on the clinical setting. It is ideal to attempt to make a specific microbiologic diagnosis by culture or nonculture methods, but often this is impractical. If a specific diagnosis cannot be made, therapy must be directed at two pathogens simultaneously, *N. gonorrhoeae* and *C. trachomatis*, because in certain high-risk groups co-infection may be present as much as 40% of the time.

The general principles of effective therapy include selection of an antibiotic that is curative with a single dose (to ensure compliance) and partner notification (so-called epitreatment). Epitreatment is best accomplished in a public health department that has the personnel and facilities to contact the sex partners of the infected person. All sex partners of patients diagnosed with *N. gonorrhoeae* should be evaluated and treated for *N. gonorrhoeae* and *C. trachomatis*

TABLE 1. **Preferred Single-Dose Regimens for the Treatment of Uncomplicated Gonococcal and Chlamydial Infections**

For Gonorrhea

Cefixime (Suprax), 400 mg PO
or
Ceftriaxone (Rocephin), 125 mg IM
or
Ciprofloxacin (Cipro),* 500 mg PO
or
Ofloxacin (Floxin),* 400 mg PO
or
Spectinomycin (Trobicin),† 2 gm IM
plus

For Chlamydia

Azithromycin (Zithromax), 1 gm PO

---

*Fluoroquinolones are contraindicated for pregnant or nursing women and for children younger than 16 years.
†Alternative regimen for patients who cannot receive beta-lactam or fluoroquinolone antibiotics.

infections if their last sexual contact with the patient was less than 60 days before onset of symptoms or diagnosis of infection in the patient. If the patient's last sexual intercourse was more than 60 days before onset of symptoms or diagnosis, the patient's most recent sex partner should be treated. Patients should be instructed to avoid sexual intercourse until therapy is completed and symptoms have resolved.

Table 1 lists the recommended single-dose treatment regimens for uncomplicated urogenital and rectal *N. gonorrhoeae* and *C. trachomatis* infection. The response rate in gonococcal pharyngitis may be less than 90%; nonetheless, the same regimens are recommended. A beta-lactamase–stable cephalosporin remains the drug of choice for gonorrhea, with a fluoroquinolone as an acceptable alternative. Spectinomycin (Trobicin) is another useful alternative in select circumstances. Azithromycin (Zithromax) is the only single-dose regimen available for *C. trachomatis* infection. Alternative oral regimens for chlamydia include 1-week courses of doxycycline, 100 mg twice daily; ofloxacin (Floxin), 300 mg twice daily; or erythromycin base, 500 mg four times daily.

Patients with uncomplicated gonorrhea who are treated with a recommended regimen need not return for a test of cure. Patients who have symptoms that persist after treatment should be evaluated with a culture for *N. gonorrhoeae*, and any positive result should be tested for antimicrobial susceptibility. Most recurrent infections are due to reinfection rather than to treatment failure, indicating a need for improved patient education and epitreatment.

Pelvic Inflammatory Disease and Disseminated Gonococcal Infection

PID is almost always a polymicrobial infection in which *N. gonorrhoeae* may be only one of the causative bacteria. Thus, antibiotic regimens should be relatively broad spectrum to cover urogenital flora such as aerobic gram-negative bacilli and anaerobes,

as well as *C. trachomatis*. Because of the the severe sequelae of infection, it is best to have a low threshold for treatment of PID, and, if compliance is an issue or severe clinical disease is present, patients should be hospitalized. Table 2 lists several possible inpatient and outpatient treatment regimens for PID.

Hospitalization is recommended for initial therapy of patients with DGI, especially when compliance is an issue, the diagnosis is uncertain, and complications such as purulent synovial effusions are present. Initial therapy is with ceftriaxone (Rocephin) 1 gram intramuscularly (IM) or intravenously (IV) every 24 hours with concurrent therapy for presumptive *C. trachomatis*, given as a single dose of azithromycin (Zithromax), 1 gram orally (PO). For patients who cannot receive beta-lactam antibiotics, ciprofloxacin (Cipro), 400 mg, or ofloxacin (Floxin), 400 mg IV every 12 hours, or spectinomycin 2 grams IM every 12 hours is recommended. Parenteral therapy should be continued for 24 to 48 hours after clinical improvement, whereupon an outpatient regimen of cefixime (Suprax), 400 mg twice daily; ciprofloxacin (Cipro), 500 mg PO twice daily; or ofloxacin, (Floxin) 400 mg PO twice daily, should be given to complete 1 full week of treatment. *C. trachomatis* is adequately treated if a 1-week course of a fluoroquinolone is used to treat DGI. Patients with gonococcal meningitis or endocarditis require therapy for a longer duration, and treatment should be undertaken in consultation with an expert.

GONOCOCCAL INFECTIONS IN NEONATES AND CHILDREN

Gonorrhea in the neonate results from vertical transmission from an infected mother to the newborn via exposure to infected cervical exudate at the time of birth. It is an acute illness that usually presents

TABLE 2. **Treatment of Pelvic Inflammatory Disease***

Inpatient regimens†
  Cefotetan (Cefotan), 2 gm IV q 12 h or cefoxitin (Mefoxin), 2 g IV q 6 h **plus** Doxycycline, 100 mg IV or PO q 12 h
  or
  Clindamycin (Cleocin), 900 mg IV q 8 h **plus**
  Gentamicin, 2 mg/kg IV loading dose, then 1.5 mg/kg q 8 h; single daily dosing of 7 mg/kg may be substituted
  or
  Ofloxacin (Floxin),‡ 400 mg IV q 12 h **plus**
  Metronidazole (Flagyl), 500 mg IV q 8 h
Outpatient Regimens
  Ceftriaxone (Rocephin), 250 mg IM once **or**
  Cefoxitin (Mefoxin), 2 gm IM plus probenicid, 1 gm PO in a single dose **plus**
  Doxycycline 100 mg PO twice/d for 14 d **plus**
  Metronidazole (Flagyl), 500 mg PO bid for 14 d

---

*Treatments are listed in order of preference.
†Inpatient regimens should be continued for at least 48 hours after the patient demonstrates clinical improvement, after which doxycycline 100 mg orally twice daily should be continued to complete a total of 14 days of treatment.
‡Fluoroquinolones are contraindicated for pregnant or nursing women and for children younger than 16 years.

within 2 to 5 days after birth. The most common manifestation of neonatal gonorrhea is ophthalmia neonatorum, a condition that is rare in the United States owing to the nearly universal use of ocular prophylaxis in newborns. Treatment of gonococcal ophthalmia neonatorum is with a single dose of ceftriaxone (Rocephin), 25 to 50 mg per kg IV or IM, not to exceed a total dose of 125 mg. More serious manifestations of neonatal infection with *N. gonorrhoeae* are sepsis (DGI), including arthritis and meningitis, and inflammation at sites of fetal monitoring (e.g., scalp abscess). Treatment is with daily doses of ceftriaxone (Rocephin), 25 to 50 mg per kg IV or IM, in consultation with an expert in the field. Infants born to mothers who have untreated gonorrhea are at risk for infection and should be treated prophylactically. The recommended regimen is the same as is recommended for ophthalmia neonatorum.

After the neonatal period, sexual abuse is the most common cause of gonococcal infection in preadolescent children. Vaginitis is the most common manifestation in sexually abused children. Anorectal and pharyngeal involvement is often present and frequently asymptomatic. Because of the legal implications of *N. gonorrhoeae* infection in a child, only standard culture procedures should be used because nonculture methods (DNA probes, immunoassays) are not approved by the Federal Drug Administration for use in children. All specimens should be obtained in conjunction with the appropriate legal authorities in case legal proceedings are necessary. The treatment for children who weigh more than 45 kg is the same as for an adult (Table 1); children who weigh less than 45 kg should receive ceftriaxone (Rocephin), 125 mg IM in a single dose. Co-treatment for *C. trachomatis* should be reserved only for children who have positive chlamydial test results.

NONGONOCOCCAL URETHRITIS

method of
HEATHER SELMAN, M.D., and
PHILIP HANNO, M.D.
*Temple University Hospital and
   University of Pennsylvania
Philadelphia, Pennsylvania*

Urethritis is an inflammation of the urethra, usually manifested by burning on urination, urethral discomfort or itching, meatal erythema, and mucoid or purulent urethral discharge. In some cases, the presence of urethral discharge may be evident only before the first morning void as meatal crusting or staining of the underwear. Asymptomatic infections occur as well. Urethritis is one of the most common problems in ambulatory medicine. Risk factors include unprotected intercourse with multiple sexual partners and change of sexual partners within 3 months. Sexual partners are often not examined and treated, because nongonococcal infections are infrequently reported to health authorities. For this reason, the incidence of nongonococcal urethritis (NGU) continues to rise.

NGU urethritis is defined as urethral inflammation not caused by *Neisseria gonorrhoeae*. Causes in men include infections with *Chlamydia trachomatis* in 23 to 55% of patients, *Ureaplasma urealyticum* in 20 to 40%, and *Trichomonas vaginalis* in 2 to 5%. Symptoms usually appear between 1 and 5 weeks after unprotected intercourse with a partner infected with these organisms. Herpes simplex virus and human papillomavirus have been implicated as well, as has yeast. Postgonococcal urethritis is defined as NGU occurring after effective treatment for gonococcal urethritis while simultaneous infection with *C. trachomatis* has been missed. A noninfectious form of urethritis can result from foreign bodies, soaps, shampoos, vaginal douches, spermicidal agents, catheters, urethral instrumentation, and manual stimulation. A cause is not always found.

NGU may be seen in the systemic diseases Stevens-Johnson syndrome and Wegener's granulomatosis. Reiter's syndrome, with arthritis and uveitis, follows 1 to 4% of cases of NGU. Epididymitis is another possible complication. Transmission of the human immunodeficiency virus (HIV) is increased two- to fivefold in association with other sexually transmitted diseases, and testing for HIV infection and syphilis should be recommended to patients with NGU. Female partners of patients with chlamydial infections are at risk for pelvic inflammatory disease, with possible subsequent ectopic pregnancies or infertility secondary to fallopian tube scarring.

Urethritis in women may be caused by *N. gonorrhoeae* or *C. trachomatis*. Although a urethral discharge is not often present in women, dysuria may occur. The physician often incorrectly presumes the presence of a bladder infection. Urinalysis may show pyuria, but cultures for routine urinary pathogens will be negative.

DIAGNOSIS

NGU is diagnosed by the presence of 5 or more polymorphonuclear leukocytes per oil immersion field on a gram-stained smear of the urethral discharge, an intraurethral swab specimen, or the first 10 mL of the patient's voided urine. The diagnosis of infectious urethritis is made by positive culture of these samples, although sampling of the urethral epithelium specifically (from 2 to 4 mm inside the urethra) must be performed to diagnose chlamydial infection. Preliminary results become available within 2 to 3 days. The inflammation is shown to be localized to the urethra by the presence of a significantly greater number of white blood cells in the first voided urine sample compared with a midstream urine specimen or that obtained after prostatic massage. The patient should be examined in the morning before voiding if urethral inflammation is suspected but cannot be detected.

TREATMENT REGIMENS

Both the patient and any sexual partners should receive treatment. Sexual partners should be treated if they were last exposed to the symptomatic patient within 30 days of the onset of symptoms or within 60 days of diagnosis in the asymptomatic patient. The most recent sexual partner should be treated if the last sexual intercourse preceded these times. Patients and partners should abstain from sexual intercourse during treatment and until both are free of symptoms and signs.

Any of the following drugs can be used as a first-line agent: doxycycline, 100 mg twice a day (bid) by mouth for 7 days; or azithromycin (Zithromax), 1 gram by mouth in a single dose; or tetracycline, 500 mg by mouth four times daily for 7 days. As alternative agents, erythromycin ethylsuccinate, 800 mg by mouth four times daily for 7 days (or 400 mg four times daily for 14 days); erythromycin base, 500 mg by mouth four times daily for 7 days (or 250 mg by mouth four times daily for 14 days); or ofloxacin (Floxin), 300 mg by mouth twice daily for 7 days, may be used. Erythromycin is the agent of choice during pregnancy and lactation. Treatment recommendations remain the same for patients with HIV infection.

FOLLOW-UP CARE

Patients should return if their symptoms persist or recur after therapy. They should be re-treated with the original regimen if they did not comply initially or if they were reinfected by an untreated sex partner. Otherwise, a wet mount of a urethral swab should be performed and the specimen sent for culture for *T. vaginalis*. If results are positive, definitive treatment consists of metronidazole (Flagyl), 2 grams by mouth in a single dose, or clotrimazole suppositories, 100 mg per vagina daily for 2 weeks during pregnancy. If results are negative, an alternative regimen is used for 14 days to treat possible infection with tetracycline-resistant *U. urealyticum*, which occurs in 6 to 10% of cases. Evaluation of sexual partners may help identify an underlying infectious cause of the urethritis.

Physical examination and a diminished urinary flow rate may suggest clinically significant structural abnormalities as the cause of chronic urethritis in approximately 10% of patients. Such abnormalities can be further evaluated by endoscopy of the lower urinary tract. They include urethral strictures, urethral diverticula, meatal stenosis, condyloma, foreign bodies, and periurethral abscesses. Bacteriuria and prostatitis may also cause chronic urethritis and may necessitate longer courses of therapy (4 to 6 weeks).

DONOVANOSIS
(GRANULOMA INGUINALE)

method of
PAUL M. BENSON, M.D.
Walter Reed Army Medical Center
Washington, D.C.

Donovanosis (granuloma inguinale) is an indolent, genital ulcerative disease caused by the pleomorphic gram-negative bacillus *Calymmatobacterium granulomatis*. The disease is rare in the United States; fewer than 10 cases were reported to the Centers for Disease Control and Prevention in 1997. Worldwide, most cases are reported from India, Papua New Guinea, China, South Africa, and Brazil

and among the aborigines in Australia. The peak incidence of disease is in sexually active adults between the ages of 20 to 40. The chronic genital ulcerations may facilitate transmission of human immunodeficiency virus (HIV), which is a significant public health concern in endemic areas. Both sexual and nonsexual modes of transmission have been reported. Infants may acquire the disease during delivery through an infected birth canal. Children and sexually inactive persons presumably acquire the disease from direct or indirect contact with infectious exudates.

The incubation period is highly variable, ranging from 1 to 4 weeks, but it may be as long as 1 year. Single or multiple nontender papules arise in the genital area and then ulcerate to form bright red, exuberant, velvety lesions with a clean, nonpurulent surface and rolled borders. In females, lesions are located most often on the labia but may also develop within the vagina or on the cervix. In males, lesions occur on the prepuce, frenulum, and coronal sulcus. Homosexual males have perianal and penile lesions associated with anal intercourse. The painless lesions expand slowly over weeks to months and can reach an enormous size, leading to extensive destruction of genital and perirectal tissue. Cervical disease may spread deeply into pelvic tissues or disseminate hematogenously to other organs. Extensive cervical involvement during pregnancy may lead to fatal hemorrhage at the time of delivery. The inguinal lymphatics are usually uninvolved, but subcutaneous lesions in this area produce inguinal swelling known as *pseudobuboes*, which may erode through the overlying skin. Complications include phimosis, urethral stenosis, genital elephantiasis, lymphedema, and the development of squamous cell carcinoma in long-standing untreated disease.

Extragenital lesions occur in 5% of patients and may involve the mouth, nongenital skin, the lungs, the liver, the spleen, and bone. Extragenital disease can occur by autoinoculation. However, most cases of systemic disease, which can be fatal, occur through hematogenous dissemination from a primary genital infection. Patients with visceral disease often have symptoms of fever, night sweats, and weight loss.

The diagnosis is based on history, clinical findings, and the demonstration of typical intracellular bacilli (Donovan bodies) on a properly stained crush preparation or tissue biopsy. Tissue is obtained by incision from the advancing rolled border. One portion of the biopsy is submitted in formalin for routine processing and special stains. A small portion is placed between two clean microscope slides, crushed, and then smeared across the slides. The air-dried smear is then stained with Wright or Giemsa stain. The organisms are found as coccobacilli with characteristic bipolar staining (appearance of a closed safety pin) within macrophages.

Laboratory culture on artificial media, antibiotic sensitivity studies, serologic tests, and skin test antigens are not commercially available.

TREATMENT

Recommended treatment includes doxycycline (Vibramycin, Monodox), 100 mg twice daily for at least 3 weeks; trimethoprim-sulfamethoxazole* (Bactrim DS, Septra DS), 160/800 mg twice daily for 3 weeks; or erythromycin,* 500 mg four times a day for 3 weeks. Treatment should be continued until all le-

---

*Not FDA approved for this indication.

sions have healed. Treatment failures resulting from antibiotic resistance or noncompliance are common. Azithromycin* (Zithromax), 1.0 gram weekly for 4 weeks (outpatients) or 500 mg daily for 7 days (inpatients), has shown great promise in field trials in Australia. Azithromycin therapy has been so successful that it is now recommended in Australia as first-line therapy for donovanosis.

---

*Not FDA approved for this indication.

LYMPHOGRANULOMA VENEREUM

method of
PAUL M. BENSON, M.D.
Walter Reed Army Medical Center
Washington, D.C.

Lymphogranuloma venereum (LGV) is a sexually transmitted disease endemic in Africa, India, Southeast Asia, and South America. It is caused by the obligate intracellular organism *Chlamydia trachomatis*. Only the serovars (immunotypes) L1, L2, and L3 cause LGV. In the United States, 113 cases of lymphogranuloma venereum were reported to the Centers for Disease Control and Prevention in 1997. The acute stages of the disease are more common in males; the highest incidence is in the 15- to 40-year-old age group. Late complications are seen more often in women. Infection with the L2 serovar may cause an acute, symptomatic proctocolitis in people who practice receptive anal intercourse. These symptoms may mimic those of inflammatory bowel disease. Infection with the L1 serovar is rare in the United States and is usually acquired from sexual contacts overseas.

The disease course is divided into three clinical stages: (1) a transient, primary genital ulcerative phase; (2) a secondary stage of painful and occasionally suppurative inguinal or pelvic lymphadenopathy; and (3) a rare tertiary phase known as the *anorectogenital stage*, consisting of perirectal abscesses, fistula formation, rectal strictures, chronic perineal lymphedema, and genital elephantiasis. The tertiary stage is a consequence of persistent untreated infection.

The incubation period ranges from 3 to 12 days but may be as long as 6 weeks. The primary lesion, which is often asymptomatic, consists of one or more small painless papules, vesicles, or shallow ulcerations on the glans penis or the mucous membranes of the vulva, vagina, cervix, or rectum. The lesions heal spontaneously within several days.

The primary stage is followed in 2 to 6 weeks by the development of tender, enlarged, firm, and matted lymph nodes (buboes). The adenopathy is unilateral in two thirds of cases. Patients with enlarged nodes above and below the inguinal ligament (Poupart's ligament) have a highly diagnostic indentation at the site of the ligament known as the *groove sign*. The adenopathy may be associated with fever, malaise, arthralgias, and myalgias. Less commonly, pneumonitis, hepatitis, or perihepatitis (Fitz-Hugh–Curtis syndrome) develops. Systemic symptoms occur when there is lymphatic spread of organisms from anal or upper cervicovaginal lesions. With penile, vulvar, and some anal infections, the inguinal and femoral nodes are enlarged. In women, the deep pelvic lymph nodes are often involved, which results in low back or pelvic pain. Affected lymph nodes may become fluctuant; about one third of cases progress to spontaneous rupture.

The diagnosis is based on history, clinical findings of inguinal adenopathy (especially in a male), and confirmatory serologic tests. The primary lesion is often inapparent to the patient if present in the vagina or rectum. The second-stage lymphadenopathy can mimic symptoms of cat-scratch disease, syphilis, and chancroid. A lymph node biopsy is not practical in most outpatient settings, but when performed, it yields findings suggestive of LGV. Laboratory isolation of chlamydiae is difficult, expensive, and infrequently done. Tests that the laboratory may perform include (1) a complement fixation test (LGV-CF), in which a rise of 1:64 or greater is seen in 50% of patients; (2) the microimmunofluorescence titer, which is usually high in LGV (titers exceed 1:512) but has broad cross-reactivity with other *C. trachomatis* serovars; (3) the enzyme-linked immunosorbent assay (ELISA); and (4) the polymerase chain reaction (PCR) for chlamydial DNA. In clinical practice, a positive complement fixation titer (1:64 or greater) with a supportive history and physical findings remains the best diagnostic approach. In other types of chlamydial infections, the complement fixation titers are usually 1:16 or less.

TREATMENT

The Centers for Disease Control and Prevention currently recommend oral doxycycline (Vibramycin, Monodox), 100 mg twice daily for 21 days. Erythromycin* and sulfisoxazole* (Gantrisin), 500 mg four times daily for 21 days, are alternative agents if doxycycline is not tolerated or is contraindicated. Erythromycin is the preferred drug for infections during pregnancy and lactation. The treatment regimen is the same for persons infected with the human immunodeficiency virus (HIV), but these patients should be monitored closely. Treatment failures have been reported with tetracycline. Fluctuant lymph nodes may necessitate aspiration or surgical drainage through intact skin to prevent spontaneous rupture or to relieve symptoms.

---

*Not FDA approved for this indication.

SYPHILIS

method of
MICHAEL AUGENBRAUN, M.D.
State University of New York—Health Science Center at Brooklyn
Brooklyn, New York

Syphilis is a complex infectious disease with both acute and chronic manifestations caused by the spirochete *Treponema pallidum*. Like other diseases caused by spirochetes, such as Lyme disease, the natural history of syphilis is characterized by chronologic progression through well-characterized stages.

Syphilis has a long and fascinating history in the annals of medicine. Debate persists as to whether the disease was described in pre-Columbian civilizations of either the old or new worlds. It is clear, however, that sometime after 1492 the disease appeared dramatically and then spread rapidly through Europe. These early descriptions of syphilis suggest its consequences were more severe than those familiar to clinicians in the 20th century. The protean manifestations of this disease have led it to be labeled "the great imitator."

BIOLOGY

T. pallidum is one of a number of organisms in its genus. Some are capable of causing disease: *T. pallidum pertenue* (yaws), *T. carateum* (pinta), and *T. pallidum endemicum* (bejel or endemic syphilis). Other treponemes are considered nonpathogenic and may inhabit the human body as commensals. Treponemes cannot be cultured on ordinary media. By light microscopy they can be visualized only under polarized light. Under such conditions these organisms appear white against a darkened background (hence the term *darkfield* microscopy) and have the classic corkscrew helical shape.

TRANSMISSION AND EPIDEMIOLOGY

Although syphilis can be acquired through exposure in a variety of ways, the predominant modes of transmission are congenital and sexual. The incidence of disease in the United States has waxed and waned since the 1940s, when useful epidemiologic data were first compiled. Starting in the mid-1980s and through the early 1990s, the numbers of cases rose significantly as a result of a confluence of events, including an urban crack cocaine epidemic and diminished funding for sexually transmitted disease (STD) control programs. The incidence of syphilis has since diminished dramatically throughout the United States, although pockets of disease persist and flare in certain urban areas and in the southeastern part of the country. Reports in the medical literature of unusual clinical manifestations of syphilis in patients coinfected with the human immunodeficiency virus (HIV) have raised serious concerns about the adequacy of currently recommended therapies and about the reliability of diagnostic strategies in these patients. There are data suggesting that syphilis, like other forms of genital ulcer disease, can enhance the transmission of HIV.

CLINICAL MANIFESTATIONS

The development of the genital chancre is the hallmark of primary syphilis. The incubation period after exposure to *T. pallidum* usually lasts 3 to 90 days. Chancres may also develop anywhere contact has occurred (e.g., the anal canal, the mouth). They are classically characterized as indurated and nontender. Single lesions are the rule, although multiple lesions may be seen. Inguinal (regional) lymphadenopathy is also usually present. Moist lesions are infectious. Serous material expressed from their surface is rich in treponemes, and this clinical material is optimal for study with darkfield microscopy. Lesions of primary syphilis heal spontaneously, even in the absence of therapy. This takes place approximately 3 to 6 weeks after the appearance of the lesions.

Sometime during the development of the clinical manifestations of primary syphilis, treponemes spread throughout the body via the bloodstream and the lymphatics. Within a variable period after the appearance of the chancre, the signs and symptoms of secondary syphilis develop. These may be quite varied. The most common finding is a maculopapular rash on the palms and soles. Systemic symptoms such as fever, malaise, headache, sore throat, lymphadenopathy, myalgias, and arthralgias also occur. Highly infectious, moist lesions known as condyloma lata may appear in intertriginous areas and on mucosal surfaces. As in the case of the chancre of primary-stage disease, the signs and symptoms of secondary syphilis resolve even without therapy.

After the resolution of secondary syphilis, the disease enters a latent phase in which organisms presumably survive but do not cause active disease. For a period of time that is ill defined but is thought to last up to 4 years, the symptoms of secondary syphilis may recur. For the purpose of guiding therapy, a period of 1 year after the resolution of early-stage syphilis is considered the "early latent" phase. At some time beyond the clinical manifestations of these early stages of disease and a variable period of latency, about one third of untreated patients develop late-stage disease: neurosyphilis, cardiovascular syphilis, or gummatous syphilis. This can happen decades after infection. Neurosyphilis can be symptomatic or asymptomatic. The meninges or brain parenchyma may be involved. Cognitive, sensory, ocular, or otic symptoms may occur.

DIAGNOSIS

When possible, darkfield microscopy of serous material from moist lesions of primary and secondary syphilis can be diagnostic. More often the lack of a culturable organism, the difficulty obtaining material for darkfield examination, and the frequent "latent" nature of disease may make syphilis difficult to diagnose. Since the beginning of the 20th century, clinicians have relied on the use of serologic tests both as screening measures and as confirmation of clinically suspected disease. Serologic testing for syphilis requires two sequential examinations. The patient's serum is initially screened for antibodies to *T. pallidum* with antigenic material similar to the lipoidal antigens present on the surface of the treponeme. A positive test result is indicated by the visible aggregation of particulate matter when the patient's serum and test reagents are mixed. Tests performed in this manner are collectively referred to as nontreponemal serologic tests (NTSTs). The first of these was the Venereal Diagnostic Reagin Laboratory (VDRL) test. Modifications in this technique suitable for commercial distribution include the rapid plasma reagin (RPR) and the automated reagin test (ART). Although sensitive, these tests are often nonspecific. A false-positive test result, often referred to as a biologic false-positive (BFP), may occur in elderly patients, in pregnant patients, after vaccination, in patients with autoimmune diseases, and in patients infected with HIV. Reactive NTSTs are reported as serial dilutions of serum (e.g., 1:1, 1:2, 1:4, 1:8). They must be confirmed with tests for *T. pallidum*–specific antibodies. Fluorescence or hemagglutination indicates reactivity. Examples of these types of tests include the fluorescent treponemal antibody absorption test (FTA-ABS) and the microhemagglutination assay–*T. pallidum* (MHA-TP), collectively referred to as treponemal serologic tests (TSTs). These tests are more expensive and labor intensive in operation than the NTSTs and are not recommended for screening.

The NTST results rise and fall with the activity of disease, with or without therapy. Results are highest during secondary-stage syphilis. It is expected that with successful resolution of infection, this titer will become nonreactive after some period of time. In the majority of patients with syphilis, the TST remains reactive for life, regardless of the activity of disease. Serologic tests can also be performed on cerebrospinal fluid (CSF) for the diagnosis of neurosyphilis, for which they are moderately sensitive and quite specific. To date, the VDRL is the only NTST standardized for this application. CSF evaluation should be considered for any patient with (1) serologic evidence of syphilis and neurologic or psychiatric symptoms, (2) HIV infection and latent syphilis, or (3) serologic treatment failure. Abnormal CSF parameters such as increased protein levels and increased numbers of lymphocytes may also be suggestive of neurosyphilis even when the CSF-VDRL is nonreactive.

TREATMENT

Syphilis is one of the few remaining infectious diseases for which penicillin is considered the treatment of choice (Table 1) and in which the phenomenon of drug resistance has not been documented. Most of the studies on which current treatment regimens are based were conducted decades ago and did not apply standards of scientific rigor that would be considered necessary today. Despite this, experience with currently recommended regimens suggests that they are effective. Tetracyclines and macrolides appear to also have effect against *T. pallidum*, but there is much less clinical experience with these agents.

Special Considerations

Pregnancy. All pregnant patients with syphilis should receive penicillin therapy appropriate for the patient's stage of syphilis. Nonpenicillin alternatives may not be used. Pregnant patients with syphilis who are allergic to penicillin should be skin tested according to established protocols and, if found to be allergic, should undergo desensitization according to established protocols.

HIV Infection. Although some reports suggest that HIV-infected patients develop aggressive forms of syphilis unresponsive to usually recommended courses of therapy, no large-scale study has confirmed this. It appears that most HIV-infected patients respond appropriately to therapy recommended for HIV-uninfected patients and that the

TABLE 1. Recommended Therapy for Syphilis*

Primary, Secondary, and Early Latent Syphilis
Benzathine penicillin, 2.4 million U IM once
Alternatives:
  Doxycycline, 100 mg orally bid for 14 days
  Tetracycline, 500 mg orally qd for 14 days
  Erythromycin, 500 mg orally qid for 14 days

Late Latent Syphilis or Latent Syphilis of Unknown Duration
Benzathine penicillin, 2.4 million U IM once weekly for 3 consecutive weeks (total, 7.2 million U)
Alternatives:
  Doxycycline, 100 mg orally bid for 28 days
  Tetracycline, 500 mg orally qid for 28 days

Tertiary Syphilis (Gummatous or Cardiovascular Syphilis)
Benzathine penicillin G, 2.4 million U IM once weekly for 3 consecutive weeks

Neurosyphilis
Aqueous crystalline penicillin G, 18–24 million U IV qd as 3–4 million U every 4 hours for 10–14 days
Alternatives:
  Procaine penicillin, 2.4 million U IM qd for 10–14 days plus probenecid, 500 mg orally qid for 10–14 days

*Abridged from the Centers for Disease Control and Prevention 1998 Guidelines for Treatment of Sexually Transmitted Diseases. MMWR 47:28–49, 1998.

clinical manifestations do not differ substantially. It has been recommended that HIV-infected patients with late latent syphilis or latent syphilis of unknown duration undergo CSF evaluation to rule out asymptomatic neurosyphilis. Serologic follow-up after therapy, important for all patients, should be assiduously conducted in HIV-infected patients.

Serologic Follow-up. Whether NTSTs should revert to nonreactive status after therapy and over what time frame this should occur remains an area of debate. It is safe to say that rising titers after therapy are suggestive of treatment failure or reinfection. NTST results should fall by two dilutions anytime from 6 months to a year after successful therapy for early syphilis and up to 2 years after successful therapy for latent syphilis. Retreatment or evaluation for possible neurosyphilis should be considered for treatment failures.

Diseases of Allergy

ANAPHYLAXIS AND SERUM SICKNESS

method of
STEPHEN F. KEMP, M.D.
The University of Mississippi Medical Center
Jackson, Mississippi

ANAPHYLAXIS

Anaphylaxis is a potentially life-threatening immunologic reaction that results from the sudden release of mast cell–derived and basophil-derived mediators into the circulatory system. Signs and symptoms of anaphylaxis may occur alone or in combination (Table 1). Urticaria and angioedema are the most common manifestations (>90% in retrospective series), and the absence of either should prompt a physician to question the diagnosis of anaphylaxis. Anaphylaxis usually develops rapidly, often within 5 to 30 minutes, but some agents, such as aspirin, may not produce signs or symptoms until hours after exposure.

The true incidence of anaphylaxis is probably underestimated because it is not a reportable disease. One episode of anaphylaxis, related primarily to drug reactions, has been reported for every 2700 hospitalized subjects. Insect stings are probably responsible for at least 50 fatalities per year in the United States. Elevated postmortem tryptase levels have been reported in 12% of otherwise healthy adults who died suddenly and in at least 40% of victims of sudden infant death syndrome. These elevations in postmortem tryptase level, a highly specific serum marker for mast cell activation, suggest that anaphylaxis was responsible for many of these fatalities.

Pathophysiology

The chemical mediators that cause anaphylaxis are preformed and released from granules (histamine, tryptase, and others) or are generated from membrane lipids (prostaglandin D_2, leukotrienes, and platelet-activating factor) by the activated mast cell or basophil. When these mediators are released by immunologic mechanisms, reactions are termed *anaphylactic*; when the mediators are released by nonimmunologic mechanisms, the reactions are called *anaphylactoid*.

Histamine exerts its pathophysiologic effects via both H_1 and H_2 receptors. Flushing, hypotension, and headache are mediated by both H_1 and H_2 receptors, whereas tachycardia, pruritus, rhinorrhea, and bronchospasm are associated only with H_1 receptors.

Increased vascular permeability during anaphylaxis can produce a shift of 50% of intravascular fluid to the extravascular space within 10 minutes. This dramatic shift of effective blood volume causes compensatory catecholamine release and activates the renin-angiotensin-aldosterone system. These internal compensatory responses produce variable effects during anaphylaxis. Some patients experience abnormal elevations in their peripheral vascular resistance, indicating maximal vasoconstriction, whereas others have depressed systemic vascular resistance despite elevated catecholamine levels.

Agents that Cause Anaphylaxis

Many different agents have been reported to cause anaphylaxis (Table 2). Beta-lactam antibiotics are the most common cause of anaphylaxis from any source. Latex allergy has become a particularly important cause of anaphylaxis since it was first described in the 1980s. Approximately 7 to 10% of health care professionals and 28 to 67% of persons with spina bifida may have allergic symptoms when exposed to medical equipment or other products, such as condoms, that contain latex. These symptoms may manifest as anaphylaxis or as contact urticaria or angioedema, which may indicate a risk of anaphylaxis for those individuals on subsequent respiratory or mucosal exposure. Anaphylaxis may be caused by murine monoclonal antibodies, used to diagnose or treat cancer; by stings from imported fire ants, a long-standing problem in the southern United States that appears to be spreading as the insect adapts to colder weather conditions; and by streptokinase, used to treat ischemic heart disease. Crustaceans and peanuts appear to cause most episodes of food-induced anaphylaxis.

A similarly diverse group of agents has been asso-

TABLE 1. **Clinical Signs and Symptoms of Anaphylaxis**

Cutaneous: Urticaria, angioedema, diffuse erythema, generalized pruritus
Respiratory: Tachypnea, bronchospasm, laryngeal or tongue edema, dysphonia
Cardiovascular: Tachycardia, hypotension, angina, cardiac arrhythmias
Gastrointestinal: Nausea, emesis, diarrhea, abdominal cramps, dysphagia
Other: Rhinitis, conjunctivitis, uterine cramps, headache, dizziness, syncope, blurred vision, seizure

TABLE 2. **Representative Agents that Cause Anaphylaxis**

Hormones: Insulin, hydrocortisone
Animal or human proteins: Equine serum (antivenin), seminal fluid, protamine sulfate, monoclonal antibodies
Enzymes: Chymopapain, streptokinase
Venoms: Imported fire ants, wasps, hornets, yellow jackets, bees, others
Animal emanations: Cat, dog, others
Allergen extracts and vaccines: Pollen, mold, dust mite, others
Foods: Eggs, milk, fish, crustaceans, tree nuts, peanuts, soybean, others
Latex
Medications: Penicillin, cephalosporin, insulin, others
Ethylene oxide gas on dialysis tubing
Angiotensin-converting enzyme inhibitor administered during renal dialysis with sulfonated polyacrylonitrile (AN69), cuprophane, or polymethylmethacrylate (PMMA) dialysis membranes
Polysaccharides: Dextran, iron dextran
Hydatid cyst rupture

Modified from Kemp SF, deShazo RD: Anaphylaxis and anaphylactoid reactions. *In* Lockey RF, Bukantz SC (eds): Allergens and Allergen Immunotherapy, 2nd ed (revised and expanded). New York, Marcel Dekker, 1999, pp 533–555.

ciated with anaphylactoid reactions (Table 3). Radiocontrast media not only cause direct release of mediators from mast cells and basophils but also activate the complement and coagulation cascades. Nonsteroidal anti-inflammatory agents may cause acute anaphylactoid reactions in individuals with or without a history of asthma. Physical stimuli, including cold and exercise, can also cause anaphylactoid reactions in some individuals. Angiotensin-converting enzyme (ACE) inhibitors may potentially increase the risk for severe episodes of anaphylaxis because they prevent angiotensin II mobilization, a compensatory physiologic mechanism activated during anaphylaxis.

Special Syndromes of Anaphylaxis

Exercise-induced anaphylaxis (EIA) occurs with prolonged strenuous exercise and is usually accompanied by a short prodrome of cutaneous warmth and generalized pruritus. It may occur only when certain foods (such as celery) or medications (such as aspirin) are ingested before exercise. Exercise avoidance re-

TABLE 3. **Representative Agents that Cause Anaphylactoid Reactions**

Nonsteroidal anti-inflammatory agents: Aspirin, ibuprofen, others
Diagnostic agents: Radiocontrast media
Opiates
Muscle relaxants: Tubocurarine, succinylcholine
Cold: Cold urticaria
Exercise
Intravenous gamma globulin

Modified from Kemp SF, deShazo RD: Anaphylaxis and anaphylactoid reactions. *In* Lockey RF, Bukantz SC (eds): Allergens and Allergen Immunotherapy, 2nd ed (revised and expanded). New York, Marcel Dekker, 1999, pp 533–555.

mains the best treatment. Subjects with EIA should learn how to self-administer epinephrine and preferably should exercise with a partner educated about EIA and how to treat it.

Idiopathic anaphylaxis is a syndrome of repeated anaphylactic episodes for which no cause can be determined despite extensive evaluation. Two large retrospective series suggest that 20 to 33% of all anaphylactic episodes are idiopathic. Fatalities are rare.

Special Considerations

Individuals on beta-adrenergic antagonists (e.g., metoprolol [Lopressor]) may be more likely to experience severe reactions marked by profound hypotension, severe bronchospasm, and paradoxical bradycardia that persists despite treatment with epinephrine. Dosage increases of beta-agonists (e.g., isoproterenol [Isuprel]) up to 80-fold are necessary experimentally to overcome beta-receptor blockade.

Depending on the report, 0 to 20% of subjects who experience anaphylaxis have recurrent or biphasic episodes. Signs and symptoms experienced during the recurrent phase of anaphylaxis may be equivalent to or worse than those seen in the initial reaction, and they may appear up to 8 hours after apparent remission. Persistent anaphylaxis—anaphylactic episodes that last from 5 to 32 hours—may also occur.

Neither biphasic nor persistent anaphylaxis can be predicted from the severity of the initial phase of anaphylaxis. Systemic corticosteroids given during the initial phase of anaphylaxis may not prevent biphasic or persistent anaphylaxis. Because life-threatening manifestations may recur, it may be necessary to monitor subjects for at least 12 hours after apparent recovery from anaphylaxis.

Differential Diagnosis

Several disorders share systemic features with anaphylaxis. The vasovagal reaction perhaps is the most likely consideration in the differential diagnosis of anaphylaxis. This reaction can often be distinguished from anaphylaxis by the following characteristics: The pulse rate is slow rather than rapid, the blood pressure is usually normal or elevated rather than decreased, and the skin is typically cool and pale rather than warm and flushed. Tachycardia is the rule in anaphylaxis, but it may be absent in subjects with atrial conduction defects or in subjects who take sympatholytic medications. Systemic mastocytosis, a disease characterized by mast cell proliferation in multiple organ systems, usually features urticaria pigmentosa (brownish macules that transform into wheals when they are stroked) and recurrent episodes of flushing, tachycardia, pruritus, headache, abdominal pain, diarrhea, or syncope. Myocardial ischemia may cause sudden collapse and may be associated with an irregular pulse. Cardiac risk factors are usually present. A pulmonary embolism may manifest with dyspnea, tachycardia, and chest discomfort that is often pleuritic. An elevated alveolar-arterial gradient may suggest the diagnosis.

Specific signs and symptoms may occur by themselves in other disorders. Patients with hereditary angioedema, for example, have episodes of typically painless, nonpruritic edema of the extremities, which may be associated with laryngeal edema or abdominal pain. Factitious anaphylaxis is a psychiatric disorder characterized by repeated, self-induced episodes of anaphylaxis. Undifferentiated somatoform idiopathic anaphylaxis likewise is a psychiatric disorder in which subjects report symptoms mimicking idiopathic anaphylaxis, but objective findings are absent and the subjects meet diagnostic criteria established by the American Psychiatric Association's *Diagnostic and Statistical Manual of Mental Disorders*, fourth edition, for undifferentiated somatoform disorder.

Management of Anaphylaxis

A sequential approach to the management of anaphylaxis is outlined in Table 4. Assessment and maintenance of the ABCs of basic life support (airway, breathing, and circulation) are necessary before other management steps for life-threatening anaphylaxis are taken. Further treatment for anaphylaxis depends on the severity of the reaction because inappropriate treatment may potentially be as hazardous as the reaction itself. Subjects are monitored continuously to facilitate the prompt detection of any therapeutic complications.

Injectable epinephrine is used in all cases of anaphylaxis to restore vasomotor tone and to prevent further release of harmful chemical mediators. All subsequent therapeutic measures depend on the initial response to epinephrine. Fatalities during witnessed anaphylaxis have usually resulted from delay in epinephrine administration and from severe respiratory complications. In a retrospective review of six fatal and seven nonfatal episodes of food-induced anaphylaxis in children and adolescents, all patients who survived had received epinephrine before or within 5 minutes of developing severe respiratory

TABLE 4. **Treatment of Anaphylaxis**

Immediate Measures

- Aqueous epinephrine 1:1000, 0.3–0.5 mL (0.01 mL/kg in children, max 0.3 mL/dose) SC or IM. Repeat as necessary every 15–20 min (×2) to control symptoms and sustain blood pressure
- Aqueous epinephrine 1:1000, 0.1–0.3 mL in 10 mL of normal saline (1:100,000) IV over several minutes and repeat as necessary for unresponsive anaphylaxis. A 1:10,000 dilution for IV infusion may be necessary.

General Measures

- Place subject in recumbent position, and elevate lower extremities.
- Establish and maintain airway (endotracheal tube or cricothyrotomy may be required).
- Administer oxygen.
- Establish venous access with normal saline IV for fluid replacement. If severe hypotension exists, rapid infusion of volume expanders is necessary (saline or colloid solutions).
- Place a venous tourniquet above the reaction site to decrease absorption of the antigen.

Specific Measures

- Aqueous epinephrine 1:1000, 0.1–0.3 mL at the reaction site will delay antigen absorption.
- Diphenhydramine (Benadryl) 5 mg/kg/d in divided doses with maximum daily dosage of 300 mg for children and 400 mg for adults.
- For bronchospasm, nebulized beta-agonist albuterol (Ventolin, Proventil) 1.25–2.5 mg (0.25–0.5 mL of 5% solution) in 3 mL of saline. Repeat as needed.
- Aminophylline 5 mg/kg over 30 min IV if not responding to inhaled beta agonist. *Note:* Adjust dosage based on age, concomitant medications, or current use of theophylline
- If hypotension persists, dopamine 400 mg in 500 mL D5W should be administered IV at 2–20 μg/kg/min with the rate titrated to maintain adequate blood pressure
- Cimetidine (Tagamet) 300 mg or ranitidine (Zantac) 150 mg administered IV over 10–15 min may also be useful. Rapid IV administration of cimetidine may cause hypotension, but ranitidine may be diluted to 20 cc and injected as a bolus over 5 min
- Glucagon 1–5 mg IV over 5 min and followed by an infusion, 5–15 μg/min, may be useful when a beta blocker complicates anaphylaxis
- Glucocorticosteroids, such as methylprednisolone 1–2 mg/kg for 24 h, are usually not helpful in acute anaphylaxis but may be useful in delayed-onset or protracted anaphylaxis

Specific Measures for Idiopathic Anaphylaxis

Reaction	Treatment
Acute	Epinephrine, 0.3 mL of 1:1000 solution SC
	Prednisone, 60 mg PO
	Antihistamine, such as hydroxyzine (Atarax), 25 mg PO
	Proceed to the nearest emergency department or contact physican for further instructions
Infrequent	Treat same as for acute reactions
Frequent and severe	Prednisone, 60–100 mg PO for 1 wk or until signs and symptoms are controlled
	Continuous oral antihistamine (such as hydroxyzine, 25 mg tid)
	Continuous oral sympathomimetic agent (such as albuterol, 2 mg tid, or ephedrine, 25 mg tid)
	When all signs and symptoms are controlled, convert to alternate-day prednisone 60–100 mg, cautiously tapering by no more than 5 mg/mo

Modified from Kemp SF, deShazo RD: Anaphylaxis and anaphylactoid reactions. *In* Lockey RF, Bukantz SC (eds): Allergens and Allergen Immunotherapy, 2nd ed (revised and expanded). New York, Marcel Dekker, 1999, pp 533–555.

symptoms. None of the subjects who died had received epinephrine before severe respiratory symptoms. Laryngeal edema necessitates early endotracheal intubation to facilitate ventilation and also to avoid intubation difficulty once laryngeal edema becomes severe. Epinephrine may potentially be given endotracheally if intravenous access is difficult to obtain. H_1 and H_2 antagonists, corticosteroids, and volume expanders can be infused once intravenous access is established.

Oxygen should be administered to patients with anaphylaxis who require multiple doses of epinephrine, who have protracted anaphylaxis, or who have pre-existing hypoxemia or myocardial dysfunction. Arterial blood gas determination or continuous pulse oximetry should regulate oxygen therapy. Inhaled $beta_2$ agonists (e.g., albuterol [Ventolin]) may be administered for any bronchospasm refractory to epinephrine.

The patient who takes beta-adrenergic antagonists may not respond to the usual doses of epinephrine administered during anaphylaxis, and higher doses of epinephrine may cause predominantly alpha-agonist effects. In such situations, volume expansion with isotonic fluids and administration of glucagon is recommended. Glucagon may potentially reverse refractory hypotension and bronchospasm in any subject in anaphylactic shock. Glucagon directly activates adenyl cyclase and completely bypasses the beta-adrenergic receptor. Therefore, beta-blockers do not influence its actions. Protection of the airway is particularly important in obtunded patients who receive glucagon because this medication may cause nausea and vomiting and these patients have an increased risk of aspiration.

Prevention of Anaphylaxis

Basic principles for the prevention of future anaphylactic episodes in high-risk individuals are outlined in Table 5. As in all allergic diseases, avoidance and prevention are crucial to the management of anaphylaxis. Agents causing anaphylaxis must be identified when possible, and subjects should be instructed how to minimize future exposure to these agents. Beta-adrenergic antagonists, including a number of topical ophthalmic medications, should be discontinued if substitutions are feasible. Alternatives to ACE inhibitors may potentially be helpful because ACE inhibitors curtail angiotensin II mobilization, a compensatory physiologic mechanism activated during anaphylaxis. More clinical data, however, are needed. Monoamine oxidase inhibitors may also pose a relative risk during anaphylaxis because they interfere with the degradation of epinephrine and make its usage more hazardous.

All persons at high risk for recurrent anaphylaxis should carry epinephrine kits and know how to administer them. An EpiPen is a spring-loaded, pressure-activated syringe with 0.3 mg of epinephrine. It is simple to use and injects through clothing. Two EpiPens are often prescribed together because more

---

TABLE 5. Preventative Measures for Subjects at High Risk for Anaphylaxis

General Measures
- Identification of causes of anaphylaxis and those individuals at risk for future episodes
- Avoidance of antigenic exposure
- Individuals at high risk for anaphylaxis should receive syringes of self-injectable epinephrine and MedicAlert bracelets or chains
- Optimal management of asthma and coronary artery disease
- Substitution of other agents for beta-adrenergic antagonists, angiotensin-converting enzyme inhibitors, and monoamine oxidase inhibitors whenever possible
- Slow, supervised administration of agents suspected of causing anaphylaxis, orally if possible, and if no alternatives are available

Specific Measures*
- Pharmacologic prophylaxis (e.g., radiocontrast media)
- Short-term desensitization† (e.g., penicillin, trimethoprim-sulfamethoxazole [Bactrim, Septra], insulin)
- Allergen immunotherapy‡ (e.g., Hymenoptera venoms, imported fire ant whole-body vaccines)

*Should be used only in an appropriately monitored setting where anaphylactic reactions can be managed effectively.
†Performed by repeated oral or parenteral administration of the medication in increasing doses over several hours to induce transient but sustained tolerance that will enable a full therapeutic course.
‡Accomplished by repeated, low-dose subcutaneous administration of allergenic vaccines at regularly scheduled intervals for several years.
Modified from Bochner BB, Lichtenstein LM: Anaphylaxis. N Engl J Med 324:1785–1790, 1991.

---

than one injection may be necessary. An EpiPen Jr., which delivers 0.15 mg of epinephrine, is appropriate for children who weigh less than 30 kg or for patients who have a co-morbid condition, such as coronary artery disease, which might be affected adversely if full-dose epinephrine is administered. The Ana-Kit contains a syringe with two 0.3-mg doses of epinephrine. Compliance with instructions to carry epinephrine kits must be assessed periodically because many patients forget to carry them.

The potential for anaphylaxis under some circumstances may be determined by skin tests. An example is the risk for allergic reactions to penicillin. The immunochemistry of most drugs and biologic agents is not well defined, however, and reliable in vivo or in vitro testing is unavailable for most agents.

There are many situations in which it is medically necessary to administer an agent known to cause anaphylaxis to individuals at high risk. Numerous protocols have been developed to prevent or reduce the severity of an anticipated anaphylactic episode. All protocols should be conducted in a setting in which anaphylaxis, should it occur, can be managed properly. These protocols recommend pretreatment with corticosteroids and antihistamines to prevent or reduce the severity of a reaction; preferably oral administration of gradually increasing doses of the offending medication over a period of several hours (short-term challenge and desensitization); or long-term desensitization via immunotherapy injections. Venom immunotherapy essentially eliminates the risk of a serious reaction after repeated insect sting and is the treatment of choice to prevent anaphylaxis from Hymenoptera (e.g., yellow jacket) stings. Similarly, immunotherapy with whole-body vaccines of imported fire ants appears to be effective treatment to prevent anaphylaxis associated with imported fire ant stings.

SERUM SICKNESS

Serum sickness is a syndrome characterized by fever, malaise, and an urticarial and/or morbilliform rash, which is often preceded by pruritus and erythema. Arthralgias or arthritis (mainly large joints), lymphadenopathy, abdominal pain (emesis or melena are possible), nephritis, neuropathy, or vasculitis (cutaneous or systemic) may occur in some cases. Cutaneous vasculitis, also known as "hypersensitivity vasculitis," is often manifested by palpable purpura, which most commonly are found on the lower extremities of ambulatory individuals or on the buttocks or sacral region of bedridden patients. These purpuric lesions reflect the leakage of erythrocytes into the skin from inflamed postcapillary venules. Systemic vasculitis may occur in association with connective tissue diseases, infection, or malignancy.

Many agents may produce serum sickness (Table 6). The most common cause of serum sickness today is immune complex–mediated drug hypersensitivity. Serum sickness generally develops 6 to 21 days after the culprit medication is started, but it can occur within 12 to 48 hours in individuals who previously have been sensitized to the medication. Heterologous antisera (often equine or murine) and hyperimmune serum globulins are also capable of producing serum sickness.

Pathogenesis and Laboratory Abnormalities

Low quantities of circulating immune complexes are formed regularly in all healthy individuals. These immune complexes are either excreted by the kidneys or cleared by monocytes and macrophages in the liver and spleen. It is hypothesized that serum sickness results when a drug acting as a hapten binds to plasma protein and antibodies are generated in response to the drug-protein complex. When large quantities of soluble immune (antigen-antibody) complexes fix to receptors in the vascular endothelium of body tissues, the complement system is activated. Complement fragments attract and activate neutrophils, which release proteases that induce tissue injury. The urticaria of serum sickness probably results from immune complex necrotizing vasculitis and complement activation, which generates anaphylatoxins and induces mast cell degranulation. It is probable that IgE-dependent mechanisms are also operative in some individuals. Laboratory abnormalities include an elevated erythrocyte sedimentation rate, leukopenia (acute phase), occasional plasmacytosis, and depressed serum concentrations of C3, C4, and total hemolytic complement (CH_{50}). Slight albuminuria, hyaline casts, and microscopic hematuria may also be present.

Treatment

Removal or stoppage of the offending antigen, when known, is recommended. Serum sickness is usually self-limited and is rarely life-threatening when the culprit drug or heterologous protein is removed. Symptoms generally resolve over 2 to 4 weeks as the body clears the immune complexes. No controlled treatment trials for serum sickness have been conducted. Long-acting, less-sedating antihistamines such as cetirizine (Zyrtec), loratadine (Claritin), or fexofenadine (Allegra) generally control urticaria. Corticosteroids (e.g., prednisone, 0.5 to 1 mg per kg daily) may prove helpful for severe symptoms. Improvement usually occurs within 72 hours, at which time the corticosteroid dosage may be tapered over 2 to 3 weeks as symptoms permit. The antihistamine is continued for an additional week and then slowly discontinued. Skin tests with heterologous antisera are performed routinely to avoid anaphylaxis to heterologous serum on future administration.

ASTHMA IN ADOLESCENTS AND ADULTS

method of
JONATHAN CORREN, M.D.
University of California, Los Angeles
Los Angeles, California

Bronchial asthma has been estimated to afflict 3 to 5% of the adult population. Despite advances in therapy, there have been gradual increases in both the prevalence of asthma as well as the mortality caused by this chronic disease. Recently, there have been international efforts aimed at improving physician diagnosis and evaluation of asthma, appropriate use of medications, and patient education. The diagnostic evaluation of patients with asthma is discussed here along with management strategies to provide optimal care.

TABLE 6. **Representative Agents that Cause Serum Sickness**

Medications: Beta-lactam antibiotics, sulfonamides, ciprofloxacin (Cipro), metronidazole (Flagyl), streptomycin, allopurinol (Zyloprim), carbamazepine (Tegretol), phenytoin (Dilantin), methimazole (Tapazole), propylthiouracil, thiazide diuretics, propranolol (Inderal), others
Heterologous (animal-derived) antisera:
Horse: Snake and spider venom, tetanus, botulism, diphtheria
Horse or rabbit: Antilymphocyte globulin
Mouse: Monoclonal antibodies
Homologous (human-derived) antisera: Cytomegalovirus, hepatitis B, rabies, tetanus, perinatal $Rh_0(D)$

OVERVIEW OF PATHOPHYSIOLOGY

Asthma is a chronic lower airway disease characterized physiologically by reversible airways obstruction and non-specific bronchial hyperresponsiveness. Histologically, alterations of the airways include an increase in mucus secretions, desquamation of the epithelium, mucosal and submucosal edema, basement membrane thickening, smooth muscle hyperplasia, and inflammatory cell infiltration. Cellular inflammation, particularly with eosinophils and lymphocytes, is now thought to underlie airway hyperresponsiveness in asthma and has been found to correlate significantly with asthma severity.

Chronic asthma has also been associated with long-term alterations in airway structure, known as airway remodeling. These changes, the most prominent of which is basement membrane thickening, are probably the result of long-standing bronchial inflammation.

EVALUATION

Appropriate therapy for asthma requires differentiation of this syndrome from other respiratory diseases, accurate categorization of severity, and evaluation of potential triggers.

Differential Diagnosis

Symptoms of asthma usually occur on an intermittent basis and include wheezing, chest tightness, dyspnea, and cough. In some patients, cough may be the principal complaint and may occur mainly at night. When making the initial diagnosis, it is important to obtain a chest radiograph to rule out parenchymal lung or cardiac abnormalities and spirometry to document the severity and reversibility of airways obstruction. In adolescents and young adults, the physician should be alert to the possibility of laryngeal dysfunction as the cause of wheezing, particularly if chest symptoms are unresponsive to bronchodilators. In older adults, cardiac asthma, infiltrative lung disease, and airway tumors need to be considered in the differential diagnosis, especially when cough and/or dyspnea are the predominant symptoms.

Evaluation of Severity and Pattern of Symptoms

The National Asthma Education and Prevention Program (NAEPP) has recommended that asthma treatment be tailored according to indicators of disease severity (Table 1). Importantly, this classification system is based on the frequency and intensity of symptoms as well as on objective measures of pulmonary function.

Asthma symptoms may have important seasonal and diurnal variations. Although the majority of patients have perennial symptoms, a significant subset have seasonal exacerbations. Asthma often worsens during the night, causing interruptions in sleep or increased symptoms on awakening in the morning. An increase in nocturnal symptoms is often the first indication of an asthma exacerbation.

Precipitating and/or Aggravating Factors

Potential triggers responsible for increased symptoms of asthma include environmental factors, infections, concomitant medical conditions, orally ingested substances, and physical stimuli.

Allergens. Airborne allergens are the most important environmental factors that contribute to chronic, persistent asthma in adolescents and adults younger than 45 years of age. Significant causes of perennial symptoms include animal danders, house dust mites, cockroaches, and indoor molds (such as *Aspergillus* and *Penicillium* species). Asthma occurring on a seasonal basis is usually due to either a plant-derived pollen or an outdoor mold (such as *Cladosporium* or *Alternaria* species). The workplace can also harbor specific allergens that may be related to substances used in production (e.g., baker's wheat) or contamination of the facility (e.g., mold in the ventilation system). Because of the importance of aeroallergens in precipitating asthma, allergy skin testing or in vitro blood tests (e.g., radioallergosorbent test [RAST]) should be performed for relevant allergens in all patients with asthma. The results of these tests are critical in establishing an effective program of allergen avoidance.

Upper Airway Disease. Allergic rhinitis is present in up to 90% of adults with asthma, and appropriate management has been shown to improve asthma symptoms, bronchial hyperresponsiveness, and pulmonary function. Upper respiratory tract infections, including both viral respiratory infections and bacterial sinusitis, can cause significant exacerbations of bronchial asthma. Acute sinusitis should always be carefully considered in patients presenting with persistent purulent rhinorrhea (>10 days) after a typical viral infection. Similarly, in asthmatics with chronic symptoms of headache, facial fullness, mucopurulent nasal discharge or postnasal drip, chronic sinus disease should be evaluated using plain radiography or computed tomography and treated aggressively when identified.

Concomitant Illnesses/Hormonal States. Gastroesoph-

TABLE 1. **Classification of Asthma Severity**

Category	Symptoms	Nocturnal Symptoms	Lung Function
Step 4: severe persistent	Continual symptoms Limited physical activity Frequent exacerbations	Frequent	FEV_1/PEFR ≤ 60% of predicted
Step 3: moderate persistent	Daily symptoms Daily use of beta$_2$-agonist Exacerbations ≥2 times per week	>1× per week	FEV_1/PEFR 60–80% of predicted
Step 2: mild persistent	Symptoms >2 times per week, <1 time per day	>2 times per month	FEV_1/PEFR ≥80% of predicted
Step 1: mild intermittent	Symptoms ≤2 times per week Asymptomatic between exacerbations	≤2 times per month	FEV_1/PEFR ≥80% of predicted

Abbreviations: FEV_1 = fraction of expiratory volume in 1 second; PEFR = peak expiratory flow rate.

ageal reflux disease may present as symptoms with heartburn or may manifest strictly as increased cough or wheezing in patients with asthma. Effective medical treatment may have significant beneficial effects on asthma. Changes in estrogen levels that occur premenstrually or during pregnancy are commonly associated with transient worsening of asthma. Other endocrine alterations (e.g., hypothyroidism) have been implicated in cases of asthma refractory to usual medical therapy.

Foods/Additives. Oral ingestants play a limited role in triggering symptoms of asthma. Whereas IgE-mediated allergy to food proteins infrequently contributes to asthma, food additives have been shown to be provocative factors in some patients. Sulfites, which are used as preservatives in white wine and dried fruit, have been shown to cause bronchospasm in up to 10% of adults with asthma.

Drugs. Aspirin and other nonsteroidal anti-inflammatory agents may elicit severe bronchospasm in approximately 10% of asthmatics, often but not limited to those with histories of nasal polyposis and chronic sinusitis. Beta-adrenergic blockers (both orally and ophthalmically) may increase wheezing in many patients and should therefore be avoided.

Physical Stimuli. Exercise can cause bronchospasm in up to 80% of asthmatics, and in many patients it is the sole trigger of asthma symptoms. Cold air appears to worsen this phenomenon in most patients, whereas in others the extremes of relative humidity may influence the intensity of bronchospasm.

TREATMENT

Once the level of asthma severity and potential triggers have been established, therapy should be initiated. Treatment modalities for asthma include allergen avoidance strategies, pharmacotherapy, and allergen immunotherapy (hyposensitization).

Allergen Avoidance Strategies

A number of environmental control measures have been proven to effectively reduce daily exposure to indoor allergens. These avoidance measures should be instituted only after careful documentation of IgE-mediated sensitivity and frequent exposure to relevant allergens.

House Dust Mite. Mites are microscopic insects that are ubiquitous in many parts of the United States and particularly thrive in areas with warm, humid climates during the summer. The principal reservoirs for mites include pillows, bedding, mattresses, upholstered furniture, and carpeting. Importantly, mite allergens cling to large, heavy particles of dust, causing them to settle out quickly after they have been disturbed by sitting on a bed or chair. Clinical studies have established that mite numbers and allergen levels are most effectively lowered by washing of bedding in hot (>130°C) water, placement of impervious encasings over the pillow and mattress, and removal of bedroom carpeting. HEPA filters and anti-mite sprays for carpeting have not been shown to consistently reduce mite allergen levels in dust or to significantly improve asthma symptoms due to dust mite allergy.

Animal Allergens. Allergens from animal pelts, particularly cats, are most successfully reduced by removing the animal from inside the home environment. This must be followed by a very thorough cleaning, along with removal or replacement of the carpeting in the home. Short of these measures, it is very difficult to lower the amount of airborne cat allergen. Steam-cleaning the carpeting and use of a HEPA filter, with the cat left inside the house, have not been shown to significantly reduce asthma symptoms caused by cat allergen.

Mold. Evidence of indoor mold growth should be investigated by all patients with asthma. Clues that suggest mold growth include dark or colored spots on the ceilings, walls, or floors; mildew in the shower stall, under sinks, in closets or in the basement; and musty odors in closed spaces inside the home. Elimination of mold from a home requires thorough cleaning; removal and replacement of damaged carpeting, plaster, or wood; and correction of water leaks in the foundation, roof, or plumbing.

Cockroaches. Cockroach infestation should be suspected if droppings are found in the home. Elevated levels of cockroach allergen may be found throughout the home, including the bedroom, because allergen is tracked onto carpeting from shoes. Effective eradication may be best accomplished by commercial exterminators.

Pharmacotherapy

The NAEPP guidelines outline a stepwise approach to asthma treatment based on disease severity (Table 2). This approach recommends that medications be given in adequate doses to gain rapid control of symptoms and should later be reduced to the minimal level required to maintain control. The new approach also differentiates between medications that are used for long-term control of asthma versus medications that are to be used for rapid relief of acute symptoms. The goals of therapy should include prevention of symptoms, reduction in frequency and severity of exacerbations, maintenance of normal (or near-normal pulmonary function), maintenance of normal activity levels, and minimization of medication side effects.

Maintenance (Controller) Medications

Maintenance medications are to be taken on a regular, daily basis and should be used in all patients with persistent asthma. This group of asthma medications includes inhaled (and occasionally oral) corticosteroids, leukotriene modifiers, long-acting beta$_2$-agonists and theophylline.

Inhaled Corticosteroids. Corticosteroid aerosols effectively reduce airway inflammation and have been shown to improve lung function and reduce bronchial hyperresponsiveness. These agents are the most effective maintenance treatment available for most patients with asthma and are the preferred choice of therapy for patients with mild to moderate persistent symptoms. Importantly, these agents are

TABLE 2. Stepwise Approach for Use of Asthma Maintenance Medications*

Category	Maintenance Medication
Step 4: severe persistent	• Inhaled corticosteriod (high dose) *plus* • Long-acting beta₂-agonist *or* sustained-release theophylline; consider both agents in combination if needed If needed, consider: • Leukotriene inhibitor If needed, consider • Oral corticosteroid taken on alternate days in lowest possible dose
Step 3: moderate persistent	• Inhaled corticosteroid (medium dose) *or* • Inhaled corticosteroid (low dose) plus long-acting beta₂-agonist *or* sustained-release theophylline
Step 2: mild persistent	• Inhaled corticosteroid (low dose)† *or* • Cromolyn *or* • Nedocromil *or* • Leukotriene inhibitor *or* • Sustained-release theophylline
Step 1: mild intermittent	• No maintenance medication needed

*Patients at all severity levels should use short-acting inhaled beta₂-agonists for relief of acute symptoms.
†Preferred medication in this category.

most effective when started early after the diagnosis of asthma and may help prevent long-term airway remodeling associated with irreversible changes in lung function.

Asthma symptoms will usually begin to improve within several days of starting inhaled corticosteroids. Once symptoms and pulmonary function have been stabilized over a period of 2 to 3 months, the corticosteroid dose may be slowly tapered every 2 months as tolerated. Even the most severe asthmatics can now be managed primarily with inhaled corticosteroids, and very few patients require oral corticosteroids on a maintenance basis.

A growing number of corticosteroid aerosols are available in the United States, and the dosing varies depending on the specific product (Table 3). All of the agents have been shown to be effective when administered as two doses per day, and data suggest that some stable patients may be well controlled with a single daily dose. Most of the available agents are available as metered-dose inhalers with the exception of budesonide (Pulmicort), which is delivered by means of a dry-powder inhaler. Pharmacy formularies, efficacy issues, and patient preference will dictate which aerosol is optimal in a given patient.

The most common side effects of inhaled corticosteroids occur locally in the upper airway. Oral candidiasis (thrush) occurs in as many as 30% of patients but can be effectively prevented by using a holding chamber and by rinsing the mouth after inhalation. Dysphonia occurs commonly in patients treated with high doses of inhaled corticosteroids; holding chambers may be helpful in preventing this complication. Reflex cough has been occasionally noted with all of the preparations and may be reduced by use of a holding chamber, by slowing the rate of inspiration, or by premedicating with an inhaled beta₂-agonist.

Because inhaled corticosteroids are administered in very small doses and there is extensive first-pass hepatic metabolism of the swallowed portion of drug, the systemic effects of these medications are relatively minor. Hypothalamic-pituitary-adrenal axis function has been studied intensively with many of the available inhaled corticosteroids and there does not appear to be significant adrenal suppression when these drugs are used in recommended doses. More sensitive assays (e.g., 24-hour integrated serum cortisol levels) have demonstrated significant changes in cortisol production, but the clinical significance of these findings is uncertain. Most importantly, clinical adrenal insufficiency has not been noted with chronic use of corticosteroid aerosols. Of greater concern have been reports describing a significant, dose-dependent reduction in bone mineral content associated with inhaled corticosteroid use. Postmenopausal female patients may be most at risk

TABLE 3. Daily Doses of Inhaled Corticosteroids*

Drug	Low Dose	Medium Dose	High Dose
Beclomethasone dipropionate (Vanceril)	168–504 μg	504–840 μg	>840 μg†
42 μg/puff	4–12 puffs	12–20 puffs	>20 puffs
84 μg/puff	2–6 puffs	6–10 puffs	>10 puffs
Budesonide (Pulmicort)	200–400 μg	400–600 μg	>600 μg†
200 μg/dose	1–2 inhalations	2–3 inhalations	>3 inhalations
Flunisolide (AeroBid)	500–1000 μg	1000–2000 μg	>2000 μg†
250 μg/puff	2–4 puffs	4–8 puffs	>8 puffs
Fluticasone propionate (Flovent)	88–264 μg	264–660 μg	>660 μg
44 μg/puff	2–6 puffs		
110 μg/puff	2 puffs	2–6 puffs	>6 puffs
220 μg			>3 puffs
Triamcinolone acetonide (Azmacort)	400–1000 μg	1000–2000 μg†	>2000 μg†
100 μg/puff	(4–10 puffs)	(10–20 puffs)	(>20 puffs)

*Some dosages may be outside product labeling.
†Exceeds dosage recommended by the manufacturer.
Modified from National Asthma Education and Prevention Program, Expert Panel Report 2: Guidelines for the Diagnosis and Management of Asthma. Washington, DC, U.S. Department of Health and Human Services, National Heart, Lung, and Blood Institute, NIH Publication No. 97-4051, p. 88.

for these effects because of the normal changes in estrogen that accompany aging. Therefore, inhaled corticosteroid doses should always be tapered to the lowest level required to maintain control of symptoms and pulmonary function.

Cromones. Inhaled cromolyn sodium (Intal), and nedocromil (Tilade), are potent mast cell stabilizers that also have mild anti-inflammatory effects. These drugs are most commonly employed as preventative treatments before a short-term allergen exposure or exercise. When used as maintenance therapy for mild persistent asthma, cromolyn metered-dose inhaler 2 puffs four times daily, and nedocromil metered-dose inhaler 2 puffs four times daily, are equally effective in reducing asthma symptoms and improving peak flow rates. However, the clinical effects of cromolyn and nedocromil in chronic asthma are less predictable than the response to inhaled corticosteroids. Although limited data from controlled trials have demonstrated that cromolyn may be effective in patients with both allergic and nonallergic asthma, it has been my clinical experience that it is most effective in atopic patients. The safety profiles of both of these agents are excellent, with no significant systemic toxicities. Therefore, it is worth trying either cromolyn or nedocromil as maintenance treatment in patients who are at significant risk for systemic effects of inhaled corticosteroids (growing adolescents, postmenopausal women, and patients with pre-existing osteoporosis) or who have difficult-to-manage local side effects (e.g., dysphonia) from corticosteroids.

Leukotriene Modifiers. Currently available agents include zafirukast (Accolate) and montelukast (Singulair), which are sulfidopeptide leukotriene receptor antagonists, and zileuton (Zyflo), which is a 5-lipoxygenase inhibitor. All of these drugs have been shown to improve asthma symptoms and to cause variable improvements in pulmonary function. In addition, they have all been shown to significantly reduce bronchoconstriction caused by exercise. Although the NAEPP guidelines suggest that these drugs may be considered as alternatives to low-dose inhaled corticosteroids for patients with mild persistent asthma, further studies are needed before their exact role in asthma can be defined. The leukotriene inhibitors may be most useful when added to inhaled corticosteroids as an adjunctive agent, particularly in patients who are aspirin intolerant.

Important differences in dosing and side effects do exist between the available leukotriene inhibitors. Montelukast (10 mg) and zafirlukast (20 mg) are administered once and twice daily, respectively. Zileuton (600 mg) must be dosed four times daily initially, but once symptoms are controlled the dose may be tapered to twice daily over 2 to 3 months. With respect to adverse effects, zileuton has been associated with hepatic transaminase elevation in approximately 3% of patients, and it has therefore been recommended that liver function tests be done when using this drug. Both zafirlukast and montelukast have been linked to small numbers of cases of Churg-Strauss syndrome. The most likely explanation for this association may be the unmasking of Churg-Strauss syndrome after the withdrawal of oral corticosteroids during treatment with zafirlukast and montelukast.

Long-acting Beta₂-Agonists. Both inhaled salmeterol (Serevent), and oral, sustained-release preparations of albuterol (Proventil Repetabs), provide long-acting bronchodilation and are important adjuncts to anti-inflammatory therapy. Both inhaled and oral agents are effective for reducing nocturnal symptoms of asthma, and inhaled salmeterol has been shown to block exercise-induced bronchospasm. Several studies have demonstrated that the addition of salmeterol to a regimen of low-dose inhaled corticosteroids is more effective than doubling the dose of the corticosteroid. These agents should not be used as the sole therapy for asthma, and it is important to reinforce the importance of continuing anti-inflammatory treatment. On an equally important note, these long-acting drugs should never be used to treat acute symptoms or exacerbations of asthma.

Typical of beta₂-agonists, these drugs may cause tachycardia, palpitations, and skeletal muscle tremor. In some cases, these side effects may be severe enough to warrant discontinuation of the drug. Use of a holding chamber will reduce oral-pharyngeal deposition of these drugs and potentially reduce systemic side effects as well as maximize pulmonary deposition. As a general rule, these drugs should be used cautiously in patients with ischemic heart disease and/or arrhythmias.

Theophylline. Theophylline is an effective bronchodilator that also appears to possess a variety of anti-inflammatory properties when steady-state serum concentrations are maintained between 5 and 15 µg per mL. In the current NAEPP guidelines, sustained-release theophylline is considered to be an alternative form of maintenance therapy for mild persistent asthma, particularly when cost of medications is an issue. However, many clinical trials have demonstrated that sustained-release preparations of theophylline are significantly less effective than inhaled corticosteroids in patients with persistent symptoms, have more side effects, and require monitoring of serum drug levels. Similar to leukotriene modifiers and long-acting beta₂-agonists, the most important role for theophylline is as an adjunct to inhaled corticosteroids.

Even at therapeutic doses, theophylline may cause nausea, headache, and central nervous system stimulation. When serum theophylline concentrations excede 20 µg per mL, tachyarrhythmias and seizures may occur. Therefore, routine monitoring is critical, particularly when the patient is taking other medications that may alter the metabolism of theophylline. As with long-acting beta₂-agonists, theophylline should be used very carefully in patients with cardiac disease.

Oral Corticosteroids. Fortunately, aggressive use of inhaled corticosteroids in combination with long-acting beta₂ agonists, sustained-release theophylline, and/or leukotriene inhibitors has markedly reduced the need to treat patients chronically with oral corticosteroids. For patients who continue to have significant asthma symptoms and frequent exacerbations despite this approach, maintenance usage prednisone or methylprednisolone (Medrol) may be necessary. In general, the lowest possible dose should be given on an alternate-day schedule (1 day on, 1 day off).

A variety of anti-inflammatory and cytotoxic medications, including troleandomycin, methotrexate, gold, intravenous immunoglobulin, dapsone, and hydroxychloroquine, have been used in selected severe patients to reduce the need for oral corticosteroids. Results from clinical trials have revealed significant potential toxicities with many of these agents and have not consistently demonstrated improvements in asthma. Therefore, these therapies should be considered experimental and reserved for use in specialized centers.

Reliever Medications

When asthma symptoms occur despite regular use of a maintenance therapy, medications for quick relief are indicated. These drugs include beta$_2$-agonists, ipratroprium bromide (Atrovent), and oral corticosteroids.

Short-acting Beta$_2$-Agonists. Short-acting beta$_2$-agonists, such as albuterol and pirbuterol (Maxair), cause prompt bronchodilation (within 15 to 30 minutes) and are the drug of choice for treating acute symptoms of asthma. Patients with mild intermittent asthma (symptoms less than 2 days per week) usually only require treatment with an inhaled beta$_2$ agonist used on an as-needed basis. Similarly, patients who experience asthma only with exercise may be adequately managed by premedicating with an inhaled beta$_2$-agonist 15 to 20 minutes before exercise. In patients with persistent asthma, regularly scheduled, daily use of short-acting beta$_2$-agonists has not been shown to improve asthma control and these agents should be used strictly for relief of acute symptoms.

Beta$_2$-agonists may cause tremor, palpitations, and racing heartbeat, particularly when these agents are used on an intermittent basis. The single R-isomer of albuterol, when available, has been shown to result in a reduced incidence of these side effects with similar or greater efficacy.

Anticholinergics. Ipratropium bromide is a quaternary derivative of atropine and has been shown to cause variable bronchodilation in patients with asthma and in general is not as effective as inhaled beta$_2$-agonists. It has minimal, if any, systemic side effects and may be used as an acute reliever in the few patients who cannot tolerate inhaled beta$_2$-agonists. Ipratropium has also been shown to provide additive bronchodilation to inhaled beta$_2$-agonists in severe asthma exacerbations.

Allergen Immunotherapy

Allergen avoidance and pharmacotherapy are the cornerstones of treatment for all patients with asthma. However, in many patients allergens are not easily avoided (i.e., pollen and mold) and medications may not be entirely effective. Allergen immunotherapy, or hyposensitization therapy, has been used for many years in patients with both seasonal and perennial allergic asthma and can be a very important adjunct to other treatments. Incremental doses of specific allergens are injected subcutaneously on a regular basis, resulting in immunologic tolerance to those proteins. A large number of double-blind, pla-

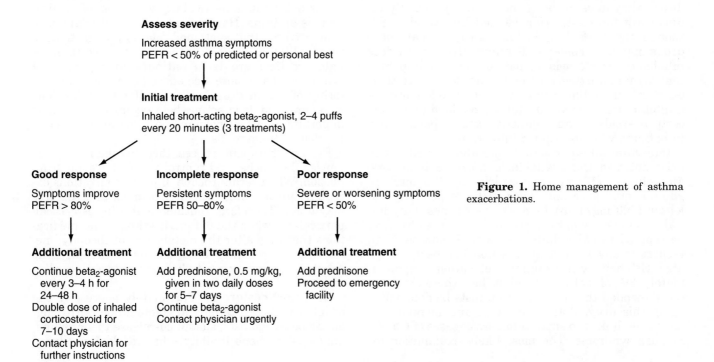

Figure 1. Home management of asthma exacerbations.

cebo-controlled trials have demonstrated that immunotherapy effectively reduces asthma symptoms in patients sensitive to pollen allergens, house dust mites, cat dander, and *Alternaria* and *Cladosporium* molds. Importantly, the efficacy of immunotherapy is dose dependent, and low doses have been shown to be equivalent to placebo.

As in allergen avoidance, effective immunotherapy is based on a patient having a well-documented sensitivity to the allergen in question (using skin tests or RAST), frequent exposure to the allergen, and a history of asthma symptoms related to the allergenic exposure. Immunotherapy should be considered in patients with asthma when (1) asthma symptoms are inadequately controlled with environmental control measures and medications; (2) medication side effects develop; (3) medications with potential long-term adverse effects (oral corticosteroids or high-dose inhaled corticosteroids) are required to control symptoms; (4) patients are interested in a therapy that may modify the natural history of their asthma; and (5) symptoms are present for at least 4 months per year. Patients will often note improvement in their symptoms during the first 6 to 12 months of therapy, although some patients will not experience benefits until a maintenance dose of extract has been administered for several months (approximately 18 months of treatment). Studies with both seasonal pollen and house dust mites have demonstrated that long-lasting benefits are more likely if immunotherapy is given for at least 3 years.

Local areas of induration may occur after immunotherapy injections but rarely limit the dose of allergen that can be administered to the patient. Because potentially serious systemic allergic reactions do occur with 0.5% of injections, all immunotherapy should be administered at a medical facility equipped to treat anaphylaxis. Because reactions usually occur within 20 minutes after an injection, patients should be instructed to wait this period of time in the clinic. Patients with poorly controlled asthma ($FEV_1 < 70\%$ of predicted) are at higher risk for systemic reactions, and immunotherapy should be avoided in these patients. In addition, immunotherapy should not be started in patients receiving oral or topical beta-adrenergic blockers because they may not respond optimally to epinephrine used to treat immunotherapy reactions.

MONITORING DISEASE ACTIVITY AND HOME TREATMENT OF EXACERBATIONS

Optimal control of asthma requires daily assessment of symptoms, paying particular attention to nocturnal asthma and need for inhaled $beta_2$-adrenergic agonists. Home monitoring of peak expiratory flow rates (PEFR) is suggested in patients with moderate-to-severe asthma or histories of sudden, severe exacerbations.

Based on the patient's clinical symptoms and PEFR values, a home treatment plan can be initiated that one hopes will control the patient's symptoms and reduce the need to seek medical attention at an acute care facility. If asthma symptoms increase acutely and the PEFR drops to less than 50% of the patient's personal best or his or her predicted value, the patient should administer a short-acting inhaled $beta_2$-agonist up to three doses (Fig. 1). If there has been a good acute response to a supplemental $beta_2$ agonist (PEFR > 80%), the attack may simply be dealt with by doubling the dose of the patient's inhaled corticosteroid for 7 to 10 days. If the response has been intermediate (PEFR 50–80%), prednisone, 0.5 mg/kg, in two daily doses should be given for 5 to 7 days (without tapering) and the patient's physician should be contacted urgently. If the response has been poor (PEFR < 50%), oral corticosteroids should be initiated as just described and the patient should be seen emergently at a physician's office or emergency facility.

ASTHMA IN CHILDREN

method of
WALTER TORDA, M.D.
Harvard Vanguard Medical Associates
Boston, Massachusetts
Harvard Medical School
Boston, Massachusetts

Asthma is the most common chronic illness in children. It has not only a great influence on their social and personal development but also significant direct and indirect costs. Asthma is commonly underdiagnosed and undertreated. Despite a rapidly developing understanding of its pathophysiology and pathogenesis, the incidence and morbidity of asthma are increasing, especially in African Americans, Puerto Ricans, and children living in poverty. The diagnosis of asthma should be considered for all children with recurrent cough, chronic cough, or exercise intolerance with or without wheezing.

DEFINITION

The definition of asthma continues to evolve. The American Thoracic Society in 1962 defined bronchial hyperreactivity as the central feature of asthma. The understanding of bronchial hyperreactivity has become more sophisticated. It is now recognized that there are both early and late phases of bronchospasm reflecting this bronchial hyperreactivity. The early phase, mediated primarily by histamine, that occurs at the time of exposure to a stimulus is responsive to bronchodilators. The late phase of reactivity occurs hours after exposure, is mediated primarily by leukotrienes and cytokines, and is responsive to anti-inflammatory therapy. The current definition of the National Heart, Lung, and Blood Institute (1995) emphasizes inflammation as the central feature of asthma. Asthma, of any severity, is defined as a "chronic inflammatory airway disease mediated by many cells and cellular elements."

Inflammation is the feature that underlies episodic symptoms. Inflammation underlies bronchial hyperreactivity and is responsible for the sub–basement membrane fibrosis that leads to decreased pulmonary function in later life. The implications for therapy are clear. If asthma is considered an episodic disease, treatment should be directed at definitive management of exacerbations to prevent airway inflammation and subsequent steroid dependence. The concept of asthma, of any severity, as a chronic inflammatory disease implies a different approach to therapy. Chronic anti-inflammatory therapy is intended to control airway inflammation, minimize airway hyperreactivity, and prevent subendothelial fibrosis. The goal is to achieve a normal childhood, maximize lung growth, and optimize pulmonary function.

EPIDEMIOLOGY

The prevalence of asthma in children (those under 18 years of age) is 7.2%, which is 41% higher than the 5.1% incidence in the general population. Approximately 5 million children have asthma, including an estimated 1.3 million children under 5 years of age. The incidence of asthma in Puerto Rican children is one and a half times higher than that in whites, and their mortality rate is five times that of white children. African American children have an incidence of asthma that is 24% higher than that among white children and a mortality rate that is three times that of white children. More than 5000 Americans per year die of asthma.

Children with asthma miss approximately 1 week of school each year, a total of 10 million school days per year. This is three times the rate of school absences of children without asthma.

Childhood asthma occurs at a higher rate in boys than in girls, with a maximum predominance at puberty. This may reflect the smaller caliber of airways in boys until puberty.

Atopy in general correlates with asthma, and IgE level reflects airway inflammation. Sensitization to indoor allergens (dust mites, cockroaches, mold, and pets, especially dogs and cats) correlates with the development of asthma. There is also a higher incidence of atopy in boys than in girls. A family history of asthma is correlated with the development of asthma, as are prenatal exposure to tobacco smoke, exposure to second-hand smoke, advanced maternal age, prematurity, and peripheral blood (and endobronchial) eosinophilia early in life.

PATHOPHYSIOLOGY

The primary physiologic abnormality in asthma is airway obstruction. Obstruction occurs throughout the tracheobronchial tree and results in increased resistance to airflow. Poiseuille's law describes this; resistance to flow is directly proportional to the length of the tube and to the fourth power of the radius. Small changes in airway caliber result in large changes in the resistance to flow. Changes in airway caliber are more significant in the peripheral lung and in small children compared with teenagers because a given change represents a larger proportional change in a small airway than it does in a large airway. The lumens of the airways become obstructed by contraction of the peribronchial smooth muscle and by airway inflammation with subsequent edema and hypersecretion.

Airway inflammation involves mast cell activation, inflammatory cell infiltration (eosinophils, macrophages, neutrophils, and TH$_2$ lymphocytes), edema, denudation and disruption of the bronchial epithelium, sub–basement membrane collagen deposition, goblet cell hyperplasia, and hypertrophy, hyperplasia, and contraction of the peribronchial smooth muscle.

Activated mast cells release a variety of preformed and newly formed mediators of inflammation. Preformed mediators such as histamine and proteases are responsible for immediate bronchospasm, the early-phase reaction. Leukotrienes, prostaglandins, and platelet-activating factor are synthesized upon activation of the mast cell. They are involved in the late phase of bronchial reactivity. In addition, cytokines are formed that promote the differentiation and chemotaxis of inflammatory cells. Mast cells promote the formation of more mast cells by releasing cytokines, including interleukin (IL)–4 and IL-5, which promote the differentiation and chemotaxis of eosinophils, the formation of TH$_2$-type lymphocytes, and the formation of more mast cells.

Eosinophils and lymphocytes infiltrate into the airway wall and the surrounding adventitial tissues. Eosinophils are the hallmark of inflammation in asthma. They secrete mediators thought to be central to bronchial hyperreactivity. The eosinophil releases proteins such as eosinophilic cationic protein and eosinophil peroxidase, which are active in damaging the respiratory epithelium and other airway cells. Activated macrophages produce a number of inflammatory products and are important in promoting eosinophil growth and differentiation.

Macrophages also produce substances that are involved in the growth and regulation of TH$_2$ lymphocytes. TH$_2$ lymphocytes in turn produce IL-3, IL-4, and IL-5 and express chemokine receptors. In addition, mediators released by structural cells such as airway epithelial cells drive the inflammatory response. The release of these mediators encourages hypertrophy, hyperplasia, and contraction of peribronchial smooth muscle, the transformation of the airway epithelium from an orderly stratified columnar arrangement into a dysplastic and thickened arrangement, deposition of collagen below the basement membrane, glandular hyperplasia and hypersecretion, and a state of enhanced contractility that promotes airway hyperreactivity.

Once this process has been initiated, it is self-perpetuating and self-amplifying.

CLINICAL MANIFESTATION

Asthma is so common that it must be considered for all infants and children who present with recurrent episodes of cough, persistent cough, chronic cough, wheeze, exercise intolerance, or nocturnal cough. Often, review of the medical record will reveal repeated episodes of bronchiolitis, bronchitis, or pneumonia. Asthma can develop at any age, although the differential diagnosis varies with the developmental stage.

It is common, in children, for asthma to manifest initially with persistent cough after a viral respiratory tract infection. Typically these children have an extended period of cough followed by repeated episodes of persistent cough with or without wheeze. These episodes commonly become chronic and repetitive. They are usually perceived by the family as frequent colds that "go right to the chest." Several clinical features make the diagnosis of asthma more likely: nocturnal increase in cough, peripheral eosinophilia, family history of asthma, and atopy.

Exercise intolerance is another common presentation. This is expressed in different ways at different ages; infants who cough or wheeze when they laugh, cry, or feed (although gastroesophageal reflux needs to be excluded); toddlers who cough whenever they go to the playground or have a tantrum; and children who cough, wheeze, or have dyspnea when they run. Cold, dry air tends to worsen these symptoms. One must differentiate here between true exercise-induced asthma and exercise intolerance due to asthma that is not adequately controlled.

Seasonal cough and wheeze are strongly suggestive of asthma. It usually takes 3 or 4 years to have sufficient exposure to pollens to become sensitized. Pollen allergy is seasonal; environmental allergy (sensitization to dust mites, mold, cockroaches, pets) is not. Viral illness and exposure to cold, dry air are also seasonal.

Features such as failure to thrive, cyanosis while feeding, vomiting while feeding, clubbing, or failure to respond to appropriate treatment argue against asthma as a diagnosis.

Many of these children will "outgrow" their asthma, but there are no clear predictors of which children will do so. Atopy, a family history of atopy, perinatal tobacco smoke exposure, low birth weight, and prematurity are associated with persistent disease.

We know that asthma severity can vary over time. One pattern is the symptomatic infant or child who has a decrease in symptoms after the adolescent growth spurt. This suggests "dysanapsis," that is, small airways compared with lung volume. This results in a functional obstruction. These children are initially symptomatic, but, as they go through their adolescent growth spurt, the airways increase in caliber so that they are commensurate with lung volume. It is important to remember that these teens may continue to have chronic inflammation and should be treated appropriately.

DIFFERENTIAL DIAGNOSIS

Infants who cough or wheeze repeatedly probably have asthma. Several other entities need to be considered, although they are relatively uncommon; tracheal stenosis, laryngotracheomalacia, bronchial stenosis, compression of the trachea (most commonly by a vascular anomaly, e.g., vascular ring), bronchiolitis, bronchopulmonary dysplasia, tracheoesophageal fistula, gastroesophageal reflux, cystic fibrosis, immunodeficiency, and congenital heart disease with pulmonary edema. Toddlers share this differential diagnosis but in addition may have foreign body aspiration, tracheal compression by tumor or lymph nodes, and allergic rhinitis and/or sinusitis.

Children are more likely to have symptoms in response to a viral illness, but a larger percentage of all attacks are triggered by allergy as children get older. Immunodeficiency, especially IgG subclass deficiency, needs to be considered.

DIAGNOSIS

The history helps to characterize the illness in the child and the impact on the family. There are a number of areas to explore, but the intention is to determine the disease onset, frequency, persistence, progress, intensity, and chronicity and the impact on the development of the child and family.

Symptoms. Does the child cough, wheeze, or have another manifestation of airway obstruction, such as shortness of breath, chest tightness, or air hunger?

Pattern of Symptoms. Are the symptoms chronic or episodic? Is there a season, or do they occur year round? What is the frequency and duration of symptoms? Is there diurnal variation?

Precipitating Factors. Common factors include viral respiratory illness, exercise (including feeding in infants, laughing or crying at any age), environmental antigens (dust mites, cockroaches, mold, pets, pollen), irritant exposure (tobacco, strong odors, air pollution), changes in the weather, foods, or preservatives (sulfites).

Progress of the Disease. What was the age of onset versus age at diagnosis? Was there early airway injury, intubation and ventilation, bronchopulmonary dysplasia, or parental smoking? Have the symptoms improved or worsened over time? Has the child been treated in emergency room settings? Has the child been hospitalized, been in the intensive care unit, or been intubated?

Management. What is the current pharmacologic management? Are peak flows determined and recorded? What is the personal best value, and which meter was it determined on? What is the intermeasurement variability? Is there a written management plan? Is there a written rescue plan? How often is the child in the yellow zone? How often is the child in the red zone?

Risk Factors for Respiratory Failure. Is there a history of sudden severe exacerbation, intubation for asthma, or intensive care unit admission? Have there been two or more admissions for asthma in the past year? Have there been more than three emergency room visits in the last year? Has there been a hospitalization or emergency room visit in the last month? Is there use of more than two beta-agonist inhalers per month? Is there current or recent use of systemic corticosteroids? Does the child have difficulty in perceiving the severity of exacerbations? Are there comorbid conditions? Is there serious psychiatric disease or psychosocial dysfunction? Is the patient or family in a low socioeconomic status? Is there illicit drug use? Is there sensitivity to *Alternaria*?

Family History. Is there a history of asthma, allergy, eczema, nasal polyp, rhinitis, or sinusitis in close relatives?

Environmental History. Are there smokers in the home? Are there pets? Is there use of a humidifier? Is there carpet over concrete? Are there wood-burning stoves or fireplaces or a gas range?

Impact on Family. How many episodes of unscheduled care have there been? How frequent are these episodes? Have there been life-threatening exacerbations? How many days of school has the child missed? How many days of work has the parent missed? Is there limitation of activity? What is the impact of asthma and its treatment on family routines? What is the economic impact of asthma on the family?

PHYSICAL EXAMINATION

Inspection. Is there cyanosis or clubbing? Is there symmetry of the thorax, flaring of the costal margins, or hyperinflation of the chest? Is there use of accessory muscles or respiration, especially the sternocleidomastoid muscle? Are there retractions, especially tracheosternal (supersternal or superclavicular), or nasal flaring? What is the timing of thoracic respiratory excursions (a thoracic lag suggests obstruction; paradoxical motion suggests severe obstruction)?

Palpation. Is there thoracic motion? Is the thoracic motion symmetric? Is there tactile fremitus?

Auscultation. Are there adventitious sounds? What is the inspiratory to expiratory (I:E) ratio? Is there egophony or whispered pectoriloquy?

Percussion. Is there hyperresonance? Is percussion symmetric?

LABORATORY EXAMINATION

Objective measures of pulmonary function are extremely helpful to establish the initial diagnosis of asthma, follow up the course of the disease, and monitor the effectiveness of therapy. Monitoring of lung function is especially important for those children who have difficulty in perceiving the severity of their symptoms, because these children are at increased risk of respiratory failure.

Spirometry

Spirometry can be performed on children after they are about 5 years old. The National Asthma Education and Prevention Project recommends spirometry at the time of initial diagnosis, after treatment and symptoms stabilize, and at least every 1 or 2 years. Spirometry can assess the degree of airway obstruction and exclude restrictive lung disease. Spirometry can evaluate the relative involvement of small airways and more precisely determine the degree of large airway involvement. Spirometry performed before and after adequate doses of bronchodilator helps to determine the success of therapy, as does comparison of spirometric data over time. Reversibility, the improvement of pulmonary function after bronchodilator administration, aids in the assessment of therapy and is particularly useful to evaluate the adequacy of current therapy as well as guide changes in therapy. Inspiratory flow volume loops can exclude laryngospasm masquerading as asthma.

Peak Flows

Although spirometry is the "gold standard" in the evaluation of lung function, it is not essential for the routine monitoring of asthma, nor is it practical as a home measurement. Peak flow is a simple, quantitative, and reproducible measure of large airway function and is adequate for routine monitoring of all but severe persistent asthma. Peak flowmeters are inexpensive tools that are useful in the longitudinal care of all persistent cases of asthma; they are not intended to be diagnostic tools. Peak flowmeters are not interchangeable; measurements should ideally be made with the same unit or, at a minimum, with another of the same make and model. Peak flow is an effort-dependent measure; children usually need to be about 5 years of age to reliably use a peak flowmeter. Patients require careful instruction in the use of peak flowmeters as well as periodic checks of their technique. Home monitoring of peak flows allows the anticipation of exacerbations, often before symptoms begin. Home measurement of peak flow aids in long-term monitoring, communication with the family, and construction of a detailed rescue plan that matches the intensity of intervention to the degree of obstruction.

Bronchoprovocation

When asthma is suspected but spirometry values are normal, spirometry can be performed before and after a stepwise challenge with methacholine, exercise, or cold air. This should be done only by experienced clinicians in an appropriate medical facility.

Radiography

Chest x-ray films can exclude pneumonia, but atelectasis can easily be interpreted as infiltrate. In asthma, increased bronchial markings, peribronchial cuffing, and fluid in the fissures are frequently seen. These are the radiographic correlates of increased work of breathing. These findings are caused by shifts of fluid into the interstitium caused by the increased negative intrathoracic pressure that is required to breathe against increased resistance to flow. X-ray films are important in the diagnosis of pneumothorax and should be obtained from asthmatic persons with chest pain, especially if there is accompanying dyspnea or hypoxia.

Sinus radiographs can rule in sinusitis as the cause of an exacerbation or difficulty in management. Because plain films miss up to 20% of maxillary sinusitis, they cannot exclude the diagnosis. Computed tomography is the definitive noninvasive study.

An upper gastrointestinal tract series is helpful in the initial evaluation of tracheal compression or gastroesophageal compression, although computerized tomography and pH probes are the definitive studies.

Other Tests

Eosinophil counts reflect bronchial reactivity and can be a useful parameter to study longitudinally. Extremely high eosinophil counts and IgE levels raise the question of allergic bronchopulmonary aspergillosis, especially if the child has a positive skin test for *Aspergillus*. Central bronchiectasis and elevated IgE or IgG against *Aspergillus fumigatus* are diagnostic.

Determination of total immunoglobulins and IgE subclasses is useful to exclude immunodeficiency in children who have frequent exacerbations triggered by illness. The radioallergosorbent test is a tool in the evaluation of atopy but should not replace a thorough allergy investigation.

TREATMENT

The goal of therapy is to achieve a normal childhood in the face of a chronic illness. Normalization of childhood activity minimizes the impact on both cognitive and emotional development as well as on family function. Good control of asthma normalizes lung function, prevents recurrent exacerbations, and prevents chronic symptoms. This implies control of the underlying inflammation. Control of the chronic inflammation minimizes airway remodeling and maximizes lung growth and function. Normal lung growth in childhood will maximize lung function after the completion of lung growth in middle to late adolescence and throughout adult life. Successful management implies optimal pharmacotherapy and a customized care plan. Customization improves child and family involvement in designing the management strategy, thereby enhancing adherence and satisfaction.

Pharmacotherapy

Optimal pharmacotherapy is based on control of the chronic inflammation. In infants and children with symptoms more than twice a week, this means the use of inhaled steroids or inhaled nonsteroidal anti-inflammatory drugs. Early aggressive use of inhaled steroids has been shown to increase pulmonary function and to do so to a greater extent than was achieved with delayed use. Symptoms as they occur are managed with inhaled beta$_2$ agonists, anticholinergics, and systemic steroids.

Because most of the agents used in the treatment of asthma are inhaled, care must be taken with their delivery. Infants are in general treated with nebulized agents. It is important to provide a high-efficiency nebulizer (LCD, by Pari; Circulaire, by Westmed) and an appropriate mask size such as the Pari Baby. Administration by "blow by" is not adequate, as the losses into the room are overwhelming. Inhaled steroids are not available for nebulization in the United States, so that if inhaled steroids are required a spacer with a facemask (such as the Aerochamber or Optichamber) must be used. There is a literature that supports the effective use of masked spacers in this age group. Toddlers become more able to cooperate with a masked spacer, and the use of metered dose inhalers with spacers is much less disruptive of normal life than is the use of compressor-driven nebulizers. Children clearly can use spacers, and once they are able to control their breathing, a conventional spacer, one without a mask, can be used.

Children often benefit from a collapsing holding chamber such as the Inspirease. Older children need more mobility, and once they are able to coordinate hand and breath, a compact spacer, such as the Aerochamber, can often be used. Inhaled asthma drugs are increasingly available as dry powder inhalers. Although these delivery systems are quite efficient, they are extremely technique dependent. Their use must be carefully taught, and they may not be suitable for children under 5 years of age.

Controllers

Chromones

Cromolyn (Intal) and nedocromil (Tilade) are both anti-inflammatory drugs, although they are not as effective as inhaled corticosteroids. They both can be used prophylactically before exercise or unavoidable allergen exposure. They inhibit both the early and the late phases of bronchial reaction. They appear to work by blocking the chloride channels. Cromolyn stabilizes the mast cell inhibiting histamine release and degranulation. It also suppresses the activation of eosinophils, monocytes, and neutrophils. Nedocromil inhibits the release of both histamine and prostaglandin D from the mast cell. It decreases eosinophil survival and the mobilization of eosinophils and neutrophils. It blocks the release of cytotoxic proteins from the eosinophil and of neuropeptides from structural cells.

Anti-inflammatory effects are relatively weak and take up to 2 weeks to develop with nedocromil and 8 weeks with cromolyn. Nedocromil is available only in a metered-dose inhaler and can be administered on a two (bid), three (tid), or four (qid) times a day basis. Cromolyn is available as a solution for use in both a nebulizer and a metered-dose inhaler; however, the nebulized dose is 20 mg compared with the 1 mg per puff from the metered-dose inhaler, and the drug's activity is dose dependent. Nedocromil is more effective than cromolyn for nonallergic asthma. Both drugs have a good safety profile, but patient response is less predictable than with inhaled steroids. Approximately 20% of patients find the taste of nedocromil unacceptable.

Corticosteroids

Inhaled steroids have an extremely broad spectrum of activity. They affect virtually every cell involved in the inflammation of the airway: eosinophils, mast cells, macrophages, mucous glands, neutrophils, smooth muscle cells, and T lymphocytes. Steroids are extremely lipophilic, enter the cell, and bind to corticosteroid receptors. These receptor complexes enter the nucleus, bind to the genes, and influence transcription. Corticosteroids directly inhibit most of the cells involved in airway inflammation. They also reduce the number of inflammatory cells and inhibit the exudation of plasma and the secretion of mucus. In addition to their anti-inflammatory effects, they up-regulate beta-adrenergic receptors. Corticosteroids have been shown to reduce the risk of hospitalization, improve pulmonary function, decrease airway hyperresponsiveness, and probably attenuate and perhaps reverse airway remodeling. They decrease the derivatives of arachidonic acid (prostaglandins, thromboxanes, cytokines, and leukotrienes) as well as the acute-phase reactants.

The effects of inhaled steroids begin after 24 to 48 hours but do not reach their peak for 2 to 4 weeks. Oral steroids up-regulate beta-adrenergic receptors after one or two hours, but their anti-inflammatory activity is not seen for 8 to 12 hours. Inhaled steroids have few proven adverse effects: cough, dysphonia, and thrush. They may affect growth, but this has not been proven. Steroids have an extensive deactivation by first-pass metabolism in the liver; however, pulmonary and buccal absorption bypasses this. Spacers and rinsing after inhalation are important to maximize the dose delivered to the lung from a metered dose inhaler, to minimize local side effects, and to minimize systemic absorption.

There are several strategies that help minimize the steroid dose required. Start therapy intensively and "step down" once control has been established. Add theophylline (Slo-bid caps, Theo-Dur tabs), a long-acting beta agonist such as salmeterol (Serevent), or a leukotriene inhibitor such as montelukast (Singulair) to inhaled steroid therapy. All of these strategies have been demonstrated to work. There is relatively little practical experience with leukotriene inhibitors for children under age 6 years or with long-acting beta agonists with children less than age 6 years.

Leukotriene Modifiers

Leukotriene modifiers seem to improve lung function, decrease symptom score, and reduce exercise-induced bronchospasm. Their long-term safety and efficacy have not been unequivocally established. Their effect on airway remodeling is unknown.

There are two classes of leukotriene modifiers. Zileuton (Zyflo) is a competitive inhibitor of 5-lipoxygenase, the enzyme responsible for the synthesis of leukotriene A$_4$ from arachidonic acid. Zileuton has been associated with reversible liver toxicity. Zileuton has not been approved for use by children younger than 12 years of age. Zafirlukast (Accolate) and montelukast (Singulair) competitively inhibit the binding of leukotriene D$_4$ to its receptor. Both of these drugs may be associated in rare cases with the development of eosinophilic vasculitis (Churg-Strauss syndrome). Zafirlukast is taken two times a day and is approved for patients aged 12 years and older. Montelukast is taken once a day, is available as a chewable tablet, and is approved for ages 6 years and over. Although the National Asthma Education and Prevention Project considers this class of drugs as an alternative therapy for mild persistent asthma, more research is needed to establish their role in therapy. They are particularly useful as part of the treatment of severe exercise-induced asthma, as an ancillary drug to reduce the inhaled steroid dose required for control, or in noncompliant families.

Methylxanthines

Theophylline is a mild to moderate bronchodilator and may have some mild anti-inflammatory activity. It is used as an adjuvant therapy in combination with inhaled anti-inflammatory drugs. It is particularly useful for controlling nocturnal symptoms. It has been shown to reduce the dose of inhaled steroid required for control even at a low dose.

Long-Acting Beta Agonists

The principal action of beta agonists is to relax airway smooth muscle. The long-acting beta agonist salmeterol has a duration of action of at least 12 hours. Their role is as an adjuvant to inhaled anti-inflammatory therapy. They are particularly effective in the control of nocturnal symptoms and exercise-induced asthma alone or in combination with a leukotriene modifier. Rebound airway hyperreactivity can be demonstrated with their regular use as a single agent. It is essential that these drugs not be used to control exacerbations.

Relievers

Beta$_2$-Agonists

Short-acting beta$_2$-agonists—albuterol (Ventolin, Proventil), terbutaline (Bricanyl), or pirbuterol (Maxair)—are the drugs of choice in the management of asthma exacerbations and in the prevention of exercise-induced bronchospasm. There is rebound hyperreactivity associated with their regular use. Scheduled use of these agents has been associated with decreased control. The use of more than four canisters a year, excluding prophylactic use, has been associated with an increased risk of hospitalization. The use of more than one canister per month has been associated with increased mortality. Scheduled use is not recommended. When used on an as-needed basis, these agents improve control; if they need to be used consistently more than twice a week to relieve

symptoms, there may be an inadequate anti-inflammatory regimen or poor compliance with the planned regimen.

Anticholinergics

Ipratropium bromide (Atrovent) is a quaternary derivative of atropine; because it does not cross the blood-brain barrier it does not have atropine's side effects. It is not clear if ipratropium bromide adds to the long-term control of asthma. There is evidence of enhanced bronchodilatation when ipratropium bromide is combined with beta$_2$-agonists in the treatment of asthma exacerbations. This effect increases with the severity of the exacerbation.

CONTROL OF CONTRIBUTING FACTORS

All children with persistent asthma deserve an investigation of their atopic status. This can start with environmental surveys and questions about seasonal symptoms or symptoms that develop in special circumstances. Children with positive histories deserve further investigation with radioallergosorbent testing or referral to an allergist for definitive evaluation. Rhinitis and sinusitis are important co-morbid conditions. They are more common in atopic children and are associated with poorer control of asthma. Non-sedating antihistamines, nasal chromones, nasal steroids, and appropriate antimicrobial therapy are important ancillary treatments of these co-morbid conditions.

Irritant exposure causes significant morbidity. Exposure to tobacco smoke, strong scents, wood stoves, fireplaces, or gas ranges is associated with increased asthma symptomatology.

Gastroesophageal reflux is associated with asthma, although its cause is not clear. It may provoke asthma exacerbations, or the increased work of breathing in an exacerbation of asthma may induce reflux. A trial of antireflux therapy is indicated if the history suggests reflux or if reflux is demonstrated objectively.

Intercurrent illnesses can be minimized by influenza and pneumococcal immunizations when appropriate.

PARTNERSHIP

Adherence, control, and satisfaction are maximized if a strong partnership between provider and patient or family can be established. Partnerships can be promoted if treatment goals are shared and if written treatment and rescue plans are formulated that consider the family dynamics. Treatment plans must be practical in terms of cost, frequency, and ease of administration. To promote adherence, treatment plans must produce clear improvements in functional status as well as minimize adverse effects. Written treatment plans improve communication, especially if they are based on objective measures of lung function. Positive reinforcement for success in asthma control and compliance with the written plan enhances adherence. Education enhances partnership if it is helpful to the family. Initial educational efforts should be directed at training in the mechanical aspects of care: spacer use, peak flowmeter use, the appropriate use of controllers and relievers, and the appropriate use of the rescue plan. Education can then advance to pathophysiology, natural history, pharmacotherapy, child development, and family dynamics as they relate to asthma and asthma control.

CLASSIFICATION OF SEVERITY

There are two considerations in the classification of asthma severity: the severity of the child's asthma and the severity of the exacerbations. Children with any level of severity can have life-threatening exacerbations.

Asthma exacerbations occur along a spectrum of severity. In mild exacerbations children are alert. Although symptomatic, these children can speak in whole sentences. They may be tachypneic or tachycardic, but there are neither retractions nor use of accessory muscles of respiration. There may or may not be wheezing, but the I:E ratio is 1:1 or 1:1.5. The peak flows are 70% of personal best or more, and the transcutaneous oxygen saturation (SaO_2) level is over 95% on room air.

Children who are having moderate exacerbations tend to prefer to sit and to speak in phrases. They are tachypneic and tachycardic. There is tracheosternal retraction and chest hyperexpansion, and respiration is primarily abdominal. There is usually wheezing, and the I:E ratio is 1:2 or 1:3. The SaO_2 level is 91% to 95%, and the peak flow is 50% to 70% of their personal best.

Children with severe exacerbations sit leaning on their elbows to aid in hyperinflation of their chests. They speak in single words or perhaps in phrases. They have deep tracheosternal retractions and may have nasal flaring. These children have I:E ratios of 1:3 or more; shorter ratios are caused by prolongation of the inspiratory phase and suggest imminent respiratory failure. There is prominent wheezing, and its absence is a cause for concern. These children are tachycardic and profoundly tachypneic. Their peak flow is less than 50% of their personal best, and their SaO_2 level is less than 90%.

Children in imminent respiratory failure have alterations in their mental status. They may not be wheezing, and their I:E ratio may be 1:1 but they have paradoxical respiratory excursions. They cannot execute a peak flow maneuver.

The staging of exacerbations in infants is more difficult and depends on activity level. The presence of tracheosternal retraction correlates with peak flows that are approximately 50% of personal best, and nasal flaring correlates with peak flows of 40% of personal best. The progress of the I:E ratio is the same, as is the presence or absence of wheezing. The presence of post-tussive emesis suggests distress.

SaO_2 level is useful in this group, although it is technically more difficult to obtain.

TREATMENT OF ACUTE ASTHMA EXACERBATIONS

Hypoxia is a stimulus to bronchoconstriction. When the SaO_2 level is less than 93% to 95% or if there is a clinical suspicion of hypoxia, the nebulizer should be run off an oxygen source. The recommended initial treatment is albuterol at 0.15 mg per kg with a range of 0.5 to 1.0 cc (2.5 to 5.0 mg). This dose may be repeated at 20-minute intervals. If there is not good response after three doses, the child should be transferred to an emergency room. If the child struggles against the nebulizer, terbutaline (Bricanyl) can be administered subcutaneously at a dose of 0.01 cc/kg (0.3 cc max) and repeated at 20-minute intervals.

Epinephrine can be used at the same dose and interval, but it produces more adverse effects and must be followed with a long-acting agent (e.g., terbutaline, Sus-Phrine). On the other hand, if anaphylaxis is a possibility, epinephrine at 0.01 cc per kg (0.3 cc max) is the drug of choice. Ipratropium bromide should be added to the nebulized albuterol at a dose of 1.25 cc and repeated three times, especially with moderate or severe exacerbations. Prednisone or prednisolone should be given early in the intervention at a dose of 2 mg per kg per dose bid for 1 or 2 days, then once daily, usually for a total of 3 to 10 days.

Early administration takes advantage of the upregulation of beta-adrenergic receptors. There is no data-driven maximum dose, and toxicity in short bursts is primarily gastrointestinal. If the child is unable to retain the oral steroid, parenteral steroids can be used. Dexamethasone sodium phosphate at 0.2 mg per kg has a long half-life, which makes it inappropriate for ongoing use, but in the acute setting it provides sustained activity from a single dose. Acute treatment should be continued until the child is comfortable, the I:E ratio is 1.0 to 1.5, the wheezing is improved, the retractions have resolved, the peak flow is more than 70% of personal best, and the SaO_2 level is 93% to 95%. Hypercapnea is a concern if an SaO_2 level greater than 93% cannot be attained. These children should be transferred to an emergency room where treatment can be continued and arterial blood gas measurements obtained. Children who cannot mount a peak flow on presentation should immediately get high-flow humidified oxygen, parenteral terbutaline, and parenteral steroids. Emergency transport, preferably by a transport team, for definitive evaluation and treatment should be arranged.

LONG-TERM MANAGEMENT OF ASTHMA IN CHILDREN

The use of peak flows can improve outcomes, especially when the patient's personal best effort is used as a reference value. Peak flow shows a diurnal variation and is lowest in the morning. Long-term monitoring is best based on measurements taken in the morning before the administration of medicines. Because of diurnal variation, the personal best can be established by measurement of the peak flow in the early afternoon. It is often helpful to measure peak flows in the morning before medicine is taken and in the early afternoon after administration of a bronchodilator for 2 or 3 weeks periodically to establish both the personal best and the intermeasurement variability. On occasion it may be necessary to treat with oral steroids for a week or two to establish the personal best peak flow. Peak flows can guide the management of exacerbations both at home and in the physician's office or emergency room. A written treatment plan given to the parents that is keyed to the child's peak flow can facilitate home management. Written treatment plans are often based on a traffic light metaphor. Green (peak expiratory flow rate [PEFR] >80% of personal best) is go, take your routine medications. Yellow (PEFR 50% to 80% of personal best) is caution, take a rescue medicine. Red (PEFR <50% of personal best) is stop, this is a medical alert, take your rescue medicine and call for medical advice.

Asthma severity has been characterized as intermittent, mild persistent, moderate persistent, and severe persistent by the National Asthma Education and Prevention Project. All asthmatic persons should have access to short-acting beta$_2$ agonists for symptomatic relief, but consumption should be monitored as an indicator of control. Prescriptions should be written for a limited number of units with one or two refills for all but severe persistent asthma. Therapy should be initiated one step above the actual severity step, and once control is attained, therapy should be stepped down.

Persons with intermittent asthma have symptoms less than twice a week and have nocturnal symptoms less than twice a month. Their peak flow or forced expiratory volume in 1 second (FEV$_1$) in the morning before taking inhalers should be 80% of personal best or more, and their intermeasurement variability should be less than 20%. These children probably do not require daily controller medication. They should use albuterol, terbutaline, or pirbuterol (Maxair) on an as-needed basis. Their severity classification should be stepped up if they require a beta agonist two or more times a week to treat symptoms as opposed to exercise prophylaxis.

People with mild persistent asthma have symptoms three to six times a week and have nocturnal symptoms three or four times a month. Their morning peak flow or FEV$_1$ should be greater than 80% of their personal best, but intermeasurement variability may be 20% to 30%. Therapy is usually started with cromolyn 1 amp four times per day (qid) to three times per day (tid) or nedocromil 4 puffs bid. Other options are beclomethasone dipropionate (Beclovent, Vanceril), 42 μg per puff, 2 to 8 puffs divided once or twice daily, or Vanceril DS, 84 μg per puff, 1 to 4 puffs divided once or twice daily. Triamcinolone ace-

tate (Azmacort) 4 to 8 puffs divided once or twice daily should be considered as an alternative, particularly if the patient or family is not compliant with spacers. Another option at this step is montelukast 5 mg once a day.

People with moderate persistent asthma have symptoms daily but not continually. They have nocturnal symptoms five or more times a month. Their morning peak flow or FEV$_1$ is between 60% and 80% of their personal best, and there is more than 30% intermeasurement variability. Appropriate therapeutic options are nedocromil 4 puffs bid or beclomethasone 84 μg per puff divided bid or budesonide (Pulmicort Turbuhaler) dry powder inhaler 1 to 2 puffs divided bid or triamcinolone acetate (Azmacort) 8 to 12 puffs divided bid, especially for children of families who will not comply with spacers. The addition of sustained-release theophylline (capsules or tablets) at 10 mg per kg per day divided bid or salmeterol xinafoate 1 to 2 puffs bid or once daily (in the morning if exercise symptoms predominate and in the evening if nocturnal symptoms predominate) or montelukast 5 mg once daily may permit a reduction in steroid dose.

People with severe persistent asthma have continual symptoms and frequent nocturnal symptoms. Their morning peak flow or FEV$_1$ is less than 60% of their personal best, and there is greater than 30% intermeasurement variability. Appropriate therapy at this step is budesonide dry powder inhaler at doses over 2 puffs divided bid or fluticasone (Flonase) 110 μg per puff more than 4 puffs divided bid 220 μg per puff more than 2 puffs divided bid. As in moderate persistent asthma, the addition of theophylline, salmeterol xinafoate, or montelukast may enhance control or minimize the dose of inhaled steroid required for control. Alternate-day or even daily oral steroids may be required for control.

Once control is established and sustained, therapy can be stepped down gradually to establish the minimum therapy required for control. Therapy can be stepped down at 2- or 3-month intervals. Ongoing peak flow monitoring and periodic spirometry are useful in guiding step-down decisions. Regular follow-up visits are recommended every 6 months for stable mild persistent asthma and every month or more for unstable severe persistent asthma. Therapy may need to be intensified temporarily to regain control after an exacerbation.

INDICATIONS FOR REFERRAL TO AN ASTHMA SPECIALIST

Children with severe asthma and young children with moderate persistent asthma should be referred to an asthma specialist. Children under 3 years of age with mild persistent asthma may benefit from consultation and co-management. Children who have had life-threatening exacerbations should be referred for consultation or co-management. Children who are difficult to manage, take more than two bursts of oral steroids a year, have more than two emergency room visits or one hospitalization per year, or are not meeting the goals of therapy after 3 to 6 months should be referred to a specialist. Children who are unresponsive to therapy should also be referred.

Referral is also appropriate for additional education or testing or when the diagnosis is complicated by other conditions (e.g., sinusitis, nasal polyps, severe rhinitis, vocal cord dysfunction, aspergillosis, gastroesophageal reflux). Referral to an allergist is appropriate for detailed environmental evaluation, skin testing, and consideration of immunotherapy.

ALLERGIC RHINITIS CAUSED BY INHALANT FACTORS*

method of
FUAD M. BAROODY, M.D.
The University of Chicago
Pritzker School of Medicine
Chicago, Illinois

Allergic rhinitis has a prevalence in the general population of approximately 20%. The incidence peaks in the teenage years and young adulthood and typically persists for 30 to 40 years before gradually improving. Men and women are equally affected and there is no apparent ethnic predilection. In addition to affecting the nasal passages, allergic rhinitis is associated with asthma and sinusitis, thus increasing the morbidity related to this disease. Of the approximately 40 million Americans with allergic rhinitis, approximately 40% seek medical help and many more resort to over-the-counter medications, resulting in a health care expenditure of several billion dollars each year in the United States.

After sensitization of the nasal mucosa to a certain allergen, subsequent exposure leads to cross-linking of specific IgE receptors on mast cells and their resultant degranulation, with the release of a host of inflammatory mediators, such as histamine, that are in large part responsible for allergic nasal symptoms. Although initially thought to involve recurrent episodes of mast cell degranulation, it has become clear that allergic rhinitis is characterized by inflammation of the nasal mucosa with a prominent role played by eosinophils, T cells, and basophils and their inflammatory products, including mediators and cytokines. These inflammatory changes lower the threshold of mucosal responsiveness and amplify it to a variety of specific and nonspecific stimuli. Our understanding of these events prompted a change in management of this prevalent disease.

HISTORY

The classic symptoms of allergic rhinitis are recurrent episodes of sneezing, pruritus of the nose, palate, throat, eyes, and ears, clear rhinorrhea, and nasal congestion after exposure to the offending allergen. Severe congestion may be associated with loss of smell and usually manifests as a loss of taste. Systemic symptoms include general malaise, fatigue, irritability, and insomnia. Allergic rhinitis can be classified as seasonal, perennial, or episodic. Seasonal allergic rhinitis is defined by symptoms that occur at the

*Supported in part by grant AI 01236 from the National Institutes of Health, Bethesda, Maryland.

same time every year during exposure to seasonal allergens (ragweed, grasses, and tree pollens). Perennial allergic rhinitis, defined by nasal symptoms for more than 2 hours per day and for more than 9 months of the year, occurs when allergies develop to house dust mites, indoor molds, animal danders, and cockroaches, or when a person acquires sensitivities to multiple seasonal allergens. Episodic rhinitis refers to symptoms on exposure to allergens that are not normally present in the environment, such as pets in somebody else's house. Inquiring about the occurrence of symptoms during vacations, at the workplace, or on a change in the patient's personal environment, such as moving to a new house, may provide clues to the etiologic agent. Once allergic symptoms are present, they may be exacerbated by irritants such as strong odors or perfumes, tobacco smoke, paint, newspaper ink, soap powders, and air pollutants.

It is important to elicit a possible family history of allergic disease during the interview. Atopy, the predisposition to respond to environmental allergens with the production of specific IgE antibodies, is present in only 13% of children when neither parent is atopic, in contrast to 29% if one parent or sibling is atopic and 47% when both parents are atopic.

PHYSICAL EXAMINATION

A complete ear, nose, and throat examination is essential in the work-up of every patient suspected of having allergic rhinitis and is useful in ensuring the absence of other problems rather than in confirming the diagnosis (Table 1).

TABLE 1. **Differential Diagnosis of Rhinorrhea and Nasal Obstruction**

Allergic rhinitis: Seasonal, perennial.
Nonallergic rhinitis
　Perennial (vasomotor): Constant symptoms of profuse, clear rhinorrhea and nasal congestion without correlation to specific allergen exposure or signs of atopy.
　Cold air–induced: Nasal congestion and rhinorrhea on exposure to cold, windy weather. Occurs in both allergic and nonallergic people.
　Nonallergic rhinitis with eosinophilia syndrome: Most often seen in adults and characterized by eosinophilia on nasal smears with negative testing for specific allergens.
Infectious rhinitis: Bacterial, viral, fungal, granulomatous (sarcoidosis, Wegener's granulomatosis).
Drug-induced rhinitis: Oral contraceptives, reserpine derivatives, hydralazine hydrochloride, topical decongestants (rhinitis medicamentosa), beta blockers (eye drops).
Mechanical obstruction
　Septal deviation: Common and might exacerbate nasal obstruction in allergic rhinitis.
　Foreign body: Unilateral purulent nasal discharge is the usual manifestation of a foreign body and resolves after removal.
　Choanal atresia or stenosis: Bilateral choanal atresia is usually diagnosed early in life, but unilateral choanal atresia or stenosis can go unnoticed for several years. Easily diagnosed by nasal endoscopy and axial computed tomography of the mid-facial skeleton.
　Adenoid hypertrophy: Common cause of nasal obstruction in children.
　Others: Encephaloceles, lacrimal duct cysts.
Neoplastic
　Benign: Polyps, nasopharyngeal angiofibroma, inverted papilloma.
　Malignant: Adenocarcioma, squamous cell carcinoma, esthesioneuroblastoma, lymphoma, rhabdomyosarcoma.

The ear examination may show otitis media with effusion, suggesting nasopharyngeal problems. Examination of the face may show puffiness of the eyelids and periorbital cyanosis, usually due to venous stasis secondary to chronic nasal obstruction, and often referred to as "allergic shiners." Localized facial tenderness on palpation, especially in conjunction with purulent anterior or posterior nasal discharge, is a sign of sinusitis. A nasal speculum, or an otoscope with a large nosepiece, is used to inspect the nasal cavities. The inferior turbinates are often described as being pale, bluish, edematous, and coated with thin, clear secretions, but it is important to remember that there really is no single pathognomonic appearance of the nasal mucosa in allergic rhinitis. Unilateral purulent drainage in a child suggests a foreign body or, less commonly, unilateral choanal atresia. For better examination of the nasal cavity, and in cases in which the existence of a pathologic process not readily accessible to anterior rhinoscopy is suspected, endoscopy should be performed after decongestion. This is usually done with a flexible fiberoptic instrument, takes less than 5 minutes, causes minor discomfort, and is well tolerated by adults and children older than 5 years of age.

DIAGNOSTIC TESTS

The two most common tests used to confirm the diagnosis of allergic rhinitis are skin testing and in vitro testing for serum levels of specific IgE antibodies. Both tests are effective for the diagnosis of allergic rhinitis. Although clear-cut seasonal allergic rhinitis that responds well to treatment rarely warrants such evaluation, defining causative allergens in perennial disease is difficult without careful history and diagnostic testing. Establishing the offending allergens facilitates avoidance counseling.

Skin Testing

Testing begins with puncture testing, whereby a small drop of concentrated allergen is placed on the skin (usually the volar surface of the forearm or the back), and a minute quantity is introduced into the dermis with a sharp object. Positive responses occur within 10 to 15 minutes and produce a characteristic raised central area of induration (wheal), with a surrounding zone of erythema (flare). The response is graded by comparison with a positive histamine response, and a negative control with the diluent for the allergen extracts is also included to control for nonspecific reactivity to the vehicle. In the presence of significant suggestive history, negative puncture tests are usually confirmed by intradermal tests, which are more sensitive. In an intradermal test, a small (0.01- to 0.05-mL) quantity of dilute allergen is injected into the superficial dermis and the same wheal-and-flare responses are observed and graded in comparison with a positive histamine control. Most H$_1$-receptor antagonists should be withheld for 2 days before skin testing except astemizole, which needs to be withheld for up to 6 weeks because of its long half-life. Advantages of skin testing include greater sensitivity, the rapidity with which results can be obtained, and low cost. Disadvantages include inability to perform the test in patients with dermatologic problems, poor tolerance in children, the inhibitory effect of certain ingested drugs such as antihistamines on skin test reactivity, and the possibility of systemic reactions.

In Vitro IgE Measurements

Drawing blood for the measurement of specific IgE can circumvent some of the disadvantages of skin testing. False-positive results may occur if patients have elevated IgE levels in their sera because of nonspecific binding. False-negative test results may also result from inhibition by IgG antibodies with similar affinities, such as in patients on immunotherapy. Data comparing results of skin testing and the radioallergosorbent assay in allergic subjects suggest a good correlation between the two, with a higher sensitivity for skin testing.

Therefore, both determinations of specific IgE levels and skin testing are useful in the diagnosis of allergic disorders, but their results should always be interpreted in the context of clinical symptomatology. Testing is performed with a panel of allergens that are prevalent in the area in addition to allergens that seem relevant from the history, such as cat and dog dander and cockroach particles. A positive test alone, however, does not confirm the diagnosis of allergic rhinitis in the absence of supporting clinical history.

Nasal Cytology

Nasal cytology can be performed to evaluate inflammatory cells in nasal secretions. Nasal swabs, scrapings, and blown secretions are the preferred methods of sampling. Secretions are spread on slides, allowed to dry, and stained with a modified Wright's stain, which allows the identification of epithelial cells, mononuclear cells, eosinophils, and polymorphonuclear cells. This technique is most useful in the acutely ill patient for whom the differential diagnosis includes allergic or infectious rhinitis. The presence of numerous eosinophils (>5 to 10% eosinophils per high-power field) helps the clinician make the diagnosis of allergic rhinitis, whereas numerous polymorphonuclear cells suggests an infectious etiology. Another advantage is that in the patient with nonallergic rhinitis with eosinophilia syndrome, a skin test for common allergens is negative but a nasal smear demonstrates numerous eosinophils. It is important to identify patients with this disorder because they respond well to intranasal corticosteroids.

THERAPEUTIC OPTIONS

Avoidance

Total avoidance of offending allergens, although often impossible, is the most effective treatment for allergic rhinitis and should be the starting point of treatment. Knowing the offending allergens is crucial in planning avoidance strategies. In the case of perennial rhinitis, avoidance is usually aimed at indoor allergens, such as house dust mites, indoor molds, and pets. Washing bedding twice a week with hot water (>130°F) kills house dust mites, and vacuuming mattresses and pillows or encasing them in plastic covers also decreases exposure to this allergen. Because house dust mites and molds thrive in moist environments, attempts should be made to reduce this factor by avoiding rug shampooing and dehumidifying damp areas of the house. In addition to the allergens found in their dander, pets can indirectly contribute to exposure by bringing outdoor allergens into the house on their coats.

Outdoor allergens, such as grasses, trees, or weeds, are more difficult to control, and patients should be instructed to avoid activities that increase exposure, such as lawn mowing, outdoor picnics, and driving with the car windows open. For indoor control, keeping windows closed and installing a high-efficiency particulate air filter on central air conditioning may prove helpful.

Antihistamines

H_1-receptor antagonists, which achieve their effects by competing with histamine for the H_1 receptor, are the most frequently used medications in the treatment of allergic rhinitis (Table 2). The older antihistamines, such as diphenhydramine, are lipophilic and cross the blood-brain barrier, causing sedation and decreased performance. These compounds have varying degrees of anticholinergic and sedating side effects and, if applied topically, some have local anesthetic effects. Although these properties might contribute to their therapeutic efficacy, they are also responsible for their adverse side effects. Studies in children have shown that allergic rhinitis affects school performance and that treatment with a nonsedating antihistamine improves performance more than does placebo, but treatment with a sedating antihistamine actually worsens performance in these children. The newer nonsedating antihistamines, such as fexofenadine (Allegra), astemizole (Hismanal), and loratadine (Claritin), are less lipophilic,

which reduces their ability to cross the blood-brain barrier and decreases their sedating and anticholinergic side effects. Cetirizine (Zyrtec) is a new antihistamine that is labeled as sedating by the FDA but seems to cause less central nervous system dysfunction than classic antihistamines in comparative studies. An intranasal antihistamine, azelastine (Astelin), a phthalazinone derivative, is available in the United States for the treatment of allergic rhinitis. Its efficacy is comparable with that of other antihistamines and it does not cause somnolence, but a sensation of altered taste occurs immediately after use. Antihistamines are effective in inhibiting sneezing, itching, ocular symptoms, and rhinorrhea associated with allergic rhinitis, but have a negligible effect in controlling nasal congestion. These agents are more useful for the treatment of episodic and seasonal allergic rhinitis than for perennial rhinitis, in which congestion is a more prominent complaint. Balancing the decreased sedative effect of the newer antihistamines with their higher cost, compared with the classic agents, is a practical clinical problem.

Decongestants

Both topical and systemic decongestants act by alpha-adrenergic stimulation and cause vasoconstric-

TABLE 2. **Commonly Used Antihistamines**

Chemical Name	Trade Name	Formulation	Dose, Adults	Dose, Pediatric
Old (sedating) H_1-receptor antagonists				
Chlorpheniramine	Chlor-Trimeton	Tabs: 2, 4, 8,* 12* mg; Syrup: 2 mg/5 mL	4 mg q 4–6 h; 8–12 mg bid	0.35 mg/kg/24 h in 3–4 divided doses
Brompheniramine	Dimetane	Tabs: 4, 8,* 12* mg; Elixir: 2 mg/5 mL	4 mg q 4–6 h; 8–12 mg bid	0.35 mg/kg/24 h in 3–4 divided doses
Diphenhydramine	Benadryl	Caps: 25, 50 mg; Elixir: 12.5 mg/5 mL; Syrup: 6.25 mg/5 mL	25–50 mg q 6 h	5 mg/kg/24 h in 3–4 divided doses
Clemastine	Tavist	Tabs: 1.34, 2.68 mg; Syrup: 0.67 mg/5 mL	1.34 mg bid or q 4 h; 2.68 mg qd or tid	0.67 mg bid
Promethazine	Phenergan	Tabs: 12.5, 25, 50 mg; Syrup: 6.25, 25 mg/5 mL; Supp: 12.5, 25, 50 mg	12.5–50 mg qid	1 mg/kg/24 h; ½ dose before bedtime and 2¼ doses during the day
Hydroxyzine	Atarax, Vistaril	Tabs: 10, 25, 50, 100 mg; Susp: 10, 25 mg/5 mL	25–50 mg q 4–6 h	2 mg/kg/24 h in 4 divided doses
Azatadine	Optimine	Tabs: 1 mg	1–2 mg bid	NA
Cyproheptadine	Periactin	Tabs: 4 mg; Syrup: 2 mg/5 mL	4 mg tid–qid	0.25 mg/kg/24 h in 3–4 divided doses
New (nonsedating) H_1-receptor antagonists				
Astemizole	Hismanal	Tabs: 10 mg	≥12 y: 10 mg qd	NA
Azelastine spray	Astelin	Nasal solution 0.1%, 137 µg/spray	≥12 y: 2 sprays/nostril bid	NA
Cetirizine	Zyrtec	Tabs: 5, 10 mg; Syrup: 5 mg/5 mL	≥12 y: 5–10 mg qd	6–11 y: 5–10 mg qd
Fexofenadine	Allegra	Caps: 60 mg	≥12 y: 60 mg bid	NA
Loratadine	Claritin	Tabs: 10 mg; Syrup: 1 mg/mL; Reditabs: 10 mg (rapidly disintegrating tabs)	≥12 y: 10 mg qd	6–11 y: 10 mg qd
	Claritin D 12 HOUR	Extended-release tabs: 5 mg loratadine, 120 mg pseudoephedrine sulfate	≥12 y: 1 tab bid	NA
	Claritin D 24 HOUR	Extended-release tabs: 10 mg loratadine, 240 mg pseudoephedrine sulfate	≥12 y: 1 tab qd	NA

*Timed release.
Abbreviations: q = every; qd = once daily; bid = twice daily; tid = three times daily; qid = four times daily; NA = not available.

tion and a reduction of nasal blood supply and the volume of blood in the sinusoids, thereby increasing the patency of the nasal cavities. Topical decongestants can be either catecholamines (e.g., phenylephrine) or imidazoline derivatives (e.g., xylometazoline [Otrivin] or oxymetazoline [Afrin]), have a rapid onset of action, and are usually more efficacious than systemic decongestants. Although they do not have systemic side effects, continued use of these agents leads to progressively shorter duration of action, until almost continuous application provides no relief; this condition is known as *rhinitis medicamentosa*. Therefore, their use in allergic rhinitis should be limited to facilitating the penetration of intranasal steroids in cases in which severe congestion precludes it, allowing proper physical examination, and facilitating sleep during severe rhinitic exacerbations.

The commonly used oral decongestants, pseudoephedrine hydrochloride and phenylpropanolamine hydrochloride, do not cause rhinitis medicamentosa but are not as effective as their topical counterparts. The usual dose of pseudoephedrine hydrochloride is 15 mg for children 2 to 5 years of age, 30 mg for children 6 to 12 years of age, and 60 mg every 6 hours for adults. Phenylpropanolamine has pharmacologic properties and potency similar to those of pseudoephedrine. These agents are used most frequently in combination preparations with different antihistamines, and the combination has an enhanced effect in controlling nasal congestion. Many are available as over-the-counter preparations. The most commonly reported side effects of these medications are insomnia and irritability, which can be seen in as many as 25% of patients. An overdose of these agents causes hypertension, nervousness, renal failure, arrhythmias, psychosis, strokes, and seizures. They should therefore be administered with caution to patients with hypertension, heart disease, seizure disorders, and hyperthyroidism, and to those receiving monoamine oxidase inhibitors.

Anticholinergics

The volume of secretions in patients with rhinitis appears to be secondary to increased parasympathetic activity that is competitively antagonized by intranasal ipratropium bromide, which has no systemic effect. Thus, this agent is useful in the treatment of patients in whom rhinorrhea is the predominant complaint. It is often used in combination with other therapies such as antihistamines and intranasal steroids. Ipratropium nasal spray (Atrovent) is available in a 0.03% concentration for clinical use for allergic and nonallergic rhinitis in adults and children 12 years of age or older (2 sprays [42 μg] per nostril two to three times daily). Its main side effects are nasal irritation, bleeding, and excessive dryness, which occur in 5 to 10% of patients and can usually be circumvented by decreasing the dosage.

Cromolyn Sodium

Cromolyn sodium is available over the counter as a 4% solution for intranasal use (Nasalcrom) in adults and children 6 years of age and older and has been shown to be clinically effective in the treatment of allergic rhinitis. Its mode of action, initially believed to be mast cell stabilization, remains unclear. It is most effective when started before the onset of symptoms and has to be administered four to six times daily (5.2 mg per actuation; 1 spray per nostril four to six times a day), causing patient compliance problems. Its safety profile, however, makes it an attractive treatment, especially in children. When effective, its potency parallels that of antihistamines but is less than that of intranasal steroids.

Glucocorticosteroids

These agents are among the most potent treatments available for allergic rhinitis. The known side effects of systemic steroids have led to the development of intranasal preparations that are much safer and have an efficacy that equals, or exceeds, that of their oral counterparts. Systemic steroids are best reserved for patients who present in the middle of the pollen season with total nasal obstruction leading to sleep disturbance. A short course of systemic steroids starting with 30 mg of prednisone daily for 3 days, 20 mg for 3 days, and 10 mg for 3 days is effective in relieving nasal obstruction. A short course of systemic steroids is also useful in reducing the nasal obstruction associated with rhinitis medicamentosa and facilitates weaning patients from topical decongestants.

Several intranasal corticosteroid preparations are available for use in patients with allergic rhinitis, and these agents are the most efficacious pharmacologic therapy available for this entity (Table 3). Intranasal corticosteroids are highly effective in reducing all symptoms of allergic rhinitis, including nasal congestion, rhinorrhea, sneezing, and itching in most patients, and available data suggest that they are more effective than oral antihistamines. Their superior efficacy is related to their anti-inflammatory effects and resultant reductions of inflammatory cells and mediators in the nasal mucosa after use. Intranasal corticosteroids do not improve the eye symptoms that often accompany allergic rhinitis, however, and adjunctive treatment with antihistamines or topical medications might be needed to control these symptoms. In clinical use, it is important to titrate the dose of these agents according to the degree of the patient's symptoms. It is also important to inform the patient that both the onset and cessation of activity will be slow, unlike antihistamines and decongestants, although some studies have shown differences from placebo within 12 hours. It is therefore best to start treatment a week or so before the beginning of the pollen season in patients with known seasonal allergic rhinitis.

Treatment should be started with the recom-

TABLE 3. **Intranasal Steroid Preparations**

Chemical Name	Trade Name	Formulation	Dose/Actuation	Age	Recommended Dosage
Beclomethasone dipropionate	Beconase inhalation aerosol or Vancenase Pockethaler	Propellant	42 μg	≥12 y	1 spray/nostril bid to qid (168–336 μg daily)
				6–12 y	1 spray/nostril tid (252 μg daily)
	Beconase AQ nasal spray	Aqueous, 0.042%	42 μg	≥12 y	1–2 sprays/nostril bid (168–336 μg daily)
				6–12 y	1–2 sprays/nostril bid (168–336 μg daily)
	Vancenase AQ	Aqueous, 0.042%	42 μg	≥6 y	1–2 sprays/nostril bid (168–336 μg daily)
	Vancenase AQ 84 μg	Aqueous, 0.084%	84 μg	≥6 y	1–2 sprays/nostril qd (168–336 μg daily)
Triamcinolone acetonide	Nasacort	Propellant, aqueous	55 μg	≥12 y	2 sprays/nostril qd (220 μg daily)
				6–11 y*	2 sprays/nostril qd (110–220 μg daily)
Budesonide	Rhinocort	Propellant	32 μg	≥6 y	2 sprays/nostril bid or 4 sprays/nostril in AM (256 μg daily)
Flunisolide	Nasalide	0.025% solution	25 μg	>14 y	2 sprays/nostril bid to tid (200–300 μg daily)
	Nasarel			6–14 y	1 spray/nostril tid (150 μg daily) 2 sprays/nostril bid (200 μg daily)
Fluticasone propionate	Flonase	0.05% nasal spray (aqueous)	50 μg	4 y to adolescent	1 spray/nostril qd (100 μg daily)
				Adults	2 sprays/nostril qd (200 μg daily)
Mometasone furoate	Nasonex	Aqueous	50 μg	≥12 y	2 sprays/nostril qd (200 μg daily)

*Not FDA approved for children younger than 12 years of age.
Abbreviations: qd = once daily; bid = twice daily; tid = three times daily.

mended dosage and the patient re-evaluated in 2 weeks. During this visit, the nose should be examined for signs of local irritation due to the drug or mechanical trauma from the applicator itself, and the patient's response to treatment should be assessed. If a favorable clinical response is reported, the dose of intranasal corticosteroids can be lowered, keeping in mind the load of allergen in the environment, with the aim of reaching the minimal dose that provides symptomatic relief. Many of the available preparations allow once-a-day administration. Local nasal irritation, the principal side effect of intranasal steroids, occurs in approximately 10% of patients and the incidence of epistaxis with different preparations ranges from 4 to 8%. Septal perforations, although rare, have been reported. These irritative symptoms are more common with the freon-propelled preparations than with the aqueous preparations. *Candida* overgrowth in the nose is rare. Controlled clinical studies have shown that intranasal corticosteroids may cause a reduction in growth velocity in pediatric patients, and this effect has been observed in the absence of laboratory evidence of hypothalamic-pituitary-adrenal axis suppression, suggesting that growth velocity is a more sensitive indicator of systemic corticosteroid exposure in pediatric patients. The long-term effects of this reduction in growth velocity, including the final impact on adult height

and the potential for catch-up growth after discontinuation of treatment, have not been adequately studied. It has therefore been recommended that the growth of pediatric patients receiving intranasal corticosteroids should be monitored regularly (every 3 to 6 months) with an accurate instrument (stadiometer) by trained staff in a consistent way.

Leukotriene Modifiers

Because leukotrienes are generated in allergic rhinitis, the effects of inhibitors of the 5-lipoxygenase pathway and leukotriene receptor antagonists have been investigated. Use of these agents has shown a reduction in nasal congestion, rhinorrhea, and sneezing in patients with allergic rhinitis, and although they are available as oral preparations in the treatment of asthma, they have been used in subjects with allergic rhinitis with some success. Examples of these agents and their doses as indicated for use in patients with asthma include the receptor antagonists montelukast sodium (Singulair), 10 mg daily in adults and children at least 15 years of age and 5 mg daily in children 6 to 14 years of age, and zafirlukast (Accolate), 20 mg twice daily in adults and children at least 12 years of age; and the 5-lipoxygenase inhibitor zileuton (Zyflo), 600 mg four times a day in adults and children 12 years of age and older.

Immunotherapy

Immunotherapy involves the repeated administration of increasing doses of antigen extract in an attempt to alter patients' immunologic responses and improve their symptoms. It is usually reserved for patients who find it difficult to avoid allergens and who have not responded adequately to pharmacologic treatment. The treatment offers relief, but the onset of action is slow, with improvement starting within 12 weeks and increasing over a period of 1 to 2 years after treatment. Most regimens begin with once- to twice-weekly subcutaneous injections of a low concentration of the allergen extract that is gradually increased until a maintenance dose is reached. This treatment is highly specific and is effective only for the allergens administered, making it important to identify carefully all allergens responsible for the patient's symptoms before embarking on treatment. Most clinicians recommend that therapy be continued for 2 to 3 years after the patient's symptoms are well controlled during seasonal exposure. Immunotherapy causes local and systemic adverse reactions that have included death (risk estimated at one fatality for every 2 million injections), and therefore special precautions need to be taken in patients with asthma, and a waiting period of 20 minutes after the administration of the injection is recommended for all patients, with longer intervals (30 minutes) appropriate for high-risk patients. Treatment should be administered by professionals trained in the use of immunotherapy and in an office setting ready to handle anaphylaxis and administer cardiopulmonary resuscitation. Mild systemic reactions such as urticaria, bronchospasm, and hypotension occur frequently, and local reactions at the site of injection are common. Immunotherapy is probably best for patients with perennial rhinitis because they are symptomatic throughout the year and are willing to undergo prolonged treatment.

Management of the Pregnant Patient with Allergic Rhinitis

Concerns for the fetus complicate treatment of allergic rhinitis during pregnancy because none of the medications available has been definitely proved to lack fetal effects. Immunotherapy is judged safe if no systemic reactions develop, and these are more frequent during initiation of therapy and seasonal exposures. Therefore, it is advised not to start immunotherapy and to lower the maintenance dose during the pollen season during pregnancy. Among the antihistamines, tripelennamine is judged safest, whereas others may increase the risk of congenital malformations and should be avoided. Cromolyn has not been associated with danger during pregnancy and oral steroids pose minimal risk to the fetus. Harm from intranasal steroids has not become evident and they are widely used during gestation.

STRATEGY FOR THE TREATMENT OF ALLERGIC RHINITIS

After the diagnosis of allergic rhinitis is made by proper history and physical examination and the offending allergens confirmed by skin or blood testing, the first recommendation for therapy is avoidance. If that is not completely successful in alleviating the symptoms, pharmacologic treatment usually starts with an antihistamine with or without a decongestant, especially in patients with seasonal disease. Cromolyn sodium is an alternative to antihistamines as an initial treatment in these patients. If these treatments fail, or the disease requires daily treatment such as in patients with perennial disease, intranasal corticosteroids should be introduced. Eye drops or antihistamines can be used to supplement intranasal steroids in the patients who complain of eye irritation, and intranasal ipratropium can be added in patients who complain of persistent rhinorrhea. The decision to start immunotherapy is based on the preferences of both the patient and the treating physician. As a general rule, however, pharmacotherapy is probably more appropriate for patients who are affected only during one season of the year. When allergies lead to perennial symptoms, the choice between daily medications and once- or twice-weekly injections might be easier to make, leading more patients in this group to select immunotherapy for treatment. When pharmacologic treatment is successful, the minimum therapy required to provide optimal symptomatic relief should be maintained. In cases in which pharmacologic treatment does not lead to symptomatic improvement, other causes of the symptoms, such as complicating sinusitis, should be investigated and treated.

ALLERGIC REACTIONS TO DRUGS

method of
SANDRA KNOWLES, B.Sc.Pharm., and
NEIL H. SHEAR, M.D.
*Sunnybrook and Women's College Health
    Sciences Center and the University of Toronto*
Toronto, Canada

Adverse drug reactions (ADRs) are not uncommon, occurring in approximately 30% of hospitalized patients. Within the realm of ADRs, there are both predictable and unpredictable reactions. Predictable reactions comprise the majority of ADRs and include those reactions that are dose related and based on the pharmacologic action of the drug. In contrast, unpredictable reactions, which include allergic and idiosyncratic reactions, are not dose related (Fig. 1). Although most patients who develop an ADR complain of being "allergic" to the drug, only 10 to 25% of all ADRs are actually allergic.

Unfortunately, many patients with an "allergic" history are often denied the drug or drugs in question without adequate assessment of the actual ADR. To assist clinicians in the evaluation of these patients, we have developed a systematic and logical approach to aid in the man-

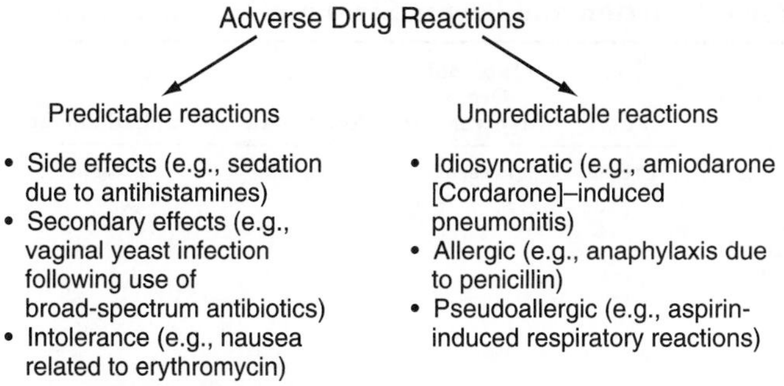

Adverse Drug Reactions

Predictable reactions

- Side effects (e.g., sedation due to antihistamines)
- Secondary effects (e.g., vaginal yeast infection following use of broad-spectrum antibiotics)
- Intolerance (e.g., nausea related to erythromycin)

Unpredictable reactions

- Idiosyncratic (e.g., amiodarone [Cordarone]–induced pneumonitis)
- Allergic (e.g., anaphylaxis due to penicillin)
- Pseudoallergic (e.g., aspirin-induced respiratory reactions)

Figure 1. Classification of adverse drug reactions.

agement of an ADR (Table 1). This approach works for most types of ADRs, including allergic and idiosyncratic reactions. Analysis of ADRs should be done for patients with acute drug-induced disease processes as well as for patients with a remote history of an ADR.

To solve complex problems in patients with histories suggestive of ADRs, a multidisciplinary clinic was formed at our institution. The team of the Drug Safety Clinic comprises specialists in the fields of clinical immunology and allergy, dermatology, internal medicine, clinical pharmacology, and clinical pharmacy. The Drug Safety Clinic attempts to provide all individual patients and their physicians with appropriate and relevant information on the suspected ADR (including drugs to avoid and drugs that could be safely taken), as well as undertaking research projects and conducting educational seminars.

DIAGNOSIS

A 20-year old white man developed a fever (39°C) and pruritic erythematous skin eruption approximately 3 weeks after starting phenytoin (Dilantin) for a seizure disorder. Laboratory tests revealed increased liver transaminase levels (aspartate transaminase, 452 IU per liter; alanine transaminase, 355 IU per liter); all other laboratory results were within normal limits.

The correct diagnosis is one of the key elements in the assessment of a patient with a possible allergic reaction. Although many patients state that they are "allergic" to a specific medication, a detailed history is needed to sort through those reactions that are simply drug intolerances or an expected pharmacologic drug effect or those that could be considered to be allergic. For example, gastrointestinal intolerance is a common complaint of patients on

TABLE 1. **Steps in the Approach to a Suspected Adverse Reaction**

Bedside Management
Clinical diagnosis
Analysis of drug exposure
Differential diagnosis

Treatment
Initiation of treatment strategies

Future Management
Literature search
Confirmation
Advice to the patient
Reporting to licensing authorities and/or manufacturer

erythromycin. However, these patients should not be labeled as "allergic" but rather as erythromycin intolerant; in fact, newer macrolides such as clarithromycin (Biaxin) and azithromycin (Zithromax) are often well tolerated by this group of patients. Unfortunately, many patients are unable to remember specific details regarding their adverse reaction. In these cases, especially when drug therapy is severely compromised, efforts should be made to obtain original notes from hospitals to document details regarding the adverse reaction.

Allergic reactions can manifest themselves through any organ system. Urticaria, angioedema, shortness of breath, and hypotension are classic descriptors of an IgE-mediated reaction, typified by anaphylaxis. Because many allergic reactions manifest as dermatologic eruptions, the diagnosis of a cutaneous eruption will serve as a broad example for allergic reactions.

Reactions in the skin can be diagnosed at two different levels. In general, these are based on the determination of a specific morphology (e.g., exanthematous, urticarial, blistering, or pustular) and the absence or presence of a fever (Table 2).

The development of a fever in conjunction with a rash, as with Mr. J. L., should alert the clinician to a possible diagnosis of a hypersensitivity syndrome reaction (HSR). A triad of fever, rash (ranging from an exanthematous eruption to Stevens-Johnson syndrome/toxic epidermal necrolysis), and internal organ involvement is characteristic of HSRs. Most commonly, the liver is involved, although other organ systems such as the kidney or lung could also be affected; the patient may be symptomatic or asymptomatic.

DRUG EXPOSURE

In addition to the phenytoin (Dilantin), Mr. J. L. had been using lorazepam (Ativan) as needed (prn) for 2 weeks at bedtime. He denied the use of over-the-counter or herbal preparations.

Drug reactions often occur in complicated clinical scenarios that include exposures to multiple agents. It is important that a detailed history be obtained for evaluation of an adverse drug reaction. This includes as much detail regarding the dosage, onset of reaction, rechallenge, and dechallenge. A history of prior exposure to the drug and to related compounds is also of interest, because if the drug has been tolerated numerous times in the past, an ADR is unlikely and alternative causes should be explored. However, a prior exposure to a drug may act as a sensitizer, inducing a reaction on re-exposure to the drug.

Although new drugs started within the preceding 6 weeks of an ADR are important, one should also look for medications that were used intermittently, including over-the-counter preparations and herbal/naturopathic remedies. For example, fixed drug eruptions can be caused by many different medications; however, over-the-counter preparations, including dimenhydrinate (Gravol), are often implicated in the development of these lesions. In addition, although many people are using herbal remedies, they may not admit to their use during a medication history inquiry. However, these medications are also prone to causing allergic reactions. For complex medication histories, it is recommended that a "time line" be developed for drug exposure analysis. The "time-line" should encompass all drugs administered and provide information on symptoms experienced by the patient.

Allergic reactions are often classified as immediate

TABLE 2. Clinical Features of Hypersensitivity Syndrome Reaction and Serum Sickness–Like Reaction

Reaction	Cutaneous Eruption	Commonly Implicated Drugs	Fever	Internal Organ Involvement	Arthralgia	Lymphadenopathy
Hypersensitivity syndrome reaction	Exanthematous eruption Exfoliative dermatitis Pustular eruptions Erythema multiforme/Stevens-Johnson syndrome/toxic epidermal necrolysis	Aromatic anticonvulsants (i.e., phenobarbital, phenytoin [Dilantin], carbamazepine [Tegretol]) Lamotrigine (Lamictal) Sulfonamide antibiotics Dapsone Allopurinol (Zyloprim) Minocycline (Minocin)	Present	Present	Absent	Present
Serum sickness–like reaction	Urticaria Exanthematous eruption	Antibiotics, especially cefaclor (Ceclor)	Present	Absent	Present	Present

(within an hour of drug administration), accelerated (less than 48 hours), or delayed. Although most delayed reactions (e.g., exanthematous eruption after antibiotic administration) occur within 7 to 10 days of drug administration, hypersensitivity syndrome reactions can occur within 2 to 6 weeks of drug initiation. As well, drug-induced lupus has been reported in some patients after 2 years of drug use. This is important because the delay in onset of symptoms may not alert the clinician to the causative drug, causing delay in proper diagnosis and subsequent treatment (specifically drug discontinuation).

The onset of HSR occurs between 2 and 6 weeks after initiation of therapy; however, in patients who have been previously exposed, the onset can occur within days. Mr. J. L. started to develop symptoms within 3 weeks after initiation of phenytoin (Dilantin).

DIFFERENTIAL DIAGNOSIS

Investigations for various viral infections (e.g., viral hepatitis, mononucleosis) yielded negative results for Mr. J. L.

The third step in diagnosing an allergic reaction involves an evaluation of the differential diagnosis of the reaction. For example, differential diagnoses for a dermatologic eruption can include viral exanthems (e.g., infectious mononucleosis, parvovirus B19 infection), bacterial infections, Kawasaki disease, collagen vascular disease, and neoplasia.

Viruses can often complicate the diagnosis of a dermatologic eruption by "imitating" a drug-induced reaction or by "interacting" with a drug to cause a reaction. A prime example of this is the ampicillin-induced rash associated with infectious mononucleosis. Sixty to 100% of patients with infectious mononucleosis who are administered ampicillin will develop a typical exanthematous eruption. However, rechallenge with ampicillin once the infectious process has cleared will not result in a dermatologic eruption. Another example of a drug-virus interaction is the large percentage (up to 60%) of patients with human immunodeficiency virus (HIV) infection who develop an adverse reaction while on a sulfonamide antibiotic. Obviously, the use of an antibiotic should be carefully assessed in any patient with a concomitant viral infection. This would help to curtail the rise in antibiotic resistance as well as decrease the number of patients who are falsely denied an antibiotic class simply because of a virus-drug interaction.

Other relevant factors to consider in the differential diagnosis include the presence of an underlying condition (e.g., heart disease, atopy/asthma), vasovagal stimulation (especially with local anesthetics on injection), and psychological factors. Preliminary work at the Drug Safety Clinic suggests that some patients with "multiple drug allergies" may actually have an underlying panic disorder. Symptoms of panic include palpitations, sweating, trembling, chest discomfort, nausea, and chills or hot flashes. These symptoms are characteristic for some patients with "multiple drug allergies." Management of these patients is aimed at treating their underlying panic disorder.

The differential diagnosis of HSR includes other cutaneous drug reactions, acute infections, lymphoma, collagen vascular diseases, and serum sickness–like reaction (SSLR). The main distinguishing features between SSLRs and HSRs are the development of arthralgias and the lack of internal organ involvement with SSLRs. Mr. J. L. did not have symptoms consistent with SSLR.

INITIATION OF TREATMENT STRATEGIES

Phenytoin (Dilantin) is discontinued. Mr. J. L. is started on a topical corticosteroid and an oral antihistamine for control of his pruritus. Treatment with prednisone is also initiated. Symptoms completely resolve in 4 days; his liver transaminase levels return to normal within 5 days.

In patients with an acute reaction, appropriate treatment strategies must be initiated. A detailed discussion of the management of the various adverse drug reactions is beyond the scope of this article.

In most patients who develop an adverse event, discontinuation of the suspected drug is recommended. The treatment of anaphylaxis includes epinephrine, oxygen, antihistamines, and corticosteroids. Corticosteroids are often administered for patients with a hypersensitivity syndrome reaction. For symptomatic relief of a mild cutaneous reaction, topical corticosteroids and/or antihistamines may be helpful.

Literature Search

Documentation of a particular drug and event in the literature may clarify a patient's case. This includes information on onset and duration of the reaction, use of diagnostic tests such as skin testing, and use of alternative non–cross-reacting drugs. It is often surprising how much information case reports can provide. For example, a patient with leukocytoclastic vasculitis was started on azathioprine (Imuran); within 15 days of initiation, she developed a fever. Azathioprine was discontinued, and an evaluation for sepsis was negative. Azathioprine was restarted 5 days later. After a single dose, fever, nausea and vomiting, diarrhea, hypotension, tachycardia, and oliguria developed. However, within 24 hours of drug discontinuation, all signs and symptoms abated. A review of case reports in the literature showed that most commonly a fever and gastrointestinal symptoms occurred on initial presentation. However, as in our case, on azathioprine rechallenge, the reaction was generally more severe and, on occasion, life threatening.

Various sources should be consulted, including textbooks, medical journals (often assessed through MEDLINE or other similar services), and the pharmaceutical manufacturers. In addition, large ADR databases such as the FDA Medwatch program in the United States or the Health Protection Branch ADR program in Canada can be accessed for further information.

HSR occurs most commonly with aromatic anticonvulsants (phenytoin [Dilantin], phenobarbital, and carbamazepine [Tegretol]), lamotrigine (Lamictal), sulfonamide antibiotics, allopurinol, dapsone, and minocycline (Minocin).

Confirmation

Because Mr. J.L. requires an anticonvulsant, he is referred to the Drug Safety Clinic. The lymphocyte toxicity assay was "positive" in this patient for phenytoin (Dilantin), phenobarbital, and carbamazepine (Tegretol).

Whenever possible, it is important to confirm causality between drug and reaction. This involves an evaluation of each potential cause, including all medications and nondrug causes. There are several causality assessment tools available; however, unless used for research purposes, most of these are either cumbersome to administer or do not provide enough detailed information to establish causation.

In vivo or in vitro testing can aid in the diagnosis of an allergic reaction. The in vivo diagnostic tests that are available for allergic reactions include oral rechallenge, skin testing, and patch testing. In vitro testing, although posing less potential risk for the patient, is often used only for research purposes. Examples include a radioallergosorbent assay, a lymphocyte transformation test, and a cytotoxicity assay.

Patch testing is used to confirm contact dermatitis, fixed drug eruptions in approximately 35% of cases, and other delayed dermatologic erup-

tions. Patch testing is performed with the drug in a suitable, nonirritant concentration and vehicle that is then applied to the skin under hypoallergenic occlusive tape. At 48, 72, and, occasionally, 96 hours the sites are inspected for pruritus, vesiculation, and erythema.

An *oral provocation test* is used when the patient's history is vague, the drug is deemed essential, and the risk of eliciting a reaction is known, is considered manageable, and does not exceed the perceived benefit of subsequent treatment with the drug. For example, it may be considered acceptable to challenge a patient with a history of headaches and pruritus who requires long-term aspirin prophylaxis for cardiovascular disease to aspirin whereas it would be unethical to challenge a person who experienced symptoms consistent with an anaphylactic reaction to penicillin. As well, drug rechallenges should not be used if a serious reaction such as Stevens-Johnson syndrome or toxic epidermal necrolysis previously occurred. In general, at the Drug Safety Clinic, drug rechallenges are performed with the use of a 10th of the dose, followed by a full dose 1 hour later. The patient is then observed for another 2 to 3 hours.

In patients who develop nonspecific symptoms during drug rechallenge (e.g., headache, pruritus, shortness of breath without any change in pulmonary function testing), we use a double-blind placebo-controlled technique (N-of-1 trial) for evaluation of the patient's reaction. These patients are generally extremely anxious and, in many cases, develop similar reactions to unrelated medications. Usually a placebo or a drug is administered on a weekly basis and the patient is observed for 3 hours; the patient, physician, and nurse are not aware of the order of the doses. A total of three placebo and three drug doses are administered. All signs and symptoms are recorded during this time. At the end of the 6- to 8-week period, the code is broken. We have found that many patients actually develop "reactions" during the placebo phase of the trial.

Desensitization is another form of drug rechallenge. Desensitization is the administration of a drug to an individual in whom drug allergy has been established. Minute quantities of the drug are administered and the dose is gradually increased until a full therapeutic dose is reached. Desensitization protocols have been described for a variety of drugs, including beta-lactam antibiotics, allopurinol, sulfonamide antibiotics (especially in the setting of HIV infection), and aspirin. Desensitization protocols for most antibiotics (an exception is sulfonamide antibiotics) are generally administered over 6 to 8 hours, with doses given every 15 to 30 minutes. For most other drugs, desensitization protocols have been developed that range from 2 to 50 days. In general, the slower the desensitization protocol, the more successful the desensitization is likely to be. Reactions can manifest themselves during the desensitization protocol. Some clinicians may elect to continue the desensitization and "treat through" the reaction, or alternatively, the dose is decreased and subsequent increases are done more slowly. Although desensitizations are useful for patients who require immediate therapy with the drug, once the drug is discontinued the patient is once again at risk for the development of the reaction on reexposure to the drug. However, if low doses of the drug are continued on a daily basis, as in the case of patients who undergo aspirin and allopurinol desensitizations, this will theoretically prevent reactions from occurring during treatment.

Skin tests, usually composed of both prick and intradermal tests, are used primarily for confirmation of IgE-mediated allergic reactions. High-molecular-weight drugs, such as vaccines and insulin, are complete antigens and are reliable skin testing materials. However, for most low-molecular weight compounds, reactive metabolites or drug-antigen complexes have not been identified, and skin testing is generally not helpful as a diagnostic test. The exceptions to this include penicillin, local anesthetics, and agents used during general anesthesia (e.g., muscle relaxants and induction agents).

The beta-lactam antibiotics (i.e., penicillins, cephalosporins, monobactams, and carbapenems) remain one of the major problems in drug allergy. The overall incidence of adverse reactions to the beta-lactam antibiotics is between 1 and 20%, with the majority of reactions being dermatologic. Penicillin skin testing with major and minor determinants is useful for confirmation of an IgE-mediated immediate hypersensitivity reaction to penicillin. At the Drug Safety Clinic, a negative skin test is usually followed by a two-dose oral challenge with penicillin. In addition, many patients are then challenged with the culprit beta-lactam antibiotic. Although early studies indicated that cross-reactions among penicillins and cephalosporins occurred in 15 to 20% of patients, clinical experience and evidence suggest that cross-reactions among the beta-lactam antibiotics probably occur in less than 1% of patients.

Although many patients report an allergy to local anesthetic agents, true allergic reactions are extremely rare, comprising less than 1% of all adverse local anesthetic reactions. Patients who usually experience vasovagal reactions, toxic reactions due to inadvertent intravascular injection, side effects from epinephrine, or psychomotor responses, including hyperventilation, are often labeled local anesthetic "allergic." However, despite reassurances that their reactions are not true "allergy" reactions, patients' risk perception remains extremely high and they will refuse subsequent local anesthetic administration. Skin testing with local anesthetic agents followed by a full-dose subcutaneous challenge (Table 3) is

TABLE 3. Local Anesthetic Skin Testing

Prick Testing: Full Strength with Preservative

Histamine (positive control)
Normal saline (negative control)
Bupivacaine (Marcaine 0.5%)
Lidocaine (Xylocaine) with preservative
Lidocaine (Xylocaine) without preservative
Mepivacaine (Carbocaine)
Prilocaine (Citanest)
Articaine (Ultracaine)

Intradermal Testing: 1:100

Normal saline
Bupivacaine (Marcaine 0.5%)
Lidocaine (Xylocaine) with preservative
Lidocaine (Xylocaine) without preservative
Mepivacaine (Carbocaine)
Prilocaine (Citanest)
Articaine (Ultracaine)

Subcutaneous Cumulative Challenge

Using specific local anesthetic that caused initial reaction, 0.3 mL, 0.7 mL, and 1.0 mL are sequentially administered

---

remarkably helpful in these patients to overcome their "fear" of local anesthetics. We have administered a visual analogue scale to assess patients' risk perception before and after skin testing. Patients with a high initial risk perception benefit greatly by skin testing and challenge. However, patients with a moderate initial risk perception do not show decreases in their measured concern.

The *lymphocyte toxicity assay* (LTA) is an in vitro drug metabolite toxicity system that uses murine hepatic microsomes as a source of cytochrome P-450, which are incubated with the drug in question to generate reactive metabolites. Human lymphocytes are used as surrogate, peripheral target cells to investigate individuals susceptible to drug toxicity. Lymphocytes are used because they are readily accessible, do not contain the enzymes that produce toxic metabolites from the parent drug, and contain detoxification enzymes (e.g., epoxide hydrolases). If the cells are susceptible to damage by reactive metabolites, this cytotoxicity can be quantified by a variety of methods. The LTA has been used extensively for sulfonamide antibiotics and the aromatic anticonvulsants (i.e., carbamazepine [Tegretol], phenobarbital, and phenytoin [Dilantin]). However, the lymphocyte toxicity assay is expensive and cumbersome to perform; currently it is being used only in certain research centers.

Advice to the Patient

On the basis of the results of the lymphocyte toxicity assay and the advice from the Drug Safety Clinic, Mr. J. L.'s physician elected to start him on valproic acid.

The patient must be provided with information regarding the ADR. This includes the drug involved in the reaction (if known), the patient's predisposition to possible recurrence on exposure to the drug, potential cross-reaction to other drugs (e.g., aspirin and nonsteroidal anti-inflammatory drugs), and genetic predisposition of family members, if applicable. The patient should also be advised to enroll in the MedicAlert program. An example of poor communication regarding an ADR is demonstrated in the following case.

A 44-year-old man underwent general anesthesia for penile prosthesis revision. He reported no known allergies. Three minutes after induction, hypotension and erythema were noted, and the patient was treated appropriately for anaphylaxis. Further investigation revealed that two previous surgeries were complicated by hypotension; however, no information was communicated to the patient. At the Drug Safety Clinic, skin testing to various anesthetic agents was done, and the patient had a positive thiopental (Pentothal) result. He underwent subsequent general anesthesia uneventfully.

No genetic basis has been found for most allergic reactions, including penicillin-allergic reactions. However, for HSRs, SSLRs to cefaclor, and serious dermatologic reactions (e.g., Stevens-Johnson syndrome and toxic epidermal necrolysis), the risk in first-degree relatives of patients who have had reactions is substantially higher, and counseling of family members is a crucial part of the assessment of the HSR.

Approximately 75% of patients who experience an HSR with an aromatic anticonvulsant (e.g., phenytoin [Dilantin], phenobarbital, carbamazepine [Tegretol], or primidone [Mysoline]) will develop a similar reaction to the other aromatic anticonvulsants. Other anticonvulsants (e.g., valproic acid, benzodiazepines, gabapentin [Neurontin]) have not been shown to be cross-reactive with the aromatic anticonvulsants. Whereas HSR with anticonvulsants is estimated to occur in 1 in 1,000 to 1 in 10,000 exposures, first-degree relatives of an afflicted individual may have a risk that approaches 1 in 4.

Mr. J. L.'s sister and parents were brought in for counseling and informed of the increased risk.

Reporting

Because of the severity of the reaction, the information was reported to the manufacturer as well as the health regulatory agency in Canada.

ADRs should be reported to local and national organizations and manufacturers, especially if the ADR is a serious event, is an unexpected reaction, or involves recently marketed drugs. Through the use of voluntary postmarketing surveillance programs, adverse events can be identified to determine whether further monitoring is required or whether a product labeling change or even drug removal from the market is required.

ALLERGIC REACTIONS TO INSECT STINGS

method of
DAVID F. GRAFT, M.D.
Park Nicollet Clinic
Minneapolis, Minnesota

The normal response to an insect sting is transient redness, pain, and itching at the sting site. A large local reaction occurs in 10% of people and consists of swelling greater than 5 cm in diameter that persists for longer than 24 hours. For example, a sting on the hand may produce swelling of the hand and entire forearm.

Systemic allergic reactions resulting from the stings of insects of the order of Hymenoptera (honeybees, yellow jackets, hornets, wasps, and imported fire ants) affect 1% of the U.S. population and may be mild, with only cutaneous symptoms (pruritus, urticaria, angioedema), or more severe, with potentially life-threatening symptoms (laryngeal edema, bronchospasm, hypotension). Approximately 50 deaths per year are attributed to insect sting in the United States. Only one or two occur in children; the number of deaths increases gradually with age, reaching 10 deaths per year for each 10 years of life for persons aged 40 to 49, 50 to 59, and 60 to 69 years. The true incidence of insect sting–related fatalities may be even higher because sudden deaths on the golf course or at poolside may be ascribed mistakenly to heart attacks or strokes. Patients with insect sting hypersensitivity often alter their lifestyles, work patterns, and leisure activities to avoid future stings.

ACUTE MANAGEMENT

Treatment recommendations for large local reactions include antihistamines and application of ice packs to and elevation of the affected limb. A short course of prednisone (0.5 to 1 mg per kg per day [20 mg twice daily for adults] for 5 days), especially if initiated immediately after the sting, may be the best treatment for massive local reactions. Sting sites should be kept clean; imported fire ant stings are especially easily infected.

Patients with anaphylaxis require careful observation. A subcutaneous or intramuscular injection of epinephrine (1:1000) at a dose of 0.3 to 0.5 mL (in children, 0.01 mL per kg; maximum, 0.3 mL) is the cornerstone of management and often is sufficient to terminate a reaction. This may be repeated in 10 to 15 minutes if necessary. Patients with a history of cardiac disease warrant careful monitoring. An oral antihistamine such as diphenhydramine hydrochloride (Benadryl), 12.5 to 50 mg, is also usually given. It may lessen urticaria or other cutaneous symptoms, but in more serious or progressive reactions its use should not delay the administration of epinephrine.

Intravenous epinephrine, 1:100,000, given slowly should be considered for patients with anaphylactic shock who are not responding to previous therapy. Diphenhydramine hydrochloride may also be administered parenterally (50 mg in adults every 4 hours; 5 mg per kg per 24 hours in divided doses every 4 to 6 hours [maximum, 50 mg per dose in children]) for more serious reactions.

Inhaled sympathomimetic agents such as isoproterenol (Isuprel) or albuterol (Ventolin) may decrease bronchoconstriction but do not address other systemic manifestations such as shock. Aminophylline may be helpful if bronchoconstriction persists after administration of epinephrine. Severe reactions often necessitate treatment with oxygen, H_2 antagonists such as cimetidine (Tagamet), volume expanders, and pressor agents. Corticosteroids such as prednisone (0.5 to 1 mg per kg per 24 hours) are commonly used, but their delayed onset of action (4 to 6 hours) limits their effectiveness in the early stages of treatment. Intubation or tracheostomy is indicated for severe upper airway edema that does not respond to therapy. Allergic reactions are generally more severe in patients who take beta-blocking drugs. Furthermore, reactions in these patients may be more difficult to treat because beta-blockers impede the response to epinephrine and other sympathomimetic medications. Glucagon, 2 to 5 U given over 2 minutes intravenously, may be helpful in this clinical situation.

Systemic reactions commencing more than several hours after a sting are generally mild. Most are easily managed with oral antihistamines and observation. On occasion, anaphylaxis may be prolonged or biphasic. Close observation and continued treatment are essential in these situations. The administration of corticosteroids as early in treatment as feasible may help to diminish later symptoms.

DECREASING FUTURE REACTIONS

Preventing Stings

Future stings can be avoided by taking common sense precautions to significantly reduce exposure. Because many stings in children occur when they step on a bee, shoes should always be worn outside. Hives and nests around the home should be exterminated. Good sanitation should be practiced because garbage and outdoor food, especially canned drinks, attract yellow jackets. Perfumes and dark floral-patterned clothing should be avoided.

Emergency Epinephrine

To encourage prompt treatment, epinephrine is available in emergency kits for self-administration (Table 1). These are used by insect sting–allergic people immediately after the sting in order to "buy time" to get to a medical facility. The Ana-Kit contains a preloaded syringe that can deliver two 0.3-mL doses of epinephrine. Incremental doses may also

TABLE 1. Epinephrine Injection Kits for Emergency Self-treatment of Systemic Reactions to Insect Stings

Injection Kit	Dosage
EpiPen*	Delivers 0.3 mL 1:1000 (0.3 mg of epinephrine)
EpiPen Jr.*	Delivers 0.3 mL 1:2000 (0.15 mg of epinephrine)
Ana-Kit†	Delivers two doses of 0.3 mL 1:1000 (total, 0.6 mg of epinephrine)

*The EpiPen and EpiPen Jr. are spring-loaded automatic injectors and are distributed by Dey Laboratories, Port Washington, New York.

†Ana-Kit is capable of delivering fractional doses and is distributed by Hollister-Stier Laboratories, Spokane, Washington.

From Graft DF: Insect stings. In Gellis SS, Kagan BM (eds): Current Pediatric Therapy, 13th ed. Philadelphia, WB Saunders, 1990, pp. 673–675.

be given. The physician who prescribes this kit must provide thorough instruction and must be confident that the patient can perform the injection procedure. These kits can be confusing to nonmedical personnel, and some patients have a tremendous fear of needles. A practice self-injection with saline resolves this issue. The EpiPen (0.3 mg of epinephrine) and EpiPen Jr. (0.15 mg of epinephrine) offer a concealed needle and a pressure-sensitive spring-loaded injection device that make them suitable for patients and families who are uncomfortable with the injection process. The Epipen EZ and Epipen EZ Jr. were slight modifications that utilized an injector button; at the time of this writing, they have been recalled and it is uncertain if they are going to be reissued.

Medihaler-Epi (10 to 30 inhalations; 1.6 to 4.8 mg of epinephrine) may also be used to achieve therapeutic levels of epinephrine in plasma and may be especially helpful for laryngeal edema and bronchospasm. Patients who are receiving maintenance injections of venom immunotherapy are advised that emergency self-treatment will probably not be required. However, they should have the kit available if they are far from medical facilities. The wearing of a MedicAlert bracelet or medallion (MedicAlert Foundation International, 2323 Colorado Avenue, Turlock CA 95382) is also advised.

Venom Immunotherapy

The clinical history is the key to determining the need for venom immunotherapy (Table 2). A careful history discloses the type, degree, and time course of symptoms and often reveals the culprit insect. A patient who has experienced a sting-induced systemic reaction should be referred to an allergist, who will perform skin tests with dilute solutions of honeybee, yellow jacket, yellow hornet, white-faced hornet, and Polistes wasp venoms. Radioallergosorbent testing (RAST) cannot replace venom skin testing but may provide additional information. Whole-body extract materials were used before 1979 to diagnose and treat insect allergy, but they were shown to be ineffective, and venoms supplanted their use. To date, fire ant venom has only been available in small

TABLE 2. **Selection of Patients for Venom Immunotherapy**

Sting Reaction	Skin Test/RAST	Venom Immunotherapy
1. Systemic, non–life-threatening (child): immediate, generalized, confined to skin (urticaria, angioedema, erythema, pruritus)	+ or −	No
2. Systemic, life-threatening (child): immediate, generalized, may involve cutaneous symptoms but also respiratory (laryngeal edema or bronchospasm) or cardiovascular (hypotension/shock) symptoms	+	Yes
3. Systemic (adult)	+	Yes
4. Systemic	−	No
5. Large local (>2 inches [5 cm] in diameter; >24 hours)	+ or −	No
6. Normal (<2 inches [5 cm] in diameter; <24 hours)	+ or −	No

Abbreviations: RAST = Radioallergosorbent test; + = positive; − = negative.
From Graft DF: Insect stings. *In* Gellis SS, and Kagan BM (eds): Current Pediatric Therapy, 13th ed. Philadelphia, WB Saunders, 1990, pp. 673–675.

research quantities. Fortunately, the fire ant whole-body extract materials seem more potent than those previously available for other Hymenoptera species and have been successfully used for skin testing and treatment.

If the reaction was severe (potentially life-threatening symptoms of bronchospasm, laryngeal edema, and shock) and the venom test result is positive, immunotherapy with the appropriate venom or venoms is commenced. Because the recurrence rate in children with a history of milder cutaneous reactions is only 10%, venom treatment is not required. Patients with large local reactions or negative skin test results also are not candidates for venom therapy.

Increasing amounts of venom or whole-body extracts for fire ant–induced anaphylaxis are given weekly for several months until the patient can tolerate a venom dose equivalent to one or more insect stings. Venom injections are given every 4 weeks during the first year of treatment, and then the interval can be extended to 6 weeks. Venom therapy is highly effective, protecting 97% of patients from reactions to challenge stings administered in-hospital (the risk of an allergic reaction for untreated insect sting–allergic persons is probably about 60%). The disadvantages of venom treatment include cost and systemic and local reactions to injections. No long-term side effects have been reported. Patients should be informed of the possible risks and closely observed for 30 minutes or more after each injection. Injections should be administered only in settings where adequate means of treating systemic reactions are available.

In about 25% of patients, negative skin test results develop after 3 to 5 years of treatment, and these patients may be able to discontinue therapy. Furthermore, a 5-year course of venom injections is probably sufficient for the majority of patients; patients who have very severe reactions constitute the major exceptions. A position paper on discontinuation of venom immunotherapy was published by the American Academy of Allergy Asthma and Immunology in the *Journal of Allergy and Clinical Immunology*, Vol. 101, pp 573–575, 1998.

Section 12

Diseases of the Skin

ACNE VULGARIS AND ROSACEA

method of
DONALD P. LOOKINGBILL, M.D.
Mayo Medical School and Mayo Clinic
  Jacksonville
Jacksonville, Florida

Acne affects most teenagers as well as many people in their twenties and thirties. The pathogenesis involves androgen stimulation of sebum production; keratinous obstruction of the sebaceous follicle outlet, leading to accumulation of keratin and sebum with the formation of open and closed comedones (i.e., blackheads and whiteheads); and bacterial *(Propionibacterium acnes)* colonization of the trapped sebum, inciting an inflammatory reaction that produces inflammatory papules, pustules, nodules, and cysts. Most therapeutic measures are directed toward diminishing outlet obstruction and bacterial colonization.

TREATMENT OF ACNE

Most of my acne patients are treated with a combination of topical and systemic agents, specifically a topical retinoid and a topical benzoyl peroxide in combination with an oral antibiotic. I instruct patients to apply their topical preparations to the entire area affected by acne (e.g., the entire face) rather than to isolated spots, explaining that the therapy not only treats existing lesions but also helps prevent the development of new ones. At the initial visit, I discuss the importance of diet, washing, and not picking the lesions. Because there is no evidence to implicate specific foods in the pathogenesis of acne, I do not recommend any dietary restrictions, except for suggesting a nutritious well-balanced diet. Acne cannot be washed away, but twice-daily facial cleansing with a washcloth is recommended. Specific acne cleansers are not necessary. Most acne patients pick at their lesions, which increases the chances for scarring. I vigorously discourage this practice. Patients must understand that results from therapy require time. I usually schedule the first follow-up visit in 2 months and, thereafter, see patients at 2- to 4-month intervals.

Topical Therapy

The most commonly used topical agents are retinoids, benzoyl peroxides, and topical antibiotics.

Topical Retinoids

Topical retinoids are vitamin A derivatives that act primarily on the abnormal follicular keratinization.

These agents are most effective in the treatment of comedones and can be used as monotherapy for the uncommon patient with pure comedonal acne. Two topical retinoids are approved for acne. Tretinoin is now available in formulations (e.g., Retin-A Micro 0.1% Cream) that cause less irritation than the original Retin-A preparations. Adapalene (Differin gel) is the other topical retinoid that is less irritating and slightly more efficacious than the original Retin-A products. Topical retinoids are used daily, usually at bedtime.

Although retinoids do not truly photosensitize, sunlight may add to the skin irritation that topical retinoids may cause. Use of a sunscreen is advised at times of sun exposure. Because topical retinoids are expensive, their use is usually confined to the face.

Benzoyl Peroxide

Benzoyl peroxide affects both the follicular keratinization and the *P. acnes* bacteria. It can be used as a single agent for patients with mild acne. There are many benzoyl peroxide preparations on the market. Some are over-the-counter products, and others require a prescription. Preparations are available in concentrations of 2.5%, 5%, and 10%. Most are gels, some of which are less drying than others. For example, Desquam-E (E for emollient) gel was developed to be less drying than Desquam-X, and Persa-Gel-W (W for water) and Benzac-W gel are less drying than their parent formulations. Therapy is usually initiated with a 5% concentration and applied in the morning to the entire facial area. For patients with acne of the upper trunk, benzoyl peroxide may also be used at night on these areas.

Like topical retinoids, benzoyl peroxide may cause irritation of the skin, but this effect usually becomes less troublesome with continued use. In rare cases, a patient may develop an allergic reaction to benzoyl peroxide. Allergic reactions last for many days after discontinuing the drug, unlike the usual time of 1 or 2 days for simple irritation. If allergy occurs, the patient should never again use benzoyl peroxide preparations. All patients should be advised that benzoyl peroxide bleaches colored fabrics, such as bedding and articles of clothing, that come in contact with it.

Topical Antibiotics

Topical antibiotics exert their effect on the *P. acnes* bacteria. The two major drugs in use are erythromycin (A/T/S, EryDerm, Erycette, Staticin, T-Stat), which is available in gels, solutions, and saturated swabs, and clindamycin (Cleocin-T), available in a gel, solution, and lotion. I prescribe these agents primarily for patients with mild to moderately severe inflammatory acne who fail to respond to benzoyl peroxide or who are unduly irritated by it.

Topical Combinations

A combination of 5% benzoyl peroxide and 3% erythromycin in a topical gel (Benzamycin) is superior to either of the agents used singly. It must be kept refrigerated, and it is moderately expensive.

Azelaic Acid

Azelaic acid (Azelex cream, 20%) was introduced to the American market for the treatment of acne. It is no more efficacious than the agents listed above. It can help to lighten hyperpigmented lesions, however, and this feature may be useful in the treatment of patients with acne and postinflammatory hyperpigmentation.

Acne Washes

Acne washes are convenient for treatment of large areas of acne, particularly the chest and back. The two agents that I prescribe are benzoyl peroxide washes (Desquam-X Wash, Benzac-W Wash) and chlorhexidine (Hibiclens). Both agents are effective against the *P. acnes* organism, but chlorhexidine is much less expensive.

Systemic Therapy

Systemic Antibiotics

Antibiotics act on the bacteria involved in acne. They may also have anti-inflammatory effect. Typically, I start patients on twice-daily therapy for the first 2 months. If the acne is well controlled at that point, the antibiotics are tapered over the next several months while maintaining topical therapy. Some patients require long-term antibiotic therapy, and bacterial resistance to a specific antibiotic can develop. Changing to an alternative drug is often useful. Bacterial resistance occurs most frequently with erythromycin and least frequently with minocycline, but it is increasing in frequency with all of the antibiotics used in acne.

Tetracycline is the antibiotic most frequently prescribed. It is inexpensive and usually well tolerated. For most patients, the usual starting dose is 500 mg twice daily. Patients should be instructed to take the medication on an empty stomach, because food (particularly dairy products) interferes with its absorption. Side effects from tetracycline are uncommon. Vaginal candidiasis may develop in women, particularly those who take birth control pills. Tetracycline has been suggested to reduce the efficacy of birth control pills, but this has not been proven. However, if a physician or patient is concerned about this possible interaction, erythromycin is a safe alternative. Photosensitivity rarely occurs during tetracycline use.

Erythromycin is also used for acne, although, as mentioned, bacterial resistance has become a problem that limits its usefulness in many patients. Erythromycin preparations are somewhat more expensive than tetracycline but still moderately priced. The standard starting dose is 500 mg twice daily. Gastrointestinal side effects are more frequent than with tetracycline, but if this is a problem, many erythromycin preparations can be taken with meals.

If tetracycline and erythromycin fail, alternative antibiotics can be considered. Doxycycline and minocycline, 100 to 200 mg daily, may be somewhat more effective than tetracycline, but doxycycline occasionally causes photosensitivity and minocycline is very expensive and also rarely causes drug-induced hepatitis or lupus. Trimethoprim-sulfamethoxazole (Bactrim) is efficacious, but side effects are of concern, including severe rashes and rare cases of agranulocytosis. Clindamycin had been more commonly used in the treatment of acne before cases of pseudomembranous colitis limited its use.

Retinoids

The development of 13-*cis*-retinoic acid (Accutane) revolutionized the treatment of severe, therapy-resistant acne. This agent profoundly shrinks sebaceous glands and reduces follicular hyperkeratinization. Other therapies primarily control the acne process until the patient "outgrows it," but Accutane induces long-term (sometimes indefinite) remissions in many patients. Its use is generally restricted to nodulocystic acne, severe papulopustular acne, scarring acne, and debilitating acne in patients who have not responded to the treatment modalities previously discussed. The drug is prescribed in a dose of 1 mg per kg daily for 20 weeks. During the first month, some patients notice a flare of their disease. Accordingly, I recommend starting the drug at half dosage for the first month and advancing to the full dose after that as tolerated.

Side effects are numerous. Of most concern is the teratogenic effects of this and all other retinoids. Therefore, it must be used with great caution in women of childbearing age. The manufacturer of the drug provides an informational kit that includes consent forms for women contemplating this therapy. Women must be using effective birth control measures, and a pregnancy test must be performed before initiating therapy and at monthly intervals thereafter. It is critical that physicians and patients who use Accutane be fully aware of its teratogenic risk and carefully follow the guidelines outlined for its use in women.

Other side effects are associated with the use of Accutane. Frequent side effects include chapped lips, red and dry skin, dry eyes (therefore, contact lenses may not be tolerated), and dryness of the nose, sometimes accompanied by nosebleeds. Less frequently, patients may develop severe headaches due to pseudotumor cerebri, muscle or joint aching, fatigue, hair loss, and a multitude of other reactions. Because retinoids can increase plasma lipids, blood levels should be monitored.

Accutane is taken for 20 weeks; after a 20-week course of Accutane, most patients are clear of acne, and many remain so for an indefinite period. Those who relapse do so slowly over the course of months to years. Relapses are usually milder than the initial condition and can usually be managed with standard therapy. Occasionally, repeated courses of Accutane are needed. Accutane is expensive.

Hormonal Therapy

Because androgens stimulate sebum production, antiandrogen therapy has been used for acne, but it is reserved mainly for women with androgen excess in whom standard therapy has failed. Women may be suspected of androgen excess if their acne is resistant to therapy or if they have accompanying hirsutism or irregular menses. For such women, I order a free and total testosterone test to screen for ovarian hypersecretion and a serum dehydroepiandrosterone sulfate level for adrenal androgen excess. For mild increases in testosterone level, estrogen therapy (i.e., birth control pills) may be used, but, because the progestin in some birth control pills can have androgenic activity, an estrogen product with low androgen effect should be selected, for example, Ortho Tri-Cyclen. This birth control pill is also now FDA approved for the treatment of acne: Women using this product experience a 50% improvement in acne after 6 months of treatment. Mild elevations of the adrenal androgen dehydroepiandrosterone sulfate can be treated with a low-dose corticosteroid (e.g., 2.5 mg of prednisone) taken at bedtime.

Antiandrogens have occasionally been used for treating acne. Cyproterone acetate is available in Europe but not in the United States. In the United States, spironolactone (Aldactone) has been used for this purpose in a dosage of 25 to 50 mg twice daily. This agent can improve acne, but women must use birth control measures (preferably birth control pills) simultaneously because of the theoretical risk of feminizing a developing male fetus by exposure to spironolactone. Other side effects of spironolactone include breast tenderness and break-through bleeding.

Accutane and hormonal therapy are not first-line choices for the treatment of acne. Most patients respond quite satisfactorily to topical agents and systemic antibiotics.

TREATMENT OF ROSACEA

Rosacea is an acneiform condition that affects middle-aged patients. It is characterized by papules and pustules occurring on a background of erythema and telangiectasia of facial skin. The process tends to affect mainly the middle third of the face, from forehead to chin. Comedones are not typically present. Some patients with rosacea develop the thickened skin and enlarged sebaceous glands of rhinophyma.

Topical Therapy

Tretinoin and benzoyl peroxide preparations may aggravate the erythema and are usually not prescribed. Topical antibiotics can be helpful. Topical metronidazole (MetroGel or MetroCream) applied twice daily is the most effective topical therapy for rosacea. It is applied for several months and then tapered. Recurrences are common, and re-treatment can be safely instituted.

Systemic Therapy

As in acne vulgaris, systemic antibiotics are effective in treating rosacea. Lower dosages can often be used, for example, tetracycline in a dose of 500 mg daily. After the first month, the dosage can often be lowered and the drug ultimately discontinued. Recurrences are common, and repeated courses of antibiotics may be needed. Antibiotics are also helpful to treat the blepharitis and keratitis that are occasionally associated with rosacea.

Rosacea that fails to respond to the above measures may be treated with daily low-dose (0.5 mg per kg) isotretinoin (Accutane) for a 20-week course. Results are usually good, but recurrences are common.

Surgical Therapy

Medical treatment has a limited effect on erythema and no impact on telangiectasia. If desired, telangiectasias can be treated with electrosurgery or laser therapy. Rhinophyma may be treated with curettage, dermabrasion, or laser therapy.

HAIR DISORDERS

method of
THOMAS N. HELM, M.D.
State University of New York at Buffalo
Williamsville, New York

Hair has no vital physiologic function, but hair is important in our self image and heavily influences our concept of beauty and aesthetics. Hair disorders may be classified as problems of hair loss, too much hair, or hair shaft abnormalities (Table 1). Hair growth changes over time. When we are born, we have fine hairs over our bodies known as lanugo hairs. The lanugo hair is shed, and terminal hairs develop. On the scalp, terminal hairs have an active hair matrix situated in the fat that gives rise to a hair shaft surrounded by an inner root sheath and an outer root sheath. The outer root sheath is continuous with the surrounding epidermis. The hair matrix is very metabolically active, and mitotic figures are encountered on histologic examination. Hairs go through various well-defined stages of growth. Unlike the hair of other animals, human hair growth is not synchronized. At any time, hairs on the scalp are in different phases. The active growth phase is known as the anagen phase. The anagen phase usually lasts approximately 3 years. After this 3-year growth phase, hair growth ceases, and there is an upward retrac-

TABLE 1. **Hair Disorders: Classification**

Hair Loss

Noninflammatory

PATTERNED

Androgenic alopecia
Traction
Hair shaft abnormalities

NONPATTERNED

Telogen effluvium
Androgen effluvium (toxic exposure)

Inflammatory

SCARRING

Lupus erythematosus
Lichen planopilaris
Autoimmune blistering disease
Infections (e.g., dissecting cellulitis of the scalp)
Trauma
Neoplasms

NONSCARRING

Alopecia areata
Psoriasis

Too Much Hair

- Ethnic and racial hair growth
- Hirsutism due to androgenic excess

Hair Shaft Abnormalities

Exogenous injuries to the hair
- Trichorrhexis nodosa
Irregularities of the hair shaft
- Monilethrix
- Pseudomonilethrix
- Bubble hair
Genetic abnormalities
- Trichothiodystrophy
- Monilethrix
- Ectodermal dysplasia

---

tion of the hair shaft. A hyaline basement membrane surrounds the hair root. The hair then enters the telogen phase. Telogen hairs are shed after approximately 3 months; and when examined grossly, telogen hairs have a nonpigmented bulb at the end. About 10% of hairs at any one time are in the telogen phase, and almost 90% of hairs are in the anagen phase. The human scalp has more than 100,000 hairs. When a patient presents with a hair abnormality, a number of questions need to be assessed. These include the pattern of remaining hairs, the duration of the hair problem, and the presence or absence of symptoms such as itching, discomfort, and any associated skin lesions (Table 2).

NONINFLAMMATORY DIFFUSE HAIR LOSS

Telogen Effluvium

One of the most common causes of diffuse noninflammatory hair loss is telogen effluvium. Telogen

TABLE 2. **Points to Consider When Evaluating Hair Loss**

Duration of hair loss
Pattern of hair loss
Associated symptoms (e.g., redness or itching)
Associated skin lesions

TABLE 3. **Medicines That Can Cause Telogen Effluvium**

Angiotensin-converting enzyme inhibitors
Anticoagulants
Anticonvulsants
Antithyroid drugs
Beta blockers
Birth control pills
Calcium channel blockers
Cholesterol-lowering agents
Cimetidine
Lithium
Nonsteroidal anti-inflammatory agents
Retinoids
Salicylates

---

effluvium represents an abnormality of the hair growth cycle. Hairs in an anagen phase abruptly switch into the telogen mode. After 6 to 16 weeks from the triggering insult, a precipitous hair shed is noted. Thirty to 40% of scalp hair can be lost, and the clinical findings may be very impressive or relatively subtle. Common culprits for telogen effluvium include major surgery, childbirth, crash diets, nutritional deficiencies, malabsorption, systemic disease, thyroid abnormalities, iron deficiency, and drugs. The most common types of drugs implicated include beta blockers, birth control pills, calcium channel blockers, nonsteroidal anti-inflammatory agents, retinoids, salicylates, and angiotensin-converting enzyme inhibitors. Many other drugs may at times cause telogen effluvium (Table 3). Telogen effluvium gradually subsides over several months and hair regrows. Many patients will show a fine regrowth of hair in areas of shedding but may still be bothered because the hair is of little cosmetic value given its short size. Patients must be reassured that with time adequate hair growth will take place. If history and examination are not helpful in identifying an underlying cause, screening laboratory studies may be indicated (Table 4).

Anagen Effluvium

Anagen effluvium represents an abrupt cessation of anagen hair growth. Immediate hair loss occurs, and there is usually complete recovery once the triggering factor is removed. The most common example of this is the hair shedding encountered after treatment with a chemotherapeutic agent. Methotrexate, vinblastine, vincristine, doxorubicin, daunorubicin, cytarabine, cyclophosphamide, bleomycin, and etopo-

---

TABLE 4. **Laboratory Studies for Telogen Effluvium**

Complete blood cell count
Serum electrolyte level
Ferritin level
Thyroid-stimulating hormone level
Serum dihydroepiandrosterone sulfate level
Free testosterone level

side are common culprits. Poisoning with arsenic, bismuth, borax, or thallium can also give rise to an anagen effluvium. Instead of hairs switching from the anagen to the telogen phase, anagen hairs abruptly stop growing because of the metabolic effect on the hair matrix, and hairs are shed. When hairs are examined under the microscope, they have a jagged or tapered end (so-called pencil-point hairs). Hair loss is noted over the entire scalp, but hairs that are not in an active anagen phase (e.g., eyelashes and eyebrows) are spared. Once the triggering cause is removed, hair regrowth can be expected. It may take several months for adequate regrowth to occur.

Loose anagen syndrome describes a defect in the hair follicle inner root sheath. Hairs are easily shed even with brushing or pulling and seem "not to grow" because of the consistent shedding. No treatment is available for this structural problem, although in some affected individuals the condition seems to improve at puberty.

Patterned Noninflammatory Hair Loss

The most common cause for patterned hair loss is androgenic alopecia. "Androgenic alopecia" is a term for hair loss that is genetically predetermined. In androgenic alopecia, hair follicles are exquisitely sensitive to circulating androgens and in predetermined areas, such as the crown and vertex of the scalp, progressive miniaturization of hair follicles occurs. Terminal hairs are transformed into vellus hairs in areas of hair thinning. Sebaceous lobules increase in size, and biopsy reveals miniaturized follicles in the skin.

In men, hair thinning begins after puberty. Approximately one fourth of men aged 25 have some degree of clinically apparent androgenic alopecia. Bitemporal recession and balding over the vertex are most common. Coarse hairs may develop at the temples and along the sideburns and are referred to as "whisker hairs." In women, the frontal hair line is often spared and there is loss of hair in the crown area. In many instances there is a strong family history of baldness.

The treatment for androgenic alopecia is difficult. Topical minoxidil solution has been shown to be of benefit. Two percent minoxidil can be applied twice daily and will stimulate the development of terminal hairs and androgenic anagen phase. Finasteride (Propecia), at a dosage of 1 mg daily, has also been shown to stimulate hair growth. Finasteride is helpful in preventing further hair loss and yields significant clinical improvement when compared with placebo in maintaining terminal hair counts. Finasteride may lower prostate-specific anagen (PSA) levels, and care must be taken to screen individuals to ensure that no underlying prostatic problem is overlooked in individuals on this therapy. The current recommendation is that the PSA level be doubled to give a more accurate reflection of the "true value" in individuals on finasteride. Finasteride does not seem to be effective in women, according to initial studies. Other treatment options that may be of value include oral spironolactone and surgical approaches, such as hair transplantation surgery. Individuals with darker or curly hair seem to benefit more from surgical approaches.

When hair loss is associated with signs of androgen excess (e.g., acne, weight gain, menstrual irregularities), evaluation is warranted to evaluate the possibility of underlying endocrinopathy, such as polycystic ovary disease, adrenal hyperplasia, or androgen-producing tumors of the ovaries. Laboratory studies that should be considered include determination of free and total testosterone, dehydroepiandrosterone sulfate, and cortisone levels and perhaps a dexamethasone suppression test.

Traction alopecia is caused by trauma or manipulation of the scalp. Traction may be patterned depending on the cause of injury to the scalp. If hairs are tightly braided, hair loss occurs along the frontal and temporal areas of the scalp.

Trichotillomania is due to pulling and tugging on hairs as part of a psychiatric condition. Hairs are usually lost in the crown area, and a fringe area on the anterior scalp is spared. Hairs are only 1 to 2 cm in length and are plucked as soon as they are long enough to be pulled or tugged.

Some hair shaft abnormalities such as autosomal dominant monilethrix cause hairs to break easily. This may be associated with more pronounced hair loss of the vertex area and can mimic androgenic alopecia.

INFLAMMATORY HAIR LOSS

Inflammatory hair loss can be evaluated and classified into scarring and nonscarring varieties. Often scarring can be identified clinically, but sometimes scarring and destruction of follicular units can be only ascertained by biopsy. Biopsy is therefore very helpful when inflammatory hair loss is suggested. Hair loss is typically patchy and irregular.

Nonscarring Inflammatory Hair Loss

Alopecia areata is a common and yet idiopathic cause of inflammatory nonscarring hair loss. Alopecia areata presents as smooth areas of hair loss that are often round or oval. Areas are asymptomatic but occasionally may be associated with mild itching or discomfort. No redness is noted on the skin, nor do pustules develop. The most important differential diagnosis for alopecia areata is fungal infection of the scalp, which is usually associated with scaling, erythema, and pustule formation. Biopsy or culture will help clarify the diagnosis.

Alopecia areata may be associated with other autoimmune abnormalities, such as autoimmune thyroid disease and vitiligo, as well as connective tissue diseases, such as lupus erythematosus. Most cases of alopecia areata do not require treatment. Most localized lesions will remit on their own. When lesions are more widespread, intralesional injections of corticosteroids are of greatest benefit in stimulating regrowth. Intralesional triamcinolone acetonide (Kenalog) at concentrations ranging from 2.5 to 5 mg per mL may be administered every 3 to 4 weeks with a small-gauge needle as an intradermal injection. Topical corticosteroids may be of value, and other topical agents that may be of benefit in some instances include anthralin as well as minoxidil. Systemic agents such as prednisone and cyclosporine (Sandimmune)* will lead to hair regrowth but are not advised because they are toxic when used for long-term therapy. If hair growth is established and these agents are withdrawn, hair loss occurs, and patients may develop a dependency on these medicines. Because alopecia areata itself does not lead to any serious medical consequence, it is difficult to justify the long-term administration of a medicine with many known serious side effects.

Traction Alopecia/Trichotillomania

Traction alopecia and trichotillomania are due to injury to the scalp from exogenous causes. Traction may result from hair styling (e.g., corn row braids) and other types of braiding practices or from wearing gear on the scalp, such as Walkman radios. Rubbing and friction over time cause damage to the hair shaft and impair hair growth. Some individuals under psychological duress may pull, rub, or pick at the hair incessantly, leading to hair breakage and hair injury. In these instances, hair shaft fragments may be found in the dermis and are surrounded by an inflammatory infiltrate. Early on this process is nonscarring and can be reversed. If long-standing, permanent damage to the hair shaft may result. Identifying and avoiding the underlying cause may be of value. In trichotillomania, psychological evaluation is mandatory. Agents such as fluoxetine (Prozac) or pimozide (Orap) may be required to control this manifestation of an obsessive and compulsive psychological disorder.

Psoriasis and Inflammatory Skin Diseases

Although most dermatoses on the scalp are not associated with substantial hair loss, psoriasis and seborrheic dermatitis as well as other dermatoses may be associated with a temporary shedding of hair. The mechanism is not entirely clear but may relate to a telogen effluvium stimulated by the underlying dermatosis. Other cutaneous clues help in establishing a diagnosis. For example, in cases of psoriasis, scaly plaques may be found over the extensor surfaces and behind the ears.

Inflammatory Scarring Hair Loss

Infections

Tinea infection is a common cause of inflammatory hair loss. Dermatophytes such as *Trichophyton rubrum, T. tonsurans, and Microsporum audouinii* infect the skin and then move down the hair shaft, where they destroy hair follicles. Hairs may break off and give a "black dot" appearance. Pustules and erythema develop, and the hair loss progresses. If the process is not controlled early on, the inflammatory infiltrate may lead to permanent damage of the hair follicle and lasting hair loss. Boggy and edematous suppurative areas of tinea infection are referred to as kerion. Biopsy or culture will help establish the diagnosis. Topical antifungal agents are not efficacious for tinea capitis because reliable penetration is not achieved around the hair follicle. Oral agents such as griseofulvin (Gris-PEG), ketoconazole (Nizoral), itraconazole (Sporanox), fluconazole (Diflucan), and terbinafine (Lamisil) are all of value. In children, the greatest experience has been with the use of fluconazole elixir or itraconazole elixir. Itraconazole is, however, not FDA approved at this time for use in children.

Dissecting Cellulitis of the Scalp

Dissecting cellulitis is a disorder most common in African-Americans. The cause is not known, but use of topical oils and scalp treatments may predispose to the development of pustules and abscesses that spread underneath the skin surface, damaging hairs. If this is not appropriately treated early on, lasting hair loss develops. Incision and drainage, use of oral antibiotics such as tetracycline or ampicillin, and use of isotretinoin (Accutane)* may all be of value.

Lupus Erythematosus

Cutaneous lupus may manifest itself in many different ways. Acute lupus manifests as a malar rash, and chronic lupus (discoid lupus erythematosus) presents as erythematous scaly plaques with atrophy and hair loss. Biopsy reveals thickening of the basement membrane zone and increased mucin in the skin as well as destruction of follicular units. Early on, topical corticosteroids may arrest the inflammatory process. The use of sunscreens and sun protection is important because sun stimulates the development of discoid lupus. In cases in which topical treatments are not effective, antimalarials such as hydroxychloroquine or chloroquine* are of value. Systemic corticosteroids may be warranted in extensive cases of discoid lupus when widespread scarring must be prevented.

Lichen Planopilaris

Lichen planopilaris is a variant of lichen planus. This idiopathic condition may be associated with lichen planus elsewhere on the body or present simply as oval pink-red to violaceous papules and plaques on the scalp. Lichen planopilaris may lead to lasting hair loss. The treatment is similar to that for cutaneous lupus. Topical corticosteroids, intralesional corticosteroids, and hydroxychloroquine* are the mainstays of therapy.

---

*Not FDA approved for this indication.

*Not FDA approved for this indication.

Too Much Hair Ethnic Variation

Many patients present with the complaint of excessive body or facial hair. Often this relates to ethnic variation. Asians have relatively little facial and body hair, whereas individuals from Middle Eastern countries have a greater degree of body hair. Often reassurance is all that is required. Unfortunately, because of the high premium placed on good looks and the image presented in the media, the beauty of less body and facial hair in women is emphasized in our culture and many individuals may seek treatment. Treatment of unwanted hair consists of electrolysis in which galvanic current is used to damage the hair bulb of unwanted follicles and impede further hair growth. Laser hair removal is also effective, but generally more expensive. Laser hair removal may be more lasting, but long-term data to prove this are not yet available.

Hirsutism

If there is increased body hair in a women in a pattern more typical of a man, the diagnosis of hirsutism is likely. Androgen-dependent growth occurs on the upper lip, chin, cheeks, central chest, and lower abdomen. This may be associated with virilization such as masculine body habitus, clitoral hypertrophy, and amenorrhea. The dehydroepiandrosterone sulfate and testosterone levels may be increased. Excessive secretion of androgens from the ovary or adrenal glands may occur, or there may be excessive stimulation by pituitary tumors. Polycystic ovary disease (Stein-Leventhal syndrome) is associated with hirsutism in almost half of cases. Cushing's disease, acromegaly, and prolactin-secreting adenomas are all possible culprits as well. If appropriate testing has ruled out serious underlying pathology, wax, depilatories, and epilation by laser treatment may all be considered. Spironolactone (Aldactone)* and cyproterone acetate* are also useful agents.

HAIR SHAFT ABNORMALITIES

Acquired Hair Shaft Abnormalities

Split ends, hair breakage, and damage may occur through the many cosmetic treatments given to hair. The frequent use of hair dryers can cause damage to the hair shaft in which hairs will have bubbles within them (e.g., bubble hair deformity). Exposure to ultraviolet light, detergents, and other factors may also lead to the development of split ends. Rarely, hair shaft abnormalities such as uncombable hair may be acquired. Identifying the causes of hair shaft abnormality and avoidance of these traumatic insults to the hair lead to improvement in many cases.

Hereditary Hair Shaft Disorders

Hereditary hair shaft disorders are uncommon but important to recognize. Some disorders such as

Menkes' kinky hair disorder are associated with defects in copper metabolism and are associated with hypothermia, seizures, and early death. Trichothiodystrophy represents an abnormality in the sulfur bond formation in hairs and is associated with brittle hairs that break and may have a spangled appearance or a twisted architecture when analyzed under the microscope. Microscopic examination of hair shafts by a dermatopathologist or dermatologist will allow for accurate diagnosis. No treatments are likely to be of value in these hereditary abnormalities.

CONCLUSION

Many abnormalities of hair growth and development are encountered in clinical practice. The identification of the pattern and history allows for accurate diagnosis in the overwhelming majority of cases. Nonscarring patterned loss is likely to be due to androgenic alopecia. Localized nonscarring hair loss may be due to alopecia areata. The presence of pustules and broken hairs suggests an infectious etiology.

CANCER OF THE SKIN

method of
THOMAS E. ROHRER, M.D.
Boston University Medical Center
Boston, Massachusetts

Skin cancer is the most common cancer in the world. More than 1 million new cases of skin cancer are diagnosed each year in the United States. This equals the annual rate for all other cancers combined. It is estimated that one in every seven Americans will develop skin cancer. Here the concentration is on basal and squamous cell carcinoma, the two most common forms of skin cancer. Melanoma is covered elsewhere in this section.

Basal cell carcinoma (BCC) is the most common form of skin cancer, comprising approximately 80% of all skin cancers. The majority of the others (15%) are squamous cell carcinoma (SCC). Strong laboratory and clinical evidence suggest that the most common cause of these skin cancers is sun exposure. Ultraviolet (UVA and UVB) radiation from the sun induces skin cancer formation by both direct damage to DNA and by suppression of the immune response. Significant UV radiation from the sun can create pyrimidine dimers in DNA and mutations in the *p53* tumor suppressor gene. The damage to the *p53* suppressor gene decreases immune surveillance and allows a sun-damaged cell with pyrimidine dimers to survive. From this damaged cell a "bad" or "weak" cell line reproduces. Further UV insults to this weak cell line, even many years later, may then initiate an actual tumor cell line to develop and replicate. This is what is known as the "two- [or multiple-] hit theory," and it is the most likely mechanism for skin cancer formation.

Significant exposure to ionizing radiation (such as radiotherapy) may also lead to the formation of skin cancer. Other less common etiologic factors include chronic ulcers, burn scars, certain serotypes of human papillomavirus,

---

*Not FDA approved for this indication.

long-term immunosuppression (usually organ transplant recipients), and exposure to arsenic and coal tar derivatives. All of these less common causes tend to lead to SCC rather than BCC formation. In addition, certain genetic diseases such as xeroderma pigmentosa, basal cell nevus syndrome, and albinism lead to a significantly increased risk of skin cancer.

Basal cell carcinoma, the most common cancer in the country, is predominantly seen in the middle-aged and elderly population. However, the incidence of basal cell carcinoma is increasing in the younger population. Almost all basal cell carcinomas occur in sun-exposed areas, the face being the most common location. People with fair skin, light-colored hair, and blue eyes and those who do not tan easily have an increased risk, owing to their lack of natural protection from the sun. Clinically, most BCCs appear initially as a small erythematous or clear papule (raised). In time, classic features of a BCC include a raised pearly or clear border, central depression, and small telangiectases running through the papule. Other subtypes of basal cell carcinoma include pigmented (dark colored), morpheaform (may appear as depressed scar), and multicentric superficial (typically expanding erythematous scaling plaque, and flat). Although BCCs grow very slowly, if not removed they may invade subcutaneous fat, muscle, nerve, cartilage, and bone. Metastatic potential for BCC is extremely low, estimated at less than 0.005%.

Cutaneous SCC, the second most common form of skin cancer, also typically occurs on sun-exposed areas of those with little natural protection from the sun. Although BCC is five times more common than SCC, SCC is more common in chronic wounds, burn scars, immunocompromised hosts, darkly pigmented patients, and those exposed to arsenic or coal tar derivatives. It is also more common than BCC in certain locations, such as the lower lip and dorsal hand. Clinically, SCC usually begins on sun-damaged skin as a small erythematous papule and slowly expands in size. Although SCC may have central depression and necrosis like BCC, it usually does not have the pearly border or associated telangiectasia. Frequently, SCC develops in preexisting actinic keratoses. Although only 2 to 10% of actinic keratoses develop into SCCs, one study reported that 44% of metastatic SCCs developed from pre-existing actinic keratoses.

Although the overall risk of metastases from SCC is low (<5%), certain lesions have a considerably higher risk. Those that are greater than 2 cm in diameter or 4 mm in depth, those that arise from ulcers, recurrences, those with perineural invasion, and those occurring in immunocompromised hosts all have a higher metastatic risk. Tumors at certain sites such as the mucous membrane and periauricular area also have an increased risk of metastasis. Early detection and complete eradication are therefore warranted.

There are many therapeutic options for removing these types of skin cancer. Treatment must be tailored to the individual patient.

TREATMENT OPTIONS

Liquid Nitrogen or Cryotherapy

Liquid nitrogen is a readily available cryogen with a boiling point of −195.6°C that may easily be stored in an office setting. When tissue is exposed to this cold cryogen, cell death occurs from rapid crystal formation, exposure to high electrolyte concentration in surrounding fluids, recrystallization during thawing, and ischemia due to vascular damage. Caution must be used when treating with liquid nitrogen because certain structures, such as melanocytes, nerves, hair follicles, and vascular endothelial cells are more sensitive to freezing than other tissue. Although liquid nitrogen is typically used in the treatment of benign and premalignant lesions, some experienced physicians have used it to treat BCCs and SCCs. Tumor cells may be lethally damaged when frozen twice to a temperature of −20°C. Special thermocouple electrodes must be used to precisely measure the temperature and ensure adequate treatment. Cryotherapy is not frequently used to treat skin cancer because it is a "blind method" of destruction. There is no histologic confirmation of complete destruction of the malignancy.

Electrodesiccation and Curettage

Electrodesiccation employs heat generated by a high-voltage, low-amperage current to destroy tissue. In electrodesiccation and curettage, a curette (a semi-sharp spoon-shaped "knife") is first scraped across the tumor while the surrounding skin is stabilized by the opposite hand. Because BCC and SCC tumor cells are held together less tightly than normal skin tissue, these tumors tend to almost scoop out. Because the tactile difference is lost with adipose tissue, this technique should not be used if the tumor extends into the subcutaneous tissue. When the bulk of the tumor has been curetted out, the area is then treated with electrodesiccation. The heat created by electrodesiccation destroys approximately 1 mm of surrounding tissue. This sequence is then repeated two more times in succession. The bulk of the tumor is removed with the first curettage, and the subsequent procedures give it a 3-mm margin. Studies have shown that experience plays a significant role in the cure rate after electrodesiccation and curettage.

Because there is no histologic confirmation of tumor eradication, this is another method of blind destruction and should be used only for benign, premalignant, or low-risk malignant lesions. Patients with certain pacemakers are not candidates for this procedure because the current can interfere with some devices. Wounds after this procedure are left to granulate in and heal by second intention. Depending on the location, this may take several weeks and often leaves an irregular, white, depressed scar with less than optimal cosmesis.

Radiation Therapy

The use of radiation in the treatment of skin cancers has decreased markedly over the past 25 years, owing to the increased understanding of the risks associated with ionizing radiation and the popularization of Mohs' micrographic surgery (MMS). Although radiation has a good cure rate of most skin cancers, it has several disadvantages. To begin with, it is a known cause of skin cancer. Patients receiving radiation to treat one lesion often develop others years later in the radiation field. In addition, it is a method of blind destruction, and when skin cancers do recur after radiation, they often come back in a more aggressive form. Radiation treatment for skin cancers varies between 4000 to 7000 cGy broken up over multiple treatments a week for several weeks (average of 6). This form of treatment is now typically reserved for elderly patients who are not surgical candidates for various reasons.

Laser Surgery

Although carbon dioxide and erbium:YAG lasers may be used as ablative or cutting tools to remove skin cancers, they offer no real advantage. In fact, wounds created by carbon dioxide laser have been shown to heal more slowly than those created by a scalpel. Premalignant lesions, superficial BCCs, and SCC in situ may be effectively treated with the ablative mode of these lasers, which may be used on patients who have certain pacemakers and are unable to use electrocoagulation.

An exciting new technology, photodynamic laser therapy, is now being used experimentally on superficial BCC and SCC in situ. A porphyrin derivative that is a potent photosensitizer is administrated either topically or intravenously to the tumor area. The tumor cells selectively uptake the porphyrin derivative and retain it, while the surrounding normal tissue clears the substance. A laser or high-intensity light source is then used to activate the photosensitizer in the tumor cells and destroy them. Although this method has not been successful in treating any deeper malignancies, investigation is ongoing.

Surgical Excision

The most common treatment for BCC and SCC is standard elliptical excision. In most cases, a standard 3- or 4-mm margin is taken around the clinically evident tumor, and the wound is converted into an elliptical shape and sutured closed. A significant benefit of this procedure is the production of tissue for histologic evaluation and margin control. Unfortunately, it is difficult to evaluate the clinical margin of some BCCs and SCCs. In those cases, histologic evaluation usually detects the residual tumor and further excision is done at a later date. The cure rate of most nonmelanoma skin cancers is over 90% with standard surgical excision, and cosmesis is usually very good.

Mohs' Micrographic Surgery

MMS offers the highest cure rate (98 to 99%) and sacrifices the least amount of normal tissue possible. Instead of guessing at the true margin of a tumor, with MMS, very thin layers are removed sequentially under the direction of a microscope and reviewed immediately by the surgeon/pathologist. The first layer is taken just around the clinically evident tu-

mor and marked for proper orientation. Keeping the orientation, the tissue is immediately processed with special horizontal sections and then reviewed by the Mohs surgeon while the patient waits. Because the tissue has been kept in proper orientation, if tumor is noted on histologic evaluation, the precise location on the patient is known and another thin layer of tissue is immediately taken at that specific location. This process is continued until all of the margins are clear. In this manner the entire tumor is removed (giving it the high cure rate) and as much normal tissue as possible has been preserved. Knowing the tumor has been completely removed also gives the surgeon the confidence to perform a more complicated repair, such as a flap or graft. With standard excision, it may take up to a week to get a pathology report back, and the confidence level is less than that with the special horizontal sectioning with the Mohs technique.

MMS is, however, time and labor intensive and is therefore reserved for only certain tumors. The most common indications include (1) recurrent tumors, (2) large tumors, (3) tumors with indistinct clinical margins, (4) tumors with more aggressive histologic subtypes, and (5) those occurring on cosmetically sensitive areas such as the central face and periauricular area. For these tumors, MMS is the treatment of choice.

CUTANEOUS T CELL LYMPHOMAS

method of
GARY S. WOOD, M.D., and
SETH R. STEVENS, M.D.
Case Western Reserve University/University Hospitals of Cleveland, and Louis Stokes Department of Veterans Affairs Medical Center Cleveland, Ohio

CLASSIFICATION

Virtually every subtype of T cell lymphoma has been reported to involve the skin either primarily or secondarily; however, the principal types of primary cutaneous T cell lymphomas (CTCLs) include mycosis fungoides (MF), CD30+ large cell, CD30− large cell, pleomorphic small/medium cell, and subcutaneous panniculitic variants (Table 1). Other T cell lymphomas involving the skin, including the human T cell lymphotropic virus type I (HTLV-I) retrovirus-associated adult T cell leukemia/lymphoma, tend to present as systemic disease. This discussion focuses on MF because together with its leukemic variant, the Sézary syndrome (SS), it accounts for the clear majority of primary cutaneous cases (about two thirds). It must be acknowledged, however, that the designation "primary" as applied to CTCLs in general is used in a clinical rather than biologic context. Studies employing sensitive molecular biologic assays for T cell clonality have shown that at least some cases of early MF, apparently confined to the skin, contain tumor cells in clinicopathologically normal lymph nodes, blood, and marrow. Therefore, it may be more correct from the standpoint of tumor biology to regard

TABLE 1. **Classification of Primary CTCLs**

CTCL Type	Proportion of Primary CTCLs	5-Year Survival
MF and variants	70%	85%
SS	<5%	<50%*
CD30⁺ large cell	13%	90%
CD30⁻ large cell	7%	15%
Pleomorphic small/medium cell	4%	60%
Subcutaneous panniculitic	<1%	Low†
Miscellaneous	<1%	Variable

*Five-year survival depends on criteria used to define SS and may be as low as 10%.
†Median survival reportedly less than 3 years, but cases are rare.

CTCLs as neoplasms of the so-called skin-associated lymphoid tissue (SALT), which is composed of lymphoid cells and immune accessory cells that traffic between the skin and peripheral lymphoid tissues through the blood and lymph. In this context, CTCLs can be thought of as proliferative disorders of a T cell circuit rather than solely the skin.

STANDARD DIAGNOSIS AND STAGING METHODS

The evaluation of CTCL patients begins with a thorough clinical history and physical examination. Key elements of the history include the pace and nature of disease development, the presence or absence of spontaneous regression of lesions, prior therapy, and ingestion of drugs that have been associated with pseudolymphomatous skin eruptions that can mimic CTCLs (e.g., anticonvulsants, antihistamines, and other agents with antihistaminic properties). The review of systems should establish whether lymphoma-associated constitutional symptoms are present (e.g., fever of unknown origin, night sweats, weight loss, and fatigue). In addition to general aspects, the physical examination should document the type and distribution of skin lesions and whether there is lymphadenopathy, hepatosplenomegaly, or edema of extremities (a potential sign of lymphatic obstruction). Histopathologic analysis of representative lesional skin biopsy specimens is the primary means of confirming the clinical diagnosis. Biopsy specimens should be deep enough to include the deepest portions of the cutaneous lymphoid infiltrates because these areas often exhibit the most diagnostic features. Routine blood tests include a complete blood cell count, differential review, and general chemistry panel. A "Sézary prep" is used to assess peripheral blood involvement (see later). Internal nodal and visceral involvement by lymphoma is generally assessed with chest radiography and computed tomography of the chest, abdomen, and pelvis. These radiologic studies are generally not needed for patients with early forms of MF (nontumorous skin lesions without evidence of extracutaneous involvement by physical examination); however, they are usually obtained during the work-up of other types of CTCL. Putative extracutaneous involvement should be confirmed by biopsy if relevant to clinical management. The role of immunopathologic and molecular biologic assays in the diagnosis and staging of CTCLs is discussed later.

MYCOSIS FUNGOIDES/SÉZARY'S SYNDROME (MF/SS) AND VARIANTS

Clinical Features

MF classically manifests as erythematous, scaly, variably pruritic, flat patches or indurated plaques, often favoring the most sun-protected areas. There may be progression to cutaneous tumors and involvement of lymph nodes or viscera, although this does not occur generally as long as the skin lesions are reasonably well controlled by therapy. SS presents as total body erythema and scaling (erythroderma), generalized lymphadenopathy, hepatosplenomegaly, and leukemia. Large plaque parapsoriasis is essentially the patch phase of MF. Lesions may exhibit poikiloderma (atrophy, telangiectasia, and mottled hyperpigmentation and hypopigmentation) and have then been referred to as "poikiloderma atrophicans vasculare." Follicular mucinosis refers to a papulonodular eruption in which hair follicles are infiltrated by T cells and contain pools of mucin. In hairy areas, this may result in alopecia. Follicular mucinosis may exist as a lesional variant of MF or as a clinically benign entity (by itself or in association with other lymphomas). Pagetoid reticulosis presents as a solitary or localized, often hyperkeratotic plaque containing atypical T cells frequently confined to a hyperplastic epidermis. Some regard it as a variant of unilesional MF, whereas others believe it to be a distinct entity. Tumor d'emblée MF is an outmoded concept used in the past to refer to cases of "MF" that presented as cutaneous tumors in the absence of patches or plaques. Most experts now prefer to classify such cases as other forms of CTCL depending on their histopathologic features.

Histopathologic and Cytologic Features

A well-developed plaque of MF contains a bandlike, cytologically atypical lymphoid infiltrate in the upper dermis that infiltrates the epidermis as single cells and cell clusters known as Pautrier's microabscesses. The atypical lymphoid cells exhibit dense, hyperchromatic nuclei with convoluted, cerebriform nuclear contours and scant cytoplasm. The term "cerebriform" comes from the brainlike ultrastructural appearance of these nuclei. In more advanced cutaneous tumors, the infiltrate extends diffusely throughout the upper and lower dermis and may lose its epidermotropism. In the earlier patch phase of disease, the infiltrate is sparser and lymphoid atypia may be less pronounced. In some cases, it may be difficult to distinguish early patch MF from various types of chronic dermatitis. The presence of lymphoid atypia and absence of significant epidermal intercellular edema (spongiosis) helps to establish the diagnosis of early MF. Involvement of lymph nodes by MF begins in the paracortical T cell domain and may progress to complete effacement of nodal architecture by the same type of atypical lymphoid cells that infiltrate the skin. These cells can be seen in low numbers in the peripheral blood of many MF patients; however, those with SS develop gross leukemic involvement, usually defined as more than 5 to 10% of the total leukocyte count or greater than 1000 tumor cells per mm³. These cells are known as Sézary cells and are traditionally detected by manual review of the peripheral blood smear (the so-called Sézary prep).

Immunophenotyping

Cellular antigen expression is usually assessed by frozen section immunoperoxidase methods for tissue biopsy specimens and by flow cytometry for blood specimens. Almost all cases of MF/SS begin as phenotypically and functionally mature CD4⁺ T cell neoplasms of the skin-associated lymphoid tissue (SALT). As such, they express the SALT-associated homing molecule cutaneous lymphocyte antigen (CLA) as well as most mature T cell surface antigens, with the exception of CD7, which is often absent and probably reflects their derivation from a CD4⁺ CD7⁻ normal T cell subset. As disease progresses, the tumor cells often dedifferentiate and lose one or more mature T cell markers such as CD2, CD3, or CD5. Most cases express the alpha/beta form of the T cell receptor. At least in advanced cases, the cytokine profile is consistent with the TH₂ subset of CD4⁺ T cells (i.e., production of interleukin [IL]–4, IL-5, and IL-10 rather than TH₁ cytokines such as IL-2 and interferon-γ). Expression of the high-affinity IL-2 receptor (CD25, TAC) ranges widely, with most cases showing a variable minority of lesional CD25⁺ cells. MF cases that are CD8⁺ or express the gamma/delta T cell receptor occur occasionally. In addition to tumor cells, MF/SS lesions contain a minor component of immune accessory cells (Langerhans cells and macrophages) and CD8⁺ T cells with a cytolytic phenotype. This presumed "host response" correlates positively with survival and tends to decrease as lesions progress. Furthermore, a favorable response to therapy such as photopheresis appears to correlate with normal levels of circulating CD8⁺ cells.

Molecular Biology

MF/SS is a monoclonal T cell lymphoproliferative disorder. Southern blotting or polymerase chain reaction (PCR)–based assays demonstrate monoclonal T cell receptor gene rearrangements. The greater sensitivity of PCR assays allows the demonstration of dominant clonality even in most early patch lesions of MF. In fact, these assays sometimes detect dominant clonality in lesional skin showing only chronic dermatitis histopathologically. These cases are termed "clonal dermatitis" and may represent the earliest manifestation of MF because several have progressed to histologically recognizable MF within a few years. In addition to aiding initial diagnosis, gene rearrangement analysis has also facilitated staging and prognosis. Because some patients without MF/SS can have low levels of circulating Sézary-like cells and because not all cases of peripheral blood involvement in MF/SS exhibit morphologically recognizable tumor cells, the demonstration of dominant clonality has proven to be a useful diagnostic adjunct. The same holds true for assessing lymph node involvement. In fact, T cell receptor gene rearrangement analysis of MF/SS lymph nodes has been shown to be more sensitive than histopathology and to be prognostically relevant.

Miscellaneous Assays

Several other laboratory assays have been reported to be of value for facilitating the diagnosis of MF/SS, including determination of nuclear contour index using electron microscopy, assessment of cellular DNA content, and detection of chromosomal abnormalities through cytogenetics, in situ hybridization, or competitive genomic hybridization. However, these methods are not used widely because they are too nonspecific, costly, labor intensive, or arcane.

TNM Staging of MF/SS

Although there have been several methods proposed that use a weighted extent approach to more accurately determine MF/SS tumor burden, the gold standard is still the TNM system detailed in Tables 2 and 3. Table 2 shows the TNM classification relevant to MF/SS, and Table 3 shows how this information is used to determine the stage of disease. The prognostic relevance of this staging system has been documented in numerous studies and helps guide the selection of therapies. For example, early stage MF is the most amenable to control with topically directed treatments whereas advanced MF/SS with extracutaneous involvement usually requires systemic therapies or topical/systemic combinations.

TABLE 2. **TNM Classification of MF/SS**

Skin—T
T0—Clinically and/or histopathologically suspicious lesions
T1—Patches and/or plaques; <10% body surface area
T2—Patches and/or plaques; ≥10% body surface area
T3—Tumors with/without other skin lesions
T4—Generalized erythroderma

Lymph Nodes—N
N0—Not clinically enlarged; histopathologically negative
N1—Clinically enlarged; histopathologically negative
N2—Not clinically enlarged; histopathologically positive
N3—Clinically enlarged; histopathologically positive

Peripheral Blood—B
B0—Atypical cells <5% of leukocytes
B1—Atypical cells ≥5% of leukocytes

Visceral Organs—M
M0—Absent
M1—Present

Based on Bunn PA, Lamberg SI: Report of the Committee on Staging and Classification of Cutaneous T-Cell Lymphomas. Cancer Treat Rep 63:725–728, 1979.

TABLE 3. **TNM Staging System for MF/SS**

Stage	Skin	Lymph Nodes	Viscera
IA	T1	N0	M0
IB	T2	N0	M0
IIA	T1, T2	N1	M0
IIB	T3	N0, N1	M0
III	T4	N0, N1	M0
IVA	T1–T4	N2, N3	M0
IVB	T1–T4	N0–N3	M1

Based on Lamberg SI, Bunn PA: Cutaneous T-cell lymphomas. Summary of the Mycosis Fungoides Cooperative Group–National Cancer Institute Workshop. Arch Dermatol 115:1103–1105, 1979. Copyright 1979, American Medical Association.

Treatment

Rather than "cure," which is attained in less than 10% of cases, the goal of MF/SS therapy is to reduce the impact of the skin disease on quality of life. For most patients, this is achieved by reducing pain, itch, and infection and improving clinical appearance. Appearance is affected by the disfigurement of the eruption as well as by the profound degree of scale shedding seen in some patients. Because the natural history of early-stage MF predicts a virtually normal life span, the goal of treatment must be directed at quality of life. For more advanced stages, prolongation of life expectancy may be a reasonable treatment goal.

Regardless of presentation, relief of symptoms should be addressed early. For dryness and scaling, the use of emollient ointments is indicated. These include petrolatum, Aquaphor, and commercially available shortening such as Crisco (an inexpensive alternative). For modest dryness, creams (e.g., Nivea, Cetaphil, Eucerin) can be adequate and more acceptable to patients. Mild superfatted soaps such as Dove and Oil of Olay are recommended. Soap substitutes such as Cetaphil are also acceptable. Pruritus can be addressed with oral agents such as hydroxyzine (Atarax) or diphenhydramine (Benadryl), 2 to 5 mg per kg per day, divided into four daily doses. Antipruritics work better when used on a regular basis rather than on an as-needed basis. Nonsedating antihistamines tend to be less effective. Measures to reduce dryness also help to reduce pruritus. Secondary infection needs to be treated with appropriate antibiotics. Their selection is guided by results of skin cultures but usually involves coverage of gram-positive organisms.

Phototherapy

Two main phototherapeutic regimens are used to treat CTCL. Ultraviolet B (290–320 nm) radiation can be used for patients with patches but not plaques or tumors. Our expectation is that 70% of such patients will achieve total clinical remission. Median time to achieve this response will be 5 months. Another 15% will achieve partial remission. Psoralen–ultraviolet A photochemotherapy (PUVA) uses oral methoxypsoralen (Oxsoralen), 0.6 mg/kg, as a photo-sensitizer before UVA (320–400 nm) exposure. Sixty-five percent of patients with patch or plaque disease will achieve complete remissions, and 30% will have partial responses to this modality. For the majority of patients, maximal responses will be achieved within 3 months, and after 5 months it is unlikely that further improvement will be gained. Limitations of these modalities include actinic damage, photocarcinogenesis, retinal damage (if eyes are not protected), and the inconvenience of getting to phototherapy centers. PUVA also has the risk of nausea and a theoretical risk of cataract induction without proper eye protection.

Topical Therapy

Like phototherapeutic regimens, topical therapies are appropriate for disease confined to the skin (stage I). Topical corticosteroids are frequently used for CTCL, often before diagnosis. Fifty percent of patients will achieve complete remission, and 40% will have partial remission. We use this modality infrequently as primary therapy, owing to frequent, early relapse and the belief that the systemic nature of even early-stage CTCL is inadequately addressed by topical corticosteroids. However, we do find topical corticosteroids useful as a means to relatively quickly ameliorate severe signs and symptoms and as an adjuvant therapy in combination with other primary treatments.

Mechlorethamine (nitrogen mustard, HN_2)* is applied topically in either an aqueous solution or in an ointment, such as Aquaphor. The aqueous form is prepared at home and involves a daily dose totaling 10 mg in 60 mL water. The ointment form is prepared by a pharmacist in 1-pound lots at a concentration of 10 mg per 100-gram ointment. Only the amount of ointment needed to apply a thin layer is used. Either formulation is usually applied at bedtime to the entire skin surface (excluding the head unless it is also involved) and then showered off every morning using soap and water. Results are similar to those from PUVA. Advantages include therapy at home and availability in all regions of the country. Disadvantages are daily preparation (aqueous form only), daily application, and possible allergic contact dermatitis (more common with the aqueous preparation). Maximal efficacy is expected within 6 months. Mild "flares" of disease may occur during the first few months of treatment and probably represent inflammation of subclinical skin lesions, analogous to the clinical accentuation of actinic damage during topical therapy with 5-fluorouracil (Efudex).

Carmustine (BCNU)* is applied to the total skin surface as an alcoholic/aqueous solution (10 to 20 mg in 60 mL). Complete responses are seen in 85% of patients with stage IA disease (< 10% involvement) and 50% of patients with stage IB disease (> 10% involvement). Another 10% of patients will obtain partial responses. Advantages include those noted with nitrogen mustard and reports of success with

*Not FDA approved for this indication.

application only to lesional skin. Disadvantages include skin irritation followed by telangiectasia formation and possible bone marrow suppression necessitating blood monitoring.

Radiotherapy

Conventional radiotherapy for mycosis fungoides therapy has been used for approximately 100 years. We find it useful in the treatment of isolated, particularly problematic lesions such as recalcitrant tumors or ulcerated plaques. In addition to benefit from the photons delivered by radiotherapy, electron beam therapy (0.4 Gy per week for 8 to 9 weeks) is also useful for CTCL therapy. Approximately 85% complete response rate of skin disease with a median duration of 16 months is expected with electron beam therapy. An advantage is an excellent rate of complete response. Disadvantages include limited access to required equipment and expertise and cutaneous toxic effects, such as alopecia, sweat gland loss, radiation dermatitis, and skin cancers. As with other skin-directed therapy, benefit for internal disease is limited. Cumulative toxicity also limits the number of courses a patient may receive. Localized electron beam therapy is also useful for treating cases of limited extent MF and in treating selected problematic MF lesions in patients who are otherwise responding to therapy.

Apheresis-Based Therapy

Leukapheresis and particularly lymphocytapheresis (6000 to 7000 mL of blood treated, thrice weekly initially, then according to response) have been used in the treatment of SS patients. Benefit has been reported in several case reports and small case series; however, response rates are not possible to determine. Photopheresis (extracorporeal photochemotherapy [ECP]) describes an apheresis-based therapy in which circulating lymphocytes are first exposed to a psoralen (either orally or extracorporeally), then exposed to UVA extracorporeally. In contrast to leukapheresis, in which leukocytes are discarded, all cells are returned to the patient's circulation during photopheresis. Response rates in erythrodermic patients are 33 to 50%, and median survival for SS patients is prolonged from 30 months to more than 60 months.

Cytokine Therapy

Interferon alfa 2a or 2b* (1 to 100 × 10⁶ units) is given subcutaneously or intralesionally every other day to once weekly. Response rates are approximately 55%, with complete response in 17% of patients. Advantages include relative ease of delivery. Disadvantages include anorexia, fever, malaise, leukopenia, and risk of cardiac dysrhythmia. Because interleukin-12 can restore immune responses in vitro and has shown promise in phase 1 and 2 clinical trials, the utility of this cytokine in the treatment of MF/SS is worthy of further exploration.

Tumor-Associated Antigen-Directed Therapies

Various specific tumor-associated antigens have been targeted with antibody-based therapy. The response rate has typically been low and response durations short. Less specific targets are CD4, CD5, and IL-2 receptors. Of this class of agent, the most promising is denileukin diftitox (ONTAK, DAB$_{389}$ IL-2, 9 to 18 µg per kg per day intravenously on 5 consecutive days, every 3 weeks). This agent is a fusion protein combining IL-2 and diphtheria toxin. Thus, cells bearing the IL-2 receptor (present in the lesions of at least half of MF patients) bind and internalize the drug. Inside the cell the toxin portion of the molecule disrupts protein synthesis, leading to cell death. Approximately 10% of patients achieve complete responses, and total response rates of near 40% have been reported. Half of responders and 20% of nonresponders experienced decreased pruritus. Adverse events include capillary leak syndrome, flu-like symptoms, and allergic reactions.

Systemic Chemotherapy

Various regimens of single-agent and multiagent chemotherapy have been used in the treatment of MF/SS. Oral methotrexate, chlorambucil (Leukeran),* with or without prednisone, and etoposide (VePesid)* have shown activity. The best response has been in erythrodermic patients treated with methotrexate (5 to 125 mg weekly), who have shown a 58% response rate. The use of multiagent regimens is controversial because of the small number of patients treated with any given regimen. There is even some evidence that for some populations of CTCL patients, survival may in fact be reduced. For individual patients, however, cyclophosphamide (Cytoxan), doxorubicin (Adriamycin),* vincristine (Oncovin),* and prednisone (CHOP) can provide some short-term palliation. In some cases, CHOP has successfully eradicated large cell transformation of MF and returned patients to their more clinically indolent patch/plaque baseline disease. Idarubicin* in association with etoposide, cyclophosphamide, vincristine, prednisone, and bleomycin (Blenoxane)* (VICOP-B) has demonstrated response rates of 80% (36% complete response rate) for patients with stage II through IV disease and 84% for MF patients, with a median duration of response greater than 8 months. Other regimens have been used with more modest success.

Several purine nucleoside analogues have been used for CTCL treatment, including erythrodermic variants. These include 2-chlorodeoxyadenosine* (response rate of 28%), 2-deoxycoformycin (pentostatin,* response rate of 39%), and fludarabine. Toxicities include pulmonary edema, bone marrow and immune suppression, and neurotoxicity.

Retinoids

Retinoids have activity in MF/SS, alone and in combination with other therapies, such as interferon

---

*Not FDA approved for this indication.

*Not FDA approved for this indication.

alfa or PUVA (the latter combination is referred to as Re-PUVA). Arotinoid,* etretinate (Tegison),† and 13-*cis*-retinoic acid (Accutane)† have variable efficacy, and we tend to use them in conjunction with other modalities. A newer RXR retinoid, Targretin,* is under investigation for use in MF and has an overall response rate of about 40%. Disadvantages of retinoid therapy include signs of vitamin A toxicity, one of the most problematic being hyperlipidemia.

Miscellaneous Therapies

Various other therapies have been tried for MF/SS with modest success. Autologous bone marrow transplantation led to complete remission in some patients; however, in most reports and our experience, these remissions are shortlived. Cyclosporine A (Sandimmune)† has been used for MF/SS. Transient improvement is followed by worsened survival due to immunosuppression and is not a recommended therapy. Thymopentin (TP-5)‡ has been reported to give excellent results in SS patients (40% complete response, 35% partial response with median duration of responses of 22 months). The lack of follow-up reports in the past decade leaves the status of this therapy in question.

Selection of Therapy for MF/SS

Initial choices among conventional treatments depend on the type of lesions and the stage of disease. Disease subsets are listed followed by recommended initial treatments in parentheses: unilesional or localized MF (local radiation therapy), patch MF (UVB, PUVA, HN₂), patch/plaque MF (PUVA, HN₂), thick plaque/tumor MF (electron beam radiation therapy), erythrodermic MF/SS (photopheresis), and nodal/visceral MF/SS (interferon alfa, ONTAK, experimental systemic therapies, systemic chemotherapy). Second-line therapeutic choices often involve retinoids or cytokines, usually in combination with primary modalities. Midpotency topical corticosteroids, such as 0.1% triamcinolone cream or ointment, are useful adjuncts to many different therapies. The optimal use of newer therapeutic agents in various subtypes and stages of MF/SS is still being established.

MF/SS-ASSOCIATED LYMPHOPROLIFERATIVE DISORDERS

Patients with MF/SS are at increased risk for the development of large T cell lymphomas, lymphomatoid papulosis, and Hodgkin's disease. Molecular biologic analysis has shown that these disorders and MF share the same clonal T cell receptor gene rearrangement when they arise in the same individual. As a consequence, they are considered to be subclones of the original MF tumor clone. The development of large T cell lymphoma in a patient with MF/

---

*Not available in the United States.
†Not FDA approved for this indication.
‡Investigational drug in the United States.

SS is referred to as "large cell transformation of MF." This occurs in up to about 20% of cases in some series and is associated with a median survival of only 1 to 2 years. Half of these large T cell lymphomas are CD30⁺; however, the generally favorable prognosis of primary CD30⁺ CTCL does not extend to these secondary forms of CD30⁺ lymphoma. These patients are usually treated with systemic chemotherapy such as CHOP or with experimental systemic therapies appropriate for advanced stage CTCL. Lymphomatoid papulosis presents as recurrent, usually generalized crops of spontaneously regressing erythematous papules that can exhibit crusting or vesiculation before resolution. Histopathologically, lesions contain a mixed cell infiltrate, including large atypical T cells that resemble either Reed-Sternberg cells and their mononuclear variants (so-called type A) or large MF-type cells (so-called type B). Type A cells are CD30⁺. A "type C" form is also recognized in which there are sheets of type A cells histologically mimicking CD30⁺ large T cell lymphoma but differing from it on clinical grounds. Patients with lymphomatoid papulosis sometimes respond to tetracycline or erythromycin (500 mg orally twice daily), presumably on the basis of anti-inflammatory activity. Most cases will improve within 1 month with low-dose methotrexate (10 to 20 mg orally every week). PUVA phototherapy given three times a week is another therapeutic option.

Treatment of Non MF/SS CTCLS

In most cases, non MF/SS CTCLs are treated with radiation therapy (with or without complete surgical excision) if they are localized or with various multiagent systemic chemotherapy regimens if they are generalized. The role of other agents remains to be defined, except that studies have proven that methotrexate (10 to 40 mg orally every week) is effective therapy for most cases of primary cutaneous CD30⁺ large T cell lymphoma.

PAPULOSQUAMOUS DISEASES

method of
ANN G. MARTIN, M.D., and
JESSICA N. MEHTA, M.D.
Washington University School of Medicine
St. Louis, Missouri

The papulosquamous diseases include conditions sharing the feature of papules or plaques capped by scale. Table 1 lists the papulosquamous diseases most encountered by dermatologists. Although these conditions may morphologically appear similar, the etiology and natural progression of disease vary widely. Often, a skin biopsy is necessary for accurate diagnosis, because the histopathology of these conditions is the distinguishing feature when clinical signs are not fully developed. A variety of papulosquamous diseases are discussed here.

TABLE 1. **Papulosquamous Diseases**

Psoriasis	Parapsoriasis
Lichen planus	Secondary syphilis
Pityriasis rosea	Cutaneous T cell lymphoma*
Pityriasis rubra pilaris	Cutaneous lupus*
Seborrheic dermatitis	Tinea corporis*
Pityriasis lichenoides chronica	

*Discussed elsewhere.

PSORIASIS VULGARIS

Psoriasis is a chronic inflammatory disease of the skin affecting 1 to 3% of the population in North America. This condition can affect persons of any age from infants to the elderly but usually has an age at onset between 20 and 30 years. The etiology of psoriasis is unknown, but certain trigger factors have been identified. These include skin injury, streptococcal infections, stress, cold weather, alcohol, smoking, and obesity. Certain drugs have also been implicated in psoriasis including beta blockers, nonsteroidal anti-inflammatory agents, lithium, and antimalarial agents.

The lesions of psoriasis are characterized by rapid keratinocyte turnover. Whereas normal skin cells turn over in 1 month, psoriatic skin turns over in 4 days, resulting in silvery scale. Another feature is inflammation in the dermis accompanied by dilated capillary loops. Psoriasis has been associated with HLA-B13, HLA-B17, HLA-Cw6, HLA-Bw16, and HLA-Bw37. One third of psoriasis patients have relatives with the disease.

Clinical Features

There are four common and distinct types of psoriasis vulgaris. Plaque-type psoriasis is the most prevalent form. In this relapsing and remitting condition, the lesions are round or oval, well circumscribed, erythematous, and dry, with a silvery white scale overlying the papule or plaque. Lesions usually occur on the scalp, nails, extensor surfaces of the extremities, elbows, knees, and sacral region. The eruption is symmetrical but varies from small macules with thin scale to large plaques with thick scale. One characteristic feature of the disease is the Koebner reaction, in which lesions form at sites of skin injury (i.e., burns, scratches). The Auspitz sign is pinpoint bleeding that occurs when a psoriatic scale is forcibly removed. The fingernails and toenails should be examined for typical psoriatic changes. These include distal onycholysis, oil spots, and pits. Approximately half of all psoriasis patients have joint complaints. Most patients suffer from metacarpophalangeal and interphalangeal involvement, whereas a very few have ankylosing spondylitis.

Guttate psoriasis is characterized by smaller psoriatic lesions 2 to 5 mm in diameter. This condition usually follows a streptococcal pharyngitis and can often be treated with antibiotics. Pustular psoriasis can be localized, involving only palms and soles, or

generalized. The generalized form can be fatal. The pustules may coalesce, forming lakes. Systemic involvement can be serious, and problems such as high fevers and hepatitis occur. Systemic retinoids are the drugs of choice in this condition. Erythrodermic psoriasis is the fourth broad category and is characterized by erythema and shedding of scales. This is a life-threatening condition, owing to generalized exfoliation, hypothermia, and hypoalbuminemia.

Treatment

Three treatment modalities can be used for psoriasis: topical, ultraviolet (UV) light, and systemic therapies. The risks and benefits of a treatment plan must be weighed against the disease severity. Duration of disease, previous treatment, and age of patient must also be considered. The nature of this disease is that recurrences are almost inevitable. Stress, infections, skin injury, and climate changes can affect expression of the disease. These exacerbating factors, as well as obesity, alcohol use, and smoking should be explained to the patient. Keeping the skin well lubricated with moisturizers is basic to any treatment plan.

Topical corticosteroids are first-line therapy for most psoriasis patients. The least potent preparation that provides results is preferable. Initially, a 2-week course of twice-daily applications of a potent (group II) or superpotent (group I) topical corticosteroid is given followed by a twice- to thrice-weekly application schedule to maintain remission. Excess use of topical corticosteroids should be avoided because of the possibility of tachyphylaxis. For this reason, topical vitamin D and topical retinoids are also finding a niche in first-line treatment of this disease. Facial lesions should receive only group VI and VII strength corticosteroids. The axilla, groin, and genital regions are also more susceptible to side effects and should not be treated with superpotent corticosteroids. The most frequently encountered local side effects of topical corticosteroid therapy are atrophy, telangiectasia, infections, and striae formation.

A newer topical psoriasis treatment is calcipotriene (Dovonex). This vitamin D analogue suppresses keratinocyte proliferation. With twice-daily usage, results may be visible in 8 weeks. Combining this therapy with topical corticosteroids can decrease the time to lesion clearing and decrease skin irritation. A rare side effect of calcipotriene is hypercalcemia. This has only been noted if more than 100 grams per week of the drug was applied.

Tazarotene (Tazorac) gel is the first topical retinoid approved for use in psoriasis. The gel is cosmetically appealing to patients, and remissions from disease are longer lasting as compared with topical corticosteroids alone. A large percentage of patients suffer skin irritation, erythema, and pruritus, but combining this therapy with topical corticosteroids and emollients can increase the efficacy and help reduce these unpleasant side effects. Time spent in patient education increases efficacy of this product. Tazarotene can be used on up to 20% of the body surface area and should be confined to plaques only. Adding tazarotene to UVB therapy results in greater efficacy and reduced time to clearing than either treatment alone.

Despite the undesirable effects of odor and staining, tar preparations are effective for treating scalp psoriasis and limited plaque psoriasis. The Goeckerman technique for psoriasis treatment employs a 2 to 5% tar solution applied to lesions daily. In addition, a daily crude coal tar bath is taken; excess tar is removed with vegetable oil, and UV light is given. Much success has been achieved with this regimen in resistant psoriasis.

Anthralin (Drithocreme) is another effective, nontoxic treatment for psoriasis that has enjoyed more popularity in Europe than in the United States. The medication is left on the plaques for 15 minutes to 24 hours, depending on the type of preparation and tolerance to skin irritation. Brown staining of the skin is a common unpleasant side effect that disappears in 2 to 3 weeks. Complete clearing of well-defined thick plaques can be achieved in 1 month, and prolonged remissions are often possible.

Phototherapy

For many patients, exposure to strong sunlight is enough to improve most psoriatic lesions. In winter months, however, most patients are unable to receive enough natural sunlight and they find that phototherapy with UVA or UVB light can be effective for their disease. UVB (290 to 320 nm) is often used for widespread small plaque psoriasis. This therapy is given by a skilled nurse three to five times per week. The amount given is measured in joules and should produce a mild erythema after each treatment. Improvement is usually noted in 6 weeks. Psoralens (methoxsalen [Oxsoralen]) with UVA (PUVA), 320 to 400 nm, is a standard treatment of choice in generalized large plaque psoriasis. Psoralens, taken orally, sensitizes the patient to UVA light. This medication is given at a dose of 0.6 mg per kg, 1½ hours before exposure to UV light. Treatment is usually given three times a week, with increasing doses of UVA as tolerated by the patient. Clearance of psoriatic lesions can be expected in 5 to 6 weeks. Maintenance PUVA of once-monthly treatments can help prolong remission of disease.

For either form of phototherapy, side effects must be considered. If the dose of UVA or UVB is increased too quickly, a blistering burn will result. High cumulative doses of UV light increase the risk of actinic keratoses, premature skin aging, squamous cell carcinoma, and basal cell carcinoma. The use of systemic retinoids, such as acitretin (Soriatane), along with PUVA has reduced the total UV light exposure necessary to achieve clearance of lesions as well as the length of time to remission.

Systemic Therapy

Several systemic medications are available for treatment of psoriasis. In patients whose disease is usually well controlled with topical agents or phototherapy, a course of antibiotics can often quell a sudden exacerbation. Infections are a common precipitant of psoriatic lesions. In these cases, antibiotics can be used for management.

Methotrexate is the systemic therapy used for severe plaque psoriasis unresponsive to other therapies. Other indications include psoriatic arthritis, severe pustular psoriasis, and erythrodermic psoriasis. Normal liver and kidney function must be confirmed before beginning methotrexate, and the patient may not abuse alcohol, be immunocompromised, or have active infections. Usually, the medication is given as a single weekly dose of 7.5 to 20 mg. The cumulative dose of methotrexate must be monitored carefully and a liver biopsy performed after each 1.5 grams of the drug has been given. Routine laboratory tests for complete blood cell count and liver and kidney functions should also be obtained. After 80% clearance, the dose of methotrexate often can be reduced to 7.5 to 10 mg per week. If the psoriasis returns at the lower dose, other treatment modalities should be considered. Frequent side effects with methotrexate are anorexia, headaches, nausea, and vomiting. Laboratory abnormalities most often noted are thrombocytopenia and leukopenia. Hepatic necrosis or cirrhosis is rare but has been the cause of death in several patients. Pregnancy is also a contraindication to this dihydrofolate reductase inhibitor, owing to the increase incidence of neural tube defects. Psoriasis can also be treated with oral retinoids. Since the early 1980s, etretinate was the retinoid used most often. In 1998, however, etretinate was discontinued, owing to the very long total elimination time of 400 days. Acitretin has replaced etretinate because of its efficacy and total elimination time of only 10 days. Retinoids are particularly useful for severe plaque psoriasis, pustular psoriasis, and hand and foot involvement. If acitretin is used alone, a dose of 25 to 50 mg per day is usual. When combined with PUVA, the dose is reduced and the total UVA light needed for clearing is significantly lower than with PUVA alone. Results are typically visible in 6 weeks. Side effects include dry mucous membranes, elevated serum lipid levels, photophobia, and musculoskeletal discomfort. The most important adverse event is teratogenicity, and precautions must be taken to avoid pregnancy during the use of any retinoid.

The immunosuppressive cyclosporine has been shown to be effective in severe recalcitrant, inflammatory psoriasis. It has been has been approved for this indication in the form of Neoral. Well-documented side effects include hypertension and nephrotoxicity. At a low dose of 3 mg per kg per day for a short period of time, cyclosporine can successfully be used to achieve remission, which can then be maintained through the use of less toxic therapies such as PUVA.

LICHEN PLANUS

Lichen planus is an inflammatory, pruritic disease of unknown etiology characterized by small flat-topped, polygonal papules with a violaceous hue. The surface of the lesions is slightly scaly with gray-white streaks called Wickham's striae. This disease predominantly affects the flexor surfaces of the forearms and also selects the anterior lower leg, dorsal hands, and medial thighs. The buccal mucosa is frequently affected in a reticulated pattern or with pinpoint, white papules. Lichen planus can also affect the genital mucosa and nails. Scalp lesions can occur, occasionally resulting in scarring alopecia.

Although the classic description of lichen planus was just described, a wide variety of lesions may be seen. These include atrophic lichen planus, hypertrophic lichen planus, ulcerative lichen planus, follicular lichen planus, and hepatitis-associated lichen planus. Oral lesions may be erosive or bullous, making diagnosis difficult. Certain drugs have been implicated in the development of lichen planus, including antimalarial agents, angiotensin-inhibiting inhibitors, penicillamine, quinidine, gold, thiazides, methyldopa, phenothiazines, and tetracyclines.

Treatment is symptomatic, and usually only corticosteroid preparations are necessary. Ruling out drug-induced lichen planus is the first priority. Initially, a potent (group II) or superpotent (group I) topical corticosteroid is applied twice daily for 2 weeks. For hypertrophic lesions, intralesional corticosteroid injections can be more effective. Oral lesions are best treated with a corticosteroid benzocaine (Orabase) compound. For extensive generalized lichen planus, a 2- to 4-week tapering course of prednisone beginning at 40 mg can be used. Alternative therapies that have been explored are griseofulvin,* oral and topical retinoids, and PUVA. Most recently, subcutaneous enoxaparin (Lovenox),* a low-molecular-weight anticoagulant, has been used for recalcitrant lichen planus with some success.

PITYRIASIS ROSEA

Pityriasis rosea is an acute inflammatory exanthem characterized by scaly, pruritic, oval, and maculopapular lesions scattered over the trunk and extremities. The condition begins with a large herald patch followed by the striking development of oval lesions that run along the lines of cleavage, forming a Christmas tree–like pattern. The rash involves the trunk most often and spares sun-exposed areas. Frequently, the patient will experience a prodrome of nausea, anorexia, and arthralgias before the development of the rash, supporting the viral etiology for the condition. Much evidence has pointed to human herpesvirus 7 as the etiologic agent.

Treatment is symptomatic, because the disease runs its natural course in 4 to 16 weeks. In rare instances, the exanthem may last 6 months. UVB treatments can expedite lesion clearing. Topical corticosteroids and oral antihistamines can be used for symptomatic relief. Occasionally, oral corticosteroids may be needed for severe extensive cases.

PITYRIASIS RUBRA PILARIS

Pityriasis rubra pilaris usually begins with scale and erythema of the scalp. It then progresses to yellowish pink, scaly patches and follicular papules on the neck, trunk, and extensor surfaces of the extremities. The palms and soles are affected by solid hyperkeratosis. The papules are the most diagnostic feature because they have a hair imbedded in the horny central plug. The skin is usually involved symmetrically with islands of sparing within the patches and papules. Nails are also involved by becoming brittle with increased tendency to break. Pityriasis rubra pilaris may be congenital or acquired. In the acquired type, the condition may last approximately 3 years. The juvenile form is chronic with poor prognosis for involution.

Topical and oral therapies are needed to control this chronic condition. Emollients such as Lac-Hydrin help control scaling. Isotretinoin (Accutane)* is the treatment of choice at doses of 1 to 2 mg per kg per day. Careful monitoring of serum lipids and liver enzymes and a complete blood cell count must be performed. Women should be counseled about reliable birth control methods because of the teratogenicity of isotretinoin. Although topical corticosteroids are not useful in this condition, a monthly injection of intramuscular triamcinolone (Kenalog) is usually very effective.

SEBORRHEIC DERMATITIS

Seborrheic dermatitis is a common, chronic skin disorder characterized by loose, greasy scales on a reddish patch of skin. This condition is thought to be caused by the yeast *Pityrosporum ovale (Malassezia furfur),* which colonizes areas with a large number of sebaceous glands, such as the scalp, forehead, nasolabial folds, and upper trunk. The disease may affect infants in the form of cradle cap. After infancy, the disease is rarely seen until after puberty, suggesting the hormonal influence on sebaceous glands as a factor promoting this condition.

Various treatments are available for seborrheic dermatitis. An antifungal medication should be used that has activity against yeast. In infants, shampoo containing selenium sulfide is very effective. Adults find faster cure rates by using ketoconazole (Nizoral) or a similar topical medication daily for 2 to 3 weeks. The intermittent biweekly use of a selenium sulfide–containing product can prevent recurrence of the condition.

PITYRIASIS LICHENOIDES CHRONICA

Pityriasis lichenoides chronica is an erythematous, scaly, macular eruption that usually appears insidiously on the trunk, thighs, and arms. The lesion may persist for months to years. A skin biopsy may be necessary to differentiate this condition from psoriasis or secondary syphilis.

UVB treatment can help speed recovery; however,

---

*Not FDA approved for this indication.

*Not FDA approved for this indication.

PUVA is even more effective. Severe cases have been treated successfully with methotrexate.

PARAPSORIASIS

Two patterns of parapsoriasis exist: small plaque and large plaque. Small plaque parapsoriasis includes lesions between 1 and 5 cm in diameter that are slightly atrophic, brown or yellowish red, oval, scaly patches. The borders are sharply defined and regular. This eruption can persist for years without progression or resolution.

Large plaque parapsoriasis lesions are between 5 and 15 cm in diameter and similar in description to small plaque lesions. Ten percent of these cases progress to cutaneous T cell lymphoma.

Both types of lesions are characterized by epidermal atrophy and are usually located on the trunk. Small plaque disease has not been found to progress to cutaneous T cell lymphoma.

Treatment is accomplished with the use of topical corticosteroids and phototherapy. Small plaque disease can be treated easily with topical corticosteroids and biannual follow-up. Occasionally, phototherapy is necessary for complete remission.

The large plaque variant is best treated by PUVA alone or combined with topical corticosteroids. A skin biopsy should be performed for accurate diagnosis to rule out cutaneous T cell lymphoma. PUVA should be continued even after lesions have receded for 6 months. Repeat biopsy may be necessary with the development of new plaques to check for progression to lymphoma.

SECONDARY SYPHILIS

Secondary syphilis must be considered in the differential diagnosis of papulosquamous disorders. The lesions can appear anywhere on the body and are usually scaly, slightly pigmented papules. Papules on the palms and soles are very suggestive of secondary syphilis. The eruption occurs 6 to 8 weeks after the primary chancre of syphilis and extends in just a few days. The exanthem is usually asymptomatic. Lymphadenopathy may also be appreciated.

Penicillin remains the treatment of choice for syphilis. If the disease has been present for less than a year, a single intramuscular injection of 2.4 million units of penicillin G is sufficient. If the disease has been present for more than 1 year, three weekly intramuscular injections of 2.4 million units of penicillin G are recommended. In penicillin-allergic patients, oral tetracycline or erythromycin* can be used. The most recent guidelines from the Centers for Disease Control and Prevention should be consulted before treatment is rendered.

---

*Not FDA approved for this indication.

AUTOIMMUNE CONNECTIVE TISSUE DISORDERS

method of
DANIEL J. WALLACE, M.D.
Cedars-Sinai/UCLA School of Medicine
Los Angeles, California

LUPUS ERYTHEMATOSUS

Lupus erythematosus (LE) is a pleomorphic disorder capable of involving the skin and any organ system. A prototypic autoimmune disease, susceptibility genes predisposing toward lupus are activated by chemicals in the environment, physical trauma, emotional stress, excessive ultraviolet light exposure, and microbes, among other factors. The classifications of LE are

1. Chronic cutaneous (discoid) lupus erythematosus (CLE): The diagnosis is based on skin biopsy material showing hyperkeratosis, follicular plugging, dermal atrophy, liquefaction or vacuolar degeneration of the epidermal basal layer, and lymphocytic inflammation in a patient who does not fulfill the American College of Rheumatology criteria for systemic lupus erythematosus (SLE).

2. Subacute cutaneous lupus erythematosus (SCLE): This form presents with red macules or papules that develop into scaly papulosquamous (psoriaform) or annular polycyclic plaques. Unlike CLE, lesions heal without scarring. SCLE occurs in 9% of patients with SLE and 20% with CLE.

3. Systemic lupus erythematosus: Patients can have cutaneous features of LE but also have systemic disease. Some of these features include Raynaud's phenomenon, mucosal ulcerations, malar rash, bullae, pigment changes, urticaria, alopecia, livedo reticularis, cutaneous vasculitis, purpura, and petechiae.

4. Drug-induced lupus erythematosus: More than 70 pharmaceutical agents produce drug-induced LE, which tends to spare the skin.

5. Mixed connective tissue disease (MCTD): Patients fulfill criteria for SLE and another autoimmune disorder but have a positive antibody to ribonucleoprotein (anti-RNP). Cutaneovascular features, especially Raynaud's phenomenon, are common. If anti-RNP is absent, the patient has a *crossover* or *overlap* syndrome.

Nonmedication Therapy

Patient education is vital. LE can become serious if patients ignore certain simple lifestyle and counseling precepts. Ultraviolet light from the sun should be avoided because it flares the disease. Individuals who are going to be outside for more than 5 minutes should wear sun-protective clothing (broad brimmed hats, long sleeves) or clothing that has a sun protection factor (SPF) of 30 in the weave (Solumbra) and try to accomplish their outdoor obligations in the early morning or early evening. Increased vigilance is necessary at higher altitudes. There are suggestions that alfalfa sprouts should be avoided and that eating fish may be beneficial. Patients with fatigue should pace themselves, with periods of activity alternating with periods of rest. Sun-sensitizing drugs, especially sulfa antibiotics, can flare the disease and should be avoided. Wigs can be worn by patients with impressive hair loss; camouflage makeups cover up unsightly lesions. The Arthritis Foundation and the Lupus Foundation of America publish useful tracts and provide support services to help patients minimize stress and improve coping. Joint pain is treated with moist heat, and general conditioning exercises that minimize the development muscle atrophy or osteoporosis should be done.

Raynaud's phenomenon responds to biofeedback and relaxation techniques as well as cold avoidance and protective gloves or mittens. Moisturizing soaps, lotions, and ointments such as Dove, Alpha-Keri lotion, or Vaseline Intensive Care make dry skin more comfortable, especially in those with concurrent Sjögren's syndrome.

Topical and Local Therapy

Sunscreens should block ultraviolet A (UVA) and B (UVB) light. The SPF rating system applies only to ultraviolet B radiation. Some brands, such as Shade UVA Guard and Ti-Screen, apply to both UVA and UVB. An SPF of at least 15 is recommended. LE lesions can be treated with topical steroids. There are two types: fluorinated and nonfluorinated steroids. The latter are used for mild lesions and are available over the counter as hydrocortisone. Creams are only 20% absorbed, and ointments are 80% absorbed by the skin but are much gloppier. No fluorinated steroid should be applied to the face for more than 2 weeks because it can induce cutaneous atrophy and telangiectasias. Fluorinated steroids range widely in strength from the middle range triamcinolone to potent clobetasol (Temovate) or betamethasone (Diprolene) proprionates. Aggressive lesions can be approached with occlusive dressings (Cordran tape) or intralesional injections of steroid compounds.

Occasionally, cutaneous lesions are treated with laser or excision. Some long-term CLE lesions may evolve into a skin cancer.

Therapy for Cutaneous Lesions

If appropriate physical measures and topical or intralesional therapy do not adequately clear cutaneous lesions, I use systemic therapy. Patients with SLE usually benefit from systemic therapy, as do most patients with CLE or SCLE, especially if the lesions are below the neck.

Antimalarial Therapy

Antimalarials are the agents of choice in managing cutaneous lupus. Three preparations are used: hy-droxychloroquine (Plaquenil), chloroquine (Aralen),* and quinacrine (Atabrine). The latter is available from compounding pharmacists. Antimalarials have disease-modifying actions and are capable of suppressing lupus in the long term. They have multiple mechanisms of action beneficial to lupus patients. By raising the pH of the cytoplasm, antimalarials turn off inflammatory pathways germane to autoimmunity. They also decrease the surface areas available for cell signaling by invaginating cell surface receptor sites. Additionally, antimalarials impart a photoprotective effect, lower serum cholesterol level by 15% (which is important if the patient is also on cholesterol-raising corticosteroids), improve Sjögren's syndrome (seen in 20% of patients with LE), decrease the risk of thromboembolic complications from antiphospholipid antibodies (seen in 10% with SLE and 5% with CLE), and diminish fatigue.

Hydroxychloroquine is usually the first agent of choice. We usually start with 200 mg a day for 2 weeks and increase to 400 mg a day thereafter. Patients begin to feel better in 2 to 3 months, with maximal relief obtained after 1 year. For children or adults not of normal size or stature, the recommended dosing is 5 mg per kg per day. Approximately 10% of patients encounter gastrointestinal upset, headache, flulike aching, or a rash during the first 2 weeks. For these individuals, the dose can be kept at 200 mg daily (it simply takes longer to work), and we have found that many of these symptoms disappear if the patient switches to the brand name preparation Plaquenil. The most important side effect of hydroxychloroquine is eye toxicity; the agent can produce macular and retinal pigmentation, which produces scotoma. The statistical risk of this is 3% if a lupus patient takes the drug for 10 years, and it is almost always reversible. Therefore, ophthalmologic screening evaluations are advised at 6-month intervals. Almost all reported cases of eye toxicity from hydroxychloroquine occurred in patients taking more than 7 mg per kg per day or those in renal failure.

Chloroquine is used infrequently in the United States. Much more potent than hydroxychloroquine, chloroquine is effective within 1 month but has a 10% risk of producing eye toxicity at 10 years that is not always reversible. I restrict this drug to patients with severe cutaneous disease who cannot wait the 2 to 3 months to start improving with hydroxychloroquine. In these situations, I usually prescribe 250 to 500 mg a day for 1 month and either taper its dose to three times a week or switch to hydroxychloroquine. Patients taking chloroquine have a 1 in 100 risk of having lower blood counts and abnormal liver tests or muscle toxicity as opposed to less than 1 in 1000 when taking hydroxychloroquine. Patients are usually maintained on hydroxychloroquine for 2 to 3 years and then tapered off it by 100 mg every 6 months. Approximately 30 to 50% of CLE patients require long-term, chronic maintenance therapy.

During World War II, 3 million Allied troops took

*Not FDA approved for this indication.

quinacrine daily as part of a malarial prophylaxis regimen. Serendipitously, some soldiers with mild lupus or rheumatoid arthritis noted improvements in their condition. Quinacrine is available from 2000 compounding pharmacists in the United States. I prescribe 25 to 100 mg a day for patients with CLE who cannot take a chloroquine preparation due to eye concerns (quinacrine does not affect the retina), who might benefit from the synergistic actions of it with a chloroquine preparation, or who have profound fatigue or cognitive impairment (quinacrine is an effective cortical stimulant). Patients start to respond in 2 to 4 weeks. Although generally well tolerated, quinacrine can cause loose stools and mild gastrointestinal cramping (for which I add Pepto-Bismol) and a yellow stain on the skin (which is present in most people taking more than 50 mg a day and can be attractive or appear as a sickly, yellow jaundice). These effects disappear with the drug's discontinuation. I check blood counts monthly for quinacrine patients for the first 6 months (and every 3 months thereafter) because 1 patient in 50,000 may develop an aplastic or hypoplastic anemia. In nearly every circumstance, marrow hypoplasia is preceded by a lichen planus-like rash, so the appearance of any new nonlupus rashes in patients taking this agent warrants immediate cessation of therapy.

Retinoids

Retinoid derivatives are particularly useful for SCLE and refractory CLE rashes. These agents are sun sensitizing and very teratogenic, and they must be used carefully. Isotretinoin (Accutane)* and acitretin (Soriatane)* can be prescribed in doses of 40 mg twice a day for 2 weeks or 20 mg a day, respectively, followed by a slow taper. If a response is not noted within 2 weeks, the drugs are discontinued. These agents are not disease modifying and should be used concurrently with antimalarials.

Antileprosy Drugs

Diaminodiphenylsulfone (Dapsone)* is the agent of choice for bullous lupus and is very effective for lupus panniculitis (profundus). I first prescribe 25 mg twice a day and then double the dose after 2 weeks if the patient has a negative screen for glucose-6-phosphate dehydrogenase deficiency. Clofazimine (Lamprene)* is a quinacrine-like agent (which even produces the same yellow stain) that may be successful for refractory cutaneous lesions after 2 to 3 months of 100 mg a day. Finally, thalidomide* recently became available on a restricted basis. In doses of 100 mg at bedtime, this teratogenic agent has no systemic effects on lupus and produces a peripheral neuropathy in 10% of users. Although quite effective for resistant cutaneous lesions, thalidomide stops working soon after it is discontinued, and concurrent antimalarial therapy is advised.

Corticosteroids

Acute cutaneous lupus lesions respond dramatically to prednisone in doses of 40 to 60 mg a day

within 1 to 2 weeks. Occasionally, pulse intravenous doses of several hundred milligrams of methylprednisolone (Solu-Medrol) may be useful. Chronic corticosteroid therapy is rarely needed if only cutaneous disease is present. If lesions return while the patient is on doses of 10 to 15 mg a day, immunosuppressive therapies should be considered for steroid-sparing purposes.

Immune Suppressive Regimens

Patients with severe refractory cutaneous disease who have no evidence of systemic activity may benefit from topical nitrogen mustard* or BCNU,* which are available from compounding pharmacists. Occasionally, azathioprine (Imuran; 100 to 200 mg a day),* methotrexate (10 to 25 mg a week),* or monthly pulse doses of cyclophosphamide (Cytoxan; 750 mg per M^2 intravenously monthly)* for 6 months are used. Because lupus of the skin is rarely life- or organ-threatening, these agents should be used infrequently and cautiously.

Specific Approaches for Cutaneous Lupus Subsets

Oral ulcerations are treated with buttermilk or hydrogen peroxide gargles, systemic therapy for lupus, and steroid impregnated with a dental gel (Kenalog in Orabase). SCLE lesions are treated with antimalarials and retinoids; bullous or panniculitis is treated with antileprosy drugs. Intralesional injections, minoxidil (Rogaine) solution, and cysteine-containing shampoos may diminish hair loss. DCNB therapy is indicated for alopecia totalis. Urticarial lupus responds to antiallergy regimens in addition to lupus therapy.

Therapies for Cutaneovascular Disease

Raynaud's phenomenon is approached with cold avoidance, use of mittens or gloves when exposed to cold, and biofeedback. Calcium channel blockers such as nifedipine (Procardia XL) 30 to 90 mg a day are used if the skin breaks down and for painful fingers and toes or discomfort in the ear lobe, tongue, or tip of the nose. In certain circumstances, nitroglycerin paste, alpha-adrenergic blocking agents (alpha-methyldopa [Aldomet]), or vasodilators (prazosin [Minipress]) are prescribed. Digital gangrene is a serious, infrequent complication. A variety of parenteral prostaglandin derivatives (e.g., (alprostadil [Prostin VR], epoprostenol [Flolan]) can often salvage an extremity or digit. No specific therapy for livedo reticularis is necessary.

DERMATOMYOSITIS

Inflammatory myositis on an autoimmune basis may also affect the skin. Although histologically sim-

---

*Not FDA approved for this indication.

*Not FDA approved for this indication.

ilar to CLE and primarily occurring in sun-exposed areas, dermatomyositis has a distinct distribution. In adults, a heliotropic-like lesion is frequently present around the eyes, and Gottron's papules may be found on the dorsal surfaces of the hands. There are many types of inflammatory myositis; those that involve the skin include

1. Childhood dermatomyositis, which is characterized by subcutaneous calcifications
2. Adult dermatomyositis, which frequently overlaps with lupus, scleroderma, and rheumatoid arthritis
3. Malignancy-associated dermatomyositis
4. Amyopathic dermatomyositis, when serum muscle enzymes and electrical muscle studies are normal

General Treatment Approaches

Children with dermatomyositis often develop atrophy and contractures. Skin lesions and calcinosis may play a role in accelerating disabling features. I initiate vigorous physical and nutritional measures to prevent deformity and debility. No acceptable treatments are available for the dramatic calcinosis universalis frequently observed in childhood dermatomyositis, although there is a suggestion that 300 mg of diltiazem (Cardizem)* per day is worth a therapeutic trial. The skin should be moisturized with emollients (e.g., Eucerin, Aquaphor, Vaseline), and excoriations from pruritus can be ameliorated with sedating antihistamines (e.g., diphenhydramine [Benadryl] 50 mg) at bedtime and nonsedating ones during the day (e.g., loratadine [Claritin] 10 mg).

Adults should undergo an evaluation to exclude an underlying malignancy. Blood chemistry panels, chest x-ray films, tumor markers (e.g., carcinoembryonic antigen, alpha-fetoprotein), bone scans, comprehensive gynecologic evaluation, and a gastrointestinal tract series are appropriate because the only way to treat this form of dermatomyositis is to treat the underlying malignancy. Patients with amyopathic dermatomyositis may develop an inflammatory muscle disorder, and muscle enzymes should be obtained every few months.

Specific Therapies

Hydroxychloroquine* is the intervention of choice for the rash of dermatomyositis. Prescribed as for lupus (see previous section), it is not effective if an underlying malignancy is present. Its application may not be necessary if inflammatory myositis necessitates corticosteroid therapy because that therapy also eliminates the rash. Corticosteroids may be used short term for amyopathic dermatomyositis, or until an antimalarial becomes effective. Patients with rashes refractory to antimalarials and steroids frequently respond to methotrexate* in doses of 10 to 25 mg per week.

---

*Not FDA approved for this indication.

SCLERODERMA

Scleroderma, or systemic sclerosis, is an autoimmune disorder manifested by tight skin. A confluence of autoantibody-mediated inflammation, increased cross-linking of collagen, endothelial cell hyperreactivity-mediated vascular changes, and abnormal T cell regulation, there are many forms of this frustrating disorder:

1. *Morphea* is usually found in children and consists of a localized patch of scleroderma.
2. *Linear scleroderma* consists of a streak or band of tight skin and usually found in children.
3. *Limited scleroderma,* or CREST syndrome (calcinosis, Raynaud's phenomenon, esophagitis, sclerodactyly, telangiectasias), is the most common form of scleroderma. Tight skin does not extend beyond the wrist, and organ involvement is limited to the gastrointestinal tract and lungs.
4. *Diffuse scleroderma,* or progressive systemic sclerosis, includes widespread tight skin and organ involvement; 50% of patients with diffuse scleroderma survive 7 years.
5. *Mixed connective tissue disease* or *overlap syndromes* are usually manifested with a scleroderma gut, Raynaud's phenomenon, sclerodactyly with features of inflammatory myositis, rheumatoid arthritis, or lupus.
6. *Environmental/drug-induced scleroderma* could be caused by organic solvents, drugs such as bleomycin, or graft-versus-host reactions, and tight skin can be seen in a variety of areas (e.g., truncal scleroderma from pentazocine injections).

The following discussion is limited to the cutaneous manifestations of scleroderma.

General Approaches

The first approach for a patient newly diagnosed with scleroderma is to stage the process to assess what is involved where. For example, if occult lung involvement is present in a patient with tight digits, treatment would be directed toward the lungs, which would indirectly help the skin. Raynaud's phenomenon is near universal in scleroderma, and its management was discussed in the previous section. Emollients and moisturizing agents keep the scleroderma patient's skin well lubricated, and anti-itching remedies (listed earlier) are also used. Physical therapy and occupational therapy, as well as evaluation by a hand specialist, may prevent contractures and deformity. Telangiectasias rarely cause any clinical problems, but unsightly lesions can be treated with CO_2 laser therapy. Biofeedback and smoking cessation are important interventions for vascular and autonomic aspects of the disease. Surgical sympathectomy is temporarily effective for severe Raynaud's phenomenon with digital compromise; unfortunately, patients usually become worse within a few months. Intravenous prostaglandin derivatives (see earlier) are recommended.

Medications

Medications are rarely needed for morphea and linear scleroderma because they are usually self-limited processes that run their course over a few years. Some reports have suggested that d-penicillamine (Cuprimine),* in doses of 250 mg per day (raised monthly by 125 mg per day until 1000 mg per day is reached or a response is seen), are beneficial. A recent double-blind controlled study suggested that this agent may not be as promising as originally hoped. Tight skin has the best chance of being loosened if it is treated aggressively within the first 2 years after diagnosis. A variety of interventions, including methotrexate (10 to 25 mg per week),* photopheresis, alpha-interferon (injected three times a week),* and cyclosporine (3 mg per kg per day),* may be of modest benefit for sclerodactyly. Prednisone, aminobenzoate (Potaba),* colchicine,* and chlorambucil* are not helpful; cyclophosphamide* may retard pulmonary involvement. The most promising agent in development is relaxin, a hormone made by the uterus during labor to make it easier to expel a fetus. Stem cell transplantation is currently being studied.

---

*Not FDA approved for this indication.

CUTANEOUS VASCULITIS*

method of
CAROL A. LANGFORD, M.D., M.H.S., and
MICHAEL C. SNELLER, M.D.
*National Institute of Allergy and Infectious
Diseases, National Institutes of Health
Bethesda, Maryland*

The term "cutaneous vasculitis" can have a broad range of possible interpretations, and to date there is no standard terminology that is universally accepted. Other names that are often used to describe this entity include leukocytoclastic vasculitis, necrotizing vasculitis, and hypersensitivity vasculitis. For the purposes of this article, cutaneous vasculitis is defined broadly as inflammation of the blood vessels within the dermis. As such, cutaneous vasculitis is not one specific disease but rather a cutaneous manifestation that can occur in a wide range of settings (Table 1). Although cutaneous vasculitis may occur idiopathically, in over 70% of cases an inciting agent or underlying illness can be identified. Recognition of these processes is critical because management of the underlying condition also usually becomes the basis for treating the cutaneous vasculitis. In addition, treatment of presumptive idiopathic cutaneous vasculitis can mask or worsen an associated illness, delaying diagnosis and potentially placing the patient at risk.

---

*All material in this chapter is in the public domain, with the exception of any borrowed figures or tables.

TABLE 1. Clinical Spectrum of Cutaneous Vasculitis

Exogenous agents
  Medications
    Prescription drugs
    Over-the-counter agents
    Alternative therapies
  Foods
  Chemicals
Infection
  Hepatitis C virus infection
  Bacterial endocarditis
  Other bacterial, viral, and fungal infections
Malignancy
Connective tissue diseases
  Systemic lupus erythematosus
  Rheumatoid arthritis
  Sjögren's syndrome
  Inflammatory myopathies
  Scleroderma
  Relapsing polychondritis
Primary systemic vasculitides
  Henoch-Schönlein purpura
  Wegener's granulomatosis
  Microscopic polyangiitis
  Polyarteritis nodosa
  Churg-Strauss syndrome
Miscellaneous
  Behçet's disease
  Cryoglobulinemia
  Inflammatory bowel disease
  Primary biliary cirrhosis
  Retroperitoneal fibrosis
  Alpha$_1$-antitrypsin deficiency
  Celiac disease
  Urticarial vasculitis
  Erythema elevatum diutinum
Idiopathic cutaneous vasculitis

TREATMENT OF CUTANEOUS VASCULITIS ASSOCIATED WITH AN UNDERLYING DISEASE OR EXOGENOUS AGENT

The appropriate course of treatment for cutaneous vasculitis will be determined by the setting in which it is occurring (Figure 1). The systemic vasculitides are among the most significant associations to rule out because these diseases can affect other organs and have the potential for morbidity or even mortality. If cutaneous vasculitis is part of an active systemic vasculitis syndrome, then treatment will be based on the nature and severity of the extracutaneous manifestations. Cutaneous vasculitis can also occur in association with other underlying illnesses, such as malignancies, infections, or a connective tissue disease (see Table 1). In these settings, treatment of the underlying condition often leads to resolution of the vasculitis.

Exogenous antigens have been implicated in up to 15% of cases of cutaneous vasculitis. Medications, specifically the antibiotics, nonsteroidal anti-inflammatory drugs (NSAIDs), antihypertensives, and antiarrhythmics are the most frequently associated agents. Generally, if the cutaneous vasculitis is related to a medication, it will resolve in 2 to 3 weeks after drug discontinuation, but the episode can last

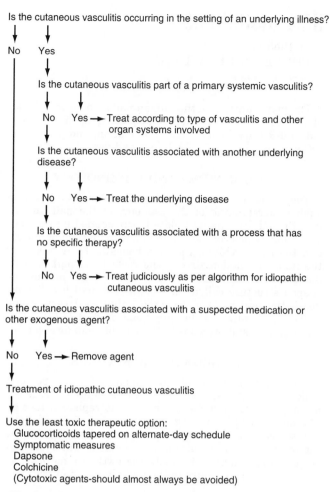

Is the cutaneous vasculitis occurring in the setting of an underlying illness?

No   Yes

Is the cutaneous vasculitis part of a primary systemic vasculitis?

No   Yes → Treat according to type of vasculitis and other organ systems involved

Is the cutaneous vasculitis associated with another underlying disease?

No   Yes → Treat the underlying disease

Is the cutaneous vasculitis associated with a process that has no specific therapy?

No   Yes → Treat judiciously as per algorithm for idiopathic cutaneous vasculitis

Is the cutaneous vasculitis associated with a suspected medication or other exogenous agent?

No   Yes → Remove agent

Treatment of idiopathic cutaneous vasculitis

Use the least toxic therapeutic option:
  Glucocorticoids tapered on alternate-day schedule
  Symptomatic measures
  Dapsone
  Colchicine
  (Cytotoxic agents-should almost always be avoided)

Figure 1. Algorithm for the treatment of cutaneous vasculitis.

longer or even be recurrent without reintroduction of the drug. In such instances, judicious use of the strategies outlined later may be considered.

TREATMENT OF IDIOPATHIC CUTANEOUS VASCULITIS

The diagnosis of idiopathic cutaneous vasculitis (ICV) should be made only after the presence of a specific exogenous antigen, infectious process, associated illness, or systemic vasculitis has been ruled out by appropriate diagnostic studies. In general, patients with ICV have been found to have an excellent long-term outcome. Although the possibility of progression to a systemic vasculitis must always be kept in mind, this occurs infrequently. Even so, it is important to repeatedly seek out emerging features that might suggest systemic disease by history, examination, and intermittent laboratory screening.

The course of ICV is extremely individual between patients, ranging anywhere from a single brief episode to multiple protracted recurrences. Spontaneous remissions of ICV happen frequently. The severity of symptoms experienced by individual patients is also highly variable, and it is appreciated that some patients will have significant discomfort. However, the

side effects of various treatments must be carefully weighed and the use of potentially toxic regimens should be avoided if at all possible.

The main principle behind treating ICV should be to use the least toxic yet effective therapy. Aggressive immunosuppressive regimens that include glucocorticoids and cytotoxic agents are important and often necessary in treating a systemic vasculitis involving a major organ. However, these regimens are frequently ineffective in treating ICV and they can be associated with considerable toxicity. Although a vast number of different treatments have been tried in patients with ICV, the efficacy for almost all of these therapies has not been firmly established. This is largely due to the difficulty of studying a process that has such a variable course. There is currently no uniformly effective and safe treatment for ICV.

In patients with painful lesions, measures to decrease discomfort are important. This can include the use of acetaminophen and NSAIDs. In addition to symptomatic improvement, it is possible that NSAIDs may also have a direct therapeutic role by reducing inflammation. Narcotic analgesics must be prescribed with care because ICV can be a chronic problem. However, selected patients may receive benefit from short-term use of such agents especially at the time of acute exacerbations. For lesions that are pruritic or urticarial, antihistamines may provide some relief. Local care and elevation of the affected region when possible is important in relieving discomfort and preventing skin breakdown. Should ulceration occur, meticulous care is necessary to prevent superinfection, which may further slow the healing process.

Glucocorticoids are often used in the treatment of ICV. The optimal glucocorticoid regimen has not been determined. One approach is to begin with a "burst" of prednisone starting at a dose of 1 mg per kg per day (up to 60 mg daily given as a single morning dose) that is tapered to discontinuation over 2 to 3 weeks. For patients who develop recurrent lesions, a more prolonged alternate-day prednisone tapering schedule can be used. For example, prednisone is initially started at 1 mg per kg per day (up to 60 mg daily) and continued for 1 to 2 weeks. After that time, the prednisone would be tapered to an every-other-day schedule by 6 to 8 weeks and ultimately discontinued after 3 to 4 months. Glucocorticoids have many potential toxicities and side effects, including infection, osteoporosis, avascular necrosis, hyperglycemia, hypertension, impairment of healing, myopathy, mood disturbance including psychosis, increase in appetite and weight, striae, and acne. Preventive interventions to lessen the risk of osteoporosis must be considered in all instances. The use of alternate-day dosing of glucocorticoids has substantial advantages with regard to side effects, in particular the risk of infection.

Dapsone,* 50 to 200 mg per day, has been found to be helpful in erythema elevatum diutinum and has

---

*Not FDA approved for this indication.

also been applied to the treatment of ICV. Before dapsone therapy is undertaken, patients should be screened for glucose-6-phosphate dehydrogenase (G6PD) deficiency because affected patients develop profound hemolysis. Even in the absence of G6PD deficiency, hemolysis is the most common adverse effect of dapsone treatment. Because this and other cytopenias can occur, the Dermatology Advisory Committee of the Food and Drug Administration recommends that complete blood cell counts be performed weekly for the first month, monthly for 6 months, and semiannually thereafter. Less frequent side effects include peripheral neuropathy, psychosis, nephrotoxicity, cholestasis, and hypoalbuminemia.

Colchicine,* 0.6 mg one to three times a day, has been used in ICV and is preferred by some authors as a first-choice agent over glucocorticoids. In one double-blind study, however, the use of colchicine failed to show a benefit. Colchicine is contraindicated in patients with bone marrow disease, renal insufficiency, or hepatic impairment. The main side effects of colchicine are gastrointestinal, with diarrhea, nausea, and vomiting limiting the dose in some patients. Less frequent but more severe side effects include bone marrow suppression, nervous system toxicity, hepatic failure, and alopecia.

The cytotoxic agents that have been most frequently used in ICV include methotrexate, azathioprine, and cyclophosphamide. These are all potent immunosuppressive drugs that have substantial toxicity. As such, their use should be reserved for very select cases in which patients have severe disease that is unresponsive to other measures or when glucocorticoids are unable to be tapered. When their use is believed to be appropriate, methotrexate or azathioprine should be the primary cytotoxic agents to be considered. Cyclophosphamide should rarely if ever be used to treat ICV. Although it remains the cytotoxic agent of choice in patients with immediately life-threatening systemic vasculitis, its efficacy in treating ICV is unknown. In one study, cyclophosphamide was found to have no beneficial effect in four of six patients with ICV. In addition, cyclophosphamide is potentially very toxic, with side effects including bone marrow suppression, infection, permanent infertility, cystitis, bladder cancer, and myeloproliferative disease. In a series of patients with Wegener's granulomatosis who were treated with daily cyclophosphamide, 42% experienced treatment-related morbidity. In this study, 6% of cyclophosphamide-treated patients developed transitional cell carcinoma of the bladder, which by Kaplan-Meier estimates may increase to 16% at 15 years after first exposure. Therefore, as well as having the potential for immediate toxicity, cyclophosphamide can have long-term side effects that may occur many years after the drug is discontinued. Given the favorable outcome of patients with ICV, the use of cyclophosphamide in such circumstances is rarely if ever justified.

*Not FDA approved for this indication.

NAIL DISORDERS
method of
PHOEBE RICH, M.D.
Portland, Oregon

The main function of the human nail is to protect the tip of the digit. Nails also assist in picking up fine objects, aid in dexterity, balance, and ambulation, and provide an esthetic appearance for the hands and feet.

NAIL ANATOMY AND TERMINOLOGY

The physician treating nail disorders should have a thorough understanding of the anatomy of the nail and its growth pattern. The nail plate is surrounded by the perionychium, which consists of proximal and lateral nail folds, and the hyponychium, the area beneath the free edge of the nail. The nail matrix is the root of the nail, and its distal portion is visible on some nails as the half-moon–shaped structure called the *lunula*. The nail bed lies beneath the nail plate and contains the blood vessels and nerves. The cuticle is the horny end product of the proximal nail fold and attaches to the nail plate to form a seal.

NAIL GROWTH AND KINETICS

Nails grow at a rate of approximately 0.1 mm per day, which means that it takes about 4 to 6 months to regenerate a fingernail and 8 to 12 months to replace a toenail. The nail matrix is the germinative portion of the nail and is responsible for the formation of the nail plate. Injury to the matrix usually results in a permanent nail dystrophy such as a split nail. Conversely, regrowth of a normal nail can occur after an injury to the nail plate or nail bed.

INFECTIOUS NAIL DISEASES

Fungi, bacteria, and viruses can cause infectious nail disorders (Table 1).

Onychomycosis (Nail Fungal Infection)

Onychomycosis includes nail infection by dermatophyte fungi (tinea unguium), yeasts such as *Candida albicans*, and nondermatophyte molds. Fungal infections of the nails are common worldwide without racial predilection. Some persons may have a genetic predisposition to develop chronic onychomycosis. Other factors that may increase the development of onychomycosis are humidity, heat, trauma, diabetes mellitus, and underlying tinea pedis.

Onychomycosis is the most common nail disorder, representing 40% of all nail disorders and 30% of all cutaneous fungal infections. It is often asymptomatic but in some patients may cause pain, limit mobility, and interfere with manual dexterity. Onychomycosis is frequently overdiagnosed. Nonfungal nail conditions such as psoriasis can be indistinguishable from onychomycosis; therefore, it is important not to rely on clinical inspection alone to diagnose fungal infections of the nail. A potassium hydroxide (KOH) preparation or fungal culture should be performed to confirm the clinical diagnosis.

There are four subtypes of onychomycosis that are

TABLE 1. **Differential Diagnosis of Nail Disorders**

Condition	Physical Examination and History	Laboratory Findings	Management
Onychomycosis	Hyperkeratosis of nail bed, yellow-brown discoloration, onycholysis; usually chronic	KOH positive; culture positive	Systemic or topical antifungal therapy
Paronychia, acute	Red, warm, tender nail; often follows injury to nail fold	Positive bacterial culture, usually *Staphylococcus*	Systemic antibiotic
Paronychia, chronic	Boggy, swollen, red, inflamed nail folds; usually occurs in people whose jobs involve wetness	Pus is KOH positive, and culture is positive for *C. albicans*	Anti-*Candida* therapy, topical or systemic
Psoriasis	Usually associated with cutaneous psoriasis; pitting, onycholysis, splinter hemorrhages, nail bed hyperkeratosis	KOH negative	Topical or intralesional steroids
Lichen planus	Ridging early; can eventuate in scarring and pterygium formation	KOH negative	Systemic, topical, or intralesional steroids
Melanoma	Pigmented band in the nail that widens or darkens	Biopsy nail bed or matrix, depending on site of pigment	Wide excision
Squamous cell carcinoma	Hyperkeratosis, onycholysis, melanomychia	Biopsy lesion	Excision; sometimes Mohs' surgery
Habit tic	Usually thumbs; horizontal parallel groove lines on nail plates. History of manipulating nail folds	KOH negative	Explain cause to patient; occasionally wrap nail
Mucous cyst	Occurs on proximal nail fold and over DIP joint	Mucin expressed from punctured lesion	Excision; repeated liquid nitrogen; intralesional cortisone

Abbreviations: KOH = potassium hydroxide; DIP = distal interphalangeal.

named according to their pattern of involvement of the nail unit. *Distal subungual onychomycosis* (DSO) is so named because the site of invasion is the distal nail bed and progression is distal to proximal. Nail bed hyperkeratosis and yellow-brown discoloration are usually present, with eventual crumbling and disintegration of the nail plate. The most common dermatophytes are *Trychophyton rubrum* and *T. mentagrophytes,* although others also can be seen. Distal subungual onychomycosis of the toenails is usually associated with tinea pedis. When it occurs in fingernails it is often associated with scaling of the palm of the affected hand and both feet. The organism on the hands is usually *T. rubrum.*

Proximal subungual onychomycosis (PSO) is quite rare in people with intact immune systems. It occurs when the organisms invade the nail plate proximally. The causative organism is usually a dermatophyte. The clinical presentation is that of white or yellow discoloration on the ventral surface of the nail plate, beginning at the proximal nail fold and extending distally.

White superficial onychomycosis (WSO) is characterized by white discoloration on the surface of the toenail, which can be easily scraped away with a blade. Because it is superficial in location, it can be treated topically. In most cases the causative organism of WSO is *T. mentagrophytes*. Finally, true *candida onychomycosis* occurs in a rare condition called *chronic mucocutaneous candidiasis*. Normally, *Candida* is not a good invader of nail plate keratin, but can involve the nail folds and nail bed (see "Chronic Paronychia").

Onychomycosis from Molds

Nondermatophyte molds are a rare cause of onychomycosis, and their role in the pathogenesis of onychomycosis is somewhat controversial. The most common mold isolated from diseased nails is *Scopulariopsis brevicaulis*.

Treatment of Onychomycosis

The therapy for onychomycosis should be tailored to the type of infection and to individual patient needs (Table 2). Because onychomycosis is frequently overdiagnosed, it is important to demonstrate fungus

TABLE 2. **Treatment of Onychomycosis**

Generic	Trade	Course
Itraconazole	Sporanox	Continuous: 200 mg q d for 12 wk Pulse: 200 bid 1 wk/mo for 2 mo for fingernails, 3 mo for toes
Terbinafine	Lamisil	Continuous: 250 mg q d for 6 wk (fingernail), 12 wk (toenail) Pulse: 250 bid 1 wk/mo for 3 mo
Fluconazole*	Diflucan	300 mg q wk until nails are clinically clear 6 to 12 mo
Griseofulvin	Gris-PEG	500 mg bid for 1 yr or until nails clear

*Not FDA approved for this indication.

by KOH preparation or culture before systemic antifungal therapy is begun. Except in the case of white superficial onychomycosis, topical antifungal therapy is rarely curative. Griseofulvin has largely been replaced by two new oral antifungal medications, itraconazole (Sporanox) and terbinafine (Lamisil), approved by the FDA for the treatment of onychomycosis. Another oral antifungal drug, fluconazole (Diflucan), is also used successfully for toenail fungus, but it is not approved by the FDA for the indication of onychomycosis. These new antifungal drugs shorten treatment duration and minimize side effects in the treatment of onychomycosis. It is incumbent on the physician treating onychomycosis with systemic antifungal medications to ensure that the proper diagnosis has been made. In addition, the physician should be aware of any potential drug-drug interactions and monitor for medication side effects (see Table 2).

Paronychia

Paronychia is defined as infection or inflammation of the nail folds. It can be acute or chronic, based on the pathogenesis and organism.

Acute Paronychia

Acute paronychia results from a bacterial infection of the nail folds. It usually follows some kind of trauma to the nail folds such as overaggressive manicuring or injury. The most common bacterial agents in acute paronychia are *Staphylococcus aureus* and *Pseudomonas* species. Treatment is similar to that for other bacterial infections of the skin and includes draining and administering a systemic antibiotic.

Chronic Paronychia

Chronic paronychia causes swollen, red, tender, boggy nail folds. It occurs most frequently in people whose jobs involve wetness or in those whose hands are exposed to solvents and chemicals. Initially there is separation of the cuticle and nail folds from the nail plate, followed by the formation of a potential space for various microbes to invade, especially *C. albicans*.

Treatment of chronic paronychia includes drying of the area around the nail folds and application of anticandidal agents. In cases of severe inflammation, topical or intralesional steroids along with oral anticandidal medications can be used. It is important to educate the patient about avoiding excessive water and chemical exposure.

The most common virus found in nail disorders is the human papillomavirus (HPV), which causes subungual and periungual warts. Warts around the nail can be difficult to treat. It is important to remember that certain HPV strains (e.g., HPV 16 and 18) are oncogenic, and the physician should be alert for the possibility of malignant degeneration in warts that have been present for many years.

DERMATOLOGIC DISEASES THAT AFFECT THE NAILS

Psoriasis

Psoriasis occurs in 2 to 3% of the population, and between 10% and 50% of those with psoriasis have nail involvement. Psoriasis of the nails is an unsightly condition, which can have an emotional impact on people who work with their hands.

Psoriasis of the nails has a variety of clinical manifestations, depending on the site of the nail unit involved. Nail plate pitting is due to involvement of the matrix; onycholysis, subungual hyperkeratosis, and yellow discoloration ("oil drop sign") result from nail bed psoriasis. Psoriasis of the nail is often indistinguishable clinically from fungal infection of the nail. Clinical inspection of other areas of the body that are psoriasis prone (elbows, knees, scalp, gluteal cleft) and negative KOH examination and fungus culture can provide clues to the diagnosis of psoriasis of the nails. Approximately 5% of patients with psoriasis have psoriasis limited to the nails, a situation that poses a diagnostic challenge.

Treatment of psoriasis of the nails can be difficult at times; however, nail psoriasis often clears as cutaneous psoriasis improves. Topical steroids may be helpful in mild cases, but results are usually disappointing in severe psoriatic involvement of the nails. Intralesional steroids (triamcinolone [Kenalog], 2.5 to 5.0 mg per mL) injected into the proximal nail folds overlying the nail matrix are generally more helpful, although not always welcomed by the patient. Psoralens plus ultraviolet A (PUVA) and grenz ray are sometimes beneficial in severe cases. A dermatologist should be consulted for these treatments.

Lichen Planus

Lichen planus is a relatively uncommon disorder that can affect the skin and nails. When it occurs in the nails, it is characterized by onychorrhexis (longitudinal ridging), and it can rapidly destroy the nail matrix, leading to scarring of the nail plate. The end stage of lichen planus of the nails is destruction of the matrix so that portions of the nail fail to grow. The resultant defect is called a *pterygium* and is characterized by areas of scarring where the nail fold adheres to the nail bed. Treatment for lichen planus is challenging, and potent topical corticosteroids with or without occlusion should be tried. Intralesional triamcinolone (2.5 mg per cc) injected into the proximal nail fold) can be tried, and systemic steroids are sometimes necessary for the treatment of rapidly destructive lichen planus of the nails.

NEOPLASTIC NAIL CONDITIONS

Pigmented Lesions of the Nail

Pigmented lesions of the nail are the most important nail condition and should be taken seriously. It is impossible to know without a biopsy whether a pigmented band in the nail is a benign melanocytic nevus, reactive melanocytic hyperplasia, or a melanoma.

Malignant Melanoma

Malignant melanoma of the nail unit is rare, accounting for only 1 to 4% of melanomas. Although 20% of these are amelanotic, containing little or no pigment, most start as a solitary longitudinal pigmented band in the nail. The band usually widens and darkens over time, and frequently there is leaching of pigment into the proximal nail fold (Hutchinson's sign). The most commonly involved nails are the great toe and thumb. More than 25% of patients give a history of trauma to the digit, which in some cases is the cause of a delay in seeking medical attention. There are many benign causes of longitudinal pigmented bands in the nail, including melanocytic nevus, certain medications, and even as a normal occurrence in patients with deeply pigmented skin; but any solitary pigmented band that widens, darkens, or otherwise alters the nail plate needs further evaluation. The onus is on the physician to be certain that a pigmented band or spot on the nail is not a melanoma.

Early detection and wide surgical excision are essential. When there is doubt about the diagnosis, referral to a dermatologist and biopsy of nail bed, nail matrix, or surrounding tissue are indicated. Once the diagnosis of malignant melanoma is confirmed, referral to an oncologic surgeon experienced in the management of malignant melanoma is mandatory.

Other cutaneous neoplasms are occasionally seen in the nail unit. Both basal cell carcinoma and squamous cell carcinoma occur rarely in the nail bed. A benign painful tumor that is often seen in a subungual location is a glomus tumor, an encapsulated tumor of the arteriovenous anastomosis in the nail bed. These tumors may be seen beneath the nail as a red or blue discoloration, but the main distinguishing feature is pain, which may be spontaneous or associated with cold. A benign bony growth called an *exostosis* can occur subungually, usually beneath the toenail, and often after trauma to the digit.

OTHER COMMON NAIL DISORDERS

Habit Tic Disorder

Habit tic disorder is a common disorder that is self-induced and characterized by horizontal parallel ridges in the nail plate. It results from frequent repetitive manipulation of the cuticle and nail fold overlying the matrix. The thumb is the most commonly involved digit. Once the cause of the problem is explained to the patient, the cure is simply a matter of leaving the nail alone.

Digital Mucous Cyst

Mucous cysts are the most common tumor of the digit and usually occur on the dorsal surface of the finger between the nail folds and the distal interphalangeal joint. They are not true cysts because they lack a cystic lining and are more accurately called *focal mucinosis*. They often cause a longitudinal groove in the nail plate because they press on the matrix and cause a defect in the nascent nail plate. These lesions can be evacuated after being punctured with a needle; however, they often re-form. Injection with triamcinolone 2.5 mg per mL is often helpful. Occasionally, they connect to the joint space, in which case surgical excision is necessary.

Nail Changes in Systemic Disease

Some nail findings provide helpful clues for the diagnosis of systemic disorders. A few nail signs are specific for underlying medical problems. Nail fold telangiectasias are associated with connective tissue disorders such as systemic lupus erythematosus and dermatomyositis. Clubbing is associated with pulmonary and gastrointestinal disorders. Other much less specific nail signs such as splinter hemorrhages may be seen in subacute bacterial endocarditis but are more commonly seen in trauma to the nail.

KELOIDS

method of
MARLENE S. CALDERON, M.D., and
WARREN L. GARNER, M.D.
University of Michigan Medical Center
Ann Arbor, Michigan

Keloids are abnormal overgrowths of connective tissue, usually occurring at the site of skin trauma. They are distinct from hypertrophic and other scars and are characterized by their propensity to extend beyond the boundary of the original injury. Keloid scars rarely regress and can become disfiguring and pendulous. They occur most often in dark-skinned persons and demonstrate a familial predisposition. Areas of skin tension, such as those overlying the presternum and deltoid muscles, are commonly affected. Other sites of skin injury on the earlobes and upper arms, from piercing and vaccination, can also develop keloids.

ETIOPATHOGENESIS

The etiopathogenetic mechanism for keloid scars is unknown. Histologically, keloids demonstrate the presence of excessive, broad eosinophilic collagen fibers and overabundant mucinous ground substance, with low fibroblast density. Biochemically, increased procollagen and messenger RNA synthesis by keloid fibroblasts correlates with increased collagen synthesis. Collagenase activity is also increased, but the rate of collagen synthesis exceeds the rate of degradation, with resultant net collagen deposition. Many growth factors, such as transforming growth factor β, epidermal growth factor, and platelet-derived growth factor, have been implicated in the pathogenesis of keloid scars, but other factors such as wound tension, chronic inflammation, and immune response also probably play a role. The precise mechanism at the cellular and molecular levels continues to be investigated.

TREATMENT

No consistently effective treatment for keloid scars exists. Prevention is best. Unnecessary procedures in susceptible persons should be avoided. Currently, the treatment of keloids can be divided into three types: nonsurgical treatment, surgical treatment, and combination treatment.

Nonsurgical Treatment

Corticosteroids

Intralesional corticosteroid injection is the most common treatment for keloids. The specific mechanism of action is unknown, but the clinical result is decreased collagen and inflammation. Used alone, intralesional corticosteroids provide effective relief of signs and symptoms, such as redness and pruritus, in most patients. The effect on size and appearance of the scars is variable. The technique is useful for the treatment of isolated earlobe keloids. The injections, using triamcinolone acetonide (Kenalog, 10 mg/mL) in a 50:50 mixture with 1% lidocaine, are often quite painful. The dense composition of the keloid scar makes the injection difficult. Side effects including tissue atrophy and hypopigmentation can be minimized with careful injection within the scar to avoid extravasation of the solution into adjacent normal tissues. Systemic response is rare and can be avoided by timing injections at 4- to 6-week intervals.

Silicone Gel Sheeting

Silicone gel sheeting is a simple, painless, and easy treatment, with few side effects. It is especially useful for children, who often cannot tolerate the pain of steroid injections. The mechanism of action is unclear, but wound hydration, temperature, and occlusion may be important factors in its effectiveness. Most lesions demonstrate lessening of hardness, elevation, and itching with use of silicone gel sheeting. The sheeting is cut 1 to 2 cm larger than the involved area, and the dressing is applied directly to the scar and worn for 12 to 24 hours per day. This treatment continues for 3 to 6 months or until the desired change in appearance is achieved. From 80 to 85% of keloids treated with this modality will demonstrate significant improvement.

Interferon

Intralesional injection of interferon gamma-1b (Actimmune)* has been studied as a treatment for keloid scars. This lymphokine down-regulates collagen synthesis and theoretically can moderate the development of abnormal and excessive scars. The treatment is expensive, and the dosing regimens have yet to be standardized, but the results with limited trials are encouraging. Few local side effects have been demonstrated, but occasional systemic effects such as headache, muscle ache, and malaise have been reported at high doses. This promising new therapy continues to be investigated.

Surgical Treatment

Primary Excision

Surgical excision alone is complicated by recurrence rates of from 50 to 80%. Surgical excision as a primary treatment without adjuvant radiation, pressure, or steroids has a limited role. Strict adherence to gentle surgical technique, avoidance of wound tension, and limited usage of subcutaneous absorbable sutures helps to minimize the rate of recurrence. Carbon dioxide laser ablation creates less local tissue trauma and less bleeding than "sharp" surgical excision. However, no data suggest that this technique is more effective than standard excision.

Cryoablation

Cryosurgery with hand-held liquid nitrogen sprays is most effective on new keloids, i.e., less than 2 years old. Keloid scars are treated with two or three freeze-thaw cycles per session, and the treatments are repeated at 1-month intervals. Side effects include hypopigmentation and skin atrophy.

Combination Treatment

Surgery with Steroids

Many studies have demonstrated the effectiveness of intraoperative and postoperative intralesional corticosteroid injections for the treatment of recalcitrant keloids. Triamcinolone acetonide is injected into the wound before wound closure, followed by serial intralesional injections for up to 6 months postopera-

---

*Not FDA approved for this indication.

tively. Although effective, this protocol is not well tolerated by patients. As many as two thirds of patients drop out owing to the inconvenience and pain of frequent follow-up injections. Recurrence rates range from 10 to 50% with this modality.

Surgery with Irradiation

The role of irradiation in the treatment of keloid scars is primarily as a postoperative adjuvant. Postoperative irradiation has been reported to be as successful in treating recurrent keloid scars as intralesional steroid injections. Radiotherapy is much better tolerated and requires fewer follow-up visits. A single postoperative dose of 1000 cGy has decreased the recurrence rate to 12.5%. Hyperpigmentation is seen in as many as two thirds of patients. There is a theoretical risk of malignancy, but the actual incidence of carcinogenesis in several large series is zero.

Surgery with Pressure

The use of pressure earring devices after excision of earlobe keloids has been reported to be an effective treatment. Pressure earrings must be worn continuously for 6 to 12 months to be effective. Pressure therapy in other anatomic locations has not been as effective for preventing keloids.

SUMMARY

Currently, the best approach to the treatment of severe keloids is surgical excision with steroid injections or low-dose radiation therapy. Combination therapy demonstrates better response rates and lower recurrence rates than with other treatment modalities alone, but no therapy is consistently effective. Results with agents such as interferon-γ that specifically target collagen synthesis are encouraging. As research clarifies the mechanisms of abnormal wound healing, new treatments will be investigated, and a cure for keloid scars may be discovered.

WARTS

method of
KAREN E. ZANOL, M.D.
University of Missouri Health Sciences Center
Columbia, Missouri

Warts are caused by human papillomavirus infection. They are common among children and young adults, with a prevalence of 10 to 20% in this population. Although we have multiple treatment options, none has been shown to eradicate the virus, and persistence of virus in a subclinical state probably accounts for the high rate of recurrence. Long-term cure rates for any treatment modality rarely exceed the expected rate of natural resolution.

Warts are generally asymptomatic but may become painful in an area subject to trauma, such as the sole of the foot. Two thirds of all warts resolve spontaneously within 2 years without any treatment, but many patients desire treatment because of perceived disfigurement. Choice of treatment modality depends on the age of the patient and the size, location, and number of warts.

Diagnosis is usually straightforward; however, plantar warts may be difficult to distinguish from calluses or clavi (corns) without paring. Warts have visible thrombosed capillaries or pinpoint areas of bleeding after paring with a No. 15 blade. Clavi show only a central core of translucent skin.

Diagnosis should be questioned and a biopsy taken when a solitary wart does not respond to treatment. Squamous cell carcinoma or even melanoma can appear very much like verrucae, especially on the fingers and soles of the feet.

Wart resolution seems ultimately dependent on the function of the cellular immune system. The treatment of verrucae in patients with impaired cellular immunity can be challenging.

STANDARD THERAPY

Keratolytics

Topical application of keratolytic preparations is inexpensive and effective but requires daily application over 6 to 12 weeks. A preparation containing 17% salicylic acid, with or without 17% lactic acid, is applied to warts daily after soaking and paring. The best time for treatment is immediately after bathing when the thickened stratum corneum overlying the wart may be easily removed with a pumice stone or callus file. Salicylic acid is also available in a 40% plaster (Mediplast) that is applied directly to the wart and left on overnight. The primary difficulty with this therapy is getting the medicated patch to stay in place. If it slips away from the wart, surrounding healthy skin is irritated.

Topical keratolytics, used properly over 12 weeks, result in cure rates of 70 to 80% of hand warts and 80% of simple plantar warts. This is a very popular method of treatment for children because it is less painful than most other treatments. Success of the treatment does, however, require a motivation of the parent and child.

Cryotherapy

Freezing warts with liquid nitrogen is the most common method of office-based wart removal. It is reliably effective in 70 to 80% of patients, relatively well tolerated, and generally free of serious complications when used carefully. It is favored over other, more destructive modalities such as electrocautery and surgery because cryotherapy is less likely to result in permanent scarring.

Liquid nitrogen can be applied using a cotton swab or a spray device. If a cotton-tipped applicator is used, the swab is dipped into a Styrofoam cup containing liquid nitrogen. A new swab is used for each application because papillomavirus can survive in liquid nitrogen and can be transmitted on the swab. The wart and a 1- to 2-mm margin of surrounding skin are frozen with a 30- to 45-second freeze-to-thaw time either once or twice, depending on the thickness of the wart. This is associated with immediate burning, stinging pain that lasts about 5 minutes. Dull, throbbing pain may continue for several hours, but this is usually relieved by over-the-counter analgesics. Patients are warned about blister formation that may become hemorrhagic. Infection is extremely unusual. Patients are instructed to leave the blister intact. If it is very painful, it may be drained, but the roof should be left in place as a natural dressing. The most common complication is hypopigmentation.

Particular caution is warranted when freezing over the digital nerves or nail matrices. These structures can be damaged if freezing is too aggressive. Cryotherapy is contraindicated in patients with conditions associated with cold intolerance such as Raynaud's disease.

Cure rates with cryotherapy drop if the interval between treatments is too long. Treating every 2 to 3 weeks until normal skin markings return is optimal. Patients may be asked to use keratolytics between treatments to potentiate therapy.

RESISTANT WARTS

Immunotherapy

Dinitrochlorobenzene (DNCB) is a potent contact sensitizer that is quite effective in treating resistant or widespread warts. It is particularly helpful when extensive periungual warts are present and there is increased risk of inducing permanent nail dystrophy or excessive pain with cryotherapy. The patient is sensitized on normal skin of the same limb as the warts (usually forearms or medial ankles) with 2% DNCB. Most patients will develop an allergic contact dermatitis in the area of application. When sensitization is successful, the chemical is applied directly to the warts on subsequent visits spaced 3 weeks apart. Warts disappear over an average of four to six treatments. This treatment is well tolerated by children with multiple warts. It is not painful, but bothersome allergic contact dermatitis may occur around warts. Patients are given topical steroids to have on hand should this become a problem.

Although this is an effective, well-tolerated, and painless procedure, multiple office visits (five to eight) are generally required. Another source of concern has centered around the fact that the chemical has a positive Ames test for mutagenicity. There is no evidence that DNCB constitutes any real danger, but this concern has led many to reserve its use for particularly resistant or widespread wart disease. Contact immunotherapy may also be accomplished with other chemicals such as diphenylcyclopropenone and squaric acid. These chemicals produce negative results in Ames test, but cure rates are somewhat lower.

Bleomycin

Bleomycin (Blenoxane)* is an antibiotic type of chemotherapeutic agent injected in small quantities into resistant warts. Bleomycin sulfate at 0.5 to 1.0 U per mL is injected directly into the wart with a 30-gauge needle or is introduced with multiple punctures of a bifurcated vaccination needle after topical application. This treatment is highly effective, and wart resolution is usually accomplished in one to three treatments. Because patients commonly experience significant pain on injection, we reconstitute bleomycin in 1% lidocaine. The total volume of the injection varies with wart size and is limited to 2 to 3 mL (1.5 U) per visit. Because serious complications such as persistent Raynaud's disease and localized tissue necrosis may result, it is recommended that only experts experienced in its application use this technique.

Laser Treatments

Of the numerous lasers that have been used for removal of resistant warts, the CO_2 laser has been used the most. It offers a great degree of precision in tissue destruction and enjoys excellent short-term cure rates. Unfortunately, the long-term follow-up studies available show no fewer recurrences with laser therapy than with other destructive techniques. It is also expensive and permanent scarring is very common, particularly after treatment of hand warts. Careful protective equipment is required because intact human papillomavirus DNA has been recovered from the CO_2 laser plume during wart treatment.

Other lasers including the 585-nm flashlamp-pulsed tunable-dye laser and, more recently, the erbium-YAG laser have been used for the treatment of warts. None of these lasers provides improvements in short- or long-term cure rates over conventional therapies, and their use is very expensive.

FLAT WARTS

Because flat warts are indeed almost flat, it is easy to damage surrounding normal skin with conventional wart treatments; thus, a different approach is needed. Tretinoin (Retin-A) cream 0.05% or 0.1% applied daily will induce the mild inflammatory reaction needed to clear flat warts. Use of sunscreen is very important during treatment because ultraviolet light exposure reliably spreads flat warts. If response has been poor after 6 to 10 weeks of tretinoin cream and sunscreen, daily application of 1 to 2% 5-fluorouracil (Efudex, Fluoroplex)* cream can be added. Excessive irritation is the primary complication of topical 5-fluorouracil cream, but persistent hyperpigmentation has also been reported. Very light application of liquid nitrogen to flat warts may also be considered in resistant cases.

ADDITIONAL THERAPIES

Cantharidin

Cantharidin (Cantharone) is a chemical derived from the blister beetle. It causes a bulla just under

---

*Not FDA approved for this indication.

*Not FDA approved for this indication.

the epidermis and is generally painless to apply. For this reason, it has a valuable place in the treatment of warts in children. It is applied in the office after paring, and treatment requires several office visits. The most problematic complication of this therapy is the potential formation of a ring of new warts surrounding the original wart.

Trichloroacetic Acid

Trichloroacetic acid in varying concentrations, usually 10 to 50%, causes tissue destruction on application and can be used for wart treatment. Penetration is difficult to control, however, and ulceration, pain, and scarring are common.

Cimetidine

There has been some enthusiasm over the past few years about the systemic use of cimetidine (Tagamet)* for the treatment of warts in children. Careful meta-analysis of the available data to this point fails to show any benefit of this approach.

Suggestion

No discussion of the treatment of common warts would be complete without mention of the great power of suggestion. Studies suggest that it is more helpful with children than with adults and probably explains the effectiveness of folk remedies. It can be used along with any wart treatment by simply telling the patient with confidence that his or her warts will be gone after a specified period of treatment.

---

*Not FDA approved for this indication.

CONDYLOMA ACUMINATUM

method of
CHARLES L. HEATON, M.D.
University of Cincinnati College of Medicine
Cincinnati, Ohio

Genital warts constitute the most common viral problem associated with sexually transmitted diseases. Between 35% and 50% of the sexually active population aged 15 to 30 years are known to be infected with one of the numerous human papillomaviruses (HPV) found on the genitalia, and approximately 60% of the sexual partners of individuals with genital warts have clinical disease. Virtually all sexual partners have HPV DNA present when a polymerase chain reaction is performed on exfoliative cells from the reproductive tract. To put this into perspective, genital warts are three times more common than herpes simplex in the sexually active population. More ominous is the increasing association of HPV with not only benign genital lesions but also genital and cervical malignancies and respiratory and cutaneous squamous cell carcinomas.

Evidence for the role of HPV in malignant oncogenesis is compelling although still largely circumstantial. Epide-miologically, HPV types 16 and 18 are routinely found in cervical dysplasia and cervical in situ neoplasm arising in sexually active populations. Approximately 90% of genital cancers contain HPV type 16, 18% contain HPV type 18, and 20% contain other HPV types. Only 1% of genital carcinomas are free of HPV.

Transmission of these viruses is through exfoliated epithelial cells, which may come from the urethra, cervix, vagina, anus, rectum, mouth, respiratory tract, or skin. Seminal fluid from some individuals has been shown to contain HPV, and crusts and scales on fomites may also serve as reservoir and vector.

The spectrum of clinical expression of infection varies from a brown macule to a small papule to a collection of papules called a *plaque* to cauliflower-like lesions that are quite large. The cutaneous macular brown lesions often herald bowenoid papulosis or carcinoma in situ. Rapidly growing tumors and extensive expression of clinical warts suggest immunosuppression on the part of the host. Frequently, organ transplant recipients and well-advanced AIDS patients express widespread wart virus infection.

Careful examination of women with external genital warts is mandatory. Frequently, women will have cervical involvement if there are external genital warts. It is important to examine the cervix of all women who have male sex partners with genital warts because almost invariably they are also infected. It is recommended that these women have Pap smears at least twice a year.

Pediatric wart infections involving genital and oral warts have for many years been considered to be a sign of sexual abuse. That concept is still debated extensively. It is estimated that no more than 25% of children with warts on oral and genital mucosa have in fact been sexually molested. It is now known that infection can be gained from mothers with asymptomatic cervical infection. Inoculation may occur at the time of delivery, with the child expressing the infection later in life. Other sources of infection may include the hands of caregivers. The clinician should carefully evaluate the family to be certain that no child molestation has occurred. This is often best accomplished by skilled social workers.

TREATMENT

Therapy for genital warts is not curative. Current treatment programs may make the patient more socially acceptable, restore and improve normal function, or relieve unpleasant symptoms. Therapy does not significantly lower epithelial viral load.

The evaluation for the selection of wart therapy should include the location of the clinical tumor, its prior response to therapies if any, the extent of the clinical tumor, and the immune status of the patient. Remember that pregnant women are at risk because of their impaired immune status, and the choice of therapy may damage the unborn fetus. Age, disease status of the patient, and current drug therapy all impact on not only the choice of therapy but also the final outcome of therapy.

Remember also that latent infection with HPV is the rule no matter how well the patient is treated or how pleasing the cosmetic outcome may be. *Recurrence is to be expected.* Treatment does not eradicate the virus.

Therapy is focused on decreasing tumor burden,

TABLE 1. **Limitations of Therapy for Condyloma Acuminatum**

Type of Treatment	Recurrence Rate (%) at 3 Mo
Simple excision	12
Electrosurgery	9
Laser surgery	14
Cryosurgery	40
Trichloroacetic acid (80% solution)	40
Podophyllin (40% solution)	50
Podophyllotoxin (Condylox 0.5%)	33
5-Fluorouracil (1% Efudex cream)*	100
Bleomycin (Blenoxane) (1 U/mL intralesional)*	50 (after one injection)
Interferon (alpha, beta, and multispecies)	30
Imiquimod (Aldara cream 5%)	Not applicable (70% of women and 33% of men have responded after 16 wk of therapy; only 2% recurred at 1 yr)
Contact sensitizers (squaric acid dibutyl ester and dinitrochlorobenzene)*	No reliable data

*Not FDA approved for this indication.

increasing the patient's cellular immune response, normalizing the rate and quality of cell proliferation in the tissue, and controlling viral spread. Tumor burden is decreased by debulking the tumor. The cellular immune response may be raised through the use of topical contact sensitizers such as squaric acid dibutyl ester and dinitrochlorobenzene and with the use of intralesional interferons and other immune modifiers.

Normalization and quality of cell proliferation can be modified with the use of vitamin A and vitamin A analogues such as Accutane and Acetretin,* bleomycin,† 5-fluorouracil,† and idoxuridine, but *none of these drugs should be used by pregnant women.* Control of viral spread is difficult. Counseling and the use of barriers during sex may be partially effective. The therapeutic limitations shown in Table 1 have been observed.

The data in Table 1 confirm the observation that most treatments do little more than make the patient more comfortable and cosmetically more appealing. They do not destroy the viruses nor do they permit unprotected sex. Transmission of the virus is still possible from cosmetically normal individuals. Virtually all sexual partners will be infected if barrier protection is not used with each and every sexual contact.

The history of therapy for genital warts is discouraging. I still prescribe the standard treatments of podophyllin for filiform warts and trichloroacetic acid and liquid nitrogen for plaque and papular warts.

*Not available in the United States.
†Not FDA approved for this indication.

I no longer use 5-fluorouracil because of the high recurrence rate associated with its use. Surgery is occasionally used but requires local anesthetics that are not always acceptable. I encourage all patients to have regular genital examinations and make it clear that no visible wart does not mean the absence of wart virus. I suggest to all women patients that they obtain a Pap test at least twice a year.

When patients can afford this treatment, I first débride the area with one of the standard chemical or surgical procedures and then offer imiquimod cream 5% (Aldara) three times a week for 16 weeks. It is hoped this combination will lower the viral population and minimize further recurrence.

MELANOCYTIC NEVI
(Moles)

method of
ALAN S. BOYD, M.D.
Vanderbilt University
Nashville, Tennessee

Melanocytic nevi are among the most common lesions arising on the skin and one of the most often submitted for histopathologic analysis. Although most of these tumors are benign and straightforward, there are occasions when they are troubling both clinically and pathologically. The average person has up to 50 nevi, a number that is affected by several factors, including genetics and amount of sun exposure during youth. Most moles arise during childhood or adolescence and reach a peak in the third decade.

Nevi are formed by nevus cells (nevomelanocytes), which are believed to develop from melanocytes within the epidermis. As the patient ages, the nevus cells drop off into the dermis, eventually forming a flesh-colored or slightly pigmented tumor known as an *intradermal nevus.* Other more uncommon variants are thought to form from aggregates of cells within the dermis.

Removal of nevi is usually for one of four reasons. The most prevalent scenario is that a nevus has become larger, symptomatic, unusually pigmented, or changed in some manner that is worrisome to the patient or clinician. Because some nevi have the capacity to become malignant (melanoma), evaluation of these specimens by a dermatopathologist is imperative. Other lesions are removed because they have become irritated or will become irritated by clothing such as waistbands and bra straps. Some moles are excised for cosmetic reasons, and, finally, some are removed to evaluate their histopathologic features and thereby develop a threshold for removal of other nevi.

TYPES OF NEVI

Junctional Nevus

Junctional nevi are most often present in young persons. They arise on almost any cutaneous surface, including the mucous membranes and nail beds. Lesions are brown to dark brown or black and usually measure no more than 6 mm in diameter. Most are round to oval, have well-demarcated borders, and are symmetrical. Some may be slightly raised with an accentuation of the skin cleavage lines, but most are flat.

Histologically, the proliferation of melanocytes is confined to the epidermis. Nests of cells are often present at the tips of the rete ridges and are usually uniform in size and configuration. The surrounding keratinocytes may be excessively pigmented. The cells display no evidence of atypia or pleomorphism, and their proliferation shows symmetry.

Compound Nevus

It is believed that as patients age junctional nevi become compound nevi. These lesions are slightly raised to pedunculated and light brown. They are round to oval with regular borders.

Nevus cells are present in the epidermis and upper dermis. Melanin may be seen in the epidermis and dermal nevus cells but usually to a lesser extent than in junctional nevi. Atypia is not present, and mitotic figures are lacking. The proliferation is, again, symmetrical.

Intradermal Nevus

Intradermal nevi are most often present in older adults. They are flesh colored and dome shaped. Most are 6 mm or smaller, but some may become much larger. Some contain hairs, and the surface, while usually smooth, may be verrucous or papillomatous and hyperkeratotic.

The proliferating nests of cells are confined to the dermis alone. Pigment production is uncommon but may be seen in the uppermost melanocytes. As the cells descend into the dermis, they become smaller and more ovoid. Atypical nevomelanocytes are very rare and if present should prompt consideration of previous irritation or inflammation or the beginnings of a melanoma.

Dysplastic Nevus

The subject of dysplastic nevi is controversial. These lesions are present in less than 10% of the populace as a whole but are found in much greater numbers in persons who sporadically develop a melanoma and persons with melanoma in their family. As such, they are considered markers for persons at greater risk for melanoma. These lesions have had various names, including *Clark's nevus, nevus with architectural and cytologic atypia,* and *B-K mole.* Patients with dysplastic nevi tend to have a greater number of moles, often more than 100. In addition, their nevi are variably sized and shaped.

Dysplastic nevi usually arise on the trunk but may also be found on the buttocks, breasts, and scalp. Individual lesions are usually 4 to 12 mm in diameter and asymmetrical. Their borders are irregular and may be difficult to visualize. A "fried egg" appearance is common, with a central raised papule and a surrounding flat component. They are light to dark brown with complex pigmentation. The topography is altered, often showing a cobblestone or pebbled appearance.

The histologic features are broken down into two components. Architecturally, the epidermis may be lentiginous, the nests of cells vary in size and shape often with bridging between adjacent rete ridges, and the lesion proliferates asymmetrically. A "shoulder phenomenon" is often present with nests of melanocytes confined to the epidermis proliferating beyond the margins of the dermal component of nevus cells. Cytologically, cells are often spindled and epithelioid. The nests may show retraction artifact from the epidermis. Nuclear atypia, including nuclear enlargement, pleomorphism, and hyperchromatism, is present. Nucleoli may be prominent. Nests of cells often display a "dusty" cytoplasm with large melanin granules. Mild fibrosis around the nests of cells is typical, as is a mild inflammatory infiltrate of lymphocytes and prominent vascularity.

Blue Nevus

Blue nevi have traditionally been divided into two categories. The common blue nevus usually arises on the hands and feet, is more prevalent in women, occurs in childhood, and is a dome-shaped blue to black papule. Most tumors are less than 10 mm in diameter. The cellular blue nevus is usually present on the scalp, head and neck, and buttocks. Lesions are a color similar to that of common blue nevi but are often larger.

Pathologically, spindle-shaped melanocytes and melanin-laden tissue macrophages are present in the dermis. The epidermis is not involved. Mild dermal fibrosis is often present. Melanocytes may aggregate around adnexal structures and can infiltrate smooth muscles and nerves. Proliferation is symmetrical and may extend deeply into the dermis.

Spitz's Nevus (Spindle and Epithelioid Cell Nevus)

Spitz's nevi were previously thought to represent a melanoma arising in childhood. Subsequent studies, however, have shown them to have a benign behavior, and radical excisions around these tumors are unwarranted. Most lesions arise on children or adolescents and more often in females. Spitz's nevi commonly occur on the face and lower extremities. Tumors are red to pink and hairless.

The histologic features of Spitz's nevi are often startling. The proliferation of cells is symmetrical with clearly demarcated borders. The epidermis may be hyperkeratotic with retraction spaces around the nests of cells. Kamino bodies, which are apoptotic melanocytes, are characteristically present in the epidermis. The nevus cells display epithelioid features with some spindling and usually very pleomorphic features. Mitotic figures, however, are rare. As the nevus cells descend into the dermis, the cells tend to become smaller with less atypia ("maturational effect") and to infiltrate between the strands of collagen.

Congenital Nevus

By definition, congenital nevi are present at birth or noticed shortly thereafter. These are uncommon lesions and are divided into small (<1.5 cm), medium (1.5 to 19.9 cm) and large (>20.0 cm) sizes. Most congenital moles are of the small variety and occur in about 1% of births. Larger lesions are rare and tend to arise on the buttocks or in the "bathing suit" area. Lesions may be flat to raised with a rugose or pebbly feel. The color is usually homogenous and ranges from tan to dark black. Hair growth is common. Satellite lesions away from the main body of the lesion are often present.

The histologic features of congenital nevi often depend on the site of biopsy and the age of the patient. Lentiginous epidermal proliferation is common. Within the dermis the nests of cells may form an interstitial pattern with involvement of adnexal structures, nerves, and blood vessels. The superficial-most nevus cells may show pleomorphic cytologic features, but an increased number of mitoses, particularly if some are atypical, suggests that malignant degeneration may have taken place.

TREATMENT

The majority of nevi may be left alone and do not require any therapy. When they are removed, the most common method is the shave biopsy or shave excision. After anesthetic has been injected, the tumor is excised in a tangential fashion with a razor blade or scalpel blade. Hemostasis is achieved with clotting agents such as aluminum chloride. This technique often leaves some nevus cells behind, and a regrowth or repigmentation of the scar may occur. It is possible to remove all the nevus cells, but this usually requires a deep "saucerization" of the area with a cosmetically unacceptable concave scar.

Suspicious lesions, particularly those believed to be a melanoma, should not be removed with a shave excision because the deep aspects of the tumor may not be visible. The prognosis of melanomas depends largely on their measured depth of dermal invasion, and a superficial shave excision may compromise that evaluation. Surgical excision is recommended with appropriate closure of the wound.

Nevi should never be destroyed with liquid nitrogen (or other cryosurgical methods) or electrocautery. Not only does this often result in a cosmetically unappealing scar, but it does not allow for histologic evaluation of the tissue specimen.

MELANOMA

method of
IRA DAVIS, M.D.
New York Medical College
Valhalla, New York

Melanoma, the most common skin cancer after basal and squamous cell carcinoma, is the deadliest of the three most common skin cancers. More than 40,000 cases are diagnosed and more than 7000 deaths are noted yearly. It is estimated that 1 of every 75 persons born in the year 2000 will develop melanoma.

DIAGNOSIS

Early detection is paramount in minimizing the mortality and morbidity associated with melanoma. The ABCDs of melanoma are helpful in diagnosing atypical lesions: *a*symmetry, *b*order irregularity, *c*olor variation, and *d*iameter greater than 6 mm. Early melanoma may lack these features. Pigmented lesions that increase in size or change color or shape should be addressed. The most common early symptom is pruritus. Late signs and symptoms include tenderness, bleeding, and ulceration.

Particular patient populations should be closely followed. Risk factors include Fitzpatrick skin type I and II, the presence of atypical nevi, large congenital nevi, and actinic skin changes. A personal history of melanoma, a family history of melanoma or atypical nevi, or a history of significant past sun exposure should arouse the concern of the physician.

The physician should note the location, size, surface change, border, and symmetry of pigmented lesions.

TABLE 1. **Suggested Margins of Excision**

Thickness (mm)	Excision Margin (cm)
In situ	0.5–1.0
0–1	1.0
1–2	1–2
2–4	2
>4	2–3

Biopsy

Suspicious lesions require a biopsy to establish a diagnosis. Because the thickness of the melanoma determines the treatment, excisional biopsy of the complete lesion is the preferred method. The specimen should include some subcutaneous fat. The excision should be oriented to allow for primary closure of the subsequent wide excision if this becomes necessary. An alternative method is saucerization, which is a deep shave biopsy that includes subcutaneous fat. This procedure requires no sutures and heals by second intention.

In certain cases, because of the size or anatomic location, the complete lesion cannot be removed. An incisional or punch biopsy can be performed in these cases. The biopsy should include the darkest and/or thickest portion of the lesion. Occasionally, multiple areas of the lesion may require sampling. This method does not increase the risk of metastases.

Shave biopsy should not be used on a presumed melanoma because the lesion will be transected.

TREATMENT

Margin of Excision

Suggested margins of excision are noted in Table 1. Excision margins depend on the thickness of the melanoma. Selective lymphadenectomy (see later) should be done before the definitive wide excision of the melanoma. The National Institutes of Health consensus development panel recommends 0.5 cm for in situ melanoma. The World Health Organization melanoma cooperative trial found that a 1-cm margin was adequate for lesions less than or equal to 2 mm in thickness. However, there was a small possibility of local recurrence with no impact on survival with these margins. Therefore, for lesions of 1 to 2 mm in thickness a 2-cm margin is preferable to avoid relapse. A 1-cm margin is appropriate in anatomically restricted areas. These guidelines result in primary closure in 90% of patients.

Guidelines are meant to be a framework. Variations on the margins of the excision may depend on certain prognostic factors, such as ulceration, anatomic location, and regression.

The excision should be oriented to allow for primary closure if possible. If feasible, the long axis should be oriented along the lymph drainage pathway to remove microsatellites. Excision should go down to but not include the muscular fascia.

Mohs' micrographic surgery or modifications of this technique using permanent horizontal sections may be useful for head and neck, hands and feet, and recurrent melanomas as well as melanomas greater than 2 cm in diameter.

Elective Lymph Node Dissection

Intraoperative lymphatic mapping and selective lymphadenectomy (SLN), a technique initially developed by Morton, allows for examination of the sentinel node as representative of the complete draining lymph node basin. This spares a complete lymph node dissection. The technique requires injection of a vital blue dye and radiocolloid at the site of the melanoma. The dye and the radiocolloid travel through the lymphatics to the draining lymph nodes. The sentinel node can then be visually and radioactively identified and removed. More than 98% of the time, the sentinel node can be correctly identified. If the node is positive for melanoma, then a complete lymph node dissection can be performed.

Sentinel lymphadenectomy is presently undergoing a randomized trial to see if the procedure results in a survival benefit. In the interim, certain patients may benefit from this procedure. Patients with melanomas greater than 1.0 mm in thickness should undergo this procedure to identify those with positive nodes who may benefit from interferon alfa-2b adjuvant therapy. Other patients in which this procedure should be considered are male patients with primary trunk lesions and patients with tumor thickness of 0.76 to 1.0 mm. These patient populations have a 9% and 5% incidence of occult nodal metastases, respectively. In addition, certain prognostic factors associated with thin melanomas (<0.76 mm) should warrant treatment of these lesions in a more aggressive manner with SLN. These patients include male patients with Clark level III (invasion fills and expands the papillary dermis), ulcerated primary lesions, lesions that exhibit regression, and axial melanomas.

In light of the advent of sentinel lymphadenectomy, the role for elective lymph node dissection will be limited if randomized studies confirm the results of previous work. Elective lymph node dissection (ELND) should still be performed in patients in whom SLN is not possible, such as those who have undergone wide excision of their primary melanoma as well as in places where SLN is not readily available. On the basis of the Intergroup Melanoma Surgical Trial of ELND for melanomas 1.0 to 4.0 mm (intermediate thickness), patients with lesions 1.1 to 2.0 mm thick and those patients who are younger than 60 years of age were noted to have a survival benefit.

Staging and Follow-up

Initial evaluation of the patient should include a thorough history and physical examination. Examination of the entire skin and mucous membranes and palpation of the lymph nodes (head and neck, axillary, supraclavicular, inguinal, and femoral nodes) should be performed. The history and physical examination should also address organ systems in which metastases commonly occur (neurologic-brain, musculoskeletal-bone, gastrointestinal-liver). Initial liver function tests and chest radiography may prove useful even if negative to serve as a baseline. It is likely that routine laboratories and chest radiography provide little additional value. Patients with local-regional disease (limited nodal metastases, satellites, and local recurrence) should have a complete blood cell count, liver function tests, chest radiography, and computed tomography (CT) of the abdomen. These tests may serve as a baseline and identify false-positive findings. CT of other body areas should be performed only if the area of disease is in or adjacent to that particular anatomic area (i.e., pelvic CT if recurrence below the waist). Patients with distant metastases may be staged with magnetic resonance imaging of the brain and CT of the chest and abdomen as well. If the primary tumor is below the waist or symptoms dictate, pelvic CT also should be done.

Suggested follow-up for various melanoma scenarios are offered in Table 2. Follow-up should include a thorough physical examination of the skin and lymphatics. Visceral metastases are not usually detected on physical examination. Chest radiography will detect pulmonary metastases. Gastrointestinal and brain metastases are usually found on the basis of review of systems (symptoms). Follow-up CT scans should be based on clinical findings. Patient education in the recognition of melanoma (ABCDs), self-examination, and sun protection should be done or reinforced at each visit.

Adjuvant Therapy

Interferon alfa-2b (Intron A) prolonged relapse-free survival and overall survival for patients with tu-

TABLE 2. **Follow-up Guidelines**

Tumor Thickness	Physical Examination	Blood Chemistry	Chest Radiograph
1 mm Negative nodes	Q 6 mo × 2 y, then annually	Annually × 5 y, then q 2 y	Annually × 5 y, then q 2 y
1–4 mm Negative nodes	Q 4 mo × 3 y, then q 6 mo × 2 y, then annually	Q 8 mo × 3 y, then annually × 2 y, then q 2 y	Annually × 5 y, then q 2 y
>4 mm Negative nodes	Q 4 mo × 3 y, then q 6 mo × 2 y, then annually	Q 8 mo × 3 y, then annually	Q 6 mo × 2 y, then annually
Positive nodes	Q 3–4 months × 5 y, then annually	Q 6–8 mo × 2 y, then annually	Q 6–8 mo × 2 y, then annually

mors larger than 4.0 mm as well as those patients with nodal disease. A recent multicenter study in a larger number of patients did not show a survival benefit in the group treated with interferon alfa-2b. Other treatments that are under clinical investigation and can be offered to those with intermediate thickness lesions or nodal disease include isolated arterial perfusion for primary and in-transit metastases of extremity lesions, adjuvant chemotherapy and adjuvant biological therapy (interferon alfa), or immunonologically active agents (vaccines). Patients with metastatic disease to distant areas may be enrolled in similar treatments. In addition, palliative therapy consisting of regional lymphadenectomy, radiation therapy, or isolated resection of metastatic lesions may be beneficial.

PREMALIGNANT LESIONS

method of
HEIDI A. WALDORF, M.D.
Waldorf Dermatology & Laser Associates, P.C.
Nanuet, New York

Mount Sinai School of Medicine
New York, New York

Recognition of and appropriate therapy for premalignant skin neoplasms are crucial aspects of any skin examination. Early removal of certain lesions can reduce the morbidity and mortality associated with malignant transformation. In addition, identification of high-risk individuals allows for the institution of preventive regimens, including vigilant sun protection, patient self-examination, and routine dermatologic surveillance.

PREMALIGNANT NEOPLASMS OF KERATINOCYTES

The epidermis is composed predominantly of keratinocytes. Under light microscopy, distinctive layers are visible: the basal, squamous, granular, and cornified layers. The cuboidal basal cells of the basal layer proliferate, migrate outward, and ultimately differentiate into the spinous squamous cells of the squamous layer. As these squamous cells advance into the granular layer, they continue the process of terminal differentiation. The cells flatten, assemble a series of keratins critical for cornification, and ultimately lose their nuclei and cellular organelles in the cornified layer. This stratum corneum varies in thickness: It is thinnest on the eyelids and thickest over the palms and soles. These cells are lost as the epidermis replaces itself every 12 to 14 days.

Keratinocytes are particularly vulnerable to short wavelength ultraviolet B radiation (UVB, 290 to 320 nm). These are the "burning rays" that, in susceptible individuals, cause severe erythema, edema, blistering, and desquamation. Chronic exposure induces mutagenesis in the keratinocyte DNA, the first step in carcinogenesis. The most common premalignant lesions seen as a result are actinic (or solar) keratoses (AK). Pathology reveals pleomorphic keratinocytes in the basal layer and disordered cornification (hyperkeratosis, increased layers, parakeratosis, retention of nuclei). Clinically, AKs present as dry, rough, scaly, erythematous macules and papules, usually less than 1 cm in diameter, on sun-exposed skin. There may be slight tenderness or pruritus. Clinical variants include pigmented AKs, hyperkeratotic AKs and cutaneous horns. Actinic cheilitis refers to AKs of the lip. Fair-skinned individuals with high occupational or recreational sun exposure are most often affected. AKs are generally first noted in the fourth and fifth decades of life, but are seen in younger individuals with significant sun exposure.

Although early AKs can spontaneously disappear if UVB exposure is limited, most remain for years. The average rate of malignant transformation into squamous cell carcinoma is estimated to be about 1%; however, a malignancy rate of 50% is reported in hyperkeratotic AKs. Large population studies indicate that the majority of patients diagnosed with cutaneous squamous cell carcinoma have coexisting AKs. Thus, treatment of AKs is medically indicated.

Surgical therapies for AKs include cryosurgery, electrodesiccation, curettage, shave excision, dermabrasion, laserabrasion, or chemical ablation (e.g., with trichloracetic acid). The goal of these destructive methods is to remove the involved epidermis. Care must be taken to avoid hypopigmentation and scarring. For extensive areas of AKs, topical chemotherapy with local application of 5% 5-fluorouracil cream or lotion is an effective nonsurgical option. Because clinical and subclinical lesions will be targeted, patients must be warned that redness, crusting, and peeling will be severe during therapy. Recalcitrant lesions should be excised to rule out foci of malignancy. Particular care should be taken of lesions of the lip because of the higher incidence of metastases from squamous cell carcinoma in that location. Arsenic-induced keratoses on the dorsal hands mimic AKs and should be treated similarly.

Human papillomavirus (HPV) also has its primary cutaneous effect on keratinocytes. Although most mucocutaneous manifestations of HPV are benign, a subset has malignant potential. HPV-associated carcinomas are more common in immunocompromised patients such as human immunodeficiency virus (HIV)-positive individuals and organ-transplant recipients. Epidermodysplasia verruciformis is a rare familial disorder of cell-mediated immunity associated with HPV-induced carcinomas on predominantly sun-exposed skin. Certain HPV DNA genotypes, including 16, 18, 31, and 35, are associated with increased risk of squamous cell carcinoma. Condyloma acuminata are cauliflower-like, pedunculated, or sessile papillomas of the oropharynx and anogenital areas that may contain high-risk HPV genotypes. Because of oncogenic potential, cervical and intra-anal examination is indicated for affected individuals and their sexual partners.

Bowenoid papulosis consists of dome-shaped,

rough, pigmented, or skin-toned papules, each a few millimeters in diameter that occur singly or in groups on the penile shaft or vulva. High-risk HPV genotypes can be isolated from these lesions. Spontaneous resolution is common; however, pathology reveals cellular atypia, and progression to squamous cell carcinoma may occur.

Oral leukoplakia is a white patch or plaque on a mucous membrane that cannot be rubbed off. Pathology reveals various degrees of epithelial dysplasia and disordered epithelial maturation. Instigating factors include viral disease (HPV or Epstein-Barr virus), chronic irritation, and tobacco use. Oral hairy leukoplakia is a variant seen in HIV-positive individuals. Oral florid papillomatosis is a variant presenting as multiple micropapules. Biopsy is necessary to confirm the diagnosis.

On nonmucosal skin, HPV-induced squamous cell carcinomas can mimic the thick keratotic papules of common warts (verruca vulgaris). This is especially true of periungual lesions. Treatment modalities for condyloma and verruca include surgical or chemical destruction and immunotherapy. Recalcitrant lesions should be biopsied to rule out carcinoma. HPV typing of specimens is available by in situ hybridization for high-risk individuals.

Porokeratosis is a familial disorder of keratinization characterized by single or multiple, erythematous to brown, hyperkeratotic papules and plaques defined by a sharply demarcated peripheral ridge. Malignant degeneration to squamous cell carcinoma or basal cell carcinoma is not infrequent. Treatment of porokeratosis involves surgical destruction, topical chemotherapy (5-fluorouracil), and topical or oral retinoids.

PREMALIGNANT NEOPLASMS OF MELANOCYTES

Melanocytes are dendritic cells, normally found in the basal layer of the epidermis, that produce pigment. On average, there is 1 melanocyte per 10 keratinocytes. Exposure to ultraviolet radiation increases the number of melanocytes and their melanin-producing activity. Both short wavelength UVB and longer wavelength UVA (tanning or "aging" rays, 320 to 400 nm) are melanogenic. Chronic exposure induces DNA damage in melanocytes.

A melanocytic nevus is a collection of melanocytes in nests. These nests can be intraepidermal (junctional nevus), intradermal (dermal nevus), or both (compound nevus). Clinically benign melanocytic nevi are small (usually less than 5 mm in diameter) symmetric, homogeneously pigmented papules with well-defined borders. Ultraviolet radiation stimulates changes in existing nevi and the production of new nevi.

Dysplastic (Clark's) nevi (DN) differ from common melanocytic nevi in their atypical clinical appearance: irregular pigmentation, ill-defined borders, and/or large size. Pathology reveals various degrees of intraepidermal melanocytic dysplasia. It is contro-

versial if DN are individually precursors of malignant melanoma; however, it is clear that patients with single or multiple DN have a higher lifetime risk of developing malignant melanoma. The risk of melanoma in individuals with familial DN syndrome can reach 100%. A Spitz's nevus, previously called juvenile melanoma, presents most commonly as an erythematous or yellow-orange papule on the face, trunk, or extremity in children. Spitz's nevi should be treated like dysplastic nevi with severe atypia and excised completely.

Congenital nevi (CN) appear at birth or within the first 2 years of life. They are common, seen in approximately 1% of newborns. Most are less than 3 cm in diameter and are singular. The risk of malignant degeneration in CN is proportional to the size. Small (less than 1.5 cm in diameter) to medium (1.5 to 20 cm) sized congenital nevi have an estimated lifetime risk for development of melanoma of between 1 and 5%. For giant congenital nevi (>20 cm) such as those covering entire anatomic units, the risk is greater than 6%. Although prepubertal metastatic melanoma is extremely rare, most reported cases have been associated with large CN.

Management of nevi vis-à-vis the risk of malignant degeneration is based on their clinical appearance, location, patient age, and personal and family history. Nevi that are atypical in appearance (the ABCDEs: Asymmetry, Border irregularity, Color change or irregularity, Diameter greater than 5 mm, Enlarging) should be surgically excised. The threshold for excision is lower for patients with a personal or family history of malignant melanoma or when the suspicious lesion is in a location that is difficult for the patient to see during self-examination. Patients with dysplastic nevus syndrome for whom excision of all suspicious lesions is not practical are studied with serial photographs and dermatologic skin examinations at short intervals. Histologic specimens revealing severe atypia or unusual changes should be re-excised to ensure clear margins. Generally, CNs are excised before puberty and when the patient is old enough to undergo surgery under local anesthesia. CN in cosmetically or functionally sensitive areas and giant CN, for which full excision is not possible or carries a high risk of morbidity or mortality, should be followed up closely and suspicious areas of pigmentation or texture change biopsied.

MISCELLANEOUS PREMALIGNANT LESIONS

Nevus sebaceous of Jadassohn is an appendageal neoplasm that consists of mature sebaceous glands, apocrine glands, and small hair follicles. Clinically it appears at birth or early childhood as a yellow, linear, verrucous papule or plaque most commonly on the scalp. It is generally removed before puberty because of the risk of malignant degeneration, most commonly to basal cell carcinoma (5 to 7%). Squamous cell carcinoma, apocrine carcinoma, and malignant eccrine poroma have also been reported in nevus sebaceous.

Parapsoriasis is a premalignant expression of mycosis fungoides (cutaneous T cell lymphoma). Parapsoriasis is classified as small plaque, large plaque, and pityriasis lichenoides. The first two variants present clinically as oval, faintly erythematous or yellow patches or thin plaques with fine "cigarette paper"–like scale. Patients may be asymptomatic or complain of pruritus. Pityriasis lichenoides presents as generalized polymorphous papules: scaly, erythematous papules become vesicular, hemorrhagic, and necrotic. Diagnosis of parapsoriasis is made based on biopsy results. Treatment modalities include lubrication, topical corticosteroids, and phototherapy. Parapsoriasis can persist for years unchanged. The goal of therapy is to prevent or delay progression to mycosis fungoides. Patients should have frequent skin examinations and undergo another biopsy if the morphology changes. Approximately 10 to 30% of large plaque parapsoriasis patients develop mycosis fungoides.

Lichen sclerosus et atrophicus is a nonviral disease of the vulva (kraurosis vulva) or penile prepuce and glans (balanitis xerotica obliterans). It appears as severely pruritic, sharply demarcated, ivory or porcelain-white, atrophic patches and plaques, which can extend onto perineal, perianal, and inguinal skin. The risk of squamous cell carcinoma in these areas is estimated to be between 3 and 6%.

PATHOLOGY

As discussed, differentiation of benign, premalignant, and malignant mucocutaneous lesions is based on histopathology. An experienced dermatopathologist, trained in both dermatology and pathology, is invaluable to the dermatologic clinician. Superficial keratinocytic lesions can generally be biopsied by curettage or shaving. Care should be taken, however, to include dermis in the specimen for evaluation to rule out progression to carcinoma. When there is doubt, a full-thickness specimen is easily obtained with a punch biopsy. Melanocytic and lymphocytic neoplasms are better biopsied with punch excisions. Small- to medium-sized pigmented lesions are often excised in full to avoid sampling error.

BACTERIAL DISEASES OF THE SKIN

method of
V. ANTOINE KELLER, M.D., and
RONALD LEE NICHOLS, M.D.

Tulane Medical School
New Orleans, Louisiana

The spectrum of bacterial diseases of the skin ranges from superficial, localized, easily recognized and easily treated skin eruptions to deep, aggressive, gangrenous, or necrotizing infections that might seem innocuous at first but quickly become life-threatening. The prompt recognition and treatment of these infections is paramount in limiting the morbidity and mortality caused by these entities. A healthy respect for the aggressiveness of gangrenous and necrotizing infections of the skin and soft tissues is developed by first harboring a high index of suspicion to provide early recognition and appropriate treatment before overwhelming clinical infection occurs.

COMMON SKIN AND SOFT TISSUE INFECTIONS

Impetigo

Impetigo is the most common bacterial infection of the skin. It is highly contagious and can occur at any age from infancy to adulthood but is most commonly seen in preschool-aged children. There are two classic forms of impetigo: nonbullous and bullous. Both forms have a predominantly staphylococcal etiology, although they present with different morphologic characteristics.

Nonbullous (crusted) impetigo can be recognized by the development of a serous, yellow-brown exudate, which dries into a golden crust. Lesions rarely elicit pain but can be associated with erythema and pruritis. They are most common on exposed areas such as the hands, feet, and legs and are often associated with a traumatic event such as an insect bite or laceration. Crusted impetigo is usually associated with a heavy mixed flora of both staphylococci and streptococci.

The bullous variety usually presents as a rapidly spreading papule, which may progress to a thin-walled vesicle if the lesion is infected with coagulase-positive *Staphylococcus aureus*, an organism that produces an exfoliative toxin. These lesions are most common in warm, moist areas of the body. Predisposing factors include warm ambient temperatures, humidity, poor hygiene, and crowded living conditions.

Treatment of impetigo begins with eradication of the environmental factors thought to be influential in the development of the process. Aggressive lesion débridement with mesh gauze sponges or brushes and antibacterial soap is encouraged, as is special attention to hygiene and disinfection of towels and bedding. Topical antibiotic treatment with mupirocin (Bactroban) has been effective in mild to moderate cases. In more extensive cases, oral systemic antibiotic therapy with a penicillinase-resistant synthetic penicillin (oxacillin) is the treatment of choice (Table 1). Erythromycin should not be used in communities that have a high incidence of resistant staphylococcal strains. Patients should be treated for at least 7 days. If no improvement is seen, lesions should be cultured and antibiotics adjusted appropriately.

Systemic complications from impetigo are very uncommon. Cellulitis has occurred, but is usually susceptible to systemic antibiotic therapy. Septicemia and staphylococcal scalded skin syndrome are exceedingly rare complications of impetigo, and, when they occur, systemic therapy is indicated.

TABLE 1. **Suggested Antibiotic Therapy for Gram-Positive Bacterial Isolates**

Isolate	Drugs of Choice		Alternative Parenteral
	Oral	*Parenteral*	
Group A beta-hemolytic *Streptococcus*	Penicillin G or V Erythromycin	Penicillin G Ampicillin/sulbactam (Unasyn) Ticarcillin/clavulanate (Timentin)	First-generation cephalosporin
Staphylococcus aureus (methicillin sensitive)	Penicillinase-resistant synthetic penicillin (Oxacillin)	First-generation cephalosporin Clindamycin Oxacillin	Azithromycin (Zithromax) Clarithromycin (Biaxin) Erythromycin
Staphylococcus aureus (methicillin resistant)		Vancomycin ± gentamicin ± rifampin	Levofloxacin (Levaquin) Trovafloxacin (Trovan)
Clostridial species	Penicillin G Clindamycin (Cleocin) Metronidazole (Flagyl)	Penicillin G Clindamycin Metronidazole	Doxycycline (Vibramycin)

Folliculitis

Folliculitis is a pyoderma that arises within a hair follicle. When this infection extends beyond the hair follicle, the process is known as a furuncle or boil. These lesions occur most frequently in the moist areas of the body and in areas subject to friction and perspiration. Host factors known to predispose one to folliculitis include obesity, blood dyscrasias, defects in neutrophil function, immune deficiency states (such as diabetes, transplant-related immunosuppression, and acquired immunodeficiency syndrome), and treatment is with corticosteroids or cytotoxic agents. The offending organism in most immunocompetent patients is usually coagulase-positive staphylococcus *(S. aureus)*; however, when immunosuppression impairs host defenses, gram-negative organisms (*Klebsiella, Enterobacter,* and *Proteus* species) can be involved.

Successful treatment of folliculitis depends on correcting the predisposing factors that promote the development of this condition. For patients with localized disease, topical wound care, including antibiotics such as mupirocin, is effective. Patients with furunculosis or multiple lesions should be treated with orally administered systemic antibiotics that are effective against *S. aureus*. Any fluctuant nodules or masses should be incised and drained, and recurrent disease deserves extended treatment.

Cellulitis

Cellulitis is an acute infection of the skin and underlying soft tissues. It commonly begins as a hot, red, edematous, sharply defined eruption and may progress to lymphangitis, lymphadenitis, and, in severe cases, necrotizing fasciitis and gangrene. Cellulitis usually occurs in the setting of local skin trauma from insect bites, abrasions, surgical wounds, contusions, and other cutaneous lacerations. Immunosuppressed patients are particularly susceptible to the progression of cellulitis to regional or systemic infections, and these patients should be treated aggressively with systemic antibiotics, drainage, and débridement where appropriate.

Initial presentation is that of a rapidly expanding, tender, erythematous, firm area of skin. An ascending lymphangitis may be present, especially in cellulitis of an extremity, and regional lymphadenopathy is common. Systemic signs and symptoms can eventually evolve and, when present, mandate hospitalization and treatment with systemic antibiotics. Offending organisms are most commonly group A beta-hemolytic *Streptococcus* species and *S. aureus*.

Treatment of localized processes is with oral antibiotics (see Table 1). If fever, septicemia, or other signs of advancement of the localized process to deeper tissues are present, the patient should be admitted to the hospital for blood and wound cultures, parenteral antibiotics (see Table 1), and observation. If a prompt response is not noted after parenteral antibiotic treatment, surgical exploration of the involved area may be indicated to rule out the presence of necrotic or gangrenous tissue. Immunosuppressed patients or patients with recurrent cellulitis should be extensively examined to exclude chronic sources of infection, and these patients should be treated with parenteral antibiotics until the cellulitis resolves, followed by 7 to 10 days of oral antibiotics.

Abscess

Signs and symptoms such as dolor, rubor, calor, and tumor often denote an abscess. Loss of function associated with fluctuance may also indicate abscess formation. Localization of purulent fluid necessitates surgical drainage and local wound care. The administration of oral or parenteral antibiotic therapy should be determined by the physician after results of wound cultures and sensitivities are obtained, but should not be used routinely after incision and drainage of localized abscesses.

LIFE-THREATENING SKIN AND SOFT TISSUE INFECTIONS

Group A Beta-Hemolytic Streptococcal Gangrene

Group A beta-hemolytic streptococcal gangrene is an extremely rapidly progressing skin and soft tissue infection commonly caused by group A beta-hemolytic streptococci. These organisms secrete hemolysins and streptolysins O and S, which are cardiotoxic, leukocidic, and responsible for the characteristic hemolysis. Gangrene results when the cutaneous blood vessels thrombose, and this finding is often associated with intense local pain. The involved skin is initially erythematous and indurated but, if treatment is delayed, quickly evolves to contain hemorrhagic blebs with focal necrotic zones. The potential for extensive tissue loss and mortality exists, especially if treatment is delayed. Therefore, prompt, aggressive tissue débridement and antibiotic therapy are necessary for a favorable outcome (see Table 1).

Synergistic Necrotizing Cellulitis

Synergistic necrotizing cellulitis (SNC) is an extremely aggressive, often lethal, polymicrobial infection of the skin and soft tissues, which exhibits progressive invasion superficial to fascial planes. This condition may arise out of an initially benign process with very little indication of the impending severity of the condition. The initial lesion in the skin is typically an erythematous, tender pustule or abscess with a small area of necrosis. The benign appearance of this lesion belies the widespread and aggressive tissue destruction that has occurred beneath it.

Direct inspection through skin incisions reveals extensive gangrene of the superficial tissues and fat that very rarely involves the underlying fascia and muscles. These lesions characteristically exude a thin, brown, malodorous discharge, which contains mixed flora with abundant polymorphonuclear leukocytes on Gram's stain. Crepitance, caused by the accumulation of gas in the tissue produced by facultative and/or obligate anaerobes, can be palpated in 25% of patients and mandates immediate attention.

The most common site of involvement is the perineum, which is involved in 50% of patients with SNC. Predisposing factors include perirectal abscess and ischiorectal abscess, both of which may track to the deeper structures of the pelvis, leading to abscess formation and subsequent septicemia. The thigh and leg are involved in approximately 40% of patients. This infection can occur after amputation and is usually associated with diabetes mellitus (75% of cases) and/or peripheral vascular disease (50% of cases). The relative immunosuppression and poor circulation that accompany these significant causes of morbidity are also responsible for upper extremity and neck SNC, which account for the remaining 10% of cases.

SNC is commonly caused by mixed flora originating in the gastrointestinal tract. Of the aerobes, coliforms are the most prevalent (*Escherichia coli, Klebsiella, Proteus*), and anaerobic flora include *Bacteroides, Peptostreptococcus, Clostridium*, and *Fusobacterium*. The primary treatment modality is aggressive débridement of nonviable skin and subcutaneous tissues. This may involve several operations and dressing changes under general anesthesia, which should be performed until all necrotic tissue is removed. Rotation or free myocutaneous flaps and split-thickness skin grafting may cover areas of tissue loss when necessary. If the perineum is involved, fecal diversion by colostomy may be necessary to facilitate healing. Empiric parenteral antibiotics effective against polymicrobial gram-positive and gram-negative aerobic and anaerobic flora are also a mainstay of therapy; however, to reduce the emergence of resistant organisms, antibiotic coverage must be modified as soon as culture and susceptibility testing reveal specific offending organisms (Table 2).

Clostridial Myonecrosis ("Gas Gangrene")

Clostridial myonecrosis is a destructive infectious process of muscle associated with infections of the skin and soft tissues. It is often associated with local crepitance and systemic signs of toxemia, which are caused by the anaerobic, gas-forming bacilli of the *Clostridium* species. This infection most often occurs after abdominal operations on the gastrointestinal tract; however, penetrating trauma, such as gunshot wounds, and frostbite can expose muscle, fascia, and subcutaneous tissues to these organisms. Common to all of these conditions is an environment containing tissue necrosis, low oxygen tension, and sufficient nutrients of amino acids and calcium to allow germination of clostridial spores and production of the lethal alpha toxin.

Clostridia are gram-positive, spore-forming, obligate anaerobes that are widely found in soil contaminated with animal excretia. They have also been isolated from the human gastrointestinal tract and skin, most importantly from the perineum and oropharynx. *Clostridium perfringens* is the most common isolate (present in 80% of cases), and is among the fastest growing clostridial species, having a gen-

TABLE 2. **Suggested Parenteral Antibiotic Therapy for Mixed Infections**

Organisms	Primary Choice
Aerobic: Must include an agent effective against anaerobic organisms	Amikacin (Amikin)
	Ceftriaxone (Rocephin)
	Ciprofloxacin (Cipro)
	Tobramycin (Nebcin)
	Levofloxacin (Levaquin)
	Aztreonam (Azactam)
	Gentamicin (Garamycin)
Anaerobic: Must include an agent effective against aerobic organisms	Chloramphenicol (Chloromycetin)
	Metronidazole (Flagyl)
	Clindamycin (Cleocin)
Aerobic/anaerobic coverage	Ampicillin/sulbactam (Unasyn)
	Piperacillin/tazobactam (Zosyn)
	Meropenem (Merrem)
	Ticarcillin/clavulanic acid (Timentin)
	Ceftizoxime (Cefizox)
	Cefoxitin (Mefoxin)
	Imipenem/cilastatin (Primaxin)
	Trovafloxacin (Trovan)

eration time, under ideal conditions, of approximately 8 minutes. This organism produces collagenases and proteases that cause widespread tissue destruction as well as alpha toxin, which is associated with the high mortality of clostridial myonecrosis. The alpha toxin causes extensive capillary destruction and hemolysis, leading to necrosis of the muscle and overlying fascia, skin, and subcutaneous tissues.

Historically, clostridial myonecrosis was a disease associated with battle injuries, but presently, 60% of cases now occur after trauma—50% of these after automobile accidents, and the remainder after crush injuries, industrial accidents, and gunshot wounds. Mortality can be the result of a failure to recognize that clostridial infection is under way, which leads to a delay in the débridement of devitalized tissues. Patients often complain of a sudden onset of pain at the site of trauma or their surgical wound, increasing rapidly in severity, and extending beyond the original borders of the wound. The skin initially becomes edematous and tense; its pale appearance progresses to a magenta hue. Hemorrhagic bullae are common, as is a thin, watery, foul-smelling discharge. Gram's stain examination of wound discharge reveals abundant gram-positive rods with a paucity of leukocytes.

The diagnosis of gas gangrene is based on the appearance of the muscle upon direct visualization by surgical exposure because many of the changes are not apparent when inspected through a small traumatic wound. Initially, the muscle is pale, edematous, and unresponsive to stimulation. As the disease process continues, the muscle becomes frankly gangrenous, black, and extremely friable. This is, however, a very late event and is often accompanied by septicemia and shock. Despite profound hypotension, renal failure, advancing crepitance, and fever, these patients may be remarkably alert and extremely sensitive to their surroundings. They feel their impending doom and often panic just before slipping into toxic delirium and eventually coma.

The clinical features should arouse suspicion early in the course, so the disease can be recognized and aggressive surgical débridement can be undertaken. Gas in the wound is a relatively late finding, and by the time crepitance is appreciated the patient may be near death. Approximately 15% of blood cultures are positive, but this too is a late finding. Serum creatinine kinase levels, although relatively nonspecific, are always elevated in cases with muscle involvement.

The mortality rate of gas gangrene is as high as 60%. It is highest in cases involving the abdominal wall and lowest in those affecting the extremities. Among the signs that prognosticate a poor outcome are leukopenia, thrombocytopenia, hemolysis, and severe renal failure. Myoglobinuria is common and can contribute significantly to worsening renal function. Frank hemorrhage may also be present and is a harbinger of disseminated intravascular coagulation.

Successful treatment of this life-threatening infection depends on early recognition and débridement of devitalized and infected tissues. Hyperbaric oxygen and systemic antibiotics are also important adjuncts. Surgical intervention should include wide débridement of all necrotic tissue and amputation if extremities are involved. Hyperbaric oxygen (100% O_2 at 3 atm) has been reported to reduce associated tissue loss and mortality; however, the mainstay of treatment is surgical débridement, and this should never be delayed to arrange for hyperbaric oxygen treatments. A parenteral antibiotic is directed toward the offending organism (see Table 1). Cardiovascular collapse mandates intravenous fluid resuscitation and may require large volumes. Failure to adequately resuscitate these patients compromises therapy by limiting oxygen delivery and antibiotic distribution to the affected tissues and may promote progression to multisystem organ failure.

A less life-threatening form of this disease is known as clostridial cellulitis. In this process, the bacterial tissue invasion is primarily superficial to the fascial layer without muscle involvement. Prompt recognition and treatment, as described earlier, can reduce morbidity and mortality.

Necrotizing Fasciitis

Necrotizing fasciitis is an aggressive soft tissue infection involving the fascia with extensive undermining and tracking along anatomic planes. This process usually occurs in patients with significant comorbidity such as diabetes mellitus or peripheral vascular disease, but it is also seen in obese or malnourished patients and in intravenous drug abusers. Cellulitis is a frequent occurrence, and progressive necrosis of the underlying subcutaneous tissue results from thrombosis of the perforating vessels. Classically associated with group A beta-hemolytic streptococci and staphylococci, the disease may now be caused by a variety of organisms, including aerobic streptococci, staphylococci, and coliforms, as well as anaerobic *Peptostreptococcus* and *Bacteroides*. Ninety percent of these infections are polymicrobial in etiology, and it is common to culture up to 15 organisms from the fascial planes involved with this infection.

Necrotizing fasciitis most commonly evolves from a benign-appearing skin lesion (80% of cases). Minor abrasions, insect bites, injection sites, and perirectal abscesses have all been implicated. Rare cases have been reported in women with Bartholin's gland abscess, from which the infection has spread to fascial planes of the perineum and thigh. The remaining 20% of patients have no visible skin lesion. Surgical procedures, especially bowel resections and penetrating trauma, can be complicated by superficial wound infections that evolve into necrotizing fasciitis. The infection commonly involves the buttocks and perineum, which result from untreated perirectal abscesses or decubitus ulcers; intravenous drug abusers commonly participate in "skin popping," which leads to infections of the upper extremities. The idiopathic form, commonly known as "spontaneous necrotizing fasciitis," is particularly dangerous due to the frequent delay in diagnosis.

The initial presentation is that of a slowly advancing cellulitis that progresses to a firm, tense, woody feel of the subcutaneous tissues. This entity may be distinguished from other aggressive anaerobic soft tissue infections (i.e., synergistic necrotizing cellulitis) by the brawny, pale, erythematous appearance of the skin overlying subcutaneous tissues that are unyielding, making fascial planes and muscle groups indistinguishable on palpation. Often a broad erythematous tract along the route of the underlying fascial plane can be discerned through the skin. If an open wound exists, probing the edges with a blunt instrument permits ready dissection of the superficial fascia well beyond the wound margins, and this is the most important diagnostic feature of necrotizing fasciitis. On direct inspection, the fascia is swollen and dully gray on appearance, with stringy areas of fat necrosis. A thin, brown exudate can be expressed from the wound, and frank purulent drainage is rare. These wounds are remarkably insensate when found and mandate immediate débridement.

As with other gangrenous soft tissue infections, the most important component of the treatment plan is aggressive, total débridement of all devitalized and necrotic tissue. This may often necessitate frequent operations and dressing changes. Wide débridement and parenteral antibiotics have a profound effect on survival, and limited or staged débridement has no place in the treatment of this very aggressive, life-threatening infection. Parenteral antibiotics (see Table 2) should be directed against the polymicrobial aerobic and anaerobic microorganisms isolated from these infections. Every effort should be made to quickly identify the offending organisms, and antibiotic therapy should be changed accordingly.

There is a rarely reported monomicrobial form of this disease known as *idiopathic necrotizing fasciitis* (INF). When erythema, induration, and warmth occur without trauma or other obvious cause for the infection, one must consider this entity, as it often arises without any obvious portal of entry. Misdiagnosis and delay in diagnosis are common (this disease is often mistaken for arthritis), and are associated with significant morbidity and mortality. Surgical exploration with débridement of infected and necrotic tissue, in addition to systemic antibiotic therapy directed toward the aerobic *Streptococcus*, can result in decreased morbidity and mortality (see Table 1).

SPECIAL CIRCUMSTANCES

Fournier's Gangrene

Necrotizing fasciitis that originates as a necrotic black area on the scrotum of male patients most often has a cryptogenic origin. In the authors' experience, Fournier's gangrene occurs more commonly without a predisposing event or after routine, uncomplicated hemorrhoidectomy. Less commonly, this condition has occurred after urologic manipulation or as a late complication of deep anorectal suppuration. Fournier's gangrene is characterized by necrosis of the skin and soft tissues of the scrotum and/or perineum associated with a fulminant, painful, and severely toxic infection. Definitive diagnosis is made by identification of a necrotic black area on the scrotum associated with local and systemic signs of infection. Left untreated, death ensues from uncontrolled, severe systemic sepsis and multiple organ failure. Prompt recognition and treatment can minimize tissue loss, specifically the skin and soft tissues of the scrotum and perineum, and may prevent complete loss of genitalia.

The infection is often polymicrobial, as with necrotizing fasciitis, with several species of aerobic and anaerobic bacteria predominating. Successful treatment is, again, based on early recognition and vigorous surgical débridement, often including diversion of the fecal stream. Empirical treatment is appropriate until results of culture and susceptibility testing are available (see Table 2). The therapeutic benefit of hyperbaric oxygen treatments remains to be proved and should only be used as an adjunct to surgical débridement at this time.

Ecthyma Gangrenosum

Occasionally, hospitalized patients with overwhelming pseudomonal septicemia develop a patchy dermal and subcutaneous necrosis. Although sepsis caused by *Pseudomonas aeruginosa* is often indistinguishable from other types of gram-negative sepsis, a characteristic skin lesion may develop with erythematous macular eruptions that quickly become bullous with central ulceration and necrosis. This lesion may resemble a decubitus ulcer with the characteristic black eschar. There are usually multiple lesions occurring in different stages of development, which may concentrate on the extremities or the gluteal region. These lesions may be distinguished from the lesions of pyoderma gangrenosum (a noninfectious dermatosis) by their association with clinical signs of infection (i.e., fever and leukocytosis) in addition to the isolation of *P. aeruginosa* from culture of the lesion. Treatment is primarily by administration of antimicrobial therapy (see Table 2) and by débridement of multiple lesions (in selected patients), which may lessen the bacterial burden, perhaps allowing greater antibiotic efficacy.

Sea Water Infections

Infections caused by *Vibrio vulnificus* and *Aeromonas hydrophilia* can be extremely aggressive, with necrosis often occurring within hours and necessitating rapid, wide débridement. Although infections caused by these organisms cannot be differentiated from those caused by mixed infections, a history of exposure to sea water and the rapidity with which the infection spreads often suggest the true etiology of the infection. The antibiotics of choice for *V. vul-*

nificus infection is doxycycline or tetracycline and an aminoglycoside. In cases with impaired renal function, chloramphenicol may be used.

CONCLUSION

The wide range of soft tissue infections caused by bacteria may be distinguished by their wide variety of presenting signs and symptoms and body location and by the time course of the pathologic processes unique to each. Early, prompt recognition is of paramount importance to the effective treatment plan, which most often includes aggressive surgical débridement and specific antimicrobial therapy. This approach can minimize tissue damage and promote recovery.

VIRAL SKIN INFECTIONS

method of
JESSICA L. SEVERSON, M.D.
University of Texas Medical Branch
Galveston, Texas

and

MONICA L. McCRARY, M.D.
Medical College of Georgia
Augusta, Georgia

HERPES SIMPLEX VIRUSES

Etiology and Epidemiology

Orolabial herpes, more commonly known as cold sores or fever blisters, is usually due to herpes simplex virus type 1 (HSV-1). Eighty to 90% of the population is seropositive for antibodies to HSV-1. Genital herpes is usually caused by herpes simplex virus type 2 (HSV-2), although it is not uncommonly due to HSV-1. The prevalence of HSV-2 seropositivity in the United States has increased by 30% in the past two decades. Forty-five million people (1 in every 5) older than 12 are seropositive, according to the Centers for Disease Control and Prevention.

Pathogenesis

The herpes simplex viruses are spread by direct contact with the infectious agent present in lesions, skin, mucosal surfaces, and mucosal secretions. Dormancy is established in sensory nerve ganglion until reactivation. Recurrences may be triggered by physical or emotional stress, fever, exposure to ultraviolet light, skin damage such as chapping or abrasion, immune suppression, or fatigue. Most recurrences are subclinical; others fail to progress beyond the prodrome or papule stage. First-episode primary genital herpes occurs in seronegative individuals 7 to 10 days after initial exposure to the virus. First-episode nonprimary genital herpes occurs in a seropositive individual. These patients have had a previous exposure to the virus but only later (months or years later) develop clinical evidence of genital herpes.

The transmission of genital herpes continues to be studied. Asymptomatic shedding of the virus occurs on 5 to 50% of days sampled by viral culture in the genital area. The transmission rate is 5 to 10% per year, with females acquiring the virus at a higher rate than males. Previous HSV-1 seropositivity is thought not to decrease the acquisition of HSV-2 as once thought but contribute to asymptomatic primary infection with the virus because of circulating antibodies for HSV-1. The majority of these people seropositive for HSV-2 have never had a recognized clinical outbreak of genital herpes. However, after education about genital herpes, the majority of these seropositive people will then recognize outbreaks.

The only way for complete prevention of transmission of genital herpes is sexual abstinence. Condoms only protect what they cover, but are an important aspect of prevention. Sexual abstinence during an outbreak is important owing to increased virus present, but asymptomatic shedding still exists. Antiviral suppression in the source partner is being investigated to determine the effect on HSV-2 transmission to the seronegative susceptible partner.

Clinical Manifestations

Prodromal signs and symptoms of an HSV outbreak may include fever, chills, malaise, myalgias, fatigue, headache, as well as localized lymphadenopathy, pain, burning, itching, tingling, and swelling. The herpetic lesions then progress from erythema to papule, vesicle, ulcer, and finally crusting if the lesion is in an area of keratinized skin. The outbreak may consist of single or multiple lesions. Primary cases are usually more severe than subsequent recurrences and may even result in urinary retention. Primary orolabial infection with HSV can present as herpetic gingivostomatitis in children and young adults. Sore throat and fever develop, as well as painful vesicles and ulcers on the tongue, palate, gingiva, buccal mucosa, and lips. Healing time averages 7 to 14 days without treatment and 3 to 7 days with early treatment. Some patients may even abort an outbreak altogether by initiating treatment with an oral antiviral drug during the prodrome. Recurrences may vary from once or twice per month to once every few years.

Diagnosis

Diagnosis may be aided by sampling vesicles for viral culture, direct fluorescent antibody, or polymerase chain reaction. Serologic testing via Western blot is 99% sensitive and specific for HSV antibodies. Enzyme-linked immunosorbent assay cannot reliably distinguish between the two herpes simplex viruses because of cross-reacting antibodies. An increase in IgM in relation to IgG can distinguish between a true primary infection and a nonprimary first episode of genital herpes.

Treatment (Table 1)

Oral acyclovir has shown efficacy in healing the lesions of herpes labialis, although topical acyclovir cream has had inconsistent results and further studies are being conducted. Oral valacyclovir (1 gram per day orally or 500 mg twice a day orally) has been shown to prevent HSV outbreaks after full facial laser resurfacing, although further studies are needed to confirm these findings and define an optimal dosing regimen. Topical penciclovir (Denavir) is the only antiviral agent approved by the U.S. Food and Drug Administration (FDA) for treatment of herpes labialis in immunocompetent persons. Lesions, pain, and viral shedding resolve more quickly with use of penciclovir. The side effects are comparable to those of a placebo.

Oral antiviral drugs are safe and effective for episodic treatment as well as suppression of recurrent genital herpes. Acyclovir, famciclovir, and valacyclovir therapy shorten the duration and severity of the signs and symptoms of recurrent genital herpes. Valacyclovir is the L-valyl ester of acyclovir, and famciclovir is the oral prodrug of penciclovir. Acyclovir and penciclovir are competitive inhibitors of viral DNA polymerase, which results in termination of viral replication. Antiviral suppression results in complete absence of outbreaks in the majority of patients. Others experience fewer and milder recurrences. Suppressive therapy reduces asymptomatic viral shedding by 95%. The side effect profile of these antiviral drugs matches that of placebo. Headache, nausea, and abdominal pain are the most common complaints. With such safe and effective treatment, many patients believe their genital herpes is merely a nuisance.

Lobucavir is a broad-spectrum nucleoside analogue found safe and superior to placebo in healing recurrent genital herpes and resolution of pain. Cidofovir (Vistide), a nucleoside analogue of deoxycytidine monophosphate, had significant antiviral effect on lesions of recurrent genital herpes in initial studies. Further studies with these agents are ongoing. Vaccines, both preventive and therapeutic, are also in clinical trials.

Interrelationships Between HSV and Human Immunodeficiency Virus

Genital herpes is the most frequent sexually transmitted disease among human immunodeficiency virus (HIV)–seropositive persons. HSV-2 seroprevalence is 81% in HIV-positive homosexual or bisexual men. Co-infection of HSV and HIV may result in both stimulation and suppression of the systemic immune response. Repeated activation of T lymphocytes due to HSV, as well as HSV-induced immunosuppression, may add to HIV susceptibility and progression of HIV disease. On the other hand, HIV-induced immunosuppression results in alterations in the natural history of HSV. More severe HSV outbreaks and more frequent viral shedding is common in HIV/HSV co-infection compared with non-HIV infection. Treatment of HSV can be more challenging in the HIV-infected patient. Increased dosing of anti-

TABLE 1. **Antiviral Treatments for Herpes Simplex Virus and Varicella Zoster Virus**

Viral Disease	Drug	Dosage
Herpes Simplex Virus		
Orolabial herpes		
Recurrence	Penciclovir (Denavir)	1% cream applied q 2 h for 4 days
Genital herpes		
First episode	Acyclovir (Zovirax)	400 mg PO tid or
		200 mg PO 5×/d for 7–10 days
	Valacyclovir (Valtrex)	1 gram PO bid for 7–10 days
	Famciclovir (Famvir)*	250 mg PO tid for 7–10 days
Recurrence	Acyclovir	400 mg PO tid for 5 days
	Valacyclovir	500 mg PO bid for 5 days
	Famciclovir	125 mg PO bid for 5 days
Chronic suppression	Acyclovir	400 mg PO bid
	Valacyclovir	500 mg PO bid or qd for ≤9 outbreaks/y
	Famciclovir	250 mg PO bid
Immunocompromised	Acyclovir	5 mg/kg IV q 8 h for 7–14 days or
		400 mg PO 5×/d for 7–14 days
Neonatal	Acyclovir	10 mg/kg IV q 8 h for 10–21 days
Varicella Zoster Virus		
Varicella	Acyclovir	20 mg/kg (800 mg max) PO qid for 5 days
Zoster	Acyclovir	800 mg PO 5×/d for 7–10 days
	Valacyclovir	1 gm PO tid for 7 days
	Famciclovir	500 mg PO tid for 7 days
Adult immunocompromised	Acyclovir	10 mg/kg IV q 8 h for 7 days
Pediatric immunocompromised	Acyclovir	500 mg/m² IV q 8 h for 7–10 days

*Not FDA approved for this indication.

viral drugs may be required, and the HIV population has an increased incidence of acyclovir-resistant HSV. In addition, disruption of the epithelial barrier and inflammation of HSV genital ulcers appear to increase the risk of HIV transmission.

These interrelationships have compelling implications for HIV control efforts, and intervention of these virus–virus interactions may have modulatory effects on progression of HIV infection. A survival benefit is seen when acyclovir is added to an HIV-positive patient's medical regimen. Further evidence suggests that HSV suppression with acyclovir indirectly lowers HIV viral load, which is important in predicting disease progression and response to anti-retroviral therapy.

Other HSV Infections

Although primarily oral or genital, HSV may infect any area of the body. Herpetic whitlow occurs on fingers when exposed to oral mucosa without glove protection. Herpes gladiatorum occurs in contact sports such as wrestling when direct skin-to-skin contact occurs with an athlete with active skin lesions. Lumbosacral herpes is often misdiagnosed as shingles until recurrence becomes apparent from the patient's history. Herpetic sycosis of the beard area and folliculitis have been reported in patients with follicular, painful vesicles that are unresponsive to antibacterial or antifungal treatment. Eczema herpeticum is a widespread infection with HSV in an individual with an underlying skin disorder such as atopic dermatitis. Erythema multiforme, classically presenting as erythematous papules that develop into target lesions and mucosal ulcerations, can appear with each recurrent episode of herpes. Neonatal herpes mostly results from intrapartum acquisition of HSV, which can lead to death or severe neurodevelopmental disability. The incidence of neonatal infection is 2 to 13.8 cases per 100,000 live births. Twenty-five percent of infants who contract herpes at delivery will develop disseminated herpetic infection, which has a 40% mortality rate despite antiviral therapy.

VARICELLA ZOSTER VIRUS

Etiology and Epidemiology

Varicella zoster virus (VZV) is the third human herpesvirus. It is the cause of varicella, more commonly known as chickenpox, and its reactivation results in zoster, also known as herpes zoster and shingles. More than 90% of the population has been infected with VZV. Twenty percent of those infected with VZV will develop shingles. Incidence and severity of the infection increase with patient age.

Pathogenesis

Initial infection with VZV is spread by respiratory droplets and contact with vesicular fluid. A person is considered contagious until the last vesicle crusts. A person with zoster cannot infect another with zoster but can infect another with chickenpox if the susceptible individual comes into direct contact with vesicular fluid. Everyone infected with VZV has the potential to develop zoster. VZV, similar to HSV, has the capacity to invade and replicate in the central nervous system and establish latency in the dorsal root ganglion. The stimulus for reactivation is similar to HSV as well. Immunologic status and stress, both emotional and physical, are often linked to the development of zoster.

Clinical Manifestations

Chickenpox consists of a generalized exanthem of simultaneously occurring pruritic macules, papules, vesicles, and crusts. The lesions are located centrally and on the proximal extremities. A low-grade fever and malaise are typical. Secondary bacterial infection is the most common complication of varicella in children. In adults, pneumonia may develop and has a 10 to 30% mortality.

Patients with zoster often have prodromal symptoms of pain, numbness, tingling, and/or itching before the appearance of classic vesicles with an erythematous base. Pain can be severe enough to prompt such misdiagnoses as myocardial infarction or surgical abdomen. It is described as burning, aching, and/or lancinating. The outbreak typically follows a unilateral dermatomal distribution. It is bilateral in 4% of patients, and recurrences in immunocompetent patients occur in 1 to 5% of cases, with 50% of these recurring in the same dermatome. Occasionally, cutaneous dissemination, defined as 20 or more vesicles outside primary or adjacent dermatomes, may occur. This is most common in immunocompromised individuals. Other complications of zoster include postherpetic neuralgia, ophthalmic zoster, motor paralysis, secondary bacterial infection, pneumonitis, encephalitis, and hepatitis. Postherpetic neuralgia, which is pain after the rash resolves, increases with patient age; and pain may continue for months or even years. Ophthalmic zoster has a 20 to 70% chance of involving the eye, causing problems ranging from conjunctivitis to blindness.

Diagnosis

The same diagnostic techniques used for HSV can be used for VZV, and often a careful history and physical examination are all that is needed. A history of recurrences is important because a patient with "shingles on the buttocks that keeps coming back" is caused by HSV until proven otherwise. This distinction affects treatment (i.e., dosage) and patient counseling regarding spread of the infection.

Prevention

Varicella is the leading cause of vaccine-preventable death in the United States; yet only about 26%

of children receive the varicella vaccine (Varivax). Varivax was approved in March 1995 and is recommended by the American Academy of Pediatrics for all children 12 months of age and older. One dose is recommended for children 12 months to 13 years of age, and two doses, with a 4- to 8-week interval, are recommended for those older than 13. Seroconversion of children after one dose of Varivax is 97%, and it gives 95% protection against severe disease. The live, attenuated vaccine is contraindicated in the immunocompromised, those with a family history of immunodeficiency, those with anaphylaxis to neomycin, and pregnant women. Side effects include injection site tenderness in 20 to 30% of patients, a transient rash in 5 to 10%, and, rarely, a fever of 102°F or greater. Studies are being done to determine if a "booster" immunization 4 to 6 years after the primary vaccine is necessary. Also, the vaccine is being tested in older individuals to boost their natural immunity to VZV and prevent zoster.

Varicella-zoster immunoglobulin is recommended for passive immune prophylaxis of the immunocompromised if exposure to the virus occurs without previous varicella infection or vaccination. It should also be considered in neonates whose mothers develop varicella 5 days before delivery until 2 days after delivery and in susceptible pregnant women exposed to VZV.

Treatment

Antiviral treatment for varicella (see Table 1) is usually not necessary for healthy children, but acyclovir may be used for immunocompromised patients and adults. Early treatment is vital for shingles, however. By the time vesicles are seen on the skin, active replication of the virus exists. Acyclovir, valacyclovir, or famciclovir treatment results in decreased duration of pain and healing time of cutaneous lesions. Valacyclovir and famciclovir also decrease the duration and severity of postherpetic neuralgia. Multiple treatments are available for postherpetic neuralgia. It is best if patients are treated early with an antiviral agent to decrease the severity and duration of pain. Other treatment options for postherpetic neuralgia include analgesics, narcotics, amitriptyline (Elavil),* capsaicin (Zostrix-HP), and nerve blocks. Recently, gabapentin (Neurontin) was found effective in treatment of pain and sleep interference associated with postherpetic neuralgia. Mood and quality of life also improved with this treatment. Gabapentin is lipophilic, penetrates the blood-brain barrier, and appears to involve GABA receptor binding.

EPSTEIN-BARR VIRUS

Human herpesvirus 4 (HHV-4) or Epstein-Barr virus (EBV) is associated with such diseases as infectious mononucleosis, African Burkitt's lymphoma,

nasopharyngeal carcinoma, oral hairy leukoplakia in patients with the acquired immunodeficiency syndrome, lymphoma and lymphoproliferative diseases in immunocompromised patients, and chronic fatigue syndrome. In infectious mononucleosis, the virus is spread by saliva, giving it the name "kissing disease." Clinical symptoms consist of a prodrome of headache, malaise, and fever for 3 to 5 days before the onset of a sore throat and posterior cervical lymphadenopathy. Other findings may include a gray-white exudative tonsillitis, red petechiae at the border of the hard and soft palates, splenomegaly, and hepatomegaly. An exanthem that is macular, maculopapular, morbilliform, urticarial, vesicular, petechial, or erythema multiforme–like develops on the trunk and upper extremities in 3 to 16% of patients. If patients are treated with a penicillin derivative such as ampicillin, the likelihood of the rash is increased fivefold. The rash may last a week, then desquamate. Patients may tolerate ampicillin after the EBV infection has cleared. Initially, granulocytopenia occurs, followed in 1 week by a lymphocytic leukocytosis with atypical lymphocytes. A positive monospot test or increased titers of heterophile antibodies (>1:112) may be detected by 4 weeks after onset of the illness. Ten percent of patients are heterophile negative, and children younger than 4 years of age have a high false-positive rate, so EBV-specific antibodies are needed for a definitive diagnosis. Treatment is symptomatic.

CYTOMEGALOVIRUS

Most people are infected with human herpesvirus type 5 or cytomegalovirus (CMV). It remains in a latent stage and is typically symptomatic only in neonates or the immunocompromised. The virus is found in urine, tears, breast milk, feces, semen, cervical secretions, blood, and saliva. After initial reactivation, viremia occurs, followed by infection of the vascular endothelium, an exanthem, vasculitis, and ulcerations. Relative sparing of epithelium exists because the virus prefers endothelial and ductal cells. Basophilic intranuclear inclusions, or "owl's eyes," are pathognomonic and are seen in urine, blood, and throat cultures.

Congenital CMV is the major infectious cause of mental retardation and deafness in the United States. Dermal hematopoiesis results in purpuric macules and papules leading to the term "blueberry muffin baby." Immunocompromised patients may have multiple skin lesions ranging from vesicles to verrucous plaques as well as CMV retinitis, colitis, and esophagitis. Probably the most specific skin finding in CMV is perianal ulcerations. In addition, in healthy patients a CMV mononucleosis-like syndrome with urticarial or morbilliform eruptions has been reported. Cidofovir, foscarnet, and ganciclovir are approved for treatment of CMV infections.

EXANTHEM SUBITUM

Exanthem subitum, also called roseola infantum and sixth disease, is due to human herpesvirus type

---

*Not FDA approved for this indication.

6 (HHV-6). It is a mild, self-limited disease, usually occurring in children aged 6 months to 2 years. High fever for 3 to 5 days is followed by 2- to 3-mm discrete rose-pink macules or maculopapules that blanch and may be tender. The trunk is affected first, followed by the neck and extremities. Also seen are periorbital edema (Berliner's physical sign) and petechiae of the soft palate. Treatment is symptomatic.

HUMAN HERPESVIRUS TYPE 7

Human herpesvirus type 7 (HHV-7) was isolated in 1990. Primary infection occurs during childhood, but its association with human disease has not been definitive. Some cases of roseola infantum have been linked to HHV-7, and HHV-7 DNA has been found in patients with pityriasis rosea during an outbreak, but not after recovery or in controls. The significance of these findings is not yet known.

HUMAN HERPESVIRUS TYPE 8

The eighth human herpesvirus (HHV-8) is postulated to be a latent virus that is associated with Kaposi's sarcoma lesions during immunosuppressed states. Kaposi's sarcoma manifests as mucocutaneous violaceous papules, nodules, plaques, and edema. HHV-8 DNA has also been found in patients with carcinomas, body cavity–based lymphomas, pemphigus vulgaris, and pemphigus foliaceus. The significance of these findings in not known. Treatment options include cryosurgery, chemotherapy (chlorambucil,* cyclophosphamide,* vinblastine, or actinomycin*), radiotherapy, interferon, electrodesiccation, laser therapy, and cidofovir.

HUMAN PARVOVIRUS B19

A benign childhood exanthem, erythema infectiosum or fifth disease, is caused by a single-stranded DNA virus, parvovirus B19, a member of the Parvoviridae. The virus is transmitted through respiratory secretions mainly in children aged 4 to 15 years. The peak incidence is in the spring and winter. Headache, chills, and mild constitutional symptoms are followed 7 days later by a "slapped-cheek" appearance, which is a bright red rash on the cheeks with circumoral pallor. One to 4 days later, an erythematous maculopapular rash with a lacelike reticular pattern may be seen on the proximal extremities. Treatment is symptomatic.

POXVIRUSES

Molluscum contagiosum virus is a DNA virus of the poxvirus family. It affects children, sexually active adults, and immunocompromised individuals. It is mostly a benign, asymptomatic disease but can be troublesome in 5 to 18% of HIV-infected individuals. The virus is spread by direct person-to-person con-

tact as well as by fomites. Molluscum contagiosum manifests as dome-shaped papules with an umbilicated center that can be found anywhere on the body. Curdlike material from the papules can be extracted, stained, and observed under the microscope, where Henderson-Paterson bodies, or large intracytoplasmic inclusion bodies, are seen to aid in the clinical diagnosis. Multiple treatments are available, including tretinoin (Retin-A),* cantharidin (Cantharone), excision, curettage, electrodesiccation, oral griseofulvin,* topical fluorouracil (Efudex),* acyclovir ointment,* carbolfuchsin, cryotherapy, cimetidine,* topical mupirocin (Bactroban),* oral isotretinoin, intralesional interferon, 30% trichloroacetic acid peel, topical and systemic psoralen with ultraviolet A, and electron irradiation. Topical and intravenous cidofovir, which has broad-spectrum anti-DNA virus activity, has shown significant improvements in HIV-infected patients. Further studies are being conducted.

Orf, or ecthyma contagiosum, is a zoonotic infection endemic in sheep and goats. Infection causes nodules on the mouth and nose of animals that can spread to humans. The virus is quite hardy, living on fomites for extended periods of time. In humans, the virus typically affects the right index finger with single to multiple 1.5- to 5.0-cm papules or nodules. The infection heals slowly in about 35 days after proceeding through papule, target, regenerative, papillomatous, and finally regression stages. Diagnosis is by history and physical examination. Treatment is symptomatic.

Milker's nodule is a zoonotic infection that is endemic among cows, in which it is termed "pseudocowpox." When transmitted to humans, it causes macules on the finger, hand, or forearm that progress to papules, then targetoid papulovesicles that erode and crust. The lesions are asymptomatic and heal in approximately 4 weeks. Again, diagnosis is by history and physical examination, and treatment is symptomatic.

COXSACKIEVIRUSES

Hand-foot-and-mouth disease is associated with several coxsackieviruses, especially A16, in the family Picornaviridae. The infection is spread by the oral or fecal-oral route. A prodrome of malaise, low-grade fever, anorexia, abdominal pain, or respiratory symptoms is followed by painful oral lesions. Red macules progress from 1- to 3-mm to 2-cm vesicles with an erythematous base. Soon, shallow yellow-gray ulcerations surrounded by a red halo develop on the hard palate, tongue, and buccal mucosa. On the extremities an exanthem of macules and papules develops into gray vesicles with an erythematous base. Healing occurs in about 1 week. Diagnosis is by physical examination, and treatment is symptomatic.

---

*Not FDA approved for this indication.

*Not FDA approved for this indication.

PARASITIC DISEASES OF THE SKIN

method of
DONALD J. MIECH, M.D.
Marshfield Clinic
Marshfield, Wisconsin

Because of the many dermatologic manifestations of parasitic diseases, it is important to be aware of the major groups of organisms as noted in Table 1. Many of these conditions are confined to tropical parts of the world, but the prevalence of international travel should alert one to incorporating recent travel locations into the medical history. The major parasites discussed include helminths, protozoa, ectoparasites, and *Diptera* species.

PROTOZOA

The protozoa infections most likely to result in skin manifestations include leishmaniasis, which is discussed in the chapter on infectious diseases, and amebiasis. Amebae are single-cell organisms that invade the intestinal tract and may affect other tissues such as liver or lung. *Entamoeba histolytica* is one of the organisms that most commonly affects humans. The skin can be involved by direct extension from the intestinal tract, hepatic abscesses, or direct contact with infected material. Particularly susceptible patients are those with decreased cell-mediated immunity. A nonspecific ulcerated granuloma develops at the cutaneous site and must be distinguished from other infectious granulomas and syphilis. Trophozoites may be identified at the edge of an ulcer or in biopsy material.

The treatment of choice for cutaneous and intestinal disease is metronidazole (Flagyl), 750 mg orally or intravenously three times a day for 10 days. Metronidazole is generally well-tolerated. This can be followed by iodoquinol (Yodoxin), 650 mg three times daily for 20 days. For patients intolerant of the above medications, chloroquine phosphate, 1.0 grams per day for 2 days followed by 0.5 grams per day for 2 to 3 weeks, can also be effective.

HELMINTHIC INFECTIONS

Cercarial Dermatitis

Helminthic infections most commonly fall under the nematode (roundworm) designation, although one of the trematodes (flukes) is common in freshwater lakes in the United States. This nonhuman schis-

TABLE 1. **Skin Parasites and Their Treatment**

Class	Causative Organism	Predominant Clinical Manifestations	Dermatologic Manifestations	Treatment
Protozoa	*Entamoeba histolytica*	Amebic dysentery, liver abscess	Amebiasis cutis	Metronidazole (Flagyl), 750 mg q 8 h PO for 5–10 d
	Leishmania	See chapter on leishmaniasis, pp. 88–91		
Helminths	*Schistosoma* species	Schistosomiasis	Cercarial dermatitis (swimmer's itch)	Symptomatic
	Ancylostoma braziliense		Cutaneous larva migrans, creeping eruption	Topical 10% thiabendazole (Mintezol) suspension bid for 2 d
	Strongyloides stercoralis	Strongyloidiasis	Urticaria, larva currens	Thiabendazole (Mintezol) 25 mg/kg q 12 h for 2 d; ivermectin (Stromectol)* 200 µg/kg single dose
	Ancylostoma duodenale	Hookworm	Ground itch, dew itch, uncinarial dermatitis	Mebendazole (Vermox), 100 mg PO q 12 h for 3 d
	Dracunculus medinensis	Dracunculiasis	Guinea worm	Symptomatic care, surgical removal
	Loa loa	Loiasis	Migratory angioedema (Calabar swellings)	Diethylcarbamazine (Hetrazan), 6 mg/kg/d PO for 21 d: use escalating drug regimen
	Onchocerca volvulus	Onchocerciasis (river blindness)	Onchodermatitis, onchocercosis, river blindness, coastal erysipelas	Ivermectin* 150 µg/kg PO as a single dose each 6 mo for up to 15 yr
Arachnida Ectoparasite	*Sarcoptes scabiei*	Scabies	Scabies	5% permethrin cream (Elimite), 10% crotamiton (Eurax), ivermectin (Stromectol)* 200 µg/kg
	Pediculus humanus	Head lice		1% permethrin (Nix), pyrethrin (RID), gamma-benzene hexachloride (lindane)
	Phthirus pubis	Pubic lice		
Myiasis	*Dermatobia hominis*	Myiasis	Furuncle with opening to the surface of the skin	Débridement, petrolatum (Vaseline), and pork fat

*Ivermectin is presently indicated only for oncocerciasis and strongyloidiasis of the gastrointestinal tract.

tosome penetrates the human skin in the free-living cercarial stage. There have been at least 20 species of these organisms implicated. The cercariae are found on cool lake water surfaces, where they attach to the skin of swimmers, hence the names *cercarial dermatitis* or *swimmer's itch*. This most frequently occurs in freshwater lakes in the northern part of the United States in early summer, but a similar eruption is seen in some of the saltwater beaches off the Atlantic and Gulf Coasts.

The affected individual will shortly notice itching, a prickling sensation that may result in a diffuse erythematous macular, papular, or even vesicular eruption for 24 to 48 hours. Only exposed skin is affected. Treatment is symptomatic with antihistamines or antipruritic lotion such as camphor menthol containing sarna lotion.

Other treatments are mainly preventive. The hosts of schistosomes are infected snails and water fowl, and treatment of the lakes with copper sulfate or sodium pentachlorphenate will eradicate the infected snail.

Creeping Eruption (Larva Migrans)

The nematode larvae of *Ancylostoma braziliensis*, commonly known as dog or cat hookworm, usually causes cutaneous larvae migrans or creeping eruption. The lesions are serpiginous linear papules produced by the burrowing larvae, which commonly develop on the feet or other areas that are exposed to sand or soil contaminated by dog or cat feces. Commonly picked up on the beach in tropical or semitropical areas, the eruption usually progresses about 1 to 2 cm per day. Treatment is usually very effective with 10% formulated thiabendazole (Mintezol) suspension or ointment applied at least twice daily for 2 to 3 days or until the lesions resolve.

Strongyloidiasis Stercoralis (Larva Currens)

Strongyloidiasis stercoralis often causes an eruption similar to that of larva migrans, but the migration is much more rapid, up to 10 cm per day. Hence, the name *larva currens* is given to this form of creeping eruption. It is often accompanied by diarrhea and infection of the proximal bowel.

Ivermectin (Stromectol), 150 to 200 µg per kg as a single dose, is now indicated for gastrointestinal strongyloidiasis and has been reported to be very effective in larva currens. Thiabendazole can be administered systemically, 25 mg per kg twice daily for 2 days, although the treatment has been associated with nausea, vomiting, and vertigo. Albendazole (Albenza),* 400 mg, has also been reported effective, although the present indication for this medication is for certain tapeworm infections.

---

*Not FDA approved for this indication.

MYIASIS

Cutaneous myiasis is produced by invasion in human tissue by the larvae of Diptera species, which include the human botfly. *Dermatobia hominis* is a common cause of furuncular myiasis. The eggs of the botfly or blowfly are deposited in open wounds or orifices (such as nostrils), and the larvae infect the skin, usually causing areas of inflammation with at least one opening to the surface.

Sometimes the larvae can be expressed through the opening, or the opening can be enlarged surgically and the larvae can be removed with forceps. (It might be noted that the larvae have been employed to débride necrotic tissue in some instances.) Pork fat, or bacon, has classically been used to allow migration of the larvae out of the infected site, but petrolatum (Vaseline) is applied over the skin opening, causing the larvae to migrate to the surface for air.

ECTOPARASITES

Scabies is a pruritic eruption caused by the human mite *Sarcoptes scabiei*. This organism is most frequently acquired through close personal contact, but can also be picked up from infected clothing or bedding where the mite can remain viable for up to 3 days. The female mite burrows into the stratum corneum and deposits her eggs, which mature in approximately 2 weeks. The patient, however, is often asymptomatic for up to 1 month before the pruritic (especially at night) papules begin to develop. These papules have a predilection for the web spaces of the fingers, hypothenar eminence of the wrist, elbows, knees, waist, and medial thighs. In infants, they can often occur on the hands and feet and even in the scalp, where they may be also found in the immunocompromised host.

There are usually only about 6 to 12 mites on the skin at any time, and the scrapings from burrows where a small, black dot is seen will most likely reveal the organism microscopically. Because burrows are seen in only 30% of patients, intact papules or papulovesicles with the same black dot often aid in the diagnosis of the condition. Because many patients have had the condition for several months, it may be mistaken for eczema. Sites of predilection, history of nocturnal pruritus, and contact history may also assist in making the diagnosis. A severe variant of scabies, known as Norwegian scabies, has been seen in the immunocompromised host or institutionalized individual. These people have widespread, crusted lesions and large numbers of mites on their skin.

Treatment of choice has switched from lindane (gamma-benzene hexachloride [Kwell]) 1% lotion to permethrin (Elimite) 5% cream. Crotamiton (Eurax), which has a scabicidal effect, also helps reduce pruritus and can be applied as needed to especially pruritic and involved areas. Ivermectin, although not specifically indicated for scabies, has been reported to be very effective in some refractory cases of Norwegian scabies and scabies in some immunocompromised patients.

For topical treatment, it is also important to have the patient apply the medications to subungual fingernail areas. It is important to eradicate the mite from the environment by washing recently used clothing, underwear, bedding, and towels. Treatment of contacts is also important even if they are asymptomatic. The patient should be reassured that a scabies diagnosis does not necessarily mean that they are "unclean." Often vigorous rubbing and scrubbing is one of the most effective ways of spreading the mite over the skin. I have seen a number of fastidiously clean patients with widespread scabies who were devastated when they learned of the diagnosis.

PEDICULOSIS

There are three main types of lice that commonly infect humans. In contrast to scabies, which burrow in the stratum corneum, the louse usually lives on the surface of the skin, particularly on hairs where the eggs (nits) are laid. One can assess the length of time the patient has had lice from the position of the nit on the hair shaft because the egg is laid where the hair emerges from the skin. *Phthirus pubis* (pubic louse) and *Pediculosis capitis* (head louse) eggs are deposited on the hair shaft, and *Pediculosis hominis* (body louse) has eggs that are deposited in the clothing and therefore is more of a problem in the unkempt person who does not change clothing. The nits and lice can easily be seen with a $10 \times$ hand lens. Head lice are a particular problem among school children because sometimes many members of a class are affected.

A single treatment of 1% permethrin (Nix) cream has a high cure rate, which is estimated to be 98%. Pyrethrins (RID) and lindane 1% can also be used, but should be repeated in 7 days because of poor ovicidal activity. Nits can also be removed with a fine-toothed comb or forceps.

For pubic lice, the treatment is also permethrin cream (Elimite)* 5%, but lindane or Nix can also be used. It is important to note that pubic lice can also affect body and axillary hair and even eyelashes. Eyelashes can be treated with petrolatum to the eyelashes three to five times a day or by applying erythromycin* 2% ointment three times a day for 3 days. Eyelash nits can also be removed with a fine forceps.

Body lice are eliminated by washing clothing in hot water and heat drying the clothing for at least a half hour or by dry cleaning. The adult lice feed on covered areas of skin such as waist and necklines and produce pruritic and indurated lesions. Excoriations often lead to secondary bacterial infection, which may need topical or systemic antibiotic treatment and sometimes antihistamines for the itching.

---

*Not FDA approved for this indication.

FUNGAL DISEASES OF THE SKIN

method of
CATHERINE C. NEWMAN, M.D.
University of Texas Medical Branch
Galveston, Texas

The superficial fungal infections—dermatophytosis, candidiasis, and tinea versicolor—often have typical clinical features; however, they may be simulated by other inflammatory skin diseases. Therefore, mycologic confirmation with potassium hydroxide preparation or culture, or both, should always be sought to ensure the most effective management, especially because the newer antifungal medications are expensive and have potential serious side effects and drug interactions.

DERMATOPHYTOSIS

The dermatophytes are a class of fungi that live in the stratum corneum of humans or animals and in soil. Although there are many species, most infections in the United States are due to five species: *Trichophyton rubrum, Trichophyton tonsurans, Trichophyton mentagrophytes, Microsporum canis,* and *Epidermophyton floccosum.*

Dermatophytosis of the scalp, tinea capitis, is the most common fungal infection of children and is most often due to *T. tonsurans.* Clinical findings can vary from slight scaling suggestive of seborrheic dermatitis to scaling patches or plaques with broken hairs to kerion formation with marked edema and the presence of exudate. In Europe and in some cities of the United States, the most common cause of scalp infections is *M. canis,* which normally infects dogs and cats. This organism causes positive fluorescence of hairs on Wood's light examination. *T. tonsurans* does not.

Oral therapy is required to treat tinea capitis. The drug of choice is griseofulvin. The dosage of microsized griseofulvin (Grifulvin V, Grisactin, Fulvicin U/F) is 15 to 20 mg per kg per day for a minimum of 6 weeks.* The suspension form must be given in higher doses at 20 mg per kg per day.* Patients who cannot tolerate griseofulvin or do not respond can be treated with itraconazole (Sporanox),† 3 to 5 mg per kg per day, or terbinafine (Lamisil).† Children weighing less than 20 kg should receive terbinafine, 62.5 mg per day (one fourth of a tablet); those weighing 20 to 40 kg should receive 125 mg per day (one half of a tablet); and those weighing more than 40 kg should receive 250 mg per day. The length of treatment for itraconazole and terbinafine is still under debate but will probably be 2 to 4 weeks. The oral solution of itraconazole contains cyclodextrin and probably should not be used in children. Selenium sulfide shampoo (Selsun Blue) or ketoconazole shampoo (Nizoral) will reduce the spread of infectious spores. All members of the patient's family need to be screened for infection to prevent recurrences.

---

*Exceeds dosage recommended by the manufacturer.
†Not FDA approved for this indication.

Dermatophytosis of nonhairy skin, or tinea corporis, is characterized by scaling patches or plaques with sharp margins. Infections due to *M. canis* frequently result in multiple lesions and tend to be more inflammatory. Chronic infections are most commonly due to *T. rubrum*. Tinea cruris of the inguinal folds occurs frequently in athletes or those who work outdoors in hot, humid climates. Tinea cruris and solitary lesions respond well to topical treatment with any of the imidazoles: clotrimazole (Lotrimin, Mycelex), miconazole (Micatin, Monistat), econazole (Spectazole), ketoconazole (Nizoral), oxiconazole (Oxistat), sulconazole (Exelderm) or ciclopirox (Loprox). If over-the-counter antifungal agents are ineffective, a fungicidal topical allylamine such as naftifine (Naftin), terbinafine (Lamisil), or butenafine (Mentax) should be considered. The treatment of choice for extensive infection, for those due to multiple inoculation, or for those involving the hair follicles is oral griseofulvin, microsized, 500 mg twice daily for 4 to 6 weeks. The ultramicrosized griseofulvin dose is 250 mg twice daily for 1 month. Infections resistant to both griseofulvin and ketoconazole have responded to topical naftifine or terbinafine. The new oral agents itraconazole (Sporanox),* 200 mg twice daily for 1 to 2 weeks, or terbinafine (Lamisil),* 250 mg daily for 2 to 4 weeks, are effective.

The most common dermatophyte infections in adults are those of the feet and nails. There are three variants of tinea pedis: the interdigital type, the inflammatory type, with vesicles involving the toes or the instep; and the plantar hyperkeratotic variety with slight redness and itching but marked thickening and scaling of the skin of the sole. Dermatophytes occasionally produce chronic disease of the palmar skin, and the disease is usually unilateral. The common toe web infections and the inflammatory form usually respond well to topical treatment for 4 to 6 weeks with the imidazole, allylamine, or ciclopirox creams mentioned earlier. Recurrences are common and require either intermittent therapy or prophylactic use of an antifungal powder (tolnaftate [Tinactin], undecylenic acid [Desenex], or miconazole [Zeasorb-AF]. Chronic infections should be treated with oral microsized griseofulvin, 500 mg twice daily for 4 weeks. The topical allylamines naftifine and terbinafine are often effective in the more resistant infections. The new oral agents itraconazole* and terbinafine* are effective in the same dose schedules as for tinea corporis.

Dermatophytosis of the nails (onychomycosis, or tinea unguium) is common and often responds poorly to treatment. The most common form is distal subungual onychomycosis, characterized by separation of the nail from the nail bed, subungual scaling and thickening, and discoloration of the nail. Infections of the fingernails respond reasonably well (60 to 70%) to oral microsized griseofulvin, 500 mg twice daily for 6 to 8 months, but the cure rate for toenails is poor even with up to 24 months of therapy and avul-

sion of the nails. Frequent clipping and filing of the infected nail, with application of a topical allylamine (naftifine or terbinafine) twice daily after bathing or after brief soaking in warm water, will sometimes result in a cure. The approval of itraconazole and terbinafine for nail infections due to dermatophytes now allows much more effective therapy. Itraconazole (Sporanox) should be given in a dosage of 200 mg daily (3 months for toenails, 2 months for fingernails). The pulse dose schedule is more economical for infected toenails.* Pulse dose itraconazole is 200 mg twice daily for 1 week and then no dosing for 3 weeks. Three pulses are repeated for toenail infection, and two pulses are repeated for fingernail infection. The dosage of oral terbinafine (Lamisil) is 250 mg per day. Fingernails are treated for 2 months and toenails for 3 months. The package inserts for itraconazole and terbinafine recommend laboratory monitoring if the agents are used for more than 1 month or in patients with liver disease. The optimal dosing for fluconazole has not been established. The section of the package insert regarding drug interactions should be consulted and patients specifically warned to avoid itraconazole and drugs metabolized by the cytochrome P-450 3A enzyme system, such as warfarin, terfenadine, astemizole, anti–human immunodeficiency virus (HIV) protease inhibitors, midazolam, triazolam, vinca alkaloids, calcium channel blockers, lovastatin, simvastatin, cisapride, cyclosporine, digoxin, or quinidine. Anticonvulsants and antimycobacterial agents may decrease itraconazole plasma concentrations. Terbinafine (Lamisil) has fewer drug interactions than itraconazole.

The serious side effects of oral antifungal agents are uncommon but include drug-induced hepatitis, neutropenia, and skin eruptions such as erythema multiforme and toxic epidermal necrolysis. These eruptions can last for several weeks because the drug reservoirs are in tissue for long periods. Terbinafine has been reported to cause taste disturbance as well as hepatitis and neutropenia.

Superficial white onychomycosis is exhibited as white spots on the dorsum of the nail plate and responds well to any of the topical antifungal agents mentioned earlier. Proximal subungual onychomycosis, with whitish discoloration of the proximal nail, occurs most frequently in persons who have HIV infection or who are otherwise immunosuppressed, and it requires oral therapy.

CANDIDIASIS

Cutaneous candidiasis is usually due to *Candida albicans,* a yeast normally found in the gastrointestinal tract. The most common forms of infection involve the skin folds. It is characterized by redness, superficial erosion, satellite pustules, and itching or pain in the skin folds. Predisposing factors such as obesity, diabetes, immunosuppression, excessive sweating, and treatment with antibiotics or systemic

---

*Not FDA approved for this indication.

*Not FDA approved for this indication.

corticosteroids are frequently noted in the patient's history. Cutaneous candidiasis usually responds well to topical treatment with any of the imidazoles (e.g., clotrimazole [Lotrimin]) applied twice daily for 2 weeks. Chronic candidal paronychia necessitates prolonged therapy with frequent applications of imidazoles (clotrimazole solution) or nonspecific remedies such as 4% thymol in ethanol or sulfacetamide lotion. This regimen is followed by ensuring hand drying and limiting irritant or allergic contact dermatitis.

TINEA VERSICOLOR

Tinea versicolor is due to the lipophilic yeast *Malassezia furfur,* which is normally found in small quantities on the skin. Overgrowth of this organism produces discrete and confluent, slightly scaly patches or plaques on the upper trunk and proximal part of the arms. It occurs most frequently in young adults during the summer and in hot, humid climates. The involved skin can be slightly hyperpigmented or, more commonly, hypopigmented. The treatment of choice is selenium sulfide, (Selsun) shampoo, 2.5% applied with water to the scalp, neck, upper trunk, and extremities for 10 minutes daily for 1 week. The pigmentary changes may persist for weeks to months. Alternative treatments include the use of ketoconazole shampoo in the same way or ketoconazole cream twice daily. In extensive or resistant cases, oral ketoconazole, 400 mg in a single dose or 200 mg per day for 10 days, is effective. Terbinafine (Lamisil)* 1% cream or spray is also effective, but oral terbinafine is not.

---

*Not FDA approved for this indication.

DISEASES OF THE MOUTH

method of
HENRY W. RANDLE, M.D., Ph.D.
Mayo Clinic Jacksonville
Jacksonville, Florida
Mayo Medical School
Rochester, Minnesota

and

GAYLE L. McCLOSKEY, M.D.
Mayo Graduate School of Medicine
Rochester, Minnesota

Oral mucous membranes are specialized, thin membranes that lack a thick, horny layer (except on the dorsum of the tongue and hard palate), making them susceptible to physical and chemical injuries. They may be the site of allergic, infectious, metabolic, nutritional, or systemic disorders. Patients may present with congenital anomalies or benign or malignant tumors of the oral mucous membranes.

Most oral malignancies are related to lifestyle and environmental factors, including chronic irritation from excessive use of alcohol and tobacco (including smokeless), dental and denture irritations, poor oral hygiene, solar radiation (carcinoma of the lower lip), syphilis, human immunodeficiency virus infection, and iron deficiency (Plummer-Vinson syndrome).

GENERAL MEASURES

For optimal treatment of oral disease, poor dental hygiene must be corrected. Control of periodontal disease is the starting point for providing good oral hygiene. The physician must insist that plaques, calculus, periodontitis, caries, ill-fitting dental appliances, and malocclusion are treated by a dentist. The patient must have an adequate oral intake of fluoride and must regularly clean with a toothbrush and fluoride toothpaste, dental floss, and perhaps an irrigating instrument such as a Water Pik. In addition to toothbrushing and oral rinsing, tongue cleaning is essential.

Bad breath or bad taste may reflect oral sepsis or excessive dryness. Halitosis may indicate a more serious pathologic condition, but most bad breath usually stems from the oral cavity, generally the dorsum of the tongue. Bacterial action on proteins creates volatile sulfur compounds, which have been linked to halitosis. Adequate hydration must be maintained, with frequent mouthwashes immediately before and after meals and several times during the day. There are many commercially available mouth rinses, but some of these, especially ones with alcohol, can be drying or irritating to an already inflamed mouth.

Topical anesthesia is sometimes necessary to relieve discomfort and pain before eating. Swishing ½ teaspoon of viscous lidocaine (Xylocaine) per 2 teaspoonfuls of water around the mouth for 2 or 3 minutes or the direct application of full-strength viscous lidocaine to the painful site with a cotton-tipped applicator is effective. An alternative would be equal parts of kaolin pectin (Kaopectate) and elixir of diphenhydramine (Benadryl) used as a mouthwash before eating. Swallowing this preparation will give an added sedative effect in anxious patients. A soothing combination that can be prepared by the pharmacist includes hydrocortisone powder, diphenhydramine elixir, nystatin suspension, and other ingredients that may include doxycycline suspension or lidocaine. Coating the mouth with magnesium hydroxide (Milk of Magnesia) or aluminum- or magnesium-containing antacids (Maalox) can relieve discomfort. When anesthetic agents are used, the patient must be cautioned against traumatizing the oral tissues during eating.

For inflammatory and ulcerative diseases, the diet should be limited to cool bland soups, milk shakes, and ice cream. Hard, hot, acid, sharp, irritating foods should be avoided, as should tobacco. These measures often provide dramatic relief of oral disease. In addition, any associated systemic disorder should be identified and managed or treatment may fail.

LESIONS OF THE LIPS

Lip lesions that require medical attention may occur at or shortly after birth.

Cleft Lip and Cleft Palate

Craniofacial deformities, with cleft lip and cleft palate being the most common, can vary from a small depression to extensive, deforming, and mutilating abnormalities that involve the nostrils, hard and soft palates, tongue, and mandible. There may be associated anomalies of other organ systems. Extensive anomalies require long-term management and rehabilitation by specialized teams of pediatricians, plastic surgeons, oral surgeons, pedodontists, dentists, speech therapists, and counselors specializing in long-term management of these defects. Specially designed nipple and palatal obturators are important for feeding and for prevention of nasal aspiration and ear infection. Cleft lip repair is usually undertaken at about 10 weeks of age, but palatal surgery is deferred until later, when speech begins to develop.

Vascular Lesions

Capillary and cavernous hemangiomas may involve the lips as well as other oral structures. Because hemangiomas of infancy have a tendency to regress, treatment is generally limited to situations in which the patient has impaired function; however, in some patients, psychosocial factors may indicate treatment. Consultation with a surgeon for treatment with a pulsed-dye laser may be indicated for the first few months of life. Management is otherwise supportive and requires careful evaluation and frequent re-examination. Residual scarring may require some reconstructive surgery; this is generally done at approximately 5 years of age for capillary hemangiomas and at puberty for cavernous hemangiomas. Covermark makeup by Lydia O'Leary or Dermablend makeup effectively conceals small lesions. Rapid growth of such lesions, especially when vital functions of organs are compromised, requires intervention. Hemangiomas regress with corticosteroid therapy, both oral and intralesional, which should be administered and monitored by a specialist. Interferon alfa-2a* (Roferon-A) has been used in the treatment of hemangiomas. Radiotherapy, if used, must be of such quality and quantity that the teeth buds and bone centers are not harmed. There is also the risk of developing certain malignancies after radiotherapy for skin hemangiomas. Surgical intervention and cryosurgery with liquid nitrogen probes are alternative therapies.

Lymphangiomas are rare tumors of the lips and tongue and may require radical surgical intervention. Venous ectasias (lakes) are common among the elderly. No treatment is required, but they may be destroyed by tunable dye laser for cosmetic reasons.

*Not FDA approved for this use.

Small telangiectases occur on the lips in patients with scleroderma and hereditary hemorrhagic telangiectases (Osler-Weber-Rendu disease). If these disorders are suspected, a general examination should be performed.

Recurrent Herpes Simplex

Recurrent herpes simplex is a common disease of the lips. After the initial infection, the virus stays in the trigeminal ganglion and recurrences are possible throughout life. They frequently appear at times of illness but may appear at any time. Topical acyclovir (Zovirax) ointment may be applied every 3 hours while the patient is awake when the first sign or symptom of lesions develops in the immunocompetent patient. Penciclovir (Denavir) cream 1% may be applied for 4 days every 2 hours while the patient is awake. Acyclovir, famciclovir (Famvir), and valacyclovir (Valtrex) have been used in various oral doses, but they are not officially approved for herpes simplex of the lips.

Cheilitis

Redness and alternating areas of dryness, flaking, and vesiculation are common to most forms of cheilitis. Physical trauma resulting from wind, sunlight, cold, lip licking, tics, and desiccation causes desquamation. White petrolatum (Vaseline) is helpful for mild to moderate cheilitis. For more severe inflammation, the application of a corticosteroid such as 0.1% triamcinolone acetonide ointment (Aristocort, Kenalog) usually is effective.

Further occurrences may be prevented by application of zinc oxide paste, photoprotective lip balm such as PreSun Lip Protection, or petrolatum. The dry and desquamating lips of severely ill patients should be greased with petrolatum.

Contact Cheilitis

Contact cheilitis affects women more often than men, and the vesiculation often extends to the adjacent skin. This usually is caused by lipstick (perfume, dyes, or the base), lip salves, and food. Elimination of the offending agent and the use of topical corticosteroids are helpful. Cinnamaldehyde is a common offending agent. Patch testing may be indicated to identify and eliminate the offending agent.

Angular Cheilitis

This condition is usually due to a low-grade intertrigo from drooling (such as occurs with ill-fitting dentures), with or without candidiasis. Local treatment with an ointment containing nystatin (Mycostatin) or both nystatin and triamcinolone acetonide (Mycolog II ointment) and drying measures (to prevent macerations) are helpful. The buccal mucosa should be examined to be certain there is no additional evidence of candidiasis.

Actinic Cheilitis

Actinic cheilitis is a premalignant lesion seen predominantly on the vermilion of the lower lip in men who have spent considerable time outdoors. The lesions most likely to be dysplastic or neoplastic are those with heavy keratinization, erosion, ulceration, and erythema. One should perform a biopsy on lips with any of these changes for histopathologic examination to exclude malignancy. For mild actinic cheilitis, cryotherapy with liquid nitrogen and the spray technique with a thaw time of 60 to 90 seconds is rapid and effective and gives a good cosmetic result. An alternative would be topical application of 5-fluorouracil (Efudex), 5% cream applied to the vermilion two times a day for about 3 weeks or until erosion of the affected area is produced. This method is effective but may be exceedingly painful. Electrosurgery is more likely to produce excessive scarring. For moderate to severe actinic cheilitis, vaporization by carbon dioxide laser gives an excellent functional and cosmetic result. Surgical excision of the vermilion closed by advancement of the labial mucosa is an alternative. All persons with actinic cheilitis should protect the lips with a photoprotective lip balm and have periodic examinations for possible development of squamous cell carcinomas.

Squamous cell carcinomas of the lip (usually lower) are treated surgically by wedge excision and primary reconstruction, occasionally combined with an upper or complete neck dissection, depending on the staging and histologic differentiation of the tumor. Recent studies show Mohs' surgery with a mucosal advancement flap yields excellent cure rates, and it also spares as much of the uninvolved tissue as possible.

Cheilitis Glandularis Apostematosa

This uncommon entity is the result of inflammation and irritation of the mucous glands along the exposed surface of the lower lip and is manifested by numerous pinhead-sized openings of the ducts of the mucous gland and enlargement of the lips. Cleaning of the lips with tap water on arising usually is sufficient to remove accumulated debris. Protection of these tissues from the sun and wind with a photoprotective lip balm applied during the day does much to relieve symptoms. The disease tends to be self-limited and disappears spontaneously after a few years. In severe cases, plastic surgery of the lower lip may be helpful.

Factitial Cheilitis

Continual licking or biting should be suspected in obsessive neurotic patients who present with non-healing lesions.

Cheilitis may occur in scarlet fever, hereditary polymorphic light eruption, Kawasaki disease (mucocutaneous lymph node syndrome), erythema multiforme, glucagonoma syndrome, and, less commonly, discoid lupus erythematosus. It is present in nearly all patients receiving oral retinoids (either isotretinoin [Accutane] or acitretin [Soriatane]).

WHITE LESIONS OF THE MOUTH

All white hyperkeratotic lesions of the mouth should be studied by biopsy unless an infection (thrush) or other obvious cause is recognized. The lesions should be classified histopathologically as benign, dysplastic, or malignant, and the patient should be treated and followed appropriately.

The diagnosis of leukokeratosis should be reserved for white lesions that show no dyskeratosis on histopathologic examination. These lesions are benign white plaques usually caused by trauma such as cheek biting, irritation or tobacco, sharp margins of carious teeth, ill-fitting dental appliances, or "aspirin burns." Correction of dental abnormalities, good oral hygiene, and avoidance of tobacco are frequently followed by considerable improvement. The chronic cheek chewer is helped by a mouthguard appliance worn at night to prevent chewing while sleeping.

Leukoplakia and Carcinomas

"Leukoplakia" is a descriptive term meaning white patch, but usually it implies a premalignant condition. Biopsy reveals cellular dysplasia, and this lesion shows a tendency toward malignant transformation into squamous cell carcinoma. Preliminary studies on chemoprevention suggest that retinoids may be effective in suppressing oral carcinomas, but this is not considered standard practice. Isotretinoin,* 1 to 2 mg per kg of body weight per day for 3 months, may cause regression of leukoplakia. Many lesions show marked clearing within 6 weeks after irritating factors are removed. Resistant plaques may be destroyed by cryosurgery. Frequent re-evaluations are important. Any change, especially induration, ulceration, or the development of erythroplasia-like areas, is an indication for additional biopsies. Because leukoplakia lesions of the tongue and floor of the mouth show the greatest potential for malignant transformation, they should be excised promptly.

Early detection of malignancy is important because the 5-year survival rate is 90% for small locally confined tumors. Patients with advanced disease have a 5-year survival of less than 50%. Other potential precancers or cancers of the oral cavity that require consideration of biopsy include hyperkeratotic, papillomatous, verrucous lesions; chronic ulcers that do not heal within 2 to 3 weeks; lesions that do not resolve after potential injury is eliminated; tissue enlargement that cannot be attributed to trauma or bacteria; pigmented lesions; cysts; and painful or enlarging bony lesions.

More than 90% of intraoral cancers are squamous cell carcinomas. They are treated by two major modalities: surgical excision and radiotherapy, either singly or in combination. These carcinomas grow locally, with invasion spreading along lymphatic channels to regional nodes. Treatment decisions are based

---

*This use of isotretinoin is not listed in the manufacturer's official directive.

on prognosis as predicted by the TNM (tumor, node, metastasis) staging system. Side effects of treatment must be considered for each individual patient. Radiotherapy results in xerostomia and stomatitis and is adversely affected when there is bone or muscle involvement. Surgical therapy has made many advancements as a result of improved use of reconstructive techniques. Chemotherapy generally is used for palliation.

Advanced disease does not do well, and the key to successful management is early detection. Oral neoplasms traditionally have been diseases of old men, but trends are showing an increase in the number of female oral cancer patients.

Rehabilitation is enhanced by the use of a prosthesis designed by a maxillofacial prosthodontist. A speech pathologist may assist in speech recovery and swallowing, two of the most important postoperative concerns. If extensive deformities occur, psychological assistance may be required during the first 2 years after operation, emphasizing the importance of a multidisciplinary approach to oral cancer treatment.

Smoker's Keratosis of the Palate (Leukokeratosis Nicotine Palati)

Enlargement of palatal mucous glands and dilation of their ducts produce papules with a central red spot on a grayish white, wrinkled palatal mucosa. These occur predominantly on the hard palate in pipe smokers. Cessation of smoking leads to gradual resolution of the problem. Another form of papillary hyperplasia of the palate is due to dentures. These papillae may be removed by light curettage with a sharp curet. Persistent lesions should undergo biopsy.

Lichen Planus

Lichen planus may resemble leukoplakia with painful erosions and ulcerations, particularly on the buccal mucosa and tongue. To exclude malignancy, histopathologic examination of a biopsy specimen may be helpful. If a biopsy specimen is taken, part should be sent for direct immunofluorescence studies. Patients with erosive and atrophic forms seek medical help because of pain. Drug-induced lichenoid reactions should be excluded and usually clear when the drug is discontinued. Chronic hepatic disease and hepatitis C virus are sometimes associated, especially with the erosive form of oral lichen planus. Contact allergy can aggravate or induce oral lichen planus, and patch testing may be indicated.

Good oral hygiene, as stressed earlier, should be strongly encouraged for all persons with oral lichen planus. Dental plaques may promote flares. These lesions frequently are colonized by yeast (Candida). If these organisms are identified, anticandidal therapy should be instituted, as described elsewhere in this article. Treatment is with class I to II topical corticosteroids, ointment or gel, two to three times per day after breakfast, dinner, and at bedtime. Once the condition is under control, the medication may be tapered. Direct application of the gel capsule contents of cyclosporine (Neoral) capsules* is a convenient and effective treatment modality. Griseofulvin,* in doses of 250 mg of the ultramicrosize (Grisactin Ultra), two times daily for 6 to 12 weeks, is effective in about 50% of cases. If conservative measures have failed, oral prednisone may be needed at 40 to 80 mg per day for up to 2 weeks with tapering. A single intramuscular injection of 40 to 60 mg of triamcinolone acetonide (Kenalog) may be given for temporary relief. One also may consider corticosteroid-sparing agents such as azathioprine (Imuran),* systemic cyclosporine, or retinoids.*

Candidiasis (Thrush)

White plaques may be localized or may involve the intraoral tissues diffusely. They may extend into the esophagus or may affect the corners of the lips, producing maceration and fissures (perlèche). To confirm the diagnosis, plaques are removed by scraping and the material is examined microscopically in 10% potassium hydroxide.

Dilute hydrogen peroxide mouth rinses soothe the oral discomfort. A lozenge of clotrimazole (Mycelex troche), 10 mg, dissolved in the mouth five times each day for 14 days may be used. Lesions in infants and young children may be removed carefully by a cotton-tipped applicator dipped into a nystatin suspension (Mycostatin oral suspension). Anticandidal creams such as clotrimazole (Lotrimin, Mycelex) applied under the dentures or at the corners of the mouth are effective. Extensive disease is best treated with fluconazole (Diflucan) at 100 mg per day for 7 days.

Other White Lesions

Fordyce spots are sebaceous glands that appear clinically as 1- to 3-mm whitish papules on the lips and buccal mucosa. These are asymptomatic and require no treatment except to reassure the patient that the process is neither malignant nor premalignant. There are several uncommon disorders that may produce white lesions in the mouth. Darier's disease causes whitish "cobblestone" papules on the buccal or palatal mucosa. The lesions in this autosomal dominantly inherited disorder are benign and do not require treatment. Another autosomal dominant disorder is the white sponge nevus. If this disorder is suspected, a biopsy specimen should be taken, and the histopathologic examination will reveal thickened mucosa with characteristic features. The lesions are asymptomatic and do not undergo malignant degeneration; therefore, no treatment is indicated. An appreciation of this disorder is important so that it can be distinguished from other white lesions of the oral cavity.

---

*This use of cyclosporine, griseofulvin, azathioprine, and retinoids is not listed in the manufacturers' official directives.

Two other rare inherited syndromes are pachyonychia congenita and dyskeratosis congenita. These rare disorders consist of opaque white or grayish white plaques on the dorsum of the tongue or the buccal mucosa along with associated cutaneous features. Oral lesions in dyskeratosis congenita may become malignant and should be removed surgically if they become irritated, ulcerated, or thickened. The whitish lesions in pachyonychia carry no risk of malignant transformation. Leukoedema forms whitish lines on the buccal mucosa and is considered a variant of normal. The white lines disappear when the mucosa is stretched, and this is diagnostic.

EROSIVE, ULCERATIVE, AND VESICULOBULLOUS LESIONS

Various inflammatory diseases may produce vesicles, bullae, erosions, and ulcers in the oral mucosa. Vesicles and bullae are quite friable and are easily eroded in the mouth, producing erosions and ulcers. Diagnosis frequently must be confirmed by histopathologic or immunopathologic examination (or both). Tissue situated adjacent to the primary lesion (perilesional tissue) should be studied by biopsy because this specimen is more likely to provide diagnostic material than is lesional tissue.

Aphthous Stomatitis

This common disorder of multiple, shallow, recurrent, painful ulcerations can be of three types: (1) minor aphthous ulcers, the most common type, which recur in crops of 1 to 5 lesions, are less than 1 cm in diameter each, and usually affect the lips, buccal mucosa, mucobuccal and mucolabial sulci, and tongue; (2) major aphthous ulcers, which are greater than 2 cm in diameter, begin as solitary nodules, and subsequently destroy deeper tissue, resulting in scarring that affects the movable oral mucosa and posterior mucosal surfaces; and (3) herpetiform ulcers, which are recurrent, multiple (10 to 100), shallow, pinpoint lesions 1 to 2 mm in diameter that may affect any part of the mucosa. The cause for any of the three types is not known, although autoimmune mechanisms are suspected.

Nutritional deficiencies of vitamin B_{12}, folate, and iron may be present, and persons with these deficiencies may respond to replacement therapy. For most patients, however, treatment of these lesions represents a challenge to both the physician and the patient, and it is necessary to be optimistic and to have several approaches available.

Correctable causes such as nutritional deficiencies should be sought. If there are none, an attempt should be made to decrease oral trauma. Local cleansing, good oral hygiene, avoidance of irritants, and pain relief measures, as discussed previously, are fundamental. Patients should avoid sharp-surfaced foods such as peanuts, popcorn, potato chips, and tacos. They should use soft-bristled toothbrushes and brush the teeth carefully, avoiding banging the toothbrush into the buccal mucosa. Efforts should be made to decrease dental trauma by correcting dentures or sharp-edged teeth, and patients should avoid talking while chewing. During flare-ups of the condition, certain foods should be eliminated from the diet, such as spices, citrus fruits, and acidic foods that aggravate the lesions. Specific foods such as chocolate, nuts, and strong cheeses should also be avoided, if these are recognized as precipitating bouts of aphthous stomatitis.

If a few lesions are present, 0.1% triamcinolone acetonide in emollient dental paste (Kenalog in Orabase), applied by gently pressing against the mucosa with the fingertip several times each day, is the first choice of treatment and is effective for many patients. Fluocinonide (Lidex gel) is an alternative.

Escharotics such as silver nitrate can be applied to early lesions and may decrease pain. These agents should not be used for late lesions, however, because they will only increase the amount of tissue necrosis. An elixir made of diphenhydramine (60 mL of Benadryl elixir) and fluocinolone acetonide solution (20 mL of Synalar) may be used as a mouthwash, 1 teaspoonful three times each day.

A short course of systemic corticosteroids (prednisone, 60 mg) orally for 7 days followed by 30 mg orally for 7 days is indicated for patients with persistent or major types of aphthous stomatitis. Alternatives include colchicine,* 0.6 mg twice daily, and dapsone,* 25 to 100 mg per day.

Behçet's Syndrome

Behçet described the classic tri-symptom complex of recurrent oral ulcers, ocular inflammation, and genital ulcerations. These may be accompanied by other systemic manifestations. When neurologic deficits are present, the mortality rate is high; therefore, these patients require a general examination and frequent follow-up visits.

Colchicine,† 0.6 mg two times each day as suppressive therapy, or systemic corticosteroids may be helpful for individual episodes but do not alter the natural course of the disease. Severe complications have been managed with cytotoxic drugs† such as azathioprine, cyclophosphamide, chlorambucil, dapsone, or methotrexate.

Herpes Simplex

Prevention of eliciting factors such as fever, sunburn, windburn, and trauma by photoprotective lip balms should be stressed. Aspirin may be used to decrease fever and inflammation.

Acyclovir (Zovirax) is the most researched and used antiviral agent with activity against herpesvi-

---

*This use of colchicine and dapsone is not listed in the manufacturers' official directives.

†This use of colchicine, azathioprine, cyclophosphamide, chlorambucil, dapsone, and methotrexate is not listed in the manufacturers' official directives.

rus infections. Acyclovir, 200 mg orally five times a day for 10 days, is suggested for herpes simplex infections in primary herpetic gingivostomatitis. Topical anesthesia with lidocaine (Xylocaine), viscous 2% applied directly to lesions with cotton swabs, may help to relieve local symptoms.

Erythema Multiforme

Many stimuli have been implicated in precipitating these shallow, painful lip and oral ulcerations. If possible, these agents should be identified and eliminated. For patients with recurrent erythema multiforme due to herpes simplex infections, measures to prevent these infections should be used (see "Herpes Simplex"). Oral acyclovir should be used as soon as infection is identified. Herpes simplex virus–associated erythema multiforme is a recurrent disease, and in children it may be unresponsive to oral or topical acyclovir. Frequent recurrences of this disease process may require prophylactic treatment with acyclovir.

For mild cheilitis, fluocinonide gel 0.05% (Lidex gel) is applied three to four times daily. Alternatives are white petrolatum (Vaseline) or bacitracin ointment. For painful mucosal erosions, frequent mouthwashes are recommended with cetylpyridinium (Cēpacol) diluted 1:4 with water several times daily. A soothing mixture of 1:1 Kaopectate plus diphenhydramine elixir (Benadryl) or viscous lidocaine diluted 1:4 with water may alleviate pain if held in the mouth for 2 to 3 minutes. If there is any evidence of secondary infection, erythromycin, 1 gram per day, can be given for several days. Severe lesions are managed with systemic corticosteroids (prednisone, 60 mg daily) until the disease is controlled, at which point drug dosage is slowly reduced over 3 weeks.

Pemphigus and Pemphigoid

Oral lesions (blisters or ulcers) may be the precipitating manifestation in patients who have pemphigus vulgaris. They may occur in bullous and cicatricial pemphigoid (benign mucous membrane pemphigoid). For histopathologic and direct immunofluorescent studies, biopsy specimens should be taken of any persistent, erosive, ulcerative, or bullous lesions. An early diagnosis facilitates early treatment and may prevent widespread disease.

Treatment of pemphigus vulgaris and bullous pemphigoid is discussed elsewhere in this text. Cicatricial pemphigoid is a chronic condition that may respond to dapsone* in doses of 50 to 150 mg per day. A trial of therapy for 3 months or longer should be given. Acute episodes may respond to short courses of prednisone, 60 mg per day tapered over 3 weeks. Cyclophosphamide (Cytoxan)* or azathioprine (Imuran)* is reserved for severe cases refractory to the medicines previously listed. Patients with this condition

---

*This use of dapsone, cyclophosphamide, and azathioprine is not listed in the manufacturers' official directives.

should be monitored by an ophthalmologist, because blindness may result.

Other Causes of Oral Ulcerations

There are other causes of oral ulcerations. Mucositis and ulceration constitute significant problems in patients receiving chemotherapy. Soothing mouthwashes and supportive care, as discussed previously, should be used in these patients. Systemic infections such as blastomycosis, histoplasmosis, cryptococcosis, tuberculosis, syphilis, leprosy, and other chronic infections may present as chronic ulcerative lesions of the mouth. Actinomycosis may form multiple sinus tracts in the skin adjacent to the mouth. Gonorrhea of the oral mucosa presents a fiery red appearance with scattered white pseudomembranes. Leishmaniasis may cause red, granulating, capillary configurations with ulceration and fibrosis of the mucosa. Treatment is indicated elsewhere in this text for specific types of infections. Hand, foot, and mouth diseases caused by the coxsackievirus may produce small red vesicles or ulcers in the oral mucosa that last from 1 to 6 days without specific therapy.

Leukokeratotic, atrophic, inflammatory, erythematous, ulcerative, and hemorrhagic plaques may be seen in both systemic lupus erythematosus and discoid lupus erythematosus, primarily of the buccal and palatal mucosa. Histologic examination and direct immunofluorescence methods confirm the diagnosis.

Symptomatic local therapy as for lichen planus, especially the application of the topical steroid 0.05% fluocinonide (Lidex gel) five to six times each day, for 10 to 14 days, is soothing, but ultimate resolution of lesions depends on systemic control of the lupus erythematosus. Hydroxychloroquine (Plaquenil), 200 mg twice daily, is effective for severe oral involvement. Severe mucosal ulcers may be a component of other multisystem diseases, such as the hypereosinophilic syndrome, neutropenia, ulcerative colitis, or regional enteritis, so virtually any nonhealing mouth ulcer should prompt a general examination.

LESIONS OF THE GINGIVA AND PERIODONTAL MEMBRANES

Gingival Hyperplasia

Localized enlargement of the gums may be evidence of a periodontal abscess, malignancy, or a hyperplastic growth caused by local irritating factors. Plaque and calculus deposits and faulty dental restorations should be corrected.

Generalized enlargement of the gums may be seen in various inherited conditions as well as in some patients who take phenytoin (Dilantin) or cyclosporine (Neoral). Careful dental prophylaxis should begin as soon as phenytoin is started because occurrence of the hyperplasia does not justify cessation of drug therapy. The condition can be managed by removing excessive gingival tissues surgically. Afterward, the construction of a positive-pressure mouth-guard may reduce the regrowth of tissue.

Diffuse gingival enlargement may occur with leukemic infiltrates. Hemorrhage is the complicating factor, and surgery is contraindicated in these patients. Gentle cleansing of the teeth with a Water Pik may be helpful in reducing irritation from dental deposits. If hemorrhage occurs, topical homeostatic agents such as Gelfoam may be applied.

Huge granular magenta gingiva and interdental papillae with diffuse petechial markings are characteristic of Wegener's granulomatosis.

Epulides

Epulides are localized "lumps on the gums" and may be of giant cell or fibrous type, or they may be pyogenic granulomas that result from irritation or inflammatory change on the gingival margin. To exclude malignant processes, one should do a histopathologic examination.

Removal of the irritant may suffice for treatment. However, a more rapid result is obtained by surgical removal of the hyperplastic and fibrotic tissue.

Gingivitis and Periodontitis

Patients with these common inflammatory reactions involving the supporting structures of the teeth should be promptly referred to the dentist for removal of plaques and calculus to prevent infection of gingiva and tooth surfaces. Appropriate preventive measures include supplemental intake of fluorides and prevention of dental plaque formation by the daily use of dental floss and proper toothbrushing techniques.

Acute Necrotizing Ulcerative Gingivitis (Vincent's Disease, Trench Mouth)

This acute bacterial (fusospirochetal) infection is usually localized in the marginal gingival tissue, presenting as painful, punched-out erosions in debilitated patients with pre-existing gingival disease. Oral penicillin V, 250 mg four times each day for 4 or 5 days, is the antibiotic of choice. Erythromycin and metronidazole (Flagyl) are alternatives. As discussed previously, mouth rinses with warm, dilute hydrogen peroxide should be used for the first few days, and necrotic tissue should be removed by gently swabbing with a cotton swab moistened with hydrogen peroxide. After the acute phase, the patient's dentist should correct any periodontal disease. Smoking and stress are aggravating factors.

Chronic Desquamative Gingivitis

The cause of this diffuse erythema of the marginal and attached gingiva with desquamation and occasional vesicle formation is obscure. It is usually a manifestation of various disorders, such as lichen planus, cicatricial pemphigoid, or pemphigus vul-

garis. A biopsy including direct immunofluorescence should be performed to establish an accurate diagnosis, with subsequent appropriate systemic disease treatment. If there is no evidence of a systemic problem, then topical medication is often helpful. Regular lavage with soothing washes as well as the frequent application of a topical corticosteroid such as fluocinonide (Lidex gel 0.05%) for several days to a dry field (this should be gently massaged into the inflamed area with the fingertips) may reduce inflammation.

Pericoronitis

An inflammatory reaction may develop around erupting third molars (wisdom teeth). Gums may become infected, and antibiotic treatment is necessary. Removal of the offending tooth or teeth is necessary for relief.

Eruption Cysts

The redness and swelling of the mucosa that may accompany the eruption of teeth may be treated by making an incision in the overlying tissue. Topical anesthetic ointments may be necessary to relieve discomfort in children. Aspirin can be used for its analgesic effect.

Dental Sinus

A dental sinus may develop from an apical abscess and present near the infected tooth intraorally or in the skin, most commonly on the face below the inferior border on the mandible or in the lateral part of the neck. These findings should prompt consideration of radiographic investigation of the dental arches. Treatment involves extraction of the infected tooth and excision of the sinus tract if it fails to heal. Successful root canal procedures often lead to spontaneous resolution of the sinus and its manifestations on the skin.

LESIONS PECULIAR TO THE TONGUE

Hairy Leukoplakia

Oral hairy leukoplakia is an asymptomatic white plaque with a hairy-appearing surface usually located on the lateral margin of the tongue and occasionally on the buccal mucosa. It is associated with both the Epstein-Barr virus and human papillomavirus. Its appearance is a poor prognostic sign because acquired immunodeficiency syndrome (AIDS) develops in a significant proportion of patients within a few months of onset. Temporary regression may be achieved with oral acyclovir (Zovirax),* 800 mg four times daily.

---

*This use of acyclovir is not listed in the manufacturer's official directive.

Geographic Tongue (Glossitis Areata Migrans, Benign Migratory Plaque, Wandering Rash of the Tongue, and Pityriasis Linguae)

The cause of this rapid shedding and growing of the papillae on the tongue is not known, although it is occasionally seen in patients with psoriasis or Reiter's disease. The patient may be reassured that this is a harmless, recurrent, self-limited condition that usually requires no therapy but may persist for years. For patients who have associated symptoms of burning and discomfort or who are concerned about the appearance, topical tretinoin 0.05% (Retin-A liquid)* applied with a cotton swab two times daily for several days may be used, but it is painful. A topical corticosteroid may alleviate symptoms. Soothing measures, such as the use of topical anesthetics and avoidance of excessively hot or spicy food, are recommended.

Scrotal Tongue

This fissuring of the tongue is a congenital anomaly that usually occurs as an isolated finding; however, it is important to consider because it is an occasional occurrence in Down, Sjögren's, and Melkersson-Rosenthal syndromes. No treatment is required, but local hygiene measures should be encouraged because these deep narrow fissures may act as sites of irritation and infection, which can lead to halitosis.

Black Hairy Tongue

Elongation and hyperplasia of the filiform papillae of the tongue, discolored brown or black by pigment-producing oral flora, may occur in association with antibiotics, smoking, radiotherapy, or chronic hyperplastic candidiasis.

In most instances, brushing the tongue with a soft-bristled toothbrush and dilute hydrogen peroxide solution is satisfactory. Topical triamcinolone acetonide (Kenalog) applied twice daily after wiping the tongue dry may alleviate this condition. Resistant cases may be treated with local anesthesia with viscous lidocaine (Xylocaine), the elongated papillae carefully snipped away with sharp scissors, and the area painted with 15% trichloroacetic acid. Several treatments usually are required. Antibiotics, smoking, chewing tobacco, and all oral irritants should be avoided.

Smooth Tongue

The absence or atrophy of the filiform papillae of the anterior two thirds of the tongue is seen in many nutritional deficiency states, such as Plummer-Vinson syndrome, pellagra, and pernicious anemia, and in the malabsorption states of sprue and celiac disease. Treatment of the underlying disease process is indicated.

Infection with *Candida* may lead to atrophy of the filiform papillae. Treatment of this is discussed in the section entitled "White Lesions of the Mouth."

Macroglossia

Various conditions may lead to an enlarged tongue. Tumors, infectious processes, metabolic processes (especially amyloidosis), and conditions such as angioneurotic edema, superior vena cava syndrome, and sarcoidosis should be suspected.

Median Rhomboid Glossitis

A depressed area on the dorsum of the tongue that is red and sharply demarcated from the adjacent white-pink papillary surface may be of a developmental origin or may represent a response to chronic infection by *Candida*. These lesions respond poorly to topical treatment, but oral fluconazole (Diflucan) or ketoconazole (Nizoral) may be tried if *Candida* is present. If the lesion does not have the typical appearance sufficient for diagnosis or if it does not respond to therapy, biopsy may be done to exclude carcinoma. If chronic irritation becomes a problem, surgical excision of the rhomboid lesion may be performed.

OTHER PAINFUL LESIONS OF THE MOUTH

Sore mouth may be an idiopathic condition or may be caused by ill-fitting dentures, drug reaction, irritant or allergic reaction, nutritional deficiency, or a psychoneurotic state. A specific diagnosis is often difficult, but an investigation should be done to exclude organic causes.

Glossodynia

The condition of a painful burning tongue is usually idiopathic and occurs almost exclusively in middle-aged and elderly women with a normal-appearing tongue. It is generally attributed to a psychoneurotic condition. However, the disease is not limited to this population.

A diagnostic investigation should consider organic causes such as diabetes mellitus; pernicious anemia; deficiencies of folic acid, zinc, and iron; xerostomia; denture sore mouth; candidiasis; stomatitis medicamentosa; trigeminal neuralgia; vascular thrombosis; and hypoestrogenism. These secondary glossodynias frequently have an associated abnormal morphology of the tongue or symptoms such as loss or perversion of the sense of taste. If no organic cause is found, the patient should be reassured that the problem is not malignant or serious. If this is not acceptable, amitriptyline (Elavil), 25 to 75 mg at bedtime, may be used. Good dental hygiene and adequate nutrition

---

*This use of tretinoin is not listed in the manufacturer's official directive.

should be maintained. Occasionally, psychiatric consultation is indicated.

Contact Stomatitis

The mucous membranes are less susceptible to irritant and allergic sensitization than is the skin. Removal of the offending agent is ideal, but frequently it is difficult to identify. A wide variety of contactants must be removed with the hope that a careful history and clinical examination will identify the source of the problem. Routine patch testing is occasionally helpful.

Elimination of potential irritants such as aspirin; strong mouthwashes; hot, spicy, and citrus foods; commercial dentifrices; chewing gum; candy; and lozenges is necessary. Cheilitis may be treated with cool tapwater compresses and the application of a topical fluorinated corticosteroid (such as Lidex gel 0.05%) and protective ointments. Gargling with 5 mL of diphenhydramine (Benadryl elixir) or Magic Mary's Mouthwash may give symptomatic relief.

The condition of atypical gingivostomatitis, in which the patient presents with fire-engine red gingiva, is frequently caused by gum chewing. Elimination of gum chewing frequently resolves the problem.

Denture Sore Mouth

This condition is most common in postmenopausal women and is attributed to bone loss in the jaw, which alters the fit of dentures. It is frequently compounded by *Candida* infections. Removal of the dentures every night and application of anticandidal cream such as clotrimazole (Lotrimin, Mycelex) to the oral mucosa and denture are often helpful. Construction of a new denture may be necessary.

Drugs frequently are associated with alteration in the mucosa and may cause sore mouth. Gingival hyperplasia may occur in patients using phenytoin (Dilantin) or cyclosporine (Neoral); mouth ulcers may result from cytotoxic drugs; antibiotics can cause black hairy tongue or overgrowth of *Candida*; gold or penicillamine therapy may produce a lichen planus–like stomatitis under the tongue; local burns may be produced by aspirin; and various drugs may cause xerostomia.

Oral Burns

Mild thermal, electrical, and chemical burns of the lips, tongue, and palate are usually minor and heal uneventfully in 1 week. Use of one of the local anesthetic preparations previously discussed relieves pain and promotes healing.

Xerostomia

Dryness of the mouth is a sign of impaired salivary gland function and may be temporary or permanent. Transient causes include emotional stress, drugs such as anticholinergic compounds and antihista-mines, excessive mouth breathing, and sialolithiasis. There is atrophy of the salivary glands with age and after radiotherapy to the head and neck. These changes are irreversible. If none of these is apparent or if keratoconjunctivitis sicca is present, a general evaluation should be performed to look for systemic disorders such as Sjögren's syndrome, scleroderma, rheumatoid arthritis, diabetes mellitus, lupus erythematosus, sarcoidosis, paraproteinemias, and malignancies.

Treatment of xerostomia is difficult. If the cause is a drug, it may not be practical to withdraw the medication. If the problem is salivary gland atrophy, there is no effective way to increase saliva production, although chewing sugarless gum, lemon slices, or sugar-free sweets may stimulate saliva production. Symptomatic relief may be obtained by frequent sips of water or a saliva substitute (Xero-Lube, Salivart).

Dental caries often occur rapidly in patients with xerostomia; therefore, good oral hygiene, prompt referral to a dentist, and intermittent fluoride treatments are necessary. Oral candidiasis can be a problem and must be treated.

OTHER BENIGN TUMORS

Melanocytic Nevi

Pigmented nevi of all types may be seen in the mucosa, including lentigos and blue, junctional, compound, and dermal nevi. Excision to exclude the possibility of melanoma is appropriate treatment.

Occasionally, bluish brown macules located on the posterior gingiva and adjacent buccal mucosa (amalgam tattoos), which represent the submucosal inclusion of amalgam particles inoculated traumatically, may be mistaken for melanocytic nevi. These metallic particles may be identified by soft tissue radiographic films, and no treatment is indicated.

Oral Pigmentation

Other oral pigmentary problems of systemic importance include those resulting from heavy metal exposure (bismuth and mercury cause black lines at the gingival margin, and lead and silver leave a diffuse grayish color on the gingiva), ingestion of antimalarial agents or phenothiazine, Addison's disease, hemochromatosis, neurofibromatosis, and Peutz-Jeghers syndrome. If there is any evidence of these disorders, the patient should undergo a general evaluation. Physiologic, asymptomatic pigmentation is common in the oral mucosa of black patients.

Mucocele

Mucous cysts are most commonly located on the lower lip and represent the reaction of oral mucous glands to obstruction of the duct carrying the mucoid secretion to the mucosal surface. They may be produced by trauma or infection. Because these usually lack a true cyst wall, excision may result in the development of further cystic lesions because healing may obliterate other ducts in the area that were severed in the surgical procedure. An alternative form of therapy is cryosurgery with a liquid nitrogen probe, although this may require more than one treatment. Persistent lesions may be incised and the enlarged glandular tissue carefully teased and squeezed out through the opening. The base should not be desiccated because this may promote recurrence.

Fibromas and Papillomas

These pedunculated, fibrous, and benign epithelial neoplasms can occur anywhere in the mucosa and can be removed by simple excision.

Warts

Verruca vulgaris and condyloma acuminatum may occur on the vermilion border or the oral mucosa. Simple excision may be done and histologic studies performed if there is any possibility of verrucous carcinoma. Light electrodesiccation and curettage during local anesthesia are usually successful. Cryosurgery with a liquid nitrogen probe may give excellent results. Areas of treatment should not be sutured because this may deposit the virus along the suture tract and result in additional lesions.

These are intraepithelial growths, and deep, destructive measures are not warranted. Multiple verrucae on the lips and oral mucosa should suggest Cowden's syndrome.

Torus Palatinus and Mandibularis

These are benign, simple bony growths on the hard palate or lingual surface of the mandible. Surgical removal may be performed when a prosthetic appliance is necessary.

OTHER MALIGNANT TUMORS

The majority of oral cancers are squamous cell carcinomas (more than 95%). Most others are adenocarcinomas arising from minor salivary glands. Definitive treatment is surgical. These are radioresponsive but probably not radiocurable. Melanomas are rare and usually advanced when diagnosed and are treated by radical excision. Other unusual primary oral tumors include lymphoma, fibrosarcoma, rhabdomyosarcoma, liposarcoma, neurofibrosarcoma, angiosarcoma, Kaposi's sarcoma, and granular cell tumor. Basal cell carcinoma may occasionally involve the mucosa of the lip as an extension from the skin surface. Mucosal basal cell carcinoma is probably an extraosseous ameloblastoma. Therapy depends on the histologic differentiation, location, and size of tumor. One percent of oral malignancies are metastatic from the breast, lung, kidney, thyroid, prostate, and occasionally other sites. Most occur in the mandi-

ble and are usually asymptomatic. Current therapeutic modalities are insufficient, and the prognosis of these patients is generally poor.

VENOUS LEG ULCERS

method of
DAVID J. MARGOLIS, M.D. M.S.C.E.
Center for Epidemiology and Biostatistics
Philadelphia, Pennsylvania

Chronic wounds of the lower extremity afflict a significant proportion of the population. The prevalence of lower extremity wounds in the adult population is between 0.18% and 1.3%. Venous leg ulcers account for 40 to 70% of all lower extremity chronic wounds. A disproportionate number of individuals with venous leg ulcers are elderly (88% are older than 60 years) or female (3:1). It has been estimated that between 500,000 and 1 million Americans have venous leg ulcers. Between 1990 and 1992, there were an estimated 1.3 million outpatient visits for venous leg ulcers in the United States. These wounds are associated with feelings of fear, social isolation, anger, depression, and resentment.

CLINICAL FEATURES

A venous leg ulcer is a wound of the lower extremity. Most frequently the wound extends to the deep dermis. This wound most commonly occurs on the "gaiter" area of the leg, which is located between the upper two thirds of the calf and one inch below the malleolus. Individuals with venous leg ulcers tend to have distinctive clinical signs and symptoms, such as limb dermatitis, lipodermatosclerosis, varicose veins, limb edema, and painful "tired" legs. Limb dermatitis is best described as a red weepy patch of skin on an edematous lower extremity. It may be painful or itchy. Lipodermatosclerosis is a patch of skin on an edematous or previously edematous lower extremity that can range in color from red to purple to brown. The skin itself is hard and indurated. Lipodermatosclerosis can be very painful. Although patients with venous dermatitis and lipodermatosclerosis may not have an ulcer, they still have a lower limb venous disorder.

The clinical diagnosis of a venous leg ulcer is made in any individual with a chronic wound in the gaiter area of the lower extremity, with other clinical signs compatible with venous abnormalities (e.g., varicose veins, venous blush, lipodermatosclerosis), who has an adequately functioning lower limb arterial system (e.g., ankle brachial index >0.80, presence of a palpable distal limb pulse). It is, of course, possible that the clinical diagnosis of a venous leg ulcer actually represents a spectrum of diseases that manifest as a common clinical syndrome that, as a group, can be treated and prevented with similar therapies. Supplemental testing to evaluate the venous functioning of a patient's lower extremity can be important. These tests include air, photo or water plethysmography, duplex ultrasonography, and invasive venous pressure monitoring. When these tests are ordered, it is important to request that the technician evaluate the anatomy or functioning of the venous system and not just evaluate the lower extremity for a deep venous thrombosis.

ETIOLOGY

Individuals with venous leg ulcers or disease are believed to have chronic ambulatory venous hypertension. During ambulation, in an individual with a properly functioning venous system, the pressure in the superficial venous system falls toward zero. In an individual with venous disease, superficial venous pressure is elevated during ambulation to as high as 40 to 100 mm Hg.

The reason that patients with ambulatory venous hypertension develop venous associated wounds or skin problems is not clear. Several models have been generated to explain the tissue damage that results in wounds. The most popular models concern the deposition of pericapillary fibrin in the small venules surrounding the ulcers, the trapping of inflammatory cells within the venules surrounding the ulcers resulting in the liberation of proteolytic enzymes, and the trapping of essential growth factors by macroglobulins within the venules and dermis surrounding the ulcers. None of these models has been fully validated by experimental evidence. Central to all of these models, however, is an alteration in venous hemodynamics of the lower limb resulting in abnormally elevated ambulatory venous pressure. Successfully addressing ambulatory venous hypertension appears to be a key ingredient to most therapies, and therefore most successful therapies use some form of lower limb compression to reduce the elevated ambulatory venous pressures.

TREATMENT

Over the past 2000 years, multiple therapies have been proposed for the treatment of venous leg ulcers. Hippocrates (circa 400 BC) wrote about the treatment of venous disease. In AD 1363, Guy de Chauliac was the first to recommend lower limb compression. The most popular form of bandage for venous leg ulcers was introduced by P. G. Unna in 1885 and has not been substantially improved. This form of lower limb compression is gauze impregnated with zinc and fitted to the patient's leg. Although not appreciated by Unna, the essential component of this technique is the compression of the lower limb afforded by this bandage, not the zinc. Lower limb compression is still the standard of care for patients with venous leg ulcers. In fact, this treatment was recently supported by two extensive literature reviews.

Limb compression can be applied with a multilayered bandage (e.g., wound dressing, and then to the full lower limb roll gauze, Unna boot, and a self-adherent crepe bandage), an Unna boot, a limb compression garment or stockings that generate at least 20 mm Hg pressure, or a limb compression pump. It is my belief that a multilayered compression bandage changed weekly is the best treatment. Very few studies, however, have demonstrated a significant and reproducible advantage of any method of lower limb compression over another. Unfortunately, the use of lower limb compression is not always successful. At best, after 24 weeks of therapy between 30% and 60% of lower limb ulcers heal. Most, if not all, patients with dermatitis and lipdermatosclerosis also improve with limb compression.

In addition to limb compression, which treats the cause of the wound (i.e., ambulatory venous hyper-
tension), the wound and periwound area must also be treated. This includes gentle cleansing of the wound, a moist wound dressing, and care and protection of the periwound. Periwound care includes treating the dermatitis with a moisturizer, such as petroleum jelly, and protecting the skin from maceration due to wound exudate with products such as zinc paste. Débridement of necrotic tissue and systemic or topical treatment for tissue infection may also be required.

With the advent of biotechnology, several novel and new treatments have been introduced. Although most of the studies that evaluate these new treatments have not been published, the Food and Drug Administration did recently approve the use of a cultured skin equivalent for the treatment of venous leg ulcers and the use of a recombinant growth factor for the treatment of diabetic neuropathic foot ulcers. Health care providers have also used horse chestnut extract, prostaglandin inhibitors, aspirin,* pentoxifylline (Trental),* stanozolol (Winstrol),* and several other agents to treat venous leg ulcers. The general consensus is that these products have not been well demonstrated to heal more wounds than standard care. Finally, several surgical therapies have been developed to treat lower limb venous disorders. The success of many of these techniques varies and may be dependent on the surgeon's skill.

PREVENTION

It is a common belief that venous leg ulcers can be successfully prevented with the use of compression stockings. These stockings help prevent edema formation and reduce ambulatory venous hypertension. For example, in a retrospective chart review it was found that the risk of recurrence for an individual with a recently healed venous leg ulcer who did not use a compression stocking was 100% in 3 years, but among individuals who did use a compression stocking the risk of recurrence was 29% over 5 years. In a recent randomized clinical trial of individuals with deep venous thrombosis, those who were randomized to compression stockings had a statistically significant decreased incidence of post-thrombotic syndrome, including venous ulceration.

CONCLUSION

The ambulatory care setting is ideal for treating a patient with a venous leg ulcer. Before commencing treatment, however, it is important to correctly differentiate a venous leg ulcer from other causes of leg ulcer (e.g., arterial insufficiency, atypical infections, diabetic neuropathic foot ulcer, and pyoderma gangrenosum). Wounds that do not heal in a reasonable period of time should be re-evaluated, a tissue biopsy considered, and perhaps a referral made to a specialist. Wounds that are least likely to respond within 6 months of care with a limb compression bandage are

---

*Not FDA approved for this indication.

more than 10 cm² and more than 12 months of age before treatment commences.

PRESSURE ULCERS

method of
DAVID R. THOMAS, M.D.
Saint Louis University
St. Louis, Missouri

A pressure ulcer is the visible evidence of pathologic changes in blood supply to the dermal and underlying tissues, usually due to compression of the tissue over a bony prominence.

A differential diagnosis of ulcer type is critical to treatment. Chronic ulcers of the skin include arterial ulcers, venous stasis ulcers, diabetic ulcers, and pressure ulcers. A classic presentation aids the diagnosis. For example, arterial ulcers occur in the distal digits or over a bony prominence, diabetic ulcers occur in regions of callous formation, and venous stasis ulcers on the lateral aspect of the lower leg. However, atypical presentations may occasionally obscure the etiology. The treatment of these various causes differs considerably. This discussion is limited to the treatment of pressure ulcers and should not be used to treat other types of ulcers.

Seven principles of management guide treatment of pressure ulcers. The chief cause of these ulcers is pressure applied to the tissues that compromises blood flow. Therefore, the first treatment principle is to relieve pressure. Pressure relief can be obtained by positioning the patient frequently at a fixed interval so as to relieve pressure over the compromised area. Turning and positioning may be difficult to achieve, owing to a patient's self-positioning or to medical treatments that interfere with the ability to position the patient. Because of this difficulty, a number of medical devices have been designed in an attempt to relieve pressure. These devices can be classified as static or dynamic. Static devices include air-, gel-, or water-filled containers that reduce the tissue-surface interface. Dynamic devices use a power source to fill compartments with air that support the patient's weight or that alternate the pressure on different areas of the body. A static device should be chosen when the patient has good bed mobility. A dynamic device should be used when the patient cannot self-position in bed.

Results of reported clinical trials do not favor one device over another. The choice should be based on durability, ease of use, and patient comfort. A simple check for "bottoming out" should be done for all devices. This is done by inserting a hand palm upward under the patient's sacrum between the device and the bed surface. If there is not an air column between the patient and the bed surface, the device is ineffective and should be changed. No device is effective in reducing heel pressure, the second most common site for pressure ulcers. Bridging with pillows is effective in reducing heel pressure in immobile patients; patients with high bed mobility may require boot devices to elevate the heel off the bed surface. Patients who fail to improve or who have multiple pressure ulcers should be considered for a dynamic type device, such as a low–air loss bed or air-fluidized bed.

The second principle of pressure ulcer therapy is to assess pain. Pressure ulcers do not always result in pain, particularly in insensate patients. However, some pressure ulcers do result in pain and should be aggressively treated. Oral or parenteral pain medications should be used to control symptoms.

The third principle of ulcer therapy is to assess nutrition and hydration. Pressure ulcers occur in sicker individuals in whom nutrient intake may be reduced by coexisting illness. Increased intake of protein (1.2 to 1.5 gram per kg per day) has been associated with higher healing rates. Achievement of high protein intake may be difficult owing to anorexia of aging or anorexia associated with coexisting diseases. Adequate calories, adjusted for stress (30 to 35 kcal per kg per day), should be prescribed. Adequate dietary intake should provide adequate vitamins and minerals. No difference in healing rates has been associated with supertherapeutic doses of vitamin C or zinc. If adequate dietary intake is compromised, a supplemental vitamin/mineral prescription including recommended daily allowances from the Food and Drug Administration should be considered. Adequate hydration can be maintained with 30 mL per kg per day of water. The decision to institute enteral feeding in patients with pressure ulcers who are unable to maintain adequate oral intake should not be undertaken lightly. The decision to use enteral feeding must consider the patient's wishes, the overall goal of care, and the complications of enteral feeding. In several studies, the long-term result of enteral feeding has been associated with poorer outcomes in patients with pressure ulcers.

The fourth principle of pressure ulcer management requires removing necrotic debris. Phagocytosis removes necrotic debris naturally. Accelerating the rate of removal may shorten healing time. Options include sharp surgical débridement, mechanical débridement with gauze dressings, application of exogenous enzymes, or autolytic débridement under occlusive dressings. Choose surgical débridement if the ulcer is infected. Surgical débridement is the fastest method but may remove some viable tissue, cause discomfort, and is the most expensive method, especially if done in an operating room. Applying moist gauze that is allowed to become adherent to the ulcer bed by drying is a form of débridement. When the dry dressing is removed, nonselective tissue removal occurs. This method can be associated with discomfort, may delay healing while débridement is in progress, and is often defeated when the dressing is remoistened before removal. Enzymatic débridement can digest necrotic material. Enzymes evaluated in pressure ulcer trials include streptokinase/streptodornase (SK/SD) combination, collagenase, trypsin, and papain. Most enzyme preparations are nonselective, resulting in some damage to fibroblasts or epithelial cells. Enzymatic débridement is slower, can be associated with discomfort, and should be limited in duration until a clean wound bed is obtained. Autolytic débridement is achieved by allowing autolysis under an occlusive dressing. Both enzymatic and autolytic débridement may require 2 to 6 weeks to achieve a clean wound bed. Unless clinically infected, heel ulcers are better left undébrided because they occur in poorly vascularized tissues.

The fifth principle of pressure ulcer management is to maintain a moist wound environment. Maintaining a moist wound environment has been associated with more rapid healing rates compared with dressings that are allowed to dry. Continuously moist saline gauze is the historical standard dressing for stage II through IV pressure ulcers. Care must be taken to change the gauze frequently to prevent drying, because this may delay healing. Newer wound dressings provide a low moisture vapor transmission rate (MVTR), a measure of how quickly the dressing allows drying. An MVTR of less than 35 grams of water vapor per square meter per hour is required to maintain a moist wound environment. Woven gauze has an MVTR of 68 grams per square meter per hour and impregnated gauze has an MVTR of 57 grams per square meter per hour. By comparison, hydrocolloid dressings have an MVTR of 8 grams per square meter per hour. Dressings with a low MVTR provide a healing environment that encourages granulation tissue formation and epithelialization.

The use of occlusive-type dressings has been shown to be more cost effective than gauze dressings, primarily due to a decrease in nursing time for dressing changes. Occlusive dressings can be divided into broad categories of polymer films, polymer foams, hydrogels, hydrocolloids, alginates, and biomembranes. Each has advantages and disadvantages. No single agent is perfect. The choice of a particular agent depends on the clinical circumstances. Nonpermeable polymers can be macerating to normal skin. Polymer films are not absorptive and may leak, particularly when the wound is highly exudative. Most films have an adhesive backing that may remove epithelial cells when the dressing is changed. Hydrogels are hydrophilic polymers that are insoluble in water but absorb aqueous solutions. They are poor bacterial barriers and are nonadherent to the wound. Because of their high specific heat, these dressings are cooling to the skin, aiding in pain control and reducing inflammation. Most of these dressings require a secondary dressing to secure them to the wound. Hydrocolloid dressings are complex dressings similar to ostomy barrier products. They are impermeable to moisture and bacteria and are highly adherent to the skin. Hydrocolloid dressings have accelerated healing 40% compared with moist gauze dressings. They are particularly suited for areas subject to urinary and fecal incontinence. Their adhesiveness to surrounding skin is higher than some surgical tapes, but they are nonadherent to wound

tissue and do not damage epithelialization of the wound. The adhesive barrier is frequently overcome in highly exudative wounds. Hydrocolloid dressings cannot be used over tendons or on wounds with eschar formation. Alginates are complex polysaccharide dressings that are highly absorbent in exudative wounds. This high absorbency is particularly suited to exudative wounds. Alginates are nonadherent to the wound, but if the wound is allowed to dry, damage to the epithelial tissue may occur with removal. The biomembranes are very expensive and not readily available.

Stage I and II pressure ulcers can be managed with a polymer film or hydrocolloid dressing. Stage III and IV ulcers may require a wound filler, such as a calcium alginate or moist gauze, to obliterate deadspace and decrease anaerobic colonization.

Electrotherapy has been used for stage III and IV pressure ulcers unresponsive to conventional therapy. Several clinical trials suggest that electrotherapy is likely to be effective. Hyperbaric oxygen, ultrasound, and infrared, ultraviolet, and low-energy laser irradiation have insufficient data to recommend their use currently. No data support the use of systemic vasodilator, hemorrheologics, serotonin inhibitors, or fibrolytic agents in the treatment of pressure ulcers. Topical agents such as zinc, phenytoin, aluminum hydroxide, honey, sugar, yeast, aloe vera gel, or gold have not been demonstrated to be effective in clinical trials. Growth factors have shown promising early results but have not been approved for use in pressure ulcers.

Because the theory of augmenting ulcer healing under the newer dressings suggests that wound fluid contains favorable healing factors, it is important not to change the dressings too frequently. Unless the wound fluid seeps from under the dressing, the dressing should not be changed more often than every 3 to 7 days.

The sixth principle of pressure ulcer treatment is to encourage granulation tissue formation and promote re-epithelialization. Wound healing factors and growth factors are under investigation for their effect in healing pressure ulcers. It is important not to negatively affect granulation and epithelial tissue. A number of wound cleaners and antiseptics have been shown to be toxic to fibroblasts and epithelial tissues, including benzalkonium chloride (Zephiran), povidone-iodine (Betadine) solution, Dakin's solution, hydrogen peroxide, Granulex, Hibiclens, and pHisoHex. For pressure ulcers, use of these agents should be only for infected ulcers and strictly limited in duration.

The seventh principle of pressure ulcer management is to control infection. Quantitative microbiology alone is a poor predictor of clinical infection in chronic wounds. All pressure ulcers are colonized with bacteria, usually from skin or fecal flora. The presence of microorganisms alone (colonization) does not indicate an infection in pressure ulcers. The diagnosis of infection in chronic wounds must be based on clinical signs—erythema, warmth, pain, edema, odor, fever, or purulent exudate. In the presence of clinical signs of infection, enteral or parenteral antibiotics should be used. In ulcers that are not progressing toward healing, an empirical trial of a topical antimicrobial may be considered, although the data are inconclusive.

ATOPIC DERMATITIS

method of
ADELAIDE A. HEBERT, M.D., and
KHANH NGUYEN, M.D.
University of Texas Medical School at Houston
Houston, Texas

DEFINITION

Atopic dermatitis is a chronic skin disorder that involves recurrent episodes of pruritus, xerosis, and lichenification. Frequently, patients with this condition have a family and personal history of asthma and allergic rhinitis. This skin condition usually begins between 3 months to 5 years of age, is characterized by a waxing and waning course, and has numerous physical or psychological triggers. Table 1 lists criteria for diagnosing atopic dermatitis. Table 2 lists the differential diagnosis for atopic dermatitis.

TABLE 1. Major and Minor Criteria for Diagnosis of Atopic Dermatitis

Must Have at Least Three Major Criteria
Pruritus
Typical morphology and distribution—a bilaterally symmetrical dermatitis usually involving the flexures of the arms, legs, and neck
Chronic or chronically relapsing dermatitis
Personal or family history of atopy (asthma, allergic rhinitis, eczema)
Must Have at Least Three Minor Criteria
Xerosis
Ichthyosis (palmar hyperlinearity, keratosis pilaris)
Immediate (type 1) skin test reactivity
Early age at onset
Tendency toward cutaneous skin infections (esp. *Staphylococcus aureus* infection and herpes simplex), impaired cell-mediated immunity
Tendency toward chronic hand and foot dermatitis
Nipple eczema
Cheilitis
Recurrent conjunctivitis
Dennie-Morgan infraorbital line
Keratoconus
Periorbital darkening
Facial pallor centrally with peripheral facial erythema
Pityriasis alba
Anterior neck folds
Itch when sweating
Intolerance to wool and lipid solvents
Perifollicular accentuation
Food intolerance
Course influenced by environment or emotional factors
White dermatographism, delayed blanch

From Roth HL: Atopic dermatitis. *In* Rakel RE (ed): Conn's Current Therapy. Philadelphia, WB Saunders Co, 1998, p 837.

TABLE 2. Differential Diagnosis for Atopic Dermatitis

Seborrheic dermatitis	Tinea/fungal infection
Contact dermatitis	Psoriasis
Drug eruption	Mycosis fungoides

POSSIBLE MECHANISM

The underlying pathology for atopic dermatitis may result from an increased release of histamine and IgE and from disequilibrium between the Th_1 and Th_2 T lymphocyte system.

TREATMENT

At the initial visit, the physician should explain to the patient that atopic dermatitis is a chronic disease that cannot be cured. Compliance with general dry skin care and medical treatment as necessary may allow patients long intervals without active skin disease.

Nonmedical Therapy

A patient with atopic dermatitis has chronically dry skin and must follow a good xerotic skin care therapy throughout the year; following this regimen will decrease the numbers of episodes of active disease. The patient may bathe daily with a gentle bar soap such as Cetaphil, Caress, and unscented Dove or with a soap-free liquid cleanser such as Cetaphil or Aquanil. Warm (not hot) water should be used, and the patient should not spend long periods of time soaking. Immediately after bathing, the patient should apply an emollient all over. In general, the greasier an emollient, the better it moisturizes. Ointments such as Vaseline and Aquaphor are excellent moisturizers; however, some patients find them unacceptably heavy and they are not suitable in warm, humid weather. Most patients prefer creams such as Eucerin and Lubriderm, although these may not be adequately moisturizing in cold weather. An emollient should be applied at least twice a day all year round; and during periods of active skin disease, multiple applications may be necessary.

As important as faithful attention to good skin care habits is the avoidance of trigger factors. Probably the most important trigger is cold, dry weather; patients with atopic dermatitis may benefit during these times from an indoor humidifier and by minimizing outdoor activities. Avoidance of hot, humid weather may also be necessary because these conditions can cause sweat retention, irritation, and pruritus. Secondary bacterial infection often exacerbates atopic dermatitis and has to be treated with topical or oral antibiotics. Other trigger factors include noncompliance with therapy, woolen clothing, animal dander, house dust, tobacco smoke, and emotional stress. Ideally, clothing should be made of 100% cotton. Patients should also keep their fingernails trimmed short to minimize bacterial infection from excoriation.

Medical Therapy

Mild Case

The current mainstay of treatment is topical corticosteroids. These agents have an anti-inflammatory and antipruritic effect. Generally, they should be applied to affected areas after bathing, and an emollient should then be applied on top of the corticosteroid preparation. Topical corticosteroids alone do not provide adequate hydration and must be used with an emollient.

There is a wide variety of topical corticosteroids, ranging from potent, class I agents, to the mild, over-the-counter class VII agents, such as 1% hydrocortisone. All have an adequate half-life in the skin such that there is no additional benefit to more than twice-daily application of these agents. Corticosteroid ointment penetrates thick, lichenified plaques better and contains fewer preservatives than do cream formulations. Although not as potent as ointment counterparts, creams are generally better tolerated and are more suitable during humid weather. A thin layer of the agent should be applied twice daily in a cephalocaudad direction. The physician should regularly inspect treated areas for signs of corticosteroid-induced skin atrophy such as telangiectasia, purpura, and skin thinning. The more potent the topical corticosteroid, the higher the risk of cutaneous atrophy; there is almost no risk with 1% hydrocortisone.

For mild cases, we use low- to mid-potency topical corticosteroids such as 0.05% desonide (DesOwen, class VI) or 0.2% hydrocortisone valerate (Westcort, class V). If there is little response, we will then use mid-potency agents, such as 0.1% triamcinolone, twice daily. Unlike the other topical corticosteroids, this agent is available in large quantities, such as a 1-pound jar, at a reasonable price. If active disease continues, we then use a potent agent such as 0.05% betamethasone dipropionate (Diprolene, class I) or 0.05% fluocinonide (Lidex, class II). These agents are very potent and probably provide adequate therapy with once-daily dosing; the patient may use additionally a less potent topical corticosteroid or a tar as the second agent. These potent topical corticosteroids carry a risk of cutaneous atrophy and even systemic absorption and should be used for more than 2 weeks consecutively only in special, well-supervised circumstances. As soon as the atopic dermatitis starts to improve, tapering of dosage should be done with a lower potency agent on a twice-daily or even once-daily basis. Tachyphylaxis does occur, and the patient should discontinue topical corticosteroid therapy soon after active disease has resolved. If the atopic dermatitis is resistant to a prolonged course of potent topical corticosteroid, a completely different treatment modality should be considered.

Certain body areas are more susceptible to corticosteroid-induced atrophy. There will be an occasional patient with severe atopic dermatitis on the face. We generally do not use topical corticosteroids more potent than 2.5% hydrocortisone in this area, and try to taper down to 1% hydrocortisone as quickly as possible. As mentioned later, other agents such as tar or (soon) topical tacrolimus may be very helpful in this area.

Atopic dermatitis of the scalp can be treated with a tar shampoo, such as T/Gel or PolyTar. A 1% hydrocortisone solution (such as Texacort) can be left on overnight. More potent agents such as 0.05% fluocinonide (Lidex) or 0.05% clobetasol propionate (Temovate) scalp solutions may be left on overnight but should not be used for more than 2 weeks continuously. For atopic dermatitis on the eyelid, we use 0.05% dexamethasone sodium phosphate (Decadron) ophthalmic solution, which is safe if accidentally spread to the eye surface. The maximum duration of use is 2 weeks. The axillary and intertriginous areas are also very vulnerable to corticosteroid atrophy and should be treated as described earlier for the face.

Alternatives to topical corticosteroids are tar preparations. Over-the-counter products include Estar 5% gel, Tegrin 1% cream, Elta Lite Tar lotion, Balnetar liquid, Neutrogena T-Derm tar emollient, and MG-217 2% ointment. Physicians may order the formulation of crude, cold tar in concentrations ranging from 1 to 20%, usually in a petrolatum base. A more cosmetically acceptable, although less efficacious, product is LCD (Liquor Carbonis Detergens), which is a refined tar; this agent can be mixed by pharmacists in various concentrations. Tar can have a good therapeutic effect, but the onset of action is slower and it may stain bathtubs, clothing, towels, and so on. Patients may use tar as a corticosteroid-sparing agent, for example, by applying the tar product at night and the topical corticosteroid in the morning after bathing. There may be a synergistic effect because the mechanism of action of tar is different from that of topical corticosteroids.

Pruritus often accompanies active episodes of atopic dermatitis. During these periods, scheduled antihistamines are necessary and the dosage depends on the age and weight of the patient. Generally, during an active episode, we will use an oral antihistamine scheduled every 6 hours. A sedating antihistamine such as hydroxyzine (Atarax) and diphenhydramine (Benadryl) probably work best. Patients must be warned of the danger of driving and other such activities while acclimatizing to the sedative effect. Some patients will prefer the nonsedating antihistamine such as a morning dose of loratadine (Claritin), although these agents may not be as antipruritic. Such patients may then take an evening dose of a sedating antihistamine. The tricyclic antidepressant doxepin (Sinequan), although not approved for this indication, has a much greater antipruritic effect but also carries the side effects typical of this class of drug. A dose of 10 mg three times daily or 25 to 50 mg nightly is usually effective in controlling the itching.

Moderate Case

Therapy for moderately severe atopic dermatitis may include phototherapy and is administered in a phototherapy unit, usually in a dermatologist's office. Patients with lupus, porphyria, prior history of cutaneous malignancies, and on photosensitizing medications should not receive this therapy. We usually administer suberythremogenic dosages of ultraviolet light B (UVB) on an every-other-day basis. Daily treatment is not advisable because signs of burning may not appear until 24 hours later. We increase the dose of UVB gradually at each treatment session. Most patients start to respond after 12 to 14 sessions. Once remission is achieved, the frequency of therapy is tapered over the next 3 to 4 weeks. During a phototherapy session, the patient must wear protective eyewear and shield the face and genitalia (unless those areas are affected). Patients will continue their normal dry skin care routine and other topical therapy as well.

For moderate to severe, chronic cases of atopic dermatitis, we use combination UVA/UVB therapy, which can be administered in the same phototherapy unit. In one study of this therapy by Jekler and Lark, significant clinical improvement with a concomitant reduction in corticosteroid use occurred in 8 weeks or less and was more efficacious than broad-band UVB. UVB at 311 nm also demonstrated effectiveness in managing this type of atopic dermatitis.

For patients with very itchy, dry, widespread atopic dermatitis and for patients with erythrodermic atopic dermatitis, we use triamcinolone 0.1% cream wet wrap therapy one to three times daily (Table 3). This therapy is soothing and may help the patient sleep well for the first time in weeks. This modality can be used in conjunction with phototherapy. Tapering of therapy begins with decreasing the frequency of wrapping or by not wrapping the improved areas. Our nurses perform wet wrap therapy in clinics and also teach patients how to do it at home; thus the initial care is both therapeutic and educational for the family and the patient.

Many patients with atopic dermatitis are colonized with *Staphylococcus aureus*, which may drive the disease even without clinical evidence of cutaneous infection. Some patients may benefit from a 2- to 3-week course of an appropriate oral antibiotic, such as dicloxacillin (Dynapen) or cephalexin (Keflex), both given at 250 to 500 mg four times daily. Cephalexin is usually the preferred liquid formulation because of better taste and ease in calculating pediatric dosages based on weight. An alternative medication that requires fewer doses is azithromycin (Zithromax), which is available in liquid and pill formulations. Use of intranasal muciprocin (Bactroban) to eliminate colonization in the nares may be necessary.

Severe Case

During the treatment of seemingly unresponsive atopic dermatitis, the physician should periodically reconsider the original diagnosis. A skin biopsy may be necessary to rule out other entities listed in Table 2.

Patients with very severe chronic atopic dermatitis and erythrodermic atopic dermatitis may be candidates for oral corticosteroid therapy. Treatment with oral corticosteroids should be considered the last therapeutic resort when all other modalities have proven inadequate. The systemic side effects are well known; and in patients with coexisting conditions such as diabetes, hypertension, and immunosuppression, systemic corticosteroids should be used with even more caution. Unfortunately, many patients treated with oral corticosteroids will subsequently be less willing to use other therapies. Oral therapy of 2 weeks or less causes little suppression of the hypothalamus-pituitary-adrenal (HPA) axis. A longer course requires tapering to finish; the function of the HPA may be abnormal for 1 year after discontinuation. A typical dose of prednisone is 1 to 2 mg per kg per day. Every-other-day dosing is preferable.

Hypersensitivity to certain food types may exacerbate atopic dermatitis in a small number of cases. The most common food types in children are eggs (nearly 50% of cases), cow's milk, soy, wheat, peanut, and fish. Dietary elimination of the responsible food, with the aid of a dietitian, may lead to improvement in these patients in 1 to 2 months.

Acute Flare

The sudden onset of cold, dry weather is a very common cause for acute exacerbation of chronic atopic dermatitis. Patients present with worsened pruritus, excoriation, intense erythema, and juicy and weeping pustules. To dry out the weeping exudate, wet compresses (soaked in plain water or germicidal aluminum acetate [Burow's] solution) may be applied for 10 minutes, two to three times daily. One can make Burow's solution by dissolving one aluminum acetate (Domeboro) effervescent tablet or packet in 1 pint of tepid water. For control of increased inflammation, the patient can use a more potent topical corticosteroid or wet wrap therapy, if necessary. The physician can increase the dosage or frequency of sedating antihistamine as needed for pruritus.

Another common cause of an acute flare is cutaneous bacterial infection. Typical findings are weeping, crusting pustules. In addition to above therapy, such patients can generally be started on an appropriate oral antibiotic for 7 to 10 days while awaiting the results of bacterial culture and sensitivity. For lim-

---

TABLE 3. **How to Apply Corticosteroid Wet Wrap Dressings**

Skin should be cleansed.
Apply triamcinolone acetonide 0.1% cream all over the body, except head, axillae, or groin.
Apply hydrocortisone 1% cream to face, axillae, or groin (if affected).
Apply thin, warm, wet cotton towels to the entire body, except the head.
Cover the body with a thermal blanket for 1 hour.
Remove towels.
Apply moisturizer all over in a head-to-toe direction.
Repeat two or three times daily.

ited areas of impetiginization, muciprocin ointment or cream alone may be sufficient.

Experimental

Current experimental drugs include interferon gamma, phosphodiesterase inhibitors, and photopheresis. UVA1 (340 to 400 nm) has been shown to reduce acute flares of atopic dermatitis and has been proposed for prophylactic therapy for atopic dermatitis. In recent trials, we have found topical tacrolimus (FK 506), a derivative of cyclosporine, to be at least as effective as potent topical corticosteroids. Tacrolimus has produced dramatic improvement in cases of atopic dermatitis resistant to other therapies, with minimal immediate side effects. Studies on ascomycin macrolactam (SDZ ASM 981) have also shown promise in the treatment of moderate atopic dermatitis. Long-term side effects remain unknown.

ERYTHEMA MULTIFORME, STEVENS-JOHNSON SYNDROME, AND TOXIC EPIDERMAL NECROLYSIS

method of
JEAN-CLAUDE ROUJEAU, M.D.
Hôpital H Mondor, Université Paris XII,
Créteil, France

ERYTHEMA MULTIFORME

Erythema multiforme (EM) is an acute, self-limited, feverish eruption characterized by its clinical pattern: papular, iris, or target cutaneous lesions mainly located on the extremities. Mucous membrane erosions are frequent, usually restricted to the lips and the mouth. Because of the different demographic characteristics of the patients, distinct patterns and distributions of the skin lesions, different pathologies, and distinct causes, EM should be separated from Stevens-Johnson syndrome and toxic epidermal necrolysis.

EM is characterized by a spontaneous resolution in 1 to 6 weeks, but is frequently (30 to 50%) recurrent. Rarely recurrences overlap, leading to "continuous" or "persistent" EM. Mouth erosions may strongly impair the quality of life of patients with recurrent or continuous disease.

Drug eruptions are sometimes reported as erythema multiforme when some of the circinate lesions resemble targets, but in my experience true typical EM is rarely, if ever, caused by drugs. The principal cause of EM is infection with herpes simplex virus (HSV), which explains 30 to 70% of all cases. Many other infectious agents can induce occasional cases, especially *Mycoplasma pneumoniae.* Most recurrent cases occur 1 to 10 days after a bout of recurrent herpes. Fragments of viral DNA, but not infective HSV, can be detected in EM lesions. EM is thought to result from an immunologic reaction to proteins produced in the skin by the viral DNA.

Management of Acute Attacks

Even in cases obviously related to HSV, acyclovir is not effective after EM has developed. When *M. pneumoniae* infection is suspected (e.g., with cough, atypical pneumonia), I prescribe erythromycin even though there is no demonstration that it shortens the course of EM.

Treating attacks of EM with a short course of systemic corticosteroids is still very popular. Based only on retrospective analyses of series, available evidence suggests that corticosteroids shorten the duration of fever and eruption but result in similar lengths of hospitalization by increasing the risk of complications. In addition, some authorities believe that corticosteroids may increase the rate of recurrences in herpes-related cases. I consider therefore that systemic corticosteroids should not be used.

Topical antiseptics can be used on skin blisters. Erosions in the mouth are treated with mouth rinses and topical analgesics (viscous lidocaine). The most severely affected patients may require enteral nutrition through a nasogastric tube.

Prevention of Recurrences

Sun protection, including sunscreens with a protection index of at least 15, prevents recurrences of labial herpes and should be recommended for herpes-related EM.

For patients with an interval of several days between herpes and EM, beginning oral acyclovir (Zovirax) 200 mg five times a day for 5 days at the onset of herpes sometimes prevents the occurrence of EM. When this fails, continuous treatment with oral acyclovir should be considered. Because asymptomatic herpes may precipitate EM, a few patients without clinical evidence of herpes may also benefit from acyclovir. I prescribe acyclovir 400 mg twice daily for 6 to 12 months for all patients with frequent (four or more per year) recurrences of EM. The treatment is efficient in two thirds of patients who adhere to it strictly.

The new antiviral agents valacyclovir (Valtrex) and famciclovir (Famvir) have not been studied for recurrent EM. Because of their better bioavailability, they can be expected to be at least as effective as acyclovir with a more convenient oral dosage. When acyclovir does not avoid recurrences, the same treatments can be proposed as for continuous EM (dapsone,* antimalarials, azathioprine (Imuran),* cyclosporine (Sandimmune),* and thalidomide*).

Treatment of Continuous EM

A course of acyclovir should be tried, but it is often ineffective in my experience. Systemic corticosteroids

---

*Not FDA approved for this indication.

suppress the disease but are never my first choice because recurrences on dose tapering lead to long-term use and side effects. Dapsone, antimalarials, azathioprine, and cyclosporine have been proposed. In my experience, thalidomide 100 mg once a day for 1 month and then decreased to 50 mg a day for a few months always induced a remission of persistent EM.

STEVENS-JOHNSON SYNDROME AND TOXIC EPIDERMAL NECROLYSIS

Stevens-Johnson syndrome (SJS) and toxic epidermal necrolysis (TEN) are rare but severe diseases, most often related to adverse drug reactions and characterized by an acute and widespread destruction of the epithelium of skin and mucous membranes with blisters and erosions. SJS has limited detachment of the epidermis (less than 10% of the body surface area [BSA]). TEN has detachment on more than 30% of the BSA. Overlapping cases of SJS and TEN have detachment between 10 and 30% of the BSA.

SJS and TEN are clinically distinct from erythema multiforme, a disease with a much better prognosis. They have distinct causes and mandate different management strategies.

Death rates of patients with SJS (5%) or TEN (25 to 40%) are higher than for burns of similar extent because of frequent lesions of epithelium in the bronchial or gastrointestinal tract. Epidermal detachment above 30% of the BSA, age more than 50 years, elevated blood urea, and pulmonary lesions indicate a poor prognosis.

Several pieces of evidence linking the death of keratinocytes to cytotoxic T lymphocytes and cytokines provide a rationale for treatment with systemic corticosteroids, immunosuppressive drugs, and anticytokines. The difficulty to predict the final extent of detachment when patients are seen early and the rarity of the diseases contribute to the persistence of controversies about treatment.

Treatments Aimed at Halting Disease Progression

Withdrawal of the suspected causative drug(s) should be done as soon as possible. The death rates of patients with SJS or TEN were lower when the causative drugs with short elimination half-lives were withdrawn no later than the day when blisters or erosions first occurred.

Low mortality rates observed in patients treated in dermatology or allergy wards with corticosteroids were interpreted as supporting a beneficial effect of such therapy. On the other hand, several studies done in burn units with patients with detachment involving large areas found that patients treated with corticosteroids had a worse prognosis. In one burn unit, the death rate for severe TEN fell from 66 to 33% after withdrawal of steroid therapy as the only change in treatment. Taken together, these data,

though uncontrolled, suggest that corticosteroids should be avoided in the most severe case, a conclusion shared by many authorities in the field.

Four publications reported that plasmapheresis induced a halt in the progression of TEN in a total of 12 patients. I stopped using plasmapheresis after seeing no alteration in the progression of skin lesions or in the general status of six consecutive patients with early TEN.

Cyclophosphamide (Cytoxan)* in high intravenous doses and oral cyclosporine (Sandimmune)* have been administered to a few patients, respectively, with claimed benefits. As these agents were usually administered after an ineffective treatment with corticosteroids for several days, their usefulness remains doubtful.

One patient appeared to benefit from treatment with pentoxifylline (Trental),* a drug suppressing the production of tumor necrosis factor alpha. (TNF-α). With the same rationale of inhibiting TNF-α production, thalidomide was tested in a double-blind placebo-controlled trial. The trial was interrupted after inclusion of 25 patients because of an unexpectedly high mortality rate that turned to be related to thalidomide.

High doses intravenous immunoglobulins were used in a short series of TEN cases on the basis of their ability to inhibit fas-fas ligand-mediated apoptosis.

In conclusion, I consider that to date no other treatment than symptomatic should be used for patients with SJS or TEN.

Symptomatic Treatment

Management of patients must be undertaken as soon as possible in an intensive care unit or a burn unit. Medical transport requires particular attention to the skin.

The main principles of symptomatic therapy are the same as for major burns and include fluid replacement, anti-infectious therapy, aggressive nutritional support, warming of environmental temperature, and skin care with appropriate dressings.

Ocular lesions require daily examination by an ophthalmologist. Antiseptic and/or antibiotic eye drops are instilled every hour or two, and developing synechiae are disrupted by a blunt instrument.

Prevention and Future Use of Drugs

Patients should be advised to avoid re-exposure to the suspected causative drug. The few published cases of recurrences were all attributed to the same generic drug or to compounds chemically closely related (e.g., aromatic anticonvulsants). Therefore, there is no rationale for restricting the use of all classes of high-risk drugs.

---

*Not FDA approved for this indication.

BULLOUS DISEASES

method of
NEIL J. KORMAN, PH.D., M.D.
Case Western Reserve University
Cleveland, Ohio

Blisters in the skin may be caused by infections (including bacterial, viral, and fungal etiologies), allergic hypersensitivity reactions (including erythema multiforme and allergic contact dermatitis), metabolic disorders (including porphyria cutanea tarda and diabetes mellitus), inherited genetic defects (including the epidermolysis bullosa group of diseases), and immunologically mediated blistering skin diseases. In the current discussion, I focus on the immunologically mediated blistering diseases, listed in Table 1, which are among the most intriguing, well-characterized, and sometimes serious skin diseases known.

Until the early 1950s, there was little understanding of the features that distinguished blistering diseases and all major blistering disease fell under the category of *pemphigus*. Since then, there has been an enormous increase in our knowledge of these blistering diseases. This knowledge is derived from advances in histopathology and the development of the immunofluorescence technique, as well as from more recent basic advances in protein chemistry and molecular biology. In this article, I discuss the major clinical features, appropriate diagnostic evaluations, and therapeutic approaches to patients with autoimmune bullous diseases. It is important to point out that most therapeutic regimens are based on clinical experience and that there are very few controlled clinical trials for the treatment of the autoimmune blistering diseases.

PEMPHIGUS

Clinical Manifestations and Diagnosis

Pemphigus is a group of autoimmune blistering skin diseases characterized by blister formation within the epidermis due to acantholysis, the loss of cohesion between epidermal cells. In pemphigus vulgaris, the more common type, the blister occurs in the suprabasilar region (an area just above the basal keratinocytes), whereas in pemphigus folia-

TABLE 1. **Autoimmune Blistering Skin Diseases**

Pemphigus
  Pemphigus vulgaris
  Pemphigus foliaceous
  Pemphigus vegetans
  Pemphigus erythematosus
Paraneoplastic pemphigus
Pemphigoid
  Bullous pemphigoid
  Cicatricial pemphigoid
  Herpes (pemphigoid) gestationis
Epidermolysis bullosa acquisita
Dermatitis herpetiformis
Linear IgA bullous disease
  Adult linear IgA bullous disease
  Chronic bullous disease of childhood
Bullous lupus erythematosus

---

ceous the blister occurs in a subcorneal location (an area just below the stratum corneum). The lesions of pemphigus vulgaris consist of flaccid blisters on either normal-appearing or erythematous skin. The lesions usually start in the oropharynx and then spread to involve the trunk, the head and neck, and intertriginous areas including the axilla and groin. Patients with severe disease may have involvement of other mucosal surfaces, including laryngeal, esophageal, conjunctival, vulvar, and rectal surfaces. The involvement of the oral cavity can become extensive, and the pain of denuded mucous membranes can be very severe, causing poor oral intake of solids and liquids that may lead to malnutrition if left untreated. Pemphigus foliaceous manifests with erythema, scaling, and crusting localized to the face, scalp, and upper trunk. Patients with pemphigus foliaceous, unlike those with pemphigus vulgaris, rarely have mucous membrane involvement.

Routine skin biopsies for pemphigus should be performed from early skin lesions to demonstrate the characteristic histology of acantholysis. Direct immunofluorescence biopsy should be performed on normal-appearing or erythematous nonbullous perilesional skin and reveal cell surface deposits of IgG and the third component of complement. The IgG deposits in the skin occur because of the presence of a circulating IgG antibody that is targeted to keratinocyte cell surface antigens. These IgG antibodies are found in most patients with pemphigus and are detected by the indirect immunofluorescence technique. The antibody titer tends to correlate roughly with the degree of disease activity. Autoantibodies in pemphigus vulgaris target a 130,000 Dalton molecular weight protein, desmoglein III, and the autoantibodies in pemphigus foliaceous target a closely related 160,000 molecular weight Dalton protein, desmoglein I. There is compelling evidence from animal studies that the autoantibodies in both major types of pemphigus are capable of reproducing the clinical, histologic, and immunopathologic features of pemphigus.

Therapy

Before glucocorticosteroids became available in the 1950s, the mortality rate from pemphigus ranged from 60% to 90%. With the use of immunosuppressive agents along with corticosteroids, the mortality rate has decreased to the 5% to 10% range. All patients with pemphigus vulgaris require systemic therapy with glucocorticosteroids to clear the circulating antibodies. Pemphigus foliaceous patients tend to have a more benign course, can often be treated with lower dosages of glucocorticosteroids, and occasionally respond to topical steroid therapy alone.

Patients with pemphigus are generally treated with prednisone at 1 to 2 mg per kg, depending on disease severity, with tapering toward an every other day dosage within a 1- to 3-month period as the disease allows. Short-term and long-term toxicities of prednisone are numerous and include gastrointestinal bleeding, diabetes mellitus, cataracts, osteoporosis, increased risk of infection, and central nervous system changes. Every effort should therefore be made to minimize the dosage of systemic glucocorticosteroids and to switch to every other day dosing as soon as is feasible.

Immunosuppressive agents, most commonly cyclophosphamide and azathioprine, are used for their steroid-sparing effects. Cyclophosphamide (Cytoxan)* appears to be the more effective of the two, but it has numerous toxicities, including bone marrow suppression, hemorrhagic cystitis, bladder fibrosis, sterility, alopecia, and an increased risk of malignancy. The major toxicities of azathioprine (Imuran)* include bone marrow suppression, hepatotoxicity, and increased risk of malignancy. Monitoring of patients treated with these immunosuppressive agents should include frequent blood counts, urinalyses, and liver function testing. Other therapies used as steroid-sparing agents in pemphigus include dapsone,* the combination of tetracycline and niacinamide,* hydroxychloroquine (Plaquenil),* gold,* cyclosporine (Sandimmune),* and, recently, mycophenolate mofetil (CellCept).* Patients with the most severe disease may be treated with the combination of systemic glucocorticosteroids and immunosuppressive agents along with plasmapheresis.

PARANEOPLASTIC PEMPHIGUS

Clinical Manifestations and Diagnosis

Paraneoplastic pemphigus is an autoimmune syndrome with features of both pemphigus vulgaris and erythema multiforme. Patients have numerous ocular and oral blisters and erosions along with generalized skin lesions that may resemble toxic epidermal necrolysis, lichen planus, bullous pemphigoid, or erythema multiforme. Paraneoplastic pemphigus occurs in the setting of an underlying malignancy, usually lymphoreticular in origin. It is rapidly progressive, leading to death in most patients who have an associated malignant neoplasm, but may resolve in patients who have an associated benign neoplasm that is surgically removed.

Histologic features of both pemphigus vulgaris and erythema multiforme may be present. Immunofluorescence studies show the presence of circulating and tissue-bound IgG antibodies in paraneoplastic pemphigus that bind to the cell surface of stratified squamous epithelia in a pattern indistinguishable from pemphigus antibodies. The same circulating IgG antibodies also recognize the cell surface of simple epithelia such as liver and heart, in contrast to pemphigus IgG antibodies, which only recognize the cell surface of stratified squamous epithelia. The circulating antibodies in paraneoplastic pemphigus recognize a complex of five skin structural proteins. The etiology of this severe mucocutaneous disease is poorly understood; it may result from the combination of both a cellular and humoral immune response to tumor antigens that also have overlapping reactivity to normal components of skin and other epithelia.

Therapy

Patients are treated very aggressively with high-dose glucocorticosteroids along with immunosuppressive agents, unfortunately often with unimpressive results. The best treatment for patients who have an associated benign tumor is surgical removal of the tumor. The majority of patients with paraneoplastic pemphigus, however, have associated malignant tumors, and there are no known effective therapies.

BULLOUS PEMPHIGOID

Clinical Manifestations and Diagnosis

Bullous pemphigoid is characterized by tense blisters that occur on normal-appearing skin or on an erythematous base and is most commonly seen in older persons. Blisters typically are found on the flexor surfaces of the arms and legs, axilla, groin, and abdomen. Oral lesions are seen in a minority of patients, and the lesions are usually transient. Patients may also present with urticarial plaques that may evolve into blisters.

The histology reveals a subepidermal blister with an inflammatory infiltrate that often is eosinophil rich but may also contain lymphocytes, histiocytes, or neutrophils. Direct immunofluorescence studies performed on normal-appearing or erythematous nonbullous perilesional skin reveal linear basement membrane zone deposits of IgG and the third component of complement in the majority of patients. Indirect immunofluorescence studies performed with salt split skin reveal that patients with bullous pemphigoid have circulating IgG antibodies that bind to the epidermal side of salt split skin.

Therapy

The management of patients with bullous pemphigoid is dictated by the degree of involvement and the rate of disease progression. Patients with localized disease may be managed with potent topical steroids. I treat patients with bullous pemphigoid who have mild generalized disease with low-dose prednisone,* and those whose disease is more significant are usually treated with moderate-dose prednisone. Patients with contraindications to systemic steroid therapy may be treated with dapsone,* a combination of tetracycline* and nicotinamide,* or immunosuppressive agents such as azathioprine.* Younger patients with bullous pemphigoid who have contraindications to systemic steroids are often treated with tetracycline and nicotinamide. I reserve azathioprine for older patients with more significant disease due to the probable increased risk of malignancy in patients treated with azathioprine.

*Not FDA approved for this indication.

*Not FDA approved for this indication.

Patients with bullous pemphigoid who have very significant disease are often successfully managed with moderate-dose prednisone along with azathioprine. As the disease comes under control, the prednisone is tapered to every other day and then discontinued. Treatment with azathioprine alone is continued for another 3 to 6 months, and then, when the disease is quiescent, the azathioprine is discontinued. Cyclophosphamide* is also used in the treatment of older patients with bullous pemphigoid as a steroid-sparing agent along with systemic corticosteroids. Due to its more severe toxicity profile than that of azathioprine, however, cyclophosphamide is reserved for use by only those patients who have extensive disease and who have not responded to or have not been able to tolerate azathioprine. Other treatments that have been utilized as steroid-sparing agents by patients with moderate to severe disease with varying degrees of success include cyclosporine, chlorambucil,* methotrexate,* and, recently, mycophenolate mofetil.*

CICATRICIAL PEMPHIGOID

Clinical Manifestations and Diagnosis

Cicatricial pemphigoid is a chronic subepidermal blistering disease involving primarily mucosal surfaces including, in decreasing order of frequency, the oropharynx and nasopharynx, conjunctiva, larynx, genitalia, and esophagus. Morbidity and mortality are caused by the scarring that results from recurrent lesions. Cutaneous involvement occurs in about one fourth of patients.

An important criterion that differentiates cicatricial pemphigoid from bullous pemphigoid is the prominent scarring that is seen in cicatricial pemphigoid. In bullous pemphigoid, lesions are largely found on the skin, whereas in cicatricial pemphigoid lesions are largely mucosal. Clinical features should therefore be used to differentiate between these two entities. Histology and immunofluorescence studies show findings similar to those seen in bullous pemphigoid, with the exception that patients with cicatricial pemphigoid may have IgA antibodies found in the skin and circulating in the blood in addition to the IgG response seen in bullous pemphigoid.

Therapy

Cicatricial pemphigoid is a chronic disease, and treatment regimens are dictated by the organs involved. Patients with involvement limited to the nasopharynx or oropharynx should be treated with topical or intralesional steroids, short bursts of oral corticosteroids, or dapsone. If the eyes, esophagus, or larynx becomes involved, the anticipated morbidity can be severe, including blindness and asphyxiation, and aggressive therapy with systemic corticosteroids and immunosuppressive agents is warranted. Cyclo-

*Not FDA approved for this indication.

phosphamide has been very effective in the treatment of patients with severe involvement, and the majority of patients go into remission after 18 to 24 months of treatment with systemic corticosteroids and cyclophosphamide.

HERPES GESTATIONIS

Clinical Manifestations and Diagnosis

Herpes gestationis is a pruritic, nonviral, subepidermal blistering disease of women that occurs during or shortly after pregnancy. Typical lesions include urticarial papules and plaques with polycyclic wheals that evolve into vesicles and bullae. Lesions start periumbically in 80% to 90% of patients and later spread to involve the entire abdomen, buttocks, and extremities. The disease may occur during any trimester of pregnancy as well as postpartum, but the most common time of onset is the second or third trimester. Although herpes gestationis usually resolves within weeks to months of parturition, patients may have recurrences in subsequent pregnancies. Exacerbations of disease can occur between pregnancies after ingestion of oral contraceptives or other hormonal stimuli.

Histologic examination of a blister reveals a subepidermal blister with eosinophils. Direct immunofluorescence reveals linear deposits of C3 at the basement membrane in all patients along with linear deposits of IgG in some patients. Indirect immunofluorescence studies reveal that most patients have the "herpes gestationis factor," a circulating IgG that avidly fixes complement.

Therapy

The goals of treatment for herpes gestationis are to control pruritus, suppress new lesion formation, and care for sites of blisters and erosions. Occasional patients with mild disease respond to potent topical corticosteroids used twice daily along with ingestion of oral antihistamines. The majority of patients with herpes gestationis, however, require treatment with moderate doses of systemic glucocorticosteroids. These patients should be treated with a single morning dosage of prednisone with incremental tapering as tolerated. Corticosteroids should be used carefully during pregnancy, but extensive experience with pregnant asthmatic women suggests minimal risks if they are properly monitored. I always recommend that patients with herpes gestationis be managed by an obstetrician skilled in high-risk obstetrics, and the newborn should be monitored for signs of adrenal insufficiency.

EPIDERMOLYSIS BULLOSA ACQUISITA

Clinical Manifestations and Diagnosis

Epidermolysis bullosa acquisita (EBA) is a chronic subepidermal blistering disease that may present with generalized inflammatory blisters that can be clinically indistinguishable from bullous pemphigoid or noninflammatory trauma-induced acral blisters, leading to scarring and milium formation. The inflammatory and noninflammatory phases of the disease may occur separately, in combination, or may evolve from one into the other.

Histopathologic studies reveal a subepidermal blister, often with a neutrophilic infiltrate when inflammatory and free of infiltrate when noninflammatory lesions are studied. Direct immunofluorescence reveals linear basement membrane deposits of IgG in all patients as well as linear deposits of C3 in many patients. Circulating IgG anti–basement membrane zone antibodies are found in about half of these patients, and they are directed against type VII collagen and bind to the dermal side of salt split skin. The course of EBA tends to be chronic and protracted with rare remissions.

Therapy

EBA is the most difficult to treat of all the autoimmune blistering diseases. Patients who present with inflammatory blistering disease may show some response to medications used to treat other blistering diseases, such as systemic corticosteroids, dapsone,* azathioprine,* and cyclophosphamide.* Many patients are quite steroid resistant, however, and relatively high dosages may be required to obtain even a partial response. Dapsone is occasionally of value for these patients.

Cyclosporine has been found to be very useful in the treatment of EBA. The original studies utilized high dosages of cyclosporine* up to 9 mg per kg, and, in these patients, although there was rapid clinical improvement, numerous toxicities occurred that required discontinuation of therapy. Recently patients were treated with cyclosporine at 5 to 6 mg per kg with very good clinical responses. Due to numerous side effects, including nephrotoxicity, hypertension, hepatotoxicity, gingival hyperplasia, hypertrichosis, and tremor, treatment with cyclosporine must be very carefully monitored. Another therapy that has been found to be of value in the treatment of EBA is extracorporeal photopheresis.

DERMATITIS HERPETIFORMIS
Clinical Manifestations and Diagnosis

Dermatitis herpetiformis is an intensely pruritic, chronic blistering disease of the skin that occurs most commonly in the second to fourth decades of life. The primary lesions are small, tense vesicles that tend to be symmetrically distributed over the elbows, knees, and buttocks. Due to the extreme pruritus, it is uncommon to see patients with intact vesicles because the vesicles have usually been scratched off prior to presentation. Sometimes the pruritus precedes the onset of new lesions by several hours, allowing the patient to predict where new lesions may occur. Biopsy of an early lesion of dermatitis herpetiformis

reveals small subepidermal clefts with accumulation of neutrophils in the neighboring dermal papillae. Biopsy of normal-appearing perilesional skin for direct immunofluorescence reveals granular deposits of IgA at the dermal papillary tips.

Most patients with dermatitis herpetiformis have an associated subclinical gluten-sensitive enteropathy, and most express the HLA-B8/DRw3 haplotype. Most patients do not manifest overt gastrointestinal symptoms, but if a biopsy of the small bowel is performed it will reveal blunting of the intestinal villi with a lymphocytic infiltrate in the lamina propria. These gastrointestinal changes are potentially reversible if the patient is placed on a gluten-free diet. If the patient stays on the gluten-free diet for several years, the skin disease may improve or sometimes even be fully controlled.

Therapy

The most effective therapy is dapsone, which is beneficial in almost all patients. The major toxicities of dapsone include hemolysis, methemoglobinemia, and agranulocytosis. Patients should be screened for glucose-6-phosphate dehydrogenase deficiency because use of dapsone by such a patient leads to severe hemolysis. Patients need to be followed up with regular blood counts. Dapsone requirements may be decreased by following a gluten-free diet, but this diet must be maintained for many months before benefit may be realized. Because a gluten-free diet can be very difficult to follow, it is important that patients be counseled by an experienced dietician. As dermatitis herpetiformis is a chronic disease, patients must take dapsone and/or remain on their gluten-free diet indefinitely to remain under control.

LINEAR IgA BULLOUS DERMATOSIS
Clinical Manifestations and Diagnosis

Linear IgA bullous dermatosis is a subepidermal blistering disease that until recently was considered a variant type of dermatitis herpetiformis. Clinical lesions consist of papulovesicles or blisters along with urticarial plaques, and sometimes the patients may have an arcuate pattern with a "cluster of jewels" grouping of blisters. Lesions of the oral mucous membranes are frequently seen. Occasionally ocular involvement with subsequent scarring may occur similar to that found in cicatricial pemphigoid. Patients with linear IgA bullous disease do not have any gastrointestinal disease, do not have an increased frequency of the HLA-B8/DRw3 phenotype, and do not benefit from a gluten-free diet. Linear IgA bullous disease may occur with increased frequency in patients older than 60 years of age, but it may be seen throughout adulthood, and a blistering disease found in children known as *chronic bullous disease of childhood* is the childhood counterpart of linear IgA bullous disease.

The histology of linear IgA bullous disease can be

---

*Not FDA approved for this indication.

indistinguishable from that of dermatitis herpetiformis, or some patients may show neutrophils along the entire epidermal basement membrane zone, in contrast to dermatitis herpetiformis, where the neutrophils tend to be limited to the dermal papillae. Direct immunofluorescence studies obtained from normal-appearing perilesional skin reveal linear basement membrane zone deposits of IgA. Indirect immunofluorescence studies performed on salt split skin often reveal a low titer circulating IgA antibody that usually binds to the epidermal side of salt split skin.

Therapy

Most patients with linear IgA disease respond to dapsone.* Some patients may require the addition of systemic glucocorticosteroids to achieve control of the disease. Rare patients who have ocular disease must be treated aggressively with systemic glucocorticosteroids and cyclophosphamide to control the disease and prevent ocular scarring.

BULLOUS SYSTEMIC LUPUS ERYTHEMATOSUS

Clinical Manifestations and Diagnosis

Bullous systemic lupus erythematosus is a blistering skin disease occurring in the setting of a patient with systemic lupus erythematosus. It occurs in a small minority of patients with systemic lupus erythematosus and is characterized by vesicles, urticarial papules, and plaques that may resemble either bullous pemphigoid or dermatitis herpetiformis.

The histology of these lesions is very characteristic, showing features similar to those of dermatitis herpetiformis with dermal papillary microabscesses of neutrophils. Routine direct immunofluorescence testing reveals the presence of linear or granular deposits of IgG, IgA, IgM, and C3 at the epidermal basement membrane zone. Indirect immunofluorescence studies reveal the presence of circulating IgG antibodies that bind to the dermal side of salt split skin in a pattern indistinguishable from that of epidermolysis bullosa acquisita antibodies.

Therapy

Bullous eruption of systemic lupus erythematosus is usually treated with dapsone* with very good results. Most patients are eventually able to discontinue therapy without recurrence of the disease.

---

*Not FDA approved for this indication.

CONTACT DERMATITIS

method of
ERIN M. WARSHAW, M.D.
*Minneapolis Veterans Affairs Medical Center
Minneapolis, Minnesota*

ETIOLOGY

There are two types of contact dermatitis: allergic and irritant. Irritant contact dermatitis is by far the most common type and is due to harsh chemicals such as acids, solvents, and strong soaps. The skin of any individual exposed to such chemicals will develop erythema, burning, itching, and/or dermatitis. This is not an allergic reaction because no immunologic sensitization occurs. A common form of irritant dermatitis is irritant hand dermatitis. This occurs in individuals whose occupation or hobby requires frequent hand washing with harsh soaps and/or exposure to various solvents. Occupations at particular risk include health care workers, housewives, janitorial staff, mechanics, hairdressers, and machinists.

There are two types of cutaneous allergic sensitization: type I and type IV. Contact urticaria is an immediate, type I, IgE-mediated reaction that occurs from exposure to certain allergens such as latex rubber products, fish, seafood, meats, and some vegetables, especially onions. Contact urticaria results in immediate urticarial wheals, erythema, or pruritus at the epidermal or mucosal site of contact. Generalized cutaneous reactions, asthma, or anaphylaxis may also be associated. Diagnosis of contact urticaria is made by history, radioallergosorbent test (RAST), prick testing, and/or use testing. Because anaphylaxis and death have been reported from prick and use tests, it is prudent to have resuscitation equipment available.

Allergic contact dermatitis is a delayed, type IV, cell-mediated allergic reaction. This is typically a pruritic erythematous eruption, which may be vesicular or bullous, occurring 24 to 72 hours after exposure to the offending allergen. Reaction to poison ivy is a typical example. Common allergens include nickel in costume jewelry or clothing, rubber additives (carbamates, mercaptobenzothiazoles, and thiurams), lanolin, neomycin, formaldehyde-releasing chemicals, and components of black hair dye. An extensive occupational and personal history is required to help elucidate possible exposures.

DIAGNOSIS

Diagnosis of allergic contact dermatitis is made by patch testing. This involves the application of allergens in specific concentrations to the patient's back. These are secured with tape and worn for 48 hours. Patches are then removed, locations marked, and reactions graded. A second reading is done at 72–168 hours; this delayed reading is important because many antigens can take longer to elicit reactions. Patch testing is usually done by a dermatologist with a special interest in contact dermatitis who has ready access to hundreds of standardized allergens. A pre-packaged screening patch test kit with 24 common allergens (True Test [GlaxoWellcome]) is available.

TREATMENT

Treatment of contact dermatitis generally involves four components: (1) avoidance of irritants and allergens, (2) alleviation of pruritus, (3) treatment of inflammation, and (4) restoration of normal skin barrier. Pruritus may be controlled by antihistamines such as diphenhydramine (Benadryl) or hydroxyzine (Atarax); newer less-sedating antihistamines such as cetirizine (Zyrtec), loratadine (Claritin), and fexofenadine (Allegra) are also helpful. Doxepin (Sinequan) at night (25–100 mg) is especially helpful for refractory pruritus.

Corticosteroids are the mainstay of treatment for contact dermatitis. Systemic corticosteroids are reserved for the most severe cases and may be administered orally (prednisone, 40 to 60 mg tapered over 3 weeks). Because delayed-type allergic reactions are persistent, it is important to taper the dose over 3 weeks; rebound dermatitis will occur if the dose of systemic corticosteroids is tapered sooner. Corticosteroids may also be given intramuscularly (triamcinolone acetonide [Kenalog] or betamethasone acetate [Celestone]). Of course, the contraindications and side effects of systemic corticosteroids must be carefully considered.

Most cases of contact dermatitis can be controlled with topical corticosteroids. Solutions are best used for hair-bearing areas such as the scalp, whereas creams or ointments are used for rest of the body. Creams contain many additives, some of which can cause allergic contact dermatitis, so whenever possible ointments are preferable. Mild corticosteroids include hydrocortisone (0.5 to 2.5%, Hytone). Moderate-strength corticosteroids include hydrocortisone valerate (Westcort), desonide (Tridesilon and DesOwen), and hydrocortisone butyrate (Locoid). Potent topical corticosteroids include desoximetasone (Topicort), fluocinonide (Lidex), and amcinonide (Cyclocort). Superpotent corticosteroids are reserved for the worst cases and should only be used for short periods of time; they include betamethasone dipropionate (Diprolene), diflorasone diacetate (Psorcon), halobetasol propionate (Ultravate), and clobetasol propionate (Temovate). Mild preparations are designed for use on the face, groin, and axillae. Stronger corticosteroids may produce atrophy, telangiectasia, and striae as well as adrenal axis suppression. The risks and benefits of such treatments must be considered, especially if used over a long period of time.

Restoration of the normal skin barrier with aggressive and prolonged moisturization is an important component of treating irritant or allergic contact dermatitis. Application of a thick cream or ointment several times a day is extremely helpful; products with few potential allergens and irritants include petroleum jelly, Vanicream, and Cetaphil. If daytime duties preclude such use of moisturizers, aggressive moisturization can be accomplished overnight by moistening the body area with water, applying a thick layer of moisturizer, and occluding the area with gloves or plastic wrap. Such therapy may need to be continued for a prolonged period of time until the normal skin barrier is restored.

SKIN DISEASES OF PREGNANCY

method of
KATHY SCHWARZENBERGER, M.D.
Medical University of South Carolina
Charleston, South Carolina

Skin changes are common during pregnancy and can reflect hormonal, metabolic, and immunologic changes or simply the physical changes that occur during the months of gestation. Several skin disorders occur specifically during or around pregnancy, and their recognition may be important for appropriate management.

PRURITIC URTICARIAL PAPULES AND PLAQUES OF PREGNANCY

Diagnosis

Pruritic urticarial papules and plaques of pregnancy (PUPPP), also known as *polymorphic eruption of pregnancy,* is the most common specific dermatosis of pregnancy. This intensely itchy eruption typically occurs in the third trimester of pregnancy. PUPPP most frequently affects primagravidas, and recurrences in successive pregnancies are rare. In some cases, symptoms do not develop until the postpartum period. No recurrence of symptoms is expected with subsequent use of oral contraceptives or during menstruation.

PUPPP characteristically begins with small, itchy red papules on the mid-abdomen, frequently within striae distensae. A small halo of pallor may surround the papules. Lesions, if edematous, may become vesicular; the presence of large vesicles or bullae, however, should suggest other diagnoses, including herpes gestationis. Papules coalesce into large, urticarial plaques on the abdomen, buttocks, and thighs. The arms, forearms, and breasts are less frequently involved, and the face is relatively spared. Palms and soles are rarely involved. Itching is often intense and may interfere with sleep. There are no associated systemic symptoms.

The cause of PUPPP is unknown. PUPPP can occur in otherwise uncomplicated pregnancies and is not associated with adverse outcome in mother or child. The diagnosis of PUPPP can usually be made on clinical grounds alone, and it should be distinguished from similar conditions, including allergic contact dermatitis, urticaria, drug eruptions, viral exanthems, and scabies. Skin biopsy should be performed if the diagnosis is unclear. Histologic findings in PUPPP are nonspecific. Typically, there is a superficial to mid-dermal lymphohistiocytic infiltrate, often with dermal edema and eosinophils, and mild epidermal spongiosis. Immunofluorescence studies on skin and serum have been consistently nonspecific and in most cases are negative.

Treatment

Most symptoms resolve spontaneously within a few days of delivery, although the intensity of itching usually requires intervention before then. Aggressive topical application of corticosteroids (triamcinolone acetonide 0.1% cream, pregnancy category C; fluocinonide 0.05% cream [Lidex], pregnancy category C) three to six times a day* to affected skin may relieve the itching and promote resolution of skin lesions. In severe cases, oral corticosteroids (prednisone, preg-

---

*Exceeds dosage recommended by the manufacturer.

nancy category B, in doses up to 20 to 40 mg a day) are needed. Once clinical improvement is seen, the dose can be tapered to every 2 to 3 days until the lowest effective dose is determined, or until it can be discontinued without recurrence.

If use of systemic corticosteroids is prolonged, the need for "stress-dose" peripartum steroids should be discussed with the mother's obstetrician. Similarly, there is a risk of neonatal adrenal suppression with prolonged maternal use of systemic steroids, and the pediatrician should be alerted to the situation. Oral antihistamines (diphenhydramine hydrochloride (Benadryl), pregnancy category B, 25 mg up to qid; or hydroxyzine hydrochloride (Atarax), pregnancy category C, 25 mg up to qid are less effective than corticosteroids in management of the itching of PUPPP. Their sedative effect, however, may help women whose extreme pruritus prevents sleep.

HERPES GESTATIONIS

Diagnosis

The term "herpes gestationis" is perhaps unfortunate, as this relatively rare, autoimmune blistering disease is in no way related to the viral infection its name suggests. The alternative term "pemphigoid gestationis" has been proposed. Herpes gestationis, along with PUPPP, is one of the few specific dermatoses of pregnancy. Herpes gestationis can occur anytime during pregnancy, but usually begins between the fourth and seventh months. Symptoms may not, however, initially develop until the immediate postpartum period, when flares of otherwise controlled disease may also occur. Symptoms usually subside within several weeks of parturition but may recur during successive pregnancies, during menstruation, or with subsequent use of oral contraceptives.

Herpes gestationis is a polymorphic eruption consisting of extremely itchy papules, vesicles and/or bullae, urticarial plaques, and erosions. Lesions frequently begin on the abdomen, and any area of skin can be involved, although mucous membranes are usually spared. In mild cases, lesions may be limited to a few itchy papules or vesicles; in more severe cases, however, involvement may be widespread. Itching is usually intense. Symptoms are limited to the skin, and there are no associated systemic problems.

Infants born to mothers with herpes gestationis may have similar skin lesions; however, these are usually self-limited and require only supportive care. Controversy has surrounded the issue of fetal outcome because early reports suggested an increased risk of fetal mortality during affected pregnancies. More recent studies, however, have not confirmed this, although there appears to be a potential risk for prematurity or low birth weight in infants born to affected mothers. Close fetal-maternal monitoring during affected pregnancies is warranted.

Understanding of the immunopathogenesis of herpes gestationis has provided the basis for specific diagnostic testing. Skin biopsy specimens from affected skin show subepidermal blistering, edema, and a superficial and deep perivascular infiltrate consisting of mixed inflammatory cells with eosinophils. Specific diagnosis is obtained from immunofluorescence studies on perilesional skin that reveal linear deposition of the third component of complement (C3), with or without IgG, along the dermoepidermal junction. These findings result from the autoimmune development of complement-fixing antibodies directed against a specific cell adhesion molecule in the skin. In a small percentage of cases, these autoantibodies can be detected in serum by indirect immunofluorescence studies. Epidemiologic studies have shown an increased incidence of certain HLA types in affected mothers, suggesting a genetic component to the disease.

Treatment

Herpes gestationis should be treated in consultation with a dermatologist familiar with autoimmune bullous diseases. Many therapies used to treat similar conditions in nonpregnant individuals are contraindicated in pregnancy. In most cases, systemic corticosteroids are required to control symptoms and suppress blister formation. Prednisone in doses of 20 to 60 mg a day may be started once the diagnosis is made and the dose adjusted until the disease is controlled. When active blistering has stopped and healing has begun, the dose may be gradually tapered by 5 to 10 mg every week until the lowest effective dose is determined by recurrence of symptoms.

Patients should be monitored postpartum for disease exacerbation; no "prophylactic" increase, however, is recommended for the skin alone. Use of peripartum "stress-dose" steroids may be considered by the obstetrician if use of systemic steroids has been prolonged, and the possibility of adrenal insufficiency in the newborn should be remembered. Corticosteroids can be gradually tapered off over several weeks to months, depending on the dosage required to control the disease. Mild cases may respond to aggressive application of topical corticosteroids applied three to six times a day* (triamcinolone acetonide 0.1% cream, pregnancy category C; fluocinonide 0.05% cream, pregnancy category C). Rarely, severe disease necessitates the postpartum use of other immunosuppressant agents such as azathioprine.

Skin care is essential, especially in the presence of multiple blisters or erosions. Aggressive débridement of blisters should be avoided. Nonadherent dressings (Telfa) coated with petrolatum or antibiotic ointment may be applied to open areas of skin to promote healing. Skin should be watched for possible infection and treated appropriately. Long-term sequelae are not expected, although affected women should be made aware of the potential for recurrences.

---

*Exceeds dosage recommended by the manufacturer.

IMPETIGO HERPETIFORMIS

Diagnosis

Impetigo herpetiformis is better termed "generalized pustular psoriasis of pregnancy." This extremely rare, severe form of pustular psoriasis usually occurs late in pregnancy when minute pustules develop on erythematous skin, frequently in a symmetrical distribution on flexural skin. Lesions spread centrifugally and may involve large areas of the body. Associated systemic symptoms of fever, nausea, vomiting, and diarrhea may be present. Severe hypoalbuminemia and symptomatic hypocalcemia may result, and maternal deaths have been reported. Placental insufficiency has been linked with increased fetal morbidity and mortality. The diagnosis of impetigo herpetiformis is made with skin biopsy, which shows characteristic changes of pustular psoriasis.

Treatment

Immediate consultation with a dermatologist is indicated. Treatment is complicated because most therapies used outside of pregnancy, including methotrexate, systemic retinoids, and phototherapy, are contraindicated in pregnancy. Systemic corticosteroids are usually required, and prednisone (pregnancy category B) up to 60 mg a day may be needed to control the disease. The drug must be tapered slowly to avoid flaring of the disease. Alternative therapy should be considered postpartum. Because of the associated problems, close monitoring with high-risk obstetrics is mandatory.

PRURITUS GRAVIDARUM

Diagnosis

Alternatively termed "prurigo gravidarum," pruritus gravidarum is thought to result from intrahepatic cholestasis and may be accompanied by elevation of transaminases and/or alkaline phosphatase. The condition is characterized by intense localized or generalized itching in the absence of specific skin lesions. Excoriations may result from scratching. Jaundice may follow onset of pruritus in severe cases. Symptoms usually start late in pregnancy, and recurrences in subsequent pregnancies are common. Some reports have suggested an increased incidence of prematurity or low birth weight in children of affected mothers.

Treatment

Treatment is symptomatic because itching usually remits within a few days after delivery. Topical application of antipruritic lotions (hydrocortisone 1% with pramoxine HCl 1% [Pramosone]), pregnancy category C, topical corticosteroids, or emollients may provide symptomatic relief. Oral antihistamines may or may not be helpful. Use of cholestyramine (Questran) has been suggested.

PRURITUS ANI AND VULVAE

method of
MICHAEL J. ADLER, M.D.
Oregon Health Sciences University
Portland, Oregon

Perineal pruritus (PP) of short duration is most commonly caused by anorectal disease, irritant or allergic contact dermatitis, or infections and infestations. Retained fecal matter profoundly irritates the perianal region and may result from diarrhea, poor hygiene, sphincter incontinence, or accumulation on irregular surfaces, such as hemorrhoids, anal fissures, or papillomas. To combat this, some patients overcleanse with soaps or bleaches, exacerbating the irritant dermatitis. Allergic contact dermatitis may further compound the problem, developing after use of topical products containing neomycin, bacitracin, fragrances, anesthetics, or various preservatives.

Patch testing to suspected allergens often yields a specific diagnosis. To help identify dermatophyte or candidal infection, any perineal erythema or scaling should be tested with a KOH examination and culture. In children, perianal erythema may also represent pinworm infestation or streptococcal infection. Scabies rarely remains isolated to the perineum but should be considered in the appropriate clinical setting. Vaginal smears help identify *Trichomonas* or bacterial vaginosis (*Gardnerella*). Dry epithelial tissues of perimenopausal or postmenopausal women often become irritated and subsequently pruritic.

Chronic PP presents a more challenging evaluation because secondary changes of lichenification or lichen simplex chronicus (LSC) may obscure the primary cause. In LSC, thickened skin and accentuated skinfolds occur in response to chronic rubbing or scratching. A habitual "itch-scratch-itch" cycle develops, often after the primary cause has resolved. These skin changes may mask or mimic other inflammatory skin conditions, including psoriasis, seborrheic dermatitis, lichen planus, or lichen sclerosis et atrophicus. Biopsy of persistent lesions establishes a diagnosis and helps exclude squamous cell carcinoma or extramammary Paget's disease. Application of 3% to 5% acetic acid for 1 to 2 minutes (aceto-whitening) helps to identify suspected human papillomavirus. Colposcopy or proctoscopy allows exclusion of internal papillomavirus infection. Systemic causes of pruritus generally do not present with isolated perineal involvement, but may occasionally be due to diabetes, uremia, liver disease, or hematologic malignancies.

THERAPY

Proper perineal hygiene is critical for successful management of PP. After each bowel movement or soiling, white, unscented toilet paper should be used to gently cleanse the area. Patients often use this as a chance to aggressively scratch, so a gentle approach should be emphasized. Tucks pads or Balneol may help with drying but can sometimes irritate. Cool water rinses should follow cleansing, followed by application of bland, occlusive emollients such as Vaseline, zinc oxide paste, or an ointment-based topical steroid if appropriate (see later). Loose-fitting cotton undergarments minimize irritation by lessening perspiration.

Although controversial, dietary changes are occasionally recommended. Methylxanthine-containing foods such as chocolate and caffeine can decrease anal sphincter tone and lead to increased incontinence. Highly acidic entities such as tomatoes, citrus fruits, or vitamin C supplements may increase the irritancy of stool. Some physicians recommend that patients avoid each of these substances until the pruritus improves and add them back one at a time weekly as tolerated.

Infectious causes of PP generally respond to an appropriate antimicrobial or antiparasitic agent. *Candida* may be an exception, frequently causing recurrent infection in certain women, patients taking antibiotics for other conditions, or immunosuppressed individuals. Weekly maintenance therapy with topical clotrimazole (Gyne-Lotrimin) or oxiconazole (Oxistat) often suffices, but some patients require weekly or monthly suppression with oral fluconazole (Diflucan), 150 to 200 mg per dose.

Perhaps more than anything else, successful treatment of chronic PP hinges on controlling LSC. Although education regarding the habitual nature of LSC often helps, the "itch-scratch-itch" cycle needs to be broken, generally with the help of topical steroids. For thick lesions of LSC, begin with ultrapotent steroids such as clobetasol (Temovate) or halobetasol (Ultravate) bid for 2 to 4 weeks, changing to triamcinolone (Aristocort, Kenalog) or desonide (DesOwen) for another 1 to 4 weeks once the pruritus improves to help minimize the risk of corticosteroid-induced skin atrophy. Topical antihistamines such as diphenhydramine (Benadryl) or doxepin (Zonalon) are generally ineffective and may induce contact allergy. Topical local anesthetics like pramoxine (Prax, Tronothane, Pramosone) or preparations containing counterirritants such as phenol or menthol often help in mild cases. Sedating agents such as hydroxyzine (Vistaril, Atarax) 10 to 50 mg, doxepin (Sinequan) 10 to 50 mg, or amitriptyline (Elavil) 25 to 50 mg may be taken at night to reduce nocturnal rubbing and scratching.

Education about LSC allows patients to understand the critical role scratching plays in their condition. Patience must also be emphasized because the skin changes of LSC may take 4 to 6 weeks to normalize, even after the last scratch.

URTICARIA AND ANGIOEDEMA

method of
CLIVE E. H. GRATTAN, M.D.
West Norwich Hospital
Norwich, Norfolk, England

Urticaria is a common skin disorder, characterized by transient plasma leakage with many possible causes, that may have a substantial impact on a patient's quality of life. Dermal edema is called a "wheal"; subcutaneous or submucosal involvement is known as "angioedema." Angioedema is most commonly recognized by swelling of the lips or eyelids, but it may affect any part of the skin or mouth. The gut may also be affected in C1 esterase inhibitor deficiency. Certain types of urticaria may progress to anaphylaxis when very severe, and urticaria is nearly always a feature of anaphylaxis.

Plasma exudation from capillaries and postcapillary venules is usually mediated by histamine and other vasoactive mediators released from mast cells, but mechanisms involving activation of the complement, fibrinolytic, and kinin pathways may be important in special circumstances.

DIAGNOSIS

It is usually possible to classify urticaria into five main groups on the clinical presentation, supported by challenge tests, skin biopsy, and blood tests where appropriate, although the groups are not mutually exclusive.

Ordinary Urticaria. This is the most common type of urticaria. Recurrent wheals may last up to 24 hours but sometimes as little as 1 to 2 hours in patients with mild or partially controlled disease. They subside without bruising. When severe, the attacks may be associated with systemic symptoms such as shivering, aching, and lassitude, but long-term complications do not occur. Angioedema is common. Ordinary urticaria is often subdivided into acute and chronic, depending on how long it has been present. Acute urticaria (resolving within days or weeks) may be triggered by minor viral infections or allergy (e.g., nuts, shellfish, fish, or fruit). Immediate hypersensitivity reactions involving the binding of an allergen to allergen-specific IgE on mast cells appears to be very uncommon in chronic ordinary urticaria in which the cause often remains uncertain. Between 30% and 50% of these "idiopathic" cases have histamine-releasing autoantibodies directed against the Fc fragment of receptor-bound IgE or the high-affinity IgE receptor (FcεRI) itself and may therefore be autoimmune. There is currently no routine laboratory test for these functional autoantibodies, but injecting autologous serum intradermally to look for a wheal response is a fairly specific and sensitive screening test.

Physical Urticarias. The diagnosis can usually be suspected from the history because the wheals appear within minutes of the stimulus application and fade within an hour, except in delayed pressure urticaria in which wheals develop several hours after pressure and last up to 24 hours. Anaphylaxis may occur. Physical urticarias are defined by the nature of the triggering stimulus, which may be light stroking (symptomatic dermographism), sustained pressure (delayed pressure urticaria), a rise in core temperature usually with sweating (cholinergic urticaria), ultraviolet radiation (solar urticaria), cold (cold urticaria), heat (localized heat urticaria), stress (adrenergic urticaria), water (aquagenic urticaria), and vibration (vibratory angioedema). More than one physical stimulus may be necessary for wheals in some patients (summation urticaria), and this can cause diagnostic difficulties when doing challenge tests in the clinic. Physical urticarias may coexist with ordinary urticaria. An association between delayed pressure urticaria and chronic idiopathic urticaria is well recognized.

Angioedema Without Wheals. Whenever angioedema occurs without wheals C1 esterase inhibitor deficiency must be considered. Although an uncommon cause of angioedema, its recognition is essential because swellings of the airway can be fatal and it may present as an acute abdomen if the bowel is involved. C1 inhibitor deficiency can be defined by laboratory tests and the two hereditary types treated effectively. Angioedema due to an angiotensin-converting enzyme (ACE) inhibitor may present months after starting therapy, and a relationship with the drug may not be obvious.

Urticarial Vasculitis. This systemic disease tends to be diagnosed by rheumatologists rather than dermatologists because joint symptoms often predominate. Patients may also show evidence of renal, gastrointestinal, pulmonary, or central nervous system involvement. The skin manifestation ranges from wheals that are indistinguishable from chronic ordinary urticaria to papules, erythema multiforme–like plaques, and angioedema. The diagnosis should be suspected if individual wheals persist for more than 2 days or show hemorrhage. They may cause burning discomfort rather than itch. Skin biopsy shows a small vessel vasculitis and is essential to confirm the diagnosis. The erythrocyte sedimentation rate (ESR) is often raised, and there may be evidence of early complement pathway activation and immune complex formation. Serum IgG antibodies to C1q are found in some patients. Hypocomplementemic urticarial vasculitis tends be associated with more severe systemic complications, including nephritis. Urticarial reactions seen after administration of blood products are also due to immune complex deposition in the skin.

Contact Urticaria. Contact urticaria usually presents little diagnostic difficulty because the stimulus for mast cell degranulation (often of plant or animal origin) elicits an immediate wheal at the site of contact. Immunologic and nonimmunologic mechanisms are recognized.

TREATMENT

The cause of urticaria should be removed whenever possible, and nonspecific aggravating factors, such as heat, stress, and alcohol, should be minimized. Aspirin and nonsteroidal anti-inflammatory drugs should in general be avoided, although tolerance may develop with repeated exposures. Specific exclusion diets are appropriate for acute urticaria due to food allergens (e.g., nuts, celery) but tend to be unhelpful unless a precipitant is obvious from the history. Strict avoidance of pseudoallergens, including natural salicylates, benzoates, azo dyes, and sulfites may help some patients with unremitting chronic ordinary urticaria. Oral challenge with a food additive series has seldom been informative in my experience. Disease associations with ordinary urticaria, such as thyroid disease, sinus or dental abscesses, and symptomatic *Helicobacter pylori* infection, should be sought.

Pharmacologic options are summarized in Table 1. Antihistamines are the mainstay of treatment for all patterns of urticaria except C1 inhibitor deficiency and urticarial vasculitis. Although mast cell stabilizing drugs theoretically offer the most rational approach to therapy of the mast cell–mediated urticarias, they tend to be disappointing. A recent report that leukotriene antagonists may help aspirin-sensitive chronic urticaria is interesting. Immunosuppressive therapies should be reserved for patients with very severe autoimmune urticaria.

Ordinary Urticaria

Antihistamines should be taken regularly at full doses. Five effective and well-tolerated nonsedating

TABLE 1. **Pharmacologic Therapy for Urticaria**

Mediator antagonists and inhibitors
  Antihistamines
    H_1 receptor antagonists (nonsedating, sedating, or combinations of both)
    Combination of an H_1 receptor antagonist with an H_2 receptor antagonist
  Nonsteroidal anti-inflammatory drugs*†
Mast cell stabilizers
  Ketotifen (antihistamine with properties of cromolyn sodium)
  Nifedipine (modifies calcium flux)
  Terbutaline (increases intracellular cyclic adenosine monophosphate)
Therapies for C_1 esterase inhibitor deficiency
  Tranexamic acid, Σ-aminocaproic acid (antifibrinolytics)
  Stanozolol, danazol (attenuated androgens)
  C1 esterase inhibitor concentrate (steam-treated lyophilized human blood product)
  Fresh-frozen plasma
Epinephrine
Oral corticosteroids*†
Immunosuppressive protocols
  Plasmapheresis*‡§
  Intravenous immunoglobulin‡
  Cyclosporine‡
Miscellaneous
  Dapsone*
  Colchicine*
  Hydroxychloroquine*

*Urticarial vasculitis.
†Delayed pressure urticaria.
‡Severe autoimmune chronic urticaria.
§Solar urticaria.

H_1 antagonists are available: acrivastine, astemizole, fexofenadine, loratadine, and terfenadine. Cetirizine (Zyrtec), a metabolite of hydroxyzine, is classed as a minimally sedating antihistamine. Acrivastine is not licensed for urticaria in the United States but is available as a combination product with pseudoephedrine (Semprex D). Astemizole (Hismanal) differs from the others in having a notably longer half-life (1–3 days for the parent drug, 12 days for the active metabolite) and a longer onset of action. It is taken as a 10-mg daily dose. Adverse effects include appetite stimulation and weight gain in some individuals. Administration should be avoided in patients with hepatic impairment or QT interval prolongation and those taking macrolides (e.g., erythromycin) or azole antifungal agents (ketoconazole [Nizoral] and itraconazole [Sporanox]) because ventricular arrhythmias have been reported. The same applies to terfenadine (Seldane), 60 mg twice daily, which was the first nonsedating antihistamine to be developed. It has now been withdrawn from the United States but is still available in some countries. Its active metabolite, fexofenadine (Allegra), 180 mg daily appears to be devoid of adverse cardiac effects and is effective for chronic urticaria, but comparative studies are not yet available. Loratadine (Claritin) is taken as a 10-mg daily dose and has a relatively short half-life (12 hours for the parent drug, 19 hours for the metabolite). Cetirizine (Zyrtec), 10 mg daily, is also short acting and may have clinically useful inhibitory effects on eosinophil migration.

Combining a nonsedating with a sedating antihistamine at night—such as hydroxyzine (Atarax, Vistaril), 10 to 50 mg, diphenhydramine (Benadryl), 25 to 100 mg, or chlorpheniramine (Chlor-Trimeton), 4 to 12 mg—can be helpful for patients whose sleep is disturbed by urticaria. Tricyclic antidepressants with potent H_1 antagonist properties, such as doxepin (Sinequan),* 10 mg three times daily, can be as effective as sedating antihistamines in this respect, but anticholinergic side effects, including blurred vision and dry mouth, can be a problem at higher doses. Addition of an H_2 receptor antagonist, such as ranitidine (Zantac),* 150 mg two times daily, or cimetidine (Tagamet),* 400 mg twice daily, sometimes improves urticaria control in patients who respond insufficiently to H_1 antagonists alone. H_2 antagonists are ineffective as monotherapy and may even aggravate urticaria.

A drug with mast cell–stabilizing properties should be considered if urticaria symptoms cannot be controlled with antihistamines alone. Nifedipine (Adalat, Procardia),* 10 to 20 mg three times daily, has been shown to be useful as monotherapy and in combination with antihistamines. It may be appropriate when hypertension coexists but should preferably be given in a sustained-release formulation because of recent concerns about the long-term safety of short-acting calcium antagonists in hypertension. Ketotifen† is a sedating antihistamine said to resemble sodium cromoglycate (cromolyn sodium [Gastrocom]) that may be beneficial for refractory urticaria. Sodium cromoglycate itself has not been shown to benefit chronic urticaria patients, probably because of its poor absorption from the bowel, although it may offer some protection against adverse reactions to foods. Oral beta agonists, such as terbutaline (Brethaire),* tend to cause unwanted palpitations and tremor at therapeutic doses for urticaria.

Prednisolone, 40 to 50 mg per day for 3 to 5 days, may lessen the severity and shorten the duration of acute urticaria when taken with an antihistamine. "Second-line" therapies for chronic urticaria, including systemic corticosteroids and immunosuppressive protocols, should be reserved for patients with severe refractory disease. Long-term corticosteroids should not be used in the routine management of chronic urticaria because their adverse effects nearly always outweigh their benefits when they are administered for months or years. Open studies of plasmapheresis and intravenous immunoglobulin in chronic urticaria have shown short- and long-term benefits in severely affected patients with histamine-releasing autoantibodies, but these therapies are expensive and not without risk. Controlled studies have confirmed the effectiveness of cyclosporine (Sandimmune)* at 4 mg per kg per day in selected chronic autoimmune urticaria patients with severe disease responding poorly to antihistamines.

Epinephrine is indicated for the emergency treatment of severe acute urticarial reactions associated with anaphylaxis and can be lifesaving for severe upper airway angioedema not due to C1 inhibitor deficiency. It must be used with caution in patients with hypertension and ischemic heart disease. Patients can be taught to self-administer 0.5 mL of 1:1000 epinephrine by subcutaneous or intramuscular injection.

A wide range of other therapies including warfarin anticoagulation, photochemotherapy, relaxation therapy, methotrexate, tranexamic acid, and leukotriene receptor antagonists have been reported to be beneficial in chronic urticaria but need to be substantiated with controlled studies.

Physical Urticarias

Many patients find antihistamines helpful in conjunction with lifestyle changes for the treatment of physical urticarias. Delayed-pressure urticaria presents the most difficult therapeutic problem because antihistamines are usually ineffective. Indomethacin,* 25 to 50 mg three times daily, may be used with success, but the response is unpredictable when delayed pressure is associated with chronic ordinary urticaria, which may be worsened by nonsteroidal anti-inflammatory drugs. Oral corticosteroids offer the most effective treatment but need to be taken at relatively high doses to maintain control. Anecdotal reports suggest that sulfasalazine* (Azulfidine) at 0.5 to 4.0 grams per day can be an effective alternative to corticosteroids. Solar urticaria has been treated successfully with plasmapheresis, photochemotherapy, and narrow waveband ultraviolet B phototherapy desensitization programs. Desensitization therapy for cold urticaria is of greater theoretical interest than practical value.

C1 Esterase Inhibitor Deficiency

Treatment of hereditary C1 esterase inhibitor deficiency should be titrated to the patient's well-being rather than inhibitor levels, which tend to correlate poorly with clinical disease activity. Some patients with little measurable inhibitor nevertheless remain attack free and do not need maintenance drug therapy. Type 1 disease (inhibitor levels are reduced to 5 to 30% of normal) and type II disease (normal antigenic levels of inhibitor that is dysfunctional) should be managed in the same way. Patients with the type II variant remain able to produce small amounts of functional as well as the dysfunctional inhibitor in response to attenuated androgens.

The antifibrinolytic drugs tranexamic acid (Cyklokapron)* 0.5 to 1.5 gram twice daily, and epsilonaminocaproic acid (Amicar),* 8 to 10 grams daily, are effective for long-term prophylaxis in many patients but contraindicated by a history of thromboembolic

---

*Not FDA approved for this indication.
†Not available in the United States.

*Not FDA approved for this indication.

disease. Regular ophthalmic examinations and monitoring of liver function are recommended with tranexamic acid. Stimulation of endogenous C1 inhibitor production by the attenuated androgens stanozolol (Winstrol) and danazol (Danocrine)* is now the treatment of choice except during pregnancy. Menstrual irregularities and mild virilizing effects such as hirsutism can be minimized by maintaining the dose as low as possible. The initial dose of danazol is 200 to 600 mg daily, but many patients can be controlled on as little as 200 mg daily 5 days a week. Liver function needs to be checked periodically. Stanozolol (Winstrol), 2.0 to 10 mg daily, may be used to control attacks, reducing the dosage to 2.5 mg three times weekly for maintenance if possible.

Short-term prophylaxis for patients undergoing traumatic procedures such as dental work or intubation may be achieved with antifibrinolytic drugs or inhibitor replacement with purified C1 esterase inhibitor concentrate infusion† or fresh-frozen plasma (FFP) if the concentrate is unavailable. Angioedema attacks should be treated in an emergency with purified C1 esterase inhibitor concentrate infusion† or FFP. Theoretically FFP, which contains the substrates for activated C1, C2, and C4, as well as C1 esterase inhibitor could cause an initial worsening of the angioedema, but in practice this is not a problem. There is no place for the prophylactic or emergency use of antihistamines. Patients with upper airway obstruction or dysphagia should be hospitalized without delay because they may require intubation or tracheostomy. Elderly patients presenting with acquired C1 esterase inhibitor deficiency should be investigated and treated for an underlying paraproteinemia.

Urticarial Vasculitis

There are no ideal treatments for this uncommon systemic disease. Antihistamines are widely used for the urticarial component but often disappointing because histamine is not the major mediator of the edema. Systemic corticosteroids (initially prednisolone, 0.5 mg per kg per day) may be required to suppress disease activity and prevent relapse. Because in the majority of patients urticarial vasculitis follows a chronic but benign course, it is preferable to explore alternative therapies to minimize long-term adverse effects. Some patients may obtain help from indomethacin,* 25 to 50 mg three times daily, dapsone,* 50 to 150 mg per day, colchicine,* 0.5 mg two to three times daily, and hydroxychloroquine (Plaquenil),* 200 to 400 mg daily. Patients taking dapsone must be monitored for anemia, which can be rapid and severe if they are deficient in glucose-6-phosphate dehydrogenase. Treatment with immunosuppressive agents including plasmapheresis, pulsed cyclophosphamide (Cytoxan), azathioprine

---

*Not FDA approved for this indication.
†Available in the United Kingdom on a named patient basis from Immuno, Vienna, Austria.

(Imuran), and gold should be given under the supervision of clinicians experienced in the use of these agents.

ACKNOWLEDGMENT

Claire Blyth, Pharmacist, West Norwich Hospital, Norwich, England, gave helpful advice on the manuscript.

PIGMENTARY DISORDERS

method of
CHRISTY A. LORTON, M.D.
Perrysburg, Ohio

The four pigments primarily responsible for normal skin color are oxygenated hemoglobin, reduced hemoglobin, carotenoid, and melanin. Of these, melanin is the major determinant of skin color. Disorders of pigmentation can be caused by at least three mechanisms: (1) an enhanced or diminished production of melanin by the melanocyte, (2) an increase or decrease in the number of melanocytes, and (3) an abnormal location of melanin and/or melanocytes within the dermis. The clinical result is either decreased pigment (hypopigmentation) or increased pigment (hyperpigmentation).

HYPERPIGMENTATION

Ultraviolet Light–Induced Hyperpigmentation (Suntan)

The constitutive or baseline skin color is genetically determined. It is independent of extrinsic factors such as exposure to sunlight. Facultative skin color is the inducible darkening of the skin that most often follows exposure to ultraviolet radiation. Suntan results from two different mechanisms. Longwave ultraviolet light (type A [UVA], 320 to 400 nm) causes immediate darkening of pigment. This occurs within 15 to 30 minutes after exposure and disappears within hours. It is probably caused by an oxidative change in the pre-existing melanin molecules. Immediate tanning is responsible for the bronzing of the skin that most individuals observe after intense exposure to summer sunlight.

Shortwave ultraviolet light (type B [UVB], 290 to 320 nm) produces sunburn and delayed tanning. Delayed tanning is often much darker than the immediate type and is caused by proliferation of melanocytes, as well as enhanced production of melanin. It takes 3 to 4 days to develop and lasts for many weeks.

Both longwave ultraviolet light and shortwave ultraviolet light contribute to photoaging, and both increase the risk of developing skin cancers. Both types of ultraviolet light are responsible for the mottled hyperpigmentation and wrinkling that are observed on heavily exposed areas of the skin such as the face, neck, and dorsum of the hands. Exposure to ultraviolet radiation in tanning parlors also hastens the process of photoaging and wrinkling and possibly increases the risk of developing skin cancers.

Treatment

The patient must recognize that sun-induced pigmentation can be reversed only by avoiding exposure of the skin to all forms of ultraviolet light. Many physical sunblocks are available that reflect ultraviolet light and protect the skin well. Clothing such as tightly woven outerwear or hats, which can be very elegant, are excellent protectants. Physical sunblocks such as zinc oxide, calamine, talc, titanium dioxide, and kaolin are opaque and act to scatter and reflect light. Most preparations, which are available commercially in skin tints to match the complexion or in microsized dispersions that rub in easily, are now cosmetically and socially acceptable. For individuals who are unusually sensitive to sunlight and who desire to enjoy outdoor activities, these sunblocks are essential.

Chemical sunscreens function in a different way. They absorb ultraviolet light in the UVB and/or UVA range. Para-aminobenzoic acid (PABA), PABA esters, salicylates, and cinnamates absorb radiation in the UVB range. Although PABA esters are used extensively in sunscreens, the use of PABA has been limited because of its potential to cause allergic reactions. Benzophenone derivatives absorb radiation mainly in the UVA range. The ideal broad-spectrum sunscreen contains an agent that absorbs UVB and an agent that absorbs UVA.

Two factors should be considered when choosing a sunscreen: the skin protection factor (SPF) and the substantivity. The SPF is the ratio of the minimal sunburn (UVB) dose of sunlight on chemically protected skin to that on unprotected skin. At the beginning of summer (June 21), the average unprotected person burns after 15 to 20 minutes of direct exposure to the sun at noontime. A sunscreen with SPF 2 absorbs half of the UVB striking the skin. Therefore, it takes twice as long to burn the treated skin (30 to 40 minutes of exposure on June 21). An SPF of 15 to 30 (which requires 15 to 30 times more UVB to burn the skin) is considered to be adequate protection against UVB radiation.

The substantivity of the sunscreen is its ability to withstand sweating and water immersion. Table 1 gives examples of current commercially available sunscreens with SPFs equal to or greater than 15 that also have good to excellent water and sweat resistance. Ideally, all sunscreens should be reapplied after prolonged swimming or heavy sweating.

Postinflammatory Hyperpigmentation

A variety of inflammatory conditions and infections (Table 2) cause hyperpigmentation of the skin, usually called *postinflammatory hyperpigmentation*. The dyschromia follows the pattern and distribution of the original disease, but its intensity is not necessarily related to the degree of the previous inflammation. Postinflammatory hyperpigmentation is common and rather persistent in darkly pigmented people. It is caused by stimulation of melanocytes to produce excessive amounts of melanin. If the melanin remains in the epidermis, the color of the skin appears to be deep tan to dark brown. Often the inflammation is associated with disruption of the dermal-epidermal barrier. Melanin is then deposited in the upper dermis. When brown melanin is located in the dermis, its color appears to be slate gray or bluish.

Treatment

Epidermal forms of hyperpigmentation may respond to treatment with bleaching agents. Dermal hyperpigmentation does not respond to any medical treatment and usually is permanent. It is important, therefore, to determine whether the pigmentation has mainly an epidermal or a dermal component. Examination of the patient with a Wood's lamp (black light) in a totally dark room can facilitate this evaluation. Epidermal melanin turns almost black when viewed with the Wood lamp. In contrast, dermal pigmentation, when observed with a Wood's lamp, is not visible to the examiner, and the blemishes on the patient's skin disappear.

Optimal management of the primary underlying skin problem is essential for treatment and prevention of further hyperpigmentation. If the hyperpigmentation is primarily epidermal, the patient may benefit from various topical modalities, which are discussed in the following section along with treat-

TABLE 1. **Partial List of Sunscreens That Have Good to Excellent Substantivity**

Brand Name Sunscreens (SPF)	Active Ingredients
PreSun (15 or 29)	Octylmethoxycinnamate, oxybenzone, octylsalicylate
Solbar (15 or 50)	Octylmethoxycinnamate, oxybenzone, octrocrylene (SPF 50)
Coppertone Sport (15 or 30)	p-Methoxycinnamate, oxybenzone, ethylhexyl salicylate
Neutrogena Sunblock (25)	Octylmethoxycinnamate, oxybenzone, octylsalicylate
Water Babies (45)	p-Methoxycinnamate, oxybenzone, ethylhexyl salicylate, homosalate
Banana Boat Ultra (30)	p-Methoxycinnamate, oxybenzone, ethylhexyl salicylate

TABLE 2. **Common Causes of Postinflammatory Hyperpigmentation**

Exanthems	Acne
Drug eruptions	Tinea versicolor
Lichen planus	Cutaneous lupus
Atopic dermatitis	Psoriasis
Trauma, burns	Lichen simplex chronicus
Herpes zoster	Pityriasis rosea
Ashy dermatosis	Fixed drug eruption

ment for other disorders of epidermal hyperpigmentation.

Melasma (Chloasma)

Melasma ("mask of pregnancy") is a common patchy, irregular, tan to brown pigmentation that is usually located on the face of women. It occurs in women who are taking oral contraceptives or who are pregnant. It usually fades slowly after the termination of either event and is exacerbated by exposure to sunlight. It also occurs in women who are not taking birth control pills or whose last pregnancy occurred many years earlier. Occasionally, it occurs in men. Melasma is caused by increased epidermal melanization, although in some patients there is a moderate amount of dermal pigment as well. In these latter individuals, treatment can never return the skin entirely to its normal appearance.

Freckles (Ephelides)

Freckles first appear in childhood in individuals who have fair complexions and who are genetically of Celtic or northern European ancestry. Freckles fade in the winter and become more prominent after exposure to sunlight. Middle-aged and older adults usually lose some or all of their freckles.

Solar Lentigines

Solar or senile lentigines are dark brown macules, usually 1 to 3 cm in diameter, that occur on the chronically sun-exposed surfaces of elderly individuals, especially on the dorsum of the hands or on the face. They are commonly misnamed "liver spots." In contrast to freckles and melasma, they do not fade in the winter but persist throughout the calendar year. They must be distinguished from lentigo maligna or seborrheic keratoses.

Treatment

Patients with these sun-induced pigmentary disorders must avoid further unprotected exposure to sunlight. This should be stressed as the most important part of their therapy. Sunscreens or sunblocks help to prevent further pigmentary abnormalities.

There is considerable individual variation in the response to treatment, but in general, most patients will respond to one or a combination of preparations. Most bleaching medications must be applied conscientiously, often for 6 to 12 months, to achieve optimal results.

Various bleaching medications are available that contain hydroquinone, either in an over-the-counter 2% concentration (Esoterica, Porcelana) or a 3% (Melanex) or 4% (Eldopaque Forte, Solaquin Forte) strength by prescription. Hydroquinone suppresses pigmentation, probably by blocking the activity of tyrosinase, the enzyme primarily involved in melanin synthesis. Side effects from hydroquinone are rare but include mild skin irritation. At higher concentra-

tions, colloid milia, dermal pigmentation, or both have been reported. The addition of a mild corticosteroid cream (hydrocortisone 1 to 2.5%) increases the effectiveness of the hydroquinone and possibly reduces the frequency of skin irritation. Caution must be exercised when prescribing corticosteroids for prolonged periods. On the face, steroids can cause telangiectasia, atrophy, or acneiform lesions. The more potent fluorinated corticosteroids should not be used on the face except under special circumstances. On the arms and trunk, potent topical steroids can cause striae. These are irreversible.

Tretinoin cream (Retin-A, Renova)* can also be used in conjunction with hydroquinone and/or mild corticosteroids to decrease epidermal hyperpigmentation. There has been a great deal of interest in the use of tretinoin alone to remove pigmentation associated specifically with photoaging. Tretinoin can be irritating to the skin and can cause erythema, desquamation, and soreness. To minimize the side effects, the following approach is suggested. Therapy should be initiated with 0.025 or 0.05% tretinoin applied at bedtime twice weekly for 1 to 2 weeks, then three times weekly for a few more weeks, followed by nightly applications. Thereafter the concentration of the cream can be increased to 0.1% if tolerated by the patient. Alternatively, the patient can begin nightly with Renova, which is tretinoin in an emollient cream.

The application of alpha-hydroxy acids (AHAs) can be used to improve hyperpigmentation, whether postinflammatory, melasma, or lentigines. Glycolic acid and lactic acid are the two most common agents used in products, most of which are available over the counter. AHAs appear to work by altering corneocyte cohesion, which results in desquamation and dispersion of melanin granules. Clinical lightening of the skin is observed after several weeks of application of skin lotions or creams containing 8 to 15% concentration of AHA. In higher concentrations, glycolic acid is used in serial skin peel systems to treat hyperpigmentation.

Topical 20% azelaic acid cream (Azelex)* causes skin lightening, possibly by inhibition of hyperactive melanocytes and by interfering with tyrosinase. The effect of tretinoin with azelaic acid is additive. A good combination approach would be to use a tretinoin cream at night and azelaic acid cream in the morning.

There are other modalities for treating localized pigmented spots such as freckles or solar lentigines. Gentle freezing with liquid nitrogen can decrease the amount of color. Melanocytes are particularly susceptible to destruction by this treatment. One must avoid causing necrosis of the skin or blistering. Dark-skinned patients should not have lesions frozen except in special circumstances because of the risk of permanent depigmentation.

Trichloroacetic acid (TAC) is another agent that is effective for solar lentigines or other localized

---

*Not FDA approved for this indication.

patches of pigmentation but is generally not useful in dark-skinned individuals. Aqueous TAC in strengths ranging from 15 to 75% is used as a peeling agent alone or in combination with Jessner's solution (resorcinol, lactic acid, and salicylic acid in an ethanol solution). An alternative to the aqueous solution is the TAC masque, which is a chelated TAC in a creamy clay formula. TAC must be used with extreme caution because it is a highly reactive chemical that can cause epidermal necrosis, delayed healing, and scarring. In the hands of the experienced physician, these peels can be done safely and effectively to improve dyschromia.

Systemic Causes of Hyperpigmentation

Generalized hyperpigmentation is associated with many systemic disorders. Usually the color is due to melanin, for example, in Addison's disease. Metabolic, nutritional, or endocrine disorders should be considered in patients with widespread or diffuse hyperpigmentation. Generalized hyperpigmentation can also be caused by drugs or heavy metals. A partial list of these disorders and drugs is given in Table 3.

Treatment

Treatment for hyperpigmentation caused by systemic disorders is directed at correcting the underlying disease or discontinuing the medication.

HYPOPIGMENTATION

Vitiligo

Vitiligo is a common acquired depigmenting disorder that occurs in about 1% of the general population. It is characterized by white (depigmented) patches on the skin. Only about 5% of affected individuals have a positive (primary family) history of vitiligo. About 15% of patients with vitiligo have thyroid disease, and 5% have diabetes mellitus. Rarely, the patient with vitiligo has Addison's disease, pernicious anemia, or other endocrine disorders.

There are two types of vitiligo. In the generalized form, the white patches are spread over the body. In the second form, segmental vitiligo, the patches are limited to localized areas (e.g., one half of the face, an entire arm, or one leg). Segmental vitiligo usually does not follow dermatomes. In either type of vitiligo,

TABLE 3. **Systemic Causes of Hyperpigmentation**

Metabolic Conditions	Drugs and Metals
Hemochromatosis	Mercury
Porphyria cutanea tarda	Silver
Addison's disease	Arsenic
Vitamin B deficiency	Gold
Pellagra	Antimalarial agents
Scleroderma	Minocycline
Acanthosis nigricans	Phenothiazines
Pregnancy	Beta carotene

the white patches generally appear spontaneously without a pre-existing rash. The depigmented areas are completely devoid of epidermal melanin and melanocytes. The cause of vitiligo is not known. Although vitiligo is commonly assumed to be an autoimmune disease, depigmentary disorders in several animal models that resemble human vitiligo suggest that the disorder may have a biochemical basis.

Treatment

The physician should be aware of the strong psychosocial impact that vitiligo has on the patient and should be prepared to provide reassurance, explanation, and appropriate referral to support groups, consultants, or psychiatrists as needed. For most people, vitiligo is a devastating disfigurement.

For certain individuals, the use of cosmetics or stains to conceal the more apparent vitiligo is all that is desired. Cover Mark and Dermablend are two opaque types of makeup that some patients find helpful. Stains or self-tanning products that contain dihydroxyacetone can be used to tint the depigmented areas so that they are less obvious.

Judicious use of broad-spectrum sunscreens is recommended for three reasons. First, the areas of vitiligo burn more easily than normal skin when exposed to sunlight. Second, sunburn injury can extend the depigmentation, a process called Koebner's phenomenon. Third, exposure to sunlight induces darkening of the surrounding normal-appearing skin and causes accentuation of the cosmetic disfigurement.

Repigmentation requires regrowth of melanocytes into the white epidermis. Unfortunately, melanocytes do not migrate more than a few millimeters from the edge of a lesion. Thus, successful repigmentation requires the presence of hair bulbs from which melanocytes can be stimulated to migrate into the surrounding white skin. Skin on the dorsa of the hands or distal to the ankles repigments poorly because this skin lacks sufficient numbers of hair bulbs.

The most effective method of treatment for vitiligo is photochemotherapy. It requires a motivated patient who is committed to prolonged therapy. It is intended for patients older than 10 years of age who are neither pregnant nor lactating. There must be no history of a photosensitivity disorder. If a collagen vascular disorder is suspected, an antinuclear antibody level and other evaluations should be obtained before starting photochemotherapy.

Psoralen (available as 8-methoxypsoralen [Oxsoralen-Ultra]) is a potent photosensitizer in combination with UVA (PUVA). PUVA therapy for vitiligo takes 6 to 24 months and must be given two times a week in gradually increasing dosages. The patient must be given careful instruction in the proper use of protective glasses that block out UVA, which might damage the eyes and lead to cataract formation. The patient must also avoid unprotected sunlight exposure for 24 hours after taking the psoralen because of the increased photosensitivity.

Topical PUVA is intended for the treatment of limited areas of vitiligo. Skin treated with topical psoralen is extremely sensitive to sunlight and UVA. Even inadvertent exposure of the treated skin through car windows for a few minutes can cause painful second-degree burns. Topical psoralen should be prescribed only by physicians thoroughly acquainted with its safe use.

Topical mild steroid creams such as hydrocortisone, 2.5% applied once daily, often treat vitiligo successfully. The medication must be applied for 6 to 12 months. The patient should be observed carefully to prevent damage to the skin from steroids. Caution must be used when applying steroids around the eyes. Patients with vitiligo probably should have a baseline eye examination that is repeated yearly if they are receiving PUVA or applying steroids around the eyes.

For patients with extensive (more than 50%) vitiligo, careful consideration should be given to total depigmentation of the remaining pigmented skin. This is accomplished by application of 20% monobenzyl ether of hydroquinone twice daily for a period of weeks to years. The medication is applied until depigmentation is complete. This medication causes irreversible destruction of melanocytes. This procedure should be done only after the patient gives careful consideration and consent. Patients need to understand that the depigmentation is permanent. They will always be sensitive to sunlight. However, the cosmetic result is gratifying.

Postinflammatory Hypopigmentation

Many of the same inflammatory disorders or infections that cause postinflammatory hyperpigmentation can also cause hypopigmentation. The most common causes are eczema, atopic dermatitis, tinea versicolor, secondary syphilis, chickenpox, and psoriasis. Pityriasis alba is a mild form of dermatitis that is common in children. It is characterized by hypopigmented patches with fine scales. Although most commonly noted on the face, it can also affect the arms, thighs, or trunk.

Treatment

Unlike postinflammatory hyperpigmentation, postinflammatory hypopigmentation usually resolves slowly over time. Hydrocortisone, 2.5% in a cream or lotion applied twice daily, may accelerate repigmentation.

Idiopathic Guttate Hypomelanosis

Idiopathic guttate hypomelanosis is a common condition characterized by hypopigmented, confetti-like macules on the extremities. These macules can also occur on the trunk and, rarely, on the face. The condition occurs in all races but is more noticeable in darker skinned or tanned people. It must be distinguished from vitiligo. The cause of idiopathic guttate hypomelanosis is not known, although sunlight is thought to be a contributing factor. There is a reduc-

tion in the number of melanocytes in the pale macules.

Treatment

The patient should always apply a broad-spectrum sunscreen and avoid excessive sun exposure. This prevents further sun damage and avoids accentuating the hypomelanosis by darkening the surrounding skin.

SUNBURN

method of
VINCENT A. DELEO, M.D.
St. Luke's/Roosevelt Hospital Center
New York, New York

The most commonly observed response to solar radiation is the wounding response called *sunburn*. Over one half of the population of the United States report having experienced at least one such response of a serious, blistering nature before adulthood. All except the most darkly complexioned persons report some milder forms of the response during childhood and adolescence.

Sunburn presents clinically as erythema with or without edema. With sufficient dose of radiation, vesicles and bullae, a second degree burn, may develop. The severity of the response depends on the dose of radiation and the individual's genetically determined "skin type" (Table 1). Skin type depends primarily on an individual's inherent melanin pigmentation. Lighter complexioned individuals with lower skin types, I and II, develop sunburn with small doses achieved in short periods of sun exposure. Even the most darkly pigmented type V or VI individuals develop a response if the dose is large enough. The skin feels warm to the touch and the affected individual experiences pain and discomfort. Pruritus may also be present. If sufficient body surface area is involved, the individual may experience systemic symptoms of weakness, chills, fever, and dehydration. The most severe cases may need hospitalization.

The timing of the development of the signs and symptoms of sunburn may be variable. Reactions usually begin 3 to 6 hours after exposure and become maximal at 24

TABLE 1. **Human Skin Types**

Type	Reaction to Sun	Example
I	Always burns easily, never tans	Red-haired, freckled
II	Always burns easily, tans minimally	Fair-skinned, blue eyed
III	Burns moderately, tans gradually	Darker Caucasian
IV	Burns minimally, tans always	Mediterranean
V	Rarely burns, tans profusely	Middle Eastern, Latin American, light-skinned African American
VI	Never burns, tans deeply	Dark-skinned African American

TABLE 2. **The Solar Spectrum**

Range	Wavelength (nm)
X-rays	<10
Ultraviolet (UV)	10–400
UVC	10–290
UVB	290–320
UVA	320–400
Visible	400–800
Infrared	>800

hours. The response then gradually fades over 1 to 3 days. In some cases, the response may be biphasic, with an immediate response of a mild erythema that quickly fades followed by the delayed phase as described above.

The initial, inflammatory, response of a sunburn is followed by a reparative one in which the skin develops desquamation and increased pigmentation, known as *tanning*.

The portion, or spectrum, of solar radiation responsible for sunburn falls within the ultraviolet (UV) range (Table 2). The ultraviolet spectrum ranges between 10 and 400 nm, between x-rays and the visible spectrum (400 and 800 nm). The UV spectrum has classically been divided into three ranges, based on biologic effects: UVA, 320 to 400 nm; UVB, 290 to 320 nm; and UVC, 10 to 290 nm. UVC radiation is completely absorbed by the ozone layer and so does not interact with skin in the natural setting. Natural sunburn is due primarily to UVB radiation, with a minor component due to UVA radiation. The peak of erythemal effectiveness or the peak action spectrum for sunburn lies just short of 300 nm. Radiation throughout the UV from artificial light sources, however, can induce inflammation in human skin. The efficiency with which such radiation induces erythema varies widely. Furthermore, there are other differences in timing and dose-response kinetics of the inflammation induced by other wavelengths (Table 3). UVC-induced erythema peaks early at 6 hours, fades quickly, and has a relatively flat dose-response curve. It is slightly more efficient at inducing a minimal erythema (minimal erythema dose) than UVB. It can only be produced by artificial sources. Such radiation is present in small amounts in home sunlamps and is very carcinogenic.

Pure UVB-induced inflammation is much like natural solar sunburn, as might be expected, because it is primarily responsible for the natural response. UVA is 1000 times less efficient than UVB at inducing minimal erythema. Its response begins immediately, peaks in 6 to 12 hours, fades quickly, and has a very flat dose-response curve, meaning that it is much less likely even in large doses to induce blistering. Because there is about 10 times as much UVA as UVB radiation in natural solar radiation, even though it is relatively inefficient at erythemal production, UVA does play a role in natural sunburn. This is particularly so

for erythema that develops through a sunscreen, which allows long exposures, because sunscreens are relatively more efficient at blocking UVB than UVA radiation.

Approximately 1 million Americans go to tanning salons every day to obtain an artificial tan. Tanning salon light sources have a relatively larger percentage of UVA than natural sunshine. Although some salons claim to use light sources that emit only UVA radiation, almost all such sources produce significant UVB as well. Radiation from these units is capable of inducing erythema and even blistering burns. Because of the spectrum of the radiation obtained in salons, patients may present with sunburns that have some features of UVA erythema.

Histologically, sunburned skin is characterized by necrotic, apoptotic keratinocytes called *sunburn cells*. These occur in solar sunburns and in those induced by UVB, but not to a great extent in skin irradiated with UVA. A dermal inflammatory infiltrate is present with edema, degranulated mast cells, and dilated superficial dermal vessels.

The mechanism by which UV radiation induces inflammation in human skin is complex and still poorly understood. Radiation in the UVC and UVB range is absorbed by DNA and leads to production of photoproducts, primarily pyrimidine dimers and 6-4 photoproducts. UVA radiation also causes DNA damage but of the strand break type rather than dimer formation. Changes with all ranges of radiation also occur at sites other than the nucleus, such as in membrane-associated signaling systems with phosphorylation of membrane receptors and activation of kinase cascades. This leads to the activation of phospholipases and cyclooxygenases with eicosanoid production, cytokine release and production, and histamine release from mast cells. These soluble mediators lead to the erythema and edema that are seen clinically. An initial inhibition of DNA synthesis is followed by an induction of synthesis that heralds the repair phase of the response, resulting in thickening of the epidermis and desquamation or sunburn "peeling."

Sunburns are uncomfortable, usually not of great severity, and resolve rather quickly. The damage induced by such insult can, however, be long lived. Multiple sunburns is a epidemiologic risk factor for the development of melanoma, particularly when the burns occurred in childhood and adolescence.

TREATMENT

The best treatment for a sunburn, of course, is prevention. In fact, very little can be done once the sunburn has occurred. Therapy is primarily supportive. Mild to moderate reactions can be treated with cool soaks, topical corticosteroids, and, because of their anti-cyclooxygenase activity as well as their analgesic effects, systemic nonsteroidal anti-in-

TABLE 3. **Erythema Response to Ultraviolet (UV) Radiation**

	Solar Radiation	UVA	UVB	UVC
Relative dose	1	1000	1	0.5–1
Minimal erythema dose	15–30 min noonday summer sun	30–60 J/cm²	30–60 mJ/cm²	15–30 mJ/cm²
Timing (hr)				
Onset	4–6	<1	6	4
Peak	24	6–12	24	6
Fade	72	24	72	12–36

flammatory agents. Topical products containing Benadryl and anesthetics should be avoided because they can cause contact allergy. Itching responds to soporific doses of antihistamines, which may have to be used only at bed time. Persons with severe reactions with fever and dehydration sometimes require hospitalization for supportive care. Although systemic corticosteroids are frequently utilized for sunburn, there is no good evidence that they are beneficial. If blisters develop into erosions, they should be kept clean to avoid secondary bacterial infection.

Prevention of sunburn requires education of the population. Such educational efforts must begin in early childhood. To accomplish this, parents must understand the short-term and long-term dangers of excessive sun exposure. Populations at special risk for photodamage, that is, types I and II complexioned individuals and individuals with a family history of skin cancer, melanoma and atypical mole syndrome should receive greatest attention. Prevention consists of a "sun sensible" program. This includes avoidance of exposure between the hours of 10 AM and 4 PM, when solar radiation is most intense; wearing clothing, including broad brimmed hats, whenever possible to limit skin exposure; and wearing a sunscreen of sun protection factor (SPF) 15 or higher on sun-exposed skin when more than minimal exposure is anticipated.

Sunscreens are tested and labeled according to FDA guidelines. The SPF indicates the protectiveness of the product and appears on the labels of all sunscreens sold in the United States. The SPF is determined by exposing the skin of volunteers to solar-simulated radiation with and without the sunscreen. The amount of radiation necessary to produce erythema in sunscreen-protected skin is divided by the amount of radiation necessary to produce the same response in unprotected skin. This ratio is the SPF. Essentially, if a product has an SPF of 10, an individual who wears the product will be able to tolerate 10 times as much exposure as he or she could without the product and develop the same degree of erythema. Thus, if a type I person who normally develops a minimal pinkness in the skin after 15 to 30 minutes of exposure wears an SPF 10 sunscreen, he or she will be able to tolerate 150 to 300 minutes of exposure with similar result.

Some sunscreens also carry a rating of substantivity. The water resistant SPF indicates that the screen will maintain its effectiveness after 40 minutes of water immersion. The water proof SPF indicates that the screen will remain active after 80 minutes of immersion. Patients should be instructed, however, to reapply the sunscreen after excessive sweating or prolonged water exposure because these ratings are laboratory based and may not mimic true beach or pool conditions.

Physicians must be the educators of their patients about the dangers of sun exposure. Instructions for avoidance of sunburn and long-term effects of excessive solar exposure should be part of routine preventive care. A "sun sensible" approach, as outlined here, should be utilized. It should be stressed that sun tanning is damaging and that tanning in tanning salons is at least as damaging as tanning with natural solar exposure.

Section 13

The Nervous System

ALZHEIMER'S DISEASE

method of
DAVID A. BENNETT, M.D.
Rush–Presbyterian–St. Luke's Medical Center
Chicago, Illinois

Alzheimer's disease is one of the most common chronic conditions of older persons. Overall, it affects about 1 in 10 Americans older than the age of 65. Occurrence of the disease is strikingly related to age, affecting about 15% of those between the ages of 75 and 84 and about half of those older than the age of 85. Between 4 and 5 million people in the United States currently have the disease. Because the number of people in the United States older than 65 is the most rapidly growing segment of the population, the number of people with the disease is projected to triple by the middle of the 21st century, making Alzheimer's disease a public health problem of truly staggering proportions. Keeping current with changes in the diagnosis, treatment, and care of persons with Alzheimer's disease can be difficult. The Alzheimer's Disease Education and Referral (ADEAR) Center, a service of the National Institute on Aging, is an excellent source of up-to-date information (electronic mail address: adear@alzheimers.org; website: http://www.alzheimers.org).

DIAGNOSIS

Many patients and family members accept memory loss and confusion as a consequence of aging. Likewise, many physicians do not look for or recognize dementia. Therefore, most persons with the disease do not come to medical attention; as few as one in five persons with Alzheimer's disease has actually been diagnosed by a physician, making it among the most underrecognized chronic conditions of older persons.

Evaluating a person for dementia involves determining whether there has been a meaningful loss of cognitive function relative to a previous level of performance. Evidence should be obtained from the patient and/or a knowledgeable informant and documented by mental status testing. A diagnosis of Alzheimer's disease, by far the most common cause of dementia in the aged, requires progressive loss of memory and other cognitive functions. Alzheimer's disease has often been thought of as a diagnosis of exclusion. However, other common conditions (e.g., stroke, Parkinson's disease) do not protect one from getting Alzheimer's disease. Thus, the diagnosis of Alzheimer's disease should be one of inclusion: that is, does the person have a syndrome consistent with Alzheimer's disease, regardless of the presence of other coexisting illnesses?

Typically, Alzheimer's disease begins with the insidious onset of memory loss. Family members may notice memory difficulties from day-to-day life events. Patients frequently repeat questions, forget phone messages and appointments, or get lost driving. Bills may not be paid. Patients may lose weight because they no longer shop, or cook, or eat. Initially, deficits are unapparent to casual observers, and patients may carry on brief, pleasant, and socially appropriate conversations. As the disease progresses, word-finding difficulties become obvious and judgment becomes poor. Patients may fall prey to fraud. Managing a checkbook becomes impossible. Patients may become disoriented as to time, day, and season.

It is crucial that all complaints of cognitive difficulties be taken seriously, whether they are provided directly by the patient, through a family member, or suspected by the physician during the course of a routine evaluation of other conditions. The incorporation of a brief mental status measure into the routine examination of older persons will greatly facilitate this aim. Patients will frequently reach medical attention with problems other than memory. Sleep disturbance, hallucinations, paranoia, and physical aggression may prompt an evaluation. The discontinuation of hobbies and community activities, along with sleep disturbances and weight loss, may suggest depression. Motor disturbances, especially gait disturbances and slowness of movement, may suggest Parkinson's disease. Typically, the cognitive deficits are relentlessly progressive; behavioral, affective, and motor signs become more common as the disease advances. Patients with Alzheimer's disease are at greater risk of hospitalization, institutionalization, and death than are persons without Alzheimer's disease.

NONPHARMACOLOGIC MANAGEMENT

Management of someone with Alzheimer's disease requires patience, compassion, and skills beyond the sophisticated therapies that characterize much of modern medical practice. The physician must care for a person with a disease that frequently changes the patient's personality and is usually relentlessly progressive; the physician must enlist the aid and ensure the cooperation of distraught family members whose own lives are often in turmoil if the patient is to be kept in a stimulating and supportive environment. The judicious use of pharmacotherapy for cognitive dysfunction and behavioral disturbances in Alzheimer's disease should be accompanied by a strong effort to provide education and support for the patient, the family, and the caregivers.

Social services include adult day care programs, respite care programs, nursing home special care units, and hospice services. County social service agencies, often with federal assistance, may provide funding for some of these services. The Alzheimer's Association has information regarding services available within specific catchment areas. There are now more than 200 local chapters; a list can be obtained from the Alzheimer's Association National Office

(919 North Michigan Avenue, Suite 1000, Chicago, Illinois 60611-1676; by phone, 800-272-3900 and 312-335-8700; by fax, 312-335-1110; by electronic mail, info@alz.org; or by website, http://www.alz.org).

Adult day care programs provide a wide range of activities aimed at different levels of client impairment and interests. Most cater to persons with moderate to severe disease. There is some evidence that these activities slow loss of physical function and delay placement into institutional long-term care. Day care also provides respite to the caregiver. There are also inpatient and outpatient respite care programs. Most take patients for periods of days to weeks on a planned basis. Some will take patients for crisis intervention. There is anecdotal evidence that the respite provided to the caregiver delays placement of the patient into institutional long-term care.

Special care units for dementia care are now available in many nursing homes. The content of these programs vary greatly, but most aim to a provide more stimulating environment and reduce the use of physical and chemical restraints. As with adult day care, there is some evidence that they slow loss of physical function.

Hospice care is also increasingly available for patients if a decision is made to limit aggressive medical intervention. Some hospice programs specialize in dementia patients. Many patients can contribute to economic and medical decisions regarding their own care. Therefore, physicians and families should discuss the diagnosis and its implications in a straightforward, honest, and supportive manner with patients as early as possible. Patients may be competent to execute a valid power of attorney, which gives another person legal authority to make decisions regarding the patient's health or estate. Many states require a durable power of attorney for it to remain valid in the event the patient becomes incompetent. Living wills and living trusts must also be initiated at a time when the patient is competent. Guardianship must be imposed if a patient is no longer competent and legal authority for decisions regarding his or her health or estate must be granted to another person. This requires that the patient be declared incompetent by a court, with the court subsequently appointing a guardian.

TREATMENT OF COGNITIVE FUNCTION

Dementia typically evolves over many years. For much of this time, the patient is not totally disabled and is more functional in a familiar and stable environment. There are many areas in which intervention can improve quality of life for both the patient and the caregiver. Although the disease is defined by its effect on cognitive function, affective and behavioral disturbances and motor signs may be the targets of intervention. Finally, there are interventions aimed at altering the course of the disease, including reducing disability, institutionalization, caregiver stress, and death.

Acetylcholine is the neurotransmitter of several central nervous system neuronal circuits. One circuit projects from the basal forebrain to the hippocampus and parts of the cerebral cortex. Agents that augment this system have been under investigation for the treatment of Alzheimer's disease for more than 20 years. The investigations have followed four basic strategies: (1) administering a precursor of acetylcholine synthesis, (2) stimulating acetylcholine release, (3) inhibiting the enzyme that catalyzes acetylcholine degradation, and (4) mimicking the action of acetylcholine at the cholinergic receptor. Of these, inhibition of acetylcholinesterase rapidly hydrolyzes acetylcholine to choline and acetic acid and has met with the most success. Inhibiting acetylcholinesterase prolongs the action of acetylcholine in the synapse, allowing for more effective transmission. Two acetylcholinesterase inhibitors, tacrine (Cognex) and donepezil (Aricept), have been approved by the Food and Drug Administration (FDA) for the symptomatic treatment of Alzheimer's disease. Several others, including metrifonate, physostigmine, and rivastigmine, are under investigation and may be approved in the future.

For a medication to be approved by the FDA for the symptomatic treatment of Alzheimer's disease, efficacy must be demonstrated with two end points in two phase III clinical trials, including a performance-based measure of cognitive abilities and a global functional assessment. The Alzheimer's Disease Assessment Scale—Cognitive (ADAS-Cog; range 0 to 70) is a commonly used performance test. On average, a person with Alzheimer's disease declines about 8 points per year on this scale. The effect size sought after in clinical trials has been a difference of about 4 points between the treatment group and the placebo group, that is, an effect size equivalent to about 6 months of disease progression.

Tacrine (Cognex) was the first acetylcholinesterase inhibitor to be approved for the treatment of Alzheimer's disease. With a duration of action of about 6 hours, the drug must be given four times daily. Several double-blind, placebo-controlled studies have documented a small, but significant, improvement in cognitive function, about 2 points on the ADAS-Cog over 12 weeks, with 40 mg four times daily for 12 to 30 weeks. Unfortunately, up to half of the persons on tacrine in these studies had to discontinue the drug due to side effects, including asymptomatic hepatotoxicity, nausea, vomiting, and diarrhea. Because of the relatively high frequency of hepatotoxicity, the manufacturer's recommendation is to slowly increase the dose of tacrine, checking serum transaminase levels weekly. For patients with mild to moderate Alzheimer's disease, the dosage should start at 10 mg four times a day and then increased to 20 mg four times a day, then to 30 mg four times a day, and finally to 40 mg four times a day. Increases should take place at 6-week intervals. Thus, it takes about 4 months to achieve a stable dose. The drug should be discontinued if transaminase levels rise above three times the upper limit of normal. Because of the limited benefit, the risk of side effects, and the difficulty of use, tacrine has already been supplanted by newer agents.

Donepezil (Aricept) was the second acetylcholinesterase inhibitor to be approved for the treatment of Alzheimer's disease. Donepezil has several advantages over tacrine, including a longer half-life and fewer side effects. Because of its longer half-life, the drug can be administered once per day. In double-blind, placebo-controlled studies, donepezil has been administered at doses of either 5 mg or 10 mg per day for 12 to 24 weeks. About 85% of subjects taking 5 mg, and 70% of subjects taking 10 mg completed the studies. Side effects, including nausea, vomiting, and diarrhea, were mild and limited. There were no significant elevations of serum transaminase levels. Both dosages of 5 mg per day and 10 mg per day were superior to placebo, with an effect size similar to that of tacrine—about 3 points on the ADAS-Cog over 24 weeks. Although the 10-mg dose was not clearly better than the 5-mg dose, the higher dose is recommended because the response to cholinesterase inhibitors, in general, tends to be dose dependent. For patients with mild to moderate Alzheimer's disease, the dosage should start at 5 mg per day for 1 month and then increased to 10 mg per day if the 5-mg dose is tolerated.

The overall effect size of both tacrine and donepezil is small, which makes it difficult to clearly determine their efficacy on an individual patient basis. Consensus regarding recommendations for discontinuation of these drugs has been elusive. On one hand, because the trials were aimed at detecting improvement of cognitive function, it has been advocated that if improvement cannot be documented in 24 to 30 weeks, the drug should be discontinued. In contrast, because there are few alternatives, others recommend that in the absence of significant side effects, the drugs should be continued until the subject becomes severely impaired. This debate is likely to continue until the discovery of agents with robust and reproducible effects that can clearly be determined on a patient-by-patient basis or the demonstration that a particular agent actually slows deterioration.

Ergoloid mesylates (Hydergine) has been available in the United States for the treatment of a variety of conditions, including dementia, for decades and is extensively used worldwide. Its mechanism of action is unclear, but it appears to effect several central nervous system receptor systems. Numerous trials of Hydergine have been conducted. Overall, there may be a small benefit of the drug at doses of up to 7.5 mg per day, although the results of the larger and more rigorous double-blind, placebo-controlled clinical trials have been negative.

Extracts of *Ginkgo biloba* are among the most commonly prescribed drugs in Europe and are used for a variety of conditions, including progressive degenerative dementia. Four *Gingko* preparations* have been used in clinical trials, differing only by the amount of ginkgo flavone glycosides. Several studies have reported small benefits of the *Gingko biloba* extract Egb 761 for Alzheimer's disease. High rates of dropout and loss to follow-up in the largest and most recent double-blind, placebo-controlled study, however, preclude a definitive conclusion regarding the efficacy of the *Gingko biloba*. The lack of clear efficacy, combined with the small magnitude of the effect and the potential for side effects either alone or when used with commonly used anticoagulants such as aspirin, suggests that it is premature to recommend it to patients with Alzheimer's disease.

TREATMENTS AFFECTING DISEASE COURSE

Vitamin E* and selegiline (Eldepryl)* have been investigated as agents to slow the progression of Alzheimer's disease because of their ability to scavenge free radicals and potentially reduce cellular damage from oxidative stress. In a novel double-blind, placebo-controlled study, the ability of these agents to delay time to one of several end points was evaluated in a 2 × 2 factorial design. Three study arms were compared with placebo: vitamin E alone, selegiline alone, and vitamin E and selegiline. The outcomes included time to any one of several end points, including loss of activities of daily living, progression to a more severe stage of disease, institutionalization, and death. Compared with placebo, all three regimens were equally efficacious in delaying time to one of the end points by about 25%. Secondary analyses examining the effect of vitamin E and selegiline on cognitive outcomes were not significant. This raises the possibility that the effect was not specific to Alzheimer's disease. Vitamin E, 1000 IU twice daily, is now frequently being recommended for persons with Alzheimer's disease. Other antioxidants are under investigation.

TREATMENT OF BEHAVIORAL DISORDERS

A variety of neuropsychiatric disturbances are common among persons with Alzheimer's disease. Among these, psychotic features, depression, insomnia, and aggression may require and respond to psychopharmacologic intervention. Before ascribing behavioral problems to Alzheimer's disease, it is important to exclude the possibility of a coexisting medical condition as the underlying cause of the behavioral disturbances.

Psychotic Features

Psychotic features such as auditory or visual hallucinations or misperceptions and delusions are common in Alzheimer's disease. These features of the

---

*Not FDA approved for this indication.

disease are more common in more advanced disease, are more common in persons who also exhibit parkinsonian signs, and appear to be associated with a more rapid disease course. Risperidone (Risperdal) is the treatment of choice if these symptoms are disruptive, because the risk extrapyramidal side effects is lower than conventional high-potency neuroleptics. Sedation and orthostatic hypotension are the main side effects. As little as 0.25 mg per day may be beneficial.

Depression

Depressive symptoms are common in Alzheimer's disease. However, the vegetative signs typical of major depression such as poor appetite, early morning awakening, reduced energy level, inability to concentrate, restlessness and agitation, and loss of interest in favorite activities can result from impaired cognitive function in the absence of dysphoria. Thus, the diagnosis of major depression in the setting of Alzheimer's disease can be problematic. The presence of dysphoria often clarifies the diagnosis. Alternatively, fluctuating vegetative signs may also suggest concomitant depression. Because of its side effect profile, a selective serotonin reuptake inhibitor is the agent of choice: sertraline (Zoloft) at a starting dose of 12.5 mg per day; paroxetine (Paxil) at a starting dose of 5 mg per day; or fluoxetine (Prozac) at a starting dose of 5 mg per day. These agents can cause sedation, but anticholinergic effects are less common than with the use of second-line agents, such as nortriptyline (Pamelor) at a starting dose of 10 mg per day. Doses should be increased slowly, with careful attention to orthostatic hypotension and cardiac arrhythmia.

Insomnia

Insomnia and alterations of the sleep/wake cycle are common in Alzheimer's disease. If related to depression, they should be treated accordingly. Otherwise, one should first ensure that the patient is awake and active during the day. Day care or other activities that ensure this and relieve the caregiver should be considered. If the patient is awake and active during the day and is still not sleeping at night, low-dose thioridazine (Mellaril), 10 mg or 25 mg each evening, is a good first-line treatment.

Aggression

Aggression, in the form of physical acts such as hitting, biting, and scratching can be a major problem in patients with Alzheimer's disease, leading to physical and/or pharmacologic restraints. Verbally aggressive behavior involving threats or obscenities also occurs. Long-term management with risperidone (Risperdal) is the treatment of choice. Episodes of acute aggression will often pass without medication if the patient is in a safe environment and can be left alone. Otherwise, haloperidol (Haldol), 2 mg once or twice as a loading dose, can be used to avoid an emergency department visit. This should be followed by 0.5 mg per day, or the patient should be switched to risperidone.

INTRACEREBRAL HEMORRHAGE

method of
ADRIAN J. GOLDSZMIDT, M.D.
Sinai Hospital
Baltimore, Maryland

and

LOUIS R. CAPLAN, M.D.
Beth Israel Deaconess Medical Center
Boston, Massachusetts

Intracerebral hemorrhage (ICH) affects nearly 40,000 Americans yearly. ICH accounts for 10 to 15% of strokes in the United States, and these patients have a poorer prognosis than those with ischemic stroke. Mortality from ICH is 35 to 50% at 30 days, and only 10 to 20% of patients resume independent living. Diagnosis and treatment of ICH are important components of neurologic practice.

ETIOLOGY

Half of spontaneous ICH is attributable to arterial hypertension. Hypertensive hemorrhages typically occur in specific areas: the putamen, thalamus, subcortical white matter, cerebellum, and pons. Two mechanisms are responsible: (1) rupture of small penetrating arteries damaged by chronic hypertension and aging and (2) sudden blood pressure increases causing rupture of arterioles unaccustomed to high blood pressure. Congenital or acquired vascular anomalies such as aneurysms and arteriovenous malformations account for 25% of ICH. Cerebral amyloid angiopathy is a leading cause of ICH, particularly in older patients. Amyloid angiopathy is seen in 10% of people at age 70, but in 60% of people older than 90. Bleeding diathesis, tumors, vasculitis, and drugs (especially cocaine and amphetamines) are other frequent causes (Table 1). Aging, African-American heritage, previous strokes, anticoagulation, coronary artery disease, alcohol abuse, and diabetes mellitus increase the risk for ICH.

CLINICAL FEATURES

Neurologic signs and symptoms vary depending on the location and size of the hemorrhage. About 50% of patients have headache, nausea, and vomiting. Most patients present with focal neurologic deficits, with smoothly progressive deterioration over minutes to hours; in 33%, the deficit is maximal at onset without further progression. Most ICH occurs during routine daily activities. Only 10% of patients note symptoms on awakening, which is less often than occurs in ischemic stroke. In another 10%, ICH is associated with physical or emotional stress.

Depressed level of consciousness may be found in 50% of patients with ICH, and coma is a sign of poor prognosis. Coma occurs in about 20% of patients at presentation. In pontine or thalamic hemorrhage, coma is caused by involvement of the reticular activating system. In lobar hemorrhage, depressed consciousness is due to midline shift from mass effect.

TABLE 1. **Etiologies of Spontaneous Intracerebral Hemorrhage**

Arterial Hypertension

Aneurysms

Saccular
Infective
Traumatic
Neoplastic

Vascular Malformations

Arteriovenous malformations
Capillary telangiectasias
Cavernous angiomas
Venous malformations

Bleeding Diatheses

Leukemia
Thrombocytopenia
Disseminated intravascular coagulation
Polycythemia
Hyperviscosity
Hemophilia
Hypoprothrombinemia
Afibrinogenemia
Clotting factor deficiencies
von Willebrand's disease
Sickle cell anemia
Anticoagulant therapy
Thrombolytic therapy

Cerebral Amyloid Angiopathy

Arteritis / Arteriopathies

Infective vasculitis
Multisystem vasculitis
Isolated central nervous system angiitis
Moyamoya disease

Drug Related

Amphetamines
Cocaine
Phenylpropanolamine
Pentazocine (Talwin)-pyribenzamine
Phencyclidine
Heroin
Monoamine oxidase inhibitor

Intracranial Tumors

Primary malignant or benign
Metastatic

Cerebral Venous Occlusion

Miscellaneous

After carotid endarterectomy
After neurosurgical procedures
After spinal anesthesia
Postmyelography
Cold related
Lightning stroke
Heat stroke
Fat embolism
After painful dental procedures
Protracted migraine
Methanol intoxication

Adapted from Biller J, Shah MV: Intracerebral hemorrhage. *In* Rakel RE (ed): Conn's Current Therapy 1997. Philadelphia, WB Saunders Co, 1997, p 877.

Seizures occur in less than 10% of ICH, but are much more common with lobar hemorrhage, approaching 25% of patients. Overall, seizures are much more likely with supratentorial hemorrhages. Patients who do not have seizures at onset are unlikely to develop seizures.

COMMON SYNDROMES

The most common site for ICH is the putamen, accounting for 33% of all hemorrhages. Typical signs include contralateral hemiplegia with sensory impairment, hemianopia, contralateral gaze paresis, and aphasia (dominant hemisphere) or neglect (nondominant hemisphere). Enlarging putaminal hemorrhages can spread medially into the internal capsule, caudate nucleus, and lateral ventricle, or laterally into the insula.

Lobar hemorrhages are usually due to hypertension or amyloid angiopathy. They occur in the subcortical white matter, and the clinical syndromes resemble those seen with ischemic infarction in the involved territory. Seizures are common.

Thalamic hemorrhages account for 20% of ICH. Posterolateral thalamic hemorrhages are most common, and patients present with sensory deficits and mild hemiparesis. Small hemorrhages in the anterior thalamus can disrupt frontal lobe connections, resulting in abulia, with impaired memory, hemiparesis, and minimal sensory loss. Vertical gaze palsy is due to pressure on the adjacent midbrain tectum. Aphasia may be seen in dominant hemisphere thalamic ICH, whereas nondominant lesions produce neglect. Medial thalamic ICH produces a markedly depressed level of consciousness, with subsequent abulia and difficulty making new memories.

Cerebellar hemorrhage occurs in 8% of patients. The hemorrhages are usually in the dentate nucleus. Vermian hemorrhages are less frequent. Compression or extension into the fourth ventricle is common. Patients may be drowsy, with nuchal rigidity and headache. Ipsilateral ataxia and hypotonia are present, but hemiparesis and hemisensory loss are absent. Conjugate gaze palsy or sixth nerve palsy and ipsilateral facial weakness may be seen. Pupils tend to be small and reactive. Rapid clinical deterioration from brain stem compression may occur. Death may result from medullary compression by cerebellar tonsillar herniation. Mortality is higher for patients who are comatose at presentation; however, decreased responsiveness may be due to hydrocephalus and can be reversed with prompt ventricular drainage.

Pontine hemorrhages are nearly as common as cerebellar hemorrhages, usually at the junction of the basis pontis and tegmentum. This area receives blood from paramedian pontine perforating vessels from the basilar artery. The hematoma can extend rostrally into the midbrain or rupture into the fourth ventricle. Findings include quadriplegia, pinpoint pupils, horizontal gaze palsies, and coma. Weakness may initially be asymmetrical before progressing to quadriplegia. Respiratory abnormalities, including Cheyne-Stokes respirations, are common. Lateral pontine tegmental hemorrhages, which occur in areas supplied by penetrators from short circumferential branches of the basilar artery, produce crossed hemisensory loss, ataxia, and oculomotor deficits, as well as ipsilateral cranial nerve signs. The pupils may be asymmetrical, with ipsilateral meiosis.

Caudate hemorrhages account for 4% of ICH. These can rupture into the ventricle, and dissect laterally into the internal capsule and putamen or inferiorly into the diencephalon. With intraventricular spread, there is headache, vomiting, and mental status changes with few motor or sensory signs. Hemorrhages that dissect posterolaterally may be difficult to distinguish from primary putaminal hemorrhages. Those that dissect posteroinferiorly cause a Horner's syndrome from hypothalamic involvement and vertical gaze paresis from thalamic involvement.

DIAGNOSIS

Thorough history taking and examination are important to diagnosis. History of hypertension, drug and alcohol ingestion, systemic diseases, and coagulopathies should be sought. Unenhanced computed tomography (CT) scanning remains the safest, most sensitive method available to identify and localize ICH (Table 2). CT findings of subarachnoid or intraventricular hemorrhage, abnormal intracranial calcification, and prominent vascular structures should prompt further evaluation for an underlying structural abnormality. Younger patients, especially those without hypertension, should also be further studied. Magnetic resonance imaging is an important tool for identifying vascular malformations and tumors and may be better than cerebral angiography in detecting cavernous angiomas. Angiography may reveal an aneurysm, moyamoya disease, vasculitis, or arteriovenous malformation.

MEDICAL TREATMENT

Despite the morbidity associated with ICH, there are no good studies documenting widespread efficacy for medical or surgical treatment modalities; therefore, there is tremendous variability in treatment. All patients should be admitted to the hospital, ideally to an intensive care or stroke unit, where blood pressure monitoring and frequent neurologic assessment can occur. Immediate assessment of ventilation is important, with intubation for obtunded patients who are at increased risk for aspiration.

Coagulation defects should be corrected. For patients receiving warfarin, subcutaneous vitamin K (10 mg) and fresh-frozen plasma, 20 mL per kg,

should be administered. For patients receiving heparin, protamine (1 mg intravenously for each 100 units of heparin infused in the previous 2 hours, but no more than 50 mg per 10 minutes) should be infused. Patients with hemophilia require therapy with factor VIII to achieve a level of 80 to 100% of normal; immediate neurosurgical evaluation may also be needed. Patients with thrombocytopenia require platelet transfusion. Thrombolytic-associated bleeding necessitates administration of 10 units of intravenous cryoprecipitate. Fresh-frozen plasma, 20 mL per kg, may also be needed. Aminocaproic acid (Amicar), 5 grams over 30 to 60 minutes followed by 1 gram per hour intravenously, may be used for continued bleeding.

Blood pressure management is crucial. Maintaining adequate blood pressure prevents ongoing or recurrent bleeding while preserving cerebral perfusion. Patients with systolic pressures greater than 180 mm Hg or mean arterial pressure (MAP) greater than 130 mm Hg should be treated. The goal is to maintain cerebral perfusion pressure at 70 to 100 mm Hg, which can be achieved with a MAP of 100 to 130 mm Hg. Antihypertensive agents should have rapid effects, be easily adjustable, and not have adverse effects on cerebral blood flow or intracranial pressure. For moderate blood pressure elevations, intravenous labetalol (Normodyne), 10 to 20 mg intravenously, may be used, with repeated doses given until an effect is achieved. For severe blood pressure elevations, nitroprusside 0.2 µg per kg per minute, titrated up or down every 5 to 10 minutes by similar increments, is recommended.

Patients with neurologic deterioration, signs of herniation, or respiratory depression should be intubated. Some patients may require intracranial pressure monitoring for optimal management. Hyperventilation (lowering the Pco_2 to 25 to 30 mm Hg) is the fastest way to decrease intracranial pressure. Hyperosmolar therapy is with mannitol, 1 gram per kg over 20 to 30 minutes, followed by 0.25 to 0.5 gram per kg every 4 to 6 hours. Serum osmolality should be monitored. Head elevation (15 to 30 degrees) promotes venous drainage. Hypo-osmolar solutions increase edema and should be avoided. Corticosteroids are associated with increased complications without clear benefit and are not recommended.

Prophylactic anticonvulsants should be considered for cases of lobar hemorrhage. Phenytoin (Dilantin), 18 mg per kg intravenously at a maximum of 50 mg per minute, or fosphenytoin (Cerebyx), 18 mg per kg phenytoin equivalents at a maximum of 150 mg per minute, may be given. Patients with ICH are also at risk for deep venous thrombosis, and pneumatic compression stockings are recommended. Frequent turning and variable pressure mattresses reduce the risk of decubitus ulcers.

TABLE 2. **Laboratory and Radiologic Evaluation in Intracerebral Hemorrhage**

All Patients
1. Complete blood count with platelet count
2. Prothrombin time, international normalized ratio, partial thromboplastin time
3. Erythrocyte sedimentation rate
4. Blood glucose
5. Serum alkaline phosphatase, glutamic oxaloacetic transaminase, calcium, blood urea nitrogen, creatinine
6. Urinalysis
7. Chest roentgenogram
8. Electrocardiogram
9. Unenhanced cranial computed tomography (CT)

Selected Patients
1. Blood cultures
2. Drug screen
3. Antinuclear antibodies assay
4. Sickle cell screen
5. Hemoglobin electrophoresis
6. Serum fibrinogen, fibrin split products, serum viscosity
7. Thrombin time, reptilase time, bleeding time
8. Type and screen
9. Human immunodeficiency virus antibody
10. Contrast-enhanced cranial CT
11. Magnetic resonance brain imaging
12. Cerebral angiography

Adapted from Biller J, Shah MV: Intracerebral hemorrhage. *In* Rakel RE (ed): Conn's Current Therapy 1997. Philadelphia, WB Saunders Co, 1997, p 879.

SURGICAL TREATMENT

Indications for surgical treatment of ICH remain controversial, without data to support clear indications for surgery. Patients with massive hemorrhage who are in a coma are not likely to benefit. Patients with putaminal hemorrhages that rupture into the ventricle also do poorly regardless of treatment modality; for deteriorating patients with moderate ICH, without ventricular spread, surgery should be considered. Young patients with lobar hemorrhage who deteriorate during observation should also be considered for surgery. Patients with thalamic hemorrhage rarely need surgery, except ventricular drainage for hydrocephalus. Patients with small ICHs who are fully conscious do best with medical therapy.

Patients with cerebellar hemorrhage greater than 3 cm in diameter, or those with smaller hemorrhages and deterioration, should be treated surgically. Brain stem compression and ventricular obstruction may be rapidly fatal, but completely reversible with early surgery.

Research is under way to evaluate whether early surgical intervention or newer, less invasive modalities such as stereoscopic or endoscopic surgery may be beneficial in some cases. Stereotactic irrigation with thrombolytic agents is also being investigated.

ISCHEMIC CEREBROVASCULAR DISEASE

method of
PATRICK D. LYDEN, M.D.
University of California, San Diego,
Stroke Center
San Diego, California

About 730,000 strokes occur per year, of which about 85% will be ischemic. Stroke is the leading cause of adult disability in America and the third leading cause of death. Stroke takes a toll on the victim as well as on the family and caretakers. The most common risk factors for stroke include hypertension, smoking, age, diabetes, history of prior stroke, history of cardiac conditions (especially atrial fibrillation), and lipid disorders. Reduction of these risk factors is associated with a reduced incidence of stroke. Alcohol is associated with risk of hemorrhage in a dose-dependent manner; the risk of alcohol for ischemic stroke remains to be determined.

STROKE PREVENTION

Patients may seek medical attention before they have any warning symptoms. Significant carotid stenosis in this setting is defined as greater than 60% narrowing. Carotid ultrasonography may be ordered after a contralateral stroke, because a physician heard a bruit, or before major peripheral surgery. Thus, although the patient has had no premonitory symptoms, the physician is faced with a decision regarding further management: does carotid endarterectomy prevent stroke in the asymptomatic patient? There have been several large trials of carotid endarterectomy for asymptomatic carotid stenosis

with controversial findings. At the moment the consensus seems to be that for very carefully selected patients the procedure is more effective than medical prevention therapy alone. Selected patients must be free of cardiac disease, which means that in most cases there will be a considerable preoperative evaluation.

Patients with atrial fibrillation benefit from antithrombotic therapy. Warfarin (Coumadin) is preferred, although aspirin is effective. The consensus recommendation is that the international normalized ratio be kept between 2.0 and 3.0 in most patients with atrial fibrillation. Patients with no other risk factors (e.g., hypertension, congestive heart failure, atrial enlargement) may be managed on 325 or 650 mg of aspirin per day. Patients younger than 55 years old with no other comorbidities (e.g., lone atrial fibrillation) may be managed without an antithrombotic treatment.

Patients must be considered for surgery after a transient ischemic attack or minor completed stroke. Large studies have proven that if the carotid stenosis is greater than 70%, as measured by a residual lumen method from an angiogram, then aspirin plus surgery is more effective than medical therapy alone. For patients with lesser degrees of stenosis there is still some benefit to surgery, although the results are not as dramatic. As in the situation of asymptomatic disease, the patient must be evaluated for cardiac risks before carotid surgery. Whether angiography can be replaced by high-resolution carotid duplex ultrasound or by magnetic resonance angiography is determined in individual medical centers.

There are new antiplatelet agents that may be more effective, or cause fewer side effects, than aspirin. Ticlopidine (Ticlid), 250 mg orally twice daily, is a reasonable alternative. Similarly, clopidogrel (Plavix), 75 mg per day orally, is effective. These drugs should not be used as first-line therapy unless the patient is known to be intolerant of aspirin. The cholesterol-lowering agents may reduce the incidence of stroke in patients with normal cholesterol who have suffered a myocardial infarction.

ACUTE TREATMENT

Thrombolysis

The most important development in the care of stroke patients has been the advent of thrombolytic therapy. Several preliminary studies were done by the National Institute of Neurologic Disorders and Stroke (NINDS) with t-PA (alteplase [Activase]) to determine that a dose of 0.9 mg of t-PA per kg was safe if given within 3 hours of the onset of stroke. Then two large-scale confirmatory studies were conducted. The European Cooperative Acute Stroke Study (ECASS) tested 1.1 mg of t-PA per kg intravenously within 6 hours of stroke onset versus placebo. There was no benefit seen in favor of treatment when data from all patients were included in the analysis. However, when a target population was analyzed separately, after excluding patients in whom there had been violations of the study protocol, there was a clear and persuasive benefit attributable to t-PA therapy. Unfortunately, in the excluded patients there were several brain hemorrhages. Thus, it was concluded from ECASS that although t-PA may be safe and effective if given within 6 hours of stroke onset, it could not be given to patients who had early computed tomographic findings of edema. These conclusions had to be validated in a further trial. The ECASS II study was completed in 1998; patients with early, subtle CT findings of ischemia were excluded, as well as patients with "severe" strokes. In this study, although the t-PA patients benefited, the results were not statistically significant because the favorable response rate was very high in both placebo and t-PA–treated groups.

In December 1995, the NINDS Stroke Trial investigators published another study of thrombolysis for stroke: patients received 0.9 mg of t-PA per kg within 3 hours of stroke symptoms beginning. Unlike ECASS, in the NINDS trial there was scrupulous attention to blood pressure management: patients were not enrolled if their blood pressure remained elevated above 185/110 mm Hg after gentle antihypertensive treatment. Similarly, after randomization and treatment, patients received sufficient blood pressure management to maintain their blood pressure below 185/90 mm Hg. In the intention-to-treat analysis there was a clear and persuasive benefit attributable to t-PA treatment on four different stroke scales, even though there were more hemorrhages in the t-PA–treated patients. Subsequent analysis of the NINDS data revealed that all subgroups of patients responded to t-PA, including patients with different subtypes of stroke, patients with a range of stroke severity, and patients of all ages. Several follow-up papers have elucidated important points: the benefits from t-PA may be detected up to 1 year after stroke; t-PA is highly cost effective; it may be given to a patient with even the most severe stroke because, although the overall prognosis is poor, results are still better with t-PA treatment. In parallel to the t-PA studies, there were three trials of streptokinase for acute stroke that were all terminated because of excessive bleeding and deaths. At this time streptokinase is not acceptable for intravenous thrombolysis of acute stroke patients.

Putting together all of the results of the thrombolytic stroke trials, it is now clear that t-PA is safe and effective for stroke patients if the NINDS protocol is followed to the letter. The inclusion and exclusion criteria, summarized in Table 1, should be consulted before treating a patient. A dose of 0.9 mg/kg is used, giving 10% as a bolus; the remainder is infused in over 60 minutes. Initially, brain computed tomography must be done to rule out hemorrhage. Early, subtle signs of ischemia that subsume less than one third of the territory of the middle cerebral artery indicate patients who are the most likely to benefit from t-PA. Patients with more severe findings on CT should be carefully considered. The treating physi-

TABLE 1. t-PA for Acute Stroke

Patient Selection

- Patients must be treated within 3 hours of acute ischemic stroke symptom onset
- Obtain baseline computed tomography to rule out intracranial hemorrhage, subarachnoid hemorrhage
- Consider risk/benefit: in patients with major early infarct signs on computed tomography (e.g., substantial edema, mass effect, or midline shift)
- Consider risk/benefit: in patients with severe neurologic deficit (e.g., NIH Stroke Scale > 22) at presentation. An increased risk of intracranial hemorrhage may exist.

Contraindications

- More than 3 hours from acute ischemic stroke symptom onset
- Rapidly improving minor or major stroke (i.e., transient ischemic attack)
- Intracranial hemorrhage on computed tomography or by history
- Suspicion of subarachnoid hemorrhage despite negative head computed tomography
- Recent intracranial surgery or serious head trauma or recent previous stroke (in past 3 months)
- Uncontrolled hypertension at time of treatment (e.g., > 185 mm Hg systolic or > 105 mm Hg diastolic)
- Seizure at the onset of stroke
- Active internal bleeding (e.g., gastrointestinal, urinary) within 21 days
- Intracranial neoplasm, arteriovenous malformation, aneurysm
- Glucose < 50 or > 400 mg/dL
- Lumbar puncture within 7 days, major surgery within 14 days
- Arterial puncture at noncompressible site
- Acute myocardial infarction or post–myocardial infarction pericarditis
- Known bleeding diathesis, including but not limited to:

  Current use of oral anticoagulants (e.g., warafin sodium) with prothrombin time > 15 seconds
  Administration of heparin within 48 hours preceding the onset of stroke and have an elevated activated partial thromboplastin time at presentation
  Platelet count < 100,000/mm³

Adapted from the NINDS t-PA Stroke Trial Protocol and the Activase Package Insert, Genentech, South San Francisco.

cian must know the precise time of stroke onset to be less than 3 hours before initiation of t-PA treatment. If the patient awoke with symptoms, then the onset time is when the patient went to bed or was last known to be deficit free. Initial blood work must be sent for prothrombin time, partial thromboplastin time, glucose, and platelet count. The glucose must be known before treatment, but the other studies are not needed unless the patient is taking warfarin or heparin. If an unexpected, abnormal value returns during the t-PA infusion, the drug is terminated. After thrombolysis, patients must be observed carefully for signs and symptoms of bleeding. Blood pressure should be checked frequently, meaning most such patients will be admitted to a direct observation unit for 24 hours (Table 2). Invasive procedures should be limited during this period. Any change in neurologic status should prompt repeat computed tomography of the brain to check for hemorrhage. Heparin, warfarin, and antiplatelet agents should be held for 24 hours after t-PA.

TABLE 2. **Blood Pressure Control Guidelines When Using rt-PA for Stroke**

Monitor blood pressure every 15 minutes before treatment, every 15 minutes for 2 hours after treatment, then every 30 minutes for 6 hours, then every hour up to 24 hours after treatment.

One to two doses of IV labetalol 10 to 20 mg over 1 hour and/or nitroglycerin paste may be given before thrombolysis.

If these measures do not bring blood pressure down to < 185/110 mm Hg and keep it down, the patient should not be treated with rt-PA.

After thrombolysis, keep blood pressure below 185/110 mm Hg using labetolol or nipride as necessary.

Adapted from the NINDS t-PA Stroke Study Group Protocol Guidelines

General Care

Despite the lack of controlled clinical trials, there are a number of symptomatic therapies that may benefit stroke patients. All stroke victims are dehydrated and should be started on normal saline. The rate and the total volume of infusion are tailored to each specific patient, after considering the probable volume loss, age, history of congestive heart failure, and renal status. Assuming the patient is not actively suffering congestive heart failure, 250 mL of normal saline is generally administered over the first hour, followed by 125 mL per hour. Other electrolytes, such as potassium, calcium, or magnesium, are added as dictated by the initial chemistries. Next I ensure that the patient is as close to normoglycemic as feasible. If the initial blood sugar (laboratory or finger stick) is greater than 160 mg per dL, I administer regular insulin; the dose is based on the patient's prior history and use of insulin. If the initial blood sugar value is less than 60 mg per dL, I administer 50% dextrose. It is important to keep the blood sugar between these limits throughout the first few days after stroke to avoid exacerbating cerebral ischemic lactic acidosis associated with hyperglycemia, or worsening of cellular energy failure associated with hypoglycemia. Finally, there is a negative effect of hyperthermia on experimental stroke subjects; I prescribe 650 mg of acetaminophen administered orally or per rectum every 4 hours for any temperatures over 38°C.

There is no consensus regarding the appropriate management of blood pressure after stroke. Acutely lowering blood pressure after ischemic stroke may augment the ischemia and worsen outcome. On the other hand, during hypertension there is reactive vasoconstriction, which may worsen ischemia. Hypertensive crisis may manifest as focal findings and altered sensorium, requiring urgent lowering of blood pressure; and current protocols require normal blood pressure in the stroke patient before administering thrombolytic treatment for acute ischemia. Considerable further research is needed in this area, and only limited guidelines can be formulated at present. I try to maintain the blood pressure below 185/95 mm Hg in most ischemic stroke patients, unless there is evidence that the patient routinely endures very high blood pressures.

Edema begins immediately after cerebral ischemia but does not reach a maximum until 2 to 4 days after onset. Intracranial pressure does not begin to rise, or adversely affect the patient, until edema increases the intracranial volume beyond the brain's compensation mechanisms: elderly patients with cerebral atrophy tolerate greater amounts of edema than younger patients. Rarely do massive strokes cause such an increase in intracranial volume within the first few hours of onset. During the first 12 to 24 hours after stroke, therefore, physicians at my institution generally do not administer antiedema therapy, other than to raise the head of the patient to 30 degrees. Although unproven to be effective, stroke edema may be treated with intravenous mannitol, 1 gram per kg bolus followed by 0.25 gram per kg every 1 or 2 hours until the edema resolves. No convincing data exist to support the use of corticosteroids early in the course of ischemic stroke.

It is important to prevent complications of stroke, including pneumonia, deep venous thrombosis, and stasis skin ulcers. At my institution, physicians try to mobilize stroke patients very early and generally begin physical and occupational therapy in the first 48 hours. We prefer heparin, 5000 units subcutaneously twice daily, for deep venous thrombosis prophylaxis, along with 325 mg of aspirin orally or rectally daily. Oral feeding should be held until a swallow study or other maneuver verifies airway protection.

Some physicians continue to recommend anticoagulation for acute completed stroke. Intravenous heparin has no benefit after acute stroke and is perhaps harmful, except in certain specific conditions, notably ventricular thrombus after transmural myocardial infarction, progressing basilar occlusion, and possibly atrial fibrillation. A very large, multicenter, adequately powered trial has been conducted of heparin and aspirin for stroke therapy (International Stroke Trial [IST]): in the high-dose treatment group, patients received 12,500 units of heparin subcutaneously twice per day. There was a trend toward harm in the group of patients who received heparin. However, this effect was not demonstrable in the low-dose group, that is, those who received 5,000 units of heparin subcutaneously twice daily. In fact, subgroup analysis showed that patients who received a low dose of heparin and 325 mg of oral aspirin daily appeared to do the best of all subgroups, but they were not statistically significantly better than the placebo-treated group. Low-molecular-weight heparin or heparinoids also have not proven to be effective in very large, well-designed, placebo-controlled, multicentered studies. Furthermore, the rate of recurrent stroke was the same in placebo and actively treated patients and was much lower than previously believed in these large studies. Therefore, the rationale for anticoagulant therapy, either as treatment or to prevent recurrence, is not supported by the evidence.

DIAGNOSTIC TESTING

The purpose of diagnostic testing after stroke is to find ways to reduce the risk of recurrent stroke. Testing includes, at a minimum, brain computed tomography and vascular imaging. I prefer to obtain an ultrasonogram of the carotid arteries within 12 hours of admission to look for treatable stenosis. If operable disease is found, and confirmed, surgery is planned but delayed until the patient has recovered from the stroke and undergone a reasonable cardiac work-up. The use of cerebral angiography and magnetic resonance imaging in the routine stroke patient is controversial: the desire for greater diagnostic accuracy must be balanced against the probability of finding something that will change the planned therapy or outcome. Newer imaging technology, such as diffusion weighted magnetic resonance imaging, single-photon emission computed tomography, and spiral computed tomographic angiography, has yet to prove beneficial in terms of improving patient outcome, but such studies are ongoing. If clinical findings dictate, detailed evaluation of the clotting system may be undertaken, but this should not be done routinely.

REHABILITATION OF THE STROKE SURVIVOR

method of
RICHARD D. ZOROWITZ, M.D.
University of Pennsylvania
Philadelphia, Pennsylvania

Stroke remains one of the most serious neurologic problems in the United States today. It is the leading cause of serious, long-term disability in the United States and is also the leading cause for admission to nursing homes or extended-care facilities. Approximately 4.0 million stroke survivors live in this country. Of patients who survive a stroke past 30 days, 50% are still alive after 7 years, and 33% live 12 years or more. The estimated cost of stroke totals $43.3 billion per year, of which $15.0 billion is lost in productivity due to mortality and morbidity.

Comprehensive rehabilitation may improve the functional abilities of the stroke survivor, despite age and neurologic deficit, and decrease long-term patient care costs. Although motor recovery occurs in predictable patterns (Table 1) and may plateau 3 to 6 months after stroke, functional recovery may continue for up to several years. Approximately 80% of stroke survivors may benefit from

TABLE 1. Synergy Patterns of Motor Recovery

Extremity	Pattern	Components
Upper	Flexor	Shoulder flexion, adduction, internal rotation; elbow flexion; wrist flexion; finger flexion
	Extensor	Shoulder, elbow, wrist, finger extension
Lower	Flexor	Hip flexion, adduction; knee flexion; ankle dorsiflexion
	Extensor	Hip, knee extension; ankle plantar flexion

TABLE 2. Techniques of Stroke Rehabilitation

Author/Type	Theory
Conventional	Range of motion/strengthening Compensatory strategies Mobility/activity of daily living training
Bobath (NDT)	Suppress synergistic movement Facilitate normal movement
Knott, Voss (PNF)	Suppress normal movement Facilitate defined mass movement
Brunnstrom	Facilitate synergistic movement
Rood	Modify movement with cutaneous sensory stimulation
Biofeedback	Modifies function using volitional control and auditory, visual, sensory cues
Forced-use paradigm	Immobilization of unaffected extremity forcing use of affected extremity
Electrical stimulation	Random or coordinated contraction of muscles

Abbreviations: NDT = neurodevelopmental therapy; PNF = proprioceptive neuromuscular facilitation.

rehabilitation in acute, subacute, skilled nursing, day hospital, outpatient, or home care environment. Ten percent of patients achieve complete spontaneous recovery within 8 to 12 weeks, and 10% of patients receive no benefit from any treatment. The functional outcome of appropriate stroke survivors appears to be better after admission to acute stroke rehabilitation units rather than subacute or nursing home units. Yet, third-party payers increasingly are sending stroke survivors to less intensive and less costly rehabilitation programs.

Stroke rehabilitation involves a transdisciplinary, holistic approach that addresses medical, functional, and psychosocial issues. The team may include a physiatrist (physician specializing in rehabilitation), rehabilitation nurse, physical therapist, occupational therapist, speech-language pathologist, social worker, psychologist, vocational counselor, family, and the patient. Therapy uses components of conventional methods and neurophysiologic theories (Table 2). The team meets periodically to evaluate the stroke survivor, to document functional gains, and to set short- and long-term goals. The stroke survivor often meets with the team to review functional progress, to confirm discharge plans, and to discuss any problems. The family participates in therapy sessions in preparation to oversee patient care at home.

Researchers are gaining a better understanding of the physiologic basis of functional recovery. Functional imaging (e.g., functional magnetic resonance imaging, single photon emission computed tomography, positron emission tomography) is demonstrating that neurons not usually utilized during normal movement (i.e., areas surrounding infarcts, in ipsilateral homologous sites, and in supplementary motor areas) are activated when rehabilitation strategies are applied in the stroke survivor. Medications such as dextroamphetamine, methylphenidate (Ritalin), and bromocriptine (Parlodel) appear to modify noradrenergic or dopaminergic systems, thus facilitating motor recovery and initiation or quality of movement or speech. Acupuncture also is emerging as a potential means to improve and maintain motor recovery and quality of life.

MOBILITY AND LOCOMOTION

Probably the most important priority of the stroke survivor is ambulation. Prerequisites for ambulation include the ability to follow commands; adequate trunk control for sitting and standing; minimal or no contractures of the hip flexor, knee flexor, and ankle plantar flexor muscles; and adequate muscle strength required to stabilize the hip and knee joints. The hip extensor muscles are the most important muscles used in ambulation because they provide stability to the hip and knee.

Gait training begins by teaching transfers to the bed, mat, and wheelchair. The patient must be able to bear weight consistently on the affected extremity. Standing balance must be maximized using visual, proprioceptive, or labyrinthine cues. The patient is taught the most optimal gait pattern in and out of the parallel bars and on stairs, ramps, and curbs. Orthoses (i.e., braces) and assistive devices are used to correct gait deviations and may decrease energy expenditure during gait. No energy differential exists between the use of plastic or metal orthoses. Harnesses to provide partial body weight support may assist in promoting motor recovery and increasing velocity of gait.

Falls during transfers or ambulation can be a disincentive to attaining mobility goals or can produce frank injury, such as hip fracture. Falls are most common in stroke survivors with right-hemisphere lesions that result in left-sided neglect, anosognosia, and impulsivity. Other factors such as use of psychotropic drugs, severity of disability as reflected by urinary incontinence, or decline in mental status have been associated with falls. Stroke survivors who are more likely to fall also may be more depressed, less socially active, and have more stressed caregivers.

Stroke survivors who have limited or no ability to ambulate may require wheelchairs for mobility. The seat should be narrow enough to allow operation of the hand rim with the unaffected arm and low enough to allow propulsion with the unaffected leg. Arm rests should be designed to permit seating at tables. Arm and leg rests should be removable to make transfers easier. Lightweight or electric chairs may be issued to patients with cardiac or other severely debilitating conditions.

ACTIVITIES OF DAILY LIVING

Stroke survivors usually do not place the same degree of importance on activities of daily living (ADLs) as they place on ambulation. Yet, in many cases, teaching ADLs may be more difficult than teaching ambulation because the affected upper limb is less functional than the affected lower limb. Performance of ADLs requires visual, cognitive, perceptual, and coordination skills in addition to range of motion, motor strength, and sensation. Occasionally, tendon lengthening or transfer procedures may improve functional status by correcting muscle imbalance, spasticity, or instability. Apraxia, poor memory skills, left-sided neglect, or loss of sensory function may render the affected arm useless. Poor prognostic factors for upper extremity function include onset of

upper extremity movement greater than 2 to 4 weeks, absence of voluntary hand movement greater than 4 to 6 weeks, prolonged flaccid period, and severe proximal spasticity.

Patients can be taught one-handed techniques to perform feeding, grooming, dressing, bathing, and writing with the nondominant unaffected limb. The affected limb can be trained as a stabilizer or gross assist. The unaffected arm can be immobilized, thus forcing the affected arm to be more active in function activity. Adaptive equipment augments the abilities of the hemiplegic patient in feeding, bathing, dressing, and grooming. Velcro closures and straps may allow easier donning and doffing of clothing, splints, and slings. Occupational therapists may fabricate devices customized to the needs of the patient and are limited only by their imaginations and technical skills.

Driving may be an important goal for some stroke survivors. Occupational therapists administer predriving evaluations that test basic cognitive skills needed for driving: memory, spatial organization, attention, concentration, and reaction times. Driving skills are tested in simulators or behind-the-wheel with licensed instructors. Adaptive aids, such as spinner knobs and accelerator extenders, may be incorporated to compensate for motor deficits. Three fourths of stroke survivors with left-hemisphere lesions are able to pass a driving test, but 50% of stroke survivors with right-hemisphere lesions fail driving tests because of cognitive and perceptual deficits.

Approximately one third of stroke survivors younger than age 65 are able to return to work. To return to work, patients with left-hemisphere strokes must demonstrate adequate verbal, cognitive, and language deficits, whereas patients with right-hemisphere strokes must have adequate ambulation skills, use of left upper extremity, and abstract reasoning skills. Vocational assessments may include neuropsychologic and driving evaluations, functional capacity evaluations, work hardening, and on-site evaluations.

SPEECH-LANGUAGE DISORDERS

Speech and language disorders may be diagnosed by both formal testing and conversational interaction. Impaired content of speech suggests an aphasia or cognitive-communication impairment. Aphasias are characterized by decreased word finding or syntax, word substitutions, and errors in understanding conversational questions or statements. They are classified as nonfluent (Broca's, transcortical motor), characterized by slow, telegraphic style of delivery; fluent (Wernicke's, conduction, anomic, transcortical sensory), characterized by rapid style with paraphasias or neologisms; and global, which involve all modes of speech and may be fluent or nonfluent.

Cognitive-communication impairments usually are associated with right-hemisphere dysfunction. They are characterized by decreased concentration, attention, memory, and orientation; confusion; confabulation; concrete or irrelevant thinking; or vague language. Associated functional problems may include unilateral neglect, constructional and dressing apraxias, anosognosia, and impairments in safety awareness and judgment.

Impaired acoustic features of speech may indicate apraxias or dysarthrias. Apraxias are characterized by inconsistent errors either in programming the positioning of the speech musculature (oral) or in sequencing muscle movements for articulation of volitional speech (verbal). Dysarthric stroke survivors present with consistent errors in articulation, decreased normal resonance or phonation, or problems with volume or breath control.

Therapy generally focuses on teaching compensatory strategies and self-correction of errors. Exercises of the oral, lingual, buccal, and laryngeal musculature may increase physiologic support for speech. Facilitation techniques are thought to recruit right-hemisphere areas that enhance verbal output. Alternative communication techniques and augmentative communication devices may be used as long as apraxia and comprehension deficits do not interfere with their use. Family education is essential to increase the awareness of the deficits and discuss prognosis. Patients with global aphasias usually have a poor prognosis, whereas those with conduction aphasias and anomias often have a complete recovery. The prognosis of apraxic stroke survivors is improved when oral apraxias and aphasias are absent. Persistent cognitive-communication problems may cause an otherwise independent patient to require 24-hour supervision.

COMMON MEDICAL COMPLICATIONS

Every stroke survivor admitted to the rehabilitation unit must be considered for secondary prophylaxis of stroke. Aspirin remains the standard treatment for completed thrombotic or lacunar strokes. Warfarin (Coumadin) is the appropriate treatment after embolic strokes or when significant intracranial stenosis or hypercoagulable states are identified. Ticlopidine (Ticlid) or clopidogrel (Plavix) may be chosen for recurrent strokes in patients on aspirin therapy or when warfarin therapy is contraindicated. Dipyridamole (Persantine)* is being reconsidered as a possible prophylactic treatment. Cholesterol-lowering agents also have been demonstrated to have direct stroke prophylactic properties. Folate is used as adjunctive therapy in strokes due to homocysteinemia. Secondary prophylaxis of hemorrhagic stroke includes control of etiologic factors, such as hypertension or hypocoagulable states.

Deep venous thrombosis (DVT) may occur in 30 to 60% of stroke survivors. Clinical signs and symptoms, such as pain, swelling, and warmth of the extremity, are at best marginally diagnostic. Clinical suspicion should be raised in the nonambulatory

hemiplegic stroke survivor. Noninvasive testing, such as duplex ultrasonography and impedance plethysmography, is a routine part of diagnosis. Stroke survivors at risk for DVT should be given compression stockings, pneumatic compression, and/or subcutaneous heparin, 5000 units every 8 to 12 hours. Prophylaxis may be discontinued once the stroke survivor is ambulating consistently in or out of the parallel bars. Treatment of DVT includes anticoagulation for 3 months or insertion of an inferior vena cava filter.

Proper positioning of the stroke survivor will prevent multiple complications. Positioning in the bed and wheelchair can prevent both flexion contractures and traction neuropathy. Dependent patients should be turned every 2 hours in bed. Wheelchair seats should be provided with appropriate cushions to decrease the incidence of pressure sores. Affected extremities can be elevated with pillows, footrests, and elevated arm rests to prevent edema. Retrograde massage or placement of an Isotoner glove may prevent or reduce edema of the affected hand.

Strokes may disinhibit the reflex mechanisms for emptying the bowels, and sensation or cognitive impairments may prevent control of defecation. Diets should include adequate fluids and fiber. Patients should be toileted after meals to take advantage of the gastrocolic reflex. Stool softeners and bowel stimulants may be prescribed as necessary. Patients who remain incontinent may require a suppository or enema every 1 to 2 days to prevent incontinence at socially inappropriate times. Persistent bowel incontinence for more than 4 weeks usually is a poor predictive indicator.

A variety of voiding disorders may be observed after stroke. Reversible causes, such as urinary tract infection, fecal impaction, and reduced mobility, should be evaluated and treated. Postvoid residuals should be measured by ultrasonography or catheterization to assess the degree of bladder emptying. Symptoms of urinary incontinence, frequency, and urgency should be noted. Patients with voiding dysfunction should be referred for urodynamic studies to characterize the voiding disorders and to determine appropriate intervention. Toileting every 2 to 4 hours during the day and fluid restriction after dinner may prevent incontinence in a majority of patients. External catheters may decrease the incidence of enuresis. Intermittent or indwelling catheterization may be indicated in patients with areflexic bladders.

Swallowing dysfunction, or dysphagia, may occur in up to one third of patients with cortical or brain stem lesions. Dysphagia should be suspected in patients with impaired cognition, nasal regurgitation, coughing, "gurgly" voice, or impaired cough associated with absence of bilateral gag reflex. After evaluation by a speech-language pathologist, a videofluorographic swallowing study of liquids, purees, and solids can be undertaken to identify swallowing disorders and organize a treatment plan. Changes in diet, head positioning, or other compensatory strategies may be incorporated to prevent aspiration pneumonitis. Stimulation of the anterior faucial arches

---

*Not FDA approved for this indication.

may help to initiate an impaired or absent pharyngeal swallow. Nonoral feedings by gastrostomy or jejunostomy may be necessary if oral caloric intake is not adequate to meet nutritional needs.

Almost three fourths of stroke survivors will experience at least one episode of shoulder pain within the first year after stroke. Shoulder pain most commonly is correlated with limited range of motion, especially external rotation. Other causes of shoulder pain include brachial plexopathy, shoulder trauma, bursitis, tendinitis, adhesive capsulitis, rotator cuff tear, heterotopic ossification, and complex regional pain syndrome. A diagnosis often may be determined from a physical examination alone, but radiographs, electromyography, bone scans, or magnetic resonance imaging may support clinical findings. Pain may be relieved with appropriate use of nonsteroidal anti-inflammatory agents, corticosteroids, tricyclic antidepressants, carbamazepine (Tegretol), gabapentin (Neurontin),* narcotics, electrical nerve stimulation, muscle or nerve blocks, local injections, or sympathectomy. Range of motion exercises, along with proper positioning of the limb using orthoses and supports, have been credited with a decrease in the number of pain complaints.

Another type of poststroke pain is known as the poststroke central pain syndrome, which usually occurs as a result of a lesion in the thalamus. The sensation of "thalamic" pain consists of a burning or other unpleasant sensation when an area on the body is stimulated. The most common treatments available today include antidepressant medications such as tricyclic or serotonin-specific reuptake inhibiting antidepressants, but also include antiseizure medications (e.g., phenytoin [Dilantin],* carbamazepine, gabapentin), mexiletine (Mexitil),* and narcotics. Modalities that may relieve poststroke central pain include transcutaneous electrical nerve stimulators or dorsal column stimulators.

Spasticity is a common complication that occurs as a result of enhanced excitatory synaptic input, reduced inhibitory synaptic input, or changes in intrinsic electrical properties of the neuron. Modalities used to treat spasticity include ice, electrical stimulation of antagonist muscles, and splinting. Dantrolene (Dantrium) reduces spasticity peripherally by reducing the release of calcium from the sarcoplasmic reticulum of muscle cells. Tizanidine (Zanaflex), a central alpha$_2$-receptor agonist, decreases the release of excitatory amino acids in spinal motor neurons. Baclofen does not have a role in cerebral spasticity. Diazepam (Valium) is unsuitable for patients with cerebral spasticity because of its sedating properties. Phenol or botulinum toxin (Botox) blocks can inhibit spasticity in individual or groups of muscles up to 3 to 6 months. Intrathecal baclofen may have a role in certain stroke survivors. If contractures inhibit function or cause significant pain, tendon releases or transfers may re-establish normal joint alignment. When surgery is performed to release contractures,

spasticity management must be initiated postoperatively to prevent recurrence of contractures.

Depression may occur in 25 to 79% of stroke survivors, but fewer than 5% receive psychotherapeutic or medical intervention. Depression may be related to mourning the loss of function or to the alteration of function of catecholamine-containing neurons. Lesion site has not been correlated with the incidence of poststroke depression.

Issues of sexual functioning rarely are addressed with stroke victims. Patients generally are fearful of causing another stroke from sexual activity. Cardiac limitations should be discussed, and medications should be reviewed. Couples should be encouraged to experiment with sexual techniques and positions and to communicate their needs to each other.

CONTINUITY OF CARE

Physiatric care should be provided throughout the continuum of rehabilitation care. Patients should return to their primary practitioners for routine medical care but should be seen by a physiatrist 1 month after discharge and periodically thereafter. Blood pressure and weight should be taken, and medications should be reviewed. Progress of mobility and ADLs should be reviewed and validated by a family member. Psychosocial issues should be discussed. All equipment should be inspected, and the patient should be able to demonstrate his or her home exercise program. A neurologic examination should be performed, including gait with appropriate assistive devices and orthoses. Most importantly, time should be allowed for questions. Good communication between the physiatrist, the patient, and the family will facilitate optimal care and provide the patient with the opportunity to reach his or her maximal functional potential.

SEIZURES AND EPILEPSY IN ADOLESCENTS AND ADULTS

method of
BASSEL ABOU-KHALIL, M.D.
Vanderbilt University Medical Center
Nashville, Tennessee

Seizures are the clinical manifestations, including signs and symptoms, of an abnormal, excessive, usually hypersynchronous electrical discharge of neurons generally originating in the cerebral cortex. Most seizures (except for status epilepticus) are brief events lasting seconds to minutes. Seizure manifestations can vary greatly depending on where the discharge originates, where it spreads in the brain, how fast it spreads, and how far it spreads. They include clouding or loss of consciousness, alteration of behavior, altered sensory perceptions, and involuntary movements.

Epilepsy is a condition characterized by recurrent unprovoked seizures. At least two spontaneous seizures are nec-

---

*Not FDA approved for this indication.

essary to diagnose epilepsy. Recurrent seizures provoked by metabolic derangements (e.g., hyponatremia or hypoglycemia), toxins (e.g., cocaine), or withdrawal from alcohol should not lead to the diagnosis of epilepsy. The diagnosis of seizures and epilepsy should not be the diagnostic end point. Seizures and epilepsy can result from a great variety of genetic or acquired causes. Underlying treatable causes, such as tumors or infections, should always be investigated.

A good history is the most important diagnostic tool in seizures and epilepsy. A description of events has to be obtained not only from the patient but also from a reliable observer, because patients are often not aware of what happens during seizures. The history should include precipitating factors, premonitory symptoms and signs, mode of onset, temporal progression of manifestations, duration, and mode of termination of the events. Past medical history and family history may help in identifying risk factors or etiology. The neurologic examination helps identify possibly related functional abnormalities.

Seizures and epilepsy are common and can start at any age. The overall incidence of epilepsy is 44 new cases per 100,000 person-years. The incidence is high in the neonatal period, decreases during the first three decades of life to become fairly stable between 30 and 60, then rises sharply after age 60 to the highest in life. The chance of developing epilepsy is 1.2% by age 24, 3% by age 74, and 4.4% by age 85. Nearly 10% of people experience at least one seizure.

DIAGNOSTIC ALTERNATIVES

Many paroxysmal events or disorders can mimic seizures and epilepsy. These can be physiologic or psychogenic in origin.

Physiologic

Syncope is common, and it is a common imitator of epilepsy. It affects more than 3% of people older than age 30. Its incidence is highest in the elderly, but it is also common in adolescents and young adults. Syncope is due to a transient global reduction in cerebral blood flow and most commonly results from decreased cardiac output, decreased blood volume, decreased peripheral resistance, or combinations of these problems. A cardiac origin is more common in older individuals. In adolescents and young adults, syncope is most often neurally mediated (commonly known as vasovagal, reflex, or neurocardiogenic syncope). Provocation can be from nociceptive stimuli, strong emotions, or rapid emptying of a distended bladder. Neurocardiogenic syncope is more likely to occur in the upright posture. There is commonly a prodrome of nausea, cold sweat, lightheadedness, and blurring or graying of vision that constitutes the elements of presyncope, and pallor is frequently observed. This prodrome is usually longer than the aura that may precede epileptic seizures. Recovery is much faster with syncope, unless there was significant associated head trauma (particularly in the elderly). Up to 90% of syncope is associated with motor activity (predominantly brief multifocal myoclonus that lasts a few seconds). This is to be distinguished from epileptic tonic-clonic activity, which is longer in duration and synchronous on the two sides. Although syncope with myoclonic activity has been termed "convulsive syncope," the myoclonic activity is not accompanied by a cortical discharge on the electroencephalogram (EEG) and most probably originates in the brain stem. The EEG shows progressive slowing leading to generalized attenuation, with rapid reversal in association

with recovery. Rarely, epileptic seizures can lead to bradycardia and syncope. Also, syncope can rarely precipitate true epileptic seizures.

Other physiologic paroxysmal events include systemic disorders such as *hypoglycemia* or other toxic/metabolic disturbances affecting consciousness or behavior. *Hyperventilation* can produce dizziness, paresthesias (particularly perioral and in fingers), and altered consciousness. Hyperventilation in the clinic can be a simple test to reproduce symptoms.

A number of neurologic disturbances can imitate seizures and epilepsy. *Migraine* can be preceded by positive visual or somatosensory symptoms, vertigo, or confusion; and occasionally headache may be absent (migraine equivalents). However, migraine symptoms tend to have a more gradual onset and a longer duration. *Transient ischemic attacks* are usually characterized by negative symptoms and signs (i.e., loss of function, such as numbness, visual loss, weakness), whereas seizures most often produce positive phenomena (e.g., paresthesias, hallucinations, involuntary motor activity). *Transient global amnesia* typically manifests after age 40, with isolated amnesia lasting several hours. *Drop attacks* are sudden falls with preserved consciousness. They are most common in the elderly; and though they have multiple causes, they often remain unexplained. *Movement disorders* can be paroxysmal, but seizures may also manifest with abnormal movements, particularly ictal dystonia. Alteration of consciousness, brief duration (seconds to minutes), and persistence or worsening in sleep will favor seizures. *Sleep disorders* commonly manifest as paroxysmal manifestations, and some forms of epilepsy can also be sleep related. Parasomnias such as sleep walking, sleep talking, or night terror arise from deep (slow wave) sleep, whereas seizures more often arise in light sleep. Rapid eye movement (REM) behavior disorder arises from an abnormal REM sleep in which inhibition of motor activity is impaired. Narcolepsy includes sleep attacks, cataplexy (loss of tone with emotion or startle), hallucinations on falling asleep or waking up, and sleep paralysis (inability to move on waking up).

Psychogenic

Psychogenic seizures (also called pseudoseizures, pseudoepileptic seizures, nonepileptic seizures, or nonepileptic psychogenic events) are episodes of alteration in movements, in responsiveness, or in sensory or cognitive experience that resemble epileptic seizures in some respects but that are purely emotional and lack a concomitant cerebral electrical discharge. Patients are commonly referred after they fail treatment for epilepsy. Psychogenic seizures may account for an estimated 20 to 30% of patients referred for intractable seizures. However, the incidence or prevalence of psychogenic seizures in the general population is unknown. Although they have been reported from 4 to 77 years, the mean age at onset is 20 to 29 years, with a female predominance of about 75%.

The clinical manifestations of psychogenic seizures are very variable and represent a continuum. There may or may not be a reported aura. The onset is often gradual. It is always in waking, even when the patient appears asleep. Clinical features often include motor manifestations, but collapse or altered responsiveness may be the only manifestations. Less frequently, only subjective experiences are reported; the diagnosis of psychogenic seizures is difficult to establish in such instances. Many clinical features have been used to diagnose psychogenic attacks and help distinguish them from epileptic seizures. Features that help distinguish psychogenic seizures from generalized tonic-clonic seizures include out-of-phase upper and lower extremity movements, side-to-side head movement, and forward pelvic thrusting. Other clinical features suggestive of psychogenic seizures include the following:

A gradual onset
"Preictal" behavioral changes
"Pseudo-sleep" before seizure onset
Discontinuous seizure activity
Prolonged duration ("pseudostatus epilepticus" is common)
Gradual cessation
Absence of postictal state
High seizure frequency
Excessive variability in ictal manifestations
Nonphysiologic progression
Eye closure during unresponsiveness
Eye fluttering
Resistance to eye opening
Vocalizations consisting of gagging, retching, gasping, screaming, crying, or moaning
Retained consciousness and recollection of events with bilateral jerking activity
Precipitation of typical attacks by suggestion
Emotional display during events (e.g., weeping)
The presence of an emotional trigger
The occurrence of events only in the presence of others

No feature alone is definitive, but a combination of the features just noted can improve the ability to distinguish psychogenic from epileptic seizures. Incontinence, tongue biting, and self-injury during attacks are more common in epilepsy but are reported by some patients with psychogenic seizures. An elevated serum prolactin level 15 to 30 minutes after a seizure suggests an epileptic basis; however, a normal level does not exclude an epileptic basis and is frequently seen with frontal lobe seizures, which can be hardest to distinguish from psychogenic seizures. Prolonged EEG-video monitoring is usually necessary for the definitive diagnosis of psychogenic seizures and exclusion of epilepsy. Ten to 20% of patients with psychogenic seizures also have epilepsy. Psychogenic seizures are a conversion symptom. However, the underlying psychopathology may vary remarkably among patients. A history of childhood sexual or physical abuse is commonly obtained. Depression is also common and is important to identify and treat.

Other psychogenic manifestations that can mimic seizures include *panic attacks, dissociative states,* and *episodic dyscontrol* (with impulsively violent behavior). *Rage attacks* are highly unlikely to be epileptic. Ictal or postictal violence is rare and is not usually directed.

CLASSIFICATION OF SEIZURE TYPE

Classification is necessary because seizures vary greatly in their manifestations. The observation that certain therapies are effective against some seizure types and not others further emphasizes the need to classify seizures before treating them. The International Classification of Seizures is based on both clinical and EEG characteristics of seizures. The latest classification has been used since 1981 (Table 1). The major subdivision of seizures into partial or generalized is based on seizure onset. Seizures are termed "partial" if there is either clinical or EEG evidence indicating onset in part of one hemisphere. *Simple partial seizures* are partial seizures that do not affect consciousness or responsiveness. *Complex partial seizures* are associated

TABLE 1. Abbreviated International Classification of Epileptic Seizures

I. Partial (Focal, Local) Seizures
   A. Simple partial seizures (with motor signs, with somatosensory or special sensory symptoms, with autonomic symptoms or signs, or with psychic symptoms)
   B. Complex partial seizures
      1. With impairment of consciousness at onset
      2. Simple partial onset followed by impairment of consciousness
   C. Partial seizures evolving to generalized tonic-clonic convulsions (GTC)
      1. Simple evolving to GTC
      2. Complex evolving to GTC (including those with simple partial onset)
II. Generalized Seizures (convulsive or nonconvulsive)
   A. Absence seizures
      1. Absence seizures
      2. Atypical absence seizures
   B. Myoclonic seizures
   C. Clonic seizures
   D. Tonic seizures
   E. Tonic-clonic (GTC) seizures
   F. Atonic seizures
III. Unclassified Epileptic Seizures

with alteration of consciousness or responsiveness. *Partial seizures that become secondarily generalized* are also classified as partial. Partial seizures vary greatly in their manifestations depending on site of seizure origin and pattern and extent of seizure spread.

Generalized seizures tend to be more homogeneous in their manifestations even though they can vary a lot in their severity. Seizures are called "generalized" if they start simultaneously in both hemispheres, without evidence of focal onset by either clinical or electrophysiologic data. *Generalized absence seizures* are characterized by brief loss of awareness or responsiveness and on EEG show generalized 2.5- to 4-Hz spike-and-wave activity. *Typical absence seizures* start abruptly and terminate abruptly, with no postictal phase. They may be associated with minor motor components such as automatisms, blinking, slight twitching, decreased tone, or increased tone. *Atypical absence seizures* may have a more gradual onset or termination, can have more prominent motor activity, tend to be associated with a slower spike-and-wave discharge, and are more likely to occur in neurologically impaired individuals. *Generalized tonic-clonic seizures* are characterized by loss of consciousness at onset and a sudden tonic muscular contraction that evolves into generalized clonic (rhythmic jerking) activity. The clonic activity is initially fast, and the frequency of the jerks decreases before the seizure stops. When respiratory muscles are involved there may be a cry and cyanosis during the tonic phase and rhythmic grunting during the clonic phase. There may be tongue biting and urinary incontinence. *Generalized myoclonic seizures* are brief sudden contractions that may be generalized or confined to a group of muscles or even a single muscle. They can be single and isolated or repetitive in a cluster. Consciousness is usually preserved. Some forms of myoclonus are not epileptic. Myoclonic seizures usually have a concomitant discharge on the EEG. *Generalized clonic seizures* are characterized by repetitive rhythmic clonic jerks, without an initial tonic component. *Generalized tonic seizures* manifest with a muscular contraction that may vary in duration, severity, and the parts of the body involved. The muscular contractions are more sustained than they are in myoclonic seizures. If the contraction is prolonged, the seizure may resemble the tonic phase of a tonic-clonic seizure. *Generalized atonic seizures* are characterized by a sudden decrease in muscle tone, which is variable in severity and extent so that there may simply be a slight head drop or an abrupt fall to the ground.

To help classify seizures correctly, evidence for focal seizure onset should be sought, such as the presence of an aura, initial focal sensory symptoms, or focal motor signs. In the classification of seizures, a commonly encountered problem of differential diagnosis is between complex partial seizures and generalized absence seizures. Absence seizures have no aura, a short duration (typically less than 15 seconds), and no postictal confusion. They also tend to occur frequently, several times a day. Complex partial seizures may or may not have an aura, but they typically have a duration of more than 30 seconds. Postictal confusion or tiredness occurs commonly. The seizure frequency varies but is most commonly several times a month. Hyperventilation in the clinic can easily reproduce absence seizures in the untreated patient, but complex partial seizures are not usually precipitated.

The International Classification of Seizures applies to individual seizure types. Patients often have more than one seizure type. They are often identified as having one type of epilepsy, or an epileptic syndrome. An epileptic syndrome is characterized by a cluster of features usually occurring together, including types of seizures, age at onset, family history, response to drugs, and prognosis. In the 1989 International Classification, the epilepsies are subdivided into two main broad categories: partial (localization-related, focal, local) and generalized (Table 2). Most patients will have either partial or generalized seizure

types. Those who have both belong to a third category. Within each category there are three subcategories: idiopathic, symptomatic, and cryptogenic epilepsies. Idiopathic epilepsies are not caused by any acquired insult and therefore are genetically determined. In these epilepsies there is usually not any associated neurologic impairment, unless it is secondary to the seizures or their therapy. Symptomatic epilepsies are acquired as a result of a known insult (e.g., head injury, brain malformation, small tumor, or infarct), and cryptogenic epilepsies are those in which an acquired cause is suspected but not identified. The partial symptomatic and cryptogenic epilepsies are further classified based on anatomic location of the epileptogenic focus where the seizure discharge originates. The most common are temporal lobe epilepsies, followed by frontal, then occipital and parietal, epilepsies. Temporal lobe epilepsies are most often amygdalohippocampal.

The potential benefit of epilepsy classification is illustrated in the following two examples of epileptic syndromes: benign partial epilepsy with centrotemporal spikes of childhood and juvenile myoclonic epilepsy. *Benign partial epilepsy with centrotemporal spikes of childhood* or *benign rolandic epilepsy* is one of the most common idiopathic epilepsies of childhood. Its age at onset is 3 to 13 years with a peak at 9 to 10 years, and it has a male predominance. The seizures are brief, hemifacial motor, with frequent associated somatosensory symptoms, usually nocturnal, and commonly associated with secondary generalization. The EEG shows blunt high-voltage centrotemporal spikes that are activated by sleep and that tend to spread or shift between the two sides. In this condition the prognosis is excellent. Seizures are easily controlled with medications, and the epilepsy is outgrown before 15 to 16 years. This condition should be contrasted to *juvenile myoclonic epilepsy* in which the age at onset is most commonly between 12 and 18 years. Myoclonic seizures are necessary for the diagnosis. Approximately 90% of patients have generalized tonic-clonic seizures, which tend to start with a series of jerks in rapid succession (as a result these have been termed "clonic-tonic-clonic" seizures), and approximately one third have generalized absence seizures. Seizures occur mainly in the morning after awakening and are precipitated by sleep deprivation. The EEG typically shows 4- to 6-Hz generalized spike-and-wave discharges interictally and during myoclonic jerks. In juvenile myoclonic epilepsy more than 90% of patients can achieve complete seizure control with appropriate therapy. However, this is a life-long condition. Seizures recur in most patients if seizure medications are withdrawn. Recognizing the epileptic syndrome in these two conditions is essential for both short-term and long-term treatment decisions and for prognostication.

The current classification of epilepsies and epileptic syndromes is not final. In the last several years a number of new idiopathic syndromes have been described that are not listed in the current classification. These include autosomal dominant nocturnal frontal lobe epilepsy, familial temporal lobe epilepsy, familial partial epilepsy with variable foci, partial epilepsy with auditory features, benign familial infantile convulsions, rolandic epilepsy with speech dyspraxia (all idiopathic partial epileptic syndromes with presumed autosomal dominant inheritance), and generalized epilepsy with febrile seizures plus (an idiopathic generalized epileptic syndrome). In addition, the genetic defect for some of these epilepsies is being defined, which may eventually provide a reliable diagnostic test. Another limitation of the current classification is that it

TABLE 2. **Abbreviated International Classification of the Epilepsies**

I. Localization-Related (Focal, Local, Partial) Epilepsies and Syndromes
    A. Idiopathic (with age-related onset): benign neonatal familial convulsions; benign neonatal convulsions; benign myoclonic epilepsy in infancy; childhood absence epilepsy; juvenile absence epilepsy; juvenile myoclonic epilepsy; epilepsy with generalized tonic-clonic seizures on awakening; other generalized idiopathic epilepsies; epilepsies with seizures precipitated by specific modes of activation (reflex epilepsies)
    B. Symptomatic
    C. Cryptogenic
        Temporal: amygdalo-hippocampal, lateral temporal
        Frontal: supplementary motor, cingulate, anterior frontopolar, orbitofrontal, dorsolateral, opercular, motor cortex
        Parietal
        Occipital
II. Generalized Epilepsies and Syndromes
    A. Idiopathic (with age-related onset): benign childhood epilepsy with centrotemporal spikes; childhood epilepsy with occipital paroxysms; primary reading epilepsy
    B. Cryptogenic or symptomatic: West syndrome; Lennox-Gastaut syndrome; epilepsy with myoclonic astatic seizures; epilepsy with myoclonic absences
    C. Symptomatic
III. Epilepsies and Syndromes Undetermined Whether Focal or Generalized
    A. With both generalized and focal seizures
    B. Without unequivocal generalized or focal features
IV. Special Syndromes: Situation-Related Seizures (Gelegenheitsanfälle)

does not account for the possible coexistence of genetic and acquired factors in the same patient.

ETIOLOGY

The classification of seizure types and of the epileptic syndrome should be followed by a search for etiology. Possible causes are numerous. Epilepsy can be purely genetically determined without associated neurologic disturbances (idiopathic) or can be secondary to a variety of conditions, including perinatal hypoxia, developmental brain disorders, head injury, infection (encephalitis, meningitis), tumors, stroke, degenerative disease, vascular malformations, and genetic disorders (e.g., tuberous sclerosis, ceroid lipofuscinosis, Lafora's disease). The past medical history and family history may provide insight into the etiology. The examination may occasionally provide focal neurologic findings or other clues to the etiology.

Every adolescent or adult with newly diagnosed epilepsy should have an EEG and undergo magnetic resonance imaging (MRI) of the brain (unless it is already very clear that we are dealing with an idiopathic epileptic syndrome). The standard EEG will show hyperventilation, photic stimulation, drowsiness, and sleep. In general, the 20-minute standard EEG will be an interictal recording (absence seizures are a notable exception because they are easily induced by hyperventilation) and may record nonspecific abnormalities (e.g., slow wave activity or asymmetry of the background) or specific epileptiform discharges (e.g., sharp waves, spikes, or spike-and-wave complexes). The initial EEG may be normal in up to 50% of patients with epilepsy. If indicated, repeat EEG may improve the yield of specific epileptiform discharges to 90%, but there is little additional benefit after four recordings. The EEG should be used only to support a clinical diagnosis of epilepsy and to help with the seizure and epileptic syndrome classification, not to make the diagnosis independently. A brain MRI is the imaging modality of choice in epilepsy investigation. It should be obtained even if the patient has already had computed tomography in the emergency department. In fact, the computed tomography should usually be omitted if the MRI can be obtained early. Brain MRI will identify most mass lesions and vascular malformations. Many centers now have MRI protocols for epilepsy that help identify even subtle cortical developmental malformations and hippocampal sclerosis (which is one of the most common epileptogenic lesions). Blood studies for evaluation of electrolytes and testing of hepatic and renal function may be indicated with acute seizures, and a spinal tap may be necessary if a central nervous system infection is suggested.

Additional investigations, such as prolonged EEG-video monitoring, are indicated only if the seizures are unusual in their characteristics or resistant to treatment. Functional neuroimaging with positron emission tomography (PET) or single-photon emission computerized tomography (SPECT) is reserved for epilepsy resistant to medical therapy, in which surgical treatment is being considered.

THERAPY

Treatment with an antiepileptic drug (AED) is usually indicated when epilepsy is diagnosed. There is evidence that uncontrolled seizures may produce cell loss in certain regions of the brain, and irreversible brain damage is well described with status epilepticus. The appropriate classification of seizures and epilepsies should help in the choice of the initial AED (Table 3). Between 1993 and 1998, five new AEDs were approved for the treatment of epilepsy. These AEDs are generally still not indicated for initial therapy, but additional studies and experience may change this position.

Treatment should begin with one AED (the most effective and safest for the seizure type). There are several advantages to monotherapy, including simpler pharmacokinetics, easier assessment of efficacy, absence of interactions, less adverse experiences, lower cost, better compliance, and, at times, even higher efficacy. Although some AEDs such as phenytoin (Dilantin) can be started immediately at the predicted maintenance dose, most need to be started

TABLE 3. **Antiepileptic Drug (AED) Efficacy in Some Seizure Types***

| | Partial Seizures | Generalized Seizures | | |
		Tonic-Clonic	Absence	Myoclonic
Classic AEDs				
Phenytoin (Dilantin)	1	1	NE	NE
Carbamazepine (Tegretol, Carbatrol)	1	1	NE	NE
Valproate, divalproex (Depakote)	1–2	1	1	1
Phenobarbital	3	2	NE	NE†
Primidone (Mysoline)	3	3	NE	NE†
Ethosuximide (Zarontin)	NE	NE	1	NE†
Clonazepam (Klonopin)	4	4	2	2
New AEDs				
Felbamate (Felbatol)	Effective	Effective	Effective	Effective
Gabapentin (Neurontin)	Effective	?Effective	NE	NE
Lamotrigine (Lamictal)	Effective	Effective	Effective	?Effective
Topiramate (Topamax)	Effective	Effective	?Effective	?Effective
Tiagabine (Gabitril)	Effective	?Effective	NE	NE

NE = not effective.
*The numbers indicate the rank of each drug as a choice for the particular seizure type. The new AEDs are still not generally indicated as a first choice for monotherapy. A question mark indicates that efficacy has not been completely established.
†May be partially effective in some instances.

at a low dose and titrated slowly (Table 4). The initial target dose may be sufficiently effective, but in many or even most instances, higher doses will be necessary. The most commonly used doses listed in the table can definitely be exceeded, and a maximum dose is not listed. If the seizures are not controlled, the dose can then be increased gradually until seizures stop or until side effects appear. The clinical response should be the primary guide in treatment, although plasma AED levels can be used to help explain lack of response or adverse experiences. Trough steady-state levels are the most useful, but peak levels may be more useful to assess intermittent symptoms of toxicity. If there is partial benefit and no significant adverse effects after reaching a steady state, then the AED can be titrated beyond the suggested plasma levels. However, small dose increments should be used when in the therapeutic range. If side effects occur without seizure control, the AED must be returned to a dose that was well tolerated, and a second drug must be considered. The second drug is then added with the expectation that the first will be later discontinued (after the second drug reaches the therapeutic range), with attempts to maintain monotherapy when the classic antiepileptic drugs are used. It is very important to be aware of pharmacokinetic properties of the AEDs used (Table 5). For example, one of the most widely used AEDs, phenytoin, has nonlinear or saturable kinetics, such that as the dose is increased plasma levels rise disproportionately, particularly after reaching the lower end of the therapeutic range (Figure 1). By using increments of 100 mg it may be possible to bypass the therapeutic zone into toxic blood levels. The use of 30-mg capsules or 50-mg tablets can help in accurate titration of the dose to an effective level. Physicians should also be familiar with the adverse effect profile of AEDs (Table 6). Patient reports of adverse experiences should be taken seriously, and seizure control should not come at the expense of normal function and well-being.

If monotherapy with one to three of the classic antiepileptic drugs fails, combination therapy can be used. This creates a potential for interactions that needs to be watched for (Tables 7 and 8). Carbamazepine, phenytoin, phenobarbital, and primidone are inducers of liver enzymes and will reduce plasma levels of AEDs metabolized by the cytochrome P-450 system, such as valproate. Valproate and felbamate inhibit the metabolism of some AEDs. Interactions may also occur in protein binding. When used in combination, phenytoin and valproate, which are both highly protein bound, compete for protein binding. As a result a greater proportion of phenytoin will be unbound, and the patient may be toxic with an apparently therapeutic or even subtherapeutic total phenytoin level. Unbound phenytoin levels are necessary in this situation, because they also are in low protein states. Some combinations appear particularly effective, with lower doses required and even possible synergism. This may be true of the combinations of valproate and lamotrigine and valproate and

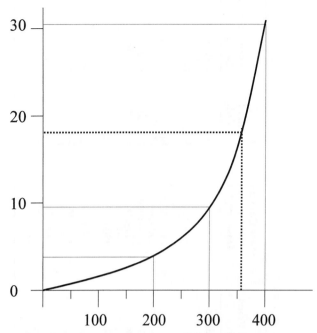

Figure 1. Illustration of the nonlinear pharmacokinetics of phenytoin. A dose of 300 mg produced a plasma level of 9 μg per mL, with incomplete seizure control. Increasing the dose by 100 mg to 400 mg per day produced clinical toxicity with a plasma level of 31 μg per mL. In this patient a dose of 360 mg per day produced complete seizure control with a plasma level of 18 μg per mL (dark dotted line).

felbamate for resistant generalized epilepsies. Combinations of more than two AEDs should be avoided.

Carbamazepine and phenytoin are the drugs of choice for initial treatment of partial seizures. Extended-release carbamazepine preparations (Tegretol XR and Carbatrol) are preferred because they allow twice-daily dosing and reduce plasma level fluctuations. Valproate may be considered the first choice in some instances, such as co-morbidity of epilepsy and migraine (valproate is effective against both). Ethosuximide (Zarontin) is the drug of choice for generalized absence seizures, but it is not effective against other seizure types. If generalized absence seizures coexist with another seizure type, valproate is the drug of choice. Valproate is therefore the drug of choice in most idiopathic generalized epilepsies, including juvenile myoclonic epilepsy, and is an important agent in symptomatic generalized epilepsies. Phenytoin, carbamazepine, phenobarbital, and primidone are not effective against absence seizures, whereas valproic acid and clonazepam have a wide spectrum of efficacy. Because phenobarbital, primidone, and clonazepam are sedating, they should not be used as first-line AEDs. In addition, tolerance often develops with clonazepam; hence, it should generally be considered a temporary agent.

Among the new antiepileptic drugs, felbamate has a wide spectrum of efficacy in both partial and generalized seizures. It is also approved for monotherapy. However, as a result of the risk of aplastic anemia and liver failure, it is indicated only after other medi-

TABLE 4. **Doses and Therapeutic Plasma Levels of AEDs**

AED	Specific Comments	Starting Dose (mg/d)	Initial Target Dose (mg/d)	Time to Reach Initial Target Dose	Most Common Maintenance Dose (mg/d)	Optimal Schedule	Target Plasma Level (μg/mL)
Phenytoin	Can be loaded intravenously (best using the prodrug fosphenytoin)	300 (200 in elderly)	Same	Immediate	300–400	bid	8–25 (unbound: 0.8–2.5)
Carbamazepine	Preferably use extended-release formulations	200	400–600	1 wk	800–1600	bid	4–12
Valproate, divalproex	Intravenous preparation available	250–500	500–1000	3–7 d	750–1500*	bid	50–130
Phenobarbital	Parenteral preparation available	30–60	60	2–4 wk	100–180	qhs	15–40
Primidone		50–125	750	4–6 wk	750–1000	bid–tid	4–12
Ethosuximide		250	750	1–2 wk	750–1000	bid–tid	50–100
Clonazepam		0.5	1–2	2–4 wk	2–6	bid–tid	0.02–0.08
Felbamate		1200 (600 bid)	2400–3600	2 wk	3600	1200 (bid–tid)	40–100
Gabapentin		300–400	900–1200	1–3 d	2400–3600	tid	>2†
Lamotrigine	With enzyme-inducing AED	50 (25 bid)	300	4 wk	400–800	bid	>1†
	With valproate	12.5	100–150	8 wk	150–200	bid	>1†
	With other AEDs or monotherapy	25	200	6 wk	200–400	bid	>1†
Topiramate		25–50	200	4–8 wk	200–400	bid	?
Tiagabine		4	24–32	5–7 wk	24–64	bid–tid	?

*In monotherapy. Higher doses are frequently necessary when used with enzyme-inducing AEDs.
†The therapeutic range is not well established, particularly with respect to toxic levels.

TABLE 5. **Pharmacokinetic Properties of AEDs**

AED	Absorption/Bioavailability	Protein Binding	Metabolism (% metabolized)	Autoinduction	Half-life (h)	Excretion
Phenytoin	>90%	90%	Liver (95%) Nonlinear kinetics	No	7–42 (mean: 22)*	Urine + feces
Carbamazepine	75–85%	75%	Liver (>95%)	Yes	6–20 (mean: 12)	Urine + feces
Valproate, divalproex	>90%	90%	Liver (>96%)	No	5–15 (mean: 8)	Urine
Phenobarbital	>90%	45%	Liver	No	65–110 (mean: 96)	Urine + feces
Primidone	>90%	<20%	Liver	No	8–15	Changed to phenobarbital
Ethosuximide	>90%	<10%	Liver (>80%)	No	30–60 (mean: 40)	Urine
Clonazepam	>80%	86%	Liver	No	30–40	Urine
Felbamate	>90%	25%	Liver (50%)	No	18–24†	Urine
Gabapentin	50–60%	0%	Not metabolized	No	5–8	Urine
Lamotrigine	>98%	55%	Liver (90%)	Slight	12–70‡	Urine
Topiramate	≥80%	15%	Liver (20–50%)	No	20–30†	Urine
Tiagabine	≥89%	96%	Liver (98%)	No	2–9†	Feces + urine

*The half-life is longer with toxicity.
†The half-life is shortened by enzyme-inducing AEDs.
‡Half-life is 12 hours with enzyme-inducing AEDs, 70 hours with valproate, and 24 hours with monotherapy.

TABLE 6. **Most Limiting Adverse Effects or Most Concerning (Usually Idiosyncratic) Toxicity of AEDs***

AED	Common or Limiting Adverse Effects	"Idiosyncratic" Toxicity
Phenytoin	Dizziness, ataxia, drowsiness	Rash, lymphadenopathy
Carbamazepine	Dizziness, blurred vision, ataxia, nausea	Rash, other hypersensitivity
Valproate, divalproex	Weight gain, hair loss, tremor, fatigue, nausea	Liver failure, pancreatitis (rare)
Phenobarbital	Drowsiness, depression	Rash, connective tissue disorders
Primidone (Mysoline)	Dizziness, drowsiness, depression	Connective tissue disorders
Ethosuximide (Zarontin)	Nausea, drowsiness	Blood dyscrasias
Clonazepam (Klonopin)	Drowsiness, depression, ataxia	
Felbamate (Felbatol)	Nausea, insomnia, headache, weight loss	Aplastic anemia (~1/5,000), liver failure (~1/10,000)
Gabapentin (Neurontin)	Drowsiness, dizziness	
Lamotrigine (Lamictal)	Dizziness, headache	Rash
Topiramate (Topamax)	Cognitive impairment, confusion, drowsiness	Agitation, psychosis
Tiagabine (Gabitril)	Dizziness, drowsiness, fatigue	Encephalopathy, psychosis

*There is great variability among patients in tolerability of AEDs, and in the type and pattern of side effects with any AED.

TABLE 7. **AED Interactions: Effects of Other Drugs on AEDs of Interest (Partial Listing Only)**

AED	Drugs That Increase AED Plasma Level		Drugs That Decrease AED Plasma Level	
	Other AEDs	Other Drugs	Other AEDs	Other Drugs
Phenytoin	Felbamate*	Cimetidine, disulfiram, isoniazid, propranolol, propoxyphene, sulfonamides, amiodarone, phenothiazines	Phenobarbital, valproate†	Antacids, rifampin, folic acid, chronic alcohol
Carbamazepine		Erythromycin and related antibiotics,* propoxyphene,* fluoxetine, isoniazid, cimetidine, verapamil, diltiazem	Phenytoin, phenobarbital, primidone, felbamate‡	
Valproate	Felbamate	Aspirin, chlorpromazine	Phenytoin, carbamazepine, phenobarbital, primidone, lamotrigine	Rifampin
Phenobarbital	Valproate*	Propoxyphene, chloramphenicol		
Primidone		Isoniazid	Phenytoin, carbamazepine§	
Ethosuximide			Phenytoin, carbamazepine, phenobarbital, primidone	
Clonazepam			Carbamazepine, phenobarbital	
Felbamate			Phenytoin, carbamazepine, phenobarbital, primidone	
Gabapentin	No interactions	No interactions	No interactions	No interactions
Lamotrigine	Valproate*	Sertraline	Phenytoin, carbamazepine, phenobarbital, primidone	
Topiramate, tiagabine			Phenytoin, carbamazepine, phenobarbital, primidone	

*Particularly clinically important interactions.
†May reduce total phenytoin level; does not reduce unbound phenytoin.
‡Reduces carbamazepine level but may cause toxicity through increase in epoxide metabolite.
§Increases conversion of primidone to phenobarbital.

TABLE 8. **AED Interactions: Effects of AEDs of Interest on Other Drugs (Partial Listing)**

AED	AED Increases Plasma Level of	AED Decreases Plasma Level of
Phenytoin, carbamazepine, phenobarbital, primidone		Hormonal contraceptives,* warfarin,* dexamethasone,* cyclosporine,* other agents metabolized by the cytochrome P-450 system* (including a number of AEDs listed in Table 7)
Valproate	Lamotrigine,* phenobarbital*	
Ethosuximide, clonazepam	No significant interactions	No significant interactions
Felbamate	Valproate, phenytoin*	Carbamazepine†
Gabapentin	No interactions	No interactions
Lamotrigine, topiramate, tiagabine	No significant interactions	No significant interactions

*Particularly clinically important interactions.
†Increases concentration of the epoxide metabolite, which may cause symptoms of toxicity.

cations fail. The other new AEDs appear to have a favorable safety profile, and generally have fewer interactions than the classic AEDs. Gabapentin (Neurontin) has very few adverse effects and no significant interactions. It is indicated as adjunctive therapy for partial-onset seizures. Although its use in monotherapy has not yet been approved by the U.S. Food and Drug Administration, it may be an appropriate first choice in the elderly or patients on multiple other medications, in whom interactions need to be avoided. Lamotrigine (Lamictal) has a wide spectrum of efficacy and is an excellent alternative in patients with generalized epilepsy, such as juvenile myoclonic epilepsy, who are unable to tolerate valproate. However, its efficacy against myoclonic seizures is not established. It has been approved for use in monotherapy. It tends to be less sedating than older AEDs and should be considered in individuals unable to tolerate other AEDs because of sedation. Topiramate (Topamax) is also approved as adjunctive treatment in patients with partial-onset seizures; however, there is strong evidence that it has a wide spectrum of efficacy against partial and generalized seizure types. Tiagabine (Gabitril) is approved as an adjunctive treatment for partial-onset seizures.

Several AEDs may become available by the year 2001. The list includes zonisamide (Zonegran), vigabatrin (Sabril), oxcarbazepine (Trileptal), and levetiracetam (Kepra). All appear effective against partial-onset seizures. Zonisamide is reported effective against progressive myoclonus epilepsies, a group of difficult-to-treat symptomatic generalized epilepsies. Oxcarbazepine offers efficacy similar to carbamazepine but has less adverse effects and less interactions. Levetiracetam appears to have a wide spectrum of efficacy and an excellent pharmacokinetic and safety profile.

AED Withdrawal in Patients Who Have Become Seizure-Free

Once seizures are controlled, therapy should preferably be continued for at least 2 years. Withdrawal of AED therapy can be considered after 2 to 5 years of seizure freedom, depending on the risk of recurrence for the individual patient. Sixty to 75% of patients who are free of seizures for 2 to 4 years on AEDs will remain seizure free after AED withdrawal. Factors associated with a greater risk of seizure recurrence include remote symptomatic etiology, presence of a structural lesion, abnormal neurologic examination, abnormal EEG with epileptiform discharges or slow activity, and age at onset in adolescence. Patients with juvenile myoclonic epilepsy have a high seizure recurrence rate and should not be withdrawn from AED therapy. AED withdrawal should be very gradual over several weeks to months. Most recurrences will occur in the first 6 to 12 months after AED discontinuation.

Special Situations

Single Seizures. Long-term AED therapy is generally not indicated for single *provoked* seizures (e.g.,

seizures caused by transient metabolic aberration or acute trauma). The risk of seizure recurrence after a single *unprovoked* seizure is estimated at 40%. The risk increases with abnormal neurologic status and abnormal EEG. Other factors may also play a role. If the neurologic examination, neuroimaging studies, and EEG are normal, the risk of recurrence is close to 20%. The decision to give long-term treatment with AEDs should be individualized and made after discussion with the patient weighing risk of seizure recurrence against risk of treatment. Once a second seizure has occurred, the risk of recurrence is 70% or more and treatment should generally be initiated.

Women with Child-Bearing Potential. Enzyme-inducing drugs such as carbamazepine and phenytoin reduce the effectiveness of oral contraceptives. A higher-dose contraceptive may then be necessary in such patients. The risk of birth defects is increased twofold to threefold in infants of mothers with epilepsy treated with AEDs. Exposure in the first 5 weeks of gestation is the most important in the genesis of these defects. Folic acid supplementation during pregnancy reduces the risk of birth defects. Because a considerable proportion of pregnancies are unplanned and are discovered after the fourth week of gestation, all women with epilepsy who have child-bearing potential should be treated with folic acid, 1 to 2 mg per day.

Pregnant Women. All classic AEDs are associated with an increased risk of birth defects. However, spina bifida is seen more specifically in 2% or more of infants exposed to valproate and 1% of infants exposed to carbamazepine in polytherapy. Other birth defects seen with AED exposure include cleft lip/cleft palate and cardiovascular, skeletal, gastrointestinal, and urogenital malformations. Birth defects are less likely to occur with monotherapy and with lower AED plasma levels. Approximately 94% of pregnancies nevertheless lead to normal infants. Limited data suggest that gabapentin and lamotrigine may be safer for use in pregnancy than older drugs. During pregnancy, seizure frequency may change and AED levels need to be monitored more closely, particularly close to the time of delivery, when generalized tonic-clonic seizures may be harmful to the fetus.

The Elderly. The elderly have a high incidence of epilepsy. They deserve special treatment consideration because of physiologic changes such as reduced creatinine clearance, decreased albumin level, and decreased hepatic drug metabolism. The elderly are also more sensitive to AED adverse effects, particularly those related to the central nervous system (CNS). In addition, they have a greater likelihood of concomitant disease and concomitant medications. For many of the AEDs, lower doses and a slower titration may need to be used. Potential CNS adverse effects should be monitored. In patients treated with phenytoin, unbound levels should be monitored. AEDs with fewer interactions such as gabapentin or lamotrigine should be considered in patients on multiple other drugs.

Status Epilepticus. Status epilepticus, a condition of recurrent or continuous seizure activity, can occur with any seizure type but is most serious if it is generalized convulsive (with partial or generalized onset). It is a medical emergency. Brain damage can occur if seizure activity is not controlled within 20 minutes. The treatment (Table 9) includes maintenance of a patent airway and intravenous administration of lorazepam (Ativan) and fosphenytoin (Cerebyx), which is a phenytoin prodrug that is water soluble and less irritating to the veins than phenytoin. General anesthesia is indicated if seizure activity remains uncontrolled (see Table 8). The use of neuromuscular blockers is inappropriate because they do not stop the seizure activity in the brain (which is the cause of brain damage).

In patients with recurrent status epilepticus, home treatment with rectal diazepam gel (Diastat), 10 to 20 mg, should be considered before transfer to an emergency facility.

Acute Repetitive Seizures. These are cluster, serial, crescendo, or sequential seizures that can be the prelude to status epilepticus. They can be precipitated by stress, sleep deprivation, fever, infections, medication changes, or missed medication doses or may simply follow a cyclical pattern. Rectal diazepam gel (Diastat), 10 to 20 mg, is effective in arresting these seizures and preventing emergency department visits.

Refractory Epilepsy

The aim of treatment should be to eliminate seizures completely. Complete seizure control with AEDs is easier to accomplish in the idiopathic epilepsies. Cryptogenic and symptomatic epilepsies are

TABLE 9. **Treatment of Generalized Convulsive Status Epilepticus**

1. Assess cardiorespiratory function and monitor breathing, heart rate, blood pressure, and oxygenation.
2. Establish intravenous access; draw blood for glucose, electrolytes, AED levels (if appropriate).
3. Start an infusion with normal saline. Give thiamine, 100 mg IV, followed by 50 mL of 50% glucose (unless glucose concentration is normal or high).
4. Give lorazepam up to 10 mg IV (maximum rate: 2 mg/min).
5. Give fosphenytoin (Cerebyx), 20 mg/kg IV, at a maximum rate of 150 mg/min, unless the status is due to alcohol withdrawal or a transient metabolic or toxic cause.
6. If the seizure activity is still not controlled after 20 minutes from onset of treatment, intubate and ventilate and give an additional 10 mg/kg of fosphenytoin.
7. For continuing status epilepticus, place patient under general anesthesia. Electroencephalographic monitoring is a must at this point. Propofol (Diprivan), a short-acting rapidly reversible agent, has become the anesthetic of choice (1–2 mg/kg then 3–10 mg/kg/h). Alternatively, give pentobarbital, 15 mg/kg, then 1–3 mg/kg/h to obtain a burst suppression pattern on the electroencephalogram.
8. Obtain diagnostic tests* if needed after the seizure activity has been controlled.
9. Treat the cause of status epilepticus (e.g., infection).

*Computed tomography, magnetic resonance imaging, lumbar puncture.

more often refractory to medical therapy. Responsiveness to therapy may also depend on the seizure type. Typical generalized absence and primary generalized tonic-clonic seizures are usually easily controlled, whereas atypical absence and generalized tonic seizures, which tend to occur in neurologically impaired individuals, are notoriously difficult to stop. Among partial seizures, secondarily generalized seizures come under control more easily than simple partial and complex partial seizures. Thirty-five to 50% of patients with cryptogenic or symptomatic epilepsies continue to have seizures despite optimal therapy. Although addition of one of the new AEDs can help reduce seizure frequency or severity in many patients refractory to the classic antiepileptic drugs, only a modest proportion ($\leq 10\%$) of these patients will achieve complete seizure control.

Before it is assumed that the epilepsy is refractory, a number of remediable causes of apparent intractability should be considered. *Suboptimal AED use* can result in continued seizures for a number of causes: levels not pushed to maximum tolerated, long interval between doses in an AED with a short half-life, toxicity that may paradoxically produce an increase in seizures, or polytherapy interactions resulting in decreased AED efficacy. *Physiologic factors* that can precipitate breakthrough seizures include stress, sleep deprivation, or fever and concurrent illness. *Patient factors* include poor compliance, alcohol or drug abuse, and co-medication. Finally, intractability may occur because of *incorrect seizure diagnosis,* with an inappropriate AED for the seizure type, or the seizures being altogether nonepileptic.

If the epilepsy is truly refractory, the patient should generally be referred to a specialized epilepsy center where alternative therapies can be considered (Figure 2). The *ketogenic diet* is a strict high-fat, low-protein, and very low-carbohydrate diet that is usually initiated with a fast to achieve ketosis. The diet is most effective in children with generalized epilepsy. Some patients may be able to reduce or eliminate concomitant AEDs. *Hormonal therapy* (progesterone) may help some women with exacerbation of seizures in relation to the menstrual period or ovulation. The *vagus nerve stimulator* is the first device to be approved for epilepsy. It is indicated in refractory partial epilepsy, but mounting evidence suggests that is also effective in refractory generalized epilepsy. Thirty to 50% of patients benefit, with reduced seizure frequency, milder and shorter seizures, or a shorter postictal phase. Because this is a palliative treatment, it should be reserved for patients who are not candidates for epilepsy surgery.

Surgery

Epilepsy surgery should be considered only in patients who are resistant to medical therapy. The most popular approach, which aims at curing the epilepsy, involves resection of the epileptogenic focus. The best candidates are patients with temporal lobe epilepsy, particularly those with right-sided foci. A multidisci-

Partial Epilepsy   Generalized Epilepsy

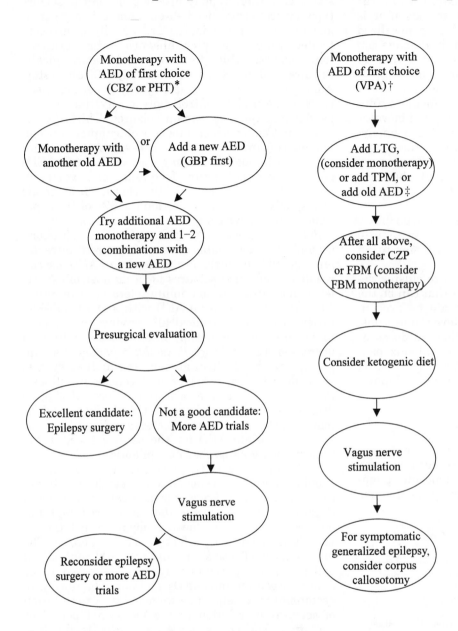

Figure 2. The author's suggested pathways in the treatment of established epilepsy. Arrows suggest the next step for refractory seizures. Avoid using more than two antiepileptic drugs (AEDs). Added AEDs that are not effective should be tapered and discontinued. If the diagnosis is not entirely certain, EEG-video monitoring is indicated before the second or third step. CBZ = carbamazepine; PHT = phenytoin; VPA = valproate; GBP = gabapentin; LTG = lamotrigine; TPM = topiramate; FBM = felbamate; CZP = clonazepam. *Valproate can be considered in certain instances. †Ethosuximide is the drug of choice for pure absence seizures. ‡If the refractory seizure type is absence, ethosuximide can be added. Phenytoin or carbamazepine can be added if the refractory seizure type is generalized tonic-clonic or generalized tonic.

plinary presurgical evaluation for localization of the epileptogenic focus and prediction of outcome should include prolonged EEG-video monitoring, brain MRI, PET, neuropsychological testing, and the intracarotid sodium amobarbital procedure (Wada test). In appropriate candidates for temporal lobectomy, complete freedom from disabling seizures can be accomplished in 70 to 80%. Localization of extratemporal foci is often challenging, and the surgical results are less good, with approximately 50% becoming free of disabling seizures. One AED is usually continued for 2 years after surgery. Some patients continue to require AED therapy to remain seizure free.

If the epileptogenic zone is in proximity to functional cortex (e.g., language or motor cortex), surgery should be preceded by mapping of cortical function

and fine localization of the epileptogenic zone by means of implanted subdural grid electrodes. If the epileptogenic zone includes functional cortex, multiple subpial transections can be used. This is an approach that disconnects cortical horizontal fibers, thereby isolating epileptogenic cortex or preventing seizure spread, without interrupting the vertical functional units.

Patients with symptomatic generalized or multifocal epilepsy may be candidates for corpus callosotomy, which is a palliative procedure. It can make seizures milder or more focal. It is most often performed in two steps, starting with a two-thirds anterior callosotomy. Complete section may not be necessary. The best results are in patients with seizures manifesting as drop attacks.

EPILEPSY IN INFANTS AND CHILDREN

method of
W. EDWIN DODSON, M.D.
Washington University School of Medicine
St. Louis, Missouri

Seizures are symptoms of abnormal brain function. The treatment of children with seizures starts with trying to identify treatable causes and then treating them specifically. When seizures persist or when specific therapy is not available, antiepileptic drugs are used. However, before moving to antiepileptic drug therapy, it is important to exclude nonepileptic paroxysmal behavioral disturbances.

NONEPILEPTIC CONDITIONS OFTEN CONFUSED WITH SEIZURES

To avoid misuse of antiepileptic drugs, the first step is to separate out nonepileptic paroxysmal pediatric conditions from seizures. Nonseizure alterations of behavior are fairly common in children and have many causes. For example, abrupt reductions in cardiac output that cause cerebral ischemia result in unconsciousness with or without convulsive movements. In toddlers (children aged 18 to 36 months), the most common cause of episodic unconsciousness is breath-holding spells that are behavioral, not epileptic. Causes of nonepileptic paroxysmal behaviors are summarized in Table 1.

Benign neonatal myoclonus is the most common nonepileptic disorder that is confused with seizures in newborns and young infants. This causes repetitive muscle jerks during sleep or on awakening. The electroencephalogram (EEG) is normal. Episodes are noticed most often after feeding while the infant is falling asleep. No treatment is indicated.

Breath-holding spells affect up to 20% of toddlers and young children. The blue or cyanotic episodes result from the child's holding his or her breath while beginning to cry. The key to diagnosis is recognizing the child's angry response to frustration or pain that precedes the episode. The treatment is to modify the caretaker's behavior so that the child's breath-holding behavior is not reinforced. Although prolonged breath-holding can result in seizures, the treatment should be behavioral modification unless there is clear evidence that the child also has epilepsy. Pallid spells are actually vasovagal episodes.

TABLE 1. Nonepileptic Paroxysmal Disorders

Breath holding
  Blue
  Pallid
Migraine variants
  Benign paroxysmal torticollis
  Benign paroxysmal vertigo
Cardiogenic cerebral ischemia
  Disorders with prolonged QT interval
  Sick sinus syndrome
Movement disorders
  Benign neonatal myoclonus
  Paroxysmal choreoathetosis
  Hyperexplexia
Sleep disorders (parasomnias)

EVALUATION OF THE CHILD WITH SEIZURES

The approach to treating seizures includes the following steps: (1) characterize the episode; (2) investigate for a treatable cause and treat it if one is found; (3) administer antiepileptic drugs based on the type of seizure and/or type of epilepsy; and (4) follow-up for response and possible drug side effects.

If a cause can be identified, specific treatment sometimes is curative and limits the need for antiepileptic drug therapy. Seizures in children are caused by both neurologic and systemic disorders. Neurologic causes include brain malformations, trauma, metabolic, infectious, toxic, vascular, or neoplastic conditions. However, approximately 75% of cases are idiopathic, except in newborns where a cause for neonatal seizures can be found in a majority. For children who are being evaluated acutely because of ongoing or frequently recurrent seizures, the following blood tests for systemic abnormalities should be considered: glucose, electrolytes, calcium and magnesium, and blood urea nitrogen. When fever, mental status change, or signs of meningeal irritation are present, a lumbar puncture should be considered. A brain imaging test, preferably magnetic resonance imaging, should be obtained if any of the following features are present: a focal or partial seizure, focal neurologic deficit or abnormal development, recent head trauma, or if the seizure(s) lasted more than 5 minutes.

Children who are suspected of having seizures should have an EEG. The two key questions to answer with the EEG are whether epileptiform discharges are present and, if so, is the pattern of the discharges localized (focal) or generalized? When interpreting the results of an EEG, remember that although the EEG is usually abnormal during a seizure, it may be normal between seizures. Thus, a normal EEG does not rule out epilepsy.

TREATMENT

Antiepileptic drugs are the mainstay of treating childhood epilepsy. However, drug therapy usually is not recommended until the child has had at least two seizures. This applies even to those cases in which the EEG reveals epileptic features. In all cases the seizure type needs to be identified because it is the basis for drug selection.

Drug Selection Based on Descriptive Classification of Seizure Types

There are two levels of descriptive classification. These include (1) the patient's seizure type and (2) the patient's type of epilepsy or epileptic syndrome. Classified according to the International Classification, seizure types indicate which antiepileptic drug to prescribe (Table 2). An eyewitness's description of the seizure provides the best information. Whereas the misdiagnosis of episodic staring is at the root of frequent treatment errors, the differential diagnostic features of daydreaming, absence seizures, and complex partial seizures are summarized in Table 3.

Initiation of Drug Therapy

Antiepileptic drugs should be started at low or low average doses, which are then increased slowly until

TABLE 2. **Drug Selection According to Seizure Types Based on the International Classification of Epileptic Seizures**

Seizure Type	Effective Drugs
I. Partial Seizures	
A. Simple partial	CBZ, PHT, LTG, TPM, VPA
B. Complex partial	CBZ, PHT, LTG, TPM, VPA, PRM
C. Secondarily generalized	VPA, CBZ, LTG, TPM, PB, PHT, GBP
II. Generalized Seizures	
A. Absence seizures	ETX, VPA, LTG, ACT
B. Myoclonic	VPA, TPM, KLO, ACT, PRM
C. Clonic	CBZ, PB, PHT
D. Tonic	TPM, PHT, VPA,
E. Tonic-clonic	VPA, CBZ, TPM, PHT, GBP, PB
F. Atonic	VPA, TPM, LTG, ETX, KLO, ACT
III. Unclassified Epileptic Seizures	
IV. Status Epilepticus	See Table 5

ACT = acetazolamide (Diamox); CBZ = carbamazepine (Tegretol); ETX = ethosuximide (Zarontin); GBP = gabapentin (Neurontin); KLO = clonazepam (Klonipin); LTG = lamotrigine (Lamictal); PB = phenobarbital (Luminal); PHT = phenytoin (Dilantin); PRM = primidone (Mysoline); TPM = topiramatae (Topamax); VPA = valproic acid (Depakene, Depakote).

seizures are prevented or intolerable side effects occur. If mild side effects occur when the dose is being increased, often a small backstep in dose or pause in the escalation will allow the child to adapt to the drug. In this process, remember that each time the dose is changed it takes five half-lives for the drug concentration to reach a steady state (Table 4). For this reason, the drug is not expected to be fully efficacious until sufficient time has passed. When starting antiepileptic drugs, it is important to counsel the child and the caregiver about this issue.

When counseling families about antiepileptic therapy, several key pieces of information need to be covered. First, the family needs to be warned about mild, transient side effects that are likely when the

TABLE 3. **Differentiation of Daydreaming from Partial Complex and Absence Seizures**

Feature	Absence	Complex Partial	Day Dreaming
Altered consciousness	Yes	Yes	No
Aura	No	Maybe	No
Automatisms	Yes	Yes	No
Duration	<30 sec	>30 sec	Variable
Postictal state*	No	Maybe	No
Precipitated by HV	Yes	Usually not	No
Ictal EEG	3 Hz S-W	Focal spikes	Normal
Medications	ETX, VPA, LTG	CBZ, PHT, LTG	None

HV = hyperventilation, S-W = spike and wave EEG pattern; ETX = ethosuximide (Zarontin); VPA = valproic acid (Depakene, Depakote); LTG = lamotrigine (Lamictal); CBZ = carbamazepine (Tegretol); PHT = phenytoin (Dilantin).

*The term "postictal state" refers to symptoms of exhaustion that sometimes occur after a seizure and include sleepiness, confusion, lethargy, and often headache.

drug is started. Second, they need to be told when to expect that the drug will be fully active so that if seizures occur before that time, they will not abandon treatment prematurely. Third, they need to be advised about serious adverse effects and instructed either to stop the medication and/or to contact the physician right away. Fourth, pill reminder boxes are recommended for all patients with epilepsy.

Assessment of Patient Response and Dosage Adjustment

The goal of treatment is the prevention of seizures without adverse drug effects. Although drug concentration measurements and improvements in the EEG are adjuncts to patient management, they are no substitute for the clinical assessment of the patient. So-called therapeutic drug levels are only loose indicators as to those antiepileptic drug concentrations at which patients begin to respond or manifest adverse effects (see Table 4). If the child's seizures are completely prevented at concentrations below the recommended range, the dose is adequate and should not be increased simply because of the level. Similarly, if the dose has been progressively escalated and produces seizure control without adverse effects, the dose should not be reduced just because the drug level exceeds the recommended range.

If one antiepileptic drug is ineffective after being raised to doses that cause intolerable side effects, it should be replaced by a second medication. If the second drug administered alone (monotherapy) is ineffective, treatment with two drugs (polytherapy) should be considered. However, when seizure control has not been attained after two medications, referral to an epilepsy specialist is in order.

Discontinuation of Antiepileptic Drug Therapy

Stopping unnecessary antiepileptic drugs is an essential aspect of treating childhood epilepsy. It avoids later drug-related concerns such as teratogenicity and effects on bone and mineral metabolism and endocrine function. When seizures are controlled for a year or more, the possibility of stopping antiepileptic drugs should be posed.

The chance of successfully withdrawing drug therapy is optimal when the following conditions are met: seizures were generalized, the child's development and neurologic examination were normal, the seizures were idiopathic, and the EEG has reverted to normal. Whereas failure to meet these conditions does not contraindicate trying to discontinue drug therapy, the chance of success decreases when there is evidence of underlying brain disease such as focal seizures or neurologic abnormalities.

The following are guidelines for discontinuing antiepileptic drugs:

1. Devise a plan with the family for getting emergency care in the unlikely event that the child has a

TABLE 4. **Useful Information for Administering Antiepileptic Drugs**

Drug	T$_{1/2}$ Range (h)	Time to Reach Stable Levels (wk)	Maintenance Dosage Range (mg/kg/d)	Therapeutic Range (μg/mL)
Carbamazepine	8–36	1–6	10–40	4–12
Clonazepam	16–60	1–2	0.1–0.3	0.04–0.07
Ethosuximide	15–68	1–2	10–75†	45–100
Felbamate	12–18	1	30–60†	Undefined
Gabapentin*	5–7	1	20–50	Undefined
Lamotrigine	22–26	1	2–5	Undefined
Methsuximide	18–30	1	10–20	10–20
Phenobarbital	37–126	2–3	1–5	10–30
Phenytoin	3–100	2	4–12	10–20
Topriamate	12–18	1	3–8	Undefined
Valproic acid	4–18	½	10–70†	50–100

*Not FDA approved for this indication (only adults).
†Exceeds dosage recommended by the manufacturer.

prolonged seizure. The discontinuation process should not be scheduled for a time when the family intends to travel afar. In the event of a prolonged seizure, the child should be taken to a facility equipped to treat pediatric emergencies.

2. Provide a schedule for withdrawing the medication over a reasonable time period.

3. Advise the resumption of the previous dose of medication if a brief seizure occurs, but request that the child's physician be notified so that follow-up can be arranged.

Most drugs such as valproate, phenytoin, or carbamazepine can be discontinued over a 6-week period or less. Drugs that need to be discontinued more slowly include benzodiazepines and barbiturates. Stopping benzodiazepines usually takes 6 months or longer because of the risk of provoking seizures.

Adjunctive Therapies for Childhood Epilepsy

Severe forms of childhood epilepsy do not respond to antiepileptic drugs but may respond to other treatments, such as adrenocorticotropic hormone (ACTH), in the case of infantile spasms, or to the ketogenic diet in severe generalized epilepsies such as Lennox-Gastaut syndrome. Surgical resection of the epileptic focus is an option for children with refractory epilepsy and partial seizures. Children with epilepsy due to approachable brain lesions should be considered for surgery in a timely fashion because epilepsy caused by brain lesions tends to resist drug treatment, resulting in frequent severe seizures that impede development. Although these therapies are needed infrequently and patient selection is complex, they should be explored in collaboration with an epilepsy specialist.

Epileptic Syndromes (Type of Epilepsy)

Approximately half the cases of childhood epilepsy can be categorized into an epileptic syndrome. Although syndromes are age-specific manifestations of epilepsy, a child may progress from one syndrome to another as he or she gets older. Syndromes are nonspecific in relation to etiology, and most have several causes. Some syndromes such as infantile spasms occur on both symptomatic and idiopathic bases; others (e.g., febrile seizures) are by definition idiopathic.

Febrile Seizures

Febrile seizures are diagnosed by exclusion. They are usually benign and do not necessitate treatment unless they result in convulsive status epilepticus. They also happen to be the most common cause of status epilepticus in young children. The two principal consequences of febrile seizures are recurrent febrile seizures and an increased risk of later epilepsy. The younger the child, the greater the chance of recurrences. For this reason, some authorities recommend prophylactic treatment for children who have a febrile seizure before age 18 months because in this group the risk of subsequent febrile seizures exceeds 50%.

Effective therapies for preventing febrile seizures include intermittently administered benzodiazepines and continuously administered valproate or phenobarbital. Orally administered diazepam (Valium), 0.33 mg per kg every 8 hours during fever, reduces the risk of recurrence by more than two thirds. Diazepam solutions for rectal administration (Diastat) in doses of 0.5 mg per kg given when fever occurs, are also effective. However, rectal diazepam administration is usually unnecessary unless seizures are prolonged (more than 5 minutes) or frequently repeated. Once the mainstay of febrile seizure prophylaxis, continuous phenobarbital administration has fallen out of favor because of side effects. Phenytoin and carbamazepine are ineffective, and although temperature-reducing interventions such as antipyretic administration or tepid baths seem logical, they have not been shown to reduce the chance of febrile seizures.

Absence Seizures in Childhood Absence Epilepsy (Petit Mal Epilepsy) and in Juvenile Myoclonic Epilepsy (JME)

Effective drugs in childhood absence epilepsy include ethosuximide (Zarontin), valproic acid (Depa-

TABLE 5. **Medications for Treating Convulsive Status Epilepticus**

Drug*	Route	Pediatric Dose	Adult Dose
Lorazepam	IV	0.05–0.5 mg/kg	0.1 mg/kg at 2 mg/min
		1–4 mg	4–8 mg
Diazepam	IV	0.1–1.0 mg/kg	10 mg
Diazepam	PR	0.5 mg/kg (maximum dose-20 mg)	
Phenytoin	IV	20 mg/kg over 20 min	15–20 mg/kg at 50 mg/min
Fosphenytoin†	IV	20 mg/kg of PE at 150 mg/min	20 mg/kg of PE‡ at 150 mg/min
Additional dose phenytoin		10 mg/kg at 1 mg/kg/min	10 mg/kg
Phenobarbital	IV	20 mg/kg	20 mg/kg at 50–75 mg/min

		Prime Dose	Continuous Infusion
Refractory Convulsive Status Epilepticus			
Midazolam		0.2 mg/kg	0.75–10 µg/kg/min
Propofol		2 mg/kg	2–10 mg/kg/h
Pentobarbital		10–15 mg/kg	0.5–1.0 mg/kg/h§

*Note that all of these agents can produce apnea and/or hypotension. Intensive supportive care, skilled nursing, and frequent monitoring of vital signs are essential aspects of treating status.

†Because of safety considerations fosphenytoin is replacing phenytoin for intravenous administration but is very expensive. For this reason it has not replaced intravenous phenytoin in all situations. Some clinicians reserve fosphenytoin for administration via peripheral intravenous routes and give phenytoin via central lines when they are available.

‡PE = phenytoin equivalents. Fosphenytoin is prescribed in phenytoin equivalents.

§Pentobarbital infusion is associated with a high risk of hypotension.

kote), and lamotrigine (Lamictal).* Although benzodiazepines such as clonazepam (Klonopin) are effective, frequent adverse effects of sedation, irritability, and dysphagia render them undesirable in this otherwise benign condition. The carbonic anhydrase inhibitor acetazolamide (Diamox) is also a valuable adjunct but is rarely needed. Valproic acid is preferred if the child also has generalized tonic-clonic seizures. However, families need to be advised about the rare possibility of valproate-associated hepatotoxicity.

The clinical manifestations of childhood absence epilepsy and JME overlap considerably in young children because both conditions cause absence seizures in the middle childhood years and because the EEG patterns are often identical. The elements of JME include absence seizures, myoclonic jerks often involving the neck, and generalized tonic-clonic seizures. All of the drugs that work in childhood absence epilepsy work in JME except ethosuximide. Therefore, valproic acid is the drug of first choice in JME.

Severe Pediatric Epilepsies: Infantile Spasms (West's Syndrome) and Lennox-Gastaut Syndrome

Infantile spasms and Lennox-Gastaut syndrome are the most common types of severe childhood epilepsy and have disastrous effects on development. Children with these types of severe epilepsy should be managed in collaboration with a specialist.

In the United States, most authorities recommend ACTH† for infantile spasms. When ACTH is initiated within 1 month of the onset of the spasms, it is most effective. Recommended doses are 40 to 80 IU of

ACTH gel or 150 IU per m² per day. ACTH is preferred over corticosteroids, but dose equivalents of 2 mg per kg per day of prednisone have been administered when ACTH injections were not feasible. Because children who respond to ACTH do so within the first 2 weeks, ACTH should be abandoned if the child does not respond in a timely fashion because the risk of a lethal complication increases with time. Overall, ACTH treatment should be limited to no more than 4 to 6 weeks. Among patients to whom ACTH has been given for 10 months or longer, the mortality rate exceeds 5%.

The drug vigabatrin (Sabril) is effective in children with symptomatic infantile spasms due to tuberous sclerosis. Although this compound has not been approved by the Food and Drug Administration, importation of limited amounts of the drug that were purchased abroad has been allowed on humanitarian grounds. The major troublesome side effect of concern is permanent constriction of visual fields, which has been suspected in approximately one third of adults treated chronically.

Conventional antiepileptic drugs have also been used to treat infantile spasms, although the probability of success is lower than with ACTH or vigabatrin. Potent antiepileptic drugs such as topiramate (Topamax), phenobarbital (Luminal), or clonazepam (Klonopin) have been used effectively in some children.

Lennox-Gastaut syndrome is similar to infantile spasms in that it is notoriously difficult to treat. Drugs that have been found effective in controlled randomized trials include topiramate and lamotrigine, but these rarely prevent all of the child's seizures. Felbamate (Felbatol) helps in some cases but should be considered as a last resort, owing to the potential adverse effects of aplastic anemia and fatal hepatotoxicity. Lamotrigine needs be instituted

*Not FDA approved for this indication (only adults).

†Not FDA approved for this indication.

slowly to minimize the chance of the Stevens-Johnson syndrome.

A major problem in treating children with the Lennox-Gastaut syndrome is that the diagnosis often is obscure when the child first begins having convulsions. When anticonvulsants such as carbamazepine, phenytoin, and phenobarbital are prescribed in this setting, they can provoke frequent astatic and/or atypical absence seizures. If this happens, the offending drug should be replaced by valproic acid or by one of the effective drugs listed earlier. If the child does not respond to medication, the ketogenic diet should be tried.

Convulsive Status Epilepticus

There are several effective approaches to treating status epilepticus in children, but the general principles are the same no matter which drugs are chosen. In so far as possible drugs should be given intravenously. When the intravenous line is inserted, blood should be obtained for the immediate measurement of glucose among other blood tests. If hypoglycemia cannot be ruled out, glucose should be given without delay. Furthermore, it is essential to have a plan of action to stop the seizures as quickly as possible: any reasonable plan is better than no plan at all.

The most popular approach is to begin with the lorazepam (Ativan) followed by fosphenytoin (Cerebyx) if there is concern that the seizures might recur (Table 5). Diazepam (Valium) used to be given first and is effective but short acting. Lorazepam is now preferred because it is longer acting. Other benzodiazepines, such as midazolam (Versed),* are also effective. Refractory convulsive status can be treated with anesthetic doses of phenobarbital, midazolam, propofol, or pentobarbital.

---

*Not FDA approved for this indication.

ATTENTION-DEFICIT/HYPERACTIVITY DISORDER

method of
TIMOTHY E. WILENS, M.D.
*Massachusetts General Hospital and
    Harvard Medical School*
Boston, Massachusetts

Attention-deficit hyperactivity disorder (ADHD used in this report refers to previously used definitions including hyperkinesis and ADD with or without hyperactivity) is the most common emotional, cognitive, and behavioral disorder pediatricians, family physicians, neurologists, and psychiatrists treat in children. It is a major clinical and public health problem because of its associated morbidity and disability. Epidemiologic studies indicate that ADHD is prevalent throughout the world, with consensus that from 4 to 9% of youth and up to 4% of adults have the disorder. Follow-up studies of ADHD children into adolescence and early adulthood indicate that ADHD frequently persists and is associated with significant psychopathology, school and occupational failure, and peer and emotional difficulties. Although previously thought to remit in early adolescence, ADHD is now seen as a chronic condition continuing into adolescence in approximately three fourths of cases and into adulthood in approximately half of childhood cases. These higher persistence findings are related to more recent information indicating that whereas many of the overt hyperactive-impulsive symptoms diminish over time, most attentional problems continue and are correlated with later difficulties. For example, in one study, 90% of ADHD adults presenting for treatment endorsed functionally impairing inattentive symptomatology. Predictors of ADHD persistence include prominent hyperactivity or impulsivity, aggression, co-occurring psychiatric and learning disorders, and a family history of ADHD.

DIAGNOSIS

The diagnosis of ADHD is made by careful clinical history applying criteria from the fourth edition of American Psychiatric Association's *Diagnostic and Statistical Manual of Mental Disorders* (DSM-IV), which is available in a user-friendly primary care version. Young persons with ADHD are characterized by a considerable degree of inattentiveness, distractibility, impulsivity, and often hyperactivity that is inappropriate for the developmental stage of the child. Other common symptoms include low frustration tolerance, shifting activities frequently, difficulty organizing, and daydreaming. These symptoms are usually pervasive; however, they may not all occur in all settings. Children with predominantly inattention may have more difficulties in school and in completing homework but not manifest difficulties with peers or family. Conversely, children with excessive hyperactive or impulsive symptoms may perform acceptably academically but have difficulties at home or in situations of less guidance and structure. Adults tend to present with prominent attentional difficulties affecting work, schooling, and relationships. ADHD adults frequently also manifest residua of impulsivity (intrusiveness, impatience) and hyperactivity (fidgetiness, restlessness).

Children, adolescents, and adults who have the cognitive features of the disorder (e.g., inattention, distractibility, shifting activities) but lack hyperactive or impulsive features are considered to have ADHD. Previously anchored by overactivity and impulsivity, connected to brain dysfunction and damage, the disorder has been reconceptualized based on *impaired cognition* as a core feature. Hence, depending on what symptoms predominate, the *DSM-IV* recognizes three subtypes of ADHD: a combined subtype (50 to 75% of cases), a predominantly inattentive subtype (20 to 30%), and a predominantly hyperactive-impulsive subtype (<15%).

Although not diagnostic, rating scales, checklists, and neuropsychiatric batteries may be helpful in providing evidence for the disorder and accompanying co-morbid conditions. Rating scales such as the Conners can be useful in assessing and monitoring school performance. Although neuropsychological testing is not relied on to diagnose ADHD, it may serve to identify particular weaknesses within ADHD or specific learning disabilities co-morbid with ADHD.

More than half of youth with ADHD are at risk for the development of co-occurring psychiatric disorders. The disruptive disorders are the best established co-morbid conditions, including oppositional (40 to 60% of ADHD cases) and conduct disorders (10 to 20%). More recently,

ADHD co-morbidity with anxiety (30 to 40%), depression (20 to 30%), and bipolar disorder (<20%) has been recognized. For example, whereas only a minority of ADHD individuals develop bipolar illness, an excess of ADHD is found in depressed (20 to 30%) and bipolar youth (50 to 90%). Persons with ADHD and its associated co-morbid conditions also are at a significant risk for higher rates and earlier ages at onset of cigarette smoking and alcohol and drug abuse.

Males are more commonly affected with ADHD than females, although underidentification in girls remains a major concern. ADHD females share with their male counterparts prototypical features of the disorder, such as inattention, impulsivity, and hyperactivity; high rates of school failure; and high levels of familiality. Compared with boys, girls with ADHD have lower rates of disruptive behavior, including conduct and oppositional disorders—common manifestations of ADHD in youth.

Although its precise neural and pathophysiologic substrate remains unknown, an emerging literature suggests the presence of abnormalities in frontal networks or frontal-striatal dysfunction. Studies have generally shown reduced corpus callosum and caudate volumes and reduced prefrontal cortex and anterior cingulate activity, although imaging studies have failed to demonstrate reversal in baseline abnormalities in ADHD adults with stimulant administration. Dopaminergic dysfunction in particular, and norepinephrine indirectly, appear to be important in the underlying neurochemistry of ADHD. Data from family-genetic, twin, and adoption studies as well as segregation analysis suggest a genetic origin for some forms of the disorder. Molecular genetic studies have implicated the dopamine D2 and D4 receptors and the dopamine transporter as candidate genes; there is evidence that in one third of ADHD subjects a repeat 7 polymorphism exists at the intramembrane region of the D4 receptor, affecting its ability to link with the intracellular potentiation of the neuronal impulse.

TREATMENT

The management of ADHD includes consideration of two major areas: nonpharmacologic (educational remediation, individual and family psychotherapy) and pharmacotherapeutic. Support groups for ADHD are an invaluable and inexpensive way for families to learn about ADHD and resources available for their children or themselves. Support groups can be accessed by calling an ADHD hotline or large support group organization (i.e., CHADD) or by using the Internet.

Specialized educational planning based on the child's difficulties is necessary in a majority of cases. Identification of co-morbid learning disorders, found in approximately one third of ADHD youth, should translate into the development of appropriate remediation plans. Parents should be encouraged to work closely with the child's school guidance counselor, who can provide direct contact with the child as well as valuable liaison with teachers and school administration. The school psychologist can be helpful in providing cognitive testing as well as assisting in the development and implementation of the individualized education plan. Educational adjustments should be considered in ADHD youth with difficulties

in behavioral or academic performance. Increased structure, predictable routine, learning aids, resource room time, and checked homework are among typical educational considerations in these youth. Similar modifications in the home environment should be undertaken to optimize the child's ability to complete homework. Frequent parental communication with the school about the child's progress is essential.

Focused therapies incorporating cognitive-behavioral features have been reportedly effective in children, adolescents, and adults with ADHD; however, the benefit of these treatments independent of pharmacotherapy has yet to be determined. Behavioral modification with the child and parents is useful in cases of co-occurring disruptive behaviors, inflexibility, anxiety, or outbursts. More traditional insight-oriented psychotherapy should be considered in ADHD cases with evidence of self-esteem issues, adjustment problems, or depression. Social skills remediation for improving interpersonal interactions and coaching for improving organization and study skills are useful adjuncts to treatment.

Pharmacotherapy

Medications remain a mainstay of treatment for ADHD (Table 1). In fact, multisite studies support that medication management of ADHD is the most important variable in outcome in the context of multimodal treatment. The stimulants, antihypertensives, and antidepressants comprise the available agents for ADHD.

Stimulants. The psychostimulants are considered first-line agents for ADHD based in part on their extensive efficacy and safety data. Stimulants are sympathomimetic drugs that increase intrasynaptic catecholamines (mainly dopamine) by inhibiting the presynaptic reuptake mechanism and releasing presynaptic catecholamines. The most commonly used compounds in this class include methylphenidate (Ritalin), dextroamphetamine (Dexedrine), amphetamine compound (Adderall), and magnesium pemoline (Cylert). Methylphenidate and dextroamphetamine are both short-acting compounds, with an onset of action within 30 to 60 minutes and a peak clinical effect usually seen between 1 and 2 hours after administration lasting 2 to 5 hours. The amphetamine compounds (Adderall) and sustained-release preparations of methylphenidate and dextroamphetamine are intermediate-acting compounds with an onset of action within 60 minutes and a peak clinical effect usually seen between 1 and 3 hours after administration maintained for up to 8 hours.

Despite the findings on efficacy of the stimulants, studies have also reported consistently that typically one third of ADHD individuals do not respond or cannot tolerate this class of agents. Although methylphenidate is by far the best studied stimulant, the literature suggests more similarities than differences in response to the various available stimulants. However, based on marginally different mechanisms of

TABLE 1. **Medications Used in Attention-Deficit/Hyperactivity Disorder**

Generic Medication	Brand Name	Daily Dose (mg/kg)	Common Adverse Effects
Stimulants			All age groups
Methylphenidate	Ritalin	1.0–2.0	Insomnia, decreased appetite, weight loss, moodiness
Amphetamines		0.3–1.5	Possible reduction in growth velocity with chronic use
Dextroamphetamine	Dexedrine		Rebound phenomena
Amphetamine compound	Adderall		
Methamphetamine	Desoxyn		
Magnesium pemoline	Cylert	1.0–3.0	Same as other stimulants Hepatitis
Antidepressants			All age groups Dry mouth, constipation
Tricyclics			
Imipramine	Tofranil	2.0–5.0	Weight loss
Desipramine	Norpramin		Vital sign and electrocardiographic changes
Nortriptyline	Pamelor	1.0–3.0	
Bupropion	Wellbutrin	3–6	Irritability, insomnia, seizure risk Contraindicated in bulimics
Venlafaxine	Effexor	0.5–3	Nausea Sedation
Antihypertensives			Juveniles only
Clonidine	Catapress	3–10 µg/kg	Sedation, depression, confusion Rebound hypertension Dermatitis with patch
Guanfacine	Tenex	30–100 µg/kg	Similar to clonidine but less sedation

action, some patients who lack a satisfactory response or manifest adverse effects to one stimulant may respond favorably to another. Stimulants should be initiated at the lowest available dosing once daily and increased every 3 to 4 days until a response is noted or adverse effects emerge. Typically, parameters for upward daily dosing of the stimulants are 1.5 mg per kg per day for the amphetamines, 2 mg per kg per day for methylphenidate, and 3 mg per kg per day for pemoline.

Predictable short-term adverse effects include reduced appetite, insomnia, edginess, and gastrointestinal upset. Pemoline may rarely cause hepatitis; hence, patient education about the symptoms of early hepatic dysfunction and infrequent liver function tests are advised. There are a number of controversial issues related to chronic stimulant use. Although stimulants may produce anorexia and weight loss, their effect on ultimate height is less certain. Initial reports suggested that there was a persistent stimulant-associated decrease in growth in height in children, but other reports have failed to substantiate this finding, and still others question the possibility that growth deficits may represent maturational delays related to ADHD itself rather than to stimulant treatment. Stimulants may precipitate or exacerbate tic symptoms in ADHD children. There is evidence that up to one third of children with tics may have worsening of their tics with stimulant exposure. Despite case reports of stimulant misuse, there is a paucity of scientific data supporting that stimulant-treated ADHD children abuse their medication; however, data suggest that diversion of stimulants to non-ADHD youth continues to be a concern. Recent studies indicate that pharmacotherapy of ADHD

(mainly stimulants) in children *reduces* substance abuse in midadolescence.

Antidepressants. The antidepressants are generally considered second-line drugs of choice for ADHD. The tricyclic antidepressants (TCAs)*—imipramine (Tofranil), desipramine (Norpramin), and nortriptyline (Pamelor, Aventyl)—block the reuptake of neurotransmitters, including norepinephrine. TCAs are effective in controlling abnormal behaviors and improving cognitive impairments associated with ADHD across the lifespan, but less so than the majority of stimulants. The TCAs are particularly useful in stimulant failures, or when oppositionality, anxiety, tics, or depressive symptoms co-occur within ADHD. Dosing of the TCAs is started with 25 mg daily and titrated upward slowly to a maximum of 5 mg per kg per day (2 mg per kg per day for nortriptyline). Although immediate relief can be seen, a lag of 2 to 4 weeks to maximal effect is common. Typical adverse effects include dry mouth, constipation, sedation, and weight gain. Four deaths in ADHD children treated with desipramine have been reported; however, independent evaluation of these cases has failed to support a causal link. Because minor increases in heart rate and the ECG intervals are predictable with TCAs, ECG monitoring at baseline and at therapeutic dose is suggested but not mandatory.

Bupropion (Wellbutrin)* is an antidepressant with indirect dopamine and noradrenergic effects. This agent has been shown effective for ADHD in controlled trials of children and an open trial in adults. Given its utility in reducing cigarette smoking, improving mood, lack of monitoring requirements, and

---

*Not FDA approved for this indication.

paucity of adverse effects, bupropion is often used as an initial agent for patients with complex ADHD who also are substance abusers or have an unstable mood disorder. On the basis of anecdotal reports of anti-ADHD effectiveness at low dosing in a minority of patients, it is recommended that the treatment be initiated at 37.5 mg and titrated upward every 3 to 4 days up to 300 mg in younger children and to 450 mg in older children or adults. Adverse events include activation, irritability, insomnia, and, rarely, seizures.

Although the serotonin reuptake inhibitors (i.e., Prozac, Zoloft) are not useful for ADHD, because of their noradrenergic reuptake inhibition, venlafaxine (Effexor) appears to have mild efficacy for ADHD. Monoamine oxidase inhibitors (MAOIs)* have been shown effective in juvenile and adult ADHD. The response to treatment is rapid, and standard antidepressant dosing is often necessary. A major limitation to the use of MAOIs is the potential for hypertensive crisis (treatable with verapamil) associated with dietetic transgressions with tyramine-containing foods such as most cheeses and interactions with prescribed, illicit, and over-the-counter drugs (pressor amines, most cold medicines, and amphetamines).

Antihypertensives. The antihypertensives clonidine (Catapress)* and guanfacine (Tenex)* are used to treat the hyperactive-impulsive symptoms of ADHD. Clonidine is a relatively short-acting compound with usual daily dose ranges from 0.05 to 0.4 mg. Guanfacine is longer acting and less potent than clonidine with usual daily dose ranges from 0.5 to 3 mg. The antihypertensives have been used for the treatment of ADHD as well as associated tics, aggression, and sleep disturbances, particularly in younger children. Although sedation is more commonly seen with clonidine, both agents may cause depression and rebound hypertension. The combination of clonidine plus methylphenidate has been implicated in the deaths of four children; however, many mitigating and extenuating circumstances were operative, making these findings uninterpretable. Cardiovascular monitoring (vital signs, electrocardiography) remains optional.

Combined pharmacologic approaches can be used for the treatment of co-morbid ADHD, as augmentation strategies for patients with insufficient response to a single agent, for pharmacokinetic synergism, and for the management of treatment emergency adverse effects. Examples include the use of an antidepressant plus a stimulant for ADHD and co-morbid depression (e.g., fluoxetine [Prozac] plus methylphenidate), the use of clonidine to ameliorate stimulant-induced insomnia, and the use of a mood stabilizer plus an anti-ADHD agent to treat ADHD co-morbid with bipolar disorder.

Unfortunately, there are a number of individuals who either do not respond to, or are intolerant of the adverse effects of, medications used to treat their ADHD. Youth who are nonresponders to one stimu-

lant should be considered for another stimulant trial. If two stimulant trials are unsuccessful, bupropion and the tricyclic antidepressants are reasonable second-line agents. Antihypertensives may be useful for younger children or those with prominent hyperactivity, impulsivity, and aggressiveness. MAOIs and cognitive activators such as donepezil (Aricept)* may be considered for refractory youth. Combined pharmacologic regimens including stimulants plus antidepressants or antihypertensives may accentuate the response to monotherapy and/or treat co-morbid conditions (i.e., ADHD plus depression or anxiety).

In summary, there is increasing recognition that ADHD is a heterogeneous disorder that persists in a number of cases into adult years. The scope of co-morbidity has expanded to include not only conduct and oppositional defiant disorder but also mood, anxiety, and substance use disorders. Emerging findings support a genetic and neurobiologic basis for ADHD with catecholaminergic dysfunction as a central finding. An extensive literature supports the effectiveness of pharmacotherapy not only for the core behavioral symptoms of ADHD but also improvement in linked impairments, including cognition, social skills, and family function. Similarities between juveniles and adults in the characteristics, biology, and pharmacologic responsivity of ADHD support the continuity of the disorder across the lifespan.

---

*Not FDA approved for this indication.

GILLES DE LA TOURETTE SYNDROME

method of
JEFFREY SVERD, M.D.
Sagamore Children's Psychiatric Center
New York State Office of Mental Health
Dix Hills, New York

Once considered rare, Gilles de la Tourette syndrome is increasingly recognized as a common hereditary neuropsychiatric spectrum disorder characterized by childhood or adolescent onset of motor and vocal tics and obsessive-compulsive behaviors. The fourth edition of the American Psychiatric Association's *Diagnostic and Statistical Manual (DSM-IV)* defines a tic as a sudden, rapid, recurrent, nonrhythmic, stereotyped motor movement or vocalization. This definition applies best to simple tics that are abrupt and myoclonic-like. Dystonic tics, which are also considered simple tics, are characterized by slower and more sustained muscle contractions. Simple motor tics include eye blinking, eye darting movements, head and arm jerks, facial twitches, and abrupt mouth opening. Dystonic motor tics include head tilts, sustained elevation of the shoulders, and sustained mouth opening. Motor tics are also defined as patterned sequences of coordinated involuntary movements. This definition is best applied to complex motor tics.

Some complex motor tics, however, may appear purposeful, and voluntary and some compulsive behaviors may be difficult to distinguish from complex motor tics. For example, about 50% of patients with Tourette's syndrome (TS) describe the experience of an urge to tic or the experience

---

*Not FDA approved for this indication.

of a variety of localized dysphoric sensations that precede and are often relieved by the performance of the tic. Because these motor behaviors may be compelled by the experience of an involuntary sensation, a number of TS experts suggest the terms "semivoluntary" or "unvoluntary" to more accurately describe the nature of some complex motor tics. Examples of complex motor tics include hair out of the eyes head tic, face touching, object touching, obscene gestures, finger and object smelling, hopping, skipping, knuckle cracking, and neck cracking.

Vocal tics include throat clearing, sniffing, grunts, barking sounds, clicking and squeaking. Complex vocal tics include whistling, belching, echolalia, and palialalia, the repeating of one's own utterances sometimes in a whisper. Corprolalia, the involuntary utterance of obscenities, occurs in less than 20% of TS patients.

The diagnosis of TS requires the presence of motor and one or more vocal tics that appear simultaneously or at different times during the illness. Tics must be present throughout a period of more than 1 year. "Transient tic disorder" refers to motor or vocal tics with a duration of less than 1 year, and "chronic tic disorder" refers to the presence of motor or vocal tics, but not both, for more than 1 year. *DSM-IV*, in contrast to its predecessors *DSM-III* and *DSM-III-R*, stipulates that tics must cause significant distress or impairment in important areas of functioning to meet criteria for the diagnosis of a tic disorder. The *DSM-IV* category of tic disorder not otherwise specified, however, allows for diagnosis of tic symptoms that do not meet criteria for other tic disorders. Chronic tic disorder and a significant portion of transient tic disorders are genetic variants of TS and thus represent milder forms of TS. Tics characteristically wax and wane in frequency and severity, fluctuate over time, are suppressible for periods of time, and may be exacerbated by stress and self-consciousness and attenuated during absorbing activity.

The syndrome occurs throughout the world, and its characteristics are similar across cultures. Because of more thorough case ascertainment and recent epidemiologic studies, it has been suggested that the prevalence of TS and tics is far greater than previously realized. One study conducted in a single school district reported that 1 in 169 children had TS (1 in 95 boys and 1 in 759 girls) and that 1 in 45 boys and 1 in 379 girls had some symptoms of TS not meeting strict criteria for the diagnosis of TS. About 25% of children in special education had tics, and in another study 65% of the children in special education categorized as emotionally and behaviorally disordered had tics. One study estimated that the prevalence of all tic disorders combined was 4.2%, with an approximately 2:1 ratio for boys to girls, and other studies conducted with mainstream school populations reported prevalence estimates for TS of 3% and 6% for tics.

The average age of onset of tics is about 7 years. Studies of the natural history of tic disorder suggests maximal severity of tics occurs between ages 8 and 12 years, that tics ameliorate with age, and that approximately one third of cases remit during adolescence or early adulthood, one third show significant improvement in symptoms, and the remaining third are symptomatic throughout early adulthood and middle age. Current data suggest that the prognosis for tic symptoms is more favorable than previously thought.

THE ASSOCIATED SPECTRUM OF NEUROPSYCHIATRIC DISORDER

Research conducted since the late 1950s on the accompanying psychiatric symptoms in patients with TS and their relatives provides support for the hypothesis that a significant relationship exists between tic disorder and a wide array of neuropsychiatric disturbances. Among the psychiatric symptoms and disorders frequently present in patients with TS are attention deficit hyperactivity disorder (ADHD), learning and behavioral problems, antisocial and temper problems, mood and anxiety disorders, sleep disorder, self-injurious behavior, inappropriate sexual behavior, alcohol and substance abuse, gambling, eating disorder, paranoid thinking, and hallucinatory experience. In addition, significant associations between TS and autistic disorder and TS and sudden infant death syndrome have been reported. A number of studies indicated that the severity of chronic tics is a clinical indication of complex psychopathology.

There is general consensus that a significant subgroup of obsessive-compulsive disorder is a genetic expression of TS. From 30% to 60% of patients with TS have obsessive thoughts and compulsive rituals, and 30% to 90% of clinical populations have been reported to have ADHD. High rates of tic disorder in children referred for ADHD have also been reported. My experience is that most children referred for ADHD show evidence of mild tic disorder that goes unrecognized by family and clinicians. There is agreement that at least a portion of ADHD is a result of TS.

GENETICS AND NEUROBIOLOGY

Early studies of the mode of genetic transmission of TS and chronic tics suggested that an autosomal dominant trait with reduced penetrance was the most likely mode of inheritance. Linkage analysis to determine if a known genetic marker occurs more often in carriers than in noncarriers, however, has not been successful, and more than 90% of the genome has been excluded. As a result, more complex modes of inheritance are being entertained. A polygenic model of inheritance suggests that the presence of multiple genetic defects, affecting multiple central nervous system neurotransmitter systems, each contributing a small, but additive, effect is responsible for the diverse neuropsychiatric phenotype associated with TS. Psychiatric disorder and tics are conceptualized as the result of the chance convergence of multiple genetic defects inherited from maternal and paternal sides of the family (bilineal transmission).

The genetic defects proposed to contribute to the pathophysiology of TS and co-morbid disturbance involve the metabolism of dopamine, serotonin, norepinephrine, and other neurotransmitter systems such as glutamate and gamma-aminobutyric acid (GABA). For example, different allelic forms of the D_2 and D_3 dopamine receptor genes, the dopamine beta-hydroxylase gene, and the dopamine transporter gene are among the defects implicated in the dopamine system, and genetic defects in the serotonin system have been reported and include abnormalities in the serotonin 1A receptor gene and two polymorphisms in the tryptophan 2,3-dioxygenase gene.

Clinical evidence implicates the basal ganglia and related corticothalamic brain regions as the site of abnormalities in TS, and neuroanatomical and neurobiological studies provide evidence for the involvement of cortico-striato-thalamo-cortico circuits (CTSC). The functioning of these neuronal circuits involves complex interactions of neurotransmitters, including dopamine, serotonin, glutamate, and GABA. Noradrenergic influences from the brain stem may influence the activity of some of the CSTC circuits. One neuroimaging study reported a high correlation between differences in D_2 receptor binding in the head of the caudate in identical twins discordant for tic severity, which supported a relationship between hypersensitivity of D_2 receptors and tic severity.

Up-regulation of dopa decarboxylase, the enzyme responsible for converting dopa to dopamine, and elevated availability of dopamine transporters in the caudate nucleus have been reported. Neuroimaging studies have documented abnormal sizes of structure within the basal ganglia and a reduction in basal ganglia volume associated with decrease in glucose metabolism and cerebral blood flow. Finally, a number of studies have reported an association between group A beta-hemolytic streptococcal infection and the development of tics, TS, and obsessive-compulsive disorder. This phenomenon has been termed *pediatric autoimmune neuropsychiatric disorder associated with strep infections*. Further study of this hypothesis is required.

TREATMENT

The decision to treat tics depends on their severity and impact on various aspects of the patient's life. Assessment is made of the effects of tics on family, peer, and social relationships, school and job functioning, and the individual's sense of physical and psychological comfort. The mere presence of tics does not require treatment, and sometimes a correct diagnosis is sufficient. Because patients with tic disorder may experience an array of psychiatric symptoms, assessment for the presence of past and current psychiatric symptoms is important. Evaluation of children and adolescents should include particular attention to the possible presence of symptoms of ADHD and learning difficulties.

When it is determined that treatment of tics is necessary, neuroleptic medications, primarily haloperidol (Haldol),* fluphenazine (Prolixin),* and pimozide (Orap),* are favored. These medications, which are dopamine antagonists, have been proven effective in controlled studies. Haloperidol was first used to treat TS in 1961 and has been reported to improve 60% to 80% of patients treated. Treatment is begun with 0.25 mg given at bedtime and raised by 0.25 mg every 4 days. Patients and family are informed of potential side effects and assessment of drug response and side effects is made by phone contact and office visits after treatment is begun. Dosage is slowly titrated upward (often more slowly than every 4 days) until symptoms are reduced by approximately 70% without adverse effects. Effective dosages range from 1.5 to 10 mg and are given in divided doses as the dose is increased. Higher doses may be required by some patients.

Because symptoms vary, titration of the dose over time permits detection, reduction, or remission of symptoms so that the lowest possible dose is used. Fifty percent of patients develop adverse effects, which can be managed successfully, and approximately 25% of patients may be unable to tolerate the side effects. Haloperidol treatment may be associated

with a number of side effects. The possible emergence early in treatment of dystonic reactions such as oculogyric crisis is explained to families, and the risk is reduced when small doses of an anticholinergic are added. I often prescribe benztropine mesylate (Cogentin) 0.5 mg once or twice daily as the dose of haloperidol approaches 1.5 mg daily.

If acute dystonia develops, intravenous benztropine completely reverses the reaction, and an oral antiparkinsonian medication is added or the dose is increased and haloperidol treatment is continued sometimes at a lower dose. Doses of benztropine up to 6 mg may be used. Other parkinsonian-like side effects may be managed by neuroleptic dose reduction or addition of anticholinergic or stimulant medications. Tremors, muscle rigidity, shuffling gait, drooling, akathisia, and akinesia are examples. Akathisia consists of motor restlessness, pacing, and skin sensations, and akinesia consists of tiredness, apathy, loss of motivation, depression, and joint and muscle aches. Cognitive impairment consisting of memory and attention problems may result in decline in school and job functioning. All of the above adverse effects may be counteracted by use of stimulant or anticholinergic medication and/or haloperidol reduction. Other side effects include sedation and drowsiness and the anticholinergic effects of the anticholinergic and neuroleptic medications such as constipation, dry mouth, and mydriasis.

Fluphenazine and pimozide are as effective as haloperidol and have a similar spectrum of side effects although sedation and extrapyramidal effects may occur less frequently. Although pimozide has been shown to potentially increase the QT interval, a number of TS experts have not found significant electrocardiographic (ECG) alterations. Some clinicians choose to monitor treatment with baseline and periodic ECGs and discontinue treatment if the QT interval is prolonged. Treatment with fluphenazine and pimozide is started with low doses (0.5 to 1 mg; and 1 mg, respectively) followed by increments of the same dose every 5 days. The maximum recommended dose of pimozide for children is 10 mg daily and for adults it is 20 mg daily. The effective dose range for fluphenazine is between 2 and 15 mg daily.

Clonidine (Catapres),* an alpha$_2$-adrenergic receptor agonist, is frequently used to treat children with ADHD and TS. Early studies suggested efficacy of clonidine in suppressing tics; however, the limited controlled study that has been conducted has not uniformly established efficacy, and there is insufficient evidence to demonstrate its efficacy in the treatment of ADHD and aggressive behavior. Most recently the reports of significant cardiovascular toxicity associated with its use alone or in combination with methylphenidate (Ritalin) has led to concern about its widespread use. Of greatest concern is clonidine's potential to produce hypotension, bradycardia, and ECG abnormalities and noradrenergic overdrive and hypertension subsequent to its abrupt

---

*Not FDA approved for this indication.

*Not FDA approved for this indication.

withdrawal. Exercise-related syncope has also been associated with its use.

Recent reports of accidental overdose associated with the use of the transdermal patch are of additional concern. The latter results from compromise of the integrity of the patch membrane, resulting in excess clonidine absorption. Cutting the patch to accommodate slower dosage increase is therefore not recommended.

A number of TS experts believe that many patients derive benefit from clonidine. In my view, cautious use may be justified if patients are unresponsive to other pharmacotherapeutic interventions and/or salutary effects of the medication on tic symptoms and behavior disorder are clearly evident. Physicians who choose to use clonidine should be thoroughly aware of the cardiovascular toxicities of the drug and should obtain baseline cardiovascular evaluation and periodic assessment of pulse, blood pressure, and ECG. Further systematic research and clinical experience is needed in the use of clonidine.

Clonidine treatment is initiated at 0.05 mg daily and increased weekly by 0.05 mg doses. Daily doses not to exceed 0.5 mg are given in three to four divided doses. The transdermal patch is supplied in 0.1-mg, 0.2-mg, and 0.3-mg doses applied weekly and beginning at the 0.1-mg dose for the first week. Sedation, headache, and dry mouth are additional side effects. Oral clonidine discontinuation must be gradual to prevent rebound hypertension. Allergic and contact dermatitis occur in 42% of patients treated with the transdermal patch.

Use of the psychostimulants for the treatment of children with co-morbid tic disorder and ADHD has been controversial because of the belief that the stimulants exacerbate or provoke emergence of tics in vulnerable individuals. The results of double-blind placebo-controlled studies of methylphenidate and clinical follow-up treatment do not support this long-held belief, and methylphenidate may be safely used by most patients with ADHD and tics. I do not hesitate to use methylphenidate as the first-line treatment for ADHD in children with tics or TS and follow the same procedure when treating ADHD children who are not diagnosed with tics.

Although little controlled study exists for the other stimulants, my clinical impression is that pemoline and dextroamphetamine are tolerated well; however, a definitive statement cannot be made until controlled study is undertaken. For other co-morbid psychiatric symptoms, TS patients derive benefit from the same psychotropic medications used to treat depression, obsessive-compulsive disorder, and other anxiety disorders. The use of serotonin reuptake inhibitors in combination with neroleptics may result in increased risk for drug-induced parkinsonism.

HEADACHE

method of
ELIZABETH LODER, M.D.
Harvard Medical School and Spaulding
Rehabilitation Hospital
Boston, Massachusetts

GENERAL CONSIDERATIONS AND DIAGNOSIS

Headache is a leading cause of visits to physicians. Over half of patients with headache initially consult their primary care provider; less than one fourth see a neurologist or headache specialist. Because headache is very common and its causality is debated, however, clinicians in nearly every patient care specialty can expect to be consulted at some time by patients with headache and will benefit from a broad general understanding of the optimal approach to this common complaint. There is consensus that primary headache disorders are not properly diagnosed or treated, and recent studies have demonstrated the significant social, economic, and financial burdens of suboptimally treated headache.

Headaches can be divided into primary and secondary headache disorders. In the primary headache disorders of migraine, tension-type, and cluster headache, headache itself is the problem. These headaches are increasingly recognized as biological, genetically based functional disorders of the nervous system. Secondary headache disorders are those in which the headache is due to some underlying cause, such as meningitis, malignancy, or infection. There are myriad causes of secondary headache, and appropriate treatment of the underlying disorder generally improves or eliminates the headache. Detailed discussion of the secondary headache disorders is beyond the scope of this article.

Only 1 in 250,000 patients who present with a chief complaint of headache are found to have a secondary cause of headache. Almost all patients have one of three benign headache disorders: migraine, tension-type, or cluster headache. These should not be viewed as diagnoses of exclusion to be arrived at only after exhaustive testing has ruled out other less common and more ominous possibilities. Rather, migraine, tension-type, and cluster headache are clinical diagnoses based on simple, well-validated exclusion and inclusion criteria developed by the International Headache Society (IHS). The criteria were initially developed to aid in conducting clinical trials of headache treatment, and it is important to understand their limitations. In particular, these criteria have high specificity (negative in patients who do not have the disorder) but low sensitivity (positive in those with the disorder) to ensure that patients enrolled in clinical trials are highly likely to have the condition under study. Experienced clinicians often make a presumptive diagnosis based on fewer criteria and proceed with treatment.

Familiarity with the typical patterns of migraine, tension-type, and cluster headache will be more than repaid by improved diagnostic certainty and efficiency in clinical practice. In addition to the patterns outlined by IHS criteria, other factors such as a stable headache pattern over time, association with hormonal fluctuations, and resolution with sleep are reassuring that a headache is benign.

Although many patients and physicians are initially concerned about the possibility of a serious cause of headache such as a brain tumor or aneurysm, in most cases a careful history and physical examination are enough to rule out those alternatives. Because serious causes of headache are rare and the primary headache disorders are common, for patients whose presentation lacks worrisome features it is more productive to focus on ruling in the diagnosis of a primary headache disorder. Generally speaking, the patient with a normal physical and neurologic examination and a history consistent with one of the patterns of benign headache should not be subjected to further diagnostic testing. Rather, efforts should be directed at instituting appropriate treatment for the diagnosis and testing reserved for patients who do not respond as expected to such treatment.

Multiple studies have demonstrated that the diagnostic yield of imaging studies in this situation is extremely low. For patients whose headaches meet criteria for migraine and who have a normal neurologic examination, only 0.4% of imaging studies are positive for any abnormality, and the majority of those "abnormalities" are such things as "white, bright spots" with no clinical or therapeutic implications. Very often, a scan with such a finding only serves to increase, rather than decrease, patient anxiety. The electroencephalogram (EEG) has no utility in the diagnosis of headache. Many patients and physicians fail to appreciate that one of the most helpful "tests" for headache disorders is the passage of time: A patient whose headache pattern and neurologic status has been normal over a period of years is extremely unlikely to have a life-threatening cause for the headaches.

Patients with worrisome features of headache, such as onset after age 50 years, headache associated with abnormal examination findings, or headaches unresponsive to treatment require a more thorough workup and perhaps referral to an appropriate specialist. It is worth mentioning that such popular ideas as "sinus" headaches or headaches due to allergy are usually mistaken. Most of those patients actually have migraine and benefit from treatment for that disorder.

THE HEADACHE HISTORY AND PHYSICAL EXAMINATION

A carefully obtained headache history is often sufficient to confidently make a diagnosis of one of the benign headache disorders, which will be corroborated by a subsequent normal neurologic and physical examination. Anxious family members may accompany the patient to the consultation and can be useful in verifying the description of the headache, related disability, and treatment trials, but the history should be obtained from the patient whenever possible. Questions should focus on the frequency and severity of headaches, age at onset, development over time and associated features, triggers, and relieving factors. Previous diagnostic tests and treatment trials should be recorded, including, when possible, the dosage of and length of time a particular agent was used. Leading questions should be avoided if possible, and patients should be encouraged to discuss whatever hidden fears or ideas they may have about the headaches. Patient recall of headache frequency and severity is commonly inaccurate. Information from one of a number of common *headache diaries* is very helpful in making an accurate headache diagnosis and in planning and assessing the response to treatment interventions.

Although many patients, with a minimum of prompting, give a history that is clearly consistent with criteria for one of the major headache disorders, some patients are poor historians or offer vague, conflicting, or difficult-to-recognize stories. Often the headache problem is long-standing, and the patient arrives with extensive diagnostic records, multiple imaging studies, and lists of failed treatment attempts. In these cases, an invaluable technique is to ask the patient to describe the pattern of headaches *when they began* (often many years ago) rather than to focus on the current, usually confusing, headache presentation. Very often the history of the initial headache will be easily recognized as the more pure form of one of the major headache disorders, before behavioral factors, medication overuse, and learned behavior intervened to obscure the diagnosis.

MIGRAINE

Migraine headaches affect approximately 20% of the population and are three times more common in females than in males. Women with migraine tend to have more frequent and more severe headaches than do men with migraine. Incidence peaks in the late teens and early twenties, but the disorder is not uncommon in children, for whom vomiting and abdominal symptoms may be more prominent than the headache. The severity of migraine waxes and wanes through the life cycle, but for most patients it is a chronic disorder. Although the frequency and severity of migraine typically improve as patients grow older, migraine may remain a problem well into old age.

Contrary to popular opinion, migraine is more common in lower socioeconomic groups, perhaps because the burden of migraine renders patients less able to compete effectively in society, school, and the workplace, leading to the phenomenon known as "downward socioeconomic drift." In addition, migraine sufferers in lower socioeconomic groups are more likely to be exposed to many of the trigger or aggravating factors that precipitate the onset or increase the severity of the disorder in those who inherit a genetic vulnerability to it. Patients in lower socioeconomic groups are often less aware that treatment options for migraine exist and may not have regular access to health care. They are particularly likely to seek care episodically through emergency rooms or walk-in clinics for especially severe bouts of headache, where they may be branded "drug seeking" and the treatable disorder of migraine goes unrecognized.

Because migraine is not a life-threatening disorder, the disability it causes has been underappreciated. This in turn has led to less than aggressive treatment and to the development of significant occupational and personal limitations over a lifetime, some of them iatrogenic. Although migraine is not itself life-threatening, many of the treatments for it can be. The development of addiction to nonspecific barbiturate or narcotic medications, gastric bleeding from overuse of anti-inflammatory medications, and end-stage renal disease from analgesic nephropathy are all too common in headache patients. Primary care providers are in an ideal position to diagnose and intervene early in the course of this illness and prevent much of its long-term morbidity.

MIGRAINE

The Pattern

Migraine is a relatively long headache, lasting between 4 and 72 hours when untreated or suboptimally treated. Although full-blown attacks are at least moderate to severe in intensity, many patients will have other *forme fruste* attacks that are mild and lack all the recognizable characteristics of migraine. If treatment for these milder attacks is necessary, the treatments employed for more severe migraine attacks will be effective.

In its pure form, migraine is an episodic disorder. Between headaches, the patient feels well and functions normally. If the disorder is poorly treated or complicated by analgesic overuse and rebound headache, patients who begin with episodic migraine can develop a mild to moderate, featureless chronic headache pattern with superimposed exacerbations that are clearly migrainous. This situation is termed *transformed migraine* and can be differentiated from chronic tension-type headache by obtaining a careful chronologic history of headache development in which it will become clear that the daily headache pattern evolved over the years from initial episodic migraine. When the overuse of medication is eliminated (a difficult and protracted process for most patients) the earlier, episodic headache pattern will generally be restored and specific antimigraine medications will be more effective for the headache episodes.

The pain of a fully developed migraine headache is usually described by patients as throbbing or pounding. Patients may use descriptive terms such as "a little man pounding inside my head." A common misconception is that migraine pain *must* be unilateral. In fact, the pain is often, though not always, unilateral. Many migraine patients experience generalized pain on the top of the head or in the posterior aspect of the head or neck. Although patients often report that their headaches are usually on a particular side, it is not worrisome or uncommon for the headache to switch sides. In fact, this switching of sides is generally considered to be an indication of the benign underlying mechanism of migraine in contrast to the headache attributable to a fixed structural lesion that is unvarying in location.

Nausea and vomiting are often features of migraine (hence the old-fashioned term "sick headache," almost always a reference to migraine). These may be present early in the headache, but more commonly begin and increase in intensity as the headache progresses. Successful early treatment may prevent these symptoms from appearing at all.

Barium studies of the gastrointestinal tract have shown that gastric stasis precedes the development of nausea in most migraine patients. It is important to remember that this stasis may impede the absorption of oral treatments for migraine. The use of prokinetic agents such as metoclopramide (Reglan) or cisapride (Propulsid) may improve absorption of oral medications for migraine. In fact, one study showed that metoclopramide plus a large dose of an aspirin-like drug was equivalent in efficacy to oral sumatriptan (Imitrex). In other situations, the early development of prominent nausea or vomiting mandates treatment by another route, either parenteral or rectal. Nasal spray formulations of some migraine medications seem to be at least partly absorbed through the gastrointestinal tract, after they drip down the oropharynx and are swallowed, so may not be optimal when severe nausea and vomiting are present. Nausea and vomiting are often very prominent features of migraine in children and adolescents and decrease in intensity and sometimes disappear altogether as patients grow older.

Photophobia and phonophobia, as well as osmophobia, are also noticeable migraine features for many patients. These may be present to some degree even between attacks, and exposures to bright light, loud noise, or strong odors may be powerful triggers for the onset of migraine in some patients. Physical activity during a migraine commonly aggravates the headache. Often even mild exertion causes an increase in headache intensity and, for some patients, can precipitate headaches. Those patients benefit from "warm up" exercises and gradual onset of activity. In refractory cases, a dose of a beta blocker or nonsteroidal anti-inflammatory medication 1 hour before activity will prevent the exercise-induced headache from occurring.

From 10 to 15% of patients with migraine have migraine with aura. In the usual case, some type of focal neurologic sign or symptom develops gradually over 30 to 60 minutes and then fades away as the headache begins. The most common aura involves some type of visual phenomenon, often photopsia (bright flashes of light) or the appearance of jagged lines or castle-like outlines (fortification spectra). These begin in the periphery of the visual field and spread toward the midline before fading away. Less commonly, patients experience complete loss of vision, numbness, tingling, weakness, or confusion. Many patients have a prodrome of vague signs and symptoms such as yawning, fatigue, elation, or a mild sensation of being less mentally alert, which cannot technically be classified as aura. Patients do not always have aura with every headache, but when it occurs it is generally stereotyped from attack to attack. Thus, it is unexpected for a patient to have a visual aura with one attack and weakness with the next. As patients age, aura may occur without the subsequent headache. In some patients, the unexpected nature of the aura is more alarming than the attack itself—worth remembering before assuming that every patient is in the office seeking relief from only the headache.

Basilar migraine, in which headache is associated with signs or symptoms of brain stem dysfunction, and hemiplegic migraine, which as the name implies is associated with hemiplegia, are rare. Familial hemiplegic migraine is an autosomal dominant disorder, and the diagnosis mandates a history of similar attacks in a first-degree relative. This particular disorder has been linked to an abnormality on chromosome 19. The genetics of "garden-variety" migraine have not yet been determined, but it seems inescapable that it will turn out to be a heterogeneic disorder.

Patients who have aura often worry that their aura symptoms place them at risk for the development of stroke. Although there does seem to be an increased relative risk of stroke in migraine patients, particularly those with aura, the elevation in absolute risk attributable to migraine is low; other risk factors such as smoking, hypertension, and elevated cholesterol or triglyceride levels are much more powerful. In theory, patients who have prolonged or complicated aura may benefit from the prophylactic use of neuroprotective calcium channel blockers or platelet inhibition with low-dose aspirin, but no studies have yet addressed this question.

Treatment

General Considerations

For all patients whose headaches are severe enough to come to medical attention, nonpharmacologic treatment techniques should be employed. These techniques can minimize, although not often eliminate, the need for medication and allow medication to work more effectively. For most patients, efforts should be made to identify and avoid or modify environmental trigger factors that increase the risk of attacks.

The underlying cause of migraine has not been completely determined, but it seems clear that genetic factors operate to determine an individual's *headache threshold*. In these persons there is a predisposition to develop a migraine headache in response to any one or a combination of environmental trigger factors. Common triggers of this headache response in susceptible individuals include lack of sleep or variation in sleep habits, skipping meals, physical or emotional stress, and hormonal fluctuations, especially a fall in estrogen levels such as occurs before the menstrual period, after childbirth, during the pill-free week of oral contraceptive (OC) use, or with an interrupted dosing regimen of hormone replacement therapy (HRT).

Although it is common for one trigger to seem most important in a particular case (e.g., hormonal factors in women with menstrual-associated migraine), it is never the case that a single trigger is responsible for causing all of a particular patient's headaches. Most migraine patients find that many factors affect their susceptibility to headache. Some triggers may be too weak individually to affect headaches, but can be important when acting in concert with other triggers. Thus, a patient with menstrual-associated migraine may develop headaches in response to lack of sleep only during the time of month when hormonal factors are also operative. Patients should be strongly discouraged from developing the idea that their headaches would cease if they only had their ovaries removed or found the one environmental toxin, allergen, or malaligned vertebra that is "causing" their headaches.

It cannot be overemphasized that for most migraine patients, emotional stress is a trigger, rather than a cause, of headaches. Patients who avoid emotional stress when possible or learn relaxation techniques to help deal with stress frequently improve, but they do not stop having migraine attacks. Patients for whom emotional stress is a prominent trigger do well with simple relaxation techniques, yoga, aerobic exercise, or formal training in biofeedback techniques. When stress is recognized as a trigger, these treatments should be started early and used in combination with other treatments rather than reserved for later, more severe stages of illness when they will be less effective. The expectation is that they will augment, not supplant the need for, other therapies, including medication. It is helpful to point out to patients that emotional stress is a known trigger of worsening in such clearly biologically based illnesses as angina pectoris, asthma, and diabetes mellitus.

Although the role of specific dietary factors in triggering migraine has not been carefully studied, anecdotal, poorly validated lists abound of foods and substances to be avoided by the migraine patient. It is important to appreciate the poor quality of the evidence for most of these recommendations and to forgo making patients fearful or overly cautious about their diet. In particular, the common practice of handing patients long lists of foods they should avoid is to be condemned. Many of these lists contain such common dietary staples as "dairy products" or "citrus fruits." The long-term health implications of proscribing such foods for young, healthy patients, many of whom are women in their childbearing years, should be carefully considered. More reasonable is for patients to keep food and headache diaries in an attempt to isolate foods that seem to play a role in triggering specific attacks. Patients can then experiment with eliminating the suspect item from their diet for a few weeks, then reintroduce it, and see if headache attacks correlate in any way with intake of that food item.

The association between migraine and psychiatric disorders has long been a controversial and contentious subject, often pitting polarized patient views ("I'm depressed because I have these horrible headaches") against those of the physician ("you have headaches because you are depressed"). In fact, epidemiologic evidence suggests that the relationship between psychiatric disorders and migraine is *bidirectional*. This implies that underlying central nervous system abnormalities, perhaps disturbances in serotonergic mechanisms, predispose patients to develop one or both disorders. In other words, neither one can be said to cause the other (although they certainly influence the course and response to treatment of the other disorder), but susceptibility to both is due to a third, shared etiologic factor.

There is clear and compelling evidence that patients with migraine, especially migraine with aura, are at increased risk of developing depression, anxiety disorders, and panic attacks. Recognition and treatment of these co-morbid disorders usually simplify the treatment of migraine, but rarely eliminate the attacks. The co-morbid occurrence of disorders such as depression and anxiety or panic may tip the balance in favor of one treatment that can beneficially affect both disorders, such as a tricyclic antidepressant. It can also suggest avoidance of therapies such as beta blockers, which may aggravate depression, or dictate caution with medications such as barbiturate-containing analgesics or opioids, which may be particularly prone to overuse by patients with affective illness.

Abortive Treatment

Essentially all patients whose migraines come to medical attention at some point during their illness require abortive medication to modify or stop an attack of headache. Despite the nausea and vomiting associated with migraine, patients have a strong preference for oral medications. Use of an antiemetic or prokinetic agent such as metoclopramide before or with an oral drug often allows this route of administration despite nausea.

In the past, abortive treatment of migraine was limited to symptomatic treatment with agents such as barbiturate-containing medications (Fiorinal, Fioricet, Phrenelin, Esgic) or opioids that modified the pain but caused unwanted sedation. These drugs are also potentially habit forming and cause drug-induced rebound headache in many patients when used on a daily basis, even in small amounts. Milder analgesics such as nonsteroidal anti-inflammatory agents, isometheptene/dichlorophenazone (Midrin), or acetaminophen have proved and remain useful for mild attacks but are not powerful enough for severe attacks and have also been implicated in analgesic rebound headache. An over-the-counter combination of acetaminophen, aspirin, and caffeine (Excedrin Migraine) recently obtained an indication for treatment of mild migraine, but the clinical trials excluded patients with nausea or vomiting, and its usefulness for many patients is limited. Semispecific agents such as ergotamine (Cafergot, Wigraine, Ercaf) are useful for many patients, but often cause nausea and vomiting, which discourage their use early in an attack or require the addition of antiemetics that have their own set of side effects, particularly sedation. Semispecific agents do have the advantage of being available in oral, sublingual, and suppository formulations, usually in combination with caffeine. Agents that contain caffeine produce analgesic rebound headache more readily than other drugs, and their use more than two or three times a week should be strongly discouraged.

Dihydroergotamine (DHE-45) is an older drug that has always been underappreciated. Although related to ergotamine, it is less likely to cause nausea and has a long half-life with a very low recurrence rate. For years it was available only in a parenteral formulation, which largely limited its use to emergency and office settings. Recently it has been introduced in a nasal spray formulation (Migranol), but technical problems make it cumbersome to use and its onset of action is quite slow. Parenteral DHE, however, remains an excellent choice for emergency treatment of migraine.

The last decade has seen a major advance in the treatment of migraine with the development of the triptans, agonists at the serotonin 1B and 1D receptor subtypes. Agonist activity at these receptor sites seems to augment the natural inhibitory system for migraine. The triptans are specific, targeted antimigraine agents with unprecedented efficacy against the entire symptom complex of migraine. Sumatriptan (Imitrex) was the first in this class. Subcutaneous sumatriptan is available in an easy to use autoinjector, which delivers a 6-mg dose of the drug. From 70 to 80% of patients in clinical trials experienced improvement in headache (from moderate or severe to mild or none at 1 hour). As of this writing, parenteral sumatriptan remains the gold standard against which other drugs are judged. Sumatriptan is also available in nasal spray formulations of 20 and 5 mg. This form of delivery has not proved as popular as expected, perhaps because of a prolonged and unpleasant bitter taste noted by many patients. The oral form of the drug is available in the United States in 25-mg and 50-mg tablets. Fifty milligrams has proved to be the optimal dose for the majority of patients, although up to 100 mg per dose can be given. Doses should be separated by at least 2 hours. Use should not exceed more than 300 mg oral, 2 nasal sprays, or 2 injections of the subcutaneous form per 24 hours. Many patients want to have more than one version of the drug available: Parenteral administration is necessary when the patient awakens with a well-established headache with vomiting, whereas the more convenient and acceptable oral formulations are preferred for other headaches that develop slowly.

Although an excellent drug, sumatriptan has limitations. Headache recurrence is a problem for up to 30% of patients, low oral bioavailability may be related to a lack of consistent response, and chest or neck pain has proved troublesome for some patients, although serious cardiac side effects have been uncommon.

Newer triptans, all in only oral formulations, have recently been introduced, each of which offers some theoretic advantage over sumatriptan in certain settings. Zolmitriptan (Zomig) is available in 2.5-mg and 5-mg tablets and may offer improved efficacy over oral sumatriptan. It has been shown to be equally effective in treating migraine associated with menses and regular migraine attacks. Its activity at the 1A receptor may account for its tendency to aggravate or cause nausea in some patients. The dose of zolmitriptan can be repeated every 2 hours as needed. The maximum daily dose of zolmitriptan should not exceed 10 mg.

Naratriptan (Amerge) is available in 1-mg and 2.5-mg tablets. Its 2-hour efficacy is significantly lower than that of all other oral triptans. Although the dose can be repeated if needed after 2 hours, the long half-life means that many patients may not need to redose, making this drug useful for patients with slow to start but prolonged headaches.

Rizatriptan (Maxalt) is the most recently introduced triptan, and it is available in 5-mg and 10-mg tablets. It is the only triptan also available as an orally disintegrating wafer, which offers convenience for patients who cannot swallow pills or do not have easy access to water. Comparative trials suggest that rizatriptan has an advantage over zolmitriptan and naratriptan in time to relief of headache. The drug can be repeated as needed every 2 hours with a maximum dose of 30 mg per 24 hours. There is an interaction with propranolol (but no other beta blocker), which mandates a reduction in rizatriptan dose to 5 mg and 15 mg per 24 hours for patients on propranolol.

No evidence suggests that any triptan offers a safety advantage over the others when they are used in pharmacologically equivalent doses. The perceived safety advantages of some of the new drugs likely stems from their recent introduction to the market or from the decision to market a low dose version of a drug. All of the triptans can constrict coronary arteries in vivo, and it is to be expected that, given the passage of time, reports will be received of adverse cardiac events occurring in association with use of the all of the triptans. These drugs should not be used by patients with known coronary artery disease and should be used with caution by patients who have risk factors for coronary artery disease. In practice, this means that judgments need to be made, with the patient, about whether the benefits of the triptans outweigh the potential risks in an individual situation. Although there has been a great deal of publicity about the cardiac side effects of the triptans, not enough attention has been paid to the long-term morbidity associated with overuse of barbiturate-containing and other nonspecific headache medications.

Overuse of triptans has not been convincingly associated with rebound headache, although anecdotal reports of this complication exist. The reasons to avoid daily use are that the safety of daily use has never been established in clinical trials and that the expense of these drugs is considerable. Combining different triptans can be done but as a rule should be discouraged because this can be confusing for some patients and has not been assessed in carefully done trials. Combination of triptans and ergotamines should be avoided; labeling suggests an interval of 24 hours between these medications.

Many managed care organizations have begun to advocate a "step care" approach to abortive migraine treatment, with patients required to fail therapy with simple analgesics, nonspecific analgesics, and semispecific drugs before being allowed to use the relatively more expensive triptans. This economically driven approach fails to consider the cost to the patient of unsuccessful therapy as well as potential patient dropout from treatment and the expense of emergency room visits made necessary by suboptimal treatment. For this reason, most headache experts encourage the use of "stratified care" in which the individual patient's headache frequency, headache severity, and other factors are considered in the decision about treatment.

Prophylactic Treatment

The goal of prophylactic treatment of migraine is to reduce headache frequency and intensity and to render abortive therapy more effective. Prophylaxis should be considered for patients with more than two headaches a week and for those who do not respond adequately to abortive treatment. The advent of specific and highly effective abortive treatment for migraine has reduced the need for prophylaxis for many patients.

Although it is still common for managed care organizations and even some headache experts to recommend prophylaxis for any patient with more than two headaches a month, in practice this is rarely desirable. Most patients dislike the idea of taking medication daily, particularly if they have highly effective abortive treatment for their headaches. In addition, even the most effective prophylactic agents reduce headache frequency by more than 50% for only 50 to 60% of patients. All prophylactic agents cause significant side effects for some patients. Many of the commonly used prophylactic agents are used "off label," with no FDA indication for migraine.

It is particularly important to remember that sodium valproate (Depakote), although a highly effective antimigraine agent, is associated with neural tube defects. Most migraine patients are women in their childbearing years, and for this population sodium valproate should not be considered a first-line drug for prophylaxis in view of the risk of unintended pregnancy.

A common reason for failure of prophylactic medication is the use of an inadequate dose of the drug for an inadequate length of time. Because many patients experience relief of headaches at low doses, many of the drugs should be started at a low dose and gradually increased. About 6 to 8 weeks are necessary to judge the effect of a particular dose, and headache diaries should be kept to aid in evaluation. Monotherapy is preferable, but combinations of drugs can work synergistically. Studies are lacking to guide determination of optimal length of therapy. Most experts favor continuing an effective prophylactic regimen for at least 6 months. Many patients wish to continue beyond that time, but those who are anxious to be off medication can after 6 months taper the dose slowly and monitor headache patterns, restarting or increasing the dose if necessary. Clinically, tachyphylaxis to prophylaxis appears to occur in some patients, but there has been no systematic evaluation of regimens that might avoid or minimize this problem.

Another reason for failure or reduced effectiveness of both prophylactic and abortive medications for migraine is overuse of short-acting abortive medications. No treatment for migraine works well when these drugs are overused. This situation often develops insidiously, and it is frequently difficult for the patient to recognize and accept the contribution of medication overuse to their situation. Patients often underestimate their use of short-acting abortive medications, and a headache diary is useful to alert them to the problem.

It is worth the effort early in headache treatment to avoid the pattern of daily use of abortive medication because there is no easy way of managing the problem once it occurs. Discontinuation of the problematic medication usually restores the prior episodic headache pattern, but only after the passage of weeks or months. Because of this slow improvement, it is difficult to convince the patient to refrain from use of the offending medication. Various strategies such as the use of repetitive doses of intravenous DHE, substitution of mild sedative or anxiolytic medications, or the use of steroids to suppress the headache can be helpful. Some patients require hospitalization for gradual withdrawal of the abortive medication. (This is mandatory for safe withdrawal from large amounts of barbiturate-containing medications.)

Prophylactic Therapy in Special Situations

Most women with migraine note some association of headache with their menstrual periods. In some cases, these menstrual-associated headaches are longer or more resistant to treatment than headaches occurring at other times of the month. Although for many women standard abortive treatment suffices, women whose menstrual periods are regular and whose headaches occur in predictable relation to the period can benefit from perimenstrual "mini-prophylaxis" of headache. Nonsteroidal anti-inflammatory drugs are most commonly employed in this manner and are typically given in scheduled doses beginning 1 to 2 days before the expected onset of headache and continued for its expected duration (e.g., flurbiprofen [Ansaid], 100 mg tid for 3 to 5 days perimenstrually). Other prophylactic agents can be tried in this manner, or the dose of one already used can be increased perimenstrually. One open-label trial found benefit from sumatriptan 25 mg tid used perimenstrually by patients with menstrual-associated migraine.

TENSION-TYPE HEADACHE

The Pattern

Tension-type headache is best thought of as a relatively featureless, mild headache. It is described as a tight, band-like pressure sensation and is not associated with pronounced nausea, vomiting, or sensitivity to light or noise. In contrast to migraine, it is often improved by physical activity or alcohol, and it responds well to simple analgesics or rest. For these reasons, patients with episodic tension-type headache rarely come to medical attention.

Pure, isolated chronic tension-type headache, in which headache is present more than 15 days per month, is uncommon; more often it coexists with superimposed episodes of migraine. It is important to distinguish this pattern, by a careful history, from transformed migraine. Patients with chronic tension-type headache suffer significant disability, despite the moderate nature of the pain. The unrelenting, chronic nature of the discomfort is often more wearing than intermittent, more intense bouts of pain.

Treatment

General Considerations

Tension-type headache has been less well-studied than migraine, and considerable controversy exists among experts as to its cause and treatment. Many view it as part of a headache continuum, with migraine at one end and tension-type headache at the other, and advocate treating it as migraine. Others continue to believe it is associated with muscle tension or psychopathology despite evidence that many patients whose headaches meet criteria for tension-type headache cannot be shown to have elevated muscle tension or excess rates of psychiatric disorders or emotional tension. In fact, migraine patients as a group have higher levels of muscle tension and psychiatric problems than do patients with tension-type headache.

Abortive Treatment

Most patients with tension-type headache obtain relief from simple analgesics such as aspirin or isometheptene (Midrin). When headaches are infrequent, the use of these medications is harmless, but when headache frequency is above two or three attacks a week there is a danger of inducing analgesic rebound headache. For these patients, the use of abortive treatments should be limited and prophylaxis considered. One recent study found the triptans to be as useful for patients whose headaches meet criteria for tension-type headache as for those whose headaches are migrainous. The use of barbiturate-containing or opioid medications to treat tension-type headache should be discouraged for all of the reasons reviewed in the discussion of migraine.

Prophylactic Treatment

Few studies of prophylaxis for tension-type headache exist. Most clinicians prescribe the tricyclic antidepressants or sodium valproate, but support exists for the traditional migraine prophylactic agents as well, including beta blockers. Nonpharmacologic prophylaxis with aerobic exercise and biofeedback is also useful and should be emphasized for most patients. There is no evidence that psychiatric treatment is useful or should be recommended for patients without co-morbid psychiatric diagnoses.

CLUSTER HEADACHE

The Pattern

Cluster headache is rare, occurs most commonly in men, and is often misdiagnosed. The average primary care provider may encounter one or two cases in a career. Once one is familiar with its unmistakable pattern, however, it is difficult to miss. This is a gratifying illness to treat because it, of all the primary headache disorders, responds most readily to prophylactic treatment.

The term *cluster* derives from the tendency of this headache to occur daily for periods of several weeks or months and then disappear for months or years. These cluster episodes often appear at characteristic times of the year (particularly around the vernal and autumnal equinoxes) and occur from 1 to 8 times a day. The propensity of these headaches to occur at exactly the same time each day has led to use of the term "alarm clock headache." The headache itself is located behind one eye and is described as a steady, intense pain that builds quickly to a crescendo and lasts 15 minutes to 3 hours. This short but excruciating headache is accompanied by some kind of ipsilateral autonomic sign such as lacrimation, conjunctival injection, ptosis, or nasal stuffiness. During (but not between) cluster episodes, individual attacks can be brought on by ingestion of even small amounts of alcohol and are frequently triggered by the onset of rapid eye movement sleep. Patients are commonly wild with pain during an attack and have been known to become violent or bang their heads against a wall.

Treatment

General Considerations

Patients with cluster headache are often misdiagnosed as having sinus problems, dental problems, or serious intracranial pathology. Many have undergone sinus surgery, tooth extractions, and multiple imaging studies. Not a few have been diagnosed as having migraine and treated ineffectively for that disorder. Patients with cluster headache may be more likely than the general population to abuse nicotine and/or alcohol. No evidence exists to suggest that psychopathology plays a role in cluster headache, and there is no justification for dietary or lifestyle modifications other than abstinence from alcohol.

Abortive Treatment

Because cluster headache develops rapidly, is very short, and is extremely severe, abortive treatment must work rapidly and be highly effective. Only subcutaneous sumatriptan and inhalation of oxygen can be considered first-line abortive treatments for most patients with cluster headache.

Sumatriptan is approved by the FDA for treatment of cluster headache and should be given in its subcutaneous form; oral and even nasal spray formulations do not work quickly enough to be acceptable treatment for most patients. Oxygen (100%) administered at a flow rate of 10 to 12 liters per minute via a nonrebreather mask for 10 to 15 minutes provides relief for 70 to 80% of patients, an efficacy comparable with that of subcutaneous sumatriptan. Both treatments can be used by patients at home, obviating trips to the emergency department. Because these two treatments are very effective, the use of parenteral narcotics should rarely be necessary.

Prophylactic Treatment

In contrast to migraine, for which prophylaxis is indicated for only a subset of patients, virtually all patients with cluster headache should be offered prophylactic medication. For all but a few patients, prophylactic agents will, within 1 week, eliminate or dramatically reduce the number of headaches. Patients should continue the drug for the expected duration of the cluster episode. In most cases, it is desirable to discontinue the drug once the cluster episode is past, but restart it immediately when the next episode commences.

THE REFRACTORY HEADACHE PATIENT

Misdiagnosis, psychiatric co-morbidity, and inadequate trials of treatment account for many cases of seeming refractoriness to treatment and should be vigorously sought when headaches do not respond as expected to therapy. For some patients, however, it is the case that current medical knowledge and therapy are simply inadequate. It is rare, though, that those patients cannot be helped to cope better with the effects of their illness. The goals of therapy should shift from cure to management, and avoidance of further iatrogenic harm, for example, from drug addiction or overuse, should be paramount. Some patients profit from involvement in a chronic pain management program that emphasizes improvement in function and minimizes reliance on medication. A subset of truly refractory patients may benefit from maintenance therapy with long-acting opioid medications; generally that course of treatment should be decided upon with the aid of a physician experienced in the treatment of refractory pain and headache.

EPISODIC VERTIGO

method of
RONALD J. TUSA, M.D., PH.D.
University of Miami
Miami, Florida

"Dizziness" is an imprecise term used to describe a variety of symptoms, including vertigo, lightheadedness, dysequilibrium, motion sickness, and nausea. Each of these symptoms has a different pathophysiologic mechanism and significance. In this discussion the focus is on episodic vertigo, which is the illusion of movement of self or environment from sudden change in tonic neural activity in the vestibular-cortical pathway (labyrinth/eighth nerve/vestibular nucleus/vestibular thalamus/vestibular cortex). Briefly discussed are episodic lightheadedness, motion sickness, and dizziness from bilateral vestibular loss. Table 1 lists the most common disorders of episodic vertigo, the prevalence of each disorder in 1300 patients evaluated, and the treatment. A discussion of each of these disorders follows.

TABLE 1. **Summary of Manifestations of Episodic Vertigo (Based on 1300 Patients)**

Disorder	Prevalence	Duration	Treatment
Benign paroxysmal positional vertigo	37%	Seconds	Acute: Canalith repositioning maneuver Chronic: Brandt-Daroff habituation
Acute vestibular neuritis, labyrinthitis, Ramsay-Hunt syndrome	15%	Days	Acute: promethazine, prednisone, acyclovir* (Ramsay Hunt syndrome) Chronic: Vestibular rehabilitation
Migraine	13%	Minutes	Acute: Sleep Chronic: Avoid foods with tyramine; therapy with beta blocker if necessary
Panic attack, hyperventilation, chronic anxiety	11%	Minutes	Acute: Alprazolam (Xanax) Chronic: Reassurance, stress reduction, selective serotonin reuptake inhibitor
Bilateral vestibular deficit	9%	Days	Chronic: Vestibular rehabilitation
Meniere's syndrome	6%	Days	Acute: promethazine or meclizine (Antivert) Chronic: <2 mg Na diet/day, diuretic, surgery if necessary
Orthostatic hypotension or intolerance	5%	Seconds	Chronic: Reduce antihypertensives, salt load, fludrocortisone, midodrine
Stroke	2%	Days	Acute: Bed rest, ondansetron (Zofran)* if necessary Chronic: Physical therapy
Motion sickness	1%	Minutes–hours	Acute: Dimenhydrinate (Dramamine) or scopolamine patch (Transderm-Scop) Chronic: Avoid visual-vestibular mismatch

*Not FDA approved for this indication.

ACUTE VESTIBULAR NEURITIS, LABYRINTHITIS, AND RAMSAY HUNT SYNDROME

Clinical Features

Acute vestibular neuritis, labyrinthitis, and Ramsay Hunt syndrome manifest as intense vertigo, nausea, and dysequilibrium that persist for days. After a few days the symptoms begin to resolve and the patient is left with a dynamic deficit (vertigo and dysequilibrium induced by rapid head movements) that can last for weeks to months until central compensation occurs.

Vestibular neuritis behaves very much like Bell's palsy and is believed to frequently represent a reactivated dormant herpes infection in Scarpa's ganglia, which innervates the labyrinth. It is preceded by a common cold 50% of the time. The prevalence of vestibular neuritis peaks at 40 to 50 years of age.

Labyrinthitis can be classified as serous (viral) or suppurative (bacterial). Viral infection presumably invades the membranous labyrinth through a hematogenous route. Bacterial infection gains access to the perilymphatic space within the labyrinth and produces a purulent inner ear infection. The route of bacterial spread may be from the middle ear through a bony fistula in the otic capsule or, more commonly, from the cerebrospinal fluid (meningitis) through the cochlear aqueduct or internal auditory canal. Patients with bacterial labyrinthitis are seriously ill and have severe auditory and vestibular impairment when compared with patients with serous labyrinthitis. Acute or chronic ear infections can also cause labyrinthitis as a result of toxins and noxious enzymes entering the inner ear.

Ramsay Hunt syndrome is due to varicella-zoster and is a variant of vestibular neuritis with multiple cranial nerves involved. It primarily causes facial paresis, tinnitus, hearing loss, and a vestibular defect. It can also involve cranial nerves V, IX, and X. The incidence is 20 per million per year.

Diagnosis

All three disorders cause an acute unilateral vestibular defect. Spontaneous horizontal and torsional nystagmus occurs, and the caloric test is markedly reduced on the side of the defect. Vestibular neuritis and viral labyrinthitis are distinguished from each other based on hearing preservation; if there is significant hearing loss (frequently with tinnitus), it is labeled labyrinthitis; otherwise it is labeled vestibular neuritis. Viral cultures are not necessary, because their results do not alter treatment. Ramsay Hunt syndrome can also be diagnosed by clinical examination (unilateral vestibular defect, hearing loss, and facial weakness). A Tzanck smear of vesicles in the external auditory canal will identify multinucleated giant cells. Serologic confirmation can be made through enzyme-linked immunosorbent assay or IgM (varicella zoster virus IgM).

Treatment

Management of acute vertigo from vestibular neuritis or labyrinthitis varies depending on how many days have elapsed since the onset (Table 2). The patient is admitted to the hospital only if extreme dehydration is present from vomiting (rarely necessary) or if a central disorder is suspected. Blood studies including a fluorescent treponemal antibody absorption test and erythrocyte sedimentation rate should be obtained to rule out otic syphilis and vasculitis. An audiogram should be obtained if the patient

TABLE 2. **Management of Acute Vertigo**

Days 1 to 3

Administer vestibular suppressants
Prescribe bed rest (hospitalize if patient is dehydrated or central defect is suspected)
Perform laboratory tests; if central defect is suspected, obtain computed tomography or magnetic resonance imaging of head

After Day 3

Stop vestibular suppressants
Prescribe vestibular adaptation exercises
Perform laboratory tests:
    Audiogram (obtain immediately if Meniere's disease is suspected)
    Caloric
    Blood work (rheumatoid factor, sedimentation factor, antinuclear antibody, fluorescent treponemal antibody absorption) if vascular cause is suspected

complains of hearing loss. Vestibular suppressant medications can be employed for symptomatic treatment. I prescribe promethazine (Phenergan), 25 mg intramuscularly, in the office at the onset of severe vertigo, and then send the patient home for 3 days of bed rest with Phenergan suppositories to be taken as needed (Table 3). This medication causes sedation and reduces nausea. It should be used for 1 week or less because the acute phase of the disorder is self-limited. Prednisone during the first 10 days of the attack may shorten the course of the illness. In Ramsay Hunt syndrome, treatment initiated within 3 to 7 days with prednisone and acyclovir (Zovirax),* or other antiherpes agents, may improve recovery and reduce facial nerve degeneration and hearing loss. The patient should be seen again in a few days to make certain the symptoms are resolving. After 1 week it is important to stop the vestibular suppressants and refer the patient for vestibular rehabilitation. At this time the patient usually no longer has

*Not FDA approved for this indication.

spontaneous vertigo but does have a dynamic deficit in which vertigo and unsteadiness occur during head movements. This dynamic deficit can be repaired only by vestibular adaptation. To facilitate vestibular adaptation, the patient is encouraged to move the head while viewing a stimulus (Table 4). In addition, the patient is given exercises to improve postural control, at first while standing still and then with head and body movement through space. The patient usually improves faster and more completely if these exercises are coordinated by a physical therapist trained in vestibular rehabilitation.

BENIGN PAROXYSMAL POSITIONAL VERTIGO

Clinical Features

Patients with benign paroxysmal positional vertigo (BPPV) usually complain of vertigo that lasts less than 1 minute. It usually occurs in the morning when the patient arises or turns over in bed. It may also occur when the patient lies down in bed or moves the head back. After a bad attack, the patient frequently complains of dysequilibrium that lasts for several hours. BPPV is usually idiopathic, but it can also occur after head trauma, labyrinthitis, and ischemia in the distribution of the anterior inferior cerebellar artery. The pathophysiologic mechanism for BPPV is usually due to portions of otoconia from the utricle that are misplaced and free floating in the posterior semicircular canal (canalithiasis). Occasionally, it is due to otoconia attached to the cupula of this canal (cupulolithiasis). Both of these conditions inappropriately cause the afferents from the posterior semicircular canal to discharge after the head stops moving backward.

Diagnosis

The diagnosis is secured by eliciting a torsional-upbeat nystagmus associated with vertigo during the

TABLE 3. **Medications for Dizziness**

Drug Type	Drug Example	Indications	Dosage
Antiviral	Acyclovir (Zovirax)	Ramsay Hunt syndrome	400 mg 5×/day × 10 days
Antianxiety	Alprazolam (Xanax)	Panic attacks	0.25 mg q 8 h prn for up to 1 wk
Antihistamine	Dimenhydrinate (Dramamine)	Motion sickness	50 mg prn
Mineralocorticoid	Fludrocortisone (Florinef)	Orthostatic hypotension	0.1–0.6 mg q day
Antihistamine and anticholinergic	Meclizine (Antivert or Bonine)	Acute vertigo from Meniere's disease, vestibular neuritis	25–50 mg q 6 h × 3 days maximum
Vasopressor	Midodrine (ProAmatine)	Orthostatic hypotension	5–10 mg tid
Serotonin antagonist	Ondansetron (Zofran)	Severe nausea from central vertigo	4 mg q 8 h for 3 days
Selective serotonin reuptake inhibitor	Paroxetine (Paxil)	Panic attacks, hyperventilation, anxiety	10–20 mg q am
Anti-inflammatory	Prednisone	Acute vestibular neuritis, labyrinthitis, Ramsay Hunt syndrome	60 mg q day, then taper over 10 days
Phenothiazine	Promethazine (Phenergan)	Acute vestibular neuritis, labyrinthitis, Ramsay Hunt syndrome	25 mg PO, IM, suppository q 6 h
Beta blocker	Propranolol (Inderal LA)	Migraine	40–80 mg bid
Anticholinergic	Scopolamine patch (Transderm Scop)	Motion sickness	1 patch for 3 days

TABLE 4. **Vestibular Rehabilitation for Patients with Loss of Vestibular Function**

Exercises to Enhance the Vestibular-Ocular Reflex

Tape a business card on the wall in front of you so that you can read it. Move your head back and forth sideways, keeping the words in focus. Move your head faster, but keep the words in focus. Continue to do this for 1–2 minutes without stopping, several times a day. Repeat the exercise, moving your head up and down. After this exercise can be easily accomplished, try to read portions of the newspaper or pages in a book while oscillating the head for 1–2 minutes several times a day.

Exercises to Improve Static Balance

1. Stand with your feet placed as close together as possible with both hands touching the wall to help maintain balance. Take your hand off the wall for longer and longer periods of time while maintaining your balance.
2. Stand with feet placed shoulder-width apart with eyes open, looking straight ahead at a target (an "X") on the wall. Slowly narrow your base of support by moving your feet closer together. Start with your feet apart, then feet together, then one foot slightly forward but still next to the other, and then heel to toe (one foot directly in front of the other). You should change your foot position 1 inch at a time. Hold each position for 15 seconds and then move on to the more difficult exercise. This exercise can be performed with arms outstretched, with arms close to the body, or with arms folded across the chest. The exercise can also be repeated with eyes closed, at first intermittently and then continuously, all the while making a special effort to mentally visualize the surroundings.
3. Practice standing on a cushioned surface. Progressively more difficult tasks might be done on a hard floor (linoleum, wood), thin carpet, shag carpet, thin pillow, or sofa cushion. Graded-density foam can also be purchased.
4. Stand with your feet as close together as possible. Then turn your head to the right and left horizontally while looking straight ahead at a target (an "X") on the wall for 1 minute without stopping. The size of your head movement should be approximately ±30 degrees. As you improve, you can move your head more rapidly (always seeing clearly) and can move your feet closer together to make the exercise more difficult.

Exercises to Improve Dynamic Postural Stability

1. Practice walking with a more narrow base of support. You can do this first by touching the wall for support and then gradually lessening touching to only intermittently and then not at all.
2. Walk close to a wall, turning your head to the right and to the left while walking. You should try to focus on different objects while you walk. As you improve, try to turn your head more often and faster, always seeing clearly. Try the same exercise moving your head up and down.
3. Practice turning around while you walk, at first making a large circle but gradually making smaller and smaller turns. Be sure to practice turning in both directions.
4. Practice standing and then walking on ramps, either with a firm surface or with a more cushioned surface.
5. Play catch, at first without much movement but then being required to move in order to catch the ball. Try walking and tossing a ball while you walk.
6. Practice walking through an obstacle course. The course should include different surfaces, turns, small and large steps, and curbs or stairs. You can also walk this course while carrying a heavy bag or while playing catch.
7. Out in the community, practice walking in a mall before it is open and therefore while it is quiet; practice walking in the mall while walking in the same direction as the flow of traffic; walk against the flow of traffic. Try walking up and down the aisles of a grocery store without a cart. Try walking in a grocery store while turning your head from side to side.

Hallpike-Dix test (Figure 1A, B) when the affected ear is inferior. The nystagmus usually has a latency of 3 to 20 seconds, fatigues in less than 1 minute, and habituates with repeat maneuvers.

Treatment

BPPV is best treated by a maneuver that moves the otoconia out of the posterior semicircular canal and back into the utricle. I use primarily a single treatment approach modified from Epley, which is now generally referred to as the canalith repositioning maneuver (see Figure 1). Total remission or significant improvement from BPPV occurred in 90% of patients treated with this maneuver. Complications from the canalith repositioning maneuver are rare. During the procedure, a Hallpike-Dix maneuver is first performed toward the side of the affected ear and the head is kept down for 1 minute. Then the head is rotated toward the unaffected side and the patient is rolled over onto this side until the face is pointed down. The patient is kept in this position for 1 minute. With the head deviated toward the unaffected side, the patient then slowly sits up. To make certain the debris does not move back toward the cupula the patient is fitted with a soft collar and

told not to bend over or look up or down for 1 day. In addition, he or she is told to sleep sitting up during this period. For the subsequent 5 days the patient is allowed to lie down, but only on the unaffected side. After 7 days the patient is re-evaluated to make certain the maneuver worked. It is unclear what happens to the free-floating otoconia after the treatment, but presumably it is reabsorbed into the calcium matrix in the utricle. If the initial treatment does not work, then the patient is re-treated. In patients who cannot tolerate sleeping upright for 1 to 2 days, I use a different maneuver described by Brandt and Daroff. In this maneuver, the patient sits on a table sideways, rotates the head 45 degrees horizontally, and then rapidly lies on his or her side in the opposite direction and waits until the vertigo has resolved or for 10 seconds (Figure 2). The patient then rapidly sits up and waits for the same period of time. The movement is then repeated in the opposite direction. This is repeated 5 to 10 times and performed once or twice a day. Unlike the single treatments described earlier, this treatment usually takes 1 to 2 weeks before symptoms resolve. The maneuver works either by habituation or by dislodging debris from the cupula of the posterior semicircular canal. Vestibular suppressant drugs do not have a role in

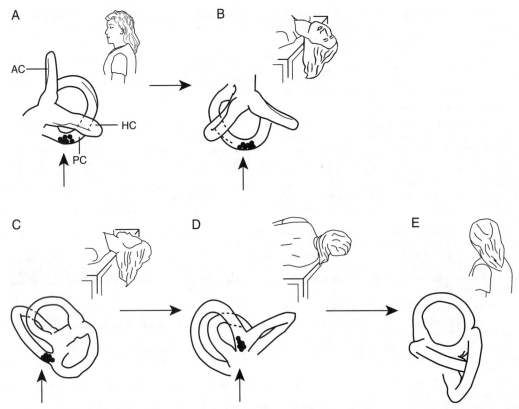

Figure 1. Hallpike-Dix test and Canalith repositioning maneuver for BPPV. In the Hallpike-Dix test, the patient sits on the examination table with the head turned 45 degrees horizontally *(A)*. The head and trunk are quickly brought straight back "en bloc" so that the head is hanging over the edge of the examination table by 20 degrees *(B)*. Nystagmus is looked for and the patient is asked if he or she has vertigo. Although not shown in the figure, the patient is then brought up slowly to a sitting position with the head still turned 45 degrees and nystagmus is looked for again. This test then is repeated with the head turned 45 degrees in the other direction. This figure also shows movement of free-floating otoconia in the left posterior semicircular canal *(large black arrows)* during the Hallpike-Dix test. In this example, the patient would have nystagmus and vertigo when the test is done on the left side but not when the test is done on the right side.

In the canalith repositioning maneuver the patient is first moved from sitting *(A)* into the Hallpike-Dix position with the head turned 45 degrees toward the affected side *(B)*. After 1 minute, the patient's head is turned so the opposite ear is down *(C)*. After 1 minute he or she is rolled onto the shoulder with the nose pointed 45 degrees down *(D)*. After 1 minute, the patient sits up, keeping the head turned while coming into the sitting position *(E)*. The patient is then asked to keep the head upright for the next 24 hours to allow the otoconia to incorporate back into utricle. Because the otoconia will move whenever the head is moved during this maneuver, the patient should be advised to expect vertigo to occur several times during the treatment. Some patients only experience vertigo during the initial movement into the Hallpike-Dix position.

the treatment of BPPV unless the patient refuses to do the treatment because of excessive vertigo and nausea.

MENIERE'S SYNDROME

Clinical Features

An attack of Meniere's syndrome usually consists of a roaring sound (tinnitus), ear fullness, hearing loss, and vertigo, which lasts for hours to days. With repeat attacks, a sustained low-frequency sensorineural hearing loss (SNHL) and constant tinnitus usually develops. The mechanism is decreased reabsorption of endolymph in the endolymphatic sac. This can be idiopathic or occur after ear trauma or viral infection.

Diagnosis

The diagnosis depends on documenting fluctuating hearing loss on audiograms.

Treatment

Restricting the diet to 2 grams or less of sodium can significantly reduce the frequency of Meniere's attacks. Some patients require the additional use of a diuretic. Acetazolamide (Diamox) may be the optimal diuretic because this drug may decrease osmotic pressure within the endolymph, but chlorthalidone (Hygroton) and other diuretics have also been found to be quite effective. Less proven prophylactic therapy includes elimination of alcohol and caffeinated products (including chocolate). During acute attacks the patient is treated the same as for any other attack of acute vertigo (promethazine or meclizine). Vestibular exercises are usually not necessary because the patient recovers quite quickly. If medical therapy may not control the disease, surgery to relieve the pressure or destroy the labyrinth can be done. Endolymphatic shunts may be used; however, they are not always effective or may stop working after a few years. Labyrinthectomy is appropriate in

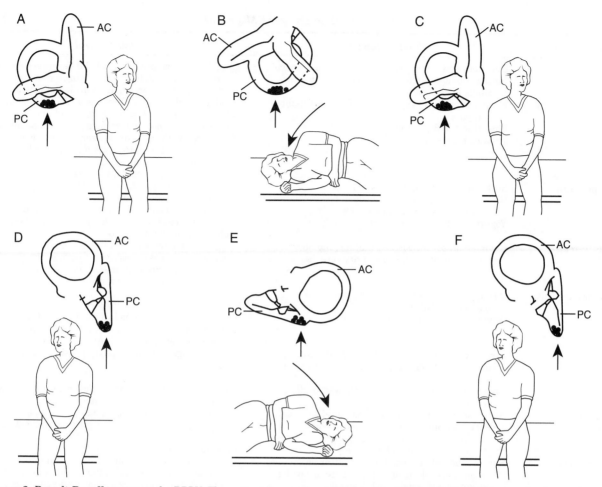

Figure 2. Brandt-Daroff treatment for BPPV. The patient is moved quickly into the sidelying position and stays in that position until the vertigo stops or for 30 seconds. The patient then sits up and again waits for the vertigo to stop. The patient then repeats the movement to the opposite side, stays there for 30 seconds, and sits up. The entire treatment is repeated five times, one to three times a day until the patient has 2 days in a row with no vertigo. This figure shows the effect of this treatment for right posterior canal BPPV.

patients in whom there is a severe pre-existing hearing loss on the side of the defective labyrinth and no evidence of disease on the other side. Vestibular neurectomy is used in patients in whom hearing is preserved.

MIGRAINE

Clinical Features

Migraine is a common but poorly recognized cause for spells of dizziness. Spells usually last 4 to 60 minutes and may or may not be associated with a headache.

Diagnosis

The International Headache Society (IHS) criteria can be helpful for the diagnosis of migraine. Because this is a diagnosis of exclusion, the diagnosis is secured with a positive response to treatment.

Treatment

Spells of vertigo due to migraine respond to the same types of treatment as those used for headaches.

After the diagnosis is established and the patient is reassured, I give the patient a handout listing the risk factors and foods that may precipitate an aura (Table 5). I encourage them to avoid hypoglycemia by eating every 6 to 8 hours, avoid nicotine, avoid or reduce exogenous estrogen, and try to maintain a regular sleep schedule. Beta blockers are among the most effective prophylactic drugs for vertigo due to migraine if strict avoidance of the risk factors does not significantly reduce these spells.

MOTION SICKNESS

Clinical Features

Motion sickness consists of episodic dizziness, fatigue, pallor, diaphoresis, excessive salivation, nausea, and occasionally vomiting induced by passive locomotion (e.g., riding in a car) or motion in the visual surroundings while standing still (e.g., viewing a large-screen movie that contains significant motion). Motion sickness is believed to be due to a sensory mismatch between visual and vestibular cues. Patients with migraine disorder are particu-

TABLE 5. **Diet to Prevent Migraine**

Food Class	Foods Allowed	Foods to Avoid
Beverages	Decaffeinated coffee, fruit juice, club soda, noncola soda. Limit caffeine sources to 2 cups per day (coffee, tea, cola)	Chocolate, cocoa, certain alcoholic beverages (red wine, port, sherry, Scotch, bourbon, gin); excessive aspartame (no more than 24 oz/day of diet drink)
Meats, fish, poultry	Fresh or frozen turkey, chicken, fish, beef, lamb, veal, pork Eggs (limit to 3 per week) Tuna or tuna salad	Aged, canned, cured, or processed meats, including ham or game, pickled herring, salad and dried fish; chicken liver, bologna; fermented sausage; any food prepared with meat tenderizer, soy sauce, or brewer's yeast; any food containing nitrates or tyramine (smoked meats, including bacon, sausage, ham, salami, pepperoni, hot dogs)
Dairy products	Milk: Homogenized, 2%, or skim Cheese: American, cottage, farmer, ricotta, cream, Canadian, processed cheese slice Yogurt (limit ½ cup per day)	Buttermilk, sour cream, chocolate milk Cheese: Stilton, bleu, cheddar, mozzarella, cheese spread, Roquefort, provolone, Gruyère, Muenster, feta, parmesan, brie, brick, camembert types, cheddar, Gouda, Romano
Breads, cereals	Commercial bread, English muffins, melba toast crackers, bagels; all hot and dry cereals	Hot, fresh, homemade yeast bread; bread or crackers containing cheese; fresh yeast coffee cake, doughnuts, sourdough bread; any product containing chocolate or nuts
Potato or substitute	White potato, sweet potato, rice, macaroni, spaghetti, noodles	None
Vegetables	Any except those to avoid	Beans such as pole, broad, lima, Italian, fava, navy, pinto, garbanzo; snow peas, pea pods, sauerkraut, onions (except for flavoring), olives, pickles
Fruit	Any except those to avoid; limit citrus fruits to ½ cup per day (1 orange); limit banana to ½ per day	Avocados, figs, raisins, papaya, passion fruit, red plums
Soups	Cream soups made from foods allowed in diet, homemade broth	Canned soup, soup or bouillon cubes, soup base with yeast or monosodium glutamate (read labels)
Desserts	Any cake or cookies without chocolate, nuts, or yeast; any pudding or ice cream without chocolate or nuts; flavored gelatin	Any product containing chocolate, including ice cream, pudding, cookies, cake, and pies; mincemeat pie
Sweets	Sugar, jelly, jam, honey, hard candy	Chocolate candy or syrup, carob
Miscellaneous	Salt in moderation, lemon juice, butter or margarine, cooking oil, whipped cream, white vinegar, commercial salad dressings	Pizza, cheese sauce, monosodium glutamate in excessive amounts (including Chinese food and Accent), meat tenderizer, seasoned salt, yeast, yeast extract; mixed dishes (including macaroni and cheese, beef Stroganoff, cheese blintzes, lasagna, frozen TV dinners); chocolate, nuts (including peanut butter); all nonwhite vinegars; anything fermented, pickled, or marinated

larly prone to motion sickness, especially during childhood.

Diagnosis

The diagnosis is based on history. Symptoms are often reproduced when exposed to a moving full-field visual target.

Treatment

Treatment consists of reassurance, reduction of circumstances that cause sensory mismatch, and medication if necessary. Intramuscular promethazine immediately relieves 90% of individuals compared with a resolution of symptoms over 72 to 96 hours in untreated individuals. Dimenhydrinate (Dramamine) or scopolamine patch (Transderm-Scop) can also be used to treat motion sickness when patients are exposed to motion-sickness situations for extended periods (seasickness).

ORTHOSTATIC HYPOTENSION OR INTOLERANCE

Clinical Features

Symptoms can range from lightheadedness when the patient first stands up to chronic fatigue, mental slowing, dizziness, nausea, and impending syncope. Common causes include medications (diuretics, antihypertensive medications, tricyclic antidepressants), prolonged bed rest, neurogenic causes (autonomic neuropathy from diabetes, amyloid, multisystem atrophy, Parkinson's disease), and idiopathic causes.

Diagnosis

Diagnosis is made based on history and results of clinical examination. Blood pressure is recorded after the patient is supine for 10 minutes. Blood pressure is repeated when the patient stands up. If there is a drop in systolic pressure by 20 mm Hg or more associated with symptoms, a diagnosis of orthostatic hypotension is suggested. If the patient is only symptomatic, then orthostatic intolerance is suggested.

Treatment

Treatment begins with removal of potentially offending drugs, if possible, and rehydration, if necessary. Salt and fluid intake should be increased. The patient is asked to sleep with the head elevated to reduce supine hypertension. If necessary, fludrocortisone (Florinef), 0.1 to 0.6 mg per day, is used. If this fails, then midodrine (ProAmatine), 10 mg three times a day, is given. In a double-blind, placebo-controlled study, midodrine significantly increased standing systolic blood pressure by 22 mm Hg and decreased orthostatic dizziness, fatigue, and weakness.

BILATERAL VESTIBULAR DEFICIT

Clinical Features

Ototoxicity is still a common cause of bilateral vestibular hypofunction, and gentamicin (Garamycin) is the most common culprit. The incidence of ototoxicity may be as high as 20% in high-risk patients (those with renal failure, the elderly, and those concomitantly taking furosemide [Lasix]). Ototoxicity can occur idiosyncratically in some individuals, but it is ototoxic in all individuals if peak or trough serum levels are above normal (>10 mg per liter and >2 mg per liter, respectively), the daily dose exceeds 5 mg per kg, or the total dose exceeds 10 days and is above 50 mg per kg. Furosemide and vancomycin are not ototoxic but enhance the ototoxic properties of gentamicin. Patients with bilateral vestibular deficits primarily complain of imbalance, not hearing loss or vertigo. They also may complain of oscillopsia (i.e., having the illusion the world is bouncing while they are walking).

Diagnosis

The clinical examination can be very helpful in the diagnosis of bilateral vestibular or static unilateral vestibular defects. These patients frequently have refixation saccadic eye movements after head thrust owing to a decrease in the vestibulo-ocular gain. In addition, bilateral lesions usually result in more than a four-line elevation in visual acuity during 2-Hz head oscillation. The diagnosis of a bilateral vestibular defect can be confirmed with an absent caloric response.

Treatment

Treatment of bilateral vestibular defects should include avoidance of all ototoxins that may cause further permanent peripheral vestibular damage (gentamicin, streptomycin, tobramycin, quinine, cisplatin) and avoidance of drugs that may transiently impair balance (sedatives, antianxiety agents, anti-epileptics, and antidepressants). Vestibular rehabilitation is very helpful for these patients (see Table 4). For bilateral defects, these vestibular adaptation exercises can be used to improve the gain of any remaining vestibular function and they enhance other reflexes such as the cervico-ocular reflex. In addition, these exercises facilitate the substitution of other ocular motor systems to improve gaze stability.

PANIC ATTACKS, HYPERVENTILATION, AND CHRONIC ANXIETY

Clinical Features

Panic attacks are an anxiety disorder that causes intense fear or discomfort that reaches a crescendo within 10 minutes and is frequently associated with dizziness, nausea, shortness of breath, and sweating. It may occur unexpectedly or be situational. It may be initiated by an organic cause of vertigo such as BPPV, especially in patients with a positive family history for panic attacks. Hyperventilation associated with chronic anxiety can also manifest as vague complaints of dizziness.

Diagnosis

Helpful diagnostic criteria can be found in the fourth edition of the American Psychiatric Association's *Diagnostic and Statistical Manual of Mental Disorders*. Usually, panic attacks are associated with shortness of breath or chest tightness and paresthesias.

Treatment

The selective serotonin reuptake inhibitors (SSRI) can be used for panic disorder. I usually prescribe paroxetine (Paxil) or sertraline (Zoloft),* which may be an ideal medication because it is non–habit forming and many patients with panic disorder have concomitant depression. Alprazolam (Xanax) can be used sporadically if attacks are infrequent. Behavioral modification is also effective.

STROKE

Clinical Features

Vertigo may occur from infarcts in the thalamus or posterior fossa when vestibular pathways are involved. The labyrinthine artery originates from the anterior inferior cerebellar artery (AICA) 85% of the time. Thus, an AICA syndrome may manifest with just peripheral vestibular signs if the labyrinth artery is solely involved (vertigo, nausea, vomiting, hearing loss, and tinnitus). Central signs will occur if the dorsolateral brain stem or cerebellar branches of the AICA are involved (dysarthria, peripheral fa-

---

*Not FDA approved for this indication.

cial palsy, trigeminal sensory loss, Horner's syndrome, dysmetria, contralateral temperature, and pain sensory loss). The posterior inferior cerebellar artery (PICA) perfuses the posterior inferior cerebellum (cerebellar branch) and the dorsolateral medulla. Infarcts in the brain stem branches result in Wallenberg's syndrome (crossed sensory signs, ipsilateral lateropulsion, ataxia, Horner's sign, nystagmus, and vertigo). Nystagmus may be pure torsion or mixed torsion and horizontal. When the nystagmus contains a horizontal component, it reverses direction on gaze toward the lesion side, unlike nystagmus from peripheral vestibular lesions. In this syndrome, vertigo occurs from involvement of the vestibular nucleus.

Diagnosis

The diagnosis is based on the results of the clinical examination aided by magnetic resonance imaging of the head.

Treatment

Bed rest for a few days should be initiated because most stroke-induced vertigo is due to a vertebrobasilar event. Ondansetron (Zofran) may also be appropriate for patients with severe vertigo and nausea, but currently this drug is only approved for chemotherapy-induced nausea. Vestibular rehabilitation is appropriate for AICA infarcts that involve the labyrinth. Recovery may be incomplete if the cerebellum and inputs to the cerebellum are involved in the stroke. Risk factors for future stroke should be reduced.

MENIERE'S DISEASE

method of
MICHAEL D. SEIDMAN, M.D.
Henry Ford Health System
West Bloomfield, Michigan

Meniere's disease is a debilitating inner ear disorder of unknown etiology having the clinical spectrum of episodic vertigo, fluctuating hearing loss, tinnitus, and pressure or fullness in the ears. Estimates of the number of Meniere's sufferers in the United States range from 3 to 5 million, with 100,000 new cases diagnosed each year. Variations of the classic form of Meniere's disease include cochlear Meniere's disease, in which aural symptoms are present without vertigo, and vestibular Meniere's disease, in which vertigo is present without the aural symptoms.

Overdistention of the membranous labyrinth due to excessive endolymph (EL) is believed to be the basis of Meniere's disease. The endolymphatic sac (ELS) is assumed to play a vital role in EL volume regulation. Possible pathogenic mechanisms underlying Meniere's disease include fibrosis and loss of fluid-transporting epithelia in the ELS, altered glycoprotein metabolism, allergy, viral etiology, calcium regulatory alteration, and immune-mediated inner ear disease. The degree of endolymphatic hydrops (ELH) may depend on residual function of the ELS and the state of balance of local ion transport in the cochlea.

It is thought that ELH damages and distorts the cochlear duct and sensory nerve endings (hair cells). Electrocochleography (ECoG) provides an objective means to record stimulus-dependent, electrophysiologic potentials of the cochlea and auditory nerve, through an electrode placed in the vicinity of the round window membrane. An enlarged negative summating potential and summating potential/action potential (SP/AP) ratio on ECoG is used by some clinicians in the diagnosis of ELH. The use of long-tone burst stimuli, especially at 1000 Hz, improves the diagnostic sensitivity of ECoG in patients with suspected ELH. The primary diagnostic criterion is the clinical manifestation of the just-mentioned symptoms.

TREATMENT

Sixty to 80% of patients with Meniere's disease appear to respond to conservative treatment by systemic medication, dietary, and allergy regimens. However, there is no strong statistical evidence that medication alters the natural history of the disease. Many patients who appear to improve are merely experiencing fewer disabling attacks of vertigo. Although the vertigo is gone, the acute attacks are exchanged for some form of chronic, often disabling, dysequilibrium. In addition, the hearing loss and tinnitus may progress. Bilateral Meniere's disease is reported to develop in 8 to 80% of patients but averages 20%.

Management Goals

The challenge is to enhance the salvage rate of systemic treatment failures by using procedures that minimize the destruction of residual hearing and balance function. The ideal treatment plan not only addresses the acute and short-term symptomatic relief of vertigo but also attempts to preserve or improve long-term auditory and vestibular function. Given the incidence of bilateral involvement, both ears should be checked periodically through audiovestibular testing and perhaps ECoG. Symptoms attributed to the "problem ear" may actually be coming from the "good ear."

Acute and Short-Term Management

Symptomatic relief of vertigo is a goal of short-term management. Some attacks of violent vertigo occur without warning. Others occur with a prodrome of aural fullness and tinnitus on one side. The vertigo attack ensues, with a concomitant or sequential loss of auditory sensitivity. An irritative nystagmus can usually be documented. The patient is often nauseated, experiences occasional vomiting, and often has significant exacerbation of dysequilibrium and vertigo with changes in body position.

The management of acute episodes of vertigo varies with the severity as well as the frequency of such attacks. In general, the patient should be confined to bed rest and rehydrated with intravenous fluids.

For the control of more severe attacks, droperidol (Inapsine) can be administered intravenously if the patient is carefully monitored in the hospital or emergency department. On an outpatient basis, 0.5 to 1.0 mL of droperidol can be given intramuscularly every 4 to 6 hours along with 0.4 to 0.6 mg of atropine subcutaneously or intramuscularly. The patient requires observation for 1 hour after administration of these agents. Although it is unusual for a second dose to be required, this medication can be repeated every 4 to 6 hours in a 24-hour period. Another approach for vestibular suppression is to use 5 mg of diazepam (Valium) intravenously, slowly titrated up to 20 mg. This can be administered over a 4- to 12-hour period, with an initial dose of 0.4 to 0.6 mg of atropine along with a possible second dose. If there is significant nausea and vomiting, a 10-mg prochlorperazine maleate suppository (Compazine) or ondansetron hydrochloride (Zofran) can be used.

For less violent attacks of vertigo, one injection of atropine with 5 mg of diazepam can be given intramuscularly. This can be followed with 5 mg of diazepam taken orally four times a day. With rest and stress reduction, this may be sufficient to bring the vertigo under control.

Long-Term Management

Before embarking on a long-term treatment plan, confirmation of a definitive diagnosis through an audiovestibular battery, including neuroradiologic testing, is extremely important. Medical treatment should be undertaken for all patients before any surgical intervention. Patient compliance with medical treatment should be emphasized. The patient should be reassured that the vertigo can likely be controlled with one of the treatment alternatives.

Systemic Medical Management

Low-Salt Diet. Although a no-salt diet is not necessary, 1000 to 1500 mg of sodium or less per day is suggested.

Diuretics. The patient should take 25 to 50 mg of hydrochlorothiazide (HydroDIURIL) orally, each morning, with a potassium-rich food such as orange juice. Another alternative is furosemide, 20 mg daily, with potassium chloride. Potassium levels should be monitored and supplemented as clinically indicated. This may help to reduce systemic extracellular fluid volume and secondarily to reduce intralabyrinthine fluid/pressure.

Vestibular Suppression. To establish adequate blood levels, 2 mg of diazepam, or a low dose (0.25) of alprazolam (Xanax), two times a day, could be given. This is an effective oral vestibular suppressant. The muscle relaxant and stress-reduction properties of such drugs are often greatly appreciated by patients and may also be helpful in breaking the cycle of periodic recurrences. It is usually unnecessary to use any of these drugs for more than 2 to 3 months. This regimen appears to be more effective than the commonly prescribed meclizine (Antivert, Bonine) in a dosage ranging from 12.5 to 25 mg three times per day, which would be the second choice. Transdermal scopolamine (Transderm-Scop) is rarely effective as a peripheral end organ vestibular suppressant, but it is an excellent adjunct when motion intolerance is also a complaint. These medications reduce the process of central compensation and can prolong the time for balance recovery; thus, judicious short-term use is recommended.

Vasodilators and Various Other Systemic Medical Regimens. Nylidrin hydrochloride (Arlidin),* histamine sulfate,* beta histine hydrochloride (Serc),* nicotinic acid, lipoflavonoids, zinc sulfate, and a variety of medical therapies may be helpful in individual cases, but with the exception of Serc, their overall efficacy in controlled studies has not been corroborated.

Corticosteroid Bursts. Intermittent and infrequent trials of systemic corticosteroids (1 mg/kg for 7 days), monitored by means of baseline and post-treatment audiovestibular/ECoG, may be helpful in patients with immune-mediated inner ear disorders, but systemic side effects or other medical problems could limit this option.

Vestibular Rehabilitation. With satisfactory compliance, a general vestibular exercise program may effectively reduce vestibular dysfunction. This works by fatiguing the positional component of asymmetrical peripheral end organ misinformation through adaptation and central compensation mechanisms.

Complimentary/Alternative Medicine. Some patients prefer more alternative options. There are several herbs that may have a beneficial effect on vertigo. These include ginkgo biloba (must be highly purified extract: 24% ginkoflavonoids/ginkoglycoids). The German Commission has noted that doses of 120–240 mg twice a day are appropriate. Several other herbs, including ginseng, blessed thistle, hawthorne, and gotukola, may be of some help.

In addition, a combination of ingredients called vertigoheel or Cocculus Compositum has been shown in a double-blinded, randomized, placebo-controlled study to be very effective at vertigo control.

Many other forms of complementary/alternative therapies (CAM), including nutritional therapies, acupuncture, chiropractic, homeopathic, cranial sacral therapy, massage therapy, and St. John's neuromuscular therapy, may have some benefit. Many other CAM therapies may or may not provide relief.

Avoidance. Caffeine, alcohol, tobacco, salt, sugars, and stress all tend to exacerbate Meniere's disease. In addition to dietary considerations, a general aerobic/cardiovascular exercise program may be helpful.

Reassurance. The patient should understand that improvement is possible.

Systemic Medical Treatment Failure

Systemic medical treatment failure is characterized by a recurrence of inner ear symptoms, particularly vertigo, despite adequate patient compliance. When compliance with the recommended treatment program is good, a 3-month trial is considered sufficient; when compliance is only fair, a 6-month trial may be necessary. If patient compliance is nil after the 3-month trial, it is unlikely that compliance will

---

*Not available in the United States.

improve with further attempts at medical treatment. It is important to watch for patients who are "better," that is, in whom attacks of vertigo are fewer and less severe, but who are still experiencing chronic dysequilibrium and possibly progressive sensorineural hearing loss. The degree of disability at work and in social situations should be assessed and considered when evaluating systemic medical treatment failure. It should be determined whether vertigo or sensorineural hearing loss is the primary basis for further treatment intervention, and the status of the patient's other ear should be considered.

Minimally Invasive Procedures

Numerous physicians in the United States and abroad are delivering medications to the round window area of the middle ear to treat inner ear disease. Various methods are being used, including intratympanic, Gelfoam, and catheter delivery. Gentamicin (Garamycin) has been the mainstay for intratympanic treatment of Meniere's disease, but corticosteroids and other medications have also been used. Reported success rates for vertigo control with intratympanic gentamicin range from 80 to 96%, and the incidence of hearing loss typically ranges from 14 to 42%. The amount and frequency of intratympanic gentamicin administration, as well as the treatment end point, varies greatly among cited reports in the literature.

Catheters such as the Round Window µ Cath (RWµCath) and Round Window E-Cath (RWE-Cath) (IntraEAR, Inc, Greenwood Village, Colorado) allow for site-specific delivery of medicine to the round window. The tip of these catheters fits snugly in the round window niche, locking in place, to create a fluid transfer space between the catheter tip and the round window membrane. Without removing the catheter, the physician can alter (add, subtract, or change) the medicine being delivered at any time. A micropump can also be connected to the inflow lumen for continuous infusion of medicine and controlled microdosing regimens. The RWE-Cath includes a built-in platinum electrode for recording ECoG before, during, and after the delivery of medicine to provide immediate objective electrophysiologic feedback to enhance the treating physician's ability to titrate therapy and potentially reduce cochlear damage.

Low-dose gentamicin through the RWµCath and the RWE-Cath adds significant control and accuracy to gentamicin treatment. Data support that low-dose gentamicin through the RWµCath and RWE-Cath controls the symptoms of Meniere's disease without significantly damaging vestibular or auditory function.

Invasive Procedures

Nondestructive Surgical Treatments

A myriad of conservative nondestructive surgical approaches to inner ear endolymphatic hydrops problems are routinely performed in attempts to alter or improve inner ear function. When one considers the large number of ELS procedures available and commonly used, it becomes apparent that there is no consensus regarding the best approach. In general, ELS surgery can provide improvement of vertigo in 70% of patients who have failed medical treatment, with a slight opportunity for hearing stabilization or improvement.

Destructive Surgical Treatments

Destructive procedures should be considered only when more conservative procedures have failed. Except in unusual cases, performing a destructive procedure as the first, irrevocable surgery after medical treatment failure is not routinely advocated. The most common destructive procedures are vestibular nerve section (VNS), which ablates balance but preserves existing hearing, and labyrinthectomy, which purposely destroys both auditory and vestibular function.

If the patient's hearing is 50 dB or better, with 50% or better speech discrimination, VNS may be performed to eliminate vertigo and preserve hearing. VNS eliminates or significantly reduces vertigo in over 90% of the cases. If the vertigo is not controlled, the most likely cause is not Meniere's disease but may be undiagnosed bilateral Meniere's disease or incomplete surgical division of the vestibular nerve from the cochleovestibular nerve.

If the hearing loss is more severe (there is a greater than 50-dB loss and less than 50% discrimination), a transmastoid labyrinthectomy will improve vertigo in 95% of patients and eliminate any residual hearing.

Meniere's disease is a complex disorder that is typically well controlled with appropriate dietary adjustments and medical management. In the 20 to 40% of patients whose symptoms cannot be controlled, there are multiple surgical options that are typically quite effective at symptom improvement. A wide spectrum of surgical options are available, from minimally invasive round window direct drug delivery to purposely nondestructive ELS surgery and then on to VNS and labyrinthectomy, which are purposely destructive and are considered major surgery, often involving neurosurgical cooperation.

VIRAL MENINGITIS AND ENCEPHALITIS

method of
VINODH NARAYANAN, M.D.
*University of Pittsburgh and
Children's Hospital of Pittsburgh
Pittsburgh, Pennsylvania*

Viral meningitis (aseptic meningitis) and encephalitis are relatively common disorders. They are especially common in the pediatric population.

CLINICAL FEATURES

Viral meningitis is a benign condition in which the infection and inflammation is limited to the meninges. In an adult or older child, this is an acute illness with fever, headache, and stiff neck. Other symptoms that may be present include general malaise, nausea, vomiting, photophobia, and pain on eye movement. The patients may be in great discomfort but are not typically critically ill, in contrast to patients with bacterial meningitis. In infants and young children (who often present with fever, lethargy, and anorexia or vomiting), the clinical differentiation between bacterial meningitis and viral meningitis may be impossible, and one has to rely on cerebrospinal fluid (CSF) analysis and the results of bacteriologic cultures to guide therapy.

Encephalitis is a more serious illness than aseptic meningitis and implies that the infection involves parenchymal cells of the brain. Very often these patients also have signs of meningeal irritation and thus may be more appropriately diagnosed as having meningoencephalitis. The symptoms and signs that distinguish encephalitis from pure meningitis are seizures, alteration of the level of consciousness, focal neurologic deficits, and increased intracranial pressure.

Lumbar puncture and examination of the CSF are crucial in the evaluation of the patient with fever and symptoms suggesting a central nervous system infection. It is important to measure the opening pressure when performing the lumbar puncture, and this should be done with the patient relaxed and the patient's legs extended. The CSF usually shows an elevated cell count, predominantly lymphocytes, with a mild to moderate elevation of protein, and normal glucose. For a patient with suspected meningitis, there is usually no contraindication to undergo the lumbar puncture. For a patient presenting with fever and a seizure or altered state of consciousness, however, a contrast-enhanced computed tomography (CT) scan is often obtained before lumbar puncture, primarily to detect a mass lesion such as an abscess or subdural empyema. Magnetic resonance imaging (MRI) of the brain is important in cases of suspected encephalitis, as this may indicate the extent and severity of parenchymal disease. Electroencephalography (EEG) should be done as soon as the patient is stabilized, as it may reveal a pattern (PLEDS: periodic lateralized epileptiform discharges) consistent with type 1 herpes simplex virus (HSV-1) encephalitis.

DIFFERENTIAL DIAGNOSIS

One can usually distinguish between viral and bacterial meningitis (except in young infants) by clinical features and CSF findings. Patients with bacterial meningitis are critically ill, with systemic signs of septicemia (very high fever, lethargy, hypotension). The CSF contains predominantly neutrophils, with an elevated protein and low glucose concentration. A lymphocytic CSF pleocytosis, however, may be seen in partially treated infections (otitis media, sinusitis) with a secondary meningitis or a parameningeal focus of infection. Fungal meningitis should be considered in immunocompromised patients, especially when the CSF protein is moderately elevated.

Lyme disease, caused by the tick-borne spirochete *Borrelia burgdorferi,* needs to be considered, especially in the Northeast and Mid-Atlantic states. Neurologic symptoms are preceded by a typical rash (erythema chronicum migrans) at the site of the tick bite. Cranial neuropathies (facial weakness) are frequent in Lyme-associated meningitis. Aseptic meningitis and acute encephalopathy are an unusual complication of cat-scratch disease (caused by *Bartonella henselae*). A red papule appears at the site of the scratch or bite, with a low-grade fever and regional adenopathy. Neurologic symptoms may appear acutely with altered consciousness, combative behavior, headache,

and seizures. Diagnoses of Lyme disease and cat-scratch disease are based on serologic tests or polymerase chain reaction (PCR) of serum and spinal fluid.

Pulmonary infections with *Mycoplasma pneumoniae* may be complicated by neurologic symptoms, including aseptic meningitis, encephalitis, myelitis, and signs of brain stem involvement. As it is difficult to culture the organism from CSF, it is difficult to discern if parenchymal involvement is due to direct infection or to an autoimmune reaction triggered by the infection.

Noninfectious disorders to consider for a patient with presumed aseptic meningoencephalitis are acute drug intoxication and metabolic disorders. Although fever is not a typical feature, drug intoxication may cause muscular rigidity and a secondary elevation in temperature. Mitochondrial disorders have many different neurologic presentations and may be mistaken for acute encephalitis (e.g., HSV). Carcinomatous meningitis may also present as an aseptic meningitis, although CSF glucose values are usually depressed and cytology is typically positive.

VIROLOGY

Many viruses have been associated with meningitis and encephalitis, although some generally cause a benign aseptic meningitis (enteroviruses) and others cause a more invasive encephalitis (HSV and arboviruses). The summer and early fall are periods of peak occurrence of enterovirus and arbovirus infections. HSV encephalitis, on the other hand, occurs sporadically, whereas lymphocytic choriomeningitis is more common in the winter. Other clues to the cause of meningoencephalitis include travel to specific parts of the world, camping outdoors, exposure to animals, or a specific rash.

Enteroviruses (coxsackieviruses A and B, echovirus, and enterovirus) account for most cases of viral meningitis. The virus is shed in the gastrointestinal tract and is transmitted usually by fecal contamination, accounting for outbreaks in families and day care centers. Enterovirus infections can cause fever, nonspecific respiratory illness, diarrhea, conjunctivitis, carditis, and a variety of rashes. Although recovery from enteroviral meningitis is usually complete, rarely these viruses may cause a focal encephalitis or be associated with acute cerebellar ataxia. The specific organism may be recovered by viral culture of nasal, oral, or rectal swabs. Among the enteroviruses, echovirus and coxsackievirus B are the most common causative agents of aseptic meningitis. Poliovirus and mumps virus may also cause meningitis, but these have become uncommon in the United States because of immunization.

Adenovirus infection, ranging from pharyngitis to pneumonitis and conjunctivitis, is a common cause of respiratory illness in children, especially in the late winter and spring. Central nervous system involvement is rare, but when it occurs it is usually an encephalitis in the setting of a severe respiratory disease. Recovery of virus from body fluids, combined with a rise in specific antibody titer, supports this diagnosis. Severe, and sometimes fatal, cases of encephalitis have been associated with adenovirus type 7.

Lymphocytic choriomeningitis virus is an uncommon cause of aseptic meningitis, the infection being acquired from mice or hamsters. Patients may develop fever, malaise, coryza, and leukopenia or thrombocytopenia, with CSF demonstrating an intense mononuclear pleocytosis.

Central nervous system infections by arboviruses are usually severe encephalitides. These viruses are transmitted to humans by arthropods (ticks or mosquitoes), occur in specific geographic domains, and are most common in the summer and early fall; the occurrence of clinical cases is determined by rainfall or changes in animal host populations. Eastern encephalitis virus (found in the eastern half of the United States can cause a fulminant and severe encephalitis, with death or severe disability. Western encephalitis, found in the western two-thirds of the United States, can be severe, but is rarely fatal. St. Louis encephalitis virus is the most widespread and most common cause of epidemic viral encephalitis in the United States while Japanese encephalitis is the leading cause of neurologic disease in the world. California (La Crosse strain) encephalitis virus is most often associated with disease in the Midwest.

Of the herpesviruses, type 1 (HSV-1) is the most frequent cause of sporadic fatal viral encephalitis. Primary infection may result in gingivostomatitis, pharyngitis, or respiratory disease and disseminated infection in immunocompromised individuals. After primary infection, a state of latency may be established within the nervous system (e.g., sensory ganglia) followed by reactivation at a later date. Acute encephalitis may be the result of primary infection or reactivation of latent infection. The frontal and temporal lobes are most often affected and show areas of necrosis, hemorrhage, and inflammation. Symptoms are typical of encephalitis (fever, headache, and meningismus) and the frontotemporal pathology. Typical signs include personality change, hallucinations, focal seizures, hemiparesis, aphasia, and rapid progression of the encephalopathy. Early in the course of disease, the CSF may show an increase in neutrophils, but later there is a mononuclear pleocytosis. EEGs often reveal either periodic sharp discharges or slow wave complexes. MRI (with contrast enhancement) is a sensitive technique to visualize the early pathologic changes. Brain biopsy as a diagnostic test for herpes simplex encephalitis has largely been replaced by PCR for viral DNA. This is sensitive and specific and can differentiate between the different HSVs.

MANAGEMENT

The first decision that must be made in the emergency setting, after cardiorespiratory stabilization, is whether to initiate treatment with broad-spectrum antibacterial agents. This decision is made based on the seriousness of the patient's illness and the results of the blood count and CSF examination.

If HSV encephalitis is suspected, based on clinical presentation, imaging studies, and EEGs, then treatment with intravenous acyclovir should be initiated. The dose of acyclovir (Zovirax) is 1500 mg per m² per day or 30 mg per kg per day, divided every 8 hours, and it should be continued for 14 to 21 days. If the course of the patient and the CSF PCR result do not support the diagnosis of HSV encephalitis, then the acyclovir treatment may be stopped. Renal function should be monitored in these patients, as the dose needs to be decreased in patients with renal impairment.

Seizures should be controlled with parenteral anticonvulsants such as phenytoin (Dilantin), phenobarbital, or lorazepam (Ativan). In patients who are unresponsive or heavily sedated, continuous EEG monitoring may be the only way to detect changes in the neurologic state or nonconvulsive status epilepticus. This should be aggressively treated and may

require the pharmacologic induction of coma by pentobarbital infusion. The syndrome of inappropriate antidiuretic hormone (SIADH) is a frequent finding in children with meningoencephalitis, and thus serum electrolytes need to be monitored closely. This usually responds to fluid restriction, but may require the careful use of hypertonic saline infusions or diuretics.

Cerebral edema (either focal or diffuse) is often seen in encephalitis and may lead to increased intracranial pressure (ICP). In patients who are obtunded or comatose, it may be critical to directly monitor ICP with a dural pressure transducer. Treatment of elevated ICP may include intubation and hyperventilation to maintain arterial P_{CO_2} in the range of 25 to 30 mm Hg, intravenous infusion of mannitol (initial dose 1.0 to 2.0 gram per kg as 20% solution given over 30 minutes), and dexamethasone (1 to 2 mg per kg loading dose, followed by 1 to 1.5 mg per kg per 24 hours maintenance divided every 6 hours) treatment.

LONG-TERM SEQUELAE

Aseptic meningitis is usually a benign illness from which the patients recover completely. With the more invasive encephalitides, there may be quite extensive brain injury and associated long-term sequelae. Decreased level of consciousness, signs of brain stem pathology (abnormal oculocephalic responses), and MRI changes suggestive of extensive parenchymal involvement predict a poor neurologic outcome. HSV encephalitis may result in focal frontal or temporal lobe necrosis and thus cause cognitive or memory impairment, behavioral changes, and epilepsy. Diffuse cystic encephalomalacia can also be seen with adenovirus and Eastern equine encephalitis infections. Patients with severe encephalitis may benefit greatly from an intensive rehabilitation program.

MULTIPLE SCLEROSIS

method of
MARIKO KITA, M.D., and
DONALD E. GOODKIN, M.D.
*University of California, San Francisco /
Mount Zion Multiple Sclerosis Center*
San Francisco, California

Multiple sclerosis (MS) is an idiopathic, chronic, demyelinating disease of the central nervous system. Affecting more than 350,000 people in the United States, it is the most common medical cause of neurologic disability in young adults in the northern hemisphere. Since 1996, three immunomodulatory medications have been approved by the U.S. Food and Drug Administration (FDA) for the treatment of MS and several others are under investigation. MS is now considered to be a treatable disease. In September 1998, the National Multiple Sclerosis Society issued a Disease Management Consensus Statement emphasizing the importance of early intervention (Table 1).

TABLE 1. Guidelines on Disease Management from The National Multiple Sclerosis Society

1. Initiation of therapy is advised as soon as possible after a definite diagnosis of MS and determination of a relapsing course.
2. Patient's access to medication should not be limited by the frequency of relapses, age, or level of disability.
3. Treatment is not to be stopped during evaluation for continuing treatment.
4. Therapy is to be continued indefinitely, unless there is clear lack of benefit, intolerable side effects, new data that reveal other reasons for cessation, or better therapy is available.
5. All three agents should be included in formularies and covered by third-party payers so that physicians and patients may determine the most appropriate agent on an individual basis.
6. Movement from one immunomodulating drug to another should be permitted.
7. Most concurrent medical conditions do not contraindicate use of any other therapies.

As such, physicians who may encounter MS patients early in their course, neurologists and non-neurologists alike, have an ever-important role in impacting the care of their MS patients. Here we summarize new definitions for the clinical patterns of MS, the role of magnetic resonance imaging (MRI) in monitoring disease progression in MS, the approved and off-label disease-modifying treatments for MS, and special considerations in the continued management of MS patients.

CLINICAL COURSE

The diagnosis of MS is based on recurrent symptoms and demonstration of signs referable to the white matter tracts within the central nervous system that cannot otherwise be explained. The initial manifestation of the disease typically involves an abrupt onset of symptoms, which often include disturbances of balance, gait, or coordination; impaired vision; weakness; fatigue; altered sensations; bowel, bladder, or sexual dysfunction; or impaired cognition. The various clinical courses of MS can be divided into four groups: relapsing-remitting (RRMS), secondary progressive (SPMS), primary progressive (PPMS), and relapsing progressive (RPMS). Figure 1 illustrates variations of these consensus definitions for clinical courses of disease activity. Initially, approximately 85% of patients are diagnosed with RRMS, a course characterized by relapses of neurologic dysfunction followed by some degree of improvement or remission. These disease-modifying medications, interferon (IFN)–β-1a (Avonex), IFN-β-1b (Betaseron), and glatiramer acetate (Copaxone) are approved for treatment of RRMS. Approximately 50% of patients with RRMS will later convert to an SPMS clinical course within 10 years of initial symptoms. In these patients the gradual progression of disability may or may not be superimposed on relapses. Fifteen percent of patients are initially diagnosed with PPMS. These patients experience gradual but progressive disability from onset without remission. A final and uncommon pattern, RPMS, describes those patients who experience progression of disability from onset with occasional superimposed relapses. RPMS may, in fact, represent a subset of PPMS patients.

PPMS can be distinguished from RRMS by clinical course as well as by histopathologic and radiologic characteristics. In contrast to patients with RRMS, patients with PPMS are older at onset and there appears to be little

gender predilection. Histopathologically, PPMS lesions have fewer perivascular inflammatory cuffs and less leukocytic infiltration extending into the surrounding white matter. Radiologically, patients with PPMS also experience fewer gadolinium-enhanced MRI lesions than patients with RRMS when monitored with monthly MRI sessions. On average, there is a lower intracranial T2-weighted focal lesion burden in PPMS, but there are more diffuse abnormalities within the white matter of the brain and spinal cord.

Patients with SPMS may be divided into two groups: those who do and those who do not experience relapses. The MRI characteristics and histopathology of patients with SPMS who experience frequent relapses are similar to those of patients with RRMS. In contrast, the MRI characteristics and histopathology of patients with SPMS who do not experience frequent relapses are more similar to those of patients with PPMS.

MEASURING DISEASE ACTIVITY WITH MRI

MRI is the most sensitive measure of disease activity in MS. The earliest event in the formation of a new MS lesion appears to be a disturbance of vascular permeability. This event is visualized on MRI as focal extravasation of gadolinium from blood vessels into the brain parenchyma. MS plaques are also evident on T2-weighted images. More than 90% of patients with clinically definite MS enrolled in controlled clinical trials manifest three or more T2-weighted lesions on MRI. In placebo recipients, total T2-weighted lesion area increases, on average, by 5 to 10% annually. Because subclinical activity can be demonstrated on serial MRIs of the brain and spinal cord, the number of new gadolinium-enhancing and T2-weighted lesions is

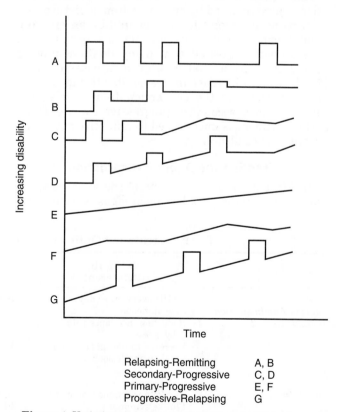

Relapsing-Remitting	A, B
Secondary-Progressive	C, D
Primary-Progressive	E, F
Progressive-Relapsing	G

Figure 1. Variations in consensus definitions for clinical course of multiple sclerosis.

commonly used as an efficacy outcome when screening promising therapies in phase III controlled clinical trials.

Total volume of T2-weighted lesion load does not consistently correlate with degree of neurologic disability. There are several possible explanations for this poor correlation. First, T2-weighted lesions may reflect largely reversible edema and inflammation. Thus, abnormal signal intensity on T2-weighted images does not distinguish between focal edema, inflammation, demyelination, or axonal loss. Second, the clinical consequence of T2-weighted lesions may be determined to a greater extent by lesion location than by total lesion "burden." For instance, a demyelinating lesion in the optic nerve might produce visual loss, whereas a lesion in the deep white matter of the parietal lobe might be asymptomatic. Finally, microscopic abnormalities may not be visualized by conventional MRI.

Preliminary evidence from magnetization transfer imaging and quantitative MRI suggests that the partially reversible acute episodes of neurologic impairment in relapsing forms of MS result from largely reversible inflammation and edema, whereas the increasing disability in progressive forms of MS results from irreversible axonal loss, demyelination, and gliosis. These differences have implications for early treatment and for developing new treatments for primary and secondary progressive MS. Promising new magnetic resonance techniques, including quantitative MRI, magnetic transfer imaging, apparent diffusion coefficients, and proton magnetic resonance spectroscopic imaging, may better distinguish reversible edema and inflammation from irreversible demyelination, axonal loss, and gliosis and may eventually be used to assess treatment efficacy in progressive forms of MS.

TREATMENT

There exists considerable evidence that demyelination is accompanied by or results from a disturbance of immune function, likely triggered by an environmental exposure in a genetically susceptible host. It has been suggested that demyelination may be accompanied by axonal loss, even in cases of early MS. A gradual increase in irreversible tissue damage probably explains the conversion from a relapsing remitting to a secondary progressive course. Thus, early treatment is encouraged to minimize sustained progression of disability.

Treating the Acute Exacerbation

An MS exacerbation consists of the appearance of new, or worsening of old, clinical signs or symptoms lasting longer than 24 hours. It should be distinguished from a "pseudo-exacerbation" or worsening of old signs/symptoms as a result of concurrent infection or fever. Corticosteroids are the mainstay in the treatment of acute exacerbations, but there is currently no consensus regarding dose, route of administration, length of treatment, or necessity of taper for MS relapses. Corticosteroids shorten the duration of clinical exacerbations, and preliminary data suggest bimonthly pulses of intravenous methylprednisolone delay time to onset of sustained progression of disability. Our current practice is to treat exacerbations that impair activities of daily living with 1 gram of intravenous methylprednisolone each day for 3 days. Patients who worsen on withdrawal of intravenous methylprednisolone are tapered with oral prednisone from a dose of 60 mg each day over 10 to 14 days.

Treatment of RRMS

The management of patients with RRMS has been advanced by the approval and availability of disease-modifying agents IFN-β-1a (Avonex) and IFN-β-1b (Betaseron) and glatiramer acetate (Copaxone). Each of these agents reduces annualized exacerbation rates by approximately 33%, and both IFN-β-1a and IFN-β-1b reduce the number of new MRI lesions. Data from phase III trials of these agents indicate that Avonex significantly delays time to onset of sustained progression of disability. Although neutralizing antibodies to both IFN-β-1a and IFN-β-1b may be detected after 6 months of treatment, the relationship between these antibodies and clinical efficacy is not sufficiently robust to guide treatment decisions. These treatment options are generally well tolerated, and the similarities and differences between them are summarized in Table 2.

Although not currently approved for use in MS, there is evidence that immune globulin intravenous (IGIV) (Polygam) reduces annualized exacerbation rates when given at a dose of 0.15 to 0.2 gram per kg per month for up to 2 years compared with placebo. The effect of IGIV on sustained progression of disability has not been confirmed. At higher doses (1 gram per kg per day for 2 consecutive days each

TABLE 2. **Treatment Options for Relapsing-Remitting Multiple Sclerosis**

	IFN-β-1b (Betaseron)	IFN-β-1a (Avonex)	Glatiramer Acetate (Copaxone)
Dose	8 MIU every other day	6 MIU per week	20 mg per day
Route of Administration	Subcutaneous	Intramuscular	Subcutaneous
Treatment Effects	Reduction in relapse rate by 30%	Reduction in relapse rate by 30%	Reduction in relapse rate by 30%
	Decrease in new gadolinium-enhancing lesions	Decrease in new gadolinium-enhancing lesions	Decrease in new gadolinium-enhancing lesions
		Delay in time to onset of sustained progression of disability	
Side Effects	Skin site reactions (common)	Skin site reactions (rare)	Skin site reactions (rare)
	Flulike symptoms	Flulike symptoms	Systemic panic-like attack
Synthesis	Recombinant *Escherichia coli*	Cultured cell lines	Synthetic polymer

month for 6 months) of IGIV, patients have been shown to develop fewer new gadolinium-enhancing lesions. However, this dose of IGIV is frequently associated with side effects, such as eczema, headache, and nausea. Thromboembolic events have also been reported in patients receiving IGIV at these doses.

Although the mechanisms of action of IGIV responsible for a treatment effect in MS are not known, several explanations are possible. IGIV from large pools of normal donors may (1) contain anti-idiotypic antibodies that exert regulatory effects on antibody production and lymphocyte activity; (2) reduce autoaggressive macrophages by blocking Fc receptors; (3) act as a receptor for activated complement components, thereby preventing their attachment to the oligodendrocyte surface and myelin proteins; and (4) down-regulate inflammatory cytokine production. IGIV may therefore be a potentially useful agent in the treatment of MS patients who fail IFN-β-1a, IFN-β-1b, or glatiramer acetate therapy. The limited availability and cost of IGIV currently restrict its widespread use.

Therapeutic Options for Patients with SPMS

The definition for RRMS was changed after approval of IFN-β-1a and IFN-β-1b and glatiramer acetate. Before 1996, patients who experienced complete recovery from relapses were categorized as having RRMS and patients who did not experience complete recovery from relapses were categorized as having "relapsing progressive" MS. Collectively, these categories were referred to as "relapsing forms of MS." In 1996 the category for relapsing progressive MS was discarded and RRMS was redefined to included patients who experienced acute relapses with or without complete recovery, and secondary MS was defined to include those patients who had progression of disability between episodes. Because patients in routine clinical follow-up are not always examined shortly after a relapse, it is probable that some patients with "relapsing progressive MS" who were enrolled in the Betaseron, Avonex, and Copaxone trials actually met criteria for the new definition for SPMS. This point is best illustrated by comparing the disease course between attacks in Figure 1*B* (RRMS) and 1*D* (SPMS). Thus, the change in definitions for the clinical types of MS should not be used as an excuse to deny access of IFN-β-1a or IFN-β-1b or copolymer I to SPMS patients with frequent relapses. Nonetheless, there are currently no approved treatment options for secondary progressive forms of MS. Several promising therapies are frequently prescribed off-label and are described in the following sections.

Interferon β

The results of the European phase III trial of IFN-β-1b in SPMS patients reported in *The Lancet* on November 4, 1998, indicate a clear reduction in exacerbations, time to onset of sustained progression of disability, and number of new MRI lesions in interferon recipients. These treatment effects were observed in SPMS patients who did and did not experience superimposed relapses. A similar trial of IFN-β-1a is ongoing in the United States and Canada, and IFN-β is already approved for use in SPMS in Europe. We expect IFN-β-1b will eventually be approved for treatment of SPMS in the United States.

Our preferred treatment for patients with SPMS who experience frequent exacerbations is IFN-β-1b. Once it is approved for use in SPMS, we will also prescribe IFN-β for patients with SPMS unaccompanied by relapses. There may be a role for MRI when making treatment decisions in SPMS patients who experience infrequent relapses. Specifically, IFN-β may be an appealing treatment option for SPMS patients who experience new MRI lesions in the absence of clinical exacerbations. We evaluate patients treated with IFN-β every 3 to 6 months and continue treatment for those who experience a reduction in annualized exacerbation rate and no progression of disability. Patients who continue to experience frequent exacerbations are usually switched to copolymer I. If patients experience sustained progression of disability while on IFN-β or copolymer I, we discontinue either drug and initiate therapy with methotrexate or intravenous methylprednisolone, as described next.

Methotrexate

Low-dose (7.5 mg) weekly oral methotrexate, has been shown to delay progression of disability in SPMS patients, an effect more pronounced in measures of upper extremity function. It has also been shown to have a positive effect on total progression of T2-weighted lesions. The relevant mechanisms of action of methotrexate include anti-inflammatory activities, suppression of proinflammatory cytokine interleukin (IL)–1, and antagonism of histamine-induced IFN-γ secretion by cytotoxic T cells.

Although low-dose, weekly oral methotrexate is not approved for use in MS, the observed treatment effect, modest toxicity, ready availability, and limited cost make it likely that many patients with progressive disease will seek and gain access to this therapy. Treatment decisions under such circumstances should be individualized and optimally should follow consultation with a physician who is experienced in the care of patients with MS and who is thoroughly familiar with the administration procedures, pharmacokinetics, potential drug interaction, and adverse effects known to occur with methotrexate.

We currently consider methotrexate as a first off-label treatment option for patients with SPMS who do not experience frequent exacerbations or for those SPMS patients with frequent relapses who continue to experience frequent exacerbations or sustained progression of disability despite treatment with IFN-β or copolymer I. Methotrexate, 7.5 mg, is administered orally each week and supplemented with folic acid, 1 mg, administered orally each day. The cost of therapy is approximately $50 each month. Methotrexate recipients should be instructed to avoid alcohol, aspirin, or nonsteroidal inflammatory agents because of potential hepatotoxicity. Because methotrexate is an abortifacient, it should not be used by women who are pregnant or attempting to become pregnant. All methotrexate recipients are monitored with determination of serum aspartate aminotransferase and alanine aminotransferase levels and a complete blood cell count each month. Hepatotoxicity, anemia, and neutropenia are uncommon and rarely necessitate cessation of therapy. Gastritis is observed occasionally and may be avoided by ingesting medication with food. Methotrexate recipients are examined every 3 months, and we continue this therapy in the absence of sustained progression of disability or intolerable drug-related adverse events. If methotrexate recipients experience sustained progression of disability, they are given the option of bimonthly pulses of methylprednisolone.

Methylprednisolone

In a dose comparison study, bimonthly intravenous pulses of methylprednisolone, 500 mg each day for 3 days, followed by a 10-day tapering course of oral methylprednisolone delayed time to onset of sustained progression of disability. The optimal dose and route of administration of methylprednisolone still need to be determined and efficacy confirmed in a phase III controlled clinical trial. The relevant mechanisms of action of corticosteroids in MS include reduction in abnormal vascular permeability, induction of monocytopenia, inhibition of metalloproteinases secreted by activated lymphocytes, and reduction in proinflammatory cytokines, including IL-1, IL-3, IL-6 through IL-8, tumor necrosis factor, and IFN-γ.

We treat SPMS patients who fail methotrexate treatment with bimonthly intravenous methylprednisolone, 500 mg per day, for 3 days without a corticosteroid taper. The cost of therapy is approximately $400 every other month. Methylprednisolone recipients are monitored with serum sodium and potassium determinations and a complete blood cell count each month. The drug is generally well tolerated, although insomnia, weight gain, acne, euphoria, and depression may be problematic. Patients undergo neurologic evaluation every 3 months, and treatment is continued in the absence of sustained progression of disability or intolerable drug-related adverse events.

Mitoxantrone

Mitoxantrone (Novantrone)* is a cytotoxic agent that intercalates DNA and inhibits the enzyme topoisomerase H. The drug exerts a potent immunosuppressive effect by directly reducing the number of B cells and by inhibiting T cell helper function and augmenting T cell suppressor function. It is 10 times more potent than cyclophosphamide in inhibiting experimental allergic encephalomyelitis, an animal model of MS. Intravenous mitoxantrone in two doses

(5 mg per m² and 12 mg per m²) has been studied in RRMS and SPMS patients in Europe, and preliminary results suggest that it has positive treatment effects on relapse rate, progression of disability, T2-weighted lesion load, and number of new gadolinium-enhancing lesions. Treatment is generally well tolerated, and the most common side effects include nausea, vomiting, reversible leukopenia, and alopecia. No significant cardiac toxicity has been observed. The final results of this study are pending, and mitoxantrone appears to be a promising treatment in SPMS.

Other Therapies

Patients who continue to experience gradual progression of disability despite methotrexate, bimonthly pulses of methylprednisolone, or mitoxantrone may be candidates for more aggressive treatments with agents such as 2-chlorodeoxyadenosine (cladribine [Leustatin])* or cyclophosphamide (Cytoxan).*

2-Chlorodeoxyadenosine (cladribine) is a purine nucleoside that selectively targets lymphoid cells both dividing and at rest. It has previously been shown to stabilize or modestly improve average neurologic impairment and disability scores; and in a more recent trial, subcutaneous cladribine demonstrated a profound reduction (90%) of gadolinium-enhancing lesions, but no effect was seen in terms of change in the scores or time to confirmed progression of disability. Final results of this trial are pending. Although the medication is well tolerated, severe lymphopenia persists for as long as 2 years. None of our cladribine recipients has experienced other drug-related adverse events. A 4-month course of therapy costs approximately $6000. The relevant mechanisms of action of cladribine are not known but may relate to drug-induced persistent lymphopenia. Cladribine remains under study in the treatment of MS, and a consensus protocol has not been established. Because of the significant potential for unwanted marrow suppression and possible complications of anemia, bleeding, and opportunistic infections, it may be most prudent to restrict the use of cladribine to research centers with strict approved protocols.

Cyclophosphamide is an alkylating agent with potent cytotoxic and immunosuppressive effects and is widely used in the treatment of neoplastic and autoimmune disorders. Modest benefit has been demonstrated in stabilizing disability in patients with progressive MS. The toxicities of cyclophosphamide have been well characterized and include alopecia, hemorrhagic cystitis, leukopenia, myocarditis, pulmonary interstitial fibrosis, and infertility. As such, cyclophosphamide should be considered only for carefully selected progressive patients with very active disease who have not responded to other less toxic alternatives.

---

*Not FDA approved for this indication.

*Not FDA approved for this indication.

Treatment of PPMS

PPMS is the remaining clinical pattern of MS for which there is no approved or promising therapy. There is only one ongoing controlled clinical trial of treatment (IFN-β-1a) for PPMS, and trials with glatiramer acetate and mitoxantrone are ongoing. In the absence of a rigorous controlled clinical trial for patients with PPMS, it remains unclear how to treat this form of the disease. The results of these ongoing and planned controlled clinical trials for PPMS are awaited with interest.

Other Considerations in the Management of MS Patients

The manifestations of MS are variable and can range from a benign disorder to a rapidly progressive debilitating illness. Complications of MS may affect multiple organ systems and necessitate profound adjustments in lifestyle and expectations for patients as well as their families. Focus on a multidisciplinary approach to the care of MS patients is desirable. Such a team generally includes the primary care physician, neurologist, psychologist, psychiatrist, nurse, occupational and physical therapist, and social worker.

Depression

Affective disorders and anxiety disorders are common in MS, and patients with MS are at increased risk for suicide. Patients should be asked directly about their emotional symptoms on a regular basis in consideration for early medical or psychotherapeutic intervention. When considering medical treatment for depression, one should take into account other symptoms the patient may be experiencing, such as fatigue, bladder symptoms, or chronic pain, because this may affect the choice of antidepressant. An otherwise unwanted side effect such as urinary retention with anticholinergic effects of the tricyclic antidepressants may prove beneficial in a patient with a spastic bladder. Amitriptyline (Elavil) may be started at a dose of 25 mg at bed time, increasing by 25 mg every week as tolerated, for a target dose of 75 to 100 mg each night. For patients with concurrent fatigue, fluoxetine (Prozac) at 10 to 20 mg per day can be helpful.

Patients with MS can also experience inappropriate laughter or crying as a result of bilateral disruption of subcortical pathways. For some, reassurance that this does not represent depression and is relatively common is sufficient. For those in whom these symptoms are bothersome or unacceptable, a trial of amitriptyline, at doses ranging from 10 to 75 mg per day, or fluoxetine, 20 mg per day, may be helpful.

Fatigue

Fatigue is extremely common in MS, but the mechanisms underlying fatigue in MS are poorly understood. The fatigue experienced by MS patients appears to be different from that in depression and sleep disorders, and it remains a very difficult symptom to treat. We recommend a combination of pharmacotherapy and behavioral changes. Patients appear to benefit from regimented sleep schedules with dedicated nap times. Amantadine (Symmetrel)* in doses of 100 mg once or twice daily is effective in about 50% of patients. Alternative pharmacotherapies include pemoline (Cylert),* 37.5 mg, or fluoxetine hydrochloride (Prozac),* 10 to 20 mg, once or twice daily.

Spasticity

Spasticity results from interruption of inhibitory influences on anterior horn cells that can occur with lesions of the brain, spinal cord, and brain stem. It is associated with increased muscle tone, weakness, hyperreflexia, extensor plantar responses, and spontaneous muscle spasms. Painful tonic spasms in the limbs may be spontaneous but are often triggered by voluntary movement, tactile stimulation, or noxious stimuli, or may occur in the setting of an infection such as a decubitus ulcer or urinary tract infection.

Before initiating therapy for spasticity it is important to consider the degree of leg weakness. Patients with spasticity may demonstrate profound hip flexor weakness, relying on the stability of their leg stiffness to ambulate. Treatment of spasticity in these patients may potentially result in increasing disability with loss of ambulation. On the other hand, some patients with spasticity maintain fairly good strength, and the limb stiffness limits their ambulatory capacity. Treatment of spasticity in these patients would be desirable to enable an improved gait.

Oral baclofen (Lioresal) is our first-line treatment for spasticity in MS. Therapy is initiated at 5 mg once daily, increasing by 5 mg every 3 days as tolerated. Most patients require and tolerate total doses of 30 to 80 mg per day, although the lowest dose providing symptomatic relief should be used. Doses exceeding 80 mg per day are usually poorly tolerated, resulting in symptoms of weakness, drowsiness, and leg swelling. Liver and renal function should be monitored routinely during treatment. Abrupt cessation of baclofen is contraindicated and has been associated with seizures and psychosis.

Although monotherapy for symptom management in MS is desirable, in some instances oral baclofen alone may be insufficient. For these patients, adding diazepam (Valium), 1 to 2 mg, or clonidine (Catapres),* 0.1 to 0.2 mg, two to three times per day may enhance the effectiveness of baclofen. An alternative monotherapy is tizanidine (Zanaflex), a centrally acting alpha₂-adrenergic agonist. We find that this treatment is most helpful for nocturnal leg spasms. Treatment is initiated at 2 to 4 mg daily, increasing by 2 to 4 mg at weekly intervals to target doses of 8 mg once to three times daily, titrating to effect. Sedation is fairly common and can be an undesirable side effect. Because of risks of hepatotoxicity, bimonthly liver panel assessment is recommended for the first

---

*Not FDA approved for this indication.

6 months and periodically thereafter. No controlled trials have been done to investigate combination therapy with tizanidine and baclofen. Dantrolene sodium (Dantrium) may also be effective in alleviating spasticity, but because it acts peripherally, inhibiting myofibril contraction, it invariably produces weakness, which limits its usefulness in MS patients. Treatment can be initiated at 25 mg per day, increasing as needed and tolerated to a maximum of 100 mg per day. Hepatotoxicity is a common and potentially fatal adverse side effect, and liver function tests should be done on a biweekly basis.

For patients who experience severe debilitating spasticity unresponsive to oral agents, baclofen can be administered intrathecally by a subcutaneous pump. This route of administration delivers a four-fold higher concentration of baclofen in the cerebrospinal fluid and is very successful in alleviating spasms. Complications relate to surgical implantation of the pump, mechanical dysfunction of the pump, and infection.

Any medical treatment of spasticity should be accompanied by a regimen of physical therapy. Daily muscle stretching exercises, both passive and active, are important adjuncts in the treatment of limb spasticity and are necessary to avoid formation of limb contractures.

Bladder/Bowel Symptoms

Symptoms of urinary urgency, frequency, hesitation, retention, and incontinence occur in up to 80% of MS patients. Treatment of bladder symptoms should begin with an assessment of the underlying dysfunction. Urinary frequency, urgency, and subsequent urge incontinence usually result from a spastic detrusor muscle. Urinary retention and hesitation result from sphincter dyssynergia, with incomplete relaxation of internal and external sphincters during detrusor contraction. Patients with urinary symptoms should undergo urinalysis to rule out underlying infection, and this should be followed by assessment of postvoid residual urine volumes.

Patients voiding less than 200 mL with residual volumes of less than 100 mL likely have detrusor spasticity. For these patients, oxybutynin chloride (Ditropan), in doses of 2.5 to 5 mg two to three times a day, can be helpful. Therapeutic alternatives include propantheline bromide (Pro-Banthine),* at a dose of 15 mg three to four times per day, or hyoscyamine sulfate (Levsin),* 0.125 to 0.375 mg every 4 hours, as needed. Side effects are due to the anticholinergic effects of these drugs and most commonly include dry mouth and constipation. Tolterodine (Detrol), 2 mg twice daily, appears to be better tolerated with fewer anticholinergic side effects. Patients who void more than 500 mL but have postvoid residual volumes more than 100 mL likely have a hypotonic detrusor muscle, whereas those with postvoid residuals more than 100 mL likely have superimposed sphincter dyssynergia. In our experience, the most

effective option for these patients is oxybutynin chloride, 2.5 mg once to three times daily, combined with intermittent self-catheterization. In those patients for whom self-catheterization is problematic (limited manual dexterity, visual symptoms), a 2-week trial of terazosin (Hytrin),* 5 mg once or twice daily, may promote bladder emptying.

Pain Syndromes

Acute facial pain, chronic dysesthesias, paroxysmal limb pain, painful tonic spasms, and musculoskeletal pain can occur in up to 85% of MS patients. Acute pain may take the form of trigeminal neuralgia (brief, lancinating pains usually in the distribution of the second and third divisions of the trigeminal nerve), Lhermitte's phenomenon (shooting pains down the spine and into the limbs with neck flexion), and painful dysesthesias. The pain is responsive to carbamazepine (Tegretol), 100 to 200 mg two to three times per day, increasing as necessary. Alternatives include gabapentin (Neurontin)* at doses of 300 to 400 mg three times daily, titrating as needed; phenytoin (Dilantin),* 100 to 200 mg two or three times daily; or baclofen, 10 to 30 mg one to three times daily.

Chronic pain in MS typically takes the form of chronic dysesthesias described as burning, deep aching, or tingling. First-line agents include tricyclic antidepressants (amitriptyline, 25 to 150 mg per day) and carbamazepine. Alternatively, gabapentin and phenytoin may be successful. In recalcitrant pain syndromes, referral to a pain center is recommended.

Because of problems of limited mobility in some MS patients, musculoskeletal pain syndromes are very common. This may take the form of radiculopathies, commonly sciatic, lumbosacral pain or limb stiffness. Over-the-counter nonsteroidal anti-inflammatory agents may be beneficial. However, increased physical activity with participation in regular exercise programs through physiotherapy, aquatherapy, yoga, and so on are recommended to all of our MS patients.

Paroxysmal Symptoms

Paroxysmal symptoms may range from brief sensory symptoms to more prolonged dystonic spasms. These spasms should be distinguished from flexor spasms associated with spasticity. They may appear in patients who have little or no spasticity and are typically prolonged, painful spasms that may affect a limb or face and may spread anatomically to cross the midline, lasting up to 2 minutes. Paroxysmal symptoms may be elicited by hyperventilation or triggered by movement or stimulation of a limb. They respond to carbamazepine* and phenytoin* in doses previously described.

*Not FDA approved for this indication.

---

*Not FDA approved for this indication.

ACQUIRED MYASTHENIA GRAVIS

method of
JANICE M. MASSEY, M.D.
Duke University Medical Center
Durham, North Carolina

Myasthenia gravis (MG) is an acquired autoimmune disease of the neuromuscular junction. Fatigable, fluctuating muscle weakness is characteristic of MG. It may be associated with the presence of a thymoma or other autoimmune diseases. Therapy is aimed at modulating the immune response.

MG is the most common and best understood immune-mediated disorder of neuromuscular transmission. There is immunologic attack of the postsynaptic membrane of the muscle end plate that reduces the number of functional acetylcholine receptors from either loss of structural integrity or blockade. Fluctuating, fatigable weakness of muscles under voluntary control produces the symptoms of MG, which vary based on involvement of specific muscle groups. Patients may have symptoms and signs only late in the day or after exertion. Thus, the diagnosis may be delayed, unrecognized, or presumed psychiatric in origin, particularly if the patient is examined early in the day.

EPIDEMIOLOGY

Disease incidence rates are estimated to be between 2.1 and 14.7 per million population per year, whereas prevalence rates range between 7.7 and 175 per million population. Prevalence rates appear to be increasing as the population ages. There is a bimodal distribution of onset based on gender. Females commonly have onset in the second and third decades, whereas men are most often affected in the seventh and eighth decades. Previously, women constituted a larger proportion of the population, but this distinction is changing as the population has increased in age. In the United States, incidence and prevalence are proportionately higher in the African-American population. After age 50, the incidence increases in men and women.

CLINICAL MANIFESTATION

Acquired MG may begin at any age and most often affects women. Virtually all patients have ocular symptoms, most frequently intermittent diplopia and ptosis, often as the initial symptom or developing within 1 to 2 years of onset of MG. Patients are usually acutely aware of diplopia because vision is disturbed, although those with mild ocular disease may repeatedly change eyeglasses in an attempt to correct blurred vision. Ocular symptoms are typically present toward the end of the day or after extensive reading, driving after dark or in bright sunlight, or working at a computer terminal. Past photographs may show progressive ptosis, changes in the smile, or other changes in facial expression.

Difficulty chewing, speaking, or swallowing is the initial symptom in about 20% of patients. Difficulty chewing may be mistakenly diagnosed as temporomandibular joint disease or dental disease.

Respiratory insufficiency as the initial manifestation is rare. Limb muscle weakness as the initial symptom is uncommon. Generalized fatigue or malaise, without accompanying specific dysfunction referable to an activity or muscle group, is rare. Infrequently, weakness at onset involves a focal or limited group of muscles, such as finger extension, neck flexion or extension, hip flexion, or asymmetrical masseter weakness.

Precipitating Events

Initial symptoms may occur during a systemic illness (especially hypothyroid or hyperthyroid dysfunction) or viral upper respiratory tract infection. Weakness may first be apparent after the patient receives general anesthesia, neuromuscular blocking agents, aminoglycoside antibiotics, antiarrhythmic cardiac agents, beta-blocking agents, penicillamine, interferon, radiologic contrast agents, or corticosteroid medications (Table 1). Manifestation during pregnancy or the immediate postpartum period also occurs. Exposure to extreme heat or undue stress may also unmask symptoms.

Signs

FACIAL APPEARANCE

Many patients have a characteristic facial appearance. The head may be held slightly extended to compensate for both ptosis and medial rectus muscle weakness. The brows are elevated in an attempt to lift the lids. Despite the frontalis contraction, ptosis is usually apparent and often asymmetrical. The globe of the eye may protrude because of weakness of the extraocular muscles. With blinking or eyelid closure, the sclera may not be completely covered owing to weakness of the orbicularis oculi muscles. A weak face may have a paucity of expression and droop bilaterally. The smile may develop a horizontal or snarling appearance.

OCULAR MUSCLES

Most patients have ocular involvement. A number of ocular signs have been described. Eyelid ptosis is usually asymmetrical and may vary throughout the period of observation. Asking the patient to close and relax the eyelids for 30 to 60 seconds may improve ptosis, whereas sustained upgaze may exacerbate ptosis. Pupillary responses are normal. Typically, the pattern of extraocular muscle weakness is asymmetrical, is not isolated to innervation by one cranial nerve, and fluctuates. If ptosis and extraocular muscle dysfunction are unilateral or if the pattern of weakness is consistent with a lesion of one or more individual cranial nerves, there should be concern about another diagnosis. The weakest extraocular muscles are usually the medial rectus followed by the superior rectus and lateral rectus muscles. With sustained upgaze of 30 to 60 seconds, there may be fatigue of the medial rectus or the elevator muscles, producing or exacerbating diplopia, and the lid elevators

TABLE 1. **Drugs That May Produce Exacerbation of Myasthenia Gravis**

- Aminoglycoside antibiotics
- Beta-blocking agents
- Botulinum toxin
- Calcium channel blockers
- Interferon
- Muscle relaxants, curare-like agents
- Magnesium salts
- Procainamide
- Quinidine, quinine
- Radiographic contrast agents
- Penicillamine—(Cuprimine) contraindicated
- Corticosteroids may initially produce worsening of myasthenia gravis

may fatigue, producing worsening ptosis. With sustained lateral gaze, fatigable weakness of the medial or lateral rectus may be noted. Also with attempted lateral gaze, the adducting eye may not move while the abducting eye demonstrates nystagmus, with the nystagmoid movements becoming coarser as lateral rectus muscle weakness fatigues. This has been termed a pseudointernuclear ophthalmoplegia and may be mistaken for brain stem abnormality.

Virtually all patients have weakness of eyelid closure.

OROPHARYNGEAL MUSCLES

Weakness of the facial, palatal, masticatory, and/or tongue muscles may produce difficulties with chewing, swallowing, speaking, or breathing. The presence of oropharyngeal weakness is a serious sign and generates concern about protection of the airway. There may be difficulty controlling secretions or aspiration when attempting to drink. Posterior pharyngeal muscle weakness may collapse the upper airway.

Facial muscle involvement is evident when there is weakness of eyelid closure and inability to whistle, pucker, or hold air in the cheeks. Palpebral fissures may be widened because of weakness of the lower facial muscles. The smile may be transverse or produce a myasthenic snarl.

Speech may be initially nasal but become unintelligible with prolonged speaking. Hoarseness or low volume is unusual. Tongue involvement may be demonstrated by weak protrusion into the cheek or inability to lift the tongue to reach the top of the upper lip. It may be atrophic with "triple furrowing."

Weakness of the muscles of mastication may have been present for a long time before weakness of jaw closure is noted. When masseter weakness exists, the patient may hold the mouth shut with the hand. Swallowing difficulties occur from weakness of the lower facial muscles, the tongue, or the muscles of the posterior pharynx. Coughing after drinking or eating suggests aspiration, and there may even be difficulty with controlling secretions. Some patients find that turning the head or tucking the chin close to the neck improves swallowing. When the palatal and posterior pharyngeal muscles are weak, there may be nasal regurgitation of liquids with swallowing.

LIMB MUSCLES

In mild disease, neck flexor muscle involvement may be the only manifestation of generalized weakness. Neck flexor muscles are more frequently weak than the neck extensor muscles, although rare patients have isolated neck extensor weakness at presentation. Whereas any limb or truncal muscles may be weak, certain patterns of weakness are characteristic. In general, upper extremity muscles are weaker than muscles of the lower limb. In the upper extremity, deltoid and wrist/finger extensor muscles are most commonly involved and the triceps is more likely to be weak than the biceps. In the lower extremity, the foot dorsiflexors may be the only detectable weak muscle, followed in frequency by hip flexor muscles. The hamstring, gastrocnemius, and quadriceps muscles are less often involved.

Fatigability of muscle strength with repeated testing is usually a significant feature of MG.

MYASTHENIC CRISIS

Respiratory distress in MG can occur precipitously in a patient with recent worsening of symptoms, especially if oropharyngeal muscles are involved. Respiratory support is required when the patient cannot achieve a negative inspiratory force of -20 cm H_2O, a tidal volume of 4 mL per kg, and a breathing capacity three times the tidal volume, or when the forced vital capacity is less than 15 mL per kg. Measurement of respiratory function may be falsely abnormal if facial weakness precludes an airtight seal on the mouth device. Respiratory distress may also occur if the upper airway collapses and prevents air movement. Immediate intubation is then necessary.

COURSE

Without treatment the disease progresses in most patients. In those whose initial manifestations are only ocular, two thirds developed generalized disease, most within the first year. Only 14% have weakness that clinically remained restricted to extraocular muscles after 2 years. The course may be marked by variations in symptoms with periods of spontaneous improvement, particularly early in the disease. Untreated patients may show fluctuations early in the disease followed by progression of severity and involvement of more muscle groups. In the era before definitive treatment for MG, mortality was 25 to 30%. Mortality rates significantly decreased for patients with onset of disease after 1960, owing to improved treatment. After many years, untreated patients may develop fixed weakness with atrophic muscles.

ASSOCIATED DISEASES

A number of diseases have been described in association with MG. Many of these are recognized as autoimmune disorders. Diabetes mellitus may be present even before treatment with corticosteroids. Thyroid disease and pernicious anemia are common, whereas rheumatoid arthritis, pancytopenia, thrombocytopenia, and systemic lupus erythematosus occur infrequently. In 10 to 15% of patients with MG, a thymoma is present. Most thymomas are benign; only rarely are they malignant.

DIFFERENTIAL DIAGNOSIS

Conditions confused with MG include chronic progressive external ophthalmoplegia, cavernous sinus lesions, amyotrophic lateral sclerosis, myotonic dystrophy, polymyositis, Lambert-Eaton myasthenic syndrome, and congenital myasthenic syndromes. Very rarely, MG and polymyositis coexist.

Comparison of Diagnostic Tests in MG

In patients with clinical weakness limited to ocular muscles, SF-EMG is abnormal in 95% of studies whereas RNS is abnormal in only 48%. The sensitivity of both RNS and AChR-Ab was higher for patients with increasing severity of clinical involvement. However, SF-EMG was abnormal in 100% of studies in the same groups. With only ocular or mild generalized weakness, RNS and AChR-Ab testing have the lowest diagnostic yield. Unfortunately, the diagnosis is clinically less evident in this group of patients. SF-EMG is most useful in confirming or excluding the diagnosis for patients in whom RNS and AChR-Ab are normal. SF-EMG is not necessary for diagnosis if a significant decrement is found on RNS.

DIAGNOSTIC TESTS

Edrophonium (Tensilon) Test

The diagnosis is supported by improvement of strength after administration of an anticholinesterase drug. Intravenous edrophonium (Tensilon), 0.15 to 0.2 mg per kg, provides a rapid assessment of improvement. There should be unequivocal demonstrable improvement of strength to judge the test results as positive. The effects of edrophonium are transient, usually less than 10 minutes in duration, but rarely may last longer. Side effects include increased tearing, salivation, muscle fasciculations, and abdominal cramps. Caution should be exercised for patients with cardiac disease because bradycardia and even cardiac arrest can occur. Intravenous administration of atropine, 0.4 mg, can reverse the side effects. A placebo also may be given, but it is difficult to truly "blind" the test.

Longer-acting anticholinesterase agents such as neostigmine (Prostigmin)* 1.5 mg intramuscularly, may also be used. The action of intramuscular neostigmine begins in 15 to 30 minutes and lasts up to 3 hours. Use of a longer-acting agent allows more time for observation of the response and is particularly useful in infants and children (neostigmine, 0.1 to 0.2 mg IM).

Electrodiagnostic Testing

Routine nerve conduction studies and electromyography are usually unrevealing in disorders of neuromuscular transmission (NMT). The techniques of repetitive nerve stimulation (RNS) studies and single fiber electromyography (SF-EMG) are often necessary for diagnostic purposes. Additionally, characterization of presynaptic versus postsynaptic disorders of neuromuscular transmission is dependent on the pattern of RNS abnormality. Whereas electrodiagnostic tests are often used to confirm the clinical diagnosis of neuromuscular junction abnormality, there are some patients in whom the clinical picture is confusing and these tests are the only means to determine the presence of abnormal neuromuscular transmission.

Acetylcholine Receptor Antibodies

The presence of serum binding antibodies to human acetylcholine receptors (AChR) is highly specific for the diagnosis of MG. In 74% of patients with MG, serum antibodies to human AChR are present. Of those patients without elevated AChR-Ab, the disease may be less severe and more often restricted to the ocular muscles. The antibody level is not predictive of response to therapy. Virtually all patients with thymoma have elevated AChR-Ab levels.

TREATMENT

There is no distinct agreement among experts in the field about the therapeutic options available for patients with MG. No therapy has been demonstrated efficacious by rigorous controlled studies. The art of providing care for patients with MG lies in deciding when to and when not to treat aggressively. A number of factors influence the decision process. The rate of progression along with the severity and distribution of the weakness are the most important considerations for immediate therapeutic decisions. Long-term therapy is also influenced by age, gender, presence of coincidental disease, and response to previous therapy.

*Not FDA approved for this indication.

Cholinesterase Inhibitors

Cholinesterase inhibitors provide symptomatic improvement for most patients with MG for a period of time. Often, they are used as the initial therapy. This group of drugs impedes the hydrolysis of acetylcholine at the neuromuscular junction. There is no alteration of the immunologic activity involved in the genesis of the disease symptoms. Treatment with cholinesterase inhibitors is rarely effective alone. Some patients are very sensitive to these drugs and develop side effects at quite low doses.

Pyridostigmine bromide (Mestinon) and neostigmine bromide (Prostigmin) may be the most commonly used agents. The initial dosage of pyridostigmine bromide is 15 to 60 mg every 4 to 6 hours. Neostigmine bromide, 7.5 to 15 mg every 4 to 6 hours, may be used. For intramuscular administration, neostigmine, 1.5 mg, is the better choice. The dosage and dose interval may be adjusted based on clinical observation to allow maximal response. For patients with oropharyngeal weakness, the dose should be timed to maximize strength during meals (usually 30 minutes before eating). The minimum dose interval should be no less than every 3 to 4 hours.

The most common side effects are gastrointestinal hyperactivity and increased oral and upper respiratory secretions. The increase in oral secretions may be problematic in the patient already having swallowing or respiratory difficulty. Bronchospasm and bradycardia can occur especially with higher doses. When excessive drug is administered or if the patient is extremely sensitive to cholinesterase inhibitors, worsening weakness may occur. The occurrence of such cholinergic-induced weakness often parallels development of the side effect of diarrhea.

Thymectomy

The relationship between the thymus and the pathogenesis of MG is not precisely understood. Often the thymus is enlarged with histologic evidence of thymic hyperplasia with germinal centers.

Although a prospective blinded study has never been performed, there is general agreement that thymectomy (Table 2) is indicated for selected pa-

TABLE 2. **Advantages and Disadvantages of Thymectomy for Myasthenia Gravis**

Advantages
- Sustained improvement in > 50%
- Excludes possibility of thymoma
- No known long-term side effects

Disadvantages
- Perioperative complications
- Unpredictable onset of response
- Unpredictable extent of response
- Complete long-term remission is rare
- Response not as frequent in elderly
- Expensive

TABLE 3. **Treatment of Myasthenia Gravis with Corticosteroids**

Advantages
- Rapid improvement
- Improvement in most patients
- Combination therapy with other immunosuppressants
- Familiar to physicians, easy to use
- Inexpensive

Disadvantages
- Steroid side effects
- Chronic administration
- Requires close monitoring

tients younger than age 60 years with generalized weakness. Thymectomy for virtually all patients with thymoma is indicated. After age 60, the thymus is largely replaced with fat, which may account for less benefit from thymectomy. Median sternotomy with cervical exploration allows maximal removal of all thymic tissue. Patients with significant weakness chosen for thymectomy should be treated preoperatively with either plasmapheresis or immunosuppression. Onset and extent of improvement are unpredictable, but any weakness that is persistent 1 year after thymectomy is unlikely to remit without additional therapy. Over 50% of those patients undergoing thymectomy have sustained improvement. The surgery excludes the presence of unsuspected thymoma or development of thymoma. In experienced hands, there are no known long-term side effects of thymectomy.

Immunosuppressant Drugs

Each of the immunosuppressant drugs has the potential to produce improvement of weakness from MG. All forms of immunosuppression carry the risk of increased infection and may incur added risk for the development of malignancy. In addition, each drug also has significant individual potential side effects. Thus, the decision to choose one or more of these drugs should be made cautiously with consideration for both short- and long-term outcomes for the patient. A patient with long-standing, mild, predominantly ocular weakness might not be best treated with aggressive immunosuppression, whereas a patient with rapidly progressive oropharyngeal musculature weakness would be best treated with immunosuppression.

Except for the corticosteroids, all of the immunosuppressant drugs are expensive, a fact that occasionally precludes their use.

Corticosteroids

The first immunosuppressant agents used in the treatment of MG were the corticosteroids* (Table 3). Most patients improve with corticosteroid therapy.

Administration of high-dose daily prednisone (60 to 80 mg per day) results in predictable rapid improvement, often producing complete reversal of weakness. Institution of this regimen is often followed within the first 1 to 3 weeks by an exacerbation of weakness. Although in most patients this worsening can be managed by administration of cholinesterase inhibitors or pretreatment with plasmapheresis, they should be admitted to a hospital for institution of high-dose prednisone while monitoring for any worsening oropharyngeal weakness that might compromise respiratory function. Once improvement is clearly established, the stable patient is safe for discharge. Some physicians attempt to avoid this exacerbation by administration of a low dose with gradual increments. The difficulty with this approach is that one cannot predict the timing of such worsening and any worsening seen during the incrementing phase may be from either corticosteroid-induced exacerbation or worsening of the disease, which are indistinguishable. Once there is maximal improvement of strength, the corticosteroid dose is gradually tapered over months to several years with frequent observation for signs of return of weakness. Many patients require long-term maintenance low-dose corticosteroid therapy to prevent return of myasthenic weakness. Corticosteroid therapy may be used in combination with other immunosuppressive agents.

Potential side effects of corticosteroid therapy are significant and numerous and include weight gain with cushingoid features, skin changes, cataracts, gastrointestinal ulcers, changes in affect, and increased susceptibility to diabetes mellitus, hypertension, osteoporosis, and infection.

Azathioprine

Azathioprine (Imuran),* a purine antimetabolite, is a relatively weak immunosuppressive drug with a delayed onset of effect (Table 4). At a dose of 2 to 3 mg per kg per day, improvement in strength begins after 2 to 8 months, and the effect may not be maximal until 12 to 24 months. At this dose, side effects are usually very mild and consist of bone marrow suppression, macrocytosis, or elevated levels of liver enzymes. Close monitoring of blood counts and liver enzymes is necessary. Side effects are usually reversible by reducing or discontinuing the drug. Fifteen to 20% of patients have an idiosyncratic response within the first month characterized by flulike symptoms, gastrointestinal symptoms, and even rash. The drug must be discontinued.

The long-term effects of azathioprine are not clearly known, but there is some concern of an increased risk of malignancy.

If corticosteroids are contraindicated, azathioprine can be used as an initial definitive therapy. It also may be used in combination with corticosteroids, thus allowing more complete improvement often with a lower dose of corticosteroid.

---

*Not FDA approved for this indication.

*Not FDA approved for this indication.

TABLE 4. **Treatment of Myasthenia Gravis with Azathioprine (Imuran)**

Advantages
- Well tolerated by most
- Sustained improvement
- Simple to use
- Side effects different than for corticosteriods

Disadvantages
- Slow onset of improvement
- Side effects: bone marrow suppression, macrocytosis, liver enzyme elevation
- Idiosyncratic response in 15% precludes usage
- Chronic administration
- Close monitoring
- Expensive

TABLE 5. **Role of Plasmapheresis in Myasthenia Gravis**

Advantages
- Rapid improvement
- No long-term side effects known

Disadvantages
- Short duration of improvement
- Vascular access
- Metabolic derangement: hypocalcemia, hypoalbuminemia
- Expensive

Role
- Adjunctive therapy
- Preoperative preparation
- To reduce corticosteroid exacerbations
- During myasthenic crisis
- When other therapy fails

Cyclosporine

Cyclosporine (Neoral)* is a potent immunosuppressive and immunomodulating agent that inhibits amplification of T lymphocyte immune responses. Cyclosporine has been used effectively for patients refractory to other forms of therapy. At a dose of 3 to 6 mg per kg per day, given in divided doses 12 hours apart, blood trough levels of 100 to 150 μg per liter are usually attained and correspond with clinical improvement. Side effects most commonly encountered include nephrotoxicity, hypertension, and interaction with a host of other common medications. In addition to monitoring renal function and blood pressure, maintenance of therapeutic cyclosporine levels is necessary to prevent toxicity.

Cyclophosphamide

Cyclophosphamide (Cytoxan)* is also a potent immunosuppressive agent. It has been used to treat patients who are refractory to other forms of therapy. A dose of 3 to 5 mg per kg per day is used and may be preceded with an initial intravenous dose of 200 mg daily for 5 days. Side effects that necessitate close monitoring include leukopenia, hemorrhagic cystitis, gastrointestinal symptoms, anorexia, and alopecia. After a therapeutic effect is achieved, the dose may be successfully lowered.

Plasmapheresis

Plasmapheresis (plasma exchange) is an effective short-term therapy for patients with severe weakness (Table 5). It is particularly useful in the setting of recent exacerbation, in preparation for surgery, and to offset the exacerbation seen with initiation of corticosteroid therapy. The mode of action is presumed to be removal of circulating pathogenic elements such as AchR-Ab and immune complexes. However, even patients with seronegative MG improve with plasma exchange. The goal is removal of 2 to 3 liters of plasma three times a week until improvement in strength reaches a plateau.

The onset of improvement is rapid, often beginning after the third exchange. Improvement lasts 6 to 8 weeks. Complications from the procedure include hypotension, cardiac arrhythmia, altered clotting mechanisms, hypoalbuminemia, hypocalcemia, and difficulty with vascular access.

Intravenous Immunoglobulin

A number of small series of patients have been reported to improve after administration of high doses of intravenous human immune globulin (IGIV).* Doses of 2 grams per kg over 2 to 5 days are associated with onset of improvement often within the first week and persisting for weeks to months. Minor side effects are the most common and include headache, chills, and fever. These may be treated symptomatically. Transient leukopenia is usually seen. Aseptic meningitis, renal failure, and stroke are uncommon. A growing number of cases of transmitted hepatitis C have been reported.

The exact mechanism of action is poorly understood. Before administering IVIG, patients should be screened for selective IgA deficiency because an anaphylactic reaction to the IgA in IgG preparations can occur.

Pregnancy

Similar to that of other neurologic diseases, the course of MG may change during pregnancy. The influence of pregnancy on MG is variable, but some women worsen during this time. MG should have no deleterious effect on the uterine smooth muscle. Frequent examination during the pregnancy to observe for worsening is important.

When there is significant weakness, the treatment plan is more complicated than in the nonpregnant patient to avoid increasing risks to both the fetus and the mother. There are also several challenging therapeutic problems unique to this group. Frequent emesis in the early months of pregnancy may interfere with absorption of any oral medication. Marked

*Not FDA approved for this indication.

*Not FDA approved for this indication.

changes in blood volume and renal clearance occur. The changing hormonal patterns may also exert some influence on MG. In women with respiratory compromise, the growing fetus may further restrict diaphragmatic movement. Magnesium sulfate for the treatment of pregnancy-induced hypertension can exacerbate weakness in MG and should be avoided. Postpartum exacerbation, particularly when acute, may also pose a problem.

Cholinesterase inhibitors have been used in pregnancy. Uterine contractions are usually not associated with oral cholinesterase inhibitors. The dosage must be adjusted frequently because there are ongoing changes in blood volume and renal clearance. When possible, one aims to avoid immunosuppressive drugs. For those patients planning pregnancy, if the disease severity allows, these drugs should be minimized or discontinued to avoid potential adverse effects on the fetus. However, this is not always possible, owing to disease severity; and respiratory compromise may pose a greater risk to both fetus and mother than treatment with immunosuppressant drugs. Infrequently, corticosteroid therapy has been associated with mild fetal defects. Azathioprine is also potentially teratogenic, although there are reports of its use without fetal risk in other autoimmune diseases and in patients with transplants.

Progressive or significant weakness may be adequately controlled with cholinesterase inhibitors and plasmapheresis. There is concern that circulating hormones crucial to the integrity of the pregnancy are removed by plasmapheresis. Hypotension must be avoided and may be less if the procedure is performed with the patient in the left lateral decubitus position. Late in the pregnancy, the obstetrician may recommend fetal monitoring during plasmapheresis.

Because the effect of thymectomy is not immediate, there is no advantage to incur the added risk of surgery during pregnancy. The safety of IGIV therapy for MG in pregnancy has not been established.

CONCLUSION

The clinical assessment of the patient's history and examination is the most crucial element in determining the presence of MG. The edrophonium test and acetylcholine receptor antibody titers are useful in confirmation of the diagnosis. In addition, electrophysiologic tests are valuable aids in the clinical assessment of patients with suspected disease. RNS is the most widely used technique to assess the integrity of neuromuscular transmission but may be normal in many patients. Among the techniques used to assess abnormality of neuromuscular transmission, SF-EMG is the most sensitive. All diagnostic tests are most reliable when potential pitfalls are known and when the results are interpreted in relation to the overall clinical setting.

Once the diagnosis is confirmed, patients with ocular signs and symptoms should be watched closely during the first 3 years for evidence of generalized weakness. If the patient has only ocular signs, man-

TABLE 6. **Approach to Treatment: Generalized Myasthenia Gravis**

Onset Before Age 60
- Thymectomy; pretreat with plasmapheresis, cholinesterase inhibitors
- If response unsatisfactory before or after thymectomy, consider high-dose daily prednisone and/or other immunosuppressive agents if necessary.

Onset After Age 60
- Prednisone, azathioprine, or other immunosuppressant drugs
- Cholinesterase inhibitors as needed for symptomatic improvement
- Plasmapheresis for severe exacerbations
- Consider thymectomy in some

agement with cholinesterase inhibitors may be adequate. Occasionally, low doses of corticosteroids or even azathioprine may be selected if the ocular dysfunction is unresponsive to cholinesterase inhibitors. For those patients with generalized weakness (Table 6), if they are middle-aged or younger and in good health, thymectomy should be considered, particularly if there is suspicion of a possible thymoma. If those patients have marked weakness, pretreatment with plasmapheresis or immunosuppression to produce improvement before thymectomy reduces complications.

In choosing a specific treatment plan for an individual patient, the potential risks versus potential benefits should be considered. Pregnant patients present unique therapeutic dilemmas. Corticosteroids and azathioprine have been used most extensively in the medical treatment of MG, whereas other immunosuppressant drugs may be beneficial but likely have greater potential risks. There is no reliable relationship of any laboratory test and the response to therapy. Thus, the clinical course must be used to determine therapy and assess response.

TRIGEMINAL NEURALGIA
method of
ROBERT M. LEVY, M.D., PH.D.
Northwestern University Medical School
Chicago, Illinois

CLINICAL PRESENTATION

The pain of trigeminal neuralgia is sometimes described as the most severe and debilitating pain ever experienced. Also known as tic douloureux, trigeminal neuralgia usually presents as a sharp, lancinating pain in the face. Each episode of pain is remarkably brief, lasting as short as a fraction of a second, but several such episodes can follow in rapid succession. The pain follows the sensory distribution of one or more of the major branches of the trigeminal nerve. Most commonly affected is the third (mandibular) division, whereas the second (maxillary) division pain is somewhat less frequently affected. First (ophthalmic) division pain is rather unusual but unique in some of the therapeutic issues it presents because this nerve also supplies critical sensation to the cornea. Pain not uncommonly involves more than one division of the trigeminal nerve.

The pain is almost always unilateral, although bilateral trigeminal neuralgia can occur. It frequently begins spontaneously. Characteristic of trigeminal neuralgia, however, are cutaneous triggers for the pain. Touching of the face while shaving or by cold air, talking, chewing, and brushing one's teeth can all serve to trigger the pain. Thus, patients with active trigeminal neuralgia will often lose weight from not eating or demonstrate poor facial hygiene as a result of their efforts to prevent the pain.

Trigeminal neuralgia is most often found in patients older than 60 years of age, although it can develop in individuals of any age. There is a smaller group of patients about the age of 30 who develop trigeminal neuralgia most often in association with multiple sclerosis. Trigeminal neuralgia is slightly more common in women and on the right side of the face.

ETIOLOGY AND DIAGNOSIS

Neurologic examination of the patient with trigeminal neuralgia is usually normal, with the exception of touch-evoked pain when triggers are activated. The presence of neurologic deficits such as sensory loss are suggestive of other pathologies. While in its pure form, trigeminal neuralgia may be straightforward to recognize, there are related pain syndromes of the face that may be difficult to distinguish and for which different treatment responses may be expected. Thus, trigeminal neuralgia exists on one end of a spectrum of facial pain disorders.

Trigeminal neuralgia is characterized by the absence of sensory deficit and the absence of any pain between short episodes of lancinating pain. Closely related is atypical trigeminal neuralgia; patients suffering from the atypical form of this disorder may have a constant burning or dysesthetic pain superimposed on which are the lancinating episodes of sharp pain. Trigeminal neuropathic pain, a clearly distinct entity, results from trauma to the trigeminal nerve or its branches, although the source of this trauma is not always recognized. Trigeminal neuropathic pain is characterized by an area of altered facial sensation, and the pain is usually experienced within this area of abnormal sensation. The pain tends to be constant and burning, aching or crawling, and not characterized by the "electric shocks" frequently described in trigeminal neuralgia. Finally, at the other end of the facial pain spectrum, is atypical facial pain. Atypical facial pain is thought by many to represent a psychologic disorder. There is no known physiologic mechanism for atypical facial pain and, as would be expected, neurologic examination is often either normal or the findings are not physiologically explained. On psychological testing, patients often demonstrate depression, somatization, and other behaviors related to psychological distress. When other facial pain syndromes have been ruled out, the diagnosis of atypical facial pain must be entertained and psychological therapy is almost always indicated in this setting.

The cause of trigeminal neuralgia, in the majority of cases, appears to be cross compression of the trigeminal nerve entry zone to the brain stem by an aberrant loop of a blood vessel. With aging, intracranial blood vessels can become ectatic and atherosclerotic. As a consequence of these processes, most commonly a loop of the superior cerebellar artery (SCA) or the anterior inferior cerebellar artery (AICA) compresses the trigeminal nerve root entry zone. The pulsatile compression of the nerve is thought to

result in demyelination and thus in trigeminal neuralgia. Less commonly, a large vein is believed to cause nerve compression whereas no compressive pathology is found in a small percentage of cases. In the setting of multiple sclerosis, this demyelination is primary and results from demyelinating plaques developing within the nerve or its immediate central projections. Rarely, brain stem strokes can result in trigeminal neuralgia.

The diagnosis of trigeminal neuralgia is largely made on clinical grounds. High-resolution magnetic resonance imaging can often demonstrate vascular cross-compression of the trigeminal nerve root entry zone. The most important reason to perform neuroimaging studies is to rule out other causes of facial pain, such as an intracranial tumor resulting in mass effect on the trigeminal nerve.

TREATMENT

Medical Therapy

Medical therapy for trigeminal neuralgia has been expanded significantly in the past few decades; most patients will get excellent relief with pharmacotherapy. Traditionally, carbamazepine (Tegretol) is chosen for initial therapy. Pain relief in response to carbamazepine therapy may be diagnostic of trigeminal neuralgia in and of itself. A starting dose of 100 mg twice daily is usually chosen, with dose escalation by 200 mg per day every 3 days until such time as pain relief is obtained or unacceptable side effects such as lethargy, gait ataxia, or dizziness develop. It is important to follow serum carbamazepine levels, liver function test results, and white blood cell counts to avoid toxicity. Although most patients' pain is well controlled in doses of less than 1000 mg, dose escalation to much higher levels is necessary in some patients.

The introduction of gabapentin (Neurontin)* has been a significant advance in the therapy for trigeminal neuralgia. With a similar mechanism of action to that of carbamazepine, gabapentin is almost as efficacious but with profoundly fewer side effects. Therapy is typically begun with 300 mg three times a day. The dose is escalated at weekly intervals until pain is controlled or a maximum dose of about 3000 mg per day is reached.

Baclofen (Lioresal)* may be a valuable adjunctive agent for the treatment of trigeminal neuralgia. Initially, patients are given 10 mg three times a day. This dose is slowly escalated as tolerated to a maximum of about 120 mg per day.† Patients may complain of lethargy, sedation, dizziness, or unsteadiness on their feet; with the similar side effect profile to carbamazepine, baclofen may be poorly tolerated in elderly patients.

Inadequate therapeutic response with a single agent may also be improved with the use of amitriptyline (Elavil).* Although commonly recognized as a tricyclic antidepressant, amitriptyline has significant analgesic properties and may be effective as a sec-

---

*Not FDA approved for this indication.
†Exceeds dosage recommended by the manufacturer.

ond-line agent or in combination with carbamazepine or gabapentin. Amitriptyline therapy is usually begun at 25 to 50 mg at night with slow dose escalation to 150 mg at night. With late evening dosing, the sedative anticholinergic side effect is used as a sleeping aid. Amitriptyline therapy is not infrequently limited by excessive sedation, dry mouth, or urinary dysfunction. If pharmacotherapy with amitriptyline is to be used in the long term, periodic evaluations of serum levels, complete blood cell counts, and liver function tests are advised.

Surgical Therapy

In patients intolerant of the side effects of pharmacotherapy, or in patients in whom pharmacotherapy has failed to control the pain of trigeminal neuralgia, surgical therapy can be profoundly effective. The surgical approaches to this disorder include open microvascular decompression, percutaneous radiofrequency lesioning, glycerol trigeminal rhizolysis, and balloon microcompression and stereotactic radiosurgery.

Microvascular decompression of the trigeminal nerve is the only therapy to directly address the presumed cause of this disorder. This procedure involves general anesthesia and entry to the posterior fossa by way of a craniectomy. Under the magnification and illumination afforded by the operating microscope, the trigeminal nerve root entry zone into the brain stem is identified. The offending blood vessel loop is also identified, and frequently the nerve is found to be indented and discolored at the site of cross-compression. The blood vessel loop is repositioned, if possible, and a small sponge is inserted between the blood vessel and the nerve; it is often fixed into place using a biologic adhesive. This procedure has been reported to have about a 90% success rate in eliminating the pain of trigeminal neuralgia; recurrence of the pain is unusual, with an average time to recurrence of about 15 years. The procedure involves a craniotomy, however; and risks, although uncommon, include cranial nerve or brain stem injury. This procedure is most often recommended in patients younger than 65 years of age and in those with good general medical health.

Percutaneous radiofrequency rhizolysis, also known as RF lesioning, is performed while patients are awake but sedated. A needle is advanced under fluoroscopic guidance through the skin of the cheek to the foramen ovale through which the trigeminal nerve exits the skull. Stimulation mapping of the nerve and ganglion is then performed to ensure that the appropriate division of the nerve is in contact with the electrode tip. The electrode tip is then heated using radiofrequency current, and a lesion is created. The success rate of this procedure is roughly 85%. The procedure may be repeated should the pain recur; the average time to recurrence is 3 to 4 years. Some degree of numbness in the affected trigeminal distribution is expected as part of the procedure.

Percutaneous glycerol rhizolysis involves a similar cannulation of the foramen ovale under fluoroscopic guidance. Once cerebrospinal fluid is obtained, the needle position is confirmed by the injection of contrast material. With the patient in the sitting position, a small volume (about 0.3 mL) of neurolytic anhydrous glycerol is instilled into the trigeminal cistern. Percutaneous balloon microcompression is performed by inserting a balloon catheter through a percutaneous trocar to the region of the trigeminal ganglion. The balloon is inflated while the patient is under general anesthesia, resulting in a compression injury. These procedures are somewhat less specific and less vigorous than the radiofrequency approach, with an average time to recurrence of 1.5 to 2 years, although they less frequently produce facial numbness.

Finally, the use of stereotactic radiosurgery, with either linear accelerator or gamma knife–based systems, has been proposed as a treatment for trigeminal neuralgia. This procedure involves the application of a stereotactic headframe, performance of stereotactic magnetic resonance imaging, and the precise delivery of focused radiation to the trigeminal nerve as it traverses the subarachnoid space. Preliminary results suggest that stereotactic radiosurgery may be an effective alternative for the treatment of trigeminal neuralgia, although it is probably not as efficacious as microvascular decompression or percutaneous radiofrequency rhizolysis. Developmental work is under way to better define the techniques and indications for stereotactic radiosurgical treatment of trigeminal neuralgia.

OPTIC NEURITIS

method of
ROY W. BECK, M.D., PH.D.
Jaeb Center for Health Research
Tampa, Florida

CLINICAL MANIFESTATIONS AND VISUAL COURSE

The term "optic neuritis" describes a set of clinical signs and symptoms that are assumed to be produced by inflammation of the optic nerve.

The diagnosis of optic neuritis rests on clinical grounds. Patients developing idiopathic or multiple sclerosis (MS)–related optic neuritis are usually between the ages of 15 and 45 years. Visual loss is acute but may progress for 7 to 10 days. Progression for a longer time is possible but should make the clinician suspicious of an alternative cause. Pain usually exacerbated by eye movement may precede or coincide with visual loss. It generally lasts less than 2 weeks. Visual acuity is reduced in most cases but varies from a mild reduction to severe loss (no light perception possible). Color vision is impaired in almost all cases and is often impaired out of proportion to acuity. The classic visual field defect has been said to be a central scotoma; however, almost any type of visual field defect is possible. A relative afferent pupillary defect will be detectable in almost all unilateral cases. If such a defect is not present, a pre-existing optic neuropathy in the fellow eye should be suspected. This is not uncommon in MS, in which subclinical demyelination may occur without visual symptoms. The optic disk may appear normal (retrobulbar neuritis) or swollen (papillitis) in optic neuritis, and clinical features are similar regardless. In a small percentage of cases, optic neuritis will simultaneously affect both eyes.

Regardless of the degree of impairment of vision, visual function in most cases of optic neuritis begins improving 1 to several weeks after the onset without any treatment. Approximately 80% of patients will recover to a visual acuity of 20/20 or better, and 95% will have vision of 20/40 or better. Even with good recovery of acuity, however, there are frequently residual deficits in color vision, contrast sensitivity, light brightness sense, and stereopsis that may be disabling. A relative afferent pupillary defect and optic disk pallor are usually still detectable, and the visually evoked potential latency almost always remains prolonged.

Optic neuritis recurs in approximately 20% of cases. With each succeeding episode in an eye, the chances for visual recovery decrease. However, even with two episodes in an eye, the probability of recovering to 20/20 is still about 75%, and few eyes suffer severe permanent visual loss.

DIFFERENTIAL DIAGNOSIS AND ETIOLOGY

There are a number of possible causes of optic neuritis, but in many cases a specific cause cannot be discerned. The pathogenesis of optic neuritis is generally considered to be immune-mediated demyelination of the optic nerve. Similarities between optic neuritis and MS in incidence, cerebrospinal fluid findings, magnetic resonance imaging (MRI) abnormalities, histocompatibility data, family history, and various clinical features suggest that in many cases optic neuritis may be a forme fruste of MS. Brain MRI is abnormal in about 35% of patients with optic neuritis who have no history or signs suggestive of MS. Of patients with abnormal brain MRI, about 40% will develop MS within 5 years, whereas of patients with normal brain MRI, about 15% will develop MS within 5 years. Among patients with normal brain MRI, certain features of the optic neuritis are associated with a very low 5-year risk of MS: no pain, optic disk edema particularly if severe, and the presence of retinal exudates or optic disk hemorrhage.

In a small percentage of cases, primary demyelination is not the cause, and another cause such as syphilis, sarcoidosis, Lyme disease, other infections, or a viral or postviral syndrome is identified. A viral or postviral syndrome is a common cause in children (Table 1). A special form of optic neuritis, called neuroretinitis, can also occur in any of these inflammatory disorders as well as with cat-scratch disease caused by *Bartonella henselae*. Neuroretinitis is

characterized by optic disk swelling associated with formation of a "star figure" composed of lipid exudate in the macula.

In addition to optic neuritis, other possible causes of an acute optic neuropathy include anterior ischemic optic neuropathy (AION), sinus disease (mucocele), vasculitis, and infiltration of the nerve with a carcinomatous, lymphoreticular, or granulomatous process. AION generally affects individuals older than 50, but there is considerable overlap in clinical features with the anterior form of optic neuritis (papillitis). One differentiating feature is that pain typically occurs in optic neuritis and is uncommon in AION. A compressive lesion such as meningioma or glioma generally produces gradual visual loss over weeks to months, and differentiation from the acute visual loss of optic neuritis is usually clear-cut. However, craniopharyngioma and pituitary apoplexy (hemorrhage into a pituitary tumor) occasionally produce fairly rapid loss that could mimic optic neuritis. Other unlikely possibilities for an optic neuropathy include nutritional and toxic processes, which almost always affect both eyes to some degree, and Leber's hereditary optic neuropathy.

DIAGNOSTIC WORK-UP

Further testing is not mandatory if the patient's clinical course is typical for optic neuritis (young adult with sudden visual loss with progression of symptoms of 1 week or less accompanied by pain on eye movement, with visual improvement beginning within 1 month, with either a swollen or normal optic disk but no more than a minimal vitreous cellular reaction, and with no history of a systemic disease that might produce optic neuritis). Brain MRI frequently shows signal abnormalities consistent with MS in patients who have clinically isolated optic neuritis. The need to obtain an MRI to assess for signs of MS is a topic of debate. If in the future a treatment is demonstrated to have long-term benefit in preventing or delaying MS, then obtaining an MRI to evaluate for signs of MS may be imperative. Until that time, the decision as to whether brain MRI should be performed to assess for signs of MS must be made on an individual patient basis.

If the course is atypical, then brain MRI is warranted as well as obtaining blood tests (antinuclear antibodies, rapid plasma reagin) and a chest radiograph. Additional work-up including the performance of a lumbar puncture will need to be decided for each patient. Cerebrospinal fluid changes in optic neuritis are similar to those in MS in general. Elevations in IgG and oligoclonal banding have been reported in 24 to 55% of optic neuritis patients.

TREATMENT

Either use of intravenous corticosteroids or no treatment is an appropriate management option for a patient with a first episode of typical optic neuritis. Oral prednisone in standard doses should not be used. The Optic Neuritis Treatment Trial (ONTT), funded by the National Eye Institute of the National Institutes of Health, demonstrated that intravenous corticosteroids followed by oral prednisone (250 mg every 6 hours of intravenous methylprednisolone [Solu-Medrol] for 3 days followed by oral prednisone, 1 mg per kg per day for 11 days) sped visual recovery but provided no lasting benefit to vision. This treatment also reduced the rate of new neurologic events

TABLE 1. **Causes of Optic Neuritis***

Most Common	Less Common	Least Common
Multiple sclerosis	Postviral	Syphilis, Lyme disease, or other infections
		Sarcoidosis
		Collagen-vascular (autoimmune) disorders
		Adjacent inflammation of paranasal sinuses or orbit

*When a cause can be identified.

consistent with MS, but this beneficial effect also was not long lasting, abating after about 2 years. Oral prednisone (1 mg per kg per day for 14 days) did not convey these benefits and was associated with an increased rate of recurrences of optic neuritis. Untreated (placebo-treated) patients showed a delay in visual recovery of 2 to 4 weeks compared with the intravenous-treated patients but ended up with equivalent vision. Thus, there is no clear-cut recommendation as to whether optic neuritis should be treated with intravenous corticosteroids. A reasonable approach is to discuss the potential short-term benefits of treatment and the possible side effects with the patient and decide with him or her as to whether therapy should be given. If the patient has a relative contraindication to corticosteroids, such as diabetes mellitus, it may be prudent to not treat. Specific circumstances in which we generally advocate treatment include (1) cases in which the patient has only one eye or in which the fellow eye has poor vision, (2) a previous episode of optic neuritis treated with corticosteroids in which there was good recovery, and (3) disabling or persistent periocular pain. When intravenous corticosteroids are prescribed, it seems reasonable to prescribe treatment as 1 gram per day for 3 days as an outpatient in a controlled environment. Whether this should be followed by a course of oral prednisone, as in the ONTT, is left to physician discretion.

Systemic corticosteroids may be extremely valuable in treating the rare cases of optic neuritis associated with certain systemic inflammatory disorders, such as sarcoidosis and systemic lupus erythematosus. The early use of corticosteroids in patients with these conditions may avert profound, irreversible visual loss. Similarly, patients with optic neuritis caused by syphilis, Lyme disease, cat-scratch disease, or other rare infections may benefit, both visually and systemically, from early and aggressive use of systemic antibiotics.

GLAUCOMA

method of
LOUIS B. CANTOR, M.D.
Indiana University Department of
Ophthalmology
Indianapolis, Indiana

Glaucoma is a group of diseases of the eye that have in common characteristic changes in the optic nerve with associated visual field loss. Glaucoma may therefore be thought of as an optic neuropathy for which many causes may exist. The glaucomas may be classified in a variety of ways. The most common classification of glaucoma today is based on whether the iridocorneal drainage angle of the eye is open or closed and whether the elevated intraocular pressure in the eye can be traced to a specific disease or process (secondary glaucoma) or not (primary glaucoma). Therefore, there is open or closed angle glaucoma, which

may subsequently be divided into primary or secondary forms.

The most common form of glaucoma is what is termed *adult-onset primary open angle glaucoma* (POAG). This form of glaucoma accounts for approximately two thirds of all cases of glaucoma in the western world. In different populations other forms of glaucoma may be more common. For example, primary angle closure glaucoma is more common in the Asian population than in persons of European descent.

Among individuals with POAG there are also known to be racial differences in how the disease presents and responds to therapy. The literature has shown that in the African-American population, there is a greater risk of developing glaucoma; generally worse damage at initial presentation or diagnosis; a poorer response to medical, laser, or surgical therapy; and higher rates of blindness from the disease. Risk factors other than race known to be associated with an increased risk of glaucoma include elevated intraocular pressure, older age, and family history. Potential risk factors that have been thought to be associated with an increased risk of glaucoma such as myopia, diabetes, and hypertension are not found consistently in different studies.

At present we do not understand those factors that may lead to damage to the optic nerve. From several epidemiologic studies as well as through time-proven clinical observation, elevated intraocular pressure (IOP) is known to be a primary risk factor for glaucoma. Not all eyes with elevated IOP, however, develop glaucomatous damage, and conversely there is no low level of IOP at which damage may not occur. Statistically, the mean IOP in the population is approximately 16 mm Hg, with a range from about 10 to 21 mm Hg ($\pm$ 2 SD). The majority of individuals with an IOP greater than 21 mm Hg will not develop glaucoma, and approximately 30% to 50% of those with glaucomatous optic nerve damage or visual field loss in the population will have an IOP less than 21 mm Hg. These findings certainly implicate other factors in the pathogenesis of glaucoma besides IOP, though at this time these other factors are poorly understood, and treatment of glaucoma primarily involves therapeutic interventions to lower the IOP. There is a growing body of evidence that compromised blood flow to the eye and specifically to the optic nerve may be involved in causing glaucomatous optic neuropathy. Autoimmune phenomena, collagen disorders, and other factors may also play an important role in some individuals with glaucoma.

Since the mid-1990s, there have been more new therapeutic agents introduced for the treatment of glaucoma than over the prior 20 years. In the following discussion I review these new agents and how they are affecting glaucoma therapy. I also review the current status of glaucoma laser and incisional surgery.

GLAUCOMA MEDICAL THERAPY

Beta-Adrenergic Antagonists

Beta-adrenergic antagonists have been the "gold standard" for glaucoma therapy since the introduction of timolol in the late 1970s. The beta-adrenergic antagonists may be divided into two classes: nonselective and beta$_1$-selective. These agents reduce the IOP by decreasing aqueous production. Of the nonselective agents, we have the longest clinical experience with timolol (Timoptic). This agent may be used topically in the eye either once or twice daily and is available as either a 0.25% or 0.5% solution or in a new formulation of gellan gum (Timoptic-XE) that prolongs the ocular residence time and reduces systemic absorption, thus allowing once-daily use. Timolol solution is also available as either timolol maleate or hemihydrate.

Levobunolol (AKBeta, Betagan) is another nonselective agent and has the longest half-life of the drugs in this class owing to its active metabolite dihydrolevobunolol. This agent is available as a 0.25% or 0.5% solution and is effective given once daily. Carteolol (Ocupress) is another nonselective beta-adrenergic antagonist, but one that also has intrinsic sympathomimetic activity (ISA). This activity may afford an increased measure of systemic safety and also decreases the adverse effects that all beta-adrenergic antagonists may have on the systemic lipid profile. All agents in this class adversely affect serum lipids by lowering high-density lipoprotein levels and increasing low-density lipoprotein levels. Carteolol's adverse effect on the lipid profile is less than that of the other nonselective beta-adrenergic antagonists, which may be important for individuals at high risk for heart disease, such as postmenopausal women who are not on hormone replacement therapy. Metipranolol (OptiPranolol) is another agent in this class that has an IOP-lowering ability similar to that of timolol when used twice daily.

The only selective beta-adrenergic antagonist available for glaucoma therapy is betaxolol (Betoptic). Betaxolol is a beta$_1$-selective antagonist and therefore has a lower risk of compromising pulmonary function than the nonselective agents. Betaxolol is available as a 0.25% suspension and is used twice daily.

The primary drawback of the beta-adrenergic antagonists is their risk of systemic side effects. These agents are generally well tolerated topically except for variable burning and stinging and occasional ocular allergy. These drugs, as a class, have a wide variety of potential systemic side effects that limit their usefulness in many patients. Beta-adrenergic antagonists can induce bronchospasm, bradycardia, or heart block and lower blood pressure. In addition, these agents may induce impotence in males, lead to confusion, reduce affect, or induce hallucinations, among other potential side effects.

Alpha-Adrenergic Agonists

Adrenergic agonists have been available for glaucoma therapy for over four decades. Recent advances in this class with the development of a highly selective alpha$_2$ agonist have altered their use significantly, and these agents may now be considered for primary therapy. Epinephrine (Epifrin) and its prodrug dipivalyl epinephrine (dipivefrin [Propine]) are nonselective alpha-adrenergic agonists whose use is declining. These agents are effective in lowering the IOP in 50% to 60% of patients; however, their use was often limited by lack of efficacy and the occur-

rence of an allergic reaction to the medication. Apraclonidine (Iopidine) was the first relatively selective alpha$_2$ agonist developed for treatment of glaucoma. Its use for chronic glaucoma therapy, however, was limited owing to a high incidence of tachyphylaxis and the development of a toxic follicular conjunctivitis in up to 40% of patients.

Brimonidine tartrate (Alphagan) is the newest alpha$_2$-adrenergic agonist developed for glaucoma therapy. This agent is highly alpha$_2$-selective. Alpha$_2$ effects are the desired effects in glaucoma therapy. These effects include IOP reduction and neuroprotection. Alpha$_1$ effects in the eye include mydriasis, lid retraction, and vasoconstriction, none of which is desired in glaucoma treatment. Brimonidine tartrate is available as a 0.2% solution and has been shown in studies up to 3 years long to have an efficacy in lowering IOP similar to that of timolol when used twice daily. The most common ocular side effect is a follicular conjunctivitis, which occurs in 10% to 12% of individuals. Systemic side effects include dry mouth, lethargy, and occasional hypotension.

Parasympathomimetic Agents

The parasympathomimetic agents have the longest history of usage for glaucoma compared with the other classes. The use of these agents as a class is decreasing, however, especially with the introduction of the newer agents. Pilocarpine (Pilocar) and similar drugs are direct-acting cholinergic agents. Available in many forms and concentrations, these agents reduce IOP by increasing outflow from the eye.

Use of these agents is limited primarily by the frequent dosing requirements (three to four times daily) and ocular side effects such as blurred vision, dimming of vision, miosis, and eye discomfort. Indirect-acting cholinergic agents are also available. These agents are anticholinesterase inhibitors and have limited indications today.

Carbonic Anhydrase Inhibitors

Oral carbonic anhydrase inhibitors (CAIs) have been available for glaucoma therapy since the 1950s. These agents are very effective in lowering the IOP by reducing aqueous production. These agents, however, have been associated with a wide variety of sulfonamide and other side effects that have complicated their usage. Recently, topically effective CAIs were developed. Dorzolamide (Trusopt) was the first available topical CAI for glaucoma therapy, followed by brinzolamide (Azopt). Both of these agents demonstrate clinical efficacy in lowering IOP that is generally less than that obtained with timolol. For monotherapy, three-times-daily dosing is required. For adjunctive therapy in combination with other agents, twice-daily dosing may be sufficient. Recently, a combination product consisting of both timolol and dorzolamide was approved for use in the United States as a twice-daily agent.

The primary benefit of the topical agents is their

relative safety and better tolerance compared with the oral CAIs. Most of the side effects associated with this class of agents are dose related and include fatigue, depression, nausea, and paresthesias, among others. These side effects, though still certainly seen with the topical agents, occur with a lower frequency and severity. Sulfonamide reactions, which are non–dose related and idiosyncratic, such as aplastic anemia, are still a concern. Renal stones may also be associated with the use of these agents.

Prostaglandin Analogues

The newest class of agents introduced for glaucoma is the prostaglandin analogues. Latanoprost (Xalatan) is currently the only available prostaglandin $F_{2\alpha}$ analogue approved for use in the United States. This agent has shown superior efficacy once daily when compared with twice-daily timolol in clinical trials of 6 months' duration. The once-daily dose can have significant positive effects with regard to compliance. Poor compliance is perhaps the most common reason for failure of medical therapy in glaucoma.

Concern about ocular side effects and the relatively short-term nature of the clinical trials led to the approval of this agent as adjunctive therapy to maximum tolerated medical therapy or when other agents have failed or not been tolerated. The initial concern was that this agent was noted to cause increased pigmentation of the iris over time in some patients. The scope of this problem remains under study; however, some aspects of this complication are beginning to be understood. It appears from animal models in the primate that this change in iris pigmentation is due to an increase in melanin granules within the iris melanocytes and not to an increase in number or proliferation of melanocytes. To date no abnormal cellular growth has been documented. In human eyes the risk of increased iris pigmentation is related to the baseline iris color. People with blue or brown eyes are at low risk, while those with hazel or green irides are at highest risk. Other ocular side effects such as cystoid macular edema and uveitis have also been reported. The incidence of these complications also appears to be low to date, and these problems are most likely to be seen in high-risk eyes such as in patients with a history of previous uveitis, recent surgery, or diabetes.

The introduction of the newer agents (brimonidine, latanoprost, topical CAIs, and the combination of timolol and dorzolamide) has begun to alter glaucoma medical therapy dramatically. Although topical beta-adrenergic antagonists remain the initial choice for primary therapy for many clinicians, brimonidine and latanoprost are beginning to compete for this role. Combination therapy, which is required by approximately 50% of glaucoma patients, is being simplified and compliance improved by agents requiring fewer doses per day or fewer total number of different drops. In addition, new research will be adding more new agents to the armamentarium of glaucoma therapy.

GLAUCOMA LASER SURGERY

Laser surgery has a variety of applications in different forms of glaucoma, both open and closed angle. In general, laser energy may be directed either at improving outflow through the trabecular meshwork to lower the IOP in open angle glaucoma or at relieving pupillary block within an eye with angle closure, allowing the aqueous fluid to pass from the posterior into the anterior chamber. Various types of laser systems may be used, including argon, diode, krypton, and neodymium:yttrium-aluminum-garnet (Nd:YAG).

Laser Trabeculoplasty

In eyes with an open angle, laser energy may be directed into the trabecular meshwork, which is the principal site for outflow of aqueous from the eye. By a mechanism that remains incompletely understood, the flow of aqueous through the drainage system may be enhanced, thereby lowering the IOP. Argon laser trabeculoplasty (ALT) has been traditionally used after medical therapy has been tried or has failed, but before incisional glaucoma surgery. Recent studies have suggested that this therapy may be used earlier in the course of the disease or perhaps even as initial therapy.

The Glaucoma Laser Trial (GLT) and the GLT Follow-up Study (GLTFS) concluded that initial ALT was at least as effective as initial therapy with topical medications. Unfortunately, the medical therapy as defined in this multicenter national trial is now obsolete, given the changes in glaucoma medical therapy. The studies still confirmed the relative safety of the laser surgery, however, and still do at least support its use for initial or early therapy in selected patients. ALT is most successful in eyes with POAG, pigmentary glaucoma, or pseudoexfoliative glaucoma and not in eyes with angle closure, inflammation, neovascularization, or previous trauma. ALT is most effective in older patients and in general is not recommended for individuals under 50 years of age unless they have pigmentary glaucoma.

In those for whom ALT is indicated, the success rate in lowering the IOP is approximately 75% over 2 to 3 years. ALT does not replace the use of glaucoma eye drops for IOP control, and it is usually necessary to continue the topical medications. Unfortunately, the effect of the laser often wanes over time, and retreatment is much less effective than the initial treatment. In 50% of eyes that have undergone ALT, further therapy or surgery is necessary within 5 years.

Laser Iridotomy

In angle closure there is commonly blockage of aqueous flow from the posterior into the anterior chamber, where normal drainage occurs through the trabecular meshwork. This abnormality of aqueous humor dynamics is termed *pupillary block,* as the fluid cannot flow normally through the pupil. This blockage can be relieved with a procedure called a *laser iridotomy*. This procedure creates a small hole through the peripheral iris, allowing communication between the anterior and posterior chambers, and is most often performed with an Nd:YAG laser. A laser iridotomy reduces or eliminates the risk of acute or chronic angle closure in most eyes predisposed to angle closure. Some eyes have other causes of angle closure that are not relieved by an iridotomy. In addition, even some eyes with typical pupillary block continue to have or develop IOP elevations owing to damage to the trabecular meshwork while the pupillary block was present before the iridotomy.

There is now evidence that laser iridotomy may be beneficial for some eyes with pigmentary glaucoma or pigment dispersion. In this disorder there may be "reverse" pupillary blockage, in which excess aqueous becomes trapped in the anterior chamber relative to the posterior chamber. The iridotomy, by allowing free fluid flow between the anterior and posterior chambers, relieves any blockage and allows the iris to assume a more normal anatomic position that decreases the risk of pigment loss.

Laser Peripheral Iridoplasty

Individual eyes with angle closure may not respond to laser iridotomy owing to an anatomic abnormality of the eye. For these eyes, the laser may be applied to the peripheral iris in order to shrink it, which results in its being pulled away from the iridocorneal angle. Most commonly this procedure is performed with the argon laser.

INCISIONAL GLAUCOMA SURGERY

Trabeculectomy

Trabeculectomy is the most common filtering procedure for glaucoma. The surgery aims to create a permanent fistula between the anterior chamber of the eye and the subconjunctival space. When the procedure is successful, a filtering bleb is established beneath the upper eyelid involving the superior conjunctiva. In uncomplicated cases, the success rate of this operation is approximately 75 to 80%, which decreases to less than 50% in eyes that have undergone prior surgery or that have chronic inflammation. The introduction of antifibrosis agents such as 5-fluorouracil* and mitomycin (Mutamycin)* has improved the success rates to better than 90% in uncomplicated eyes and to 75% to 80% in most eye with risk factors for failure of the surgery. In the majority of cases it is no longer necessary to use glaucoma drops after surgery.

Complications of surgery are numerous over time, and the risk of complications is increased with the use of the antifibrosis regimens mentioned earlier. Although early postoperative complications are of great concern (e.g., wound leaks, hypotony, hemor-

*Not FDA approved for this indication.

rhage, infection, cataract progression) it is the more long-term complications that are increasingly problematic. In particular, the risk of endophthalmitis is present for life. Any patient who has undergone glaucoma surgery should regard any red eye or conjunctivitis as an ocular emergency and see a physician as soon as possible. If an intraocular infection was developing, the loss of just a few hours could mean the loss of the eye.

Glaucoma Tube Shunt Procedures

In eyes that have either failed standard glaucoma filtering surgery or for which standard surgery is unlikely to succeed owing to the nature of the eye, an artificial plastic tube may be implanted to act as an aqueous shunt between the anterior or posterior chamber and the subconjunctival space. The tube shunts the fluid from the eye to a reservoir that is attached to the eye near or behind the equator of the globe beneath the conjunctiva. There are several available shunt designs.

Cyclodestructive Procedures

Cyclodestructive procedures decrease the IOP by destroying the part of the ciliary body in which the aqueous fluid is produced. The decrease in fluid production may lower the IOP but may also be associated with other ocular complications. The normal function of the eye depends on a certain amount of continuous fluid production, without which the eye will atrophy. Newer laser technology has improved the safety of this procedure; however, most surgeons will consider a cyclodestructive procedure only after several attempts at standard surgery or tube shunting have been performed or in an eye with poor visual potential.

ACUTE FACIAL PARALYSIS
(Bell's Palsy)

method of
BRUCE J. GANTZ, M.D., and
PETER C. WEBER, M.D.
The University of Iowa Hospitals and Clinics
Iowa City, Iowa

"Bell's palsy" and "idiopathic facial paralysis," have been synonymous terms for acute facial paralysis of unknown etiology. Research has clarified the etiology of this common disorder. Studies by Murakami and coworkers have identified herpes simplex virus type 1 (HSV-1) as the active infectious agent in idiopathic facial paralysis. Their research demonstrated that 11 of 14 subjects undergoing facial nerve decompression during the acute phase of the illness displayed DNA fragments of HSV-1 in perineurial fluid. Another group of researchers has identified HSV-1 DNA in a temporal bone section in the region of the geniculate ganglion in a patient who had died 6 days after the onset of Bell's palsy of other causes. These two independent pieces of evidence strongly support the concept that the facial paralysis known as Bell's palsy is caused by a viral infection that induces an inflammatory edema within the facial nerve. The neural conduction block that causes the voluntary facial paralysis is secondary to the constrictive size of the bony fallopian canal that houses the facial nerve as it traverses the temporal bone. An animal model of Bell's palsy has also been developed by inoculating the auricles and tongues of mice with herpes simplex virus, providing further evidence that a viral infection is an important cause in this disease. Together, this information provides more than circumstantial support for a herpes simplex viral etiology of Bell's palsy, first postulated by McCormick in 1972. A review by Schirm and Mulkens states that the Murakami study was "... so well-controlled that it provides conclusive evidence that the reactivation of HSV genomes from the geniculate ganglia is the most important cause of Bell's palsy."* This section highlights the epidemiology, clinical manifestation, evaluation, and treatment of Bell's palsy, taking into account the new information regarding etiology.

EPIDEMIOLOGY

The prevalence of Bell's palsy is approximately 30 cases per 100,000 individuals, thus making it the most common cause of unilateral facial paralysis. There appears to be no sex predilection, and the ages range from infant to elderly, with manifestation in the fifth and sixth decades of life most common. Right- and left-side facial palsy occurs equally. Recurrence may be unilateral or contralateral in up to 10% of patients but should alert the physician to perform a rigorous examination to rule out other causes. Pregnancy triples the risk, whereas hypertension and diabetes mellitus are associated with only a small increase in incidence. Roughly 10% have a familial orientation, and 70% relate an upper respiratory tract infection preceding the onset.

Recovery begins within 3 weeks for 85% of the patients, with full recovery occurring in 6 months. Only 4 to 6% of patients will experience severe deformity with minimal return of facial movement, but 10 to 15% of patients will be troubled with asymmetrical movement, mass movement of all branches when closing the eye, or movement of the mouth. Some cases may demonstrate total inability to close the eye. Identification of this poor recovery group must be accomplished within 2 weeks of the onset of complete paralysis. Delay beyond 2 weeks renders the patient with residual facial dysfunction for the rest of his or her life.

EVALUATION

A detailed history is mandatory for any patient with facial paralysis. Date of onset, duration of associated symptoms, and other precipitating factors are important to document. Many patients report an antecedent viral illness 7 to 10 days before the onset of paralysis. Description of otalgia associated with skin and auricular blebs or blisters is not Bell's palsy but rather herpes zoster oticus (Ramsay Hunt syndrome), which is treated best with antiviral agents (valacyclovir [Valtrex]). The facial paralysis in Bell's palsy may be abrupt or worsen over 2 to 3 days, but it is not slowly progressive over weeks to months. Patients with Bell's palsy do not complain of facial twitching, decreased

hearing, otorrhea, severe otalgia, or balance dysfunction. It is equally important to rule out recent trauma, tick bites, or current ear infections.

Physical examination should confirm a facial paralysis of all branches. If the forehead is intact, a central etiology is of concern, whereas involvement of a single branch indicates a parotid tumor or trauma. The middle ear, tympanic membrane, and external canal should be normal. No aural or oral vesicular lesions should be seen. The parotid gland is palpated bimanually to ensure against a deep lobe tumor. All other cranial nerves should function normally, including cranial nerve V, even though patients may complain of vague facial numbness.

Audiometric evaluation is necessary for every patient. Unilateral hearing loss or acoustic reflex decay is suggestive of a cerebellopontine angle tumor and an indication for further retrocochlear evaluation. If vestibular complaints are present, an electronystagmogram is performed.

Radiographic studies are important in patients with facial paralysis. It is not necessary, however, to obtain expensive imaging studies on all patients with acute facial paralysis immediately. Imaging studies are obtained immediately if the signs and symptoms are not compatible with Bell's palsy or if no return of facial motion is observed at 5 to 6 months. Both high-resolution computed tomography and magnetic resonance imaging with gadolinium are useful. Computed tomography will allow better visualization of the fallopian canal and associated temporal bone structures. Magnetic resonance imaging can demonstrate inflammatory changes associated with Bell's palsy as well as tumors. Imaging studies are not essential in patients with classic symptoms of Bell's palsy.

ELECTRODIAGNOSIS

Electroneurography (ENoG) and voluntary electromyography (EMG) are the two electrical diagnostic tests used most often to assess facial paralysis. ENoG can estimate the amount of severe nerve fiber degeneration from a minor injury or conduction block, such as neurapraxia. It takes approximately 3 days for wallerian degeneration to occur after severe injury; therefore, ENoG is not performed until more than 3 days after total paralysis. Electrical testing is not employed if a patient exhibits paresis, because the presence of even minimal voluntary motion after 3 days indicates minor injury, with full recovery to be expected.

ENoG uses an evoked electrical stimulus to activate the facial nerve as it exits the temporal bone at the stylomastoid foramen. Resulting facial movement generates a compound muscle action potential (CMAP) that can be measured with surface electrodes. The amplitude of the CMAP biphasic response correlates with the number of remaining stimulatable fibers. The CMAP from the paralyzed side can be compared with the CMAP of the normal side. A percentage of functioning or degenerated nerve fibers can then be calculated. Degeneration of 90% or more of the fibers indicates poor recovery in more than 50% of patients. Conversely, if 90% of degeneration is not obtained by 2 weeks, a good prognosis is indicated. In addition to the percent of degeneration, the time course to get to 90% degeneration is important. Patients reaching 90% degeneration within 5 days have a far worse prognosis than those who exhibit 90% degeneration in 2 to 3 weeks.

If the ENoG demonstrates 100% degeneration and no CMAP is discernible, then voluntary EMG testing is performed. EMG measures voluntary motor activity: The patient is asked to make forceful contractions, and the single

---

*Schirm J, Mulkens PS: Bell's palsy and herpes simplex virus. APMIS 105:815–823, 1997.

motor unit action potentials are recorded. Because all nerve fibers must synchronously depolarize to generate a CMAP, no response may be seen on ENoG, even when polyphasic potentials (a sign of regenerating nerve fibers) are noted on EMG. ENoG is also not of benefit in long-standing facial paralysis (>3 weeks) because of polyphasic potentials when degeneration and regeneration are occurring. ENoG is not a useful diagnostic test for tumors for similar reasons.

TREATMENT PROTOCOLS

The management of patients with idiopathic facial paralysis depends on a number of variables. An overview of our treatment protocol is seen in the flowchart in Figure 1. This chart is a general guide. Alterations may be made on an individual basis depending on specific circumstances.

Patients with so-called paresis and seen within the initial week of onset are treated with oral corticosteroids and antiviral medication. Prednisone is usually prescribed at 60 to 80 mg per day for 7 days without tapering, and the recommended dosage of valacyclovir is 500 mg three times a day for 7 days. Patients are re-evaluated within 5 days to assess the progress of the disease. Patients coming to medical attention more than 14 days after onset are followed with only intermittent examinations. If during the course of treatment complete flaccid paralysis ensues, the patient is managed according to the acute paralysis protocol (see Figure 1).

Patients coming to medical attention with complete paralysis within the first 14 days are started on oral prednisone, 60 to 80 mg per day, and valacyclovir, 500 mg three times a day. ENoG is obtained on the third day after the onset of paralysis. If degeneration is less than 90%, medical management is continued for a full 7 days. ENoG testing is then repeated every other day until 2 weeks have elapsed from the date of onset of total paralysis. If more than 90% neural degeneration is appreciated, then surgical decompression of the internal auditory canal, labyrinthine segment, and tympanic portion of the facial nerve through a middle cranial fossa approach is recommended. Decompression is considered only if more than 90% degeneration occurs within 2 weeks after the onset of complete paralysis. Surgical decompression of the facial nerve in Bell's palsy has been controversial since it was reported in 1932. Decompression of the mastoid segment of the nerve has been shown to provide no benefit to severely degenerated facial nerves compared with the natural history of the disease. Decompression of the nerve medial to the geniculate ganglion, including the meatal foramen, through a middle cranial fossa craniotomy, has been reported to improve the facial nerve return in severely degenerated nerves. We have reported a series of subjects with severely degenerated facial nerves that were decompressed through the middle fossa surgical exposure. Ninety-one percent of decompressed subjects exhibited normal or near-normal return of facial function 6 months after the onset of their paralysis. Control subjects electing not to undergo decompression exhibited normal or near-normal facial function in only 42% of the cases. This study demonstrated that surgical decompression of the meatal foramen and labyrinthine segment of the facial nerve in severely degenerated cases of Bell's palsy was strongly statistically significant and provides improved return of facial function, compared with those with similar neural degeneration not decompressed. Surgical decompression through the middle fossa more than 2 weeks after the onset of paralysis provided results similar to the control group and did not result in improved facial function.

If ENoG demonstrates 100% degeneration, voluntary EMG is performed to confirm that complete wallerian degeneration has occurred. EMG testing is also performed if patients come to medical attention more than 3 weeks after the onset of paralysis. EMG testing will demonstrate nerve regeneration with polyphasic potentials.

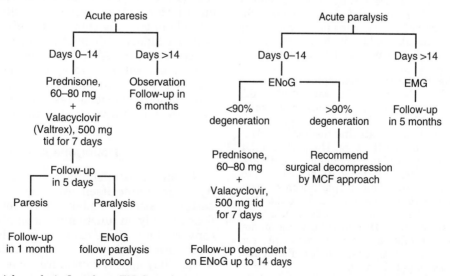

Figure 1. Acute facial paralysis flow-chart. ENoG = electroneurography; EMG = electromyography; MCF = middle cranial fossa.

Preventive eye care is mandatory for all patients with Bell's palsy. Failure to keep the eye moist (with drops during the day and ointment/moisture chamber at night) may result in corneal abrasions and ulcers.

Bell's palsy invariably demonstrates some improvement by 6 months.

If no movement is identified 6 months after the onset of paralysis, the original diagnosis of Bell's palsy should be questioned and imaging studies, to rule out a neoplastic process, must be performed.

PARKINSON'S DISEASE

method of
JOSEPH H. FRIEDMAN, M.D.
Memorial Hospital of Rhode Island
Pawtucket, Rhode Island

The term *parkinsonism* is a generic term for akinetic-rigid syndromes. These disorders include Parkinson's disease (PD), drug-induced parkinsonism, and a variety of other conditions that may mimic PD. It is interesting that James Parkinson, whose description of the syndrome is arguably the best ever written, recognized neither the akinesia nor the rigidity that are now considered core features required for diagnosis. It is also rarely noted that Parkinson recognized the limits of his clinical observations that had no pathological correlation. In the foreword to his monograph, he observed that his attempt to identify a single disease might be undercut in the future by autopsy evidence. And it has been. Advances in pathology revealed many diagnostic categories for parkinsonian syndromes. More important perhaps have been genetic breakthroughs demonstrating that inherited forms of PD, a single pathologically characterized entity, have more than a single genetic cause. Meanwhile the etiology of sporadic PD, the most common form of PD, remains a mystery.

PD is defined in life by clinical criteria. There is no diagnostic test to confirm the diagnosis. Imaging studies are performed only to exclude other diagnoses such as tumor, stroke or hydrocephalus, so that patients with uncomplicated symptoms that are straightforward require no diagnostic studies. The cardinal features required for diagnosis of PD are three of the following four: hypokinesia (akinesia and bradykinesia); rigidity (with or without cogwheeling); tremor at rest; and posture (stooped), balance, and gait abnormalities.

Rigid patients have increased resistance to passive movement that is often "cogwheeling" or ratchet-like. Akinetic patients have a paucity of spontaneous movements; some are unconscious, like blinking and swallowing, and others are nonautomatic, like scratching the head, shifting weight in a chair, and crossing the legs. The parkinsonian posture typically is stooped. Balance is impaired, and walking deteriorates with shortened stride, flattened foot strike, and reduced armswing. With advancing parkinsonism, people turn en bloc: that is, in one piece, using more than one step, without pivoting. Tremor at rest occurs in 80% of patients with idiopathic PD (IPD) and is very uncommon in other parkinsonian conditions, so that tremor at rest, while not diagnostic of parkinsonism, helps distinguish IPD from other causes of parkinsonism.

The diagnosis of parkinsonism may be difficult early in the disease, especially in the elderly, because normal aging produces slowness, stooped posture, and a mildly parkinsonian gait. Only time may reveal whether a pathological condition is present. The diagnosis of IPD is most secure in patients who have a resting tremor, hypokinesia, which develops before significant problems with gait and balance, coupled with a degree of asymmetry, that is, one side more affected than the other. The distinctions between IPD and other forms of parkinsonism are important primarily for prognosis. None of the PD-like disorders have recognized therapies. They are treated with the usual medications used for PD, but only occasional patients show benefit and this is usually less than with PD.

The principles of therapy rest on facts and disputed theories. Accepted as facts are (1) there is no cure for PD; (2) long-term complications of levodopa (Larodopa) therapy occur in the majority of patients within 3 to 5 years; (3) dopamine agonists are less likely than levodopa to produce dyskinesias or fluctuations if patients were not previously treated with levodopa; (4) treatment with a dopamine agonist necessitates the addition of levodopa within 1 to 3 years; and all PD patients under a physician's care will end up taking levodopa and will then continue on it for the rest of their lives.

Controversial issues are (1) levodopa is toxic and might hasten the disease progression; (2) selegiline may slow disease progression and reduce mortality; (3) selegiline may increase mortality; (4) dopamine agonists may retard disease progression; (5) dopamine agonists may have different benefits and side effects based on their differential effects on dopamine receptor subtypes; (6) the development of dyskinesias and clinical fluctuations is related to the dose and duration of levodopa exposure; (7) the development of dyskinesias and clinical fluctuations is related to disease severity and duration; and (8) the development of levodopa-induced fluctuations is due to the pulsatile nature of levodopa therapy.

DRUGS FOR TREATING PD (Table 1)

Levodopa

Levodopa has been the major drug for treating PD since the late 1960s. It works by increasing dopamine secretion by the remaining dopaminergic neurons in the pars compacta of the substantia nigra. It works on all the motor signs of the illness but is least reliable in treating tremor. It is given in combination with carbidopa (Sinemet), which reduces the incidence of nausea. All PD patients end up taking this drug, most within 3 to 4 years despite attempts to use alternative drugs. It causes dyskinesias and "fluctuations" (variable responses) in the majority of patients within 5 years of initiation.

Dopamine Agonists

Dopamine agonists have the pharmacologic activity of dopamine itself. Although this sounds like a better treatment modality than levodopa because it does not rely on functioning dopaminergic neurons to convert the inactive drug to an active form, it is not. Dopamine agonists do not work if levodopa does not work. They appear to require some dopamine tone in order to have any effect. Early in the disease they

TABLE 1. **Drugs Used in the Treatment of Parkinson's Disease***

Drug	Target Symptoms	Mechanism of Action	Side Effects
Levodopa (Larodopa)	All major motor symptoms	Increases dopamine secretion	Nausea, vivid dreams, drowsiness, OH, hallucinations, psychosis
Levodopa and carbidopa (Sinemet)			
Dopamine agonists			
Bromocriptine (Parlodel)	All major motor symptoms	Dopamine agonist	Hallucinations, psychosis, OH, vivid dreams, nausea
Pergolide (Permax)			
Pramipexole (Mirapex)			
Ropinirole (Requip)			
Anticholinergic agents			
Benztropine (Cogentin)	Tremor, rigidity, drooling	Anticholinergic	Dry mouth, constipation, urinary retention, amnesia, delirium, blurred vision, psychosis
Biperiden (Akineton)			
Procyclidine (Kemadrin)			
Trihexiphenidyl (Artane)			
Amantadine (Symmetrel)	All major symptoms; dyskinesias	Glutamate antagonist	Pedal edema, livedo reticularis, hallucinations, psychosis
MAO-b inhibitor			
Selegiline (Eldepryl)	Enhances levodopa's duration of action	MAO-b inhibition: breakdown of dopamine	OH, dry mouth, potentiates levodopa side effects, insomnia
COMT inhibitors			
Tolcapone (Tasmar)‡ Entacapone†	Enhances levodopa's activity and duration	COMT inhibition	Diarrhea, hepatitis, potentiates levodopa side effects

*All medications are for symptom relief only. None has been shown to slow disease progression.
†Not available in the United States.
‡Requires biweekly monitoring of liver enzymes.
Abbreviations: OH = orthostatic hypotension; MAO-b = Mono amine oxidase b; COMT = catechol-O-methyltransferase.

are as effective as levodopa, but after 1 to 3 years efficacy usually wears off despite increasing doses and levodopa needs to be added. These drugs have a much higher incidence of acute side effects, particularly orthostatic hypotension and behavioral disturbance, than levodopa. They also must be initiated at a low dose followed by cautious titration so that benefits are usually not seen for weeks.

Anticholinergic Agents

Drugs that block acetylcholine appear to ameliorate PD by acting on interneurons in the basal ganglia that are controlled by dopamine-secreting neurons. Anticholinergics are inexpensive but have a high incidence of side effects. They work best on tremor and rigidity but do not help slowness, gait, or balance.

Glutamate Antagonist

Amantadine (Symmetrel), an antiviral compound, is helpful for all symptoms of PD at 100 mg bid. It recently has been shown to reduce drug-induced dyskinesias in PD at 300 to 400 mg per day. It is a well-tolerated medication that does not appear to have a dose-response curve. Amantadine's mechanism of action is unclear.

Monoamine Oxidase b and Catechol-O-Methyltransferase Inhibitors

Most dopamine secreted at the synaptic cleft is taken up by the neurons that secreted it. Some of the

chemical, however, is broken down by two enzymes, monoamine oxidase b (MAO-b) and catechol-O-methyltransferase (COMT). Drugs that block these enzymes therefore prolong the action of dopamine. They enhance the action of levodopa. In so doing they make each dose last longer and increase the potency of each dose as well. The clinical result is longer "on" periods in the fluctuating patient but increased, more prolonged dyskinesias. The COMT inhibitors produce an effect within the first few hours. Selegiline (Eldepryl) takes a few days to work. It is usually necessary to reduce levodopa when these drugs are started. By themselves, none of these drugs produces significant symptomatic benefit.

Tolcapone (Tasmar), a COMT inhibitor, necessitates biweekly testing of liver enzymes for the first year, followed by less frequent testing.

WHEN TO START THERAPY

The first question is when to institute therapy. The answer depends on where one stands with regard to the unsettled questions on PD management. If one believes selegiline slows disease progression, then, of course, each patient gets placed on this drug at the very earliest development of symptoms or signs. It is my opinion, shared by most, but not all, experts that no medication has been shown to slow PD progression. I therefore do not start with selegiline for mildly affected patients. If a patient has only mild symptoms, few significant signs, and does not like to take medications, the choice is easy. No medications are started, and the patient is told to exercise, particularly to walk at least 30 minutes daily. If the patient is bothered by the symptoms, then the decision to institute drug therapy is balanced against the potential problems of adverse drug reactions. Finally, some patients minimize their condition and maintain an unrealistic view of their disability, often viewing their slowness and immobility as a normal concomitant of aging. They are reluctant to add additional medications to their often complex drug regimens for hypertension, diabetes, and heart disease. These patients must often be cajoled into taking new medications. I strongly encourage patients who have a significant risk of falling to begin taking levodopa immediately.

In general, most specialists, myself included, approach patients differently by age. With younger patients one is more concerned about long-term side effects, whereas older patients generate more concern for early adverse drug effects.

All patients require counseling on the importance of exercise, maintenance of as normal a lifestyle as possible, the need for socialization and avoidance of giving in to ever more restrictive and reclusive habits, the benefits of PD support groups, the fact that they are not alone, and that PD is a common disorder, affecting the famous (Pope John Paul II, Billy Graham, Janet Reno, Michael J. Fox, and Yasir Arafat) and rich as well as themselves. In addition, many patients require reassurance that PD is different from Alzheimer's disease, Lou Gehrig's disease (ALS), and perhaps some other eponymic diseases with which it is confused. Very importantly, patients must be told that progression occurs over months to years, not days or weeks. Many patients confuse PD and multiple sclerosis and worry that they may wake up one day to find themselves suddenly disabled.

INTRODUCTION OF THE DRUG THERAPY

Drug therapy is a highly individualized process in PD. Different patients who look fairly similar may be treated quite differently by the same neurologist as a result of several factors that include lifestyle, physical and coping abilities, immediate-term versus long-term needs, ability to afford medication, family support, emotional state, intellectual function, the existence of other medical conditions, and possibly other factors as well. What follows is therefore a guide and not a rule book.

For patients under the age of 60 years and for the "physiologically young" patient between ages 60 and 70, I usually initiate treatment with a dopamine agonist unless the main problem is tremor, in which case I often try an anticholinergic, first prescribing a low dose and increasing weekly. There are no data to suggest significant differences among pergolide (Permax), pramipexole (Mirapex), and ropinirole (Requip) in terms of benefits or side effects. All three seem to have some benefits over bromocriptine in terms of the duration of response and the prolongation of the

time until levodopa needs to be added. All three are comparable in cost and are considerably less extensive than bromocriptine in the United States, although not in Europe.

The main question in initiating any drug for the symptomatic treatment of PD is how high to titrate the dose. With carbidopa-levodopa (C-L) (Sinemet), the decision is usually easier than with dopamine agonists because the response is much quicker. C-L is usually started at 25/100 mg given tid with meals. If the drug is tolerated without nausea, the dosing is usually moved to before meals because it is absorbed better, both by the gut and the brain, if there is no excess protein in the blood; the dose should be slowly raised until benefit is seen. If no benefit ensues by the time 1 gm of levodopa is taken in a 24-hour period, it is unlikely that higher doses will prove beneficial and the drug should be stopped. Most patients improve within a few days, some with the first dose.

If 25/100 tid is insufficient, I increase to 1½ tablets tid for a week and then 2 tablets tid for a week, then 25/250 tid for a week, and then 25/250 qid. If, on the other hand, a patient becomes nauseated on 25/100 tid with meals, I try ½ tablet once daily and increase by ½ tablet increments to a full tablet tid. When even tiny doses produce nausea, I add extra carbidopa, which is obtained free of charge from Merck Pharmaceuticals. If adding carbidopa does not eliminate the nausea, I have the patient obtain domperidone* from Canada. This is an antiemetic that does not cross the blood-brain barrier. I then prescribe the extra carbidopa 25 mg plus domperidone 10 mg with each dose.

When assessing the response to treatment, keep in mind that tremor does not always respond to medications. Slowness and rigidity do reliably respond so that the assessment should focus on target symptoms such as ease of standing up from a chair, speed of doing chores, and shuffling gait. Many patients will report a lack of response because their tremor is unchanged but readily note that they can now get out of their car unassisted, use buttons and zippers, and perform a variety of tasks that could not be done before. Patients who do not respond to C-L rarely respond to a dopamine agonist so these drugs are not worth trying when levodopa fails.

When initiating a dopamine agonist for the mild, young PD patient, I usually follow the drug company's guidelines for pramipexole and ropinirole, but start pergolide at 0.125 mg tid and increase by this amount after 1 week. Because each patient responds differently, the question becomes how high to go.

It is not adequate merely to prescribe an arbitrary dose of a drug simply because it is tolerated. Symptomatic therapy must produce benefits, which means that the dose of whichever drug is started must be pushed to a level at which there is a therapeutic response without significant side effects.

Other choices for initiation of therapy are occasion-

---

*Not available in the United States.

ally indicated. For physicians who believe selegiline shows disease progression, it is the treatment for patients who do not require symptomatic therapy as it produces almost no benefit when used without levodopa. For patients with tremor only and who are younger (younger than 60 years of age), an anticholinergic may be used. Amantadine, which is generally the best tolerated of all PD medications, often loses its benefit within a few months when used as the only medication rather than as a supplement so that it is not usually a good choice for the first drug. COMT inhibitors do not help patients unless they are concurrently taking C-L and should therefore never be used as the initial drug.

ADVANCING DISEASE

Because PD is always progressive, all patients worsen over time, but the rate of progression is highly variable. Occasional patients remain relatively stable on a small, fixed dose of medication for several years. As patients progress, two different types of problems emerge. One is disease worsening. Despite taking levodopa and an agonist, the patient's walking slows, posture stoops more, balance declines, or, less commonly, tremor worsens. The second general problem is a variable response to the drug. This latter problem occurs with levodopa and not when a dopamine agonist or any other drug is the only one used. With levodopa, patients develop "wearing off" in which the drug works for an increasingly shorter period or has a variable response in which some levodopa doses produce no benefit while others last for short or long periods of time.

When a dopamine agonist is employed first, patients have a stable response to the drug and only rarely develop drug-induced movement disorders like dyskinesias or dystonia. After 1 to 3 years, however, most patients develop progressive parkinsonism despite increasing doses of the agonist, leading to use of levodopa. After a "moderate" dose of the agonist has been reached, levodopa is begun, using the C-L dose of 25/100 tid. The drug may initially be given at mealtimes and then moved to about 30 minutes before meals, taken on an empty stomach.

If levodopa was the initial drug and the patient declines, then the options include increasing the levodopa, from one tablet to 1½ tablets at each dose (the pills are scored), or adding a dopamine agonist, adding amantadine, or adding a COMT inhibitor. Selegiline is indicated only to increase the duration of the levodopa response. For a "younger" patient I generally add a dopamine agonist. I believe this is usually the most helpful approach and allows for dose titration both immediately and over the next several years. The initial dose is low and is titrated up weekly, as indicated. In general, dose changes can be made via telephone contact rather than office visits.

For a declining older and frailer patient, for whom there are greater concerns over the risk/benefit ratio considering that much of the patient's slowness and balance dysfunction could be age related and not due to PD, hence not amenable to drug treatment, I frequently add amantadine. The advantage of this drug is that it is generally better tolerated than dopamine agonists and requires little or no dose titration. It either works quickly or can be stopped in a week or two.

Anticholinergics are used only for tremor or drooling. They cause dry mouth and constipation in almost all patients and frequently cause bladder retention, memory impairment, blurred vision, or confusion. The elderly are at greater risk for all of these side effects.

THE FLUCTUATING PATIENT

Despite a lot of research, little is understood about the mechanism of "over" and "under" response to levodopa. Within 5 years, more than half of PD patients treated with levodopa develop some drug-related complication. These vary from the mild dyskinesia to the severe and incapacitating "on-off" or "yo-yo" affect. *Dyskinesia* refers to a chorea-athetoid movement disorder induced by PD medications that may affect any body part, on one side or on both. With high doses of levodopa this can be seen early, but with the usual low to medium doses typically used, these develop over a few years. These are not perceived by the patient, when mild, and are perceived as "fidgets" by the family. Dyskinesias are not a problem per se, but indicate a developing "sensitivity" toward dopamine stimulation.

The first type of fluctuation seen is "wearing off," in which the response to a dose of levodopa winds down before the next dose is taken. In mild disease a single dose of C-L produces a clinical effect lasting about 6 hours, although the serum half life is only 90 minutes. With advancing disease, presumably due to decreased numbers of nigral neurons resulting in a decreased storage capacity, the duration of the response diminishes. There are several options for coping with this. One can add an additional dose and decrease the spacing. I usually go to four doses taken every 4 hours (e.g., 7-11-3-7). Another approach is to use Sinemet CR, the long-acting formulation of C-L. This preparation has a long action as the result of slow absorption. It therefore takes a long time for each dose to produce an effect, generally about 90 to 120 minutes, in contrast to a regular C-L dose. (This long lag time may be offset in the first morning dose by using a standard C-L dose plus a sustained-release preparation.) The other options are to add a dopamine agonist, or to add selegiline or a COMT inhibitor, which block the degradation of dopamine.

With the exception of wearing off, other fluctuations are almost always associated with dyskinesias. Most commonly patients are dyskinetic when having a good response to their medication and akinetic when "off." These fluctuations may be predictable or unpredictable and may or may not be understandable. For example, a patient may consistently have bad mornings and good afternoons without any apparent explanation or may be "good" from 9 to 12 and 3 to 6 and be "off" the rest of the day. A great deal of effort is required with these patients. Generally, I try to prescribe one of the dopamine agonists, as these provide a stable plasma level and stable clinical response, and combine it with frequent low doses of C-L. The usual problem with increasing doses of the anti-PD medication is that they worsen the dyskinesias unless levodopa is reduced. Amantadine at doses of 300 to 400 mg per day, in contrast to the earlier used doses of 200 mg per day, has been shown to reduce dyskinesias even as it improves function during "off" times.

SPECIAL PROBLEMS

Certain motor problems in PD deserve special mention as they may be approached differently depending on the status of the rest of the disease. For example, a patient with minimal evidence of PD except for tremor may be treated differently than a more advanced patient with a similar tremor.

Tremor

Tremor is the parkinsonian sign that is least predictable in its response to drugs. Some patients respond to all drugs, while some respond to nothing short of brain surgery (which is almost 100% effective). Levodopa is the most reliable drug for tremor, followed by dopamine agonists, anticholinergics, and amantadine, in that order. Levodopa and the dopamine agonists work on the same patients, so that if levodopa fails to control tremor it is unlikely that agonists will. Anticholinergics and amantadine, however, work via different mechanisms and may prove successful when levodopa fails and vice versa. Propranolol (Inderal) has been proven also to be helpful in controlled clinical trials, although I have rarely seen it help patients who have failed the usual anti-PD medications. When all else fails, clozapine, the atypical antipsychotic drug, has been extremely effective in some cases.

The only positive thing one can say about tremor is that patients whose tremor is the major symptom of the disease typically have a more benign course.

Speech

Retrospective studies suggest that the dysarthria of PD does not respond well to medication changes. This is generally the case, but hypophonia does occasionally improve. Poor articulation and stuttering rarely benefit from medication adjustment. The most beneficial intervention is speech therapy, but this requires the patient to practice the exercises regularly.

Drooling

Drooling occurs as the result of diminished automatic or unconscious swallowing, leading to saliva pooling in the throat and eventually dribbling out when the mouth opens due to flexed posture and gravity. Sometimes improving motor function in general leads to better swallowing and less drooling. Anticholinergics help by reducing salivation but frequently cause equal distress from an overly dry mouth. Central acting anticholinergics like benztropine (Cogentin) and trihexphenidyl (Artane) are especially useful when other PD problems also need attention, such as tremor. When memory and cognitive function is impaired, peripherally acting anticholinergics like oxybutynin may be used. Paradoxically, chewing gum and sucking candies, which increase salivation, may reduce drooling by increasing swallowing. This is obviously the easiest and most benign approach. Patients should be told to use sugar-free candy and gum to offset the formation of dental caries.

TREATMENT OF SOME NONMOTOR ASPECTS

In some patients, more disability is caused by nonmotor problems that frequently occur in PD. Although depression and dementia are well known to occur in PD, less well recognized are fatigue, constipation, autonomic dysfunction (hypotension, bladder, and sexual dysfunction), and skin and sleep disorders.

Depression

Depression occurs in about 50% of people with PD. Although the question of whether this high prevalence reflects a reaction to the diagnosis or an intrinsic aspect of basal ganglia disease has not been convincingly answered, a number of reports suggest that PD patients respond as well to antidepressant drugs as age-matched nonparkinsonian depressed patients. Reports on antidepressant efficacy in PD have been surprisingly sparse, but include beneficial responses to tricyclics (TCAs), buproprion, and the selective serotonin reuptake inhibitors (SSRIs).

Identifying depression in PD is not always easy because many of the signs used for identifying depression such as reduced facial expression, psychomotor retardation, insomnia, and soft speech are features of all PD patients. Fatigue, weight loss, and diminished initiative are common as well. I usually rely heavily on the patient and family's own assessment of mood and functional decline that I believe is out of proportion to the motor dysfunction. The main and most difficult distinction is between depression and abulia. The latter is a frontal lobe syndrome in which patients, usually demented, fail to feel emotion. They are not sad or upset, they are empty. Their families suffer while they do not. They sit in front of the TV, uncomplaining, not paying attention, falling asleep intermittently throughout the day.

Depression treatment is relatively straightforward once a drug has been chosen. Experts on PD are split between TCAs and SSRIs. Some favor the latter because of their lack of side effects and hence the tolerability of effective doses without need for a lengthy titration phase. There are no data to support the use of one SSRI over another. There is concern that occasional PD patients suffer worsening motor function on the SSRI and rare reports of parkinsonism caused by an SSRI. There is also concern for a serious interaction between an SSRI and selegiline, the MAO-b inhibitor. It is not clear that this does occur, and many patients have taken the two drugs together without mishap. Low doses of any antidepressant should be the initial dose, and titration should take place after 2 weeks in order to allow time for improvement.

Electroconvulsive therapy (ECT) is generally reserved for the treatment of refractory severe depression. It is given in the form of one seizure every 2 to 3 days for a total of 8 to 15 seizures. The advantages of ECT are that it has a higher success rate than any other form of depression therapy and it usually conveys motor benefits, even in advance of its psychiatric benefits. The motor benefits usually wane, though, within a few days and are never sustained. The mood benefits last longer but need to be maintained with antidepressant medications. Reports on "maintenance ECT" for PD, in which the benefits of ECT are maintained by single seizures given every 2 to 4 weeks, have rarely been published. I strongly endorse the use of ECT for selected patients. These are severely depressed, nondemented or mildly demented patients who have failed to respond to medications. Some patients become confused after ECT. This usually lasts for only a few hours, but may last long enough to preclude the effectiveness of ECT.

Psychosis

Hallucinations, typically visual and usually benign, occasionally auditory, occur in 20% to 30% of drug-treated patients. Often these symptoms are buried and not discussed unless asked about specifically because patients are afraid they will be considered "crazy." When patients have insight into these and can readily distinguish real from imagined images there is no need for intervention unless anti-PD medications can be reduced. When delusions complicate the picture, and these tend to be either paranoid or jealous, treatment is almost always required. The first approach is to taper and discontinue as many psychoactive drugs as possible. Usually the anti-PD medications are reduced in this order: anticholinergics, selegiline, amantadine, dopamine agonists, COMT inhibitors, and then levodopa. When motor function has declined to the lowest tolerable level and psychosis persists, then an atypical antipsychotic is added because these have little or no propensity to worsen parkinsonism. Thus far clozapine has been proven to have these effects, and a small body of data supports the use of quetiapine as well.

Fatigue

Fatigue is a common problem in PD that has been poorly studied. It may arise from poor sleeping at night, depression, or medications or as the direct result of the PD itself. Its treatment has never been studied. I have found stimulants to sometimes be helpful, starting with dextroamphetamine 10 mg in the morning and increasing slowly. Obviously cardiac status needs to be factored in, but patients generally tolerate low doses quite well and the drug does have mild beneficial actions on motor function as well.

SURGERY

Although the surgical treatment of PD has advanced dramatically in recent years, it is still only rarely indicated (Table 2). Treatment is with either ablation or deep brain simulators. The thalamus is the target for tremor only. The internal segment of the globus pallidum and the subthalamic nuclei are the targets for patients with severe fluctuations, generally with intolerable dyskinesias when "on" and severe disability when "off."

TABLE 2. **Surgical Treatments of Parkinson's Disease**

Procedure*	Location	Effects
Lesions		
Thalamotomy	Lesion of contralateral thalamus	Excellent relief of tremor and rigidity; no improvement in speed or dexterity
Pallidotomy	Lesion of internal globus palladum	Excellent relief of drug-induced dyskinesias; improvement of clinical fluctuations; moderate benefit in "off" function
Deep brain stimulation†		
Thalamic, contralateral thalamus		Excellent relief of tremor and rigidity
Globus pallidum, internal globus pallidum		Excellent relief of drug-induced dyskinesias; improvement of clinical fluctuations; moderate benefit in "off" function
Subthalamic nucleus, bilateral subthalamic nucleii		Excellent relief of drug-induced dyskinesias; excellent improvement in "off" function; improved clinical fluctuations; improved gait

*These procedures do not slow disease progression.
†Stimulator adjustments do not offset disease worsening over time.

Thalamus

Thalamic surgery improves contralateral tremor in almost all PD patients. The standard treatment until recently has been the thalamotomy, in which a lesion is placed via stereotactic neurosurgery. The patient is awake when the lesion is made. If the tremor persists the hole is enlarged. A device that provides constant electrical stimulation has supplanted the ablative approach. A thin electrode is permanently planted in the thalamus and connected to the stimulator, which is placed in the chest. Because this procedure does not improve slowness or dexterity, it does not significantly improve function. The morbidity rate is low.

Globus Pallidum

Pallidotomy has been proven to be very helpful for improving function in some PD patients. Its effects are predominantly on reducing drug-induced dyskinesias and dystonia. It is mildly beneficial in improving "off" period function but has little effect on speech, balance, or freezing, which are often debilitating aspects of PD unresponsive to medication adjustment. It works bests for young patients who have asymmetrical disease, with one side very dyskinetic when the other side just becomes functional, especially if the patient fluctuates. Thus, after pallidotomy the patient, no longer being intolerant on one side of the body, can be treated with more medication. Pallidal stimulation appears to be replacing pallidotomy, and both procedures may be supplanted by subthalamic nucleus stimulation, which appears to be better for suppressing dyskinesias and tremor and for improving "off" period gait problems.

Subthalamic Nucleus

Bilateral subthalamic stimulation appears, as of the end of 1998, to be the procedure of choice for patients with uncontrollable clinical fluctuations who can walk unassisted at some times. Although subthalamic nucleus strokes cause hemiballismus, stimulation of the area, which simulates an ablation, actually reduces drug-induced dyskinesias and dystonia while improving slowness, tremor, and gait.

Caveats

It must be noted that surgery does not alter disease progression. Like medication, it is a symptomatic therapy only. Also like medication, surgical treatments also fail to improve the most advanced cases, those who are unable to walk at any time. Although surgical treatments do not cause dementia, they seem to worsen it if present so that moderate dementia or worse is a contraindication. Finally, surgery does not help patients who fail to respond to levodopa; patients with atypical parkinsonism do not benefit from these surgeries.

PERIPHERAL NEUROPATHIES

method of
PHILIP G. McMANIS, M.D.
University of Sydney
Sydney, Australia

The peripheral nervous system has afferent (sensory) and efferent (motor) components. Most peripheral nerves consist of mixed motor and sensory nerve fibers (axons) that can be affected in isolation or together. Nerve fibers that make up the peripheral nerves are of various diameters and can be classified into large myelinated, small myelinated, and small unmyelinated fibers. Most motor axons are large myelinated fibers, but sensory axons can be of any of the types mentioned. Large-diameter sensory axons carry information about vibration and joint position, whereas small-diameter sensory axons transmit information about pain and temperature. The autonomic nerves consist of small unmyelinated fibers. Disorders of the peripheral nervous system may affect some or all of these fiber types. If involvement is selective, a distinctive clinical syndrome results (Table 1).

A useful way of approaching peripheral neuropathies is to place patients into one of several diagnostic categories based on the distribution of nerves affected, the type of nerve fiber involved, and the time course of the disease (see Table 1). This allows a problem-based approach to the evaluation of peripheral neuropathies and minimizes unnecessary testing. The process does not depend on the results of laboratory testing of the peripheral nerves and begins with a careful and thorough history, with particular attention to other illnesses, toxin exposures, habits, and medications. The types of motor, sensory, and autonomic symptoms need careful documentation. The findings on clinical examination supplement this information, which then allows the classification of the type of peripheral neuropathy. When approaching the problem in this way, one should remember that diabetes can cause any of these categories of neuropathy.

DISTAL SYMMETRIC SENSORIMOTOR NEUROPATHY

Sometimes called "glove and stocking" neuropathy, distal symmetric sensorimotor neuropathy is the most commonly encountered form of peripheral neuropathy. Many different conditions produce this pattern of distal muscle wasting and weakness with decreased or absent tendon reflexes and loss of sensation. In general, these are "dying back" or "axonal" neuropathies, but some demyelinating neuropathies manifest in the same way. If the cause of the neurop-

TABLE 1. **Diagnostic Categories of Peripheral Neuropathies**

Distal symmetrical sensorimotor neuropathy ("glove and stocking")
Polyradiculoneuropathy
Mononeuritis multiplex
Large-fiber sensory neuropathy
Small-fiber sensory and autonomic neuropathy
Motor neuropathy

athy is found, the treatment is directed toward managing the underlying disease or eliminating the offending drug or toxic agent.

About 60% of patients with this clinical syndrome will be found to have diabetes mellitus or an inherited neuropathy. In a further 30% the cause cannot be identified.

Hereditary Neuropathies

As many as 30% of undiagnosed neuropathies are eventually found to be familial, and it is important to look for the clues to hereditary neuropathies before undertaking an expensive diagnostic work-up. The presence of pes cavus, clawed toes, and scoliosis together with a youthful age at onset or very long-standing symptoms is strongly suggestive of hereditary neuropathy. If possible, family members should be examined and sometimes tested with electromyography in an attempt to identify subclinical neuropathy in relatives. The inherited neuropathies may be axonal or demyelinating and are sometimes associated with other abnormalities of the nervous system (Table 2).

Patients can be given genetic counseling regarding the likelihood that their progeny will develop the disorder. They can also be informed about the prospective severity of their disease and counseled about suitable employment. Treatment can be offered to a few patients with inherited neuropathies; some of them have a peculiar predisposition to developing pressure palsies, and measures can be taken to avoid situations likely to produce these and to treat them if they occur. This disorder has been shown to be due to a deletion in the gene encoding a peripheral myelin protein (PMP-22). Another group may inherit a polyradiculoneuropathy and have elevated cerebrospinal fluid protein levels. This group obtains considerable benefit from prednisone therapy.

Neuropathies with Predominant Axonal Degeneration

Most distal sensorimotor neuropathies are caused by primary axonal degeneration. At times the same

TABLE 2. **Inherited Peripheral Neuropathies**

Hereditary motor and sensory neuropathies
   (Charcot-Marie-Tooth disease)
Type I (demyelinating; three subtypes)
Type II (axonal)
Type III (severe demyelinating; Dejerine-Sottas disease)
Type IV (Refsum's disease; phytanic oxidase deficiency)
Type V (with spastic paraplegia)
Type VI (with optic atrophy)
Type VII (with retinitis pigmentosa)
Fabry's disease
Hepatic porphyrias
Giant axonal neuropathy
Neuroaxonal dystrophy
Neuropathies associated with central nervous system
   myelin disorders
   Adrenomyeloneuropathy
   Metachromatic leukodystrophy
   Krabbe's disease

---

clinical picture can be produced by a demyelinating neuropathy, and nerve conduction studies may be very helpful in differentiating between these groups. In axonal degeneration, the amplitude of the evoked motor or sensory response is low (or absent), whereas conduction velocities are relatively unaffected. In demyelinating neuropathies, there is a prominent reduction in nerve conduction velocities, sometimes with conduction block, together with marked prolongation of distal latencies and F wave latencies, but amplitudes are relatively spared.

Metabolic and Endocrine Disorders

DIABETES MELLITUS

In diabetes mellitus, the neuropathy may be predominantly axonal, demyelinating, or angiopathic. Some diabetics present with mononeuritis multiplex, whereas others present with predominant involvement of either large or small nerve fibers (see later). The most common form of diabetic neuropathy is a mild to moderate distal sensorimotor neuropathy, which is almost invariably present in patients with long-standing non–insulin-dependent diabetes. This is frequently asymptomatic, although patients may describe mild distal tingling or numbness.

The aim of treatment is to obtain the best possible control of the blood sugar level. If this cannot be achieved with diet alone or with oral hypoglycemic agents, then insulin therapy may be indicated. Caution should be exercised when insulin treatment is first begun, however, because rapid normalization of the blood glucose level may cause the acute onset of severe painful tingling and hypersensitivity of the extremities. Thus, a gradual reduction in the elevated blood sugar level may be preferable to a rapid change.

It has been shown that pancreas transplantation is beneficial in diabetic peripheral neuropathy, even when strict glycemic control has failed to help.

UREMIA

The neuropathy associated with renal failure follows a pattern typical of distal neuropathies, with distal loss of strength and sensation and decreased reflexes. One notable feature, however, is that unpleasant sensory symptoms are pronounced; patients complain of unpleasant pulling or drawing sensations in the legs together with burning or tingling discomfort in the feet. Frequent cramps and restless legs may appear during the development of the neuropathy.

Uremic neuropathy occurs only in end-stage renal failure. Treatment of the neuropathy depends on correction of the chronic metabolic abnormalities, but hemodialysis is generally not effective in relieving the symptoms and may even fail to prevent progression. On the other hand, renal transplantation is almost always followed by a significant improvement in the neuropathy. This may influence the choice of treatment for patients with severe uremic neuropathy.

OTHER METABOLIC DISORDERS

A peripheral neuropathy may be seen in acromegaly. In this condition, nerves are edematous and are susceptible to compression. Patients may present with carpal tunnel syndrome or ulnar nerve compression at the elbow. In the absence of focal compressions, the neuropathy is usually mild. A dramatic improvement in symptoms may occur after hypophysectomy or suppression of growth hormone production.

Distal sensorimotor neuropathy may also occur in rare disorders such as porphyria and recurrent hypoglycemia secondary to an insulinoma. Both of these are predominantly motor neuropathies and tend to affect the upper extremities before the lower. Porphyric neuropathy may produce greater weakness in proximal muscles than in distal muscles and is characteristically associated with autonomic disturbances, abdominal pain, and neuropsychiatric symptoms. Again, the treatment is directed at the underlying disease process.

Drugs and Toxins

DRUGS

Many drugs are known to cause a peripheral neuropathy. Some medications do this only rarely, whereas peripheral neuropathy is expected when other agents are used (Table 3). The pattern of disease is variable: some agents produce a mild distal sensory neuropathy, whereas others lead to a generalized motor neuropathy, sometimes affecting proximal and upper limb muscles more than distal lower limb muscles (e.g., chloroquine). Megadose pyridoxine causes a severe and often irreversible dorsal root ganglionopathy. It is essential that a careful drug history be obtained from any person with neuropathy so that suspect drugs can be discontinued.

TOXINS

Toxins that cause peripheral neuropathy are predominantly heavy metals (lead, mercury, arsenic, thallium), hexacarbons (e.g., *n*-hexane, methyl *n*-bu-

TABLE 3. **Drugs That Cause Peripheral Neuropathy**

Drugs That Frequently Cause Neuropathy
Amiodarone (Cordarone)
Isoniazid
Misonidazole*
Platinum antineoplastic drugs
Megadose pyridoxine
Thalidomide
Vinca alkaloids
Drugs That Occasionally Cause Neuropathy
Chloramphenicol
Chloroquine
Colchicine
Dapsone
Disulfiram
Phenytoin (Dilantin)
Nitrofurantoin (Macrodantin)
Metronidazole (Flagyl)
Gold salts

*Not available in the United States.

tyl ketone), and industrial agents (e.g., acrylamide monomer, carbon disulfide, methyl bromide, trichloroethylene, organophosphates). Most toxic agents produce a typical pattern of neuropathy: symptoms are very symmetrical and begin in the feet, the severity and rate of proximal progression being dose related. Upper limbs are affected later in the course. Sensory nerves are more affected than motor fibers. The patient complains of distal burning and tingling together with prominent hypersensitivity. Examination reveals impaired sensation. The sensory deficit may be very mild relative to the symptoms in milder cases. Weakness is not a prominent feature early in the course or in mild to moderate toxic neuropathy. Exceptions to this pattern include glue sniffer's neuropathy, which is due to the long-term inhalation of *n*-hexane, and lead neuropathy. Both produce predominantly motor abnormalities. In addition, lead intoxication may result in a mononeuritis multiplex picture, with often preferential involvement of the upper extremities.

Treatment of these neuropathies depends on the identification of the toxin. Recovery generally follows the withdrawal of the causative agent but is slow and frequently incomplete. Specific therapy is available for metal poisoning (arsenic, lead, mercury, thallium); this is best and most safely treated with D-penicillamine. The usual dose is 250 mg four times daily, and therapy should continue until urinary excretion of the metal returns to the normal range.

LEAD

In adults, lead intoxication generally causes an axonal neuropathy, whereas in children it usually causes a demyelinating neuropathy in association with encephalopathy and anemia. Although lead is ubiquitous in the environment, lead neuropathy is now a rare disease because of the awareness of the toxic nature of lead and the institution of effective precautions to minimize lead exposure. Nevertheless, lead neuropathy may still occur in certain groups exposed to high lead concentrations, especially those in lead-working industries. Children with pica may ingest lead-containing paint from old houses, but lead-intoxicated children usually present with the encephalopathy rather than the neuropathy.

The clinical picture is one of a motor neuropathy mainly affecting upper limbs, often in the pattern of a mononeuritis multiplex. Wrist drop is a prominent feature, but sensory symptoms are virtually absent. Lead-poisoned children are more likely to have a symmetrical distal motor neuropathy. A hypochromic microcytic anemia with basophilic stippling of red blood cells is almost always present. The optimal method of treatment is controversial, but, as with other metal intoxications, most cases of lead neuropathy can be treated safely and effectively with oral D-penicillamine.

Vitamin Deficiencies and Alcoholic Neuropathy

ALCOHOLIC NEUROPATHY

Alcoholics frequently develop a sensorimotor neuropathy characterized by distal muscle wasting and weakness with prominent sensory symptoms. Hypersensitivity and burning discomfort in the soles of the feet are frequent complaints, and calf tenderness is often present. Examination reveals distal lower limb weakness with absent ankle jerks and mild to moderate reduction of all sensory modalities. The upper extremities are relatively spared. The skin over the legs is often thin, pigmented, and shiny. Although a direct toxic effect of alcohol on nerve cannot be completely excluded, it is more likely that the nerve damage is due to nutritional deficiencies, especially a lack of thiamine and other B group vitamins. Alcoholic neuropathy occurs in the setting of grossly abnormal dietary intake; heavy drinkers who maintain a satisfactory diet rarely develop peripheral neuropathy. For these reasons, treatment of the neuropathy consists of a balanced high-protein diet with B vitamin supplements. The recommended daily vitamin doses are 100 mg of thiamine, 50 mg of pyridoxine, 100 mg of niacin, 10 mg of riboflavin, and 10 mg of pantothenic acid. Abstinence from alcohol should be encouraged, as this is likely to lead to an improvement in diet.

VITAMIN B$_{12}$ DEFICIENCY

In contrast to the vitamin deficiency syndromes seen in alcoholics and others, lack of vitamin B$_{12}$ is not caused by reduced dietary intake. In most cases the condition is due to an inability of the gut to absorb the vitamin, resulting from an autoimmune disease that reduces the production or blocks the action of intrinsic factor, or to other forms of malabsorption. This substance is essential for the absorption of vitamin B$_{12}$. Examination of patients with vitamin B$_{12}$ deficiency reveals prominent loss of vibration and joint position sense in the lower limbs. This often results in a sensory ataxia. Because weakness and reflex changes appear later in the course, the presence of neuropathy may be masked by a concurrent myelopathy. Treatment consists of intramuscular injection of B$_{12}$ and must be continued indefinitely. The usual dose is 1000 μg five times the first week followed by the same dose once a month.

OTHER B GROUP VITAMIN DEFICIENCIES

Other nutritional neuropathies are rarely due to a single vitamin deficiency. Patients with neuropathy due to poor diet usually have other evidence of malnourishment, such as loss of fat and muscle bulk. These patients have clinical signs similar to those seen with alcoholic neuropathy and should be treated the same way, with a balanced diet and supplementary vitamins.

Pellagra is a vitamin deficiency syndrome consisting of diarrhea, dermatitis, and dementia. These symptoms respond to treatment with niacin. On occasion a peripheral neuropathy occurs in conjunction with the classic triad, but it is rarely responsive to niacin supplementation. In these cases, the neuropathy will improve with pyridoxine and other B group vitamins. In the United States, pellagrins are usually alcoholics, and vitamin supplements should be given in doses similar to those recommended for alcoholic neuropathy except that the niacin dose should be increased to 100 mg three times daily.

Deficiencies of three other B group vitamins—thiamine, pantothenic acid, and pyridoxine—are also thought to produce a peripheral neuropathy. As a rule, these are seen only as part of a general nutritional deficiency, except for pyridoxine deficiency. This substance may be specifically deficient in some patients during treatment with the antituberculosis drug isoniazid. The deficiency causes a neuropathy characterized by a symmetrical numbness and tingling in the feet followed by burning pains and calf tenderness. It has been shown that the neuropathy results from markedly increased excretion of pyridoxine and that it can be prevented by the administration of pyridoxine in a dose of 50 to 100 mg daily.

Patients with peripheral neuropathy of unknown cause rarely benefit from the indiscriminate use of vitamins. In particular, large doses of B$_6$ (pyridoxine) can cause a very severe sensory neuropathy that responds only slowly (if at all) to withdrawal of the vitamin. Dorsal root ganglion cells may be irreversibly damaged. Patients taking vitamin supplements should be advised to adhere to recommended dosage regimens.

Neoplasms

Neoplasia is associated with several different neuropathic syndromes, including large-fiber sensory neuropathy, acute pandysautonomia, subacute neuropathy resembling Guillain-Barré syndrome, and other demyelinating neuropathies. The most common form, however, is a mild, chronic, distal sensorimotor peripheral neuropathy. This can be detected in many cancer patients if specifically sought but does not often cause significant symptoms, partly because it commonly appears during the terminal stages of cancer. Improvement with treatment of the underlying neoplasm has not been documented except in the case of solitary plasmacytomas of bone and osteosclerotic myeloma. Irradiation of these tumors may result in improvement of the neuropathy.

Infections

Although uncommon in the United States, leprosy is the most frequent cause of peripheral neuropathy worldwide. It is the lepromatous, rather than the tuberculoid, form of the disease that causes neuropathy. Because the organism (Mycobacterium leprae) grows best at temperatures lower than body core temperature, it is the cooler parts of the body that are most affected, such as fingers, toes, cheeks, and the tip of the nose.

Most patients with human immunodeficiency virus (HIV) infection develop a peripheral neuropathy. This is most commonly a small-fiber neuropathy, although some patients have Guillain-Barré syndrome, often at the time of seroconversion. Lyme disease may cause a polyradiculoneuropathy or mononeuritis multiplex. Cytomegalovirus infections are associated with a painful lumbosacral plexus neuropathy or polyradiculopathy similar to that caused by diabetes.

Neuropathies with Predominant Demyelination

Neuropathies with primary demyelination of the peripheral nerves commonly manifest with the clinical pattern of polyradiculoneuropathy. The prototypes of this pattern are acute and chronic inflammatory demyelinating polyradiculoneuropathy (see later discussion). In these conditions, proximal and sometimes trunk and cranial muscles are weak. Less commonly, some patients with a distal sensorimotor neuropathy are found to have primary demyelination or mixed demyelination and axonal degeneration on pathologic examination of the nerves. The clinical symptoms and signs may be indistinguishable from those of distal sensorimotor neuropathies with primary axonal degeneration. Electromyography, however, may be very helpful, as outlined previously, and the cerebrospinal fluid protein level is more likely to be elevated in demyelinating neuropathies.

Acromegaly

In acromegaly, the distal sensorimotor neuropathy is frequently accompanied by entrapment neuropathies, particularly median nerve compression in the carpal tunnel. The nerves are edematous and often palpably enlarged. Hypophysectomy is followed by a rapid and complete recovery from the neuropathy.

Hypothyroidism

Hypothyroid patients may develop a severe demyelinating neuropathy that mainly affects large sensory fibers. Clinically there is distal sensory loss, particularly of proprioception and vibration, whereas loss of strength is minimal. There may be an associated proximal myopathy, and cerebellar degeneration may combine with the proprioceptive loss to produce severe ataxia. Cerebrospinal fluid protein level is usually elevated. Treatment with thyroid hormone replacement leads to a complete resolution of the neuropathy.

Paraproteinemia

Patients with paraproteinemias who develop neuropathy may present with a distal sensorimotor neuropathy or with a polyradiculoneuropathy. Most patients with an abnormal serum protein level have a monoclonal gammopathy of undetermined significance (MGUS), and only a minority have myeloma, amyloidosis, or Waldenström's macroglobulinemia. About 10% of MGUS patients develop neuropathy, and it is thought that the paraprotein contains antibodies directed against peripheral nerve myelin in these cases, especially myelin-associated glycoprotein (MAG) and P zero. Most of these antibodies are IgM immunoglobulins, which tend to produce a demyelinating peripheral neuropathy. Occasionally IgG and IgA paraproteins occur, and these are more likely to cause axonal degeneration. The neuropathy in patients with myeloma and macroglobulinemia is often associated with amyloid deposits in nerves. The clinical picture in these cases is of a predominantly sensory peripheral neuropathy, unlike that in primary amyloidosis, which causes a small-fiber neuropathy with prominent autonomic dysfunction.

An unusual form of myeloma with osteosclerotic bone lesions (osteosclerotic myeloma) has a strong association with neuropathy, either the distal sensorimotor form or a polyradiculoneuropathy. Patients with this form of neuropathy also have a high incidence of endocrine abnormalities such as hirsutism, hypogonadism, gynecomastia, and skin pigmentation. Bony lesions may be solitary or multiple and either sclerotic or mixed lytic and sclerotic. The acronym POEMS is used to describe this condition (peripheral neuropathy, organomegaly, endocrine disturbances, m protein, and skin changes).

Treatment of the paraproteinemic neuropathies seen with macroglobulinemia or multiple myeloma is difficult, as there is no therapy available for amyloid infiltration. The treatment of the underlying disorder with prednisone and melphalan or chlorambucil may help if the paraprotein itself is neurotoxic. On the other hand, the neuropathy of osteosclerotic myeloma often improves with excision or irradiation of the bony lesions. The response is not as good in patients with widespread disease. The treatment of the neuropathy of MGUS is still being evaluated in clinical trials, but prednisone, immunosuppressive agents, intravenous infusions of high-dose immunoglobulins (IGIV),* and plasma exchange all hold promise. The relative safety and efficacy of plasma exchange and IGIV suggest that these modalities should be tried as initial therapy. Some groups recommend prednisone in the high doses used to treat chronic inflammatory demyelinating polyradiculoneuropathy (120 mg and 7.5 mg on alternate days, gradually tapering to a low maintenance dose over several months). Others use a combination of prednisone with melphalan or chlorambucil (Leukeran)* and manage patients who fail to respond with plasma exchange or IGIV.

Other Demyelinating Neuropathies

Diabetes may result in demyelination of peripheral nerves, as already discussed. Sarcoidosis can produce a demyelinating distal sensorimotor neuropathy but more commonly manifests with the picture of mononeuritis multiplex or polyradiculoneuropathy. Lead causes a demyelinating neuropathy in children. Multifocal conduction block motor neuropathy (see later discussion) and hereditary neuropathy associated with a predisposition to the development of pressure palsies are associated with focal areas of demyelination.

POLYRADICULONEUROPATHY

The next major group of peripheral neuropathies consists of disorders that produce a clinical picture

---

*Not FDA approved for this indication.

of a polyradiculoneuropathy. These may be acute, subacute, or chronic. Although sensory and motor fibers are usually involved together, weakness is much more prominent than sensory complaints. Nerve roots and proximal portions of nerves are frequently affected, resulting in proximal limb, trunk, and cranial nerve involvement. Weakness may be severe and life-threatening. Tendon reflexes are universally hypoactive or absent. Minor abnormalities of sensation can often be detected. Examination of the cerebrospinal fluid usually reveals a high protein level with normal cell counts, and nerve conduction studies show marked slowing of conduction in most cases.

Acute Inflammatory Demyelinating Polyradiculoneuropathy

Often called Guillain-Barré syndrome, acute inflammatory demyelinating polyradiculoneuropathy is abrupt in onset and rapidly progressive. There is often a precipitant such as preceding viral infection, vaccination, or bee sting, and the syndrome may be seen in association with diseases such as infectious mononucleosis, *Campylobacter jejuni* and HIV infections, viral hepatitis, sarcoidosis, lymphoma, and leukemia. The clinical picture is of a rapidly ascending weakness of all four extremities, which frequently progresses to involve respiratory, facial, and bulbar muscles. Sphincter muscles are invariably spared. Sensory loss is usually mild but in some patients may be the dominant feature of the illness. Autonomic neuropathy may be present and in some cases may be severe and life-threatening with sustained or paroxysmal tachycardia or hypertension.

The most important aspect of treatment for this disorder is early diagnosis and admission to the hospital, because mild weakness may progress to respiratory failure within hours. The respiratory function and pulse rate must be monitored closely, and assisted ventilation should begin if the vital capacity falls below 1 liter. Meticulous pulmonary hygiene must be maintained. Physical therapy to prevent contractures should begin early, and great care should be taken to avoid complications of prolonged bed rest such as decubitus ulcers and hypostatic pneumonia. If tachycardia or sustained hypertension develops, propranolol should be given. Paroxysmal fluctuations in blood pressure generally require a combination of alpha and beta blockers.

Recovery often begins 1 to 3 weeks after onset, and in these cases the prognosis for recovery is good. Patients whose illness continues to progress for more than 6 weeks are more likely to have a chronic or relapsing course. Some patients will have a severe axonal (instead of demyelinating) neuropathy and may have a very prolonged illness with incomplete recovery after months or years. This syndrome has been called acute motor axonal neuropathy (AMAN).

Specific therapy is now available for Guillain-Barré syndrome. Steroids are no longer used, as studies show no benefit from corticosteroids or adrenocortico-

tropic hormone, and one trial documented a slower recovery in patients treated with prednisone. Steroids also reduce the patient's resistance to respiratory and urinary infection. Most physicians use either plasmapheresis (2 to 3 liter exchanges, two to three treatments for mild disease or 4 to 5 treatments for more severe disease), or IGIV* (0.4 g per kg per day for 5 days) in the management of this condition. Treatment is based on the proposal that weakness is caused by demyelination and conduction block produced by circulating antibodies. If this is so, plasma exchange should be effective because the antibodies would be removed by the procedure. High-dose IGIV works by bulk displacement of pathogenetic antibodies from myelin. Patients undergoing plasma exchange or given IGIV improve more rapidly and have shorter hospital stays than untreated patients. Problems with these therapies are the expense, the inconvenience to the patient, and the potential for anaphylactic reactions to the products used to replace the serum. There is a risk of viral infection with the use of pooled blood products. Treatment is not recommended for the patient with mild or resolving neuropathy.

Chronic Inflammatory Demyelinating Polyradiculoneuropathy

In chronic inflammatory demyelinating polyradiculoneuropathy, the initial rate of progression is slower than that in Guillain-Barré syndrome. The time to maximum disability is greater than 6 weeks in most cases and may be 1 year or more in some. There is rarely a history of an antecedent illness or other precipitating factor. Other features differentiating the two disorders include nerve thickening, more prominent sensory symptoms, and a more protracted course, sometimes with spontaneous remissions and relapses, in chronic inflammatory polyradiculoneuropathy. Clinical symptoms and signs are otherwise similar; evidence of a generalized neuropathy with proximal weakness is essential to the diagnosis of both. The cerebrospinal fluid protein level is elevated, and nerve conduction velocities are slowed in both disorders, although these abnormalities are more common and more marked in the chronic form.

Despite the apparent similarities, it is important to distinguish chronic inflammatory demyelinating polyradiculoneuropathy from Guillain-Barré syndrome because the response to treatment is different. Evidence strongly suggests a definite benefit from prolonged prednisone therapy in the chronic form. For moderate to severe disease, a trial of at least 3 months is indicated. Prednisone is given in doses of 120 mg and 7.5 mg on alternate days initially. If a response occurs, the doses are slowly tapered over 9 months, but if there is no beneficial effect after 2 months, the prednisone is reduced more rapidly. For patients with less severe disease, the potential benefit must be weighed against the risks of long-term

---

*Not FDA approved for this indication.

corticosteroid therapy such as infection, cataracts, and elevated blood sugar level. Plasmapheresis has been shown in a double-blind sham-controlled clinical trial to be beneficial. It therefore should be considered in the management of patients with severe disease unresponsive to conventional treatment. Similarly, IGIV* is effective in inducing and maintaining a remission in the disorder. An occasional patient is unresponsive to all conventional therapy but improves with a combination of plasmapheresis and IGIV.

Before a diagnosis of chronic inflammatory polyradiculoneuropathy can be made, certain conditions that mimic this disorder must be excluded. A similar clinical picture with increased cerebrospinal fluid protein level may be seen in diabetes, sarcoidosis, various neoplastic disorders (especially lymphoma, POEMS, and other paraproteinemic neuropathies), and some of the hereditary neuropathies. Evidence of these diseases should be sought by careful clinical examination, including testing of relatives and appropriate laboratory tests.

MONONEURITIS MULTIPLEX

Mononeuritis multiplex is a distinctive pattern of peripheral nerve disease characterized by marked asymmetry of limb involvement and is the result of damage of individual peripheral nerves rather than diffuse disease. The nature and distribution of symptoms are determined by the nerves that are affected.

Mononeuritis Multiplex of Gradual Onset

The most common cause of a slowly progressive mononeuritis multiplex is entrapment or pressure palsies of multiple nerves. Many of the peripheral nerves are vulnerable at well-known sites, such as the median nerve in the carpal tunnel, the ulnar nerve at the elbow, the radial nerve in the upper arm, and the peroneal nerve at the fibular head. When these nerves are chronically compressed, symptoms can be alleviated in most cases by surgery and avoidance of activities known to compress these nerves. If damage to axons has been severe, however, recovery will be slow and incomplete.

Several medical conditions predispose the patient to the development of pressure palsies. In rheumatoid arthritis, bony deformities may result in chronic nerve compression, and surgery may be necessary to correct the deformity or move the nerve to a less vulnerable site. Hypothyroidism and acromegaly are associated with multiple focal neuropathies, and correction of the hormonal abnormalities leads to rapid symptomatic relief. Amyloidosis may cause local pressure palsies by infiltrating tight compartments. This is most common in the carpal tunnel. Surgical decompression relieves the compressive neuropathy, but there is currently no effective treatment for amyloidosis. Mononeuritis multiplex is also one of the

most common manifestations of sarcoidosis involving the nervous system and is often associated with large areas of sensory loss over the trunk. This probably represents involvement of thoracic nerve roots. Nerve lesions in sarcoidosis tend to worsen slowly and then recover gradually, but prednisone therapy is usually warranted, as it is believed to abbreviate the course of neuropathy and to prevent new lesions from appearing. The recommended dose is 60 mg daily with gradual tapering to 15 mg daily. This dosage should be maintained for several months and then tapered slowly.

Lead neuropathy is currently a rare disorder but typically manifests as a mononeuritis multiplex with a predilection for the radial nerves. Treatment is discussed in the section on demyelinating neuropathies.

Mononeuritis Multiplex of Abrupt Onset

When a patient develops a flurry of individual nerve lesions, with each one evolving almost overnight, the underlying process is usually a vasculitis. Typically, the onset of paralysis is preceded by severe pain and paresthesias, which are often more distressing than the weakness that follows. The clinical picture is easily recognized, and the diagnosis can be confirmed by sural nerve biopsy. Even if this nerve is not involved clinically, the pathologic changes of the underlying angiopathy can almost always be demonstrated. Nerve tissue has low metabolic demands and a richly anastomotic blood supply, so angiopathic changes must be extensive before nerve infarction develops.

Many diseases are known to produce this pattern of disease: polyarteritis nodosa and Churg-Strauss syndrome, rheumatoid arthritis, systemic lupus erythematosus, Sjögren's syndrome, diabetes, Wegener's granulomatosis, cryoglobulinemia, and cranial arteritis. With the exception of diabetes and cryoglobulinemia, these conditions are treated with high doses of prednisone, 60 to 100 mg daily for 2 weeks and then 100 mg on alternate days. Disease progression sometimes occurs on this schedule, so cyclophosphamide (Cytoxan), 2 mg per kg, is often added (this use not listed by the manufacturer). A high fluid intake is recommended to avoid hemorrhagic cystitis, and regular checks of the blood count and platelet count, blood sugar level, and blood pressure are essential for patients following this drug regimen. The use of cyclophosphamide may permit a lower corticosteroid dose than would otherwise be necessary, and weaning from steroids can often be started earlier.

The management of diabetic mononeuritis multiplex is essentially the same as for other types of diabetic neuropathy discussed previously. Cryoglobulinemia causes nerve infarction by occluding vessels with proteins that precipitate on exposure to cold. Essential (idiopathic) cryoglobulinemia is best dealt with by simple avoidance of cold exposure, but that due to cryoglobulins produced in plasma cell dyscrasias as paraproteins often needs more aggres-

---

*Not FDA approved for this indication.

sive treatment. This is usually directed toward the cause of the paraprotein, but in some cases plasma exchange can be of great benefit in decreasing the total amount of the cryoglobulin.

LARGE-FIBER SENSORY NEUROPATHY

Some peripheral neuropathies cause selective dysfunction of the largest nerve fibers. This produces an easily recognizable clinical syndrome resulting from the loss of proprioceptive sense that travels in these large fibers. Patients with this disorder have a severe sensory ataxia in darkness or with eyes closed. Examination shows disproportionate loss of vibration and joint position sense with relative preservation of pain, temperature, and touch sensations. The inability to sense the position of the joints may cause pseudoathetosis, or "searching" movements of fingers and toes, particularly when the individual is attempting to maintain a specified posture.

Neoplastic Sensory Neuropathy

In some patients with carcinoma, a slowly progressive large-fiber neuropathy occurs and may antedate the diagnosis of the cancer by up to 3 years. The associated malignancy is almost always an oat cell carcinoma of the lung, but occasional instances of other primary lung neoplasms or carcinoma of the cecum or esophagus are found. The usual symptoms are peripheral numbness and tingling associated with clumsiness and falls due to the sensory ataxia. Treatment of the neoplasm does not appear to influence the course of this neuropathy. In most cases, the symptoms are due to disease of the dorsal root ganglia ("paraneoplastic sensory neuronopathy").

Drug-Associated Sensory Neuropathy

The long-term abuse of nitrous oxide can produce a large-fiber neuropathy with sensory ataxia. This is usually found in medical personnel with ready access to the drug but has also been reported with the inhalation of nitrous oxide from canisters used to prepare whipped cream. Cessation of the abuse is generally followed by improvement, but a residual deficit may persist. Large doses of pyridoxine (vitamin B_6) can lead to a severe large-fiber sensory neuropathy. Clioquinol, a drug once commonly used for travelers' diarrhea, is thought to be the cause of a degenerative disorder of spinal cord and optic nerves known as subacute myelo-optic neuropathy. An associated large-fiber neuropathy has been described but not clearly documented.

Other Large-Fiber Neuropathies

Some of the classic causes of large-fiber neuropathies are discussed in earlier sections. These include hypothyroidism, which is associated with a demyelinating large-fiber neuropathy that is exquisitely re-sponsive to replacement therapy, and diabetes mellitus, which can cause selective damage to large sensory fibers as well as other types of peripheral neuropathy. Vitamin B_{12} deficiency produces a large-fiber neuropathy, but the peripheral abnormalities are often overshadowed by the presence of myelopathy. IgM paraproteinemia is sometimes associated with a large-fiber neuropathy, and treatment rarely leads to improvement. Idiopathic subacute sensory neuronopathy may affect the upper limbs more than the lower limbs and can be difficult to distinguish from neoplastic sensory neuropathy. The treatment of these disorders is described in the appropriate sections.

SMALL-FIBER SENSORY AND AUTONOMIC NEUROPATHY

The clinical picture in small-fiber sensory and autonomic neuropathy can sometimes cause diagnostic confusion because pain and discomfort may be severe in the absence of the usual clinical signs of neuropathy. The main complaints are intense pricking, tingling, and burning pains in the feet and sometimes in the hands. Symptoms of autonomic nervous system dysfunction are also common and consist of postural dizziness, bloating, diarrhea, and impotence in males. Severe autonomic neuropathy may cause urinary and fecal incontinence. Examination reveals normal distal strength and reflexes, whereas sensory testing shows marked impairment of pain and temperature sensation with preserved joint position and vibration sense. Electromyography is often completely normal in the beginning but may show mild abnormalities with progression.

Diabetes

Diabetic neuropathy is seen most commonly in insulin-dependent juvenile diabetics. Adult diabetics whose blood sugar level is normalized rapidly with insulin may also develop a neuropathy with prominent positive sensory symptoms that may be associated with a less severe dysautonomia. The prognosis for recovery from the painful symptoms is good with satisfactory control of the blood glucose level, but recovery from autonomic neuropathy is unusual.

Amyloidosis

The next largest group of patients with small-fiber neuropathy consists of patients with primary amyloidosis. These patients are usually middle-aged or elderly males with postural syncope, impotence, constipation, bladder disturbances, and impaired sweating. Examination shows decreased pain and temperature sensation. About 90% are found have an abnormal protein band with immunoelectrophoresis of serum and urine. Amyloid deposits can also be found in abdominal fat, in peripheral nerves, and in rectal neurons. There is no effective treatment available for this condition, although the use of colchicine has been described. Amyloidosis secondary to myeloma, macroglobulinemia, or chronic inflammation does not often produce this type of neuropathy.

Other Small-Fiber Neuropathies

Occasionally, small-fiber neuropathy occurs in patients with lung cancer. In these cases, the autonomic failure may be severe, with complete anhidrosis and marked postural hypotension, and peripheral nerve symptoms may be absent. Treatment of the malignancy has been reported to improve the autonomic function. Rare hereditary neuropathies such as Fabry's disease, Tangier disease, and hereditary sensory neuropathy type 1 can manifest with dysautonomia and the sensory symptoms. Autonomic function may be prominent in acute inflammatory demyelinating polyradiculoneuropathy.

MOTOR NEUROPATHY

Acute motor axonal neuropathy is described in an earlier section. A syndrome of selective motor axonal neuropathy associated with multiple conduction blocks on nerve conduction studies has been recognized in the last few years. Affected patients may have fasciculations and severe proximal and distal wasting and weakness—features suggestive of amyotrophic lateral sclerosis. In some instances, the tendon reflexes are preserved or brisk, making it difficult to separate the two disorders on clinical grounds. This problem emphasizes the need for careful nerve conduction studies in patients with peripheral nerve disease.

Lead intoxication, the hepatic porphyrias (acute intermittent porphyria, variegate porphyria, and coproporphyria), and diphtheria can all cause selective motor peripheral neuropathies. Some patients with IgM paraproteinemia have a purely motor syndrome.

TREATMENT OF PERIPHERAL NEUROPATHY

In many instances there is no specific treatment for a particular type of neuropathy. It is important to keep in mind the value of general supportive measures to alleviate symptoms. Range-of-motion exercises to prevent joint contractures and braces and splints for weakened muscle groups are often invaluable in maintaining mobility. Patients with severe lower extremity weakness or sensory loss often benefit considerably from the stability provided by a cane. The importance of protection and care of insensitive feet, particularly in the patient with diabetes, cannot be overemphasized. Patients should be instructed to trim their toenails with great care and to be fastidious about foot hygiene. Any fungal or bacterial infection mandates prompt medical attention. The need for well-fitting shoes should also be emphasized. In addition, patients should be warned that the lack of

sensation makes their feet more susceptible to damage from frostbite in winter.

Patients with peripheral neuropathy severe enough to confine them to bed (e.g., Guillain-Barré syndrome) are at risk for deep vein thrombosis and respiratory complications. Care should be taken to prevent these complications or to treat them promptly if they arise.

TREATMENT OF PAINFUL NEUROPATHIES

Pain is a prominent feature in some peripheral neuropathies and can be the most distressing part of the disease. The quality of the pain is usually an intense burning or pricking sensation and is often associated with marked hypersensitivity to light touch. Some patients complain of deep-seated aching and pulling sensations or tightness. Certain neuropathies are more prone to produce these sensations than others: the worst offenders are generally axonal degenerations, particularly alcoholic and uremic neuropathies; metal intoxications; and the small-fiber neuropathies of diabetes and Fabry's disease. Pain is often severe in nerve infarction resulting from angiopathy and in the neuropathy produced by some drugs, such as gold and vincristine (Oncovin). In addition, some patients with very little clinical evidence of neuropathy complain of prominent positive symptoms but do not have the marked loss of pain and temperature sensation and the dysautonomia that characterize small-fiber neuropathies. These patients probably have an idiopathic minimal sensory neuropathy.

Treatment of these symptoms can be challenging, as they often do not respond well to conventional analgesics, and there is a real risk of the development of drug dependence. Mild symptoms can be relieved by soaking the extremities in cool tap water (about 15°C) for 20 minutes. If this is done late in the evening and combined with 600 to 900 mg of aspirin orally, the patient may be able to sleep undisturbed. When more severe symptoms are present, phenytoin (Dilantin)* or carbamazepine (Tegretol)* can be tried in standard anticonvulsant doses. Amitriptyline (Elavil),* 25 mg in the morning and 50 mg at night, sometimes provides very effective relief, although anticholinergic drugs should be used with caution by the elderly, for whom there is a significant risk of delirium and autonomic side effects. Mexiletine (Mexitil),* 300 to 900 mg daily in divided doses, is effective in some patients. An electrocardiogram should be obtained to avoid giving this drug to patients with heart block or myocardial disease. Capsaicin creams (0.025% or 0.075%), applied sparingly three or four times a day, often relieve pain after the initial burning wears off. Transcutaneous nerve stimulation is often effective at the outset, but the benefit is often transient.

---

*Not FDA approved for this indication.

ACUTE HEAD INJURIES IN ADULTS

method of
SHARON B. MARSHALL, M.D., and
LAWRENCE F. MARSHALL, M.D.
University of California, San Diego
San Diego, California

Despite a rather dramatic reduction in vehicular accidents and related death and disability, trauma remains the leading cause of death and disability for Americans younger than the age of 45 years. Head injury is responsible for more than half of those deaths, making it a public health problem of epidemic proportions. Hospital admission rates for the entire spectrum of head injury in the United States remain at approximately 200 per 100,000 Americans per year. Approximately 10% of these patients die.

The term *head injury* covers a broad spectrum and includes patients who have

1. *Minor head injury (80%):* Defined as a transient loss of consciousness. This is usually followed by recovery over several weeks or months.

2. *Moderate head injury (10%):* Defined by an impairment of consciousness. Focal deficits are more common, and recovery is more prolonged.

3. *Severe head injury (10%):* Defined as those patients who are in a coma for at least 24 hours. In this group, the mortality rate since the late 1980s has remained at approximately one third for those who reach the hospital alive. Most are left with at least some residua, while a small percentage remain in a persistent vegetative state for the remainder of their lifetime.

The care of the head-injured patient, whether the injury is mild, moderate, or severe, depends on a well-organized system of diagnosis, triage, and care. The development of sophisticated emergency medical service (EMS) systems in the United States has resulted in dramatic improvements in care in many regions. The increasing recognition that shock and hypoxia play a major role in the outcome in patients with severe head injury has been a major impetus for improvements in the quality of care during the prehospital phase and for the development of appropriate systems of rapid evacuation and transport. As the majority of closed head injuries in the United States occur as a result of vehicular trauma, regional planning must take into account the quality of trauma care within regional hospitals and their proximity to roadways. In urban areas where open injuries, particularly gunshots, remain a leading cause of death and disability from brain injury, increasing emphasis has been placed on attempts at prevention through regulation of firearms and by defining central urban locations for trauma centers.

The introduction of computed tomography (CT) revolutionized neurologic surgery in general and neurotraumatology in particular. To take a patient with what appears to be a relatively trivial injury to a hospital that does not have such facilities is inappropriate. Thus, it is important that patients be transported to facilities that have competent emergency facilities, neurosurgical care, operating rooms, anesthesia, and emergent CT capabilities available on a 24-hour basis.

PATHOPHYSIOLOGY OF ACUTE BRAIN INJURY

Head injury covers a wide spectrum of severity from trivial to immediately fatal. Almost ubiquitous to all patterns of injury are injuries to the axons, which is called *diffuse axonal injury.* In patients who have had only transient losses of consciousness, white matter damage is usually seen in the brain stem, the fornix, and the deep white matter. In patients with much more severe brain injury, massive shearing of the white matter in a variety of locations is common. This is usually associated with profound disability, a persistent vegetative state, or death.

In addition to damage to the white matter, injuries to neurons occur primarily from secondary insults such as ischemia, hypoxia, and hypercapnia. These result in inadequate substrate delivery and acidosis, which, if not rapidly reversed, results in cell death. In addition, in patients with more severe head injuries, particularly those occurring in individuals whose head is not protected by a helmet, intracranial hemorrhages of the extradural, subdural, or intracerebral type occur in approximately 35%.

As the severity of injury increases, patients usually have a variety of types of tissue damage, including *contusion,* which refers to blood mixed into the tissues of the brain, diffuse axonal injury, and hematomas as described above. The combination of these processes often results in brain swelling. Brain swelling has recently been shown to be primarily due to an increase in the water content of the cells, which is called *cytotoxic edema.* In addition, increases in brain-blood volume as a result of vasomotor paralysis also occur. This is because the normal response of the cerebrovasculature, to maintain a constant flow over a wide variety of systemic blood pressures, is progressively lost as head injury becomes more severe. It is important, therefore, to understand that maintenance of normal blood pressures and, therefore, cerebral perfusion is critically important in the management of patients, particularly those with severe head injuries.

Metabolic regulation of blood flow is also a critical issue for the more severely injured. The accumulation of CO_2, which results in a lowered pH, produces vasodilatation, which clearly exacerbates problems of increased intravascular volume. Hyperventilation, however, which has frequently been used as both an acute and chronic treatment, may have deleterious effects. This is particularly true if the CO_2 is reduced to below 30 mm Hg for long periods because a secondary ischemia due to vasoconstriction can be produced. Hyperventilation for a short period, however, when intracranial hypertension is likely to be present, such as instances when pupillary abnormality has developed, is not only acceptable, but is recommended. Hyperventilation on a more chronic basis, however, is to be discouraged.

TREATMENT

Minor Head Injury

The overwhelming majority of patients who suffer head injury have only a mild or minor injury. These are characterized by a transient loss of consciousness, usually 5 minutes or less, followed by amnesia for the event and, perhaps, for a period of time before their injury. Patients who are alert and awake when they arrive at the emergency room, have an entirely normal neurologic examination, and no headache may be discharged.

For patients in whom a state of normal alertness has been reached, but there is still confusion, a CT scan is necessary to rule out the possibility of a developing intracranial hematoma. Patients who are particularly at risk are those with fractures, and fractures are more common in patients whose head was unprotected at the time of injury. Thus, helmets, particularly for bicyclists, motorcyclists, and horseback riders, offer a great deal of protection. CT scanning is also mandatory for any patient whose injury is thought to be minor yet the patient's state of alertness has not rapidly returned.

The likelihood of an intracranial hematoma is much less than 1 per 100 in patients whose Glasgow Coma Scale (GCS) score (Table 1) is 15 and the patient is alert. Of patients whose GCS score is 13, approximately 10% have a lesion that potentially requires surgical intervention. Thus, these patients should be kept in the hospital and have an additional CT scan within 12 to 24 hours to rule out the possibility of an expanding mass lesion. It is inappropriate to discharge a patient who has an abnormal CT scan from an emergency department. One should not rely on family members to watch a patient with an identified hematoma. The use of head injury sheets for families should be limited only to those instances when the injury is thought to be trivial.

As the frequency of anticoagulation for cardiac and atherosclerotic cerebrovascular disease increases, more patients who are at increased risk of developing intracranial hematoma are being seen. These patients should have their anticoagulation reversed and be observed for a minimum of 24 hours after injury to be certain a delayed hematoma does not develop.

Finally, delayed intracranial hematomas are much more common in older persons. It is strongly recommended that older patients be kept in the hospital for a minimum of 48 hours if they have any abnormality on CT scan.

Moderate and Severe Head Injury

The initial priority in the treatment of patients with moderate and severe head injuries is to be certain that normal oxygenation is maintained and that the systolic blood pressure not be allowed to fall below 100 to 110 mm Hg. There is substantial evidence that shock, even for a brief period of time, results in much worse outcomes than if it is never present. Every attempt should be made to maintain the arterial oxygen saturation at greater than 96% to avoid hypoxia. In patients who are deteriorating in the field, endotracheal intubation with mild to moderate hyperventilation to reduce the $Paco_2$ to a range of 28 to 32 is also recommended. Significant blood loss should be replaced with blood and not just isotonic crystalloid solutions.

Serial neurologic assessment, from the initial visit in the field throughout the patient's hospital stay, is mandatory. The GCS along with assessment of the pupils is optimal. Once the patient is in or has been transferred to a hospital capable of taking care of patients with significant head injury, an initial primary survey should be conducted to identify all life-threatening injuries and to assess the level of consciousness of the patient. Occasionally, a muscle relaxant must be used in the field to ensure the airway. The last GCS score, before paralyzation, is used to further classify the patient's severity of injury.

Cervical spine radiographs should be obtained and must visualize from C1 to T1. Spine instability must be assumed until the patient can be examined or CT scanning has been done to rule out bony disruption or subluxation should plain radiographs be inadequate.

Early CT scanning in patients with moderate and severe head injuries (defined as a GCS score of 3 to 12) is essential. Approximately one in four patients with an acute severe head injury requires craniotomy for evacuation of an intracranial hematoma. Generally, in patients whose likelihood of salvageability is high, blood clots larger than 25 mL need to be removed, particularly those adjacent to the temporal lobe. Conversely, in the extremely old patient or those with Alzheimer's disease, surgical intervention is probably almost always inappropriate.

INTENSIVE CARE UNIT MANAGEMENT

The modern management of the severely head-injured person necessitates the use of an intracranial pressure (ICP) monitor so that the ICP can be longitudinally followed. A ventricular catheter has the advantage of allowing for cerebrospinal fluid drainage in addition to pressure measurements. If the ventricles are too small to be entered, however, a fiberoptic monitoring device is very useful.

The fundamental objective of intensive care unit management is to restore the patient to a physiologic milieu optimal for brain recovery. The major features of this management are to keep the ICP below 20 mm Hg and the mean arterial pressure (MAP) above 80 if at all possible. This results in a cerebral perfusion pressure (CPP) of greater than 60 mm Hg (MAP minus ICP), which is essential to ensure adequate brain perfusion. Elevation of the head of the bed may improve cerebral perfusion and venous drainage.

TABLE 1. **Glasgow Coma Scale**

Eyes open	Never	1
	To pain	2
	To speech	3
	Spontaneously	4
Best verbal response	None	1
	Garbled	2
	Inappropriate	3
	Confused	4
	Oriented	5
Best motor response	None	1
	Extension	2
	Abnormal flexion	3
	Withdrawal	4
	Localizes pain	5
	Obeys commands	6
Total Score		___

Points are assigned in each category for the patient's best response to stimuli (e.g., sternal rub in the apparently comatose patient). The minimum score is 3 (completely unresponsive); the maximum is 15 (no apparent mental status deficits).

Severely head-injured patients are administered phenytoin (Dilantin) for a period of 7 days. If a patient has seizures after the first 24 hours, anticonvulsant therapy is maintained for a minimum of 6 months. H$_2$ blockers are now used universally to reduce the risk of stress ulcer, and sequential pneumatic compression devices are applied to the lower extremities. Enteral nutrition can be begun as soon after injury as is feasible, almost always within 48 hours with an objective of 1800 to 2400 kcal per day.

MANAGEMENT OF INTRACRANIAL HYPERTENSION

The most common cause of death after severe head injury is intracranial hypertension. Major efforts must be made to try to maintain the ICP below 20 mm Hg. A staircase approach to the management of elevated ICP is usually applied (Table 2).

Sudden elevations of ICP in patients with evidence on the first CT scan of either a contusion or a small subdural or epidural hematoma mandate immediate rescanning. A follow-up CT scan is routinely performed in such patients to detect the 25% whose initial lesion enlarges sufficiently to need surgery.

When the ICP can be controlled below 20 mm Hg in the absence of major sedation and muscle relaxants, the ICP monitor can be removed and patients weaned from mechanical ventilation.

COMPLICATIONS

Complications frequently occur in the severely head injured, particularly those who also have significant intracranial injuries. These complications include, but are not limited to, the following:

1. Pneumonia occurs in approximately 40% of comatose, intubated, head-injured patients and necessitates treatment with broad-spectrum antibiotics until the organism and appropriate sensitivities are identified.

TABLE 2. **Stepwise Approach to Management of Elevated Intracranial Pressure**

1. All physiologic and hemodynamic parameters normalized
   a. Pco$_2$ 35 ± 2 mm Hg
   b. Po$_2$ > 80 mm Hg
   c. Mean arterial pressure 100 ± 10 mm Hg
   d. Central venous pressure (CVP) 6 − 15 cm H$_2$O
   e. Core temperature 36°C
2. Systemic neuromuscular paralysis (vecuronium [Norcuron] or pancuronium [Pavulon])
3. Narcotic sedation (morphine or fentanyl)
4. Intermittent cerebrospinal fluid (CSF) drainage
5. Mannitol (25–50 gm)
   a. Not used if serum osmolality exceeds 315 mOsm
   b. Urine output replaced milliliter per milliliter with isotonic saline solution
6. Furosemide (Lasix) (40 mg q 4 h)
   a. Not used if serum osmolality exceeds 315 mOsm
7. Pentobarbital to achieve electroencephalographic burst suppression
8. Propofol to reduce intracranial pressure
9. Moderate hypothermia (32°–33°C for 24 h)

2. Atelectasis and pneumothorax are also common complications not only of the primary injury but also of the use of mechanical ventilation.

3. Approximately 15% of severely head-injured patients develop hydrocephalus, which mandates shunting.

4. A number of patients develop heterotopic ossification and, occasionally, decubitus ulcers if skin care is not optimal.

5. Spastic contractures, which were very common before the modern era of head injury management, are much less or rarely seen and can be prevented with aggressive physical therapy.

6. The risk of deep venous thrombosis and pulmonary embolism is a real one. After the first 48 hours of injury, many units use not only compression stockings but also low-dose heparin and, occasionally, the placement of caval filters to prevent this dreaded complication.

SEQUELAE AND PROGNOSIS

Minor Head Injury

The overwhelming majority of patients who have suffered minor head injury recover quite well within 3 to 6 months. Approximately 15% of patients who have suffered a minor head injury that has resulted in no CT scan abnormality have long-term residua. These include behavioral problems, such as easiness to anger, depression, and hostility, and cognitive problems, particularly with memory, concentration, and abstract thinking.

It is not uncommon for patients with minor injuries to have headache in the postoperative period with approximately one half still complaining of headache 3 months after injury. These headaches often respond to propranolol (Inderal), in doses of 30 to 60 mg daily, or occasionally to calcium channel blocking agents.

Severe Head Injury

Patients who have suffered severe head injuries almost always have some sequelae. In addition to the behavioral problems noted for patients with minor head injury, much more severe cognitive difficulties are the rule rather than the exception. The abilities to concentrate, attend to a task, and particularly to perform any task with distractions in the environment are often severely impaired. Significant depression, loss of libido, and loss of behavioral control are also common problems that may take many months or years to resolve.

Because the frequency of survival of severely head-injured patients is much greater than it was before, the neuropsychological problems increasingly are seen by a wide variety of practitioners, not just neurosurgeons or psychiatrists. Many of these patients can be helped by a program of intervention by a neuropsychologist skilled in the assessment and treatment of patients with acute brain injury and by the judicious use, in those who are depressed, of antidepressants such as fluoxetine (Prozac). With appropriate support and intervention, many of these patients can lead productive lives after very severe injuries.

PEDIATRIC HEAD INJURY

method of
FERNANDO STEIN, M.D., and
JOSE A. CORTES, M.D.

Texas Children's Hospital and Baylor College of Medicine
Houston, Texas

Typically, head trauma in children is closed and mild to moderate. Head injury is a frequent problem encountered by primary care physicians. After a child is injured, the caregivers usually contact the physician by telephone first.

The majority of cases of head injury in children do not require any diagnostic imaging, and even fewer necessitate hospitalization. The emphasis of this chapter is on mild to moderate head injury, because most cases of pediatric head trauma fall into this category.

Head injury has been classified as mild, moderate, and severe. Mild head injury is divided into two categories:

Low risk: Glasgow Coma Scale (GCS) score of 15 without acute radiologic abnormality

High risk: GCS score of 13 to 14 or GCS score of 15 with acute radiologic abnormality, both with a period of unconsciousness of less than 20 minutes

Moderate head injury is defined as a GCS score of 9 to 12, or of 13 to 14 with a mass effect or lesion on computed tomography (CT) scan. Severe head injury is defined as a GCS score of less than 8.

The classic criteria have been based on the GCS score (Table 1). However, other elements of judgment such as the degree of concussion or the duration of loss of consciousness have been used (Table 2). The GCS score has not been validated for children younger than 5 years old.

In the simplest analysis, mild to moderate head injury is any head trauma that did not cause coma.

TABLE 1. Glasgow Coma Scale Score

Eye Opening Response	Score
Spontaneous	4
To verbal command	3
To pain	2
None	1
Motor Response	
Obeys verbal commands	6
Localizes pain	5
Withdraws to pain	4
Decorticate posture	3
Decerebrate posture	2
None	1
Verbal Response	
Oriented	5
Confused	4
Inappropriate words	3
Incomprehensible sounds	2
None	1

TABLE 2. Classification of Concussion

Grade	Symptoms
0	Not stunned or dazed. Later headache and difficulty in concentration.
1	Stunned or dazed. No loss of consciousness or amnesia. Sensorium clears in less than 1 minute.
2	Clouding, not loss of consciousness, tinnitus, amnesia. Confused or dizzy.
3	Loss of consciousness for less than 1 minute, never comatose.
4	Loss of consciousness for more than 1 minute, without coma. Hyperexcitable, confused, or dizzy afterward.

Adapted and modified from Nelson WE, Glieck JH, Jane JH, Hawthorne P: Athletic head injuries. J Natl Athletic Trainers Assn 19:95–102, 1984.

EPIDEMIOLOGY

Each year an estimated 2 per 1000 children sustain a head injury. Common causes are falls, sports accidents, and child abuse.

At all ages, the male/female ratio is 2:1 for head trauma. In children younger than 2 years of age, falls and abuse are responsible for the majority of injuries. Motor vehicle–related injuries are more common in older children.

Eighty percent of children who sustain a head injury are not hospitalized. Close to 12% of children are hospitalized for fewer than 3 days, and only about 8% who are considered to have severe head injury are hospitalized for more than 3 days. Mild to moderate head injuries account for 93% of all hospital admissions for head injury, whereas severe head injuries account for only 7%.

PATHOPHYSIOLOGY

Brain injury occurs in two phases: primary and secondary. The primary injury is the damage sustained at the time of impact. It is proportional to the magnitude, duration, and velocity of the applied mechanical force. The brain may become distorted, leading to axonal injuries.

Secondary injury is the neuronal damage caused by the pathophysiologic consequences of the primary injury, such as decreased cerebral blood flow, cerebral hypoxia, brain swelling, and uncoupling of energy-substrate ratios. Systemic complicating factors that include hyperthermia and hypotension also aggravate secondary injury. The main goal of therapy is to limit secondary injury to allow maximal functional recovery.

EVALUATION

The majority of children sustain mild to moderate head injury and are not hospitalized. Normally, the family calls the physician first, inquiring whether the child with the injured head should be examined. This is the first decision that has to be made. Of the patients who are examined by a physician, more than 75% receive only a physical examination and require no imaging. Strict office policies on what to ask and what answers to give to parents or caregivers during the initial telephone contact need to exist so that there can be a consistent and disciplined approach to the evaluation of the child with head trauma.

The initial telephone interview will determine whether the child needs to be examined, whether the child can be transported safely by the parents to the office or to an emergency center, and whether the child needs to be transported to an emergency center by an ambulance. In determining who should be examined, it is necessary to establish as clearly as possible the mechanism of the injury. If the injury involves the generation of high velocity, the child should be examined.

A child should be examined by a physician if any of the following is present:

History of loss of consciousness for more than 1 minute
Vomiting more than twice
Lethargy lasting more than 30 minutes
Severe persistent headache, confusion, weakness, incoordination, abnormal gait, or slurred speech
Swelling over a body part other than the head
Fall from height greater than an adult waist
High-velocity injury (bicycle, skateboard)
High-velocity projectile injury with loss of consciousness (baseball, softball, stone)
Blood coming from the ear or bruising behind the ear
Loss of a previously mastered developmental milestone
Parental desire to have the child examined

If the child is not evaluated in the office, specific instructions must be given regarding what to look for and when to call. Obviously, the availability of a telephone has to be ascertained. No analgesics other than acetaminophen or ibuprofen should be used.

If no imaging studies were indicated after the child's evaluation, a "head injury sheet" should be given to the family. The physician should determine whether the family has a reliable form of transportation immediately available.

IMAGING IN HEAD INJURY

The most important objective in the patient evaluation after head trauma is to identify whether the child has sustained an intracranial injury as opposed to a skull fracture.

Skull Films

This technique is useful only in identifying skull fractures or radiopaque lesions. Patients who present with low-risk criteria such as headache, scalp hematoma, or scalp laceration have been studied systematically with skull radiograph and CT of the head. In 7035 cases in 31 hospitals, no intracranial injuries were discovered in any low-risk patient. Therefore, no intracranial pathology would have been missed by excluding the skull radiograph.* Skull fractures can be identified by CT scan of the head.

Computed Tomography

A CT scan of the head is the imaging modality of choice and is recommended in all head trauma patients who exhibit any of the following:

A GCS score lower than 14
Persistent vomiting after 1 hour of injury
Loss of consciousness for more than 1 minute
Deteriorating mental status, focal neurologic deficit, and seizure
High-velocity injury with history of loss of consciousness for an undetermined amount of time

*N Engl J Med 316:84–91, 1987.

Depressed skull fracture
Penetrating head injury
Unwitnessed head injury (relative indication)

CT is not indicated in minor injuries when there is a GCS score of 15, without loss of consciousness, without focal neurologic signs, and without clinical evidence of a depressed skull fracture.

CT scanning without contrast medium enhancement is an important tool to define any surgical lesion that should be treated promptly. This technique allows visualization of epidural and subdural hematomas, intraventricular and subarachnoid hemorrhage, skull fractures, and cerebral edema.

Magnetic Resonance Imaging

Magnetic resonance imaging (MRI) is superior for visualizing diffuse axonal injury and subarachnoid hemorrhage and for detecting traumatic hematomas of varying ages. It is not the imaging modality of choice in emergencies, because it is time consuming and it requires heavy sedation in younger children and uncooperative adolescents.

MANAGEMENT

The patient should be admitted to a hospital that can offer definitive care. The hospital should offer pediatric intensive care services and, ideally, neurointensive care for the patient who needs neurosurgical interventions. Although initially the child may show few or no symptoms, a neurosurgeon must be available with the necessary support services if an intracranial hemorrhage or an increase in intracranial pressure (ICP) develops. These services include a 24-hour blood bank, anesthesia, clinical laboratory, and neuroimaging availability. The reason for this is obvious: transporting a patient with these symptoms to another hospital once a problem has developed increases morbidity and mortality. An interhospital transport should be provided by medical personnel trained in pediatric intensive care with experience in the care of critically ill and injured children. If the mentioned services are not available, the transport should take place as soon as possible.

Mild to Moderate Head Injury

The child who sustained a mild head injury and who did not require hospitalization will need close observation from a responsible adult for 24 to 48 hours. During this time the caregiver should keep the child at home in a quiet environment. The child must be prohibited from working or playing hard, from riding a bicycle or skateboard, and from driving any vehicle. The child should be awakened every 2 hours and checked for arousal abnormalities for the first night. If during the observation period, the child develops one or more of the "signs of danger" (Table 3), the observer must call a physician or the emergency center immediately for further recommendations. If the child does not develop any of the symptoms in Table 3 during the first 24 hours after head injury, the child can be allowed to return to normal activities.

TABLE 3. **Signs of Danger Requiring Immediate Contact with Physician**

The child does not wake up as usual.
The child is sleepy at unusual times.
The child has seizures.
The child vomits more than six times in 24 hours.
The child has problems with coordination.
The child has a bad headache that does not go away.
The child experiences a change in the visual pattern.
The child seems confused and does not act normally.
When the observer thinks that the child's condition has changed.

If the decision was made to hospitalize a child with mild to moderate head injury, the anticipation should be that some interventions may become necessary such as intensive monitoring and/or care. The hospitalization purpose is to watch closely for the need for interventions, and therefore services such as those mentioned previously must be available.

Severe Head Injury

In children who sustained severe head injury, defined as a GCS score of 8 or less, the following five items are crucial for brain protection:

1. Maintaining adequate oxygenation and ventilation
2. Maintaining adequate blood pressure and perfusion (a single episode of hypotension after head injury worsens prognosis significantly)
3. The prevention and treatment of cerebral edema
4. Adequate monitoring and general supportive care (probably the single most effective group of interventions)
5. Immediate availability of neurosurgery, anesthesia, neuroimaging, and full laboratory and intensive care capabilities

Securing the airway and providing appropriate oxygenation as well as ventilation are universally accepted. The provision of prophylactic hyperventilation has not been proved scientifically as beneficial for the prevention of cerebral edema. The liberal use of osmotic diuretics without regard to the circulating blood volume of the child may prove hazardous, although it is frequently necessary to use these agents for the treatment of cerebral edema. The prevention of hypotension is considered paramount to avoid further neurologic injury. Well-documented studies show that elevation of body temperature more than 102°F is detrimental; therefore, meticulous attention should be paid to the prevention of fever in this type of children. From the surgical standpoint the most frequently needed interventions are the drainage of hematomas and elevation of fractures.

Intracranial Pressure Measurements

Children who have traumatic brain injury with brain swelling generally need to be monitored for increases in ICP. The most commonly used devices are the intraventricular cannula and the intraparenchymal monitor. Intradural and epidural monitors are still used in some institutions. Patients who sustain ICP elevations have impairment of cerebral blood flow and therefore worsening of neurologic injury.

The cerebral perfusion pressure should be maintained above 50 mm Hg in younger children and above 70 mm Hg in adolescents and young adults.

Published clinical experience indicates that ICP monitoring and control may improve outcome and help determine prognosis and that ICP can be reduced by drainage of cerebrospinal fluid. ICP monitoring can help in the early detection of an expanding intracranial mass lesion.

Barbiturate therapy is effective in the setting of uncontrollable ICP refractory to all other conventional medical and surgical treatments. This kind of therapy should be provided in the critical care unit with the appropriate systemic monitoring.

Nutritional support of the head-injured patient should be instituted as early as possible, because poor nutrition worsens outcome.

PROGNOSIS AND COMPLICATIONS

Few criteria allow us to predict the clinical outcome in a head-injured patient. However, the GCS score carries a relationship with recovery, disability, and mortality. There is direct correlation of the degree of disability with duration of coma after head injury (Figure 1).

Postconcussion Syndrome

Postconcussion syndrome is a combination of affective, somatic, and cognitive complaints that follow head injury. Although the literature has questioned its existence, well-controlled studies have shown that more than 50% of the patients blindly interviewed reported symptoms (Figure 2). Most of the somatic complaints tend to decrease or disappear within 3 months of the injury, whereas the affective and cognitive complaints tend to remain for a longer period of time. This period of time for the majority of cases seems to be 6 to 9 months.

Post-traumatic Epilepsy

Post-traumatic epilepsy (PTE) is a condition of recurrent seizures that occur without cause other than an enduring physiologic abnormality of the brain that is the result of trauma. Ninety percent of post-traumatic seizures occur within the first 2 years after the injury. PTE has been classified into early PTE (occurring within 7 days after the event) and late PTE (occurring more than 7 days after the event). Immediate seizures (PTE that occurs during the first 24 hours) constitute 50 to 80% of all cases of early PTE.

The pathogenesis of PTE has been associated with pathophysiologic findings of bruised parenchyma with leptomeningeal thickening and the subsequent

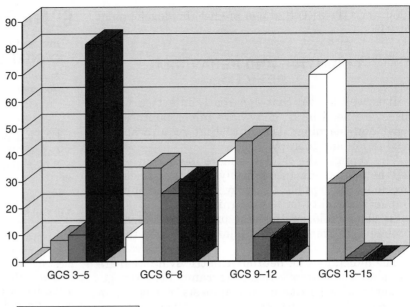

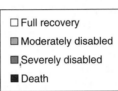

Figure 1. Outcome related to Glasgow Coma Scale (GCS) score.

deposition of hemosiderin. Gliosis, neuronal loss, and microglial reaction determine the formation of scars that act as a focus for seizures. A single seizure at the time of injury increases the risk of post-traumatic epilepsy 10-fold.

Treatment Guidelines

1. A generalized seizure at the time of injury should be treated with a long-acting anticonvulsant.
2. The prophylactic administration of anticonvulsants has been proved in double-blind and placebo-controlled studies to be ineffective in prevention of PTE.

3. The current recommendation is that patients with mild to moderate head injury who have had a seizure at the time of injury or are considered at risk for PTE should receive phenytoin (Dilantin) for the first 7 days after injury. Treatment is then stopped and the patient kept on seizure precautions. If seizures develop, appropriate medication should be started.

There are no reliable objective tests (electroenceph-

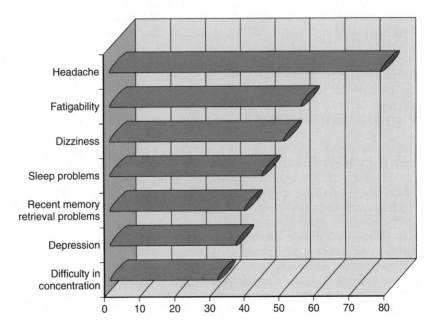

Figure 2. Associated symptoms of postconcussion syndrome.

alogram, CT, MRI) that can predict the development of PTE.

COGNITIVE AND BEHAVIORAL DEFICITS

It is well known that apparently intact survivors of severe head injury may have minor neurobehavioral and learning disabilities that require special evaluation and therapy.

The younger the child, the more likely that injury will be permanent. Incompletely myelinated neurons are more susceptible to injury. Early head injuries impair the ability for new learning.

In older children the best predictor of cognitive problems is amnesia after injury for longer than 7 days.

The indications for neuropsychiatric evaluation are patients who suffered from intracranial hemorrhage, patients with post-traumatic amnesia of more than 24 hours' duration, patients with postconcussion syndrome of more than 3 months' duration, and patients with PTE.

The most common language problem is word retrieval, in which the child is unable to name an object. Other language problems include difficulty writing from dictation, problems with organizing thoughts, difficulty understanding multiple-step commands, and decreased speed with information processing. Cognition problems include lack of attention and concentration, distractibility, short-term memory impairment, and difficulty with logical reasoning. The problems tend to abate over time. Persistent neurobehavioral deficits for moderately and severely injured children resolve over 3 years of follow-up, with a rapid rate of improvement during the first year and then a negligible rate of change.

REHABILITATION

Children of school age who sustain a moderate head injury that keeps them from being able to attend school for a period of time longer than 3 to 4 weeks have an interruption of social life and an interruption of academic life. Frequently there are unrealistic expectations and poor understanding on the part of the parents and teachers about the consequences of brain injury of this magnitude, and there is a very high frequency of academic and social failure. A negative behavioral response is displayed by the child, and when the causative problem is coupled with the misinterpretations of teachers, parents, and friends that this response represents a behavioral issue, many of these children fail academically.

These children are not mentally retarded. What they need is a mainstream experience in a creative mix. This includes a learning disabilities resource room at the school or individual tutoring according to their needs. Appropriate ancillary services such as speech, physical, and occupational therapy are highly recommended as well as counseling for both parents, teachers, and friends.

BRAIN TUMORS

method of
DANIEL H. LaCHANCE, M.D.
Mayo Clinic / Mayo Foundation
Rochester, Minnesota

and

PETER K. DEMPSEY, M.D.
Lahey Clinic
Burlington, Massachusetts

The general concept of brain tumors loosely encompasses a group of neoplasms that may arise from diverse cellular structures in the cranium and may affect the function of the central nervous system (CNS). Although glial tissue neoplasms constitute the most commonly encountered and most feared tumors, neoplastic transformation can occur in neurons, the meninges, vasculature, primitive notochord, primitive neuroectoderm, choroid, ependyma, pineal, pituitary, cranial nerves, and primary or metastatic lymphocytes. Neoplasms metastatic from other sites are also among the most common brain tumors. Clinical presentations are, therefore, diverse and depend primarily on the age of the patient and the primary histology and location of the tumor. Management generally employs a limited number of modalities, but treatment plans are highly specific and depend heavily on the age of the patient and the tumor histology and location.

CLASSIFICATION AND PRESENTATION

A general approach to brain tumors considers lesions as extra-axial, intra-axial (within brain or spinal cord) but well demarcated, or intra-axial and infiltrative.

Extra-axial tumors are usually well circumscribed with benign histology. Clinical presentation is directly related to the nervous system structures immediately adjacent to the lesion. In childhood, craniopharyngioma and pineal region tumors are most common, whereas in adulthood meningioma, accounting for 18 to 20% of all cranial tumors, and acoustic neuroma are commonly encountered. Craniopharyngioma arises from remnants of squamous epithelium in the region of the sella. Growth failure, hypothalamic and pituitary failure, visual loss, and, less commonly, hydrocephalus are the major management issues. Pineal region tumors arise from primary pinocytes, primitive germ cells, primitive neuroectoderm, and, rarely, glial cells. Presentation varies with histology but includes obstructive hydrocephalus, dorsal midbrain dysfunction, and meningeal seeding with cranial nerve, spinal cord, and nerve root dysfunction. Meningiomas are generally benign tumors arising from cells within the arachnoid layer of the meninges. They can occur anywhere along the neuroaxis but commonly appear over the convexities or at the skull base. Meningiomas are often encapsulated, making separation from the surrounding brain and surgical resection possible. Involvement of anatomic structures such as blood vessels or cranial nerves can cause problems. Approximately 7% of meningiomas have malignant features with substantial invasiveness and potential for metastasis. Subtypes of meningiomas may have receptors for estrogen or progesterone, which may explain the slight female predominance of these tumors. Acoustic neuromas are more properly called vestibular schwannomas, as they arise from Schwann cells on the vestibular portion of cranial nerve

VIII. These tumors usually manifest with hearing loss, although tinnitus and disequilibrium occur. Surgical resection is the treatment of choice, and, with present microsurgical techniques, facial nerve function can be preserved nearly 100% of the time.

Intra-axial well-circumscribed tumors are usually also of very different histologies in adults and children. Although most of these lesions are radiographically distinct, few are so well circumscribed as to lend themselves to complete microscopic surgical excision, and adjunctive therapy is often necessary depending on malignant growth potential. A typical example is ependymoma. This tumor often occurs in childhood. It arises from ependyma in the fourth ventricle and has a tendency to recur at the primary site and along cerebrospinal fluid (CSF) pathways. A childhood tumor with low growth potential arises from astrocytes. Juvenile pilocytic astrocytoma is an easily identifiable histologic subtype of glial tumor that, unlike all its other glial counterparts, is primarily noninfiltrating. In young children, the cerebellum is the likely site of occurrence; in older children and younger adults, the diencephalon around the third ventricle and, less commonly, brain stem are usual locations. Presentation is often heralded by the effects of large cystic structures on nearby regions of the brain.

The most common well-circumscribed intraparenchymal lesion is a metastasis. Spread to the brain is usually hematogenous. Occurrence is primarily in adults. Location in the cortex is often at the junction of gray matter and white matter, but any area of the neuroaxis, including the pituitary and spinal cord, may be affected, and frequency of occurrence in any one particular region is generally proportional to the size of that region. Presentation is directly related to the particular CNS region affected. The mass lesion itself does not usually cause symptoms directly except as may be related to its proclivity to cause seizures by way of particular location (temporal and frontal lobes) or hemorrhage by way of particular histologies (melanoma, choriocarcinoma, renal cell carcinoma). Usually, symptoms relate primarily to the sometimes massive extent of edema in adjacent brain tissue. Dysfunction is most often directly related to the size and location of brain affected and to the extent to which mass effect compresses nearby structures, occupies intracranial space, and causes increase in intracranial pressure. Primary lung tumors and tumors metastatic to lung frequently herald brain metastasis, which presumably is related to direct access to systemic arterial circulation. Besides primary lung tumors, melanoma and breast, renal, and colorectal carcinomas account for 85% of metastasis.

A few less common intra-axial well-circumscribed lesions in adults deserve special mention, as accurate diagnosis and direct surgical management are extremely important to long-term outcome. Central neurocytoma and colloid cysts are lesions that may occur in the region of the foramen of Monro and may manifest with the sudden development of potentially life-threatening hydrocephalus. Neurocytoma is a monomorphic clear cell lesion with no anaplastic features that appears to be of neuronal origin. Colloid cysts are nonenhancing cystic structures composed of primitive neuroepithelial cells with minimal growth potential. Another lesion of primary neuronal origin is the ganglioglioma. Discovered mainly in frontal and temporal lobes, it may be responsible for years of medically refractory epilepsy in some patients. Other uncommon entities such as dysembryoplastic neuroepithelial tumor and pleomorphic xanthoastrocytoma may be similarly responsible for years of poorly controlled seizures. Complete surgical excision of these lesions is sometimes possible, often resulting in dramatic reduction in seizure frequency. Hemangioblastoma is a highly vascular, angioblastic, nonanaplastic lesion often associated with large cysts, primarily in the cerebellum and, less commonly, in the spinal cord. When this tumor occurs in an individual younger than 50, 10 to 40% of the cases may be associated with von Hippel–Lindau disease, an autosomal dominant disorder with incomplete penetrance associated with retinal angiomas, renal and pancreatic cysts, and, most important, hypernephroma.

Infiltrative neoplasms of the CNS are primarily primitive neuroectodermal tumors (PNET) or of glial origin. Medulloblastoma and brain stem astrocytomas occur primarily in children, whereas supratentorial gliomas occur mainly in adults. Astrocytic tumors and PNETs behave very differently, and management principles are accordingly very different. In medulloblastoma, histologic subtyping is of no prognostic significance, but the extent of local and meningeal disease at diagnosis, extent of surgical resection, patient age, and local and craniospinal axis radiation dose are major determinants of survival. Glial neoplasms are usually of astrocytic or oligodendrocytic origin. On occasion, the two cell types may be mixed in a single lesion. Survival depends on a number of factors, but tumor grade is most important. The grading system of glial tumors can often cause confusion. The two most commonly accepted systems use either a three- or four-tiered scale, with grade I tumors being more indolent with longer survival and the highest grade tumors (grade III/III or grade IV/IV), commonly known as glioblastoma multiforme (GBM), being most aggressive. Middle-grade tumors—anaplastic astrocytoma (AA) and anaplastic oligodendroglioma (AO)—have fewer malignant histologic features with a more favorable prognosis than that of glioblastoma. In most classification systems, the degree of anaplasia and the presence or absence of vascular proliferation and necrosis are the main determinants of grade and prognosis.

Brain stem gliomas are almost always of astrocytic origin. Histologic subtype seems to vary with location. Dorsal midbrain and medullary lesions are usually low grade and can often be excised from the medullary region or watched, with the possible exception of surgical management of hydrocephalus, in the case of a dorsal midbrain lesion. Pontine and ventral midbrain astrocytomas are almost always highly anaplastic and uniformly fatal. Recent intensive accelerated and hyperfractionated radiotherapy schemes have been of no benefit.

In adults, survival with astrocytic tumors is highly dependent not only on histology but also on age and general and neurologic performance status (Table 1). In general, low-grade and anaplastic tumors occur in younger adults. Glioblastoma may occur at any age but is predominant in older adults. Low-grade tumors progress by increasingly extensive infiltration, often with minimal clinical symptoms. With time, dedifferentiation to a more aggressive histology is the main determinant of survival. Anaplastic astrocytoma and glioblastoma manifest clinically with the effects of destruction of brain parenchyma; infiltration of surrounding brain, often to a distance of several centimeters; and, most significantly, extensive associated edema. The size of the tumor and the extent of associated edema often generate significant mass effect. Seizures may be a presenting or secondary feature of each histologic grade but may be the only clinical consequence of low-grade lesions. Recent observations suggest that anticonvulsants do not prevent the development of seizures that occur in up to 25% of patients with GBM.

Table 1. **Glioma Survival Statistics**

	Median (months)	2 Years	5 Years	10 Years
AA, age <50, KPS = 100, no neurologic deficit	58	76%	20–30%	?
GBM, age <50, KPS = 90–100	18	35%	5–6%	?
GBM, age >50, KPS = 90–100	11	15%	? 0	
GBM, age >50, KPS <70, neurologic deficit	5	4%	? 0	
Low-grade astrocytoma	60			25–30%
Oligodendroglioma, age 20–59			56%	32%

Abbreviations: AA = anaplastic astrocytoma; GBM = glioblastoma multiforme; KPS = Karnofsky performance status.

DIAGNOSIS

Computed Tomography

The advent of computed tomography (CT) in the mid-1970s revolutionized diagnosis and treatment of CNS neoplasms. Late-generation CT scans not only show parenchymal lesions but are also capable of delineating vascular structures. Three-dimensional volumetric reconstructions of the brain are possible with newer scanners. CT remains the initial radiographic tool in the management of most patients with brain tumors. The speed and ubiquity of CT scanners allow for any patient with signs or symptoms of neurologic compromise to be evaluated quickly. The administration of intravenous iodinated contrast allows for demonstration of blood-brain barrier breakdown. The neovascularity of rapidly growing tumors results in permeable vascular membranes, allowing the contrast agent to "leak" out into the parenchyma, showing up as an increased density on the image.

Magnetic Resonance Imaging

Magnetic resonance imaging (MRI) has further expanded the visualization of the structure and function of the brain. Often after the presence of a neoplasm is established with CT, MRI is employed to better define the lesion. Valuable data regarding anatomic location and proximity to neural and vascular structures can be obtained with MRI. Later generation scanners also provide information regarding function of the brain. Perfusion imaging indicates blood flow to regions of the brain and can often distinguish between areas of necrosis and tumor growth. Functional MRI can localize motor, visual, and speech regions of the brain and can be used in preoperative planning.

TREATMENT

Despite imaging advances, the first step in the management of most patients with CNS neoplasms is to obtain tissue for diagnosis.

Surgery: Craniotomy

As outlined previously for extra-axial or intra-axial well-circumscribed lesions, surgery is not only diagnostic but definitive therapy. Surgery appears to have a clear role in the treatment of symptomatic, superficially located, solitary metastatic tumors. A distinct benefit has been measured in patients who underwent surgical resection followed by radiation therapy as opposed to those undergoing irradiation alone. Craniotomy for resection of infiltrative glial tumors is usually reserved for superficially located tumors with evidence of mass effect. Debulking the tumor mass is often helpful in both providing a histologic diagnosis and relieving symptoms of elevated intracranial pressure (headache, nausea, and vomiting). Debate exists over the value of cytoreduction in the treatment of these lesions. Proponents believe that reducing the tumor burden will allow for greater success with subsequent radiation therapy and chemotherapy. Potential complications with craniotomy are generally quite low in incidence and include bleeding, infection, neurologic injury (coma, stroke, death), and the generation of seizures. The risk of these complications, not to mention additional hospitalization, may not be justified by the potential benefit. Surgical resection is not an ideal treatment for an infiltrative neoplasm. It is difficult, if not impossible, to detect where the tumor margin ends and normal tissue begins. In addition, tumor cells may migrate several centimeters along white matter pathways, including the corpus callosum, making complete resection impossible.

Surgery: Image Directed

For deep-seated tumors in eloquent areas of the brain, stereotactic biopsy has been a valuable technique. Commonly, this is done with a guiding device (stereotactic frame) attached to the outer table of the skull with pins and local anesthesia. Imaging with CT or MRI is obtained; a target is selected and its location measured relative to this frame. The frame then serves as a platform for guiding a biopsy needle to the selected target. This can usually be accomplished with local anesthesia, through a small burr hole. Diagnostic samples are obtained more than 90% of the time. The limitation of stereotactic biopsy comes from small sample size. This can occasionally lead to sampling error, in which a portion of the tumor with less aggressive histologic features is obtained, leading to a diagnosis of a lower grade neoplasm. In addition, stereotactic biopsy does not allow for treatment of mass effect. In poor–surgical risk patients, however, stereotactic biopsy is preferred.

Techniques have been developed that allow stereotactic guidance to be used during a conventional craniotomy. This allows the surgeon to have imaging information during the procedure and helps to improve localization and resection. Several medical centers have incorporated intraoperative MRI scanners, which provide real-time imaging during the surgery. The cost of these units as well as the necessary modifications to the surgical and anesthesia equipment is prohibitive for most institutions at this time.

Radiation Therapy

Photon irradiation from linear accelerators is derived from an accelerated beam of electrons striking tungsten and emitting photons. These particles create free radicals and can disrupt cellular functions, damage DNA, and induce apoptosis. Mitotically active cells are most prone to radiation injury. Normal cells are capable of repair processes that can restore cell integrity after damage by radiation. Tumor cells are often deficient in such repair mechanisms. The efficacy of radiotherapy lies in the exploitation of this difference, mainly through fractionation (the daily delivery of small doses of radiation), which allows normal cells to repair while tumor cells are unable to do so.

Radiation therapy is generally well tolerated by patients. The most noticeable side effects are alopecia and fatigue. Women usually have return of hair growth after treatment, whereas hair growth in men is more variable. Fatigue often occurs toward the end of radiotherapy and can persist for several weeks. Late effects of radiation, including necrosis, memory dysfunction, loss of higher cognitive functions, and hypothalamic failure, can occur months to years after treatment and are generally irreversible. The risk of the most serious consequence of standard radiotherapy, radiation necrosis, is about 5%.

Radiation treatment protocols are determined by tumor type. Malignant gliomas are usually treated with a dose approaching 6000 centigray (cGy). Initially, the tumor and a generous margin are covered, with the treatment volume focusing on the tumor location as the cumulative dose increases. The daily fraction is usually 200 cGy, administered over a 5- to 6-week period. In contrast, metastatic tumors to the brain are treated with whole-brain radiation to a typical dose of 3000 cGy, usually in a smaller number of fractions.

Stereotactic Radiosurgery

Stereotactic radiosurgery is a single-session radiation treatment in which a small, well-defined intracranial target is treated. Either a gamma knife or a modified linear accelerator is used. Both methods are similar in that the tumor is localized with stereotactic techniques and the radiation is precisely delivered to the specified target. Owing to the high degree of accuracy in targeting and the rapid fall-off of radiation dose, a tumoricidal dose can be delivered to the lesion, while normal brain structures a few millimeters away are spared. The two techniques differ in that gamma radiation from radioactive cobalt 201 is used in the gamma knife and in that conventional photon radiation is used in the linear accelerator. The gamma unit is devoted solely to the treatment of brain lesions, whereas the linear accelerator is more versatile. The major limitation of this technique is the volume of the tumor that can be irradiated. If the lesion is larger than 3.5 to 4 cm in maximal diameter, irradiation of surrounding structures be-

comes too great, with potentially severe radiation injury to normal brain structures a result.

Radiosurgery can be used either as a boost to conventional, fractionated radiation or as a single treatment. Tumors often resistant to conventional radiation, such as melanoma, seem to be particularly sensitive to single-treatment radiosurgery. Gliomas, with no well-defined margin, are not ideally treated with radiosurgery. Nevertheless, radiosurgery in addition to fractionated radiation may offer some benefit in slowing the rate of local recurrence in small-volume gliomas.

Chemotherapy

Chemotherapy for brain tumors has been generally considered adjunctive therapy for highly aggressive and infiltrating neoplasms. Scattered small series have been reported for treatment of meningioma with agents such as actinomycin* (Cosmegen),* tamoxifen (Nolvadex),* and mifepristone (RU486†). Carboplatin* has been used with some success in juvenile pilocytic astrocytoma. Medulloblastoma, germ cell tumors, and lymphomas have proved to be highly sensitive to a variety of chemotherapeutic agents, with significant survival impact. Alkylating agent chemotherapy probably produces a small increase in the number of 1-year and 18-month survivors with GBM and may have a somewhat greater impact for AA. BCNU (carmustine), or a combination of procarbazine (Matulane),* CCNU (lomustine), and vincristine (Oncovin) (PCV),* is a standard therapy. In the last few years, the characterization of oligodendroglioma with both low-grade and anaplastic histologies has taken on major importance, as 75 to 80% of lesions appear to be chemosensitive to a variety of drugs, especially variants of PCV. It remains yet to be determined how this affects survival.

Unfortunately, a great deal of time and effort in therapeutic trials of a number of agents over 20 years since the first published report of the impact of BCNU on survival in malignant glioma has produced little therapeutic advance. Promising avenues in current clinical trials include the placement of polymer wafers impregnated with chemotherapeutic agents intraoperatively, a variety of gene therapy approaches, new approaches to blood-brain barrier disruption, new chemotherapeutic agents such as topoisomerase inhibitors, and metabolic pathway inhibitors such as merimistat and tamoxifen.

Treatment of Symptoms

Day-to-day therapeutic issues are important in the management of brain tumor patients. Neurologic deficits can have major impact on quality of life, and standard rehabilitation strategies may play a major role in maximizing performance. The need to address spiritual and psychosocial concerns is often of para-

---

*Not FDA approved for this indication.

†Not yet approved for use in the United States.

mount importance in developing a specific treatment program. Social service input is invaluable. Some patients derive tremendous help from each other in organized support groups. Depression is often a significant problem, and appropriate pharmacotherapy should be offered early. Fatigue is common, especially during and after radiotherapy. Stimulants such as pemoline (Cylert) and protriptyline (Vivactil)* may be useful.

A number of specific medical issues are important in patient management. Seizures may present significant morbidity. Special concerns in brain tumor patients include propensity for adverse drug interactions and a higher incidence of postictal neurologic deficit. The proper and reserved use of corticosteroids cannot be overemphasized. Lowest effective doses for

---

*Not FDA approved for this indication.

management of associated brain edema should be monitored constantly. Cushingoid side effects and steroid myopathy can sometimes become severe. Many patients with brain tumors, especially those with neurologic deficit and immobility, are at risk for deep vein thrombosis and pulmonary emboli. Recent reports have suggested that the risk of tumor bleeding with use of anticoagulants is not as high as was once feared, and anticoagulation should be considered in appropriate cases.

Finally, the process of death and dying should not be ignored. Hearing patients' fears and concerns and responding to them can be of great value to patients, their families, and caregivers. Hospice groups are available in many locations and can be exceedingly helpful in managing the final phase of illness in many patients with malignant brain tumors.

The Locomotor System

RHEUMATOID ARTHRITIS

method of
WILLIAM S. WILKE, M.D.
The Cleveland Clinic Foundation
Cleveland, Ohio

Rheumatoid arthritis (RA) is a chronic inflammatory disease with a variable course. Some patients with symmetrical polyarthritis who satisfy the American College of Rheumatology criteria for RA but are rheumatoid factor (RF)–negative have a mild disease with a remitting course. Indeed, many of these patients may not have classic RA but some other process, such as "postinfectious" arthritis. The majority of patients in whom RF is positive will eventually demonstrate radiographic damage and experience disability without treatment. Not only does the disease cause swelling, deformity, cartilage loss, juxta-articular bony erosions, muscular atrophy, and tendon contractions and possible dissolution, but it can also involve extra-articular structures (Table 1). Studies have demonstrated that RA also decreases life expectancy.

STRATEGY FOR TREATMENT

A large number of drugs are now available for the treatment of RA. These can be classified as drugs that have been demonstrated in controlled trials to solely improve signs and symptoms and drugs that have been shown in long-term prospective trials to modify disease outcome and are referred to as disease-modifying antirheumatic drugs (DMARDs). Nonsteroidal anti-inflammatory drugs (NSAIDs), while providing symptom relief, have not been shown to favorably modify the outcome of disease. Corticosteroids, alternatively, have been demonstrated to decrease radiographic progression compared with placebo. A large number of other agents have also been demonstrated to have the potential for long-term disease modification (Table 2). The physician who oversees the care of patients with RA must be very familiar with demonstrated physiologic mechanisms of benefit, time course to onset of action, potential adverse effects, and potential interactions if these agents are given simultaneously.

Long-term prospective and retrospective series have demonstrated that the pyramid model of therapy for RA often fails to control disease activity and prevent long-term disability. Alternative approaches have been suggested, but none has been fully embraced by the American College of Rheumatology or by the majority of rheumatologists. One method of treatment that seems logical and should result in better outcome is a goal-oriented treatment.

Arguably, information already exists about disease characteristics that allows stratification of rheumatoid disease as benign or progressive at the time of initial diagnosis. This information includes both (1) prognostic indicators, such as the presence and titer of RF, DRB1-shared epitopes, and older age, and (2) process signs and symptoms, which include initial high number of involved joints, early initial radiographic deterioration, and elevated acute phase reactants. Initial introduction of disease-modifying treatment is crucial for patients with these indicators because joint damage appears to occur early in disease in all patients and be accelerated in this subset. One series of 42 RA patients with a median symptom duration of 4 months demonstrated erosions detected by magnetic resonance imaging in 47%. In another study, the 75 representative patients among 137 patients who were initially treated with the combination of oral gold and NSAIDs or NSAIDs alone for the first 8 months, at which time oral gold was added, were observed 5 years later. Early outcome at 1 year clearly favored initial treatment with oral gold. Of interest, at 5 years, differences between the two groups in outcome measures were maintained and still favored early initiation of oral gold. This prospective study suggested that early treatment with disease-modifying agents influenced disease outcome for many years.

Disease-modifying agents have been demonstrated in prospective studies to decrease the number of swollen and tender joints and decrease the acute phase response. If reduction of these measures favorably influences outcome in RA, then the primary goal of therapy should be to maintain these process measures at their lowest possible value. In fact, modification of these measures has been demonstrated to influence outcome, allowing classification of these measures as both process and prognostic factors. In

TABLE 1. **Extra-articular Rheumatoid Arthritis**

Organ/System	Manifestations
Skin	Rheumatoid nodules, palpable purpura, and vasculitic ulcers
Lung	Interstitial inflammation and fibrosis
Eyes	Scleritis and episcleritis
Vascular	Vasculitis with mononeuritis multiplex and bowel infarction
Neurologic	Carpal and tarsal tunnel syndrome Cervical cord damage due to atlantoaxial or other cervical subluxation

TABLE 2. Overview of Symptom-Modifying Antirheumatic Drugs

Agent	Effective Dosage (Route of Administration)	Time to Onset of Action (Weeks)	Relative Efficacy	Relative Toxicity	Comments
Auranofin (Ridaura)	3–9 mg/d (oral)	8–16	+	+ + +	Gastrointestinal toxicity common; marginal efficacy
Azathioprine (Imuran)	75–150 mg/d (oral)	6–12	+ + +	+ + +	Reasonably effective; lingering concerns about malignancy limit usefulness
Cyclosporine (Sandimmune)	2–5 mg/kg/d (oral)*	6–16	+ + +	+ + +	Renal toxicity is universal; expensive
Hydroxychloroquine (Plaquenil Sulfate)	200–400 mg/d (oral)	12–24	+ +	+	Modest efficacy, minimal toxicity
Leflunomide (Arava)	100 mg loading dose; 20 mg/d (oral)	4–8	+ + + +	+ +	Low frequency of cytopenia
Methotrexate	5–25 mg/wk (intramuscular, subcutaneous, oral)	3–8	+ + + +	+ +	Excellent efficacy/toxicity ratio
Minocycline (Dynacin)	100–200 mg/d (oral)	6–12	+	+ +	Weak efficacy; for mild disease
Parenteral gold (Myochrysine)	25–50 mg/wk loading (intramuscular)	12–20	+ + +	+ + + +	Excellent short-term efficacy; toxicity is common, effect wanes with time
Penicillamine (Depen)	250–1000 mg/d (oral)	8–16	+ +	+ + +	Relatively unfavorable efficacy/toxicity ratio
Sulfasalazine (Azulfidine)	1000–3000 mg/d (oral)	4–12	+ + +	+ +	Excellent short-term efficacy; reasonably well tolerated
TNFα-Fc fusion protein (Enbrel)	25 mg twice weekly (subcutaneous)	2–4	+ + + +	+	Very safe, very expensive

TNFα = tumor necrosis factor-alpha.
*Exceeds dosage recommended by the manufacturer.
Adapted from Wilke WS, Cash JM: The use of slower-acting (class III) symptom-modifying anti-rheumatic drugs in rheumatoid arthritis. Clin Immunother 4:306, 1996.

a 3-year prospective study of 149 patients, the magnitude of the acute phase response and the number of swollen joints during therapy predicted the degree of radiographic damage. Of interest, joint tenderness during therapy was a better predictor of ultimate physical disability. Many other prospective series have demonstrated that when acute phase reactants are normalized by therapy, RA patients show significantly less radiographic progression versus patients in whom acute phase reactants remained elevated.

Remission should be the ultimate goal of therapy but is very difficult to achieve. When the body of prospective series is analyzed, "near-remission," which requires normalization of acute phase reactants and a swollen-tender joint count maintained at 5 or below during treatment, predicts a favorable outcome. This kind of disease control has been demonstrated both with methotrexate (MTX, Rheumatrex) alone and in patients treated with the combination of sulfasalazine (SSZ, Azulfidine), MTX, and hydroxychloroquine (HDC, Plaquenil).

A parallel for this kind of goal-oriented therapy exists in the treatment model for hypertension. Reduction of blood pressure to certain goal values has been demonstrated to favorably modify long-term outcome. If one antihypertensive medication marginally decreases blood pressure but does not achieve goal pressures, another medication is substituted or added to the treatment protocol until the goal is achieved. Once the goal is achieved, antihypertensive medications are not slowly withdrawn because such withdrawal invariably leads to higher blood pressure. As in hypertensive therapy, once control is achieved for patients with RA, treatment should be maintained constant for the long term, unless otherwise dictated by adverse effects.

NONSTEROIDAL ANTI-INFLAMMATORY DRUGS

Pain control must also be an initial therapeutic goal, because without such control patients may become discouraged and noncompliant. NSAIDs represent one alternative to provide pain control.

The primary mechanism of action of available NSAIDs is down-regulation of the cyclooxygenase (COX) enzyme system. Unfortunately, prostaglandins produced by the action of this system are both proinflammatory (COX-2) and gastroprotective (COX-1). Inhibition of the local production of gastroprotective prostaglandins results in significant gastrointestinal adverse effects that are most prominent in patients with a history of previous peptic ulcer disease and in those who are age 65 or older. Although some agents, which include nabumetone (Relafen) and etodolac (Lodine), are associated with less gastrointestinal adverse effects, they may be marginally less effective. Meloxicam,* celecoxib (Celebrex), and rofecoxib (Vioxx), which primarily inhibit COX-2 and spare COX-1, represent the first of many more acceptable

NSAIDs. Of importance, agents that primarily inhibit COX-2 have been demonstrated to be only safer, not more effective.

Alternative analgesics include acetaminophen and tramadol (Ultram), which can be given in doses as high as 100 mg four times daily. Because up to 25% of patients with RA also have signs and symptoms of fibromyalgia, and because tricyclic antidepressant medications have been demonstrated to provide analgesia for patients with diabetic neuropathy or other chronic pain syndromes, the judicious use of amitriptyline (Elavil),* trazodone (Desyrel),* or doxepin (Sinequan),* given in small doses (10 to 50 mg) 1 hour before bed can be useful. For treatment of pain, I prefer to prescribe acetaminophen and, if indicated, doxepin, as "base" analgesic therapy and ask the patient to use a tolerated NSAID intermittently for disease flares or when activities of daily living dictate, such as a golf outing or shopping trip. It is important to remember that if patients must rely on analgesic medications to function at an expected level, control of disease with specific antirheumatic agents may not be appropriately robust. When NSAID medications are used continuously, the addition of misoprostol (Cytotec) or other gastroprotective agents is indicated for most.

INDIVIDUAL AGENTS

Corticosteroids

Proscription against oral/systemic corticosteroid treatment has been based on at least two premises: (1) that these agents are significantly more dangerous than other agents, and (2) that such treatment is not disease modifying and only controls symptoms. Interleukin-6 (IL-6), which is elevated in inflammatory diseases such as RA, stimulates osteoclastic bone resorption. Corticosteroids have been demonstrated to decrease IL-6 in RA and improve calcium metabolism in bone. Furthermore, in a meta-analysis of nine carefully conducted prospective studies of corticosteroid therapy, short-term improvement of tender and swollen joints, grip strength, and erythrocyte sedimentation rate was demonstrated and was equal to or superior to that obtained with all other DMARDs. A double-blind controlled trial by Kirwan and others has confirmed the findings of trials from the 1950s that demonstrated that treatment with corticosteroids improved radiographic outcome.

All of this information suggests that the short-term use of corticosteroids can be appropriate therapy for RA. Data beyond 1 year, however, are inconclusive, and caution regarding long-term treatment with systemic corticosteroids is suggested.

I find systemic corticosteroid treatment useful in at least three circumstances: At the time of diagnosis, patients with at least six swollen tender joints, and elevated acute phase reactants, respond very well to prednisone, 0.1 mg per kg (5 to 7.5 mg), given in

---

*Not FDA approved for this indication.

*Not FDA approved for this indication.

the morning as "bridge therapy," anticipating later effects of other prescribed treatment. At the time of disease flare, for a patient who has otherwise experienced control of disease, bolus corticosteroids (80 to 160 mg of intramuscular methylprednisolone) can obviate the need to raise the dose of existing DMARDs or add yet another to the treatment program. Finally, long-term therapy is occasionally necessary. This occurs when despite treatment with multiple DMARDs used at their highest tolerated doses, significant disease activity remains. In this circumstance, small doses of prednisone (2.5 to 5 mg each morning) can be surprisingly effective and are clearly excessive DMARD therapy sparing.

Although studies have demonstrated some favorable effects of corticosteroids on bone metabolism in patients with inflammatory disease, all patients who take short-term or long-term corticosteroids should be given extra calcium and extra vitamin D to prevent osteoporosis. In addition, information from bone densitometry should be available in all corticosteroid-treated postmenopausal women, most other females, and older males. A variety of treatments are now available and include cyclical etidronate (Didronel), daily nasal calcitonin (Miacalcin), and daily alendronate (Fosamax). Although alendronate is best studied, the need for early morning fasting and upright posture after taking the drug to prevent esophageal damage limits usefulness for some patients. Estrogen has been shown to reduce the degree of osteoporosis in corticosteroid-treated postmenopausal women and should be added to any osteoporosis protocol if the patient does not have a history of breast cancer. Concomitant progestin supplementation should always be given to women who have not undergone hysterectomy.

Less controversial is the use of corticosteroids for local joint injection. This is usually necessary during the course of therapy when one or two joints are more symptomatic than others. The treating physician should always inquire about new activities, injury, fever, night sweats, rash, recent dental procedures, and any other recent infection before considering injection. If there is any question of sepsis, only aspiration should be done and injection reconsidered when the results of bacterial cultures have returned. Repeated injections of the same joints should be limited to once or twice a year. If repeated injections are necessary, diagnoses other than RA (osteoarthritis, crystal-induced arthritis, ligamentous or meniscal damage/deterioration) should be sought.

When injection is performed, sterility should be observed. All patients should be questioned about allergic reactions to iodine or lidocaine. Skin analgesia can be provided by intradermal lidocaine injection with a 25-gauge needle or with fluoroethyl spray. A long-acting corticosteroid such as triamcinolone hexacetonide can be combined with lidocaine for injection of the knees and shoulders. I would suggest that only rheumatologists or physicians who have been specifically instructed in the procedure inject ankles, elbows, wrists, or the small joints of the fingers.

Methotrexate

The short- and long-term efficacies of MTX are well established. It is given once weekly, generally at a dose of 7.5 to 15 mg taken by mouth. Intramuscular therapy is indicated for patients who experience gastrointestinal adverse effects or in whom poor absorption is suspected. Ameliorative effects are experienced within 4 weeks by most patients and plateau at approximately 6 months. Nearly 80% of treated patients will experience moderate to excellent symptomatic benefit from treatment, but remission is rare.

Although MTX is one of the safest DMARDs, many patients will experience adverse effects during the course of treatment. The most common adverse effects—nausea, vomiting, mouth ulcers, and mild alopecia—occur in approximately 10% of patients. A smaller percentage of patients may develop fatigue, headaches, and/or arthralgias in the 24 hours after the dose of MTX. I prescribe folic acid, 1 to 2 mg per day, for all patients to limit "nuisance" toxicity. Macrocytosis can also occur due to folate inhibition. However, serious hematologic reactions are usually associated only with renal insufficiency or concomitant treatment with other antifolate medications such as sulfa-containing antibiotics.

Hepatic fibrosis and cirrhosis have been reported in a minority of patients taking MTX and are associated with alcohol use, obesity, diabetes mellitus, and renal insufficiency. It is important that treated patients abstain from alcoholic beverages to limit this risk. Acute lung toxicity has been reported to occur in up to 5% of treated patients, although this estimate may be high. Patients come to medical attention with relatively acute (2 to 3 days) cough, fever, and severe shortness of breath and demonstrate bilateral pulmonary infiltrates on the chest radiograph. Withdrawal of MTX, supportive care, and, in some cases, short-term high-dose corticosteroid therapy, usually control this adverse effect. A few deaths, however, have been reported. Pulmonary toxicity can occur at any time during treatment and with any weekly dose of MTX.

Although early studies of MTX-treated patients with psoriasis and uterine cancer failed to show evidence of oncogenesis, reports of B cell pseudolymphomas and lymphomas, which often remit when MTX is withdrawn, suggest that rare malignancies may indeed be associated with MTX therapy.

If an excessive dose of MTX is taken, leucovorin calcium should be given immediately to limit serious toxicity. Folinic acid (leucovorin) can be given chronically in equal milligram doses approximately 12 hours after the dose of MTX to control severe nausea or mouth ulcers that might otherwise threaten continued therapy. If a substantial dose of folinic acid is given simultaneously with MTX, it will reverse efficacy.

Because MTX blood levels are almost entirely dependent on renal excretion, the most important laboratory monitoring test during therapy is determination of the serum creatinine level. Elevated levels of serum creatinine represent a serious, relative contraindication to the use of MTX. Other tests that should be performed initially every 2 to 4 weeks include those for liver enzymes and albumin and a complete blood cell count (CBC). Because histologic evidence of liver toxicity is associated with the frequency of abnormal liver enzyme elevations rather than any isolated elevation, liver enzyme elevations that persist for 2 to 3 months must be investigated. In my experience, NSAIDs are often responsible. I discontinue the NSAID and repeat the liver enzyme testing in 2 weeks. If enzyme levels are still elevated, investigation for hepatitis B and C is indicated, as is liver biopsy, if MTX therapy is to be continued.

Gold Compounds

Parenteral gold is available in two forms: sodium aurothiomalate (Myochrysine) and aurothioglucose (Solganol). Both forms are equally effective, but aurothioglucose may be more toxic. The clinical efficacy of injectable gold has been called into question. However, it is very clear that a subset of patients (young women with early disease?) experience significant disease control and/or remission with gold therapy. In comparative studies, injectable gold has shortterm efficacy that is comparable to MTX. Unfortunately, long-term studies suggest that gold loses its effectiveness over time.

The protocol for parenteral gold administration requires a test dose of 10 mg given on week 1, 25 mg on week 2, and 50 mg thereafter. If a response has not occurred after a total dose of 1 gram, further treatment is unlikely to be beneficial. After a therapeutic effect is achieved, the dosage interval can be lengthened to 2 weeks and eventually 4 weeks.

Parenteral gold is one of the more toxic treatments for RA. Rashes occur in approximately 15% of patients and vary from small, eczematous patches to sometimes life-threatening epidermolysis and exfoliative dermatitis. Nitritoid reactions characterized by flushing and tachycardia occur in a small percentage of patients given sodium aurothiomalate.

Renal toxicity occurs in 10 to 20% of patients given gold and is manifested by proteinuria. If identified early, proteinuria eventually clears without clinically significant long-term renal damage. Pulmonary toxicity, enteropathy that is manifest by severe diarrhea, and thrombocytopenia with agranulocytosis occur in a small percentage of patients.

Patients receiving gold should be questioned about rashes and other adverse effects at each weekly visit. In addition, a weekly CBC and urinalysis are also necessary.

Oral gold (auranofin [Ridaura]) administered in a dose of 3 mg up to three times daily has been demonstrated in controlled trials to be more effective than placebo and in comparative trials to have efficacy similar to HDC. Many patients experienced treatment-limiting diarrhea when full doses of oral gold were given. Patients tolerating oral gold should be followed with regular CBC determinations.

Sulfasalazine

Sulfasalazine is effective when given orally in dosages of 1.5 to 3.0 grams per day in divided doses. Within 4 to 12 weeks, most patients experience some improvement.

Gastrointestinal complaints (especially diarrhea), rashes, and rare cases of thrombocytopenia complicate SSZ treatment. These adverse effects are usually encountered during the first 3 months of therapy. Close monitoring of the CBC during initial therapy is therefore recommended.

Penicillamine

Penicillamine (Depen, DPN) was initially recommended for treatment of gold failure in RA. It may be given at an initial dose of 250 mg per day with monthly escalation to a maximum of 1000 mg per day. Most patients experience some improvement at a dose of 500 mg per day.

Adverse effects with DPN are dose related. They include diarrhea and rashes. Thrombocytopenia and leukopenia can occur in up to 10% of patients. Glomerulonephritis can also occur, especially during initial therapy. Unique to DPN, reversible autoimmune syndromes, including myasthenic neuromuscular disease, lupus-like syndrome, polymyositis, and Goodpasture's syndrome, have been reported.

A CBC and urinalysis are indicated every 2 to 4 weeks during initial DPN therapy. Historical evidence for any aforementioned autoimmune disease must also be sought at each visit.

Hydroxychloroquine

Antimalarial drugs have been used to treat rashes and RA for at last 45 years. The safest among them is the 4-aminoquinolone derivative HDC. It is given orally as 200 to 400 mg per day, not to exceed 6 mg per kg per day. Response to therapy is delayed for 3 to 6 months with a plateau at approximately 9 months.

Antimalarial drugs are very well tolerated. Rashes, pigmentary change, and diarrhea occur in 1% to 2% of treated patients. Corneal deposits can occur and are an indication of excessive dose. Dose reduction is curative.

Severe retinopathy, a result of deposition of HDC in the retina, producing the characteristic "bull's-eye" lesion, can eventually diminish vision but rarely occurs. In the most recent studies, less than 1% of patients treated with standard doses for 5 years experienced this adverse effect. A baseline eye examination is recommended for patients 60 years or older. The need for frequent eye examinations thereafter is becoming controversial; however, because it has been demonstrated that retinal lesions are reversible if they are detected early, yearly eye examinations are probably indicated.

Cyclosporine

Cyclosporine (Sandimmune, Neoral),* a fungus-derived peptide, was first developed to prevent rejection of organs after transplant. It has been demonstrated to be efficacious and relatively well tolerated in a number of well-designed prospective double-blind studies.

The initial dose of cyclosporine should not exceed 2.5 mg per kg per day. This dose can be slowly escalated to 5 mg per kg as dictated by disease activity. Most patients experience some improvement of disease within 3 to 6 weeks after initiation.

Adverse effects from cyclosporine are in large measure due to its effect on the kidney. It decreases renal perfusion in a dose-related fashion that can result in blood pressure elevation and fluid retention with dependent edema. Because NSAIDs can produce similar renal toxicity, they should be avoided in patients taking cyclosporine. In high doses (10 mg per kg per day), cyclosporine stimulates interstitial cell growth, which can produce interstitial fibrosis of the kidney and chronic renal insufficiency.

Before initiating cyclosporine, I obtain a baseline creatinine clearance for future reference. Serum creatinine should be determined every 2 to 4 weeks during initial therapy. In addition, blood pressure must be assiduously monitored. Patients must be warned to avoid over-the-counter pain medicines such as ibuprofen or naproxen.

Azathioprine

The dosage range for azathioprine (AZA, Imuran) is 1 to 2.5 mg per kg per day. Effect on disease is seen within 6 to 12 weeks. Diarrhea and mild hematologic problems occur commonly during AZA therapy. Some experts now suggest that an assay for the enzyme thiopurine methyltransferase be performed before therapy. Patients with this enzyme deficiency are at high risk of cytopenia from AZA, and treatment should be avoided.

Debate remains regarding lymphoma and AZA. A case-control study demonstrated that AZA-treated patients were at a slightly higher risk of developing lymphoma versus RA patients treated with other medications.

During the initial weeks of therapy a CBC should be obtained every 2 to 4 weeks. The dose of AZA should be reduced by 50 to 75% if patients are taking concomitant allopurinol (Zyloprim) for hyperuricemia.

Minocycline

Minocycline (Dynacin, Minocin)* is a tetracycline antibiotic that has been demonstrated to be superior to placebo for the treatment of RA. The efficacy of

minocycline is not robust, and it may be less than that of HDC and/or oral gold. The recommended dosage is 100 mg twice daily. Beneficial effects are delayed for approximately 6 weeks. Adverse effects include rash and nausea in less than 10% of treated patients.

Alkylating Agents

Three alkylating agents have been used for the treatment of RA and include oral cyclophosphamide (Cytoxan),* oral chlorambucil (Leukeran),* and intravenous nitrogen mustard (Mustargen).* Because of severe acute toxicities, gonadal toxicities, and a clear increased risk of future oncogenesis when these agents are used chronically, they are recommended only for the treatment of severe extra-articular manifestations of disease such as vasculitis.

Soluble Tumor Necrosis Factor-α Receptor–Fc Fusion Protein

There is compelling evidence to support a crucial role for tumor necrosis factor-α (TNF-α) in the pathogenesis of RA. The receptors for TNF-α are found on many cells, including polymorphonuclear leukocytes. When TNF binds to these receptors, proinflammatory events occur. Down-modulation of these proinflammatory events is accomplished when neutrophils shed the extracellular portion of the cell-bound TNF-α receptors, which become soluble. The soluble receptors then bind to soluble TNF, preventing TNF from binding to cell receptors and initiating inflammation.

A form of TNF receptor, fused to the Fc fragment of human immunoglobulin G1 (Enbrel), has been approved for treatment of RA and is prescribed as 25 mg, given subcutaneously twice weekly. In the most convincing clinical trial, 180 patients with refractory RA received subcutaneous injection of placebo or one of three doses of the fusion protein (0.25, 2, or 16 mg per m² of body surface area) twice weekly for 3 months. The results of treatment were published in the *New England Journal of Medicine* in July 1997. Of great importance, at 3 months, patients receiving the highest dose of the fusion protein experienced a 61% reduction in the number of tender or swollen joints.

The onset of action occurs quickly, within a few weeks. In addition, TNF-α is responsible for a variety of dysphoric symptoms in patients with connective tissue disease, including fatigue. Those symptoms also improved very quickly. Of great importance, acute adverse events are limited to mild injection-site reactions without "systemic" adverse effects. Because this recombinant TNF inhibitor is a "normal" constituent of plasma, induction of antiglobulin response has not been observed. Although TNF participates in control of infection, to date the use of this and other anti-TNF agents has not resulted in a statistically significant increase in the frequency of infection. Of theoretical concern, TNF plays a role in

---

*Not FDA approved for this indication.

*Not FDA approved for this indication.

neoplastic surveillance. Whether inhibition will lead to a higher frequency of neoplasm will be known only after careful, prospective long-term follow-up.

Leflunomide

Leflunomide (LEF, Arava) is an isoxazole immunomodulatory agent that inhibits an enzyme involved in the de novo synthesis of pyrimidine. This action may be the basis of its antiproliferative and antirheumatic activity. It is supplied as a loading dose of 100 mg given every day for the first 3 days of therapy and then as 20-mg doses given once daily thereafter. When I combine this agent with other drugs such as MTX, I avoid the initial loading dose and begin with 20 mg each day. Most patients experience improvement of disease within 6 weeks of beginning therapy. Improvement plateaus at 3 months.

Liver enzyme elevations have occurred in up to 10% of patients but usually resolve during continued treatment. Although thrombocytopenia has been reported among 7 of approximately 500 cases followed for at least 1 year, leukopenia has not been seen. Oncogenesis is always a concern when antiproliferative agents are used, but, to date, no increased incidence of acute malignancy has been reported.

SPECIFIC RECOMMENDATIONS FOR TREATMENT

The best drugs to treat RA should demonstrate long-term safety as well as continued efficacy. Comparative meta-analyses have been performed and show that the safest drugs are HDC, MTX, and SSZ and that the most efficacious drugs are MTX, SSZ, and AZA. Because MTX is both very safe and efficacious, it should be used as first-line therapy for most patients with RA. However, rare, significant toxicity from MTX, including acute pulmonary pneumonitis, limits its usefulness for patients with very mild disease. The relative safety of HDC suggests that it should be given as first-line therapy for essentially all patients with RA.

Patients with very mild disease, defined as normal acute phase reactants and five or fewer swollen/tender joints, might be treated initially with acetaminophen, intermittent NSAIDs, and HDC. For elderly patients with ophthalmologic problems such as macular degeneration, oral gold represents an alternative to HDC.

Patients with mild elevation of acute phase reactants and more than five swollen/tender joints at presentation should be considered for the combination of MTX and HDC with or without low-dose prednisone and without chronic NSAIDs. This combination might also be selected for patients whose disease was initially mild but did not respond to HDC or oral gold alone. For patients who do not wish to take MTX because they do not wish to abstain from alcoholic beverages, SSZ represents an alternative.

Patients with more severe disease defined as high acute phase reactants (Westergren sedimentation rate $\geq$ 60 mm per hour) and 10 or more swollen/tender joints are candidates for more potent DMARD combinations. These include the combination of (1) HDC, SSZ with MTX or (2) HDC, cyclosporine with MTX. Both of these combinations have been shown to perform effectively with only mild toxicity compared with their component drugs used alone. Often these patients also need initial prednisone treatment at a dose of 5 to 7.5 mg per day. Alternative combinations for this subset include MTX and parenteral gold with low-dose corticosteroids or the combination of AZA, MTX, and HDC with low-dose prednisone. When patients with moderate disease fail to respond to MTX with HDC, these more potent combinations are also indicated.

The combination of penicillamine (Cuprimine) and HDC should be avoided because this combination was less effective than penicillamine alone in controlled trials.

The newcomers to our armamentarium, TNF-α inhibitor fusion protein and LEF, have been demonstrated to be safe when combined with MTX and to provide at least additive disease control. They represent "add-on" therapy for patients who do not respond to the combinations already suggested, or might represent alternatives when there are contraindications to the use of MTX. For instance, TNF-α inhibitor fusion protein might be substituted for MTX for patients with renal insufficiency and LEF might be used in patients who did not wish to abstain from alcoholic beverages or have demonstrated adverse effects such as cytopenia when treated with MTX.

What some authorities consider overtreatment might be the best treatment. Once disease is controlled, the natural reflex is to attempt to decrease medications to limit toxicity. Studies suggest that a majority of patients will experience flare of disease if medications are reduced or withdrawn once control has been achieved. Re-treatment may not return the patient to the same level of ability and disease control achieved before the flare. I recommend that when patients are well controlled on a particular regimen, that regimen should be maintained unless adverse effects occur. The one exception to this rule is prednisone. If, as the dose of prednisone is decreased or prednisone is discontinued, disease flares, an additional agent or an increased dose of an agent already present is indicated.

Office Follow-up

There are three kinds of information that are equally important and that must be obtained at each clinic visit. Information that both reflects the process of disease and prognosis includes the number of swollen/tender joints and the magnitude of acute phase reactants. Of the acute phase reactants, C-reactive protein is a better indicator of acute disease activity and the Westergren sedimentation rate is a better indicator of long-term damage. Other measures that can help to characterize disease activity include the duration and severity of morning stiffness, the severity of chronic pain, and the time from arising to the onset of afternoon fatigue. Morning stiffness and time to afternoon fatigue have been shown to best reflect sleep duration and architecture. Because both active disease and concomitant co-morbidity such as osteoarthritis and fibromyalgia might contribute to sleep difficulties, morning stiffness and afternoon fatigue do not necessarily directly measure RA disease activity.

Radiographs of the hands and feet should be obtained at the initial visit. If there is any question of continued disease progression, these radiographs should be repeated and compared with baseline films. Other outcome measures include grip strength and some measure of the patient's ability to perform activities of daily living, such as the modified Stanford Health Assessment Questionnaire Disability Index (HAQ-DI).

Outcome measures must be recorded. I prefer preprinted sheets for follow-up visits so that these elements can be recorded regularly and uniformly. If performed conscientiously, a moderate complete picture of the patient's progress or lack thereof will be available. It will then be apparent over time that if grip strength shows a downward trend and the HAQ-DI is rising, a change of therapy will be indicated. It is difficult to provide appropriate medical care for RA patients without this kind of orderly record.

ALTERNATIVE THERAPIES

Forty-two percent of the population of the United States uses some form of alternative medical therapy each year, and most studies show that the prevalence is steadily increasing. In my practice, at least half of my RA patients ask about alternative therapies at each visit. Although copper bracelets and pyramids do indeed partake of quackery, antibiotic therapy for RA was until 1995 considered unsavory. When the treating physician is ignorant about alternative therapies, patient communication is hampered. Alternatively, although one must keep an open mind, it should not be so open that as one nods in assent, one's brains spill out.

Controlled trials have demonstrated that high doses (1200 IU per day) of vitamin E reduce pain in RA, that fish oil (1.8 gm eicosapentaenoic and 0.9 mg docosahexaenoic acid)* reduces stiffness and number of tender joints, that zinc sulfate,* 220 mg three times daily, reduces the number of tender and swollen joints, and that fasting improves most RA symptoms. Prospective, nonblinded studies have demonstrated that food elimination diets clearly identify certain foods, such as dairy products, which when eliminated, improved symptoms in a subset of patients. Given the studies demonstrating beneficial effects of oral tolerance with type 2 collagen, these observations do not seem farfetched. Hard science shows that *Tripterygium wilfordi* Hook-f, a vine-like

plant indigenous to China, exerts powerful suppressive effects on the human immune system and down-regulates TNF-α, IL-6, and IgG secretion from B cells.

When I am asked about alternative therapies, I suggest that patients try fish oil and vitamin E because they have been demonstrated to improve symptoms of RA and are likely to improve general health. I also tell my patients that if certain foods seem to worsen symptoms of arthritis, those foods should be avoided. When asked about other treatments such as magnets, electrical fields, or various herbs, I simply admit ignorance and suggest that one of the adverse effects associated with these treatments is lightening of the wallet. If the patient has not experienced meaningful improvement of symptoms after 6 weeks of an alternative therapy, I suggest that he or she discontinue spending money on it. I also ask the patient to tell me about all alternative treatments he or she wishes to take so that I can attempt to discover whether that treatment is safe or might interact with existing therapy.

SURGICAL MEASURES

Despite our best efforts, some patients have such severe disease that control is impossible without risking unacceptable adverse effects. In other patients, simultaneous osteoarthritis or crystal-induced arthritis complicates the clinical picture. Surgery is a welcome and necessary alternative.

Severe foot pain due to dorsal subluxation at the proximal interphalangeal joints is best treated by metatarsal head resection with realignment of the toes. In general, all metatarsal heads should be resected at one procedure. Painful, damaged ankles and feet often respond to arthrodesis. Although after the procedure, ankle movement may be limited, pain is controlled.

Total joint replacement has revolutionized the treatment of osteoarthritis and can be very helpful for patients with RA. Total knee replacement gives best results in patients who have good bone stock and who have not been exposed to chronic corticosteroid treatment. Replacement of the metacarpophalangeal joints and wrist replacement have been variably successful. These procedures do reduce pain and realign the hand and digits for better function, but strength is usually not improved. Total joint replacement of the shoulder relieves pain but often does not improve motion or function. Replacement surgery for elbows and ankles has not been successful in the past and is generally discouraged.

Patients with joint prostheses are at least theoretically more susceptible to septic arthritis and should be afforded antibiotic prophylaxis when undergoing dental and surgical procedures and endoscopies.

Proliferative dorsal tenosynovitis of the extensor tendons of the hands can result in rupture of the tendons. Prophylactic tenosynovectomy should be considered for patients whose disease is otherwise well controlled. Carpal tunnel release can also be

---

*Not FDA approved for this indication.

very helpful for patients with chronic median nerve compression despite systemic disease control.

Patients with RA face many risks in the perioperative period. Cervical spine involvement is common and can affect the stability of C1–C2, owing to loosening of the transverse alar and apical ligaments. Loosening can result in subluxation of C2 on C1 during neck flexion, causing spinal cord compression by the odontoid. Spinal cord injury has been reported in these patients after manipulation of the neck for intubation during general anesthesia. Thus, it is important to evaluate the stability of C1–C2 before surgery.

Symptoms of cervical cord disease include paresthesias, numbness, and electric shocks in the upper extremities when the neck is moved. Weakness in the lower extremities or long track signs can also occur. Finally, if the neck is very unstable, occipital paresthesias are common. If these symptoms are not present, I ask my patients to flex their necks so that their chins rest against their chest. I then inquire about symptoms. If they are able to perform this maneuver, it is unlikely that they have meaningful C1–C2 instability. Still, some experts recommend that all patients with RA have lateral cervical radiographs taken in extension and flexion before surgery and consider a distance of 3.0 mm between the atlas and the odontoid at flexion to indicate some instability. Subluxation producing a distance of 9 mm or greater is associated with a high incidence of cord compression. If any instability is found, anesthesia should be notified.

The cricoarytenoid joints can become inflamed and ankylotic, thereby reducing vocal cord movement and subluxating the vocal cord in adduction. Ankylosis makes intubation difficult or impossible. In one study, 26% of RA patients in an outpatient clinic had cricoarytenoid disease. Patients with involvement of these joints may have hoarseness in the morning that parallels early morning stiffness, pain on talking, a sense of fullness in the throat, or pain that radiates to the ears. Constant hoarseness is an indication of chronic subluxation. RA patients with these symptoms should undergo indirect laryngoscopy before surgery.

Patients who receive chronic corticosteroid treatment should be given stress doses of corticosteroids during the perioperative period, and the presurgical dose should be started immediately after surgery. Symptoms of hypotension, weakness, confusion, and nausea in the perioperative period can be caused by sepsis or primary cardiopulmonary difficulties, but in my experience they are regularly due to inadvertent discontinuation of chronic, daily corticosteroid treatment. MTX should be discontinued 1 week before surgery and reintroduced 2 weeks (skip 2 doses) after surgery. Other DMARDs are usually continued throughout the perioperative period.

THE ROLE OF EXERCISE

Obesity, muscle weakness, and muscle atrophy are common in patients with RA, much of it due to inactivity. Prospective series have demonstrated that patients with functional class 2 or 3 disease not only are able to participate in home exercise programs but also experience clinically significant improvement in mood, fatigue, physical capacity, and pain perception. Some studies have demonstrated fewer swollen joints and higher hemoglobin levels when patients participate in strength and aerobic exercise programs.

All programs should be tailored to individual patient needs. This often means that initial exercises are directed at stretching and improving range of motion of large joints. Once this is accomplished, low-impact walking, a stationary bicycle, cross-country skiing machines, and endurance swimming all have their place. Endurance of type-I muscle fibers will be increased if patients are able to reach a goal of continuous activity of the involved muscles maintained for 20 to 30 minutes three times each week. I tell all of my patients that an exercise that causes mild muscle pain is not dangerous; however, any activity that results in swelling of a joint 24 hours later must be modified.

FUTURE THERAPY

Therapy with any single agent, including the newest members of our armamentarium, LEF and TNF-α fusion protein, produce remission in only a small percentage of patients. As new agents are introduced, they not only will have to perform well as monotherapy but also will have to be compatible with existing background therapies and offer at least the potential of additive benefit, if not synergy. Among the most likely candidates to emerge is the de novo purine synthesis inhibitor mycophenolate mofetil (CellCept) and the specific biological IL-1 receptor antagonist anakinra (Antril). As these and other agents are rationally combined with specific TNF-α inhibitors or pyrimidine synthesis inhibitors (MTX, AZA, LEF), they may be able to provide early remission or near-remission for a significant proportion of treated patients. Long-term, open, comparative trials of these combinations will be necessary to discover the ultimate safety and effectiveness of this approach.

JUVENILE RHEUMATOID ARTHRITIS

method of
SUZANNE L. BOWYER, M.D.
Indiana University School of Medicine
Indianapolis, Indiana

"Juvenile rheumatoid arthritis" (many clinicians now prefer the term "juvenile idiopathic arthritis" to differentiate the condition from adult rheumatoid arthritis) is defined as arthritis that lasts 6 weeks or more in a child younger than 16 years of age at onset. With an incidence of 13.9 per 100,000 and a prevalence of 134 per 100,000, it affects between 35,000 and 99,000 children in the United States, making it the most common of the rheumatic dis-

TABLE 1. **Subtypes of Juvenile Rheumatoid Arthritis**

Name	Usual Age at Onset	Joints Affected	Associated Findings	Prognosis
Pauciarticular (oligoarticular)	2–4 years	Four or fewer	>50% ANA positive Rarely RF positive 20% develop uveitis	50% remission at 1 year. May develop polyarticular involvement and a more severe course
Polyarticular	2–4 years	Five or more	50% ANA positive 15% RF positive 5% develop uveitis	Chronic arthritis lasting 10–15 years. About 25% can be quite severe.
Systemic	Any age	Any number	Systemic features: fever, rash, lymphadenopathy, hepatosplenomegaly, pericarditis, and pleural effusion No ANA or RF Uveitis rare	50% remission at 1 year. The rest have chronic disease, with 25% developing end-stage arthritis. Death in 1%.

ANA = antinuclear antibody; RF = rheumatoid factor.

eases of childhood. There are three subtypes of JRA that are differentiated by the number of joints involved and the presence or absence of systemic features during the first 6 months of symptoms (Table 1). Within each subtype there are children who have mild, moderate, and severe symptoms; therefore, although a general course of treatment for JRA can be outlined, the treatment of each individual child must be tailored to his or her symptoms and the severity of the underlying arthritis.

Arthritis treatment in children is multidisciplinary with the following major components:

1. Medication to decrease inflammation
2. Stretching and splinting to preserve range of motion of involved joints
3. Exercise to maintain strength in the muscles surrounding affected joints
4. A proper balance between rest and exercise
5. Good nutrition with special attention to calcium intake and avoidance of fad diets
6. Attention to normal development, including family and peer interactions and school function
7. Prevention of long-term disability from uveitis, joint contractures, muscle atrophy, and limb length discrepancies

MEDICATIONS

The medications used to treat JRA are divided into first-line agents, second-line agents, immunosuppressive agents, and biologicals. Medications, dosing schedules, and strengths available are listed in Table 2.

First-Line Agents

Nonsteroidal Anti-inflammatory Agents

Nonsteroidal anti-inflammatory agents (NSAIDs) represent first-line therapy for children with arthritis. They decrease inflammation by inhibiting the synthesis of prostaglandins. Overall, they are well tolerated by most children. Half of the children who respond to NSAIDs do so after 2 weeks and two thirds by a month; thus if a patient has minimal response, it may be advantageous to change to another NSAID after a month. Four NSAIDs are approved for use in children:

Ibuprofen. Ibuprofen is the weakest of the NSAIDs but is also the one with the fewest gastrointestinal side effects. Now available over the counter in both pill and liquid form, it is often the first NSAID for children with joint pain or swelling. Its three-times-a-day dosing interval makes it less desirable for long-term use, however.

Naproxen. Naproxen is the easiest medication to administer to children with arthritis because it is available in a liquid preparation that has a twice-daily dosing interval. According to surveys, pediatric rheumatologists in the United States consider naproxen the NSAID of first choice for the treatment of JRA. It has a unique side effect in addition to those common to all of the NSAIDs: pseudoporphyria, a blistering rash that heals with shallow pitted scars, most common in very fair-skinned children.

Tolmetin (Tolectin). Tolmetin is available as a tablet with a three-times-a-day dosing interval, making it harder to administer to small children. The tablet is not bitter, but it can be crushed and mixed with various foods.

Indomethacin (Indocin). Indomethacin* is the strongest of the prostaglandin inhibitors and also is hardest on gastric mucosa and the renal vasculature. It also has more central nervous system effects than the other NSAIDs. Indomethacin is most often used in HLA-B27–associated arthritides and in children with systemic-onset JRA.

Salicylates

Although aspirin remains one of the best drugs for inflammation on the market, its many side effects, the association with Reye's syndrome, and the need for four-times-a-day dosing have caused it to fall out of favor. Two salicylate-containing preparations are still occasionally used to treat children with arthritis: choline salicylate/magnesium salicylate (Trilisate)* and salsalate (Disalcid).* These preparations are easier on the stomach than aspirin and have longer dosing intervals. They do not affect platelets in the same way as aspirin and are much less likely to

*Not FDA approved for this indication.

TABLE 2. **Medications Available to Treat Arthritis in Children**

Medication	How Supplied	Dose Range	Interval	Major Side Effects	Laboratory Monitoring
NSAIDs					
Ibuprofen (Motrin, Advil, Nuprin)	Liquid: 100 mg/5 mL Tablets: 200, 400, 600, 800 mg Chewables: 50, 100 mg	30–40 mg/kg/d	tid	Gastrointestinal distress, renal, hepatic	q 4–6 months
Naproxen (Naprosyn)	Liquid: 125 mg/5 mL Tablets: 250, 375, 500 mg	10–15 mg/kg/d	bid	Same as ibuprofen + pseudoporphyria	Same as above
Tolmetin (Tolectin)	Tablet: 200 mg, 600 mg Capsule: 400 mg	20–30 mg/kg/d	tid	Same as ibuprofen but more gastrointestinal distress	Same as above
Indomethacin (Indocin)	Liquid: 25 mg/5 mL Capsule: 25, 50 mg SR capsule: 75 mg	1–3 mg/kg/d	tid	Same as tolmetin + headaches	Same as above
Salicylates					
Aspirin	Tablets: 325, 500 mg Baby aspirin: 81 mg	70–100 mg/kg/d	qid	Gastrointestinal, renal, hepatic, tinnitus, caries, associated with Reye's syndrome	Same as above
Choline magnesium salicylate (Trilisate)	Liquid: 500 mg/5 mL Tablet: 500, 750 mg, 1000 mg Capsule: 500 mg	Same as above	tid	Same as above	Same as above
Salsalate (Disalcid)	Tablet: 500, 750 mg	Same as above	bid	Same as above	Same as above
Methotrexate	Tablets: 2.5 mg Parenteral: 25 mg/mL (IV, IM, SC); may give parenteral form orally to young children	10–20 mg/m² or 0.3–0.6 mg/kg	Weekly	Gastrointestinal, hepatic, bone marrow suppression, immunosuppression, teratogenicity	q 6 weeks
Sulfasalazine (Azulfadine)	Tablets: 500 mg	40–60 mg/kg/d; maximum: 3 gm	bid	Gastrointestinal, hepatic, rash, allergic reactions, Stevens-Johnson, bone marrow suppression, associated with Reye's syndrome	q 3 months
Hydroxycholoroquine (Plaquenil)	Tablets: 200 mg	5 mg/kg/d	Daily	Retinopathy, nausea, rash	Eye exams q 6 months
Azathioprine (Imuran)	Tablets: 50 mg	1–2.5 mg/kg/d*	Daily	Immunosuppression, bone marrow suppression, gastrointestinal, hepatic, malignancy	Monthly
Cyclophosphamide (Cytoxan)	IV	0.5–1 gm/m²	Monthly	Immunosuppression, bone marrow suppression, nausea, hair loss, hemorrhagic cystitis, hypogamma-globulinemia, infertility, malignancy	q 2 weeks
Cyclosporine (Neoral, Sandimmune)	Liquid: 100 mg/mL Gelcaps: 25, 100 mg Gelcaps: 25, 50, 100 mg	2–5 mg/kg/d*	bid	Hypertension, renal, immuno-suppression, malignancy	Weekly, then monthly
IGIV	IV	1–2 gm/kg	Monthly	Allergic reactions, headaches, risk of blood-borne disease	?
Etanercept (Enbrel)	SC	0.4 mg/kg; maximum: 25 mg	Twice weekly	Irritation at injection site, ? increased frequency of infection	?

*Exceeds dosage recommended by the manufacturer.

955

exacerbate asthma in sensitive asthmatics. All of the salicylate preparations can be dangerous in patients with systemic-onset JRA. Patients with systemic-onset disease can develop an unusual reaction to certain medications that can be fatal. This reaction begins with a generalized erythroderma and may be associated with vasculitis and disseminated intravascular coagulation. Salicylates must be used with extreme caution, if at all, in patients with systemic JRA.

Corticosteroids

The use of corticosteroids in JRA falls into the following four categories:

Intra-articular Injection. In children with pauciarticular JRA and involvement of one or two joints, injection of the affected joints can lead to long-term remission in 50% of the patients so treated. For this reason, some clinicians choose to use an intra-articular corticosteroid as first-line therapy in children with pauciarticular disease, bypassing the use of NSAIDs. In children with polyarticular joint involvement, injection can be used if one joint is swollen out of proportion to the others or if the child is developing a flexion contracture around the joint. Corticosteroid injection can prevent and reverse the development of flexion contractures and decrease the development of limb length discrepancies in children who have knee involvement. Triamcinolone hexacetonide (Aristospan Intra-articular) is the preferred drug. Its crystalline structure prolongs its action in the joint but can cause subcutaneous atrophy.

Topical. Topical corticosteroid preparations such as prednisolone acetate (Pred Forte) are used in children with JRA who have uveitis.

Intravenous. Steroid "pulse" therapy (methylprednisolone [Solu-Medrol], 30 mg per kg [maximum 1 gram]), given intravenously over 1 hour, can be useful in selected children with systemic JRA to treat severe systemic symptoms and minimize daily steroid dosing. The dose may be repeated 3 days in a row, but, in some patients, one pulse is given every 1 to 2 weeks. Side effects are minimal and usually consist of facial flushing and a metallic taste during the infusion. Occasional patients experience an increase in blood pressure.

Oral. Rarely, patients with severe systemic or polyarticular disease may require long-term oral corticosteroid use, but efforts must be made to keep the dose as low as possible. The inability to taper corticosteroid therapy is an indication to start second-line therapy and/or immunosuppressive medications.

Second-Line Agents

Second-line medications are started for the following indications:

1. NSAIDs ineffective after 3 months
2. Progressive contractures and disability despite appropriate NSAID therapy at 2 months

3. Inability to taper corticosteroids in children with systemic and polyarticular JRA
4. The clinician's impression that this is severe, potentially crippling arthritis

It is not appropriate to wait to use second-line agents until the patient shows signs of joint space narrowing on radiographs or other signs of permanent joint damage. These medications are rarely used in children with pauciarticular disease.

Methotrexate

Methotrexate (MTX)* has become the number one second-line agent used in children with JRA, on the basis of its demonstrated effectiveness, ease of administration, and favorable side effect profile. Although it is a powerful inhibitor of dihydrofolate reductase, in the low doses used for the treatment of arthritis, different mechanisms of action seem to be involved. Use of the drug in teenagers necessitates special counseling: It is a known teratogen, and effective birth control is essential. Also, patients on MTX cannot use alcohol because it increases the chance of liver damage. MTX has not been shown to be carcinogenic.

The MTX dose is advanced in 2.5-mg increments every 2 to 3 weeks with careful laboratory monitoring. Above 10 to 15 mg per dose, the drug is not reliably absorbed by mouth, and many clinicians switch to parenteral administration if they choose to increase the dose beyond this level. Subcutaneous injection is as effective (and less painful) than intramuscular injection. NSAID therapy is continued during MTX treatment.

Sulfasalazine (Azulfidine)

Sulfasalazine* consists of an antibiotic (sulfapyridine) linked to a salicylate molecule (5-aminosalicylic acid). Although it is not as effective as MTX, it may be useful for patients intolerant of MTX or for whom the issue of alcohol use or teratogenicity is critical. Sulfasalazine's side effects limit its use in about a third of patients. It is a salicylate preparation, and patients may be at risk for Reye's syndrome. Vaccination for chickenpox before starting this medication and yearly influenza vaccine can help to minimize this risk.

Sulfasalazine, like other salicylates, can cause severe reactions in patients with systemic-onset JRA.

Hydroxychloroquine (Plaquenil Sulfate)

This medication is thought to work by interfering with lysosomal function. Although widely used in systemic lupus erythematosus and adult RA, hydroxychloroquine has little effect by itself in JRA. It is usually used as part of a combination regimen: NSAID + MTX + hydroxychloroquine.

---

*Not FDA approved for this indication (only in adults).

Gold and Penicillamine

Gold* and penicillamine,* in common usage in the 1980s as second-line agents for the treatment of JRA, are rarely used now, having been supplanted by MTX.

Immunosuppressive Agents

For patients with severe systemic-onset JRA or for polyarticular JRA patients who have not responded to the first- and second-line medications, immunosuppressive medications may be used.

Azathioprine (Imuran)

Azathioprine* is a purine analogue that inhibits nucleic acid synthesis. It is rarely used except in patients with severe systemic disease in whom treatment with multiple other medications has failed.

Cyclophosphamide (Cytoxan)

Cyclophosphamide* is an alkylating agent that has been used since the 1970s to treat lupus in a regimen of 500 mg to 1 gram per m² per month. It has been used in similar doses with varying dosing intervals to treat life-threatening systemic-onset JRA.

Cyclosporine (Sandimmune)

This medication is a powerful inhibitor of T cell function. It is used in patients with severe polyarticular and/or systemic JRA and seems to work best in combination with MTX.

Biologicals

Intravenous Immune Globulin (IGIV)

IGIV* may be effective in selected patients with systemic or polyarticular JRA. Its mechanism of action is uncertain, and IGIV is extremely expensive to administer. If it is given for JRA, improvement should be noted within 4 to 6 months. Currently there is a widespread shortage of IGIV, and, given the weak evidence for its effect in JRA, it is indicated only for the rare patient who cannot tolerate MTX or sulfasalazine.

Anti–Tumor Necrosis Factor (TNF) Agents

Two anti-TNF drugs have been approved by the U.S. Food and Drug Administration: infliximab (Remicade),* a TNF receptor blocker used for Crohn's disease, and etanercept (Enbrel), a soluble TNF-α receptor fusion protein approved for treatment of rheumatoid arthritis. Etanercept was studied in 69 children, and in 74% their condition improved. It can be given simultaneously with NSAIDs and MTX and can result in further symptomatic improvement in patients who are already on MTX. This drug is indicated only in patients with severe disease in whom all standard therapy has failed.

*Not FDA approved for this indication.

PHYSICAL AND OCCUPATIONAL THERAPY

The long-term outcome of untreated JRA includes flexion contractures of the affected joints, weakness and atrophy of the muscles surrounding these joints, and, in the most severely affected joints, decrease in joint space, erosions, and, ultimately, bony fusion. Physical and occupational therapy are necessary to prevent these events. There must be a balance between rest and exercise. Severely affected children may need to take a nap during the day to conserve energy, but constant rest would lead to rapid development of deformities. Even during flares of arthritis exercise is important: inflamed joints can be gently stretched and taken through range-of-motion exercises. Warm baths in the morning when joints are most stiff and later in the day before doing exercises can be helpful in loosening joints to get maximum effect from the stretching. Ice packs can be helpful in relieving the pain of an acutely swollen joint. During times of active arthritis, it may be necessary to splint involved joints, especially at night, to keep them in good position for function and to prevent contractures from developing. Sturdy foot orthotics may be necessary to keep sore ankles from developing a valgus deformity.

When the inflammation has subsided, splint wearing may be tapered off and muscle strengthening can be done. Efforts must constantly be directed to strengthening extensors and preventing flexion contractures. It is absolutely essential that limbs be kept as strong and as straight as possible, even if joints have severe destructive arthritis. It is possible to replace hips and knees, but only if there is adequate muscle strength and range of motion to make the operation feasible. If a child with JRA is allowed to sit in a wheelchair all day, irreversible hip and knee flexion contractures will develop, muscles will atrophy, and the bones will become so osteopenic that surgery will never be an option, and the child will be unable to ambulate without a wheelchair for life. Usually intermittent visits to a physical or occupational therapist expert in the care of children with JRA coupled with a daily home exercise program supervised by the parent is adequate to prevent deformity.

SURGERY

Surgery can help to correct deformities that develop as a result of severe arthritis, but it is far better to be aggressive with medications and physical therapy to prevent such deformities in the first place! Surgical procedures that can be useful in selected patients include soft tissue releases, arthroscopic synovectomy, derotational osteotomy, joint fusion, and epiphyseal stapling. Total hip and knee replacement can be done as long as the patient has adequate muscle strength and does not have severe flexion contractures.

NUTRITION

It is important for children with a chronic condition like JRA to eat a healthy well-balanced diet. Although appetite in general may be poor in JRA patients, it is especially important to optimize the intake of calcium. Studies have shown that children with JRA tend to develop osteopenia as a result of chronic inflammation and disuse. Adequate intake of calcium and a daily multivitamin can help prevent this. Despite claims from tabloid newspapers, no one diet has ever been shown in double-blind testing to improve rheumatoid arthritis in children or adults. It is important that children not be given a rigidly restricted diet, because they need adequate calories for development.

EYE EXAMINATIONS

Patients with antinuclear antibody–positive pauci-articular-onset JRA are most at risk for eye disease. Current recommendations call for slit-lamp examination every 3 months for this population and less frequently for children with polyarticular or systemic-onset disease. Treatment of uveitis ranges from corticosteroid eye drops and mydriatics for mild disease to parenteral MTX for severe disease.

NORMAL DEVELOPMENT

It is important for children with arthritis to have expectations similar to those of their siblings. They need to have chores at home that are appropriate for their abilities and need reasonable discipline. They should attend school daily, although modifications may be necessary to enable them to get through the day. Such modifications may include having an extra set of books at home, being released from class 5 minutes early to be able to negotiate the halls before they are packed with children, having a key to the school elevator, clustering classes in one floor or one section of the building, and assigning a "buddy" to help take notes in class and open milk cartons during lunch. Children with JRA should not be excused from gym but should be in an adaptive physical education program. If this service cannot be provided, the child should be expected to do his or her assigned occupational or physical therapy exercises during time allotted for gym. Schools employ physical and occupational therapists, and their services should be used.

ANKYLOSING SPONDYLITIS

method of
C. M. DE GEUS-WENCESLAU, M.D., and
A. S. RUSSELL, M.B., B. CHIR.
University of Alberta
Edmonton, Alberta, Canada

DEFINITION

Ankylosing spondylitis (AS) is primarily a chronic inflammatory disease of the axial skeleton (sacroiliac joints and spine), although peripheral joints may be involved, and it is associated, especially in the vertebrae, with a tendency toward bony ankylosis. Another feature of the disease is enthesitis, which is inflammation at sites of bony insertions for tendons and ligaments.

HISTORY

AS was not clearly recognized as a clinical entity until the 1890s by Bechterew, Strumpell, and Marie; however, in 1693, Connor provided the first pathologic description of AS that was based on skeletal remains from France. Whether the disease was present in ancient times remains controversial. One difficulty is distinguishing AS from diffuse idiopathic skeletal hyperostosis and other causes of intervertebral fusion.

EPIDEMIOLOGY AND GENETICS

The prevalence of AS in white people is 0.1 to 0.2%. It is lower in Asians and black people, which relates to the frequency of the human leukocyte antigen HLA-B27. It is a familial disease: first-degree relatives of patients with AS have a risk of spondylitis of 5 to 10%, and when they carry the susceptibility antigen HLA-B27, the risk is doubled. A negative test virtually excludes the development of familial AS. Genetic factors seem to be responsible for most of the susceptibility to AS, and the search for additional specific loci is ongoing. Although HLA-B27 is the major genetic susceptibility factor in AS, HLA-B60 and, to a minor extent, HLA-DR1 have also been shown to predispose to AS. AS is more frequent in males; a ratio of 2:1 to 3:1 is seen in clinical studies, whereas in epidemiologic studies the sex ratio is nearly equal. AS is often described as primary or secondary, the latter designation meaning associated with another disease, such as Reiter's syndrome, inflammatory bowel disease, and psoriasis (especially psoriatic arthritis). It seems that at least in some patients the relationship is genetic; thus, not only do patients with Crohn's disease have a higher prevalence of AS but so do their relatives. The relationship to the inflammatory bowel disease is clearly not cause and effect; that is, the AS is not secondary to inflammatory bowel disease but is associated with it.

CLINICAL FEATURES

The disease usually begins at 15 to 30 years of age with an insidious onset of pain in the lower back and/or buttocks, sometimes radiating down to the legs as far as the knee. A cardinal feature is stiffness and pain after resting, which is most evident after getting out of bed. Characteristically, unless modified by treatment, this stiffness may last 1 or 2 hours and is relieved by moderate exercise. In contrast, although patients with mechanical back dysfunction may feel some temporary stiffness in the morning, their symptoms are generally aggravated by exercise. In about 10% of patients, the onset is abrupt and may more closely mimic sciatica; if the onset is associated with trauma, the diagnosis can easily be missed. Other patients present with a peripheral (i.e., nonaxial) arthritis, and the diagnosis of AS is made because of the characteristic distribution of joint disease (large joints predominating), with either an associated history of back problems or physical or radiologic signs of AS. The most important peripheral joint involved is the hip. This is associated with a worse prognosis. AS beginning in childhood presents typically as an oligoarticular disease with enthesitis and frequent hip involvement. This juvenile-onset form of AS is also associated with a worse prognosis and is relatively more common in developing countries.

The disease may spread proximally to involve the joints of the dorsal spine; involvement here is often associated with referred anterior thoracic pain of a deep, gripping quality on one or both sides. We have seen several patients admitted to the hospital with a suspected myocardial infarction based on this manifestation. Other joints that may be involved are the manubriosternal, sternoclavicular, and symphysis pubis (although the last is usually associated with radiologic features only). In addition, plantar fasciitis is common, and symptoms may be seen at the insertion of the tendo Achillis or hamstrings.

Physical examination, even in the early stages, often reveals a stiff back, which is most obvious by assessing lumbar flexion using the Schober test, in which a measured 10-cm segment up from the L5–S1 junction should expand at least 4 cm on full forward flexion. Restricted movement is especially impressive in the absence of acute symptoms, because severe pain, such as acute sciatica, may also decrease the range of movement. It is important not to use the ability to touch the toes as a measure of back flexion because mobile hips can often mask a marked decrease in lumbar spine flexion. Schober's test is used to follow the course of disease in a patient. A loss of the lumbar lordosis is often seen at an early stage but is not a necessary feature. The decreased lumbar flexion and the early loss of lumbar lordosis are probably due to involvement of the facetal joints of the lumbar spine. Although the first radiologic signs and manifestations are usually in the sacroiliac joints, there is no clinical test of sacroiliac function that is reliable. Also, because the joint is so deeply buried, tenderness over the sacroiliac joints is *not* a feature of AS. Involvement of the dorsal spine is manifested as reduced rotation and reduced chest expansion (less than 1 inch at the nipple line). As the disease progresses, a more obvious stoop may be noted with a progressive dorsal kyphosis. This stoop can be best assessed by the distance from occiput to wall: the individual stands erect with heels and buttocks against the wall and attempts to have the occiput also in contact with the wall, as it should be, when looking straight ahead.

RADIOLOGY

The cardinal feature is sacroiliitis, which is manifested by sclerosis, erosions, and, later, fusion of the sacroiliac joints. These findings on the sacroiliac joint are usually symmetrical. Other features are erosions of the anterior vertebral margin ("shining corners"), leading to squaring of the anterior surface of lumbar vertebrae; syndesmophytes, initially best seen at the thoracolumbar junction; and apophyseal fusion. These changes normally progress from below upward but may skip areas completely. Syndesmophytes (ossification of the outer layers of the annulus fibrosis of the disk) in AS are bilateral and thin, ascending the spine in a symmetrical fashion to produce a bamboo appearance. Bone scans have been used to try to detect inflammation of the sacroiliac joints but with variable success. Computed tomography (CT) of the sacroiliac joint or magnetic resonance imaging (MRI) is more sensitive than radiographs to detect early sacroiliitis but should be used only for those few patients whose conventional radiographs give normal or equivocal results.

DIAGNOSIS

The diagnosis of AS requires relevant symptoms, that is, back pain with morning stiffness and, usually, associated sacroiliitis. Some patients with a typical history may (rarely) have a normal radiologic appearance. They have a forme fruste of AS, which can be most easily recognized if they have relatives with the full-blown disease. A diagnosis of "possible AS," is, however, quite permissible, and treatment can be instituted on this basis. If after 1 or 2 years there is no radiologic progression, the physician can be confident that, although inflammation may be present, radiologic change is unlikely to occur.

Laboratory tests are of little value in the diagnosis or management of the disease except to exclude other disorders. The erythrocyte sedimentation rate is often normal. Ninety percent of patients are HLA-B27–positive, but because this is found in 5 to 15% of most white populations, it is of no value in making the diagnosis. Indeed, the overwhelming majority of individuals with HLA-B27 (i.e., more than 95%) do *not* have AS.

COMPLICATIONS

Eyes. Acute nongranulomatous, unilateral anterior uveitis occurs in 25 to 40% of patients. Both eyes may be involved but usually at different times. The patient presents with ocular pain, redness, photophobia, and blurred vision. Patients should be warned of the possibility of this complication at the outset and to seek immediate medical advice on developing a painful red eye. Prompt management (topical mydriatics and corticosteroids) is critical for an uncomplicated outcome.

Heart. AS may be associated with aortic ring dilatation and regurgitation and with conduction disturbances in less than 5% of patients. Conduction disturbances (e.g., atrioventricular blocks, bundle branch block, fascicular block, and Wolff-Parkinson-White syndrome) may be intermittent, and can be seen independently of aortic ring involvement. The prevalence of aortic incompetence and conduction abnormalities in AS increases with disease duration, presence of peripheral arthritis, and uveitis.

Echocardiographic studies have demonstrated myocardial wall involvement in AS, especially abnormalities in diastolic function, but the clinical significance remains unclear.

Lungs. Apical pulmonary fibrosis has been described, but it is very rare; indeed, apical shadows in AS are still probably more likely to be due to tuberculosis than to the AS itself. As restriction of chest wall movement occurs, some reduction in vital capacity is seen, but a compensatory increase in diaphragmatic excursion prevents any serious problems from this restriction. On the other hand, if a severe kyphosis—or even worse, a kyphoscoliosis leading to ventilation/perfusion imbalance—develops, progressive pulmonary dysfunction may occur.

Osteoporosis and Spinal Fractures. Vertebral osteoporosis is observed in AS, and fractures of the spine occur with relatively minor trauma and are associated with substantial mortality and neurologic damage. Fractures in the cervical spine are the most common, usually at the C5–6 or C6–7 level. One should exclude the possibility of a spinal fracture in any patient with AS who complains of sudden neck or back pain, after even mild trauma.

Secondary Renal Amyloidosis and Cauda Equina Syndrome. Both of these are very rare complications of AS; however, renal amyloidosis should be considered in the differential diagnosis of proteinuria in a patient with AS.

TREATMENT

The mainstay of therapy is exercise to achieve and retain spinal mobility. Strengthening of spinal extensors, chest expansion, and breathing exercises are important. Along with this goes advice regarding posture, sleeping positions, and so forth. Patient education about the disease is essential to elicit the patient's commitment for long-term cooperation through exercise. The Arthritis Foundation in the United States, the Arthritis Society in Canada, and the British Society of Rheumatology all produce useful pamphlets that describe the clinical features and treatment programs for AS. The patient should be encouraged to lead as normal a lifestyle as possible, including participation in sporting activities. On the other hand, once spinal fusion has occurred, that is, after many years of disease, the spine becomes more susceptible to fracture with sudden stresses, and contact sports should be excluded. Swimming is the ideal exercise.

Anti-inflammatory medication, usually one of the nonsteroidal anti-inflammatory drugs (NSAIDs), is effective in most patients for relieving pain and stiffness and thereby improving mobility and allowing effective exercise. Some patients, once they achieve an active exercise program, may require only minimal drug treatment. In others, the disease remains steadily active; in still others, it fluctuates year to year. In most patients the NSAIDs are roughly equivalent to each other, although many physicians use indomethacin (Indocin) in a dose of 75 to 150 mg per day.

Remittive agents have been used for AS, especially sulfasalazine* (Azulfidine): 0.5 to 1.5 gram twice daily. The beneficial results on axial involvement are controversial; however, sulfasalazine does seem to have some impact in the subgroup of AS patients with peripheral arthritis.

A new therapeutic approach for patients with severe, unresponsive inflammatory back pain is CT-guided intra-articular injection of the sacroiliac joint with a long-acting corticosteroid. Studies have shown clinical benefit lasting for months.

Treatment of osteoporosis may also be of importance in reducing the risk of spinal fractures in AS.

One uncontrolled study of pamidronate (Aredia),* a biphosphonate given intravenously, showed beneficial effects in decreasing overall axial symptoms.

Radiotherapy is an older approach for severe unresponsive disease. The risks of this modality remain, but with lower doses and therapy carefully focused on only those areas with demonstrable activity (via bone scan), it has a helpful role in patients intolerant of other approaches. It has also been used for painful heels (due to calcaneal periostitis or Achilles tendon inflammation) when there has been no response to conservative treatment.

PROGNOSIS

Once the diagnosis is made in a young patient, in the absence of complicating features such as inflammatory bowel disease or hip involvement, the prognosis should be good. If a patient is diagnosed at an early enough stage and faithfully follows an exercise program and, if necessary, an anti-inflammatory regimen, effective disease control should be possible in most subjects. In patients with severe hip disease, remittive therapy might be begun earlier because of the poor prognosis. Prosthetic hip replacements may be necessary and usually have a good outcome, although there is a small risk of clinically important heterotopic ossification. In addition, spondylitis associated with inflammatory bowel disease tends to be more severe and more difficult to control than is uncomplicated spondylitis. The emphasis again must be on exercise. Taking anti-inflammatory agents to relieve discomfort is by itself insufficient.

TEMPOROMANDIBULAR DISORDERS

method of
MAJOR M. ASH, JR., D.D.S., M.D.
University of Michigan School of Dentistry
Ann Arbor, Michigan

Temporomandibular disorders (TMD) are a heterogeneous group of disturbances involving primarily the masticatory muscles and/or temporomandibular joint (TMJ) and, in some instances, other muscles of the head and neck as well. Depending on the disorder and its severity, diagnostic criteria for TMD include the following:

1. *Myalgia* of the masticatory muscles (including the lateral pterygoid), often with palpation tenderness of the anterior temporalis and masseter muscles, which may lead to jaw dysfunction with limited range of movement (e.g., opening < 40 mm)
2. *Pain* (acute/chronic), which may be present in and around the TMJ with/without internal derangement and/or adhesions and can interfere with range of motion (e.g., opening < 35 mm to 5 to 10 mm). Pain and/or dysfunction may also relate to sprain/strain from trauma, capsulitis/synovitis, degenerative joint diseases (e.g., arthritis with arthralgia), and collagen vascular diseases. Pain and dysfunction may also be caused by systemic diseases with local manifestations (e.g., Sjögren's syndrome, systemic lupus erythematosus, ankylosing spondylitis, psoriasis, gout, Lyme disease, and fibromyalgia).
3. *TMJ sounds* (clicking, crepitus) on jaw movement, which correspond loosely to various degrees of internal derangement (e.g., disk displacement with reduction and episodic catching on opening). There are no sounds without disk reduction (e.g., "closed lock").
4. *Headaches*, which may be present at the time of TMD and subside after effective treatment of TMD (e.g., tension-type [TTH] that arise from disorders of oromandibular structures such as the teeth, jaws, muscles of mastication, TMJ, or adjacent structures). Headaches with TMD may also be central in origin (e.g., causative factors such as psychosocial stress, anxiety, depression, delusion, and drug overdose for TTH). Other types of headache must be considered in a differential diagnosis.

The subjective symptoms of TMD that patients have in common vary considerably within and between patients in severity, causal factors, time of onset, duration, response to

---

*Not FDA approved for this indication.

therapy, and subsidence and recurrence of TMD symptoms. Abatement of symptoms after initial treatment may be unrelated to a therapy thought at first to be highly successful.

TERMINOLOGY AND SIGNIFICANCE

Internal derangement implies a biomechanical interference with the smooth gliding action of a TMJ: an abnormal relationship of the disk to the condyle, including various forms of disk displacement (e.g., anterior, lateral, medial). However, internal derangement appears to be much more complicated than simply disk displacement; therefore, disk displacement may not be the major cause of TMJ arthralgia. This shift in thinking away from believing that disk displacement is the major or only factor in internal derangement has focused attention on inflammation, changes in joint lubrication and synovial fluid, joint loading, effusion, adhesions, and degenerative osteoarthritic processes. Some of the reasons for this shift in emphasis are listed below:

1. Disk position is not necessarily related to pain.
2. Osteoarthritic changes may follow or precede disk displacement or be unrelated or related casually.
3. Almost 70% of autopsy specimens show derangement, but significant symptoms appear in only 4% of the living.
4. Arthroscopy and arthrocentesis with lavage of the superior joint compartment in closed lock can re-establish normal mouth opening in some patients.
5. Many magnetic resonance images show abnormal positions of the disk without clinical symptoms.

The cause of disk displacement remains controversial but does not appear to be significantly associated with age, gender, missing teeth, or dentures. Although the causes of internal derangement are speculative, chronic trauma of both soft and hard structures (e.g., chronic traumatic TMJ arthritis) associated with bruxism and clenching has been proposed.

Oromandibular dysfunction (OMD) is a collective term created by the International Headache Society (IHS) for problems involving the muscles of mastication, TMJ, and related structures. Some of the criteria relate to pain, limitation of jaw movement, TMJ noise, "locking," and bruxing and clenching of the teeth. This term is used in the IHS classification in place of such terms as myofascial pain-dysfunction and craniomandibular dysfunction. The term "OMD" is not widely accepted, but the practitioner who must assess concurrent headache and TMD should be familiar with the nosology of the IHS as it relates to OMD for better communication.

Occlusal dysfunction refers to functional and/or structural disturbances of the masticatory system that are related to occlusion (e.g., inability to bring teeth together in any of the normal jaw positions because of the teeth or occlusal relations).

A number of biomechanical interocclusal devices are used in the treatment of TMD. They can be categorized into posterior partial coverage splints, anterior partial coverage splints, pivots, full-coverage stabilization splints, and repositioning devices (e.g., functional orthopedic appliances). With the exception of the stabilization splint, control of occlusal stability is not maintained. An occlusal bite plane splint is a stabilization type device with cuspid rise that covers all the teeth (usually maxillary). It is used as a reversible form of occlusal therapy in the treatment of some forms of TMD and bruxism. It provides for occlusal stability and muscle relaxation, prevents trauma to the teeth, and, if designed correctly, provides relief of symptoms for a majority of the patients with a temporomandibular disorder. It constitutes one of the reversible forms of therapy for TMD. A nightguard is a name given to an appliance that is worn at night to protect against the adverse effects of clenching and bruxism during sleep. If it is worn during the day, it is called a biteguard. These appliances are generally made of hard, processed clear acrylic and have the form of an occlusal bite plane splint. A mouthguard is a protective device made of a soft resilient material that covers both maxillary and mandibular teeth. It is used primarily in contact sports and not generally recommended for treatment of TMD except on a very short-term basis (7 to 10 days) because it does not stabilize the occlusion. Some orthotic or functional orthopedic appliances (e.g., Clark "Twin Block," Herbst, and Summer/Westesson devices) are used in the treatment of TMD to advance the mandible with the idea of reducing anterior disk displacement. Because of the positional change in the mandible, expansion of the arches and movement of the teeth into occlusion and/or reconstruction of the occlusion may be necessary. After active treatment, an orthotic appliance must be used at night to maintain the position unless retrodiskal tissues become organized (fibrosed) to form a pseudodisk.

Although at one time the treatment of TMD with anterior repositioning devices seemed almost universal, the failure rate caused by attempting to reposition the disk even in displacements other than reducing anterior displacement, difficulties of maintaining the therapeutic position of the condyle, the need for comprehensive orthodontics and/or occlusal reconstruction, and the need for an orthotic appliance at night led to a decrease in the use of these devices. Studies suggest that anterior repositioning is most successful when limited to patients with anterior reducing disk displacement. This would seem to rule out repositioning for other forms of disk displacement. Thus, an accurate picture of where the disk is located is necessary for the chance of effective repositioning treatment.

In the report of a National Institute of Health (NIH) Technology Conference (1996) it was held that therapies that permanently alter the patient's occlusion cannot be recommended on the basis of current data. This statement would relate to repositioning devices as well as occlusal adjustment. If this position were to be maintained without reservation, it might be expected that research grants in the area would be reduced in favor of behavioral treatment for TMD management. Unfortunately, there were few proponents of other forms of therapy present and a very good prospective longitudinal study on occlusal adjustment was seemingly ignored. The panel invited by the NIH seemed to take the position that there is no significant involvement of occlusion as a causal factor in TMD. This position is, as said by many others, contrary to widespread clinical dental opinion.

Myofascial pain-dysfunction (MPD) is a term that has been around for some time, but its meaning is redefined with time by new or additional criteria. Initially, the term focused on treatment of emotional stress, which was considered to cause symptoms involving muscles with jaw dysfunction related to muscles and not the disk(s). In one survey (1993) of American Dental Association members it was indicated that 15% of the specialists treating MPD did so with anterior positioning. MPD for the survey was defined as "bilateral or unilateral muscle pain of four months or longer duration." Perhaps those who treat MPD as disk derangement conclude that displacement is found in most patients with MPD.

CHARACTERISTICS AND SEVERITY OF SYMPTOMS

The characteristics and severity of symptoms of TMD can be classed as to type, severity, and frequency: about one third of patients with TMD have episodic, mild to relatively severe myalgia; about one fifth have internal derangement with reducing disk displacement, some with mild to severe pain on displacement and reduction, even with clicking; approximately 1 in 10 patients have varying degrees of relatively severe pain often combined with headache with internal derangement without reduction; and fewer than 1 in 10 of TMD patients have overt degenerative joint disease (DJD): primary osteoarthritis with episodic or acute arthralgia for months or arthritis without arthralgia (due to aging, trauma, and idiopathic factors). About a third of the patients with TMD have some variation or combination of the other categories.

Pain associated with TMD is typically episodic pain. As already suggested, improvement from treatment may be due to the effects of treatment, the placebo effect, or regression to the mean (i.e., if the average patient seeks treatment when the pain is at its peak, then the pain will decrease toward its characteristic level whether or not treatment is provided). Because of the latter two factors, improvement in pain after initiating a treatment with unproven efficacy may not necessarily be due to the treatment itself.

When pain is unrelieved for a long period of time (e.g., 4 to 6 months or more), patients can develop changes in their psychological and behavioral status, especially if the initiating causal factors have been removed or have not recurred. Whether pyschological disorders in chronic pain are a consequence of persistent pain or whether pre-existing physiologic disorders predispose to the chronic pain sometimes associated with TMD has not been determined. For example, substance abuse or depression may reflect the absence of significant relief of pain in TMD.

Although the number of patients who have chronic pain associated with TMD appears to be small compared to the number of patients with TMD, some patients can be considered to be chronic pain patients and their management is beyond the scope of simple counseling in the office of the general practitioner. Ineffective treatment should not be prolonged to the point of causing a patient with persistent pain to develop the characteristics of the chronic pain patient.

Dysfunctional chronic pain is a subset of illness behaviors inconsistent with dental/medical documented findings (i.e., persistent pain without recognizable nociceptive input). Changes occurring in emotional status include mood and behavioral changes associated with depression, such as helplessness, demoralization, and social isolation. Thus, there are some patients that exhibit psychological and emotional problems beyond that which might be considered consistent with the objective findings. Only a relatively few TMD patients have behavioral disturbances manifested by social isolation, an inability to carry on daily living, an increased reliance or dependence on medications or even addictive drugs, and an overuse of traditional health care resources.

DIAGNOSIS

The diagnosis of TMD is based primarily on the clinician's assessment of the patient and, when indicated, other appropriate procedures (e.g., radiography, magnetic resonance imaging [MRI]). The confounding aspects of adhesions and arthrotic degeneration limit diagnostic certainty based on the clinical examination alone. Tomography, MRI, and arthrography are generally reserved for making decisions on irreversible forms of therapy (e.g., anterior repositioning and TMJ surgery). Radiographs of the TMJ (preferably transcranial oblique) are not used routinely and, except in a litigious environment, are taken only when it is suspected that significant arthritis is present. Thus, TMJ imaging is not generally indicated for the diagnosis of most forms of TMD. Diagnostic aids, other than those included in the clinical examination, are not usually indicated (e.g., laboratory tests). Unless there are specific reasons for them (e.g., history of arthritis with arthralgia and swelling of TMJ), radiographs are not generally indicated for initial diagnosis and therapy, except as already considered.

Treatment uncertainty is usually reflected in diagnostic uncertainty. The cause of TMD is considered to be multifactorial even when the primary diagnosis appears to be certain (e.g., ankylosing spondylitis). Other factors enter into the nature of the problem that may have a bearing on treatment (e.g., absence of protrusive jaw movement, lateral movements, cheek and tongue biting, and whether the disease is progressive). If chronic pain is present and associated with psychological disorders, referral to an appropriate medical specialist is in order.

The evaluation of psychosocial dimensions in TMD is not often necessary beyond that found in appropriate screening materials and indications of interrelated chronic pain and psychosocial problems. This interrelationship is not always determined until after failure of initial treatment.

The differential diagnosis of TMD may require evaluation of painful disorders of the head and neck that involve peripheral and central mechanisms (e.g., musculoskeletal disorders [arthralgia, myalgia], neurogenic inflammation such as facial migraine, and peripheral neuropathic pain [trigeminal neuralgia]). It is apparent that joint pain and dysfunction may relate to systemic inflammatory disease with primarily joint involvement, autoimmune disorders, infections, granulomatous vasculitis, trauma, and crystalline arthropathies. Therefore, an evaluation of a patient with TMD may require more than the completion of a medical history form. The complex nature of pain may give rise to diagnostic uncertainty leading to the unfortunate dilemma of undertreatment, overtreatment, or no treatment at all. The continuation of ineffective treatment can lead to chronic pain and its systemic effects. In some respects, TMD is similar to the problem of diagnosing and treating low back pain.

TREATMENT

Initial Treatment

Most patients with TMJ/muscle dysfunction are treated initially with one or more types of conservative/reversible forms of therapy, including pharmacologic regimens (e.g., nonsteroidal anti-inflammatory drugs), physiotherapy (e.g., moist heat, exercises), counseling by the dentist about causal factors, restriction of "chewy" foods, and stabilization occlusal bite plane splints when indicated. When a patient does not respond to reversible treatment and the severity of pain interferes significantly with quality of life, re-evaluation of the diagnosis should be undertaken and other forms of treatment considered. Stabilization occlusal bite plane splints have been found to be very effective for TMJ and/or muscle disorders, including some cases of locking and dislocation. Physiotherapy, exercises, and the use of a stabilization splint to reduce loading, especially with bruxism, are always necessary to reduce the incidence of repeated episodes of locking.

Irrespective of the device used, many joint noises are difficult to control. Control of joint noises is not a good indicator of the success of TMD therapy.

Behavioral/Educational Modalities

Biobehavioral therapy used in the treatment of TMD includes biofeedback, relaxation, hypnosis, patient education, and cognitive behavioral interventions (e.g., stress management and modification of negative or maladaptive behavioral and emotional patterns for coping with persistent TMD pain). Some of the current conservative therapies include some biobehavioral treatment (e.g., physical therapy, exercise, control of bruxism, clenching, diet [chewy foods]) and control of other aggravating factors in TMD.

For the relatively few patients with persistent pain who *cannot* (not *will not*) benefit from further treatment, intervention by professional medical specialists should be considered. The term *cannot* means the patient is no longer psychologically capable of coping with the stress of pain. Such individuals have the diagnostic probability of being in chronic pain.

Occlusal Adjustment

A comprehensive occlusal adjustment is not recommended as treatment for active TMD. It is recommended that gross occlusal interferences be adjusted to the extent possible, especially when there are faulty restorative interferences and/or when the appropriate design of an occlusal bite plane splint would be compromised if an extruded tooth is not adjusted. Attempts to adjust completely to centric relation contact with painful joints and muscles is useless and counterproductive. In the case of faulty restorations and extruded teeth, the adjustment is conditionally reversible.

Changing Treatment

When there is failure of reversible therapy because of any significant lack of progress in pain control, even in the presence of an objective basis for pain and dysfunction, an absence of apparent psychosocial problems, and a reasonable diagnostic certainty of the nature of the TMD, then it is time to make a decision about a change to another form of treatment. Thus, when various forms of reversible treatment do not satisfy the needs of a relatively few but important subset of patients, a stepwise change in TMD therapy becomes a studied option of available therapies:

Intervention by behavioral medical specialists for psychosocial problems

Anterior mandibular repositioning with comprehensive orthodontics and/or occlusal reconstruction

Arthroscopic lysis and lavage, arthrocentesis, modified condylotomy

These modalities all have their advocates who consider a particular therapy to be successful in the treatment of TMD. However, no form of therapy provides success for every patient.

Treatment Decisions

The process of deciding which patient may be helped by one of the options may require additional methods of evaluation (e.g., MRI to determine the presence of a transverse position of the TMJ disk, evaluation by medical specialists for systemic disease or psychosocial problems). Under conditions of pain, the human factor may be the most significant aspect in making a decision about additional treatment. In the absence of pain, the degree of dysfunction may be most important if it interferes significantly with the quality of life and occupation (e.g., opening the mouth wide enough to sing opera). It is recognized that without pain many patients over time and with physical therapy can regain mouth opening sufficiently wide to function quite well.

A significant point in the decision to change to irreversible therapy may also come when a patient *will* not (not *cannot*) tolerate any longer his or her pain and dysfunction irrespective of its actual severity and desires another form of treatment after a complete understanding of risk, potential benefits, and cost factors of the intervention proposed. Whatever the form of more aggressive therapy considered, whether mandibular repositioning or surgery (e.g., arthroscopy, arthrocentesis, or partial condylotomy), the potential risks and probability of success should be understood by the patient. Some of the indications for the use of anterior repositioning devices are listed below:

Persistent pain/dysfunction remains after reasonable period of reversible therapy.

The patient does not have significant psychosocial problems.

The patient is aware that comprehensive occlusal restoration and/or comprehensive orthodontics may be necessary.

A diagnosis of anterior (not transverse) disk displacement has been made (e.g., MRI) to rule out other displacements of the disk.

Arthroscopic or surgical procedures are not indicated.

The patient needs correction of class II malocclusion.

There is a need for occlusal restorative therapy.

If the symptoms abate significantly after 5 to 7 days with use of the anterior repositioning device, it would be reasonable to consider "stepping the mandible back" by adjustment of the orthotic appliance. However, if symptoms return when attempting to "walk-back" the mandible, or there is no reduction in posterior open bite created by mandibular advancement, orthodontic and/or restorative therapy will probably be necessary to maintain the "therapeutic" position of the disk. The general use of repositioning appliances is diminishing because of the examination and appropriate screening questionnaire and, when indicated, the results of referrals to medical specialists. There is also agreement that a large majority of patients with TMD should be treated initially by noninvasive and reversible therapy because of the high success rate of this approach and because of the increased cost and risk factors involved in nonreversible forms of therapy. The recommended modalities include medication (e.g., nonsteroidal anti-inflammatory drugs), physiotherapy, behavioral modification when a problem, removal of gross occlusal interferences, and appliance therapy (i.e., appropriate design and adjustment of a stabilization occlusal bite plane splint).

When noninvasive reversible treatment is not effective, more determined, perhaps more aggressive (irreversible) forms of treatment may be needed for relief of pain and/or dysfunction. The objectives of this second phase of irreversible treatment have much in common with an initial phase of therapy: management of pain and dysfunction, reduction of inflammation, control of adverse joint loading, and treatment of internal derangement, including adhesions.

Irreversible forms of therapy using anterior mandibular repositioning for anterior reducing disk displacement only appears to have reasonable success. However, the need to treat the induced malocclusion and maintain the disk in a therapeutic position makes a cost/risk/benefit comparison with other irreversible, invasive procedures such as surgery (e.g., arthroscopic lavage and lysis of adhesions, arthrocentesis, pressure injections, and modified condylotomy) difficult to assess without comparison data based on randomized clinical trials for the two different forms of therapy.

Initial noninvasive reversible therapy is successful 80 to 90% of the time, perhaps because many of the patients who receive that form of treatment would have managed without any treatment ultimately. The 12 to 15% of patients who need more aggressive (irreversible) therapy are more difficult to treat with a decreasing probability of success, especially if psychosocial problems develop.

Surgical Procedures

If pain is not caused by disk displacement, but is intracapsular in origin, then surgery should be considered. The generally accepted indication for TMJ surgery is when pain and dysfunction are not resolved by adequate nonsurgical therapy. For a closed lock, initial treatment may include manual manipulation. However, the problem may not be just disk displacement; arthrotic degeneration may be present as well and prevent reduction and mainte-

nance of improved function. The choice of surgery should include consideration as to which is least invasive and yet most effective. Closed lock is not caused invariably by disk displacement; fibrous adhesions may also cause restricted opening. In cases in which mandibular manipulation is not effective, surgical procedures are indicated, except where any surgery is not accepted by or possible for a patient. Arthroscopy for elimination of adhesions and for débridement or arthrocentesis for closed lock are acceptable forms of therapy when indicated.

BURSITIS, TENDINITIS, MYOFASCIAL PAIN, AND FIBROMYALGIA

method of
THOMAS W. JAMIESON, M.D.
Uniformed Services University of the Health Sciences
Bethesda, Maryland

BURSITIS

Bursae are subcutaneous spaces lined with synovial membranes that secrete fluid to allow smooth and nearly frictionless motion among muscles, ligaments, tendons, bones, and skin. Some bursae are present at birth and are constant throughout life, whereas others are "formed" in response to repetitive physical pressure (e.g., bursae under metatarsal heads that may occur in rheumatoid arthritis). Although there are approximately 150 bursae in the body, most are not likely to be of pathologic significance. Bursal inflammation may be a clinical problem, however, in a few predictable anatomic sites: the subacromial bursa of the shoulder, olecranon bursa at the elbow, iliopsoas bursa near the hip, trochanteric-subtrochanteric bursae below the hip, gastrocnemiosemimembranous bursa of the knee, and retrocalcaneal bursa of the heel.

Subacromial bursitis is usually secondary to inflammatory lesions of the rotator cuff or bicipital tendon, both of which are anatomically contiguous to the bursal floor. Subacromial bursitis causes severe pain in all planes of movement but usually is worse with abduction and internal-external rotation movements. Subacromial bursitis should be distinguished from the more frequently encountered tendinitis problems of the shoulder, as the latter are more indolent and longer tolerated by patients. Subacromial bursitis causes prompt and severe pain and is distinguished on physical examination from the tendinitis overuse syndromes.

The olecranon bursa overlies the distal portion of the triceps tendon and the olecranon of the ulna. With inflammation, swelling is seen at the point of the elbow and pain may be present. If so, it occurs most typically with resisted extension of the arm (i.e., with increased tension in the adjacent triceps tendon). If pain is present, particularly with accompanying skin erythema, suspicion of an infection or a crystal-induced process is heightened and a bursal aspiration is indicated. Presumably, bacteria can access the olecranon bursa through the skin even without a visible skin wound. Typically, septic olecranon bursitis is seen in manual laborers and in alcohol abusers; chronic obstructive pulmonary disease patients may also be disproportionately affected. Hemorrhagic olecranon bursitis may be seen in uremic patients undergoing dialysis.

The iliopsoas bursa overlies the hip capsule (lateral to the femoral blood vessels, between the iliopsoas muscle and the anterior surface of the hip joint). The iliopsoas bursa is large (about 6 × 3 cm) and may communicate with the hip joint in select patients. Most often the iliopsoas bursa becomes symptomatic in a patient with predicate hip pathology (often osteoarthritis) and may manifest as an enlarging inguinal mass with pressure on adjacent tissues. These protruding bursae may be confused with a hernia, hydrocele, adenopathy, or psoas abscess. Computed tomography or magnetic resonance imaging scan is diagnostically useful and will demonstrate a well-defined water density mass in the appropriate anatomic site, often with a concurrent hip joint effusion.

The trochanteric bursae, several in number, overlie the lateral hip region. The largest and most important structure lies between the gluteus maximus and the tendon of the gluteus medius muscles. Patients usually complain of a deep, dull, aching pain in the lateral hip area, but half also describe anterolateral proximal lower extremity pain radiating to the knee, often worsening with activity and sometimes disturbing sleep. Differential diagnostic considerations here may include herniated nucleus pulposus of L3–4 (i.e., with symptoms in the L-4 nerve root distribution), spinal stenosis, or an entrapment neuropathy (i.e., meralgia paresthetica).

Distention of the gastrocnemiosemimembranous bursa (Baker's cyst) often is a subclinical finding. Baker's cysts may be present and not palpable and may be palpable but not of clinical significance. In inflammatory knee conditions there is usually communication with the knee joint and a one-way synovial fluid flow into the bursa. If dissection or rupture of a Baker's cyst occurs, differentiation from deep vein thrombophlebitis can be difficult ("pseudothrombophlebitis"). Diagnostic ultrasonography is sensitive in detecting the presence of an intact Baker's cyst, but it becomes less reliable when bursal dissection or rupture into the calf occurs. Associated thrombophlebitis must be definitively excluded by venography or reliable, noninvasive means before accepting knee cyst–related phenomena as the sole cause of calf-foot pain and swelling.

Between the calcaneus bone and the Achilles tendon lies the retrocalcaneal bursa. Symptoms in the area of this bursa may be mistaken for Achilles tendinitis, and care should be taken to differentiate these conditions. A swollen retrocalcaneal bursa commonly will show bulging on the medial and lateral sides of the Achilles tendon. The swollen bursa may be extremely sensitive to pressure on direct palpation and with dorsiflexion of the foot. (Caution regarding the introduction of corticosteroid agents in the vicinity of the Achilles tendon is discussed in the treatment section later.)

TENDINITIS

Common sites of tendon inflammation are the frequently used tendons of the upper extremities where they pass over bony prominences. Although the rotator cuff refers generically to a collection of four muscles about the shoulder, it is specifically the supraspinous muscle that is most commonly involved in tendinitis, perhaps owing to the stress resulting from humeral impingement against the coracoacromial arch. Patients note pain subacromially and laterally over the shoulder with abduction of the arm. Bicipital tendinitis affects the long head of the biceps muscle and characteristically causes shoulder pain anteriorly and over the bicipital groove (particularly with flexion of the shoulder against resistance, elbow extended, and forearm supinated).

Lateral epicondylitis at the elbow ("tennis elbow") results from inflammation and degeneration of extensor tendons of the forearm, particularly the extensor carpi radialis brevis, with eventual fibrous adherence to the capsule of the lateral elbow. Contracture of the wrist extensor muscles then chronically pulls on the capsule, producing pain about 2 cm distal to the lateral epicondyle. Medial epicondylitis ("golfer's elbow") similarly produces pain at the origin of the flexor muscles of the wrist, distal to the medial epicondyle.

The dorsum of the wrist contains six compartments through which numerous tendons glide. Although an inflammatory process may affect any of these, inflammation of the abductor pollicis longus and extensor pollicis brevis tendons in the first compartment (i.e., most radial) may result in a lack of smooth excursion of the enclosed tendons, a condition known as de Quervain's disease (stenosing tenosynovitis). Patients describe pain at the radial aspect of the wrist, especially with pinch gripping. Palpation of the tendons in the anatomic "snuff box" area may reveal swelling compared with the uninvolved side.

TREATMENT OF BURSITIS AND TENDINITIS

Immobilization of an inflamed musculoskeletal part, whether partial or complete, is an important adjunct in management and helps to expedite and optimize chances for recovery. The exception to this general rule is with tendinitis or bursitis of the shoulder, where immobilization may foster development of a "frozen" shoulder and, except for brief periods (e.g., 24 to 48 hours), should be avoided. Splints are especially useful in epicondylitis of the elbow ("elbow band") and in de Quervain's disease of the thumb. Ice during the acute phase and moist heat during the chronic phase are useful, and nonsteroidal anti-inflammatory drugs (NSAIDs) are helpful in many cases. The choice of a specific NSAID is not critical, but all such agents should be given in ample doses and with food (ideally in the middle of a meal) to lessen the risk of gastropathy. An enteric-coated aspirin preparation, 975 mg every 8 hours; naproxen (Naprosyn), 250 to 500 mg twice daily; and oxaprozin (Daypro), 1200 mg once a day, are representative examples. For patients with a bleeding diathesis, persons on warfarin (Coumadin) therapy, or those otherwise unable to tolerate the standard NSAIDs, possible treatment options include a nonacetylated salicylate (e.g., Trilisate or Disalcid) or a course of a centrally acting synthetic analgesic such as tramadol (Ultram), 50 to 100 mg every 6 hours as needed.

Physical therapy, ultrasonography, or hydrotherapy has application in many cases but is most important in shoulder tendinitis or bursitis, in which there is greater risk of permanent compromise in range of motion. Acute tendinitis or bursitis may render such severe pain, however, that physical therapy intended to augment range-of-motion function becomes impractical or ignored. In such a clinical setting, selective local anesthetic-corticosteroid injections are often valuable. The anatomic area is cleaned with povidone-iodine (Betadine) and alcohol, and an ethyl chloride spray may be applied as a topical anesthetic. Selection of corticosteroid is based on the extent of symptoms and, for practical reasons, the relative depth of involved tissue pathology owing to the potential for soft tissue atrophy (especially likely with synthetic fluorinated preparations such as triamcinolone). Consideration should be given to the relative solubility and potency when selecting a corticosteroid preparation (or combination) for soft tissue injection. Medium-potency agents include prednisolone sodium phosphate and prednisolone tebutate; these agents are useful at superficial injection sites. A high-potency fluorinated corticosteroid, such as triamcinolone hexacetonide (Aristospan Intra-articular, slow onset but prolonged duration of action) should be used only for injection of deep structures or for intra-articular injections, to minimize the danger of leakage to the skin with resultant atrophy and/or depigmentation of skin. Ideal technique favors injection near the affected tendon but not directly into the structure itself. A frequently used narrow tendon, such as the bicipital tendon, may be prone to rupture with direct injection; the Achilles tendon and surrounding areas should not be directly exposed to corticosteroid agents because this structure is inherently weak and prone to tear. Although more than a single corticosteroid injection may not be necessary to modify a soft tissue pain syndrome, caution should be taken not to exceed three injections in the same anatomic site over a 12-month period. Under sterile conditions, the incidence of iatrogenic infection with soft tissue injection is extremely low. A patient with glucose intolerance may have a transient effect from local corticosteroid injection. A period of reduced activity of 24 to 48 hours is best to optimize therapeutic results.

Surgical attention is seldom necessary in tendinitis or bursitis, but with structural rupture or recalcitrance to full conservative measures, surgical excision or repair may become a consideration.

Patients with recurrent symptoms must be instructed to avoid provocative or aggravating activities that strain susceptible anatomic structures by overuse. Warm-up and stretching exercises should always precede aerobic conditioning activities.

MYOFASCIAL PAIN

In the nomenclature of soft tissue pain syndromes, "myofascial pain" infers regional discomfort, often with a discernible soft tissue focus palpable on physical examination and radiating pain with modest pressure (4 kg) ("trigger zone"). The development of an anatomic trigger zone may result from trauma (of even minimal severity) or from overuse. Although often post-traumatic, or ostensibly autonomous, myofascial pain may also occur in systemic illnesses. The lack of gross "swelling" should not mislead the physician to conclude that the patient has no "sensation of swelling." The importance of a careful and "hands-on" physical examination cannot be overstated in this setting. Documentation of palpable soft tissue abnormalities is obviously important, but assessment of joint range of motion (passive and active), possible joint hypermobility, and subtle synovial warmth and/or thickening is useful whether any abnormalities are, in fact, present.

Myofascial pain appears to be distinct from the condition of fibromyalgia. Unlike the generalized pain and fatigue of fibromyalgia, and the disproportionate female preponderance of fibromyalgia patients, the condition of myofascial pain shows negligible gender variation, stiffness that is regional rather than generalized, and pain that is more focused and less whole bodied.

FIBROMYALGIA

Fibromyalgia is a common pain amplification syndrome characterized by generalized chronic pain (longer than 3 months in duration), stiffness, gelling, and fatigue. Typically, patients are women of middle age with predictable tender points on physical examination and a disturbed sleep pattern such that they awaken nonrefreshed from sleep (a nonrestorative sleep pattern). The most frequently affected anatomic sites in fibromyalgia include (bilaterally) at the occiput, low cervical region, midpoint of the trapezius, supraspinatus at the medial border of the scapula, second ribs at costochondral junctions, 2 cm distal to the lateral epicondyles of the elbow, gluteal area in the upper-outer quadrants of the buttocks, 2 cm posterior to the greater trochanter, and at the medial fat pads of the knees proximal to the joint line. Predictable features of fibromyalgia (100% incidence) include generalized pain for at least 3 months and widespread local tenderness at 11 or more of the aforementioned 18 anatomic sites; characteristic features (greater than 75% incidence) are fatigue, sleep disturbance, and morning stiffness; common features (greater than 25% incidence) may be headache, paresthesias, psychologic abnormality, subjective swelling, and functional disability.

The diagnosis of fibromyalgia is based on a characteristic history, the exclusion of systemic diseases that may cause musculoskeletal pain (e.g., rheumatoid arthritis, systemic lupus erythematosus, inflammatory muscle disease, polymyalgia rheumatica, and hypothyroidism), the finding of nonarticular tender points with an essentially normal joint examination, and a normal laboratory profile (i.e., complete blood count, acute phase response, and thyroid functions). Occasionally, a low titer of antinuclear antibody is found but in the absence of an obvious cause such as connective tissue disease or a drug-induced effect.

The pathophysiology of fibromyalgia is not well understood, although an association with psychologic abnormalities has been suggested. There may be a subgroup of fibromyalgia patients with significant coexisting psychologic problems, especially depression, and there appears to be an increased incidence of depression in first-degree relatives of fibromyalgia patients. Most patients with fibromyalgia, however, are not depressed.

The most characteristic sleep abnormality in fibromyalgia is the loss of "slow wave" deep sleep with a relative loss of the restorative phase of sleep. Sleep apnea may be seen disproportionately in male patients with fibromyalgia, and polysomnography is a reasonable consideration for selected patients. The natural history of fibromyalgia is not established definitively. Although symptoms may be chronic, perhaps lasting 10 to 15 years or longer, a majority of patients show symptomatic improvement when fully informed and optimally managed.

Fibromyalgia may occur following motor vehicle accidents or other trauma. Although some have suggested that no scientific data support a causality link between soft tissue trauma and the development of fibromyalgia, it seems presumptuous to rule out completely any possible linkage between trauma and fibromyalgia when so little is definitively understood about the latter condition itself. Patients who develop neck, upper back, or upper extremity pain after automobile trauma may have experienced sudden extreme movements of the cervical spine ("whiplash") and may stretch an individual nerve root with impingement or a herniated disk. Some patients may continue to complain of soft tissue pain a year or more after traumatic injury yet have no objective evidence of neurologic pathology or radiographic abnormalities. A diagnostic-prognostic paradigm is not easily applied to the work-up, disposition, or compensatory claims of post-traumatic nonarticular pain patients. Although doubtlessly there are self-serving motives in some cases, it would seem reckless to categorically discount or dismiss the potential problems patients may encounter in the post-traumatic setting.

TREATMENT

Proper management of fibromyalgia must begin with a definite diagnosis and assurance regarding the noncrippling nature of the process. Physician-patient dialogue is essential for the initiation of an effective treatment program, and printed educational material, including that from the Arthritis Foundation, often is also useful. Pharmacologic intervention is used most effectively in attempting to rectify the underlying sleep abnormality. Favorable results often are seen by instituting amitriptyline (Elavil),* 10 mg 2 hours before bedtime with increments of 10 mg every 2 weeks if necessary, not to exceed 75 mg total dose. These are not, of course, antidepressant dosages of amitriptyline, and depression is usually not the pathologic focus of managing fibromyalgia. A concurrent morning dose of a selective serotonin reuptake inhibitor such as paroxetine (Paxil), 20 mg, may be useful in depressed patients. The improvement of sleep pattern with the resulting attenuation or amelioration of pain symptoms is the single most

_____
*Not FDA approved for this indication.

important application of pharmacology in fibromyalgia. Cyclobenzaprine (Flexeril),* 10 mg at bedtime, may also be useful in improving sleep patterns. Owing to their similar side effects, though, antidepressants and muscle relaxants should not be prescribed concurrently. NSAIDs sometimes are helpful as analgesics but not as the sole drug used to alleviate the symptoms of fibromyalgia. Generally, NSAIDs should be minimally utilized.

For selected patients, tender point injections with corticosteroids or lidocaine may be useful. A reasonable injection regimen is 1 to 2 mL of 1% lidocaine or the same amount of lidocaine plus a corticosteroid. The total amount of corticosteroid administered (to all sites in total) should not exceed 40 mg of methylprednisolone or the equivalent, and tender points should not be injected more frequently than once a month or a maximum of three times a year. Synthetic fluorinated corticosteroid agents are not recommended for soft tissue injection owing to the potential atrophy of subcutaneous tissues and depigmentation of skin at the injection site.

Nonpharmacologic modalities, including meditation, relaxation techniques, and biofeedback, may be useful in lessening tension. Physical fitness training resulting in cardiovascular conditioning is beneficial. Patients should select the aerobic activity of their choice (walking, running, swimming, bicycling) and commit themselves to incorporate such activity into their routine daily schedules three to five times per week. Patients must start slowly and advance their workouts gradually, and exercise periods should not become an "inner competition" but remain relaxing and not unduly stressful. A caring physician can provide important psychologic support for most patients, but in a few select cases the help of a psychologist or psychiatrist may be necessary.

_____
*Not FDA approved for this indication.

OSTEOARTHRITIS

method of
LARISSA ROUX, M.D., and
MATTHEW H. LIANG, M.D., M.P.H.
*Harvard Medical School and Brigham and
   Woman's Hospital*
Boston, Massachusetts

Osteoarthritis (OA) is an acquired, noninflammatory, musculoskeletal disorder that results from cartilage degradation without adequate regeneration. It commonly affects the distal and proximal interphalangeal (DIP and PIP) joints, the first carpometacarpal joints, hips, knees, and cervical or lumbar spine. Reported prevalence rates of OA vary widely between specific joints, but 90% of the U.S. population older than 65 years of age has radiographic evidence of disease. The DIP and PIP joints are most commonly affected radiographically (63 to 84% in people older than 55 years), but are symptomatic only in 2 to 4%. The hip (6 to 14%) and knee (3 to 6%) are the second and third most commonly radiographically affected joints and are symptomatic in 1% and 10 to 30%, respectively, in the same age group. A number of risk factors have been identified for this disease entity, with age the predominant one for all sites of OA. In addition, for weight-bearing joints, such as the knee and hip, obesity can be a predisposing factor. Tasks associated with repetitive trauma, particularly at the DIP and PIP joints of the hand and, to a lesser extent, at the knee, may also potentiate this disease. Last, bony fracture involving the articular surface, or knee meniscectomy, may result in future development of OA. Secondary OA is the result of mechanical incongruity of joints, which can be congenital or can result from trauma, infection, inflammation, or endocrine abnormalities.

Increased understanding of the etiology and pathophysiology of OA has opened up possible therapeutic options. Under normal circumstances, cartilage remodeling is characterized by an equilibrium between cartilage matrix degradation and chondrocyte-mediated synthesis of type II collagen and glycosaminoglycans. When cartilage degradation exceeds its regeneration, progressive erosion and fissuring of cartilaginous joint surfaces result. Although aging is strongly associated with the incidence of OA, the composition, water content, genetic expression (chondroitin sulfate epitope 846), and degradative enzymatic activity differ between osteoarthritic and aging cartilage. This suggests that although age may somehow (e.g., reduced functional chondrocyte density) predispose people to cartilage degradation, OA is acquired rather than simply a consequence of aging. The synthesis-degradation equilibrium of cartilage is also affected by soluble factors such as matrix metalloproteinases, proinflammatory cytokines, cytokine inhibitors, growth factors, as well as certain oncogenes, and all of these may be targets for new therapies.

DIAGNOSIS

The diagnosis of OA is a clinical one and one of exclusion because there are no biologic markers or associated diagnostic laboratory abnormalities. The cardinal radiographic features of OA that must all be present for diagnosis are early unequal joint space narrowing (<4 mm in the hip), osteophytes, juxta-articular sclerosis ("eburnation"), and subchondral bone cysts. However, radiographs are confirmatory and not useful for following patients because there is such a poor relationship between radiographic findings and symptoms. Other diagnoses must be entertained with atypical presentations of joint pain, even in the presence of radiographic OA changes. These include (1) pain in a joint not usually affected by OA; (2) the presence of neuromotor or vascular symptoms; (3) acute onset of symptoms; (4) severe pain at rest; (5) marked signs of inflammation, and systemic or constitutional signs or symptoms; and (6) evidence of synovitis. Tenderness elicited by direct palpation of a tendon or bursa suggests an alternate etiology, such as tendonitis or bursitis. Prolonged morning stiffness and systemic symptoms are more in keeping with rheumatic illnesses (such as rheumatoid arthritis, lupus, or polymyalgia rheumatica). Finally, intense joint inflammation suggests sepsis or a crystalline disease.

Osteoarthritis typically presents with joint pain, stiffness, and loss of motion, the severity and implications of which are specific to the affected joint. Early disease is characterized by localized joint pain of insidious onset that worsens with activity. In more advanced disease, pain is present with any joint loading and occasionally at night. "Gel phenomenon," or stiffness after prolonged inactivity, usually does not exceed 30 minutes. The precise cause of the symptoms is not known, and the possibilities include low-grade synovitis, joint capsule distention, periosteal elevation from bony proliferation, ischemia of subchondral bone, muscle spasm, and ligament or tendon strain.

Physical findings of osteoarthritic joints may include bony enlargement, crepitus, diminished range of motion, pain with passive motion, and joint line tenderness and malalignment.

Hand

Absence of objective synovitis and presence of bony proliferation in the small joints of the hand characterize OA involvement of the hand. Patients present with aching and stiffness of fingers, worsened by repetitive finger use. Bony enlargements are known as Bouchard's nodes around the PIP joints and Heberden's nodes around the DIP joints.

Hip

The earliest abnormality detected in hip OA is restricted range of motion, with limited internal rotation (<35 degrees) and abduction (<45 degrees) the predominant effects. As the disease progresses, the hip may become flexed and foreshortened. Patients often complain of pain in the groin or over the greater trochanter. Symptoms are aggravated by excessive weight bearing and prolonged immobility. The earliest radiographic finding is unequal narrowing of the joint space.

Knee

Osteoarthritic involvement of the medial and lateral compartments of the knees and of the patellofemoral joint is common. Affected people present with pain on weight bearing or anterior knee pain, respectively. OA of the patellofemoral joint is exacerbated particularly by descending stairs (more so than by climbing stairs). Both are worse with rising from a sitting position. Joint space narrowing is best visualized on weight-bearing radiographs in medial or lateral compartment views or with skyline views in patellofemoral disease.

Spine

The lower cervical (C6-7) spine and the lower lumbar (L-3 to S-1) spine are most commonly affected. Pain is often poorly localized. Muscle spasm and stiffness often accompany it, and restricted range of motion develops with progression of disease. In advanced disease, with encroachment of intervertebral foramina by osteophytes and intervertebral disk space narrowing, nearby nerves may be impinged and a patient may present with predominantly neurologic symptoms. Localized tenderness, paraspinal muscle spasm, and crepitus can be noted on physical examination. In the neck, extension and lateral bending and rotation are the first motions to be limited. In the lower back, severe loss of motion does not occur until very late in the disease process.

MANAGEMENT

General Considerations

The goals of therapy are to decrease pain, to maintain or improve joint function, and to educate the patient and family about the disease and its therapeutic options. How this disease affects a patient's life, as perceived by the patient, will be a critical guide in managing his or her care. In addition, the natural history of the disease at the affected joint is of particular importance. For example, OA of the fingers tends to be less progressive than that of weight-bearing joints.

Prevention

Approximately 17 million Americans have OA, and this figure is expected to increase as the population ages. Furthermore, the trend of increasing sports injuries in a more recreationally athletic population will likely increase the incidence of OA. These trends make population approaches to the prevention of OA of paramount importance. Particular attention should be given in primary care settings to the identification and modification of risk factors for occupational and athletic joint injury, such as repetitive, unsupported motion, poor conditioning, and poor technique.

Cognitive and Behavioral Control of Arthritis Pain

Pain intensity and extent of disability correlate poorly with radiographic severity of OA, implying potential avenues for application of biopsychosocial approaches. Studies demonstrate that highly motivated patients and those with favorable rational thinking indices have significantly lower levels of pain and psychological distress, and better overall health. Psychoeducational interventions are effective in reducing pain, disability, and medication and health resource utilization. Studies including spouses in cognitive behavior therapy have demonstrated the importance of social factors in perception of pain.

Biomechanical Factors

Initial approaches to medical management of OA focus on unloading the involved joint and strengthening associated periarticular muscle groups. Reduced joint loading on weight-bearing joints may result from weight loss or the use of aids, such as a cane in the contralateral hand, crutches, or appliances such as heel or insole wedges, as indicated. In determining what devices might best meet the needs of the patient, it is also imperative to assess his or her physical environment. Potential aids to daily living, such as increasing chair height, elevating toilet seats, and eliminating stairs, may improve function and reduce pain. Even modest weight loss can dramatically lower joint-loading forces. Adjustment of work activities and posture and strengthening of equal but opposing muscle groups are useful adjuncts in joint load distribution.

Exercise regimens in patients with OA have discernible benefits. Fitness walking reduces pain and disability over the short term, and fitness in general is associated with improved all-cause mortality rates. Strength in periarticular muscle groups is a critical determinant of joint stability and alignment, and knee extensor weakness has been implicated as a predictor of incident OA. Continued exercise in people with mild to moderate OA does not damage cartilage and may in fact slow the progression of disease. For acute episodes of musculoskeletal pain, cold applied to the joint may reduce symptoms. For subacute pain, the application of heat, superficially or deeply, is preferable to raise the pain threshold and to facilitate muscle relaxation.

Pharmacotherapy

Analgesics

Acetaminophen (up to 4 grams per day) is first-line therapy for OA of the hip and knee. Acetaminophen has the same efficacy as nonsteroidal anti-inflammatory drugs (NSAIDs) in OA with an excellent side effect profile, especially in elderly patients. It acts centrally, thereby elevating the pain threshold. It has no anti-inflammatory properties at therapeutic doses. Acetaminophen is metabolized in the liver. Hepatotoxicity occurs with massive overdose or in people with underlying liver disease, but is otherwise very well tolerated. Opioids can be added to analgesic regimens in OA for short periods.

Nonsteroidal Anti-inflammatory Drugs, Including Cyclooxygenase-2 Inhibitors

These agents exert their anti-inflammatory and adverse effects through cyclooxygenase (COX) inhibition. It has been difficult to demonstrate significant differences in efficacy among the different agents in this class; their toxicity has been the subject of considerable study. NSAID-induced gastropathy, the most common complication of NSAID use, can present simply as dyspepsia or, more seriously, as ulceration and perforation of the gastrointestinal (GI) tract. The elderly are more prone to NSAID-induced GI ulceration, and endoscopic evidence of this complication is seen in up to 20% of users. Ibuprofen and diclofenac (Voltaren) are the safest, whereas piroxicam (Feldene) and azapropazone* are the most ulcerogenic. Aspirin is more ulcerogenic than other NSAIDs. Although all NSAIDs inhibit platelet adhesion and hence may potentiate GI bleeding and perforation, administration of misoprostol (Cytotec; stabilized prostaglandin E) with NSAIDs reduces the incidence of GI complications. Acute renal insufficiency, also more commonly seen in the elderly, can be hemodynamically mediated or the result of idiosyncratic tubular interstitial disease. Indomethacin has the most pronounced central nervous system effects. Hepatotoxicity is a reported side effect of diclofenac. Aseptic meningitis is a rare toxicity of ibuprofen and sulindac. Finally, skin reactions, central nervous system disturbances, and interference with diuretics and antihypertensives are also recognized.

A new class of NSAIDs appear to have the same

---

*Not available in the United States.

analgesic and anti-inflammatory effects, but preferentially inhibit the COX-2 isoform of the COX enzyme. The specificity of COX-2 inhibition reduces GI ulceration compared with conventional NSAIDs, but whether it will also reduce GI bleeding or perforation is not known. The only available COX-2 agent, celecoxib (Celebrex), is more expensive than NSAIDs already available.

Chondroprotective Agents

Glucosamine (up to 1500 mg daily), an aminomonosaccharide, is a substrate in the production of glycosaminoglycans and proteoglycans in articular cartilage. Although some studies suggest that it may provide pain relief, reduce tenderness, and improve mobility in osteoarthritic patients, the improvement in symptoms is generally delayed compared with conventional OA medications. Glucosamine is claimed to slow or reverse cartilage destruction, but no data are available.

Chondroitin sulfate 4 and 6 (800 to 1200 mg daily) are glycosaminoglycans that have in vitro inhibitory effects on proteoglycan and collagen metabolism, and stimulate matrix synthesis. Early randomized trials have demonstrated good tolerance, functional impairment reduction of 50% at 1 year, and joint structure modulation reflected by improved intra-articular space measurements.

Intra-articular Therapy

Intra-articular injection of corticosteroids (Kenalog, Depo-Medrol) can be useful in the adjunctive management of OA. Injection may provide relief of synovitis or inflamed Heberden's nodes. With large, painful, inflammatory effusions of osteoarthritic knees, arthrocentesis followed by injection of steroids and topical anesthetic agents may provide greater symptomatic relief, presumably as a result of suppression of synovial inflammation.

Hyaluronic acid (HA), a polysaccharide, is a prototype glycosaminoglycan that is normally produced by chondrocytes and synoviocytes. In OA, HA becomes depolymerized, resulting in diminished viscoelasticity and increased susceptibility to cartilage injury. In vitro, exogenous HA stimulates further HA synthesis, inhibits synthesis of various inflammatory mediators, alters leukocyte behavior, and protects against cellular damage by oxygen free radicals. A blinded, randomized trial of intra-articular purified avian HA injection (20 mg per week for 3 weeks) demonstrated sustained pain relief, comparable with that with naproxen use, with fewer adverse reactions but at considerably higher cost.

Chondrocyte transplantation with cartilage cells genetically engineered to produce growth factors has been explored, with the idea that areas of cartilage loss could be restored by new chondrocytes. So far, clinical benefit has not been demonstrated.

Surgery

Patients with intractable pain and disability from structural damage should be considered for surgical intervention. Surgical options include arthroscopy, osteotomy, and arthroplasty. Surgical removal of loose bodies and fragments can be accomplished through arthroscopy. Tibial osteotomy can result in symptomatic relief in patients with varus angulation less than 10 degrees and good ligamentous support. It may delay the time for total joint arthroplasty, but the rehabilitation process is long. Joint replacement is considered with severe pain and end-stage structural disease. Results of arthroplasty are better if profound muscle weakness has not set in so that postoperative rehabilitation is possible. Co-morbidity and functional status should be assessed before recommendation for arthroplasty. Pain relief is achieved in more than 90% of patients who undergo total joint replacement of the knee or hip. Approximately 2% of patients undergo revisional surgery. Operative mortality rates range from 0.5 to 1.9%. Complications include loosening of the prosthesis, infection, and dislocation.

POLYMYALGIA RHEUMATICA AND GIANT CELL ARTERITIS

method of
GREGORY C. GARDNER, M.D.
University of Washington School of Medicine
Seattle, Washington

Polymyalgia rheumatica and giant cell arteritis began to emerge separately as clinical syndromes in the 1930s. Their recognition has been aided by the increasing life expectancy in the industrialized nations because most of the cases occur in the sixth and seventh decades of life. The relationship between polymyalgia rheumatica and giant cell arteritis was recognized in the late 1950s, and in literature from Scandinavia the term *polymyalgia arteritica* has been used due to the co-occurrence of the two diseases. Approximately 10% of people who present with clinically pure polymyalgia rheumatica develop giant cell arteritis weeks to years later, whereas up to 50% of people with giant cell arteritis have coexisting polymyalgia rheumatica. Both syndromes are common in people of Northern European ancestry and less common among Asians and rare among Africans.

DIAGNOSIS

The symptoms of polymyalgia rheumatica often begin abruptly. Stiffness in shoulder and hip regions after a period of inactivity is the most prominent symptom and can be so profound that patients report rolling themselves out of bed in the morning. *Polymyalgia* is a misnomer because the pathophysiology involves synovitis/tenosynovitis of proximal joints and tendons as documented by synovial biopsy and magnetic resonance imaging scans. Other symptoms include loss of sense of well-being, fever, and joint swelling. Up to 20% of patients have discernible synovitis in knees, wrists, or hand joints that may be confused with rheumatoid arthritis. Synovitis/tenosynovitis around the shoulder may lead to rotator cuff tendonitis or adhesive capsulitis.

Patients with giant cell arteritis generally present with headache. It is usually severe and localized to temporal or occipital regions. Other symptoms include transient visual changes (blurring, transient visual loss, diplopia), scalp tenderness, jaw claudications, dysphagia, fever, and weight loss. If peripheral vessels are involved, there may be claudications of the arms or legs. The most feared manifestation is blindness.

The sedimentation rate is often elevated over 100 mm per hour, although on occasion (up to 10% in some series) sedimentation rate may be normal. Mild anemia and mild elevation in liver function tests are not uncommon. Polymyalgia rheumatica is a clinical diagnosis aided by the presence of an elevated sedimentation rate while temporal artery biopsy is useful for confirmation of giant cell arteritis. It is helpful to have as large a biopsy specimen as possible (up to 4 cm) and to obtain multiple histologic sections due to the skip nature of the pathology.

TREATMENT

Polymyalgia rheumatica often responds dramatically to low-dose prednisone in doses of 10 to 20 mg per day. Response usually occurs within 24 to 48 hours and always within 1 week. Splitting the initial dose (e.g., 10 mg in the morning and 2.5 to 5 mg in the evening) more adequately addresses the morning stiffness and avoids having to use larger doses. After 4 to 6 weeks at the response dose, begin a slow taper by no more than 1 mg per week. If symptoms return during the taper, the dose can be increased by 1 to 2 mg per day; it is not necessary to return to the initial response dose. Check the sedimentation rate at 3 weeks after treatment initiation to document a reduction but follow symptoms rather than the sedimentation rate for tapering purposes. Once the dose has reached 5 to 7 mg per day, the taper should be 1 to 2 mg per month. It is important to remember that corticosteroids do not cure polymyalgia but simply suppress the inflammation until the disease goes away. Knowing this, some patients are willing to endure mild symptoms and take less medicine.

Approximately 60% to 70% of patients can stop corticosteroids by 2 years, although a few patients have symptoms for up to 10 years. Data from the Mayo Clinic suggest that 10% of patients have a relapse after resolution of disease. Steroid-sparing medications include hydroxychloroquine (Plaquenil Sulfate) and methotrexate. Physical therapy may be needed for associated rotator cuff tendonitis or adhesive capsulitis. Attention to corticosteroid osteoporosis is important for polymyalgia rheumatica and critical for giant cell arteritis. Patients with polymyalgia rheumatica should be aware of the symptoms of temporal arteritis and instructed to call with concerning symptoms.

Giant cell arteritis necessitates high-dose corticosteroids, mainly to prevent blindness. Doses of 40 to 60 mg per day are standard and should be divided initially. Response is usually as rapid as with polymyalgia rheumatica. After 4 to 6 weeks, a taper by 10% of current dose per week should be started with the goal of getting the patient down to 5 to 7 mg per day. Once corticosteroids are started, blindness is unusual. Patients with visual symptoms or jaw claudications at presentation should take low-dose aspirin as well as corticosteroids. It is rare to restore vision once it is lost, but high-dose corticosteroids (i.e., 1000 mg methylprednisolone [Solu-Medrol] IV each day × 3) should be tried. It is important to not chase the sedimentation rate. Check it at 3 weeks of therapy to document a decrement, but recheck only with a reoccurrence of symptoms. Use symptoms as a guide to tapering rather than the sedimentation rate. The disease usually lasts no more than 2 years, and relapse after disease resolution is rare. Methotrexate has been used as a steroid-sparing agent.

OSTEOMYELITIS

method of
DAVID W. HAAS, M.D.
Vanderbilt University School of Medicine
Nashville, Tennessee

Osteomyelitis (infection of bone) causes substantial morbidity worldwide. Management depends on the causative pathogen, the route by which bacteria gained access to bone, local and systemic host immune factors, and patient age. Radiographic imaging and nonspecific blood tests may suggest the diagnosis, but invasive tissue sampling usually is necessary to identify the specific organism. Knowledge of relative activities and pharmacokinetics of individual drugs, supported by animal models, has largely dictated antibacterial regimens. Definitive therapy often necessitates combined medical and surgical interventions.

PATHOPHYSIOLOGY

Bone infection arises either by hematogenous seeding or by contiguous spread that includes traumatic or surgical inoculation of bacteria. The presence of orthopedic hardware may complicate either scenario. In children older than 1 year of age, hematogenous osteomyelitis usually begins in a long bone metaphysis, typically the distal femur or proximal tibia. Once established, infection causes infarction of the endosteum, allowing pus to penetrate to the subperiosteal space. The detached periosteum gradually produces new bone. In contrast, hematogenous osteomyelitis in adults usually involves the vertebrae, sternoclavicular and sacroiliac joints, or symphysis pubis, where it first involves subchondral bone, then spreads to the joint space. In vertebral osteomyelitis, this causes sequential destruction of the end plate, adjoining disk, and contiguous vertebral body. Infection also has a tendency to arise in sites of previous, often minor trauma.

Osteomyelitis from contiguous spread may involve virtually any traumatized bone. Although healthy bone resists infection, injury from local inflammation or trauma may allow microorganisms to thrive. In diabetic patients, osteomyelitis may complicate decubitus ulcers or vascular insufficiency. Neuropathy allows unappreciated trauma to cause cutaneous ulceration, and poor perfusion impairs immune defenses and healing. Bacterial infection is a dreaded complication of prosthetic joint replacement. Once bacteria adhere to orthopedic hardware, they resist killing by antimicrobials and host immunity.

A functional definition of chronic osteomyelitis is refractoriness to cure by antimicrobials alone. The transition from acute to chronic osteomyelitis is heralded by bacterial attachment to functionally inert substrata. The time necessary to establish refractory infection depends on route of infection. Hematogenous vertebral osteomyelitis can usually be cured by antimicrobials alone, largely because sequestra are slow to form. In contrast, prosthetic implant infection may be "chronic" (i.e., refractory) from inception. When trauma leads to sequestrum formation, refractoriness to medical therapy also develops rapidly. Chronic osteomyelitis usually necessitates surgical débridement for cure.

MICROBIOLOGY

Virtually any pathogenic bacteria may cause osteomyelitis under appropriate circumstances. The identity of the likely causative organism depends on how bacteria gained access to bone, and the local epidemiology. This explains why bacteriology differs between diabetic foot osteomyelitis and prosthetic joint infection, and between nosocomial and community-acquired infections.

Staphylococcus aureus has a predilection for causing osteomyelitis, especially hematogenous infection. Contamination of open trauma by soil causes indolent osteomyelitis due to *Clostridia, Bacillus,* or *Nocardia* species; fresh-water contamination favors *Aeromonas* or *Plesiomonas* infection; *Salmonella* osteomyelitis may complicate sickle cell disease; *Pasteurella multocida* osteomyelitis may follow cat bites. When a sharp object (e.g., a nail) passing through a shoe into the foot produces osteomyelitis, the organism is usually *Pseudomonas aeruginosa,* which thrives in innersoles. *Pseudomonas* also causes most cases of invasive otitis externa in diabetic patients. This manifests with ear pain and purulent discharge, and may cause extensive bony destruction. Osteomyelitis due to anaerobic bacteria usually results from contiguous spread of polymicrobial infection. Anaerobes rarely cause hematogenous osteomyelitis. Diabetic foot osteomyelitis is typically polymicrobial, with gram-negative and gram-positive aerobic and anaerobic bacteria present.

RADIOLOGIC EVALUATION

There is confusion regarding the radiologic approach to osteomyelitis, with too much emphasis often placed on radiographic imaging. No technique can absolutely confirm or exclude osteomyelitis, and the impact of a misleading radiographic finding dictates the relative importance of a technique's sensitivity versus its specificity. When the therapeutic implication is great, no study may be sufficiently accurate to guide therapy. Imaging studies should be thought of as providing information that may support clinical suspicion.

A simple plain film should be the initial study for most cases. Cortical destruction and periosteal new bone formation strongly suggest osteomyelitis, and further studies may be unnecessary. Unfortunately, plain films are not sensitive and will not show abnormality until 2 or more weeks after the patient's initial symptoms appear in children (often much longer in adults).

Bone scanning with ^{99m}Tc-diphosphonate detects areas of osteoblastic activity and increased vascularity. Soft tissue inflammation causes increased uptake during the first 5 minutes after injection, which normalizes or remains diffuse at 3 hours. In contrast, osteomyelitis causes persistent focal enhancement. Thus, delayed images better differentiate bone from soft tissue uptake. Unfortunately, bone scans are limited by low specificity, even with delayed images. In clinical practice, most scans interpreted as "consistent with osteomyelitis" probably do not represent osteomyelitis. Any inflammation or new bone formation may increase uptake. In the diabetic foot, sterile osteoarthropathy causes enhancement, whereas vascular insufficiency may prevent radioisotope accumulation in infected bones. Nevertheless, bone scans in general are quite sensitive. A normal scan makes osteomyelitis very unlikely.

Indium 111 leukocyte scintigraphy is more specific for infection, but much less sensitive than bone scanning. In addition, osteomyelitis is difficult to distinguish from soft tissue inflammation, and marrow-containing skeleton may enhance with ^{111}In-labeled leukocytes. White blood cell scanning may not detect indolent infection, the situation in which imaging would be most helpful.

An advantage of both computed tomography (CT) and magnetic resonance imaging (MRI) is that bone and soft tissues are evaluated simultaneously. CT is good for visualizing sequestra (islands of dead bone), which may guide surgery because sequestrum removal is necessary for cure. MRI does not image crystalline hydroxyapatite, but rather soft tissues and fluid around and within bone. Replacement of marrow by inflammatory tissue is easily visualized. However, soft tissue inflammation may cause nearby bone marrow to enhance, even in the absence of osteomyelitis. MRI is the best modality for detection of spinal infection. Typical findings are decreased signal intensity of vertebral bodies and disk spaces on T1-weighted images with blurring of the margin between body and disk, and increased intensity of the disk and adjacent vertebral bodies on T2-weighted images.

In patients with back pain, the pattern of radiographic changes helps distinguish between osteomyelitis, degenerative disease, and neoplasia. During hematogenous osteomyelitis, seeding first involves the vertebral end plate. Infection extends into the disk space early during infection and later to the adjacent vertebral body. In contrast, metastatic tumor typically destroys the vertebral bodies but spares the disks. Unlike osteomyelitis, the uninfected degenerated disk shows decreased signal intensity on T2-weighted MRI.

Invariably, initial publications describing the usefulness of imaging modalities are more encouraging than results achieved in clinical practice. Thus, the accuracy of newer techniques may be overestimated. The predictive value of any study also decreases in more complicated clinical situations.

NONSPECIFIC BLOOD TESTS

Noninvasive tests that are sometimes useful include the erythrocyte sedimentation rate (ESR) and C-reactive protein. Both tests have low sensitivity and specificity. In the patient without a prior history of osteomyelitis, these tests are most helpful when infection is unlikely. For example, in patients with persistent low back pain but without historical clues to suggest vertebral osteomyelitis, a normal ESR is reassuring. Conversely, a markedly elevated ESR suggests the need for further evaluation. The C-reactive protein, like the ESR, is an acute-phase reactant. The primary difference between these tests is that an elevated C-reactive protein has a shorter half-life (e.g., after surgery) than the ESR.

MICROBIOLOGIC DIAGNOSIS

The gold standard for diagnosing osteomyelitis is histopathologic and microbiologic examination of bone, but this is not necessary in every case. Abundant neutrophils are highly suggestive; a positive culture confirms the diagnosis and guides antimicrobial therapy. Although a sinus tract would seem a ready source for culture, in most cases deep surgical isolates do not correlate with bacteria cultured from the overlying sinus tract. A possible exception is when *S. aureus* is isolated in pure culture from a sinus tract that overlies osteomyelitis, in which case this organism is also likely to be present in the underlying bone. In general, open biopsy is preferred for microbiologic diagnosis.

Is there any value to culturing diabetic foot ulcers? Comparisons of deep surgical cultures (obtained through intact skin) versus superficial swabs, curettage, and needle aspiration in diabetic patients show poor concordance. Antimicrobial choices are usually made empirically. Nevertheless, if methicillin-resistant *S. aureus* is isolated from superficial cultures, an antimicrobial active against this pathogen should probably be included. It is occasionally difficult to culture fastidious or atypical pathogens, and negative cultures do not exclude osteomyelitis.

TREATMENT

General Considerations

When treating chronic osteomyelitis, the ultimate goal must be determined. In some cases, attempting cure would so adversely effect quality of life that chronic suppressive antibacterials or another, less aggressive approach is preferred. If microbiologic cure is pursued, then sequestra and foreign material should be removed, if possible, because bacterial adherence to necrotic bone, metal, or plastic dramatically compromises antimicrobial efficacy. If this is not done, failure rates after even prolonged courses of antimicrobials are high.

In addition to surgical débridement, patients should receive prolonged courses of antimicrobials, typically for 6 weeks or longer. As a rule, bactericidal antibiotics are preferred, although bacteriostatic antibiotics do not inevitably fail. Some clinicians monitor serum bactericidal titers to predict the efficacy of long-term antibiotic therapy, but this test is not widely available. Serial determinations of the ESR or C-reactive protein are also helpful. An ESR that rises after an initial decline, or remains elevated, suggests persistent infection. Finally, plain radiographs may be taken at later intervals to confirm healing. Given limitations of current tests, resolution of signs and symptoms may indicate response to therapy about as well as more sophisticated techniques. In some cases, the patient relapses months or years after apparent cure.

Antimicrobial Therapy

No comparative clinical trial has definitively established the best regimen for osteomyelitis in adults. Rigorous trials are difficult to perform because of different surgical techniques, clinical situations, pathogens, and the need for years of follow-up to demonstrate cure. Animal models have therefore been developed to compare antimicrobial efficacy.

In a rabbit model of osteomyelitis, vancomycin cured only 10% of staphylococcal infections. Combining rifampin with vancomycin, as well as with other agents, increased cure rates to nearly 100%. Clindamycin also performed very well as monotherapy. However, routine rifampin use is strongly discouraged, and this agent should not be used as monotherapy because resistant organisms will emerge. Despite its poor performance in animal models, vancomycin is commonly used for methicillin-resistant (and occasionally methicillin-susceptible) staphylococcal osteomyelitis, with failure rates not dramatically different from those for other drugs.

Treatment of chronic osteomyelitis usually demands high doses of antimicrobials administered for extended periods of time, usually at least 6 weeks. Some clinicians prefer "induction" with intravenous agents (or oral agents of equivalent efficacy) for 6 weeks, followed by more prolonged oral therapy. In some cases, residual infection may be sterilized by this continued oral therapy, although the superiority of this approach is uncertain.

There are many alternative antibiotic regimens for osteomyelitis (Table 1). For methicillin-resistant staphylococci, vancomycin (Vancocin) is preferred. When relapse is likely, rifampin (Rifadin) administered two or three times daily may be added (see Table 1). Because rifampin induces metabolism of many drugs, great caution must be exercised when it is initiated or discontinued. If oral therapy for methicillin-resistant staphylococcal infection is indicated, rifampin plus minocycline (Minocin) is recommended, assuming susceptibility to both agents. For streptococcal infection, ceftriaxone (Rocephin) is preferred because of once-daily dosing. This may be followed by oral amoxicillin (Amoxil; 500 mg orally every 6 hours), which is inexpensive and well tolerated. For enteric gram-negative bacilli, ceftriaxone is also reasonable. However, some Enterobacteriacae (e.g., *Enterobacter* species) may develop resistance to third-generation cephalosporins during therapy. Some oral fluoroquinolones, including ciprofloxacin (Cipro), ofloxacin (Floxin), and levofloxacin (Levaquin), are active against most gram-negative aerobes and achieve reasonable bone concentrations, making these acceptable oral alternatives. If the organism is susceptible to trimethoprim-sulfamethoxazole (Bactrim or Septra), this provides inexpensive therapy, which may be given for many months. For *P. aeruginosa*, oral ciprofloxacin may perform as well as parenteral regimens, although administering ciprofloxacin with ceftazidime (Fortaz, Tazidime) initially is probably more effective than monotherapy.

Effective oral regimens for staphylococcal osteomyelitis are needed. A regimen combining rifampin with a fluoroquinolone has shown promise, but controlled studies are needed to confirm its efficacy for selected patients. Noncompliance with oral therapy limits its use in many patients. Failure to reliably adhere to therapy may lead to relapse, with greater overall morbidity.

Ideally, therapy of diabetic foot osteomyelitis should be guided by deep tissue culture. It is unclear

TABLE 1. **Antimicrobial Therapy for Bacterial Osteomyelitis in Adults**

Organism	Regimen*	Comments
Staphylococci		
Methicillin sensitive	Nafcillin (Unipen) ± rifampin (Rifadin)	Rifampin is usually unnecessary.
	Oxacillin (Prostaphlin) ± rifampin (Rifadin)	Rifampin is usually unnecessary.
	Cefazolin (Ancef, Kefzol) ± rifampin (Rifadin)	Rifampin is usually unnecessary.
	Clindamycin (Cleocin)	Alert patient about possible colitis.
Methicillin resistant	Vancomycin (Vancocin) ± rifampin (Rifadin)	Use vancomycin if no effective alternative. Rifampin is usually unnecessary.
Streptococci	Ceftriaxone (Rocephin)	Once-daily dosing is advantageous.
Enterococci		
Ampicillin sensitive	Ampicillin (Omnipen, Principen) ± gentamicin (Garamycin)	Consider gentamicin during first 2 weeks.
Ampicillin resistant	Vancomycin (Vancocin) ± gentamicin (Garamycin)	Consider gentamicin during first 2 weeks.
Enterobacteriaciae	Ciprofloxacin (Cipro)	Avoid simultaneous oral Mg^{2+}, Fe^{2+}, or Al^{2+}.
	Ofloxacin (Floxin)	Avoid simultaneous oral Mg^{2+}, Fe^{2+}, or Al^{2+}.
	Levofloxacin (Levaquin)	Avoid simultaneous oral Mg^{2+}, Fe^{2+}, or Al^{2+}.
	Ceftriaxone (Rocephin)	Once-daily dose advantage over IV options.
Pseudomonas aeruginosa	Ceftazidime (Fortaz, Tazidime) ± ciprofloxacin (Cipro)	May be superior to monotherapy.
	Ciprofloxacin (Cipro)	Convenient oral regimen.
	Ceftazidine (Fortaz, Tazidime) ± tobramycin (Nebcin)	Risk of ototoxicity and nephrotoxicity.
Anaerobes	Clindamycin (Cleocin)	Usually given IV, but also effective orally.
	Metronidazole (Flagyl)	Active only against strict anaerobes.

* Dosages: cefazolin (2 gm IV q8h); ceftriaxone (2 gm IV q24h); ciprofloxacin (750 mg PO q12h); clindamycin (900 mg IV q8h); gentamicin (5 mg/kg/day IV); levofloxacin (500 mg PO q24h); metronidazole (500 mg PO q8h); nafcillin (2 gm IV q4–6h *or* 500 mg/h IV by constant infusion); ofloxacin (400 mg PO q12h); oxacillin (2 gm IV q4–6h *or* 500 mg/h IV by constant infusion); rifampin (if <50 kg, give 300 mg PO q12h; if 50–75 kg, give 300 mg PO q8h; if >75 kg, give 600 mg PO q12h); tobramycin (5 mg/kg/day IV).

how aggressive surgery should be in such patients. In some cases, aggressive surgery may actually hasten amputation. Empirical therapy is often used for less severe cases. Broad-spectrum antimicrobials active against gram-positive and gram-negative aerobes and anaerobes are preferred.

Surgical Management

The latest surgical approaches to osteomyelitis include aggressive soft tissue management and bony reconstruction. In many cases, cure depends more on surgical skill than antimicrobial choice. Marginal surgical excision usually is necessary for cure, but in some cases this may cause major functional loss. Physicians should therefore consider partial excision or chronic suppression in selected cases. Local or systemic host immunocompromise predicts an increased risk of failure. This, along with knowledge of patient lifestyle and functional demands, guides choices between cure or suppression, salvage or amputation.

Local Antibacterial Delivery

Systems for local delivery of antibacterials to bone may overcome limited penetration of systemic agents into poorly vascularized tissues. Antibacterial-loaded polymethylmethacrylate (PMMA) bone cement beads are sometimes used to maintain and sterilize dead space after surgery for chronic osteomyelitis. Antibiotics mixed with liquid PMMA become suspended in the cement as it polymerizes. Aminoglycosides elute most effectively from PMMA, whereas vancomycin elutes much less well. To avoid systemic toxicity in

adults, no more than 17.5 gram of gentamicin or tobramycin should be added to PMMA beads. A disadvantage of using PMMA beads is the need for subsequent surgical removal. Many clinicians consider antibiotic-impregnated cement beads to be adjunctive, rather than a substitute for systemic antimicrobials.

Hyperbaric Oxygen

Hyperbaric oxygen (HBO) has not been definitely shown to be effective for treating chronic osteomyelitis. Nevertheless, there are theoretical reasons why HBO might be beneficial. The greatest potential benefit may be to increase tissue vascularity and enhance bone and soft tissue healing. However, without controlled studies, HBO cannot be recommended for the routine management of osteomyelitis.

COMMON SPORTS INJURIES

method of
BRADFORD H. STILES, M.D.
University of California, San Diego, and Kaiser Permanente San Diego Medical Center San Diego, California

Sports injuries can be classified as either acute (traumatic) or chronic (overuse). Whereas acute injuries usually are caused by a single event, overuse injuries result from the cumulative effects of repetitive microtrauma to muscles and tendons, ligaments, cartilage, and bone. Patients with overuse injuries usually complain of an insidious onset of symptoms that worsen with certain activities.

TABLE 1. **PRICE-MM Management Guidelines**

Protection—avoiding aggravating activity through activity modification or immobilization
Rest—rest from abuse; can be "relative rest" with continued activity that does not aggravate condition
Ice—most effective anti-inflammatory modality; can limit inflammation, decrease edema, and minimize spasm; should be limited to 20 minutes per hour
Compression—limits edema; can be combined with ice in the form of a cold elastic wrap
Elevation—assists in limiting edema; must be above the level of the heart
Medications—includes nonsteroidal anti-inflammatory medications (ibuprofen 200–800 mg q8h, naproxen 250–500 mg q12h); usually function more as analgesics; use as anti-inflammatories is controversial
Modalities—physical therapy, including range-of-motion exercises followed by progressive resistance exercises, electrical stimulation, iontophoresis, and ultrasound therapies

As with any medical problem, diagnosis begins with a thorough history, with attention on the mechanism of injury, if known. This alerts the examiner to potentially serious conditions and helps to avoid common pitfalls. A thorough examination of the injured area helps define the diagnosis further. The joints above and below the injured joint or area should always be examined as well because referred pain is not rare, and external forces damaging one joint may travel up structures such as bone and exit at another joint, leading to further damage. Neurovascular status should always be ascertained with acute injuries.

With most benign, nonemergent musculoskeletal injuries, treatment begins with the PRICE-MM mnemonic (*protection*, *rest*, *ice*, *compression*, *elevation*, *medications*, and *modalities*; Table 1).

MOST COMMON SPORTS INJURIES

Fortunately, the most common sports injuries are minor. Muscle contusions can be a consequence of nearly all sports activities and are characterized by inflammation, hemorrhage, and usually some restriction in the range of motion of the subtended joint. In the acute setting, the amount of hemorrhage in a severely contused muscle should be minimized by keeping the muscle in a stretched position and by the application of ice packs. Large intramuscular hematomas necessitate longer healing periods and may be complicated by myositis ossificans.

Open wounds to the skin (abrasions and lacerations) are also common and usually easily treated. Abrasions should be cleansed and dressed with antibiotic ointment and a dry sterile dressing. Lacerations should be vigorously irrigated to reduce the chance of infection ("the solution to pollution is dilution"), and most can be closed primarily with adhesive strips, sutures, or a skin-bonding agent. The patient's tetanus status should be ascertained and updated as needed.

Injured ligaments are called *sprains*, and injured muscles and tendons are referred to as *strains*. Both sprains and strains can be categorized into three grades. Grade I injuries involve only a few fibers and produce pain on stressing but no joint laxity or loss

of strength. Grade II injuries involve a tear of a significant number of fibers and are involved with laxity and loss of strength, most often secondary to pain. Both grade I and II injuries can usually be treated conservatively following the PRICE-MM guidelines. Rehabilitation through physical therapy is often important for proper healing, and the general time course for complete recovery is 8 to 10 weeks. Grade III injuries are defined as complete tears of either ligaments or muscles, the latter usually at the musculotendinous junction. Initial management of these injuries is the same as for grade I and II injuries, but surgical repair is sometimes required, and early referral should be considered.

SHOULDER INJURIES

The shoulder girdle is a complex structure formed by three joints (glenohumeral or true shoulder joint, acromioclavicular [AC] joint, and sternoclavicular joint) and one articulation (scapulothoracic). These structures work in concert to allow a wide, multidirectional range of motion. The rotator cuff is made up of four muscles: the supraspinatus, infraspinatus, teres minor, and subscapularis (the SITS muscles). In addition to being primary movers of the shoulder joint, the rotator cuff muscles also act as active stabilizers, maintaining the humeral head on the glenoid of the scapula.

Acute strains in the rotator cuff tendons can occur with upper extremity distraction injuries, and overuse injuries can occur with repetitive overhead motions as in throwing or swimming. Pain with resisted external or internal rotation of the humerus or with resistance to a downward force on the arms as they are held at 90 degrees of abduction and 30 degrees of forward flexion with the thumbs pointing downward (empty can test) helps confirm the diagnosis. Treatment involves relative rest, icing, and strengthening exercises. If the offending activities are continued, the rotator cuff muscles become fatigued and lose strength, thereby allowing the humeral head to translate superiorly with overhead motions. An impingement syndrome results as the rotator cuff, primarily the supraspinatus tendon, becomes repetitively pinched between the humeral head and the acromion. The patient usually demonstrates a painful arc between 60 to 120 degrees of abduction. If not treated early, tears of the supraspinatus may result from attrition. Radiographs may be useful to identify a subacromial spur that can impede recovery. Treatment includes avoiding activities that reproduce the pain, oral nonsteroidal anti-inflammatory drugs (NSAIDs) for recent injuries, and subacromial injection of corticosteroid for chronic cases. Rehabilitation exercises to increase flexibility first and strength second are also needed for recovery. These exercises should be continued after recovery is complete to help prevent recurrences.

Injuries to the glenoid labrum can occur acutely, usually from a direct blow to the arm causing the humeral head to impact against the glenoid, or may manifest with a chronic pain pattern from repetitive use, typically seen in throwing athletes. The superior labrum is more commonly involved (SLAP lesion: *s*uperior *l*abrum, *a*nterior and *p*osterior). The patient may complain of a clicking sensation in the shoulder that is somewhat painful, and overhead activities reproduce the pain. Plain radiographs are usually negative, and gadolinium-enhanced magnetic resonance imaging or computed tomographic arthrography is often needed to confirm the diagnosis. Initial treatment should follow the PRICE-MM regimen, but persistent symptoms despite proper treatment should lead to referral to a specialist because surgical repair is often required in these injuries.

Shoulder dislocations occur at the glenohumeral joint. A forced abduction and external rotation can result in an anterior-inferior dislocation (most common) of the humeral head from the glenoid. Reduction is easiest in the first several minutes after the injury before swelling and spasm have set in. Neurovascular status should be documented before and after reduction, and radiographs should be obtained to ensure adequate reduction and rule out an associated fracture. First-time dislocations are usually treated with reduction and maintenance in a sling for 3 weeks. Rehabilitation exercises are begun early, with pendular exercises first, followed by a strengthening program. The recurrence rate in young athletes is high, and repetitive shoulder dislocations lead to chronic instability. Surgical intervention may then be required.

Shoulder separations occur at the AC joint and involve injury to the AC and coracoclavicular ligaments. The mechanism of injury is usually a direct blow to the lateral shoulder, as in a fall with an adducted arm. Several types of AC separations have been described. In first- and second-degree separations, there is still some integrity of the supporting ligaments, and radiographs may show slight displacement of the distal clavicle. Treatment involves a sling for comfort, ice, and early range-of-motion exercises. In third-degree (and higher) injuries, the AC and coracoclavicular ligaments are completely disrupted, resulting in significant disruption of the AC joint. The treatment of third-degree AC separations begins with immobilization, but referral to an orthopedic surgeon should be made because the definitive treatment may necessitate surgery.

ELBOW INJURIES

Lateral epicondylitis ("tennis elbow") and medial epicondylitis ("golfer's elbow") are common overuse sports injuries. Lateral epicondylitis is a painful tendinitis of the common extensor tendon at the lateral epicondyle and is common in patients involved in racquet sports. Poor technique, especially in the backhand stroke, is a common cause. Patients often complain of lateral elbow pain with picking up objects such as a cup of coffee, which can be reproduced on examination with resisted wrist extension. Medial epicondylitis is a painful tendinitis of the common

flexor/pronator origins at the medial epicondyle and is common in racquet sports, bowling, and golf. Treatment of both entities is conservative, with rest, ice, massage, and counterforce bracing. The role of NSAIDs is controversial. An aggressive stretching and strengthening program, however, is the cornerstone to recovery and prevention. Corticosteroid injections for recalcitrant cases of lateral epicondylitis can be effective. An analysis of the patient's swing and form by the local "pro" is also helpful to correct any underlying mechanical faults.

Throwing athletes are at risk for injury to the ulnar collateral ligament due to repetitive valgus stress of the elbow. Medial elbow pain with overhead throwing combined with point tenderness and laxity on examination confirm the diagnosis. Treatment may be conservative, with the PRICE-MM regimen followed by formal rehabilitation. In highly competitive athletes, however, these measures are not as successful, and those wishing to continue to throw often need surgical reconstruction.

"Little Leaguer's elbow" describes a spectrum of overuse injuries in the elbow of a skeletally immature athlete. Treatment begins with cessation of throwing and icing. Continued throwing or failure to recognize the problem may lead to complications such as osteochondritis dissecans. Referral to a specialist should be made for any young throwing athlete with persistent elbow pain if the practitioner is not knowledgeable about this type of injury.

WRIST AND HAND INJURIES

The wrist is easily injured when an athlete falls onto an outstretched hand. Careful history and examination help differentiate minor wrist sprains from more problematic injuries. Fracture of the scaphoid is the most common wrist fracture in the athlete, and delay in diagnosis is associated with a high complication rate. A history consistent with a mechanism of injury combined with tenderness in the anatomic snuffbox on the dorsoradial wrist warrants special attention. If initial radiographs are negative, the wrist should be immobilized in a thumb spica cast, and the patient brought back in 10 to 14 days for reexamination and new radiographs, at which time a fracture may be more evident.

Persistent wrist pain after an injury, despite conservative measures, may be indicative of a ligamentous disruption with resultant instability. Point tenderness over specific carpal ligaments and negative standard radiographs lend support to this diagnosis. A few special provocative examination techniques and special radiographic views (clenched fist, radial and ulnar deviation) may also help. Most of these injuries necessitate surgical correction and should be referred to a hand surgeon.

Forced abduction and dorsiflexion of the thumb at the metacarpophalangeal joint may result in a tear of the ulnar collateral ligament, a condition commonly referred to as gamekeeper's or skier's thumb. Radiographs should be obtained before stressing the joint to rule out an associated avulsion fracture that may become displaced with manipulation. The distinction between partial and complete ligament tears is important. Complete tears are suspected when there is a 30-degree difference in laxity at the metacarpophalangeal joint with stress testing compared with the uninjured side. Complete tears necessitate early surgical correction, whereas partial tears may be treated with a thumb spica cast for 4 weeks, followed by rehabilitation and continued splinting during athletic endeavors.

Mallet finger is frequently seen in ball sports and results from a direct blow to the extended finger. Disruption of the extensor tendon over the distal interphalangeal joint results in a lack of full active extension. Radiographs are needed to rule out an associated fracture or any subluxation. Simple mallet finger may be treated with continuous splinting of the distal interphalangeal joint in extension for 6 to 8 weeks.

Simple dorsal dislocations of the proximal interphalangeal joints of the fingers without associated fractures may by treated with reduction, followed by extension block splinting for 3 weeks. Volar proximal interphalangeal dislocations are less common but often more complex. Postreduction splinting in extension for 6 weeks is required, but referral to a hand surgeon is often required because malrotation problems are frequent. Simple capsular strains of the proximal interphalangeal joints ("jammed finger") may be treated with buddy taping to the adjacent finger until symptoms have resolved.

KNEE INJURIES

Most knee injuries can be initially managed using the PRICE-MM regimen, but early follow-up is required for a more thorough examination after the acute inflammation has lessened. Crutches may be needed initially until the athlete can ambulate without significant pain. Most diagnoses can be made by the history and physical examination, although radiographs are usually obtained to rule out associated injuries or fractures.

The medial collateral ligament is the most commonly injured ligament in the knee, with injury resulting from a direct blow to the lateral knee (valgus stress). Tenderness and edema over the ligament combined with painful laxity on valgus testing confirm the diagnosis. Isolated medial collateral ligament strains usually heal with conservative measures. Grade I and II strains are treated symptomatically. Grade III strains usually necessitate functional bracing with a hinged knee brace for 4 to 6 weeks with appropriate rehabilitation. Surgery is indicated for grossly unstable injuries.

Anterior cruciate ligament tears may result from direct blows to the knee or from noncontact mechanisms, such as a violent twisting injury with a planted foot, or from landing from a jump. The athlete often recalls feeling a "pop" in the knee, and swelling usually occurs within the first few hours.

Diagnosis is confirmed with a positive Lachman test (excessive anterior translation of the tibia on the femur with the knee at 30 degrees of flexion). Radiographs are obtained to rule out associated fracture. Grade I and II injuries can be treated with functional rehabilitation. Grade III injuries are more common, however, and are treated with early bracing and rehabilitation with surgical consultation for reconstruction.

Meniscus tears are the result of a forceful twisting injury or sudden change in direction, common scenarios in sports. A history of such an injury with knee swelling several hours later and complaints of clicking or locking or inability to fully extend the knee suggest a meniscal injury. Initial treatment is with the PRICE-MM protocol with protected weight bearing. Most often, however, the symptoms of recurrent effusion, pain, and inability to perform a full squat persist, and surgical correction is required.

Patellofemoral pain syndrome is a malalignment of the patellar extensor mechanism that produces increased loads on the patellofemoral joint, usually the lateral facet. It is more common in women, and patients complain of worsening pain with activity, especially walking down stairs. They may also relate a history of increased pain with walking after a prolonged sitting period (theater sign). Radiographs should include lateral and sunrise views of both knees to check for patellar positioning. Rehabilitation exercises focusing on stretching of the hamstrings and quadriceps and on strengthening of the vastus medialis obliquus are the key to recovery and prevention.

Iliotibial band syndrome is an overuse injury seen in long-distance runners and cyclists. It is caused by friction between the distal iliotibial band and the lateral femoral epicondyle and causes pain over the lateral knee. Tenderness over the lateral epicondyle of the femur just above the joint line is a common finding. Treatment begins with rest, ice, NSAIDs, and an aggressive stretching program. Recalcitrant cases may necessitate a steroid injection into the underlying bursa.

LEG INJURIES

Medial periostalgia, or "shin splints," is a common overuse injury seen in runners. It is a benign entity but must be distinguished from a more problematic stress fracture. It most often occurs after a recent increase in training activities, as do stress fractures. Patients with medial periostalgia, however, often complain of pain that persists after cessation of exercise, even when not weight bearing. The tenderness of medial periostalgia tends to be diffuse along the medial border of the tibia, whereas stress fractures manifest with more point-specific tenderness. Plain radiographs are often negative in both cases, and a bone scan can help differentiate the two, with periostalgia showing a diffuse increased uptake as opposed to the more focal increased uptake of a stress fracture. Treatment of medial periostalgia includes the

PRICE-MM regimen. Orthotics may be of benefit to athletes with gait disturbances. Training modification is also required. Tibial stress fractures are treated with limitation of activity to promote healing. An anterior cortical stress fracture in the mid-third of the tibia as evidenced by a radiolucent line on the lateral radiograph (the so-called "dreaded black line") is likely to progress to complete fracture and should be treated with non–weight bearing and referral to an orthopedic surgeon.

FOOT AND ANKLE INJURIES

Lateral ankle sprains from inversion injuries are the most common injury in running and jumping sports. They are usually classified as grade I, a partial tear of the anterior talofibular ligament with no instability; grade II, a tear of the anterior talofibular and intact or partial tear of the calcaneofibular ligament with a positive drawer (anterior translation of the talus) sign; and grade III, complete tears of the anterior talofibular and calcaneofibular ligaments with positive drawer and positive talar tilt (excessive subtalar motion) tests. These injuries can be associated with proximal fibula (Maisonneuve) and fifth metatarsal metaphyseal (Jones) fractures, and these areas should be checked for tenderness. Radiographs are mandatory for any patient with malleolar tenderness or the inability to bear weight. Treatment is with the PRICE-MM guidelines, with weight bearing as tolerated, usually with support such as an Air Cast or Cam Walker. Crutch or cane support is sometimes required early in treatment. Rehabilitation focuses on early range-of-motion, followed by strengthening and then proprioception exercises.

Plantar fasciitis has an insidious onset and is a common cause of heel pain in athletes involved in running sports. Pain and tenderness usually center around the plantar fascial origin on the medial calcaneal tubercle, but may be anywhere along the plantar fascia. Pain with the first few steps in the morning is pathognomonic. Improper shoe wear and biomechanical imbalances are usually the cause. Treatment focuses on stretching of the plantar fascia and correction of underlying gait abnormalities with orthotics. Posterior night splints that keep the foot in mild dorsiflexion can help reduce symptoms. Recalcitrant cases often benefit from corticosteroid injection.

"Turf toe" is described as a hyperflexion injury to the first metatarsophalangeal joint with injury to the plantar plate. The resulting pain, especially with the toe-off phase of gait, can be debilitating. Treatment follows PRICE-MM guidelines with subsequent taping. More severe cases may necessitate a stiff-soled shoe for 2 to 4 weeks.

Morton's neuroma is seen in runners and is most common in the web space between the third and fourth toes. A vague forefoot pain that gradually progresses to a burning sensation with radiating pain to the toes is the usual history. A painful, palpable click with compression of the metatarsal heads can be elicited on examination. Treatment consists of a metatarsal pad placed just proximal to the metatarsal heads or orthotics with a metatarsal pad. NSAIDs can also be effective. If symptoms persist, corticosteroid injection is an option. Surgical resection is sometimes required.

Section 15

Obstetrics and Gynecology

ANTEPARTUM CARE

method of
FAITH JOY FRIEDEN, M.D.
Englewood Hospital and Medical Center
Englewood, New Jersey
Mt. Sinai School of Medicine
New York, New York

Pregnancy offers the health care provider a window of opportunity to positively influence the health of today's women and tomorrow's children. Although the cornerstone of treatment during this unique time period is antepartum care, the ideal time to begin is before conception. At a preconception visit, a basic history should be obtained and a physical examination performed, along with a risk assessment. Special areas of concern include pre-existing maternal medical conditions, medication use, family history of birth defects, carrier screening for inherited diseases, occupational hazards, and recreational drug use, including cigarettes and alcohol. This visit provides an opportunity to determine susceptibility to infectious diseases, such as toxoplasmosis, cytomegalovirus infection, varicella, rubella, and human immunodeficiency virus (HIV) infection, and to vaccinate as appropriate. When risk factors are identified, the patient can be advised of the potential consequences. In some situations (such as uncontrolled diabetes, recent vaccination, recent viral infection, or potentially teratogenic exposure), pregnancy can be postponed until the risk factor is managed and the risk reduced.

ROUTINE CARE

Normal Duration of Pregnancy

Human pregnancy has a duration of 280 days (40 weeks). By convention, duration is measured from the first day of the last menstrual period to the expected delivery date. The count is based on the occurrence of ovulation on day 14 of a 28-day menstrual cycle and therefore reflects menstrual weeks, not conceptional weeks.

Initial Prenatal Visit

At the initial prenatal visit, a thorough history is obtained, including age, menstrual history, prior obstetric history, past medical and surgical history, family history, genetic screening, medication or drug use, and history of exposure to infections (e.g., tuberculosis, hepatitis B, genital herpes, HIV infection, sexually transmitted diseases). Any risk factors identified should be addressed and incorporated into the plan of care for the pregnancy. Certain obstetric conditions, such as prior preterm birth, recurrent pregnancy loss, or pre-eclampsia remote from term, have been associated with a relatively high recurrence risk compared with that in women with no such history.

Medical conditions, such as diabetes, hypertension, lupus, asthma, or a seizure disorder, must be stabilized as quickly as possible. When counseling the pregnant woman with an underlying medical disorder, we must consider the effects of the medical condition on a pregnancy and the effects of pregnancy on the woman's health. We also must weigh the risk of medication compared with the risks of not treating the condition. The general rule of thumb is that the best thing for a healthy baby is a healthy mother. Many medications are available that are not known to incur any increased risk of birth defects above the background risk in the general population.

The initial physical examination should include a general physical examination as well as a pelvic examination. The prepregnancy height and weight are recorded, along with the initial vital signs. It is important to perform a thorough examination at this time because many women have not had a physical examination before becoming pregnant. Also, at subsequent prenatal visits, less emphasis is placed on nonobstetric areas in the absence of complaints. The pelvic examination should include assessment of the cervix, uterus size, and adnexa, as well as a clinical impression of the adequacy of the pelvis. At this time, a Papanicolaou smear and culture for gonorrhea and chlamydial infection are done.

The initial laboratory evaluation includes blood studies for blood type, Rh and antibody screen, hemoglobin and hematocrit, and serologic tests for hepatitis B, rubella, and syphilis. Urine is checked for protein and glucose, and a sample is sent for culture. The American College of Obstetricians and Gynecologists (ACOG) recommends that all pregnant women receive counseling about HIV and that testing be recommended as part of routine prenatal care. In some states, health care providers are required by law to offer HIV testing to all pregnant women. Depending on the patient's ethnic background or family history, it may be appropriate to send blood for hemoglobin electrophoresis (to check for sickle cell or thalassemia trait) or carrier testing for other inherited disorders (such as Tay-Sachs and cystic fibrosis).

Follow-up Prenatal Visits

In general, prenatal visits are repeated every 4 weeks until 28 weeks of pregnancy, then every 2 to 3 weeks until 36 weeks, and then weekly until delivery. Of course, this should be individualized to the patient, and more frequent visits may be appropriate. The purpose of each prenatal visit is to assess maternal and fetal well-being. Therefore, in a systematic fashion at each visit, the patient's weight and blood pressure are recorded, along with the presence or absence of edema. A urine dipstick test is performed to check protein and glucose levels. The height of the uterine fundus is measured, and fetal heart tones are recorded. Usually, the fetal heart rate can be auscultated with a Doppler device by 12 weeks. The patient is also asked about the perception of fetal movement, which is usually apparent by 20 weeks.

Subsequent Laboratory Evaluations

Specific assessments of maternal and fetal well-being are performed throughout pregnancy, as appropriate to the gestational age. At approximately 16 weeks, patients are offered biochemical marker screening, also known as maternal serum alpha-fetoprotein or triple screen. This test increases the detection of certain fetal abnormalities, such as open fetal defects and certain chromosomal abnormalities. Further laboratory evaluations are performed at 28 weeks, including a glucose challenge test for gestational diabetes, assays for hemoglobin and hematocrit, and blood antibody screening and repeat testing for syphilis, if indicated. If the patient is Rh negative and unsensitized, she should receive Rh immunoglobulin (RhoGAM) at this time. At 35 to 37 weeks, a vaginal and rectal culture can be obtained for group B *Streptococcus,* in anticipation of possible treatment at delivery.

Nutrition in Pregnancy

Pregnant women should increase their daily caloric intake by approximately 300 kcal. Total weight gain should be 25 to 35 pounds for women of normal prepregnancy weight with a singleton gestation. Pregnant women should receive 30 mg of ferrous iron supplements daily. Folic acid supplementation is advised both on a hematologic basis and to decrease certain birth defects. The amount found in prenatal vitamins (1 mg) is sufficient for most women. For women at increased risk for neural tube defects, however, the recommended dose is 4 mg of folate starting before conception and continuing through the 12th week of gestation.

Common Complaints

Nausea and vomiting frequently complicate early pregnancy. Nonpharmacologic remedies include frequent small feedings and avoidance of spicy foods. Several medications have been used as well, including diphenhydramine (Benadryl), metoclopramide (Reglan), prochlorperazine (Compazine), promethazine (Phenergan), and trimethobenzamide (Tigan). One of the newer treatment modalities that has met with considerable success is continuous infusion of metoclopramide via a subcutaneous infusion pump.

Heartburn is a frequent problem, which occurs owing to relaxation of the esophageal sphincter with reflux of gastric contents into the lower esophagus. Patients should avoid spicy foods and lying completely flat. Antacids may be helpful, especially in liquid form that coats the lining of the esophagus.

Constipation occurs as a result of smooth muscle relaxation and delayed bowel transit time. It can usually be treated successfully with dietary modification, incorporating increased fruits, vegetables, and water. Stool softeners may also be helpful.

ENVIRONMENTAL HAZARDS AND EXPOSURES

When considering the teratogenic potential of an exposure, the physician must keep in mind the 3% background risk of major birth defects in the general obstetric population. Only a small percentage of birth defects can actually be linked to a known agent. Examples include such infectious agents as rubella virus and *Toxoplasma gondii;* drugs such as alcohol, thalidomide, and isotretinoin; chemicals such as lead, organic mercury, and organic solvents; and physical agents such as ionizing radiation and hyperthermia.

PRENATAL DIAGNOSIS

The purpose of prenatal diagnosis is to gather information with which to optimize medical care and to enable the patient to make informed reproductive decisions. Our responsibility as health care providers is to assess the risks unique to each pregnancy, convey that information to the patient, and guide her through the testing process while allowing her to choose a course of action that is right for her. This "nondirective" approach, based on the principle of patient autonomy, is critical to the process of genetic counseling and prenatal diagnosis.

Carrier Screening

There are several autosomal recessive disorders that occur with increased frequency in certain ethnic groups. Carrier detection should be offered whenever one or both expectant parents belong to the group at increased risk. The most frequently encountered of these conditions are Tay-Sachs disease in the Ashkenazi Jewish population, sickle cell disease in the African-American population, and the thalassemias in people of Mediterranean and Asian descent. Cystic fibrosis is the most common serious autosomal recessive disorder in the Caucasian population. The role of routine testing for carrier detection is controversial, however, owing to the over 700 different known mutations, the relatively high false-negative rate in certain populations, and the resultant difficulty in post-test counseling.

Biochemical Marker Screening

As previously mentioned, maternal serum screening is offered at approximately 16 weeks of gestation. This test generally evaluates three markers, namely, alpha-fetoprotein (AFP), human chorionic gonadotropin, and unconjugated estriol. AFP is produced by the fetus and is present in high concentrations in the amniotic fluid and, to a lesser extent, in maternal serum. Elevated levels of maternal serum AFP have been associated with open neural tube defects, ventral wall defects, renal abnormalities, multiple gestation, certain skin disorders, maternal tumors, fetal demise, placental abnormality, and otherwise unexplained adverse perinatal outcome. Low levels of maternal serum AFP have been associated with Down syndrome. The addition of the other two markers enhances the detection rate from 25% with AFP alone to approximately 60% with all three. Analysis of all three is especially useful for younger women, who might not otherwise pursue prenatal diagnosis. In the event of an abnormal result, patients are offered ultrasonography for confirmation of gestational age and for anatomic survey. They also have the option of amniocentesis for direct assessment of the fetal chromosomes and AFP level.

Amniocentesis and Chorionic Villus Sampling

Genetic amniocentesis is the most commonly performed invasive prenatal diagnostic procedure. It is generally performed at 15 to 20 weeks. Although it is performed under ultrasound guidance with sterile technique, it still carries a pregnancy loss rate attributable to the procedure of approximately 0.5%. The amniotic fluid is sent to a laboratory for fetal karyotyping and AFP determination, although other specific genetic testing can also be performed.

An alternative to traditional amniocentesis is chorionic villus sampling (CVS), which allows for a first-trimester diagnosis. CVS can be performed at 10 to 12 weeks with a transabdominal or transcervical approach. It should be noted that the pregnancy loss rate is approximately 0.8% higher with CVS than with traditional amniocentesis, according to a large multicenter trial conducted by the National Institute of Child Health and Human Development. Another drawback is that AFP cannot be measured in villi. It is conceivable, therefore, that an amniocentesis might be necessary later to evaluate an elevated maternal serum AFP level. Subsequent amniocentesis could also be indicated to clarify an ambiguous CVS finding, which occurs in approximately 1% of cases.

Fetal Blood Sampling

There are times when it becomes necessary to sample fetal blood directly for rapid karyotyping, evaluation for fetal infection, or prenatal diagnosis of platelet disorders. This technique of accessing fetal blood via the umbilical cord is known as *percutaneous umbilical blood sampling*. This procedure has an estimated fetal loss rate of 1% to 2%.

ANTEPARTUM TESTING

Ultrasonography

There are a variety of noninvasive techniques for evaluating fetal health. The most powerful tool in our armamentarium, and perhaps the most controversial, is diagnostic ultrasonography. Ultrasound technology has fundamentally altered the practice of obstetrics and refined the art of prenatal diagnosis. Its clinical utility is under constant scrutiny, analysis, and expansion. Although there is an academic controversy as to whether routine ultrasound screening is useful or cost-effective in low-risk pregnancies, this tool is almost universal in the United States. Therefore, the safety, indications, and testing terminology must be well understood by the health care team.

At present, exposure to diagnostic ultrasound imaging is not associated with any harmful biologic effects. Studies of in utero exposure have found no significant differences between exposed offspring and their nonexposed siblings. It is still incumbent on every ultrasound practitioner to keep energy exposures "as low as reasonably achievable" (the ALARA principle).

In 1984, the National Institutes of Health released a list of 27 indications for ultrasonography during pregnancy. These include gestational age determination, assessment of fetal growth, vaginal bleeding, suspected amniotic fluid abnormality, abnormal biochemical screening, history of previous congenital anomaly, and guidance for invasive procedures.

Most pregnancy ultrasound studies can be described as basic, comprehensive, or limited. A basic examination provides the following information: fetal number, presentation, documentation of cardiac activity, placental location, assessment of amniotic fluid volume, assessment of gestational age, survey of fetal anatomy for gross malformations, and evaluation for maternal pelvic masses.

A comprehensive ultrasound examination is indicated for a fetus at increased risk, as determined by history, clinical evaluation, or prior ultrasound examination. It is usually performed at approximately 20 weeks of gestation and encompasses a more detailed anatomic survey and therefore demands a higher level of expertise than that for the basic scan.

A limited examination is desirable under certain circumstances when only a specific or urgently needed bit of information is sought. Such circumstances include ultrasound guidance for amniocentesis, confirmation of fetal cardiac activity, confirmation of fetal presentation, placental localization in the presence of bleeding, and biophysical profile testing.

Nonstress Test

The nonstress test is a simple, noninvasive method of monitoring fetal well-being by recording fetal heart rate patterns along with the maternal perception of fetal movement. It is based on the premise that the heart rate of a nonacidotic or neurologically depressed fetus accelerates in response to fetal movement. If two or more accelerations of 15 beats per minute, lasting for 15 seconds, are present in a 20-minute period, then the test is considered "reactive" or normal. The major pitfall of this test is the high false-positive rate because "non-reactivity" is more likely to be associated with a fetal sleep cycle than with actual central nervous system depression.

Biophysical Profile

Biophysical profile testing combines multiple biophysical parameters to assess fetal well-being in an attempt to more accurately identify the compromised fetus. It is composed of the nonstress test and four parameters evaluated by ultrasonography, namely, fetal breathing movement, fetal body movement, fetal tone, and amniotic fluid volume.

MEDICAL COMPLICATIONS

Diabetes Mellitus

Diabetes in pregnancy encompasses two very different groups of women: diabetic women who become pregnant and pregnant women who become diabetic. The former group, although smaller in number, is more significant in terms of the impact on a pregnancy. Preconception counseling is most important for this group. With a two- to fourfold increase in the risk of major malformations in infants of diabetic mothers, congenital malformations are the most important cause of perinatal loss in these pregnancies. The organ systems most frequently affected are the cardiovascular, skeletal, and central nervous systems. It has been demonstrated repeatedly that excellent glycemic control at the time of conception and organogenesis can dramatically reduce this risk. Fetal overgrowth due to maternal hyperglycemia can be another complication; delivery of excessively large infants occurs up to 10 times more often in diabetic women than in the nondiabetic population. If maternal blood glucose levels are not controlled adequately, these newborns are also subject to metabolic derangements, including hypoglycemia, magnesium deficiency, and hyperbilirubinemia, as well as respiratory distress and polycythemia. When the diabetes is associated with vasculopathy, such as nephropathy or retinopathy, then the fetus is at risk for intrauterine growth restriction.

Therefore, it is essential that diabetic women maintain meticulous glycemic control, adhering to an appropriate diet and monitoring blood glucose levels from four to seven times daily. Target values are fasting glucose levels of 60 to 90 mg/dL and 1-hour postprandial values of 120 to 140 mg/dL. In addition, it is useful to evaluate the glycosylated hemoglobin levels of these women, which indicate the overall level of control for the preceding 6 weeks. Fetal well-being is assessed with ultrasonography and echocardiography in the second trimester and with nonstress tests and biophysical profile examinations in the third trimester. Owing to the increased risk of adverse perinatal outcome in these pregnancies, delivery is usually recommended at term, as soon as fetal lung maturity is ensured.

Approximately 3% of pregnant women develop carbohydrate intolerance, or gestational diabetes, during the latter part of pregnancy. Because roughly half of these women have no identifiable risk factors, it is good practice to screen all pregnant women for this condition at 28 weeks with the 1-hour 50-gram oral glucose challenge test. If this result is elevated, then the 3-hour 100-gram oral glucose tolerance test is performed. Gestational diabetes is subsequently diagnosed in approximately 15% of women who screen positive. The mainstay of management is diet with self-monitoring of blood glucose level, in most cases four times daily (fasting and 1 hour after meals). If the target glucose values cannot be reached and maintained with this regimen, then insulin therapy may be necessary. Although carbohydrate intolerance should resolve after delivery, gestational diabetic patients should know that they have a 50% chance of becoming diabetic later in life.

Hypertension

Hypertensive disorders of pregnancy complicate approximately 6% of pregnancies in the United States and rank second only to thromboembolic disease as a cause of maternal mortality. In addition, there is an impact on perinatal outcome, attributable to both intrauterine effects of the condition and preterm delivery for worsening maternal disease.

Normally, first-trimester blood pressure reflects the baseline value. It should fall somewhat during the second trimester and return to baseline values in the third trimester. Therefore, it is imperative to check a pregnant woman's blood pressure at each prenatal visit to establish her baseline and to identify any changes, especially in the third trimester, that may indicate a pathologic process.

SURGERY IN PREGNANCY

When the physician is faced with the decision of whether a pregnant woman should undergo an operation, the risks of surgery must be weighed against the risks of conservative management, keeping in mind that the sequelae of nonintervention could actually be more severe in a pregnant patient. If surgery is performed, a general rule of thumb is to minimize uterine manipulation to minimize the risk for preterm labor. Cesarean section should be reserved for obstetric indications.

Appendicitis is the most common nonobstetric emergency that occurs during pregnancy. The diagnosis is complicated by the overlap of the symptoms of appendicitis with some common symptoms in pregnancy. In addition, the position of the appendix becomes higher as pregnancy advances, making it more difficult to pinpoint the source of the pain. Maternal and fetal complications are directly associated with advanced disease and delay in treatment. Therefore, once acute appendicitis is suspected in pregnancy, emergency surgery should be performed. To lower maternal and fetal morbidity, we accept a higher negative exploration rate than in the nonpregnant population.

Gallbladder disease is the second most common nonobstetric surgical condition in pregnancy, usually presenting with right upper quadrant pain, nausea, and vomiting. Medical management includes bedrest, no oral feedings, intravenous fluids for hydration, and antibiotics. When attacks are recurrent or if the patient develops an acute abdomen, cholecystectomy should be performed.

TRAUMA IN PREGNANCY

Trauma and violence are the leading causes of death in women of reproductive age. The first priority when encountering a pregnant trauma victim is treatment and stabilization of the woman. Only then should attention be directed to the fetus. Pregnancy should not alter the necessary evaluation and treatment. It cannot be overstated that necessary radiographic studies should be performed without delay, with efforts made to minimize the dose to the lower abdomen. A systematic approach to evaluation should be utilized, consisting of the "ABCs": airway, breathing, and circulation. There are some considerations unique to pregnancy. The patient should be tilted or wedged in the left lateral position, thus deflecting the uterus off the inferior vena cava and aorta. The pregnant trauma victim requires a greater volume of blood replacement to maintain her cardiovascular integrity than a nonpregnant patient. In gestations beyond 20 weeks, electronic monitoring for uterine contractions, as well as fetal heart rate, is helpful in evaluation for placental abruption and other injury.

Motor vehicle accidents are a significant source of trauma and death, especially when the victim is ejected from the car. The three-point lap belt/shoulder harness restraint is superior to the lap belt alone in preventing maternal and fetal injury.

Perhaps the most insidious form of trauma in pregnancy is domestic violence. The actual incidence is not known, but it is estimated that nearly one fourth of women in the United States are abused by a current or former partner sometime in their lives. Because obstetricians are the primary care providers for many women, they are in a unique position to identify women who are victims of abuse and to offer them help. If an abusive relationship is identified, then the woman should be encouraged to leave the violent situation, and she should be referred to appropriate agencies to protect herself and her children.

OBSTETRIC COMPLICATIONS

Preterm Birth

Preterm birth, occurring before the completion of 37 weeks of gestation, complicates 9% of all births in the United States and accounts for 75% of the neonatal deaths that are not due to congenital malformations. Despite the advent of new diagnostic and therapeutic modalities, the preterm birth rate has not changed since the late 1950s. This may be largely due to the multifaceted nature of this problem.

Approximately one third of such births are iatrogenic in that they are indicated because of medical or obstetric disorders that place the mother or fetus at increased risk, such as hypertension, diabetes, hemorrhage, or intrauterine growth restriction. The remaining two thirds are attributed to preterm labor, preterm premature rupture of membranes, and cervical incompetence. Some current therapies directed at early diagnosis and treatment include home uterine activity monitoring, tocolytic therapy, ultrasonographic measurements of cervical length, and assays of fetal fibronectin levels in cervicovaginal secretions. When preterm birth is imminent, delivery in a setting with appropriate neonatal intensive care available optimizes perinatal outcome.

Prolonged Pregnancy

A postdate or post-term pregnancy is defined as one that has reached 42 weeks after the last menstrual period. Perinatal morbidity and mortality increase dramatically after 40 weeks and especially after 42 weeks. Possible maternal complications include an increased incidence of cesarean section, hemorrhage, and trauma due to fetal macrosomia. Potential problems of these neonates include birth trauma from macrosomia and meconium aspiration. Good outcomes can be expected with accurate dating, careful fetal surveillance, and intervention when indicated.

Multiple Gestations

The incidence of twinning in the United States is approximately 1.2% of all pregnancies. With the increased use of assisted reproduction technologies, the incidence of higher order multiple gestations (triplets and higher) is approximately 0.3%. These pregnancies pose special concerns for management of the mother as well as the fetuses.

Increased maternal risks include an increased strain on the cardiovascular system, pulmonary edema, pre-eclampsia, anemia, complications related to tocolysis, and delivery complications. The greatest fetal risk is that of prematurity. In addition, when identical twin fetuses have a single placenta and a shared placental circulation, there is a significant risk for twin-twin transfusion syndrome, a potentially fatal complication of twinning. Early diagnosis of multiple gestations, frequent check-ups to monitor maternal health, serial ultrasound examinations to assess fetal growth and well-being, reduced maternal activity level, prompt treatment of preterm labor, close intrapartum surveillance, and appropriate neonatal personnel in the delivery room all contribute to optimizing the outcome of these pregnancies.

INFECTIONS

Certain perinatal infections, such as toxoplasmosis, cytomegalovirus infection, human parvovirus B19 infection, rubella, varicella, and syphilis, have a potential for teratogenicity or fetal loss. Some infections have the potential for other adverse perinatal sequelae. For example, vertical transmission of hepatitis B has been demonstrated. Group B beta-hemolytic *Streptococcus,* although a frequent component of vaginal flora, is one of the most common and dangerous perinatal pathogens in susceptible newborns, mandating intrapartum prophylaxis in high-risk settings. Genital herpes can colonize newborns during passage through an infected birth canal. Chorioamnionitis, or bacterial infection of the amniotic cavity and membranes, is an important cause of perinatal morbidity and mortality, best treated with intrapartum antibiotics and delivery. There is increasing evidence that exposure to such intrauterine infection may be associated with an increased risk of cerebral palsy.

Special attention must be paid to HIV infection, which is estimated to complicate 7000 pregnancies per year in the United States. HIV testing should be offered to all pregnant women in light of the findings of the landmark study Pediatric AIDS [acquired immunodeficiency syndrome] Clinical Trials Group 076. This study demonstrated a significant reduction in mother-to-infant transmission of the virus, from 26% in the placebo group to 8% in the group taking zidovudine (ZDV) (Retrovir). According to this protocol, prophylactic ZDV therapy is given to HIV-positive women starting at 14 weeks and continued throughout pregnancy in an oral dose of 100 mg five times daily. During labor, it is given intravenously in a 1-hour loading dose of 2 mg per kg of maternal body weight, followed by a continuous infusion of 1 mg per kg of maternal body weight every hour until delivery. The neonate is then given ZDV syrup at a dose of 2 mg per kg body weight every 6 hours for the first 6 weeks of life.

Other risk factors may affect perinatal transmission. Prolonged fetal exposure to ruptured membranes, fetal scalp sampling, fetal scalp electrodes, and any other fetal abrasions should be avoided. Breast-feeding is contraindicated for HIV-positive women because this also increases transmission.

There are new multiple antiretroviral regimens for the treatment of HIV infection and AIDS. Although data are limited on their use in pregnancy, the drugs should be administered as necessary for the life and well-being of the mother and certainly should not be avoided, especially after the first trimester, when organogenesis is completed.

FETAL THERAPY

With improved prenatal diagnosis and the resultant opportunity for antenatal therapy, the concept of the fetus as a patient has emerged. Fetal therapy has taken two main forms, pharmacologic manipulation of the fetal environment via maternal medication that crosses the placenta and the exciting and challenging new frontier of fetal surgery. Perhaps the most frequently utilized form of in utero therapy is maternal administration of betamethasone (Celestone),* a corticosteroid, for the purpose of accelerating fetal lung maturity when delivery is anticipated before 34 weeks of gestation. The recommended dosage is 12 mg given by intramuscular injection for 2 doses, 24 hours apart. Maternally administered antiarrhythmics, such as digoxin, are useful in treating certain fetal cardiac arrhythmias that, if left untreated, may lead to fetal congestive heart failure. Another striking example of in utero drug therapy is the use of dexamethasone* in pregnancies at risk for congenital adrenal hyperplasia to prevent the external genital masculinization of affected female fetuses.

When fetal anemia is suspected as a cause of fetal hydrops, such as in cases of certain congenital infections or hemolytic disease due to Rh or other maternal blood group antibodies, the fetal circulation can be accessed through percutaneous umbilical blood sampling. This allows for measurement of the fetal hematocrit, as well as direct intravascular fetal transfusion. A few fetal treatment centers in the country have used fetal surgery successfully to treat such conditions as obstructive uropathy, congenital diaphragmatic hernia, and spina bifida.

ETHICAL ISSUES

As medical technology advances, it inevitably raises new questions regarding when and how to apply the technology in clinical practice. Ethical principles require full disclosure of the diagnosis, prognosis, and management alternatives. The wishes of the pregnant woman, who still retains autonomy, must always be respected. An even more perplexing ethical question is how to handle fetal-fetal conflicts, such as in the case of twins with competing interests, when surgery or delivery of the affected twin will jeopardize the unaffected one. Such cases are optimally managed by carefully balancing these concerns and striving for the safety of both fetuses.

Given all the facets of antepartum care discussed, it is clear why physicians who care for pregnant

---

*Not FDA approved for this indication.

women play a pivotal role in guiding them through this most important time.

ECTOPIC PREGNANCY

method of
BRYAN D. COWAN, M.D.
University of Mississippi
Jackson, Mississippi

The incidence of hospital admissions for ectopic pregnancy in the United States has been tracked since 1970. During this time, both the incidence and number of ectopic pregnancies have increased almost linearly. Currently, the rate of ectopic pregnancy is estimated to be approximately 20 per 1000 live births (2%). Depending on the source and methods used to track this condition, ectopic pregnancy is rated as the third or fourth leading cause of maternal mortality in the United States and is the leading cause of maternal death during the first trimester. Fortunately, deaths due to ectopic pregnancy have decreased since the 1970s and are now estimated to occur at a rate of approximately 0.8 per 1000 ectopic pregnancies, or 14 per 100,000 live births. Nonetheless, 20 to 50 women die annually from the complications of ectopic pregnancy. Risk factors associated with ectopic pregnancy are principally related to acquired pelvic abnormalities. As a rule, patients with acquired risk for ectopic pregnancy have a fivefold (10%) risk of ectopic pregnancy (Table 1). However, one unique condition is associated with a 50% risk for ectopic pregnancy (prior sterilization). The recognition of this high occurrence of ectopic pregnancy requires special concern and evaluation for patients with abdominal/pelvic pain after sterilization.

DIAGNOSIS

Before the development of sensitive biochemical screening tests and sonography, clinical signs and symptoms were the only tools for evaluation of suspected ectopic pregnancies. Today, modern strategies use biochemical screening and pelvic visualization to evaluate both symptomatic and asymptomatic patients known to be at risk for ectopic pregnancy. Nonetheless, clinicians must be familiar with the signs and symptoms of ectopic pregnancy. When symptoms occur during the development of an ectopic pregnancy, pain accompanies nearly 100% of them. Unfortunately, abdominal/pelvic pain is common in women of reproductive age and is seen frequently in the emergency and office settings. Thus, it is critical to consider the possibility of pregnancy in women of reproductive age who seek medical attention for evaluation of pain regardless of the

TABLE 1. Risk Factors for Ectopic Pregnancy

Risk Factor	Approximate Incidence
General population	2%
Pelvic infection	10%
Previous tubal surgery	10%
Previous ectopic pregnancy	10%
Prior sterilization	50%
Gamete technologies	5%

TABLE 2. Minimal Human Chorionic Gonadotropin in Normal Pregnancy

Interval Day	Minimum Human Chorionic Gonadotropin
1	33%
2	66%
3	110%
4	175%
5	255%

Modified from Kadar in Caldwell BV, Romero R: A method of screening for ectopic pregnancy and its indications. Obstet Gynecol 58:162–166, 1991.

patient's reported sexual, contraceptive, or menstrual history.

Pregnancy is confirmed by measurement of urinary or serum human chorionic gonadotropin (hCG). Although we commonly describe this test as "beta hCG," this is a reference to old methodology by which the beta subunit of hCG was specifically tested. Current clinical assays measure intact hCG to provide a true measurement of the hCG molecule. Pregnancy testing, whether urine or serum, is widely available and inexpensive. To complement the nominal results from hCG testing (pregnant or not pregnant), hCG quantitation can substantially improve our ability to assess early gestational complications. During the first 40 days of pregnancy, hCG rises geometrically and on average doubles every 2 days. In general, 90% of patients with normal hCG increments have a normal intrauterine gestation, and patients with abnormal or low hCG increments have an abnormal gestation in approximately 75 to 80% of cases. Unfortunately, abnormal hCG increments cannot distinguish between an ectopic gestation and an impending intrauterine spontaneous abortion. In addition, the assignment of "normal" or "abnormal" hCG increments should not be based on an average hCG doubling time. The clinically important information is the minimal increment associated with normal pregnancies. Kadar (1981) described minimal increments associated with normal pregnancies at intervals from 1 to 5 days (Table 2). For example, an hCG increment of 66% or more in 2 days would be consistent with a normal pregnancy. An hCG increment below these established thresholds is considered abnormal.

In addition to biochemical screening with hCG, multiple retrospective case series analyses have suggested that ectopic pregnancy can be predicted from a single progesterone measurement. Evidence from these reports provides wide ranges for the best discriminatory serum progesterone levels. Like hCG, serum progesterone cannot discriminate between an intrauterine and an ectopic pregnancy.

Measurements of hCG or serum progesterone in the evaluation of patients with suspected ectopic pregnancy are classified as predictive, but not diagnostic. Confirmation of ectopic pregnancy is established by visualizing a gestational sac in an extrauterine location. This can be accomplished by sonography, surgery, or histopathologic evaluation.

To aid in the evaluation of ectopic pregnancy, hCG measurements have been used to establish a "discriminatory" zone. Serum progesterone does not demonstrate similar efficacy. When hCG concentrations are at or above a discriminatory zone (between 1000 and 2000 mIU per mL, depending on the reference preparation of hCG measurements and the sophistication of the sonography equipment), the observer expects to see an intrauterine gestation. When sonography fails to detect an intrauterine gestation at or above the discriminatory hCG zone, a presumptive diagnosis of ectopic pregnancy is correct in more than 90% of cases. Nonetheless, twin gestations, clinical variations, differences in observer skills, and laboratory errors contribute to a low but troubling rate of false interpretations. Other methods of confirmation include endometrial biopsy, uterine curettage, and surgery. Usually, these tools are used when a diagnosis must be urgently established to evaluate the symptomatic patient.

TREATMENT

Three options are available for the treatment of confirmed or presumed ectopic pregnancy. Variables that influence selection include patient symptoms, physician preferences, and patient acceptance. The three treatment options are surgery, cytotoxic chemotherapy (almost universally methotrexate), and expectant management.

Trends in surgical treatment of ectopic pregnancy show that an increasing number of patients are treated with laparoscopy. Nonetheless, whether surgery is performed by laparotomy or laparoscopy, the best evidence suggests that most patients are treated with nonconservative salpingectomy. Conservative surgery involves creating a salpingostomy on the tube and removing only the gestational sac, or segmental resection of a small portion of tube that contains the gestational sac. After salpingostomy, the risk of persistent trophoblast ranges from 2 to 7%. Therefore, these patients should have hCG concentrations measured until the value is below pregnancy levels.

The decision to perform laparoscopy or laparotomy is influenced by the state of the patient and physician preference. The decision to perform conservative versus extirpative surgery depends on the damage evoked by the ectopic pregnancy on the ipsilateral tube, the location of the ectopic pregnancy, the status of the contralateral tube, and the patient's future desire for pregnancy.

Despite the enthusiasm for medical chemotherapy, the critical factor that determines suitability for this treatment is the absence of pain. Ectopic pregnancy produces pain from either distention of the fallopian tube or spillage of blood into the peritoneum. Because 20 to 50 days is required for complete resolution after methotrexate therapy (depending on the initial hCG titer), patients with clinically important pain must be classified as having "impending rupture" and are not considered candidates for methotrexate. However, those patients with confirmed or presumed ectopic pregnancy who have no clinically important pain can be treated with methotrexate. Criteria for use of methotrexate have been suggested by the American College of Obstetricians and Gynecologists (Table 3). These criteria (and others) suggest that the ectopic pregnancy should be small and that the patient should be clinically stable and desire a future pregnancy.

There are over 12 protocols reported that administer a wide variety of methotrexate doses using three different routes of administration. There are no ran-

TABLE 3. **Recommended Selection Criteria for Medical Therapy for Ectopic Pregnancy**

Indications include the following:
  Ectopic gestational sac size <3 cm
  Desire for future fertility
  Stable or rising human chorionic gonadotropin levels, with peak values below 15,000 mIU/mL
  Tubal serosa intact
  No active bleeding
  Ectopic pregnancy fully visualized at laparoscopy
  Selected cases of cervical and cornual pregnancy
  No cardiac activity in the gestational sac
Contraindications to chemotherapy include the following:
  Poor patient compliance
  History of active hepatic or renal disease
  Presence of fetal cardiac activity
  Abnormal serum creatinine or aspartate aminotransferase
  Active peptic ulcer disease
  Blood leukocyte count of <3000 cells/mm³ or a platelet count of <100,000 cells/mm³

From ACOG Technical Bulletin 150, December, 1990.

domized, clinical trials comparing the efficacy of one medical treatment protocol with another. Two treatment protocols are the most popular. Single-dose methotrexate involves 50 mg per m² as a single dose, followed by the assessment of hCG concentrations. Repeat methotrexate is administered if the hCG concentration 7 days after methotrexate is not 20% lower than the hCG concentration obtained 4 days after methotrexate. With this treatment protocol, the original treatment success rate was 92 to 94%. However, subsequent studies with this regimen have reported lower success rates that range between 65 and 82%. An alternative treatment protocol uses 1 mg/kg on alternate days. Treatment efficacy from this protocol has also been reported at 92 to 94%.

Finally, expectant management has been used in selected patients. Women with known ectopic pregnancies have been observed, and in nearly 70%, the ectopic pregnancy resolved without intervention. Unfortunately, there are few criteria to select for observation, but one of the criteria may be falling hCG levels in patients who have no or limited pain.

Most studies reporting fertility outcome after treatment of ectopic pregnancy demonstrate a pregnancy rate of approximately 50 to 55%. This applies equally to both medical and surgical therapies. However, no controlled trials have been performed to determine if one therapy is superior.

VAGINAL BLEEDING IN THE THIRD TRIMESTER

method of
DONNA D. JOHNSON, M.D., and
J. PETER VanDORSTEN, M.D.
Medical University of South Carolina
Charleston, South Carolina

During pregnancy, the uterus receives approximately 25% of the cardiac output or approximately

1500 mL of blood per minute. Consequently, an obstetric hemorrhage in the third trimester can have disastrous results for the mother as well as the fetus. The physician must be able to implement support for the maternal cardiovascular system quickly, develop a differential diagnosis to ascertain the source of bleeding, and then provide the best treatment for the mother and fetus.

The first issue is basic life support for the mother: airway, breathing, circulation. Most patients with a third trimester hemorrhage do not have any airway or breathing difficulties, but administering oxygen (6 to 8 liters by face mask) may forestall the onset of maternal tissue hypoxia and increase oxygen delivery to the fetus. Maintaining adequate intravascular volume is more problematic. Intravenous access should be established immediately with two 18-gauge or larger intravenous catheters to facilitate transfusion of blood products if necessary.

The average pregnant woman can tolerate a 15% volume loss (1000 mL) without any hemodynamic alteration. With a 20 to 25% volume loss (1200 to 1500 mL), the pregnant patient demonstrates mild tachycardia, slightly increased respiratory rate, and orthostatic hypotension. However, the only change in the patient's blood pressure may be a more narrow pulse pressure. With a 30 to 35% volume loss (approximately 2 liters), the patient becomes overtly hypotensive and markedly tachycardic (120 to 160 beats per minute). When the volume deficit exceeds 40% (2.5 liters), the patient may have no discernible blood pressure or pulse in the extremities. Unless volume therapy is quickly initiated, circulatory collapse and cardiac arrest soon follow. Monitoring urine output with a Foley catheter can provide important clinical information. As renal perfusion declines, urine output often decreases before changes in the patient's hemodynamic parameters are noted. In addition, the physician must be mindful of other underlying medical conditions, such as preeclampsia, anemia, or cardiovascular disease, that could alter the response to hemorrhage.

To assess quickly the potential complication of disseminated intravascular coagulopathy, a blood specimen should be drawn into a red-top tube. If the blood firmly clots within 7 minutes, the patient is not yet coagulopathic. In addition, a type and cross-match, a complete blood count, platelet count, prothrombin time, and partial thromboplastin time should be obtained. In Rh-negative patients, a Kleihauer-Betke test should be ordered and Rh immune globulin administered accordingly. Arterial blood gas analysis can also be useful in managing antepartum hemorrhage. Oxygen tension is usually normal, but the pH, carbon dioxide, and bicarbonate values usually reflect some degree of metabolic acidosis, which may or may not be compensated. A base deficit of −6 to −8 indicates shock and the need for aggressive fluid and blood replacement. Base excesses of greater than −8 usually precede cardiovascular collapse.

The clinician should initially estimate the amount of blood the patient has lost and develop a plan for volume replacement. Volume replacement can be started with crystalloid solutions such as lactated Ringer's or 0.9% normal saline. In general, 3 mL of a crystalloid solution replaces the volume of approximately 1 mL of whole blood. One milliliter of colloid solutions, such as hetastarch or albumin, replaces the volume of 1 mL of whole blood. Although both crystalloids and colloids may be used for volume expansion and improved circulation, neither is a substitute for the oxygen-carrying capacity of maternal red blood cells. Consequently, the physician may consider a blood transfusion earlier than in the nonpregnant state to maintain adequate oxygen delivery to the placenta and fetus.

Although whole blood is the ideal therapy for an antepartum hemorrhage, blood component therapy is normally the only option. One unit of packed red blood cells is expected to increase the maternal hemoglobin by 1 gram per dL. If a transfusion is needed urgently, type-specific blood can be safely administered to a patient with a known negative antibody screen with minimal transfusion risk. Platelets and fresh frozen plasma should be administered for clinical evidence of disseminated intravascular coagulopathy. However, prophylactic transfusion with fresh frozen plasma and platelets is no longer recommended.

Only after the mother has been stabilized should the physician focus attention on fetal well-being. All too often, impaired fetal status is diagnosed before the mother has been stabilized. Not only is the fetus delivered unnecessarily by cesarean section, but the maternal health also is further jeopardized by rushing an unstable patient to surgery. Apparent fetal distress often resolves with adequate maternal resuscitation.

The final step in managing third trimester bleeding is determining the etiology. After the initial assessment of the patient and fetus, ultrasonography should be performed to determine placental location. If the relationship between the placental edge and the internal os is not well visualized, a transvaginal probe may be used carefully. A skilled sonographer should be able readily to detect a placenta previa. Visualization of an abruptio placentae, however, is much more difficult. A large retroplacental clot must be present before an abruption is detectable by ultrasonography. Occasionally, a chorionic separation at the edge of the placenta may suggest a retroplacental clot.

A placenta previa is usually associated with painless vaginal bleeding and occurs in 1 in 250 live births. Once the diagnosis of placenta previa is made, management options depend on the gestational age, the amount of bleeding, fetal condition, and fetal presentation. At term, a major hemorrhage (≥750 mL) or nonreassuring fetal status after adequate maternal volume resuscitation should prompt the physician to consider an urgent cesarean delivery. Management decisions are more difficult in the preterm patient. With a stable mother and fetus, the obstetrician may consider an amniocentesis to determine fetal lung maturation between 34 and 37 weeks of gestation before proceeding to delivery. With immaturity or gestational age less than 34 weeks, expectant management is reasonable. In the face of uterine activity and prematurity, tocolytics with either magnesium sulfate or indomethacin may be considered. Although beta-mimetics have been used, the associated tachycardia complicates maternal evaluation. Corticosteroid administration to enhance fetal lung development is warranted in patients at less than 34 weeks' gestation. Maternal blood transfusion to maintain the hematocrit greater than 30% provides a margin of safety in expectantly managed patients.

Historically, a double setup has been advocated to determine the possibility of a vaginal delivery. With current high-resolution sonography, we rarely use a double setup. However, a double setup may be useful in patients with a marginal placenta previa or a very-low-lying placenta. Otherwise, a cesarean section should be the choice of delivery. The type of uterine incision depends on the fetal lie and the position of the previa. For back-down transverse fetal lie or anterior complete previa, we prefer a low vertical uterine incision. For a posterior previa and all other presentations at term, we prefer a low transverse uterine incision.

The obstetrician should be aware that a placenta previa is associated with a higher incidence of placenta accreta, especially if the patient has an anterior previa and has undergone one or more prior cesarean sections. Ideally, the patient can be evaluated antenatally by ultrasonography or magnetic resonance imaging to determine if the placenta invades the myometrium. If either modality suggests a placenta accreta, the positive predictive value is high. However, the detection rate is low (approximately 50%), and the depth of invasion of the placenta into the myometrium is underestimated through these radiographic techniques. If a placenta accreta is diagnosed before surgery, blood loss can be reduced if the placenta is left in situ while cesarean hysterectomy is performed.

Management of a placental abruption depends on the degree of placental separation. Grade 1 abruption is associated with minimal uterine bleeding and uterine activity, no signs of hypovolemia, and reassuring fetal status. In a term patient, we consider oxytocin (Pitocin) augmentation because of concern that the abruption may extend. In the preterm patient with uterine activity, tocolysis may be considered. We follow the same guidelines for tocolysis as for the management of a placenta previa. Grade 2 abruption is associated with mild to moderate uterine bleeding, frequent uterine contractions or tetanic uterine contractions, a 20 to 25% volume loss, and evidence of early disseminated intravascular coagulopathy. The fetal heart rate pattern is usually nonreassuring. If vaginal delivery is imminent, it is the preferred mode of delivery. However, a cesarean delivery often must be performed because of impaired fetal status remote from delivery. In a patient with early disseminated intravascular coagulopathy, the surgeon should con-

sider a vertical skin incision because this incision is more hemostatic than a Pfannenstiel incision. Grade 3 abruption is associated with moderate to severe uterine bleeding, maternal hypotension, and fetal death in utero. As with all classifications of abruption, the bleeding may be concealed. The mother must receive vigorous volume replacement with packed red blood cells, platelets, and fresh frozen plasma after the appropriate laboratory test samples have been drawn. A vaginal delivery is the preferred mode of delivery. A cesarean delivery is rarely indicated and should be performed only if the physician cannot maintain adequate maternal blood volume.

A rare cause of vaginal bleeding is vasa previa. This condition occurs when the placenta has a velamentous cord insertion and the vessels cross the internal cervical os. The vessels can rupture with either spontaneous or artificial rupture of membranes. Because all of the blood is fetal in origin, abrupt changes in the fetal heart rate tracing occur. The obstetrician must have a high index of suspicion to diagnosis this cause of vaginal bleeding. Immediate delivery by cesarean section is warranted, and the pediatric team must be ready to provide volume resuscitation to the infant after birth. Under the best circumstances, perinatal morbidity and mortality rates are high.

Although abruptio placentae and placenta previa account for most of the significant vaginal bleeding in the third trimester, other causes should be considered. The patient may have lower genital tract trauma, cervical cancer, or leiomyoma. In such cases, the same principles of maternal and fetal evaluation should be observed. However, treatment needs to be individualized on the basis of the source of vaginal bleeding.

HYPERTENSIVE DISORDERS OF PREGNANCY

method of
JOHN T. REPKE, M.D.
University of Nebraska Medical Center
Omaha, Nebraska

Hypertension, of one type or another, may be expected to complicate up to 10% of human pregnancies. Although in the United States pulmonary embolism is the leading cause of maternal mortality, hypertensive disorders of pregnancy remain the leading cause of maternal mortality worldwide and, either directly or indirectly, remain one of the leading causes of perinatal morbidity and mortality. With respect to pregnancy, three generic forms of hypertension are generally described: chronic hypertension, pre-eclampsia, and gestational hypertension.

Chronic hypertension is hypertension that existed before the pregnancy whether or not antihypertensive therapy was initiated. Pre-eclampsia is a disease characterized by hypertension, proteinuria, and edema that appear in the latter half of pregnancy in an otherwise healthy, nonhypertensive woman. Gestational hypertension, also known as *pregnancy-induced hypertension* or *transient hypertension of pregnancy,* is the occurrence of hypertension in the latter half of pregnancy in an otherwise nonhypertensive woman but without the other clinical manifestations associated with pre-eclampsia. Because of the different roles that each of these diagnoses may play in the clinical management of pregnant women, the conditions are considered as separate entities. Of course, overlap may occur, and these cases present unique challenges to the clinician.

DEFINITIONS AND CLASSIFICATION

The Sixth Report of The Joint National Committee on Prevention, Detection, Evaluation, and Treatment of High Blood Pressure defines hypertension as a systolic blood pressure of 140 mm Hg or greater and a diastolic pressure of 90 mm Hg or greater or the maintenance of normal blood pressure through the use of antihypertensive medication. This committee also recognized that blood pressures taken in a clinic setting tend to be higher than those blood pressures taken as part of a home blood pressure monitoring program and consider home-monitored blood pressures in excess of 135/85 mm Hg to be elevated.

In addition, The American College of Obstetricians and Gynecologists recognizes the same blood pressure parameters as being indicative of pre-eclampsia when the other criteria for this disease have been met. Previous inclusion of systolic blood pressure rises of 30 mm Hg above baseline or diastolic blood pressure rises of 15 mm Hg above baseline has largely been abandoned, although there is not unanimity of agreement on this point.

MEASUREMENT OF BLOOD PRESSURE

Whether the problem is chronic hypertension or pre-eclampsia, many clinical decisions are based on the absolute measurement of blood pressure. The Joint National Committee on Prevention, Detection, Evaluation, and Treatment of High Blood Pressure concluded that blood pressure measurement should begin after at least 5 minutes of rest. An appropriate-sized blood pressure cuff should be utilized, and the first and fifth Korotkoff's sounds should be used to make blood pressure determinations. An important point must be made, however, with respect to blood pressure measurement during pregnancy. Blood pressures should be measured with patients in the seated position and the sphygmomanometer placed at the level of the heart. Ideally, on a first visit, blood pressure should be measured in both upper extremities. In hospitalized patients, blood pressure may be measured with the patient in the semirecumbent position. Of note, however, is that left-sided blood pressures should not be used to rule in or out the diagnosis of a hypertensive disorder whether or not the patient is pregnant.

CHRONIC HYPERTENSION

Chronic hypertension occurs in 5 to 10% of the adult population. More than 90% of cases will be essential hypertension, with the remaining 10% being secondary hypertension, including but not limited to hypertension from renal disease, endocrine disorders, or collagen-vascular diseases. The diagnosis of chronic hypertension is made with the criteria mentioned previously.

Diagnosis

Chronic hypertension during pregnancy is generally characterized by its occurrence in older, multiparous patients, with recognition of hypertension in the first trimester and in general with persistence post partum. The diagnosis of chronic hypertension is easier to make in the nonpregnant state or in the first trimester. Blood pressures in the middle trimester of pregnancy are generally reduced, and so a blood pressure that is seemingly in the normal range at the middle trimester may in fact be elevated for an individual patient. This underlines the importance of preconception care and early prenatal care.

The importance of establishing a diagnosis of chronic hypertension is not only to give the patient optimal treatment during pregnancy but also to recognize the potential increased risk of certain medical complications of pregnancy that occur in the setting of underlying chronic hypertension. Such risks include an increased incidence of pre-eclampsia superimposed on chronic hypertension as well as an increased risk of abruptio placentae.

There are additional high-risk characteristics that one may identify during prenatal care. Women over the age of 40 years, women who have had hypertension for more than 15 years, and women who present in early pregnancy with uncontrolled hypertension are at increased risk for an adverse pregnancy outcome. Complicating underlying systemic illnesses such as diabetes, cardiac disease, and collagen vascular diseases also predispose to adverse pregnancy outcome. In fact, patients who have uncontrolled hypertension in the first trimester have a one in two chance of developing pre-eclampsia, a perinatal mortality rate approaching 25%, and an incidence of intrauterine growth restriction that approaches 50%. In addition, the risk of premature separation of the placenta, or abruptio placentae, is increased and may occur in up to 10% of pregnancies complicated by chronic hypertension, although it is not clear whether this risk is influenced by the use of antihypertensive medication.

Management

The initial management of the pregnant patient with chronic hypertension includes a thorough evaluation. Ideally, such an evaluation should be done before conception. This allows the most flexibility of testing, the most realistic appraisal of baseline blood pressure, and the most comprehensive counseling with respect to the risks of pregnancy. Preconception evaluation also allows the health care provider an opportunity to adjust antihypertensive medications, when indicated, to those medications more suited to continuation during pregnancy.

Initial patient evaluation includes a complete history and physical examination and a baseline laboratory evaluation that can be used for comparison as pregnancy progresses. These baseline studies should include electrolytes, serum creatinine, a urinalysis, and an electrocardiogram. If screening for hyperlipidemia has not previously been done, this should also be accomplished at this time. Of course, during this evaluation every attempt should be made to eliminate identifiable causes of hypertension and thus, via exclusion, establish a diagnosis of essential hypertension.

Pharmacotherapy

Once the initial evaluation has been completed, a decision must be made as to whether pharmacotherapy is indicated. Although the long-term benefits of pharmacotherapy for mild to moderate hypertension have clearly been established, their utility and their benefit in pregnancy remains controversial. Blood pressures of up to 150/100 mm Hg may be well tolerated during pregnancy without apparent adverse maternal or fetal effects.

Initial therapy should be aimed at lifestyle modification. Attention to diet and exercise may result in moderate reductions in blood pressure. Nonpharmacologic measures to lower blood pressure, such as calcium supplementation, have been reported with largely favorable, but nevertheless mixed, results. When a decision has been made to proceed with pharmacotherapy, it should be recognized that the primary benefit of pharmacotherapy is to reduce the acute effects of hypertension on the mother. It has not been established that pharmacotherapy of chronic hypertension during pregnancy favorably influences perinatal outcome, the incidence of intrauterine growth restriction, the incidence of superimposed pre-eclampsia, or the perinatal mortality rate.

When pharmacotherapy is chosen, methyldopa (Aldomet) remains the most widely used drug for the treatment of hypertension during pregnancy because it is the drug that has been most extensively evaluated during pregnancy and has an established safety record for both mother and fetus. Recommended doses for antihypertensive therapy during pregnancy are given in Table 1. Alternative pharmacotherapy includes beta blockers, specifically labetalol (Normodyne, Trandate) and, in selected cases, calcium channel blockers. Beta blockers compare quite favorably with methyldopa when their use is confined to the latter third of pregnancy. There has been some suggestion of an association between beta-blocker therapy and intrauterine growth restriction, specifically with the beta blocker atenolol (Tenormin), but this should only alert the clinician to the need for close monitoring of fetal growth and should not contraindicate the use of these agents in clinically appropriate circumstances. Beta blockers are relatively contraindicated for diabetics or individuals with reactive airway disease.

Calcium channel blockers are effective and probably safe, although they are generally not used as first-line therapy in pregnancy. Oral hydralazine (Apresoline) is rarely used for the management of chronic hypertension in pregnancy as there are better choices available. More controversial is the issue of continued diuretic drugs during pregnancy. In patients who have been maintained on long-standing diuretic therapy, pregnancy does not absolutely contraindicate continuation of diuretic therapy, or at least thiazide diuretic therapy. Loop diuretics, such as furosemide (Lasix), are best discontinued during pregnancy unless absolutely indicated.

Worthy of special mention are the angiotensin-converting enzyme (ACE) inhibitors. Although very effective agents in the management of chronic hypertension, these drugs are contraindicated for use during pregnancy. Fetal renal dysplasia, neonatal renal failure, and decreased fetal calvarium calcification have all been described when these agents have been used during pregnancy. There is also evidence that ACE inhibitors negatively affect uterine blood flow and can increase fetal mortality. Similar precautions apply to the use of the newer angiotensin II receptor antagonists, which are Food and Drug Administration category C in the first trimester and category D in the second and third trimesters.

Fetal Surveillance

Whether taking antihypertensive drugs or not, patients with chronic hypertension during pregnancy require more intense fetal surveillance in the third trimester. Although no strict guidelines exist and fetal monitoring protocols should be tailored to the individual patient, my approach has been to begin

TABLE 1. **Medical Treatment of the Pregnant Hypertensive Woman**

Drug	Usual Dose	Disadvantages
First-line agents		
Methyldopa (Aldomet)	250 mg tid to 500 mg qid	Rare: drug-induced hepatitis, positive Coombs' test
Beta-blockers: labetalol (Normodyne, Trandate)	100 mg bid to 300 mg qid	Possible: decreased fetal growth, fetal bradycardia
Second-line agents		
Hydralazine (Apresoline)	50 mg qid to 100 mg tid	Postural hypotension, edema, lupus-like syndrome
Calcium-channel blockers		
Nifedipine (Procardia)		Maternal hypotension, uteroplacental insufficiency, IUGR
Diuretics: furosemide (Lasix)		Maternal hypovolemia, decreased placental perfusion
ACE inhibitors: enalapril (Vasotec)		Fetal oliguria, renal failure, death

Abbreviations: ACE = angiotensin-converting enzyme; IUGR = intrauterine growth restriction.

weekly nonstress testing, including amniotic fluid index determinations, at 32 weeks of gestation. Fetal growth should be monitored closely with either clinical examination or ultrasonography, depending on patient body habitus. Additional surveillance utilizing umbilical artery Doppler velocimetry or mid-trimester uterine artery Doppler evaluation may be of some value, although these techniques are still considered investigational. Post partum, the initial assessment must include determination of whether antihypertensive therapy continuation is necessary and then selection of a drug that may be used for long-term hypertension management.

Gestational Hypertension

Gestational hypertension is worthy of special mention only to reassure clinicians that in and of itself this entity poses no increased risk to mother or fetus. Because approximately one in five women with gestational hypertension (transient hypertension of pregnancy) will go on to develop superimposed pre-eclampsia, however, close surveillance is required, and consideration of delivery at 39 weeks of gestation with a cervical examination favorable for induction of labor may be a prudent course of action. Because of incompletely studied effects of gestational hypertension on fetal-placental function, surveillance of patients with a diagnosis of gestational hypertension is prudent from the time that the diagnosis is made until delivery.

PRE-ECLAMPSIA

Pre-eclampsia is defined as the occurrence of hypertension, proteinuria, and edema after the 20th week of pregnancy in a previously normotensive woman with no underlying medical illnesses. Pre-eclampsia is largely diagnosed on the basis of blood pressure and proteinuria because these are more objectively determined. Hyperuricemia, although an important marker for this disease, is not part of the current diagnostic criteria. It has, however, been utilized as a diagnostic criterion in the past. Hypertension, as described earlier, is defined as a blood pressure in excess of 140 mm Hg systolic or 90 mm Hg diastolic on two consecutive occasions measured at least 6 hours apart in a woman not taking antihypertensive medication. Proteinuria is defined as more than 300 mg of protein excreted in 24 hours, or more than 1+ on dipstick test, in two consecutively voided specimens. It is important to note that approximately 15% of patients with trace or negative urinary protein on dipstick test do, in fact, have in excess of 300 mg of protein in a 24-hour collection.

Pathophysiology

The etiology of pre-eclampsia remains unknown. Previous hypotheses have included such things as electrolyte imbalances, maternal malnutrition, and a circulating toxin—hence the name *toxemia of pregnancy.* Although the etiology remains unknown, the pathogenesis of pre-eclampsia is currently thought to involve a process of uteroplacental ischemia, possibly secondary to disordered trophoblast invasion during implantation, with resultant vascular endothelial cell damage. This endothelial cell damage may account for all of the clinical signs and symptoms associated with pre-eclampsia, including but not limited to intravascular volume constriction, increased vascular tone, edema, capillary leak syndrome, and, in severe cases, activation of the coagulation system. Cardiac output is also altered in pre-eclamptic patients, although there remains some controversy as to how cardiac output is affected in pre-eclampsia. In all probability, pre-eclamptic patients are capable of exhibiting either increased or decreased cardiac output depending on other disease parameters.

Unlike many diseases, pre-eclampsia is characterized by having only two categories: mild pre-eclampsia and severe pre-eclampsia. Mild pre-eclampsia was defined earlier. Patients are thought to have severe pre-eclampsia if their blood pressure remains persistently above 160 mm Hg systolic or 110 mm Hg diastolic; if they have nephrotic proteinuria in excess of 3 grams of protein excreted per 24 hours (several sources define ranges from 3 to 5 grams of protein excreted per 24 hours in this category; hence, the range is given); persistent oliguria; and a series of clinical signs and symptoms including but not limited to right upper quadrant or epigastric pain, central nervous system dysfunction including blurred vision, scotomata, severe headaches, or altered sensorium, the occurrence of pulmonary edema and cyanosis, and the occurrence of eclampsia. Eclampsia is defined as the occurrence of a grand mal tonic-clonic seizure in the setting of pre-eclampsia and in the absence of underlying neurologic disease.

Atypical forms of pre-eclampsia may also lead to classification of the disease as severe. The most notable of these is the so-called HELLP syndrome, consisting of *h*emolysis, *e*levated *l*iver enzymes, and *l*ow *p*latelets.

Prevention

Much work has been devoted to prevention of pre-eclampsia. These strategies have focused on a variety of therapies, the most popular of which currently are low-dose aspirin therapy (40 to 150 mg per day) and calcium supplementation (2 grams elemental calcium per day in four divided doses). Both of these approaches are perhaps best suited for those women thought to be at high risk for developing pre-eclampsia (Table 2). Recently however, a completed randomized clinical trial by the National Institute of Child Health and Human Development failed to demonstrate the efficacy of low-dose aspirin in preventing pre-eclampsia in four specifically identified high-risk groups. These high-risk groups included women with diabetes, women with chronic hypertension, women with a history of pre-eclampsia, and women with multiple gestations.

TABLE 2. **High-Risk Factors for the Development of Pre-eclampsia**

Diabetes mellitus
Chronic hypertension
Multiple gestation
Previous pre-eclampsia
Autoimmune disease (e.g., systemic lupus erythematosus)
Antiphospholipid syndrome
Hyperlipidemia

Another recent trial investigating calcium supplementation for healthy low-risk primigravidas was also disappointing in that it failed to demonstrate a statistically significant reduction in the incidence of pre-eclampsia in the calcium-supplemented group. Unlike with aspirin, a similar trial of calcium supplementation, and of equal size, in high-risk women has not been performed to date. Other preventive strategies have included zinc supplementation, magnesium supplementation, folic acid supplementation (in an effort to reduce plasma homocysteine levels), and administration of omega-3 fatty acids (fish oil) and/or other antioxidants (e.g., ascorbic acid, alpha tocopherol). At this time, none of these preventive strategies has been conclusively demonstrated to prevent pre-eclampsia across all populations of pregnant women.

Currently, I recommend utilization of calcium supplementation at a level of 2 grams of elemental calcium per day in four divided doses to be administered to those women who are at increased risk for the development of pre-eclampsia, as defined in Table 2. In all of the studies of calcium supplementation published to date, no adverse side effects of this approach have been reported.

Management

The management of pre-eclampsia remains a challenge for the clinician. Previous strategies were simple and easy to follow and centered on whether a woman had pre-eclampsia and whether her disease was mild or severe. In the past, severe pre-eclampsia was an indication for immediate delivery. More recently, however, studies have demonstrated a potential role for the conservative management of severe pre-eclampsia when it occurs remote from term. This type of management should occur in a tertiary center under the direct supervision and care of a fetal-maternal medicine specialist. Conservative management is attempted with the goal of maximizing the benefit for the fetus by allowing continued gestation and fetal lung maturation, with a reduction in neonatal morbidity and mortality. There are no direct maternal benefits to this approach, but there are those that could be perceived as indirect benefits based on the potential benefits to the woman's unborn child.

Management of Mild Preeclampsia

Once a diagnosis of mild pre-eclampsia is made, patients should be hospitalized and evaluated. If the pregnancy is preterm, and after a period of initial evaluation, consideration may be given to either close ambulatory monitoring of such patients or continued hospitalization until delivery. After 37 completed weeks of gestation, patients with mild pre-eclampsia should be considered candidates for delivery, especially if the cervical examination is favorable for induction of labor. Patients being expectantly managed with mild pre-eclampsia should have their platelet count and liver enzymes checked twice weekly and should also have fetal surveillance consisting of at least a nonstress test and amniotic fluid index two times per week. More complete ultrasound evaluations of the fetus for growth should be performed if clinically indicated.

In general, antihypertensive therapy for mild pre-eclampsia is not indicated. If blood pressures rise to a level that is dangerous from the perspective of maternal cerebrovascular accident risk, then antihypertensive therapy may be initiated, but this should be done in conjunction with a plan for expeditious delivery as this patient would now be categorized as having severe disease. In general, it is not my clinical practice to initiate antihypertensive medication in the management of mild pre-eclampsia.

Management of Severe Pre-eclampsia

Severe pre-eclampsia is a potentially life-threatening emergency. All patients with severe pre-eclampsia should be managed, when feasible, in a tertiary care setting. Severe pre-eclampsia can be unpredictable in its course and may become fulminant quite rapidly. All severe pre-eclamptic patients beyond 34 weeks of pregnancy should be expeditiously delivered. Between 32 and 34 weeks, there is room for clinical judgment on the part of the managing perinatologist as to how expeditiously delivery must be accomplished. Before 32 weeks and certainly before 30 weeks, consideration may be given to expectant management as discussed previously, provided that full informed consent is obtained from the patient and that both mother and fetus are stable enough to allow for consideration of expectant management (Table 3).

HELLP Syndrome

The HELLP syndrome remains an enigma for practicing obstetricians. Although generally considered to be a variant of pre-eclampsia, up to one third of patients with signs and symptoms of HELLP syndrome may not, at the time of diagnosis, have evidence of hypertension or proteinuria. Nevertheless, this syndrome is considered as part of the spectrum of the disease of pre-eclampsia and should be managed accordingly.

The occurrence of HELLP syndrome in general necessitates making plans for expeditious delivery. An exception to this may be a patient with minimal elevation of transaminases, thrombocytopenia but with a platelet count of more than 100,000/mm³, and no clinical symptoms. A diagnosis of HELLP syn-

TABLE 3. **Guidelines for Expedited Delivery and Conservative Management of Severe Pre-eclampsia Remote from Term**

Management	Clinical Findings
Maternal guidelines	
Expedited delivery (within 72 h)	One or more of the following
	Uncontrolled severe hypertension*
	Eclampsia
	Platelet count <2 × upper limit of normal with epigastric pain or right upper quadrant tenderness
	Pulmonary edema
	Compromised renal function†
	Persistent severe headache or visual changes
Conservative management	One or more of the following
	Controlled hypertension
	Urinary protein >5000 mg/24 h
	Oliguria (<0.5 mL/kg/h) that resolves with routine fluid or food intake
	AST or ALT >2 × upper limit of normal without epigastric pain or right upper quadrant tenderness
Fetal guidelines	
Expedited delivery (within 72 h)	One or more of the following
	Fetal distress as indicated by fetal heart rate tracing or biophysical profile
	Amniotic fluid index ≤2
	Ultrasonographically estimated fetal weight ≤5th percentile
	Reverse umbilical artery diastolic flow
Conservative management	One or more of the following
	Biophysical profile ≥6
	Amniotic fluid index >2
	Ultrasonographically estimated fetal weight >5th percentile

*Blood pressure persistently ≥160 mm Hg systolic or ≥110 mm Hg diastolic despite maximum recommended doses of two antihypertensive medications.
†Persistent oliguria (<0.5 ml/kg/h) or a rise in serum creatinine of 1 mg/dL over baseline levels.
Abbreviations: AST = aspartate aminotransferase; ALT = alamine aminotransferase.

drome requires hospitalization of the patient immediately and, when stable, transfer to a tertiary institution. These patients should be given magnesium sulfate, and continuous maternal and fetal surveillance should be initiated. HELLP syndrome is frequently confused with a variety of other illnesses, including but not limited to cholestasis, immune thrombocytopenia, viral illness, acute fatty liver of pregnancy, and autoimmune disease (Table 4). Patients with HELLP syndrome may also be at increased risk for cerebrovascular accident based on their coagulopathy and based on data suggesting that pre-eclamptic patients may have a disordered capacity for cerebral autoregulation.

It is my practice to aggressively control blood pressure in patients with HELLP syndrome. Some experts have suggested continuous administration of dexamethasone for the amelioration of HELLP syndrome in an effort to prolong pregnancy, and some have even suggested utilization of plasmapheresis for the management of HELLP syndrome, the latter more specifically for postpartum HELLP syndrome. Neither of these approaches has been widely accepted, and further studies are needed to determine if in fact there is a place for such management approaches in the treatment of this disease.

Intrapartum Management

Once a decision for delivery has been made, the mainstay of management in pre-eclampsia is to control blood pressure and to prevent progression of this

TABLE 4. **Clinical Characteristics of HELLP Syndrome, Thrombotic Thrombocytopenic Purpura (TTP), Hemolytic-Uremic Syndrome (HUS), and Acute Fatty Liver of Pregnancy (AFLP)**

Characteristics	HELLP	TTP	HUS	AFLP
Primary organ involved	Liver	Neurologic	Renal	Liver
Gestational age	2nd and 3rd trimester	2nd trimester	Post partum	3rd trimester
Platelets	↓	↓	↓	Nl/↓
PT/PTT	Nl	Nl	Nl	↑
Hemolysis	+	+	+	−/+
Glucose	Nl	Nl	Nl	↓
Fibrinogen	Nl	Nl	Nl	↓↓
Creatinine	Nl/↑	↑	↑↑	↑

Abbreviations: ↓ = decreased; ↑ = increased; Nl = normal value; + = present; − = absent; PT = prothrombin time; PTT = partial thromboplastin time.

disease to eclampsia. The latter goal is accomplished by the utilization of magnesium sulfate. Magnesium sulfate may be administered as a 4- to 6-gram bolus over 15 minutes followed by a continuous infusion at a rate of 2 grams per hour (Table 5).

Controversy in the past has centered on magnesium sulfate's efficacy as an anticonvulsant. Two large-scale randomized clinical trials have demonstrated magnesium sulfate's superiority in this clinical setting over both phenytoin and diazepam. Patients receiving magnesium sulfate must be monitored very closely. Patellar reflexes should be 1+, and there should be no evidence of respiratory depression, with a respiratory rate being maintained above 12 per minute. More rarely, arrhythmias may occur with magnesium sulfate therapy. If there is evidence of acute magnesium toxicity, this may be treated by administering 1 gram of calcium chloride or calcium gluconate intravenously.

Because of the statistical probability of seizures in the postpartum period, I recommend continuation of magnesium sulfate therapy for at least 24 hours after delivery. The most common sign of disease reversal is a brisk diuresis. In certain circumstances, continuation of magnesium sulfate therapy for greater than 24 hours may be warranted. It is rare that patients who are otherwise healthy will require invasive hemodynamic monitoring for the management of pre-eclampsia, but when utilized, this should be done only by personnel experienced in critical care obstetric medicine.

ECLAMPSIA

Rarely, pre-eclampsia will progress to eclampsia. This is an obstetric and medical emergency. The hallmarks of management are to protect the patient from injury and to protect her airway. Eclampsia has a very predictable course, and, in general, aggressive anticonvulsant treatment is not needed. The mainstays of therapy, other than what I have mentioned earlier, include allowing the convulsion to abate, resuscitating the mother with fluids and oxygen, and waiting for fetal resuscitation to occur. The course is very predictable, with uterine hypertonus occurring

TABLE 5. Magnesium Sulfate Administration for Seizure Prophylaxis

Intramuscular (IM)	Intravenous (IV)
10 gm (5 IM deep in each buttock)*	6-gm bolus over 15 min
5 gm IM deep q 4 h, alternating sides	1–3 gm/h by continuous infusion pump*
	May be mixed in 100 mL crystalloid; if given by IV push, make up as 20% solution; push at maximum rate of 1 gm/min (usual rate 150 mg/min)
	40 gm MgSO$_4$ · 7H$_2$O in 1000 mL lactated Ringer's; run at 25–75 mL/h (1–3 gm/h)*

*Made up as 50% solution.

TABLE 6. Management of Eclampsia

Protect maternal airway; prevent patient injury
Wait for convulsion to abate
Maternal resuscitation
   Maximum oxygenation (mask or endotracheal oxygen)
   Intravenous access and judicious hydration
Fetal resuscitation
   Maternal oxygen, left lateral positioning
   Continuous fetal heart rate monitoring
Maternal postictal assessment
   Complete blood count, platelets, electrolytes, glucose, calcium, magnesium, toxin screen, blood type, and antibody screen
   Careful neurologic examination
   Cervical examination
Magnesium sulfate prophylaxis for subsequent seizures
Formulate delivery strategy
Avoid "stat" cesarean section

during the convulsion and increased contractility and resting tone lasting from 3 to 15 minutes after cessation of seizure activity. During this time, initial fetal bradycardia is the norm. Gradual recovery should occur as the mother is resuscitated, and, in general, most of these patients will be able to undergo vaginal delivery after appropriate stabilization and reassessment of their anticonvulsant medication.

Emergency cesarean section is best avoided, as neither mother nor fetus may be a suitable candidate for operative delivery during the acute event (Table 6). In cases in which seizures occur despite adequate anticonvulsant therapy, consideration should be given to initiating further neurologic assessment, possibly including imaging studies of the central nervous system to rule out other etiologies for seizure activity. There is no consensus as to whether magnetic resonance imaging is superior to computed tomography in this setting, and the decision of which method to employ may be largely institutional, based on experience and availability and, to a lesser degree, cost.

POSTPARTUM MANAGEMENT

With the current trend toward shorter hospital stays, postpartum management of pre-eclampsia assumes a new importance. A syndrome of late postpartum pre-eclampsia and eclampsia has been described. Patients with a diagnosis of pre-eclampsia, when discharged from the hospital, should be carefully educated about the signs and symptoms of pre-eclampsia and impending eclampsia, such as headache, progressive shortness of breath, visual disturbances, or epigastric pain. These and other signs or symptoms suggestive of pre-eclampsia should prompt immediate referral into the hospital for evaluation and further management. The long-term prognosis for patients with uncomplicated pre-eclampsia or eclampsia, even when the disease is severe, is quite good.

OBSTETRIC ANESTHESIA

method of
MARIE E. MINNICH, M.D.
Penn State Geisinger Health System
Danville, Pennsylvania

Obstetric anesthesia is a subspecialty of anesthesiology involved with the care of the pregnant woman throughout the duration of her pregnancy. In this article, emphasis is placed on the care of the healthy, non–high-risk patient during labor, delivery, and the initial postpartum period. Topics discussed include the physiologic changes of pregnancy, anesthetic techniques available for labor and delivery, and complications of those techniques. There are several excellent texts of obstetric anesthesia for those interested in further information concerning anesthesia for normal and high-risk pregnancies.

PHYSIOLOGIC CHANGES OF PREGNANCY

Physiologic changes of pregnancy influence the risks and benefits of various anesthetic techniques applicable to both vaginal and cesarean deliveries. These physiologic changes expose the parturient to potentially serious complications from anesthesia. Increased gastric acid production, decreased gastric emptying, and decreased lower esophageal sphincter tone are changes that result in an increased risk of pulmonary aspiration of gastric contents. The anesthesia-related maternal mortality rate has decreased from 2.7 per 100,000 to approximately 0.6 per 100,000, with many of these deaths related to pulmonary aspiration or inability to secure the airway during administration of general anesthesia. This is one important reason to have qualified and experienced anesthesia providers available for the care of the parturient. It must be emphasized that even though not risk free, current obstetric analgesic and anesthetic techniques are safe and effective and can enable the parturient to participate in her delivery to a much greater extent than the use of heavy sedation and general anesthesia, which were commonly used in the past.

Several major changes occur during pregnancy that influence anesthetic techniques and outcomes. Mucosal swelling of the upper airway and trachea as well as increased breast mass and anteroposterior diameter of the chest wall result in an increased risk of obstructed airway, bleeding, and inability to intubate the trachea. These factors in conjunction with increased O_2 consumption and decreased functional residual capacity (FRC) place the patient at risk of rapidly developing hypoxemia when apnea occurs. Early in pregnancy, arterial CO_2 drops to 30 to 32 mm Hg with concurrent decreases in bicarbonate stores that allow the normal parturient to maintain a pH of 7.4. The pregnant patient, therefore, has substantially less buffering capacity.

Intravascular volume increases by approximately 40% at term. A physiologic anemia is caused by the greater increase in plasma volume compared with cellular components. This increase in blood volume allows the healthy parturient to tolerate the blood loss of vaginal or cesarean delivery without developing symptoms of hypovolemia. Cardiac output increases throughout pregnancy and reaches its peak immediately after the delivery of the placenta. Owing to the expanding size of the uterus during the late second and third trimesters, the parturient at more than 24 weeks of gestation is at risk for developing aortocaval compression (supine hypotension syndrome).

Decreased placental perfusion and fetal heart rate changes may result with or without maternal hypotension. Approximately 10% of mothers at term develop overt hypotension and symptoms of inadequate central nervous system perfusion (e.g., dizziness, presyncope, nausea) when placed in the supine position. Exacerbation of these symptoms occurs during hemorrhage or other hypovolemic states and during sympathetic blockade. To prevent or ameliorate symptoms associated with aortocaval compression, all parturients beyond 24 weeks of gestation should avoid lying supine. This is especially critical during labor and after initiation of any sympathetic blockade.

The gastrointestinal system also undergoes major changes during pregnancy. Gastric acid volume production increases and gastric emptying is delayed. Gastroesophageal reflux is common in the parturient. These factors place parturients at risk for passive regurgitation of stomach contents and potential pulmonary aspiration. This risk occurs with depression of protective airway reflexes (e.g., induction of general anesthesia, heavy sedation, high spinal blockade). Labor and administration of narcotics further delay emptying of stomach contents.

Physiologic changes that occur in the central and peripheral nervous systems result in greater sensitivity to general and local anesthetics, sedatives, and narcotics. Sensitivity to the toxic effects of these agents increases. Bupivacaine (Marcaine, Sensorcaine) is known to have greater cardiac toxicity than other commonly used local anesthetics. Vigilance in the use of bupivicaine is imperative.

LABOR ANALGESIA

Nonpharmacologic Techniques

There are several nonpharmacologic techniques that can be beneficial to expectant mothers either alone or in combination with pharmacologic interventions. These techniques include psychoprophylaxis, breathing exercises, position changes, water (e.g., showers, whirlpool), hypnosis, and use of support persons. Expectant mothers who attend childbirth preparation classes are exposed to and encouraged to practice these techniques.

Interventions such as acupuncture and transcutaneous electrical nerve stimulation (TENS) have been used with varying degrees of success. TENS and acupuncture are not routinely taught during childbirth education and preparation. These techniques require specialized training and equipment not immediately available at all institutions. None of these techniques can provide the level of analgesia comparable to that provided by regional anesthesia. The techniques may, however, provide adequate control for some patients and are certainly a useful adjunct to regional analgesia.

Intravenous Sedatives and Narcotics

Agents such as barbiturates, phenothiazines, and benzodiazepines do not possess analgesic properties but may be used in early labor to decrease anxiety. These agents may be used to augment the effectiveness of intravenous narcotics. Sedatives and narcotics have been shown to depress newborn respiration

995

and are best avoided in the latter stages of labor. In addition, dosages sufficient to control the pain of labor are likely to depress maternal respiratory drive and airway reflexes, thereby increasing the risk of aspiration. Other side effects of narcotics include decreases in gastric emptying and nausea. The most commonly used narcotics are fentanyl (Sublimaze), meperidine (Demerol), and morphine. The agonist-antagonist nalbuphine (Nubain) is also used. Sedatives are commonly administered as bolus doses. Narcotics may be administered as intermittent bolus doses or through patient-controlled analgesia pumps.

Regional Techniques

Continuous Lumbar Epidural (Peridural) Analgesia

This is perhaps the most commonly used regional technique to provide labor analgesia. The extent of blockade may range from analgesia without motor blockade to an anesthetic level sufficient to proceed with a surgical delivery. This is easily accomplished by changing the local anesthetic or its concentration. The level of analgesia or anesthesia can be varied as labor progresses.

Epidural analgesia for labor is usually provided by an epidural catheter in the lumbar epidural space. Maintenance of analgesia is commonly by continuous infusion of local anesthetics with or without lipid-soluble narcotics. The concentration of local anesthetic used is sufficiently dilute to prevent marked motor blockade in most individuals. If the pain of labor is not controlled with dilute local anesthetics, one can either increase the rate of infusion or provide boluses of a more concentrated local anesthetic.

The agents most commonly used to establish epidural blockade are bupivacaine (Sensorcaine, Marcaine), lidocaine (Xylocaine), 2-chloroprocaine (Nesacaine), and, more recently, ropivacaine (Naropin). The pharmacologic profile of bupivacaine and ropivacaine is favorable for labor analgesia as these agents provide greater sensory blockade than motor blockade. One of the most common infusions for maintenance of labor analgesia is bupivacaine 0.125%, often in combination with small amounts of lipid-soluble narcotics (e.g., fentanyl 1 to 2 µg per mL). At this concentration, bupivacaine provides analgesia with minimal motor blockade. Ropivacaine is used similarly. During the second stage of labor and especially at the expulsive stage, a bolus of a more concentrated local anesthetic provides adequate perineal anesthesia. This is especially true for repair of an episiotomy or laceration. If necessary, anesthesia can be rapidly established to provide for comfortable placement of vacuum or forceps for an assisted vaginal delivery.

Although bupivacaine 0.125% does not cause marked motor blockade, the patient must be restricted to bed when blockade with this solution is established. Investigators have studied the effectiveness of solutions of bupivacaine in the range of 0.04% to 0.06% in combination with lipid-soluble narcotics

(e.g., fentanyl 1 µg per mL) and/or epinephrine 1.25 µg per mL. These solutions are administered by pumps, allowing patient-controlled analgesia (i.e., programmed continuous infusions plus patient administered boluses). Ultradilute concentrations such as these provide substantial (though not always complete) analgesia for most patients without any demonstrable motor blockade. This allows the mother to maintain her mobility for an extended period during labor despite having epidural analgesia. Many patients are sufficiently comfortable, prefer the sense of control, and can be maintained on the ultradilute solution until delivery. Others may require more concentrated solutions, necessitating restriction to bed during the latter portion of labor. Patient acceptance of the ultradilute solutions and patient-controlled analgesia is high. Many patients prefer the more active role that these solutions provide. Expulsive efforts are not inhibited with these solutions.

Most practitioners prefer to establish epidural analgesia in a nonaugmented labor after the cervix is dilated 5 cm, as blockade established in the latent phase may slow labor. In induced or augmented labors, however, epidural analgesia may be established earlier if the patient's comfort is not adequately maintained by other techniques. To establish epidural blockade, aseptic preparation of the lumbar area, a specially designed epidural needle, and a catheter if continuous infusion is planned are needed. After the catheter is placed, to prevent untoward effects, it is important to determine that it has not been placed in either a blood vessel or the subarachnoid space. Before injection, one should aspirate the catheter and then inject only small amounts of local anesthetic at a time. Between injections, one must assess for symptoms of intravenous or subarachnoid injections before the next bolus or establishment of a continuous infusion. It is important to note that a catheter may "migrate" into a vessel or the subarachnoid space during the maintenance phase of epidural analgesia. It is important that experienced anesthesia providers be available to assess for adequacy of blockade and misadventures of the epidural catheter.

Spinal (Subarachnoid/Intrathecal) Analgesia

Provision of spinal analgesia is more commonly known as the classic saddle block. When used alone with local anesthetics, this technique is of limited duration (unless one is willing to do repeated spinal punctures). It is associated with significant motor blockade, making expulsive efforts difficult and incurring a risk for development of spinal headache.

Newer developments in regional anesthesia use intrathecal injection of highly lipid-soluble narcotics such as fentanyl and sufentanil (Sufenta). These agents by themselves provide excellent analgesia for the visceral pain associated with the first stage but are not sufficient for the somatic pain of the second stage of labor. The onset of action is very rapid, usually less than 5 minutes. The duration of action, however, is limited, with a range of 60 to 100 minutes. For mothers experiencing a rapidly progressing labor, these agents can be combined with a pudendal block for the second stage of labor. Some practitioners include small doses (2.5 mg) of bupivacaine with the narcotic discussed previously.

It is important to realize that the use of these narcotic agents is not risk free. Review of recent literature reveals side effects such as hypotension, severe pruritus, fetal bradycardia and decreased heart rate variability, and maternal respiratory depression.

Currently the use of subarachnoid narcotics is most commonly applied in conjunction with the placement of an epidural catheter to provide continuous analgesia as the effects of the subarachnoid narcotic wane. This is discussed next.

Combined Spinal-Epidural Analgesia

Combined spinal and epidural analgesia takes advantage of the rapid onset of intense analgesia provided by intrathecal injection and the continuous analgesia of the epidural catheter technique. It is accomplished through a single skin puncture with a specially designed spinal needle that is placed through an epidural needle. After the selected lipid-soluble narcotic is injected into the intrathecal space, the spinal needle is removed and the epidural catheter is inserted through the epidural needle. This technique is especially useful if the patient desires labor analgesia provided by ultradilute solutions of local anesthetics as noted earlier. After the epidural catheter is placed, analgesia is maintained with a pump, as noted previously.

ANESTHESIA FOR CESAREAN SECTION

Regional Anesthesia Techniques

Both epidural and spinal techniques are excellent ways to provide anesthesia for cesarean delivery. Each can be used for elective or urgent delivery. These techniques provide for an alert mother who has a greater sense of participation in the birth of her infant. They also decrease pulmonary aspiration risk to the mother. These techniques are contraindicated in patients with active hemorrhage, coagulopathy, infection at the site of intended needle placement, or sepsis, and when the mother refuses anesthesia. As previously discussed, establishment of regional anesthesia is associated with an increased risk of aortocaval compression syndrome owing to sympathetic blockade.

Epidural Anesthesia

Epidural anesthesia for cesarean section may be established immediately before surgery or with an indwelling catheter that has been placed previously for labor analgesia. If a catheter is present, local anesthetic of sufficient concentration for surgical anesthesia (e.g., lidocaine 1.5% or 2% with epinephrine 1:200,000, bupivacaine 0.5%, or 2-chloroprocaine 3%) is injected to establish surgical anesthesia to a der-

matomal level of minimally T-6, preferably T-4 or higher. Surgical anesthesia can be obtained within 15 minutes in an urgent situation if labor analgesia has been maintained by continuous lumbar epidural analgesia.

To establish a surgical anesthetic level in a patient who has not had epidural analgesia maintained for labor takes additional time. The length of time depends on the local anesthetic chosen and ranges from 25 to 50 minutes. The technique of placing an epidural for cesarean section is similar to that of placing an epidural catheter for labor. It is essential to have an indwelling intravenous catheter of sufficient gauge (preferably 16 gauge) to provide the ability to hydrate the patient rapidly. Uterine displacement must be maintained before delivery of the infant.

Spinal Anesthesia

Spinal anesthesia provides the ability to establish excellent surgical anesthesia in rapid fashion. The technique is associated with less risk of local anesthetic toxicity as the dosages used are much smaller than those required to establish epidural anesthesia. Spinal anesthesia is established by placement of a spinal needle into the subarachnoid space in the lumbar region. The most commonly used local anesthetics are bupivacaine 0.75% in D8.25W, tetracaine 1% in D10W, and lidocaine 5% in D7.5W. Recent discussions in the anesthesia literature raise the possibility of neurotoxicity of intraspinal hyperbaric lidocaine. Some practitioners have abandoned the use of this agent while additional research into this area is completed. The duration of effective surgical anesthesia depends on the agent chosen. As with epidural anesthesia, a large-bore intravenous catheter is desirable.

Combined Spinal-Epidural Anesthesia

On occasion, the anesthesiologist may desire the rapid establishment of surgical anesthesia afforded by spinal injection but is unwilling to accept the limited duration of the technique. In these cases, the combined technique described earlier can provide the advantages of both techniques with little additional time needed.

With all regional techniques, the patient may perceive pulling or pressure despite an adequate level of anesthesia. These sensations tend to be less with spinal anesthesia and can be lessened further with the administration of intraspinal (subarachnoid or epidural) fentanyl when either technique is used. If these sensations are unpleasant for the mother, intravenous sedative or analgesic agents in small amounts may be administered. The anesthesia practitioner must be extremely vigilant, however, as these agents may cause respiratory depression and loss of airway reflexes. If small quantities of intravenous agents are not sufficient to provide adequate analgesia, general anesthesia with endotracheal intubation should be established.

General Anesthesia

General anesthesia should be used only when regional anesthesia is contraindicated. Maternal risk of major morbidity is higher with general anesthesia than with regional anesthesia. As discussed earlier, much of the risk of general anesthesia lies in the difficulty in establishing the airway and in aspiration pneumonia. Although these risks are not eliminated with regional anesthesia, they are lessened substantially. It should be noted that infants born after induction of general anesthesia tend to have a lower Apgar score at 1 minute compared with those infants born of mothers undergoing regional anesthesia. By 5 minutes, however, the effects of general anesthesia have dissipated and the Apgar scores of infants are equivalent. The lower Apgar score at 1 minute represents, not necessarily asphyxia, but rather the effects of general anesthesia on the newborn.

Although the anesthesiologist should examine the parturient's airway before induction of any anesthesia, inspection is especially important before the induction of general anesthesia. If there is evidence that intubation of the trachea will be difficult, either general anesthesia should be avoided or the airway should be secured before induction of general anesthesia.

In addition, techniques to reduce the likelihood of aspiration pneumonia should be used. These include the oral administration of the nonparticulate antacid sodium citrate, preoxygenation of the mother before intravenous induction of anesthesia, and maintenance of cricoid pressure until endotracheal intubation has been ensured. As with regional anesthesia, one must ensure that aortocaval compression is minimized by left uterine displacement.

Although there are numerous intravenous induction agents that may be used, the most common agent to establish general anesthesia is thiopental (Pentothal). Thiopental is used in conjunction with a muscle relaxant to facilitate intubation of the trachea. Most anesthesiologists use succinylcholine (Anectine) to establish rapid muscle paralysis. As noted earlier, cricoid pressure should be maintained until endotracheal intubation has been established. This pressure must be maintained by someone other than the anesthetist performing the intubation. General anesthesia is then maintained by use of inhaled agents until the infant is delivered. Some anesthesiologists elect to use nitrous oxide 50% and oxygen 50%; others administer low concentrations of more potent inhaled anesthetics such as isoflurane (Forane), enflurane (Ethrane), or halothane in oxygen. After delivery of the infant is complete, the level of anesthesia is deepened with intravenous and/or inhaled agents as necessary. After completion of the surgery, the patient is allowed to awaken until airway reflexes and consciousness have returned sufficiently to enable safe removal of the endotracheal tube.

Postoperative Analgesic Techniques

Administration of preservative-free morphine in the epidural or subarachnoid space provides 18 to 24 hours of good analgesia after cesarean delivery under regional anesthesia. The dosage used in the epidural space ranges from 2.5 to 5 mg compared with a range of 0.2 to 0.3 mg in the subarachnoid space. The common side effects of morphine administered in this manner include pruritus, nausea, vomiting, and urinary retention. An uncommon, but potentially harmful, side effect is central respiratory depression, which can occur 10 to 14 hours after administration of the morphine. For this reason, it is important that vital signs, including respiratory rate, be checked hourly for 24 hours after neuraxially administered morphine.

Postoperative analgesia is best maintained by intravenous patient-controlled analgesia pumps for patients who have had general anesthesia. This technique is associated with good analgesia, high patient satisfaction, and lower total doses of narcotics than intermittent intramuscular or intravenous narcotic administration.

COMPLICATIONS ASSOCIATED WITH ANESTHESIA

Complications of Regional Techniques

One of the most frequent complications of regional anesthesia is hypotension. The development of hypotension can be ameliorated or prevented by hydration of the parturient before spinal or epidural anesthesia is established and maintenance of left uterine displacement after the regional block is placed. If hypotension persists despite these maneuvers, intravenous ephedrine is used to return blood pressure to an adequate level while hydration is continued.

The local anesthetics are agents that reversibly inhibit action potentials from being propagated in any excitable tissue, including cardiac and central nervous tissues, as well as the peripheral nerves. Local anesthetic toxicity, including seizures and cardiac arrest, can occur if doses of local anesthetic intended for the epidural space are inadvertently administered into any vessel.

High or "total" spinal anesthesia may occur with intended subarachnoid block or when local anesthetic doses intended for the epidural space are actually placed in the subarachnoid space. This may result in profound hypotension, circulatory collapse, and central respiratory inhibition. High spinal anesthesia may occur during initial establishment of the epidural anesthesia or during the maintenance phase if the epidural catheter migrates into the subarachnoid space. All bolus doses of local anesthetics should be administered in a fractionated manner while the physician watches for signs of intravenous or subarachnoid administration of local anesthetics to decrease both the likelihood and the severity of these complications.

Should either intravenous or subarachnoid injection of local anesthetics result in any of these complications, maintenance of airway and breathing (usually requiring endotracheal intubation) and circulation (with hydration, vasopressors, and cardiopulmonary resuscitation as necessary) are critically important. Avoidance of these complications is preferable to treatment of them.

Partial or complete failure of epidural or spinal anesthesia is an infrequent complication. This can be the result of an inability to properly locate the needle into the epidural or spinal space, too small a dosage of local anesthetic, or, in the case of epidural anesthesia, a laterally placed epidural catheter. These complications may require the procedure to be repeated or a general anesthetic to be used, depending on circumstances.

Post–dural puncture headache can be associated with spinal anesthesia or with inadvertent dural puncture during attempted epidural placement. Recent advances in spinal needle design and the common use of smaller gauge, pencil point needles have decreased the frequency and severity of headache after spinal anesthesia. Post–dural puncture headache is much more frequent after inadvertent dural puncture during epidural catheter placement. The incidence of inadvertent dural puncture during epidural catheter placement is uncommon (1% to 5%, depending on the skill of the anesthetist). Post–dural puncture headache associated with inadvertent dural puncture approaches 85%, however, and frequently mandates treatment other than hydration. The most common and effective treatment is an epidural blood patch with aseptically obtained autologous blood.

Nerve injury is uncommonly caused by regional anesthesia techniques. Most nerve injuries are position or birth related but are falsely associated with regional anesthesia.

Complications of General Anesthesia

Hypoxic injury due to the inability to secure the maternal airway and pulmonary aspiration of gastric contents are the two most feared complications of general anesthesia. Either of these complications can be associated with severe morbidity or mortality. Prevention or amelioration of these complications was discussed. Other complications that can occur during general anesthesia include dental damage and recall of events during surgery due to maintenance of light levels of anesthesia, especially before delivery of the infant.

POSTPARTUM CARE

method of
R. SCOTT RUSHING, M.D., and
JAMES A. THORP, M.D.
Obstetrix of Missouri and Kansas, St. Luke's Hospital, and University of Missouri at Kansas City
Kansas City, Missouri

NORMAL PUERPERIUM EVENTS

The puerperium, or postpartum period, begins immediately after delivery of the placenta and arbitrarily ends 6 weeks later. The uterus begins its involution immediately after expulsion of the placenta. It decreases on average from a gravid weight of 1000 to 500 grams within 1 week and returns to its prepregnant size by 4 to 6 weeks post partum. Postpartum vaginal bleeding, or lochia rubra, decreases in flow to a reddish-brown discharge within the first 3 to 4 days after delivery. This is followed by a mucopurulent and often malodorous discharge, lochia serosa, which lasts an average of 2 to 3 weeks. A sudden increase in vaginal bleeding often occurs between 7 and 14 days post partum, and this results from shedding the eschar at the site of placental implantation.

There are many hemodynamic changes that occur immediately after delivery of the infant and placenta. One third of the blood volume increment achieved during pregnancy is lost within 3 days of delivery. The majority of this loss of volume occurs within 1 hour of delivery. The average blood loss is commonly underestimated, and for an uncomplicated vaginal or cesarean delivery it is 500 or 1000 mL, respectively. There occurs a significant shifting of fluids from extravascular to intravascular spaces during the first week post partum. A significant physiologic diuresis occurs between the second and fifth days after delivery and is often exaggerated with pre-eclampsia.

"Afterpains," often worse in multiparas, are caused by uterine contractions as involution occurs. These pains are most evident during suckling as oxytocin is released and the uterine contractions intensify. These afterpains usually diminish or resolve within 1 week. Nonsteroidal anti-inflammatory drugs such as ibuprofen, 600 to 800 mg every 6 hours, provide significant relief.

MANAGEMENT OF THE PUERPERIUM

Observation. The most common complications of the puerperium are postpartum hemorrhage and genital tract infection. Therefore, careful observation is recommended for 24 to 48 hours in patients undergoing a vaginal delivery and 72 to 96 hours in patients undergoing a cesarean delivery. The vital signs should be taken every 15 minutes for the first hour after the delivery, every 30 minutes for the next 2 hours, and then every 4 hours for the remaining 24 hours. The amount of postpartum vaginal bleeding should also be monitored very closely. Pads and sheets should be weighed to accurately quantify the blood loss if the amount of bleeding becomes worrisome.

Perineal Care. For most vaginal deliveries the requirement for analgesic agents is minimal. Acetaminophen or nonsteroidal anti-inflammatory agents are usually sufficient. Occasionally, with more severe lacerations and/or episiotomy, a mild narcotic such as codeine or oxycodone may be used. Ice packs to the perineum and sitz baths can relieve discomfort and hasten the recovery of the perineum. Prolapsed hemorrhoids are frequently seen as a source of perineal pain. Corticoid suppositories, local analgesic sprays, or emollients may be useful in relieving discomfort. Stool softeners should be given to patients who have a third- or fourth-degree laceration/episiotomy.

Immunizations. Before discharge, the rubella vaccine should be given to patients who are not immune. The nonimmunized Rh-negative woman who has delivered an Rh-positive infant should undergo testing (fetal screen and Kleihauer-Betke) to document that one vial of Rh immune globulin is sufficient.

Contraception. Oral contraceptives can be started within 1 to 2 weeks post partum in nonlactating mothers; a delay of 4 weeks in breast-feeding mothers reduces the risk of lactation suppression. Medroxyprogesterone acetate (Depo-Provera) or the progesterone-only contraceptive pill may be initiated immediately post partum without effect on the quality and/or quantity of breast milk.

Breast Care and Lactation. Breast engorgement usually occurs by the third postpartum day and may be accompanied by a "milk fever" for 24 hours. Ice packs, a tight-fitting bra, and ibuprofen effectively treat this condition in the non–breast-feeding patient. Pharmacologic lactation suppressants are no longer recommended, because of undesirable side effects. Breast-feeding should be encouraged because of the following benefits: improved infant nutrition, increased infant resistance to infections, decreased expense, convenience, and enhanced mother-infant bonding. Frequent feeding and alternating sides help relieve engorgement discomfort in breast-feeding patients. Cracked and painful nipples can be helped with proper positioning and allowing the nipples to air-dry between feedings. Mastitis is characterized by unilateral breast erythema, pain, fever, and myalgias. Breast-feeding and oral antibiotic therapy are continued as indicated; penicillin V (Pen-Vee K), 500 mg four times a day, and dicloxacillin (Dynapen), 500 mg four times a day, are reasonable options. If *Candida* infection is suspected, then nystatin (Mycostatin) should be applied to the breast and the infant treated for oral thrush.

COMPLICATIONS OF THE PUERPERIUM

Hemorrhage

Postpartum hemorrhage can occur immediately after delivery of the infant and/or placenta or may be delayed for several hours after delivery. It may be defined as a blood loss of 1000 mL after a vaginal delivery, 1500 mL after a cesarean birth, or 500 mL in the first 12 to 24 hours of the puerperium. Although the incidence of this complication is only 4% for vaginal deliveries and 6% for cesarean deliveries, it accounts for 35% of maternal deaths caused by bleeding during pregnancy. Once hemorrhage is recognized, the cause must quickly be determined so that the most appropriate therapy can be immediately implemented. The most common causes of postpartum hemorrhage in order of decreasing frequency are atony, genital tract lacerations, and retained placental tissue. Less common causes of hemorrhage are an inverted uterus, placenta accreta, placenta previa, and uterine rupture. Two large-bore intravenous lines should be started, blood products made available, coagulation studies ordered, and the vital signs closely monitored.

If atony is suspected, a bimanual examination with vigorous uterine massage is necessary. Occasionally, large clots in the lower uterine segment can inhibit uterine contractions and cause continued bleeding; therefore, manual removal of the clots is indicated. Pharmacologic intervention should be initiated immediately when atony is suspected. Oxytocin (Pitocin), 20 to 40 µL per liter of crystalloid, should be started at a rate of 200 mL per hour. Refractory bleeding can be treated with additional drugs, including the following: 15-methyl ester of prostaglandin $F_{2\alpha}$ (Hemabate), 0.25 mg, can be given intramuscularly; misoprostol (Cytotec), 400 µg, may be given orally or rectally; and methylergonovine (Methergine), 0.20 mg, can be given intramuscularly in patients without a history of hypertension.

If the uterus is well contracted but there is persistent bleeding, other causes such as genital tract laceration, retained placenta, or uterine rupture should be considered and appropriate interventions taken. If retained placenta is found, then manual extraction alone or with curettage should be performed with an anesthesiologist in attendance. If pharmacologic intervention and/or curettage is unsuccessful, then other therapeutic options should be considered, including uterine packing, uterine artery embolization, O'Leary stitch, hypogastric artery ligation, and hysterectomy.

Infection

There are several causes of a postpartum infection or fever: endomyometritis, urinary tract infection, wound/episiotomy infection, atelectasis, pneumonia, deep venous thrombosis, pelvic thrombophlebitis, engorged breasts, mastitis, drug reaction, and autoimmune disease. A thorough history and physical examination will usually identify the source of the postpartum infection. Laboratory studies commonly ordered to assist in diagnosis include a urinalysis, complete blood cell count with differential, chest radiography, and, occasionally a deep venous Doppler study. Transcervical endometrial cultures are usually not helpful.

Endomyometritis is the most common infection in the puerperium. This polymicrobial infection occurs in 2% of vaginal deliveries and in 10 to 15% of cesarean deliveries. It is diagnosed by fever and uterine tenderness, often accompanied by a foul-smelling discharge. A postpartum fever is defined as a temperature of more than 100.4°F on two occasions separated by at least 4 hours, excluding the first 24 hours after delivery. Traditionally, this infection is treated with gentamicin (Garamycin), 1.5 mg per kg loading dose and then 1.0 mg per kg every 8 hours, and clindamycin (Cleocin), 900 mg every 8 hours. Alternative regimens include single-agent treatment with cefotetan (Cefotan), 1 to 2 grams intravenously every 12 hours, or ampicillin/sulbactam (Unasyn), 3 grams every 6 hours. If first-line therapies are unsuccessful, then triple therapy with ampicillin (2 grams intravenously every 6 hours), gentamicin, and clindamycin is given. When the patient is pain free and afebrile for at least 48 hours the antibiotics are discontinued. Follow-up oral antimicrobial therapy has no proven value.

If a patient fails to respond to aggressive antimicrobial therapy over 3 to 4 days, then pelvic or ovarian vein thrombosis or other less likely causes should be considered. Pelvic imaging with computed tomography, magnetic resonance imaging, and ultrasonography may sometimes be helpful. Therapeutic intravenous heparin is recommended for septic pelvic or ovarian vein thrombosis.

Deep Venous Thrombosis/Pulmonary Embolism

Pregnancy and the puerperium are considered "hypercoagulable states." Deep venous thrombosis (DVT) occurs in about 1 in 400 deliveries. More common in patients who have undergone cesarean section, it is characterized by leg and/or calf tenderness, swelling, erythema, and/or warmth. Venography, previously the gold standard for diagnosis, has been largely replaced by Doppler plethysmography. Full heparinization is the recommended treatment. Pulmonary embolism (PE) occurs in 15% to 24% of untreated DVTs and in 5% of treated DVTs. The mortality rate for untreated PE is approximately 30%. Signs of PE may include chest discomfort, shortness of breath, tachypnea, apprehension, an increased alveolar-arterial gradient, and an abnormal ventilation/perfusion scan. A pulmonary angiogram is the most sensitive test, but because of its invasiveness, it is used only when the clinical suspicion is high and the ventilation/perfusion scan is indeterminate.

Vulvar/Vaginal Hematoma

This complication is often discovered after the patient complains of excessive perineal pain. The majority of these lesions can be managed conservatively with ice packs, analgesia, and observation. If the hematoma is of sufficient size to cause urinary retention, a Foley catheter should be placed temporarily. If the hematoma becomes infected or causes hemodynamic compromise, then surgical drainage is warranted.

Postpartum Blues/Depression/Psychosis

After childbirth, women can experience a spectrum of psychological reactions. The mild and transient "maternity blues" is experienced by 50 to 70% of patients. Common symptoms are tearfulness, irritation, insomnia, negative feelings toward the infant, restlessness, anxiety, and feeling melancholy over the loss of the gestational relationship. The "blues" usually lasts for no longer than 10 days. No therapy is indicated other than reassurance and support. The incidence of postpartum major depression is between 8% and 15%. Many view postpartum depression as a prolonged and more severe case of the "blues." The signs and symptoms do not differ from depression in nonpregnant patients but are difficult to differentiate from normal postpartum symptoms (e.g., sleeplessness, weight loss, change in appetite). The patient may also have suicidal ideation, ambivalence toward the infant, and a feeling of guilt. Postpartum depression was historically treated with tricyclic antidepressants, but studies have demonstrated that the selective serotonin reuptake inhibitors (SSRIs) are equally effective and have fewer side effects. Postpartum psychosis can manifest as a schizophrenic or manic-depressive reaction. Patients often are delusional, confused, and disoriented. The psychosis may last as long as 2 to 3 months and necessitates immediate consultation with a psychiatrist.

HOSPITAL DISCHARGE

Before discharge it is important to recognize that the patient's vaginal bleeding is decreasing and that she is hemodynamically stable. The patient should be tolerating a regular diet and be able to care for herself and her newborn. Discharge medications usually include prenatal vitamins, an iron supplement, and analgesics for perineal or incisional discomfort. The patient is encouraged to abstain from sexual intercourse for 4 to 6 weeks or until vaginal bleeding ceases. A 6-week return appointment is usual for vaginal deliveries. After cesarean delivery, a 1- to 2-week appointment for an incision evaluation is also common. The patient is encouraged to telephone the health care provider if she experiences an increase in pain, significant vaginal bleeding, or a temperature greater than 100.4°F.

RESUSCITATION OF THE NEWBORN
method of
CARACIOLO J. FERNANDES, M.D.
Baylor College of Medicine
Houston, Texas

A normal delivery, culminating in the birth of a healthy full-term infant, is the wish of most pregnant women. Although many variables are beyond one's control, attempts to fulfill this wish require that a person skilled in basic neonatal resuscitation be present at every delivery. To be able to deliver the highest standard of care, the caregiver must understand perinatal physiology and the principles of resuscitation and have mastered the necessary technical skills. The Neonatal Resuscitation Program sponsored by the American Academy of Pediatrics/American Heart Association presents a logical, coordinated approach to neonatal resuscitation and is highly recommended for anyone involved in the delivery room care of the newborn.

PERINATAL PHYSIOLOGY

In utero, the placenta is the organ of respiration and the lungs are filled with fluid. Because the lung does not function to oxygenate the blood in utero, oxygenated blood from the placenta, entering the right atrium through the inferior vena cava, is shunted through the foramen ovale into the left side of the heart and distributed to the brain and peripheral circulation. The right side of the heart primarily receives blood with a lower oxygen content, which is ejected into the pulmonary artery and then diverted through the ductus arteriosus to the aorta rather than the high-resistance lungs. This blood is then distributed to the placenta through the aorta and umbilical arteries to receive oxygen and nutrients and to release carbon dioxide and waste products.

At birth the newborn transitions from an intrauterine to extrauterine environment, in which the lung is the organ of respiration. With the newborn's first few breaths, certain cardiopulmonary adaptations rapidly occur that make this transition successful. First, the lungs expand as they are filled with gas; fetal lung fluid gradually leaves the alveoli by moving into the extra-alveolar interstitium and is eventually cleared by lung lymphatic vessels. At the same time, the pulmonary vascular resistance decreases rapidly and pulmonary blood flow correspondingly increases. These changes are associated with an increase in the partial pressure of oxygen in the alveoli and arterial circulation from the fetal level (approximately 25 mm Hg) to 50 to 70 mm Hg. With clamping of the umbilical cord, the systemic vascular resistance increases. Even though the foramen ovale and ductus arteriosus remain anatomically open, the decrease in pulmonary vascular resistance and the increase in systemic vascular resistance effectively reverse the direction of blood flow through these two shunt pathways. However, if pulmonary vascular resistance remains elevated, blood shunts right-to-left through the foramen ovale and ductus arteriosus, mimicking the fetal circulatory pathways and impairing oxygen delivery. Hypoxia, acidosis, and hypothermia are common causes of elevated pulmonary vascular resistance; hence, it is apparent that attention to prevention of hypoxia, acidosis, and hypothermia at birth will help ensure a smooth transition to normal postnatal circulation.

Fortunately, the first few breaths of most newborns are effective and allow the cardiopulmonary adaptations previously discussed to take place. However, some infants are asphyxiated in utero and are born with ineffective respiratory efforts, which lead to hypoxia and acidosis and make these adaptations difficult.

Human newborns respond to asphyxia by a short period of increased respiratory effort followed by *primary apnea,* during which spontaneous respiration can be restored by tactile stimulation. However, if the asphyxial episode continues, the newborn develops irregular gasping respiration, decreasing heart rate and blood pressure, and then lapses into *secondary apnea.* Now the newborn is unresponsive to stimulation and will only respond to positive-pressure ventilation. The longer the delay in resuscitation, the longer it will take for spontaneous respiration to occur. Because the fetus may experience asphyxia in utero, primary and secondary apnea may occur in utero. Therefore, if a newborn is born apneic, differentiation between primary and secondary apnea is not possible and it must be assumed that the newborn is in secondary apnea and that positive-pressure ventilation should be initiated.

PREPARATION

Preparation is the first step in effective neonatal resuscitation. Because newborns requiring resuscitation are often born in hospitals where most infants are born healthy, it is essential to ensure that personnel adequately skilled in neonatal resuscitation be present at every delivery, whether or not perinatal problems are anticipated. At deliveries where a normal, healthy infant is expected, one person (e.g., physician, nurse, respiratory therapist) who has the skills to perform a complete neonatal resuscitation must be present. If this person is also caring for the mother, another person who is capable of initiating and assisting with neonatal resuscitation must be present. It is inappropriate to have someone "on call" to provide neonatal resuscitation because this may cause unnecessary delay. At high-risk deliveries in which an infant with respiratory depression is likely to be born, two persons not involved in the care of the mother must be readily available, one of whom must be skilled in endotracheal intubation and the administration of medications. If time permits, the problems and plans for care of the infant should be discussed with the parents.

Equipment needed for resuscitation (Table 1) should be present in every delivery area and routinely checked to ensure that all equipment is working properly. When the antepartum or intrapartum history suggests that an asphyxiated infant may be born, all equipment should be immediately accessible. One should check quickly to ensure that (1) the radiant warmer is heating, (2) oxygen is flowing through the tubing, (3) the suction apparatus is functioning properly, (4) the resuscitation bag and mask can provide an adequate seal and generate pressure, and (5) the laryngoscope light source is functional. Several minutes into the resuscitation of a cyanotic infant is not the time to realize that the valve to the oxygen source was never opened or that the laryngoscope light is dim. For multiple gestations, a full complement of equipment and personnel is needed for each infant. It should be remembered that exposure to blood and other body fluids is inevitable in the delivery room, and universal precautions should always be practiced. If the delivery room is not close to the nursery, a transport incubator (with a portable oxygen supply/ventilator and battery-operated heat source) is required.

INITIAL STEPS OF RESUSCITATION

Although there are certain aspects of neonatal resuscitation that make it unique, the so-called ABCs (*a*irway, *b*reathing, *c*irculation) of resuscitation in any age group still apply. Most infants will respond to airway management and the initiation of positive-pressure ventilation if needed. Chest compressions and medications rarely are necessary. This also applies to medically complicated infants such as those prenatally detected to have complex congenital heart disease or hydrops fetalis. During resuscitation, it is of paramount importance to continually evaluate the patient to decide what the next step of the resuscitation algorithm will be.

One very important aspect of newborn resuscitation that is unique is the importance of temperature

TABLE 1. **Equipment and Supplies for Resuscitation**

Environment

Radiant warmer (with temperature probe)
Blankets, towels (warm)
Wall clock with sweep second hand

Suction

Bulb syringe
Suction catheters (Nos. 6, 8, 10 French)
Regulated wall suction
Meconium aspiration devices

Airway Management

Stethoscope
Oxygen
Flowmeter
Oxygen tubing
Infant resuscitation bag (with pressure relief valve and
    manometer)
Masks (premature and infant sizes)
Laryngoscope (with extra batteries)
Size No. 0 and No. 1 laryngoscope blades
Endotracheal tubes (Nos. 2.5, 3.0, 3.5—all uncuffed)
Stylets

Vascular Access

Umbilical catheters (Nos. 3.5 and 5 French)
Umbilical catheterization tray
Syringes (1, 3, 5, 10, 20, and 60 mL)
Needles (various gauges from 25 to 18)
Stopcocks
Suture (3-0 or 4-0 silk)
Sterile saline (10 mL)
IV catheters
IV tubing
Umbilical tape

Medications

Epinephrine (1:10,000)
Naloxone (Narcan) (1 mg/mL or 0.4 mg/mL)
IV solutions (normal saline, 10% dextrose)
Sodium bicarbonate (4.2%, 0.5 mEq/mL)
Albumin (5%)
Sterile water

Miscellaneous

Gloves (sterile and nonsterile)
Masks, with eye shield
Quick reference card for ages and weight

control. Simply keeping the newborn warm decreases morbidity more than the other components of resuscitation. In fact, paying attention to temperature should come before the ABCs.

Cold stress in the newborn leads to increased oxygen consumption and increased metabolic demands, which further complicate resuscitation of the asphyxiated newborn. This is especially true in very-low-birth-weight infants. The newborn's large surface area relative to body mass and poor insulating ability (decreased body fat, particularly in preterm infants) accelerate heat loss. Placing the newborn under a prewarmed radiant heat source and quickly drying the newborn with a prewarmed towel or blanket can minimize heat loss. Any wet blankets or towels should be removed from under the infant, or evaporative heat loss will continue. Drying of the infant also has an added benefit of providing gentle stimulation,

which may aid in the onset of spontaneous respiration.

It also is important not to allow the newborn to become too warm. An infant should not be left on a radiant warmer on manual control for more than a few minutes before servo-controlled temperature regulation is initiated. The control temperature should be set properly (at approximately 36.5°C). It is important to know how the warmer and temperature probe work, to ensure their proper functioning.

Establishment of an open airway is accomplished by placing the newborn on his or her back with the neck in a neutral to slightly extended position on a flat radiant warmer bed. The neck should not be hyperextended or flexed, and the warmer bed should not be in the Trendelenburg position, as was once recommended. If needed, a rolled blanket or towel may be placed under the shoulder, extending the head slightly. The newborn should now be in the best position to maintain an open airway.

When the infant has been correctly positioned, the mouth and nose should be quickly suctioned with either a bulb syringe or mechanical suction device. The material in the mouth should be suctioned first to decrease the risk for aspiration should the infant gasp. Deep suctioning of the esophagus and stomach or prolonged suctioning is contraindicated because it can produce a vagal response, leading to apnea and bradycardia. Suctioning should be limited to 3 to 5 seconds. This time limit, in addition to the avoidance of deep suctioning, will decrease the risk of vagal-induced apnea or bradycardia. Unfortunately, deep and prolonged suctioning maneuvers are common, preventable mistakes, which often cause bradycardia and lead to more intervention.

The next step is to provide tactile stimulation. The infant has already been dried and suctioned, which in many cases is sufficient tactile stimulation to initiate respiration. If not, there are two safe and appropriate ways to provide additional tactile stimulation: (1) briefly slapping or flicking the soles of the feet and (2) rubbing the infant's back. Other actions such as slapping the newborn's back or buttocks or blowing cool oxygen or air into the newborn's face can result in unnecessary bruising and hypothermia. Tactile stimulation should not be prolonged. The time elapsed from placing the newborn under the warmer to positioning, suctioning, and providing additional tactile stimulation should be no more than 15 to 20 seconds. During this time period, the adequacy of the infant's respiration and the heart rate should be assessed. Apnea noted at birth must be assumed to be secondary apnea; therefore, if apnea persists, then positive-pressure ventilation should be initiated.

The initial steps of warming, positioning, suctioning, and stimulation are applied in every newborn delivery. The remaining guidelines to resuscitation depend on evaluation of the infant while performing those initial steps of resuscitation. Apgar scores are of little value to the pediatrician or neonatologist at the delivery. Continued need for resuscitation depends on three clinical signs: (1) respiratory effort, (2) heart rate, and (3) color.

If the infant demonstrates a regular, effective breathing pattern after tactile stimulation, the heart rate is checked next. If the infant is gasping, is apneic, or has ineffective respiration, positive-pressure ventilation should be given. When respiratory effort has been evaluated and the appropriate action taken, if needed, the heart rate is monitored. If the heart rate is more than 100 beats per minute, the infant's color is evaluated. If the heart rate is less than 100 beats per minutes, even if the infant has spontaneous respiration, positive-pressure ventilation is begun. The heart rate can be monitored by auscultation or palpation of the pulse in the umbilical cord; for the less experienced, it is generally more prudent to auscultate (although not for longer than 6 seconds). Monitoring of the heart rate determines the extent of resuscitation, as is discussed later. The infant's color should be evaluated next. Peripheral cyanosis (acrocyanosis) is common in the newborn, but central cyanosis is abnormal. Central cyanosis involves the entire body, including the mucous membranes. If central cyanosis is present in a newborn with adequate respiration and a heart rate of more than 100 beats per minute, free-flowing oxygen should be administered. Oxygen at a flow rate of 5 liters per minute should be delivered through an oxygen hose held steadily (not waved back and forth) one-half inch from the infant's nares. This will deliver approximately 80% inspired oxygen to the infant. The infant should receive a high concentration of oxygen until he or she turns pink; then oxygen should be gradually withdrawn to the degree that the newborn can maintain a pink color.

MECONIUM-STAINED AMNIOTIC FLUID

Another situation unique to the resuscitation of the newborn is that of meconium-stained amniotic fluid. Thin, watery meconium-stained fluid has not been proven to contribute to increased perinatal morbidity, and specific management of these infants is probably unnecessary. However, thick and particulate meconium-stained amniotic fluid can lead to meconium aspiration syndrome, with or without persistent pulmonary hypertension. To minimize this risk, the newborn's mouth, pharynx, and nose should be suctioned with a No. 10 French catheter by the obstetrician as the newborn's head is delivered and before the shoulders are delivered. After delivery, the newborn should be placed under a radiant warmer and, before drying, any remaining meconium should be suctioned from the hypopharynx. The trachea should then be suctioned under direct vision. This is best accomplished by intubating with an endotracheal tube and applying suction (no more than 100 mm Hg) to a special meconium aspiration device attached to the endotracheal tube as the tube is withdrawn. Passing a suction catheter through the endotracheal tube is inappropriate, because it may be too small to

suction particulate meconium. Re-intubation followed by repeat suctioning should be performed until all meconium is removed, provided the infant's condition remains stable. Free-flowing oxygen should be provided with all intubation attempts, to minimize the risk of hypoxia. It is important to monitor the heart rate continuously, because positive-pressure ventilation may have to be initiated before all the meconium can be removed from the trachea. Gastric contents should be suctioned to evacuate any meconium swallowed, and thus prevent the possibility of later regurgitation and aspiration. However, this should only be done after resuscitation is completed and the infant's condition is stable.

POSITIVE-PRESSURE VENTILATION

Positive-pressure ventilation is the single most valuable therapeutic technique for resuscitating a newborn. Unfortunately, it also is the technique requiring the most skill and practice to apply correctly. Although anesthesia bags may be used, they are technically more difficult to master to effectively use to deliver the higher pressures sometimes required to resuscitate a sick newborn. A self-inflating resuscitation bag is preferable and should be equipped with a face mask and oxygen reservoir, which enables the bag to deliver a higher concentration of oxygen (90 to 100%). Without the oxygen reservoir, the self-inflating bag is unable to deliver a high concentration of oxygen. The flow of oxygen through the tubing should be increased to 5 to 8 liters per minute and be connected to the oxygen inlet on the resuscitation bag. The self-inflating bags have a pressure-release valve, commonly called a pop-off valve, that usually releases at 25 to 35 cm H_2O pressure. It often is necessary to occlude this pop-off valve to generate a sufficient amount of pressure to effectively ventilate a newborn's nonaerated lungs, especially with the first few breaths. With the pop-off valve occluded, care should be taken not to overventilate the newborn because this may cause a pneumothorax. A pressure manometer should always be used in conjunction with the bag to allow monitoring of the pressures generated and minimize the risk of inadvertent overdistention of the lung. Masks come in different shapes and sizes, with or without cushioned rims. The mask should be positioned to cover the chin, mouth, and nose but not the eyes.

For effective bag-and-mask ventilation, the infant should be in the correct position for an open airway, with the neck in a neutral to slightly extended position. The ventilator should stand in a position so as not to obstruct the view of the newborn's chest. The mask is placed over the infant's face, and light downward pressure is applied while squeezing the edges of the mask to form a seal between the mask and the infant's face. Large amounts of downward pressure are not required. Constant re-evaluation is necessary to ensure that the seal between the face and the mask is adequate and that chest expansion occurs with each assisted ventilation. If chest expansion is inadequate, the most common problem is an inadequate face/mask seal. Another common problem is blockage of the infant's airway by improper positioning or secretions. It may be necessary to reposition the infant or suction the infant's mouth and nose. If a good face/mask seal is obtained and airway patency maintained, then increasing the pressure may be necessary to expand the chest. Pressures of 20 to 40 cm H_2O are often required in infants with respiratory conditions that decrease lung compliance. The infant should be ventilated at a rate of 40 to 60 times per minute. After 15 to 30 seconds of effective bag-and-mask ventilation, the heart rate is determined. If the heart rate is more than 100 beats per minute and spontaneous, effective respiration has begun, then bag-and-mask ventilation can be gradually decreased, free-flowing oxygen provided, and continuation of effective respiration observed for. If the heart rate is 60 to 100 beats per minute and increasing, bag-and-mask ventilation is continued. If the heart rate is 60 to 100 but not increasing, the adequacy of the ventilation should be reassessed. If the heart rate remains less than 80 beats per minute, chest compressions should be begun. If the heart rate is less than 60 beats per minutes, the adequacy of ventilation is again assessed for and chest compressions are begun immediately. The need for establishing effective positive-pressure ventilation before initiating chest compressions cannot be overly emphasized, and failure to establish adequate face/mask seal is an extremely common (and preventable) cause of failing to establish effective positive-pressure ventilation.

CHEST COMPRESSIONS

Chest compressions are performed on the lower one third of the sternum, located between an imaginary line drawn between the nipples and the xiphoid process. Pressure should not be applied directly over the xiphoid. There are two methods for compressing the chest: (1) the thumb method and (2) the two-finger method. The thumb technique involves encircling the infant's body with both hands and placing the thumbs on the sternum and the fingers under the infant. Extreme caution should be used in stabilizing the fingers under the infant's back; flexing the fingers can injure the newborn's spine. The thumbs are used to compress the sternum. In the two-finger method, the physician uses the tips of the first two fingers or the middle and ring finger placed in a perpendicular position over the lower sternum. Only the fingertips rest on the chest and pressure is applied directly downward. Obviously, long fingernails preclude use of this method. The fingertips need to remain in contact with the sternum at all times; there should be no thumping of the sternum. Pressure sufficient to depress the sternum ½ to ¾ inch is used. The Neonatal Resuscitation Program suggests interposing chest compressions with ventilation in a 3:1 ratio. This amounts to 90 compressions and 30 breaths per minute. Therefore, the ventilation rate

during chest compressions is lower than the 40 to 60 range recommended when chest compressions are not being performed. The heart rate is evaluated every 30 seconds, and chest compressions are continued until the heart rate is more than 80 beats per minute.

ENDOTRACHEAL INTUBATION

Endotracheal intubation is indicated when prolonged positive-pressure ventilation is required or bag-and-mask ventilation is deemed ineffective. It is also indicated in the special circumstance of infants born with thick or particulate meconium in the amniotic fluid or in the case of congenital diaphragmatic hernia. Intubation is a skill that takes practice and becomes easier to do with experience.

At least two people are required for endotracheal intubation. The second person prepares the tape for securing the tube in place, administers free flow oxygen during the attempt, monitors the heart rate, limits the time of the attempt to no more than 20 seconds, assesses if the attempt is successful, helps determine the appropriateness of the position of the tube, and helps secure the tube in place. In preparation for intubation, the laryngoscope should be equipped with a No. 0 blade for premature infants and a No. 1 blade for full-term infants (although many skilled intubators find a No. 0 blade sufficient for full-term infants as well). The light source should be checked to see that it is functional. Then the proper-sized endotracheal tube is selected based on the newborn's weight. A 2.5-mm (internal diameter) size is appropriate for infants weighing less than 1.0 kg, a 3.0-mm size is used for infants weighing 1.0 to 2.0 kg, and a 3.5-mm sized endotracheal tube is appropriate for infants weighing more than 2.0 kg. Use of a stylet is optional but is not really necessary. If a stylet is used, care should be taken to ensure that the tip of the stylet does not protrude beyond the tip of the endotracheal tube and that the stylet is easily removable once in the tube. Mechanical suctioning (not to exceed 100 mm Hg) should be available as well as free-flowing oxygen to provide a high concentration of oxygen during the procedure to minimize hypoxia. The resuscitation bag and mask are kept at the bedside for use between intubation attempts and for connecting to the endotracheal tube after intubation is accomplished.

The infant is placed in the proper position with the head midline with the neck slightly extended. The laryngoscope handle is held in the left hand, irrespective of handedness of the operator; the infant's head is stabilized with the right hand, and the blade is inserted between the tongue and palate until the tip of the blade rests in the vallecula. The glottis is visualized by lifting the entire blade in a direction parallel to the length of the laryngoscope handle. The laryngoscope is never used like a lever, as in a "prying" or "can opener" type of maneuver. Once the glottis is in view, the endotracheal tube is inserted with the right hand until the vocal cord guideline (the heavy black line near the tip of the tube) is at the level of the vocal cords. Another guideline for positioning the endotracheal tube is to add "6" to the infant's weight in kilograms, then tape the endotracheal tube at that number of centimeters at the gum. The endotracheal tube is held securely until it is taped into position. Equal breath sounds are listened for bilaterally in the axillae, and then a chest radiograph is obtained to confirm the tube position. The position that the tube is taped at should be recorded, because this is useful for repositioning later and for determining if the tube has inadvertently shifted in position.

Often one is so elated at successfully passing the tube that one fails to pay attention to the distance that it is inserted. Much harm can come from having an endotracheal tube inserted too far. If the endotracheal tube is inserted too far, it can rest in the right mainstem bronchus, causing poor oxygen and carbon dioxide exchange and overdistention of that lung segment, possibly leading to pulmonary interstitial emphysema and pneumothorax. In the premature infant, extra care should be taken to ensure proper endotracheal tube placement because the "6 plus weight in kilograms" rule may be less reliable; the tube may need to be inserted to a shorter length. To ensure against esophageal intubation, auscultation for air entering the stomach is done and gastric distention is observed for. This usually becomes apparent because secretions will enter the endotracheal tube and the newborn will fail to respond clinically.

MEDICATIONS

Medications are rarely needed for resuscitation in the newborn. Ventilation with 100% oxygen is usually sufficient. However, in the newborn whose heart rate remains less than 80 beats per minute despite adequate ventilation with 100% oxygen and effective chest compressions of more than 30 seconds, or in the newborn with no heart rate, medications should be administered. The initial medication administered usually is epinephrine. Epinephrine increases cardiac output by increasing the heart rate and myocardial contractility and increases blood pressure by causing peripheral vasoconstriction. It should be given rapidly either intravenously or through the endotracheal tube in a dose of 0.1 to 0.3 mL per kg of the 1:10,000 solution. The intravenous route is preferred, because plasma concentrations through the endotracheal route are sometimes low. However, intravenous access often has not been established when the first dose of epinephrine is required, so it may be preferable to give the higher recommended dose when it is administered through the endotracheal route. During this time, umbilical venous access can easily be established in any infant by inserting a catheter in the umbilical vein 2 or 3 cm so that the catheter tip is below the liver. The umbilical vein is the single, large, thin-walled vessel usually in the 12 o'clock position when looking at the infant with the head at the top. Thereafter, all medications

are preferably given by this route. Epinephrine may be repeated every 5 minutes if the heart rate remains less than 100 beats per minute. (Epinephrine should never be given in the umbilical artery.)

If there is no response to epinephrine, one should suspect metabolic acidosis. This is also a good time to reassess adequacy of ventilation and to check that 100% oxygen is being administered. In this case, sodium bicarbonate is indicated in a dose of 2 mEq per kg intravenously. Intracranial hemorrhage has been associated with the use of bicarbonate in animal studies. To reduce that risk, sodium bicarbonate in the commercially available 4.2% solution (0.5 mEq per mL) should be given slowly over a minimum of 2 minutes, not to exceed a rate of 1 mEq per minute. Hypovolemia must also be considered if there is no response to the administration of epinephrine and bicarbonate. Hypovolemia that manifests in the newborn is usually a known event (e.g., umbilical cord accidents, placenta previa) and is indicated by pallor and poor perfusion despite a normal pH and P_{O_2}, and weak pulses despite a good heart rate. A dose of 10 mL per kg of volume expander should be given intravenously, slowly. In the premature infant at risk for intracranial hemorrhage, this volume should always be given slowly over at least 30 minutes. However, in the asphyxiated, hypovolemic full-term infant it may be necessary to administer the volume over 5 to 10 minutes. It is essential to monitor the heart rate and discontinue medications once the heart rate is more than 100 beats per minute.

In the instance of an infant born with respiratory depression to a mother who received narcotics within 4 hours of delivery, naloxone, 0.1 mg per kg, given rapidly is indicated. When needed, naloxone may be given through the endotracheal tube, intravenously, intramuscularly, or subcutaneously. It should not be given if the mother has a narcotic dependency, because this may precipitate a drug withdrawal syndrome in the infant. The infant who receives naloxone should be observed, because the narcotic causing the respiratory depression may have a longer duration of action than the naloxone, whose duration of action is 1 to 4 hours.

Successful neonatal resuscitation requires communication between the resuscitation team and obstetric staff, advance preparation, and skilled and knowledgeable personnel. The attainment of these objectives is an easily achievable and laudable goal for all hospitals catering to pregnant women. I strongly recommend all delivery room personnel complete the Neonatal Resuscitation Program offered by the American Academy of Pediatrics/American Heart Association in an effort to improve their individual and group competence.

CARE OF THE HIGH-RISK NEONATE

method of
DIANNE J. ALBRECHT, M.D.
Louisiana State University School of Medicine
New Orleans, Louisiana

and

DAVID A. CLARK, M.D.
Albany Medical College
Albany, New York

DELIVERY ROOM MANAGEMENT

Neonatal Resuscitation

An adequately prepared for and properly performed resuscitation is of paramount importance in providing the high-risk neonate optimal chances for a good outcome. Anticipation of the high-risk delivery is the first step in this process. In addition, adequate preparation and supplies should be available for the distressed neonate in all facilities where such deliveries could occur (e.g., obstetric observation areas and emergency departments). All health professionals who care for patients in areas where newborns are cared for should participate in the Neonatal Resuscitation Program (NRP), which is sponsored by the American Heart Association in conjunction with the American Academy of Pediatrics, and should have regular updates, reviews, and drills on the subject matter. Further information regarding the specifics of neonatal resuscitation can be found in the article on neonatal resuscitation.

Transition Physiology

At birth, the infant must rapidly make the transition from fetal to extrauterine circulation. In order for this to happen, a number of physiologic changes must take place. In the fetal circulatory system, the relatively oxygenated blood from the placenta flows through the umbilical vein and ductus venosus, into the inferior vena cava, and through the foramen ovale and then enters the systemic circulation. Relatively unoxygenated blood returns from the body through the superior vena cava at the right atrium and then through the pulmonary artery, where it is shunted via the ductus arteriosus to the descending aorta and on to the umbilical arteries, back to the placenta. With the birth process and clamping of the umbilical cord, the systemic pressure increases. Concomitantly the newborn takes its first breaths with clearing of the fetal lung fluid, and the pulmonary pressure begins to fall. The formerly patent ductus arteriosus, under the influence of multiple factors (including increasing arterial oxygen content), begins to close, thereby further encouraging blood flow through the newborn's lungs.

In certain situations, this transition does not occur smoothly, and the clinician needs to be especially alert to this possibility. For instance, infants delivered by cesarean section may have delayed clearing of fetal lung fluid, which leads to tachypnea. Other substances in the lungs such as meconium or maternal blood may interfere with adequate ventilation, as may pulmonary immaturity in the preterm infant, which leads to surfactant deficiency. Infants with congenital heart disease also may not be capable of easily making the transition from fetal to neonatal circulation.

Transition Assessment and Apgar Scores

A quantitative and fairly universally used method of assessing the infant's adaptation to extrauterine life is the Apgar score, developed by Dr. Virginia Apgar. This score is composed of five components: heart rate, respiratory effort, muscle tone, reflex irritability and skin color (Table 1). After delivery and initial resuscitation measures, the score is calculated at 1 minute and then again at 5 minutes of age.

The 1-minute score can be viewed as a reflection of how the infant tolerated the birth process and immediate resuscitation efforts. The 5-minute score reflects the infant's ongoing adaptation and responses to resuscitation. An Apgar score of 7 or higher is usually thought to be "normal"; 2 or less is thought of as severely depressed. Also, when the Apgar score is less than 6 at 5 minutes, a 10-minute score may be calculated.

It is also important to note that in less mature infants, especially those who are extremely immature, the muscle tone and reflex irritability components may be less accurate merely as a reflection of gestational age.

NEWBORN ASSESSMENT

History

A complete copy of the mother's pregnancy, labor, and delivery records, as well as any pertinent medi-

TABLE 1. **Components of the Apgar Score**

Component	0	1	2
Heart rate	Absent	<100 beats per minute	>100 beats per minute
Respiratory effort	Apneic	Shallow, irregular, gasping	Vigorous cry
Reflex irritability	Absent	Grimace	Active avoidance
Muscle tone	Flaccid	Weak, passive	Active movement
Skin color	Pale, cyanotic	Pale, acrocyanotic	Pink

From Gowen CW Jr: Care of the high-risk neonate. *In* Rakel RE: Conn's Current Therapy 1995. Philadelphia, WB Saunders Co., 1995, p. 964.

cal history, should be available to the pediatrician or neonatologist either before or at the time of the infant's birth. There should also be adequate communication between the obstetrician and personnel assuming care of the newborn. Necessary components of the maternal history are listed in Table 2.

TABLE 2. **Components of the Maternal History**

Routine Prenatal Care

Ages of the mother and father
Marital status
Last menstrual period
Estimated date of confinement
Onset of prenatal care
Prepregnancy weight and weight gain during pregnancy

Previous Pregnancies

Number
Outcome of each
Previous prenatal, intrapartum, neonatal complications

Prenatal Maternal Laboratory Studies

Blood type and Rh
Antibody screen
HBsAg
HIV antibody

Underlying Maternal Systemic Illnesses

Pregnancy-Related Illnesses

Maternal Medications

Steroids
Tocolytics
Antibiotics
Sedatives, analgesics, anesthetics

Maternal Substance Use/Abuse

Tobacco
Alcohol
Marijuana, cocaine
Amphetamines, heroin, methadone
Phencyclidine (PCP)

Prenatal Fetal Laboratory Studies

Alpha-fetoprotein
Bacterial, viral cultures
Amniotic fluid lung maturity studies
Fetal chromosome studies

Fetal Status

Number
Ultrasound results
Time of rupture of membranes
Cord injuries/prolapse
Results of fetal heart rate monitoring
Maternal bleeding: placenta previa, abruption
History of oligohydramnios or polyhydramnios
Meconium staining

Delivery

Premature labor (use of tocolytics)
Method of delivery
Presentation
Use of instrumentation: forceps, vacuum

Preferred Method of Feeding

Desire for Circumcision

Abbreviations: HBsAg = hepatitis B surface antigen; HIV = human immunodeficiency virus.

Adapted from D'Harlingue A, Durand D: Recognition, stabilization, and transport of the high-risk newborn. *In* Klaus M, Fanaroff A (eds): Care of the High-Risk Neonate, 4th ed. Philadelphia, WB Saunders Co., 1993, pp 62–85.

Intrauterine Growth, Physical Maturity, and Gestational Age Assessment

Crucial to any examination of the newborn is an assessment of intrauterine growth and gestational age. The New Ballard score (see Figure 1) is probably the most common tool in aiding the examiner along those lines. It is widely used and can be applied to infants older than 20 weeks of gestational age. It is commonly done with the initial postdelivery examination and is a part of the nursing admission protocol in many nurseries. However, the neuromuscular evaluation section is more appropriately performed at a follow-up examination within 24 hours of delivery. The birth process itself is stressful for the infant; in addition, medications given to the mother during labor and delivery may also affect the newborn (e.g., leading to alterations in tone) and produce a falsely low score.

In addition to assessment of gestational age and maturity, infant growth parameters are compared to standardized growth charts. On the basis of the 90th and 10th percentiles, newborns are categorized as appropriate for gestational age (AGA), small for gestational age (SGA), or large for gestational age (LGA). Infants are classified in terms of weight with regard to gestational age: preterm (less than 37 weeks), full-term (38 to 42 weeks), and post-term (greater than 42 weeks). Each category has associated possible problems that may be associated and these are shown in Figure 2.

Neonates can also be classified according to birth weight as follows: normal birth weight is 2500 grams or more; low birth weight (LBW) is less than 2500 grams; very low birth weight (VLBW) is less than 1500 grams.

Physical Examination

A quick physical examination is usually performed in the delivery room and enables discovery of most major malformations as well as further clues to any problems the infant may be having in terms of adapting to extrauterine life.

A second physical examination is usually performed in the nursery and includes a complete set of vital signs. At the neonatal assessment more than at any other time, observation plays a major role in the physical examination. The newborn's color, tone, level of activity, and general responsiveness to the environment are very important. In general, neonates are best examined in the following order: observation, auscultation, and palpation, followed by the systematic head-to-toe approach with its attendant manipulations. Listed next are some findings that may be noted at the initial physical examination.

Head. Inspection and palpation of the head should be performed, and any bruising or abnormality of shape should be noted. Significant molding of the head can result from intrauterine or vaginal positioning and pressure during labor. The anterior and posterior fontanelles should also be palpated, as should

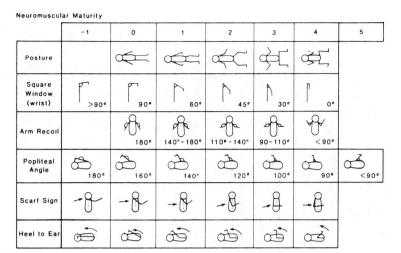

Figure 1. Expanded New Ballard Score. (From Ballard JL, Khoury JC, Wedig K, et al: New Ballard Score, expanded to include extremely premature infants. J Pediatr *119:*417–423, 1991.)

Physical Maturity

	-1	0	1	2	3	4	5
Skin	sticky friable transparent	gelatinous red, translucent	smooth pink, visible veins	superficial peeling &/or rash. few veins	cracking pale areas rare veins	parchment deep cracking no vessels	leathery cracked wrinkled
Lanugo	none	sparse	abundant	thinning	bald areas	mostly bald	
Plantar Surface	heel-toe 40-50mm:-1 <40mm:-2	>50mm no crease	faint red marks	anterior transverse crease only	creases ant. 2/3	creases over entire sole	
Breast	imperceptible	barely perceptible	flat areola no bud	stippled areola 1-2mm bud	raised areola 3-4mm bud	full areola 5-10mm bud	
Eye/Ear	lids fused loosely:-1 tightly:-2	lids open pinna flat stays folded	sl. curved pinna; soft; slow recoil	well-curved pinna; soft but ready recoil	formed &firm instant recoil	thick cartilage ear stiff	
Genitals male	scrotum flat, smooth	scrotum empty faint rugae	testes in upper canal rare rugae	testes descending few rugae	testes down good rugae	testes pendulous deep rugae	
Genitals female	clitoris prominent labia flat	prominent clitoris small labia minora	prominent clitoris enlarging minora	majora & minora equally prominent	majora large minora small	majora cover clitoris & minora	

Maturity Rating

score	weeks
-10	20
-5	22
0	24
5	26
10	28
15	30
20	32
25	34
30	36
35	38
40	40
45	42
50	44

the suture lines. Because of the widespread use of transvaginal intrauterine monitoring, the scalp should also be inspected for puncture marks or lacerations that may serve as a later nidus for infection. The presence of a caput succedaneum, which is a subcutaneous collection of edema, should be noted and differentiated from a cephalhematoma, which is a true subperiosteal hemorrhage and does not cross suture lines.

Eyes. The eyes are best examined shortly after delivery, and this examination may prove difficult for the clinician because eyelids may be edematous, either from delivery or from the chemical conjunctivitis that sometimes develops with application of antimicrobial agents to the eyes. In spite of this, an ophthalmoscopic examination should be performed to document the presence of the "red reflex." Findings associated with an abnormal light reflex include cataracts (which suggest a metabolic or an infectious process) glaucoma and retinoblastoma. Conjunctival hemorrhages are a common finding on the neonatal eye examination, especially in infants delivered vaginally.

Ears. The shape, size, and position of the ears should be noted, because "low-set" ears may accompany certain malformation sequences. This can be determined by imagining a line from the outer corner of the infant's eye to the occipital prominence. If the upper attachment of the ear is below this line, the ears are said to be "low-set." The examiner is cautioned, however, to take into consideration the amount of molding that may be present for a particular infant's head. Anterior ear "pits" and skin tags are also common findings.

Nose. Flaring of the ala nasi may be indicative of respiratory distress, although transitioning newborns may be expected to have some degree of nasal flaring. The patency of the nares should be ascertained; in fact, newborns with choanal atresia or choanal stenosis may exhibit respiratory distress in the delivery room, as newborns are primarily nose breathers. The passage of a feeding tube through both nares into the hypopharynx is routinely done to check for atresia or stenosis.

Mouth. Evaluation of the oral cavity is done to detect palatal clefts or natal teeth. The infant should also be observed crying, because cranial nerve VII palsies are a fairly common finding in association

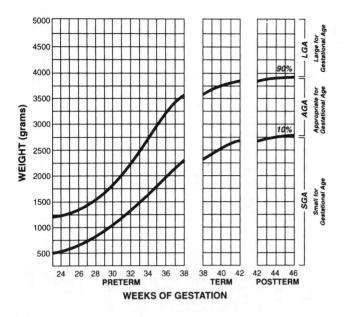

Term LGA	Preterm LGA	Post-term LGA
Birth trauma Hypoglycemia Transposition of the great vessels	Hypoglycemia Hyperbilirubinemia Birth injury Infant of diabetic mother Hypocalcemia Hyperviscosity Congenital anomalies	Birth trauma Polycythemia Hypoglycemia Meconium aspiration Pneumothorax
Term AGA	Preterm AGA	Post-term AGA
Lowest Risk	Respiratory distress syndrome Hypothermia Hypoglycemia Hyperglycemia Hyperbilirubinemia Hyponatremia Hypocalcemia Apnea Infection CNS hemorrhage	Pneumothorax Meconium aspiration Hypoglycemia
Term SGA	Preterm SGA	Post-term SGA
Hypothermia Hypoglycemia Meconium aspiration Polycythemia Malnutrition Congenital infection Congenital anomalies Maternal addiction	Hypothermia Hypoglycemia Anemia Asphyxia Hyperbilirubinemia Hypocalcemia Malnutrition Congenital infection Congenital anomalies	Polycythemia Hypoglycemia Congenital anomalies Dysmaturity

Figure 2. Neonatal morbidity risk. (Adapted from Lubchenco LO, Searls DT, Brazie JV: Neonatal mortality rate: Relationship to birthweight and gestational age. J Pediatr *81*:818, 1972; reprinted with permission from Coen RW, Koffler H: Primary Care of the Newborn, published by Little, Brown and Company, Boston, 1987, p 60.)

with forceps compression of the nerve or with a traumatic passage through the birth canal.

Neck. The infant's neck should be checked for any clefts, sinuses, or masses. The trachea should be in the midline. The sternocleidomastoid muscle may be injured at birth, and this may lead to limited range of motion. In addition to this, intrauterine positioning may have contributed to congenital torticollis. The clavicles should be palpated to detect fractures, especially in large infants.

Chest and Cardiovascular Examination. The infant should be observed in the quiet state; any intercostal, supraclavicular, substernal, or subcostal retractions should be noted. Presence and spacing of the nipples should also be noted. The examiner can then proceed to auscultation of the lungs and of heart sounds. The normal newborn heart rate is 120 to 160 beats per minute, with a range of 80 to 180 beats per minute. Heart sounds should be best heard over the left sternal border. The examiner should note the presence of any murmurs. A closing ductus arteriosus may lead to a transient continuous murmur, but more serious pathology may not be accompanied by any murmur at all. Pulses should be palpated in all extremities (this may be done concomitantly with examination of the extremities, as described later).

The respiratory rate of the newborn is usually between 40 to 60 breaths per minute. Depending on the timing of the physical examination, rales may be heard and may be indicative of unabsorbed lung fluid. Such rales should be noted and monitored, but in the otherwise healthy-appearing infant, they are usually of little concern. Other than that, the breath sounds should be symmetrical.

Abdomen. The abdomen should appear symmetrical and nondistended. The liver can usually be palpated in the newborn at about 2 cm below the right costal margin. The spleen is usually not palpable. The kidneys are fairly easy to palpate at the first examination and can be felt to be about 2.0 to 2.5 cm in length with deep palpation. If a mass is detected on first examination, further work-up is warranted; it should be kept in mind that the majority of abdominal masses detected in the newborn period are of renal origin. The umbilicus should be examined, and the presence of meconium staining should be noted. Two arteries and one vein should also be noted in the cord.

Genitalia. The male infant should be examined for the presence of hypospadias or epispadias, and both testes should be palpable in the scrotum. The female infant usually has notably enlarged labia majora. In addition to this, common benign findings include a vaginal mucosal tag or a creamy white vaginal discharge.

Anus. The anus should be examined externally for patency and location.

Spine. The back should be carefully examined for sinus tracts, sacral dimpling, or meningomyeloceles. The hyperpigmented mongolian spot is a common, prominent finding in darker pigmented populations.

Extremities. Pulses may be palpated during examination of the extremities, if not already done as part of the cardiovascular examination. Anomalies of the digits, including the presence of extra digits and syndactyly, are fairly common, as is talipes (clubfoot). Intrauterine positioning may cause a bowing of the legs and pronation of the feet. As a general rule, if the feet can be brought into normal position by gentle pressure, they are probably normal and the abnormality will resolve spontaneously. The hips should be checked for dislocation.

Skin. The newborn skin can manifest a variety of findings, including mottling, harlequin color change, and erythema toxicum, to name a few, the descriptions of which are beyond the scope of this article. Those findings should be noted for follow-up evaluation.

Neurologic Examination. The neurologic assessment of the infant is best performed by close observation during other parts of the physical examination. Much information is gathered concerning the infant's state of alertness, responsiveness to examination, and general tone and posture. In addition to this, the primitive reflexes such as the Moro reflex, palmar grasp, rooting, and sucking should be evaluated.

In general, a thorough and complete physical examination of the newborn, especially the healthy full-term infant, can be done in 5 to 10 minutes. Many "abnormal" findings are merely normal variants or the after-effects of the somewhat traumatic birth process and will resolve with the passage of time. Parents, especially first-time parents, may need reassurance about many of these, such as prominent cranial molding, conjunctival hemorrhages, and the numerous "benign" neonatal skin findings.

Transport

An ideal situation allows identification of the high-risk neonate before delivery and thus allows optimal time for planning of transportation. In all cases, it could seem to be beneficial to transport the unborn fetus in utero. However, many high-risk deliveries occur without warning, and so the need may arise to transport an unstable infant to a tertiary or regional neonatal intensive care unit (NICU). Most regional units have a complete neonatal transport team (usually with both ground and air transportation capabilities) and have a neonatologist available 24 hours a day to provide phone consultation and assistance in the care of the newborn before and during the transport. The transport team is usually tailored to the needs of the particular infant and may include a nurse, a respiratory therapist, a neonatal nurse practitioner, and/or a physician.

GENERAL MANAGEMENT

Laboratory Assessment

The immediate laboratory assessment of the sick newborn is performed in accordance with the suspected cause of problems. A complete blood cell count (CBC) with differential and platelets is almost universally obtained because this provides a baseline hematocrit if there are concerns with anemia or polycythemia; it can also give some clue as to whether infection may be playing a role in the particular infant's pathologic process. Blood cultures are also done fairly early if the suspicion of sepsis exists. If there is extreme concern over the possibility of anemia, as in cases of placentae abruptio or maternal bleeding, most nurseries have the capability of performing a "spun hematocrit" on site. A dip stick test is also usually performed soon after birth because the infant's blood glucose level may be lowered from the stress of the delivery and from any resuscitation measures that may have been necessary. Infants usually tolerate a blood glucose level of 40 mg per dL or higher, although this value would indicate a need for either the initiation of enteral feedings or intravenous fluids in a timely manner. The healthy infant born to a healthy mother can be expected to have serum chemistry profiles reflective of the mother's for the first 24 hours after birth. However, in the extremely immature infant or in the infant in whom the possibility of metabolic derangement exists (e.g., an infant of a diabetic mother or of a mother maintained on magnesium sulfate before delivery), it may be useful to check baseline laboratory findings before the 24-hour mark is reached. These findings may include serum electrolytes, blood urea nitrogen (BUN), creatinine, calcium, magnesium, and possibly serum bilirubin concentrations if a hemolytic process is suspected or anticipated.

To identify maternal-fetal red blood cell antigen incompatibilities, it is also common for the infant's blood type to be determined and Coombs' test to be performed (in many nurseries, these tests are performed on cord blood as a standing order on admission).

Fluid and Electrolytes

Many factors influence the balance of fluid, electrolytes, and glucose levels in preterm and sick neonates. A few guidelines can be laid out, but it is of paramount importance to take into consideration the underlying pathologic process when fluids and electrolytes are administered. For instance, the needs of a 4000-gram infant born at term with meconium aspiration and subsequent persistent pulmonary hypertension of the newborn (PPHN) would be vastly different from those of the extremely immature 500-gram infant with respiratory distress syndrome (RDS).

In general, fluids in our institution are initiated as follows: On day 1 (date of birth), infants weighing less than 1.0 kg are started on 5% dextrose in water at a rate of 100 to 120 mL per kg per day. Infants born weighing between 1.0 kg and 1.5 kg are usually started on 10% dextrose in water at 80 to 100 mL per kg per day, and those weighing more than 1.5 kg are started on 10% dextrose in water at a rate of 80 mL per kg per day. Weight is the most accurate means of assessing a neonate's fluid status in the first days of life, and a loss of about 1 to 2% of body weight per day typically occurs over the first 3 to 4 days. The intravenous fluid rate is usually advanced by about 20 to 30 mL per kg per day up to a maximum of 180 mL per kg per day in larger infants and 150 mL per kg per day in infants for whom fluid overload may be a concern (i.e., with possibility of patent ductus arteriosus).

Fluid requirements are sometimes increased in situations involving extreme immaturity or skin breakdown, excessive environmental temperatures (as with radiant warmers or phototherapy), or "third spacing"–type losses or losses from the gastrointestinal tract. Many of these losses are not unexpected and can be taken into account when daily plans are made.

As mentioned previously, the neonate's electrolytes generally reflect those of the mother unless certain extenuating factors apply (extreme prematurity, for instance). Maintenance sodium (2 to 3 mEq per kg per day) and maintenance potassium (1 to 2 mEq per kg per day) are usually added after 24 hours; potassium is added after urine output and renal function are ensured. The serum electrolytes are then usually monitored at least daily and more frequently if the infant's condition is unstable.

Serum sodium levels are considered within normal range at 130 to 150 mEq per dL and potassium is considered normal at 3.5 to 5.5 mEq per dL. Hypocalcemia is generally defined as a serum calcium level of less than 7.0 mg per dL in a preterm infant or less than 8.0 mg per dL in a full-term infant. Treatment is with 100 to 200 mg per kg of calcium gluconate given either as a slow infusion over 20 to 30 minutes or added into the daily intravenous fluids.

Nutrition

Parenteral Nutrition

In those infants too small or unstable to consider oral feedings, parenteral nutrition is usually begun on the second or third day of life. Total volume is usually maintained according to plans (as discussed earlier); some adjustments sometimes have to be made for medication volumes, fluid balances, need for blood product replacement, and so forth. Glucose for parenteral infusion likewise is planned and adjusted according to what the neonate had been receiving in intravenous fluids. If long-term parenteral alimentation is foreseen, glucose concentrations may be increased daily up to 12% when administered peripherally and up to 20 to 25% when administered through a central vessel. Infants are monitored periodically for hyperglycemia, especially as concentrations are be advanced. Protein infusion is commonly started at 0.5 gram per kg per day and gradually increased to 2.5 to 3.0 grams per kg per day. Attention is paid here to a rising BUN or the presence of metabolic acidosis. Fat infusion is also started at 0.5 gram per kg day and increased to 2.5 to 3.0 grams per kg day gradually. Serum triglyceride levels are usually monitored at least weekly, because fat metabolism may vary. It is usually safe to advance both fat and protein in increments of 0.5 gram per kg day. Vitamins and trace elements are also provided daily. The usual caloric goal is 120 kcal per kg per day, although some infants may begin to gain weight with as little as 80 kcal per kg per day.

Enteral Nutrition

In infants well enough to tolerate oral feedings, these are initiated as soon as possible, usually by the second or third day of life as ventilatory status permits. For the small, immature infant, breast milk or a preterm whey-predominant formula is usually started at 40 mL per kg per day (or 5 mL per kg per feeding on a 3-hour schedule) by nipple or gavage as tolerated. Especially with the small preterm infants (<1500 grams), feeding tolerance is monitored closely, in regard to both undigested food and episodes of vomiting and stooling patterns. At least one stool is expected to occur daily, and all stools are tested for blood. Feedings are usually discontinued or advancement is postponed if residuals occur or if there is a deviation from the normal stooling pattern, because both these occurrences can be markers for impending necrotizing enterocolitis.

Again, the caloric goal for adequate weight gain is 120 kcal per kg per day. The volume to provide this for the growing premature or full-term infant is 180 mL per kg per day. Smaller premature infants and those at risk for bronchopulmonary dysplasia may be limited to 150 mL per kg per day, and this may be supplied as a more calorie-dense formula so that adequate caloric intake is supplied. Breast milk for preterms is usually supplemented with human milk fortifier for adequate supplies of electrolytes and minerals.

Thermoregulation

Attention to temperature control is one of the most important immediate concerns with the high-risk infant at delivery. Small premature infants have an increased surface area in relation to weight and a lack of subcutaneous fat stores and so are more prone to cold stress. Hypothermia in the large, stressed infant can predispose to development of metabolic acidosis and contribute to the development of PPHN. For those reasons, among others, strict attention should be paid to delivering the infant into a relatively warm environment (delivery room temperature of 24° to 27°C) and placing under a preheated radiant warmer. The infant is then dried, and a cap should be placed on the head, because this is one of the greatest sources of heat loss for the newborn. In the NICU, the sick infant is usually cared for under a radiant warmer because this provides optimal access to the infant. A double-walled incubator may also be used for this purpose in some nurseries and is used in most units for the growing stable infant. The neonate's temperature is maintained in the range of 36.5° to 37.5°C in order to permit normal body temperature for a minimum expenditure of energy. This is termed the "neutral thermal environment" and varies with gestational age, size, and chronological age of the infant.

Blood Pressure Support

Hypotension is a problem common to both ill preterm infants and full-term newborns. Infants who have suffered acute blood loss at delivery either with placenta previa or with placentae abruptio may require volume replacement at delivery. This is usually best accomplished by inserting an umbilical venous line under sterile conditions in the delivery room and infusing 5% albumin as a bolus volume expander. For infants in whom the need for blood is suspected before delivery, such as infants with erythroblastosis fetalis, most blood banks have type O-negative blood available for emergency release.

Normal blood pressure varies with gestational and chronological age. A general rule for the immediate neonatal period is that the mean arterial blood pressure should equal the gestational age of the infant (e.g., an infant of 25 weeks' gestation may be expected to have a mean arterial pressure of 25 mm Hg). If decreased blood pressure remains a problem after adequate volume expansion, dopamine may be administered. The usual method is to start at 5 μg per kg per minute and titrate upwards to a maximum of 20 μg per kg per minute until desired blood pressure is achieved.

Respiratory Support

Ventilator management is complex, and strategies vary according to institution, mode of therapy, and, most important, the neonate's underlying pathologic process. The general goal is to provide for optimal oxygen and carbon dioxide levels in the blood while minimizing the risks of oxygen toxicity and barotrauma. Many infants with mild RDS, pneumonia, and tachypnea of the newborn can be managed with humidified oxygen provided by means of an oxygen hood or tent. All infants needing oxygen therapy or ventilatory support of any kind should be placed on cardiorespiratory monitoring and transcutaneous pulse oximetry. The goal is for arterial blood gases to have a pH in the range of 7.30 to 7.45, a carbon dioxide partial pressure (Pco_2) of 35 to 50, and an oxygen partial pressure (Po_2) of 60 to 90 (different disease states may warrant adjusting these parameters; e.g., in the infant with PPHN, the goal is hyperventilation and alkalosis). Neonates needing ventilatory support are usually started on conventional ventilation with a time-cycled, pressure-limited standard ventilator. Some tertiary centers may place very small preterm infants on high-frequency oscillators as an initial therapy; this type of ventilation is also used variably with air leak syndromes, PPHN, and congenital diaphragmatic hernia (CDH) before repair. In addition to these modalities, extracorporeal membrane oxygenation (ECMO) is used in some institutions to manage PPHN and CDH patients. Volume-cycled ventilators are commonly used to manage chronically ventilated older infants, and nitric oxide is used as an investigational drug as a means of managing pulmonary hypertension.

SPECIAL PROBLEMS OF THE HIGH-RISK NEONATE
Neurologic

Seizures

Seizure activity in the neonatal period, especially in the extremely premature infant, often does not manifest as the stereotypical tonic-clonic activity seen in older patients. Seizures in neonates can be classified as myoclonic, clonic, tonic, and subtle. Subtle seizures include tonic eye deviation, sucking movements of the mouth, and bicycling- and swimming-type movements of the extremities, along with autonomic or vascular changes. Apnea may also be a manifestation of seizure activity in the newborn. The causes of seizures include central nervous system (CNS) pathologic processes (such as intraventricular hemorrhage or hypoxic-ischemic encephalopathy), congenital anomalies leading to CNS malformation, metabolic problems (e.g., hypoglycemia, hypocalcemia), and infectious causes (meningitis and encephalitis). It is often difficult to distinguish jitters from seizure activity, and an electroencephalogram is obtained if seizure activity is thought to be likely. Management includes initiation of anticonvulsant therapy; phenobarbital is the usual drug of first choice, and other agents usually include phenytoin or lorazepam. It is important to correct the underlying problem and to provide supportive therapy.

Intraventricular Hemorrhage

Periventricular-intraventricular hemorrhage is one of the most common concerns in caring for the sick preterm newborn. It is estimated that 25 to 40% of infants born at less than 34 weeks' gestation may have some evidence of intracranial bleeding documented on computed tomography or ultrasonography of the head; the incidence is inversely proportional to the gestational age. Most such hemorrhages occur in the first few days of life, and more than 95% occur by the end of the first week. Signs and symptoms vary according to the severity of the hemorrhage but are generally nonspecific and may include seizure activity, hypotension, need for increasing ventilatory support, or more subtle signs such as a drop in hematocrit or decreased muscle tone and activity. Often the least severe hemorrhages are diagnosed on routine screening cranial ultrasonographic studies 1 week after birth in infants born at 34 weeks' gestation or less. In managing the premature infant at risk for periventricular or intraventricular hemorrhage (PVH-IVH), the focus is on prevention with the goal of minimal stimulation, the avoidance of rapid administration of intravenous fluids, and attention to electrolyte and acid-base balance. Once an intracranial hemorrhage has occurred, the treatment is supportive with the management of attendant complications (e.g., seizures or posthemorrhagic hydrocephalus). Prognosis varies with severity of the hemorrhage.

Periventricular Leukomalacia

Periventricular leukomalacia is a lesion of white matter that is increasingly diagnosed today, probably as ultrasonographers become more adept at the imaging of the infant brain. Risk factors are essentially the same as those associated with PVH-IVH and include fetal distress, immaturity, hypoxia, and alterations in cerebral blood flow. The lesion consists of ischemic necrosis of periventricular white matter with possible progression to cavitation, cyst formation, and subsequent enlargement of ventricles. Ultimate outcomes differ but may include spastic diplegia and variable degrees of intellectual involvement.

Hypoxic-Ischemic Encephalopathy

Hypoxic-ischemic encephalopathy is commonly a problem of full-term or post-term infants who have undergone either prepartum, intrapartum, or perinatal asphyxial brain insult. The underlying cerebral pathologic process is brain edema and swelling with possible accompanying intraventricular hemorrhage. Management is supportive, with seizure control and ventilatory support as necessary. Long-term outcomes are variable, but many of these infants have severe intellectual and motor defects.

Respiratory

Respiratory Distress Syndrome

RDS, or hyaline membrane disease, can occur in full-term and preterm infants and is the result of decreased amounts of or inadequate function of pulmonary surfactant. The incidence is thought to be about 1% of all live births and about 10% of infants delivered prematurely. The incidence also can be said to vary inversely with gestational age; the majority of cases are in infants born at less than 30 weeks' gestation. Major risk factors include prematurity, perinatal asphyxia, and maternal diabetes.

Treatment is aimed primarily at prevention, with obstetric attention to successfully managing preterm labor. At-risk mothers are commonly placed on bed rest, are hydrated, and are given tocolytics such as magnesium sulfate or terbutaline. The administration of glucocorticoids to the mother, especially if done more than 24 hours before delivery, greatly helps enhance fetal lung maturity and has probably been the most important factor in decreasing the incidence of RDS. Once an infant with RDS is delivered, therapy is aimed at providing adequate ventilation and oxygenation while minimizing barotrauma and oxygen toxicity. Artificial surfactant replacement therapy is undertaken in ventilated infants with RDS either prophylactically (e.g., in the delivery room) or once the infant has been moved to the NICU. Surfactant therapy may be repeated every 6 hours up to a total of 4 doses, depending on the clinical condition of the infant and the individual product used.

Bronchopulmonary Dysplasia (BPD)

Chronic lung disease of varying degrees is the outcome of approximately 3 to 5% of newborns with RDS. BPD is classically defined as the ongoing need for oxygen therapy more than 28 days after birth; however, pulmonary changes may be seen radiographically much earlier than that, usually by days 5 to 7 after birth, and may include atelectasis alternating with areas of overdistention or pulmonary

interstitial emphysema. Treatment again is aimed at prevention with aggressive weaning from ventilatory support and attention to fluid status. In spite of the widespread use of prenatal steroids, surfactant replacement therapy, and aggressive, careful pulmonary management, the incidence of BPD has not been seen to decrease over the years. This may, however, be a reflection of survival of the more immature, and thus at-risk, infants than a failure of therapy modalities.

Apnea of Prematurity

Apnea is one of the most common problems of premature infants and may occur at some point in up to 50% of infants born before 34 weeks' gestation. Apnea is classically defined as a cessation of breathing that lasts longer than 20 seconds. However, even shorter episodes may pose a problem for the immature neonate and may be accompanied by bradycardia (heart rate less than 80 beats per minute) and desaturation. Premature infants, as well as full-term infants, may also manifest periodic breathing in which 5- to 10-second intervals of apnea alternate with fairly rapid breathing, and this may be considered normal in most cases.

Apnea of prematurity is a diagnosis of exclusion, and in any infant with new-onset apnea, it must first be ascertained that there is no underlying cause. Apnea may be associated with infection, metabolic disease, intraventricular hemorrhage, hyperthermia, and seizures. Once the etiology is determined, the severity and frequency of episodes is taken into consideration. If episodes are infrequent or mild, the infant may respond to tactile stimulation. More frequent or severe episodes may necessitate oxygen therapy or ventilatory support. Theophylline, as an artificial stimulant, may also be helpful in some infants and is usually given either enterally or parenterally in a loading dose followed by a maintenance dose. Serum levels should be monitored because infants may metabolize the drug differently. Therapeutic levels for theophylline are generally said to be in the range of 7 to 10 mg per dL. Side effects most often include jitteriness and tachycardia, but seizures are also possible at high levels. True apnea of prematurity is a function of immature respiratory control, and the majority of infants outgrow this by 34 to 35 weeks' gestational age. If this is the case, theophylline may be discontinued, although monitoring of the infant should be continued at least 7 days before planned discharge. In infants with more severe, persistent episodes, it may be necessary to consider home monitoring if all else is going well with the infant and if the parents are capable of performing such monitoring. Home monitoring, however, has not been shown to lower the incidence of sudden infant death syndrome, and this should be discussed with the parents.

Pulmonary Hypertension

PPHN is a disorder primarily of full-term and post-term infants, although it occasionally occurs in premature infants as well. Affected infants have severe, persistent elevation of pulmonary pressures to levels equal to or higher than systemic pressures, leading to right-to-left shunting of blood through the patent ductus arteriosis and foramen ovale. This in turn leads to hypoxemia, acidosis, and respiratory distress, which further enhances pulmonary vasoconstriction. The cause is probably multifunctional, but certain precipitating events are known to place infants at increased risk, including fetal distress with passage of meconium or meconium aspiration syndrome, sepsis, metabolic derangements (e.g., hypoglycemia, hypocalcemia), and hypothermia. In certain cases, no underlying problem can be found, and the condition is said to be idiopathic PPHN. Treatment is aimed at alleviating the cyclic progress to hypoxemia and pulmonary vasoconstriction and correcting the underlying cause if one has been identified.

PPHN must also be differentiated at the outset from congenital cyanotic heart disease. Along these lines, an echocardiogram is almost universally obtained as part of the initial work-up. Other laboratory work usually includes serum chemistry profiles, a CBC with differential, and blood cultures. Infants are placed on nothing-by-mouth (NPO) status, with intravenous fluids and antibiotics as appropriate to cover for possible sepsis. (Blood pressure support is generally undertaken in an attempt to increase septemic pressures beyond those of the pulmonary circulation.) It may be very difficult, from a ventilatory standpoint, to manage these infants, who often require a high inspired oxygen concentration and high ventilator pressures. Some centers choose to hyperventilate these neonates with the goal of respiratory alkalosis. Other possible therapy modalities in patients with refractory pulmonary hypertension include ECMO and the use of a high-frequency oscillating ventilator (HFOV). The use of nitric oxide is under investigation in some centers.

Cardiac

Patent Ductus Arteriosus

Although the right-to-left shunt through the patent ductus arteriosus is an integral part of the fetal circulation, it may become a problem for the preterm infant. In infants weighting less than 1500 grams, a patent ductus arteriosis may become significant in up to 20 to 30% and the incidence varies inversely with gestational age. Hemodynamically significant patent ductus arteriosis with left-to-right shunt in these infants usually manifests itself by days 3 to 10 after birth and often becomes apparent during attempts to wean the preterm infant from ventilatory support. Clinical signs suggestive of a patent ductus arteriosis may include a pulse pressure greater than 20 mm Hg, an "active" or hyperdynamic precordium, and "bounding" or especially vigorous pulses. Some infants may have a systolic murmur, but this is not a reliable sign because the murmur is caused by turbulence of blood flow, and a large, open ductus arterious may not cause a murmur. Metabolic acidosis is also sometimes found, along with pink-tinged pulmonary secretions and a need for increasing respiratory support or failure to continue weaning as expected. Diagnosis is made through echocardiography. Treatment is aimed initially at prevention, with fluids restricted to approximately 150 mL per kg per day. However, once a significant patent ductus arteriosis is documented, treatment is with indomethacin initially. If pharmacologic closure does not occur, surgical ligation may be necessary.

Congenital Heart Disease

Congenital heart disease occurs in approximately 8 in every 1000 live births. Depending on the lesion, problems may be obvious at birth or shortly thereafter. Classically, right-sided heart lesions (pulmonary stenosis, pulmonary atresia, tricuspid atresia), transposition of the great vessels, and severe tetralogy of Fallot manifest fairly early as the patent ductus arteriosus begins to close. A cardiac lesion should be suspected in any infant with persistent cyanosis, congestive heart failure, or a heart murmur either alone or in combination with the previous two factors. A murmur, however, is not always present with congenital heart disease. Other lesions may manifest later in the first week of life with the onset of respiratory distress and a shock-like appearance. Affected infants are often initially thought to be septic. Lesions that may manifest this way include aortic stenosis, coarctation of the aorta, and hypoplastic left heart syndrome. Still other lesions such as ventriculoseptal defect may manifest even later with the onset of congestive heart failure. Diagnosis is through echocardiography and, possibly, cardiac catheterization. Treatment is aimed at stabilization, pharmacologic management of the ductus arteriosis with prostaglandins if necessary, and transfer to a regional center for consultation with a cardiologist and cardiothoracic surgeon.

Gastrointestinal

Necrotizing Enterocolitis

Necrotizing enterocolitis is an inflammatory disease of the bowel that is predominantly seen in, but is not limited to, premature infants; infants with birth weights of less than 1500 grams are especially at risk. The etiology is commonly said to be multifactorial; the general consensus is that malabsorption, microbial agents, gut immaturity, and altered microcirculation all may play a role in the development of this devastating disease. The incidence varies widely by center; some centers have a large number of yearly cases, whereas others may have none at all. Several studies indicate that on average, 10% of infants weighing between 501 and 1500 grams are affected.

Prevention is by far the most important factor in limiting the disease, and an awareness of risk factors is necessary for achieving this goal. Antenatal and intrapartum risk factors include prematurity, prolonged rupture of membranes, history of maternal intrapartum hemorrhage or maternal cocaine use, perinatal asphyxia, and low Apgar scores. Postnatal factors may include polycythemia, patent ductus arteriosis, umbilical vessel catheters, and infection. Breast milk is thought to afford some protection, even in the tiniest infants, when all other factors are equal and feedings are started and advanced appropriately.

Signs and symptoms may be nonspecific initially and may include temperature instability, increasing or new-onset apnea and/or bradycardia, respiratory distress, jaundice, and lethargy. Infants may also first exhibit signs of feeding intolerance, including vomiting, gastric residuals, and abdominal distention. Hematest and/or Clinitest may yield positive findings for stools, or stools may be grossly bloody from the outset. Increased eosinophil numbers may also be seen in peripheral blood smears.

Any infant in whom the suspicion of necrotizing enterocolitis arises should have an immediate and thorough physical examination, with special attention to the abdominal examination. The infant's history should be reviewed in terms of risk factors and recent feeding and stooling patterns. If a diagnosis of necrotizing enterocolitis is seriously entertained at this point, enteral feedings should be withheld and intravenous fluid and broad-spectrum antimicrobial therapy initiated. An orogastric tube is inserted for decompression. Laboratory studies at this time should include a CBC with differential, along with blood, urine, cerebrospinal fluid, and stool cultures as appropriate; other laboratory studies may include a baseline chemistry profile and a blood gas study. Abdominal films should also be obtained at this point. The infant may need respiratory and circulatory support, as well as blood product replacement. Radiographs and laboratory work may need to be repeated as often as every 4 to 6 hours until the infant is stable.

Medical management of necrotizing enterocolitis is usually sufficient and includes continuing NPO status, parenteral nutrition, and antibiotic coverage for 10 to 14 days. However, surgical consultation is usually obtained at the outset, and the infant is monitored by the surgeon and neonatologist during the acute phase of the illness. Indications for surgery include evidence of perforation or gut necrosis, which necessitates resection.

Hematologic

Anemia

Anemia is a fairly common problem in newborns and is of special concern in the infant being cared for in a NICU. The consideration of anemia in the neonatal period must first take into account the gestational age of the infant and the fact that the normal range is wider during this period than at any other time in life. The clinician must also take into consideration the changes in the newborn's hematopoietic system that takes place at birth and in the ensuing 2 to 3 months. In general, anemia in the full-term infant is said to occur when the venous hemoglobin is less than 13 mg per dL and the hematocrit is less than 40%. Thereafter, the full-term newborn can be expected to show a decreasing hematocrit until the nadir is reached at 6 to 12 weeks of postnatal age. The preterm infant can be expected to reach its nadir somewhat earlier, and this is both for iatrogenic reasons (e.g., blood sampling) and a result of physiologic factors. The causes of anemia are varied and include obstetric blood loss (mother-to-fetus transfusions, twin-to-twin transfusions, or placentae abruptio), hemolytic processes, and decreased red blood cell production (rare). Evaluation of the anemic infant begins with a thorough family, obstetric, and immediate postpartum history. Laboratory evaluation includes a CBC, Coombs' test, and other more specific tests according to the infant's history and clinical condition. The need for transfusion therapy is based on the infant's condition and the underlying etiology of the anemia.

Polycythemia

Polycythemia is defined as a central hematocrit greater than 65 to 70%. Common causes include delayed clamping of the umbilical cord (delayed clamping of the cord by 30 to 60 seconds my increase the infant's hematocrit by as much as 25%), mother-to-fetus or fetus-to-fetus transfusion, and maternal conditions such as hypertension or diabetes. Polycythemia places the infant at risk for red blood cell "sludging" in small capillaries and possibly for respiratory distress, necrotizing enterocolitis, or adverse CNS events. In the asymptomatic infant with central hematocrit greater than 70% or in the symptomatic neonate with hematocrit greater than 65%, a partial exchange transfusion with a crystalloid or colloid solution is performed to lower the hematocrit to around 50%. Phlebotomy alone is never employed as a means of lowering the hematocrit because it may cause acute, severe hyperemia.

Hyperbilirubinemia

Hyperbilirubinemia in jaundice is the most common problem dealt with in the newborn nursery. Clinically, jaundice becomes apparent at a bilirubin level of approximately 5 mg per dL and is seen to occur in about 75% of full-term newborns during the first several days of life. It is even more common in the preterm population. Hyperbilirubinemia occurs in the newborn period as a result of a number of factors, including decreased hepatic metabolism of bilirubin, increased enterohepatic circulation, and an increased circulating red blood cell mass with shortened survival time of the cells (70 to 80 days, in contrast to the normal adult red blood cell life of 120 days). Physiologic jaundice is usually observed to peak on or before day 4 after birth in full-term infants and by day 7 in preterm infants. Nonphysiologic jaundice occurs during the first 24 hours after, is prolonged, peaks at more than 12 mg per dL, or is observed in conjunction with other abnormal signs or symptoms in the infant. Laboratory tests should always include the blood type of both mother and infant, Coombs' test, and the infant's CBC with a reticulocyte count in addition to total and direct (or conjugated) serum bilirubin levels. Phototherapy is started when total serum bilirubin levels reach 12 to 15 mg per dL in the full-term infant.

Infectious Disease

Sepsis

Sepsis or suspected sepsis remains one of the most commonly dealt problems in the neonatal intensive care setting. The incidence of neonatal infections is commonly reported as 1 to 10 per 1000 live births; the incidence is higher in premature infants. Because of the relatively immunocompromised state of the newborn, and especially of the premature infant, a high index of suspicion is usually maintained in regard to this diagnosis.

Early-onset sepsis usually manifests within the first 72 hours of life and is probably acquired in utero or during the birth process. There is an increased risk associated with prolonged rupture of membranes (especially more than 24 hours after rupture), premature rupture of membranes, prolonged labor, multiple obstetric procedures, fetal distress, maternal fever or infection, and foul-smelling amniotic fluid. Organisms to be considered include group B *Streptococcus* species, *Listeria* species, *Escherichia coli*, other gram-negative enterics, *Haemophilus influenzae*, *Gonococcus* species, herpesviruses, and *Candida* species.

Late-onset sepsis manifests after the first 72 hours of life and is probably acquired postnatally. A subset of this would be nosocomial disease, the diagnosis of which is often entertained in infants in the NICU. Risk factors include male sex, preterm delivery, meconium aspiration syndrome, and congenital malformations. Any other conditions that may lead to invasive procedures, such as placement of intravenous lines, umbilical catheters, central lines, or endotracheal intubation, also place the infant at risk for the subsequent development of infection and sepsis. Organisms to be considered are *Staphylococcus* species, *E. coli, Pseudomonas,* streptococci, *Proteus* species, *Klebsiella* species, and *Candida* species.

Signs and symptoms of neonatal sepsis and/or meningitis are very often nonspecific and may include any of the following: color change, lethargy, poor feeding, temperature instability, cyanosis, tachycardia, hypotension, disordered glucose metabolism (hypoglycemia or hyperglycemia), or evidence of new-onset or worsening respiratory distress.

Evaluation of the infant with suspected sepsis must be undertaken immediately and begins with a thorough physical examination. Cultures are obtained and should include blood, cerebrospinal fluid, urine, stool, and tracheal aspirate as appropriate. A CBC with differential and platelet count, serum chemistry profiles, urinalysis, blood gas determinations, and chest and abdominal radiographs are also obtained.

Management of these infants involves the rapid initiation of broad-spectrum antimicrobial therapy (see Table 3). In early- and late-onset primary sepsis,

TABLE 3. **Antibiotics for Neonatal Infection**

Type of Infection	Age	Dose (IV or IM) (mg/kg/dose)	Interval
Ampicillin (For use in suspected sepsis and meningitis)			
Suspected sepsis	<1 week	50	q 12 h
Meningitis	<1 week	100	q 12 h
Suspected sepsis	>1 week	50	q 8 h
Meningitis	>1 week	100	q 8 h
Cefotaxime (Claforan) (For use with gram-negative meningitis and sepsis, e.g., *Escherichia coli, Haemophilus influenzae, Klebsiella,* and *Pseudomonas*)			
	Preterm infants <1 week	50	q 12 h
	Preterm infants >1 week	50	q 8 h
	Term infants <1 week	50	q 8 h
	Term infants >1 week	50	q 6 h
Gentamicin (Garamycin) (Loading dose: 4 mg/kg/dose IV (preferred) or IM, *first dose only.* This includes anuric infants—one-time dose.)			
	<30 weeks	2.5	q 24 h
	30–37 weeks	2.5	q 18 h
	38–42 weeks	2.5	q 12 h
Vancomycin (Vancocin) (For use with *Staphylococcus aureus* or *S. epidermidis* infection)			
	<29 weeks	18*	q 24 h
	30–36 weeks	15*	q 12 h
	37–44 weeks	10*	q 8 h
	>45 weeks	10*	q 6 h

*IV only.
Abbreviations: IV = intravenous; IM = intramuscular.
Modified from Koffler H: Care of the high-risk neonate. *In* Rakel RE: Conn's Current Therapy 1994. Philadelphia, WB Saunders, 1994, p 1025.

the initial treatment is either (1) ampicillin and gentamicin or (2) a cephalosporin. The initial treatment of a suspected nosocomial sepsis is with vancomycin and gentamicin. Further antimicrobial choices or changes in initial regimen are dictated by culture results and specific organisms' sensitivities. Additional management includes general supportive measures with correction of hypotension, of anemia, and of fluid, electrolyte, and glucose disturbances, as well as respiratory support as needed.

Special Considerations

Multiple Congenital Anomalies

Major congenital malformations are defined as those that have cosmetic, medical or surgical significance and are known to occur in up to 2 to 3% of live births. These may have been diagnosed prenatally and are therefore expected by the parents, or they may be unexpected by both parents and physicians. In either situation, emotional support and counseling of the parents are extremely important. The infant should be stabilized as quickly as possible and transported to a regional perinatal center for further evaluation, care, and development follow-up if needed.

Surgical Emergencies

As in the case of the infant with congenital malformations, the neonate with a surgical emergency such as congenital diaphragmatic hernia, gastrointestinal obstruction, abdominal wall defect, tracheoesophageal fistula, or neural tube defect is stabilized as quickly and efficiently as possible in preparation for transfer to a regional neonatal center for correction of the specific lesion. Again, whether the emergency is unexpected or not, the parents need emotional support and information about their newborn's condition.

DISCHARGE PLANNING

Good discharge planning with any high-risk neonate essentially begins with admission. Parents should be well informed about their child and his or her disease state and should be updated daily on the infant's status and the plans of the health care team. Parents should be made to feel comfortable in seeking information concerning their newborn; for an infant expected to have lengthy hospital stays, the parents should be involved in the infant's physical care as much as possible. As home discharge nears, extensive teaching as to any necessary equipment may be needed, and most perinatal centers allow parents to "room-in" with their infant before discharge. The home situation is usually reviewed by social services, and a needs assessment is performed. Adequate follow-up by a designated primary care pediatrician must be ensured before discharge, and communication must be established between the pediatrician and the neonatologist, pediatric surgeon, or any pediatric subspecialists involved. Continuity

of care for these neonates is of paramount importance.

NORMAL INFANT FEEDING

method of
JAMES L. SUTPHEN, M.D., PH.D., and
ANA ABAD-SINDEN, M.S., R.D.
The University of Virginia
Charlottesville, Virginia

BREAST-FEEDING

Breast-feeding is preferable to formulas for the full-term infant. Breast milk protein is of high biologic value and provides a low renal solute load. The presence of the saturated fatty acids in the 2 position of the triglycerides and the action of lipase enhance fat digestibility. Lactose, the predominant form of carbohydrate in human milk, enhances calcium and mineral absorption. Milk from a well-nourished healthy woman provides adequate levels of almost all micronutrients.

Although breast-feeding is a natural act, it is not totally instinctive. Women who wish to breast-feed should be encouraged to do so and should receive procedural instruction during the prenatal and early postnatal period. Successful breast-feeding depends on supportive obstetric, pediatric, and nursing care. Parental attitudes, including those of the father, should be discussed during the prenatal period. A breast examination should be conducted to identify problems with the nipple, areola, or breast itself. Several manipulation techniques such as nipple rolling, as well as the wearing of a breast shield, can help flat or inverted nipples become more everted. Sometimes an infant with a strong, healthy suck can bring out inverted nipples. Breast care should also be addressed with emphasis on the avoidance of strong soaps or ointments on the nipples. Sufficient lubrication for the areola and nipples is provided by the glands of Montgomery during pregnancy and lactation.

The mother should have the opportunity to nurse her infant as soon as possible after the delivery. Feedings initially should be offered every 2 to 4 hours and adjusted according to infant demand. For a proper grasp and seal, the nipple should be drawn up against the roof of the infant's mouth with the tongue stroking the bottom of the nipple. The infant's lips should almost completely surround the areola while the jaw applies pressure, forcing the milk out through the pores in the nipple during the act of suckling. The infant should be allowed to suck for at least 4 to 5 minutes, at which time the mother can break the seal by inserting a clean finger in the corner of her infant's mouth. The infant should then be offered the second breast. A normal healthy infant should demonstrate appropriate rooting, grasping, and suckling behaviors. Gradually the feeding period will increase, taking up to 10 minutes or more on each side by the third postpartum day.

Bottle-feeding should not be offered to an infant during the first 2 weeks until lactation is well established. Because bottle-feeding requires a different tongue and jaw motion, introducing it too early could lead to nipple confusion. Moreover, an infant who bottle feeds may take less from the breast, especially when an entire feeding is substituted with a bottle feeding. This leads to decreased milk production.

Successful lactation also depends on the establishment of the letdown reflex. To establish letdown, a mother should be encouraged to relax and establish a comfortable nursing environment. If letdown does not proceed, the woman should be encouraged to massage her breast in a circular pattern with her fingertips to help promote the emptying of her breasts through an external means. Awareness of letdown can be felt in a variety of ways, such as through tingling sensations during nursing, uterine contractions, or thirst.

Monitoring the breast-fed infant involves checking feeding frequency, number of wet diapers, and weight gain. During the first few weeks of life, the breast-fed infant will nurse at least 6 times a day, but more frequently 8 to 12 times a day, and will produce 6 to 8 wet diapers per day. The infant should regain birth weight by 3 weeks of age. As the infant becomes older and requires more milk, there will be an increased emptying and sucking stimulation, which will promote increased milk production. For the older infant who has been introduced to solid foods, the nursing interval may lengthen with a simultaneous shortening of the nursing period, resulting in less milk production.

The quantity and quality of human milk are affected by maternal diet and nutritional status. The lactating mother needs approximately 500 to 600 kcal extra and 20 extra grams of protein per day. Precise needs depend on maternal age, metabolism, and activity, as well as duration of lactation and number of infants being breast-fed. A balanced, varied diet consisting of four servings of milk or milk products, two servings of meat or high-protein meat substitutes, four servings of fruits and vegetables, including a source of vitamins A and C, and four servings of breads and cereals should promote adequate nutritional support. As traces of anything consumed can show up in breast milk, foods suspected of causing infantile colic or congestion should be gradually eliminated from the diet, one at a time, to identify if the food is indeed causing the symptoms.

Woman who anticipate returning to work should be encouraged to continue breast-feeding. Woman who work part-time may be able to breast-feed totally; full-time working mothers may be able to provide their infant's nutritional needs by various combinations of breast milk, stored breast milk, or supplemental formula feedings. Women who wish to feed their infants breast milk while they are working need to express their milk with a breast pump. Breast pumps have a funnel-shaped flange that comes in

contact with the nipple and removes the milk by suction. Breast milk not intended for immediate use should be properly stored for maintenance of its safety and nutritional quality. Breast milk can be safely frozen in new plastic bags or disposable liners from baby bottles and then thawed under cold running water. To ease the transition, the infant should be offered a bottle a few times a week before the mother returns to work.

Common deterrents to successful breast-feeding include lack of maternal confidence, incorrect nursing techniques, improper positioning of the infant's lips onto the areola, and maternal stress caused by fatigue, inadequate nutrition, or postpartum depression. Breast problems such as engorgement, sore nipples, and infections also prevent successful lactation. Appropriate emptying of the engorged breast via manual expression and nursing often can help alleviate maternal discomfort. Painful or cracked nipples may be caused by improper positioning of the infant on the breast or consistent nursing in the same position. Dry heat is quite effective in healing sore nipples, and changing nursing positions can vary nipple stress points. Mastitis or a localized breast infection produces systemic flulike symptoms. Nursing on the unaffected side to promote letdown, followed by manual expression or nursing on the affected side is often effective. A 10-day course of an appropriate antibiotic may be prescribed to minimize recurrence.

Certain drugs are contraindicated for the mother's use while nursing, such as radioactive agents, antimetabolites, atropine, metronidazole, and tetracycline, and others are viewed as potentially harmful if used inappropriately. Prolonged breast-feeding beyond the sixth month to the exclusion of other important nutrient sources has been associated with infant malnutrition and iron deficiency. The introduction of solid foods, including iron-fortified cereals, between the fourth and six months and gradual reduction in breast milk intake through the first year provide the appropriate nutrient blend to meet an infant's nutritional needs.

FORMULA-FEEDING

The decision to breast-feed is a personal one and should be reached with freedom from guilt or pressure. Information on formula-feeding as an acceptable substitute should be provided by the physician or health care professional in the event that the decision not to breast-feed is made. In the developed world the advantages of breast-feeding relative to formula-feeding are less pronounced, assuming a clean water supply is available. The usual reason for instituting formula-feedings is parental preference. Occasionally, parents will prefer to substitute formula-feeding completely when the mother returns to work.

When bottle-feeding is initiated, parents may find that infants have marked preferences for different commercially available nipples. Before abandoning one type of nipple, the parents should be certain that the hole in the nipple is adequately patent. There is little reason to recommend one style of bottle over another, although advantages are claimed by manufacturers. When the infant is fed, there should be few distractions, and the parents should be discouraged from making rapid or jerking motions during feeding. Children should be fed in a semi-inclined position. Supine feeding and bottle propping should be discouraged, as they could promote aspiration of the formula. When bottle-feeding is initiated, it is reasonable to involve the father in the feeding. There is no reason to isolate feeding as a strictly maternal duty. The mother's work schedule is often as demanding as the father's. We suggest that mothers and fathers share responsibility for night-time feedings as well.

All formulas are available as a liquid or powdered concentrate or as a ready-to-feed form. Formula should be prepared with a clean water supply. Parents may prefer to use boiled water for this purpose. If the water supply is a public treated water supply in the United States, there is little advantage provided by boiling. Other water sources, however, probably should be boiled. After each feeding, equipment should be washed in hot soapy water with a bottle and nipple brush, followed by rinsing in hot water. If an automatic dishwasher is used, the heated drying cycle should be used.

Before feeding, the formula should be warmed. It is convenient to do this in a pan of warm water, but it is faster to use a microwave oven. Different microwave ovens heat at dramatically different rates. Parents who microwave should be cautioned that the temperature of the formula may exceed that of the glass or plastic bottle. It is, therefore, advisable to test the actual temperature of the formula before feeding the baby.

During feedings, the infant should be periodically burped. It is best to do this by supporting the child in a sitting position with one hand holding both the chest and the lower chin. The back is gently tapped and rubbed, and occasionally the infant may be moved up and down or gently side to side to facilitate the passage of air from the stomach. This process requires considerable practice but is absolutely essential. Finally, it is best to warn parents that normal infants often spit even when burping is done adequately. Therefore, several washable blankets and towels should be within reach in the area where infants are fed.

Cow's Milk Formula

In the United States, there are several cow's milk protein formulas (Table 1). For the full-term normal infant, there is little advantage of one over the other. In fact, infants generally accept these formulas interchangeably. Therefore, parents are best advised to look for the lowest price in the their local market. Lactofree is a cow's milk formula that is lactose free and is designed for use specifically for lactose intolerance. Although this condition is frequently suspected

after gastroenteritis, more often infants can tolerate lactose, even in the face of mild diarrhea. Malnutrition, age less than 6 months, and dehydrating diarrhea are risk factors for clinically significant postenteropathy transient lactose intolerance. In this situation, a lactose-free formula may be useful. In addition to Lactofree, the soy and protein hydrolysate formulas do not contain lactose.

Soy Formula

Soy formula provides protein from soy. The carbohydrate component is derived from corn syrup solids and sucrose in various combinations. These formulas are intended to be used when there is proven cow's milk protein sensitivity or lactose intolerance. The absorption of calcium in soy formula is adequate but less than with cow's milk formula. Full-term infants fed soy milk grow at rates equal to those fed cow's milk formulas. It is best for parents to try once or twice to reintroduce cow's milk formula to be certain that there is indeed an allergy or intolerance to cow's milk. If there is a true allergy to cow's milk, it is not uncommon for allergies to develop to soy milk as well. If this is the case, a protein hydrolysate formula should be used.

Protein Hydrolysate Formula

Protein hydrolysate formulas generally are somewhat less palatable than soy or cow's milk formulas (see Table 1). The major distinction between currently available hydrolysate formulas is that Pregestimil and Alimentum contain a portion of their fat as medium-chain triglycerides. Any of the formulas may be used when there is proven allergy to both cow's milk and soy protein. Pregestimil and Alimentum are more extensively hydrolyzed. With more extensive hydrolysis the protein should be theroretically less allergenic.

If formulas containing medium-chain triglyceride are clearly producing improved weight gain for a child, the physician should begin a preliminary investigation into the etiology of possible fat malabsorption (e.g., sweat test). Generally, even infants who have severe cow's or soy milk sensitivity will ultimately be able to accept cow's milk. It may take several months or even years for tolerance to develop; however, more often by 1 year of age the other protein sources can be safely introduced.

Evaporated Milk Formula

Evaporated milk formula was at one time popular in the United States. These formulas are now discouraged for many reasons. The renal solute load is unacceptably high. The vitamin content is not standardized and is often inadequate, and the amounts of protein and phosphorus are excessive.

TABLE 1. Infant Formulas*

Formula	kcal/mL	gm/mL			Nutrient Source (gm/mL)				Comments
		Cho	Fat	Pro	Cho	Fat	Pro		
Standard									
Enfamil 20	0.67	0.069	0.038	0.015	Lactose	Palm olein, soy, coconut, sunflower	Whey, casein	60:40 ratio	
Enfamil 24	0.80	0.084	0.045	0.018	Lactose	Palm olein, soy, coconut, sunflower	Whey, casein	60:40 ratio	
Gerber 20	0.67	0.069	0.038	0.015	Lactose	Soy, coconut oil	Whey, casein	18:82 ratio	
Lactofree	0.67	0.069	0.037	0.015	Corn syrup solids	Palm olein, soy, coconut, sunflower	Whey, casein	For lactose intolerance	
Similac 20	0.67	0.072	0.036	0.015	Lactose	High oleic safflower, coconut, soy oil	Whey, casein	48:52 ratio	
Similac 24	0.80	0.085	0.043	0.022	Lactose	High oleic safflower, coconut, soy oil	Whey, casein	48:52 ratio	
Carnation Good Start	0.67	0.073	0.034	0.016	Lactose, maltodextrin	Palm olein, soy oil, coconut, safflower	100% whey	Partially hydrolyzed whey	
Carnation Follow-Up	0.67	0.088	0.027	0.017	Maltodextrin, corn syrup solids	Palm olein, soy oil, coconut, safflower	Whey, casein	For infants >4 mo and started on solids	
Soy-based									
Prosobee 20	0.67	0.068	0.036	0.020	Corn syrup solids	Palm olein, soy, coconut, sunflower	Soy protein and L-methionine	For milk protein allergy/lactose intolerance	
Isomil 20	0.67	0.068	0.037	0.018	Corn syrup, sucrose	High-oleic safflower, coconut, soy oil	Soy protein and L-methionine	For milk protein allergy/lactose intolerance	
Carnation Alsoy	0.67	0.074	0.033	0.018	Maltodextrin, sucrose	Palm olein, soy oil, coconut, safflower	Soy protein isolate	For milk protein allergy/lactose intolerance	
Specialized									
Nutramigen	0.67	0.090	0.026	0.019	Corn syrup, tapioca	Palm olein, soy, coconut, sunflower	Casein hydrolysate	For allergy to intact protein	
Pregestimil	0.67	0.091	0.028	0.019	Corn syrup, tapioca	Corn (20%), MCT (55%), soy (12.5%), sunflower (12.5%)	Casein hydrolysate, amino acids	For generalized malabsorption	
Portagen	0.67	0.074	0.030	0.022	Corn syrup, lactose, and sucrose	MCT (88%), corn oil (12%)	Sodium caseinate	For long-chain fatty acid malabsorption	
Alimentum	0.67	0.068	0.038	0.019	Tapioca, sucrose	MCT (50%), soy, safflower	Casein hydrolysate, amino acids	For generalized malabsorption	
Neocate	0.67	0.078	0.030	0.021	Corn syrup solids	MCT (35%), canola, high-oleic sunflower	Free amino acids	For severe protein allergy	

*Infant formula osmolality ranges from 200 to 360.
Abbreviations: Cho = cholesterol; MCT = medium-chain triglyceride; Pro = protein.

Juices

Although fruit juices, especially apple juice, are popular in the United States, they have little or no nutritional value for infants. They are primarily a source of sugar and little else. Some infants develop a "sweet tooth" as a result and begin to drink less formula. Excessive juice intake can lead to diarrhea. Moreover, fruit juices promote tooth decay, especially for the child who continually drinks them. We prefer water as an additional fluid source and avoid apple juice.

Formula Volume

Infants are generally started on 1 to 2 ounces of formula per feeding. The frequency initially should be every 2 to 4 hours. Gradually the frequency should be decreased to every 4 hours and the volume slowly increased to 6 to 8 ounces per feeding. When the infant is consuming 800 to 1000 mL of formula per day, it is reasonable to introduce solid foods. Generally, this occurs somewhere between 4 and 6 months of age. If the infant attains this goal earlier and is not obese or the child of obese parents, it is acceptable to introduce solids earlier.

Earlier introduction is also sometimes necessary for infants who are adjusting or rechanneling their linear growth curve from a low percentile to a higher percentile. This rechanneling is common in the first year of life, and, if the growth velocity is extremely rapid, it is not uncommon for formula-feedings to become inadequate before the usual time of 4 to 6 months. The same can be said of breast-feeding in this situation. If the infant or the parents are obese, early feeding of solids should be discouraged.

Solid Foods

Solid foods can be made by grinding regular foods in a baby food grinder, or they may be purchased in prepared form. If parents elect to prepare their own solid foods, they should be warned that the feedings should be well pureed because a coarse texture may be unacceptable to an infant. Generally, infants do not switch to home-prepared solids if they have first been introduced to ready-made solids.

Solid foods are difficult to feed before 4 months of age, as the extrusion reflex of the tongue makes it difficult for the infant to consume them. Parents should be cautioned that the infant will inevitably spit out a small amount in the course of learning how to swallow from a spoon. This does not mean that the infant does not tolerate that particular food.

Solid feedings are progressed along a common (but unproven) schedule. Cereal is started first, followed by yellow vegetables and fruits, then green vegetables, and then finally meats. No mixed foods are provided until the components of the mixture have been previously introduced. No more than one new food should be introduced every 3 to 7 days so that food intolerances may be detected. We generally discourage the feeding of strained egg yolks and strained desserts at any age. The concentrated cholesterol in the former and sugar in the latter are unnecessary and potentially harmful.

Cow's Milk

Whole cow's milk feedings should not be introduced before 9 to 12 months of age. There is evidence that allergy to cow's milk protein may be more common if it is introduced too early. Late introduction of whole cow's milk decreases the tendency toward iron deficiency anemia seen with early introduction. When parents introduce cow's milk, they should be cautioned against using skim milk, which has been shown to cause nutritional deficiencies when given to infants who are younger than 6 months of age and consume little solid food. Two percent fat cow's milk is adequate for infants over 1 year of age who are consuming an adequate amount of solid foods. In fact, for families with atherosclerotic heart disease, 2% is preferable. The use of 2% milk is undesirable if limited solid foods are being consumed or if the child is underweight.

VITAMIN AND MINERAL SUPPLEMENTS

Infants should receive supplemental iron by the age of 6 months. This can be given most easily in the form of iron-fortified cereals. Alternatively, iron-fortified formula is available. Fluoride drops should be given to infants who live in an area where the water supply does not contain fluoride. Infants who are formula-fed require no additional vitamin supplements. Infants who are breast-fed probably require no vitamin supplements as well, assuming that the mother's diet is adequate.

There is a relatively low concentration of vitamin D in human milk. Rickets is very uncommon in full-term infants who are breast-fed, however, especially if solid foods are introduced at the usual time and there is adequate exposure to sunlight and adequate maternal vitamin D intake. If this is not the case, 400 IU of vitamin D should be provided daily to the infant.

DISEASES OF THE BREAST

method of
ARMANDO E. GIULIANO, M.D., and
PETER J. BOSTICK, M.D.
John Wayne Cancer Institute
Santa Monica, California

BENIGN BREAST DISORDERS

Common benign breast disorders include fibrocystic disease, fibroadenoma of the breast, nipple discharge, breast abscess, fat necrosis, and disorders of the augmented breast. One of the most important aspects of managing patients with these lesions is to exclude the possibility of malignancy.

Fibrocystic Disease

Fibrocystic disease is the most frequent benign or malignant lesion of the breast. It usually occurs in women 30 to 50 years of age, and estrogen is considered a causative factor. There are a wide variety of pathologic entities that encompass the term "fibrocystic disease" or "mammary dysplasia." The microscopic findings of this disorder include cysts, papillomatosis, adenosis, fibrosis, and ductal epithelial hyperplasia. Only lesions with proliferative changes, especially with atypia, represent a true risk factor for developing breast cancer. This entity is best not considered a disease because it occurs in most young women and is probably a variant of the normal response to fluctuating hormones.

Fibrocystic disease often manifests as a painful mass that may increase in size during the premenstrual phase of the menstrual cycle. Fluctuation in size of a breast mass and cyclic breast pain are common in this condition. Multiple or bilateral masses are often noted. A mass from fibrocystic disease is frequently indistinguishable from carcinoma. Mammography may not be helpful because the breast tissue in young women is too radiodense to permit a worthwhile study. Ultrasonography can be used to differentiate a cystic from a solid mass.

The diagnosis of fibrocystic disease must be established before determining the treatment of this disorder. Usually the history and physical examination are all that are necessary to make a diagnosis. Fine-needle aspiration may be performed on a discrete mass. If no fluid is obtained or the fluid is bloody, or the mass persists or recurs at any time during follow-up, excision of the mass is necessary to rule out carcinoma. The breast pain may be relieved after fine-needle aspiration of a cyst. The pain can also be managed by avoiding trauma and wearing a brassiere that gives good support and protection. Hormone therapy (danazol [Danocrine], 100 to 200 mg twice daily orally) is not recommended because it does not cure the condition and is associated with significant side effects (e.g., acne, edema, hirsutism). The role of caffeine consumption in the development and treatment is controversial. Some studies suggest that vitamin E and decreased caffeine consumption are associated with improvement of the breast pain. Most patients require only reassurance that they do not have cancer to feel remarkable relief.

Fibroadenoma of the Breast

Fibroadenomas are benign neoplasms that occur most commonly in adolescents and young women. This disorder does not usually occur in postmenopausal women unless they are on hormonal therapy. Multiple tumors are encountered in 10 to 15% of cases. Fibroadenomas are characteristically round, rubbery, discrete, mobile, and less than 5 cm in diameter. Fibrocystic disease or carcinoma of the breast must be considered in the differential diagnosis in women older than the age of 30. Fine-needle aspiration or ultrasonography can identify a cystic lesion. If the diagnosis of fibroadenoma is made by fine-needle aspiration, no further treatment is necessary. In some cases, excision of the mass with histologic examination is necessary for both diagnosis and treatment.

Cystosarcoma phyllodes, although rarely malignant, is a fibroadenoma-like tumor that has the potential to grow rapidly. Treatment of both benign and malignant lesions is by local excision with a rim of normal tissue. In some cases the tumor may be so large that a simple mastectomy is required. Lymph node dissection is not necessary for the malignant form of this disease, because the sarcomatous portion of the tumor will usually metastasize directly to the lungs and not the lymph nodes. A fibroadenoma that is enlarging should be excised to rule out cystosarcoma phyllodes.

Nipple Discharge

Nipple discharge in the nonlactating breast is usually caused by nonmalignant conditions such as fibrocystic disease with ectasia of the ducts (most common), intraductal papilloma, endocrine disorders (prolactinoma, hypothyroidism), medications (phenothiazines, estrogen), or infectious causes. However, in some situations breast carcinoma must be ruled out. Important characteristics of the nipple discharge include (1) the nature of the discharge (serous, bloody, or other), (2) whether it is unilateral or bilateral, (3) whether discharge is spontaneous or must be expressed, (4) whether discharge is produced by pressure at a single site or by general pressure on the breast, (5) the presence of single or multiple duct discharge, (6) association with or without a mass, (7) the relation to menses, (8) whether it is premenopausal or postmenopausal, (9) and whether the patient is taking hormonal medications.

The most common cause of unilateral, spontaneous serous or serosanguineous discharge is intraductal papilloma and, occasionally, intraductal cancer. Cytologic examination and ductography may identify malignant cells or a filling defect, respectively. However, negative findings on cytology do not rule out cancer, and excision of the bloody ductal system is recommended whether or not a filling defect is identified by ductography. The duct and mass if present should be excised. Spontaneous multiple, unilateral or bilateral, green or brownish duct discharge, in premenopausal women is often due to fibrocystic disease. Under these conditions, if a mass is present, it should be removed. Milky discharge can be caused by oral contraceptive agents, estrogen replacement therapy, phenothiazines, prolactinoma, or hypothyroidism. With oral contraceptives or estrogen the discharge can also be clear or serous and usually involves multiple ducts. The cause of the nipple discharge can be determined by obtaining serum levels of prolactin and thyroid-stimulating hormone and the discontinuation of these medications. If the nipple discharge persists and is from a single duct, exploration should be considered, but without blood the cause is rarely malignancy. Purulent discharge may be caused by a subareolar abscess and necessitates excision of the abscess and related lactiferous sinus. If a nonbloody discharge cannot be localized and there is no palpable mass, the patient should be reexamined every 3 to 4 months for a year and then routinely observed.

Breast Abscess

Staphylococcus aureus is the most common organism that occurs in a breast abscess of a lactating woman. If the abscess is in its early stages, antibiotics such as dicloxacillin or oxacillin, 250 mg four times daily for 7 to 10 days, can be administered. However, if progressive local or systemic signs of infection develop, the abscess should be drained and nursing stopped. In young, nonlactating women, a subareolar abscess may occur, although rarely. Excision of the involved duct(s) is often necessary to prevent recurrence. In these women, inflammatory carcinoma must always be considered as a cause of the signs of inflammation. Therefore, findings suggestive of abscess in the nonlactating breast are an indication for incision and biopsy of any indurated tissue if the inflammation does not resolve rapidly on antibiotics.

Fat Necrosis

Fat necrosis can occur as a result of trauma to the tissue, which incites an inflammatory response. In only about half of cases, however, is a traumatic event recalled. Fat necrosis can also occur after segmental mastectomy and radiation therapy. With this condition, a mass develops with skin or nipple retraction that is indistinguishable from carcinoma. At times the entire mass should be excised to rule out carcinoma, but usually the history and a fine-needle aspiration will enable the patient to be carefully observed.

Disorders of the Augmented Breast

The concerns associated with breast implants include capsular contraction with subsequent breast deformity, inability to detect early breast cancer, and the development of autoimmune disease associated with silicone implants. Breast augmentation is performed by placing implants in the subcutaneous tissue or under the pectoralis muscle. Capsular contraction or scarring around the implant occurs in 15 to 25% of patients. In some cases this necessitates removal of the implant and capsule because of the firmness and distortion that develops in the breast. Mammography is less able to detect early lesions of breast cancer in patients with implants for augmentation. However, local recurrence after breast reconstruction is usually cutaneous or subcutaneous and is easily detectable by palpation. If a cancer develops, the options of mastectomy, breast-conserving therapy, and adjuvant therapy should be given for the same indications as for women who have no implants. There are no clinical data proving an increased incidence of connective tissue disorders in patients with silicone gel breast implants. The Mayo Clinic performed a retrospective cohort study that showed no increased incidence of autoimmune disorders among women with silicone implants. However, the U.S. Food and Drug Administration, in 1992, concluded that additional preclinical and clinical studies were necessary to establish the safety of silicone breast implants. They advised women in whom the implant had ruptured or who have symptoms suggestive of autoimmune disorder to discuss with a physician the risks and benefits of surgical removal of the implant. More recently, a panel of experts concluded there was no scientific evidence relating autoimmune disease to implants.

PRIMARY BREAST CANCER

Incidence and Risk Factors

The American Cancer Society predicts that one of every eight or nine American women will develop breast cancer during her lifetime. The breast is the second most common site of cancer in women (the skin is most common) and is second to lung cancer as a cause of death from cancer among women.

Factors associated with increased risk of breast cancer include (1) race, (2) age, (3) family history of breast cancer, (4) genetic mutations, (5) previous history of breast or uterine cancer, (6) menstrual history and hormone use, and (7) age at first pregnancy. In the United States, breast cancer is more common in white women, although the incidence is increasing in nonwhite women. Only about 2% of breast cancers occur in women younger than the age of 30. Women whose mothers or sisters had breast cancer are three to four times more likely to develop breast cancer than is the general population. This risk is further increased if the disease occurred in two or more first-degree relatives, involved both breasts, or occurred premenopausally. However, for over 90% of breast cancer patients there is no family history of breast cancer.

An increased risk in the development of breast cancer has been associated with mutations involving the *BRAC1* and *BRAC2* genes, the *TP53* gene (tumor suppressor gene), and the ataxia-telangiectasia gene. The *BRAC1* gene, which is located on chromosome 17, has been shown to be mutated in families with early-onset breast and ovarian cancer. Women with the *BRAC1* gene mutation have an estimated 85% life-time risk of developing breast cancer. Genetic testing is commercially available but is highly controversial because of the management and social issues that arise in patients identified with the mutation. A woman who has had cancer in one breast is at risk of developing contralateral disease at a rate of 1 to 2% per year. Women with uterine cancer are at increased risk of developing breast cancer when compared with the general population. In addition, women with breast cancer are also at increased risk of developing uterine cancer. Women who began menarche before age 12 or had a late natural menopause after age 50 are also at increased risk of developing breast cancer. Nulliparous women and women whose first full-term pregnancy was after age 35 have a 1.5 times higher incidence of developing this disease than does the general population.

Women at increased risk of developing breast cancer should be taught the techniques of self-examination and be observed carefully by a physician. Those with a strong family history of breast cancer should be counseled and given the option of genetic testing. Tamoxifen (Nolvadex) has been shown to decrease the incidence of breast cancer among high-risk women. The management of high-risk women with bilateral mastectomy seems to lower their risk of breast cancer in nonrandomized trials. Considerable counseling is necessary when advising women at high risk of their treatment options.

Early Detection of Breast Cancer

SCREENING FOR BREAST CANCER

Screening programs require both physical examination and mammography to obtain the highest yield. These programs identify about 10 cancers for every 1000 women older than the age of 50 and approximately 2 cancers per 1000 women younger than age 50. Approximately 80% of these women will have negative axillary nodes at the time of surgery, and about 85% of such women will survive at least 5 years.

The frequency of breast examination is determined by the age of the patient. Breast self-examination should be performed monthly in all women older than the age of 20. Premenopausal women should perform the examination 7 to 8 days after the menstrual period begins. Women 20 to 40 years of age should have a breast examination by a physician every 2 to 3 years, and those older than the age of 40 should have yearly breast examination.

The current recommendations of screening mammography are age related. In young women with dense breasts, mammography is less sensitive than in older women with fatty breasts. The policy of the National Cancer Institute has been that there is no agreement about the role of screening mammography for women aged 40 to 49. However, two Swedish trials that had shown a 13% decrease in breast cancer mortality (not statistically significant) later showed a statistical advantage for screening women in their 40s. A meta-analysis similarly showed a statistical survival advantage for screened women in this age group with longer follow-up. On the basis of these findings, in March 1997, the National Cancer Advisory Board recommended that women aged 40 to 49 with average risk factors should have screening mammography every 1 to 2 years and that women at higher risk should seek expert advice on when to begin screening. The American Cancer Society, as a result of these findings, recommended screening every year for asymptomatic women starting at age 40. For women aged 50 to 69, randomized controlled trials have strongly supported routine screening in this age group. The efficacy of screening in women older than 70 is difficult to determine because of the very few women over 70 screened.

SELF-EXAMINATION

Most women do not practice self-examination, and it is controversial whether it improves patient outcome. However, self-examination is clearly not harmful. Women who are older than the age of 20 should be instructed by their physician to examine their breasts monthly. In premenopausal women this should be performed 7 to 8 days after the menstrual period begins. Initially, the breast should be inspected in the standing position before a mirror. With the hands at the sides, overhead, and pressed firmly on the hips to contract the pectoralis muscles, any masses, areas of asymmetry, and skin dimpling of the breast are noted. Next, in the supine position, each breast should be examined with the fingers of the opposite hand. This examination can also be performed while bathing or showering.

PHYSICAL EXAMINATION

The symptoms associated with breast cancer include breast mass (most common), nipple discharge, erosion, retraction, enlargement or itching of the nipple, generalized hardness, and enlargement or shrinking of the breast. Less frequently, the patient may have an axillary mass or arm swelling without a palpable breast mass. Breast pain is rarely caused by cancer, but it may call attention to a mass that is malignant. Symptoms indicating systemic metastases are back or bone pain, weight loss, dyspnea, and jaundice.

Inspection of the breast is the first part of the physical examination and should be carried out with the patient sitting, arms at sides, and then overhead. Axillary and supraclavicular lymphadenopathy should be palpated with the patient sitting. Palpation for breast masses should be performed with the patient both seated and supine with the arm abducted. Palpation should be performed in a clocklike as well as a horizontal stripping motion. Skin changes, consisting of retraction, dimpling, edema, and redness, or asymmetry of the breast is suspicious for malignancy. One or two movable, nontender lymph nodes in the axilla and less than 5 mm in diameter are generally insignificant. However, firm or hard nodes larger than 1 cm in diameter usually contain metastases. Matted or fixed axillary nodes to the skin or deep structures represent advanced disease. Firm or hard nodes in the supraclavicular fossa of any size are suggestive of malignancy. A breast mass that is hard and has poorly delineated margins is suggestive of breast cancer. Associated skin and nipple changes further increase the probability that the mass is

malignant. A small lesion detected by the patient but not felt by the examiner may be further assessed by mammography, ultrasonography, or repeat physical examinations at 2- to 3-month intervals.

MAMMOGRAPHY

Mammography is the most common method used for detecting early breast cancer. Indications for mammography include (1) to screen women at high risk for developing breast cancer; (2) to screen women before a cosmetic operation or biopsy of a mass for an unsuspected cancer; (3) to evaluate both breasts when a diagnosis of breast cancer has been established; (4) to evaluate an ill-defined mass or suspicious change in the breast; (5) to search for an unknown primary tumor in a woman who has axillary lymph node metastases; and (6) to follow these women after they have been treated with breast-conserving surgery and irradiation or mastectomy with reconstruction.

Clustered polymorphic microcalcifications are the most common mammographic abnormality associated with this disease. These calcifications are grouped together, numbering 5 to 8 with a branched or V- or Y-shaped configuration. Mammographic mass densities and areas of architectural distortion are identified with breast cancer. These lesions may or may not be associated with microcalcifications. However, patients with a dominant or suggestive mass palpated on physical examination must undergo biopsy despite mammographic findings. Mammography is not a substitute for biopsy because it may not detect cancer in women with very dense breasts.

High-quality screening and diagnostic mammography is dependent on communication and documentation between the patient and the referring and interpreting physicians. The patient should be informed of the technique and the need for breast compression, which is uncomfortable. The mammography facility should be informed in writing of abnormal physical examination findings. All mammography reports should be communicated in writing to the patient as well as the health care provider.

Currently, ultrasonography is the most useful adjunct to mammography in assessing breast lesions. Ultrasonography can distinguish between solid and cystic lesions and is particularly useful in young women with dense breast tissue. More recently, the utility of magnetic resonance imaging (MRI) and positron emission tomography (PET) in detecting breast cancer has been examined. Although these new imaging modalities may be used in special circumstances (e.g., an unknown primary tumor), it is unlikely that they will be used for routine imaging for detection of early breast cancer.

Diagnostic Tests

The treatment of breast cancer should never be undertaken without an unequivocal histologic or cytologic diagnosis of cancer. The safest course is to sample all suspicious masses found on physical examination or mammography. However, lesions thought to be definitely cancerous are benign in about 60% of cases, and about 30% of lesions thought to be malignant are benign. In general, a breast mass should not be followed without histologic diagnosis. An exception may be in premenopausal women with a nonsuspicious mass presumed to be fibrocystic disease. However, if this mass does not completely resolve within one or two menstrual cycles, it must be sampled.

The methods of obtaining a biopsy include fine-needle aspiration, large-needle (core needle) biopsy, open biopsy, mammographic stereotactic biopsy, and mammographic localization biopsy. *Fine-needle aspiration* is performed by using a small (usually 22-gauge) needle to aspirate cells from a breast tumor. This technique requires a skilled cytopathologist. The false-negative rate is as high as 10% in some series. The incidence of false-positive findings is extremely low, ranging from 1 to 2%. *Large-needle (core needle) biopsy,* which entails the use of a large cutting needle, removes a core of tissue for histologic examination. Similar to the technique of fine-needle aspiration, a sampling error can occur because of improper positioning of the needle. If the fine-needle aspiration or core biopsy is negative, or atypical, and the clinical diagnosis or breast imaging studies are suspicious for cancer, open biopsy must be performed. *Open biopsy* under local anesthesia is performed as a separate procedure before deciding on definitive treatment. *Computerized mammographic stereotactic biopsy* is performed in lesions or suspicious abnormalities noted on mammography alone. Under mammographic guidance, a biopsy needle can be inserted into the lesion in the mammographer's suite and a core of tissue for histologic examination or cells for cytology can be examined.

Some suspicious mammographic abnormalities noted on mammogram alone cannot be assessed by stereotactic biopsy because of the location of the lesion in the breast (especially very posterior lesions). In these cases, *mammographic localization biopsy* is performed by obtaining a mammogram in two perpendicular views and placing a needle or hook wire near the abnormality. After mammography confirms the position of the needle, the abnormality can be localized and excised. It is essential to obtain a mammogram of the specimen to confirm that the mammographic abnormality was excised.

Staging

The American Joint Committee on Cancer and the International Union Against Cancer have previously described the TNM (tumor, regional lymph nodes, distant metastases) staging system for breast cancer. The extent of disease evident from physical findings and preoperative studies is used to determine its clinical stage.

Histopathologic Types

Histologically there are numerous subtypes of breast cancer. In general, breast cancer arises from the epithelial lining of the large or intermediate-sized ducts (ductal) or from the epithelium of the terminal ducts of the lobules (lobular). The cancer may be invasive or in situ. Most cancers arise from the intermediate ducts and are invasive (invasive ductal, infiltrating ductal), and most histologic types are merely subtypes of invasive (medullary, colloid, tubular, papillary) ductal cancer. Ductal carcinoma that has not invaded the extraductal tissue is intraductal or ductal carcinoma in situ. Associated invasive cancers are present in 1 to 3% of ductal carcinomas. Lobular carcinoma may be invasive or in situ. Lobular carcinoma in situ (LCIS) is a risk factor, and an invasive cancer develops in either breast in at least 20% of cases. Histologic subtypes have only a slight bearing on prognosis, except for in situ cancers that lack the ability to metastasize.

Special Clinical Forms of Breast Cancer

IN SITU CARCINOMA

Noninvasive cancer can occur in the ducts or lobules. Ductal carcinoma in situ (DCIS) is a premalignant lesion, whereas lobular carcinoma in situ (LCIS) is a tumor marker indicating patients at increased risk for breast cancer. DCIS is usually unilateral and most likely progresses to invasive cancer if untreated. Patients with LCIS are at increased risk of developing breast cancer in either breast.

DCIS can be treated by total mastectomy or breast conservation with wide excision with or without radiation therapy. LCIS is managed by observation or rarely by bilateral mastectomy in those patients unwilling to accept the increased risk of developing breast cancer. In situ cancer should not metastasize to the lymph nodes unless there is an occult invasive cancer, and therefore an axillary dissection is not indicated for patients with in situ carcinoma.

BILATERAL BREAST CANCER

Bilateral breast cancer occurs in less than 1% of cases, but there is a 5 to 8% incidence of later occurrence of a second breast cancer. Bilateral breast cancer is found more commonly in familial breast cancer, in women younger than age 50, and when the histopathology is lobular. The incidence of a second breast cancer increases about 1% a year. Mammography should always be performed before primary treatment to search for a second cancer in the opposite breast.

PAGET'S DISEASE OF THE BREAST

Paget's carcinoma occurs in about 1% of all breast cancers and is frequently misdiagnosed. There is often a delay in both diagnosis and treatment because these lesions are frequently treated as dermatitis or bacterial infections. The ducts of the nipple epithelium are infiltrated, but gross nipple changes are minimal and a tumor mass may not be palpable. The first symptom is often itching or burning of the nipple, with superficial erosion or ulceration. Biopsy of the erosion or ulceration should be performed to confirm the diagnosis.

BREAST CANCER DURING PREGNANCY OR LACTATION

Only 1 to 2% of all breast cancers occur during pregnancy. There is often a delay in diagnosis and treatment because of the physiologic changes that may obscure the lesion. Pregnancy (or lactation) is not a contraindication to operation, and treatment should be based on the stage of the disease as in the nonpregnant (or nonlactating) woman. Breast-conserving surgery, radiation therapy, and even chemotherapy may be performed usually after delivery of the infant.

INFLAMMATORY CARCINOMA

Inflammatory carcinoma occurs in 3% of all cases of breast cancer and is the most malignant form. The patient comes to medical attention with a rapidly growing mass and skin that is edematous and erythematous. There is often no distinct mass because the tumor infiltrates the involved breast diffusely. If an infection is suggested but the lesion does not respond rapidly to antibiotics (1 to 2 weeks), a biopsy that includes the skin must be performed. Inflammatory carcinoma is rarely curable because metastases have already occurred at the time of presentation in most cases. Mastectomy is usually not performed unless the patient has responded to radiation therapy and chemotherapy and has no evidence of metastatic disease.

MALE BREAST CANCER

The incidence of breast cancer in men is about 1% of that in women. The prognosis of this disease is worse in men than in women even when matched by stage of disease. The patient usually comes to medical attention with a hard, ill-defined, nontender mass that may or may not be accompanied by gynecomastia. Systemic metastases usually exist at the time of initial presentation. Surgical and adjuvant treatment should be chosen by the same criteria as in women with the disease. Tamoxifen treatment in patients with estrogen-receptor positive tumors is indicated.

CURATIVE TREATMENT

Curative treatment is possible for patients with stage I and II disease. In those with more advanced disease (stage III and IV disease), only palliation can be achieved in most cases. The principal determinants of primary therapy are the extent of disease and its biologic aggressiveness. Legislation in numerous states requires physicians to inform patients of alternative treatment methods in the management of breast cancer.

Breast-Conserving Therapy

The National Surgical Adjuvant Breast Project (NSABP) showed that disease-free survival rates were similar for patients treated by partial mastectomy plus axillary dissection followed by radiation therapy and for those treated by modified radical mastectomy (total mastectomy plus axillary dissection). Patients were randomized into one of three arms in the NSABP trial: (1) lumpectomy plus whole-breast irradiation, (2) lumpectomy alone, and (3) total mastectomy. All patients underwent axillary lymph node dissection. Tumor size was as large as 4 cm. The local recurrence rate was highest among patients with lumpectomy alone. However, there was no difference in overall or disease-free survival among the three treatment groups. This study, as well as the Milan trial and several nonrandomized trials, showed that lumpectomy and axillary dissection with postoperative radiation therapy is as effective as modified radical mastectomy for the management of patients with stage I and II breast cancer.

Tumor size is a major determinant of the feasibility of breast conservation. Relative contraindications to breast conservative therapy include large tumor size, multifocality, involvement of the nipple or overlying skin, or fixation to the chest wall. However, the patient, not the surgeon, must ultimately decide what is cosmetically acceptable.

Axillary dissection is important in staging the disease, preventing axillary recurrences, and planning additional therapy. More recently, sentinel lymphadenectomy (SLND) has been developed as a minimally invasive technique that accurately stages the axillary basin. SLND identifies the first node (sentinel node) in the lymphatic basin to receive metastases from the primary tumor. Studies have indicated that if the sentinel node does not contain tumor than the chance of the remaining lymph nodes having metastases is small. These early results suggest that sentinel node biopsy may replace axillary dissection for staging and treatment in histopathologically node-negative women.

Current Recommendations

The NIH 1990 consensus stated that breast-conserving surgery with radiation is the preferred treatment in patients with early-stage breast cancer. However, breast conservative therapy appears underused because modified radical mastectomy has been the standard of care for most patients with breast cancer. This operation removes the entire breast, overlying skin, nipple, and areolar complex, as well as the underlying pectoralis fascia with the axillary lymph nodes in continuity. Radical mastectomy, which removes the underlying pectoralis muscle, is rarely indicated. Axillary node dissection is not necessary for noninfiltrating cancers, because nodal metastases are rarely present. Breast reconstruction, either immediately or delayed, should be discussed with patients who choose or require mastectomy.

Radiation therapy after partial mastectomy consists of 5 to 6 weeks of five daily fractions to a total dose of 5000 to 6000 cGy. Some radiotherapists use a boost dose, but the value of this is controversial. Radiation is not routinely given to patients who have undergone modified radical mastectomy, because clinical trials have failed to show a survival benefit in patients receiving radiation to the chest wall after undergoing a total mastectomy. However, two randomized trials from Denmark and Canada have renewed interest in radiation therapy after mastectomy because these studies demonstrate not only reduced recurrence rates but also improved survival in premenopausal node-positive women who received radiation therapy and chemotherapy versus chemotherapy alone.

Adjuvant Systemic Therapy

Chemotherapy or hormonal therapy is recommended for most patients with curable breast cancer. Although surgery and radiation therapy treat local-regional disease, adjuvant systemic therapy seeks to eliminate occult metastatic disease.

Many clinical trials have assessed the benefit of various chemotherapeutic regimens in the adjuvant setting for breast cancer patients. The most extensive experience is with the cyclophosphamide (Cytoxan), methotrexate, and fluorouracil (CMF) regimen. These studies have demonstrated that all women with positive axillary nodes definitely benefit from adjuvant chemotherapy. Other trials using different combinations of agents, such as doxorubicin (Adriamycin) plus cyclophosphamide (AC), have also demonstrated the benefit of adjuvant chemotherapy in patients with positive axillary nodes. Promising new agents are emerging as possible successors or supplements to these standard regimens. The most notable of these is paclitaxel (Taxol), a member of the taxanes. One study has shown that AC combined with paclitaxel had a statistically significant benefit at 4 years compared with patients who did not receive paclitaxel.

The addition of hormonal therapy to chemotherapy

TABLE 1. **Adjuvant Chemotherapy for Premenopausal and Postmenopausal Women***

Axillary Nodal Involvement	Estrogen Receptors	Adjuvant Systemic Therapy (Premenopausal)	Adjuvant Systemic Therapy (Postmenopausal)
Yes	Positive	Combination chemotherapy	Tamoxifen
Yes	Negative	Combination chemotherapy	Combination chemotherapy
No	Positive	Tamoxifen	Tamoxifen
No	Negative	Combination chemotherapy	Combination chemotherapy

*Summary of National Institutes of Health Consensus Conference, June 18–21, 1990.

in the adjuvant setting may improve the outcome in breast cancer patients. Although tamoxifen has been the recommended treatment for postmenopausal women with estrogen receptor–positive tumors, an NSABP trial showed that tamoxifen plus chemotherapy lowered the recurrence rates more than tamoxifen alone in postmenopausal women with estrogen receptor–positive tumors.

The length of time adjuvant therapy must be administered appears to be shorter than previously recommended. One study that compared 6 versus 12 cycles of postoperative CMF found 5-year disease-free survival rates to be comparable. One NSABP study showed that 5 years of treatment with tamoxifen may be superior to 10 years of adjuvant treatment with tamoxifen.

Several studies of adjuvant therapy in node-negative women have now been published and show a beneficial effect of adjuvant chemotherapy or tamoxifen in delaying recurrence and improving survival. A number of protocols, including CMF with leucovorin rescue as well as tamoxifen alone, have increased disease-free survival times.

The current recommendations for adjuvant chemotherapy are summarized in Table 1. In addition to the tumor status of the axillary lymph nodes, other prognostic factors being used to determine the need for adjuvant therapy include tumor size, estrogen and progesterone receptor status, oncogene expression, histologic type, ploidy status, lymphatic or vascular invasion, and nuclear grade.

There are several issues to address regarding the use of adjuvant therapy in breast cancer patients. Some of the questions include timing and duration of adjuvant chemotherapy, which chemotherapeutic agents should be applied for which subgroup of patients, how best to coordinate adjuvant chemotherapy with postoperative radiation therapy, the use of combinations of hormonal therapy and chemotherapy, and the value of prognostic factors other than hormone receptors in predicting response to adjuvant therapy. In addition, the role of neoadjuvant therapy, given before resection of the primary tumor, needs to be further addressed. Early neoadjuvant studies indicate that a complete response in vivo before operation is associated with improvement in survival.

Palliative Therapy

Radiation Therapy

Locally advanced cancers with or without metastases that are causing pain, ulceration, or other symp-

toms can be treated by radiation therapy. Neoadjuvant therapy should be considered in patients with locally advanced breast cancer who have no evidence of distant metastases. The field of radiation should include the entire breast and axillary, supraclavicular, and internal mammary nodes. Radiation therapy can also be used to palliate patients with chest wall recurrences, bony metastases, and acute spinal cord compression.

Hormone Therapy

Endocrine therapy may slow the progression of metastatic disease. This effect can be achieved by blocking hormone receptor sites, inhibiting hormonal synthesis, or ablating organs involved in hormone synthesis. Choice of therapy is based on menopausal status. In the premenopausal patient with metastatic disease, tamoxifen is the primary hormonal therapy of choice. A new tamoxifen analogue, toremifene (Fareston), is being evaluated as an alternative to tamoxifen as primary hormonal therapy. The two drugs have similar efficacy and side effects, but the long-term effects of toremifene are unknown. Randomized clinical trials have shown no significant difference in the survival or response between tamoxifen therapy and bilateral oophorectomy. Premenopausal women with metastatic disease that initially responds to tamoxifen or oophorectomy but subsequently relapses may respond to aminoglutethimide (Cytadren)* or megestrol acetate (Megace) as secondary or tertiary hormonal therapy. These agents result in a medical adrenalectomy or hypophysectomy, therefore replacing the need for surgical ablation. Patients who respond initially to oophorectomy but experience relapse should receive tamoxifen. Those patients who do not respond to either tamoxifen or oophorectomy should be treated with chemotherapy. In the postmenopausal patient with metastatic disease, tamoxifen is the initial therapy of choice. Postmenopausal women who initially respond to tamoxifen but later progress could be given diethylstilbestrol or megestrol acetate. Postmenopausal patients who do not respond to tamoxifen should be given cytotoxic drugs (AC or CMF). Aromatase inhibitors (aminoglutethimide) is an alternative in postmenopausal women who fail to respond to tamoxifen.

Chemotherapy

Chemotherapy should be considered for the treatment of metastatic breast cancer if visceral metasta-

---

*Not FDA approved for this indication.

ses are present, hormonal therapy is unsuccessful, or disease progression has occurred, or if the primary tumor is estrogen receptor negative. Combination regimens containing doxorubicin (Adriamycin) have been shown to be most effective. More recently, paclitaxel (a taxoid agent) has been shown to be very effective for patients with breast cancer. It is usually given after failure of combination chemotherapy for metastatic disease or relapse shortly after completion of adjuvant chemotherapy. Studies now suggest that paclitaxel is beneficial as both a first-line agent and as an adjuvant systemic agent, in combination with doxorubicin (Adriamycin) and cyclophosphamide. Docetaxel (Taxotere) is another taxoid that has shown promise for treatment of patients with anthracycline-resistant tumors. Both agents are currently being used after treatment with anthracyclines in patients with advanced disease as well as in adjuvant and neoadjuvant settings. High-dose chemotherapy with autologous bone marrow or stem cell transplantation has gained widespread interest for the treatment of metastatic breast cancer. This form of therapy has significant morbidity and is very expensive. Although complete response rates are considerably better than conventional chemotherapy, median survival and overall survival rates do not appear to be different between the two methods. No randomized controlled clinical trial has been published that compares conventional chemotherapy with high-dose chemotherapy followed by stem cell support. A study is underway to evaluate these two options in a controlled prospective manner.

PROGNOSIS

The prognosis of breast cancer patients can be determined by the stage of disease. Those patients with disease localized to the breast have a much more favorable outcome compared with patients with metastases to the axillary lymph nodes. In addition, as the number of nodes involved increases, an adverse effect on survival is seen. Other factors that help to determine prognosis include hormone-receptor status, DNA ploidy, S-phase, *HER-2/neu* oncogene expression, epidermal growth factor, and cathepsin D levels. None of these prognostic factors is as effective as lymph node metastases in predicting outcome. The histologic subtype (e.g., medullary, tubular, lobular, colloid) of invasive breast cancers appears to have little significance on prognosis. The role of anti-HER2 antibody (Herceptin) in patients with metastatic breast cancer who overexpress the *HER-2/neu* oncogene is being assessed in clinical trials. Results of a large, multinational phase III trial of Herceptin added to chemotherapy significantly increased time to progression and response rate compared with chemotherapy alone.

Five-year statistics do not accurately predict the final outcome in breast cancer patients. The mortality rate of patients with this disease exceeds that of age-matched normal controls for nearly 20 years. When cancer is localized to the breast the clinical cure rate is 75 to 90%. When axillary lymph nodes are involved with tumor, the 5-year survival decreases to 40 to 50% and at 10 years to about 25%.

FOLLOW-UP CARE

Patients treated for breast cancer should be followed for life to detect recurrences and observe the opposite breast for a second primary carcinoma. Most recurrences, both local and distant, tend to occur within the first 3 years. During this period the patient should be examined every 3 to 4 months. The patient is then examined every 6 months up until 5 years and every 6 to 12 months after 5 years. The patient should examine her own breast monthly, and a mammogram should be obtained annually.

RECURRENCE

The incidence of local recurrence is related to characteristics of the primary tumor, axillary lymph node tumor status, and the initial local breast therapy. Patients with locally advanced breast cancers and with axillary lymph node metastases have an increased risk of local recurrence. When the axillary nodes are not involved and the tumor is small, the local recurrence rate is about 5%, but the rate is as high as 25% when the tumor is large or multiple nodes contain metastases. Factors that may affect the rate of local recurrence in patients who have a partial mastectomy include multifocal cancer, in situ tumors, positive resection margins, chemotherapy, and radiation therapy. Any suspicious nodule or skin lesions of the chest wall should be sampled. An isolated lesion can be treated by excision and radiation therapy. If multiple lesions are present, chest wall radiation to include the parasternal, supraclavicular, and axillary nodal regions should be performed. Patients with local recurrence after mastectomy should undergo a metastatic work-up to search for evidence of metastases. If there is no evidence of disease beyond the chest wall and regional nodes, irradiation for cure or complete local excision should be attempted. After partial mastectomy, local recurrence may not have as serious a prognostic significance as after mastectomy. Completion of the mastectomy should be done for local recurrence after partial mastectomy. Systemic chemotherapy or hormonal treatment should be used for women who develop disseminated disease or those in whom local recurrence occurs after total mastectomy.

ENDOMETRIOSIS

method of
DAVID ADAMSON, M.D.
Fertility Physicians of Northern California
Palo Alto, California

Endometriosis is an enigmatic disease affecting about 7% of reproductive-aged women—approximately 5 million

Americans. Most of these women do not know that they have endometriosis, although many may suffer significant symptoms ranging from pelvic pain to infertility. Because our understanding of the clinical presentation, diagnosis, and management of endometriosis has improved dramatically in the past few years, physicians can now provide better care for patients who may suffer from this potentially debilitating and chronic disease.

DEFINITION

Endometriosis is the presence of endometrial tissue, consisting of endometrial glands and stroma, in ectopic locations. This tissue reacts to estrogen and progesterone. The usual location is in the pelvis, but endometriosis has also been found in omentum, small intestine, appendix, anterior abdominal wall, surgical scars, diaphragm, lung, urinary tract, and musculoskeletal and neural systems. The tissue can be very diverse histologically and can appear to be proliferative, secretory, or menstrual.

PREVALENCE AND INCIDENCE

The prevalence and incidence of endometriosis depend on the population of women studied. The range is 1 to 50% depending on the surgical series. It has been reported to occur in 10 to 15% of women undergoing diagnostic laparoscopy, 2 to 5% of women undergoing tubal sterilization, 30 to 40% of infertile women having laparoscopy, and 14 to 53% of women with pelvic pain.

PATHOGENESIS AND PATHOPHYSIOLOGY

There are several theories that attempt to describe the pathogenesis of endometriosis. The most popular are retrograde menstruation through the fallopian tubes, metaplasia, activation of embryonic rests of müllerian tissue, hematogenous and lymphatic spread, or direct placement in wounds. Each of these and other possible etiologies may contribute variably to endometriosis in different patients. Altered immunity may also play a role.

There are numerous factors that appear to affect whether a woman will have this disease, the severity of the disease, symptoms, and response to treatment. These factors include genetics (an affected sister or mother doubles the risk), hormonal status (higher estrogen levels and prolonged heavy menses increase risk), lifestyle (low weight and smoking reduce risk by decreasing estrogen levels), contraceptive use (oral contraceptives possibly reduce progression of disease), obstetric history (pregnancy and lactation reduce risk), anatomic factors (cervical stenosis increases risk), treatment history (prior medical or surgical treatment reduces risk), race, and possibly exposure to environmental toxins, especially those that are estrogenic.

Endometriosis is thought to cause reproductive dysfunction by resulting in cyclic bleeding at the time of menses that leads to an inflammatory reaction, fibrosis, and adhesions. This may cause distorted anatomy, endocrinopathies, such as increased prostaglandin production, altered pelvic physicochemical milieu, abnormally functioning immune system, interference with sperm function, and possibly an altered process of embryo implantation. It is certain there is an association between endometriosis and pain and endometriosis and infertility. A cause and effect relationship has been reasonably established for all stages of disease, including minimal, mild, moderate, severe, and different types of associated lesions, including endometriomas, adhesions, and invasive disease.

CLINICAL PRESENTATION

Endometriosis manifests primarily as pelvic pain in about 50% of patients, infertility in about 25%, pain and infertility in about 25%, and ovarian endometrioma in less than 5% of cases. There is also a large incidence of asymptomatic disease, from 1 to 40%. Endometriosis may occur anytime after puberty, including adolescence.

Pain symptoms of endometriosis often do not correlate well with severity of disease. Pain may occur as a result of secretion of irritating factors (e.g., histamine), adhesions that cause scarring or retraction, leaking endometriomas, compression of other visceral structures (e.g., bowel), compression of uterosacral nodules, and/or invasion of the urinary or gastrointestinal tract. Endometriosis is associated with infertility in patients with all stages of disease. Patients who have endometriomas, extensive endometriosis lesions and/or adhesions, or extensive invasive disease have a poorer prognosis than patients without these lesions. Endometriosis may also be associated with intraluminal fallopian tube pathology. Studies overall do not support an association between endometriosis and increased spontaneous abortion rates.

Endometriosis lesions occur throughout the pelvis. They tend to be more frequently in the posterior cul-de-sac and the ovary and less frequently on the fallopian tubes. Endometriosis is almost certainly a progressive disease, but the rate of progression and the nature of lesions vary from patient to patient.

Adhesions develop as a result of the inflammatory process caused by long-standing endometriosis, with more extensive and dense adhesions developing over time. Complete cul-de-sac obliteration can result from long-standing invasive and adhesive disease or may result from abnormal müllerian development.

DIAGNOSIS

The diagnosis of endometriosis is suggested by several symptoms, including dysmenorrhea, dyspareunia (especially with aching following coitus), dyschezia, dysuria, mittelschmerz, or focal or generalized pelvic pain. Hematuria and hematochezia may also be symptoms of endometriosis. About 30% of patients with endometriosis do not have any pain. Signs of endometriosis include tenderness or nodularity in the posterior cul-de-sac, especially on the uterosacral ligaments, anterior cul-de-sac nodularity, adnexal masses from endometriomas, and reduced mobility or fixation of the pelvis due to pelvic adhesions. The location of tenderness often corresponds to the location of the pain. Pelvic examination should be performed at the time of menses because disease is more easily identified at that time.

Tests that may assist in the diagnosis of endometriosis include ultrasonography to evaluate the adnexa for endometriomas and the uterus for myomas or adenomyosis. CA 125 may occasionally be helpful in studying the course of endometriosis after diagnosis and treatment, but the high false-positive and false-negative rates give it little utility in the initial diagnostic work-up.

Currently the only definite test for pelvic endometriosis is diagnostic laparoscopy. Biopsy of lesions may sometimes be necessary to confirm the diagnosis of endometriosis and should always be performed if the surgeon is uncertain of the diagnosis. Preoperative consultations with gastroenterologists, urologists, general surgeons, or other specialists as indicated should be scheduled to help ensure that laparoscopy produces maximum benefits for the patient.

The differential diagnosis includes pelvic inflammatory disease, ectopic pregnancy, adenomyosis, myomas, benign ovarian tumors, malignant ovarian tumors (rare), hernias, abdominal wall trigger points, interstitial cystitis, irritable bowel syndrome, pelvic pain of undetermined etiology, and normal pelvis. It should be emphasized to patients that diagnosis mandates laparoscopy but that endometriosis is not always found at laparoscopy even when it has been suggested by the history, physical examination, and preoperative testing. The degree of pain frequently does not correlate with the extent of disease, but pain does seem to be present more often when the patient has invasive, nodular lesions or endometriomas.

It has been estimated that the diagnosis of endometriosis has been missed in more than 7% of patients, and the extent of disease has been underestimated in as many as 50% of patients. Subtle lesions can be missed even by experienced laparoscopists. Other lesions such as old suture, ovarian cancer, carbon deposits from prior laser surgery, and hemangiomas may look like endometriosis. The surgeon must recognize the classic powder burn or blueberry lesion; white scar tissue that may be older, less endocrinologically active disease; clear or slightly brown-colored papillary lesions; or strawberry or flame-like lesions that are more recently developed and have more endocrinologic, immunologic, and inflammatory activity. Peritoneal pockets may also be associated with endometriosis.

LAPAROSCOPY

Indications

Indications for laparoscopy to diagnose endometriosis include infertility of more than 1 year duration without other symptoms or possibly after 6 months if the patient has symptoms or is older than 35 years. Evaluation for other female factors and sperm quality should be performed before laparoscopy. Patients with pelvic pain that has not responded after 3 months of nonsteroidal anti-inflammatory drugs (NSAIDs) and/or 3 months of oral contraceptives are candidates for laparoscopy. Patients with an adnexal mass suspected of being an endometrioma should have laparoscopy if the lesion does not resolve by 3 months or sooner if there are concomitant symptoms such as pain or other factors that make surgery appropriate.

Contraindications

Contraindications to surgery include multiple repeat operations at short intervals to treat lesions. If appropriate surgery is performed, it is uncommon for endometriotic lesions to recur within a few months. Repeat surgery for adhesiolysis is indicated for selected patients, usually those with infertility. Repeated surgery may occasionally be indicated after 1 to 2 years if symptoms recur and are not treatable with medical therapy. Laparoscopy may be repeated to perform gamete intrafallopian transfer in selected patients. Surgery should not be performed in patients with unacceptably high medical or surgical risks. Laparoscopy should not be performed in patients at high risk for bowel injury unless an open technique or a technique designed to avoid bowel injury is utilized. Laparotomy is an appropriate approach for many surgeons when laparoscopy may be too hazardous or the surgeon may not have the requisite skills or facilities to perform operative laparoscopy.

MANAGEMENT OPTIONS

Managing the patient with endometriosis requires evaluation of her reproductive goals. She may be a teenager desiring future pregnancy, a woman planning immediate pregnancy, or a woman who has completed her childbearing and/or does not desire future pregnancy. Patients may present with undiagnosed pelvic pain or pain associated with recurrence of endometriosis after prior treatment. The objectives of therapy are to remove or destroy implants, relieve symptoms, maintain or restore fertility, and avoid or delay recurrence of the disease. Several management options are available.

No Treatment

No treatment does include expectant management and/or limited use of analgesics and NSAIDs. These may be especially helpful for women with dysmenorrhea associated with endometriosis.

Medical Treatment

Medical therapy can consist of oral contraceptives (OCs), progestins, danazol, or gonadotropin-releasing hormones (GnRH) agonists. OCs can be given cyclically, but many patients do better with continuous active-ingredient tablets for 3 months, followed by withdrawal, and then repetition. Monophasic OCs are superior to triphasic OCs. The best dosage to begin is usually 35 μg of ethinyl estradiol, but this can be decreased if the patient is symptomatic with headaches or increased for break-through bleeding. Norethindrone, 0.35 to 5.0 mg daily, may be added if the patient is still symptomatic with bleeding. Transdermal estradiol (Estraderm) 0.05 mg or 0.1 mg twice weekly may also be used if this is better tolerated. Treatment lasts 3 to 6 months. Progestins (Provera),* 30 mg every day, alone suppress gonadotropin secretion and ovarian function, but can be associated with break-through bleeding, mastalgia, bloating, weight gain, and depression. They may be useful for a few women who cannot tolerate OCs. Treatment is relatively inexpensive.

Danazol (Danocrine), 200 to 400 mg twice a day, is an ethisterone derivative that functions primarily by suppressing follicle-stimulating hormone (FSH) and luteinizing hormone (LH) from the pituitary gland, thereby creating a hypoestrogenic state. Danazol is

---

*Not FDA approved for this indication.

also associated with androgenic side effects, however, including weight gain, vasomotor instability (hot flushes), muscle cramps, acne, edema, hirsutism, reduced breast size, vaginitis, and sweating. It is contraindicated during pregnancy and lactation and in women with undiagnosed abnormal genital bleeding or markedly impaired hepatic, renal, or cardiac function. These pharmacologic effects are reversed within 2 months of discontinuing treatment.

GnRH agonists are synthetic decapeptides. Nafarelin acetate (Synarel), 200 μg nasal spray used twice a day, is a superactive, hydrophobic stimulatory analogue of GnRH that is 200 times more potent than naturally occurring GnRH and is delivered in a metered nasal spray pump. Leuprolide acetate (Lupron Depot) is usually given as a single monthly 3.75-mg intramuscular injection. The GnRH agonists result in an initial stimulation of the pituitary gland with release of FSH and LH and a consequent increase in serum estradiol levels to approximately 100 pg per mL. Continued used of GnRH agonists, however, leads to down-regulation and desensitization of the pituitary gland after 7 to 14 days and the inability to release FSH and LH. This produces hypoestrogenemia (estradiol less than 40 pg per mL) and resultant amenorrhea, which permits regression of endometriosis and relief of symptoms. The GnRH agonists do not have any known direct effects on the ovary. Treatment costs approximately $2,400 for 6 months.

Side effects include hot flashes in about 90% of patients, decreased libido, vaginal dryness, headaches, emotional lability, and insomnia. Cardiovascular and liver enzyme parameters show favorable changes relative to danazol. The major concern with GnRH agonists is the loss of bone density, about 3 to 8%, which occurs over 6 months of drug therapy, with a 2 to 3% loss persisting about 1 year after treatment. The FDA and others' consensus is that this loss is not clinically significant in women who have no evidence of bone disease, and it is not generally necessary to perform an evaluation of bone density before initiating treatment. Although only one 6-month course of GnRH agonist is FDA approved, studies have shown that 3 months of treatment, both initially and from subsequent retreatment if symptoms recur, is as effective as 6 months of treatment and is associated with less bone loss. Patients should generally undergo dual photon absorptiometry and have normal bone density before GnRH agonist retreatment, and they should be fully informed of the potential risks. Subsequent symptoms may also be treated with OCs, danazol, and/or surgery.

Hot flushes can be effectively managed with norethindrone (Aygestin), 2.5 mg per day. Higher doses of norethindrone may provide some protection against bone loss, but have an unfavorable side effect profile for liver and cardiovascular systems, and patients are often very symptomatic. Low doses of estrogen (Premarin, 0.625 mg per day) have also been used as "add-back" therapy to reduce bone loss and show some promise. More recently, add-back therapy for 6 to 12 months with norethindrone, 2.5 mg, and

alendronate (Fosamax), 10 mg per day, has been suggested, along with calcium, 1000 mg per day. However, the long-term efficacy of such add-back therapy and its effect on the therapeutic efficacy of the GnRH agonist is still being evaluated.

Surgical Treatment

Diagnostic laparoscopy provides a relatively safe and simple method of diagnosing endometriosis. When appropriate, operative laparoscopy enables treatment to be initiated and possibly completed at the same time. Surgical therapy is usually conservative, consisting of excision, laser vaporization, or electrosurgical fulguration of endometriosis. Adjunctive procedures such as salpingo-ovariolysis may also be performed. Additional, occasionally indicated, but still controversial procedures for pain include uterosacral nerve ablation and, for severe midline dysmenorrhea, presacral neurectomy. In cases of advanced disease, radical surgery comprising hysterectomy and/or bilateral salpingo-oophorectomy may be required. Laparoscopic treatment of endometriosis mandates a surgeon who is familiar with the pathophysiology of endometriosis and who can integrate this knowledge with surgical judgment and technique.

Medical and surgical treatment modalities sometimes have the same results, but surgical treatment completed at the time of diagnosis has a distinct advantage over medical therapy because of decreased time, cost, and side effects. The patient can also be spared a second operation (laparotomy) if operative laparoscopy can be performed at the time of diagnosis. Operative laparoscopy offers several advantages to laparotomy, primarily because of better visualization, less tissue trauma, and much shorter recovery time. Tactile sense, however, is less than that which can be obtained digitally at laparotomy.

It is more important to give the patient the best operation possible in the particular surgeon's hands rather than to compromise by performing a poor operation at laparoscopy. The guiding surgical principle is complete removal of all endometriosis lesions, fibrosis, and adhesions, including those needing deep dissection. The prevention of postoperative adhesions is based primarily on meticulous surgical technique.

Combined Treatments

Laparoscopic treatment of endometriosis may sometimes be combined with medical therapy involving danazol or GnRH agonists. The purpose of combined treatment is to improve treatment success or facilitate surgical procedures.

Preoperative medical treatment suppresses ovulation so that functional cysts are not present or confused with endometriosis. Metastatic or extensive superficial disease is suppressed and becomes atrophic. The reduced vascularity in the pelvis may result in reduced inflammation and postoperative adhesions, although this has not been proved. There may be a slight reduction in endometrioma size. Other uses of GnRH agonists before surgery include reduction of symptoms, increased time for adequate preoperative evaluation, easier scheduling of surgery, and even delay or avoidance of surgery for a woman nearing menopause. Potential disadvantages of preoperative medical treatment include the changed appearance of endometriosis, which might make it more difficult to diagnose; drug cost and side effects; delay of diagnosis; and delay in attempting pregnancy. Postoperative medical treatment with GnRH agonists may be indicated if complete resection of disease has not been accomplished, for treatment of microscopic or metastatic disease, or for treatment of pain.

Preoperative or postoperative treatment is usually given for 2 to 6 months, but 3 months is adequate for most patients. A very successful treatment approach is to use OCs continuously for 2 to 3 months, withdraw for 1 week, and repeat the 2 to 3 months of treatment. This cycle can be continued even to menopause or to the time of attempting pregnancy. It is the most cost-effective approach for many patients.

The approach to each patient must be individualized depending on her symptoms, signs, age, type and extent of disease, and desire for fertility. Many patients prefer no treatment or medical treatment before surgery. Surgery, however, is often the most appropriate approach. Most patients prefer to retain as many of their reproductive organs as possible, but for some oophorectomy and/or hysterectomy is a better option. Laparoscopy is generally the preferred surgical approach, but laparotomy may be appropriate for some patients, especially those requiring extirpation of large endometriomas, extensive enterolysis, enterostomy, or bowel resection. Alternatives to treatment, or treatment in combination with surgery, such as the use of GnRH agonists preoperatively to treat severe endometriosis, should be considered.

It is critical that physicians recognize the degree to which endometriosis can physically and emotionally disrupt patients' lives and provide comprehensive understanding and an empathetic management approach. Attention to a healthy lifestyle with respect to diet, exercise, sleep, and stress reduction through mind-body techniques can be very helpful. Psychological support through information can be obtained from organizations such as the Endometriosis Association (414-355-2200), RESOLVE (617-623-1156), and the American Society of Reproductive Medicine (205-978-5000). Personal or group counseling may also be helpful, especially for the patient with chronic pain. Some patients may seek nontraditional and unproven approaches to treatment such as acupuncture, herbal medicine, or special diets.

Management in these chronic, complex situations should focus on alleviation of symptoms and improved quality of life. A comprehensive evaluation of gastrointestinal, genitourinary, musculoskeletal, neurologic, and psychological systems may be indicated. Referral to a pain clinic may be helpful for further treatment, including biofeedback strategies, nerve blocks, psychotherapy, or other pain management techniques. Treatment of reactive depression is often necessary and often mandates a multidisciplinary approach. A comprehensive long-range treatment approach needs to be individualized for each patient. A complete cure can sometimes only be achieved by total hysterectomy and bilateral salpingo-oophorectomy.

COMPARISON OF TREATMENT OUTCOMES

Pain

No treatment or mild analgesics or NSAIDs may be entirely appropriate for many young patients with minimal symptoms or for women who have just completed a course of medical treatment. Women who remain symptomatic with minimal or mild pain may frequently be successfully treated with cyclic OCs, and this treatment should be attempted by most women. For women who have persistent pain, treatment with progestins, danazol, or GnRH agonists have similar efficacy, with approximately 80 to 90% of patients having significant relief.

In one study that is representative of those in the literature, nafarelin acetate (Synarel) at both high (400 µg bid) and low (200 µg bid) doses, as well as danazol (Danocrine 400 mg bid), provided significant relief of several types of pain associated with endometriosis during 6 months of daily treatment (Table 1). This beneficial effect persisted after the end of drug treatment, but by 6 months after treatment was completed, approximately two-thirds of patients had experienced a return of dysmenorrhea; however, pelvic pain was reported by only about one-half and dyspareunia by about one-third of subjects. Dysmenorrhea returns with menses and presumably the cyclic release of endometrial prostaglandins. Generalized pelvic pain and dyspareunia may depend on the re-establishment of endometrial implants. Patients with severe disease or large endometriomas tend to have an earlier recurrence. Danazol and GnRH agonists should not be used in the treatment of endometriosis unless the diagnosis has been confirmed with laparoscopy.

Laparoscopy and laparotomy are also effective in the treatment of pelvic pain, with approximately 90% of patients showing significant clinical improvement after complete resection of disease. Approximately 90% should have good symptom relief at 5 years and 50% at 10 years if the disease is completely resected. Patients with more severe disease are at higher risk of recurrence than those with mild disease.

Hysterectomy is the definitive treatment for patients with recurrent or intractable pain associated with endometriosis. In young women of reproductive age, removal of one or both ovaries is controversial even though the ovaries are the most common site of endometrial implants and the growth of endometrial implants is driven by cyclic ovarian activity. An ovarian cystectomy for endometrioma is usually the most appropriate approach. If a hysterectomy is war-

TABLE 1. **Reports of Specific Types of Pain in Patients with Laparoscopically Diagnosed Endometriosis Treated with Nafarelin Acetate or Danazol**

Treatment	Dysmenorrhea (%)			Dyspareunia (%)				Pelvic (%)		
	No.	Absent	Present	No.	Absent	Present	Not Reported	No.	Absent	Present
Nafarelin 800 µg	45			26				40		
Admission		0	100		0	100	0		0	100
Treatment*		100	0		62	31	8		65	35
Post-treatment†		36	64		62	35	4		45	55
Nafarelin 400 µg	45			31				37		
Admission		0	100		0	100	0		0	100
Treatment*		98	2		65	32	3		57	43
Post-treatment†		33	67		71	29	0		49	51
Danazol	34			23				28		
Admission		0	100		0	100	0		0	100
Treatment*		94	6		70	17	13		64	36
Post-treatment†		50	50		65	30	4		50	50

All subjects reported pain on admission.
*Treatment was continued for 6 months.
†Post-treatment period was 6 months follow-up.
From Adamson GD, Kwei L, Edgren RA: Pain of endometriosis: Effects of nafarelin and danazol therapy. Int J Fertil *39(4)*:215–217, 1994.

ranted, all remaining endometriosis lesions should be removed at the same time.

Hysterectomy combined with oophorectomy for endometriosis results in a very high probability of "cure." There is a small recurrence rate in the range of 5 to 8%, but it is clear that such recurrence can occur. This may be due to residual endometriosis, recurrent endometriosis, ovarian remnant syndrome, adhesions, or other nongynecologic problems. This recurrence rate may be reduced by meticulous resection of all endometriosis at the time of hysterectomy and by oophorectomy at the time of hysterectomy. Postoperatively, hormone replacement therapy can probably be started immediately.

Infertility

For minimal and mild disease, a prospective randomized study has demonstrated that laparoscopic treatment of endometriosis results in higher pregnancy rates at 9 months than no treatment. The pregnancy rate by 3 years is not different for no treatment, laparoscopy, and laparotomy when 3-year estimated cumulative life table pregnancy rates are calculated (Table 2). Likewise, no treatment or surgery is superior to medical treatment for minimal and mild endometriosis associated with infertility. Meta-analysis has also shown that there is no statistically significant difference in crude pregnancy rates between no treatment and medical treatment (Fig. 1). Therefore, no treatment is appropriate for selected young patients with minimal or mild disease and short duration of infertility, although superior pregnancy rates can be achieved with laparoscopic surgery. Controlled ovarian hyperstimulation with clomiphene citrate (Clomid, Serophene), 100 mg every day from cycle day 3 to 7, or gonadotropins (Pergonal, Humegon, Repronex, Gonal-F, Follistim) and intrauterine insemination improve pregnancy rates in this group.

Medical treatments for minimal and mild endometriosis result in at best negligible improvement in ultimate pregnancy rates and are associated with additional cost and undesirable side effects. Medical treatment merely delays the possibility of pregnancy by the duration of the therapy. Medical therapy alone should never be used to treat minimal and mild endometriosis when the only symptom is infertility.

Preoperative medical therapy should probably be reserved for patients with severe symptomatology, to facilitate surgery scheduling when necessary, or for patients with known severe disease when medical treatment may allow for a better pelvic milieu for reconstructive surgery. It is unknown what, if any, effect preoperative medical treatment has on subsequent pregnancy rates. Postoperative medical treatment may be indicated for patients with severe re-

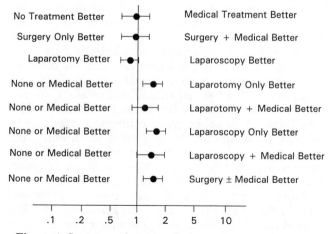

Figure 1. Summary of meta-analysis estimates of relative risk of pregnancy (point estimate and 95% confidence interval): Different endometriosis treatment comparisons. (From Adamson GD, Pasta DJ: Surgical treatment of endometriosis-associated infertility: Meta-analysis compared with survival analysis. Am J Obstet Gynecol *171*[6]:1488–1505, 1994.)

TABLE 2. **Estimated Cumulative Life Table Pregnancy Rates by Treatment Group for Different Stages of Endometriosis**

| | Entire Patient Population | | | | | | Endometriosis-Only Subset | | | | | |
| | No. | No. Pregnant in 3 y | Pregnant (%) | | | No. | No. Pregnant in 3 y | Pregnant (%) | | |
			1 y	2 y	3 y			1 y	2 y	3 y
Minimal/Mild										
No treatment	15	10	53.3 ± 12.9*	66.7 ± 12.2	66.7 ± 12.2	13	9	61.5 ± 13.5	69.2 ± 12.8	69.2 ± 12.8
Medical treatment	44	20	26.5 ± 7.2	53.0 ± 8.9	62.3 ± 9.3	32	13	25.6 ± 8.4	47.7 ± 10.2	55.2 ± 11.2
Laparoscopy	241	122	43.6 ± 3.5	59.6 ± 3.8	67.8 ± 4.1	134	70	45.5 ± 4.7	60.4 ± 5.1	70.3 ± 5.4
Laparotomy	46	28	55.7 ± 7.9	65.6 ± 7.9	74.3 ± 8.1	13	6	38.0 ± 15.1	50.4 ± 16.4	64.5 ± 16.8
Moderate/Severe‡										
Laparoscopy	120	52	29.1 ± 4.5	50.8 ± 5.6	62.2 ± 6.2	48	25	32.2 ± 7.5	70.0 ± 9.0	82.0 ± 8.5
Laparotomy	102	37	23.8 ± 4.5	36.7 ± 5.3	44.4 ± 5.6	15	5	20.0 ± 10.3	26.7 ± 11.4	33.3 ± 12.2

*Values are estimates ± SE.
‡Eleven patients treated nonsurgically have been excluded from the entire patient population. Three patients treated nonsurgically have been excluded from the endometriosis-only subset.
From Adamson GD, Hurd SJ, Pasta DJ, Rodriguez BD: Laparoscopic endometriosis treatment: Is it better? Fertil Steril 1993 *59(1)*:35–44, 1993.

fractory pelvic pain or in whom disease has not been completely extirpated but should be avoided whenever possible in infertility patients because of the inability to conceive while taking the medication. Postoperative medical treatment does not improve pregnancy rates (see Fig. 1). Overall, the available data do not support the routine perioperative use of GnRH agonists or other hormonal therapies, but these may be of value for selected patients.

A recent review of laparoscopic treatment of endometriosis reported pregnancy rates for minimal and mild disease after laparoscopic electrocoagulation of 64% and 52%, respectively. Treatment with CO_2 laser vaporization was reported to result in a 59% pregnancy rate for minimal and 58% for mild disease. The author's experience is reflected in Table 2. It is not known whether patients with extensive and/or invasive peritoneal disease alone will have pregnancy rates higher or lower than those reported in these studies. Surgical treatment is required for more advanced endometriosis with invasive nodular disease, endometriomas, and adhesions.

Infertile women with endometriosis can be treated at laparoscopy if the equipment and skill of the surgeon permit. In every analysis, laparoscopy group pregnancy rates were equal to or higher than those with other treatment options whether it was in the entire population (n = 579), the endometriosis-only subset with at least one normal tube and fimbria and normal male (n = 258), patients with minimal or mild endometriosis, or in patients with moderate or severe endometriosis. Furthermore, even when significant variables were controlled for, laparoscopy group pregnancy rates were equal to or higher than those with other treatments.

The assisted reproductive technologies of in vitro fertilization and gamete intrafallopian transfer can be used effectively to treat infertile patients with endometriosis after failed prior treatment. They are also sometimes appropriate for older women with extensive endometriosis and/or adhesions who do not have pelvic pain or endometriomas and for whom the prognosis following surgery would be limited. Patients with minimal or mild endometriosis undergoing an assisted reproductive technique have similar rates as those of patients in other diagnostic

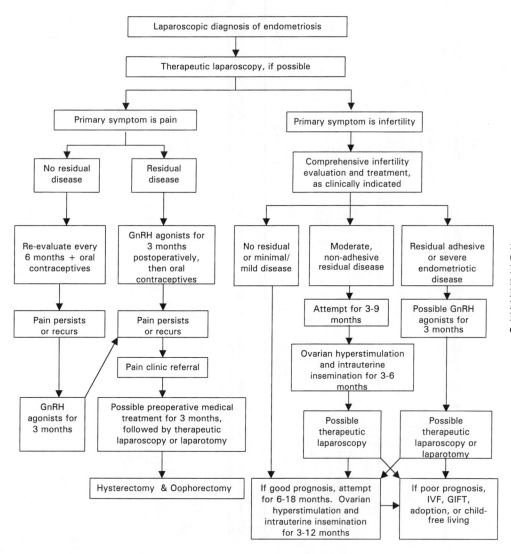

Figure 2. Postlaparoscopy management of endometriosis. (Modified from Adamson GD: Laparoscopic treatment of endometriosis. *In* Adamson GD, Martin DC [eds]: Endoscopic Management of Gynecologic Disease. Philadelphia, Lippincott-Raven, 1995, pp 147–187.)

categories. Those with moderate or severe disease probably have slightly reduced pregnancy rates possibly due to reduced ovarian response to gonadotropins secondary to endometriomas or prior ovarian surgery. Pregnancy rates depend on patient age, ranging from about 35% per cycle at age 30 years to 15% per cycle at age 40 years.

Endometriomas

Endometriomas cannot be successfully treated medically and if left untreated are thought generally to enlarge and potentially destroy more ovarian tissue and/or cause pelvic pain and reduced fertility. Surgical removal can be accomplished at least as well at laparoscopy as at laparotomy by an experienced surgeon. Postoperative pregnancy rates are approximately 40 to 50% by 2 years. Most, if not all, surgeons favor complete ovarian cystectomy as opposed to less extirpative procedures, such as cyst drainage or coagulation of the endometrioma cyst wall, both of which are associated with higher recurrence rates. Recurrence rates are approximately 10 to 20% after cystectomy. Oophorectomy is rarely indicated except for a nonfunctional ovary or for older women who have completed their childbearing.

ALGORITHM FOR MANAGEMENT OF ENDOMETRIOSIS

Laparoscopy is necessary to diagnose endometriosis. Whether the patient's symptoms are pain or infertility, surgical treatment involving complete laparoscopic resection of the disease should be performed at the time of diagnosis if the surgeon is capable of so doing. The only exception to this approach is the young woman with infertility as her only symptom and extensive superficial peritoneal and/or ovarian disease. Treatment of such lesions may increase pregnancy rates but also may result in pelvic adhesions. Patients with pain should generally receive OCs postoperatively. For infertility patients, controlled ovarian hyperstimulation and intrauterine insemination postoperatively for 3 to 6 months with clomiphene and/or 3 to 6 months with gonadotropins will increase pregnancy rates.

When adequate surgical extirpation of the disease, can be achieved, no further postoperative medical treatment is indicated (except for OCs) for patients with either pain or infertility. If pain recurs, GnRH agonists should usually be the first line of treatment. For infertile patients who fail to conceive, a second-look laparoscopy at 6 to 18 months may be indicated, with possibly gamete intrafallopian transfer performed at the same time. If extensive endometriosis, adhesions, or tubal abnormalities are found, in vitro fertilization should be considered within 0 to 12 months after surgery.

If the patient does not have operative laparoscopy at the time of diagnosis or has incomplete resection of endometriosis, patients with pain have the option of a repeated laparoscopy or laparotomy, most likely by a more experienced surgeon specializing in endometriosis, or use of GnRH agonists or danazol for 3 to 6 months. GnRH agonists are generally preferred because of their more favorable side effect profile. Failure to manage pain with surgical and/or medical treatment should result in referral to pain specialists for a comprehensive approach to the pain. Such an option should be discussed with the patient at her first consultation and integrated into the treatment plan.

For infertility patients who have not had operative resection or inadequate resection, minimal and mild disease (no adhesions, no invasive lesions, no endometriomas) need no further treatment. Patients with moderate or advanced disease should be referred for laparoscopy or occasionally laparotomy. Medical treatment should not be used.

Infertile patients who do not conceive within approximately 6 to 15 months should have a repeated laparoscopy for treatment and/or assisted reproductive technologies such as in vitro fertilization and/or gamete intrafallopian transfer (Fig. 2), depending on the patient's age and other infertility factors.

THE FUTURE

We have much to learn about endometriosis. More detailed evidence-based meta-analysis and prospective randomized studies are being performed to help improve the clinical guidelines. Basic research currently underway should give us a better understanding of beta$_3$ integrins and immunology and hopefully lead to new therapeutic approaches. An international study to determine the genetic basis of endometriosis is currently underway and hopefully will lead to much more successful treatments in the years ahead.

DYSFUNCTIONAL UTERINE BLEEDING

method of
TIMOTHY R. YEKO, M.D., and
JERYL NATOFSKY, M.D.
University of South Florida, College of Medicine
Tampa, Florida

DEFINITION AND PATHOPHYSIOLOGY

Dysfunctional uterine bleeding (DUB) refers to abnormal uterine bleeding that cannot be attributed to an organic pathologic condition. It is considered a diagnosis of exclusion, and therefore other potential causes need to be ruled out before the designation of this diagnosis. The term "dysfunctional" is applied because it is inferred that DUB is due to a dysfunction of the normal hormonal control of menstruation. Strictly speaking, in cases of DUB the endometrium is responding to the appropriate ovarian steroid hormone (estrogen and progesterone) signals, but under circumstances in which these signals are no longer functioning in a normal cyclic fashion. Hence, DUB is most frequently associated with anovulation that produces unopposed estrogen stimulation of the endometrium. Less frequently, DUB can occur in women with ovulatory cycles, but in this setting abnormal bleeding occurs because the uterus is exposed to progesterone stimulation that is deficient (inadequate corpus luteum), erratic (oligoanovulatory cycles), or prolonged because of a persistent corpus luteum cyst. Others speculate that the typical regular but heavy menses (menorrhagia) seen with ovulatory DUB is a result of an imbalance in prostanoid synthesis that inhibits vasoconstriction and platelet aggregation in the endometrium.

Familiarity with the physiology of normal menstrual bleeding is necessary to understand the endometrial sequelae of anovulation. The normal menstrual cycle is produced by the sequential and coordinated effects of estrogen and progesterone on the endometrium. During the first 2 weeks of the menstrual cycle, the functional layer of the endometrium proliferates in response to increasing levels of estradiol produced by the growing follicle. After ovulation, progesterone becomes the dominant steroid and is secreted by the corpus luteum for the remaining 2 weeks of the luteal phase of the menstrual cycle. Progesterone stops further endometrial growth and converts the proliferative endometrium into a secretory endometrium that is necessary for embryo implantation. If pregnancy does not occur, progesterone levels drop precipitously because of the self-limited 14-day life span of the corpus luteum. In response to the withdrawal of progesterone, the functional layer of the endometrium is sloughed, producing a typical menses lasting 3 to 5 days. In contrast, in the pathologic state of anovulation, a corpus luteum does not form, progesterone is not secreted, and the endometrium is exposed to prolonged periods of unopposed estrogen. The result is excessive proliferation and endometrial growth that outgrows its blood supply. Varying degrees of necrosis lead to asynchronous tissue breakdown and episodes of irregular bleeding. These bleeding episodes can range from mild intermenstrual spotting to prolonged, heavy bleeding leading to potentially life-threatening anemia.

To define abnormal uterine bleeding, it is necessary to define normal menstrual flow. The mean interval between menses is 28 days, with an interval of 21 to 35 days being within the norm. The mean duration of menstrual flow is 4 days, menses lasting longer than 7 days being abnormal. Average menstrual blood loss is 35 mL, with 95% of women losing less than 60 mL of blood during each menses. Menstrual blood loss greater than 80 mL is considered abnormal and may lead to iron deficiency anemia. It is important for patients to document the frequency, duration, and amount of flow in a menstrual diary. Objective criteria, including hemodynamic instability and anemia, are most useful in judging the severity of the condition because subjective estimates of menstrual blood loss are unreliable. Decisions regarding management should be based on severity of anemia as well as chronicity of the bleeding episodes as documented in the menstrual diary.

DUB is most commonly seen during the postmenarchal and premenopausal extremes of a woman's reproductive years; this is due to anovulatory cycles that commonly occur during these times, when the pubertal hypothalamic–pituitary–ovarian axis is still immature and, later, as the premenopausal ovary begins to undergo senescence. In adolescent girls within the first 4 years after menarche, 25% of menstrual cycles are anovulatory. These girls begin to have normal ovulatory cycles as their hypothalamic–pituitary–ovarian axis predictably reaches complete maturity in the mid- to late teens. However, 5% of women remain in a state of anovulation throughout their reproductive years. Besides DUB, these women frequently have other complaints associated with chronic anovulation, including infertility, hirsutism, hyperinsulinemia, and poly-

cystic-appearing ovaries on ultrasonography. Obesity, emotional stress, and supplements containing ginseng, herbal roots, and phytoestrogens can also exacerbate DUB in some women.

DIFFERENTIAL DIAGNOSIS AND WORK-UP

DUB is the most common cause of abnormal vaginal bleeding, and anovulation is the most common cause of DUB. Therefore, documentation of the ovulatory status by menstrual history, basal body temperature monitoring, a serum progesterone, or an endometrial biopsy should be done early in the work-up. Other primary causes of abnormal vaginal bleeding, however, must be considered and ruled out in accordance with each patient's clinical presentation. Table 1 lists the diagnostic tests, including clinical evaluation, laboratory tests, ultrasonography, and endometrial biopsy, that are useful in excluding other causes of abnormal vaginal bleeding. All patients should have a history and physical examination, pregnancy test, and complete blood count. A simple office pipelle endometrial biopsy should be performed in patients with risk factors for endometrial hyperplasia and cancer, including a long history of anovulation, obesity, diabetes, hypertension, and age older than 30 years. Coagulopathies are rare in the general population, but are present in 20% of adolescent girls who come to the emergency room with acute heavy menstrual bleeding. Therefore, in adolescents and women with a history of easy bruising suggesting a bleeding disorder, a platelet count, prothrombin time, and a partial prothrombin time should be ordered.

Vaginal ultrasonography should be reserved for patients with a history or physical examination positive for a structural abnormality and for any patient with a normal examination but whose DUB is resistant to hormonal management. Particularly in the latter circumstance, women with ovulatory cycles, a normal pelvic examination, and menorrhagia may harbor lesions in the endometrial cavity, such as polyps and submucosal leiomyomas, in up to 30% of cases. These lesions are best evaluated with the use of sonohysterography, which is a sonographic image of the uterus obtained after transcervical instillation of saline to outline the endometrial cavity. This simple, 5-minute office procedure has virtually eliminated the use of the much more invasive and costly technique of hysteroscopy.

TREATMENT

Once the diagnosis of DUB has been established, treatment depends on the severity of anemia and whether the patient's hemodynamic condition is stable or unstable. For patients with acute, life-threatening bleeding in which there may be either a severe anemia or hemodynamic instability, hospitalization is required. Before initiating hormonal treatment, systemic treatment for blood loss should be administered, including intravenous fluids and blood as needed. Laboratory tests should include a complete blood count with platelets, a coagulation profile, and a pregnancy test. Once the patient is stabilized and pregnancy has been ruled out, attention can be directed toward therapy to stop the bleeding. Uterine curettage is an effective means of immediately stopping uterine bleeding due to DUB. Several high-dose hormonal regimens also stop or reduce bleeding to a manageable level within 24 hours of administration.

TABLE 1. **Evaluation for Organic Causes of Abnormal Vaginal Bleeding**

Cause	Applicable Diagnostic Work-up			
	Basic*	Ultrasound	Endometrial Biopsy	Other
Abnormalities of pregnancy				
Threatened, missed, or incomplete abortion	+	+		
Tubal pregnancy	+	+		
Gestational trophoblastic disease	+	+	+	
Malignancy				
Endometrial adenocarcinoma	+		+	
Functional ovarian neoplasm	+	+		
Cervical	+			Pap smear
Vaginal and fallopian tube—rare	+	+		
Infection				
Endometritis	+		+	Genital cultures
Cervicitis	+			Genital cultures
Vaginitis	+			Genital cultures
Benign uterine and cervical lesions				
Uterine leiomyoma	+	+		
Endometrial hyperplasia	+		+	
Endometrial or endocervical polyp	+	+		
Cervical erosion	+			
Traumatic vaginal lesion	+			
Foreign body (IUD)	+	+		
Coagulation disorders				
Von Willebrand disease	+			Coagulation profile
Idiopathic thrombocytopenic purpura	+			
Endocrinopathies				
Thyroid disease	+			Thyroid-stimulating hormone
Hyperprolactinemia	+			Prolactin
Organ failure				
Liver cirrhosis	+			Liver function tests
Kidney failure	+			Renal function tests
Exogenous steroid or phytoestrogen use	+			

*Basic evaluation includes a history and physical examination, pregnancy test, and complete blood count.

Table 2 outlines three hormonal therapies: a high-dose conjugated estrogen (Premarin) regimen, a high-dose progestogen (Provera) regimen, and a combination high-dose estrogen and progestogen regimen with oral contraceptive pills (OCPs). The high-dose oral progestogen regimen is useful in avoiding the troublesome side effects such as severe nausea and vomiting sometimes experienced by patients taking both the high-dose estrogen and OCP regimens. With each of these regimens, relief of bleeding usually occurs within the first 24 to 48 hours. Each regimen includes a subsequent short, 10- to 14-day course of either a synthetic progestogen such as medroxy-progesterone acetate or an OCP to stabilize the endometrium and prepare it for a withdrawal period. Functionally, this produces what has been termed a "medical curettage." Once the acute episode of bleeding resolves, these patients should be placed on a regimen of OCPs or cyclic Provera, 10 mg daily for 14 days each month. This regulates the menstrual cycle, prevents endometrial hyperplasia, and, in the case of women using OCPs, provides contraception. If none of these hormonal regimens is successful a uterine curettage should be performed.

In adolescents and adults with von Willebrand disease, desmopressin acetate (DDAVP), a synthetic an-

TABLE 2. **High-Dose Hormone Regimens for the Treatment of Acute Dysfunctional Uterine Bleeding**

High-Dose Hormonal Regimen	Dose Schedules	
	First 24 Hours	Subsequent Treatment
Conjugated estrogen	Premarin 25 mg IV repeated q4h for 12 h or until bleeding stops	Cyclic Provera 10 mg PO daily × 14 d each month versus cyclic OCPs
Medroxyprogesterone acetate*	Provera 5–10 mg PO q2h for 24 h or until bleeding stops	Provera 20 mg PO daily × 10 d, followed by either cyclic Provera 10 mg × 14 d each month versus cyclic OCPs
OCP (35 µg ethinyl estradiol)	2–4 tablets/d × 5 d	Cyclic OCPs

*Exceeds dosage recommended by the manufacturer.
Abbreviation: OCP = oral contraceptive pill.

alogue of arginine vasopressin, can be used to treat DUB by increasing coagulation factor VIII. It can be self-administered by nasal spray, 150 to 300 µg, has a rapid onset within 30 minutes, and lasts up to 48 hours.

In patients with complaints of mild and more chronic bleeding episodes, medical therapy is aimed at cycle regulation, prevention of endometrial hyperplasia, and avoidance of surgery. The most commonly used treatment is low-dose (20 to 35 µg of ethinyl estradiol) OCPs, which induce endometrial atrophy and reduce menstrual blood loss by 50% after 3 months of treatment. They also provide the secondary benefits of reducing the acne and hirsutism that are frequent complaints in anovulatory women with polycystic ovaries and ovarian hyperandrogenism. Although all OCPs provide these benefits, only Ortho Tri-Cyclen (which contains norgestimate) is FDA approved for the treatment of acne. Patients who are not candidates for OCP use may be treated with cyclic Provera, 10 mg orally for 14 days each month. Administration of nonsteroidal anti-inflammatory agents is also useful in reducing blood loss by up to 30%. Ibuprofen, 400 mg, can be given every 4 to 6 hours during each day of menses. Finally, the progesterone-releasing intrauterine device Progestasert can significantly reduce menstrual blood loss by up to 80% and remains hormonally active for 7 years. If medical therapy fails or the patient does not desire chronic medical therapy, conservative or definitive surgical therapy with endometrial ablation or hysterectomy, respectively, may be offered.

AMENORRHEA

method of
OWEN K. DAVIS, M.D.
Weill College of Medicine of Cornell University
New York, New York

Amenorrhea is most simply defined as the absence or cessation of menstrual bleeding in women of reproductive age. Physiologic causes of amenorrhea include pregnancy, lactation, menopause, and constitutional delay of puberty. Pathologic causes of amenorrhea, which are the focus of this article, include a variety of structural abnormalities and endocrinopathies.

By convention, amenorrhea has been designated as either primary or secondary. Primary amenorrhea is defined as the failure of menstrual function to commence (menarche) by age 16 years in general or by the age of 14 years in the absence of normal secondary sexual characteristics (e.g., growth, thelarche [breast development] and pubarche [growth of pubic hair]). Secondary amenorrhea is defined as the cessation of menstrual bleeding for a period of at least 3 months in a woman who has previously menstruated. Clearly, these definitions, while useful as guidelines, should not be rigidly applied; it would be both unnecessary and inappropriate to defer the clinical evaluation of a 13-year-old girl manifesting obvious stigmata of Turner's syndrome (45,XO gonadal dysgenesis). Furthermore, although certain abnormalities absolutely preclude the occurrence

of menarche (uterine agenesis, complete androgen insensitivity in a genotypic male), there is nonetheless considerable overlap in the causes of primary and secondary amenorrhea (e.g., central nervous system [CNS] tumors) that limits the validity of strict categorization.

The diagnosis and treatment of amenorrhea based on clinical presentation and the methodical application of targeted laboratory testing and imaging modalities are discussed in this article.

PHYSIOLOGY OF MENSTRUATION

Menstruation is the cyclic vaginal efflux of blood and tissue resulting from the sloughing of the functional strata of the endometrium. The menstrual cycle is entrained by a finely balanced interplay of the various components of the reproductive axis, including the CNS/hypothalamus, the adenohypophysis, the gonads (ovaries), and the outflow tract (uterus and vaginal canal). Hence, a functional or structural lesion at any point along this axis may result in the symptom of amenorrhea.

Briefly, neurons in the arcuate nucleus of the basal hypothalamus secrete the decapeptide gonadotropin-releasing hormone (GnRH) in a pulsatile fashion. This releasing factor is transported via the portal circulation of the pituitary stalk to the gonadotroph cells of the anterior pituitary, which in turn elaborate corresponding pulses of the gonadotropins follicle-stimulating hormone (FSH) and luteinizing hormone (LH) into the peripheral circulation. These gonadotropins in turn stimulate the steroidogenic cells of the ovarian follicular apparatus (specifically, the theca and granulosa cells), resulting in the orderly maturation of the follicle, which culminates in ovulation and formation of the corpus luteum.

The endometrium is one of the principal targets of the ovarian steroid hormones estradiol and progesterone. Proliferation of the endometrium and induction of its progesterone receptors are dependent on estrogen (estradiol), whereas the secretory transformation of the endometrium, which is critical for embryonic implantation, results from the postovulatory secretion of progesterone by the corpus luteum. It is clinically salient to reiterate and emphasize that progesterone will not act on endometrium that has not previously been estrogen primed. Unless implantation and pregnancy ensue, the corpus luteum regresses (luteolysis) within a mean interval of 14 days, and it is the resulting cyclic withdrawal of progesterone that directly leads to the breakdown and sloughing of the endometrium. The normal efflux of menstrual blood in turn requires patency of the cervical canal, vagina, and introitus.

In short, a significant intrinsic or acquired physiologic or anatomic perturbation at any point along this reproductive axis (hypothalamus, pituitary, ovaries, uterus/outflow tract) can result in the clinical manifestation of amenorrhea. An adequate diagnostic algorithm must therefore methodically assess the integrity and interplay of these various compartments.

HISTORY AND PHYSICAL EXAMINATION

In most cases a thorough history and physical examination will direct the clinician to the appropriate major diagnostic category; adjunctive laboratory and dynamic testing and in some instances imaging techniques should provide a definitive diagnosis. The clinician should ascertain whether the patient is presenting with primary or secondary amenorrhea. In the presence of previous menstrual function, a history of the regularity and frequency of prior cycles, any prior pregnancies, contraceptive use, and onset and duration of amenorrhea should be obtained. The patient should be queried regarding her medical and surgical history.

Various drugs can impede menstrual cyclicity (e.g., oral contraceptives, antidopaminergic agents, opioids, antineoplastic agents), and surgery can compromise ovarian function (e.g., ovarian cystectomies) or the integrity of the outflow tract (e.g., dilatation and curettage, cervical conization). A CNS-linked etiology may be suggested by a history of headaches, visual changes, galactorrhea (milky nipple discharge), significant weight loss, psychological stress, or intensive exercising. Gonadal failure is suggested by a history of vasomotor symptoms (hot flashes/flushes) and chronic anovulation by symptoms and signs of androgen excess (hirsutism, acne). Congenital or acquired outflow obstruction may result in cyclic pelvic pain and molimina in the absence of visible bleeding (cryptomenorrhea).

The physical examination should commence with the determination of vital signs, height, and weight and an assessment of body habitus. Hypertension in a sexually immature patient with primary amenorrhea could reflect 17-hydroxylase deficiency; systolic hypertension in the upper extremities can occur in the setting of coarctation of the aorta, which may accompany Turner's syndrome. Bradycardia is often manifest in patients with anorexia nervosa or hypothyroidism. Obesity is frequent in patients with polycystic ovary syndrome and severe weight loss in women with anorexia nervosa. Short stature is a hallmark of Turner's syndrome.

The clinical examination should particularly focus on the presence, absence, or discordance of secondary sexual characteristics. Normal breast development depends on current or past exposure to estrogens (gonadal function), and normal pubic and axillary hair growth indicates both adequate levels of gonadal and/or adrenal androgens and the presence of functional androgen receptors. Mature breast development in the absence of pubic hair, for example, points to a likely diagnosis of complete androgen insensitivity (testicular feminization). A male-pattern distribution of sexual hair (hirsutism) is characteristic of syndromes of androgen excess, including polycystic ovary syndrome. If galactorrhea is elicited on breast examination, a diagnosis of hyperprolactinemia is strongly suggested.

The pelvic examination is of particular importance in patients presenting with primary amenorrhea. A bulging, imperforate hymen is one form of outflow obstruction. A blind vaginal pouch or dimple without a palpable uterus on bimanual rectal-abdominal examination suggests uterine agenesis (Mayer-Rokitansky-Kuster-Hauser syndrome) in a genotypic female or an androgen receptor defect or enzyme deficiency in a genotypic male (e.g., complete androgen insensitivity or, less frequently, 17-hydroxylase deficiency). The uterus is absent in the latter instances, as the fetal gonads (testes) elaborate müllerian-inhibiting substance. The pelvic examination should also exclude the presence of an adnexal mass.

CLINICAL EVALUATION AND MANAGEMENT

The following diagnostic algorithm is presented as a general outline and should be appropriately modified by the specific clinical circumstances determined by the history and physical examination. Where the possibility exists, pregnancy should always be ruled out at the outset by peripheral assay for beta-human chorionic gonadotropin. The evaluation of both primary and secondary amenorrhea should initially include measurement of thyroid function (specifically including thyroid-stimulating hormone [TSH]) and a prolactin level, regardless of the presence or absence of galactorrhea, as approximately one third of women with hyperprolactinemia do not manifest galactorrhea.

Primary hypothyroidism (suggested by an elevated TSH) may cause amenorrhea directly or via hyperprolactinemia incited by the stimulation of pituitary lactotrophs by excess thyrotropin-releasing hormone. Primary hypothyroidism in the United States most commonly results from autoimmunity (Hashimoto's disease) and should be treated with thyroid hormone replacement (e.g., levothyroxine sodium [Synthroid]). An elevated prolactin level should always be retested, preferably in the morning.

The amenorrhea associated with hyperprolactinemia is due to the central inhibition of pulsatile GnRH secretion. In the setting of a normal TSH level, confirmed hyperprolactinemia should be evaluated with hypothalamic/pituitary imaging, preferably by means of magnetic resonance imaging or computed tomography. Among the more common causes of excess prolactin secretion are functioning pituitary adenomas and, less frequently, other mass lesions compressing the pituitary stalk (e.g., craniopharyngiomas). Hyperprolactinemia may be idiopathic, iatrogenic (e.g., dopamine antagonists, phenothiazines), or, less commonly, due to chronic renal failure or ectopic secretion by bronchogenic tumors.

Irrespective of whether the patient has a pituitary adenoma, the preferred treatment of hyperprolactinemia is generally medical (prolactinomas are benign, and recurrence rates after surgical resection are high). Treatment is indicated because of the risks of the resulting hypoestrogenism (e.g., osteoporosis) and frequently for the restoration of fertility. A dopamine agonist such as bromocriptine (Parlodel) may be administered at an initial night-time dosage of 1.25 mg per os (PO) for 3 days, increased to 2.5 mg per day and subsequently titrated by increments of 2.5 mg at 2-week intervals as necessary for normalization of the prolactin level, which is generally followed by prompt resumption of menses. Common side effects include postural hypotension and gastrointestinal upset; the tablets may be administered vaginally* if poorly tolerated by mouth.

After excluding pregnancy, thyroid disease, and hyperprolactinemia, a progestational challenge may be undertaken to assess the level of endogenous estrogen and the integrity of the outflow tract. Progestin is commonly administered as a single dose of intramuscular progesterone in oil (200 mg) or a 5-day oral course of medroxyprogesterone acetate (Provera), 10 mg per day. A positive response to a progestational challenge is the documentation of withdrawal bleeding, generally ensuing within a few days to 1 week.

---

*Not in the product labeling.

Here, any degree of vaginal bleeding warrants a diagnosis of chronic anovulation with adequate endogenous estrogen (recall that endometrial responsiveness to progestin requires estrogen priming) and further demonstrates a competent outflow tract.

In this setting, the most common diagnosis is polycystic ovarian syndrome. Classically, thus affected women manifest secondary amenorrhea with varying degrees of obesity and signs of androgen excess (hirsutism, acne); further laboratory work-up frequently reveals an LH:FSH ratio exceeding 2.5:1. Management of chronic anovulation depends on the patient's immediate reproductive goals. If pregnancy is not desired, cyclic progestin-withdrawal bleeding should be elicited to counter the propensity toward developing endometrial hyperplasia or carcinoma secondary to unopposed estrogen. This may be achieved by the use of a low-dose combination oral contraceptive or periodic (e.g., monthly) administration of medroxyprogesterone acetate, 10 mg for 10 days.

If pregnancy is desired, successful induction of ovulation may be achieved in approximately 80% of cases through the oral administration of clomiphene citrate (Clomid, Serophene), starting at 50 mg per day for 5 days and increasing by increments of 50 mg per day up to a dosage of 150 to 200 mg per day. When anovulation is unresponsive to treatment with clomiphene citrate, monitored daily intramuscular injections of menopausal gonadotropins (Pergonal, Humegon, Repronex), subcutaneous recombinant FSH (Gonal-F Follistim), or, less commonly, laparoscopic ovarian drilling may be employed. It should be noted that a progestational challenge, in and of itself, will occasionally trigger ovulation in an anovulatory patient: here, withdrawal bleeding will occur 14 days after the challenge.

When the progestational challenge fails to elicit withdrawal bleeding in a nonpregnant patient, the broad differential diagnosis includes either inadequate endogenous estrogen production (hypogonadism) or an anatomic or functional abnormality of the outflow tract. In cases of primary amenorrhea, the physical examination alone should generally suffice to diagnose the latter (e.g., imperforate hymen, transverse vaginal septum, vaginal or uterine agenesis, testicular feminization).

An imperforate hymen or vaginal septum can be surgically excised. In women with vaginal agenesis, a sexually functional vagina can be created through either the use of graduated dilators or surgical creation of a neovagina. When the diagnosis is unclear, consideration may be given to repeating the progestational challenge after priming with an exogenous estrogen, such as oral conjugated estrogens (Premarin), 1.25 mg per day for 21 days, with the addition of oral medroxyprogesterone acetate, 10 mg for each of the last 5 days of estrogen administration.

Patients with hypogonadism will bleed in response to the combination of estrogen and progesterone (hormone replacement), whereas patients with an outflow abnormality will not. Acquired outflow dysfunction in women with secondary amenorrhea may be due to destruction or scarring of the endometrium (Asherman's syndrome) as a consequence of prior surgical manipulation (dilatation and curettage, metroplasty, myomectomy) or uterine infection (pelvic tuberculosis, schistosomiasis). Asherman's syndrome is generally confirmed through hysterosalpingography revealing multiple intrauterine synechia or obliteration of the cavity and may be treated surgically (e.g., via hysteroscopic lysis of the adhesions followed by high-dose estrogen). Cervical stenosis is a relatively uncommon cause of acquired outflow obstruction that results from scarring of the cervical canal after procedures such as cervical conization for the treatment of dysplasia.

A positive response to estrogen priming followed by progestin withdrawal suggests hypogonadism with hypoestrogenemia. This may be due either to gonadal failure or secondarily to CNS or pituitary dysfunction. At this point, measurement of FSH and LH levels is indicated; this should be performed at least 2 weeks after the administration of exogenous steroids to avoid pituitary suppression. Elevated gonadotropins (e.g., FSH >40 mIU per mL) are indicative of gonadal failure (hypergonadotropic hypogonadism).

In cases of primary amenorrhea, this may be due to karyotypic abnormalities such as Turner's syndrome (monosomy X), other forms of gonadal dysgenesis, or, rarely, 17-hydroxylase deficiency in a genotypic male or female (lack of sex steroids secondary to an enzyme defect). The presence of a Y cell line (pure XY gonadal dysgenesis or Y-mosaicism) generally mandates extirpation of the gonads to avoid the risk of gonadal malignancies, including gonadoblastomas and dysgerminomas. A growth spurt and development of secondary sexual characteristics may be promoted by the daily administration of low-dose estrogens (0.3 mg of conjugated equine estrogens [Premarin] or 1 mg of micronized oral estradiol-17-beta [Estrace]) in conjunction with a progestin (5 mg of medroxyprogesterone acetate) for 12 days of each month. Once final height has been achieved, a combined oral contraceptive may be used to maintain secondary sexual characteristics and to avoid the long-term sequelae of hypoestrogenism.

In cases of secondary amenorrhea, gonadal failure (i.e., premature menopause) may be iatrogenic (gonadal surgery, antineoplastic therapy), autoimmune, idiopathic, or due to mosaic gonadal dysgenesis (e.g., 46,XX/45,XO); karyotyping is indicated for women under 30 years of age to rule out the presence of a Y chromosome given the associated risk of gonadal malignancy. Treatment in these cases may include standard menopausal hormone replacement or administration of a combined oral contraceptive. Although pregnancies can occasionally occur in this setting, the most effective treatment for such patients desiring fertility is in vitro fertilization with donated oocytes.

If gonadotropin levels are low or normal in the setting of hypoestrogenemia (hypogonadotropic hypogonadism), the defect resides in the CNS-pituitary compartment and may be functional, for example, the disruption of pulsatile GnRH secretion that may accompany weight loss, exercise, stress, and eating disorders (anorexia nervosa, bulimia) or due to CNS tumors or lesions, pituitary infarction (Sheehan's syndrome after postpartum hemorrhage), or isolated GnRH deficiency (Kallmann's syndrome). The evaluation of these patients should include hypothalamic and pituitary magnetic resonance imaging or computed tomography to diagnose a possible neoplasm (adenomas, craniopharyngiomas).

Constitutional pubertal delay is a physiologic cause of delayed sexual development and primary amenorrhea and is a diagnosis of exclusion; here, expectant management is appropriate. Treatment of other disorders should optimally correct the specific underlying etiology (e.g., weight gain, exercise moderation, surgical or medical therapy for a structural lesion). Otherwise, clinical management entails correction of the hypoestrogenemia through hormone replacement (e.g., oral contraceptives) or ovulation induction when pregnancy is desired (injectable gonadotropins or pulsatile intravenous or subcutaneous administration of GnRH, the latter being efficacious only in women with intact pituitary function).

DYSMENORRHEA

method of
CHRISTINE W. JORDAN, M.D.
Lakeside Hospital
Metairie, Louisiana

and

ANDREW M. KAUNITZ, M.D., and
DEBORAH S. LYON, M.D.
University of Florida Health Science Center /
Jacksonville
Jacksonville, Florida

Primary dysmenorrhea is defined as menstrual discomfort occurring in ovulatory women without pelvic pathology. Usually, the pain is colicky, midline lower abdominal pain that may radiate to the thighs and lower back. It typically begins just before the onset of menstrual flow, peaks in less than 24 hours, and resolves within 3 days. It may also be associated with systemic symptoms, such as headache, nausea/vomiting, diarrhea, and backache. Primary dysmenorrhea affects over half of postpubescent females, generally within 6 months to 1 year after menarche, as regular ovulation starts. Without treatment, 10% of women with this condition are disabled for up to 3 days each month. Some women experience improvement of symptoms after childbirth. Most women with primary dysmenorrhea can be managed effectively by primary care providers.

Secondary dysmenorrhea is menstrual pain related to pelvic pathology and frequently begins later in reproductive life. Conditions most frequently associated with secondary dysmenorrhea include uterine leiomyomata ("fibroids"), endometriosis, adenomyosis, pelvic inflammatory disease/chronic salpingitis, and cervical and endometrial polyps. Other causes of secondary dysmenorrhea include congenital and acquired müllerian anomalies resulting in outflow tract obstruction and use of an intrauterine device. The pain of secondary dysmenorrhea, usually noted to be midline plus one or both lower quadrants, starts before menstrual flow, continues throughout menstruation, and persists after the flow has ceased. Dyspareunia, which may worsen with menses, commonly accompanies this condition. The pelvic examination of a patient with secondary dysmenorrhea may reveal uterine and/or adnexal tenderness, fixed uterine retroflexion, uterosacral nodularity, or a pelvic mass. In contrast, the pelvic examination of a patient with primary dysmenorrhea should not demonstrate tenderness, masses, or any other pathologic changes.

In ovulatory women, endometrial production of prostaglandin $F_{2\alpha}$ ($PGF_{2\alpha}$) increases in the late luteal phase. Release of $PGF_{2\alpha}$ causes sensitization of myometrial nerve endings, uterine contractions, and local ischemia. Prostaglandin-synthetase inhibitors reduce the synthesis of

TABLE 1. **Prescription NSAIDs for Dysmenorrhea**

Drug (by Class)	Brand Name	Dosage
Anthranilic Acid		
Mefenamic acid	Ponstel	500 mg stat, then 250 mg q 6 h
Meclofenamate*	**Meclomen**	**100 mg q 8–12 h**
Phenylpropionic Acid		
Ibuprofen*†	**Motrin**	**400 mg q 4 h/800 mg q 8 h**
Ketoprofen*	Orudis	50 mg q 6–8 h
Oxaprozin	Daypro	600–1200 mg q 24 h
Arylacetic Acid		
Naproxen sodium*	**Anaprox**	**550 mg stat, then 275 mg q 6–8 h**
Naproxen†	**Naprosyn**	**500 mg stat, then 250 mg q 6–8 h**
	Naprelan	375 mg and 500 mg controlled-release tablets, 2 tablets PO q 24 h
Fenoprofen	Nalfon	200–600 mg q 6 h
Phenylalkanoic Acid		
Flurbiprofen	Ansaid	100 mg q 8–12 h
Phenylacetic Acid		
Indomethacin†§	Indocin	25–50 mg q 6–8 h
Diclofenac potassium	Cataflam	50–100 mg stat, then 50 mg q 8 h
Pyranocarboxylic Acid		
Etodolac	Lodine	300 mg q 6–8 h‡
Oxicam		
Piroxicam§	Feldene	20 mg q 24 h
Salicylates§		
Salsalate	Salflex	500–1000 mg q 8 h
Choline magnesium trisalicylate†	Trilisate	1 gm q 8 h
Diflunisal	Dolobid	500 mg q 12 h
Cyclooxygenase-2 Inhibitors		
Celecoxib	Celebrex	100–200 mg q 12 h

Most commonly used drugs are listed in **boldface.**
*Peak in 30 to 60 minutes; most commonly used because of faster pain relief.
†Available in suspension form.
‡Exceeds dosage recommended by the manufacturer.
§Piroxicam, indomethacin, and salicylates are not considered first-line agents because of high incidence of gastrointestinal (GI) upset, diarrhea, and GI bleeding.

TABLE 2. **Over-the-Counter NSAIDs for Dysmenorrhea**

Drug (by Class)	Brand Name	Dosage
Phenylpropionic Acid **Ibuprofen***	**Advil, Motrin IB, Nuprin, Haltran, Midol IB, generic**	**200 mg, 1–2 tablets q 4–6 h**
Ketoprofen*	Actron, Orudis KT	12.5 mg, 1–2 tablets q 4–6 h
Arylacetic Acid **Naproxen sodium***	**Aleve, generic**	**220 mg, 2 tablets stat, then 220 mg q 8–12 h**
Salicylates Aspirin	Bayer, Bufferin, Ecotrin, generic	650 mg q 4 h

Most commonly used drugs are listed in **boldface.**
*Fast onset of action.

$PGF_{2\alpha}$ by inhibiting cyclooxygenase, the enzyme that converts arachidonic acid to cyclic endoperoxides. Thus, a reasonable first approach to treating dysmenorrhea is to advise use of the nonsteroidal anti-inflammatory drug (NSAID) ibuprofen, which is the least expensive of all the NSAIDs and is available over the counter. Ibuprofen reduces menstrual pain by decreasing the $PGF_{2\alpha}$ levels in the menstrual fluid and reducing intrauterine pressure. The fenamates are the most effective class of NSAIDs for treating menstrual pain, with 90% of patients reporting excellent pain relief. Fenamates not only inhibit prostaglandin synthetase but also decrease the activity of already synthesized prostaglandins. Continuous, rather than as-needed use of NSAIDs, beginning with the onset of symptoms, may treat dysmenorrhea more effectively. A new category of NSAIDs, cyclooxygenase-2 inhibitors, provides a therapeutic alternative for patients with peptic ulcer disease or other gastrointestinal disturbances. These should not be first-line agents, however, because of expense. See Tables 1 and 2 for a complete listing of drugs effective in treating dysmenorrhea.

TREATMENT

For patients desiring pregnancy, NSAIDs are the mainstay of therapy for dysmenorrhea. For patients who do not wish to conceive, combination oral contraceptive pills (OCs) and depot medroxyprogesterone acetate (DMPA) (Depo-Provera) provide highly effective pain relief and, if desired, protection from pregnancy. Both of these agents suppress ovulation, preventing the late luteal phase increase in prostaglandin production. The use of these contraceptive agents also results in decreased menstrual flow. Three consecutive cycles of OCs are necessary before their effectiveness can be determined. Initially combining NSAIDs with OCs is appropriate, as the NSAIDs typically provide relief during the initial cycle of use. Any low-dose (less than 50 µg estrogen) combination OC should be acceptable if no contraindications to OC use are present. If dysmenorrhea persists, the frequency of menses may be reduced by prolonging the duration of active OC use to 42 or 63 consecutive active tablets rather than the conventional 21.

DMPA (150 mg every 3 months) suppresses ovulation and endometrial growth. Most women bleed or spot intermittently after the first injection or two but then develop oligomenorrhea or amenorrhea with continued use. Over half of all women using DMPA for 1 year (4 injections) experience amenorrhea. The irregular bleeding associated with DMPA tends to be very light and is typically not associated with significant dysmenorrhea. Patients counseled about these expected menstrual changes tend to be more compliant with continued therapy. DMPA is an excellent choice for the patient with contraindications to use of OCs, including smokers over age 35 years, as well as those with a history of thromboembolism, active liver disease, or coronary artery disease. DMPA also avoids the OC-related problems of nausea and noncompliance. Patients desiring fertility should be counseled about DMPA's prolonged duration of action, with ovulation returning on average 9 to 10 months after the last injection.

Patients unable to achieve relief from their dysmenorrhea after a 6- to 12-month trial of NSAIDs, OCs, DMPA, or some combination of these should be referred to a gynecologist to further investigate for possible pelvic pathology and to consider the need for diagnostic laparoscopy and hysteroscopy. In 20% of such women, no evidence of pelvic pathology is noted. If such women have completed childbearing, hysterectomy can be considered.

PREMENSTRUAL SYNDROME

method of
M. L. ELKS, M.D., Ph.D
Morehouse School of Medicine
Atlanta, Georgia

Premenstrual syndrome (PMS), a constellation of symptoms occurring premenstrually and remitting soon after the onset of menses, varies in prevalence depending on the definition of spectrum and severity of symptoms. Common symptoms include swelling and bloating, fluid retention, breast tenderness, mood swings, irritability and tension, anxiety, crying spells, anger, appetite changes, fatigue, sleep disturbance, headache, abdominal pain and bloating, and back pain (Table 1). If PMS is defined broadly to include modest breast tenderness or swelling, fluid retention, or other changes in the days preceding menses, essentially 90 to 100% of women experience such changes at some time during their reproductive years. If the definition is limited to significant swelling and pain, significant depression, anxiety, or mood lability, sufficient to cause noticeable and problematic interference with daily activities, the incidence falls to 1 to 3%, depending on the survey. Although often attributed to a "hormone imbalance," the elegant studies of Schmidt and others have demonstrated convincingly that those individuals significantly impacted by narrowly defined PMS have a normal hormonal ebb and flow and an abnormal and reproducible symptom response to these normal hormonal changes.

ETIOLOGY

PMS, by definition, occurs only in women with biphasic menstrual cycles—that is, an intact hormonal system with a follicular phase of estrogen secretion and a luteal phase of progesterone and estrogen secretion with decline of hormones in the late premenstrual phase. A uterus is not necessary for PMS; functioning ovaries are. PMS type complaints can occur with oral contraceptives, with use of progestational agents, and with the hormonal fluxes of fertility treatments, but these would not be true PMS. The abolition of PMS symptoms with the abrogation of cyclic hormone fluxes by use of luteinizing hormone–releasing hormone (LHRH) analogues confirms the biologic role of the hormones in the genesis of the symptoms, and careful studies comparing affected and unaffected cycling women have shown no differences in the hormonal profiles, including estrogen, progesterone, androgen, aldosterone, luteinizing hormone, and follicle-stimulating hormone levels. Thus, there is an abnormal response to a normal sex hormone milieu.

It is well recognized that breast tissue is strongly impacted by the normal hormonal cycle, and the cyclic stimulation is cited as the cause of the breast swelling and tenderness. Progesterone has aldosterone-antagonist qualities, and there is normally a rise in aldosterone in the second phase of the cycle. This and the impact of estrogen on the angiotensin-renin system are cited as the underlying mechanism of the fluid retention, weight gain, and

bloating of the luteal phase (although no consistent differences in these systems have been seen in affected women). Progesterone and its derivatives can impact neurochemistry and cause somnolence. Progesterone also relaxes smooth muscle, which may lead to the constipation, abdominal swelling, bloating, and weight gain. Progesterone alters the central setpoint for body temperature and may lead to changes in diurnal rhythms and sleep. Muscle and joint achiness can occur from fluid retention and swelling and/or insufficient deep sleep. Headaches may be due to fluid retention, tension, or insufficient sleep.

Estrogen is recognized to have complex effects on mood and sense of well-being, but the mechanism is unclear. Direct metabolism to centrally active catechol estrogens has been observed, but the role of this or the interaction of estrogens with other neurochemical balances is unclear. Some researchers believe that the unopposed (by progesterone) rise in estrogen in the follicular phase causes a relative euphoria that could raise the spirits of a depressed individual (that is, we are seeing "midcycle euphoria" in a person whose basal state is depression, rather than premenstrual depression in a euthymic individual). The excellent response to low doses of selective serotonin reuptake inhibitors (SSRIs) including fluoxetine (Prozac) and sertraline (Zoloft) suggests a strong role of hormonal impact on neuroendocrine balance in the etiology of the mood swings, fatigue, irritability, anxiety, appetite changes, and tension. Although there are no published genetic studies, a strong familial predisposition for PMS has been long noted by practitioners and patients.

The role of calcium deficiency is unclear. Low calcium is a cause of weakness, fatigue, irritability, and a loss of sense of well-being, but the relationship to mood lability, depression, pain, and bloating is less clear.

APPROACH TO THE PATIENT WITH PMS

The evaluation and management of PMS requires a careful and sensitive history and evaluation. It is often the case that the patient will present with a self-diagnosis of PMS, and it is the role of the physician to determine if this is the case and to assess for other maladies common to the reproductive years that may be mislabeled as PMS. Anemia, thyroid dysfunction, endometriosis, depression, anxiety disorders, menopause, exacerbation of another underlying chronic condition, and insufficient sleep patterns are not uncommonly diagnosed in those with a presenting complaint of "PMS." The assessment of PMS is also made more complex by a broad public awareness of the term but a misunderstanding of its meaning. There is a widespread misconception that all women are emotionally labile, especially *during* the menstrual flow. (*Premenstrual* changes abate with the onset of flow.) In addition, it is not uncommon for affected women to be concerned not about the illness per se but rather how their altered activity, energy, moods, and behavior affect their families and/or coworkers. Thus, the first challenge for the physician in taking a history is to carefully delineate the spectrum of symptoms, the periodicity specifically in relationship to the timing of the menstrual flow, and the concerns of the individual with respect to roles and functions. Use of a menstrual symptom calendar can be helpful in the diagnosis as well as in following treatment in selected patients. A prior or current history of sexual, physical, or verbal abuse is more common in women with severe PMS (but also affects one in seven women overall). Explicit recovery of prior forgotten abuse is not necessary for a good therapeutic response, however.

The social and psychological impacts on a diagnosis of

TABLE 1. **Symptoms of Premenstrual Syndrome**

Psychological

Irritability
Tension
Mood swings
Crying spells
Depression
Anger and hostility

Somatic

Headaches
Abdominal pain and bloating
Back pain
Achiness
Breast tenderness and swelling
Fluid retention
Ankle or hand swelling
Weight gain

Miscellaneous

Increased appetite
Carbohydrate craving
Other cravings
Fatigue
Increased or decreased sleep

PMS are very complex. On the one hand, there is significant cultural impact on the diagnosis. Rates of incidence of PMS vary considerably in world cultures and are increased in those cultures with strong negative views of the menstrual process. In America, PMS appears to be a more socially acceptable diagnosis than depression or anxiety disorder, and insurance coverage can also be better in some plans. These issues impact the incidence and presentation of the condition.

In America, many women work the "second shift," having full-time jobs outside the home but also retaining most of the household duties. It is not uncommon in taking a history of a patient with complaints of PMS to hear complaints of difficulty keeping up with a list of duties and responsibilities that would wear out anyone. Studies suggest that women commonly need 8 to 9 hours of sleep nightly but that average sleep is only 6 to 7 hours. Eating disorders, poor and variable diets, excessive stress, and lack of regular exercise are common. Thus, an important aspect of the evaluation and management of PMS includes an inventory of current health practices, diet, and work and sleep schedules with advice on a healthier regimen, if warranted. Controlled studies have not shown a therapeutic benefit to dietary, exercise, or vitamin regimens, but these are often cited as helpful in surveys of women with mild PMS who have not sought medical attention. (Usual recommendations are a low salt, low fat, low simple-sugar, high complex-carbohydrate diet, ample in fresh fruits and vegetables, and 30 minutes of aerobic exercise daily.)

Exacerbation of underlying conditions in the late luteal (premenstrual) phase of the cycle is well documented and should not be considered PMS. Some women with asthma, seizure disorders, depression, anxiety disorders, diabetes, and other conditions experience exacerbation, a worsening of control, or a change in medication requirements at this time in the cycle. Some such individuals experience improved or more stable control of the condition with use of combined oral contraceptives or, in more severe circumstances, abolition of the cycle by use of LHRH analogues. In rare circumstances, severe cyclic exacerbations, combined with other indications, have been considered appropriate reasons for ablative surgery, including hysterectomy/bilateral ovariectomy. It is wise to confirm the role of hormonal fluxes in the symptom pattern by demonstrating amelioration by "medical ovariectomy" with LHRH analogues before such surgery.

On physical examination, particular attention should be devoted to signs of thyroid dysfunction or anemia. A careful pelvic examination is warranted to assess periodic pain because individuals with endometriosis and dysmenorrhea (and sometimes chronic pelvic inflammatory disease) not uncommonly present with a complaint of "PMS" when they have periodic menstrual pain. Depending on the nature of the history and examination, more extensive evaluation for these diagnoses should be considered in appropriate patients. Unless there are data, a thyroid-stimulating hormone determination or thyroid profile is warranted and a hematocrit and complete blood cell count should be considered. An automated chemistry profile including electrolyte levels, liver function tests, and creatinine and glucose levels should be considered. If the patient has perimenopausal symptoms, such as hot flashes, interrupted sleep, irregular flow, and so forth, a determination of follicle-stimulating hormone to confirm menopause may be warranted. Sex hormone levels are normal in women with PMS, so hormonal profiles are rarely warranted.

The lay and Internet literature available on PMS is abundant and relatively consistent. As with many chronic symptomatic conditions, many of the therapeutic recommendations from such sources focus on lifestyle (e.g., diet, exercise, rest) and use of over-the-counter products (e.g., nonsteroidal anti-inflammatory agents, vitamins, calcium supplements, herbs). Many patients will have tried these products before consultation. Surveys suggest that a large proportion of women with menstrually related symptoms successfully deal with the problem by increasing exercise, avoiding salt and/or simple carbohydrates, and taking vitamins. Published studies of the use of supplements have shown little or no effect except the very important study by Thys-Jacobs in 1998 demonstrating a 48% versus 30% reduction in symptoms scores by the third cycle in women receiving 3000 mg of calcium carbonate in two divided doses daily (1200 mg elemental calcium) versus those receiving placebo. Because of the widespread availability of this information, careful history of the prior therapeutic maneuvers of the patient is very important in assessment.

THERAPEUTICS

The therapeutic approach to the patient with PMS should be individualized and symptom focused. After the findings of a thorough history and physical examination have defined the symptom pattern, external impacts and factors, health habits, and prior self-treatment efforts and have eliminated alternative diagnoses, the role of lifestyle factors and the available medical therapies should be discussed (Table 2). Patients with inadequate sleep patterns, overwork, inappropriate diets, excessive stress, and insufficient exercise should be counseled on improved habits. Unless the patient has already tried the calcium supplements, these should be tried (calcium carbonate, 1500 mg twice a day). Most women's diets are also deficient in magnesium as well as calcium, and magnesium supplements can be added (magnesium oxide, 800 mg twice a day). Vitamin supplements, in particular 100 mg per day of vitamin B_6 or high-potency vitamin B complex with vitamin C, have been recommended, but there is no documented efficacy. This can be combined with specific symptomatic treatment on an as-needed basis. For those experiencing considerable fluid retention, swelling, and bloating, judicious use of mild diuretics, such as low-

TABLE 2. **Premenstrual Syndrome: Helpful Lifestyle Changes**

Diet
  Low in fat (less than 30%), low in simple sugars
  High in complex carbohydrates
  Increased fresh vegetables, fruits
  Avoid salt and sodium
Exercise
  30 minutes daily of aerobic exercise, at least 3 hours
    before bedtime
Meditation
  20–30 minutes daily of meditation, yoga, or other
    relaxation exercise
Rest
  8–9 hours of sleep daily
Stress reduction
  Simplify lifestyle
  Avoid "superwoman" syndrome

dose triamterene/thiazide (Dyazide) combinations for a few days a month can be of benefit. Scheduled alprazolam (Xanax), 0.5 mg four times a day, has shown benefit in some studies, but the habit-forming potential of this agent on a regular basis causes many practitioners to prefer to prescribe other benzodiazepines on a limited basis for episodes of anxiety, tension, or difficulty sleeping (such as lorazepam [Ativan], 0.5 mg every 6 hours, as needed for anxiety and 1 to 2 mg orally at bedtime as needed for sleep for 3–5 days).

For those whose problems include severe mood swings, irritability, crying, depression, inattention, fogginess, fatigue, excessive sleep, hostility, anger outbursts, and similar symptoms, SSRIs may be of particular benefit. These agents (such as 20 mg of fluoxetine or 100 to 150 mg of sertraline daily for 6 to 12 months) would be the agents of choice in individuals whose symptoms have not been adequately controlled after a trial of calcium. Some individuals respond to low doses (such as 10 mg of fluoxetine daily or 50 mg of sertraline). Cyclic use, starting at midcycle, also appears to be helpful for many (taking the agents for the last 7 to 14 days of the cycle). Progesterone in various forms, including oral synthetic analogues and natural hormone by means of vaginal suppositories, has not been shown to be of benefit for PMS in most studies (and may cause PMS symptoms in some women). Some women find their symptoms improve on oral contraceptives, but more find that oral hormones exacerbate or have no effect on their symptoms, and controlled studies have not shown benefit. They are not a part of the usual therapeutic approach but can be useful in selected cases.

In approaching the therapy for PMS, it is important to note that most controlled studies of 1 to 3 months' duration show a strong placebo response of around 30%. This placebo response may decline after 3 to 6 months. In addition, the month-to-month pattern and severity of symptoms varies considerably, so careful baseline data and long-term follow-up may be necessary to confirm a good response to an intervention. Careful and detailed symptom calendars are very helpful in following patients but are difficult for most patients to maintain. Although many practitioners discuss symptom calendars at the initial evaluation, they are most helpful in the management of patients who see no improvement after 3 to 6 months of intervention. They are of use both therapeutically in monitoring the response to treatment as well as diagnostically in revealing patterns consistent with alternative diagnoses.

If symptoms remain severe after several cycles of such therapies and the symptom calendar confirms a regular menstrual pattern (ovulatory) and a late luteal timing of symptoms, then a trial of LHRH analogues to ablate the hormonal fluxes should be considered (with and without "add back" estrogen or estrogen/progesterone). If this is helpful, then the role for surgical ablation (ovariectomy or hysterectomy/ovariectomy) can be considered on an individual basis.

Treatment of PMS has been very frustrating for the patient and the practitioner. It is very important to recognize that current therapeutic options can be expected to produce a significant improvement in symptoms for almost all patients but may take several cycles to reach full effect. They usually work best in a patient-centered approach that also addresses stress and lifestyle issues. It is also important to recognize the significant month-to-month variability of symptoms and the strong impact of stress and external factors on symptom severity and interference with activities. It is often a condition that is not cured but is endured until remission with menopause.

MENOPAUSE

method of
MURRAY A. FREEDMAN, M.D.
Medical College of Georgia
Augusta, Georgia

The average age of menopause is 51.4 years, and more than 30 million women in the United States will spend the last third of their lives in an estrogen-deficient state. Although the cessation of menses is a natural event, the consequences of this deficiency state are devastating to some women. Estrogen deficiency qualifies as a bona fide endocrinopathy, just like thyroid or adrenal insufficiency, that results in gland failure (ovary), hormone deficiency (estrogen), and pathologic events, such as genitourinary atrophy and osteoporosis. Hormone replacement therapy (HRT) prevents or ameliorates the pathologic process associated with this deficiency.

Estrogen replacement therapy (ERT) not only improves the rates of morbidity and mortality experienced by postmenopausal women, it affects quality-of-life issues. The healthy woman who enters menopause today has a life expectancy well into her ninth decade, and vitality and infirmity are as important to her as any putative risk of breast cancer. Every woman should develop her own risk/reward profile and then determine the applicability of various lifestyle modifications, such as ERT, antioxidants, exercise, and diet modification.

Whereas "menopause" refers to the cessation of menses, the term "perimenopause" is perhaps more useful for referring to the epoch in a woman's life when she undergoes the transition from reproductive to nonreproductive life, and the term "postmenopausal" for the years that follow. Such a distinction has merit because many women become symptomatic (i.e., experience hot flushes) before the onset of amenorrhea, and others begin to have irregular menses during the perimenopausal years. These women would derive considerable benefit from the institution of low-dose oral contraceptive (OC) therapy during perimenopause. This technology remains greatly underused in healthy perimenopausal women because of unfounded fears that the "pill" causes cardiovascular disease, as well as a lack of appreciation of the many noncontraceptive benefits associated with long-term use of OCs, such as the 50% decline in both endometrial and ovarian cancer. Just as with OCs, the putative risks associated with ERT keep many patients from gleaning the benefits that accrue with treatment. It is estimated that only 25% to 35% of postmenopausal women are taking ERT, yet there continues to be a large subset of high-risk postmenopausal women for whom therapy would be beneficial. Each patient should assess her potential risks and benefits and then decide whether estrogen replacement therapy is right for her.

ONCOGENIC POTENTIAL OF HORMONE REPLACEMENT THERAPY

Before the numerous areas of recognized benefits associated with ERT are described, the oncogenic potential of exogenous hormone administration should be addressed because of the considerable and unwarranted anxiety it fosters among the public.

Uterus

There was an increased incidence of endometrial adenocarcinoma during the 1970s associated with the use of unopposed estrogen in women with intact uteri. With the addition of the appropriate dosage of progestogens (ERT is then referred to as HRT), however, there is no risk of estrogen therapy inducing endometrial cancer, and there is even some evidence to suggest that HRT actually reduces the normal background incidence of uterine neoplasia. In women who have undergone a hysterectomy, the necessity of adding progestogen therapy to ERT is obviated.

Breast

In spite of 30 years of epidemiologic study, there is no detectable significant increase in the overall incidence of breast cancer in women who use HRT compared with those who do not. Some studies have shown a slightly increased risk (risk ratio, 1.3) with 10 or more years of use, but this may be attributable to the estrogen users having more mammograms and drinking more alcohol compared with nonusers. The risk also disappeared after discontinuing estrogen therapy, suggesting some observation bias. Because all of the studies to date have been observational instead of randomized clinical trials, no definitive conclusion can be drawn. It can be stated with certainty, however, that if there is risk for breast cancer associated with HRT, it is minimal. It is reassuring that women in whom breast cancer develops while taking HRT have better survival rates than do nonusers in whom breast cancer develops. Theory suggests that estrogen therapy might stimulate the growth of nonpalpable breast cancers; therefore, mammograms should be performed routinely before initiating HRT. On the other hand, administering estrogen to women who have been treated successfully for either breast or uterine cancer is associated with increased survival rates compared with similarly staged patients with cancer in whom hormone therapy has been withheld. The improved survival rates do not represent an antineoplastic effect of HRT, but rather the significant beneficial effects of estrogens, such as reduced mortality from coronary heart disease.

To summarize the oncogenic potential of HRT on the breast, although there is no scientific evidence that the appropriate use of estrogens induces cancer, there is concern that estrogens might stimulate cancer cell growth. For this reason, women at increased risk of breast cancer, (i.e., those with several first-degree relatives who have had breast cancer) should be cautioned that they are genetically at increased risk for development of breast cancer, but that taking estrogen will not increase that risk.

SYSTEMIC BENEFITS OF HORMONE REPLACEMENT THERAPY

Cardiovascular Disease

Adverse effects of ERT/HRT on the cardiovascular system are typically limited to rare, idiosyncratic reactions, excessive dose, or other confounding factors. Any minor adverse cardiovascular effects pale in comparison with the benefits of HRT, and because 50% of women in the United States die from cardiovascular disease, the cardioprotective effect of estrogen is one of the most compelling advantages that all postmenopausal women should consider. Patients with risk factors for cardiovascular disease, such as coronary atherosclerosis or diabetes mellitus, receive even more benefit from ERT than do women without these risk factors.

HYPERTENSION

Postmenopausal use of ERT is normally associated with a slight decrease in blood pressure. Women with high blood pressure derive even more benefit from ERT than do normotensive women because hypertension predisposes them to an increased risk of heart disease. In the rare patient who becomes hypertensive because of an increase in renin substrate secondary to oral estrogen, nonoral therapy can be used to avoid the first-pass effect and minimize any adverse hepatoglobulin change.

DIABETES

Because of their predisposition to cardiovascular events, especially premature coronary artery disease, diabetic patients derive particular benefit from HRT. The benefit is not associated with any significant change in the "area under the curve," and people with diabetes actually experience improved insulin sensitivity with HRT. As with hypertensive women, those with diabetes are at risk for cardiovascular disease and demonstrate a greater benefit from ERT than do "normal" women.

VENOUS THROMBOEMBOLISM

There is a small group of patients who are at risk for thromboembolism when taking exogenous estrogen. Such thrombophilic patients may reduce their risk somewhat by using low-dose, nonoral estrogens to minimize potential hepatoglobulin alteration induced by exogenous estrogen. Because the incidence of thromboembolism with HRT is so rare, it is not cost effective to screen for this predisposition (i.e., by checking for Leiden factor V, protein S or C deficiency, or antithrombin III deficiency) before initiating therapy. Inquiring about a family history of thrombophilia, however, is prudent because a positive family history is an indication for screening. On the other hand, a history of previous thrombophlebitis does not necessarily contraindicate HRT. A history documenting thrombophilic phenomena in association with one or more of Virchow's triad (hypercoagulability, intimal damage, or stasis) does not constitute a contraindication to HRT in the future.

CORONARY ARTERY DISEASE

Since 1984, more women than men have died from cardiovascular disease, and the risk of coronary artery disease increases alarmingly after loss of ovarian function at any age. Although numerous factors contribute to an increased risk of cardiovascular disease (e.g., smoking, weight gain, adverse lipid profiles, and estrogen deficiency), replacement of estrogen in postmenopausal women is associated with a 60% reduction in the risk of cardiovascular disease. The most widely acknowledged benefit has been the alteration in serum lipoproteins: a significant increase in high-density lipoprotein cholesterol (HDL-C), a decrease in low-density lipoprotein cholesterol (LDL-C), and a decrease in total cholesterol. It is estimated, however, that non-lipid-mediated changes are responsible for approximately 70% of the cardioprotective effects associated with estrogen administration.

Evidence indicates that ERT is just as effective as statin therapy for treating hyperlipidemias. Furthermore, there is evidence that estrogen lowers lipoprotein(a), although it increases triglycerides. There is also evidence that estrogen administration provides benefit by increasing production of prostacyclin, increasing fibrinolysis, and decreasing fibrinogen and plasminogen activator inhibitor. Further protective effects with estrogen administration include maintaining production of endothelial-derived relaxing factor and reducing production of endothelin, a powerful vasoconstrictor, resulting in reduced coronary spasm. Estrogen therapy is associated with increased nitric oxide production, reduced thromboxane A_2, and increased release of prostaglandin I_2. The consensus is that the antioxidant properties of estrogen are associated with decreased oxidized LDL-C particle deposition in the arterial wall. Although the addition of progestogens, especially medroxyprogesterone acetate (MPA; Provera), may blunt estrogen's beneficial effects on lipoproteins and slightly but adversely alter vasoactivity in the arterial wall, the overall cardioprotective effect of HRT is maintained.

The risk of myocardial infarction has been reduced by 50% in women treated with estrogens compared with that of nonusers. The Nurses' Health Study, a particularly respected epidemiologic study that includes 59,000 postmenopausal nurses, revealed a 60% reduction in cardiovascular disease among current ERT users. Most of the patients in the Nurses' Health Study and in other U.S. studies were using conjugated equine estrogens (CEE; Premarin), whereas most European studies involved estradiol valerate (Delestrogen). Four cohort studies using comparative angiographic data have demonstrated a statistically significant reduction in the rate of coronary artery atherosclerosis and mortality associated with estrogen use. It appears that the women who derive the greatest benefit from estrogen therapy are those with cardiovascular disease, and current use is associated with considerably greater protection than past use. These findings support the positive vasoactive effect of ERT.

Osteoporosis

Sophisticated bone densitometry has allowed confirmation of the strong relationship between loss of bone mass and declining levels of circulating estrogen in postmenopausal women. Numerous epidemiologic studies have confirmed the clinical utility of ERT/HRT by demonstrating reduced fracture rates in estrogen users compared with nonusers. Calcium supplementation and weight-bearing exercise are adjunctive measures in reducing bone loss, but even a combination of the two does not adequately prevent bone loss in estrogen-deficient women.

Approximately 30 million women older than 50 years of age in the United States are at increased risk for osteoporosis. Fractures occur most commonly in the vertebrae, hip, and wrist, and it is estimated there are over 300,000 hip fractures each year among postmenopausal women in the United States. There is a 50% lifetime risk for a 50-year-old, white woman suffering at least one osteoporotic fracture. Of those elderly patients who fracture a hip, 20% die within 6 months of the fracture, and almost 50% who survive become either infirm or an invalid. Because these women are asymptomatic before the actual fracture, osteoporosis has been referred to as the "silent epidemic" in postmenopausal women.

Predisposing factors include early menopause, white race, reduced weight for height, family history of osteoporosis, low-calcium diet, high caffeine and alcohol intake, cigarette smoking, sedentary lifestyle, and administration of either thyroid replacement or corticosteroid therapy.

Although not cost effective as a routine screening procedure before the initiation of ERT/HRT, dual energy x-ray absorptiometry may have utility in the decision-making process for patients who might be reluctant to initiate estrogen therapy but in whom low bone mass is suspected. Follow-up bone densitometry also may be useful in high-risk patients because it has been demonstrated that as much as 10% to 15% of patients on adequate HRT may continue to lose bone mass. Patients whose bone density measurements exceed 2 standard deviations below the peak bone mass are at significant risk for fractures and should consider adjunctive therapy. Preliminary data confirm that the combination of estrogen and alendronate (Fosamax), the only approved bisphosphonate for the prevention and treatment of osteoporosis, is efficacious in patients who continue to lose bone mass on either drug alone.

Because estrogen has so many other significant benefits, it remains the optimal choice for prevention of osteoporosis in postmenopausal women. The timely administration of estrogen prevents the rapid loss of trabecular bone from the vertebral column that accompanies menopause. Even after long-term, irreversible loss of bone, the initiation of estrogen therapy is beneficial because it not only prevents further loss but often promotes increased bone mass. The discontinuation of ERT results in the resumption of the rapid bone loss that occurs initially with ovarian failure. Recommendations include the initiation of therapy whenever estrogen levels decline and the indefinite continuation of therapy to maintain bone density. The addition of progestogens in patients with an intact uterus does not have a deleterious effect on estrogen's ability to maintain bone density.

Genitourinary Atrophy

Genitourinary atrophy is the least-publicized but most inevitable consequence of estrogen deficiency. The only FDA-approved indications for ERT are in the prevention/treatment of vasomotor symptoms, osteoporosis, and genital atrophy. The vagina and urethra are both derived from the urogenital sinus, and the highest concentration of estrogen receptors in the body is in this area. Because of the exquisite sensitivity of the genitourinary structures to estrogen, the postmenopausal woman is particularly susceptible to sexual dysfunction and genital atrophy. It is estimated that approximately 40% of institutionalized women in the United States have urinary incontinence, and 50% of women attending menopausal clinics list sexual dysfunction as one of their three primary complaints. Urethral competence (continence) depends on the integrity and quality of the urethral epithelium, connective tissue, musculature, and vasculature, all of which derive a positive impact from ERT in postmenopausal women. Fifty percent of all postmenopausal patients with incontinence who are treated with a combination of ERT and alpha-adrenergic stimulation (e.g., phenylpropanolamine [Entex]) report subjective improvement of urinary incontinence. All postmenopausal women with urinary incontinence should be offered medical therapy before surgery because many women, even some with genuine stress urinary incontinence, may experience subjective improvement and elect not to have surgery.

The integrity of the vaginal epithelium is maintained by both estrogen and coital activity. Furthermore, vaginal lubrication in the postmenopausal woman is greatly improved with estrogen therapy. This positive epithelial response can be maintained by surprisingly small amounts of topically applied estrogen. Postmenopausal women usually enjoy an enhanced arousal phase of the sexual response cycle with ERT, but because estrogens are associated with increased serum hormone binding globulin, some women experience diminished libido because of a decrease in "free" testosterone. Estrogen-replete women who fail to show an improvement in their sexuality with estrogen alone may find androgen therapy in addition to ERT to be particularly beneficial. Because of the abrupt loss of ovarian androgen with oophorectomy, postoperative patients often benefit from the replacement of both estrogen and androgen. Although psychosocial factors are the primary determinant of female sexuality, hormone replacement plays a critical role in preventing genital atrophy and in complementing sexual desire and arousal. Because genital atrophy is inevitable and yet amenable to therapy, its prevention or treatment certainly deserves consideration.

Central Nervous System

Osteoporosis and Alzheimer's disease (AD) are two of the most common causes for which older women become institutionalized. Although ERT has not been approved for the prevention or treatment of AD, estrogens have a positive impact on this neurodegenerative disease, which affects 50% of people older than 85 years of age. Numerous independent epidemiologic studies demonstrate significant delay in the onset or progression of AD in estrogen-treated women as well as a positive, consistent correlation between dose and duration of therapy. Data also indicate that estrogens both promote and preserve neuron growth in tissue culture.

A number of placebo-controlled, double-blinded, crossover studies have documented the efficacy of estrogen in treating vasomotor symptoms and improving rapid eye movement sleep. The increased psychometric scores in women taking ERT may represent part of this "domino effect," but it may actually be a more direct effect of the hormone on the brain. Part of estrogen's role in cognition and mood enhancement includes increased cerebral blood flow, prolonged neuron viability, protection against hypoglycemia, and modulation of neurotransmitter activity.

HORMONE REPLACEMENT THERAPY: ESTROGENS, PROGESTOGENS, ANDROGENS

Estrogens

The most commonly used "natural" estrogens include CEE (Premarin), micronized estradiol (Estrace), estropipate (Ortho-Est), esterified estrogen (Estratab), and transdermal estradiol (the "patch"). Ethinyl estradiol, a totally synthetic estrogen, is used in all of the commonly prescribed low-dose OC preparations. The introduction of raloxifene (Evista), a selective estrogen receptor modulator (SERM), broadens the therapeutic options of ERT to include nonsteroidal estrogens as a clinically approved modality (see later).

Most of the adverse side effects associated with estrogen therapy are primarily dose-related phenomena. The lowest-dose OCs contain 20 μg of ethinyl estradiol and are too potent for use in HRT: they induce adverse side effects such as nausea and breast tenderness. Use of a new, lower-dose transdermal application of ethinyl estradiol in combination with norethindrone may avoid some of the gastrointestinal side effects associated with oral preparations. Most of the epidemiologic data gathered since the early 1950s have been with the 0.625 mg of CEE, which remains the most commonly used reference dose for clinical application of ERT in menopausal women. Doses equivalent to 0.625 mg of CEE include estropipate preparations at a dose of 0.625 to 1.25 mg, micronized estradiol at a dose of 1 mg, and esterified estrogen at a dose of 0.625 mg. The transdermal patch equivalent is 0.05 mg of estradiol.

Transdermal administration of estradiol has the potential advantage of maintaining constant levels of circulating estrogen and avoiding the first-pass effect on the liver to minimize gastrointestinal and enzymatic changes. Unfortunately, as much as 20% of patients who use "patch" therapy in warm climates experience skin irritation with the transdermal system.

The desired therapeutic effect of circulating estrogen can be achieved with the use of various equivalent doses of ERT, but specific situations may dictate preference for one system of administration over another. For example, oral estrogens more favorably affect HDL-C and LDL-C, but transdermal estrogens have a potential advantage for a patient with a history of a thromboembolic event. Long-acting estrogens in the form of injectable or subdermal application are useful primarily in combination with nonoral androgen therapy. Locally applied vaginal estrogens (creams or rings) have the advantage of providing high local levels of estrogen while avoiding a systemic level of estrogen sufficient to cause endometrial proliferation.

The standard dose for preventing osteoporosis and genitourinary atrophy, providing cardiovascular protection, and deriving the central nervous system benefits associated with ERT is 0.625 mg of CEE or the equivalent. Vasomotor symptoms may necessitate higher initial doses of estrogen, but once flushes are controlled, a lower dose is usually sufficient. Genital atrophy can be prevented with much lower doses of vaginally applied estrogen because the vaginal epithelium and subcutaneous tissue are exquisitely sensitive to estrogen and local absorption is excellent.

The SERMs have proved to be a useful therapeutic modality. Tamoxifen (Nolvadex), the first SERM introduced, was marketed as a chemoprophylactic agent for patients with breast cancer. It was found to act as an estrogen antagonist on breast tissue but as an estrogen agonist on the uterus and bone. The second SERM to be marketed, raloxifene, was approved for the prevention of osteoporosis and has also been shown to have chemoprophylactic properties similar to those of tamoxifen: a 50% or greater reduction in the incidence of breast cancer is associated with its use. Compared with tamoxifen, raloxifene provides the additional advantage of not stimulating the endometrium. Although raloxifene is effective in preventing bone loss and improving lipid profiles, the natural estrogens may have a greater protective effect on the cardiovascular and skeletal system. Long-term studies are necessary to assess the full impact of SERMs on fracture rates and coronary heart disease.

Selective estrogen receptor modulators are an attractive alternative to the conventional forms of HRT for patients unduly concerned about breast cancer and those who abhor the continuation or resumption of menses. Raloxifene lacks estrogen's efficacy in ameliorating vasomotor symptoms, and it remains to be seen whether other central nervous system benefits accrue with its use. The "designer estrogen" of the future will provide antagonist activity on the breast and endometrium while maintaining the current benefits on the cardiovascular, skeletal, genitourinary, and central nervous systems.

Progestogens

The term "progestogen" includes compounds that exhibit progestogenic activity when administered orally, transdermally, or injectably. The natural progestogens are the C21 progesterone derivatives: MPA, megestrol, and micronized progesterone. The synthetic progestogens are referred to as "progestins" and include norethindrone (Micronor), norethindrone acetate (Aygestin), and norgestrel (Ovrette). The progestins are 19-nortestosterone derivatives and possess minimal androgenic activity, so they potentially affect lipoproteins and endometrial proliferation slightly more than natural progestogens. The typical doses of progestogens to provide endometrial protection with ERT are 5 to 10 mg of MPA, 0.7 to 1 mg of norethindrone, and 200 mg of micronized progesterone for 12 to 14 days per cycle.

Androgens

Androgen production begins to decline at approximately 30 years of age. Some postmenopausal women, especially those subjected to surgical castration, may experience symptoms and derive benefit from androgen replacement therapy. Women with decreased libido in spite of adequate ERT often benefit from the addition of androgen therapy. There is also the potential benefit of androgen replacement therapy in estrogen-replete patients with recurrent headaches, mastalgia, recalcitrant flushes, osteopenia, hypertriglyceridemia, or refractory malaise and fatigue. Available preparations include esterified estrogens in combination with 1.25 or 2.5 mg of methyltestosterone (Estratest), depo-injectable forms of estrogen plus androgen (Depo-Testadiol), and subcutaneous pellets of both estrogen and androgen. Because of the delicate balance between the therapeutic efficacy of androgens and adverse side effects (principally mild hirsutism and acne), androgen administration should be initiated with the lowest effective dose.

Administration of Hormone Replacement Therapy

Almost without exception, all patients can derive some benefit from HRT, but therapy should be individualized with specific goals in mind. Patients who have intact uteri and take ERT require adequate endometrial protection with progestogen therapy, either cyclically or on a continuous daily basis. In cyclic therapy, most patients continue to have withdrawal bleeding up to 65 to 70 years of age. Bleeding typically begins on completion of the progestogen each cycle, usually day 14 or 15 of the month (Figure 1). Some patients who initiate continuous combined estrogen-progestogen therapy may experience amenorrhea primarily, whereas others may bleed intermittently for several months after starting therapy. This bleeding usually ceases within 3 to 6 months. Patients without a uterus are given progestogen only if they have had endometriosis, or after adequate therapy for low-grade endometrial adenocarcinoma.

In the United States, progestogen therapy is usu-

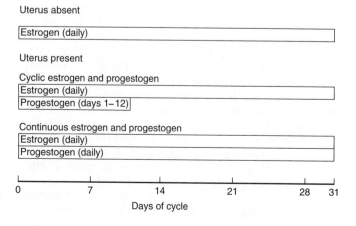

Figure 1. Hormone replacement regimens.

ally given orally, and MPA is the most commonly prescribed formulation. Some women who experience side effects with MPA (i.e., bloating, mood dysphoria, or breast tenderness) may decrease the dose from 10 to 5 mg without compromising endometrial protection. Women who remain intolerant to MPA have used 0.7 µg to 1 mg of norethindrone without difficulty. More recently, an oral micronized progestogen (Prometrium), as well as a vaginal gel (Crinone) have been approved for use and, when used for the typical 12 to 14 days per cycle, provide adequate endometrial protection. Bleeding sometimes begins during the last day or two of progestogen therapy, and this is not considered pathologic.

Because there is no proven advantage to interrupting its therapy, estrogen is administered daily. The effective dose of 0.625 mg of CEE or the equivalent is normally tolerated without adverse effect, although occasionally patients may experience nausea, headache, or breast tenderness on initiation of ERT. These patients may find transdermal estrogen more tolerable. Women who have been hypoestrogenic for many years are often extremely sensitive to ERT and require initiation of estrogen at exceedingly low doses before advancing to full therapeutic doses. Patients unduly sensitive to ERT represent a specific niche for raloxifene because it rarely causes nausea and does not cause breast tenderness.

Calcium (1000 mg in estrogen-replete women and 1500 mg in estrogen-deficient women) and weight-bearing exercise are important adjuncts in maintaining bone density. Neither one alone nor the two in combination, however, provides adequate protection against bone loss without estrogen. Estrogen is the essential ingredient in eliminating bone resorption and, when used in conjunction with adequate exercise and calcium, lower doses of estrogen are efficacious in preventing bone loss.

Measurement of circulating levels of estrogen during ERT or HRT is of little clinical utility, and gonadotropin values rarely suppress to premenopausal levels with normal HRT. Serum estradiol levels are considered therapeutic as long as they remain in the range of 40 to 50 pg per mL, which is the level attained with a standard 0.625-mg dose of CEE or the equivalent. This level of estrogen administration is associated with all of the benefits typically ascribed to ERT, although slightly higher levels of estrogen therapy may be necessary initially to control vasomotor symptoms.

Patients receiving HRT should be monitored with routine mammography, Papanicolaou (Pap) smears, blood chemistry at appropriate intervals (particularly lipoprotein levels and thyroid-stimulating hormone), and periodic colon evaluation. In the absence of abnormal uterine bleeding, there is no need for endometrial sampling. Rare circumstances may necessitate validating serum estrogen levels, such as in patients with persistent hot flushes in spite of the administration of adequate doses of HRT.

Hormone replacement therapy should commence whenever the consequences of estrogen deficiency are demonstrable. A common scenario involves sleep disturbance and hot flushes in patients who are still experiencing cyclic bleeding. Low-dose OCs for the nonsmoking perimenopausal patient are particularly useful because they allow suppression of endogenous gonadotropin and provide adequate cycle control, along with the many noncontraceptive benefits of OCs.

Hormone replacement therapy should be continued indefinitely unless there is some adverse event. Preventing and treating genital atrophy remains a lifelong indication because all of the consequences of estrogen deficiency begin anew once therapy is discontinued. The only absolute contraindications to estrogen therapy include breast cancer, active liver disease, or thromboembolic phenomena. Many authorities believe that the benefits of estrogen far exceed any putative risks, even in patients who have previously received adequate treatment for early-stage breast cancer.

CONCLUSION

There is tremendous benefit in preventing the potential consequences of estrogen deficiency. The transition from reproductive to nonreproductive life affords health care providers the ideal opportunity to counsel and educate women about menopause, and we should meet the obligation to affect patients' lifestyles in a positive way with enthusiasm. ERT has a tremendously beneficial effect on the cardiovascular and skeletal systems: a 50% decrease in coronary heart disease and an equally protective role in reducing osteoporotic fractures. Data suggest that ERT has a demonstrative effect in delaying the onset of AD and improving cognitive function. New, encouraging data suggest a benefit in reducing age-related macular degeneration, a positive effect on diabetes mellitus, diminished tooth loss, and a 50% reduction in the rate of colon cancer, the third most common neoplasm in women. Genital atrophy, the least-publicized but most inevitable consequence of estrogen deficiency, is of no benefit to any patient and remains the consequence most amenable to therapy. It is not simply the improved morbidity and mortality associated with ERT that matters to women; the enhancement in quality of life is equally important.

More than 35 years of observational studies serve as evidence that estrogen neither induces breast cancer nor adversely affects its outcome. That fact not withstanding, in a woman with a strong family history or in whom oncogenic potential remains a concern, raloxifene offers the added benefit of chemoprophylaxis. On the other hand, the risk profile for a woman with factors predisposing her to cardiovascular, skeletal, or central nervous system disorders may actually dictate that ERT would be therapeutic and therefore indicated. Therapy must be individualized; each patient should assess her own risk/benefit ratio.

Compliance continues to be a problem because of patient fears about breast cancer and their disdain for uterine bleeding. Allaying anxiety and educating patients about the many therapeutic options available today will enhance compliance. We must now tailor the use of HRT to accommodate each patient's individual needs. With all that is known about the science of HRT, the new challenge is in the art.

VULVOVAGINITIS

method of
MAURIZIO MACCATO, M.D.
Baylor College of Medicine
Houston, Texas

Vulvovaginitis is one of the most common gynecologic disorders. It has both infectious and noninfectious causes. The most common infectious causes include several different species of yeasts, *Trichomonas vaginalis,* and *Gardnerella vaginalis* with its associated proliferation of anaerobic bacteria. Reaction to an inflammatory agent is a common noninfectious vulvovaginitis, referred to as *contact vulvovaginitis.* In the postmenopausal woman, atrophic vaginitis is the most common noninfectious cause of vaginitis. In prepubertal girls, *Neisseria gonorrhoeae,* group A betahemolytic streptococcus *(Streptococcus pyogenes),* other bacteria, pinworms, and foreign bodies in the vagina are also possible causes of vaginitis.

DIAGNOSIS

Proper therapy of this condition is based on the careful determination of the etiologic agent. The history and physical examination provide clues as to the cause of the vaginitis. Confirmation of such suspicion is generally obtained by straightforward laboratory tests that can be performed, in the majority of cases, directly in the office of the practitioner. The evaluation of the patient should include a menstrual history, especially from postmenopausal women, for whom development of symptoms may be associated with a significant decrease in estrogen level. The sexual history and the history of use of feminine hygiene products or of medications such as antibiotics, oral contraceptives, or immunosuppressive agents should be obtained. The pelvic examination is vital to determine the correct type of vaginitis.

It is important to point out that in most cases the history and physical examination alone should not be relied on to make the definitive diagnosis because there is a significant degree of overlap between the signs and symptoms associated with the various types of vaginitis. Therefore, the etiologic agent should be confirmed by laboratory testing, as discussed in the following section.

MONILIAL VULVOVAGINITIS

General Considerations

One of the most common causes of infectious vulvovaginitis is a yeast, usually *Candida albicans.* Other organisms are *Candida glabarata* and *Candida tropicalis.* A handful of case reports of less common yeasts have appeared in the literature. *Candida albicans* is responsible for more than 90% of all cases of yeast vaginitis. Itching is the most common symptom

associated with vulvovaginal candidiasis. An unusual odor is not a prominent feature of this vaginitis. The physical examination reveals a discharge that is usually white and clumpy. Plaques of secretions may be adherent to the mucous membrane of the vagina, and, on their removal, a reddened and irritated base is noted.

The confirmatory test for vulvovaginal candidiasis is the examination of the discharge by wet mount or KOH preparation. A drop of vaginal secretion is suspended in a drop of saline, and this is examined under the microscope. The identification of yeast in the wet mount confirms the diagnosis suspected on clinical grounds. The examination of a drop of vaginal fluid suspended in a solution of 10% KOH may help in identification of the yeast by lysing epithelial cells. The pH of the vaginal discharge is usually normal (i.e., less than 4.5). The so-called whiff test is negative. In this test, the application of 10% KOH to a sample of the vaginal discharge does not release the amine odor characteristic of bacterial vaginosis. It should be noted that in approximately 30% of patients with vulvovaginal candidiasis, the examination of the discharge for yeast forms by wet mount will not reveal the presence of either cellular or hyphal forms. Therefore, in the presence of the appropriate signs and symptoms (i.e., a normal pH and a negative whiff test), it is reasonable to assume that the symptoms are caused by yeast, and an adequate antifungal therapy may be prescribed. Culture of the vaginal secretion for yeast is another method to confirm the diagnosis.

Recurrent monilial vulvovaginitis is a vexing problem for both patients and physicians. The cause of such recurrent infections is frequently unclear. Therapy for the sexual partner is rarely associated with a decrease in the rate of recurrence. It is possible that the source of the patient's continued colonization of the vagina may be the lower gastrointestinal tract. Unfortunately, therapy of the gastrointestinal tract with oral antifungal agents does not reliably decrease the incidence of recurrent infection. Therapy of such infection is frequently based on long-term suppression of the causative agents of the vaginitis, as discussed in the following section.

Treatment

First-line therapy for vulvovaginal candidiasis are vaginal creams containing an antifungal agent, most frequently of the imidazole class. Common topical drugs are summarized in Table 1. The two alternative agents (boric acid gelatin capsules, 600 mg intravaginally twice daily for 2 weeks, and gentian violet used as a 1% aqueous solution) have been used with success, especially in the treatment of species of *Candida* other than *C. albicans.* Gentian violet is an aniline dye that is mutagenic and has been associated with possible teratogenic effects, and it is therefore seldom used.

Oral antifungal agents include ketoconazole (Nizoral), fluconazole (Diflucan), and itraconazole (Spor-

TABLE 1. **Topical Agents Used in the Initial Therapy of Fungal Vulvovaginitis**

Generic Name	Trade Name
Miconazole	Monistat-7
Clotrimazole	Gyne-Lotrimin, Mycelex-7
Butoconazole	Femstat
Terconazole	Terazol-3
Tioconazole	Vagistat-1
Nystatin	Mycostatin
Alternatives	
Gentian violet (1% aqueous solution)	
Boric acid (gelatin capsules)	

anox). All three have demonstrated activity against vulvovaginal candidiasis. They have not, at this point, been considered as first-line therapy because of their systemic effects. In particular, ketoconazole has been associated with liver dysfunction in some patients. The role of the oral antifungal agents may be found in long-term suppression of recurrent candidal vaginitis in specific patients. They may also have a role in the prevention of infection in patients with immunodeficiencies.

BACTERIAL VAGINOSIS

General Considerations

On physical examination, bacterial vaginosis is characterized by a grayish discharge, which is at times profuse and associated with an amine odor. Itching is generally not a significant problem. The examination of the discharge on a wet mount reveals epithelial cells that have bacteria adherent to them, which are the so-called clue cells. If bacterial vaginosis is not complicated by other infections (e.g., trichomoniasis, gonorrhea or chlamydia, or pelvic inflammatory disease), white blood cells will be rare in the wet mount. The performance of a whiff test on the discharge will reveal the characteristic fishy odor of amines. The pH of the vaginal discharge is usually greater than 4.7. Although the microbiology of bacterial vaginosis is exceedingly complex, the presence of *G. vaginalis* and an increased number of anaerobic bacteria and a decrease in the number of *Lactobacillus* appears to be the dominant characteristic of the microbiology of the vagina affected by bacterial vaginosis. The condition has been linked to increased risk of postpartum endometritis, postsurgical pelvic infections, and preterm labor.

Treatment

With the above-noted changes in microbiology, the therapy of bacterial vaginosis hinges on the use of antibiotics that decrease the number of anaerobic organisms and are effective against *G. vaginalis*. The use of metronidazole (Flagyl) has been advocated. Metronidazole can be administered either as an oral agent at a dose of 500 mg twice daily for 1 week or as an intravaginal cream (MetroGel). Other agents that have demonstrated efficacy in the conditions are clindamycin (Cleocin), either orally or intravaginally (as a 2% cream), and amoxicillin-clavulanic acid (Augmentin).* Amoxicillin-clavulanic acid also is effective against *G. vaginalis,* an organism that is only partially susceptible to Flagyl. The advantage of intravaginal versus systemic therapy with metronidazole or clindamycin is the reduction in the risk of possible side effects from these agents, especially diarrhea with clindamycin and an Antabuse effect with metronidazole. With the use of amoxicillin-clavulanic acid, it is wise to anticipate the possible development of yeast overgrowth in the vagina.

The problem of chronic recurrent bacterial vaginosis again is the subject of much current research. It appears that the treatment of the sexual partner in recurrent bacterial vaginitis may decrease the risk of recurrence.

TRICHOMONIASIS

General Considerations

T. vaginalis is the flagellate protozoan responsible for the development of *Trichomonas* vaginitis. The organism is both species specific and site specific. It causes a vaginitis with a profuse, greenish, malodorous discharge. The patient usually complains of pruritus and possibly dyspareunia and dysuria. Irritation of the cervix often leads to punctate lesions in the cervix, giving it the characteristic appearance of a so-called strawberry cervix, often best appreciated on colposcopy. The vulva and vagina may appear erythematous and edematous.

The pH of the vaginal discharge is about 4.5, and, because of a proliferation of anaerobic organisms, the whiff test is again positive. Motile *T. vaginalis* are usually easily identified on wet mount of the discharge. The organism may be cultured as well in Diamond's media. Trichomoniasis is almost invari-

---

*Not FDA approved for this indication.

TABLE 2. **Characteristics of Vaginal Infections**

	Vaginal Discharge	Symptoms	Wet Mount	pH
Fungal	White, sometimes curdy	Itching	Budding yeast, pseudohyphae	<4.5
Bacterial vaginosis	Gray, homogeneous	Malodorous discharge	Clue cells	>4.5
Trichomoniasis	Greenish, sometimes frothy	Malodorous discharge, itching	Trichomonads, white blood cells	>4.5

From Maccato M: Vulvovaginitis. *In* Conn's Current Therapy. Philadelphia, FA Davis, 1995, pp 1006–1008.

ably a sexually transmitted condition. Treatment of the partner, therefore, is indispensable to prevent reinfection. On rare occasions, however, the transmission of *Trichomonas* by nonsexual methods has been demonstrated. It has also been noted that *Trichomonas* may remain asymptomatic for long periods of time. Recurrent trichomoniasis is usually related to failure of adequate therapy of all sexual partners involved. On rare occasions, it may be secondary to the presence of true resistance to metronidazole of the organism. Table 2 summarizes the characteristics of the most common vaginal infections.

Treatment

The current recommended treatment for trichomoniasis is oral metronidazole (Flagyl). The dose of metronidazole varies from 250 mg orally three times a day for 1 week to 500 mg twice a day for 1 week or a single oral dose of 2 grams. It appears that 250 mg orally three times a day may have a slightly higher cure rate than the single dose of 2 grams. The decision of which regimen to use should be based on the requirements of the specific patient and the likelihood of adequate compliance of the patient to the various regimens. Again, it is important to ensure treatment of all sexual partners.

Strains of *T. vaginalis* resistant to metronidazole have been identified. In these cases, the use of combined oral and intravaginal metronidazole or intravenous metronidazole has been advocated. It has been observed that clotrimazole (Mycelex) used intravaginally provides some relief of the symptoms. The therapy, however, is not curative. The use of a vaginal douche with 20% sodium chloride has been used with some success as well. It is important to remember that metronidazole has an Antabuse-like effect and, therefore, while the patient is on therapy with metronidazole she should avoid alcohol. Metronidazole also is not recommended during the first trimester of pregnancy because of concerns about mutagenicity. No teratogenetic effect, however, has ever been described in humans, even when it was used in the first trimester.

POSTMENOPAUSAL PATIENTS

Atrophic vaginitis has to be included in the differential diagnosis of vaginitis in postmenopausal women. The symptoms reported include burning, dyspareunia, and, at times, vaginal spotting. The diagnosis is suspected because of the absence of identifiable infectious disease etiologies for the vaginitis in the presence of a hypoestrogenic state. On wet mount, a large number of white blood cells are noted.

The therapy involves the supplementation of estrogen either orally or intravaginally. It is important to remember that the hypoestrogenic vagina has a pH of greater than 5.0. Vaginal and vulval pruritus also are commonly associated with malignancies of the vulva, and, therefore, evaluation of the patients for such a possibility is imperative.

PREMENARCHEAL GIRLS

In premenarcheal girls the etiology of vaginitis may not be confined to the same organisms discussed earlier. *Neisseria gonorrhoeae, Streptococcus pyogenes, Shigella,* and other bacteria may all be associated with the development of vaginitis. In this population it is, therefore, useful to routinely obtain cultures of the vaginal discharge. The presence of a foreign body in the vagina is also a frequent finding in young girls presenting with vaginitis. Therefore, careful inspection of the vagina for such an occurrence is important. Therapy of this type of vaginitis is based on the etiologic agents.

CHLAMYDIA TRACHOMATIS INFECTION

method of
KIMBERLY A. WORKOWSKI, M.D.
Emory University
Atlanta, Georgia

and

CAROLYN M. BLACK, PH.D.
Centers for Disease Control and Prevention
Atlanta, Georgia

Chlamydia trachomatis infection is the most commonly reported infectious disease in the United States, accounting for an estimated 4 million infections annually. In most instances, the initial lower genital tract infection is asymptomatic and hence difficult to recognize clinically. Undetected infections can cause serious sequelae, including pelvic inflammatory disease, infertility, ectopic pregnancy, and chronic pelvic pain. In addition, chlamydial infection increases the risk for acquiring human immunodeficiency virus infection, and pregnant women infected with *C. trachomatis* can infect their infants during delivery. Thus, as a leading cause of pelvic inflammatory disease and infertility, chlamydial infections are an important threat to women's reproductive health.

EPIDEMIOLOGY

Although the prevalence of genital chlamydial infection has ranged from 2 to 30% in various settings, precise epidemiologic data are not available because screening programs are targeted at women only and reporting practices vary across states and municipalities. However, in 1997, 526,653 chlamydial infections were reported to the Centers for Disease Control and Prevention from 49 states, the District of Columbia, and New York City. Demographic factors associated with an increased risk of chlamydial infection include young age, nonwhite race, multiple sexual partners, single marital status, concurrent gonorrhea, and nonbarrier contraceptive methods (Table 1). Transmission rates vary, depending on the presence of symptoms in the index case and whether the sexual encounter is casual or repeated. Studies using DNA amplification techniques indicate that the frequencies of transmission of chlamydial infection by infected men and women are equivalent at 68%.

TABLE 1. **Demographic Risk Factors**

Age <19 y
Nonwhite race
Multiple sexual partners
Single marital status
Nonbarrier contraceptive use

BIOLOGY

Chlamydiae are obligate intracellular parasites that infect squamocolumnar epithelial cells, causing damage from replication of the organism as well as from the resultant inflammatory response. Chlamydiae are distinguished from all other microorganisms on the basis of their unique life cycle in which two different phases of highly specialized morphologic forms are adapted to either intracellular or extracellular environments. *C. trachomatis* is one of the four species in the genus *Chlamydia*. *C. trachomatis* can be differentiated into 18 serovars based on monoclonal antibody-based typing assays. Serovars A, B, Ba, and C are associated with endemic trachoma, serovars D to K with genital tract disease, and L_1 to L_3 with lymphogranuloma venereum. *C. trachomatis* can be further differentiated by molecular subtyping methods that are based on the sequence of the major outer membrane protein gene.

CLINICAL MANIFESTATIONS

Cervicitis

Clinical recognition of chlamydial cervicitis depends on a high index of suspicion based on history and careful examination, because most women are asymptomatic (Table 2). Findings suggestive of chlamydial infection include easily induced endocervical bleeding, mucopurulent endocervical discharge, and hypertrophic ectopy. A Gram stain of endocervical secretions from women with chlamydial cervicitis usually shows more than 30 polymorphonuclear leukocytes per $1000\times$ field.

Urethritis

Although urethral symptoms may develop in women with chlamydial infection, most women with urethral infection do not have dysuria or urinary frequency.

However, chlamydial urethritis should be suspected in young women with dysuria lasting more than 7 to 10 days, lack of hematuria, presence of suprapubic tenderness, use of birth control pills, and sterile pyuria.

Among heterosexual men, chlamydial infections are usually urethral and up to 50% are asymptomatic. When symptoms do occur, they are indistinguishable from those of gonorrhea (urethral discharge or pyuria). Chlamydial urethritis is presumptively diagnosed by history, urethral discharge, and the presence of four or more polymorphonuclear leukocytes per oil immersion field of Gram-stained urethral smear or pyuria noted on urinalysis.

Endometritis and Salpingitis

In the absence of appropriate treatment, the proportion of women with cervical chlamydial infection in whom upper genital tract infection (endometritis, salpingitis, pelvic peritonitis) develops is thought to be significant. Histologic evidence of endometritis is present in approximately 50% of women with mucopurulent cervicitis and almost all of those with salpingitis. The presence of endometritis in women with chlamydial cervicitis correlates with a history of intermenstrual bleeding. One study showed that 30% of women with both gonococcal and chlamydial infections and treated only for gonorrhea subsequently had salpingitis. Studies of the long-term complications of salpingitis underscore the impact of so-called silent infections. Infertility due to obstructed fallopian tubes and ectopic pregnancy have been correlated with serologic evidence of chlamydial infection.

Perihepatitis

Studies suggest that *C. trachomatis* is more commonly associated with perihepatitis than is *Neisseria gonorrhoeae*. Perihepatitis should be suspected in women with right upper quadrant pain, fever, nausea and vomiting, and salpingitis.

Neonatal Infection

The attack rate of chlamydial conjunctivitis in infants varies from 18 to 50%, and that of chlamydial pneumonitis from 3 to 18%. Chlamydial pneumonitis is clinically indistinguishable from pneumonitis caused by other pathogens. Other infant infections thought to be caused by *C. tracho-*

TABLE 2. **Spectrum of *Chlamydia trachomatis* Infections in Women**

Diagnosis	Clinical Criteria	Diagnostic Criteria	
		Presumptive	*Confirmatory*
Mucopurulent cervicitis	Mucopurulent cervical discharge, cervical ectopy and edema, easily induced endocervical bleeding	Cervical Gram stain ≥30 polymorphonuclear leukocytes/1000× field (nonmenstruating women)	Culture, laboratory tests that detect antigen (cervix) or nucleic acid (cervix or urine)
Acute urethral syndrome	Dysuria—frequency >7 d; new sexual partner	Pyuria, no bacteriuria	Culture, laboratory tests that detect antigen or nucleic acid (cervix, urethra, urine)
Pelvic inflammatory disease	Lower abdominal pain, adnexal tenderness, mucopurulent cervical discharge	Cervical mucopus	Culture, laboratory tests that detect antigen or nucleic acid (cervix, endometrium, fallopian tube, urine)
Perihepatitis	Right upper quadrant pain, nausea, vomiting, fever, salpingitis	Cervical mucopus	*C. trachomatis* serology indicative of acute infection

matis include otitis media, bronchiolitis, and vulvovaginitis.

DIAGNOSTIC TESTING

The most sensitive and specific methods used to diagnose chlamydial infections are nucleic acid amplification tests. At present, only the nucleic acid amplification tests offer noninvasive methods (urine testing) for screening asymptomatic people. However, nucleic acid amplification tests are expensive and not yet widely available; therefore, nonamplification methods based on DNA probe hybridization or antigen detection methods offer reasonable but less sensitive alternatives. Antigen detection methods include a fluorescent monoclonal antibody for direct visualization of the organism or enzyme immunoassays. In patients in whom sexual assault or abuse is suspected, or when legal consequences may result, diagnosis of chlamydial infections should be performed by culture. Isolation rates depend on strict sample handling, transport, and culture procedures. Therefore, specimens should be immediately placed in specific transport media and shipped overnight under refrigeration, or frozen at $-70°C$ if specimens cannot be delivered to the laboratory within 24 hours of collection. The sensitivities of the various tests are as follows: nucleic acid amplification tests, 85 to 90%; DNA probe hybridization, 70%; enzyme immunoassay, 50 to 70% depending on the manufacturer; and direct fluorescent antibody tests, 70 to 80% depending on the laboratory. Culture sensitivity varies widely but is generally 70 to 80% in very highly qualified laboratories, and substantially lower in many other laboratories. Because of their lower specificities, in populations in which the prevalence of chlamydial infection is below 5%, the positive predictive value of nonculture, nonamplification tests may be less than 50%. Confirmatory testing can be performed with direct fluorescent antibody tests (for enzyme immunoassay screening tests), competitive probes (for DNA probe hybridization screening tests), or a test that uses a different technology than the screening test to confirm the initial result. There is no need to confirm the commercially available nucleic acid amplification tests (polymerase chain reaction test [Roche, Indianapolis, IN], ligase chain reaction test [Abbott, Abbott Park, IL], transcription-mediated amplification test [Gen-Probe, San Diego, CA]) because of their high specificity (99.6%).

TREATMENT

The recommended treatment regimen for uncomplicated chlamydial urethral, endocervical, and rectal infections is azithromycin* (Zithromax) in a single 1-gram dose or doxycycline (Vibramycin), 100 mg twice daily for 7 days (Table 3). Azithromycin offers the advantage of single-dose therapy with proven efficacy in comparative trials with doxycycline in the treatment of uncomplicated chlamydial infections. Alternative regimens include a 7-day regimen of ofloxacin (Floxin), 300 mg twice daily; erythromycin base, 500 mg four times daily; or erythromycin ethylsuccinate, 800 mg four times daily. To minimize transmission of infection and the risk of reinfection, treated patients should be instructed to abstain from sexual intercourse for 7 days after single-dose therapy or until

*Not FDA approved for this indication.

TABLE 3. Treatment Regimens for Uncomplicated Urethral, Endocervical, or Rectal Chlamydial Infections

Recommended regimens
  Azithromycin* (Zithromax) 1 gm PO in single dose
  or
  Doxycycline (Vibramycin) 100 mg PO bid for 7 d
Alternative regimens
  Erythromycin base 500 mg PO qid for 7 d
  or
  Erythromycin ethylsuccinate 800 mg PO qid for 7 d
  or
  Ofloxacin (Floxin) 300 mg PO bid for 7 d
In pregnancy
  Erythromycin base 500 mg PO qid for 7 d
  or
  Amoxicillin* 500 mg PO tid for 7 d

*Not FDA approved for this indication.

completion of a 7-day regimen, and until all of their sex partners are cured.

Pregnant women with chlamydial infection should not be treated with doxycycline, ofloxacin, or erythromycin estolate. Although preliminary data indicate that azithromycin may be safe and effective, data are insufficient to recommend the routine use of azithromycin in pregnancy. Recommendations for treatment in pregnancy include a 7-day regimen of either erythromycin base, 500 mg four times daily, or amoxicillin,* 500 mg three times daily. Alternative regimens for pregnant patients include erythromycin base, 250 mg four times daily for 14 days; erythromycin ethylsuccinate, 800 mg four times daily for 7 days or 400 mg four times daily for 14 days; or azithromycin, 1 gram in a single dose.

Although a routine test of cure during the immediate post-treatment period is not recommended for patients treated with the standard treatment regimens, retesting should be considered at least 3 weeks after completion of an alternative regimen. A nonculture test for confirming organism eradication conducted sooner than 3 weeks after completion of therapy could produce a false-positive result because of the presence of residual antigen or nucleic acid.

In addition, screening for other sexually transmitted diseases should be considered, along with referral of the sexual partner for evaluation and treatment.

*Not FDA approved for this indication.

PELVIC INFLAMMATORY DISEASE

method of
JOHN C. PETROZZA, M.D., and
WARNER K. HUH, M.D.
*New England Medical Center and Tufts
  University School of Medicine
Boston, Massachusetts*

Pelvic inflammatory disease (PID) is most commonly known as inflammation of the upper genital tract caused by an infectious etiology. PID may involve multiple sites, including the fallopian tubes (i.e., salpingitis), the ovaries (i.e., oophoritis), and the endometrium (i.e., endometritis) and thus is often considered as a generalized term without a precise definition. Microorganisms that have ascended to the upper genital tract from colonization of the cervix most often cause PID. Many clinicians prefer to use the term "salpingitis" because this type of infection is the most common manifestation of PID and because many of the long-term effects of PID result directly from tubal distortion and destruction. The term "chronic pelvic inflammatory disease" has been largely abandoned because the long-term sequelae, including abdominopelvic adhesions and hydrosalpinges, are usually bacteriologically sterile; exceptions to this include actinomycotic and tubercular infections.

Pelvic inflammatory disease continues to be a significant health concern in the United States. Statistics indicate that at least one million women per year are treated for acute salpingitis in the United States. Moreover, 250,000 to 300,000 women are hospitalized each year with acute salpingitis. There are over 2.5 million office visits per year for salpingitis in the United States, and approximately 100,000 to 150,000 surgeries performed annually for treatment of acute salpingitis.

Of all sexually active women in the United States, those aged 15 to 19 years old have the highest rate of PID, and the rate of hospitalization for PID is inversely proportional to age. The estimated overall cost of treatment of women with PID is from $700 million to $3 billion annually. This estimate does not factor in the treatment of the long-term consequence of PID, including infertility, ectopic pregnancy, chronic pelvic pain, and dyspareunia. No less than one fourth of women with a history of PID have long-term sequelae of PID, and the risk is proportional to the number of episodes of PID.

ETIOLOGY

Pelvic inflammatory disease is caused by organisms that have colonized the endocervix and ascended into the upper genital tract. Many cases of PID are caused by sexually transmitted organisms, including *Neisseria gonorrhoeae* and *Chlamydia trachomatis*; however, it is well known that the infectious etiology of PID can be polymicrobial as well. In patients with PID, gonococci and chlamydiae can be isolated from the endocervix in 25 to 50% and 22 to 47% of cases, respectively. Neither organism, however, is identified from the endocervix in one third of patients with PID. In contrast, *N. gonorrhoeae* and *C. trachomatis* are isolated from the upper genital tract in only 28% and 23% of cases, respectively. Gram-negative and anaerobic organisms are isolated from the upper genital tract in at least 65% of cases. Commonly identified gram-negative and anaerobic organisms include *Escherichia coli*, *Klebsiella* species, *Proteus* species, *Peptostreptococcus* species, *Bacteroides fragilis*, and *Bacteroides biviens*. In patients with acute PID, peritoneal fluid and tubal cultures frequently grow anaerobic species, and a significant percentage of these cultures do not grow *N. gonorrhoeae* or *C. trachomatis*.

Other microorganisms, including *Mycoplasma hominis*, *Ureaplasma urealyticum*, and *Mycoplasma genitalium*, have been implicated in PID. However, this issue continues to be controversial and there is no significant difference in the rates of isolation from the cervices of patients with PID and matched, sexually active control subjects. Mycoplasmas also have been infrequently isolated from peritoneal and tubal cultures in patients with acute PID. In rarer cases, respiratory organisms, including *Haemophilus*

influenzae, group A streptococci, and pneumococci have been shown to colonize the endocervix and ultimately cause PID. Bacterial vaginosis organisms, including *Gardnerella vaginalis*, have been implicated in PID; the mechanism of infection is thought to be secondary to enzymatic breakdown of the cervical mucus barrier from the complex alteration in the vaginal flora, resulting in ascending spread of pathogenic organisms. Finally, *Actinomyces israelii* is classically isolated in women with PID and concurrent intrauterine device (IUD) use and, as stated previously, *Mycobacterium tuberculosis* is seen in rare, chronic cases of PID.

Most cases of PID (>99%) are caused by ascending pathogenic organisms; however, there have been cases secondary to both hematogenous and lymphatic spread. Again, at least 80% of cases are spontaneous, with the remaining fraction secondary to uterine procedures, including dilation and curettage, IUD placement, and endometrial biopsy.

RISK FACTORS

One of the most significant risk factors for PID is a prior history of PID. A second significant risk factor is sexual activity with multiple partners. It is well known that women with multiple sexual partners have a fourfold increased risk for development of PID; the risk is mainly attributed to women who have multiple partners in a short period of time rather than multiple monogamous relationships. Other risk factors include exposure to sexually transmitted diseases and, possibly, IUD use; however, the risk associated with IUDs is most significant immediately postinsertion and minimal with appropriate screening and counseling. Finally, adolescents are at a significant risk for development of acute PID; 15- to 19-year-olds are the most vulnerable.

Multiple studies indicate that oral contraceptive pills reduce the risk of PID. The exact mechanism is unknown but is thought to be secondary to thickening of the cervical mucus or decreased duration and amount of menses, resulting in decreased opportunities for organisms to ascend the genital tract. In addition, it is well known that oral contraceptive pills cause endometrial atrophy. Barrier contraceptive methods with spermicides are thought to be protective only when used correctly and appropriately. Tubal ligations decrease the risk of PID significantly, but there have been numerous reports of PID after tubal ligations, both in the immediate postoperative period and the long term.

DIAGNOSIS

The diagnosis of PID is often based on clinical symptoms, which include fever, leukocytosis, lower abdominal pain/tenderness, cervical mucopus, cervical motion tenderness, and adnexal tenderness. However, there is marked, wide variation in the signs and symptoms of PID, which makes clinical diagnosis very difficult. In a study by Jacobson and Westrom, 26.5% of patients with clinical PID had a normal-appearing pelvis on laparoscopy. Conversely, 65% had true acute salpingitis, demonstrating that rigid clinical criteria can overdiagnose PID over one third of the time. Multiple women may come to medical attention with very subtle symptoms or no symptoms at all. A delay in diagnosis and treatment may ultimately contribute to the long-term sequelae of acute PID.

Because it is not possible laparoscopically to diagnose all suspected cases of PID, the following clinical guidelines have been established for the diagnosis of PID. Patients need to have all of the following: history of lower abdominal pain or presence of lower abdominal tenderness, cervical motion tenderness, and adnexal tenderness. Also, patients need to have at least one of the following: temperature greater than 38.0°C, mucopurulent cervicitis, leukocytosis greater than 10,500 cells per mm³, erythrocyte sedimentation rate greater than 20 mm per hour, presence of adnexal mass on exam or sonography, and positive cervical cultures. These clinical criteria have not been subjected to adequate clinical trials and are regarded strictly as guidelines. Thus, the clinician should have a high index of suspicion so that acute salpingitis can be diagnosed and treated early. The differential diagnosis should include ectopic pregnancy, ruptured ovarian cyst, ovarian torsion, urinary tract infection, pyelonephritis, diverticulitis, gastroenteritis, and appendicitis.

Multiple tests are available for the diagnosis of gonorrhea from the endocervix. Gram stains are diagnostic in only 60% of cases. Culture on Thayer-Martin medium or DNA ligase probes are acceptable methods for diagnosis of gonorrhea. The diagnosis of endocervical chlamydial infection can also be made by culture with the use of McCoy cells; however, this type of culture is technically difficult and expensive. Direct fluorescent antibody and enzyme-linked immunosorbent assay chlamydial tests are helpful in the diagnosis of chlamydial infection, with a sensitivity and specificity greater than 90%. DNA ligase probes have superlative sensitivity and specificity, provide rapid diagnosis of chlamydial infection, and can be used concurrently to diagnose gonorrhea on the same swab. Patients should also be offered human immunodeficiency virus testing, a pregnancy test, and other sexually transmitted disease testing (e.g., syphilis and hepatitis). The partner should be tested and treated as well.

Other diagnostic modalities for PID include sonography and endometrial biopsy. Sonography is particularly helpful in the diagnosis of a tubo-ovarian abscess, and endometrial biopsy is a reasonable alternative to laparoscopy, with a reported 90% correlation between histologic endometritis and laparoscopically diagnosed salpingitis. Some authorities believe that ultrasonography is indicated only if the patient fails to show an adequate response to antimicrobial therapy in the first 48 to 72 hours. One other test that is thought to increase the specificity of the diagnosis of PID is an elevated C-reactive protein. Finally, as described previously, laparoscopy provides definitive diagnosis of acute PID.

TREATMENT

Treatment should provide broad-spectrum coverage of the most likely pathogenic organisms, including *N. gonorrhoeae*, *C. trachomatis*, anaerobes, gram-negative bacteria, and streptococci. Goals of treatment should also include resolution of symptoms and prevention of the long-term inflammatory sequelae of PID. Several regimens have been shown to be effective in treating patients and obtaining both a clinical and microbiologic cure in randomized clinical trials; however, very few studies have investigated the cure of infection in both the fallopian tubes and endometrium and the incidence of long-term complications, including infertility and ectopic pregnancy. There are no data directly comparing the efficacy of parenteral versus oral therapy and outpatient versus inpatient therapy. The decision for hospitalization is based on the clinical judgment of the health care provider. However, certain scenarios mandate inpatient treatment, including pregnancy, failure to respond to oral antimicrobial therapy, inability to tolerate or follow an outpatient regimen, severe illness including nausea, vomiting, and high fever, presence of a tubo-ovarian abscess, potential surgical emergencies, concern regarding future fertility, and immunodefi-

TABLE 1. **1998 Centers for Disease Control and Prevention Guidelines for Parenteral Treatment of Pelvic Inflammatory Disease**

Regimen A
  Cefotetan (Cefotan) 2 gm IV q12h, *or*
  Cefoxitin (Mefoxin) 2 gm IV q6h
     plus
  Doxycycline 100 mg IV or PO q12h
Regimen B
  Clindamycin (Cleocin) 900 mg IV q8h
     plus
  Gentamicin loading dose IV or IM (2 mg/kg body weight)
    followed by a maintenance dose (1.5 mg/kg) q8h. Single daily
    dosing may be substituted.

Parenteral therapy may be discontinued 24 hours after a patient improves clinically, and continuing oral therapy should consist of doxycycline 100 mg PO bid or clindamycin 450 mg PO qid to complete a total of 14 days of therapy. When a tubo-ovarian abscess is present, many health care providers use clindamycin rather than doxycycline because clindamycin provides more effective anaerobic coverage.

TABLE 2. **1998 Centers for Disease Control and Prevention Guidelines for Oral Treatment of Pelvic Inflammatory Disease**

Regimen A
  Ofloxacin (Floxin) 400 mg PO bid for 14 d
     plus
  Metronidazole (Flagyl) 500 mg PO bid for 14 d
Regimen B
  Ceftriaxone (Rocephin) 250 mg IM once, *or*
  Cefoxitin (Mefoxin) 2 gm IM plus Probenecid 1 gm PO in a
    single dose concurrently once, *or*
  Other parenteral third-generation cephalosporin (e.g.,
    ceftizoxime [Cefizox] or cefotaxime [Claforan])
     plus
  Doxycycline 100 mg PO bid for 14 d

TABLE 3. **Alternative Parenteral Therapy for Pelvic Inflammatory Disease**

Regimen A
  Ofloxacin (Floxin) 400 mg IV bid
     plus
  Metronidazole (Flagyl) 500 mg IV tid
Regimen B
  Ampicillin/sulbactam (Unasyn) 3 gm IV qid
     plus
  Doxycycline 100 mg IV or PO bid
Regimen C
  Ciprofloxacin (Cipro) 200 mg IV bid, *or*
  Trovafloxacin (Trovan) 300 mg IV qd,
     plus
  Doxycycline 100 mg IV or PO bid, *or*
  Metronidazole (Flagyl) 500 mg IV tid

TABLE 4. **Alternative Oral Treatment of Pelvic Inflammatory Disease**

Ofloxacin 400 mg PO bid for 14 d, *or*
Trovafloxacin 200 mg qd for 14 d
plus
Metronidazole 500 mg PO bid for 14 d

ciency. The patient must be reexamined within 48 hours of treatment and receive inpatient parenteral therapy if not improved. Table 1 lists the 1998 Centers for Disease Control and Prevention (CDC)-recommended parenteral therapies for PID, and Table 2 lists the 1998 CDC-recommended oral therapies for PID. Alternative regimens are listed in Tables 3 and 4.

Most studies using parenteral treatment are based on continuation of therapy for 48 hours after the onset of clinical improvement, but this period of time is not based on any evidence. Switching to oral therapy can be safely done in many circumstances after 24 hours of treatment. Most clinicians aggressively treat tubo-ovarian abscesses with at least 24 hours of inpatient parenteral antibiotics, and if the patient demonstrates significant clinical improvement, treatment can be switched to home parenteral therapy.

If patients fail to respond adequately to treatment, either additional imaging studies, including sonography, or laparoscopy must be entertained to make a diagnosis and provide surgical therapy (i.e., drainage of abscesses) when appropriate. Finally, identification and treatment of the partner is critical to the success of treatment.

LEIOMYOMATA

method of
A. F. HANEY, M.D.
Duke University Medical Center
Durham, North Carolina

Uterine leiomyomata are the most common tumors of the female genital tract and likely the most common soft tissue tumors in the entire body. Approximately 200,000 hysterectomies and 20,000 myomectomies are performed annually in the United States because of leiomyomata. They can reach very large size with few if any symptoms, and, alternatively, relatively small leiomyomata can cause massive uterine bleeding and pain. Although leiomyomata represent one of the most frequent indications for gynecologic surgery, their incidence far exceeds the frequency of clinical problems attributable to them, with estimates as high as 40% of women having identifiable leiomyomata in their uterus at menopause.

CLINICAL PRESENTATION

The reasons that leiomyomata come to clinical attention vary, and the symptoms depend on tumor location as well as size. Excessive uterine bleeding, increasing dysmenorrhea, and generalized pelvic pain or pressure may ulti-

mately be present, but noncyclic pelvic pain is a very late symptom of leiomyomata. Leiomyomata may rapidly enlarge during pregnancy and undergo necrosis, causing a great deal of pain in pregnancy. As the size of the leiomyomata and the total uterine volume increase, the adjacent pelvic viscera may be compressed, causing urinary frequency, constipation, and dyspareunia. The location and size of the leiomyomata generally determine the symptoms (Table 1).

The impact of leiomyomata on reproduction is less clear. Intracavitary and large submucosal leiomyomata are most likely causally related to infertility. With intramural leiomyomata, the relationship is more tenuous, and all other potential causes should be considered. Removal of submucosal and large intramural leiomyomata has been associated with improved outcome in infertile women undergoing assisted reproductive technologies such as in vitro fertilization. If the clinical problem is repeated miscarriage, preterm labor, or intrauterine growth restriction or the leiomyomata are large, preconceptional removal of intramural leiomyomata may be appropriate.

ANATOMIC FEATURES

Leiomyomata represent benign estrogen-responsive smooth uterine muscle tumors originating as monoclonal expansions of myometrial cells. The histology is virtually identical to that of normal myometrium. The cellularity is highly variable, and there are often interspersed areas of fibrosis and occasional calcifications. Leiomyomata grow in a spherical fashion with a clear demarcation from the surrounding normal myometrium. The blood supply is uniformly peripheral at the interface with the normal myometrium and not separate vascular pedicles. With rapid growth, the center may undergo necrosis and be replaced by fibrous tissue.

A rare leiomyosarcoma is encountered and may be grossly indistinguishable from typical leiomyomata. The histologic criteria for malignancy are increased numbers of mitoses on permanent sections and cellular pleomorphism. Because of the difficulty identifying mitoses on frozen section microscopy, an intraoperative diagnosis cannot be made with confidence. Leiomyosarcomas are estimated to comprise 0.1% of uterine tumors in reproductive-age women and in 1.7% of women undergoing hysterectomy for leiomyomata in their 60s. These tumors should be considered benign in premenopausal women, with pathologic examination of all specimens required.

DIAGNOSTIC STUDIES

Most leiomyomata are detected on pelvic examination with the uterus being enlarged and irregular. A pelvic ultrasound examination can distinguish leiomyomata from ovarian masses, which are usually cystic, and the proximity to the endometrial cavity can usually be demonstrated by identifying the endometrial stripe. Simultaneously injecting saline into the endometrial cavity (sonohysterography) can easily delineate intracavitary and submucous lei-

TABLE 1. **Location of Leiomyomata**

Serosal	Intracavitary
Intramural	Cervical
Submucosal	Parasitic

omyomata. Hysterosalpingography is often used if the patients are infertile and in whom a large but otherwise normal endometrial cavity is often noted when the uterus is enlarged. Occasionally, localized adenomyosis can be difficult to distinguish from leiomyomata, and magnetic resonance imaging (MRI) may be helpful as adenomyosis is less well demarcated.

GENETIC INHERITANCE PATTERN

More than 40% of first-degree female relatives of women with leiomyomata will develop them sometime during their lifetime. In addition, while leiomyomata are common in all races, African-American women undergoing hysterectomies have increased numbers of leiomyomata, which are larger in size. The familial pattern seems most consistent with a multifactorial genetic inheritance pattern and not simple mendelian genetics. Aside from noting that the disease is familial, there is little clinical predictability.

MOLECULAR MECHANISMS AND GENETIC DYSREGULATION

Leiomyomas are monoclonal neoplasms, representing a situation in which etiologic genetic mutations are likely. Cytogenetic studies of individual leiomyomas reveal that approximately one-third have some type of clonal chromosomal aberration. Undoubtedly, neoplastic myometrial cells represent a complex interaction of factors involving sex steroid responses altered by genetic mutations, resulting in the dysregulation of autocrine growth factors. Abnormal expression of a variety of individual genes has been observed in individual leiomyomata, but there is no consensus regarding a single predominant error. Similarly, dysregulation of protooncogenes has been noted, but the molecular evidence does not suggest a progression from benign leiomyomata to leiomyosarcoma. In the coming years, molecular geneticists will undoubtedly unravel the mechanisms of this pathologic transformation and provide opportunities for therapeutic intervention.

INFLUENCE OF SEX STEROIDS

There is little doubt that the growth of leiomyomata is related to gonadal steroids as leiomyomata (1) are not noted before puberty, (2) typically regress after menopause, (3) possess sex steroid receptors, (4) often dramatically enlarge during pregnancy, and (5) can be made to shrink in size with medically induced hypogonadism. There is no evidence that higher or aberrant patterns of ovarian steroid secretion contribute to the development of leiomyomata. The use of oral contraceptives has not been demonstrated to be associated with an increased incidence of leiomyomata. Similarly, treatment of postmenopausal women with hormone replacement therapy rarely is associated with growth. For clinical purposes, withholding hormone replacement therapy for fear of stimulating leiomyomata in otherwise appropriate candidates for treatment is not rational given the well-documented benefits of hormone replacement. Special note should be made of postmenopausal women with breast cancer taking tamoxifen because tamoxifen can be associated with growth of leiomyomata.

TREATMENT GOALS

Because a variety of treatment options exist (Table 2), it is important to clearly establish the goal of

TABLE 2. **Clinical Therapeutic Options**

Surgical
Myomectomy
Abdominal
Vaginal
Laparoscopic
Hysterectomy
Vaginal
Abdominal
Medical
Gonadotropin-releasing hormone agonists

therapy. Simply because leiomyomata are present does not indicate that they will cause symptoms in the future, and observation is all that is necessary. When the symptoms are mild, nonsteroidal antiinflammatory agents and oral contraceptives are prescribed, and often the symptoms will improve sufficiently to avoid further intervention. The use of continuous progestins should be discouraged, as their main side effect is irregular bleeding.

Many leiomyomata have limited growth potential and will remain static in size until menopause. The critical issues are whether future reproduction is desired and how close is menopause. As simple hysterectomy is curative, this is an attractive option when maintenance of reproduction is not desired. When the preservation of future childbearing is desired, a myomectomy is the primary choice. Many women today desire the preservation of the uterus even in the absence of any intention of future childbearing. This remains controversial because, if only the tumors are removed, there is a high frequency of recurrence.

MEDICAL TREATMENT OF LEIOMYOMATA

Many agents have been considered for medical suppression, including progestins, androgens, gestrinone,* estrogen antagonists, and progestin antagonists. None of these, however, has been proven to be clinically beneficial; only suppressing ovarian steroid production with a gonadotropin-releasing hormone agonist (GnRH agonist) has proved useful (Table 3). The volume of the leiomyomata typically decreases by 40%, but this is somewhat misleading as most physicians consider the diameter to be the most clini-

---

*Not available in the United States.

TABLE 3. **Available Gonadotropin-Releasing Hormone Agonists**

Leuprolide acetate (Lupron Depot)
3.75 mg IM q mo
11.25 mg IM q 3 mo
Nafarelin acetate (Synarel)*
200 µg intranasally bid
Goserelin acetate (Zoladex)*
3.6 mg SC monthly

*Not FDA approved for this indication.

cally useful measurement and the diameter decreases much less than the volume.

The induction of hypogonadism cannot be sustained for a prolonged interval because of the significant associated side effects, such as vasomotor hot flashes, accelerated bone loss, genital tract atrophy, and loss of the cardiovascular benefits of estrogenization. Approximately 1% of the bone mass is lost for every month of hypoestrogenism, and the hot flashes can be very debilitating. Although most of the bone mass is regained if the therapy is limited to 6 months, longer intervals of therapy may result in a permanent lowering of the age-adjusted bone mineral density. Unfortunately, the leiomyomata most often return to the pretreatment size rapidly after stopping therapy, and the symptoms recur.

The real question is what is the goal of medical therapy? The main indications for using a GnRH agonist are to stop heavy bleeding and to reverse anemia before surgery or temporarily delay surgery to correct other medical problems posing a surgical risk. Although reduced intraoperative blood loss and shortened operative time by preoperative use of a GnRH agonist are often espoused as benefits, there exist scant data to support this contention. Indeed, the softening of small intramural leiomyomata leads to the possibility that they will not be palpated during a myomectomy and increases the probability that some tumors will be missed. The simultaneous administration of low doses of estrogen and progestin, so-called add-back therapy, relieves symptoms but has not been demonstrated to be as efficacious as GnRH-agonist alone.

MYOMECTOMY

If leiomyomata are intracavitary, a hysteroscopic resection is the most cost-effective method of removal. Submucosal leiomyomas that protrude into the endometrial cavity can also be removed via hysteroscopic resection. When the bulk of the tumor is not protruding into the endometrial cavity, however, an abdominal approach is necessary. The goal of a myomectomy is to remove all the identifiable leiomyomata with the least distortion of the genital tract. The women should wait 2 to 3 months before attempting pregnancy to allow the uterine incisions to heal and to minimize the potential for myometrial scar disruption during pregnancy.

Significant intraoperative blood loss is frequently encountered, and myomectomy at the time of cesarean section is particularly hazardous because of the increased vascularity during pregnancy. Careful attention to surgical blood loss, applying tourniquets on vascular pedicles, and using an intraoperative blood salvage apparatus can reduce the net blood loss. Intramyometrial injection of vasopressin has been advocated by some surgeons, but there is a risk that bleeding will occur postoperatively. These steps, coupled with preoperative correction of anemia and autologous blood storage, reduce the need for homologous transfusion.

Another risk of myomectomy is the development of postoperative adhesions. Minimizing the amount of surgical trauma, making incisions on the anterior uterine surface and covering the uterine incisions with surgical barriers have significantly reduced this problem. Once the myometrium has incurred a surgical injury to a significant portion of the uterine wall, an elective cesarean section is recommended, as the incision may not be capable of withstanding the force of a prolonged labor without rupture.

ENDOSCOPIC PROCEDURES

With improvements in endoscopic surgery, it was logical that intracavitary and submucous leiomyomata would be removed or resected via hysteroscopy. This technique utilizes a hysteroscopic resectoscope, but careful preoperative selection and a high level of surgical skill are necessary. Preoperative shrinkage of the leiomyoma by the use of a GnRH agonist may often be helpful. In addition, care must be taken to avoid excessive intravascular absorption of the distending medium.

Similar improvements directed toward laparoscopic myomectomy have also been made. It is clear that pedunculated and smaller (<8 cm in diameter) serosal or superficial intramural leiomyomata can be removed via laparoscopy, but the surgery is lengthy and difficult and should be undertaken by only the most experienced endoscopic surgeons. Closure of the uterine incisions is difficult, and there have been several reports of spontaneous uterine rupture during pregnancy after laparoscopic myomectomy. This suggests that even careful attention to incisional closure by skilled endoscopic surgeons will not prevent uterine rupture. In the absence of long-term safety studies, laparoscopic myomectomy should be an infrequently performed procedure, primarily when subsequent reproduction is not anticipated.

Attempts at killing cells within leiomyomata, myolysis, and thereby shrinking the tumor have been made. This can be accomplished by repetitive insertion of either monopolar or biopolar electrodes into the tumor at a laparoscopy (i.e., electromyolysis). Similarly, interstitial laser hyperthermia can also be accomplished by insertion of a fiber laser. A similar technique with a cyroprobe for a thermal injury is termed *cryomyolysis*. All these techniques, however, cause a variable amount of cellular injury that can be very painful in the postoperative interval. No data are available on these techniques regarding long-term efficacy, complications, and persistence/recurrence rates. As a result of these concerns, intralesional destructive techniques should be considered experimental until these issues are clarified by comparative clinical trials.

UTERINE ARTERY EMBOLIZATION

When menometrorrhagia is the primary problem and the surgical risks judged unacceptable, embolization of the uterine arteries has been advocated to deprive the uterus along with the leiomyomata their blood supply. Although this approach has been useful as a palliative measure for women with unremitting bleeding caused by advanced cervical cancer, its safety and efficacy for women with leiomyomata remain to be clarified, particularly for women wishing to retain fertility.

RECURRENCE OF LEIOMYOMATA

When all of the palpable leiomyomata have been surgically removed, the rate of recurrence has been variably reported up to 60%, depending on the length of follow-up. Undoubtedly, the technical skill to remove all the identifiable leiomyomata is critically important and will influence the rate of apparent recurrence. The typical time frame for a clinically significant recurrence is 3 to 5 years. Women should clearly understand that myomectomy provides an opportunity to reproduce and does not "cure" the problem, as they have an inherited predisposition to leiomyomata. No long-term data are available regarding recurrence risk with destructive procedures or with uterine artery embolization.

SUMMARY

Leiomyomata represent the most common gynecologic tumors and are almost invariably benign. They can cause a variety of symptoms, including menometrorrhagia, pain, reproductive problems, and compression of adjacent pelvic viscera. They have a complex genetic inheritance pattern, and the therapeutic choices depend on the goals of therapy. Hysterectomy is most often used for definitive treatment, and myomectomy is used when preservation of childbearing potential is desired, albeit with a high recurrence risk. Although GnRH agonists will reduce the volume of the leiomyomata, the severe side effects and prompt recurrences make these agonists useful only for short-term goals such as reversing anemia, shrinking an intracavitary tumor, or decreasing the size of the uterus.

CANCER OF THE ENDOMETRIUM

method of
MARY L. GEMIGNANI, M.D., and
RICHARD R. BARAKAT, M.D.

Memorial Sloan-Kettering Cancer Center
New York, New York

Carcinoma of the endometrium is the most common gynecologic malignancy. It is estimated that, in 1999, there were 37,400 new cases and 6,400 deaths attributed to this malignancy in the United States. Currently, endometrial adenocarcinoma is the fourth most common cancer in females, ranking behind breast, bowel, and lung cancers, and ranks as the seventh leading cause of death attributable to cancer in women.

The majority of women, 75%, are postmenopausal at the time of diagnosis, with less than 5% of women diagnosed under the age of 40 years. Seventy-five percent of all cases are confined to the endometrium at the time of diagnosis. Endometrial cancer was initially staged clinically in 1971, with a revision to a more accurate surgical staging system in 1988. In all but the most medically compromised patients, surgical staging requires the removal of the uterus. The increasing use of minimal-access surgery, including laparoscopically assisted vaginal hysterectomy and lymph node sampling for staging and treatment, has been investigated.

EPIDEMIOLOGY

The incidence of endometrial carcinoma is highly dependent on age, with a median age at diagnosis of 63 years. Twenty-five percent of women are premenopausal at diagnosis, and only 5% are younger than 40 years of age. Most women present to their doctors with postmenopausal bleeding. The greater the age of the patient at the time of postmenopausal bleeding, the higher the risk that endometrial cancer is the cause.

Classic risk factors are based on the effects of unopposed estrogen and include obesity, diabetes, hypertension, chronic anovulation, estrogen-secreting tumors, early menarche, and late menopause, as well as exogenous unopposed estrogens. Administration of unopposed estrogen is associated with a fourfold to eightfold increased risk of developing endometrial cancer (Table 1).

DIAGNOSIS AND SCREENING

Endometrial cancer is usually diagnosed in its early stages because most women report postmenopausal or abnormal vaginal bleeding to their physicians. Initial evaluation in the physician's office should include a pelvic examination, Papanicolaou smear, and endometrial sampling. It is preferable to perform both endocervical and endometrial sampling to evaluate possible cervical extension and/or to exclude the possibility of a primary endocervical adenocarcinoma. When an endometrial sampling cannot be performed in the office or insufficient endometrial tissue is obtained, a dilatation and curettage should be performed in the operating room. It is for this group of women that additional testing with ultrasonography or hysteroscopy may provide useful information.

The role of screening for endometrial cancer has not yet been established and screening is therefore generally not recommended.

TAMOXIFEN AND ENDOMETRIAL CANCER

The U.S. Food and Drug Administration first approved the nonsteroidal antiestrogen tamoxifen (Nolvadex) for the treatment of patients with breast cancer in 1978. Most

TABLE 1. **Risk Factors**

Risk Factor	Relative Risk
Obesity	1.9–11
Parous vs. nulliparous	0.1–0.9
Late menopause	1.7–2.4
Diabetes mellitus	1.3–2.7
Estrogen replacement therapy	1.6–12
Hypertension	1.2–2.1

recently, it has also been approved as a chemopreventive agent for healthy women at risk for developing breast cancer. Tamoxifen is believed to exert its main effect by blocking the binding of estrogen to the estrogen receptor. Although primarily an antiestrogen, tamoxifen may also exhibit some mild estrogenic effects, particularly in the endometrium.

One of the most significant complications of long-term tamoxifen use is the possible development of endometrial cancer. A 7.5-fold increased risk of developing endometrial cancer with tamoxifen use was noted in the National Surgical Adjuvant Breast and Bowel Project (NSABBP) B-14 trial, which randomized women with estrogen receptor–positive, node-negative, invasive breast cancer to tamoxifen versus placebo. Eighty-eight percent of those tamoxifen-associated endometrial cancers were FIGO stage I. Women receiving tamoxifen should be encouraged to undergo annual gynecologic evaluation, which should include endometrial sampling in the presence of abnormal vaginal bleeding.

STAGING AND SURGICAL TREATMENT

Since 1980, treatment and staging for endometrial cancer has undergone many changes. Endometrial cancer was initially staged clinically in 1971, with a revision to a more accurate surgical staging system in 1988 (Table 2). This revision incorporated many of the prognostic factors reported in two large prospective staging trials conducted by the Gynecologic Oncology Group (GOG) in 1984 and 1987. The GOG studied the pathologic features of the tumor (e.g., grade and histologic subtype) and depth of myome-

TABLE 2. **International Federation of Gynecology and Obstetrics 1988 Surgical Staging for Carcinoma of the Corpus Uteri**

Stage	
I	
IA grade 123	Tumor limited to endometrium
IB grade 123	Invasion to less than one-half of endometrium
IC grade 123	Invasion to more than one-half of endometrium
II	
IIA grade 123	Endocervical glandular involvement only
IIB grade 123	Cervical stromal invasion
III	
IIIA grade 123	Tumor invades serosa and/or adnexa and/or positive peritoneal cytology
IIIB grade 123	Vaginal metastases
IIIC grade 123	Metastases to pelvic and/or para-aortic lymph nodes
IV	
IVA grade 123	Tumor invasion of bladder and/or bowel mucosa
IVB grade 123	Distant metastases, including intra-abdominal and/or inguinal lymph nodes
Degree of differentiation	
G1	5% or less of a nonsquamous or nonmorular solid growth pattern
G2	6%–50% of a nonsquamous or nonmorular solid growth pattern
G3	More than 50% of a nonsquamous or nonmorular solid growth pattern

From Pettersson F (ed): Annual Report on the Results of Treatment in Gynecologic Cancer, Vol 20. Stockholm, International Federation of Gynecology and Obstetrics, 1988, with permission.

trial invasion and correlated these factors with lymph node metastases. Deep myometrial invasion and higher grade were both associated with a higher rate of lymph node metastases. These features can be used to assign patients with clinical early-stage endometrial cancer to low-risk or high-risk groups and to determine which patients will benefit from an extended surgical staging procedure.

The traditional approach for staging and treatment is an exploratory laparotomy through a midline incision, total abdominal hysterectomy, bilateral salpingo-oophorectomy, peritoneal washings, and, for patients with selected high-risk factors, sampling of pelvic and para-aortic nodes. Surgical exploration is most often performed through a midline incision that allows access to the upper abdomen and diaphragm. Cytologic washings are obtained upon entering the abdomen. After careful exploration of the abdominal cavity, including the omentum and peritoneal surfaces, an extrafascial hysterectomy and bilateral salpingo-oophorectomy is performed. The histologic diagnosis and grade is often known by a sampling of the endometrium performed preoperatively. Intraoperatively, the depth of myometrial invasion can be determined by gross inspection of the opened uterus or by frozen section if no obvious deep invasion is seen. In patients with grade 3 histologic type, deep (>50%) myometrial invasion, suspected adnexal involvement, extrauterine disease, or extension to uterine isthmus, pelvic and para-aortic lymph node sampling is performed. Lymph nodes that are visibly or palpably enlarged should also be removed.

Vaginal hysterectomy has often been cited as the simplest and least morbid approach to hysterectomy, with similar treatment outcomes in patients with clinical stage I endometrial cancer. It is often used as an alternative to an abdominal approach in obese and high-surgical-risk patients. Laparoscopically assisted vaginal hysterectomy offers an attractive alternative, as it allows exploration of the abdominal cavity and procurement of peritoneal washings, as well as lymph node sampling, if necessary. The laparoscopic approach also provides a faster recovery. Published reports have shown advantages to the laparoscopic approach, including reductions in both length of stay and hospital charges.

Laparoscopically assisted surgical staging is feasible for select groups of patients. It is not known, however, whether it is applicable to all patients with clinical stage I disease. Patients with intra-abdominal adhesions and obese patients may not be candidates. Para-aortic lymph node sampling is also technically more difficult laparoscopically. The GOG is currently performing a randomized trial to compare the laparoscopically assisted vaginal hysterectomy approach to a traditional abdominal hysterectomy in patients with clinical stage I disease.

POSTOPERATIVE THERAPY AND ADJUVANT TREATMENT

The approach to postoperative treatment of patients with endometrial cancer is based on prognostic factors. Patients with grade 1 or 2 lesions confined to the endometrium (stage IA) are considered low risk and do not appear to benefit from adjuvant radiation. Patients with stage IB or stage IC, endocervical glandular (IIA) or stromal (IIB) involvement, are considered to be at intermediate risk. Patients with endometrial cancer limited to the uterus with less than 50% myometrial invasion (stage IB) and no other adverse features are offered vaginal brachytherapy at our institution. Other patients in this intermediate group are offered vaginal brachytherapy and whole-pelvic radiation. Radiation therapy is begun approximately 6 to 8 weeks after surgery.

The GOG recently completed protocol 99, a randomized trial of no additional treatment versus 5040 cGy of pelvic radiotherapy in patients with intermediate-risk endometrial cancer. Most of the recurrences in the no-treatment arm were pelvic or vaginal and were salvaged with radiation therapy. Thus, the study did not show any survival benefit to adjuvant radiation: 96% of patients who received adjuvant radiation were alive at 3 years compared with 89% of patients who did not receive radiation initially. Moreover, toxicity was greater in the pelvic radiation group. Based on these findings, further studies of intermediate-risk group patients are needed, particularly to address the question of whether vaginal brachytherapy alone would offer the greatest therapeutic benefit in this group.

Patients with extrauterine disease, intraperitoneal spread, or disease metastatic to retroperitoneal lymph nodes are considered high risk. Patients with metastases to only pelvic lymph nodes benefit from whole-pelvic radiation therapy. Para-aortic lymph node sampling is important for this group of patients, as approximately 40% of patients with aortic node metastases can be salvaged with adjuvant treatment. Extended-field radiation therapy is recommended. Patients with completely resected intraperitoneal disease are candidates for whole-abdominal radiation therapy with a pelvic boost. The GOG is currently comparing whole-abdominal radiation with combination chemotherapy with cisplatin and doxorubicin in patients with stage III or IV disease and less than 2 cm of residual after surgery.

The significance of positive peritoneal washing with no evidence of extrauterine disease is unclear. Many authors have reported on whole-abdominal radiation, intraperitoneal chromic phosphate, or oral progestins.

TREATMENT OF RECURRENT DISEASE

The treatment of recurrent disease is often based on the histologic subtype and grade of the original tumor as well as on the estrogen and progesterone receptor status. Treatment is usually with cytotoxic chemotherapy or hormonal agents. Hormonal agents such as megestrol acetate (Megace) or medroxy-

progesterone acetate (Provera)* are often used, with response rates ranging from 15% to 40%. Tamoxifen has also been used, with response rates of approximately 22%. Because of their low toxicities and good tolerance levels, hormonal agents are usually the first-line treatment. Long-term responses have been reported. Doxorubicin (Adriamycin) is the most active agent in patients with advanced endometrial cancer, with an overall response rate of 26%. Paclitaxel (Taxol) also appears promising, with the GOG demonstrating a 36% response rate to this agent.

POSTOPERATIVE SURVEILLANCE

The follow-up for patients with endometrial cancer includes close surveillance in the first 3 years after surgery because most recurrences occur in this period. Patients should undergo semiannual pelvic examinations during the first 3 years, then annually thereafter. Although obtaining routine Pap smears at each visit does not appear to improve the outcome of patients with isolated vaginal recurrences, annual Pap smears are recommended, at least during the first 3 years. Serial CA-125 determinations should only be performed in patients with elevations at diagnosis or those with known extrauterine disease. Postoperative surveillance should also include a complete physical examination as well as health maintenance, including annual mammography and assessment of stool guaiac.

There is no evidence in the literature that surveillance with routine chest radiographs improves survival. Because the majority of all recurrences are symptomatic, patient education regarding the signs and symptoms of recurrent disease should be incorporated into a surveillance program. Diagnostic tests can then be targeted toward the symptoms.

ESTROGEN REPLACEMENT THERAPY

The postoperative use of supplemental estrogen as treatment for menopausal symptoms and prophylaxis against osteoporosis and heart disease appears to be safe, although small numbers of patients have been evaluated. In retrospective reports, a total of 122 patients with stage I disease received postoperative estrogen. Of these, only one patient had a tumor recurrence. The patients in these reports were not randomized. It appears, however, that survival is not decreased by the postoperative use of estrogen by patients with early-stage disease. The American College of Obstetricians and Gynecologists Committee Opinion concluded that for women with a history of endometrial carcinoma, estrogens could be used for the same indications as for any other woman except that the selection of appropriate candidates should be based on prognostic indicators and the risk the patient is willing to assume. A randomized trial is currently being conducted by the GOG to conclu-

---

*Not FDA approved for this indication.

sively prove the safety of estrogen replacement therapy for this group of patients.

CANCER OF THE UTERINE CERVIX

method of
CHARLES LEVENBACK, M.D.
The University of Texas M. D. Anderson Cancer Center
Houston, Texas

INCIDENCE

The incidence of cervical cancer varies throughout the world, but in many regions it is the leading cause of cancer death in women. In the United States there were an estimated 13,700 new cases and 4700 deaths in 1998, in comparison with more than 200,000 new cases of breast cancer in 1998. The incidence for the general female population in the United States is 2.5 in 100,000, but it is as high as 43 in 100,000 among Vietnamese women. The incidence for Hispanic women is 16.2 in 100,000 and for African-American women, 13.2 in 100,000.

The introduction of the Papanicolaou (Pap) smear in the 1940s led to a dramatic reduction in mortality from cervical cancer in well-screened populations and an increase in the detection of carcinoma in situ. In the United States, deaths from cervical cancer have remained steady in the 1980s and 1990s. Today in the United States, 50% of patients with cervical cancer have never been screened, and another 10% have not been screened in the past 5 years.

PATHOGENESIS AND RISK FACTORS

One feature of cervical cancer that distinguishes it from other cancers is that it resembles a sexually transmitted disease. Many epidemiologic studies have found an association between sexual behavior of both men and women and the risk for development of cervical cancer. With over 90% of cervical tumors demonstrating human papillomavirus (HPV) DNA, researchers believe that infection with HPV is a likely causative agent. HPV genes E6 and E7 incorporate into the host's genetic material, which results in malignant transformation. HPV has many subtypes, some of which are associated with carcinoma in situ and invasive disease more often than others. HPV infection, however, is probably only one factor involved in the development of cervical cancer. Diet, contraceptive methods, and smoking have also been linked to cervical cancer in women with and without HPV infections. In addition, the timing of HPV infection may be important. In the years after menarche, the cervical epithelium undergoes metaplasia, a process by which glandular epithelium is transferred to squamous epithelium. This is apparently a vulnerable period, and coitus during this time increases the risk for cervical cancer. Primary prevention efforts should be directed at postponing the onset of sexual activity, especially since it was discovered that barrier contraceptives may not provide adequate protection against HPV infection.

PAP SMEAR SCREENING

The American Cancer Society recommends that women begin to undergo annual Pap smear screening at 18 years of age or at the onset of sexual activity. If a woman has three consecutive normal smears and is at low risk for cervical cancer, then a longer interval may be selected. Risk factors for continuing annual screening include known infection with HPV or the human immunodeficiency virus, history of an abnormal Pap smear, or high-risk sexual behavior by either the patient or her partner(s). Because sexual partners may change and because of other health benefits associated with annual physical examination, most primary care physicians continue to recommend annual Pap smears. Women older than 65 years of age and those who have had a hysterectomy should also continue to have annual checkups that include a Pap smear.

A single Pap smear has a false-negative rate of up to 20%. Fortunately, the natural progression from preinvasive to invasive cancer is slow, and the probability of three consecutive false-negative tests is very low. Recent douching, poor sampling technique, poor fixing technique, laboratory errors, and interpretation errors by the cytopathologist or clinician all contribute to false-negative results.

EVALUATION OF AN ABNORMAL PAP SMEAR

In 1998, a panel of experts recommended standardizing the nomenclature used to report Pap smear results. This standard has become known as The Bethesda System (TBS). All Pap smears should be reported in TBS terminology, and all providers performing Pap smears should be familiar with all TBS categories (Table 1).

Abnormal Pap smears are evaluated by colposcopy. Colposcopy is a difficult procedure to perform, and dedicated training is necessary for developing the appropriate skills. Colposcopic findings should be clearly recorded in the medical record, usually with an annotated drawing and a clear indication about whether the study was satisfactory. Any abnormal lesions should be sampled for biopsy. All patients, even those with no visible lesion, should undergo endocervical curettage. If there is a lesion visible to the naked eye, colposcopy is not necessary; however, a biopsy should be performed immediately.

TREATMENT OF INTRAEPITHELIAL NEOPLASIA

If colposcopy and directed biopsies rule out the possibility of invasive disease, then treatment for intraepithelial neoplasia can be initiated. Several

TABLE 1. **International Federation of Gynecology and Obstetrics (FIGO) Staging System for Carcinoma of the Cervix Uteri (1995)**

Stage	Description
Stage 0	Carcinoma in situ, intraepithelial carcinoma
Stage I	The carcinoma is strictly confined to the cervix.
Stage IA	Invasive cancer identified only microscopically. All gross lesions even with superficial invasion are Stage IB cancers. Invasion is limited to measured stromal invasion with maximum depth of 5 mm and no wider than 7 mm.*
Stage IA$_1$	Measured invasion of stroma no greater than 3 mm in depth and no wider than 7 mm
Stage IA$_2$	Measured invasion of stroma greater than 3 mm and no greater than 5 mm in depth, and no wider than 7 mm
Stage IB	Clinical lesions confined to the cervix or preclinical lesions greater than stage IA
Stage IB$_1$	Clinical lesions no greater than 4 cm in size
Stage IB$_2$	Clinical lesions greater than 4 cm in size
Stage II	The carcinoma extends beyond the cervix but has not extended to the pelvic wall. The carcinoma involves the vagina but not as far as the lower third.
Stage IIA	No obvious parametrial involvement
Stage IIB	Obvious parametrial involvement
Stage III	The carcinoma has extended to the pelvic wall. On rectal examination, there is no cancer-free space between the tumor and the pelvic wall. The tumor involves the lower third of the vagina. All cases with a hydronephrosis or nonfunctioning kidney are included unless they are known to be due to other causes.
Stage IIIA	No extension to the pelvic wall
Stage IIIB	Extension to the pelvic wall or hydronephrosis or nonfunctioning kidney
Stage IV	The carcinoma has extended beyond the true pelvis or has clinically involved the mucosa of the bladder or rectum. A bullous edema as such does not permit a case to be allotted to stage IV.
Stage IVA	Spread of the growth to adjacent organs
Stage IVB	Spread to distant organs

Comments

Notes about the staging:

Stage IA carcinoma should include minimally microscopically evident stromal invasion as well as small cancerous tumors of measurable size. Stage IA should be divided into those lesions with minute foci of invasion visible only microscopically as stage IA$_1$ and macroscopically measurable microcarcinoma as stage IA$_2$, to gain further knowledge of the clinical behavior of these lesions. The term *IB occult* should be omitted.

The diagnosis of both stage IA$_1$ and IA$_2$ cases should be based on microscopic examination of removed tissue, preferably a cone, which must include the entire lesion. The lower limit of stage IA$_2$ should be measurable macroscopically (even if dots need to be placed on the slide before measurement), and the upper limit of stage IA$_2$ is given by measurement of the two largest dimensions in any given section. The depth of invasion should not be more than 5 mm taken from the base of the epithelium, either surface or glandular, from which it originates. The second dimension, the horizontal spread, must not exceed 7 mm. Vascular space involvement, either venous or lymphatic, should not alter the staging but should be specifically recorded, because it may affect treatment decisions in the future.

Lesions of greater size should be classified as stage IB. As a rule, it is impossible to estimate clinically whether a cancer of the cervix has extended to the corpus. Extension to the corpus should therefore be disregarded. A patient with a growth fixed to the pelvic wall by a short and indurated but not nodular parametrium should be allotted to stage IIB. It is impossible at clinical examination to decide whether a smooth and indurated parametrium is truly cancerous or only inflammatory. Therefore, the case should be placed in stage III only if the parametrium is nodular on the pelvic wall or if the growth itself extends to the pelvic wall.

The presence of hydronephrosis or nonfunctioning kidney due to stenosis of the ureter by cancer permits a case to be allotted to stage III even if, according to the other findings, the case should be allotted to stage I or stage II.

The presence of bullous edema, as such, should not permit a case to be allotted to stage IV. Ridges and furrows in the bladder wall should be interpreted as signs of submucous involvement of the bladder if they remain fixed to the growth during palpation (i.e., examination from the vagina or the rectum during cystoscopy). A finding of malignant cells in cytologic washings from the urinary bladder requires further examination and biopsy from the wall of the bladder.

*The depth of invasion should not be more than 5 mm taken from the base of the epithelium, either surface or glandular, from which it originates. Vascular space involvement, either venous or lymphatic, should not alter the staging.

Adapted from Shepard JH: Staging announcement: FIGO staging of gynecologic cancers: Cervical and vulva. *Int J Gynecol Cancer* 5:319, 1995.

modalities can be used to treat intraepithelial neoplasia, including cryotherapy, loop electrosurgical excision procedure (LEEP), and laser vaporization. A randomized trial at The University of Texas M. D. Anderson Cancer Center found no difference in patients with squamous lesions regarding persistence of disease, recurrence, or complications treated with the three previously mentioned modalities.

If invasive disease has not been ruled out by colposcopy and directed biopsies, then a conization is required. Indications for cone biopsy are (1) cytologic or histologic suspicion of invasion, (2) endocervical curettage positive for dysplasia, (3) significant discordance between cytologic, histologic, and colposcopic findings, and (4) microinvasion on biopsy. Conization is both diagnostic and, for some patients, therapeutic. Cone biopsy can be performed as an outpatient procedure with the use of LEEP or laser vaporization. For both techniques, experience on the part of the clinician is necessary to reduce the cautery artifact at the margins. Conization may also be performed in the operating room under general anesthesia, especially if a deep cone is required or if the procedure is being repeated because of positive margins.

MICROINVASION

Clearly, there is a group of patients with squamous carcinomas and minimal stromal invasion who have essentially no risk of metastatic disease. The most commonly used clinical definition of microinvasion, provided by the Society of Gynecologic Oncologists, is less than 3 mm invasion, negative cone biopsy margins, and no lymphatic vascular invasion. Patients meeting these criteria may be treated with simple hysterectomy. There are small published series of patients with microinvasive squamous carcinoma successfully treated with cone biopsy alone to preserve fertility. There is no agreed-on definition of microinvasive adenocarcinoma of the cervix.

HISTOLOGY

At least 80% of invasive cancers of the cervix are squamous carcinomas, and the available survival and response data refer primarily to these patients. Next most common are adenosquamous carcinomas and adenocarcinoma. Adenocarcinomas have a wide range of malignant potential. Metastases are rare in patients with grade 1 adenocarcinoma, whereas even small high-grade adenocarcinomas are associated with increased treatment failure.

Small cell cancers make up less than 5% of cervical cancers and have a high mortality rate. Most authorities now recommend multimodality treatment for patients with these tumors.

MANIFESTATIONS OF INVASIVE CERVICAL CANCER

Abnormal vaginal bleeding is the most common presenting symptom of cervical cancer. Bleeding after coitus may be a prominent sign in patients with exophytic tumors. On speculum examination, the tumor is visible, and a biopsy should be obtained without delay. Patients with endophytic tumors may have continuous bleeding. The tumor may not be visible and may not be palpable on vaginal examination only. Rectovaginal examination is a mandatory aspect of the evaluation of patients with known or suspected cervical cancer. Endocervical curettage is diagnostic.

Pain is a prominent symptom in patients with more advanced disease. Hip, buttock, and sciatic pain are usually signs of pelvic wall involvement. Ureteral obstruction is usually asymptomatic, but it can result in flank pain.

STAGING

Staging of cervical cancer is clinical because patients are treated with radiation therapy and never undergo surgery. The palpatory findings are crucial and should be documented in the medical record with an annotated drawing. The radiation oncologist and gynecologic oncologist should confirm each other's findings when appropriate. In rare cases, an examination under anesthesia is necessary to clarify the findings. Liver and renal laboratory tests, chest radiography, and intravenous pyelography are parts of the basic staging work-up. Barium enema, plain radi-

ography, bone scan, liver and spleen scan, cystoscopy, and proctoscopy are allowed where suspicion of metastases warrants. Other tests, such as computed tomography, magnetic resonance imaging, and lymphangiography, may be performed; however, because they are not available in many areas of the world where cervical cancer is very common, they are not used to upstage disease. Lymphangiography is the best study for evaluating lymph nodes because it reveals their internal architecture. Studies that rely on size criteria only, such as computed tomography, are confounded by false-positive results because of inflammation and anatomic variation. Unfortunately, lymphangiography also is not widely available, and can be painful and complicated by lymphangitis.

TREATMENT OF INVASIVE CERVICAL CANCER

Definitive surgical treatment for invasive cervical cancer is radical hysterectomy and pelvic lymphadenectomy. Radical hysterectomy should be performed only by personnel with appropriate clinical privileges, usually a gynecologic oncologist. Radical hysterectomy includes removal of the uterus, cervix, upper vagina, parametrium, and paravaginal tissue to obtain adequate margins around the cervix.

A small number of centers have been pioneering radical trachelectomy, which spares the uterine fundus in patients with small primary tumors. Successful pregnancies have been reported after this procedure.

Cervical cancer was the first cancer to be cured with radiation therapy. Treatment is initiated with external-beam radiation to parallel opposed fields encompassing the pelvic lymph nodes for a total of 40 Gy. With modern high-energy equipment, skin complications are nonexistent. Modern brachytherapy allows a high dose of radiation to be delivered to the cervix, which itself is relatively radioresistant. Two intracavitary treatments are given 2 weeks apart. The entire course should take approximately 7 weeks, and treatment should be delayed only if absolutely necessary.

Acute radiation complications such as diarrhea and cystitis usually are self-limited and easy to treat. Late complications such as radiation enteritis, sigmoiditis, proctitis, stricture, fistula obstruction, or even perforation are difficult to treat. Radiation enteritis frequently can be managed with low-residue diet and antimotility agents; however, some patients require surgery. The risk of one of these serious complications is less than 5% for patients with small tumors, but this rate increases with larger tumors treated at higher doses of radiation.

Most studies indicate that the 5-year survival rate for patients with stage IB_1 disease treated with radical hysterectomy or pelvic irradiation ranges from 80 to 90%. Survival decreases as tumor size and stage increase. The 5-year survival rate for patients with stage III cervical cancer is 30 to 50%. These data underscore the importance of screening and early detection.

Patients with advanced cervical cancer should receive chemoradiation. In February 1999, the National Cancer Institute issued a clinical alert recommending chemoradiation based on five studies that all found chemoradiation to be superior to irradiation alone in various subgroups of patients. In a randomized trial sponsored by the Radiation Therapy Oncology Group, patients with primary tumors greater than 5 cm in diameter were treated with pelvic irradiation and 5-fluorouracil, cisplatin (Platinol), or extended-field irradiation. Chemoradiation resulted in a nearly 50% reduction in mortality at 5 years compared with radiation therapy alone.

Finally, a note of caution for primary care providers: published data show that many radiation oncologists' treatment plans do not meet the accepted standards for treating patients with cervical cancer. Patients and providers should seek a radiation oncologist who regularly treats cervical cancer, even when this means the inconvenience of travel to a referral center.

LONG-TERM FOLLOW-UP

Primary care physicians commonly perform follow-up for patients treated with cervical cancer. A study at the M. D. Anderson Cancer Center revealed that Pap smears rarely detected recurrence not suggested by symptoms or detected on physical examination. On the other hand, chest radiographs can detect asymptomatic recurrence, and the median survival for patients with isolated pulmonary metastases was significantly longer than for patients with abdominal or pelvic recurrences, which suggests that patients with pulmonary metastases can benefit from treatment. Current follow-up recommendations are a pelvic examination every 6 months for 5 years, a Pap smear and chest radiograph once a year, except years 2 through 4, when a chest radiograph should be obtained twice each year.

RECURRENT DISEASE

Most patients with recurrent cervical cancer die, usually within 12 months of relapse. Pelvic recurrence after radical hysterectomy is curable if the tumor volume is small. Central pelvic recurrences after pelvic irradiation can be cured with pelvic exenteration, which is an ultraradical operation necessitating the removal of the bladder, the rectum, or both, along with the reproductive organs.

Pelvic recurrence in the irradiated field that is unresectable is catastrophic. The response rate to various chemotherapeutic agents is approximately 5%. Pelvic sidewall recurrence is very painful, and patients usually require high doses of opioid analgesics to remain comfortable. The assistance of an expert in symptom management is very helpful to oncologists and nononcologists at this point.

Over 60 chemotherapy agents have been described in the literature as treatment of recurrent cervical cancer. Cisplatin remains the gold standard because of its relatively low toxicity and high response rates. Approximately 50% of patients treated with cisplatin have stabilization of disease or a response. A complete response is rare, and long-term remission is extremely rare. The median survival after the start of chemotherapy is between 6 and 9 months.

TUMORS OF THE VULVA

method of
BHAGIRATH MAJMUDAR, M.D.
Emory University School of Medicine
Atlanta, Georgia

The vulva is a common site for both benign and malignant primary tumors. Metastatic tumors, on the other hand, are distinctly uncommon. A clinical approach to vulvar neoplasms should include a complete clinical history and a thorough and careful examination of the vulva, vagina, and inguinal and perianal areas. The colposcope can provide extra help, but a hand magnifying lens usually suffices. The spectrum of tumors and tumor-like conditions seen in the vulva are summarized in Table 1.

DIAGNOSIS

Because a wide variety of tumors and tumor-like conditions occur in the vulva, the diagnostic approach should encompass all the possibilities. The cytology of vulvar lesions, although often not obtained, can be very helpful in establishing the diagnoses of infectious conditions such as those listed in Table 1 (e.g., melanoma, squamous cell carcinoma). Cytologic studies are most helpful when performed as a first diagnostic step before the lesion is manipulated. A fine-needle aspiration biopsy, although not usually used by clinicians, can establish the diagnosis in a variety of benign and malignant tumors of the vulva and detect inguinal lymph node metastasis.

Vulvar biopsies can be performed in the office and may establish a specific diagnosis in a large number of cases. Clinically malignant dark pigmented lesions in young women may represent metastatic choriocarcinoma. A biopsy may cause intractable hemorrhage and therefore should be avoided until after human chorionic gonadotropin (hCG) determination. All biopsy specimens should generally include the lesion, its margin, and adjacent uninvolved tissue. A 4-mm punch biopsy can be surprisingly diagnostic in a number of instances. After the biopsy is obtained, the tissue specimen should be properly oriented on a piece of filter paper or paper towel. Gauze pieces are undesirable. A proper orientation is vital for correct histologic interpretation because tangential or oblique cuts may render the biopsy nondiagnostic or may even lead to a mistaken diagnosis.

A 4 to 5% acetic acid may unmask clinically invisible lesions such as human papillomavirus (HPV) infection and vaginal intraepithelial neoplasia (VIN) and facilitate identification of the correct biopsy site. The complete clinical history and findings should be furnished to the pathologist to obtain maximal benefit of the diagnostic procedure.

Some infections can mimic vulvar tumors. Condyloma acuminatum caused by HPV is borderline between infec-

TABLE 1. **Tumors and Tumor-like Conditions of the Vulva**

Infections mimicking tumors
  Condyloma acuminatum
  Granuloma inguinale
  Fungal infections
  Molluscum contagiosum
  Herpes simplex
  Bartholin's abscess
  Others
Benign solid tumors
  Epidermal origin
    Acrochordon
    Seborrheic keratosis
    Nevus
  Dermal appendage origin
    Adenoma
    Sebaceous adenoma
  Mesodermal origin
    Fibroma
    Lipoma
    Neurofibroma
    Leiomyoma
    Granular cell tumors
    Hemangioma
    Pyogenic granuloma
    Lymphangioma
    Angiokeratoma
    Angiomyxoma
    Angiomyofibroblastoma
  Bartholin's and vestibular gland origin
    Adenofibroma
    Mucous adenoma
  Urethral origin
    Caruncle
    Prolapse of the urethral mucosa
  Ectopic breast origin
    Fibroadenoma
Benign cystic tumors
  Epidermal origin
    Epidermal inclusion cysts
    Pilonidal cysts
  Dermal appendage origin
    Sebaceous cysts
    Hidradenoma
    Fox-Fordyce disease
    Syringoma

Embryonic remnant origin
  Mesonephric (Gartner's) cysts
  Paramesonephric (müllerian) cysts
  Urogenital sinus cysts
  Cysts of canal of Nuck (hydrocele)
  Adenosis
  Cysts of supernumerary mammary glands
  Dermoid cysts
Bartholin's gland origin
  Duct cysts
  Abscess
Urethral and paraurethral origin
  Paraurethral (Skene's duct) cysts
  Urethral diverticula
Miscellaneous origin
  Endometriosis
  Liquefied hematoma
Primary malignant tumors
  Epithelial tumors of the skin and mucosal origin
  Squamous cell origin
    Squamous cell carcinoma
    Verrucous carcinoma
  Basal cell carcinoma
  Melanoma
  Adenocarcinoma
    Paget's disease
    Skin appendage
  Malignant tumors of the urethra and Bartholin's gland
    Squamous cell carcinoma
    Adenocarcinoma
    Adenoid cystic carcinoma
    Adenosquamous carcinoma
    Transitional cell carcinoma
  Carcinoma and sarcoma of ectopic breast tissue
  Soft tissue sarcomas
    Embryonal rhabdomyosarcoma
    Leiomyosarcoma
    Malignant fibrous histiocytoma
    Epithelioid sarcoma
Metastatic tumors
  Melanoma
  Choriocarcinoma
  Cervical carcinoma
  Endometrial carcinoma
  Tubo-ovarian carcinoma
  Breast carcinoma
  Others

Modified from Kaufman RH, Faro S (eds): Benign Diseases of the Vulva and Vagina, 4th ed. St. Louis, Mosby–Year Book, 1994, pp 168, 268.

tion and neoplasm. The latter further envelops a spectrum of benign, premalignant, locally invasive, and frankly malignant neoplasms. These categories are expressed as condyloma acuminatum, VIN, verrucous carcinoma, and squamous cell carcinoma. The distinguishing clinical features of each category are generally easy to define but may occasionally be subtle and result in a delayed or missed diagnosis of underlying malignancy.

All condylomata that exhibit sudden rapid growth, bleeding, or clinical symptoms and those that appear large, flat, sitting tightly on a broad-based surface, fungating, or fixed to the underlying tissue should be generously biopsied from multiple sites to rule out malignancy. Verrucous carcinoma is locally destructive but appears histologically benign. Squamous cell carcinoma in a condylomatous lesion is diagnosed by multiple biopsies that include surface and underlying stroma. Granuloma inguinale and herpes simplex virus can sometimes be very necrotizing and simulate malignancy. Molluscum contagiosum may provide a clue to

a possibly underlying condition of acquired immunodeficiency virus. It can be diagnosed clinically and the diagnosis confirmed by cytologic studies with or without biopsy.

BENIGN TUMORS OF THE VULVA

A wide spectrum of benign solid and cystic tumors involve the vulva. These tumors can be classified on the basis of the tissue of origin, embryologic derivation, morphologic findings, or gross appearance. Clinically they can be subdivided into solid and cystic tumors.

Benign Solid Tumors

The most common of the benign solid tumors affecting the vulva are the acrochordon (often called fibroepithelial polyp), fibroma, lipoma, neurofibroma, granular cell tumor, and solid tumors arising in the Bartholin and vestibular glands. Angiomyxoma can sometimes be large and aggressive and recurrent after removal. Angiomyofibroblastoma, on the other hand, is cured by local excision. Granular cell tumors can be multicentric in genital, nongenital, and visceral locations. Rarely they may behave in a malignant fashion in spite of structural benignancy. When the diagnosis is in doubt or a vulvar tumor is causing discomfort, the tumor should be widely excised either in the office with local anesthesia or in the hospital with general anesthesia. Wide local excision with primary closure of the defect is all that is needed.

Benign Cystic Tumors

The most common cystic tumors involving the vulva are the epidermal inclusion cyst, cystic hidradenoma, developmental cysts of urogenital sinus, paramesonephric duct, mesonephric duct, and Bartholin's duct.

The hidradenoma is often a confusing tumor for clinicians as well as pathologists. It may be confused with a primary or metastatic adenocarcinoma of the vulva. The distinction is made on the basis of clinical features and the characteristic microscopic pattern of the tumor as well as the absence of nuclear atypia and multilayering of cells. This tumor is easily removed in the office by local excision under local anesthesia. It usually does not recur.

Bartholin's duct cyst and abscess are seen in approximately 2% of new gynecologic patients. The cysts arise within the duct system of Bartholin's gland. Occlusion of the duct usually occurs near the opening of the main duct into the vestibule. Most cysts involve only the main duct and thus are unilocular, although occasionally one or more loculi lie deep in the main cyst. The majority of patients with small Bartholin's duct cysts are asymptomatic. If the cyst becomes infected or enlarged, the patient may experience discomfort and pressure, especially during coitus and when walking.

Treatment under these circumstances is best managed by marsupialization. The incision for marsupialization should be made medial enough so that the new orifice of the duct is located close to the original opening of Bartholin's duct into the vestibule. An incision 4 to 6 cm in length is made extending through the wall of the cyst. After evacuation of the contents, the lining of the cyst is sewn to the mucosal and skin surfaces with interrupted fine, absorbable sutures. If a Bartholin's cyst is partly or completely solid and occurring in an older patient, the possibility of underlying malignancy should be considered.

An acute Bartholin's duct abscess may arise primarily or may occur in the presence of a previous Bartholin's duct cyst. Culture of the contents of an abscess reveals a wide spectrum of organisms. The chief symptom of a Bartholin's duct abscess is pain and tenderness over the affected gland. The rapidity of development and the extent of involvement depend on the size of the infected cyst and the virulence of the infectious agent. Objective signs include unilateral swelling over the site of the affected gland, redness of the overlying skin, and frequently edema of the surrounding labia. An acute Bartholin's gland abscess usually requires surgical therapy, but local application of heat in the form of hot, wet dressings or sitz baths may promote spontaneous drainage within 72 hours. If treatment is begun early enough with a broad-spectrum antibiotic, formation of an abscess can occasionally be prevented. Incision and drainage of the abscess can be accomplished in the physician's office.

MALIGNANT NEOPLASMS OF THE VULVA

Both intraepithelial and invasive neoplasms are found in the vulva. The International Society for the Study of Vulvar Diseases has classified intraepithelial neoplastic disorders of the vulva skin and mucosa as follows:

1. Squamous (may include HPV changes)
   A. Vulvar intraepithelial neoplasia–1 (VIN-1) (mild dysplasia)
   B. VIN-2 (moderate dysplasia)
   C. VIN-3 (severe dysplasia; carcinoma in situ)
2. Other
   A. Paget's disease
   B. Melanoma, level 1

A comparison of the cases recorded between 1973 to 1976 and 1985 to 1987 shows that the incidence of VIN-3 has nearly doubled (Sturgeon and colleagues). During the same period, however, the incidence of invasive carcinoma remained stable. Sturgeon and colleagues reported that the incidence of VIN-3 increased from 1.1 to 2.1 cases per 100,000 women-years. The largest increase occurred in white women younger than 35 years. The peak incidence of in situ carcinoma decreased in time from women older than 54 years to women between the ages of 35 and 54 years.

Several possible factors may explain the increased incidence of this disease and its occurrence at a younger age. Heightened awareness of neoplasia on the part of the physician plays some role in its more frequent diagnosis. Similarly, vulvar self-examination by patients and in the general population brings many asymptomatic and early lesions to medical attention. Associated with this factor is an increasing tendency to perform biopsies on questionable lesions. A third factor is the increased occurrence of viral infections involving the lower genital tract.

The association of HPV with the development of lower genital tract neoplasia is now well accepted. Whereas most condylomata acuminata of the lower genital tract are associated with infection by HPV-6 and HPV-11, squamous cell carcinoma of the vulva is most often associated with HPV-16. It has been postulated, however, that possibly two forms of invasive squamous cell carcinoma of the vulva are seen.

One is observed most often in younger women whose lesions morphologically resemble changes seen with intraepithelial neoplasia, who smoke, and whose tumors have a high association with HPV infection. The other type of cancer is seen more often in older women with a more well-differentiated type of squamous cell carcinoma, who do not smoke, and whose lesions are infrequently associated with HPV infection.

The diagnosis of VIN must be established by biopsy before treatment is undertaken. The lesions are often multifocal, and if this is the case several biopsy specimens should be taken from different sites to establish that the lesion is in fact intraepithelial and not invasive.

Treatment of VIN-3

Opinion regarding management of intraepithelial squamous cell carcinoma of the vulva has changed radically since about 1980. The treatment should be individualized on the basis of location and extent of the lesion. Wide local excision, cryosurgery, local chemotherapy, and laser surgery have all been tried with variable results.

If wide local excision is chosen as the method of treatment, the entire lesion should be surgically removed, taking with it at least 0.5 to 1 cm of normal tissue. Frozen sections should be taken from the distal margins of the excised tissue to be certain that there is no residual disease. If disease is noted along the margins of the excised tissue, further skin and mucosa should be removed until the margins are free of disease. Recurrence of disease is related to the presence or absence of free margins, HPV type reinfection, and immunologic status of the patient. When extensive VIN-3 is present, wide local excision is preferred and may consist of performance of a wide superficial skinning vulvectomy. The skin and a small amount of subcutaneous tissue are removed, leaving the bulk of the vulvar structures intact. The defect can often be closed primarily, but it will occasionally be necessary to use a skin graft to adequately cover the denuded vulvar surfaces. If the disease extends into the anal canal, it is necessary to remove the anal mucosa up to the level of the pectinate line. The rectal mucosa can then be undermined and pulled down to cover the defect.

The use of the carbon dioxide laser to treat VIN is becoming increasingly popular. It is an excellent tool for the treatment of this disease, especially when localized. Before this approach is used, however, an occult invasive carcinoma must be excluded by adequate biopsies. Lesions demonstrating thickening of the tissues or those that appear ulcerated are better treated by excision than by the laser. When the laser is used, the lesion and the surrounding 0.5 to 1 cm of normal tissue should be ablated down to a depth of 1 to 3 mm, depending on the location of the lesion. On skin surfaces, the ablation should be carried down to a depth of 3 mm to remove any possible disease that has extended into the superficial skin appendages. A depth of destruction to 1 mm is adequate on mucosal surfaces.

The primary complications observed after laser therapy to the vulva are pain, bleeding, and discharge. Usually, the degree of pain is related to the area of the vulva treated and to the depth of treatment. The pain usually becomes most severe 4 to 5 days after therapy and may persist for another 5 to 10 days. Analgesics and warm sitz baths are of value in alleviating the symptoms.

Paget's disease of the vulva requires surgical treatment (wide local excision) similar to that for squamous cell carcinoma in situ. Paget's disease of the anogenital skin can be associated with underlying malignancy of skin adnexa, Bartholin's gland, urethra, anus, rectum, or breast. The surgical excision has to be appropriately modified. Intraepidermal and dermal migration of Paget's cells often occurs; thus, an adequate margin of normal-appearing tissue must be removed. When the disease involves large areas of the vulva, a wide superficial vulvectomy can be performed. This is carried out in the form of a skinning vulvectomy with removal of the skin and underlying adnexal structures, leaving the subcutaneous fat in place. If an underlying adnexal or invasive carcinoma is found, a second procedure consisting of a more extensive vulvectomy and inguinal-femoral lymphadenectomy should be performed.

Invasive Malignant Neoplasms of the Vulva

Invasive malignant vulvar tumors are classified in Table 1. The most common of the malignant tumors is squamous cell carcinoma with an annual incidence of 1.5 cases per 100,000 women in the United States. This most often presents as a raised granular tumor on the vulva but may also be seen as a thickened white plaque or granular ulceration. Invasive squamous cell carcinoma is often seen in association with VIN and occasionally with lichen sclerosus, which in the past led to the concept that lichen sclerosus was a precursor of invasive carcinoma. The likelihood that an individual with lichen sclerosus will ultimately develop invasive carcinoma of the vulva, however, is less than 5%. HPV infection (especially HPV-16) may also be associated with invasive squamous cell carcinoma of the vulva. In addition to the presence of a mass, the patient symptomatically often complains of pruritus, bleeding from the vulva, discharge, and occasionally pain. The diagnosis is established on the basis of a biopsy.

Treatment of Invasive Malignant Neoplasms

Treatment to a large extent depends on the stage of disease. Also of importance is an understanding of the method of spread of vulvar carcinoma. This is by direct extension and through the lymphatics to the ipsilateral inguinal and femoral lymph nodes. From here, the cancer may spread to the contralateral groin nodes and/or to the deep pelvic lymph nodes. Centrally located lesions are more apt to involve lymph nodes bilaterally because of the criss-crossing of lymphatics in the median line.

Surgical staging also plays a role in the decision as to appropriate therapy. The International Federation of Gynecology and Obstetrics (FIGO) staging system for carcinoma of the vulva is surgically accomplished and is as follows:

Stage 0: Carcinoma in situ; intraepithelial carcinoma

Stage I: Tumor confined to the vulva and/or perineum, 2 cm or less in greatest dimension, nodes are negative

Stage II: Tumor confined to the vulva and/or perineum, more than 2 cm in greatest dimension, nodes are negative

Stage III: Tumor of any size with

1. Adjacent spread to the lower urethra and/or the vagina, or the anus, and/or

2. Unilateral regional lymph node metastasis

Stage IVA: Tumor invades any of the following: upper urethra, bladder mucosa, rectal mucosa, pelvic bone, and/or bilateral regional node metastasis

Stage IVB: Any distant metastasis, including pelvic lymph nodes

Before treatment is planned, the patient should be carefully evaluated for the presence of distant metastasis, although this is highly unlikely in a stage I or II lesion. Certainly, a preoperative chest radiograph, bone scan, and computed tomographic scan of the pelvis looking for enlarged lymph nodes should be performed, especially in those individuals with suspected stage III and IV diseases.

Although radical vulvectomy with bilateral femoral-inguinal lymph node dissection was in the past considered the standard of care for all invasive carcinomas of the vulva, this is no longer true today. Treatment is individualized and based on the knowledge of the natural spread of vulvar carcinoma. The latter includes clinical staging, gross and microscopic features of the tumor, and angiolymphatic invasion.

Stage 1 Carcinoma

For a tumor localized to one side of the vulva, a partial deep vulvectomy with ipsilateral groin node dissection is considered adequate treatment. This allows preservation of much of the normal vulvar anatomy and is also associated with less postoperative morbidity than is radical vulvectomy. In the tumor excision at least a 2- to 3-cm margin of normal skin should be removed surrounding the tumor, and the subcutaneous fat should be excised down to the fascia. The distance between the tumor and the surgical margin is a significant predictor of local recurrence. If there is no evidence of spread to the groin lymph nodes, no further therapy is required. If positive nodes are found, however, contralateral lymph nodes should be removed, or the ipsilateral and contralateral groin could be treated with external beam radiotherapy. The deep pelvic nodes should also re-

ceive radiation therapy. In the presence of a midline lesion, a bilateral inguinal-femoral lymph node dissection should be performed. After surgical excision of the lesion and groin lymph nodes, suction drainage should be left in place until the drainage has decreased to a minimal amount.

Levenbach and colleagues have suggested injecting isosulfan blue solution (0.5 mL) into the tumor margin before the lymph node dissection. The dye is transported by lymphatic vessels to the lymph nodes, turning them a deep blue. This allows the easy identification of the sentinel node. Frozen sections can then be taken, and if no tumor is identified, it is not necessary to remove the deep nodes. The diagnosis of minimal lymph node metastasis can be augmented by use of polyclonal keratin antibody.

Stage II Disease

Depending on the size of the tumor, an operative procedure similar to that recommended for stage I disease can be carried out for stage II disease. Occasionally, however, when the lesion is of larger size, it is necessary to perform a complete deep vulvectomy to remove the entire tumor along with an adequate margin of normal tissue. When this is done, the inguinal and femoral lymph nodes are removed through separate groin incisions. To close a large defect, it is often necessary to swing skin flaps with attached subcutaneous fat to cover the defect.

Stage III Disease

Stage III disease that has spread to the lower urethra and vagina is also treated by vulvectomy with removal of the lower portion of the urethra and/or vagina to allow at least a 2-cm margin of normal tissue. When the anus is involved with the tumor, it may be necessary to perform a vulvectomy with abdominoperineal resection while removing the anus. Bilateral inguinal and femoral lymph nodes could be removed through separate groin incisions. It is occasionally necessary to use a full-thickness skin flap with the gracilis muscle to cover a large vulvar defect that cannot be covered by a "rhomboid" flap.

Radiotherapy may decrease the size of a large, bulky lesion to the point at which a less radical excision is required.

Stage IV Disease

Therapy for stage IV vulvar carcinoma must be individualized. Depending on whether there is evidence of distant metastasis, local palliative excision with or without radiation therapy is used. In the absence of distant metastasis, patients are managed as described for stage III disease.

VERRUCOUS CARCINOMA

Verrucous carcinoma, previously also called giant condyloma of Buschke-Lowenstein, presents as a large, irregular cauliflower-like lesion. It locally invades the vulvar tissue without metastasis. Like condylomata acuminata, it has been found to be associated with HPV-6. It is very important to inform the pathologist of the verrucous carcinoma as a clinical possibility; otherwise multiple and repeated biopsies will be reported as fragments of benign squamous epithelium showing no evidence of malignancy. This is because the verrucous carcinoma retains a deceptively benign microscopic appearance despite local invasion. The lesion also needs to be distinguished from invasive squamous cell carcinoma, which will show dysplastic squamous epithelium in an invasive background.

The treatment of verrucous carcinoma generally consists of wide local excision. If enlarged, suspicious lymph nodes are palpated, fine-needle aspiration followed by groin dissection should be performed. Radiation therapy is contraindicated in the management of this tumor because doing so frequently transforms it into an aggressive, anaplastic tumor.

BASAL CELL CARCINOMA

Basal cell carcinoma usually arises as a solitary, ulcerated lesion with raised, round, pearly edges. If left untreated, this lesion will continue to destructively invade the vulvar tissues. Only rarely does basal cell carcinoma metastasize. Squamous cell carcinoma having basaloid features should be diagnosed as such because of its metastatic potential.

Treatment consists of wide local excision of the neoplasm. It is not necessary to perform a regional lymph node dissection because spread to the lymph nodes is extremely rare.

MELANOMA

Melanoma occurs as a primary vulvar lesion uncommonly. When it does occur, however, early diagnosis is mandatory if cure is to be achieved. Prognosis is directly related to the depth of tumor invasion. Several methods for microstaging melanoma have been proposed. The staging systems of Clark and of Breslow are most commonly used by the pathologist. They are listed in Table 2.

The diagnosis is established with a biopsy. The microstaging is determined after excision of the neoplasm. As a site, genital melanoma is prognostically unfavorable. Education of patients for vulvar self-examination and immediate attention to symptomatic nevi may curb that poor outlook.

Level 1 and 2 melanomas have an extremely good prognosis. Melanoma that extends into the subcutaneous fat carries with it an almost hopeless outlook.

TABLE 2. **Methods for Microstaging Melanoma**

Clark's Levels	Breslow's Levels (Modified)
1. Intraepithelial	<0.76 mm
2. Into papillary dermis	0.76–1.49 mm
3. Fills papillary dermis	1.50–2.49 mm
4. Into reticular dermis	2.50–3.99 mm
5. Into subcutaneous fat	≥4 mm

Tumors invading less than 1 mm can be treated by wide local excision and removal of the underlying subcutaneous fat. When the level of invasion is deeper than 1 mm, a wide radical excision of the neoplasm is recommended along with ipsilateral inguinal-femoral lymph node removal. The lymph node dissection is more prognostic than therapeutic because, once spread to the regional lymph nodes has occurred, the prognosis is extremely poor regardless of additional adjunctive therapy that is attempted.

BARTHOLIN'S GLAND CARCINOMA

The diagnosis of Bartholin's gland carcinoma is established when the neoplasm is localized to the region of Bartholin's gland and there is histologic evidence that Bartholin's gland structures are contiguous with the tumor. In addition, the skin overlying the neoplasm should be intact. Suspicion of a malignant neoplasm of Bartholin's gland should be aroused when the postmenopausal woman suddenly develops what is thought to be a Bartholin's duct abscess or cyst. Another finding that should arouse suspicion is the presence of a solid mass developing in this region. Bartholin's gland carcinomas are managed in a manner similar to that for invasive squamous cell carcinoma of the vulva.

SOFT TISSUE SARCOMA

Soft tissue sarcomas are extremely rare. They usually present as rapidly growing solid tumors. The diagnosis is made on the basis of biopsy or histologic examination of the surgical specimen. Therapy consists primarily of wide local excision. Radiotherapy is of little use in the management of most vulvar sarcomas. Sarcoma botryoides characteristically may present as a urogenital polypoid lesion in children. It should be promptly diagnosed followed by surgery, radiation, and chemotherapy.

METASTATIC TUMORS

Metastatic tumors are uncommon tumors of the vulva. By the time a metastasis takes place in the vulva, the primary site of the tumor is generally obvious. In young women, gestational choriocarcinoma can be evident by metastasis while the primary tumor is still silent. In general, metastatic tumors to the vulva carry a dismal prognosis.

CONTRACEPTION

method of
KATHRYN M. ANDOLSEK, M.D., M.P.H.
Duke University Medical Center
Durham, North Carolina

More than 60 million women in the United States are currently between 15 and 44 years of age, the major reproductive period of their lives. Thirty percent do not need contraception because they are sterile, pregnant, postpartum, attempting to become pregnant, or are not or never have been sexually active. Most of the remaining women who do not desire a pregnancy use contraception. The percentage of sexually active women *not* using a contraceptive method declined by one-third between 1982 and 1995. Nonetheless, more than 3 million unintended pregnancies occur each year in the United States. Nearly half of the unintended pregnancies (47%) occur in the 3 million women who do not use contraception.

The average couple who desires "the average number of two children" needs to practice some method of contraception for at least 20 years. Generally, several methods of contraception are used at different times. The clinician, therefore, cannot merely assess and counsel a contraceptive choice at a single point in time, but must provide ongoing support, effectively manage side effects, evaluate for impediments to use, and help couples evaluate their options.

Contraception has been used for centuries. The most common methods have been variations of the condom, vaginal pessaries, coitus interruptus, or abortion. It was illegal in the United States to write for or to mail information about contraceptive devices until the 1940s and in some states to provide contraceptive information to unmarried women until the 1970s.

CHOOSING A CONTRACEPTIVE METHOD

Ideally, the contraceptive method should be chosen by a couple. The "perfect contraceptive" should be safe, effective, inexpensive, always available, acceptable to both partners, easy to use, reversible, lack side effects, and include noncontraceptive benefits (such as protection from sexually transmitted disease). In reality, many contraceptive decisions are made by the woman. There is usually no "perfect method" but rather compromises among these criteria (Table 1).

ASSESSING CONTRACEPTIVE EFFICACY

Men are essentially fertile all the time. Women are fertile for no more than 24 to 36 hours each menstrual cycle. Because sperm are viable for no more than 48 hours, couples are fertile at most 4 to 5 days each menstrual cycle window; contraception is thus needed only during this portion of the cycle. It is challenging, however, to determine which 4 to 5 days are the fertile period. The efficacy of contraceptive methods is calculated as the number of pregnancies per 100 woman years, or the number of pregnancies experienced by 100 fertile sexually active women who use a given method for a year. Efficacy of various methods are compared with the outcome of couples who use no method. The use of no method results in 85 pregnancies among 100 women over 1 year. The use of no method is 15% effective (some couples are infertile) and has an 85% failure rate.

Efficacy is further categorized as theoretical (perfect use) and actual (typical use). The first measure of efficacy is the method efficacy that estimates the true effectiveness of the method if it is used correctly and consistently with each act of intercourse. It is represented as the number of unintended pregnancies per 100 women that occur during the first year of use. Methods are used by couples, however, and couples rarely use a method perfectly. A more realistic measure of efficacy is the usual or typical efficacy rate. This value is generally derived from studies of actual us-

ers. The typical use is influenced by a couple's fertility, motivation, risk-taking attitude, frequency of intercourse, ability to use and continue the method, and use of backup methods.

RISKS AND BENEFITS OF CONTRACEPTIVE METHODS

For women under 45 years of age, almost all forms of contraception result in less morbidity and mortality than would a pregnancy. Women older than 35 years of age who smoke cigarettes have a greater risk from oral contraception than from pregnancy. Women with chronic medical conditions (such as hypertension, diabetes, heart disease, and some collagen vascular diseases) may have higher morbidity and mortality from certain contraceptive methods than do healthier women. They may also, however, have a higher risk from pregnancy and pregnancy-related complications as well.

Some contraceptives offer noncontraceptive benefits in addition to their contraceptive effect. Barrier methods (such as the male and female condoms) may decrease the risk of common sexually transmitted diseases such as chlamydia, gonorrhea, and the human immunodeficiency virus (HIV). The incidence of some cancers may be reduced. Dysmenorrhea, acne, and iron deficiency anemia can be decreased in many users of oral contraceptives.

MAKING EVERY VISIT AN OPPORTUNITY FOR CONTRACEPTIVE ASSESSMENT

Every visit provides an ideal opportunity to inquire about a patient's reproductive status and sexual activity. The U.S. Preventive Services Task Force rates counseling about effective contraceptive methods a "B" recommendation, which indicates that there is at least fair clinical evidence supporting its use in practice. Even if uninterested in contraception, all sexually active patients can be assessed for their risk of sexually transmitted disease. If at risk, they can be counseled regarding safe sex practices, including abstinence, the benefits from condoms and how to use them effectively, and the risk of hepatitis B. Screening at-risk patients for sexually transmitted diseases such as gonorrhea, chlamydia, syphilis, hepatitis B, and HIV is recommended. Papanicolaou smears can be obtained to screen for cervical dysplasia. Sexually active patients who are interested in achieving a pregnancy may benefit from preconception assessment and recommendations such as folic acid supplementation.

ABSTINENCE

The only 100% effective contraceptive, if used 100% of the time, is abstinence. In reality, abstinence may be difficult to practice.

FERTILITY AWARENESS

Fertility awareness attempts to determine the few fertile days each cycle. The couple then avoids genital relations during that time. As the scientific understanding of ovulation has increased, this method has become more precise.

Women generally ovulate approximately 14 days before the start of their period. The use of "calendar" rhythm—predicting by extrapolating the "fertile"

Text continued on page 1084

TABLE 1. Advantages and Disadvantages of Various Contraceptive Methods

Method	Advantages	Disadvantages	Contraindications	Comments	% of Women Experiencing Unintended Pregnancy Within First Year	
					Typical Use	*Perfect Use*
No method but sexually active					85	
Abstinence	The only 100% effective method No associated risks (i.e., STDs) No financial costs	High rate of failure	None	Clinician should support patient's and partner's decision; discuss other sexual intimate options that do not risk pregnancy or STDs; patients may benefit from specific role playing to think through discussion with their partners and their partners' specific responses Adolescents may be more open to abstinence once they have had intercourse and satisfied their curiosity	?	0
Fertility awareness and periodic abstinence	Acceptable to some religions that find other contraceptive methods objectionable "Reversible" in that it can be used to conceive as well as not to conceive	Usually requires classes to learn method (which may not be available widely) Both partners need to communicate and be committed to it 7–15 abstinent days required each cycle			25	
Natural family planning	No hormones, chemicals, or instruments used No costs beyond initial classes unless home kits are used to detect ovulation					
Calendar rhythm		Cannot be used by women with irregular periods Many conditions put off menstrual timing by 2–3 d, even in women with "regular" cycles, making it unreliable Woman must be able to monitor and interpret temperature and mucus characteristics	Irregular menses	Least reliable of all fertility awareness methods		9
Sympathothermal						3
Lactational amenorrhea	Some contraceptive benefit if exclusively breast-fed baby suckles no less than every 4 h for the first 6 months postpartum or until bleeding occurs	Any supplementation or disruption in feeding pattern can lower efficacy	Another method should be started once menstruation occurs, frequency or duration of feeding lowers, supplemental feeding started, or baby >6 mo old HIV-positive mother should not breast-feed if other safe feeding methods available	Only 50% of U.S. mothers breast-feed; advice should be combined with breast-feeding counseling Milk expression by pump is not an effective substitution; suckling disrupts pulsatile gonadotropin release HIV is transmitted in breast milk	0.5–1.5	
Withdrawal/coitus interruptus		Depends on trust and "control" of partner Failure rate 18% but better than no contraceptive at all No protection against STDs		No reinsertion of penis after ejaculation unless partner washes penis with soap and water and urinates fully Consider backup emergency contraception	19	4

Method	Advantages	Disadvantages	Comments	Contraindications	Typical use failure (%)	Perfect use failure (%)
Douching	Some reduction in fertility; no difference between commercial preparations and home-prepared water and vinegar; unknown risks					
Spermicidal products	Accessible to couples Reversible Up to 25% protection against STDs such as gonorrhea and chlamydia (*not* HIV) Increase efficacy of barrier methods	Suppositories and tablets dissolve in less than 30 minutes; effective for ≤1 h Creams, jellies, gels (for use with diaphragm) place high up in the vagina, 10–60 min before coitus Vary in consistency and percentage of active ingredient May raise risk of HIV (due to irritation)	Cream provides better coverage than gels Use 10–60 min before intercourse; use additional dose if ≥1 h between application and intercourse or repeated intercourse Leave in place >6 h after intercourse No douching for >6 h after use	Hypersensitivity to spermicidal products	26	6
Sponges Parous Nulliparous	Lowers incidence of candidiasis Continuous protection for 24 hours	No current U.S. manufacturer	Moisten with 2 tbsp water before insertion Can order from Canada (http://www.birthcontrol.com)		40 20	20 9
Condoms	Accessible to couples Some STD protection (perhaps 50%), including HIV, GC, chlamydia; less for HPV and HSV "Reversible" May decrease cervical cancer by 50% Counseling to promote condoms for STD/HIV protection also increases proportion of women using other contraceptive methods and women using other contraceptive methods who use them consistently Male participation Few side effects	Partner dependent Condom may "break" (1/100 episodes); may slip (5/100 episodes) (mainly due to error in use and not from product) Leakage, 3.5% Animal-based products do not protect against HIV May decrease sensitivity/spontaneity Oil-based preparations that impair latex condom efficacy: Butoconazole, miconazole, ticonazole, conjugated estrogens (cream), estradiol (cream), baby oil, butter, cocoa butter, cold cream, mineral oil, hand lotion, massage oil, petroleum jelly, vegetable oil, shortening, suntan oil, rubbing alcohol	Brands trade off reliability/strength vs less thickness to enhance sexual stimulation Counseling may improve consistency and help partners negotiate use Lubrication and reservoir tip lowers risk of breakage Safe lubricants: Egg white, glycerine, Nonoxynol-9, saliva, water, aloe-9, KY Jelly, Astroglide, Gynol II Prepair, Probe, Ramses Personal Lubricant	Latex allergy Hypersensitivity to spermicidal products Do not use male and female condoms together	14	3
Female condom	Three varieties available Not latex, so no problem if latex allergic Can use oil-based products	Does not contain spermicide Cannot be used with male condom	Remove immediately after intercourse and before standing Unproven STD benefit (though, theoretically, should provide some)		21	5

Table continued on following page

TABLE 1. **Advantages and Disadvantages of Various Contraceptive Methods** *Continued*

Method	Advantages	Disadvantages	Contraindications	Comments	% of Women Experiencing Unintended Pregnancy Within First Year	
					Typical Use	*Perfect Use*
Diaphragm	Several varieties; available in sizes from 50 to 100 mm in 2.5-mm and 5.0-mm increments "Reversible" Some STD protection Some protection from cervical dysplasia	Must be used with spermicidal products Risk of TSS if worn >24 h Higher incidence of urinary tract infection (times 2) Less efficacy with increased intercourse Damaged by oil-based lubricants (see Condoms) Repeat dose of spermicidal product for repeated intercourse	Most cause latex allergy Hypersensitivity to spermicidal products History of TSS Abnormal anatomy (may preclude use)	For parous women, diaphragm more effective than sponge or cap May be inserted up to 8 h before intercourse Should be left in place 6-8 h after last coitus Should be refit yearly and after pregnancy, miscarriage, abortion, pelvic surgery, or weight change of >10 lb Used with spermicidal product If recurrent UTIs, try smaller diaphragm or different rim or change to different method TSS symptoms: Sudden high fever, vomiting, diarrhea, dizziness, faintness, weakness, sore throat, aching muscles and joints, sunburn-like rash	20	6
Cervical cap Parous	"Reversible" Spermicide not necessary but improves efficacy Continuous protection for 48 h	Hypersensitivity to spermicidal products Damaged by oil-based lubricants (see Condoms) Should not be worn >48 h	Latex allergy History of toxic shock syndrome		40	26
Nulliparous	Additional spermicide not necessary with repeated intercourse	Abnormal anatomy may preclude use Not widely available Few clinicians trained in use About 6% of women cannot be fitted			20	9
IUDs	Most cost effective contraception when used >2 yr No increase in endometrial cancer Infections usually occur within the first 20 d; incidence, 0.3% Can be inserted at any time of menstrual cycle Can prevent and treat Asherman's syndrome Works primarily to decrease fertilization; does not interfere with lactation	Uterine perforation possible but rare Expulsion rate 2%–10% within the first year Higher risk expulsion with nulliparity, severe dysmenorrhea, abnormal menstrual blood flow After one expulsion, 30% risk of second If woman becomes pregnant, 50% risk SAB; 25% lower risk if IUD removed early If woman becomes pregnant, 5% risk of ectopic pregnancy Slight increased risk of PID in first few weeks after insertion	Distortion of uterine cavity; polyps, leiomyomata, etc. Active PID See individual IUDs, later	Although labeling says nulliparous women should not receive, can be used if risks are carefully discussed and alternatives excluded Prophylactic antibiotics for SBE recommended at IUD insertion if valvular heart disease (not mitral valve prolapse) Nulliparity not a contraindication Treat vaginal infection before placement; treat vaginal yeast infection before insertion Although pre-insertion doxycycline* 200 mg or azithromycin (Zithromax)* 500 mg PO, 1 h before insertion has been used to attempt to reduce the rate of infection, this has not been consistently demonstrated in studies		

Copper T 380A	Effective for 10 years Can be used as emergency contraception First year failure rate, 0.6% Reduces risk of ectopic pregnancy by 90%	If pregnancy occurs, it is more likely ectopic Increased bleeding, spotting, infertility risks	Pregnancy Active or history of PID Genital actinomycosis STD risk Uterine or cervical malignancy Postpartum endometriosis or infected abortion (within 3 months) Immunosuppressed women Acute vaginitis or cervicitis, uterine cavity distortion, uterine malignancy, unresolved Pap or abnormal pap smear STD risk Undiagnosed abnormal gynecologic bleeding Wilson's disease Copper allergy Presence of previous IUD that has not been removed	Postpartum: Needs to be inserted within 10 minutes of delivery or at 6–8 wk Special care to avoid perforation Immunosuppressed women (steroid treatment, HIV/AIDS) need careful weighing of risks/benefits; may increase risks for transmission to partner and for PID Patient needs access to follow-up	0.8 0.6
Progesterone T	Decreases menstrual flow (50%) Decreases dysmenorrhea	6–10 times increased risk of ectopic pregnancy than with Copper T 380A Requires annual reinsertion	Pregnancy Active or history of PID Genital actinomycosis History of pelvic surgery, which increases ectopic risk Uterine cavity <6 cm, >10 cm STD risk Uterine or cervical malignancy History of ectopic pregnancy Postpartum endometriosis or infected abortion within 3 months Acute vaginitis or cervicitis Immunosuppression Undiagnosed abnormal gynecologic bleeding Incomplete uterine involution after childbirth Previously inserted IUD still in place	Primarily useful if woman only desires 1 year of contraception	2.0 1.5
Levonorgestrel IUD (LNg 2)*	Decreases PID Treats amenorrhea Can be used to treat menorrhagia				0.3 0.3

Table continued on following page

TABLE 1. **Advantages and Disadvantages of Various Contraceptive Methods** *Continued*

Method	Advantages	Disadvantages	Contraindications	Comments	% of Women Experiencing Unintended Pregnancy Within First Year	
					Typical Use	*Perfect Use*
Combined oral contraceptive pill	"Reversible" Decreases endometrial cancer, ovarian cancer, ovarian cysts, benign breast disease, ectopic pregnancy, PMS, dysmenorrhea, hirsutism, acne, PID, uterine fibroids, endometriosis, menstrual flow, TSS Increases bone mass Decreases 1/750 hospitalizations per year, lowers risk of rheumatoid arthritis No risk of DM with current low dose estrogens and progestins	Certain medications may lower hormonal level of OCs: ampicillin, rifampin (the most evidence), griseofulvin, tetracycline, barbiturates, phenobarbital, phenytoin, primidone; not apparently true for penicillin and cephalosporins in dosages commonly used for women with acne May lower anticoagulation effect of warfarin, enhance benzodiazepine effect, reduce prednisolone clearance May increase levels of certain drugs: TCAs, insulin, ibuprofen, oral hypoglycemics, cyclosporine, 10%–30% break-through bleeding first month, antipsychotic medications 3% post pill amenorrhea Slight increase in blood pressure among some women (only 42:100,000 hypertension patients attributed to OC use) Increases chlamydial infections No STD protection Small increased risk of breast cancer (but cancers are less advanced)	Active liver disease Hepatic adenomas Jaundice with pregnancy or OC use Thrombophlebitis Active or history of thromboembolic disorders (CVA, PE, DVT) Cardiovascular disease (severe CHF predisposes to thrombus) Coronary occlusion, polycythemia vera Cerebrovascular disease Known or suspected breast cancer Undiagnosed abnormal gynecologic bleeding Symptomatic gallbladder disease Breast-feeding (?) Cigarette smoking if >45 yr Women who smoke and are >35 yr should be counseled regarding greater risk Some conditions may worsen with OC use, and combined OCs may not be able to be used; women could try OC with lower estrogen or progesterone-only OC. These conditions include diabetes mellitus, hypertension, migraine headaches, fibrocystic breast disease Women with well-controlled diabetes or hypertension and triglycerides <750 mg/dL on OCs, inactive liver disease, history of pregnancy-induced hypertension, or gestational DM may use OCs with close follow-up	Sickle cell disease (sickle C disease or sickle cell), uterine leiomyoma, or before elective surgery no longer contraindications Grapefruit juice will increase ethinyl estradiol concentration Cancer reduction ↓ Ovarian cancer → 30% ≥4 yr → 60% ≥5 yr → 80% ≥12 yr Endometrial cancer → 40% ≥2 yr → 60% ≥4 yr Benefit persists after OC use stops No significant fetal risk if inadvertent pregnancy, no effect on height of adolescents Discontinue estrogen-containing pills 4 weeks before major surgery Add condoms if STD protection needed Early pill warning signals: abdominal pain, chest symptoms (cough, shortness of breath), eye problems (vision loss or blurring), severe leg pain, headache Effect on cervical cancer unclear	5	0.1
Progestin-only pill	"Reversible" May be tolerated by women who cannot tolerate or have contraindication to estrogen Compatible with lactation	Amenorrhea Spotting Do not take with carbamazepine, phenobarbital, phenytoin, primidone, rifampin (will lower OC efficacy)	Undiagnosed abnormal gynecologic bleeding Pregnancy Active liver disease Liver tumors Breast cancer	Must be used at same time of day each day If break-through bleeding persists, consider NSAIDs, combined OCs, or 10–13 d of oral estrogen		0.5

Emergency contraception	Useful backup method Pregnancies that occur have no increased risk of congenital abnormalities No evidence of increased ectopic pregnancy risk Can use pills for ≤72 h after unprotected intercourse; copper IUD ≤5 d	Nausea, 30%–50% Vomiting, 15%–25%	Women with most hormonal contraindications can usually tolerate for short duration as emergency method	Exclude possibility that patient is already pregnant More successful the sooner it is initiated 10%–15% have change in next menstrual period (amount, duration, timing) Routine antinausea or antiemetic 1 h before first dose may help Need to offer regular contraception; woman should use backup contraceptive for the remainder of the cycle, then a regular method with next menstrual cycle Preven kit combines urine pregnancy test and 4 contraceptive tablets Consider including antiemetic, consider prescribing prospectively for women who do not use contraception or those who use methods with high failure rates Progestin-only pills associated with decreased nausea and vomiting	Decreases pregnancy rate by 75%
Injected DMPA	"Reversible" 150 mg IM effective for 12 weeks Can be used postpartum May lower endometrial cancer risk No change in clotting parameters Useful if effective, temporary contraceptions needed (isotretinoin [Accutane], waiting for vasectomy) Lowers risk of endometrial cancer, ovarian cancer, PID, ectopic pregnancy, anemia, and pain due to endometriosis Lowers risk sickle cell crisis Lowers seizure frequency in women with seizure disorders	Contraceptive effects persist 4 mo to >1 yr (>85% conceive within 18 months), not related to duration of use Menstrual disturbance 50% develop amenorrhea with >1 yr use Weight gain 5 + lb 1st year; 16 2nd year Bloating, dizziness, mood changes, palpitations; depression, breast tenderness, headache LDL and total cholesterol may increase Lowers HDL Unknown effect on bone No STD protection Cramps Acne May decrease libido Overweight women have lower efficacy May increase risk of later osteoporosis for adolescents (unlike Norplant or OCs)	Pregnancy Acute liver disease or tumors Known or suspected breast cancer Undiagnosed abnormal gynecologic bleeding Hypersensitivity to the drug (thrombophlebitis or thromboembolic disorders are listed on the package, but women may be treated cautiously) Avoid in women who desire rapid return of fertility	150 mg IM q 12 wk, IM in gluteal or deltoid muscle using 21 or 23 gauge needle within 5 d of onset of menses and negative pregnancy test. If given beyond this time, back-up contraceptive for 2–4 wk If break-through bleeding persists, consider NSAIDs, combined OCs, or 10–13 d of oral estrogen Do not massage over injection site Have allergic emergency support available Injectable norethindrone not available in the United States	0.3 0.3

Table continued on following page

TABLE 1. **Advantages and Disadvantages of Various Contraceptive Methods** *Continued*

Method	Advantages	Disadvantages	Contraindications	Comments	% of Women Experiencing Unintended Pregnancy Within First Year	
					Typical Use	*Perfect Use*
Norplant (Levonorgestrel implants)	Effective for 5 years Reversible "immediately" (within 24 hours of insertion) Lowers risk of endometrial cancer, ovarian cancer, PID, ectopic pregnancy, anemia, and pain due to endometriosis No demonstrated risk of breast or cervical cancer No change in cholesterol, glucose, blood coagulation, or liver function tests Effective for 5 years	Weight gain (5 lb) Higher rate of pregnancy in women >154 lb; less a problem since 1991 Requires surgical removal and insertion Higher initial costs (approx. $350 for materials, $150 for insertion) Less effective with carbamazepine, phenytoin, phenobarbitol, rifampin Increased risk of ectopic pregnancy if the woman becomes pregnant Most women have menstrual irregularity, generally more bleeding days with less total blood loss Not as reliable with women of higher weights; failure rates are increased 0.2%–1.0% to 5% in women ≥70 kg Not reliable in last year of use	Active liver disease or tumors Active thrombophlebitis Known or suspected breast cancer Undiagnosed abnormal gynecologic bleeding Pregnancy Hypersensitivity to the drug	Each implant contains 36 mg levonorgestrel, released 85 µg/d 0–9 mo 35 µg/d 9–18 mo 30 µg/d >18 mo Decreased ovulation in at least half the cycles Norplant Foundation (800-760-9030) may provide financial help for disadvantaged women For persistent irregular bleeding, consider 1.25 mg conjugated estrogen (or equivalent) × 1 wk Testing "suitability" with DMPA or progestin-only OC does not make sense. The hormones and fluctuations in levels *differ*	0.05	0.05

Sterilization Female	No compliance needs Single decision Safe, mortality rate 1–2/100,000 (anesthesia, sepsis, hemorrhage), complications <1%	6% regret (regret related to inadequate counseling, age <30 yr, post partum, and change in marital status or relationships) Failure rate, 1/250 post partum Failure rate, 1/400 interval 1% of women choose to reverse Reversibility difficult and expensive (success rate 43%–88%); assisted reproductive technologies frequently required Serious morbidity (major infection or organ injury), 1.5%–9% Minor morbidity (wound infection), 6%–11% No STD protection	Failure increases with young women, bipolar technique, error (30%–50%) 5.5 pregnancies: 1000 over 10 yr Provide counseling or options to minimize regret If pregnancy occurs, one-third are ectopic; patient should be assumed to have ectopic pregnancy unless proven otherwise Serum progesterone may decrease No proven change in menstrual patterns	.55 0.5–1.9 (within 10 yr)
Male	Single decision Most cost-effective method Complications, <3% Failure rate, 0.1%–4% Compared with tubal ligation: less expensive, fewer complications and surgical risks, shorter recovery time, less time away from work, no long-term health risks, outpatient procedure	Complications: hematoma; spermatocele; congestive epididymitis; 1/2 to 2/3 men develop sperm antibodies, significance unknown (does not correlate with health risks); testicular discomfort; infection; granuloma; failure Reversibility difficult and expensive (success rate, 16%–79%; usually >50%) No STD protection	Success of reversal related to length of time from procedure; overall success rate, 50%; 30% if after 10 yr No impact on prostate cancer Fewer complications with "no scalpel" method Not sterile until >20 ejaculations Requires microscopic evaluation for sperm	0.15 0.10

*Not available in the United States.

Abbreviations: STDs = sexually transmitted diseases; HIV, human immunodeficiency virus; GC, gonococcus; HPV = human papillomavirus; HSV = herpes simplex virus; UTI, urinary tract infection; TSS, toxic shock syndrome; SAB = significant asymptomatic bacteriuria; SBE = subacute bacterial endocarditis; PMS = premenstrual syndrome; OCs, oral contraceptives; TCA = tricyclic antidepressant; CVA = cardiovascular accident; PE = pulmonary embolism; DVT = deep vein thrombosis; CHF = chronic heart failure; DM = diabetes mellitus; ↓ = decreased; IUD = intrauterine device; NSAIDs = nonsteroidal anti-inflammatory drugs; DMPA = depomedroxyprogesterone acetate; LDL = low-density lipoprotein; HDL = high-density lipoprotein; IM = intramuscular.

period based on the last several months cycle lengths—is not reliable. Only 16% of cycles are 28 days in length. Most women do not have consistently regular cycles. Even those who do frequently deviate 2 to 3 days from their previous cycle.

The sympathothermal methods of natural family planning take advantage of predictable changes in a woman's physiology that coincide with ovulation. *Thermal* refers to the predictable temperature elevation associated with progesterone level. Before ovulation, temperature falls approximately 0.3°F from the usual baseline. It then rises to approximately 0.5° to 1.0°F and remains elevated for 12 to 16 days. The basal body temperature must be taken in the morning just before arising, eating, drinking, and smoking and at the same time each day. Many conditions affect the basal body temperature. A febrile illness can cause confusion. Alcohol consumption can cause a temperature increase. Pharmacies stock nonprescription kits that measure urine luteinizing hormone (LH). Women can predict the day of ovulation by testing their first morning urine specimen. These cost $40 or more per cycle.

Sympatho refers to other predictable physiologic changes associated with ovulation. These include Mittelschmerz's pain (pain in the area of an ovary at midcycle), changes in the cervix, and moliminal symptoms (breast tenderness). The easiest to discern, however, is the change in cervical mucus. To learn this method a woman and her partner should attend classes. They will learn to recognize the mucus changes, interpret their significance, understand the days that require abstinence, and gain confidence with the method. Semen, vaginitis, the use of vaginal creams, pregnancy, and breast-feeding cause changes that couples need to be able to recognize.

COITUS INTERRUPTUS AND WITHDRAWAL

Coitus interruptus and withdrawal involve the withdrawal of the man's penis from the vaginal canal before ejaculation. Failures occur with lack of clear communication, the inability of the man to withdraw at this time of sexual activity, and, because they are present in the pre-ejaculatory fluid, sperm release before withdrawal.

SPERMICIDES

Hundreds of compounds have been used to kill or inactivate sperm without causing irritation or toxicity to the partners. Spermicidal contraceptives can be used alone or in combination with condoms, diaphragms, or cervical caps. Spermicides reduce the risk of acquiring sexually transmitted diseases somewhat but probably offer no protection against HIV. Spermicides are available as gels, creams, jellies, foam, film, and suppositories. Most have nonoxynol-9 or octoxynol-9 as the active ingredient. Creams may have a higher concentration of the spermicide, but no clinical trials comparing the efficacy of one product with another have been done. Scents and flavors are "cosmetic," with no impact on spermicidal effectiveness. Either partner may develop a hypersensitivity reaction to these products.

CONDOMS

Condoms are popular because they are widely accessible and provide some protection against sexually transmitted diseases. Animal-based condoms do not protect against HIV. The addition of spermicidal products increases their efficacy.

The female condom became available in the early 1990s. The most common has two flexible rings on each end of a polyurethane tube. The one ring inserts into the vagina similarly to a diaphragm, and the other end remains at the vulva. The female condom has been demonstrated to prevent the transmission of HIV in laboratory studies, but clinical trials have not been conducted. Male and female condoms should not be used together. Because of breakage, slippage, and inconsistency of use, couples should be aware of emergency contraception.

DIAPHRAGM

Most diaphragms are soft latex barriers that fit between the area just under the symphysis pubis and the posterior fornix. They act as a physical barrier to keep sperm from entering the cervix. They are used with a spermicidal product that provides additional protection. The spermicidal cream or gel is applied to the rim of the diaphragm, and this diaphragm inserted up to 2 hours before intercourse. Products that affect latex integrity should be avoided. If intercourse is repeated during the same sexual encounter, additional spermicide is inserted *without* removing the diaphragm. The diaphragm should be left in place at least 6 to 8 hours after intercourse. It can be removed and cleaned with regular soap and water. A diaphragm should not be left in place more than 24 hours.

Several kinds of diaphragms are available, including a coil spring, flat spring, arcing spring, and hinged spring. A proper fit is essential. Clinicians can estimate the size by measuring the distance between the introitus to the cervix on vaginal examination. The largest diaphragm that corresponds to this measurement should be selected to try initially. There should be no sensation of tightness or pressure. The diaphragm should be checked after the woman coughs or performs a Valsalva maneuver. If it is too small it will become displaced. If it is too large it may protrude from the introitus. The woman should be instructed about insertion and removal and given time to demonstrate success with these skills before she leaves the office. The couple should be made aware of emergency contraception if the diaphragm breaks or becomes displaced.

CERVICAL CAP

The cervical cap is much smaller than the diaphragm, fits snugly over the cervix, and is held in place by suction. Its availability is limited, and many clinicians are unfamiliar with it. In the United States only the Prentif Cavity Rim Cervical Cap is available.

ORAL CONTRACEPTIVE PILLS

Oral contraceptives (OCs) combine an estrogen with a progesterone or contain just a progesterone. Combined oral contraceptive pills act primarily through inhibition of ovulation. The progestin exerts the major contraceptive effect by inhibiting LH, thereby inhibiting ovulation, altering tubal peristalsis, and thickening cervical mucus. The estrogen decreases follicle-stimulating hormone and potentiates progesterone effects.

There are many combined OC varieties available. Most are "monophasic," with a fixed dose of estrogen (usually 20 to 50 μg of ethinyl estradiol) and a fixed dose of one of several progesterone products (levonorgestrel, norethindrone, desogestrel, norgestrel, norgestimate). "Biphasic" pills have a constant dose of estrogen combined with one of two different doses of progesterone, with a lower dose for the first half of the cycle and a higher dose for the second half of the cycle to more closely mimic a woman's normal progesterone levels. "Triphasic" pills have a fixed concentration of estrogen and three different increasing concentrations of progesterone. Biphasic and triphasic pills were developed to decrease the incidence of progesterone-related side effects and break-through bleeding. One available OC varies the dose of estrogen throughout the cycle. Three different doses of estrogen are combined with a single fixed dose of progesterone (Estrostep 21).

Progestin-only pills contain one of two types of progesterone. Progestin-only OCs are less effective than combination OCs. They must be taken at the same time of day each day. If the pill is delayed by more than 3 hours, a backup method of contraception should be used for 48 hours. Menstrual periods may be irregular or absent.

The risk of thromboembolism is related to duration of use, with decreasing risk over time. It is not dose related, so that lower dose estrogen pills do not decrease the thrombotic risk.

In the mid-1990s, some European studies reported an increased risk of deep vein thrombophlebitis and other thromboembolic diseases among women who used the newer progesterone products gestodene* or desogestrel. These progestins had been developed because they caused fewer androgenic side effects. Since these early reports, a reanalysis of the studies has refuted this interpretation. There is currently no compelling evidence to suggest avoiding these progestins.

*Not available in the United States.

Although OC pills are generally contraindicated for women over 35 years of age who continue to smoke, newer OCs with low estrogen or newer progesterones are associated with less heart disease risk than older pills.

The relationship between OC use and breast cancer continues to be debated. Data from the Nurses Cohort Study revealed no increased breast cancer risk for women over 40 years of age who used OCs before a full-term pregnancy. Younger women had a slightly increased risk.

The presence of some chronic medical conditions can influence the choice among estrogen-containing OCs, progestin-only OCs, or the use of other methods (Table 2). Many common medications can affect estrogen-containing OCs. The progesterone-only OCs may be a better option. Women taking OC pills experience common symptoms that may need management (Table 3).

There is no evidence that women taking OCs require intermittent month-long pill-free "holidays." They also do not need to wait 3 months between discontinuing OCs and then attempting to conceive.

INJECTABLE PROGESTIN

Depomedroxyprogesterone acetate provides 12 weeks of contraception. Fertility typically returns in 4 to 9 months, but may take as long as 18 months.

SUBDERMAL IMPLANTABLE PROGESTIN CONTRACEPTIVE

Subdermal implantable progestin, the Norplant System, consists of six flexible elastic capsules. Each is 34-mm long and 2.4 mm in diameter. They release 50 to 80 μg per day of levonorgestrel the first year and 30 to 50 μg per day the next 4 years. This is one fourth to one tenth the progestin of typical combined OCs.

EMERGENCY CONTRACEPTION

Emergency contraception includes OC pills and the copper T intrauterine device (IUD). Many people are not aware of these options, although they have been proven to be cost effective and the likelihood of conception is decreased by 75%. Emergency contraception prevents pregnancy, hinders or delays ovulation, but does not appear to interrupt or disrupt an already established pregnancy. It may alter the sperm or ova transport. In 1997, the U.S. Food and Drug Administration established that seven currently available oral contraceptives can be safely and effectively used as emergency contraception. Their use could potentially prevent half of the estimated 3.5 million unintended pregnancies that occur annually. Although emergency contraception can be used up to 72 hours after unprotected intercourse, it is much more efficacious the sooner it is begun. Common regimens include

TABLE 2. **Impact of Common Medical Conditions on the Choice of an Oral Contraceptive**

Medical Condition	Impact on Contraceptive Choice
Migraine headache without neurologic symptoms	Consider low-dose estrogen or progesterone-only pill; if headaches persist, use nonhormonal method
Migraine headache with neurologic symptoms	Avoid estrogen-containing OCs
Seizure disorder	OCs do not change seizure threshold; with drug interaction between some anticonvulsants and hormones in OCs, the level of hormone may "decrease" with increased risk of contraceptive failure
Diabetes mellitus	Effect of OCs generally not clinically significant; lower dose estrogen OCs and progestin-only OCs acceptable with close follow-up; otherwise, choose nonhormonal method
Hypertriglyceridemia	Combined low-dose OC acceptable if triglycerides <750 mg/dL; consider progestin-only pills
Thrombotic event	Consider progestin-only contraceptive or other contraceptive; avoid estrogen
Mitral valve prolapse	OCs acceptable
Hypertension	In nonsmoking women, low-dose OCs or progestin-only OCs can be used and blood pressure monitored
Chronic heart failure	Avoid estrogen-containing OCs
Severe cardiovascular disease for those over age 35 yr with mild to moderate cardiovascular disease	Individualize therapy, but generally OCs are contraindicated
History of DVT, CVA, PE	Estrogen-containing OCs contraindicated
SLE with vasculitis	Contraindication to OCs; progestin-only contraceptive, barrier methods, and IUDs good alternate choices
SLE without vasculitis	Estrogens may exacerbate or ameliorate symptoms of SLE; cautious monitoring of patient if low-dose OC chosen
Perimenopausal women	Nonsmoking women can use OCs until menopause; to determine if menopausal, serum FSH level determined the fifth day of the week of menses while taking OCs; if FSH >25 mIU/mL, probably menopausal and consider changing to hormone replacement therapy (if desired)
Breast-feeding	Consider progestin-only OCs because they do not affect milk production

Abbreviations: OCs = oral contraceptives; DVT = deep vein thrombosis; CVA = cardiovascular accident; PE = pulmonary embolism; SLE = systemic lupus erythematosus; IUDs = intrauterine devices; FSH = follicle-stimulating hormone.

TABLE 3. **Management of Some Common Symptoms Women Experience While Taking Oral Contraceptives**

Symptom	Management Strategy
Amenorrhea	Check pregnancy test; consider higher estrogen or lower progestin pill
Breath-through bleeding	Expect BTB in the first 3 mo (10% of women); the progesterone norgestrel may cause less BTB; rule out pregnancy. If BTB persists, consider higher dose progestin or estrogen pill
Hair growth Male pattern baldness Acne	These are generally androgenic effects due to the progestin content. Consider changing to OC with a low androgenic potential (such as desogestrel or norgestimate)
Nausea	Consider decreasing the estrogen content; take the OC before sleep
Elevated blood pressure	BP rise on OC is usually <5 mm Hg. The risk of increasing BP increases with age; it generally resolves within 3 mo of discontinuing the pill. If BP increases, consider lower progestin pill
Weight gain	Inconsistent effect; consider lower estrogen and lower progestin content OC
Breast soreness	Change to pill with decreased estrogen; vitamin E 400 IU PO bid
Fluid retention	Change to pill with decreased estrogen
Depression	Generally progestin related; consider lower progestin or different progestin; pyridoxine 25–50 mg q d
Fatigue	Generally progestin related; change to different progestin or decreased dose
Missed pill	If one missed pill, take two pills the next day and continue the rest of the pack as normal If two missed pills in first 2 wk of the cycle, take two pills each day for 2 d; finish the pack as usual, but use a backup method of contraception If two pills are missed in the third week or more pills are missed, discard the current pack, start a new pack, and use a backup method of contraception for 7 d
Perimenopausal	Check serum FSH on the fifth days of menses; if >25 mIU/L, then probably menopausal and can change to HRT (if desired)
Inadvertent pregnancy on OCs	Stop the OCs. Teratogenic effect probably overstated in the past
Stopping the pill to become pregnant	>50% will become pregnant in 3 months; 80% in 1 yr Remember to use folic acid supplement 0.4 mg q d as OCs can cause folic acid depletion and preconception folic acid supplementation decreases the incidence of neural tube defects Do not need to wait 3 mo until attempt to conceive

Abbreviations: BTB = break-through bleeding; OCs = oral contraceptives; BP = blood pressure; FSH = follicle-stimulating hormone; HRT = hormone replacement therapy.

Ovral,* 2 tablets; repeat in 12 hours
Nordette,* 4 tablets; repeat in 12 hours
Levlen,* 4 tablets; repeat in 12 hours
Alesse,* 5 tablets; repeat in 12 hours

Other options are

LoOvral,* 4 tablets; repeat in 12 hours
Triphasill,* 4 tablets; repeat in 12 hours
Tri Levlen,* 4 tablets; repeat in 12 hours

Diethylstilbestrol (DES)* 25 to 50 mg every day for 5 days has been used in the past but has an unacceptably high rate of nausea. Danazol (Danocrine)* use has been abandoned because of lack of efficacy. Because vomiting is likely in one fifth of users, an antiemetic such as meclizine can be taken an hour before the OCs. Many clinicians include a prescription for an antiemetic and an extra dose of the medication in case the patient vomits. Emergency OC is of such short duration and limited dose that it is not thought to pose a major risk for women at risk of stroke, deep vein thrombosis, or cardiovascular disease who otherwise are not candidates for combination OCs. Women who truly should avoid estrogen completely can use the progestin-only pills or the copper T IUD. When progestin-only pills are indicated, 20 Ovrette* tablets are used within 48 hours of unprotected intercourse and the dose repeated in 12 hours. Compared with combination pills for emergency contraception, progestin-only pills are equally efficacious and cause less nausea and vomiting.

To be effective, the copper IUD must be inserted within 5 days of unprotected intercourse. When used in this way, the copper IUD most probably affects implantation.

In September 1998, the PREVEN Emergency Contraceptive Kit was approved by the FDA. Washington state allowed its pharmacies to make it available without prescription. The kit combines a pregnancy test with four tablets that combine 0.25 mg levonorgestrel and 0.05 mg ethinyl estradiol.

INTRAUTERINE DEVICES

IUDs are the most widely used reversible contraceptive method worldwide. In the United States, however, less than 1% of women use IUDs. Two varieties are currently available in the United States. The Copper T 380A IUD is a polyethylene T. The stem is wrapped with copper wires, and its arms are partially covered by copper tubing. It has two white monofilament threads. The progesterone-releasing IUD is made of plastic. The plastic contains progesterone designed to be released at a rate of 65 μg per day for 1 year. It has two blue-black monofilament threads.

IUDs are thought to work through preventing fertilization by creating a sterile inflammation in the endometrium. The inflammation is spermicidal and

*Not FDA approved for this indication.

prevents viable sperm from reaching the fallopian tubes. The failure rate is highest in the first year of use. Low-risk women are at low risk of developing a pelvic inflammatory disease or infertility from the IUD. It was once thought that IUDs were best placed during a woman's menses. There are no data to support this practice, and the expulsion rate is lower if placed after day 11 of the menstrual cycle. Table 4 provides directions on placement of the IUD. Table 5 outlines management for patients with common IUD situations.

STERILIZATION

Tubal ligation (occlusion) is the most commonly used contraception method in the United States. Although reasonably effective, pregnancies do occur and may occur more than 10 years after the procedure. The failure rate for all tubal occlusion methods is 1.85%. The failure rates vary, however, from 0.7 to 5.4% depending on the technique used. Unipolar coagulation and postpartum partial salpingectomy result in the lowest cumulative failure rates; however, unipolar coagulation results in the most deaths

TABLE 4. **Steps for Intrauterine Device (IUD) Placement**

1. Exclude contraindications, and discuss risks and benefits
2. Exclude pregnancy
3. Perform pelvic examination to exclude vaginitis and identify uterine position
4. Obtain cultures for chlamydia and gonorrhea*
5. Obtain Pap smear
6. Advise women to take nonsteroidal anti-inflammatory medication 1–2 h before procedure
7. Obtain and document informed consent
8. Set up instruments on a sterile field
9. Insert speculum to localize cervix
10. Clean cervix with antiseptic
11. Consider a paracervical block for patients with cervical stenosis
12. Apply tenaculum to anterior lip of cervix; straighten the axis of the uterus with gentle traction on the tenaculum for steps 13 and 16
13. Measure uterus with sound, and note depth of cavity
14. Load device through sterile packaging
15. Set stop/flange to depth indicated by sound
16. Insert IUD
17. Release IUD
18. Remove insertion device
19. Cut strings to 1–2 cm from cervical os and note length in chart
20. Remove tenaculum
21. Observe for bleeding; pressure or silver nitrate will generally control bleeding
22. Remove speculum
23. Have patient check string length herself
24. Discharge patient with appointment for position check of string and review of side effects after first postinsertion menses
25. Discuss management of spotting and mild cramping and follow-up

*Not all authorities recommend pre-insertion cultures, but currently this is the position of American College of Obstetricians and Gynecologists.
Adapted from Canavan TP: Appropriate use of the intrauterine device. Am Fam Phys 58(9):2080, 1998.

TABLE 5. **Common Situations in Use of Intrauterine Devices (IUDs)**

Common Situations	Treat with IUD in Place	Remove IUD	Comments
Cramping/bleeding (no signs/symptoms of infection)	X		Nonsteroidal anti-inflammatory drug; evaluate for infection if persists
Patient develops candidal infection, vulvovaginitis, bacterial vaginosis	X		Treat with indicated medications
Vaginitis, trichomonal vaginitis/cervicitis	X		Treat with indicated medications
Patient develops asymptomatic gonorrhea or chlamydia	X		Treat with indicated medications
Simple endometritis (uterine tenderness without adnexal tenderness)	X		Doxycycline 100 mg bid × 14 d; if endometritis does not resolve, remove IUD
Pelvic inflammatory disease (adnexal or cervical motion tenderness)		X	
Patient will not practice safe sex		X	A different contraception should be chosen
Partially expelled IUD		X	Expulsion should be suspected with cramping, vaginal discharge, lengthening of the string, or patient's partner feels a plastic device protruding from the cervix
			Expulsion rate decreases the later in cycle IUD is inserted; replacement IUD inserted after expulsion is less likely to be expelled
Pregnancy with IUD in place		X	Rule out ectopic; if intrauterine pregnancy occurs, 60% risk of SAB; 30% risk of SAB if IUD removed
String cannot be felt or visualized			Ultrasound to evaluate if IUD still present and within uterus
Uterine perforation		X (surgically)	Usually perforation occurs at time of insertion
Actinomyces on Pap smear		X	If actinomycosis is reported on Pap smear in asymptomatic woman with IUD, some clinicians would leave IUD in place unless evidence of upper tract disease is present; some would prescribe 2-wk course of penicillin

Abbreviation: SAB = spontaneous abortion.

due to bowel injury. Spring clip application and bipolar coagulation are associated with the highest cumulative failure rates. Postpartum tubal ligation has a failure rate of 1 per 250 procedures compared with 1 per 400 for those done at other times. Because many of these pregnancies are ectopic, *all women with tubal sterilizations who have symptoms or signs of pregnancy should be considered as having an ectopic pregnancy until proven otherwise.*

Counseling is essential. Six percent of women regret their decision. Regret is more likely in women under 30 years of age and those who had postpartum sterilizations. Couples should understand that this sterilization is a permanent method of contraception. Although reversals are possible, they are costly, not always reimbursed by insurance, and not uniformly successful.

For details about vasectomy, see Table 1.

SPECIAL POPULATIONS

Some populations present unique issues in contraception counseling.

Adolescents

Clinicians should be knowledgeable concerning state law regarding contraceptive counseling and prescribing for adolescent patients. In most states, sexually active adolescents can consent to contraception and screening for sexually transmitted diseases without parental permission. In reality, it is helpful to encourage adolescents to discuss their decision-making with their families. Abstinence, if chosen, should be accompanied by specific negotiating strategies to use with their partners and facilitate peer support of their decision. Adolescents frequently are excellent candidates for OCs because they are usually at low risk and may benefit from the noncontraceptive benefits such as more regular periods, less dysmenorrhea, and improvement in acne. IUDs are generally avoided. The use of condoms to enhance contraceptive efficacy and to provide some protection from STDs should be discussed, as should the availability of emergency contraception. Clinicians should also be aware that coerced sex in this age group, especially in girls under 15 years of age, is prevalent.

Postpartum Women

Ovulation can occur within 3 to 4 weeks postpartum and frequently before the first menses. Over two thirds of couples resume sexual relations within the first postpartum month and 90% within the second. Contraception should be initiated either immediately postpartum or within the first 2 to 3 weeks. Many couples use more than one method during the first postpartum year as the woman's physiology, contraceptive risks, and needs change.

Breast-feeding Women

Lactation itself provides a contraceptive benefit. Lactational amenorrhea is highly reliable for 6 months in women who exclusively breast-feed at least every 4 hours and have no menstruation. Spermicides and condoms are excellent initial choices. IUDs are less likely to be expelled if inserted within 10 minutes after placental delivery. Insertion after 10 minutes and up to 6 weeks increases the risk of expulsion. The IUD should be inserted at 6 to 8 weeks postpartum, if not immediately.

Fertility awareness methods require different interpretations as the predictability of symptoms and signs in breast-feeding women may be less reliable. Basal body temperatures are not reliable if sleep disruption occurs. The general anesthesia required for tubal ligation can disrupt lactation both chemically and due to separation from the infant. Progestin methods (Norplant, progesterone IUDs, Depo Provera, and progestin-only pills) are not recommended immediately postpartum because the abrupt decrease of natural progesterone 2 to 3 days postpartum triggers lactogenesis. Theoretically, a high dose of progestin might interfere with this process. Recommendations to delay these methods until 6 weeks postpartum are based on theoretical concerns and animal studies.

Use of combined OCs by breast-feeding mothers is controversial. Although there is no direct harm to infants, breast milk composition changes and its supply decreases. Experts vary in their recommendation to not use OCs at all while breast-feeding to only cautiously initiating them 2 to 3 months or 6 months postpartum.

Barrier methods are acceptable, although the diaphragm and cap may be difficult to fit until 4 to 6 weeks post partum.

Postpartum Non–Breast-feeding

If not breast-feeding, most women have a menstrual period within 4 to 6 weeks of delivery. Two thirds of these cycles are ovulatory, but this cycle and the next few cycles may be accompanied by a deficient corpus luteum. Fertility should be assumed and couples provided with counseling and protection. Combined OCs theoretically should be withheld until 2 weeks postpartum to minimize the impact on the physiologic peak of thrombotic complications immediately postpartum. Progestin-only OCs can be initiated immediately. Within the first postpartum week, good choices are male and female sterilization (couples should wait to confirm absence of sperm following male sterilization), Norplant, and Depo Provera. Spermicidal products, IUDs, and diaphragms are used the same as for breast-feeding women.

Perimenopausal Women

Nonsmoking women without a medical contraindication can safely continue using OCs until menopause. Many have this need because fertility, although decreased, can extend into a woman's late 40s and even early 50s. Because of the regular withdrawal bleeding, it is sometimes difficult to determine when women are going through menopause. For details about management, see Table 5.

WOMEN WITH DISABILITIES

The presence of disabilities may influence the contraceptive choice in women. See Stifel EN, Anderson J: Contraception. *In* Rosenfeld JA: Women's Health in Primary Care. Baltimore, Williams & Wilkins, 1997 (Table 10.2.10)

Section 16

Psychiatric Disorders

ALCOHOL-RELATED PROBLEMS

method of
ROBERT G. BATEY, M.D.

*John Hunter Hospital and University of
Newcastle
Newcastle, New South Wales, Australia*

Alcohol-related problems continue to contribute to a high percentage of patients seeking medical treatment in general practice, in hospital outpatient practice, and in hospital wards. Alcohol abuse leads to a wide range of medical problems, and alcohol dependence creates specific problems requiring appropriate intervention. Up to 15% of patients seen in family practice and up to 20% of patients in hospitals have an alcohol problem requiring at least minimal intervention to minimize the risk of major problems in the future. In the general population, between 3% and 5% of the adult male population have a serious drinking problem. Women are less affected, although evidence suggests that rates in males and females are converging.

ASSESSING LEVELS OF HARM

Alcohol consumption has been conveniently divided into three levels, aiding a discussion of risk attributable to alcohol intake. Safe drinking in males and females has been defined as fewer than four standard drinks, or 40 grams of alcohol, per day for males and two standard drinks, or 20 grams of alcohol, per day for women. Alcohol consumption at or below this level is regarded as safe, although it is still stressed that alcohol-free days are important in maintaining good health. Alcohol consumption of more than four standard drinks per day for men or two standard drinks for women is regarded as hazardous drinking, and it is associated with a significant risk of alcohol-related problems.

HARMFUL DRINKING

Harmful drinking is defined as hazardous drinking associated with evidence of alcohol-related harm. A list of medical problems associated with excessive alcohol consumption is shown in Table 1.

Above and beyond the medical disorders associated with heavy regular alcohol intake, individuals may develop the alcohol dependence syndrome.

ALCOHOL DEPENDENCE SYNDROME

The alcohol dependence syndrome is increasingly well defined but remains poorly understood. It is characterized by a series of major features, which include the following:

A stereotyped narrow pattern of drinking
A subjective awareness of a loss of control with repeated attempts to control the excessive alcohol intake

An increasing importance of drinking over and above other things, leading to impairment in work, family relationships, and personal responsibility
A pharmacologic tolerance to alcohol that results in an increased capacity to drink without showing significant signs of intoxication
Repeated withdrawal symptoms (e.g., nausea, tremor, irritability, anxiety, and sleep disturbance)
Relief of withdrawal symptoms by drinking
A rapid reinstatement of pathologic drinking after a period of abstinence

It is usual to identify three or more of these features before diagnosing a full alcohol dependence syndrome, but any one of the features is of importance in the evaluation of a heavy drinker. Dependence ranges from mild to severe, and those most severely dependent are more likely to have major medical problems. With increasing dependence comes increasing tolerance, with some individuals able to consume 400 grams of alcohol per day without showing major signs of impaired neurologic function to standard testing. The more severe the dependence, the more likely an individual is to exhibit withdrawal features on sudden cessation of alcohol.

Physicians of every specialty group need to be aware of the multivariate manifestations of alcohol abuse. Alcohol is a toxic chemical, and regular use can lead to a variety of organ damage as well as creating problems because of its effect on central nervous system function. Table 1 highlights the various manifestations of the damage associated with excessive alcohol use, and these issues are discussed briefly.

It is extremely important for general practitioners, physicians, and surgeons to recognize that early intervention in the history of alcohol abuse can lead to better clinical outcomes. Treatment begun when patients have well-entrenched drinking habits and medical disorders associated with alcohol abuse are less likely to achieve success. The importance of early intervention and of the role of the generalist in defining this problem cannot be overemphasized.

MEDICAL PROBLEMS OF ALCOHOL ABUSE

Multiple organ systems are affected in the heavy drinker. As indicated in Table 1, patients may seek medical attention with symptoms ranging from the effects of hypertension to the effects of alcohol on the gastrointestinal tract, producing nausea, vomiting, or diarrhea. This wide-ranging medical effect of alcohol demands that a concise but accurate alcohol history be taken on all patients seeking medical attention. It is only as alcohol is recognized as a major cause of illness that there will be significant effort directed to reducing alcohol abuse as a cause of morbidity. Furthermore, it is only as the many manifestations of alcohol abuse are recognized that early intervention will become standard practice.

TABLE 1. **Alcohol-Related Problems**

Medical Problems	*Muscle Problems*	**Psychiatric Problems**
Gastrointestinal Disorders	Rhabdomyolysis	Suicide
Reflux esophagitis	Chronic proximal myopathy	Parasuicide
Gastritis	*Hematologic Disorders*	Alcohol withdrawal delirium
Bleeding peptic ulcers	Anemia	Dementia
Vomiting	Iron deficiency	Korsakoff's psychosis
Diarrhea	Folate deficiency	Anxiety
Alcoholic liver disease	Macrocytosis	Depression
Alcohol-related fatty liver	Thrombocytopenia	**Social Problems**
Alcoholic hepatitis	*Immune System Problems*	Financial difficulty
Alcoholic cirrhosis	Impaired lymphocyte function	Marital conflict
Portal hypertension (esophageal varices)	Hyperglobulinemia	Absenteeism (especially Mondays)
Pancreatitis	*Metabolic Disorders*	Unemployment
Cardiovascular Problems	Obesity	**Legal Problems**
Hypertension	Gout	Drunk driving
Cardiomyopathy	Hypertriglyceridemia	Assault
Arrhythmias	Diabetes	Homicide
Respiratory Problems	Testicular failure	Domestic violence
Sleep apnea	Hyperestrogenism	Trauma
Pneumonia	Pseudo-Cushing's syndrome	Falls
Pulmonary abscess	*Pregnancy-Related Problems*	Fractures
Tuberculosis	Lower birth weight	Head injuries
Neurologic Problems	Fetal alcohol syndrome	Industrial accidents
Peripheral neuropathy	Second trimester abortion	Drownings
Wernicke-Korsakoff syndrome	*Carcinoma Risk*	Domestic fires
Subdural hematoma from trauma	Increased incidence of	Motor vehicle accidents
Cerebellar degeneration	Oropharyngeal cancer	
Marchiafava-Bignami syndrome	Esophageal cancer	
Central pontine myelinolysis	Colonic cancer	
	Breast cancer	

SOCIAL PROBLEMS OF ALCOHOL ABUSE

An individual growing up with major social problems may well turn to alcohol use to ease some of these. Alternatively, individuals who become dependent on alcohol may become affected by a variety of social problems. In either case, those dealing with people with impaired social backgrounds need to be conscious of the role alcohol may be playing in the lives of their patients. Addressing social issues can facilitate an individual's ability to deal with the problem of excessive alcohol intake. Table 1 highlights the various social difficulties that may result from or lead to alcohol dependence.

FAMILY PROBLEMS

Many individuals with an alcohol problem fail to come to therapeutic centers for advice, but the family members come requesting help for the affected individual. Often it is only appropriate to deal with the family member who makes contact, hoping that this will lead the patient to seek help. Addressing the specific needs of family may be enough to induce the alcohol-dependent to seek help with his or her problem. Family members of an alcohol-dependent individual may be at risk of violence within the home and even of life-threatening situations. The individual may also experience quite marked psychiatric symptoms, which can lead to suicide and parasuicidal attempts.

THE DIAGNOSIS—WHAT DIAGNOSIS?

The high frequency of high alcohol problems in clinical practice demands an ongoing effort to encourage physi-cians to diagnose these problems early. Levels of suspicion of alcohol use in a variety of social, family, and medical problems have increased, but they need to increase further.

History of Alcohol Use

It is imperative that time is devoted to obtaining a history of alcohol consumption. When suspicion exists that alcohol consumption may be playing a role in the individual's presentation, then care must be taken to ensure that a sound doctor-patient relationship is established. Very few individuals will admit to hazardous levels of alcohol consumption on a first visit to a medical practitioner. Because many patients may not return, it is important that every effort is made to obtain as accurate a history as possible at the first visit. When one is seeking to document a high alcohol intake, it is often possible to overestimate the amount of consumption in an attempt to allow the patient to admit to heavy intake. For example, if it is clear that an individual spends many hours of the week in a club or hotel drinking with friends, it might be appropriate to suggest that he or she could be drinking 20 standard drinks a day. The patient will often say, "Oh no, I only drink 15." Sometimes the person may be emboldened to indicate that 20 is really not much at all and will admit to a higher level of intake. When suspicion exists and the history is not appropriate, it is worth making a further appointment to see the individual, at which time the results of several blood tests can be shared and a further effort made to obtain a reasonable estimate of alcohol intake. When an individual is not forthcoming, it may be appropriate to seek help from family members or from others known to the patient. Sometimes a visit to the individual's home may be required. The dividing of drinking levels into harmful and hazardous requires that some quantitation of intake be made in all individuals being evaluated for drinking problems.

In history taking it is important to determine the importance of alcohol to the individual's daily existence. The points highlighted in the definition of the Alcohol Dependence Syndrome need to be evaluated in a history. When time is limited or when an individual is unwilling to give much information, the use of the CAGE questionnaire (Table 2), a series of four questions that can indicate a dependence on alcohol, can be used.

Medical History

It is important to question patients about symptoms that may result from heavy alcohol intake (see Table 1). A family history be taken because there is a significant component to alcohol dependence. Those with a major genetic component to their own alcohol dependence often come to medical attention early with excessive drinking, a feature from early teenage years. These individuals often come to medical attention with trauma and legal problems.

Alcohol Dependence

If three or more of the criteria of alcohol dependence syndrome are present, moderate or severe alcohol dependence exists.

Examination

All patients should undergo a full medical examination, seeking evidence of central nervous system damage that may render a history less reliable and examining other systems for the disorders listed in Table 1. Of particular importance, the physician should examine for the following:

Hypertension and obesity (alcohol is responsible for up to 30% of essential hypertension)
Evidence of trauma
Evidence of liver disease
Signs of withdrawal, with anxiety, sweating, and tachycardia being common features
Evidence of intoxication, ataxia, and disinhibition
Evidence of neurologic injury, including peripheral neuropathy and memory loss extending to the Wernicke-Korsakoff psychosis

Investigations

A number of investigations can be used to confirm the existence of an alcohol problem and to define the medical problems present.

Full Blood Cell Count. This will provide evidence of anemia, and the mean corpuscular volume is often elevated. Anemia can result from gastrointestinal hemorrhage or from nutritional deficiencies associated with the poor diet of the heavy drinker. Severe liver disease can lead to anemia, and in these situations spur cells are commonly seen on the blood film. The mean corpuscular volume is commonly elevated in regular drinkers, and a mean corpuscular volume of more than 100 fL should suggest alcohol abuse.

Liver Function Tests. Liver function tests not only can document the presence of significant liver disease but also can act as an early marker of alcohol excess, with a raised gamma-glucamyltransferase level being a useful marker. In hospital populations, elevation of gamma-glucamyltransferase levels lacks specificity; but in the community a raised gamma-glucamyltransferase value will commonly indicate excess alcohol intake.

Blood Alcohol Levels. Measuring blood alcohol these days may demand consent from the patient. The presence of a level of alcohol above 0.05% in the morning does indicate heavy alcohol intake the previous evening and can be used as a discussion point in further history taking. Blood alcohol levels can often be significantly higher than suspected from a clinical examination in the dependent individual. This reflects both neuroadaptation and hepatic metabolic adaptation to the regular presence of high levels of alcohol.

Carbohydrate Deficient Transferrin (CDT). The measurement of CDT has been shown to provide sensitive and specific information in individuals consuming more than 60 grams per day of alcohol. The test is not appropriate for screening general populations. When CDT is present in a heavy drinker, it does indicate regular daily intake. The test results return to normal 2 to 3 weeks after alcohol cessation and are thus able to detect problems for much longer than blood alcohol measures.

MANAGEMENT

Management of alcohol-dependent patients is determined by the stage they have reached in their problem drinking. Those with medical problems need specific attention directed to their medical condition. By using this as a means to bring the patient back to a clinic on a number of occasions it is often possible to engage them in further discussion of their alcohol problem. At Westmead Hospital, Sydney, New South Wales, it was found that attendance at the medical clinic was always significantly higher than at clinics specifically designed for counseling or psychotherapy. It is important to stress the critical role of the medical practitioner in moving a patient from contemplating addressing the alcohol dependence to actually doing something about it.

In dealing with the dependent patient it is important to determine if psychiatric co-mobidity is a major feature. If this is the case, attention to the psychiatric disorder must be given or other interventions will fail to achieve abstinence. Often a psychiatric evaluation is required in the complex patient to ensure that appropriate management strategies are put in place.

Early Intervention Strategies

A number of papers during the 1980s documented the value of providing brief advice and counseling

---

TABLE 2. **The CAGE Questionnaire**

Over the past 12 months have you ever:
1. Felt you should **C**ut down your drinking?
2. Been **A**nnoyed by anyone commenting on your drinking?
3. Felt **G**uilty about your drinking?
4. Needed an **E**ye opener to get started?

sessions to individuals identified as drinking at harmful levels. At this stage of their problem with alcohol, patients have no significant cognitive impairment, are often socially competent, and thus able to make adjustments to their lifestyle, given appropriate information about the risks they face if they continue heavy drinking.

My practice is to identify the heavy drinker and have him or her discuss the problems with a counselor, who may spend 15 to 30 minutes going through the issues of alcohol toxicity, risks of organ damage, and ways and means of reducing alcohol intake.

In this process it is important to outline the benefits of reducing alcohol intake while highlighting the issues that may make this decision a little more difficult. Patients may need to make significant changes to their social life to avoid situations in which drinking would automatically occur, but if given support over a period of months it is often very rewarding to see the changes that can be made.

In those with medical problems it is appropriate to use measures of liver function, hematologic function, and psychologic functioning to indicate that the decision to reduce alcohol has led to improvements in these various tests. Positive feedback from improving tests proves that it is a very valuable resource in managing the heavy drinker.

Managing Withdrawal States

Many patients will need treatment for their alcohol withdrawal before they can undergo further treatment for problem drinking. Home detoxification has become more accepted for those with a supporting person with them. Ceasing alcohol should be accompanied by the use of a sedative to minimize risk of withdrawal seizures in the heavy drinker. Moderate levels of intake do pose a small but real risk of complications during withdrawal, but the presence of a supportive person can allow safe drug-free withdrawal in most.

Admission to a nonmedical or medical facility may be required for some patients. Medication for major withdrawal is now largely diazepam (Valium) in a dose regulated by the use of an alcohol withdrawal scale. Thiamine is administered routinely to minimize the risk of Wernicke-Korsakoff syndrome.

Alcohol Dependence

Managing alcohol dependence remains a complicated process because our understanding of the dependence syndrome remains inadequate. It is evident that even the most dependent patient can overcome the problem and lead a life free of the need to consume alcohol. Individuals with social support are more likely to achieve abstinence than those who have to try on their own. Evidence from major works such as those of Vaillant in the 1970s is that if individuals can develop a lasting relationship with a significant other or if they take up a significant religious commitment, they are more likely to achieve

abstinence than those who do neither. Alcoholics Anonymous continues as an organization that helps more individuals than any other therapeutic modality available to the dependent population. Alcoholics Anonymous does achieve significant abstinence rates by providing a stable environment, personal support, and a belief system that an individual can adhere to firmly as he or she seeks to give up the alcohol dependence.

If an individual absolutely refuses Alcoholics Anonymous at the first and second encounters, it is important to stress that other therapies are available, ranging from behavioral modification strategies for those who are not severely dependent with neurologic damage to psychotherapeutic approaches. Psychotherapy can be directed to the individual or the family. An individual with significant cognitive impairment usually is unable to benefit from the rigors of psychotherapeutic approaches.

It is important to seek to match individuals with the treatment options available, and in any city it is appropriate for those dealing with patients who have significant alcohol problems to be aware of what treatment modalities can be offered. Therapies that aim at control of drinking are of some value in populations of dependent individuals, but it is of interest that most truly dependent individuals quickly find that abstinence is a more practical goal for them to seek than is control drinking.

It is important that if an individual refuses a particular treatment in the first instance, it is appropriate to have him or her return for follow-up visits while seeking to encourage reconsideration of decisions made during earlier consultations.

Long-Term Follow-up

It is important to continue observing individuals with a dependence problem. The fact that an individual is concerned about the outcome of a dependent patient means much to them and can be a therapeutic intervention in its own right. Dependence is a long, drawn-out process, and abstinence is a tenuous situation. By seeing individuals with a dependence problem on a regular basis, preemptive actions can be taken to minimize the risks of changes in the person's environment that may lead him or her back to compulsive drinking. Patients who have been abstinent for 20 years can relapse quickly to heavy drinking if they find themselves alone, under stress, or unable to find help in a crisis. Practitioners can provide that help in critical times.

DRUG ABUSE

method of
LESLIE K. JACOBSEN, M.D., and
THOMAS R. KOSTEN, M.D.
Yale University School of Medicine
New Haven, Connecticut

Abuse of and dependence on illicit substances are among the most prevalent psychiatric disorders. The

1996 National Institute on Drug Abuse Household Survey estimated that 13 million people in the United States were current illicit drug users. The 1988 Surgeon General's Report indicated that relapse rates for abusers of most substances range between 80 and 90%. Those who are able to remain abstinent for long periods usually do so only after many failed attempts at quitting. Thus, substance abuse and addiction are pervasive and tenacious problems.

With the third revised and fourth editions of the *Diagnostic and Statistical Manual of Mental Disorders,* emphasis has shifted toward loss of control over substance use and disruption of normal activities in defining all addictions. Tolerance, or reduction in drug effect with repeated use, and symptoms and signs of a characteristic withdrawal syndrome on abrupt cessation of drug use are no longer required for the diagnosis of addiction. Treatment must focus beyond initial detoxification and address relapse prevention, bearing in mind that successful treatment often is preceded by multiple failures. Often referral to specialized clinics or treatment facilities is required. Although some medications reduce craving and/or abuse of some substances, postdetoxification treatment programs generally also include a psychosocial component geared toward helping addicts shift from the drug-abusing lifestyle and culture toward being constructive members of their families and society. Vigorous treatment of co-morbid psychiatric conditions, including mood, anxiety, and psychotic disorders, is also a key component of relapse prevention.

An important cornerstone of both emergency department management and postdetoxification treatment of substance abuse is accurate drug testing. Abusers of substances may not be willing or able to reliably inform caregivers of the identity of the substances they have used. Furthermore, in some individuals, abuse of certain substances can trigger symptoms that mimic other psychiatric disorders, such as schizophrenia. Although blood drug levels are more closely related to brain levels and represent stronger evidence of recent use, urine is usually the preferred biofluid for drug detection testing, as drug levels are higher in urine than in blood. For Department of Health and Human Services Substance Abuse and Mental Health Services Administration certification, laboratories are required to screen samples for amphetamines, cannabinoids, cocaine, opioids, and phencyclidine. Additional substances commonly screened for include barbiturates, benzodiazepines, methadone, propoxyphene, methaqualone, and ethanol. Substances usually not screened for include lysergic acid diethylamide (LSD), fentanyl, psilocybin, methylenedioxymethamphetamine (MDMA), methylenedioxyamphetamine (MDA), and other designer drugs.

COCAINE

The 1996 National Institute on Drug Abuse Household Survey estimated that 1.75 million people in the United States currently use cocaine. Cocaine is taken intransally ("snorting"), intravenously (when combined with heroin this is referred to as "speed balling"), or by smoking of cocaine freebase or "crack" cocaine (freebase prepared with sodium bicarbonate). Although substance abuse is generally more common in males, this male dominance is less for crack cocaine, in part owing to the frequent use of crack in drugs-for-sex exchanges. An association between cocaine abuse and human immunodeficiency virus (HIV) infection has been observed.

Because cocaine is a stimulant, its acute subjective effects include intense euphoria and alertness, grandiosity, and anxiety. These effects rapidly give way to dysphoria as the drug is metabolized and excreted, leading to the binge pattern of usage that is commonly seen, where the drug is used repeatedly until either the supply or the user is exhausted. Intense usage can lead to pervasive anxiety states, which can be treated with lorazepam (Ativan), 2 mg orally or 1 mg intramuscularly (IM), and psychotic symptoms, including paranoid ideation and auditory, visual, or tactile hallucinations. These latter symptoms can be treated with haloperidol (Haldol), 5 mg orally or 2.5 mg IM. Large doses of cocaine can lead to atrial and ventricular arrhythmias, hypertension, myocardial infarction, cerebrovascular accidents, and seizures.

Withdrawal from cocaine after heavy, prolonged use may involve dysphoric mood, vivid dreams, insominia or hypersomnia, increased appetite, and psychomotor retardation. This constellation of symptoms may be accompanied by suicidal ideation, which should prompt close observation and formal psychiatric consultation.

Common therapeutic goals of all treatment approaches for cocaine abuse include keeping the abuser in treatment, disrupting the binge cycle, and preventing relapse. Crack and freebase abusers tend to drop out of treatment at a higher rate than abusers of other forms of cocaine. Psychosocial rehabilitation, including behavioral treatment that reinforces cocaine-free urine tests, can be effective in preventing relapse and, when relapse occurs, reducing its severity. Given the rapidity with which cocaine is metabolized, use of a sensitive assay for screening urine samples is important.

The tricyclic antidepressants and serotonin reuptake inhibitors have been shown to be effective in some, but not all, double-blind studies in initiation of abstinence and reduction of craving for cocaine. Depressed cocaine abusers may be especially responsive to desipramine (Norpramin).* Because there may be a 2- to 3-week delay before patients experience a reduction in target symptoms from antidepressants, dropout rates are high. Both of the dopamine-agonist agents amantadine (Symmetrel)* and bromocriptine (Parlodel)* have been found to be effective in reducing craving and cocaine abuse, although not consistently. Amantadine has fewer side effects than bromocriptine. Mood stabilizing agents,

---

*Not FDA approved for this indication.

such as lithium and carbamazepine (Tegretol), have not been found to be effective in the treatment of cocaine abuse.

AMPHETAMINES AND DESIGNER STIMULANT DRUGS

Amphetamines, which include dextroamphetamine (Dexedrine), methylphenidate (Ritalin), and pemoline (Cylert), are not as frequently abused as cocaine, but rates of abuse of these substances are increasing. These drugs are usually taken orally; however, the methamphetamine ("ice") form of amphetamine can be taken intravenously or intranasally or by smoking. The effects of methamphetamine in particular are similar to those of cocaine except that they are approximately 10 times longer in duration. Acute clinical management and postdetoxification treatment are also similar. Hyperpyrexia is a serious complication of methamphetamine overdose that can develop from the resulting vasoconstriction, hepatic metabolism of fat and glucose, agitation, and muscle rigidity. This can be managed with hydration, infusion of ice-cold saline, and external cooling with ice packs, sponging, and cooling blankets. If the drug has been ingested, gastric lavage and activated charcoal can be administered. Ipecac should not be used because of the risk of inducing seizures, arrhythmias, or hypertensive hemorrhages. Cardiac monitoring for arrhythmias in the setting of stimulant (cocaine or amphetamine) overdose is necessary. Significant stimulant-induced hypertension should be carefully controlled with antihypertensive agents. As with cocaine intoxication, psychotic symptoms and agitation may develop and can be treated with haloperidol; however, because of the longer half-life of methamphetamine, these symptoms may persist longer.

Transplacental exposure to stimulants, including cocaine, is associated with intrauterine growth retardation, preterm labor and premature birth, fetal distress, placental hemorrhage, decreased head circumference, neonatal anemia, and postnatal developmental abnormalities. The withdrawal syndrome associated with amphetamines is similar to that associated with cocaine.

MDMA ("Ecstasy," "E," "Adam"), MDA, and the less commonly abused methylenedioxymethamphetamine (MDME; "Eve") are amphetamine analogues with many of the effects of amphetamine and are most popular among adolescents and college students. Physiologic toxicity is relatively common at high doses of MDMA and can include cardiac arrhythmias, seizures, hyperthermia, renal failure, intracerebral hemorrhage, metabolic acidosis, and disseminated intravascular coagulation.

OPIOIDS

Opioids include natural substances, such as opium, heroin, and morphine, and synthetic substances, such as meperidine (Demerol), fentanyl (Sublimaze; "China White"), methadone (Dolophine), 1-methyl-4-phenyl-1,2,3,6-tetrahydropyridine (MPTP), and 1-methyl-4-phenyl propionoxy-piperidine tetrahydropyridine (MPPP). These drugs can be taken orally, intravenously, or intranasally or by smoking. The 1996 National Institute on Drug Abuse Household Survey estimated that 216,000 Americans currently use heroin. Although many believe that current patterns of heroin usage in the United States are endemic, Drug Abuse Warning Network data have recently shown marked increases in heroin-related emergency department visits, made chiefly by older chronic heroin users.

Opioid intoxication is associated with euphoria, analgesia, drowsiness, respiratory depression, and pinpoint pupils. Opioid overdose is associated with respiratory arrest and death. Meperidine overdose is also often associated with seizures. Treatment involves providing a patent airway and mechanical ventilation as needed and administering the opioid antagonist naloxone (Narcan). Overdoses with synthetic or longer acting opioids, such as methadone, require higher and repeated doses of naloxone, which is relatively short acting.

Onset and course of opioid withdrawal are determined by the pharmacokinetics of the particular opioid used. Subjective symptoms include restlessness, insomnia, drug craving, and anxiety. Objective signs include myalgia, vomiting, lacrimation, rhinorrhea, meiosis, diarrhea, sweating, and chills. Although opioid withdrawal is very uncomfortable, it is not associated with serious medical complications except in pregnancy, where it can precipitate spontaneous abortion or preterm labor and premature birth later in pregnancy.

The choice of treatment referral for opioid addiction should involve consideration of the extent and severity of previous opioid abuse and past treatment history. Patients with a relatively recent onset of opioid abuse and no previous treatment are optimally referred for rapid opioid detoxification, which typically involves naltrexone (ReVia) and clonidine (Catapres),* or for drug-free treatment. Patients with a long history of opioid abuse and multiple previous treatment attempts are best referred for treatment with methadone or l-α-acetyl-methadol (LAAM), another long-acting opioid. In all cases, concomitant random urine drug screening and psychosocial treatments focused on helping patients shift away from the drug-abusing lifestyle are essential. In addition, screening for HIV, hepatitis B, and tuberculosis should be offered to all intravenous drug abusers.

Pregnant heroin addicts taking methadone are less likely to experience withdrawal and receive better prenatal care and nutrition; rates of prematurity, low birth weight, and infant mortality are lower than those for pregnant heroin addicts not receiving methadone. Thus, all pregnant heroin addicts should be referred for methadone maintenance. Sixty percent of methadone-exposed neonates experience a withdrawal syndrome within 72 hours of birth, which is

*Not FDA approved for this indication.

often treated with paregoric. No long-term sequelae of prenatal methadone exposure have been noted.

SEDATIVE HYPNOTICS AND ANXIOLYTICS

The sedative hypnotics and anxiolytics include the benzodiazepines, barbiturates (e.g., secobarbital [Seconal]), the barbiturate-like hypnotics (e.g., methaqualone), and the carbamates (e.g., meprobamate [Equanil]), all of which are taken orally. These agents are available through prescription and illegal sources, are brain depressants, and in high doses can be lethal, particularly when combined with alcohol. These drugs may be used by individuals to promote sleep after abuse of cocaine or other stimulants.

Patients taking prescription sedative hypnotics or anxiolytics can become physiologically dependent such that a withdrawal syndrome is elicited on abrupt medication discontinuation, which can include sweating; tremor; autonomic hyperactivity; insomnia; nausea; vomiting; psychomotor agitation; anxiety; transient visual, tactile, or auditory hallucinations or illusions; generalized seizures; and life-threatening delirium. Physiologic dependence in the absence of unauthorized dose escalation, drug-seeking behavior, or other behavioral signs of addiction does not merit a formal diagnosis of addiction. Timing of the onset of the withdrawal syndrome after drug cessation is determined by the pharmacokinetics of the specific drug used. Shorter acting medications, such as lorazepam (Ativan) and oxazepam (Serax), produce withdrawal symptoms within 6 to 8 hours, which peak in intensity by the second day and improve substantially by the fourth or fifth day. With longer acting medications, such as diazepam (Valium) and chlordiazepoxide (Librium), withdrawal symptoms may not develop for a week, peak during the second week, and improve by the third or fourth week. Severity of withdrawal is determined by the amount of drug routinely taken. Severe withdrawal is treated with long-acting benzodiazepines (e.g., diazepam or chlordiazepoxide) and anticonvulsants such as carbamazepine* (Tegretol)* or valproate (Depakote).*

Symptoms of sedative hypnotic or anxiolytic intoxication are similar to those associated with alcohol intoxication and include behavioral disinhibition, slurred speech, nystagmus, incoordination, unsteady gait, memory or attentional impairments, and stupor or coma. Overdose may necessitate intubation and mechanical ventilation. Benzodiazepine overdose can be treated with flumazenil (Romazicon), a benzodiazepine antagonist. Postdetoxification treatment of sedative hypnotic abuse and addiction is primarily psychosocial.

PHENCYCLIDINE

Phencyclidines or phencyclidine-like substances include phencyclidine (PCP), ketamine (Ketalar, Keta-

ject), and 1-[1-2-thienyl-cyclohexyl]piperidine (TCP). These substances can be taken orally or intravenously, or they can be smoked. Phencyclidine is the most commonly abused substance of this group and is usually mixed with tobacco or marijuana and smoked. Phencyclidine abuse is most common among individuals between 20 and 40 years of age and is more common among males.

Phencyclidine intoxication is associated with rapid onset of impulsive, unpredictable behavior, psychomotor agitation, impaired judgment, and assaultiveness. In addition, nystagmus, hyperacusis, ataxia, hypertension, tachycardia, hyperthermia, dysarthria, muscle rigidity, seizures, psychotic symptoms, or coma can be seen. Although a withdrawal syndrome has not been observed in humans, dependent individuals may take phencyclidine as often as two or three times per day, despite clear social and medical sequelae of ongoing use. Heavy users do report experiencing craving for phencyclidine. Patients presenting to the emergency department with phencyclidine intoxication are often brought there by the police because of their aggressive behavior. Restraints are often necessary, along with haloperidol, 2 mg intramuscularly, and lorazepam, 1 mg intramuscularly. Because intoxicated patients may experience brief lucid periods only to return to an agitated and aggressive state, restraints should be maintained until consistent lucidity and impulse control are demonstrated.

HALLUCINOGENS

The hallucinogens include lysergic acid diethylamide (LSD), mescaline (peyote), and psilocybin mushrooms, all of which are usually taken orally. A 1996 Substance Abuse and Mental Health Services Administration household survey found that 2% of individuals over the age of 12 years had used hallucinogens in the previous month. LSD use is most prevalent in individuals between the ages of 18 and 25 years. The different hallucinogens produce similar intoxication syndromes consisting of significant anxiety or depression, ideas of reference, paranoid ideation, impaired judgment, illusions, vivid visual hallucinations, depersonalization, derealization, pupillary dilation, tachycardia, diaphoresis, blurred vision, tremor, and incoordination. Tolerance develops to the psychedelic and euphoric effects of hallucinogens, but not to their autonomic effects. Cross-tolerance has been observed between LSD and other hallucinogens. No withdrawal syndrome, however, has been demonstrated for the hallucinogens.

Management of hallucinogen intoxication is generally conservative; however, lorazepam, 1 to 2 mg orally or intramuscularly, and/or haloperidol, 2 mg orally or intramuscularly, can be administered in cases of significant agitation or distress. Hallucinogen persisting perception disorder (flashbacks) may develop in some hallucinogen users and consists of transient recurrence of perceptual disturbances experienced during previous episodes of hallucinogen in-

---

*Not FDA approved for this indication.

toxication in the absence of current hallucinogen intoxication. These episodes may remit after several months, although in some cases they have persisted for years. Persistent psychotic symptoms may develop after LSD use, although this appears to occur primarily in individuals predisposed to psychosis (e.g., by virtue of previous episodes of psychosis in the absence of drug use, family history of psychosis). Such cases merit formal psychiatric consultation and referral for psychiatric treatment.

INHALANTS

Inhalants are a heterogenous group of psychoactive substances found in gasoline, adhesives, spray paints, cleaning fluids, typewriter correction fluid, and lighter fluids. These agents are taken only by inhalation, usually by "sniffing" an open container or "huffing" a rag soaked in the substance. Because of their low cost, ease of concealment, and easy availability, inhalants are often the first psychoactive substance used by young people. In 1989 it was estimated that 7% of high school seniors had used inhalants during the previous year. In addition, evidence suggests that the prevalence of inhalant abuse among 9- to 12-year-olds is increasing. Inhalant abuse may be more common among impoverished ethnic minorities, with the exception of African Americans.

Inhalant intoxication resembles alcohol intoxication, with stimulation and disinhibition followed by depression at higher doses. In addition, dizziness, nystagmus, incoordination, slurred speech, lethargy, decreased reflexes, tremor, generalized muscle weakness, blurred vision or diplopia, and stupor or coma may be seen. An odor of the inhalant used, as well as burns resulting from the flammability of these substances, may be present. Treatment of acute intoxication is generally supportive. Physical complications of inhalant abuse include cardiac arrhythmias, which can lead to sudden death; cerebellar disease, including cerebellar atrophy; cranial neuropathies; generalized cerebral atrophy and demyelination; distal renal tubular acidosis, glomerulonephritis; hepatic disease; chemical pneumonitis; and bone marrow suppression. Thus, thorough medical evaluation is warranted.

Prenatal exposure to toluene, present in most volatile adhesives, has been associated with craniofacial and limb abnormalities, developmental delay, and behavioral deficits. Tolerance to the effects of inhalants has been reported. A withdrawal syndrome consisting of sleep disturbance, nausea, tremor, diaphoresis, abdominal and chest discomfort, and irritability developing within 24 to 48 hours of cessation of use and lasting 2 to 5 days has been observed in some chronic users. Currently, there are no efficacious medications for the treatment of inhalant abuse and addiction. Psychosocial approaches have had limited success except when treatment occurs in a residential setting and/or is court mandated.

CANNABINOIDS

Cannabinoids, specifically marijuana, are the most widely used of illegal drugs and are often the first drugs used by all cultural groups in the United States. The 1996 National Institute on Drug Abuse Household Survey estimated that there are 10.1 million regular marijuana users in the United States. Derived from the cannabis plant, marijuana consists of the dried tops and leaves of the plant, whereas hashish consists of exudate from the leaves. These substances are usually smoked, but can be ingested, such as when mixed with food. Heavy users are predominantly males between the ages of 18 and 30 years. The component primarily responsible for the psychoactive properties of cannabis is δ-9-tetrahydrocannabinol (THC).

Intoxication can be associated with euphoria, anxiety, impaired coordination, impaired judgment, sensation of slowed time, social withdrawal, conjunctival injection, increased appetite, dry mouth, and tachycardia. High doses of cannabinoids can be associated with effects similar to those of hallucinogens, including paranoid ideation, delusions, hallucinations, depersonalization, and derealization. A withdrawal syndrome associated with cannabinoid use has not been reliably demonstrated. A dependence syndrome consisting of compulsive use despite disruption of family, work, social, psychological, and physical functioning, however, does occur. Few cannabinoid users seek treatment for intoxication or dependence. Conservative treatment of intoxication is indicated. Psychosocial treatments of marijuana dependence may be associated with reduction in the frequency of marijuana use.

ANTICHOLINERGICS

Abused anticholinergics include antihistamines, such as diphenhydramine (Benadryl) and benztropine (Cogentin), and tricyclic antidepressants, such as amitriptyline (Elavil) and doxepin (Sinequan). Intoxication is associated with euphoria, delirium, visual hallucinations, mydriasis, tachycardia, hypertension, arrhythmias, increased temperature, and seizures. Treatment involves maintaining an airway and administering charcoal and a cathartic. This should be done even if a number of hours have transpired since ingestion, as anticholinergics markedly decrease gastrointestinal motility. Physostigmine can be administered for arrhythmias that do not respond to beta blockers; however, physostigmine can produce seizures, bradycardia, bronchospasm, and laryngospasm and so must be used with caution and only if the potential benefits outweigh the risks.

ANABOLIC STEROIDS

Anabolic steroid abuse has become an increasing problem among adolescent and young adult competitive sports participants and body builders. Both natural (e.g., testosterone) and synthetic (e.g., stanozolol

[Winstrol], metandienone, I17-beta-methyl-5 beta-androst-1-ene-3 alpha, 17 alpha-diol, and 18-nor-17, 17-dimethyl-5 beta-androsta-1, 13-dien-3 alpha-ol) anabolic androgenic steroids are abused. Anabolic steroids are typically injected. These substances have recently been placed on the Food and Drug Administration's list of controlled substances because of the adverse effects seen in athletes taking these drugs. Symptoms of anabolic steroid abuse include weight gain, irritability, major mood disturbance, personality disorders, and self- and other-directed aggressive behavior. Occasionally, anabolic steroid abuse has been associated with severe, aggressive criminal behavior, including homicide. Anabolic steroid abusers are more likely than nonabusers to also use alcohol, tobacco, marijuana, cocaine, hallucinogens, sedatives, opiates, amphetamines, and designer drugs. Medical complications of anabolic steroid abuse include liver neoplasms, gynecomastia, severe coronary artery disease leading to myocardial infarction, activation of the hemostatic system (which may contribute to acute vascular events), and renal cell carcinoma. In addition, a significant proportion of anabolic steroid abusers share needles, thus increasing the risk of HIV and hepatitis B transmission.

Detection of anabolic steroid abuse is most reliably accomplished by analysis of urine specimens with gas chromatography–mass spectrometry or high-resolution mass spectrometry. Educational programs that emphasize adverse anabolic steroid effects, strength training alternatives to anabolic steroid abuse, and drug refusal role play may reduce established anabolic steroid abuse and reduce the number of nonabusers who begin to abuse anabolic steroids.

NICOTINE

Approximately 37% of the general population in the United States currently uses nicotine-containing products, with 30% of this group smoking cigarettes. Between 50 and 80% of persons who currently smoke are addicted to nicotine, as manifested by their smoking to avoid withdrawal symptoms, avoidance of situations where smoking is restricted, smoking more than intended, inability to quit smoking, and continuing to smoke despite having tobacco-related illnesses such as chronic obstructive lung disease or cancer. The addiction produced by nicotine is extremely difficult to treat, with long-term abstinence rates among smokers receiving treatment for nicotine addiction being the poorest of any drug of abuse. Most alcoholics and cocaine and heroin addicts who also smoke experience greater difficulty with smoking cessation than with achieving abstinence from other addicting substances.

Nicotine acutely produces both stimulant (increased alertness) and depressant (muscle relaxation) effects. Symptoms of nicotine withdrawal develop within 24 hours of cessation of nicotine use and include dysphoric or depressed mood, insomnia, irritability, anxiety, difficulty concentrating, restlessness, decreased heart rate, and increased appetite and weight gain. These symptoms peak within 1 to 4 days and last for 3 to 4 weeks. Tobacco use also increases the risk of lung, oral, and other cancers; chronic obstructive lung disease; ulcers; cardiovascular and cerebrovascular disease; and maternal and fetal complications, including intrauterine growth retardation.

There is evidence that at least part of the drive to use nicotine-containing products is to maintain a certain blood level of nicotine. Consistent with this, nicotine replacement therapies (nicotine gum or patch) appear to help with the first phase of treatment of nicotine addiction. However, although most nicotine users are able to achieve abstinence, within 6 months most resume smoking. There appears to be a small advantage of the nicotine patch over placebo that persists for 6 to 12 months. Abstinence rates at 12 months are typically in the range of only 20%. Efforts to improve these abstinence rates include combining nicotine replacement therapy with behavioral therapy. Antidepressant therapy may be helpful when smoking cessation is accompanied by depression.

ANXIETY DISORDERS

method of
NAOMI M. SIMON, M.D., and
MARK H. POLLACK, M.D.
Massachusetts General Hospital
Boston, Massachusetts

Anxiety is common in the medical setting. It may represent a transient response to concerns about medical illness, be a symptom of a medical syndrome, emerge as a side effect of medication, or be due to use of, or withdrawal from, alcohol or other abused substances (Table 1). Primary anxiety disorders may also be present in patients in the medical setting but may manifest primarily with somatic symptoms. Anxiety may worsen the presentation and experience of medical illness, increase utilization of medical services, decrease compliance with prescribed regimens, and be a significant source of distress and disability.

Although the common presence of anxiety or fear in the medical setting may lead to its dismissal as "normal," it is important to recognize pathologic anxiety. Pathologic anxiety is distinguished by four criteria: autonomous distress not clearly due to an external cause, high intensity of symptoms, persistence over time, and development of harmful behavioral strategies (e.g., avoidance, compulsions) that impair function.

Anxiety disorders are among the most common psychiatric disorders in the general population, with almost one in four people in the United States experiencing pathologic anxiety over his or her lifetime, as reported by the National Comorbidity Survey. Patients with panic and other anxiety disorders typically present first to their primary care doctors, emergency rooms, or other medical settings; and many high utilizers of medical services have anxiety or affective disorders. Appropriate diagnosis and treatment are critical to optimize utilization of medical services and improve the patient's quality of life and overall outcome.

TABLE 1. **Common Medical Causes of Anxiety**

Cardiovascular and Respiratory	Substances
Arrhythmia	Intoxication
Cardiac ischemia	Amphetamines
Congestive heart failure	Antidepressants
Hypoxia (i.e., in COPD)	Antiparkinsonian agents
Pulmonary embolus	Caffeine
Endocrine and Metabolic	Chemotherapy
Adrenal dysfunction	Cocaine
Acute intermittent porphyria	Corticosteroids
Electrolyte abnormalities	Digitalis
Hyperparathyroidism	Neuroleptics
Hypoglycemia	Sympathomimetics
Pheochromocytoma	Theophylline
Thyroid dysfunction	Thyroid hormone
Neurologic	Withdrawal
Brain tumor	Alcohol
Cerebral anoxia	Narcotics
Delirium (toxic, metabolic, infectious)	Sedative hypnotics
Epilepsy (especially complex partial seizures)	
Migraines	
Vestibular dysfunction	

Abbreviation: COPD = chronic obstructive pulmonary disease.

DIAGNOSIS AND ASSESSMENT

Diagnosis of anxious patients in the medical setting must include consideration of organic factors, reactive or situational distress, and primary psychiatric disorders. All patients should undergo a thorough medical evaluation, including history, and relevant physical and neurologic examinations. A careful substance abuse history should be taken to consider both current abuse (e.g., caffeine, cocaine) and withdrawal (e.g., alcohol, benzodiazepines) as contributing factors. Prescribed medications must also be considered for their potential anxiogenic potential (e.g., bronchodilators). Although many medical and neurologic illnesses may underlie or contribute to anxiety symptoms (see Table 1), the extent of the work-up varies by patient age, associated symptoms and health status, medical history, and the nature of the anxiety. Physical examination and laboratory studies should be targeted to the major locus of symptomatology (e.g., prominent respiratory or cardiac symptoms).

Several factors may help distinguish an organic anxiety syndrome (i.e., anxiety secondary to a medical illness or substance) from a primary anxiety disorder, including (1) onset of anxiety symptoms after age 35 years, (2) absence of personal or family history of anxiety disorders, (3) absence of childhood anxiety difficulties, (4) absence of life stressors precipitating or contributing to the anxiety symptoms, (5) absence of avoidance behavior, and (6) poor treatment response to anxiolytic medications. Any identified medical illness or organic factor should be treated, though associated anxiety symptoms may persist and require additional specific anxiolytic interventions.

PRIMARY ANXIETY DISORDERS

Primary anxiety disorders include adjustment disorder with anxiety, panic disorder with or without agoraphobia (see later), generalized anxiety disorder, social phobia, specific phobia, obsessive-compulsive disorder, post-traumatic stress disorder, simple phobias, and anxiety disorder not otherwise specified.

Adjustment Disorder with Anxiety

Reactive or situational anxiety, diagnosed in the *Diagnostic and Statistical Manual of Mental Disorders, Fourth Edition* (DSM-IV) as Adjustment Disorder with Anxiety, involves nervousness or anxiety as a response to a situational stressor that occurs within 3 months of the onset of the stressor and causes clinically significant marked distress or impairment in social or occupational functioning.

Treatment of adjustment disorders may include psychosocial interventions, including provision of general support, psychotherapy, or specific environmental interventions targeted to the stressor (e.g., public assistance programs). Anxiety symptoms may also require symptomatic relief with anxiolytic or antidepressant medications. Although adjustment disorders are sometimes dismissed by clinicians and family members as expected reactions to distressing situations, symptomatic treatment may greatly improve the patient's quality of life and prevent the development of more severe symptomatology.

Panic Disorder (With or Without Agoraphobia)

Panic disorder is characterized by recurrent panic attacks, which initially may occur spontaneously or "out of the blue" and, over time, may develop in a number of agoraphobic situations (i.e., situations in which the patient has previously experienced a panic attack or one in which escape may be difficult or help not readily available). The symptoms associated with a panic attack usually peak within a few minutes and may last 30 minutes or more. They include a number of physical symptoms of autonomic arousal such as cardiac, respiratory, neurologic, and gastrointestinal. The patient may experience a sense of terror or fear associated with a panic attack, including concerns about dying, going crazy, or losing control. Behaviorally, the patient may feel the need to flee the setting in which the attack occurred to a more safe and familiar place or person. Agoraphobic situations include crowds, shopping malls, public transportation, bridges, tunnels, open spaces, and being at home alone. Panic disorder has its typical onset in adolescence through the third and fourth decades of life and tends to occur more frequently in women than in men. Panic disorder can be associated with marked emotional and physical disability and is associated with high rates of medical utilization, making it a critical disorder to recognize and treat in the medical setting.

Treatment (Table 2) includes the use of the antidepressants, particularly the serotonin reuptake inhibitors (SSRIs) (e.g., fluoxetine [Prozac],* paroxetine [Paxil], or sertraline [Zoloft]), tricyclic antidepressants (TCAs) (e.g., imipramine [Tofranil*]), and monoamine oxidase inhibitors (MAOIs) (e.g., phenelzine [Nardil*]), or high-potency benzodiazepines (e.g., alprazolam [Xanax], clonazepam [Klonopin]). Cognitive-behavioral therapies are also effective.

Generalized Anxiety Disorder

Generalized anxiety disorder (GAD) is defined in DSM-IV as excessive anxiety or worry that is difficult to control and occurs disproportionate to any situational factors. It should be present for a majority of days over a 6-month period and is associated with fatigue, poor concentration, restlessness or inability to relax, irritability, muscle tension, and insomnia. Although generalized anxiety symptoms may fluctuate in response to life stressors, patients

---

*Not FDA approved for this indication.

TABLE 2. **Standard Medication Treatments for Anxiety Disorders**

Medication	Initial Dose (mg)	Dose Range (mg)	Main Limitations	Indication
SSRIs				
Fluoxetine (Prozac)	5–10	10–80	SSRI side effects	PDAG, OCD,* PTSD, SP, GAD
Sertraline (Zoloft)	25	25–200	SSRI side effects	PDAG,* OCD,* PTSD, SP, GAD
Paroxetine (Paxil)	10	10–50	Sedation, SSRI side effects	PDAG,* OCD,* PTSD, SP,* GAD
Fluvoxamine (Luvox)	50	50–300	SSRI side effects	PDAG, OCD,* PTSD, SP, GAD
Citalopram (Celexa)	10	10–60	SSRI side effects	PDAG, OCD, PTSD, SP, GAD
TCAs				
Clomipramine (Anafranil)	25	25–250	Weight gain, sedation, TCA side effects	OCD,* PTSD, GAD, PDAG, ?SP
e.g., Desipramine (Norpramin), imipramine (Tofranil)	10–25	150–300	TCA side effects, jitteriness	GAD, PTSD, PDAG, ?SP
MAOIs				
e.g., Phenelzine (Nardil)	15–30	45–90	Drug and diet interactions, MAOI side effects	OCD, PTSD, SP, PDAG, ?GAD
Novel Antidepressants				
Venlafaxine (Effexor)	37.5	75–300	Jitteriness, GI distress	PDAG, ?GAD, ?PTSD, ?SP, ?OCD
Nefazodone (Serzone)	50	300–550	Sedation, GI distress	?PDAG, GAD, ?OCD, ?PTSD, ?SP
Buspirone (BuSpar)	5 tid	15–60/d	Dysphoria	GAD*
Beta Blockers				
e.g., propranolol (Inderal)	10–20	10–160/d	Depression, sedation	SP (esp. performance), PDAG (adj), GAD (adj)
Benzodiazepines				
Alprazolam (Xanax)	0.25 qid	2–10/d	Memory impairment, abuse risk, sedation discontinuation difficulties, interdose anxiety (shorter acting agents)	PDAG,* PTSD, GAD,* SP, ?PS
Clonazepam (Klonopin)	0.25 qhs	1–5.d		PDAG, PTSD, GAD,* SP
Lorazepam (Ativan)	0.5 tid	3–12/d		GAD, SP, PS, PDAG

*FDA approved.
Abbreviations: GAD = generalized anxiety disorder; PDAG = panic disorder and agoraphobia; GI = gastrointestinal; PTSD = post-traumatic stress disorder; SP = social phobia; PS = specific phobia; BDZ = benzodiazepine; MAOI = monoamine oxidase inhibitor; SSRI = serotonin reuptake inhibitor; TCA = tricyclic antidepressant; adj = adjunctive.

with GAD are described as persistent "worriers" in contrast to patients with more episodic attacks of panic disorder or situationally related phobic symptoms. GAD usually occurs co-morbid with other affective disorders. Clinicians should be particularly alert to the common presence of depressive symptoms in patients with generalized anxiety, as this would indicate the need for treatment with an antidepressant rather than with anxiolytics such as a benzodiazepine or buspirone alone.

Treatment (see Table 2) includes benzodiazepines, buspirone, antidepressants, and cognitive behavioral therapy.

Social Phobia

Social phobia is defined in DSM-IV by marked or persistent fear of embarassment or humiliation in response to situations in which the person is exposed to possible scrutiny by others. The social or performance situations nearly always bring on anxiety and possibly situational panic attacks, resulting in avoidance or marked distress that interferes with social or occupational function. Social phobia may be generalized to many social situations (i.e., meeting new people, speaking to authority figures) or occur solely in response to performance situations such as public speaking. Although "performance anxiety" is common, symptoms occurring in these situations must be intensely distressing or cause impairment to warrant a diagnosis of social phobia. Social phobia may be diagnosed in children and often presents initially in adolescence, with persistence of symptoms into adulthood.

Treatment (see Table 2) includes high-potency benzodiazepines (e.g., clonazepam), SSRIs, MAOIs, beta blockers, and cognitive behavioral therapy. MAOIs have typically been used for social phobia and are generally more effective than the tricyclics (e.g., imipramine) but, given ease of use, side effect profile, and efficacy, SSRIs are now first-line pharmacotherapy. Beta blockers are useful for performance anxiety but are not as effective for the generalized type of social phobia.

Specific Phobia

DSM-IV differentiates specific phobias from less significant, though more common fears by the excessive distress and impairment associated with the anxious response to the phobic stimulus (i.e., heights, blood/injection, airplanes, animals). Phobias frequently begin in childhood or during the middle twenties depending on type or may occur at any time in response to a traumatic event (e.g., being attacked by a dog). Predisposing factors include related traumatic events, unexpected panic attacks associated with the phobic stimulus, or transmission of information by media or from others (i.e., dramatic newspaper reports or parental warnings). In addition, there may be familial transmission by type of phobia.

Although benzodiazepines may be used on an as-needed basis to help patients tolerate the feared stimulus short term, behavior therapy (i.e., exposure and desensitization) is generally more definitive treatment.

Obsessive-Compulsive Disorder

Obsessive-compulsive disorder (OCD) is characterized by persistent, intrusive, anxiety-provoking thoughts or images (obsessions) (e.g., contamination fears) and/or driven, repetitive behaviors (compulsions) that are aimed at decreasing anxiety (e.g., handwashing, checking). The obsessions or compulsions must cause significant distress, take more than 1 hour daily, or significantly interfere with the patient's normal functioning to warrant a diagnosis of OCD. OCD is typically chronic, with onset in childhood or adolescence for males and during the twenties for females. OCD occurs in 1 to 2% of the population and has been associated with Tourette's syndrome and other tic disorders.

Treatment for OCD includes serotonergic antidepressants (i.e., SSRIs), clomipramine (Anafranil), and cognitive-behavioral therapy, including exposure and response prevention to extinguish obsessive thoughts and compulsive behaviors.

Post-traumatic Stress Disorder

To meet DSM-IV criteria, patients with post-traumatic stress disorder (PTSD) must have experienced an event involving serious injury or death, or a threat to physical integrity, to which they responded with fear, helplessness, or horror. Traumatic events may vary from a single disaster (i.e., earthquake) to more chronic, repetitive traumas (e.g., combat, childhood physical abuse). Patients persistently re-experience the trauma in some way (e.g., nightmares, flashbacks) and experience marked physiologic arousal or psychological distress to cues that remind them of the traumatic event. In addition, they have at least three psychological symptoms, including emotional detachment, decreased pleasure and interest, avoidance of reminders of the trauma, amnesia for the trauma, or a sense of a foreshortened future, and at least two symptoms of hyperarousal, including insomnia, irritable outbursts, poor concentration, hypervigilance, and easy startle. This syndrome may be acute or chronic and is quite heterogeneous in presentation. For example, some patients show more prominent depressive symptoms and withdrawal, whereas others are more angry, agitated, and suspicious.

Symptoms usually present within 3 months of the trauma but may have a delayed onset. Some patients develop chronic symptoms, although about half remit within 3 months. Population assessments have reported the lifetime incidence of PTSD to range from 1 to 14%, but rates are higher in populations exposed to serious trauma (e.g., disaster victims, combat veterans).

Pharmacologic treatment is generally directed at relief of predominant symptoms (i.e., antidepressants for depression or anxiety, anticonvulsants for agitation). The Food and Drug Administration has not indicated a specific medication for PTSD. SSRIs are often used because of their broad spectrum of activity against a range of mood, anxiety, and impulsive symptoms. Psychotherapy, including cognitive behavioral therapy, may also be helpful.

TREATMENT CONSIDERATIONS

Explanation of the diagnosis and education provided in a supportive, informative manner can in itself be quite reassuring for many patients. Therapeutic options, including pharmacotherapies and cognitive-behavioral therapy, should be reviewed. Patients started on medication should be studied closely initially in person and/or by telephone. Treatment with antidepressants or benzodiazepines should be initiated with low dose and gradually titrated upward to minimize side effects and maximize compliance. Patients with complex symptoms (often patients with PTSD, OCD, or co-morbidity) or poor initial response to medication may benefit from psychiatric referral. Anxious patients should be carefully observed for the development or presence of depressive symptoms, necessitating the administration of an antidepressant to avoid the common scenario of incomplete treatment with a benzodiazepine alone.

SSRIs are now used as first-line therapy for many anxiety disorders because of their broad spectrum of activity against most mood and anxiety disorders and their relatively favorable side effect profile. SSRIs are better tolerated than older classes of antidepressants (e.g., TCAs), yet may be associated with transient or persistent adverse effects, including nausea, gastrointestinal distress, headaches, sexual dysfunction, and sleep disturbance. SSRIs are usually administered in the morning to minimize insomnia, with the exception of paroxetine, which may be more sedating. Patients with anxiety disorders may experience an initial increase in anxiety when SSRIs are begun. To minimize this, patients initially receive lower doses (e.g., 5 to 10 mg fluoxetine*), 25 mg sertraline,* 10 mg paroxetine,* 25 mg fluvoxamine* [Luvox]) than are indicated for depression, but generally acclimate to dose increases within a week. Therapeutic levels appear similar to those for depression, although higher doses (e.g., fluoxetine 60 to 80 mg per day) may be necessary for patients with OCD and PTSD. Another technique to reduce initial increased anxiety associated with antidepressants in anxious patients is coadministration of benzodiazepines (e.g., lorazepam [Ativan], clonazepam). Benzodiazepines also provide more rapid anxiolysis during the 2- to 6-week therapeutic lag for SSRI effects. For some patients, benzodiazepines may be tapered after a few weeks when the antidepressant becomes effective, but many patients benefit from combined treatment without significant adverse effects.

Other newer agents, including venlafaxine (Effexor),* nefazodone (Serzone),* and mirtazapine (Remeron),* appear to be effective for anxious patients in clinical practice, although there is relatively little systematic data for these indications. Venlafaxine and nefazodone may cause jitteriness or anxiety during treatment initiation and thus, as with the SSRIs, should be initiated at low doses (i.e., venlafaxine 18.75 to 25 mg per day, nefazodone 50 mg per day), with gradual titration to therapeutic levels. Limited data suggest that buproprion and trazodone may not be as reliably anxiolytic as other antidepressants.

Other antidepressants, such as the TCAs and MAOIs, may be useful but have a more aversive side effect profile than the newer agents. TCAs (i.e., desipramine [Norpramin],* imipramine*) are effec-

---

*Not FDA approved for this indication.

tive for panic disorder and generalized anxiety disorder, but less so for social phobia, and are, with the exception of clomipramine, ineffective for OCD. The TCAs are also effective for depressive and anxiety symptoms associated with PTSD. Side effects of the TCAs include anticholinergic effects (e.g., dry mouth, constipation), cardiac conduction disturbance, orthostatic hypotnesion, weight gain, and sexual dysfunction. In addition, the TCAs, unlike the SSRIs, may be fatal in overdose.

MAOIs (i.e., phenelzine [Nardil]* and tranylcypromine [Parnate]*) are broadly effective for the treatment of panic disorder, social phobia, agoraphobia, OCD, PTSD, generalized anxiety, and depression. The MAOIs are less likely to cause increased anxiety at treatment initiation than are the other antidepressants, but over time may be associated with a variety of side effects, including weight gain, insomnia, edema, sexual dysfunction, and myoclonus. In addition, patients taking MAOIs must maintain a strict diet free of tyramine and avoid sympathomimetic agents (e.g., pseudoephedrine) to prevent hypertensive reactions. In addition, all physicians should be aware that MAOI-treated patients should not receive meperidine (Demerol) because of a potentially fatal interaction. Because of the higher risks associated with their use, the MAOIs are generally reserved for patients who are refractory to other interventions and are typically prescribed by psychiatrists or others experienced in their use.

Because many anxiety disorders are effectively treated with either antidepressants or benzodiazepines, the choice of initial medication involves consideration of the risks and benefits of each class of agents. Benzodiazepines act more rapidly than antidepressants, but carry a greater abuse potential, and may cause sedation, psychomotor impairment, ataxia, physical dependence, and disinhibition. They should generally be avoided by patients with organic brain impairment; elderly patients in general should be dosed cautiously and are at increased risk for adverse effects, including falls, disinhibition, and oversedation. Respiratory depression is rare, but is a concern in overdose, when benzodiazepines are combined with alcohol or other sedatives, and in patients with chronic obstructive pulmonary disease or sleep apnea. Depression, frequently co-morbid with anxiety disorders, is usually poorly responsive and may be worsened by benzodiazepines.

Pharmacokinetic properties may be used to guide benzodiazepine selection. All benzodiazepines are effective for generalized anxiety and insomnia; however, panic disorder may be more responsive to high-potency benzodiazepines (e.g., alprazolam, clonazepam). Rapid-onset, short-acting agents (e.g., alprazolam) can provide acute anxiolysis, but may have higher addictive potential, require frequent dosing, and be associated with interdose rebound anxiety. Longer acting agents (e.g., clonazepam) provide more consistent anxiolysis and require less frequent dosing. A short-acting

agent free of liver metabolites (e.g., lorazepam) can minimize drug accumulation and oversedation, particularly in the medically ill. Benzodiazepines should be initiated at low doses (e.g., alprazolam, 0.25 mg two to three times daily; clonazepam, 0.25 to 0.5 mg at bedtime) to minimize initial sedation and increased every 3 to 4 days as tolerated until therapeutic effects are achieved. Although tolerance to the anxiolytic effects of benzodiazepines is rare, patients do become physically dependent after being maintained on benzodiazepines for a few weeks. Benzodiazepine discontinuation may be difficult, and the drug should be tapered slowly to minimize rebound or withdrawal symptoms.

Buspirone (BuSpar) is an azaspirone anxiolytic with effects on serotonin and dopamine receptors. As a nonbenzodiazepine, it lacks sedative properties and abuse potential. It is primarily indicated in generalized anxiety disorder and is not effective alone for the treatment of panic disorder. Experience with buspirone in clinical practice has been variably effective, particularly in patients with prior exposure to benzodiazepines. It is not yet clear if this is due to inadequate dosing or to the lag time (several weeks) for therapeutic response.

Beta blockers are primarily indicated for "performance anxiety" (e.g., propranolol [Inderal] 10 to 40 mg per day as needed 1 to 2 hours before a performance situation) and may reduce peripheral autonomic symptoms of anxiety. They are poorly effective in preventing cognitive and affective symptoms (e.g., worry or fear) associated with anxiety, although they may be useful adjunctively to reduce physical symptoms of arousal. Atenolol (Tenormin), 25 to 100 mg per day, is also effective and may cause fewer side effects to the central nervous system, such as dysphoria and fatigue, than propranolol because it is less lipophilic.

BULIMIA NERVOSA

method of
JAMES E. MITCHELL, M.D.
Neuropsychiatric Research Institute and
University of North Dakota School of Medicine
and Health Sciences
Fargo, North Dakota

Bulimia nervosa is an eating disorder that was first described as a discrete, common diagnostic entity by Gerald Russell in 1979. The disorder is characterized by binge-eating episodes, during which the individual consumes large amounts of food in a short period of time, frequently followed by self-induced vomiting or other compensatory behaviors, such as laxative abuse.

The criteria for bulimia nervosa from the fourth edition of the American Psychiatric Association's *Diagnostic and Statistical Manual of Mental Disorders* (DSM-IV) are shown in Table 1.

Most patients with bulimia nervosa who have been described in the literature, and in particular those who have

---

*Not FDA approved for this indication.

TABLE 1. **Diagnostic Criteria for Bulimia Nervosa**

A. Recurrent episodes of binge-eating. An episode of binge-eating is characterized by both of the following:
   1. Eating, in a discrete period of time (e.g., within any 2-hour period), an amount of food that is definitely larger than most people would eat during a similar period of time and under similar circumstances.
   2. A sense of lack of control over eating during the episode (e.g., a feeling that one cannot stop eating or control what or how much one is eating).
B. Recurrent inappropriate compensatory behavior in order to prevent weight gain, such as self-induced vomiting; misuse of laxatives, diuretics, enemas, or other medications; fasting; or excessive exercise.
C. The binge-eating and inappropriate compensatory behaviors both occur, on average, at least twice a week for 3 months.
D. Self-evaluation is unduly influenced by body shape and weight.
E. The disturbance does not occur exclusively during episodes of anorexia nervosa.
   Specify type:
   • *Purging type:* During the current episode of bulimia nervosa, the person has regularly engaged in self-induced vomiting or the misuse of laxatives, diuretics, or enemas.
   • *Non-purging type:* During the current episode of bulimia nervosa, the person has used other inappropriate compensatory behaviors, such as fasting or excessive exercise, but has not regularly engaged in self-induced vomiting or the misuse of laxatives, diuretics, or enemas.

From the American Psychiatric Association: Diagnostic and Statistical Manual of Mental Disorders, 4th ed. Washington, DC: American Psychiatric Association, 1994, pp 549–550.

been the focus of treatment research, have been of the purging subtype; very little is known about nonpurging patients who engage in other types of compensatory behaviors, such as excessive exercise or fasting, although these patients are occasionally seen in clinical practice. Therefore, the focus of most of our discussion is on the purging type of bulimia nervosa.

In addition to the abnormal eating and compensatory behaviors, most of these patients can also be characterized by evidencing certain distinct psychological symptoms. In particular, most of them are very preoccupied with body weight and shape concerns, and most fear that they are or will become overweight, despite the fact that most are of normal or low weight. These symptoms are similar to those seen in anorexia nervosa, although usually not as severe.

The disorder has been described in all socioeconomic groups. It does appear, however, to be seen most commonly among women in industrialized societies in which a high positive value is placed on slimness as a model of attractiveness for young women, and where food is freely available to the general population. Prevalence studies suggest that 1 to 2% of women in such societies develop this disorder, whereas prevalence studies in preindustrial countries suggest that bulimia nervosa occurs rarely. In addition, studies suggest that eating disorders are becoming more common in the Third World and that patients in these settings may present with atypical characteristics. Data also suggest that bulimia nervosa is more common in urban than in rural areas.

The median age at onset of bulimia nervosa is around 18 years, but it can occur at any time during adolescence or young adulthood; it is rare for patients to report an age

at onset past 40 years. It is interesting that the age at onset clusters around the age of 18, this being the time when many young women are leaving home and going into the work force or to college. This crucial period of role transition seems to be a high-risk time for the development of this disorder.

DIAGNOSTIC CRITERIA

As summarized in Table 1, the hallmark of the disorder is the binge-eating episode. Although at times these episodes appear to be precipitated by discrete cues such as stressful events or unpleasant emotions, often the binge-eating episodes become an institutionalized activity, occurring usually late in the day when the individual returns home from work or school.

The caloric content of binge-eating episodes can vary dramatically, but commonly as many as 3000 to 5000 calories are consumed. The most commonly ingested binge-eating foods include those that are easily prepared and that tend to be high in fat and carbohydrates, with ice cream being the most common. These same foods tend to be avoided at times when the individual is not binge-eating.

Many individuals describe feeling "out of control" while binge-eating. After binge-eating they then engage in some compensatory behavior; this is most often self-induced vomiting. At other times they may ingest drugs as a way of attempting to precipitate weight loss, for example, large numbers of laxatives or diuretics, both of which result in a decrease in body weight through the loss of fluid rather than ingested calories. In rare instances, patients with bulimia nervosa use ipecac to induce vomiting, which is particularly dangerous given the dose-dependent cardiomyopathy that this agent can cause.

CO-MORBIDITY

Although some individuals with bulimia nervosa are relatively free of other problems, it is not uncommon to encounter co-morbid psychopathologic conditions in these patients. Most common are affective disorders, particularly recurrent depression. The prevalence of anxiety disorders has also been examined and appears high as well. Co-morbid substance abuse problems also have received considerable attention, because they markedly complicate the treatment of patients. These patients appear to be at increased risk for the abuse of both typical substances of abuse (e.g., alcohol) and atypical substances of abuse (e.g., laxatives, diuretics, diet pills, and ipecac). Screening for both types of problems should be part of a routine evaluation.

Bulimia nervosa has also been associated with certain personality disorders, particularly cluster B, axis II disorders, such as borderline personality disorder. Such individuals generally are characterized by poor insight, problems with affect regulation, impulsivity, and difficulties with interpersonal relationships.

COMPLICATIONS

Most patients with bulimia nervosa are at a relatively normal body weight, and one does not usually see the marked physical changes associated with starvation that one encounters with anorexia nervosa patients. However, despite a grossly normal body weight, many patients with bulimia nervosa evidence subtle changes suggestive of malnutrition, including, on screening laboratory examination, elevations in beta-hydroxybutyric acid and free fatty acid levels and fasting hypoglycemia. Interestingly, brain imaging studies using computed tomography or magnetic resonance imaging have demonstrated "pseudoatrophy" in some patients with bulimia nervosa, again suggesting problems with malnutrition, although the degree of atrophy is usually less severe than in anorexia nervosa.

On physical examination there are a few clues that are useful in making this diagnosis. The best area of focus is the teeth. Recurrent episodes of vomiting are associated with decalcification of the dental surfaces that are exposed to the vomitus, and the majority of patients who have been actively vomiting for more than 4 years have obvious evidence of enamel erosion. Interestingly, the amalgams or fillings are relatively resistant to the acid and therefore often project above the surface of the teeth.

Some patients with bulimia nervosa evidence salivary gland hypertrophy, often involving the parotid glands, which at times can be dramatic and which may persist intermittently for several months during recovery. Some patients with bulimia nervosa also show callus or scar formation on the dorsum of the hand or knuckles, resulting from trauma to these areas when using the hand to stimulate the gag reflex to induce vomiting.

On laboratory testing, patients with bulimia nervosa not uncommonly evidence fluid and electrolyte abnormalities. Most commonly, metabolic alkalosis, hypochloremia, and, occasionally, hypokalemia are seen. Edema generally is suggestive of laxative or diuretic abuse, both of which result in reflex fluid retention.

Many patients with bulimia nervosa have a variety of gastrointestinal complaints, including constipation, diarrhea, bloating after eating, abdominal pain, and dyspepsia. Gastric dilation and rupture have also been reported and may be the leading cause of death in these patients. Various subtle endocrine abnormalities have been described in bulimic patients.

ETIOLOGY

There are three variables that correlate highly with the development of the disorder:

1. *Female sex:* Bulimia nervosa is rare in males, who account for only 2 to 8% of the cases.

2. *Age at onset in teen to early adult years:* Bulimia nervosa seems to develop in the context of dieting during adolescence or early adulthood and rarely outside of this context.

3. *Cultural variables:* Bulimia nervosa and other similar eating disorders appear to exist almost exclusively in societies in which a high positive value is placed on slimness as a model of attractiveness and in which obesity is disparaged.

However, all three of these variables identify a very large group of girls and women, most of whom do not develop full-blown eating disorders or bulimia nervosa. The reason why some move from experimentation to ongoing problems is unclear, although genetic studies suggest there may be a genetic diathesis for the development of this disorder.

Other risk factors appear important, including a history of sexual abuse in childhood and a history of excessive weight before illness onset. It is possible that certain physiologic changes that develop in the course of the eating disorder may perpetuate the behavior. For example, studies suggest that metabolism of serotonin, a neurotransmitter involved in appetite and impulse regulation, may be abnormal in patients with bulimia nervosa. Also, elevated levels of a peptide known to increase appetite, the pancre-

atic polypeptide PYY, have been found in bulimic patients after a period of eating stability. Some bulimic patients may have impaired satiety responses, including impaired peripheral release of satiety hormones such as cholecystokinin.

DIAGNOSIS

The most important ingredient in the diagnosis of eating disorders is a high index of suspicion. Disorders of mood and eating are common enough in adolescent girls and young adult women that questions about such problems should be included in the routine evaluation of such patients. The physician should routinely inquire about the presence of binge-eating, protracted fasting, and compensatory behaviors such as self-induced vomiting. Also, it is useful to inquire about body image. A straightforward, nonjudgmental approach will increase the likelihood of a valid response.

TREATMENT

Most patients with bulimia nervosa can be successfully treated out of hospital. However, they tend to be somewhat difficult to work with for many health care professionals, and the available treatment studies suggest that they do best in structured programs that use techniques designed specially to treat this group. Hospitalization may be considered in patients who fail to respond to outpatient treatment, who are co-morbidly depressed to the point at which suicide is of concern, or for whom mental instability is a problem.

The treatment literature on bulimia nervosa has centered on the parallel development of two strategies: pharmacologic strategies, primarily using antidepressant drugs, and psychotherapy or counseling approaches.

Pharmacotherapies

Many placebo-controlled double-blind antidepressant trials of bulimia nervosa have been published, and the results are fairly consistent in showing that antidepressant drugs do have a potent and significant suppressant effect on binge-eating and purging behavior. The available studies suggest that individuals who are not depressed at baseline may respond equally well to antidepressant treatments, suggesting that the mechanism of action may be other than the antidepressant effect. Many tricyclic antidepressant compounds and monoamine oxidase inhibitors have been used experimentally. However, the serotonin reuptake inhibitors have become the agents of choice, mainly because they appear to be as efficacious as the older agents but better tolerated. The agent that has been studied in the most subjects, including in two large multicenter trials, is fluoxetine (Prozac); this drug appears to work optimally in these patients at dosages higher than those usually employed in the treatment of depression (e.g., 60 mg per day).

Although there are dramatic and significant reductions in the frequency of target eating behaviors with antidepressant treatment, and impressive improvement in symptoms of mood, many patients with bulimia nervosa remain symptomatic despite antidepressant treatment. This raises questions as to whether antidepressants are a sufficient treatment for these patients.

Several studies have examined the combined use of antidepressants and psychotherapy, and these studies suggest that, for eating disorder symptoms, certain psychotherapeutic approaches are probably superior; however, there is some evidence that on certain variables, such as depression, anxiety, and in some eating disorder symptoms, the combination is best. Therefore, consideration should be given to treatment with combined drug and psychotherapy when both are available.

Psychotherapy

Paralleling the interest in antidepressant treatment, a fairly large treatment literature on psychotherapy approaches has developed. Initial studies compared active treatments with waiting list control groups or minimal interventions, but more recently psychotherapy studies have progressed to the point at which active treatments are being compared and dismantling studies are being undertaken. The results of these studies are quite consistent in showing that cognitive behavioral therapy (CBT) techniques, delivered in either group or individual formats, appear to be as effective as or more effective than the comparison treatments that have been used. There are a number of common elements among these CBT treatments:

1. There is strong emphasis on nutritional counseling. In many of the programs patients are given a structured meal-planning system at the beginning of treatment and are strongly encouraged to eat regular, balanced meals, while treatment focuses on the problem of dietary restraint as a precipitant to binge-eating.

2. Other behavioral techniques are employed, such as examining cues associated with binge-eating and the consequences of the behavior (both positive and negative). Many of these programs also focus on cognitive restructuring techniques around weight and shape concerns and irrational beliefs about food and dieting.

3. Self-monitoring is also very useful. Research has shown that simply having patients record when and how much they are binge-eating can be very helpful in teaching them to gain control of the behavior.

4. Family involvement may be useful, particularly for younger patients who are living at home.

One other form of structured psychotherapy, interpersonal therapy, has also been shown to be effective and is being tested in two studies.

COURSE AND OUTCOME

Unfortunately, many patients with bulimia nervosa go untreated and have the illness chronically or in a chronic relapsing fashion over many years. Carefully designed research studies have shown that using structured techniques, 40 to 80% of patients with bulimia nervosa can learn to control their eating behavior during the course of a relatively short-term therapy (e.g., 3 to 4 months). However, 20 to 25% of these patients will later experience relapse, usually within 6 months after treatment. Long-term followup, at 10 to 15 years after evaluation, suggested that upward of 80% of individuals eventually improve significantly or completely recover.

DELIRIUM

method of
SUE LEVKOFF, Sc.D.
Harvard Medical School
Boston, Massachusetts

Although the diagnostic criteria for delirium have changed over the years, the core features have remained relatively unchanged. Diagnostic criteria, as identified in the *Diagnostic and Statistical Manual of Mental Disorders, Fourth Edition* (DSM-IV), include (1) disturbance of consciousness (i.e., reduced clarity of awareness of the environment) with reduced ability to focus, sustain, or shift attention; (2) a change in cognition (such as memory deficit, disorientation, language disturbance) or the development of a perceptual disturbance that is not better accounted for by a pre-existing, established, or evolving dementia; (3) rapid onset (usually hours to days) and fluctuations during the course of a day; and (4) evidence from the history, physical examination, or laboratory findings that the disturbance is caused by the direct physiologic consequences of a general medical condition.

Prevalence rates of delirium in hospitalized elderly medical patients range from 10 to 30%, with incidence rates ranging from 4 to 55%. As the numbers of elderly individuals increase, clinicians can expect to encounter delirium more frequently. Clinicians are not typically well-trained in the diagnosis, work-up, and management of delirium. This omission in training is significant, given that substantial research has documented the poor clinical outcomes associated with the syndrome, including longer hospital lengths of stay, increased risk of institutionalization upon discharge, and poorer physical function up to 6 months after hospital discharge. Moreover, the fact that large numbers of hospitalized patients have been found to be discharged with symptoms of delirium that persist for up to 6 months past hospital discharge has implications for discharge planners, who are responsible for ensuring a safe environment for patients on their return home from the hospital.

CLINICAL FEATURES

Delirium has several subtypes: the hyperactive variant, the hypoactive variant, and the mixed variant, which demonstrates features of both clinical subtypes. Research has found no differences among these groups with respect to age, sex, or presence of dementia. It is important that clinicians recognize these different subtypes because the hyperactive patient who develops the florid subtype with its accompanying psychomotor overactivity, hyperresponsiveness to stimuli, hallucinations, fear, and irritability is more likely to be diagnosed and treated than the hypoactive patient with reduced levels of psychomotor activity, alertness, and vigilance.

Although studies of the phenomenology of delirium in the elderly do not exist, it is believed that the core features of the syndrome are consistent across all age groups. Because of age-related biologic changes in the central nervous system, the elderly have a reduced reserve capacity and reduced ability to compensate for insult to homeostasis. As a result, the elderly brain is likely to show impaired function in response to stress. The symptoms of delirium can develop more insidiously in the elderly because the added impairment is superimposed on pre-existing limitations, and symptoms typically subside more slowly following treatment.

CLINICAL COURSE

The onset of delirium is rapid and occurs over a few hours or days. Often a patient first experiences symptoms during the night, after waking from a dream. The patient may become confused, inattentive, and disoriented. The patient's awareness of his or her surroundings and ability to communicate can become extremely impaired. Many patients develop olfactory and gustatory hallucinations and paranoid delusional ideas. Often, patients experience reversal of sleep patterns, being drowsy and difficult to arouse during the day and confused and agitated during the night. Although it has generally been assumed that delirium resolves within 1 to 2 weeks, research has found that symptoms can persist for up to 6 months after hospital discharge.

DIAGNOSTIC WORK-UP

Because delirium often has multiple etiologies, the work-up should include a thorough search for all potential contributing factors. Knowledge of a patient's baseline cognitive function is crucial, as the more impaired the patient, the fewer the stressors needed to precipitate delirium. Table 1 provides an overview of the known contributing factors. Medications are the most common reversible causes of delirium, with benzodiazepines, narcotics, and medications with anticholinergic side effects the most common offenders. A careful review of all medications, including both prescription and nonprescription drugs, and attention to recent additions, dose changes, and discontinuations is important. A work-up should include a careful history with the patient (when possible) and family, physical examination (including the Mini-Mental Status Examination), and medication review. Additional diagnostic testing may be necessary, depending on findings from the initial work-ups: for example, laboratory examination for complete blood count, electrolytes, glucose, calcium, magnesium, phosphate, renal function, hepatic function, and oxygen saturation; infection work-up (urinalysis, chest film, additional cultures); and selected additional testing (dementia profile, serum drug levels, toxicology, arterial blood gases, electrocardiogram, brain imaging, cerebrospinal fluid).

Table 2 demonstrates how important knowledge of a patient's prior cognitive status is to distinguish delirium from dementia. The central diagnostic feature of delirium is inattention, which can be assessed formally by forward and backward digit span or reciting the months of the year backwards. Additional key diagnostic elements for delirium are an abnormal level of consciousness (comatose, drowsy, hyperalert) and disorganized thinking (rambling, incoherent speech), which should be evident from taking a basic history. Another feature is a fluctuating course over

TABLE 1. Contributing Factors in Delirium

Therapeutic drug intoxication/withdrawal
  Psychoactive drugs
  Toxic levels of drugs
  Any drug with appropriate time course of initiation, change, withdrawal
Disorders of inadequate cerebral oxygenation
  Hypoxia
  Anemia
  Hypotension or low cardiac output
  Arteriovenous shunting states (sepsis)
Metabolic disorders
  Hypo/hypervolemia
  Electrolyte disorders (especially hyponatremia, hypercalcemia)
  Glucose disorders
  Hypercapnia
  Renal/hepatic failure
Infection and/or fever
  Pneumonia
  Urinary tract infection
  Soft tissue infections
  Others
Cardiovascular disorders
  Congestive heart failure
  Arrhythmia
  Acute myocardial infarction
Brain disorders
  Stroke
  Trauma
  Infection
  Tumors (primary and metastatic)
Severe pain
  Postoperative states
  Terminal states
Sensory deprivation/alteration
  Blindness and/or deafness
  Severe isolation
  Environmental change/loss of cues
Alcohol intoxication/withdrawal
Urinary retention/fecal impaction

minutes to hours. An acutely ill, hospitalized elderly patient with an acute change in mental status, inattention, and disorganized thinking or an abnormal level of consciousness with fluctuations almost certainly has delirium. The Confusion Assessment Method is an easy-to-use diagnostic algorithm for clinicians (Table 3).

MANAGEMENT

Management of the delirious patient requires a thorough search for and correction of all contributing factors. Although some factors, such as an offending medication, can be rectified immediately, others, such as underlying medical problems, may take longer to correct. Even with prompt reversal of contributing factors, rapid resolution of delirium does not always occur due to the existence of new exacerbants.

TABLE 2. Delirium Versus Dementia

Delirium	Dementia
Develops abruptly	Develops slowly
Reversible	Progressive
Short duration	Present for many months or years
Fluctuating consciousness	Rarely altered consciousness
Precise time of onset	Uncertain date of onset

TABLE 3. **Confusion Assessment Method (CAM) Diagnostic Algorithm**

Feature 1: Acute Onset and Fluctuating Course

This feature is usually observed by a family member or nurse and is shown by positive responses to the following questions: Is there evidence of an acute change in mental status from the patient's baseline? Did the (abnormal) behavior fluctuate during the day (i.e., tend to come and go) or increase and decrease in severity?

Feature 2: Inattention

This feature is shown by a positive response to the following question: Did the patient have difficulty focusing attention (e.g., being easily distracted) or have difficulty keeping track of what was being said?

Feature 3: Disorganized Thinking

This feature is shown by a positive response to the following question: Was the patient's thinking disorganized or incoherent, such as rambling or irrelevant conversation, unclear or illogical flow of ideas, or unpredictable switching from subject to subject?

Feature 4: Altered Level of Consciousness

This feature is shown by any answer other than "alert" to the following question: Overall, how would you rate this patient's level of consciousness (alert [normal], vigilant [hyperalert], lethargic [drowsy, easily aroused], stupor [difficult to arouse], or coma [unarousable])?

The diagnosis of delirium by CAM requires the presence of features 1, 2, and either 3 or 4.

From Inouye SK, Viscoli CM, Horwitz RI, et al: Clarifying confusion: The confusion assessment method. Ann Intern Med 113:941–948, 1990.

Because delirium may not reverse quickly even with appropriate intervention, delirious patients should be managed by an interdisciplinary team of physicians, nurses, family members, and anyone else who comes into contact with the patient. Table 4 lists the delirious patient's vulnerabilities and proposes management strategies.

The best way to manage delirium is to prevent it. Very old patients (>80 years of age); patients with sensory, cognitive, and functional impairments; and

TABLE 4. **Management of the Delirious Patient**

Vulnerability	Management
Agitated behavior	Obtain a sitter
	Allow family to stay in room
Medication side effects	Carefully review and discontinue medications
Deconditioning	Mobilize patient to chair and even ambulate, with assistance
Malnutrition	Feed patient, if necessary by hand
Failure to rehabilitate	Work with patient as tolerated, using simple repetitive tasks
Sensory deprivation	Use glasses, hearing aids
	Provide adequate (soft) lighting
	Provide clocks, calendar, radio
	Socialize as tolerated
	Allow patient to sleep when possible
Nosocomial complications	Re-evaluate carefully for
	Cardiac decompensation
	Infections, especially lung, urinary tract
	Aspiration
Incontinence/retention/ obstipation	Toilet frequently
	Careful perineal hygiene
	Monitor output carefully
	Fecal disimpaction, if necessary
	Administer gentle laxatives
Severe pain	Administer round-the-clock:
	Acetaminophen
	Local/regional analgesia
	Low-dose narcotics

those with multiple chronic medical problems and medications are at greatest risk. Especially for these high-risk patients, clinicians must attempt to prevent problems that precipitate delirium by recognizing and treating illnesses early, minimizing medicines, providing appropriate treatment environments, and attending to nutrition and mobility.

A multicomponent risk-factor intervention to prevent delirium (consisting of standardized protocols for the management of cognitive impairment, sleep deprivation, immobility, visual impairment, hearing impairment, and dehydration) has been found to successfully reduce the incidence of delirium in hospitalized older patients. In effect, the clinician should treat the delirium before it begins. It is only by understanding delirium—its clinical features, course, diagnosis, and management—that the clinician can hope to prevent it, which may be the best way of avoiding its adverse clinical, functional, and economic sequelae.

MOOD DISORDERS

method of
ELLIOTT RICHELSON, M.D.
Mayo Clinic-Jacksonville
Jacksonville, Florida

Depression is a relatively common disease that is vastly undertreated and largely treatable. It is thought to result ultimately from biochemical changes in the brain. Aside from the risk of suicide in untreated depression, this disease significantly modifies outcome for other diseases. For example, in the months after myocardial infarction, death is much more likely to occur in patients who are depressed. Pharmacologic treatment of depression is the focus of this article; however, other modalities (psychotherapy and electroconvulsive therapy [ECT]) are briefly discussed.

In most cases, depression can be effectively treated in an outpatient setting, with inpatient treatment being reserved for the more severely ill, such as those patients who are actively suicidal. In either case, the treatment modality is most likely to involve a pharmacologic agent alone or in combination with some form of psychotherapy. ECT is usually used for the patient who has failed to respond to other types of treatment (treatment-resistant patient), for the patient who is very debilitated due to lack of nourishment, or for the patient with an overwhelming desire to commit suicide.

There are 21 drugs approved by the U.S. Food and Drug Administration (FDA) for use as antidepressants; and if one goes outside the approved indication, two other drugs can be added to the list. This discussion aims to simplify the selection of an antidepressant by providing information on their pharmacologic properties.

EPIDEMIOLOGY

Depression afflicts about 5% of the adult population in the United States at any given time. In addition, 1 to 2% of the adult population has acute manic-depressive (bipolar) illness. About 30% of the adult population will suffer from at least one episode of depression at some point in their lives. Also, the lifetime probability of death by suicide in major depressive disorder has been estimated to be as high as 25%. Studies suggest that more than 50% of patients who committed suicide saw a physician during the month before death; however, these patients were not diagnosed as being depressed. Data on suicide in the United States from 1991 show that there were 30,000 reported suicides in that year. It is the eighth leading cause of death in the United States, which ranks 24th in the rate of suicide worldwide.

The risk of depression is two to three times higher among women than among men. In addition, depression is two to three times higher in first-degree relatives of depressed individuals. Days lost from work (disability days) for persons with major depression are nearly five times higher than for individuals who are not depressed. Thus, depressive illness can have major economic impact.

Depression unfortunately is underdiagnosed and undertreated. Surveys done by the National Institute of Mental Health (NIMH) show that about 70% of depressed patients do not get treatment for their disease even though 85 to 90% can be treated successfully.

About 70% of patients respond to antidepressant drug therapy and can enjoy a complete recovery from their depression. ECT can help those patients who are refractory to antidepressants (about another 20%). About 10% of depressed patients are resistant to all known forms of therapy.

DIAGNOSIS

The diagnosis of depression rests on the identification of core signs and symptoms. These include depressed mood, diminished pleasure or interest in activities, significant change in appetite or weight, alterations in sleep (insomnia or hypersomnia), psychomotor agitation or retardation, fatigue or loss of energy, inability to concentrate, indecisiveness, and thoughts of death, dying, or suicide. The clinician's index of suspicion should also be raised if a patient presents with a chief complaint of fatigue, pain, sleep disturbances, anxiety, irritability, or gastrointestinal problems. If a physical reason for these complaints is not found, the clinician should evaluate the patient for depression.

Other psychiatric disorders, such as schizophrenia, schizoaffective disorder, and anxiety disorders, may also have features of depression, which can coexist with another disorder. Many nonpsychiatric disorders can present with complaints of fatigue, insomnia, and difficulty concentrating. The differential diagnosis includes endocrinopathies (hypothyroidism, hyperparathyroidism, Cushing's and Addison's diseases), subcortical dementias (Huntington's and Parkinson's diseases), frontal lobe disease, right hemisphere stroke, occult tumors outside the brain, and infections of the brain. In addition, anemia, hypoglycemia, and hyperglycemia may simulate depression.

TREATMENT

Antidepressant Drugs

Classification

Treatment of depression is largely pharmacologic, usually in combination with some form of limited, supportive psychotherapy. The antidepressants available in the United States today include three drugs classified as monoamine oxidase inhibitors (MAOIs) (isocarboxazid [Marplan], phenelzine [Nardil], tranylcypromine [Parnate]), and 18 others (Table 1). In addition, it is likely that the FDA will soon approve the 22nd antidepressant (reboxetine [Vestra]). Until several years ago, the so-called tricyclic antidepressants (e.g., amitriptyline [Elavil], desipramine [Norpramin]) were the first-line drugs. However, with the introduction of newer compounds with more favorable side effect profiles and low toxicity in overdose, the older drugs are being prescribed less often (although the economics of health care may reverse this trend).

Until the 1970s, antidepressants approved for use in the United States could be classified into two groups: tricyclic antidepressants and MAOIs. This classification mixed structural (tricyclic) and functional (inhibition of monoamine oxidase) criteria; a classification based on either structure or activity would be better. With the introduction of some of the newer compounds (e.g., mirtazapine [Remeron]), drugs could be divided into multiple classes, complicating the picture. A simplified classification for the purpose of this review divides the antidepressants into those that are MAOIs and those that are not (the majority) (see Table 1). This functional classification eliminates the confusion in the literature from the incorrect usage of terms such as "heterocyclic," "tricyclic," and "tetracyclic." Classifying antidepressants as either tricyclic or heterocyclic is not correct. For example, doxepin [Adapin, Sinequan] is correctly classified on the basis of its structure as a heterocyclic, tricyclic antidepressant.

Clinical Pharmacology

The clinical effects of antidepressants generally do not appear until the first 1 or 2 weeks after the start of therapy. This time lag for the onset of therapeutic effects may relate to changes in sensitivity of certain neurotransmitter receptors. As a clinical rule of thumb, an adequate trial constitutes at least 6 weeks of treatment at an adequate dosage, which is often difficult to know. The wide interindividual variation in the absorption, distribution, and excretion of anti-

TABLE 1. **Pharmacokinetics, Daily Doses, and Projected Therapeutic Plasma Ranges of Antidepressants**

Drug (Generic and Trade Names)	Individual Variation in Metabolism	Elimination Half-Life, $T_{1/2}$ (h) Mean	Range	Starting Dosage* (mg/d)	Usual Daily Dose for Adults (mg)	Usual Dose Range (mg/d)	Projected† Optimal Therapeutic Plasma Range (ng/mL)
Non-Monoamine Oxidase Inhibitor Antidepressants							
Amitriptyline (Elavil)‡	10-fold	21	13–36	50	150–200	50–300	80–250§
Amoxapine (Asendin)		8	8–30‖	50	200–300	50–400	200–600¶
Bupropion (Wellbutrin)		9.8	3.9–23.1	200**	300††	100–450‡‡	
Bupropion SR (Wellbutrin SR)		21		150	150–300	100–400	
Citalopram (Celexa)		33		20	20–60	20–80	
Clomipramine (Anafril)***		32	19–37	25	50–250	75–250	
Desipramine (Norpramin)‡	10-fold	21	12–30	50	100–200	50–300	125–300
Doxepin (Adapin, Sinequan)‡	10- to 15-fold	17	8–24	50	75–150	50–300	150–250¶¶
Fluoxetine (Prozac)		87	26–220	20	20–80	20–80	
Fluvoxamine (Luvox)***		16		50	50–300†††	50–300	
Imipramine (Tofranil)‡	30-fold	28	18–34	50	75–150	50–300	150–250‡‡‡
Maprotiline (Ludiomil)		43		50	100–150	50–225	200–600
Mirtazapine (Remeron)		30	20–40	15	15–45	15–60	
Nefazodone (Serzone)		3	2–4	200	300–600	200–600	
Nortriptyline (Pamelor)‡	30-fold	36	14–79	20	75–100	30–125	50–150
Paroxetine (Paxil)		21	4–65	10	20–50	10–50	
Protriptyline (Vivactil)‡	10- to 15-fold	78	55–127	10	15–40	10–60	70–260
Reboxetine (Vestra)§§§		13		4	8–10	8–12	
Sertraline (Zoloft)		26		25	50–150	50–200	
Trazodone (Desyrel)		7	3–16	50	150–400	50–600	800–1600
Trimipramine (Surmontil)‡		13		50	100–200	50–300	150–250
Venlafaxine (Effexor)		5	2–7	37.5	75–225	75–375	
Venlafaxine XR (Effexor XR)		5		37.5	75–225	75–375	
Monoamine Oxidase Inhibitors							
Isocarboxazid (Marplan)				20§§	10–30	10–60‖‖	
Phenelzine (Nardil)		2.8	1.5–4	15	45–60	45–90§§§	
Tranylcypromine (Parnate)	4-fold	2.4	1.5–3	10	30–40	30–60	

*Dosage should be divided initially for all listed drugs, and elderly persons should be treated with about half of the usual dosage for adults.

†Only amitriptyline, imipramine, nortriptyline, and desipramine have been significantly studied for blood level versus clinical response.

‡A classic tricyclic antidepressant.

§Amitriptyline + nortriptyline.

‖Amoxapine, 8 hours; 8-hydroxyamoxapine, 30 hours.

¶Amoxapine + 8-hydroxyamoxapine; of total drug measured, amoxapine ≈ 20%; 7-hydroxyamoxapine ≈ 15%; and 8-hydroxyamoxapine ≈ 65%.

**Dose should be divided, 100 mg bid.

††The divided dose by fourth day of treatment.

‡‡Maximum recommended divided dose achieved if no response after 3 weeks at the lower dosage.

§§Dosage should be divided.

‖‖Dose should be reduced to a maintenance level of 10–20 mg daily (or less) once response begins, because of the drug's cumulative effects.

¶¶Doxepin + desmethyldoxepin.

***Not marketed in the United States as an antidepressant.

†††Divided dose above 100 mg/day.

‡‡‡Imipramine + desipramine.

§§§1 mg/kg.

Updated and modified from Richelson E: Antidepressants: Pharmacology and clinical use. *In* Karasu TB (ed): Treatments of Psychiatric Disorders. A Task Force Report of the American Psychiatric Association, Washington, DC, vol 3, pp 1773–1787, 1989, and reproduced with permission from the publisher.

depressants may explain why dosages for specific antidepressants may vary widely. In addition, drug clearance generally declines with increasing age.

Table 1 outlines the usual daily doses and projected optimal therapeutic plasma ranges of antidepressants currently available in the United States. In addition, reboxitene is included in anticipation of its becoming available shortly. Few antidepressants have rigorously defined therapeutic blood ranges. Nonetheless, one can use the projected ranges presented in Table 1 as a guide in clinical practice. For newer second-generation compounds (bupropion [Wellbutrin]; fluoxetine [Prozac]; mirtazapine [Remeron]; nefazodone [Serzone]; paroxetine [Paxil]; sertraline [Zoloft]; and venlafaxine [Effexor]), projecting a therapeutic range at this time is not possible. Two drugs listed in Table 1, clomipramine (Anafranil) and fluvoxamine (Luvox) are presently approved in the United States for treatment of obsessive-compulsive disorder but are marketed elsewhere as antidepressants.

Therapeutic drug monitoring is most readily available for the tricyclic compounds. Reasons for monitoring these drugs include assessing compliance, maximizing response, avoiding toxicity, reducing cost for the patient, and avoiding medical-legal problems.

There is a substantiated 10- to 30-fold variation in individual metabolism for some of these tricyclic compounds (see Table 1). This variation requires specific attention to individualization of drug dosages and emphasizes the need to monitor drug plasma levels to achieve an appropriate therapeutic response, particularly in the elderly patient.

The idea of a therapeutic window (i.e., a blood level range below and above which the drug is ineffective) has been thoroughly evaluated only for nortriptyline (Pamelor). Protriptyline (Vivactil) and nortriptyline, in comparison with other tricyclic antidepressants, have increased potency (see Table 1). Therefore, a smaller mean daily dose of these drugs should be prescribed. The longer elimination half-life for protriptyline may in part explain the requirement for a lower dosage.

The mean elimination half-lives of most of the antidepressants listed in Table 1 are in the 15- to 30-hour range. The half-lives of maprotiline (Ludiomil), protriptyline, and fluoxetine, however, are much longer. Consequently, these drugs not only require a longer time to achieve a steady state after initiation of treatment, but also need a longer period of observation of complications after ingestion of an overdose. Based on pharmacokinetic considerations, a rational dosing interval for an antidepressant drug is equal to its elimination half-life (see Table 1). In practice, a single daily dose is appropriate for those drugs with half-lives of around 15 hours or greater. It is

also reasonable to consider prescribing the very long half-life compounds—protriptyline, fluoxetine, and maprotiline—less frequently, especially in the elderly patient. Bupropion and venlafaxine are now available in a sustained-release and extended-release form, respectively (Wellbutrin SR and Effexor XR), allowing less frequent (once- or twice-daily) dosing than is required for the immediate-release formulations.

A pharmacokinetic rule of thumb is that it takes four to five times the elimination half-life with a constant dosing interval to achieve steady-state levels. Another pharmacokinetic rule of thumb based on the elimination half-life is that it takes four to five times this number to have greater than 90% of the drug eliminated from the body after stopping the medication. Abrupt discontinuation of drugs with elimination half-lives of around 24 hours or less can result in a withdrawal syndrome.

These agents are highly lipid soluble and therefore have a high volume of distribution. Most are also strongly bound to plasma proteins. Changes in body fat and plasma proteins with aging, therefore, can have effects on the clearance of a drug and its potency.

Basic Pharmacology (Table 2)

For the pharmacodynamic effects of antidepressants, the site of action that may be especially rele-

TABLE 2. **Some Pharmacodynamic Effects of Antidepressants**

Drug	Potency of Blockade of Transporters			Transporter Selectivity (5-HT/NE)*	Potency of Blockade of Neurotransmitter Receptors			
	5-HT	NE	DA		Histamine H_1	Muscarinic	Alpha$_1$-Adrenergic	Dopamine D_2
Amitriptyline (Elavil)	+ + + +	+ + +	+	+ + +	+ + + +	+ +	+ +	+/−
Amoxapine (Asendin)	+ + +	+ + +	+	− − −	+ +	+/−	+ +	+
Bupropion (Wellbutrin)	0	0	+ +	+ + +	0	0	0	0
Citalopram (Celexa)	+ + + +	0	0	+ + + + + +	+/−	0	0	0
Clomipramine (Anafranil)†	+ + + + +	+ + +	+	+ + + +	+ +	+ +	+ +	+
Desipramine (Norpramin)	+ + +	+ + + +	+	− − − −	+	+	+	0
Doxepin (Adapin, Sinequan)	+ + +	+ + +	0	− − −	+ + + + +	+	+ +	0
Fluoxetine (Prozac)	+ + + +	+ +	+	+ + + + +	0	0	0	0
Fluvoxamine (Luvox)†	+ + + +	+	0	+ + + + + +	0	0	0	0
Imipramine (Tofranil)	+ + + +	+ + +	0	+ + + +	+ + +	+	+	0
Maprotiline (Ludiomil)	0	+ + + +	+ +	− − − − −	+ + + +	+/−	+	+/−
Mirtazapine (Remeron)	0	0	0	− − − −	+ + + + + +	+/−	+/−	0
Nefazodone (Serzone)	+ +	+ +	+ +	+ + +	+ +	0	+ +	+/−
Nortriptyline (Pamelor)	+ + +	+ + + +	+	− − −	+ + +	+	+ +	+/−
Paroxetine (Paxil)	+ + + + + +	+ + +	+ +	+ + + + +	0	+	0	0
Phenelzine (Nardil)	0	0	0		0	0	0	0
Protriptyline (Vivactil)	+ + +	+ + + +	+	− − − −	+ +	+ +	+	0
Sertraline (Zoloft)	+ + + + +	+ +	+ + +	+ + + + + +	0	+/−	+/−	0
Reboxetine (Vestra)	+ + +	+ + + +	0	− − −	+ +	+/−	0	+/−
Tranylcypromine (Parnate)	0	0	0		0	0	0	0
Trazodone (Desyrel)	+ +	0	0	+ + + +	+ +	0	+ +	0
Trimipramine (Surmontil)	+ +	+	+	+ + + +	+ + + + +	+ +	+ +	+
Venlafaxine (Effexor)	+ + + +	+	0	+ + + +	0	0	0	0

*Ratio of potency of 5-hydroxytriptanine (5-HT) transport blockade to potency of norepinephrine (NE) transport blockade: + + + + + + means very selective for 5-HT and − − − − − means very selective for NE.

†Not marketed in the United States as an antidepressant.

Data can be compared both vertically and horizontally to find the most potent drug for a specific property and to find the most potent property for a specific drug.

DA = dopamine.

vant clinically is the synapse. By blocking transport of neurotransmitters, blocking certain neurotransmitter receptors, or inhibiting the mitochondrial enzyme monoamine oxidase, antidepressants alter the effects of neurotransmitters at synapses.

Neurons use neurotransmitters to communicate with one another and with other cell types. These small molecules, usually amino acids or their derivatives, are released from the nerve ending to interact with specific receptors on the outside surface of cells. Receptors are highly specialized proteins, which have often been molecularly cloned by researchers. These receptors are very selective in their ability to bind neurotransmitters. When the chemical messenger stimulates its receptor, the receiving neuron is changed electrically and biochemically because of the coupling of the complex of neurotransmitter and receptor to other components of the membrane in which the receptor resides. However, some receptors (e.g., nicotinic acetylcholine receptor) are ion channels, which open upon binding the neurotransmitter. Thus, this class of receptors requires no other membranal component to activate the receiving cell.

Neurons can also regulate their own activity by feedback mechanisms involving receptors on the nerve ending (autoreceptors). An example of an autoreceptor is the alpha$_2$-adrenergic receptor on noradrenergic nerve endings that modulate release of norepinephrine. When stimulated, this presynaptic receptor inhibits further release of norepinephrine.

Some biogenic amine neurotransmitters (e.g., norepinephrine, serotonin, and dopamine) are taken back into the nerve ending after release (a process called uptake, reuptake, or simply, transport). Reuptake occurs through transport proteins (transporters), which have been molecularly cloned from human and other species. This transport is a mechanism that prevents overstimulation of receptors in the synapse. Neurotransmission can be enhanced acutely by blocking this uptake with a drug. However, the blockade of uptake can ultimately diminish neurotransmission as the receptor undergoes a compensatory change and becomes less sensitive (desensitizes) to the neurotransmitter. Antidepressants of many types, probably acting by different mechanisms, can desensitize certain receptors for catecholamines and serotonin. These effects are the basis of one hypothesis of their mechanism of action. On the other hand, the therapeutic effects of the new antidepressant mirtazapine may be caused by direct blocking of presynaptic α_2-adrenergic receptors.

By blocking the postsynaptic receptor with an antagonist, the effects of the neurotransmitter can be selectively and acutely abolished. Very often with chronic blockade, the receptor undergoes another type of compensatory change and becomes more sensitive (supersensitive) to the neurotransmitter. Supersensitivity may be the mechanism of adaptation to some receptor-related side effects of certain drugs. This process may also be related to the development of tardive dyskinesia following chronic treatment with neuroleptics that block dopamine receptors.

This adaptive process may also be involved in causing the withdrawal effects that sometimes occur with abrupt cessation of some antidepressants.

Most antidepressants can block uptake of biogenic amine neurotransmitters and antagonize certain receptors. In addition, a few antidepressants inhibit the activity of monoamine oxidase, a ubiquitous enzyme that is important in the degradation of catecholamines, serotonin, and dopamine. Since this enzyme is present in mitochondria, which are found in most cells and in the nerve ending, its inhibition results in an elevation in the concentration of neurotransmitter available for release at the synapse.

Blockade of Neurotransmitter Transport

Most antidepressants are more potent at blocking transport of serotonin than transport of norepinephrine at the human transporters (see Table 2). Newer antidepressants are generally more selective and more potent than the older compounds at blocking transport of serotonin over norepinephrine (selective serotonin reuptake inhibitors [SSRIs]) (Figure 1). In addition, some antidepressants (e.g., bupropion, mirtazapine) very weakly block transport of norepinephrine, serotonin, and dopamine. Bupropion is the only antidepressant more selective in blocking uptake of dopamine (see Table 2) than other neurotransmitters. However, bupropion is more noradrenergic than dopaminergic, owing to the effects of a metabolite that is present in much higher concentrations than the parent compound. Sertraline is the most potent of the antidepressants at blocking transport of dopamine, being about as potent as methylphenidate (Ritalin). Paroxetine is the most potent blocker of uptake of serotonin, whereas the recently marketed citalopram (Celexa) is the most selective.

Selectivity cannot be equated with potency, because selectivity is derived from a ratio of potencies. In the foregoing example, citalopram is more selective (i.e., more specific) at blocking transport of serotonin than paroxetine but only about one tenth as potent as paroxetine.

Blockade of Some Neurotransmitter Receptors

Most of the newer, second-generation antidepressants are weaker than the older compounds (especially, tricyclic antidepressants) at blocking receptors for neurotransmitters. This fact predicts a side effect profile for these compounds that is different from that for older drugs.

Overall, the most potent interaction of antidepressants, especially the classic tricyclic drugs, is at the histamine H$_1$ receptor (see Table 2). Histamine is considered a neurotransmitter in the brain where, as elsewhere in the body, it causes its effects by acting at three types of receptors, histamine H$_1$, H$_2$, and H$_3$. The most recently discovered histamine receptor, H$_3$, affects the presynaptic synthesis and release of histamine and other neurotransmitters. Histamine H$_2$ receptors are present in the brain, but classically these receptors are involved with gastric acid secretion.

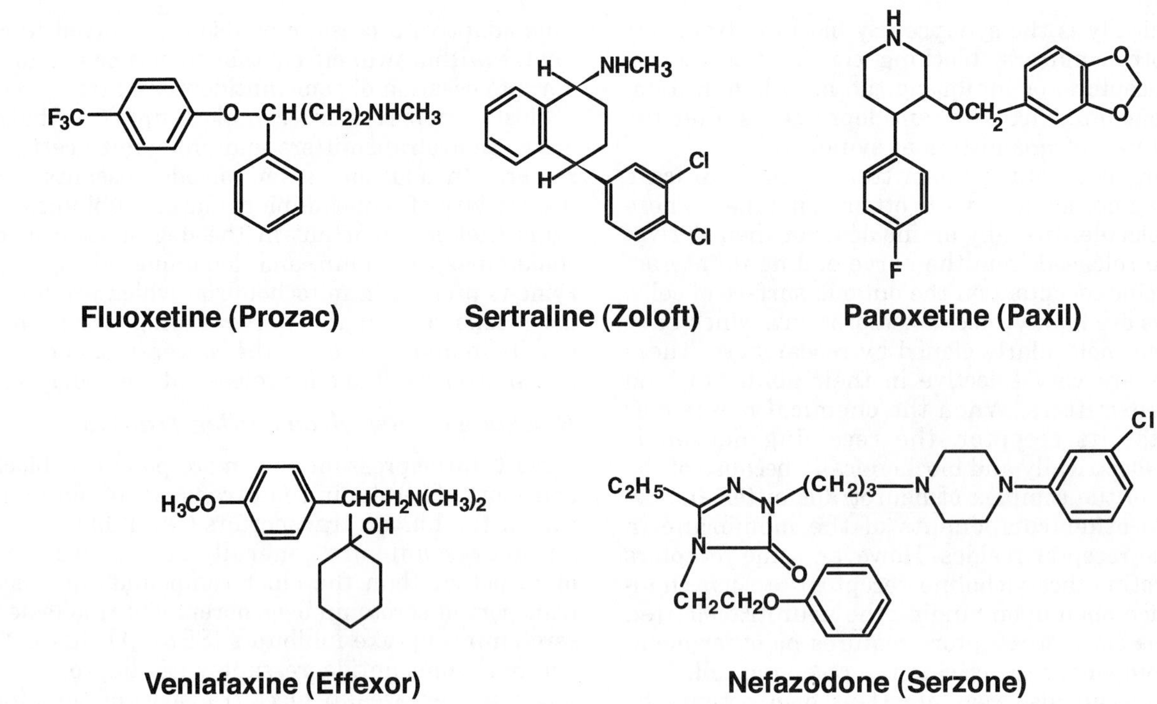

Figure 1. Some serotonin reuptake inhibitors.

Outside the nervous system, histamine H_1 receptors are involved in allergic reactions. Some antidepressants are exceedingly potent histamine H_1 antagonists (see Table 2), being more potent than all of the newer generation histamine H_1 antagonists marketed in recent years in the United States. As a result, clinicians are using them to treat allergic and dermatologic problems.

The next most potent effect of antidepressants is at the muscarinic acetylcholine receptor, which is the predominant type of cholinergic receptor in brain. In that organ they are involved with memory and learning, among other functions. In addition, some evidence suggests that these brain receptors are involved with affective illness. Antidepressants have a broad range of effectiveness at blocking human brain muscarinic receptors (see Table 2). The most potent is amitriptyline. The SSRI paroxetine is unique among the newer compounds for having appreciable antimuscarinic potency (similar to that for imipramine) (see Table 2). Studies with the molecularly cloned human muscarinic receptors, of which there are five, show that paroxetine has the highest affinity for the m3 subtype of this receptor, which is found predominantly in brain, glandular tissue, and smooth muscle. Overall, antidepressants vary little in their affinities for the five subtypes of the human muscarinic receptor.

At the alpha$_1$-adrenoreceptor, the most potent compounds, although a little weaker than the antihypertensive drug phentolamine, are likely to have clinical effects (Table 3). Antidepressants are also weak competitive antagonists of dopamine (D_2) receptors (see Table 2). The most potent compound, amoxapine

(Asendin), is a demethylated derivative of the neuroleptic loxapine (Loxitane).

MAOIs have negligible direct effects on transporters and receptors (see Table 2).

Clinical Relevance of Synaptic Pharmacology

Because all of the pharmacologic effects of these drugs occur shortly after ingestion, most of the possible clinical effects discussed here occur early in treatment. However, with chronic administration of the drug, changes may occur that can result in adaptation to certain side effects, the development of new side effects, and the onset of therapeutic effects. Table 3 lists the pharmacologic properties of various antidepressants and their possible clinical consequences. The clinician should keep in mind that the more potent the drug for a given property, the more likely it is to cause the associated effect (see Table 2).

Evidence suggests that the efficacy of antidepressants is not related to selectivity or potency for norepinephrine, serotonin, or dopamine transport blockade. These data are from clinical studies and basic studies that show the wide range of potencies of antidepressants at blocking this transport (see Table 2). On the other hand, clinical data suggest that potent transport blockade of serotonin is necessary for treatment of certain anxiety disorders including obsessive-compulsive disorder.

Transport blockade of neurotransmitters by antidepressants likely relates to certain adverse effects of these drugs and to some of their drug interactions (see Table 3). For example, serotonin transport blockade likely is the property that causes sexual side effects, seen more commonly with the SSRIs. This same property underlies the serious consequences that occur when an MAOI is combined with an antidepressant (serotonergic syndrome). In addition, researchers have reported adverse interactions between L-tryptophan, the precursor of serotonin, and fluoxetine. St. John's wort, which has become popular recently, has some monoamine oxidase activity and therefore should not be combined with an antidepressant that is a potent blocker of serotonin transport (see Table 2).

There are reports of adverse effects of fluoxetine (and other SSRIs), including extrapyramidal side effects, anorgasmia and other sexual problems, paranoid reaction, and intense suicidal preoccupation. The extrapyramidal side effects are not due to blockade of dopamine receptors, because these SSRIs are very weak at this binding site (see Table 2). Serotonin receptor antagonists (e.g., cyproheptadine [Periactin]) have been useful in treating all these side effects.

Potentiation of the effects of central depressant drugs, which cause sedation and drowsiness, is a pharmacodynamic drug interaction of antidepressants related to histamine H_1 receptor antagonism. This antagonism is probably responsible for the side effects of sedation and drowsiness. Sedation, however, may be a desired effect in patients who are agitated as well as depressed. This property may also be responsible for weight gain.

Muscarinic receptor blockade by these antidepressants may be responsible for several adverse effects (see Table 3). The relatively high affinity of paroxetine for these receptors distinguishes it from the other newer, second-generation compounds. In addition, it may explain the common complaint of dry mouth and constipation reported in some published clinical trials with paroxetine. Because elderly patients are more sensitive to the antimuscarinic side effects of drugs (see Table 3), it is best to select antidepressants that are weak in this property (see Table 2).

Alpha$_1$-adrenergic receptor blockade by antidepressants may be responsible for orthostatic hypotension, the most serious common cardiovascular effect of these drugs, which can cause dizziness and a reflex tachycardia. In addition, this property of antidepressants results in the potentiation of several antihypertensive drugs that potently block alpha$_1$-adrenergic receptors (see Table 3).

Antidepressants are weak competitive antagonists of dopamine (D_2) receptors (see Table 2). The most potent compound, amoxapine, is a demethylated derivative of the neuroleptic, loxapine (Loxitane). It is very likely that this property of amoxapine explains its extrapyramidal side effects and its ability to elevate prolactin levels. Because of this dopamine receptor blocking property, amoxapine should be reserved for patients with psychotic depression.

Antidepressants also block alpha$_2$-adrenergic re-

TABLE 3. **Pharmacologic Properties of Antidepressants and Their Possible Clinical Consequences**

Property	Possible Clinical Consequences
Blockade of norepinephrine uptake at nerve endings	Tremors Tachycardia Erectile and ejaculatory dysfunction Blockade of the antihypertensive effects of guanethidine (Esimil, which also contains hydrochlorothiazide) and guanadrel (Hylorel) Augmentation of pressor effects of sympathomimetic amines
Blockade of serotonin uptake at nerve ending	Gastrointestinal disturbances Increase or decrease in anxiety (dose-dependent) Sexual dysfunction Extrapyramidal side effects Interactions with L-tryptophan and monoamine oxidase inhibitors
Blockade of dopamine uptake at nerve ending	Psychomotor activation Antiparkinsonian effect Aggravation of psychosis
Blockade of histamine H_1 receptors	Potentiation of central depressant drugs Sedation drowsiness Weight gain
Blockade of muscarinic receptors	Blurred vision Dry mouth Sinus tachycardia Constipation Urinary retention Memory dysfunction
Blockade of alpha$_1$-adrenergic receptors	Potentiation of antihypertensive effect of prazosin (Minipress), terazosin (Hytrin), doxazosin (Cardura), labetalol (Normodyne) Postural hypotension, dizziness Reflex tachycardia
Blockade of dopamine D_2 receptors	Extrapyramidal movement disorders Endocrine changes (including hyperprolactinemia, which can lead to sexual dysfunction in males)

ceptors and 5-HT$_{1A}$ and 5-HT$_{2A}$ receptors. Usually, the blockade is weak; the exceptions are trazodone (Desyrel) and nefazodone (Serzone), which are relatively potent at these three receptors, and mirtazapine, which is relatively potent at alpha$_2$-adrenergic and 5-HT$_{2A}$ receptors.

Pharmacokinetic Drug Interactions

Drug interactions for antidepressants can be divided into two groups: pharmacokinetic and pharmacodynamic. Pharmacokinetic interactions occur when one drug affects the metabolism or protein binding of another drug. Pharmacodynamic interactions occur when one drug affects the mechanism of action of another drug. These pharmacodynamic interactions relate to the synaptic effects of antidepressants discussed previously.

The important pharmacokinetic interactions of antidepressants relate to their effects on the cytochrome P-450 system. Although we lack complete knowledge of the metabolism of many of the antidepressants, available data show that antidepressants can be substrates or inhibitors of more than one enzyme of the cytochrome P-450 system, which consists of many isozymes coded for by distinct genes. The inhibition of cytochrome P-450 2D6 enzyme by fluoxetine and its metabolite norfluoxetine is now well established. This enzyme is involved with the aromatic 2-hydroxylation of imipramine (Tofranil) and the biotransformation of many other drugs. Inhibition of cytochrome P-450 2D6 likely underlies the many reports of elevations in blood levels of other drugs used in combination with fluoxetine.

Pharmacokinetic drug interactions of antidepressants are a potential rather than a certain problem. These interactions are more likely to occur with high-risk drugs such as nefazodone at CYP 3A4; fluoxetine and paroxetine at CYP 2D6; and fluvoxamine at CYP 1A2. They are less likely to occur with low-risk drugs, such as citalopram, venlafaxine, sertraline, and probably bupropion, mirtazapine, and reboxetine. Therefore, the clinician needs to be vigilant.

Cytochrome P-450 3A4 metabolizes many drugs, including the prodrug antihistamines terfenadine (Seldane) and astemizole (Hismanal) and active compounds, such as triazolam (Halcion) and alprazolam (Xanax). Combinations of these antihistamines with potent inhibitors of this enzyme (e.g., ketoconazole [Nizoral]) can lead to fatal arrhythmias. Antidepressants that inhibit this enzyme, such as nefazodone, are contraindicated with these antihistamines. However, terfenadine has been removed from the U.S. market by the FDA because of its potential cardiotoxicity. The drug's manufacturer is now promoting the noncardiotoxic metabolite of terfenadine, fexofenadine (Allegra). In addition, astemizole was recently withdrawn in the United States for a reason similar to that for terfenadine.

Drugs metabolized by cytochrome P-450 2D6 include tricyclic antidepressants, neuroleptics, antiarrhythmics, and beta blockers. Cytochrome P-450 1A2 metabolizes some antidepressants and some neuroleptics, along with caffeine and theophylline (Aerolate and others).

Clinical Guidelines

The clinician should consider any concomitant medical disorder (Table 4), whether the patient is experiencing agitation or psychomotor retardation, and possible side effects when deciding on the appropriate choice of a drug in any particular clinical situation. Certain clinical guidelines exist for drug choice, dosage, duration, maintenance, termination, and alternatives to treatment with antidepressants (Table 5).

The first step is the appropriate choice of a drug. A history of a previous response by the patient or a family member to a particular antidepressant drug can sometimes be helpful. Starting anew, one usually chooses a more sedating drug (potent histamine H$_1$ antagonist) for patients with episodes of agitated depression and a less sedating one (weak histamine H$_1$ antagonist) for those with retarded depressive episodes. With the new antidepressant mirtazapine, sedation is usually more prominent at lower dosages, owing to counteracting mechanisms occurring at the higher dosages.

The second important guideline is the appropriate dose of medication. Most patients tolerate treatment best if the beginning dose is one fourth of the maximal usual daily dosage for adults (see Table 1). The dosage should be increased in a stepwise, divided-dose fashion every 2 to 3 days until the maximal, usual daily dose has been achieved, if tolerated. For example, for sertraline the target dose is 100 mg per day. A patient could be started on sertraline, 25 mg every day for 2 days; then 25 mg twice a day for 2 days; then 50 mg in the morning, and 25 mg in the evening for 2 days; and finally, if no very troublesome adverse effects are present, 100 mg once per day.

After 1 to 2 weeks of therapy at the target dosage, patients may take antidepressants with the longer elimination half-lives (around 15 hours or more; see Table 1) once a day at bedtime, except bupropion. Elderly patients taking the older antidepressant compounds may benefit from continuation of the divided-dose schedule, so that high blood levels (possibly leading to the adverse effect of postural hypotension or difficulty urinating) do not occur during the night when the patient may arise to eliminate. This will likely not be a problem with the newer second-generation drugs that can be given once per day (i.e., fluoxetine, sertraline, paroxetine, mirtazapine, and citalopram).

Use of MAOIs requires special considerations. These are efficacious drugs for treating depression, are well tolerated by the elderly, and should be used when a patient fails to respond to antidepressants of other classes. However, these drugs are not suitable for all patients because of the need for the patient receiving an MAOI to avoid certain foodstuffs, especially those containing tyramine, and certain drugs, especially over-the-counter cold remedies containing sympathomimetics. The clinician must make the pa-

TABLE 4. **Preferred Antidepressants When Specific Medical Disorders Coexist with Depression**

Cardiovascular Disorders

Congestive heart failure or coronary artery disease—bupropion (Wellbutrin or Zyban), citalopram (Celexa), fluoxetine (Prozac), mirtazapine (Remeron), sertraline (Zoloft), venlafaxine (Effexor)

Conduction defect—monoamine oxidase inhibitors, bupropion or fluoxetine, mirtazapine, sertraline, paroxetine (Paxil), venlafaxine

Hypertension treated with guanethidine (Esimil*) and guanadrel (Hylorel)—bupropion, trazodone (Desyrel), mirtazapine, citalopram, trimipramine (Surmontil)

Hypertension treated with prazosin (Minipress), terazosin (Hytrin), doxazosin (Cardura), labetalol (Normodyne)—venlafaxine, fluoxetine, bupropion, paroxetine, citalopram, mirtazapine, reboxetine

Hypertension treated with clonidine (Catapres), guanabenz (Wytensin), guanfacine (Tenex), or alpha-methyldopa (Aldomet)—venlafaxine, bupropion, paroxetine, fluoxetine

Untreated mild hypertension—monoamine oxidase inhibitor

Postural hypotension—venlafaxine, fluoxetine, bupropion, paroxetine, citalopram, mirtazapine, reboxetine, sertraline, protriptyline (Vivactil), desipramine (Norpramin). Avoid imipramine (Tofranil), amitriptyline (Elavil), and monoamine oxidase inhibitors.

Neurologic Disorders

Seizure disorder—monoamine oxidase inhibitor best, fluoxetine, secondary amine tricyclic (desipramine) better than tertiary amine (e.g., imipramine). Avoid maprotiline (Ludiomil), amoxapine (Asendin), trimipramine (Surmontil), and bupropion.

Organic mental disorders—venlafaxine, trazodone, bupropion, nefazodone (Serzone), citalopram, fluoxetine

Chronic pain syndrome—amitriptyline, imipramine

Migraine headaches—nefazodone, trazodone, mirtazapine, doxepin (Sinequan or Adapin), amitriptyline, trimipramine

Psychosis—antidepressant plus neuroleptic, amoxapine

Parkinsonism—amitriptyline, protriptyline, trimipramine, doxepin, bupropion, or sertraline. Avoid amoxapine.

Tardive dyskinesia—bupropion, maprotiline, mirtazapine. Avoid amoxapine.

Allergic Disorders

Mirtazapine, doxepin, trimipramine, amitriptyline, maprotiline

Gastrointestinal Disorders

Chronic diarrhea—amitriptyline, protriptyline, trimipramine, doxepin

Chronic constipation—venlafaxine, trazodone, bupropion, nefazodone, citalopram, fluoxetine

Peptic ulcer disease—doxepin, trimipramine, amitriptyline, imipramine

Urologic Disorders

Neurogenic bladder—venlafaxine, trazodone, bupropion, nefazodone, citalopram, fluoxetine

Organic impotence—nefazodone, trazodone, bupropion

Ophthalmologic Disorders (angle-closure glaucoma)—venlafaxine, trazodone, bupropion, nefazodone, citalopram, fluoxetine

*In the United States, also contains hydrochlorothiazide.

Updated and modified from Richelson E: Antidepressants: Pharmacology and clinical use. *In* Karasu TB (ed): Treatments of Psychiatric Disorders. A Task Force Report of the American Psychiatric Association, Washington, DC, Vol 3, pp 1773–1787, 1989, and reproduced with permission from the publisher.

tient aware of these important precautions when prescribing an MAOI. A convenient way to ensure that the patient has all the information in hand is to give him or her a copy of the list of "foods to avoid" in the package insert. When a patient is not willing or able to comply with these restrictions, another type of antidepressant should be prescribed.

The three antidepressant MAOIs in use in the United States are irreversible inhibitors. This means that "washout" from the drug depends not on its pharmacokinetics but rather on the synthesis of new monoamine oxidase. Reversible MAOIs are under development that promise to pose less of a problem with tyramine-containing foodstuffs.

If the patient is taking a tricyclic antidepressant or another MAOI, then this drug should be stopped for 10 days before starting a new MAOI. To be underscored in the list of drugs that should be avoided by patients taking an MAOI are meperidine (Demerol), imipramine, citalopram, clomipramine (Anafranil),

TABLE 5. **Clinical Guidelines for Use of Antidepressants**

1. Appropriate choice: Select on the basis of the profile of side effects, particularly sedative effects in agitated patients or on the basis of previous response or family history of a response to a particular antidepressant.
2. Adequate dose: Check blood level if toxicity ensues or if response is inadequate.
3. Adequate duration: Administer for a minimum of 4 months after recovery.
4. Adequate termination or maintenance: For first depressions, 4 to 5 months after recovery, taper dose gradually for 2 to 4 months and then discontinue therapy. For recurrent unipolar depression, maintain therapy with antidepressant.
5. Adequate therapy: For almost all types of depression, a combination of psychotherapy (usually, brief supportive) and antidepressants may be slightly more effective than antidepressants alone.
6. Adequate alternative: Change drug; add lithium carbonate; add thyroid hormone; add buspirone, or use electroshock therapy.

Modified from Richelson E: Antidepressants: Pharmacology and clinical use. *In* Karasu TB (ed): Treatments of Psychiatric Disorders. A Task Force Report of the American Psychiatric Association, Washington, DC, Vol 3, pp 1773–1787, 1989, and reproduced with permission from the publisher.

fluoxetine, sertraline, paroxetine, and venlafaxine. Because of the very long half-life of fluoxetine and the even longer half-life of its active metabolite, norfluoxetine, at least 5 weeks' washout is required before starting an MAOI. Some evidence suggests that this washout period should be longer.

Of the three MAOIs available in the United States (see Table 1), researchers have studied phenelzine most frequently. About 2 weeks are needed to achieve maximal inhibition of platelet monoamine oxidase when depressed patients are given phenelzine and about the same length of time is necessary to recover activity after the drug is stopped. Patients with 80% or greater inhibition of this platelet enzyme have a better antidepressant response than do those with less enzyme inhibition. Although laboratories are making measurement of platelet monoamine oxidase available, a clinically useful rule of thumb is to target a dosage of 1 mg per kg body weight per day for the patient to achieve this desired level of inhibition.

As with other antidepressants, MAOIs may be started slowly. For example, when starting a patient on phenelzine, the clinician may prescribe 15 mg the first day, 15 mg twice daily the second day, 15 mg thrice daily the third day, and so forth until the target dosage is achieved.

A treatment period of 2 to 4 weeks is usually necessary before the onset of therapeutic effects of any type of antidepressant. At the outset, the patient may need a thorough explanation of the side effects to be expected and encouragement to persist with treatment until some clinical response results. If the clinical response is inadequate after 3 to 4 weeks and the adverse effects are small, one should increase the dosage a step further. Underdosing is a common error with these drugs. As outlined previously for sertraline, one should increase the dosage another 25 to 50 mg per day; with phenelzine, one should increase the dosage another 15 mg per day. However, if poor response persists after 2 more weeks at the higher dosage or if toxicity supervenes, then plasma levels of the drug (if it is not an MAOI) may be obtained when available.

Although therapeutic plasma concentrations have been firmly established for only imipramine, nortriptyline, desipramine, and possibly amitriptyline, enough data are available for other antidepressants (other than MAOIs and the newer second-generation antidepressants bupropion, citalopram, fluoxetine, nefazodone, paroxetine, sertraline, trazodone, venlafaxine, and mirtazapine) to decide whether a dosage of a drug is adequate for problem patients or elderly patients. The projected optimal therapeutic plasma ranges presented in Table 1 for the other antidepressants are to be used only as a very rough guide.

Elderly patients are likely to require about one half the usual daily dose recommended for a younger adult and may require a slower escalation of the dosage to the maximal level because of their increased sensitivity to the adverse effects of antidepressants. However, under-dosing can be a mistake in treating elderly patients, and plasma levels should be used more often with this group to determine proper dosage. Achievement of a steady state in these patients may take longer as well.

The third guideline is adequate duration of treatment. After a complete clinical response has been achieved, therapy should be continued for at least 4 to 5 months.

The fourth important clinical guideline involves stopping antidepressant therapy or maintenance therapy for patients with recurrent illness. Four to 5 months after complete recovery, the drug dose should be tapered gradually over 2 to 4 months and then stopped. A slow taper is essential, because abrupt withdrawal of medication can predispose the patient to relapse of depressive symptoms, to uncomfortable symptoms (e.g., dysesthesias and severe sleep disturbance), or to a withdrawal syndrome. The evidence being gathered suggests that maintenance therapy with the same antidepressant without lowering the dosage should be used for those patients with recurrent unipolar depression.

The fifth clinical guideline is that adequate therapy for most types of depression should include some form of psychotherapeutic alliance between the patient and doctor at least to ensure compliance with the pharmacotherapy. This may be achieved through brief (10 to 20 minutes) supportive visits with the primary physician or, sometimes, more extensive psychotherapy. However, a combination of antidepressants and psychotherapy may be only slightly more effective than antidepressants alone.

Finally, adequate knowledge of alternative or adjunctive treatments for depression is important. This includes a change in the primary antidepressant drug to an antidepressant of a different chemical class; the addition of lithium carbonate in sufficient dosage to achieve a blood level of 0.6 to 1.0 mEq per liter; the addition of thyroid hormone (1-triiodothyronine, 25 to 50 μg/d); or the addition of buspirone.

Electroconvulsive therapy is still the most effective treatment for refractory depression and may be the treatment of choice in certain situations in which antidepressants are contraindicated, in patients at extremely high suicidal risk, or in depression with psychotic features. In this latter case, the combination of an antidepressant with a neuroleptic may be superior to either drug alone. Psychostimulants (e.g., methylphenidate [Ritalin]) may also be useful to treat depression in certain medical and surgical patients, but their efficacy in more general cases of depression is not established.

Bipolar (Manic-Depressive) Illness

This disorder, which is much less common than unipolar illness, occurs in about 1% of the general population, affecting men and women equally. Modal age at onset is 30 years. It is more frequently diagnosed in higher social classes. In about 7% of cases, a first-degree relative is affected. Acute episodes of bipolar disorder recur about every 3 to 9 years.

For the bipolar patient in a depressive phase, decisions about choice and use of an antidepressant are the same as for the unipolar depressed patient, with at least two important exceptions. First, the bipolar patient is much more likely to switch suddenly into mania during this treatment. The literature is controversial regarding whether one type of antidepressant is less likely than another to cause this switch. However, tricyclic antidepressants may induce rapid cycling in some bipolar patients.

Another exception to the treatment of the bipolar depressed patient is that this patient will very likely be medicated with a mood stabilizer as well. Lithium carbonate (Eskalith, Lithobid, Lithonate), the only medication approved by the FDA for maintenance therapy for bipolar disorder, is a mood stabilizer. However, other types of medications, such as anticonvulsants, are being used, too, as mood stabilizers.

Lithium salts are effective in the treatment of acute mania and in the prophylaxis of mania and depression. In the prophylaxis of bipolar disorder, the efficacy of imipramine plus lithium carbonate is equal to that of lithium carbonate alone. In the prophylaxis of recurrent, unipolar depression, imipramine plus lithium carbonate has similar efficacy to imipramine alone.

Salts of lithium ion have similar physiologic effects to those of sodium and potassium. Lithium ion is readily assayed in biologic fluids by flame-photometric and atomic-absorption spectrophotometric methods. Traces are found in animal tissues. It is abundant in some mineral springs, which are thought to have medicinal properties.

There is no known physiologic role for lithium ion; that is, the body appears not to require lithium ion for normal function. Lithium ion is readily absorbed in the gut and distributed throughout the body. It is concentrated in bone, thyroid, and brain. The majority is excreted in the urine. Therapeutic blood levels range from 0.6 to 1.0 mEq per liter, beyond which serious toxic effects can occur. Side effects, which may not be dose related, include tremor, edema, nausea, psoriasis, weight gain, acne, mental dulling, hypothyroidism, and nephrogenic diabetes insipidus/polyuria. Thus, before initiation of lithium therapy, patients need to have baseline laboratory tests of thyroid and kidney function, which are repeated, depending on the patient, every 4 to 6 months, during therapy.

Acute manic episodes are managed with antipsychotic drugs or divalproex sodium (Depakote), which is the only anticonvulsant drug that has received FDA approval for treatment of acute mania. Although not approved for this use by the FDA, it and other anticonvulsants (e.g., carbamazepine [Tegretol]) are being used for the prophylaxis of bipolar disorder in patients who are intolerant or nonresponsive to lithium salts. Sometimes these drugs are used in combination with one another and with lithium salts.

Acute mania can often be a very serious clinical situation, requiring hospitalization and occasionally ECT. Compliance can often be a problem with bipolar patients, who prefer to have their mood elevated above the normal range.

SCHIZOPHRENIA

method of
JOHN G. CSERNANSKY, M.D.
Washington University School of Medicine and Metropolitan St. Louis Psychiatric Center
St. Louis, Missouri

Although schizophrenia may not be the most common of psychiatric disorders, it can be the most disabling. In all cultures, approximately 1% of persons develop this disorder; men tend to have more severe symptoms and an earlier age at onset. The symptoms of schizophrenia are episodic; however, many patients do not recover sufficiently from their first episode to resume school or work. These symptoms can be categorized into three groups: (1) psychotic symptoms, such as delusions and hallucinations; (2) disorganized symptoms, such as illogical thinking and bizarre behavior; and (3) negative symptoms, such as emotional withdrawal, lack of emotional expression, and apathy. In addition, it is now widely accepted that patients with schizophrenia have substantial mood instability and cognitive deficits, including poor attention, working memory, and decision making. Although the cognitive deficits of schizophrenia rarely become as apparent to other people as those found in Alzheimer's disease, they strongly predict a poor quality of life.

Antipsychotic drugs are the cornerstone of treatment for patients with schizophrenia. For several decades, such drugs have been recognized to be effective in ameliorating positive symptoms and in preventing such symptoms to maintain periods of remission. More recently, other symptom groupings have become recognized as important targets for drug therapy. Psychosocial therapies continue to play a critical role in educating patients and their families about the illness and in maintaining compliance with drug treatment regimens.

TYPICAL VERSUS ATYPICAL ANTIPSYCHOTIC DRUGS

Much has changed since the 1980s in the drug treatment of schizophrenia. Before 1987, all available antipsychotic drugs had highly similar risks and benefits. Currently, these compounds are called typical or conventional antipsychotic agents (Table 1). Historically, they have also been termed "neuroleptics." All typical antipsychotic drugs share two major characteristics: (1) they ameliorate the psychotic and disorganized symptoms of schizophrenia, and (2) they produce a neurologic syndrome analogous to Parkinson's disease, called pseudoparkinsonism. These two actions share a common pharmacodynamic mechanism: the blockade of brain dopamine D_2 receptors. When administering typical antipsychotics, other side effects are also common due to blockade of neurotransmitter receptors other than dopamine.

In 1987, a new generation of antipsychotic drugs appeared. Clozapine (Clozaril), a dibenzepine compound, was the prototype for this new generation of drugs and has been shown to cause little or no pseudoparkinsonism and to be superior to typical antipsychotics for the treatment of psychotic symptoms, disorganized symptoms, and negative

TABLE 1. **Characteristics of Typical and Atypical Antipsychotic Drugs**

Generic Name	Trade Name	Optimal Daily Dose (in mg)
Typical		
Chlorpromazine	Thorazine	100–800
Fluphenazine	Prolixin	2–10
Haloperidol	Haldol	2–10
Loxapine	Loxitane	15–80
Mesoridazine	Serentil	25–200
Molindone	Moban	10–60
Perphenazine	Trilafon	8–64
Pimozide	Orap	2–6
Thioridazine	Mellaril	50–600
Thiothixene	Navane	6–60
Trifluoperazine	Stelazine	4–20
Atypical		
Clozapine	Clozaril	300–900
Olanzapine	Zyprexa	10–20
Quetiapine	Seroquel	200–600
Risperidone	Risperdal	2–6

symptoms, particularly in patients who are refractory to typical antipsychotic drugs. Clozapine has been shown to have mixed effects on cognition in schizophrenia patients; that is, performance on tests of cognitive function that involve speeded activities is improved, whereas performance on tests of memory and executive function is further impaired. Thus, the absence of pseudoparkinsonism during treatment with clozapine may have indirect benefits for some elements of cognition, whereas other elements are adversely affected, perhaps because of clozapine's anticholinergic properties. Finally, plasma concentrations of clozapine greater than or equal to 350 ng per mL appear to predict better therapeutic responses to this drug.

There are now several other available examples in this new generation of drugs (see Table 1). Risperidone (Risperdal), olanzapine (Zyprexa), and quetiapine (Seroquel) are commercially available, whereas ziprasidone and sertindole have not yet been approved for marketing. These atypical antipsychotic drugs are approximately equal in efficacy to typical drugs for the psychotic and disorganized symptoms of schizophrenia, whereas their efficacy for the negative symptoms of schizophrenia is superior. Like clozapine, they have reduced liability for pseudoparkinsonism. Preliminary evidence has also begun to appear to suggest that at least some of these atypical antipsychotic drugs have benefits for mood instability and cognitive impairment in patients with schizophrenia.

The atypical antipsychotic drugs differ in potency; the average daily dose of risperidone is 4 mg, whereas the average daily doses of olanzapine and quetiapine are 15 mg and 300 mg, respectively. In general, they have fewer neurologic side effects and are better accepted by patients than are the typical antipsychotic drugs. Although their half-lives are somewhat shorter than many of the typical antipsychotics, the atypical antipsychotics are most often given in once- or twice-a-day dosing.

MECHANISMS OF DRUG ACTION

All antipsychotic drugs block brain dopamine D_2 receptors to some degree. However, because of clozapine's actions at a variety of other neurotransmitter receptors, the role of other neurotransmitter systems in mediating the effects of the atypical antipsychotic drugs has been investigated with enthusiasm. Clozapine acts as an antagonist at two other dopamine receptors (D_1 and D_4), four serotonin receptors ($5\text{-}HT_{2a}$, $5\text{-}HT_{2c}$, $5\text{-}HT_6$, and $5\text{-}HT_7$), two norepinephrine receptors ($alpha_1$ and $alpha_2$), a variety of muscarinic receptors (M_1 through M_5), the histamine H_1 receptor, and the sigma receptor, with affinities equivalent to or greater than its affinity for the dopamine D_2 receptor. The most popular hypothesis regarding the explanation of clozapine's unusual benefits for schizophrenia patients is the combined blockade of $5\text{-}HT_{2a}$ and D_2 receptors. This hypothesis was originally based on an empirical comparison of antipsychotic drugs with known typical and atypical properties. However, $5\text{-}HT_{2a}$–receptor blockade may have stimulatory effects on neurons of the cerebral cortex, which may explain not only clozapine's unusual benefits for some symptom groupings but also its beneficial actions on some elements of cognition.

Several other potential mechanisms of action to explain the actions of atypical antipsychotic drugs remain under investigation. These include the blockade of dopamine receptors other than D_2, the blockade of certain subtypes of norepinephrine and muscarinic acetylcholine receptors, and the facilitation of glutamatergic transmission at *N*-methyl-D-aspartate (NMDA) receptors. Unfortunately, we still do not have a precise understanding of schizophrenia's underlying pathophysiology, and thus such hypotheses cannot be directly tested.

TREATMENT

Schizophrenia is a life-long psychiatric illness, and antipsychotic drugs must be used intermittently or continuously. Most patients with schizophrenia begin treatment with the onset of an acute psychotic episode, and the latency of clinical responses in acutely psychotic patients is highly variable. Approximately one third of patients have an amelioration of their symptoms over several days; one third improve over several weeks; and in the last third of patients, symptom amelioration may be too slow to appreciate at all, and so such patients are deemed nonresponders. Especially large doses of antipsychotic drugs have not been shown to produce more rapid clinical responses.

Continuation of treatment for patients with schizophrenia is variable in length, but it can be defined as drug treatment after the acute benefits have appeared but while the underlying episode of psychosis remains active. An indicator that the patient remains in the continuation phase of treatment is that discontinuation of drug treatment triggers almost immediate relapse. Maintenance treatment follows continuation treatment in schizophrenia. Maintenance treatment in patients with schizophrenia has broad goals, including relapse prevention, resumption of school or work activities, prevention of long-term neurologic side effects, and, more recently, the remediation of cognitive deficits. The same antipsychotic agent is usually used for all three phases of treatment. Occasionally, a more sedating antipsychotic may be used only during the acute phase of treatment to more effectively cope with the psychomotor agitation that often accompanies psychosis.

Drug Side Effects

The side effects of typical antipsychotic drugs can be divided into two categories. First, neurologic side effects, such as pseudoparkinsonism, occur because of D_2-receptor blockade in the basal ganglia. Other neurologic side effects, such as dystonia, akathisia, and tardive dyskinesia have also been linked to dopamine-receptor blockade, but with less certainty. Neuroleptic malignant syndrome, characterized by extreme rigidity, fever, and very high elevations of serum creatine kinase concentrations, is an unusual, but potentially fatal, complication of antipsychotic drug therapy and may represent an extreme form of pseudoparkinsonism.

Finally, increases in serum prolactin concentrations also occur through dopamine-receptor blockade on pituitary lactotrophs. Although some of the clinical consequences of serum prolactin elevations are known, such as loss of sexual interest and galactorrhea, others, such as osteoporosis, are only speculative.

The second category of side effects associated with use of typical antipsychotic drugs occurs through blockade of neurotransmitter receptors other than dopamine, such as acetylcholine (blurry vision, constipation, confusion, and urinary hesitancy), norepinephrine (orthostatic hypotension and sedation), and histamine (sedation). Lower potency typical antipsychotic drugs are more likely to produce such side effects. Because such drugs produce both neurologic side effects and these more nonspecific side effects, their continued use in the modern era is difficult to defend.

Atypical antipsychotic drugs, as a group, have fewer neurologic side effects than typical antipsychotic drugs. This may be the case because they tend to occupy a lower proportion of dopamine D_2 receptors (40 to 60%) than typical antipsychotic drugs (70–80%) when used in clinically optimal doses. However, atypical antipsychotic drugs, especially less potent ones, can still cause side effects not related to dopamine D_2-receptor blockade.

Treatment with clozapine has been associated with sedation, orthostatic hypotension, seizures, and sweating at night. During chronic treatment with clozapine, patients can also gain significant amounts of weight. Clozapine causes leukopenia in approximately 1% of patients treated, and for this reason, white blood cell counts must be carefully monitored during therapy. When the total white blood cell count per mm^3 of blood drops below 3000 or the granulocyte count drops below 1000 per mm^3, treatment with clozapine must be stopped and measures taken to stimulate white blood cell production and treatment of opportunistic infections.

Risperidone is the most potent of atypical antipsychotic drugs. Optimal efficacy and a lack of pseudoparkinsonism are observed when the dose of risperidone is maintained between 4 and 6 mg per day. Doses higher than this have been associated with neurologic side effects like those of typical drugs.

Risperidone can be sedating and cause orthostatic hypotension, especially during the first few days of treatment. Chronic treatment with risperidone has also been associated with weight gain.

Olanzapine is slightly less potent than risperidone. This drug has been associated with very few neurologic side effects at doses between 5 and 20 mg per day, although such side effects may be observed when daily doses in excess of 50 mg are used. Although olanzapine is a chemical analogue of clozapine, agranulocytosis has not been observed. As with both clozapine and risperidone, weight gain during chronic treatment has been observed.

Although quetiapine is the least potent of the commercially available atypical antipsychotic drugs, it has a particularly benign side-effect profile. In fact, few side effects, other than sedation, have been observed over a rather wide dose range (150 to 700 mg per day).

Practical Guidelines for the Use of Antipsychotic Drugs

Clinical research and the pharmaceutical industry have afforded clinicians a new array of more effective and safe antipsychotic drugs. However, no matter what drug the clinician may first select to treat a patient with schizophrenia, some patients will fail to respond or experience unacceptable side effects. Therefore, the following guidelines are offered as a guide for pursuing an optimal course of drug therapy (see also Table 2).

First, the patient's diagnosis is established using all available sources of clinical information. By doing so, the clinician can relate selected treatment options to studies from the research literature that match the patient's diagnosis. Rates of response and side effects documented for groups of patients with schizophrenia may not apply to patients with other psychotic disorders.

Second, a sequence of treatment options is developed in decreasing order of probable success. The clinician is better prepared when he or she faces the possibility of early treatment failure at the beginning of therapy and has considered possible alternatives. Also, this preparation allows the clinician to better educate the patient and the patient's family regarding the possible outcomes of therapy.

Third, only one drug treatment variable is changed

TABLE 2. **Guidelines for the Use of Antipsychotic Drugs**

1. Establish the patient's diagnosis using all available sources of information.
2. Develop a sequence of treatment options in decreasing order of probable success.
3. Change only one drug treatment variable at a time.
4. Allow for the gradual effects of antipsychotic drugs.
5. Use the minimum effective dose.
6. Select drug treatment options using evidence from controlled clinical trials.

at a time. Although there is usually considerable pressure to expedite the treatment of psychotic patients, rushing through multiple treatment options (e.g., changing drugs and doses simultaneously) often causes confusion. Even if the ultimate treatment regimen is successful, the clinician may not know which of the selected drugs or doses are mainly responsible for the response, and so the patient becomes committed to unnecessary drugs or doses during the maintenance phase of therapy.

Fourth, the clinician should remember that antipsychotic and most other psychotropic drugs act slowly. When increases in drug doses are too rapid, it is easy to mistake a time-dependent clinical response for a dose-dependent one.

Fifth, the minimum effective dose should be used. Higher than minimum effective doses bring avoidable side effects, and plans to decrease doses later during the maintenance phase of therapy sometimes never materialize. Relationships have been established between plasma concentrations and clinical efficacy for some antipsychotic drugs (e.g., haloperidol [Haldol] and clozapine); in such cases, blood level monitoring can be helpful in achieving optimal drug doses.

Sixth, the clinician should select antipsychotic drug treatment options based on the best available evidence from controlled clinical trials. Individual clinical experience can be helpful, but it can also be misleading. Schizophrenia, like many psychiatric disorders, can spontaneously wax and wane in severity, and such changes can be mistaken for drug-induced responses.

PANIC DISORDER

method of
MANUEL E. TANCER, M.D.
Wayne State University School of Medicine
Detroit, Michigan

Anxiety is one of the most common symptoms seen by physicians. Patients experiencing panic attacks often come to primary care physicians or emergency departments for evaluation because of the sudden and extreme somatic symptoms. Panic attacks are defined as paroxysmal episodes of marked anxiety accompanied by at least four somatic or psychosensory symptoms that reach a crescendo within 10 minutes and then dissipate. Panic attack symptoms are listed in Table 1. The most common somatic symptoms are palpitations, chest pressure or pain, difficulty catching one's breath, and dizziness.

DIAGNOSIS

Panic attacks can be a symptom of a wide range of medical conditions (e.g. hypothyroidism or hyperthyroidism, hypoxia), can be a side effect of a variety of medications or intoxication from substances of abuse (Table 2), or can be due to withdrawal from medications and substances of abuse (Table 3). It is therefore essential that the symptoms of anxiety be carefully evaluated by detailed history,

TABLE 1. **Diagnostic Criteria for Panic Attack**

A discrete period of intense fear or discomfort, starting abruptly, reaching a crescendo within 10 minutes, and associated with at least four of the following signs and symptoms:
Palpitations, pounding heart, or accelerated heart rate
Sweating
Trembling or shaking
Sensations of shortness of breath or smothering
Feeling of choking
Chest pain or discomfort
Nausea or abdominal distress
Feeling dizzy, unsteady, lightheaded, or faint
Derealization (feelings of unreality) or depersonalization (being detached from oneself)
Fear of losing control or going crazy
Fear of dying
Paresthesias (numbness or tingling sensations)
Chills or hot flushes

physical examination, and appropriate laboratory evaluation. Panic disorder must be included in the differential diagnosis of chest pain in an individual younger than 40 year of age.

In the history, attention should be paid to the use of medications (prescription and over the counter), ethanol and drug use (amounts and patterns), and caffeine use. In particular, changes in medications or medication dosages may result in panic attacks. The same is true for illicit drug use. Specifically, cocaine use may trigger panic attacks in susceptible individuals and can lead to spontaneous panic attacks in a subset of these subjects. Furthermore, many individuals with panic disorder are highly sensitive to the anxiogenic effects of caffeine. Caffeine, which is most commonly found in coffee, tea, and chocolate, is also found in a variety of over-the-counter analgesic compounds. Reduction or elimination of caffeine can sometimes be an effective therapeutic intervention. Finally, it is important to ask about herbal or over-the-counter agents in relation to possible drug interactions.

The physical examination should focus on ruling out organic causes for the presenting physical symptoms. Particular attention should be paid to the cardiac examination (given the high rates of palpitations and chest pain).

Laboratory studies should include thyroid studies to rule out hypothyroidism or hyperthyroidism, both of which are associated with panic-like symptoms. Although symptoms of panic may resemble those of hypoglycemia, the absence of a postprandial temporal pattern generally precludes the diagnosis and little information is gained from glucose tolerance testing. Electroencephalograms may be useful for patients with prominent psychosensory symptoms, especially if obtained under sleep deprivation conditions with nasopharyngeal leads.

Panic disorder is a syndrome characterized by recurrent, initially unexpected, panic attacks. At first the panic attacks come "out of the blue," but they may become situa-

TABLE 2. **Medications/Drugs Associated with Anxiety Symptoms**

Corticosteroids	Nonsteroidal anti-inflammatory agents
Antihypertensives	Birth control pills
Lidocaine	Selective serotonin reuptake inhibitors
Caffeine	Analgesics containing caffeine
Cocaine	Marijuana

TABLE 3. Withdrawal from Medications and Substances Associated with Anxiety Symptoms

Corticosteroids
Beta blockers
Opiates
Cocaine
Alcohol

tionally cued or predisposed. Panic attacks may occur at night ("nocturnal panic"). Sleep polysomnography studies have documented that nocturnal panic attacks are sudden arousals from non–rapid-eye-movement sleep. Agoraphobia, defined as the avoidance of situations and/or places associated with panic attacks, is a common complication of panic disorder and contributes significantly to its morbidity.

The diagnostic criteria for panic disorder listed in the fourth edition of the American Psychiatric Association's *Diagnostic and Statistical Manual of Mental Disorders* include (1) recurrent unexpected panic attacks and either at least 1 month worry about subsequent attacks, worry about the implications of the attack (e.g., having a heart attack or losing control), or significant change in behavior related to the attacks; (2) the absence of an organic (direct physiologic effect of a drug or medication or a general medical condition) basis for the attacks; and (3) symptoms not better accounted for by another mental disorder. The diagnosis of panic disorder can be further characterized by the presence or absence of agoraphobia.

Panic disorder has a lifetime prevalence of 3.5% of the population. Peak age at onset is between 18 and 35, although there is recognition that panic disorder can begin earlier. There is a 2:3 to 2:1 female/male ratio in the prevalence of panic disorder. Family studies have shown a fair degree of familial association, although there has been failure to replicate linkages in several genetic linkage studies. Epidemiologic samples have reported that approximately one third of individuals have had one or more panic attacks but do not seek medical attention and do not meet the diagnostic criteria for panic disorder.

Panic disorder is associated with a highly variable course of illness: some patients experience episodic symptoms and others experience chronic, unremitting symptoms. Patients with panic disorder have been reported to use increased psychiatric and general medical services, have increased rates of financial dependency and substance abuse or misuse, or experience suicidal ideation compared with persons who have never experienced them. Patients with panic disorder are at increased risk of having a major depression (either before, concurrent with, or subsequent to the onset of panic disorder), with most studies reporting 50 to 75% of persons with histories of major depression. There is also an increased risk of substance abuse in patients with panic disorder, specifically, a rate of alcohol abuse or dependence in up to 30% of patients diagnosed with panic disorder.

Given the high rates of psychiatric co-morbidity in patients with panic disorder, the presence of panic attacks in a patient should alert the clinician to look carefully for symptoms of depression, drug, and/or ethanol abuse or dependence. The presence of co-morbid conditions worsens the prognosis and often influences treatment choices.

TREATMENT

Panic disorder can be treated either with pharmacotherapy or non-medication therapies. Of the non-medication treatments, cognitive-behavioral therapy (CBT) has been shown to be the most effective form of therapy. Although a combination of pharmacologic and cognitive-behavioral treatments is effective in groups of patients suffering from panic disorder, there are patients who respond to one form of treatment but not the other. Unfortunately, there are few pretreatment predictors of who these individuals are. Few studies have systematically examined the efficacy of combined treatments on outcome. If a panic disorder patient is not showing any clinical improvement after 6 to 8 weeks with one treatment modality, a reassessment of the patient and a shift in treatment modalities is probably warranted. Patients with exclusive nocturnal panic attacks should be started on pharmacotherapy. There are no studies showing the efficacy of CBT in this patient subgroup.

Pharmacotherapy

Pharmacotherapy can be quite effective in the treatment of panic disorder, particularly in blocking the panic attacks. Antidepressant medications and high-potency benzodiazepines have been the most widely studied and used agents (Table 4). Historically, imipramine (Tofranil),* a tricyclic antidepressant, has been the "gold standard" antidepressant,

---

*Not FDA approved for this indication.

TABLE 4. Medications for the Treatment of Panic Disorder

Drug Class	Drug	Dose Range	FDA Indicated
Antidepressant			
TCA	Desipramine (Norpramin)	50–300 mg/d	No
TCA	Imipramine (Tofranil)	50–300 mg/d	No
SSRI	Fluoxetine (Prozac)	5–40 mg/d	No
SSRI	Fluvoxamine (Luvox)	25–150 mg/d	No
SSRI	Paroxetine (Paxil)	10–40 mg/d	Yes
SSRI	Sertraline (Zoloft)	25–150 mg/d	Yes
MAOI	Phenelzine (Nardil)	30–90 mg/d	No
Benzodiazepine	Alprazolam (Xanax)	1.5–6 mg/d	Yes
	Clonazepam (Klonopin)	1.5–6 mg/d	Yes
	Diazepam (Valium)	15–60 mg/d	No

TCA = tricyclic antidepressant; SSRI = selective serotonin reuptake inhibitor; MAOI = monoamine oxidase inhibitor.

and many patients respond well to the monoamine oxidase inhibitor phenelzine (Nardil). Currently, the selective serotonin reuptake inhibitors (SSRIs) are the standard first-line agents for the treatment of panic disorder, given the side effects and need for dose titration for the tricyclic antidepressants and the highly restrictive diet required and concern regarding hypertensive reactions with monoamine oxidase inhibitors. Both paroxetine (Paxil) and sertraline (Zoloft) have been approved by the U.S. Food and Drug Administration (FDA) for the treatment of panic disorder. In addition, fluoxetine (Prozac)* and fluvoxamine (Luvox)* have both been reported to be superior to placebo in the treatment of panic disorder in several well-designed trials. Antidepressants take 4 to 6 weeks for full effects to be seen. Some patients treated with SSRIs experience excessive arousal, so starting with a low dose—one fourth to one half the typical starting dose—may be necessary. If a patient does exhibit arousal or sleep disturbance from an SSRI dosed in the morning, shifting the dose to bedtime may improve sleep and minimize the arousal. One antidepressant, bupropion (Wellbutrin), and the anxiolytic agent buspirone (Buspar) are ineffective in panic disorder and should not be used.

The high-potency benzodiazepines alprazolam (Xanax) and clonazepam (Klonopin) are also FDA approved for the treatment of panic disorder. The benzodiazepines work rapidly (often within 1 week) and may be especially valuable for patients with rapidly progressing symptoms or in patients unable to tolerate antidepressant medications. Benzodiazepines should be used cautiously in individuals with histories of alcohol abuse. They should not be used as monotherapies in patients with co-morbid major depressive disorder. When benzodiazepines are used in panic disorder, it is important that they be dosed on a regular basis. Too often, they are prescribed "as needed." Patients with panic tend to wait until they experience a panic attack; they then take the benzodiazepine, which does nothing to block or decrease the attack and leaves them drowsy an hour later. The goal of treatment is to prevent the attacks from occurring.

Monotherapy with antidepressants is generally sufficient for treating patients with panic disorder, given that many patients have been experiencing symptoms for some time before the diagnosis is made. There is a subset of panic disorder patients with rapidly escalating symptoms or patients with severe symptoms who require combination pharmacotherapy, usually an SSRI combined with a benzodiazepine. After 6 to 8 weeks the antidepressant should

*Not FDA approved for this indication.

be fully effective and a gradual benzodiazepine taper can begin.

Once a patient is stabilized on medication, the optimum duration of treatment is not clear. Some patients can be tapered from the medication successfully after 9 to 12 months without panic attacks, whereas other patients will experience a recurrence of attacks during or shortly after medication reduction.

Cognitive-Behavioral Therapy

CBT can be conducted individually or in groups and is equally effective in either format. The cognitive perspective underlying CBT is that panic attacks are associated with catastrophic misinterpretations of benign stimuli (e.g., skipped heartbeat), most of which are related to immediately impending physical danger (e.g., heart attack) and/or mental catastrophe. The cognitive part of CBT involves identifying the misinterpreted thoughts and helping the patient learn more realistic appraisals of the symptoms. The behavioral perspective on panic disorder is that the extreme symptoms of the panic attack are responsible for the escape/avoidance behavior. The escape/avoidance behaviors become a conditioned response. The traditional treatment of such conditioned behavior is graduated exposure to the fearful stimuli until habituation develops. Accordingly, the behavioral component of CBT is graduated exposure to feared stimuli. CBT involves a commitment from the patient to do homework, the filling out of logs of automatic thoughts and reactions to different situations, and the motivation to place himself or herself in uncomfortable situations. In addition, clinicians are required to have experience in conducting CBT therapy. In many areas of the country, there is a paucity of such practitioners.

Patient Education

Patient education is an essential part of the treatment of patients with panic disorder. Patients should be given a definitive diagnosis and should never be told that there is "nothing wrong with them." It is also important to inform them that the antidepressants will take 4 to 6 weeks to work. Patients should be asked about avoidance behavior in addition to the frequency of panic attacks. The learned avoidance behavior may persist long after the panic attacks have ceased. For these individuals it is important to recommend gradual exposure to overcome the avoidance behavior. There are a variety of self-help books about panic disorder that can be found in most bookstores.

Physical and Chemical Injuries

BURNS

method of
ROBERT L. SHERIDAN, M.D.
*Shriners Burns Hospital, Harvard Medical
School, and Massachusetts General Hospital
Boston, Massachusetts*

As recently as 1970, patients suffering burns over more than 30% of their body surface rarely survived. Those who did survive the agony of eschar separation and protracted burn wound healing were generally crippled by the intense hypertrophic scarring and wound contraction that accompanies the spontaneous healing of deep dermal and full-thickness burn wounds. The outlook for burn patients has improved enormously since then. Today, the majority of those suffering much larger injuries not only survive but also have satisfactory long-term functional and cosmetic outcomes.

NATURAL HISTORY

The natural history of a large burn is short, measured in hours or a few days. This is because burns over large surface areas, through the release of mediators from the injured tissue, cause a diffuse capillary leak in unburned tissues and organs. The resulting hypovolemia is called burn shock and is fatal if volume depletion is not accurately corrected. Patients with smaller injuries who do not die of burn shock experience a process of eschar liquefaction, separation, wound contraction, and spontaneous healing. If wounds do not involve the full thickness of the skin, this process will result in a functionally healed wound, generally by 3 weeks. If the injury is deep dermal or full thickness, the wounds may never epithelialize, despite progressive wound contraction. This process of wound liquefaction and separation is a septic physiologic challenge that is accompanied by high fevers, malaise, and systemic illness. Wounds managed this way can also be very painful. The powerful forces of wound contraction and hypertrophic scar formation routinely cause crippling deformities in patients with extensive deep dermal and full-thickness wounds that heal spontaneously.

INITIAL EVALUATION

As burn patients enter the health care system, they should be evaluated in a systematic manner, so that their cutaneous injury does not cause clinicians to overlook other important issues.

Primary Survey

Patients should first be examined as if they have suffered a traumatic injury. The airway should be assessed first because burn patients are prone to the development of progressive facial and oropharyngeal edema, which can occlude the airway. Patients with severe facial burns and inhalation injury, particularly small children, are often best managed with prophylactic intubation. Early intubation in such circumstances is advised, because endotracheal intubation will become progressively difficult as edema becomes marked and symptomatic. Vascular access should be obtained, ideally through the percutaneous central venous route, in patients with serious burns. Intravenous fluids should be given on the basis of a predicted resuscitation requirement.

Secondary Survey

After the airway is controlled and vascular access is obtained, the patient should undergo a systematic secondary survey. It is important to obtain a clear history of the mechanism of injury, because this will prompt the clinician to suspect other non-burn injuries. Children should be evaluated for the possibility of child abuse or neglect as a contributing factor to their injuries. The neurologic status of the patient should be carefully assessed, and computed tomography should be done if the mechanism of injury suggests a head injury. This is particularly important in those with large burns who will predictably develop a progressive decrement in their level of consciousness over the first few postinjury days, rendering serial neurologic examinations suspect. The eyes should be evaluated for corneal burns before significant adnexal edema makes such an evaluation difficult. The patient should be evaluated for the possibility of an inhalation injury through examination and history. Inhalation injury is suggested if burns occurred in a closed space or if there is carbonaceous debris in the mouth or sputum. The chest should be assessed for bilateral air movement. The abdomen should be examined for distention and other injuries. A nasogastric tube should be placed in those patients with large injuries to prevent gastric distention. Burn patients are prone to virulent ulcer disease because of burn shock–related splanchnic ischemia. Prophylactic histamine receptor antagonists and antacids should be administered. Particular attention should be paid to maintaining the patient's body temperature during evaluation. Routine laboratory studies should be performed and radiographs should be obtained, depending on the mechanism of injury and the suspicion of concomitant non-burn trauma. A decision must be made regarding transfer. The American Burn Association and American College of Surgeons have a burn center verification process and a set of suggested burn transfer criteria (Table 1).

TABLE 1. **American Burn Association Burn Center Transfer Criteria**

1. Second- and third-degree burns greater than 10% total body surface area (TBSA) in patients younger than 10 or older than 50 years
2. Second- and third-degree burns greater than 20% TBSA in other age groups
3. Second- and third-degree burns that involve the face, hands, feet, genitalia, perineum, and major joints
4. Third-degree burns greater than 5% TBSA in any age group
5. Electrical burns including lightning injury
6. Chemical burns
7. Inhalation injury
8. Burn injury in patients with pre-existing medical disorders that could complicate management, prolong recovery, or affect mortality
9. Any patient with burns and concomitant trauma (e.g., fractures) in which the burn injury poses the greatest risk of morbidity or mortality. In such cases, if the trauma poses the greater immediate risk, the patient may be treated initially in a trauma center until stable before being transferred to a burn center. Physician judgment will be necessary in such situation and should be in concert with the regional medical control plan and triage protocols.
10. Hospitals without qualified personnel or equipment for the care of children should transfer children with burns to a burn center with these capabilities.
11. Burn injury in patients who will require special social/emotional and/or long-term rehabilitative support, including cases involving suspected child abuse and substance abuse

TABLE 2. **The Modified Brook Formula**

First 24 Hours

Adults and Children > 20 kg:

Ringer's lactate: 2–4 mL/kg/% burn/24 hours (first half in first 8 hours)
Colloid: none

Children < 20 kg:

Ringer's lactate: 2–3 mL/kg/% burn/24 hours (first half in first 8 hours)
Ringer's lactate with 5% dextrose: maintenance rate (approximately 4 mL/kg/h for the first 10 kg, 2 mL/kg/h for the next 10 kg and 1 mL/kg/h for weight over 20 kg)
Colloid: none

Second 24 Hours

All patients:

Crystalloid: To maintain urine output. If aqueous silver nitrate is used, sodium leaching will mandate continued isotonic crystalloid. If other topical agent is used, free water requirement is significant. Serum sodium level should be monitored closely. Nutritional support should begin, ideally by the enteral route.
Colloid: (5% albumin in Ringer's lactate):
0–30% burn: None
30–50% burn: 0.3 mL/kg/% burn/24 h
50–70% burn: 0.4 mL/kg/% burn/24 h
70–100% burn: 0.5 mL/kg/% burn/24 h

It is very important that the adequacy of perfusion of the distal extremities is ensured throughout the period of resuscitation. This is best done by serial examination. Extremity perfusion can be compromised by progressive swelling occurring within a circumferentially burned extremity, or through progressive intracompartmental muscle edema after high voltage electrical injury or extremely deep thermal burn. If perfusion is threatened, manifested by increasing firmness or coolness of the extremity, escharotomy or fasciotomy should be done to ensure continued viability of the extremity. If circumferential chest wall burns compromise ventilation, chest escharotomy should be done.

TREATMENT

Fluid Resuscitation

Patients suffering burns in excess of 30% of the body surface will predictably develop burn shock if they are not properly resuscitated.

Physiology

Mediators released by injured soft tissues cause loss of capillary integrity distant from the wound. When burns are in excess of 20% of the body surface, this phenomenon often results in intravascular volume depletion of profound degree.

Resuscitation Formulas

A number of fluid resuscitation formulas have been developed to help clinicians predict the fluid replace-

ment requirements of individual patients. However, no formula is able to accurately predict the individual requirements of specific patients. Variables affecting fluid requirements include the vapor transmission characteristics of particular wounds, the increased mediator release associated with inhalation injury, the increased requirements associated with young age, and the predictably increased capillary leak associated with delayed resuscitation. The modified Brook formula (Table 2) is a widely used starting point. The capillary leak associated with a burn injury typically abates 18 to 24 hours after injury in patients who are well resuscitated. The normalization of capillary integrity that is seen 18 to 24 hours after injury explains the decreased infusion rate recommended by most resuscitation formulas at about this time (see Table 2). It is very important to adjust resuscitation infusions so as not to overresuscitate or underresuscitate; usual resuscitation endpoints are itemized in Table 3. It is critically important that careful attention be paid to a high-quality resuscitation if reliably good outcomes are to be achieved.

Wound Management

Proper management of the burn wound is central both to survival and subsequent function.

TABLE 3. **Standard Resuscitation Endpoints**

Urine output: 0.5 mL/kg/h, 1–2 mL/kg/h in small children
Sensorium: alert
Base deficit: less than 2
Blood pressure: within adult norms; in small children, 90 plus twice the age in years is a reasonable systolic target

Wound Management Decisions

Wounds should be evaluated for size, depth, and circumferential components initially.

Subsequently, full-thickness components need to be identified, excised, and closed biologically. It is optimal if this exercise is completed during the first few days after injury, before the inevitable development of wound sepsis. Numerous aids have been developed over the years to facilitate identification of full-thickness wound components, but at present this remains a clinical skill that requires the help of an experienced examiner.

Outpatient Burn Care

Many patients can have some or all of their burn care rendered outside the hospital. Several conditions must be met for an outpatient plan of care to be considered. There should be no question of airway compromise or inhalation injury. Patients must be capable of taking oral fluids. Patients must have burns small enough such that a resuscitation requirement is not expected. Patients with circumferential burns of the extremity should be admitted for monitoring for distal perfusion as edema progresses. Patients with high- or intermediate-voltage electrical injury should be admitted for cardiac monitoring. Patients who have unequivocal full-thickness burns should be admitted for prompt surgery. It is important that patients with injuries involving abuse or neglect not be managed initially as outpatients. The patient must have a family capable of supporting the wound care and transportation needs associated with an outpatient burn program. Pain control should be addressed in a sensitive but safe way in the outpatient setting. It is essential that a specific program of frequent follow-up and wound monitoring is arranged before embarking on an outpatient plan of care. Despite this rigid set of criteria, most patients can be successfully managed in the outpatient setting.

Initial Wound Excision and Closure

Most patients with full-thickness burns of less than 40% of the body surface can undergo immediate wound excision and closure with split-thickness autografts. Patients with larger wounds may have to have this done in a series of staged procedures over the first few postinjury days, with wounds closed with allograft or another temporary wound covering material. When donor sites heal, they can be reharvested and temporary coverings replaced with permanent split-thickness autograft. These can be bloody and physiologically stressful operations but are extremely well tolerated if properly performed.

Definitive Wound Closure

After full-thickness wounds have been excised and grafted with a combination of permanent and temporary materials, temporary covers are gradually replaced with full-thickness autografts in a series of operations to achieve definitive wound closure. Also during this phase of care, wounds of small areas but high complexity are addressed. These areas include the face, ears, hands, feet, and genitalia. It is critically important to optimize closure in these important areas to achieve the best possible cosmetic and functional long-term outcome. The face and hands are closed with sheet autograft to facilitate this objective. Facial burns are grafted in cosmetic units whenever possible. Definitive wound closure with materials other than split-thickness autografts is an active area of investigation. However, at present, split-thickness autografts provide the closure of choice for most patients.

Selected Issues in Burn Critical Care

Successful management of a patient with a large burn requires significant critical care during the physiologically stressful period of initial resuscitation and wound excision as well as during periods of pulmonary dysfunction and sepsis. If the wound can be promptly closed, these needs can be minimized.

Inhalation Injury

Patients burned in structural fires may inhale the products of incomplete combustion or super-heated air, resulting in an inhalation injury. On occasion, hot liquids can be aspirated, particularly by small children, resulting in upper airway edema. The pathophysiology of inhalation injury is incompletely understood, but the clinically important sequelae include upper airway edema, necrosis and sloughing of endobronchial mucosa with obstruction of small airways, ventilation/perfusion mismatching with hypoxia, alveolar flooding with deterioration of compliance, and subsequent pulmonary infection. Management involves the provision of noninjurious supportive care while awaiting spontaneous healing and specific treatment for identified pulmonary infections. Initially, airway patency should be maintained, often requiring intubation. Subsequently, intubation and mechanical ventilation are only required for those patients with decrements in compliance or gas exchange significant enough to result in respiratory failure. Pulmonary toilet is an important component of care, given the common occurrence of small airway occlusion with secondary ventilation/perfusion mismatching and infection.

Nutritional Support

Patients with burns have increased needs for calories and protein. Predictions vary, much like the predictions of resuscitation volume requirements, but consensus is that provision of approximately one and one-half times a basal metabolic rate will be adequate caloric support, and 1.5 to 3 grams per kg per day will constitute adequate protein supplementation for most patients. The enteral route is the ideal route of support, but patients who do not tolerate enteral support because of frequent surgery or sepsis can be supported adequately by the parenteral route until enteral support is again tolerated. The adequacy of nutritional support can be monitored through serial weights, protein balance studies, and indirect calorimetry.

Septic Complications

Burn patients are prone to a number of infectious complications because of their weakened immunologic resistance. Not only do they have a cutaneous wound that compromises the barrier function of the skin, but white cell studies have also demonstrated a global impairment of function after an extensive thermal burn. The specific focus of infection can often be occult despite severe systemic symptoms. Ideally, one is vigilantly monitoring the patient, anticipating signs of looming sepsis. Protracted courses of broad-spectrum antibiotics are harmful in that they predispose to infection with resistant organisms and fungus. It is important to be able to differentiate the normal fever associated with a burn wound from the high fever and toxicity associated with sepsis.

Special Injury Considerations

Patients with electrical, chemical, and tar injuries are commonly referred to burn units for care. There are certain unique characteristics of these injuries that the clinician should be aware of.

Electrical Injury

Patients suffering high-voltage electrical injuries, greater than 1000 volts, are at risk for deep muscle damage with compartment syndrome, cardiac arrhythmias, and myoglobinuria with associated renal failure. Patients need to be monitored closely for these complications. Should intracompartmental edema manifest through distal neurologic signs and pain, prompt fasciotomy is indicated. Should pigmented urine be noted after placement of a bladder catheter, this must be cleared with crystalloid volume infusions and selective use of mannitol and loop diuretics. Patients should undergo cardiac monitoring for at least 72 hours, with the treatment of rhythm disturbances as noted. These patients often have a cutaneous injury that does not completely reflect the extent of their deep burn, thereby making resuscitation requirements more difficult to predict. Therefore, they need to be closely monitored for the adequacy of their fluid resuscitation.

Chemical and Tar Injury

Patients exposed to noxious chemicals are at risk not only for the cutaneous injury associated with chemical burn but also for systemic toxicity associated with absorption of various chemicals. Wounds should be initially copiously irrigated with water. Local poison control centers can provide valuable information facilitating management of any systemic absorption. Patients suffering hydrofluoric acid exposure (particularly concentrated forms) are at risk for life-threatening hypocalcemia, because the fluoride ion is very permeable and avidly binds to divalent cations. These patients should be treated with intravenous and subeschar calcium gluconate.

Modern thermoplastic road materials are designed to require heating up to 700° F before they liquefy. This is so they will remain solid in the hot sun on an asphalt road. When splashed with these viscous, extremely hot substances, patients suffer very deep burns. The first maneuver should be to copiously irrigate the wounds to cool the tar. The tar can be removed later, after soaking in a lipophilic solvent. Underlying wounds are generally deep and commonly require excision and grafting.

Rehabilitation, Reconstruction, and Reintegration

With increasing survival of patients with very large injuries, the need for skillful rehabilitation, reconstruction, and reintegration efforts is becoming increasingly important. It is essential that skilled therapists be members of the burn team and be involved in patient care from the time of resuscitation. Furthermore, it is optimal if patients can be followed long term by the acute burn care team to facilitate successful management of predictable long-term issues.

Rehabilitation

Rehabilitation efforts should begin at the time of admission, with splinting, range of motion exercises, and antideformity positioning. It is particularly important to pay close attention to the burned hand so that range of motion is not lost while attention is paid to higher priority issues. Each joint should be taken through a full range of motion twice daily and the hand otherwise splinted in a position of function: the metacarpophalangeal joints at 70 to 90 degrees, the interphalangeal joints in extension, the first web space open, and the wrist in 20 degrees of extension. As wound closure is achieved, passive and active strengthening programs intensify. The retention of muscle bulk is enhanced by active strengthening and proper nutrition. These rehabilitation efforts continue into the outpatient setting and are a critical component to optimizing long-term outcome. If these efforts are not followed, a predictable set of contractures will develop (Table 4).

Scar Management

The process of hypertrophic scarring is not well understood. Wounds destined to become hypertrophic are those second-degree burns that take more than 3 weeks to heal or widely meshed autografts. Wounds across areas of tension or highly elastic skin are also more prone to become hypertrophic. Small children seem to be more prone to develop hypertrophic scars. Our ability to favorably influence the development of hypertrophic scars is limited. Available tools include scar massage, compression garments, topical silicone, limited corticosteroid injections, limited topical corticosteroid applications, and surgery. None of these modalities will reliably work, but when used in com-

TABLE 4. **Predictable Contractures That Will Develop if Rehabilitation Efforts Are Not Adequate**

Anatomic Part	Typical Contracture	Keys to Prevention
Neck	Flexion contracture	Ranging, splinting with neck in neutral
Shoulder	Adduction contracture	Ranging and splinting
Elbow	Flexion contracture	Extension or rotating elbow splints
Hips	Flexion contracture, particularly in infants	Ranging, splinting, and prone positioning (in selected patients)
Knee	Flexion contracture	Ranging and extension splints
Ankle	Equinous deformity	Ranging and splinting in neutral
Hand	Dorsal contracture	Ranging and splinting with metacarpo-phalangeal joints at 70–90°

bination they can favorably influence scar development.

Reconstruction

There are a predictable set of reconstructive needs that burn patients will have, but the proper timing of these needs is often difficult to predict with certainty. Early after the acute hospitalization, if contractures interfere with function, they should be addressed surgically. It is particularly important to be sensitive to the developmental needs of small children so that normal development is not hindered by contractures. For example, if developmentally it is time for the child to develop fine motor function, it is important to correct contractures that interfere with fine hand function, even if they seem relatively minor. It is important to time reconstructive surgery so that it does not overly interfere with school, sports, work, or family activities. Often, operations that are perceived of as primarily cosmetic can have enormous psychological benefits. If such operations will help patients interact with other people, they should be given their due priority.

Reintegration

The ultimate goal of burn care is to bring the patient back, as much as possible, to the status that was held before the injury. This requires the involvement of members of the patient's family and community. Many patients will suffer the sequela of post-traumatic stress disorder after injuries of this magni·tude. If this predictable problem is addressed in a sensitive and effective way, recovery can be greatly enhanced. Today, if patients participate in a coordinated program of burn aftercare, very satisfying long-term outcomes can be expected.

CONCLUSION

The techniques now available to care for those who have suffered serious burns have come a long way since 1970, but an isolated burn intensive care unit with the principal objective of patient survival simply will not generate the quality outcomes that are now possible. Burn care today is truly a long-term multi-disciplinary effort. Even those patients suffering massive burns, if they are able to participate in such a scheme of care, can be expected to have satisfying long-term outcomes.

HIGH-ALTITUDE SICKNESS

method of
URS SCHERRER, M.D., and
CLAUDIO SARTORI, M.D.
*Centre Hospitalier Universitaire Vaudois
Lausanne, Switzerland*

High altitude is a hostile environment, characterized by normal air oxygen content but low oxygen disposal, owing to low atmospheric pressure, cold temperatures, and severe exposure to sunshine. With regard to human physiology and pathophysiology, high altitude starts at elevations above 2500 m (8000 ft), the height at which in most people arterial oxygen saturation drops below 90%. Starting at this altitude, failure to acclimatize to hypoxia can be associated with three major, and potentially fatal, medical problems: acute mountain sickness (AMS), high-altitude cerebral edema (HACE), and high-altitude pulmonary edema (HAPE). These three entities share many clinical features and may represent different degrees of severity of a common underlying pathophysiologic process.

Three principal factors favor the development of high-altitude sickness: individual susceptibility (possibly genetically determined), rapidity of the ascent (i.e., rate of ascent exceeding the rate of acclimatization), and absolute altitude itself. Exact estimates of the incidence of mountain illness are difficult to obtain. Studies indicate that at 3050 m and 4559 m, respectively, 15% and 52% of mountaineers suffer from AMS. The overall incidence of HAPE in the Alps is estimated to be about 0.2%. After a rapid ascent to 4559 m in the Swiss Alps, however, roughly 10% of the mountaineers develop HAPE, and this incidence increases to 60% in mountaineers who had suffered from HAPE before. At a comparable altitude in Nepal (4200 m) reached after a slower ascent, the incidence of HAPE among trekkers was 2%. This article summarizes the clinical presentation, the current knowledge of underlying pathophysiologic mechanisms, and the possibilities for both prevention and management of mountain sickness.

ACUTE MOUNTAIN SICKNESS

AMS is a common, benign, and generally self-limiting condition that occurs typically in healthy people who ascend rapidly to altitudes above 2500 m. Both sexes are equally affected, but children are more susceptible than elderly people. During the first 8 to 24 hours of altitude exposure, susceptible individuals suffer from a variety of symptoms, the most prominent being headache, nausea, vomiting, anorexia, lassitude, and insomnia. Headache is usually frontal, bitemporal, or occipital; and it typically worsens at

TABLE 1. **Recommendations for the Prevention and the Treatment of High-Altitude Sickness**

	Acute Mountain Sickness	High-Altitude Cerebral Edema	High-Altitude Pulmonary Edema
Prevention		Staging (2–5 days at intermediary altitude) Slow ascent (400 m/d) High-carbohydrate diet Adequate fluid intake Avoid alcohol, hypnotics, and unnecessary exertion	
	Acetazolamide (Diamox) (250 mg every 8 hours, day −1 to day 5) Dexamethasone (Decadron)* (2–4 mg every 6 hours, day 1 to day 3 then tapered over 5 days)	Dexamethasone ? (2–4 mg every 6 hours, day 1 to day 3 then tapered over 5 days)	Nifedipine* (Procardia) (30 mg slow-release/d, day −3 to day 0; then 20 mg every 8 hours for 5 to 7 days) Acetazolamide ? Dexamethasone ?
Treatment	DESCENT Paracetamol Acetazolamide (250–500 mg every 8 hours) Dexamethasone (4–8 mg every 6 hours) Hyperbaric chamber ? Oxygen ?	DESCENT Oxygen Dexamethasone* (4–8 mg every 6 hours) Hyperbaric chamber	DESCENT Oxygen Nifedipine* (20 mg every 6 hours) Hyperbaric chamber

*Not FDA approved for this indication.

night and during a Valsalva maneuver. Sleep disturbance, lightheadedness, and dizziness may complete the symptoms. Physical signs are nonspecific and may include mild peripheral fluid retention, tachycardia, and, occasionally, retinal hemorrhage. The differential diagnosis includes exhaustion, dehydration, and hypothermia.

Within the next 24 to 48 hours at high altitude, as the process of acclimatization occurs, the symptoms abate spontaneously in the majority of the subjects, but in some cases, symptoms may progress to life-threatening HACE and/or HAPE. The exact pathophysiologic mechanism is not known, but a mild cerebral edema may play a role. A low hypoxic ventilatory response predisposes to AMS.

Management

In most cases, stopping the ascent and rest are sufficient (Table 1). Acetaminophen, paracetamol, aspirin, and ibuprofen are helpful to improve headache. Prochlorperazine (Compazine) or metoclopramide (Reglan) may be used to improve the gastrointestinal upset. The carbonic anhydrase inhibitor acetazolamide (Diamox) stimulates the ventilation and improves symptoms of AMS. In patients allergic to sulfa drugs or with worsening AMS, dexamethasone (Decadron)* may be used. Descent, oxygen, and/or hyperbaria are possible, but usually not necessary, treatment alternatives. Once the symptoms have resolved, further ascent can be permitted without restrictions.

In particularly susceptible subjects, acetazolamide (side effects: mild diuresis, peripheral paresthesias, flat taste of carbonated drinks) decreases the incidence and severity of AMS. Dexamethasone* has also been used for this purpose, but rebound effects and

*Not FDA approved for this indication.

potentially serious side effects preclude its routine recommendation for the prophylaxis of AMS.

HIGH-ALTITUDE CEREBRAL EDEMA

During the second and third day at high altitude, some degree of infraclinical generalized edema is common and represents an increase in the extracellular fluid volume. In the skull, this mild edema may lead to an increase in the intracranial pressure and give rise to the symptoms of AMS. The underlying mechanism is still not clear.

HACE is characterized by the progression of the symptoms of AMS, and the appearance of truncal ataxia, severe lassitude, irrationality, hallucinations, and global neurologic defects. Focal neurologic signs are unusual. With raising intracranial pressure, there is lethargy, irregular breathing, and a progressive deterioration of the mental functions and consciousness. Once coma has developed, the disease has a very high mortality rate of up to 60%.

The cornerstone of the treatment is immediate descent, associated with oxygen (4 to 6 liters per minute). If descent is impossible or delayed, oxygen (4 to 6 liters per minute) or hyperbaria and dexamethasone should be used. Delayed treatment may result in persistent ataxia and cognitive impairment after recovery from HACE.

High-Altitude Pulmonary Edema

Rapid ascent to high altitude associated with moderate to heavy exercise, followed within the next 8 to 24 hours by symptoms of AMS, represents the characteristic clinical setting for HAPE. HAPE may, however, occur without accompanying symptoms of AMS and affect even the most experienced high-altitude mountaineers.

In most cases, HAPE occurs between 36 and 72 hours after arrival at high altitude, most often during the second night. In addition to symptoms of AMS, subjects suffer from dyspnea (often aggravated at night from decreased ventilation and, in turn, more severe hypoxemia), dry cough (eventually evolving into a productive form with frothy white or blood-tinged sputum), reduced exercise performance, chest pain, weakness, and lethargy. Physical signs include tachypnea, orthopnea, tachycardia, low-grade fever, and cyanosis. Lung auscultation may reveal crackles at the site of edema, but characteristically there exists a striking discrepancy between the paucity of the auscultatory findings and the severity of the radiographic findings. Signs of HACE may complicate the clinical picture.

The characteristic radiographic signs of HAPE are patchy infiltrates that with time and increasing severity become more homogeneous and diffusely distributed. The electrocardiogram may show signs of pulmonary hypertension. If left untreated, the clinical picture may evolve dramatically, with the patient becoming comatose; and death may occur within hours. Mortality is closely dependent on how quickly treatment is begun. If HAPE is associated with HACE, the prognosis is worse; and further deterioration and death may occur even after rapid and correct management.

Predisposing factors include a previous episode of HAPE (suggesting a possible genetic predisposition), cold exposure, physical overactivity on arrival at high altitude, recent respiratory infection, male sex, and young age. Exercise training and athletic fitness do not provide immunity against HAPE. Interestingly, the incidence of HAPE is augmented in high-altitude residents, particularly in children and young adults, when returning home from a sojourn at low altitude (reentry edema).

An exaggerated pulmonary hypertension is a hallmark of HAPE and is thought to play an important role in its pathogenesis. Both the pulmonary wedge pressure and the cardiac output are normal, excluding heart failure as a causal factor. Sympathetic vasoconstrictor overactivity and endothelial dysfunction (impaired nitric oxide release and augmented endothelin-1 release) may contribute to pulmonary hypertension in HAPE-prone subjects. The exaggerated hypoxic pulmonary vasoconstriction is thought to be uneven, leading to areas of hyperperfusion (and, in turn, alveolar fluid flooding) and hypoperfusion. There is evidence that pulmonary hypertension is not sufficient to trigger HAPE, suggesting that additional mechanisms may play a role. An impairment of the alveolar transepithelial sodium and water transport may represent a candidate mechanism.

Prediction

HAPE-susceptible subjects have a lower hypoxic ventilatory response than HAPE-resistant subjects, but there is a large overlap between groups, and such measurements do not allow the prediction of HAPE susceptibility in a given individual. Similarly, pulmonary artery pressure responses to short-term hypoxia, used both alone or in combination with the hypoxic ventilatory response, do not discriminate reliably between HAPE-resistant and HAPE-susceptible individuals.

Treatment

HAPE is a life-threatening condition best managed by descent. Other treatment options should never be considered as a substitute for rapid descent but should be used either to improve the clinical condition to facilitate descent or to gain time when descent is impossible. In this latter situation, and if available, oxygen (2 to 4 liters per minute) should be administered to improve arterial oxygenation and decrease pulmonary artery pressure. Because both oxygen administration and pressurization are effective, portable hyperbaric chambers (Gamow [USA], Certec [France]) which are lighter to carry than oxygen cylinders, are of interest (the continuous pumping necessary to maintain pressurization can be tiring, however). There may be a rebound effect on stopping hyperbaria.

Lowering of pulmonary artery pressure by pharmacologic agents has beneficial effects in HAPE. Several vasodilator agents (nifedipine [Procardia]*, hydralazine [Apresoline],* phentolamine [Regitine], nitric oxide) have been used successfully to treat HAPE under experimental conditions. Among them, nifedipine (20 mg every 8 hours) and inhaled nitric oxide (40 ppm) have proven to be effective and well tolerated.

Other pharmacologic agents have been used or proposed for the treatment of HAPE, but their beneficial effects (and lack of detrimental side effects) are not established. Morphine has vasodilator effects, but its depressor effect on respiration precludes its use in this setting. In contrast to the treatment of AMS and HACE, the efficacy of corticosteroids to treat HAPE is not established. Furosemide has no proven beneficial effects but may have severe adverse effects (i.e., severe hypotension and shock). The routine administration of antibiotics is not recommended, but they may prove beneficial to prevent infection of the waterlogged lung.

SUBACUTE AND CHRONIC MOUNTAIN SICKNESS

In subjects born at low altitude and having moved later to a highland region, and in populations residing at high altitude, two other conditions have been described. During subacute exposure of some 9 to 10 weeks to high altitude, susceptible infants and adults develop pulmonary arterial hypertension associated with signs of congestive heart failure, papilledema,

---

*Not FDA approved for this indication.

and polycythemia. Symptoms resolve spontaneously without any treatment after descent.

In susceptible highland residents, chronic mountain sickness (Monge's disease) may develop. It is characterized by a disproportionate polycythemia due to an excessive erythropoiesis. The symptoms may develop insidiously, and subjects suffer from dyspnea, headache, irritability, lassitude, loss of mental acuity, and sleep disturbances. Clinical signs include cyanosis, plethora, congested conjunctivae, finger clubbing, and signs of right ventricular hypertrophy and/or failure. If socially feasible, permanent descent to sea level is curative. Periodic venisection and long-term use of the respiratory stimulant medroxyprogesterone acetate (Provera)* help to lower the hematocrit and may be beneficial to improve the clinical picture.

*Not FDA approved for this indication.

DISTURBANCES DUE TO COLD

method of
GERALD K. BRISTOW, M.D.
University of Manitoba
Winnipeg, Manitoba, Canada

Cold-induced disturbances may be classified as generalized or localized. Generalized disturbances include accidental hypothermia and near-drowning in cold water. Localized disturbances may be classified as freezing or nonfreezing injuries. Freezing injuries include frostnip and frostbite, whereas nonfreezing injuries include chilblains, pernio, and trench (immersion) foot.

ACCIDENTAL HYPOTHERMIA

Hypothermia is defined as a core or central body temperature of less than 35°C. Core temperature is most easily and best measured in the esophagus or rectum. Accidental hypothermia may be classified as mild (30 to 35°C), moderate (25 to 30°C), and severe (less than 25°C). This simple classification has the advantage of correlating strongly with key physiologic changes as well as morbidity and mortality. Furthermore, methods of treatment, particularly rewarming techniques, can be largely based on the presenting core temperature.

Pathophysiology

Accidental hypothermia occurs whenever heat loss exceeds the ability of the body to produce an equal amount of heat. Although this may result from excessive heat loss, diminished heat production, or indeed impaired thermoregulation (Table 1), often many of these factors are involved in the pathogenesis of accidental hypothermia. There are many factors that affect the rate of cooling (Table 2). Regardless of the mechanism of cooling, those individuals with a

TABLE 1. Etiology of Accidental Hypothermia

Excessive Heat Loss
- Extremes of age
- Acute exposure
- Skin disease/burns

Diminished Heat Production
- Extremes of age
- Dehydration/malnutrition
- Endocrine disorders
    Hypopituitarism
    Hypothyroidism
- Exhaustion
- Trauma

Impaired Thermoregulation
- Brain injury/disease
- Spinal cord injury
- Alcohol/drugs
- Severe illness

greater percentage of body fat cool more slowly. Although heat loss is inversely proportional to the air or water temperature, it is important to remember that water removes heat from the body at approximately 30 times the rate of air at the same temperature. In dry exposure, as wind velocity increases so does heat loss, whereas in water exposure, heat loss increases with current velocity. Even in dry exposure, clothing, once having become wet, increases the rate of heat loss from the body.

As the core temperature drops there are widespread alterations in normal physiology. The most important of these changes occur in the musculoskeletal system, in the cardiovascular system, in metabolism and oxygen delivery, and in the central nervous system.

At a core body temperature of approximately 35°C, particularly if the hypothermia is due to a rapid heat loss such as very cold air or water exposure, fine movements of the fingers and strength in the large muscles will be much reduced. By 30°C, little strength is retained in the muscles and activity involving dexterity of the fingers has all but vanished. These changes probably represent alterations in the viscoelastic properties of tendons, ligaments, and muscles. The result of this is that although consciousness may be maintained, the ability to extricate oneself from the cold environment may be almost impossible.

The cardiovascular changes induced by hypothermia are multiple and severe and, in the final analy-

TABLE 2. Factors Affecting Rate of Cooling

- Ambient temperature
- Wind velocity
- Wet or dry exposure
- Type of clothing
- Natural insulation (fat)
- Activity
- Physical condition

sis, cause death. Initially, with cold exposure, sympathetic stimulation causes tachycardia, hypertension, and increased cardiac output. There is intense vasoconstriction of the cutaneous blood vessels with closing of the arteriovenous anastomosis in an effort to conserve heat. As the temperature decreases the hypothermia causes a reduction of myocardial contractility and cardiac output, but the blood pressure, although reduced, is relatively well maintained because of the intense vasoconstriction and increased systemic vascular resistance. Cardiac conduction velocity decreases, manifested by prolongation of the PR, QRS, and QTc intervals. The heart rate, initially a sinus tachycardia, becomes a sinus bradycardia and at approximately 30°C manifests often as atrial fibrillation with a slow ventricular response. All manner of supraventricular or ventricular ectopic activity may also be seen during the cooling process. At temperatures less than 30°C a low heart rate predominates, and at temperatures of less than 25°C imminent danger of ventricular fibrillation or asystole exists.

An interesting relationship between oxygen delivery and consumption occurs during the evolution of hypothermia. During the intense vasoconstriction induced by hypothermia there is a movement of crystalloid from the intravascular to extravascular space. This causes a rise in hematocrit and blood viscosity with an aggregation of red blood cells and ultimately sludging of blood. This sludging of blood combined with a decreased cardiac output and a leftward shift of the oxyhemoglobin dissociation curve caused by the hypothermia per se as well as a respiratory alkalosis all conspire to produce a decrease in oxygen delivery to the tissue. On the other hand, the falling temperature, once shivering has ceased, reduces the metabolic demand of the tissue in a predictable fashion. For each degree centigrade fall of body temperature, the whole-body oxygen consumption is reduced by 6 to 7%. The brain's requirement for oxygen falls at an even greater rate. Stated another way, for every 10°C reduction in the core body temperature (Q_{10}), cerebral oxygen consumption is reduced by 60 to 80%. Therefore, although oxygen delivery is severely compromised as the body temperature drops, the oxygen utilization falls even faster and, particularly for the brain, allows a significant margin of safety against hypoxia and extends the biologic survival time in the case of cardiac arrest in the hypothermic state. Simply stated, if the safe circulatory arrest time at 37°C is generally considered to be approximately 5 minutes, that would be extended to approximately 15 minutes at 27°C and 75 minutes at 17°C. Although much of the cerebral protective effect of hypothermia has been thought to have been due to the reduced cerebral requirement for oxygen, it is also likely that milder degrees of hypothermia, namely, 32 to 34°C, inhibit the release of excitatory amino acids, thus enhancing the protective effect of hypothermia, particularly at higher body temperatures.

In the otherwise healthy, undrugged, and nonin-toxicated hypothermic victim, cerebral dysfunction begins to manifest at approximately 32°C with confusion, disorientation, introversion, and amnesia. Consciousness, however, is not lost until temperatures of less than 30°C are encountered. The electroencephalogram becomes flat at approximately 19°C. When dealing with the hypothermic victim it is critical to remember that unconsciousness associated with temperatures of 30°C or greater has a cause other than the hypothermia.

Clinical Presentation

Clinical presentation depends on the core temperature of the victim. In all cases the skin is cold, and violent shivering generally occurs at temperatures greater than approximately 31°C. Unless associated with concomitant illness or injury, a conscious or shivering individual can be assumed to be warmer than 30°C whereas an individual unconscious and nonshivering can be assumed to have a core temperature of less than 30°C. The verification of the core temperature should be made with a low-reading rectal thermometer or preferably an esophageal thermistor probe or thermocouple. In the urban setting the hypothermic victim should always be examined carefully for the concomitant presence of other systemic illness or injury, including the use of alcohol and drugs.

On presentation of the hypothermic victim, the three-level severity classification in accidental hypothermia is particularly useful in formulating a prognosis. In cases of accidental hypothermia not associated with serious medical, surgical, or traumatic events, the finding of mild hypothermia (30 to 35°C) suggests a good prognosis with the victim being conscious and having a relatively stable cardiovascular system. The victims with moderate hypothermia (25 to 30°C) are invariably unconscious with an unstable cardiovascular system manifested by low blood pressure and more severe cardiac dysrhythmias. The outcome in this group is guarded. For patients with severe hypothermia (less than 25°C) the prognosis is poor because they are unconscious, are usually severely hypotensive, and manifest considerable cardiac dysrhythmias. If it has not already happened, these individuals are at imminent risk of ventricular fibrillation or asystole.

Treatment

An overview of the treatment to be provided in a health care facility is presented here as opposed to the much more limited range of options encountered in the field.

Gentle handling and moving of all hypothermic victims is essential, particularly those who are moderately or severely hypothermic. Rough handling and such interventions as tracheal intubation are capable of precipitating ventricular fibrillation or asystole in the very cold victim. An accurate core temperature should be continuously measured by a method referred to previously. In addition, continuous electrocardiographic monitoring should be undertaken. Obviously, attention to airway, breathing, and circulation takes precedence over any attempts to rewarm the victim. In virtually all cases of uncomplicated mild hypothermia and in many of the uncomplicated moderate hypothermic victims respiration and cardiovascular function are stable, although far from normal with respect to vital signs. For those victims with core temperatures below 25°C, cardiorespiratory arrest has usually occurred and standard cardiopulmonary resuscitation (CPR) should be performed. However, a prolonged (1 minute) effort should be taken to ensure that in the severely hypothermic victim no vital signs exist before instituting CPR. Because of the infrequent and shallow respirations and very slow pulse rates encountered at approximately 25°C, viability may be mistaken for cardiorespiratory arrest. The danger of premature CPR in these individuals is often the initiation of ventricular fibrillation where viability had previously existed. The severely hypothermic individual requires very little circulation, respiration, and oxygenation for tissue viability. Therefore, before initiation of CPR a concerted effort must be made to rule out a viable cardiovascular respiratory status.

All hypothermic individuals should have a large-bore intravenous line started and warm (42 to 45°C) crystalloid administered rapidly. Most hypothermic individuals are hypovolemic on presentation because of fluid shift and require several liters of fluid rapidly during the first hour of resuscitation. Routine hematology, coagulation, biochemical, and arterial blood gas studies should be undertaken soon after presentation. Although the initial hemoglobin value may be high because of the hemoconcentration due to fluid shift previously described, platelets may be quantitatively or qualitatively depressed due to the cold effect. This combined with the direct inhibition of the enzymatic reactions of the coagulation cascade by the cold may lead to coagulopathy. This may not be recognized by the measurement of the prothrombin time, partial thromboplastin time, or international normalized ratio because these tests are performed at 37°C in the laboratory, where their function would be normal. There are generally no constant biochemical abnormalities found with hypothermia per se. The arterial blood gas analysis in a patient who is hypothermic is measured in the laboratory at 37°C. It is now generally believed that the arterial blood gas values should be interpreted in the uncorrected state when making decisions regarding oxygen administration or ventilation and acid-base balance.

Because hypotension and numerous cardiac dysrhythmias are often found in moderate to severe levels of hypothermia at least, it is tempting to treat these abnormalities pharmacologically. By and large, except as noted later, this temptation should be avoided. Hypotension usually responds to fluid administration, and the cardiac dysrhythmias will in most instances resolve as body warming occurs. The danger with pharmacologic management of hypotension or cardiac dysrhythmias is that in the cold state the action and metabolism of these drugs is uncertain and may compound the problem. The only possible exception to this is the use of bretylium (Bretylol), which may be infused as a dose of 10 mg per kg in those individuals with ventricular fibrillation or ventricular tachycardia. Ventricular fibrillation or asystole, regardless of whether it is the presenting rhythm or occurs during the initial treatment of the hypothermic victim, is generally difficult to treat and usually does not respond to direct-current defibrillation or epinephrine (Adrenalin). Notwithstanding the use of bretylium once the cold heart has fibrillated or becomes asystolic a viable rhythm cannot usually be established until warming has occurred to at least several degrees warmer than that at which the heart fibrillated or becomes asystolic. This temperature is usually in the range of 28 to 30°C. This, of course, means a period of sometimes prolonged CPR or other means of supporting the circulation until the warming can be achieved.

Table 3 outlines the rewarming strategies that may be used in the hypothermic victim. The onset of treatment of hypothermia, and particularly rewarming, is often complicated by two adverse reactions. *Rewarming shock* is the often sudden deterioration in cardiovascular status, especially blood pressure, on the application of heat; and although the exact mechanism is uncertain, it has been postulated that it represents an uncovering of a relative hypovolemia or the presentation to the general circulation from the previously severely vasoconstricted extremities of metabolites, including lactic acid. The second

TABLE 3. **Rewarming Strategies**

Endogenous Rewarming
- Basal/resting metabolism
- Shivering
- Exercise

Exogenous External Rewarming
LOW-MODERATE HEAT SOURCE
- Heating pads
- Charcoal heater
- Human body
- Hot water bottles
- Radiant heat
- Piped suits
- Warmed blankets

MODERATE-HIGH HEAT SOURCE
- Forced air
- Warm water immersion

Exogenous Internal Rewarming
NONINVASIVE
- Hot food/drink
- Inhalation of heated/water saturated air/O$_2$

INVASIVE
- Warm intravenous fluids
- Arteriovenous fistula
- Peritoneal lavage
- Cardiopulmonary bypass

complication on the initiation of rewarming may be the *afterdrop of core temperature*. This is manifested by the continued fall of the core temperature by sometimes of up to 3°C after the initiation of rewarming and resuscitation. Both conductive and convective mechanisms are responsible for this, and there is now ample evidence to show that the majority of the afterdrop is probably due to reperfusion of the very cold extremities, particularly the legs, with the warmer core blood during the initial rewarming efforts. Both the rewarming shock and afterdrop phenomena are seen more commonly when the rewarming strategies are of the exogenous external variety.

For patients in mild hypothermia, endogenous rewarming would likely be sufficient; and, in fact, shivering, if present, often causes rapid rewarming, but at the expense of considerably increased oxygen consumption and discomfort to the victim. Rewarming shock and the afterdrop phenomena are less pronounced or critical in these individuals. An exogenous external rewarming method is usually chosen. Although all hypothermic victims should receive warm crystalloid infusion in the hospital setting, the mildly hypothermic victim can usually safely and effectively be reheated with forced air (approximately 42°C) administration. This has the advantage of ease of administration through units that are used routinely during surgery in the operating room to prevent or limit accidental hypothermia. Other methods of exogenous external rewarming are listed in Table 3 and may be more applicable in any given facility or indeed a prehospital setting.

Those individuals who are moderately or severely hypothermic should be rewarmed with an exogenous internal (invasive) method. Once again, warm intravenous fluids are given routinely and the use of, for instance, peritoneal lavage generally limits the afterdrop phenomenon. Peritoneal dialysate warmed to approximately 45°C delivered through a double-lumen catheter or two separate catheters, one for inflow and one for outflow, effectively transfers heat. For patients in cardiopulmonary arrest or converting to that state when treatment has been initiated, rewarming should preferably be achieved and their cardiovascular status supported with the use of cardiopulmonary bypass. Because this method may be limited in its availability, peritoneal lavage with ongoing CPR is the method of choice.

Because of the cerebral protection from ischemia afforded by hypothermia and prolongation of the biologic survival time, there is an important decision to make whether or not to initiate resuscitation. Although there is no clear-cut answer to that question because many of the victims suffer an unwitnessed cooling event and cardiac arrest, it is generally safe to say that if the core body temperature is 20°C or greater (assuming the ambient air or water temperature is considerably less than this) and if there is no evidence of rigor mortis or freezing injury that would preclude intubating the trachea, resuscitation and rewarming should be undertaken. Once undertaken, it should be continued until the patient is at least warmed to 32°C core temperature, and a failure to achieve a viable rhythm at that point may be taken as an indication of futility and the resuscitation discontinued. The traditional adage that applies to any hypothermic victim who has suffered a cardiac arrest whether immersed or not is once resuscitation has been established "no one is pronounced dead until warm and dead."

COLD-WATER NEAR-DROWNING

Cold-water near-drowning affecting mainly, but not solely, young children is the ultimate example of the ability of hypothermia to protect the brain from ischemia during prolonged cardiac arrest.

Pathophysiology

Traditionally, the explanation for this dramatic event was thought to be a combination of a rapid heat loss in the child because of the favorable body surface area to mass ratio and the effect of an operative mammalian diving reflex. The former would account for rapid cooling in the cold water, whereas the latter would cause closure of the glottis with a reservoir of oxygen in the lungs combined with redirection of the circulation away from the superficial, peripheral, and visceral areas of the body to the core, namely, heart, lung, and brain. This combination of rapid cooling and the extension of the biologic survival time based on the Q_{10} principle, combined with an enhanced oxygen reservoir for the brain, was thought to be responsible for the outcome. More recently, it has been shown that cerebral protection from global ischemia may be afforded by much lesser degrees of hypothermia through the mechanism of suppression of excitatory amino acid release (i.e., glutamate) in the cooling phase. Such cooling may occur preferentially through the skull by conduction in very cold water. As well, there is some evidence to suggest that the rapid cooling seen and ascribed to a large body surface area to mass ratio may actually be due to breathing cold water in which the lungs then act as an efficient and rapid heat exchanger to the brain.

Generally, the pathophysiologic findings are those as described for severe accidental hypothermia. When, however, aspiration and particularly breathing of cold water has occurred, additional findings appear. In these cases the effects on pulmonary mechanics, red blood cell integrity, intravascular volume, and serum electrolyte concentrations assume the clinical picture seen in fresh or salt water near drowning.

Clinical Presentation

In almost all cases the victim is a child and comes to medical attention as in severely hypothermic cardiorespiratory arrest. In most cases the incident is witnessed and a successful outcome to the resuscitation is possible if the submersion time has been 1 hour or less in near freezing water with a resultant core temperature approaching or less than 20°C. An initial core temperature greater than 20°C may be associated with a successful outcome when the immersion time has been less than 1 hour.

Treatment

Tracheal intubation with CPR is generally the initial management modality in almost all cases. Temperature and cardiac monitoring, as well as early investigative studies, are the same as those described for accidental hypothermia.

Because the initial cardiac rhythm is either ventricular fibrillation or, commonly, asystole, which is unresponsive to the usual pharmacologic or defibrillation therapies, CPR should occur coincidentally with rewarming attempts. The treatment is the same as for severe accidental hypothermia.

FROSTBITE

Of all of the localized disturbances due to the cold, frostbite is probably the most common in peace time and potentially the most serious. Although this is a freezing injury, the nonfreezing injuries include the often-serious trench foot or immersion foot, owing to prolonged exposure to nonfreezing cold water, and the often dermatologic manifestations of cold wet or dry exposure known as chilblains and pernio, respectively. The discussion here is confined to frostbite.

Pathophysiology

On exposure to freezing temperatures the digits of the hands and feet as well as the tissue of the forearms and lower extremities become exquisitely sensitive to intense vasoconstriction that occurs as part of the body temperature–conserving reaction. Frostbite in other areas of the body, including the face, is possible, but generally because of the nature of the vascular supply and often greater insulation, these body areas are less subject to at least the more severe forms of frostbite.

Frostnip describes the sequelae of intense vasoconstriction of the vessels in the toes and particularly the hands that occurs on exposure for a short time to freezing temperatures. Frostbite, on the other hand, occurs as the more prolonged exposure or exposure to a lower temperature and may be classified, as are burns, into three degrees, namely, first, second, and third. In contrast to that of frostnip, the pathophysiology in frostbite includes the intravascular and extravascular, including intracellular ice crystal formation. This may be compounded with localized hyperosmolar changes with resultant intracellular damage. In addition, endothelial damage occurs in the frostbitten digit/extremity. The damage is produced not only by the freezing process itself but also on rewarming and the attempt to establish nutritional flow.

Clinical Presentation

All degrees of frostbite, including frostnip, appear relatively benign and manifest as a digit/extremity that is white, insensate, and immobile. The difference among these entities becomes obvious on rewarming. In frostnip the digits become hyperemic after thawing, with associated paresthesia but no evidence of tissue damage or edema. In first-degree frostbite, thawing is painful and associated with hyperemia and edema of the digits. In second-degree frostbite the digits, on thawing, become hyperemic and edematous, and vesicles that are filled with a clear or straw-colored fluid appear. Third-degree frostbite, on rewarming, manifests with some areas of persistent numbness and the appearance of vesicles filled with bloody exudate.

Treatment

All degrees of frostbite, and for that matter frostnip, should be treated initially the same way: with rapid warming in a 45°C water bath. This should be done only if there is no chance of re-exposure and refreezing. Obviously, this would be the appropriate treatment once the victim has arrived at the hospital. The thawing process for frostnip and particularly in frostbite of all degrees is very painful and should be accompanied by a liberal administration of parenteral narcotics. Once thawing has taken place, the appearance of the digit/extremity, particularly the presence or absence of vesicles, and, if vesicles are present, the color of the fluid in them give a good indication as to the degree of frostbite. For first-degree frostbite the only treatment required is ongoing analgesia, elevation to reduce the edema, and protection from refreezing. When vesicle formation has occurred, liberal use of analgesics, physiotherapy after thawing, as well as elevation of the extremity should be undertaken with close observation for the appearance of blood-filled vesicles, which would indicate third-degree damage and tissue loss. Blisters should be left intact, and there should be no hurry to excise apparently dead tissue from third-degree frostbite because the process of demarcation between viable and nonviable tissue is notoriously slow and may take weeks, if not months, to evolve. Early débridement and amputation may result both in removing tissue that may have been viable and in removing too little tissue, only to have to operate again in the weeks to come.

The treatment of second- and third-degree frostbite has included many modalities over the years to try and improve blood flow to the damaged digital arteries. Treatment such as low-molecular-weight dextran and sympathectomy whether achieved medically, surgically, or by nerve block have all been tried with no obvious sustained effect. Because the tissue damage in third-degree frostbite generally leads to dry gangrene, watchful waiting is in order. A popular saying in referring to frozen digits of "freeze them in January, amputate in July" makes reasonable sense.

EFFECTS OF HEAT STRESS

method of
JEFF FAUNT, M.B.B.S.

University of Adelaide and Royal Adelaide
Hospital
South Australia, Australia

High environmental temperatures can adversely affect human health, ranging from minor discomfort to death. Heat stress causes physiologic responses in which fluid and electrolyte balance, cardiovascular regulation, and central nervous system function are progressively impaired. Heat-related illness occurs in athletes, military recruits, and outdoor workers who perform sustained activity in warm, humid environments. Seasonal heat waves can precipitate heat-related illness in individuals with compromise of thermoregulation such as elderly persons, the homeless population, and patients taking medications such as diuretics and agents with anticholinergic activity.

HEAT EDEMA

Swelling of the hands, feet, and ankles during the first days of high ambient temperatures is caused by salt and water retention. This is a temporary condition and resolves with the body's acclimatization. It is more common in women than men.

Treatment

There is no specific treatment except simple reassurance.

HEAT SYNCOPE

Heat syncope usually occurs in the setting of heat exposure and orthostatic stress, such as standing. It can occur with use of spas and saunas, especially after exercise or alcohol ingestion. Cutaneous vasodilatation, the absence of muscle venous pump activity, and moderate fluid loss due to sweating all contribute to reduced central venous return and ventricular filling volumes. Syncope is probably mediated by activation of ventricular stretch receptors due to inadequate filling, causing vagal reflex bradycardia and loss of sympathetic vasomotor tone (Bezold-Jarisch reflex).

Treatment

Treatment of heat syncope is supportive. Vital signs should be monitored and the airway protected from tongue obstruction or vomitus. Lifting the lower extremities and cooling the skin initially enhances venous return. Volume repletion may be required if orthostatic intolerance continues. Individuals with heat syncope should be asked about the role of drugs, alcohol, and history of recurrent orthostatic intolerance (which may indicate autonomic dysfunction).

HEAT CRAMPS

Heat cramps are involuntary, painful contractions of skeletal muscle. They occur in the setting of excessive sweat losses in athletes or outdoor workers. The exact mechanism of heat cramps is uncertain, although evidence supports the depletion of body sodium and chloride stores or dilutional hyponatremia related to the excessive intake of salt-free water. Other electrolytes (e.g., calcium, potassium) may also be involved.

Treatment

Replenishment of serum sodium levels with oral (0.1% NaCl solution) or intravenous (normal saline) fluids usually terminates the cramps. Heat cramps can be prevented by adequate hydration with sodium- and glucose-containing drinks.

HEAT EXHAUSTION

Heat exhaustion can occur in athletes but is also common in a variety of persons in outdoor occupations that require sustained moderate activity in warm weather. Heat exhaustion can be divided into two types: water deprivation and salt depletion. Water deprivation is characterized by dehydration, pyrexia (less than 40°C), hypernatremia with or without anxiety, renal impairment, fatigue, and impaired judgment. Salt depletion results in fatigue, headache, cramps, weakness, nausea, vomiting, and diarrhea while being normothermic with no dehydration or thirst. In practice, a pure type of heat exhaustion is rare. Examination reveals a mildly elevated heart rate, blood pressure that is low to normal, and a nonvisible jugular venous pressure. With standing, there can be a fall in systolic pressure to below 90 mm Hg. Laboratory studies reveal hemoconcentration, variable electrolyte patterns (due to electrolyte losses and hemoconcentration), and increased urine specific gravity.

Treatment

Initial treatment is similar to that for heat syncope but with active cooling and intravascular volume repletion with oral or intravenous electrolyte fluids. If intravenous fluids are required, 0.5 or 0.25 normal saline can be used because these fluids approximate the sodium concentration of "non-acclimatized" sweat. Intravenous glucose and water (5% dextrose) should preferably be avoided because hyponatremia may occur with excessive hypotonic fluid replacement. Stabilization of vital signs, normalization of orthostatic hypotension, and serum electrolyte values and urine output should guide administration of intravenous fluid therapy. Extensive investigations are usually unnecessary.

HEAT STROKE

Heat stroke is a progression in severity from heat exhaustion. It has two subgroups: (1) exertional heat stroke resulting from excessive physical exertion with or without high environmental temperature and, more commonly, (2) the "classic" form in which the individual has some compromise of thermoregulation. Examination reveals hyperthermia (rectal temperature exceeding 40°C) plus marked central nervous system impairment (ranging from delirium to coma and convulsions). The skin is warm, dry, and flushed, unless severe hypotension and shock have occurred. Vital signs are that of moderate to severe tachycardia and blood pressure that is usually low but can vary according to cardiac function and state of vasomotor tone. Patients with documented or suspected heat stroke should always be admitted for observation, because some complications may not develop for 24 to 48 hours.

Treatment

Heat stroke is a medical emergency. Treatment requires a multisystem management approach. Urgent cooling of body temperature is essential. The best method of cooling hyperthermic patients is somewhat debatable. Wet towel cooling with a fan appears acceptable, allowing good patient access. A modification is the use of water spray and a fan with the placement of ice packs in the flexures: neck, axillae, and groin (producing a cooling rate of 0.03 to 0.06°C per minute). Body immersion is still practiced, although this limits patient access and monitoring and may actually inhibit heat loss, so is a less-fa-

vored approach. This method also requires body massage in order to overcome cold-induced vasoconstriction. Cooled intravenous fluid and invasive practices such as lavage, enemas, and ice packs have been shown to have faster cooling rates (around 0.15°C per minute), but the need for such interventions is questionable. Rectal temperature must be monitored continuously to allow active cooling efforts to be discontinued when body temperature falls to 39°C. Consciousness has usually improved by this time.

The basics of airway, breathing, and circulation need monitoring. Insertion of large-bore intravenous catheter lines and use of a Foley catheter are essential. Fluid therapy should be administered carefully in small boluses of up to 500 mL to avoid circulatory overload resulting in cerebral or pulmonary edema. Urine output should be monitored carefully, and intravenous furosemide (Lasix), 40 to 80 mg, may be administered to commence diuresis. The hemodynamic state may necessitate definitive cardiovascular support with insertion of a pulmonary artery catheter to facilitate the judicious use of vasopressors (dopamine or norepinephrine) and intravenous fluids (saline). Seizures can occur, necessitating the use of intravenous diazepam (Valium) and, if the seizures persist, phenytoin (Dilantin). Antipyretic medications are of no use because their effect depends on normal hypothalamic function; in severe heat-related illness these central thermoregulatory mechanisms are impaired.

Comprehensive investigations should be ordered,

TABLE 1. **Summary of Heat-Related Illnesses**

Illness	Symptoms	Examination	Investigations	Management	Other Issues
Heat edema	Peripheral edema	Peripheral edema	None	Reassurance	None
Heat syncope	Brief loss of consciousness	None Possibly orthostatic hypotension	None	Elevate legs, restore venous return and vasomotor tone Fluid replacement and cooling of skin if needed	Possible drug effects Baroreflex disorders (if recurrent)
Heat cramps	Painful contractions of skeletal muscle	None	None	Rest Oral or IV sodium chloride	Prevention by increasing salt intake Limit salt-free water
Heat exhaustion	Fatigue, lethargy, headache, cramps, irritability, anxiety, nausea, vomiting, diarrhea	Mild confusion, dehydration, presyncope on standing Vasoconstricted—cool Active sweating, <40°C Heart rate 90–120 bpm BP usually <110 mm Hg orthostatic drop of >20 mm Hg	Basic laboratory studies including complete blood cell count, electrolytes (i.e., Na⁺, K⁺), urea, creatinine, and urinalysis	Monitor vital signs, rectal temperature Fluid replacement PO to IV to restore orthostatic blood pressure and urine output	Comprehensive investigation in those with severe hypotension or suspected prior hyperthermia
Heat stroke	Significant altered conscious state	Marked alteration in conscious state with delirium, coma Vasolidated—warm Dry or sweating, >40°C Heart rate >120 bpm BP varies—low if in shock Low vascular resistance Multisystem abnormalities	Comprehensive baseline laboratory studies including as above plus muscle and hepatic enzymes, calcium, uric acid, lactate, glucose, coagulation factors, platelets, arterial blood gases and urine for myoglobin + hemoglobin	Continuous vital signs monitoring Immediate cooling to <39°C (avoid body immersion) Initiate diuresis with loop diuretic Fluid replacement as needed to maintain blood pressure and urine output Judicious use of vasopressors or inotropic agents	Complications are rhabdomyolysis, renal failure (acute tubular necrosis), hepatic failure, disseminated intravascular coagulation, hypoglycemia

including complete blood cell count, complete biochemistry studies (Table 1), determination of creatinine kinase, coagulation studies, and evaluation of levels of lactic acid and arterial blood gases. The urine should be tested for hemoglobin and/or myoglobin. Significant complications of heat stroke include hypoglycemia, metabolic acidosis, renal failure with acute tubular necrosis, rhabdomyolysis, disseminated intravascular coagulation, and hepatic failure.

SUMMARY

The management of significant heat-related illness includes these steps:

1. Removal of the patient from the heat stress into a cool environment.
2. Ensurance of airway, breathing, and circulation.
3. Rapid cooling to obtain temperature of 39°C with ice packs in flexures, tepid sponges, and the use of a fan with close monitoring of a response.
4. Treatment of seizure activity with intravenous diazepam with or without phenytoin if seizure activity persists.
5. Judicious fluid treatment.

SPIDER BITES AND SCORPION STINGS

method of
JAMES R. BLACKMAN, M.D.
University of Washington School of Medicine
Seattle, Washington
WWAMI (Idaho/Wyoming) Office for Clinical
*   Medical Education*
Boise, Idaho

SPIDER BITES

Approximately 60 species of spiders in North America have been implicated in human bites of medical importance. Most bites are by female spiders. Deaths occur rarely and only with brown recluse and black widow envenomations. Mechanisms of injury from spider bites include dermonecrosis, development of secondary infection, neuromuscular damage, and allergic reactions (including urticaria). Children may be more likely to have greater morbidity and mortality. Hands and cutaneous areas with ample subcutaneous tissue develop more serious lesions, and individuals with underlying skin disorders may develop more extensive cutaneous reactions.

The diagnosis of spider bite is frequently very difficult to make, especially when the spider has not been seen or recovered. Because of their behavior, spiders are placed near the bottom of biting candidates. If the spider was not seen or captured close to the site of injury and at the proper time, all evidence is circumstantial. Systemic symptoms associated with the bite are suggestive of spider envenomation.

Most spider bites involving humans cause minimal medical problems. Bites result in erythema, local edema, vesiculation, and pain. Secondary infection may occur with ecchymosis, ulceration, and lymphadenopathy. Treatment includes cool soaks, soothing lotions, analgesics, and tetanus prophylaxis. Antibiotics may be necessary.

Loxoscelism (Brown Recluse) Envenomation

The most important necrotizing arachnid found in North America is the brown recluse. The brown recluse *(Loxosceles reclusa)* is found primarily in south central states, with other less toxic family members scattered throughout the rest of the country. It is absent from the Pacific Northwest. The spider has a body length of 8 to 15 mm, with a leg length of 18 to 30 mm. Color varies from fawn to dark brown with darker legs. There is a violin-shaped figure on the anterodorsal cephalothorax. The brown recluse prefers hot, dry, abandoned environments such as woodpiles, vacant buildings, rock piles, tire piles, clothes piles, and boxes. It bites defensively when trapped against the skin.

The clinical features of brown recluse envenomation are produced by both cytotoxic and hemotoxic reactions. The bite produces a brief mild stinging sensation, with mild to moderate pain appearing in 2 to 8 hours. Local and systemic reactions follow. Erythema may be followed by pustule and ulcer formations. The classic brown recluse lesion consists of a cyanotic macule or "volcano lesion" appearing several hours or days after envenomation. Healing is slow (weeks to months), and a black eschar sometimes forms. Systemic reactions include fever, chills, malaise, weakness, nausea, vomiting, joint pain, and skin rash. Intravascular coagulation produces jaundice and hematuria.

Treatment of brown recluse bites remains primarily medical. The wound should be cleaned, immobilized, and elevated (if on an extremity), and ice packs should be applied. The primary offending venom component is sphingomyelinase-D. Its activity can be reduced by cooling and is increased by heating. Therefore, erythromycin could be given to prevent infection that would result in increased wound temperature. Tetanus prophylaxis should be provided. Antihistamines may reduce pruritus. Topical steroids are useless. Immediate total wound excision should be avoided to reduce morbidity. Delayed excision of the eschar might be necessary to allow for skin grafting. Hyperbaric oxygen therapy has been used successfully in some medical centers. Overtreatment should be avoided because most lesions heal without sequelae.

In severe cases dapsone may be tried. Dapsone appears to act by inhibiting the inflammatory response through limiting neutrophil migration into the bite site. Dapsone is used in doses of 50 to 200 mg per day for 10 to 25 days. It is most effective when given early in the course of wound development. Numerous side effects have been reported, including nausea, vomiting, headache, dizziness, minor rashes, erythema nodosum, and toxic epidermal necroliasis. A hypersensitivity syndrome may develop within 2 to 6 weeks after the drug is discontinued. Serologic confirmation of brown recluse envenomation and an antivenin against sphingomyelinase-D could become available in the future. Improperly treated individuals may develop serious long-term sequelae such as poor wound healing, repeated failure of skin grafts, chronic pyoderma gangrenosum–like reactions, chronic pain, deep venous thrombosis, and chronic hand function impairment.

In the Pacific Northwest, the Hobo spider *(Tegenaria agrestis)* is the spider that causes necrotic arachnidism. Bite symptoms and findings are similar to those of the brown recluse. Therapy is the same as for brown recluse bites.

Latrodectims (Black Widow Spider) Envenomation

The female black widow spider, the primary envenomator of its species, is coal black with hourglass-shaped markings of red or yellow on the ventral surface of the abdomen. The spider is found in every state and is more common in the south and west. The black widow builds an irregularly shaped mesh close to the ground with a strong-walled funnel-shaped retreat. Its common habitats include warm and dry environments both indoors and out. Webs are found under stones, logs, and debris and in corners of abandoned and infrequently used buildings. If the spider is trapped against the skin or crushed, it will bite.

The venom contains a potent neurotoxin, alpha-latrotoxin, which is specific to nerve terminals and causes a release of massive amounts of acetylcholine at neuromuscular junctions, as well as releasing epinephrine and norepinephrine from sympathetic and parasympathetic nerve endings. Reuptake of neurotransmitters is also blocked. As a result of these neurochemical changes, the clinical manifestations of a black widow envenomation are primarily neurologic.

Pain at the bite site varies from minimal to sharp. Two small fang marks might be recognized as tiny red spots. Venom produces no local tissue reactions. Within 15 minutes to 4 hours, muscle fasciculations and spasms associated with cutaneous sweating and piloerection may occur. These findings may spread to regional muscles. Pain is intense and peaks in 2 to 3 hours and may last 12 to 48 hours. Autonomic stimulation can produce sweating, increased salivation, fever, chills, urinary retention, priapism, nausea, vomiting, ptosis, headache, hypertension, and dizziness. Reflexes can become hyperactive. Elevated white cell count, proteinuria, and hematuria can complicate the diagnosis of an acute abdomen.

The treatment of black widow spider envenomation is primarily symptomatic, focused on relieving muscle spasm. Although calcium carbonate and methocarbamol (Robaxin) have been used, they are generally considered ineffective. More useful is the provision of diazepam (Valium) and narcotics to relieve symptoms. Opioid analgesics either alone (55%) or in combination with a benzodiazepine (75%) effectively relieve most symptoms.

Treatment with black widow antivenin remains controversial, and its use has generally been restricted for severe poisonings and for pregnant women and children. More frequent use of antivenin has been recommended. After an obligatory skin test, a vial of antivenin is delivered intravenously. A second vial is seldom necessary. After infusion of antivenin, relief is often dramatic and rapid (1 hour). Antivenin administration is titrated to relief of clinical features. The rate of allergic reactions is high (9% in those who skin test negative; up to 80% of those who skin test positive). Those persons who skin test positive should be premedicated with epinephrine before antivenin administration. Patients must be watched closely for the development of anaphylaxis and serum sickness.

SCORPION STINGS

Scorpion bites are divided into two groups based on the clinical severity of envenomations. Scorpion stings other than from the bark scorpion *(Centruroides exilicauda)* produce a local reaction consisting of pain, swelling, and burning with ecchymosis. Treatment includes ice, elevation of extremity, and possibly antihistamines.

Of more importance are stings by the bark scorpion. This scorpion is less than 5 cm in length, yellow to brown in color, and may be striped. It is found under wood and ground debris and in crevices during the daytime. They may also hide in shoes, blankets, or clothing left on the floor during daylight hours as well as under common ground covers (tents).

The bark scorpion has a neurotoxic venom that may be life-threatening. This species is found mainly in Arizona, Texas, New Mexico, and California and along the northern shore of Lake Mead in Nevada.

Envenomations are graded from 1 to 4, with 1 being local pain and/or paresthesias at the site of envenomation and 4 manifesting both cranial nerve and skeletal muscle dysfunction. Local pain control (ice) and oral analgesics manage grade 1 and 2 envenomations. Tetanus immunizations may be needed. For more severe envenomations, antivenin administration may be indicated. Local poison control centers should be contacted regarding the availability of antivenin. When this antivenin is used, anaphylaxis and serum sickness should be anticipated. Envenomated individuals should be managed in the intensive care setting, and focus should be on maintenance of a clear airway. Prevention includes careful handling of firewood and other wood debris; checking of clothing, shoes, and camping gear left outside; and wearing appropriate footwear.

SNAKE VENOM POISONING

method of
BARRY S. GOLD, M.D.

Johns Hopkins University School of Medicine
Baltimore, Maryland

Snake venom poisoning is a complex type of poisoning that not only affects the bite site but may affect multiple organ systems either primarily or secondarily. An estimated 45,000 snakebites occur annually in the United States, of which about 8000 are venomous, averaging 5 to 6 deaths per year. Most deaths occur in children, the elderly, victims to whom antivenin was not administered or was delayed or given in insufficient quantities, or members of certain religious sects who handle snakes during their ceremonies. Most victims are young males, of whom 50% are intoxicated and deliberately handling or molesting the snake. Most bites occur between April and October, with the highest incidence in July and August. The most common bite site is on the extremities.

Only about 25 of the 120 species of snakes native to the United States are poisonous. At least one species of poisonous snake is found in every state except Alaska, Maine, and Hawaii. The majority of poisonous snakebites are caused by members of the family Crotalidae, or pit vipers, which includes rattlesnakes, copperheads, and cottonmouths. The coral snake (family Elapidae) is the only other native poisonous snake and accounts for fewer than 20 to 25 bites per year. About 100 bites per year occur from foreign or exotic species that are held in zoos or found in amateur and professional collections. Most deaths are due to bites of the Eastern diamondback rattlesnake *(Crotalus adamanteus),* the Western diamondback rattlesnake *(C. atrox),* various subspecies of the Western rattlesnake *(C. viridis),* and the timber rattlesnake *(C. horridus).* Deaths resulting from coral snake bite are rare. A small number of deaths occur from bites of exotic or foreign snakes imported illegally.

Pit viper venoms are complex proteins, many of which possess enzymatic activity. Although the enzymes contribute to the deleterious effects of the venom, the lethal components may be secondary to the smaller, low-molecular-weight polypeptides. The effects of pit viper venom cause local tissue damage, vascular defects, hemolysis, a disseminated intravascular coagulation (DIC)–like syndrome, and pulmonary, cardiac, renal, and neurologic defects. Coral snake venoms cause changes in neuromuscular transmission, with minimal local tissue damage.

DIAGNOSIS

A definitive diagnosis of snakebite poisoning requires identification of the snake along with signs and symptoms of envenomation. Usually the snake is not available for identification; therefore, accurate diagnosis and treatment depend on identifying symptoms and signs of snakebite poisoning. About 25% of all pit viper bites and 50% of all coral snake bites are "dry" and do not result in envenomation. Fear is the most commonly encountered reaction associated with any snakebite. Consequently, it is essential not to mistake autonomic reactions for systemic symptoms and signs from the bite, which could lead to unwarranted treatment.

The primary local clinical findings with most pit viper bites occur within 30 to 60 minutes after the bite. These consist of single or multiple fang punctures, pain, and edema, erythema, or ecchymosis of the bite site and adjacent tissues. Single or multiple punctures and scratches are commonly seen. Pain initially follows envenomation, and edema appears within 10 minutes and is rarely delayed longer than 20 to 30 minutes. Rarely, bullae may be seen. There may be signs of lymphangitis, with tender regional lymph nodes.

Frequent systemic manifestations include nausea, vomiting, perioral paresthesias, tingling of the fingertips and toes, fasciculations, lethargy, and weakness. Complaints of a rubbery, minty, or metallic taste in the mouth are frequent following bites by some species of rattlesnakes. More severe, systemic effects include hypotension, dyspnea, and altered sensorium. Coagulopathies are frequently seen following bites by rattlesnakes and may result in a DIC-like picture manifested by prolonged prothrombin time (PT) and activated partial thromboplastin time (aPTT), hypofibrinogenemia, thrombocytopenia, and abnormal fibrin degradation products. Pit viper venoms increase capillary membrane permeability, resulting in extravasation of electrolytes, colloid, and red blood cells into the envenomated site. This process may also occur in the lungs, kidneys, peritoneum, myocardium, and, rarely, the central nervous system. There may also be changes in the membranes of red blood cells, leading to hemolysis. Edema formation, hypoalbuminemia, and hemoconcentration occur initially. They are followed by pooling of blood and fluids in the microcirculation, resulting in hypovolemic shock. Renal failure may be secondary to decreased glomerular filtration rate, intravascular hemolysis, DIC, or the nephrotoxic effects of the venom components.

The ultimate severity of any venomous snakebite depends on the size and species of the snake, the amount and toxicity of venom injected, the location of the bite, first aid modalities performed, timing of definitive treatment, and underlying medical conditions in the victim, among other factors. Envenomations are graded as minimal, moderate, or severe. Minimal envenomations are localized to the bite site and demonstrate edema, erythema, or ecchymosis, unassociated with any systemic manifestations or coagulation or laboratory abnormalities. Moderate envenomations show progression beyond the bite site, significant symptoms and signs (e.g., nausea, vomiting, paresthesias, fasciculations) or mildly abnormal results of coagulation and laboratory studies. Severe envenomations show rapid progression of edema, erythema, or ecchymosis to involve the entire extremity. Systemic manifestations are severe and may include dyspnea, tachypnea, tachycardia, altered sensorium, and profound hypotension. Severe bleeding and markedly abnormal coagulation profile including PT, aPTT, hypofibrinogenemia, and thrombocytopenia (less than 20,000 cells per µL) and a DIC-like picture may result, in addition to other laboratory abnormalities.

Coral snake envenomations produce little or no pain after the bite. Occasionally, there is a delay of 8 to 24 hours before the onset of systemic manifestations. These are usually cranial nerve palsies manifested as ptosis, dysarthria, dysphagia, intense salivation, and respiratory depression.

FIELD TREATMENT

In any venomous snakebite, the victim should be moved beyond striking distance, placed at rest, reassured, kept warm, and transported to the nearest medical facility as quickly as possible. The injured part should be immobilized in a functional position below the level of the heart and all rings, watches,

1139

and constrictive clothing removed. The use of ice, tourniquets, incision and suction, or electroshock is contraindicated. A Sawyer Extractor applied directly over the fang punctures may be of value when used within the first 5 minutes of the bite and kept in place for 30 to 40 minutes. Emergency medical personnel should be advised to establish an intravenous access line on the contralateral side and to administer oxygen.

EMERGENCY DEPARTMENT TREATMENT

A rapid, detailed history should include time of the bite, description of the snake, type of field therapy, and identification of co-morbid medical conditions, allergy to horse products, or prior history of snakebite and therapy. A complete physical examination should be performed, with special emphasis on the cardiovascular, pulmonary, and neurologic systems, followed by inspection of the bite site for fang punctures or scratches. If not previously done, a venous access site should be established in the contralateral extremity. If a tourniquet or constriction band was applied, it should not be removed until venous access has been established. Baseline laboratory tests should include a complete blood count with platelets, coagulation profile (PT, aPTT, fibrinogen), electrolytes, blood urea nitrogen (BUN), serum creatinine, and urinalysis. These tests should be repeated every 4 hours for the first 12 hours and then on a daily basis. Additional tests such as blood typing and cross-match, measurement of creatine kinase level, chest radiography, and electrocardiography should be performed for moderate or severe envenomations. The envenomation should be classified as minimal, moderate, or severe based on the most severe symptom, sign, or laboratory finding noted at that time. The patient should be continuously assessed because a mild envenomation may progress rapidly to severe over a period of an hour in the absence of treatment. Circumferential measurements at several points above and below the bite site should be recorded every 15 to 20 minutes, and the advancing edge of the swelling should be marked with a pen.

Administration of antivenin is the only effective treatment for moderate to severe envenomations, along with aggressive life support in an intensive care setting. Its effectiveness is both dose and time related, with its greatest effect occurring during the first 4 hours. It is less effective after 12 hours but has been shown to reverse coagulopathies after 24 hours.

A skin test for hypersensitivity to horse serum should be performed, according to the instructions in the package insert, *only* if antivenin is to be administered. A negative result on skin testing does not preclude the possibility of an immediate hypersensitivity reaction. If the skin test is positive and the envenomation is life or limb threatening, antivenin treatment must not be delayed, and the antivenin should be administered after consultation with a regional poison control center.

The amount of antivenin (Crotalidae) polyvalent to be administered should be based on the severity and progression of local signs, systemic symptoms and signs, or results of coagulation studies. No antivenin is administered for trivial or minimal poisoning. Moderate cases require the use of 10 vials administered over 1 to 2 hours. Severe cases usually require the use of 15 vials or more. Those patients with profound circulatory collapse should initially receive 20 vials over 1 hour. Isotonic fluid administration followed by pressors is appropriate for severe hypotension. Antivenin dosage is usually lower for cottonmouth envenomations, and antivenin therapy is unnecessary in most cases of copperhead bites.

Reconstituted antivenin should initially be diluted in 250 to 1000 mL of sterile 0.9% sodium chloride or 5% dextrose and given by intravenous drip. It should initially be administered slowly at 1 mL per minute for the first 15 to 20 minutes. If there is no reaction, the remainder can be infused over 1 to 2 hours. The amount of intravenous fluids given should be reduced in pediatric and geriatric patients, except when hypovolemia or shock occurs. The initial dose of antivenin should be re-administered every 1 to 2 hours until local and/or systemic symptoms or laboratory abnormalities no longer progress or are terminated.

Antitetanus therapy should be administered when indicated. An antimicrobial drug should be given based on clinical signs of wound infection. Hypovolemic shock, often with concomitant lysis of red blood cells and platelet destruction, requires fluid and blood component replacement. Severe defects of hemostasis such as abnormal clotting or disturbance of platelets require replacement with packed red blood cells, fresh-frozen plasma, or platelets only after adequate neutralizing doses of antivenin have been given.

If a positive skin test result occurs, reassessment of the need for antivenin should be considered, along with pretreatment with an H_1 blocker (diphenhydramine) and dilution and slowing of the antivenin infusion.

Early reactions to antivenin are common and anaphylactoid (dose related), generally resulting from too-rapid infusion of the antivenin. If this occurs, the antivenin infusion should be discontinued immediately. Epinephrine, diphenhydramine (Benadryl), and ranitidine (Zantac) (or other histamine H_2 blockers) should be administered. The benefit/risk ratio should be re-evaluated before antivenin therapy is continued. In most instances, antivenin administration can be resumed after further dilution, with administration at a slower rate. Mild sedation with diazepam is indicated in all severe cases of snakebite in which respiratory depression is not a problem. Codeine may be used for moderate pain and morphine for severe pain. Acetylsalicylic acid and other NSAIDs should be avoided.

All victims of snakebite, whether venomous or nonvenomous, should be observed for at least 12 hours. Routine use of fasciotomy should be discouraged. It is usually unnecessary, and the presence of compartment pressure syndrome reflects a lack of or insufficient antivenin administration during the first 12 hours after the envenomation. Fasciotomy may be necessary when there is objective evidence of a compartment syndrome, as demonstrated by measurements of compartment pressures of greater than 30 mm Hg that is unresponsive to limb elevation and administration of mannitol (1 to 2 grams per kg) and an additional 15 vials of antivenin. The wound should be cleansed and covered with a sterile dressing and the injured extremity maintained in a functional position.

The use of corticosteroids has no proven clinical efficacy in the acute phase of envenomation and is contraindicated except in treatment of delayed reactions. Follow-up care utilizing appropriate corrective measures and exercises can prevent contractures. Within 3 to 4 days after the bite, a complete evaluation should be instituted by a physiatrist, who should perform periodic assessments of joint motion and muscle strength and girth measurements. The most frequently recognized complication of venomous snakebite treatment is serum sickness, which occurs about 7 to 14 days following the administration of antivenin. The probability of serum sickness increases with the administration of more than 5 vials of antivenin. It is usually manifested as fever, arthralgias, rash, and lymphadenopathy and responds to diphenhydramine and a rapid tapering course of prednisone.

The same principles noted for management of pit viper envenomations should be followed for coral snake envenomations; however, the Sawyer extractor should not be used. The value of other first aid measures (e.g., pressure immobilization wraps) has not been established for coral snakebites. Five vials of North American coral snake antivenin (i.e., antivenin; *Micrurus fulvius*) should be administered when a possible coral snake envenomation has occurred. If symptoms evolve, an additional 10 to 15 vials should be administered. The patient's condition should be monitored in an intensive care unit because of the potential for respiratory paralysis. Once manifested, the neurotoxic venom effects are difficult to reverse even with antivenin and may last for 3 to 6 days. There is no antivenin for the Arizona coral snake, and treatment is symptomatic because bites are rarely serious.

The local zoo is the initial place to call when a patient presents with a bite from an exotic venomous snake. All zoos maintain a list of consulting physicians, as well as the *Antivenom Index,** which lists the location and number of vials of antivenin available for exotic snakes. Regional poison control centers also maintain listings for antivenin. In all envenomations, it is wise to consult with a regional poison control center, where trained physicians and specialists in the management and treatment of snakebite are available at all times.

---

*Boyer DM (ed): Antivenom Index. Dallas, Department of Herpetology, Dallas Zoo, 1994.

MARINE ANIMAL INJURIES

method of
BRUCE W. HALSTEAD, M.D.
International Biotoxicological Center, World Life Research Institute
Colton, California

With the explosive worldwide increase in jet travel and underwater activities, there has been a corresponding increased exposure of people to hazardous marine plants and animals in both tropical and temperate zones. Military operations in these warm seas have furthered the problem. Dangerous marine animals can be grouped into four major categories: those that inflict serious bites, venomous invertebrates and vertebrates, those that are poisonous to eat, and the electric fishes. The sudden occurrence of these torrid-zone injuries may present unexpected therapeutic problems to physicians working in temperate climes. The following sections attempt to address some of these issues.

TRAUMATOGENIC FISH AND REPTILES

Among the fish and reptiles, sharks and crocodiles head the list of the feared denizens of marine waters. It is estimated that there are approximately 350 species of sharks worldwide, but only 32 species have definitely been incriminated in human attacks. The great white shark (*Carcharodon carcharias*) is the largest and heaviest of the predatory sharks. It can attain a length in excess of 21 feet and a weight in excess of 3000 pounds. Another large shark that is probably more aggressive than the great white is the tiger shark, which attains a length of approximately 18 feet, but weighs much less than the great white. Both sharks are found in tropical and temperate seas, and both may be found in inshore, shallow waters. The bite of a large shark may attain a force of 18 tons.

Other sharks that can inflict fatal bites include the mako (*Isurus oxyrinchus*), with a length up to 12 feet; the Zambesi shark or bull shark (*Carcharhinus leucas*), with a length of 12 feet; and the gray reef shark (*Carcharhinus amblyrhynchos*), with a length of 7 feet. All are found in the Indo-Pacific region. The gray reef shark has a nasty temperament, is sometimes found in large schools, may go into a feeding frenzy, and can inflict serious bites. Any shark with adequate dentition is capable of producing a fatality under suitable circumstances.

Other biting fish include the great barracuda, moray eel, and giant grouper. Most of their bites are relatively minor. One of the most dangerous of all the biting marine organisms is the saltwater crocodile (*Crocodylus porosus*), which may attain a length of over 20 feet and is found in the western Indo-Pacific and Indian Oceans. Attacks by this crocodile are usually fatal.

Most shark and crocodile bites result in massive tissue and blood loss. The victim should be removed from the water as soon as possible and administered first aid on the beach immediately. The victim should be kept warm but out of the sun, and bleeding should be controlled by manual compression. The victim should be moved to a trauma center. Bleeding must be controlled to prevent hypovolemic shock; large blood vessels can be ligated or compressed manually. Pain should be controlled with a suitable narcotic. Marine animal wounds are usually contaminated and should be surgically irrigated. Débridement is essential. The wound should be closed loosely, with drains inserted. Wounds are frequently contaminated with virulent bacteria of the genera *Vibrio, Pseudomonas, Erysipelothrix, Staphylococcus, Streptococcus,* and *Clostridium,* necessitating the use of appropriate antibiotics. Bacterial cultures of the wound are recommended. Tetanus prophylaxis is essential. All serious wounds should be treated with hyperbaric oxygen (HBO) therapy for 1 hour at 2 atmospheres of pressure absolute (ATA) in the morning and again in the afternoon for 1 to 3 weeks, depending on the extent of the wound. This treatment is important because it helps speed healing and reduces scarring.

MARINE ENVENOMATIONS

Marine animals that possess venom glands are divided into stinging invertebrates (animals without backbones) and vertebrate fish and sea snakes. All the stinging animals have one thing in common: they are equipped with a venom gland of some type. The venomous invertebrates range from sponges, which secrete irritating agents, to coelenterates such as hydroids, jellyfish, corals, and sea anemones; mollusks such as cone shells and octopuses; bristle worms and glycerid worms; and a variety of sea urchins.

Sponge dermatitis may be helped by sponging the area with vinegar. Anti-inflammatory agents and emollients such as aloe vera cream also are helpful.

Hydroid, fire coral, Portuguese man-of-war, and most jellyfish stings can be very painful but usually subside when treated symptomatically. The immediate elimination of pain can be accomplished with the application of products known as "Wipe Out," or "Wipe Away Pain." The use of emollients and anti-inflammatory agents is also helpful. A jellyfish repellent, Medu-sun, is a combination of a repellent and a sunblocker. It is 90% effective in preventing jellyfish stings. Special note should be taken of coral cuts, which can begin as minor cuts or abrasions but become seriously infected with secondary bacterial invaders. Topical application of vinegar, hydrogen peroxide, and antibacterial agents is useful. If a cellulitis ensues, systemic antibiotics may be required. The most dangerous jellyfish is the sea wasp *(Chironex fleckeri).* Stings can be fatal and treatment must be immediate. Pouring vinegar or isopropyl alcohol over the affected area inactivates any nematocysts in the adhering tentacles, which must not be touched with the bare hands. Commonwealth Serum Laboratories (Melbourne, Australia) produces an effective antivenin against *Chironex.* Anyone traveling

and diving along the northeast coast of Australia should avail themselves of this antivenin. The remainder of the treatment is symptomatic.

Some sea anemone stings, such as those of the hell's fire anemone *(Actinodendron)* and the Red Sea anemone *(Triactis),* are very painful and can ulcerate and produce a necrotic base. These anemone stings can result in a severe cellulitis that may take several months to heal. In addition to the usual treatment for coelenterate stings, HBO therapy may be necessary, with 2 ATA for 1 hour twice a day. The length of time HBO therapy is required varies with the severity of the ulcer, but it speeds healing and reduces scarring.

Cone shell envenomations may be fatal. There is no antivenin available, and treatment is symptomatic. Live cone shells should be handled with extreme care to avoid the mouth parts and the venomous teeth.

The blue-spotted octopus *(Octopus maculosus)* possesses an extremely potent venom, and its bite may be fatal. There is no antivenin available, and treatment is symptomatic.

Bristle worms can cause a very irritating dermatitis with their setae, or bristles, which are situated on the side of each segment of the body. Some of the polychaete worms have powerful jaws and can inflict painful bites. Glycerid worms can inflict painful bites with their venomous jaws. Visible setae in wounds should be removed with forceps. The smaller setae may be removed with the application of adhesive tape. Treatment is symptomatic.

Sea urchins can inflict painful wounds with their spines. *Diadema* is equipped with long spines that are venomous. Most of the spines embedded in a wound are almost impossible to remove because of the retrorse spinules covering the spines. It is usually best to leave the spines alone; after a few days, they will be absorbed into the subcutaneous tissues. Warm water soaks help. Spines embedded in a joint region may have to be surgically removed to avoid ankylosis. A granulomatous foreign tissue reaction may ultimately develop. Secondary bacterial invaders may be present, requiring antibiotic therapy. Tetanus prophylaxis is recommended. Some sea urchins, such as *Toxopneustes,* are equipped with venomous globiferous pedicellariae, which may appear to cover the outside of the sea urchin like tiny, flower-like rosettes. These are the venomous jaws, and some species have been known to produce fatalities. There is no known antivenin, and treatment is symptomatic.

There are numerous species of venomous fish, including stingrays, horned sharks, ratfish, catfish, weeverfish, scorpion fish, lionfish, stonefish, toadfish, surgeonfish, and stargazers. Stingray and stonefish stings have produced fatalities. Treatment is aimed at alleviating pain, combating the effects of the venom, and preventing secondary infections. Stonefish antivenin is available through Commonwealth Serum Laboratories in Melbourne, Australia. Otherwise, treatment is symptomatic. Fish stings should be immediately immersed in hot water (approximately 120°F) for 20 minutes. This helps attenuate the venom and the pain. Localized anesthetics may be needed. Stingray wounds usually need to be irrigated with normal saline. The integumentary sheath of the fish spine may have to be removed from the wound with forceps or by irrigating the wound. Larger wounds may require a drain until the wound heals.

Sea snake envenomations can be serious and may result in fatalities. Sea snakes are equipped with a flat, paddle-like tail and are found only in the tropical Indian and Pacific oceans, from Panama westward to the Persian Gulf. Sea snake bites do not necessarily mean that the victim has been envenomated, because sea snake fangs are short and easily dislodged. There are approximately 51 species of sea snake, but only approximately 14 of them are known to have inflicted serious envenomations. Symptoms usually appear within 6 hours after the bite. The bite is usually painless. The presence of fang marks should be determined before therapy. The venom is a myotoxin and produces a flaccid paralysis. Initial symptoms of sea snake envenomation include painful muscle movements, paralysis of the legs, trismus, and ptosis. Once symptoms begin to appear, treatment should be instituted. If no symptoms appear after 6 hours, there is probably no envenomation, and treatment is unecessary. If an envenomation has occurred, treatment with sea snake hydrophiid antivenin or elapid antivenin should be started as soon as possible. The antivenin therapy should be instituted within a maximum of 8 hours of envenomation—the sooner, the better. Complete instructions for use of the antivenin are given in the package insert.

ORAL INTOXICATIONS

Marine organisms that are poisonous to eat are divided into two major groups, the invertebrates and the vertebrates. The invertebrate intoxications include a number of types of dinoflagellate poisonings such as paralytic shellfish poisoning, amnesic, brevitoxic, and diarrhetic (okadaic) shellfish poisonings, and *Pfiesteria* poisoning. Some sea anemones are poisonous to eat. Toxic mollusks are the causal agents of abalone, callistin, cephalopod, ivory shell, scallop, turban shell, whelk, and venerupin poisonings. Mollusks are also responsible for transvectoring the dinoflagellate toxins previously mentioned. Paralytic shellfish poisoning appears to be spreading throughout the world. Most public health agencies maintain close surveillance of poisonous shellfish in endemic areas. There are no known antidotes for dinoflagellate, sea anemone, and molluskan poisonings. Fatalities are usually caused by eating shellfish that have been feeding on toxic dinoflagellates. Without treatment, the victim dies of respiratory paralysis. Treatment is symptomatic; follow the suggested treatment for ciguatera fish poisoning. Contaminated shellfish may also spread a number of viral diseases, such as

polio, hepatitis, and coxsackievirus infections, and bacterial diseases such as typhoid fever and cholera.

The sea anemone *Rhodactis*, found in Polynesia, is poisonous when eaten raw but is safe to eat when cooked. Treatment is symptomatic.

Poisonings from the echinoderms—sea urchins and sea cucumbers—are rare but may be serious. The nature of the poisons is unknown. Treatment is symptomatic.

Poisonings from the Asiatic horseshoe crab, coconut crab, spiny lobster, and a variety of tropical reef crabs may result in fatalities. The toxicity of these arthropods is unpredictable. It is suspected that in some cases the poison involved may be one of the members of the ciguatoxin complex; in other instances, tetrodotoxin may be involved. Treatment is symptomatic, and there are no specific antidotes available. Follow the suggested treament for ciguatera fish poisoning.

Poisonings from marine vertebrates are not uncommon. Intoxications from some of the tropical sharks, such as *Carcharhinus amboensis*, may be serious and cause fatalities. The Greenland shark *(Somniosus)* may be toxic when fresh but is edible when cooked.

There are approximately 400 species of tropical insular reef fishes that have been incriminated in ciguatera poisoning. Ciguatera involves a complex of poisons, some of which are among the most deadly toxins known. The poisons originate in the environment from the food chain, beginning with toxic dinoflagellates, which are ingested by herbivorous fishes that are subsequently eaten by carnivorous fishes. Ciguatera is characterized by a spectrum of neurologic disturbances, including paresthesias, motor weakness, and gastrointestinal upset. Some of the worst offenders include moray eels, barracuda, jack, and red snappers. The amount of poison in the fish varies greatly from one specimen to the next. The diagnosis of ciguatera fish poisoning is based on the symptoms, not on the appearance of the fish. Gastric lavage is used or vomiting is induced by sticking a finger down the victim's throat or by using apomorphine or ipecac. This should be done as soon as possible and should be followed by the administration of a slurry of charcoal to absorb the poison in the intestinal tract. Nausea and vomiting from the poisoning can later be controlled by using an antiemetic drug such as prochlorperazine (Compazine). Hypotension can usually be alleviated with the use of a pressor drug such as dopamine (Intropin) or dobutamine (Dobutrex). Calcium gluconate may also be helpful in treating hypotension and myocardial insufficiency. Bradycardia may be controlled with the use of atropine. Cool showers and the use of hydroxyzine (Atarax) may be helpful in relieving the pruritus. Intravenous sodium ascorbate, 25 g diluted in a 250 mL of normal saline per day for 10 days, and vitamin B complex have been used in relieving some of the effects of ciguatoxin. Mannitol provides symptomatic relief in many cases.

The fruit of the nono tree (*Morinda citrifolia* Linnaeus) has been used for centuries by South Pacific islanders to treat the symptoms of ciguatera fish and puffer poisoning. The juice of this fruit is now sold in the United States and elsewhere under the trade name of "Noni." The usual dosage is 4 to 6 ounces of the juice per day, or 4 to 6 (500-mg) tablets, divided into evenly spaced intervals. The product is nontoxic and should be tried and is available in most health food stores.

A variety of other therapies have been used, but none has been shown to be completely effective.

When catching fish in a suspect ciguatoxic region, it is advisable to seek the advice of the locals as to the edibility of the fish. The viscera (i.e., liver, gonads, and intestines) of many tropical reef fish are toxic and should not be eaten. Such ordinary cooking procedures as frying, baking, boiling, or drying do not render a fish safe to eat. If in doubt concerning the toxicity of the fish, eat only a small amount and wait for a period of several hours before eating additional quantities of the fish. Tropical moray eels frequently are toxic, may be deadly, and should not be eaten. Offshore fish in general are safer to eat than inshore reef species.

An inexpensive and reliable immunoassay stick test has been developed in Hawaii. The test measures ciguatoxin and polyether compounds, including okadaic acid. The stick test has been used commercially to a limited extent in Hawaii. It appears to be the most reliable and practical assay method available for the screening of ciguatoxic fish. Unfortunately, the stick test is not generally available in most endemic ciguatoxic regions of the world.

Scombroid poisoning involves the scombroid fish such as tuna, mackerel, skipjack, and related species. Poisonings are the result of ingesting fresh scombroid fish that have been inadequately refrigerated. A variety of bacteria are known to decarboxylate histidine to histamine in these dark-meated fish. Scombroid poisoning is not an ordinary form of bacterial food poisoning. Scombroid fishes that have a sharp, peppery taste should be discarded. This is the most common form of fish poisoning worldwide. Treatment consists of antihistamines and induction of vomiting, followed by administration of a charcoal slurry.

Puffer or fugu poisoning is caused by ingesting fish of the suborder Tetraodontoidea. These fish are also known as globefish, swellfish, swelltoads, fahaka, maki maki, porcupine fish, puffers, toados, and balloon fish. These fish contain tetrodotoxin, a fast-acting poison with a high mortality rate. The treatment is to induce vomiting as soon as possible; there is no known antidote. Follow the treatment procedure as suggested for ciguatera fish poisoning.

Marine turtles may become poisonous as a result of feeding on toxic algae. Ingestion of poisonous turtles can be fatal. There is no known antidote. Treatment is to induce vomiting, followed by administration of a slurry of charcoal. Follow the treatment procedure suggested for ciguatera fish poisoning.

Polar bear liver and kidneys may contain extremely high levels of vitamin A. Fatalities have occurred from eating polar bear viscera. Induce vomiting and administer a charcoal slurry.

ELECTRIC FISH SHOCKS

There are approximately 250 species of electric fish. Some of them are marine and others are freshwater inhabitants. The Amazonian electric eel discharges the greatest shock, which varies from 370 to 550 V, sufficient to stun a human or a horse. These shocks may be painful but usually are not fatal. No treatment is required.

ACUTE POISONINGS
method of
HOWARD C. MOFENSON, M.D.,
THOMAS R. CARACCIO, PHARM.D.,
and
JOSEPH GREENSHER, M.D.
Long Island Regional Poison Control Center
Mineola, New York

COMMON ABBREVIATIONS

ABG	=	arterial blood gas
AC	=	activated charcoal
AG	=	anion gap
ALT	=	alanine aminotransferase
AST	=	aspartate aminotransferase
AV	=	atrioventricular
BZP	=	benzodiazepine
BUN	=	blood urea nitrogen
CDC	=	Centers for Disease Control and Prevention
CNS	=	central nervous system
ECG	=	electrocardiogram
EEG	=	electroencephalogram
FDA	=	Food and Drug Administration
GABA	=	γ-aminobutyric acid
GI	=	gastrointestinal
HIV	=	human immunodeficiency virus
ICU	=	intensive care unit
MAOI	=	monoamine oxidase inhibitor
MDAC	=	multiple-dose activated charcoal
NAC	=	*N*-acetylcysteine
OSHA	=	Occupational Safety and Health Administration
$PaCO_2$	=	arterial carbon dioxide tension
PaO_2	=	arterial oxygen tension
PEEP	=	positive end-expiratory pressure

PEG = polyethylene glycol
pK$_a$ = negative logarithm of dissociation constant
PTZ = phenothiazine
SG = specific gravity
t$_{1/2}$ = half-life
Vd = volume of distribution

MEDICAL TOXICOLOGY (INGESTIONS, INHALATIONS, DERMAL AND OCULAR ABSORPTIONS)

Epidemiology

An estimated 5 million potentially toxic exposures occur each year in the United States. Poisoning is responsible for almost 12,000 deaths (including those caused by carbon monoxide) and more than 200,000 hospitalizations.

Poisoning accounts for 2 to 5% of pediatric hospital admissions, 10% of adult admissions, 5% of hospital admissions in the elderly population (older than 65 years), and 5% of ambulance calls. The largest number of fatalities resulting from poisoning are caused by carbon monoxide (CO).

Pharmaceutical preparations are involved in 40% of poisonings. The number one pharmaceutical toxic exposure is to acetaminophen. The leading pharmaceuticals causing fatalities in 1994 were the analgesics, antidepressants, sedative hypnotics or antipsychotic drugs, stimulants and street drugs, cardiovascular agents, and alcohols.

The severity of the manifestations of acute poisoning exposures varies greatly with whether the poisoning was accidental or intentional.

Nonintentional (accidental poisoning) exposures make up 60 to 65% of all poisoning exposures. The majority are acute, occur in children younger than 5 years, occur in the home, and result in no or minor toxicity. Many are ingestions of relatively nontoxic substances that necessitate minimal medical care.

Intentional (suicidal poisoning) exposures constitute 10 to 15% of exposures. Intentional ingestions are often of multiple substances and frequently include ethanol, acetaminophen, and aspirin. Suicides make up 60 to 90% of reported poisoning fatalities. About 25% of suicides are attempted with drugs.

ASSESSMENT AND MAINTENANCE OF VITAL FUNCTIONS

The initial assessment of all medical emergencies follows the principles of basic and advanced cardiac life support. The adequacy of the patient's airway, degree of ventilation, and circulatory status should be determined. The vital functions should be established and maintained. Vital signs should be measured frequently and should include body core temperature. Evaluation of vital functions should include not only rate numbers but also effective function (e.g., respiratory rate and depth and air exchange) (Table 1).

The level of consciousness should be assessed by immediate AVPU signs (alert, responds to verbal stimuli, responds to painful stimuli, or unconscious). If the patient is unconscious, the severity is assessed by the Reed classification (Table 2) or the Glasgow Coma Scale (Table 3).

If the patient is comatose, management requires administering 100% oxygen, establishing vascular access, obtaining blood for pertinent laboratory studies, and administering glucose, thiamine, and naloxone (Narcan); intubation to protect the airway should also be considered. Pertinent laboratory studies include ABGs, electrocardiography, determination of glucose and electrolyte concentrations, renal and liver tests, and for all intentional ingestions determination of the acetaminophen plasma concentration

TABLE 1. **Important Measurements and Vital Signs**

Age	BSA (m²)	Weight (kg)	Height (cm)	Pulse (bpm), Resting	Blood Pressure (mm Hg)			RR (rpm)
					Hypotension	Hypertension		
						SIGNIFICANT	SEVERE	
NB	0.19	3.5	50	70–190	<40/60	>96	>106	30–60
1–6 mo	0.30	4–7	50–65	80–160	<45/70	>104	>110	30–50
6 mo–1 y	0.38	7–10	65–75	80–160	<45/70	>104	>110	20–40
1–2 y	0.50–0.55	10–12	75–85	80–140	<47/74	>74/112	>82/118	20–40
3–5 y	0.54–0.68	15–20	90–108	80–120	<52/80	>76/116	>84/124	20–40
6–9 y	0.68–0.85	20–28	122–133	75–115	<60/90	>82/122	>86/130	16–25
10–12 y	1.00–1.07	30–40	138–147	70–110	<60/90	>82/126	>90/134	16–25
13–15 y	1.07–1.22	42–50	152–160	60–100	<60/90	>86/136	>92/144	16–20
16–18 y	1.30–1.60	53–60	160–170	60–100	<60/90	>92/142	>98/150	12–16
Adult	1.40–1.70	60–70	160–170	60–100	<60/90	>90/140	>120/210	10–16

Abbreviations: bpm = beats per minute; BSA = body surface area; NB = newborn; rpm = respirations per minute; RR = respiratory rate.
Data from Nadas A: Pediatric Cardiology, 3rd ed. Philadelphia, WB Saunders Co, 1976; Blumer JL (ed): A Practice Guide to Pediatric Intensive Care. St. Louis, CV Mosby, 1990; AAP and ACEP Respiratory Distress in APLS Pediatric Emergency Medicine Course, 1993, p 5; Second Task Force on blood pressure control in children—1987. Pediatrics 79:1, 1987; and Linakis JG: Hypertension. *In* Fleisher GR, Ludwig S (eds): Textbook of Pediatric Emergency Medicine, 3rd ed. Baltimore, Williams & Wilkins, 1993, p 249.

TABLE 2. **Classification of the Level of Consciousness**

Stage	Status	Conscious Level	Pain Response	Reflexes	Respiration	Circulation
0	Lethargic, able to answer questions and follow commands	Asleep	Arousable	Intact	Normal	Normal
I	Responsive to pain, brain stem and deep tendon reflexes intact	Comatose	Withdraws	Intact	Normal	Normal
II	Unresponsive to pain	Comatose	None	Intact	Normal	Normal
III	Unresponsive to pain, most reflexes absent, respiratory depression	Comatose	None	Absent	Depressed	Normal
IV	Unresponsive to pain, all reflexes absent, cardiovascular and respiratory depression	Comatose	None	Absent	Cyanosis	Shock

Modified from Reed CE, Driggs MF, Foote CC: Acute barbiturate intoxication: A study of 300 cases based on a physiologic system of classification of the severity of the intoxication. Ann Intern Med 37:290, 1952.

(APC). Radiography of the chest and abdomen may be useful.

The severity of a stimulant's effects can also be assessed (Table 4). The assessment should be recorded to follow the trend.

Exposure: Completely expose the patient by removing clothes and other items that interfere with a full evaluation. Look for clues to etiology in the clothes, including the hat and shoes.

Prevention of Toxin Absorption and Reduction of Local Damage

Routes

Poisoning exposure routes include ingestion (80%), dermal routes (7%), ophthalmic routes (5%), inhalation (5%), insect bites and stings (2.7%), and parenteral injections (0.3%). The effect of the toxin may be local, systemic, or both.

Local effects (skin, eyes, mucosa of respiratory or GI tract) occur in areas of contact with the poisonous substance. Local effects are nonspecific chemical reactions that depend on the chemical properties (e.g., pH), concentration, contact time, and type of exposed surface.

Systemic effects occur when the poison is absorbed into the body and depend on the dose and distribution of the toxin, and the functional reserve of the organ systems. Complications resulting from shock, hypoxia, chronic exposure, and existing illness may also influence systemic toxicity.

Delayed Toxic Action

Most pharmaceuticals are absorbed within 90 minutes. However, the patient with exposure to a potential toxin may be asymptomatic at the time of presentation for several reasons: the substance may be nontoxic, an insufficient amount of the toxin may

TABLE 3. **Glasgow Coma Scale**

Scale	Adult Response	Score	Pediatric Response (0–1 y)*
Eye opening	Spontaneous	4	Spontaneous
	To verbal command	3	To shout
	To pain	2	To pain
	None	1	No response
Motor response			
To verbal command	Obeys	6	
To painful stimuli	Localized pain	5	Localized pain
	Flexion withdrawal	4	Flexion withdrawal
	Decorticate flexion	3	Decorticate flexion
	Decerebrate extension	2	Decerebrate extension
	None	1	None
Verbal response, adult	Oriented and converses	5	Cries, smiles, coos
	Disoriented but converses	4	Cries or screams
	Inappropriate words	3	Inappropriate sounds
	Incomprehensible sounds	2	Grunts
	None	1	Gives no response
Verbal response, child	Oriented	5	
	Words or babbles	4	
	Vocal sounds	3	
	Cries or moans to stimuli	2	
	None	1	

*From Seidel J: Preparing for pediatric emergencies. Pediatr Rev 16:466–472, 1995.
Modified from Teasdale G, Jennett B: Assessment of coma and impaired consciousness. Lancet 2:81–84, 1974; and Simpson D, Reilly P: Pediatric coma scale. Lancet 2:450, 1982.

TABLE 4. **Classification of Severity of Effects of Stimulants**

Severity	Manifestations
Grade 1	Diaphoresis, hyper-reflexia, irritability, mydriasis, tremors
Grade 2	Confusion, fever, hyperactivity, hypertension, tachycardia, tachypnea
Grade 3	Delirium, mania, hyperpyrexia, tachydysrhythmia
Grade 4	Coma, convulsions, cardiovascular collapse

Modified with permission from Espelin DE, Done AK: Amphetamine poisoning. Effectiveness of chlorpromazine. N Engl J Med *278*:1361–1365, 1968. Copyright © 1968 Massachusetts Medical Society. All rights reserved.

have been involved, or a sufficient amount may not yet have been absorbed or metabolized to produce toxicity.

Absorption may be significantly delayed for several reasons:

- A drug with anticholinergic properties is involved (e.g., antihistamines, belladonna alkaloids, diphenoxylate with atropine [Lomotil], PTZs, cyclic antidepressants).
- Sustained-release and enteric-coated preparations, which have delayed and prolonged absorption, are involved.
- Concretions may form (e.g., with ingestions of salicylates, iron, glutethimide, or meprobamate) that can delay absorption and prolong the action.
- Substances must be metabolized to a toxic metabolite or time is required to produce a toxic effect on the organ system (e.g., acetaminophen, *Amanita phalloides* mushrooms, acetonitrile, carbon tetrachloride, colchicine, digoxin, ethylene glycol, heavy metals, methanol, methylene chloride, MAOIs, oral hypoglycemic agents, parathion, paraquat).

Decontamination

Decontamination procedures should be considered for an asymptomatic patient if the exposure involves potentially toxic substances in toxic amounts.

Ocular exposure should be treated immediately with water or saline irrigation for 15 to 20 minutes with the eyelids fully retracted. The use of neutralizing chemicals is contraindicated. All caustic and corrosive injuries should be evaluated with examination after instillation of fluorescein dye and by an ophthalmologist.

Dermal exposure is treated immediately with copious irrigation for 30 minutes. Shampooing the hair; cleansing fingernails, navel, and perineum; and irrigating the eyes are necessary in an extensive exposure. The clothes should be specially bagged and may have to be discarded. Leather goods can be irreversibly contaminated and must be abandoned. Caustic (alkali) exposures can require hours of irrigation. Dermal absorption can occur with, for example, pesticides, hydrocarbons, and cyanide.

Injection exposures to drugs and toxins can involve envenomation. Cold packs and tourniquets should not be used, and incision is generally not recommended. Venom extractors may be used within minutes of envenomation, and proximal lymphatic constricting bands or elastic wraps may be used to delay lymphatic flow and immobilize the extremity.

Inhalation exposure to toxic substances is managed by immediately removing the victim from the contaminated environment, by protected rescuers if necessary.

GI exposure is the most common route of poisoning. GI decontamination may be done by gastric emptying (induction of emesis, gastric lavage), adsorption by administering single or multiple doses of activated charcoal (AC), or whole-bowel irrigation. No procedure is routine; the procedure should be individualized on the basis of the patient's age, properties of the substance ingested, and time since the ingestion. If no attempt is made to decontaminate the patient, the reason should be clearly documented on the medical record (e.g., time elapsed, past peak of action, ineffectiveness, or risk of procedure).

Gastric Emptying Procedures. The procedure used is influenced by the patient's age and the procedure's effectiveness (the size of the orogastric tube used in a small child may not be large enough for adequate lavage, e.g., with iron tablets), time of ingestion (gastric emptying is usually ineffective more than 1 hour after ingestion), clinical status (asymptomatic time to peak effect has elapsed or the patient's condition is too unstable), formulation of substance ingested (regular-release, sustained-release, enteric-coated), amount ingested, caustic action, and rapidity of onset of CNS depression or stimulation (convulsions). Most studies show that only 30% (19 to 62%) of ingested toxins is removed by gastric emptying under optimal conditions. It has not been demonstrated that the procedure improved the outcome.

The clinician should attempt to obtain ample information about the patient. The intent should be determined.

The regional poison control center should be consulted for the exact ingredients and the latest management. The first-aid information on the labels of products is notoriously inaccurate, and product ingredients change.

Syrup of Ipecac–Induced Emesis. The poison control center should be called before emesis is induced.

Contraindications or situations in which induction of emesis is inappropriate include the following:

- Caustic ingestions
- Loss of airway protective reflexes—this can occur with substances that can produce rapid onset of CNS depression or convulsions
- Ingestion of high-viscosity petroleum distillates
- Significant vomiting before presentation, or hematemesis
- Age younger than 6 months
- Foreign bodies (emesis is ineffective and may lead to aspiration)
- Clinical conditions: pregnancy, neurologic impair-

ment, hemodynamic instability, increased intracranial pressure, and hypertension
- Delay in presentation (more than 1 hour after ingestion)

The presence of factors such as oral injury may interfere with administration of AC or oral antidotes. The patient cannot tolerate oral intake for a mean of 2 to 3 hours after ipecac-induced emesis.

The dose of syrup of ipecac for the 6- to 9-month-old infant is 5 mL; for the 9- to 12-month-old, 10 mL; and for the 1- to 12-year-old, 15 mL. For children older than 12 years and for adults, the dose is 30 mL. The dose may be repeated once if the child does not vomit in 15 to 20 minutes. The vomitus should be inspected for remnants of pills or toxic substances, and the appearance and odor should be documented.

Gastric Aspiration and Lavage. The contraindications are similar to those for ipecac-induced emesis. The procedure can be accomplished after the insertion of an endotracheal tube in CNS depression or controlled convulsions. The patient should be placed with the head lower than the hips in a left lateral decubitus position. The location of the tube should be confirmed by radiography, if necessary, and suctioning equipment should be available.

Contraindications to gastric aspiration and lavage include the following:

- Caustic ingestions (because of risk of esophageal perforation)
- Uncontrolled convulsions, because of the danger of aspiration and injury during the procedure
- High-viscosity petroleum distillate products
- CNS depression or absence of protective airway reflexes, which necessitates insertion of an endotracheal tube to protect against aspiration
- Significant cardiac dysrhythmias, which should be controlled
- Either significant emesis before presentation or hematemesis
- Delay in presentation (more than 1 hour after ingestion)

For adults, a large-bore orogastric Lavacuator hose or a No. 42 French Ewald tube is used. For children, a No. 22 to No. 28 French orogastric-type tube is used, but this is usually ineffective in solid ingestions (e.g., iron tablets).

The amount of fluid used for lavage varies with the patient's age and size. In general, aliquots of 50 to 100 mL per lavage are used for adults and 5 mL per kg up to 50 to 100 mL per lavage for children. Lavage fluid is 0.89% saline.

Activated Charcoal. Oral AC adsorbs the toxin onto its surface before GI absorption and interrupts enterogastric and enterohepatic circulation of toxic metabolites. AC is a stool marker, indicating that the toxin has passed through the GI tract.

AC does not effectively adsorb small molecules or molecules lacking carbon, as listed in Table 5. AC adsorption may be diminished by the concurrent

TABLE 5. Substances Poorly Adsorbed by Activated Charcoal

C—Caustics and corrosives, cyanide*
H—Heavy metals (arsenic, iron, lead, lithium, mercury)
A—Alcohols (ethanol, methanol, isopropyl) and glycols (ethylene glycol)
R—Rapid onset or absorption of cyanide and strychnine
C—Chlorine and iodine
O—Others insoluble in water (substances in tablet form)
A—Aliphatic and poorly absorbed hydrocarbons (petroleum distillates)
L—Laxatives, sodium, magnesium, potassium

*If cyanide is ingested, AC is given in large doses; 1 gm of AC adsorbs 35 mg of cyanide.

presence in the stomach of ethanol, milk, cocoa powder, or ice cream.

There are a few relative contraindications to the use of AC:

- It does not interfere with the effectiveness of NAC in acetaminophen overdose.
- It does not effectively adsorb caustics and corrosives, may produce vomiting or cling to the mucosa, and may falsely appear as a burn at endoscopy.
- It should not be given to a comatose patient without securing the airway.
- It should not be given if there are no bowel sounds.

The usual initial adult dose is 60 to 100 grams, and the dose for children is 15 to 30 grams. It is administered orally (PO) as a slurry mixed with water or by nasogastric or orogastric tube. *Caution:* The clinician must be sure the tube is in the stomach. Cathartics are not necessary.

MULTIPLE-DOSE ACTIVATED CHARCOAL. Repeated dosing with AC decreases the half-life and increases the clearance of phenobarbital, dapsone, salicylate, quinidine, theophylline, and carbamazepine. The MDAC dosage varies from 0.25 to 0.50 gram per kg every 1 to 4 hours, and continuous nasogastric tube infusion of 0.25 to 0.5 gram per kg per hour has been used to decrease vomiting.

GI dialysis involves the diffusion of the toxin from the higher concentration in the serum of the mesenteric vessels to the lower levels in the GI tract mucosal cells and subsequently into the GI lumen, where the concentration has been lowered by adsorption onto the intraluminal AC.

Complications of AC have been reported in at least a dozen cases. There are many cases of unreported pulmonary aspiration and "charcoal" lung.

Catharsis. No studies have demonstrated the effectiveness of a cathartic.

Whole-Bowel Irrigation. In whole-bowel irrigation, bowel-cleansing solutions of PEG with balanced electrolytes are used to avoid changes in body weight or electrolytes.

Indications (not approved by the FDA): The procedure has been studied and used successfully in iron overdose when abdominal radiographs revealed incomplete emptying of excess iron. There are additional implications in other ingestions, as in body packing of illicit drugs (e.g., cocaine, heroin). The procedure is to administer, PO or by nasogastric tube, the solution (GoLYTELY or Colyte), at 0.5 liter per hour in children younger than 5 years, 1 liter per hour in children aged 6 to 12 years, or 1.5 to 2 liters per hour in adolescents and adults for 5 hours. The end point is reached when the rectal effluent is clear or radiopaque materials can no longer be seen in the GI tract on abdominal radiographs.

Contraindications: These measures should not be used if extensive hematemesis, ileus, or signs of bowel obstruction, perforation, or peritonitis are present.

Dilution. Dilutional treatment is indicated for the immediate management of caustic and corrosive poisonings but is otherwise not useful. Administration of large quantities of diluting fluid—above 30 mL in children and 250 mL in adults—may produce vomiting, re-exposing the vital tissues to the effects of local damage, and possible aspiration.

Neutralization. Neutralization has not been proved to be safe or effective.

Endoscopy and Surgery. Surgery has been required in the management of body packer's obstruc-

TABLE 6. Toxic Effects of Central Nervous System Depressants*

General Manifestations	CNS Depressants
Bradycardia	Alcohols and glycols (S-H)
Bradypnea†	Anticonvulsants (S-H)
Shallow respirations	Antidysrhythmics (S-H)
Hypotension	Antihypertensives (S-H)
Hypothermia	Barbiturates (S-H)
Flaccid coma	Benzodiazepines (S-H)‡
Miosis	Butyrophenones (Syly)
Hypoactive bowel sounds	Beta-adrenergic blockers (Syly)
Frozen addict syndrome§	Calcium channel blockers (Syly)
	Digitalis (Syly)
	Opioids (O)‖¶
	Lithium (mixed)
	Muscle relaxants
	Phenothiazines (Syly)
	Nonbarbiturate, benzodiazepine sedative hypnotics (S-H)‖ (chloral hydrate, glutethimide, methaqualone, methyprylon, ethchlorvynol, bromide)
	Tricyclic antidepressants late (Syly)

*CNS depressants are cholinergics (C), opioids (O) and sedative hypnotics (S-H), and sympatholytic agents (Syly). The hallmarks of CNS depressant activity are lethargy, sedation, stupor, and coma.

†Barbiturates may produce an initial tachycardia.

‡Benzodiazepines rarely produce coma that interferes with cardiorespiratory functions.

§The "frozen addict" syndrome is due to a neurotoxin resulting from improper synthesis of an analogue of meperidine. Its manifestations are similar to those of the permanent type of parkinsonism.

‖Convulsions are produced by codeine, propoxyphene (Darvon), meperidine (Demerol), glutethimide, phenothiazines, methaqualone, and tricyclic or other cyclic antidepressants.

¶Pulmonary edema is common with opioids and sedative hypnotics.

TABLE 7. Toxic Effects of Central Nervous System Stimulants*

General Manifestations	CNS Stimulants
Tachycardia	Amphetamines (Sy)
Tachypnea and dysrhythmias	Anticholinergics (Ach)†
Hypertension	Cocaine (Sy)
Convulsions	Camphor (mixed)
Spastic coma‡	Ergot alkaloids (Sy)
Toxic psychosis	Isoniazid (mixed)
Mydriasis (reactive)	Lithium (mixed)
Agitation and restlessness	Lysergic acid diethylamide (LSD) (H)
Moist skin	Hallucinogens (H)
Tremors	Mescaline and synthetic analogues
	Metals (arsenic, lead, mercury)
	Methylphenidate (Ritalin) (Sy)
	MAOIs (Sy)
	Pemoline (Cylert) (Sy)
	Phencyclidine (H)§
	Salicylates (mixed)
	Strychnine (mixed)
	Sympathomimetics (Sy) (phenylpropanolamine, theophylline, caffeine, thyroid)
	Withdrawal from ethanol, beta-adrenergic blockers, clonidine, opioids, sedative hypnotics (W)

*CNS stimulants are anticholinergics (Ach), hallucinogens (H), sympathomimetics (Sy), and withdrawal (W). The hallmarks of CNS stimulant activity are convulsions and hyperactivity.

†Anticholinergics produce dry skin and mucosa and decreased bowel sounds.

‡Flaccid coma eventually develops after seizures.

§Phencyclidine may produce miosis.

tion, intestinal ischemia produced by cocaine ingestion, and local caustic action of iron.

Differential Diagnosis Based on Central Nervous System Manifestations of Poisoning

Neurologic parameters help in classifying and assessing the need for supportive treatment and provide diagnostic clues to the etiology. See Tables 6 through 9.

Use of Antidotes

Antidotes are available for only a relatively small number of poisons. An available antidote should be administered only after the integrity of vital functions has been established. Table 10 summarizes the commonly used antidotes, their indications, and methods of administration. The regional poison control center should be consulted for further information on these antidotes.

Enhancement of Elimination

The medical methods for elimination of absorbed toxic substances are diuresis, dialysis, hemoperfu-

TABLE 8. **Toxic Effects of Hallucinogens***

General Manifestations	Hallucinogens
Tachycardia and dysrhythmias	Amphetamines
Tachypnea	Anticholinergics
Hypertension	Carbon monoxide
Hallucinations, usually visual	Cardiac glycosides
Disorientation	Cocaine
Panic reaction	Ethanol
Toxic psychosis	Hydrocarbon inhalation: abuse or occupational
Moist skin	Lysergic acid diethylamide
Mydriasis (reactive)	Marijuana
Hyperthermia	Mescaline (peyote)
Flashbacks	Mescaline-amphetamine hybrids†
	Metals (chronic mercury, arsenic)
	Mushrooms (psilocybin)
	Phencyclidine
	Plants (morning glory seeds, nutmeg)

*There is considerable overlap in this category; however, the major hallmark manifestation is hallucinations.

†The mescaline-amphetamine hybrids are methylene dioxymethamphetamine (MDMA, Ecstasy, Adam) and methylene dioxyamphetamine (MDA, Eve), which have been associated with deaths.

sion, exchange transfusion, plasmapheresis, enzyme induction, and inhibition. Methods of increasing urinary excretion of toxic chemicals and drugs have been studied extensively, but the other modalities have not been well evaluated.

In general, these methods are needed in only a

TABLE 9. **Effects of Toxins on Autonomic Nervous System**

General Manifestations	Agents
Anticholinergic	
Tachycardia, dysrhythmias (rare)	Antihistamines
Tachypnea	Antispasmodic GI preparations
Hypertension (mild)	Antiparkinsonian preparations
Hyperthermia	Atropine
Hallucinations	Cyclobenzaprine (Flexeril)
Mydriasis (unreactive)	Mydriatic ophthalmologic agents
Flushed skin	Over-the-counter sleep agents
Dry skin and mouth	Plants (*Datura* species), mushrooms
Hypoactive bowel sounds	Phenothiazines (early)
Urinary retention	Scopolamine
Lilliputian hallucinations	Tricyclic or other cyclic antidepressants (early)
Cholinergic	
Bradycardia (muscarinic)	Bethanechol
Tachycardia (nicotinic)	Carbamate insecticides (carbaryl)
Miosis (muscarinic)	
Diarrhea (muscarinic)	Edrophonium
Hypertension (variable)	Organophosphate insecticides (malathion, parathion)
Hyperactive bowel sounds	
Excess urination (muscarinic)	Parasympathetic agents (physostigmine, pyridostigmine)
Excess salivation (muscarinic)	
Lacrimation (muscarinic)	
Bronchospasm (muscarinic)	Toxic mushrooms (*Amanita muscaria, Clitocybe* species)
Muscle fasciculations (nicotinic)	
Paralysis (nicotinic)	

minority of instances and should be reserved for life-threatening circumstances or when a definite benefit is anticipated.

Diuresis

Diuresis increases the renal clearance of compounds that are eliminated primarily by the renal route, are significantly reabsorbed in the renal tubules, and have a small volume of distribution (Vd) and low protein binding (PB). Acid diuresis is not recommended and may precipitate myoglobin in the renal tubules. Alkalization without diuresis with sodium bicarbonate ($NaHCO_3$) at 1 to 2 mEq per kg in 15 mL of 5% dextrose in water (D5W) per kg may be used in the therapy of weak acid intoxications, such as with salicylates (severe salicylate poisoning can necessitate hemodialysis) and long-acting barbiturates (LABs) (e.g., phenobarbital). Additional boluses of 0.5 mEq per kg can be administered to maintain alkalization, but blood pH values higher than 7.55 should be avoided. Many clinicians use the alkalization without the diuresis because of the danger of fluid overload.

Dialysis

Dialysis is an extrarenal means of removing certain substances from the body and can substitute for the kidneys when renal failure occurs. Dialysis is not the first measure instituted; however, it may be lifesaving later in the course of a severe intoxication. It is needed in only a minority of intoxicated patients.

Peritoneal dialysis utilizes the peritoneum as the membrane for dialysis. It is only one-twentieth as effective as hemodialysis. It is easier to use and less hazardous to the patient but also less effective in removing the toxin; thus, it is seldom used except for small infants.

Hemodialysis is the most effective means of dialysis but requires experience with sophisticated equipment. Blood is circulated past a semipermeable membrane by an extracorporeal method. Substances are removed by diffusion down a concentration gradient. Anticoagulation with heparin is necessary.

Hemodialysis is contraindicated when (1) the substance is not dialyzable, (2) hemodynamic instability (e.g., shock) is present, and (3) coagulopathy is present because heparinization is required.

The patient-related criteria for dialysis are (1) anticipated prolonged coma and the likelihood of complications, (2) renal compromise (toxin excreted or metabolized by kidneys and dialyzable chelating agents in heavy metal poisoning), (3) laboratory confirmation of lethal blood concentration, (4) lethal-dose poisoning with an agent with delayed toxicity or known to be metabolized into a more toxic metabolite (e.g., ethylene glycol, methanol), and (5) hepatic impairment when the agent is metabolized by the liver and clinical deterioration occurs despite optimal supportive medical management.

Dialyzable substances diffuse easily across the dialysis membrane and have the following characteristics: (1) a low molecular weight (less than 500 and

Text continued on page 1156

TABLE 10. **Initial Doses of Antidotes for Common Poisonings, Alphabetically Arranged**

Antidote	Use	Dose	Route	Adverse Reactions (AR) and Comments
N-Acetylcysteine (NAC, Mucomyst). Stock level to treat 70-kg adult for 24 h: seven vials, 20%, 30 mL.	Acetaminophen, carbon tetrachloride (experimental).	140 mg/kg loading, followed by 70 mg/kg q 4 h for 17 doses.	PO	Nausea, vomiting. Dilute to 5% with sweet juice or flat cola.
Atropine. Stock level to treat 70-kg adult for 24 h; 1 gm (1 mg/mL in 1 or 10 mL).	Organophosphate and carbamate pesticides.	*Child:* 0.02–0.05 mg/kg repeated q 5–10 min to maximum of 2 mg as necessary until cessation of secretions. *Adult:* 1–2 mg q 5–10 min as necessary. Dilute in 1–2 mL of 0.89% saline for endotracheal instillation. *IV infusion dose:* Place 8 mg of atropine in 100 mL of D5W or saline. Concentration = 0.08 mg/mL. Dose range = 0.02–0.08 mg/kg/h or 0.25–1 mL/kg/h. Severe poisoning may require supplemental IV atropine intermittently in doses of 1–5 mg until drying of secretions occurs.	IV or ET	Tachycardia, dry mouth, blurred vision, and urinary retention. Ensure adequate ventilation before administration.
Calcium chloride (10%). Stock level to treat 70-kg adult for 24 h: 5–10 vials, 1 gm (1.35 mEq/mL).	Hypocalcemia, fluoride, calcium channel blockers.	0.1–0.2 mL/kg (10–20 mg/kg) slow push q 10 min up to maximum of 10 mL (1 gm). Because calcium response lasts 15 min, some patients may require continuous infusion of 0.2 mL/kg/h up to maximum of 10 mL/h during monitoring for dysrhythmias and hypotension.	IV	Administer slowly with BP and ECG monitoring and have magnesium available to reverse calcium effects. **AR:** Tissue irritation, hypotension, dysrhythmias resulting from rapid injection. Contraindication: Digitalis glycoside intoxication.
Calcium gluconate (10%). Stock level to treat 70-kg adult for 24 h: 5–10 vials, 1 gm (0.45 mEq/mL).	Hypocalcemia, fluoride, calcium channel blockers, hydrofluoric acid, black widow envenomation.	0.3–0.4 mL/kg (30–40 mg/kg) slow push; repeat as needed up to maximum dose of 10–20 mL (1–2 gm).	IV	Same as for calcium chloride.
Calcium gluconate gel. Stock level: 3.5 gm.	Hydrofluoric acid.	2.5 gm of USP powder added to 100 mL of water-soluble lubricating jelly (e.g., K-Y Jelly, Lubifax) (or 3.5 gm into 150 mL). Some use 6 gm of calcium carbonate in 100 gm of lubricant. Place injured hand in surgical glove filled with gel; or apply q 4 h. If pain persists, calcium gluconate injection may be needed (following).	Dermal	Powder is available from Spectrum Pharmaceutical Company in California: 1-800-772-8786. Commercial preparation of calcium gluconate gel is available from Pharmascience in Montreal, Quebec: 514-340-1114.
Infiltration of calcium gluconate.	Hydrofluoric acid.	Dose: Infiltrate each square cm of affected dermis or subcutaneous tissue with about 0.5 mL of 10% calcium gluconate using a 30-gauge needle. Repeat as needed to control pain.	Infiltrate	
Cyanide antidote kit. Stock level to treat 70-kg adult for 24 h: two Lilly Cyanide Antidote kits.	Cyanide; hydrogen sulfide (nitrites are given only; do not use sodium thiosulfate for hydrogen sulfide). Individual portions of the kit can be used in certain circumstances (consult PCC).	Amyl nitrite: 1 crushable ampule for 30 s of every minute. Use new ampule q 3 min. May omit step if venous access is established.	Inhalation	If methemoglobinemia occurs, do not use methylene blue to correct this because it releases cyanide.

Table continued on following page

1151

TABLE 10. **Initial Doses of Antidotes for Common Poisonings, Alphabetically Arranged** *Continued*

Antidote	Use	Dose	Route	Adverse Reactions (AR) and Comments
Cyanide antidote kit. Stock level to treat 70-kg adult for 24 h; two Lilly Cyanide Antidote kits.	Cyanide; hydrogen sulfide (nitrites are given only; do not use sodium thiosulfate for hydrogen sulfide). Individual portions of the kit can be used in certain circumstances (consult PCC).	Sodium nitrite: *Child:* 0.33 mL/kg 3% solution if hemoglobin level is not known, otherwise follow tables with product. *Adult:* up to 300 mg (10 mL). Dilute nitrite in 100 mL of 0.9% saline, administer slowly at 5 mL/min. Slow infusion if fall in BP.	IV	If methemoglobinemia occurs, do not use methylene blue to correct this because it releases cyanide.
	Do not use sodium thiosulfate for hydrogen sulfide. Individual portions of the kit can be used in certain circumstances (consult PCC).	Sodium thiosulfate: *Child:* 1.6 mL/kg 25% solution; may be repeated q 30–60 min to a maximum of 12.5 gm or 50 mL in *adult.*	IV	**AR:** Nausea, dizziness, headache; tachycardia, muscle rigidity, and bronchospasm (rapid administration).
Dantrolene sodium (Dantrium). Stock level to treat 70-kg adult for 24 h: 700 mg in 35 vials (20 mg per vial).	Malignant hyperthermia.	Administer over 20 min. 2–3 mg/kg IV rapidly. Repeat loading dose q 10 min, if necessary up to a maximum total dose of 10 mg/kg. When temperature and heart rate decrease, slow the infusion to 1–2 mg/kg q 6 h for 24–48 h until all evidence of malignant hyperthermia syndrome has subsided. Follow with oral doses of 1–2 mg/kg qid for 24 h as necessary.	IV or PO	Available as 20-mg lyophilized dantrolene powder for reconstitution, which contains 3 gm of mannitol and sodium hydroxide in 70-mL vials. Mix with 60 mL of sterile distilled water without a bacteriostatic agent and protect from light. Use within 6 h after reconstituted. **AR:** Hepatotoxicity occurs with cumulative dose of 10 mg/kg; thrombophlebitis (best given in central line).
Deferoxamine (DFO, Desferal). Stock level to treat 70-kg adult for 24 h: 12 vials (50 mg per ampule).	Iron (100 mg of DFO binds 8.5–9.3 mg of iron).	IV infusion of 15 mg/kg/h (3 mL/kg/h: 500 mg in 100 mL D5W), maximum of 6 gm/d. Rates of >45 mg/kg/h if conc >1000 μg/dL.	IV preferred; avoid therapy >24 h	Hypotension (minimized by avoiding rapid infusion rates). DFO challenge test (50 mg/kg) is unreliable if negative.
Diazepam (Valium). Stock level to treat 70-kg adult for 24 h: 200 mg.	Any intoxication that provokes seizures when specific therapy is not available, for example, amphetamines, PCP, barbiturate and alcohol withdrawal, chloroquine poisoning.	*Adult:* 5–10 mg (maximum of 20 mg) at a rate of 5 mg/min until seizure is controlled. May be repeated two or three times. *Child:* 0.1–0.3 mg/kg up to 10 mg slowly over 2 min.	IV	**AR:** Confusion, somnolence, coma, hypotension. Intramuscular absorption is erratic. Establish airway and administer 100% oxygen and glucose.
Digoxin-specific Fab antibodies (Digibind). Stock level to treat 70-kg adult for 24 h: 20 vials.	Digoxin, digitoxin, oleander tea with any of the following: (1) imminent cardiac arrest or shock, (2) hyperkalemia of >5.0 mEq/L, (3) serum digoxin of >10 ng/mL (adult) or >5 ng/mL (child) at 8–12 h after ingestion in adults, (4) digitalis delirium, (5) ingestion of more than 10 mg in adult or 4 mg in child, (6) bradycardia or second- or third-degree heart block unresponsive to atropine, (7) life-threatening digitoxin or oleander poisoning.	1. *Amount (total mg) ingested known* multiplied by bioavailability (0.8) = body burden. The body burden divided by 0.6 (0.6 mg of digoxin is bound by one vial of 40 mg of Fab) = number of vials needed. 2. *If amount is unknown but the steady-state serum concentration is known in ng/mL: Digoxin:* ng/mL × (Vd = 5.6 L/kg) × wt (kg) = μg body burden. Body burden divided by 1000 = mg body burden/0.6 = number of vials needed.	IV	Administer by infusion over 30 min through a 0.22-μm filter. If cardiac arrest is imminent, may administer by bolus injection. Consult PCC for more details. **AR:** Allergic reactions (rare), return of condition being treated with digitalis glycoside.

1152

Antidote	Indication	Route	Dose	Comments
			3. *If the amount is not known,* agent is administered in life-threatening situations as 10 vials (400 mg) IV in saline over 30 min in adults. If cardiac arrest is imminent, administer 20 vials (adult) as a bolus.	
Dimercaprol (BAL in oil). Stock level to treat 70-kg adult for 24 h: 1200 mg (four ampules, 100 mg/mL 10% in oil in 3-mL ampule).	Chelating agent for arsenic, mercury, lead, antimony, bismuth, chromium, copper, gold, nickel, tungsten, and zinc.	Deep IM	3–5 mg/kg q 4 h, usually for 5–10 d.	**AR:** Local injection site pain and sterile abscess, nausea, vomiting, fever, salivation, hypertension, and nephrotoxicity (alkalize urine). Fatal dose, 20–40 mg/kg.
Diphenhydramine (Benadryl). Antiparkinsonian action. Stock level to treat 70-kg adult for 24 h: five vials (10 mg/mL, 10 mL each).	Used to treat extrapyramidal symptoms and dystonia induced by phenothiazines, PCP, and related drugs.	IV and PO	*Child:* 1–2 mg/kg IV slowly over 5 min up to maximum of 50 mg, followed by 5 mg/kg per 24 h PO divided q 6 h, up to 300 mg per 24 h. *Adult:* 50 mg IV followed by 50 mg PO qid for 5–7 d. Note: Symptoms abate within 2–5 min after IV administration.	**AR:** Dry mouth, drowsiness.
Ethanol (ethyl alcohol). Stock level to treat 70-kg adult for 24 h: three bottles 10% (1 L each).	Methanol, ethylene glycol.	IV	10 mL/kg loading dose concurrently with 1.4 mL/kg (average) infusion of 10% ethanol. (Consult PCC for more details.)	**AR:** Nausea, vomiting, sedation. Use 0.22-μmfilter if preparing from bulk 100% ethanol.
Flumazenil (Romazicon). Stock level to treat 70-kg adult for 24 h: 10 vials (0.1 mg/mL, 10 mL).	Benzodiazepines.	IV	Administer 0.2 mg (2 mL) over 30 s. (Pediatric dose not established, 0.01 mg/kg.) Wait 3 min for a response. If desired consciousness is not achieved, administer 0.3 mg (3 mL) over 30 s. Wait 3 min for response. If desired consciousness is not achieved, administer 0.5 mg (5 mL) over 30 s at 60-s intervals up to a maximal cumulative dose of 3 mg (30 mL) (1 mg in children). Because effects last only 1–5 h, if there is a response monitor carefully over next 6 h for resedation. If multiple repeated doses, consider a continuous infusion of 0.2–1 mg/h.	It is not recommended to improve ventilation. Its role in CNS depression needs to be clarified. It should not be used routinely in comatose patients. It is *contraindicated* in cyclic antidepressant intoxications, stimulant overdose, long-term benzodiazepine use (may precipitate life-threatening withdrawal), if benzodiazepines are used to control seizures, in head trauma. **AR:** Nausea, vomiting, facial flushing, agitation, headache, dizziness, seizures, and death.
Folic acid (Folvite). Stock level to treat 70-kg adult for 24 h: two 100-mg vials.	Methanol or ethylene glycol (investigational).	IV	1 mg/kg up to 50 mg q 4 h for 6 doses.	Uncommon.
Glucagon. Stock level to treat 70-kg adult for 24 h: 100 mg (10 vials, 10 units).	Beta blockers, calcium channel blockers, hypoglycemic agents.	IV	*Adult:* 5–10 mg, then infuse 1–5 mg/h. *Child:* 0.05–01 mg/kg, then infuse 0.07 mg/kg/h. Large doses up to 100 mg per 24 h have been used.	**AR:** Hyperglycemia, nausea, vomiting. Dissolve in D5W, not in 0.9% saline. Do not use diluent in package because of possible phenol toxicity.
Magnesium sulfate. Stock level to treat 70-kg adult for 24 h: approximately 25 gm (50 mL of 50% or 200 mL of 12.5%).	Torsades de pointes.	IV	*Adult:* 2 gm (20 mL of 20%) over 20 min. If no response in 10 min, repeat and follow by continuous infusion 1 gm/h. *Child:* 25–50 mg/kg initially, maintenance with 30–60 mg/kg per 24 h (0.25–0.50 mEq/kg per 24 h) up to 1000 mg per 24 h. (Dose not studied in controlled fashion.)	Use with caution if there is renal impairment.

Table continued on following page

TABLE 10. **Initial Doses of Antidotes for Common Poisonings, Alphabetically Arranged** *Continued*

Antidote	Use	Dose	Route	Adverse Reactions (AR) and Comments
Methylene blue. Stock level to treat 70-kg adult for 24 h: five ampules (10 mg per 10 mL).	Methemoglobinemia.	0.1–0.2 mL/kg of 1% solution, slow infusion, may be repeated q 30–60 min.	IV	**AR:** Nausea, vomiting, headache, dizziness.
Nalmefene (Revex). Stock level: not established.	Narcotic antagonist.	The dose for opioid overdose as bolus in adults is 0.5–1 mg q 2 min up to a total of 2 mg IV. May also be given IM or SC. In patients with renal failure, administer over 1 min. In postoperative opioid depression reversal IV 0.1–0.5 µg/kg every 2 min as needed and may repeat up to a total dose of 1 µg/kg.	IV, IM, SC	Role in comatose patients and opioid overdose is not clear. It is 16 times more potent than naloxone; duration of action is up to 8 h (half-life 10.8 h, compared with naloxone, 1 h). Clinical trials in more than 1750 patients have not shown significant adverse reactions.
Naloxone (Narcan). Stock level to treat 70-kg adult for 24 h: 3 vials (1 mg/mL, 10 mL).	Comatose patient; ineffective ventilation or adult respiratory rate <12 rpm; opioids.	In suspected overdose administer IV 0.1 mg/kg in a child younger than 5 y up to 2 mg. In older children and adults administer 2 mg q 2 min up to a total of 10–20 mg. Can also be administered into the ET tube. If no response by 10 mg, a pure opioid intoxication is unlikely. If opioid abuse is suspected, restraints should be in place before administration, initial dose 0.1 mg to avoid withdrawal and violent behavior. The initial dose is then doubled every minute progressively to a total of 10 mg. A continuous infusion has been advocated because many opioids outlast the short half-life.	IV, ET	Larger doses of naloxone may be required for more poorly antagonized synthetic opioid drugs: buprenorphine, codeine, dextromethorphan, fentanyl, pentazocine, propoxyphene, diphenoxylate, nalbuphine, new potent designer drugs, or long-acting opioids such as methadone. **Complications:** Although naloxone is safe and effective, there are rare reports of complications (in less than 1% of cases) of pulmonary edema, seizures, hypertension, cardiac arrest, and sudden death. The infusions are titrated to avoid respiratory depression and opioid withdrawal manifestations. Tapering of infusions can be attempted after 12 h and when the patient's condition has been stabilized.
Physostigmine (Antilirium). Stock level to treat 70-kg adult for 24 h: 10 ampules (2 mL each).	Anticholinergic agents (not routinely used, indicated only with life-threatening complications).	*Child:* 0.02 mg/kg slow push to maximum of 2 mg q 30–60 min. *Adult:* 1–2 mg q 5 min to maximum of 6 mg.	IV	**AR:** Bradycardia, asystole, seizures, bronchospasm, vomiting, headaches. Do not use for cyclic antidepressants.
Pralidoxime (2-PAM, Protopam). Stock level to treat 70-kg adult for 24 h: 12 vials (1 gm per 20 mL).	Organophosphates.	*Child ≤12 y:* 25–50 mg/kg maximum (4 mg/kg/min); *older than 12 y:* 1–2 gm per dose in 250 mL of 0.89% saline over 5–10 min. Maximal 200 mg/min. Repeat q 6–12 h for 24–48 h. Maximum adult dose 6 gm/d. Alternative: Main infusion 1 gm in 100 mL of 0.9% saline at 5–20 mg/kg/h (0.5–12 mL/kg/h) up to maximum 500 mg/h or 50 mL/h. Titrate to desired response. End point is absence of fasciculations and return of muscle strength.	IV	**AR:** Nausea, dizziness, headache; tachycardia, muscle rigidity, bronchospasm (rapid administration).

Antidote / Stock level	Indication	Route	Dose	Comments
Pyridoxine (vitamin B₆). Stock level to treat 70-kg adult for 24 h: four ampules (20 gm [20 vials, 10 mL each or equivalent]).	Seizures caused by isoniazid or *Gyromitra* mushrooms; ethylene glycol (investigational).	IV	Isoniazid (INH): *Unknown amount ingested:* 5 gm (70 mg/kg) in 50 mL of D5W over 5 min with diazepam 0.3 mg/kg IV at rate of 1 mg/min in child or 10 mg per dose at rate up to 5 mg/min in adults. Use different site (synergism). May repeat q 5–20 min until seizure controlled. Up to 375 mg/kg has been given (52 gm). *Known amount ingested:* 1 gm for each gram of INH ingested over 5 min with diazepam (dose above). *Gyromitra* mushrooms: 25 mg/kg for child or 2–5 gm for adult over 15–30 min to maximum of 20 gm.	After seizure is controlled, administer remainder of pyridoxine at 1 gm per 1 gm of INH or total 5 gm as infusion over 60 min. **AR:** Uncommon; do not administer in same bottle as sodium bicarbonate. For *Gyromitra* mushrooms, some use 25 mg/kg PO early when mushroom is suspected.
Sodium bicarbonate (NaHCO₃). Stock level to treat 70-kg adult for 24 h: 10 ampules or syringes (500 mEq).	Tricyclic antidepressant (TCA) cardiotoxicity (wide QRS >0.10 s, severe ventricular tachycardia, severe conduction disturbances); metabolic acidosis; phenothiazine cardiotoxicity.	IV	Ethylene glycol: 100 mg daily. 1–2 mEq/kg undiluted as a bolus. If no effect on cardiotoxicity, repeat twice a few minutes apart. An infusion of NaHCO₃ may follow to keep blood pH at 7.5–7.55 but not higher.	Monitor serum sodium and potassium and blood pH because fatal alkalemia and hypernatremia have been reported. Continuous infusion of bicarbonate by itself is of limited usefulness in setting of TCA intoxication because of delayed onset. Prophylactic NaHCO₃ has not been encouraged.
	Salicylate: To keep blood pH 7.5–7.55 (not >7.55) and urine pH 7.5–8.0. Alkalization is recommended if salicylate concentration >40 mg/dL in acute poisoning and at lower levels if symptomatic in chronic intoxication. 2 mEq/kg raises blood pH 0.2 unit.	IV	*Adult* with clear physical signs and laboratory findings of acute moderate or severe salicylism: bolus 1–2 mEq/kg followed by infusion of 100–150 mEq NaHCO₃ added to 1 L of 5% dextrose at rate of 200–300 mL/h. *Child:* Bolus same as for adult followed by 1–2 mEq/kg in infusion of 20 mL/kg/h 5% dextrose in 0.45% saline. Add potassium when patient voids. Rate and amount of the initial infusion, if patient is volume depleted: 1 h to achieve urine output of 2 mL/kg/h and urine pH of 7–8. In mild cases without acidosis and with urine pH of >6, administer 5% dextrose in 0.9% saline with 50 mEq/L or 1 mEq/kg NaHCO₃ as maintenance to replace ongoing renal losses. If acidemia and pH <7.2, add 2 mEq/kg as loading dose followed by 2 mEq/kg q 3–4 h to keep pH at 7.5–7.55. If acidemia, recommend isotonic NaHCO₃, three ampules to 1 L of D5W at 10–15 mL/kg/h or sufficient to produce normal urine flow and a urine pH of 7.5 or higher.	Monitor both urine pH and blood pH. Do not use urine pH alone to assess the need for alkalization because of the paradoxical aciduria that may occur. Adjust the urine pH to 7.5–8 by NaHCO₃ infusion. After urine output established, add potassium, 40 mEq/L.
	Long-acting barbiturates: phenobarbital, mephobarbital (Mebaral), metharbital (Gemonil); primidone (Mysoline). Note: Alkalization is not effective for the shorter- and intermediate-acting barbiturates.	IV	2 mEq/kg during the first hour or 100 mEq in 1 L of D5W with 40 mEq/L potassium at rate of 100 mL/h in adults. Adequate potassium is necessary to accomplish alkalization.	Additional NaHCO₃ and potassium chloride may be needed. Adjust the urine pH to 7.5–8 by NaHCO₃ infusion.

Abbreviations: BP = blood pressure; D5W = 5% dextrose in water; ET = by endotracheal route; INH = isoniazid; PCP = phencyclidine; PCC = poison control center; rpm = respirations per minute; USP = U.S. Pharmacopeia.

TABLE 11. Considerations for Hemodialysis or Hemoperfusion

Serious Ingestions

Immediately notify the nephrologist. Compounds that are ingested in potentially lethal doses in which rapid removal may improve the prognosis include

Amatoxins from *Amanita phalloides* mushroom: any amount with symptoms
Arsenic trioxide: 120 mg in adults
Ethylene glycol: 1.4 mL/kg 100% solution or equivalent
Methanol: 6 mL/kg 100% solution or equivalent
Paraquat: 1.5 gm in adults
Diquat: 1.5 gm in adults
Mercuric chloride: 1.0 gm in adults

Dialyzable Substances

Alcohol*	Isoniazid
Ammonia	Lithium*
Amphetamines	Meprobamate
Anilines	Paraldehyde
Antibiotics	Potassium*
Barbiturates (long-acting)*	Procainamide
Boric acid	Quinidine
Bromides*	Quinine*
Calcium	Salicylates*
Chloral hydrate*	Strychnine
Fluorides	Thiocyanates
Iodides	

Nondialyzable Substances

Anticholinergics	Glutethimide
Antidepressants (cyclic and MAOIs)	Hallucinogens
	Methyprylon (Noludar)†
Barbiturates (short-acting)	Methaqualone†
Benzodiazepines	Opioids including heroin
Digitalis and related drugs	Phenothiazines
Ethchlorvynol	Phenytoin

*Most useful.
†Controversial.

preferably less than 350); (2) a Vd of less than 1 liter per kg; (3) low PB (less than 50%); (4) high water solubility (low lipid solubility); and (5) high plasma concentration and a toxicity that correlates reasonably with the plasma concentration (Tables 11 and 12).

Hemodialysis also has a role in correcting disturbances that are not amenable to appropriate medical management. These are easily remembered by the "vowel" mnemonic:

A = refractory acid-base disturbances
E = refractory electrolyte disturbances
I = intoxication with dialyzable substances (see Tables 11 and 12)
O = overhydration
U = uremia (renal failure)

Complications of dialysis include hemorrhage, thrombosis, air embolism, hypotension, infections, electrolyte imbalance, thrombocytopenia, and removal of therapeutic medications.

Hemoperfusion

Hemoperfusion is the parenteral form of oral AC therapy. Heparinization is necessary. The patient's blood is routed extracorporeally through an outflow arterial catheter and then through a filter-adsorbing cartridge (charcoal or resin) and returned through a venous catheter. High flow rates (e.g., 300 mL per minute) through the filter are used to maximize the efficient use of the filter. Cartridges must be changed every 4 hours. Blood glucose, electrolytes, calcium, albumin, complete blood cell count (CBC), platelets,

TABLE 12. Plasma Drug Concentrations Above Which Removal by Extracorporeal Measures May Be Indicated*

Drug	Plasma Concentration	Protein Binding (%)	Vd (L/kg)	Method of Choice
Amanitine	Not available	25	1.0	HP
Ethanol	500–700 mg/dL	0	0.3	HD
Ethchlorvynol	150 µg/mL	35–50	3–4	HP
Ethylene glycol	25–50 µg/mL	0	0.6	HD
Glutethimide	100 µg/mL	50	2.7	HP
Isopropyl alcohol	400 mg/dL	0	0.7	HD
Lithium	4 mEq/L	0	0.7	HD
Meprobamate	100 µg/mL	0	NA	HP
Methanol	50 mg/dL	0	0.7	HD
Methaqualone	40 µg/dL	20–60	6.0	HP
Other barbiturates	50 µg/dL	50	0–1	HP
Paraquat	0.1 mg/dL	Poor	2.8	HP>HD
Phenobarbital	100 µg/dL	50	0.9	HP>HD
Salicylates	80–100 mg/dL	90	0.2	HD>HP
Theophylline		0	0.5	
Chronic	40–60 µg/mL			HP
Acute	80–100 µg/mL			HP
Trichloroethanol	250 µg/mL	70	0.6	HP

*In mixed or chronic drug overdoses, extracorporeal measures may be considered at lower drug concentrations.
Abbreviations: HP = hemoperfusion; HD = hemodialysis; HP>HD = hemoperfusion preferred over hemodialysis.
Modified from Winchester JF: Active methods for detoxification. *In* Haddad LM, Winchester JF (eds): Clinical Management of Poisoning and Drug Overdose, 2nd ed. Philadelphia, WB Saunders Co, 1990, pp 148–167; Balsam L, Cortitsidis GN, Fienfeld DA: Role of hemodialysis and hemoperfusion in the treatment of intoxications. Contemp Manage Crit Care 61–71, 1990.

and serum and urine osmolarity must be carefully monitored. This procedure has extended extracorporeal removal to a large range of substances that were formerly either poorly dialyzable or nondialyzable. It is not limited by molecular weight, water solubility, or protein binding. However, hemoperfusion is limited by a Vd greater than 400 liters, by plasma concentration, and by rate of flow through the filter. AC cartridges are used primarily for hemoperfusion in the United States. Analysis of studies using hemodialysis and hemoperfusion indicates that use of these techniques does not reduce morbidity or mortality substantially except in certain cases (e.g., with theophylline). Hemoperfusion may be recommended in combination with hemodialysis (e.g., for paraquat, electrolyte disturbances).

The contraindications are similar to those for hemodialysis.

The patient-related criteria for use of hemoperfusion are (1) anticipated prolonged coma and the likelihood of complications, (2) laboratory confirmation of lethal blood concentrations, (3) lethal-dose poisoning with an agent with delayed toxicity or known to be metabolized into a more toxic metabolite, and (4) hepatic impairment when an agent is metabolized by the liver and there is clinical deterioration despite optimal supportive medical management.

Limited data are available to determine which toxicities are best treated with hemoperfusion. However, hemoperfusion has proved useful in glutethimide intoxication, barbiturate overdose even with short-acting barbiturates (SABs), carbamazepine, phenytoin, theophylline, and chlorophenothane (DDT). See Tables 11 and 12.

Complications include hemorrhage, thrombocytopenia, hypotension, infection, leukopenia, depressed phagocytic activity of granulocytes, decreased immunoglobulin levels, hypoglycemia, hypothermia, hypocalcemia, pulmonary edema, and air and charcoal embolism.

Plasmapheresis

Plasmapheresis consists of removal of a volume of blood. All the extracted components are returned to the blood except the plasma, which is replaced with a colloidal protein solution. Clinical data related to guidelines and efficacy in toxicology are limited.

Supportive Care, Observation, and Therapy of Complications

The Comatose Patient or Patient with Altered Mental Status

If airway protective reflexes are absent, endotracheal intubation is indicated. If respirations are ineffective, ventilation with 100% oxygen is instituted. If a cyanotic patient fails to respond to oxygen, the presence of methemoglobinemia should be suspected. A reagent strip test for blood glucose should be performed to detect hypoglycemia and the specimen sent to the laboratory for confirmation.

Glucose. Glucose is administered if the glucose reagent strip visually reads less than 150 mg per dL. Venous rather than capillary blood should be used for the reagent strip if the patient is in shock or is hypotensive.

Hypoglycemia accompanies many poisonings, including those with ethanol (especially in children), clonidine (Catapres), insulin, organophosphates, salicylates, sulfonylureas, and the fruit or seed of a Jamaican plant called akee. If hypoglycemia is present or suspected, glucose is administered immediately as an intravenous bolus in the following doses: for a neonate, 10% glucose (5 mL per kg); for a child, 25% glucose at 0.25 gram per kg (2 mL per kg); and for an adult, 50% glucose at 0.5 gram per kg (1 mL per kg).

Thiamine. This agent is administered to avoid precipitating thiamine deficiency encephalopathy (Wernicke-Korsakoff syndrome) in alcohol abusers and in malnourished patients. The overall incidence of thiamine deficiency in ethanol abusers is 12%. Thiamine at 100 mg intravenously (IV) should be administered around the time of the glucose administration but not necessarily before the glucose, because it is more important to correct the hypoglycemia. The clinician should be prepared to manage anaphylaxis associated with thiamine allergy, but it is extremely rare.

Naloxone. This agent reverses CNS and respiratory depression, miosis, bradycardia, and decreased GI peristalsis caused by opioids acting through mu, kappa, and delta receptors.

In suspected overdose in a child younger than 5 years, naloxone is administered IV in a dose of 0.1 mg per kg up to 2 mg; in older children and adults, 2 mg should be administered every 2 minutes for 5 doses up to a total of 10 mg. Naloxone can also be administered into an endotracheal tube. If there is no response after 10 mg has been given, pure opioid intoxication is unlikely. If opioid abuse is suspected, restraints should be in place before the administration of naloxone, and it is recommended that the initial dose be 0.1 to 0.2 mg to avoid withdrawal and violent behavior. The initial dose is then doubled every minute progressively to a total of 10 mg. Naloxone may unmask concomitant sympathomimetic intoxication as well as withdrawal.

Larger doses of naloxone may be required for more poorly antagonized synthetic opioid drugs: buprenorphine (Buprenex), codeine, dextromethorphan, fentanyl, pentazocine (Talwin), propoxyphene (Darvon), diphenoxylate, nalbuphine (Nubain), new potent "designer" drugs, or long-acting opioids such as methadone.

Indications for a continuous infusion include a second dose for recurrent respiratory depression, exposure to poorly antagonized opioids, a large overdose, and decreased opioid metabolism (e.g., in impaired liver function). A continuous infusion has been advocated because many opioids outlast the short half-life ($t_{1/2}$) of naloxone (30 to 60 minutes). The naloxone infusion hourly rate is equal to the effective dose required to produce a response (improvement in ventilation and arousal). An additional dose may be required in 15 to 30 minutes as a bolus. The infusions are titrated to avoid respiratory depression and manifestations of opioid withdrawal. Tapering of infusions can be attempted after 12 hours and when the patient's condition has been stabilized.

Complications: Although naloxone is safe and effective, there are rare reports (in less than 1% of cases) of complications of pulmonary edema, seizures, hypertension, cardiac arrest, and sudden death.

Agents Whose Role Is Not Clarified

Nalmefene (Revex). This long-acting parenteral opioid antagonist, approved by the FDA, is undergoing investigation, but its role for comatose patients and in opioid overdose is not clear. It is 16 times more potent than naloxone, and its duration of action is up to 8 hours ($t_{1/2}$ of 10.8 hours, in comparison with 1 hour for naloxone).

Flumazenil (Romazicon). This agent is a pure competitive benzodiazepine (BZP) antagonist. It has been demonstrated to be safe and effective for BZP-induced sedation. It is not recommended for improving ventilation. Its role in CNS depression needs to be clarified. It should not be used routinely for comatose patients and is not an essential ingredient of the coma therapeutic regimen. It is contraindicated in cyclic antidepressant intoxications, in stimulant overdose, in long-term BZP use (may precipitate life-threatening withdrawal), if BZPs are used to control seizures, and in head trauma. There have been reports of seizures, dysrhythmias, and death in the contraindicated scenarios.

Laboratory and Radiographic Studies

Initial studies should include an ECG to assess for dysrhythmias or conduction delays (resulting from cardiotoxic medications); a chest radiograph, for aspiration pneumonia (if there is a history of loss of consciousness, unarousable state, vomiting) or noncardiac pulmonary edema; and measurement of electrolyte and glucose concentrations in the blood. The anion gap (AG) should be calculated, and acid-base and ABG profiles (if the patient has respiratory distress or altered mental status) and serum osmolality assay should be obtained. See Table 13 for appropriate testing on the basis of clinical toxicologic presentation. All laboratory specimens should be carefully labeled, timed, and dated. For potential legal cases, a "chain of custody" must be established. Assessment of the laboratory studies may give a clue to the etiologic agent.

Electrolyte, Acid-Base, and Osmolality Disturbances

Electrolyte and acid-base disturbances are evaluated and corrected. Metabolic acidosis (low pH with a low $PaCO_2$ and low HCO_3^-) with an increased AG is seen with many agents in overdose.

Metabolic Acidosis and the Anion Gap. The AG

TABLE 13. Patient Condition/Systemic Toxin and Appropriate Tests

Condition/Toxin	Tests
Comatose	Toxicologic tests (acetaminophen, sedative hypnotic, ethanol, opioids, benzodiazepines)
	Glucose, ammonia, CT, CSF analysis
Respiratory toxin	Spirometry, ABGs, chest radiography, monitor O_2 saturation
Cardiac toxin	ECG 12-lead and monitoring, echocardiogram, serial cardiac enzymes, hemodynamic monitoring
Hepatic toxin	Enzymes (AST, ALT, GGT), ammonia, albumin, bilirubin, glucose, PT, APTT, amylase
Nephrotoxin	BUN, creatinine, electrolytes (Na^+, K^+, Mg^{2+}, Ca^{2+}, PO_4^{3-}), serum and urine osmolarity, 24-h urine for heavy metals, CK, serum and urine myoglobin, urinalysis, and urinary sodium
Bleeding	Platelets, PT, APTT, bleeding time, fibrin split products, fibrinogen type and match blood

Abbreviations: ALT = alanine aminotransferase; AST = aspartate aminotransferase; CSF = cerebrospinal fluid; CT = computed tomography; GGT = γ-glutamyltransferase; PT = prothrombin time; APTT = activated partial thromboplastin time; ABGs = arterial blood gases.

is an estimate of the anions other than chloride and HCO_3^- necessary to counterbalance the positive charge of sodium. The AG gives a clue to the underlying disorder, compensation, and complications.

The AG is calculated from the standard serum electrolytes by subtracting the total carbon dioxide (which reflects the actual measured HCO_3^-) and chloride from the sodium: $Na^+ - (Cl^- + HCO_3^-) = AG$. Potassium is usually not used in the calculation because it may be hemolyzed and is an intracellular cation. The lack of an AG disturbance does not exclude a toxic basis for the disorder.

The normal gap was found to be 8 to 12 mEq per liter by flame photometry. However, a lower normal AG of 7 ± 4 mEq per liter has been determined by newer techniques (e.g., use of ion-selective electrodes or coulometric titration). Some studies have found the AG to be relatively insensitive for determining the presence of toxins.

It is important to recognize the AG toxins salicylates, methanol, and ethylene glycol because they have specific antidotes, and hemodialysis is effective in management.

A list of the potential causes of increased AG, decreased AG, or no change in AG is shown in Table 14. The most common cause of a decreased AG is laboratory error. Lactic acidosis produces the largest AG and can result from any poisoning that causes hypoxia, hypoglycemia, or convulsions.

Other blood chemistry derangements that suggest certain intoxications are shown in Table 15.

Serum Osmolal Gaps. The serum *osmolality* is a measure of the number of molecules of solute per kilogram of solvent, or mOsm per kg of water. The

TABLE 14. **Potential Causes of Metabolic Acidosis**

No Gap, Hyperchloremic	Increased Gap, Normochloremic	Decreased Gap
Acidifying agents	Methanol	Laboratory error†
Adrenal insufficiency	Uremia*	Intoxication (bromine, lithium)
Anhydrase inhibitors	Diabetic ketoacidosis*	Protein abnormal
Fistula	Paraldehyde,* phenformin	Sodium low
Osteotomies	Isoniazid	
Obstructive uropathies	Iron	
Renal tubular acidosis	Lactic acidosis†	
Diarrhea, uncomplicated*	Ethanol,* ethylene glycol*	
Dilutional hyperchloremia	Salicylates, starvation, solvents	
Sulfamylon		

*Indicates hyperosmolar situation. Studies have found that the anion gap may be relatively insensitive for determining the presence of toxins.

†Lactic acidosis caused by carbon monoxide, cyanide, hydrogen sulfide, hypoxia, ibuprofen, iron, isoniazid, ischemia, phenformin, salicylates, seizures, or theophylline.

osmolarity is solute per liter of solution, or mOsm per liter of water at a specified temperature. Osmolarity is usually a calculated value, and osmolality is usually a measured value. They are considered interchangeable when 1 liter equals 1 kilogram. The normal serum osmolality is 280 to 290 mOsm per kg. Serum for the freezing point osmolarity measurement and serum electrolyte specimens for calculation should be drawn simultaneously.

The serum osmolal gap is defined as the difference between the measured osmolality determined by the freezing point method and the calculated osmolarity determined as follows: the serum sodium value multiplied by 2 plus the BUN divided by 3 (0.1 molecular weight [MW] of BUN), plus the blood glucose value divided by 20 (0.1 MW of glucose). This gap estimate is usually within 10 mOsm of the simultaneously measured serum osmolality. Ethanol, if present, may be included in the equation to eliminate its influence on the osmolality; the ethanol concentration divided by 4.6 (0.1 of ethanol MW) is added to the equation. See Table 16.

Calculated mOsm =

$$2Na^+ + \frac{BUN\ (mg/dL)}{3} + \frac{blood\ glucose\ (mg/dL)}{20} + \frac{ethanol\ (mg/dL)}{4.6}$$

The osmolal gap is valid for a hemodynamically intact individual; it is not valid in shock and the postmortem state. Metabolic disorders such as hyperglycemia, uremia, and dehydration increase the osmolarity but usually do not cause gaps greater than 10 mOsm per kg.

A gap greater than 10 mOsm per kg suggests that unidentified osmolal-acting substances are present: acetone, ethanol, ethylene glycol, ethchlorvynol, glycerin, isopropyl alcohol, isoniazid, ethanol, mannitol, methanol, NaHCO$_3$ (1 mEq per kg raises osmolality by 2 mOsm per liter), and trichloroethane. Assessment for alcohol and glycol ingestion should be made when the degree of obtundation exceeds that expected from the blood ethanol concentration (BEC) or when other clinical conditions exist, such as visual loss (methanol), metabolic acidosis (methanol and ethylene glycol), and renal failure (ethylene glycol).

A falsely elevated osmolal gap may be produced by other low-molecular-weight un-ionized substances (acetone, dextran, dimethyl sulfoxide, diuretics, ethyl ether, mannitol, sorbitol, trichloroethane) or in conditions such as diabetic ketoacidosis, hyperlipidemia, and an excess of unmeasured electrolytes (e.g., magnesium).

False-negative results can occur when a normal osmolal gap is reported in the presence of alcohol or glycol poisoning if the parent compound is already metabolized—as, for example, when the osmolal gap is measured after a significant time has elapsed since ingestion. In alcohol and glycol intoxications, an early osmolar gap is due to the relatively nontoxic parent drug, and delayed metabolic acidosis and an increased AG are due to the more toxic metabolites.

TABLE 15. **Blood Chemistry Derangements in Toxicology**

Derangement	Toxin or Disease
Acetonemia without acidosis	Acetone or isopropyl alcohol
Hypomagnesemia	Ethanol, digitalis
Hypocalcemia	Ethylene glycol, oxalate, fluoride
Hyperkalemia	Beta blockers, acute digitalis, renal failure
Hypokalemia	Diuretics, salicylism, sympathomimetics, theophylline, corticosteroids, chronic digitalis
Hyperglycemia	Diazoxide, glucagon, iron, isoniazid, organophosphate insecticides, phenylurea insecticides, phenytoin, salicylates, sympathomimetic agents, thyroid vasopressors
Hypoglycemia	Beta blockers, ethanol, insulin, isoniazid, oral hypoglycemic agents, salicylates
Elevated CK	Amphetamines, ethanol, cocaine, phencyclidine
Elevated creatinine and normal BUN	Isopropyl alcohol, diabetic ketoacidosis

TABLE 16. **Alcohols and Glycols**

Alcohol or Glycol	1 mg/dL in Blood Raises Osmolality (mOsm/L) by	Molecular Weight	Conversion Factor*
Ethanol	0.228	40	4.6
Methanol	0.327	32	3.2
Ethylene glycol	0.190	62	6.2
Isopropanol	0.176	60	6.0
Acetone	0.182	58	5.8
Propylene glycol	Not available	72	7.2

*Example: Methanol osmolality: Subtract the calculated osmolarity from the measured serum osmolality (freezing point method) = osmolar gap × 3.2 (0.1 molecular weight) = estimated serum methanol concentration.

The serum concentration (mg per dL) =
    mOsm gap × MW of substance divided by 10.

See Table 16.

Radiographic Studies

Chest and neck radiographs are obtained to detect pathologic conditions such as aspiration pneumonia and pulmonary edema, for localization of foreign bodies, and to determine the location of the endotracheal tube.

Abdominal radiographs are obtained to detect radiopaque substances. A mnemonic for radiopaque substances seen on abdominal radiographs is CHIPES: chlorides and chloral hydrate; heavy metals (arsenic, barium, iron, lead, mercury, zinc); iodide; Play Doh, Pepto-Bismol, or phenothiazine (which does not always show up on an abdominal radiograph if already dissolved); enteric-coated tablets; sodium, potassium, and other elements in tablet form (bismuth, calcium, potassium) and solvents containing chlorides (e.g., carbon tetrachloride).

Toxicologic Studies

In the average toxicology laboratory, false-negative results occur at a rate of 10 to 30% and false-positive results at a rate of 0 to 10%.

The predictive value of a positive result is about 90%. A negative result of a toxicology screen does not exclude poisoning. The negative predictive value of toxicologic screening is about 70%. For example, the following BZPs may not be detected by routine screening tests for BZP: alprazolam (Xanax), clonazepam (Klonopin), temazepam (Restoril), and triazolam (Halcion).

The "toxic" urine screen is a qualitative urine test for several common drugs, usually substances of abuse (cocaine and metabolites, opioids, amphetamines, BZPs, barbiturates, phencyclidine). Results are usually available within 2 to 6 hours. Because these tests may vary in different hospitals and communities, the physician should determine exactly which substances are included in the toxic urine screen of the laboratory used.

The detection time is the number of days after intake of a substance during which a person would be expected to excrete detectable levels of the substance or metabolite in urine. In general, urine detection is possible for 1 to 3 days after cocaine exposure, 2 to 4 days after heroin (the presence of monoacetylmorphine is diagnostic of heroin use but is detectable for only 12 hours after use), and 2 to 4 days after phencyclidine; if use is chronic, the time is doubled.

COMMON POISONS

Acetaminophen (N-acetyl-p-aminophenol [APAP], Tylenol, called paracetamol in the United Kingdom). *Toxic mechanism:* Of therapeutic doses of APAP, less than 5% is metabolized by cytochrome P-450IIE1 to a toxic reactive oxidizing metabolite, N-acetyl-p-benzoquinonimine (NAPQI). In overdose, sufficient glutathione is not available to reduce the excess NAPQI into a nontoxic conjugate, and it forms covalent bonds with hepatic intracellular proteins to produce centrilobular necrosis and, by a similar mechanism, renal damage. *Toxic dose:* The therapeutic dosage is 10 to 15 mg per kg per dose with a maximum of 5 doses per 24 hours and a maximal total daily dose of 2.5 grams. The acute single toxic dose is greater than 140 mg per kg, possibly greater than 200 mg per kg in children. Factors affecting the cytochrome P-450 enzymes (enzyme inducers such as anticonvulsants [barbiturates, phenytoin], isoniazid, alcoholism) and factors that decrease glutathione stores (e.g., alcoholism, malnutrition, HIV infection) contribute to the toxicity of APAP. Patients with chronic alcoholism who ingest APAP at 3 to 4 grams per day for a few days can have depleted glutathione stores and require NAC therapy at blood APAP levels 50% below hepatotoxic levels on the nomogram (Figure 1). *Kinetics:* Onset of action occurs in 0.5 to 1 hour, the peak plasma concentration occurs in 20 to 90 minutes but usually 2 to 4 hours after an overdose, and the duration is 4 to 6 hours. The Vd is 0.9 liter per kg. PB is low, less than 50% (albumin); $t_{1/2}$ is 1 to 3 hours. The route of elimination is hepatic metabolism to an inactive nontoxic glucuronide conjugate and inactive nontoxic sulfate metabolite by two saturable pathways, and less than 5% is metabolized to the reactive metabolite NAPQI. In children younger than 6 years, metabolic elimination occurs to a greater degree by conjugation with the sulfate pathway, which may be hepatoprotective. *Manifestations:* The four phases of the intoxication's clinical course may overlap, and the absence of a phase does not exclude toxicity. Phase I occurs within 0.5 to 24 hours after ingestion and may consist of a few hours of malaise, diaphoresis, nausea, and vomiting, or there may be no symptoms. CNS depression or coma is not a feature. Phase II occurs 24 to 48 hours after ingestion and is a period of diminished symptoms. The liver enzymes AST (earliest) and ALT may increase as early as 4 hours or as late as 36 hours after ingestion. Phase III occurs in 48 to 96 hours, with peak liver function abnormalities at 72 to 96 hours. The degree of elevation of the hepatic enzyme values does not correlate with outcome. Recovery starts in about 4 days unless hepatic failure develops. Less than 1% of patients develop fulminant hepatotoxicity. Phase IV occurs in 4 to 14 days, with hepatic enzyme abnormalities reaching resolution. If extensive liver damage has occurred, sepsis and disseminated intra-

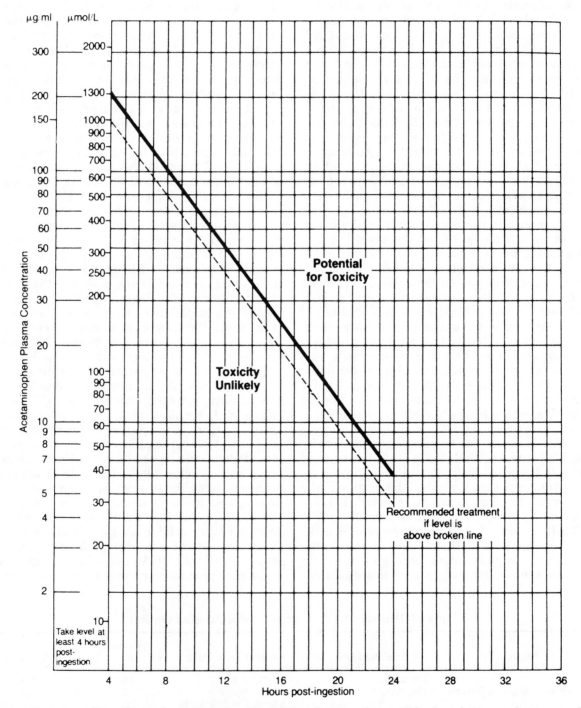

Figure 1. Nomogram for acetaminophen intoxication. Start *N*-acetylcysteine therapy if levels and time coordinates are above the lower line on the nomogram. Continue and complete therapy even if subsequent values fall below the toxic zone. The nomogram is useful only in acute, single ingestions. Levels in serum drawn before 4 hours may not represent peak levels. (From Rumack BH, Matthew H: Acetaminophen poisoning and toxicity. Reproduced by permission of Pediatrics, Vol 55, Page 871, Figure 2, Copyright 1975.)

vascular coagulation may ensue. Death can occur at 7 to 14 days. Transient renal failure may develop at 5 to 7 days with or without evidence of hepatic damage. Rare cases of myocarditis and pancreatitis have been reported.

Management: (1) For GI decontamination, emesis may be useful within 30 minutes. However, it may interfere with the retention of AC and NAC. Gastric lavage is not necessary if AC is administered early. Studies have indicated that AC is useful within 4 hours after ingestion. MDAC has not been well studied. AC does adsorb NAC if they are given together, but this is not clinically important. However, if AC must be given along with NAC, the administration of AC must be separated from that of NAC by 1 to 2 hours to avoid vomiting. Use of a saline sulfate cathartic in adults is recommended because it can enhance the activity of the sulfate metabolic pathway, which may be hepatoprotective. (2) NAC (Table 17; also see Table 10), a derivative of the amino acid cysteine, acts as a sulfhydryl donor for glutathione synthesis and may enhance the nontoxic sulfation pathway, resulting in conjugation of NAPQI. Oral NAC should be administered within the first 8 hours after a toxic amount of APAP has been ingested. NAC may be started while the results of the blood tests for the APC are awaited, but there is no advantage to giving it before 8 hours. If the APC at more than 4 hours after ingestion is above the lower line on the modified Rumack-Matthew nomogram (see Figure 1), the full 17-dose maintenance course should be continued. Repeated blood specimens should be obtained 4 hours after the initial level if it is greater than 20 μg per mL, because of unexpected delays in the peak caused by food and coingestants. An intravenous preparation (see Table 17) has been used in Europe and Canada since the late 1970s but is not approved in the United States (studies are in progress). There have been a few anaphylactoid reactions and deaths with the intravenous route. *Variations in NAC therapy:* (a) In patients with chronic alcoholism, it is recommended that NAC be administered at 50% below the lower toxic line on the nomogram. (b) If emesis occurs within 1 hour after NAC administration, the dose should be repeated. To help prevent emesis, the proper dilution from 20 to 5% NAC should be served in a palatable vehicle in a covered container with a straw. If this is unsuccessful, NAC should be administered through a nasogastric tube or a fluoroscopically placed nasoduodenal tube by a slow drip over 30 to 60 minutes. Antiemetics may be used if necessary: metoclopramide (Reglan) at 10 mg per dose IV a half-hour before NAC (in children, 0.1 mg per kg with a maximum of 0.5 mg per kg per day) or, as a last resort, ondansetron (Zofran) at 32 mg (0.15 mg per kg) by infusion over 15 minutes, repeated for 3 doses if necessary. The potential side effects of ondansetron are anaphylaxis and increases in liver enzyme values. (c) Some investigators recommend variable durations of NAC therapy, stopping the therapy if the APC becomes nondetectable in serial determinations and the liver enzymes (ALT and AST) remain normal after 36 hours. (d) Time of administration: There is a loss of efficacy if NAC is initiated more than 8 to 10 hours after ingestion, but the loss is not complete, and NAC may be initiated 36 or more hours after ingestion. Late treatment (after 24 hours) has been shown to decrease the rates of morbidity and mortality in fulminant liver failure caused by acetaminophen and other etiologic agents. (e) An extended-release caplet ("ER" is embossed on the caplet) contains 325 mg of immediate-release and 325 mg of delayed-release formulations. A single serum APAP determination 4 hours after ingestion can underestimate the dose because the extended-release formulation can yield secondary delayed peaks. In overdoses of extended-release formulation, it is recommended that additional APAP levels at 4-hour intervals after the initial level be obtained. If any peak is in the toxic zone, initiate therapy. (3) Pregnancy: It is recommended that pregnant patients with toxic plasma concentrations of APAP receive NAC therapy to prevent hepatotoxicity in both fetus and mother. The available data suggest no teratogenicity caused by NAC or APAP. (4) Chronic intoxication: Indications for NAC therapy are a history of ingestion of 3 to 4 grams for several days, elevated liver enzyme (AST and ALT) values, and chronic alcoholism or use of chronic enzyme inducers. (5) Specific support care may be needed to treat liver failure, pancreatitis, transient renal failure, and myocarditis. (6) Liver transplantation has a definite but limited role in acute APAP overdose. According to a retrospective analysis, a continuing rise in the prothrombin time (4-day peak: 180 seconds), pH less than 7.3 (2 days after overdose), serum creatinine level greater than 3.3 mg per dL, severe hepatic encephalopathy, and a disturbed coagulation factor VII/V ratio of more than 30% suggest a poor prognosis and may be indicators for hepa-

TABLE 17. **Protocol for *N*-Acetylcysteine Administration**

Route	Loading Dose	Maintenance Dose	Course Duration (h)	FDA Approval
Oral	140 mg/kg	70 mg/kg q 4 h	72	Yes
Intravenous—England, Canada	150 mg/kg over 15 min	50 mg/kg over 4 h followed by 100 mg/kg over 16 h	20	No
Intravenous—investigational in United States	140 mg/kg	70 mg/kg q 4 h	48	No

tology consultation for consideration of orthotopic liver transplantation (OLT). (7) Extracorporeal measures are not expected to be of benefit.

Laboratory investigations: The therapeutic reference range is 10 to 20 μg per mL. For toxic levels see the nomogram in Figure 1. Appropriate reliable methods for analysis are radioimmunoassay, high-performance liquid chromatography (HPLC), and gas chromatography. Spectroscopic assays often give falsely elevated values. Cross-reactions: Bilirubin, salicylate, salicylamide, diflunisal, phenols, and methyldopa increase the APAP level. Each 1 mg per dL increase in creatinine increases the APAP plasma level 30 μg per mL. Monitoring: If a toxic APAP level is present, monitor the liver profile (including AST, ALT, bilirubin, prothrombin time), serum amylase, blood glucose, CBC, platelet count, phosphate, electrolytes, bicarbonate, ECG, and urinalysis. *Disposition:* All cases of intentional ingestion require a serum APAP level obtained 4 hours or more after ingestion. Patients who ingest more than 140 mg per kg should receive therapy within 8 hours after ingestion or until the results of the APC determination 4 hours after ingestion are known.

Amphetamines (illicit methamphetamine ["ice"], diet pills, various trade names). *Analogues:* 3,4-methylenedioxymethamphetamine (MDMA; known as Ecstasy, XTC, Adam) and 3,4-methylenedioxyamphetamine (MDEA; known as Eve). Other similar stimulants are phenylpropanolamine and cocaine. *Toxic mechanism:* Amphetamines have a direct CNS stimulant effect and a sympathetic nervous system effect by releasing catecholamines from alpha- and beta-adrenergic nerve terminals but inhibiting their reuptake. Phenylpropanolamine stimulates only the beta-adrenergic receptors. *Toxic dose:* In children, 1 mg per kg dextroamphetamine; in adults, 5 mg per kg. A dose of 12 mg per kg has been reported to be lethal. *Kinetics:* Amphetamine is a weak base with a pK_a of 8 to 10. Onset of action is in 30 to 60 minutes. Peak effects occur at 2 to 4 hours. The $t_{1/2}$ is pH-dependent; it is 8 to 10 hours with acidic urine (pH less than 6.0) and 16 to 31 hours with alkaline urine (pH greater than 7.5). The Vd is 2 to 3 liters per kg. Elimination is 60% hepatic to a hydroxylated metabolite that may be responsible for psychotic effects. Excretion by the kidney is 30 to 40% at alkaline urine pH and 50 to 70% at acidic urine pH. *Manifestations:* Effects are seen within 30 to 60 minutes after ingestion. Restlessness, irritation and agitation, tremors and hyper-reflexia, and auditory and visual hallucinations occur. Dilated but reactive pupils, cardiac dysrhythmias (supraventricular and ventricular), tachycardia, and hyperpyrexia may precede seizures, convulsions, hypertension, paranoia, violence, intracranial hemorrhage, rhabdomyolysis, myoglobinuria, psychosis, and self-destructive behavior. Paranoid psychosis and cerebral vasculitis occur with chronic abuse.

Management (similar to that for cocaine): (1) Provide supportive care: blood pressure and cardiac thermal monitoring and seizure precautions. Diazepam is also administered (see Table 10). (2) GI decontamination: Administer AC and MDAC. (3) Treat anxiety, agitation, and convulsions with diazepam. If diazepam fails to control seizures, use neuromuscular blockers and monitor the EEG for nonmotor seizures. Avoid neuroleptics (PTZs and butyrophenone), which can lower the seizure threshold. (4) Cardiovascular disturbances: Hypertension and tachycardia are usually transient and can be managed by titration of diazepam. Nitroprusside may be used for hypertensive crisis; use a maximal infusion rate of 10 μg per kg per minute for 10 minutes, followed by 0.3 to 2 μg per kg per minute. Myocardial ischemia is managed by oxygen, vascular access, BZPs, and nitroglycerin. Aspirin and thrombolysis are not routinely recommended because of the danger of intracranial hemorrhage. Delayed hypotension can be treated with fluids and vasopressors if needed. Life-threatening tachydysrhythmias may respond to an alpha blocker (e.g., phentolamine at 5 mg IV for adults and 0.1 mg per kg IV for children) and a short-acting beta blocker (esmolol at 500 μg per kg IV over 1 minute for adults and 300 to 500 μg per kg IV over 1 minute for children). Ventricular dysrhythmias may respond to lidocaine or, in a severely hemodynamically compromised patient, immediate synchronized electrical cardioversion. (5) Treat rhabdomyolysis and myoglobinuria with fluids, alkaline diuresis, and diuretics. (6) Treat hyperthermia with external cooling and cool 100% humidified oxygen. (7) If focal neurologic symptoms are present, consider a diagnosis of a cerebrovascular accident and perform CT of the head. (8) Treat paranoid ideation and threatening behavior with rapid tranquilization. (9) Observe the patient for suicidal depression, which may follow intoxication and may require suicide precautions. (10) Extracorporeal measures are of no benefit.

Laboratory investigations: Monitoring: ECG and cardiac monitoring is instituted, and monitoring is also indicated for ABGs and oxygen saturation, electrolytes, blood glucose, BUN, creatinine, creatine kinase and cardiac fraction (if there is chest pain), and liver profile; evaluate for rhabdomyolysis, and check urine for myoglobin, cocaine and metabolites, and other substances of abuse. The peak plasma concentration is 10 to 50 ng per mL 1 to 2 hours after ingestion of 10 to 25 mg. The toxic plasma concentration is 200 ng per mL. Cross-reactions occur with amphetamine derivatives (e.g., methylenedioxyamphetamine derivative [MDMA], Ecstasy), brompheniramine, chlorpromazine, ephedrine, phenylpropanolamine, phentermine, phenmetrazine, ranitidine, and Vicks Inhaler (L-desoxyephedrine) and may give false-positive results. *Disposition:* Symptomatic patients should be observed in a monitored unit until the symptoms resolve and then observed for a short time after resolution for relapse.

Anticholinergic Agents. Drugs with anticholinergic properties include antihistamines (H₁ blockers); neuroleptics (PTZs); tricyclic antidepressants; antiparkinsonism drugs (trihexyphenidyl [Artane], benztropine [Cogentin]); over-the-counter sleep, cold, and hay fever medicines (methapyrilene); ophthalmic products (atropine); products of common plants including jimsonweed *(Datura stramonium)*, deadly nightshade *(Atropa belladonna)*, and henbane *(Hyoscyamus niger)*; and antispasmodic agents for the bowel (atropine derivatives). *Toxic mechanism:* By competitive inhibition, anticholinergic agents block the action of acetylcholine on postsynaptic cholinergic receptor sites. The mechanism involves primarily the peripheral and CNS muscarinic receptors. *Toxic dose:* Toxic amounts of atropine are 0.05 mg per kg in children and greater than 2 mg in adults. The minimal estimated lethal dose of atropine is greater than 10 mg in adults and greater than 2 mg in 2-year-old children. Other synthetic anticholinergic agents are less toxic, the fatal dose varying from 10 to 100 mg. *Kinetics:* The onset of action with intravenous administration occurs in 2 to 4 minutes; peak effects on salivation after an intravenous or intramuscular dose occur in 30 to 60 minutes. The onset after ingestion is in 30 to 60 minutes, peak action occurs in 1 to 3 hours, and the duration is 4 to 6 hours, but symptoms are prolonged with overdose or sustained-release preparations. *Manifestations:* Anticholinergic signs: hyperpyrexia ("hot as a hare"), mydriasis ("blind as a bat"), flushing of skin ("red as a beet"), dry mucosa and skin ("dry as a bone"), "Lilliputian-type" hallucinations and delirium ("mad as a hatter"), coma, dysphagia, tachycardia, moderate hypertension, and, in rare instances, convulsions and urine retention.

Management: (1) If respiratory failure occurs, use intubation and assisted ventilation. (2) For GI decontamination, emesis should be avoided in a patient with diphenhydramine overdose because of rapid onset of action and the possibility of seizures. Use AC if bowel sounds are present; MDAC is not recommended. (3) Control seizures with BZPs (diazepam or lorazepam). (4) Use of physostigmine (see Table 10) is not routine and is reserved for reversal of life-threatening anticholinergic effects refractory to conventional treatments. This drug should be administered with adequate monitoring and resuscitative equipment available; it should be avoided if a tricyclic antidepressant is present in the patient's system. (5) Relieve urine retention by catheterization to avoid reabsorption. (6) If cardiac dysrhythmias are present, treat supraventricular tachycardia only if the patient is unstable. Control ventricular dysrhythmias with lidocaine or cardioversion. (7) Control hyperpyrexia by external cooling. (8) Hemodialysis and hemoperfusion are not effective.

Laboratory investigations: These include ABGs (in respiratory depression), electrolytes, glucose, and ECG monitoring. Anticholinergic drugs and plants having anticholinergic effects are not routinely included in screens for substances of abuse. *Disposition:* Symptomatic patients should be observed in a monitored unit until the symptoms resolve and then observed for a short time after resolution for relapse.

Antihistamines (H$_1$-receptor antagonists). Antihistamines include the H$_1$-blocker "sedating anticholinergic" type. A single adult dose includes the following:

1. Ethanolamines: diphenhydramine (Benadryl), 25 to 50 mg (1 mg per kg in a child); dimenhydrinate (Dramamine), 50 mg; and clemastine (Tavist), 1.34 to 2.68 mg.
2. Ethylenediamines: tripelennamine (Pyribenzamine), 25 to 50 mg (1 mg per kg in a child).
3. Alkylamines: chlorpheniramine (Chlor-Trimeton), 4 to 8 mg (0.9 mg per kg in a child), and brompheniramine (Dimetane), 4 to 8 mg (0.125 mg per kg in a child).
4. Piperazines: cyclizine (Marezine), 50 mg; hydroxyzine (Atarax), 50 to 100 mg (0.6 mg per kg in a child); and meclizine (Antivert), 50 to 100 mg.
5. Promethazine (Phenergan), 12.5 to 25 mg (0.1 mg per kg in a child).

THE H$_1$-BLOCKER SEDATING ANTIHISTAMINES. Many of these agents are used in combination with other medication, such as acetaminophen, aspirin, codeine, dextromethorphan, ephedrine, phenylephrine, phenylpropanolamine, and pseudoephedrine. *Toxic mechanism:* H$_1$ sedating-type antihistamines produce blockade of cholinergic muscarinic receptors (anticholinergic action) and depress or stimulate the CNS; in large overdoses, some have a cardiac membrane–depressant effect (e.g., diphenhydramine) and cause alpha-adrenergic receptor blockade (e.g., promethazine). *Toxic dose:* For diphenhydramine, the estimated toxic oral amount in a child is 15 mg per kg, and the potential lethal amount is 25 mg per kg. In an adult the potential lethal amount is 2.8 grams. Ingestion of five times the single dose of an antihistamine is toxic. *Kinetics:* Onset is in 15 to 30 minutes to 1 hour, peak effects occur in 1 to 4 hours; PB is 75 to 80%; Vd is 3.3 to 6.8 liters per kg; and t$_{1/2}$ is 3 to 10 hours. Elimination is 98% hepatic by *N*-demethylation. Interactions with erythromycin, ketoconazole (Nizoral), and derivatives produce excessive blood levels and ventricular dysrhythmias. *Manifestations:* Exaggerated anticholinergic effects, jaundice (cyproheptadine), coma, seizures, dystonia (diphenhydramine), rhabdomyolysis (doxylamine), and, with large doses, cardiotoxic effects (diphenhydramine) may be seen. *Management and disposition* (see "Anticholinergic Agents"): NaHCO$_3$ at 1 to 2 mEq per kg IV may be useful for myocardial depression and QRS prolongation.

THE NONSEDATING SINGLE-DAILY-DOSE ANTIHISTAMINES. Single adult doses include loratadine (Claritin), 10 mg; and fexofenadine (Allegra), 60 mg. *Toxic mechanism:* These agents produce peripheral H$_1$ blockade and do not possess anticholinergic and sedating actions. They can produce prolonged QT intervals and torsades de pointes if blood levels are elevated because of impaired hepatic function or interactions with enzyme-inhibiting drugs (cimetidine, ketoconazole and derivatives, or macrolide antibiotics). Loratadine and fexofenadine have not been reported to have these drug interactions. *Toxic dose:*

An adult with an overdose of 3360 mg of terfenadine developed ventricular tachycardia and fibrillation that responded to lidocaine and defibrillation; a 1500-mg overdose produced hypotension. Cases of delayed serious dysrhythmias (torsades de pointes) have been reported with more than 200 mg of astemizole. *Kinetics:* Onset occurs in 1 hour, peak effects occur in 4 to 6 hours, and duration is greater than 24 hours. These drugs are more than 90% protein bound. Plasma $t_{1/2}$ is 3.5 hours. Metabolism is in the GI tract and liver. Only 1% is excreted unchanged, 60% in feces and 40% in urine. The chemical structure of these medications prevents entry into the CNS. *Manifestations:* Overdose produces headache, nausea, confusion, and serious dysrhythmias (e.g., torsades de pointes). *Management:* (1) Obtain an ECG and establish cardiac monitoring. Treat dysrhythmias with standard agents. Torsades de pointes is best treated with magnesium sulfate at 4 grams or 40 mL of a 10% solution given IV over 10 to 20 minutes (see Table 10) and countershock if the patient fails to respond. (2) GI decontamination with AC is advised. *Disposition:* All children who ingest nonsedating antihistamines and adults who ingest more than the therapeutic maximal dose require close cardiac monitoring for torsades de pointes for at least 24 hours. Patients receiving concurrent macrolide antibiotics or ketoconazole should not continue to take these while receiving terfenadine or astemizole. Medical evaluation is required for chronic use of this combination.

Barbiturates. Barbiturates are used as sedatives, anesthetic agents, and anticonvulsants. *Toxic mechanism:* Barbiturates are GABA agonists (they increase chloride flow and inhibit depolarization). They enhance the CNS depressant effect and depress the cardiovascular system. *Toxic dose:* (1) The SABs (including the intermediate-acting agents) and their hypnotic doses are amobarbital (Amytal), 100 to 200 mg; aprobarbital (Alurate), 50 to 100 mg; butabarbital (Butisol), 50 to 100 mg; butalbital (Sandoptal), 100 to 200 mg; pentobarbital (Nembutal), 100 to 200 mg; and secobarbital (Seconal), 100 to 200 mg. They cause toxicity at lower doses than do longer-acting barbiturates (LABs) and the minimal toxic dose is 6 mg per kg; the fatal adult dose is 3 to 6 grams. (2) The LABs include mephobarbital (Mebaral), 50 to 100 mg, and phenobarbital (Luminal), 100 to 200 mg. The minimal toxic dose of these agents is greater than 10 mg per kg; the fatal adult dose is 6 to 10 grams. A general rule is that an amount 5 times the hypnotic dose is toxic and 10 times the hypnotic dose is potentially fatal. Methohexital and thiopental are ultra–short-acting (USA) parenteral preparations and are not discussed in detail here. *Kinetics:* Barbiturates are enzyme inducers. (1) SABs are highly lipid soluble, penetrate the brain readily, and have shorter elimination times. Onset is in 10 to 30 minutes, the peak occurs in 1 to 2 hours, the duration is 3 to 8 hours. The Vd is 0.8 to 1.5 liters per kg. The pK_a is about 8. Mean $t_{1/2}$ varies from 8 to 48 hours. (2) LABs have longer elimination times and may be used as anticonvulsants. Onset is in 20 to 60 minutes, the peak occurs in 1 to 6 hours or, in an overdose, 10 hours, and the duration is greater than 8 to 12 hours. The Vd is 0.8 liter per kg. The pK_a of phenobarbital is 7.2, and alkalization of urine promotes its excretion. The $t_{1/2}$ is 11 to 120 hours. *Manifestations:* In mild intoxication, the initial symptoms resemble those of alcohol intoxication and include ataxia, slurred speech, and depressed cognition. Severe intoxication causes slow respirations, coma, and loss of reflexes (except pupillary light reflex). Hypotension (venodilatation), hypothermia, and hypoglycemia occur, and death is by respiratory arrest. Bullous skin lesions ("barb burns") over pressure points may be present. Barbiturates can precipitate an attack of acute intermittent porphyria. *Management:* (1) Establish and maintain the vital functions. Intense supportive care, including intubation and assisted ventilation, should dominate the management. All stuporous and comatose patients should have glucose, thiamine, and naloxone given IV and be admitted to the ICU. (2) GI decontamination: Avoid emesis, especially in SAB ingestions. AC followed by MDAC (0.5 gram per kg) every 2 to 4 hours, has been shown to reduce the serum $t_{1/2}$ of phenobarbital by 50%, but its effect on the clinical course is undetermined. (3) Fluid management: Administer fluids to correct dehydration and hypotension. Vasopressors may be necessary to correct severe hypotension, and hemodynamic monitoring may be needed. Observe carefully for signs of fluid overload. (4) Alkalization (ion trapping) is used for phenobarbital (pK_a 7.2) but not for SABs. $NaHCO_3$, 1 to 2 mEq per kg IV in 500 mL of 5% dextrose for adults or 10 to 15 mL per kg for children during the first hour, followed by sufficient bicarbonate to keep the urine pH at 7.5 to 8.0, enhances excretion of phenobarbital and shortens the $t_{1/2}$ by 50% (see Table 10). Diuresis is not advocated because of the danger of cerebral or pulmonary edema. (5) Hemodialysis shortens the $t_{1/2}$ to 8 to 14 hours and charcoal hemoperfusion shortens the $t_{1/2}$ to 6 to 8 hours. Both may be effective for LABs and SABs. If the patient does not respond to supportive measures or if the phenobarbital plasma concentration is greater than 150 μg per mL, both procedures may be tried to shorten the $t_{1/2}$. (6) Treat any bullae as local second-degree skin burns. (7) Treat hypothermia. *Laboratory investigations:* Most barbiturates are detected by routine drug screens and can be measured in most hospital laboratories. Monitor barbiturate levels, ABGs, and a toxicology screen, including acetaminophen and ethanol, glucose, electrolytes, BUN, creatinine, creatine kinase, and urine pH. Minimal toxic plasma levels are greater than 10 μg per mL for SABs and greater than 40 μg per mL for LABs. Fatal levels are 30 μg per mL for SABs and greater than 80 to 150 μg per mL for LABs. SABs and LABs can be detected in urine 24 to 72 hours after ingestion and LABs up to 7 days. *Disposition:* All comatose patients should be admitted to the ICU. Awake and oriented patients with an overdose of an SAB should be observed for at least 6 asymptomatic hours, and those with an overdose of an LAB, for at least 12 asymptomatic hours. In an intentional overdose, psychiatric clearance is needed before discharge. Chronic use can lead to tolerance, physical dependence, and withdrawal and necessitates follow-up.

Benzodiazepines. BZPs are used as anxiolytics, sedatives, and relaxants. *Toxic mechanism:* GABA agonists produce CNS depression and increase chloride flow, inhibiting depolarization. *Toxic dose:* In the elderly the therapeutic dose should be reduced by 50%. BZPs have an additive effect with other CNS depressants. (1) For long-acting BZPs ($t_{1/2}$ greater than 24 hours), the maximal therapeutic doses are chlordiazepoxide (Librium), 50 mg; clorazepate (Tranxene), 30 mg; clonazepam, 20 mg; diazepam (Valium), 10 mg (0.2 mg per kg for children); flurazepam (Dalmane), 30 mg; and prazepam (Centrax), 20 mg. (2) Short-acting BZPs ($t_{1/2}$ 10 to 24 hours) include alprazolam, 0.5 mg, and lorazepam, 4 mg or 0.05 mg per kg for children, which act similarly to the long-acting BZPs. (3) The BZPs that are ultra short acting ($t_{1/2}$ less than 10 hours) are more toxic and include temazepam, 30 mg; triazolam, 0.5 mg; midazolam, 0.2 mg per kg; and oxazepam (Serax), 30 mg. (4) In overdoses: Ingestions of 10 to 20 times the therapeutic dose (greater than 1500 mg of diazepam or 2000 mg of chlordiazepoxide) of long-acting BZPs have resulted in mild coma without respiratory depression. Fatalities are rare, and most patients recover within 24 to 36 hours after overdose with long- and short-acting BZPs. Asymptomatic patients who have taken nonintentional overdoses of less than five times the therapeutic dose may be observed. The USA BZP triazolam has produced respiratory arrest and coma within 1 hour after ingestion of 5 mg and death with ingestion of as little as 10 mg. Midazolam and diazepam administered by rapid intravenous injection have produced respiratory arrest. *Kinetics:* Onset of CNS depression is usually in 30 to 120 minutes, and the peak usually occurs within 1 to 3 hours with the oral route. The Vd is 0.26 to 6 liters per kg (for long-acting BZPs, 1.1 liter per kg). PB is 70 to 99%. *Manifestations:* Ataxia, slurred speech, and CNS depression may be seen. Deep coma leading to respiratory depression suggests the presence of short-acting BZPs or should prompt a search for other causes. *Management:* (1) GI decontamination: Emesis should be avoided. Gastric lavage (within 1 hour) and AC are advised if the ingestion was recent. (2) Supportive treatment should be provided, but intubation and assisted ventilation are rarely required. (3) Flumazenil (see Table 10) is a specific BZP receptor antagonist that blocks chloride flow and is an inhibitor of neurotransmitters. It reverses sedative effects of BZPs, zolpidem (Ambien), and endogenous BZPs associated with hepatic encephalopathy. It is not recommended for reversing BZP-induced hypoventilation. It should be used with caution in overdoses if there is possible BZP dependence (because it can precipitate life-threatening withdrawal), if a cyclic antidepressant is suspected, or if the patient has a known seizure disorder. *Laboratory investigations:* Most BZPs can be detected in urinary drug screens. Quantitative blood levels are not useful. The BZPs usually not detected in urinary screens include alprazolam, clonazepam, flunitrazepam,* lorazepam, lormetazepam,* midazolam, oxazepam, temazepam, and triazolam. BZPs may not be detected if the dose is less than 10 mg, elimination is rapid, or there are different or no metabolites. Cross-reactions occur with nonsteroidal anti-inflammatory drugs (NSAIDs) (tolmetin, naproxen, etodolac, and fenoprofen). *Disposition:* Comatose patients should be admitted to the ICU. If the overdose was intentional, psychiatric clearance is needed before discharge. Chronic use can lead to tolerance, physical dependence, and withdrawal.

Beta-Adrenergic Blockers (beta blockers). Beta blockers are used in the treatment of hypertension and a number of systemic and ophthalmic disorders. Lipid-soluble drugs have CNS effects, active metabolites, a longer duration of action, and interactions with other drugs (e.g., propranolol). Cardioselectivity is lost in overdoses. Intrinsic partial agonist agents (e.g., pindolol) may initially produce tachycardia and hypertension. A cardiac membrane–depressive effect (quinidine-like) occurs with overdose but not therapeutic doses (e.g., metoprolol, sotalol). The alpha-blocking effect is weak (e.g., labetalol). Properties of beta blockers include the factors listed in Table 18. *Toxic mechanism:* Beta blockers compete with the catecholamines for receptor sites and block receptor action in the bronchi and the vascular smooth muscle and myocardium. *Toxic dose:* Ingestions of more than twice the maximal recommended daily therapeutic dose are considered toxic (see Table 18). Ingestion of propranolol at 1 mg per kg by a child may produce hypoglycemia. Fatalities have been reported in adults who ingested 7.5 grams of metoprolol. The most toxic agent is sotalol, and the least toxic, atenolol. *Kinetics:* Regular release usually causes symptoms within 2 hours. Propranolol's onset of action is in 20 to 30 minutes; the peak is at 1 to 4 hours but may be delayed with coingestants and sustained-release preparations. The duration is 4 to 6 hours but may be 24 to 48 hours in overdoses and longer with the sustained-release type. With sustained-release preparations, the onset may be delayed 6 hours and the peak 12 to 16 hours; the duration may be 24 to 48 hours. The regular preparation with the longest $t_{1/2}$ is nadolol (12 to 24 hours) and with the shortest is esmolol (5 to 10 minutes). PB is variable, ranging from 5 to 93%. The Vd is 1 to 5.6 liters per kg. Atenolol, nadolol, and sotalol have enterohepatic recirculation. *Manifestations:* See toxic properties and Table 18. Lipid-soluble agents produce coma and seizures. Bradycardia and hypotension are the major clinical signs and may lead to cardiogenic shock. Intrinsic partial agonists may initially cause tachycardia and hypertension. Bronchospasm may occur in

---

*Not available in the United States.

TABLE 18. **Pharmacologic and Toxic Properties of Beta Blockers***

Name	Dose	Lipid Solubility	Intrinsic Sympatho-mimetic Activity (Partial Agonist)	Membrane-Stabilizing Effect	Cardiac Selectivity (Beta-Selective)	Alpha Blocker
Acebutolol (Sectral)	Maximum daily dose 800 mg, therapeutic plasma level 200–2000 ng/mL	Moderate	+	+	+	+
Alprenolol†	Maximum daily dose 800 mg, therapeutic plasma level 50–200 ng/mL	Moderate	2+	+	−	−
Atenolol (Tenormin)	Maximum daily dose 100 mg, therapeutic plasma level 200–500 ng/mL	Low	−	−	2+	−
Betaxolol (Kerlone)	Maximum daily dose 20 mg, therapeutic plasma level NA	Low	+	−	+	−
Carteolol (Cartrol)	Maximum daily dose 10 mg, therapeutic plasma level NA	No	+	−	−	−
Esmolol (Brevibloc) (class II antidysrhythmic, by intravenous route only)		Low	−	−	+	−
Labetalol (Trandate)	Maximum daily dose 800 mg, therapeutic plasma level 50–500 ng/mL	Low	+	±	−	+
Levobunolol (eye drops 0.25% and 0.5%)	Maximum daily dose 20 mg, therapeutic plasma level NA	No	−	−	−	−
Metoprolol (Lopressor)	Maximum daily dose 450 mg, therapeutic plasma level 50–100 ng/mL	Moderate	−	−	2+	−
Nadolol (Corgard)	Maximum daily dose 320 mg, therapeutic plasma level 20–400 ng/mL	Low	−	−	−	−
Oxprenolol†	Maximum daily dose 480 mg, therapeutic plasma level 80–100 ng/mL	Moderate	2+	+	−	−
Pindolol (Visken)	Maximum daily dose 60 mg, therapeutic plasma level 50–150 ng/mL	Moderate	3+	±	−	−
Propranolol (Inderal) (class II antidysrhythmic)	Maximum daily dose 360 mg, therapeutic plasma level 50–100 ng/mL	High	−	2+	−	−
Sotalol (Betapace) (class III antidysrhythmic)	Maximum daily dose 480 mg, therapeutic plasma level 500–4000 ng/mL	Low	−	−	−	−
Timolol (Blocadren)	Maximum daily dose 60 mg, therapeutic plasma level 5–10 ng/mL	Low	−	±	−	−

*− indicates no effect; + indicates mild effect; 2+ indicates moderate effect; 3+ indicates severe effect; ± indicates no effect or mild effect; NA indicates not available.
†Not available in the United States.

patients with reactive airway disease with any beta blocker because the selectivity is lost in overdoses. ECG changes include AV conduction delay and frank asystole. Membrane-depressant effects produce prolonged QRS and QT intervals, which may result in torsades de pointes. Sotalol produces a prolonged QT. Hypoglycemia (blocking of catecholamine counterregulatory mechanisms) and hyperkalemia may occur, especially in children.

Management: (1) Establish and maintain vital functions. Establish vascular access, obtain a baseline ECG, and institute continuous cardiac and blood pressure monitoring. Have a pacemaker available. Hypotension is treated with fluids initially, although it usually does not respond. Frequently, glucagon and cardiac pacing are needed. Cardiology consultation should be sought. (2) GI decontamination is done initially with AC and a single-dose cathartic. MDAC is recommended for symptomatic patients with ingestions of beta blockers with enterohepatic recirculation or of sustained-release preparations (no data). Gastric lavage is done at less than 1 hour after ingestion. If gastric lavage is done, use of prelavage atropine (0.02 mg per kg for a child and 0.5 mg for an adult) and cardiac monitoring is recommended. Whole-bowel irrigation should be considered in large overdoses with sustained-release preparations (although no studies have been done). (3) Cardiovascular disturbances: A cardiology consultation should be obtained. Class IA (procainamide, quinidine) and class III (bretylium) antidysrhythmic agents are not recommended. Bradycardia in asymptomatic, hemodynamically stable patients necessitates no therapy. It is not predictive of the future course. If the patient is unstable (has hypotension or high-degree AV block), use atropine (0.02 mg per kg up to 2 mg in adults), glucagon, and a pacemaker. In ventricular tachycardia, use overdrive pacing. A wide QRS interval may respond to NaHCO$_3$ (see Table 10). Torsades de pointes (associated with sotalol) may respond to magnesium sulfate (see Table 10) and overdrive pacing. Prophylactic magnesium for a prolonged QT interval has been suggested, but there are no supporting data. Do not use epinephrine, because an unopposed alpha effect may occur. Hypotension and myocardial depression are managed by correction of dysrhythmias, use of the Trendelenburg position, and administration of fluids, glucagon, and/or amrinone (Inocor). Hemodynamic monitoring may be needed to manage fluid therapy. Glucagon (see Table 10) is the initial drug of choice. It works through adenylate cyclase and bypasses catecholamine receptors, so it is not affected by beta blockers. It increases cardiac contractility and heart rate. It is given as an intravenous bolus of 5 to 10 mg* over 1 minute, followed by continuous infusion at 1 to 5 mg per hour (in children, 0.15 mg per kg followed by 0.05 to 0.1 mg per kg per hour). In large doses and in infusion therapy use D5W, sterile water, or saline as the diluent to reconstitute glucagon in place of the 0.2% phenol

diluent provided with some drugs. Effects are seen within minutes. Glucagon can be used with other agents such as amrinone. Amrinone inhibits the enzyme phosphodiesterase, which metabolizes cyclic adenosine monophosphate (AMP). A bolus of 0.15 to 2 mg per kg (0.15 to 0.4 mL per kg) is administered IV, followed by infusion of 5 to 10 µg per kg per minute. (4) Treat hypoglycemia with intravenous glucose and emergency hyperkalemia with calcium (avoid if digoxin is present), bicarbonate, and glucose. (5) Control convulsions with diazepam or phenobarbital. (6) If bronchospasm is present, give beta$_2$ nebulized bronchodilators and aminophylline. (7) Extraordinary measures include intra-aortic balloon pump support. (8) Extracorporeal measures: Hemodialysis for poisonings with atenolol, acebutalol, nadolol, and sotalol (low Vd, low PB) may be helpful, particularly with evidence of renal failure. It is not effective for intoxication with propranolol, metoprolol, or timolol. (9) Investigational: Prenalterol has successfully reversed both bradycardia and hypotension (it is not available in the United States).

Laboratory investigations: Measurement of blood levels is not readily available or useful. (For propranolol the toxic level is greater than 2 ng per mL.) Monitoring: ECG and cardiac monitoring is recommended, as well as monitoring of blood glucose and electrolytes, BUN and serum creatinine, and ABGs if respiratory symptoms are present. *Disposition:* Asymptomatic patients with a history of overdose require a baseline ECG and continuous cardiac monitoring for at least 6 hours with regular-release preparations and for 24 hours with sustained-release preparations. Symptomatic patients should be observed with cardiac monitoring for 24 hours. If seizures, abnormal rhythm, or vital signs indicate, the patient should be admitted to the ICU.

Calcium Channel Blockers. These agents are used in the treatment of effort angina, supraventricular tachycardia, and hypertension. *Toxic mechanism:* Calcium channel blockers reduce the influx of calcium through the slow channels in membranes of the myocardium, the AV nodes, and vascular smooth muscles, resulting in peripheral, systemic, and coronary vasodilatation; impaired cardiac conduction; and depression of cardiac contractility. All calcium channel blockers have vasodilatory action, but only bepridil, diltiazem, and verapamil depress myocardial contractility and cause AV block. *Toxic dose:* Any ingested amount greater than the maximum daily dose has the potential of being severely toxic. The maximum oral daily doses are as follows: for amlodipine (Norvasc), 10 mg; for bepridil (Vascor), 400 mg; for diltiazem (Cardizem), 360 mg (toxic dose greater than 2 grams), 6 mg per kg in children; for felodipine (Plendil), 10 mg; isradipine (DynaCirc), 20 mg; for nicardipine (Cardene), 120 mg; for nifedipine (Procardia), 120 mg, 0.9 mg per kg per day in children; for nimodipine (Nimotop), 360 mg; for nitrendipine (Baypress),* 80 mg; and for verapamil (Calan), 480

---

*Exceeds dosage recommended by the manufacturer.

*Not available in the United States.

mg, 4 to 8 mg per kg in children. *Kinetics:* Onset of action of regular-release preparations varies: for verapamil, 60 to 120 minutes; for nifedipine, 20 minutes; and for diltiazem, 15 minutes after ingestion. The peak effect is at 2 to 4 hours for verapamil, 60 to 90 minutes for nifedipine, and 30 to 60 minutes for diltiazem; however, the peak action may be delayed for 6 to 8 hours. The duration is up to 36 hours. With sustained-release preparations the onset is usually at 4 hours but may be delayed; the peak effect is at 12 to 24 hours; and concretions and prolonged toxicity can develop. The $t_{1/2}$ for hepatic elimination varies from 3 to 7 hours. The Vd varies from 3 to 7 liters per kg. *Manifestations:* Hypotension, bradycardia, and conduction disturbances occur 30 minutes to 5 hours after ingestion. A prolonged PR interval is an early and constant finding and may occur at therapeutic doses. Torsades de pointes has been reported. All degrees of blocks may occur and may be delayed 12 to 16 hours. Lactic acidosis may be present. Calcium channel blockers do not affect intraventricular conduction, so the QRS interval is usually not affected. Hypocalcemia is rarely present. Hyperglycemia may be present because of calcium-dependent insulin release. Mental status changes, headaches, seizures, hemiparesis, and CNS depression may occur. Calcium channel blockers may precipitate respiratory failure in patients with Duchenne's muscular dystrophy.

Management: (1) Establish and maintain vital functions. Obtain a baseline ECG, and institute continuous cardiac and blood pressure monitoring. A pacemaker should be available. Cardiology consultation should be sought. (2) GI decontamination: AC is recommended, and MDAC may be useful (no data are available). If a large sustained-release preparation is involved, MDAC for 48 to 72 hours and whole-bowel irrigation may be useful, but the effectiveness has not been investigated. (3) If the patient is symptomatic, immediate cardiology consultation should be obtained because a pacemaker and hemodynamic monitoring may be needed. (4) In the presence of heart block, atropine is rarely effective and isoproterenol may produce vasodilatation. Consider the use of a pacemaker early. (5) Treat hypotension and bradycardia with positioning, fluids, calcium gluconate or calcium chloride, glucagon, amrinone, and ventricular pacing. Calcium gluconate or calcium chloride (see Table 10): Avoid calcium salts if digoxin is present. Calcium usually reverses depressed myocardial contractility but may not reverse nodal depression or peripheral vasodilatation. Calcium chloride is used as a 10% solution at 0.1 to 0.2 mL per kg up to 10 mL in an adult, or calcium gluconate as a 10% solution at 0.3 to 0.4 mL per kg, up to 20 mL in an adult, administered IV over 5 to 10 minutes. Monitor for dysrhythmias, hypotension, and serum calcium. The aim is to increase the calcium value 4 mg per dL to a maximum of 13 mg per dL. The calcium response lasts 15 minutes, and repeated doses or a continuous calcium gluconate infusion (0.2 mL per kg per hour, up to a maximum of 10 mL per hour) may be neces-

sary. If calcium fails, try glucagon (see Table 10) for its positive inotropic or chronotropic effect or both. Amrinone, an inotropic agent, may reverse calcium channel blockers. The effective dose is 0.15 to 2 mg per kg (0.15 to 0.4 mL per kg) by intravenous bolus followed by infusion of 5 to 10 µg per kg per minute. (6) Hypotension: Fluids, norepinephrine, and epinephrine may be required for hypotension. Amrinone and glucagon have been tried alone and in combination. Dobutamine and dopamine are often ineffective. (7) Extracorporeal measures (e.g., hemodialysis and charcoal hemoperfusion) are not considered useful. (8) Patients receiving digitalis and calcium channel blockers run the risk of digitalis toxicity because calcium channel blockers increase digitalis levels. (9) Extraordinary measures such as the intra-aortic balloon pump and cardiopulmonary bypass have been used successfully. (10) Hyperglycemia does not necessitate insulin therapy.

Laboratory investigations: Specific drug levels are not easily available and are not useful. Monitor blood glucose, electrolytes, calcium, ABGs, pulse oximetry, creatinine, BUN, hemodynamics, ECG, and cardiac function. *Disposition:* With intoxications involving regular-release preparations, monitoring is indicated for at least 6 hours, and with those involving sustained-release preparations, for 24 hours after alleged ingestion. For patients with intentional overdose, psychiatric clearance is needed. Symptomatic patients should be admitted to the ICU.

Carbon Monoxide. CO is an odorless, colorless gas produced by incomplete combustion; it is an in vivo metabolic breakdown product of methylene chloride used in paint removers. *Toxic mechanism:* The affinity of CO for hemoglobin is 240 times greater than that of oxygen; it shifts the oxygen dissociation curve to the left, which impairs hemoglobin release of oxygen to tissues and inhibits the cytochrome oxidase system. *Toxic dose and manifestations:* See Table 19. CO exposure and manifestations: Exposure to 0.5% for a few minutes is lethal. Contrary to popular belief, the skin rarely turns cherry-red in the living patient. Sequelae correlate with the level of consciousness at presentation. ECG abnormalities may be noted. The creatine kinase level is often elevated; rhabdomyolysis and myoglobinuria may occur. The carboxyhemoglobin (COHb) level expresses as a percentage the extent to which CO has bound with the total hemoglobin. This may be misleading in the anemic patient. The patient's presentation is more reliable than the COHb level. In Table 19, the manifestations listed for each level are in addition to those already listed at the preceding level. Note that 0.01% = 100 parts per million (ppm). A level greater than 40% is usually associated with obvious intoxication. The COHb may not correlate reliably with the severity of the intoxication, and attempts to link symptoms to specific levels of COHb are frequently inaccurate. *Kinetics:* The natural metabolism of the body produces small amounts of COHb: less than 2% for nonsmokers and 5 to 9% for smokers. CO is rapidly absorbed through the lungs. The rate of absorption

TABLE 19. **Carbon Monoxide Exposure and Possible Manifestations**

CO in Atmosphere (%)	Duration of Exposure (h)	COHb Saturation (%)	Manifestations
<0.0035 (35 ppm)	Indefinite	3.5	None
0.005–0.01 (50–100 ppm)	Indefinite	5	Slight headache, decreased exercise tolerance
Up to 0.01 (100 ppm)	Indefinite	10	Slight headache, dyspnea on vigorous exertion; driving skills may be impaired
0.01–0.02 (100–200 ppm)	Indefinite	10–20	Dyspnea on moderate exertion; throbbing, temporal headache
0.02–0.03 (200–300 ppm)	5–6	20–30	Severe headache, syncope, dizziness, visual changes, weakness, nausea, vomiting, altered judgment
0.04–0.06 (400–600 ppm)	4–5	30–40	Vertigo, ataxia, blurred vision, confusion, loss of consciousness
0.07–0.10 (700–1000 ppm)	3–4	40–50	Confusion, tachycardia, tachypnea, coma, convulsions
0.11–0.15 (1100–1500 ppm)	1.5–3	50–60	Cheyne-Stokes respirations, coma, convulsions, shock, apnea
0.16–0.30 (1600–3000 ppm)	1.0–1.5	60–70	Coma, convulsions, respiratory and heart failure, death
>0.40 (>4000 ppm)	Few minutes		Death

Abbreviation: COHb = carboxyhemoglobin.

is directly related to alveolar ventilation. Elimination occurs through the lungs. The $t_{1/2}$ of COHb in room air (21% oxygen) is 5 to 6 hours; in 100% oxygen, 90 minutes; and in hyperbaric oxygen at 3 atmospheres of oxygen, 20 to 30 minutes.

Management: (1) Adequately protect the rescuer. Remove the patient from the contaminated area. Establish vital functions. (2) The mainstay of treatment is administration of 100% oxygen via a non-rebreathing mask with an oxygen reservoir or endotracheal tube. Give 100% oxygen to the patient until the COHb level is 2% or less. Assisted ventilation may be necessary. (3) Monitor ABGs and COHb. Determine the current COHb level and extrapolate to the COHb level at the time of exposure, using the $t_{1/2}$ COHb in different percentages of ambient oxygen (see kinetics just discussed). Note: A near-normal COHb level does not exclude significant CO poisoning, especially if measured several hours after the termination of exposure or if oxygen has been administered before the sample is obtained. (4) An exposed pregnant woman should be kept in 100% oxygen for several hours after the COHb level is almost zero because COHb concentrates in the fetus and oxygen is needed longer to ensure elimination of CO from the fetal circulation. Monitor the fetus. CO and hypoxia are teratogenic. (5) Metabolic acidosis should be treated with sodium bicarbonate only if the pH is below 7.2 after correction of hypoxia and adequate ventilation. Acidosis shifts the oxygen dissociation curve to the right and facilitates oxygen delivery to the tissues. (6) Use of the hyperbaric oxygen (HBO) chamber: The decision must be made on the basis of availability of a hyperbaric chamber, the ability to handle other acute emergencies that may coexist, extrapolated COHb level, and the severity of the poisoning. The standard of care for persons exposed to CO has yet to be determined, but most authorities recommend HBO therapy with any of the following

guidelines: (a) if HBO therapy is not readily available, a COHb greater than 40%, or if HBO therapy is readily available, COHb greater than 25%; (b) if the patient is unconscious or has a history of loss of consciousness or seizures; (c) if cardiovascular dysfunction (clinical ischemic chest pain or ECG evidence of ischemia) is present; (d) if there is metabolic acidosis; (e) if symptoms persist despite 100% oxygen therapy; (f) if the initial COHb level is greater than 15% in a child, in a patient with cardiovascular disease, or in a pregnant woman; or (g) if there are signs of maternal or fetal distress regardless of COHb level. Management of CO toxicity in infants and fetuses is a special problem because fetal hemoglobin has greater affinity for CO than does adult hemoglobin. A neurologic-cognitive examination has been used to help determine which patients with low CO levels should receive more aggressive therapy. Testing should include the following: general orientation memory testing (address, phone number, date of birth, present date) and cognitive testing (serial 7s, digit span, forward and backward spelling of three- and four-letter words). Patients with delayed neurologic sequelae or recurrent symptoms for up to 3 weeks may benefit from HBO treatment. (7) Treat seizures and cerebral edema.

Laboratory investigations: ABGs may show metabolic acidosis and normal oxygen tension. If there is significant poisoning, monitor the ABGs, electrolytes, blood glucose, serum creatine kinase and cardiac enzymes, renal function, and liver function. Obtain a urinalysis and test for myoglobinuria. Obtain a chest radiograph if there has been smoke inhalation or if use of an HBO chamber is being considered. ECG monitoring is needed especially if the patient is older than 40 years, has a history of cardiac disease, or has moderate to severe symptoms. Determine the blood ethanol level, and conduct toxicology studies on the basis of symptoms and circumstances. Monitor

COHb during and at the end of therapy. The pulse oximeter has two wavelengths and overestimates oxyhemoglobin saturation in CO poisoning. The true oxygen saturation is determined by blood gas analysis measuring the oxygen bound to hemoglobin. The co-oximeter measures four wavelengths and separates out COHb and the other hemoglobin-binding agents from oxyhemoglobin. Fetal hemoglobin has a greater affinity for CO than does adult hemoglobin, and the COHb may be falsely elevated as much as 4% in young infants. *Disposition:* Patients with no or mild symptoms (after exposures of less than 5 minutes) who become asymptomatic after a few hours of oxygen therapy and have a CO level below 10%, normal findings on physical examination and on neurologic-cognitive examination, and normal ABG parameters may be discharged but instructed to return if there are any signs of neurologic dysfunction. Patients with CO poisoning necessitating treatment need follow-up neuropsychiatric examinations.

Caustics and Corrosives. The U.S. Consumer Products Safety Commission labeling recommendations on containers for acids and alkalis indicate the potential for producing serious damage: caution (weak irritant), warning (strong irritant), danger (corrosive). Some common acids with corrosive potential are acetic acid (>50%), calcium oxide, formic acid, glycolic acid (>10%), hydrochloric acid (>10%), mercuric chloride, nitric acid (>5%), oxalic acid (>10%), phosphoric acid (>60%), sulfuric acid (battery acid) (>10%), zinc chloride (>10%), and zinc sulfate (>50%). Some common alkalis with corrosive potential include ammonia (>5%), calcium carbide, calcium hydroxide (dry), potassium hydroxide (lye) (>1%), and sodium hydroxide (lye) (>1%). *Toxic mechanism:* Acids produce mucosal coagulation necrosis and an eschar and may be systemically absorbed, but with the exception of hydrofluoric acid, they do not penetrate deeply. Injury to the gastric mucosa is more likely, although specific sites of injury for acids and alkalis are not clearly defined. Alkalis produce liquefaction necrosis and saponification and penetrate deeply. The esophageal mucosa is more likely to be damaged. Oropharyngeal and esophageal damage is more frequently caused by solids than by liquids. Liquids produce superficial, circumferential burns and gastric damage. *Toxic dose:* The toxicity is determined by concentration, contact time, and pH. Significant injury is more likely at pH values less than 2 or greater than 12, stricture at pH 14, prolonged contact time, and large volumes. *Manifestations:* The absence of oral burns does not exclude the possibility of esophageal or gastric damage. General clinical findings include stridor; dysphagia; drooling; oropharyngeal, retrosternal, and epigastric pain; and ocular and oral burns. Alkali burns are yellow, soapy, frothy lesions. Acid burns are gray-white in color and later form an eschar. Abdominal tenderness and guarding may be present if there is perforation.

Management: Bring the container; the substance must be identified and the pH of the substance, vomitus, tears, and saliva tested. *Ingestion, ocular, and dermal management:* (1) Prehospital and initial hospital management: If ingestion occurs, all GI decontamination procedures are contraindicated except for immediate rinsing, removal of the substance from the mouth, and then dilution with small amounts (sips) of milk or water. Check for ocular and dermal involvement. Contraindications to oral dilution are dysphagia, respiratory distress, obtundation, and shock. If ocular involvement occurs, immediately irrigate with tepid water for at least 30 minutes, perform fluorescein staining of the eye, and consult with an ophthalmologist. If dermal involvement occurs, immediately remove contaminated clothes and irrigate the skin with tepid water for at least 15 minutes. Consult with a burn specialist. (2) For acid ingestion, some authorities advocate placement of a small flexible nasogastric tube and aspiration within 30 minutes after ingestion. (3) The patient should receive only intravenous fluids after dilution until endoscopy consultation is obtained. (4) Endoscopy is valuable for predicting damage and the risk of stricture. The indications are controversial: Some authorities recommend its use in all caustic ingestions regardless of symptoms, whereas others are selective, using clinical features such as vomiting, stridor, and drooling and oral or facial lesions as criteria. Endoscopy is indicated for all symptomatic patients or those with intentional ingestions. Endoscopy may be done immediately if the patient is symptomatic but is usually done 12 to 48 hours after ingestion. After 72 hours there is increased risk of perforation. (5) Corticosteroids may be ineffective and are considered mainly for second-degree circumferential burns. If a corticosteroid is used, start hydrocortisone sodium succinate IV at 10 to 20 mg per kg per day within 48 hours and change to oral prednisolone at 2 mg per kg per day. Continue prednisolone for 3 weeks, and then taper the dose. (6) Provide tetanus prophylaxis. Antibiotics are not useful prophylactically. (7) An esophagogram is not useful in the first few days and may interfere with endoscopic evaluation; later, it may be used to assess the severity of damage. (8) Investigative therapy includes agents to inhibit collagen formation and the use of intraluminal stents. (9) Esophageal and gastric outlet dilatation may be needed if there is evidence of stricture. Bougienage of the esophagus has, however, been associated with brain abscess. Interposition of a colon segment may be necessary if dilatation fails to provide a passage of adequate size. *Inhalation management* requires immediate removal of the patient from the environment, administration of humid supplemental oxygen, and observation for airway obstruction and noncardiac pulmonary edema. Obtain radiographic and ABG evaluation when appropriate. Intubation and respiratory support may be required. Certain caustics produce systemic disturbances: formaldehyde, metabolic acidosis; hydrofluoric acid, hypocalcemia and renal damage; oxalic acid, hypocalcemia; phenol, hepatic and renal damage; and pitric acid, renal injury.

Laboratory investigations: If acid has been ingested, determine the acid-base balance and electrolytes. If there are pulmonary symptoms, use chest radiography, ABGs, and pulse oximetry. *Disposition:* Infants and small children should be medically evaluated and observed. Admit all symptomatic patients. Admit to the ICU if there are severe symptoms or danger of airway compromise. After endoscopy, if there is no damage, the patient may be discharged when oral feedings are tolerated. Intentional exposures necessitate psychiatric evaluation before discharge.

Cocaine (benzoylmethylecgonine). Cocaine is derived from the leaves of *Erythroxylon coca* and *Truxillo coca*. A body packer is a person who conceals many small packages of cocaine contraband in the GI tract or other areas for illicit transport. A body stuffer spontaneously ingests substances for the purpose of hiding evidence. *Toxic mechanism:* Cocaine directly stimulates CNS presynaptic sympathetic neurons to release catecholamines and acetylcholine, blocks presynaptic reuptake of the catecholamines, blocks the sodium channels along neuronal membranes, and increases platelet aggregation. Long-term use depletes the CNS of dopamine. *Toxic dose:* The maximal mucosal local anesthetic therapeutic dose is 200 mg, or 2 mL of 10% solution. Psychoactive effects occur at 50 to 95 mg; cardiac and CNS effects occur at 1 mg per kg. The potential fatal dose is 1200 mg intranasally, but death has occurred with 20 mg parenterally. *Kinetics:* See Table 20. Cocaine is well absorbed by all routes, including nasal insufflation and oral, dermal, and inhalation routes. It is metabolized by plasma and liver cholinesterase to the inactive metabolites ecgonine methyl ester and benzoylecgonine. Plasma pseudocholinesterase is congenitally deficient in 3% of the population and decreased in fetuses, in young infants, in elderly persons, in pregnant women, and in patients with liver disease. Persons with this enzyme deficit are at increased risk for life-threatening cocaine toxicity. The PB is 8.7%; the Vd, 1.2 to 1.9 liters per kg; 10% of cocaine is excreted unchanged. Cocaine and ethanol undergo liver synthesis to form cocaethylene, a metabolite with a $t_{1/2}$ three times longer than that of cocaine. This metabolite may account for some of cocaine's cardiotoxicity and appears to be more lethal than cocaine or ethanol alone. *Manifestations:* (1) CNS: euphoria, hyperactivity, agitation, convulsions, intracranial hemorrhage; (2) eye-ear-nose-throat: mydriasis, septal perforation; (3) cardiovascular: cardiac dysrhythmias, hypertension and hypotension (in severe overdose), chest pain (occurs frequently, but only 5.8% of affected patients have true myocardial ischemia and infarction); (4) hyperthermia (vasoconstriction, increased metabolism); (5) GI: ischemic bowel perforation if the drug was ingested; (6) rhabdomyolysis, myoglobinuria, and renal failure; (7) premature labor and abruptio placentae; (8) in prolonged toxicity, suspect body cavity packing; (9) mortality resulting from cerebrovascular accidents, coronary artery spasm and myocardial injury, and lethal dysrhythmias.

Management: (1) Supportive care: Blood pressure, cardiac, and thermal monitoring and seizure precautions are instituted. Diazepam is the agent of choice for treatment of cocaine toxicity with agitation, seizures, and dysrhythmias; the dose is 10 to 30 mg IV at 2.5 mg per minute for an adult and 0.2 to 0.5 mg per kg at 1 mg per minute up to 10 mg for a child. (2) GI decontamination: If cocaine was ingested, administer AC. MDAC may absorb cocaine leakage in body stuffers or body packers. Whole-bowel irrigation with PEG solution has been used in body packers and stuffers if the contraband is in a firm container. If packages are not visible on an abdominal radiograph, a contrast study and/or ultrasonography can help to confirm successful passage. PEG may desorb the cocaine from AC. Cocaine in the nasal passage can be removed with an applicator dipped in a non–water-soluble product (lubricating jelly). (3) In body packers and stuffers, secure venous access and have drugs readily available to treat life-threatening manifestations until contraband is passed in the stool. Surgical removal may be indicated if a packet does not pass the pylorus, in a symptomatic body packer, or in intestinal obstruction. (4) Cardiovascular disturbances: Hypertension and tachycardia are usually transient and can be managed by careful titration of diazepam. Nitroprusside may be used for management of hypertensive crisis. Myocardial ischemia is managed by oxygen, vascular access to administer intravenous medications, BZPs, and nitroglycerin. Use of aspirin and thrombolytic agents is not routinely recommended because of danger of intracranial hemorrhage. Dysrhythmias are usually supraventricular tachycardias and do not mandate specific management. Adenosine is ineffective. Life-threatening tachydysrhythmias may respond to phentolamine, in a dose of 5 mg given as an intravenous bolus in adults, or 0.1 mg per kg in children, at 5-

TABLE 20. **Different Routes and Kinetics of Cocaine**

Type	Route	$t_{1/2}$ (min)	Onset	Peak (min)	Duration (min)
Cocaine leaf	Oral, chew	NA	20–30 min	45–90	240–360
Hydrochloride	Insufflation	78	1–3 min	5–10	60–90
	Ingested	54	20–30 min	50–90	Sustained
	Intravenous	36	30–120 s	5–11	60–90
Freebase, crack	Smoked	—	5–10 s	5–11	Up to 20
Coca paste	Smoked	—	Unknown		

to 10-minute intervals. Phentolamine also relieves coronary artery spasm and myocardial ischemia. Electrical synchronized cardioversion should be considered for hemodynamically unstable dysrhythmias. Lidocaine is not recommended initially but may be used after 3 hours for ventricular tachycardia. Wide-complex QRS ventricular tachycardia may be treated with NaHCO$_3$ at 2 mEq per kg as a bolus. Beta-adrenergic blockers are not recommended. (5) Treat anxiety, agitation, and convulsions with diazepam. If diazepam fails to control seizures, use neuromuscular blockers and monitor the EEG for nonmotor seizures. (6) Hyperthermia: Administer external cooling and cool humidified 100% oxygen. Neuromuscular paralysis to control seizures reduces temperature. Dantrolene and antipyretics are not recommended. (7) Treat rhabdomyolysis and myoglobinuria with fluids, alkaline diuresis, and diuretics. (8) If the patient is pregnant, monitor the fetus and observe for threatened spontaneous abortion. (9) Treat paranoid ideation and threatening behavior with rapid tranquilization. Observe the patient for suicidal depression that may follow intoxication and may necessitate suicide precautions. (10) If focal neurologic manifestations are present, consider a diagnosis of cerebrovascular accident and perform CT. (11) Extracorporeal measures are of no benefit.

Laboratory investigations: Monitoring: ECG and cardiac monitoring is instituted, as is monitoring of ABGs and oxygen saturation, electrolytes, blood glucose, BUN, creatinine, creatine kinase and cardiac function if chest pain is present, liver profile, rhabdomyolysis and urine for myoglobin, and urine for cocaine and metabolites and other substances of abuse. Abdominal radiography or ultrasonography is performed for assessment in body packers. A urine sample collected more than 12 hours after cocaine intake contains little or no cocaine. If cocaine is present, it has been used within the past 12 hours. Cocaine's metabolite benzoylecgonine may be detected within 4 hours after a single nasal insufflation and as long as 48 to 114 hours after use. Intravenous drug users should have HIV and hepatitis virus testing. Cross-reactions with herbal teas, lidocaine, and droperidol may give false-positive results with some laboratory methods. *Disposition:* Patients with mild intoxication or a brief seizure that does not necessitate treatment who become asymptomatic may be discharged after 6 hours with appropriate psychosocial follow-up. If there are cardiac or cerebral ischemia manifestations, monitor in the ICU. Body packers and stuffers require ICU care until passage of the contraband.

Cyanide. Some sources of cyanide: (1) Hydrogen cyanide (HCN) is a by-product of burning plastic and wools and is produced in residential fires and salts in ore extraction. (2) Nitriles, such as acetonitrile (present in artificial nail removers), are metabolized in the body to produce cyanide. (3) Cyanogenic glycosides in the seeds of fruit stones (as amygdalin in apricots, peaches, and apples) in the presence of intestinal β-glucosidase form cyanide (the seeds are harmful only if the capsule is broken). (4) Sodium nitroprusside, the antihypertensive vasodilator, contains five cyanide groups. *Toxic mechanism:* Cyanide blocks the cellular electron transport mechanism and cellular respiration by inhibiting the mitochondrial ferricytochrome oxidase system and other enzymes. This results in cellular hypoxia and lactic acidosis. *Toxic dose:* The ingestion of 1 mg per kg or 50 mg of HCN can produce death within 15 minutes. The lethal dose of potassium cyanide is 200 mg. Five to 10 mL of 84% acetonitrile is lethal. The permissible exposure limit for volatile HCN is 10 ppm, and 300 ppm is fatal in minutes. *Kinetics:* Cyanide is rapidly absorbed by all routes. In the stomach it forms hydrocyanic acid. The PB is 60%; the Vd, 1.5 liters per kg. Cyanide is detoxified by metabolism in the liver via the mitochondrial endogenous thiosulfate-rhodanese pathway, which catalyzes the transfer of sulfur to cyanide to form irreversibly the less toxic thiocyanate, which is excreted in the urine. The t$_{1/2}$ for cyanide elimination from the blood is 1.2 hours. Cyanide is also detoxified by reacting with hydroxocobalamin (vitamin B$_{12a}$) to form cyanocobalamin (vitamin B$_{12}$). Elimination is through the lungs. *Manifestations:* HCN has the distinctive odor of bitter almonds (odor of silver polish). The clinical findings are flushing, hypertension, headache, hyperpnea, seizures, stupor, cardiac dysrhythmias, and pulmonary edema. Cyanosis is absent or appears late. Various ECG abnormalities may be present.

Management: (1) Protect rescuers and attendants. Immediately administer 100% oxygen and continue during and after the administration of the antidote. If cyanide is inhaled, remove the patient from the contaminated atmosphere. Attendants should not administer mouth-to-mouth resuscitation. (2) Cyanide antidote kit (see Table 10): The clinician must decide whether to use any or all components of the kit. The mechanism of action of the antidote kit is to form methemoglobin (MetHb), which has a greater affinity for cyanide than does the cytochrome oxidase system and forms cyanomethemoglobin. The cyanide is transferred from MetHb by sodium thiosulfate, which provides a sulfur atom that is converted by the rhodanese-catalyzed enzyme reaction (thiosulfate sulfurtransferase) to convert cyanide into the relatively nontoxic sodium thiocyanate, which is excreted by the kidney. Procedure for using the antidote kit: Step 1, use of amyl nitrite inhalant Perles, is only a temporizing measure (forms only 2 to 5% MetHb) and can be omitted if venous access is established. Administer 100% oxygen and the inhalant for 30 seconds of every minute. Use a new Perle every 3 minutes. Step 2, administration of sodium nitrite ampule, is not necessary in poisonings associated with residential fires, smoke inhalation, nitroprusside, or acetonitrile. Sodium nitrite is administered IV to produce MetHb of 20 to 30% at 35 to 70 minutes after administration. For adults, 10 mL of a 3% solution of sodium nitrite (0.33 mL per kg of 3% solution for children) is diluted to 100 mL with 0.9% saline and administered slowly IV at 5 mL per minute.

If hypotension develops, slow the infusion. Step 3, administration of sodium thiosulfate, is useful alone in smoke inhalation, nitroprusside toxicity, and acetonitrile toxicity and should not be used at all in hydrogen sulfide poisoning. For adults, administer 12.5 grams of sodium thiosulfate or 50 mL of 25% solution (for children, 1.65 mL per kg of 25% solution) IV over 10 to 20 minutes. If cyanide-related symptoms recur, repeat antidotes in 30 minutes as half of the initial dose. The dosage regimen for children on the package insert must be carefully followed. One hour after antidotes are administered, the MetHb level should be obtained and should not exceed 20%. Methylene blue should not be used to reverse excessive MetHb. (3) GI decontamination after oral ingestion by gastric lavage and AC is recommended but is not very effective (1 gram of AC binds only 35 mg of cyanide). (4) Treat seizures with intravenous diazepam. Correct acidosis with NaHCO₃ if it does not resolve rapidly with therapy. (5) Treat metabolic acidosis with NaHCO₃. (6) There is no role for the HBO chamber, hemodialysis, or hemoperfusion. (7) Other antidotes: In France, hydroxocobalamin (vitamin B₁₂ₐ) is used (it exchanges its hydroxyl with free cyanide to form cyanocobalamin). It has proved effective when given immediately after exposure in large doses of 4 grams (50 mg per kg) or 50 times the amount of cyanide in the exposure with 8 grams of sodium thiosulfate (it has FDA orphan drug approval).

Laboratory investigations: Obtain and monitor ABGs, oxygen saturation, blood lactate (which takes 0.5 hour), blood cyanide (which takes hours), hemoglobin, blood glucose, and electrolytes. Lactic acidemia, a decrease in the arterial-venous oxygen difference, and bright red color of the venous blood are manifestations of toxicity. If smoke inhalation is the possible source of exposure, obtain COHb and MetHb concentrations. The cyanide level in whole blood for a smoker is less than 0.5 μg per mL; with exposures with flushing and tachycardia, 0.5 to 1.0 μg per mL; with obtundation, 1.0 to 2.5 μg per mL; and with coma and death, greater than 2.5 μg per mL. *Disposition:* Asymptomatic patients should be observed for a minimum of 6 hours. Patients who ingest nitrile compounds must be observed for 24 hours. Patients requiring antidote administration should be admitted to the ICU.

Digitalis. Cardiac glycosides are found in cardiac medications, common plants, and the skin of *Bufo* species of toad. More than 1 to 3 mg may be found in a few leaves of oleander or foxglove. *Toxic mechanism:* Cardiac glycosides inhibit the enzyme Na⁺,K⁺-ATPase, leading to intracellular potassium loss, increased intracellular sodium-producing phase 4 depolarization, increased automaticity, and ectopy. Increased intracellular calcium and potentiation of contractility occur. Pacemaker cells are inhibited and the refractory period is prolonged, leading to AV block. Vagal tone is increased. *Toxic dose:* The digoxin total digitalizing dose is 0.75 to 1.25 mg, or 10 to 15 μg per kg in patients older than 10 years and 40 to

50 μg per kg in those younger than 2 years; 30 to 40 μg per kg at 2 to 10 years of age produces a therapeutic serum concentration of 0.6 to 2.0 ng per mL. The acute single toxic dose is more than 0.07 mg per kg, or more than 2 to 3 mg in adults; however, 2 mg in a child or 4 mg in an adult usually produces mild toxicity. Serious and potentially fatal overdoses are greater than 4 mg in a child and greater than 10 mg in an adult. Digoxin clinical toxicity is usually associated with serum digoxin levels of 3.5 ng per mL or more in adults. Patients at greatest risk of overdose include those with cardiac disease, electrolyte abnormalities (low potassium, low magnesium, low thyroxine, high calcium), or renal impairment and those receiving amiodarone, quinidine, erythromycin, tetracycline, calcium channel blockers, and beta blockers. *Kinetics:* Digoxin is a metabolite of digitoxin. With oral ingestion, onset occurs within 1 to 2 hours, peak levels occur at 2 to 3 hours, and peak effects occur at 3 to 4 hours; the duration is 3 to 4 days. In overdose, the typical onset is at 30 minutes with peak effects in 3 to 12 hours. With intoxications due to intravenous use, onset is in 5 to 30 minutes, the peak level occurs immediately, and the peak effect occurs at 1.5 to 3 hours. Elimination is 60 to 80% renal. The Vd is 5 to 6 liters per kg. The cardiac-to-plasma ratio is 30:1. The elimination t₁/₂ is 30 to 50 hours. After an acute ingestion overdose, the serum concentration does not reflect the tissue concentration for at least 6 hours or more, and steady state is reached 12 to 16 hours after the last dose. *Manifestations:* These may be delayed 9 to 18 hours. (1) GI effects: Nausea and vomiting are always present in acute ingestion and may occur in chronic ingestion. (2) Cardiovascular effects: The "digitalis effect" on the ECG consists of scooped ST segments and PR prolongation. In overdose, any dysrhythmia or block is possible, but none is characteristic. Bradycardia occurs in acute overdose in patients with healthy hearts or tachycardia with existing heart disease, or in chronic overdose. Ventricular tachycardia is seen only in severe poisoning. (3) CNS effects are headaches, visual disturbances, and colored-halo vision. (4) Potassium disturbances: Hyperkalemia is a predictor of serum digoxin concentrations greater than 10 ng per mL and is associated with a 50% mortality rate without treatment. In one review, if serum potassium was less than 5.0 mEq per liter, the survival rate was 100%; if 5 to 5.5 mEq per liter, 50% of the patients survived; and if greater than 5.5 mEq per liter, all died. Hypokalemia is commonly seen with chronic intoxication. Patients with normal digitalis levels may have toxicity in the presence of hypokalemia. (5) Chronic intoxications are more likely to produce scotoma, color perception disturbances, yellow vision, halos, delirium, hallucinations or psychosis, tachycardia, and hypokalemia.

Management: Obtain a cardiology consultation and have a pacemaker readily available. (1) GI decontamination: Use caution with vagal stimulation, and avoid emesis and gastric lavage. Administer AC; if a nasogastric tube is required for AC therapy, consider pretreatment with atropine (0.02 mg per kg for a child and 0.5 mg for an adult). MDAC may interrupt enterohepatic recirculation of digitoxin and adsorb active metabolites. (2) Digoxin-specific antibody fragment (Fab, Digibind), 40 mg, binds with 0.6 mg of digoxin and is then excreted through the kidneys. It decreases digoxin levels 50-fold. (See Table 10). Indications include life-threatening, hemodynamically unstable dysrhythmias (ventricular dysrhythmias or rapid deterioration of clinical findings); ingestions greater than 4 mg in a child and 10 mg in an adult; serum potassium greater than 5.0 mEq per liter produced by cardiac glycoside toxicity; serum digoxin toxicity (more than 10 ng per mL in adults or more than 5 ng per mL in children) 6 to 8 hours after acute ingestion; and unstable severe bradycardia or second- or third-degree block unresponsive to atropine. This agent is also useful in digitalis delirium with thrombocytopenia and in treatment of life-threatening digitoxin and oleander poisoning. Empirical digoxin-specific Fab fragment therapy may be administered as a bolus through a 22-μm filter if there is a critical emergency. If the clinical situation is less urgent, administer over 30 minutes. The empirical dose is 10 vials for adults and 5 vials or children. *Calculation of dose:* The amount (total mg) of digoxin known to have been ingested multiplied by 80% bioavailability (0.8) = body burden. If the agent was given as liquid capsules or IV, do not multiply by 0.8. The body burden divided by 0.6 (0.6 mg of digoxin is bound by 1 vial of 40 mg of Fab) = number of vials needed. If the amount is unknown but the steady-state serum concentration is known, for digoxin:

Digoxin (ng/mL) × Vd (5.6 L/kg) × weight (kg) = body burden (μg)

Body burden/1000 = body burden (mg)

Body burden/0.6 = number of vials needed

For digitoxin:

Digitoxin (ng/mL) × Vd (0.56 L/kg) × weight (kg) = body burden

Body burden/1000 = body burden (mg)

Body burden/0.6 = number of vials needed

(3) Antidysrhythmic agents and a pacemaker should be used only if Fab therapy fails. The onset of action is within 30 minutes. Complications of Fab therapy are related mainly to withdrawal of digoxin and worsening heart failure and include hypokalemia, decreased glucose levels (if glycogen stores are low), and allergic reactions (rare). Digitalis administered after Fab therapy is bound and may be inactivated for 5 to 7 days. (4) For ventricular tachydysrhythmias, correct electrolyte disturbances and administer lidocaine or phenytoin. For torsades de pointes, ad-

minister 20 mL of 20% magnesium sulfate, given IV slowly over 20 minutes, to an adult or 25 to 50 mg per kg to a child, and titrate to control the dysrhythmia. Discontinue magnesium if hypotension, heart block, or a decrease in deep tendon reflexes occurs. Magnesium should be used with caution if renal impairment is present. Ventricular pacing should be reserved for patients who fail to respond to Fab. (5) Do not use antidysrhythmics of classes IA, IC, II, and IV or agents that increase conduction time (e.g., procainamide, bretylium, diltiazem, beta blockers). Class IB drugs can be used. (6) Cardioversion should be used with caution; start at a setting of 5 to 10 joules and pretreat with lidocaine, if possible, because cardioversion may precipitate ventricular fibrillation or asystole. (7) Treat unstable bradycardia and second- and third-degree AV block with atropine. If the patient is unresponsive, use Fab. A pacemaker should be available if the patient fails to respond. Avoid isoproterenol, which causes dysrhythmias. (8) Electrolyte disturbances: Potassium disturbances are due to a shift, not a change, in total body potassium. Treat hyperkalemia (potassium level greater than 5.0 mEq per liter) with Fab only. Never use calcium, insulin, or glucose. Do not use $NaHCO_3$ concomitantly with Fab because it may produce severe life-threatening hypokalemia. Sodium polystyrene sulfonate (Kayexalate) should not be used. Treat hypokalemia with caution because this condition may be cardioprotective. (9) Extracorporeal procedures are ineffective. Hemodialysis is used for severe or refractory hyperkalemia.

Laboratory investigations: Monitor baseline ECG and continuous cardiac function and blood glucose, electrolytes, calcium, magnesium, BUN, and creatinine levels. Measure initial digoxin levels more than 6 hours after ingestion because earlier values do not reflect the tissue distribution. Obtain free (unbound) serum digoxin concentrations after Fab therapy because the free (unbound) digoxin decreases and reflects the true level. Cross-reactions: An endogenous digoxin-like substance cross-reacts in most common immunoassays (not with HPLC), and values as high as 4.1 ng per mL have been reported in newborns, in patients with chronic renal failure or abnormal immunoglobulins, and in women in the third trimester of pregnancy. *Disposition:* Consult with a poison control center and cardiologist experienced with the use of digoxin-specific Fab fragments. All patients with significant dysrhythmias, symptoms, an elevated serum digoxin concentration, or elevated serum potassium level should be admitted to the ICU. Fab and pacemaker therapy should be readily available. Asymptomatic patients with nontoxic levels should have studies repeated in 12 hours.

Ethanol (grain alcohol). See Table 21. *Toxic mechanism:* Ethanol has CNS hypnotic and anesthetic effects produced by a variety of mechanisms, including membrane fluidity and effect on the GABA system. It promotes cutaneous vasodilatation (contributing to hypothermia), stimulates secretion of gastric juice (potentially causing gastritis), inhibits secretion of

TABLE 21. **Summary of Alcohol and Glycol Features***

| Feature | Alcohol | | | Ethylene Glycol |
	Methanol	Isopropanol	Ethanol	
Principal uses	Gas line Antifreeze Sterno Windshield wiper deicer	Solvent Jewelry cleaner Rubbing alcohol	Beverage Solvent	Antifreeze Deicer
Odor	None	None	Yes	None
Specific gravity	0.719	0.785	0.789	1.12
Fatal dose	1 mL/kg, 100% mortality	3 mL/kg, 100% mortality	5 mL/kg, 100% mortality	1.4 mL/kg
Hepatic enzyme	Alcohol dehydrogenase	Alcohol dehydrogenase	Alcohol and acetaldehyde dehydrogenases	Alcohol dehydrogenase
Toxic metabolite(s)	Formate, formaldehyde	Acetone	Acetaldehyde	Glyoxylic acid, oxalate
Drunkenness	±	2+	2+	1+
Metabolic change		Hyperglycemia	Hypoglycemia	Hypocalcemia
Metabolic acidosis	4+	0	1+	2+
Anion gap	4+	±	2+	4+
Ketosis	Ketobutyric acid	Acetone	Hydroxybutyric acid	None
GI tract	Pancreatitis	Hemorrhagic gastritis	Gastritis	
Visual	Blindness, pink optic disk			
Crystalluria	0	0	0	+
Pulmonary edema				+
Renal failure				+
Molecular weight	32	60	46	62
Osmolality†	0.337	0.176	0.228	0.190

*0 indicates no effect; + indicates mild effect; ± indicates no effect or mild effect; 2+ indicates moderate effect; 4+ indicates severe effect.

†1 mL/dL of substances raises the freezing point osmolarity of serum. The validity of the correlation of osmolality with blood concentrations has been questioned. Inebriation index: methanol < ethanol < ethylene glycol < isopropanol.

the antidiuretic hormone, inhibits gluconeogenesis (potentially causing hypoglycemia), and influences fat metabolism (potentially causing lipidemia). *Toxic dose:* 1 mL per kg of absolute or 100% ethanol or 200-proof ethanol (proof defines alcohol concentration in beverages) results in a BEC of 100 mg per dL. The potentially fatal dose is 3 grams per kg for children or 6 grams per kg for adults. Children frequently have hypoglycemia at a BEC greater than 50 mg per dL. *Kinetics:* Onset of action occurs 30 to 60 minutes after ingestion, peak action is at 90 minutes on an empty stomach, and the Vd is 0.6 liter per kg. The major route of elimination (more than 90%) is by hepatic oxidative metabolism. The first step involves the enzyme alcohol dehydrogenase (ADH), which converts ethanol to acetaldehyde. The kinetics in this step are zero order at a constant rate (regardless of the level) of 12 to 20 mg per dL per hour (12 to 15 mg per dL per hour in nonalcoholic drinkers, 15 mg per dL per hour in social drinkers, 30 to 50 mg per dL per hour in alcoholics, and 28 mg per dL per hour in children). At a low BEC (less than 30 mg per dL), the metabolism is by first-order kinetics. In the second step of metabolism, the acetaldehyde is metabolized by acetaldehyde dehydrogenase to acetic acid. In subsequent steps, acetic acid is metabolized via the Krebs citric acid cycle to carbon dioxide and water. The enzyme steps are dependent on nicotinamide adenine dinucleotide, which interferes with gluconeogenesis. Only 2 to 10% of ethanol is excreted unchanged by the kidneys. BEC and amount ingested can be estimated by the following equations (SG indicates specific gravity):

$$\text{BEC (mg/dL)} = \frac{\text{amount ingested (mL)} \times \text{\% ethanol in product} \times \text{SG (0.79)}}{\text{Vd (0.6 L/kg)} \times \text{body weight (kg)}}$$

$$\text{Dose (amount ingested)} = \frac{\text{BEC (mg/dL)} \times \text{Vd (0.6 L/kg)} \times \text{body weight (kg)}}{\text{\% ethanol} \times \text{SG (0.79)}}$$

Manifestations: See Table 22. (1) Acute: BECs over 30 mg per dL produce euphoria; over 50 mg per dL, incoordination and intoxication; over 100 mg per dL, ataxia; over 300 mg per dL, stupor; and over 500 mg per dL, coma. Levels of 500 to 700 mg per dL may be fatal. Children frequently have hypoglycemia at a BEC above 50 mg per dL. (2) Patients with chronic alcoholism tolerate a higher BEC, and correlation with manifestations is not valid. A rapid interview for alcoholism uses the CAGE questions: C, Have you felt the need to *c*ut down? A, Have others *a*nnoyed you by criticizing your drinking? G, Have you felt *g*uilty about your drinking? E, Have you ever had a morning *e*ye-opening drink to steady your nerves or get rid of a hangover? Two affirmative answers indicate probable alcoholism.

Management: Inquire about trauma and disulfiram (Antabuse) use. (1) Protect from aspiration and hypoxia. Establish and maintain vital functions. The patient may require intubation and assisted ventilation. (2) GI decontamination plays no role. (3) If the patient is comatose, administer IV 50% glucose at 1 mL per kg in adults and 25% glucose at 2 mL per kg in children. Thiamine, 100 mg IV, is administered if the patient has a history of chronic alcoholism, malnutrition, or suspected eating disorders and to prevent Wernicke-Korsakoff syndrome. Naloxone has produced a partial inconsistent response and is not recommended for known alcoholics taking CNS depressants. (4) General supportive care: Administer fluids to correct hydration and hypotension; correct electrolyte abnormalities and acid-base imbalance. Vasopressors and plasma expanders may be necessary to correct severe hypotension. Hypomagnesemia is frequently present in chronic alcoholics. For hypomagnesemia, administer a loading dose of 2 grams of a 10% magnesium sulfate solution given IV over 5 minutes in the ICU with blood pressure and cardiac monitoring and have 10% calcium chloride on hand in case of overdose. Follow with constant infusion of 6 grams of 10% magnesium sulfate over 3 to 4 hours. Be cautious with magnesium administration if renal failure is present. (5) Hypothermic patients should be warmed. See general treatment of poisoning. (6) Hemodialysis may be used in severe cases when conventional therapy is ineffective (rarely needed). (7) Treat repeated or prolonged seizures with diazepam. Brief "rum fits" do not necessitate long-term anticonvulsant therapy. Repeated seizures or focal neurologic findings may warrant skull radiography, lumbar puncture, and CT of the head, depending on the clinical findings. (8) Treat withdrawal with hydration and large doses of chlordiazepoxide (50 to 100 mg) or diazepam (2 to 10 mg) IV; these may be repeated in 2 to 4 hours. Large doses of BZPs may be required for delirium tremens. Withdrawal can occur in the presence of an elevated BEC and can be fatal if untreated.

Laboratory investigations: The BEC should be specifically requested and followed. (Gas chromatography or a Breathalyzer test gives rapid reliable results if there is no belching or vomiting; enzymatic methods do not differentiate between the alcohols.) Monitor ABGs, electrolytes, and glucose; determine anion and osmolar gaps (measure by freezing point depression, not vapor pressure); and check for ketosis. See discussion of general management. The AG increases 1 mg per kg for each 4.5 mg per dL BEC. Obtain a chest radiograph to determine whether aspiration pneumonia is present. Perform renal and liver function tests and obtain bilirubin levels. *Disposition:* Clinical severity (e.g., whether intubation or assisted ventilation is needed or aspiration pneumonia is present) should determine the level of hospital care needed. Young children with significant accidental exposure to alcohol (calculated to reach a BEC of 50 mg per dL) should have BEC measured and blood glucose levels monitored for hypoglycemia frequently for 4 hours after ingestion. Patients with acute ethanol intoxication seldom require admission unless a complication is present. However, intoxicated patients should not be discharged until they are fully functional (can walk independently, talk and think coherently), have had suicide potential evaluated, have a proper environment to which they can be discharged, and have a sober escort. Extended liability means that a physician can be held liable for subsequent injuries or death of an intoxicated patient who has been allowed to sign out against medical advice. No patient with an altered mental status can sign out.

Ethylene Glycol. Ethylene glycol is found in solvents, windshield deicer, antifreeze (95%), and air-conditioning units and has contaminated imported wines. Ethylene glycol is a sweet-tasting, colorless, water-soluble liquid with a sweet aromatic aroma. *Toxic mechanism:* Ethylene glycol is oxidized by ADH to glycolaldehyde and then is metabolized to glycolic acid and glyoxylic acid. Glyoxylic acid is metabolized to oxalic acid. Ethylene glycol metabolites are metabolized via pyridoxine-dependent pathways to glycine, benzoic acid, and hippuric acid and by thiamine- and magnesium-dependent pathways to α-hydroxyketoadipic acid. The metabolites of ethylene glycol produce a profound metabolic acidosis, increased AG, hypocalcemia, deposition of oxalate crystals in tissues, and renal damage. *Toxic dose:* The ingestion of 0.1 mL of 100% ethylene glycol per kg can result in a toxic serum ethylene glycol concentration (SEGC) of 20 mg per dL, a level that necessitates ethanol therapy, the antidote. Ingestion of 3.0 mL of 100%

TABLE 22. **Clinical Signs in the Intolerant Ethanol Drinker**

Ethanol (mg/dL)	Blood (μg/mL)	Concentration* (mmol/L)	Manifestations† in Nonalcoholics
>25	>250	>5.4	Euphoria
>47	>470	>10.2	Mild incoordination, sensory and motor impairment
>50	>500	>10.8	Increased risk of motor vehicle accidents
>100	>1000	>21.7	Ataxia (legal toxic level in many localities)
>150	>1500	>32.5	Moderate incoordination, slow reaction time
>200	>2000	>43.4	Drowsiness and confusion
>300	>3000	>65.1	Severe incoordination, stupor, blurred vision
>500	>5000	>108.5	Flaccid coma, respiratory failure, hypotension; may be fatal

*Ethanol concentrations are sometimes reported as percents. Note that mg% is not equivalent to mg/dL because ethanol weighs less than water (specific gravity 0.79). A 1% ethanol concentration is 790 mg/dL and 0.1% is 79 mg/dL.
†There is a great variation in individual behavior at particular blood ethanol levels. Behavior is dependent on tolerance and other factors.

solution by a 10-kg child or 30 mL of 100% ethylene glycol by an adult produces an SEGC of 50 mg per dL (8.1 mmol per liter), a concentration that requires hemodialysis. The fatal amount is 1.4 mL of 100% solution per kg. *Kinetics:* Absorption is by dermal, inhalation, and ingestion routes. Ethylene glycol is rapidly absorbed from the GI tract. Onset is in 30 minutes to 12 hours, and the peak level usually occurs at 2 hours. Without ethanol the $t_{1/2}$ is 3 to 8 hours; with ethanol, 17 hours; and with hemodialysis, 2.5 hours. The Vd is 0.65 to 0.8 liter per kg. For metabolism, see the toxic mechanism discussion. Renal clearance is 3.2 mL per kg per minute. About 20 to 50% is excreted unchanged in the urine. The following equations can be used for calculating SEGC and the amount ingested (SG indicates specific gravity; EG is ethylene glycol):

Calculation of SEGC:

$$0.12 \text{ mL/kg of } 100\% = \text{SEGC of } 10 \text{ mg/dL}$$

$$\text{SEGC (mg/dL)} = \frac{\text{amount ingested (mL)} \times \% \text{ EG} \times \text{SG (1.12)}}{\text{Vd (0.65 L/kg)} \times \text{weight (kg)}}$$

$$\text{Amount ingested (mL)} = \frac{\text{SEGC (mg/dL)} \times 0.65 \text{ L/kg} \times \text{weight (kg)}}{\% \text{ EG} \times \text{SG (1.12)}}$$

Manifestations: Phase I: The onset is 30 minutes to 12 hours after ingestion or longer with concomitant ethanol ingestion. The patient acts inebriated at an SEGC of 50 to 100 mg per dL. Hypocalcemia, tetany, and calcium oxalate and hippuric acid crystals in the urine may be observed within 4 to 8 hours but are not always present. Early, before metabolism of ethylene glycol, an osmolal gap may be present. Later, the metabolites of ethylene glycol produce changes starting 4 to 12 hours after ingestion, including an AG, metabolic acidosis, coma, convulsions, cardiac disturbances, and pulmonary and cerebral edema. Oral mucosa and urine fluoresce under Wood's light if "antifreeze" ethylene glycol has been ingested. Phase II: After 12 to 36 hours, cardiopulmonary deterioration occurs with pulmonary edema and congestive heart failure. Phase III: In 36 to 72 hours, oliguric renal failure resulting from oxalate crystal deposition and from tubular necrosis predominates, and pulmonary edema occurs. Phase IV: Neurologic sequelae occur 6 to 10 days after ingestion. They include facial diplegia, hearing loss, bilateral visual disturbances, elevated cerebrospinal fluid (CSF) pressure with or without elevated protein and pleocytosis, vomiting, hyper-reflexia, dysphagia, and ataxia.

Management: (1) Establish and maintain the vital functions. Protect the airway and use assisted ventilation, if necessary. (2) GI decontamination has a limited role, with only gastric lavage within 30 to 60 minutes after ingestion. AC is not effective. (3) Obtain baseline serum electrolytes and calcium, glucose, ABGs, ethanol, SEGC (difficult to obtain and often takes more than 48 hours), and methanol concentrations. In the first few hours, determine the measured serum osmolality and compare it with the calculated osmolarity (see "Serum Osmolal Gaps"). (4) If seizures occur, exclude hypocalcemia and treat with intravenous diazepam. If hypocalcemic seizures occur, treat with 10 to 20 mL of 10% calcium gluconate (0.2 to 0.3 mL per kg for children) slowly IV and repeat as needed. (See Table 10.) (5) Correct metabolic acidosis with $NaHCO_3$ given IV. (6) Ethanol therapy (see Table 10): The enzyme ADH has 10 times greater affinity for ethanol than for ethylene glycol. Therefore, ethanol blocks the metabolism of ethylene glycol at BECs of 100 to 150 mg per dL. Initiate therapy if there is a history of ingestion of 100% ethylene glycol at 0.1 mL per kg, if the SEGC is more than 20 mg per dL, if there is an osmolar gap not accounted for by other alcohols or factors (e.g., hyperlipidemia) (see "Serum Osmolal Gaps"), if there is metabolic acidosis with an increased AG, or if there are oxalate crystals in the urine or positive results on fluorescence testing of urine for antifreeze, and while awaiting hemodialysis. Ethanol should be administered IV (the oral route is less reliable) to produce a BEC of 100 to 150 mg per dL. The loading dose is derived from the formula 1 mL of 100% ethanol per kg = a BEC of 100 mg per dL (which protects against metabolism of ethylene glycol). Therefore, 10 mL of 10% ethanol is administered IV concomitantly with a maintenance dose of 10% ethanol of 2.0 mL per kg per hour (alcoholic), 0.83 mL per kg per hour (nondrinker), or 1.4 mL per kg per hour (social drinker). Increase the infusion rate of 10% ethanol to 2 to 3.5 mL per kg per hour when the patient is receiving hemodialysis. (7) Hemodialysis: Obtain a nephrology consultation. Early hemodialysis is indicated if the ingestion was potentially fatal, if the SEGC is more than 50 mg per dL (some authorities recommend hemodialysis at levels of more than 25 mg per dL), if severe acidosis or electrolyte abnormalities occur despite conventional therapy, or if congestive heart failure or renal failure is present. Hemodialysis reduces the ethylene glycol $t_{1/2}$ from 17 hours with ethanol therapy to 3 hours. Continue therapy (ethanol and hemodialysis) until the SEGC is less than 10 mg per dL or undetectable, the glycolate level is undetectable, the acidosis has cleared, there are no mental disturbances, the creatinine level is normal, and the urine output is adequate. This may require 2 to 5 days. (8) Adjunctive therapy: Thiamine (100 mg per day [children 50 mg] slowly over 5 minutes IV or IM and repeated every 6 hours) and pyridoxine (50 mg IV or IM every 6 hours) have been recommended until intoxication is resolved but have not been extensively studied. Folate may be given at 50 mg IV (in children, 1 mg per kg)* every 4 hours for 6 doses. (9) Therapy with 4-methylpyrazole given PO at 15 mg per kg, followed by 5 mg per kg in 12 hours and then 10 mg per kg every 12 hours, until

---

*Exceeds dosage recommended by the manufacturer.

levels of the toxin are not detectable, blocks ADH without causing inebriation.

Laboratory investigations: Monitor blood glucose, electrolytes, urinalysis (look for oxalate ["envelope"] and monohydrate ["hemp seed"] crystals and for urine fluorescence), and ABGs. Obtain ethylene glycol and ethanol levels and determine plasma osmolarity (use freezing point depression method), calcium, BUN, and creatinine. An SEGC of 20 mg per dL is toxic (ethylene glycol levels are difficult to obtain). If possible, obtain a glycolate level. Fluorescence testing: The oral mucosa and urine (do not put in a glass tube) fluoresce under Wood's light if antifreeze ethylene glycol is present. Cross-reactions: Propylene glycol, a vehicle in many liquids and intravenous medications (phenytoin, diazepam), other glycols, and triglycerides may produce spurious ethylene glycol levels. *Disposition:* All patients who ingest significant amounts of ethylene glycol should be referred to the emergency department. If the SEGC cannot be obtained, follow-up for 12 hours, monitoring the osmolal gap, acid-base parameters, and electrolytes, is recommended to rule out development of metabolic acidosis with an AG.

Hydrocarbons. The lower the viscosity and surface tension or the greater the volatility, the greater the risk of aspiration. Volatile substance abuse has resulted in the "sudden sniffing death syndrome," most likely caused by dysrhythmias. *Toxicologic classification and toxic mechanism:* All systemically absorbed hydrocarbons can lower the myocardial threshold for development of dysrhythmias produced by endogenous and exogenous catecholamines. (1) Petroleum distillates are aliphatic hydrocarbons. Toxic dose: Aspiration of a few drops produces chemical pneumonitis, but these substances are poorly absorbed from the GI tract and produce no systemic toxicity by this route. Examples are gasoline, kerosene charcoal lighter fluid, mineral spirits (Stoddard's solvent), and petroleum naphtha. (2) Aromatic hydrocarbons are six-carbon ringed structures that produce CNS depression and, in chronic abuse, may have multiple organ effects. Examples are benzene (which in chronic intoxications produces leukemia), toluene, styrene, and xylene. The ingested seriously toxic dose is 20 to 50 mL in an adult. (3) Halogenated hydrocarbons are aliphatic hydrocarbons with one or more halogen substitutions (Cl, Br, Fl, or I). They are highly volatile and abused as inhalants. They are well absorbed from the GI tract, produce CNS depression, and have metabolites that can damage the liver and kidneys. Examples are methylene chloride (which may be converted to CO in the body), dichloroethylene (which also causes a disulfiram reaction ["degreaser's flush"] when associated with consumption of ethanol), and 1,1,1-trichloroethane (Glamorene Spot Remover, Scotchgard, typewriter correction fluid) (acute lethal oral dose is 0.5 to 5 mL per kg). (4) Dangerous additives to the hydrocarbons include those in the mnemonic CHAMP: *c*amphor (demothing agent), *h*alogenated hydrocarbons, *a*romatic hydrocarbons, *m*etals (heavy), and *p*esticides.

Exposure to these agents may warrant gastric emptying with a small-bore nasogastric lavage tube. (5) Heavy hydrocarbons have high viscosity, low volatility, and minimal GI absorption, so gastric decontamination is not necessary. Examples are asphalt (tar), machine oil, motor oil (lubricating oil, engine oil), home heating oil, and petroleum jelly and mineral oil. (7) Mineral seal oil (e.g., signal oil), found in furniture polishes, is a low-viscosity, low-volatility oil with minimal absorption that never warrants gastric decontamination. It can produce severe pneumonia if aspirated.

Management: (1) Asymptomatic patients who ingested small amounts of petroleum distillates may be observed at home by reliable caretakers for development of signs of aspiration (cough, wheezing, tachypnea, and dyspnea) with periodic telephone contact for 4 to 6 hours. (2) Inhalation of any hydrocarbon vapors in a closed space can produce intoxication. Remove the victim from the environment, and administer oxygen and respiratory support. (3) GI decontamination is not advised in ingestions of hydrocarbons that usually do not cause systemic toxicity (petroleum distillates, heavy hydrocarbons, mineral seal oil). For hydrocarbons that cause systemic toxicity in small amounts (aromatic hydrocarbons, halogenated hydrocarbons), pass a small-bore nasogastric tube (these substances are liquids) and aspirate if appropriate time has not elapsed (absorption with aromatic and halogenated hydrocarbons is complete in 1 to 2 hours) and spontaneous vomiting has not occurred. Patients with altered mental status should have the airway protected because of concern over uncontrolled vomiting. Although some toxicologists advocate ipecac-induced emesis under medical supervision instead of small-bore nasogastric gastric lavage, we do not. AC is suggested, but there are no reliable data concerning its effectiveness, and it may produce vomiting. AC may, however, be useful for adsorbing toxic additives or co-ingestants. (4) The symptomatic patient who is coughing, gagging, choking, or wheezing on arrival has probably already aspirated. Offer supportive respiratory care: maintain the airway, provide assisted ventilation, and offer supplemental oxygen with monitoring of pulse oximetry; also measure ABGs, obtain a chest radiograph and ECG, and admit to the ICU. A chest radiograph for aspiration may be positive as early as 30 minutes, and almost all are positive within 6 hours. If bronchospasm occurs, administer a nebulized beta-adrenergic agonist and intravenous aminophylline if necessary. Avoid epinephrine because of the susceptibility to dysrhythmias. If cyanosis is present that does not respond to oxygen and the PaO_2 is normal, suspect methemoglobinemia, which may necessitate therapy with methylene blue (see Table 10). Corticosteroids and prophylactic antimicrobial agents have not been shown to be beneficial. (Fever or leukocytosis may be produced by the chemical pneumonitis itself.) It is not necessary to surgically treat pneumatoceles that develop, because they usually resolve. Most infiltrations resolve spontaneously in 1 week except for lipoid pneumonia, which may last up to 6 weeks. Dysrhythmias may necessitate alpha- and beta-adrenergic antagonists or cardioversion. (5) There is no role for enhanced elimination procedures. (6) Methylene chloride is metabolized in several hours to CO. See the section on treatment of CO poisoning. Give 100% oxygen, and monitor serial COHb levels, ECG, and pulse oximetry. (7) Halogenated hydrocarbons are hepatorenal toxins; therefore, monitor liver and kidney function. NAC therapy may be useful if there is evidence of hepatic damage. (8) Investigational: Surfactant has been used for hydrocarbon aspiration in an animal study of aspirated hydrocarbons and was found to be detrimental. Extracorporeal membrane oxygenation has been used successfully in a few patients with life-threatening respiratory failure.

Laboratory investigations: Monitor ECG continuously; ABGs; liver, pulmonary, and renal function; serum electrolytes; and serial chest radiographs. *Disposition:* Asymptomatic patients with small ingestions of petroleum distillates can be managed at home. Symptomatic patients with abnormal results on chest radiograph, oxygen saturation, or ABGs should be admitted. If the patient becomes asymptomatic, oxygenation is normal, and repeated radiographs are normal, the patient can be discharged.

Iron. There are more than 100 over-the-counter iron preparations for supplementation and treatment of iron deficiency anemia. *Toxic mechanism:* Toxicity depends on the amount of elemental (free) iron available in various salts (gluconate 12%, sulfate 20%, fumarate 33%, lactate 19%, and chloride 21%, of elemental iron), not on the amount of the preparation. Locally, iron is corrosive and may cause fluid loss, hypovolemic shock, and perforation. Excessive free iron in the blood is directly toxic to the vasculature and leads to the release of vasoactive substances that produce vasodilatation. In overdose, iron deposits injure mitochondria in the liver, the kidneys, and the myocardium. The exact mechanism of cellular damage is not clear. *Toxic dose:* The therapeutic dose of elemental iron is 6 mg per kg per day. Elemental iron at 20 to 40 mg per kg per dose may produce mild self-limited GI symptoms; a dose of 40 to 60 mg per kg produces moderate toxicity; more than 60 mg per kg produces severe toxicity and is potentially lethal; and more than 180 mg per kg is usually fatal without treatment. Children's chewable vitamins with iron have from 12 to 18 mg of elemental iron per tablet or per 0.6 mL of liquid drops. These preparations rarely produce toxicity unless extremely large quantities are ingested. The following equation can be used to calculate the amount of elemental iron ingested:

$$\text{Elemental iron (mg/kg)} = \frac{\text{number of tablets ingested} \times \%\text{ elemental iron}}{\text{body weight (kg)}}$$

Kinetics: Absorption occurs chiefly in the upper small intestine, usually with iron in the ferrous $(2+)$ state absorbed into the mucosal cells, where it is oxidized to the ferric $(3+)$ state and bound to ferritin. Iron is slowly released from ferritin into the plasma to become bound to transferrin and transported to specific tissues for production of hemoglobin (70%), myoglobin (5%), and cytochrome. About 25% of iron is stored in the liver and spleen. In overdoses, larger amounts of iron are absorbed because of direct mucosal corrosion. There is no mechanism for additional elimination of iron (normal elimination is 1 to 2 mg per day) except through bile, sweat, and blood loss. *Manifestations:* Serious toxicity is unlikely if the patient remains asymptomatic for 6 hours, has a normal WBC count and glucose level and has a negative abdominal radiograph. Iron intoxication usually follows a multiphasic course. A phase may be omitted entirely. Phase I: GI mucosal injury occurs 30 minutes to 12 hours after ingestion. Vomiting starts 30 minutes to 1 hour after ingestion and is persistent. Hematemesis and bloody diarrhea, abdominal cramps, fever, hyperglycemia, and leukocytosis occur. Enteric-coated tablets may pass through the stomach without causing symptoms. Acidosis and shock can occur within 6 to 12 hours. Phase II is a latent period of apparent improvement spanning the 8 to 12 hours after ingestion. Phase III is the systemic toxicity phase (12 to 48 hours after ingestion), with cardiovascular collapse and severe metabolic acidosis. Phase IV (2 to 4 days after ingestion) is characterized by hepatic injury associated with jaundice, elevated liver enzymes, prolonged prothrombin time, and kidney injury with proteinuria and hematuria. Pulmonary edema, disseminated intravascular coagulation, and *Yersinia enterocolitica* sepsis can occur. In phase V (4 to 8 weeks after ingestion), sequelae affecting the pyloric outlet or intestinal stricture may cause obstruction or anemia secondary to blood loss.

Management: (1) GI decontamination: Induce emesis immediately in ingestions of elemental iron greater than 40 mg per kg if the patient has not already vomited. Gastric lavage with 0.9% saline is less effective than emesis because of the large size of the tablets but may be useful if chewed tablets and liquid preparations are involved. AC is ineffective. Obtain an abdominal radiograph after emesis or lavage to determine the success of gastric emptying procedures. Children's chewable vitamins and liquid iron are not radiopaque. If radiopaque iron is still present, consider whole-bowel irrigation with PEG solution (see the section on evaluation and general management). (2) In extreme cases, removal by endoscopy or surgery may be necessary because coalesced iron tablets can produce hemorrhagic infarction in the bowel and perforation peritonitis. (3) Deferoxamine (DFO) (see Table 10): About 100 mg of DFO binds only 8.5 to 9.35 mg of free iron in the serum in transit. The DFO infusion rate (the intravenous route is preferred) should not exceed 15 mg per kg per hour or 6 grams daily, but higher rates (up to 45 mg per kg per hour) and larger daily amounts have been administered and tolerated in extreme cases of iron poisoning (greater than 1000 µg per dL). The DFO-iron complex is hemodialyzable if renal failure develops. Indications for chelation therapy are any of the following: serious clinical intoxication (severe vomiting and diarrhea [often bloody], severe abdominal pain, metabolic acidosis, hypotension, or shock); symptoms that persist or become worse; estimate of elemental iron ingestion that is quite high and presence of symptoms; and serum iron (SI) levels greater than 500 µg per dL. Chelation should be performed as early as possible, within 12 to 18 hours, to be effective. Start the infusion slowly and gradually increase to avoid hypotension. Successful chelation results in a urine color change from a positive vin rosé color to a normal color. Adult respiratory distress syndrome has developed in patients receiving high doses of DFO for several days; therefore, avoid prolonged infusions over 24 hours. The end points of treatment are absence of symptoms and clearing of the urine that was originally a positive vin rosé color. In a diagnostic chelation test, DFO, 50 mg per kg in children or 1 gram in adults intramuscularly (IM), produces a vin rosé color (ferroxime-iron complex) of the urine within 3 hours. This is not a reliable test for elevated SI levels; however, obtain a baseline urine sample for comparison with subsequent specimens. (4) Supportive therapy: Intravenous bicarbonate may be needed to correct the metabolic acidosis. Hypotension and shock treatment may necessitate fluid volume expansion, vasopressors, and blood transfusions. Attempt to keep the urine output at more than 2 mL per kg per hour. Coagulation abnormalities and overt bleeding necessitate infusion of blood products and vitamin K. (5) Treatment in pregnant patients is similar to that in any others with iron poisoning. (6) Extracorporeal measures: Hemodialysis and hemoperfusion are not effective. Exchange transfusion has been used in single cases of massive poisoning in children.

Laboratory investigations: Iron poisoning produces AG metabolic acidosis. Monitor the CBC, blood glucose, SI, stools and vomitus (for occult blood), electrolytes, acid-base balance, urinalysis results and urine output, liver function tests, BUN, and creatinine. If GI bleeding occurs, obtain and match the blood type. SI measured at the proper time correlates with the clinical findings. The lavender-top Vacutainer tube contains ethylenediaminetetraacetic acid (EDTA), which falsely lowers the SI. Obtain the SI before administering DFO. SI levels at 2 to 6 hours of less than 350 µg per dL predict an asymptomatic course; levels of 350 to 500 µg per dL are usually associated with mild GI symptoms; levels above 500 µg per dL predict a 20% risk of shock and serious iron intoxication with phase III manifestations. A follow-up SI level after 6 hours may not be elevated even in severe poisoning; however, an SI level at 8 to 12 hours is useful for excluding delayed absorption from a bezoar or sustained-release preparation. Determination of the total iron-binding capacity is not a necessary study. Abdominal radiographs can visualize adult iron tablet preparations before they dissolve. A nega-

tive radiograph does not exclude iron poisoning. Iron sepsis: Patients who develop high fevers and signs of sepsis after iron overdose should have blood and stool cultures checked for *Y. enterocolitica. Disposition:* Observe the patient who is asymptomatic or has minimal symptoms for persistence and progression of symptoms or development of signs of toxicity (GI bleeding, acidosis, shock, altered mental state). A patient with mild self-limited GI symptoms who becomes asymptomatic or has no signs of toxicity for 6 hours is unlikely to have serious intoxication and can be discharged after psychiatric clearance, if needed. Patients with moderate or severe toxicity should be in the ICU.

Isoniazid (isonicotinic acid hydrazide, INH, Nydrazid). INH is a hydrazide derivative of vitamin B_3 (nicotinamide) used as an antituberculosis drug. *Toxic mechanism:* INH produces pyridoxine deficiency by doubling the excretion of pyridoxine (vitamin B_6) and by inhibiting the interaction of pyridoxal 5-phosphate (the active form of pyridoxine) with L-glutamic acid decarboxylase to form GABA, the major CNS neurotransmitter inhibitor, resulting in seizures and coma. INH blocks the conversion of lactate to pyruvate, resulting in profound lactic acidosis. *Toxic dose:* The therapeutic dose is 5 to 10 mg per kg (maximum of 300 mg) daily. A single acute dose of 15 mg per kg lowers the seizure threshold, 35 to 40 mg per kg produces spontaneous convulsions, more than 80 mg produces severe toxicity, and 200 mg per kg is an obligatory convulsant. Malnourished persons, those with a previous seizure disorder or alcoholism, and slow acetylators are more susceptible to INH toxicity. In chronic intoxication, 10 mg per kg per day produces hepatitis in 10 to 20% of patients, but doses of 3 to 5 mg per kg per day affect less than 2%. *Kinetics:* Rapid absorption from intestine occurs in 30 to 60 minutes, onset is in 30 to 120 minutes, and the peak level of 5 to 8 µg per mL is reached within 1 to 2 hours. The Vd is 0.6 liter per kg; PB is minimal. Elimination is by liver acetylation to a hepatotoxic metabolite, acetylisoniazid, which is then hydrolyzed to isonicotinic acid. Slow acetylators show a $t_{1/2}$ of 140 to 300 minutes (mean 5 hours) and eliminate 10 to 15% of the drug unchanged in the urine. Forty-five to 75% of whites and 50% of African blacks are slow acetylators and with chronic use (without pyridoxine supplements) may develop peripheral neuropathy. Fast acetylators show a $t_{1/2}$ of 35 to 110 minutes (mean 80 minutes) and excrete 25 to 30% of the drug unchanged in the urine. About 90% of Asians and patients with diabetes mellitus are fast acetylators and may develop hepatitis with chronic use. In overdose and hepatic disease, the serum $t_{1/2}$ may increase. INH inhibits the metabolism of phenytoin, diazepam, phenobarbital, carbamazepine, and prednisone. These drugs also interfere with the metabolism of INH. Ethanol may decrease the INH $t_{1/2}$ but may increase its toxicity. *Manifestations:* Within 30 to 60 minutes, nausea, vomiting, slurred speech, dizziness, visual disturbances, and ataxia are present. Within 30 to 120 minutes, the major clinical triad of severe overdose develops: (1) refractory convulsions (90% of overdose patients have one or more seizures), (2) coma, and (3) resistant severe AG lactic acidosis (secondary to convulsions), and metabolic blocks, often with pH of 6.8. Acidosis occurs after seizures.

Management: (1) Control seizures: Administer pyridoxine, 1 gram for each gram of isoniazid ingested (see Table 10). If the dose ingested is unknown, give at least 5 grams (70 mg per kg) of pyridoxine IV. Pyridoxine is administered in 50 mL of D5W or 0.9% saline over 5 minutes IV. Do not administer in the same bottle as for NaHCO₃. Repeat intravenous pyridoxine every 5 to 20 minutes until seizures are controlled. Total doses of pyridoxine up to 52 grams have been safely administered. However, patients given 132 and 183 grams of pyridoxine have developed a persistent crippling sensory neuropathy. Some authorities recommend prophylactic pyridoxine if there is a history of ingestion of 80 mg of INH per kg. Administer diazepam concomitantly with pyridoxine but at a different site. They work synergistically. Administer diazepam IV at 0.3 mg per kg slowly at rate of 1 mg per minute in children or 10 mg per dose slowly at rate of 5 mg per minute in adults. After the seizures are controlled, administer the remainder of the pyridoxine (1 gram per gram of INH), or total dose of 5 grams, as an infusion drip over 60 minutes. Do not use phenobarbital (it increases INH metabolism to toxic metabolites) or phenytoin (it interferes with INH metabolism and is not effective). (2) In asymptomatic patients or patients without seizures, pyridoxine should be considered prophylactically in gram-for-gram doses with large overdoses (80 mg per kg per dose or more) of INH (there are no supporting studies, however). (3) In comatose patients, pyridoxine administration may result in rapid regaining of consciousness. (4) Correction of the acidosis and control of the seizures may occur spontaneously with pyridoxine administration. Administer NaHCO₃ if acidosis persists. (5) GI decontamination: After the patient is stabilized, or if the patient is asymptomatic, gastric lavage may be performed after recent (less than 1 hour) ingestion, with protection of the airway if necessary. AC may be administered. (6) Hemodialysis is rarely needed because of antidotal therapy and the short $t_{1/2}$ but may be used as adjunctive therapy for uncontrollable acidosis and seizures. Hemoperfusion has not been adequately evaluated. Diuresis is ineffective.

Laboratory investigations: INH produces AG metabolic acidosis. Therapeutic levels are 5 to 8 μg per mL, and acute toxic levels are more than 20 μg per mL. Monitor the blood glucose (hyperglycemia is common), electrolytes (hyperkalemia is frequent), bicarbonate, ABGs, liver function tests (elevations occur with chronic exposure), BUN, and creatinine. *Disposition:* Asymptomatic or mildly asymptomatic patients who become asymptomatic may be observed in the emergency department for 4 to 6 hours. Larger amounts of INH may warrant pyridoxine and longer periods of observation. Patients with intentional ingestions require psychiatric evaluation before discharge. Patients with convulsions or coma should be admitted to the ICU.

Isopropanol (IP or rubbing alcohol, solvents, lacquer thinner). Coma has occurred in children sponged for fever with isopropanol. See Table 21. *Toxic mechanism:* Isopropanol is a gastric irritant. It is metabolized to acetone, a CNS and myocardial depressant. It inhibits gluconeogenesis. Normal propyl alcohol is related to isopropanol but is more toxic. *Toxic dose:* The toxic dose is 0.5 to 1 mg of 70% isopropanol per kg (1 mL of 70% isopropanol per kg produces a blood isopropyl alcohol concentration [BIPC] of 70 mg per dL). The CNS depressant effect is twice that of ethanol. *Kinetics:* Onset is within 30 to 60 minutes, and the peak effect occurs 1 hour after ingestion. Elimination is renal. Isopropyl alcohol is metabolized to acetone. The Vd is 0.6 liter per kg. The BIPC and amount ingested can be estimated by using equations in ethanol kinetics and an SG of 0.785 for isopropanol:

$$\text{BIPC (mg/dL)} = \frac{\begin{matrix}\text{amount} \\ \text{ingested} \\ \text{(mL)}\end{matrix} \times \begin{matrix}\text{\% isopropyl} \\ \text{alcohol in} \\ \text{product}\end{matrix} \times \text{SG (0.79)}}{\text{Vd (0.6 L/kg)} \times \text{body weight (kg)}}$$

$$\text{Dose (amount ingested)} = \frac{\text{BIPC (mg/dL)} \times \text{Vd (0.6 L/kg)} \times \text{body weight (kg)}}{\text{\% ethanol} \times \text{SG (0.79)}}$$

Manifestations: Ethanol-like inebriation with an acetone odor of the breath, gastritis occasionally with hematemesis, acetonuria, and acetonemia without systemic acidosis are seen. CNS depressant effects include lethargy at 50 to 100 mg per dL and coma at 150 to 200 mg per dL; ingestion of more than 240 mg per dL is potentially fatal in adults. Hypoglycemia and seizures may occur. *Management:* (1) Protect the airway with intubation and administer assisted ventilation if necessary. If the patient is hypoglycemic, administer glucose. Supportive treatment is similar to that for ethanol. (2) GI decontamination has no role. (3) Hemodialysis in life-threatening overdose is rarely needed. Consult a nephrologist if the BIPC is greater than 250 mg per dL. *Laboratory investigation:* Monitor isopropyl alcohol levels, acetone, glucose, and ABGs. The osmolal gap increases 1 mOsm per 5.9 mg per dL of isopropyl alcohol and 1 mOsm per 5.5 mg per dL of acetone. Absence of excess acetone in the blood (normal, 0.3 to 2 mg per dL) within 30 to 60 minutes or excess acetone in the urine within 3 hours excludes the possibility of significant isopropanol exposure. *Disposition:* Symptomatic patients with concentrations greater than 100 mg per dL require at least 24 hours of close observation for resolution and should be admitted. If the patient is hypoglycemic, hypotensive, or comatose, admit to the ICU.

Lead. Lead is an environmental toxin. Acute lead intoxication is rare and is usually caused by inhalation of lead, resulting in severe intoxication and often death. It may be produced by burning lead batteries or using a heat gun to remove lead paint. It also results from exposure to high concentrations of organic lead (e.g., tetraethyl lead). Chronic lead poisoning occurs most often in children 6 months to 6 years of age who are exposed in their environment and in adults in certain occupations. See Table 23. In the United States, the percentage of children 1 to 5 years of age with a venous blood lead level (VBPb) greater than 10 μg per dL decreased from 88.2% in a survey from 1976 to 1980 to 8.9% in a survey from 1988 to 1991 as a result of measures to reduce lead in the environment, particularly by reducing leaded gasoline. However, an estimated 1.7 million children between 1 and 5 years old have blood lead levels greater than 10 μg per dL, and more than 1 million workers in over 100 different occupations are exposed to lead. *Toxic dose in chronic lead poisoning:* An intake of more than 5 μg per kg per day in children or more than 150 μg per day in adults can give toxic screen levels of lead. In 1991, the Centers for Disease Control and Prevention (CDC) recommended routine screening for children. The CDC recommended a VBPb or a capillary blood lead determination for all children. In children a VBPb greater than 10 μg per dL was determined by the CDC to be a threshold of concern (it was 25 μg per dL in 1985). The average VBPb in the United States is 4 μg per dL. In occupational exposure (see Table 23) a VBPb greater than 40 μg per dL is indicative of increased lead absorption in adults. *Toxic mechanism:* Lead affects the sulfhydryl enzyme systems of the proteins, the immature CNS, the enzymes of heme synthesis, vitamin D conversion, the kidneys, the bones, and growth. Lead alters the tertiary structure of cell proteins, denaturing them and causing death. Risk factors are mouthing behavior of infants and children and excessive oral behavior (pica), living in the inner city, a poorly maintained home, and poor nutrition (e.g., low calcium and iron). Use of the CDC questionnaire is recommended at every pediatric visit. See Table 24. If any answers to the CDC questionnaire

are positive, obtain a blood screening test for lead. However, studies have suggested that to be more accurate in identifying lead exposure, the questionnaire would have to be modified for each community because it has had poor sensitivity (40%) and specificity (60%). *Sources of lead* (Table 25): (1) The primary source of lead is deteriorating lead-based paint, which forms leaded dust. Lead concentrations in indoor paint were not reduced to safer levels (0.06%) until 1978. Lead can also be produced by improper interior or exterior home renovation (scraping or demolition). (2) The use of leaded gasoline (limited in 1973) resulted in residues from leaded motor vehicle emissions. Lead persists in the soil near major highways and deteriorating homes and buildings. Vegetables grown in contaminated soil may contain lead. (3) Oil refineries and lead-processing smelters are other sources. (4) Food cans produced in Mexico contain lead solder (95% of those produced in the United States do not). (5) Lead pipes (manufactured until 1950) and pipes with lead solder (manufactured until 1986) deliver lead-containing drinking water (calcium deposits, however, may offer some protection). Water at the consumer's tap should have a lead level less than 15 ppb (parts per billion). See Table 26. (6) Occupational exposure (see Table 23): Occupational Safety and Health Administration (OSHA) standards require employers to provide showering and clothes-changing facilities for persons working with lead; however, businesses with fewer than 25 employees are exempt from regulation. The OSHA lead standard of 1978 set a limit of 60 μg per dL for occupational exposure to lead. At a blood lead level of 60 μg

TABLE 24. CDC Questionnaire: Priority Groups for Lead Screening

1. Children 6–72 mo old (was 12–36 mo) who live in or are frequent visitors to older deteriorated housing built before 1960
2. Children 6–72 mo old who live in housing built before 1960 with recent, ongoing, or planned renovation or remodeling
3. Children 6–72 mo old who are siblings, housemates, or playmates of children with known lead poisoning
4. Children 6–72 mo old whose parents or other household members participate in a lead-related industry or hobby
5. Children 6–72 mo old who live near active lead smelters, battery recycling plants, or other industries likely to result in atmospheric lead release

TABLE 23. Occupations Associated with Lead Exposure

Lead production or smelting	Instructor or janitor at firing range
Production of illicit whiskey	
Brass, copper, and lead foundries	Demolition of ships and bridges
	Battery manufacturing
Radiator repair	Machining or grinding lead alloys
Scrap handling	
Sanding of old paint	Welding of old painted metals
Lead soldering	Thermal paint stripping of old buildings
Cable stripping	
	Ceramic glaze and pottery mixing

Modified from Rempel D: The lead-exposed worker. JAMA *262*:532–534, 1989. Copyright 1989, American Medical Association.

TABLE 25. Product Lead Content by Dry Weight

Product	Lead (%)	Product	Lead (%)
Plastic additives	2.0	Construction material	0.1
Priming inks	2.0	Fertilizers	0.1
Plumbing fixtures	2.0	Toys and recreational games	0.1
Solder	0.6		
Pesticides	0.1	Curtain weights	0.1
Stained glass came	0.1	Fishing weights	0.1
Wine bottle foils	0.1	Glazes, enamels, frits	0.06
		Paint	0.06

TABLE 26. **Agency Regulations and Recommendations for Lead Content**

Agency	Specimen	Acceptable Level	Comments
CDC	Blood, child	10 μg/dL	Investigate community
OSHA	Blood, adult	60 μg/dL	Medical removal from work
OSHA	Air	50 μg/m³	PEL
	Air	0.75 mg/m³	Tetraethyl or tetramethyl
ACGIH	Air	150 μg/m³	TWA
EPA	Air	1.5 μg/m³	3-mo average
EPA	Water	15 μg/liter (ppb)	5 ppb circulating
EPA	Food	100 μg/d	Advisory
FDA	Wine	300 ppm	Plan to reduce to 200 ppm
EPA	Soil and dust	50 ppm	
CPSC	Paint	600 ppm (0.06%)	By dry weight

Abbreviations: ACGIH = American Conference of Governmental Industrial Hygienists; CDC = Centers for Disease Control and Prevention; CPSC = Consumer Products Safety Commission; EPA = Environmental Protection Agency; FDA = Food and Drug Administration; OSHA = Occupational Safety and Health Administration; PEL = permissible exposure limit (highest level over 8-h workday); ppb = parts per billion; ppm = parts per million; TWA = time-weighted average (air concentration for 8-h workday and 40-h workweek).

per dL, a worker should be removed from lead exposure and not allowed back until the level is below 40 μg per dL. Many authorities think that this level should be lower. The lead residue on workers' clothes may represent a hazard to their families. Others occupationally exposed to lead include plumbers, pipefitters, lead miners, auto repairers, shipbuilders, printers, steel welders and cutters, construction workers, and those in rubber product manufacturing. (7) Other sources are leaded pots to make molds and "kusmusha" tea. (8) Hobbies (see Table 27) associated with lead exposure include making stained glass windows, lead fish sinkers, and curtain weights, which may pose additional hazard if ingested and retained

TABLE 27. **Hobbies Associated with Lead Exposure**

Casting of ammunition
Collecting antique pewter
Collecting or painting lead toys (e.g., soldiers and figures)
Ceramics or glazed pottery
Refinishing furniture
Making fishing weights
Home renovation
Jewelry making (lead solder)
Glassblowing (lead glass)
Bronze casting
Printmaking and other fine arts (when lead white, flake white, chrome yellow pigments are involved)
Liquor distillation
Hunting and target shooting
Painting
Car and boat repair
Burning lead-painted wood
Making stained lead glass
Copper enameling

by children; imported pottery with ceramic glaze can leach large amounts of lead into acids (e.g., citrus fruit juices). (9) Some "traditional" folk remedies or cosmetics contain lead: "Azarcon por empacho" ("Maria Louisa," 90 to 95% lead trioxide), a bright orange powder (used in Hispanic culture, especially Mexican, for digestive problems and diarrhea); "Greta" (4 to 90% lead), a yellow powder for "empacho" ("empacho" refers to a variety of GI symptoms; used in Hispanic cultures, especially Mexican); "Payloo-ah," an orange-red powder for rash and fever (used in Southeast Asian cultures, especially northern Laotian Hmong immigrants); "Alkohl" (kohl, suma, 5 to 92% lead), a black powder (used in Middle Eastern, African, and Asian cultures as a cosmetic and umbilical stump astringent); "Farouk," an orange granular powder with lead (Saudi Arabian); "Bint Al Zahab," used to treat colic (Saudi Arabian); "Surma" (23 to 26% lead), a black powder used in India as a cosmetic and to improve eyesight; and "Bali goli," a round black bean that is dissolved in "grippe water" (used by Asian and Indian cultures to aid digestion). (10) Substance abuse: The synthesis of amphetamines includes lead acetate, which may not be removed before use. Lead poisoning as a result of sniffing organic lead gasoline has been reported. *Kinetics:* Absorption of lead is 10 to 15% of the ingested dose in adults; in children, up to 40% is absorbed, especially when iron deficiency anemia is present. Inhalation absorption is rapid and complete. The Vd in blood (0.9% of total body burden) is 95% in red blood cells; the $t_{1/2}$ is 35 to 40 days; $t_{1/2}$ in soft tissue, 45 days; and $t_{1/2}$ in bone (99% of the lead), 28 years. Lead is eliminated via the stool (80 to 90%); kidneys (10%; 80 μg per day); and hair, nails, sweat, and saliva. Organic lead is metabolized in the liver to inorganic lead; 9% is excreted in the urine per day. Lead passes through the placenta to the fetus and is present in breast milk. *Manifestations:* See Table 28. Adverse health effects include the following: (1) Hematologic: Lead inhibits δ-aminolevulinic acid dehydratase early in the synthesis of heme (which has been associated with CNS symptoms) and ferrochelatase (which transfers iron to ferritin for iron incorporation into protoporphyrin to produce heme); anemia is a late finding. Decreased heme synthesis starts at a VBPb of more than 40 μg per dL. Basophilic stippling occurs in 20% of persons with severe lead poisoning. (2) Neurologic: segmental demyelination and peripheral neuropathy, usually of motor type (wrist and ankle drop), occur in workers. A VBPb greater than 70 μg per dL (usually greater than 100 μg per dL) produces encephalopathy in children (a symptom mnemonic is PAINT: *p*ersistent forceful vomiting and papilledema, *a*taxia, *i*ntermittent stupor and lucidity, *n*eurologic coma and refractory convulsions, *t*ired and lethargic). Decreased cognitive abilities have been associated with a VBPb higher than 10 μg per dL; behavior problems and decreased attention span and learning abilities have been reported. IQ scores may begin to decrease at 15 μg per dL. In adults, peripheral neuropathies and "lead gum lines" at the dental border of the gingiva

TABLE 28. **Summary of Lead-Induced Health Effects in Adults and Children**

Blood Lead Level (μg/dL)	Age Group	Health Effect
>100	Adult	Encephalopathic signs and symptoms
>80	Adult	Anemia
	Child	Encephalopathy
		Chronic nephropathy (e.g., aminoaciduria)
>70	Adult	Clinically evident peripheral neuropathy
	Child	Colic and other GI symptoms
>60	Adult	Female reproductive effects
		CNS disturbances and symptoms (i.e., sleep disturbances, mood changes, memory and concentration problems, headaches)
>50	Adult	Decreased hemoglobin production
		Decreased performance on neurobehavioral tests
		Altered testicular function
		GI symptoms (i.e., abdominal pain, constipation, diarrhea, nausea, anorexia)
	Child	Peripheral neuropathy
>40	Adult	Decreased peripheral nerve conduction
		Hypertension, age 40–59 y
		Chronic neuropathy
>25	Adult	Elevated erythrocyte protoporphyrin in males
15–25	Adult	Elevated erythrocyte protoporphyrin in females
	Child	Decreased intelligence and growth
>10	Fetus/child	Preterm delivery
		Impaired learning
		Reduced birth weight
		Impaired mental ability

From Implementation of the Lead Contamination Control Act of 1988. MMWR Morb Mortal Wkly Rep *41*:288–290, 1992.

occur. Encephalopathy is rare in adults. (3) Renal nephropathy with damaged capillaries and glomeruli is seen at a VBPb greater than 80 μg per dL, but renal damage and hypertension have been observed with low VBPb values. Lead reduces excretion of uric acid, and high-level exposure is associated with hyperuricemia and "saturnine gout," Fanconi's syndrome (aminoaciduria and renal tubular acidosis), and tubular fibrosis. A linear association between hypertension and a VBPb of 30 μg per dL has been reported. (4) Reproductive system effects include spontaneous abortion, transient delay in development (catch-up age, 5 to 6 years), a decreased sperm count, and abnormal sperm morphology. Lead is transmitted across the placenta in 75 to 100% of cases and is teratogenic. (5) Metabolic: Decreased cytochrome P-450 (which alters metabolism of drugs and endogenously produced substances), decreased activation of cortisol, and decreased growth caused by interference with vitamin conversion (25-hydroxyvitamin D to 1,25-dihydroxyvitamin D) have been seen at a VBPb of 20 to 30 μg per dL. (6) Other abnormalities of thyroid, cardiac, and hepatic function occur in adults. Abdominal colic is seen in children with a VBPb greater than 50 μg per dL.

Management: The basis of treatment is removal of the source. Cases of poisoning in children should be reported to the local health department, and cases of occupational poisoning, to OSHA. Control the exposure by identifying and abating the source, improving housekeeping by wet mopping and using a high-phosphate detergent solution, allowing cold water to run for 2 minutes before using it for drinking, and planting shrubbery in contaminated soil to keep chil-

dren away. (1) GI decontamination: Lead does not bind to AC. Do not delay chelation therapy for complete GI decontamination in severe cases. Whole-bowel irrigation has been used before treatment. Some authorities recommend abdominal radiography followed by GI decontamination, if necessary, before switching to oral therapy. (2) Supportive care includes measures to deal with refractory seizures (continue antidotal therapy, diazepam, and possibly neuromuscular blockers), hepatic and renal failure, and intravascular hemolysis. Treat seizures with diazepam, followed by neuromuscular blockers if needed. (3) Chelation therapy is used for children with levels above 45 μg per dL and adults with levels above 80 μg per dL or at lower levels with a positive lead mobilization test. See Table 29. Dimercaprol (BAL, British antilewisite) is a peanut oil–based dithiol (two sulfhydryl molecules) that combines with one atom of lead to form a heterocyclic stable ring complex. It is usually reserved for cases in which VBPb is above 70 μg per dL. It chelates red blood cell–bound lead and enhances its elimination through the urine and bile. It also crosses the blood-brain barrier. About 50% of patients have adverse reactions, including an unpleasant metallic taste in the mouth, pain at the injection site, sterile abscesses, and fever. Edetate calcium disodium (EDTA, CaNa$_2$EDTA, Calcium Disodium Versenate) is a water-soluble chelator given IM (with 0.5% procaine) or IV. The calcium in the compound is displaced by divalent and trivalent heavy metals, which form a soluble complex that is stable at physiologic pH (but not at acid pH) and enhances clearance in the urine. It is usually administered IV, especially in severe cases. It must not be

TABLE 29. **Pharmacologic Chelation Therapy for Lead Poisoning**

Drug	Route	Dose	Duration	Precautions	Monitor
Dimercaprol (BAL in oil)	IM	3–5 mg/kg q 4–6 h	3–5 d	G6PD deficiency Concurrent iron therapy	AST and ALT
CaNa₂EDTA (Calcium Disodium Versenate)	IM or IV	50 mg/kg/d	5 d	Inadequate fluid intake Renal impairment	Urinalysis BUN Creatinine
D-Penicillamine (Cuprimine)	PO	10 mg/kg/d; increase to 30 mg/kg over 2 wk	6–20 wk	Penicillin allergy Concurrent iron therapy Lead exposure Renal impairment	Urinalysis BUN Creatinine CBC
2,3-Dimercaptosuccinic acid (DMSA; succimer)	PO	10 mg/kg per dose tid for 5d 10 mg/kg per dose bid for 14 d	19 d	AST and ALT elevations Concurrent iron therapy G6PD deficiency Lead exposure	AST and ALT

Abbreviations: BAL = British antilewisite; G6PD = glucose-6-phosphate dehydrogenase; AST = aspartate aminotransferase; ALT = alanine aminotransferase; BUN = blood urea nitrogen; CBC = complete blood count; EDTA = ethylenediaminetetra-acetic acid.

administered until adequate urine flow is established. It may redistribute lead to the brain; therefore, BAL is started at a VBPb exceeding 55 μg per dL in children and 100 μg per dL in adults. Phlebitis occurs at concentrations above 0.5 mg per mL. Alkalization of the urine may be helpful (see Table 10). CaNa₂EDTA should not be confused with sodium EDTA (disodium edetate), which is used to treat hypercalcemia; inadvertent use may produce severe hypocalcemia. Succimer (dimercaptosuccinic acid [DMSA], Chemet), a derivative of BAL, is an oral agent approved by the FDA in 1991 for chelation in children with a VBPb above 45 μg per dL. The recommended dose is 10 mg per kg given every 8 hours for 5 days and then every 12 hours for 14 days (see Table 10). DMSA is under investigation to determine its role in children with VBPb less than 45 μg per dL. Although not approved for adults, it has been used in adults at the same dosage. Monitor the CBC, liver transaminases, and urinalysis for toxicity. D-Penicillamine is given at 20 to 40 mg per kg per day, not to exceed 1 gram per day. It is an oral chelator used to enhance the urinary elimination of lead; it is not FDA approved and has a 10% adverse reaction rate. Succimer is preferred. D-Penicillamine is used in adults with minimal symptoms but high VBPbs. A VBPb above 70 μg per dL or clinical symptoms suggesting encephalopathy in children indicate a potential life-threatening emergency. Management should be accomplished in a medical center with a pediatric ICU by a multidisciplinary team that includes a critical care specialist, toxicologist, neurologist, and neurosurgeon, with careful monitoring of neurologic parameters, fluid status, and intracranial pressure if necessary. These patients need close monitoring for hemodynamic instability. Adequate hydration should be maintained to ensure renal excretion of lead. Monitor fluids, renal and hepatic function, and electrolytes. While measures to ensure adequate urine flow are implemented, therapy should be initi-

ated with intramuscular dimercaprol (BAL) only (25 mg per kg per day divided into 6 doses). Four hours later, a combination of a second dose of BAL given IM with CaNa₂EDTA (50 mg per kg per day) given IV as a single dose infused over several hours or as a continuous infusion is administered. The double therapy is continued until VBPb is less than 40 μg per dL. Therapy is continued for 72 hours and followed by one of two alternatives: either parenteral therapy with the two drugs (CaNa₂EDTA and BAL) for 5 days or continued therapy with CaNa₂EDTA alone if there is a good response and VBPb is below 40 μg per dL. If a report on VBPb has not been obtained, continue therapy with both BAL and EDTA for 5 days. In cases of lead encephalopathy, parenteral chelation should be continued with both drugs until the patient is clinically stable before therapy is changed. Mannitol and dexamethasone can reduce the cerebral edema, but removal of the lead is essential, and the role of these agents in lead encephalopathy is not clear. Avoid surgical decompression to reduce cerebral edema. If BAL and CaNa₂EDTA are used together, a minimum of 2 days with no treatment should elapse before another 5-day course of therapy is considered. Repeat the 5-day course with CaNa₂EDTA alone if the blood lead level remains above 40 μg per dL or in combination with BAL if it is above 70 μg per dL. If a third course is required, unless there are compelling reasons, wait at least 5 to 7 days before administration. Continue chelation therapy at all costs. After chelation therapy, a period of equilibration of 10 to 14 days should be allowed, and repeated determinations of VBPb concentrations should be obtained. If the patient is stable enough for oral intake, oral succimer at 30 mg per kg per day in three divided doses for 5 days, followed by 20 mg per kg per day in two divided doses for 14 days, has been suggested, but data are limited. Continue therapy until VBPb is less than 20 μg per dL in children or 40 μg per dL in adults. Chelators combined with lead are hemodialyzable in the event of renal failure.

Laboratory investigations: (1) A classification of blood lead concentrations in children is given in Table 30. (2) The lead mobilization test is used to determine the chelatable pool of lead. It consists of the administration of 25 mg of CaNa$_2$EDTA per kg in children or 1 gram in adults as a single dose deeply IM, with 0.5% procaine diluted 1:1, or as an infusion. Empty the bladder and collect the urine for 24 hours (3 days if there is renal impairment). A modified 8-hour collection may be obtained. If the ratio of micrograms of lead excreted in the urine to the milligrams of CaNa$_2$EDTA administered is greater than 0.6, it represents an increased lead body burden, and therapeutic chelation is indicated. However, many authorities consider this test of little importance in making the decision about chelation. The use of x-ray fluorescence of bone as an alternative to determine the lead burden is being tested. (3) Evaluate the CBC, serum ferritin, VBPb, erythrocyte protoporphyrin (greater than 35 μg per dL indicates lead poisoning as well as iron deficiency and other causes), electrolytes, serum calcium and phosphorus, urine, BUN, and creatinine. Abdominal and long bone radiographs are not routine but may be useful in certain circumstances for identifying radiopaque material in bowel and lead lines in proximal tibia (these occur after prolonged exposure in association with VBPb above 50 μg per dL). Serial VBPb measurements are obtained on days 3 and 5 during treatment, 7 days after chelation therapy, then every 1 to 2 weeks for 8 weeks, and then every month for 6 months. Stop the intravenous infusion at least 1 hour before obtaining blood for lead determination. (4) Neuropsychologic tests are difficult to conduct in young children but should be considered at the end of treatment, especially to determine auditory dysfunction. *Disposition:* All patients with VBPb above 70 μg per dL or who are symptomatic should be admitted to the hospital. If a child is hospitalized, all lead hazards must be removed from the home before the child is allowed to return. The source must be eliminated by environmental and occupational investigations. The local health department should be involved in the management of children with lead poisoning; OSHA should be involved in occupational lead poisoning. Consultation with the poison control center and/or an experienced toxicologist is necessary when chelation therapy is used. Follow-up VBPb concentrations should be obtained within 1 to 2 weeks, then every 2 weeks for 8 weeks, and then monthly for 6 months if the patient required chelation therapy. All patients with VBPb values above 10 μg per dL should undergo follow-up evaluation at least every 3 months until two serial measurements are 10 μg per dL or three serial measurements are less than 15 μg per dL.

Lithium (Li, Eskalith, Lithane). Lithium is an A-1 alkali metal whose primary use is in the treatment of bipolar psychiatric disorders. Most intoxications are chronic overdoses. One gram of lithium carbonate contains 189 mg of lithium; a regular tablet, 300 mg or 8.12 mEq; and a sustained-release preparation, 450 mg or 12.18 mEq. *Toxic mechanism:* The brain is the primary target organ of toxicity, but the mechanism is unclear. Lithium may interfere with physiologic functions by acting as a substitute for cellular cations (sodium and potassium), depressing neural excitation and synaptic transmission. *Toxic dose:* A lithium dose of 1 mEq per kg (40 mg per kg) results in a serum lithium concentration of about 1.2 mEq per liter. The therapeutic serum lithium concentration in acute mania is 0.6 to 1.2 mEq per liter; for maintenance, it is 0.5 to 0.8 mEq per liter. Serum lithium levels are usually obtained 12 hours after the last dose. The toxic dose is determined by clinical manifestations and serum levels after the distribution phase. Acute ingestion of twenty 300-mg tablets (300 mg increases the serum lithium concentration by 0.2 to 0.4 mEq per liter) in adults may produce serious intoxication. Chronic intoxication is produced by any state that increases lithium reabsorption. Risk factors that predispose to chronic lithium toxicity are febrile illness, impaired renal function, hyponatremia, advanced age, lithium-induced diabetes insipidus, dehydration, vomiting and diarrheal illness, concomitant drugs (thiazide

TABLE 30. **Classification of Blood Lead Concentrations in Children**

Blood Lead Level (μg/dL)	Classification	Recommended Interventions
<9	I	None
10–14	IIa	Community intervention Repeat blood lead determination in 3 mo
15–19	IIb	Individual case management Environmental counseling Nutritional counseling Repeat blood lead determination in 3 mo
20–44	III	Medical referral Environmental inspection and/or abatement Nutritional counseling Repeat blood lead determination in 3 mo
45–69	IV	Environmental inspection and/or abatement Nutritional counseling Pharmacologic therapy: oral succimer or parenteral CaNa$_2$EDTA Repeat q 2 wk for 6–8 wk, monthly for 4–6 mo
>70	V	Hospitalization in intensive care unit Environmental inspection and/or abatement Pharmacologic therapy: dimercaprol given IM alone initially, then dimercaprol given IM and CaNa$_2$EDTA together; repeat every week

and spironolactone diuretics, NSAIDs, salicylates, angiotensin-converting enzyme inhibitors [captopril], and selective serotonin reuptake inhibitors [SSRIs] [e.g., fluoxetine and antipsychotic drugs]). *Kinetics:* GI absorption is rapid and peaks in 2 to 4 hours after ingestion of regular-release preparations, and complete absorption occurs by 6 to 8 hours. Absorption may be delayed 6 to 12 hours after ingestion of sustained-release preparations. The onset of toxicity may occur 1 to 4 hours after acute overdose but is usually delayed because lithium enters the brain slowly. The Vd is 0.5 to 0.9 liter per kg. Lithium is not protein bound. The $t_{1/2}$ after a single dose is 9 to 13 hours; at steady state it may be 30 to 58 hours. The renal handling of lithium is similar to that of sodium: by glomerular filtration and reabsorption (80%) in the proximal renal tubules. Adequate sodium must be present to prevent lithium reabsorption. More than 90% of lithium is excreted by the kidney unchanged, 30 to 60% within 6 to 12 hours. Alkalization of the urine increases clearance. *Manifestations:* It is important to distinguish among side effects and acute, acute in a patient on chronic therapy, and chronic intoxications. Chronic is the most common and dangerous type of intoxication. (1) Side effects of lithium include fine tremor, GI upset, hypothyroidism, polyuria and frank diabetes insipidus, dermatologic manifestations, and cardiac conduction deficits. Lithium is also teratogenic. (2) Toxic effects: Patients with acute poisoning may be asymptomatic with an early high serum lithium concentration of 9 mEq per liter and deteriorate as the serum level falls 50% and lithium is distributed to the brain and the other tissues. Nausea and vomiting may begin within 1 to 4 hours, but the systemic manifestations are usually delayed several more hours. It may take as long as 3 to 5 days for serious symptoms to develop. Acute toxicity is manifested by neurologic findings, including weakness, fasciculations, altered mental state, myoclonus, hyper-reflexia, rigidity, coma, and convulsions with limbs in hyperextension. Cardiovascular effects are nonspecific and occur at therapeutic doses: flat T or inverted T waves, AV block, and prolonged QT interval. Lithium is not a primary cardiotoxin. Cardiogenic shock is secondary to CNS toxicity. Chronic intoxication is associated with manifestations at lower serum lithium concentrations. There is some correlation with manifestations, especially at higher serum lithium concentrations. See Table 31. Permanent neurologic sequelae can result from lithium intoxication.

Management: (1) Establish and maintain vital functions. Institute seizure precautions and treat seizures, hypotension, and dysrhythmias. Restore normothermia. (2) Evaluation: Examine for rigidity and signs of hyper-reflexia, and monitor hydration status, renal function (BUN, creatinine), and electrolytes, especially sodium. Inquire about use of diuretics and other drugs that increase the serum lithium concentrations, and have the patient discontinue them. If the patient has been receiving chronic therapy, discontinue the lithium. Obtain serial serum lithium

TABLE 31. **Classification of Severity of Chronic Lithium Intoxication**

Classification	Manifestations	Blood Concentration (mEq/L)*
Subacute or pretoxic	Apathy, fine tremor, vomiting and diarrhea, weakness	<1.2
Mild intoxication	Lethargy, drowsiness; hypertonia, hyperreflexia; muscle rigidity, dysarthria; ataxia, apathy, nystagmus	1.2–2.5
Moderate intoxication	Impaired consciousness; severe fasciculations; coarse tremor, severe ataxia; myoclonus, paresthesias; diabetes insipidus; electrocardiographic changes; renal tubular acidosis; paralysis, blurred vision	2.5–3.5
Severe intoxication	Muscle twitching, coma; severe myoclonic jerking; cardiac dysrhythmias; seizures, spasticity, shock	>3.5

*Plasma lithium concentrations (not an absolute correlation).
Modified from El-Mallakh RS: Treatment of acute lithium toxicity. Vet Hum Toxicol 26:31–35, 1984.

concentrations every 4 hours until the concentration peaks and there is a downward trend toward an almost therapeutic range, especially with sustained-release preparations. Monitor vital signs, including temperature and ECG, and conduct serial neurologic examinations, including those of mental status and urine output. Obtain a nephrology consultation if there is a chronic and elevated serum lithium level (above 2.5 mEq per liter), a large ingestion, or altered mental state. (3) Fluid and electrolyte therapy: An intravenous line should be established, and hydration and electrolyte balance restored. Determine the serum sodium level before administration of 0.89% saline fluid in chronic overdoses, because hypernatremia may be present as a result of diabetes insipidus. Although current evidence indicates that an initial 0.89% saline infusion (at 200 mL per hour) enhances excretion of lithium, once hydration, output, and normonatremia are established, administer 0.45% saline and slow the infusion (to 100 mL per hour). (4) GI decontamination: Gastric lavage is useful only after recent acute ingestion and is not necessary after chronic intoxication. AC is ineffective. With slow-release preparations, whole-bowel irrigation may be useful, but this has not been proved. Sodium polystyrene sulfonate, an ion exchange resin, in a dose of 15 to 50 grams PO every 4 to 6 hours, may be useful in preventing absorption and in enhancing the removal in acute massive overdoses, but it is difficult to administer. The data are based on a few uncontrolled studies. (5) Hemodialysis is the most efficient method of removing lithium from the vascular compartment. It is the treatment of choice for severe intoxication with an altered mental state and seizures and in anuric patients. Long "runs" are used until the serum lithium level is below 1 mEq per liter, because of extensive re-equilibration. Monitor the serum lithium level every 4 hours after dialysis for rebound. Repeated and prolonged hemodialysis may be necessary. Expect a lag in neurologic recovery.

Laboratory investigations: Monitor CBC (lithium causes significant leukocytosis), renal dysfunction, thyroid dysfunction (chronic intoxication), ECG, and electrolytes. Determine the serum lithium concentrations every 4 hours until there is a downward trend to near the therapeutic range. The levels do not always correlate with the manifestations but are more predictive in severe intoxication. A value above 3.0 mEq per liter with chronic intoxication and altered mental state indicates severe toxicity. Patients with a value above 9 mEq per liter after an acute overdose may be asymptomatic. *Cross-reactions:* The green-top Vacutainer specimen tube containing heparin spuriously elevates the serum lithium value by 6 to 8 mEq per liter. *Disposition:* An acute asymptomatic lithium overdose cannot be medically cleared on the basis of a single lithium level. Patients should be admitted if they have any neurologic manifestations (altered mental status, hyper-reflexia, stiffness, or tremor). Patients should be admitted to the ICU if they are dehydrated, have renal impairment, or have a high or rising lithium level.

Methanol (wood alcohol). The concentration of methanol in Sterno fuel is 4% (it also contains ethanol); in windshield washer fluid, 30%; and in gas line antifreeze, 100%. *Toxic mechanism:* Methanol is metabolized by hepatic ADH to formaldehyde and formate. Formate produces tissue hypoxia, metabolic lactic acidosis, and retinal damage. Formate is converted by folate-dependent enzymes to carbon dioxide. *Toxic dose:* The minimum toxic amount is approximately 100 mg per kg. One tablespoonful (15 mL) of 40% methanol was lethal for a 2-year-old child and can cause blindness in an adult. The lethal oral dose is 30 to 240 mL of 100% methanol (20 to 150 grams). The toxic blood methanol concentration (BMC) is above 20 mg per dL; the very serious toxic and potentially fatal level is greater than 50 mg per dL. The BMC and amount ingested can be estimated from the following equations and an SG for methanol of 0.719:

$$BMC \ (mg/dL) = \frac{\substack{\text{amount} \\ \text{ingested} \\ (mL)} \times \substack{\% \ \text{methanol} \\ \text{in product}} \times SG \ (0.719)}{Vd \ (0.6 \ L/kg) \times \text{body weight (kg)}}$$

$$\text{Dose (amount ingested)} = \frac{BMC \ (mg \ per \ dL) \times Vd \ (0.6 \ L/kg) \times \text{body weight (kg)}}{\% \ \text{ethanol} \times SG \ (0.719)}$$

Kinetics: Onset of effect can be within 1 hour but is typically delayed 12 to 18 hours by metabolism to toxic metabolites. It may be delayed longer if ethanol is ingested concomitantly. Onset may be up to 72 hours in infants. The peak blood methanol concentration occurs at 1 hour. The Vd is 0.6 liter per kg (total body water); $t_{1/2}$ is 8 hours (with ethanol blocking it is 30 to 35 hours, and with hemodialysis, 2.5 hours). For metabolism, see the section on toxic mechanism. Elimination is renal. *Manifestations:* Slow metabolism may delay onset for 12 to 18 hours in adults or longer if ethanol is ingested concomitantly. Methanol may produce inebriation, a formaldehyde odor on the breath, hyperemia of the optic disk, violent abdominal colic, "snow" vision, blindness, and shock. Later, worsening acidosis, hypoglycemia, and multiple organ failure develop; death results from complications of intractable acidosis and cerebral edema. Methanol produces an osmolal gap (early), and its metabolite formate produces AG metabolic acidosis (later). Absence of an osmolar gap or AG disturbance does not always rule out methanol intoxication.

Management: (1) Protect the airway by intubation to prevent aspiration, and administer assisted ventilation as needed. Administer 100% oxygen if needed. Consult with a nephrologist early regarding the need for hemodialysis. (2) GI decontamination procedures have no role. (3) Treat metabolic acidosis vigorously with $NaHCO_3$ at 2 to 3 mEq per kg IV. Large amounts may be needed. (4) Ethanol therapy and hemodialysis (see Table 10): Classically, ethanol therapy was started if the blood methanol concentration was above 20 mg per dL, and hemodialysis was added if the concentration was above 50 mg per dL, but values less than 25 mg per dL are currently used as an indication for hemodialysis. Ethanol therapy: ADH has 100 times greater affinity for ethanol than methanol. Therefore, ethanol blocks the metabolism of methanol at a blood methanol concentration of 100 to 150 mg per dL. Initiate therapy to block metabolism if there is a history of ingestion of 0.4 mL of 100% methanol per kg, if the blood methanol level is above 20 mg per dL or the patient has an osmolar gap that is not accounted for, or if the patient is symptomatic or acidotic with an increased AG and/or hyperemia of the optic disk. (See Table 10.) Hemodialysis: Hemodialysis increases the clearance of both methanol and formate 10-fold over renal clearance. Continue to monitor methanol levels and/or formate levels for rebound every 4 hours after the procedure. Toxicologists and nephrologists have recommended early hemodialysis at blood methanol levels greater than 25 mg per dL because it significantly shortens the course of the intoxication and provides better outcomes. Other indications for early hemodialysis are significant metabolic acidosis, electrolyte abnormalities despite conventional therapy, and the presence of visual or mental symptoms. A serum formate level greater than 20 mg per dL has also been used as a criterion for hemodialysis. If hemodialysis is used, increase the infusion rate of 10% ethanol to 2.0 to 3.5 mL per kg per hour. Obtain the BEC and glucose every 2 hours. Continue therapy with both ethanol and hemodialysis until a blood methanol level is undetectable, there is no acidosis, and there are no mental or visual disturbances. This may require 2 to 5 days. (5) Treat hypoglycemia with intravenous glucose. (6) A bolus of folinic acid and folic acid has been used successfully in animal investigations to enhance formate metabolism to carbon dioxide and water. Administer leucovorin (Wellcovorin) at 1 mg per kg up to 50 mg IV every 4 hours for several days. (7) 4-Methylpyrazole inhibits ADH and is being investigated for use in methanol and ethylene glycol poisoning (see dosage under ethylene glycol management). It has been approved for use in the United States. (8) Obtain ophthalmologic consultation initially and at follow-up.

Laboratory investigations: Methanol is detected on drug screens if specified. Monitor methanol and ethanol levels every 4 hours, electrolytes, glucose, BUN, creatinine, amylase, and ABGs. Formate levels correlate more closely than do blood methanol levels with severity of intoxication and should be obtained if possible. If methanol levels are not available, the osmolal gap × 3.2 can be used to estimate the blood methanol levels in mg per dL. *Disposition:* All patients who ingest significant amounts of methanol should be referred to the emergency department for evaluation and determination of blood methanol concentration. Ophthalmologic follow-up of all intoxications should be arranged.

Monoamine Oxidase Inhibitors. MAOIs include MAO-A inhibitors, the hydrazine phenelzine sulfate (Nardil; dose, 60 to 90 mg per day), isocarboxazid (Marplan; 10 to 30 mg per day), and the nonhydrazine tranylcypromine (Parnate; 20 to 40 mg per day). The MAO-B inhibitor selegiline (deprenyl, Eldepryl; 10 mg per day), an antiparkinsonism agent, does not have toxicity similar to that of MAO-A and is not discussed. MAOIs are used to treat severe depression. *Toxic mechanism:* MAO enzymes are responsible for the oxidative deamination of both endogenous and exogenous catecholamines. MAO-A in the intestinal wall also metabolizes tyramine in food. MAOIs permanently inhibit MAO enzymes until a new enzyme is synthesized at 14 days or later. The toxicity results from the accumulation, potentiation, and prolongation of the catecholamine action followed by profound hypotension and cardiovascular collapse. *Toxic dose:* Toxicity begins at 2 to 3 mg per kg, and fatalities occur at 4 to 6 mg per kg. Death has occurred after a single dose of tranylcypromine of 170 mg in an adult. *Kinetics:* Structurally, MAOIs are related to amphetamines and catecholamines. The hydrazine peak level occurs at 1 to 2 hours; elimination is by hepatic acetylation metabolism and excretion of inactive metabolites in the urine. The nonhydrazine peak level is at 1 to 4 hours, and elimination is by hepatic metabolism to active amphetamine-like metabolites. The onset of symptoms in overdoses is delayed 6 to 24 hours after ingestion, peak activity occurs at 8 to 12 hours, and the duration is 72 hours or longer. Peak MAOI effect occurs in 5 to 10 days,

and effects last as long as 5 weeks. *Manifestations:* (1) Acute ingestion overdose: Phase I consists of an adrenergic crisis in which onset of effects is delayed for 6 to 24 hours and the peak may not be reached until 24 hours. Initial manifestations are hyperthermia, tachycardia, tachypnea, dysarthria, transient hypertension, hyper-reflexia, and CNS stimulation. Phase II consists of neuromuscular excitation and sympathetic hyperactivity with increased temperature (above 104°F [40°C]), agitation, hyperactivity, confusion, fasciculations, twitching, tremor, masseter spasm, muscle rigidity, acidosis, and electrolyte abnormalities. Seizures and dystonic reactions may occur. The pupils are mydriatic and sometimes nonreactive, with a "ping-pong gaze." Phase III, CNS depression and cardiovascular collapse, occurs in severe overdose as the catecholamines are depleted. Symptoms usually resolve within 5 days but may last 2 weeks. Phase IV consists of secondary complications; rhabdomyolysis, cardiac dysrhythmias, multiple organ failure, and coagulopathies. (2) Biogenic interactions usually occur while therapeutic doses of MAOIs are given or shortly after they are discontinued, before the new MAO enzyme is synthesized. The onset occurs within 30 to 60 minutes after exposure. The following substances have been implicated: indirect-acting sympathomimetics (e.g., amphetamines); serotonergic drugs, opioids (e.g., meperidine, dextromethorphan), tricyclic antidepressants, and SSRIs; tyramine-containing foods (wine, beer, avocados, cheese, caviar, chocolate, chicken liver); and L-tryptophan. SSRIs should not be started for at least 5 weeks after MAOIs have been discontinued. In mild cases, usually caused by foods, headache and hypertension develop and last for several hours. In severe cases, malignant hypertension and malignant hyperthermia syndromes consisting of hypertension or hyperthermia, altered mental state, skeletal muscle rigidity, shivering (often beginning in the masseter muscle), and seizures may occur. The serotonin syndrome, which may be due to inhibition of serotonin metabolism, has clinical manifestations similar to those of malignant hyperthermia and may occur with or without hyperthermia or hypertension. (3) Clinical findings in chronic toxicity include tremors, hyperhidrosis, agitation, hallucinations, confusion, and seizures and can be confused with withdrawal syndromes.

Management: (1) MAOI overdose: GI decontamination with ipecac-induced emesis should not be used because it may aggravate the food-MAOI interaction hypertension. Use gastric lavage and AC or AC alone. If the patient is admitted to the hospital and is well enough to eat, order a nontyramine diet. Extreme agitation and seizures can be controlled with BZPs and barbiturates. Phenytoin is ineffective. Nondepolarizing neuromuscular blockers (not depolarizing succinylcholine) may be needed in severe cases of hyperthermia and rigidity. If there is severe hypertension (catecholamine-mediated), use phentolamine, a parenteral alpha-blocking agent, at 3 to 5 mg IV, or labetalol, a combination of an alpha-blocking agent and beta blocker, as a 20-mg intravenous bolus. If malignant hypertension with rigidity is present, use short-acting nitroprusside and BZP. Hypertension is often followed by severe hypotension, which should be managed with fluid and vasopressors. Caution: Vasopressor therapy should be administered at lower doses than usual because of an exaggerated pharmacologic response. Norepinephrine is preferred to dopamine, which requires release of intracellular amines. Cardiac dysrhythmias are treated with standard therapy but are often refractory, and cardioversion and pacemakers may be needed. For malignant hyperthermia, administer dantrolene (see Table 10), a nonspecific peripheral skeletal relaxing agent that inhibits the release of calcium from the sarcoplasm. Dantrolene is reconstituted with 60 mL of sterile water without bacteriostatic agents; do not use glass equipment, and protect from light and use within 6 hours. The loading dose of dantrolene is 2 to 3 mg per kg given IV as a bolus, which is repeated until the signs of malignant hyperthermia (tachycardia, rigidity, increased end-tidal carbon dioxide, and increased temperature) are controlled. The maximum total dose is 10 mg per kg to avoid hepatotoxicity. When malignant hyperthermia subsides, give 1 mg dantrolene per kg IV every 6 hours for 24 to 48 hours; then give 1 mg per kg PO every 6 hours for 24 hours to prevent recurrence. There is a danger of thrombophlebitis after peripheral dantrolene administration, and it should be given through a central line if possible. In addition, provide external cooling and correct metabolic acidosis and electrolyte disturbances. BZP can be used for sedation. Dantrolene does not reverse central dopamine blockade; therefore, give bromocriptine mesylate at 2.5 to 10 mg PO or through a nasogastric tube three times a day. Treat rhabdomyolysis and myoglobinuria with fluid diuresis, furosemide, and alkalization. Hemodialysis and hemoperfusion are of no proven value. (2) Biogenic amine interactions are managed symptomatically as for overdose. For the serotonin syndrome, cyproheptadine, a serotonin blocker, may be given at 4 mg PO every hour for 3 doses, or methysergide (Sansert) at 2 mg PO every 6 hours for 3 doses may be used, but their efficacy is not proven.

Laboratory investigations: Monitor ECG, cardiac parameters, creatine kinase, ABGs, pulse oximetry, electrolytes, blood glucose, and acid-base balance. *Disposition:* All patients who ingest more than 2 mg per kg should be admitted to the hospital for 24 hours of observation and monitoring in the ICU because the life-threatening manifestations may be delayed. Patients with drug or dietary interactions that are mild may not require admission if symptoms subside within 4 to 6 hours and they remain asymptomatic. Patients with symptoms that persist or require active intervention should be admitted to the ICU.

Opioids (narcotic opiates). Opioids are used for analgesia, as antitussives, and as antidiarrheal agents, and illicit forms (heroin, opium) are used in substance abuse. Tolerance, physical dependence, and withdrawal may develop. *Toxic mechanism:* At least four main opioid receptors have been identified. Mu is considered the most important for central analgesia and depression. Kappa and delta are predominant in spinal analgesia. The sigma receptors may mediate dysphoria. Death is due to dose-dependent CNS respiratory depression or is secondary to apnea, pulmonary aspiration, or noncardiac pulmonary edema. The mechanism of noncardiac pulmonary edema is unknown. *Toxic dose:* This depends on the specific drug, route of administration, and degree of tolerance. For therapeutic and toxic doses, see Table 32. In children, respiratory depression has been produced by 10 mg of morphine or methadone, 75 mg of meperidine, and 12.5 mg of diphenoxylate. Infants younger than 3 months are more susceptible to respiratory depression; reduce the dose by 50%. *Kinetics:* Oral onset of the analgesic effect of morphine is at 10 to 15 minutes; the effect peaks in 1 hour, and the duration is 4 to 6 hours, but with sustained-release preparations (e.g., MS Contin), the duration is 8 to 12 hours. Opioids are 90% metabolized in the liver by hepatic conjugation and 90% excreted in the urine as inactive compounds. The Vd is 1 to 4 liters per kg; PB is 35 to 75%. The typical plasma $t_{1/2}$ of opiates is 2 to 5 hours, but that of methadone is 24 to 36 hours. Morphine metabolites include morphine-3-glucuronide (M3G) (inactive) and morphine-6-glucuronide (M6G) (active) and normorphine (active). Meperidine is rapidly hydrolyzed by tissue esterases into the active metabolite normeperidine, which has twice the convulsant activity of meperidine. Heroin (diacetylmorphine) is deacetylated within minutes to the metabolite 6-monacetylmorphine (6MAM), the presence of which is diagnostic of heroin use, and morphine. Propoxyphene (Darvon) has a rapid onset, and death has occurred within 15 to 30 minutes after a massive overdose. Propoxyphene is metabolized to norpropoxyphene, an active metabolite with convulsive, cardiac dysrhythmic, and heart block effects. Symptoms of diphenoxylate (Lomotil) intoxication appear within 1 to 4 hours. It is metabolized into the active metabolite difenoxin, which is five times more active as a recurrent respiratory depressant. Death has been reported in children after a single tablet. *Manifestations:* (1) Initial or mild intoxication produces miosis, dull facial expression, drowsiness, partial ptosis, and "nodding" (head drops to chest and then bobs up). Larger amounts produce the classic triad of miotic pupils (exceptions follow), respiratory depression, and depressed level of consciousness (flaccid coma). The blood pressure, pulse, and bowel sounds are decreased. (2) The presence of dilated pupils does not exclude opioid intoxication. Some exceptions to miosis include dextromethorphan (which paralyzes the iris), fentanyl, meperidine, and diphenoxylate (rarely). Physiologic disturbances, including acidosis, hypoglycemia, hypoxia, and postictal state or those due to a co-ingestant, may also produce mydriasis. (3) Usually the muscles are flaccid, but increased muscle tone may be produced by meperidine and fentanyl (chest rigidity). (4) Seizures are rare but can occur with codeine, meperidine, propoxyphene, and

TABLE 32. **Doses, Onset, and Duration of Action of Common Opioids**

Drug	Oral Dose		Onset of Action (min)	Duration of Action (h)	Adult Fatal Dose
	Adult	*Child*			
Camphored tincture of opium (0.4 mg/mL), paregoric	25 mL	0.25–0.50 mL/kg	15–30	4–5	NA
Codeine	30–180 mg (>1 mg/kg is toxic in a child, above 200 mg in adult; >5 mg/kg fatal in a child)	0.5–1 mg/kg	15–30	4–6	800 mg
Dextromethorphan	15 mg 10 mg/kg is toxic	0.25 mg/kg	15–30	3–6	NA
Diacetylmorphine (heroin)	60 mg Street heroin is less than 10% pure	NA	15–30	3–4	100 mg
Diphenoxylate (Lomotil)	5–10 mg 7.5 mg is toxic in a child, 300 mg is toxic in adult	NA	120–240	14	300 mg
Fentanyl (Sublimaze, Duragesic transdermal)	0.1–0.2 mg	0.001–0.002 mg/kg	7–8	0.5–2	1.0 mg
Hydrocodone (Hycodan, Vicodin)	5–30 mg	0.15 mg/kg	30	3–4	100 mg
Hydromorphone (Dilaudid)	4 mg	0.1 mg/kg	15–30	3–4	100 mg
Meperidine (Demerol)	100 mg	1–1.5 mg/kg	10–45	3–4	350 mg
Methadone (Dolophine)	10 mg	0.1 mg/kg	30–60	4–12	120 mg
Morphine	10–60 mg Oral dose is six times parenteral dose; MS Contin (sustained-release)	0.1–0.2 mg/kg	<20	4–6	200 mg
Oxycodone (Percodan)	5 mg	NA	15–30	4–5	NA
Pentazocine (Talwin)	50–100 mg	NA	15–30	3–4	NA
Propoxyphene (Darvon)	65–100 mg 100 mg hydrochloride = 65 mg of napsylate, toxic at 10 mg/kg	NA	30–60	2–4	700 mg

Abbreviation: NA = not available.

dextromethorphan. Hallucinations and agitation have been reported. (5) Pruritus and urticaria caused by histamine release of some opioids or by sulfites may be present. (6) Noncardiac pulmonary edema often occurs after resuscitation and naloxone administration, especially with intravenous abuse. (7) Cardiac effects include vasodilatation and hypotension. A heart murmur in a person who is addicted to an intravenous drug suggests endocarditis. Propoxyphene can produce delayed cardiac dysrhythmias. (8) Fentanyl is 100 times more potent than morphine and can cause chest wall muscle rigidity. Some of its derivatives are 2000 times more potent than morphine.

Management: (1) Provide supportive care, particularly an endotracheal tube and assisted ventilation. Temporary ventilation may be provided by bag-valve-mask with 100% oxygen. Begin cardiac monitoring; establish intravenous access; and obtain specimens for ABGs, glucose, electrolyte, BUN, creatinine, CBC, coagulation profile, liver function determinations, a toxicology screen, and urinalysis. (2) GI decontamination: Do not induce emesis. Administer AC if bowel sounds are present. Cathartics may be needed because of opioid-induced decreased GI mobility and constipation. (3) Naloxone (Narcan) (see Table 10): If addiction is suspected, restrain the patient first; then administer 0.1 mg of naloxone and double the dose every 2 minutes until the patient responds or 10 to 20 mg has been given. If addiction is not suspected, give 2 mg every 2 to 3 minutes to total of 10 to 20 mg. It is essential to determine whether there is a complete response to naloxone (mydriasis, improvement in ventilation), because administration of this drug is a diagnostic therapeutic test. A continuous naloxone infusion may be appropriate, with the use of the "response dose" every hour. Repeated doses of naloxone may be necessary because the effects of many opioids can last much longer than that of naloxone (30 to 60 minutes). Methadone intoxication may necessitate a naloxone infusion for 24 to 48 hours. Half of the response dose may have to be repeated in 15 to 20 minutes after the infusion is started. Acute iatrogenic withdrawal on administration of naloxone to a dependent patient should not be treated with morphine or other opioids. Naloxone's effects are limited to 30 to 60 minutes (shorter than those of most opioids), and withdrawal effects subside in a short time. (4) Nalmefene (Revex), an FDA-approved long-acting (4 to 8 hours) pure opioid antagonist, is being investigated, but its role in acute intoxication is unclear. It may have a role in place of naloxone infusion but could produce prolonged withdrawal. (5) Noncardiac pulmonary edema does not respond to naloxone, and the patient requires intubation, assisted ventilation, PEEP, and hemodynamic monitoring. Fluids should be given cautiously in opioid overdose because they stimulate antidiuretic hormone. (6) If the patient is comatose, give 50% glucose (3 to 4% of comatose opioid-overdose patients have hypoglycemia) and thiamine before naloxone. If the patient has seizures unresponsive to naloxone, administer diazepam and examine for other metabolic (hypoglycemia, electrolyte disturbances) and structural disorders. (7) Hypotension is rare and should prompt a search for another cause. (8) If the patient is agitated, exclude hypoxia and hypoglycemia before considering opioid withdrawal. (9) Complications to consider include urine retention, constipation, rhabdomyolysis, myoglobinuria, hypoglycemia, and withdrawal.

Laboratory investigations: For overdoses, monitor ABGs, blood glucose, and electrolytes; obtain chest radiographs and an ECG. For drug abusers, consider testing for hepatitis B, syphilis, and HIV antibody (HIV testing usually requires consent). Blood opioid concentrations are not useful. They confirm the diagnosis (morphine therapeutic levels are 65 to 80 ng per mL; toxic levels are greater than 200 ng per mL) but are not useful for making a therapeutic decision. Cross-reactions can occur with Vicks Formula 44, poppy seeds on baked goods, and other opioids (codeine and heroin are metabolized to morphine). Naloxone in a dose of 4 mg IV was not associated with a positive enzyme multiple immunoassay technique (EMIT) urine screen at 60 minutes, 6 hours, or 48 hours. *Disposition:* If a patient responds to intravenous naloxone, careful observation for relapse and the development of pulmonary edema is required, with cardiac and respiratory monitoring for 6 to 12 hours. Patients who need repeated doses of naloxone or an infusion or who develop pulmonary edema require ICU admission and cannot be discharged from the ICU until they are symptom-free for 12 hours. With intravenous administration, complications are expected to be present within 20 minutes after injection, and discharge after four symptom-free hours has been recommended. Adults with oral overdose have a delayed onset of toxicity and require observation for 6 hours. Children with oral opioid overdose should be admitted to the hospital for 24 hours of observation because of delayed toxicity. Restrain the patient who attempts to sign out against medical advice after treatment with naloxone, at least until psychiatric evaluation.

Organophosphates and Carbamates. Sources of cholinergic intoxication are insecticides, medications (carbamates), and some mushrooms. Examples of organophosphate (OP) insecticides are malathion (Cythion; low toxicity, median lethal dose [LD_{50}] is 2800 mg per kg), chlorpyrifos (Dursban; moderate toxicity, LD_{50} is 250 mg per kg), and parathion (high toxicity, LD_{50} is 2 mg per kg); carbamate insecticides are carbaryl (Sevin; low toxicity, LD_{50} is 500 mg per

kg), propoxur (Baygon; moderate toxicity, LD_{50} is 95 mg per kg), and aldicarb (Temik; high toxicity, LD_{50} is 0.9 mg per kg). Carbamate medicinals include neostigmine and physostigmine (Antilirium). Cholinergic compounds also include the dreaded "G" nerve war weapons Tubun (GA), Sarin (GB), Soman (GB), and VX. *Toxic mechanism:* (1) OPs phosphorylate the active site on red blood cell acetylcholinesterase and pseudocholinesterase in the serum (3% of the general population have a deficiency) and other organs, causing irreversible inhibition. There are two types of OP action: direct action by the parent compound (e.g., tetraethyl pyrophosphate) and indirect action by the toxic metabolite (e.g., paraoxon or malaoxon). (2) Carbamates (esters of carbonic acid) cause reversible carbamylation of the active site of the enzymes. When a critical amount of cholinesterase is inhibited (more than 50% from baseline), acetylcholine accumulates, causing transient stimulation of conduction and, soon after, paralysis of conduction, through cholinergic synapses and sympathetic terminals (muscarinic effect), the somatic nerves, the autonomic ganglia (nicotinic effect), and CNS synapses. (3) Major differences of the carbamates from OPs: Carbamate toxicity is less severe and the duration is shorter. Carbamates rarely produce overt CNS effects (poor CNS penetration); with carbamates, the acetylcholinesterase returns to normal rapidly, so blood values are not useful even in confirming the diagnosis. With carbamates, pralidoxime, the enzyme regenerator, may not be necessary in the management of mild intoxication (e.g., carbaryl), but atropine is required. *Toxic dose:* Parathion's minimum lethal dose is 2 mg in children and 10 to 20 mg in adults. The lethal dose of malathion is greater than 1375 mg per kg (it is 1000 times less toxic than parathion) and that of chlorpyrifos is 25 grams, but such high amounts are rarely ingested. *Kinetics:* Absorption is by all routes. The onset of acute ingestion toxicity occurs as early as 3 hours, usually before 12 hours, and always before 24 hours. The onset with lipid-soluble agents absorbed by the dermal route (e.g., fenthion) may be delayed more than 24 hours after exposure. Inhalation toxicity occurs immediately after exposure. Massive ingestion can produce intoxication within minutes. The effects of the thions (e.g., parathion, malathion) are delayed because they undergo hepatic microsomal oxidative metabolism to their toxic metabolites, oxons (e.g., paraoxon, malaoxon). The $t_{1/2}$ of malathion is 2.89 hours; that of parathion is 2.1 days. The metabolites are eliminated in the urine, and the presence of *p*-nitrophenol in the urine is a clue up to 48 hours after exposure. *Manifestations:* Many OPs produce a garlic odor on the breath or in the gastric contents or the container. Diaphoresis, excessive salivation, miosis, and muscle twitching are helpful clues. (1) Early, a cholinergic (muscarinic) crisis develops and consists of parasympathetic nervous system activity. DUMBELS is a mnemonic for the manifestations of *d*efecation, cramps, and increased bowel mobility; *u*rinary incontinence; *m*iosis (mydriasis may occur in 20%); *b*ronchospasm and bronchorrhea;

excess secretion; *l*acrimation; and *s*eizures. Bradycardia, pulmonary edema, and hypotension may be present. (2) Later, sympathetic and nicotinic effects occur, consisting of *m*uscle weakness and fasciculations (eyelid twitching is often present), *a*drenal stimulation and hyperglycemia, *t*achycardia, *c*ramps in muscles, and *h*ypertension (mnemonic, MATCH). Finally, paralysis of the skeletal muscles ensues. (3) CNS effects are headache, blurred vision, anxiety, ataxia, delirium and toxic psychosis, convulsions, coma, and respiratory depression. Cranial nerve palsies have been noted. Delayed hallucinations may occur. (4) Delayed respiratory paralysis and neurologic and neurobehavioral disorders have been described after exposure to certain OPs or with dermal exposure. The "intermediate" syndrome consists of paralysis of proximal and respiratory muscles developing 24 to 96 hours after the successful treatment of OP poisoning. A delayed distal polyneuropathy has been described with certain OPs (e.g., tri-*o*-cresyl phosphate [TOCP], bromoleptophos, methomidophos). (5) Complications include aspiration, pulmonary edema, and adult respiratory distress syndrome.

Management: (1) Safeguard health care personnel with protective clothing (masks, gloves, gowns, goggles, and respiratory equipment or hazardous material suits as necessary). General decontamination consists of isolation, bagging, and disposal of contaminated clothing and other articles. Establish and maintain vital functions. Institute cardiac and oxygen saturation monitoring. Intubation and assisted ventilation may be needed. Suction secretions until atropinization drying is achieved. (2) Specific decontamination: Dermal: Prompt removal of clothing and cleansing of all affected areas of skin, hair, and eyes are indicated. Ocular: Irrigation with copious amounts of tepid water or 0.9% saline is performed for at least 15 minutes. GI: If ingestion is recent, use gastric lavage with airway protection, if necessary, and administer AC. (3) Antidotes: Atropine sulfate (see Table 10) is both a diagnostic and a therapeutic agent. Atropine counteracts the muscarinic effects but is only partially effective for the CNS effects (seizures and coma). Use preservative-free atropine (no benzyl alcohol). If the patient is symptomatic (bradycardia or bronchorrhea may be present), administer a test dose of 0.02 mg per kg for a child or 1 mg for an adult IV. If there are no signs of atropinization (tachycardia, drying of secretions, and mydriasis), immediately administer atropine at 0.05 mg per kg for a child or 2 mg for an adult every 5 to 10 minutes as needed to dry the secretions and clear the lungs. Beneficial effects are seen within 1 to 4 minutes, and the maximal effect occurs in 8 minutes. The average dose in the first 24 hours is 40 mg, but 1000 mg or more has been required in severe cases. Glycopyrrolate (Robinul) may be used if atropine is not available. Maintain the maximal dose for 12 to 24 hours; then taper it and observe for relapse. Poisoning, especially with lipophilic agents (e.g., fenthion, chlorfenthion), may necessitate weeks of atropine therapy. The alternative is a continuous infusion of 8 mg of atropine in 100 mL of 0.9% saline at a rate of 0.02 to 0.08 mg per kg per hour (0.25 to 1.0 mL per kg per hour) with additional 1- to 5-mg boluses as needed to dry the secretions. Pralidoxime chloride (2-PAM) has antinicotinic, antimuscarinic, and possibly CNS effects. Concomitant use of this agent may require a reduction in the dose of atropine (see Table 10). It acts to reactivate the phosphorylated cholinesterases by binding the phosphate moiety on the esteric site and displacing it. It should be given early before "aging" of the phosphate bond produces tighter binding. However, reports indicate that 2-PAM is beneficial even several days after the poisoning. Improvement is seen within 10 to 40 minutes. The initial dose of 2-PAM is 1 to 2 grams in 250 mL of 0.89% saline over 5 to 10 minutes, for a maximum of 200 mg per minute (in adults), or 25 to 50 mg per kg (in children younger than 12 years), for a maximum of 4 mg per kg per minute. Repeat every 6 to 12 hours for several days. An alternative is a continuous infusion of 1 gram in 100 mL of 0.89% saline at 5 to 20 mg per kg per hour (0.5 to 12 mL per kg per hour) up to 500 mg per hour, with titration to the desired response. The maximum adult daily dose is 12 grams. Cardiac monitoring and blood pressure monitoring are advised during and for several hours after the infusion. The end point is absence of fasciculations and return of muscle strength. (4) Contraindicated drugs: Do not use morphine, aminophylline, barbiturates, opioids, phenothiazine, reserpine-like drugs, parasympathomimetics, or succinylcholine. (5) Noncardiac pulmonary edema may necessitate respiratory support. (6) Seizures may respond to atropine and 2-PAM, but the effect is not consistent and anticonvulsants may be required. (7) Cardiac dysrhythmias may necessitate electrical cardioversion or antidysrhythmic therapy if the patient is hemodynamically unstable. (8) Extracorporeal procedures are of no proven value.

Laboratory investigations: Monitor chest radiograph, blood glucose (nonketotic hyperglycemia occurs frequently), ABGs, pulse oximetry, ECG, blood coagulation status, liver function, hyperamylasemia (pancreatitis has been reported), and the urine for the metabolite alkyl phosphate *p*-nitrophenol. Draw blood for red blood cell cholinesterase determination before giving pralidoxime. In mild poisoning, this value is 20 to 50% of normal; in moderate poisoning, 10 to 20% of normal; and in severe poisoning, 10% of normal (more than 90% depressed). A postexposure rise of 10 to 15% in the cholinesterase level determined at least 10 to 14 days after exposure confirms the diagnosis. *Disposition:* Asymptomatic patients with normal examination findings after 6 to 8 hours of observation may be discharged. If intentional poisoning occurred, psychiatric clearance is required for discharge. Symptomatic patients should be admitted to the ICU. Observation of patients with milder carbamate poisoning, even those requiring atropine, for 6 to 8 hours without symptoms may be sufficient to rule out significant toxicity. If workplace exposure occurred, notify OSHA.

Phencyclidine (PCP, "angel dust," "peace pill," "hog"). PCP is an arylcyclohexylamine related to ketamine and chemically related to the PTZs. It is a "dissociative" anesthetic that has been banned in the United States since 1979 and is now an illicit substance; there are at least 38 analogues. It is inexpensively manufactured by "kitchen" chemists and is mislabeled as other hallucinogens. Improperly synthesized PCP may release cyanide when heated or smoked and can cause explosions. *Toxic mechanism:* PCP action is complex and not completely understood. It inhibits neurotransmitters and causes loss of pain sensation without depressing the CNS respiratory status. It stimulates alpha-adrenergic receptors and may act as a "false" neurotransmitter. The effects are sympathomimetic, cholinergic, and cerebellar stimulation. *Toxic dose:* The usual dose in "joints" is 100 to 400 mg weight; joints or leaf mixture, 0.24 to 7.9%, 1 mg per 150 leaves; tablets, 5 mg (usual street dose). CNS effects at 1 to 6 mg are hallucinations and euphoria; 6 to 10 mg produces toxic psychosis and sympathetic stimulation, 10 to 25 mg produces severe toxicity, and more than 100 mg has resulted in fatality. *Kinetics:* PCP is a lipophilic weak base with a pK_a of 8.5 to 9.5. It is rapidly absorbed when smoked and snorted, poorly absorbed from the acid stomach, and rapidly absorbed from the alkaline medium of the small intestine. It is secreted enterogastrically and is reabsorbed in the small intestine. The onset of action when it is smoked is at 2 to 5 minutes, with a peak in 15 to 30 minutes. The onset is at 30 to 60 minutes when it is taken orally and immediate when it is taken IV. Most adverse reactions in overdose begin within 1 to 2 hours. Its duration of action at low doses is 4 to 6 hours, and normality returns in 24 hours; in large overdoses, fluctuating coma may last 6 to 10 days. The $t_{1/2}$ is 1 hour (in overdose, 11 to 89 hours). The Vd is 6.2 liters per kg, and the PB is 70%. It is eliminated by gastric secretion, liver metabolism, and 10% urinary excretion of conjugates and free PCP. Renal excretion may be increased 50% with urinary acidification. PCP concentrates in brain and adipose tissue. *Manifestations:* The classic picture is one of bursts of horizontal, vertical, and rotary nystagmus, which is a clue (occurs in 50% of cases); miosis; hypertension; and fluctuating altered mental state. There is a wide spectrum of clinical presentations: (1) Mild intoxication: A dose of 1 to 6 mg produces drunken and bizarre behavior, agitation, rotary nystagmus, and blank stare. Violent behavior and sensory anesthesia make these patients insensitive to pain, self-destructive, and dangerous. Most are communicative within 1 to 2 hours, are alert and oriented in 6 to 8 hours, and recover completely in 24 to 48 hours. (2) Moderate intoxication: A dose of 6 to 10 mg produces excess salivation, hypertension, hyperthermia, muscle rigidity, myoclonus, and catatonia. Recovery of consciousness occurs in 24 to 48 hours and complete recovery in 1 week. (3) Severe intoxication: A dose of 10 to 25 mg results in opisthotonos, decerebrate rigidity, convulsions, prolonged fluctuating coma, and respiratory failure. This category involves a high rate of medical complications. Recovery of consciousness occurs in 24 to 48 hours, with complete normality in 1 month. (4) Medical complications include apnea, aspiration pneumonia, cardiac arrest, hypertensive encephalopathy, hyperthermia, intracerebral hemorrhage, psychosis, rhabdomyolysis and myoglobinuria, and seizures. Flashbacks and loss of memory last for months. PCP-induced depression and suicide have been reported. (5) Fatalities occur with ingestions of greater than 100 mg and with serum levels higher than 100 to 250 ng per mL.

Management: Observe the patient for violent, self-destructive, bizarre behavior and paranoid schizophrenia. Patients should be placed in a low-sensory environment, and dangerous objects removed from the area. (1) GI decontamination is not effective because PCP is rapidly absorbed from the intestines. Avoid overtreating mild intoxication. Administer AC initially and MDAC every 4 hours, because PCP is secreted into the stomach even if it is smoked or snorted. Continuous gastric suction is not routine but may be useful (with protection of the airway) in severe toxicity (stupor or coma), because the drug is secreted into the gastric juice. (2) Protect patients from harming themselves or others. Physical restraints may be necessary, but use them sparingly and for the shortest time possible because they increase the risk of rhabdomyolysis. Avoid metal restraints such as handcuffs. For behavioral disorders and toxic psychosis, diazepam is the agent of choice. Pharmacologic intervention includes diazepam in a dose of 10 to 30 mg PO or 2 to 5 mg IV initially; titrate upward to 10 mg, but up to 30 mg may be required. The "talk-down" technique is usually ineffective and dangerous. Avoid PTZs and butyrophenones in the acute phase because they lower the convulsive threshold; however, they may be needed later for psychosis. Haloperidol (Haldol) administration has been reported to produce catatonia. (3) Seizures and muscle spasms are controlled with diazepam in a dose of 2.5 mg, up to 10 mg. (4) Hyperthermia (temperature above 38.5°C [101.3°F]) is treated with external cooling measures. (5) Hypertension is usually transient and does not mandate treatment. In an emergency hypertensive crisis (blood pressure above 200/115 mm Hg) use nitroprusside, 0.3 to 2 µg per kg per minute. The maximal infusion rate is 10 µg per kg per minute for only 10 minutes. (6) Acid ion–trapping diuresis is not recommended because of the danger of myoglobin precipitation in the renal tubules. (7) Rhabdomyolysis and myoglobinuria are treated by correcting volume depletion and ensuring a urine output of at least 2 mL per kg per hour. Alkalization is controversial because of PCP reabsorption. (8) Hemodialysis is beneficial if renal failure occurs; otherwise, the extracorporeal procedures are not beneficial.

Laboratory investigations: Marked elevation of the creatine kinase level may be a clue to PCP intoxication. Values of greater than 20,000 units have been reported. Monitor results of urinalysis and test urine for myoglobin with *o*-toluidine blood reagent strip. A 3+ or 4+ test result and less than 10 red blood cells per high-power field on microscopic examination suggest myoglobinuria. Measure for PCP in the gastric juice, where it is concentrated 10 to 50 times higher than in blood or urine. Monitor blood for creatine kinase, uric acid (an early clue to rhabdomyolysis), BUN, creatinine, electrolytes (hyperkalemia), and glucose (20% of intoxications involve hypoglycemia); also monitor urine output, liver function, ECG, and ABGs if there are any respiratory manifestations. PCP blood concentrations are not helpful. A level of 10 ng per mL produces excitation, 30 to 100 ng per mL produces coma, and more than 100 ng per mL produces seizures and fatalities. PCP may be detected in the urine of the average user for 10 to 14 days or up to 3 weeks after the last dose. With chronic use it can be detected for more than 1 month. The analogue of PCP may not test positive for PCP in the urine. Cross-reactions: Bleach and dextromethorphan may cause false-positive urine test results on immunoassay; doxylamine, a false-positive result on gas chromatography. *Disposition:* All patients with coma, delirium, catatonia, violent behavior, aspiration pneumonia, sustained hypertension (blood pressure above 200/115 mm Hg), or significant rhabdomyolysis should be admitted to the ICU until they are asymptomatic for at least 24 hours. If patients with mild intoxication are mentally and neurologically stable and become asymptomatic (except for nystagmus) for 4 hours, they may be discharged in the company of a responsible adult. All patients must be assessed for risk of suicide before discharge. Drug counseling and psychiatric follow-up should be arranged. Patients should be warned that episodes of disorientation and depression may continue intermittently for 4 weeks or more.

Phenothiazines and Nonphenothiazines: Neuroleptics. *Toxic mechanism:* Neuroleptics have complex mechanisms of toxicity, including (1) block of the postsynaptic dopamine receptors, (2) block of peripheral and central alpha-adrenergic receptors, (3) block of cholinergic muscarinic receptors, (4) a quinidine-like antidysrhythmic and myocardial depressant effect in large overdose, (5) a lowered convulsive threshold, and (6) an effect on hypothalamic temperature regulation. See Table 33. *Toxic dose:* Extrapyramidal reactions, anticholinergic effects, and orthostatic hypotension may occur at therapeutic doses. See Table 33 for therapeutic doses. The toxic amount is not established, but the maximum daily therapeutic dose may result in significant side effects, and twice this amount is potentially fatal. Chlorpromazine (Thorazine), the prototype, may produce serious hypotension and CNS depression at doses above 200 mg (17 mg per kg) in children and 3 to 5 grams in adults. Fatalities have been reported after ingestion of 2.5 grams of loxapine and mesoridazine and 1.5 grams of thioridazine. *Kinetics:* These agents are lipophilic and have unpredictable GI absorption. Peak levels occur 2 to 6 hours after ingestion and have enterohepatic recirculation. The mean

serum $t_{1/2}$ in phase I is 1 to 2 hours, and the biphasic $t_{1/2}$ is 20 to 40 hours. The PB is 92 to 98%. Oral chlorpromazine has onset at 30 to 60 minutes, peak effect at 2 to 4 hours, and a duration of 4 to 6 hours. With sustained-release preparations, the onset is at 30 to 60 minutes and the duration is 6 to 12 hours. The PB is 95%; the Vd, 10 to 40 liters per kg. Elimination is by hepatic metabolism, which results in multiple metabolites (some are active). Metabolites may be detected in urine months after chronic therapy. Only 1 to 3% is excreted unchanged in the urine. *Manifestations:* (1) PTZ overdose effects: Anticholinergic symptoms may be present early but are not life-threatening. Miosis is usually present (80%) if the PTZ has strong alpha-adrenergic blocking effect (e.g., chlorpromazine), but if there is strong anticholinergic activity, mydriasis may occur. Agitation and delirium rapidly progress to coma. Major problems are cardiac toxicity and hypotension. The cardiotoxic effects are seen more commonly with thioridazine and its metabolite mesoridazine. These agents have produced the largest number of fatalities in PTZ overdoses. Cardiac conduction disturbances include prolonged PR, QRS, and QT$_C$ intervals; U and T wave abnormalities; and ventricular dysrhythmias, including torsades de pointes. Seizures occur mainly in patients with convulsive disorders or with loxapine overdose. Sudden death in children and adults has been reported. (2) Idiosyncratic dystonic reactions are most common with the piperidine group. The reaction is not dose-dependent and consists of opisthotonos, torticollis, orolingual dyskinesia, and oculogyric crisis (painful upward gaze). It occurs more frequently in children and women. (3) Neuroleptic malignant syndrome occurs in patients receiving chronic therapy and is characterized by hyperthermia, muscle rigidity, autonomic dysfunction, and altered mental state. One case of this syndrome has been reported with acute overdose. (4) The loxapine syndrome consists of seizures, rhabdomyolysis, and renal failure.

Management: (1) Establish and maintain the vital functions. All patients with overdose require venous access, 12-lead ECG (to measure intervals), cardiac and respiratory monitoring, and seizure precautions. Monitor core temperature to detect a poikilothermic effect. The comatose patient may require intubation and assisted ventilation, 100% oxygen, intravenous glucose, naloxone, and 100 mg of thiamine. (2) GI decontamination: Emesis is not recommended. Gastric lavage may be useful but is not necessary if AC or a cathartic is administered promptly. MDAC has not been proved beneficial. A radiograph of the abdomen may be useful, if the PTZ is radiopaque. Haloperidol and trifluoperazine are most likely to be radiopaque. Whole-bowel irrigation may be useful when a large number of pills is visualized on a radiograph or sustained-release preparations are involved, but this modality has not been investigated for management of PTZ toxicity. (3) Treat convulsions with diazepam or lorazepam. A loxapine overdose may result in status epilepticus. If nondepolarizing neuro-

TABLE 33. **Neuroleptic Daily Doses and Properties: Comparison of Effects***

Compound/Dose	Effects				
	Antipsychotic	*Anticholinergic*	*Extrapyramidal*	*Hypotensive and Cardiotoxic*	*Sedative*
PHENOTHIAZINE					
Aliphatic†	1+	3+	2+	**2+**	3+
Chlorpromazine (Thorazine), 20–50 mg adult, dose, range 20–2000 mg per 24 h					
Promethazine (Phenergan), 25–50 mg adult dose, range 25–200 mg per 24 h					
Piperazine‡	3+	1+	3+	1+	1+
Fluphenazine (Prolixin), 2.5–10 mg adult dose, range 2.5–20 mg per 24 h					
Perphenazine (Trilafon), 4–16 mg adult dose, range 10–30 mg per 24 h					
Prochlorperazine (Compazine), 5–10 mg adult dose, range 15–40 mg per 24 h					
Trifluoperazine (Stelazine), 2–5 mg adult dose, range 15–40 mg per 24 h					
Piperidine†	1+	2+	1+	3+	3+
Mesoridazine (Serentil), 25–100 mg adult dose, range 150–400 mg per 24 h					
Thioridazine (Mellaril), 25–100 mg adult dose, range 150–300 mg per 24 h					
NONPHENOTHIAZINE					
Butyrophenone‡	3+	1+	3+	1+	1+
Haloperidol (Haldol), 0.5–5.0 mg adult dose, range 1–100 mg per 24 h					
Dibenzoxazepine‡	3+	1+	3+	1+	2+
Loxapine (Loxitane), 10–50 mg adult dose, range 60–100 mg per 24 h					
Dihydroindolone‡	3+	1+	3+	1+	1+
Molindone (Moban), 5–25 mg adult dose, range 50–225 mg per 24 h					
Thioxanthenes‡	3+	1+	3+	3+	1+
Thiothixene (Navane), 2–15 mg adult dose, range 5–80 mg per 24 h					
Chlorprothixene (Taractan), 5–60 mg adult dose, range 75–200 mg per 24 h					

*1+ indicates very low activity; 2+, moderate activity; 3+, very high activity. Bold indicates major effect. Equivalent doses: 100 mg of chlorpromazine or thioridazine = 50 mg of mesoridazine = 15 mg of loxapine or prochlorperazine = 10 mg of molindone or perphenazine = 5 mg of thiothixene = 2 mg of fluphenazine or haloperidol.
†Low antipsychotic potency.
‡High antipsychotic potency.

muscular blockade is required, use pancuronium (Pavulon) or vecuronium (Norcuron) (not succinylcholine [Anectine], which may cause malignant hyperthermia), and monitor the EEG during paralysis. (4) Dysrhythmias: Monitor with serial ECG. Treat unstable rhythms with electrical cardioversion. Avoid class IA anti-dysrhythmic drugs (procainamide, quinidine, and disopyramide). Hypokalemia predisposes to dysrhythmias and should be corrected aggressively. Supraventricular tachycardia with hemodynamic instability is treated with electrical cardioversion. The role of adenosine has not been defined. Avoid calcium channel blockers and beta blockers. QRS interval prolongation is treated with $NaHCO_3$ at 1 to 2 mEq per kg by intravenous bolus given over a few minutes. Torsades de pointes is treated with 2 grams of a 20% magnesium sulfate solution given IV over 2 to 3 minutes; if there is no response in 10 minutes, this is repeated and followed by a continuous infusion of 5 to 10 mg per minute, or an infusion of 50 mg per minute is given for 2 hours, followed by an infusion of 30 mg per minute given over 90 minutes twice a day for several days, as needed. The dose in children is 25 to 50 mg per kg initially with a maintenance dose of 30 to 60 mg per kg per 24 hours (0.25 to 0.50 mEq per kg per 24 hours), up to 1000 mg per 24 hours. Monitor serum magnesium: Ventricular tachydysrhythmias: If the patient is stable, lidocaine is the agent of choice. If the patient is unstable, electrical cardioversion is used. Heart blocks with hemodynamic instability should be managed with temporary cardiac pacing. (5) Hypotension is treated with the Trendelenburg position, 0.89% saline, and, in refractory cases or if there is danger of fluid overload, administration of vasopressors. The vasopressor of choice is the alpha-adrenergic agonist norepinephrine, 0.1 to 0.2 μg per gram per minute and titrated to response. Epinephrine and dopamine should not be used because beta-receptor stimulation in the presence of alpha-receptor blockade may provoke dysrhythmias, and PTZs are antidopaminergic. (6) Treat hypothermia or hyperthermia with external warming or cooling measures. Do not use antipyretic drugs. (7) Management of the neuroleptic malignant syndrome includes discontinuing the offending agent, aggressively reducing the temperature with passive and active cooling measures, correcting electrolyte and metabolic imbalances, and administering dantrolene sodium (see Table 10 and the section on malignant hyperthermia syndrome management). The loading dose is 2 to 3 mg per kg given IV as a bolus, and the loading dose is repeated until the signs of the syndrome (tachycardia, rigidity, and temperature elevation) are controlled. The maximum total dose is 10 mg per kg. (8) Idiosyncratic dystonic reaction can be treated with diphenhydramine at 1 to 2 mg per kg per dose given IV over 5 minutes up to a maximum of 50 mg; a response is noted within 2 to 5 minutes. Follow with oral doses for 5 to 7 days to prevent recurrence. (9) Extracorporeal measures (hemodialysis, hemoperfusion) are not effective in enhancing removal of these agents.

Laboratory investigations: Monitor ABGs, renal and hepatic function, electrolytes, blood glucose, and creatine kinase and assess for myoglobinemia in neuroleptic malignant syndrome. Most of these agents are detected by routine screens. A positive ferric chloride test of the urine occurs if there is a sufficient blood level; however, it is not specific (salicylates and phenolic compounds also produce a positive result). Quantitative serum levels are not useful in management. Cross-reactions with EMIT tests occur with cyclic antidepressants. PTZs produce false-negative results of pregnancy urine test in which human chorionic gonadotropin is used as the indicator and false-positive results of tests for urinary porphyrins, the indirect Coombs test, and urobilinogen and amylase tests. *Disposition:* Asymptomatic patients should be observed for at least 6 hours after gastric decontamination. Symptomatic patients with cardiotoxicity, hypotension, or convulsions should be admitted to the ICU and monitored for 48 hours.

Salicylates (acetylsalicylic acid, aspirin, salicylic acid). *Toxic mechanism:* The primary toxic mechanisms include (1) direct stimulation of the medullary chemoreceptor trigger zone and respiratory center; (2) uncoupling of oxidative phosphorylation; (3) inhibition of the Krebs cycle enzymes; (4) inhibition of vitamin K–dependent and –independent clotting factors; (5) alteration of platelet function; and (6) inhibition of prostaglandin synthesis. *Toxic dose:* Acute mild intoxication occurs at a dose of 150 to 200 mg per kg (tinnitus, dizziness), moderate intoxication at 200 to 300 mg per kg, and severe intoxication at 300 to 500 mg per kg (CNS manifestations). An acute salicylate plasma concentration (SPC) higher than 30 mg per dL (usually over 40 mg per dL) may be associated with clinical toxicity. Chronic intoxication occurs at ingestions of more than 100 mg per kg per day for more than 2 days because of cumulative kinetics. Methyl salicylate (oil of wintergreen) is the most toxic form of salicylate; 1 mL of 98% methyl

salicylate contains 1.4 grams of salicylate. Fatalities have occurred with ingestion of 1 teaspoonful in a child and 1 ounce in adults. It is found in topical ointments and liniments (18 to 30%). *Kinetics:* Acetylsalicylic acid is a weak acid, with a pK_a of 3.5; salicylic acid has a pK_a of 3.0. Salicylic acid is absorbed from the stomach and small bowel and dermally. Onset of action is within 30 minutes. Methyl salicylate and effervescent tablets are absorbed more rapidly. An SPC is detectable within 15 minutes after ingestion, and the peak occurs in 30 to 120 minutes but may be delayed 6 to 12 hours in large overdoses, in overdoses with enteric-coated and sustained-release preparations, and if concretions develop. The therapeutic duration of action is 3 to 4 hours but is markedly prolonged in an overdose. The $t_{1/2}$ of salicylic acid is 3 hours after a 300-mg dose, 6 hours after a 1-gram overdose, and over 10 hours after a 10-gram overdose. The Vd is 0.13 liter per kg for salicylic acid but increases as the SPC increases. PB is up to 90% for salicylic acid at pH 7.4 at a therapeutic SPC, 75% at an SPC above 40 mg per dL, 50% at an SPC of 70 mg per dL, and 30% at an SPC of 120 mg per dL. Elimination includes Michaelis-Menten hepatic metabolism by three saturable pathways: (1) glycine conjugation to salicyluric acid (75%), (2) saturable glucuronyltransferase to salicyl phenol glucuronide (10%), and (3) salicyl aryl glucuronide (4%). Nonsaturable pathways involve hydrolysis to gentisic acid (<1%), and 10% is excreted unchanged. Acidosis increases the severity by increasing the nonionized salicylate that can move into the brain cells. In the kidneys the un-ionized salicylic acid undergoes glomerular filtration, and the ionized portion undergoes secretion in proximal tubules and passive reabsorption in the distal tubules. Renal excretion of salicylate is enhanced by alkaline urine. *Manifestations:* Ingestion of concentrated topical salicylic acid preparations (e.g., Compound W) can cause caustic mucosal injury to the GI tract. The possibility of occult salicylate overdose should be considered in any patient with an unexplained acid-base disturbance. Acute overdose: (1) Minimal symptoms—tinnitus, dizziness, and difficulty hearing—may occur at a high therapeutic SPC of 20 to 30 mg per dL. Nausea and vomiting may occur immediately as a result of local gastric irritation. (2) Phase I consists of mild manifestations (1 to 12 hours after ingestion at a 6-hour SPC of 45 to 70 mg per dL). Nausea and vomiting followed by hyperventilation are usually present within 3 to 8 hours after acute overdose. Hyperventilation with an increase in both rate (tachypnea) and depth (hyperpnea) is present but may be subtle. It results in a mild respiratory alkalosis (serum pH greater than 7.4 and urine pH greater than 6.0). Some patients may have lethargy, vertigo, headache, and confusion. Diaphoresis is prominent. (3) Phase II involves moderate manifestations (12 to 24 hours after ingestion at a 6-hour SPC of 70 to 100 mg per dL). Serious metabolic disturbances including a marked respiratory alkalosis, followed by AG metabolic acidosis, and dehydration occur. The pH may be normal, elevated, or depressed, with a urine pH less than 6.0. Other metabolic disturbances may include hypoglycemia or hyperglycemia, hypokalemia, decreased ionized calcium, and increased BUN, creatinine, and lactate. Mental disturbances (confusion, disorientation, hallucinations) may occur. Hypotension and convulsions have been reported. (4) Phase III involves severe intoxication (more than 24 hours at a 6-hour SPC of 100 to 130 mg per dL). In addition to the preceding clinical findings, coma and seizures develop and indicate severe intoxication. Pulmonary edema may occur. Metabolic disturbances include metabolic acidemia (pH less than 7.4) and aciduria (pH less than 6.0). In adults, alkalosis may persist until terminal respiratory failure occurs. (5) In children younger than 4 years, a metabolic or mixed metabolic acidosis and respiratory alkalosis develop within 4 to 6 hours, because these children have less respiratory reserve and accumulate lactate and other organic acids. Hypoglycemia is more common in children. (6) Fatalities occur at a 6-hour SPC greater than 130 to 150 mg per dL and result from CNS depression, cardiovascular collapse, electrolyte imbalance, and cerebral edema. Chronic salicylism is more serious than acute intoxication, and the 6-hour SPC does not correlate with the manifestations. It usually occurs with therapeutic errors in young children or the elderly with underlying illness, and the diagnosis is delayed because it is not recognized. Noncardiac pulmonary edema is a frequent complication in the elderly. The mortality rate is about 25%. Chronic salicylate poisoning in children may mimic Reye's syndrome. It is associated with exaggerated CNS findings (hallucinations, delirium, dementia, memory loss, papilledema, bizarre behavior, agitation, encephalopathy, seizures, and coma). Hemorrhagic manifestations, renal failure, and pulmonary and cerebral edema may occur. The metabolic picture is that of hypoglycemia and mixed acid-base derangements. A chronic SPC higher than 60 mg per dL with metabolic acidosis and an altered mental state is extremely serious.

Management: Treatment is started on the basis of clinical and metabolic findings, not on the basis of salicylate levels. Continuous monitoring of the urine pH is essential for successful alkalization treatment. Always obtain an acetaminophen plasma level. (1) Establish and maintain vital functions. If the mental state is altered, administer glucose, naloxone, and thiamine in standard doses. Depending on the severity, the initial studies include an immediate and a 6-hour postingestion SPC, ECG and cardiac monitoring, pulse oximetry, urine assays (analysis, pH, specific gravity, and ferric chloride test), chest radiography, ABGs, blood glucose, electrolytes and AG calculation, calcium (ionized), magnesium, renal and liver profiles, and prothrombin time. Test gastric contents and stool for occult blood. Bismuth and magnesium salicylate preparations may be radiopaque on radiographs. A nephrologist should be consulted for moderate, severe, or chronic intoxication. (2) GI decontamination: Gastric lavage and AC are useful (each gram of AC binds 550 mg of salicylic acid) if a toxic dose was ingested up to 12 hours before because of factors with salicylism that delay absorption, such as food, enteric-coated tablets, pylorospasm, concretions, and co-ingestants. "It's never too late to aspirate salicylate." MDAC effectively reduces the $t_{1/2}$ and should be administered every 4 hours. Concretions may occur with massive (usually greater than 300 mg per kg) ingestions, and if blood levels fail to decline, prompt contrast radiography of the stomach may reveal concretions that must be removed by repeated lavage, whole-bowel irrigation, endoscopy, or gastrostomy. (3) Fluids and electrolytes (Table 34): Shock: Establish perfusion and vascular volume with 5% dextrose in 0.89% saline; then proceed with correction of dehydration and alkalization. Fluids and bicarbonate: In acute moderate or severe salicylism (see Table 34), adults should receive a bolus of 1 to 2 mEq of $NaHCO_3$ per kg followed by an infusion of 100 to 150 mEq of $NaHCO_3$ added to 500 to 1000 mL of 5% dextrose and administered over 60 minutes. Children should receive a bolus of 1 to 2 mEq of

TABLE 34. **Fluid and Electrolyte Treatment of Salicylate Poisoning**

Type of Salicylism	Metabolic Disturbance	Blood pH	Urine pH	Hydrating Solution	Amount of NaHCO₃ (mEq/L)	Amount of Potassium (mEq/L)
Mild	Respiratory alkalosis	>7.4	>6.0	5% dextrose 0.45% saline	50 (adult) 1 mEq/kg (child)	20
Moderate						
Chronic	Respiratory alkalosis	>7.4	<6.0	D5W	100 (adult)	40
Child younger than 4 y	Metabolic acidosis	<7.4			1–2 mEq/kg (child)	
Severe						
Chronic	Metabolic acidosis	<7.4	<6.0	D5W	150 (adult)	60
Child younger than 4 y	Respiratory alkalosis				2 mEq/kg (child)	
CNS depressant coingestant	Respiratory acidosis	<7.4	<6.0	D5W	100–150*	60

*Hypoventilation must be corrected.
Abbreviation: D5W = 5% dextrose in water.
Modified from Linden CH, Rumack BH: The legitimate analgesics, aspirin and acetaminophen. *In* Hansen W Jr (ed): Toxic Emergencies. New York, Churchill Livingstone, 1984, p 118.

$NaHCO_3$ per kg followed by an infusion of 1 to 2 mEq per kg added to 20 mL per kg of 5% dextrose administered over 60 minutes. Add potassium to the intravenous infusion after the patient voids. Attempt to achieve a target urine output of more than 2 mL per kg per hour and a target urine pH of more than 7. The initial infusion is followed by subsequent infusions (two to three times normal maintenance) of 200 to 300 mL per hour in adults or 10 mL per kg per hour in children. If the patient is acidotic and the serum pH is less than 7.15, an additional 1 to 2 mEq $NaHCO_3$ per kg is given over 1 to 2 hours, and persistent acidosis may necessitate $NaHCO_3$ at 1 to 2 mEq per kg every 2 hours. Adjust the infusion rate, the amount of bicarbonate, and the electrolytes to correct serum abnormalities and to maintain the targeted urine output and urinary pH. Most authorities believe that the diuresis is not as important as the alkalization or MDAC. Carefully monitor for fluid overload in those at risk of pulmonary and cerebral edema (e.g., the elderly) and because of inappropriate secretion of antidiuretic hormone. In patients with mild intoxication who are not acidotic and whose urine pH is greater than 6, administer 5% dextrose in 0.45% saline, with $NaHCO_3$ at 50 mEq per liter or 1 mEq per kg as maintenance to replace ongoing renal losses. (4) Alkalization: $NaHCO_3$ is administered to produce a serum pH of 7.4 to 7.5 and urine pH above 7. Carbonic anhydrase inhibitors (e.g., acetazolamide [Diamox]) should not be used. If the patient is acidotic, additional bicarbonate may be required. About 2 mEq per kg raises the blood pH by 0.1. In children, alkalization may be a difficult problem because of the organic acid production and hypokalemia. Hypokalemic and fluid-depleted patients cannot undergo adequate alkalization. Alkalization is usually discontinued in asymptomatic patients with an SPC below 30 to 40 mg per dL but is continued in symptomatic patients regardless of the SPC. A decreased serum bicarbonate with a normal or high blood pH indicates respiratory alkalosis predominating over metabolic acidosis, and the bicarbonate should be administered cautiously. An alkalemia (pH of 7.40 to 7.50) is not a contraindication to bicarbonate therapy because these patients have a significant base deficit in spite of the elevated blood pH. (5) Potassium is added (20 to 40 mEq per liter) to the infusion after the patient voids. In severe, late, and chronic salicylism, potassium at 60 mEq per liter may be needed. When the serum potassium level is below 4.0 mEq per liter, add 10 mEq per liter over the first hour. If the patient has hypokalemia (less than 3 mEq per liter), flat T waves, and U waves, administer 0.25 to 0.5 mEq per kg up to 10 mEq per hour. Administer potassium with ECG monitoring. Recheck the serum potassium value after each rapidly administered dose. A paradoxical urine acidosis (alkaline serum pH and acidic urine pH) indicates that potassium is probably needed. (6) Convulsions are treated with diazepam or lorazepam, but rule out hypoglycemia, low ionized calcium, cerebral edema, or hemorrhage with CT. If tetany develops, discon-

tinue the $NaHCO_3$ therapy and administer 10% calcium gluconate at 0.1 to 0.2 mL per kg. (7) Pulmonary edema management consists of fluid restriction, high forced inspiratory oxygen (FIO_2), mechanical ventilation, and PEEP. (8) Cerebral edema management consists of fluid restriction, elevation of the head, hyperventilation, osmotic diuresis, and dexamethasone. (9) Administer vitamin K_1 parenterally to correct an increased prothrombin time of more than 20 seconds and coagulation abnormalities. If there is active bleeding, administer fresh plasma and platelets as needed. (10) Hyperpyrexia is managed by external cooling measures, not antipyretics. (11) Hemodialysis is the method of choice for removing salicylates because it corrects the acid-base, electrolyte, and fluid disturbances as well. Indications for hemodialysis include acute poisoning with an SPC greater than 100 to 130 mg per dL without improvement after 6 hours of appropriate therapy; chronic poisoning with cardiopulmonary disease and an SPC as low as 40 mg per dL with refractory acidosis, severe CNS manifestations (coma and seizures), and progressive deterioration, especially in the elderly; impairment of vital organs of elimination; clinical deterioration in spite of good supportive care, repeated doses of AC, and alkalization; and severe refractory acid-base or electrolyte disturbances despite appropriate corrective measures.

Laboratory investigations: In all intentional salicylate overdoses, the acetaminophen plasma level should be determined after 4 hours. (1) Continuously monitor ECG, urine output, urine pH, and specific gravity. Every 2 to 4 hours in severe intoxication, monitor SPC, glucose (in salicylism, CNS hypoglycemia may be present despite a normal serum glucose level), electrolytes, ionized calcium, magnesium and phosphorus, AG, ABGs, and pulse oximetry. Daily, monitor BUN, creatinine, liver function tests, and prothrombin time. (2) In the *ferric chloride test,* 1 mL of boiled urine containing 2 or 3 drops of 10% ferric chloride turns purple if salicylates are present. This is a nonspecific test and is positive for ketones (if the sample is not boiled), PTZs, and phenolic compounds in urine. (3) SPC: The therapeutic value is less than 10 mg per dL for analgesia and 15 to 30 mg per dL for an anti-inflammatory effect. Mild toxicity occurs at values above 30 mg per dL (tinnitus, dizziness), severe toxicity above 80 mg per dL (CNS changes). Cross-reaction: Diflunisal (Dolobid) results in a falsely high SPC. The Done nomogram (Figure 2) has been used as a predictor of expected severity after an acute single ingestion. The nomogram is not useful for chronic intoxications; for enteric-coated aspirin ingestions; or for methyl salicylate, phenyl salicylate, or homomethyl salicylate intoxications. The blood sample for use with the Done nomogram should be obtained 6 hours or more after ingestion. *Disposition:* There are limitations of SPCs, and patients are managed on the basis of clinical and laboratory findings. Patients who are asymptomatic should be monitored for a minimum of 6 hours and longer if an ingestion of enteric-coated tablets, a massive overdose, or sus-

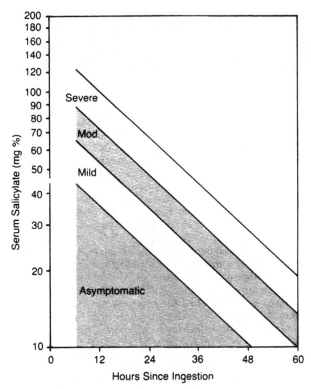

Figure 2. The Done nomogram for salicylate intoxication. For limitations of use, see *Laboratory Investigations*. (Redrawn from Done A: Salicylate intoxication: Significance of measurements of salicylate in blood in cases of acute ingestion. Reproduced by permission of Pediatrics, Vol 26, Page 800, Figure 3, Copyright 1960.)

picion of concretions is involved. Those who remain asymptomatic with an SPC below 35 mg per dL may be discharged after psychiatric evaluation, if indicated. Patients with chronic salicylate intoxication, acidosis, and an altered mental state should be admitted to the ICU. Patients with acute ingestion, an SPC below 60 mg per dL, and mild symptoms may be able to receive adequate treatment in the emergency department. Patients with moderate or severe intoxications should be admitted to the ICU.

Tricyclic and Other Cyclic Antidepressants. Traditionally, tricyclic antidepressants have been an important cause of pharmaceutical overdose fatalities (more than 100 in 1992). The mortality has been reduced from 15% in the 1970s to less than 1% in the 1990s through a better understanding of their pathophysiology and improvements in management. See Table 35. *Toxic mechanism:* The major mechanisms of toxicity of the tricyclic antidepressants are central and peripheral anticholinergic effects, peripheral alpha-adrenergic blockade, quinidine-like cardiac membrane–stabilizing action blocking the fast inward sodium channels, and inhibition of synaptic neurotransmitter reuptake in the CNS presynaptic neurons. The tetracyclic, monocyclic aminoketone dibenzoxazepine possesses convulsive activity and less cardiac toxicity in overdoses. Triazolopyridine has less serious cardiac and CNS toxicity. *Toxic dose:* The

therapeutic dose of imipramine is 1.5 to 5 mg per kg; a dose of less than 3 to 5 mg per kg may be mildly toxic; 10 to 20 mg per kg may be life-threatening, although doses of less than 20 mg per kg have produced few fatalities; more than 30 mg per kg is associated with 30% mortality; and at doses higher than 70 mg per kg, survival is rare. Doses of 375 mg in a child and as little as 500 to 750 mg in an adult have been fatal. In adults, 5 times the maximum daily dose is toxic, and 10 times the maximum daily dose is potentially fatal. Major overdose symptoms are associated with plasma concentrations above 1 μg per mL (1000 ng per mL). Relative dosage equivalents are as follows: 100 mg of amitriptyline = 125 mg of amoxapine = 75 mg of desipramine = 100 mg of doxepin = 75 mg of imipramine = 75 mg of maprotiline = 50 mg of nortriptyline = 200 mg of trazodone. See Table 35. *Kinetics:* Cyclic antidepressants are lipophilic. They are rapidly absorbed from the alkaline small intestine, but absorption may be prolonged and delayed in massive overdose owing to anticholinergic action. Onset varies from less than 1 hour (30 to 40 minutes) rarely to 12 hours. The peak serum levels are reached in 2 to 8 hours, and the peak effect is in 6 hours but may be delayed 12 hours because of erratic absorption. The clinical effects correlate poorly with plasma levels. Cyclic antidepressants are highly protein bound to plasma glycoproteins (98% at pH 7.5 and 90% at pH 7.0); the Vd is 10 to 50 liters per kg. The $t_{1/2}$ varies from 10 hours for imipramine to 81 hours for amitriptyline and 100 hours for nortriptyline. The active metabolites have considerable $t_{1/2}$ values. Elimination is by hepatic metabolism. The tertiary amines are metabolized to active demethylated secondary amine metabolites. The active secondary amine metabolites undergo 15% enterohepatic recirculation and are metabolized over a period of days to nonactive metabolites. The intestinal bacterial flora may reconstitute the active metabolites. Only 3% of an ingested dose is excreted in the urine unchanged. *Manifestations:* On arrival, previously alert, oriented patients may suddenly become comatose, have a seizure, develop hemodynamically unstable dysrhythmias within minutes, and die. Most patients with severe toxicity develop symptoms within 1 to 2 hours, but onset may be delayed 6 hours after an overdose. (1) Small overdoses produce early anticholinergic effects, agitation, and transient hypertension, which are not life-threatening. (2) Large overdoses produce depression of CNS and myocardium, convulsions, and hypotension. Death usually occurs within the first 2 to 6 hours after ingestion. (3) ECG screening tools for use in tricyclic antidepressant toxicity include QRS greater than 0.10 second (seizures are likely) and QRS greater than 0.16 second (50% of patients developed ventricular dysrhythmias—life-threatening in 20% of the cases—and seizures); a terminal 40 milliseconds of the QRS axis greater than 120 degrees in the right frontal plane; and an R wave greater than 3 mm as measured by the right arm lead. The quinidine cardiac membrane–stabilizing effect produces depres-

TABLE 35. **Cyclic Antidepressants: Daily Doses and Major Properties***

Generic Name	Adult Daily Dose (mg)	Therapeutic Range (ng/mL)	Half-life (h)	Toxicity		
				Antichol	*CNS*	*Cardiac*
TRICYCLIC ANTIDEPRESSANTS						
Major toxicity is cardiac						
Tertiary amines demethylated into secondary active amine metabolites						
Amitriptyline (Elavil)	75–300	120–250	31–46	3+	3+	3+
Imipramine (Tofranil)	75–300	125–250	9–24	3+	3+	2+
Doxepin (Sinequan)	75–300	30–150	8–24	3+	3+	2+
Trimipramine (Surmontil)	75–200	10–240	16–18	3+	3+	2+
Secondary amines metabolized into inactive metabolites						
Nortriptyline (Pamelor)†	75–150	50–150	18–93	2+	3+	3+
Desipramine (Norpramin)	75–200	75–160	14–62	1+	3+	3+
Protriptyline (Vivactil)	20–60	70–250	54–198	2+	3+	3+
NEWER CYCLIC ANTIDEPRESSANTS						
Tetracyclic agent produces a high incidence of cardiovascular disturbances and seizures						
Maprotiline (Ludiomil)	75–300	—	30–60	1+	2+	3+
Triazolopyridine, a noncyclic agent, produces less serious cardiac and CNS toxicity						
Trazodone (Desyrel)	50–600	700	4–7	1+	1+	1+
Monocyclic aminoketone produces seizures in doses >600 mg						
Bupropion (Wellbutrin)	200–400	—	8–24	1+	3+	1+
Dibenzazepine						
Clomipramine (Anafranil)	100–250	200–500	21–32	2+	2+	2+
Dibenzoxazepine produces syndrome of convulsions, rhabdomyolysis, and renal failure						
Amoxapine (Asendin)	150–300	200–500	6–10	1+	3+	2+

*Other drugs with similar structures are cyclobenzaprine (Flexeril), a muscle relaxant (similar to amitriptyline) and carbamazepine (Tegretol), an anticonvulsant (similar to imipramine); however, they cause less cardiac toxicity. 1+ indicates mild effect; 2+ indicates moderate effect; 3+ indicates severe effect.

†Not available in the United States.

Abbreviations: Antichol = anticholinergic effect; CNS = central nervous system effect (primarily seizures); Cardiac = cardiac effect.

sion of myocardium, conduction disturbances, and ECG changes. The peripheral alpha-adrenergic blockade produces hypotension.

Management: (1) Establish and maintain vital functions. Even if the patient is asymptomatic, establish intravenous access, monitor vital signs and neurologic status, obtain a baseline 12-lead ECG, and continue cardiac monitoring for at least 6 hours from admission or 8 to 12 hours after ingestion. Measure the QRS interval every 15 minutes. (2) GI decontamination: Do not induce emesis, and omit gastric lavage if AC is available. If the mental state is altered, protect the airway. AC at 1 gram per kg is recommended immediately and repeated once (0.5 mg per kg) in 4 hours. A clinical benefit of MDAC has not been demonstrated. (3) Control seizures. Alkalization does not control seizures; use diazepam or lorazepam. Status epilepticus (as may occur with amoxapine) may necessitate high-dose barbiturates or neuromuscular blockers with intravenous diazepam. If this is

not successful, paralysis is induced by short-acting, nondepolarizing neuromuscular blockers such as vecuronium, with intubation and assisted ventilation. A bolus of NaHCO$_3$ is recommended as an adjunct to correct the acidosis produced by the seizures. (4) Cardiovascular management consists of administration of NaHCO$_3$ (see Table 10). A dose of 1 to 2 mEq per kg is given undiluted as a bolus and repeated twice a few minutes apart, if needed, for sodium loading and alkalization, which increases PB. The sodium loading overcomes the sodium channel blockage and is more important than the alkalization, which increases the PB from 90 to 98%. Indications include a QRS complex greater than 0.12 second, ventricular tachycardia, severe conduction disturbances, metabolic acidosis, coma, and seizures. An infusion of NaHCO$_3$ may follow to keep the blood pH at 7.5 to 7.55. The continuous infusion by itself is of limited usefulness for controlling dysrhythmias because of its delayed onset of action. Bolus therapy is given as needed. Hyperventilation alone has been advocated, but the pH elevation is not so instantaneous and there is compensatory renal excretion of bicarbonate; therefore, it is not recommended. The combination of hyperventilation and $NaHCO_3$ has produced fatal alkalemia and is not recommended. Monitor the serum potassium (the sudden increase in blood pH can aggravate or precipitate hypokalemia), serum sodium, ionized calcium (hypocalcemia may occur with alkalization), and blood pH. (5) Specific cardiovascular complications should be treated as follows: For management of hypotension, norepinephrine, a predominantly alpha-adrenergic drug, is preferred to dopamine. Hypertension that occurs early rarely necessitates treatment. Sinus tachycardia usually does not necessitate treatment. Supraventricular tachycardia with hemodynamic instability necessitates synchronized electrical cardioversion, starting at 0.25 to 1.0 watt-second per kg, after sedation. Ventricular tachycardia that persists after alkalization mandates intravenous lidocaine or countershock if the patient is hemodynamically unstable. Ventricular fibrillation should be treated with defibrillation. Torsades de pointes is treated with 20% magnesium sulfate solution given IV, 2 grams over 2 to 3 minutes, followed by a continuous infusion of 1.5 mL of 10% solution or 5 to 10 mg per minute (see Table 10). For bradydysrhythmias, atropine is contraindicated because of the anticholinergic activity. Isoproterenol at 0.1 μg per kg per minute with caution may produce hypotension. If the patient is hemodynamically unstable, use a pacemaker. (6) Extraordinary measures such as intra-aortic balloon pump and cardiopulmonary bypass have been successful. (7) Investigational: Use of Fab specific for tricyclic antidepressants has been successful in animals. Prophylactic $NaHCO_3$ to prevent dysrhythmias is being investigated. (8) Contraindicated: Physostigmine has produced asystole. Flumazenil has produced seizures.

Laboratory investigations: Monitoring: If altered mental status or ECG abnormalities are present, obtain ABGs, institute ECG monitoring, perform chest radiography, and determine blood glucose, serum electrolytes, calcium, magnesium, BUN and creatinine, liver profile, creatine kinase, and urine output; in severe cases, hemodynamic monitoring is indicated. Levels of tricyclic and other cyclic antidepressants below 300 ng per mL are therapeutic, levels above 500 ng per mL indicate toxicity, and levels above 1000 ng per mL indicate serious poisoning and are associated with QRS widening. *Disposition:* Admission to the ICU for 12 to 24 hours is essential for any patient with an antidepressant overdose who meets any of the following criteria: ECG abnormalities (except sinus tachycardia), altered mental state, seizures, respiratory depression, or hypotension. Caution: In 25% of fatal cases the patients were alert and awake at presentation. Low-risk patients are those who do not have the preceding symptoms at 6 hours after ingestion, those who present with minor transient manifestations such as sinus tachycardia and subsequently become and remain asymptomatic for a 6-hour period, and asymptomatic patients who remain asymptomatic for 6 hours. These patients may be discharged if the ECG remains normal and they have normal bowel sounds, have AC therapy repeated once, and undergo psychiatric counseling. Children younger than 6 years with nonintentional (accidental) exposures should be referred to the emergency department for monitoring, observation, and AC therapy.

Section 18

Appendices and Index

REFERENCE INTERVALS FOR THE INTERPRETATION OF LABORATORY TESTS

method of
WILLIAM Z. BORER, M.D.
Thomas Jefferson University Hospital
Philadelphia, Pennsylvania

Most of the tests performed in a clinical laboratory are quantitative in nature. That is, the amount of a substance present in blood or serum is measured and reported in terms of concentration, activity (e.g., enzyme activity) or counts (e.g., blood cell counts). The laboratory must provide reference intervals to assist the clinician in the interpretation of laboratory results. These reference intervals comprise the physiologic quantities of a substance (concentrations, activities, or counts) to be expected in healthy persons. Deviation above or below the reference range may be associated with a disease process, and the severity of the disease process may be associated with the magnitude of the deviation. Unfortunately, a sharp demarcation rarely exists to distinguish between physiologic and pathologic values, and the time of transition between the two is often gradual as the disease process progresses.

The terms "normal" and "abnormal" have been used to describe the laboratory values that fall inside and outside the reference range, respectively. Use of these terms is inappropriate, because no good definition of normality exists in the clinical sense and because the term "normal" may be confused with the statistical term "Gaussian." Reference ranges are established from statistical studies in groups of healthy volunteers. These study subjects must be free of disease, but they may have lifestyles or habits that result in variations in certain laboratory values. Examples of these variables include diet, body mass, exercise, and geographic location. Age and gender may also affect reference values.

When the data from a large cohort of healthy subjects fit a Gaussian distribution, the usual statistical approach is to define the reference limits as two standard deviations above and below the mean. By definition, the reference range excludes the 2.5% of the population with the lowest values and the 2.5% with the highest values. Non-Gaussian distributions are handled by different statistical methods, but the result is similar in that the reference range is defined by the central 95% of the population. In other words, the probability that a healthy person will have a laboratory result that falls outside the reference

TABLE 1. Base SI Units

Property	Base Unit	Symbol
Length	meter	m
Mass	kilogram	kg
Amount of substance	mole	mol
Time	second	s
Thermodynamic temperature	kelvin	K
Electric current	ampere	A
Luminous intensity	candela	cd
Catalytic amount	katal	kat

TABLE 2. Derived SI Units and Non-SI Units Retained for Use with SI Units

Property	Unit	Symbol
Area	square meter	m^2
Volume	cubic meter	m^3
	liter	L
Mass concentration	kilogram/cubic meter	kg/m^3
	gram/liter	g/L
Substance concentration	mole/cubic meter	mol/m^3
	mole/liter	mol/L
Temperature	degree Celsius	$C = K - 273.15$

TABLE 3. Standard Prefixes

Prefix	Multiplication Factor	Symbol
yocto	10^{-24}	y
zepto	10^{-21}	z
atto	10^{-18}	a
femto	10^{-15}	f
pico	10^{-12}	p
nano	10^{-9}	n
micro	10^{-6}	μ
milli	10^{-3}	m
centi	10^{-2}	c
deci	10^{-1}	d
deca	10^1	da
hecto	10^2	h
kilo	10^3	k
mega	10^6	M
giga	10^9	G
tera	10^{12}	T

range is 1 in 20. If 12 laboratory tests are performed, the probability that at least one of the results will be outside the reference range increases to about 50%. This means that all healthy persons are likely to have a few laboratory results that are unexpected. The clinician must then integrate these data with other clinical information such as the history and physical examination to arrive at an appropriate clinical decision.

The reference intervals for many tests (especially enzyme and immunochemical measurements) vary with the method used. Accordingly, each laboratory must establish reference intervals that are appropriate for the methods used.

SI UNITS

During the 1980s a concerted effort was made to introduce SI units (le Système International d'Unités). The rationale for conversion to SI units is sound. Laboratory data are scientifically more informative when the units are based on molar concentration rather than on mass concentration. For example, the conversion of glucose to lactate and pyruvate or the binding of a drug to albumin is more easily understood in units of molar concentration. Another example is illustrated as follows:

Conventional Units

1.0 gram of hemoglobin:

- Combines with 1.37 mL of oxygen
- Contains 3.4 mg of iron
- Forms 34.9 mg of bilirubin

SI Units

4.0 mmol of hemoglobin:

- Combines with 4.0 mmol of oxygen
- Contains 4.0 mmol of iron
- Forms 4.0 mmol of bilirubin

The use of SI units would also enhance the standardization of nomenclature to facilitate global communication of medical and scientific information. The units, symbols, and prefixes employed in the International System are shown in Tables 1, 2, and 3.

Unfortunately, problems have arisen with the implementation of SI units in the United States. Their introduction in 1987 prompted many medical journals to report laboratory values in both SI and conventional units in anticipation of complete conversion to SI units in the early 1990s. The lack of a coordinated effort toward this goal has forced a retrenchment on the issue. Physicians continue to think and practice with laboratory results expressed in conventional units, and few if any American hospitals or clinical laboratories use SI units exclusively. Complete conversion to SI units is not likely to occur in the foreseeable future, but most medical journals will probably continue to publish both sets of units. For this reason the values in the tables of reference ranges in this appendix are given in both conventional units and SI units.

TABLES OF REFERENCE INTERVALS

Some of the values included in the tables that follow have been established by the Clinical Laboratories at Thomas Jefferson University Hospital, Philadelphia, Pennsylvania, and have not been published elsewhere. Other values have been compiled from the sources cited in the references. These tables are provided for information and educational purposes only. Laboratory values must always be interpreted in the context of clinical data derived from other sources including the medical history and physical examination. Users must exercise individual judgment when employing the information provided in this appendix.

Reference Intervals for Hematology

Test	Conventional Units	SI Units
Acid hemolysis (Ham test)	No hemolysis	No hemolysis
Alkaline phosphatase, leukocyte	Total score 14–100	Total score 14–100
Cell counts		
Erythrocytes		
Males	4.6–6.2 million/mm³	$4.6–6.2 \times 10^{12}$/L
Females	4.2–5.4 million/mm³	$4.2–5.4 \times 10^{12}$/L
Children (varies with age)	4.5–5.1 million/mm³	$4.5–5.1 \times 10^{12}$/L
Leukocytes, total	4500–11,000/mm³	$4.5–11.0 \times 10^{9}$/L
Leukocytes, differential counts*		
Myelocytes	0%	0/L
Band neutrophils	3–5%	$150–400 \times 10^{6}$/L
Segmented neutrophils	54–62%	$3000–5800 \times 10^{6}$/L
Lymphocytes	25–33%	$1500–3000 \times 10^{6}$/L
Monocytes	3–7%	$300–500 \times 10^{6}$/L
Eosinophils	1–3%	$50–250 \times 10^{6}$/L
Basophils	0–1%	$15–50 \times 10^{6}$/L
Platelets	150,000–400,000/mm³	$150–400 \times 10^{9}$/L
Reticulocytes	25,000–75,000/mm³ (0.5–1.5% of erythrocytes)	$25–75 \times 10^{9}$/L

Reference Intervals for Hematology *Continued*

Test	Conventional Units	SI Units
Coagulation tests		
Bleeding time (template)	2.75–8.0 min	2.75–8.0 min
Coagulation time (glass tube)	5–15 min	5–15 min
D-Dimer	<0.5 µg/mL	<0.5 mg/L
Factor VIII and other coagulation factors	50–150% of normal	0.5–1.5 of normal
Fibrin split products (Thrombo-Welco test)	<10 µg/mL	<10 mg/L
Fibrinogen	200–400 mg/dL	2.0–4.0 g/L
Partial thromboplastin time, activated (aPTT)	20–35 s	20–35 s
Prothrombin time (PT)	12.0–14.0 s	12.0–14.0 s
Coombs' test		
Direct	Negative	Negative
Indirect	Negative	Negative
Corpuscular values of erythrocytes		
Mean corpuscular hemoglobin (MCH)	26–34 pg/cell	26–34 pg/cell
Mean corpuscular volume (MCV)	80–96 µm^3	80–96 fL
Mean corpuscular hemoglobin concentration (MCHC)	32–36 g/dL	320–360 g/L
Haptoglobin	20–165 mg/dL	0.20–1.65 g/L
Hematocrit		
Males	40–54 mL/dL	0.40–0.54
Females	37–47 mL/dL	0.37–0.47
Newborns	49–54 mL/dL	0.49–0.54
Children (varies with age)	35–49 mL/dL	0.35–0.49
Hemoglobin		
Males	13.0–18.0 g/dL	8.1–11.2 mmol/L
Females	12.0–16.0 g/dL	7.4–9.9 mmol/L
Newborns	16.5–19.5 g/dL	10.2–12.1 mmol/L
Children (varies with age)	11.2–16.5 g/dL	7.0–10.2 mmol/L
Hemoglobin, fetal	<1.0% of total	<0.01 of total
Hemoglobin A$_{1C}$	3–5% of total	0.03–0.05 of total
Hemoglobin A$_2$	1.5–3.0% of total	0.015–0.03 of total
Hemoglobin, plasma	0.0–5.0 mg/dL	0.0–3.2 µmol/L
Methemoglobin	30–130 mg/dL	19–80 µmol/L
Sedimentation rate (ESR)		
Wintrobe: Males	0–5 mm/h	0–5 mm/h
Females	0–15 mm/h	0–15 mm/h
Westergren: Males	0–15 mm/h	0–15 mm/h
Females	0–20 mm/h	0–20 mm/h

*Conventional units are percentages; SI units are absolute cell counts.

Reference Intervals* for Clinical Chemistry (Blood, Serum, and Plasma)

Analyte	Conventional Units	SI Units
Acetoacetate plus acetone		
Qualitative	Negative	Negative
Quantitative	0.3–2.0 mg/dL	30–200 µmol/L
Acid phosphatase, serum (thymolphthalein monophosphate substrate)	0.1–0.6 U/L	0.1–0.6 U/L
ACTH (see Corticotropin)		
Alanine aminotransferase (ALT) serum (SGPT)	1–45 U/L	1–45 U/L
Albumin, serum	3.3–5.2 g/dL	33–52 g/L
Aldolase, serum	0.0–7.0 U/L	0.0–7.0 U/L
Aldosterone, plasma		
Standing	5–30 ng/dL	140–830 pmol/L
Recumbent	3–10 ng/dL	80–275 pmol/L
Alkaline phosphatase (ALP), serum		
Adult	35–150 U/L	35–150 U/L
Adolescent	100–500 U/L	100–500 U/L
Child	100–350 U/L	100–350 U/L
Ammonia nitrogen, plasma	10–50 µmol/L	10–50 µmol/L
Amylase, serum	25–125 U/L	25–125 U/L
Anion gap, serum, calculated	8–16 mEq/L	8–16 mmol/L
Ascorbic acid, blood	0.4–1.5 mg/dL	23–85 µmol/L
Aspartate aminotransferase (AST) serum (SGOT)	1–36 U/L	1–36 U/L
Base excess, arterial blood, calculated	0 ± 2 mEq/L	0 ± 2 mmol/L
Bicarbonate		
Venous plasma	23–29 mEq/L	23–29 mmol/L
Arterial blood	21–27 mEq/L	21–27 mmol/L

Table continued on following page

Reference Intervals* for Clinical Chemistry (Blood, Serum, and Plasma) *Continued*

Analyte	Conventional Units	SI Units
Bile acids, serum	0.3–3.0 mg/dL	0.8–7.6 μmol/L
Bilirubin, serum		
Conjugated	0.1–0.4 mg/dL	1.7–6.8 μmol/L
Total	0.3–1.1 mg/dL	5.1–19.0 μmol/L
Calcium, serum	8.4–10.6 mg/dL	2.10–2.65 mmol/L
Calcium, ionized, serum	4.25–5.25 mg/dL	1.05–1.30 mmol/L
Carbon dioxide, total, serum or plasma	24–31 mEq/L	24–31 mmol/L
Carbon dioxide tension (P$_{CO_2}$), blood	35–45 mm Hg	35–45 mm Hg
β-Carotene, serum	60–260 μg/dL	1.1–8.6 μmol/L
Ceruloplasmin, serum	23–44 mg/dL	230–440 mg/L
Chloride, serum or plasma	96–106 mEq/L	96–106 mmol/L
Cholesterol, serum or ethylenediaminetetraacetic acid (EDTA) plasma		
Desirable range	<200 mg/dL	<5.20 mmol/L
Low-density lipoprotein (LDL) cholesterol	60–180 mg/dL	1.55–4.65 mmol/L
High-density lipoprotein (HDL) cholesterol	30–80 mg/dL	0.80–2.05 mmol/L
Copper	70–140 μg/dL	11–22 μmol/L
Corticotropin (ACTH), plasma, 8 AM	10–80 pg/mL	2–18 pmol/L
Cortisol, plasma		
8 AM	6–23 μg/dL	170–630 nmol/L
4 PM	3–15 μg/dL	80–410 nmol/L
10 PM	<50% of 8 AM value	<50% of 8 AM value
Creatine, serum		
Males	0.2–0.5 mg/dL	15–40 μmol/L
Females	0.3–0.9 mg/dL	25–70 μmol/L
Creatine kinase (CK), serum		
Males	55–170 U/L	55–170 U/L
Females	30–135 U/L	30–135 U/L
Creatine kinase MB isoenzyme, serum	<5% of total CK activity	<5% of total CK activity
	<5% ng/mL by immunoassay	<5% ng/mL by immunoassay
Creatinine, serum	0.6–1.2 mg/dL	50–110 μmol/L
Estradiol-17β, adult		
Males	10–65 pg/mL	35–240 pmol/L
Females		
Follicular	30–100 pg/mL	110–370 pmol/L
Ovulatory	200–400 pg/mL	730–1470 pmol/L
Luteal	50–140 pg/mL	180–510 pmol/L
Ferritin, serum	20–200 ng/mL	20–200 μg/L
Fibrinogen, plasma	200–400 mg/dL	2.0–4.0 g/L
Folate, serum	3–18 ng/mL	6.8–41 nmol/L
Erythrocytes	145–540 ng/mL	330–1220 nmol/L
Follicle-stimulating hormone (FSH), plasma		
Males	4–25 mU/mL	4–25 U/L
Females, premenopausal	4–30 mU/mL	4–30 U/L
Females, postmenopausal	40–250 mU/mL	40–250 U/L
Gamma-glutamyltransferase (GGT), serum	5–40 U/L	5–40 U/L
Gastrin, fasting, serum	0–100 pg/mL	0–100 mg/L
Glucose, fasting, plasma or serum	70–115 mg/dL	3.9–6.4 nmol/L
Growth hormone (hGH), plasma, adult, fasting	0–6 ng/mL	0–6 μg/L
Haptoglobin, serum	20–165 mg/dL	0.20–1.65 g/L
Immunoglobulins, serum (see table of Reference Intervals for Tests of Immunologic Function)		
Iron, serum	75–175 μg/dL	13–31 μmol/L
Iron binding capacity, serum		
Total	250–410 μg/dL	45–73 μmol/L
Saturation	20–55%	0.20–0.55
Lactate		
Venous whole blood	5.0–20.0 mg/dL	0.6–2.2 mmol/L
Arterial whole blood	5.0–15.0 mg/dL	0.6–1.7 mmol/L
Lactate dehydrogenase (LD), serum	110–220 U/L	110–220 U/L
Lipase, serum	10–140 U/L	10–140 U/L

Reference Intervals* for Clinical Chemistry (Blood, Serum, and Plasma) *Continued*

Analyte	Conventional Units	SI Units
Lutropin (LH), serum		
Males	1–9 U/L	1–9 U/L
Females		
Follicular phase	2–10 U/L	2–10 U/L
Midcycle peak	15–65 U/L	15–65 U/L
Luteal phase	1–12 U/L	1–12 U/L
Postmenopausal	12–65 U/L	12–65 U/L
Magnesium, serum	1.3–2.1 mg/dL	0.65–1.05 mmol/L
Osmolality	275–295 mOsm/kg water	275–295 mOsm/kg water
Oxygen, blood, arterial, room air		
Partial pressure (PaO_2)	80–100 mm Hg	80–100 mm Hg
Saturation (SaO_2)	95–98%	95–98%
pH, arterial blood	7.35–7.45	7.35–7.45
Phosphate, inorganic, serum		
Adult	3.0–4.5 mg/dL	1.0–1.5 mmol/L
Child	4.0–7.0 mg/dL	1.3–2.3 mmol/L
Potassium		
Serum	3.5–5.0 mEq/L	3.5–5.0 mmol/L
Plasma	3.5–4.5 mEq/L	3.5–4.5 mmol/L
Progesterone, serum, adult		
Males	0.0–0.4 ng/mL	0.0–1.3 mmol/L
Females		
Follicular phase	0.1–1.5 ng/mL	0.3–4.8 mmol/L
Luteal phase	2.5–28.0 ng/mL	8.0–89.0 mmol/L
Prolactin, serum		
Males	1.0–15.0 ng/mL	1.0–15.0 µg/L
Females	1.0–20.0 ng/mL	1.0–20.0 µg/L
Protein, serum, electrophoresis		
Total	6.0–8.0 g/dL	60–80 g/L
Albumin	3.5–5.5 g/dL	35–55 g/L
Globulins		
$Alpha_1$	0.2–0.4 g/dL	2.0–4.0 g/L
$Alpha_2$	0.5–0.9 g/dL	5.0–9.0 g/L
Beta	0.6–1.1 g/dL	6.0–11.0 g/L
Gamma	0.7–1.7 g/dL	7.0–17.0 g/L
Pyruvate, blood	0.3–0.9 mg/dL	0.03–0.10 mmol/L
Rheumatoid factor	0.0–30.0 IU/mL	0.0–30.0 kIU/L
Sodium, serum or plasma	135–145 mEq/L	135–145 mmol/L
Testosterone, plasma		
Males, adult	300–1200 ng/dL	10.4–41.6 nmol/L
Females, adult	20–75 ng/dL	0.7–2.6 nmol/L
Pregnant females	40–200 ng/dL	1.4–6.9 nmol/L
Thyroglobulin	3–42 ng/mL	3–42 µg/L
Thyrotropin (hTSH), serum	0.4–4.8 µIU/mL	0.4–4.8 mIU/L
Thyrotropin-releasing hormone (TRH)	5–60 pg/mL	5–60 ng/L
Thyroxine (FT_4), free, serum	0.9–2.1 ng/dL	12–27 pmol/L
Thyroxine (T_4), serum	4.5–12.0 µg/dL	58–154 nmol/L
Thyroxine-binding globulin (TBG)	15.0–34.0 µg/mL	15.0–34.0 mg/L
Transferrin	250–430 mg/dL	2.5–4.3 g/L
Triglycerides, serum, after 12-h fast	40–150 mg/dL	0.4–1.5 g/L
Triiodothyronine (T_3), serum	70–190 ng/dL	1.1–2.9 nmol/L
Triiodothyronine uptake, resin (T_3RU)	25–38%	0.25–0.38
Urate		
Males	2.5–8.0 mg/dL	150–480 µmol/L
Females	2.2–7.0 mg/dL	130–420 µmol/L
Urea, serum or plasma	24–49 mg/dL	4.0–8.2 nmol/L
Urea nitrogen, serum or plasma	11–23 mg/dL	8.0–16.4 nmol/L
Viscosity, serum	1.4–1.8 × water	1.4–1.8 × water
Vitamin A, serum	20–80 µg/dL	0.70–2.80 µmol/L
Vitamin B_{12}, serum	180–900 pg/mL	133–664 pmol/L

*Reference values may vary, depending on the method and sample source used.

Reference Intervals for Therapeutic Drug Monitoring (Serum)

Analyte	Therapeutic Range	Toxic Concentrations	Proprietary Name(s)
Analgesics			
Acetaminophen	10–20 µg/mL	>250 µg/mL	Tylenol Datril
Salicylate	100–250 µg/mL	>300 µg/mL	Aspirin Bufferin
Antibiotics			
Amikacin	25–30 µg/mL	Peak >35 µg/mL Trough >10 µg/mL	Amikin
Gentamicin	5–10 µg/mL	Peak >10 µg/mL Trough >2 µg/mL	Garamycin
Tobramycin	5–10 µg/mL	Peak >10 µg/mL Trough >2 µg/mL	Nebcin
Vancomycin	5–35 µg/mL	Peak >40 µg/mL Trough >10 µg/mL	Vancocin
Anticonvulsants			
Carbamazepine	5–12 µg/mL	>15 µg/mL	Tegretol
Ethosuximide	40–100 µg/mL	>150 µg/mL	Zarontin
Phenobarbital	15–40 µg/mL	40–100 ng/mL (varies widely)	Luminal
Phenytoin	10–20 µg/mL	>20 µg/mL	Dilantin
Primidone	5–12 µg/mL	>15 µg/mL	Mysoline
Valproic acid	50–100 µg/mL	>100 µg/mL	Depakene
Antineoplastics and Immunosuppressives			
Cyclosporine	50–400 ng/mL	>400 ng/mL	Sandimmune
Methotrexate, high-dose, 48-h	Variable	>1 µmol/L, 48 h after dose	
Tacrolimus (FK-506), whole blood	3–10 µg/L	>15 µg/L	Prograf
Bronchodilators and Respiratory Stimulants			
Caffeine	3–15 ng/mL	>30 ng/mL	
Theophylline (aminophylline)	10–20 µg/mL	>20 µg/mL	Elixophyllin Quibron
Cardiovascular Drugs			
Amiodarone 　(obtain specimen more than 8 h after last dose)	1.0–2.0 µg/mL	>2.0 µg/mL	Cordarone
Digitoxin 　(obtain specimen 12–24 h after last dose)	15–25 ng/mL	>35 ng/mL	Crystodigin
Digoxin 　(obtain specimen more than 6 h after last dose)	0.8–2.0 ng/mL	>2.4 ng/mL	Lanoxin
Disopyramide	2–5 µg/mL	>7 µg/mL	Norpace
Flecainide	0.2–1.0 ng/mL	>1 ng/mL	Tambocor
Lidocaine	1.5–5.0 µg/mL	>6 µg/mL	Xylocaine
Mexiletine	0.7–2.0 ng/mL	>2 ng/mL	Mexitil
Procainamide	4–10 µg/mL	>12 µg/mL	Pronestyl
Procainamide plus *N*-acetyl-*p*- 　aminophenol (NAPA)	8–30 µg/mL	>30 µg/mL	
Propranolol	50–100 ng/mL	Variable	Inderal
Quinidine	2–5 µg/mL	>6 µg/mL	Cardioquin Quinaglute
Tocainide	4–10 ng/mL	>10 ng/mL	Tonocard
Psychopharmacologic Drugs			
Amitriptyline	120–150 ng/mL	>500 ng/mL	Elavil Triavil
Bupropion	25–100 ng/mL	Not applicable	Wellbutrin
Desipramine	150–300 ng/mL	>500 ng/mL	Norpramin
Imipramine	125–250 ng/mL	>400 ng/mL	Tofranil
Lithium 　(obtain specimen 12 h after last dose)	0.6–1.5 mEq/L	>1.5 mEq/L	Lithobid
Nortriptyline	50–150 ng/mL	>500 ng/mL	Aventyl Pamelor

Reference Intervals* for Clinical Chemistry (Urine)

Analyte	Conventional Units	SI Units
Acetone and acetoacetate, qualitative	Negative	Negative
Albumin		
Qualitative	Negative	Negative
Quantitative	10–100 mg/24 h	0.15–1.5 μmol/d
Aldosterone	3–20 μg/24 h	8.3–55 nmol/d
δ-Aminolevulinic acid (δ-ALA)	1.3–7.0 mg/24 h	10–53 μmol/d
Amylase	<17 U/h	<17 U/h
Amylase/creatinine clearance ratio	0.01–0.04	0.01–0.04
Bilirubin, qualitative	Negative	Negative
Calcium (regular diet)	<250 mg/24 h	<6.3 nmol/d
Catecholamines		
Epinephrine	<10 μg/24 h	<55 nmol/d
Norepinephrine	<100 μg/24 h	<590 nmol/d
Total free catecholamines	4–126 μg/24 h	24–745 nmol/d
Total metanephrines	0.1–1.6 mg/24 h	0.5–8.1 μmol/d
Chloride (varies with intake)	110–250 mEq/24 h	110–250 mmol/d
Copper	0–50 μg/24 h	0.0–0.80 μmol/d
Cortisol, free	10–100 μg/24 h	27.6–276 nmol/d
Creatine		
Males	0–40 mg/24 h	0.0–0.30 mmol/d
Females	0–80 mg/24 h	0.0–0.60 mmol/d
Creatinine	15–25 mg/kg/24 h	0.13–0.22 mmol/kg/d
Creatinine clearance (endogenous)		
Males	110–150 mL/min/1.73 m²	110–150 mL/min/1.73 m²
Females	105–132 mL/min/1.73 m²	105–132 mL/min/1.73 m²
Cystine or cysteine	Negative	Negative
Dehydroepiandrosterone		
Males	0.2–2.0 mg/24 h	0.7–6.9 μmol/d
Females	0.2–1.8 mg/24 h	0.7–6.2 μmol/d
Estrogens, total		
Males	4–25 μg/24 h	14–90 nmol/d
Females	5–100 μg/24 h	18–360 nmol/d
Glucose (as reducing substance)	<250 mg/24 h	<250 mg/d
Hemoglobin and myoglobin, qualitative	Negative	Negative
Homogentisic acid, qualitative	Negative	Negative
17-Ketogenic steroids		
Males	5–23 mg/24 h	17–80 μmol/d
Females	3–15 mg/24 h	10–52 μmol/d
17-Hydroxycorticosteroids		
Males	3–9 mg/24 h	8.3–25 μmol/d
Females	2–8 mg/24 h	5.5–22 μmol/d
5-Hydroxyindoleacetic acid		
Qualitative	Negative	Negative
Quantitative	2–6 mg/24 h	10–31 μmol/d
17-Ketosteroids		
Males	8–22 mg/24 h	28–76 μmol/d
Females	6–15 mg/24 h	21–52 μmol/d
Magnesium	6–10 mEq/24 h	3–5 mmol/d
Metanephrines	0.05–1.2 ng/mg creatinine	0.03–0.70 mmol/mmol creatinine
Osmolality	38–1400 mOsm/kg water	38–1400 mOsm/kg water
pH	4.6–8.0	4.6–8.0
Phenylpyruvic acid, qualitative	Negative	Negative
Phosphate	0.4–1.3 g/24 h	13–42 mmol/d
Porphobilinogen		
Qualitative	Negative	Negative
Quantitative	<2 mg/24 h	<9 μmol/d
Porphyrins		
Coproporphyrin	50–250 μg/24 h	77–380 nmol/d
Uroporphyrin	10–30 μg/24 h	12–36 nmol/d
Potassium	25–125 mEq/24 h	25–125 mmol/d
Pregnanediol		
Males	0.0–1.9 mg/24 h	0.0–6.0 μmol/d
Females		
Proliferative phase	0.0–2.6 mg/24 h	0.0–8.0 μmol/d
Luteal phase	2.6–10.6 mg/24 h	8–33 μmol/d
Postmenopausal	0.2–1.0 mg/24 h	0.6–3.1 μmol/d
Pregnanetriol	0.0–2.5 mg/24 h	0.0–7.4 μmol/d
Protein, total		
Qualitative	Negative	Negative
Quantitative	10–150 mg/24 h	10–150 mg/d
Protein/creatinine ratio	<0.2	<0.2

Table continued on following page

Reference Intervals* for Clinical Chemistry (Urine) *Continued*

Analyte	Conventional Units	SI Units
Sodium (regular diet)	60–260 mEq/24 h	60–260 mmol/d
Specific gravity		
Random specimen	1.003–1.030	1.003–1.030
24-hour collection	1.015–1.025	1.015–1.025
Urate (regular diet)	250–750 mg/24 h	1.5–4.4 mmol/d
Urobilinogen	0.5–4.0 mg/24 h	0.6–6.8 µmol/d
Vanillylmandelic acid (VMA)	1.0–8.0 mg/24 h	5–40 µmol/d

*Values may vary depending on the method used.

Reference Intervals for Toxic Substances

Analyte	Conventional Units	SI Units
Arsenic, urine	<130 µg/24 h	<1.7 µmol/d
Bromides, serum, inorganic	<100 mg/dL	<10 mmol/L
Toxic symptoms	140–1000 mg/dL	14–100 mmol/L
Carboxyhemoglobin, blood:	Saturation	
Urban environment	<5%	<0.05
Smokers	<12%	<0.12
Symptoms		
Headache	>15%	>0.15
Nausea and vomiting	>25%	>0.25
Potentially lethal	>50%	>0.50
Ethanol, blood	<0.05 mg/dL	<1.0 mmol/L
	<0.005%	
Intoxication	>100 mg/dL	>22 mmol/L
	>0.1%	
Marked intoxication	300–400 mg/dL	65–87 mmol/L
	0.3–0.4%	
Alcoholic stupor	400–500 mg/dL	87–109 mmol/L
	0.4–0.5%	
Coma	>500 mg/dL	
	>0.5%	>109 mmol/L
Lead, blood		
Adults	<25 µg/dL	<1.2 µmol/L
Children	<15 µg/dL	<0.7 µmol/L
Lead, urine	<80 µg/24 h	<0.4 µmol/d
Mercury, urine	<30 µg/24 h	<150 nmol/d

Reference Intervals for Tests Performed on Cerebrospinal Fluid

Test	Conventional Units	SI Units
Cells	<5/mm³; all mononuclear	<5 × 10⁶/L, all mononuclear
Protein electrophoresis	Albumin predominant	Albumin predominant
Glucose	50–75 mg/dL	2.8–4.2 mmol/L
	(20 mg/dL less than in serum)	(1.1 mmol less than in serum)
IgG	<8% of total protein	<0.08 of total protein
Children under 14	<14% of total protein	<0.14 of total protein
Adults		
IgG index		
$\left(\dfrac{\text{CSF/serum IgG ratio}}{\text{CSF/serum albumin ratio}}\right)$	0.3–0.6	0.3–0.6
Oligoclonal banding on electrophoresis	Absent	Absent
Pressure, opening	70–180 mm H₂O	70–180 mm H₂O
Protein, total	15–45 mg/dL	150–450 mg/L

*Abbreviation: CSF = cerebrospinal fluid.

Reference Intervals for Tests of Gastrointestinal Function

Test	Conventional Units
Bentiromide	6-hour urinary arylamine excretion greater than 57% excludes pancreatic insufficiency
β-Carotene, serum	60–250 ng/dL
Fecal fat estimation	
Qualitative	No fat globules seen by high-power microscope
Quantitative	<6 g/24 h (>95% coefficient of fat absorption)
Gastric acid output	
Basal	
Males	0.0–10.5 mmol/h
Females	0.0–5.6 mmol/h
Maximum (after histamine or pentagastrin)	
Males	9.0–48.0 mmol/h
Females	6.0–31.0 mmol/h
Ratio: basal/maximum	
Males	0.0–0.31
Females	0.0–0.29
Secretin test, pancreatic fluid	
Volume	>1.8 mL/kg/h
Bicarbonate	>80 mEq/L
D-Xylose absorption test, urine	>20% of ingested dose excreted in 5 h

Reference Intervals for Tests of Immunologic Function

Test	Conventional Units	SI Units
Complement, serum		
C3	85–175 mg/dL	0.85–1.75 g/L
C4	15–45 mg/dL	150–450 mg/L
Total hemolytic (CH_{50})	150–250 U/mL	150–250 U/mL
Immunoglobulins, serum, adult		
IgG	640–1350 mg/dL	6.4–13.5 g/L
IgA	70–310 mg/dL	0.70–3.1 g/L
IgM	90–350 mg/dL	0.90–3.5 g/L
IgD	0.0–6.0 mg/dL	0.0–60 mg/L
IgE	0.0–430 ng/dL	0.0–430 μg/L

Lymphocyte Subsets, Whole Blood, Heparinized

Antigen(s) Expressed	Cell Type	Percentage	Absolute Cell Count
CD3	Total T cells	56–77%	860–1880
CD19	Total B cells	7–17%	140–370
CD3 and CD4	Helper-inducer cells	32–54%	550–1190
CD3 and CD8	Suppressor-cytotoxic cells	24–37%	430–1060
CD3 and DR	Activated T cells	5–14%	70–310
CD2	E rosette T cells	73–87%	1040–2160
CD16 and CD56	Natural killer (NK) cells	8–22%	130–500

Helper/suppressor ratio: 0.8–1.8

Reference Values for Semen Analysis

Test	Conventional Units	SI Units
Volume	2–5 mL	2–5 mL
Liquefaction	Complete in 15 min	Complete in 15 min
pH	7.2–8.0	7.2–8.0
Leukocytes	Occasional or absent	Occasional or absent
Spermatozoa		
Count	60–150 × 10⁶/mL	60–150 × 10⁶/mL
Motility	>80% motile	>0.80 motile
Morphology	80–90% normal forms	>0.80–0.90 normal forms
Fructose	>150 mg/dL	>8.33 mmol/L

SELECTED REFERENCES

Drug Evaluations Annual. Chicago, American Medical Association, 1994.

Bick RL (ed): Hematology—Clinical and Laboratory Practice. St Louis, Mosby–Year Book, 1993.

Borer WZ: Selection and use of laboratory tests. *In* Tietz NW, Conn RB, Pruden EL (eds): Applied Laboratory Medicine. Philadelphia, WB Saunders Co, 1992, pp 1–5.

Campion EW: A retreat from SI units. N Engl J Med *327*:49, 1992.

Friedman RB, Young DS: Effects of Disease on Clinical Laboratory Tests, 3rd ed. Washington, DC, AACC Press, 1997.

Henry JB: Clinical Diagnosis and Management by Laboratory Methods, 19th ed. Philadelphia, WB Saunders Co, 1996.

Hicks JM, Young DS: DORA 97–99: Directory of Rare Analyses. Washington, DC, AACC Press, 1997.

Jacob DS, Demott WR, Grady HJ, et al (eds): Laboratory Test Handbook, 4th ed. Baltimore, Williams & Wilkins, 1996.

Kaplan LA, Pesce AJ: Clinical Chemistry—Theory, Analysis, and Correlation, 3rd ed. St Louis, Mosby–Year Book, 1996.

Kjeldsberg CR, Knight JA: Body Fluids: Laboratory Examination of Amniotic, Cerebrospinal, Seminal, Serous and Synovial Fluids, 3rd ed. Chicago, ASCP Press, 1993.

Laposata M: SI Unit Conversion Guide. Boston, NEJM Books, 1992.

Scully RE, McNeely WF, Mark EJ, McNeely BU: Normal reference laboratory values. N Engl J Med *327*:718–724, 1992.

Speicher CE: The Right Test: A Physician's Guide to Laboratory Medicine, 2nd ed. Philadelphia, WB Saunders Co, 1993.

Tietz NW (ed): Clinical Guide to Laboratory Tests, 3rd ed. Philadelphia, WB Saunders Co, 1995.

Wallach J: Interpretation of Diagnostic Tests: A Synopsis of Laboratory Medicine, 6th ed. Boston, Little, Brown, 1996.

Young DS: Implementation of SI units for clinical laboratory data. Ann Intern Med *106*:114–129, 1987.

Young DS: Determination and validation of reference intervals. Arch Pathol Lab Med *116*:704–709, 1992.

Young DS: Effects of Drugs on Clinical Laboratory Tests, 4th ed. Washington, DC, AACC Press, 1995.

Young DS: Effects of Preanalytical Variables on Clinical Laboratory Tests, 2nd ed. Washington, DC, AACC Press, 1997.

NEW DRUGS FOR 1998

method of
GREGORY C. TOMPKINS, PHARM.D., B.C.P.S.
Memorial Hospital Southwest
Houston, Texas

Generic Name	Trade Name (Manufacturer)	Dosage Form	Strength	Average Dosage Range	FDA Rating*	Approved Use	Approval Date	Classification
Brinzolamide	Azopt (Alcon)	Ophthalmic suspension	1%	1 drop three times daily	1-S	Treatment of elevated IOP in patients with ocular hypertension or open-angle glaucoma	April 1998	Carbonic anyhydrase inhibitor
Calfactant	Infasurf (Forest)	Intratracheal suspension	35 mg/6 mL	3 mL/kg as soon as possible after birth	1-S	Prevention of RDS in premature infants (<29 weeks of gestational age) or treatment of RDS in premature infants ≤72 hours after birth	July 1998	Lung surfactant
Candesartan	Atacand (Astra)	Tablet	4 mg, 8 mg, 16 mg, 32 mg	8–32 mg/d	1-S	Treatment of hypertension alone or in combination with other antihypertensive agents	June 1998	Angiotensin II receptor antagonist
Capecitabine	Xeloda (Roche)	Tablet	150 mg, 500 mg	2500 mg/M²/d in divided doses (q 12 h) for 2 weeks, then 1 week off	1-P	Treatment of metastatic breast cancer refractory to paclitaxel and when an anthracycline-containing regimen has failed or further treatment with anthracyclines is not an option	April 1998	Antineoplastic
Celecoxib	Celebrex (Searle)	Capsule	100 mg, 200 mg	200 mg/d	1-P	Relief of the signs and symptoms of rheumatoid and osteoarthritis in adults	December 1998	COX-2 inhibitor
Citalopram	Celexa (Forest)	Tablet	20 mg, 40 mg	20–40 mg/d	1-S	Treatment of depression	July 1998	Selective serotonin reuptake inhibitor

Table continued on opposite page

Generic Name	Trade Name (Manufacturer)	Dosage Form	Strength	Average Dosage Range	FDA Rating*	Approved Use	Approval Date	Classification
Efavirenz	Sustiva (DuPont)	Capsule	50 mg, 100 mg, 200 mg	200–600 mg/d	1-P	Treatment of HIV-1 infection in combination with other antiretrovirals	September 1998	Non-nucleoside reverse transcriptase inhibitor
Eptifibatide	Integrilin (COR Therapeutics)	Injection	20 mg/10 mL, 75 mg/100 mL	180-μg/kg bolus, then 2 μg/kg/min	1-P	Treatment of ACS, including patients to be managed medically and those undergoing PCI; treatment of patients undergoing PCI	May 1998	Glycoprotein IIb/IIIa inhibitor (anti-platelet)
Etanercept	Enbrel (Immunex)	Injection	25 mg	25 mg SC twice a week	1-P	Reduction in signs and symptoms of moderately or severely active rheumatoid arthritis in patients who have had inadequate response to other DMARDs	November 1998	Biologic response modifier
Fomivirsen	Vitravene (Isis Pharmaceuticals)	Injection (intra-vitreal)	1.65 mg in 0.25-mL vial	330 μg q 2 weeks $\times$ 2 doses, then 330 μg q 4 weeks	1-P	Local treatment of CMV retinitis in AIDS patients	August 1998	Antiviral
Leflunomide	Arava (Hoechst Marion Roussel)	Tablet	10 mg, 20 mg, 100 mg	100 mg/d $\times$ 3 d, then 20 mg/d	1-P	Treatment of active rheumatoid arthritis	September 1998	Anti-inflammatory via inhibition of pyrimidine synthesis
Lepirudin	Refludan (Hoechst Marion Roussel)	Injection	50 mg	0.4 mg/kg bolus, then 0.15 mg/kg/h as continuous infusion	1-P	For anticoagulation in patient with HIT and thromboembolic disease to prevent further events	March 1998	Thrombin inhibitor
Loteprednol	Lotemax (Bausch and Lomb)	Ophthalmic suspension	0.5%	1–2 drops in affected eye four times a day	1-S	Treatment of steroid-responsive inflammatory eye conditions	March 1998	Ophthalmic corticosteroid
Modafinil	Provigil (Cephalon)	Tablet	100 mg, 200 mg	200–400 mg/d	1-S	Treatment of narcolepsy	December 1998	Central alpha$_1$ receptor agonist
Naratriptan	Amerge (Glaxo Wellcome)	Tablets	1 mg, 2.5 mg	2.5 mg as needed; no more than 5 mg in 24 h	1-S	Treatment of acute migraine attacks, with and without aura, in adults	February 1998	Serotonin 5-HT$_1$ receptor agonist
Paricalcitol	Zemplar (Abbott)	Injection	5 μg/mL, in 1- and 2-mL vials	0.04–0.1 μg/kg every other day	1-S	Prevention and treatment of secondary hyperpara-thyroidism associated with CRF	April 1998	Synthetic vitamin D analogue
Rifapentine	Priftin (Hoechst Marion Roussel)	Tablet	150 mg	600 mg twice weekly	1-P	Treatment of pulmonary tuberculosis	June 1998	Rifamycin antibiotic
Rizatriptan	Maxalt (Merck)	Tablet	5 mg, 10 mg	5–10 mg as needed; no more than 30 mg in 24 h	1-S	Treatment of acute migraine attacks, with and without aura, in adults	June 1998	Serotonin 5-HT$_1$ receptor agonist
Sevelamer	Renagel (Geltex Pharmaceuticals)	Capsule	403 mg	2–4 capsules with each meal	1-S	Reducing serum phosphorus in ESRD	October 1998	Phosphate binder
Sildenafil	Viagra (Pfizer)	Tablet	25 mg, 50 mg, 100 mg	25–100 mg as needed; no more than 1 dose per day	1-P	Treatment of erectile dysfunction	March 1998	Impotence agent
Telmisartan	Micardis (Boehringer Ingelheim)	Tablet	40 mg, 80 mg	20–80 mg/d	1-S	Treatment of hypertension alone or in combination with other antihypertensive agents	November 1998	Angiotensin II receptor antagonist

Table continued on following page

Generic Name	Trade Name (Manufacturer)	Dosage Form	Strength	Average Dosage Range	FDA Rating*	Approved Use	Approval Date	Classification
Thalidomide	Thalomid (Celgene Corp)	Capsule	50 mg	100–300 mg/d	1-P	Acute treatment of the cutaneous manifestations of moderate to severe erythma nodosum leprosum	July 1998	Immuno-modulator
Tirofiban	Aggrastat (Merck)	Injection	250 μg/mL in 50-mL vial; 50 μg/mL in 500-mL solution for injection	0.4 μg/kg/min for 30 min, then 0.1 μg/kg/min	1-P	In combination with heparin for treatment of ACS, including patients to be managed medically and those undergoing PCI	May 1998	Glycoprotein IIb/IIIa inhibitor (antiplatelet)
Tolcapone	Tasmar (Roche)	Tablet	100 mg, 200 mg	100–200 mg three times a day	1-S	As an adjunct to levadopa and carbidopa for the treatment of Parkinson's disease	January 1998	Antiparkinsonian (Catechol-O-methyl-transferase inhibitor)
Tolterodine	Detrol (Pharmacia and Upjohn)	Tablet	1 mg, 2 mg	1–2 mg twice a day	1-S	Treatment of patients with an overactive bladder with symptoms of frequency, urgency, or urge incontinence	March 1998	Muscarinic receptor antagonist
Trastuzumab	Herceptin (Genentech)	Injection	440 mg	4 mg/kg initially, then 2 mg/kg weekly	1-P	Treatment of metastatic breast cancer with tumors overexpressing the HER2 protein	September 1998	Biologic response modifier
Valrubicin	Valstar (Anthra Pharmaceuticals)	Solution (intravesical)	40 mg/mL	800 mg administered intravesically weekly for 6 weeks	1-P	Intravesical treatment of BCG-refractory carcinoma in situ for patients who are not candidates for cystoscopy	September 1998	Antineoplastic (anthracycline)

*1 = new molecular entity; P = priority drug review; S = standard drug review.

Abbreviations: ACS = acute coronary syndrome; AIDS = acquired immune deficiency syndrome; BCG = bacillus Calmette-Guèrin; COX-2 = cyclooxygenase-2; CMV = cytomegalovirus; CRF = chronic renal failure; DMARD = disease-modifying antirheumatic drug; ESRD = end-stage renal failure; HIT = heparin-induced thrombocytopenia; HIV-1 = human immunodeficiency virus-1; IOP = intraocular pressure; PCI = percutaneous coronary intervention; RDS = respiratory distress syndrome.

NOMOGRAM FOR THE
DETERMINATION OF BODY SURFACE
AREA OF CHILDREN AND ADULTS

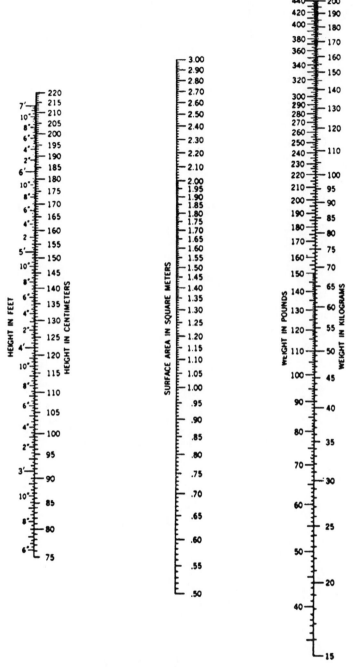

From Boothby WM, Sandiford RB: Boston Med Surg J *185*:337, 1921.

Index

Note: Page numbers in *italics* refer to illustrations; page numbers followed by t refer to tables.

Abacavir (ABC), for HIV infection, 45t, 48t
  hypersensitivity to, 47
Abdominal bloating, 12
Abdominal colectomy, with ileorectal
  anastomosis, for constipation, 20
Abdominal distention, due to rectus
  muscle relaxation, 12
Abetalipoproteinemia, acanthocytosis in,
  365
  malabsorption due to, 512
ABO incompatibility, hemolytic transfusion
  reaction due to, 459
  maternal-fetal, 388, 388t, *390*
  Rh isoimmunization and, 384
Abrasions, 975
Abruptio placentae, 987, 988
  disseminated intravascular coagulation
  in, 402, 988
Abscess, anorectal, 495
  Bartholin's duct, 1071
  breast, 1023–1024
  cutaneous, 795
  liver. See *Liver abscess.*
  lung, 203–204
  perinephric, 662
  renal, 682
  tubo-ovarian, 1059–1060
Abstinence, as contraceptive method, 1075,
  1076t
    for adolescents, 1088
  periodic, in natural family planning
    methods, 1075–1084, 1076t
    during breast-feeding, 1089
Abulia, depression vs., 922
ABVD regimen, for Hodgkin's disease,
  406–407, 407t
  side effects of, 408
AC regimen, for breast cancer, 1027
Acanthocytosis, hereditary, 365
Acarbose, for type 2 diabetes, 557t, 559
Accessory pathways, tachycardias with,
  271, 272–274
Acebutolol, for hypertension, 308t
  intoxication with, 1167t
Acetaminophen, dosage limitations on, in
  cirrhosis, 468
  for chronic fatigue syndrome, 112
  for febrile nonhemolytic transfusion reac-
    tion, 459–460
  for fever, 22
  for ischemic stroke, 852
  for migraine, 881
  for mountain sickness, 1128, 1128t
  for osteoarthritis, 969
  for pain, 2
  for painful episode in sickle cell disease,
    376, 377
  for rheumatoid arthritis, 947, 951
  for viral hepatitis, 502
  for viral respiratory infection, 214
  in analgesic combinations, 2
    for migraine, 881

Acetaminophen *(Continued)*
    for painful episode in sickle cell dis-
      ease, 376
    intoxication by, 1160–1163, *1161,* 1162t
    reference intervals for, 1210t
    with very-low-calorie diet, 588
Acetate, in parenteral nutrition solutions,
  605t
Acetazolamide, for epilepsy in infants and
  children, 868t
  for Meniere's disease, 888
  for mountain sickness, 1128, 1128t
    prophylactic, 150, 1128, 1128t
  for obstructive sleep-disordered breath-
    ing, 184
Acetic acid, for human papillomavirus
  detection, 833, 1069
  for otitis externa, 114–115
  in vulvar lesion diagnosis, 1069
Acetoacetate, reference intervals for, in
  serum, 1207t
  in urine, 1211t
Acetohexamide, for type 2 diabetes, 557t
Acetohydroxamic acid, for struvite stone
  prevention, 715
Acetone, reference intervals for, in serum,
  1207t
  in urine, 1211t
  serum concentration estimation for,
    1160t
Acetonitrile, cyanide poisoning due to,
  1173
Acetylcholine receptor antibodies, in
  myasthenia gravis, 905
Acetylcholinesterase inhibitors, for
  Alzheimer's disease, 845
Acetylcysteine, as antidote, 1151t
  for acetaminophen intoxication, 1151t,
    1162, 1162t
  for atelectasis due to mucous plugs, 171
α-*l*-Acetylmethadol, for opioid abuse, 1095
Acetylsalicylic acid. See *Aspirin;*
  Salicylates.
Achalasia, 474–475, 478
Acid hemolysis test, reference intervals for,
  1206t
Acid injury, 1171–1172
Acid phosphatase, serum, reference
  intervals for, 1207t
Acid pump inhibitors. See also specific
  drugs.
  defective iron absorption due to, 356
  for dyspepsia, 11
  for gastroesophageal reflux disease, 525–
    526
Acid-base balance. See also *Acidosis.*
  management of, in acute renal failure,
    697–698
Acidosis, in acute poisoning, 1158, 1159t
  in acute renal failure, 698
  in chronic renal failure, 704
  in malaria, 99

Acidosis *(Continued)*
  in neonate, 1006
Acitretin, cheilitis due to, 810
  for lupus erythematosus, 776
  for psoriasis, 772
Acne vulgaris, 757–759
Acoustic neuromas, 940–941
Acquired immunodeficiency syndrome
  (AIDS). See *Human immunodeficiency
  virus (HIV) infection.*
Acrivastine, for ordinary urticaria, 835
Acrodermatitis chronica atrophicans, 125t,
  126, 128t
Acromegaly, 615–617
  peripheral neuropathy in, 926, 928
  pressure palsies in, 930
Acromioclavicular separation, 976
ACTH. See *Corticotropin (ACTH).*
Actinic cheilitis, 792, 810
Actinic keratosis, 792
  squamous cell carcinoma and, 764, 792
Actinomycosis, oral ulceration in, 813
Activated charcoal, for acute poisoning,
  1148, 1148t
  for protoporphyria, 453
  for pruritus in cholestatic liver disease,
    37
Activated partial thromboplastin time,
  reference intervals for, 1207t
Activities of daily living, after stroke, 854
Acupuncture, for labor analgesia, 995
Acute phase reactants, as prognostic
  factors in rheumatoid arthritis,
  945–947
Acyclovir, for aplastic anemia, 354
  for erythema multiforme, 813, 824
  for hairy leukoplakia, 814
  for herpes simplex, 800, 800t
    in conjunctivitis, 68
    in encephalitis, 896
    in HIV infection, 53, 801
    in primary gingivostomatitis, 812–813
    in recurrent labial infection, 809
  for herpes zoster, 800t, 802
  for Ramsay Hunt syndrome, 886t
  for varicella, 71, 800t, 802
  for vertigo, 886
  for viral pneumonia, 216t
Adapalene, for acne, 757
Addiction. See also *Drug abuse;* specific
  substances.
  defined, 4, 1094
Addison's disease, 618–619, 618t
  diagnosis of, 619–620
  treatment of, 620–621
Adefovir (ADF), for HIV infection, 47, 48t
Adenocarcinoma, cervical, 1068. See also
  Cervical cancer.
  endometrial. See *Endometrial cancer.*
  esophageal, dysphagia due to, 474
  gastric, 528–530, 528t, 529t
  prostatic. See *Prostate cancer.*

Adenocarcinoma *(Continued)*
  salivary gland, 817
Adenoma, adrenal, aldosterone-producing,
    315, 634–635
  Cushing's syndrome due to, 624
  colorectal, malignant transformation of,
    532–533
  gastric, 527–528
  parathyroid, hyperparathyroidism due
    to, 627, 628
  pituitary, acromegaly due to, 615
    Cushing's syndrome due to, 622–623
    prolactin-secreting, 641–642
Adenomatous polyposis, familial, colorectal
    cancer and, 533
Adenomyosis, leiomyoma vs., 1061
Adenosine, for atrial flutter, 275t
Adenovirus infection, conjunctivitis due to,
    68
  encephalitis due to, 895
  pneumonia due to, 215, 215t, 216t
ADF (adefovir), for HIV infection, 47, 48t
Adjustment disorder with anxiety, 1099
Adjustment sleep disorder, 32
Adolescents. See also *Child(ren)*.
  asthma in. See under *Asthma*.
  contraception for, 1088
  diabetes mellitus in, 566–572. See also
    Diabetes mellitus, type 1.
  epilepsy and seizures in, 856–866. See
    also *Epilepsy; Seizures*.
  severe hypoglycemia in, in type 1 diabe-
    tes, 571
Adrenal adenoma, aldosterone-producing,
    315, 634–635
  Cushing's syndrome due to, 624
Adrenal carcinoma, Cushing's syndrome
    due to, 624
Adrenal crisis, 619, 620, 620t
Adrenal hyperplasia, aldosteronism due to,
    315, 635
  congenital, prenatal treatment of, 984
Adrenal insufficiency, 618–621, 618t–621t
  neonatal, due to maternal corticosteroid
    use, 832
  secondary, 619, 619t, 637, 640t
Adrenal scintigraphy, in aldosteronism
    diagnosis, 635
Adrenal venous catheterization, in
    aldosteronism diagnosis, 635
Adrenalectomy, for Cushing's syndrome,
    624
  for pheochromocytoma, 656
Adrenergic agonists. See *Alpha agonists;
    Beta agonists;* specific drugs.
Adrenergic blockers. See *Alpha blockers;
    Alpha/beta blockers; Beta blockers;*
    specific drugs.
α-Adrenergic receptors, antidepressants'
    action at, 1110t, 1112, 1113–1114,
    1113t
Adrenocortical insufficiency. See *Adrenal
    insufficiency*.
Adrenocorticotropic hormone. See
    Corticotropin (ACTH).
Adult respiratory distress syndrome,
    167–168
Adverse drug reactions, allergy and,
    748–749, 749, 749t. See also *Allergy,
    to drugs*.
  classification of, 749
  reporting of, 753
Aeromonas hydrophila infection, 798
Aerophagia, 12
Affective spectrum disorder, 110
Afibrinogenemia, 392

Afterpains, 999
Aggression, in Alzheimer's disease, 847
Agoraphobia, 1099, 1100t, 1121
AIDS. See *Human immunodeficiency virus
    (HIV) infection*.
Air embolism, with central catheter
    placement, 606
Air swallowing, 12
Air travel, circadian rhythm disorders due
    to. See *Jet lag*.
  in chronic obstructive pulmonary dis-
    ease, 175
Airway management. See also *Intubation*.
  in neonatal resuscitation, 1003
Akathisia, due to haloperidol, 876
Akinesia, due to haloperidol, 876
Alanine aminotransferase, serum,
    reference intervals for, 1207t
Albendazole, 544
  for ascariasis, 540t, 544
  for capillariasis, 540t, 545
  for cutaneous larva migrans, 544
  for cysticercosis, 541t, 546
  for echinococcosis, 541t, 547
  for giardiasis, 539t, 542
  for hookworm, 540t, 544
  for liver flukes, 540t
  for microsporidiosis, 539t, 543
  for pinworm, 540t, 544
  for strongyloidiasis, 805
  for trichinosis, 541t, 545
  for *Trichostrongylus* infection, 541t, 545
  for whipworm, 541t, 544
Albumin, preparations of, 458
  reference intervals for, in serum, 1207t,
    1209t
    in urine, 1211t
Albuterol, for acute bronchitis, 208
  for anaphylaxis, 727t
  for asthma, 733, 734
    in children, 740, 741
  for atelectasis due to mucous plugs, 171
  for cystic fibrosis, 176t
  for hyperkalemia in acute renal failure,
    697t
  for insect sting allergy, 754
  for pertussis, 139
Albuterol–ipratropium bromide, for chronic
    obstructive pulmonary disease, 173
Alcohol. See also *Alcohol consumption*.
  anticonvulsant interactions with, 863t
  as antidote, 1153t
    for ethylene glycol intoxication, 1178
    for methanol intoxication, 1189
  blood, as marker for excess alcohol in-
    take, 1092
    reference intervals for, 1212t
  methotrexate interaction with, 956
  serum concentration estimation for,
    1160t
Alcohol consumption, abstinence from, for
    chronic pancreatitis, 520
  in dependent persons, social support
    and, 1093
  assessing level of, 1090, 1091–1092,
    1092t
  chronic pancreatitis and, 518–519
  in type 2 diabetes, 555
  intoxication due to, 1156t, 1175–1177,
    1176t, 1177t
  limiting, for hypertension, 305
  neuropathy due to, 926–927
  obstructive sleep-disordered breathing
    and, 181
  problems related to, 1090–1093, 1091t
Alcohol dependence syndrome, 1090, 1092,
    1092t

Alcohol dependence syndrome *(Continued)*
  management of, 1092, 1093
Alcoholic liver disease, 468. See also
    Cirrhosis.
Alcoholics Anonymous, 1093
Alcuronium, for tetanus, 136
Aldicarb, 1193
Aldolase, serum, reference intervals for,
    1207t
Aldosterone, measurement of, in
    aldosteronism diagnosis, 315, 634
  reference intervals for, in plasma, 1207t
    in urine, 1211t
Aldosterone suppression test, 315, 634
Aldosteronism, 314–315, 634–635
Alendronate, adverse effects of, 599
  for osteopenia in thalassemia patient,
    372
  for osteoporosis, 595
  for osteoporosis prevention, 595
    in inflammatory bowel disease, 487
    in primary biliary cirrhosis, 468
    with corticosteroid therapy, 596, 948
    with gonadotropin-releasing hormone
      agonists, 1032
  for Paget's disease of bone, 598t, 599
Alginate dressings, for pressure ulcers,
    820
Alkali injury, 1171–1172
Alkaline phosphatase, leukocyte, reference
    intervals for, 1206t
  serum, reference intervals for, 1207t
Alkylating agents. See also specific drugs.
  DNA damage due to, acute leukemia
    and, 413
  for membranous glomerulopathy, 678
  for minimal change disease, 677–678
  for primary glomerular disease, 676
  for rheumatoid arthritis, 950
Allergic conjunctivitis, 68–69
Allergic contact dermatitis, 830–831
Allergic rhinitis, 743–748
  diagnosis of, 743–744
  postnasal drip syndrome and cough in,
    24
  treatment of, 744–748, 745t, 747t
    drugs for, 745–747, 745t, 747t
    during pregnancy, 748
    environmental control in, 744–745
    immunotherapy for, 748
Allergy, 725–755. See also *Hypersensitivity*
    entries.
  antidepressants for use with, 1115t
  asthma and, 730
    environmental control measures for,
      731
  to drugs, 748–753
    advice to patient on, 752–753
    confirmation of, 751–752
    diagnosis of, 749–750, 750t
    family member risk in, 753
    reporting of, 753
    sources of information on, 750–751
    treatment of, 750–753
  to food, atopic dermatitis and, 823
  to insect sting, 753–755, 754t, 755t
Allopurinol, azathioprine interaction with,
    578, 950
  for gout, 578
  for leishmaniasis, 91
  for tumor lysis syndrome in acute leuke-
    mia, 422
  hypersensitivity reaction to, 578
  with phlebotomy for polycythemia vera,
    446
  with very-low-calorie diet, 589

Alopecia, androgenic, 761
  traction, 761, 762
Alopecia areata, 761–762
Alosetron, for irritable bowel syndrome, 491
Alpha agonists. See also specific drugs.
  central, for hypertension, 308t, 309
  for glaucoma, 913
Alpha blockers. See also specific drugs.
  for benign prostatic hyperplasia, 688, 690t
  for hypertension, 307–309, 308t
    in type 2 diabetes, 563
  for pheochromocytoma, 655
Alpha globulin, serum, reference intervals for, 1209t
Alpha receptors, antidepressants' action at, 1110t, 1112, 1113–1114, 1113t
Alpha₂-antiplasmin deficiency, bleeding in, 392
Alpha/beta blockers. See also specific drugs.
  for hypertension, 308t, 309
Alpha-fetoprotein, maternal serum, measurement of, 980, 981
Alpha-D-galactosidase, for gaseousness, 13
Alpha-glucosidase inhibitors. See also specific drugs.
  for type 2 diabetes, 557t, 559
Alpha-hydroxyacids, for hyperpigmentation, 839
Alpha-mercaptopropionylglycine, for cystinuria, 715
Alpha-methyl-paratyrosine, for pheochromocytoma, 314
Alprazolam, antidepressant interactions with, 1114
  for anxiety disorders, 1100t, 1102
  for Meniere's disease, 893
  for panic disorder, 886t, 891, 1121t, 1122
  for premenstrual syndrome, 1047
  intoxication with, 1166
Alprenolol, intoxication with, 1167t
Alprostadil, for cutaneovascular disease in lupus erythematosus, 776
  for erectile dysfunction, 693
    in diabetes, 566
  in erectile dysfunction assessment, 692
Alteplase. See Tissue plasminogen activator (t-PA).
Altitude sickness, 1127–1130, 1128t
  cerebral edema due to, 1128, 1128t
  prevention of, 150, 1128t
  pulmonary edema due to, 1128–1129, 1128t
Aluminum, antacids containing, for mouth disease, 808
  in acute renal failure, 699
  levothyroxine interaction with, 644
  phosphate binders containing, in acute renal failure, 698
    in chronic renal failure, 704, 704t
Alveolitis, extrinsic allergic, 230–231, 231t
Alzheimer's disease, 844–847
  hormone replacement therapy and, 1050
Amalgam tattoos, 816
Amantadine, for cocaine abuse, 1094
  for fatigue in multiple sclerosis, 901
  for hiccup, 14t
  for influenza, 87
  for Parkinson's disease, 919, 919t, 921, 922
  for viral pneumonia, 216t
Ambulation, after stroke, 853–854
Ambulatory venous hypertension, after venous thrombosis, 340

Ambulatory venous hypertension (Continued)
  venous leg ulcers and, 818
Amebiasis, 56–59, 57t–59t, 539t, 542
  acute diarrhea due to, 16, 17t
  skin disease due to, 804, 804t
Ameboma, 57. See also Amebiasis.
Amenorrhea, 1040–1043
American Society of Tropical Medicine and Hygiene, 145
American trypanosomiasis, 101–102
Amifostine, for xerostomia prevention, with radioiodine therapy for thyroid cancer, 652
Amikacin, for bacterial meningitis, 105t
  for cystic fibrosis exacerbations, 179t
  for Mycobacterium avium complex infection in HIV infection, 54
  for sepsis, 63t
  reference intervals for, 1210t
Amiloride, for ascites in cirrhosis, 469
  for congestive heart failure, 294t
  for diabetes insipidus, 626t, 627
  for hypertension, 308t
  for primary aldosteronism, 635
Amino acids, in parenteral nutrition solutions, 604, 605t
  malabsorption of, congenital defects causing, 514
Aminocaproic acid, for C1 esterase inhibitor deficiency, 836–837
  for disseminated intravascular coagulation, 402
  for hemophilia, 395
  for intracerebral hemorrhage, 849
  for platelet-mediated bleeding disorders, 399
Aminoglutethimide, for breast cancer, 1028
  for Cushing's syndrome, 623, 623t
δ-Aminolevulinic acid, urine, reference intervals for, 1211t
Aminolevulinic acid dehydratase deficiency porphyria, 448t. See also Porphyria(s).
Aminophylline, for anaphylaxis, 727t
  for insect sting allergy, 754
  reference intervals for, 1210t
Amiodarone, adverse effects of, 275, 275t
  anticonvulsant interactions with, 863t
  for atrial fibrillation, 257, 258t, 259, 259t, 260
    after myocardial infarction, 323
  for atrial flutter, 275t
  for cardiac arrest, 253
  for congestive heart failure, 296
  for myocardial infarction, 322
  for ventricular premature beats, 264
  for ventricular tachycardia after myocardial infarction, 324
  reference intervals for, 1210t
  relative antiarrhythmic efficacy of, 262t
  thyroid disorders due to, 660
Amitriptyline, for chronic fatigue syndrome, 112
  for depression, 1109t
    in multiple sclerosis, 901
  for diabetic neuropathy, 565
  for fibromyalgia, 967
  for glossodynia, 815
  for hiccup, 14t
  for insomnia, 35
  for lichen simplex chronicus, 834
  for pain, 3
    in multiple sclerosis, 902
  for painful neuropathy, 932
  for rheumatoid arthritis, 947
  for stress-related tinnitus, 38

Amitriptyline (Continued)
  for trigeminal neuralgia, 909–910
  intoxication with, 1097, 1201, 1202t
  pharmacodynamic effects of, 1110t
  reference intervals for, 1210t
Amlodipine, for angina, 249
  for congestive heart failure, 296
  for hypertension, 308t, 310
  intoxication with, 1168
Ammonia nitrogen, plasma, reference intervals for, 1207t
Amnesia, post-traumatic, cognitive dysfunction and, 940
  transient global, seizure vs., 857
Amnesic shellfish poisoning, 79, 80t
Amniocentesis, 981
Amniotic fluid, analysis of, in Rh isoimmunization assessment, 385, 386
  meconium-stained, 1004
Amobarbital, intoxication with, 1165
Amoxapine, for depression, 1109t
  intoxication with, 1201, 1202, 1202t
  pharmacodynamic effects of, 1110t
Amoxicillin, for bacterial pneumonia, 212t, 213
  for Chlamydia trachomatis infection during pregnancy, 1057, 1057t
  for endocarditis prophylaxis, 301t, 303
    in mitral valve prolapse, 289, 290t
  for Helicobacter pylori infection, 11, 501, 501t
  for Lyme disease, 128t, 129t
  for osteomyelitis, 973
  for otitis media, 205, 205t, 206
    prophylactic, 206
  for pregnancy-associated urinary tract infection, 664t, 666
  for streptococcal pharyngitis, 237, 238t
  for typhoid carriage, 164
  for typhoid fever, 162–163, 163t
  rash due to, in infectious mononucleosis, 109
Amoxicillin-clavulanate, for bacterial overgrowth, 510
  for bacterial pneumonia, 212t
  for bacterial vaginosis, 1054
  for cystic fibrosis exacerbations, 179t
  for cystitis, 663, 664t
  for foot ulcer in diabetes, 566
  for laryngitis, 30
  for otitis media, 205, 205t, 206
  for pregnancy-associated urinary tract infection, 664t, 666
  for pyelonephritis in women, 664, 664t
  for typhoid fever, 162–163
AMP (amprenavir), antitubercular drug interaction with, 52
  for HIV infection, 46t, 49t
Amphetamines, for hiccup, 14t
  intoxication with, 1095, 1163
  lead in, 1184
Amphotericin B, for blastomycosis, 200t, 201
  for coccidioidomycosis, 193, 194
    with extrapulmonary dissemination, 195
  for cryptococcal meningitis in HIV infection, 52
  for fever in aplastic anemia, 354
  for histoplasmosis, 196, 197t, 198
    in HIV infection, 197t, 198, 199
  for infection in neutropenia, 419
  for leishmaniasis, 90
  for mucosal candidiasis in HIV infection, 54
  liposomal, for cryptococcal meningitis in HIV infection, 52

Amphotericin B *(Continued)*
    for leishmaniasis, 90
    premedication for, 193t, 201
Ampicillin, for bacterial meningitis,
        dosages for, 105t
    for bacterial overgrowth in diabetes, 565
    for bacterial tracheitis, 31
    for dissecting cellulitis of scalp, 762
    for endocarditis, 300t, 301
    for endocarditis prophylaxis, 301t, 303
        in mitral valve prolapse, 290t
    for epididymitis, 675
    for *Haemophilus influenzae* meningitis,
        104t
    for *Listeria monocytogenes* infection, 77t,
        79, 103t, 104t, 106
    for meningococcal meningitis, 103t, 104t,
        105
    for osteomyelitis, 974t
    for pneumococcal meningitis, 104t
    for postpartum endomyometritis, 1000–
        1001
    for pyelonephritis, 682t
        in women, 664, 664t
    for sepsis, 63t
        in neonate, 1017t, 1018
    for *Streptococcus agalactiae* meningitis,
        103t, 104t, 107
    for typhoid carriage, 164
    for typhoid fever, 162, 163t
    for urinary tract infection in girls, 667
    rash due to, in infectious mononucleosis,
        109, 802
Ampicillin-sulbactam, for laryngitis, 30
    for pelvic inflammatory disease, 1059t
    for postpartum endomyometritis, 1000
    for pyelonephritis in women, 664, 664t
    for sepsis, 63t
Amplicor, 242, 242t
Amprenavir (AMP), antitubercular drug
        interaction with, 52
    for HIV infection, 46t, 49t
Amputation, in diabetes, 566
    in frostbite, 1134
Amrinone, for beta blocker intoxication,
        1168
    for calcium channel blocker intoxication,
        1169
Amyl nitrite, in cyanide antidote kit,
        1151t, 1173
Amylase, serum, in acute pancreatitis
        diagnosis, 515
    reference intervals for, 1207t
    urine, reference intervals for, 1211t
Amylase/creatinine clearance ratio,
        reference intervals for, 1211t
Amyloidosis, peripheral neuropathy in,
        928, 931
    pressure palsies in, 930
    renal, in ankylosing spondylitis, 959
Amyotrophy, diabetic, 565
Anabolic steroids, abuse of, 1097–1098
Anagen effluvium, 760–761
Anagrelide, for polycythemia vera, 446t,
        447
Ana-Kit, 728
    for insect sting allergy, 754, 754t
Anal fissure, 493–495
Analgesia. See also *Analgesics;* specific
        drugs and classes of drugs.
    after cesarean delivery, 998
    for labor, 995–997
    patient-controlled, for painful episode in
        sickle cell disease, 376–377
Analgesics. See also *Analgesia;* specific
        drugs and classes of drugs.

Analgesics *(Continued)*
    adjuvant, 2–4
    for insomnia, 34
    nonopioid, 2
Anaphylactoid reaction, agents causing,
        726, 726t
    defined, 725
    to snake antivenin, 1140
Anaphylaxis, 725–729
    agents causing, 725, 726t
    biphasic, 726
    clinical signs and symptoms of, 725t
    differential diagnosis of, 726–727
    due to blood components, 460
    exercise-induced, 726
    factitious, 727
    idiopathic, 726
        treatment of, 727t
        undifferentiated somatoform, 727
    pathophysiology of, 725
    persistent, 726
    prevention of, 728–729, 728t
    treatment of, 727–728, 727t
        in insect sting allergy, 753–754
Ancylostoma braziliense, 544, 804t, 805
Ancylostoma caninum, 544
Ancylostoma duodenale, 540t, 544
    skin disease due to, 804t
Androgen(s). See also specific androgens.
    anabolic, abuse of, 1097–1098
    for aplastic anemia, 354
    for Fanconi's anemia, 355
    for hormone replacement therapy, 1051
Androgen excess, acne in, 759
    hair loss in, 761
    hirsutism in, 763
Androgenic alopecia, 761
Anemia, aplastic, 351–356. See also
        Aplastic anemia.
    autoimmune hemolytic, 358–363. See
        also *Autoimmune hemolytic anemia.*
    Fanconi's, 354–355
    hypoplastic, criteria for, 351
    in acute renal failure, 698, 699
    in chronic renal failure, 703
    in malaria, 95t, 99
    in multiple myeloma, 444
    in newborn, 1016. See also *Hemolytic
        disease of fetus and newborn;
        Rh isoimmunization.*
    iron deficiency, 356–358
    megaloblastic, 366–369
    nonimmune hemolytic, 363–366, 363t.
        See also specific disorders.
        acquired, 363t, 365–366
        hereditary, 363–365, 363t
    pernicious, 367–368
    sickle cell, 374, 375t. See also *Sickle cell
        disease.*
Anesthesia. See also specific drugs.
    general, for status epilepticus, 865, 865t
    local, testing for drug allergy before,
        752, 752t
    obstetric, 995–999. See also *Obstetric
        anesthesia.*
Anesthetic-corticosteroid injections, for
        bursitis or tendinitis, 965–966
    for fibromyalgia, 967
    for osteoarthritis, 970
    for rheumatoid arthritis, 948
Aneurysm, aortic, 243–245, 338, 338t
    peripheral arterial, 338–339, 338t
Angina pectoris, 247–250
    pathophysiology of, 247–248
    Prinzmetal's (variant), 247
    risk factor control in, 249–250

Angina pectoris *(Continued)*
    treatment of, 248–249
    unstable, 247, 316
Angina sine dolore, 247
Angioedema, 834–837
    hereditary, anaphylaxis vs., 727
    migratory, due to *Loa loa,* 804t
Angiography, coronary, after myocardial
        infarction, 333
    magnetic resonance, in pulmonary
        thromboembolism workup, 221
    pulmonary, in pulmonary thromboembo-
        lism workup, 220
Angiomatosis, bacillary, 157–159, 158t
Angiomyofibroblastoma, vulvar, 1071
Angiomyxoma, vulvar, 1071
Angioplasty, aortoiliac, for abdominal
        aortic occlusive disease, 246
    coronary, recanalization using, for myo-
        cardial infarction, 320–321
    for peripheral arterial occlusive disease,
        337–338
    for renal artery stenosis, 314
Angiostrongyliasis, 540t, 545
Angiotensin II receptor blockers. See also
        specific drugs.
    for hypertension, 309t, 310–311
        during pregnancy, 990
    for primary glomerular disease, 677
Angiotensin-converting enzyme inhibitors.
        See also specific drugs.
    adverse effects of, 293–294, 310
    after myocardial infarction, 330–331
    anaphylaxis and, 726, 728
    for angina, 249
    for congestive heart failure, 293–294,
        294t
    for hypertension, 309t, 310
        during pregnancy, 990, 990t
        in chronic renal failure, 702
        in mitral valve prolapse, 290
        in type 2 diabetes, 563
    for microalbuminuria in diabetes, 564–
        565
    for myocardial infarction, 322
    for primary glomerular disease, 677
Angular cheilitis, 809
Anion gap, in acute poisoning, 1158, 1159t
    reference intervals for, 1207t
Anisakiasis, 540t, 545
Ankle, sports injuries to, 978
Ankle:brachial systolic pressure indices, in
        peripheral arterial occlusive disease
        diagnosis, 337
Ankylosing spondylitis, 958–960
Anorectal abscess, 495
Anorectal fistula, 495
Anorectic agents. See also specific drugs.
    for obesity, 590–591, 591t
Anorexia nervosa, parenteral nutrition for,
        603
Anovulation, dysfunctional uterine
        bleeding with, 1037, 1038
    treatment of, 1042
Antacids, aluminum-containing, for mouth
        disease, 808
    in acute renal failure, 699
    levothyroxine interaction with, 644
    anticonvulsant interactions with, 863t
Antepartum care, 979–985. See also
        Pregnancy.
Anterior cruciate ligament tear, 977
Anterior ischemic optic neuropathy, optic
        neuritis vs., 911
Anterior repositioning devices, for
        temporomandibular disorders, 961,
        963–964

Anthralin, for psoriasis, 772
Antiandrogen therapy, for acne, 759
Antiarrhythmic agents, 262t. See also
    specific drugs and classes of drugs.
    adverse effects of, 262t, 275, 275t
        in chronic therapy, 260
    for atrial flutter, 275, 275t
    for atrial premature beats, 261
    in mitral valve prolapse, 290
    torsades de pointes due to, 279, 279
Antibiotics. See also specific drugs and
    classes of drugs.
    bile acid resin interaction with, 582
    diarrhea associated with, diagnosis of,
        15
    for acne, 757–758
    for cholera, 73, 74t
    for chronic obstructive pulmonary dis-
        ease, during hospitalization, 174–
        175
    for cutaneous bacterial infections, 795t,
        796t
    for cystic fibrosis exacerbations, 178,
        179t
    for infection in neutropenia, 419
    for infective endocarditis, 299–302, 300t
    for Lyme disease, 127, 128t–129t
    for osteomyelitis, 973–974, 974t
    for rhinosinusitis, 235
    for sepsis, 63–64, 63t
        in neonate, 1017–1018, 1017t
    in acute pancreatitis, 516
    resistance to, in otitis media pathogens,
        205
Anticholinergic agents. See also specific
    drugs.
    for irritable bowel syndrome, 491
    for Parkinson's disease, 919, 919t, 921,
        922
    intoxication with, 1097, 1150t, 1163–
        1164
Anticoagulant therapy. See also specific
    drugs.
    after ischemic stroke, 852
    after myocardial infarction, 330
    for atrial fibrillation, 258–259, 258t
    for atrial flutter, 274–275
    for brain tumor patients, 944
    for deep venous thrombosis, 340–342,
        341t, 342t
    for disseminated intravascular coagula-
        tion, 401
Anticonvulsants. See also specific drugs.
    adverse effects of, 861, 863t
    birth defects associated with, 864
    drug interactions with, 861, 863t
    during pregnancy, vitamin K deficiency
        in newborn due to, 592, 593
    for epilepsy, 860–864, 860t, 862t
        combination therapy with, 861
        dosages for, 860–861, 862t
            in infants and children, 869t
        in infants and children, 867–869, 868t,
            869t
        withdrawal of, 864
            in infants and children, 868–869
    for pain, 3
    pharmacokinetic properties of, 861, 861,
        862t
    prophylactic, with intracerebral hemor-
        rhage, 849
Antidepressants. See also specific drugs
    and classes of drugs.
    adverse effects of, 1112–1113, 1113t
    classification of, 1108
    clinical guidelines for use of, 1114–1116,
        1115t

Antidepressants (Continued)
    drug interactions of, 1114
    for anxiety disorders, 1100t, 1101–1102
    for attention-deficit/hyperactivity disor-
        der, 873–874, 873t
    for bulimia nervosa, 1104–1105
    for depression, 1108–1116, 1109t, 1110t,
        1112, 1113t, 1115t
    for insomnia, 35
    for irritable bowel syndrome, 491
    for pain, 3–4
    for panic disorder, 1121–1122, 1121t
    intoxication with, 1201–1203, 1202t
    pharmacology of, basic, 1110–1112,
        1110t, 1112
        clinical relevance of, 1112–1114,
            1113t
        clinical, 1108–1110, 1109t
        potency vs. selectivity of, 1110t, 1111
Antidotes, for acute poisoning, 1149,
    1151t–1155t
Antidromic reciprocating tachycardia, 273,
    274
Antiemetic agents, 7–8, 8t. See also
    specific drugs and classes of drugs.
Antiepileptic drugs. See Anticonvulsants;
    specific drugs.
Antifibrinolytic agents. See also specific
    drugs.
    for disseminated intravascular coagula-
        tion, 402
    for hemophilia, 395
Antifungal agents. See also specific drugs.
    adverse effects of, 807
Antiglaucoma drugs, topical, conjunctivitis
    due to, 69
Anti–glomerular basement membrane
    disease, 679
Anti-HER2 antibody, 1216t
    for breast cancer, 1029
Antihistamines. See also specific drugs.
    antidepressants as, 1110t, 1111–1112
    antifungal interactions with, 196, 198,
        200–201
    for allergic rhinitis, 745, 745t
    for atopic dermatitis, 822
    for contact dermatitis, 830
    for insomnia, 35
    for ordinary urticaria, 835–836
    for pain, 3
    for pruritus, 37
    for rhinosinusitis, 235
    H₂. See Histamine₂ blockers; specific
        drugs.
    intoxication with, 1097, 1164–1165
Antihypertensive agents, 306–311,
    308t–309t. See also specific drugs and
    classes of drugs.
    adjustments in dosage of, with very-low-
        calorie diet, 589
    causes for inadequate response to, 311t
    during pregnancy, for chronic hyperten-
        sion, 990, 990t
    for attention-deficit/hyperactivity disor-
        der, 873t, 874
    for intracerebral hemorrhage, 849
    for primary glomerular disease, 677
Antimonials, for leishmaniasis, 89, 91
Antimotility agents. See also specific
    drugs.
    for diarrhea, 16
Antioxidants, for hyperlipidemia in
    angina, 249
α₂-Antiplasmin deficiency, bleeding in, 392
Antiplatelet therapy, after myocardial
    infarction, 328, 329–330

Antipsychotic drugs. See also specific
    drugs.
    adverse effects of, 1119
    characteristics of, 1117–1118, 1118t
    for schizophrenia, 1117–1120
        guidelines for use of, 1119–1120, 1119t
    intoxication with, 1196–1198, 1197t
    mechanisms of action of, 1118
    SSRI interaction with, 877
Antireflux surgery, 526–527
Antiretroviral therapy, for HIV infection,
    43–50
    alternative dosing schedules in, 46t
    classes of drugs for, 44
    decision to begin, 43–44, 44t
    drug combinations for, 44, 45t, 46t
    failure of, 47–50
    pharmacokinetics in, 45–46
    pharmacologic and pharmacodynamic
        compatibility in, 45, 45t
    regimen adherence in, 46–47
    regimen design for, 44–46, 45t, 46t
    regimen durability in, 44–45
    secondary, 50
    therapeutic monitoring of, 47
    tuberculosis treatment and, 51, 52,
        52t
    viral drug resistance in, 45, 45t, 50
    virus genotyping and phenotyping in,
        50
Antispasmodics. See also specific drugs.
    for irritable bowel syndrome, 491, 492
Antithrombin, for disseminated
    intravascular coagulation, 401
    for thrombosis prevention, 458
Antithymocyte globulin (ATG), for aplastic
    anemia, 352, 353
    for paroxysmal nocturnal hemoglobin-
        uria, 366
Antithyroid antibodies, in chronic
    thyroiditis, 659
    in Hashimoto's thyroiditis, 642
    in subclinical hypothyroidism, 643
Anxiety. See also Anxiety disorder(s); Panic
    disorder.
    adjustment disorder with, 1099
    chronic, dizziness due to, 885t, 891
    medical causes of, 1099, 1099t, 1120,
        1120t
    pathologic, characteristics of, 1098
Anxiety disorder(s), 1098–1102
    diagnosis of, 1099
    generalized, 1099–1100, 1100t
    treatment of, 1100t, 1101–1102
Anxiolytics. See also specific drugs.
    abuse of, 1096
Aorta, acquired diseases of, 243–247
    aneurysms of, 243–245, 338, 338t
    coarctation of, 283
    infection of, 246–247
    occlusive disease of, 246
    surgery on, preoperative evaluation for,
        243
Aortic dissection, 245–246
Aortic insufficiency, with subaortic
    stenosis, 283
Aortic stenosis, 282–283
Aortic valve, bicuspid, aortic stenosis with,
    282
    coarctation of the aorta with, 283
Aorto-bifemoral bypass grafts, for
    abdominal aortic occlusive disease,
    246
Aortoenteric erosion, due to aortic
    infection, 247
Aortoiliac balloon angioplasty, for
    abdominal aortic occlusive disease,
    246

Apgar score, 1007, 1007t
Aphasias, after stroke, 854
Aphonia, 25
Aphthous stomatitis, 812
Aplastic anemia, 351–356
    classification of, 351t
    clinical features of, 351
    laboratory features of, 351–352
    mild/moderate, criteria for, 351
        treatment of, 354
    severe, criteria for, 351
    treatment of, 352–354, *352*
Aplastic crisis, in sickle cell disease, 375
Apnea, in neonate, 1002, 1003
    of prematurity, 1014
    sleep. See also *Obstructive sleep-disor-
        dered breathing.*
        defined, 180
        insomnia due to, 33, 34
Appendicitis, during pregnancy, 983
Appetite suppressants. See also specific
        drugs.
    for obesity, 590–591, 591t
Apraclonidine, for glaucoma, 913
Apraxias, after stroke, 855
Aprobarbital, intoxication with, 1165
Aqueous shunts, for glaucoma, 915
Ara-C. See *Cytarabine (ara-C).*
Arboviruses, encephalitis due to, 895–896
Arginine butyrate, fetal globin gene
        activation by, for thalassemia, 373
Arginine vasopressin. See *Vasopressin.*
Arprinocid, for toxoplasmosis, 154
Arrhythmias. See also specific
        arrhythmias.
    after myocardial infarction, 322–324,
        324t
    fetal, maternal antiarrhythmic treat-
        ment for, 984
    in antidepressant intoxication, 1201–
        1202
        treatment of, 1202–1203
    in mitral valve prolapse, 290
    in neuroleptic intoxication, 1197
Arrhythmogenic right ventricular
        dysplasia, 279
Arsenic, keratosis due to, 792
    urine, reference intervals for, 1212t
Arsenic trioxide, for acute promyelocytic
        leukemia, 420, 425
Artemether, for malaria, 99t
Artemether-benflumetol, for malaria, 96
Artemisinin, for malaria, 97t
Arterial lacerations, with central catheter
        placement, 605
Arterial occlusive disease. See also
        Atherosclerosis.
    peripheral, acute, 338
        chronic, 336–338, 336t, 337t
Arterial switch operation, for transposition
        of the great arteries, 285
Arterial thrombosis, in polycythemia vera,
        445
Arteriovenous hemofiltration, continuous,
        700, 700t
Arteritis, giant cell, 339, 970–971
    occlusive arterial disease due to, 339
Artesunate, for malaria, 97t, 99t
Arthritis, degenerative, 967–970
    diagnosis of, 968
    prevention of, 969
    treatment of, 968–970
    gouty. See *Gout.*
    in Lyme disease, 125t, 126
        treatment of, 127, 129t, 130
    rheumatoid. See *Rheumatoid arthritis.*

Arthroplasty. See *Joint replacement.*
Arytenoid adduction surgery, for vocal fold
        paralysis, 27
5-ASA (mesalamine), for inflammatory
        bowel disease, 483–484
Ascariasis, 540t, 544
Ascites, in cirrhosis, 469–470
Ascomycin macrolactam, for atopic
        dermatitis, 824
Ascorbic acid (vitamin C), blood, reference
        intervals for, 1207t
    with deferoxamine therapy, 372
    with iron supplements, 357
ASHAP regimen, for aggressive
        lymphoma, 436t, 437
Asherman's syndrome, 1042
Asparaginase, for acute lymphoblastic
        leukemia in children, 423
    for acute nonlymphocytic leukemia in
        children, 424
Aspartate aminotransferase, serum,
        reference intervals for, 1207t
Aspiration (event), lung abscess due to, 203
    of foreign body, cough due to, 23
    of meconium, 1004
    with hydrocarbon ingestion, 1179–1180
    with obstetric anesthesia, 995, 998, 999
Aspiration (procedure), gastric, for acute
        poisoning, 1148
    in breast cancer diagnosis, 1026
    in thyroid nodule evaluation, 649–650
Aspirin. See also *Salicylates.*
    after myocardial infarction, 329
    anticonvulsant interactions with, 863t
    for bursitis or tendinitis, 965
    for clotting abnormalities in type 2 diabe-
        tes, 563
    for dysmenorrhea, 1044t
    for juvenile rheumatoid arthritis, 954,
        955t, 956
    for membranous glomerulopathy, 679
    for mountain sickness, 1128
    for myocardial infarction, 319
    for niacin-induced flushing, 583
    for non–Q wave myocardial infarction,
        328
    for pain in pericarditis, 333
    for painful neuropathy, 932
    for peripheral arterial occlusive disease,
        337
    for pre-eclampsia prevention, 991
    for stroke prevention, in atrial fibrilla-
        tion, 258, 258t, 850
        secondary, 855
    for thrombotic thrombocytopenic pur-
        pura, 404
    for venous thrombosis prophylaxis after
        ischemic stroke, 852
    for viral respiratory infection, 214
    in analgesic combinations, 2
        for migraine, 881
    reference intervals for, 1210t
    with very-low-calorie diet, 588
Astemizole, antidepressant interactions
        with, 1114
    antifungal interactions with, 196, 200–
        201, 807
    for allergic rhinitis, 745, 745t
    for ordinary urticaria, 835
    for pruritus, 37
    intoxication with, 1164, 1165
Asthma, chronic obstructive pulmonary
        disease and, 171, *171*
    cough variant, 23–24, 736
    definition of, 735–736
    in adolescents and adults, 729–735

Asthma *(Continued)*
    Chlamydia pneumoniae bronchitis
        and, 208
    differential diagnosis of, 730
    home monitoring and treatment of,
        734, 735
    pathophysiology of, 730
    precipitating or aggravating factors
        for, 730–731
    severity classification for, 730, 730t
    treatment of, 731–735, 732t
        maintenance drugs in, 731–734,
            732t
        reliever drugs in, 734
    in children, 735–743
    atopy and, 736, 740
    clinical features of, 736–737
    diagnosis of, 737–738
    differential diagnosis of, 737
    epidemiology of, 736
    home monitoring in, 738, 741–742
    indications for specialist referral in,
        742–743
    pathophysiology of, 736
    precipitating factors for, 737
    severity classification for, 741
        management keyed to, 742
    treatment of, 738–741
        exacerbation management in, 741
        long-term, 741–742
        maintenance drugs in, 739–740
        partnership in, 740–741
        reliever drugs in, 740
Astrocytoma, 941, 942t, 943
Asystole. See also *Sudden cardiac death.*
    in accidental hypothermia, 1131
    treatment of, 255
Ataxia, cerebellar, in chickenpox, 70
Atelectasis, 170–171, 170t
    after head injury, 935
Atenolol, after myocardial infarction, 330
    during pregnancy, intrauterine growth
        restriction and, 990
    for anxiety disorders, 1102
    for atrial fibrillation, 257
    for atrial premature beats, 261
    for hypertension, 308t
    for hyperthyroidism, 647
    for myocardial infarction, 321–322
    for neurocardiogenic syncope in mitral
        valve prolapse, 291
    for ventricular premature beats, 263
    intoxication with, 1166, 1167t
    relative antiarrhythmic efficacy of, 262t
ATG (antithymocyte globulin), for aplastic
        anemia, 352, 353
    for paroxysmal nocturnal hemoglobin-
        uria, 366
Atheroembolism, with peripheral arterial
        aneurysm, 339
Atherosclerosis. See also *Coronary artery
        disease; Peripheral arterial disease.*
    abdominal aortic occlusive disease due
        to, 246
    angina and, 247–248
    renovascular hypertension due to, 313
    risk factors for, diabetes' interaction
        with, 553–554
        diabetes treatment directed at, 562–
            563, 562t
    in insulin resistance syndrome, 551–
        552
Atony, uterine, postpartum hemorrhage
        due to, 1000
Atopic dermatitis, 821–824. See also *Atopy.*
    diagnostic criteria for, 821t

Atopic dermatitis (Continued)
  differential diagnosis of, 821t
  treatment of, experimental, 824
    medical, 822–824, 823t
    nonmedical, 821
Atopy. See also Atopic dermatitis.
  asthma and, 736, 740
  family history and, 743
Atorvastatin, for hyperlipidemia, 581
    after myocardial infarction, 332
    in angina, 249
    in type 2 diabetes, 563
Atovaquone, for microsporidiosis, 539t, 543
  for Pneumocystis carinii pneumonia in
      HIV infection, 51
    prophylactic, 51
  for toxoplasmosis, 153–154
    in HIV infection, 156
Atovaquone-proquanil, for malaria, 96, 97t
Atrial fibrillation, 256–260
  after myocardial infarction, 323, 324t
  cardioversion in, 259–260, 259t
  conditions associated with, 257t
  manifestations of, 257, 257t
  new approaches to, 260
  preexcited, 273, 273, 274
  rate control in, 257–258, 258t
  stroke prevention in, 258–259, 258t, 850
Atrial flutter, 271, 274–276
  after myocardial infarction, 323, 324t
Atrial premature beats, 261
Atrial septal defect, 281
Atrial septostomy, balloon, for
      transposition of the great arteries, 285
Atrial switch operation, for transposition
      of the great arteries, 285
Atrial tachycardia, 271, 274–276
  after myocardial infarction, 324t
  focal, atrial fibrillation and, 260
  multifocal, 276
Atrioventricular block. See also Heart
      block.
  after myocardial infarction, 323, 324t
  causes of, 265
  clinical manifestations of, 266–267
  electrocardiographic diagnosis of, 265–
      266, 267
  natural history of, 267
  pacemaker therapy for, 268, 268t
Atrioventricular canal defect, 282
Atrioventricular dissociation, after
      myocardial infarction, 323, 324t
Atrioventricular junction, structure and
      function of, 264–265
Atrioventricular nodal artery, 264
Atrioventricular nodal reentry tachycardia,
      269, 271–272, 271, 272
Atrioventricular node, structure and
      function of, 264
Atrioventricular reentry tachycardia, 271,
      272, 273, 274
Atrioventricular septal defect, 282
Atropine, as antidote, 1151t
  for beta blocker intoxication, 1168
  for bradycardia after myocardial in-
      farction, 322
  for carbamate poisoning, 1151t, 1194
  for cardiac arrest, 255
  for digitalis intoxication, 1175
  for Meniere's disease, 893
  for mushroom poisoning, 79
  for organophosphate poisoning, 1151t,
      1194
  intoxication with, 1164
Atropine-diphenoxylate, for diarrhea in
      food-borne illness, 76

Atropine-diphenoxylate (Continued)
  for radiation enteritis, 511
Attention-deficit/hyperactivity disorder,
      871–874
  diagnosis of, 871–872
    Tourette's syndrome and, 875, 877
  treatment of, 872–874, 873t
Aura, in migraine, 879
    stroke risk and, 879–880
Auranofin, for rheumatoid arthritis, 946t,
      949, 951
Aurothioglucose, for rheumatoid arthritis,
      949
Aurothiomalate, for rheumatoid arthritis,
      946t, 949
Auspitz sign, in psoriasis, 771
Autoantibodies. See also Autoimmune
      entries.
  antithyroid, in chronic thyroiditis, 659
    in Hashimoto's thyroiditis, 642
    in subclinical thyroiditis, 643
  in ordinary urticaria, 834
Autoimmune connective tissue disorders,
      774–778. See also specific disorders.
  silicone gel breast implants and, 1024
Autoimmune disease. See also specific
      disorders.
  bullous, 826–830, 826t
  due to penicillamine, 949
Autoimmune hemolytic anemia, 358–363
  classification of, 359, 359t
  clinical diagnosis of, 359–360
  cold antibody, 359t
    clinical diagnosis of, 360
    laboratory diagnosis of, 361
    treatment of, 362–363
  drug-induced, 359, 360
    clinical diagnosis of, 360
    laboratory diagnosis of, 361
    treatment of, 363
  laboratory diagnosis of, 360–361
  treatment of, 361–363
  warm antibody, 359t
    clinical diagnosis of, 359–360
    laboratory diagnosis of, 361
    treatment of, 361–362
Autoimmune hepatitis, 469. See also
      Cirrhosis.
Autoimmune pericarditis, postinfarction,
      328
Autoimmune thrombocytopenia, 400
Autoinflation of middle ear, for otitis
      media, 206
Autolytic débridement, for pressure ulcers,
      820
Autonomic nervous system, dysfunction of,
      in mitral valve prolapse, 291
    in tetanus, 136
  toxins' effects on, 1150t
Autonomic neuropathy, 931–932
  in diabetes, 565–566
Autosplenectomy, in sickle cell disease, 380
Avascular necrosis of femoral head, in
      sickle cell disease, 379–380
AVPU mnemonic, 1145
Axillofemoral bypass grafts, for abdominal
      aortic occlusive disease, 246
Axonal degeneration, peripheral
      neuropathies with, 925–928
Axonal injury, acute, with head injury, 933
Axonal neuropathy, acute motor, 929
5-Azacitidine, fetal globin gene activation
      by, for thalassemia, 373
Azapropazone, adverse effects of, 969
Azatadine, for allergic rhinitis, 745t
Azathioprine, allopurinol interaction with,
      578, 950

Azathioprine (Continued)
  for anti–glomerular basement membrane
      disease, 679
  for autoimmune hepatitis, 469
  for bullous pemphigoid, 827–828
  for cicatricial pemphigoid, 813
  for cutaneous vasculitis, 780
  for immune thrombocytopenic purpura,
      400
  for inflammatory bowel disease, 485
  for juvenile rheumatoid arthritis, 955t,
      957
  for lupus erythematosus, 776
  for membranous glomerulopathy, 678
  for myasthenia gravis, 906, 907t
    during pregnancy, 908
  for pauci-immune glomerulonephritis,
      680
  for pemphigus, 827
  for primary glomerular disease, 676
  for rheumatoid arthritis, 946t, 950, 951
  for sarcoidosis, 225–226
  for warm antibody autoimmune hemo-
      lytic anemia, 362
Azelaic acid, for acne, 758
  for hyperpigmentation, 839
Azelastine, for allergic rhinitis, 745, 745t
Azithromycin, for atopic dermatitis, 823
  for bacillary angiomatosis, 158t
  for bacterial pneumonia, 212, 212t
  for cat-scratch disease, 158t
  for chancroid, 717
  for chlamydial infection, 719, 719t, 1057,
      1057t
    for conjunctivitis, 68
    for urethritis in men, 661
  for cryptosporidiosis, 539t, 542
  for donovanosis, 722
  for endocarditis prophylaxis, 301t, 303
  for epididymitis, 674
  for legionellosis, 217–218, 217t
  for Lyme disease, 128t
  for Mycobacterium avium complex infec-
      tion, 241
    in HIV infection, 54
  for mycoplasmal pneumonia, 216
  for nongonococcal urethritis, 721
  for otitis media, 205, 205t
  for pertussis, 139
  for psittacosis, 117–118
  for streptococcal pharyngitis, 237, 238t
  for toxoplasmosis in HIV infection, 156
  for typhoid fever, 163, 163t
  safety of, during pregnancy, 1057
AZT. See Zidovudine (AZT, ZDV).
Aztreonam, for acute pyelonephritis, 682t
  for bacterial meningitis, 105t
  for cystic fibrosis exacerbations, 179t
  for sepsis, 63t
  for typhoid fever, 163, 163t

B lymphocytes, reference intervals for,
      1213t
Babesiosis, Lyme disease with, 127, 130
  transmission of, by blood components,
      461
Bacillary angiomatosis, 157–159, 158t
Bacillary peliosis, 158, 158t
Bacille Calmette-Guérin (BCG), 242
  for travelers, 148
  intravesical therapy with, for bladder
      cancer, 708–709
Bacillus cereus infection, food-borne, 75t,
      76

Bacitracin, for bacterial conjunctivitis, 67
for erythema multiforme, 813
Back pain, 39–40
in osteoporosis, 596–597
Baclofen, for hiccup, 14–15, 14t
for tetanus, 136
for trigeminal neuralgia, 909
in multiple sclerosis, for pain, 902
for spasticity, 901, 902
Bacteremia, 61–64, 62t
Bacterial endocarditis. See *Infective endocarditis.*
Bacterial overgrowth, after gastrectomy, 513
bile salt deficiency due to, 509–510
in diabetes, 565
treatment of, 510
with jejunal diverticula, 480
Bacterial vaginosis, 1054, 1054t
Bacteriuria, asymptomatic, in elderly men, 661, 662
in elderly women, 666
in pregnancy, 664t, 666
catheter-associated, in men, 662
in women, 665
threshold for diagnosis of, 663
Bag-and-mask ventilation, in neonatal resuscitation, 1004–1005
Baker's cyst, 965
BAL. See *Dimercaprol (BAL).*
Balantidium coli infection, 539t, 543
Balloon angioplasty, aortoiliac, for abdominal aortic occlusive disease, 246
coronary, recanalization using, for myocardial infarction, 320–321
Balloon atrial septostomy, for transposition of the great arteries, 285
Balloon catheters, urethral dilation using, for anterior urethral stricture, 711
Balloon counterpulsation, intra-aortic, for cardiogenic shock, 326
for ventricular septal rupture, 327
Balloon microcompression, for trigeminal neuralgia, 910
Balloon pericardiotomy, for pericarditis, 335
Barbiturates. See also specific drugs.
for intracranial hypertension after head injury in children, 938
for migraine, 881
insomnia due to chronic use of, 32
intoxication with, 1096, 1156t, 1165–1166
Bariatric surgery, for obstructive sleep-disordered breathing, 185
Barium studies, in colorectal cancer screening, 534, 535t
in dysphagia evaluation, 477
Barrett's esophagus, 524
Bartholin's duct abscess, 1071
Bartholin's duct cyst, 1071
Bartholin's gland carcinoma, 1074
Bartonella henselae infection, 157–159, 158t
meningitis due to, 895
Basal cell carcinoma, 763–765
of mouth, 817
of nail, 783
of vulva, 1074
Base excess, arterial blood, reference intervals for, 1207t
BCG (bacille Calmette-Guérin), 242
for travelers, 148
intravesical therapy with, for bladder cancer, 708–709

BCNU (carmustine), for lupus erythematosus, 776
for mycosis fungoides, 768–769
bcr-abl gene, 426
BEACOPP regimen, for Hodgkin's disease, 407, 407t
BEAM regimen, with stem cell rescue, for indolent B cell lymphoma, 435
Beclomethasone dipropionate, for allergic rhinitis, 747t
for asthma, 732t
in children, 742
Bee sting allergy, 753–755, 754t, 755t
Beef house syndrome, 476
Beger's procedure, for chronic pancreatitis, 523
Behavioral problems, after head injury, 935
in children, 940
in Alzheimer's disease, 846–847
Behavioral therapy. See also *Cognitive-behavioral therapy.*
for insomnia, 33–34, 33t, 34t
for nocturnal enuresis, 670
for obesity, 590
for stress incontinence, 673
for temporomandibular disorders, 963
for urgency incontinence, 672
Behçet's syndrome, 812
Belching, 12
Bell's palsy. See *Facial paralysis, acute.*
Benazepril, for congestive heart failure, 294t
for hypertension, 309t
Benflumetol-artemether, for malaria, 96
Bentiromide test, reference intervals for, 1213t
Benzene, 1179
Benznidazole, for Chagas' disease, 102
Benzodiazepines. See also specific drugs.
for anxiety disorders, 1100t, 1101, 1102
for insomnia, 34
for panic disorder, 1121t, 1122
intoxication with, 1096, 1166
withdrawal from, 1096
insomnia due to, 32
Benzonatate, for cough, 24
Benzophenone derivatives, in sunscreens, 838
Benzoyl peroxide, for acne, 757, 758
Benztropine, abuse of, 1097
for dystonia due to haloperidol therapy, 876
for Parkinson's disease, 919t, 922
Bepridil, intoxication with, 1168
Berliner's physical sign, in exanthem subitum, 803
Beta agonists. See also specific drugs.
for asthma, 733, 734
in children, 740
for chronic obstructive pulmonary disease, 172, 173, *173*
for hyperkalemia in acute renal failure, 697, 697t
Beta blockers. See also specific drugs.
adverse effects of, 275t
after myocardial infarction, 330
anaphylaxis management and, 726, 728, 754
as antiarrhythmic agents, 262t
for angina, 248–249
for anxiety disorders, 1100t, 1102
for atrial fibrillation, 257, 258t
for congestive heart failure, 294t, 295
for glaucoma, 912–913
for hypertension, 307, 308t

Beta blockers *(Continued)*
during pregnancy, 990, 990t
in type 2 diabetes, 563
for hyperthyroidism, 647
for hypertrophic cardiomyopathy, 349
for myocardial infarction, 321–322
for pheochromocytoma, 655
for portal hypertension, 473
for ventricular premature beats, 263, 264
for vertigo due to migraine, 889
intoxication with, 1166–1168, 1167t
masking of hypoglycemia symptoms by, 248, 250
Beta globulin, serum, reference intervals for, 1209t
Beta-carotene, colorectal cancer and, 533
for protoporphyria, 453
serum, reference intervals for, 1208t, 1213t
Betamethasone, for atopic dermatitis, 822
to accelerate fetal lung maturity, 984
Betaxolol, for glaucoma, 913
for hypertension, 308t
intoxication with, 1167t
Bethanechol, for neurogenic bladder in diabetes, 565
Bezafibrate, for hyperlipidemia, 583
Bicarbonate, as antidote, 1150, 1155t
for antidepressant intoxication, 1202–1203
for salicylate intoxication, 1199–1200, 1199t
for acidosis, in acute renal failure, 698
in chronic renal failure, 704
for cardiac arrest, *254*
for cocaine intoxication, 1173
for cyanide intoxication, 1174
for diabetic ketoacidosis, 574
in children, 567
for hyperkalemia in acute renal failure, 697t
for neuroleptic intoxication, 1197
in neonatal resuscitation, 1006
plasma, reference intervals for, 1207t
Bicipital tendinitis, 965
Bicuspid aortic valve, aortic stenosis with, 282
coarctation of the aorta with, 283
Bifascicular block, 266. See also *Heart block.*
after myocardial infarction, 324t
Bile acid(s), serum, reference intervals for, 1208t
Bile acid sequestrants. See also specific drugs.
for hyperlipidemia, 582, 584
Bile salts, for cholelithiasis, 464
maldigestion due to deficiency of, 509–510
Bilevel positive airway pressure, nasal, for obstructive sleep-disordered breathing, 183
Bilharziasis. See *Schistosomiasis.*
Biliary cirrhosis, focal, in cystic fibrosis, 180
primary, 468. See also *Cirrhosis.*
Biliary colic, 463
Biliary drainage, bile salt deficiency due to, 509
Biliary scintigraphy, for cystic duct obstruction detection, 464
Bilirubin. See also *Jaundice.*
reference intervals for, in serum, 1208t
in urine, 1211t
removal of, in Rh isoimmunization, 387, 387t

Bilirubin oxidase, for Rh isoimmunization, 388t
Biofeedback training, for constipation, 20
Biophysical profile testing, during pregnancy, 982
Biperiden, for early dyskinesia diagnosis, 135
  for Parkinson's disease, 919t
Bipolar diathermy, for hemorrhoids, 493
Bipolar disorder, 1116–1117
  sleep in, 33
Birth control pills. See *Contraceptives, oral.*
Bisacodyl, for constipation, 19
Bismuth subsalicylate, for diarrhea, 16, 17t
  in travelers, 17, 76, 150
  for *Helicobacter pylori* infection, 501t
  for salmonellosis, 160
Bisoprolol, for congestive heart failure, 295
  for hypertension, 308t
Bisphosphonates. See also specific drugs.
  for Paget's disease of bone, 598–599, 598t
Bithionol, for liver flukes, 540t, 546
B-K mole. See *Dysplastic nevus.*
Black hairy tongue, 815
Bladder, cancer of, 708–709
  denervation of, for incontinence, 672–673
  dysfunction of, in multiple sclerosis, 902
    urinary incontinence with, 671–673
  functional capacity of, calculation of, 669
  neurogenic, antidepressants for use with, 1115t
    in diabetes, 565
  non-neurogenic, in children, 669–670
  reconstruction of, for incontinence, 673
  trauma to, 684
Bladder instability, in girls, urinary tract infections and, 668
  urinary incontinence with, 671–672
Blalock-Taussig shunt, for hypoplastic left heart syndrome, 287
  for tetralogy of Fallot, 285
  for tricuspid atresia, 286
Blastocystis hominis infection, 539t, 543
Blastomycosis, 199–201, 200t
Bleaching medications, for hyperpigmentation, 839–840
  in vitiligo treatment, 841
Bleeding. See *Hemorrhage.*
Bleeding time, reference intervals for, 1207t
Bleomycin, for aggressive lymphoma, 436t
  for Hodgkin's disease, 407t
    side effects of, 408
  for penile carcinoma, 710
  for Sézary's syndrome, 769
  for warts, 786
Blind loop syndrome, after gastrectomy, 513
Bloating, abdominal, 12
Blood, drug testing in, 1094
  fecal occult, in colorectal cancer screening, 534, 535t
  fetal, sampling of, 981, 984
  whole, for transfusion, 454
Blood components, bacterial contamination of, 461
  irradiation of, for prevention of graft-versus-host disease, 457, 460
  recent administration of, live-virus vaccine administration and, 145
  therapeutic use of, 453–458. See also *Transfusion(s).*

Blood pressure. See also *Hypertension; Hypotension.*
  age-specific reference values for, 1145t
  classification of, 303t
  goals for, in diabetes, 554, 554t
  home monitoring of, 304
  management of, after head injury in children, 938
    in hemorrhagic stroke, 849
    in ischemic stroke, 852
    in severe head injury, 934
  measurement of, 303, 989
    during pregnancy, 989
  recommendations for follow-up based on, 304t
Blue nevus, 789
Blue toe syndrome, 246
Body mass index, obesity classification using, 585–587, 586, 587, 588t, 589t
Body packers, 1149, 1172, 1173
Body surface area, age-specific reference values for, 1145t
  nomogram for, 1217
Boil, 795
Bone cement, antibacterial-loaded, for osteomyelitis, 974
Bone densitometry, in osteoporosis diagnosis, 594
Bone marrow transplantation, for acute lymphoblastic leukemia in adults, 418–419
  for acute myelogenous leukemia, 416, 417–418
  for acute nonlymphocytic leukemia in children, 424, 425
  for aplastic anemia, 352–353
  for breast cancer, 1029
  for chronic myelogenous leukemia, 429
  for Fanconi's anemia, 355
  for Sézary's syndrome, 770
  for sickle cell disease, 381
  for thalassemia, 373
Bone pain, in multiple myeloma, 441
Bordetella pertussis. See *Pertussis.*
Bordet-Gengou media, for *Bordetella* culture, 138
Boric acid gelatin capsules, for vulvovaginal candidiasis, 1053
Borrelia burgdorferi. See *Lyme disease.*
Borrelia species, laboratory identification of, 124
  relapsing fever due to, 123–125
Borrelial lymphocytoma, 125t, 126, 128t
Botfly, human, 804t, 805
Bottle-feeding, for infants, 1019–1022, 1021t
Botulinum toxin injection, for anal fissure, 494
  for esophageal dysphagia, 478
  for oropharyngeal dysphagia, 478
  for spasmodic dysphonia, 28
  for spasticity after stroke, 856
Botulism, 75t, 78
Bowel incontinence, after stroke, 855
Bowenoid papulosis, 792–793
BRAC1 gene, breast cancer and, 1024
Bradycardia, after myocardial infarction, 322–323, 324t
Brain tumors, 940–944. See also specific tumors.
  classification of, 940–941
  diagnosis of, 942
  extra-axial, 940–941
  infiltrative, 941
  intra-axial, 941
  metastatic, 941

Brain tumors *(Continued)*
  in small cell lung cancer, 191
  radiation therapy for, 943
  surgery for, 942
  treatment of, 942–944
Brandt-Daroff treatment, for benign paroxysmal positional vertigo, 887, 889
Breast, augmented, disorders of, 1024
  diseases of, 1022–1029
    benign, 1022–1024
    malignant, 1024–1029. See also *Breast cancer.*
Breast abscess, 1023–1024
Breast cancer, 1024–1029
  after Hodgkin's disease treatment, 409, 412–413
  diagnosis of, 1025–1026
  early detection of, 1024–1025
  follow-up care in, 1029
  histopathologic types of, 1026
  hormone replacement therapy and, 1048, 1052
  male, 1026–1027
  oral contraceptives and, 1085
  osteoporosis management in presence of, 596
  prognosis in, 1029
  recurrence of, 1029
  risk factors for, 1024
  screening for, 1024–1025
  special clinical forms of, 1026–1027
  staging of, 1026
  treatment of, 1027–1029, 1028t
Breast implants, breast disorders with, 1024
Breast milk. See also *Breast-feeding.*
  for high-risk neonate, 1012
  necrotizing enterocolitis and, 1016
Breast self-examination, 1025
Breast-feeding, 1018–1019. See also *Breast milk; Lactation.*
  contraception during, 1000, 1086t, 1089
  HIV transmission by, 41
  immunizations during, 148–149
  initiation of, 1000, 1018
  nutritional supplements with, 1022
  vitamin K deficiency due to, 592, 593
Breath-holding spells, seizure vs., 867
Bretylium, for cardiac arrest, 253, 254
  for ventricular arrhythmias in accidental hypothermia, 1132
Brevitoxic shellfish poisoning, 79, 80t
Brewers' yeast, with pyrimethamine therapy for toxoplasmosis, 152
Brimonidine tartrate, for glaucoma, 913
Brinzolamide, 1214t
  for glaucoma, 913
Bristle worms, 1142
British antilewisite. See *Dimercaprol (BAL).*
Brockenbrough's sign, in hypertrophic cardiomyopathy, 348
Bromides, serum, reference intervals for, 1212t
Bromocriptine, for acromegaly, 616–617
  for cocaine abuse, 1094
  for Cushing's syndrome, 623
  for hyperprolactinemia, 641, 1041
  for monoamine oxidase inhibitor overdose, 1191
  for Parkinson's disease, 919t
Brompheniramine, for allergic rhinitis, 745t
  intoxication with, 1164
Bronchitis, acute, 207–208

Bronchitis *(Continued)*
  chronic, 171, *171.* See also *Chronic ob-
      structive pulmonary disease.*
    acute exacerbation of, 208–209
    in smoker, 24
Bronchodilators. See also specific drugs
    and classes of drugs.
  for acute bronchitis, 208
  for chronic obstructive pulmonary dis-
      ease, 172–173, *173*
  for silicosis, 229
Bronchogenic carcinoma. See *Lung cancer.*
Bronchopulmonary dysplasia, 1014
Bronchoscopy, for atelectasis, 171
Brook formula, modified, for burn patient
    resuscitation, 1124, 1124t
Brucellosis, 64–67, 65t
Bubble hair deformity, 763
Buboes, in plague, 115
Bucillamine, for cystinuria, 715
Budesonide, for allergic rhinitis, 747t
  for asthma, 732t
    in children, 742
  for chronic obstructive pulmonary dis-
      ease, 173
  for inflammatory bowel disease, 484
Buffy coat method, quantitative, in
    malaria diagnosis, 96
Bulimia nervosa, 1102–1105, 1103t
Bullous dermatosis, linear IgA, 829–830
Bullous disease, autoimmune, 826–830,
    826t. See also specific diseases.
Bullous disease of childhood, chronic, 829
Bullous pemphigoid, 813, 827–828
Bullous systemic lupus erythematosus,
    830
Bumetanide, for congestive heart failure,
    294t
  for hypertension, 308t
  for volume overload in acute renal fail-
      ure, 697
Bundle branch block. See also *Heart block.*
  after myocardial infarction, 324t
  electrocardiographic diagnosis of, 266
  natural history of, 267
Bundle branch reentrant ventricular
    tachycardia, 278
Bundle of His, structure and function of,
    264–265
Bupivacaine, cardiac toxicity of, obstetric
    use and, 995
  for cesarean delivery, in epidural anes-
      thesia, 997
  in spinal anesthesia, 997
  for labor, in epidural analgesia, 996
  in intrathecal analgesia, 997
  for tetanus, 136
Buprenorphine, for pain, 4t
Bupropion, for attention-deficit/hyper-
      activity disorder, 873–874, 873t
  for chronic fatigue syndrome, 112
  for depression, 1109t
  intoxication by, 1202t
  pharmacodynamic effects of, 1110t
  reference intervals for, 1210t
Burkholderia cepacia infection, in cystic
    fibrosis, 178
Burkitt's lymphoma, 438. See also
    Lymphoma.
Burns, 1123–1127
  chemical, 1126, 1171–1172
  criteria for transfer in, 1123, 1124t
  initial evaluation in, 1123–1124, 1124t
  natural history of, 1123
  oral, 816
  reconstruction after, 1127

Burns *(Continued)*
  rehabilitation after, 1126, 1127t
  treatment of, 1124–1127
    critical care in, 1125–1126
    fluid resuscitation in, 1124, 1124t
    outpatient, 1125
    scar management in, 1126–1127
    wound management in, 1124–1125
Burow's solution, for atopic dermatitis, 823
Bursitis, 964–966
Buspirone, for anxiety disorders, 1100t,
    1102
  for depression, 1116
Busulfan, for chronic myelogenous
    leukemia, 427
  for multiple myeloma, 442
Butabarbital, intoxication with, 1165
Butalbital, in analgesic combinations, 2
  intoxication with, 1165
Butenafine, for tinea infection, 807
Butorphanol, contraindicated for chronic
    pain, 5

C1 esterase inhibitor deficiency, 836–837
  angioedema due to, 834–835
C3 (complement component), serum, in
    acute renal failure diagnosis, 696
  reference intervals for, 1213t
C4 (complement component), serum,
    reference intervals for, 1213t
Cabergoline, for acromegaly, 617
  for hyperprolactinemia, 641
Cachexia, cardiac, parenteral nutrition for,
    604
Caffeine, anorectic agent interactions with,
    591
  fibrocystic disease of breast and, 1023
  in analgesic combinations, 2
  for migraine, 881
  panic attacks due to, 1120
  reference intervals for, 1210t
Calabar swellings, 804t
Calcifediol, for secondary hyperparathy-
    roidism, 631
Calcification, ectopic, in acute renal
    failure, 698
  pancreatic, in chronic pancreatitis, 519
Calcinosis universalis, in childhood
    dermatomyositis, 777
Calcipotriene, for psoriasis, 771
Calcitonin, adverse effects of, 600
  for hypercalcemic crisis, 630
  for osteoporosis, 595–596
  for Paget's disease of bone, 598t, 599–
      600
Calcitriol, for hypoparathyroidism, 633
  for metabolic bone disease in chronic
      renal failure, 704
  for osteoporosis, 596
    prophylactic, in primary biliary cirrho-
        sis, 468
  for secondary hyperparathyroidism, 631–
      632
Calcium. See also *Hypercalcemia;*
    Hypocalcemia.
  blood pressure and, 305
  colorectal cancer and, 533
  for hypocalcemia in acute renal failure,
      698
  for osteopenia in thalassemia patient
      with iron overload, 372
  for osteoporosis, 595
  for osteoporosis prevention, 1052
    in inflammatory bowel disease, 487

Calcium *(Continued)*
  for pre-eclampsia prevention, 991, 992
  for premenstrual syndrome, 1046
  for secondary hyperparathyroidism, 631
  in acute renal failure, 698
  in intravenous solutions for infants and
      children, 608t
  in juvenile rheumatoid arthritis, 958
  in medical management of primary
      hyperparathyroidism, 630
  in parenteral nutrition solutions, 605t
  in short-bowel syndrome, 511
  levothyroxine interaction with, 644
  reference intervals for, in serum, 1208t
    in urine, 1211t
  supplement selection, 633
  with gonadotropin-releasing hormone
      agonists, 1032
Calcium acetate, for hyperphosphatemia in
    acute renal failure, 698
Calcium blockers. See *Calcium channel
    blockers;* specific drugs.
Calcium carbonate, as oral supplement,
    633
  for hyperphosphatemia in acute renal
      failure, 698
  for osteoporosis prevention in primary
      biliary cirrhosis, 468
  for premenstrual syndrome, 1046
Calcium channel blockers. See also specific
    drugs.
  adverse effects of, 310
  after myocardial infarction, 331
  antifungal interactions with, 807
  as antiarrhythmic agents, 262t
  contraindications to, 277
  for angina, 249
  for atrial fibrillation, 257, 258t
  for hypertension, 308t, 309–310
    during pregnancy, 990, 990t
    in type 2 diabetes, 563
  for hypertrophic cardiomyopathy, 349
  for non–Q wave myocardial infarction,
      328
  for primary glomerular disease, 677
  intoxication with, 1168–1169
Calcium chloride, as antidote, 1151t
  as oral supplement, 633
  for calcium channel blocker intoxication,
      1151t, 1169
  for hyperkalemia in acute renal failure,
      697
  for magnesium toxicity in pre-eclampsia,
      994
Calcium citrate, as oral supplement, 633
  for hyperphosphatemia in chronic renal
      failure, 704t
Calcium disodium edetate, for lead
    poisoning, 1185–1187, 1186t
Calcium glubionate, as oral supplement,
    633
Calcium gluconate, as antidote, 1151t
  as oral supplement, 633
  for calcium channel blocker intoxication,
      1151t, 1169
  for ciguatera poisoning, 1143
  for hyperkalemia in acute renal failure,
      697, 697t
  for hypocalcemia, in acute renal failure,
      698
    in ethylene glycol intoxication, 1178
    in neonate, 1012
  for hypoparathyroidism, 633
  for magnesium toxicity in pre-eclampsia,
      994
  for salicylate intoxication, 1200

Calcium lactate, as oral supplement, 633
Calcium-containing phosphate binders, in
chronic renal failure, 704, 704t
Calculus, urinary tract, 712–715
in primary hyperparathyroidism, 629
Calf vein thrombosis, 344, *344*. See also
Venous thrombosis.
Calfactant, 1214t
California encephalitis virus, 896
Caloric requirements, in parenteral
nutrition, 601
for high-risk neonate, 1012
Calorie-to-nitrogen ratio, in parenteral
nutrition, 601–602
Calymmatobacterium granulomatis
infection, 721–722
Campylobacter infection, food-borne, 75t,
77t, 78
Canalith repositioning maneuver, 887, *888*
Cancer. See also specific sites and types.
bladder, 708–709
breast. See *Breast cancer.*
cervical, 1066–1069, 1067t
in HIV infection, 55
lung. See *Lung cancer.*
metastatic. See *Metastasis(es).*
mouth, 810–811, 817
of lip, 810
parenteral nutrition in, 604
skin, 763–765. See also *Melanoma.*
uterine. See *Endometrial cancer.*
Candesartan, 1214t
for hypertension, 309t, 311
Candidiasis, angular cheilitis and, 809
cutaneous, 807–808
epiglottitis due to, 31
hepatosplenic, with intensive chemotherapy for leukemia, 419
in denture sore mouth, 816
in HIV infection, 54
mastitis due to, 1000
median rhomboid glossitis in, 815
nail involvement in, 781, 782
oral, 811
with inhaled corticosteroids for
asthma, 732
perineal pruritus due to, 834
vulvovaginal, 1053–1054
in HIV infection, 54
with oral lichen planus, 811
with parenteral nutrition, 606
Cannabinoids, 1097
for nausea and vomiting, 8t
Cantharidin, for warts, 786–787
Capecitabine, 1214t
Capillariasis, 540t, 545
Capillary hemangioma, lip involvement in,
809
Caplan's syndrome, 229
Capnography, in cardiac arrest
management, 255–256, *255*
Capsaicin, for diabetic neuropathy, 565
for painful neuropathy, 932
for pruritus, 36
Captopril, after myocardial infarction, 331
for congestive heart failure, 294t
for hypertension, 309t
Captopril renal flow scanning, in
renovascular hypertension diagnosis,
313
Captopril stimulation test, in primary
aldosteronism diagnosis, 634
Capture beats, in ventricular tachycardia,
276–277, *277*
Caput succedaneum, cephalhematoma vs.,
1009

Carbamates. See also specific drugs.
abuse of, 1096
intoxication with, 1193–1194
Carbamazepine, adverse effects of, 863t
birth defects associated with, 864
drug interactions with, 863t
antifungals, 196, 200
levothyroxine, 644
for diabetes insipidus, 626
for diabetic neuropathy, 565
for epilepsy, 860t, 861, 862t
in infants and children, 868t, 869t
for hiccup, 14t
for pain, 3
in multiple sclerosis, 902
for painful neuropathy, 932
for trigeminal neuralgia, 909
pharmacokinetics of, 862t
reference intervals for, 1210t
withdrawal from, 1096
Carbaryl, 1193
Carbidopa-levodopa, for parkinsonism due
to metyrosine therapy, 655
for Parkinson's disease, 918, 919t, 920
fluctuating response to, 921
for primary sleep disorders, 34
Carbohydrate, in parenteral nutrition
solutions, 604, 605t
Carbohydrate-deficient transferrin, as
marker for excess alcohol intake, 1092
Carbohydrate malabsorption, 513–514
Carbon dioxide, serum, reference intervals
for, 1208t
Carbon dioxide tension, blood, reference
intervals for, 1208t
Carbon monoxide poisoning, 1169–1171,
1170t
Carbonic anhydrase inhibitors. See also
specific drugs.
for glaucoma, 913–914
Carboplatin, for non–small cell lung
cancer, 189
for small cell lung cancer, 190
Carboxyhemoglobin, in carbon monoxide
poisoning, 1169–1171
reference intervals for, 1212t
Carcinoid tumors, gastric, 532
Carcinoma. See also specific sites and
types.
adrenal, Cushing's syndrome due to, 624
basal cell, 763–765
of mouth, 817
of nail, 783
of vulva, 1074
breast. See *Breast cancer.*
cervical, 1066–1069, 1067t
in HIV infection, 55
colorectal. See *Colorectal cancer.*
endometrial. See *Endometrial cancer.*
esophageal, dysphagia due to, 474
treatment of, 478
hepatocellular, chronic viral hepatitis
and, 506
in cirrhosis, 467
in hemochromatosis, 406
laryngeal, hoarseness due to, 27
lung. See *Lung cancer.*
metastatic. See *Metastasis(es).*
neuroendocrine, of stomach, 532
penile, 710
prostate. See *Prostate cancer.*
renal cell, 709–710
sebaceous cell, conjunctivitis due to, 69
sensory neuropathy with, 931
squamous cell. See *Squamous cell carcinoma.*

Carcinoma (Continued)
thyroid. See *Thyroid cancer.*
transitional cell, 708–709
vulvar, 1071–1074
Carcinomatous meningitis, viral
meningitis vs., 895
Cardiac arrest, 250–256. See also *Sudden
cardiac death.*
in accidental hypothermia, 1131, 1132
Cardiac cachexia, parenteral nutrition for,
604
Cardiac catheterization, in hypertrophic
cardiomyopathy assessment, 348
Cardiac rehabilitation, after myocardial
infarction, 331–332
Cardiac tamponade, 334–335, *334*
Cardiogenic shock, after myocardial
infarction, 325–326, 327t
Cardiomyopathy, dilated, causes of,
291–292
hypertrophic, 346–350. See also *Hypertrophic cardiomyopathy.*
nonischemic, ventricular tachycardia in,
278
Cardiopulmonary resuscitation, 251, *252*
in accidental hypothermia, 1132
Cardioversion, for atrial fibrillation,
259–260, 259t
after myocardial infarction, 323
for atrial flutter, 274–275
for digitalis intoxication, 1175
for neuroleptic intoxication, 1197
Cardioverter-defibrillator, implantable, for
congestive heart failure, 296
for monomorphic ventricular tachycardia, 278
for ventricular premature beats with
cardiac disease, 264
Carditis, in Lyme disease, 125t, 126
treatment of, 127, 128t
radiation, due to therapy for Hodgkin's
disease, 412
Carisoprodol, for chronic fatigue syndrome,
112
Carmustine (BCNU), for lupus
erythematosus, 776
for mycosis fungoides, 768–769
β-Carotene, colorectal cancer and, 533
for protoporphyria, 453
serum, reference intervals for, 1208t,
1213t
Carotid stenosis, 850
Carpal tunnel release, in rheumatoid
arthritis, 952–953
Carteolol, for glaucoma, 913
for hypertension, 308t
intoxication with, 1167t
Carvedilol, after myocardial infarction, 330
for congestive heart failure, 294t, 295
for hypertension, 308t
Castration, for prostate cancer, 708
Cat(s), asthma and, 731
Catecholamines. See also *Dopamine;
Epinephrine; Norepinephrine.*
plasma, in pheochromocytoma diagnosis,
314, 654
urine, reference intervals for, 1211t
Catechol-O-methyltransferase inhibitors,
for Parkinson's disease, 919, 919t, 921
Catheter(s), for middle ear drug delivery,
894
urethral dilation using, for anterior stricture, 711
Catheter ablation, for atrial fibrillation,
260
for atrial flutter, 276

Catheter ablation *(Continued)*
for reentrant tachycardia, mechanism of action of, 269, *269*
Catheter sepsis, in acute renal failure, 699
with parenteral nutrition, 606, *607*
Catheterization, bilateral adrenal venous, in primary aldosteronism diagnosis, 635
cardiac, in hypertrophic cardiomyopathy assessment, 348
urinary, bacteriuria associated with, in men, 662
clean intermittent, for urgency incontinence, 672
infection associated with, in women, 665
pyelonephritis associated with, 682
Cat-scratch disease, 157–159, 158t
meningitis in, 895
Caustic ingestion, 1171–1172
Cavernosometry, in erectile dysfunction assessment, 692
Cavernous hemangioma, lip involvement in, 809
Cefadroxil, for endocarditis prophylaxis, 301t, 303
Cefamandole, vitamin K deficiency and, 592
Cefazolin, for endocarditis, 300t
prophylactic, 301t, 303
for osteomyelitis, 974t
for staphylococcal toxic shock syndrome, 85t
Cefdinir, for streptococcal pharyngitis, 237, 238t
Cefepime, for bacterial meningitis, 105t
for cystic fibrosis exacerbations, 179t
for *Haemophilus influenzae* meningitis, 104t, 106
for infection in neutropenia, 419
for sepsis, 63t
Cefixime, for epididymitis, 674
for gonococcal infection, 719t
disseminated, 719
in men, 661
for otitis media, 205, 206
for typhoid fever, 163, 163t
Cefoperazone, for typhoid fever, 163, 163t
vitamin K deficiency and, 592
Cefotaxime, for bacterial meningitis, 105t
for *Haemophilus influenzae* meningitis, 103t, 104t, 106
for Lyme disease, 128t, 129t
for pelvic inflammatory disease, 1059t
for pneumococcal meningitis, 103t, 104t, 105
for sepsis, 63t
in neonate, 1017t
for spontaneous bacterial peritonitis in cirrhosis, 470
for typhoid fever, 163, 163t
Cefotetan, for pelvic inflammatory disease, 719t, 1059t
for postpartum endomyometritis, 1000
Cefoxitin, for diverticulitis, 482
for pelvic inflammatory disease, 719t, 1059t
Cefpirome, for typhoid fever, 163, 163t
Cefpodoxime, for bacterial pneumonia, 213
for otitis media, 205, 205t, 206
Ceftazidime, for bacterial meningitis, 105t
for cystic fibrosis exacerbations, 179t
for fever in aplastic anemia, 353
for infection in neutropenia, 419
in child, 422
for nosocomial pneumonia, 213

Ceftazidime *(Continued)*
for osteomyelitis, 973, 974t
for *Pseudomonas aeruginosa* meningitis, 104t, 106
for pyelonephritis in women, 664, 664t
for sepsis, 63t
Ceftibuten, for otitis media, 205, 206
Ceftizoxime, for pelvic inflammatory disease, 1059t
for sepsis, 63t
for typhoid fever, 163, 163t
Ceftriaxone, for bacterial conjunctivitis, 67
for bacterial meningitis, dosages for, 105t
prophylactic, 108
for bacterial prostatitis, 686
for bacterial tracheitis, 31
for chancroid, 717
for epididymitis, 662, 674, 675
for epiglottitis, 31
for gonococcal infection, 719t
disseminated, 719
in children, 720
in men, 661
in neonate, 720
for *Haemophilus influenzae* meningitis, 103t, 104t, 106
for infection in sickle cell disease, 378
for infective endocarditis, 300t, 301
for Lyme disease, 127, 128t, 129t
for osteomyelitis, 973, 974t
for otitis media, 205t, 206
for pelvic inflammatory disease, 719t, 1059t
for pneumococcal meningitis, 103t, 104t, 105
for pyelonephritis, 682t
in women, 664, 664t
for salmonellosis, 77t, 78, 161
for sepsis, 63t
for streptococcal toxic shock syndrome, 85, 85t
for typhoid fever, 163, 163t
for urinary tract infection, in girls, 667–668
in men, 661–662
for *Yersinia enterocolitica* infection, 77t
Cefuroxime, for bacterial pneumonia, 212t, 213
for laryngitis, 30
for Lyme disease, 128t
for otitis media, 205–206, 205t
for streptococcal pharyngitis, 237, 238t
in sickle cell disease, for acute chest syndrome, 377
for infection, 379
Celecoxib, 1214t
for dysmenorrhea, 1043t
for osteoarthritis, 970
for pain, 2
peptic ulcer disease and, 500
Celiac disease. See *Gluten-sensitive enteropathy.*
Celiac plexus block, for chronic pancreatitis, 520
Cellulitis, 795, 795t
clostridial, 797
dissecting, of scalp, 762
synergistic necrotizing, 81, 796, 796t
Central nervous system, in uremic syndrome, 699
infection of. See *Encephalitis; Meningitis.*
leukemia involving, 414
in children, 424
prophylaxis of, 423, 424–425

Central nervous system *(Continued)*
lymphoma involving, in HIV infection, 439
sarcoidosis involving, 227t, 228
tumors of. See *Brain tumors;* specific tumors.
Central venous access, for parenteral nutrition, 604
complications associated with, 605–606, *607*
Cephalexin, for atopic dermatitis, 823
for bacterial overgrowth, 510
with jejunal diverticula, 480
for endocarditis prophylaxis, 301t, 303
for pyelonephritis, 681t
for recurrent urinary tract infection prophylaxis in women, 664t
for streptococcal pharyngitis, 237, 238t
for toxic shock syndrome prophylaxis, 85
Cephalhematoma, caput succedaneum vs., 1009
Cephalosporins. See also specific drugs.
vitamin K deficiency and, 592
Cercarial dermatitis, 804–805, 804t
Cerebellar ataxia, in chickenpox, 70
Cerebral edema, after ischemic stroke, 852
high-altitude, 1128, 1128t
in diabetic ketoacidosis in children, 567, 568
in encephalitis, 896
with head injury, 933
in children, 938
Cerebral palsy, intrauterine infection and, 984
Cerebrospinal fluid analysis, in bacterial meningitis diagnosis, 103
in encephalitis diagnosis, 895
in viral meningitis diagnosis, 895
reference intervals for, 1212t
Cerebrovascular accident. See *Intracranial hemorrhage; Stroke.*
Cerivastatin, for hyperlipidemia, 581
Ceruloplasmin, serum, reference intervals for, 1208t
Cervical cancer, 1066–1069, 1067t
in HIV infection, 55
Cervical cap, 1078t, 1085
Cervical intraepithelial neoplasia, 1066–1067
Cervical spine instability, in rheumatoid arthritis, 953
Cervicitis, chlamydial, 1056, 1056t
treatment of, 1057, 1057t
Cesarean delivery, anesthesia for, 997–998
with placenta previa, 988
with placental abruption, 988
Cestodes, 543, 546–547. See also specific worms and diseases.
treatment of, 541t, 543–544
Cetirizine, for allergic rhinitis, 745, 745t
for ordinary urticaria, 835–836
for pruritus, 37
Cetylpyridinium, for erythema multiforme, 813
Chagas' disease, 101–102
CHAMP mnemonic, 1179
Chancroid, 717
Charcoal, activated, for acute poisoning, 1148, 1148t
for protoporphyria, 453
for pruritus in cholestatic liver disease, 37
Charcoal lighter fluid, 1179
Cheilitis, 809–810
actinic, 792, 810
contact, 809, 816

Cheilitis *(Continued)*
in erythema multiforme, 813
Cheilitis granularis apostematosa, 810
Chelation therapy, for iron overdose,
1152t, 1180–1181
for lead poisoning, 1153t, 1185–1187,
1186t
for transfusional hemosiderosis in thalassemia, 372
Chemical burns, 1126, 1171–1172
Chemotherapy. See also specific drugs and
regimens.
emesis due to, 8–10, 9t, 10t
Chest compressions, in neonatal
resuscitation, 1005
Chest pain, differential diagnosis of,
318–319
in acute myocardial infarction, 317
Chest syndrome, acute, in sickle cell
disease, 377
Chest tube drainage, for pleural effusion,
202, *202*, 203
Chickenpox, 800t, 801–802
clinical manifestations of, 70, 801
complications of, 70–71, 801
during pregnancy, 70, 71, 802
epidemiology of, 69, 801
treatment of, 71, 800t, 802
Chickenpox vaccine, 71, *140–141*, 143,
144t, 801–802
for travelers, 147t, 148
Child(ren). See also *Adolescents; Infant(s);
Neonate(s)*.
asthma in, 735–743. See also under
Asthma.
bacterial conjunctivitis treatment in, 67
bacterial meningitis treatment in, 104t,
105t
brucellosis in, 65, 65t, 66
chlamydial conjunctivitis treatment in,
68
chronic bullous disease in, 829
cold-water near-drowning in, 1133–1134
cough in, 23–24
dermatomyositis in, 777
diabetes mellitus in, 566–572. See also
Diabetes mellitus, type 1.
doxycycline use in, tooth-staining and,
166
enuresis in, 668–671
epilepsy in, 867–871. See also *Epilepsy;
Seizures*.
genital and oral warts in, sexual abuse
and, 787
gonococcal infection in, 720
head injury in, 936–940. See also under
Head injury.
Hodgkin's disease in, radiation therapy
for, 411
influenza in, 86, 87, 87t
lead poisoning in. See *Lead poisoning*.
leukemia in, 421–425. See also under
Leukemia.
Lyme disease in, 126–127
metabolic requirements for, 607
otitis media in, 204–207, 205t–207t
parenteral fluid therapy in, 607–613.
See also under *Fluids, parenteral*.
pyelonephritis treatment in, 681–682
rheumatoid arthritis in, 953–958. See
also *Rheumatoid arthritis, juvenile*.
sarcoma botryoides in, 1074
splenectomized, antibiotic prophylaxis
for, 362, 364, 371
tinea capitis treatment in, 762
ureteral injury in, 684

Child(ren) *(Continued)*
urinary tract infections in, 666–668
vaginitis in, 1055
viral respiratory infection treatment in,
214–215
Child procedure, for chronic pancreatitis,
523
Child-Pugh staging score, for cirrhosis,
466, 466t
Chinese restaurant syndrome, 78
CHIPES mnemonic, 1160
Chlamydia pneumoniae bronchitis, adult-
onset asthma and, 208
Chlamydia psittaci infection, 116–118
Chlamydia species, characteristics of, 117,
1056
Chlamydia trachomatis infection,
1055–1057
cervical, 1056, 1056t
conjunctival, 67–68, 1056
epidemiology of, 1055, 1056t
epididymal, 662, 674
gonorrhea and, 718–719, 719t
lymphogranuloma venereum due to,
722
neonatal, 67, 68, 1056–1057
pelvic inflammatory disease due to,
1056, 1056t, 1058, 1059
perihepatitis due to, 1056, 1056t
pneumonia due to, in infant, 1056
cough in, 23
treatment of, 1057, 1057t
urethral, 720
in women, 1056, 1056t
urinary tract, in men, treatment of,
661
Chloasma, 839
Chlorambucil, for chronic lymphocytic
leukemia, 431, 432
for focal segmental glomerulosclerosis,
678
for indolent B cell lymphoma, 435t
for membranous glomerulopathy, 678
for primary glomerular disease, 676
for sarcoidosis, 226
Chloramphenicol, anticonvulsant
interactions with, 863t
for bacterial meningitis, 105t
for plague, 116
for relapsing fever, 124
for Rocky Mountain spotted fever, 166,
166t
for typhoid fever, 162, 163t
resistance to, in *Haemophilus influenzae,* 106
in *Neisseria meningitidis,* 106
Chlordiazepoxide, for ethanol withdrawal,
1177
intoxication with, 1166
withdrawal from, 1096
Chlorfenthion, intoxication with, 1194
Chlorhexidine, for acne, 758
Chloride, in intravenous solutions, for
infants and children, 608t
in parenteral nutrition solutions, 605t
reference intervals for, in serum, 1208t
in urine, 1211t
2-Chlorodeoxyadenosine. See *Cladribine*.
2-Chloroprocaine, for cesarean delivery,
997
Chloroquine, for amebiasis, 58t, 59
for amebiasis cutis, 804
for cutaneous lupus, 762, 775
for malaria, 96, 96t
prophylactic, 100t, 101, 149
for porphyria cutanea tarda, 452

Chlorpheniramine, for allergic rhinitis,
745t
for ordinary urticaria, 836
for viral respiratory infection, 214
intoxication with, 1164
Chlorpromazine, anticonvulsant
interactions with, 863t
characteristics of, 1118t
for acute hepatic porphyria, 448, 448t
for hiccup, 14, 14t
intoxication with, 1196, 1197t
Chlorpropamide, for diabetes insipidus,
626
for type 2 diabetes, 557t
Chlorprothixene, intoxication by, 1197t
Chlorpyrifos, 1193
Chlorthalidone, for hypertension, 308t
for Meniere's disease, 888
Choanal atresia, differential diagnosis of,
743t, 744
Cholangiocarcinoma, in primary sclerosing
cholangitis, 468–469
Cholangiopancreatography, endoscopic
retrograde, for choledocholithiasis,
465
in chronic pancreatitis, 520
Cholangitis, primary sclerosing, 468–469.
See also *Cirrhosis*.
Cholecystectomy, for cholecystitis, 464
for cholelithiasis, 463
for gallstone pancreatitis, 517
Cholecystenteric fistula, 465
Cholecystitis, 463–465
Cholecystostomy, percutaneous, for acute
cholecystitis, 464
Choledocholithiasis, 465
Cholelithiasis. See *Gallstones*.
Cholera, 72–74, 72t, 74t
food-borne, 75t, 77, 77t
Cholera vaccine, 74, 146
Cholesteatoma, 115
Cholesterol, dietary, in type 2 diabetes,
555
high-density lipoprotein, serum, cardiovascular risk and, 579
reference intervals for, 1208t
low-density lipoprotein, goals for, in diabetes, 554, 554t, 563
pharmacologic reduction of, 581–584
for angina, 249
reference intervals for, 1208t
regulation of, 580
treatment guidelines based on, 579,
579t
serum, goals for, in diabetes, 554, 554t,
563
reference intervals for, 1208t
Cholestyramine, for bile salt
malabsorption, 510
for diarrhea in inflammatory bowel disease, 482
for hyperlipidemia, 582
for protoporphyria, 453
for pruritus in cholestatic liver disease,
37
levothyroxine interaction with, 644
Choline magnesium trisalicylate, for
dysmenorrhea, 1043t
for juvenile rheumatoid arthritis, 954–
956, 955t
Cholinergic agents. See also specific
agents.
intoxication due to, 1150t, 1193–1194
Cholinesterase inhibitors. See also specific
drugs.
for myasthenia gravis, 905

Cholinesterase inhibitors (Continued)
  during pregnancy, 908
Chondrocyte transplantation, for
  osteoarthritis, 970
Chondroitin sulfate, for osteoarthritis, 970
CHOP regimen, for aggressive lymphoma,
  436t, 437
  for indolent B cell lymphoma, 435, 435t
  for Sézary's syndrome, 769
CHOP-Bleo regimen, for aggressive
  lymphoma, 436t
  for indolent B cell lymphoma, 435
Chorioamnionitis, 984
Chorionic villus sampling, 981
Chorioretinitis, toxoplasmosis, treatment
  of, 156
Chromium deficiency, with parenteral
  nutrition, 607
Chronic fatigue syndrome, 110–113, 110t,
  111t
  infectious mononucleosis and, 109
Chronic obstructive pulmonary disease,
  171–175, 171. See also Bronchitis,
  chronic; Emphysema.
  diagnosis of, 172
  ethical issues in, 175
  management of, inpatient, 174–175,
    174t
    outpatient, 172, 172t
    stepwise pharmacotherapy in, 172–
      174, 173
  nutrition in, 175
  sleep disorders in, 175
  staging of, 172, 172t
  surgery for, 175
  ventilatory failure management in, 169–
    170
Chronic pelvic pain syndrome, 686–687
Chvostek's sign, 632
  in tetanus, 134
Cicatricial pemphigoid, 813, 828
Ciclopirox, for tinea infection, 807
Cidofovir, for herpes simplex, 800
  for laryngeal papilloma, 25
  for molluscum contagiosum in HIV infec-
    tion, 803
  for resistant herpesvirus infections in
    HIV infection, 53–54
Ciguatera poisoning, 79, 80t, 1143–1144
Cilastatin-imipenem, for pyelonephritis,
  682t
  for sepsis, 63t
Cimetidine, anticonvulsant interactions
  with, 863t
  defective iron absorption due to, 356
  for anaphylaxis, 727t
  for cystic fibrosis, 177t
  for gastrointestinal complications in
    acute renal failure, 699
  for insect sting allergy, 754
  for ordinary urticaria, 836
  for reflux-related cough, 24
  for warts, 787
Ciprofloxacin, for bacillary angiomatosis,
  158t
  for bacterial meningitis, 105t
    prophylactic, 108
  for bacterial prostatitis, 686
  for Campylobacter infection, 77t, 78
  for cat-scratch disease, 158t
  for chancroid, 717
  for cholera, 73, 74t
  for cystic fibrosis exacerbations, 179t
  for diarrhea, 17t
    in travelers, 150
  for diverticulitis, 482

Ciprofloxacin (Continued)
  for draining ear, 207t
  for ehrlichiosis, 166, 166t
  for enterotoxigenic Escherichia coli infec-
    tion, 77, 77t
  for epididymitis, 674, 675
  for gonococcal infection, 718, 719t
    disseminated, 719
    in men, 661
  for inflammatory bowel disease, 486
  for legionellosis, 217, 218
  for Mycobacterium avium complex infec-
    tion in HIV infection, 54
  for osteomyelitis, 973, 974t
  for pelvic inflammatory disease, 1059t
  for pyelonephritis, 681t, 682t
    in women, 664t
  for Q fever endocarditis, 118
  for Rocky Mountain spotted fever, 166t
  for salmonellosis, 77t, 78, 160–161
  for sepsis, 63t
  for Shigella infection, 77t
  for typhoid carriage, 164
  for typhoid fever, 163, 163t
  for urinary tract infection, in men, 661
    in women, 664t
  for Yersinia enterocolitica infection, 77t
Circadian rhythm, angina management
  and, 248
  disorders of, in travel, 150
    insomnia due to, 32, 34
    melatonin for, 35
Circumcision, penile carcinoma and, 710
Cirrhosis, 465–471
  biliary, focal, in cystic fibrosis, 180
    primary, 468
  causes of, 466, 466t
  due to methotrexate, 948
  in chronic viral hepatitis, 466, 506
    treatment of, 469
  in hemochromatosis, 405–406
  management of complications of, 469–
    471
  treatment of, 466–468, 467t
    disease-specific, 468–469
Cisapride, antifungal interactions with,
  196, 198, 200–201, 525, 807
  for bacterial overgrowth, 510
  for constipation, 19, 19t
  for dyspepsia, 11, 497
  for gaseousness, 12
  for gastroesophageal reflux, 525
    in cystic fibrosis, 179t, 180
  for gastroparesis in diabetes, 565
  for hiccup, 15
  for irritable bowel syndrome, 491
  for nausea and vomiting, 7, 8t
  macrolide interactions with, 525
Cisplatin, for aggressive lymphoma, 436t
  for AIDS-related lymphoma, 439
  for cervical cancer, 1069
  for gastric adenocarcinoma, 530
  for non–small cell lung cancer, 189
  for small cell lung cancer, 190
  for transitional cell carcinoma, 709
Citalopram, 1214t
  for anxiety disorders, 1100t
  for depression, 1109t
  monoamine oxidase inhibitor interaction
    with, 1115
  pharmacodynamic effects of, 1110t
Citrate, for hypocitraturia, 715
  toxicity due to, with massive transfu-
    sion, 461
Cladribine, for chronic lymphocytic
  leukemia, 432

Cladribine (Continued)
  for indolent B cell lymphoma, 435t
  for multiple sclerosis, 900
  for Sézary's syndrome, 769
Clarithromycin, for bacillary angiomatosis,
  158t
  for endocarditis prophylaxis, 301t, 303
  for Helicobacter pylori infection, 11, 501,
    501t
  for inflammatory bowel disease, 486
  for legionellosis, 218
  for leprosy, 92
  for Mycobacterium avium complex infec-
    tion, 241
    in HIV infection, 54
  for mycoplasmal pneumonia, 216
  for otitis media, 205
  for pertussis, 139
  for psittacosis, 118
  for streptococcal pharyngitis, 237, 238t
  for toxoplasmosis in HIV infection, 156
Clark's nevus, 789, 793
Claudication, in abdominal aortic occlusive
  disease, 246
  in occlusive peripheral arterial disease,
    336–338, 336t
Clavulanate-amoxicillin. See Amoxicillin-
  clavulanate.
Clavulanate-ticarcillin. See Ticarcillin-
  clavulanate.
Clavus(i), plantar warts vs., 785
Cleft lip, 809
Cleft palate, 809
Clemastine, for allergic rhinitis, 745t
  for viral respiratory infection, 214
    intoxication with, 1164
Clindamycin, for acne, 758
  for babesiosis, 130
  for bacterial vaginosis, 1054
  for diverticulitis, 482
  for endocarditis prophylaxis, 301t, 303
    in mitral valve prolapse, 289, 290t
  for fever in aplastic anemia, 353
  for lung abscess, 204
  for malaria, 97t
  for necrotizing skin and soft tissue infec-
    tions, 82
  for osteomyelitis, 973, 974t
  for otitis media, 205t, 206
  for pelvic inflammatory disease, 719t,
    1059t
  for Pneumocystis carinii pneumonia in
    HIV infection, 51
  for postpartum endomyometritis, 1000–
    1001
  for sepsis, 63t
  for streptococcal pharyngitis, 237, 238
  for streptococcal toxic shock syndrome,
    85, 85t
  for toxoplasmosis, 153, 155
    central nervous system, in HIV infec-
      tion, 53, 156, 157
    ocular, 156
Clinical chemistry, reference intervals for,
  on blood, serum, and plasma,
    1207t–1209t
  on urine, 1211t–1212t
Clioquinol, neuropathy due to, 931
Clobetasol, for atopic dermatitis, 822
  for lichen simplex chronicus, 834
Clofazimine, for erythema nodosum
  leprosum, 93
  for leprosy, 92
  for lupus erythematosus, 776
Clofibrate, for diabetes insipidus, 626
  for hyperlipidemia, 583

Clomiphene citrate, ovarian stimulation by, in endometriosis, 1034
  in polycystic ovarian syndrome, 1042
Clomipramine, for anxiety disorders, 1100t, 1102
  for depression, 1109t
  intoxication by, 1202t
  monoamine oxidase inhibitor interaction with, 1115
  pharmacodynamic effects of, 1110t
Clonazepam, adverse effects of, 863t
  drug interactions with, 863t
  for anxiety disorders, 1100t, 1102
  for epilepsy, 860t, 861, 862t
    in infants and children, 868t, 869t
  for panic disorder, 1121t, 1122
  for seizures in acute porphyria, 449
  intoxication with, 1166
  pharmacokinetics of, 862t
Clonidine, for attention-deficit/hyper-activity disorder, 873t, 874
  for diarrhea in diabetes, 565
  for hypertension, 308t, 309
  for opioid abuse, 1095
  for orthostatic hypotension in mitral valve prolapse, 291
  for spasticity in multiple sclerosis, 901
  for tetanus, 136
  for Tourette's syndrome, 876–877
  overdose of, with transdermal patch, 877
Clonidine suppression test, in pheochromo-cytoma diagnosis, 314, 654
Clonorchis sinensis infection, 540t, 546
Clopidogrel, after myocardial infarction, 329–330
  for non–Q wave myocardial infarction, 328
  for peripheral arterial occlusive disease, 337
  for stroke prevention, 850
    secondary, 855
Clorazepate, intoxication with, 1166
Clostridial cellulitis, 797
Clostridial myonecrosis, 81, 795t, 796–797
Clostridium botulinum infection, food-borne, 75t, 78
Clostridium difficile diarrhea, 15
Clostridium perfringens infection, food-borne, 75t, 77
  gas gangrene due to, 796–797
  hemolysis with, 366
  in acute cholecystitis, 464
Clostridium tetani infection. See Tetanus.
Clotrimazole, for Candida suppression in perineal pruritus, 834
  for candidiasis, 808, 811
    in HIV infection, 54
  for tinea infection, 807
  for trichomoniasis, 1055
Clotting factor(s). See also specific factors.
  reference intervals for, 1207t
Clotting factor concentrates, 392–394, 458
Cloxacillin, for staphylococcal toxic shock syndrome, 85t
Clozapine, adverse effects of, 1119
  characteristics of, 1117–1118, 1118t
  in Parkinson's disease, for psychosis, 923
    for tremor, 922
  mechanism of action of, 1118
Clubbing, diseases associated with, 783
CMF regimen, for breast cancer, 1027, 1028
Coagulation factor(s). See also specific factors.
  reference intervals for, 1207t
Coagulation factor concentrates, 392–394, 458

Coagulation tests, reference intervals for, 1207t
Coagulation time, reference intervals for, 1207t
Coagulopathy(ies), 390–400, 398t. See also specific disorders.
  dilutional, with massive transfusion, 461
  in acute renal failure, 699
  intracerebral hemorrhage management in, 849
  signs and symptoms of, 391
Coarctation of the aorta, 283
Coartemether, for malaria, 96
Coastal erysipelas, 804t
Cobalamin. See also Vitamin B12.
  deficiency of, dietary, 368–369
    megaloblastic anemia due to, 366–369
  supplemental, for dietary deficiency, 369
    for pernicious anemia, 367–368
Cocaine, 1094–1095
  intoxication with, 1172–1173, 1172t
  panic attacks due to, 1120
Coccidioidomycosis, 193–195, 193t
Cockroaches, asthma and, 731
Codeine, for cough, 24
  for pain in pericarditis, 334
  intoxication with, 1191, 1192t
Codeine-acetaminophen, for painful episode in sickle cell disease, 376
CODOX-M regimen, for Burkitt's lymphoma, 438
Cognitive dysfunction, after head injury, 935
  in children, 940
  after stroke, 854–855
  due to haloperidol, 876
  in Alzheimer's disease, 845–846
  in schizophrenia, 1117
Cognitive-behavioral therapy, for bulimia nervosa, 1105
  for chronic fatigue syndrome, 112
  for panic disorder, 1122
Cognitive-motor disorder, minor, HIV-associated, 55
Coitus interruptus, 1076t, 1084
Colchicine, for aphthous stomatitis, 812
  for Behçet's syndrome, 812
  for constipation, 19t, 20
  for cutaneous vasculitis, 780
  for gout, 577–578
  for urticarial vasculitis, 837
Cold, common, rhinosinusitis and, 233
Cold hemagglutinin disease, 359t
  clinical diagnosis of, 360
  laboratory diagnosis of, 361
  treatment of, 362–363
Cold hemoglobinuria, paroxysmal, 359t
  clinical diagnosis of, 360
  laboratory diagnosis of, 361
  treatment of, 363
Cold injury, 1130–1134. See also Hypothermia.
Cold urticaria, 834, 836
Colectomy, abdominal, with ileorectal anastomosis, for constipation, 20
  for colon cancer, 535–536
Colestipol, for bile salt malabsorption, 510
  for hyperlipidemia, 582
  for pruritus in cholestatic liver disease, 37
Colic, biliary, 463
Colitis, amebic. See Amebiasis.
  ulcerative. See Inflammatory bowel disease.
Collagen injections, for stress incontinence, 673

Collagenous sprue, 511
Colloid cysts, 941
Colon, diverticular disease of, 481
Colonoscopy, for cancer screening, 534, 535t
  in inflammatory bowel disease, 487
Colorectal adenoma, malignant transformation of, 532–533
Colorectal cancer, 532–537
  causes of, 532–534
  diagnosis of, 534
  epidemiology of, 532
  genetic alterations in, 533, 534, 534t
  hereditary nonpolyposis, 533–534, 534t
  management of, 535–537
  screening for, 534, 535t
    in inflammatory bowel disease, 487
  staging of, 537t
Colposcopy, in cervical cancer diagnosis, 1066
Coma, assessment of. See Glasgow Coma Scale.
  in acute poisoning, 1145–1146, 1146t
  in head injury. See Head injury, severe.
  myxedema, 644–645, 644t
  with intracerebral hemorrhage, 847
Combitube, for airway management, 253
Common cold, rhinosinusitis and, 233
Complement, serum, in acute renal failure diagnosis, 696
  reference intervals for, 1213t
  total hemolytic, reference intervals for, 1213t
Compound nevus, 789
Compression bandage, for venous leg ulcers, 818
Compression stockings, for post-thrombotic edema, 343–344
  for venous leg ulcer prevention, 818
Computed tomography (CT), for staging renal injuries in trauma victim, 683
  in acute pancreatitis diagnosis, 515
  in brain tumor diagnosis, 942
  in head injury, 933–934
    in children, 937
  spiral, in pulmonary thromboembolism workup, 220–221
  in renal calculus evaluation, 713
Concussion, aftereffects of, 938, 939, 940
  classification of, 936t
Condoms, 1077t, 1084
Condyloma, giant, of Buschke-Lowenstein, 1073–1074
Condyloma acuminatum, 787–788, 788t
  oral, 817
  oropharyngeal, 792
  vulvar, 1069–1070
Cone shell, 1142
Confusion Assessment Method, for delirium diagnosis, 1107t
Congestive heart failure. See Heart failure.
Conjunctivitis, 67–69
  chlamydial, 67–68, 1056
  gonococcal, in neonate, 67, 720
Connective tissue disorders. See also specific disorders.
  autoimmune, 774–778
  breast implants and, 1024
Consciousness, level of. See Coma; Glasgow Coma Scale.
Constipation, 18–20, 18t, 19t
  chronic, antidepressants for use in, 1115t
  during pregnancy, 980
Contact cheilitis, 809, 816
Contact dermatitis, 830–831

Contact lens–induced conjunctivitis, 69
Contact stomatitis, 816
Contact urticaria, 830, 835
Continuous arteriovenous hemofiltration, 700, 700t
Continuous positive airway pressure, for atelectasis, 170
nasal, for obstructive sleep-disordered breathing, 182–183, 182t, 183t
Continuous venovenous hemofiltration, 700, 700t
Contraception, 1074–1089. See also *Contraceptives.*
assessing efficacy of, 1075
breast-feeding and, 1000, 1086t, 1089
counseling on, 1075
emergency, 1081t, 1085–1087
for adolescents, 1088
methods of, advantages and disadvantages of, 1076t–1083t
risks and benefits of, 1075
postpartum, 1000, 1088–1089
Contraceptives, injectable depot, 1081t, 1085
oral, 1080t, 1085
anticonvulsant interactions with, 863t, 864
antifungal interactions with, 200
chronic medical conditions and, 1086t
for acne, 759
for acute porphyria, 451
for amenorrhea due to polycystic ovarian syndrome, 1042
for dysfunctional uterine bleeding, 1039, 1039t, 1040
for dysmenorrhea, 1044
for emergency contraception, 1085–1087
for endometriosis, 1031, 1033
in perimenopausal years, 1047, 1052
management of symptoms associated with, 1086t
melasma due to, 839
nipple discharge due to, 1023
pelvic inflammatory disease risk and, 1058
postpartum use of, 1000, 1086t, 1089
tetracycline and, 758
troglitazone interaction with, 559
subdermal implantable, 1082t, 1085
Contractures, after burns, 1126, 1127, 1127t
after head injury, 935
after stroke, 856
in juvenile rheumatoid arthritis, prevention of, 957
Contusions, muscle, in sports injuries, 975
with head injury, 933
Cooling, for heat stroke, 1136
Coombs' test, in Rh isoimmunization assessment, 385
reference intervals for, 1207t
Copper, hereditary defects in metabolism of, hair abnormalities due to, 763
reference intervals for, in serum, 1208t
in urine, 1211t
Coproporphyria, hereditary, 448t. See also *Porphyria(s).*
Coproporphyrin, urine, reference intervals for, 1211t
Coral, 1142
Cordocentesis, in Rh isoimmunization assessment, 385
Corn(s), plantar warts vs., 785
Corn oil, in short-bowel syndrome, 511
Corneal transplantation, rabies transmission by, 119, 120, 122

Coronary angiography, after myocardial infarction, 333
Coronary angioplasty, recanalization using, for myocardial infarction, 320–321
Coronary artery bypass, for angina, 249
Coronary artery disease. See also *Atherosclerosis.*
after Hodgkin's disease treatment, 409, 412
dilated cardiomyopathy in, 291, 292
hormone replacement therapy and, 1048–1049
migraine therapy in, 882
monomorphic ventricular tachycardia and, 277–278
pathogenesis of myocardial infarction in, 316, 317t
risk factors for, 579t
ventricular fibrillation and, 279–280
Corpus callosotomy, for epilepsy, 866
Corrosive ingestion, 1171–1172
Corticosteroid(s). See also specific agents.
bone disease due to, 487, 596
classification of, 831
drugs increasing metabolism of, 676
for allergic rhinitis, 746–747, 747t
for alopecia areata, 761–762
for ankylosing spondylitis, 960
for asthma, inhaled, 731–733, 732t
in children, 739
oral, 733–734
for atopic dermatitis, 822
for brain tumors, 944
for chronic obstructive pulmonary disease, 173, *173*
for cicatricial pemphigoid, 828
for congenital toxoplasmosis, 156
for contact dermatitis, 830–831
for cutaneous hemangiomas, 809
for cutaneous lupus, 762, 775
for cutaneous vasculitis, 779
for dermatomyositis, 777
for erythema multiforme, 824–825
for giant cell arteritis, 971
for gout, 577
for inflammatory bowel disease, 484–485
bone disease due to, 487
for juvenile rheumatoid arthritis, 956
for keloids, 784–785
for lichen planopilaris, 762
for lichen planus, 773, 811
for Meniere's disease, 893
for multiple sclerosis exacerbations, 898
for myasthenia gravis, 906, 906t
during pregnancy, 908
for mycosis fungoides, 768
for myxedema crisis, 645
for optic neuritis, 911–912
for parapsoriasis, 774
for primary glomerular disease, 675–676
for pruritic urticarial papules and plaques of pregnancy, 831–832
for psoriasis, 771
for rheumatoid arthritis, 947–948
surgery on patients using, 953
for rhinosinusitis, 235
for sarcoidosis, 225, 226–227, 228
for silicosis, 230
for thrombotic thrombocytopenic purpura, 404
for toxic epidermal necrolysis, 825
for warm antibody autoimmune hemolytic anemia, 361–362
interference by, with vitamin D therapy, 634
replacement therapy with, for adrenal crisis, 620, 620t

Corticosteroid(s) *(Continued)*
for chronic adrenal insufficiency, 620–621, 621t
safety of, during pregnancy, 748
to enhance fetal lung maturity, 988, 1014
Corticosteroid-anesthetic injections. See *Anesthetic-corticosteroid injections.*
Corticotropin (ACTH), deficiency of, in hypopituitarism, 637, 640t
ectopic secretion of, Cushing's syndrome due to, 624
for gout, 577
for infantile spasms, 870
plasma, reference intervals for, 1208t
Corticotropin stimulation test, prolonged, in adrenocortical insufficiency diagnosis, 620
short, in adrenocortical insufficiency diagnosis, 619–620
Corticotropin-releasing hormone test, in adrenocortical insufficiency diagnosis, 620
Cortisol, reference intervals for, in plasma, 1208t
in urine, 1211t
Cortisone, for paroxysmal nocturnal hemoglobinuria, 366
Co-trimoxazole. See *Trimethoprim-sulfamethoxazole (TMP-SMX).*
Cough, 22–25
reflex, with inhaled corticosteroids for asthma, 732
Cough variant asthma, 23–24, 736
Courvoisier's sign, 464
Cowden's syndrome, oral warts in, 817
COX-2 inhibitors. See *Cyclooxygenase 2 (COX-2) inhibitors.*
Coxiella burnetii infection, 118
Coxsackieviruses, meningitis due to, 895
skin infections due to, 803
Cradle cap, 773
Cramps, heat, 1135, 1136t
Craniopharyngioma, 940
optic neuritis vs., 911
Craniotomy, for brain tumor, 942
Creatine, reference intervals for, in serum, 1208t
in urine, 1211t
Creatine kinase, serum, in myocardial infarction, 318
reference intervals for, 1208t
Creatinine, serum, for glomerular filtration rate measurement, 701
in acute renal failure diagnosis, 696
reference intervals for, 1208t
urine, reference intervals for, 1211t
Creatinine clearance, for glomerular filtration rate measurement, 701–702
reference intervals for, 1211t
Creeping eruption, 544, 804t, 805
CREST syndrome, 777
Cricoarytenoid joints, in rheumatoid arthritis, 953
Cricopharyngeal myotomy, for Zenker's diverticulum with dysphagia, 478
Crocodiles, 1141–1142
Crohn's disease. See *Inflammatory bowel disease.*
Cromolyn, for allergic conjunctivitis, 68
for allergic rhinitis, 746
for asthma, 733
in children, 739, 742
for rhinosinusitis, 235
safety of, during pregnancy, 748
Crossover syndrome, lupus in, 774

Crossover syndrome *(Continued)*
  scleroderma in, 777
Crotamiton, for scabies, 804t, 805
Croup, 31, 214–215
Cruciate ligament tear, anterior, 977
Cryoglobulinemia, nerve infarction due to, 930–931
Cryomyolysis, for leiomyomata, 1062
Cryoprecipitate, 458
  for bleeding in acute renal failure, 699
  for hemolytic transfusion reaction, 459
  for hemophilia, 392–393
  for intracerebral hemorrhage, 849
  for von Willebrand disease, 395
Cryotherapy, for actinic cheilitis, 810
  for hyperpigmentation, 839
  for keloids, 784
  for mucocele, 817
  for oral warts, 817
  for skin cancer, 764
  for warts, 785–786
Cryptococcal meningitis, in HIV infection, 52
Cryptosporidiosis, 539t, 542
  food-borne, 77
Cullen's sign, in acute pancreatitis, 515
Cultures, for *Chlamydia trachomatis,* 1057
  for *Streptobacillus moniliformis,* 122
  in infective endocarditis, 299
  in pertussis diagnosis, 138
  in sepsis diagnosis, 62–63
  in typhoid fever diagnosis, 162
Curettage, for oral warts, 817
  for skin cancer, 764
  uterine, for dysfunctional uterine bleeding, 1038, 1039
Cushing's syndrome, 621–624
  causes of, 622t
  diagnosis of, 621–622
  treatment of, 622–624
CVP regimen, for chronic lymphocytic leukemia, 431
  for indolent B cell lymphoma, 435t
Cyanide, 1173–1174
  antidote kit for, 1151t–1152t, 1173–1174
Cyanosis, in newborn, 1004
Cyclizine, intoxication with, 1164
Cyclobenzaprine, for chronic fatigue syndrome, 112
  for fibromyalgia, 967
Cyclodestructive surgery, for glaucoma, 915
Cyclooxygenase 1 (COX-1), 2
Cyclooxygenase 2 (COX-2), 2
Cyclooxygenase 2 (COX-2) inhibitors, 2
  for dysmenorrhea, 1043t, 1044
  for gout, 577
  for osteoarthritis, 970
  for rheumatoid arthritis, 947
  peptic ulcer disease and, 500
Cyclophosphamide, for acute lymphoblastic leukemia in children, 423
  for aggressive lymphoma, 436t
  for anti–glomerular basement membrane disease, 679
  for aplastic anemia, 352, 353
  for breast cancer, 1027, 1029
  for bullous pemphigoid, 828
  for chronic lymphocytic leukemia, 431
  for cicatricial pemphigoid, 813, 828
  for cutaneous vasculitis, 780
  for Fanconi's anemia, 355
  for focal segmental glomerulosclerosis, 678
  for highly aggressive lymphoma, 438t
  for Hodgkin's disease, 407t

Cyclophosphamide *(Continued)*
  for immune thrombocytopenic purpura, 400
  for indolent B cell lymphoma, 435t
  for juvenile rheumatoid arthritis, 955t, 957
  for lupus erythematosus, 776
  for membranous glomerulopathy, 678
  for multiple myeloma, 442, 443
  for multiple sclerosis, 900
  for myasthenia gravis, 907
  for nerve infarction, 930
  for pauci-immune glomerulonephritis, 679–680
  for pemphigus, 827
  for primary glomerular disease, 676
  for sarcoidosis, 226, 228
  for Sézary's syndrome, 769
  for toxic epidermal necrolysis, 825
  for warm antibody autoimmune hemolytic anemia, 362
  in CHOP regimen, for aggressive lymphoma, 436t
    for indolent B cell lymphoma, 435t
    for Sézary's syndrome, 769
  in CVP regimen, for chronic lymphocytic leukemia, 431
    for indolent B cell lymphoma, 435t
Cyclospora infection, 77, 539t, 542–543
Cyclosporine, drug interactions with, 676–677
  anticonvulsants, 863t
  antifungals, 194, 196, 200, 807
  HMG-CoA reductase inhibitors, 581–582
  for aplastic anemia, 353
  for autoimmune hepatitis, 469
  for autoimmune urticaria, 836
  for epidermolysis bullosa acquisita, 829
  for focal segmental glomerulosclerosis, 678
  for inflammatory bowel disease, 485–486
  for juvenile rheumatoid arthritis, 955t, 957
  for membranous glomerulopathy, 678
  for minimal change disease, 678
  for myasthenia gravis, 907
  for oral lichen planus, 811
  for paroxysmal nocturnal hemoglobinuria, 366
  for primary glomerular disease, 676–677
  for psoriasis, 772
  for rheumatoid arthritis, 946t, 950, 951
  for sarcoidosis, 226
  for scleroderma, 778
  for Sézary's syndrome, 770
  for toxic epidermal necrolysis, 825
  for warm antibody autoimmune hemolytic anemia, 362
  gingival hyperplasia due to, 813
  gout due to, 578
  hair growth in response to, in alopecia areata, 762
  reference intervals for, 1210t
Cyproheptadine, for allergic rhinitis, 745t
  for Cushing's syndrome, 623
  for pain, 3
  for pruritus, 37
  for serotonin syndrome with MAO inhibitors, 1191
Cyproterone acetate, for acne, 759
  for hirsutism, 763
Cyst(s), Baker's, 965
  Bartholin's duct, 1071
  colloid, 941
  eruption, 814

Cyst(s) *(Continued)*
  mucous, digital, 781t, 783
  vocal fold, 25–26
Cystectomy, for bladder cancer, 709
Cysteine, urine, reference intervals for, 1211t
Cystic fibrosis, 176–180
  carrier screening for, during pregnancy, 980
  complications of, 178–180, 179t
  cough due to, 23, 25
  diagnosis of, 176
  maintenance therapy for, nutritional, 177–178, 177t
  pulmonary, 176–177, 176t
Cysticercosis, 541t, 546
Cystine, urine, reference intervals for, 1211t
Cystinuria, amino acid malabsorption in, 514
  urinary stones due to, 715
Cystitis, in girls, 668
  in men, 661–662
  in women, 663, 664t
  recurrent, in girls, 668
  in women, 664t, 665
Cystogram, in bladder injury evaluation, 684
Cystometrics, in urinary incontinence evaluation, 672
Cystosarcoma phyllodes, 1023
Cystoscopy, in urethral stricture assessment, 711
Cytarabine (ara-C), for acute lymphoblastic leukemia in children, 423
  for acute myelogenous leukemia, 416, 417
    in elderly persons, 418
  for acute nonlymphocytic leukemia in children, 424
  for aggressive lymphoma, 436t
  for central nervous system leukemia, 424
  for chronic myelogenous leukemia, 428–429
  for highly aggressive lymphoma, 438t
Cytarabine ocfosate, for chronic myelogenous leukemia, 429
Cytomegalovirus infection, 802
  in HIV infection, 53–54
  peripheral neuropathy in, 927–928
  pneumonia due to, 215, 215t, 216t
  transmission of, by blood components, 457, 461
Cytosine arabinoside. See *Cytarabine (ara-C).*

Dacarbazine, for Hodgkin's disease, 407t
Dactylitis, in sickle cell disease, 376
Dalteparin, for deep venous thrombosis prophylaxis, 222t
Danazol, for C1 esterase inhibitor deficiency, 837
  for endometriosis, 1031–1032, 1033, 1034t
  for fibrocystic disease of breast, 1023
  for immune thrombocytopenic purpura, 400
  for warm antibody autoimmune hemolytic anemia, 362
  levothyroxine interaction with, 644
Dantrolene, for malignant hyperthermia, 1152t

Dantrolene (Continued)
 in monoamine oxidase inhibitor overdose, 1191
 for neuroleptic malignant syndrome,
  1198
 for spasticity, after stroke, 856
  in multiple sclerosis, 902
 for tetanus, 136
Dapsone, for aphthous stomatitis, 812
 for brown recluse spider bite, 1137–1138
 for cicatricial pemphigoid, 813
 for cutaneous vasculitis, 779–780
 for dermatitis herpetiformis, 829
 for leprosy, 92
 for lupus erythematosus, 776
 for Pneumocystis carinii pneumonia in
  HIV infection, 51
  prophylactic, 51
 for toxoplasmosis, 153
  in HIV infection, 156
 for toxoplasmosis prophylaxis, 154
  in HIV infection, 52
 for urticarial vasculitis, 837
Darier's disease, oral lesions in, 811
Daunorubicin, for acute lymphoblastic
  leukemia in children, 423
 for acute nonlymphocytic leukemia in
  children, 424
Day care, adult, in Alzheimer's disease,
  845
Daydreaming, seizure vs., 868t
DDAVP. See Desmopressin (DDAVP).
ddC (zalcitabine), for HIV infection, 45,
  48t
ddI. See Didanosine (ddI).
De Quervain's disease, 965
Débridement, for clostridial myonecrosis,
  797
 for necrotizing fasciitis, 798
 for necrotizing skin and soft tissue infections, 82
 for pressure ulcers, 819–820
 for synergistic necrotizing cellulitis, 796
Decongestants, for allergic rhinitis,
  745–746
 for rhinosinusitis, 234
Decontamination, in acute poisoning,
  1147–1149, 1148t
Decortication, for empyema, 202, 202
Deep brain stimulation, for Parkinson's
  disease, 923–924, 923t
Deep venous thrombosis. See Venous
  thrombosis.
Deferipone, iron chelation using, for
  transfusional hemosiderosis in
  thalassemia, 372
Deferoxamine, iron chelation using, for
  iron overdose, 1152t, 1180–1181
 for transfusional hemosiderosis in thalassemia, 372
Defibrillation, for cardiac arrest, 251–253,
  252, 253
 for ventricular fibrillation after myocardial infarction, 324
 with biphasic waveforms, 256
Defibrillator. See also Cardioverter-
  defibrillator.
 automated external, 251–253, 253
 implantable atrial, 260
Degenerative joint disease, 967–970
 diagnosis of, 968
 prevention of, 969
 treatment of, 968–970
Dehydration, clinical evaluation of,
  610–611, 610t
 in cholera, categorization of, 72

Dehydration (Continued)
 in food-borne illness, 76
 in infants and children, hypernatremic,
  611, 611, 612–613
  hyponatremic, 609t, 611, 611, 612
  isotonic, 611–612, 611
  parenteral fluid therapy for, 609–613,
   610t, 611
  oral rehydration therapy for. See Oral
   rehydration therapy.
Dehydroepiandrosterone, urine, reference
  intervals for, 1211t
Delavirdine (DLV), drug interactions with,
  45
  antituberculars, 52
 for HIV infection, 46t, 47, 49t
Delirium, 1105–1107, 1106t, 1107t
Dementia, delirium vs., 1106t
 evaluation for, 845
 HIV-associated, 55
 treatment of, 845–846
Demyelinating polyradiculoneuropathy,
  inflammatory, acute, 929
  influenza vaccine and, 87
  chronic, 929–930
Demyelination, peripheral neuropathies
  with, 928
Dental appliances, for obstructive sleep-
  disordered breathing, 183–184
 for temporomandibular disorders, 961,
  962–963
Dental care, for mouth disease, 808
 in hemophilia, 396
Dental sinus, 814
Dentures, papillary hyperplasia of palate
  due to, 811
 sore mouth due to, 816
2-Deoxycoformycin, for Sézary's syndrome,
  769
Dependence, physical, defined, 4
 psychological. See also Drug abuse; specific substances.
  defined, 4
Depressants. See also specific drugs.
 central nervous system, toxic effects of,
  1149t
Depression, 1107–1116
 after stroke, 856
 chronic fatigue syndrome vs., 112
 diagnosis of, 1108
 differential diagnosis of, 1108
 epidemiology of, 1108
 fibromyalgia and, 966–967
 in Alzheimer's disease, 847
 in multiple sclerosis, 901
 in Parkinson's disease, 922–923
 insomnia and, 33
 postpartum, 1001
 treatment of, 1108–1116, 1109t, 1110t,
  1112, 1113t, 1115t
  clinical guidelines for, 1114–1116,
   1115t
Dermatitis, atopic. See Atopic dermatitis.
 cercarial, 804–805, 804t
 chronic, mycosis fungoides vs., 766
 clonal, mycosis fungoides and, 767
 contact, 830–831
  limb, 817
 otitis externa due to, 115
 seborrheic, 773
  hair loss with, 762
Dermatitis herpetiformis, 829
Dermatobia hominis, 804t, 805
Dermatographism, symptomatic, 834
Dermatomyositis, 776–777
Dermatophytosis, 806–807

Dermatophytosis (Continued)
 hair loss due to, 762
 of nails, 780, 781, 807
Desensitization, for drug allergy, 751–752
 phototherapy, for solar urticaria, 836
Designer stimulants, intoxication with,
  1095, 1163
Desipramine, for anxiety disorders, 1100t,
  1101–1102
 for attention-deficit/hyperactivity disorder, 873, 873t
 for cocaine abuse, 1094
 for depression, 1109t
 for pain, 3
 intoxication with, 1201, 1202t
 pharmacodynamic effects of, 1110t
 reference intervals for, 1210t
Desmopressin (DDAVP), for bleeding in
  acute renal failure, 699
 for diabetes insipidus, 625, 626, 626t
 for dysfunctional uterine bleeding in von
  Willebrand disease, 1039–1040
 for nocturnal enuresis, 670–671
 for platelet-mediated bleeding disorders,
  399
 for von Willebrand disease, 395
Desonide, for atopic dermatitis, 822
 for lichen simplex chronicus, 834
Desquamative gingivitis, chronic, 814
Detrusor hyperreflexia, urinary
  incontinence with, 671
Detrusor-sphincter dyssynergia, in
  children, 669–670
 in multiple sclerosis, 902
Dew itch. See Hookworms.
Dexamethasone, anticonvulsant
  interactions with, 863t
 during pregnancy with congenital adrenal hyperplasia risk, 984
 for acute chest syndrome in sickle cell
  disease, 377
 for aggressive lymphoma, 436t
 for asthma exacerbations in children,
  741
 for atopic dermatitis, 822
 for bacterial meningitis, 107–108
 for HELLP syndrome, 993
 for high-altitude cerebral edema, 1128,
  1128t
 for highly aggressive lymphoma, 438t
 for immune thrombocytopenic purpura,
  400
 for intracranial hypertension in encephalitis, 896
 for mountain sickness, 1128, 1128t
 for multiple myeloma, 442
 for nausea and vomiting, 8t
  due to chemotherapy, 9–10, 10t
 for pertussis, 139
 for secondary adrenal insufficiency, 637
 for skin disease in sarcoidosis, 227
 for spinal cord compression in multiple
  myeloma, 444
 for thyroid storm, 648
 for typhoid meningitis, 164
 prefilled syringes with, for home use in
  chronic adrenal insufficiency, 621,
  621t
 with ketoconazole, for Cushing's syndrome, 623
Dexamethasone-tobramycin, for draining
  ear, 207t
Dextroamphetamine, for attention-deficit/
  hyperactivity disorder, 872, 873t
 for fatigue in Parkinson's disease, 923
 for pain, 3

Dextroamphetamine *(Continued)*
  intoxication with, 1095, 1163
Dextromethorphan, for cough, 24
  for viral respiratory infection, 214
  intoxication with, 1191, 1192, 1192t
Dextrose, for ischemic stroke, 852
  in fluid therapy, for high-risk neonate, 1011
    for infants and children, 608
  in parenteral nutrition solutions, 604, 605t
Diabetes insipidus, 624–627, 626t
Diabetes mellitus. See also *Diabetic ketoacidosis.*
  classification of, 549–550, 550t
  diagnostic criteria for, 549–550, 550t
  due to protease inhibitors, 47
  during pregnancy, 982
  epidemiology of, 549
  gestational, 982
    screening for, 550
  hormone replacement therapy and, 1048
  in chronic pancreatitis, 521
  in cystic fibrosis, 178–180
  malignant otitis externa in, 114
  maturity-onset, of youth, genetic muta-tion in, 550
  niacin use in, 583
  oral contraceptives and, 1086t
  osteomyelitis in, 971, 972
    microbiologic diagnosis of, 973
    treatment of, 973–974
  peripheral neuropathies in, 565, 925, 931
  type 1, 566–572
    adult-onset, 575
    intercurrent illness management in, 571–572, 575–576
    outpatient care in, 571
      to avoid ketoacidosis, 575–576
    treatment of, goals of, 568
      initial, 567–568
      long-term, 568–572
  type 2, 549–566
    complications of, hemoglobin A$_{1c}$ levels and, 554
      macrovascular, 562–563, 562t
      microvascular, 563–566
    insulin resistance in, 551–552
    ketoacidosis in, 574–575
    pathophysiology of, 550–551
    screening for, 550
    treatment of, 552–566
      combination therapy in, 561–562, *562*
      for cardiovascular risk factors, 562–563, 562t
      for microvascular complications, 563–566
      goals for, 553–554, 554t
      nonpharmacologic, 554–556
      pharmacologic, 556–562, *557*, 557t, *562*
      standards of care for, 554, 555t
      team approach in, 552–553
Diabetic amyotrophy, 565
Diabetic ketoacidosis, 572–576
  during pregnancy, 574
  hospital discharge preparation in, 575
  in children, 566–567
    treatment of, 567–568
  in type 2 diabetes, 574–575
  initial evaluation of, 572–573, *573*, 573t
  treatment of, 573–574, 574t
Diabetic retinopathy, 563–564
Diacetylmorphine (heroin), intoxication with, 1095–1096, 1191, 1192t

Dialysis. See also *Hemodialysis; Peritoneal dialysis.*
  for acute poisoning, 1150–1156, 1156t
  gastrointestinal, for acute poisoning, 1148
Diaminodiphenylsulfone. See *Dapsone.*
Diaphragm (contraceptive device), 1078t, 1084
Diaphragmatic flutter, hiccup vs., 13
Diarrhea, acute, defined, 15
  differential diagnosis of, 15
    infectious, 15–18, 17t
    nutritional aspects of, 17–18
  antibiotic-associated, 15
  chronic, antidepressants for use in, 1115t
  defined, 15
  diabetic, 565
  due to parasites, diagnosis of, 15–16
  in cholera, 72
  in food-borne illness, inflammatory, 77–78
    noninflammatory, 76–77
    treatment of, 76
  in inflammatory bowel disease, selection of therapy for, 482
  in travelers, 150
    diagnosis of, 15
    prophylaxis of, 17, 150
    treatment of, 16–17, 76, 150
Diazepam, as antidote, 1152t
  for alcohol withdrawal, 1093, 1177
  for amphetamine intoxication, 1163
  for antidepressant intoxication, 1202
  for black widow spider bite, 1138
  for cocaine intoxication, 1172, 1173
  for febrile seizure prevention, 869
  for isoniazid intoxication, 1182
  for Meniere's disease, 893
  for nausea and vomiting, 8t
  for panic disorder, 1121t
  for phencyclidine intoxication, 1195
  for spasticity in multiple sclerosis, 901
  for status epilepticus, 865
    in infants and children, 870t, 871
  for tetanus, 136
  intoxication with, 1166
  withdrawal from, 1096
Dichloroethylene, 1179
Dichlorophenazone-isometheptene, for migraine, 881
Diclofenac, adverse effects of, 969
  for dysmenorrhea, 1043t
  for pain, 2
Diclofenac-misoprostol, 500
Dicloxacillin, for atopic dermatitis, 823
  for breast abscess, 1023
  for mastitis, 1000
Dicyclomine, for colonic diverticulosis, 481
Didanosine (ddI), for HIV infection, 46t, 48t
  hydroxyurea interaction with, 45, 50
  pancreatitis due to, 47
Dientamoeba fragilis infection, 539t, 543
Diet. See also *Nutrition;* specific nutrients.
  after myocardial infarction, 332
  chemically defined, for short-bowel syn-drome, 511
  colonic diverticulosis and, 481
  colorectal cancer and, 533
  diverticulitis and, 482
  for abetalipoproteinemia, 512
  for acute renal failure, 698
  for anal fissure, 494
  for aphthous stomatitis, 812
  for ascites in cirrhosis, 469

Diet *(Continued)*
  for chronic fatigue syndrome, 112
  for chronic pancreatitis, 521
  for chronic renal failure, 702–703, 704, 704t
  for cirrhosis, 468
  for congestive heart failure, 292
  for constipation, 18
  for cystic fibrosis, 177
  for dermatitis herpetiformis, 829
  for gaseousness, 12
  for gastroesophageal reflux disease, 525
  for gluten-sensitive enteropathy, 511
  for hypercalciuria, 715
  for hyperlipidemia, 580
  for hyperoxaluria, 715
  for hypertension, 305
  for inflammatory bowel disease, 486
  for irritable bowel syndrome, 491
  for juvenile rheumatoid arthritis, 958
  for Meniere's disease, 888, 893
  for mouth disease, 808
  for nephrogenic diabetes insipidus, 627
  for obesity, 588–590
  for premenstrual syndrome, 1046, 1046t
  for primary glomerular disease, 677
  for type 1 diabetes, 570
  for type 2 diabetes, 554–556
  in medical management of primary hyperparathyroidism, 630
  ketogenic, for epilepsy, 865
    in infants and children, 869, 870
  migraine and, 880, 889, 890t
  perineal pruritus and, 834
  pressure ulcers and, 819
  rheumatoid arthritis and, 952
Diethylcarbamazine, for loiasis, 804t
Diethylpropion, for obesity, 591, 591t
Diethylstilbestrol, for breast cancer, 1028
  for emergency contraception, 1087
Diffuse esophageal spasm, dysphagia due to, 475, 478
Diflunisal, for dysmenorrhea, 1043t
DiGeorge's syndrome, truncus arteriosus in, 286
Digital rectal examination, in prostate cancer screening, 706
Digitalis. See also *Digitoxin; Digoxin.*
  intoxication with, 1174–1175
Digitoxin, intoxication with, 1174–1175
  reference intervals for, 1210t
Digoxin, antifungal interactions with, 196, 200, 807
  bile acid resin interaction with, 582
  for arrhythmia in mitral valve prolapse, 290
  for atrial fibrillation, 257, 258, 258t, 259, 259t
    after myocardial infarction, 323
  for atrial flutter, 275t
  for congestive heart failure, 294t, 295–296
  for Jarisch-Herxheimer reaction in re-lapsing fever, 124
  intoxication with, 1174–1175
  reference intervals for, 1210t
Digoxin-specific Fab antibodies, for digitalis intoxication, 1152t–1153t, 1175
Dihydroergotamine, for migraine, 881
Diiodohydroxyquin. See *Iodoquinol.*
Dilated cardiomyopathy, causes of, 291–292
Diloxanide furoate, for amebiasis, 58, 58t, 59t, 539t, 542
  for diarrhea, 16

Diltiazem, anticonvulsant interactions
    with, 863t
  for angina, 249
  for atrial fibrillation, 257, 258t
  for atrial flutter, 275t
  for atrial premature beats, 261
  for childhood dermatomyositis, 777
  for hypertension, 308t, 310
  intoxication with, 1168, 1169
  relative antiarrhythmic efficacy of, 262t
Dilution, for acute poisoning, 1149
Dilutional coagulopathy, with massive
    transfusion, 461
Dimenhydrinate, for motion sickness, 886t,
    890
  intoxication with, 1164
D-Dimer, in pulmonary thromboembolism
    workup, 221
  reference intervals for, 1207t
Dimercaprol (BAL), as antidote, 1153t
  for lead poisoning, 1185–1187, 1186t
Dimercaptosuccinic acid, for lead
    poisoning, 1186–1187, 1186t
Dinitrochlorobenzene (DNCB), for warts,
    786
Diphenhydramine, as antidote, 1153t
  for neuroleptic intoxication, 1198
  for allergic reaction to blood components,
    460
  for allergic rhinitis, 745, 745t
  for anaphylaxis, 727t
    due to insect sting, 753, 754
  for aphthous stomatitis, 812
  for atopic dermatitis, 822
  for childhood dermatomyositis, 777
  for contact stomatitis, 816
  for erythema multiforme, 813
  for mouth disease, 808
  for mycosis fungoides, 768
  for nausea and vomiting, 8t
  for ordinary urticaria, 836
  for pruritic urticarial papules and
      plaques of pregnancy, 831–832
  for pruritus, 37
  intoxication with, 1097, 1164
Diphenoxylate, for diarrhea in diabetes,
    565
  intoxication with, 1191, 1192t
Diphenoxylate-atropine, for diarrhea in
    food-borne illness, 76
  for radiation enteritis, 511
Diphtheria, risk of, for travelers, 148
Diphtheria toxin–interleukin 2 fusion
    protein, for Sézary's syndrome, 769
Diphtheria toxoid. See Tetanus-diphtheria
    toxoid.
Diphtheria-tetanus-pertussis vaccines,
    135, 139, 140, 141, 144t
  in tetanus management, 135
Diphyllobothrium latum infection, 541t,
    546
Dipivefrin, for glaucoma, 913
Diplophonia, defined, 25
Dipylidium caninum infection, 541t, 546
Dipyridamole, for stroke prevention, 855
Dirithromycin, for legionellosis, 218
Disabilities, contraceptive choice and,
    source of information on, 1089
Disaccharidase inhibitors. See also specific
    drugs.
  for type 2 diabetes, 557t, 559
Discoid lupus erythematosus, 774
  hair loss in, 762
  oral lesions in, 813
  treatment of, 775–776
Disk herniation, lumbar, 40

Dislocation, of interphalangeal joints of
    fingers, 977
  shoulder, 976
Disopyramide, for atrial fibrillation, 260
  for atrial flutter, 275t
  for hypertrophic cardiomyopathy, 349
  reference intervals for, 1210t
  relative antiarrhythmic efficacy of, 262t
Dissecting cellulitis of scalp, 762
Disseminated intravascular coagulation,
    400–402
  due to hemolytic transfusion reaction,
    459
  in acute leukemia, 415
  testing for, with antepartum hemor-
    rhage, 987
  vitamin K deficiency vs., 592, 592t
  with placental abruption, 402, 988
Distal intestinal obstruction syndrome, in
    cystic fibrosis, 178, 179t
Disulfiram, anticonvulsant interactions
    with, 863t
Diuresis, for acute poisoning, 1150
Diuretics. See also specific drugs.
  bile acid resin interaction with, 582
  for congestive heart failure, 293, 294t
  for diabetes insipidus, 626–627
  for hypercalciuria, 715
  for hypertension, 307, 308t
    during pregnancy, 990, 990t
  for hypertrophic cardiomyopathy, 349
  for hypervolemia in chronic renal fail-
    ure, 704
  NSAID interference with, 293
  renal calcium handling and, 634
Divalproex, adverse effects of, 863t
  for acute mania, 1117
  for epilepsy, 860t, 862t
  pharmacokinetics of, 862t
Diverticulitis, 481–482
Diverticulum(a), alimentary tract, 479–482
  esophageal, 478, 479–480
    dysphagia due to, 474
Dizziness. See also Vertigo.
  medications for, 886t
DLV. See Delavirdine (DLV).
DNAse I, recombinant, for cystic fibrosis,
    25, 176t, 177
DNCB (dinitrochlorobenzene), for warts,
    786
Dobutamine, for cardiogenic shock after
    myocardial infarction, 326
  for ciguatera poisoning, 1143
  for congestive heart failure, 294t, 296
Docetaxel, for breast cancer, 1029
Docusate, for constipation, 19, 19t
  with opioid therapy, 5
Dolasetron, for nausea and vomiting, 8t
Domestic violence, during pregnancy, 983
  premenstrual syndrome and, 1045
Domoic acid poisoning, 79, 80t
Domperidone, for gastroparesis in
    diabetes, 565
  with carbidopa-levodopa therapy for
    Parkinson's disease, 920
Donath-Landsteiner antibodies, in
    paroxysmal cold hemoglobinuria, 361
Done nomogram, for salicylate
    intoxication, 1200, 1201
Donepezil, for Alzheimer's disease, 846
Donovanosis, 721–722
Dopamine, for anaphylaxis, 727t
  for cardiogenic shock after myocardial
      infarction, 326
  for ciguatera poisoning, 1143
  for congestive heart failure, 293, 294t,
      296

Dopamine (Continued)
  for hypotension in high-risk neonate,
    1013
Dopamine agonists. See also specific drugs.
  for Parkinson's disease, 918–919, 919t,
    921
Dopamine receptors, antidepressants'
    action at, 1110t, 1112
  clinical consequences of, 1113t, 11113
  antipsychotic drugs' action at, 1118
  neurologic side effects and, 1119
Dornase alfa, for cystic fibrosis, 25, 176t,
    177
Dorzolamide, for glaucoma, 913
Dorzolamide-timolol, for glaucoma, 913
Douching, for contraception, 1077t
Down syndrome, atrioventricular septal
    defect in, 282
Doxazosin, for benign prostatic
    hyperplasia, 688
  for chronic occlusive arterial disease due
      to blunt trauma, 339
  for chronic pelvic pain syndrome, 687
  for hypertension, 307–309, 308t
    in type 2 diabetes, 563
  for pheochromocytoma, 655
Doxepin, for atopic dermatitis, 822
  for chronic fatigue syndrome, 112
  for contact dermatitis, 830
  for depression, 1109t
  for insomnia, 35
  for lichen simplex chronicus, 834
  for ordinary urticaria, 836
  for pruritus, 36, 37
  for rheumatoid arthritis, 947
  intoxication with, 1097, 1201, 1202t
  pharmacodynamic effects of, 1110t
Doxorubicin, for aggressive lymphoma,
    436t
  for bladder cancer, 709
  for breast cancer, 1027, 1029
  for gastric adenocarcinoma, 530
  for highly aggressive lymphoma, 438t
  for Hodgkin's disease, 407t
    side effects of, 408
  for indolent B cell lymphoma, 435t
  for multiple myeloma, 442
  for recurrent endometrial cancer, 1065
  for Sézary's syndrome, 769
  for transitional cell carcinoma, 709
  in CHOP regimen, for aggressive lym-
      phoma, 436t
    for indolent B cell lymphoma, 435t
    for Sézary's syndrome, 769
Doxycycline, for acne, 758
  for amebiasis, 58–59, 59t
  for bacillary angiomatosis, 158t
  for bacterial pneumonia, 212, 212t
  for brucellosis, 64, 65, 65t, 66
  for chlamydial infection, 719, 1057,
    1057t
    for conjunctivitis, 68
  for cholera, 74t
  for chronic pelvic pain syndrome, 687
  for donovanosis, 721
  for ehrlichiosis, 166, 166t
  for enterotoxigenic Escherichia coli infec-
      tion, 77, 77t
  for epididymitis, 662, 674
  for legionellosis, 217, 217t, 218
  for Lyme disease, 127, 128t, 129t
  for lymphogranuloma venereum, 722
  for malaria, 96, 97t
    prophylactic, 100t, 101, 149
  for mycoplasmal pneumonia, 216
  for nongonococcal urethritis, 721

Doxycycline (Continued)
  for pelvic inflammatory disease, 719t, 1059t
  for plague prophylaxis, 116
  for psittacosis, 117
  for Q fever, 118
  for relapsing fever, 124
    prophylactic, 125
  for Rocky Mountain spotted fever, 165–166, 166t
  for syphilis, 724t
  for toxoplasmosis, 154
  for urinary tract infection in men, 661
  in children, tooth-staining and, 166
Dracunculus medinensis, skin disease due to, 804t
Dressings, for pressure ulcers, 820
Dressler's syndrome, 328
Driving, after stroke, 854
Dronabinol, for AIDS-related weight loss, 56
  for nausea and vomiting, 8t
    due to chemotherapy, 10
Drooling, in Parkinson's disease, 922
Drop attacks, seizure vs., 857
Droperidol, for Meniere's disease, 893
  for nausea and vomiting, 8t
Drowning, cold-water, 1133–1134
Drug(s). See Medications; specific drugs and classes of drugs.
Drug abuse, 1093–1098. See also specific substances.
  in bulimia nervosa, 1103
  lead poisoning due to, 1184
  stimulant therapy for attention-deficit/hyperactivity disorder and, 873
Drug testing, 1094, 1160
d4T (stavudine), for HIV infection, 45, 48t
DUMBELS mnemonic, 1193–1194
Dumping syndrome, after gastrectomy, 512–513
Duodenal diverticula, 480
Duodenal ulcers. See also Peptic ulcer disease.
  dyspepsia and, 496
Duodenitis, defined, 496
Dust mites, control of, for allergic rhinitis, 744
  for asthma, 731
Dysembryoplastic neuroepithelial tumor, 941
Dysentery, amebic. See Amebiasis.
  bacterial, amebiasis vs., 57, 57t
Dysfunctional uterine bleeding, 1037–1040
  defined, 1037
  differential diagnosis of, 1038, 1039t
  pathophysiology of, 1037–1038
  treatment of, 1038–1040, 1039t
Dyskeratosis congenita, 355
  oral lesions in, 812
Dyskinesia, due to Parkinson's disease treatment, 921–922
  early, tetanus vs., 135
  tardive, antidepressants for use in, 1115t
Dysmenorrhea, 1043–1044, 1043t, 1044t
Dyspepsia, 11, 496–497, 497t
  clinical approach to, 497–498, 497
  functional (nonulcer), defined, 11, 496
    irritable bowel syndrome and, 11, 488
  ulcers and, 11, 496
Dysphagia, 473–479
  after stroke, 855–856
  causes of, 473–475, 473t, 474t
  diagnosis of, 475–477, 475, 476
  treatment of, 477–478

Dysphonia. See also Hoarseness.
  muscle tension, 28–29
  spasmodic, 28
  with inhaled corticosteroids for asthma, 732
Dysplastic nevus, 789, 793
Dystonia, due to haloperidol, 876
  in neuroleptic intoxication, 1196, 1198

EAP regimen, for gastric adenocarcinoma, 530
Eastern encephalitis virus, 896
Echinococcosis, 541t, 546–547
Echocardiography, in acute myocardial infarction diagnosis, 319
  in hypertrophic cardiomyopathy diagnosis, 348
  in mitral valve prolapse, 287–288, 289
  transesophageal, for atrial thrombus identification, before cardioversion in atrial fibrillation, 259
  in pulmonary thromboembolism workup, 221
Echovirus, meningitis due to, 895
Eclampsia, 994, 994t
  defined, 991
Econazole, for tinea infection, 807
Ecthyma contagiosum, 803
Ecthyma gangrenosum, 796t, 798
Ectopic pregnancy, 985–986, 985t, 986t
  after tubal ligation, 1088
Eczema herpeticum, 801
Edema, cerebral. See Cerebral edema.
  heat, 1135, 1136t
  post-thrombotic, elastic compression for, 343–344
  pulmonary, acute, after myocardial infarction, 325, 327t
    high-altitude, 1128–1129, 1128t
  Reinke's, 26
Edetate calcium disodium, for lead poisoning, 1185–1187, 1186t
Edrophonium test, in myasthenia gravis, 904–905
Eels, electric, 1144
  toxic, 1144
Efavirenz (EFV), 1215t
  antitubercular drug interaction with, 52
  for HIV infection, 45t, 46t, 49t
  toxic effects of, 47
Ehrlichiosis, 165–166, 166t
  Lyme disease with, 127
Elbow, bursitis of, 964–965
  sports injuries to, 976
  tendinitis of, 965, 976
Electric fish, 1144
Electrical injury, 1126
Electrical stimulation, for stress incontinence, 673
  for urgency incontinence, 672
Electrocardiography, in acute myocardial infarction diagnosis, 318
  intracardiac, normal findings on, 265, 266
Electrocoagulation, for hemorrhoids, 493
Electrocochleography, in Meniere's disease diagnosis, 892
Electroconvulsive therapy, for depression, 1108, 1116
  in Parkinson's disease, 923
Electrodesiccation, for oral warts, 817
  for skin cancer, 764
Electrodiagnostic testing, in myasthenia gravis, 905

Electroencephalography, in seizure evaluation, 860
  in infants and children, 867
Electrolysis, for hair removal, 763
Electrolytes. See also specific electrolytes.
  in parenteral nutrition solutions, 604, 605t
  requirements for, for infants and children, 608, 608t
Electromyography, in facial paralysis diagnosis, 916–917
Electromyolysis, for leiomyomata, 1062
Electroneurography, in facial paralysis diagnosis, 916–917
Electrophysiologic study, in heart block evaluation, 268
  in monomorphic ventricular tachycardia, 278
Electrotherapy, for pressure ulcers, 820
Elliptocytosis, hereditary, 364
EMB. See Ethambutol (EMB).
Embolism. See also Atheroembolism; Thromboembolism.
  air, with central catheter placement, 606
  guide wire, with central catheter placement, 606
  in infective endocarditis, 299
  pulmonary. See Pulmonary embolism.
Embolization, uterine artery, for leiomyomata, 1062–1063
Emesis. See Vomiting.
Emphysema, 171, 171. See also Chronic obstructive pulmonary disease.
  chronic pulmonary histoplasmosis in, 195, 198
  surgery for, 175
Employment, after stroke, 854
  breast-feeding and, 1019
  lead exposure in, 1183–1184, 1183t, 1184t
Empyema, 202, 202
  spontaneous bacterial, in cirrhosis, 470
Enalapril, after myocardial infarction, 331
  for congestive heart failure, 294t
  for hypertension, 309t
  for primary glomerular disease, 677
Encephalitis, Japanese, 896
  vaccine for, for travelers, 147t, 148
  measles, 133
  meningitis vs., 895
  tetanus vs., 135
  tick-borne, vaccine for, for travelers, 148
  toxoplasmosis, in HIV infection, 52–53, 151
    central nervous system lymphoma vs., 55
    treatment of, 156–157
  varicella, 70
  viral, 894–896
Encephalomalacia, diffuse cystic, after viral encephalitis, 896
Encephalomyelitis, in Lyme disease, 129t
Encephalopathy, hepatic. See Hepatic encephalopathy.
  hypoxic-ischemic, in neonate, 1014
  in Bartonella henselae infection, 157
  lead, 1184–1185
    treatment of, 1186
  pertussis, 137–138
  subacute or chronic, in Lyme disease, 126, 129t
Endocardial cushion defect, 282
Endocarditis, culture-negative, antibiotics for, 300t
  causes of, 297–298, 299
  infective. See Infective endocarditis.

Endolymphatic sac surgery, for Meniere's disease, 888, 894
Endometrial cancer, 1063–1066
  breast cancer and, 1024
  diagnosis of, 1063
  epidemiology of, 1063
  follow-up in, 1065
  hormone replacement therapy and, 1048, 1063, 1063t, 1065–1066
  recurrent, treatment of, 1065
  risk factors for, 1063, 1063t
  staging of, 1064, 1064t
  tamoxifen and, 1063–1064
  treatment of, 1064–1065
Endometriomas, 1037
Endometriosis, 1029–1037
  clinical presentation of, 1030
  defined, 1030
  diagnosis of, 1030–1031
  incidence and prevalence of, 1030
  laparoscopy in, 1031, 1032
  pathophysiology of, 1030
  sources of information on, 1033
  treatment of, 1031–1033
    algorithm for, *1036,* 1037
    outcomes comparisons for, 1033–1037, *1034,* 1034t, 1035t
Endometritis. See also *Pelvic inflammatory disease.*
  chlamydial, 1056
Endomyometritis, postpartum, 1000–1001
Endophthalmitis, after glaucoma surgery, 915
Endorectal advancement flap repair, for anorectal fistula, 495
Endoscopic retrograde cholangiopancreatography, for choledocholithiasis, 465
  in chronic pancreatitis, 520
Endovascular stent placement, for abdominal aortic aneurysm, 244
Enemas, for constipation, 20
  for fecal impaction, 18–19
Energy requirements, in parenteral nutrition, 601
  for high-risk neonate, 1012
Enflurane, for obstetric anesthesia, 998
Enoxaparin. See also *Heparin, low-molecular-weight.*
  for deep venous thrombosis, 342
    prophylactic, 222t
  for femoral-popliteal vein thrombosis, 345
  for lichen planus, 773
Entamoeba dispar, 56, 542
  Entamoeba histolytica vs., 57
Entamoeba histolytica. See *Amebiasis.*
Enteral feeding. See also *Nutritional support.*
  for head injury, 935
  for high-risk neonate, 1012
  gastrostomy, nighttime, for cystic fibrosis, 178
  parenteral nutrition vs., 602
  pressure ulcers and, 819
Enteric fever, 161. See also *Typhoid fever.*
Enteritis. See also *Enterocolitis; Gastroenteritis.*
  due to chemotherapy toxicity, parenteral nutrition for, 603
  radiation, after cervical cancer treatment, 1068
    malabsorption due to, 511
    parenteral nutrition for, 603
Enterobius vermicularis infection, 540t, 544
Enterocolitis. See also *Enteritis.*

Enterocolitis *(Continued)*
  necrotizing, in newborn, 1015–1016
    with intensive chemotherapy for leukemia, 419
Enterovirus infection, meningitis due to, 895
  pneumonia due to, 215, 215t, 216t
Enthesitis, in ankylosing spondylitis, 958
Entrapment neuropathies, 930
Enuresis, childhood, 668–671
Envenomation, by marine animals, 1142–1143
  by scorpions, 1138
  by snakes, 1139–1141
  by spiders, 1137–1138
  decontamination procedures for, 1147
Enzymatic débridement, for pressure ulcers, 819–820
Eosinophilia, nonallergic rhinitis with, 743t, 744
Eosinophilia-myalgia syndrome, 81
Eosinophilic gastroenteritis, 513
Ependymoma, 941
Ephedrine, for anaphylaxis, 727t
  for hiccup, 14t
Ephelides, 839
Epicondylitis of elbow, 965, 976
Epidermodysplasia verruciformis, 792
Epidermoid cysts, vocal fold, 25–26
Epidermolysis bullosa acquisita, 828–829
Epidermophyton floccosum. See *Dermatophytosis.*
Epididymitis, 674–675
  urinary tract infection and, 662
Epidural analgesia, continuous lumbar, for labor, 996
Epidural anesthesia, complications of, 998–999
  for cesarean delivery, 997
Epiglottitis, 30–31
Epilepsy, 856–866. See also *Seizures.*
  benign rolandic, 859
  causes of, 860
  classification of, 859–860, 859t
    in infants and children, 869–871
  cryptogenic, 859, 859t
    refractory, 865
  diagnosis of, 856
  differential diagnosis of, 856–858
    in infants and children, 867, 867t
  idiopathic, 859, 859t
  in infants and children, 867–871
  juvenile myoclonic, 859, 870
  petit mal, in infants and children, 869–870
  post-traumatic, 935, 938–940
  refractory, brain tumors causing, 941
    treatment of, 865
  symptomatic, 859
    refractory, 865
  treatment of, 860–866, *866*
    adjunctive, in infants and children, 869
    anticonvulsant withdrawal in, 864
      in infants and children, 868–869
    during pregnancy, 864
    for status epilepticus, 865, 865t
      in infants and children, 870t, 871
    in elderly persons, 864
    in infants and children, 867–871
    pharmacologic, 860–864, 860t, *861,* 862t, 863t
      in infants and children, 867–868, 868t, 869t
    surgical, 865–866
      in infants and children, 869

Epinephrine, emergency kits with, 728
  for insect sting allergy, 754, 754t
  for anaphylaxis, 727–728, 727t
    due to insect sting, 753–754
  for asthma exacerbations, in children, 741
  for cardiac arrest, 253–255, *254*
  for croup, 31
  for glaucoma, 913
  for severe urticaria or angioedema, 836
  for ventricular fibrillation, after myocardial infarction, 324
  in epidural analgesia for labor, 996
  in epidural anesthesia for cesarean delivery, 997
  in neonatal resuscitation, 1006
  in pheochromocytoma diagnosis, 654
  urine, reference intervals for, 1211t
EpiPen, 728
  for insect sting allergy, 754, 754t
Episiotomy, pain management after, 999
Epoetin alfa. See *Erythropoietin.*
Epoprostenol, for cutaneovascular disease in lupus erythematosus, 776
Epsilon-aminocaproic acid, for C1 esterase inhibitor deficiency, 836–837
  for disseminated intravascular coagulation, 402
  for hemophilia, 395
  for intracerebral hemorrhage, 849
  for platelet-mediated bleeding disorders, 399
Epstein-Barr virus infection, 802
  chronic fatigue syndrome and, 110, 111
  infectious mononucleosis and, 109, 109t, 802
  transmission of, by blood components, 461
Eptifibatide, 1215t
Epulides, 814
Erectile dysfunction, 691–694
  after radical prostatectomy, 707
  antidepressants for use with, 1115t
  classification of, 692
  diagnosis of, 692–693
  in diabetes, 566
  treatment of, 693–694
Ergocalciferol, for hypoparathyroidism, 633
  for secondary hyperparathyroidism, 631
Ergoloid mesylates, for Alzheimer's disease, 846
Ergotamine, for migraine, 881
Eruption cysts, 814
Erysipelas, coastal, 804t
Erythema, due to radiation therapy for Hodgkin's disease, 411
Erythema infectiosum, 803
Erythema migrans, in Lyme disease, 125t, 126
  treatment of, 127, 128t
Erythema multiforme, 824–825
  herpes simplex–associated, 801, 813, 824
Erythema nodosum, in sarcoidosis, 227
Erythema nodosum leprosum, 93
Erythroblastosis fetalis. See *Hemolytic disease of the fetus and newborn; Rh isoimmunization.*
Erythrocyte(s), fragmentation of, hemolytic anemia due to, 366
  transfusion of. See also *Transfusion(s).*
    physiologic basis for, 455
    products for, 454–455
Erythrocyte count, reference intervals for, 1206t
Erythrocyte enzymopathies, hemolytic disease of the newborn due to, 390

Erythrocyte membrane disorders, hemolytic anemia due to, 363–365, 363t
hemolytic disease of the newborn due to, 390
Erythromycin, anticonvulsant interactions with, 863t
for acne, 757–758
for acute necrotizing ulcerative gingivitis, 814
for amebiasis, 58t
for bacillary angiomatosis, 158t
for bacterial conjunctivitis, 67
for bacterial pneumonia, 212, 213
for *Campylobacter* infection, 77t, 78
for chancroid, 717
for chlamydial infection, 719, 1057, 1057t
for conjunctivitis, 68
for urethritis in men, 661
for cholera, 73, 74t
for donovanosis, 721
for erythema multiforme, 813
for eyelash lice, 806
for gastroparesis in diabetes, 565
for legionellosis, 217, 217t
for lymphogranuloma venereum, 722
for lymphomatoid papulosis, 770
for mycoplasmal infection, 24, 216
for nongonococcal urethritis, 721
for pertussis, 23, 139
for psittacosis, 118
for relapsing fever, 124
for streptococcal pharyngitis, 237, 238t
for syphilis, 724t, 774
for tetracycline-resistant *Ureaplasma urealyticum* urethritis, 661
for toxic shock syndrome, 85t
prophylactic, 85
HMG-CoA reductase inhibitor interaction with, 581–582
prophylactic, in sickle cell disease, 380
resistance to, in acne, 758
in *Streptococcus pneumoniae*, 211
Erythromycin-sulfisoxazole, for otitis media, 205
Erythropoietic porphyria, congenital, 448t, 451–452, 452t
Erythropoietin, for anemia, in acute renal failure, 699
in chronic renal failure, 703
in multiple myeloma, 444
for porphyria cutanea tarda with end-stage renal disease, 453
for pruritus in uremia, 37
Escherichia coli infection, enterohemorrhagic (EHEC, O157:H7), food-borne, 75t, 78
enterotoxigenic (ETEC), food-borne, 75t, 77
treatment of, 77, 77t
meningitis due to, antimicrobial therapy for, 103t
ESHAP regimen, for aggressive lymphoma, 436t, 438
Esmolol, for amphetamine intoxication, 1163
for atrial fibrillation, 257, 258t
intoxication with, 1166, 1167t
Esophageal diverticula, 479–480
dysphagia due to, 474
treatment of, 478, 479
Esophageal rings, 474, 478
Esophageal spasm, diffuse, 475, 478
Esophageal varices, in cirrhosis, 467
bleeding, 470, 471–473

Esophagitis, *Candida*, in HIV infection, 54
due to radiation therapy for Hodgkin's disease, 411
pill-induced, 476
reflux. See *Gastroesophageal reflux disease.*
Esophagogastroduodenoscopy, in dyspepsia evaluation, 497–498
Esophagogastroscopy, in dysphagia evaluation, 477
Esophagus, dilation of, for dysphagia, 478
neoplasms of, 478
dysphagia due to, 474
strictures of, 474, 478
Estradiol. See also *Estrogen(s).*
for endometriosis, 1031
for hormone replacement therapy, 1050
for hypogonadism in women, 638, 640t
for osteoporosis prevention in primary biliary cirrhosis, 468
Estradiol-17β, reference intervals for, 1208t
Estriol, maternal serum, measurement of, 981
Estrogen(s). See also specific estrogens.
endometrial cancer and, 1048, 1063, 1063t, 1065–1066
for acne, 759
for atrophic vaginitis, 1055
for bleeding in acute renal failure, 699
for dysfunctional uterine bleeding, 1039, 1039t
for endometriosis, 1031, 1032
for hormone replacement therapy, 1050–1051, 1052. See also *Hormone replacement therapy.*
for hyperlipidemia, 584
for hypogonadism, 638–639, 640t, 1042
for osteoporosis, 594–595, 595t
prophylactic, with corticosteroid therapy, 948
for prostate cancer, 708
for stress incontinence, 673
growth hormone replacement and, 636–637, 640t
hyperprolactinemia and, 642
in normal menstrual cycle, 1038, 1040
levothyroxine interaction with, 644
mood and, 1045, 1050
nipple discharge due to, 1023
recurrent urinary tract infections and, 665
troglitazone interaction with, 559
urine, reference intervals for, 1211t
Estropipate. See also *Estrogen(s).*
for hormone replacement therapy, 1050
Etanercept, 1215t
for congestive heart failure, 296
for juvenile rheumatoid arthritis, 955t, 957
for rheumatoid arthritis, 946t, 950–951
Ethacrynic acid, for hypertension, 308t
Ethambutol (EMB), adverse effects of, 241
for *Mycobacterium avium* complex infection, 54, 241
for *Mycobacterium kansasii* infection, 241
for tuberculosis, 240
in HIV infection, 53t
Ethanol. See *Alcohol* entries.
Ethanolamine oleate, endoscopic therapy with, for bleeding esophageal varices, 472
Ethchlorvynol, intoxication by, 1156t
Ethinyl estradiol. See also *Estrogen(s).*
for endometriosis, 1031

Ethinyl estradiol–levonorgestrel, in emergency contraceptive kit, 1087
Ethosuximide, adverse effects of, 863t
drug interactions with, 863t
for epilepsy, 860t, 861, 862t
in infants and children, 868t, 869t
pharmacokinetics of, 862t
reference intervals for, 1210t
Ethylene glycol, intoxication by, 1156t, 1176t, 1177–1179
serum concentration estimation for, 1160t
Etidronate, for osteoporosis, 595
due to corticosteroids, 596
prophylactic, in inflammatory bowel disease, 487
for Paget's disease of bone, 598, 598t
Etodolac, for dysmenorrhea, 1043t
Etoposide, for aggressive lymphoma, 436t
for gastric adenocarcinoma, 530
for Hodgkin's disease, 407t
for non–small cell lung cancer, 189
for Sézary's syndrome, 769
for small cell lung cancer, 190, 191
Etretinate, for psoriasis, 772
Evening primrose oil, for chronic fatigue syndrome, 112
Exanthem subitum, 802–803
Excessive vasopressinase syndrome, 626
Exercise. See also *Physical therapy.*
after myocardial infarction, 331–332
anaphylaxis induced by, 726
asthma induced by, 731
in children, 736–737
for angina, 250
for ankylosing spondylitis, 959–960
for chronic fatigue syndrome, 111–112
for chronic obstructive pulmonary disease, 173
for congestive heart failure, 293
for fibromyalgia, 967
for hypertension, 305
for juvenile rheumatoid arthritis, 957
for low back pain, 39, 40
for obesity, 590
for osteoarthritis, 969
for osteoporosis prevention, 1052
for Parkinson's disease, 920
for peripheral arterial occlusive disease, 337
for rheumatoid arthritis, 953
for type 2 diabetes, 556
in hemophilia, 396
in type 1 diabetes, 570–571
migraine induced by, 879
Exercise intolerance, in children, asthma and, 736–737
Ex-Lax, for constipation, 19–20
Exostosis, subungual, 783
Extrinsic allergic alveolitis, 230–231, 231t
Eye(s), antimalarial toxicity to, 775
care of, in facial paralysis, 918
in myasthenia gravis, 903–904
sarcoidosis involving, 227, 227t
toxic exposure of, decontamination for, 1147

Fab antibodies, digoxin-specific, for digitalis intoxication, 1152t–1153t, 1175
Facial nerve decompression, for facial paralysis, 917
Facial pain, atypical, 909
Facial paralysis, acute, 915–918

Facial paralysis *(Continued)*
  electrodiagnosis of, 916–917
  epidemiology of, 916
  evaluation of, 916
  treatment of, 917–918, *917*
  in Lyme disease, 125t, 126
    treatment of, 127, 128t
  in otitis media, 207
Factor V deficiency, 392
Factor V Leiden, pulmonary
  thromboembolism and, 221
Factor VII deficiency, 392
Factor VIIa, recombinant, 394–395, 458
Factor VIII, for intracerebral hemorrhage,
  849
  reference intervals for, 1207t
Factor VIII deficiency. See also
  Hemophilias.
  genetics of, 391
  therapeutic options for, 393–394, 458
Factor IX deficiency. See also *Hemophilias.*
  genetics of, 391
  therapeutic options for, 394, 458
Factor X deficiency, 392
Factor XI deficiency, 391
Factor XII deficiency, 392
Factor XIII deficiency, 392
Falls, after stroke, 854
Famciclovir, for chronic hepatitis B, 507
  for herpes simplex, 800, 800t, 809
    in HIV infection, 53
  for herpes zoster, 71, 800t, 802
Familial adenomatous polyposis, colorectal
  cancer and, 533
Familial benign hypocalciuric hypercal-
  cemia, laboratory evaluation of,
  628–629, 628t
  parathyroid hyperplasia in, 627–628
Family planning. See also *Contraception.*
  natural, 1075–1084, 1076t
  during breast-feeding, 1089
Famotidine, for NSAID-induced ulcers,
  500
FAMTX regimen, for gastric
  adenocarcinoma, 530
Fanconi's anemia, 354–355
Fascicular tachycardia, 279
Fasciitis, necrotizing, 81, 796t, 797–798
  plantar, 978
Fasciola hepatica infection, 540t, 546
Fasciolopsis buski infection, 540t, 546
Fasting, in type 2 diabetes, 556
  rheumatoid arthritis and, 952
Fat, dietary, colorectal cancer and, 533
  in abetalipoproteinemia, 512
  in chronic pancreatitis, 521
  in chronic renal failure, 704
  in cystic fibrosis, 177
  in type 2 diabetes, 555
  fecal, estimation of, in malabsorption
    diagnosis, 508
    reference intervals for, 1213t
  in parenteral nutrition, 604, 605t
    for high-risk neonate, 1012
    requirements for, 602
Fat necrosis, of breast, 1024
Fatigue, causes of, 110
  chronic. See also *Chronic fatigue syn-
    drome.*
    idiopathic, 110
  in multiple sclerosis, 901
  in Parkinson's disease, 923
Fatty acids, essential, deficiency of, with
  parenteral nutrition, 607
  omega-3, for hyperlipidemia, 584
Fatty liver of pregnancy, acute, HELLP
  syndrome vs., 993t

Fecal fat estimation, in malabsorption
  diagnosis, 508
  reference intervals for, 1213t
Fecal impaction, 18–19
Fecal leukocyte test, in infectious
  diarrhea, 15
Fecal occult blood testing, in colorectal
  cancer screening, 534, 535t
Fedotozine, for irritable bowel syndrome,
  491
Felbamate, adverse effects of, 863t
  drug interactions with, 863t
  for epilepsy, 860t, 861–864, 862t
    in infants and children, 869t
    for Lennox-Gastaut syndrome, 870
  pharmacokinetics of, 862t
Felodipine, for hypertension, 308t, 310
  intoxication with, 1168
Femoral-popliteal vein thrombosis,
  344–345. See also *Venous thrombosis.*
Fenfluramine, for obstructive sleep-
  disordered breathing, 184
Fenofibrate, for hyperlipidemia, 583–584
  for hypertriglyceridemia in type 2 diabe-
    tes, 563
  HMG-CoA reductase inhibitor interac-
    tion with, 581–582
Fenoprofen, for dysmenorrhea, 1043t
Fentanyl, for cesarean delivery, in spinal-
  epidural anesthesia, 997
  for labor, in epidural analgesia, 996
    in intrathecal analgesia, 996–997
  for painful episode in sickle cell disease,
    376
  for tetanus, 136
  intoxication with, 1095, 1191, 1192,
    1192t
  transdermal, for pain, 4t
Fenthion, intoxication with, 1194
Ferric chloride test, for salicylate
  intoxication, 1200
Ferritin, serum, in hemochromatosis
  diagnosis, 404
  in hemochromatosis monitoring, 405
  reference intervals for, 1208t
Ferrous gluconate, for iron deficiency, 357
Ferrous sulfate, for anemia in chronic
  renal failure, 703
  for iron deficiency, 357
Fertility. See also *Infertility.*
  preservation of, with radiation therapy
    for Hodgkin's disease, 413
Fertility awareness, periodic abstinence
  with, for contraception,
    1075–1084, 1076t
  during breast-feeding, 1089
Fetal blood sampling, 981, 984
Fetal globin gene activation, for sickle cell
  disease, 381
  for thalassemia, 373
Fetal hemoglobin, affinity of, for carbon
  monoxide, 1170, 1171
  hereditary persistence of, sickle hemoglo-
    bin with, 375, 375t. See also *Sickle
    cell disease.*
  increasing levels of, for sickle cell dis-
    ease, 381
    for thalassemia, 373
  reference intervals for, 1207t
Fetal lung maturity, corticosteroids to
  enhance, 984, 1014
  with placenta previa, 988
Fetal monitoring, with antihypertensive
  therapy, 990–991
α-Fetoprotein, maternal serum,
  measurement of, 980, 981

Fetus, amphetamine exposure of, 1095
  hemolytic disease of, 383–390. See also
    *Hemolytic disease of the fetus and
    newborn; Rh isoimmunization.*
  intrauterine treatment of, 984
  toluene exposure of, 1097
Fever, 20–22
  seizures due to, 21, 869
  with head injury in children, 938
Fexofenadine, for allergic rhinitis, 745,
  745t
  for ordinary urticaria, 835
  for pruritus, 37
  intoxication with, 1164
Fiber, dietary, colonic diverticulosis and,
  481
  colorectal cancer and, 533
  diverticulitis and, 482
  for anal fissure, 494
  for constipation, 18
  for irritable bowel syndrome, 491
  for type 2 diabetes, 555
  supplemental, for anal fissure, 494
    for constipation, 19, 19t
    for irritable bowel syndrome, 491
Fibric acid derivatives. See also specific
  drugs.
  for hyperlipidemia, 583–584
Fibrin glue, for bleeding in hemophilia,
  395
Fibrin split products, reference intervals
  for, 1207t
Fibrinogen, reference intervals for, 1207t,
  1208t
Fibroadenoma, of breast, 1023
Fibrocystic disease of breast, 1023
Fibromas, oral, 817
Fibromuscular dysplasia, renovascular
  hypertension due to, 313
Fibromyalgia, 966–967
  Lyme disease and, 130
  myofascial pain vs., 966
Fibrosing mediastinitis, due to
  histoplasmosis, 195, 199
Fifth disease, 803
Filgrastim. See *Granulocyte colony-
  stimulating factor (G-CSF).*
Finasteride, for androgenic alopecia, 761
  for benign prostatic hyperplasia, 690
Fine-needle aspiration, in breast cancer
  diagnosis, 1026
  in thyroid nodule evaluation, 649–650
Fire ant sting allergy, 753–755, 754t, 755t
Fish, biting, 1141–1142
  electric, 1144
  poisonous, 79, 80t, 1143–1144
  venomous, 1142–1143
Fish oil, for hyperlipidemia, 584
  for IgA nephritis, 679
  for inflammatory bowel disease, 487
  for rheumatoid arthritis, 952
Fistula, anorectal, 495
  aortoenteric, due to aortic infection, 247
  cholecystenteric, 465
  gastrointestinal-cutaneous, parenteral
    nutrition for, 602–603
  with acute pancreatitis, 518
Fitz-Hugh–Curtis syndrome, in
  lymphogranuloma venereum, 722
Flashbacks, after hallucinogen use,
  1096–1097
  after phencyclidine intoxication, 1195
  in post-traumatic stress disorder, 1101
Flatulence, 12
Flecainide, adverse effects of, 275, 275t
  for atrial fibrillation, 260

Flecainide *(Continued)*
  for atrial flutter, 275t
  for atrial premature beats, 261
  for pain, 3
  reference intervals for, 1210t
  relative antiarrhythmic efficacy of, 262t
Fleroxacin, for typhoid fever, 163, 163t
Flexible endoscopic evaluation of
    swallowing and sensation, in
    dysphagia evaluation, 477
Fluconazole, drug interactions with, 194,
    198
  for blastomycosis, 201
  for *Candida* suppression in perineal pru-
    ritus, 834
  for candidiasis, in HIV infection, 54
    of oral cavity, 811
    vulvovaginal, 1053–1054
  for coccidioidomycosis, 193–194
    for meningitis, 195
  for cryptoccal meningitis in HIV infec-
    tion, 52
  for histoplasmosis, 197t, 198, 199
  for median rhomboid glossitis, 815
  for onychomycosis, 782, 782t
Flucytosine, for cryptoccal meningitis in
    HIV infection, 52
Fludarabine, for chronic lymphocytic
    leukemia, 431–432
  for indolent B cell lymphoma, 435, 435t
  for Sézary's syndrome, 769
Fludrocortisone, for adrenal crisis, 620
  for chronic adrenal insufficiency, 621
  for orthostatic hypotension, 886t, 891
    in diabetes, 566
    in mitral valve prolapse, 291
  with mitotane for Cushing's syndrome,
    623
Fluids, for urinary calculus prevention,
    714
  parenteral, for antepartum hemorrhage,
    987
    for burn patients, 1124, 1124t
    for diabetic ketoacidosis, 573
      in children, 567
    for heat illness, 1135, 1136, 1136t
    for high-risk neonate, 1011–1012
    for hypovolemic shock after myocar-
      dial infarction, 325
    for ischemic stroke, 852
    for volume expansion in neonate, 1006
    in acute renal failure, 697
    in infants and children, 607–613
      for dehydration, 609–613, 610t, *611*
      for maintenance, 607–609, 608t
      with abnormal losses, 608–609
Flukes, 543, 545–546. See also specific
    worms and diseases.
  treatment of, 540t, 544
Flumazenil, for benzodiazepine
    intoxication, 1096, 1153t, 1166
  in acute poisoning management, 1158
Flunisolide, for allergic rhinitis, 747t
  for asthma, 732t
Fluocinonide, for aphthous stomatitis, 812
  for atopic dermatitis, 822
  for chronic desquamative gingivitis, 814
  for erythema multiforme, 813
  for herpes gestationis, 831
  for oral lesions in lupus, 813
  for pruritic urticarial papules and
    plaques of pregnancy, 831
Fluoride, supplemental, for infant, 1022
5-Fluorouracil (5-FU), for actinic cheilitis,
    810
  for actinic keratosis, 792

5-Fluorouracil (5-FU) *(Continued)*
  for AIDS-related lymphoma, 439
  for breast cancer, 1027
  for cervical cancer, 1069
  for colorectal cancer, 537
  for gastric adenocarcinoma, 530
  for penile carcinoma, 710
  for toxoplasmosis, 154
  for warts, 786
  with trabeculectomy for glaucoma, 915
Fluoxetine, anticonvulsant interactions
    with, 863t
  for anxiety disorders, 1100t, 1101
  for bulimia nervosa, 1104
  for depression, 1109t
    in Alzheimer's disease, 847
    in multiple sclerosis, 901
  for fatigue in multiple sclerosis, 901
  for obstructive sleep-disordered breath-
    ing, 184
  for pain, 3
  for panic disorder, 1121t, 1122
  for premenstrual syndrome, 1047
  for trichotillomania, 762
  pharmacodynamic effects of, 1110t
  phentermine with, for obesity, 590
  washout required for, before MAO inhibi-
    tor therapy, 1115–1116
Fluphenazine, characteristics of, 1118t
  for diabetic neuropathy, 565
  for Tourette's syndrome, 876
  intoxication by, 1197t
Flurazepam, for insomnia, 34
  intoxication with, 1166
Flurbiprofen, for dysmenorrhea, 1043t
  for migraine, 883
Fluticasone, for allergic rhinitis, 747t
  for asthma, 732t
    in children, 742
  for chronic obstructive pulmonary dis-
    ease, 173
Flutter device, for atelectasis due to
    mucous plugs, 171
Fluvastatin, for hyperlipidemia, 581
Fluvoxamine, for anxiety disorders, 1100t,
    1101
  for depression, 1109t
  for panic disorder, 1121t, 1122
  pharmacodynamic effects of, 1110t
Folate, after splenectomy for hereditary
    spherocytosis, 364
  anticonvulsant interactions with, 863t
  as antidote, 1153t
    for ethylene glycol intoxication, 1178
  deficiency of, aphthous stomatitis due to,
    812
    megaloblastic anemia due to, 369
    during pregnancy, 980
  for elevated homocysteine in type 2 dia-
    betes, 563
  for megaloblastic anemia, 368, 369
  for short-bowel syndrome, 511
  for stroke prevention, 855
  for tropical sprue, 511
  reference intervals for, 1208t
  with anticonvulsant therapy, 864
  with drug therapy for inflammatory
    bowel disease, 483, 486
  with methotrexate for rheumatoid arthri-
    tis, 948
Folinic acid. See *Leucovorin (folinic acid)*.
Folk remedies, lead content of, 1184
Follicle-stimulating hormone, deficiency of,
    in hypopituitarism, 638–639, 640t
  in normal menstrual cycle, 1040
  measurement of, in amenorrhea evalua-
    tion, 1042

Follicle-stimulating hormone *(Continued)*
  plasma, reference intervals for, 1208t
Follicular mucinosis, mycosis fungoides
    and, 766
Folliculitis, 795
Fomivirsen, 1215t
  for cytomegalovirus infection in HIV
    infection, 53
Fontan procedure, for hypoplastic left
    heart syndrome, 287
  modified, for tricuspid atresia, 286
Food additives, asthma and, 731
Food allergy, atopic dermatitis and, 823
Food-borne illness, 74–81, 75t. See also
    specific diseases.
  acute infectious diarrhea vs., 15
  classification of, by predominant symp-
    tom, 76–81
  resources on, 74–76
Foot, sports injuries to, 978
Foot care, in diabetic neuropathy, 932
Foot disease, in diabetes, 566
Forchheimer's sign, in rubella, 131
Fordyce spots, 811
Foreign body aspiration, cough due to, 23
Formula-feeding, for infants, 1019–1022,
    1021t
Foscarnet, for cytomegalovirus infection, in
    HIV infection, 53
  for viral pneumonia, 216t
Fosinopril, for congestive heart failure,
    294t
  for hypertension, 309t
Fosphenytoin, for status epilepticus, 865,
    865t
  in infants and children, 870t
  prophylactic, with intracerebral hemor-
    rhage, 849
Fournier's gangrene, 796t, 798
4-2-1 rule, for IV fluid rate estimation for
    infants and children, 608
Fractures, in ankylosing spondylitis, 959
  in osteoporosis, 594, 596–597, 1049
  tibial stress, 978
  wrist, in athlete, 976
Freckles, 839
Free water deficit, calculation of, in
    diabetes insipidus, 624
Frey procedure, for chronic pancreatitis,
    523
Frostbite, 1134
Fructose, semen, reference intervals for,
    1213t
5-FU. See *5-Fluorouracil (5-FU)*.
Fugu (puffer fish), 79, 80t, 1144
Fundoplication, for gastroesophageal reflux
    disease, 527
Fungal infection. See also specific
    infections.
  of external ear canal, 114–115
  of nails, 780–782, 781t, 782t, 807
  of skin, 806–808
Furazolidone, for cholera, 74t
  for diarrhea, 16, 17t
  for giardiasis, 61, 61t, 538–542, 539t
Furosemide, contraindicated in
    nephrogenic diabetes insipidus, 627
  for ascites in cirrhosis, 469
  for heart failure, 294t
    after myocardial infarction, 325
  for heat stroke, 1136
  for hemolytic transfusion reaction, 459
  for hypertension, 308t
    during pregnancy, 990, 990t
  for Meniere's disease, 893
  for volume overload in acute renal fail-
    ure, 697

Furosemide (Continued)
  with transfusion therapy for pernicious anemia, 368
Furuncle, 795
Fusion beats, in ventricular tachycardia, 276, 277

Gabapentin, adverse effects of, 863t
  drug interactions with, 863t
  for epilepsy, 860t, 862t, 864
    in infants and children, 868t, 869t
  for HIV-associated peripheral neuropathy, 56
  for pain, 3
    in multiple sclerosis, 902
  for postherpetic neuralgia, 802
  for seizures in acute porphyria, 449, 451
  for trigeminal neuralgia, 909
  pharmacokinetics of, 862t
Gait training, after stroke, 854
Galactose, malabsorption of, 514
α-D-Galactosidase, for gaseousness, 13
Gallbladder disease, 463–465
  during pregnancy, 983
  in cystic fibrosis, 180
Gallium nitrate, adverse effects of, 600
  for Paget's disease of bone, 598t, 600
Gallstones, 463–465
  bowel obstruction due to, 465
  in protoporphyria, 453
  in sickle cell disease, 379
  pancreatitis due to, 517
Gamekeeper's thumb, 976–977
Gamma globulin. See also Immune globulin.
  serum, reference intervals for, 1209t
Gamma-glutamyltransferase, as marker for excess alcohol intake, 1092
  serum, reference intervals for, 1208t
Ganciclovir, for cytomegalovirus infection in HIV infection, 53
  for viral pneumonia, 216t
Ganglioglioma, 941
Gangrene, digital, in lupus erythematosus, 776
  Fournier's, 796t, 798
  gas, 81, 795t, 796–797
  hemolytic streptococcal, 81, 795–796, 795t
  in synergistic necrotizing cellulitis, 81, 796
Gardner's syndrome, colorectal cancer and, 533
Gargling, laryngitis due to, 30
Gas gangrene, 81, 795t, 796–797
Gaseousness, 11–13
Gasoline, 1179
Gastrectomy, for gastric adenocarcinoma, 530
  malabsorption after, 512–513
Gastric acid output, reference intervals for, 1213t
Gastric aspiration, for acute poisoning, 1148
Gastric banding, for obesity, 591
Gastric bypass, for obesity, 591
Gastric diverticula, 480
Gastric emptying. See also Gastroparesis.
  delayed, dyspepsia and, 11
  procedures for, in acute poisoning, 1147–1148
Gastric lavage, for acute poisoning, 1148
  for ciguatera poisoning, 1143
Gastric stapling, for obesity, 591

Gastric tumors, 527–532
Gastric varices, in cirrhosis, 467, 471
  bleeding, 472
Gastrin, serum, reference intervals for, 1208t
Gastritis, defined, 496
  in acute renal failure, 699
Gastrocnemiosemimembranous bursitis, 965
Gastroduodenal ulcers. See also Peptic ulcer disease.
  dyspepsia and, 496
Gastroenteritis. See also Enteritis.
  eosinophilic, 513
  in type 1 diabetes, 572
  infectious, irritable bowel syndrome and, 490
Gastroesophageal reflux disease, 524–527
  asthma and, 730–731
    in children, 740
  cough due to, 24
  dyspepsia and, 11
  dysphagia due to, 474, 475
    treatment of, 478
  extraesophageal symptoms of, 524
  in cystic fibrosis, 179t, 180
  laryngitis due to, 30, 31
  subglottic stenosis due to, 29
  treatment of, 525–527, 526
  vocal fold granuloma due to, 26
Gastrointestinal dialysis, for acute poisoning, 1148
Gastrointestinal tract. See also Gastric entries.
  bleeding from, from diverticula, 481
    from esophagogastric varices, 470, 471–473
    in acute renal failure, 699
    iron deficiency anemia due to, 356–357
  disease of. See also specific diseases.
    diverticular, 479–482
    malabsorption due to, 510–511
  function of, reference intervals for tests of, 1213t
  motor dysfunction of, gastroesophageal reflux and, 524
    irritable bowel syndrome and, 489
  non-Hodgkin's lymphoma of, 439–440, 530–531
  obstruction of, by colorectal cancer, 536–537
    in cystic fibrosis, 178, 179t
  perforation of, by colorectal cancer, 537
  resection of, malabsorption after, 510, 511
  stromal tumors of, 531
  toxic exposure by, decontamination for, 1147–1149, 1148t
Gastrointestinal-cutaneous fistula, parenteral nutrition for, 602–603
Gastrolaryngeal reflux. See Gastroesophageal reflux disease.
Gastroparesis, in diabetes, 565
Gastroplasty, for obesity, 591
Gastrostomy feeding, nighttime, for cystic fibrosis, 178
G-CSF. See Granulocyte colony-stimulating factor (G-CSF).
Gemcitabine, for non–small cell lung cancer, 189
Gemfibrozil, for hyperlipidemia, 583–584
  for hypertriglyceridemia in type 2 diabetes, 563
  HMG-CoA reductase inhibitor interaction with, 581–582

Gene therapy, for thalassemia, 373–374
Genitourinary tract. See Urogenital tract; specific structures.
Gentamicin, bilateral vestibular deficit due to, 891
  for bacterial conjunctivitis, 67
  for bacterial meningitis, 105t
  for brucellosis, 64, 65, 65t, 66
  for cat-scratch disease, 158t
  for cystic fibrosis exacerbations, 179t
  for diverticulitis, 482
  for draining ear, 207t
  for endocarditis, 300t, 301
    prophylactic, 301t
  for epididymitis, 675
  for Meniere's disease, 894
  for necrotizing skin and soft tissue infections, 82
  for nosocomial pneumonia, 213
  for osteomyelitis, 974, 974t
  for pelvic inflammatory disease, 719t, 1059t
  for postpartum endomyometritis, 1000–1001
  for pyelonephritis, 682t
    in women, 664, 664t
  for sepsis, 63t
    in neonate, 1017t, 1018
  for urinary tract infection, in girls, 667
    in men, 661–662
  reference intervals for, 1210t
Gentian violet, for vulvovaginal candidiasis, 1053
Geographic tongue, 815
Gestations. See also Pregnancy.
  multiple, 983–984
Giant cell arteritis, 339, 970–971
Giant condyloma of Buschke-Lowenstein, 1073–1074
Giant papillary conjunctivitis, contact lens–induced, 69
Giardiasis, 59–61, 538
  malabsorption due to, 513
  treatment of, 16, 17t, 538–542, 539t
Gilles de la Tourette syndrome, 874–877
Gingival hyperplasia, 813–814
Gingival lesions, 813–814
Gingivitis, 814
  acute necrotizing ulcerative, 814
  chronic desquamative, 814
Gingivostomatitis, atypical, 816
  herpetic, 799, 813. See also Herpes simplex.
Ginkgo biloba extract, for Alzheimer's disease, 846
Glasgow Coma Scale, 934t, 936t, 1146t
  in head injury, 934
    injury classification using, 936
    outcome and, 938, 939
Glatiramer acetate, for multiple sclerosis, 898, 898t
Glaucoma, 912–915
  antidepressants for use in, 1115t
Glenn procedure, bidirectional, for tricuspid atresia, 286
Glimepiride, for type 2 diabetes, 557t, 558
Glioblastoma multiforme, 941, 942t, 943
Glioma, optic neuritis vs., 911
  radiation therapy for, 943
  supratentorial, 941
  survival with, 941, 942t
Glipizide, for type 2 diabetes, 557t, 558
Global amnesia, transient, seizure vs., 857
Globulins. See also Immune globulin.
  serum, reference intervals for, 1209t
Globus, dysphagia vs., 475

Globus pallidus surgery, for Parkinson's disease, 923t, 924
Glomerular disease, diagnosis of, 675
  primary, 675–680. See also specific diseases.
    therapeutic options in, 675–677
Glomerular filtration rate, as measure of renal function, 701–702
Glomerulonephritis, anti–glomerular basement membrane, 679
  IgA, 679
  immune complex, 679
  membranoproliferative, 679
  pauci-immune, 679–680
  rapidly progressive, 679–680
Glomerulosclerosis, focal segmental, 678
Glomus tumor, subungual, 783
Glossitis, median rhomboid, 815
Glossitis areata migrans, 815
Glossodynia, 815–816
Glottic insufficiency, 27–28
Glucagon, as antidote, 1153t
    for beta blocker intoxication, 1168
    for calcium channel blocker intoxication, 1169
    for anaphylaxis, 727t, 728
      due to insect sting, 754
    for gastroenteritis in type 1 diabetes, 572
Glucosamine, for osteoarthritis, 970
Glucose, for ethanol intoxication, 1177
  for hyperkalemia in acute renal failure, 697, 697t
  for hypoglycemia in acute poisoning, 1157
  for opioid intoxication, 1193
  for status epilepticus, 865t
    in infants and children, 871
  malabsorption of, 514
  reference intervals for, in cerebrospinal fluid, 1212t
    in plasma, 1208t
    in urine, 1211t
Glucose effect, in acute hepatic porphyria management, 449
Glucose monitoring, home, for children, 569–570
  in type 2 diabetes, 553, 554t
Glucose tolerance, abnormal, 550, 550t
  in insulin resistance syndrome, 551
Glucose toxicity, 551
Glucose-6-phosphate dehydrogenase deficiency, 365
  hemolytic disease of the newborn due to, 390
α-Glucosidase inhibitors. See also specific drugs.
  for type 2 diabetes, 557t, 559
Glue, fibrin, for bleeding in hemophilia, 395
Glue sniffer's neuropathy, 926
γ-Glutamyltransferase, as marker for excess alcohol intake, 1092
  serum, reference intervals for, 1208t
Gluten-sensitive enteropathy, 510–511
  dermatitis herpetiformis and, 829
  impaired iron absorption in, 356
Glutethimide, intoxication by, 1156t
Glyburide, for type 2 diabetes, 557t, 558
Glycerid worms, 1142
Glycerol, for bacterial meningitis, 108
Glycerol rhizolysis, for trigeminal neuralgia, 910
Glycolic acid, for hyperpigmentation, 839
Glycoprotein IIb/IIIa receptor antagonists, after myocardial infarction, 328, 330

Glycopyrrolate, for carbamate poisoning, 1194
  for organophosphate poisoning, 1194
Glycosylated hemoglobin. See Hemoglobin A₁c.
GM-CSF. See Granulocyte-macrophage colony-stimulating factor (GM-CSF).
Goeckerman technique, for psoriasis, 772
Gold, for rheumatoid arthritis, 946t, 949, 951
  thrombocytopenia due to, 399
Golfer's elbow, 965, 976
Gonadal dysgenesis, 1042
Gonadotropin-releasing hormone, in normal menstrual cycle, 1040
Gonadotropin-releasing hormone agonists. See also Luteinizing hormone–releasing hormone analogs; specific drugs.
  for endometriosis, 1032
    surgery combined with, 1032–1033
  for leiomyomata, 1061–1062, 1061t
Gonococcal infection, 718–720, 719t
  conjunctivitis due to, 67, 720
  epididymitis due to, 662, 674
  in men, treatment of, 661
  oral ulceration in, 813
  pelvic inflammatory disease and, 718, 1058, 1059
Goserelin, for leiomyomata, 1061t
Gout, 576–578, 577t. See also Hyperuricemia.
  in acute renal failure, 698
  saturnine, 1185
Graft-versus-host disease, transfusion-associated, 457, 460
Grandmother theory of Rh sensitization, 384
Granisetron, for irritable bowel syndrome, 492
  for nausea and vomiting, 8t, 10
Granular cell tumors, vulvar, 1071
Granulocyte(s), transfusion of, 456–457
  in acute leukemia, 420
Granulocyte colony-stimulating factor (G-CSF), for aplastic anemia, 354
  for highly aggressive lymphoma, 438t
  for neutropenia, chronic, 383
    with intensive chemotherapy for leukemia, 419–420
Granulocyte-macrophage colony-stimulating factor (GM-CSF), for chronic myelogenous leukemia, 429
  for neutropenia, chronic, 383
    with intensive chemotherapy for leukemia, 419–420
Granuloma, vocal fold, 26
Granuloma inguinale, 721–722
Granulomatous prostatitis, 687
Graves' disease, 645. See also Hyperthyroidism.
  diagnosis of, 646
  treatment of, 646–648
Grepafloxacin, for legionellosis, 217, 218
Grey Turner's sign, in acute pancreatitis, 515
Griseofulvin, for onychomycosis, 782, 782t, 807
  for oral lichen planus, 811
  for tinea capitis, 762, 806
  for tinea corporis, 807
  for tinea pedis, 807
Groove sign, in lymphogranuloma venereum, 722
Ground itch. See Hookworms.
Growth delay, due to intranasal corticosteroids, 747

Growth delay (Continued)
  in sickle cell disease, 379
  intrauterine, with chronic maternal hypertension, 989
Growth hormone, deficiency of, in hypopituitarism, 636–637, 640t
  measurement of, in acromegaly diagnosis, 615
  plasma, reference intervals for, 1208t
  recombinant, for AIDS-related weight loss, 56
Growth hormone–releasing hormone, tumor secretion of, acromegaly due to, 615
Guaifenesin, for cough, 24–25
  for viral respiratory infection, 214
Guanabenz, for hypertension, 308t, 309
Guanadrel, for hypertension, 308t, 309
Guanethidine, for hypertension, 308t, 309
Guanfacine, for attention-deficit/hyperactivity disorder, 873t, 874
  for hypertension, 308t, 309
Guide wire embolism, with central catheter placement, 606
Guillain-Barré syndrome, 929
  influenza vaccine and, 87
Guinea worm, 804t
Guttate hypomelanosis, idiopathic, 841

Habit cough, 24
Habit tic disorder, nail abnormality due to, 781t, 783
Haemophilus ducreyi infection, 717
Haemophilus influenzae, antibiotic resistance in, 205
  meningitis due to, antimicrobial therapy for, 103t, 104t, 106, 107
  chemoprophylaxis of, 108
  pneumonia due to, treatment of, 212, 212t
Haemophilus influenzae type b vaccine, 140, 141, 142t, 144t
Hair disorders, 759–763
  classification of, 759, 760t
  with hair excess, 763
  with hair loss, 760–762, 760t
  with hair shaft abnormalities, 763
Hairy leukoplakia, 814
Hairy tongue, black, 815
Halitosis, 808
Hallpike-Dix test, in benign paroxysmal positional vertigo, 887, 888
Hallucinogens, 1096–1097, 1150t
Halobetasol, for lichen simplex chronicus, 834
Halofantrine, for malaria, 96, 97t
Haloperidol, characteristics of, 1118t
  for aggression in Alzheimer's disease, 847
  for cocaine-induced psychosis, 1094
  for hallucinogen intoxication, 1096
  for phencyclidine intoxication, 1096
  for Tourette's syndrome, 876
  intoxication with, 1196, 1197t
Halothane, for obstetric anesthesia, 998
Ham test, reference intervals for, 1206t
Hand, burns of, maintenance of function after, 1126
  sports injuries to, 976–977
Hand-foot syndrome, in sickle cell disease, 376
Hand-foot-and-mouth disease, 803, 813
Hansen's disease. See Leprosy.
Hantavirus, pneumonia due to, 215, 215t, 216t

Haptoglobin, reference intervals for, 1207t, 1208t

Harris-Benedict equation, for basal energy expenditure calculation, 601

Hartnup's disease, amino acid malabsorption in, 514

Hashimoto's thyroiditis, 642, 659–660

Hashish, 1097

Haverhill fever, 122

Head injury, 933–940
  classification of, 933, 936
  imaging in, 933–934
    in children, 937
  in adults, 933–936
  in children, 936–940
    complications of, 938–940, 939
    epidemiology of, 936
    evaluation of, 936–937
    prognosis in, 938–940, 939
    rehabilitation after, 940
    treatment of, 937–938
  in hemophilia, 396
  mild (minor), defined, 933, 936
    prognosis in, 935
    treatment of, 933–934
      in children, 937, 938t
  moderate, defined, 933
    treatment of, 934
      in children, 938
  pathophysiology of, 933, 936
  prognosis in, 935–936
    in children, 938–940, 939
  severe, complications of, 935
    defined, 933, 936
    prognosis in, 935–936
    treatment of, 934–935
      in children, 938
  treatment of, 933–935, 934t, 935t
    in children, 937–938

Head lice, 804t, 806

Headache, 877–884. See also Migraine.
  after dural puncture in obstetric anesthesia, 999
  after minor head injury, 935
  cluster, 883–884
  diagnosis of, 877–878
  in temporomandibular disorders, 960
  rebound, in migraine, 881
    in tension-type headache, 883
  refractory, 884
  secondary, 877
  tension-type, 883
    transformed migraine vs., 879, 883

Headache threshold, 880

Health Hints for the Tropics, 145–146

Hearing loss, tinnitus and, 38
  with otitis media, 207

Heart block, 264–268
  after myocardial infarction, 323, 324t
  antidepressants for use in, 1115t
  bifascicular, 266
    after myocardial infarction, 324t
  causes of, 265
  clinical manifestations of, 266–267
  congenital, causes of, 265
    electrocardiographic diagnosis of, 265–266, 267
    natural history of, 267
  electrocardiographic diagnosis of, 265–266, 267
  management of, 267–268, 268t
  trifascicular, 266
    after myocardial infarction, 324t

Heart disease, Chagas', 102
  congenital, 280–287. See also specific lesions.

Heart disease (Continued)
  acyanotic, with left-to-right shunt, 280–282
    with outflow tract obstruction, 282–284
  cyanotic, 284–287
    in newborn, 1015
  in ankylosing spondylitis, 959
  in sarcoidosis, 227–228, 227t
  in sickle cell disease, 379
  infiltrative, ventricular tachycardia in, 279
  ischemic. See Coronary artery disease.
  oral contraceptives and, 1086t

Heart failure, 291–297
  acute, after myocardial infarction, 324–325
  antidepressants for use in, 1115t
  causes of, 291–292
  due to transfusion, 461
  evaluation of, 292, 292t
  oral contraceptives and, 1086t
  treatment of, 292–297, 294t
  outpatient follow-up in, 293

"Heart on a string" appearance, in transposition of the great arteries, 285

Heart transplantation, for Chagas' heart disease, 102
  toxoplasmosis after, 157

Heartburn. See also Gastroesophageal reflux disease.
  during pregnancy, 980
  gastroesophageal reflux and, 524

Heat illness, 150, 1135–1137, 1136t

Heavy metal poisoning. See also Lead poisoning.
  from acidic beverages, 76
  oral pigmentation due to, 816
  peripheral neuropathy due to, 926

Helicobacter pylori infection, 500–501
  cholera and, 73–74
  diagnosis of, 501
  dyspepsia and, 11
  MALT lymphoma and, 440, 531
  peptic ulcer disease and, 500–501, 501t
  test and treat strategies for, in dyspepsia, 498, 498
  treatment of, 501, 501t

HELLP syndrome, 991, 992–993, 993t

Helminths, 538. See also Parasites; specific diseases and worms.
  intestinal, 543–547
    drugs for, 538, 540t–541t, 543–544
  skin disease due to, 804–805, 804t

Hemangioblastoma, 941

Hemangioma, capillary, lip involvement in, 809
  cavernous, lip involvement in, 809
  subglottic, dysphonia due to, 29

Hemarthrosis, hip, in hemophilia, iliopsoas hemorrhage vs., 396

Hematin, for acute hepatic porphyrias, 449

Hematocrit, reference intervals for, 1207t

Hematologic growth factors. See also specific factors.
  for aplastic anemia, 354

Hematology, reference intervals for, 1206t–1207t

Hematoma, intracranial, with minor head injury, 933–934
  with severe head injury, 934
  vaginal, postpartum, 1001
  vulvar, postpartum, 1001

Heme, for acute hepatic porphyrias, 448t, 449, 451
  for protoporphyria, 453

Heme-oxygenase inhibitors, for Rh isoimmunization, 388t

Hemochromatosis, 404–406
  porphyria cutanea tarda and, 452

Hemodialysis, for acute poisoning, 1150–1156, 1156t
  for acute renal failure, continuous, 700, 700t
    intermittent, 699–700, 700t
  for chronic renal failure, preparations for, 705

Hemofiltration, renal replacement therapy using, 700, 700t

Hemoglobin, reference intervals for, 1207t
  in urine, 1211t
  synthesis of, mechanisms of, 369

Hemoglobin A$_{1c}$, as measure of glycemic control, 553, 554t
  in children, 570
  reference intervals for, 1207t

Hemoglobin A$_2$, reference intervals for, 1207t

Hemoglobin Bart's, 370

Hemoglobin C, sickle hemoglobin with, 375, 375t. See also Sickle cell disease.
  prognosis with, 381

Hemoglobin F, affinity of, for carbon monoxide, 1170, 1171
  hereditary persistence of, sickle hemoglobin with, 375, 375t. See also Sickle cell disease.
  increasing levels of, for sickle cell disease, 381
  for thalassemia, 373

Hemoglobin H disease, 370, 373

Hemoglobin M disease, 365

Hemoglobin S, 374. See also Sickle cell disease.

Hemoglobinopathy. See also Sickle cell disease.
  hemolytic anemia due to, 365
  hemolytic disease of the newborn due to, 390

Hemoglobinuria, paroxysmal cold, 359t
  clinical diagnosis of, 360
  laboratory diagnosis of, 361
  treatment of, 363
  paroxysmal nocturnal, 365–366

Hemolytic anemia, autoimmune, 358–363. See also Autoimmune hemolytic anemia.
  nonimmune, 363–366, 363t. See also specific disorders.
  acquired, 363t, 365–366
  hereditary, 363–365, 363t

Hemolytic disease of fetus and newborn, 383–390
  due to ABO incompatibility, 388, 388t, 390
  Rh isoimmunization and, 384
  due to erythrocyte enzymopathies, 390
  due to erythrocyte membrane disorders, 390
  due to hemoglobinopathies, 390
  due to minor blood group incompatibility, 388
  due to Rh isoimmunization, 383–388. See also Rh isoimmunization.
  steps for bedside management of, 389t

Hemolytic streptococcal gangrene, 81, 795–796, 795t

Hemolytic-uremic syndrome, 366. See also Thrombotic thrombocytopenic purpura.
  causes of, 403
  HELLP syndrome vs., 993t

Hemoperfusion, for acute poisoning, 1156–1157, 1156t
Hemophilias, 390–397
  clinical classification of, 392
  comprehensive care in, 397
  genetics of, 391
  hemorrhage management in, 396–397
  inhibitors in, 391–392
    treatment in presence of, 394–395
  intracerebral hemorrhage management in, 849
  laboratory abnormalities in, 392
  pathophysiology of, 391
  preventive care in, 395–396
  sequelae of, 391–392
  sources of information on, 397
  treatment of, 392–394
    adjunctive therapies in, 395
    in patients with inhibitors, 394–395
Hemorrhage, diverticular, 481
  from esophagogastric varices, 470, 471–473
  gastrointestinal, in acute renal failure, 699
    iron deficiency anemia due to, 356–357
  iliopsoas, in hemophilia, hip hemarthrosis vs., 396
  in acute renal failure, 699
  in hemophilia, 396–397, 849
  in pancreatitis, 518
  in polycythemia vera, 445
  in sports injuries, 975
  intracranial, 847–850. See also Intracranial hemorrhage.
  postpartum, 999, 1000
  splinter, 783
  urethral, with anterior urethral stricture, 711
  vaginal, abnormal. See also Dysfunctional uterine bleeding.
    differential diagnosis of, 1038, 1039t
    during third trimester of pregnancy, 986–988
Hemorrhagic disorders. See Coagulopathy(ies); specific disorders.
Hemorrhoids, 492–493
Hemosiderosis. See Hemochromatosis; Iron overload.
Heparin, for disseminated intravascular coagulation, 401
  for femoral-popliteal vein thrombosis, 345
  for paroxysmal nocturnal hemoglobinuria, 366
  for venous thrombosis prophylaxis, 222t
    after stroke, 852, 855
  intracerebral hemorrhage due to, treatment of, 849
  low-molecular-weight. See also Enoxaparin.
    for deep venous thrombosis, 341–342, 342t
    for disseminated intravascular coagulation, 401
    for pulmonary thromboembolism, 222t, 223–224
    thrombocytopenia due to, 399
      platelet transfusions' effect in, 455
  unfractionated, for deep venous thrombosis, 340–341, 341t, 342t
    for pulmonary thromboembolism, 221, 223t
  with thrombolytic therapy, for myocardial infarction, 320
Hepatic encephalopathy, in cirrhosis, after transjugular intrahepatic portosystemic shunt placement, 470

Hepatic encephalopathy (Continued)
  management of, 470–471
  parenteral nutrition for, 603, 605, 605t
Hepatic fibrosis, due to methotrexate, 948
Hepatic flexure syndrome, 12
Hepatic hydrothorax, in cirrhosis, 470
Hepatitis, alcoholic, 468. See also Cirrhosis.
  autoimmune, 469. See also Cirrhosis.
  due to antitubercular drugs, 241
  viral, 501–507. See also specific diseases, e.g., Hepatitis A.
    acute, 502, 503t
    chronic, 503t, 505–507
    diagnostic tests for, 503t
    transmission of, by blood components, 460
      by clotting factor concentrates, 393
Hepatitis A, 502–503, 502t, 503t
  transmission of, by blood components, 460
Hepatitis A vaccine, 503
  for cirrhosis patient, 466–467
  for travelers, 146–147, 147t
Hepatitis B, 502t, 503–504
  chronic, diagnosis of, 503t, 504t, 506
    hepatocellular carcinoma and, 506
    treatment of, 507
  cirrhosis in, 469. See also Cirrhosis.
  diagnostic tests for, 503t, 504t
  hepatitis D and, 505
  transmission of, by blood components, 460
Hepatitis B immune globulin, 504
Hepatitis B vaccine, 139–141, 140, 144t, 504
  for cirrhosis patient, 467
  for travelers, 147, 147t
Hepatitis C, 502t, 504–505
  chronic, diagnosis of, 503t, 506
    hepatocellular carcinoma and, 506
    treatment of, 507
  cirrhosis in, 466, 506. See also Cirrhosis.
    treatment of, 469
  diagnostic tests for, 503t
  in thalassemia patient on chronic transfusion therapy, 370–371
  oral lichen planus and, 811
  porphyria cutanea tarda and, 452
  transmission of, by blood components, 460
Hepatitis D, 502t, 503t, 505
  transmission of, by blood components, 460
Hepatitis E, 502t, 503t, 505
Hepatitis G, 502t, 505
Hepatocellular carcinoma, chronic viral hepatitis and, 506
  in cirrhosis, 467
  in hemochromatosis, 406
Hepatoerythropoietic porphyria, 448t, 452, 452t
Hepatopulmonary syndrome, in cirrhosis, 471
Herbal compounds, dysfunctional uterine bleeding and, 1038
  for benign prostatic hyperplasia, 688
  for insomnia, 35
Herniation, lumbar disk, 40
Heroin, 1095–1096, 1191, 1192t
Herpes gestationis, 828, 832
Herpes simplex, 799–801, 800t
  chemotherapy-associated mucositis due to, in acute leukemia, 419

Herpes simplex (Continued)
  conjunctivitis due to, 68
  encephalitis due to, 896
  erythema multiforme and, 801, 813, 824
  facial nerve paralysis and, 915–916
  gingivostomatitis due to, 799, 813
  HIV infection and, 53, 800–801
  neonatal, 800t, 801, 984
  of lips, recurrent, 799, 800, 800t, 809
  oral, 812–813
  pneumonia due to, 215, 215t, 216t
Herpes zoster, 801
  acute vertigo due to, 885–886, 885t
  epidemiology of, 69, 801
  external ear involvement in, 115
  in HIV infection, 53
  ocular involvement in, 801
  treatment of, 71, 800t, 802
  varicella vaccine and, 71
Herpesvirus infections, types 1 and 2. See Herpes simplex.
  type 3. See Chickenpox; Herpes zoster; Varicella-zoster virus infection.
  type 4. See Epstein-Barr virus infection.
  type 5. See Cytomegalovirus infection.
  type 6, 802–803
  type 7, 803
  type 8, 803
    Kaposi's sarcoma and, 54, 803
Heterophile antibodies, in infectious mononucleosis, 109
Heterophyes heterophyes infection, 540t, 546
n-Hexane, neuropathy due to, 926
Hiccup, 13–15, 14t
HiDAC/MTX regimen, for highly aggressive lymphoma, 438t
Hidradenoma, vulvar, 1071
High-altitude sickness. See Altitude sickness.
High-density lipoprotein cholesterol. See Cholesterol; Hyperlipoproteinemias.
High-risk neonate. See Neonate(s), high-risk.
Hip joint, hemarthrosis of, in hemophilia, iliopsoas hemorrhage vs., 396
Hip replacement, in ankylosing spondylitis, 960
  in juvenile rheumatoid arthritis, 957
  in osteoarthritis, 970
Hirsutism, 763
His-Purkinje cells, 265
Histamine₁ blockers. See Antihistamines; specific drugs.
Histamine₂ blockers. See also specific drugs.
  defective iron absorption due to, 356
  for dyspepsia, 497
  for gastroesophageal reflux disease, 525
  for gastrointestinal complications in acute renal failure, 699
  for head injury, 935
  for NSAID-induced ulcers, 500
  prophylactic, 499
Histamine receptors, 1111–1112
  antidepressants' action at, 1110t, 1111–1112
  clinical consequences of, 1113, 1113t
Histoplasmosis, 195–199
  chronic pulmonary, 195
    treatment of, 197t, 198
  clinical features of, 195
  diagnosis of, 195–196
  disseminated, 195
    diagnosis of, 196
    treatment of, 197t, 198–199

Histoplasmosis (Continued)
  treatment of, 196–198, 197t
HIV. See Human immunodeficiency virus (HIV) infection.
HLA-B27 antigen, ankylosing spondylitis and, 958, 959
Hoarseness, 25–31
  due to developmental disorders, 29–30
  due to kinetic laryngeal disorders, 27–29
  due to laryngeal inflammation, 30–31
  due to vocal fold lesions, 25–27
Hodgkin's disease, advanced, chemotherapy for, 407
    radiation therapy for, 411
  bulky, 410
    chemotherapy for, 407–408
  chemotherapy for, 406–409, 407t
    follow-up with, 409
    late effects of, 408–409
    side effects of, 408
  early-stage, chemotherapy for, 407
    radiation therapy for, 410–411
  in children, radiation therapy for, 411
  mycosis fungoides/Sézary's syndrome and, 770
  prognostic factors in, 410
  radiation therapy for, 409–413
    after chemotherapy, 407, 408, 411
    late effects of, 412–413
    side effects of, 411–412
    strategies for, 410–411
    techniques in, 409–410
  relapsed and refractory, chemotherapy for, 408
  staging of, 406, 406t, 409
Homocysteine, blood levels of, cardiovascular risk and, 563
Homogentisic acid, urine, reference intervals for, 1211t
Homoharringtonine, for chronic myelogenous leukemia, 429
Hookworms, 540t, 544, 804t
  cutaneous larva migrans due to, 544, 804t, 805
Horder's spots, in psittacosis, 117
Hormone replacement therapy, 1050–1052, 1051. See also Estrogen(s).
  contraindications to, 1052
  endometrial cancer and, 1048, 1063, 1063t, 1065–1066
  for hyperlipidemia, 584
  for hypogonadism, 638–639, 640t, 1042
  for stress incontinence, 673
  monitoring during, 1052
  oncogenic potential of, 1048
  osteoporosis and, 594–595, 1049
  systemic benefits of, 1048–1050
House dust mites, control of, for allergic rhinitis, 744
  for asthma, 731
"Huffing," 1097
Human chorionic gonadotropin, measurement of, 981
  in ectopic pregnancy diagnosis, 985, 985t
Human herpesviruses. See Herpesvirus infections; specific viruses.
Human immunodeficiency virus (HIV) infection, 41–56
  acute retroviral syndrome in, 42–43, 42t
  chancroid and, 717
  common conditions associated with, 43t
  cryptosporidiosis in, 542
  Cyclospora infection in, 539t, 543
  diagnosis of, 43
  disseminated histoplasmosis in, 195, 197t, 198–199

Human immunodeficiency virus (HIV) infection (Continued)
  during pregnancy, 984
  epidemiology of, 41
  hairy leukoplakia in, 814
  hemolytic-uremic syndrome and, 403
  herpes simplex and, 53, 800–801
  isosporiasis in, 543
  leishmaniasis in, 88, 89, 90
  lymphoma in, 55, 439
  management of, 43–56
    antiretroviral therapy in, 43–50, 44t–46t, 48t–49t. See also Antiretroviral therapy.
    baseline medical care in, 43, 44t
    opportunistic infection management in, 50–54
  microsporidiosis in, 543
  molluscum contagiosum in, 803
  Mycobacterium avium complex infection in, 54, 241
  neoplasms in, 54–55
  neurologic disorders in, 55–56, 927
  progression of, 42, 42
  risk factors for, 43t
  strongyloidiasis in, 545
  syphilis treatment in, 724
  toxoplasmosis encephalitis in, 52–53, 151
    central nervous system lymphoma vs., 55
    treatment of, 156–157
  toxoplasmosis prophylaxis in, 154
  transmission of, 41
    in blood components, 461
    in clotting factor concentrates, 393
    vertical, 984
  tuberculosis in, 51–52, 52t, 53t
    symptoms of, 239
    treatment of, 240–241
  viral kinetics in, 41–42
  weight loss in, 56
Human papillomavirus infection, aceto-whitening for detection of, 833, 1069
  cervical, in HIV infection, 55
  cervical cancer and, 787, 1066
  genital cancer and, 787
  genital warts due to, 787
  of nails, 782
  premalignant cutaneous lesions due to, 792–793
  transmission of, 787, 788
  vulvar neoplasia and, 1071–1072
  warts due to, 785
Human parvovirus infection. See Parvovirus infection.
Human T cell lymphotropic viruses, transmission of, by blood components, 461
Humidification, for rhinosinusitis, 234
Hungry bones syndrome, hypoparathyroidism vs., 633
Hutchinson's sign, in melanoma of nail, 783
Hyaline membrane disease, 1014
Hyaluronic acid, for osteoarthritis, 970
Hydatid disease, 541t, 546–547
Hydralazine, adverse effects of, 311
  for congestive heart failure, 294, 294t
  for hypertension, 308t, 311
    during pregnancy, 990, 990t
Hydrocarbons, intoxication by, 1179–1180
Hydrocephalus, after head injury, 935
Hydrochlorothiazide, for diabetes insipidus, 626–627, 626t
  for hypertension, 308t

Hydrochlorothiazide (Continued)
  in type 2 diabetes, 563
  for Meniere's disease, 893
  for premenstrual syndrome, 1047
  for primary aldosteronism, 635
Hydrocodone, for urinary calculus, 713
  in analgesic combinations, 2
  intoxication with, 1192t
Hydrocolloid dressings, for pressure ulcers, 820
Hydrocortisone, after surgery for Cushing's disease, 622
  for adrenal crisis, 620, 620t
  for adrenal insufficiency, chronic, 621
    secondary, 637, 640t
  for atopic dermatitis, 822
  for corrosive ingestion, 1171
  for hyperpigmentation, 839
  for inflammatory bowel disease, 484–485
  for pertussis, 139
  for postinflammatory hypopigmentation, 841
  for pruritus, 36
  for vitiligo, 841
  with deferoxamine therapy, 372
Hydrocortisone-neomycin-polymyxin, for draining ear, 207t
  for otitis externa, 114
Hydrocortisone-pramoxine, for pruritus gravidarum, 833
Hydrofluoric acid exposure, 1126
Hydrogel dressings, for pressure ulcers, 820
Hydrogen breath tests, for bacterial overgrowth, 509
Hydrogen cyanide, intoxication with, 1173
Hydrogen peroxide, for acute necrotizing ulcerative gingivitis, 814
  for black hairy tongue, 815
  for thrush, 811
Hydroids, 1142
Hydromorphone, for pain, 4t
  for painful episode in sickle cell disease, 376
  intoxication with, 1192t
Hydrops fetalis. See also Hemolytic disease of the fetus and newborn; Rh isoimmunization.
  due to alpha-globin gene deletion, 370
Hydroquinone, for hyperpigmentation, 839
  in vitiligo treatment, 841
Hydrothorax, hepatic, in cirrhosis, 470
α-Hydroxy acids, for hyperpigmentation, 839
Hydroxychloroquine, for cutaneous lupus, 762, 775
  for dermatomyositis, 777
  for juvenile rheumatoid arthritis, 955t, 956
  for lichen planopilaris, 762
  for oral lesions in lupus, 813
  for porphyria cutanea tarda, 452
  for rheumatoid arthritis, 946t, 949–950, 951
  for sarcoidosis, 226, 227
  for urticarial vasculitis, 837
Hydroxycobalamin. See also Vitamin B₁₂.
  for cyanide intoxication, 1174
  for pernicious anemia, 367
17-Hydroxycorticosteroids, urine, reference intervals for, 1211t
5-Hydroxyindoleacetic acid, urine, reference intervals for, 1211t
Hydroxymethylglutaryl coenzyme A (HMG-CoA) reductase inhibitors. See also specific drugs.

Hydroxymethylglutaryl coenzyme A (HMG-CoA) reductase inhibitors *(Continued)*
  adverse effects of, 581–582
  drug interactions of, 581–582
  for hyperlipidemia, 581–582
    after myocardial infarction, 332
    in angina, 249
    in combination therapy, 584
  mechanism of action of, 581
Hydroxyurea, didanosine interaction with, 45, 50
  fetal globin gene activation by, for sickle cell disease, 381
  for chronic myelogenous leukemia, 427–428
  for leukostasis in acute leukemia, 415
  for polycythemia vera, 446, 446t
Hydroxyzine, for allergic rhinitis, 745t
  for anaphylaxis, 727t
  for atopic dermatitis, 822
  for ciguatera poisoning, 1143
  for lichen simplex chronicus, 834
  for mycosis fungoides, 768
  for ordinary urticaria, 836
  for pain, 3
  for painful episode in sickle cell disease, 377
  for pruritic urticarial papules and plaques of pregnancy, 831–832
  for pruritus, 37
  intoxication with, 1164
Hymen, imperforate, 1042
Hymenolepis nana infection, 541t, 546
Hymenoptera sting allergy, 753–755, 754t, 755t
Hyoscyamine, for bladder dysfunction in multiple sclerosis, 902
  for diurnal enuresis, 669
Hyperactivity disorder. See *Attention-deficit/hyperactivity disorder.*
Hyperaldosteronism, 314–315, 634–635
Hyperbaric oxygen, for carbon monoxide poisoning, 1170
  for clostridial myonecrosis, 797
  for high-altitude cerebral edema, 1128, 1128t
  for high-altitude pulmonary edema, 1128t, 1129
  for marine animal bites, 1142
  for necrotizing skin and soft tissue infections, 82
  for osteomyelitis, 974
  for sea anemone sting, 1142
Hyperbilirubinemia. See *Jaundice.*
Hypercalcemia, due to calcitriol therapy, for secondary hyperparathyroidism, 632
  familial benign hypocalciuric, laboratory evaluation of, 628–629, 628t
    parathyroid hyperplasia in, 627–628
  humoral, of malignancy, primary hyperparathyroidism vs., 629
  in multiple myeloma, 443
  in primary hyperparathyroidism, 628
    medical management of, 630–631
  in sarcoidosis, ketoconazole for, 226
    treatment of, 227t, 228
Hypercalcemic crisis, in primary hyperparathyroidism, 630–631
Hypercalciuria, in sarcoidosis, 227t, 228
  renal, hyperparathyroidism due to, 631
  urinary stones due to, 715
Hypercapnia, ventilatory failure with, 169
Hypercoagulability, workup for, in pulmonary thromboembolism workup, 221

Hypercortisolism. See also *Cushing's syndrome.*
  classification of, 621t
HyperCVAD regimen, for Burkitt's lymphoma, 438–439, 438t
  for mantle cell lymphoma, 438
Hypercyanotic spells, in tetralogy of Fallot, 285
Hyperemesis gravidarum, parenteral nutrition for, 603
Hyperglycemia, in acute pancreatitis, 516
  toxic effects of, in type 2 diabetes, 551
  with parenteral nutrition, 606
Hyperinsulinemia, in insulin resistance syndrome, 551
Hyperkalemia, due to massive transfusion, 461
  in acute renal failure, 697, 697t
  in chronic renal failure, 704–705
  in digitalis intoxication, 1174, 1175
Hyperkinesis. See *Attention-deficit/hyperactivity disorder.*
Hyperlipoproteinemias, 578–584. See also *Cholesterol.*
  hormone replacement therapy's effects on, 1049
  in insulin resistance syndrome, 551
  treatment of, after myocardial infarction, 322, 332
    dietary, 580
    drug combinations in, 584
    guidelines for, 578–580, 579t
    in type 2 diabetes, 562t, 563
    pharmacologic, 580–584
Hypermagnesemia, in acute renal failure, 698
Hypernatremia, dehydration with, in infant or child, 611, *611*, 612–613
  in acute renal failure, 698
  in diabetes insipidus, 625
Hyperoxaluria, urinary stones due to, 715
Hyperoxia testing, in cyanotic newborn, 284
Hyperparasitemia, in malaria, 95t, 100
Hyperparathyroidism, 627–632
  in chronic renal failure, 631, 703–704
  primary, 627–631
    causes of, 627–628, 628t
    clinical manifestations of, 628
    diagnosis of, 629
    incidence of, 627
    laboratory evaluation in, 628–629, 628t
    treatment of, 629–631
  secondary, 628t, 631–632
  tertiary, 628t, 632
Hyperphosphatemia, in acute renal failure, 698
  in chronic renal failure, 703–704
Hyperpigmentation, 837–840
  bleaching medications for, 839–840
  postinflammatory, 838–839, 838t
  systemic causes of, 840, 840t
  ultraviolet light–induced, 837–838, 838t
Hyperprolactinemia, 640–642, 640t
  amenorrhea due to, 1041
  due to antipsychotic drugs, 1119
  in acromegaly, 615
Hypersensitivity pneumonitis, 230–231, 231t
Hypersensitivity syndrome reaction, 749, 750, 750t
  drugs commonly implicated in, 750t, 751
Hypersensitivity vasculitis, 729
Hypersplenism, in cystic fibrosis, 180
Hypertension, 303–315

Hypertension *(Continued)*
  ambulatory venous, after venous thrombosis, 340
    venous leg ulcers and, 818
  antidepressants for use in, 1115t
  classification of, 303t
  due to pheochromocytoma, 653
    intraoperative management of, 656
  during pregnancy, 982, 988–994. See also *Pre-eclampsia.*
    chronic, 988, 989–991, 990t
    gestational (transient), 988, 991
    types of, 988–989
  home monitoring in, 304
  hormone replacement therapy and, 1048
  in acute renal failure, 699
  in angina, 249–250
  in chronic renal failure, 702
  in diabetes, renal disease and, 564–565
    treatment of, 562t, 563
  in insulin resistance syndrome, 551
  in mitral valve prolapse, 289, 290
  in phencyclidine intoxication, 1195
  in primary aldosteronism, 314–315, 634, 635
  initial evaluation in, 303–304, 304t
  intracerebral hemorrhage due to, 847
  intracranial. See *Intracranial hypertension.*
  malignant, in monoamine oxidase inhibitor overdose, 1191
  oral contraceptives and, 1086t
  portal, in cystic fibrosis, 180
  pulmonary, in high-altitude pulmonary edema, 1129
    in newborn, 1014–1015
  recommendations for follow-up based on initial reading in, 304t
  renovascular, 313–314
  resistant (refractory), 311–312
  risk factors in, 304t
  risk stratification in, 304t, 305t
  secondary, 312–315, 312t
  treatment of, 304–311
    algorithm for, *306*
    during pregnancy, 989–991, 990t
    goals for, 306
    in hemorrhagic stroke patient, 849
    in ischemic stroke patient, 852
    lifestyle modifications in, 304–306
    pharmacologic, 306–311, 308t–309t
      causes for inadequate response to, 311t
Hypertensive crisis, 312, 312t
  in stroke patient, 852
Hyperthermia, fever vs., 20
  malignant, in monoamine oxidase inhibitor overdose, 1191
Hyperthyroidism, 645–648
  causes of, 645, 646t
  clinical features of, 646t
  diagnosis of, 645–646
  due to amiodarone, 660
  treatment of, 646–648
    in angina management, 250
    in subacute thyroiditis, 659
Hypertriglyceridemia, oral contraceptives and, 1086t
  treatment of, guidelines for, 579–580
    in type 2 diabetes, 554, 554t, 563
Hypertrophic cardiomyopathy, 292, 346–350
  clinical manifestations of, 347
  defined, 346
  diagnostic modalities in, 348
  epidemiology of, 346

Hypertrophic cardiomyopathy (Continued)
  genetics of, 346–347
  natural history of, 348
  pathology of, 347
  pathophysiology of, 347
  physical examination in, 347–348
  treatment of, 349–350, 349t
  unusual variants of, 348–349
Hyperuricemia, 576–578. See also Gout.
  due to niacin, 583
  in acute renal failure, 698
  in lead poisoning, 1185
  in pre-eclampsia, 991
  with very-low-calorie diet, 589
Hyperuricosuria, urinary stones due to,
    715
Hyperventilation, dizziness due to, 885t,
    891
  for head injury, 933, 934
  for intracranial hypertension, in bacte-
    rial meningitis, 108
  with intracerebral hemorrhage, 849
  seizure vs., 857
Hyperviscosity, in multiple myeloma, 444
  in polycythemia vera, 445
Hypervolemia, in acute renal failure, 697
  in chronic renal failure, 704
Hypnotics. See also specific drugs and
    classes of drugs.
  abuse of, 1096
  chronic use of, insomnia due to, 32
  for insomnia, 34–35
Hypocalcemia, due to citrate toxicity with
    massive transfusion, 461
  in acute renal failure, 698
  in chronic renal failure, 703
  in ethylene glycol intoxication, 1178
  in hypoparathyroidism, 632–634, 633t
  in neonate, 1012
Hypocalciuric hypercalcemia, familial
    benign, laboratory evaluation of,
    628–629, 628t
  parathyroid hyperplasia in, 627–628
Hypocitraturia, urinary stones due to, 715
Hypofibrinogenemia, cryoprecipitate for,
    calculation of dosage for, 458
Hypoglycemia, in acute poisoning, 1157
  in malaria, 95t, 99
  in type 1 diabetes, 571
  masking of symptoms of, by beta block-
    ers, 248, 250
  recurrent, with insulinoma, peripheral
    neuropathy in, 926
  seizure vs., 857
  with parenteral nutrition, 606
Hypoglycemia-avoidance diet, for chronic
    fatigue syndrome, 112
Hypoglycemic agents. See also specific
    drugs and classes of drugs.
  oral, for type 2 diabetes, 556–560, 557,
      557t
    mechanisms of action of, 556–557,
      557
    selection of, 557–558
Hypogonadism, amenorrhea due to,
    1042–1043
  hypogonadotropic, 638–639, 640t
Hypokalemia, in primary aldosteronism,
    315, 634
    treatment of, 635
    with cobalamin therapy for pernicious
      anemia, 367
Hypomelanosis, idiopathic guttate, 841
Hyponatremia, dehydration with, in infant
    or child, 609t, 611, 611, 612
  due to treatment of diabetes insipidus,
    626

Hyponatremia (Continued)
  in acute renal failure, 698
Hypoparathyroidism, 632–634, 632t, 633t
Hypopharyngeal diverticulum, 479
  dysphagia due to, 474
  treatment of, 478, 479
Hypopigmentation, 840–841
Hypopituitarism, 635–640. See also
    specific hormone deficiencies.
  causes of, 636, 636t
  clinical picture of, 636
  treatment of, 639–640, 640t
Hypoplastic anemia. See also Aplastic
    anemia.
  criteria for, 351
Hypoplastic left heart syndrome, 286–287
Hypoprolactinemia, 639, 640t
Hypotension, in high-risk neonate,
    1012–1013
  in neuroleptic intoxication, 1197
  orthostatic, 885t, 890–891
    antidepressants for use in, 1115t
    in diabetes, 565–566
    in mitral valve prolapse, 291
  with obstetric anesthesia, 998
Hypothermia, accidental, 1130–1133,
    1130t, 1132t
  due to massive transfusion of cold blood,
    461
  neuroprotective effect of, 1131
  in cardiac arrest, 256
Hypothyroidism, 642–645
  amenorrhea due to, 1041
  atrophic, 643
  clinical manifestations of, 643
  due to radiation therapy, 643
    for Hodgkin's disease, 412
  due to radioiodine therapy, 647
  in hypopituitarism, 637–638, 640t, 645
  in hypothalamic disease, 645
  laboratory evaluation of, 643
  myxedema crisis in, 644–645, 644t
  obstructive sleep-disordered breathing
    and, 182
  peripheral neuropathy in, 928
  pressure palsies in, 930
  primary, causes of, 645–646, 645t
  subclinical, 643
    treatment of, 659
  treatment of, 643–644
    in angina management, 250
    in chronic thyroiditis, 659
    in hypopituitarism, 638, 640t
    in subacute thyroiditis, 659
Hypovolemia. See also Fluids, parenteral.
  in acute renal failure, 697
  in chronic renal failure, 705
  in neonate, 1006
  shock due to, after myocardial in-
    farction, 325
Hypoxic-ischemic encephalopathy, in
    neonate, 1014
Hysterectomy, for cervical cancer, 1068
  for endometrial cancer, 1064
  for endometriosis, 1032, 1033–1034
Hysteroscopy, for leiomyomata, 1062

Ibandronate, for Paget's disease of bone,
    599
Ibuprofen, adverse effects of, 969
  for afterpains, 999
  for cystic fibrosis, 176t, 177
  for dysfunctional uterine bleeding, 1040
  for dysmenorrhea, 1043t, 1044, 1044t

Ibuprofen (Continued)
  for fever, 22
  for juvenile rheumatoid arthritis, 954,
    955t
  for mountain sickness, 1128
  for pain in pericarditis, 333
  for painful episode in sickle cell disease,
    376
  for viral respiratory infection, 214
Ibutilide, for atrial fibrillation, 259, 259t
  after myocardial infarction, 323
Icterus. See Jaundice.
Idarubicin, for acute myelogenous
    leukemia, 416
  for aggressive lymphoma, 436t, 437
  for Sézary's syndrome, 769
IDV. See Indinavir (IDV).
Ifosfamide, for aggressive lymphoma, 436t
Ig. See Immunoglobulin entries.
Ileal conduit, after cystectomy for bladder
    cancer, 709
Ileal diverticula, 480
Ileus, gallstone, 465
  in cystic fibrosis, 178, 179t
  prolonged, parenteral nutrition for, 603
Iliac artery aneurysm, 338–339
Iliofemoral vein thrombosis, 345–346, 345.
    See also Venous thrombosis.
Iliopsoas bursitis, 965
Iliopsoas hemorrhage, in hemophilia, hip
    hemarthrosis vs., 396
Iliotibial band syndrome, 977
Imipenem, for bacterial meningitis, 106
  for bacterial pneumonia, 212t
  for cystic fibrosis exacerbations, 179t
  for fever in aplastic anemia, 353
Imipenem-cilastatin, for pyelonephritis,
    682t
  for sepsis, 63t
Imipramine, for anxiety disorders, 1100t,
    1101–1102
  for attention-deficit/hyperactivity disor-
    der, 873, 873t
  for depression, 1109t
  for irritable bowel syndrome, 492
  for nocturnal enuresis, 670
  for panic disorder, 1121–1122, 1121t
  for urinary incontinence due to bladder
    dysfunction, 672
  intoxication with, 1201, 1202t
  monoamine oxidase inhibitor interaction
    with, 1115
  pharmacodynamic effects of, 1110t
  reference intervals for, 1210t
Imiquimod, for genital warts, 788
Immune complex glomerulonephritis, 679
Immune function, reference intervals for
    tests of, 1213t
Immune globulin, for aplastic anemia, 354
  hepatitis B, 504
  intramuscular, for hepatitis A protection
      for travelers, 147t, 148
    for measles prophylaxis, 134
    for rubella prophylaxis, 131–132
  intravenous, 458
    for chronic inflammatory demyelinat-
        ing polyradiculoneuropathy, 930
    for Guillain-Barré syndrome, 929
    for immune thrombocytopenic pur-
        pura, 400
    for juvenile rheumatoid arthritis, 955t,
        957
    for multiple sclerosis, 898–899
    for myasthenia gravis, 907
    for necrotizing skin and soft tissue in-
        fections, 82

Immune globulin *(Continued)*
  for post-transfusion purpura, 399, 460
  for Rh isoimmunization, 388t
  for streptococcal toxic shock syndrome, 85, 85t
  for toxic epidermal necrolysis, 825
  for warm antibody autoimmune hemolytic anemia, 362
  measles protection provided by, 134
  rabies, 121
  Rh. See *Rh immune globulin.*
  tetanus, 135, 136
  varicella-zoster, 71, 802
Immune thrombocytopenic purpura, 400
Immunizations, 139–145. See also *specific vaccines.*
  contraindications to, 144–145
  during breastfeeding, 148–149
  during pregnancy, 145, 148
  for hemophiliac infants, 396
  for immunocompromised persons, 144–145, 149
  for travelers, 146–149, 147t
  information statements for patients, 145
  interchangeability of vaccines from different manufacturers for, 145
  late, 144
  minimal ages and intervals for, 144t
  recommended schedule for, *140–141*
  simultaneous, 145
Immunocompromised persons. See also *specific immunodeficiency states, e.g. Human immunodeficiency virus (HIV) infection.*
  immunizations for, 144–145
    for travel, 149
  toxoplasmosis in, 156–157
Immunoglobulin A (IgA), deficiency of, anaphylactic reaction to blood components in, 455, 460
  serum, reference intervals for, 1213t
Immunoglobulin A (IgA) bullous dermatosis, linear, 829–830
Immunoglobulin A (IgA) nephritis, 679
Immunoglobulin D (IgD), serum, reference intervals for, 1213t
Immunoglobulin E (IgE), measurement of, in allergic rhinitis, 744
  serum, reference intervals for, 1213t
Immunoglobulin G (IgG), reference intervals for, in cerebrospinal fluid, 1212t
  in serum, 1213t
Immunoglobulin G (IgG) index, reference intervals for, 1212t
Immunoglobulin M (IgM), serum, reference intervals for, 1213t
Immunosuppressive therapy. See also *specific drugs.*
  for aplastic anemia, 353
  for autoimmune hepatitis, 469
  for inflammatory bowel disease, 485–486
  for juvenile rheumatoid arthritis, 955t, 957
  for lupus erythematosus, 776
  for myasthenia gravis, 906–907, 906t, 907t
    during pregnancy, 908
  for primary glomerular disease, 675–677
  for sarcoidosis, 225–226
  for warm antibody autoimmune hemolytic anemia, 362
Immunotherapy, contact, for warts, 786
  for allergic rhinitis, 748
  for allergy with recurrent rhinosinusitis, 235

Immunotherapy *(Continued)*
  for anaphylaxis prevention, 728–729
  for asthma, 734–735
  for insect sting allergy, 754–755, 755t
Immunotoxic B43 pokeweed antiviral protein, for acute lymphoblastic leukemia, 425
Imperforate hymen, 1042
Impetigo, 794, 795t
  in atopic dermatitis, 823–824
  in chickenpox, 70
Impetigo herpetiformis, 833
Impotence. See *Erectile dysfunction.*
Incentive spirometry, for atelectasis, 170
Incontinence, bowel, after stroke, 855
  urinary, 671–674
    after radical prostatectomy, 707
    after stroke, 855
    hormone replacement therapy for, 1049–1050
    in children, 668–671
    overflow, 674
    paradoxical, in children, 670
    stress, 673–674
    urgency, 671–673
    with bladder dysfunction, 671–673
    with urethral dysfunction, 673–674
Indapamide, for hypertension, 308t
Indigestion. See *Dyspepsia.*
Indinavir (IDV), antitubercular drug interactions with, 52, 240
  for HIV infection, 45, 46t, 49t
  toxic effects of, 47
Indomethacin, adverse effects of, 969
  for ankylosing spondylitis, 960
  for delayed pressure urticaria, 836
  for diabetes insipidus, 626t, 627
  for dysmenorrhea, 1043t
  for gout, 577
  for juvenile rheumatoid arthritis, 954, 955t
  for patent ductus arteriosus, 1015
  for urticarial vasculitis, 837
Infant(s). See also *Child(ren); Neonate(s).*
  bacterial meningitis management in, 104t, 105t
  carbon monoxide poisoning in, 1170, 1171
  cough in, 22–23
  epilepsy in, 867–871. See also *Epilepsy; Seizures.*
  feeding of, 1018–1022
    breast, 1018–1019. See also *Breastfeeding.*
    formula, 1019–1022, 1021t
    solid food, 1022
  fever in, 21
  Glasgow Coma Scale responses in, 1146t
  ipecac dosage for, 1148
  of cobalamin-deficient mother, megaloblastic anemia in, 369
  of hemophilia carriers, preventive care in, 395–396
  parenteral fluid therapy for, 607–613. See also under *Fluids, parenteral.*
  pertussis in, 137
  pyelonephritis symptoms in, 666
  seborrheic dermatitis in, 773
  thrush in, 811
  viral respiratory infection treatment in, 214
  vitamin K deficiency in, 592
  vitamin K supplements for, 593
Infantile spasms, 869, 870
Infection(s). See also *Sepsis; specific infections.*

Infection(s) *(Continued)*
  aortic, 246–247
  bacterial, in malaria, 99
    of skin and soft tissue, 81–82, 794–799, 795t, 796t
    tracheal, 31
  drug reactions and, 750
  fungal, of external ear canal, 114–115
    of nails, 780–782, 781t, 782t, 807
    of skin, 806–808
  hemolysis due to, 366
  in acute leukemia in children, 422
  in acute renal failure, 699
  in aplastic anemia, 353
  in burn patients, 1126
  in neutropenia, 382–383
  in newborn, 1017–1018, 1017t
  in pancreatitis, 517
  in pernicious anemia, 368
  in pressure ulcers, 820–821
  in sickle cell disease, 378–379
  laryngeal, 30
  opportunistic, in HIV infection, 50–54
  Paget's disease of bone and, 597
  perinatal, 984
  peripheral neuropathy due to, 927–928
  postpartum, 1000–1001
  respiratory tract. See *Pneumonia; Respiratory tract infection.*
  sea water, 798–799
  urinary tract. See *Urinary tract infection.*
  viral, of skin, 799–803
  with intensive chemotherapy for leukemia, 419–420
Infectious mononucleosis, 108–109, 109t, 802
Infectious rhinitis, allergic rhinitis vs., 744
Infective endocarditis, 297–303
  acute, 297
  classification of, 297
  clinical manifestations of, 298–299
  culture-negative, 297, 299
    antibiotics for, 300t
  diagnosis of, 299, 299t
  epidemiology of, 297
  in brucellosis, 65t, 66
  in Q fever, 118
  in rat bite fever, 122, 123
  indications for surgery in, 302
  mitral valve prolapse and, 288
  native valve, 297, 298t
  nosocomial, 297, 298t
  organisms causing, 297–298, 298t
    antibiotics directed at, 300t
  predisposing factors for, 297, 298t
  prophylaxis for, 301t, 302–303, 302t
    in mitral valve prolapse, 289, 290, 290t
    procedures requiring, 302–303, 302t
  prosthetic valve, 297, 298t
  subacute, 297
  treatment of, 299–302, 300t
Inferior vena cava filter, for femoral-popliteal vein thrombosis, 345
  for pulmonary thromboembolism prevention, 224
Infertility, in endometriosis, 1034–1037, *1034*, 1035t
  leiomyomata and, 1060
Inflammatory bowel disease, 482–488
  ankylosing spondylitis and, 958, 960
  bone loss in, 487
  cancer surveillance in, 487
  colorectal cancer and, 533
  dietary therapy for, 486

Inflammatory bowel disease *(Continued)*
  drug therapy for, 483–486
  emotional support in, 488
  parenteral nutrition for, 603
  surgery for, 487–488
Inflammatory carcinoma of breast, 1026
Inflammatory demyelinating poly-
    radiculoneuropathy, acute, 929
  influenza vaccine and, 87
  chronic, 929–930
Infliximab, for inflammatory bowel
    disease, 486
Influenza, 85–88, 87t
  clinical manifestations of, 86
  diagnosis of, 86
  pneumonia due to, 215, 215t, 216t
  prevention of, 86–87, 87t
  treatment of, 87–88
Influenza vaccine, 86–87, 87t, 143–144
  for cirrhosis patient, 467
  for travelers, 148
INH. See *Isoniazid (INH)*.
Inhalants, abuse of, 926, 1097
Inhalation, toxic exposure by,
    decontamination for, 1147
Inhalation injury, thermal, 1125
  signs suggesting, 1123
Insect sting allergy, 753–755, 754t, 755t
Insecticides, intoxication with, 1193–1194
Insomnia, 32–35, 32t–34t
  in Alzheimer's disease, 847
Insulin, adjustments in dosage of, with
    very-low-calorie diet, 589
  for diabetic ketoacidosis, 574, 574t
    in children, 568
    in type 2 diabetes, 575
  for diabetic neuropathy, 925
  for hyperkalemia in acute renal failure,
    697, 697t
  for ischemic stroke, 852
  for type 1 diabetes, 568–570, 569t, 570t
    dosage adjustment in, after ketoacido-
      sis, 575
    with intercurrent illness, 571–572
  for type 2 diabetes, 560–561
    in combination therapy, 561, 562
  in parenteral nutrition solutions, 605,
    605t
Insulin pump, for diabetes in children, 569
Insulin resistance, ketoacidosis treatment
    in presence of, 574–575
Insulin resistance syndrome, 551–552
Insulin tolerance test, in adrenocortical
    insufficiency diagnosis, 620
Insulin-like growth factor 1, measurement
    of, in acromegaly diagnosis, 615
Insulin-like growth factor 1–binding
    protein, measurement of, in
    acromegaly diagnosis, 615
Interferon, for brucellosis, 66
  for hepatitis C and cirrhosis, 469
Interferon α, adverse effects of, 506
  contraindications to, 506
  for chronic viral hepatitis, 506–507
  for indolent B cell lymphoma, 435
  for metastatic renal cell carcinoma, 709–
    710
  for multiple myeloma, 442
  for scleroderma, 778
Interferon alfa-2a, for chronic hepatitis C,
    507
  for cutaneous hemangiomas, 809
  for laryngeal papilloma, 25
  for polycythemia vera, 446t, 447
  for Sézary's syndrome, 769
Interferon alfa-2b, for chronic hepatitis B,
    469

Interferon alfa-2b *(Continued)*
  for chronic hepatitis C, 507
  for chronic myelogenous leukemia, 427,
    427t, 428–429
  for melanoma, 791–792
  for polycythemia vera, 446t, 447
  for Sézary's syndrome, 769
Interferon beta-1a, for multiple sclerosis,
    898, 898t
Interferon beta-1b, for multiple sclerosis,
    in relapsing remitting disease, 898,
      898t
  in secondary progressive disease, 899
Interferon γ, for toxoplasmosis, 154
Interferon gamma-1b, for keloids, 784
  for leishmaniasis, 90
Interleukin 2, for metastatic renal cell
    carcinoma, 709–710
Interleukin 2–diphtheria toxin fusion
    protein, for Sézary's syndrome, 769
Interleukin 12, for Sézary's syndrome, 769
Intermediate-density lipoprotein, 580. See
    also *Cholesterol; Hyperlipoprotein-
    emias*.
Intermittent positive pressure breathing,
    for atelectasis, 170
International Society of Travel Medicine,
    145
Interphalangeal joints of fingers,
    dislocation of, 977
Intervertebral disk herniation, lumbar, 40
Intestinal flukes, 540t, 546
Intra-aortic balloon counterpulsation, for
    cardiogenic shock, 326
  for ventricular septal rupture, 327
Intracranial hematoma, with minor head
    injury, 933–934
  with severe head injury, 934
Intracranial hemorrhage, 847–850
  causes of, 847, 848t
  clinical features of, 847–848
  common syndromes of, 848
  diagnosis of, 849, 849t
  due to bicarbonate, 1006
  due to thrombolytic therapy, 320
  in hemophilia, 849
  in neonate, 1013
  rehabilitation after, 853–856, 853t. See
    also under *Stroke*.
  secondary prophylaxis of, 855
  treatment of, 849–850
Intracranial hypertension, after head
    injury, 935, 935t
  in children, 938
  benign, tinnitus due to, 38
  in bacterial meningitis, 108
  in encephalitis, 896
  with intracerebral hemorrhage, 849
Intracranial pressure. See also
    Intracranial hypertension.
  monitoring of, after head injury, 934
    in children, 938
Intradermal nevus, 788, 789
Intraocular pressure, elevated, glaucoma
    and, 912
Intrapulmonary percussive ventilation, for
    atelectasis due to mucous plugs, 171
Intrathecal analgesia, for labor, 996–997
Intrauterine device(s), 1078t–1079t, 1087
  copper T, 1079t, 1087
    for emergency contraception, 1085,
      1087
  during breast-feeding, 1089
  management of problems with, 1088t
  pelvic inflammatory disease and, 1058
  placement of, 1087, 1087t

Intrauterine device(s) *(Continued)*
  progesterone-releasing, 1079t, 1087
    during breast-feeding, 1089
    for dysfunctional uterine bleeding,
      1040
Intrauterine growth restriction, risk of,
    with chronic maternal hypertension,
    989
Intubation, for tetanus, 135
  in neonatal resuscitation, 1005–1006
  nasogastric, for acute pancreatitis, 516
  of burn patient, 1123
Inulin clearance, for glomerular filtration
    rate measurement, 701
Iodide deficiency, hypothyroidism due to,
    643
Iodoquinol, for amebiasis, 58, 58t, 59t,
    539t, 542
  for amebiasis cutis, 804
  for *Balantidium coli* infection, 539t, 543
  for *Blastocystis hominis* infection, 539t,
    543
  for *Dientamoeba fragilis* infection, 539t,
    543
Iopanoic acid, for hyperthyroidism, 647
Iothalamate clearance, for glomerular
    filtration rate measurement, 702
Ipecac, to induce vomiting, for acute
    poisoning, 1147–1148
  for mushroom poisoning, 76
  in bulimia nervosa, 1103
Ipratropium bromide, for allergic rhinitis,
    746
  for asthma, 734
    in children, 740, 741
  for chronic obstructive pulmonary dis-
    ease, 172, 173, *173*
  for rhinosinusitis, 235
Ipratropium bromide–albuterol, for chronic
    obstructive pulmonary disease, 173
Irbesartan, for hypertension, 309t, 311
Iridocyclitis, in leprosy, 94
Iridoplasty, peripheral laser, for glaucoma,
    915
Iridotomy, laser, for glaucoma, 914–915
Iris pigmentation, due to latanoprost, 914
Iron, deficiency of, 356–358
  aphthous stomatitis due to, 812
  impaired absorption of, causes of, 356
  levothyroxine interaction with, 644
  overdose of, 1180–1181
  serum, reference intervals for, 1208t
  supplemental, 357–358, 357t, 358t
    during pregnancy, 980
    for anemia in chronic renal failure,
      703
    for infant, 1022
Iron-binding capacity, serum, reference
    intervals for, 1208t
Iron chelation therapy, for iron overdose,
    1180–1181
  for transfusional hemosiderosis in thalas-
    semia, 372
Iron dextran, for anemia in chronic renal
    failure, 703
  for iron deficiency, 358, 358t
Iron overload. See also *Hemochromatosis*.
  due to chronic transfusion therapy, 461
  in thalassemia, 371–372
  with chronic heme therapy for acute por-
    phyria, 451
Irradiation. See also *Radiation* entries.
  of blood components, for prevention of
    transfusion-associated graft-versus-
    host disease, 457, 460
Irritable bowel syndrome, 488–492

Irritable bowel syndrome *(Continued)*
  definition of, 488–489
  diagnosis of, 490
  dyspepsia and, 11, 488
  management of, 490–492
  natural history of, 489
  pathophysiology of, 489–490
Irritant contact dermatitis, 830–831
Ischemic bowel disease, chronic,
    malabsorption due to, 511
Ischemic heart disease. See *Coronary
    artery disease.*
Ischemic optic neuropathy, anterior, optic
    neuritis vs., 911
Ischemic syndrome, acute, 316. See also
    Myocardial infarction.
Ischiorectal abscess, 495
Islet cell transplantation, with
    pancreatectomy, 523
Isocarboxazid, for depression, 1109t
  overdose of, 1190
Isoflurane, for obstetric anesthesia, 998
Isometheptene-dichlorophenazone, for
    migraine, 881
Isoniazid (INH), adverse effects of, 241
  anticonvulsant interactions with, 863t
  antifungal interactions with, 196
  for *Mycobacterium kansasii* infection,
    241
  for tuberculosis, 240
    in HIV infection, 53t
  for tuberculosis prophylaxis, 241–242
    in HIV infection, 52t
  intoxication by, 1181–1182
  pyridoxine deficiency due to, neuropathy
    in, 927
Isopropanol, intoxication by, 1176t, 1182
  treatment of, 1156t, 1182
  serum concentration estimation for,
    1160t
Isoproterenol, for antidepressant
    intoxication, 1203
  for cardiac tamponade, 335
  for insect sting allergy, 754
Isosorbide dinitrate, after myocardial
    infarction, 330
  for angina, 248
  for congestive heart failure, 294, 294t
Isosorbide mononitrate, after myocardial
    infarction, 330
  for angina, 248
  for prevention of variceal bleeding, 471,
    473
Isosporiasis, 539t, 543
Isotretinoin, cheilitis due to, 810
  for acne, 758–759
  for dissecting cellulitis of scalp, 762
  for intraoral leukoplakia, 810
  for lupus erythematosus, 776
  for pityriasis rubra pilaris, 773
  for prevention of second malignancies in
    lung cancer, 191
  for rosacea, 759
Isradipine, for hypertension, 308t
  intoxication with, 1168
Itraconazole, drug interactions with, 194,
    196, 200–201, 807
    HMG-CoA reductase inhibitors, 581–
    582
  for blastomycosis, 200–201, 200t
  for candidiasis, in HIV infection, 54
    vulvovaginal, 1053–1054
  for coccidioidomycosis, 193–194
  for histoplasmosis, 196–198, 197t
    in AIDS, 197t, 198–199
  for leishmaniasis, 91

Itraconazole *(Continued)*
  for onychomycosis, 782, 782t, 807
  for tinea infection, 762, 806, 807
Ivermectin, for cutaneous larva migrans,
    544
  for onchocerciasis, 804t
  for scabies, 804t, 805–806
  for strongyloidiasis, 541t, 545, 804t, 805

Janeway's lesions, 298
Japanese encephalitis, 896
Japanese encephalitis vaccine, for
    travelers, 147t, 148
Jarisch-Herxheimer reaction, in Lyme
    disease, 127
  in relapsing fever, 124
Jaundice, in acute viral hepatitis, 502
  in malaria, 99–100
  in newborn, 1016–1017
    in Rh isoimmunization, 387, 387t
Jejunal diverticula, 480
Jellyfish, 1142
Jervell and Lange-Nielsen syndrome,
    torsades de pointes in, 279
Jessner's solution, for hyperpigmentation,
    840
Jet lag, 150
  insomnia due to, 32, 34
  melatonin for, 35
Joint replacement, in ankylosing
    spondylitis, 960
  in juvenile rheumatoid arthritis, 957
  in osteoarthritis, 970
  in rheumatoid arthritis, 952
  osteomyelitis and, 971–972
Junctional nevus, 788–789
Junctional premature beats, 261
Junctional tachycardia, nonparoxysmal,
    272

Kala-azar. See *Leishmaniasis.*
Kamino bodies, in Spitz's nevus, 789
Kaolin pectin, for erythema multiforme,
    813
  for mouth disease, 808
Kaposi's sarcoma, herpesvirus type 8 and,
    54, 803
  in HIV infection, 54–55
Keloids, 783–785
Keratinocytes, premalignant neoplasms of,
    792–793
Keratolytics, for warts, 785
Keratosis, actinic, 792
    squamous cell carcinoma and, 764,
    792
  smoker's, of palate, 811
Keratosis obturans, 115
Kerion, in tinea infection, 762
Kernicterus, in Rh isoimmunization, 387,
    387t
Kerosene, 1179
Ketamine, abuse of, 1096
Ketoacidosis, diabetic. See *Diabetic
    ketoacidosis.*
Ketoconazole, drug interactions with, 194,
    196, 200–201
    HMG-CoA reductase inhibitors, 581–
    582
  for blastomycosis, 200–201
  for candidiasis, in HIV infection, 54
    vulvovaginal, 1053–1054
  for coccidioidomycosis, 193–194

Ketoconazole *(Continued)*
  for Cushing's syndrome, 623, 623t
  for histoplasmosis, 196, 197t
    in AIDS, 199
  for hypercalcemia in sarcoidosis, 226,
    228
  for leishmaniasis, 91
  for median rhomboid glossitis, 815
  for seborrheic dermatitis, 773
  for tinea infection, 762, 807
  for tinea versicolor, 808
Ketogenic diet, for epilepsy, 865
  in infants and children, 869, 870
17-Ketogenic steroids, urine, reference
    intervals for, 1211t
Ketoprofen, for dysmenorrhea, 1043t,
    1044t
Ketorolac, for allergic conjunctivitis, 68
  for urinary calculus, 713
17-Ketosteroids, urine, reference intervals
    for, 1211t
Ketotifen, for ordinary urticaria, 836
Kidney(s). See also *Renal* entries.
  functions of, 701t
    measurement of, 701–702
  trauma to, 682–684
  tuberculosis involving, 239
Kidney stones, 712–715
  in primary hyperparathyroidism, 629
Knee, sports injuries to, 977
Knee replacement, for juvenile rheumatoid
    arthritis, 957
  for osteoarthritis, 970
  for rheumatoid arthritis, 952
Koebner's phenomenon, in psoriasis, 771
  in vitiligo, 840
Koplik spots, in measles, 132

Labetalol, for hypertension, 308t, 309
    during pregnancy, 990, 990t
  for intracerebral hemorrhage, 849
  for monoamine oxidase inhibitor over-
    dose, 1190–1191
  for pheochromocytoma, 655
  for tetanus, 136
  intoxication with, 1166, 1167t
Labor analgesia, 995–997
Labyrinthectomy, for Meniere's disease,
    888–889, 894
Labyrinthitis, 885–886, 885t
Lacerations, arterial, with central catheter
    placement, 605
  in sports injuries, 975
Lachman test, for anterior cruciate
    ligament tear, 977
Lactase insufficiency, 513–514
  in infant, lactose-free formulas for, 1020,
    1021t
Lactate, blood, reference intervals for,
    1208t
Lactate dehydrogenase, serum, reference
    intervals for, 1208t
Lactated Ringer's solution, electrolyte
    composition of, 608t
Lactation. See also *Breast milk; Breast-
    feeding.*
  breast abscess during, 1023
  breast cancer during, 1026
  contraceptive benefit of, 1076t, 1089
  mastitis during, 1000, 1019
  nutritional requirements during, 1019
Lactic acid, for hyperpigmentation, 839
Lactic acidosis, due to metformin, 558
Lactose intolerance, 513–514

Lactose intolerance *(Continued)*
  in infant, lactose-free formulas for, 1020, 1021t
Lactulose, for constipation, 19
  for hepatic encephalopathy, 470, 471
Lamivudine (3TC), drug interactions with, 45
  for chronic hepatitis B, 469, 507
  for HIV infection, 45t, 48t
Lamivudine-zidovudine (AZT-3TC), for HIV infection, 48t
Lamotrigine, adverse effects of, 863t
  drug interactions with, 863t
  for epilepsy, 860t, 862t, 864
    in infants and children, 868t, 869t
  for Lennox-Gastaut syndrome, 870–871
  pharmacokinetics of, 862t
Language disorders, after head injury in children, 940
  after stroke, 854–855
Lanreotide, for acromegaly, 617
Lansoprazole, for dyspepsia, 497
  for gastroesophageal reflux disease, 525–526
  for *Helicobacter pylori* infection, 501, 501t
  for NSAID-induced ulcer, 500
    prophylactic, 499, 499t
Lanugo hair, 759
Laparoscopy, cholecystectomy using, for acute cholecystitis, 464
  for cholelithiasis, 463
  for gallstone pancreatitis, 517
  endometrial cancer surgery with, 1064
  in endometriosis, 1031, 1032
    for infertility, 1036
    for pain, 1033
  myomectomy using, for leiomyomata, 1062
Larva currens, 804t, 805
Larva migrans, cutaneous, 544, 804t, 805
Laryngitis, 30
  defined, 25
  reflux, 30, 31
Laryngomalacia, dysphonia due to, 29
Laryngopharyngeal reflux, 30, 31. See also *Gastroesophageal reflux disease.*
Larynx, cancer of, hoarseness due to, 27
  developmental disorders of, 29–30
  examination techniques for, 25
  inflammatory disorders of, 30–31
  kinetic disorders of, 27–29
Laser therapy, for actinic cheilitis, 810
  for benign prostatic hyperplasia, 691
  for glaucoma, 914–915
  for hair removal, 763
  for hemorrhoids, 493
  for keloids, 784
  for laryngeal papilloma, 25
  for leiomyomata, 1062
  for obstructive sleep-disordered breathing, 184–185
  for skin cancer, 765
  for subglottic hemangioma, 29
  for vulvar intraepithelial neoplasia, 1072
  for warts, 786
Latanoprost, for glaucoma, 914
Lateral epicondylitis of elbow, 965, 976
Latex allergy, 725
Laxatives, for constipation, 19–20, 19t
Lead. See also *Lead poisoning.*
  blood, classification of concentrations, in children, 1187t
    reference intervals for, 1212t
  urine, reference intervals for, 1212t
Lead mobilization test, 1187

Lead poisoning, 1183–1187
  acute, 1183
  follow-up in, 1187
  manifestations of, 1184–1185, 1185t
  neuropathy due to, 926, 1184
  occupational, 1183–1184, 1183t, 1184t
  screening for, 1183, 1183t
  sources of, 1183–1184, 1183t
  treatment of, 1185–1187, 1186t
Learning disorders, in attention-deficit/hyperactivity disorder, 872
Leflunomide, 1215t
  for rheumatoid arthritis, 946t, 951
Left bundle branch, 265
Left bundle branch block. See also *Heart block.*
  after myocardial infarction, 324t
  electrocardiographic diagnosis of, 266
  natural history of, 267
Left-to-right shunt, acyanotic congenital heart disease with, 280–282. See also specific lesions.
Leg, sports injuries to, 977–978
Leg pain, low back pain with, 40
Leg ulcers, in sickle cell disease, 379
  venous, 817–819
Legionellosis, 216–218, 217t
Leiomyomata, uterine, 1060–1063, 1060t, 1061t
Leiomyosarcoma, uterine, 1060
Leishmaniasis, 88–91
  oral ulceration in, 813
Lemonade, for urinary stone prevention, 715
Lennox-Gastaut syndrome, 870–871
Lentigines, senile (solar), 839–840
Lepirudin, 1215t
Leprosy, 91–94
  classification of, 91
  complications in, 93–94
  control measures for, 94
  future prospects for, 94
  patient follow-up in, 92–93
  peripheral neuropathy due to, 94, 927
  treatment of, 92
Leriche's syndrome, 246
Leucovorin (folinic acid), for aggressive lymphoma, 436t
  for AIDS-related lymphoma, 439
  for gastric adenocarcinoma, 530
  for highly aggressive lymphoma, 438t
  for isosporiasis, 543
  for methanol intoxication, 1190
  for *Pneumocystis carinii* pneumonia in HIV infection, 51
    prophylactic, 51
  for toxoplasmosis, 152
    congenital, 156
    during pregnancy, 155
    in HIV infection, 53, 156, 157
    ocular, 156
  for toxoplasmosis prophylaxis, in HIV infection, 52
  with methotrexate for rheumatoid arthritis, 948
Leukapheresis, for Sézary's syndrome, 769
Leukemia, acute, classification of, 414, 421–422
  in adults, 413–421
    causes of, 413–414
    clinical manifestations of, 414–415
    cytogenetic features of, 415, 416t
    demographics of, 414
    diagnosis of, 415
    new directions in, 420–421
    prognosis in, 415, 416t

Leukemia *(Continued)*
    supportive care for, 419–420
    treatment of, 415–419
  in children, 421–425
    diagnosis of, 421, 421t
    future directions in, 425
    prognosis in, 421–422, 422t
    treatment of, 422–425
  multiple drug resistance in, 420
  acute lymphoblastic, 416t
    Burkitt's type, 416t, 419
    classification of, 414, 421
    clinical manifestations of, 414–415
    demographics of, 414
    epidemiologic associations of, 413
    in children, 421
      prognosis in, 421, 422t
      treatment of, 422–424
    in chronic myelogenous leukemia, 427
    prognosis in, 416t
    treatment of, in adults, 418–419
  acute myelogenous, 416t
    classification of, 414
    clinical manifestations of, 414–415
    demographics of, 414
    epidemiologic associations of, 413–414
    in chronic myelogenous leukemia, 427
    prognosis in, 416t
    treatment of, 415–418, *417*
      in elderly persons, 418
  acute nonlymphocytic, classification of, 421, 422t
    in children, 421
      treatment of, 424–425
  acute promyelocytic, treatment of, 418, 420, 425
  central nervous system, 414
    in children, 424
      prophylaxis of, 423, 424–425
  chronic lymphocytic, 429–432
    diagnostic criteria for, 430, 430t
    differential diagnosis of, 430
    genetic alterations in, 429–430
    immune abnormalities in, 430
    staging of, 430, 431t
    treatment of, 431–432
  chronic myelogenous, 425–429
    causes of, 426
    clinical manifestations of, 426–427
    incidence of, 425
    molecular biology of, 426
    treatment of, 427–429
  gingival enlargement in, 814
  prolymphocytic, chronic lymphocytic leukemia vs., 430
  varicella vaccination in, 143
Leukemia cutis, 414
Leukocyte(s), fecal, in infectious diarrhea, 15
  semen, reference intervals for, 1213t
Leukocyte alkaline phosphatase, reference intervals for, 1206t
Leukocyte count, reference intervals for, 1206t
Leukocyte esterase test, in cystitis diagnosis, 663
Leukoedema, 812
Leukoencephalopathy, progressive multifocal, in HIV infection, 55
Leukokeratosis, 810
Leukokeratosis nicotine palati, 811
Leukomalacia, periventricular, in neonate, 1013–1014
Leukopenia, due to clozapine, 1119
Leukoplakia, hairy, 814
  oral, 793, 810

Leukoplakia (*Continued*)
vocal fold, 26–27
Leukostasis, in acute leukemia, in adults, 415
in children, 422
Leukotriene modifiers. See also specific drugs.
for allergic rhinitis, 747
for asthma, 733
in children, 739–740
Leuprolide, for acute porphyria, 451
for endometriosis, 1032
for irritable bowel syndrome, 492
for leiomyomata, 1061t
with cyclophosphamide therapy for primary glomerular disease, 676
Levamisole, for brucellosis, 66
for colorectal cancer, 537
Levetiracetam, for epilepsy, 864
Levobunolol, for glaucoma, 913
intoxication with, 1167t
Levodopa, for Parkinson's disease, 918, 919t
fluctuating response to, 921–922
with disease progression, 921
Levodopa-carbidopa. See *Carbidopa-levodopa.*
Levofloxacin, for acute pyelonephritis, 681t, 682t
for bacterial pneumonia, 212
for ehrlichiosis, 166t
for legionellosis, 217, 217t, 218
for osteomyelitis, 973, 974t
for Q fever, 118
for Rocky Mountain spotted fever, 166t
for tuberculosis, 240
for urinary tract infection in men, 661
Levomethadyl acetate, for opioid abuse, 1095
Levonorgestrel, subdermal implantable, for contraception, 1082t, 1085
Levonorgestrel–ethinyl estradiol, in emergency contraceptive kit, 1087
Levorphanol, for pain, 4t
Levothyroxine, drug interactions with, 644
for depression, 644
for hypothyroidism, 643–644
in chronic thyroiditis, 659
in hypopituitarism, 638, 640t
in subacute thyroiditis, 659
for myxedema crisis, 644–645
for thyroid cancer, 651
Lhermitte's phenomenon, due to radiation therapy for Hodgkin's disease, 412
in multiple sclerosis, 902
Lice, 804t, 806
relapsing fever carried by, 123–125
Lichen planopilaris, 762
Lichen planus, 772–773
nail involvement in, 781t, 782–783
oral, 811
Lichen sclerosus, invasive vulvar cancer and, 1072
Lichen sclerosus et atrophicus, 794
Lichen simplex chronicus, 833, 834
Lidocaine, derivatives of. See also specific drugs.
for pain, 3
for atrial flutter, 275t
for black hairy tongue, 815
for cardiac arrest, 253, *254*, 255
for cesarean delivery, in epidural anesthesia, 997
in spinal anesthesia, 997
for erythema multiforme, 813
for fibromyalgia, 967

Lidocaine (*Continued*)
for hiccup, 14t
for mouth disease, 808
for neuroleptic intoxication, 1197
for oral herpes simplex, 813
for rheumatoid arthritis, 948
for ventricular tachycardia after myocardial infarction, 323–324
reference intervals for, 1210t
relative antiarrhythmic efficacy of, 262t
Lidocaine-prilocaine, for pruritus, 36
Light. See also *Sunlight.*
exposure to, sleep patterns and, 34
Light therapy. See *Phototherapy.*
Limb compression, for post-thrombotic edema, 343–344
for venous leg ulcers, 818
prophylactic, 818
Limb dermatitis, 817
Lindane, for lice, 804t, 806
Linear IgA bullous dermatosis, 829–830
Liothyronine, for depression, 644
for hypothyroidism, 644
for myxedema crisis, 645
Liotrix, for hypothyroidism, 644
Lip lesions, 809–810
Lipase, deficiency of, malabsorption due to, 508–509
serum, in acute pancreatitis diagnosis, 515
reference intervals for, 1208t
Lipid disorders. See *Hyperlipoproteinemias.*
Lipodermatosclerosis, 817
Lipoprotein metabolism, 580. See also *Hyperlipoproteinemias.*
Lisinopril, after myocardial infarction, 331
for congestive heart failure, 294t
for hypertension, 309t
Listeria monocytogenes infection, food-borne, 75t, 77t, 79–81
meningitis due to, 103t, 104t, 106–107
Lithium, diabetes insipidus due to, 627
for aplastic anemia, 354
for bipolar disorder, 1117
for depression, 1116
hypercalcemia due to, 629
intoxication by, 1187–1189, 1188t
treatment of, 1156t, 1188–1189
reference intervals for, 1210t
Lithostatin, chronic pancreatitis and, 519
Lithotripsy, shock wave, for urinary calculus, 714
Litter boxes, disinfection of, 152
Little Leaguer's elbow, 976
Liver abscess, amebic, 57, 57t. See also *Amebiasis.*
diagnosis of, 58
treatment of, 59, 59t
pyogenic, amebic abscess vs., 57, 57t
Liver cancer, chronic viral hepatitis and, 506
in cirrhosis, 467
in hemochromatosis, 406
Liver disease. See also specific diseases.
alcoholic, 468. See also *Cirrhosis.*
cholestatic, pruritus in, 37
in cystic fibrosis, 179t, 180
in protoporphyria, 453
in sarcoidosis, 227t, 228
vitamin K deficiency vs., 592, 592t
Liver dysfunction, with parenteral nutrition, 606–607
Liver failure, fulminant, due to niacin, 583
in acute viral hepatitis, 502, 502t
parenteral nutrition for, 603

Liver flukes, 540t, 546
Liver spots, 839–840
Liver transplantation, for alcoholic liver disease, 468
for cirrhosis, 466, 466t
for fulminant hepatic failure, 502
for protoporphyria, 453
for viral hepatitis, 506
Living will, for Alzheimer's disease patient, 845
Loa loa, 804t
Lobucavir, for herpes simplex, 800
Lodoxamide, for allergic conjunctivitis, 68
Loose anagen syndrome, 761
Loperamide, for diarrhea, 16, 17t
in diabetes, 565
in food-borne illness, 76
in travelers, 17, 150
for irritable bowel syndrome, 491
for radiation enteritis, 511
for salmonellosis, 160
Loracarbef, for otitis media, 206
Loratadine, for allergic rhinitis, 745, 745t
for atopic dermatitis, 822
for childhood dermatomyositis, 777
for ordinary urticaria, 835
for pruritus, 37
intoxication with, 1164
Lorazepam, for anxiety disorders, 1100t, 1102
for cocaine-induced anxiety, 1094
for hallucinogen intoxication, 1096
for nausea and vomiting, 8t
for phencyclidine intoxication, 1096
for premenstrual syndrome, 1047
for status epilepticus, 865, 865t
in infants and children, 870t, 871
intoxication with, 1096, 1166
Losartan, for hypertension, 309t
Loteprednol, 1215t
Louse (lice), 804t, 806
Louse-borne relapsing fever, 123–125
Lovastatin, antifungal interactions with, 807
for hyperlipidemia, 581
after myocardial infarction, 332
levothyroxine interaction with, 644
Low-density lipoprotein cholesterol. See *Cholesterol; Hyperlipoproteinemias.*
Loxapine, characteristics of, 1118t
intoxication with, 1196, 1197t
Lucio phenomenon, in leprosy, 93
Lumbar disk herniation, 40
Lumbar puncture, in encephalitis diagnosis, 895
in meningitis diagnosis, 895
Lumbar spinal stenosis, pseudoclaudication due to, intermittent claudication vs., 336, 336t
Lumpectomy, for breast cancer, 1027
Lung(s), acute toxicity of, due to methotrexate, 948
fetal, corticosteroids to enhance maturity of, 984, 1014
with placenta previa, 988
hypoplastic, in neonatal hydrops, 386
resection of, for emphysema, 175
for non–small cell lung cancer, 187
Lung abscess, 203–204
Lung cancer, 186–192
after Hodgkin's disease treatment, 412
causes of, 186
chemoprevention of second malignancies in, 191
clinical manifestations of, 186

Lung cancer *(Continued)*
  diagnosis of, 186
  histologic classification of, 186
  neuropathy with, 931, 932
  non–small cell, staging of, 186–187, 187t
    treatment of, 187–190, 190t
  palliative care in, 191
  silicosis and, 229
  small cell, 190–192
    sensory neuropathy with, 931
  staging of, 186–187, 187t
Lung disease. See also specific diseases.
  in sarcoidosis, 226–227, 227t
  in sickle cell disease, 379
Lung flukes, 546
Lung injury, acute, transfusion-related, 460
Lung lavage, for silicosis, 230
Lung transplantation, for chronic obstructive pulmonary disease, 175
Lupus erythematosus, 774–776
  bullous systemic, 830
  classification of, 774
  cutaneous, chronic. See *Discoid lupus erythematosus.*
    hair loss in, 762
    subacute, 774, 776
  drug-induced, 774
  systemic. See *Systemic lupus erythematosus.*
  treatment of, 775–776
Lupus pernio, 227
Luteinizing hormone, deficiency of, in hypopituitarism, 638–639, 640t
  in normal menstrual cycle, 1040
  measurement of, in amenorrhea evaluation, 1042
  serum, reference intervals for, 1209t
Luteinizing hormone–releasing hormone analogs. See also *Gonadotropin-releasing hormone agonists;* specific drugs.
  for acute porphyria, 451
  for irritable bowel syndrome, 492
  for premenstrual syndrome, 1047
  for prostate cancer, 708
  with cyclophosphamide therapy, for primary glomerular disease, 676
Lutropin. See *Luteinizing hormone.*
Lyme disease, 125–130
  chronic, erroneous diagnosis of, 130
  clinical manifestations of, 125–126, 125t
  co-infection in, 127
  in children, 126–127
  laboratory testing for, 127
  meningitis in, 125t, 126, 895
    treatment of, 127, 128t
  peripheral neuropathy in, 126, 927
    treatment of, 127, 128t
  prevention of, 130
  relapsing fever vs., 124
  treatment of, 127–130, 128t–129t
Lymphadenectomy, sentinel, for breast cancer, 1027
  for melanoma, 791
  for vulvar carcinoma, 1073
Lymphadenitis, tuberculous, 239
Lymphangiomas, of lips and tongue, 809
Lymphatic drainage of intestinal tract, abnormal, malabsorption due to, 512
Lymphatic mapping, intraoperative, selective lymphadenectomy with, for breast cancer, 1027
  for melanoma, 791
  for vulvar carcinoma, 1073
Lymphocytapheresis, for aplastic anemia, 354

Lymphocytapheresis *(Continued)*
  for Sézary's syndrome, 769
Lymphocyte(s), subsets of, reference intervals for, 1213t
Lymphocyte toxicity assay, for drugs, 752
Lymphocytic choriomeningitis virus, 895
Lymphocytic thyroiditis, 642–643
Lymphocytoma, borrelial, 125t, 126, 128t
Lymphogranuloma venereum, 722
Lymphoid tissue, mucosa-associated, lymphoma of, 440, 531
  skin-associated, cutaneous T cell lymphoma and, 766, 767
Lymphoma, aggressive, treatment of, 436t, 437–438
  AIDS-related, 439
  Burkitt's, 438
  central nervous system, in HIV infection, 439
  cutaneous T cell, 765–770. See also *Mycosis fungoides; Sézary's syndrome.*
    classification of, 765–766, 766t
    diagnosis of, 766
    parapsoriasis and, 766, 774, 794
    staging of, 766
    treatment of, 770
  gastrointestinal, 439–440, 530–531
  highly aggressive, treatment of, 438–439, 438t
  Hodgkin's. See *Hodgkin's disease.*
  indolent B cell, treatment of, 434–437, 435t
  lymphoblastic, 439
  MALT, 440, 531
  mantle cell, 438
    chronic lymphocytic leukemia vs., 430
  non-Hodgkin's, 432–440
    classification of, 433, 433t
    in HIV infection, 55
    staging of, 433–434, 433t, 434t
    treatment of, 434–440, 435t, 436t, 438t
Lymphomatoid papulosis, mycosis fungoides/Sézary's syndrome and, 770
Lynch's syndrome, 533–534, 534t
Lysergic acid diethylamide (LSD), 1096–1097
Lyssaviruses, 119. See also *Rabies.*

MACOP-B regimen, for aggressive lymphoma, 436t
Macroglossia, 815
Maddrey index, 468
Magenblase syndrome, 12
Magic Mary's Mouthwash, for contact stomatitis, 816
Magnesium. See also *Hypermagnesemia.*
  blood pressure and, 305
  for myocardial infarction, 322
  for premenstrual syndrome, 1046
  for short-bowel syndrome, 511
  for ventricular tachycardia after myocardial infarction, 324
  in parenteral nutrition solutions, 605t
  reference intervals for, in serum, 1209t
    in urine, 1211t
Magnesium choline trisalicylate, for dysmenorrhea, 1043t
  for juvenile rheumatoid arthritis, 954–956, 955t
Magnesium hydroxide, for mouth disease, 808
Magnesium sulfate, for cardiac arrest, *254*
  for ethanol intoxication, 1177

Magnesium sulfate *(Continued)*
  for HELLP syndrome, 993
  for hiccup, 14t
  for seizure, in acute porphyria, 449
  for seizure prevention in pre-eclampsia, 994, 994t
  for tetanus, 136
  for torsades de pointes, 1153t
    in antidepressant intoxication, 1203
    in antihistamine poisoning, 1165
    in digitalis intoxication, 1175
    in neuroleptic intoxication, 1197
Magnetic resonance angiography, in pulmonary thromboembolism workup, 221
Magnetic resonance imaging (MRI), disease activity measurement with, in multiple sclerosis, 897–898
  in brain tumor diagnosis, 942
  in epilepsy evaluation, 860
  in hypertrophic cardiomyopathy diagnosis, 348
Malabsorption, 507–514
  after gastrectomy, 512–513
  after intestinal resection, 510, 511
  carbohydrate, 513–514
  diagnosis of, 507–508
  due to primary intestinal disorders, 510–511
  in chronic pancreatitis, 508–509, 521
  megaloblastic anemia due to, 369
Malaria, 94–101
  cerebral, 95t, 99
  clinical features of, 95, 95t
  diagnosis of, 95–96
  epidemiology of, 94
  hemolysis with, 366
  non–*P. falciparum,* drug resistance in, 96, 149–150
    management of, 96, 96t
  P. falciparum, drug resistance in, 96, 149
    mild, 96, 97t
    severe, management of, 96–101, 98t, 99t
    manifestations of, 95t
    sickle cell trait and, 374
  pathogenesis of, 95
  prevention of, 100–101, 100t, 149–150
  species causing, 94
  transmission of, by blood components, 461
Malassezia furfur, seborrheic dermatitis and, 773
  tinea versicolor due to, 808
Malathion, 1193
Maldigestion, due to bile salt deficiency, 509–510
Malignancy. See also specific sites and types.
  second, treatment-related, in Hodgkin's disease, 409, 412–413
    in thyroid cancer, 652
Malignant hypertension, in monoamine oxidase inhibitor overdose, 1191
Malignant hyperthermia, in monoamine oxidase inhibitor overdose, 1191
Malignant neuroleptic syndrome, 1119, 1196, 1198
Mallet finger, 977
Malnutrition, in chronic pancreatitis, 521
  in chronic renal failure, 704
  in surgical patient, parenteral nutrition for, 603–604
  neuropathy due to, 927
Malone antegrade continent enema, for constipation, 20

Mammary dysplasia, 1023
Mammography, 1025
  recommendations for, 1024–1025
Mandibular repositioning devices, for
    temporomandibular disorders, 961,
    963–964
Manganese, with parenteral nutrition, 605
Mania, acute, 1117
Manic-depressive disorder, 1116–1117
  sleep in, 33
Mannitol, for cerebral edema in diabetic
    ketoacidosis, 568
  for cerebral malaria, 99
  for ciguatera poisoning, 79, 1143
  for intracranial hypertension, in encepha-
    litis, 896
  with intracerebral hemorrhage, 849
  for snake bite, 1141
  for stroke edema, 852
Manometry, esophageal, in dysphagia
    evaluation, 477
Mantle field irradiation, for Hodgkin's
    disease, 410
Mantoux test, for tuberculosis, 242
Maprotiline, for depression, 1109t
  intoxication with, 1201, 1202t
  pharmacodynamic effects of, 1110t
Marijuana, 1097. See also Cannabinoids.
Marine animals, biting, 1141–1142
  electric, 1144
  poisonous, 79, 80t, 1143–1144
  venomous, 1142–1143
Mask(s), for preventing tuberculosis
    transmission, 240
Mask of pregnancy, 839
Mastectomy, for breast cancer, 1027
  prophylactic bilateral, in high risk of
    breast cancer, 1024
Mastitis, during lactation, 1000, 1019
Mastocytosis, systemic, anaphylaxis vs.,
    726
Mastoiditis, with otitis media, 207
MATCH mnemonic, 1194
Maturity-onset diabetes of youth, genetic
    mutation in, 550
Maxillofacial surgery, for obstructive sleep-
    disordered breathing, 185
Mazindol, for obesity, 591, 591t
M-BACOD regimen, for aggressive
    lymphoma, 436t
  for AIDS-related lymphoma, 439
M-BACOS regimen, for aggressive
    lymphoma, 436t, 437
Mean corpuscular hemoglobin, reference
    intervals for, 1207t
Mean corpuscular hemoglobin concen-
    tration, reference intervals for,
    1207t
Mean corpuscular volume, reference
    intervals for, 1207t
Measles, 132–134
Measles vaccine, 133–134, 143
  for travelers, 148
Measles-mumps-rubella vaccine, 132, 133,
    143
  for travelers, 147t
  schedules for, 140–141, 144t
Mebendazole, 544
  for angiostrongyliasis, 540t, 545
  for ascariasis, 540t, 544
  for capillariasis, 540t, 545
  for echinococcosis, 541t, 547
  for hookworm, 540t, 544, 804t
  for pinworm, 540t, 544
  for trichinosis, 541t, 545
  for Trichostrongylus infection, 541t, 545

Mebendazole (Continued)
  for whipworm, 541t, 544
Mebeverine, for irritable bowel syndrome,
    492
Mechanical ventilation. See Ventilation,
    mechanical.
Mechlorethamine, for Hodgkin's disease,
    407t
  for lupus erythematosus, 776
  for mycosis fungoides, 768
Meckel's diverticulum, 480–481
Meclizine, for Meniere's disease, 893
  for vertigo, 886t
  intoxication with, 1164
Meclofenamate, for dysmenorrhea, 1043t
Meconium, amniotic fluid stained by, 1004
Meconium ileus equivalent, in cystic
    fibrosis, 178, 179t
Medial collateral ligament of knee, injury
    to, 977
Medial epicondylitis of elbow, 965, 976
Medial periostalgia, 977–978
Median rhomboid glossitis, 815
Mediastinal fibrosis, due to histoplasmosis,
    195, 199
MedicAlert, 754
Medications. See also specific drugs and
    classes of drugs.
  adverse reactions to, allergy and, 748–
    749, 749, 749t. See also Allergy, to
    drugs.
    classification of, 749
    reporting of, 753
  allergic reactions to, 748–753. See also
    under Allergy.
  anagen effluvium due to, 760–761
  anxiety symptoms due to, 1120, 1120t,
    1121t
  asthma exacerbated by, 731
  autoimmune thyroiditis due to, 658t,
    660
  conjunctivitis due to, 69
  constipation due to, 18, 18t
  cutaneous vasculitis due to, 778–779
  DNA damage due to, acute leukemia
    and, 413
  erectile dysfunction due to, 692
  erythema multiforme and, 824
  gastroesophageal reflux and, 525
  hypothyroidism due to, 643
  immune hemolytic anemia due to, 359,
    360
    clinical diagnosis of, 360
    laboratory diagnosis of, 361
    treatment of, 363
  in acute hepatic porphyrias, safety of,
    449, 450t
  intoxication by, meningoencephalitis vs.,
    895
  intratympanic delivery of, for Meniere's
    disease, 894
  lichen planus due to, 773
  lupus erythematosus due to, 774
  myasthenia gravis and, 903, 903t
  new for 1998, 1214t–1216t
  ototoxic, bilateral vestibular deficit due
    to, 891
  paroxysmal symptoms in pheochromocy-
    toma due to, 653
  peripheral neuropathy due to, 926, 926t,
    931
  psoriasis due to, 771
  rhinitis due to, 743t
  scleroderma due to, 777
  serum sickness due to, 729, 729t
  sore mouth due to, 816

Medications (Continued)
  Stevens-Johnson syndrome due to, 825
  telogen effluvium due to, 760, 760t
  therapeutic monitoring of, reference
    intervals for, 1210t
  thrombocytopenia due to, 399
  thrombotic thrombocytopenic purpura
    due to, 403
  tinnitus due to, 38
  torsades de pointes due to, 279, 279
  toxic epidermal necrolysis due to, 825
Medihaler-Epi, for insect sting allergy, 754
Medium-chain triglycerides, for
    maldigestion due to bile salt
    deficiency, 509, 510
  infant formulas with, 1020, 1021t
Medroxyprogesterone, for amenorrhea due
    to polycystic ovarian syndrome, 1042
  for dysfunctional uterine bleeding, 1039,
    1039t, 1040
  for dysmenorrhea, 1044
  for hormone replacement therapy, 1051,
    1052
  for hypogonadism, 638–639, 640t, 1042
  for mountain sickness, 1130
  for obesity-hypoventilation syndrome,
    184
  for recurrent endometrial cancer, 1065
  injectable depot, for contraception,
    1081t, 1085
Medulloblastoma, 941, 943
Mefenamic acid, for dysmenorrhea, 1043t
Mefloquine, for malaria, 96, 97t
  prophylactic, 100t, 101, 149
Megacolon, in Chagas' disease, 102
Megaesophagus, in Chagas' disease, 102
Megaloblastic anemia, 366–369
Megestrol, for AIDS-related weight loss, 56
  for breast cancer, 1028
  for recurrent endometrial cancer, 1065
Meglumine antimoniate, for leishmaniasis,
    89
Melanocytes, premalignant lesions of, 793
Melanocytic nevi, 788–790, 793
  of oral mucosa, 816
Melanoma, 790–792, 790t, 791t
  congenital nevus and, 793
  dysplastic nevus and, 789, 793
  of mouth, 817
  of nail, 781, 783
  of vulva, 1074, 1074t
  sunburn and, 842
Melasma, 839
Melatonin, sleep and, 35
Meloxicam, for pain, 2
Melphalan, for multiple myeloma, 442
Membranoproliferative glomerulonephritis,
    679
Membranous glomerulopathy, 678–679
Meniere's disease, 892–894
  tinnitus in, 38
  vertigo in, 885t, 888–889, 892–893
Meningeal myelomatosis, 444
Meningioma, 940, 943
  optic neuritis vs., 911
Meningitis, bacterial, 103–108
  chemoprophylaxis of, 108
  treatment of, adjunctive therapy in,
    107–108
    antimicrobial therapy in, 103–107,
    103t–105t
    duration of, 107
    in infants and children, 104t, 105t
    in neonates, 104t, 105t, 1017–1018,
    1017t
    initial approach to, 103, 103t, 104t

Meningitis (Continued)
viral meningitis vs., 895
carcinomatous, viral meningitis vs., 895
coccidioidal, 195
cryptococcal, in HIV infection, 52
due to enteric gram-negative bacilli,
104t, 106, 107
due to NSAIDs, 969
encephalitis vs., 895
Escherichia coli, 103t
Haemophilus influenzae, antimicrobial
therapy for, 103t, 104t, 106, 107
chemoprophylaxis of, 108
in Lyme disease, 125t, 126, 895
treatment of, 127, 128t
Listeria monocytogenes, 103t, 104t, 106–
107
Neisseria meningitidis, antimicrobial
therapy for, 103t, 104t, 105–106,
107
chemoprophylaxis of, 108
Pseudomonas aeruginosa, 104t, 106
staphylococcal, 104t, 107
Streptococcus agalactiae, 103t, 104t, 107
Streptococcus pneumoniae, 103–105,
103t, 104t, 107
tetanus vs., 135
tuberculous, 239
in HIV infection, 52
typhoid, 163–164
viral, 894–896
bacterial meningitis vs., 895
Meningococcal meningitis, antimicrobial
therapy for, 103t, 104t, 105–106, 107
chemoprophylaxis of, 108
Meningococcal vaccine, before splenectomy
for hereditary spherocytosis, 364
for travelers, 147t, 148
Meniscus tears, 977
Menkes' kinky hair disorder, 763
Menopause, 1047–1053. See also Hormone
replacement therapy.
atrophic vaginitis after, 1055
contraception at, 1086t, 1089
Menorrhagia, with ovulatory dysfunctional
uterine bleeding, 1038
Menstruation, absent, 1040–1043
dysfunctional. See Dysfunctional uterine
bleeding.
iron deficiency anemia due to, 356–357
migraine associated with, 883
normal physiology of, 1038, 1040
painful, 1043–1044, 1043t, 1044t
Meperidine, abuse of, 1095
for acute hepatic porphyria, 448, 448t
for pain, 4t, 5
in pericarditis, 334
for pancreatitis, 516
for urinary calculus, 713
intoxication with, 1095, 1191, 1192t
monoamine oxidase inhibitor interaction
with, 1102, 1115
toxic metabolite of, 5
Mephenytoin, for vitamin K deficiency,
592, 593
Mephobarbital, intoxication with, 1165
Meprobamate, intoxication with, 1156t
α-Mercaptopropionylglycine, for cystinuria,
715
Mercaptopurine (6-MP), for acute
lymphoblastic leukemia in children,
423
for inflammatory bowel disease, 485
Mercury, urine, reference intervals for,
1212t
Meropenem, for bacterial meningitis, 105t,
106

Meropenem (Continued)
for Listeria monocytogenes meningitis,
107
for pneumococcal meningitis, 104t, 105
for sepsis, 63t
Mesalamine (5-ASA), for inflammatory
bowel disease, 483–484
Mescaline, 1096
Mesna, for aggressive lymphoma, 436t
for highly aggressive lymphoma, 438t
Mesoridazine, characteristics of, 1118t
intoxication with, 1196, 1197t
Metabolic acidosis, in acute poisoning,
1158, 1159t
in acute renal failure, 698
in chronic renal failure, 704
in neonate, 1006
Metabolic bone disease, in chronic renal
failure, 703–704
Metacarpophalangeal joint replacement,
for rheumatoid arthritis, 952
Metagonimus yokogawai infection, 540t,
546
Metandienone, abuse of, 1098
Metanephrines, urine, in pheochromocytoma diagnosis, 314, 654
reference intervals for, 1211t
Metastasis(es), from breast cancer,
treatment of, 1028–1029
from gastric sarcoma, 531–532
from melanoma, 791
from renal cell carcinoma, 709–710
from skin cancer, 764
from thyroid cancer, radioiodine therapy
for, 652
from transitional cell carcinoma, 709
to brain, 941
in small cell lung cancer, 191
radiation therapy for, 943
surgery for, 942
to mouth, 817
to spine, osteomyelitis vs., 972
to vulva, 1074
Metatarsal head resection, for rheumatoid
arthritis, 952
Metaxalone, for chronic fatigue syndrome,
112
Metered dose inhalers, for asthmatic
children, 739
Metformin, for type 2 diabetes, 557t,
558–559
in combination therapy, 561, 562
Methadone, during pregnancy, 1095–1096
for opioid abuse, 1095
for pain, 4t, 5
intoxication with, 1095, 1191, 1192,
1192t
Methamphetamine, for attention-deficit/
hyperactivity disorder, 873t
intoxication with, 1095, 1163
Methanol, intoxication by, 1176t,
1189–1190
treatment of, 1156t, 1189–1190
serum concentration estimation for,
1160t
Methaqualone, intoxication by, 1156t
Methemoglobin, reference intervals for,
1207t
Methimazole, adverse effects of, 646–647
for hyperthyroidism, 646–647
for thyroid storm, 648
Methosuximide, for epilepsy in infants and
children, 869t
Methotrexate, for acute lymphoblastic
leukemia in children, 423
for aggressive lymphoma, 436t

Methotrexate (Continued)
for breast cancer, 1027
for central nervous system leukemia,
424
prophylactic, 423
for cutaneous T cell lymphoma, 770
for cutaneous vasculitis, 780
for dermatomyositis, 777
for ectopic pregnancy, 986, 986t
for gastric adenocarcinoma, 530
for highly aggressive lymphoma, 438t
for Hodgkin's disease, 407t
for inflammatory bowel disease, 485
for juvenile rheumatoid arthritis, 955t,
956
for lupus erythematosus, 776
for lymphomatoid papulosis, 770
for multiple sclerosis, 899–900
for penile carcinoma, 710
for psoriasis, 772
for rheumatoid arthritis, 946t, 948–949,
951
surgery on patients using, 953
for sarcoidosis, 225, 227
for scleroderma, 778
for Sézary's syndrome, 769
for transitional cell carcinoma, 709
reference intervals for, 1210t
side effects of, 772
Methoxsalen, phototherapy using. See
Psoralen photochemotherapy.
Methyl salicylate, intoxication by, 1198
Methylbenzethonium chloride, for
cutaneous leishmaniasis, 91
Methyldopa, for cutaneovascular disease in
lupus erythematosus, 776
for hypertension, 308t, 309
during pregnancy, 990, 990t
Methylene blue, as antidote, 1154t
for mushroom poisoning, 79
Methylene chloride, 1179, 1180
Methylenedioxyamphetamine, intoxication
with, 1095, 1163
Methylenedioxyethamphetamine,
intoxication with, 1095, 1163
Methylenedioxymethamphetamine,
intoxication with, 1095, 1163
Methylergonovine, for postpartum
hemorrhage, 1000
α-Methyl-paratyrosine, for pheochromocytoma, 314
Methylphenidate, abuse of, 1095
for attention-deficit/hyperactivity disorder, 872, 873t
with Tourette's syndrome, 877
for depression, 1116
for hiccup, 14t
for pain, 3
1-Methyl-4-phenyl propionoxy-piperidine
tetrahydropyridine (MPPP), abuse of,
1095
1-Methyl-4-phenyl-1,2,3,6-tetrahydro-
pyridine (MPTP), abuse of, 1095
Methylprednisolone, for aggressive
lymphoma, 436t
for anaphylaxis, 727t
for aplastic anemia, 353
for asthma, 734
for chronic obstructive pulmonary disease, during hospitalization, 174
for fibromyalgia, 967
for giant cell arteritis, 971
for juvenile rheumatoid arthritis, 956
for lupus erythematosus, 776
for multiple sclerosis, in acute exacerbations, 898

Methylprednisolone (Continued)
    in secondary progressive disease, 900
    for optic neuritis, 911–912
    for osteoarthritis, 970
    for Pneumocystis carinii pneumonia in
      HIV infection, 51
    for primary glomerular disease, 676
    for rheumatoid arthritis, 948
    for warm antibody autoimmune hemo-
      lytic anemia, 362
    with parenteral iron, 358
4-Methylpyrazole, for ethylene glycol
    intoxication, 1178–1179
    for methanol intoxication, 1190
Methyltestosterone, for hormone
    replacement therapy, 1051
Methyltransferase deficiency, azathioprine
    metabolism in, 226
Methysergide, for serotonin syndrome with
    MAO inhibitors, 1191
Metipranolol, for glaucoma, 913
Metoclopramide, for bacterial overgrowth,
    510
    for gaseousness, 12
    for gastroesophageal reflux disease, 525
    for gastroparesis in diabetes, 565
    for hiccup, 14t
    for mountain sickness, 1128
    for nausea and vomiting, 7, 8t
      due to chemotherapy, 10
      during pregnancy, 980
    in migraine treatment, 881
    with N-acetylcysteine treatment, for acet-
      aminophen intoxication, 1162
Metolazone, for congestive heart failure,
    293, 294t
    for hypertension, 308t
    for volume overload in acute renal fail-
      ure, 697
Metoprolol, after myocardial infarction,
    330
    for atrial fibrillation, 257, 258t
    for atrial premature beats, 261
    for congestive heart failure, 295
    for hypertension, 308t
    for hyperthyroidism, 647
    for myocardial infarction, 321–322
    for pheochromocytoma, 655
    for ventricular premature beats, 263
    intoxication with, 1166, 1167t
    relative antiarrhythmic efficacy of, 262t
Metorchis conjunctus infection, 540t
Metronidazole, for acute necrotizing
    ulcerative gingivitis, 814
    for amebiasis, 58–59, 58t, 59t, 539t, 542
    for amebiasis cutis, 804, 804t
    for bacterial overgrowth, 510
      in diabetes, 565
      with jejunal diverticula, 480
    for bacterial vaginosis, 1054
    for Balantidium coli infection, 543
    for Blastocystis hominis infection, 539t,
      543
    for diarrhea, 16, 17t
    for diverticulitis, 482
    for giardiasis, 61, 61t, 513, 538, 539t
    for Helicobacter pylori infection, 11, 501,
      501t
    for hepatic encephalopathy prevention,
      in cirrhosis, 471
    for inflammatory bowel disease, 486
    for lung abscess, 204
    for osteomyelitis, 974t
    for pelvic inflammatory disease, 719t,
      1059t, 1060t
    for recurrent urethritis in men, 661

Metronidazole (Continued)
    for rosacea, 759
    for sepsis, 63t
    for tetanus, 135
    for trichomoniasis, 721, 1055
Metyrapone, for Cushing's syndrome, 623,
    623t
Metyrapone test, in adrenocortical
    insufficiency diagnosis, 620
Metyrosine, for pheochromocytoma, 655
Mexiletine, for atrial flutter, 275t
    for pain, 3
    for painful neuropathy, 932
    reference intervals for, 1210t
    relative antiarrhythmic efficacy of, 262t
Miconazole, for tinea infection, 807
Microalbuminuria, in diabetic nephrop-
    athy, 564–565
Microsporidiosis, 539t, 543
Microsporum species. See Dermato-
    phytosis.
Midazolam, antifungal interactions with,
    807
    for hiccup, 14t
    for status epilepticus in infants and chil-
      dren, 870t
    for tetanus, 136
    intoxication with, 1166
Midodrine, for orthostatic hypotension,
    886t, 891
    in diabetes, 566
Mifepristone, for Cushing's syndrome, 623
Miglitol, for type 2 diabetes, 557t, 559
Migraine, 878–883
    antidepressants for use with, 1115t
    basilar, 879
    diet and, 880, 889, 890t
    hemiplegic, 879
    oral contraceptives and, 1086t
    patterns of, 878–880
    rebound headache in, 881
    seizure vs., 857
    stroke risk in, 879–880
    transformed, tension-type headache vs.,
      879, 883
    treatment of, 880–883
      step care vs. stratified care in, 882
    triggers of, 880
    vertigo due to, 885t, 889, 890
Migratory angioedema, due to Loa loa,
    804t
Migratory plaque, benign, 815
Milk, cow's, infant formulas based on,
    1020, 1021t
    introduction of, for infants, 1022
    human. See Breast milk; Breast-feeding;
      Lactation.
Milk of magnesia, for constipation, 19, 19t
Milker's nodule, 803
Milrinone, for cardiogenic shock after
    myocardial infarction, 326
    for congestive heart failure, 294t, 296
MINE regimen, for aggressive lymphoma,
    436t, 437
Mineral oil, for constipation, 19, 19t
Mineral spirits, 1179
Mineralocorticoid excess syndromes,
    primary aldosteronism vs., 634–635
Minimal change disease, 677–678
Minocycline, for acne, 758
    for chronic pelvic pain syndrome, 687
    for leprosy, 92, 94
    for osteomyelitis, 973
    for rheumatoid arthritis, 946t, 950
    for toxoplasmosis, 154
Minor cognitive/motor disorder, HIV-
    associated, 55

Minoxidil, adverse effects of, 311
    for androgenic alopecia, 761
    for hypertension, 308t, 311
Mirtazapine, for depression, 1109t
    pharmacodynamic effects of, 1110t
Misoprostol, for constipation, 19, 19t
    for NSAID-induced ulcer prophylaxis,
      499, 499t
      in osteoarthritis, 969
      in rheumatoid arthritis, 947
    for postpartum hemorrhage, 1000
Misoprostol-diclofenac, 500
Mites, house dust, control of, for allergic
    rhinitis, 744
    for asthma, 731
Mitomycin, for bladder cancer, 709
    with trabeculectomy for glaucoma, 915
Mitotane, for adrenal carcinoma, 624
    for Cushing's syndrome, 623, 623t
Mitoxantrone, for aggressive lymphoma,
    436t
    for Hodgkin's disease, 407t
    for multiple sclerosis, 900
Mitral regurgitation, after myocardial
    infarction, 326, 327t
    in hypertrophic cardiomyopathy, 347
    in mitral valve prolapse, 288, 289
    management of, 289–290
Mitral valve, in hypertrophic
    cardiomyopathy, 347
    repair of, for mitral valve prolapse, 290
Mitral valve prolapse, 287–291
    clinical features of, 288
    complications of, 288–289
    diagnosis of, 287–288, 287t, 289
    oral contraceptives and, 1086t
    pathogenesis of, 287
    treatment of, 289–291, 289t, 290t
Mixed connective tissue disease, lupus in,
    774
    scleroderma in, 777
Modafinil, 1215t
Moexipril, for hypertension, 309t
Mohs' micrographic surgery, for lip cancer,
    810
    for melanoma, 790–791
    for skin cancer, 765
Moisture alarm, for nocturnal enuresis,
    670
Molds, asthma and, 731
    onychomycosis due to, 781
Moles, 788–790, 793
    of oral mucosa, 816
Molindone, characteristics of, 1118t
    intoxication by, 1197t
Molluscum contagiosum, 803
Mollusks, toxic, 1143
Mometasone furoate, for allergic rhinitis,
    747t
Monge's disease, 1130
Monilethrix, 761
Monilial infection. See Candidiasis.
Monoamine oxidase inhibitors. See also
    specific drugs.
    anaphylaxis and, 728
    biogenic interactions with, 1190, 1191
    clinical pharmacology of, 1109t
    drug interactions with, 1115–1116
    for anxiety disorders, 1100t, 1102
    for attention-deficit/hyperactivity disor-
      der, 874
    for depression, clinical guidelines for use
      of, 1114–1116
    for Parkinson's disease, 919, 919t
    overdose of, 1190–1191
Monoclonal gammopathy of undetermined
    significance, 440

Monoclonal gammopathy of undetermined significance *(Continued)*
  peripheral neuropathy in, 928
Mononeuritis multiplex, 930–931
Monosodium glutamate, neurologic symptoms due to, 78
Montelukast, for allergic rhinitis, 747
  for asthma, 733
    in children, 740, 742
Mood disorders, 1107–1117. See also *Bipolar disorder; Depression.*
MOPP regimen, for Hodgkin's disease, 406, 407t
Moraxella catarrhalis, antibiotic resistance in, 205
Morinda citrifolia fruit, for ciguatera poisoning, 1143–1144
Morphea, 777, 778
Morphine, for acute hepatic porphyria, 448, 448t
  for hypercyanotic spells in tetralogy of Fallot, 285
  for myocardial infarction, 319
  for pain, 4, 4t
    after cesarean delivery, 998
    in pericarditis, 334
  for painful episode in sickle cell disease, 376
  for urinary calculus, 713
  intoxication with, 1191, 1192t
Morton's neuroma, 978
Mosquitos, avoidance of, in malaria prevention, 100, 150
Motion sickness, 885t, 889–890
  prevention of, in travel, 150
Motor axonal neuropathy, acute, 929
Mountain sickness, acute, 1127–1128, 1128t
  chronic, 1130
  subacute, 1129–1130
Mouth diseases, 808–817. See also specific diseases.
  erosive, ulcerative, and vesiculobullous, 812–813
  general measures for, 808
  malignant, 810–811, 817
  pigmentary, 816
  premalignant, 810
  with white lesions, 810–812
Movement disorders, seizure vs., 857
Moxalactam, vitamin K deficiency and, 592
6-MP (mercaptopurine), for acute lymphoblastic leukemia in children, 423
  for inflammatory bowel disease, 485
M-protein, 440
  evaluation of patient with, 440, 441t
Mucinosis, focal, 781t, 783
  follicular, mycosis fungoides and, 766
Mucocele, 816–817
Mucositis, chemotherapy-associated, 813
  in acute leukemia, 419
Mucous cyst, digital, 781t, 783
Mucous plugs, atelectasis due to, 171
Mucous retention cysts, vocal fold, 25–26
Multiple endocrine neoplasia, type 1, hyperparathyroidism due to, 627
  type 2, genetic screening in, 650
    medullary thyroid carcinoma in, 649
    pheochromocytoma in, 654
Multiple myeloma, 440–444
  complications of, 443–444
  diagnosis of, 440, 441t
  peripheral neuropathy in, 928
  treatment of, 440–443, 443t

Multiple organ dysfunction syndrome, 62, 62t
  in acute pancreatitis, 516
Multiple sclerosis, 896–902
  clinical course of, 897, *897*
  management of, 898–902
    for complications, 901–902
    guidelines on, 897t
    in acute exacerbations, 898
    in primary progressive disease, 901
    in relapsing remitting disease, 898–899, 898t
    in secondary progressive disease, 899–900
  measuring disease activity in, magnetic resonance imaging for, 897–898
  optic neuritis and, 910, 911
"Multiple-hit theory" of skin cancer formation, 763
Mumps, 113
Mumps vaccine, 113. See also *Measles-mumps-rubella vaccine.*
Mupirocin, for atopic dermatitis, 823
  for impetigo, 794
Murphy's sign, 464
  sonographic, 463
Muscarinic receptor, antidepressants' action at, 1110t, 1112
  clinical consequences of, 1113, 1113t
Muscle tension dysphonia, 28–29
Mushrooms, poisoning by, 78–79, 78t
  treatment of, 76, 79, 1156t
  psilocybin, 78t, 79, 1096
Mustard procedure, for transposition of the great arteries, 285
Myasthenia gravis, 903–908
  clinical manifestations of, 903–904
  course of, 904
  diagnosis of, 904–905
  differential diagnosis of, 904
  diseases associated with, 904
  drugs associated with, 903, 903t
  epidemiology of, 903
  pregnancy and, 907–908
  treatment of, 905–908, 905t–908t
Myasthenic crisis, 904
Mycobacterium avium complex infection, 241
  disseminated, in HIV infection, 54, 241
  Whipple's disease vs., 512
Mycobacterium kansasii infection, 241
Mycobacterium leprae. See *Leprosy.*
Mycobacterium tuberculosis. See *Tuberculosis.*
Mycophenolate mofetil, for anti–glomerular basement membrane disease, 679
  for pauci-immune glomerulonephritis, 680
  for primary glomerular disease, 676
Mycoplasma infection, cough due to, 24
Mycoplasma pneumoniae infection, 215–216, 215t
  erythema multiforme and, 824
  neurologic symptoms in, 895
Mycosis fungoides, 766–770
  clinical features of, 766
  cytologic and histopathologic features of, 766–767
  immunophenotyping in, 767
  molecular biology of, 767
  staging of, 767, 767t, 768t
  treatment of, 768–770
Mycotic aneurysm, 243, 244
Myectomy, for hypertrophic cardiomyopathy, 350
Myeloma. See also *Multiple myeloma.*

Myeloma *(Continued)*
  extramedullary, 444
  osteosclerotic, 444, 928
  solitary osseous, 444
Myelomatosis, meningeal, 444
Myelo-optic neuropathy, subacute, due to clioquinol, 931
Myiasis, cutaneous, 804t, 805
Myocardial infarction, 315–328
  care after, 328–333
    drug therapy in, 329–331
    goals of, 329
    risk factor modification in, 331–333, *331, 332*
    tests and procedures in, 333
  causes of, 315–316, 316t
  clinical manifestations of, 316–318
  complications of, 322–328, 324t, 327t
  differential diagnosis of, 318–319
  in type 2 diabetes, 562
  incidence of, 315
  management of, 319–328
    adjunctive therapy in, 321–322
    reperfusion therapy for, 320–321
  non–Q wave, management of, 328
  pathogenesis of, 316, 317t
  pathophysiology after, 329
  predictors of outcome after, *331*
  Q wave, 318
    management of, 319–322, 323t
  recurrent ischemia after, 328
  right ventricular, 327, 327t
  serum enzyme levels in, 318–319
  ventricular premature beats and, 262
  ventricular remodeling after, 329
Myocardial ischemia, anaphylaxis vs., 726
  recurrent, after myocardial infarction, 328
Myocardial revascularization, for angina, 249
Myoclonus, benign neonatal, seizure vs., 867
  tinnitus due to, 38
Myofascial pain, 966
Myofascial pain-dysfunction, in temporomandibular disorders, 961
Myoglobin, serum, in myocardial infarction, 318
  urine, reference intervals for, 1211t
Myomectomy, for leiomyomata, 1062
Myonecrosis, clostridial, 81, 795t, 796–797
  synergistic nonclostridial anaerobic, 81, 796, 796t
Myositis, due to combination therapy for hyperlipidemia, 584
  due to HMG-CoA reductase inhibitors, 581–582
  necrotizing cutaneous, 81, 796, 796t
Myotomy, for hypertrophic cardiomyopathy, 349–350
Myxedema crisis, 644–645, 644t

Nadolol, for arrhythmia in mitral valve prolapse, 290
  for hypertension, 308t
  intoxication with, 1166, 1167t
Nafarelin, for endometriosis, 1032, 1033, 1034t
  for leiomyomata, 1061t
Nafcillin, for bacterial meningitis, 105t
  for bacterial pneumonia, 212t
  for bacterial tracheitis, 31
  for cystic fibrosis exacerbations, 179t
  for infective endocarditis, 300t

Nafcillin *(Continued)*
  for necrotizing skin and soft tissue infections, 82
  for osteomyelitis, 974t
  for staphylococcal meningitis, 104t, 107
  for staphylococcal toxic shock syndrome, 85t
Naftifine, for onychomycosis, 807
  for tinea infection, 807
Nail disorders, 780–783, 781t. See also specific disorders.
Nalbuphine, for pain, 5
  for painful episode in sickle cell disease, 376
Nalmefene, for opioid intoxication, 1154t, 1158, 1192–1193
Naloxone, for opioid intoxication, 1095, 1154t, 1157–1158, 1192, 1193
  for pruritus in cholestatic liver disease, 37
  in neonatal resuscitation, 1006
Naltrexone, for opioid abuse, 1095
Nandrolone, for AIDS-related weight loss, 56
  for aplastic anemia, 354
Nanophyetus salmincola infection, 540t, 546
Naphazoline, for allergic conjunctivitis, 68
Naproxen, for bursitis or tendinitis, 965
  for dysmenorrhea, 1043t, 1044t
  for juvenile rheumatoid arthritis, 954, 955t
  for pain, 2
  for urinary calculus, 713
Naratriptan, 1215t
  for migraine, 881
Narcolepsy, 857
Narcotics. See *Opioids;* specific drugs.
Nasal cytology, in allergic rhinitis diagnosis, 744
Nasal obstruction, differential diagnosis of, 743t
Nasal polyps, in cystic fibrosis, 178
Nasogastric intubation, for acute pancreatitis, 516
Nasogastric suction, fluid therapy requirements with, 609
National Hemophilia Foundation, 397
Natural killer cells, reference intervals for, 1213t
Nausea, 5–10
  causes of, 6t
  clinical findings with, 7
  defined, 5
  during pregnancy, 980
  in food-borne illness, 76
  in migraine, 879
  treatment of, 7–8, 8t
Near-drowning, cold-water, 1133–1134
Nebulizer therapy, for asthma in children, 739, 741
Necator americanus, 540t, 544
Neck dissection, for thyroid cancer, 651
Necrotizing cellulitis, synergistic, 81, 796, 796t
Necrotizing enterocolitis, in newborn, 1015–1016
  with intensive chemotherapy for leukemia, 419
Necrotizing fasciitis, 81, 796t, 797–798
Necrotizing pneumonia, 203
Necrotizing ulcerative gingivitis, acute, 814
Nedocromil, for asthma, 733
  in children, 739, 742
Nefazodone, for anxiety disorders, 1100t, 1101

Nefazodone *(Continued)*
  for chronic fatigue syndrome, 112
  for depression, 1109t
  pharmacodynamic effects of, 1110t
Neisseria gonorrhoeae, 718. See also *Gonococcal infection.*
Neisseria meningitidis meningitis, antimicrobial therapy for, 103t, 104t, 105–106, 107
  chemoprophylaxis of, 108
Nelfinavir (NFV), antitubercular drug interactions with, 52, 240
  for HIV infection, 46t, 49t
Nelson's syndrome, after bilateral adrenalectomy for Cushing's disease, 624
Nematodes, 543, 544–545. See also specific worms and diseases.
  treatment of, 543
Neomycin, allergy to, measles vaccine and, 134
  conjunctivitis due to, 69
  for hepatic encephalopathy prevention in cirrhosis, 471
Neomycin-polymyxin-hydrocortisone, for draining ear, 207t
  for otitis externa, 114
Neonate(s). See also *Child(ren); Infant(s).*
  adrenal suppression in, due to maternal corticosteroid use, 832
  assessment of, 1007–1011, 1008t, *1009, 1010*
  bacterial meningitis management in, 104t, 105t, 1017–1018, 1017t
  benign myoclonus in, 867
  chlamydial infection in, 1056–1057
    conjunctival, 67, 68, 1056
  classification of, by weight, 1008, *1010*
  conjunctivitis in, bacterial, 67
    chlamydial, 67, 68, 1056
  feeding of, 1018–1022
    breast, 1018–1019. See also *Breast-feeding.*
    formula, 1019–1022, 1021t
  gonococcal infection in, 719–720
  hemolytic disease of, 383–390. See also *Hemolytic disease of the fetus and newborn; Rh isoimmunization.*
  herpes simplex in, 800t, 801, 984
  high-risk, 1007–1018
    assessment of, 1007–1011, 1008t, *1009, 1010*
    delivery room management of, 1007, 1007t. See also *Neonate(s), resuscitation of.*
    discharge planning for, 1018
    general management of, 1011–1013
    multiple congenital anomalies in, 1018
    nutrition for, 1012
    special problems of, 1013–1018
    surgical emergencies in, 1018
    transport of, 1011
  infection in, 1017–1018, 1017t
  low-birth-weight, fluid maintenance therapy for, 609
  maternal anesthesia's effects on, 998, 1006
  methadone withdrawal in, 1095–1096
  multiple congenital anomalies in, 1018
  physiologic changes in, at birth, 1001–1002, 1007
  pyelonephritis symptoms in, 666
  resuscitation of, 1001–1006, 1007
    chest compressions in, 1005
    endotracheal intubation in, 1005–1006
    initial steps of, 1002–1004

Neonate(s) *(Continued)*
  meconium aspiration management in, 1004
  medications in, 1006
  positive-pressure ventilation in, 1004–1005
  preparation for, 1002, 1003t
  surgical emergencies in, 1018
  vitamin K deficiency in, 592
  vitamin K injection for, 593
Neostigmine, for myasthenia gravis, 905
  in myasthenia gravis diagnosis, 905
  intoxication due to, 1193
Neovagina, 1042
Nephrectomy, for renal cell carcinoma, 709
Nephritis. See *Glomerulonephritis.*
Nephrolithiasis, 712–715
  in primary hyperparathyroidism, 629
Nephrolithotomy, percutaneous, 714
Nephronia, 662
Nephroureterectomy, for transitional cell carcinoma, 709
Nerve blocks, for chronic pancreatitis, 520
Nerve war weapons, cholinergic intoxication due to, 1193
Neuritis, in leprosy, 93, 94
Neurobrucellosis, 65t, 66
Neurocytoma, central, 941
Neuroendocrine tumors, of stomach, 531t, 532
Neuroepithelial tumor, dysembryoplastic, 941
Neurofibromatosis, pheochromocytoma in, 654
Neurogenic bladder, antidepressants for use with, 1115t
  in diabetes, 565
Neuroleptic(s). See *Antipsychotic drugs;* specific drugs.
Neuroleptic malignant syndrome, 1119, 1196, 1198
Neuroma, acoustic, 940–941
  Morton's, 978
Neuroretinitis, 911
Neurosarcoidosis, 227t, 228
Neurotoxic shellfish poisoning, 79, 80t
Neurotransmitters. See also specific neurotransmitters.
  antidepressants' effects on, 1110t, 1111–1112
Neutropenia, 381–383
  in acute leukemia in children, 422
  with intensive chemotherapy for leukemia, 419–420
Nevirapine (NVP), for HIV infection, 45t, 46t, 49t
  toxic effects of, 47
Nevus(i), 793
  of oral mucosa, 816
  treatment of, 790
  types of, 788–789
  white sponge, 811
Nevus sebaceus of Jadassohn, 793–794
New Ballard Score, for neonatal assessment, 1008, *1009*
Newborn. See *Neonate(s).*
NFV (nelfinavir), antitubercular drug interactions with, 52, 240
  for HIV infection, 46t, 49t
Niacin, deficiency of, peripheral neuropathy in, 927
  drug interactions of, 583
  for alcoholic neuropathy, 927
  for hyperlipidemia, 582–583
    in combination therapy, 584

Niacin *(Continued)*
   in type 2 diabetes, 563
   side effects of, 583
Nicardipine, for hypertension, 308t
   intoxication with, 1168
Nicotine. See also *Smoking.*
   abuse of, 1098
Nicotine patch, for inflammatory bowel
      disease, 486–487
Nicotinic acid. See *Niacin.*
Nifedipine, for angina, 249
   for cutaneovascular disease in lupus ery-
      thematosus, 776
   for hiccup, 14t
   for high-altitude pulmonary edema,
      1128t, 1129
   for hypertension, 308t, 310
      during pregnancy, 990t
   for ordinary urticaria, 836
   intoxication with, 1168, 1169
Nifurtimox, for Chagas' disease, 101–102
Nimodipine, intoxication with, 1168
Nipple discharge, 1023
Nisoldipine, for hypertension, 308t
Nitrates. See also specific drugs.
   after myocardial infarction, 330
   for angina, 248
Nitrendipine, intoxication with, 1168
Nitric oxide, for high-altitude pulmonary
      edema, 1129
Nitrite dipstick test, in cystitis diagnosis,
      663
Nitrofurantoin, for urinary tract infection,
      in girls, 668
   in men, contraindicated in, 661
   in women, 664t
   pregnancy-associated, 664t, 666
Nitrogen, liquid, cryotherapy using. See
      Cryotherapy.
Nitrogen mustard. See *Mechlorethamine.*
Nitroglycerin, after myocardial infarction,
      330
   for acute heart failure, 325
   for amphetamine intoxication, 1163
   for anal fissure, 494
   for angina, 248
   for bleeding esophageal varices, 471
   for cocaine intoxication, 1172
   for cutaneovascular disease in lupus ery-
      thematosus, 776
   for myocardial infarction, 319, 321
   paradoxical response to, 319, 321
Nitroprusside, for amphetamine
      intoxication, 1163
   for cocaine intoxication, 1172
   for heart failure, 296
      after myocardial infarction, 325
   for hypertension, during surgery in pheo-
      chromocytoma, 656
   in phencyclidine intoxication, 1195
   for intracerebral hemorrhage, 849
   for pheochromocytoma crisis, 657
Nitrous oxide, for obstetric anesthesia, 998
   neuropathy due to, 931
Nocturnal hemoglobinuria, paroxysmal,
      365–366
Noise exposure, tinnitus due to, 38
Nonallergic rhinitis with eosinophilia
      syndrome, 743t, 744
Nono tree fruit, for ciguatera poisoning,
      1143–1144
Nonsteroidal anti-inflammatory drugs
      (NSAIDs). See also specific drugs.
   adverse effects of, 969
   colorectal cancer and, 533
   contraindicated in chronic renal failure,
      705

Nonsteroidal anti-inflammatory drugs
      (NSAIDs) *(Continued)*
   cyclosporine interaction with, 950
   for ankylosing spondylitis, 960
   for bursitis or tendinitis, 965
   for cutaneous vasculitis, 779
   for dysmenorrhea, 1043t, 1044, 1044t
   for gout, 577, 578
   for juvenile rheumatoid arthritis, 954,
      955t
   for low back pain, 40
   for migraine, 881, 882
   for osteoarthritis, 969–970
   for pain, 2
   for rheumatoid arthritis, 947, 951
   interference by, in loop diuretic action,
      293
   selective. See *Cyclooxygenase 2 (COX-2)
      inhibitors.*
   types of pain responsive to, 1
   ulcers due to, 498–500, 499t, 969
Nonstress test, during pregnancy, 982
Nonulcer dyspepsia, defined, 11, 496
   irritable bowel syndrome and, 11, 488
Norepinephrine, for antidepressant
      intoxication, 1203
   for cardiogenic shock after myocardial
      infarction, 326
   for hypotension in neuroleptic intoxica-
      tion, 1197
   in pheochromocytoma diagnosis, 654
   urine, reference intervals for, 1211t
Norethindrone, for endometriosis, 1031,
      1032
   for hormone replacement therapy, 1051,
      1052
Norfloxacin, for diarrhea, 17t
   for typhoid carriage, 164
   for typhoid fever, 163, 163t
   for urinary tract infection in women,
      664t
   prophylactic, for spontaneous bacterial
      peritonitis in cirrhosis, 470
Nortriptyline, for attention-deficit/hyper-
      activity disorder, 873, 873t
   for depression, 1109t
      in Alzheimer's disease, 847
   for pain, 3
   intoxication with, 1201, 1202t
   pharmacodynamic effects of, 1110t
   reference intervals for, 1210t
Norwalk virus, food-borne illness due to,
      75t, 76–77
Norwood procedure, for hypoplastic left
      heart syndrome, 287
NOVP regimen, for Hodgkin's disease, 407,
      407t
Nuclear imaging. See *Scintigraphy.*
Nucleic acid amplification tests, for
      tuberculosis, 242, 242t
Nutrition. See also *Diet; Malnutrition;*
      specific nutrients.
   during lactation, 1019
   during pregnancy, 980
   for high-risk neonate, 1012
   for infants, 1018–1022
   in acute diarrhea, 17–18, 73
   in adult respiratory distress syndrome,
      168
   in chronic obstructive pulmonary dis-
      ease, 175
   in cystic fibrosis, 177–178, 177t
   pressure ulcers and, 819
Nutritional support. See also *Enteral
      feeding; Parenteral nutrition.*
   enteral vs. parenteral, 602

Nutritional support *(Continued)*
   for burn patients, 1125–1126
   in acute pancreatitis, 517
   in acute renal failure, 698
   indications for, 602
   pressure ulcers and, 819
   requirements in, 601–602
NVP (nevirapine), for HIV infection, 45t,
      46t, 49t
   toxic effects of, 47
Nystatin, for angular cheilitis, 809
   for candidiasis, for mastitis, 1000
      in HIV infection, 54
      of oral cavity, 811

Obesity, 585–591
   classification of, 585–587, *586, 587,* 588t,
      589t
   health hazards of, 587
   in insulin resistance syndrome, 551
   obstructive sleep-disordered breathing
      and, 182
   treatment of, 587–591
      goals of, 587
      pharmacologic, 590–591, 591t
      surgical, 591
Obesity-hypoventilation syndrome, 180
   treatment of, 183, 184, 185
Obsessive-compulsive disorder, 1100t, 1101
Obstetric anesthesia, 995–999
   complications of, 998–999
   during labor, 995–997
   for cesarean delivery, 997–998
   physiologic changes of pregnancy and,
      995
Obstructive airway disease. See *Chronic
      obstructive pulmonary disease.*
Obstructive sleep-disordered breathing,
      180–186. See also *Sleep apnea.*
   consequences of, 180, 180t, 181t
   features suggesting, 181t
   legal issues in, 186
   perioperative airway management in,
      185
   treatment of, conservative, 181–182,
      181t
      medical, 181t, 182–184
      surgical, 181t, 184–185
Occlusal appliances, for temporomandibu-
      lar disorders, 961, 962–963
Occlusal dysfunction, in temporomandibu-
      lar disorders, 961
Occlusive arterial disease. See also
      Atherosclerosis.
   peripheral, acute, 338
      chronic, 336–338, 336t, 337t
Occupational therapy, for juvenile
      rheumatoid arthritis, 957
Octopus, 1142
Octreotide, for acromegaly, 617
   for bleeding esophageal varices, 471
   for cryptosporidiosis, 542
   for Cushing's syndrome, 623, 624
   for diarrhea in diabetes, 565
Octylonium bromide, for irritable bowel
      syndrome, 492
Odynophagia, dysphagia vs., 475
Ofloxacin, for bacterial prostatitis, 686
   for chlamydial infection, 719, 1057,
      1057t
   urethral, in men, 661
   for cystitis in women, 664t
   for draining ear, 207t
   for epididymitis, 674, 675

Ofloxacin *(Continued)*
  for gonococcal infection, 719t
    disseminated, 719
    in men, 661
  for legionellosis, 217, 218
  for leprosy, 92, 94
  for nongonococcal urethritis, 721
  for osteomyelitis, 973, 974t
  for pelvic inflammatory disease, 719t,
    1059t, 1060t
  for pyelonephritis, 681t, 682t
    in women, 664t
  for sepsis, 63t
  for typhoid fever, 163, 163t
  for urinary tract infection in men, 661
Olanzapine, adverse effects of, 1119
  characteristics of, 1118, 1118t
Olecranon bursitis, 964–965
Oligodendroglioma, 941, 942t, 943
Oliguria, renal function evaluation in, 609
Olsalazine, for inflammatory bowel
  disease, 483
Omega-3 fatty acids, for hyperlipidemia,
  584
Omeprazole, defective iron absorption due
  to, 356
  for dyspepsia, 497
  for gastroesophageal reflux disease, 525–
    526
  for *Helicobacter pylori* infection, 501,
    501t
  for hiccup, 15
  for NSAID-induced ulcer, 500
    prophylactic, 499, 499t
  for reflux-related cough, 24
  for tetanus, 136
Onchocerciasis, 804t
Ondansetron, for hiccup, 14t
  for Hodgkin's disease, 408
  for irritable bowel syndrome, 492
  for Meniere's disease, 893
  for nausea and vomiting, 8t
    due to chemotherapy, 9–10
  for severe central vertigo, 886t, 892
  with *N*-acetylcysteine treatment for acet-
    aminophen intoxication, 1162
Onychomycosis, 780–782, 781t, 782t, 807
Oophorectomy, for breast cancer, 1028
  for endometriosis, 1034
Ophthalmia neonatorum, chlamydial,
  67–68, 1056
  gonococcal, 67, 720
Ophthalmoplegia, pseudointernuclear, in
  myasthenia gravis, 904
Opioids. See also specific drugs.
  abuse of, 1095–1096
  adverse effects of, 4–5
  for black widow spider bite, 1138
  for chronic pancreatitis, 520
  for cutaneous vasculitis, 779
  for diabetic neuropathy, 565
  for labor analgesia, 995–996
  for pain, 4–5, 4t
  intoxication with, 1191–1193, 1192t
    naloxone for, 1157–1158
  neonatal respiratory depression due to,
    1006
  perioperative, in obstructive sleep-disor-
    dered breathing, 185
  prescribing principles for, 4–5, 4t
  receptors for, 1191
  types of pain responsive to, 1
Opisthorchis viverrini infection, 540t, 546
Opium tincture, intoxication with, 1192t
Optic neuritis, 910–912, 911t
Optic neuropathy, acute, differential
  diagnosis of, 911

Oral appliances, for obstructive sleep-
  disordered breathing, 183–184
  for temporomandibular disorders, 961,
    962–963
Oral cavity lesions. See *Mouth diseases;*
  specific diseases.
Oral provocation testing, for drug allergy,
  751
Oral rehydration therapy, for cholera, 72t,
  73
  for diarrhea, 16, 17
  for food-borne illness, 76
  for salmonellosis, 159–160
  for travelers' diarrhea, 150
Orchiectomy, for prostate cancer, 708
Orchitis, in leprosy, 94
  in mumps, 113
Orf, 803
Organophosphate poisoning, 1193–1194
Orlistat, for obesity, 591, 591t
Ornidazole, for diarrhea, 16
Ornithosis, 116–118
Oromandibular dysfunction, 961
Oropharyngeal dysphagia, causes of,
  473–474, 473t
  treatment of, 477–478
Orthodromic reciprocating tachycardia,
  271, 272, 273, 274
Orthostatic hypotension, 885t, 890–891
  antidepressants for use in, 1115t
  in diabetes, 565–566
  in mitral valve prolapse, 291
Osler's nodes, 298
Osmolal gaps, serum, in acute poisoning,
  1158–1160, 1160t
Osmolality, serum, defined, 1158
  reference intervals for, 1209t
  urine, reference intervals for, 1211t
Osmolarity, defined, 1159
Osmophobia, in migraine, 879
Ossification, heterotopic, after head injury,
  935
Osteoarthritis, 967–970
  diagnosis of, 968
  prevention of, 969
  treatment of, 968–970
Osteodystrophy, renal, 703–704
Osteomalacia, due to aluminum in chronic
  renal failure, 704
  in cirrhosis, prevention of, 467t
  osteoporosis vs., 594
Osteomyelitis, 971–974
  diagnosis of, 972–973
  organisms causing, 972
  painful episode vs., in sickle cell disease,
    376
  pathophysiology of, 971–972
  treatment of, 973–974, 974t
Osteopenia, defined, 594
  due to transfusional hemosiderosis in
    thalassemia, 372
Osteoporosis, 593–597
  approach to patient in, 597
  corticosteroid-induced, 487, 596
    prevention of, in rheumatoid arthritis,
     948
  defined, 594
  diagnosis of, 594
  fractures in, 594, 596–597, 1049
  hormone replacement therapy and, 594–
    595, 1049
  in ankylosing spondylitis, 959, 960
  in cirrhosis, prevention of, 467t, 468
  in cystic fibrosis, 180
  in inflammatory bowel disease, 487
  in multiple myeloma, 441

Osteoporosis *(Continued)*
  in primary hyperparathyroidism, 629
  management of, 594–596, 595t
  risk factors for, 593–594, 593t
  vertebral deformity and back pain in,
    596–597
Otitis, tinnitus due to, 38
Otitis externa, 114–115
Otitis media, 204–207, 205t–207t
Ototoxicity of medications, bilateral
  vestibular deficit due to, 891
Otovent, middle ear autoinflation with, for
  otitis media, 206
Overlap syndrome, lupus in, 774
  scleroderma in, 777
"Owl's eye" inclusions, in cytomegalovirus
  infection, 802
Oxacillin, for breast abscess, 1023
  for impetigo, 794
  for infective endocarditis, 300t
  for osteomyelitis, 974t
  for staphylococcal toxic shock syndrome,
    85t
Oxaluria, urinary stones due to, 715
Oxamniquine, for schistosomiasis, 540t,
  546
Oxandrolone, for AIDS-related weight loss,
  56
Oxaprozin, for bursitis or tendinitis, 965
  for dysmenorrhea, 1043t
Oxazepam, intoxication with, 1166
  withdrawal from, 1096
Oxcarbazepine, for epilepsy, 864
Oxiconazole, for *Candida* suppression in
  perineal pruritus, 834
  for tinea infection, 807
Oxprenolol, intoxication with, 1167t
Oxybutynin, for bladder dysfunction, 672
  in multiple sclerosis, 902
  for diurnal enuresis, 669
  for Parkinson's disease, 922
Oxycodone, for pain, 4t
  in analgesic combinations, 2
  for urinary calculus, 713
  intoxication with, 1192t
Oxygen partial pressure, arterial blood,
  reference intervals for, 1209t
Oxygen saturation, arterial blood,
  reference intervals for, 1209t
Oxygen therapy, for anaphylaxis, 728
  for antepartum hemorrhage, 987
  for carbon monoxide poisoning, 1170
  for chronic obstructive pulmonary dis-
    ease, 173–174, 175
    air travel and, 175
  for cluster headache, 884
  for high-altitude cerebral edema, 1128,
    1128t
  for high-risk neonate, 1013
  for myocardial infarction, 321
  for obstructive airway disease, problems
    in, 169
  for obstructive sleep-disordered breath-
    ing, 184
  for pulmonary edema, after myocardial
    infarction, 325
    due to altitude, 1128t, 1129
  hyperbaric. See *Hyperbaric oxygen.*
  in neonatal resuscitation, 1004
Oxymetazoline, for viral respiratory
  infection, 214
Oxymetholone, for aplastic anemia, 354
  for Fanconi's anemia, 355
Oxytocin, for postpartum hemorrhage,
  1000

Pacemaker, for beta blocker intoxication,
  1168

Pacemaker (Continued)
  for calcium channel blocker intoxication, 1169
  for heart block, 268, 268t
  for hypertrophic cardiomyopathy, 349
  for sinus bradycardia after myocardial infarction, 322–323
Pachyonychia congenita, oral lesions in, 812
Paclitaxel, for aggressive lymphoma, 438
  for breast cancer, 1027, 1029
  for non–small cell lung cancer, 189
  for recurrent endometrial cancer, 1065
  for small cell lung cancer, 190
Pagetoid reticulosis, mycosis fungoides and, 766
Paget's disease of bone, 597–600
  approach to patient in, 600
  diagnosis of, 598
  treatment of, 598–600, 598t
Paget's disease of breast, 1026
Paget's disease of vulva, 1072
Pain, 1–5
  after stroke, 856
  assessment of, 1–2
  atelectasis due to, 170
  back, 39–40
    in osteoporosis, 596–597
  bone, in multiple myeloma, 441
  chest, differential diagnosis of, 318–319
    in myocardial infarction, 317
  chronic, antidepressants for use with, 1115t
    defined, 1
  facial, atypical, 909
  in chronic pancreatitis, 508–509, 519, 519t
    as indication for surgery, 521
    treatment of, 520–521
  in endometriosis, 1030
    treatment of, 1033–1034, 1034t
  in irritable bowel syndrome, 491
  in migraine, 879
  in multiple sclerosis, 902
  in osteoarthritis, cognitive and behavioral control of, 969
  in pericarditis, 333–334
  in peripheral neuropathies, 932
  in rheumatoid arthritis, 947
  in temporomandibular disorders, 960, 962
  in trigeminal neuralgia, 908–909
  insomnia due to, 32, 34
  leg, low back pain with, 40
  myofascial, 966
  neuropathic, 1
    treatment of, 2–4
  pressure ulcers and, 819
  treatment of, 2–5
    nonmedicinal approaches to, 5
  types of, 1–2
  with urinary calculus, 712, 713
Painful episodes, in sickle cell disease, 376–377
PAINT mnemonic, 1184
PAIR procedure, for echinococcosis, 547
Palate, cleft, 809
  papillary hyperplasia of, due to dentures, 811
  radiofrequency volumetric tissue reduction of, for obstructive sleep-disordered breathing, 185
  smoker's keratosis of, 811
Pallidotomy, for Parkinson's disease, 923t, 924
Pamidronate, adverse effects of, 599

Pamidronate (Continued)
  for ankylosing spondylitis, 960
  for hypercalcemic crisis, 630–631
  for multiple myeloma, 442
  for osteopenia in thalassemia patient with iron overload, 372
  for osteoporosis due to corticosteroids, 596
  for Paget's disease of bone, 598–599, 598t
Pancoast tumors, 188
Pancreas transplantation, for diabetic neuropathy, 925
Pancreatectomy, for chronic pancreatitis, 509, 523
Pancreatic duct, endoscopic stent placement in, for chronic pancreatitis, 523
Pancreatic duct drainage, for chronic pancreatitis, 522–523
Pancreatic enzymes, replacement of, for chronic pancreatitis, 508–509, 520, 521
  supplemental, for cystic fibrosis, 177, 177t
Pancreatic insufficiency, endocrine. See Diabetes mellitus.
  exocrine, in chronic pancreatitis, 521
Pancreatic pseudocyst, 517–518
Pancreatic stone protein, chronic pancreatitis and, 519
Pancreaticoduodenectomy, for chronic pancreatitis, 523
Pancreaticojejunostomy, lateral, for chronic pancreatitis, 522–523
Pancreatitis, acute, 514–518
  assessment of severity of, 515–516, 516t
  causes of, 514, 514t
  classification of, 514–515
  diagnosis of, 515
  management of, 516–518, 517t
  pathogenesis of, 514
  biliary, 465
  "burned-out," 521
  chronic, 518–524
    causes of, 518–519, 518t
    classification of, 518, 518t
    diagnosis of, 508, 519–520
    malabsorption in, 508–509
    treatment of, 508–509, 520–524
      medical, 520–521
      surgical, 521–524, 521t, 522t
  classification of, 518, 518t
  didanosine-associated, 47
  due to antimonial therapy, 89
  in cystic fibrosis, 180
  obstructive, 519
  parenteral nutrition for, 604
  risk of, triglycerides and, 579–580
  tropical, 519
Pancuronium, for neuroleptic intoxication, 1197
  for tetanus, 136
Panencephalitis, subacute sclerosing, 133
Panic disorder, 1099, 1120–1122
  diagnostic criteria for, 1120–1121, 1120t
  dizziness due to, 885t, 891
  drug allergies and, 750
  mitral valve prolapse and, 288, 291
  treatment of, 1099, 1100t, 1121–1122, 1121t
Pantothenic acid, for alcoholic neuropathy, 927
Pap smear, cervical cancer screening using, 1066, 1067t

Papaverine, for erectile dysfunction, 693
  in diabetes, 566
  in erectile dysfunction assessment, 692
Papillary muscle infarction, mitral regurgitation due to, 326, 327t
Papilloma(s), intraductal, nipple discharge due to, 1023
  laryngeal, 25
  oral, 793, 817
Papillomatosis, oral florid, 793
Papillomavirus. See Human papillomavirus infection.
Papulosquamous diseases, 770–774, 771t. See also specific diseases.
Para-aminobenzoic acid, in sunscreens, 838
Para-aortic field radiation, for Hodgkin's disease, 410
Paracentesis, for ascites in cirrhosis, 469, 470
Paracetamol. See Acetaminophen.
Paragonimus westermani infection, 546
Paralytic shellfish poisoning, 79, 80t, 1143
Paranasal sinuses, disease of, asthma and, 730
  in cystic fibrosis, 178, 179t
  healthy function of, 231, 232
  inflammation involving. See Rhinosinusitis.
Paraneoplastic pemphigus, 827
Parapsoriasis, 774, 794
  cutaneous T cell lymphoma and, 766, 774, 794
Paraquat, 1156t
ParaSight F antigen-capture test, in malaria diagnosis, 96
Parasites. See also specific diseases.
  intestinal, 537–547
    classification of, 538
    diagnosis of, 15–16, 538
    treatment of, 538–547, 539t–541t
  malabsorption due to, 513
  skin disease due to, 804–806, 804t
Parasomnias, seizure vs., 857
Parathion, 1193
Parathyroid adenoma, hyperparathyroidism due to, 627, 628
Parathyroid hormone, elevated. See also Hyperparathyroidism.
  differential diagnosis of, 628t
  for hypoparathyroidism, 634
  for osteoporosis, 596
Parathyroid hyperplasia, hyperparathyroidism due to, 627–628
Parathyroidectomy, for primary hyperparathyroidism, 629–630
  for tertiary hyperparathyroidism, 632
Paregoric, intoxication with, 1192t
Parenteral nutrition. See also Nutritional support.
  complications of, 605–607
  components of, 604–605, 605t
  delivery of, 604
  for high-risk neonate, 1012
  for inflammatory bowel disease, 486
  in adults, 600–607
  indications for, 602–604, 602t
  initiation of, 605
  monitoring of, 605
  requirements in, 601–602
Paricalcitol, 1215t
Parinaud's oculoglandular syndrome, 157
Parkinsonism, 918. See also Parkinson's disease.
  antidepressants for use in, 1115t
  due to metyrosine therapy for pheochromocytoma, 655

Parkinsonism (*Continued*)
  idiopathic Parkinson's disease vs., 918
Parkinson-plus syndromes, dysphonia in, 28
Parkinson's disease, 918–924
  diagnosis of, 918
  dysphonia in, 28
  treatment of, drugs for, 918–919, 919t
    introduction of, 920–921
    special problems in, 922–923
    surgical, 923–924, 923t
    when to start, 919–920
    with disease progression, 921
Paromomycin, for amebiasis, 58, 58t, 59, 59t, 539t, 542
  for cryptosporidiosis, 539t, 542
  for *Dientamoeba fragilis* infection, 539t, 543
  for giardiasis, 61, 61t, 539t, 542
  for leishmaniasis, 90, 91
Paronychia, 781t, 782, 808
Parotid swelling, differential diagnosis of, 113
Paroxetine, for anxiety disorders, 886t, 1100t, 1101
  for depression, 1109t
    in Alzheimer's disease, 847
    in fibromyalgia, 967
  for pain, 3–4
  for panic disorder, 891, 1121t, 1122
  monoamine oxidase inhibitor interaction with, 1115
  pharmacodynamic effects of, 1110t
  phentermine with, for obesity, 590
Paroxysmal cold hemoglobinuria, 359t
  clinical diagnosis of, 360
  laboratory diagnosis of, 361
  treatment of, 363
Paroxysmal nocturnal hemoglobinuria, 365–366
Partial thromboplastin time, activated, reference intervals for, 1207t
Parvovirus infection, aplastic crisis in sickle cell disease and, 375
  erythema infectiosum due to, 803
  transmission of, by blood components, 461
    by clotting factor concentrates, 393
    by fresh-frozen plasma, 457
Patch testing, for allergic contact dermatitis, 830
  for drug allergy, 751
Patellofemoral pain syndrome, 977
Patent ductus arteriosus, 281–282, 1015
Pautrier's microabscesses, in mycosis fungoides, 766
Pediculosis, 804t, 806
Pefloxacin, for typhoid fever, 163, 163t
Peliosis, bacillary, 158, 158t
Pellagra, peripheral neuropathy in, 927
Pelvic field irradiation, for Hodgkin's disease, 410
Pelvic floor dyssynergia, 20
Pelvic floor rehabilitation, for stress incontinence, 673
  for urgency incontinence, 672
Pelvic inflammatory disease, 1057–1060
  causes of, 1058
  chlamydial, 1056, 1056t, 1059
  diagnosis of, 1058–1059
  gonococcal, 718, 1058, 1059
  risk factors for, 1058
  treatment of, 719, 719t, 1059–1060, 1059t, 1060t
Pelvic pain syndrome, chronic, 686–687
Pemoline, abuse of, 1095

Pemoline (*Continued*)
  for attention-deficit/hyperactivity disorder, 873, 873t
  for fatigue in multiple sclerosis, 901
  for pain, 3
Pemphigoid, 827–828
  oral lesions in, 813
Pemphigus, 826–827
  herpesvirus type 8 and, 803
  oral lesions in, 813
  paraneoplastic, 827
Penbutolol, for hypertension, 308t
Penciclovir, for herpes simplex, 800, 800t, 809
Penectomy, for penile carcinoma, 710
Penicillamine, for cystinuria, 715
  for lead poisoning, 1186, 1186t
  for neuropathy due to metal poisoning, 926
  for rheumatoid arthritis, 946t, 949, 951
  for scleroderma, 778
Penicillin(s). See also specific drugs, e.g., *Amoxicillin*.
  for acute necrotizing ulcerative gingivitis, 814
  for bacterial meningitis, dosages for, 105t
  for infective endocarditis, 300t, 301, 302
  for *Listeria monocytogenes* meningitis, 103t, 104t, 106
  for Lyme disease, 128t, 129t
  for mastitis, 1000
  for meningococcal meningitis, 103t, 104t, 105
  for necrotizing skin and soft tissue infections, 82
  for pneumococcal meningitis, 104t
  for pneumococcal pneumonia, 212, 212t
  for rat bite fever, 123
  for relapsing fever, 124
  for streptococcal pharyngitis, 237, 238, 238t
  for streptococcal toxic shock syndrome, 85, 85t
  for *Streptococcus agalactiae* meningitis, 103t, 104t, 107
  for syphilis, 724t, 774
  for tetanus, 135
  for toxic shock syndrome prophylaxis, 85
  for Whipple's disease, 512
  prophylactic, after splenectomy, in hereditary spherocytosis, 364
    in thalassemia, 371
    in warm antibody autoimmune hemolytic anemia, 362
    in sickle cell disease, 380
  resistance to, in *Neisseria meningitidis*, 105–106
    in rat bite fever organisms, 123
    in *Streptococcus pneumoniae*, 103–105, 211
  testing for allergy to, 752
Penile erection. See also *Erectile dysfunction*.
  physiology of, 691–692
Penile island flap, with substitution urethroplasty, for anterior stricture, 712
Penile prosthesis, for erectile dysfunction, 693–694
Penis, carcinoma of, 710
  surgical reconstruction of, 694
  trauma to, 685
Pentamidine, for leishmaniasis, 90
  for *Pneumocystis carinii* pneumonia in HIV infection, 51

Pentamidine (*Continued*)
  for *Pneumocystis carinii* prophylaxis, in aplastic anemia, 353
    in HIV infection, 51
Pentazocine, contraindicated for chronic pain, 5
  for pain in pericarditis, 334
  intoxication with, 1192t
Pentetic acid clearance, for glomerular filtration rate measurement, 702
Pentobarbital, for status epilepticus, 865t
  in infants and children, 870t
  intoxication with, 1165
Pentostatin, for Sézary's syndrome, 769
Pentoxifylline, for alcoholic hepatitis, 468
  for peripheral arterial occlusive disease, 337
  for toxic epidermal necrolysis, 825
Peptic ulcer disease, 496–501
  antidepressants for use in, 1115t
  clinical approach to, 497–498, *497*
  dyspepsia and, 11, 496
  Helicobacter pylori infection in, 500–501, 501t
  NSAID-induced, 498–500, 499t, 969
Percussion, for atelectasis due to mucous plugs, 171
Performance anxiety, 1100, 1100t, 1102
Pergolide, for hyperprolactinemia, 641
  for Parkinson's disease, 919t, 920
  for primary sleep disorders, 34
Perianal abscess, 495
Pericardial effusion. See also *Pericarditis*.
  hemodynamic changes due to, 334, *334*
  treatment of, 334–335
Pericardial window, for pericarditis, 335
Pericardiocentesis, for pericarditis, 334, 335
Pericardiotomy, balloon, for pericarditis, 335
Pericarditis, 333–336
  after myocardial infarction, 328
  causes of, 333t
  constrictive, 335
  due to radiation therapy for Hodgkin's disease, 412
  in acute renal failure, 699
  in chronic renal failure, 335–336
  pain management in, 333–334
Pericoronitis, 814
Peridural analgesia, for labor, 996
Perihepatitis, chlamydial, 1056, 1056t
Perinephric abscess, 662
Periodic limb movement disorder, 33, 34
Periodontal lesions, 813–814
Periodontitis, 814
Periostalgia, medial, 977–978
Peripheral arterial disease, 336–339. See also *Atherosclerosis*.
  acute occlusion in, 338
  aneurysmal, 338–339, 338t
  chronic occlusive, 336–338, 336t, 337t
Peripheral neuropathy(ies), 924–932
  acute motor axonal, 929
  classification of, 924, 924t
  distal symmetric sensorimotor, 924–928
  hereditary, 925, 925t
  HIV-associated, 55–56, 927
  in diabetes, 565, 925, 931
  in leprosy, 94, 927
  in Lyme disease, 126, 927
    treatment of, 127, 128t
  in renal failure, 699, 925
  large-fiber sensory, 931
  motor, 932
  painful, treatment of, 932

Peripheral neuropathy(ies) (Continued)
small-fiber sensory and autonomic, 931–932
treatment of, 932
with axonal degeneration predominant, 925–928
with demyelination predominant, 928
with mononeuritis multiplex pattern, 930–931
with polyradiculopathy pattern, 928–930
Peritoneal dialysis, for acute poisoning, 1150
for acute renal failure, 700, 700t
for chronic renal failure, preparations for, 705
Peritoneal lavage, for accidental hypothermia, 1133
for pancreatitis, 517
Peritonitis, spontaneous bacterial, in cirrhosis, 470
Perlèche, 811
Permethrin, for lice, 804t, 806
for scabies, 804t, 805
Pernicious anemia, 367–368
Perphenazine, characteristics of, 1118t
intoxication by, 1197t
Pertussis, 23, 137–139
Pertussis vaccines, 139, 140, 141, 144t
contraindications and precautions for, 144, 145
Pessary, for stress incontinence, 673
Petrolatum, for cheilitis prevention, 809
for erythema multiforme, 813
Petroleum distillates, intoxication by, 1179
Petroleum naphtha, 1179
Peyote, 1096
pH, arterial blood, reference intervals for, 1209t
semen, reference intervals for, 1213t
urine, reference intervals for, 1211t
pH monitoring, esophageal, in dysphagia evaluation, 477
Pharyngitis, causes of, 236
streptococcal, 236–238, 238t
Phencyclidine, 1096, 1195–1196
Phenelzine, for anxiety disorders, 1100t, 1102
for depression, 1109t, 1116
for panic disorder, 1121t, 1122
overdose of, 1190
pharmacodynamic effects of, 1110t
Phenobarbital, adverse effects of, 863t
drug interactions with, 200, 644, 863t
for epilepsy, 860t, 861, 862t
in infants and children, 868t, 869t
for Rh isoimmunization, 388t
for status epilepticus in infants and children, 870t
intoxication with, 1156t, 1165
pharmacokinetics of, 862t
prophylactic, in severe malaria, 97
reference intervals for, 1210t
Phenol injection, for spasticity after stroke, 856
Phenothiazines. See also specific drugs.
anticonvulsant interactions with, 863t
intoxication with, 1196–1198, 1197t
Phenoxybenzamine, for pheochromocytoma, 314, 655
Phentermine, drug interactions with, 591
for obesity, 590–591, 591t
Phentolamine, for amphetamine intoxication, 1163
for cocaine intoxication, 1172–1173

Phentolamine (Continued)
for erectile dysfunction, 693
in diabetes, 566
for hypertension during surgery in pheochromocytoma, 656
for monoamine oxidase inhibitor overdose, 1190
for pheochromocytoma, 314
for pheochromocytoma crisis, 657
in erectile dysfunction assessment, 692
Phenylephrine, for viral respiratory infection, 214
Phenylpropanolamine, anorectic agent interactions with, 591
for allergic rhinitis, 746
for stress incontinence, 673
intoxication with, 1163
Phenylpyruvic acid, urine, reference intervals for, 1211t
Phenytoin, adverse effects of, 863t
drug interactions with, 863t
antifungals, 196, 200
levothyroxine, 644
for epilepsy, 860t, 861, 862t
in infants and children, 868t, 869t
post-traumatic, 939
for head injury, 935
for hiccup, 14t
for pain, 3
in multiple sclerosis, 902
for painful neuropathy, 932
for status epilepticus in infants and children, 870t
gingival hyperplasia due to, 813–814
pharmacokinetics of, 861, 861, 862t
prophylactic, with intracerebral hemorrhage, 849
reference intervals for, 1210t
Pheochromocytoma, 314, 653–657
clinical features of, 653–654
determining location of, 654–655
diagnosis of, 654
epidemiology of, 654
familial syndromes with, 654
in pregnancy, 657
malignant, treatment of, 656–657
prognosis in, 657
treatment of, 655–657
Pheochromocytoma crisis, 657
Philadelphia chromosome, 426
Phlebotomy, for hemochromatosis, 404–405
for polycythemia vera, 445–446
for porphyria cutanea tarda, 452
Phlegmon, 662
Phobia, specific, 1100, 1100t
Phonophobia, in migraine, 879
Phosphate. See also Hyperphosphatemia.
dietary, in chronic renal failure, 703–704, 704t
for diabetic ketoacidosis, 574
in children, 568
for primary hyperparathyroidism, 630
in parenteral nutrition solutions, 605t
reference intervals for, in serum, 1209t
in urine, 1211t
Phosphate binders, in acute renal failure, 698
in chronic renal failure, 704, 704t
Phosphodiesterase inhibitors. See also specific drugs.
for angina, 249
Phospholipid-rich Russell Viper Venom Time, in hypercoagulability workup, 221
Photochemotherapy. See Psoralen photochemotherapy.

Photocoagulation, for diabetic retinopathy, 564
for hemorrhoids, 493
Photodynamic laser therapy, for skin cancer, 765
Photopheresis, for scleroderma, 778
Photophobia, in migraine, 879
Phototherapy, desensitization using, for solar urticaria, 836
for atopic dermatitis, 822–823
for bilirubin removal in Rh isoimmunization, 387
for mycosis fungoides, 768
for neonatal jaundice, 1017
for pruritus, 37
for psoriasis, 772
with psoralen pretreatment. See Psoralen photochemotherapy.
Phthirus pubis, 804t, 806
Physical abuse, during pregnancy, 983
premenstrual syndrome and, 1045
Physical dependence, defined, 4
Physical therapy. See also Exercise.
for bursitis or tendinitis, 965–966
for juvenile rheumatoid arthritis, 957
for low back pain, 39
Physostigmine, for anticholinergic intoxication, 1097, 1154t, 1164
for mushroom poisoning, 79
intoxication due to, 1193
Phytohemagglutinin, for aplastic anemia, 354
Phytonadione, for vitamin K deficiency, 592–593
Pigmentary disorders, 837–841
of mouth, 816
Pilocarpine, for glaucoma, 913
Pimozide, characteristics of, 1118t
for Tourette's syndrome, 876
for trichotillomania, 762
Pindolol, for hypertension, 308t
intoxication with, 1166, 1167t
Pineal region tumors, 940
Pinworm, 540t, 544
Piperacillin, for cystic fibrosis exacerbations, 179t
for sepsis, 63t
Piperacillin-tazobactam, for nosocomial pneumonia, 213
for sepsis, 63t
Pirbuterol, for asthma, 734
in children, 740
Piroxicam, adverse effects of, 969
for dysmenorrhea, 1043t
for pain, 2
Pituitary adenoma, acromegaly due to, 615
Cushing's syndrome due to, 622–623
prolactin-secreting, 641–642
Pituitary apoplexy, after irradiation for acromegaly, 616
optic neuritis vs., 911
Pityriasis alba, 841
Pityriasis lichenoides, 794
Pityriasis lichenoides chronica, 773–774
Pityriasis linguae, 815
Pityriasis rosea, 773
herpesvirus type 7 and, 803
Pityriasis rubra pilaris, 773
Placenta, retained, postpartum hemorrhage due to, 1000
Placenta accreta, 987
Placenta previa, 987–988
Placental abruption, 987, 988
disseminated intravascular coagulation in, 402, 988
Plague, 115–116

Plague vaccine, 116
  for travelers, 147t, 148
Plantar fasciitis, 978
Plasma, derivatives of, for infusion, 458
  for disseminated intravascular coagulation, 402
  fresh-frozen, 457
    for C1 esterase inhibitor deficiency, 837
    for hemolytic transfusion reaction, 459
    for intracerebral hemorrhage, 849
    for severe bleeding in vitamin K deficiency, 593
  virus inactivation methods used on, 457, 458
Plasmacytoma. See *Myeloma.*
Plasmapheresis, for acute poisoning, 1157
  for anti–glomerular basement membrane disease, 679
  for aplastic anemia, 354
  for chronic inflammatory demyelinating polyradiculoneuropathy, 930
  for Guillain-Barré syndrome, 929
  for HELLP syndrome, 993
  for myasthenia gravis, 907, 907t
    during pregnancy, 908
  for renal failure in multiple myeloma, 443
  for thrombotic thrombocytopenic purpura, 403
  for toxic epidermal necrolysis, 825
  for warm antibody autoimmune hemolytic anemia, 362
Plasmodium species, 94. See also *Malaria.*
Platelet(s), for transfusion, 455–456. See also *Transfusion(s), platelet.*
  in clot formation, 397
Platelet count, reference intervals for, 1206t
Platelet-mediated bleeding disorders, 397–400, 398t. See also specific disorders.
  clinical manifestations of, 397–398
  laboratory evaluation of, 398
  treatment of, 398–400
Pleural effusion, 201–203
  atelectasis due to, 171
  tuberculous, 203, 239
Pleurodesis, for malignant pleural effusion, 203
Plicamycin, for Paget's disease of bone, 598t, 600
Pneumococcal infection. See *Streptococcus pneumoniae infection.*
Pneumocystis carinii infection, in HIV infection, 51
  prophylaxis of, in aplastic anemia, 353
Pneumonectomy, for non–small cell lung cancer, 187
Pneumonia, after head injury, 935
  bacterial, 209–213
    causes of, 209–210
    clinical presentation of, 210
    diagnosis of, 210–211
    host factors in, 210
    treatment of, 211–213, 212t
  chlamydial, in infant, 23, 1056
  in acute renal failure, 699
  in chickenpox, 70
  in coccidioidomycosis, 194–195
  in plague, 115–116
  Legionella, 216–218, 217t
  mycoplasmal, 215–216, 215t
    neurologic symptoms in, 895
  necrotizing, 203
  nosocomial, causes of, 210

Pneumonia *(Continued)*
  treatment of, 213
  viral, 215, 215t, 216t
Pneumonitis, hypersensitivity, 230–231, 231t
  radiation, due to therapy for Hodgkin's disease, 412
Pneumothorax, after head injury, 935
  with central catheter insertion, 605
Podagra, in gout, 576
POEMS syndrome, 444, 928
Poikiloderma atrophicans vasculare, in mycosis fungoides, 766
Poisoning. See also specific poisons.
  acute, 1144–1203
    delayed effects in, 1146–1147
    differential diagnosis of, based on CNS effects, 1149, 1149t–1150t
    epidemiology of, 1145
    management of, 1145–1160
      antidotes in, 1149, 1151t–1155t
      decontamination in, 1147–1149, 1148t
      elimination enhancement in, 1149–1157
      in patient with altered mental status, 1157–1158
      initial assessment in, 1145–1146, 1146t
      laboratory tests in, 1158–1160, 1158t–1160t, 1212t
      prevention of toxin absorption in, 1146–1149
      radiographic studies in, 1160
  drug, meningoencephalitis vs., 895
  peripheral neuropathy due to, 926
Pokeweed antiviral protein, for acute lymphoblastic leukemia, 425
Polar bear viscera, vitamin A poisoning from, 1144
Poliovirus vaccines, *140,* 142, 144t
  for travelers, 147t, 148
Poloxamer 188, for sickle cell disease, 381
Polychaete worms, 1142
Polycystic ovarian syndrome, amenorrhea due to, 1042
Polycythemia, in newborn, 1016
Polycythemia vera, 445–447, 446t
Polyethylene glycol, for constipation, 19, 19t
  for intestinal obstruction in cystic fibrosis, 178, 179t
  whole-bowel irrigation with, for acute poisoning, 1148–1149
Polymer film dressings, for pressure ulcers, 820
Polymethylmethacrylate bone cement, antibacterial-loaded, for osteomyelitis, 974
Polymorphic eruption of pregnancy, 831–832
Polymyalgia rheumatica, 970–971
Polymyxin-neomycin-hydrocortisone, for draining ear, 207t
  for otitis externa, 114
Polymyxin-trimethoprim, for bacterial conjunctivitis, 67
Polyp(s), adenomatous, colorectal, malignant transformation of, 532–533
  nasal, in cystic fibrosis, 178
  vocal fold, 26
Polypectomy, for gastric adenoma, 528
Polyradiculopathies, 928–930
Polysaccharide-iron complex, for iron deficiency, 357–358
Polytef injection, for vocal fold paralysis, 27

Polytef patch, for ventricular free wall rupture, 328
Pontiac fever, 217
Popliteal artery aneurysm, 339
Porokeratosis, 793
Porphobilinogen, urine, reference intervals for, 1211t
Porphyria(s), 447–453, 448t
  acute hepatic, prevention of attacks in, 450t, 451
    safety of drugs and chemicals in, 449, 450t
    treatment of, 448–451, 448t
  acute intermittent, 448t
  ALA dehydratase deficiency, 448t
  chronic cutaneous, 448t
    treatment of, 451–453, 452t
  congenital erythropoietic, 448t, 451–452, 452t
  hepatoerythropoietic, 448t, 452, 452t
  peripheral neuropathy in, 926
  variegate, 448t
Porphyria cutanea tarda, 448t, 452–453, 452t
Porphyrins, urine, reference intervals for, 1211t
Portal hypertension, in cystic fibrosis, 180
Portosystemic shunt, transjugular intrahepatic, for variceal bleeding, 470, 472
Portuguese man-of-war, 1142
Positive end-expiratory pressure, in adult respiratory distress syndrome, 168
Positive-pressure ventilation, in neonatal resuscitation, 1004–1005
Postcholecystectomy syndrome, functional disorder and, 12
Postconcussion syndrome, 938, *939,* 940
Postherpetic neuralgia, 801, 802
Postnasal drip syndrome, cough due to, 22, 24
  in child, 23, 24
Postpartum care, 999–1001
Postpartum thyroiditis, 642–643, 658t, 659
Poststroke central pain syndrome, 856
Post-thrombotic syndrome, 340
Post-traumatic stress disorder, 1100t, 1101
Postural drainage, for atelectasis due to mucous plugs, 171
  for lung abscess, 204
Potassium. See also *Hyperkalemia; Hypokalemia.*
  for diabetic ketoacidosis, 573–574
    in children, 567–568
  for hypokalemia due to cobalamin therapy, 367
  for salicylate intoxication, 1199t, 1200
  in intravenous solutions, for high-risk neonates, 1012
    for infants and children, 608, 608t
  in parenteral nutrition solutions, 605t
  reference intervals for, in serum, 1209t
    in urine, 1211t
  requirements for, for infants and children, 608, 608t
    for low-birth-weight infant, 609
  supplemental, for hypertension, 305
    with very-low-calorie diet, 588
Potassium citrate, for urinary stone prevention, 715
Potassium hydroxide preparation, in candidiasis diagnosis, 1053
Potassium iodide, for thyroid storm, 648
Potassium magnesium citrate, for urinary stone prevention, 715
Potassium phosphate, for hypercalciuria, 715

Pott's disease, 239
Power of attorney, for Alzheimer's disease patient, 845
Poxviruses, skin infections due to, 803
Pralidoxime, for carbamate poisoning, 1194
  for organophosphate poisoning, 1154t, 1194
Pramipexole, for Parkinson's disease, 919t, 920
  for primary sleep disorders, 34
Pramoxine-hydrochlorothiazide, for pruritus gravidarum, 833
Pravastatin, for hyperlipidemia, 581
  after myocardial infarction, 332
Prazepam, intoxication with, 1166
Praziquantel, for cysticercosis, 541t, 546
  for flukes, 540t, 546
  for schistosomiasis, 540t, 546
  for tapeworms, 541t, 546
Prazosin, for cutaneovascular disease in lupus erythematosus, 776
  for hypertension, 307–309, 308t
    in type 2 diabetes, 563
  for pheochromocytoma, 655
Prednisolone, for asthma exacerbations, in children, 741
  for bursitis or tendinitis, 966
  for corrosive ingestion, 1171
  for ordinary urticaria, 836
  for paroxysmal nocturnal hemoglobinuria, 366
  for sarcoidosis, 225, 227
  for subacute thyroiditis, 658–659
  for urticarial vasculitis, 837
Prednisone, after adenectomy for acromegaly, 616
  for acute exacerbation of chronic bronchitis, 209
  for acute lymphoblastic leukemia in children, 423
  for aggressive lymphoma, 436t
  for allergic rhinitis, 746
  for anaphylaxis, 727t
    due to insect sting, 754
  for anti–glomerular basement membrane disease, 679
  for aphthous stomatitis, 812
  for asthma, 734, 735
    in children, 741
  for atopic dermatitis, 823
  for autoimmune hepatitis, 469
  for bullous pemphigoid, 827–828
  for chronic adrenal insufficiency, 621
  for chronic inflammatory demyelinating polyradiculoneuropathy, 929–930
  for chronic lymphocytic leukemia, 431, 432
  for chronic obstructive pulmonary disease, 173
  for cicatricial pemphigoid, 813
  for contact dermatitis, 831
  for cutaneous vasculitis, 779
  for eosinophilic gastroenteritis, 513
  for erythema multiforme, 813
  for erythema nodosum leprosum, 93
  for facial paralysis, 917
  for Fanconi's anemia, 355
  for focal segmental glomerulosclerosis, 678
  for herpes gestationis, 828, 832
  for histoplasmosis, 198
  for Hodgkin's disease, 407t
  for hypercalcemia in multiple myeloma, 443
  for hypersensitivity pneumonitis, 230, 231

Prednisone (Continued)
  for IgA nephritis, 679
  for immune thrombocytopenic purpura, 400
  for impetigo herpetiformis, 833
  for indolent B cell lymphoma, 435t
  for infantile spasms, 870
  for infectious mononucleosis, 109
  for inflammatory bowel disease, 484
    bone disease due to, 487
  for insect sting allergy, 753, 754
  for juvenile rheumatoid arthritis, 956
  for lichen planus, 773
  for lupus erythematosus, 776
  for membranoproliferative glomerulonephritis, 679
  for membranous glomerulopathy, 678
  for minimal change disease, 677
  for multiple myeloma, 442, 443
  for multiple sclerosis, 898
  for myasthenia gravis, 906
  for nerve infarction, 930
  for nerve involvement in sarcoidosis, 930
  for neuropathy due to paraproteinemia, 928
  for ocular toxoplasmosis, 156
  for optic neuritis, 911–912
  for oral lichen planus, 811
  for otitis media with effusion, 206
  for pain in pericarditis, 334
  for pauci-immune glomerulonephritis, 679–680
  for pemphigus, 826–827
  for *Pneumocystis carinii* pneumonia in HIV infection, 51
  for polymyalgia rheumatica, 971
  for primary glomerular disease, 675–676
  for pruritic urticarial papules and plaques of pregnancy, 831–832
  for reversal reaction in leprosy, 93–94
  for rheumatoid arthritis, 947–948, 951
  for serum sickness, 729
  for Sézary's syndrome, 769
  for trichinosis, 545
  for vertigo, 886, 886t
  for warm antibody autoimmune hemolytic anemia, 362
  hair growth in response to, in alopecia areata, 762
  in CHOP regimen, for aggressive lymphoma, 436t
    for indolent B cell lymphoma, 435t
    for Sézary's syndrome, 769
  in CVP regimen, for chronic lymphocytic leukemia, 431
    for indolent B cell lymphoma, 435t
  with radioiodine therapy for Graves' disease, 648
Pre-eclampsia, 991–994, 992t, 993t
  defined, 988–989, 991
  management of, 992–994, 993t, 994t
    postpartum, 994
  pathophysiology of, 991
  prevention of, 991–992
  risk of, 992t
    with chronic hypertension, 989
Preexcitation syndrome, *271*, 272–274, *273*
Pregnancy, 979–985
  acetaminophen intoxication during, 1162
  acute fatty liver of, HELLP syndrome vs., 993t
  acute porphyria and, 451
  allergic rhinitis management during, 748
  amebiasis treatment during, 59
  anticoagulant therapy during, 341

Pregnancy (Continued)
  anticonvulsant therapy during, 864
  asymptomatic bacteriuria during, 664t, 666
  benzimidazole use during, 544
  blastomycosis during, 200
  breast cancer during, 1026
  brucellosis treatment during, 64, 65t, 66
  carbon monoxide poisoning during, 1170
  chickenpox during, 70, 71
  Chlamydia trachomatis infection during, 1057, 1057t
  cocaine intoxication during, 1173
  coccidioidomycosis during, 194
  diabetes development during, 982
    screening for, 550
  diabetes insipidus during, 626
  diabetes management during, 982
  diabetic ketoacidosis and, 574
  ectopic, 985–986, 985t, 986t
    after tubal ligation, 1088
  environmental hazards during, 980
  ethical issues in, 984–985
  fetal health evaluation during, 981–982
  fetal therapy during, 984
  genetic counseling and prenatal diagnosis during, 980–981
  genital warts during, 787, 788
  giardiasis during, 61, 538, 542
  HIV infection and, 984
  Hodgkin's disease treatment during, 408
  hyperprolactinemia treatment during, 642
  hypertensive disorders of, 982, 988–994. See also *Hypertension, during pregnancy; Pre-eclampsia.*
  hyperthyroidism during, 648
  immunizations during, 145, 148
    measles, 133–134
    rubella, 132
  in hypogonadotropic hypogonadism, 638
  infections during, 984
  lead poisoning during, 1185
  leiomyoma symptoms during, 1060
  Listeria monocytogenes infection during, 79
  Lyme disease during, 127, 129t
  mask of, 839
  medical complications in, 982
  methadone use during, 1095–1096
  methotrexate use during, 772
  myasthenia gravis during, 907–908
  nausea and vomiting in, treatment of, 8
  obstetric complications in, 983–984
  opioid withdrawal during, 1095
  pheochromocytoma during, 657
  physiologic changes of, anesthetic techniques and, 995
  polycythemia vera during, 447
  prolonged, 983
  pulmonary thromboembolism workup during, 220
  pyelonephritis during, 666, 680
    treatment of, 681–682
  relapsing fever during, 124
  retinoid use during, 758, 772
  routine care during, 979–980
  rubella during, 131
  screening for antithyroid antibodies in, 659
  skin diseases of, 828, 831–833
  spironolactone use during, 759
  surgery during, 982–983
  syphilis treatment during, 724
  thrombotic thrombocytopenic purpura during, 403, 404

Pregnancy (Continued)
thyroid hormone replacement during, 644
toxoplasmosis during, 151, 155
trauma during, 983
urinary tract infection in, 664t, 665–666
vaginal bleeding during third trimester of, 986–988
vertical HIV transmission in, 41
vitamin K deficiency during, 592, 593
with mutiple fetuses, 983–984
Pregnanediol, urine, reference intervals for, 1211t
Pregnanetriol, urine, reference intervals for, 1211t
Premature beats, 260–264
atrial, 261
junctional, 261
ventricular, 262–264
after myocardial infarction, 324t
Premature birth, 983. See also Neonate(s), high-risk.
apnea in, 1014
Premenstrual syndrome, 1044–1047, 1045t, 1046t
Prenalterol, for beta blocker intoxication, 1168
Prenatal care, 979–985. See also Pregnancy.
Presbylarynx, 28
Pressure earring devices, for keloids, 785
Pressure palsies, 930
Pressure ulcers, 819–821
after head injury, 935
Preterm birth, 983. See also Neonate(s), high-risk.
apnea with, 1014
Priapism, in sickle cell disease, 378
PRICE-MM management, for sports injuries, 975, 975t
Prilocaine-lidocaine, for pruritus, 36
Primaquine, for malaria, 96, 96t
prophylactic, 149–150
for Pneumocystis carinii pneumonia in HIV infection, 51
Primidone, adverse effects of, 863t
drug interactions with, 863t
for epilepsy, 860t, 861, 862t
in infants and children, 868t
pharmacokinetics of, 862t
reference intervals for, 1210t
Prinzmetal's angina, 247
Probenecid, for gout, 578
for pelvic inflammatory disease, 1059t
for syphilis, 724t
for typhoid carriage, 164
Procainamide, for atrial fibrillation, 259, 259t, 260
after myocardial infarction, 323
for atrial flutter, 275t
for cardiac arrest, 253, 254
for wide complex tachycardia, 277
reference intervals for, 1210t
relative antiarrhythmic efficacy of, 262t
Procainamide–N-acetyl-p-aminophenol, reference intervals for, 1210t
Procarbazine, for Hodgkin's disease, 407t
Prochlorperazine, for ciguatera poisoning, 1143
for food-borne illness, 76
for Meniere's disease, 893
for mountain sickness, 1128
for nausea and vomiting, 8t
due to chemotherapy, 10t
in acute viral hepatitis, 502
intoxication by, 1197t

Proctitis, chlamydial, treatment of, 1057, 1057t
Procyclidine, for Parkinson's disease, 919t
Progestational challenge test, in amenorrhea assessment, 1041–1042
Progesterone. See also Progestins; specific progestins.
effects of, 1045
for epilepsy, 865
for hormone replacement therapy, 1051
in normal menstrual cycle, 1038, 1040
measurement of, in ectopic pregnancy diagnosis, 985
serum, reference intervals for, 1209t
Progestins. See also specific progestins.
contraceptive methods based on, 1079t, 1080t–1082t, 1085, 1087
during breast-feeding, 1089
for endometriosis, 1031
for hormone replacement therapy, 1051–1052
subdermal implantable, for contraception, 1082t, 1085
Progressive massive fibrosis, in silicosis, 229
Progressive multifocal leukoencephalopathy, in HIV infection, 55
Proguanil, for malaria prophylaxis, 100t, 101, 149
Proguanil-atovaquone, for malaria, 96, 97t
Prolactin, serum. See also Hyperprolactinemia.
reference intervals for, 1209t
Prolactinoma, 641–642
Promethazine, for allergic rhinitis, 745t
for food-borne illness, 76
for motion sickness, 890
for nausea in acute viral hepatitis, 502
for vertigo, 886, 886t
for viral respiratory infection, 214
intoxication with, 1164, 1197t
Propafenone, adverse effects of, 275, 275t
for atrial fibrillation, 259, 259t, 260
for atrial flutter, 275t
for atrial premature beats, 261
relative antiarrhythmic efficacy of, 262t
Propantheline, for bladder dysfunction in multiple sclerosis, 902
Propionibacterium acnes colonization, in acne, 757
Propofol, for status epilepticus, 865t
in infants and children, 870t
Propoxur, 1193
Propoxyphene, anticonvulsant interactions with, 863t
intoxication with, 5, 1191, 1192, 1192t
Propranolol, anticonvulsant interactions with, 863t
for acute hepatic porphyria, 448, 448t
for anxiety disorders, 1100t, 1102
for atrial fibrillation, 257, 258t
for esophagogastric varices in cirrhosis, 467
for headache after minor head injury, 935
for hypertension, 308t
for hyperthyroidism, 647
in subacute thyroiditis, 659
for migraine, 886t
for pheochromocytoma, 655
for tetanus, 136
for thyroid storm, 648
for tremor in Parkinson's disease, 922
intoxication with, 1166, 1167t, 1168
reference intervals for, 1210t
relative antiarrhythmic efficacy of, 262t

Propranolol (Continued)
rizatriptan interaction with, 882
Propylene glycol, serum concentration estimation for, 1160t
Propylthiouracil, adverse effects of, 646–647
for hyperthyroidism, 646–647
for thyroid storm, 648
Prostaglandin E₁. See Alprostadil.
Prostaglandin F₂α, for postpartum hemorrhage, 1000
in dysmenorrhea, 1043–1044
Prostate cancer, 705–708
diagnosis of, 706
staging of, 706
treatment of, 706–708
Prostatectomy, for benign prostatic hyperplasia, 691
for prostate cancer, 706–707
stress incontinence after, 673
Prostate-specific antigen, in prostate cancer screening, 706
Prostatic hyperplasia, benign, 687–691
diagnosis of, 688
epidemiology of, 687
pathophysiology of, 687–688
symptoms of, 688, 689
treatment of, 688–691, 690, 690t, 691t
Prostatitis, 685–687
recurrent urinary tract infection with, 662, 686
Prostatodynia, 685–686
Protamine, heparin reversal with, for intracerebral hemorrhage, 849
Protease inhibitors. See also specific drugs.
antifungal interactions with, 807
antitubercular drug interactions with, 51, 52, 52t, 240–241
for HIV infection, in combination regimens, 45t, 46t
resistance profiles of, 45, 45t
mechanism of action of, 44
toxic effects of, 47
Protein, dietary, in acute renal failure, 698
in chronic renal failure, 702–703, 704
in nephrogenic diabetes insipidus, 627
in primary glomerular disease, 677
pressure ulcers and, 819
in parenteral nutrition, 601
for high-risk neonate, 1012
malabsorption of, congenital defects causing, 514
reference intervals for, in cerebrospinal fluid, 1212t
in serum, 1209t
in urine, 1211t
requirements for, for burn patients, 1125
in parenteral nutrition, 601
Protein C concentrate, for thrombosis prevention, 458
Protein hydrolysate formula, for infant feeding, 1020, 1021t
Protein/creatinine ratio, urine, reference intervals for, 1211t
Proteinuria. See also Microalbuminuria.
due to gold therapy, 949
in glomerular disease, 675
in pre-eclampsia, 991
Prothrombin, deficiency of, 392
genetic mutation in, pulmonary thromboembolism and, 221
Prothrombin complex concentrates, for hemophilia, 393, 394
for severe bleeding in vitamin K deficiency, 593
Proton pump inhibitors. See also specific drugs.

Proton pump inhibitors *(Continued)*
  defective iron absorption due to, 356
  for dyspepsia, 11
  for gastroesophageal reflux disease, 525–526
Protoporphyria, 448t, 452t, 453
Protozoa, 538. See also *Parasites; specific diseases.*
  intestinal, 538–543
    drugs for, 538, 539t
  nonpathogenic, 543
  skin disease due to, 804, 804t
Protriptyline, for chronic fatigue syndrome, 112
  for depression, 1109t
  for obstructive sleep-disordered breathing, 184
  intoxication by, 1202t
  pharmacodynamic effects of, 1110t
Provocation testing, oral, for drug allergy, 751
Pruritic urticarial papules and plaques of pregnancy, 831–832
Pruritus, 35–37, 35t, 36t
  perineal, 833–834
Pruritus gravidarum, 833
Pseudoachalasia, 474–475
Pseudobuboes, in donovanosis, 721
Pseudoclaudication, intermittent claudication vs., 336, 336t
Pseudocowpox, 803
Pseudocyst, pancreatic, 517–518
Pseudodiverticulosis, esophageal intramural, 480
Pseudoephedrine, anorectic agent interactions with, 591
  for allergic rhinitis, 746
  for stress incontinence, 673
  for viral respiratory infection, 214
Pseudointernuclear ophthalmoplegia, in myasthenia gravis, 904
Pseudomonas aeruginosa infection, antibiotic-resistant, 205
  ecthyma gangrenosum due to, 798
  in cystic fibrosis, 177, 178
  meningitis due to, antimicrobial therapy for, 104t, 106
Pseudomonas infection, malignant otitis externa due to, 114
Pseudoparkinsonism, due to antipsychotic drugs, 1117, 1119
Pseudoporphyria, due to naproxen, 954
Pseudoseizures, epilepsy vs., 857–858
Psilocybin mushrooms, 78t, 79, 1096
Psittacosis, 116–118
Psoralen photochemotherapy, extracorporeal, for Sézary's syndrome, 769
  for lymphomatoid papulosis, 770
  for mycosis fungoides, 768
  for parapsoriasis, 774
  for pruritus, 37
  for psoriasis, 772, 782
  for vitiligo, 840–841
Psoriasis, 771–772
  during pregnancy, 833
  hair loss with, 762
  nail involvement in, 781t, 782
Psychiatric disorders, 1090–1122. See also specific disorders.
  attention-deficit/hyperactivity disorder and, 871–872
  migraine and, 880–881
  temporomandibular disorders and, 962
  Tourette's syndrome and, 875
Psychogenic cough, 24
Psychogenic seizures, epilepsy vs., 857–858

Psychological dependence. See also *Drug abuse; specific substances.*
  defined, 4
Psychosexual therapy, for erectile dysfunction, 693
Psychosis, antidepressants for use in, 1115t
  in Alzheimer's disease, 846–847
  in Parkinson's disease, 923
  LSD use and, 1097
  postpartum, 1001
Psychotherapy, for bulimia nervosa, 1105
  for depression, 1116
  for irritable bowel syndrome, 491, 492
Psyllium, for constipation, 19, 19t
Pterygium, in lichen planus of nails, 783
Pubic lice, 804t, 806
Puerperium, care during, 999–1001
Puestow's operation, for chronic pancreatitis, 522–523
Puffer fish poisoning, 79, 80t, 1144
Pulmonary angiography, in pulmonary thromboembolism workup, 220, 221
Pulmonary edema, acute, after myocardial infarction, 325, 327t
  high-altitude, 1128–1129, 1128t
Pulmonary embolism, 218–224
  anaphylaxis vs., 726–727
  atelectasis due to, 170–171
  oral contraceptives and, 1086t
  postpartum, 1001
  prevention of, 222t
    after head injury, 935
  screening for, 218, 219t
  treatment of, 221–224, 222t, 223t, *224*
  workup for, 218–221, 219t, 220t
Pulmonary hypertension, in high-altitude pulmonary edema, 1129
  in newborn, 1014–1015
Pulmonary rehabilitation program, 173
Pulmonary stenosis, 283–284
Pulseless electrical activity. See also *Sudden cardiac death.*
  treatment of, 255, 256
Pupillary block, in glaucoma, 914–915
Purified protein derivative, tuberculosis testing with, 242
  in HIV infection, 51
Purpura, immune thrombocytopenic, 400
  post-transfusion, 399–400, 460
  thrombotic thrombocytopenic, 402–404, 402t. See also *Hemolytic-uremic syndrome.*
    HELLP syndrome vs., 993t
    platelet transfusions' effects in, 455
Purpura fulminans, in chickenpox, 71
Pyelography, intravenous, for staging renal injuries in trauma victim, 683
  in renal calculus evaluation, 713
Pyelonephritis, 680–682, 681t, 682t
  catheter-associated, 682
  complications of, 682
  during pregnancy, 666, 680
  emphysematous, 682
  in girls, 667–668
  in infants, symptoms of, 666
  in men, 661–662
  in women, 663–665, 664t
  treatment of, 681–682, 681t
Pyoderma gangrenosum, ecthyma gangrenosum vs., 798
Pyrantel pamoate, for ascariasis, 540t, 544
  for hookworm, 540t, 544
  for pinworm, 540t, 544
  for *Trichostrongylus* infection, 541t, 545
Pyrazinamide (PZA), adverse effects of, 241

Pyrazinamide (PZA) *(Continued)*
  for tuberculosis, 240
    in HIV infection, 53t
  for tuberculosis prophylaxis in HIV infection, 52t
Pyrethrins, for lice, 804t, 806
Pyridostigmine, for myasthenia gravis, 905
Pyridoxine, deficiency of, neuropathy due to, 927
  for alcoholic neuropathy, 927
  for elevated homocysteine in type 2 diabetes, 563
  for ethylene glycol intoxication, 1155t, 1178
  for isoniazid intoxication, 1155t, 1182
  for mushroom poisoning, 79, 1155t
  for tuberculosis, 240
  neuropathy due to, 926, 927, 931
Pyrimethamine, for isosporiasis, 539t, 543
  for *Pneumocystis carinii* pneumonia in HIV infection, 51
    prophylactic, 51
  for toxoplasmosis, 152, 154–155
    congenital, 156
    during pregnancy, 155
    in HIV infection, 53, 156–157
    ocular, 156
  for toxoplasmosis prophylaxis, 154
    in heart transplant recipients, 157
    in HIV infection, 52
Pyrimethamine-sulfadoxine, for malaria, 96, 97t
  for toxoplasmosis, 153
Pyropoikilocytosis, hereditary, 364
Pyruvate, blood, reference intervals for, 1209t
Pyruvate kinase deficiency, 365
Pyuria, detection of, 663
PZA. See *Pyrazinamide (PZA).*

Q fever, 118
Quetiapine, adverse effects of, 1119
  characteristics of, 1118, 1118t
Quinacrine, for diarrhea, 16
  for giardiasis, 61, 61t, 513, 538, 539t
  for lupus erythematosus, 775–776
  U.S. sources for, 61
Quinapril, for congestive heart failure, 294t
  for hypertension, 309t
Quinidine, antifungal interactions with, 807
  for atrial flutter, 275t
  for hiccup, 14t
  for malaria, 97, 99t
  reference intervals for, 1210t
  relative antiarrhythmic efficacy of, 262t
Quinine, for babesiosis, 130
  for malaria, in mild disease, 96, 97t
    in severe disease, 97–99, 99t
Quinolones. See also specific drugs.
  for salmonellosis, 160–161

Rabies, 119–122
  clinical management of, 120–122
  clinical manifestations of, in humans, 120
  epidemiology of, 119
  infection control in, 122
  laboratory diagnosis of, 120
  molecular virology, 119–120
  pathogenesis of, 120

Rabies *(Continued)*
  postexposure prophylaxis of, 121
  pre-exposure prophylaxis of, 120–121
Rabies immune globulin, 121
Rabies vaccine, 121
  for travelers, 147t, 148
Radiation, chronic myelogenous leukemia
    and, 426
  thyroid cancer and, 648
Radiation therapy, carditis due to, 412
  enteritis due to, 1068
    malabsorption due to, 511
    parenteral nutrition for, 603
  for acromegaly, 616
  for aggressive lymphoma, 437
  for ankylosing spondylitis, 960
  for brain tumor, 943
  for breast cancer, 1027, 1028
    for recurrence, 1029
  for central nervous system leukemia,
      424
    prophylactic, 423
  for cervical cancer, 1068
  for colorectal cancer, 536, 537
  for Cushing's disease, 622–623
  for cutaneous hemangiomas, 809
  for endometrial cancer, 1065
  for extramedullary plasmacytoma, 444
  for Fanconi's anemia, 355
  for Hodgkin's disease. See under *Hodg-
    kin's disease.*
  for indolent B cell lymphoma, 434
  for keloids, 785
  for lytic bone lesions in multiple my-
    eloma, 441
  for mycosis fungoides, 769
  for oral cancer, 811
  for pheochromocytoma, 657
  for prostate cancer, 707–708
  for skin cancer, 764–765
  for solitary osseous plasmacytoma, 444
  for spinal cord compression in multiple
    myeloma, 444
  for thyroid cancer, 652. See also under
    Radioiodine therapy.
  hypothyroidism due to, 412, 643
  pneumonitis due to, 412
Radiculoneuritis, in Lyme disease, 125t,
    126
  treatment of, 127, 128t
Radiofrequency ablation. See *Catheter
  ablation.*
Radiofrequency rhizolysis, for trigeminal
    neuralgia, 910
Radiofrequency volumetric tissue
    reduction of the palate, for obstructive
    sleep-disordered breathing, 185
Radioiodine therapy, for hyperthyroidism,
    647–648
  for thyroid cancer, 651–652
    complications of, 652
    thyroid hormone replacement and, 644
    tumor resistance to, 653
Radionuclide imaging. See *Scintigraphy.*
Raloxifene, for hormone replacement
    therapy, 1051
  for hyperlipidemia, 584
  for osteoporosis, 595
Ramipril, for congestive heart failure, 294t
  for hypertension, 309t
  in mitral valve prolapse, 290
Ramsay Hunt syndrome, 115, 885–886,
    885t
Ranitidine, for anaphylaxis, 727t
  for cystic fibrosis, 177t
  for dyspepsia, 497

Ranitidine *(Continued)*
  for gastroesophageal reflux disease, 525
  for gastrointestinal complications in
    acute renal failure, 699
  for *Helicobacter pylori* infection, 501,
    501t
  for NSAID-induced ulcer, 500
    prophylactic, 499
  for ordinary urticaria, 836
  for reflux-related cough, 24
Ranson's criteria, in acute pancreatitis,
    515–516, 516t
Rapid eye movement behavior disorder,
    seizure vs., 857
Rat bite fever, 122–123
Raynaud's phenomenon, in lupus
    erythematosus, 775, 776
  in scleroderma, 777–778
Reboxetine, for depression, 1109t
  pharmacodynamic effects of, 1110t
Rechallenge, in drug allergy, 751–752
Reciprocating tachycardia, antidromic,
    273, 274
  orthodromic, *271, 272,* 273, 274
Rectal cancer, 536. See also *Colorectal
  cancer.*
Rectal examination, digital, in prostate
    cancer screening, 706
Red blood cells. See *Erythrocyte* entries.
Reentrant tachycardia, atrioventricular,
    271, 272, 273, 274
  atrioventricular nodal, *269,* 271–272,
    271, 272
  bundle branch, 278
  mechanism of, 269, *269*
  sinoatrial node, 270–271, *271*
Reference intervals, 1205–1206
  for cerebrospinal fluid tests, 1212t
  for clinical chemistry, on blood, serum,
    and plasma, 1207t–1209t
    on urine, 1211t–1212t
  for gastrointestinal function tests, 1213t
  for hematology, 1206t–1207t
  for immunologic function tests, 1213t
  for semen analysis, 1213t
  for therapeutic drug monitoring, 1210t
  for toxic substances, 1210t
  tables of, 1206, 1206t–1213t
Reflux, gastroesophageal. See
    Gastroesophageal reflux disease.
  vesicoureteral, 667
    pyelonephritis and, 680
Regan-Lowe media, for *Bordetella* culture,
    138
Regurgitation, vomiting vs., 5
Rehabilitation, after head injury in
    children, 940
  after stroke, 853–856, 853t. See also un-
    der *Stroke.*
  cardiac, after myocardial infarction,
    331–332
  for burn patients, 1126, 1127t
  pelvic floor, for stress incontinence, 673
    for urgency incontinence, 672
  pulmonary, 173
  vestibular, 886, 887t
    for bilateral vestibular deficit, 887t,
      891
    for Meniere's disease, 893
Rehydration, oral. See *Oral rehydration
  therapy.*
  parenteral, for infants and children,
    609–613, 610t, *611*
Reinke's edema, 26
Relapsing fever, due to *Bartonella
  henselae,* 158

Relapsing fever *(Continued)*
  due to *Borrelia* species, 123–125
Relaxation, for chronic fatigue syndrome,
    112
Relaxin, for scleroderma, 778
Renal abscess, 682
Renal amyloidosis, in ankylosing
    spondylitis, 959
Renal artery stenosis, renovascular
    hypertension and, 313
  screening for, 313
  treatment of, 314
Renal artery thrombosis, after trauma,
    683
Renal cell carcinoma, 709–710
Renal disease. See also specific diseases.
  end-stage, in diabetes, 564–565
    in porphyria cutanea tarda, 453
    progression from chronic renal failure
      to, 705
  hypertension due to, 312–313
  in lead poisoning, 1185
  in sickle cell disease, 379
Renal failure, acute, 694–700
  approach to patient with, 695–697,
      696t
  causes of, 694–695, 694t
  complications of, 698–699
  due to hemolytic transfusion reaction,
      459
  in malaria, 95t, 99
  management of, 697–700
  parenteral nutrition for, 603
  prevention of, 695
  recovery from, 700
  replacement therapy for, 699–700,
      699t, 700t
  chronic, 701–705
  causes of, 701, 701t
  complications of, 703–705
  epidemiology of, 701
  hyperparathyroidism in, 631, 703–704
  treatment of, 702–705
  in acute pancreatitis, 516
  in multiple myeloma, 443
  parenteral nutrition solutions for, 605,
      605t
  peripheral neuropathy in, 699, 925
Renal hypercalciuria, hyperparathyroidism
    due to, 631
Renal replacement therapy. See also
    specific modalities.
  for acute renal failure, 699–700, 699t,
      700t
  for chronic renal failure, 705
Renal stones, 712–715
  in primary hyperparathyroidism, 629
Renal transplantation, for chronic renal
    failure, 705
  in multiple myeloma, 443
Renin activity, plasma, measurement of, in
    primary aldosteronism diagnosis, 634
Renovascular hypertension, 313–314
Repaglinide, for type 2 diabetes, 557t, 558
  in combination therapy, 561, 562
Reperfusion therapy, for myocardial
    infarction, 320–321
Reproduction, assisted, in endometriosis,
    1036–1037
Reserpine, for hypertension, 308t, 309
Respiratory distress syndrome, adult,
    167–168
  in neonate, 1014
Respiratory disturbance index, 180
Respiratory failure, acute, 167–170
  in acute pancreatitis, 516

Respiratory failure *(Continued)*
mechanical ventilation for. See *Ventilation, mechanical.*
Respiratory insufficiency, parenteral nutrition in, 604
Respiratory quotient, in caloric needs calculation, 601
Respiratory syncytial virus, pneumonia due to, 215, 215t, 216t
Respiratory tract infection, lower. See also *Pneumonia.*
cough due to, in infant, 23
upper, asthma and, 730
cough due to, 22
in child, 23
viral, 213–215
Respite care, for Alzheimer's disease, 845
Restless legs syndrome, 33, 34
Resuscitation, cardiopulmonary, 251, *252*
in accidental hypothermia, 1132
for burn patients, 1124, 1124t
of newborn, 1001–1006. See also under *Neonate(s).*
Retching, defined, 5
Reteplase. See *Tissue plasminogen activator (t-PA).*
Reticulocyte count, reference intervals for, 1206t
Reticulosis, pagetoid, mycosis fungoides and, 766
Retinitis, cytomegalovirus, in HIV infection, 53
toxoplasmosis, 156
all-*trans*-Retinoic acid. See *Tretinoin.*
13-*cis*-Retinoic acid. See *Isotretinoin.*
Retinoic acid syndrome, 418
Retinoids. See also specific drugs.
adverse effects of, 758–759
for acne, systemic, 758–759
topical, 757
for lupus erythematosus, 776
for mycosis fungoides, 769–770
for psoriasis, 772
Retinopathy, diabetic, 563–564
due to hydroxychloroquine, 775, 949–950
in sickle cell disease, 379
Retrocalcaneal bursitis, 965
Retroviral syndrome, acute, 42–43, 42t
Retroviruses. See also *Human immunodeficiency virus (HIV) infection.*
transmission of, by blood components, 461
Reverse transcriptase inhibitors. See also specific drugs.
antitubercular drug interactions with, 51, 52, 52t
for HIV infection, in combination regimens, 45t, 46t
resistance profiles of, 45, 45t
mechanism of action of, 44
Rewarming, for accidental hypothermia, 1132–1133, 1132t
for frostbite, 1134
Reye's syndrome, chickenpox and, 70, 71
with salicylate therapy for juvenile rheumatoid arthritis, 954, 956
RFB. See *Rifabutin (RFB).*
Rh immune globulin, 384–385
during pregnancy, 980
for immune thrombocytopenic purpura, 400
postpartum administration of, 999–1000
with antepartum hemorrhage, 987
Rh isoimmunization, 383–388
incidence of, 384

Rh isoimmunization *(Continued)*
management of, maternal-fetal, 385–386, *386*
postnatal and neonatal, 386–388, 387t, 388t
modulating factors for, 384
pathogenesis of, 384
prevention of, 384–385
risk for, 384
Rheumatoid arthritis, 945–953
extra-articular, 945t
juvenile, 953–958
classification of, 954t
eye disease in, 958
medications for, 954–957, 955t
normal development in, 958
nutrition in, 958
physical and occupational therapy for, 957
surgery for, 957
pressure palsies in, 930
treatment of, alternative therapies in, 952
disease-modifying drugs in, 945–947
drugs used in, 946t, 947–951
exercise in, 953
future directions in, 953
specific recommendations for, 951–952
strategy for, 945–947
surgical, 952–953
Rheumatoid factor, reference intervals for, 1209t
Rhinitis, allergic. See *Allergic rhinitis.*
differential diagnosis of, 743t
infectious, allergic rhinitis vs., 744
nonallergic, differential diagnosis of, 743t
with eosinophilia, 743t, 744
Rhinitis medicamentosa, 234, 746
Rhinophyma, in rosacea, 759
Rhinosinusitis, 231–236
acute, 232, *233*, 233t
recurrent, 232, *233*, 233t
treatment of, 235
chronic, 232, *232*, *233*, 233t
pathogens causing, 233
treatment of, 235
classification of, 232, *233*, 233t
diagnostic algorithm for, *234*
pathogens causing, 232–233
signs and symptoms of, 232t
subacute, 232, 233t
treatment of, 233–236
surgical, 236, 236t
Rhizolysis, for trigeminal neuralgia, 910
Rhythm method, for contraception, 1075–1084, 1076t
during breast-feeding, 1089
Ribavirin, for chronic hepatitis C, 506–507
for viral pneumonia, 216t
Riboflavin, for alcoholic neuropathy, 927
Riedel's thyroiditis, 660
RIF. See *Rifampin (RIF).*
Rifabutin (RFB), for *Mycobacterium avium* complex infection, 54, 241
for toxoplasmosis, 154
for tuberculosis in HIV infection, 51, 52, 53t, 240, 241
prophylactic, 52t
Rifampin (RIF), adverse effects of, 241
anticonvulsant interaction with, 863t
antifungal interaction with, 194, 196, 200
antiretroviral interaction with, 51, 52t, 240–241
for bacterial meningitis, 105t

Rifampin (RIF) *(Continued)*
prophylactic, 108
for brucellosis, 64, 65, 65t, 66
for cat-scratch disease, 158t
for ehrlichiosis, 166, 166t
for infective endocarditis, 300t, 301, 302
for legionellosis, 217, 217t
for leprosy, 92, 94
for *Mycobacterium kansasii* infection, 241
for osteomyelitis, 973, 974t
for pneumococcal meningitis, 104t, 105
for Q fever, 118
for streptococcal pharyngitis, 238
for tuberculosis, 240
in HIV infection, 53t
for tuberculosis prophylaxis, in HIV infection, 52t
levothyroxine interaction with, 644
Rifapentine, 1215t
for tuberculosis, 240
Right bundle branch, 265
Right bundle branch block. See also *Heart block.*
after myocardial infarction, 324t
electrocardiographic diagnosis of, 266
Right ventricular dysplasia, arrhythmogenic, 279
Right-to-left shunts, in congenital heart disease, 284–287
Rimantadine, for influenza, 87
for viral pneumonia, 216t
Ringer's solution, lactated, electrolyte composition of, 608t
Risedronate, adverse effects of, 599
for Paget's disease of bone, 598t, 599
Risperidone, adverse effects of, 1119
characteristics of, 1118, 1118t
for behavioral disorders in Alzheimer's disease, 847
Risus sardonicus, in tetanus, 134
Ritonavir (RTV), drug interactions with, 45
antitubercular agents, 52
for HIV infection, 46t, 49t
River blindness, 804t
Rizatriptan, 1215t
for migraine, 881–882
Rocky Mountain spotted fever, 165–166, 166t
Rodenticide poisoning, 592, 593
Rofecoxib, peptic ulcer disease and, 500
Romano-Ward syndrome, torsades de pointes in, 279
Ropinirole, for Parkinson's disease, 919t, 920
Ropivacaine, for labor analgesia, 996
Rosacea, 759
Rose spots, in typhoid fever, 161
Roseola infantum, 802–803
Rosiglitazone, for type 2 diabetes, 559–560
Rotator cuff strains, 975
Rotator cuff tendinitis, 965
Rotavirus vaccine, *140*, 142–143
Roth's spots, 298
Round window, drug delivery to, for Meniere's disease, 894
RTV. See *Ritonavir (RTV).*
RU486 (mifepristone), for Cushing's syndrome, 623
Rubber band ligation, for hemorrhoids, 493
Rubella, 130–132
Rubella vaccine, 132. See also *Measles-mumps-rubella vaccine.*
postpartum administration of, 999

Rubeola. See *Measles*.

Sacral stimulation, for urgency incontinence, 672
Sacroiliitis, in ankylosing spondylitis, 959
Saddle block, for labor, 996
St. John's wort, 1113
St. Louis encephalitis virus, 896
Salicylates. See also specific drugs.
  for juvenile rheumatoid arthritis, 954–956, 955t
  intoxication by, 1156t, 1198–1201, 1199t, *1201*
  reference intervals for, 1210t
Salicylic acid, for warts, 785
Saline, nasal, for rhinosinusitis, 234
Salivary glands, adenocarcinoma of, 817
  impaired function of, 816
    due to irradiation, 411, 412, 652
Salmeterol, for asthma, 733
  in children, 740, 742
  for chronic obstructive pulmonary disease, 173, *173*
Salmon calcitonin. See *Calcitonin*.
Salmonella typhi. See also *Typhoid fever*.
  drug resistance in, 162
Salmonellosis, 75t, 159–161, 160t
  aortic infection in, 246–247
  prevention and control of, 161
  treatment of, 77–78, 77t, 159–161, 160t
Salpingectomy, for ectopic pregnancy, 986
Salpingitis. See also *Pelvic inflammatory disease*.
  chlamydial, 1056
Salpingo-oophorectomy, for endometrial cancer, 1064
  for endometriosis, 1032, 1033
Salpingostomy, for ectopic pregnancy, 986
Salsalate, for dysmenorrhea, 1043t
  for juvenile rheumatoid arthritis, 954–956, 955t
Saquinavir (SQV), antitubercular drug interaction with, 52
  for HIV infection, 45, 46t, 49t
Sarcoidosis, 224–228
  peripheral neuropathy in, 928
  pressure palsies in, 930
  treatment of, by involved organ, 226–228, 227t
    drugs used for, 225–226
  ventricular tachycardia in, 279
Sarcoma. See also specific sites and types.
  of stomach, 531–532
  of vulva, 1074
Sarcoma botryoides, 1074
Sarcoptes scabiei, 804t, 805–806
Sargramostim. See *Granulocyte-macrophage colony-stimulating factor (GM-CSF)*.
Saucerization, for melanoma excision, 790
Saw palmetto, for benign prostatic hyperplasia, 688
Saxitoxin poisoning, 79, 80t, 1143
Scabies, 804t, 805–806
Scalp, dissecting cellulitis of, 762
Scars, from burns, 1126–1127
  keloid, 783–785
Schilling test, in pernicious anemia diagnosis, 367
Schistosomiasis, 540t, 545–546
  prevention of, 150–151
  skin disease due to, 804–805, 804t
Schizophrenia, 1117–1120
  sleep disturbance in, 33

Schizophrenia *(Continued)*
  treatment of, 1118–1120, 1119t
Schober test, in ankylosing spondylitis, 959
School, adjustments at, for head-injured child, 940
  in attention-deficit/hyperactivity disorder, 872
  in juvenile rheumatoid arthritis, 958
Schwachman-Diamond syndrome, 355
Schwannomas, vestibular, 940–941
Scintigraphy, adrenal, in aldosteronism diagnosis, 635
  biliary, for cystic duct obstruction detection, 464
  in acute myocardial infarction diagnosis, 319
  in osteomyelitis evaluation, 972
  in pheochromocytoma localization, 654–655
  in thyroid nodule evaluation, 650
  somatostatin receptor, in detection of ACTH-secreting tumor, 624
  ventilation/perfusion, in pulmonary thromboembolism workup, 218, 220t
Scleroderma, 777–778
  dysphagia due to, 475, 478
Sclerosing cholangitis, primary, 468–469. See also *Cirrhosis*.
Sclerotherapy, for bleeding esophageal varices, 472
  for hemorrhoids, 493
Scombroid poisoning, 79, 80t, 1144
Scopolamine, for Meniere's disease, 893
  for motion sickness, 886t, 890
  for nausea and vomiting, 7, 8t
Scopulariopsis brevicaulis, onychomycosis due to, 781
Scorpions, 1138
Scrofula, 239
Scrotal island flap, for substitution urethroplasty with anterior stricture, 712
Scrotal tongue, 815
Scrotum, trauma to, 685
Sea anemones, envenomation by, 1142
  poisoning from eating, 1143
Sea cucumbers, 1143
Sea snakes, 1143
Sea urchins, envenomation by, 1142
  poisoning from eating, 1143
Sea wasp, 1142
Sea water infections, 798–799
Seafood poisoning, 79, 80t, 1143–1144
Sebaceous cell carcinoma, conjunctivitis due to, 69
Seborrheic dermatitis, 773
  hair loss with, 762
Secobarbital, intoxication with, 1165
Secretin test, reference intervals for, 1213t
Secretin-pancreozymin test, for pancreatic insufficiency, 508
Sedatives. See also specific drugs and classes of drugs.
  abuse of, 1096
  for labor analgesia, 995–996
  perioperative, in obstructive sleep-disordered breathing, 185
  withdrawal of, insomnia due to, 32
Sedimentation rate, reference intervals for, 1207t
Seizures, 856–866. See also *Epilepsy*.
  absence, 858, 859
    in infants and children, 869–870
    treatment of, 860t, 861
  after head injury, 935, 938–940

Seizures *(Continued)*
  antidepressants for use with, 1115t
  atonic, 859
  classification of, 858–859, 858t
  clonic, 858
  diagnosis of, 856
    in infants and children, 867
  differential diagnosis of, 856–858
    in infants and children, 867, 867t
  due to brain tumors, 941, 944
  due to heat stroke, 1136
  febrile, 21, 869
  generalized, 858–859, 858t
  in acute porphyria, 448t, 449–450
  in antidepressant intoxication, 1202
  in eclampsia, 994, 994t
  in ethanol intoxication, 1177
  in ethylene glycol intoxication, 1178
  in isoniazid intoxication, 1182
  in lead poisoning, 1185
  in meningoencephalitis, 896
  in neonate, 1013
  in neuroleptic intoxication, 1196–1197
  in salicylate intoxication, 1200
  myoclonic, 858
  oral contraceptives and, 1086t
  partial, 858, 858t, 859
  prevention of, in pre-eclampsia, 994, 994t
  psychogenic, epilepsy vs., 857–858
  single, 864
  tonic, 858–859
  tonic-clonic, 858
  with intracerebral hemorrhage, 848
Selective estrogen receptor modulators. See also specific drugs.
  for hormone replacement therapy, 1050–1051
Selective serotonin reuptake inhibitors (SSRIs). See also specific drugs.
  for anxiety disorders, 1100t, 1101
  for chronic fatigue syndrome, 112
  for depression in Parkinson's disease, 922–923
  for irritable bowel syndrome, 491
  for pain, 3–4
  for panic disorder, 1121t, 1122
  for postpartum depression, 1001
  insomnia due to, 35
  neuroleptic interaction with, 877
  phentermine with, for obesity, 590–591
Selegiline, for Alzheimer's disease, 846
  for Parkinson's disease, 919, 919t, 921
  selective serotonin reuptake inhibitor interaction with, 923
Selenium sulfide, for seborrheic dermatitis, 773
  for tinea capitis, 806
  for tinea versicolor, 808
Semen analysis, reference intervals for, 1213t
Sengstaken-Blakemore tube, with Minnesota modification, for bleeding esophageal varices, 472
Senile lentigines, 839–840
Senna, with opioid therapy, 5
Senning procedure, for transposition of the great arteries, 285
Sensation, gastrointestinal motility and, in irritable bowel syndrome, 489–490
Sensorimotor neuropathy, 924–928
  in diabetes, 565, 925
  in renal failure, 699, 925
Sentinel lymphadenectomy, for breast cancer, 1027
  for melanoma, 791

Sentinel lymphadenectomy *(Continued)*
for vulvar carcinoma, 1073
Sepsis, 61–64, 62t
catheter, in acute renal failure, 699
with parenteral nutrition, 606, *607*
diagnosis of, 62–63
in newborn, 1017–1018, 1017t
parenteral nutrition for, 604
treatment of, 63–64, 63t
Septal reduction therapy, for hypertrophic
cardiomyopathy, 349
Septic shock, 62, 62t
Serotonin, antidepressants' effects on
transport of, clinical consequences of,
1112–1113, 1113t
Serotonin antagonists. See also specific
drugs.
type 3, for nausea and vomiting, 7, 8t
due to chemotherapy, 9–10, 10t
Serotonin receptors, antidepressants'
effects at, 1114
Serotonin syndrome, due to biogenic
interaction with MAO inhibitors, 1190,
1191
Sertraline, anticonvulsant interactions
with, 863t
for anxiety disorders, 1100t, 1101
for depression, 1109t, 1114, 1116
in Alzheimer's disease, 847
for panic disorder, 891, 1121t, 1122
for premenstrual syndrome, 1047
levothyroxine interaction with, 644
monoamine oxidase inhibitor interaction
with, 1115
pharmacodynamic effects of, 1110t
phentermine with, for obesity, 590
Serum sickness, 729, 729t
after snake bite treatment, 1141
hypersensitivity syndrome reaction vs.,
750, 750t
Sevelamer, 1215t
Sexual abuse, of child, genital and oral
warts and, 787
gonococcal infection and, 720
premenstrual syndrome and, 1045
Sexual function. See also *Erectile
dysfunction.*
after stroke, 856
Sexually transmitted diseases, 717–724.
See also specific diseases.
epididymitis due to, 674–675
pelvic inflammatory disease and, 1058
six Cs of treating patients with, 674
Sézary's syndrome, clinical features of, 766
immunophenotyping in, 767
leukemia in, 767
molecular biology of, 767
staging of, 767, 767t, 768t
treatment of, 768–770
Sharks, bites of, 1141–1142
poisoning from eating, 1143
Shave biopsy, for nevus, 790
Sheehan's syndrome, 639
Shellfish poisoning, 79, 80t, 1143
Shigellosis, 75t, 77t, 78
Shin splints, 977–978
Shingles. See *Herpes zoster.*
Shock, burn, 1124
cardiogenic, after myocardial infarction,
325–326, 327t
hypovolemic, after myocardial infarction,
325
rewarming, 1132–1133
septic, 62, 62t
Shock wave lithotripsy, for urinary
calculus, 714

Short-bowel syndrome, malabsorption due
to, 511
parenteral nutrition for, 603
Shoulder, bursitis of, 964
sports injuries to, 975–976
tendinitis of, 965
Shoulder pain, after stroke, 856
Shoulder replacement, in rheumatoid
arthritis, 952
Shunts, aqueous, for glaucoma, 915
in congenital heart disease, left-to-right,
280–282
right-to-left, 284–287
transjugular intrahepatic portosystemic,
for variceal bleeding, 470, 472
Shy-Drager syndrome, dysphonia in, 27
SI units, 1205t, 1206
Sibutramine, for obesity, 591, 591t
in type 2 diabetes, 555–556
Sickle cell anemia, 374, 375t. See also
Sickle cell disease.
Sickle cell disease, 374–381
carrier screening for, during pregnancy,
980
clinical manifestations of, 374–380
acute, 375–379
chronic, 379–380
diagnosis of, 374, 375t
pathophysiology of, 374
preventive care and health maintenance
in, 380
prognosis in, 381
treatment of, 380–381
Sickle cell trait, 374, 375t. See also *Sickle
cell disease.*
Sickle hemoglobin C, 375, 375t. See also
Sickle cell disease.
prognosis with, 381
Sickle β-thalassemia, 375, 375t. See also
Sickle cell disease.
Sickle–hereditary persistence of fetal
hemoglobin, 375, 375t. See also *Sickle
cell disease.*
Sigmoidoscopy, in colorectal cancer
screening, 534, 535t
Sildenafil, 1215t
for erectile dysfunction, 693
contraindications to, 249
in diabetes, 566
Silicone gel breast implants, connective
tissue disorders and, 1024
Silicone gel sheeting, for keloids, 784
Silicoproteinosis, 229
Silicosis, 228–230
Silver nitrate, for aphthous stomatitis, 812
Simvastatin, antifungal interactions with,
807
for hyperlipidemia, 581
after myocardial infarction, 332
Singultus, 13–15, 14t
Sinoatrial node reentrant tachycardia,
270–271, *271*
Sinus(es), paranasal. See *Paranasal
sinuses.*
Sinus bradycardia, after myocardial
infarction, 322–323, 324t
Sinus tachycardia, 270
Sinus tract, dental, 814
Sixth disease, 802–803
Skier's thumb, 976–977
Skin, decontamination of, after toxic
exposure, 1147
Skin cancer, 763–765. See also *Melanoma.*
Skin disease(s), 757–843. See also specific
disorders.
bacterial, 81–82, 794–799, 795t, 796t

Skin disease(s) *(Continued)*
bullous autoimmune, 826–830, 826t
fungal, 806–808
in sarcoidosis, 227, 227t
malignant, 763–765. See also *Melanoma.*
of pregnancy, 831–833
papulosquamous, 770–774, 771t
parasitic, 804–806, 804t
pigmentary, 837–841
premalignant, 792–794
viral, 799–803
Skin grafts, for burns, 1125
Skin protection factor of sunscreens, 838,
843
Skin testing, for coccidioidomycosis, 193
for drug allergy, 752, 752t
for insect sting allergy, 754–755, 755t
for tuberculosis, 242
in HIV infection, 51
in allergic rhinitis, 744
SLAP lesion, 976
Sleep apnea. See also *Obstructive sleep-
disordered breathing.*
defined, 180
insomnia due to, 33, 34
Sleep deprivation, obstructive sleep-
disordered breathing and, 181
Sleep disorders. See also *Insomnia.*
adjustment, 32
in chronic obstructive pulmonary disease, 175
in fibromyalgia, 966, 967
seizure vs., 857
Sleep hygiene, 32, 33–34, 34t
Sleep hypopnea, defined, 180
Sleep restriction therapy, for insomnia, 33
SM. See *Streptomycin (SM).*
Small cell carcinoma, cervical, 1068. See
also *Cervical cancer.*
of lung, 190–192. See also *Lung cancer.*
sensory neuropathy with, 931
Smallpox vaccine, 146
Smoker's keratosis of the palate, 811
Smoking, 1098
chronic myelogenous leukemia and, 426
cough due to, 24
hypertension and, 305–306
laryngeal cancer and, 27
lung cancer and, 186
Reinke's edema and, 26
second malignancies and, in small cell
lung cancer, 191
second-hand, cough due to, in child, 23
Smoking cessation, after myocardial
infarction, 333
for chronic obstructive pulmonary disease, 172, 172t
Snakes, 1139–1141
sea, 1143
"Sniffing," 926, 1097
Social phobia, 1100, 1100t
Social support, for Alzheimer's disease
patients and families, 844–845
for attention-deficit/hyperactivity disorder patients and families, 872
for brain tumor patients, 944
in Parkinson's disease, 920
in recovery from alcohol dependence,
1093
Sodium. See also *Hypernatremia;
Hyponatremia.*
dietary, in chronic renal failure, 704
in cirrhosis, 468, 469
in congestive heart failure, 292
in hypercalciuria, 715
in hypertension, 305

Sodium *(Continued)*
  in Meniere's disease, 888, 893
  in nephrogenic diabetes insipidus, 627
  in primary glomerular disease, 677
  estimation of deficit of, in dehydrated
    child, 609t, 611
  fractional excretion of, calculation of,
    609, 609t
    in acute renal failure, 696
  in intravenous solutions, for high-risk
    neonate, 1012
    for infants and children, 608, 608t
  in parenteral nutrition solutions, 605t
  reference intervals for, in serum, 1209t
    in urine, 1212t
  requirements for, for infants and chil-
    dren, 608, 608t
    for low-birth-weight infant, 609
Sodium ascorbate, for ciguatera poisoning,
    1143
Sodium bicarbonate. See *Bicarbonate.*
Sodium channel blockers, 262t. See also
    specific drugs.
Sodium chloride, for heat cramps, 1135,
    1136t
  for orthostatic hypotension in mitral
    valve prolapse, 291
Sodium chloride douche, for trichomoni-
    asis, 1055
Sodium citrate, for acidosis in chronic
    renal failure, 704
Sodium fluoride, for osteoporosis, 596
Sodium iodide, for thyroid storm, 648
Sodium ipodate, for hyperthyroidism, 647
  for thyroid storm, 648
Sodium nitrite, in cyanide antidote kit,
    1152t, 1173–1174
Sodium phenylbutyrate, fetal globin gene
    activation by, for thalassemia, 373
Sodium polystyrene sulfonate, for
    hyperkalemia, in acute renal failure,
    697, 697t
    in chronic renal failure, 705
  for lithium intoxication, 1188
Sodium stibogluconate, for leishmaniasis,
    89
Sodium tetradecyl sulfate, endoscopic
    therapy with, for bleeding esophageal
    varices, 472
Sodium thiosulfate, in cyanide antidote
    kit, 1152t, 1174
Sodoku, 122–123
Soft tissue infections, bacterial, 81–82,
    794–799, 795t, 796t
Soft tissue sarcoma, of vulva, 1074
Sokal scores, in chronic myelogenous
    leukemia, 427t
Solar keratosis, 792
  squamous cell carcinoma and, 764, 792
Solar lentigines, 839–840
Solar urticaria, 834, 836
Somatostatin, for acute pancreatitis, 517
  for chronic pancreatitis, 520
Somatostatin receptor scintigraphy, in
    detection of ACTH-secreting tumor,
    624
Somatotropin. See *Growth hormone.*
Sonohysterography, in dysfunctional
    uterine bleeding evaluation, 1038
  in leiomyoma diagnosis, 1060–1061
Sorbitol, for constipation, 19, 19t
Sotalol, adverse effects of, 275, 275t
  for atrial fibrillation, 260
  for atrial flutter, 275t
  for atrial premature beats, 261
  for ventricular premature beats, 264

Sotalol *(Continued)*
  intoxication with, 1166, 1167t, 1168
  relative antiarrhythmic efficacy of, 262t
Soy formula, for infant feeding, 1020,
    1021t
Sparfloxacin, for legionellosis, 217, 218
  for Q fever, 118
  for tuberculosis, 240
Spasmodic dysphonia, 28
Spasticity, after stroke, 856
  in multiple sclerosis, 901–902
Specific gravity, urine, reference intervals
    for, 1212t
Spectinomycin, for gonococcal infection,
    719, 719t
Speech disorders, after stroke, 854–855
  in Parkinson's disease, 922
Speech therapy, for oropharyngeal
    dysphagia, 477–478
Spermicides, 1077t, 1084
Spherocytosis, hereditary, 363–364
Sphincteroplasty, for chronic pancreatitis,
    523
Sphincterotomy, for anal fissure, 494
  for chronic pancreatitis, 523
Spider bites, 1137–1138
Spinal analgesia, for labor, 996–997
Spinal anesthesia, complications of,
    998–999
  for cesarean delivery, 997
Spinal cord, compression of, in multiple
    myeloma, 444
  injury to, in rheumatoid arthritis, 953
  subacute combined degeneration of, in
    pernicious anemia, 368
Spinal fractures, in ankylosing spondylitis,
    959
  in osteoporosis, 594, 596–597
Spinal stenosis, lumbar, pseudoclaudica-
    tion due to, intermittent claudication
    vs., 336, 336t
Spinal-epidural analgesia, combined, for
    labor, 997
Spinal-epidural anesthesia, combined, for
    cesarean delivery, 997
Spine, cervical, instability of, in
    rheumatoid arthritis, 953
Spiramycin, for toxoplasmosis, 153
  congenital, 156
  during pregnancy, 155
Spirillum minus infection, 122–123
Spirometry, for asthma diagnosis in
    children, 738
  incentive, for atelectasis, 170
Spironolactone, for acne, 759
  for congestive heart failure, 293, 294t
  for Cushing's syndrome, 624
  for hirsutism, 763
  for hypertension, 308t
  for primary aldosteronism, 315, 635
Spitz's nevus, 789, 793
Splanchnicectomy, for chronic pancreatitis,
    523–524
Splenectomy, for aplastic anemia, 354
  for chronic lymphocytic leukemia, 431
  for hereditary spherocytosis, 364
  for Hodgkin's disease, 409
  for immune thrombocytopenic purpura,
    400
  for sickle cell disease, 376
  for thalassemia, 371
  for warm antibody autoimmune hemo-
    lytic anemia, 362
Splenic flexure syndrome, 12
Splenic sequestration, in sickle cell
    disease, 375–376

Splenomegaly, platelet-mediated bleeding
    disorders with, 399
Splinter hemorrhages, 783
Sponge (contraceptive device), 1077t
Sponge (marine animal), 1142
Sports injuries, 974–978
  PRICE-MM management for, 975, 975t
Sprains, 975
  ankle, 978
Sprue, celiac. See *Gluten-sensitive
    enteropathy.*
  collagenous, 511
  tropical, 511
Sputum examination, in pneumonia
    diagnosis, 211
Squamous cell carcinoma, actinic keratosis
    and, 764, 792
  cervical, 1068. See also *Cervical cancer.*
  cutaneous, 763–765
  esophageal, dysphagia due to, 474
  human papillomavirus infection and,
    792, 793
  laryngeal, hoarseness due to, 27
  of lip, 810
  of nail, 781t, 783
  oral, 810–811
  vulvar, 1072–1073
Squamous cell papilloma, laryngeal, 25
SQV (saquinavir), antitubercular drug
    interactions with, 52
  for HIV infection, 45, 46t, 49t
SSRIs. See *Selective serotonin reuptake
    inhibitors (SSRIs);* specific drugs.
Stanford V regimen, for Hodgkin's disease,
    407, 407t
Stanozolol, abuse of, 1097–1098
  for C1 esterase inhibitor deficiency, 837
Staphylococcal toxic shock syndrome, 83
  diagnostic criteria for, 83–84, 84t
  treatment of, 84, 85t
Staphylococcus aureus infection, atopic
    dermatitis and, 823
  food-borne, 75t, 76
  meningitis due to, antimicrobial therapy
    for, 104t, 107
  of skin, 794–795, 795t
Staphylococcus epidermidis meningitis,
    antimicrobial therapy for, 104t
Statins. See *Hydroxymethylglutaryl
    coenzyme A (HMG-CoA) reductase
    inhibitors;* specific drugs.
Status epilepticus, 865, 865t
  in infants and children, 870t, 871
Stavudine (d4T), for HIV infection, 45, 48t
Steatorrhea. See also *Malabsorption.*
  in chronic pancreatitis, 508–509, 521
Steeple sign, in bacterial tracheitis, 31
Stem cell rescue, high-dose chemotherapy
    with, for aggressive lymphoma,
    437–438
  for breast cancer, 1029
  for Hodgkin's disease, 408
  for indolent B cell lymphoma, 435
  for multiple myeloma, 441–442
Stenosing tenosynovitis, 965
Stent, endovascular, for abdominal aortic
    aneurysm, 244
  pancreatic duct, for chronic pancreatitis,
    523
  ureteral, for urinary calculus, 714
  urethral, for anterior urethral stricture,
    711–712
    for benign prostatic hyperplasia, 690–
    691
Stereotactic surgery, for acromegaly, 616
  for brain tumor, 942, 943

Stereotactic surgery (Continued)
for breast lesion biopsy, 1026
for Cushing's disease, 622–623
for trigeminal neuralgia, 910
Sterilization, ectopic pregnancy risk after, 985
for contraception, 1083t, 1087–1088
Steroids. See also Corticosteroid(s); specific drugs.
anabolic, abuse of, 1097–1098
Stevens-Johnson syndrome, 825
Stick test, for toxic fish screening, 1144
Stiff-man syndrome, tetanus vs., 135
Stimulants. See also specific drugs.
designer, intoxication with, 1095, 1163
for attention-deficit/hyperactivity disorder, 872–873, 873t
for pain, 3
insomnia due to, 32
toxic effects of, 1149t
classification of severity of, 1147t
Stimulus control therapy, for insomnia, 33, 33t
Stingray, 1142–1143
Stockings, compression, for post-thrombotic edema, 343–344
for venous leg ulcer prevention, 818
Stoddard's solvent, 1179
Stokes-Adams attack, due to complete heart block, 267
Stomach. See Gastric entries.
Stomatitis, aphthous, 812
contact, 816
Stomatocytosis, hereditary, 364–365
Stonefish, 1142–1143
Stool antigen test, for amebiasis diagnosis, 57, 57t
for giardiasis diagnosis, 60
Strains, in sports injuries, 975
Streptobacillus moniliformis infection, 122–123
Streptococcal infection, group A beta-hemolytic, in chickenpox, 70
of skin and soft tissue, 81, 795–796, 797–798
treatment of, 82, 795t
Tourette's syndrome and, 876
group B beta-hemolytic, perinatal, 984
Streptococcal pharyngitis, 236–238, 238t
food-borne, 81
Streptococcal toxic shock syndrome. See under Toxic shock syndrome.
Streptococcus agalactiae meningitis, antimicrobial therapy for, 103t, 104t, 107
Streptococcus pneumoniae infection, antibiotic resistant, 205, 211–212
otitis media treatment in, 206
in sickle cell disease, 378–379
prophylaxis of, 380
meningitis due to, antimicrobial therapy for, 103–105, 103t, 104t, 107
pneumonia due to, treatment of, 212, 212t
Streptococcus pneumoniae vaccines, polysaccharide, 144
before splenectomy, in hereditary spherocytosis, 364
in thalassemia, 371
in sickle cell disease, 380
protein-conjugate, for otitis media prevention, 206
Streptokinase, for myocardial infarction, 320
for paroxysmal nocturnal hemoglobinuria, 366

Streptokinase (Continued)
for pulmonary thromboembolism, 223t, 224
Streptomycin (SM), for brucellosis, 64, 65, 65t
for infective endocarditis, 301
for plague, 116
for rat bite fever, 123
for tuberculosis in HIV infection, 52, 53t
for Whipple's disease, 512
Stress, chronic fatigue syndrome and, 111, 112
in chronic adrenal insufficiency, corticosteroids for, 621, 621t
irritable bowel syndrome and, 489, 491
migraine and, 880
tinnitus and, 38
Stress fractures, tibial, 978
Stroke, hemorrhagic. See Intracranial hemorrhage.
in atrial fibrillation, prophylaxis of, 258–259, 258t, 850
in sickle cell disease, 377–378
ischemic, 850–853
medical complications after, 855–856
migraine and, 879–880
oral contraceptives and, 1086t
rehabilitation after, 853–856, 853t
activities of daily living in, 854
continuity of care in, 856
medical complication management in, 855–856
mobility and locomotion in, 853–854
motor recovery patterns in, 853t
speech-language disorders in, 854–855
secondary prophylaxis of, 855
vertigo due to, 885t, 891–892
Strongyloidiasis, 541t, 544–545
skin disease due to, 804t, 805
Strychnine poisoning, tetanus vs., 135
Styrene, 1179
Subacromial bursitis, 964
Subacute combined degeneration of the spinal cord, in pernicious anemia, 368
Subacute sclerosing panencephalitis, 133
Subarachnoid analgesia, for labor, 997
Subclavian artery stenosis, 336–337
Subclavian thrombosis, with parenteral nutrition, 606
Subglottic hemangioma, dysphonia due to, 29
Subglottic stenosis, dysphonia due to, 29
Substance abuse. See Drug abuse; specific substances.
Substantivity of sunscreens, 838, 838t, 843
Subthalamic nucleus stimulation, for Parkinson's disease, 923t, 924
Subungual exostosis, 783
Succimer, for lead poisoning, 1186–1187, 1186t
Succinylcholine, for obstetric anesthesia, 998
for tetanus, 136
Sucralfate, levothyroxine interaction with, 644
NSAID-induced ulcers and, 499
Sudden cardiac death, 250–256
advanced care in, 253–255, 254
assessment of risk for, after myocardial infarction, 322
capnography in, 255–256, 255
cardiopulmonary resuscitation in, 251, 252
chain of survival for, 250–251, 252
defibrillation in, 251–253, 252, 253
in hypertrophic cardiomyopathy, 348, 350

Sudden cardiac death (Continued)
in mitral valve prolapse, 288, 290
innovations in management of, 256
with asystole or pulseless electrical activity, 255
Sudden sniffing death syndrome, 1179
Sufentanil, for labor analgesia, 996–997
Suggestion, for warts, 787
Suicide, depression and, 1108
poisoning and, 1145
Sulbactam-ampicillin. See Ampicillin-sulbactam.
Sulconazole, for tinea infection, 807
Sulfacetamide, for candidal paronychia, 808
Sulfadiazine, for toxoplasmosis, 154–155
congenital, 156
during pregnancy, 155
in HIV infection, 53
ocular, 156
Sulfadoxine, for toxoplasmosis during pregnancy, 155
Sulfadoxine-pyrimethamine, for malaria, 96, 97t
for toxoplasmosis, 153
Sulfamethoxazole-trimethoprim. See Trimethoprim-sulfamethoxazole (TMP-SMX).
Sulfasalazine, for ankylosing spondylitis, 960
for delayed pressure urticaria, 836
for inflammatory bowel disease, 483
for juvenile rheumatoid arthritis, 955t, 956
for rheumatoid arthritis, 946t, 949, 951
Sulfisoxazole, for lymphogranuloma venereum, 722
for otitis media prophylaxis, 206
Sulfisoxazole-erythromycin, for otitis media, 205
Sulfonamides. See also specific drugs.
anticonvulsant interactions with, 863t
conjunctivitis due to, 69
for toxoplasmosis, 152–153
in HIV infection, 156–157
Sulfonylureas. See also specific drugs.
antifungal interactions with, 196
for type 2 diabetes, 557t, 558
in combination therapy, 561–562
Sulindac, adverse effects of, 969
Sumatriptan, contraindicated in angina, 250
for cluster headache, 884
for migraine, 881, 882
Sunblocks, 838
Sunburn, 841–843, 841t, 842t
Sunlight, classification of skin response to, 841t
flat warts and, 786
herpes-related erythema multiforme and, 824
hyperpigmentation due to, 837–838, 838t
idiopathic guttate hypomelanosis and, 841
irritation due to, with topical therapy for acne, 757
lupus erythematosus and, 762, 774–775
melanocyte response to, 793
premalignant skin lesions and, 792
protection from, 150, 838, 838t, 843
skin cancer and, 763, 842
spectrum of, 842, 842t
therapy using. See Phototherapy.
Sunscreens, 150, 838, 838t, 843

Sunscreens (Continued)
in lupus erythematosus, 775
in vitiligo, 840
Sunstroke, prevention of, 150
Suntan, 837–838, 838t
Superantigens, in toxic shock syndrome, 83
Superficial femoral vein ligation, for femoral-popliteal vein thrombosis, 345
Superior sulcus tumors, 188
Superwarfarin poisoning, 592, 593
Supine hypotension syndrome, during pregnancy, 995
Support groups. See Social support.
Supraspinatus strain, 975
Supraspinatus tendinitis, 965
Supraventricular tachycardia, 269–276. See also under Tachycardia.
Surfactant therapy, for neonatal respiratory distress syndrome, 1014
Surgery, parenteral nutrition in preparation for, 603–604
Swallowing, flexible endoscopic evaluation of, 477
problems with. See Dysphagia.
Sweat tests, in cystic fibrosis diagnosis, 176
Sweet's syndrome, 414
Swimmer's ear, 114
Swimmer's itch, 804–805, 804t
Sycosis, herpetic, 801
Sympathectomy, for Raynaud's phenomenon, 777
Sympathothermal methods, for contraception, 1076t, 1084
during breast-feeding, 1089
Syncope, heat, 1135, 1136t
in mitral valve prolapse, 291
seizure vs., 857
vasovagal, anaphylaxis vs., 726
Syndrome of inappropriate antidiuretic hormone, in meningoencephalitis, 896
Syndrome X (angina variant), 247
Syndrome X (insulin resistance syndrome), 551–552
Synergistic necrotizing cellulitis, 81, 796, 796t
Syphilis, 722–724, 724t
cutaneous manifestations of, 774
transmission of, by blood components, 461
Systemic inflammatory response syndrome, 62, 62t
Systemic lupus erythematosus, bullous, 830
maternal, congenital heart block and, 265
oral contraceptives and, 1086t
oral lesions in, 813
treatment of, 775–776

T lymphocytes, reference intervals for, 1213t
Tachycardia, 269–280
antidromic reciprocating, 273, 274
atrial, 271, 274–276
after myocardial infarction, 324t
focal, atrial fibrillation and, 260
multifocal, 276
atrioventricular nodal reentry, 269, 271–272, 271, 272
atrioventricular reentry, 271, 272, 273, 274
bundle branch reentrant ventricular, 278

Tachycardia (Continued)
fascicular ventricular, 279
in Wolff-Parkinson-White syndrome, 271, 272–274, 273
junctional, nonparoxysmal, 272
nodal, 270–272, 271
orthodromic reciprocating, 271, 272, 273, 274
reentrant, mechanism of, 269, 269
sinoatrial node reentrant, 270–271, 271
sinus, 270
supraventricular, 269–276
after myocardial infarction, 324t
classification of, 269–270, 270, 270t
ventricular tachycardia vs., 276–277, 277
ventricular, 276–280
after myocardial infarction, 323–324, 324t
bundle branch reentrant, 278
defined, 276
idiopathic left (fascicular), 279
monomorphic, 277–279
after myocardial infarction, 323–324, 324t
polymorphic, 273, 279, 279
after myocardial infarction, 324, 324t
supraventricular tachycardia vs., 276–277, 277
wide complex, acute management of, 277
common causes of, 273
differentiation of origin of, 276–277, 277
with accessory pathways, 271, 272–274
Tacrine, for Alzheimer's disease, 845–846
Tacrolimus, antifungal interactions with, 196
for atopic dermatitis, 824
for autoimmune hepatitis, 469
HMG-CoA reductase inhibitor interaction with, 581–582
reference intervals for, 1210t
Taenia saginata infection, 541t, 546
Taenia solium infection, 541t, 546
Takayasu's arteritis, 339
Talc pleurodesis, for malignant pleural effusion, 203
Tamoxifen, endometrial cancer and, 1063–1064
for breast cancer, 1028, 1028t
prophylactic, 1024
for hormone replacement therapy, 1050–1051
for osteoporosis in breast cancer patients, 596
for recurrent endometrial cancer, 1065
leiomyoma and, 1061
Tamsulosin, for benign prostatic hyperplasia, 688
for chronic pelvic pain syndrome, 687
Tapeworms, 543, 546–547
treatment of, 541t, 543–544
Tar injury, 1126
Tar preparations, for atopic dermatitis, 822
for psoriasis, 772
Tardive dyskinesia, antidepressants for use in, 1115t
Targretin, for Sézary's syndrome, 770
Tattoos, amalgam, 816
Tay-Sachs disease, carrier screening for, during pregnancy, 980
Tazobactam-piperacillin, for nosocomial pneumonia, 213

Tazobactam-piperacillin (Continued)
for sepsis, 63t
3TC. See Lamivudine (3TC).
Tears, artificial, for allergic conjunctivitis, 68
Teeth. See Dental entries.
Teflon injection, for vocal cord paralysis, 27
Teflon patch, for ventricular free wall rupture, 328
Telangiectasias, nail fold, diseases associated with, 783
of lips, in systemic disease, 809
Telmisartan, 1215t
Telogen effluvium, 760, 760t
Temazepam, for insomnia, 34
intoxication with, 1166
Temperature, body. See also Fever; Hyperthermia; Hypothermia.
measurement of, 20–21
Temperature control, for high-risk neonate, 1012
in neonatal resuscitation, 1002–1003
Temporal arteritis, 339, 970–971
Temporomandibular disorders, 960–964
clinical features of, 962
diagnosis of, 960, 962
terminology of, 961
treatment of, 962–964
Tendinitis, 965–966, 976
Tennis elbow, 965, 976
Tenosynovectomy, prophylactic, in rheumatoid arthritis, 952
Tenosynovitis, stenosing, 965
Tensilon test, in myasthenia gravis, 904–905
Tension dysphonia, 28–29
Terazosin, for benign prostatic hyperplasia, 688
for bladder dysfunction in multiple sclerosis, 902
for chronic pelvic pain syndrome, 687
for hypertension, 307–309, 308t
in type 2 diabetes, 563
for pheochromocytoma, 655
Terbinafine, adverse effects of, 807
for onychomycosis, 782, 782t, 807
for tinea infection, 762, 806, 807
for tinea versicolor, 808
Terbutaline, for asthma in children, 740, 741
Terfenadine, antidepressant interactions with, 1114
antifungal interactions with, 196, 200–201, 807
for ordinary urticaria, 835
for pruritus, 37
intoxication with, 1164, 1165
troglitazone interaction with, 559
Testes, leukemia involving, in children, 424
Testosterone, for AIDS-related weight loss, 56
for erectile dysfunction, 693
for hypogonadotropic hypogonadism, in men, 639, 640t
in women, 638
plasma, reference intervals for, 1209t
Tetanus, 134–136
Tetanus immune globulin, 135, 136
Tetanus toxoid. See also Diphtheria-tetanus-pertussis vaccines; Tetanus-diphtheria toxoid.
after injury, 135
in primary tetanus prophylaxis, 135
Tetanus-diphtheria toxoid, 140

Tetanus-diphtheria toxoid *(Continued)*
  for travelers, 147t, 148
  in tetanus management, 135
Tetracaine, for cesarean delivery, 997
Tetracycline(s). See also specific drugs,
    e.g., *Doxycycline.*
  for acne, 758
  for amebiasis, 58t
  for bacterial overgrowth, 510
    in diabetes, 565
    with jejunal diverticula, 480
  for *Balantidium coli* infection, 539t, 543
  for cholera, 73, 74t, 77t
  for *Dientamoeba fragilis* infection, 539t,
    543
  for dissecting cellulitis of scalp, 762
  for *Helicobacter pylori* infection, 501t
  for Lyme disease, 128t
  for lymphomatoid papulosis, 770
  for nongonococcal urethritis, 721
  for plague, 116
    prophylactic, 116
  for psittacosis, 117
  for rat bite fever, 123
  for relapsing fever, 124
  for rosacea, 759
  for syphilis, 724t, 774
  for tropical sprue, 511
  for Whipple's disease, 512
Tetralogy of Fallot, 284–285
Tetrodotoxin poisoning, 79, 80t, 1144
Thalamic surgery, for Parkinson's disease,
    923t, 924
Thalassemia, 369–374
  alpha, 370, 373
  beta, 369–370
    sickle hemoglobin with, 375, 375t. See
        also *Sickle cell disease.*
  carrier screening for, during pregnancy,
    980
  diagnosis of, 370
  intermedia, 370
    treatment of, 372–373
  major, 370–372, 371t
  pathophysiology of, 369–370
  treatment of, 370–374, 371t
Thalassemia trait, 370
  iron deficiency anemia vs., 357
Thalidomide, 1216t
  for erythema multiforme, 825
  for erythema nodosum leprosum, 93
  for lupus erythematosus, 776
Theater sign, in patellofemoral pain
    syndrome, 977
Theophylline, for angina, 249
  for apnea of prematurity, 1014
  for asthma, 733
    in children, 740, 742
  for chronic obstructive pulmonary dis-
      ease, 173, *173*
    during hospitalization, 174
  intoxication by, 1156t
  reference intervals for, 1210t
Therapeutic drug monitoring, reference
    intervals for, 1210t
Thiabendazole, adverse effects of, 545
  for angiostrongyliasis, 540t, 545
  for cutaneous larva migrans, 544, 804t,
    805
  for strongyloidiasis, 541t, 545, 804t, 805
Thiamine, for alcoholic neuropathy, 927
  for ethanol intoxication, 1177
  for ethylene glycol intoxication, 1178
  for neuroleptic intoxication, 1196
  for opioid intoxication, 1193
  for status epilepticus, 865t

Thiamine *(Continued)*
  in acute poisoning management, 1157
  in alcohol withdrawal management,
    1093
Thiazolidinediones. See also specific drugs.
  for type 2 diabetes, 557t, 559–560
1-[1–2-Thienyl-cyclohexyl]piperidine (TCP),
    abuse of, 1096
Thiethylperazine, for nausea and vomiting,
    8t
Thiopental, for obstetric anesthesia, 998
Thioridazine, characteristics of, 1118t
  for insomnia in Alzheimer's disease, 847
  intoxication with, 1196, 1197t
Thiotepa, for bladder cancer, 709
Thiothixene, characteristics of, 1118t
  intoxication by, 1197t
Thirst, in diabetes insipidus management,
    625
Thoracentesis, diagnostic, in pneumonia,
    211
Thoracoscopy, video-assisted, for empyema,
    202, *202*
Thoracostomy, for pleural effusion, 202,
    202, 203
Throat culture, in pharyngitis diagnosis,
    237
Thrombectomy, venous, 343, 343t
  for iliofemoral vein thrombosis, 346
Thromboangiitis obliterans, 339
Thrombocythemia, in polycythemia vera,
    445
Thrombocytopenia, autoimmune, 400
  causes of, 397, 398t
  clinical manifestations of, 397–398
  drug-induced, 399
  heparin-induced, 341, 399
    platelet transfusions' effect in, 455
  intracerebral hemorrhage treatment in,
    849
  treatment of, 398–400
  with massive transfusion, 461
Thrombocytopenic purpura, immune, 400
  thrombotic, 402–404, 402t. See also
      Hemolytic-uremic syndrome.
    HELLP syndrome vs., 993t
    platelet transfusions' effect in, 455
Thromboembolism, oral contraceptives
    and, 1085
  pulmonary. See *Pulmonary embolism.*
  venous, hormone replacement therapy
      and, 1048
Thrombolytic agents. See also specific
    drugs.
  for deep venous thrombosis, 342, 342t
  for disseminated intravascular coagula-
      tion, 402
  for iliofemoral vein thrombosis, 345–346
  for ischemic stroke, 850–851, 851t, 852t
  for myocardial infarction, 320
  for pulmonary thromboembolism, 223t,
    224
Thrombophlebitis, Baker's cyst vs., 965
  septic, with parenteral nutrition, 606
Thrombosis, abnormalities promoting, in
    insulin resistance syndrome, 551
  in polycythemia vera, 445
  oral contraceptives and, 1086t
  renal artery, after trauma, 683
  subclavian, with parenteral nutrition,
    606
  vena caval, with parenteral nutrition,
    606
  venous. See *Venous thrombosis.*
Thrombotic thrombocytopenic purpura,
    402–404, 402t. See also *Hemolytic-
    uremic syndrome.*

Thrombotic thrombocytopenic purpura
    (Continued)
  HELLP syndrome vs., 993t
  platelet transfusions' effect in, 455
Thrush, 811. See also *Candidiasis.*
  in HIV infection, 54
Thymectomy, for myasthenia gravis,
    905–906, 905t
Thymol, for candidal paronychia, 808
Thymoma, myasthenia gravis and, 904,
    906
Thymopentin, for Sézary's syndrome, 770
Thyroglobulin, reference intervals for,
    1209t
Thyroid cancer, 648–653
  anaplastic, treatment of, 651
  causes of, 648–649
  classification of, 649, 649t
  clinical manifestations of, 649–650
  follow-up care in, 652–653
  medullary, 649
    surgery for, 651
  radioiodine therapy for, thyroid hormone
      replacement and, 644
  staging of, 650, 650t
  treatment of, adjuvant, 651–652
    surgical, 650–651
Thyroid nodules, evaluation of, 649–650
Thyroid storm, 648
Thyroid tissue, desiccated, for
    hypothyroidism, 644
Thyroidectomy, for hyperthyroidism, 648
  for thyroid cancer, 650
  prophylactic, in multiple endocrine neo-
      plasia type 2, 650
Thyroiditis, 657–660
  acute (suppurative), 657–658, 658t
  atrophic, 659
  chronic (autoimmune), 658t, 659–660
  clinical features of, 658t
  diagnostic tests in, 658t
  drug-induced, 658t, 660
  Hashimoto's, 642, 659–660
  lymphocytic, 642–643
  postpartum, 642–643, 658t, 659
  Riedel's, 660
  silent, 658t, 659
  subacute, 643, 658–659, 658t
Thyroid-stimulating hormone. See
    Thyrotropin.
Thyroplasty, for vocal fold paralysis, 27
Thyrotoxicosis. See *Hyperthyroidism.*
Thyrotropin, deficiency of, in
    hypopituitarism, 637–638, 640t
  serum, reference intervals for, 1209t
  suppression of, for thyroid cancer, 651
Thyrotropin alfa, in residual thyroid
    cancer detection, 653
Thyrotropin-releasing hormone, reference
    intervals for, 1209t
Thyroxine, bile acid resin interaction with,
    582
  serum, reference intervals for, 1209t
L-Thyroxine. See *Levothyroxine.*
Thyroxine-binding globulin, reference
    intervals for, 1209t
Tiagabine, adverse effects of, 863t
  drug interactions with, 863t
  for epilepsy, 860t, 862t, 864
  pharmacokinetics of, 862t
  porphyrogenic effect of, 449–451
Tibial osteotomy, for osteoarthritis, 970
Tibial stress fractures, 978
Tic(s), in Tourette's syndrome, 874–875
  treatment of, 876–877
Tic disorder(s), habit, nail abnormality due
    to, 781t, 783

Tic disorder(s) *(Continued)*
  Tourette's syndrome and, 875
Tic douloureux. See *Trigeminal neuralgia.*
Ticarcillin, for cystic fibrosis
    exacerbations, 179t
  for sepsis, 63t
Ticarcillin-clavulanate, for cystic fibrosis
    exacerbations, 179t
  for diverticulitis, 482
  for pyelonephritis, 682t
  for sepsis, 63t
Tick-borne encephalitis vaccine, for
    travelers, 148
Tick-borne relapsing fever, 123–125
Ticlopidine, after myocardial infarction,
    329
  for stroke prevention, 850, 855
Tiludronate, adverse effects of, 599
  for Paget's disease of bone, 598t, 599
Timolol, for glaucoma, 912–913
  for hypertension, 308t
  intoxication with, 1167t
Timolol-dorzolamide, for glaucoma, 913
Tinea capitis, 762, 806
Tinea corporis, 807
Tinea cruris, 807
Tinea pedis, 807
Tinea versicolor, 808
Tinidazole, for amebiasis, 539t, 542
  for diarrhea, 16, 17t
  for giardiasis, 61, 538, 539t
Tinnitus, 37–39, 38t
Tiopronin, for cystinuria, 715
Tirofiban, 1216t
Tissue plasminogen activator (t-PA),
    catheter administration of, for
    iliofemoral vein thrombosis, 346
  for ischemic stroke, 850–851, 851t, 852t
  for myocardial infarction, 320
  for paroxysmal nocturnal hemoglobin-
    uria, 366
  for pulmonary thromboembolism, 223t,
    224
Tizanidine, for spasticity, after stroke, 856
  in multiple sclerosis, 901–902
Tobacco. See *Smoking.*
Tobramycin, for bacterial conjunctivitis, 67
  for bacterial meningitis, 105t
  for complications of cystic fibrosis, 176t,
    177, 179t
  for osteomyelitis, 974, 974t
  for sepsis, 63t
  reference intervals for, 1210t
Tobramycin-dexamethasone, for draining
    ear, 207t
Tocainide, reference intervals for, 1210t
Tocolysis, for placenta previa, 988
Tolazamide, for type 2 diabetes, 557t
Tolbutamide, for type 2 diabetes, 557t, 558
Tolcapone, 1216t
  for Parkinson's disease, 919, 919t
Tolerance, defined, 4
Tolmetin, for juvenile rheumatoid
    arthritis, 954, 955t
Tolterodine, 1216t
  for bladder dysfunction, 672
  in multiple sclerosis, 902
Toluene, 1179
  prenatal exposure to, 1097
Tongue lesions, 814–815
Tongue reduction surgery, for obstructive
    sleep-disordered breathing, 185
Tooth. See *Dental* entries.
Tophi, in gout, 576, 577
Topiramate, adverse effects of, 863t
  drug interactions with, 863t

Topiramate *(Continued)*
  for epilepsy, 860t, 862t, 864
    in infants and children, 868t, 869t
  pharmacokinetics of, 862t
Topotecan, for small cell lung cancer, 190
Toremifene, for breast cancer, 1028
Torsades de pointes, 279, *279*
  due to nonsedating antihistamines,
    1164–1165
  in antidepressant intoxication, 1203
  in digitalis intoxication, 1175
  in neuroleptic intoxication, 1197
Torsemide, for congestive heart failure,
    294t
  for hypertension, 308t
Torus mandibularis, 817
Torus palatinus, 817
Tourette's syndrome, 874–877
Toxemia of pregnancy. See *Pre-eclampsia.*
Toxic epidermal necrolysis, 825
Toxic shock syndrome, 82–85, 84t, 85t
  staphylococcal, 83
    diagnostic criteria for, 83–84, 84t
    treatment of, 84, 85t
  streptococcal, diagnostic criteria for, 83–
    84, 84t
    group A, 83
    group B, 83, 85
    soft tissue infection and, 81
    treatment of, 84–85, 85t
Toxic substances. See also *Poisoning;*
  specific substances.
  reference intervals for, 1212t
Toxoplasmosis, 151–157
  congenital, 155–156
  during pregnancy, 151, 155
  ocular, 156
  prevention of, 151–152
  treatment of, 152–157
    drugs used for, 152–154
    failure of, 152
    regimens for, 154–157, 154t
Toxoplasmosis encephalitis, in HIV
    infection, 52–53, 151
  central nervous system lymphoma vs.,
    55
  treatment of, 156–157
t-PA. See *Tissue plasminogen activator
    (t-PA).*
Trabeculectomy, for glaucoma, 915
Trabeculoplasty, laser, for glaucoma, 914
Trace elements, in parenteral nutrition,
    604–605
  for high-risk neonate, 1012
Tracheitis, bacterial, 31
Trachelectomy, for cervical cancer, 1068
Tracheostomy, for obstructive sleep-
    disordered breathing, 185
Traction alopecia, 761, 762
Traction diverticulum, 479
Tramadol, for bursitis or tendinitis, 965
  for chronic fatigue syndrome, 112
  for rheumatoid arthritis, 947
Trandolapril, for hypertension, 309t
Tranexamic acid, for C1 esterase inhibitor
    deficiency, 836–837
  for hemophilia, 395
Transcutaneous electrical nerve
    stimulation, for labor analgesia, 995
Transferrin, carbohydrate-deficient, as
    marker for excess alcohol intake, 1092
  reference intervals for, 1209t
Transferrin saturation, in hemochroma-
    tosis diagnosis, 404
Transfusion(s), 453–458
  acute lung injury due to, 460

Transfusion(s) *(Continued)*
  adverse reactions to, 458–461, 459t. See
    also *Transfusion reactions.*
  congestive heart failure due to, 461
  exchange, for hyperparasitemia in ma-
    laria, 100
    for neonatal polycythemia, 1016
    for Rh isoimmunization, 387
  fetal, in Rh isoimmunization manage-
    ment, 385–386
  for acute leukemia, 420
  for antepartum hemorrhage, 987, 988
  for aplastic anemia, 353
  for cerebrovascular accident in sickle cell
    disease, 378
  for cold hemagglutinin disease, 362
  for drug-induced immune hemolytic ane-
    mia, 363
  for paroxysmal nocturnal hemoglobin-
    uria, 366
  for pernicious anemia with cardiac de-
    compensation, 368
  for sickle cell disease, 380
  for thalassemia, 370–371, 371t
    iron overload due to, 371–372
  for warm antibody autoimmune hemo-
    lytic anemia, 361
  graft-versus-host disease due to, 457,
    460
  granulocyte, 456–457
    in acute leukemia, 420
  immune system modulation by, 460
  infectious complications of, 459t, 460–
    461
  iron overload due to, 371–372, 461
  massive, complications of, 461
  neonatal, in Rh isoimmunization man-
    agement, 387
  platelet, alloimmunization to, 420, 456
    prevention of, 454
    for acute leukemia, 420
    for aplastic anemia, 353
    for hemolytic transfusion reaction, 459
    for intracerebral hemorrhage, 849
    for leukostasis in acute leukemia, 415
    for platelet-mediated bleeding disor-
      ders, 398
    immune thrombocytopenia after, 399–
      400, 460
    indications for, 455
    products for, 455–456
    refractoriness to, 456
    procedure for, 453–454
    purpura after, 399–400, 460
  red blood cell, physiologic basis for, 455
    products for, 454–455
Transfusion reactions, 459–460, 459t
  allergic, 460
    washed red cells to prevent, 454–455
  febrile nonhemolytic, 459–460
    leukocyte-reduced red cells to prevent,
      454
  hemolytic, 459
  septic, 461
Transient global amnesia, seizure vs., 857
Transient ischemic attack, seizure vs., 857
Transit tests, in constipation diagnosis, 18
Transitional cell carcinoma, 708–709
Transjugular intrahepatic portosystemic
    shunt, for variceal bleeding, 470, 472
Transplantation, bone marrow. See *Bone
    marrow transplantation.*
  chondrocyte, for osteoarthritis, 970
  corneal, rabies transmission by, 119,
    120, 122
  heart, for Chagas' heart disease, 102

Transplantation *(Continued)*
  toxoplasmosis after, 157
  islet cell, with pancreatectomy, 523
  liver. See *Liver transplantation.*
  lung, for chronic obstructive pulmonary
    disease, 175
  pancreas, for diabetic neuropathy, 925
  renal, for chronic renal failure, 705
    in multiple myeloma, 443
  stem cell. See *Stem cell rescue.*
Transposition of the great arteries, 285
Transsphenoidal surgery, for acromegaly,
    615–616
  for Cushing's disease, 622
  for prolactinoma, 641–642
Transurethral procedures, for benign
    prostatic hyperplasia, 690–691
  for bladder cancer, 708
Tranylcypromine, for anxiety disorders,
    1102
  for depression, 1109t
  overdose of, 1190
  pharmacodynamic effects of, 1110t
Trastuzumab, 1216t
  for breast cancer, 1029
Trauma, anterior urethral stricture due to,
    710
  aphthous stomatitis due to, 812
  clostridial myonecrosis and, 797
  during pregnancy, 983
  fat necrosis of breast due to, 1024
  fibromyalgia and, 967
  head. See *Head injury.*
  in leprosy, 94
  osteoarthritis and, 968
  repetitive, chronic occlusive arterial dis-
    ease due to, 339
  sports, 974–978
    PRICE-MM management for, 975,
      975t
  to genitourinary tract, 682–685
Travel, 145–151
  by air, circadian rhythm disorders due
    to. See *Jet lag.*
    in chronic obstructive pulmonary dis-
      ease, 175
  care after return from, 151
  diarrhea in, 150
    diagnosis of, 15
    prophylaxis of, 17
    treatment of, 16–17, 76
  general advice for, 150–151
  immunizations for, 146–149, 147t
  malaria prophylaxis for, 100–101, 100t,
    149–150
  medical kits for, 146
  pre-travel advice for, 146
Trazodone, for chronic fatigue syndrome,
    112
  for depression, 1109t
  for insomnia, 35
  for rheumatoid arthritis, 947
  intoxication with, 1201, 1202t
  pharmacodynamic effects of, 1110t
Trematodes, 543, 545–546. See also
    specific worms and diseases.
  treatment of, 540t, 544
Tremor, essential, dysphonia due to, 29
  in Parkinson's disease, 922
Trench mouth, 814
Treponema pallidum infection. See
    Syphilis.
Tretinoin, for acne, 757
  for acute promyelocytic leukemia, 418,
    425
  for geographic tongue, 815

Tretinoin *(Continued)*
  for hyperpigmentation, 839
  for warts, 786
Triamcinolone, for allergic rhinitis, 747t
  for alopecia areata, 762
  for aphthous stomatitis, 812
  for asthma, 732t
    in children, 742
  for atopic dermatitis, 822
    wet wrap dressings with, 823, 823t
  for black hairy tongue, 815
  for bursitis or tendinitis, 966
  for cheilitis, 809
  for digital mucous cyst, 783
  for gout, 577
  for herpes gestationis, 832
  for juvenile rheumatoid arthritis, 956
  for keloids, 784–785
  for lichen planus, of mouth, 811
    of nails, 783
  for lichen simplex chronicus, 834
  for osteoarthritis, 970
  for pityriasis rubra pilaris, 773
  for pruritic urticarial papules and
    plaques of pregnancy, 831
  for pruritus, 36
  for psoriasis of nails, 782
  for rheumatoid arthritis, 948
Triamterene, for congestive heart failure,
    294t
  for hypertension, 308t
  for premenstrual syndrome, 1047
Triangle of Koch, 264
Triazolam, antidepressant interactions
    with, 1114
  antifungal interactions with, 807
  for insomnia, 34
  intoxication with, 1166
Trichinosis, 541t, 545
Trichloroacetic acid, for black hairy
    tongue, 815
  for hyperpigmentation, 839–840
  for warts, 787
1,1,1-Trichloroethane, 1179
Trichloroethanol, intoxication by, 1156t
Trichomoniasis, 1054–1055, 1054t
  urethral, 720, 721
Trichophyton species. See *Dermatophy-
    tosis.*
Trichostrongylus infection, 541t, 545
Trichothiodystrophy, 763
Trichotillomania, 761, 762
Trichuriasis, 541t, 544
Tricuspid atresia, 285–286
Tricyclic antidepressants. See also specific
    drugs.
  antihistamine effects of, 1111–1112
  for anxiety disorders, 1100t, 1101–1102
  for attention-deficit/hyperactivity disor-
    der, 873, 873t
  for chronic fatigue syndrome, 112
  for dyspepsia, 11
  for gaseousness, 13
  for insomnia, 35
  for irritable bowel syndrome, 491
  for obstructive sleep-disordered breath-
    ing, 184
  for pain, 3
  for pruritus, 37
  intoxication with, 1097, 1201–1203,
    1202t
Trifascicular block, 266. See also *Heart
    block.*
  after myocardial infarction, 324t
Trifluoperazine, characteristics of, 1118t
  intoxication with, 1196, 1197t

Trifluridine, for herpes simplex
    conjunctivitis, 68
Trigeminal neuralgia, 908–910
  in multiple sclerosis, 902
Trigeminal neuropathic pain, 909
Trigger zone, 966
Triglycerides. See also *Hypertriglycer-
    idemia.*
  malabsorption due to impaired transport
    of, 512
  medium-chain, for maldigestion due to
    bile salt deficiency, 509, 510
    infant formulas with, 1020, 1021t
  serum, goals for, in diabetes, 554, 554t
    reference intervals for, 1209t
    treatment guidelines based on, 579–
      580
Trihexyphenidyl, for Parkinson's disease,
    919t, 922
Triiodothyronine, for depression, 1116
  serum, reference intervals for, 1209t
Trimethaphan camsylate, for tetanus, 136
Trimethoprim, for *Pneumocystis carinii*
    pneumonia in HIV infection, 51
  for urinary tract infection, in girls, 668
    in women, 663, 664t
Trimethoprim-polymyxin, for bacterial
    conjunctivitis, 67
Trimethoprim-sulfamethoxazole (TMP-
    SMX), after splenectomy for
    thalassemia, 371
  contraindicated in cobalamin deficiency,
    368
  for acne, 758
  for bacterial meningitis, 105t
  for brucellosis, 64, 65, 65t, 66
  for catheter-associated bacteriuria in
    women, 665
  for cat-scratch disease, 158t
  for cholera, 74t, 77t
  for chronic bacterial prostatitis, 686
  for *Cyclospora* infection, 77, 539t, 543
  for cystic fibrosis exacerbations, 179t
  for diarrhea, 16, 17t
  for donovanosis, 721
  for enterotoxigenic *Escherichia coli* infec-
    tion, 77, 77t
  for epididymitis, 662, 675
  for isosporiasis, 539t, 543
  for *Listeria monocytogenes* infection, 77t,
    79–81, 104t, 106
  for osteomyelitis, 973
  for otitis media, 205, 205t
  for pertussis, 139
  for plague prophylaxis, 116
  for *Pneumocystis carinii* pneumonia in
    HIV infection, 51
  for *Pneumocystis carinii* prophylaxis, in
    aplastic anemia, 353
    in HIV infection, 51
  for pyelonephritis, 681t, 682t
    in women, 664, 664t
  for salmonellosis, 78, 161
  for *Shigella* infection, 77t
  for spontaneous bacterial peritonitis pro-
    phylaxis in cirrhosis, 470
  for toxoplasmosis, 153
  for toxoplasmosis prophylaxis, 154
    in HIV infection, 52
  for typhoid carriage, 164
  for typhoid fever, 163, 163t
  for urinary tract infection, in girls, 668
    in men, 661–662
    in women, 663, 664, 664t
    prophylactic, in diabetes, 565
  for Whipple's disease, 512

Trimetrexate, for *Pneumocystis carinii* pneumonia in HIV infection, 51
for toxoplasmosis, 153
Trimipramine, for depression, 1109t
intoxication by, 1202t
pharmacodynamic effects of, 1110t
Tripelennamine, intoxication with, 1164
safety of, during pregnancy, 748
Triptans. See also specific drugs.
for migraine, 881–882
for tension-type headache, 883
Trismus, in tetanus, 134
Trisulfapyrimidines, for toxoplasmosis, 154–155
congenital, 156
Trochanteric bursitis, 965
Troglitazone, drug interactions with, 559
for type 2 diabetes, 557t, 559
in combination therapy, 561, 562
Tropical pancreatitis, 519
Tropical sprue, 511
Tropisetron, for nausea and vomiting, 8t
Troponins, cardiac-specific, serum levels of, in myocardial infarction, 318–319
Trousseau's sign, 632
Trovafloxacin, for bacterial pneumonia, 212
for legionellosis, 217, 217t, 218
for pelvic inflammatory disease, 1059t, 1060t
for Q fever, 118
for toxoplasmosis, 154
Truncus arteriosus, 286
Trypanosomiasis, American, 101–102
TSH. See *Thyrotropin.*
Tubal ligation, for contraception, 1083t, 1087–1088
Tube thoracostomy, for pleural effusion, 202, *202,* 203
Tuberculosis, 238–242
chemoprophylaxis of, 241–242
classification of, 240
drug resistance in, 240, 242
extrapulmonary, 239
in HIV infection, 51–52, 52t, 53t
symptoms of, 239
treatment of, 240–241
in infant, cough due to, 23
miliary, 239
pleural effusion in, 203, 239
progress in fight against, 239
public health department services in, 242
silicosis and, 229–230
symptoms of, 239
tests for, 242, 242t
in HIV infection, 51
transmission of, 239–240
treatment of, 240–241
Tuberous sclerosis, infantile spasms in, 870
Tubo-ovarian abscess, 1059–1060
Tumor(s). See also specific sites and types.
brain. See *Brain tumors.*
colorectal, 532–537. See also *Colorectal cancer.*
in HIV infection, 54–55
of nails, 781t, 783
of stomach, 527–532
of vulva, 1069–1074, 1070t
benign, 1070–1071, 1070t
diagnosis of, 1069–1070
malignant, 1070t, 1071–1074
peripheral neuropathy due to, 927
sensory neuropathy with, 931
skin, malignant, 763–765. See also *Melanoma.*

Tumor(s) *(Continued)*
premalignant, 792–794
Tumor d'emblée, mycosis fungoides and, 766
Tumor lysis syndrome, in acute leukemia, 416, 422
in highly aggressive lymphomas, 438
Tumor necrosis factor-α receptor antibody, for inflammatory bowel disease, 486
Tumor necrosis factor-α receptor fusion protein. See *Etanercept.*
Turf toe, 978
Turtles, poisonous, 1144
TWAR agent, bronchitis due to, adult-onset asthma and, 208
"Two-hit theory" of skin cancer formation, 763
Tympanostomy, office, for otitis media prevention, 206
tube placement with, for otitis media with effusion, 206–207
Typhlitis, with intensive chemotherapy for leukemia, 419
Typhoid fever, 161–165
carriers of, management of, 164
clinical manifestations of, 161–162
complications of, 162
treatment of, 163–164
diagnosis of, 162
epidemiology of, 161
management of, 162–164, 163t
prevention of, 164–165, 164t
Typhoid fever vaccines, 164–165, 164t
for travelers, 147t, 148
Typhus vaccine, 148

Ulcer(s), aphthous, 812
gastroduodenal. See also *Peptic ulcer disease.*
dyspepsia and, 496
leg, in sickle cell disease, 379
venous, 817–819
NSAID-induced, 498–500, 499t, 969
oral, 812–813
pressure, 819–821
after head injury, 935
Ulcerative colitis. See *Inflammatory bowel disease.*
Ulcerative gingivitis, acute necrotizing, 814
Ulnar collateral ligament injury, at elbow, 976
at thumb, 976–977
Ultrasonography. See also *Echocardiography; Sonohysterography.*
during pregnancy, 981–982
in acute renal failure evaluation, 697
in breast lesion assessment, 1025
in Rh isoimmunization assessment, 385
renal, in urinary tract infection evaluation in children, 667
transrectal, in rectal cancer assessment, 536
Ultraviolet light. See *Sunlight.*
Ultraviolet light therapy. See *Phototherapy.*
Umbilical blood sampling, percutaneous, 981, 984
Umbilical venous access, in neonatal resuscitation, 1006
Unstable hemoglobin disease, 365
Upper airway resistance syndrome, 180
Urate, reference intervals for, in blood, 1209t

Urate *(Continued)*
in urine, 1212t
Urea, plasma, reference intervals for, 1209t
Urea breath test, for *Helicobacter pylori* infection, 498, 501
Urea nitrogen, serum, reference intervals for, 1209t
Ureaplasma urealyticum infection, urethral, 720, 721
tetracycline-resistant, 661
Urease test, rapid, for *Helicobacter pylori* infection, 501
Uremia. See also *Renal failure.*
pericarditis in, 335–336
peripheral neuropathy in, 699, 925
pruritus in, 37
Uremic syndrome, 698–699
Ureter(s), ectopic, 670
trauma to, 684
Ureteral cancer, 708, 709
Ureteral stent, for urinary calculus, 714
Ureteral stones. See *Urolithiasis.*
Ureterectomy, for ureteral cancer, 709
Ureteroscopy, for urinary calculus, 714
Urethra, bleeding from, with anterior urethral stricture, 711
dilation of, for anterior urethral stricture, 711
dysfunction of, incontinence with, 673–674
male, divisions of, 710, *710*
open reconstruction of, for anterior stricture, 712
trauma to, 684–685
Urethral stent, for anterior urethral stricture, 711–712
for benign prostatic hyperplasia, 690–691
Urethral stricture, anterior, 710–712, *710*
Urethritis, chlamydial, in men, 1056
in women, 1056, 1056t, 1057, 1057t
in men, 661, 1056
nongonococcal, 661, 720–721
noninfectious, 720
postgonococcal, 720
Urethrography, retrograde, in urethral injury evaluation, 685
in urethral stricture assessment, 711
Urethroplasty, substitution, for anterior urethral stricture, 712
Urethrotomy, direct vision internal, for anterior urethral stricture, 711
Urinalysis, in acute renal failure evaluation, 695–696, 696t
in renal calculus evaluation, 713
Urinary catheterization, bacteriuria associated with, in men, 662
clean intermittent, for urgency incontinence, 672
infection associated with, in women, 665
pyelonephritis associated with, 682
Urinary diversion, after cystectomy for bladder cancer, 709
Urinary incontinence. See under *Incontinence.*
Urinary sphincter, artificial, for stress incontinence, 673
Urinary tract infection. See also specific type, e.g., *Cystitis.*
bacterial, in men, 661–662
in women, 662–666
clinical syndromes of, 663–666
medications used for, 664t
pathogenesis of, 662–663
catheter-associated, 665

Urinary tract infection *(Continued)*
epididymitis with, 675
in elderly women, 666
in girls, 666–668
pregnancy-associated, 664t, 665–666
recurrent, in women, 664t, 665
prostatitis and, 686
urinary stones associated with, 715
Urine, alkalinization of, for acute
poisoning, 1150
for porphyria cutanea tarda, 452–453
clinical chemistry reference intervals for,
1211t–1212t
drug testing in, 1094, 1160
free water loss in, calculation of, in diabetes insipidus, 624–625
normal volume of, fluid therapy requirement calculation and, 609
specimen collection, in prostatitis diagnosis, 686
in pyelonephritis diagnosis, 680–681
Urobilinogen, urine, reference intervals
for, 1212t
Urodynamic studies, in incontinence
evaluation, 671
Urogenital atrophy, hormone replacement
therapy and, 1049–1050
vaginitis due to, 1055
Urogenital tract. See also specific
structures.
malignancies of, 705–710
trauma to, 682–685
ultrasonography of, in urinary tract infection evaluation in children, 667
Urokinase, for iliofemoral vein thrombosis,
345
for paroxysmal nocturnal hemoglobinuria, 366
for pulmonary thromboembolism, 223t,
224
Urolithiasis, 712–715
in primary hyperparathyroidism, 629
Uroporphyrin, urine, reference intervals
for, 1211t
Ursodeoxycholic acid, for cholelithiasis,
464
for hepatobiliary disease in cystic fibrosis, 179t, 180
for primary biliary cirrhosis, 468
for primary sclerosing cholangitis, 468
Urticaria, 834–837, 835t
contact, 830, 835
due to blood components, 460
Uterine artery embolization, for
leiomyomata, 1062–1063
Uterus, carcinoma of. See *Endometrial
cancer.*
leiomyomata of, 1060–1063, 1060t, 1061t
leiomyosarcoma of, 1060
Uveitis, in ankylosing spondylitis, 959
in juvenile rheumatoid arthritis, 958
Uvulopalatopharyngoplasty, for obstructive
sleep-disordered breathing, 184–185

Vacuum constriction device, for erectile
dysfunction, 693
VAD regimen, for multiple myeloma, 442
Vaginal agenesis, 1042
Vaginal atrophy, hormone replacement
therapy and, 1049–1050
vaginitis due to, 1055
Vaginal bleeding, abnormal. See also
Dysfunctional uterine bleeding.
differential diagnosis of, 1038, 1039t

Vaginal bleeding *(Continued)*
during third trimester of pregnancy,
986–988
Vaginal hematoma, postpartum, 1001
Vaginal septum, 1042
Vaginitis, 1053–1055, 1054t
Candida, 1053–1054
in HIV infection, 54
Vaginosis, bacterial, 1054, 1054t
Vagus nerve stimulator, for epilepsy, 865
Valacyclovir, for facial paralysis, 917
for herpes simplex, 800, 800t, 809
for herpes zoster, 71, 800t, 802
Valproic acid, adverse effects of, 863t
birth defects associated with, 864
drug interactions with, 863t
for absence seizures in infants and children, 869–870
for epilepsy, 860t, 861, 862t
in infants and children, 868t, 869t
for hiccup, 14t
for migraine, 882
for pain, 3
pharmacokinetics of, 862t
reference intervals for, 1210t
withdrawal from, 1096
Valrubicin, 1216t
for bladder cancer, 709
Valsartan, for hypertension, 309t
Vancomycin, for bacterial meningitis,
dexamethasone interaction with,
107
dosages for, 105t
for bacterial pneumonia, 212, 212t
for endocarditis, 300t, 301, 302
prophylactic, 301t, 303
for fever in aplastic anemia, 353
for necrotizing skin and soft tissue infections, 82
for osteomyelitis, 973, 974t
for pneumococcal meningitis, 103t, 104t,
105
for sepsis, 63t
in neonate, 1017t, 1018
for staphylococcal meningitis, 104t, 107
for staphylococcal toxic shock syndrome,
85t
reference intervals for, 1210t
resistance to, 419
Vanillylmandelic acid, urine, reference
intervals for, 1212t
Variceal ligation, endoscopic, for bleeding
esophageal varices, 472
Varicella vaccine, 71, *140–141,* 143, 144t,
801–802
for travelers, 147t, 148
Varicella-zoster immune globulin, 71, 802
Varicella-zoster virus infection, 69–71,
800t, 801–802. See also *Chickenpox;
Herpes zoster.*
Varices, esophagogastric, in cirrhosis, 467
bleeding, 470, 471–473
Variegate porphyria, 448t. See also
Porphyria(s).
Vasa previa, 988
Vasculitis, cutaneous, 778–780, 778t, *779*
hypersensitivity, 729
mononeuritis multiplex due to, 930
urticarial, 835, 837
Vasectomy, 1083t
Vasodilators. See also specific drugs.
adverse effects of, 311
for hypertension, 308t, 311
Vasopressin, for bleeding esophageal
varices, 471
for diabetes insipidus, 625, 626t

Vasopressin *(Continued)*
for diverticular bleeding, 481
Vasovagal reaction, anaphylaxis vs., 726
VBM regimen, for Hodgkin's disease, 407,
407t
Vecuronium, for neuroleptic intoxication,
1197
for tetanus, 136
Vegetarians, dietary cobalamin deficiency
in, 368–369
Vena cava filtration, for femoral-popliteal
vein thrombosis, 345
for pulmonary thromboembolism prevention, 224
Vena caval thrombosis, with parenteral
nutrition, 606
Venlafaxine, for anxiety disorders, 1100t,
1101
for attention-deficit/hyperactivity disorder, 873t, 874
for chronic fatigue syndrome, 112
for depression, 1109t
monoamine oxidase inhibitor interaction
with, 1115
pharmacodynamic effects of, 1110t
Venom immunotherapy, 754–755, 755t
Venous access, central, for parenteral
nutrition, 604
complications associated with, 605–
606, *607*
umbilical, in neonatal resuscitation,
1006
Venous duplex scan of lower extremities,
in pulmonary thromboembolism
workup, 218, 220t
Venous ectasias, 809
Venous leg ulcers, 817–819
Venous thrombectomy, 343, 343t
for iliofemoral vein thrombosis, 346
Venous thromboembolism, hormone
replacement therapy and, 1048
Venous thrombosis, 339–346
after stroke, 855
anticoagulation for, 340–342, 341t, 342t
calf vein, 344, *344*
elastic compression for lower extremity
edema with, 343–344
femoral-popliteal, 344–345
iliofemoral, 345–346, *345*
in polycythemia vera, 445
natural history of, 339–340
oral contraceptives and, 1086t
postpartum, 1001
prophylaxis of, 222t
after head injury, 935
after stroke, 849, 852, 855
thrombectomy for, 343, 343t, 346
thrombolytic therapy for, 342, 342t
treatment strategies for, 344–346, *344,
345*
Venovenous hemofiltration, continuous,
700, 700t
Ventilation, bag-and-mask, in neonatal
resuscitation, 1004–1005
intrapulmonary percussive, for atelectasis due to mucous plugs, 171
mechanical, avoiding atelectasis in, 171
discontinuation of, ethical issues in,
175
for high-risk neonate, 1013
in adult respiratory distress syndrome, 168
in obstructive airway disease with ventilatory failure, 169–170
noninvasive, in chronic obstructive pulmonary disease, 174

Ventilation (Continued)
in hypercapnic ventilatory failure, 170
weaning from, 170
Ventilation/perfusion scanning, in pulmonary thromboembolism workup, 218, 220t
Ventilatory failure, 168–170
Ventricular fibrillation, 279–280. See also Sudden cardiac death.
after myocardial infarction, 324, 324t
in accidental hypothermia, 1131, 1132
in antidepressant intoxication, 1203
pharmacologic treatment for, 253–255, 254
Ventricular free wall rupture, after myocardial infarction, 327–328
Ventricular premature beats, 262–264
after myocardial infarction, 324t
Ventricular septal defect, 280–281
Ventricular septal rupture, after myocardial infarction, 326–327, 327t
Ventricular tachycardia, 276–280. See also under Tachycardia.
Verapamil, anticonvulsant interactions with, 863t
for arrhythmia in mitral valve prolapse, 290
for atrial fibrillation, 257, 258t
contraindications to, 274, 277
for atrial flutter, 275t
for atrial premature beats, 261
for hypertension, 308t, 310
intoxication with, 1168–1169
relative antiarrhythmic efficacy of, 262t
Verotoxins, hemolytic-uremic syndrome and, 366, 403
Verruca vulgaris. See Warts.
Verrucous carcinoma, of vulva, 1073–1074
Vertebral fractures, in ankylosing spondylitis, 959
in osteoporosis, 594, 596–597
Vertigo, acute, 885–886, 885t, 886t
benign paroxysmal positional, 885t, 886–888, 888, 889
episodic, 884–892, 885t
in anxiety disorders, 885t, 891
in bilateral vestibular deficit, 885t, 891
in Meniere's disease, 885t, 888–889, 892–893
in migraine, 885t, 889, 890t
in motion sickness, 885t, 889–890
in orthostatic hypotension, 885t, 890–891
stroke-induced, 885t, 891–892
Very-low-density lipoprotein, 580. See also Cholesterol; Hyperlipoproteinemias.
Vesicoureteral reflux, 667
pyelonephritis and, 680
Vesiculobullous lesions, of mouth, 812–813
Vestibular deficit, bilateral, 885t, 891
Vestibular nerve section, for Meniere's disease, 894
Vestibular neuritis, acute, 885–886, 885t
Vestibular rehabilitation, 886, 887t
for bilateral vestibular deficit, 887t, 891
for Meniere's disease, 893
Vestibular schwannomas, 940–941
Vibrio cholerae, 72. See also Cholera.
laboratory isolation of, 73
O139 (Bengal) strain of, 74
Vibrio parahaemolyticus, food-borne illness due to, 75t, 78
Vibrio vulnificus infection, 798–799
VICOP-B regimen, for Sézary's syndrome, 769

Vidarabine, for herpes simplex conjunctivitis, 68
Vigabatrin, for infantile spasms, 870
for seizures in acute porphyria, 449
Vinblastine, for Hodgkin's disease, 407t, 408
for non–small cell lung cancer, 189
for transitional cell carcinoma, 709
Vinca alkaloids. See also specific drugs.
antifungal interactions with, 807
Vincent's disease, 814
Vincristine, for acute lymphoblastic leukemia in children, 423
for aggressive lymphoma, 436t
for chronic lymphocytic leukemia, 431, 432
for highly aggressive lymphoma, 438t
for Hodgkin's disease, 407t
for immune thrombocytopenic purpura, 400
for indolent B cell lymphoma, 435t
for multiple myeloma, 442
for Sézary's syndrome, 769
in CHOP regimen, for aggressive lymphoma, 436t
for indolent B cell lymphoma, 435t
for Sézary's syndrome, 769
in CVP regimen, for chronic lymphocytic leukemia, 431
for indolent B cell lymphoma, 435t
Vinegar. See Acetic acid.
Vinorelbine, for non–small cell lung cancer, 189
Visceral hypersensitivity, irritable bowel syndrome and, 489–490
Viscosity, blood, in multiple myeloma, 444
in polycythemia vera, 445
serum, reference intervals for, 1209t
Vital signs, age-specific reference values for, 1145t
Vitamin(s). See also specific vitamins.
in parenteral nutrition, 604–605
for high-risk neonate, 1012
supplemental, for cystic fibrosis, 177, 177t
in short-bowel syndrome, 511
Vitamin A, colorectal cancer and, 533
serum, reference intervals for, 1209t
supplemental, for cystic fibrosis, 177, 177t
for measles, 133
Vitamin B₁. See Thiamine.
Vitamin B₂ (riboflavin), for alcoholic neuropathy, 927
Vitamin B₆. See Pyridoxine.
Vitamin B₁₂. See also Cobalamin; Hydroxycobalamin.
deficiency of, aphthous stomatitis due to, 812
neuropathy due to, 927
for elevated homocysteine in type 2 diabetes, 563
for tropical sprue, 511
malabsorption of, after intestinal resection, 510
in chronic pancreatitis, 508
serum, reference intervals for, 1209t
supplemental, in short-bowel syndrome, 511
Vitamin C (ascorbic acid), blood, reference intervals for, 1207t
with deferoxamine therapy, 372
with iron supplements, 357
Vitamin D. See also Calcifediol; Calcitriol; Ergocalciferol.
deficiency of, hyperparathyroidism due to, 631

Vitamin D (Continued)
in chronic renal failure, 703, 704
for osteopenia in thalassemia patient with iron overload, 372
for osteoporosis, 595
prophylactic, in inflammatory bowel disease, 487
supplemental, for infant, 1022
Vitamin E, colorectal cancer and, 533
lipid-lowering effects of, 332
supplemental, for Alzheimer's disease, 846
for cystic fibrosis, 177, 177t
for fibrocystic disease of breast, 1023
for rheumatoid arthritis, 952
in abetalipoproteinemia, 512
Vitamin K, deficiency of, 592–593, 592t
for salicylate intoxication, 1200
supplemental, for cystic fibrosis, 177t
warfarin reversal with, for intracerebral hemorrhage, 849
with parenteral nutrition, 605
Vitiligo, 840–841
Vocal fold lesions, hoarseness due to, 25–27
Vocal fold paralysis, 27–28
Vocal nodules, 26
Voice therapy, for spasmodic dysphonia, 28
for vocal fold polyps, 26
for vocal nodules, 26
Voiding dysfunction, 669–670
after stroke, 855
treatment of, 668
urinary tract infection and, 667
Volume homeostasis. See also Fluids, parenteral.
in acute renal failure, 697
in chronic renal failure, 704, 705
Volume ventilation, nasal, for obesity hypoventilation syndrome, 183
Volvulus, in Chagas' disease, 102
Vomiting, 5–10
causes of, 6t
chemotherapy-induced, 8–10, 9t, 10t
clinical findings with, 7
defined, 5
during pregnancy, 980
parenteral nutrition for, 603
in bulimia nervosa, 1103, 1104
in food-borne illness, 76
in migraine, 879
induced, for acute poisoning, 1147–1148
for ciguatera poisoning, 1143
mechanisms stimulating, 5
physiologic consequences of, 5–7
treatment of, 7–8, 8t
Von Hippel–Lindau disease, hemangioblastoma in, 941
pheochromocytoma in, 654
renal cell carcinoma in, 709
Von Willebrand disease, categorization of, 392
clinical bleeding pattern in, 391
dysfunctional uterine bleeding in, 1039–1040
genetics of, 391
laboratory abnormalities in, 392
pathophysiology of, 391
treatment of, 395
Von Willebrand factor, in thrombotic thrombocytopenic purpura, 403
in von Willebrand disease, 391
Vowel mnemonic, 1156t
Vulva, tumors of, 1069–1074, 1070t. See also specific tumors.
benign, 1070–1071, 1070t

Vulva *(Continued)*
  diagnosis of, 1069–1070
  malignant, 1070t, 1071–1074, 1074t
Vulvar hematoma, postpartum, 1001
Vulvar intraepithelial neoplasia,
  1071–1072
Vulvectomy, for vulvar carcinoma, 1073
  for vulvar intraepithelial neoplasia, 1072
Vulvovaginitis, 1053–1055, 1054t

Waldenström's macroglobulinemia,
  peripheral neuropathy in, 928
Wallenberg's syndrome, 892
Wandering rash of the tongue, 815
Warfarin, after myocardial infarction, 330
  anticonvulsant interactions with, 863t
  antifungal interactions with, 194, 196,
    807
  bile acid resin interaction with, 582
  fibrate interaction with, 584
  for congestive heart failure, 296
  for deep venous thrombosis, 341
    prophylactic, 222t
  for disseminated intravascular coagula-
    tion, 401
  for paroxysmal nocturnal hemoglobin-
    uria, 366
  for pulmonary thromboembolism, 223,
    223t
    treatment of toxicity due to, *224*
  for stroke prevention, in atrial fibrilla-
    tion, 258–259, 258t, 850
    secondary, 855
  intracerebral hemorrhage due to, treat-
    ment of, 849
  vitamin K deficiency due to, 592
Warts, 785–787, 793. See also *Condyloma
  acuminatum.*
  genital, 787–788, 788t
  oral, 817
Water loss. See also *Dehydration.*
  calculation of, in diabetes insipidus,
    624–625
Water requirements, for infants and
  children, calculation of, 608, 608t
  for low-birth-weight infant, 609
Webs, congenital laryngeal, 29–30
Wegener's granulomatosis, gingival
  enlargement in, 814
Weight loss, after myocardial infarction,
  332–333
  AIDS-related, 56

Weight loss *(Continued)*
  for hypertension, 305
  for obesity, 587–591, 591t
  for obesity-hypoventilation syndrome,
    185
  for obstructive sleep-disordered breath-
    ing, 182, 185
  in type 2 diabetes, 555–556
Western encephalitis, 896
West's syndrome, 869, 870
Wet mount, in vulvovaginitis diagnosis,
  1053, 1054, 1054t
Wheelchair, for stroke survivor, 854, 855
Whiff test, in vulvovaginitis diagnosis,
  1053, 1054
Whipple's disease, 512
Whipple's procedure, for chronic
  pancreatitis, 523
Whipworm, 541t, 544
White lesions of mouth, 810–812
White sponge nevus, 811
Whitlow, herpetic, 801
Whole-bowel irrigation, for acute
  poisoning, 1148–1149
Whooping cough. See *Pertussis.*
Wickham's striae, in lichen planus, 773
Williams' syndrome, aortic stenosis in, 283
Wintergreen oil, intoxication by, 1198
Withdrawal, anxiety symptoms due to,
  1121t
  from alcohol, 1093, 1177
  from anxiolytics, 1096
  from cocaine, 1094
  from inhalants, 1097
  from nicotine, 1098
  from opioids, 1095
    due to naloxone for intoxication, 1192
  from sedatives, 1096
    insomnia due to, 32
Wolff-Parkinson-White syndrome, *271,
  272–274, 273*
Wood's lamp examination, for postinflammatory hyperpigmentation evaluation,
  838
Wrist, sports injuries to, 976
Wrist replacement, in rheumatoid
  arthritis, 952

Xanthoastrocytoma, pleomorphic, 941
Xerostomia, 816
  due to salivary gland irradiation, in
    Hodgkin's disease, 411, 412

Xerostomia *(Continued)*
  in thyroid cancer, 652
Xylene, 1179
Xylometazoline, for viral respiratory
  infection, 214
D-Xylose absorption test, reference
  intervals for, 1213t

Yeast infection. See *Candidiasis.*
Yellow fever vaccine, 146, 147t
Yersinia enterocolitica infection, food-
  borne, 75t, 78
  treatment of, 77t
  in iron overdose, 1180, 1181
Yersinia pestis. See *Plague.*

Zafirlukast, for allergic rhinitis, 747
  for asthma, 733
    in children, 740
Zalcitabine (ddC), for HIV infection, 45,
  48t
Zaleplon, for insomnia, 34
Zanamivir, for viral pneumonia, 216t
ZDV. See *Zidovudine (AZT, ZDV).*
Zenker's diverticulum, 479
  dysphagia due to, 474
  treatment of, 478, 479
Zidovudine (AZT, ZDV), for HIV infection,
  45t, 48t
  drug interactions with, 45
  for prevention of vertical HIV transmis-
    sion, 984
  toxic effects of, 47
Zidovudine-lamivudine (AZT-3TC), for HIV
  infection, 48t
Zileuton, for allergic rhinitis, 747
  for asthma, 733
    in children, 739–740
Zinc deficiency, with parenteral nutrition,
  607
Zinc oxide, for cheilitis prevention, 809
Zinc sulfate, for rheumatoid arthritis, 952
Zoledronate, for Paget's disease of bone,
  599
Zolmitriptan, for migraine, 881
Zolpidem, for insomnia, 34
Zonisamide, for epilepsy, 864
Zoster. See *Herpes zoster.*

ISBN 0-7216-7225-6

90071

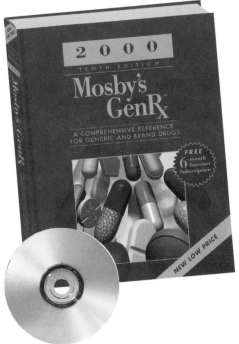

Process Immediately for 30-Day Trial!

|||||

BUSINESS REPLY MAIL
FIRST-CLASS MAIL   PERMIT NO. 7135   ORLANDO FL

POSTAGE WILL BE PAID BY ADDRESSEE

NO POSTAGE
NECESSARY
IF MAILED
IN THE
UNITED STATES

BOOK ORDER FULFILLMENT DEPT
HARCOURT HEALTH SCIENCES
11830 WESTLINE INDUSTRIAL DRIVE
SAINT LOUIS MO 63146-9988

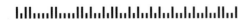